PRINCIPLES AND PRACTICE OF

INFECTIOUS DISEASES

THIRD EDITION

PRINCIPLES AND PRACTICE OF
INFECTIOUS DISEASES

THIRD EDITION

Edited by

GERALD L. MANDELL, M.D.
Professor, Department of Internal Medicine
Owen R. Cheatham Professor of the Sciences
Head, Division of Infectious Diseases
University of Virginia School of Medicine
Charlottesville, Virginia

R. GORDON DOUGLAS, JR., M.D.
E. Hugh Luckey Distinguished Professor in Medicine
Chairman, Department of Medicine
Cornell University Medical College
Physician-in-Chief
The New York Hospital
New York, New York

JOHN E. BENNETT, M.D.
Head, Clinical Mycology Section
Laboratory of Clinical Investigation
National Institute of Allergy and Infectious Diseases
National Institutes of Health
Bethesda, Maryland

CHURCHILL LIVINGSTONE
New York, Edinburgh, London, Melbourne

Library of Congress Cataloging-in-Publication Data

Principles and practice of infectious diseases / edited by Gerald L.
Mandell, R. Gordon Douglas, Jr., John E. Bennett. — 3rd ed.
p. cm.
Includes bibliographies and index.
ISBN 0-443-08686-9 (single volume)
ISBN 0-443-08710-5 (two-volume set)
1. Communicable diseases. I. Mandell, Gerald L. II. Douglas, R.
Gordon (Robert Gordon), date. III. Bennett, John E. (John
Eugene), date.
[DNLM: 1. Communicable Diseases. WC 100 P957]
RC111.P78 1990
616.9—dc20
DNLM/DLC
for Library of Congress 89-15734
CIP

Distributed in the United Kingdom by Churchill Livingstone, Robert Stevenson House, 1–3 Baxter's Place, Leith Walk, Edinburgh EH1 3AF, and by associated companies, branches, and representatives throughout the world.

Accurate indications, adverse reactions, and dosage schedules for drugs are provided in this book, but it is possible that they may change. The reader is urged to review the package information data of the manufacturers of the medications mentioned.

The Publishers have made every effort to trace the copyright holders for borrowed material. If they have inadvertently overlooked any, they will be pleased to make the necessary arrangements at the first opportunity.

Acquisitions Editor: *Beth Kaufman Barry*
Assistant Editor: *Leslie Burgess*
Copy Editor: *David Terry*
Production Designer: *Charlie Lebeda*
Production Supervisor: *Jocelyn Eckstein*

Printed in the United States of America

First published in 1990

CONTENTS

CONTRIBUTORS

N. FRANKLIN ADKINSON, M.D.
Professor, Department of Medicine, Johns Hopkins University School of Medicine; Physician-in-Charge, Asthma and Allergy Clinics, Baltimore, Maryland

ROBERT H. ALFORD, M.D.
Clinical Professor, Department of Medicine, Vanderbilt University School of Medicine; Medical Director, Park View Medical Center, Nashville, Tennessee

DAVID M. ALLEN, M.D.
Senior Fellow in Infectious Diseases, Department of Medicine, Cornell University Medical College; Assistant Attending Physician and Chief Medical Resident, Department of Medicine, The New York Hospital, New York, New York

VINCENT T. ANDRIOLE, M.D.
Professor, Department of Medicine, Yale University School of Medicine; Attending Physician, Yale-New Haven Hospital, New Haven, Connecticut

MICHAEL A. APICELLA, M.D.
Professor of Medicine and Microbiology, Department of Medicine, State University of New York at Buffalo School of Medicine, Buffalo, New York

GORDON L. ARCHER, M.D.
Professor, Departments of Medicine and Microbiology/Immunology, Virginia Commonwealth University Medical College of Virginia School of Medicine, Richmond, Virginia

DONALD ARMSTRONG, M.D.
Professor, Department of Medicine, Cornell University Medical College; Chief, Infectious Disease Service, and Director, Microbiology Laboratory, Memorial Sloan-Kettering Cancer Center, New York, New York

LARRY M. BADDOUR, M.D.
Associate Professor, Department of Medicine, University of Missouri—Columbia School of Medicine, Columbia, Missouri

CAROL J. BAKER, M.D.
Professor, Departments of Pediatrics and Microbiology and Immunology, and Head, Section of Pediatric Infectious Diseases, Baylor College of Medicine, Houston, Texas

J. RICHARD BARINGER, M.D.
Professor and Chairman, Department of Neurology, University of Utah School of Medicine, Salt Lake City, Utah

KENNETH J. BART, M.D.
Agency Director for Health, Agency for International Development, Office of Health, Bureau for Science and Technology, Washington, D.C.

JOHN G. BARTLETT, M.D.
Professor, Department of Medicine, and Chief, Division of Infectious Diseases, Johns Hopkins University School of Medicine, Baltimore, Maryland

STEPHEN G. BAUM, M.D.
Professor, Department of Medicine, Mount Sinai School of Medicine of the City University of New York; Director, Department of Medicine, Beth Israel Medical Center, New York, New York

EDWIN H. BEACHEY, M.D.
Professor, Departments of Medicine and Microbiology and Immunology, and Chief, Division of Infectious Diseases, University of Tennessee College of Medicine; Associate Chief of Staff, Department of Research and Development, Veterans Administration Medical Center, Memphis, Tennessee

JOHN E. BENNETT, M.D.
Head, Clinical Mycology Section, Laboratory of Clinical Investigation, National Institute of Allergy and Infectious Diseases, National Institutes of Health, Bethesda, Maryland

KENNETH W. BERNARD, M.D., D.T.M. & H.
Medical Epidemiologist, International Health Program Office, Centers for Disease Control, Atlanta, Georgia; Consultant, Departments of Public Health Policy and Tropical Medicine, Peace Corps, Washington, D.C.

ROBERT F. BETTS, M.D.
Professor, Department of Medicine, University of Rochester School of Medicine and Dentistry; Attending Physician, Department of Medicine, Strong Memorial Hospital, Rochester, New York

ALAN L. BISNO, M.D.
Professor, Department of Medicine, University of Miami School of Medicine; Chief, Department of Medical Service, Miami Veterans Administration Medical Center, Miami, Florida

NEIL R. BLACKLOW, M.D.
Professor, Department of Medicine, and Director, Division of Infectious Diseases, University of Massachusetts Medical School, Worcester, Massachusetts

MARTIN J. BLASER, M.D.
Addison B. Scoville Professor of Medicine and Director, Division of Infectious Diseases, Department of Medicine; Professor, Department of Microbiology, Vanderbilt University School of Medicine, Nashville, Tennessee

WILLIAM BONNEZ, M.D.
Assistant Professor, Department of Medicine, University of Rochester School of Medicine and Dentistry; Attending Physician, Department of Medicine, Strong Memorial Hospital, Rochester, New York

RICHARD C. BOUCHER, M.D.
Professor, Department of Medicine, University of North Carolina at Chapel Hill School of Medicine, Chapel Hill, North Carolina

WILLIAM R. BOWIE, M.D.
Professor, Department of Medicine, University of British Columbia Faculty of Medicine, Vancouver, British Columbia, Canada

JOHN M. BOYCE, M.D.
Associate Professor, Department of Medicine, Brown University Program in Medicine; Associate Director, Infectious Diseases Section, Miriam Hospital, Providence, Rhode Island

PHILIP S. BRACHMAN, M.D.
Director, Epidemiology Program Office, Department of Health and Human Services, Centers for Disease Control, Atlanta, Georgia

BARRY D. BRAUSE, M.D.
Clinical Associate Professor, Department of Medicine, Cornell University Medical College; Associate Attending Physician, Department of Medicine, The New York Hospital for Special Surgery, New York, New York

ROBERT B. BREITENBUCHER, M.D.
Associate Professor, Department of Medicine, and Former Director, Division of Geriatric Medicine, University of Minnesota Medical School, Minneapolis, Minnesota

ARTHUR E. BROWN, M.D.
Associate Professor of Clinical Medicine and Clinical Pediatrics, Department of Medicine and Pediatrics, Cornell University Medical College; Attending Physician, Infectious Disease Service, Memorial Sloan-Kettering Cancer Center; Associate Attending Pediatrician, Department of Pediatrics, The New York Hospital, New York, New York

RALPH T. BRYAN, M.D.
Medical Epidemiologist, Parasitic Diseases Branch, Division of Parasitic Diseases, Centers for Disease Control, Atlanta, Georgia

RICHARD E. BRYANT, M.D.
Professor, Department of Medicine, and Director, Division of Infectious Disease, Oregon Health Sciences University School of Medicine, Portland, Oregon

WARD E. BULLOCK, M.D.
Professor, Department of Internal Medicine, and Director, Division of Infectious Disease, University of Cincinnati College of Medicine; Attending Physician, University of Cincinnati Medical Center, Cincinnati, Ohio

JAMES E. BURNS, M.D.
Department of Pediatrics, Division of Infectious Diseases, University of Virginia School of Medicine, Charlottesville, Virginia

LARRY M. BUSH, M.D.
Clinical Assistant Professor, Department of Medicine, Medical College of Pennsylvania, Philadelphia, Pennsylvania

THOMAS BUTLER, M.D.
Professor and Chief, Division of Infectious Diseases, Department of Internal Medicine, Texas Tech University Health Sciences Center School of Medicine, Lubbock, Texas

CHARLES C. J. CARPENTER, M.D.
Professor, Department of Medicine, Brown University Program in Medicine; Physician-in-Chief, Miriam Hospital, Providence, Rhode Island

THOMAS R. CATE, M.D.
Professor, Department of Medicine, Baylor College of Medicine, Houston, Texas

RICHARD E. CHAISSON, M.D.
Assistant Professor, Departments of Medicine and Epidemiology, Johns Hopkins University School of Medicine; Director, AIDS Service, Johns Hopkins Hospital, Baltimore, Maryland

MARY E. CHAMBERLAND, M.D., M.P.H.
Medical Epidemiologist, Surveillance and Evaluation Branch, AIDS Program, Centers for Disease Control, Atlanta, Georgia

STANLEY W. CHAPMAN, M.D.
Associate Professor, Department of Medicine, University of Mississippi School of Medicine; Chief, Medical Service and Infectious Diseases Section, Veterans Administration Medical Center, Jackson, Mississippi

ANTHONY W. CHOW, M.D., F.R.C.P.(C.)
Professor, Department of Medicine, and Head, Division of Infectious Diseases, University of British Columbia Faculty of Medicine; Head, Department of Medicine, Vancouver General Hospital, Vancouver, British Columbia, Canada

GORDON D. CHRISTENSEN, M.D.
Associate Professor, Departments of Medicine, Microbiology, and Immunology, University of Missouri-Columbia School of Medicine, Columbia, Missouri; Clinical Investigator, Research Service, Harry S. Truman Hospital, Columbia, Missouri

JEFFREY D. CHULAY, M.D., D.T.M. & H.
Associate Professor, Department of Medicine, Uniformed Services University of the Health Sciences F. Edward Hébert School of Medicine, Bethesda, Maryland; Chief, Department of Immunology, Walter Reed Army Institute of Research, Washington, D.C.

MARY LOU CLEMENTS, M.D., M.P.H.
Associate Professor, Department of International Health, Johns Hopkins University School of Hygiene and Public Health; Associate Professor, Department of Medicine, Johns Hopkins University School of Medicine; Director, Johns Hopkins University Center for Immunization Research, Baltimore, Maryland

C. GLENN COBBS, M.D.
Professor, Department of Medicine, and Director, Division of Infectious Diseases, University of Alabama School of Medicine, Birmingham, Alabama

MYRON S. COHEN, M.D.
Associate Professor, Departments of Medicine and Microbiology and Immunology, University of North Carolina at Chapel Hill School of Medicine, Chapel Hill, North Carolina

ROBERT B. COUCH, M.D.
Professor, Department of Medicine, and Chairman, Department of Microbiology and Immunology, Baylor College of Medicine, Houston, Texas

JAMES W. CURRAN, M.D., M.P.H.
Director, AIDS Program, and Associate Director for AIDS, Center for Infectious Diseases, Centers for Disease Control, Atlanta, Georgia

CARLOS DEL RIO, M.D.
Senior Associate, Department of Medicine, Emory University School of Medicine; Chief Resident, Department of Medicine, Crawford W. Long Memorial Hospital, Atlanta, Georgia

PETER DENSEN, M.D.
Associate Professor, Department of Internal Medicine, University of Iowa College of Medicine, Iowa City, Iowa

ROGER M. DES PREZ, M.D.
Professor, Department of Medicine, Vanderbilt University School of Medicine; Chief, Medical Service, Veterans Administration Medical Center, Nashville, Tennessee

RICHARD D. DIAMOND, M.D.
Professor, Departments of Medicine and Biochemistry, Boston University School of Medicine; Head, Section of Infectious Disease, Evans Memorial Department of Clinical Research, University Hospital, Boston, Massachusetts

CHARLES A. DINARELLO, M.D.
Professor, Departments of Medicine and Pediatrics, Tufts University School of Medicine; Staff Physician, Department of Medicine, New England Medical Center Hospital, Boston, Massachusetts

WILLIAM E. DISMUKES, M.D.
Professor and Vice-Chairman, Department of Medicine, University of Alabama School of Medicine; Director, Medical House Staff, University of Alabama Medical Center, Birmingham, Alabama

WILLIAM O. DOBBINS III, M.D.
Professor, Department of Internal Medicine, University of Michigan Medical School; Associate Chief of Staff for Research, Veterans Administration Medical Center, Ann Arbor, Michigan

JAY F. DOBKIN, M.D.
Associate Professor of Clinical Medicine, Department of Medicine, Columbia University College of Physicians and Surgeons; Medical Director, AIDS Center, Presbyterian Hospital, New York, New York

BRADLEY N. DOEBBELING, M.D.
Fellow Associate, University of Iowa Hospitals and Clinics, Iowa City, Iowa

RAPHAEL DOLIN, M.D.
Professor, Department of Medicine, and Director, Division of Infectious Diseases, University of Rochester School of Medicine and Dentistry; Head, Infectious Disease Unit, and Attending Physician, Department of Medicine, Strong Memorial Hospital, Rochester, New York

GERALD R. DONOWITZ, M.D.
Associate Professor, Department of Internal Medicine, and Associate Director, Hematology-Oncology Unit, University of Virginia School of Medicine, Charlottesville, Virginia

R. GORDON DOUGLAS, JR., M.D.
E. Hugh Luckey Distinguished Professor in Medicine and Chairman, Department of Medicine, Cornell University Medical College; Physician-in-Chief, The New York Hospital, New York, New York

J. STEPHEN DUMMER, M.D.
Associate Professor, Departments of Medicine and Surgery, University of Pittsburgh School of Medicine, Pittsburgh, Pennsylvania

HERBERT L. DuPONT, M.D.
Mary W. Kelsey Professor of the Medical Sciences, The University of Texas Medical School at Houston; Interim Chairman, Department of Internal Medicine, Director, Program in Infectious Diseases, and Interim Clinical Chief of the Internal Service, The Hermann Hospital, Houston, Texas

DAVID T. DURACK, M.B., D. PHIL.
Professor, Departments of Medicine and Microbiology and Immunology, and Chief, Division of Infectious Diseases, Duke University School of Medicine, Durham, North Carolina

JOHN E. EDWARDS, JR., M.D.
Professor, Department of Medicine, University of California, Los Angeles, UCLA School of Medicine, Los Angeles, California; Chief, Division of Infectious Diseases, Harbor-UCLA Medical Center, Torrance, California

MORVEN S. EDWARDS, M.D.
Associate Professor, Department of Pediatrics, Baylor College of Medicine, Houston, Texas

BARRY I. EISENSTEIN, M.D.
Professor and Chairman, Department of Microbiology and Immunology, and Professor, Department of Internal Medicine, University of Michigan Medical School, Ann Arbor, Michigan

JERROLD J. ELLNER, M.D.
Professor, Department of Medicine, Case Western Reserve University School of Medicine; Director, Division of Infectious Diseases, University Hospitals, Cleveland, Ohio

STANLEY FALKOW, PH.D.
Professor, Departments of Medicine and Microbiology and Immunology, Stanford University School of Medicine, Stanford, California

GUO-DONG FANG, M.D.
Associate Professor, Department of Medicine, Beijing Union Medical College, Beijing, China

BARRY M. FARR, M.D.
Associate Professor, Department of Medicine, University of Virginia School of Medicine, Charlottesville, Virginia

W. EDMUND FARRAR, M.D.
Professor, Department of Medicine, Medical University of South Carolina College of Medicine, Charleston, South Carolina

ANTHONY S. FAUCI, M.D.
Director, National Institute of Allergy and Infectious Diseases, National Institutes of Health, Bethesda, Maryland

STEPHEN M. FEINSTONE, M.D.
Medical Officer, Hepatitis Viruses Section, Laboratory of Infectious Diseases, National Institute of Allergy and Infectious Diseases, National Institutes of Health, Bethesda, Maryland

ROBERT FEKETY, M.D.
Professor, Department of Internal Medicine, and Head, Division of Infectious Diseases, University of Michigan Medical School; Chief, Adult Infectious Diseases Service, University Hospital, Ann Arbor, Michigan

BERNARD N. FIELDS, M.D.
Adele Lehman Professor and Chairman, Department of Microbiology and Molecular Genetics, and Professor, Department of Medicine, Harvard Medical School, Boston, Massachusetts

SYDNEY M. FINEGOLD, M.D.
Professor, Departments of Medicine and Microbiology, and Immunology, University of California, Los Angeles, UCLA School of Medicine; Associate Chief of Staff, Research and Development Service, Wadsworth Veterans Administration Medical Center, Los Angeles, California

GERALD W. FISCHER, M.D.
Professor, Department of Pediatrics, Uniformed Services University of the Health Sciences F. Edward Hébert School of Medicine, Bethesda, Maryland

DANIEL B. FISHBEIN, M.D.
Medical Epidemiologist, Viral and Rickettsial Zoonoses Branch, Division of Viral and Rickettsial Diseases, Center for Infectious Diseases, Centers for Disease Control, Atlanta, Georgia

L. NEAL FREEMAN, M.D.
Fellow in Ophthalmic Plastic and Reconstructive Surgery, Department of Ophthalmology, University of California, San Francisco, School of Medicine, San Francisco, California

JOHN I. GALLIN, M.D.
Director, Intramural Research Program, National Institute of Allergy and Infectious Diseases, and Senior Investigator, Bacterial Diseases Section, Laboratory of Clinical Investigation, National Institutes of Health, Bethesda, Maryland

HARRY A. GALLIS, M.D.
Associate Professor, Department of Internal Medicine, Duke University School of Medicine, Durham, North Carolina

ROBERT C. GALLO, M.D.
Chief, Laboratory of Tumor Cell Biology, National Cancer Institute, National Institutes of Health, Bethesda, Maryland

WALTER R. GAMMON, M.D.
Professor, Department of Dermatology, University of North Carolina at Chapel Hill School of Medicine, Chapel Hill, North Carolina

JEFFREY A. GELFAND, M.D.
Associate Professor, Department of Medicine, Tufts University School of Medicine; Physician, Department of Medicine, New England Medical Center, Boston, Massachusetts

ANNE A. GERSHON, M.D.
Professor, Department of Pediatrics, and Director, Division of Pediatric Infectious Diseases, Columbia University College of Physicians and Surgeons, New York, New York

PETER GILLIGAN, M.D.
Associate Professor, Departments of Microbiology and Immunology and Pathology, University of North Carolina at Chapel Hill School of Medicine, Chapel Hill, North Carolina

ALAN PAUL GLOMBICKI, M.D.
Assistant Professor, Department of Medicine, Baylor College of Medicine; Medical Director, Liver Transplant Unit, Texas Medical Center, Houston, Texas

ELLIE J. C. GOLDSTEIN, M.D.
Associate Clinical Professor, Department of Medicine, University of California, Los Angeles, UCLA School of Medicine, Los Angeles, California; Director, R. M. Alden Research Laboratory, Santa Monica Hospital Medical Center, Santa Monica, California

ROBERT A. GOODWIN, JR., M.D.
Professor Emeritus, Department of Medicine, Vanderbilt University School of Medicine, Nashville, Tennessee

W. RICHARD GREEN, M.D.
Professor, Department of Ophthalmology, and Associate Professor, Department of Pathology, Johns Hopkins University School of Medicine; Chief, Eye Pathology Laboratory, Johns Hopkins Hospital, Baltimore, Maryland

JOHN E. GREENLEE, M.D.
Professor, Department of Neurology, University of Utah School of Medicine; Chief, Neurology Service, Veterans Administration Medical Center, Salt Lake City, Utah

WILLIAM B. GREENOUGH III, M.D.
Professor, Department of Medicine, Johns Hopkins University School of Medicine, and Professor, Department of International Health, Johns Hopkins University School of Hygiene and Public Health, Baltimore, Maryland

DIANE E. GRIFFIN, M.D.
Professor, Departments of Medicine and Neurology, Johns Hopkins University School of Medicine, Baltimore, Maryland

DIETER H. M. GRÖSCHEL, M.D.
Professor, Departments of Pathology and Internal Medicine, and Director, Division of Clinical Microbiology, University of Virginia School of Medicine, Charlottesville, Virginia

DAVID I. GROVE, M.D.
Director of Postgraduate Medical Education, Sir Charles Gairdner Hospital, Nedlands, Western Australia

RICHARD L. GUERRANT, M.D.
Professor, Department of Internal Medicine, and Head, Division of Geographic Medicine, University of Virginia School of Medicine, Charlottesville, Virginia

JACK M. GWALTNEY, JR., M.D.
Professor, Department of Internal Medicine, and Head, Division of Epidemiology and Virology, University of Virginia School of Medicine, Charlottesville, Virginia

ASHLEY T. HAASE, M.D.
Professor and Head, Department of Microbiology, University of Minnesota Medical School, Minneapolis, Minnesota

CAROLINE BREESE HALL, M.D.
Professor, Departments of Pediatrics and Medicine, University of Rochester School of Medicine and Dentistry, Rochester, New York

WILLIAM J. HALL, M.D.
Professor of Medicine and Pulmonology, Department of Medicine, University of Rochester School of Medicine and Dentistry; Chairman, Department of Medicine, Rochester General Hospital, Rochester, New York

MARGARET A. HAMBURG, M.D.
Special Assistant to the Director, National Institute of Allergy and Infectious Diseases, National Institutes of Health, Bethesda, Maryland

W. LEE HAND, M.D.
Professor, Department of Medicine, and Director, Division of Infectious Diseases, Emory University School of Medicine; Chief, Infectious Diseases Section, Veterans Administration Medical Center, Atlanta, Georgia

H. HUNTER HANDSFIELD, M.D.
Professor, Department of Medicine, University of Washington School of Medicine; Director, Sexually Transmitted Disease Control Program, Seattle-King County Department of Public Health, Seattle, Washington

GAVIN HART, M.D., M.P.H.
Clinical Associate Professor, Department of Medicine, Flinders University School of Medicine; Director, STD Control Branch, South Australian Health Commission, Adelaide, South Australia

BARRY J. HARTMAN, M.D.
Associate Professor of Clinical Medicine, Department of Medicine, Cornell University Medical College; Associate Attending Physician, Department of Medicine, The New York Hospital, New York, New York

R. J. HAY, D.M., F.R.C.P.
Reader in Clinical Mycology, Department of Clinical Sciences, London School of Hygiene and Tropical Medicine; Consultant Dermatologist, Department of Microbial Diseases, St. Johns Hospital for Diseases of the Skin, London, England

FREDERICK G. HAYDEN, M.D.
Associate Professor, Departments of Internal Medicine and Pathology; Stuart S. Richardson Professor, Department of Internal Medicine; and Associate Director, Clinical Microbiology Laboratory (Virology), University of Virginia School of Medicine, Charlottesville, Virginia

CRAIG R. HEIM, M.D.
Associate Professor, Department of Medicine, Vanderbilt University School of Medicine; Attending Physician, Department of Medicine, Vanderbilt University Hospital, Nashville, Tennessee

FREDERICK P. HEINZEL, M.D.
Assistant Professor, Department of Medicine, University of California, San Francisco, School of Medicine, San Francisco, California

DAVID K. HENDERSON, M.D.
Associate Director for Quality Assurance and Hospital Epidemiology, Office of the Director, Clinical Center; Hospital Epidemiologist, Clinical Center; Investigator, Laboratory of Clinical Investigation, National Institute of Allergy and Infectious Diseases, National Institutes of Health, Bethesda, Maryland

J. OWEN HENDLEY, M.D.
Professor, Department of Pediatrics, and Head, Division of Pediatric Infectious Diseases, University of Virginia School of Medicine, Charlottesville, Virginia

JOHN E. HERRMANN, PH.D.
Associate Professor, Departments of Medicine and Molecular Genetics and Microbiology, University of Massachusetts Medical School, Worcester, Massachusetts

ERIK L. HEWLETT, M.D.
Professor, Departments of Internal Medicine and Pharmacology, and Head, Division of Clinical Pharmacology, University of Virginia School of Medicine, Charlottesville, Virginia

DAVID R. HILL, M.D.
Assistant Professor, Department of Medicine, University of Connecticut School of Medicine, Farmington, Connecticut

ALAN R. HINMAN, M.D., M.P.H.
Director, Center for Prevention Services, Centers for Disease Control, Atlanta, Georgia

MARTIN S. HIRSCH, M.D.
Professor, Department of Medicine, Harvard Medical School; Physician, Department of Medicine, Infectious Diseases Unit, Massachusetts General Hospital, Boston, Massachusetts

SHALOM Z. HIRSCHMAN, M.D.
Professor, Department of Medicine, and Director, Division of Infectious Diseases, Mount Sinai School of Medicine of the City University of New York, New York, New York

MONTO HO, M.D.
Professor and Chairman, Department of Microbiology; Professor, Department of Medicine; and Chief, Division of Infectious Diseases, University of Pittsburgh School of Medicine, Pittsburgh, Pennsylvania

GARY S. HOFFMAN, M.D.
Expert, Laboratory of Immunoregulation, National Institute of Allergy and Infectious Diseases, National Institutes of Health, Bethesda, Maryland

F. BLAINE HOLLINGER, M.D.
Professor, Departments of Medicine, Virology, and Epidemiology, and Head, Hepatitis and AIDS Research Units, Baylor College of Medicine, Houston, Texas

KING K. HOLMES, M.D., PH.D.
Professor and Vice Chairman, Department of Medicine, University of Washington School of Medicine, Physician-in-Chief, Harborview Medical Center, Seattle, Washington

JAY H. HOOFNAGLE, M.D.
Director, Division of Digestive Diseases and Nutrition, and Senior Investigator, Liver Diseases Section, National Institutes of Diabetes and Digestive and Kidney Diseases, National Institutes of Health, Bethesda, Maryland

EDWARD W. HOOK, M.D.
Professor and Chairman, Department of Internal Medicine, University of Virginia School of Medicine; Physician-in-Chief, University of Virginia Hospitals, Charlottesville, Virginia

EDWARD A. HOROWITZ, M.D.
Assistant Professor, Departments of Medicine and Medical Microbiology, Creighton University School of Medicine, Omaha, Nebraska

JAMES M. HUGHES, M.D.
Clinical Assistant Professor, Department of Medicine, Emory University School of Medicine; Deputy Director, Center for Infectious Diseases, Centers for Disease Control, Atlanta, Georgia

KARL M. JOHNSON, M.D.
Visiting Professor, Department of Tropical Medicine, Tulane University School of Public Health and Tropical Medicine, New Orleans, Louisiana; Consultant, Pharmaceutical Research and Development, Big Sky, Montana

RICHARD T. JOHNSON, M.D.
Dwight D. Eisenhower Professor, Department of Neurology, and Professor, Departments of Microbiology and Neuroscience, Johns Hopkins University School of Medicine, Baltimore, Maryland

WARREN D. JOHNSON, JR., M.D.
Professor, Department of Medicine, and Chief, Division of International Medicine, Cornell University Medical College; Attending Physician, Department of Medicine, The New York Hospital, New York, New York

THOMAS C. JONES, M.D.
Adjunct Professor, Department of Medicine, Cornell University Medical College, New York, New York; Head, Department of Allergy and Infectious Diseases, Sandoz, Ltd., Basle, Switzerland

ALLEN B. KAISER, M.D.
Associate Professor and Vice Chairman for Clinical Affairs, Department of Medicine, Vanderbilt University School of Medicine, Nashville, Tennessee

DENNIS L. KASPER, M.D.
Edward H. Kass Professor, Department of Medicine, Harvard Medical School; Co-Director, Channing Laboratory, Brigham and Women's Hospital, and Chief, Division of Infectious Diseases, Beth Israel Hospital, Boston, Massachusetts

MICHAEL KATZMAN, M.D.
Assistant Professor, Department of Medicine, Pennsylvania State University College of Medicine, Hershey, Pennsylvania

DONALD KAYE, M.D.
Professor and Chairman, Department of Medicine, Medical College of Pennsylvania; Chief, Department of Medicine, Hospital of the Medical College of Pennsylvania, Philadelphia, Pennsylvania

LOUIS V. KIRCHHOFF, M.D., M.P.H.
Assistant Professor, Department of Internal Medicine, University of Iowa College of Medicine; Staff Physician, Department of Veterans Affairs Medical Center, Iowa City, Iowa

JEROME O. KLEIN, M.D.
Professor, Department of Pediatrics, Boston University School of Medicine; Director, Division of Pediatric Infectious Diseases, Maxwell Finland Laboratory for Infectious Diseases, Boston City Hospital, Boston, Massachusetts

FREDERICK A. KLIPSTEIN, M.D.
Professor, Departments of Medicine and Microbiology, University of Rochester School of Medicine and Dentistry; Attending Physician, Department of Medicine, Strong Memorial Hospital, Rochester, New York

MICHAEL R. KNOWLES, M.D.
Associate Professor, Department of Medicine, University of North Carolina at Chapel Hill School of Medicine, Chapel Hill, North Carolina

SCOTT KOENIG, M.D., PH.D.
Senior Investigator, National Institute of Allergy and Infectious Diseases, National Institutes of Health, Bethesda, Maryland

JOHN N. KRIEGER, M.D.
Associate Professor, Department of Urology, University of Washington School of Medicine; Attending Surgeon, Department of Urology, University Hospital and Harborview Medical Center; Consultant, Division of Urology, Seattle Veterans Administration Medical Center, Seattle, Washington

CALVIN M. KUNIN. M.D.
Professor, Department of Internal Medicine, Ohio State University College of Medicine; Attending Physician, Department of Internal Medicine, Ohio State University Hospital, Columbus, Ohio

F. MARC LaFORCE, M.D.
Professor, Department of Medicine, University of Rochester School of Medicine and Dentistry; Physician-in-Chief, Genesee Hospital, Rochester, New York

WILLIAM J. LEDGER, M.D.
Professor, Department of Obstetrics and Gynecology, Cornell University Medical College; Obstetrician and Gynecologist-in-Chief, The New York Hospital, New York, New York

JAMES R. LEHRICH, M.D.
Associate Professor, Department of Neurology, Harvard Medical School; Director, Neurology Ambulatory Unit, Department of Neurology, Massachusetts General Hospital, Boston, Massachusetts

PHILLIP I. LERNER, M.D.
Professor, Department of Medicine, Case Western Reserve University School of Medicine; Chief, Division of Infectious Diseases, Mt. Sinai Hospital, Cleveland, Ohio

MATTHEW E. LEVISON, M.D.
Professor, Department of Medicine, and Chief, Division of Infectious Diseases, Medical College of Pennsylvania, Philadelphia, Pennsylvania

PAUL S. LIETMAN, M.D.
Professor of Medicine, and Director, Division of Clinical Pharmacology, Johns Hopkins University School of Medicine, Baltimore, Maryland

NATHAN LITMAN, M.D.
Associate Professor, Department of Pediatrics, Albert Einstein College of Medicine of Yeshiva University; Assistant Chief of Service and Associate Director, Department of Pediatrics, Montefiore Medical Center, Bronx, New York

JACOB A. LOHR, M.D.
Professor, Vice Chairman, and Chief, Department of Pediatrics, University of Virginia School of Medicine, Charlottesville, Virginia

JAMES E. LOYD, M.D.
Assistant Professor, Department of Medicine, Vanderbilt University School of Medicine, Nashville, Tennessee

ROB ROY MacGREGOR, M.D.
Professor, Department of Medicine, and Chief, Division of Infectious Diseases, University of Pennsylvania School of Medicine, Philadelphia, Pennsylvania

EL SHEIKH MAHGOUB, M.D.
Professor, Department of Medical Microbiology and Parasitology, University of Khartoum School of Medicine, Khartoum, Sudan

ADEL A. F. MAHMOUD, M.D., PH.D.
John H. Hord Professor and Chairman, Department of Medicine, Case Western Reserve University School of Medicine; Physician-in-Chief, University Hospitals of Cleveland, Cleveland, Ohio

GERALD L. MANDELL, M.D.
Professor, Department of Internal Medicine; Owen R. Cheatham Professor of the Sciences; and Head, Division of Infectious Diseases, University of Virginia School of Medicine, Charlottesville, Virginia

THOMAS J. MARRIE, M.D.
Professor, Department of Medicine, Dalhousie University Faculty of Medicine; Head, Division of Infectious Diseases, Victoria General Hospital, Halifax, Nova Scotia, Canada

MICHAEL A. MARTIN, M.D.
Assistant Professor, Department of Medicine, University of Maryland School of Medicine; Hospital Epidemiologist, University of Maryland Hospital, Baltimore, Maryland

HENRY MASUR, M.D.
Professor, Department of Medicine, George Washington University School of Medicine, Washington, D.C.; Chief, Department of Critical Care Medicine, Clinical Center, National Institutes of Health, Bethesda, Maryland

GLENN E. MATHIESEN, M.D.
Assistant Professor, Department of Medicine, University of California, Los Angeles, UCLA School of Medicine, Los Angeles, California; Physician Specialist, Department of Medicine, Olive View Hospital, Sylmar, California

KENNETH H. MAYER, M.D.
Associate Professor, Department of Medicine, and Director, AIDS Program, Brown University Program in Medicine, Providence, Rhode Island; Chief, Division of Infectious Disease, Memorial Hospital, Pawtucket, Rhode Island

ROBERT E. McCABE, M.D.
Assistant Professor, Department of Medicine, University of California, Davis, School of Medicine, Davis, California; Chief, Infectious Diseases Section, Veterans Administration Medical Center, Martinez, California

J. BRUCE McCLAIN, M.D.
Associate Professor, Department of Clinical Medicine, Uniformed Services University of Health Sciences F. Edward Hébert School of Medicine, Bethesda, Maryland; Infectious Disease Officer, Walter Reed Army Institute of Research, Washington, D.C.

PETER J. McDONNELL, M.D.
Assistant Professor, Department of Ophthalmology, University of Southern California School of Medicine, Los Angeles, California

ZELL A. McGEE, M.D.
Professor, Departments of Medicine and Pathology, and Director, Center for Infectious Diseases, Division of Diagnostic Microbiology and Immunology, University of Utah School of Medicine, Salt Lake City, Utah

JOHN E. McGOWAN, JR., M.D.
Professor, Departments of Medicine and Pathology and Laboratory Medicine, Emory University School of Medicine; Director, Clinical Microbiology Section, Grady Memorial Hospital, Atlanta, Georgia

KENNETH McINTOSH, M.D.
Professor, Department of Pediatrics, Harvard Medical School; Chief, Division of Infectious Diseases, The Children's Hospital, Boston, Massachusetts

ANTONE A. MEDEIROS, M.D.
Professor, Department of Medicine, Brown University Program in Medicine; Chief, Division of Infectious Disease, Miriam Hospital, Providence, Rhode Island

MARILYN A. MENEGUS, M.D.
Associate Professor, Departments of Microbiology and Immunology; Pathology; and Pediatrics; Director, Clinical Microbiology Laboratories, University of Rochester School of Medicine and Dentistry, Rochester, New York

FRANÇOISE MEUNIER, M.D.
Chief, Division of Infectious Diseases and Microbiology Laboratory; Research Associate, Fund for Medical Scientific Research, Institute Jules Bordet, Brussels, Belgium

JOEL D. MEYERS, M.D.
Professor, Division of Infectious Diseases, Department of Medicine, University of Washington School of Medicine; Member and Head, Program in Infectious Diseases, Fred Hutchinson Cancer Research Center, Seattle, Washington

DENNIS J. MIKOLICH, M.D.
Clinical Assistant Professor, Department of Medicine, Brown University Program in Medicine, Providence, Rhode Island

JOHN F. MODLIN, M.D.
Associate Professor, Department of Pediatrics, Johns Hopkins University School of Medicine, Baltimore, Maryland

ROBERT C. MOELLERING, JR., M.D.
Shields Warren-Mallinckrodt Professor of Clinical Research, and Professor, Department of Medicine, Harvard Medical School; Physician-in-Chief, New England Deaconess Hospital, Boston, Massachusetts

THOMAS P. MONATH, M.D.
Chief, Division of Virology, U.S. Army Medical Research Institute of Infectious Diseases, Fort Detrick, Frederick, Maryland

E. RICHARD MOXON, M.D.
Professor, Department of Paediatrics, Oxford University Faculty of Medicine; Head, Department of Paediatrics, John Radcliffe Hospital, Headington, Oxford, England

MAURICE A. MUFSON, M.D.
Professor and Chairman, Department of Medicine, Marshall University School of Medicine; Associate Chief of Staff, Research and Development Section, Veterans Administration Medical Center, Huntington, West Virginia

DANIEL M. MUSHER, M.D.
Professor, Department of Medicine, Baylor College of Medicine; Chief, Infectious Diseases Section, Veterans Administration Hospital, Houston, Texas

THEODORE E. NASH, M.D.
Medical Officer and Senior Scientist, Laboratory of Parasitic Diseases, National Institute of Allergy and Infectious Diseases, National Institutes of Health, Bethesda, Maryland

JOHN M. NEFF, M.D.
Professor, Department of Pediatrics, and Associate Dean, University of Washington School of Medicine; Medical Director, The Children's Hospital and Medical Center; Seattle, Washington

HAROLD C. NEU, M.D.
Professor, Departments of Medicine and Pharmacology, Columbia University College of Physicians and Surgeons; Hospital Epidemiologist, Department of Epidemiology, Presbyterian Hospital, New York, New York

CHARLES H. NIGHTINGALE, PH.D.
Research Professor, University of Connecticut School of Pharmacy, Farmington, Connecticut; Vice President, Hartford Hospital, Hartford, Connecticut

CARL W. NORDEN, M.D.
Professor, Department of Medicine, University of Pittsburgh School of Medicine; Head, Division of Infectious Disease, Montefiore Hospital, Pittsburgh, Pennsylvania

SANDRA NORRIS, Pharm. D.
President, DataMed Scientific Communications, Inc., New York, New York

STEVEN M. OPAL, M.D.
Assistant Professor, Department of Medicine, Brown University Program in Medicine, Providence, Rhode Island; Hospital Epidemiologist and Infectious Disease Consultant, Memorial Hospital, Pawtucket, Rhode Island

WALTER A. ORENSTEIN, M.D.
Director, Division of Immunization, Center for Prevention Services, Centers for Disease Control, Atlanta, Georgia

MICHAEL N. OXMAN, M.D.
Professor, Departments of Medicine and Pathology, University of California, San Diego, School of Medicine; Chief, Infectious Diseases Section, Veterans Administration Medical Center, San Diego, California

RICHARD D. PEARSON, M.D.
Associate Professor, Departments of Internal Medicine and Pathology, University of Virginia School of Medicine, Charlottesville, Virginia

JAMES E. PENNINGTON, M.D.
Clinical Professor, Department of Medicine, University of California, San Francisco, School of Medicine, San Francisco, California; Director, Department of Medical Research, Cutter Biological, Berkeley, California

PHILLIP K. PETERSON, M.D.
Professor, Department of Medicine, University of Minnesota Medical School—Minneapolis; Director, Section of Infectious Diseases, Hennepin County Medical Center, Minneapolis, Minnesota

WILLIAM A. PETRI, JR., M.D.
Lucille P. Markey Scholar and Assistant Professor, Departments of Internal Medicine and Microbiology, University of Virginia School of Medicine, Charlottesville, Virginia

PHILIP A. PIZZO, M.D.
Head, Infectious Disease Section, and Chief, Pediatric Branch, National Cancer Institute, National Institutes of Health, Bethesda, Maryland

MATTHEW POLLACK, M.D.
Professor, Department of Medicine, Uniformed Services University of the Health Sciences F. Edward Hébert School of Medicine, Bethesda, Maryland

STEPHEN R. PREBLUD, M.D.
Surveillence, Investigation, and Research Branch, Division of Immunization, Center for Prevention Services, Centers for Disease Control, Atlanta, Georgia

D. RAOULT, M.D.
Unité des Rickettsies, Laboratoire de Bacteriologie-Sérologie-Virologie, Groupe Hospitalier de la Timone; Directeur, Centre National de Référence des Rickettsioses, Marseille, France

JONATHAN I. RAVDIN, M.D.
Associate Professor, Departments of Internal Medicine and Pharmacology, University of Virginia School of Medicine, Charlottesville, Virginia

RICHARD C. REICHMAN, M.D.
Associate Professor, Departments of Medicine and Microbiology and Immunology, University of Rochester School of Medicine and Dentistry; Attending Physician, Department of Medicine, Strong Memorial Hospital, Rochester, New York

MICHAEL F. REIN, M.D.
Professor, Department of Internal Medicine, University of Virginia School of Medicine, Charlottesville, Virginia

MARVIN S. REITZ, JR., PH.D.
Investigator, Laboratory of Tumor Cell Biology, Division of Cancer Etiology, National Cancer Institute, National Institutes of Health, Bethesda, Maryland

DAVID A. RELMAN, M.D.
Postdoctoral Fellow, Departments of Microbiology, Immunology, and Medicine, Standford University School of Medicine, Stanford, California

JACK S. REMINGTON, M.D.
Professor, Department of Medicine, Stanford University School of Medicine, Stanford, California; Chairman, Department of Immunology and Infectious Diseases, and Marcus A. Krupp Research Chair, Palo Alto Medical Foundation, Palo Alto, California

ANGELA RESTREPO M., PH.D.
Head, Mycology Laboratory, and Investigator, Corporacion para Investigaciones Biológicas, Medellín, Colombia

HERBERT Y. REYNOLDS, M.D.
Professor and Chairman, Department of Medicine, Pennsylvania State University College of Medicine, Hershey, Pennsylvania

NORBERT J. ROBERTS, JR., M.D.
Associate Professor, Department of Medicine, University of Rochester School of Medicine and Dentistry; Attending Physician, Strong Memorial Hospital, Rochester, New York

WILLIAM S. ROBINSON, M.D.
Professor, Department of Medicine, Stanford University School of Medicine, Stanford, California

RICHARD K. ROOT, M.D.
Professor and Chairman, Department of Medicine, University of California, San Francisco, School of Medicine, San Francisco, California

DANIEL ROTROSEN, M.D.
Senior Staff Fellow, Bacterial Diseases Section, Laboratory of Clinical Investigation, National Institute of Allergy and Infectious Diseases, National Institutes of Health, Bethesda, Maryland

ALFRED J. SAAH, M.D., M.P.H.
Associate Professor, Department of Epidemiology, Johns Hopkins University School of Hygiene and Public Health, and Associate Professor, Department of Medicine, Johns Hopkins University School of Medicine, Baltimore, Maryland

MERLE A. SANDE, M.D.
Professor and Vice Chairman, Department of Medicine, University of California, San Francisco, School of Medicine; Chief, Medical Service, San Francisco General Hospital, San Francisco, California

W. EUGENE SANDERS, JR., M.D.
Professor and Chairman, Department of Medical Microbiology, and Professor, Department of Medicine, Creighton University School of Medicine; Attending Physician, Department of Medicine, Veterans Administration Medical Center and St. Joseph Hospital, Omaha, Nebraska

JAY P. SANFORD, M.D.
Professor, Department of Medicine; President and Dean, Uniformed Services University of the Health Sciences F. Edward Hébert School of Medicine, Bethesda, Maryland

MARIA C. SAVOIA, M.D.
Assistant Adjunct Professor, Department of Medicine, University of California, San Diego, School of Medicine; Acting Chief, Department of Medicine, San Diego Veterans Administration Medical Center, San Diego, California

WILLIAM SCHAFFNER, M.D.
Professor and Chairman, Department of Preventive Medicine, and Professor, Department of Medicine, Vanderbilt University School of Medicine, Nashville, Tennessee

W. MICHAEL SCHELD, M.D.
Professor, Departments of Internal Medicine and Neurosurgery, University of Virginia School of Medicine, Charlottesville, Virginia

STEPHEN C. SCHIMPFF, M.D.
Professor, Departments of Medicine and Oncology, University of Maryland School of Medicine; Executive Vice President, University of Maryland Medical System, Baltimore, Maryland

CHARLES J. SCHLEUPNER, M.D.
Associate Professor, Department of Internal Medicine, University of Virginia School of Medicine, Charlottesville, Virginia; Chief, Infectious Diseases Section, Veterans Administration Medical Center, Salem, Virginia

ROBERT T. SCHOOLEY, M.D.
Associate Professor, Department of Medicine, Harvard Medical School; Assistant Physician, Infectious Disease Unit, Massachusetts General Hospital, Boston, Massachusetts

G. TOM SHIRES, M.D.
Lewis Atterbury Stimson Professor and Chairman, Department of Surgery, Cornell University Medical College; Surgeon-in-Chief, The New York Hospital, New York, New York

RICHARD L. SIMMONS, M.D.
George Vance Foster Professor and Chair, Department of Surgery, University of Pittsburgh School of Medicine; Chief of Surgery, Presbyterian-University Hospital, Pittsburgh, Pennsylvania

W. ANDREW SIMPSON, M.D.
Associate Professor, Departments of Medicine and Microbiology and Immunology, University of Missouri—Columbia School of Medicine, Columbia, Missouri

JAMES W. SMITH, M.D.
Professor, Department of Internal Medicine, University of Texas Health Science Center at Dallas Southwestern Medical School; Chief, Infectious Diseases Section, Veterans Administration Medical Center, Dallas, Texas

ROSEMARY SOAVE, M.D.
Assistant Professor, Departments of Medicine and Public Health, Cornell University Medical College; Assistant Attending Physician, Department of Medicine, The New York Hospital, New York, New York

JACK D. SOBEL, M.D.
Professor, Department of Medicine, and Chief, Division of Infectious Diseases, Wayne State University School of Medicine, Detroit, Michigan

ANASTACIO DE QUEIROZ SOUSA, M.D.
Assistant Professor, Department of Medicine, Federal University of Ceara, Fortaleza, Brazil

CAROL A. SPIEGEL, Ph.D., A.B.M.M.
Director, Clinical Microbiology Laboratory, University of Wisconsin Hospital and Clinics, Madison, Wisconsin

HAROLD C. STANDIFORD, M.D.
Professor, Department of Medicine, University of Maryland School of Medicine; Chief, Infectious Diseases Section, Veterans Administration Medical Center, Baltimore, Maryland

ALLEN C. STEERE, M.D.
Professor, Department of Medicine, and Chief, Department of Rheumatology and Immunology, Tufts University School of Medicine, Boston, Massachusetts

NEAL H. STEIGBIGEL, M.D.
Professor, Department of Medicine, Albert Einstein College of Medicine of Yeshiva University; Head, Division of Infectious Diseases, Montefiore Medical Center, Bronx, New York

DAVID A. STEVENS, M.D.
Professor, Department of Medicine, Stanford University School of Medicine, Stanford, California; Chief, Division of Infectious Diseases, Department of Medicine, Santa Clara Valley Medical Center; Principal Investigator, Infectious Diseases Research Laboratory, Institute for Medical Research, San Jose, California

MARK STOECKLE, M.D.
Assistant Professor, Department of Medicine, Cornell University Medical College; Attending Physician, Department of Medicine, The New York Hospital; Adjunct Faculty Member, Laboratory of Molecular Oncology, Rockefeller University, New York, New York

STEPHEN E. STRAUS, M.D.
Head, Medical Virology Section, Laboratory of Clinical Investigation, National Institute of Allergy and Infectious Diseases, National Institutes of Health, Bethesda, Maryland

STEPHEN A. STREED, M.S., C.I.C.
Manager, Epidemiology Systems, University of Iowa Hospital and Clinics, Iowa City, Iowa

ALAN M. SUGAR, M.D.
Associate Professor, Department of Medicine, Boston University School of Medicine, Boston, Massachusetts

BARRETT SUGARMAN, M.D.
Professor, Departments of Medicine, Microbiology, and Public Health, and Chief, Division of Infectious Diseases, Michigan State University College of Human Medicine, East Lansing, Michigan

MORTON N. SWARTZ, M.D.
Professor, Department of Medicine, Harvard Medical School; Chief, Department of Infectious Diseases, Massachusetts General Hospital, Boston, Massachusetts

ROBERT V. TAUXE, M.D.
Chief, Epidemiology Section, Enteric Diseases Branch, Division of Bacterial Diseases, Center for Infectious Diseases, Centers for Disease Control, Atlanta, Georgia

DAVID TAYLOR-ROBINSON, M.D.
Head, Division of Sexually Transmitted Diseases, MRC Clinical Research Centre, Harrow, Middlesex; Research Director, Jefferies Research Wing of the Praed Street Clinic, St. Mary's Hospital, London, England

MICHAEL G. THRELKELD, M.D.
Fellow, Department of Medicine, University of Alabama School of Medicine, Birmingham, Alabama

EDMUND C. TRAMONT, M.D.
Colonel, United States Army Medical Department; Professor, Department of Medicine, and Chief, Division of Infectious Diseases, Uniformed Services University of the Health Sciences F. Edward Hébert School of Medicine, Bethesda, Maryland; Associate Director, Walter Reed Army Institute of Research, Washington, D.C.

CARMELITA U. TUAZON, M.D.
Professor, Department of Medicine, and Director, Division of Infectious Disease, George Washington University School of Medicine and Health Sciences, Washington, D.C.

KENNETH L. TYLER, M.D.
Associate Professor, Department of Neurology-Neuroscience, Harvard Medical School; Assistant Neurologist, Department of Neurology, Massachusetts General Hospital, Boston, Massachusetts

DAVID E. VAN REKEN, M.D.
Clinical Associate Professor, Department of Pediatrics, Indiana University School of Medicine, Indianapolis, Indiana

PAUL A. VOLBERDING, M.D.
Associate Professor, Department of Medicine, and Chief, AIDS Activities Division, University of California, San Francisco, School of Medicine, San Francisco, California

KENNETH F. WAGNER, D.O.
Associate Professor, Department of Internal Medicine, Uniformed Services University of the Health Sciences F. Edward Hébert School of Medicine, Bethesda, Maryland; Senior Research Physician, HIV Research Program, Henry M. Jackson Foundation for the Advancement of Military Medicine, Bethesda, Maryland; Attending Physician, Department of Internal Medicine, Naval Hospital, Bethesda, Maryland, and Walter Reed Army Medical Center, Washington, D.C.

FRANCIS A. WALDVOGEL, M.D.
Professor, Department of Medicine, Faculty of Medicine, University of Geneva Medical School; Physician-in-Chief, Department of Medicine, Clinique Médicale Thérapeutique, University Hospital, Geneva, Switzerland

D. H. WALKER, M.D.
Professor and Chairman, Department of Pathology, University of Texas Medical School at Galveston, Galveston, Texas

PETER D. WALZER, M.D.
Professor, Department of Internal Medicine, University of Cincinnati College of Medicine; Chief, Division of Infectious Diseases, Department of Medical Services, Veterans Administration Medical Center, Cincinnati, Ohio

JOHN W. WARREN, M.D.
Associate Professor, Department of Medicine, and Head, Division of Infectious Diseases, University of Maryland School of Medicine, Baltimore, Maryland

KENNETH S. WARREN, M.D.
Professor, Department of Medicine, New York University School of Medicine; Adjunct Professor, Rockefeller University; Director for Science, Maxwell Communication Corporation, The Maxwell Foundation, New York, New York

RONALD G. WASHBURN, M.D.
Assistant Professor, Department of Medicine, Bowman Gray School of Medicine of Wake Forest University, Winston-Salem, North Carolina

JOHN A. WASHINGTON II, M.D.
Chairman, Department of Microbiology, The Cleveland Clinic Foundation, Cleveland, Ohio

PEYTON E. WEARY, M.D.
Professor and Chairman, Department of Dermatology, University of Virginia School of Medicine, Charlottesville, Virginia

DAVID J. WEBER, M.D., M.P.H.
Assistant Professor, Department of Medicine, University of North Carolina at Chapel Hill School of Medicine, Chapel Hill, North Carolina

CYNTHIA S. WEIKEL, M.D.
Assistant Professor, Department of Medicine, Johns Hopkins University School of Medicine, Baltimore, Maryland

MICHAEL E. WEISS, M.D.
Postdoctoral Fellow, Department of Medicine, Johns Hopkins University School of Medicine, Baltimore, Maryland

RICHARD P. WENZEL, M.D.
Professor, Department of Internal Medicine, and Director, Division of Clinical Epidemiology, University of Iowa College of Medicine; Hospital Epidemiologist, University of Iowa Hospitals and Clinics, Iowa City, Iowa

RICHARD J. WHITLEY, M.D.
Professor, Departments of Pediatrics and Microbiology, University of Alabama School of Medicine, Birmingham, Alabama

BARBARA BRAUNSTEIN WILSON, M.D.
Assistant Professor, Department of Dermatology, University of Virginia School of Medicine, Charlottesville, Virginia

CHRISTOPHER B. WILSON, M.D.
Professor, Department of Pediatrics, and Head, Division of Immunology and Rheumatology, University of Washington School of Medicine; Associate, Division of Infectious Disease, Children's Hospital and Medical Center, Seattle, Washington

BRIAN WISPELWEY, M.D.
Assistant Professor, Department of Internal Medicine, University of Virginia School of Medicine, Charlottesville, Virginia

MARTIN S. WOLFE, M.D.
Clinical Professor, Department of Medicine, George Washington University School of Medicine and Health Science, and Clinical Associate Professor, Department of Medicine, Georgetown University School of Medicine; Director, Traveler's Medical Service of Washington, Washington, D.C.

SHELDON M. WOLFF, M.D.
Endicott Professor and Chairman, Department of Medicine, Tufts University School of Medicine; Physician-in-Chief, New England Medical Center Hospital, Boston, Massachusetts

DAVID J. WYLER, M.D.
Professor, Department of Medicine, Tufts University School of Medicine; Physician and Director, Travelers' Health Service, Boston, Massachusetts

LOWELL S. YOUNG, M.D.
Clinical Professor, Department of Medicine, University of California, San Francisco, School of Medicine; Chief, Division of Infectious Diseases, Pacific Presbyterian Medical Center, and Director, Kuzell Institute for Arthritis and Infectious Diseases, Medical Research Institute of San Francisco, San Francisco, California

VICTOR L. YU, M.D.
Professor, Department of Medicine, University of Pittsburgh School of Medicine; Chief, Infectious Disease Section, Veterans Administration Medical Center, Pittsburgh, Pennsylvania

ROGER W. YURT, M.D.
Associate Professor and Vice Chairman, Department of Surgery, Cornell University Medical College; Director, Trauma Center, The New York Hospital, New York, New York

DORI F. ZALEZNIK, M.D.
Assistant Professor, Department of Medicine, Harvard Medical School; Hospital Epidemiologist, Division of Infectious Diseases, Beth Israel Hospital, Boston, Massachusetts

STEPHEN H. ZINNER, M.D.
Professor, Department of Medicine, Brown University Program in Medicine; Director, Infectious Diseases Section, Department of Medicine, Roger Williams General Hospital; Consultant in Infectious Disease, Rhode Island Hospital, Veterans Administration Medical Center, Miriam Hospital, and Women and Infants Hospital, Providence, Rhode Island

PREFACE TO THE THIRD EDITION

This expanded and extensively rewritten third edition reflects the immense changes that have occurred in the field of infectious diseases in the five years since the second edition of *Principles and Practice of Infectious Diseases* was published. The authors have met the challenge of providing accurate, up-to-date information relative to the science and practice of infectious diseases. All of the chapters have been revised, rewritten, and updated. Many new authors have been added to the roster of outstanding clinician-scientists, and chapters have been added to thoroughly cover important new aspects of our specialty.

Part I of the book considers basic principles important for the diagnosis and management of infectious diseases. New chapters in this section include A Molecular Perspective of Microbial Pathogenicity; Evaluation of the Patient with Suspected Immunodeficiency; Mechanisms of Antibiotic Resistance; β-Lactam Allergy; and Quinolones. New additions to Part II, which covers Major Clinical Syndromes, include The Acutely Ill Patient with Fever and Rash; Cystic Fibrosis; Infections with Prostheses in Bones and Joints; Slow Infections of the Central Nervous System; and an extensive coverage of the acquired immunodeficiency syndrome that includes epidemiology and prevention, immunology, clinical manifestations, diagnostic tests for HIV infection, therapy, and vaccines.

Newly recognized pathogens discussed in Part III, Infectious Diseases and Their Etiologic Agents, include papillomaviruses; reovirus and orbivirus; parvoviruses; retroviruses including the lentiviruses, human immunodeficiency viruses types 1 and 2, the oncoviruses, and human T-cell leukemia virus types I and II; prions; TWAR; *Borellia burgdorferi*; cat scratch disease agent; microsporidia; and *Ehrlichia* species. Finally, new considerations under Part IV, Special Problems, include HIV nosocomial infections; infections in bone marrow recipients; infections in solid organ transplant recipients; infections in patients with spinal cord injuries; and infections in the elderly.

We are immensely pleased with the superb job our publisher, Churchill Livingstone Inc., has done in producing the third edition. Special thanks go to Leslie Burgess, David Terry, and Beth Barry for their tireless devotion to excellence.

Gerald L. Mandell, M.D.
R. Gordon Douglas, Jr., M.D.
John E. Bennett, M.D.

PREFACE TO THE FIRST EDITION

Infectious diseases traverse the usual boundaries established by medical specialists. All organ systems may be involved, and all physicians caring for patients may have to deal with infected patients. The format of this book was chosen with the intent that it would contain the necessary information to aid the practitioner in the understanding, diagnosis, and treatment of infectious diseases. Thus, internists, family or general practitioners, pediatricians, surgeons, obstetrician-gynecologists, urologists, residents and fellows in training, medical students, hospital infection control personnel, and clinical microbiologists should find the book a valuable reference.

In planning this book the editors considered several different patterns of organization. The system adopted allows the reader to approach an infected patient three different ways: (a) by major clinical syndrome, (b) by specific etiologic organism, and (c) by host characteristics for patients who are compromised.

Principles and Practice of Infectious Diseases consists of four major parts. The book may be perused as a whole, or individual chapters may be examined when the reader is concerned with a specific problem. Part I covers the basic principles necessary for a clear understanding of the concepts of diagnosis and management of infectious disease. Chapters dealing with microbial virulence factors, host defense mechanisms, the epidemiology of infectious diseases, and the clinician and the microbiology laboratory are included. In addition, there is a comprehensive discussion of anti-infective chemotherapy.

Part II considers major clinical syndromes. The syndromes are described, followed by a discussion of the potential etiologic agents, evaluation of differential diagnostic possibilities, and an outline of presumptive therapy. All major infectious diseases are discussed in this part of the book.

Part III describes all important pathogenic microbes for man and the diseases they cause. The pathogen is classified and described, the epidemiology is discussed, clinical manifestations are listed, and specific information on therapy and prevention is presented. The most comprehensive discussion of a disease entity can be found by reading about both the etiologic agent and the clinical syndrome. Thus, a comprehensive treatment of pneumococcal pneumonia could be found in reading the appropriate sections of the chapters on acute pneumonia and *Streptococcus pneumoniae*. We attempted to make the chapters dealing with etiologic agents and those dealing with syndromes complete. Therefore some repetition was unavoidable.

The final section, Part IV, covers special problems in infectious diseases including nosocomial infections, infections in impaired hosts, immunizations, and protection of travelers.

The editors are grateful to our expert contributors. These physicians are the world's leaders in their fields, and they diligently prepared carefully written, well-referenced "state of the art" chapters. Our secretaries were skillful and meticulous in their attention to the complexities of assembling *Principles and Practices of Infectious Diseases*. John de Carville, executive editor of John Wiley & Sons, encouraged, cajoled, and advised us from the formative steps all the way through to completion. Lastly, and perhaps most important, we are grateful to our wives and children for putting up with interminable editorial work and meetings.

Gerald L. Mandell, M.D.
R. Gordon Douglas, Jr., M.D.
John E. Bennett, M.D.

PRINCIPLES AND PRACTICE OF

INFECTIOUS DISEASES

THIRD EDITION

BASIC PRINCIPLES IN THE DIAGNOSIS AND MANAGEMENT OF INFECTIOUS DISEASES

PART I

SECTION A. MICROBIAL VIRULENCE FACTORS

1. TOXINS AND OTHER VIRULENCE FACTORS

ERIK L. HEWLETT

Although humans are continually exposed to a vast array of microorganisms in the environment, only a small proportion of those microbes are capable of interacting with the host in such a way that infection and disease result. The capacity to cause disease is determined by the production of a variety of virulence factors by the infecting organism. Although it was once thought that all microorganisms elicit their adverse effects on hosts by elaboration of toxins, it is now clear that the pathogenetic process is complex and represents a well-orchestrated sequence of events in which many microbial components are required.

The first step in this process is the initial interaction of host and parasite. The adherence of microorganisms to host surfaces or tissues is now recognized to be highly specific and essential for subsequent events in the pathogenetic process to occur.[1] The specificity, mechanisms, and pathogenetic significance of bacterial attachment will be addressed in Chapter 2.

For some bacteria, the attachment to a mucosal surface represents the final destination. These bacteria, such as *Vibrio cholerae, Bordetella pertussis,* and some *Escherichia coli,* remain attached to the mucosa and exert their ill effects by cell contact and/or elaboration of toxins that interact with adjacent or distant cells. For many other organisms, however, the attachment process represents only the establishment of a beachhead from which tissue penetration and/or cell invasion can be launched. Organisms such as *Salmonella, Shigella,* and *Yersinia* penetrate the anatomic barriers of the host and either enter cells or disseminate within the body. In order to survive under these conditions all of these organisms have special virulence factors that enable them to avoid or disarm host defenses. Some are true toxins, in the classic sense, that kill, damage, or alter the function of host cells, but others such as staphylococcal protein A and the polysaccharide capsule of a variety of bacteria provide protection without being directly harmful to individual cells.

Survival and continued proliferation of the infecting organisms are often accompanied by the production of toxins, that is, protein molecules capable of adversely affecting cells or tissues of the host. In some cases, these toxins only enhance the development of the disease process, whereas in others they are the sine qua non in that they appear to be totally responsible for the manifestations of disease. Examples in this latter group include diphtheria, cholera, tetanus, and botulinum toxins.

Finally, one of the following three outcomes results: (*1*) The proliferation of organisms and production of toxic products impair the host to such an extent that the host dies. (*2*) A state of relative equilibrium is reached with the establishment of a chronic infection. (*3*) Host defense mechanisms, with or without the aid of exogenous factors such as antibiotics, supervene, and the infecting organism is cleared. It is of note that in some cases elimination of the causative organism may not be sufficient to terminate the disease process because toxin effects or immunologic reactions may persist in the absence of microbes.

The remainder of this chapter is devoted to the role of bacterial toxins and other components such as virulence factors. Additional information on each example cited herein can be obtained from the chapters on specific causative organisms.

TOXINS

Classification and Structure of Toxins

The word *toxin* is derived from the Greek *toxikon,* bow poison, referring to poisonous material placed on arrows by Greek warriors. The implication of this choice of terms is that the bacterium produces a molecule that it "releases" to affect host cells at a distance. The term was first used by Roux and Yersin to describe the factor released into the culture medium by *Corynebacterium diphtheriae* that caused the death of recipient animals.[2] Subsequently, many toxins have been identified, and confusion has arisen concerning the terminology used to describe and classify different toxins. Exotoxin was previously used to refer to toxins produced by and released from gram-positive bacteria during growth, whereas endotoxin was used for the intracellular and cell-associated toxic components of gram-negative organisms, including the lipopolysaccharide component that now bears the name endotoxin. Because gram-negative bacteria are now recognized to elaborate classic protein toxins, it seems prudent that the term *exotoxin* be used for bacterial products that are protein in nature, are released from the bacterium during exponential growth, and are toxic for target cells or experimental animals. As noted earlier, this definition excludes protein toxins that are intracellular and released only with lysis of the bacterial cells (intracellular or cell-associated toxins), gram-negative bacterial lipopolysaccharide, and bacterial virulence factors that may be involved in attachment, local or systemic dissemination, and acquisition of nutrients but that possess no capacity for direct toxicity to the host.

Although exotoxins occur in many forms, there is a general structural model to which a number of the important exotoxins conform (Table 1). According to the A-B model described by Gill, each of these toxins is composed of a binding (B) domain, component, or subunit portion and an enzymatic (A) portion, which is responsible for the toxic effect once inside the cell.[12] Isolated A subunits are enzymatically active but lack binding and cell entry capability and thus have no biologic activity (the ability to intoxicate intact cells). Isolated B subunits, on the other hand, may bind to target cells and even block the action of holotoxin, but they are, in most instances, nontoxic and biologically inactive.

Other criteria by which toxins may be classified are their cellular or tissue target of action (i.e., enterotoxins, neurotoxins, leukotoxins), their mechanisms of action (ADP-ribosylating toxins, adenylate cyclase toxins, etc., Table 1), their major biologic effects (dermonecrotic toxin, edema-producing toxin, hemolytic toxin, lymphocytosis-promoting toxin), and the establishment of their contribution to the pathogenicity of the disease process (Table 2). Quite clearly the difficulties associated with describing and classifying these bacterial products reflect limitations in our knowledge of their production, target cell interaction, mechanism of action, and clinical significance. The available information on these aspects of bacterial toxins is discussed below.

Control of Synthesis and Release of Toxins

There are many variations in the genetic regulation of toxin production.[12] For example, both regulatory and structural genes

TABLE 1. Properties of A-B Type Bacterial Toxins

Toxin	*Organism*	*Genetic Control*	*Subunit Structure*	*Target Cell Receptor*	*Enzymatic Activity*	*Biologic Effects*
Anthrax toxins	*B. anthracis*	Plasmid	Three separate proteins (EF, LF, PA)[a]	Unknown, probably glycoprotein	EF is a calmodulin-dependent adenylate cyclase; LF enzyme activity is unknown	EF + PA: increase in target cell cAMP level, localized edema; LF + PA: death of target cells and experimental animals
Bordetella adenylate cyclase toxin	*Bordetella* species	Chromosomal	A-B[b]	Unknown, probably glycolipid	Calmodulin-activated cyclase	Increase in target cell cAMP level; modified cell function or cell death
Botulinum toxin	*C. botulinum*	Phage	A-B[c]	Possibly ganglioside (GD_{1b})	None known	Decrease in peripheral, presynaptic acetylcholine release; flaccid paralysis
Cholera toxin	*V. cholera*	Chromosomal	A-5B[d]	Ganglioside (GM_1)	ADP ribosylation of adenylate cyclase regulatory protein, G_s	Activation of adenylate cyclase, increase in cAMP level; secretory diarrhea
Diphtheria toxin	*C. diphtheriae*	Phage	A-B[e]	Probably glycoprotein	ADP ribosylation of elongation factor II	Inhibition of protein synthesis; cell death
Heat-labile enterotoxins[f]	*E. coli*	Plasmid	Similar or identical to cholera toxin			
Pertussis toxin	*B. pertussis*	Chromosomal	A-5B[g]	Unknown, probably glycoprotein	ADP ribosylation of signal-transducing G proteins	Block of signal transduction mediated by target G proteins
Pseudomonas exotoxin A	*P. aeruginosa*	Chromosomal	A-B	Unknown, but different from diphtheria toxin	Similar or identical to diphtheria toxin	
Shiga toxin	*S. dysenteriae*	Chromosomal	A-5B[h]	Glycoprotein or glycolipid	RNA *N*-glycosidase	Inhibition of protein synthesis, cell death
Shiga-like toxins	*Shigella* species, *E. coli*	Phage	Similar or identical to shiga toxin			
Tetanus toxin	*C. tetani*	Plasmid	A-B[c]	Ganglioside (GT_1 and/or GD_{1b})	None known	Decrease in neurotransmitter release from inhibitory neurons; spastic paralysis

[a] The binding component (known as protective antigen [PA]) catalyzes/facilitates the entry of either edema factor (EF) or lethal factor (LF).[3]
[b] Apparently synthesized as a single polypeptide with binding and catalytic (adenylate cyclase) domains.[4]
[c] Holotoxin is apparently synthesized as a single polypeptide and cleaved proteolytically as diphtheria toxin; subunits are referred to as L: light chain, A equivalent; H: heavy chain, B equivalent.[5,6]
[d] The A subunit is proteolytically cleaved into A_1 and A_2, with A_1 possessing the ADP-ribosyl transferase activity; the binding component is made up of five identical B units.
[e] Holotoxin is synthesized as a single polypeptide and cleaved proteolytically into A and B components held together by disulfide bonds.[7]
[f] The heat-labile enterotoxins of *E. coli* are now recognized to be a family of related molecules with identical mechanisms of action.[8]
[g] The binding portion is made up of two dissimilar heterodimers labeled S2-S3 and S2-S4 that are held together by a bridging peptide, S5.[9]
[h] Similar subunit composition and structure to cholera toxin.[10]

TABLE 2. Categorization of Bacterial Toxins according to Their Relative Contribution to Disease Pathogenesis

Well-studied toxin with a clear role as a major effector
- Diphtheria toxin
- Botulinum toxin
- Tetanus toxin
- Enterotoxins
  - Cholera toxin
  - *E. coli* heat-labile toxin (LT)
  - *E. coli* heat-stable tosin (ST_a)
  - Staphylococcal enterotoxin (neurotoxin)
  - Clostridial enterotoxin

Well-studied toxin with a contributory role
- Anthrax toxins (edema factor, lethal factor, protective antigen)
- *Pseudomonas* exotoxin A

Well-studied toxin with a probable, but unproven role
- Pertussis toxin and *Bordetella* extracytoplasmic adenylate cyclase
- *Shigella* (shiga) toxin
- Streptolysin O and other streptococcal toxins
- Other clostridial toxins (including *C. difficile* cytotoxin)
- Cholera-like enterotoxins produced by *Salmonella, Klebsiella, Aeromonas,* and *Citrobacter*
- Yersinia toxins
- Other staphylococcal toxins (toxic shock syndrome toxin, TSST-1)

for toxin synthesis and release may be chromosomal in location, as is the case for cholera toxin.[13] Production of the family of immunologically and functionally homologous heat-labile toxins of *E. coli,* on the other hand, is plasmid mediated.[13] The structural gene for diphtheria toxin is located on a β-phage, but toxin synthesis is inhibited by excess iron, apparently through interaction with a factor of bacterial origin.[7] The structural gene for tetanus toxin is located on a large (75 kilobase [kb]) plasmid.[14] The pertussis toxin gene is present in three *Bordetella* species but is expressed only in *B. pertussis* due to mutations in the promoter region of the gene in *B. parapertussis* and *B. bronchiseptica.*[15,16] Finally, the gene for staphylococcal enterotoxin may be either chromosomal or plasmid in location, but its production is regulated by genes on a plasmid.[17]

The question of how large proteins such as toxins are exported from the bacterial cell has been clarified by analysis of DNA sequences. There are two major hypotheses to explain the mechanism, the signal hypothesis and the membrane trigger hypothesis.[18] Many of the classic exotoxins are synthesized with an NH-terminal signal or leader sequence consisting of a few (1–3) charged amino acids and a stretch (14–20) of hydrophobic amino acids.[19] The signal sequence may bind and be inserted into the cytoplasmic membrane during translation such that the polypeptide is secreted while being synthesized. The signal peptide is then cleaved, which leaves the intact toxin molecule free in the periplasm. Alternatively (membrane trigger hypothesis), the protein may be synthesized intracytoplasmically. Subsequent binding via the leader sequence to the cytoplasmic membrane may cause a conformational change allowing the protein to traverse the membrane with or without the help of pores or transport molecules. The synthesis and release of some toxins such as *E. coli* hemolysin clearly entail a process requiring the products of multiple genes involved in processing and/or transport.[20] Some multicomponent toxins such as cholera toxin have their subunits secreted separately; they are then assembled in the periplasmic space. In gram-negative organisms, however, the outer membrane provides an additional barrier for escape of periplasmic protein molecules.

Middledorp and Witholt have proposed that some toxins such as *E. coli* heat-labile toxin may not be released but rather delivered to target cells while contained in vesicles of the outer membrane.[21] These vesicles would possess outer membrane-associated attachment factors enabling them to act as "bombs" capable of interacting with and possibly entering target cells to release their contents of toxin.

Attachment and Entry of Toxins

Some toxins such as the hemolytic phospholipases are bacterial exoenzymes that appear to interact with the external surface of host cell membranes by catalyzing their specific reactions and thereby eliciting their toxic effects without cell entry.[22] A number of toxins, however, act on intracellular substrates and thus require cell entry to be effective. Most of these conform to the A-B model described earlier[11] and have binding components that interact with specific receptors on the target cells such as the sialogangliosides GM_1 for cholera toxin, GT_1 for tetanus toxin, and probably GD_{1b} for botulinum toxin.[23] The relatively wide distribution of FM_1 ganglioside among cell types accounts for the apparent lack of specificity of cholera toxin in vitro. The specificity of the effect of cholera toxin during infection (secretory diarrhea), however, is due to the localization of the organisms and the toxin to the intestinal tract. Pertussis toxin has been shown to interact with sialic acid-containing glycoproteins,[23,24] which also must be widespread since most cells are sensitive to intoxication by pertussis toxin. Diphtheria toxin and *Pseudomonas* exotoxin A, on the other hand, catalyze the identical reaction intracellularly[7,25] and are both distributed systemically, yet the resultant disease processes are quite distinct. The differences between the two appear to reside, at least in part, at the level of target cell specificities.[26]

There are several different mechanisms by which the A subunits of A-B toxins enter the target cell. In each case, however, a large protein molecule must insert into or cross the lipid bilayer.[27] In some cases such as diphtheria toxin, there appears to be binding to a surface receptor, uptake into an endocytotic vesicle, and acidification of that vesicle so as to result in a conformational change that enables a part of the toxin molecule to traverse the membrane.[7] The final step in diphtheria toxin translocation is energy requiring and dependent upon membrane potential and a proton gradient.[28] A part of this process can be mimicked in vitro with diphtheria toxin B subunit, which makes artificial membranes permeable to small ions.[29] *Pseudomonas* exotoxin A appears to be internalized somewhat differently, by endocytosis into coated pits and vesicles.[27]

Often toxins with identical enzymatic mechanisms also enter cells by separate and distinct pathways. Adenylate cyclase toxins from *Bordetella pertussis* and *Bacillus anthracis* both catalyze the production of cAMP from host intracellular ATP stores.[4] Anthrax toxin (edema factor plus protective antigen [EF + PA]) enters by receptor-mediated endocytosis, whereas pertussis adenylate cyclase toxin has a different entry mechanism to traverse the cell membrane directly.[30] For many toxins such as pertussis toxin, tetanus toxin, and others, putative receptors have been identified, but the entry mechanisms remain a mystery.

Mechanism of Toxin Action and Role in Clinical Disease

As noted earlier, bacterial toxins can be categorized according to our concept of their relative contribution to the disease process with which they are associated (Table 2). In this section, individual toxins and families of toxins will be discussed by that classification scheme. The criteria indicating a major pathogenic role for a particular toxin include (*1*) production of the toxin by pathogenic organisms and not by avirulent ones, (*2*) avirulence of organisms specifically lacking the toxin, (*3*) protection against disease by antibody against the toxin, and (*4*) the ability of purified toxin to mimic the disease.[31]

Diphtheria Toxin. One of the most extensively studied of all toxins is that produced by β-phage–infected *C. diphtheriae*.[7] It is the prototype ADP-ribosylating toxin that inhibits cellular protein synthesis by catalyzing the transfer of ADP-ribose from nicotinamide adenine dinucleotide (NAD) to elongation factor II.[7] This single enzymatic reaction, which is responsible for the systemic toxicity in clinical diphtheria, does not occur in individuals infected with nontoxigenic strains. The widespread control of diphtheria with the use of diphtheria toxoid attests to the dominant role of this toxin both in the establishment of infection and in the systemic manifestations of disease. As noted in Table 1, exotoxin A of *Pseudomonas aeruginosa* catalyzes the identical reaction but is associated with a disease process quite different from diphtheria. These differences are felt to be due to different tissue (Target cell) specificities of the toxins[26] and to the fact that exotoxin A is only one of a number of virulence factors involved in *Pseudomonas*-induced disease.[32]

Tetanus Toxin. In contrast to diphtheria, immunization with tetanus toxin has no effect on the establishment of infection with *Clostridium tetani*. The resultant antibody response does, however, totally prevent the disease process of clinical tetanus, the major effector role of tetanus toxin. The toxin exhibits selectivity for neural tissue, being taken up at myoneural junctions and transported by retrograde axonal flow to alpha motoneuron synapses. It crosses the synapse where it acts presynaptically to impair inhibitory neurotransmitter release.[5] The toxin specificity is attributed to its binding domain, which interacts with cell surface ganglioside (GT_1 or GD_{1b}). Tetanus toxin can, however, at high enough concentrations cause the inhibition of acetylcholine release at the myoneural junction and flaccid paralysis equivalent to that elicited by botulinum toxin.[33] There are also structural homologies between the two toxins, which suggests that they may act by a similar, as yet unknown intracellular mechanism and may be derived from a common ancestral gene.[34] While tetanus toxin is not known to affect non-neuronal cells clinically, it can inhibit exocytosis when injected into adrenal chromaffin cells.[35] Furthermore, tetanus toxin causes the inhibition of lysozyme secretion from human macrophages and is associated with reduced protein kinase C activity.[36,37] Such studies provide a new approach for study of the mechanism of tetanus toxin action in vitro.

Botulinum Toxin. Botulinum toxin is among the most potent toxins known, with a human lethal dose (toxin type A) of approximately 1 ng/kg.[38] "Botulinum toxin" consists of a family of seven immunologically distinct molecules, most of which cause flaccid paralysis by inhibiting myoneural junction acetylcholine release.[6] The mechanism of this neurotoxic activity is unknown, but a related toxin from *C. botulinum*, botulinum C2 toxin, possesses ADP-ribosyl transferase activity, with G-actin as the target substrate.[39]

The classic presentation of clinical botulism results from the ingestion of preformed toxin in improperly prepared foods. A subacute intoxication can occur in infants (infant botulism) harboring *C. botulinum* in their gastrointestinal tracts.[40] In most cases the low-level toxin absorption results in listlessness and hypotonia, but the course can be fulminant, and infant botulism has been proposed as a cause of sudden infant death syndrome.[40]

Cholera Toxin and Escherichia coli Heat-Labile Toxin. Cholera and *E. coli* heat-labile enterotoxin (LT) are discussed together because their structures are similar and their mechanisms of action appear to be identical.[41] It has been recognized recently, however, that the heat-labile enterotoxins of *E. coli* represent a more heterogeneous group, with some (type II) being nonimmunologically cross-reactive and interacting with a different receptor despite operating by an apparently identical mechanism of action.[8] Cholera toxin and the LTs promote isotonic intestinal secretion by catalyzing the ADP ribosylation of the B-subunit of the stimulatory guanine nucleotide protein G_s.[41] This covalent modification causes semipermanent activation of the cellular adenylate cyclase and increased cAMP accumulation. While these enterotoxins reproduce the secretory diarrhea when administered experimentally, it is clear that multiple other bacterial components such as attachment factors, mucinase, etc., are required for establishment of infection and perhaps toxin delivery in order for the disease process to occur.

Enterotoxin effects can be prevented by the addition of specific antibody to toxin in animal assay systems,[42] but the use of parenteral toxoid immunization has been largely unsuccessful. The combination of killed whole *Vibrio cholerae* organisms and purified nontoxic B-subunit administered orally has shown limited efficacy in vaccine trials.[43] Genetically engineered vaccines consisting of organisms that produce inactive toxin are being evaluated for oral use at present.[44] Related enterotoxins are produced by a variety of other gram-negative organisms such as *Klebsiella, Salmonella, Aeromonas,* and *Plesiomonas,* but the incidence of diarrhea caused by these organisms and the roles of such toxins in that disease are unknown.

Escherichia coli Heat-Stable Toxin. A separate enterotoxin produced by *E. coli* causes diarrhea in humans. This heat-stable toxin, referred to as ST_a or ST-I, is a peptide of 18 or 19 amino acids.[45] It causes secretory diarrhea by promoting the activation of intestinal particulate guanylate cyclase and increasing cyclic guanosine monophosphate (GMP) levels in the jejunum and ileum.[46] Unlike cholera toxin and LT, ST_a exhibits striking target cell specificity with little activity in extraintestinal tissues.[47] The molecule is poorly immunogenic alone, but antitoxin antibody may develop against hybrid toxins in which St_a is covalently linked to LT B-subunits.[48] As with LT, other bacterial species such as *Yersinia enterocolitica,* non-01 *Vibrio cholerae,* and *Citrobacter freundii* can produce homologous molecules that are of unknown significance.[49]

There is a second heat-stable enterotoxin of *E. coli,* ST_b or ST-II, that is not a human pathogen but produces diarrhea in piglets by a noncyclic nucleotide mechanism.[50]

Toxins of Bordetella pertussis. *Bordetella pertussis,* the causative agent of whooping cough, produces several toxins that have striking effects in experimental systems and are hypothesized to be major contributors to the pathophysiology of the disease process. Pertussis toxin, also known as lymphocytosis-promoting factor, histamine-sensitizing factor, or islet-activating protein, is expressed only by *B. pertussis,* although a silent gene is present in *B. parapertussis*.[16] Pertussis toxin acts by ADP ribosylating several members of the family of guanine nucleotide-binding G proteins involved in cellular signal transduction.[9] The result of this covalent modification is inhibition of G protein function and consequently interruption of the signal from the receptor to inhibition of adenylate cyclase, activation of phospholipase, or modulation of ion channels.[9,51] Although pertussis toxin is clearly a virulence factor for *B. pertussis* and a protective antigen,[52,53] its role in clinical pertussis remains unclear. In contrast to tetanus and botulinum toxins, pertussis toxin can be given to human volunteers (1 μg/kg iv) without adverse effects.[54]

Bordetella species also produce an adenylate cylcase toxin that can enter target cells to catalyze the production of cAMP from endogenous ATP.[4] This toxin is also a virulence factor for *B. pertussis*[52] and is believed to contribute to both the evasion of host defenses by the organism and damage to the respiratory mucosa.[55]

Anthrax Toxins. *Bacillus anthracis* produces three toxin components that are novel in their interaction with cells.[3] None of the three components, edema factor (EF), lethal factor (LF), or protective antigen (PA) has toxin activity alone. Edema factor is a calmodulin-dependent adenylate cyclase analogous to *Bordetella* adenylate cyclase toxin and when combined with PA is able to enter target cells to increase cAMP levels.[3] Lethal factor when combined with PA is lethal for macrophages and experimental animals by unknown mechanisms.[56] Protective antigen serves as the binding subunit to facilitate the entry of either EF or LF into target cells. Protective antigen is so named because it is an important PA in anthrax vaccine. The genes for all three toxin components are located on plasmids.[57]

Shiga and Shiga-like Toxins. *Shigella dysenteriae* 1 produces a toxin, shiga toxin, that is responsible for a variety of biologic activities in experimental animals including neurotoxicity, enterotoxicity, and cytotoxicity.[58] The toxin conforms to the A-B model, with a subunit structure similar to cholera toxin (i.e., A-5B).[10] The A subunit causes inhibition of protein synthesis by enzymatic inactivation of 60S ribosomes within the target cell by a process (RNA *N*-glycosidase) analogous to that employed by ricin.[59,60] Despite the striking effects of shiga toxin in vitro, definition of its role in clinical shigellosis remains circumstantial.[61]

A family of related molecules designated shiga-like toxins (previously vero toxins) have been demonstrated in other *Shigella* species and *E. coli*.[10] These toxins have been implicated in enteropathogenic (EPEC)- and enterohemorrhagic (EHEC)-mediated disease as well as hemolytic–uremic syndrome.[10] Those shiga-like toxins that are neutralized by antishiga toxin serum are designated SLT-I, while those which are not immunologically cross-reactive are SLT-II.[10] As with other toxins, the genetic regulation is different in the different organisms; the shiga toxin gene in *S. dysenteriae* is chromosomal, while production of shiga-like toxin in *E. coli* is phage mediated.[62]

Other toxins. The list of toxins discussed in the preceding sections is, by no means, all inclusive. It is, however, representative of those toxins that are most extensively characterized with regard to their roles in pathogenesis. Additional toxins include toxins A and B of *Clostridium difficile,* which appear to be involved in psuedomembranes colitis but by unknown mechanisms.[63] There are other toxins, such as the heterogeneous group of molecules known as hemolysins, which are also important virulence factors. One group (i.e., *C. perfringens* α toxin) possesses phospholipase C activity and produces hemolysis by cleavage of membrane phospholipids on target cells.[63a] Another group (some of which are activated by sulfhydryl reagents) appear to act by inserting into host cell membranes. Examples include streptolysins S and O, staphylococcal α-toxin, and *E. coli* hemolysin.[64–65a] The hemolysins from intracellular pathogens such as *Shigella flexneri* and *Listeria monocytogenes* are virulence factors that are postulated to aid the organism in its disruption of phagosome membranes during entry into the cytoplasm.[65b,65c] Most hemolysins are also cytolytic for other host cells such as leukocytes. While there are many other toxins that have been identified, their contributions to the diseases caused by the respective organisms is, in many cases, uncertain.

OTHER VIRULENCE FACTORS

In contrast to toxins, "other virulence factors" are, by definition, not toxic to target cells. Although bacterial virulence is often quantitated by the number of organisms required to kill 50 percent of challenged experimental animals (LD_{50}), any single nontoxin virulence factor alone is likely to have little or no effect on a host animal. In most cases, the pathophysiologic process requires the concerted action of a variety of microbial products, including those involved in attachment (see Chapter 2), entry into the host and dissemination, acquisition of nutrients, proliferation, avoidance of host defenses, and production of tissue damage.[66] A loss of virulence in association with elimination of a specific bacterial component is strongly supportive of a major role for that factor in the pathogenic process. Production of one or more putative virulence factors by avirulent strains, however, does not mean that they are not, in fact, virulence factors. Because infection and disease result from a carefully orchestrated sequence of events, single factors are often inadequate to promote the development of disease without their supporting cast.

Many virulence factors do possess specific biologic activities that interfere with normal host function to the advantage of the microbe.[67,68] The discussion of these other virulence factors will focus on those responsible for circumventing major host defenses such as anatomic barriers, serum (humoral) factors, and phagocytic cells (Table 3). The examples are primarily those of pathogenic bacteria, and the reader is referred to specific reviews for information on viral and parasitic virulence mechanisms.[66,69,70] It is important to note that the current understanding of virulence mechanisms is frequently incomplete and there are many factors that have been demonstrated to be major virulence determinants yet have no biologic or biochemical activity yet identified.[67] Examples include the V protein and W lipoprotein of *Yersinia* species[68] and the Vi antigen of *Salmonella* species,[71] which have been postulated to contribute to cell invasion and avoidance of host clearance mechanisms. This deficiency in the knowledge of pathogenesis is being overcome by molecular biologic approaches to define the structure of these antigens and their role in the disease process.[72]

Virulence Factors for Overcoming Anatomic Barriers

The first line of host defense against microorganisms is the anatomic barrier of skin and mucous membranes. These "external" surfaces are colonized by normal flora, which in itself provides a barrier against the uncontrolled proliferation of potentially pathogenic bacteria. Thus, in order for pathogens to survive and proliferate to sufficient to numbers to cause disease, they must compete successfully with the other microorganisms present. Many bacteria produce bacteriocins, which are toxins directed at other microbes.[73] These products provide an adaptive advantage, and some even exhibit activity against host cells such as mononuclear phagocytes, which further explains their contribution to microbial virulence.[74]

Although many organisms are able to enter the body through skin disrupted by laceration, abrasion, a puncture wound, or an insect bite, there are no bacteria known to be capable of penetrating intact skin. In contrast, some parasites such as cercariae of *Schistosoma mansoni* and larvae of *Strongyloides stercoralis, Ancylostoma duodenale,* and *Necator americanus* do have this capability (direct penetration of intact skin), which represents a major mechanism for entry into the host.

Many bacteria gain access to the body through breaks in the mucosa of the respiratory, gastrointestinal, or genitourinary tracts and thus are not truly "invasive." In contrast, invasive organisms such as *Salmonella typhimurium, Shigella flexneri, Yersinia enterocolitica,* and some *Escherichia coli* strains have a special capacity for the penetration of intact cells.[72,75–78] When administered by the oral route, wild-type *S. flexneri* organisms are lethal for guinea pigs, whereas noninvasive mutants are without effect.[75] The importance of other virulence factors, however, is illustrated by the full virulence (lethality) of the noninvasive mutants when administered intraperitoneally to mice.[75] This process, which may be the sine qua non of virulence for these organisms, occurs by a poorly understood process.

Invasive strains of *E. coli* are restricted to a few serotypes and have been shown to share surface determinants with invasive shigellae, which suggests that these components may be involved in the invasion process.[75,76] In vitro models of invasiveness have been developed with the use of tissue culture cells, which allows for the screening of many strains for the invasiveness trait.[77,78] With this approach, large (>100 megadalton) plasmids have been demonstrated to be associated with invasiveness in several organisms.[72,79–81]

Bacterial proteins with a variety of enzymatic activities such as protease, hyaluronidase, neuraminidase, elastase, collagenase, and mucinase have been postulated to contribute to cell invasion. While these products are certainly contributory to virulence factors for many bacteria, their role appears to be in facilitating local tissue spread of the organisms rather than the primary invasion event.

Virulence Factors for Avoiding or Disrupting Humoral Defenses

One secondary line of defense against microbial infections is provided by humoral factors such as antibody, complement, complement-activated mediators, and an assortment of other soluble host proteins such as clotting factors, B-lysin, and transferrin. Several organisms have mechanisms that impair antibody production at different sites in the multistep process. These include induction of suppressor cells,[82] blockade of antigen processing,[83] and inhibition of lymphocyte mitogenesis.[84] Other bacteria possess antiphagocytic capsules that either prevent the binding of opsonic antibodies or allow them to penetrate the capsule and bind but prevent subsequent interaction with phagocytic cell receptors.[85]

While there is little complement present on mucosal surfaces, antibody such as secretory IgA may be active against microorganisms even before invasion. In response to this protective measure of the host, several organisms including *Neisseria gonorrhoeae, Streptococcus pneumonia,* and *Haemophilus influenzae* produce IgA-specific proteases that cleave and inactivate the secretory antibody.[86,87] Similarly, the ability of organisms to elaborate factors that modify or degrade serum components such as fibrin, heparin, and clotting factors is recognized to be associated with increased virulence. The binding of the F_c domains of host immunoglobulin by staphylococcal protein A is postulated to represent a protective mechanism. The production of protein A by a variety of virulent and avirulent staphylococcal strains, however, has prevented adequate assessment of this possibility.

One of the bacterial traits most clearly associated with virulence or systemic infections is resistance to the lytic effect of serum. It has long been recognized that most blood stream isolates are serum resistant.[88] This observation explains why the *N. gonorrhoeae* isolates from patients with disseminated disease are serum resistant while those isolated only from the genital tract are predomiantly serum sensitive.[89] The serum lytic

TABLE 3. Other Virulence Factors[a] and Their Activities

Penetration of anatomic barriers
Bacteriocins
Direct skin penetration activity
Mucosal invasiveness traits
Connective tissue-disrupting enzymes
Disruption or avoidance of humoral factors
Antibody-degrading enzymes
Enzymes that disrupt other humoral factors (fibrinolysin)
Serum resistance
Avoidance or inactivation of phagocytic cells
Components resulting in impaired phagocytosis
Factors preventing oxidative burst
Molecules preventing phagosome–lysosome fusion
Surfaces that are resistant to lysosomal enzymes

[a] Adherence factors are excluded here but are discussed in Chapter 2.

effect in gram-negative organisms is complement-mediated but can be activated by either of two pathways. Many organisms entering the blood stream activate complement by the classic pathway in an antibody-dependent manner and are lysed by the membrane attach complex (C_{5b}-C_9).[88–90] In contrast, some organisms are direct activators of the alternative pathway, but their killing may be enhanced by an antibody-mediated amplification.[91] Antibodies involved in both of these processes arise from prior exposure to the organisms or reflect cross-reactivity with antigens from common organisms in the environment.[92] Several mechanisms appear to be involved in serum resistance including (*1*) a failure to activate complement, (*2*) shedding of molecules that activate the system, (*3*) blockade of activation before the formation of C_{5b}-C_9, and (*4*) formation of a nonlytic complex.[93] In addition, some bacteria and parasites have been shown to invade host cells by using complement deposited on their surfaces to facilitate interaction with target cell complement receptors.[93a,93b] The structure and quantity of lipopolysaccharide (LPS) on the surface of gram-negative organisms, including that absorbed from the medium, may contribute to resistance.[94] Plasmids encoding some outer membrane proteins may enhance virulence by virtue of the binding of LPS to the induced surface components.[95] In other cases, serum resistance is mediated by masking of sensitive surface antigens by K antigens,[90,96] nonbactericidal blocking antibodies,[97] or sialic acid residues.[91] The latter modification creates a surface that is poor in its ability to activate the alternative pathway of complement.[91,93]

Nontoxin Virulence Factors Directed at Phagocytic Cells

Microbes that have penetrated the protection of anatomic barriers meet another main line of the host defenses, phagocytic cells including polymorphonuclear leukocytes, monocytes, and macrophages. The phagocytosis and killing of microorganisms are part of a specific sequence of events consisting of (*1*) attraction of the phagocyte in a chemotactic gradient of bacterial products, (*2*) movement of the phagocyte to the site, (*3*) contact between the organism and the phagocyte, (*4*) phagocytosis (ingestion), (*5*) development of an oxidative burst, (*6*) fusion of the phagosome and lysosome with degranulation of lysosomal contents, and (*7*) death and degradation of the ingested organism (see Chapter 7).[66,98] In the evolution of virulence mechanisms, microbes have developed methods to elude, inactivate, or ignore each of these steps.[98,99]

Parasites are particularly adept at disguising their surfaces to avoid recognition by immune effector cells.[100] Similarly, an array of microorganisms resists phagocytosis by protective surface components such as capsular polysaccharide or other antigens.[101–103] The capsule of *Bacteroides fragilis* is not only antiphagocytic but also plays a major role in the induction of abscess formation by this organism.[101] Other pathogenic parasites and bacteria such as *Toxoplasma gondii, Leishmania* sp., *Legionella pneumophila,* and *Listeria monocytogenes* either do not elicit or actively suppress the oxidative response associated with surface contact and phagocytosis.[102–104] In addition, many organisms produce enzymes such as catalase, glutathione peroxidase, and superoxide dismutase that destroy the reactive oxygen species generated in the oxidative burst, or they are individually resistant to those reactive lethal molecules.[103,104] Still other organisms survive intracellularly by inhibiting phagosome–lysosome fusions.[105] Several mycobacteria appear to do so by increasing phagocyte cAMP concentrations to inhibitory levels.[106] Finally, microbes such as *Mycobacterium leprae, Salmonella enteritidis* serotype *typhimurium,* and *Leishmania* sp. survive despite phagosome–lysosome fusion and degranulation, apparently by virtue of innate resistance to the lysosomal enzymes.[105,107] Although the mechanisms of these microbial defensive actions are largely unknown, it is clear that they play a major role in the establishment of intracellular infections.

Finally, as mentioned earlier, there are a number of recognized characteristics of microorganisms that are associated with virulence but are of unknown pathophysiologic significance such as the presence of large plasmids,[108] The complete understanding of the pathogenetic process and the role of these additional factors awaits future research efforts.

REFERENCES

1. Beachey EH, ed. Bacterial Adherence. London: Chapman & Hall; 1980:1.
2. Roux E, Yersin A. Contribution a l'étude de la diphtherie. Ann Inst Pasteur. 1988;2:629.
3. Leppla SH. *Bacillus anthracis* calmodulin-dependent adenylate cyclase: Chemical and enzymatic properties and interactions with eucaryotic cells. Adv Cyclic Nucleotide Prot Phos Res 1984;17:189.
4. Hewlett EL, Gordon VM. Adenylate cyclase toxin of *Bordetella pertussis*. In: Wardlaw AC, Parton R, eds. Pathogenesis and Immunity in Pertussis. Chichester, England: John Wiley & Sons; 1988:193.
5. van Heyningen S. Tetanus toxin. In: Dorner F, Drews J, eds. Pharmacology of Bacterial Toxins. IEPT Section 119. Oxford: Pergamon Press; 1986:549.
6. Sakaguchi G. *Clostridium botulinum* toxins. In: Dorner F, Drews J, eds. Pharmacology of Bacterial Toxins. IEPT Section 119. Oxford: Pergamon Press; 1986:519.
7. Uchida T. Diphtheria toxin. In: Dorner F, Drews J, eds. Pharmacology of Bacterial Toxins. IEPT Section 119. Oxford: Pergamon Press; 1986:693.
8. Holmes RK, Twiddy EM, Neill RJ. Recent advances in the study of heat-labile enterotoxins of *Escherichia coli*. In: Takeda Y, Minatoni, eds. Bacterial Diarrheal Diseases. Boston: Martinus Nijhoff Publishing; 1985:125.
9. Ui M. The multiple biological activities of pertussis toxin. In: Wardlaw AC, Parton R, eds. Pathogenesis and Immunity in Pertussis. Chichester, England: John Wiley & Sons; 1988:121–145.
10. O'Brien AD, Holmes RK. Shiga and shiga-like toxins. Microbiol Rev. 1987;51:206.
11. Gill DM. Seven toxic peptides that cross cell membranes. In: Jeljaszewicz J, Wadstrom T, eds. Bacterial Toxins and Cell Membranes. New York: Academic Press; 1978:291.
12. Maas WK. Genetic aspects of toxigenesis in bacteria. In: Dorner F, Drews J, eds. Pharmacology of Bacterial Toxins. IEPT Section 119. Oxford, Pergamon Press; 1986:17.
13. Betley MJ, Miller VL, Mekalanos JJ. Genetics of bacterial enterotoxins. Annu Rev Microbiol. 1986;40:577.
14. Finn CW, Silver RP, Habig WH, et al. The structural gene for tetanus neurotoxin is on a plasmid. Science. 1984;224:881.
15. Locht C, Keith JM. Pertussis toxin gene: Nucleotide sequence and genetic organisation. Science. 1986;232:1258.
16. Arico B, Rappuoli R. *Bordetella parapertussis* and *Bordetella bronchiseptica* contain transcriptionally silent pertussis toxin genes. J Bacteriol. 1987; 169:2847.
17. Dyer DW, Iandolo JJ. Plasmid-chromosomal transition of genes important in staphylococcal enterotoxin B expression. Infect Immun. 1981;33:450.
18. Randall LL, Hardy SJS. Export of protein in bacteria. Microbiol Rev. 1984;48:290.
19. Oliver D. Protein secretion in *Escherichia coli*. Annu Rev Microbiol. 1985;39:615.
20. Cavalieri SJ, Bohach GA, Snyder IS. *Escherichia coli* α-hemolysin: Characteristics and probable role in pathogenicity. Microbiol Rev. 1984;48:326.
21. Middeldorp JM, Witholt B. K88-mediated binding of *Escherichia coli* outer membrane fragments to porcine intestinal epithelial cell brush borders. Infect Immun. 1981;31:42.
22. Mollby R. Bacterial phospholipases. In: Jeljaszewicz J, Wadstrom T, eds. Bacterial Toxins and Cell Membranes. New York: Academic Press; 1978:367.
23. Eidels L, Proia RL, Hart DA. Membrane receptors for bacterial toxins. Microbiol Rev. 1983;47:596.
24. Sekura RD, Zhang Y-L, Quentin-Millet M-JJ. Pertussis toxin: Structural elements involved in the interaction with cells. In: Sekura RD, Moss J, Vaughan M, eds. Pertussis Toxin. Orlando, FL: Academic Press; 1985:45.
25. Iglewski BH, Kabat D. NAD-dependent inhibition of protein synthesis by *Pseudomonas aeruginosa* toxin. Proc Natl Acad Sci USA. 1975;72:2284.
26. Middlebrook JL, Dorland RB. Response of cultured mammalian cells to the exotoxins of *Pseudomonas aeruginosa* and *Corynebacterium diphtheriae:* Differential cytotoxicity. Can J Microbiol. 1977;23:183.
27. Middlebrook JL, Dorland RB. Bacterial toxins: Cellular mechanisms of action. Microbiol Rev. 1984;48:199.
28. Hudson TH, Scharff J, Kimak MAG, et al. Energy requirements for diphtheria toxin translocation are coupled to the maintenance of a plasma membrane potential and a proton gradient. J Biol Chem. 1988;263:4773.
29. Kagan BL, Finkelstein A, Colombini M. Diphtheria toxin fragment forms large pores in phospholipid bilayer membranes. Proc Natl Acad Sci USA. 1981;78:4950.
30. Gordon VM, Leppla SH, Hewlett EH. Inhibitors of receptor-mediated endocytosis block the entry of *Bacillus anthracis* adenylate cyclase toxin but

not that of *Bordetella pertussis* adenylate cyclase toxin. Infect Immun. 1988;56:1066.
31. McDonel JL, Dorner F, Drews J. The role of toxins in bacterial pathogenesis. In: Dorner F, Drews J, eds. Pharmacology of Bacterial Toxins. IEPT Section 119. Oxford: Pergamon Press; 1986:1.
32. Pollack M, Young LS. Protective activity of antibodies to exotoxin A and lipopolysaccharide at the onset of Pseudomonas aeruginosa septicemia in man. J Clin Invest. 1979;863:276.
33. Habermann E, Dreyer F, Bigalke H. Tetanus toxin blocks the neuromuscular transmission in vitro like botulinum A toxin. Naunyn Schmiedebergs Arch Pharmacol. 1980;311:33.
34. Eisel U, Jaransch W, Goretzki K, et al. Tetanus toxin: Primary structure, expression in *E. coli* and homology with botulinum toxins. EMBO J. 1986;5:2495.
35. Penner R, Neher E, Dreyer F. Intracellularly injected tetanus toxin inhibits exocytosis in bovine adrenal chromaffin cells. Nature. 1986;324:76.
36. Ho JL, Klempner MS. Tetanus toxin inhibits secretion of lysosomal contents from human macrophages. J Infect Dis. 1985;152:922.
37. Ho JL, Klempner MS. Diminished activity of protein kinase C in tetanus toxin-treated macrophages and in spinal cord of mice manifesting generalized tetanus intoxication. J Infect Dis. 1988;157:925.
38. Gill DM. Bacterial toxins: A table of lethal amounts. Microbiol Rev. 1982;46:86.
39. Aktories K, Barmann M, Ohishi I, et al. Botulinum C2 toxin ADP-ribosylates actin. Nature. 1986;322:390.
40. Arnon SS. Infant botulism. Annu Rev Med. 1980;31:541.
41. Moss J, Vaughan M. Mechanism of action of choleragen and *E. coli* heat-labile enterotoxin: Activation of adenylate cyclase by ADP-ribosylation. Mol Cell Biochem. 1981;37:75.
42. Pierce NF, Cray WC Jr, Sacci JB Jr. Oral immunization of dogs with purified cholera toxin, its B-subunit or a crude culture filtrate of *Vibrio cholerae:* Evidence for synergistic protection by antitoxic and anti-bacterial mechanisms. Infect Immun. 1982;37:687.
43. Clemens JD, Harris JR, Sack DA, et al. Field trial of oral cholera vaccines in Bangladesh: results of one year of follow-up. J Infect Dis. 1988;158:60.
44. Levine MM, Kaper JB, Herrington D, et al. Volunteer studies of deletion mutants of *Vibrio cholerae* prepared by recombinant techniques. Infect Immun. 1988;56:161.
45. Greenberg RN, Guerrant RL. *E. coli* heat-stable enterotoxin. In: Dorner F, Drews J, eds. Pharmacology of Bacterial Toxins. IEPT Section 119. Oxford: Pergamon Press; 1986:115.
46. Hughes JM, Murad F, Cherry B, et al. Role of cyclic GMP in the action of heat-stable enterotoxin of *Escherichia coli.* Nature. 1978;271:755.
47. Guerrant RL, Hughes JM, Chang B, et al. Activation of rat and rabbit intestinal guanylate cyclase by the heat-stable enterotoxin of *Escherichia coli:* Studies of tissue specificity, potential receptors and intermediates. J Infect Dis. 1980;142:220.
48. Klipstein FA, Engert RF, Clemens JD, et al. Vaccine for enterotoxigenic *Escherichia coli* based on synthetic heat-stable toxin cross-linked to the B subunit of heat-labile toxin. J Infect Dis. 1983;147:318.
49. Guarino A, Caparo G, Malamisura B, et al. Production of *Escherichia coli* ST_a-like heat-stable enterotoxin by *Citrobacter freundii* isolated from humans. J Clin Microbiol. 1987;25:110.
50. Kennedy DJ, Greenberg RN, Dunn JA, et al. Effects of *Escherichia coli* heat stable enterotoxin ST_b on intestines of mice, rats, rabbits and piglets. Infect Immun. 1984;46:639.
51. Fain JN, Wallace MS, Wojcikiewics RJH. Evidence for involvement of guanine nucleotide-binding regulatory proteins in the activation of phospholipases by hormones. FASEB J 1988;2:2569.
52. Weiss AA, Hewlett EL, Myers GA, et al. Pertussis toxin and extracytoplasmic adenylate cyclase as virlence factors of *Bordetella pertussis.* J Infect Dis. 1984;150:219.
53. Sato Y, Izumiya K, Dato H, et al. Role of antibody to leukocytosis-promoting factor hemagglutinin and to filamentous hemagglutinin in immunity to pertussis. Infect Immun. 1981;31:1223.
54. Toyota T, Kai Y, Kakizaki M, et al. Effect of islet-activating protein (IAP) on blood blucose and plasma insulin in healthy volunteers (phase 1 studies). Tohoku J Exp Med. 1980;130:105.
55. Weiss AA, Hewlett EL. Virulence factors of *Bordetella pertussis.* Annu Rev Microbiol. 1986;40:661.
56. Friedlander AM. Macrophages are sensitive to anthrax lethal toxin through an acid-dependent process. J Biol Chem. 1986;201:7123.
57. Robertson DL, Leppla SH. Molecular cloning and expression in *Escherichia coli* of the lethal factor gene of *Bacillus anthracis.* Gene. 1986;44:71.
58. Keusch GT, Donohue-Rolfe A, Jacewicz M. *Shigella* toxin and the pathogenesis of shigellosis. In: Microbial Toxins and Diarrheal Disease. Ciba Foundation Symposium 112. London: Pitman; 1985:193.
59. Reisbig R, Olsnes S, Eiklid K. The cytotoxin activity of *Shigella* toxin. Evidence for catalytic inactivation of the 60S ribosomal subunit. J Biol Chem. 1981;256:8739.
60. Obrig TG, Morgan TP, Colinas RJ. Ribonuclease activity associated with the 60S ribosome-inactivating proteins ricin A, phytolaccin and Shiga toxin. Biochem Biophys Res Commun. 1985;130:879.
61. Cantey RJ. Shiga toxin—an expanding role in the pathogenesis of infectious diseases. J Infect Dis. 1985;151:766.
62. O'Brien AD, Newland JW, Miller SF, et al. Shiga-like toxin-converting phages from *Escherichia coli* strains that cause hemorrhagic colitis or infantile diarrhea. Science. 1984;226:694.
63. Chang WT, Bartlett JH, Sullivan NM, et al. *Clostridium difficile* toxin. In: Dorner F, Drews J, eds. Pharmacology of Bacterial Toxins. IEPT Section 119. Oxford: Pergamon Press; 1986:571–580.
63a. Mollby R: Bacterial phospholipases. In: Jeljaszewicz J, Wadstrom T, eds. *Bacterial Toxins and Cell Membranes.* New York: Academic Press; 1978:367.
64. Alouf JE. Streptococcal toxins (streptolysin O, streptolysin S, erythrogenic toxin). In: Dorner F, Drews J, eds. Pharmacology of Bacterial Toxins. IEPT Section 119. Oxford: Pergamon Press; 1986:635–692.
65. Freer JH, Arbuthnott JP. Toxins of *Staphylococcus aureus.* In: Dorner F, Drews J, eds. *Pharmacology of Bacterial Toxins.* IEPT Section 119. Oxford: Pergamon Press; 1986:581–634.
65a. Cavalieri SJ, Bohach GA, Synder IS. *Escherichia coli* α-hemolysin: Characteristics and probable role in pathogenicity. Microbiol Rev. 1984;48:326.
65b. Clerc PL, Ryter A, Mounier J, et al. Plasmid-mediated early killing of eucaryotic cells by *Shigella flexneri* as studied by infection of J774 macrophages. Infect Immun. 1987;55:521.
65c. Portnoy DA, Jacks PS, Hinrichs DJ. Role of hemolysin for the intracellular growth of *Listeria monocytogenes.* J Exp Med. 1988;167:1459.
66. Mims CA. The Pathogenesis of Infectious Disease. London: Academic Press; 1987.
67. Smith H. Biochemical challenge of microbial pathogenicity. Bacteriol Rev. 1968;32:164.
68. Brubaker RR. Mechanisms of bacterial virulence. Annu Rev Microbiol. 1985;39:21.
69. Sweet C, Smith H. Pathogenicity of influenza virus. Microbiol Rev. 1980;44:303.
70. Fields BN, Greene MI. Genetic and molecular mechanisms of viral pathogenesis: Implications for prevention and treatment. Nature. 1982;300:19.
71. Hornick RS, Greisman SE, Woodward TE, et al. Typhoid fever: Pathogenesis and immunologic control. N Engl J Med. 1970;283:686.
72. Falkow S, Small P, Isberg R, et al. A molecular strategy for the study of bacterial invasion. Rev Infect Dis. 1987;9(Suppl 5):5450.
73. Smith HW, Huggins MB. Further observations on the association of the colicine V plasmid of *Escherichia coli* with pathogenicity and with survival in the alimentary tract. J Gen Microbiol. 1976;92:335.
74. Aguerro ME, Cabello FC. Relative contribution of Col V plasmid and K1 antigen to the pathogenicity of *Escherichia coli.* Infect Immun. 1983;40:359.
75. Labre EH, Schneider H, Magnani TJ, et al. Epithelial cell penetration as an essential step in the pathogenesis of bacillary dysentery. J Bacteriol. 1964; 88:1503.
76. DuPont HL, Formal SB, Hornick RB, et al. Pathogenesis of *Escherichia coli* diarrhea. N Engl J Med. 1971;285:1.
77. Maki M, Gronroos P, Vesikari T. In vitro invasiveness of *Yersinia enterocolitica* isolated from children with diarrhea. J Infect Dis. 1978;138:677.
78. Giannella RA, Washington O, Gemski P, et al. Invasion of HeLa cells by *Salmonella typhimurium:* A model for study of invasiveness of *Salmonella.* J Infect Dis. 1973;128:69.
79. Zink DL, Feeley JC, Wells JG, et al. Plasmid-mediated tissue invasiveness in *Yersinia enterocolitica.* Nature. 1980;283:224.
80. Hale TL, Sansonett PJ, Schad PA, et al. Characterization of virulence plasmids and plasmid-associated outer membrane proteins in *Shigella flexneri, Shigella sonnei,* and *Escherichia coli.* Infect Immun. 1983;40:340.
81. Harris JR, Wachsmuth IK, Davis BR, et al. High-molecular weight plasmid correlates with *Escherichia coli* enteroinvasiveness. Infect Immun. 1982; 37:1295.
82. Garzelli C, Colizzi V, Campa M, et al. Depression of contact sensitivity by *Pseudomonas aeruginosa*–induced suppressor cells which affect the induction phase of immune response. Infect Immun. 1979;26:4.
83. Baugh RE, Musher DM. Aberrant secondary antibody response to sheep erythrocytes in rabbits with experimental syphilis. Infect Immun. 1979; 25:133.
84. Higerd TB, Vesole DH, Goust J-M. Inhibitory effects of extracellular products from oral bacteria on human fibroblasts and stimulated lymphocytes. Infect Immun. 1978;21:567.
85. Wilkinson BJ, Sisson SP, Kim Y, et al. Localization of the third component of complement on the cell wall of encapsulated *Staphylococcus aureus* M: Implications for the mechanism of resistance to phagocytosis. Infect Immun. 1979;26:1159.
86. Kilian M. Bacterial enzymes degrading human IgA. In: Robbins JR, Hill JC, Sadoff JC, eds. Seminars in Infectious Disease. v. 4. Bacterial Vaccines. New York: Thieme-Stratton; 1982:213–8.
87. Male C. *Streptococcus pneumoniae* and *Haemophilus influenzae* IgA_1, proteases and their possible role in pathogenesis. In: Robbins JB, Hill JC, Sadoff JC, eds. Seminars in Infectious Disease. v. 4. Bacterial Vaccines. New York: Thieme-Stratton; 1982:219–24.
88. Roantree RJ, Rantz LA. A study of the relationship of the normal bactericidal activity of human serum to bacterial infection. J Clin Invest. 1960;39:72.
89. Schoolnik GK, Buchanan TM, Holmes KK. Gonococci causing disseminated gonococcal infection are resistant to the bactericidal action of normal human sera. J Clin Invest. 1976;58:1163.
90. Frank M, Joiner K, Hammer C. The function of antibody and complement in the lysis of bacteria. Rev Infect Dis. 1987;9(Suppl 5):5537.
91. Fearon DT, Austen KF. The alternative pathway of complement: A system for host resistance to microbial infection. N Engl J Med. 1980;303:259.

92. Glode MP, Robbins JB, Liu TY, et al. Cross antigenicity between capsular polysaccharides of group C *Neisseria meningitidis* and *Escherichia coli* K92. J Infect Dis. 1977;135:94.
93. Joiner KA. Complement evasion by bacteria and parasites. Annu Rev Microbiol. 1988;42:201.
93a. Wozencraft AO, Sayers G, Blackwell JM: Macrophage type 3 complement receptors mediate serum-independent binding of *Leishmania donovani*. J Exp Med. 1986;164:1332.
93b. Payne NR, Bellinger-Kawahara C, Horwitz MA: Phagocytosis of *Legionella pneumophilia* is mediated by human monocyte complement receptors: J Exp Med. 1987;166:1377.
94. Allen RJ, Scott GK. Comparison of the effects of different lipopolysaccharides on the serum bactericidal reactions of two strains of *Escherichia coli*. Infect Immun. 1981;31:831.
95. Nilins AM, Savage DC. Serum resistance encoded by colicin V plasmids in *Escherichia coli* and its relationship to the plasmid transfer system. Infect Immun. 1984;43:547.
96. Howard CJ, Glynn AA. The virulence for mice of strains of *Escherichia coli* related to the effects of K antigens on their resistance ot phagocytosis and killing by complement. Immunology. 1971;20:767.
97. McCutchan JS, Katzenstein D, Norquist D, et al. Role of blocking antibody in disseminated gonococcal infection. J Immunol. 1978;121:1884.
98. Densen P, Mandell GL. Phagocyte strategy vs microbial tactics. Rev Infect Dis. 1980;2:817.
99. Quie PG. Perturbation of the normal mechanisms of intraleukocytic killing of bacteria. J Infect Dis. 1983;148:189.
100. Sher A, Hall BF, Vadas MA. Acquisition of murine major histocompatibility complex gene products by schistosomula of *Schistosoma mansoni*. J Exp Med. 1978;148:46.
101. Zalezwik DF, Kasper DL. The role of anaerobic bacteria in abscess formation. Annu Rev Med. 1982;33:217.
102. Wilson CW, Tsai V, Remington JS. Failure to trigger the oxidative metabolic burst by normal macrophages. J Exp Med. 1980;151:328.
103. Murray HW. How protozoa evade intracellular killing. Ann Intern Med. 1983;98:1016.
104. Murray HW, Nathan CF, Cohn ZA. Macrophage oxygen-dependent antimicrobial activity IV. Role of endogenous scavengers of oxygen intermediates. J Exp Med. 1980;152:1601.
105. Goren MB. Phagocyte lysosomes: Interactions with infectious agents, phagosomes, and experimental perturbations in function. Annu Rev Microbiol. 1977;31:507.
106. Lowrie DB, Aber VR, Jackett PS. Phagosome lysosome fusion and cyclic adenosine 3′:5′ monophosphate in macrophages infected with *Mycobacterium lepraemurium*. J Gen Microbiol. 1979;110:431.
107. Lewis DH, Peters W. The resistance of intracellular *Leishmania* parasites to digestion by lysosomal enzymes. Ann Trop Med Parasitol. 1977;71:295.
108. Elwell LP, Shipley PL. Plasmid-mediated factors associated with virulence of bacteria to animals. Annu Rev Microbiol. 1980;34:465.
109. Welch RA, Dellinger EP, Minshew B, et al. Haemolysin contributes to virulence of extraintestinal *E. coli* infections. Nature. 1981;294:665.
110. Macrina FL. Molecular cloning of bacterial antigens and virulence determinants. Annu Rev Microbiol. 1984;38:193.

2. MICROBIAL ADHERENCE

LARRY M. BADDOUR
GORDON D. CHRISTENSEN
W. ANDREW SIMPSON
EDWIN H. BEACHEY

The process by which microbes bind to surfaces is known as *adherence*. In 1908 Guyot first recognized that certain bacteria bind to erythrocytes, a process resulting in hemaglutination.[1] In 1935, ZoBell and Allen examined bacterial adherence in marine environments.[2] Medical interest in bacterial adherence dates to 1955 when Duguid and coworkers began a series of publications relating filamentous bacterial surface structures to intestinal cell adherence by certain gram-negative bacilli.[3–9] In the 1970s, Gibbons and van Houte reported that the selective attachment of bacteria to various oral surfaces resulted in dental disease.[10,11] Microbial adherence has been recently reviewed in several books,[12,16] monographs,[17–19] and articles.[20–22] Understanding this literature requires familiarity with the terms defined below:

1. *Adhesins*. Adhesins are microbial surface molecules or organelles that function to bind the organism to a surface.[6]
2. *Capsules*. Capsules are a subclass of extracellular polymeric substances that are generally polysaccharide in nature. Capsules cling closely to the surface and have a distinct outer margin. In general, capsules inhibit phagocytosis and adherence, although there are many exceptions.[23,24]
3. *Extracellular polymeric substances*. Extracellular polymeric substances are usually polysaccharides, may include slime or capsules, and are roughly synonymous with the extracellular glycocalyx.
4. *Fibrillae*. Fibrillae are the fine "hairy" structures on bacterial cells that are irregular in size and structure.[22]
5. *Fimbriae*. Fimbriae (or pili) are nonflagellar filamentous structures on bacterial cells that have a regular structure and diameter. Generally but not exclusively, they function as adhesins.[3]
6. *Glycocalyx*. The glycocalyx is the superficial polysaccharide-containing structure on the external surface of cells.[25] It includes the cuticle of invertebrates, cell walls of plants, epithelial cell basement membrane, intercellular cement, the carbohydrate-rich surface of mammalian cells,[26] and the carbohydrate-rich surface of prokaryotic cells.[21] It may be subdivided into the intrinsic glycocalyx, which is required for cell viability, and the extracellular or extraneous glycocalyx, which is not required for cell viability.[26] An overlap in definitions should be noted, see for example, definitions 2, 3, 9, and 12.
7. *Lectin*. Lectins are carbohydrate-binding proteins of nonimmune origin that agglutinate cells or precipitate polysaccharides or glycoproteins.[27]
8. *Ligand*. A ligand is a molecule that exhibits specific binding to a complementary substrate molecule.
9. *Mucous gel*. The mucous gel is the viscous layer composed of mucins, a class of glycoproteins, produced by specialized cells that cover animal mucosal surfaces.[28] It is equivalent to the extracellular glycocalyx.
10. *Sex pili*. Traditionally, sex pili are a subclass of fimbriae that bind prokaryotic cells to each other for the conjugative transfer of genetic information.[9,22]
11. *Receptors*. Receptors are the complementary substrate molecules that bind specific ligands or adhesins.
12. *Slime*. Slime is a subclass of extracellular polymeric substances that is generally polysaccharide in composition. Slime loosely associates with the bacterial surface and has an indistinct margin. Generally, slime mediates the nonspecific attachment of a bacterium to a surface in a slimy layer.[23,24]
13. *Substratum*. The substratum is the surface to which a cell binds.

THE ADHERENCE PROCESS

All immersed objects attract suspended particles, including microbes, to their surfaces. The colloidal theories of Derjaguin and Landau and of Verwey and Overbeek (DLVO theory) describe this attraction by postulating that two positions of thermodynamic stability exist near a submerged surface. (For a more complete discussion of the DLVO theory and the following material, see refs. 22, 29–34.) A variety of long-range nonspecific weak interactions that include gravitation, chemotaxis, London–van der Waals forces, electrostatic forces, and surface tension, for example, attract particles to surfaces (Fig. 1). At closer range, however, London–van der Waals repulsion and steric hindrance repel particles from the surface. In addition, if the particles share the same charge as the surface, which is the rule when negatively charged prokaryotic cells bind to negatively charged eukaryotic cells, charge repulsion between like charges strongly repels the particles from the surface. As a re-

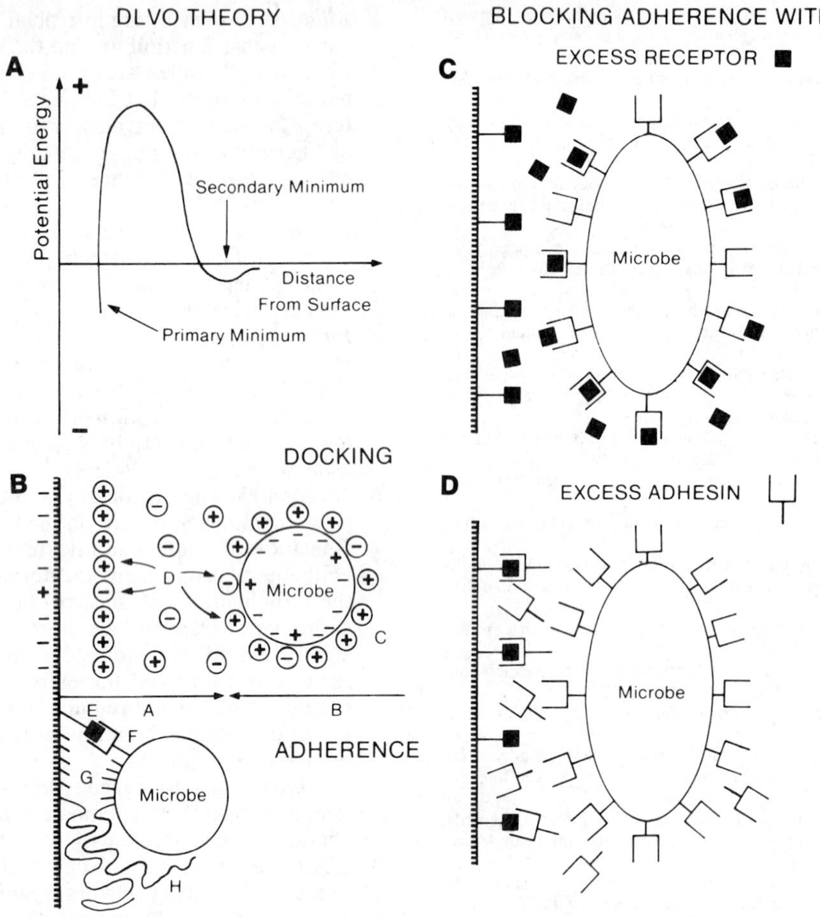

FIG. 1. (**A**) Illustration of the DLVO theory. Shown are the two points of low potential energy that lead to the association and attachment of soluble particles to surfaces. The low-energy point closest to the surface is the primary energy minimum; it is separated by a high-energy barrier from an additional point further away from the surface known as the secondary energy minimum. The precise shape and amplitude of this energy curve varies with local conditions, but the energy level of the secondary minimum is always higher than the energy level of the primary minimum. (**B**) The top portion of Fig. B shows a microbe surrounded by a charge field near a surface. This is the first stage in the attachment of a microbe to a surface in which the microbe "docks" at the surface by entering the secondary energy minimum. The particle is propelled into the secondary energy minimum by physical and chemical forces of repulsion and attraction, thereby resulting in the nonspecific and reversible adsorption of the particle to the surface. In this case, the adsorbed microbe also has an adhesin that extends beyond the surrounding charge field. The close proximity of the adsorbed microbe to the surface allows the adhesin to come into contact with surface structures. If a complementary surface structure is present, the adhesin binds to the surface receptor in a lock-and-key manner, drawing the microbe across the high-energy barrier and into the primary energy minimum. This process of microbial adherence is illustrated in the bottom portion of Fig. B. The microbe is now permanently attached to the surface. Adherence can be blocked by flooding the microbe with soluble receptors (**C**) or by flooding the surface with soluble adhesins (**D**).

sult, the forces of attraction and repulsion counterbalance each other, loosely holding the particle at the "secondary minimum" position just off the surface (Fig. 1). We refer to the concentration of particles at the secondary minimum as *adsorption* or *docking*. Characteristically, adsorption is a reversible process; particles may desorb as well as adsorb. If the particle overcomes the forces of repulsion, stronger but short-range forces of attraction bind the particle closely to the surface. These stronger, short-range forces include covalent, hydrogen, ionic, and hydrophobic binding. The DLVO theory describes this binding as the *primary minimum* (Fig. 1); particles held in this position are essentially irreversibly bound to the surface.

We refer to the process whereby particles leave the secondary minimum and enter the primary minimum as *adherence*. The energy barrier separating the secondary minimum from the primary minimum can be broached by several means. In a water environment such as on a mucosal surface, microbial surface hydrophobicity promotes the close association of microbes with lypophilic regions of eukaryotic cell membranes (see also below). In addition, many microbes excrete or extracellularly synthesize polymeric compounds such as "slime." The substrate adsorbs these compounds, which in turn embed the organism and "glue" it onto the surface. Perhaps the area of greatest interest is in the adhesive surface structures (adhesins) of microbes. Because of their smaller size, these adhesins are not subject to the forces of repulsion on the same scale as the microbe and can bridge the gap between microbe and substrate. These "bridging" adhesins include adhesive organelles and adhesive molecules or "ligands."

Generally, adhesins recognize only particular molecular conformations (receptors), and binding to these receptors is considered to be specific. The situation is analogous to the specific binding of an antigen by an antibody or a carbohydrate by a lectin. Indeed, in a very general sense, these two examples represent specific adherence systems. The former mediates the binding of a particle to a phagocyte; the latter mediates the binding of a commensal bacterium to a plant. The latter also mediates the binding of bacteria to epithelial cells as well as to phagocytes.[35] We can conclude that the binding is specific in any given circumstance if adherence is blocked by the following

1. A large excess of isolated receptor (or receptor analogue) or isolated adhesin (or adhesin analogue) (Fig. 1)
2. Specific chemical or enzymatic treatment of the microbe or substrate
3. Specific antireceptor or antiadhesin antibody

If the adhesin binds the organism to a wide variety of substrata, the binding is considered *nonspecific*. This term, however, is misleading. Many systems that appear superficially to be nonspecific are, in fact, quite specific. The reason is that all solid surfaces when exposed to fluids instantaneously adsorb macromolecules onto their surfaces, a process referred to as *conditioning*. These adsorbed molecules may, in turn, serve as receptors for microorganisms to bind to the surface.

Some authors describe a third stage in microbial surface colonization called *coaggregation*. In this stage, the microbe uses the same general processes involved in surface adherence, but rather than binding to a solid surface, the organism binds to other adherent organisms. Coaggregation allows for the accumulation of thick colonies of microorganisms on a surface.

Bacterial adherence is the first stage of bacterial invasion. To the microorganism's disadvantage, the same mechanisms that promote tissue adherence also may promote adherence to and ingestion by phagocytes. To overcome this potential liability, pathogenic microbes alter their surface characteristics by three general means. First, an organism may stop producing its adhesins and leave future generations with a surface free of adhesive structures. This can take place in response to environmental conditions (environmental regulation) or by switching on and off the adhesin gene (phase variation). Second, an organism may cover the adhesins with a capsule. Capsules, which for bacteria tend to be polysaccharides, also have some nonspecific functions. They increase the negative-charge density on the particle's surface and thereby increase the like-charge repulsion force. Capsules tend to be hydrophilic and cover surfaces that tend to be hydrophobic; capsules may mask surface structures that are antigenic or complement activating. Finally, pathogenic microbes can alter their surface by adsorbing host proteins. By covering adhesive, antigenic, or complement-activating sites, these proteins further "encapsulate" the organism's surface and immunologically confuse host defenses.

Examples of Microbial Adherence Mechanisms

Table 1 lists microorganisms that appear to rely upon adherence mechanisms to colonize and infect mammalian tissues. The specifics of the adherence process vary considerably from organism to organism, but the overall principles remain the same. Rather than discuss all the entries on Table 1, we will concentrate upon a few systems that exhibit certain basic principles, beginning with *Streptococcus pyogenes* as a paradigm of the adherence process.

Adherence Paradigm: Lipoteichoic Acid, a Streptococcal Adhesin. A fine irregular fuzz, or *fibrillae*, covers the streptococcal surface. Fibrillae bind streptococci to human epithelial cells[123,124] (Fig. 2) and are composed of M protein, lipoteichoic acid (LTA),[123] and other unidentified substances.

Because LTA is an amphipathic surface molecule that binds to virtually all eukaryotic cells, it makes an excellent candidate for a streptococcal adhesin.[125–127] An ester bond links LTA's hydrophilic polyglycerolphosphate "backbone" to its hydrophobic glycolipid "tail." The molecule is found with its tail buried in the bacterial cytoplasmic membrane of most gram-positive bacteria. LTA has a variety of biologic activities, mostly inflammatory in nature, all of which depend upon the integrity of the hydrophobic tail.

We might expect that in the native state the biologically active tail would be unavailable for binding, but apparently this is not so. The streptococcus constantly leaks LTA into the surrounding media,[128] and LTA can complex with M protein.[129] This suggests that as the LTA crosses the cell wall it might complex with surface proteins and make an about-face, thereby exposing the hydrophobic moiety.[8,129] Observations in support of this include the following: (*1*) the streptococcal cell wall is fatty acid rich,[130] (*2*) the unencapsulated streptococcal surface is very hydrophobic,[131,132] (*3*) the surface hydrophobicity is sensitive to proteolysis,[131,133] (*4*) the surface hydrophobicity correlates with surface LTA,[133] and (*5*) the selective inactivation of the hydrophobic tail converts the hydrophobic streptococcal surface into a hydrophilic one.[131]

As noted previously, hydrophobic surfaces promote prokaryotic–eukaryotic cell contact. In this regard, LTA's contribution to surface hydrophobicity and ultimately to bacterial adherence is important. Nevertheless, hydrophobic interactions are general processes and cannot by themselves explain the specificities of streptococcal adherence. For example, streptococcal cutaneous strains preferentially bind to cutaneous epithelial cells.[134] Furthermore, rheumatogenic strains bind preferentially to pharyngeal cells of rheumatic heart disease patients,[135] and streptococci bind to adult buccal epithelial cells but not to neonatal epithelial cells.[136] Finally, bound streptococci exhibit a highly nonuniform topographic distribution on epithelial cells, thus indicating the existence of privileged binding sites.[137] The specificity of this cellular attachment indicates that specific bacterial adhesins interact with specific cellular receptors. There is evidence that LTA also functions as one of these adhesins: LTA blocks streptococcal adherence to epithelial cells,[123,125,126,134] as does antibody to LTA.[123] Lipopolysaccharide from *Escherichia coli* and *Serratia marcescens,* streptococcal somatic antigens (M protein, C carbohydrate, and peptidoglycan sonicate), and M-type-specific and group A-specific antisera do not block adherence.[123] The inhibitory activity of LTA resides in its hydrophobic tail because the hydrophobic backbone alone (deacylated LTA) cannot block streptococcal adherence.[125]

Cellular binding of LTA is highly specific. For example, buccal epithelial cells from newborn infants bind only half as much LTA as do cells from 3-day-old infants and from adults.[126] Furthermore, LTA binds 10 times greater to right-side-out red blood cell (RBC) ghosts than to inside-out RBC ghosts,[138] thus indicating that LTA binds to a receptor on the exterior of the RBC rather than simply intercalating its tail into the lipid cell membrane. Finally, LTA binds to a single population of binding sites (receptors) on neutrophilic leukocytes,[139] RBCs,[140] platelets,[141] lymphocytes,[142] and oral epithelial cells.[126]

Fibronectin is a ubiquitous adhesive glycoprotein that also binds LTA, but not deacylated LTA,[143] via fatty acid receptors in a manner entirely analogous to albumin's binding of LTA.[144] Streptococci will bind soluble and surface-fixed fibronectin,[88] and fibronectin inhibits the adherence of streptococci to epithelial cells.[88] As we might expect, LTA but not deacylated LTA blocks the binding of fibronectin to streptococci.[88]

Previous work demonstrated that group A streptococci incubated in the presence of sublethal concentrations of penicillin released their surface LTA.[128] At the same time, the streptococci lost their ability to bind to oral epithelial cells.[145] More recent studies have examined the formation and release of LTA–fibronectin complexes from streptococcal surfaces in the presence of sublethal concentrations of penicillin.[146,147] The binding of fibronectin to penicillin-exposed streptococci decreased, and this decrease corresponded to a loss of LTA. Radiolabeling experiments using [^{3}H] fibronectin and antisera to LTA showed that cells of *S. pyogenes* that had been incubated in penicillin released the radiolabeled fibronectin and antiserum to LTA precipitated most of the released fibronectin. Examination of the fibronectin molecule has shown that *S. pyogenes* and *S. aureus* bind to the NH_2-terminal region of the fibronectin

TABLE 1. Partial List of Pathogenic and Commensal Microorganisms with Adherence Mechanisms

Microbe	*Adhesin*	*Receptor (Carrier)*	*Reference*
Viruses			
Orthomyxovirus (influenza)	Hemagglutinin	Sialic acid	36, 37
Picornavirus (poliovirus, rhinovirus, coxsackievirus)	Capsid protein	Four receptor "families"	36, 37
Adenovirus	Fiber protein	?	36, 37
Togavirus (Sindbis, Semliki Forest)	Glycoprotein spike	Phospholipid or cholesterol?	36, 37
Rhabdovirus (vesicular stomatitis virus)	Sialic acid residue on glycoprotein spike	Phospho- or glycolipid	36, 37
Intracellular bacteria and mycoplasma			
Chlamydia	Cell surface lectin	*N*-acetyl-D-glucosamine	38, 39
Mycoplasma			
M. gallisepticum	Tip structure	Sialic acid (glycophorin)	40
M. pneumoniae	Protein P-1 on tip structure	Sialic acid	40–42
Aerobic gram-negative bacilli			
Escherichia coli	Type I fimbriae	D-Mannose (Tamm-Horsfall glycoprotein)	43, 44
	K88 fimbriae	GM_1 ganglioside	18, 45
	K99 fimbriae	Galp-β(1–4)-GLcp-β(1–1)-ceramide	18, 46
	CFA/1 fimbriae	GM ganglioside	18, 47
	CFA/2 fimbriae	?	18
	987P fimbriae	Glycoprotein	48–51
	F41 fimbriae	?	52, 53
	PCF8775 fimbriae	?	54–56
	P fimbriae	P blood group glycolipid	57, 58
Enterobacteriaceae (*Salmonella, Shigella, Klebsiella, Citrobacter, Morganella, Aeromonas*)	Type I fimbriae	D-Mannose	59–63
Klebsiella aerogenes	Type III fimbriae	?	62
Serratia marcescens	Type III fimbriae	?	62
Proteus			
P. mirabilis	Fimbriae, type IV fimbriae	?	62, 64
P. vulgaris	Fimbriae	?	64
Providencia	Fimbriae	?	64, 65
Yersinia enterocolitica	Two types of fimbriae	?	66, 67
Pseudomonas aeruginosa	Fimbriae	?	68, 69
Pasteurella multocida	Fimbriae	*N*-acetyl-D-glucosamine	70
Bordetella pertussis	Fimbriae	?Sterol	71–73
Hemophilus influenzae	Fimbriae	?	74, 75
Vibrio cholera	Fimbriae	?	76
	Cholera lectin	?Protein	77, 78
Legionella pneumophila	Fimbriae	?	79
Aerobic gram-negative cocci			
Neisseria			
N. meningitidis	Fimbriae	?	80, 81
N. gonorrhoeae	Fimbriae	GD_1 ganglioside	62, 82
	Type II outer membrane	?	82, 83
	Protein	?	83
Moraxella	Fimbriae	?	62

(*Continued*)

structure.[148–150] Unlike *S. pyogenes, S. aureus* cells bind to an additional site close to the cell attachment region. It should be noted that the streptococci may not always be recognized by cell surface receptors such as fibronectin because their adhesin may be masked either by hyaluronate capsules[151] or by adsorbed host proteins once the organisms invade deeper tissue.[152]

Adhesive Organelles. As opposed to *S. pyogenes*, many organisms use a specific adhesive organelle, fimbriae (or pili), to mediate adherence. The archetypical fimbria is type I, or common fimbriae, and is expressed by most Enterobacteriaceae (Table 2). Originally recognized for their hemagglutinin properties, these adhesins enable the bacterium to attach to most of the protozoal, fungal, and animal cells and cell products so far tested. Characteristically, D-mannose, methyl-α-D-mannoside, yeast mannan, and other D-mannose derivatives inhibit this attachment.[174,175] As such, type I fimbriae from different genera exhibit close structural but limited antigenic similarities.[176] The precise oligosaccharide receptor also varies between genera.[177] Typically, bacteria have 50–400 of these filaments projecting from their surface. The filaments radiate outward from where their hydrophobic tips initiate contact with other cells and substrata. The phenotypic expression of type I fimbriae switches on and off from bacterial generation to bacterial generation (phase variation) so that under any given cultural condition a proportion of the bacterial population will always be fimbriated and nonfimbriated.[9,178] Although these organelles aid saprophytic and commensal bacterial colonization, their importance in pathogenicity remains controversial because many pathogenic Enterobacteriaceae do not express type I fimbriae.[9] However, almost all possess the ability to produce fimbriae.

Fimbria-mediated attachment is exemplified by *E. coli*. The organisms are richly endowed with fimbriae and may simultaneously exhibit several different kinds.[176,179–181] The structure and function of many of these fimbriae have only been partially characterized. The best described fimbriae fall into three groups: the common fimbriae, the enteric colonization fimbriae of enterotoxigenic E. coli (ETEC), and the P fimbriae of uropathogenic *E. coli* (Table 2).

Similar to other Enterobacteriaceae, most but not all strains of *E. coli* express type I fimbriae under appropriate cultural conditions.[9] They enable the organism to attach to almost all human tissues including white blood cells, buccal epithelial cells, enterocytes, uroepithelial cells, and uromucoid (Tamm-Horsfall glycoprotein). Although we would expect type I fimbriae to promote the colonization of epithelial surfaces by pathogenic *E. coli*,[18] investigators have not found type I fimbriae to be associated with ETEC diarrhae.[182] On the other hand, animal studies suggest that there is a role for type I fimbriae in the pathogenesis of urinary tract infections.[108,183,184] Rene and Silverblatt[185] reported an association between pyelonephritis in

TABLE 1. (Continued)

Microbe	Adhesin	Receptor (Carrier)	Reference
Aerobic gram-positive bacilli			
Corynebacterium renale	Fimbriae	?	84, 85
Aerobic gram-positive cocci			
Staphylococcus aureus	Lipotechoic acid (LTA)	?	86
Staphylococcus epidermidis	Slime	?	87
Streptococcus			
S. pyogenes	LTA-M protein complex		
	Fibrillae		88, 89
S. mitior			
S. salivarius			
S. mutans, groups C and G	?	?	90, 91
S. mutans	Glucosyltransferase and glucan-binding protein	Glucan	92–96
	Cell surface lectin	Galactose	97
S. sanguis	LTA, fibrillae	Salivary agglutinin	98, 99
	Cell surface lectin	Galactose, on *Actinomyces viscosus*	100
	Binding protein	*A. viscosus*	100
	Binding protein	Dental pellicle	101
S. salivarius	Cell surface lectin	Galactose, on *Veillonella alcalescens*	102, 103
	Binding protein	?	102
	Glucosyltransferase	Glucan	104
S. agalactiae	Protein	*N*-acetyl-D-glucosamine	105, 106
Enterococcus			
E. faecalis	Fimbriae	?	107
Anaerobic bacteria			
Bacteroides fragilis	Capsular polysaccharide	?	108
Eikenella corrodens	?	Galactose	109
Actinomyces			
A. viscosus	Fimbriae	Galactose on *S. sanguis*	100, 110
	Fimbriae	*S. sanguis*	100, 110
	Fimbriae	Dental pellicle	111
	Glucan-binding protein	Glucan	112
A. naeslundii	Fimbriae	Galactose on *S. sanguis*	100
	Fimbriae	*S. sanguis*	100
	Fimbriae	Dental pellicle	111
	Fimbriae	Epithelial cells	113
Spirochetes			
Treponema pallidum	P_1, P_2, P_3	Fibronectin	114, 115
Fungi			
Candida albicans	Mannan	?	116, 117
Protozoa			
Plasmodium			
P. falciparum	Apical complex	*N*-acetyl-D-glucosamine (glycophorin)	118, 119
P. vivax	Apical complex	Duffy blood group antigen	118
Entamoeba histolytica	Cell surface lectin	*N*-acetyl-glucosamine	120, 121
Giardia lamblia	Gripping disk	Mechanical	122

humans and type I fimbriated *E. coli*. They also noted a specific immune response to type I fimbriae in their infected patients.[185] Swedish investigators, however, have not found an association between urinary tract infection and type I fimbriae.[57,186] These organelles may be more important in the initiation of a urinary tract infection than in its persistence.[187] Type I fimbriated organisms have a particularly high affinity for the uromucoid that bathes the urinary tract.[43] This could encourage bacterial colonization, or alternatively, by entrapment and excretion uromucoid may actually be a nonspecific host defense against type I fimbriated bacteria.[188]

Enterotoxigenic *E. coli* cause traveler's diarrhea and infant diarrhea in humans and neonatal enteric colibacillosis of piglets, calves, and lambs. ETEC bacteria possess plasmids that code for the production of either or both heat-stable (ST) or heat-labile (LT) enterotoxin. The enterotoxin, in turn, causes a secretory diarrhea. Genetic manipulations demonstrate that the production of an enterotoxin alone is not sufficient for pathogenicity. The organism must also have an adhesin that binds the organism to the enterocyte so that the toxin can be expeditiously delivered to the target tissue.[189–192] These adhesins, or colonization factors, are fimbriae that exhibit host specificity. For example, the K88 fimbriae determine organ specificity (anterior portion of the small intestine) and host specificity (neonatal pigs).[193,194] Furthermore, the different antigenic types of K88, namely K88ab, K88ac, and K88ad, bind to different piglet phenotypes.[195] A number of colonization factors for human and animal ETEC strains have been described in addition to those listed in Table 2.[18,182] Unlike type I fimbriae, the agglutination is not inhibited by mannose; thus arises the term *mannose-resistant* adherence. Other common properties of this group include plasmid location of the fimbrial gene (generally not on the same plasmid as the enterotoxin gene), phenotypic expression of fimbriation at body temperature (37°C) but not at room temperature (18°C), and confinement of fimbriation to certain serogroups.[9,18] Despite these common functional properties, this is actually a heterogenous group. The fimbriae have different hemagglutinin patterns, mucosal receptors, antigens, and primary and quaternary structures (Table 2).[18,196] Human and animal studies indicate that the enteric colonization fimbriae mediate specific enterocyte adherence that is saturable, inhibited by homologous but not heterologous purified fimbriae, and inhibited by homologous but not heterologous antifimbrial antibodies.[53,197–200] Veterinary studies demonstrate an 80–100 percent protection of neonatal animals passively immunized by the ingestion of colostrum from mothers vaccinated with purified fimbriae of the homologous type.[200,201]

P fimbriae refers to a class of antigenically distinct (designated F-7 through F-12) uropathogenic *E. coli* adhesins that share the common property of agglutinating human RBCs carrying the ubiquitous P blood group antigen, which consists of globoseries glycolipids.[169] Characteristically, this agglutination is mannose resistant, but it is inhibited by the isolated and purified P blood group substance or by a synthetic Galα(1–4)Galβ-

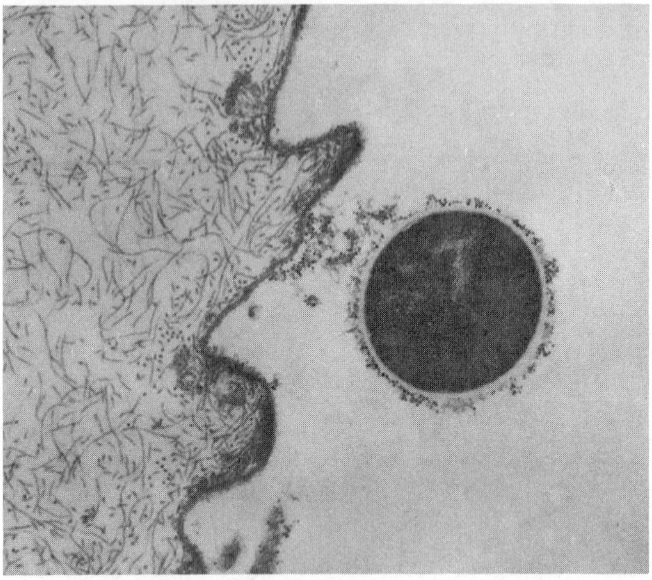

FIG. 2. Transmission electron micrograph of an ultrathin section of human buccal epithelial cells incubated with a suspension of *Streptococcus pyogenes* and treated first with rabbit antibody to fibronectin and then with ferritin-conjugated goat antibody to rabbit IgG. An *S. pyogenes* cell (center) is seen associated with an epithelial cell coated with ferritin particles, which indicates the presence of fibronectin. The rim of ferritin-labeled antibody around the bacterium appears to be due to the acquisition of fibronectin from epithelial cell surfaces during incubation.

ceramide derivative.[57,58,166,176,202] Coating a substrate with the natural or synthetic glycolipid promotes attachment of P fimbriated bacteria. The P antigen, the minimum structural determinant being a digalactose Galα(1–4)Galβ residue, is not only present on human RBCs but is also present on the kidney tissues of humans and mice (but not rats).[203] P. fimbriae are at least a marker for pyelonephritogenic *E. coli* that bind to human and mouse uroepithelial cells in a mannose-resistant but globoside-sensitive manner.[167,176] P-specific adherence is most commonly seen in collections of pyelonephritogenic *E. coli* strains[57,164,186] and is also frequently present in collections of cystitis and asymptomatic bacteruria strains.[57,164,186] In comparison, it is a rare finding in collections of fecal *E. coli* isolates. In an elegant study performed in mice, Swedish and U.S. investigators used genetically manipulated *E. coli* strains as tools to determine the importance of fimbriae in murine urinary tract infections. The P fimbriae served to localize the organism to the upper urinary tract, whereas both P fimbriae and common fimbriae localized the organism to the mouse bladder.[183]

The P fimbriae specificity determines the host specificity of these organisms. CBA mice have a higher concentration of P antigen than do BALB/c mice. CBA mice are also more predisposed to P-fimbriated *E. coli* experimental pyelonephritis than are BALB/c mice.[183] There is similar evidence that humans with high concentrations of P antigen are also particularly predisposed to pyelonephritis.[183,204] Thus, P fimbriae join the enteric colonization fimbriae as host-specific adhesins. P fimbriae also share with enteric colonization fimbriae the properties of serogroup restriction[179] and temperature-dependent expression of fimbriae.[205] P fimbriae, on the other hand, appear to be closely related to type I fimbriae. Both have chromosomal genetic codes,[165] and they share considerable primary structure homology[206] and similar quaternary structure.[168]

Another fimbrial type on *E. coli*, termed S fimbriae, is characterized by its specific binding to sialyl galactosides on human erythrocytes and is associated with *E. coli* serotype 018:K1:H7, which is commonly isolated from infants with meningitis and septicemia.[170–173,207–212] The major erythrocyte receptor for S-fimbriated *E. coli* is the NeuAcα(2–3)Galβ(1–3)GlcNac sequence of the *O*-linked oligosaccharide chains of glycophorin A.[173] S fimbriae, serum resistance, and hemolysin production are operative virulence factors of *E. coli* strains in the rat pyelonephritis model.[207] Binding sites for S fimbriae of *E. coli* to frozen sections of human kidney include epithelial and vascular endothelial cells.[208] The genetic determinant coding for the S-fimbrial adhesin has been cloned, and analysis of the DNA sequences are highly conserved in their coding and flanking regions and are identical, except for small alterations, in uropathogenic (06:K+) and meningitis (018:K1, 083:K1) strains.[209,210]

Recent data from the infant rat model examining the pathogenesis of *E. coli* bacteremia and meningitis are particularly intriguing and support a virulence role of S fimbriae.[211] Inocula subpopulations of strain IH3080, 018:K1:H7 organisms that contain S fimbriae, were the most virulent in this animal model as compared with subpopulations with type I fimbriae or nonfimbriated isolates. Fimbrial phase variation to the type S fimbriated forms was observed in all body fluids 6 hours after injection, while nonfimbriated forms were seen 1 hour after challenge, which led the investigators to speculate on the role of phase variation in establishing serious infections in this animal model. Moreover, three different cell types of the neonatal rat brain demonstrated specific binding sites for S fimbriae of *E. coli.*[212]

Tip Location of Fimbrial Adhesin Proteins. Until recently it was thought that the sugar binding sites of bacterial fimbriae were located within the major structural subunits. While this may be true for some fimbriae, new evidence suggests that the sugar binding sites of several fimbrial types (e.g., type I, P and S) reside in minor proteins that represent only 1/100–1000 of the total structural protein. That a protein other than the major subunit was involved was first shown by insertion and deletion mutation analyses of fimbrial clones. Mutants producing morphologically normal fimbriae that were nonadhesive lacked certain minor proteins. By using a combination of specific antibodies and gold-conjugated protein A as probes, the adhesin proteins of type I, P and S fimbriae were shown to be located at the tips of the respective organelles.[213–216a] Further studies of type I fimbriae have revealed that the antigenic structure of the adhesin protein of type I fimbriae is more highly conserved than is that of the major structural protein among different strains of *E. coli*. The vaccine implications of these findings are obvious; vaccines prepared from the shared adhesin proteins should be broadly protective against many strains of *E. coli* and perhaps other gram-negative bacillary infections.

Adherence as a Means of Toxin Delivery. The pathogenesis of cholera parallels the pathogenesis of diarrhea by ETEC; however, the adherence mechanisms are entirely different. Certain *Vibrio cholerae* biotypes, namely, classic and El Tor, colonize the human small intestine where they release an enterotoxin (choleragen). When the choleragen comes into contact with the host intestinal mucosa, it stimulates host adenyl cyclase and results in a secretory diarrhea. As with diarrhea caused by ETEC, the key to this chain of events is the successful delivery of toxin to the target cell.[217] Although we cannot be sure of the precise means by which the vibrios associate with the human intestinal mucosa in vivo, in vitro and animal model studies conducted primarily by Freter and Jones indicate a multistep process.[218] An overlying blanket of mucus (mucous gel) blocks contact between luminal bacteria and intestinal mucosa.[76,219,220] Vibrios possess flagella that can propel them through the mucous gel, providing that the organism can also follow a chemotactic gradient to the intestinal surface.[219] Nonmotile[219,221,222] or nonchemotactic[219,223] mutant vibrios are avirulent unless they spontaneously revert and recover their locomotive powers.[219,222] Having arrived at the mucosal surface, the organism

TABLE 2. Characteristics of Some *Escherichia coli* Fimbrial Adhesins

	Fimbrial Classes												
	Common	*Host Specific*											
		Enteropathogenic				*Uropathogenic*							
										PCF8775			
Characteristic	*Type 1*	*K88*	*K99*	*987P*	*F-41*	*CFA/I*	*CFA/II: CS1, CS2, CS3*	*CFA/III*	*AF/R1*	*CS4/CS6*	*CS5/CS6*	P. fimbriae *(F-7 to F-12 and Others)*	*S*
Host	Animals Plants Bacteria Fungi	Pigs	Calves Lambs Pigs	Pigs	Calves Lambs Pigs	Humans	Humans	Humans Mice Rabbits	Rabbits	Humans		Humans	Humans Rats
Target cells	Procarytoic cells, eucarytoic cells	Enterocytes, brush border membranes			Enterocytes	Uroepithelial cells							Uroepithelial cells, vascular endothelial cells
Serogroup restricted?	No	Yes	Yes	Yes	Yes	Yes	Yes	Yes	Yes	Yes		Yes	Yes
Phenotypic expression	Phase variation	Temperature dependent	Temperature dependent	Phase variation	Temperature dependent	Temperature dependent	Temperature dependent	Temperature dependent	Temperature dependent	Temperature dependent		Temperature dependent	Phase variation
Genetic control	Chromosomal	Plasmid		Chromosomal			Plasmid					Chromosomal	Chromosomal
Agglutination													
Yeast cells	MS	0	0	0	0	0	0	—	—	—	—	0	0
Human RBC	MS	0	0	0	MR	MR	0	0	0	MR	MR	MR	MR
Guinea pig RBC	MS	MR	0	0	MR	0	0	—	0	0	MR	0	—
Horse RBC	MS	0	MR	0	MR	0	0	—	—	—	—	0	—
Sheep RBC	MS	0	MR	0	MR	0	0	—	—	—	—	0	—
Chicken RBC	—	MR	0	0	0	MR	MR	—	0	—	—	0	—
Bovine RBC	—	0	0	0	0	MR	MR	0	0	MR	MR	0	—
Structure													
Shape	Tubular	Filament	Helical filament	Tubular	Filament	Filament	Filament	—	Filament	—		Tubular	Tubular
Diameter	7.0 nm	2.1 nm	4.8 nm	7.0 nm	3.2 nm	3.2 nm	3.2 nm	—	5 nm	7 nm		5–7 nm (variable with type)	5–7 nm
Subunit molecular weight	17,100	27,540	18,500	20,000	29,500	15,058	13,000	18,000	19,000	—		17,000–22,000	17,000
References	44, 153	18, 154	18, 155	18, 48	18, 52, 53	18, 156	18	157, 158	159–163	54–56		57, 165–169	170–173

Abbreviations: MS: mannose-sensitive agglutination; MR: mannose-resistant agglutination; 0: no agglutination; (—): no data available.

firmly adheres to the brush border membranes of the intestinal epithelium, first by the nonflagellar end and then sideways.[76] The adhesin that mediates this attachment appears to be fimbriae (see below). The adherence is specific,[224] temperature dependent,[225] and time dependent;[76,226] requires divalent cations;[225] and is saturable.[76,226,227] In animal models characterized by bowel stasis, the organisms disengage from the mucosa after 7–16 hours;[76,228] if bowel flow is unimpeded, however, adherence remains constant.[227] Adherence to intestinal epithelial tissue is closely but not absolutely linked to vibrio motility.[222,224,226,228] Generally, nonmotile organisms do not adhere, even if compacted upon the intestinal mucosa.[222] *Vibrio cholerae* produces one or more hemagglutinins, and hemagglutination correlates with intestinal epithelial adherence.[222,225] Mannose[222] and fucose[222] inhibit hemagglutination and intestinal epithelial cell adherence (although some investigators question the latter[229]). Recently, Finkelstein and Hanne[77] and Finkelstein et al.[78] found a multifunctional cholera surface protein (cholera lectin) with the properties of hemagglutination, hydrophobicity, and protease activity. Antibodies to this material block *V. cholerae* adherence to intestinal epithelial cells, which suggests it may be the long-sought cholera adhesin.[77,78] Booth and colleagues, using cultured human intestinal epithelial cells, demonstrated correlations between adhesion of *V. cholerae* and expression of hemagglutinin activity.[230] This in vitro system had been used previously to examine adherence mechanisms of enterotoxigenic *E. coli*.[231,232] Key studies recently demonstrated that the same gene product (*tox R*) is (*1*) required for production of a pilus colonization factor that is encoded by the *tcp A* gene and is important in intestinal colonization; (*2*) controls the production of cholera toxin by regulating the activity of the *ctx* operon, the transcriptional unit that encodes for cholera toxin; (*3*) and is necessary for the expression of an outer-membrane protein encoded by the *ompll* gene.[233,234] This "coupling" of enterotoxicity and colonization where the same regulatory gene controls the transcription of multiple virulence factors of *V. cholerae* is fascinating pathogenetically.[233] In a similar vein, linkage of the genes for toxin and adhesive antigen production on a plasmid has been shown in enterotoxigenic *E. coli* strains of human[56,236–239] and animal[240] origin.

Multiple Adhesins. In the preceding sections, we have taken the simplistic approach—that each microbe has its own variety of adhesin and that the display of the adhesin directly determines the adherence of the microbe. A microorganism, however, is not necessarily limited to one adhesin system, particularly since having two or more systems could be advantageous to the organism. A fastidious organism could increase both the specificity and range of its adherence by simultaneously and differentially using more than one adhesin. In the following discussion of *N. gonorrhoeae*, two surface structures determine the adherence of gonococci to tissues and also influence the antigenicity of the bacterial surface and its resistance to host defenses. The first structure is a fimbrial adhesin referred to as gonococcal pili (P); the second structure is a protein component of the outer membrane known as protein II (P.II). The expression or nonexpression of both of these structures is independently subject to spontaneous change through a process of phase variation. Both structures are also susceptible to spontaneous antigenic and functional changes.[241]

Gonococcal infections begin with bacterial adherence to mucous-secreting cells of the urogenital tract.[82,242,243] The attachment is species[244] and host[242,245] specific. Organisms freshly isolated from the male urethral mucosa generally produce small, high-domed, opaque colonies; after several transfers on fresh media, however, a variety of other colonial forms develop. Swanson demonstrated that this polymorphism reflects a change in piliation and P.II under in vitro conditions[246] (Fig. 3). Gonococci with pili (P+ and P.II+) produce small, high-domed colonies, whereas cells without pili (P−) produce low,

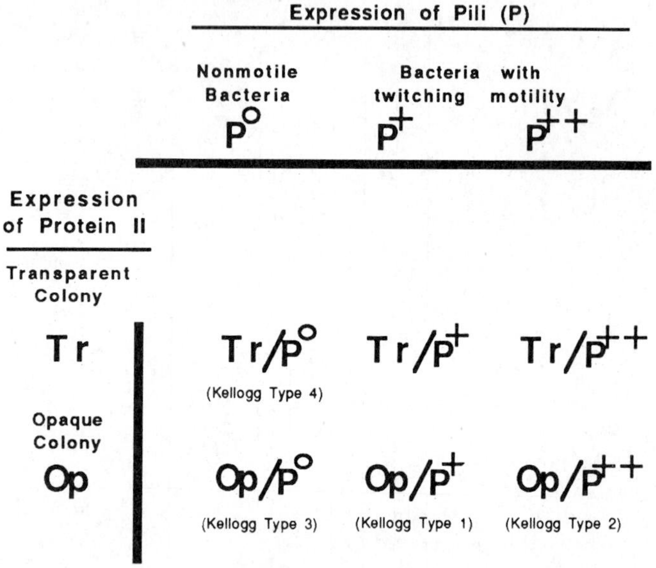

FIG. 3. The variety of colonial forms exhibited by *Neisseria gonorrhoeae* are organized on this chart according to the expression of two adhesins: pili and protein II. Gonococci without pili are nonmotile (P°), while gonococci with varying amounts of pili demonstrate twitching motility (P^{+} and P^{++}). Most forms of protein II cause gonococci to aggregate and result in opaque (Op) colonies. If the gonococci do not produce protein II (or produce certain varieties of protein II), the cells do not aggregate, and the colony appears translucent (Tr). The independent expression of these two adhesins results in four to six colonial forms with different virulence properties.

broad colonies.[246] Particular types of P.II, on the other hand, cause the gonococci to adhere to one another, thereby resulting in highly aggregated opaque (Op) colonies.[246] Other types of P.II or the complete absence of P.II cause the organisms to grow separately and result in translucent (Tr) colonies.[246,247] Since both pili and opaque forms of P.II are conserved, the course of a natural gonococcal urethritis must select for these proteins.

We know that pili function as adhesins since cells with pili adhere better than do cells without pili.[248,249] Furthermore, purified pili preferentially adhere to human cells of buccal and genital (sperm, vaginal epithelium, fallopian tube mucosa) origin over a variety of other human cells (e.g., RBCs polymorphonuclear [PMN] leukocytes, and tissue culture cells.[250,251] This adherence has pH and temperature optimums and is saturable and promoted by multivalent ions (particularly ferric).[250,251] Anti-pilus antibodies are naturally present in the vaginal fluid of infected patients, and these antibodies inhibit gonococcal adherence.[252] This inhibition, however, is much greater for homologous than for heterologous strains, thus indicating that pili exhibit antigenic variation.[253] Spontaneous antigenic variation has also been observed in the course of natural infections.[247,254] This antigenic variation arises spontaneously from rearrangements of the pili gene,[255,256] which results in structural[257] and functional variation[258] along with antigenic variation. Despite this variability, different gonococcal pili have identical amino acid sequences that are shared at the aminotermini with the fimbriae of *Neisseria meningitidis, Moraxella nonliquifaciens*, and *Pseudomonas aeruginosa*.[259]

P.II actually includes a family of outer-membrane proteins that are structurally related[260] but antigenically[261] and functionally distinct.[83] For example, one particular P.II promotes gonococcal adherence to PMN leukocytes, whereas another P.II discourages it.[83] Individual P.II also influence antimicrobial resistance.[83] In general, P.II protects the gonococci from the lytic effect of serum[83] and promotes gonococcal adherence to buccal[83] and vaginal[262] epithelial cells. This adherence is selective. Opaque strains do not adhere as well to RBCs[83] and fallopian tube mucosa[82] as do transparent strains. Clones with different amounts and types of P.II arise spontaneously through the course of an infection[247,263] or its transmission.[264] Certain anatomic sites (male urethra) and metabolic conditions (cervical isolates from women at the midmenstrual cycle) seem to select for the expression of P.II, whereas other sites (fallopian tube) and metabolic conditions (cervical isolates from women during menses or from women using oral contraceptives) appear to exclude strains of P.II.[82,263] Even though pili are conserved under each of these conditions, they also undergo spontaneous antigenic and functional variation. Taken together, this evidence indicates that the quantitative and qualitative differential expression of P.II and pili enable the gonococci to infect and exploit a wide variety of human microenvironments by determining to which tissues the organism will adhere and its ability to repel host defenses.

Polymicrobial Adherence. So far, we have examined the topic of bacterial adherence by emphasizing the deployment and use of adhesins by individual pathogens as they launch their assault on the host. A much more common and wider application of bacterial adherence is in the coordination and construction of polymicrobial communities on surfaces. The best-studied example of this is in the microbiology of the human oropharynx.[10,11]

Infections of the gums and the teeth afflict more humans than do any other infectious disease. The causative agents are indigenous to our mouths and persist in that environment despite the constant scrubbing of our oral tissues by salivation and mastication. In the past, we ascribed this persistence to the organism's growth rate, that is, rapidly growing organisms replenish their losses and remain in place, whereas slowly growing organisms simply wash away.[10] Gibbons and Van Houte changed this concept by introducing evidence that the selective adherence of bacteria to the oral tissues determines the pattern of their oral colonization.[10] Abnormal conditions that accentuate or change this pattern, such as a sucrose-rich diet, result in dental disease.

Dental plaque, the provoking agent of dental disease, includes the bacterial accumulations in the crevices between tooth and gum (subgingival or supragingival plaque) and over the tooth's enamel surfaces (coronal plaque). By fixing bacteria onto oral surfaces, plaque allows microbial digestive and toxic products to cause dental dimineralization (caries) and mucosal inflammation (periodontitis and gingivitis). These bacterial accumulations should not be construed as amorphous conglomerates of random components. Rather, they represent microbial climax communities whose precise composition and organization varies in a predictable manner with certain factors such as oral location, host diet, and salivary secretions. For example, subgingival plaque is organized along three zones: the organisms next to the tooth are gram-positive, the organisms next to the gum are spirochetes and other motile bacteria, and the organisms in between are gram-negative.[10]

Specific molecular interactions dictate the plaque architecture. The interactions include bacterial cell to dental surface, bacterial cell to homologous cell, bacterial cell to heterologous cell, and bacterial cell to extracellular substance.[11] Extracellular substances are either host derived, such as secretory IgA, or bacterial derived, such as extracellular polymeric substances. Referred to as the plaque matrix, these substances give the bacterial biomass structural integrity in addition to influencing its overall design. Extracellular substances also play a role in anchoring the microbial plaque to the dental surface. As we mentioned earlier, all immersed solids adsorb dissolved materials to their surfaces. The teeth are no exception. A variety of salivary products of host and bacterial origin such as high-molecular-weight glycoproteins (salivary mucins), lysozyme, salivary agglutinins, IgA, fibronectin, and bacterial extracellular polymeric substances coat the dental surface and form a biofilm, or *pellicle*.[10,11,90] Consequently, these adsorbed substances function as either specific bacterial receptors or adherence blockers, thereby dictating the microbial composition of the adherent plaque. Two factors determine pellicle composition: first, hydroxyapatite, the major constituent of dental enamel, selectively adsorbs certain compounds such as acidic glycoproteins and acidic proteins. Second, the quality and quantity of various salivary constituents such as agglutinins and immunoglobulins vary greatly from person to person.[265–267]

The primary microbial constituents of dental plaque are streptococci (*S. mutans, S. mitis, S. mitior, S. sanguis,* and *S. salivarius*), actinomyces (*A. viscosus, A. naeslundii*), and veillonellae, but the microbial membership also includes *Lactobacillus, Neisseria, Bacteroides, Fusobacterium, Capnocytophaga, Actinobacillus, Selenomonas,* and *Campylobacter*, to name only a few.[10,11] The ecologic interactions among the oral bacteria, tissues, and secretions are far too complex and controversial to be discussed here. Instead, we will concentrate upon the proposed adherence mechanisms of three microorganisms—*S. mutans, S. sanguis,* and *A. viscosus*—as an illustration of the intricacies of plaque construction.

Streptococcus mutans produces dental caries in experimental animals only if the animals are fed a sucrose-rich diet. Curiously, when grown in vitro, the addition of sucrose—but not other carbohydrates—to laboratory media enables *S. mutans* to coat the media container with an adhesive layer of bacteria. This artificial plaque has attracted considerable attention because its form resembles dental plaque and because a similar processs in vivo could explain the association of dental caries with *S. mutans* and sucrose.[10,96] In sucrose media, *S. mutans* extracellular enzymes synthesize a number of polysaccharides, including glucans and fructans, that form part of the dental pellicle and the plaque matrix. The glucans may function as adhesins and bind *S. mutans* cells to each other through surface glucosyltransferases (GT)[95] and glucan-binding proteins (GBP),[92,94] which essentially act as cell surface lectins (or adhesins). *Streptococcus mutans* constantly release GT into the surrounding media where the GT remains active, creates more glucan, and perhaps further enmeshes the *S. mutans* and other bacteria.[10] As a component of the dental pellicle, glucan also functions as a receptor binding the *S. mutans* to the dental enamel[93] via GT and GBP. It appears, however, that a variety of other mechanisms may play a greater role in the adherence of *S. mutans* to teeth.[95] For example, hydroxyapatite adsorbs streptococci via cell surface teichoic acid in vitro and could thus bind the cells in vivo.[268] Furthermore, *S. mutans* adheres to pellicle proteins such as fibronectin[90] and to salivary agglutinins,[10] and antibodies to serotype antigens are known to interfere with adherence.[269] In a similar manner, a cell surface galactose-specific lectin binds *S. mutans* to pellicle carbohydrates, further tying the organisms to the dental surface.[97]

Streptococcus mutans dental adherence does not take place independently of other bacteria. Organisms such as *A. viscosus* can also bind to *S. mutans*-generated glucan via their own cell surface GBP.[112] If the microbe lacks GBP such as in the case of most *S. sanguis* strains, the organism may still bind to the glucan by adsorbing to its surface GT released from *S. mutans*.[270] *S. sanguis* and *A. viscosus* coaggregate, which further illustrates the complexity of dental plaque architecture. *Actinomyces viscosus* binds to *S. sanguis* surface carbohydrate by a fimbrial lactose-sensitive lectin[110,271,272] and by lactose-resistant fimbriae.[100] Isolation of phage-resistant mutants has allowed investigators to observe a functional relationship between phage receptors of *A. viscosus* and coaggregation.[273,274] Continuation of these studies should allow delineation of the molecular mechanisms involved in these interactions. The lactose-resistant fimbriae also appear to bind *A. viscosus* to the dental pellicle.[111] Recent work by Gibbons and Hay[275] suggests that both proline-rich proteins and statherin may act as pellicle receptors for *A. viscosus*. An interesting finding in these studies was that the proline-rich proteins apparently undergo a confirmational change upon binding to hydroxyapatite that allows the *A. viscosus* to recognize "hidden molecular segments" on these receptors.[275] *Streptococcus sanguis* seems to bind to the dental surface by mechanisms similar to *S. mutans*[90,93,276] and to possess fibrillae that bind salivary agglutinins, further fixing the organism to the dental plaque.[98,99] The sum of these adherence mechanisms, along with others that we have not described, is a tightly knit and highly organized microbial community. The host's secretions, diet, and tissues determine the array of exposed bacterial receptors, which in turn, guide the dental plaque architecture and composition by promoting the adherence of particular bacteria.

Receptor Specificity. The presence of microbial receptors on host tissue is just as much a determinant of microbial infectivity as is the microbe's display of adhesins. If the host does not express the correct receptor, binding and subsequent colonization and infection cannot take place. The host's display of microbial receptors may be genetically determined or subject to later modification or induction. These host receptors fall into two categories—cell surface sugar residues of the glycocalyx and cell surface proteins.

Table 1 demonstrates that, so far, sugar moieties are the primary residues identified as microbial receptors. Whereas many simple sugars are listed as receptors, more precisely, these receptors represent the simplest molecular structures exhibiting receptor activity. In actuality, these sugars are submolecular components of larger structures that function as the true receptor; the saccharide is simply the active site. The precise orientation of the sugar moiety on the molecule and the presence of neighboring submolecular structures primarily determines the specificity of the adhesin–receptor interaction. For example, Firon et al.[44] recently demonstrated that the combining site for *E. coli* contains a hydrophobic region and is in a form to best receive a D-mannose-containing trisaccharide, Manα(1–3)Manβ(1–4)GlcNac. The best receptor–fimbriae fits that they obtained were with short oligomannoside chains linked to a carrier molecule by *N*-glycoside.[44] Carrier molecules for sugar-specific receptors are either glycoproteins (e.g., glycophorin for *Mycoplasma gallisepticum*,[40] and *Plasmodium falciparum*[119], and Tam-Horsfall protein[43] and erythrocyte glycoprotein[227] for *E. coli* type I fimbriae) or glycolipids (e.g., the gangliosides: GM_1 for K88 fimbriae,[18] GM_2 for K99 and CFA/1 fimbriae,[18,47] GD_1 for *N. gonorrhoeae*,[62] and the glycolipid P blood group antigens for P fimbriae.[58])

As opposed to the variety of sugar-specific receptors, only one protein, fibronectin, has been promoted as a microbial receptor. Fibronectin has attracted considerable interest since it binds a variety of gram-positive cocci (*S. aureus*,[278–281] S. pyogenes,[89] *S. mutans*,[90] S. salivarius,[90] *S. mitior*,[90] and groups C and G streptococci[91]) rather than one or two selected microbial species. This binding is truly multivalent because different fragments of the fibronectin molecule bind different bacteria.[88,89] Fibronectin does not bind as well to gram-negative bacteria,[89,280] which suggests that one of fibronectin's functions is to fix gram-positive bacteria rather than gram-negative bacteria to the cell surface. Woods et al. first suggested that fibronectin functions as a modulator of the human oral microecology by selectively promoting gram-positive coccal adherence over gram-negative bacillary adherence.[282,283] They noted that by using trypsin they could digest cell-bound fibronectin and thereby increase the adherence of *P. aeruginosa* to oral epithelial cells. Fibronectin on the oral mucosa is confined to the exposed epithelial surface.[284] By scraping the buccal epithelium, Abraham et al.[285] found two populations of cells. One population was coated with fibronectin and probably represented superficial cells; a second population was not coated with fibronectin and may have been deeper, unexposed cells. The fibronectin-coated cells bound *S. pyogenes* but not *E. coli* and *P. aeruginosa*, whereas the uncoated cells could not bind *S. pyogenes* but did bind *E. coli* and *P. aeruginosa*.[285] These observations tie in with the well-known clinical observation that certain patients (hospitalized, ill, aged) have predominantly gram-negative bacilli colonizing their oropharynx rather than the usual gram-positive cocci seen in healthy people.[286] Whether this change is due to salivary proteases[282,283] or diminished fibronectin levels in oral secretions[90,287] remains to be determined.[288] Since the aged and infirm are also subject to gram-negative bacillary pneumonias, it does suggest that fibronectin protects the host from certain infections by selectively influencing the oral microecology toward less invasive organisms.

Nonspecific Adherence. Even though the stereospecific interlocking of complementary microbial and host surface molecules characterizes the infection process, we should bear in mind that, in microbiology, host–pathogen interactions are special cases. Microbes can and do adhere to a wide range of animate and inanimate surfaces in a very nonspecific manner. For example, the human parasite *S. pyogenes* not only adheres to human epithelial cells but also to the surface of hydrocarbon droplets.[289,290] The hydrocarbon-degrading saprophyte *Acinetobacter calcoaceticus* RAG-1, on the other hand, binds to human epithelial cells in addition to its normal habitat of hydrocarbon droplets.[289,290] Furthermore, if a RAG-1 variant loses the ability to adhere to hydrocarbon droplets, it also loses the ability to adhere to epithelial cells.[289] This demonstrates that certain common adherence mechanisms mediate the binding of many different kinds of microbes to many different substrata. Less attention has been paid in the medical literature to these nonspecific processes since they do not directly select for the host. Nevertheless, nonspecific processes such as hydrophobicity are important for their ability to potentiate more specific adherence processes and promote the colonization and infection of inanimate foreign bodies such as indwelling medical devices.

Hydrophobicity. Since the human host is an aqueous environment, suspended particles with hydrophobic surfaces, such as microbes, will tend to leave the water phase and associate with host tissues. The earlier cited example of bacterial adherence to hydrocarbon droplets is, itself, an indirect measurement of microbial surface hydrophobicity,[289–291] as are hydrophobic interaction chromatography[182,229,292–295] and phase partition studies.[296–298] Microorganisms determined to be hydrophobic by these means have a greater tendency to adhere to animal tissues than do hydrophilic particles. The microbial expression of hydrophobicity, like other adherence mechanisms, changes with the stage of growth,[229,289] in response to environmental[229] or genetic influences, and by display of adhesive structures.[299] For example, the streptococcal adhesin LTA[131,300] and the *E. coli* adhesins type I fimbriae,[182] CFA fimbriae,[301] and K88 fimbriae[294] have hydrophobic properties that increase the organisms's hydrophobicity and its tissue adherence. At the same time, the surface hydrophobicity and in vitro adherence vary greatly among *E. coli* strains with type I fimbriae.[302] Several authors have suggested that hydrophobicity promotes more specific binding by bringing the two surfaces together and stabilizing their juxtaposition so that specific interactions between complementary molecules can take place.[229,294,303] In this regard, Falkowski and colleagues[304] have provided evidence that there may be a hydrophobic binding domain for *E. coli* adherence to epithelial cells.

Adherence of Bacteria to Medical Devices. Microbial colonization and infection of medical devices probably do not depend upon specific substrate receptors but likely proceed through more nonspecific means. We know that the engineering and composition of the surfaces of various devices encourage or discourage microbial colonization. Studies of the in vitro adhesion of various microorganisms to urinary catheters,[305] prosthetic vascular grafts,[306] suture material,[307] myringotomy tubes,[308] and intravascular catheters[309,310] indicate that the device's roughness,[307–309] chemical composition,[305,310–313] and hydrophobicity[311,314,315] increase microbial colonization. More recent studies[316] of coagulase-negative staphylococci treated with antimicrobial agents measured hydrophobicity and showed an excellent correlation with adherence of these organisms to plastic tissue culture plates in vitro. This suggests that this adherence depends heavily on hydrophobic surface moieties. The precise method of microbe-to-device binding is unknown for most of these situations. In the case of coagulase-negative staphylococcal adherence to plastic catheters, however, the situation appears analogous to Fletcher's investigations into the formation of microbial slime layers on marine solid surfaces. Fletcher's study organism, a marine pseudomonad, bound to surfaces such as polystyrene and glass by producing extracellular adhesive polymeric substances.[317] In a similar manner, some but not all strains of coagulase-negative staphylococci bind in vitro to plastic, glass, and intravascular catheters in a slime layer consisting of polysaccharides.[87,318–321] Epidemiologic and animal studies suggest that this slime plays a role in the pathogenesis of coagulase-negative staphylococccal foreign-body infections.[87,318,322–324] Consistent with these findings are the observations of Bayston and Penny[325] and others[326–328] that, upon removal from the patient, cerebrospinal fluid shunts and intravascular catheters are covered with coagulase-negative staphylococci enmeshed in a slimy or mucoid deposit. Moreover, recent clinical evidence[329,330] demonstrates that medical treatment failures and shunt complications are more likely to occur in cerebrospinal fluid shunt infections due to slime-producing coagulase-negative staphylococci as compared with strains that fail to produce slime.

ANTIADHESIVE THERAPY

Now that a number of adhesin–receptor systems have been identified, workers are using this knowledge to design antiadhesive prophylactic strategies that interdict the infectious process before it begins.[331] Three areas of investigation to develop effective prophylactic strategies have included (*1*) immunization, including both passive and active vaccines, (*2*) antimicrobial therapy, and (*3*) novel antiadhesive therapies.

The identification and purification of bacterial adhesins have enabled the production of adhesin vaccines that could provide the host with long-lasting protection. In order to be effective, however, vaccine-generated antibodies must be released near the susceptible tissue and be able to block bacterial attachment. If the adhesin is characterized by antigenic variation (such as in *N. gonorrhoeae* fimbriae) or has multiple forms (as in *E. coli* fimbriae), then the successful vaccine will have to evoke an immune response to common epitopes of antigenic variants or be manufactured as a multivalent vaccine that includes all adhesin forms. These last two points have been the major stumbling blocks in the current efforts to produce effective antiadhesive vaccines. The recent discovery that some of the fimbrial types contain structurally conserved adhesion proteins[216] may overcome some of these obstacles; a vaccine prepared from a single adhesin protein may be protective against a broader variety of bacteria bearing fimbriae exhibiting the same sugar binding specificity.

Immunization experiments in humans demonstrated excellent vaccine efficacy against diarrhea caused by enterotoxigenic *E. coli*.[332] None of the 10 volunteers who previously received the lyophilized milk immunoglobulins that had been prepared from the colostrum of cows immunized with several *E. coli* virulence antigens developed diarrhea after an oral challenge with *E. coli* H10407. In contrast, 9 of 10 control volunteers who received an immunoglobulin concentrate with no anti-*E. coli* activity had diarrhea.

Bacterial adherence to tissues can be blocked by antibiotics. Subinhibitory concentrations of antibiotics poison a variety of biologic functions and result in profound effects upon the bacterial surface and adherence capabilities. These effects may be used to prevent bacterial adherence and infection, particularly if the host is only transiently and predictably at risk such as in the prophylaxis against bacterial endocarditis.

The effect of antibiotics on adherence is neither predictable nor readily explained. Some strains of *S. pyogenes*,[331] *S. mutans*,[333] *A. naeslundii*,[333] and *E. coli*[334] exhibit decreased adherence when grown in subinhibitory concentrations of penicillin. This antibiotic causes resting-phase *S. pyogenes* organisms to leak their adhesin, LTA, into the surrounding medium and become less adherent.[128] *Escherichia coli*, on the other hand, loses its fimbriae and mannose-sensitive adherence when grown in sublethal concentrations of various antibiotics including streptomycin.[123,331,335] Eisenstein et al.[336] noted that one streptomycin-resistant isolate of *E. coli* retained its fimbriation despite a concurrent loss in its adherence ability when the organisms were grown in streptomycin. Examination by electron microscopy indicated that the functionless fimbriae were twice the length of normal fimbriae.[336] Taken together, these reports indicate that sublethal antibiotics may induce the leakage of preformed adhesins from resting cells, suppress the formation or expression of adhesins in growing cells, or induce the formation of functionally aberrant forms. Alternatively, antibiotics may cause the organism to reveal hidden adhesins or induce adhesin formation.

In addition to the traditional therapeutic modalities of antibiotics and vaccination, novel approaches to the prophylaxis of infectious diseases may become possible through knowledge of the specific adherence mechanisms involved. Aronson et al. reasoned that mannose and its derivatives would act as receptor analogues and block the attachment of type I fimbriated *E. coli* to mouse bladder epithelial cells.[184] To test this hypothesis, they instilled *E. coli* with either the receptor analogue, α-methylmannoside or the control α-methylglucoside into mouse bladders. Animals receiving the receptor analogue had far fewer episodes of cystitis than did animals receiving the control carbohydrate. Receptor analogue therapy may become complicated if the receptor analogue binds to the cell and functions as a cell surface receptor or if the receptor analogue also blocks attachment of the bacterium to professional phagocytes. Bar-Shavit et al.[337] demonstrated that when type I fimbriated organisms were instilled into the peritoneal cavity of mice along with mannose the virulence of the organisms was accentuated. The alternative approach, using chemical modification of the surface, was elegantly demonstrated by Parsons et al.[338–340] They noted that the natural glycosaminoglycan layer covering the urinary bladder mucosa prevented the adherence of bacteria. Stripping the bladder of the cover increased bacterial adherence, but covering the denuded surface with natural (heparin) or synthetic glycoaminoglycans once again protected it from bacterial adherence.

ACKNOWLEDGMENTS

The authors would like to thank the following individuals who provided key suggestions in the revision of this chapter: Drs. Joel B. Baseman, James P. Duguid, Richard A. Finkelstein, Madilyn Fletcher, Anthony G. Gristina, Richard E. Isaacson, Kevin Marshall, Itzak Ofek, Barrett Sugarman, and John Swanson. We are also indebted to Susan Selig for reference review and Pamela Swann for her untiring efforts in the preparation of the chapter revision.

REFERENCES

1. Guyot G. Uber die bakterielle hemagglutination. Zbt Bakt Abt I Orig. 1908;47:640–53.
2. Zobell CE, Allen EC. The significance of marine bacteria in the fouling of submerged surfaces. J Bacteriol. 1935;29:239–51.
3. Duguid JP, Smith IW, Dempster G, et al. Non-flagellar filamentous appendages (''fimbriae'') and haemagglutinating activity in *Bacterium coli*. J Pathol Bacteriol. 1955;70:335–48.
4. Duguid JP, Gillies RR. Fimbriae and adhesive properties in dysentery bacilli. J Pathol Bacteriol. 1957;74:397–411.
5. Duguid JP, Gillies RR. Fimbriae and haemagglutinating activity in *Salmonella, Klebsiella, Proteus* and *Chromobacterium*. J Pathol Bacteriol. 1958;75:519–20.
6. Duguid JP. Fimbriae and adhesive properties in klebsiella strains. J Gen Microbiol. 1959;21:271–86.
7. Duguid JP, Anderson ES. Fimbriae and adhesive properties in salmonellae. J Pathol Bacteriol. 1966;92:107–38.
8. Duguid JP, Anderson ES. Terminology of bacterial fimbriae, or pili, and their types. Nature. 1967;215:89–90.
9. Duguid JP, Old DC. Adhesive properties of Enterobacteriaceae. In: Beachey EH, ed. Bacterial Adherence (Receptors and Recognition). v. 6. ser. B. New York: Chapman & Hall; 1980:184–218.
10. Gibbons RJ, van Houte J. Bacterial adherence and the formation of dental plaques. In: Beachey EH, ed. Bacterial Adherence (Receptors and Recognition). v. 6. ser. B. New York: Chapman & Hall; 1980:60–104.
11. van Houte J. Bacterial adherence and dental plaque formation. Infection. 1982;10:252–60.
12. Beachey EH, ed. Bacterial Adherence (Receptors and Recognition). v. 6. ser. B. New York: Chapman & Hall; 1980.
13. Berkeley RCW, Lynch JM, Melling J, et al. Microbial Adhesion to Surfaces. Chichester, England: Ellis Horwood; 1980.
14. Bitton G, Marshall KC. Adsorption of Microorganisms to Surfaces. New York: John Wiley & Sons; 1980.
15. Marshall KC. Interfaces in Microbial Ecology. Cambridge, MA: Harvard University Press; 1976.
16. Elliot K, O'Connor M, Whelan J. Adhesion and Microorganisms Pathogenicity, Ciba Foundation Symposium 80. London: Pitman Medical; 1981.
17. Beachey EH, Eisenstein BI, Ofek I. Bacterial Adherence in Infectious Diseases, Current Concepts. Kalamazoo, MI: Upjohn; 1982.
18. Gaastra W, de Graaf FK. Host-specific fimbrial adhesins of noninvasive enterotoxigenic *Escherichia coli* strains. Microbiol Rev. 1982;46:129–61.
19. Smith H. Microbial surfaces in relation to pathogenicity. Bacteriol Rev. 1977;41:475–500.
20. Beachey EH. Bacterial adherence: Adhesin–receptor interactions mediating the attachment of bacteria to mucosal surfaces. J Infect Dis. 1981;143:325–45.
21. Costerton JW, Geesey GG, Cheng K-J. How bacteria stick. Sci Am. 1978;238:86–95.
22. Jones GW. The attachment of bacteria to the surface of animal cells. In: Reissig JL, ed. Microbial Intereactions (Receptors and Recognition). v. 3. ser. B. London: Chapman & Hall; 1977:139–76.
23. Geesey GG. Microbial exopolymers: Ecological and economic considerations. Am Soc Microbiol News. 1982;48:9–14.
24. Ward JB, Berkeley RCW. The microbial cell surface and adhesion. In: Berkeley RCW, Lynch JM, Melling J, et al, eds. Microbial Adhesion to Surfaces. Chichester, England: Ellis Horwood; 1980:48–60.
25. Bennet HS. Morphological aspects of extracellular polysaccharides. J Histochem Cytochem. 1963;11:14–23.
26. Ito S. Structure and function of the glycocalyx. Fed Proc. 1969;28:12–25.
27. Goldstein IJ, Hughes RC, Monsigny M, et al. What should be called a lectin? Nature. 1980;285:66.
28. Freter R. Mechanisms of association of bacteria with mucosal surfaces. In: Elliot K, O'Connor M, Whelan J, eds. Adhesion and Microorganism Pathogenicity, Ciba Foundation Symposium 80. London: Pitman Medical; 1981:36–55.
29. Marshall KC, Stout R, Mitchell R. Mechanism of the initial events in the sorption of marine bacteria to surfaces. J Gen Microbiol. 1971;68:337–48.
30. Fletcher M, Latham MJ, Lynch JM, et al. The characteristics of interfaces and their role in microbial attachment. In: Berkeley RCW, Lynch JM, Melling J, et al, eds. Microbial Adhesion to Surfaces. Chichester, England: Ellis Horwood; 1980:67–78.
31. Grieg RG, Jones MN. The possible role of steric forces in cellular cohesion. J Theor Biol. 1976;63:405–9.
32. Grieg RG, Jones MN. Mechanisms of intercellular adhesion. Biosystems. 1977;9:43–55.
33. Rutter PR, Vincent B. The adhesion of micro-organisms to surfaces: Physico-chemical aspects. In Berkeley RCW, Lynch JM, Melling J, et al, eds. Microbial Adhesion to Surfaces. Chichester, England: Ellis Horwood; 1980:79–92.
34. Tadros RF. Particle surface adhesion. In Berkeley RCW, Lynch JM, Melling J, et al, eds. Microbial Adhesion to Surfaces. Chichester, England: Ellis Horwood; 1980:93–116.
35. Ofek I, Sharon N. Lectinophagocytosis: A molecular mechanism of recognition between cell surface sugars and lectins in the phagocytosis of bacteria. Infect Immun. 1988;56:539–47.
36. Meager A, Hughes RC. Virus receptors. In: Cuatrecasas P, Greaves MF, eds. Receptors and Recognition, v. 4, ser. A. London: Chapman & Hall; 1977:143–59.
37. Crowell RL, Lonberg-Holm K. Viral Attachment and Entry Into Cells. Washington DC: American Society for Microbiology; 1986.
38. Levy NJ. Wheat germ agglutinin blockage of chlamydial attachment sites: antagonism by *N*-acetyl-D-glucosamine. Infect Immun. 1979;25:946–53.
39. Levy NJ, Moulder JW. Attachment of cell walls of *Chlamydia psittaci* to mouse fibroblasts (L cells). Infect Immun. 1982;37:1059–65.
40. Razin S, Kahane I, Banai M, et al. Adhesion of mycoplasms to eukaryotic cells. In: Elliot K, O'Connor M, Whelan J, eds. Adhesion and Microorganism Pathogenicity, Ciba Foundation symposium 80. London: Pitman Medical; 1981:98–106.
41. Krause DC, Baseman JB. Inhibition of *Mycoplasma pneumoniae* hemadsorption and adherence to respiratory epithelium by antibodies to a membrane protein. Infect Immun. 1983;39:1180–6.
42. Krause DC, Leith DK, Baseman JB. Reacquisition of specific proteins confers virulence in *Mycoplasma pneumoniae*. Infect Immun. 1983;39:830–6.
43. Chick S, Harber MJ, Mackenzie R, et al. Modified method for studying bacterial adhesion to isolated uroepithelial cells and uromucoid. Infect Immun. 1981;34:256–61.
44. Firon N, Ofek I, Sharon N. Interaction of mannose-containing oligosaccharides with the fimbrial lectin of *Escherichia coli*. Biochem Biophys Res Commun. 1982;105:1426–32.
45. Laux DC, McSweegan EF, Williams TJ, et al. Identification and characterization of mouse small intestine mucosal receptors for *Escherichia coli* K-12 (K88ab). Infect Immun. 1986;52:18–25.
46. Smit H, Gaastra W, Kamerling JP, et al. Isolation and structural characterization of the equine erythrocyte receptor for enterotoxigenic *Escherichia coli* K99 fimbrial adhesion. Infect Immun. 1984;46:578–84.
47. Faris A, Lindahl M, Wadstrom T. GM_2-like glycoconjugate as possible erythrocyte receptor for the CFA/I and K99 hemagglutinins of enterotoxigenic *Escherichia coli*. FEMS Microbiol Lett. 1980;7:265–9.
48. Isaacson RE, Richter P. *Escherichia coli* 987P pilus: Purification and partial characterization. J Bacteriol. 1981;146:784–9.
49. Dean EA, Isaacson RE. In vitro adhesion of piliated *Escherichia coli* to small intestinal villous epithelial cells from rabbits and the identification of a soluble 987P pilus receptor-containing fraction. Infect Immun. 1982;36:1192–8.
50. Dean EA, Isaacson RE. Purification and characterization of a receptor for the 987P pilus of *Escherichia coli*. Infect Immun. 1985;47:98–105.
51. Dean EA, Isaacson RE. Location and distribution of a receptor for the 987P pilus of *Escherichia coli* in small intestines. Infect Immun. 1985;47:345–8.
52. de Graaf F, Frits K, Roorda I. Production, purification, and characterization of the fimbrial adhesive antigen F41 isolated from calf enteropathogenic *Escherichia coli* strain B41M. Infect Immun. 1982;36:751–8.
53. Morris JA, Thorns C, Scott AC, et al. Adhesion *in vitro* and *in vivo* associated with an adhesive antigen (F41) produced by a K99 mutant of the reference strain *Escherichia coli* B41. Infect Immun. 1982;36:1146–53.
54. Thomas LV, Cravioto A, Scotland SM, et al. New fimbrial antigenic type (E8775) that may represent a colonization factor in enterotoxigenic *Escherichia coli* in humans. Infect Immun. 1982;35:1119–24.
55. Thomas LV, McConnell MM, Rowe B, Field AM. The possession of three novel coli surface antigens by enterotoxigenic *Escherichia coli* strains positive for the putative colonization factor PCF8775. J Gen Microbiol. 1985;131:2319–26.
56. Thomas LV, Rowe B, McConnell MM. In strains of *Escherichia coli* 0167 a single plasmid encodes for the coli surface antigens CS5 and CS6 of putative colonization factor PCF8775, heat-stable enterotoxin, and colicin IA. Infect Immun. 1987;55:1929–31.
57. Leffler H, Svanborg-Eden C. Glycolipid receptors for uropathogenic *Escherichia coli* on human erythrocytes and uroepithelial cells. Infect Immun. 1981;34:920–9.
58. Svenson SB, Hultberg H, Kallenius G, et al. P-fimbriae of pyelonephritogenic *Escherichia coli*: Identification and chemical characterization of receptors. Infection. 1983;11:61–7.
59. Fader RC, Duffy LK, Davis CP, et al. Purification and chemical characterization of type 1 pili isolated from *Klebsiella pneumoniae*. J Biol Chem. 1982;257:3301–5.
60. Korhonen TK, Lounatmaa K, Ranta H, et al. Characterization of type 1 pili of *Salmonella typhimurium* LT2. J. Bacteriol. 1980;144:800–5.
61. Mirelman D, Altmann G, Eshdat Y. Screening of bacterial isolates for mannose-specific lectin activity by agglutination of yeast. J Clin Microbiol. 1980;11:328–31.
62. Pearce WA, Buchanan TM. Structure and cell membrane-binding properties of bacterial fimbriae. In: Beachey EH, ed. Bacterial Adherence (Receptors and Recognition). v. 6. ser. B. New York: Chapman & Hall, 1980:289–344.
63. Pruzzo C, Debbia EA, Satta G. Identification of the major adherence ligand of *Klebsiella pneumoniae* in the receptor for coliphage T7 and alteration of *Klebsiella* adherence properties by lysogenic conversion. Infect Immun. 1980;30:562–71.
64. Old DC, Adegbola RA. Haemagglutinins and fimbriae of *Morganella, Proteus,* and *Providencia*. J Med Microbiol. 1982;15:551–64.
65. Old DC, Scott SS. Hemagglutinins and fimbriae of *Providencia* spp. J Bacteriol. 1981;146:404–8.
66. Maclagan RM, Old DC. Hemagglutinins and fimbriae in different serotypes and biotypes of *Yersinia enterocolitica*. J Appl Bacteriol. 1980;49:353–60.
67. Old DC, Robertson J. Adherence of fimbriate and non-fimbriate strains of

Yersinia enterocolitica to human epithelial cells. Microbiol Immunol. 1981;25:993–8.
68. Sastry PA, Pearlstone JR, Smillie LB, et al. Amino acid sequence of pilin isolated from *Pseudomonas aeruginosa* PAK. FEBS Lett. 1983;151:253–6.
69. Woods DE, Straus DC, Johanson WG Jr, et al. Role of pili in adherence of *Pseudomonas aeruginosa* to mammalian buccal epithelial cells. Infect Immun. 1980;29:1146–51.
70. Glorioso JC, Jones GW, Rush HG, et al. Adhesion of type A *Pasteurella multocida* to rabbit pharyngeal cells and its possible role in rabbit respiratory tract infections. Infect Immun. 1982;35:1103–9.
71. Muse KE, Collier AM, Baseman JB. Scanning electron microscopic study of hamster tracheal organ cultures infected with *Bordetella pertussis*. J Infect Dis. 1977;136:768–77.
72. Morse JH, Morse SI. Studies on the ultrastructure of *Bordetella pertussis*. I. Morphology, origin, and biological activity of structures present in the extracellular fluid of liquid cultures of *Bordetella pertussis*. J Exp Med. 1970;131:1342–57.
73. Sato Y, Sato H, Izumiya K, et al. Role of antibody of filamentous hemagglutinin in immunity to pertussis. In: Robbins JB, Hill JC, Sadoff JC, eds. Bacterial Vaccines (Symposium on Infectious Diseases). New York: Thieme; 1981:380–5.
74. Lampe RM, Mason EO Jr, Kaplan SL, et al. Adherence of *Haemophilus influenzae* to buccal epithelial cells. Infect Immun. 1982;35:166–72.
75. Pichichero ME, Loeb M, Anderson P, et al. Do pili play a role in pathogenicity of *Haemophilus influenzae* type B? Lancet. 1982;2:960–2.
76. Nelson ET, Clements JD, Finkelstein RA. *Vibrio cholerae* adherence and colonization in experimental cholera: Electron microscopic studies. Infect Immun. 1976;14:527–47.
77. Finkelstein RA, Hanne LF. Purification and characterization of the soluble hemagglutinin (cholera lectin) produced by *Vibrio cholerae*. Infect Immun. 1982;36:1199–208.
78. Finkelstein RA, Boesman-Finkelstein M, Holt P. *Vibrio cholera* hemagglutinin/lectin/protease hydrolyzes fibronectin and ovomucin: F. M. Burnet revisited. Proc Natl Acad Sci USA. 1983;80:1092–5.
79. Rodgers FG, Greaves PW, Macrae AD, Lewis MJ. Electron microscopic evidence of flagella and pili on *Legionella pneumophila*. J Clin Pathol. 1980;33:1184–8.
80. Stephens DS, McGee ZA. Attachment of *Neisseria meningitidis* to human mucosal surfaces: Influence of pili and type of receptor cell. J Infect Dis. 1981;143:525–32.
81. Salit IE, Morton G. Adherence of *Neisseria meningitidis* to human epithelial cells. Infect Immun. 1981;31:430–5.
82. Swanson J. Adhesion and entry of bacteria into cells: A model of the pathogenesis of gonorrhea. In: Smith H, Skehel JJ, Turner MJ, eds. The Molecular Basis of Microbial Pathogenicity, Dahlem Konferenzen. Weinheim: Verlag Chemie GmbH; 1980:17–40.
83. Lambden PR, Heckels JE, James LT, et al. Variations in surface protein composition associated with virulence properties in opacity types of *Neisseria gonorrhoeae*. J Gen Microbiol. 1979;114:305–12.
84. Sato H, Yanagawa R, Fukuyama H. Adhesion of *Corynebacterium renale, Corynebacterium pilosum*, and *Corynebacterium cystitidis* to bovine urinary bladder epithelial cells of various ages and levels of differentiation. Infect Immun. 1982;36:1241–5.
85. Honda E, Yanagawa R. Pili-mediated attachment of *Corynebacterium renale* to mucous membrane of urinary bladder of mice. Am J Vet Res. 1978;39:155–8.
86. Carruthers MM, Kabat WJ. Mediation of staphylococcal adherence to mucosal cells by lipoteichoic acid. Infect Immun. 1983;40:444–6.
87. Christensen GD, Simpson WA, Bisno AL, et al. Adherence to slime-producing strains of *Streptococcus epidermidis* to smooth surfaces. Infect Immun. 1982;37:318–26.
88. Simpson WA, Beachey EH. Adherence of group A streptococci to fibronectin on oral epithelial cells. Infect Immun. 1983;39:275–9.
89. Simpson WA, Hasty DL, Mason JM, et al. Fibronectin-mediated binding of group A streptococci to human polymorphonuclear leukocytes. Infect Immun. 1982;37:805–10.
90. Babu J, Simpson WA, Courtney HS, et al. Interaction of human plasma fibronectin with cariogenic and non-cariogenic oral streptococci. Infect Immun. 1983;41:162–8.
91. Switalski LM, Ljungh A, Ryden C, et al. Binding of fibronectin to the surface of group A, C, and G streptococci isolated from human infections. Eur J Clin Microbiol. 1982;1:381–7.
92. Germaine GR, Schachtele CF. *Streptococcus mutans* dextransucrase: Mode of interaction with high-molecular-weight dextran and role in cellular aggregation. Infect Immun. 1976;13:365–72.
93. Liljemark WF, Schauer SV. Competitive binding among oral streptococci to hydroxyapatite. J Dent Res. 1977;56:157–65.
94. McCabe MM, Hamelik RM, Smith EE. Purification of dextran-binding protein from cariogenic *Streptococcus mutans*. Biochem Biophys Res. Commun. 1977;78:273–8.
95. Staat RH, Langley SD, Doyle RJ. *Streptococcus mutans* adherence: Presumptive evidence for protein-mediated attachment followed by glucan-dependent cellular accumulation. Infect Immun. 1980;27:675–81.
96. Wenham DG, Davies RM, Cole JA. Insoluble glucan synthesis by mutansucrase as a determinant of the cariogenicity of *Streptococcus mutans*. J Gen Microbiol. 1981;127:407–15.
97. Gibbons RJ, Qureshi JV. Inhibition of adsorption of *Streptococcus mutans* strains to saliva-treated hydroxyapatite by galactose and certain amines. Infect Immun. 1979;26:1214–7.
98. Hogg SD, Embery G. Blood-group reactive glycoprotein from human saliva interacts with lipoteichoic acid on the surface of *Streptococcus sanguis* cells. Arch Oral Biol. 1982;27:261–8.
99. Hogg SD, Handley PS, Embery G. Surface fibrils may be responsible for the salivary glycoprotein-mediated aggregation of the oral bacterium *Streptococcus sanguis*. Arch Oral Biol. 1981;26:945–9.
100. Kolenbrander PE. Isolation and characterization of coaggregation detective mutants of *Actinomyces viscosus, Actinomyces naeslundii*, and *Streptococcus sanguis*. Infect Immun. 1982;37:1200–8.
101. Liljemark WF, Bloomquist CG. Isolation of a protein-containing cell surface component from *Streptococcus sanguis* which affects its adherence to saliva-coated hydroxyapatite. Infect Immun. 1981;34:428–34.
102. Weerkamp AH, Jacobs T. Cell wall-associated protein antigens of *Streptococcus salivarius*: Purification, properties, and function in adherence. Infect Immun. 1982; 38:233–42.
103. Weerkamp AH, McBride BC. Identification of a *Streptococcus salivarius* cell wall component mediating coaggregation with *Veillonella alcalescens* V-1. Infect Immun. 1981;32:723–30.
104. McCabe RM, Donkersloot JA. Adherence of *Veillonella* species mediated by extracellular glucosyltransferase from *Streptococcus salivarius*. Infect Immun. 1977;18:726–34.
105. Bagg J, Poxton IR, Weir DM, et al. Binding of type 111 group B streptococci to buccal epithelial cells. J Med Microbiol. 1982;15:363–72.
106. Broughton RA, Baker CJ. Role of adherence in the pathogenesis of neonatal group B streptococcal infection. Infect Immun. 1983;39:837–43.
107. Handley PS, Jacob AE. Some structural and physiological properties of fimbriae of *Streptococcus faecalis*. J Gen Microbiol. 1981;127(Pt 2):289–93.
108. Onderdonk AB, Moon NE, Kasper DL, et al. Adherence of *Bacteroides fragilis* in vivo. Infect Immun. 1978;19:1083–7.
109. Yamazaki Y, Ebisu S, Okada H. *Eikonella corrodens* adherence to human buccal epithelial cells. Infect Immun. 1981;31:21–7.
110. Revis GJ, Vatter AE, Crowle AJ, et al. Antibodies against the Ag2 fimbriae of *Actinomyces viscosus* T14V inhibit lactose-sensitive bacterial adherence. Infect Immun. 1982;36:1217–22.
111. Clark WB, Webb EL, Wheeler TT, et al. Role of surface fimbriae (fibrils) in the adsorption of *Actinomyces* species to saliva-treated hydroxyapatite surfaces. Infect Immun. 1981;33:908–17.
112. Bourgeau G, McBride BC. Dextran mediates interbacterial aggregation between dextran-synthesizing streptococci and *Actinomyces viscosus*. Infect Immun. 1976;13:1228–34.
113. Ellen RP, Walker DL, Chau KH. Association of long surface appendages with adherence related functions of the gram-positive species *Actinomyces naeslundii*. J Bacteriol. 1978;134:1171–5.
114. Thomas DD, Baseman JB, Alderette JF. Fibronectin mediates *Treponema pallidum* cytadherence through recognition of fibronectin cell-binding domain. J Exp Med. 1985;161:514–25.
115. Thomas DD, Baseman JB, Alderette JF. Putative *Treponema pallidum* cytadhesins share a common functional domain. Infect Immun. 1985;49:833–5.
116. Maisch PA, Calderone RA. Role of surface mannan in the adherence of *Candida albicans* to fibrin-platelet clots formed in vitro. Infect Immun. 1981;32:92–7.
117. Sandin RL, Rogers AL, Patterson RJ, et al. Evidence for mannose-mediated adherence of *Candida albicans* to human buccal cells in vitro. Infect Immun. 1982;35:79–85.
118. Howard RJ, Miller LH. Invasion of erythrocytes by malaria merozoites: Evidence for specific receptors involved in attachment and entry. In: Elliott K, O'Connor M, Whelan J, eds. Adhesion and Microbial Pathogenicity, Ciba Foundation Symposium 80. Tunbridge Well, England: Pitman Medical; 1981:202–14.
119. Jungery M, Pasvol G, Newbold CI, et al. A lectin-like receptor is involved in invasion of erythrocytes by *Plasmodium falciparum*. Proc Natl Acad Sci USA. 1983;80:1018–22.
120. Kobiler D, Mirelman D. Lectin activity in *Entamoeba histolytica* trophozoites. Infect Immun. 1980;29:221–5.
121. Kobiler D, Mirelman D. Adhesion of *Entamoeba histolytica* trophozoites to monolayers of human cells. J Infect Dis. 1981;144:539–46.
122. Erlandsen SL, Chase DG. Morphological alterations in the microvillous border of villous epithelial cells produced by intestinal microorganisms. Am J Clin Nutr. 1974;27:1277–86.
123. Beachey EH, Ofek I. Epithelial cell binding of group A streptococci by lipoteichoic acid on fimbriae denuded of M protein. J Exp Med. 1976;143:759–71.
124. Ellen RP, Gibbons RJ. Parameters affecting the adherence and tissue tropisms of *Streptococcus pyogenes*. Infect Immun. 1974;9:85–91.
125. Ofek I, Beachey EH, Jefferson W, et al. Cell membrane-binding properties of group A streptococcal lipoteichoic acid. J Exp Med. 1975;141:990–1003.
126. Simpson WA, Ofek I, Sarasohn C. Characteristics of the binding of streptococcal lipoteichoic acid to human oral epithelial cells. J Infect Dis. 1980;141:457–62.
127. Wicken AJ, Knox KW. Biological properties of lipoteichoic acids. In: Schlessinger D, ed. Microbiology. Washington, DC: American Society for Microbiology; 1977:360–365.
128. Alkan ML, Beachey EH. Excretion of lipoteichoic acid by group A strep-

tococci: Influence of penicillin on excretion and loss of ability to adhere to human oral epithelial cells. J Clin Invest. 1978;61:671–7.
129. Ofek I, Simpson WA, Beachey EH. Formation of molecular complexes between a structurally defined M protein and acylated or deacylated lipoteichoic acid of *Streptococcus pyogenes*. J Bacteriol. 1982;149:426–33.
130. Hill MJ, James AM, Maxted WR. Some physical investigations of the behaviour of bacterial surfaces. X. The occurrence of lipid in the streptococcal cell wall. Biochim Biophys Acta. 1963;75:414–24.
131. Ofek I, Whitnack E, Beachey EH. Hydrophobic interactions of group A streptococci with hexadecane droplets. J Bacteriol. 1983;154:139–45.
132. Tylewska S, Hjerten S, Wadstrom T. Contribution of M protein to the hydrophobic surface properties of *Streptococcus pyogenes*. FEMS Microbiol Lett. 1979;6:249–53.
133. Miorner H, Johansson G, Kronvall G. Lipoteichoic acid is the major cell wall component responsible for surface hydrophobicity of group A streptococci. Infect Immun. 1983;39:336–43.
134. Alkan M, Ofek I, Beachey EH. Adherence of pharyngeal and skin strains of group A streptococci to human skin and oral epithelial cells. Infect Immun. 1977;18:555–7.
135. Selinger DS, Julie N, Reed WP, et al. Adherence of group A streptococci to pharyngeal cells: A role in the pathogenesis of rheumatic fever. Science. 1978;201:455–7.
136. Ofek I, Beachey EH, Eyal F, et al. Postnatal development of binding of streptococci and lipoteichoic acid by oral mucosal cells of humans. J Infect Dis. 1977;135:267–74.
137. Beachey EH, Simpson WA, Ofek I. Interaction of surface polymers of *Streptococcus pyogenes* with animal cells. In: Berkeley RCW, Lynch JM, Melling J, et al, eds. Microbial Adhesion to Surfaces. London: Ellis Horwood; 1980:389–405.
138. Chiang TM, Alkan ML, Beachey EH. Binding of lipoteichoic acid of group A streptococci to isolated human erythrocyte membranes. Infect Immun. 1979;26:316–21.
139. Courtney H, Ofek I, Simpson WA, et al. Characterization of lipoteichoic acid binding to polymorphonuclear leukocytes of human blood. Infect Immun. 1981;32:625–31.
140. Beachey EH, Dale JB, Simpson WA, et al. Erythrocyte binding properties of streptococcal lipoteichoic acids. Infect Immun. 1979;23:618–25.
141. Beachey EH, Chiang TM, Ofek I, et al. Interaction of lipoteichoic acid of group A streptococci with human platelets. Infect Immun. 1977;16:649–54.
142. Beachey EH, Dale JB, Grebe S, et al. Lymphocyte binding and T-cell mitogenic properties of group A streptococcal lipoteichoic acid. J Immunol. 1979;122:189–95.
143. Simpson WA, Beachey EH. Adherence of group A streptococci to fibronectin on oral epithelial cells. Infect Immun. 1983;39:275–9.
144. Courtney HS, Simpson WA, Beachey EH. Binding of streptococcal lipoteichoic acid to fatty-binding sites on human plasma fibronectin. J Bacteriol. 1983;153:763–70.
145. Phillips GN Jr, Flicker PF, Cohen C, et al. Streptococcal M protein: alpha-helical coiled-coil structure and arrangement on the cell surface. Proc Natl Acad Sci USA. 1981;78:4689–93.
146. Nealon TJ, Beachey EH, Courtney HS, et al. Release of fibronectin-lipoteichoic acid complexes from group A streptococci with penicillin. Infect Immun. 1986;51:529–35.
147. Stanislawski L, Courtney HS, Simpson WA, et al. Hybridoma antibodies to the lipid-binding site(s) in the amino-terminal region of fibronectin inhibits binding of streptococcal lipoteichoic acid. J Infect Dis. 1987;156:344–9.
148. Mosher DF, Proctor RA. Binding and factor XIIIa-mediated cross-linking of a 27-kilodalton fragment of fibronectin to *Staphylococcus aureus*. Science. 1980;209:927–9.
149. Kuusela P, Vartio T, Vuento M, et al. Binding sites for streptococci and staphylococci in fibronectin. Infect Immun. 1984;45:433–6.
150. Hasty DL, Courtney HS, Simpson WA, et al. Immunochemical and ultrastructural mapping of the gelatin-binding and cell-attachment regions of human plasma fibronectin with monoclonal antibodies. J Cell Sci. 1986;81:125–41.
151. Whitnack E, Bisno AL, Beachey EH. Hyaluronate capsule prevents attachment of group A streptococci to mouse peritoneal macrophages. Infect Immun. 1981;31:985–91.
152. Whitnack E, Beachey EH. Antiopsonic activity of fibrinogen bound to M protein on the surface of group A streptococci. J Clin Invest. 1982;69:1042–5.
153. Davis CP, Avots-Avotins AE, Fader RC. Evidence for a bladder cell glycolipid receptor for *Escherichia coli* and the effect of neuraminic acid and colominic acid on adherence. Infect Immun. 1981;34:944–8.
154. Klemm P. The complete amino-acid sequence of the K88 antigen, a fimbrial protein from *Escherichia coli*. Eur J Biochem. 1981;117:617–27.
155. de Graaf FK, Klemm P, Gaastra W. Purification, characterization, and partial covalent structure of *Escherichia coli* adhesive antigen K99. Infect Immun. 1980;33:877–83.
156. Klemm P. Primary structure of the CFA-1 fimbrial protein from human enterotoxigenic *Escherichia coli* strains. Eur J Biochem. 1982;124:339–48.
157. Honda T, Khan MM, Takeda Y, et al. Grouping of enterotoxigenic *Escherichia coli* by hydrophobicity and its relation to hemagglutination and enterotoxin productions. FEMS Microbiol Lett. 1983;17:273–6.
158. Honda T, Arita M, Miwatani T. Characterization of new hydrophobic pili of human enterotoxigenic *Escherichia coli*: A possible new colonization factor. Infect Immun. 1984;43:959–65.
159. Cheney CP, Formal SB, Schad PA, et al. Genetic transfer of a mucosal adherence factor (R1) from an enteropathogenic *Escherichia coli* strain into a *Shigella flexneri* strain and the phenotypic suppression of this adherence factor. J Infect Dis. 1983;147:711–23.
160. Berendson R, Cheney CP, Schad PA, et al. Species-specific binding of purified pili (AF/R1) from the *Escherichia coli* RDEC-1 to rabbit intestinal mucosa. Gastroenterology 1983;85:837–45.
161. Sherman PM, Houston WL, Boedeker EC. Functional heterogeneity of intestinal *Escherichia coli* strains expressing type 1 somatic pili (fimbriae): Assessment of bacterial adherence to intestinal membranes and surface hydrophobicity. Infect Immun. 1985;49:797–804.
162. Inman LR, Cantey JR, Formal SB. Colonization, virulence, and mucosal interaction of an enteropathogenic *Escherichia coli* (strain RDEC-1) expressing shigella somatic antigen in the rabbit intestine. J Infect Dis. 1986;154:742–51.
163. Sherman PM, Boedeker EC. Pilus-mediated interactions of the *Escherichia coli* strain RDEC-1 with mucosal glycoproteins in the small intestine of rabbits. Gastroenterology 1987;93:734–43.
164. Kallenius G, Mollby R, Svenson SB, et al. Occurrence of P-fimbriated *Escherichia coli* in urinary tract infections. Lancet. 1981;2:1369–72.
165. Hull RA, Gill RE, Hsu P, et al. Construction and expression of recombinant plasmids encoding type 1 or D-mannose-resistant pili from a urinary tract infection *Escherichia coli* isolate. Infect Immun. 1981;33:933–8.
166. Klemm P, Orskov I, Orskov F. Isolation and characterization of F-12 adhesive fimbrial antigen from uropathogenic *Escherichia coli* strains. Infect Immun. 1983;40:91–6.
167. Korhonen TK, Vaisanen V, Kallio P, et al. The role of pili in the adhesion of *Escherichia coli* to human urinary tract epithelial cells. Scand J Infect Dis. 1982;33(Suppl):26–31.
168. Korhonen TK, Vaisanen V, Saxen H, et al. P-antigen–recognizing fimbriae from human uropathogenic *Escherichia coli* strains. Infect Immun. 1982;37:286–91.
169. Orskov I, Orskov F, Birch-Andersen A, et al. O, K, H and fimbrial antigens in *Escherichia coli* serotypes associated with pyelonephritis and cystitis. Scand J Infect Dis. 1982;33(Suppl):18–25.
170. Korhonen TK, Valtonen MV, Parkkinen J, et al. Serotypes, hemolysin production, and receptor recognition of *Escherichia coli* strains associated with neonatal sepsis and meningitis. Infect Immun. 1985;48:486–91.
171. Parkkinen J, Finne J, Achtman M, et al. *Escherichia coli* strains binding to neuraminyl 2-3 galactosides. Biochem Biophys Res Commun. 1983;111:456–61.
172. Korhonen TK, Vaisanen-Rhen V, Rhen M, et al. *Escherichia coli* fimbriae recognizing sialyl galactosides. J Bacteriol. 1984;159:762–6.
173. Parkkinen J, Rogers GN, Korhonen T, et al. Identification of the O-linked sialyloligosaccharides of glycophorin A as the erythrocyte receptors for S-fimbriated *Escherichia coli*. Infect Immun. 1986;54:37–42.
174. Sharon N, Ofek I. Mannose specific bacterial surface lectins. In Mirelman D, ed. Microbial Lectins. New York: John Wiley & Sons; 1986:55–81.
175. Sharon N. Bacterial lectins, cell-cell recognition and infectious diseases. FEBS Lett. 1987;217:145–57.
176. Korhonen TK, Leffler H, Svanborg-Eden C. Binding specificity of piliated strains of *Escherichia coli* and *Salmonella typhimurium* to epithelial cells, *Saccharomyces cerevisiae* cells and erythrocytes. Infect Immun. 1981;32:796–804.
177. Firon N, Ofek I, Sharon N. Carbohydrate-binding sites of the mannose-specific fimbrial lectins of enterobacteria. Infect Immun. 1984;43:1088–90.
178. Brinton CC Jr, Buzzell A, Lauffer MA. Electrophoresis and phage susceptibility studies on a filament-producing variant of the *E. coli* B bacterium. Biochim Biophys Acta. 1954;15:533–42.
179. Czirok E, Orskov I, Orskov F. O:K:H:F serotypes of fimbriated *Escherichia coli* strain isolated from infants with diarrhea. Infect Immun. 1982;37:519–25.
180. Jann K, Schmidt G, Blumenstock E, et al. *Escherichia coli* adhesion to *Saccharomyces cerevisiae* and mammalian cells: Role of piliation and surface hydrophobicity. Infect Immun. 1981;32:484–8.
181. Klemm P. Fimbrial colonization factor CFA/1 protein from human enteropathogenic *Escherichia coli* strains. FEBS Lett. 1979;108:107–10.
182. Bergman MJ, Updike WS, Wood SJ, et al. Attachment factors among enterotoxigenic *Escherichia coli* from patients with acute diarrhea from diverse geographic areas. Infect Immun. 1981;32:881–8.
183. Hagberg L, Hull R, Hull S, et al. Contribution of adhesion to bacterial persistence in the mouse urinary tract. Infect Immun. 1983;40:265–72.
184. Aronson M, Medalia O, Schori L, et al. Prevention of *E. coli* colonization of the urinary tract by blocking bacterial adherence with methyl alpha-D-mannopyranoside. J Infect Dis. 1979;139:329–32.
185. Rene P, Silverblatt FJ: Serological response to *Escherichia coli* pili in pyelonephritis. Infect Immun. 1982;37:749–54.
186. Hagberg L, Jodal U, Korhonen TK, et al. Adhesion, hemagglutination, and virulence of *Escherichia coli* causing urinary tract infections. Infect Immun. 1981;31:564–70.
187. Ofek I, Mosek A, Sharon N, Mannose-specific adherence to *Escherichia coli* freshly excreted in the urine of patients with urinary tract infections, and of isolates subcultured from the infected urine. Infect Immun. 1981;34:708–11.
188. Orskov I, Orskov F, Birch-Andersen A. Comparison of *Escherichia coli* fimbrial antigen F7 with type 1 fimbriae. Infect Immun. 1980;27:657–66.
189. Jones GW, Rutter JM. Role of the K88 antigen in the pathogenesis of neo-

natal diarrhea caused by *Escherichia coli* in piglets. Infect Immun. 1972;6:918–27.
190. Sellwood R. *Escherichia coli*-associated porcine neonatal diarrhea: Antibacterial activities of colostrum from generally susceptible and resistant sows. Infect Immun. 1982;35:396–401.
191. Smith HW, Huggins MB. The influence of plasmid-determined and other characteristics of enteropathogenic *Escherichia coli* on their ability to proliferate in the alimentary tracts of piglets, calves and lambs. J Med Microbiol. 1978;11:471–92.
192. Smith HW, Linggood MA. Observations on the pathogenic properties of the K88, Hly and Ent plasmids of *Escherichia coli* with particular reference to porcine diarrhoea. J Med Microbiol. 1971;4:467–85.
193. Sellwood R, Gibbons RA, Jones GW, et al. Adhesion of enteropathogenic *Escherichia coli* to pig intestinal brush borders: The existence of two pig phenotypes. J Med Microbiol. 1975;8:405–11.
194. Smith HW, Halls S. Observations by the ligated intestinal segment and oral inoculation methods in *Escherichia coli* infections in pigs, calves, lambs and rabbits. J Pathol Bacteriol. 1967;93:499–529.
195. Bijlsma IG, de Nijs A, Frik JF. Adhesion of *Escherichia coli* to porcine intestinal brush borders by means of serological variants of the K88 antigen. Antonie van Leeuwenhoek. 1981;47:467–8.
196. de Graaf FK, Roorda I. Production, purification and characterization of the fimbrial adhesive antigen F41 isolated from calf enteropathogenic *Escherichia coli* strain B41M. Infect Immun. 1982;36:751–8.
197. Cheney CP, Boedeker EC. Adherence of an enterotoxigenic *Escherichia coli* strain, serotype 078:H11, to purified human intestinal brush borders. Infect Immun. 1983;39:1280–4.
198. Isaacson RE, Fusco PC, Brinton CC, et al. In vitro adhesion of *Escherichia coli* to porcine small intestinal epithelial cells: Pili as adhesive factors. Infect Immun. 1978;21:392–7.
199. McNeish AS, Turner P, Fleming J, et al. Mucosal adherence of human enteropathogenic *Escherichia coli*. Lancet. 1975;2:946–8.
200. Wilson MR, Hohmann AW. Immunity to *Escherichia coli* in pigs. Adhesion of enteropathogenic *Escherichia coli* to isolated intestinal epithelial cells. Infect Immun. 1974;10:776–82.
201. Nagy B, Moon HW, Isaacson RE, et al. Immunization of suckling pigs against enterotoxigenic *Escherichia coli*-induced diarrheal disease by vaccinating dams with purified pili. Infect Immun. 1978;21:269–74.
202. Kallenius G, Mollby R, Svenson SB. Identification of a carbohydrate receptor recognized by uropathogenic *Escherichia coli*. Infection. 1980;8(Suppl 3):288–93.
203. Hagberg L, Engberg I, Freter R, et al. Ascending, unobstructed urinary tract infection in mice caused by pyelonephritogenic *Escherichia coli* of human origin. Infect Immun. 1983;40:273–83.
204. Lomberg H, Jodal U, Eden CS, et al. P_1 blood group and urinary tract infection. Lancet. 1981;1:551–2.
205. Kallenius G, Mollby R. Adhesion of *Escherichia coli* to human periurethral cells correlated to mannose-resistant agglutination of human erythrocytes. FEMS Microbiol Lett. 1979;5:295–9.
206. Klemm P, Orskov I, Orskov F. F-7 and type 1-like fimbriade from three *Escherichia coli* strains isolated from urinary tract infections: Protein chemical and immunological aspects. Infect Immun. 1982;36:462–8.
207. Marre R, Hacker J, Henkel W, et al. Contribution of cloned virulence factors from uropathogenic *Escherichia coli* strains to nephropathogenicity in an experimental rat pyelonephritis model. Infect Immun. 1986;54:761–7.
208. Korhonen TK, Parkkinen J, Hacker J, et al. Binding of *Escherichia coli* S fimbriae to human kidney epithelium. Infect Immun. 1986;54:322–7.
209. Hacker J, Schmidt G, Hughes C, et al: Cloning and characterization of genes involved in production of mannose-resistant, neuraminidase-susceptible (X) fimbriae from a uropathogenic 06:K15:H31 *Escherichia coli* strain. Infect Immun. 1985;47:434–40.
210. Ott M, Hacker J, Schmoll T, et al. Analysis of the genetic determinants coding for the S-fimbrial adhesin (*sfa*) in different *Escherichia coli* strains causing meningitis or urinary tract infections. Infect Immun. 1986;54:646–53.
211. Saukkonen KMJ, Nowicki B, Leinonen M. Role of type 1 and S fimbriae in the pathogenesis of *Escherichia coli* 018:K1 bacteremia and meningitis in the infant rat. Infect Immun. 1988;56:892–7.
212. Parkkinen J, Korhonen TK, Pere A, et al. Binding sites in the rat brain for *Escherichia coli* S fimbriae associated with neonatal meningitis. J Clin Invest. 1988;81:860–5.
213. Moch T, Hoschutzky H, Hacker J, et al. Isolation and characterization of the alpha-sialyl-beta-2,3-galactosyl-specific adhesin from fimbriated *Escherichia coli*. Proc Natl Acad Sci USA. 1987;84:3462–6.
214. Lindberg F, Lund B, Johansson B, et al. Localization of the receptor-binding protein adhesin at the tip of the bacterial pilus. Nature. 1987;328:84–7.
215. Abraham SN, Goguen JD, Sun D, et al. Identification of two ancillary subunits of *Escherichia coli* type 1 fimbriae by using antibodies against synthetic oligopeptides of *fim* gene products. J Bacteriol. 1987;169:5530–6.
216. Hanson MS, Brinton CC Jr. Identification and characterization of *E. coli* type 1 pilus tip adhesion protein. Nature. 1988;332:265–8.
216a. Abraham SN, Sun D, Dale JB, et al. Conservation of the D-mannose-adhesion protein among type I fimbriated members of the family *Enterobacteriaceae*. Nature. 1988;336:682–4.
217. Chitnis DS, Sharma KD, Kamat RS. Role of bacterial adhesion in the pathogenesis of cholera. J Med Microbiol. 1982;15:43–51.
218. Jones GW. The adhesive properties of *Vibrio cholerae* and other *Vibrio* species. In Beachey EH, ed. Bacterial Adherence. New York: Chapman & Hall; 1980:219–49.
219. Freter R, Allweiss B, O'Brien PCM, et al. Role of chemotaxis in the association of motile bacteria with intestinal mucosa: In vitro studies. Infect Immun. 1981;34:241–9.
220. Schrank GD, Verwey WF. Distribution of cholera organisms in experimental *Vibrio cholera* infections: Proposed mechanisms of pathogenesis and antibacterial immunity. Infect Immun. 1976;13:195–203.
221. Guentzel MN, Berry LJ. Motility as a virulence factor for *Vibrio cholerae*. Infect Immun. 1975;11:890–7.
227. Jones GW, Freter R: Adhesive properties of *Vibrio cholerae*: Nature of the interaction with isolated rabbit brush border membranes and human erythrocytes. Infect Immun. 1976;14:240–5.
223. Freter R, O'Brien PCM, Macsai MS. Role of chemotaxis in the association of motile bacteria with intestinal mucosa: In vivo studies. Infect Immun. 1981;34:234–40.
224. Freter R, Jones GW. Adhesive properties of *Vibrio cholerae*: Nature of the interaction with intact mucosal surfaces. Infect Immun. 1976;14:246–56.
225. Jones GW, Abrams GD, Freter R. Adhesive properties of *Vibrio cholerae*: Adhesion to isolated rabbit brush border membranes and hemagglutinating activity. Infect Immun. 1976;14:232–9.
226. Bhattacharjee JW, Srivastava BS. Adherence of wild-type and mutant strains of *Vibrio cholerae* to normal and immune intestinal tissue. Bull WHO. 1979;57:123–8.
227. Spira WM, Sack RB. Kinetics of early cholera infection in the removable intestinal tie–adult rabbit diarrhea model. Infect Immun. 1982;35:952–7.
228. Srivastava R, Sinha VB, Srivastava BS. Events in the pathogenesis of experimental cholera: Role of bacterial adherence and multiplication. J Med Microbiol. 1980;13:1–9.
229. Kabir S, Ali S. Characterization of surface properties of *Vibrio cholera*. Infect Immun. 1983;39:1048–58.
230. Booth BA, Dyer TJ, Finkelstein RA. Adhesion of *Vibrio cholerae* to cultured human cells. In: Advances in Research on Cholera and Related Diarrheas. Tokyo: KTK Scientific Publishers. In press.
231. Bergman MJ, Updike WS, Wood SJ, et al. Attachment factors among enterotoxigenic *Escherichia coli* from patients with acute diarrhea from diverse geographic areas. Infect Immun. 1981;32:381–8.
232. Bergman MJ, Evans DG, Mandell GL, et al. Attachment of *E. coli* to human intestinal epithelial cells: A functional in vitro test for intestinal colonization factor. Trans Assoc Am Physicians 1978;91:80–9.
233. Miller VL, Taylor RK, Mekalanos JJ. Cholera toxin transcriptional activator ToxR is a transmembrane DNA binding protein. Cell. 1987;48:271–9.
234. Taylor RK, Miller VL, Furlong DB, et al. Use of *phoA* gene fusions to identify a pilus colonization factor coordinately regulated with cholera toxin. Proc Natl Acad Sci USA. 1987;84:2833–7.
235. Betley MJ, Miller VL, Mekalanos JJ. Genetics of bacterial enterotoxins. Annu Rev Microbiol. 1986;40:577–605.
236. Smith HR, Cravioto A, Willshaw GA, et al. A plasmid coding for the production of colonization factor antigen I and heat-stable enterotoxin in strains of *Escherichia coli* of serogroup 078. FEMS Microbiol Lett. 1979;6:255–60.
237. McConnell MM, Smith HR, Field AM, et al: Plasmids coding for colonization factor antigen I and heat-stable enterotoxin production isolated from enterotoxigenic *Escherichia coli*: Comparison of their properties. Infect Immun. 1981;32:927–36.
238. Penaranda ME, Mann MB, Evans DG, Evans DJ. Transfer of an ST:LT:CFA/II plasmid into *Escherichia coli* K12 strain RRI by co-transformation with PSC301 plasmid DNA. FEMS Microbiol Lett. 1980;8:251–4.
239. Smith HR, Scotland SM, Rowe B. Plasmids that code for production of colonization factor antigen II and enterotoxin production in strains of *Escherichia coli*. Infect Immun. 1983;40:1236–9.
240. Harnett NM, Gyles GL. Linkage of genes coding for heat-stable enterotoxin, drug resistance, K99 antigen, and colicin in bovine and porcine strains of enterotoxigenic *Escherichia coli*. Am J Vet Res. 1985;46:428–33.
241. Sparling PF, Cannon JG, So M. Phase and antigenic variation of pili and outer membrane protein II of *Neisseria gonorrhoeae*. J Infect Dis. 1986;153:196–201.
242. Johnson AP, Taylor-Robinson D, McGee ZA. Species specificity of attachment and damage to oviduct mucosa by *Neisseria gonorrhoeae*. Infect Immun. 1977;18:833–9.
243. Watt PJ, Ward ME. Adherence to *Neisseria gonorrhoeae* and other *Neisseria* species to mammalian cells. In: Beachey EH, ed. Bacterial Adherence (Receptors and Recognition). v. 6. ser B. New York: Chapman & Hall; 1980:251–88.
244. McGee ZA, Melly A, Gregg CR, et al. Virulence factors of gonococci: Studies using human fallopian tube organ cultures. In: Brooks GF, Gotschlich EC, Holmes KK, et al, eds. Immunobiology of *Neisseria gonorrhoeae*. Washington, DC: American Society for Microbiology; 1978:258–62.
245. Johnson AP, Clark JB, Osborn MF, et al. A comparison of the association of *Neisseria gonorrhoeae* with human and guinea pig genital mucosa maintained in organ cultures. Br J Exp Pathol. 1980;61:521–7.
246. Swanson J. Studies on gonococcus infection. XII. Colony color and opacity variants of gonococci. Infect Immun. 1978;19:320–31.
247. Zak K, Diay J-L, Jackson D, et al. Antigenic variation during infection with *Neisseria gonorrhoeae*: Detection of antibodies to surface proteins in sera of patients with gonorrhea. J Infect Dis. 1984;149:166–74.
248. McGee ZA, Johnson AP, Taylor-Robinson D. Pathogenic mechanisms of

Neisseria gonorrhoeae: Observations on damage to human fallopian tubes in organ culture by gonococci of colony type 1 or type 4. J Infect Dis. 1981;143:413–22.

249. Trust TJ, Lambden PR, Watt PJ. The cohesive properties of variants of *Neisseria gonorrhoeae* strain P9: Specific pilus-mediated and non-specific interactions. J Gen Microbiol. 1980;119:179–87.
250. Buchanan TM, Pearce WA, Chen KC. Attachment of *Neisseria gonorrhoeae* pili to human cells and investigations of the chemical nature of the receptor for gonococcal pili. In: Brooks GF, Gotschlich EC, Holmes KK, et al, eds. Immunobiology of *Neisseria gonorrhoeae*. Washington DC: American Society for Microbiology; 1978:242–9.
251. Pearce WA, Buchanan TM. Attachment role of gonococci pili. J Clin Invest. 1978;61:931–43.
252. Tramont EC, Ciak J, Boslego J, et al. Antigenic specificity of antibodies in vaginal secretions during infection with *Neisseria gonorrhoeae*. J Infect Dis. 1980;143:23–31.
253. Tramont EC. Specificity of inhibition of epithelial cell adhesion of *Neisseria gonorrhoeae*. Infect Immun. 1976;14:593–5.
254. Swanson J, Robbins K, Barrera O, et al. Gonococcal pili variants in experimental gonorrhea. J Exp Med. 1987;165:1344–57.
255. Bergstrom S, Robbins K, Koomey JM, et al. Piliation control mechanisms in *Neisseria gonorrhoeae*. Proc Natl Acad Sci USA. 1986;83:3890–4.
256. Segal E, Hagblom P, Seifert HS, et al. Antigenic variation of gonococcal pilus involves assembly of separated silent gene segments. Proc Natl Acad Sci USA. 1986;83:2177–81.
257. Lambden PR. Biochemical comparison pili from variants of *Neisseria gonorrhoeae* P9. J Gen Microbiol. 1982;128:2105–11.
258. Lambden PR, Robertson JN, Watt PJ. Biological properties of two distinct pilus types produced by isogenic variants of *Neisseria gonorrhoeae* P9. J Bacteriol. 1980;141:393–6.
259. Hermodson MA, Chen KCS, Buchanan TM. *Neisseria* pili proteins: Amino-terminal amino acid sequences and identification of an unusual amino acid. Biochemistry. 1978;17:442–5.
260. Heckels JE. Structural comparison of *Neisseria gonorrhoeae* outer membrane proteins. J Bacteriol. 1981;145:736–42.
261. Diaz JL, Heckels JE. Antigenic variation of outer membrane protein II in colonial variants of *Neisseria gonorrhoeae* PA. J Gen Microbiol. 1982;128:585–91.
262. Forslin L, Danielsson D. In vitro studies of the adherence of *Neisseria gonorrhoeae* and other urogenital bacteria to vaginal and uroepithelial cells, with special regard to the menstrual cycle. Gynecol Obstet Invest. 1980;11:327–40.
263. James JF, Swanson J. Studies on gonococcus infection. XIII. Occurrence of color/opacity colonial variants in clinical cultures. Infect Immun. 1978;19:332–40.
264. Duckworth M, Jackson D, Zak K, et al. Structural variations in pili expressed during gonococcal infection. J Gen Microbiol. 1983;129:1593–6.
265. Gahnberg L, Olsson J, Krasse B, et al. Interference of salivary immunoglobulin A antibodies and other salivary fractions with adherence of *Streptococcus mutans* to hydroxyapatite. Infect Immun. 1982;37:401–6.
266. Malamud D, Appelbaum B, Kline R, et al. Bacterial aggregating activity in human saliva: Comparisons of bacterial species and strains. Infect Immun. 1981;31:1003–6.
267. Rosan B, Malamud D, Appelbaum B, et al. Characteristic differences between saliva-dependent aggregation and adhesion of streptococci. Infect Immun. 1982;35:86–90.
268. Ciardi JE, Rolla G, Bowen WH, et al. Adsorption of *Streptococcus mutans* lipoteichoic acid to hydroxyapatite. Scand J Dent Res. 1977;85:387–91.
269. Hamada S, Slade DH. Adherence of serotype e *Streptococcus mutans* and the inhibitory effect of Lancefield group E and *S. mutans* type e antiserum. J Dent Res. 1976;55:65.
270. Hamada S, Torii M, Kotani S, et al. Adherence of *Streptococcus sanguis* clinical isolates to smooth surfaces and interaction of the isolates with *Streptococcus mutans* glucosyltransferase. Infect Immun. 1981;32:364–72.
271. Heeb MJ, Costello AH, Gabriel O. Characterization of a galactose-specific lectin from *Actinomyces viscosus* by a model aggregation system. Infect Immun. 1982;38:993–1002.
272. McIntire FC, Crosby LK, Vatter AE. Inhibitors of coaggregation between *Actinomyces viscosus* T14V and *Streptococcus sanguis* 34: Beta-galactosides, related sugars, and anionic amphipathic compounds. Infect Immun. 1982;36:371–8.
273. Tylenda CA, Enriquez E, Kolenbrander PE, et al. Simultaneous loss of bacteriophage receptor and coaggregation mediator activities in *Actinomyces viscosus* MG-I. Infect Immun. 1985;48:228–33.
274. Delisle AL, Donkersloot JA, Kolenbrander PE, et al. Use of lytic bacteriophage for *Actinomyces viscosus* T140 as a probe for cell surface components mediating intergeneic coaggregation. Infect Immun. 1988;56:54–9.
275. Gibbons RJ, Hay DI. Human salivary acidic proline-rich proteins and statherin promote the attachment of *Actinomyces viscosus* L47 to apatite surfaces. Infect Immun. 1988;56:439–45.
276. Rolla G, Robrish SA, Bowen WH. Interaction of hydroxyapatite and protein-coated hydroxyapatite with *Streptococcus mutans* and *Streptococcus sanguis*. Acta Pathol Microbiol Scand [B]. 1977;85:341–6.
277. Giampapa CS, Abraham SN, Chiang TM, et al. Isolation and characterization of a receptor for type 1 fimbriae of *Escherichia coli* from guinea pig erythrocytes. J Biol Chem. 1988;263:5362–7.
278. Doran JE, Raynor RH. Fibronectin binding to protein A-containing staphylococci. Infect Immun. 1981;33:683–9.
279. Espersen F, Clemmensen I. Isolation of a fibronectin-binding protein from *Streptococcus aureus*. Infect Immun. 1982;37:526–31.
280. Kuusela P. Fibronectin binds to *Streptococcus aureus*. Nature. 1978;276:718–20.
281. Proctor RA, Mosher DF, Olbrantz PJ. Fibronectin binding to *Staphylococcus aureus*. J Biol Chem. 1982;257:14788–94.
282. Woods DE, Straus DC, Johanson WG Jr, et al. Role of salivary protease activity in adherence of gram-negative bacilli to mammalian buccal epithelial cells in vivo. J Clin Invest. 1981;68:1435–40.
283. Woods DE, Straus DC, Johanson WG Jr, et al. Role of fibronectin in the prevention of adherence of *Pseudomonas aeruginosa* to buccal cells. J Infect Dis. 1981;143:784–90.
284. Zetter BR, Daniels TE, Quadra-White C, et al. LETS protein in normal and pathological human oral epithelium. J Dent Res. 1979;58:484–8.
285. Abraham SN, Beachey EH, Simpson WA. Adherence of *Streptococcus pyogenes, Escherichia coli* and *Pseudomonas aeruginosa* to fibronectin-coated and uncoated epithelial cells. Infect Immun. 1983;41:1261–8.
286. Valenti WM, Trudell RG, Bentley DW. Factors predisposing to oropharyngeal colonization with gram negative bacilli in the aged. N Engl J Med. 1978;298:1108–11.
287. Simpson WA, Courtney H, Beachey EH. Fibronectin—a modulator of the oropharyngeal bacterial flora. In: Microbiology 1982. Washington, DC: American Society for Microbiology; 1982:346–7.
288. Woods DE. Role of fibronectin in the pathogenesis of gram-negative bacillary pneumonia. Rev Infect Dis. 1987;9(Suppl 4):386–90.
289. Rosenburg M, Perry A, Bayer EA, et al. Adherence of *Acinetobacter calcoaceticus* RAG-1 to human epithelial cells and to hexadecane. Infect Immun. 1981;33:29–33.
290. Rosenberg M, Gutnick D, Rosenberg E. Adherence of bacteria to hydrocarbons: A simple method for measuring cell surface hydrophobicity. FEMS Microbiol Lett. 1980;9:29–33.
291. Olsson J, Westergren G. Hydrophobic surface properties of oral streptococci. FEMS Microbiol Lett. 1982;15:319–23.
292. Kihlstrom E, Edebo L. Association of viable and inactivated *Salmonella typhimurium* 395 MS and MR 10 with HeLa cells. Infect Immun. 1976;14:851–7.
293. Perers L, Andaker L, Edebo O, et al. Association of some enterobacteria with the intestinal mucosa of mouse in relation to their partition in aqueous polymer two-phase systems. Acta Pathol Microbiol Scand [B]. 1977;85:308–16.
294. Smyth CJ, Jonsson P, Olsson E, et al. Differences in hydrophobic surface characteristics of porcine enteropathogenic *Escherichia coli* with or without K88 antigen as revealed by hydrophobic interaction chromatography. Infect Immun. 1978;22:462–72.
295. Tylewska SK, Wadstrom T, Hjerten S. The effect of subinhibitory concentrations of penicillin and rifampicin on bacterial cell surface hydrophobicity and on binding to pharyngeal epithelial cells. J Antimicrob Chemother. 1980;16:292–4.
296. Colleen S, Hovelius B, Wieslander A, et al. Surface properties of *Staphylococcus saprophyticus* and *Staphylococcus epidermidis* as studied by adherence tests and two-polymer, aqueous phase systems. Acta Pathol Microbiol Scand [B]. 1979;87:321–8.
297. Gerson DF, Akit J. Cell surface energy, contact angles and phase partition. II. Bacterial cells in biphasic aqueous mixtures. Biochim Biophys Acta. 1980;602:281–4.
298. Stendahl O, Tagesson C, Edebo M. Partition of *Salmonella typhimurium* in a two-polymer aqueous phase system in relation to liability to phagocytosis. Infect Immun. 1973;8:36–41.
299. Ohman L, Normann B, Stendahl O. Physicochemical surface properties of *Escherichia coli* strains isolated from different types of urinary tract infections. Infect Immun. 1981;32:951–5.
300. Miorner H, Myhre E, Bjorck L, et al. Effect of specific binding of human albumin, fibrinogen, and immunoglobulin G on surface characteristics of bacterial strains as revealed by partition experiments in polymer phase systems. Infect Immun. 1980;39:879–85.
301. Faris A, Wadstrom T, Freer JH. Hydrophobic adsorptive and hemagglutinating properties of *Escherichia coli* possessing colonization factors, antigen (CFA/I or CFA/II), type 1 pili or other pili. Curr Microbiol. 1981;5:67–72.
302. Sherman PM, Houston WL, Boedeker EC. Functional heterogeneity of intestinal *Escherichia coli* strains expressing type I somatic pili (fimbriae): Assessment of bacterial adherence to intestinal membranes and surface hydrophobicity. Infect Immun. 1985;49:797–804.
303. Nesbitt WE, Doyle RJ, Taylor KG. Hydrophobic interactions and the adherence of *Streptococcus sanguis* to hydroxyapatite. Infect Immun. 1982;38:637–44.
304. Falkowski W, Edwards M, Schaeffer AJ. Inhibitory effect of substituted aromatic hydrocarbons on adherence of *Escherichia coli* to human epithelial cells. Infect Immun. 1986;52:863–6.
305. Sugarman B. Adherence of bacteria to urinary catheters. Urol Res. 1982;10:37–40.
306. Sugarman B. In vitro adherence of bacteria to prosthetic vascular grafts. Infection. 1982;10:9–14.
307. Sugarman B, Musher D. Adherence of bacteria to suture materials (41141). Proc Soc Exp Biol Sci. 1981;167:156–60.

308. Karlan MS, Skobel A, Grizzard M, et al. Myringotomy tube materials: Bacterial adhesion and infection. Otolaryngol Head Neck Surg. 1980;88:783–94.
309. Locci R, Peters G, Pulverer G. Microbial colonization of prosthetic devices. III. Adhesion of staphylococci to lumina of intravenous catheters perfused with bacterial suspensions. Zentralbl Bakteriol Mikrobiol Hyg. 1981;172:300–7.
310. Sheth NK, Rose HD, Franson TF, et al. In vitro quantitative adherence of bacteria to intravascular catheters. J Surg Res. 1983;34:213–8.
311. Hogt AH, Feijen J, Dankert J, et al. Adhesion of *Staphylococcus epidermidis* and *Staphylococcus saprophyticus* onto FEP-Teflon and cellulose acetate. In: Proceedings of International Conference on Biomedical Polymers. London: Biological Engineers Society; 1982:39–47.
312. Rotrosen D, Gibson TR, Edwards JE Jr. Adherence of *Candida* species to intravenous catheters. J Infect Dis. 1983;147:594.
313. Gristina AG. Biomaterial-centered infection: Microbvial adhesion versus tissue integration. Science. 1987;237:1588–95.
314. van Loosdrecht MCM, Lyklema J, Norde W, et al. Electrophoretic mobility and hydrophobicity as a measure to predict the initial steps of bacterial adhesion. Appl Environ Microbiol. 1987;53:1898–1901.
315. van Loosdrecht MCM, Lyklema J, Norde W, et al. The role of bacterial cell wall hydrophobicity in adhesion. Appl Environ Microbiol. 1987;53:1893–7.
316. Schadow KH, Simpson WA, Christensen GD. Characteristics of adherence to plastic tissue culture plates of coagulase-negative staphylococci exposed to subinhibitory concentrations of antimicrobial agents. J Infect Dis. 1988;157:71–7.
317. Fletcher M. Adherence of marine micro-organisms to smooth surfaces. In: Beachey EH, ed. Bacterial Adherence (Receptors and Recognition). New York: Chapman & Hall; 1980:345–74.
318. Christensen GD, Simpson WA, Beachey EH, et al. Adherence to pathogenic *Streptococcus epidermidis* to smooth surfaces and to catheters implanted in mice (abstract). In: Proceedings of the 22nd Interscience Conference on Antimicrobial Agents and Chemotherapy. Washington, DC: American Society for Microbiology; 1982:649.
319. Peters G, Locci R, Pulverer G. Adherence and growth of coagulase-negative staphylococci on surfaces of intravenous catheters. J Infect Dis. 1982;146:479–82.
320. Peters G, Schumacher-Perdreau F, Jansen B, et al. Biology of *S. epidermidis* extracellular slime. In: Pulverer G, Quie PG, Peters G, eds. Pathogenicity and clinical significance of coagulase-negative staphylococci. Stuttgart: Gustav Fischer Verlag; 1987:15–32.
321. Tojo M, Yamashita N, Goldmann DA, et al. Isolation and characterization of a capsular polysaccharide adhesin from *Staphylococcus epidermidis*. J Infect Dis. 1988;157:713–22.
322. Christensen GD, Simpson WA, Bisno AL, et al. Experimental foreign body infections in mice challenged with slime-producing *Staphylococcus epidermidis*. Infect Immun. 1983;40:407–10.
323. Baddour LM, Smalley DL, Kraus AP Jr, et al. Comparison of microbiologic characteristics of pathogenic and saprophytic coagulase-negative staphylococci from patients on continuous ambulatory peritoneal dialysis. Diagn Microbiol Infect Dis. 1986;5:197–205.
324. Christensen GD, Baddour LM, Simpson WA. Phenotypic variation of *Staphylococcus epidermidis* slime production in vitro and in vivo. Infect Immun. 1987;55:2870–7.
325. Bayston R, Penny SR: Excessive production of mucoid substance in staphylococcus SIIA: A possible factor in colonisation of Holter shunts. Dev Med Child Neurol. 1972;14(Suppl 27):25–8.
326. Peters G, Locci R, Pulverer G. Microbial colonization of prosthetic devices. II. Scanning electron microscopy of naturally infected intravenous catheters. Zentralbl Bakteriol Mikrobiol Hyg. 1981;173:293–9.
327. Franson TR, Sheth NK, Rose HD, et al. Scanning electron microscopy of bacteria adherent to intravascular catheters. J Clin Microbiol. 1984;20:500–5.
328. Marrie TJ, Costerton JW. Scanning and transmission electron microscopy of in situ bacterial colonization of intravenous and intra-arterial catheters. J Clin Microbiol 1984;19:687–93.
329. Younger JJ, Christensen GD, Bartley DL, et al. Coagulase-negative staphylococci isolated from cerebrospinal fluid shunts: Importance of slime production, species identification, and shunt removal to clinical outcome. J Infect Dis. 1987;156:548–54.
330. Diaz-Mitoma F, Harding GKM, Hoban DJ, et al. Clinical significance of a test for slime production in ventriculoperitoneal shunt infections caused by coagulase-negative staphylococci. J Infect Dis. 1987;156:555–60.
331. Beachey EH, Eisenstein BI, Ofek I. I. Adherence of bacteria: Prevention of the adhesion of bacteria to mucosal surfaces: Influence of antimicrobial agents. In: Eickenberg HU, Hahn H, Opferkuch W, eds. The Influence of Antibiotics on the Host Parasite Relationship. Munich: Springer-Verlag; 1982:171–82.
332. Tacket CO, Losonsky G, Link H, et al. Protection by milk immunoglobulin concentrate against oral challenge with enterotoxigenic *Escherichia coli*. New Engl J Med. 1988;318:1240–3.
333. Peros WJ, Gibbons RJ. Influence of sublethal antibiotic concentrations on bacterial adherence to saliva treated hydroxyapatite. Infect Immun. 1982;35:326–34.
334. Vosbeck K, Handschin H, Menge EB, et al. Effects of subminimal inhibitory concentrations of antibiotics on adhesiveness of *Escherichia coli in vitro*. Rev Infect Dis. 1979;1:845–51.
335. Ofek I, Beachey EH, Eisenstein BI, et al. Suppression of bacterial adherence by subminimal inhibitory concentrations of beta-lactam and aminoglycoside antibiotics. Rev Infect Dis. 1979;1:832–7.
336. Eisenstein BI, Ofek I, Beachey EH. Loss of lectin-like activity in aberrant type 1 fimbriae of *Escherichia coli*. Infect Immun. 1981;31:792–7.
337. Bar-Shavit Z, Ofek I, Goldman R, et al. Mannose residues on phagocytes as receptors for the attachment of *Escherichia coli* and *Salmonella typhi*. Biochem Biophys Res Commun. 1977;78:455–60.
338. Parsons CL, Mulholland SG, Anwar H. Antibacterial activity of bladder surface mucin duplicated by exogenous glycosaminoglycan (heparin). Infect Immun. 1979;24:552–7.
339. Parsons CL, Pollen SS, Anwar H, et al. Antibacterial activity of bladder surface mucin duplicated in the rabbit bladder by exogenous glycosaminoglycan (sodium pentosanpolysulfate). Infect Immun. 1980;27:876–81.
340. Parsons CL, Stauffer C, Schmidt JD. Bladder-surface glycosaminoglycans: An efficient mechanism of environmental adaptation. Science. 1980;208:605–7.

3. A MOLECULAR PERSPECTIVE OF MICROBIAL PATHOGENICITY

DAVID A. RELMAN
STANLEY FALKOW

The study of microbial pathogenicity at the molecular level has altered the way we view the host–parasite relationship and forced the redefinition of some commonly used terms. Infection, infectious disease, and virulence have been defined and used in numerous and sometimes misleading ways. The essential feature of most infections, however, is the successful multiplication of a microbe on or within a host. This process is often of benefit to both participants. Thus, following birth, human exposure to a myriad of microorganisms leads to the establishment of a protective microbial flora, stimulates the immune system, and in addition, provides small amounts of human accessory growth factors. The human participants in these infections are most often asymptomatic or exhibit subclinical signs but are generally better off for their encounter with the infecting organism(s). It is probably fair to say that this is the usual outcome of most infections.

The term *infectious disease* applies when signs and symptoms result from infection and its associated damage or altered physiology. A *pathogen* is usually defined as any microorganism that has the capacity to cause disease. Yet not all pathogens have an equal probability of causing disease in the same host population. *Virulence* provides a quantitative measure of pathogenicity, or the likelihood of causing disease. For example, encapsulated pneumococci are more virulent than are nonencapsulated pneumococci, and type b encapsulated *Haemophilus influenzae* organisms are more virulent than are other *H. influenzae* capsular types. Virulence factors refer to the properties, i.e., gene products, that enable a microorganism to establish itself on or within a host of a particular species and enhance its potential to cause disease.

If one is to examine microbial pathogenicity in detail, it is useful to distinguish "principal" pathogens, which *regularly* cause disease in some proportion of susceptible individuals with apparently *intact* specific and nonspecific defense systems, from other potentially pathogenic microorganisms. Certain microorganisms do not meet this definition of a principal pathogen because they do not regularly cause disease in individuals with intact host defenses. *Pseudomonas aeruginosa* is a good example. This microorganism does not usually cause disease in people with intact host defense systems; yet it can clearly cause devastating disease in many hospitalized and immunocompromised patients. It is probable that virtually any microorganism with a capacity for sustained multiplication in humans can cause disease more readily in individuals with underlying chronic disease or who are otherwise compromised. The common term *opportunist* suits this category of pathogen well. One could extend this argument to say that, for most organisms classified as principal pathogens, for example, *Staphylococcus aureus* and the pneumococcus, there must be some impairment or local breakdown of the normal host defense mechanisms in order for these bacteria to cause disease. On the other hand, it seems clear that the capacity of certain microorganisms to cause disease in seemingly uncompromised human hosts on a regular basis reflects some fundamental difference in their virulence capabilities as compared with opportunists or nonpathogens.

THE ATTRIBUTES OF MICROBIAL PATHOGENS

To be successful a pathogen must find an appropriate host niche and multiply there. Disease is arguably only an inadvertent outcome of microbial multiplication. To cause infection, a microorganism must possess an interactive group of complementary genetic properties, sometimes coregulated, that promote its interaction with a particular host. For a given microorganism these genetic traits define unique attributes[1] that enable it to follow a common sequence of steps used by organisms that are successful in establishing infection or subsequent disease. These traits are reflected as phenotypes for which one or more genes and their gene products may be responsible. Elegant molecular techniques, many devised only since 1980, have permitted the identification, isolation, and characterization of many of these genes and their products. Precise manipulation of the pathogen's genome has led to the determination of the roles for some of these putative virulence factors.

An initial step required of a pathogen is for it to gain access to the host in sufficient numbers. Gaining access to a potential host requires that the microorganism not only make contact with an appropriate surface but also then reach its unique niche or microenvironment on or within the host. This requirement is not trivial. Some pathogens must survive for varying lengths of time in the external environment. Others have evolved an effective and suitable means of transmission. To accomplish this goal the infecting microbe may make use of chemotactic properties and adhesive structures, or adhesins, that mediate binding to specific eukaryotic cell receptors.[2] Pre-existing microorganisms, the normal flora, provide competition against establishment of the newcomer; in addition, the latter must adapt, at least temporarily, to the particular nutrient environment in which it now finds itself.

Normal host defense mechanisms pose the next and most difficult set of obstacles to the arriving pathogen. For any set of specific host defenses an individual pathogen may have devised a unique and distinctive counterstrategy. Some of the best known mechanisms for countering host defenses include the use of an antiphagocytic capsule and the elaboration of toxins and microbial enzymes that act on host immune cells and destroy anatomic barriers. In addition, microorganisms may employ subtle mechanisms to avoid or even subvert host defenses, including immunoglobulin-specific protease, iron sequestration mechanisms, or coating themselves with host proteins so as to confuse the immune surveillance system. Examples of these mechanisms include the production of IgA1 protease by *H. influenzae,* the use of receptors for iron-saturated human transferrin and lactoferrin by *Neisseria gonorrhoeae,* and the coating of *Treponema pallidum* with human soluble fibronectin. Antigenic variation and intracellular invasion are other common strategies used by successful pathogens to avoid immune detection.

The ability to multiply is a characteristic of all living organisms. Whether the pathogen's niche in the relevant host be intracellular or extracellular, mucosal or submucosal, within the blood stream or within a privileged anatomic site, the pathogen will have evolved a distinct set of biochemical tactics to achieve this goal. The success of a pathogen, indeed of any microorganism, is measured by the degree with which it can survive, usually with multiplication, upon reaching its specific niche.

Thus, the outcome of the events just described is determined by the degree to which the pathogen has perpetuated itself and by the nature of the relationship it has established with its host. The result may be altered host physiology, tissue damage, and even clinical manifestations of disease. Death of the host is a rare event and one that must be viewed as most often detrimental to both parties involved! The more usual outcome is sufficient multiplication of the pathogen to ensure its establishment within the host (transient or long-term colonization) or its successful transmission to a new susceptible host.

Why do some pathogens cause disease more readily than others do? The strategy used for multiplication on or within the host often defines fundamental differences between pathogens that commonly cause disease and those that do not. If a microorganism succeeds by multiplying within deep fascial planes, it is far more likely to cause disease than is a nontoxinogenic microorganism that is content to grow on a mucosal surface. If a microorganism has evolved a means to nullify or destroy phagocytic cells in order to multiply successfully, it is more likely a disease-causing pathogen. Furthermore, an organism that can reach and multiply in privileged anatomic sites away from the competitive environment of skin and some mucosal surfaces is likely to disrupt homeostasis in the host and cause disease. Commensal organisms are content to multiply just enough, in the midst of competing microflora, to persist but not damage the host's self-preserving homeostatic mechanisms. It is important to emphasize that a microorganism exceptionally equipped to cause infection may be an unexceptional pathogen and only infrequently, if ever, cause clinically manifested disease.

Why are some organisms like *Pseudomonas aeruginosa* only opportunists despite their impressive array of virulence factors? An organism has no presupposition about the state of the host defenses when it encounters a human host. For opportunistic pathogens that state is the main determinant of whether disease will be the outcome of their interaction with the host. This reflects the fact that these organisms may lack an effective means to overcome normal host defense mechanisms. Opportunists may be very adept at establishing an infection, but because of their preferred growth locale, e.g., the mucosal surface, and preferred growth conditions, e.g., a microaerophilic environment, they may have limited growth opportunities outside of their restricted niche in an unimpaired individual. As a result, disease may be only a rare consequence of the host–microbe encounter.

Pathogens were once viewed as organisms, largely unadapted to their hosts, that elaborated potent toxins or other powerful aggressive factors that caused the signs and symptoms of disease. The current view is that a microbial pathogen is a highly adapted organism that follows a strategy for survival requiring multiplication on or within another living organism. Occasionally this survival strategy produces overt damage to the host. Of course, some infectious diseases occur predominantly in dramatic epidemic form, arguing against the evolution of a balanced host-parasite relationship; however, in many such epidemics there are mitigating circumstances that involve herd immunity and other underlying social, economic, and political issues that impinge upon this relationship. Furthermore, some of the most serious infectious diseases occur when humans are infected by microorganisms that prefer and are better adapted to another mammalian host.

THE CLONAL NATURE OF BACTERIAL PATHOGENS

Pathogenicity is not a microbial trait that has appeared by chance. Instead, particular microbial strains and species have evolved to carry very specific arrays of virulence-associated genes. By examining the genetic organization of pathogens, opportunists, and nonpathogenic bacteria one can now begin to understand the origins of pathogenicity.

Techniques used in the study of genetic relatedness include primary protein or nucleic acid sequence comparisons and DNA hybridization methods. A technique gaining widespread use is multilocus enzyme electrophoresis by which chromosomal structure or genotype is deduced from the electrophoretic mobility variations in a number of common metabolic enzymes.[3] The grouping of strains according to electrophoretic type assumes the absence of selective pressure favoring any particular electrophoretic enzyme variant. On the other hand, it avoids comparisons of phenotype, i.e., gross observable characteristics of a microbe, which can be unreliable. When these techniques are employed, a consistent finding emerges concerning the population structure of microorganisms.

Most natural populations of microorganisms consist of a number of discrete clonal lineages with preserved genotypes.[4] This finding implies that the rates of recombination of chromosomal genes between different strains of the same species and between different bacterial species are very low. At first view, this may seem somewhat unexpected since there exist well-established naturally occurring mechanisms for horizontal genetic exchange between and within species, including transformation, transduction, and conjugation. But bacteria are haploid creatures. If horizontal transfer of genetic material and subsequent recombination were frequent occurrences, one would expect to see homogenization of bacterial species and little specialization. In fact, the opposite is true. Bacterial species have remained discrete and distinct taxonomic entities.[5] This is because the bacterial chromosome is a highly integrated and coadapted entity that has resisted rearrangement.

Analysis of natural populations of *Escherichia coli*[4,6] as well as other species with pathogenic potential including *Salmonella* sp.,[7] *Neisseria meningitidis, Bordetella pertussis, H. influenzae, Legionella* sp., and *Streptococcus* sp.[8] has revealed the prominent representation of a relatively few clones. In fact, most cases of serious disease may be caused by a small proportion of the total number of extant clones that constitute a pathogenic bacterial species (Table 1). For example, from 104 distinct *H. influenzae* type b clones identified in natural populations, only 6 are commonly recovered from patients with invasive disease. The differences between pathogenic and nonpathogenic clones of the same species should provide considerable insight into the virulence mechanisms of these microorganisms. It has been noted that, in many instances, the proper unit of study in bacterial pathogenicity is not a phenotypic trait such as biotype or serotype but rather the clone. Phenotypic traits do not correlate directly with genotype and do not distinguish one clonal lineage from another. Indeed, in some extreme cases all members of a species such as *Shigella sonnei* or *Bordetella pertussis* belong to the same electrophoretic type or small group of closely related types. Although it is true of most that have been studied, not all pathogenic bacterial species reveal this pattern of clonal organization. Two notable exceptions are *Neisseria gonorrhoeae* and *Pseudomonas aeruginosa,* which appear to use chromosomal recombination to increase their genetic diversity. In addition, while the members of the genus *Salmonella* are largely clonal, there is evidence indicating that some diversity seen among members of the same serogroup can be best explained by horizontal genetic transmission rather than by the presence of numerous discrete clonal subpopulations.

Clonal analysis using multilocus enzyme electrophoresis has generated other important conclusions concerning the evolution of bacterial species and pathogenic strains in particular. The study of *E. coli* populations in the human intestinal tract indicates that only a small number of clonal lineages persist while numerous unrelated cell lines appear and disappear.[4] The nonrandom association of particular versions of different genes within a distinct clone has led to speculation that this species has evolved, not by means of accumulated random recombinational events, but by "random sampling" of clonal populations from the environment with periodic selection and extinction. *Escherichia coli* urinary tract pathogens causing symptomatic disease in humans are even less genetically diverse than are *E. coli* strains found in the intestinal flora or those that cause asymptomatic urinary tract colonization.[4]

PLASMIDS, PHAGES, INSERTION ELEMENTS AND PATHOGENICITY

The study of natural populations of bacteria suggests that the genetic potential for pathogenicity within a bacterial species has arisen among a small number of unrelated clones. It has arisen through means that do not compromise the genetic individuality of the organism or its unique place in nature but nonetheless in a fashion that provides the microbe with genetic and biochemical flexibility for a competitive environment. How might this have happened? Although periodic selection of mutant clones may play some role in the evolution of pathogenesis, it does not explain many of the differences seen between pathogenic and nonpathogenic clones of the same species.

A number of separate observations indicate that microbes frequently carry virulence-associated genes on mobile genetic elements.[1] Bacteriophages and extrachromosomal elements such as bacterial plasmids are supplements to the bacterial genome that allow a microbe to maintain the integrity of its chromosome and still increase its genetic diversity. Some of these mobile elements are able to enter a wide variety of host organisms and may facilitate the transfer of genes that have been selected for their ability to function in diverse genetic backgrounds.[10] Clinicians are painfully aware that genes encoding

TABLE 1. Proportion of Certain Infectious Diseases Caused by Common Bacterial Clonal Types

Species	Total number of Clonal Types Identified	Number of Clonal Types Commonly Isolated from Cases of Disease	Percentage of Disease Due to Common Clonal Types
B. bronchiseptica	21	3	87
B. parapertussis	1	1	100
B. pertussis	2	2	100
H. influenzae type b			
North America	104	6	81
Europe	60	3	78
L. pneumophila			
Global	50	5	52
Wadsworth VA Hospital	10	1	86
N. meningitidis			
serogroups B and C (clone families)	192	7	85
S. sonnei	1	1	100

(Modified from Selander et al.,[9] with permission.)

TABLE 2. Examples of Plasmid and Phage-Encoded Virulence Determinants

Organism	Virulence Factor	Biologic Function
Plasmid-encoded		
Enterotoxigenic *E. coli*	Heat labile, heat-stable enterotoxins (LT, ST)	Activation of adenyl/guanylcyclase in the small bowel, which leads to diarrhea
	CFA/I and CFA/II	Adherence/colonization factors
Extraintestinal *E. coli*	Hemolysin	Cytotoxin
Shigella sp. and enteroinvasive *E. coli*	Gene products involved in invasion	Induces internalization by intestinal epithelial cells
Yersinia sp.	Adherence factors and gene products involved in invasion	Attachment/invasion
B. anthracis	Edema factor, lethal factor, and protective antigen	Edema factor has adenylcyclase activity
S. aureus	Exfoliative toxin	Causes toxic epidermal necrolysis
C. tetani	Tetanus neurotoxin	Blocks the release of inhibitory neurotransmitter, which leads to muscle spasms
Phage-encoded		
C. diphtheriae	Diphtheria toxin	Inhibition of eukaryotic protein synthesis
S. pyogenes	Erythrogenic toxin	Rash of scarlet fever
C. botulinum	Neurotoxin	Blocks synaptic acetylcholine release which leads to flaccid paralysis
Enterohemorrhagic *E. coli*	Shigalike toxin	Inhibition of eukaryotic protein synthesis

(Data from Elwell et al.,[11] Kopecko et al.,[12] and Falkow et al.[13])

antibiotic resistance are efficiently disseminated among different microbial species in nature by such means. The presence of virulence factors in pathogenic bacteria is also associated with the presence of plasmids,[11,12] transposons, and bacteriophages to a striking degree, both in gram-positive and gram-negative species (Table 2).

Comparisons of pathogenic and nonpathogenic representatives of a single genus or species usually demonstrate the nonpathogens to be totally devoid of genetic sequences encoding the pathogenic trait(s). Inactive mutational variants or portions of virulence-associated genes infrequently occur in nonpathogenic strains of the same species. Not uncommonly, virulence-specific sequences are bounded by repeated DNA segments, some of which represent known insertion elements. This suggests that these virulence genes were once associated with a mobile genetic element or that these genes formerly occupied another chromosomal locale in either the same species or another microorganism all together. Thus, it often seems that microbes gain pathogenic potential through the inheritance of unique genetic information. Acquisition of an adhesin, toxin, or serum-resistance factor might dictate that a previously nonpathogenic organism will cause disease in a host that had previously been insusceptible.

Plasmids, transposons, and phages provide bacteria with the potential for relatively rapid adaptation to an unfavorable, changing, or new environment. Although these mobile genetic elements are often dispensable to the host bacterium, they are typically conserved over substantial periods of time within diverse cell lineages.[14] This is hardly surprising if the mobile element enables the organism to multiply successfully in a host. Often the mobile element carries multiple virulence-associated genes as a coadapted block. When such gene blocks are accompanied by a separate self-regulatory system that is responsive to a changing microbial environment, they influence the pathogenic potential even more.

THE REGULATION OF BACTERIAL PATHOGENICITY

All bacteria respond to environmental changes with metabolic alterations. A successful host–parasite relationship demands that a pathogen be capable of sensing its local host environment; it must distinguish between conditions favorable to rapid growth and those that are threatening and require a protective response. Consequently, regulating the expression of virulence factors is an additional, yet essential complication of a pathogenic microbe's life. When it first encounters a host, a pathogen must adapt dramatically to its changed environment. A study of the environmental regulation of microbes should recognize biases that arise from the peculiarities of laboratory culture conditions. These conditions may be inappropriate or irrelevant to the natural environments encountered by a microorganism. Given these limitations, some studies indicate that bacteria may be found in a "viable but nonculturable state" in their natural external environment.[15] *Vibrio cholerae,* for example, is thought to persist in this state in brackish estuaries and other saline aquatic environments, sometimes associated with the chitinous exoskeleton of various marine organisms.[16–18] Transition from this milieu to the contrasting environment of the human small intestinal lumen must be accompanied by substantial genetic regulatory events.

Less dramatic changes in the surrounding environment affect the expression of the determinants of virulence. Some pathogens, e.g., *B. pertussis, V. cholerae, E. coli, Shigella* sp., and *Yersinia* sp., regulate their virulence determinants in response to changes in temperature, ionic conditions, pH, and iron and other metal concentrations. Other microbial pathogens periodically vary prominent antigenic components of their surface and, by so doing, may avoid the host immune response, e.g., *N. gonorrhoeae, Borrelia recurrentis,* and *Trypanosoma brucei.*

The number of well-characterized virulence regulatory systems is rapidly increasing. At the same time relatively little is known about both the specific environmental signals to which these systems respond and the rationale for these responses in the human host. The examples of regulation of bacterial virulence factors that are provided below illustrate two common themes for the response of prokaryotes to their environmental stimuli. First, the mechanism for transducing environmental signals typically involves a two-component regulatory system that acts on gene expression, usually at the transcriptional level. Such systems make use of similar pairs of proteins; one protein of the pair has a transmitter domain and may act as a sensor of environmental stimuli, whereas the other has a receiver domain and acts as the regulator. The first of these proteins transmits a signal to the second, usually by means of phosphorylation. The second protein, upon receiving this signal, may regulate the expression of a variety of genes. Systems of this type control, for example, the permeability properties of the *E. coli* cell envelope in response to osmotic stimuli (*envZ*/*omp*R), motor control involved in *E. coli* chemotaxis (*che*A/*che*Y), the switch from vegetative growth to sporulation by *Bacillus subtilis* (an unidentified sensor/*spo*OA), and even the ability of the soil bacterium *Agrobacterium tumefaciens* to induce tumors in susceptible plant cells in response to plant wound exudates (*vir*A/*vir*G). The *tox*R gene of *V. cholerae* and the *vir* region of

B. pertussis share several features common to these systems, but they also retain significant differences.

The coordinated control of pathogenicity illustrates a second common feature of bacterial regulation, i.e., the *regulon.* A regulon is a group of operons controlled by a common regulator, usually a protein activator or repressor. This regulator may, in some cases, also be a receiver protein in a two-component system as described above. A regulon provides a means by which many genes can respond in concert to a particular stimulus. At other times the same genes may respond independently to other signals. The concept of a regulon is integral to the study of bacterial physiology. However, only recently has it been appreciated that microbial virulence determinants can be under the control of such a global regulatory network (Table 3).

Bordetella pertussis synthesizes a group of surface-associated or extracellular products that are responsible for the pathologic and clinical findings of pertussis. These products include pertussis toxin, filamentous hemagglutinin, adenylate cyclase, and fimbrial protein. A *trans*-acting regulatory locus, *vir,*[20] positively controls the coordinate expression of these virulence factors. In the few situations that have been studied *vir* activates expression at the level of transcription. The deduced amino acid sequence of genes within the *vir* locus demonstrates homologies to known transmitter and receiver domains in proteins of the two-component regulatory system; however, the exact mechanisms by which the *vir* proteins act are as yet unknown. Twenty or more unlinked chromosomal genes of *B. pertussis* and their gene products are involved in this global regulatory scheme.

The *vir* region mediates spontaneous phase variation and phenotypic modulation, both of which represent oscillation between full expression of all factors and a complete lack thereof. Phenotypic modulation occurs in response to environmental stimuli including temperature. At 37°C the full array of *vir*-regulated genes is expressed, while at 30°C these genes are silent. This regulatory response probably allows *B. pertussis* to cope with the diverse local conditions of the human upper respiratory mucosal surface, its natural site of infection.

Reversible regulation by temperature of the expression of virulence genes is a feature common to several bacterial pathogens, including enteropathogenic and uropathogenic *E. coli* (K-88 and K-99 fimbriae, pyelonephritis associated pilus (Pap) fimbriae, and K-1 capsular antigen), *Shigella* sp. (invasiveness and shiga toxin), and *Yersinia* sp. (virulence-associated determinants including a low calcium response and outer membrane proteins). Temperature-responsive regulation in *Shigella* sp. depends upon another *trans*-acting genetic locus, *vir*R, which exerts a negative regulatory effect upon a number of both chromosomal and plasmid virulence-associated genes.[21]

The regulation of the expression of virulence determinants by *Vibrio cholerae* also illustrates the use of a global regulatory protein that, in this case, serves a dual function. The *tox*R gene product is a transmembrane, DNA-binding protein that can activate transcription of the genes encoding cholera toxin, pilus colonization factor, and specific outer membrane proteins.[22] The *tox*R protein is also thought to sense a variety of other environmental regulatory signals including osmolarity, amino acid concentration, temperature, and pH.[23] At the level of amino acid sequence as well, the *tox*R protein contains features of both sensor and regulator proteins from the two-component sensory transduction system. The combination of these features into one protein may lead to an increased specificity of action.

Antigenic variation in *Salmonella typhimurium* and *Neisseria gonorrhoeae* provide examples of alternative molecular mechanisms, i.e., DNA rearrangements, that mediate the regulation of the expression of virulence factors. *Salmonella typhimurium* varies an immunodominant antigen by alternating between the expression of two different flagellin genes, H1 and H2. The mechanism for this form of variation has been well characterized: inversion of a 995 basepair (bp) chromosomal DNA sequence orients a promoter such that transcription of the H2 flagellin gene occurs together with that of a gene encoding a *trans*-acting repressor of the H1 gene.[24] The opposite orientation allows relief of H1 gene repression and prevents transcription of H2. Inversion is catalyzed by the *hin* gene product. It promotes site-specific recombination between the 14 bp inverted repeats that flank the invertible segment. In this manner, *S. typhimurium* avoids the host antibody response directed against it.

Pili are essential for virulence of the gonococcus in the human host, probably as a result of their role in adherence to the mucosal target surface.[25] They also elicit a specific local and systemic host antibody response.[26] Intermittent production of pili as well as variation in the antigenic type of pilus may be strategies used by the gonococcus to avoid the host immune response. The molecular mechanisms behind these strategies are complex. In general terms, phase and antigenic variation results from DNA rearrangements that move pilin-related sequences scattered around the gonococcal chromosome (in silent *pil*S loci) to the expression site (*pil*E locus).[27] Numerous different pilus types may be expressed by derivatives of a single *N. gonorrhoeae* strain. Gene conversion and other recombination mechanisms may be involved. Among other microbial pathogens DNA rearrangements account for the antigenic variation of variant surface glycoproteins of *Trypanosoma brucei*[28] and the antigenic variation of variable major proteins in *Borrelia* sp.[29] A DNA rearrangement is also associated with the expression of type I pili in *E. coli.*

THE IDENTIFICATION AND CHARACTERIZATION OF VIRULENCE GENES

The characterization of microbial pathogenicity at the molecular level begins with the identification of a virulence-associated phenotype. This may come from clinical observation, epidemiologic investigation, or the use of a model system that reliably reproduces the microbial phenotype in a manner similar to that seen in the natural infection. Traditionally, a virulent strain was compared with a naturally occurring avirulent variant. Such variants, however, may have complex genotypic alterations in-

TABLE 3. Examples of Bacterial Virulence Regulatory Systems

Organism	*Regulatory Gene(s)*	*Environmental Stimuli*	*Regulated Functions*
E. coli	ND	Temperature	Pyelonephritis-associated pili
	fur	Iron concentration	Shigalike toxin, siderophores
B. pertussis	*vir*	Temperature, ionic conditions, nicotinic acid	Pertussis toxin, filamentous hemagglutinin, adenylate cyclase, others
V. cholerae	*tox*R	Temperature, osmolarity, pH, amino acids	Cholera toxin, pili, outer membrane proteins
Yersinia sp.	*lcr* loci	Temperature, calcium	Outer membrane proteins
	ND	Temperature	Adherence, invasiveness
Shigella sp.	*vir*R	Temperature	Invasiveness
S. aureus	*agr*	ND	Alpha toxin, toxic shock syndrome toxin 1, protein A

Abbreviation: ND: not determined.
(Data from Miller et al.[19])

volving multiple genetic loci. The comparison of strains of naturally occurring virulent and nonvirulent organisms may be even more confounding since we now understand that they may represent entirely different clones.

Analysis using mutant strains of identical genetic background is a more desirable approach to the definition of virulence phenotypes. The goal is to define a single, well-defined genetic lesion that alters a recognizable phenotype and then test the effect of this alteration on the pathogenicity or virulence of the organism in an appropriate model system. The use of insertional elements, e.g., antibiotic-resistant transposons, as mutational agents is an attractive means of accomplishing this aim. Transposons are pieces of DNA that are able to translocate from one genomic site to another. Insertion into a gene usually disrupts its function. Transposons have the advantage of marking the mutagenized genetic locus with a new selectable phenotype, typically antibiotic resistance. The development of broad host range plasmid vectors carrying well-defined transposons has extended this method of analysis to a number of pathogenic species for which a method of genetic manipulation was not previously available.[30] Consequently, the comparison of organisms with identical genetic backgrounds, differing only in a single, defined mutation, is employed widely to identify putative virulence genes. Once identified, more precise characterization of such genes and the identification of the gene products usually follow.

Molecular cloning has been the method preferred by many investigators in recent years to isolate specific virulence genes and to modify them in a precise way.[31] A description of the methodologies available for the isolation and characterization of virulence genes is outside the scope of this discussion; however, it may be useful to point out several basic approaches.

Single genes are usually isolated by screening a "library" of overlapping pieces of a fragmented microbial genome that have been inserted into an appropriate plasmid or bacteriophage vector, which is then introduced into a carrier microorganism, typically *E. coli* K-12. In some instances only a few hundred carrier organisms bearing such recombinant molecules need to be examined to screen effectively an entire, average-sized bacterial genome.[32] Typical strategies for screening a genomic library may or may not depend upon expression of the cloned gene of interest by the carrier organisms.

Genes encoding putative virulence determinants may not express their gene products in the *E. coli* carrier strain, either because the product is lethal to the cell or because the appropriate mechanisms for transcription or translation are not available. Screening techniques based upon hybridization with DNA probes avoid the need for expression of the cloned gene, although not the possible lethal effects of expression. These probes may derive from previously isolated genes known to be homologous to the gene of interest,[33] from an oligonucleotide corresponding to the N-terminal amino acid sequence of the gene product,[34] or from DNA flanking an insertion element that has been used to mutagenize the gene in the original host.[30] In the case of the last method, DNA flanking a transposon-marked gene can be easily isolated by screening an initial genomic library for a clone with the appropriate antibiotic resistance phenotype.[35]

Screening recombinant clones for the presence of a cloned gene whose product is stable and expressed at adequate levels is often accomplished by using labeled antibodies directed against the gene product. Although transcription and translation of the cloned gene and stability of the gene product may be enhanced by special expression vectors,[36] appropriate antibodies are not always available. In some cases a recombinant host expressing the cloned gene will display a corresponding phenotype that can be exploited for screening purposes: expression of the cloned *inv* locus from *Yersinia pseudotuberculosis* confers on the *E. coli* host an ability to invade certain types of cultured eukaryotic cells in vitro.[37] The carrier organisms bearing the recombinant clones, once intracellular, are uniquely resistant to the killing effect of gentamicin, which acts only on extracellular bacteria.

To isolate the cloned gene on a DNA fragment of minimal size the boundaries of the gene must be mapped on the initial recombinant vector insert. Transposon mutagenesis may be used for this purpose. The smallest restriction endonuclease fragment that carries the virulence-associated gene is then subcloned. Further characterization at this point includes introducing specific mutations in the gene and defining their effect on a function of its protein product. Site-directed mutagenesis,[38] rapid DNA sequencing,[39] and in vitro coupled transcription–translation of plasmid-encoded proteins[40,41] are techniques that facilitate such analyses. Final proof, however, that the cloned and characterized gene is associated with pathogenicity requires its return to the strain of origin and that certain criteria be met.

ASSOCIATION OF GENES WITH VIRULENCE: PROOF BY A MOLECULAR FORM OF KOCH'S POSTULATES

Technical advances have brought about a proliferation of reports describing the cloning and sequencing of genes thought to be involved in microbial pathogenicity. At the same time these advances have dramatized the need for defined criteria by which genes may be assigned a role in pathogenesis. In a manner analogous to Koch's original postulates these criteria must include the return of the putative causal agent (the cloned virulence-associated gene, mutated or intact) to the host of origin. Unless one can demonstrate an effect on pathogenicity by this kind of controlled genetic manipulation, causality with respect to virulence has not been proved. Just as the original Henle-Koch postulates have provided a reference point for later revised criteria of microbial causality,[42] the criteria outlined below best serve as guidelines, in this case, for an experimental approach to the molecular genetic basis of pathogenicity.

A molecular form of Koch's postulates[43] can be stated as follows: (*1*) The phenotype or property under investigation should be associated significantly more often with pathogenic members of a genus or pathogenic strains of a species than with nonpathogenic members or strains. (*2*) Specific inactivation of the gene or genes associated with the suspected virulence trait should lead to a measurable decrease in virulence. If inactivation of the gene has taken place in a cloned copy carried by a recombinant host, then this mutated gene must be exchanged for the wild-type copy of the gene in the host of origin; the latter must suffer a loss of virulence following the exchange. (*3*) Restoration of full pathogenicity should accompany replacement of the mutated version of the gene with the wild-type version in the strain of origin.

Technical limitations often face the investigator who wishes to apply these postulates to an organism poorly characterized from a genetic standpoint. The ability to exchange alleles in the organism under investigation is crucial because it allows a virulence-associated gene to be studied in an isogenic background. Until recently this was an impossible task with the respiratory tract pathogen *Bordetella pertussis*. Although the complementation of chromosomal mutations was possible by using recombinant multiple-copy plasmids, there was no easy means of replacing a chromosomal gene with a cloned copy, thereby avoiding a multiple gene dose effect. The construction of a suicide vector, pRTP1,[44] provided a solution to this problem and illustrates some of the principles by which this kind of problem can be approached in other organisms.

Homologous recombination is the process by which a segment of DNA replaces an equivalent segment elsewhere that has identical or nearly identical nucleotide sequences. Enzymes that catalyze DNA repair and synthesis mediate this process. Cloned genes, carried into the strain of origin on plasmid vectors, are exchanged for the analogous chromosomal version of the same genes by means of homologous recombination. A suicide plasmid cloning vector can be used for this purpose. Such vectors carry DNA sequences responsible for transfer of the plasmid to a broad range of hosts so that the plasmid can be mated, by conjugation, into a variety of gram-negative organisms. A suicide plasmid also carries *E. coli* DNA sequences that allow it to replicate in this gram-negative organism but not many others. pRTP1 is such a plasmid vector that can be transferred to *B. pertussis* but cannot replicate there. When conjugation is performed in the presence of an antibiotic that selects for the presence of the suicide plasmid, the plasmid becomes recombined into the recipient organism's chromosome because of the homology with the cloned gene copy in the plasmid. Subsequent antibiotic selection against the presence of the suicide plasmid causes a second recombinational event to occur that results in excision of the plasmid and replacement of the original *B. pertussis* chromosomal gene copy with that carried by the plasmid. In this way, chromosomal virulence genes can be modified in a directed fashion.

Another difficulty in the application of a molecular form of Koch's postulates is similar to a problem that faced Koch in his own day: finding an appropriate animal model system. This is a problem that limits the study of microbial pathogenesis as much as any other. It does little good to return a carefully constructed virulence gene mutation to the original strain if there is no way to evaluate its effect on a particular virulence phenotype. A model must duplicate relevant pathology commonly observed in the normal host. The animal host must become consistently infected by using a natural route. Clearly, a model of this sort does not exist for many pathogens. At the same time, it should be remembered that exposure to a known human pathogen does not uniformly lead to disease in all humans.

The postulates just outlined are meant to provide principles by which one may study the genes and gene products associated with microbial pathogenesis. This kind of approach can also be used to analyze the internal structure of these genes and the corresponding functional domains of the encoded proteins.

UNDERSTANDING VIRULENCE: CLINICAL CORRELATIONS AND APPLICATIONS

Do these concepts of microbial pathogenicity have a practical impact on the practice of clinical infectious diseases? It is already apparent that studies of microbial pathogenicity at the molecular level have made substantial contributions to our understanding of the epidemiology, clinical manifestations, diagnosis, and immunoprophylaxis of infectious diseases.

Infectious disease epidemiology hinges upon clear definition of the clinical problem under study and, moreover, precise identification of the etiologic agent. Molecular techniques, including multilocus enzyme electrophoresis and diagnostic DNA probe hybridization, provide for both sensitive and specific detection of putative pathogens and a means for establishing relationships among multiple isolates of the same species. As a result, seemingly unrelated cases occurring during an outbreak have been connected; similarly, geographically or temporally distinct outbreaks have been linked to the same pathogenic clone. Molecular techniques have been employed in other epidemiologic investigations to study transmission mechanisms and the role of avirulent microbial variants in the spread of disease.

Multilocus enzyme electrophoresis has been used in epidemiologic investigation to define clonal relationships among pathogens in numerous outbreaks. These include *E. coli* 0157:H7 strains associated with hemorrhagic colitis and hemolytic uremic syndrome,[45] *N. meningitidis* strains causing epidemic disease,[46] and *Bordetella* sp. isolated from diverse hosts at different times and locations[47]; all demonstrate the prevalence of a relatively few distinct clonal lineages.

Specific DNA probes are available for an increasing number of microbial pathogens.[48] Probes linked to nonradioactive detection systems are readily applied to field investigations and are widely used in laboratory diagnosis. By creating DNA probes that detect sequences encoding virulence factors, investigations of outbreaks and field surveillance work can precisely target the presumed pathogen. One of the first examples of this approach was the detection of enterotoxinogenic *E. coli* by colony hybridization with a probe for the LT gene.[49] DNA probes offer the ability to detect sexually transmitted disease agents, for example, directly in clinical specimens.[50] The recent development of a *Y. pestis*-specific DNA probe allows rapid in situ detection of this pathogen in its normal host vector, the rat flea.[51] In addition, DNA probes have been used for strain identification in epidemiologic investigations: analysis of Swedish *C. diphtheriae* isolates from recent years by using a probe against a specific multicopy transposable DNA insertion element has linked most epidemic diphtheria cases to a single clonal strain and provided important information about the epidemiology of this disease.[52]

One of the most exciting technical advances in recent years is the development of the polymerase chain reaction (PCR) for amplification of a DNA sequence.[53] When using this technique it is possible to detect the presence of a single target DNA sequence in a sample of 10^5 cells. This should greatly benefit epidemiologic investigations that depend upon the screening of environmental material for a presumed pathogen. Other molecular techniques that are commonly used in infectious disease epidemiology include plasmid analysis[54] and restriction endonuclease analysis.[55] Recent investigations into the spread of chloramphenicol-resistant *Salmonella newport* in the food chain[54] and an outbreak of *Legionella* sp. prosthetic valve endocarditis[55] illustrate the usefulness of these methods.

The clinical manifestations of numerous infectious diseases are more readily understood as a result of the molecular analysis of microbial virulence factors. Methods by which genes encoding virulence determinants can be isolated, modified, and returned to the original strain have been described earlier. Further techniques are available to create specific internal mutations within these genes, e.g., site-directed mutagenesis.[38] In this manner, not only can virulence factors be correlated with specific manifestations of disease, but particular protein domains can be correlated with specific biologic activities. This kind of analysis is currently underway for the ADP-ribosylating protein pertussis toxin.[56]

Improvements in the diagnosis of infectious diseases have followed in step with many of the advances in epidemiologic investigation. In particular, DNA probe technology and PCR amplification techniques seem destined to have major impacts on diagnosis. The list of pathogens for which there are diagnostic DNA probes is already quite substantial.[48] Polymerase chain reaction amplification is quickly finding numerous applications, including the detection of human immunodeficiency virus sequences in clinical specimens.[57] As these two techniques become simplified and more widely used, it will be increasingly important to distinguish target sequences that are virulence associated from those that are not.

The application of molecular techniques and theory to infectious disease therapeutics and prophylaxis is in its infancy.[58] As virulence factors for essential steps in pathogenesis are identified in individual pathogens, it should be possible to interfere with their function. For example, one might design competitive inhibitors of microbial adherence factors or invasion-promoting proteins.[59] As they become better characterized, manipulation of global virulence regulatory systems may have therapeutic value. New acellular or recombinant live attenuated vaccines will likely result from the identification of immunoprotective antigens with molecular approaches. A growing understanding of microbial pathogenesis at the molecular level is expected to foster these kinds of practical developments. The result should be a more informed and effective approach to the detection and treatment of infectious diseases.

REFERENCES

1. Falkow S, Small P, Isberg R, et al. A molecular strategy for the study of bacterial invasion. Rev Infect Dis. 1987;9:450–5.
2. Jones GW, Isaacson RE. Proteinaceous bacterial adhesins and their receptors. CRC Crit Rev Microbiol. 1983;10:229–60.
3. Selander RK, Caugant DA, Ochman H, et al. Methods of multilocus enzyme electrophoresis for bacterial population genetics and systematics. Appl Environ Microbiol. 1986;51:873–84.
4. Selander RK, Caugant DA, Whittam TS. Genetic structure and variation in natural populations of *Escherichia coli*. In: Neidhardt FC, ed. *Escherichia coli* and *Salmonella typhimurium*. Washington, DC: American Society for Microbiology; 1987:1625–48.
5. Ochman H, Wilson AC. Evolutionary history of enteric bacteria. In: Neidhardt FC, ed. *Escherichia coli* and *Salmonella typhimurium*. Washington, DC: American Society for Microbiology; 1987:1649–54.
6. Ochman H, Selander RK. Evidence for clonal population structure in *Escherichia coli*. Proc Natl Acad Sci USA. 1984;81:198–201.
7. Beltran P, Musser JM, Helmuth R, et al. Toward a population genetic analysis of *Salmonella:* Genetic diversity and relationships among strains of serotypes *S. choleraesuis, S. derby, S. dublin, S. enteriditis, S. heidelberg, S. infantis, S. newport,* and *S. typhimurium*. Proc Natl Acad Sci USA. 1988;85:7753–7.
8. Selander RK, Musser JM, Caugant DA, et al. Population genetics of pathogenic bacteria. Microbial Pathogenesis. 1987;3:1–7.
9. Selander RK, Musser JM. The population genetics of bacterial pathogenesis. In: Iglewski BH, Clark VL, eds. Molecular Basis of Bacterial Pathogenesis. Orlando, FL: Academic Press. In press.
10. Campbell A. Evolutionary significance of accessory DNA, elements in bacteria. Annu Rev Microbiol. 1981;35:55–83.
11. Elwell LP, Shipley PL. Plasmid-mediated factors associated with virulence of bacteria to animals. Annu Rev Microbiol. 1980;34:465–96.
12. Kopecko DJ, Formal SB. Plasmids and the virulence of enteric and other bacterial pathogens (Editorial). Ann Intern Med. 1984;101:260–2.
13. Falkow S, Portnoy DA. Bacterial plasmids—an overview. Clin Invest Medicine. 1983;6:207–12.
14. Mercer AA, Morelli G, Heuzenroeder M, et al. Conservation of plasmids among *Escherichia coli* K1 isolates of diverse origins. Infect Immun. 1984;46:649–57.
15. Roszak DB, Colwell RR. Survival strategies of bacteria in the natural environment. Microbiol Rev. 1987;51:365–79.
16. Huq A, Small EB, West PA, et al. Ecological relationships between *Vibrio cholerae* and planktonic crustacean copepods. Appl Environ Microbiol. 1983;45:275–83.
17. Tamplin ML, Colwell RR. Effects of microcosm salinity and organic substrate concentration on production of *Vibrio cholerae* enterotoxin. Appl Environ Microbiol. 1986;52:297–301.
18. Perez-Rosas N, Hazen TC. In situ survival of *Vibrio cholerae* and *Escherichia coli* in tropical coral reefs. Appl Environ Microbiol. 1988;54:1–9.
19. Miller JF, Mekalanos JJ, Falkow S. Coordinate regulation and sensory transduction in the control of bacterial virulence. Science. 1989;243:916–22.
20. Weiss AA, Falkow S. Genetic analysis of phase change in *Bordetella pertussis*. Infect Immun. 1984;43:263–9.
21. Maurelli AT, Sansonetti PJ. Identification of a chromosomal gene controlling temperature-regulated expression of *Shigella* virulence. Proc Natl Acad Sci USA. 1988;85:2820–4.
22. Miller VL, Taylor RK, Mekalanos JJ. Cholera toxin transcriptional activator *tox*R is a transmembrane DNA binding protein. Cell 1987;48:271–9.
23. Miller VL, Mekalanos JJ. A novel suicide vector and its use in construction of insertion mutations: Osmoregulation of outer membrane proteins and virulence determinants in *Vibrio cholerae* requires *tox*R. J Bacteriol. 1988; 170:2575–83.
24. Simon M, Zieg J, Silverman M, et al. Phase variation: Evolution of a controlling element. Science. 1980;209:1370–4.
25. McGee ZA, Johnson AP, Taylor-Robinson D. Pathogenic mechanisms of *Neisseria gonorrhoeae:* Observations on damage to human fallopian tubes in organ culture by gonococci of colony type 1 or type 4. J Infect Dis. 1981;143:413–22.
26. McChesney D, Tramont EC, Boslego JW, et al. Genital antibody response to a parenteral gonococcal pilus vaccine. Infect Immun. 1982;36:1006–12.
27. Seifert HS, So M. Genetic mechanisms of bacterial antigenic variation. Microbiol Rev. 1988;52:327–36.
28. Borst P. Discontinuous transcription and antigenic variation in trypanosomes. Annu Rev Biochem. 1986;55:701–32.
29. Meier JT, Simon MI, Barbour AG. Antigenic variation is associated with DNA rearrangements in a relapsing fever borrelia. Cell. 1985;41:403–9.
30. Weiss AA, Hewlett EL, Myers GA, et al. *Tn*5-induced mutations affecting virulence factors of *Bordetella pertussis*. Infect Immun. 1983;42:33–41.
31. Macrina FL. Molecular cloning of bacterial antigens and virulence determinants. Annu Rev Microbiol. 1984;38:193–219.
32. Collins J. *Escherichia coli* plasmids packageable in vitro in lambda bacteriophage particles. Methods Enzymol. 1979;68:309–26.
33. Pearson GDN, Mekalanos JJ. Molecular cloning of *Vibrio cholerae* enterotoxin genes in *Escherichia coli* K-12. Proc Natl Acad Sci USA. 1982;79:2976–80.
34. Livey I, Duggleby CJ, Robinson A. Cloning and nucleotide sequence analysis of the serotype 2 fimbrial subunit gene of *Bordetella pertussis*. Mol Microbiol. 1987;1:203–9.
35. Stibitz S, Weiss AA, Falkow S. Genetic analysis of a region of the *Bordetella pertussis* chromosome encoding filamentous hemagglutinin and the pleiotropic regulatory locus *vir*. J Bacteriol. 1988;170:2904–13.
36. Shatzman AR, Rosenberg M. Expression, identification, and characterization of recombinant gene products in *Escherichia coli*. Methods Enzymol. 1987;152:661–73.
37. Isberg RR, Falkow S. A single genetic locus encoded by *Yersinia pseudotuberculosis* permits invasion of cultured animal cells by *Escherichia coli* K-12. Nature. 1985;317:262–4.
38. Botstein D, Shortle D. Strategies and applications of in vitro mutagenesis. Science. 1985;229:1193–201.
39. Sanger F, Nicklen S, Coulson AR. DNA sequencing with chain-terminating inhibitors. Proc Natl Acad Sci USA. 1977;74:5463–7.
40. Frazer AC, Curtiss R. Production, properties and utility of bacterial minicells. Curr Top Microbiol Immunol. 1975;69:1–84.
41. Sancar A, Hack AM, Rupp WD. Simple method for identification of plasmid-coded proteins. J Bacteriol. 1979;137:692–3.
42. Evans AS. Causation and disease: The Henle-Koch postulates revisited. Yale J Biol Med. 1976;49:175–95.
43. Falkow S. Molecular Koch's postulates applied to microbial pathogenicity. Rev Infect Dis. 1988;10(Suppl):274–6.
44. Stibitz S, Black W, Falkow S. The construction of a cloning vector designed for gene replacement in *Bordetella pertussis*. Gene. 1986;50:133–40.
45. Whittam TS, Wachsmuth IK, Wilson RA. Genetic evidence of clonal descent of *Escherichia coli* 0157:H7 associated with hemorrhagic colitis and hemolytic uremic syndrome. J Infect Dis. 1988;157:1124–33.
46. Caugant DA, Froholm LO, Bovre K, et al. Intercontinental spread of a genetically distinctive complex of clones of *Neisseria meningitidis* causing epidemic disease. Proc Natl Acad Sci USA. 1986;4927–31.
47. Musser JM, Hewlett EL, Peppler MS, et al. Genetic diversity and relationships in populations of *Bordetella* spp. J Bacteriol. 1986;166:230–7.
48. Tenover FC. Diagnostic deoxyribonucleic acid probes for infectious diseases. Clin Microbiol Rev. 1988;1:82–101.
49. Moseley SL, Huq I, Alim AR, et al. Detection of enterotoxigenic *Escherichia coli* by DNA colony hybridization. J Infect Dis. 1980;142:892–8.
50. Horn JE, Quinn T, Hammer M, et al. Use of nucleic acid probes for the detection of sexually transmitted infectious agents. Diagn Microbiol Infect Dis. 1986;4(Suppl):101–9.
51. McDonough KA, Schwan TG, Thomas RE, et al. Identification of a *Yersinia pestis*-specific DNA probe with potential for use in plague surveillance. J Clin Microbiol. 1988;26:2515–9.
52. Rappuoli R, Perugini M, Falsen E. Molecular epidemiology of the 1984–1986 outbreak of diphtheria in Sweden. N Engl J Med. 1988;318:12–4.
53. Saiki RK, Gelfand DH, Stoffel S, et al. Primer-directed enzymatic amplification of DNA with a thermostable DNA polymerase. Science. 1988;239:487–91.
54. Spika JS, Waterman SH, Hoo GW, et al. Chloramphenicol resistant *Salmonella newport* traced through hamburger to dairy farms. N Engl J Med. 1987; 316:565–70.
55. Tompkins LS, Roessler BJ, Redd SC, et al. *Legionella* prosthetic-valve endocarditis. N Engl J Med. 1988;318:530–5.
56. Black WJ, Munoz JJ, Peacock MG, et al. ADP-ribosyltransferase activity of pertussis toxin and immunomodulation by *Bordetella pertussis*. Science 1988;240:656–9.
57. Ou CY, Kwok S, Mitchell SW, et al. DNA amplification for direct detection of HIV-1 in DNA of peripheral blood mononuclear cells. Science. 1988;239:295–7.
58. Engleberg NC, Eisenstein BI. The impact of new cloning techniques on the diagnosis and treatment of infectious diseases. N Engl J Med. 1984;311:892–901.
59. Isberg RR, Voorhis DL, Falkow S. Identification of invasin: A protein that allows enteric bacteria to penetrate cultured mammalian cells. Cell. 1987;50:769–78.

SECTION B. HOST DEFENSE MECHANISMS

4. GENERAL OR NONSPECIFIC HOST DEFENSE MECHANISMS

EDMUND C. TRAMONT

General or nonspecific host defense mechanisms refer to a formidable array of host resistance factors that interfere with a microorganism's ability to invade and/or harm its host. The protective effects are due to innate resistance (i.e., intact skin) or are stimulated by the invading organism. In contrast to antibodies, they are not specifically directed against the invading organism (i.e., cytokines). These mechanisms are an important first encounter for a microorganism with its host and often represent the initial response elicited by the host. Because of their general nature, these nonspecific host defense mechanisms are difficult to quantitate, and because they are so efficient, they are often taken for granted (Table 1). Taken as a whole, the effect of this first line of defense is impressive; taken individually, each mechanism or factor is of a much smaller magnitude and much less dramatic than are responses that confer resistance to a specific infectious agent (i.e., antibodies).

NORMAL INDIGENOUS MICROBIAL FLORA

A microorganism in most cases must gain access into or onto the host in order to develop a particular relationship with that host (a preformed toxin such as that produced by *Clostridium botulinum* would be an exception). This host–parasite relationship may be *symbiotic*, *commensal*, or *parasitic*, depending upon the particular situation that is being described. For example, *Escherichia coli* is a commensal organism in the gastrointestinal tract, but it is a parasite in the lung. Certain organisms always behave in a predictable fashion. In humans, the rabies virus is always considered a pathogen, whereas the lactobacillus seldom is. From the point of view of the microorganism, the better adapted it becomes to exist in a symbiotic or commensal relationship with its host, the better its chances for survival.

The normal commensal flora plays an important role in protecting the host from microbial invasion by "pathogenic" organisms.[1] Mechanisms of this protection include the following: (*1*) competition for the same nutrients (interference), (*2*) competition for the same receptors on host cells (tropism), (*3*) production of bacteriocins, that is, bacterial products that are toxic to other organisms, usually of the same species, (*4*) continual stimulation of the immune system to maintain low but constant levels of class II histocompatibility (DR) molecule expression on macrophages and other accessory cells,[2] and (*5*) stimulation of cross-protective immune factors such as the so-called natural antibodies.

The ultimate effect of the first three protective mechanisms is to limit the quantity or dominance of any one species of organism. For example, broad-spectrum antibiotic therapy decreases the concentration of all sensitive bacteria in the gut. When the antibiotic therapy is stopped, a rebound results and the gut is repopulated, but to the advantage of the faster-growing aerobic Enterobacteriaceae over the slower-metabolizing anaerobes. A disproportion therefore is created that may be reflected in "rebound bacteremia," especially in immunocompromised hosts.[2] We might favorably influence the development of commensal flora in this case by stopping all antibiotics that have an anaerobic spectrum 24–36 hours before stopping aminoglycoside antibiotics that lack an anaerobic spectrum to allow anaerobic organisms to reestablish a competitive foothold.[3] Other examples include the purposeful recolonization of *Staphylococcus aureus* carriers with the relatively avirulent S. aureus strain 502A and the repopulation of gut flora with lactobacilli or normal fecal flora.

The microbial flora harbored by the host can be divided into two groups: (*1*) normal resident flora that is regularly found and, if disturbed, prompty reestablishes itself and (*2*) a transient flora that may colonize the host for periods ranging from hours to weeks but does not permanently establish itself.

The normal microbial flora that can be isolated from sites of the body are listed in Table 2. Certain organisms characteristically colonize certain sites (tropism). This is obviously taken into consideration when deciding whether a particular organism is behaving in a pathogenic fashion. Bacteria and fungi make up the great majority of commensal and symbiotic organisms. Mycoplasmas and viruses are much less prevalent. The presence of a member of the herpesvirus family usually reflects activation of latency rather than true colonization of mucosal surfaces. Protozoa are also less ubiquitous than bacteria and fungi, almost always reside in the gastrointestinal tract, and are more prevalent in underdeveloped countries.

The species that make up the normal flora are obviously influenced by environmental factors such as diet, sanitary conditions, air pollution, and hygienic habits. For example, lactobacilli are common intestinal commensals whenever dairy products make up a significant proportion of the dietary intake; protozoa are common intestinal inhabitants of those living where sanitation is poor; and a patient with underlying chronic bronchitis is more likely to harbor *Haemophilus influenzae* in the tracheobronchial tree.

The normal flora is also influenced by hormones. Premenarchal and postmenopausal vaginal flora differ significantly from that present during the childbearing period.

However, perhaps the ultimate effect of the normal flora on the immune system is to keep it "primed" and thus more rapid and efficient in its response to invading microorganisms. Antigens must be presented to the immune system in an ordered and specified way. T cells recognize antigens only after they

TABLE 1. Factors Contributing to Host Nonspecific Resistance to Infection

Normal indigenous microflora
Genetic factors
Natural antibodies
Morphologic integrity
Normal excretory secretions and flow
Phagocytosis
Natural killer (NK) cells
Nutrition
Non-antigen-specific immune response
Fibronectin
Hormonal factors

The views of the author do not purport to reflect the position of the Department of the Army or the Department of Defense (para 4–3. AR 360–5).

TABLE 2. Microorganisms That Commonly Colonize Healthy Human Body Surfaces (Normal Flora)

Skin	
Bacteria	
Staphylococcus epidermidis	+ + + +[a]
Diphtheroids	
Corynebacterium spp.	+ + + +
Propionibacterium acnes	+ + + +
Staphylococcus aureus	+ +
Streptococcus spp. including *S. pyogenes*	+
Peptococcus	+
Mycobacterium spp.	+
Bacillus spp.—soil or free-living bacteria	+
Acinetobacter	±
Enterobacteriaceae	±
Pseudomonas spp.	±
Fungi	
Malassezia furfur	+ + + +
Candida spp.	+
Mouth and oropharynx[b]	
Bacteria	
Streptococcus spp.	
St. mitus	+ + + +
Non-group A *Streptococcus*	+ +
St. pneumoniae	+ +
St. pyogenes	+
St. salivarius	+ + + +
Anaerobic gram-negative spp.	
Veillonella spp.	+ + + +
Bacteroidaceae spp.	+ +
Fusobacterium spp.	+ + + +
S. epidermidis	+ + +
Treponema spp.	+ + +
Lactobacillus spp.	+ +
Neisseria spp.	+ +
N. meningitidis	+
Nonpathogenic (*N. sicca*, etc.)	+ +
Haemophilus spp.	+
H. influenzae, non-group B	+
H. influenzae, group B	+
H. parainfluenzae	+
Anaerobic streptococci and micrococci	+
Peptococcus	+
Peptostreptococcus	+
Mycoplasma	±
Actinomycetes	+
S. aureus	+
Enterobaciaceae	±
Fungi	
Yeasts	
Candida spp. (*C. albicans*)	+ +
Virus	
Herpes simplex	±
Nose	
Bacteria	
Staphylococcus spp.	
S. epidermidis	+ + + +
S. aureus	+ +
Neisseria spp.	+
Streptococcus spp.	+ +
St. pneumoniae	+
St. pyogenes	+
Haemophilus spp.	+
Outer ear	
Bacteria	
S. epidermidis	+ + + +
Pseudomonas spp.	+
St. pneumoniae	±
Enterobacteriaceae	+
Conjunctivae	
Bacteria	
S. epidermidis	+ + +
Haemophilus spp.	+
S. aureus	+
Streptococcus spp.	±
St. pneumoniae	±
Group A streptococci	±
Neisseria spp.	±
Moraxella spp.	±
Enterobacteriaceae	±

(Continued)

TABLE 2. (Continued)

Esophagus and stomach	
Bacteria	
Low numbers of (10^4/ml)	
Surviving bacteria from upper respiratory tract and food	+
Mycobacterium spp.	+
Small intestine	
Bacteria	
Lactobacillus spp.	+ + +
Mycobacterium spp.	+ +
Enterobacteriaceae	+ +
S. aureus	±
Enterococcus	+ +
Gram-negative anaerobic spp.	+ + +
Bacteroides spp.	+ +
Clostridium spp.	+ +
Large intestine (95% or more of species are obligate anaerobes)	
Bacteria	
Gram-negative anaerobes	
Bacteroidaceae spp.	+ + + +
Fusobacterium spp.	+ + + +
Gram-positive anaerobes	
Peptococcus spp.	+ + + +
Peptostreptococcus spp.	+ + + +
Enterobacteriaceae	+ + + +
E. coli	+ + + +
Klebsiella spp.	+ + +
Proteus spp.	+ + +
Enterococcus	+ +
Lactobacillus	+ + +
Clostridium spp.	+ + + +
C. perfringens	+ + +
C. welchii	+ + +
Streptococcus spp.	+ +
Group B streptococci	±
Pseudomonas spp.	+
Aeromonas spp.	±
P. aeruginosa	
Alcaligenes spp.	+
Acinetobacter spp.	+
S. epidermidis	+
S. aureus	+
Campylobacter spp.	±
Arizona spp.	±
Mycobacterium spp.	+
Actinomycetes	+
Treponema spp.	+
Virus	
Adenovirus (in children)	±
Fungi	
Yeasts, especially *Candida* spp.	±
Protozoa[c]	
Giardia lamblia	±
Liver, gallbladder, pancreas (normally sterile or low numbers of anaerobic organisms)	
Vagina	
Bacteria	
Mycoplasma spp.	±
Ureaplasma urealyticum	±
Döderlein's bacillus	+ + + +
Lactobacillus spp.	+ + + +
Gram-positive anaerobic spp.	+ + +
Peptococcus	+ +
Peptostreptococcus	+
Bifidobacterium	+
Propionibacterium	+
Clostridium spp.	+ +
Streptococcus spp.	+
Enterococcus	+
S. epidermidis	+
Mobiluncus spp.	+
Diphtheroids	+ +
Gram-positive anaerobic spp.	+ +
Veillonella spp.	+
Bacteroidaceae	+
Gardnerella vaginale	+
Acinetobacter	+
Enterobacteriaceae	±
Neisseria spp.	±

(Continued)

TABLE 2. (Continued)

Fungi	
Candida spp.	++
Torulopsis spp.	+
Actinomycetes	+
Protozoa	
Trichomonas vaginalis	±
External genitalia and anterior urethra	
Bacteria	
Mycoplasma spp.	±
Ureaplasma urealyticum	±
"Skin flora"	++++
Fusobacterium spp.	+
Gram-negative anaerobe spp.	+
Mycobacterium spp.[d]	++
Peptostreptococcus	+
Enterococcus	+
Enterobacteriaceae	±
Acinetobacter	±
Protozoa	
Trichomonas vaginalis	±

[a] Relative frequency of isolation: ++++, almost always present; +++, usually present; ++, frequently present; +, occasionally present; ±, rarely present.
[b] The presence of teeth affects the normal flora and anerobic organisms, *Fusobacterium* and *Treponema* being less prevalent in edentulous people.
[c] Protozoa are more prevalent in the intestines of people living in underdeveloped countries.
[d] Mycobacteria are particularly common in the smegma of uncircumcised boys and men.

are displayed on the surface of a macrophage (or other antigen-presenting cell) in physical association with a class II histocompatibility (DR) molecule. Normally, 75–85 percent of circulating monocytes in adults maintain relatively high levels of DR molecule expression. DR expression is much lower on monocytes in human newborns,[2] neonatal mice, and germ-free animals.[4] Thus, the constant stimulation by the host's indigenous microbial flora maintains the high level of DR molecule expression on macrophages and perhaps other antigen-presenting cells, and this serves to keep the immune system primed. This modulation is due, at least in part, to low-level production of γ-interferon, interleukin-4, and other cytokines by activated T cells (see below).

TISSUE TROPISMS AND HEREDITARY FACTORS

Receptors exist on tissues that permit the attachment of microorganisms. The attachment of a microorganism to a receptor is dependent upon the presence of a complementary ligand or adhesin on that microorganism.[5] (see Chapter 2). The ligand and the receptor vary independently as to their specificity—a receptor binding to one or many different organisms (ligands), a ligand binding one or many different receptors. Thus, most organisms preferentially colonize certain tissues and spare others. This phenomenon is referred to as *tissue tropism*. For example, influenza virus and mycoplasmas preferentially adhere to respiratory epithelial cells, *E. coli* and *Vibrio cholerae* to intestinal cells, and *Streptococcus mutans* to tooth enamel; also, gram-positive organisms more readily attach to heart valves than do gram-negative organisms.[6] *Treponema pallidum*, on the other hand, binds to many different tissue receptors, and untreated late syphilis may involve any organ.

Receptors on host cells may change. For example, there is evidence to suggest that viral illness may affect tissue tropisms of the oropharynx to allow easier colonization by gram-negative organisms.[7] Also, urinary epithelial cells from people prone to develop urinary tract infections support the attachment of urinary pathogens over urinary epithelial cells from healthy people.[8] The genetics of tissue tropisms are unknown. The role of these factors in determining susceptibilities of a host to a particular infection is obviously important.

The relationship of genetic factors to susceptibilities to infectious agents has been appreciated for many years.[9,10] Infections have been one of the strongest selective pressures in human evolution. The devastating effects of tuberculosis, measles, and smallpox on the native American populations was tantamount to genocide. Conversely, the protective effects of sickle cell trait on the outcome of falciparum malaria are well known.

Histocompatible antigens have been linked to a predisposition to some infectious complications. The HLA-B27 and reactive arthropathy or Reiter syndrome was one of the earliest associations that was recognized. There is evidence of HLA-linked determinants in tuberculoid leprosy,[11] acute glomerulonephritis,[12] paralytic poliomyelitis,[13,14] and responsiveness to antigenic stimulus.[15] The list is destined to grow. Genetic influences on other infectious processes are not as well understood.

Natural Antibodies

Natural antibodies are specific antibodies found in healthy people without a previous history of a compatible infection. These antibodies are of great importance in the immunity to many bacteria, especially encapsulated bacteria such as *Neisseria meningiditis* and *H. influenzae*, type b.

These antibodies are stimulated by colonization in the oropharynx, gut, or elsewhere of organisms sharing cross-reactive (cross-protective) antigens.[15] However, these antibodies are not always beneficial. There are data to suggest that specific serum IgA antibodies to *N. meningitidis* may predispose an otherwise immune person to become susceptible by preferentially attaching to the organism, thus blocking the beneficial bactericidal effect of the protective IgG and IgM antibodies.[16] The blood group antibodies are a consequence of colonization in the gut of microorganisms bearing cross-reactive antigens.

NATURAL BARRIERS TO THE ENTRY OF MICROORGANISMS INTO THE BODY

The morphologic integrity of the body surface is an important and effective first line of defense.

Skin and Mucous Membranes

The intact skin forms a very effective mechanical barrier to invasion by microorganisms. Since very few organisms have the innate ability to penetrate the skin, they must gain access by some physical means such as by an arthropod vector, a primary skin lesion such as eczema, trauma, a surgeon's incision, or an intravenous catheter. The papovavirus (warts) is an exception.

The specific antimicrobial properties of skin have not been exhaustively studied. However, the relative dryness or desiccating effect of skin, the mild acidity (acid mantle, pH 5–6), and the normal skin flora act in concert to form an effective prohibitive environment. Inflamed skin is more permeable to water and therefore leads to greater colonization. It has been speculated that oily skin may retard evaporation of water, resulting in increased numbers of organisms. The acidity of the skin results from the breakdown of lipids into fatty acids. Sebum contains few esterified fatty acids, but the normal skin flora partially hydrolyzes the triglycerides, thereby liberating fatty acids. Desquamation of skin scales also aids in the elimination of microorganisms.

The mucous membranes support a larger number of microorganisms but also offer mechanical resistance. Also, the mucosal surfaces are bathed in secretions with antimicrobial properties. For example, cervical mucus, prostatic fluid, and tears have been shown to be toxic to a large variety of microorganisms. One of the more potent antimicrobial substances is lysozyme, which is found in every local secretion. It is an enzyme that lyses bacteria by splitting the muramic acid B-(1–4)-*N*-acetylglucosamine linkage in the bacterial cell wall and is especially effective against gram-positive organisms. Local secretions also contain specific immunoglobulins, principally IgG and secretory IgA (which act primarily to block the attachment of organisms to host cells [ligands]) and significant amounts of iron-binding proteins. The importance of iron for microorganisms is well recognized, and all fluids that are potentially exposed to microbes are enriched with iron-binding proteins.[17]

Respiratory Tract

The respiratory tract has formidable antimicrobial defense mechanisms.[18] First, the inhaled particles must survive and penetrate the aerodynamic filtration system of the upper airway and tracheobronchial tree. The airflow in these areas is quite turbulent, causing large particles to impact on the mucosal surfaces. Humidification of the incoming air causes hydroscopic organisms to increase in size, thus aiding phagocytosis.

Once deposited, the mucociliary blanket transports the invading offender away from the lung. Coughing obviously aids this expulsion. This system is amazingly efficient: 90 percent of deposited material is cleared in less than 1 hour. In addition, the bronchial secretions contain various antimicrobial substances (e.g., lysozyme).

Once a particle reaches the alveoli, physical expulsion becomes much less effective, and the alveolar macrophage and tissue histiocytes play a more prominent role in protecting the host. When the lungs become inflamed, they are aided by the influx of polymorphonuclear leukocytes and monocytes, which become even more efficient when specific immune mechanisms such as opsonins are present.

Like all defense mechanisms, these nonspecific mechanisms can be overcome by the introduction of large numbers of invading organisms (e.g., contaminated respirator), particularly when exposed over an extended period of time. Furthermore, their effectiveness is decreased by air pollutants (e.g., cigarette smoke), mechanical respirators, tracheostomy, concomitant infection, and allergenic agents.

Intestinal Tract

The acid pH of the stomach, the antibacterial effect of the various pancreatic enzymes, and bile and intestinal secretions are effective antimicrobial factors. Peristalsis and the normal loss of epithelial cells also act to purge the intestinal tract of harmful microorganisms. Alteration of these parameters can lead to increased susceptibility of the host to infection. For example, *Salmonella* and tuberculosis infections are more common in achlorhydric patients, and slowing peristalsis with belladonna or opium alkaloids prolongs symptomatic shigellosis.[19] Intubated patients treated with inhibitors of gastric acid secretion have a higher incidence of aspiration pneumonia.

Normal bowel flora competition (10^{12} organisms per gram of feces) plays an extremely important protective role. Altering this flora with broad-spectrum antibiotics can lead to overgrowth with inherently pathogenic organisms (e.g., *Salmonella typhimurium*) or suprainfection with ordinarily commensal organisms (e.g., *Candida albicans*). The interfering competitive capacity of the normal flora can be overcome by large numbers of virulent organisms. For example, the rate of development of salmonellosis has been directly related to the number of *Salmonella* organisms ingested.[20]

Genitourinary Tract

Urine is normally sterile. The factors that contribute to the ability of the urinary tract to resist infection are quite complex. Urine may be bactericidal for some strains of bacteria. This is mostly due to the pH of the urine, but factors such as urea and other solutes may play a role.

The lower urinary tract is flushed with urine four to eight times each day, eliminating potential pathogenic organisms unless they are capable of firmly attaching to epithelial cells of the urinary tract, such as *N. gonorrhoeae* and certain strains of *E. coli*. The length of the male urethra (20 cm in the adult) also provides protection, and bacteria seldom gain access to the bladder in men unless introduced by instrumentation. The female urethra is much shorter (5 cm in the adult and more readily traversed by microorganisms, which may be one reason why urinary tract infections are 14 times more common in women than in men. The hypertonic state of the kidney medulla presents an unfavorable milieu for most microorganisms. Tamm-Horsfall protein is a glycoprotein produced by the kidneys and excreted in large amounts in urine (approximately 50 mg/liter). Certain bacteria avidly bind to it, suggesting that it prevents them from gaining a foothold in the urinary tract, thereby acting as a natural host defense mechanism against colonization and subsequent infection.[21]

The vagina has a unique mechanism of protection. Under hormonal influence, especially estrogens, the vaginal epithelium contains increased amounts of glycogen that Döderlein's bacilli and other commensals metabolize into lactic acid. *Döderlein's bacilli* is an all-encompassing term used to describe acidogenic gram-positive rods residing in the vagina. Normal vaginal secretions contain up to 10^8 of such bacteria per milliliter. Thus an acid environment that is unfavorable to most pathogenic bacteria is established. The vaginal secretions of women with nonspecific vaginitis are usually characterized by an elevated pH.

The Eye

Constant bathing of the eyes by tears is an effective means of protection. Foreign substances are continually diluted and washed away via the tear ducts into the nasal cavity. Tears also contain large amounts of lysozyme and other antimicrobial substances.[22]

NONSPECIFIC ASPECTS OF THE IMMUNE SYSTEM

The immune system is modulated by a large number of regulatory mediators known as *cytokines* (see Chapter 8), which act through a complicated bidirectional feedback network similar to the endocrine system to influence other cells, especially lymphoid cells and cells of the neuroendocrine system.

Cytokines

Cytokines are hormone-like polypeptides that are produced during the initial response to an invading foreign agent (microorganism) and participate in a variety of cellular responses, including modulation of the immune system (Fig. 1). They are produced by a growing list of different cells, but principally by macrophages and activated lymphocytes (Table 3). Many of the generalized symptoms (morbidity) associated with infections are attributable to this cytokine cascade (e.g., fever, sleepiness, muscle aches and pain) (Fig. 1). Unlike antibodies, whose chemical composition is specifically determined by the stimulating antigen, the chemical composition of cytokines is constant and independent of the stimulating antigen.[23]

Cytokines are usually named for the cell that produces them (e.g., lymphokines, monokines). Most cytokines have more than one biologic property and share a number of overlapping functions (Table 4). This is probably why no single disease state has ever been traced to a deficiency or overproduction of any single cytokine and why their individual functions could not be discerned until the recent advances in molecular biologic techniques were made. As foreign agents (e.g., toxins, microbial products) trigger the immune system, a non-antigen-specific cascading release of cytokines ensues, acting in concert to increase resistance to invading microorganisms (and neoplastic cells). Cytokines thus form the first line of defense of the immune system and their impact is a prelude to specific immune responses.

There is a constant low-level background sentinel-like activity that helps to maintain the host's steady state of good immunologic health. This steady-state background activity may be either diminished or augmented (i.e., dysregulated). For example, persons who are immunocompromised for any reason have their immune "thermostat" set much lower and/or their level of maximal response dampened; therefore, the efficiency of their response is clearly hampered. This can be measured clinically by examining their *cellular immune status*, although all components of the immune system are adversely affected.[24] The most convenient means to measure the state of one's cellular immune system is with skin tests.[25]

In the United States, end-stage cancer, renal disease, human immunodeficiency virus (HIV) infection (acquired immune deficiency syndrome, AIDS), liver disease, and alcoholism are the most common underlying illnesses resulting in diminished cellular immune responsiveness. Worldwide, malnutrition is the leading cause.[26,27] This is especially evident in malnourished children, who have increased susceptibility to and severity of several infections. These include life-threatening bacterial in-

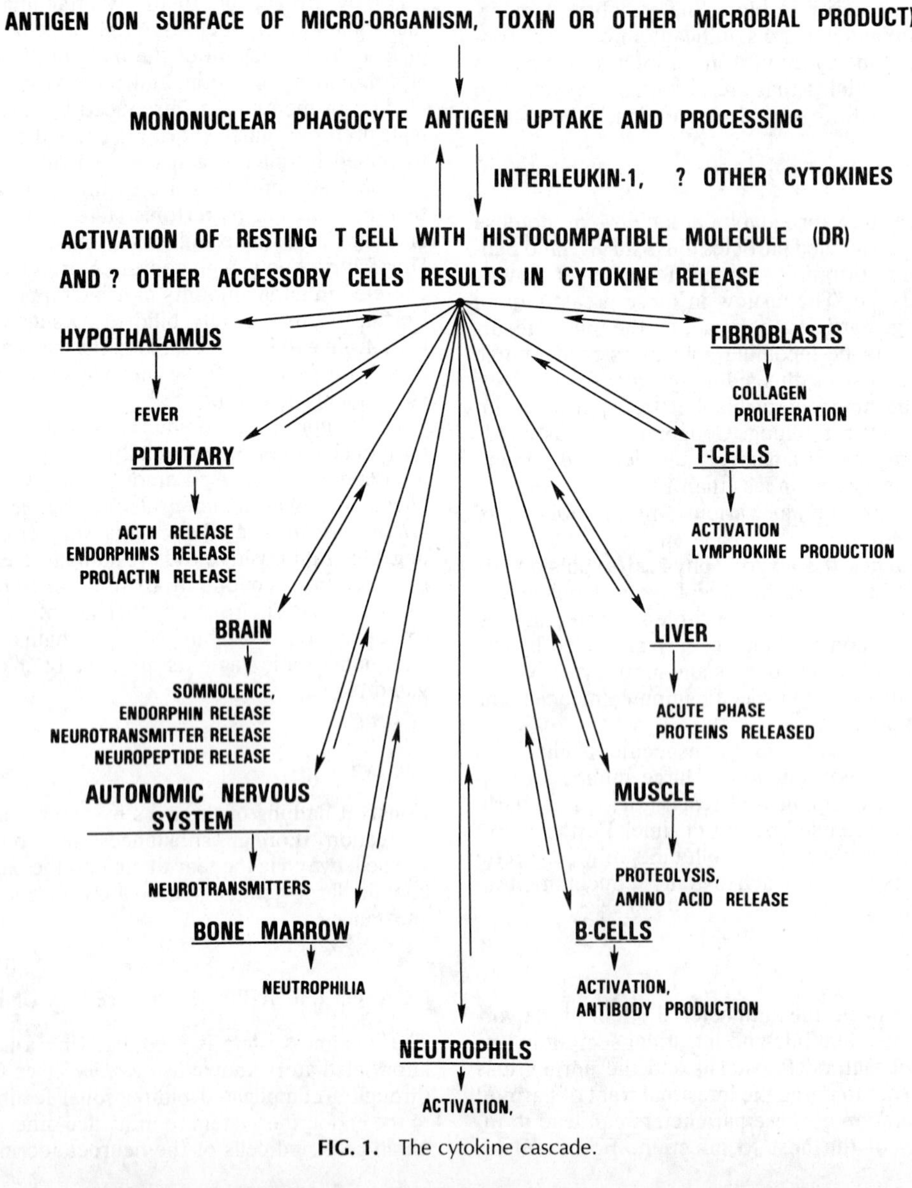

FIG. 1. The cytokine cascade.

TABLE 3. Cell Sources of Cytokines

Monocytes/macrophages
Lymphocytes
Langerhan cells
Histiocytes
Keratinocytes/epithelial cells
Corneal cells
Gingival epithelium
Melanocytes
Astrocytes
Microglial cells
Gliomal cells
Hypothalamus
Fibroblasts
Synovial cells
Neutrophils
Endothelial cells

fections of the middle ear, pervasive dental carries, and common childhood diseases, especially measles.[28]

Acute Phase Response

An easily recognized augmented non-antigen-specific response referred to as the *acute phase response* is a generalized but remarkably consistent host reaction that develops irrespective of the local or systemic nature of the inciting microorganism. It is mediated through an increased release of various cytokines, particularly interleukin-1 and tumor necrosis factor α (cachectin).[29,30]

Fever is the most obvious sign of the acute phase response and is the result of the action of cytokines, particularly interleukin-1, tumor necrosis factor, and α-interferon on the thermoregulatory center (hypothalamus) of the brain. The beneficial vs. detrimental effects of fever on the host have long been debated.[31] However, its role in upregulating the initial phase of an immune response appears to be critical (see Chapter 39).

An increase in the number and immaturity of circulating neutrophils is another readily demonstrated response (see Chapter 7) and is a direct consequence of the effect of cytokines, especially interleukin-1 and colony-stimulating factors, on the bone marrow. Other cytokines are involved in the activation of the neutrophils[31a] and promote and stimulate the colony formation of the various cell lines.

A decrease in serum iron and zinc and an increase in ceruloplasmin have long been recognized as components of the acute phase response. The virulence of many microorganisms is enhanced by increased availability of iron, and this has led to speculation that the host redistributes iron by an increased release of transferrin in an attempt to withhold this critical metal from the invader.[17] Furthermore, all normal mucosal secretions contain iron-binding proteins, suggesting a host defense mechanism to starve colonizing organisms. For example, gonococci disseminate most often in women during menstruation, a time when these organisms are exposed to increased amounts of free iron.

Zinc appears to be involved in wound healing, improves lymphocyte responsiveness, is required for hepatic RNA polymerase activity (increased during infection), and is implicated in the synthesis of protein, including acute phase globulins by the liver. Zinc also has been shown to affect phagocytosis. Thus, a deficiency of zinc, which is not stored in the body, influences the effectiveness of the immune response and aids with tissue repair.[25a]

The effects of the increased level of ceruloplasmin are not well understood, but it possibly increases the oxidation of catecholamines and therefore indirectly affects the redistribution of bood to vital organs.

During the acute phase response, the liver decreases albumin synthesis but dramatically increases the synthesis of other proteins, such as haptoglobin, complement components, amyloid A protein, C-reactive protein,[32] and certain protease inhibitors like α1-antitrypsin, α2-macroglobulins, and glycoproteins. Some of these derangements become quite prominent as the chronicity of the infection develops, (e.g., the decreased serum albumin levels noted in certain chronic infections).

A number of other systemic derangements are also evident during the acute phase response. These include increased production of thyroid-stimulating hormone, vasopressin, insulin, and glucagon, as well as a profound catabolism of muscle protein as a result of oxidation of amino acids from skeletal muscles. Prolonged infection results in muscle wasting, which can be clearly evident within days. Increased oxygen and caloric demands because of fever also contribute to this negative nitrogen balance. The increased circulating amino acids may be utilized by cells of the immune system.

Cytokines, especially interleukin-1 and tumor necrosis factor, also induce sleepiness through their effects on the central nervous system, a common host response leading to reduced energy demands.

The exact effects of cytokines on the brain and hypothalamus have not yet been fully elucidated. The release of ACTH, endorphins, prolactin, neurotransmitters, and growth hormone are induced by cytokines.[33] As the infectious process progresses, this nonspecific cytokine-driven response is augmented by the development of specific immunologic responses.[34]

Taken as a whole, this initial nonspecific response appears to be quite efficient and effective. The overlapping functions of the cytokines and their far-flung effects appear to be an evo-

TABLE 4. Biologic Properties of Cytokines Involved in the Non-Antigen-Specific Immune Response

Cytokine	*Biologic Properties*
Interleukin-1	Activates resting T cells; induces the acute phase response and sleep; stimulates the pituitary gland, ACTH, endorphin, prolactin release; stimulates the synthesis of other cytokines, collagen, and collagenases; activates macrophages; mediates inflammation; primes neutrophils.
Tumor necrosis factor α (cachectin)	Induces the acute phase response, sleep; is cytotoxic for some tumor cells; stimulates the synthesis of other cytokines, collagen, and collagenase; activates macrophages; mediates inflammation; primes neutrophils.
Interleukin-2	Induces cytokine synthesis; activates cytotoxic lymphocytes; is growth factor for activated T cells.
Interleukin-3	Growth factor for multilineage (pluripotent) cells and mast cells.
Interleukin-4	Growth factor for activated B cells, resting T cells, and mast cells; induces DR expression on B cells; enhances cytotoxic T cells; activates macrophages.
Interleukin-5	B-cell differentiating and growth factor; eosinophil differentiation.
Interleukin-6	B-cell maturation factor (stimulates antibody formation).
γ-Interferon	Induces class I and class II molecule (DR) on cells. Induces other antigens on cells; activates macrophages; enhances natural killer cell activity; enhances and inhibits other cytokines; exerts antiviral activity.
α- and β-Interferon	Exerts antiviral activity; augments natural killer cell activity; induces fever; induces class I antigen expression; inhibits protein synthesis.
Granulocyte–macrophage colony-stimulating factor (CSF)	Promotes growth of neutrophil, eosinophil, and monocyte bone marrow colonies; activates PMNs and macrophages. Primes neutrophil.
Granulocyte colony-stimulating factor (GSF)	Promotes growth of neutrophil colonies.
Macrophage colony-stimulating factor (MSF)	Promotes growth of macrophage colonies.

lutionary development resulting in effective backup systems that improve the host's chances of surviving in a potentially hostile environment. However, dysregulation can and does occur. For example, it may be the critical underlying defect leading to septic shock.[35,36]

Stress. There are studies that suggest that there is a link between mental state and susceptibility to infections,[37] and a growing body of evidence demonstrating a relationship between stress and immune function.[33,38,39]

Fibronectin. Fibronectin is a large molecular weight glycoprotein found in plasma and on cell surfaces. It mediates nonspecific clearance of bacterial and nonbacterial particulates such as fibrinogen–fibrin complexes, fragments of damaged cells, collagen debris, and altered platelets. It also covers the receptors of surface cells, blocking the attachment of many organisms, such as *Pseudomonas aeruginosa*, but it also enhances the binding of other organisms, such as *S. aureus*, to host cells.[40]

Hormones. Increased ACTH production occurs during the acute phase response and appears to augment the host's survival potential. The depressive effects of excess corticosteroids on inflammation and cellular immunity are well known. Estrogen affects the lining of the vagina, resulting in increased nonspecific resistance. Pregnant women develop weaker cell-mediated immune responses,[41] which may account for the severity of certain viral infections such as poliomyelitis and influenza. There is also speculation that the increased severity of influenza pneumonia in pregnant women may be due to increased pulmonary venous pressure. Certain other acute bacterial infections appear to be more serious during pregnancy. For example, group A β-hemolytic streptococci and *N. gonorrhoeae*, organisms that ordinarily colonize mucosal surfaces, are more prone to disseminate in the last trimester of pregnancy.

Phagocytosis. Microorganisms that enter the lymphatics, lung, or blood stream are engulfed by a variety of phagocytic cells, among them polymorphonuclear cells, wandering macrophages, and fixed macrophages (histiocytes). Phagocytosis that occurs independently of the action of opsonins is related to the contact angle between the microorganism and the surface upon which it rests, and therefore is most efficient when organisms are trapped in small tissue spaces (e.g., alveoli) as compared to smooth open surfaces (e.g., synovium).[42]

The reticuloendothelial system refers to a functional concept whereby mononuclear phagocytic cells in the blood, lymphoid tissue, liver, spleen, lung, bone marrow, and other tissues remove particulate matter from the lymph and blood stream. An example of a dramatic deleterious consequence of failure of this system occurs in asplenics (surgical or nonfunctional), whose blood stream is invaded by encapsulated bacteria such as pneumococci.

Natural Killer (NK) cells are interferon-induced leucocytes capable of recognizing cell surface changes, especially on virally infected cells. The NK cells bind to and lyse these target cells.[42a]

Age

The very young and the elderly are more susceptible to infection than persons in other age groups. The underlying defects, however, are usually different. Young children are at particular risk after their maternal antibody disappears and before they have had time to stimulate their own antibody production. This is particularly evident in acute infections with encapsulated organisms, especially *N. meningitidis* and *H. influenzae*.[44]

In the elderly, there is a functional decline in cell-mediated immunity. There is also a diminution in the physiologic functions of certain organ systems such as the lung.[45] Taken together, their reserve is severely taxed.

Complement. Complement refers to a group of upwards of 20 serum components that interact with each other in an orderly fashion and are referred to as the complement cascade. Although most often activated in conjunction with specific immunity through the classical pathway, complement can be spontaneously activated by the surface of some microorganisms and lyse them through the alternative complement pathway. Complement lyses microbial cells by destroying the cell wall.[46]

Inflammation. Inflammation is a complex reaction that directs elements of the immune system into sites of injury or infection. It is manifest by an increase in the local blood supply and capillary permeability that allows chemotactic peptides, especially the complement fragment C5a, to reach the site of irritation. Migration of polymorphonuclear leukocytes and later mononuclear cells (macrophages) to the site follows. Other consequences include local edema and fibrin deposition, which acts to limit the spread of infection. Other mediators of inflammation include cytokines and derivatives of arachidonic acids, including prostaglandins, thromboxanes, and leukotrienes.

REFERENCES

1. Mackowiak PA. The normal microbial flora. N Engl J Med. 1982;307:83–6.
2. Stiehm ER, Sztein MB, Steeg PS, et al. Deficient antigen expression on human cord blood monocytes. Reversal with lymphokines. Clin Immunol Immunopathol. 1984;30:430–6.
3. Quiot HR, van der Meer JW, Van Furth R. Selective antimicrobial modulation of human microbial flora: Infection prevention in patients with decreased host defense mechanisms by selective elimination of potentially pathogenic bacteria. J Infect Dis. 1981;143:644–54.
4. Steinman RM, Nogueira N, Witmer MD, et al. Lymphokine enhances the expression and synthesis of 1a antigens on cultured mouse peritoneal macrophages. J Exp Med. 1980;152:1248–61.
5. Beachley EH. Bacterial adherence: Adhesion–receptor interactions mediating the attachment of bacteria to mucosal surfaces. J Infect Dis. 1981;143:325.
6. Gould RC, Rameriez-Randa H, Holmes RK, et al. Adherence of bacteria to heart valves. J Clin Invest. 1978;56:1364.
7. Ramirez-Ronda CH, Fuxench-Lopez Z, Nevarez M. Increased pharyngeal bacterial colonization during viral illness. Arch Intern Med. 1981;141:1599.
8. Svanburg-Eden C, Jodal V. Attachment of E. coli to urinary sediment epithelial cells from urinary tract infection prone to healthy children. Infect Immun. 1979;26:837.
9. Kaslow RA, Shaw S. The role of histocompatibility antigens (HLA) in infection. Epidemiol Rev. 1981;3:90.
10. Whisnant JK, Rogentine N, Gradmick MA, et al. Host factors and antibody response to Haemophilus influenzae type B meningitidis and epiglottitis. J Infect Dis. 1976;133:488.
11. Van Eden W, de Vries RRP, Mehra NK, et al. HLA segregation of tuberculoid leprosy: Confirmation of the DR2 marker. J Infect Dis. 1980;141:693.
12. Sasazuki I, Hayose R, Wanto I, et al. HLA and acute poststreptococcal glomerulonephritis. N Engl J Med. 1979;301:1184.
13. Zander H, Gross-Wilde H, Kuntz B, et al. HLA-A -B, and -D antigens in paralytic poliomyelitis. Tissue Antigens. 1979;13:310.
14. de Vries RRP, Kreeftenberg HG, Loggen HG, et al. In vitro responsiveness to vaccinia virus and HLA. N Engl J Med. 1979;297:692.
15. Schneerson R, Robbins JB. Induction of serum haemophilus influenzae type b capsular antibodies in adult volunteers fed cross reacting Escherichia coli 075:K100:H5. N Engl J Med. 1975;292:1093.
16. Griffiss JM. Bactericidal activity by IgA of lytic antibody in human convalescent sera. J Immunol. 1975;114:1779.
17. Weinberg ED. Iron Witholdings: A defense against infection and neoplasia. Physiol Rev. 1984;64:65–102.
18. Green GM. In: Defense of the lung. Am Rev Respir Dis. 102:691, 1970.
19. Dupont HL, Hornick RB. Adverse effect of Lomotil therapy in shigellosis. JAMA. 1973;226:1525.
20. Hornick RB, Greisman SE, Woodward TE, et al. Typhoid fever: Pathogenesis and immunologic control. N Engl J Med. 1970;283:686.
21. Israde V, Darabi A, McCracken GH. The role of bacterial virulence factors and Tamm-Horsfall protein in the pathogenesis of *E. coli* urinary tract infections in infants. Am J Dis Child. 1987;147:1230–4.
22. Golden B, ed. Ocular Inflammatory Diseases. Springfield, Ill.: Charles C. Thomas, 1974.
23. Dinarello CA, Mier JW. Lymphokines. N Engl J Med. 1987;317:940–5.
24. Blackburn GL. Nutritional assessment and support during infection. Am J Clin Nutr. 1977;30:1943.

25. MacLean LD. Delayed type hypersensitivity testing in surgical patients. Surg Gyn Obs. 1988;166:285–293.
25a. Powanda MC. Changes in body balances of nitrogen and other key nutrients. Am J Clin Nutr. 1977;30:1254.
26. Corman LC. The relationship between nutrition, infection and immunity. Med Clin North Am. 1985;69:519–31.
27. Keenan RA, Moldawer H, Yang RD, et al. An altered response by peripheral leukocytes to synthesize or release leukocyte endogenesis mediator in critically ill, protein-malnourished patients. J Clin Lab Med. 1982;100:844–56.
28. Gordon JE, Scrimshan NS: Infectious disease in the malnourished. Med Clin North Am 1970;54:1495.
29. Dinarello CA. Interleukin-1 and the pathogenesis of the acute-phase response. N Engl J Med. 1984;311:1413–7.
30. Beutler B, Cerami A. Cachectin: More than a tumor necrosis factor. N Engl J Med. 1987;316:379–85.
31. Dinarello CA, Wolff SM. Molecular basis of fever in humans. Am J Med. 1981;72:799–819.
31a. Sullivan GW, Carper HT, Sullivan JA, et al. Both recombinant interleukin-1 (Beta) and purified human monocyte interleukin-1 prime human neutrophils for increased oxidative activity and promote neutrophil spreading. J Leukocyte Biol. 1989; Press.
32. Pepys MB, Baltz ML. Acute phase proteins with special reference to C-reactive protein and related proteins (pentaxins) and serum amyloid A protein. Adv Immunol. 1983;34:141–211.
33. Breder CD, Dinerello CA, Saper CB. Interleukin-1: Immuno-reactive innervation of the human hypothalamus. Science. 1988;240:321–3.
34. Rouse BT, Nordey S, Martin S. Antiviral cytotoxic T lymphocyte induction and vaccination. Rev Infect Dis. 1988;10:16–33.
35. Michie HR, Manogue KR, Spriggs DR, et al. Detection of circulating tumor necrosis factor after endotoxin administration. N Engl J Med. 1988;318:1481–6.
36. Tracey KJ, Lowry SF, Cerami A. Cachectin: A hormone that triggers acute shock and chronic cachexia. J Infect Dis. 1988;157:413–20.
37. Goetzl EJ, ed. Neuromodulation of immunity and hypersensitivity. J Immunol. 1985;135(Suppl):739–863.
38. Stein M, Keller SE, Schleifer SJ: Stress and immunomodulation: The role of depressive and neuroendocrine function. J Immunol. 1985;135(Suppl):827–33.
39. Pert CB, Ruff MR, Weber RJ, et al. Neuropeptides and their receptors: A psychosomatic network. J Immunol. 1985;135(Suppl):820–6.
40. Proctor RA. Fibronectin: A brief overview of its structure, function and physiology. Rev Infect Dis. 1984;9:S317–21.
41. Weingerg ED. Pregnancy—associated depression of cell-mediated immunity. Rev Infect Dis. 1984;6:814–31.
42. Van Oss CJ, Gillman CF. Phagocytosis as a surface phenomenon. I. Contact angles and phagocytosis of nonopsonized bacteria. J Reticuloendothel Soc. 1972;12:283.
43. Herberman RB. Immunoregulation and natural killer cells. Mol Immunol. 1982;19:1313–1321.
44. Goldschneider I, Gotschlich EC, Artenstein MS. Human immunity to the meningococcus. J Exp Med. 1969;129:1307.
45. Saltzman RL, Peterson PK. Immunodeficiency of the elderly. Rev Infect Dis. 1987;1127–39.
46. Frank MM. Complement. In: Samter M, Immunological Diseases. 4th ed. Boston: Little Brown; 1987:247–61.

5. ANTIBODIES

FREDERICK P. HEINZEL
RICHARD K. ROOT

Defense against infections involves nonspecific mechanisms mediated by mucocutaneous barriers, the phagocytic and complement systems, and responses that are specifically determined by the antigenic structures on invading microorganisms. The humoral immune response refers to that mediated by antibodies, i.e., immunoglobulins with binding specificity for microbial or other antigens. Such antibodies may be instrumental in aiding the host to eradicate the organism, directly or indirectly, as protection against subsequent challenge with the same organisms (immunity); in the diagnosis of infection by acting as a highly specific marker for the presence of a given organism; or in the pathogenesis of certain features of some infections (e.g., immune complex-mediated tissue injury). The mechanisms of antibody development and the essential features of the specific humoral immune response will be reviewed as they relate to these events. In addition, disorders of the antibody-forming capacity will be discussed.

IMMUNOGLOBULIN STRUCTURE

All antibodies are complex glycoproteins known as immunoglobulins. Although all normal immunoglobulins can be presumed to be capable of binding antigens, the term antibody is reserved for those immunoglobulins for which a target antigen has been identified. To date five major classes of immunoglobulins have been recognized and characterized: immunoglobulins G (IgG), M (IgM), A (IgA), D (IgD), and E (IgE). IgG immunoglobulins are made up of four subclasses and comprise 75 percent of the total in serum; IgA, 15 percent, with two subclasses; IgM, 10 percent, IgD, 0.2 percent; and IgE, only 0.004 percent. Of the four IgG subclasses, IgG_1 comprises the majority (approximately 80 percent of total IgG). These concentrations may be indicative of their relative importance to host defenses against infection, as will be discussed below. The chemical properties that permit this classification are summarized in Table 1, their metabolic properties in Table 2, and their biologic activities in Table 3 (for reviews see Refs. 1–4).

Regardless of class, every immunoglobulin molecule has the same basic unit structure, consisting of two longer peptide chains known as "heavy" or H-chains bound by disulfide bridges to two shorter peptide chains known as "light" or L-chains (Fig. 1). Depending on immunoglobulin class and subclass, a variable number of disulfide bridges bind the H-chains to each other, with the one closest to the amino terminus located in a region of the molecule known as the "hinge." Insertion of the disulfide bonds from the L-chains into this region theoretically permits, on antigen binding, their free rotation together with the corresponding amino-terminal segment of the H-chain.

On the basis of amino acid sequence, L-chains can be placed into one of two groups, known as "kappa" and "lambda." A single monomeric immunoglobulin molecule has two κ- or two λ-chains, never one of each. Each light chain has a chemically "constant" and "variable" region. The variable region is located at the amino terminus and is so named because it has an amino acid sequence that varies with different antibody molecules. This variability provides the basis of antibody specificity for different antigenic targets and comprises an intimate portion

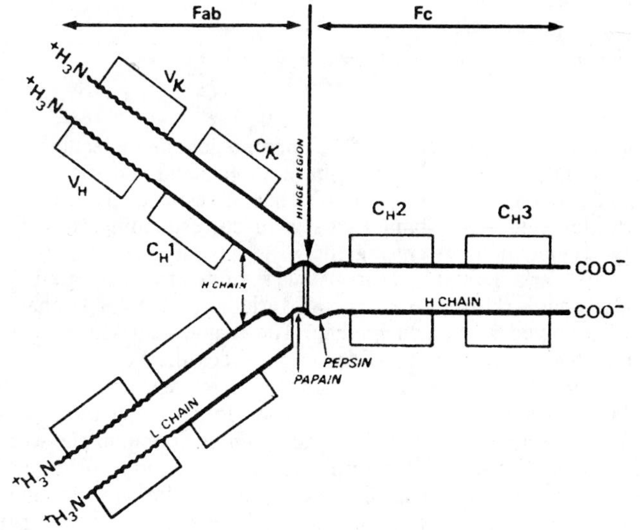

FIG. 1. A simplified model for an IgG_1 (κ) human antibody showing the four-chain basic structure and domains. V, variable region; C, constant region; vertical arrow, the hinge region; thick lines, H- and L-chains; thin lines, disulfide bonds. (From Stites et al.,[323] with permission.)

TABLE 1. Chemical Properties of Human Immunoglobulins

	IgG	*IgA*	*IgM*	*IgD*	*IgE*
Basic structure	Monomer	Monomer[a] Dimer[b]	Pentamer	Monomer	Monomer
Molecular weight	150,000	160,000[a] or 400,000[b]	900,000	180,000	190,000
Sedimentation coefficient(s)	6–7	7[a]	19	7–8	8
H-chain class	γ	α	μ	δ	ϵ
Subclass	$\gamma_1, \gamma_2, \gamma_3, \gamma_4$	α_1, α_2	μ_1, μ_2		
L-chain type	κ and λ	κ and λ	κ and λ	κ and λ	κ and λ
Molecular formula	γ_2L_2	α_2L_2[a] or $(\alpha_2L_2)_2$ SC J[c]	$(\mu_2L_2)_5J$	δ_2L_2	ϵ_2L_2
Electrophoretic mobility	γ	Fast γ and β	Fast γ to β	Fast γ	Fast γ

[a] Properties that belong to the monomeric form of IgA.
[b] Properties that belong to the dimeric form of IgA.
[c] Properties of secretory IgA. SC, secretory component; K, J-piece; a J-piece is also found in pentameric serum IgA.

TABLE 2. Metabolic Properties of Immunoglobulins

	IgG	*IgA*	*IgM*	*IgD*	*IgE*
Serum level mean (range) (mg/dl)	989 (600–1600)	200 (60–330)	100 (45–150)	3	0.008
Total body pool mean (range) (mg/kg)	1030 (570–2050)	210	36	1.1	0.01
Synthesis rate mean (range) (mg/kg/day)	36 (20–60)	28	2.2	0.4	0.004
Plasma half-life mean (range) (days)	21 (14–28)	5.9	5.1	2.8	2.4
Fractional turnover rate mean (range) (%/day)	6.9 (4.3–9.8)	24.0	10.6	37.0	72.0
Fraction in plasma[a] mean (range)	0.52 (0.32–0.64)	0.55	0.74	0.75	0.51

[a] This fraction represents the portion of the total immunoglobulins of each class that is found in the plasma.
(Adapted from Wells,[322] with permission.)

TABLE 3. Biologic Properties of Antibodies by Immunoglobulin Class

	IgG	*IgA*	*IgM*	*IgD*	*IgE*
Complement activation					
Classical pathway	++	0	++++	0	0
Alternative pathway	+	+	+	+	+
Opsonic activity	++++	0	+[a]	0	0
Lytic activity[a]	++	0	++++	0	0
Inhibition of bacterial adherence	+	+++	+	?	?
Viral neutralization	+++	+++	++	?	?
Reaginic activity	0	0	0	0	++++
Placental transfer	++++	0	0	0	0

[a] Through activation of complement after combining with cellular antigens.

of the antigen-binding site of the immunoglobulin molecule. The constant regions of L-chains have similar and specific amino acid sequences for all κ- and λ-chains, respectively. The disulfide bridges that bind L-chains to corresponding H-chains insert near the constant region.

One variable and three constant regions have been defined in H-chains.[2] Like L-chains, the variable regions of H-chains are involved in antigen binding. The amino acid sequence of the constant regions of H-chains provides the basis for class specificity of each immunoglobulin and is consistent within a class and subclass (isotype). It also provides the structural basis of the biologic functions of each immunoglobulin class, as mediated by the carboxy terminal or "Fc" region of the molecule (see below). The variable regions of immunoglobulins make them antigenically unique with respect to each other (idiotypes).

Soluble IgG, IgE, and IgD exist in serum and tissues as monomers. However, other immunoglobulins may polymerize or associate with nonimmunoglobulin accessory proteins. IgM is found in its monomeric form on the surface of B lymphocytes[5] but exists in serum as a pentamer. Whereas serum IgA is monomeric, IgA found on mucosal surfaces ("secretory") is largely dimeric. Polymeric IgM and IgA are linked, via disulfide bonds, with a 15 kD protein called J-chain[6] (Fig. 2). The J-chain is produced by B lymphocytes and is probably required to initiate polymerization and cellular secretion of IgM and dimeric IgA. No other function for the J-chain is currently known. Secretory component is another protein uniquely associated with mucosal IgA or IgM. It is synthesized by epithelial cells and serves as a membrane receptor for serum polymeric IgA or IgM, facilitating endocytosis, transport, and secretion of the immunoglobulin onto the mucosal surface.[7]

IMMUNOGLOBULIN METABOLISM AND DISTRIBUTION

The distribution and metabolism of the different immunoglobulin classes have been studied by a number of investigators (see

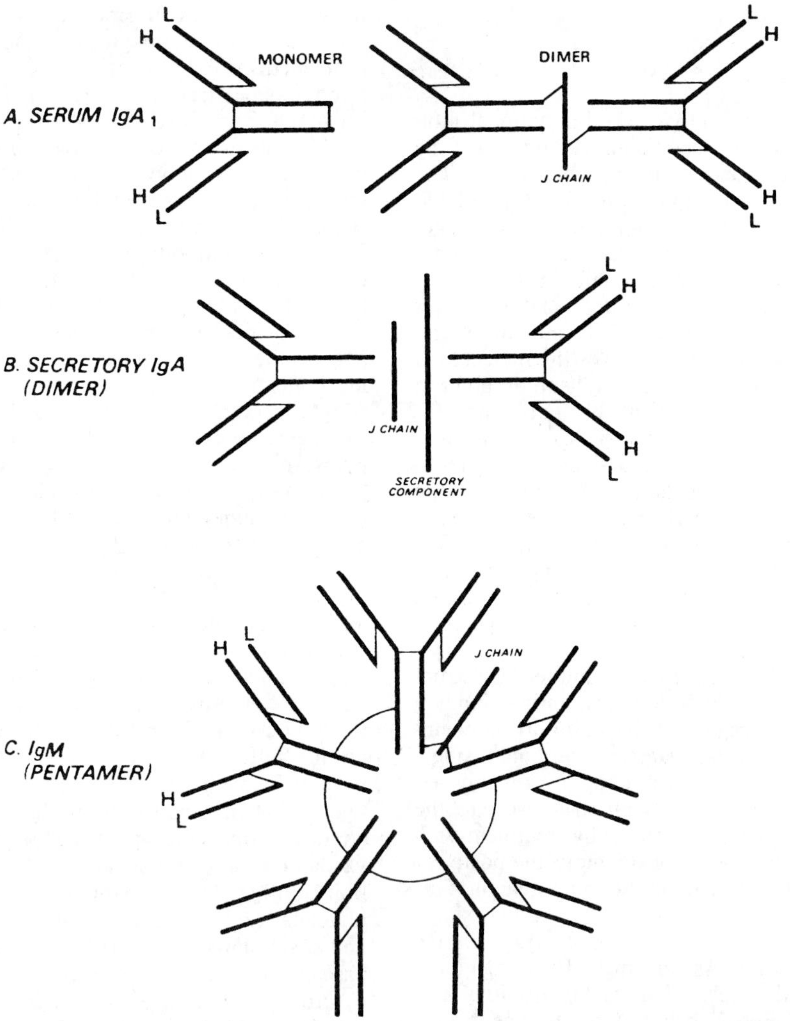

FIG. 2. Highly schematic illustration of polymeric immunoglobulins. Polypeptide chains are represented by lines; disulfide bonds linking different polypeptide chains are represented by thin lines. (From Stites et al.,[323] with permission.)

Refs. 8–10 for reviews). As noted in Table 2, under normal conditions both serum concentrations and the total body pool of IgG (in particular IgG) average 5 to 20 times higher than those of IgA and IgM and 1000 to 100,000 times higher than IgD and IgE, respectively. The differences in amounts of the separate immunoglobulin classes reflect differing rates of both synthesis and catabolism. These have been measured by infusing small amounts of radiolabeled immunoglobulin into normal subjects and measuring their clearance from the circulation. For example, the rates of synthesis of plasma IgA and IgG are almost identical (approximately 30 mg/kg/day); however, catabolic rates for IgA are almost fivefold higher. IgM is synthesized at one-tenth the rate of either IgA or IgG (approximately 2 mg/kg/day) and is catabolized four times as fast. Similarly, synthesis rates for IgE and IgD are low, and catabolic rates are high. A limitation of all of these studies is that they provide information only on those immunoglobulins that readily gain access to the circulation after production. At present there are no corresponding data for secretory immunoglobulins.

Using the same techniques of infusion of radiolabeled immunoglobulins, the intravascular vs. extravascular distribution of the immunoglobulins has been calculated. Approximately 50 percent of IgG, IgA (serum), and IgE is intravascular, compared with 75 percent of IgM and IgD. Thus the body pool of IgG is not only large, but it is well distributed in extravascular locations, particularly in lymphatic fluid.[11] IgG is the only immunoglobulin class to be actively transported across the placenta.[12] In contrast to the prevailing situation in the circulation, more IgA than IgG is isolated from saliva, tears, human colostrum or milk, and gastrointestinal secretions. In addition, secretory IgA is largely dimeric subclass IgA_2, whereas serum IgA is monomeric and mostly of the IgA_1 subclass.[13] These observations reflect the local production of secretory IgA_2 by plasma cells located beneath the lamina propria of the gut and serum IgA_1 by plasma cells in the bone marrow. During inflammation the secretions contain significantly higher amounts of IgG, as well as complement components, due to increased exudation from serum.[14]

These findings indicate that the major operational site of IgA in host defense against infection is on mucosal surfaces. IgM would appear to be involved primarily in intravascular defenses, particularly during the early phases of infection before the IgG antibody response develops. IgG, by virtue of its large amount, wide distribution, and penetration into inflamed tissues, is capable of operating in both the intravascular location and at tissue sites of active infection. The presence of long-lived IgG antibodies against many organisms can be correlated most closely with active "immunity" against these species or their toxins (see below). How these molecules can participate in host defense against infection will be discussed below.

FUNCTIONAL PROPERTIES OF IMMUNOGLOBULINS

Structure–Function Correlations

Immunoglobulins with antibody activity are bifunctional molecules: one function is to bind to specific antigenic targets; the other is to elicit a biologic response on the part of the host. The nature of this response will be determined by the type of immunoglobulin bound to the antigen and its interaction with specific host cells as well as with the serum complement system.

Through enzymatic cleavage of immunoglobulin molecules, the underlying structures that govern the bifunctional properties have been identified and characterized.[2,3] Treatment of immunoglobulins with the enzyme papain cleaves the molecule at the amino-terminal side of the inter-H-chain disulfide bond in the hinge region, thereby yielding two identical "Fab" (antigen-binding) fragments and a third "Fc" (crystallizable) fragment (Fig. 1). Each Fab fragment consists of a single complete L-chain and the variable and one constant (C_Hl) domain of the amino-terminal portions of a single H-chain. The two peptide H-chains are bound to each other by a single interchain disulfide bridge. The Fc fragment consists of the remaining portion of the two H-chains, also bound together by interchain disulfide bridges and the carboxy-terminal region of the immunoglobulin molecule.

By virtue of specific amino acid sequences and tertiary structure contained within the "variable" domains, antigen binding occurs at the amino-terminal region of the Fab portion of immunoglobulin molecules. Each Fab fragment can bind a single antigenic determinant. The affinity of binding presumably depends upon the degree of "fit" of antigen structure into the binding site.[15] Cleavage of immunoglobulins by treatment with the enzyme pepsin results in a break of the molecule posterior to the inter-H-chain disulfide bridge or the hinge region. This results in a single large $F(ab)_2'$ fragment (i.e., the two single Fab fragments joined together by the disulfide bridge linking the H-chains (pFc fragments). As do single Fab fragments, $F(ab)_2'$ molecules also bind antigens and display affinities similar to the parent molecule. Both Fab and $F(ab)_2'$ fragments lack the capacity to generate certain critical biologic activites of intact immunoglobulins; such activities are contained within the Fc region.

The structure of the hinge region varies considerably between immunoglobulin classes and may determine some of the functions of the molecule. For instance, the short, inflexible hinge region of IgG_4 is predicted to hinder Fc portion accessibility to C1q (complement) and may account for the poor complement-fixing characteristics of IgG_4.[16] Similarly, the great length and flexibility of the hinge region in IgD may be important for effective cross-linking of membrane-bound IgD with antigen.[17]

The Fc fragment cannot bind antigens; however, it is because of the molecular characteristics of this region that certain subclasses of immunoglobulins possess the ability to bind C1q and to initiate activation of C1 of the complement system or to bind to and affect critical cells in the host immune or inflammatory system.[3,18]

Effects of Antibody Binding to Fc Receptors on Cells

Cells involved in the immune or inflammatory response possess surface molecules that can bind Fc portions of immunoglobulins (Fc receptors). These have been operationally demonstrated usually using aggregates of immunoglobulins or Ig-coated erythrocytes; monoclonal antibodies are also available that inhibit function or identify the presence of specific classes of Fc receptors.[19]

Considerable heterogeneity in isotope affinity, cellular distribution, and function of these receptors exists (Table 4). Three classes of Fc receptors for IgG (FcRI, -II, and -III) are recognized; all bind IgG_1 and IgG_3 with much higher affinity than IgG_2 or IgG_4.[20] FcRI binds monomeric IgG with high affinity, is expressed on monocytes and some neutrophils, and provides a mechanism for attachment to, and lysis of, appropriate antibody-coated target cells (antibody-dependent cell cytotoxicity—ADCC).[21] FcRII has low affinity for monomeric IgG but binds antigen–antibody complexes effectively. This receptor is expressed on monocytes, neutrophils, eosinophils, B lymphocytes, and platelets; receptor function differs on phagocytes and B cells. Cross-linking of FcRII on the surface of phagocytic cells by antigen–antibody complexes induces phagocytosis, discharge or lysosomal contents, and superoxide anion generation.[22] The binding of aggregated IgG or antigen–antibody complexes to B-cell Fc receptors inhibits the subsequent activation and proliferation of these cells and may serve as a feedback mechanism to prevent antibody-excess states.[23] The third class of IgG receptor is FcRIII (or FcRlo), which is present on macrophages, neutrophils, and cytotoxic lymphocytes. On phagocytes, this receptor binds and removes circulating immune complexes and is implicated in the clearance of Ig-coated blood cells during immune cytopenias.[24] FcRIII is also expressed on large granular lymphocytes (LGL) and CD3+ T cells with ADCC activity. FcR on these cells is required for antibody-directed cytotoxocity.[25] Certain of these IgG Fc receptors stimulate release of potent vasoactive and chemoattractant substances (PGE_2, LTC_4, and LTB_4) when bound to aggregated IgG.[26] This response may contribute to inflammation induced by immune complexes deposited in tissue.

Two classes of IgE receptor have been characterized. High-affinity FcR is present on mast cells and basophils and is important in mediating anaphylactic responses to allergenic antigen.[27] When receptor-bound IgE is cross-linked with antigen, an intracytoplasmic signal is generated that results in release of vasoactive amines and arachidonic acid derivatives. Low-affinity FcR_ϵ (CD23) is expressed on macrophages, eosinophils, platelets, and T and B lymphocytes.[28] FcR_ϵ on macrophages and eosinophils is involved in IgE-directed cytotoxicity against parasites.[29–31] In the presence of specific IgE, platelets possess cytotoxic activity against *Schistosoma mansoni*; this requires that antigen-specific IgE link the parasite to platelet FcR_ϵ.[32,33] The mechanisms of platelet cytotoxic behavior are not yet understood. T cells bearing FcR_ϵ are implicated in the regulation of IgE production, presumably via the secretion of IgE-binding proteins that promote or suppress IgE synthesis.[34]

In a similar fashion, T cells that express Fc receptors for IgA, IgD, IgM, and IgG may have analogous isotype-specific regulatory functions.[35,36] The release of heavy-chain binding factors for isotypes other than IgE has been described.[37] T lymphocytes bearing receptors for IgM possess "helper cell" activity and promote the production of IgG synthesis.[38] However, the expression of these surface antigens on T cells is inconstant; the presence of CD4 and CD8 membrane proteins has proven more reliable as a phenotypic marker.[38,39] Recently, IgA Fc receptors capable of mediating phagocytosis have been described on mucosal neutrophils and on circulating monocytes.[40–42]

Complement Fixation

The Fc regions of the immunoglobulin molecules have differing capabilities for binding to C1q and thus activating the classical complement pathway through assembly of the C1qrs molecular complex. On a molecular basis, IgM is the most effective in this regard, perhaps in part due to its pentameric structure.[4] IgG_1 and IgG_3 are more active than the other IgG subclasses in C1q binding and activation.[3,18] None of the other immunoglobulin subclasses are capable of classical pathway activation; however, aggregates of IgA, IgE, and IgD may activate the alternative pathway, perhaps because of their high substitution with sugar residues.[4] IgG bound to sialic acid moieties on nonac-

TABLE 4. Immunoglobulin Fc Receptors: Distribution and Function

Type	*Synonyms*	*Cellular Distribution*	*Function*
IgG Fc receptors ($IgG_1/IgG_3 \gg IgG_2/IgG_4$)			
Fcγ RI	High affinity[a] MoAb: 32	Monocytes[b]	Antibody-mediated cytotoxicity
Fcγ RII (CD_w 32)	Low affinity MoAb: IV.3, KuFc 79	Monocytes, neutrophils, eosinophils, B lymphocytes, platelets	Antibody-mediated cytotoxicity, phagocytosis, lysosomal discharge, superoxide anion generation, regulation of immunoglobulin production
Fcγ RIII (CD 16)	Low affinity MoAb: 3G8, 4F7, Leu11, B73, VEP13	Macrophages, neutrophils, large granular lymphocytes (LGL), T lymphocytes	Phagocytosis, removal of immune complexes, ADCC
IgE Fc receptors			
Fcε R (high affinity)		Mast cells, basophils	Degranulation, leukotriene production if cross-linked by IgE bound to antigen
Fcε R (low affinity) (CD 23)		T lymphocytes, B lymphocytes, macrophages, eosinophils, platelets	Regulation of IgE production, ADCC, phagocytosis
IgA Fc receptors			
Fcα R		T lymphocytes, monocytes, neutrophils[b]	Mediates phagocytosis and regulation of IgA production

[a] High affinity for monomeric IgG; low-affinity receptors bind immune complexes. MoAb, monoclonal antibodies specific for receptor.
[b] Inducible on neutrophils with cytokine treatment.

tivating bacteria may also trigger alternative pathway activation.[43,44]

ROLE OF ANTIBODIES IN PROTECTION AGAINST INFECTION

After binding to specific microbial antigens and depending on the immunoglobulin class, antibodies can either enlist the effector cells of the host or can activate the complement system or both to assist in the eradication of infecting organisms. The success of this defense system depends greatly on the efficacy with which these coordinated systems complete this task. There is no evidence to indicate that viable organisms that are in an intracellular location can be selectively reached or modified by extracellular antibody or complement without destroying the host cell as well. Thus if tissue damage is to be limited, the primary protective role of these factors must be directed against pathogens when they are in an extracellular location. Specific antibodies can be involved in this process by promoting the following:

1. Opsonization of organisms for ingestion and destruction by phagocytic cells
2. Cell-free lysis of susceptible organisms by the complement system
3. Neutralization of toxins
4. Inhibition of attachment of organisms to host cells
5. Inhibition of the infectivity of extracellular viruses (virus neutralization)

Once pathogens are in an intracellular location, they are, in most circumstances, in a sanctuary where they are protected against the action of antibodies and complement. They may then serve as a source of chronic antigenic stimulation for more antibody production, as well as for activation of the cellular immune system (see Chapter 8). In addition, organisms may modify the surface properties of cells that they invade so that an antibody response occurs against these infected cells. Antibodies directed against cells harboring organisms may be destroyed by an ADCC reaction. A potential role for IgE antibodies in protection of hosts from parasitic infections that uses none of these mechanisms has recently been postulated. In this section the various mechanisms outlined will be discussed as they apply to different species of infecting microorganisms.

Opsonization

To describe the role that serum factors play in promoting the ingestion of staphylococci by polymorphonuclear leukocytes, Wright and Douglas in 1903 coined the term "opsonin" from the Greek opsono meaning "I prepare victuals for."[45] Opsonization thus refers to the process by which organisms or other particles are coated by antibodies and/or complement or other factors and thereby are prepared for "recognition" and ingestion by phagocytic cells. The efficacy of this process as a mechanism of defense against infection depends on (*1*) the ability of specific antibodies, complement, and other proteins to promote these events, (*2*) the presence and phagocytic capacity of host polymorphonuclear leukocytes, monocytes, and macrophages, and (*3*) the susceptibility of organisms to intracellular killing, once ingested. These latter two areas will be subjects for discussion in Chapters 7 and 8. In their classic investigations with staphyloccoci, Wright and Douglas observed that some, but not all of the opsonic activity or normal serum was lost with heating.[45] Heat-labile and heat-stable components of the serum opsonic system were defined and for most organisms are now known to involve a role largely for antibody or complement, respectively. In addition, recent evidence indicates that for some organisms fibronectin[46] or C-reactive protein[47,48] may be opsonic.

Complement serves as an opsonin when the cleavage products of C3 convertase activity, C3b or C3bi, are deposited on the particle or cellular surface and engage the complementary CR1 or CR3 receptors on polymorphonuclear (PMN) and macrophage cell membranes.[49] The mechanisms by which these events occur are discussed in detail in Chapter 6. Antibodies bound to organism surfaces may be opsonic either indirectly through their ability to activate the complement system, directly through binding to Fc receptors on phagocytes for IgG, IgA, or IgE, or by a combination of both mechanisms.

Experiments utilizing C3b or IgG coated erythrocytes indicated that phagocytosis was triggered when the IgG FcR was engaged, with the C3b receptor serving as an adherence ligand only.[50,51] While antibody and complement often function synergistically in promoting opsonization in phagocytes, a requirement for dual receptor involvement is not essential for microbial ingestion. A number of organisms can be readily opsonized in serum that contains no measurable immunoglobulins.[52–56] For example, protein A-positive strains of staphylococci are often more effectively opsonized in agammaglobulinemic than in normal serum.[54] Protein A serves as an antiopsonic factor in normal serum by binding the Fc portion of IgG[54,57]; conversely, in agammaglobulinemic serum it can activate C1 directly.[54] Similarly, opsonization and ingestion of some strains of group B streptococci[58] and *Escherichia coli*[59] may proceed by direct activation of the classical complement pathway without a role for antibodies. Thus the requirements for both antibody and complement to serve as components in the opsonization process vary considerably from species to species and even from strain to strain of microorganisms.

Physicochemical factors between particles and phagocytes other than engagement of specific complement and Fc receptors may affect opsonization and phagocytosis. Encapsulated as opposed to "rough" bacteria have differences in surface charge. Rough organisms have a hydrophobic surface charge and can often be ingested without opsonization. A hydrophobic surface charge on encapsulated organisms develops upon opsonization with antibody and complement.[60–63] Binding of IgG and C3 to the surface of salmonellae allows these organisms to fuse with artificial liposomes that contain no specific receptors for IgG and C3.[64] Finally, some organisms also contain surface lectins that bind to glycoproteins on phagocytes, thereby promoting adherence and ingestion.[65]

Opsonic antibodies are almost invariably of the IgG_1, IgG_3, or IgM classes, corresponding to the specificity of FcR on phagocytes for IgG_1 and IgG_3 and the ability of these antibodies to activate the complement system.[66,67] With the exception of mucosal phagocytes, which display functional Fc receptors for IgA, IgA antibodies are not opsonic.[40] In fact, IgA antibodies bound to the surface of microorganisms may block the binding of complement-fixing IgM or IgG.[68] IgE antibodies may bind metazoan parasites to macrophages or platelets, as discussed above,[20–33] and in this sense are "opsonic"; however, most such organisms are too large to be ingested by phagocytes.

Identified microbial targets for opsonizing antibodies include capsular polysaccharides,[49,56,58,67,69–72] M protein of group A streptococci,[73] and peptidoglycans.[74] Purified polysaccharides of pneumococci,[75] meningococci, group B streptococci,[76] and *Haemophilus influenzae*[77] are normally effective immunogens in all but young infants and have been used as subunit antigens in vaccines that generate opsonizing (pneumococci, streptococci) or opsonizing plus lytic activity (meningococci, *H. influenzae*). Administration of IgG obtained from normal or specifically immunized subjects prevents recurrent bacterial infections in patients with hypogammaglobulinemia through provision of specific opsonins.[78–80] Antipseudomonal hyperimmune globulin works through a similar mechanism.[81] While opsonic antibodies can be demonstrated against viruses[82,83] and fungi,[84–86] their role in defense against infection with these organisms is uncertain. Opsonic antibodies are thus most effective against organisms that are rapidly destroyed by phagocytes upon ingestion, i.e., "obligate extracellular parasites."

Lysins

Antibodies that can initiate the activation of the complement system through the terminal component membrane attack mechanism can cause lysis of susceptible organisms or cells. Microbial susceptibility is usually unique to gram-negative bacterial species[87,88] and to some viruses[83]; the initiating antibodies are of the IgM or IgG classes. Gram-negative enteric organisms causing bacteremia are often resistant to lysis by complement in contrast to the commensal gut flora.[88] Bactericidal antibodies that operate through the complement system play a major role in protection against infections with *Neisseria* sp. and *H. influenzae* type B. It should be emphasized that it is not entirely clear in all cases whether antibodies that initiate the membrane attack system of complement are also opsonic or whether separate immunoglobulin molecules are involved in the respective responses. With respect to gram-positive species, coating of organisms with complement does not cause lysis but may render them more susceptible to intracellular killing[89] or to the lytic action of lysozyme.[90]

Finally, infections of target cells with some viruses may lead to an antibody response that destroys infected cells by lysis in the presence of complement.[83] The importance of this mechanism in vivo in the control of viral infections remains to be confirmed.

Toxin-Neutralizing Antibodies

The demonstration by Roux and Yersin in 1888 that the virulence of *Corynebacterium diphtheriae* was due to the production of a protein exotoxin led to development of the first successful treatment and prevention of a bacterial infection by the use of passive and active immunization. The function of antibodies contained in an equine antiserum or developed actively in the human host by immunization with formalinized diphtheria toxoid is to bind to circulating or locally produced toxin and to prevent either its attachment to receptor sites or host target cells or its entry into the cells. Since the mechanism of action of the toxin in inhibiting cellular protein synthesis depends on passage of the active "A" fragment into the cytosol of the target cell, inhibition of binding (by the "B" fragments) or entry of the A fragment blocks the toxic effect.[91] The presence of neutralizing antibodies in the immunized host may be detected in vivo by a negative reaction in the Schick test, which measures the local reaction to an intracutaneous injection of toxin.[92] These antibodies are predominantly of the IgG class. Similar principles apply to passive and active antitoxic therapy of tetanus, botulism, and histotoxic clostridial infections and will be discussed in more detail in the chapters dealing with these organisms.

It is difficult to identify a specific toxigenic mechanism in the pathogenesis of disease caused by most other organisms; however, the role of endotoxin in the production of the shock syndrome seen with gram-negative infections has been extensively studied.[93] Immunization of animals[94,95] and perhaps humans[96] with mutant bacteria that are deficient in all or most polysaccharides in the terminal and core portions of their endotoxins ("Re" mutants) provides broad protection against lethal infection with a variety of gram-negative bacteria. Furthermore, in nonimmunized human hosts, survival from bacteremic gram-negative infection can be correlated with the presence of antibodies that react with Re lipopolysaccharides.[97] Passive immunization with serum obtained from normal individuals vaccinated with a "rough" mutant *E. coli* J5 decreased the morbidity and mortality of gram-negative sepsis in a hospitalized patient population.[96,98] Passively administered monoclonal antibodies directed against surface epitopes of J5 *E. coli* are protective against lethal gram-negative sepsis in animals[99] and are currently undergoing trial in man. The precise mechanism of this protective effect is currently under active investigation; the data suggest that it operates not through an opsonic effect of the antibodies[100] but rather through "detoxification" of the LPS.

Adherence-Inhibiting Antibodies

The capacity of bacteria to colonize the mucosal surfaces of human and other mammalian hosts is dependent in part on their ability to adhere to the epithelial and endothelial cells that form their lining. The role of adherence in the pathogenicity of various bacterial species has been recently reviewed.[101] For example, M proteins and lipoteichoic acids in group A streptococci project from the cell walls in fimbria that adhere to the oral mucosa.[102] Pili of pathogenic gonococcal strains promote adherence to mucosal cells and leukocytes while inhibiting phagocytosis.[103] Nonpathogenic strains of gonococci lack pili and do not adhere to cells; they are promptly phagocytized and killed. Enteric bacteria that cause diarrhea have an adherence-promoting "intestinal colonization factor."[104] Organisms that lack this factor cannot cause diarrhea even if they contain pathogenic enterotoxins. The pathogenicity of gram-negative enteric organisms in urinary tract infections can be correlated with pili that adhere to mucosal carbohydrates such as mannose or galactose dimers.[105,106]

Secretory IgA may contain antibodies that bind to these adherence-promoting factors and block their ability to attach to cellular receptors.[106–108] This constitutes a major protective mechanism for IgA against infection by pathogenic bacteria and perhaps other species on mucosal surfaces.[101,109] Proteases that cleave the hinge region of IgA or IgA_2 and that block adherence-inhibiting activity may be important virulence factors in some bacteria.[109] IgG antibodies may also block adherence by similar mechanisms, but the relatively low concentration of IgG in secretions and on mucosal surfaces does not support a major role for IgG in this phenomenon.

Viral Neutralization

Antibodies of the IgG, IgM, or IgA (including secretory IgA) classes have been described that inhibit (i.e., neutralize) the ability of extracellular viruses to infect their target cells (see Refs. 83 and 110 for reviews). Fixation of classical pathway complement components, in particular C4b, to the virus may aid in the neutralization process.[83,111–113] Infection of cells may be inhibited by antibodies because the virus does not fix to key cell membrane targets, or because of interference with entry or uncoating.[110,114] The development of neutralizing antibodies is instrumental in limiting the capacity of viruses to spread from an extracellular focus to an intracellular location, whether it be from a mucosal surface or by a hematogenous route.

The production of neutralizing antibody is synonymous with immunity against infection with viruses causing the common childhood exanthems or polio.[110] It should be emphasized that neutralizing antibodies can only aid against viruses that have a cell-free location in their spread ("type II" transfer). Those that are spread directly from one cell to another ("type I" transfer) are not likely to be directly neutralized in the presence of antibody (e.g., human immunodeficiency virus [HIV], herpesvirus). Cellular immune mechanisms become much more important in controlling infection caused by these viruses as well as in inhibiting viruses in an intracellular location. These mechanisms may involve a cooperative role for antibody, as noted below.[83,115]

Antibody-Dependent Cell-Mediated Cytotoxicity

Certain viruses may cause changes in the surface properties of infected target cells that lead to the development of an antibody response directed against the infected cell. Lysis of the infected cell may be achieved by the combined action of antibody and complement[83] or by the antibody-directed binding of effector "killer" lymphocytes, neutrophils, or macrophages via their Fc regions to the altered target cell (ADCC).[116–118] Cytotoxic lymphocytes possess cytoplasmic granules that contain serine proteinases similar to the complement proteins. These are discharged onto the target cell surface and assemble into membrane-bound complexes that induce osmotic lysis in a fashion akin to complement.[119,120]

IgE and Parasitic Infections

Immune mechanisms against parasites are only partially understood. Cellular immunity appears to play a major role in the containment of infections caused by protozoa. A role for humoral immunity in some protozoan infections is suggested by the high frequency of chronic intestinal giardiasis in patients with primary hypogammaglobulinemia.[121] In addition, *Pneumocystis carinii* infections may occur spontaneously in patients with isolated hypogammaglobulinemia.[122] The exact mechanisms of protection by antibodies in these infections remains to be ascertained.

Helminthic infections, particularly those that have a tissue invasive phase, are often associated with both eosinophilia and elevated levels of IgE.[123] Eosinophils are capable of destroying schistosomules in the presence of immune serum by binding to the surface of the organism and discharging their lysosomal granules.[30,31,124,125] The nature of the antibody promoting binding appears to be IgG, which can act in concert with complement to mediate the cytotoxic effect.[22,126,127] Similarly, cytophilic IgE may play a role in macrophage-dependent and platelet-dependent killing of schistosomes by serving as a ligand between the organism and the cells.[33,128]

The binding of antigen to IgE on mast cells and basophils triggers their degranulation with the release of a variety of amines that act on smooth muscle or affect vascular permeability.[27] It has been suggested that local amine release may be a protective mechanism in the gut to aid in expelling worms.[129] Increased vascular permeability may enhance the delivery of cells and serum components to local sites of infestation to participate in an attack on the parasite. In support of these suggestions, basophils and mast cells can be observed in gut mucosa at the site of invasion by nematodes in experimental infections.[130] Furthermore, treatment with drugs that inhibit histamine activity may impair elimination of the worms.[129,130] Definition of antiparasitic host defense mechanisms remains an important area for future investigation.

IMMUNOGLOBULIN GENETICS

Antibody diversity is created by a process of random genetic recombination that takes place in immunoglobulin genes during the early development of B lymphocytes. An estimated 10^8 possible antigen-binding specificities (idiotypes) result from the variable joining of 1100 component genes contained in the germ line DNA of all B-cell precursors.[131–133] Similar mechanisms have proved central to the generation of diversity in another immunologically important class of molecules, the T-cell receptor.[134] Certain constant portions of the immunoglobulin gene have also been incorporated into a large variety of surface receptor and identity proteins, such as the mixed major histocompatibility complexes (MHC). This aggregate of related genes thus constitutes an "immunoglobulin supergene family."[135] Beyond explaining the mechanism underlying antibody diversity, these observations have also provided understanding of antibody isotypic switching and affinity maturation during the course of repeated immune responses.

The gene complexes encoding the two light chains of immunoglobulin reside on separate chromosomes, with the genes for κ constant (C_κ) and variable regions (V_κ) on chromosome 22 and the genes for λ constant (C_λ) and variable (V_λ) regions on chromosome 2. There are several hundred V DNA segments and 5–10 short joining (J) segments contained in each light chain gene complex. The κ complex has one C_κ gene and the λ complex has six or more C_λ genes. During B-cell maturation, one of the light chain complexes undergoes recombination, a process whereby a single V and J segment will joint with a C_λ gene. Together, these form a single linear array, which constitutes the mature light chain gene. Both V and J DNA contribute to the final variable region of the light chain; therefore the number of possible V regions is the product of the numbers of V and J segments. Additional diversity is created through the inaccuracy of the joining process and the resultant random choice of amino acids at the splice site. Only one of the four light chain complexes present in each B cell (one κ and λ complex for each set of parental chromosomes) will undergo rearrangement at a time. The other gene complexes are activated only if a functional recombination does not occur, but are "turned off" for the life of the cell otherwise.

The genes of the heavy chain complex rearrange in a fashion that is similar in principle to light chain recombination. The heavy chain complex consists of about 1000 V_H genes and 4 J_H segments located on chromosome 14 (Fig. 3). In addition, there are 10 or more short, diversity-generating (D_H) segments. One of each is joined together in the order V-D-J during rearrange-

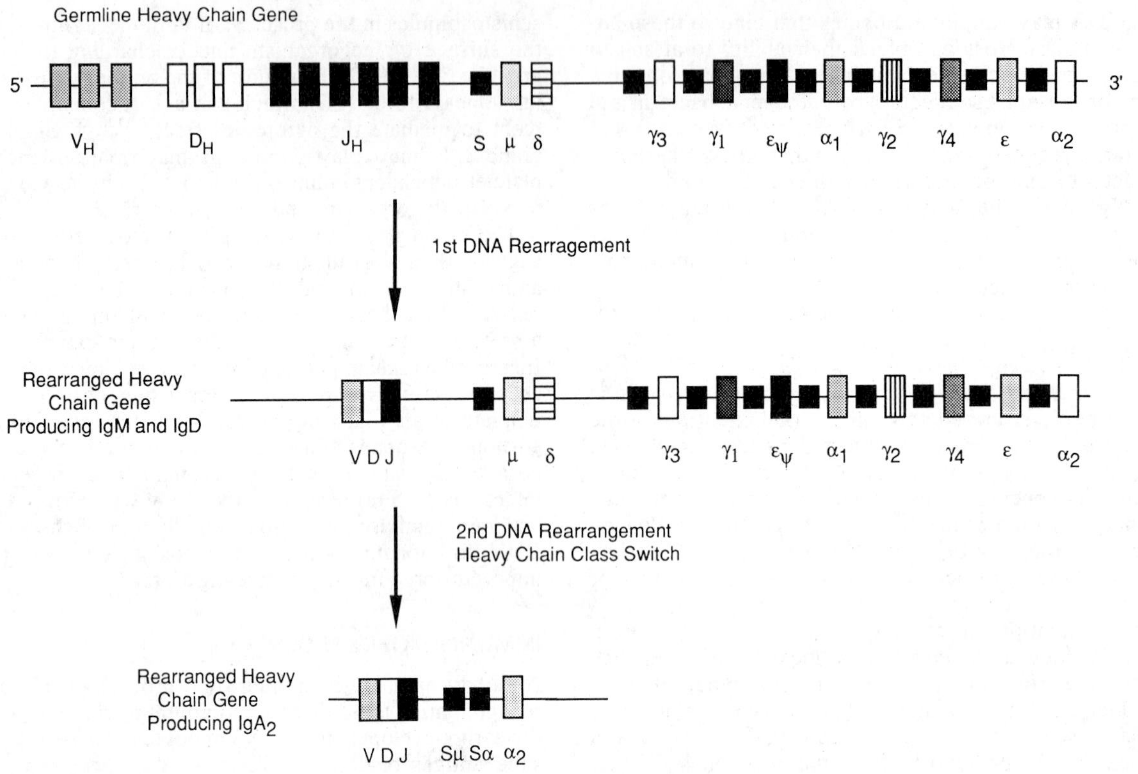

FIG. 3. Schematic illustration showing how immunoglobulin heavy chain genes recombine to create antibody diversity. During the first DNA rearrangement, single units from each set of variable (V_H), diversity (D_H), and joining (J_H) segments are joined together (VDJ) to form an active variable region gene. RNA transcribed from the variable region through the proximal heavy chain constant regions (μ and δ) generates either IgM or IgD heavy chains, depending on RNA processing. A second DNA rearrangement is illustrated to show the juxtaposition of the same variable region gene to a switch site (S) immediately before the α_2 constant region. Intervening genes are deleted. Transcription of the recombined gene results in production of IgA_2 heavy chain with unaltered antigen specificity. (Adapted from Waldmann et al.,[324] with permission.)

ment, and this combination encodes the mature heavy chain variable gene. The addition of D segments increases the potential number of combinations. The rearranged variable gene is linked with an available C_H gene to form the complete heavy chain gene. The C_H genes are arranged in linear fashion, in the following order: C_μ, C_δ, $C_{\gamma3}$, $C_{\gamma1}$, $C_{\epsilon\psi}$, $C_{\alpha1}$, $C_{\gamma2}$, $C_{\gamma4}$, C_ϵ, and $C_{\alpha2}$ (the $C_{\epsilon\psi}$ gene is a nonfunctional duplication of the C_ϵ gene). The rearranged variable region gene is initially joined with the C_μ and C_δ genes. The length of DNA encompassing the variable gene and both heavy chain genes is transcribed into messenger RNA. Splicing of the RNA transcript then determines whether IgM or IgD, or both, are produced.[136] Later, during B-cell differentiation, the variable gene can be spliced into proximity with distal heavy chain genes at defined "switch" regions; the intervening DNA is excised. The completed heavy chain gene, whatever the isotype, is capable of producing both membrane-bound and soluble immunoglobulin. This is regulated by the inclusion or deletion of a short segment of RNA encoding a 40-residue hydrophobic "tail" that promotes anchorage in the plasma membrane of the B cell.[137]

The structure of the heavy chain complex explains how isotypic switches occur during B-cell differentiation. The order of C_H genes approximates the order of appearance of isotypes during maturation of B cells. IgM and IgD are the first classes to be produced and are replaced by IgG, IgE, or IgA during subsequent differentiation. B cells producing the latter immunoglobulin classes have not been observed to revert to earlier isotypes. This is understandable given the order of heavy chain genes and the fact that they are deleted during recombination. The antigen-binding specificity is preserved during isotypic switches, as there is no alteration of the variable genes for heavy and light chains. It is unclear if a switch to distal genes occur in one step or via multiple, transient recombinations with intervening genes. The mechanisms that control isotypes switches are also not well understood, although T-cell products may play key roles in augmenting IgE or IgA production from stimulated B cells.[34,37] Thus B cell production of IgA in the intestinal lymphoid tissue may reflect the presence of IgA-promoting T cells ("switch cells").

In summary, antigen-binding diversity is generated through the recombination of diverse V, D, and J sequences, the inexact junction of these segments, and the combination of V_H and V_L regions that occurs during final assembly of the immunoglobulin molecule. However, a fourth mechanism can create further diversity after recombination has taken place; this occurs via somatic mutation of the variable regions. Comparisons of immunoglobulin gene sequences before and after secondary antigen challenges demonstrate single base pair mutations in previously rearranged variable regions of light and heavy chains. These mutations occur at frequencies considerably greater than those observed for constant region genes.[138,139] Mutations resulting in greater immunoglobulin affinity for a specific antigen may therefore generate a B cell more easily activated to proliferate and to produce that antibody. This will result in selection of higher-affinity antibodies during repeated cycles of immune stimulation with a single antigen, so-called "affinity maturation."

CELLULAR MECHANISMS IN ANTIBODY PRODUCTION

Antibodies must be produced promptly in response to the introduction of foreign protein and polysaccharide antigens on microbial invaders. There is need for economy and specificity in this response. The humoral immune response to infection must therefore direct antibodies to the relevant antigens, prevent self-directed responses, and control the classes of antibodies produced. When the need is past, the antibody response must be attenuated and a pool of memory cells reserved to allow brisk and specific recall of immunoglobulin production for future needs. Not surprisingly, intricate control mechanisms have evolved to serve this immunologic mandate. These mechanisms depend on the participation of three major cellular components: B cells, T cells, and accessory cells.

B cells are bone marrow-derived lymphocytes responsible for manufacturing antibody. The cardinal feature of mature B cells is the expression of surface-bound immunoglobulin with single antigen specificity and the ability of the cells to secrete soluble immunoglobulin of the same specificity when the cells are stimulated by antigen.[140,141] The antigen binds to surface immunoglobulin and triggers a series of chemical reactions and ionic events that stimulate the B cell into proliferative and antibody secretory activity; this initial signaling event is termed "activation." A subsequent proliferative phase precedes terminal differentiation of the B cell into the antibody-secreting plasma cells (for reviews see Refs. 142–144).

Thymus-derived or T lymphocytes are mononuclear cells, also derived from hematopoietic stem cells, that undergo precursor growth and maturation in the thymus.[144,145] T cells do not display surface Ig but instead express an antigen-binding protein, the T-cell receptor (TcR), which belongs to the immunoglobulin gene "family" and which derives clonal specificity through the same diversity-generating rearrangements as occur in B cells.[134] T-cell receptors are not secreted but remain associated on the T-cell membrane. Binding of specific antigen to the TcR also initiates a cascade of activation events, inducing T cells to proliferate and differentiate along a variety of functional lines. Unlike B cells, which bind to soluble, intact antigen, T-cell receptors recognize antigen that is displayed on accessory cell surfaces in close proximity with (perhaps even bound to) the class II histocompatibility antigen (HLA-DR). T cells additionally displaying the CD4 surface marker (OKT4, Leu3), participate or "help" in the activation or differentiation of B cells and are broadly referred to as T-helper cells.[39,146] This participation occurs in the form of either direct cell-to-cell contact or in the production of soluble immunoregulatory proteins called lymphokines, which are received via specific receptors on the target B cell. Another subset of T cells, which displays the surface CD8 marker (OKT8, Leu2), includes some cells that can inhibit B-cell antibody production.[147] The suppression may be specific for a single antigen response or may serve to limit production of selected or all subclasses of immunoglobulin. The mechanisms of suppression are heterogenous and poorly understood in humans but may function via elaborated antigen-specific inhibitory proteins.[148]

Accessory cells constitute the third group of cells important to activation of B cells; the best known and studied accessory cells are blood monocytes and tissue macrophages, but this group also includes dendritic cells, endothelial cells, and Langerhans cells.[149,150] These cells continually monitor the internal milieu through endocytosis and display of available proteins, in partially digested form, on their cell surface for T-cell scrutiny. An important feature of the accessory cell is the presence on its membrane of MHC class II antigen.[151] These surface proteins constitute the HLA-D (DR, DP, DQ) antigens in humans. When T-cell receptors recognize foreign antigen in close association with MHC, a TcR–antigen–MHC trimolecular complex is formed, and the lymphocyte receives the first of several signals necessary for activation to occur. Mature T cells only express TcR that recognizes the unique host MHC antigen—"MHC restriction." Accessory cells assist in B-cell activation by both direct and indirect means. B-cell activation is assisted by the presence of interleukin-1 (IL-1), which is produced by many types of accessory cells.[152] Accessory cells may indirectly participate in B-cell function by activating T cells, which produce many of the activation, growth, and differentiation factors required for B-cell development.[153,154] B cells are also capable of functioning as accessory cells to T lymphocytes. Soluble antigen can be specifically bound to surface Ig of B cells, internalized by endocytosis, and presented on the surface in conjunction with MHC antigen in a form recognizable by T cells.[155]

Ontogeny of B Cells

B cells, as well as T cells and the cells of hematopoiesis, are derived from pluripotent stem cells. Precursor, or pre-B cells develop in the fetal liver until the time of birth, when B-cell production shifts to the bone marrow. In this location, stem cells continuously produce new B cells throughout life; the daily yield is estimated to be more than one billion cells.[142] Proliferation and maturation of pre-B cells are supported by growth factors produced by stromal cells in the marrow microenvironment.[154,156] Pre-B cells are defined as B cells prior to the expression of surface Ig.[142] It is at this stage that immunoglobulin gene rearrangement takes place. The first gene to undergo recombination is the heavy chain complex; therefore IgM heavy chains are the first Ig products detectable in the cytoplasm of the pre-B cell. Light chains appear next when successful recombination takes place. When both light and heavy chains are present in the cytoplasm, Ig is assembled and displayed on the cell membrane, cell proliferation ceases, and the B-cell phenotype, as defined by the presence of surface Ig, is apparent. With further maturation, B cells express first IgM and then both IgM and IgD surface antibodies. Expression of other Ig isotypes occurs after activation and differentiation of the B cell.

Other important surface molecules on mature B cells include complement receptors and Fc receptors. The complement receptor CR1, which binds the proteins C3b and C4b, is expressed on the cell membrane of B cells.[157] CR2, which binds C3d, occurs only on B cells and is the receptor for Epstein-Barr virus.[158] Cross-linked C3d ligand binds to its receptor and promotes B-cell growth; soluble C3d inhibits B-cell growth.[159] A variety of Fc receptors have been described on B cells; many of these receptors are specific for a single isotype and are implicated in regulation of antibody production. In general, binding of the Fc portion of immunoglobulin to the B-cell FcR inhibits cellular functioning and may function to prevent antibody overproduction. Class II MHC is displayed on mature B cells and is enhanced when B cells are activated by antigen or IL-4. Possession of this surface complex allows B cells to function as accessory cells to T cells. A subpopulation of human B lymphocytes express the T-cell marker CD5 (Leu1), which may identify B cells committed to produce rheumatoid factor antibody.[160]

B-Cell Activation

There are many different activating signals, and B cells may require a specific combination and sequence of stimulations or signals before cell division can occur (for reviews, see Refs. 142 and 161). In general, activation may be antigen-specific or -nonspecific (polyclonal activation). The activation pathway can be additionally categorized according to the need for the presence of T cells (T-dependent) or activation in the absence of T cells (T-independent activation).

The central event in antigen-specific B-cell activation is the binding of antigen to surface Ig at a time when the B cell has matured sufficiently.[17] Antigen binding early in B-cell development generates an inhibitory signal and results in B-cell unresponsiveness to further stimulation.[162] This mechanism may function to ensure tolerance to host antigens that are present during early B-cell development. If no early inhibitory signal is received, the B cell activates when antigen cross–links surface

Ig and initiates a series of intracellular molecular events. Phospholipids of the cellular membrane are cleaved by phospholipase C to form inositol polyphosphates and diacylglycerol, which are potent intracellular second messengers. These molecules induce increases in intracellular calcium and mediate activation of functionally important proteins that prompt the cell to synthesize RNA and enter G_1 of the cell cycle. Activation of the cell also results in the expression of receptors for various growth factors, including IL-2, IL-4, transferrin, and B-cell stimulatory factor (BSF)-2.[163–165] Binding of these receptors with the appropriate growth factor initiates the proliferative phase of the B-cell response.

Antigen-specific B-cell activation (Fig. 4) can occur in the absence of T cells upon stimulation with certain antigens, usually polysaccharides that consist of repeating subunits; these are referred to as T-independent antigens.[166] These include polysaccharide molecules derived from the capsules of pathogenic bacteria such as *H. influenzae* and *Streptococcus pneumoniae*. The dependence of B-cell activation on the polymeric nature of these antigens suggests that extensive cross-linking of surface Ig is an important feature for T-independent B-cell responses. Such cellular responses are only T-independent in that T-cell contact is not required for activation. T-cell products are probably necessary for proliferation and maturation of B cells into plasma cells after activation occurs; the T cells involved need not be antigen-specific or matched for DR antigen. Activation of this pathway results in the appearance of B cells producing only certain isotypes of immunoglobulin.[167] Normal humans challenged with pneumococcal capsular polysaccharide vaccine, for instance, develop an antibody response consisting largely of IgG_2 molecules,[168] whereas T-dependent protein vaccines, such as tetanus toxoid, elicit IgG_1 subclass production.[167] In addition, secondary antibody responses to protein antigen tend to be greater than those following polysaccharide antigen immunization.[169] Polysaccharide vaccines therefore have been conjugated with protein antigens to increase the variety and magnitude of the antibodies produced during immunization.[169] In hosts devoid of T cells, B-cell activation occurs but results in a diminished antibody response, wholly of the IgM isotype.[166]

T-dependent B-cell activation (Fig. 4) largely requires contact of B and T cells—"cognate" activation.[170] B cells ingest and process antigen bound to surface immunoglobulin and present the immunogen in conjunction with B cell MHC protein.[171] Antigen-specific T-cell receptors on CD4+ cells recognize this molecular combination and prompt binding of T and B cells. The bicellular complex is stabilized by nonspecific interactions between CD4 on the T cell with nonpolymorphic portions of the B cell MHC molecules. The cellular adhesion molecule LFA-1 is also a necessary factor for cellular binding.[172,173] The T-cell receptor does not necessarily identify the same portion or epitope of the antigen recognized by B-cell surface antibody. This interaction is the probable molecular equivalent of the classic description of hapten-carrier cooperation.[174] The intimate binding of T and B cells provides greater opportunity for delivery of activation signals in either direction, and it is likely that each member of the pair simultaneously activates the other. The production of lymphokines by the T cell would then assist in subsequent proliferation and maturation of the B cell, even when contact is severed.

Cognate B-cell activation seems to be the major pathway responsible for formation of antibodies directed toward protein antigens, as patients who lack LFA-1 (and therefore do not form T:B cell complexes) produce only small quantities of specific antibody following vaccination with protein antigens, such as

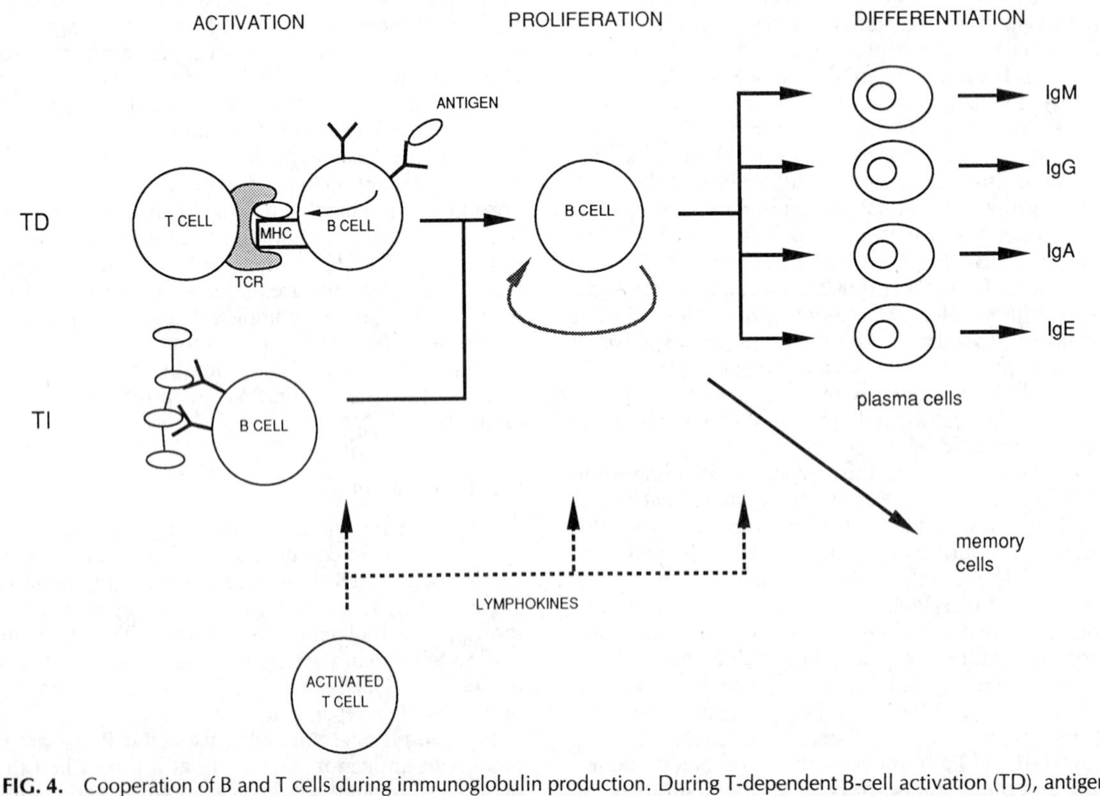

FIG. 4. Cooperation of B and T cells during immunoglobulin production. During T-dependent B-cell activation (TD), antigen binds to antibody receptors on antigen-specific B cells and is internalized, processed, and displayed on the B-cell surface in conjunction with the major histocompatibility complex antigen (MHC). T-helper cells bearing antigen-specific T-cell receptor (TCR) recognize the antigen–MHC complex and stimulate B-cell activation. During T-independent B-cell activation (TI), surface Ig is cross-linked by polymeric antigen, resulting in B-cell activation without T-cell contact. Either pathway of activation results in repeated cycles of B-cell proliferation, followed by differentiation of B cells into Ig-secreting plasma cells or long-lived memory cells. All stages of B-cell function are influenced by lymphokines secreted by activated T cells (dashed line).

tetanus toxoid, pertussis toxin, diphtheria toxin, purified protein derivative of tuberculin (PPD), and influenza vaccine.[173] However, these patients generate antibody to T-independent antigens, such as mannan and isohemagglutinin polysaccharides.

Other types of activation occur upon exposure to nonspecific mitogens of B cells, such as phorbol esters and lipopolysaccharide (LPS), which bypass the need for binding with surface antibody and directly activate regulatory proteins in the cell.[161] B cells can also be nonspecifically activated with anti-IgM/IgD immunoglobulin or with staphylococcal protein A, which are capable of multivalent binding of human Ig. These reagents activate B cells in a polyclonal fashion that may not be physiologic but that provides useful models for in vitro experimentation.[175]

The activated B cell next enters a proliferative phase that amplifies, by clonal expansion of antigen-specific cells, the quantity of antibody produced. Whatever the mode of activation, the subsequent proliferative phase is dependent on the presence of B-cell growth factors.[153,154] Several of these factors have been isolated and cloned, allowing for careful functional studies (Table 5). Many of these factors are not functionally restricted to B-cell stimulation, as IL-2 and IL-4 also induce T-cell proliferation, nor is their action on B cells specific for a single stage: IL-4 is capable of supporting activation, proliferation, and differentiation. The expression of regulatory surface molecules, such as membrane IgD, CR2, and MHC, diminishes during proliferation and subsequent differentiation of the activated cells.

One outcome of growth and differentiation of B cells is that they become nondividing plasma cells within 3–4 days after initial activation of the cell. The plasma cell is evolved for the single purpose of producing large quantities of immunoglobulin. The cytoplasm is crowded with ribosomes and a massive golgi apparatus, displacing the nucleus into its characteristic eccentric location. Certain other activated B cells are differentiated into long-lived memory cells that are capable of rapidly producing mature antibody isotypes upon restimulation with antigen.[142,143] Because IgM is the isotype first expressed by activated B cells, it constitutes the first class of antibody to be observed in the serum following primary antigenic challenge. IgM levels peak at 5–7 days after exposure and decline thereafter. IgG antibodies first appear at 7–14 days following antigenic exposure, consistent with the longer time necessary for B cells to differentiate into IgG-synthesizing cells. Secondary antigenic exposures, by virtue of pre-existing memory B cells, produce prompt IgG responses. The association of IgM with acute exposure has importance in the serodiagnosis of certain infections.

Control mechanisms have evolved to direct the type of antibodies produced by the fully differentiated B cell. Certain T-cell lymphokines function as B-cell differentiation factors and influence isotype commitment during maturation (Table 5). For example, the lymphokine IL-4 induces experimentally activated murine B-cell populations to preferentially produce IgG_1 and IgE.[176] This interaction may be central to the elevated levels of IgE in mammals infected with helminths, as has been shown in experimental *Nippostrongylus nipponensis* infection.[177] Interferon–γ, in contrast, is antagonistic to IL-4 isotype selection and separately induces the production of other Ig classes.[178] Similarly, IL-5 augments IgA secretion from activated B cells.[179]

In addition to producing these characterized lymphokines, T cells secrete heavy chain binding factors that can either augment or inhibit the production of certain immunoglobulin isotypes. The best characterized of these bind IgE or IgA. IgE binding factors are produced by CD4+ T lymphocytes that possess surface receptors for the Fc portion of IgE ($Fc_\epsilon R$).[39] The binding factor has stimulatory or inhibitory activity, depending on the state of glycosylation. A similar network regulating IgA synthesis has been proposed. T cells bearing IgA Fc receptors ($Fc_\alpha R$) have been indentified that also secrete factors that bind and regulate IgA production. The increased numbers of $Fc_\alpha R+$ T cells in the intestinal lymphoid tissue may therefore account for the increased production of IgA in that location.[37] Peyer's patch T cells also produce increased amounts of IL-5, which may additionally stimulate IgA production.[180,181]

B cells are also subject to various inhibitory mechanisms that prevent self-directed immune responses or excessive immunoglobulin synthesis. Inhibitory networks that act on B cells at different stages of development have been described. Tolerance to self-antigen may occur during early B-cell development and result from the selective deletion of self-reactive B-cell clones. An excess of foreign antigen may accomplish the same result—"immune paralysis."[182] At a second level, mature B-cell function can be actively inhibited by suppressor T cells. These cells suppress antibody production in either an antigen-specific or -nonspecific fashion and may act either directly on B cells or on other, antibody-promoting T cells. The exact suppressor mechanism is poorly characterized, partly because of its complexity. Although the effector cell in the suppressor circuit is typically CD8+, interactions with CD4+ cells may be required, and the final inhibitory signal may be mediated by soluble suppressor factors.[147,148,183]

Antibody production may also be regulated by other immunoglobulins that specifically recognize the variable region of the first, or idiotypic antibody. These anti-idiotypic antibodies have been observed during native immune responses and are speculated to modulate antibody production.[182,184] Because the variable region of anti-idiotype antibodies may mimic the original antigen epitope, these immunoglobulins have been used as experimental vaccines.[185,186] Finally, circulating antibodies or immune complexes may provide an inhibitory signal to B cells by binding to surface Fc receptors, an interaction that suppresses B-cell activation and development.[17,23]

TABLE 5. Cytokine Involvement in B-Cell Activation, Proliferation and Antibody Secretion

Cytokine	*Synonyms*	*Cell of Origin*	*Effect on B Cell*
Interleukin-1 (α and β)	Lymphocyte activating factor	Macrophages, B cells	Activation and proliferation
Interleukin-2	T-cell growth factor	T cells	Proliferation
Interleukin-4	(BSF-1, BCGF I)	T cells, mast cells	Activation (increases HLA-DR, CD 23), proliferation, differentiation (stimulates IgE production)
Interleukin-5	(BCGF II, TRF)	T cells	Differentiation (stimulates IgA production)
Interleukin-6	BSF-2, hybridoma growth factor, IFN-β_2	Fibroblasts, T cells, macrophages	Proliferation, differentiation
$BCGF_{low}$		T cells	Proliferation
γ-Interferon	Macrophage activating factor	T cells	Proliferation, differentiation (inhibits IL-4 action)

Abbreviations: BSF: B-cell stimulatory factor; BCGF: B-cell growth factor; TRF: T-cell replacing factor; HLA: human leukocyte antigen; CD: common determinant.

Diagnosis of Disease

With organisms that may be difficult to identify by standard culture methods, the identification of a specific humoral immune response may be instrumental in the diagnosis of infection. This technique is particularly useful in the diagnosis of viral infections, since most laboratories are not equipped to grow the organisms in tissue culture. A high IgM response is characteristic of most acute or recrudescent viral infections, whereas the presence of IgG antibodies can only be correlated with established, chronic, quiescent, or resolved infection.[187]

Tissue Injury

Chronic antigenic stimulation of B lymphocytes results in the production of large amounts of polyclonal antibodies (polyclonal gammopathy), as well as the related production of immune complexes and rheumatoid factor. Polyclonal gammopathy is the most commonly recognized disorder of serum immunoglobulin levels and is associated with a large number of infectious, neoplastic, and inflammatory states.[188] Prolonged activation of antigen-specific B and T cells is hypothesized to result in the nonspecific recruitment of ''bystander'' B-cell clones, many of which produce autoantibodies or antibody to unrelated antigens. Several chronic infectious diseases induce a polyclonal gammopathy, as exemplified by infective endocarditis.[189,190] Although IgG responses predominate, helminthic infections additionally induce elevated levels of polyclonal IgE.[191] Certain viruses, such as Epstein-Barr virus,[192] interact directly with B cells to stimulate polyspecific antibody generation during acute infection. Polyclonal gammopathy can be a prominent feature of symptomatic infection with HIV (see Chapter 108).

Antibody and antigen bind together to form immune complexes. Circulating immune complexes are apparent during many infectious processes, but are clinically significant in only a minority of patients.[193,194] The pathologic potential of immune complexes depends on size, valency, charge characteristics, and site of formation of the complex.[193] Immune complexes can initiate a cascade of proinflammatory events through interaction with Fc receptors on phagocytic cells or by activating complement. Binding of immune complexes to Fc receptor induces granulocytes to discharge lysosomal contents and generate reactive oxidative products. Macrophages are similarly stimulated by immune complexes to produce proinflammatory agents such as IL-1 and arachidonic acid derivatives.[195] Immune complexes containing IgM or IgG can also activate the classical pathway of complement and generate C3a and C5a, which contribute to inflammatory responses through their chemotaxic and anaphylatoxic properties.

Immune complex-mediated damage is most evident in the wide spectrum of glomerular disease that complicates the course of various acute and chronic infections. The prototypic lesion is that of poststreptococcal glomerulonephritis, which is caused when bacterial antigen–antibody complexes are deposited in the glomerular capillary wall. Local damage is presumably mediated by complement and mesangial cell products triggered by the immobilized complexes.[196] Immune complex glomerulonephritis is also associated with infections that cause prolonged antigenemia, such as infective endocarditis,[189] ventriculoatrial shunt infections (''shunt nephritis''),[193] and hepatitis B.[197]

Rheumatoid factors are IgM or IgG antibodies distinguished by their specificity for the Fc portion of autologous IgG.[198] A population of Leu1+ B cells may be uniquely evolved for rheumatoid factor synthesis.[160] IgM rheumatoid factors are normal products of secondary humoral immune reactions. Production only becomes pathologic when prolonged and elevated levels result.[198,199] Molecular analysis has shown that the genes encoding the variable (antigen-binding) portions of rheumatoid factor light chains are highly conserved during B-cell ontogeny, so that remarkable homology is evident in rheumatoid factors elicited from different individuals or from different B-cell hybridomas.[200] This degree of conservation suggests that important immune functions may be served by rheumatoid factor, a teleologic argument supported in part by animal studies.[201] For example, the opsonizing and cytolytic capacity of complement-nonreactive IgG may be increased when bound to an IgM molecule that efficiently activates the classical pathway of complement.[200] Rheumatoid factor may also improve the antigen-binding performance of low-affinity IgG by increasing valency. Finally, rheumatoid factor may facilitate the removal of soluble immune complexes by accelerating complement activation on the complex and thus promoting uptake by complement receptor-bearing phagocytes. Rheumatoid factor production accompanies polyclonal B-cell activation and immune complex formation and is frequently present during prolonged infection. No direct pathologic role is usually evident. When rheumatoid factor associates with circulating antigen–antibody complexes, cryoglobulins may result.[193] The mixed cryoglobulinemia that accompanies chronic infection is usually benign, but has been associated with hypersensitivity vasculitis and severe glomerulonephritis during hepatitis B infection.[202]

Certain infectious agents are hypothesized to induce autoimmunity because they share antigenic determinants with host tissue—''molecular mimicry.''[203] For instance, streptococcal M proteins share determinants with myocardial sarcolemma proteins,[204] *Klebsiella pneumoniae* epitopes cross react with HLA-B27,[205] and monoclonal antibodies against any of several viruses bind to several different normal human tissues.[206] Although circulating antibodies that are cross-reactive with these antigens have been recognized in some patients, these instances of molecular mimicry have not yet proven to be causal in the pathogenesis of autoimmune disease.

IMMUNOGLOBULIN AND ANTIBODY DEFICIENCY STATES

Interference with any of the stages of antigen processing, cellular proliferation, or regulation of the formation of immunoglobulins or specific antibodies may lead to a deficiency of the humoral immune responses. The consequences to the host may range from a loss of function of a specific antibody or immunoglobulin class to all classes depending on the nature of the defect. The loss of the IgG class has the most serious effects when compared with the other classes. A variety of disorders that involve the humoral immune system as it relates to antibody formation or action have been described and are indicated in Table 6 (for reviews see Refs. 207–209).

When the capacity to develop IgM or, in particular, IgG antibodies is lacking, then the host is unable to generate specific antibody-mediated serum opsonic, lytic, or neutralizing activities as they relate to these molecules. The serum of agammaglobulinemic patients is not capable of fixing complement by the classical pathway unless C1 is activated by an non-immunoglobulin-dependent mechanism; the ability to activate the complement system through the alternative pathway is retained, however. The end result of such deletions in the host defense system is the development of recurrent infections involving encapsulated bacteria and, to a lesser extent, gram-negative organisms in which opsonic and lytic defenses are important. These infections often involve the sinopulmonary tract, and the causative organisms may enter the blood stream with subsequent wide dissemination to other sites.[210] Thus patients who have unusually severe or recurrent infections with pneumococci, streptococci, *H. influenzae*, or meningococci should be examined carefully for possible defects in humoral immunity.

Even though the development of neutralizing antibodies of the IgG class is the hallmark of measurable long-standing protection against reinfection by specific viruses,[187] with some important exceptions[211–213] unusually severe disseminated or re-

TABLE 6. Disorders Involving the Humoral Immune System

	Consequences to Host Defense
Primary	
Pure antibody-mediated B-cell disorders	
X-linked hypogammaglobulinemia	Major[a]
Transient hypogammaglobulinemia of infancy	Variable[b]
Common variable hypogammaglobulinemia	Major
X-linked immunodeficiency with hyper-IgM	Major
Selective IgA deficiency	Minor[c]
Selective IgM deficiency	Minor
Selective deficiency of IgG subclasses	Variable
Mixed antibody-mediated (B-cell) and cell-mediated (T-cell) immunodeficiency disorders	
Severe combined immunodeficiency disease	Major
Nezelof syndrome	Major
Ataxia–telangectasia	Variable
Wiskott-Aldrich syndrome	Major
Short-limbed dwarfism	Major
Episodic lymphocytopenia with lymphotoxin	Major
Secondary to another disease or therapy	
Pure (B-cell) disorders	
Multiple myeloma	Major
Waldenström's macroglobulinemia	Variable
Heavy chain disease	Major
Chronic lymphocytic leukemia	Major
Some lymphomas	Major
Nephrotic syndrome	Variable
Splenectomy	Variable
Mixed disorders	
Cytotoxic therapy	Variable
Corticosteroid therapy	Variable
Severe burns	Major
Graft-vs.-host disease	Variable
Intestinal lymphangiectasia	Major
Acquired immunodeficiency syndrome	Major

[a] Antibody and/or cellular immune deficiency is routinely so severe that major infections result.
[b] Deficiency of antibodies or cellular immunity varies from patient to patient.
[c] Most patients have no significant increase in susceptibility to infection.

current viral infections are not characteristic of most patients with immunoglobulin deficiency. This finding suggests that cellular immune mechanisms may play a more important role in limiting the extent and severity of viral infection than do humoral mechanisms, a point substantiated by the observation that patients who are deficient in cellular immunity are at great risk for serious viral infections.

Likewise, the humoral immune deficiencies are not particularly associated with recurrent or severe fungal or parasitic infections, with two exceptions: patients who are hypogammaglobulinemic may develop pneumonia due to *P. carinii* or may be plagued with recurrent severe intestinal giardiasis.[121,122] Gastrointestinal giardiasis in patients with dysgammaglobulinemia or hypogammaglobulinemia may lead to prolonged malabsorption. In patients with acquired hypogammaglobulinemia, a peculiar nodular hyperplasia of lymphoid tissues in the submucosa of the small intestine may be seen with giardiasis.[121,210] Malabsorption may occur in humorally deficient patients in the absence of giardiasis, however, and has been associated with a sprue-like histologic pattern on intestinal biopsy specimens.[210,214] Treatment of such patients with replacement immunoglobulin theory may not only reduce the susceptibility to infection but may also reverse the malabsorption syndromes. This suggests that the intestinal mucosal changes may be related to chronic low-grade bacterial infection. When antibodies such as serum IgA function to clear or block environmental antigens, their loss may result in undesirable allergic responses. IgA deficiency is accompanied by a high rate of atopic disorders.

Clinical Features

Table 6 lists the major immunodeficiency disorders affecting the synthesis or function of antibody. They have been classified into primary diseases or secondary disorders, which represent complications of other disease states or therapy.

Primary Disorders: Pure Antibody Deficiency. X-LINKED HYPOGAMMAGLOBULINEMIA. Originally described by Bruton in 1952,[215] this represents the first immunodeficiency disorder to be characterized. The genetic origin of this disorder has been mapped to a locus on the long arm of the X chromosome.[216] Possession of this genotype in males results in defective maturation of B cells as a result of abortive heavy chain assembly.[217] As a consequence, B cells and plasma cells are absent from lymphoid tissue and bone marrow. Due to passive transfer of maternal IgG, affected infants are usually asymptomatic until 5–6 months of age, at which time maternal antibodies are almost completely cleared from the system.[218] The hypogammaglobulinemia will then usually manifest as recurrent middle ear, sinopulmonary, and gastrointestinal tract infections with or without complicating bacteremia, meningitis, and cellulitis.[219] Less commonly, such patients may not develop these recurrent infections until later in childhood, when they have other disorders such as chronic conjunctivitis, dental caries, or malabsorption. Because of severe pulmonary infection some patients may have bronchiectasis by the time hypogammaglobulinemia in diagnosed. Severe enteroviral infections are characteristic of this group of patients. Echovirus, in particular, is associated with a prolonged meningoencephalitis or a disseminated infection producing a dermatomyositis-like syndrome.[212,220,221] Other patients may have a chronic recurring type of arthritis syndrome that can resemble rheumatoid arthritis; *Mycoplasma* and *Ureaplasma* have been isolated from the joint fluid of some of these patients.[222,223] The futility of serodiagnosis makes it likely that additional viral complications are underrecognized. Mortality commonly occurs in the second or third decade and results from chronic pulmonary disease or from disseminated viral infections.

A diagnosis of this disease is made by demonstrating that there is a marked absence or deficiency of all five immunoglobulin classes. IgG levels in particular are usually less than 200 mg/dl, a level below which antibody-dependent serum opsonization is severely affected. These patients are incapable of antibody formation after specific antigenic stimulation. Biopsy specimens from appropriate tissues will demonstrate a complete absence of plasma cells in the germinal centers of lymph nodes and the lamina propria of the gut. An absence of circulating B cells, with normal or elevated levels of circulating T cells, is also characteristic.[224] Cellular immunity is completely intact.[218] Related syndromes include X-linked hypogammaglobulinemia with isolated growth hormone deficiency[225] and autosomal recessive hypogammaglobulinemia.[208]

Historically, replacement IgG was provided by intramuscular gammaglobulin. However, the limited volume tolerable by this route of delivery made normalization of serum IgG levels unrealistic. Immunoglobulin preparations for intravenous injection are now available that can be administered in quantities that result in normal serum IgG levels.[226,227] These preparations are 95–99 percent IgG, with trace quantities of IgA, IgM, IgD, and IgE; the half-life of the delivered IgG is variable but averages about 20 days. Maintenance doses start at 200 mg/kg in monthly infusions, but may need to be increased up to 500 mg/kg/month to achieve protection. A comparative study has shown that a higher-dose regimen resulted in improved pulmonary function. The incidence of acute infection diminished when serum levels were 500 mg/dl or higher.[228]

Intravenous immunoglobulin is typically well tolerated and can be self-administered at home after appropriate training of the patient or family. About 3–12 percent of patients experience fever, chills, headache, myalgia, and nausea with infusion.[226] When symptoms are severe enough, pretreatment with acetaminophen, antihistamines, or hydrocortisone is justified in order to reduce these side effects.[229] A few cases of non-A, non-B hepatitis have been transmitted by intravenous immunoglobulin, apparently due to contamination of isolated lots of infusate.[227] Otherwise the infectious risk of intravenous immunoglobulin is very small; no known instances of HIV transmission from IgG have occurred. In addition to immunoglobulin replacement therapy, specific infections must be treated with appropriate antimicrobials. The efficacy of maintenance prophylactic antimicrobials in the long-term management of these patients is questionable, and this practice may lead to superinfections with resistant bacteria.

TRANSIENT HYPOGAMMAGLOBULINEMIA OF INFANCY. This is an exaggerated form of the normal reduction in serum IgG levels that occurs at approximately 5–6 months of age.[208,230] In normal infants, serum IgG levels may fall to as low as 350 mg/dl before such patients begin to generate substantial amounts of IgG antibody from their own plasma cells. Occasionally the onset of IgG synthesis is delayed, resulting in a pathologically significant decrease in its level for a period of time. As a result, the patients may be subjected to the same type of infections as children with X-linked hypogammaglobulinemia. Suggested mechanisms for a delay in IgG production include immaturities in macrophage function,[231,232] reduced T-helper cells,[233] or exaggerated suppressor function.[234] Because of a risk of active infection, these children should not receive immunizations with live virus vaccine until a normal immunocompetency has been established.[235] Treatment with immune serum globulin is required when these patients are symptomatic with infection, but concern exists that such treatment may suppress subsequent production of endogenous immunoglobulin.[236]

COMMON VARIABLE UNCLASSIFIABLE IMMUNODEFICIENCY. This disorder is also called "acquired" hypogammaglobulinemia and appears to have a familial pattern, although the mechanism of inheritance has not been clearly established.[208,237] This disease is usually not apparent until the age of 15–35 years. Affected persons appear to have an unusually high frequency of autoimmune disorders in addition to an increased susceptibility to pyogenic infections.[210] While IgG levels are invariably below 250 mg/dl in symptomatic patients, and the levels of other immunoglobulins are also very low, this pattern is less pronounced or consistent when compared with that of patients with X-linked hypogammaglobulinemia. They also differ from these subjects in having detectable B cells in the peripheral circulation. However, the numbers of mature plasma cells in lymphoid tissues are decreased, consistent with a defect in B-cell maturation and differentiation. This disorder is probably heterogenous with respect to pathogenesis. Increased T-suppressor numbers and function[225,238] or reduced T-helper cell activity[239] have been described; other patients have intrinsic B-cell defects. A very few patients have anti-B-cell antibodies.

The disease affects men and women with approximately equal frequency. Its manifestation is often more subtle than that of X-linked hypogammaglobulinemia, with many patients merely experiencing an increased number or severity of sinopulmonary infections. Other patients may have chronic bacterial conjunctivitis, severe malabsorption, or a rheumatoid arthritis-like disorder. Systemic lupus erythematosus, idiopathic thrombocytopenia purpura, dermatomyositis, hemolytic anemia, or pernicious anemia have been described in some. In contrast to patients with X-linked hypogammaglobulinemia, many patients with acquired hypogammaglobulinemia have significant lymphadenopathy, splenomegaly, and intestinal lymphoid nodular hyperplasia rather than absence of lymphatic tissue.[210,221,235] Histologic examination of the lymph nodes reveals a marked accumulation of macrophages, immature B cells, and both CD4+ and CD8+ T cells.[206,208] The treatment of patients with the acquired form is similar to that of those with X-linked hypogammaglobulinemia. Successful treatment results in amelioration of infections as well as lymphadenopathy and splenomegaly.[206] In addition, affected patients may require therapy for associated autoimmune disorders. Some patients who have been appropriately treated have survived for a long time. Besides acute infection, a major complication appears to be chronic lung disease. An increased incidence of malignant disease has also been noted.[235,237] For patients with increased suppressor cell activity, cimetidine treatment has resulted in increased production of immunoglobulin.[240]

HYPER-IGM WITH IGG DEFICIENCY. A syndrome characterized by high IgM levels and very low IgG and IgA levels has been described. In most patients the inheritance appears to be sex-linked, and the manifestation is characterized by recurrent pyogenic infections.[241] There is an apparent inability of B cells and their successor plasma cells to form IgG and IgA after initial IgM and IgD synthesis. A deficiency in the heavy chain gene switch mechanism is thus suggested and may be caused by the absence of switch T cells in these patients.[242] This syndrome can be separated diagnostically from the other disorders by the characteristic increase in serum IgM concentrations, with low-to-absent levels of IgA and IgG. Treatment is similar to that of the other hypogammaglobulinemic disorders outlined above.

SELECTIVE IGA DEFICIENCY. This is the most common immunodeficiency disorder, with an incidence of about 1:600 in the normal population.[243] Whereas the majority of people with IgA deficiency are clinically normal, it is clear that this defect predisposes to a variety of diseases including (*1*) recurrent sinopulmonary infections, (*2*) atopy, (*3*) gastrointestinal tract disease, (*4*) autoimmune disorders (e.g., systemic lupus erythematosus, rheumatoid arthritis, pernicious anemia), and (*5*) malignancy (diffuse histiocytic lymphona or gastrointestinal carcinoma).[243–245] These clinical manifestations are probably due to the absence of protective IgA on mucosal surfaces and the loss of serum IgA blocking antibody directed against environmental antigens.[246] Affected patients have markedly reduced levels of IgA in both serum (< 5 mg/dl) and secretions, with normal or increased values of the other immunoglobulin classes. Most patients have decreases in both IgA_1 and IgA_2. Cellular immune functions and B- and T-cell numbers are usually normal. Some patients with IgA deficiency also have decreased levels of IgG_2, IgG_4, and/or IgE, indicative of a more generalized disorder affecting isotypic switching of immunoglobulins and further contributing to the heterogeneity of clinical manifestations.[247,248] A few of these cases may be caused by deletions of heavy chain genes.[249,250] These patients should not receive immune serum globulin therapy, since IgG levels are normal-to-elevated, and dangerous anaphylactic responses to transfused IgA may ensue. Similarly, treatment with plasma or blood may lead to anaphylactic transfusion reactions because of IgE antibodies to IgA in the recipient's circulation.[251] No effective replacement therapy is yet available; therefore treatment is directed primarily at complications.

SELECTIVE IGM DEFICIENCY. This is a rare disorder. Affected patients exhibit a susceptibility to autoimmune diseases or to severe infection with organisms that have polysaccharide capsules.[252] Cellular immunity is intact, and other classes of immunoglobulins are synthesized normally. The pathogenesis is unknown, but antibody production to T-independent antigens is impaired. Treatment is preventive and directed toward the complicating infections. No replacement therapy is available, except possibly with plasma.

SELECTIVE DEFICIENCY OF IGG SUBCLASSES. Isolated deficiency of IgG_1 is very rare and results in total IgG levels that are reduced, since this subtype accounts for approximately 70 percent of the IgG class. Patients with this disorder experience an increased incidence of infections with encapsulated bacteria, like hypogammaglobulinemic patients.[253] The pathogenesis is not known. Replacement gammaglobulin therapy is usually effective in reducing the incidence of infections.

The use of sensitive and specific IgG subclass immunoassays has uncovered selective deficiencies of IgG_2 and IgG_4, often coexisting with IgA and IgE deficiencies, in patients suffering from recurrent bacterial infections.[247,254] In most cases, the total levels of IgG were in the normal range. IgG_2 deficiency has been linked to impaired antibody responses to polysaccharide vaccines.[255]

MIXED DISORDERS WITH ANTIBODY DEFICIENCY. A number of primary immunodeficiency disorders have been described in which both antibody production and cellular immunity are impaired. Affected patients are susceptible to severe, recurrent, and often fatal infections with all classes of organisms, including obligate extracellular parasites as well as organisms that are capable of intracellular survival. They have both impaired antibody formation as well as defects in cellular immunity.

COMBINED IMMUNODEFICIENCY OF INFANCY. This is the most severe of the mixed immunodeficiency disorders and is discussed in Chapter 8 as well. Described inheritance patterns are either sex-linked or autosomal recessive. Typical patients are markedly lymphopenic and lack both B and T cells in their lymph nodes, thymus, or blood[208,209]; other patients exhibit only immature T-cell precursors in their circulation.[224,256] Normal immunologic competence has been restored in some patients by bone marrow transplantation, consistent with a stem cell defect.[257] About one-half of the patients with the autosomal recessive form of severe combined immunodeficiency lack enzymatic activities involved in adenosine nucleoside metabolism.[258] Adenosine deaminase deficiency causes lymphocyte depletion by allowing toxic levels of deoxyadenosine triphosphate to accumulate in the cells of these patients. Transfusion of normal erythrocytes to patients with adenosine deaminase deficiency has resulted in immunologic and clinical improvement,[259] based on the fact that the nucleosides pass freely through cell membranes, enter the erythrocytes, and are there metabolized by donor enzyme. Bone marrow transplantation is curative and the treatment of choice if a suitable donor is available.[260] A related metabolic cause of severe immunodeficiency in childhood is purine–nucleoside phosphorylase deficiency.[258,261] This rare syndrome similarly results in accumulations of nucleotides, which are selectively toxic for T cells. In contrast to the other forms of severe combined immunodeficiency, B-cell numbers and serum immunoglobulin levels may be normal in this disorder.

CELLULAR IMMUNODEFICIENCY WITH ABNORMAL IMMUNOGLOBULIN SYNTHESIS: NEZELOF SYNDROME. A variety of patients have been described who have marked impairments in cellular immunity with variable depression of antibody-forming capacity. They are grouped loosely under the eponym of "Nezelof syndrome," unless other characteristic features permit a different classification.[262] No specific genetic pattern can be demonstrated, and both affected males and females have been described. On a pathogenetic basis, it has been suggested that the defect in immunoglobulin synthesis is a consequence of the loss of function of the helper T-cell population, although this notion requires further definition. In contrast to the patients described above with severe combined immunodeficiency, most affected patients have lymphoid hypertrophy and hepatosplenomegaly, with macrophage infiltration and granuloma formation. Circulating B and T cells are usually normal in number, and immunoglobulin levels may be normal or reduced. Markedly depressed cellular immunity is characteristic, and most patients are incapable of mounting a humoral immune response to new antigens, although evidence of prior antibody formation may be found (e.g., isohemagglutinins).

WISKOTT-ALDRICH SYNDROME. This is an X-linked recessive disorder in which both cellular immunity and antibody synthesis are impaired. In contrast to Nezelof syndrome, affected patients also have thrombocytopenia and chronic eczematoid dermatitis. The precise mechanism involved in the defect in this syndrome is unknown, although a specific glycoprotein is missing from the surface of platelets and lymphocytes in these patients.[263] Affected patients have normal numbers of B and T cells. Immunoglobulin levels are in the low-normal range; however, patients have a characteristic difficulty in the synthesis of antibodies to T-independent antigens (e.g., polysaccharides).[264,265] They have major problems due to severe infection with encapsulated bacteria such as the pneumococcus and *H. influenzae*, since they cannot generate opsonic antibody against these organisms. Patients have had both the hematologic and immunologic abnormalities corrected by bone marrow transplantation.[266]

ATAXIA-TELANGIECTASIA. Patients with this neurologic disorder have variable deficiencies of IgG, IgA, and/or IgE levels, decreased humoral immune responses to new antigens, and diminished cellular immunity.[267,268] These findings suggest the existence of abnormal T-lymphocyte function affecting both IgA and IgE synthesis and immunity to cellular antigens. This disease may be caused by deficient DNA repair mechanisms, and chromosomal damage near the T-cell receptor and immunoglobulin genes may contribute to the immune defects.[269,270] Selective deficiencies of IgG_2 in this syndrome may be associated with chronic infections.[271] No effective treatment has been devised for the immune disorders in this disease.

OTHER COMBINED IMMUNODEFICIENCIES. There are a variety of other disorders of combined immunodeficiency, as outlined in Table 6. As far as the infectious complications are concerned, their manifestations are similar to those already described. For a more detailed description the interested reader is referred to several reviews.[147,208,209] The syndrome of hyper-IgE with eosinophilia, deficient chemotaxis, and recurrent staphylococcal infections is described in more detail in Chapter 7. Evidence supports the concept that this is due to a T-cell immunoregulatory defect involving impaired control of IgE synthesis as well as the production of a neutrophil chemotactic inhibitor.[272]

Humoral Deficiency Secondary to Other Diseases or Treatment. PURE B-CELL DISORDERS. Certain disorders may characteristically impair the humoral immune response as one of their central features. Accordingly, affected patients may develop severe or recurrent infections with organisms that are similar to those seen in hypogammaglobulinemic states. Two major types of disorders are seen: (*1*) those that affect immunoglobulin or antibody synthesis, and (*2*) those that increase the rate of immunoglobulin catabolism. Prime examples of the former are seen in a variety of malignant conditions affecting the lymphoreticular or hematopoietic systems.[273] Some patients with certain types of lymphoma, lymphosarcoma, thymoma, or chronic lymphocytic leukemia will be incapable of production of one or more classes of immunoglobulins and will become hypogammaglobulinemic.[274,275] Such abnormalities could be due to a primary involvement of the B-cell system in unregulated proliferation without maturation or increased suppressor activity. Besides treatment of the primary disease, such patients may benefit from regular administration of intravenous immunoglobulin.[275a] Conversely, patients with primary immunodeficiencies, in particular those involving the T-lymphocyte system, have a higher incidence of hematopoietic and lymphatic malignancies.[276]

In multiple myeloma, Waldenstrom's macroglobulinemia, and the various "heavy chain diseases," overproduction of a given class or subcomponent of an immunoglobulin occurs because of unregulated expansion and production of these proteins by a malignant clone of plasma cells or their precursors. When intact, the immunoglobulins produced in these diseases characteristically bear only a single L-chain type and have no effective antibody activity.[277] The expansion of the malignant plasma cell pool occurs at the expense of normal cells and diminishes the activity of the latter. In addition, disordered immunoregulation has been reported in myeloma.[278] Infections with encapsulated and gram-negative bacteria are prominent in these patients.[274,279,280] Immune serum globulin therapy is of little help, since catabolic rates of immunoglobulins are increased (particularly in the case of IgG myeloma),[8] and little additive effect of exogenous IgG can be defined.[281]

Immunoglobulin catabolism is also increased in some patients with severe burns,[282] protein-losing enteropathies,[8] or the nephrotic syndrome.[8,283] In burned patients, immunoglobulins are lost excessively into the burn site, whereas gastrointestinal or urinary tract losses of IgG are responsible for hypogammaglobulinemia in the other disorders. Treatment of the primary disease process will bring about a reversal of these conditions. Therapy with immune serum globulin may be desirable but is of no proven benefit.

SPLENECTOMY. The spleen performs several important host defense functions. As a phagocytic filter it can nonspecifically survey and present intravascular antigen to the large numbers of T and B cells that reside in or transit through this lymphoid organ.[284] It removes senescent or defective red blood cells, including those infected with intraerythrocytic parasites during malaria or babesiosis.[285,286] Although the liver may contain a greater total mass of phagocytic cells, the spleen is more efficient at removing poorly or unopsonized pathogens.[287] The spleen is also an important site of IgM production and memory B-cell differentiation during primary humoral responses. In particular, it is responsible for generating antibody responses to polysaccharide antigens.[288]

Some splenectomized patients are susceptible to severe infections with pneumococci, other streptococci, *H. influenzae*, meningococci, and the capnophilic gram-negative bacterium DF-2.[289] They are also susceptible to severe infection with *Babesia microttii*.[286] These infections are particularly prominent when splenectomy is performed in children for congenital hemolytic anemia[290] or Hodgkin's disease[291] and in some adults within the first 3 years after an incidental or post-traumatic splenectomy.[292] Sickle cell patients, who are functionally asplenic following infarction of that organ, also suffer from an increased incidence and severity of pneumococcal, *Haemophilus*, and meningococcal infections.[293] The increased susceptibility to infection in these patients have been attributed to the removal or dysfunction of an organ important for the clearance of intravascular organisms, to poor antibody responses to capsular polysaccharides, and to deficient serum opsonizing activity. Impaired antibody formation may be the central factor responsible for the observed serum opsonizing defects.[294] Tuftsin is an immunoglobulin-derived tetrapeptide produced in the spleen that stimulates phagocyte cell functions. Tuftsin levels are decreased following splenectomy and may also contribute to immunoincompetence.[295]

The improvement in intravascular clearance of organisms or foreign cells with specific immunization of splenectomized subjects[296,297] indicates that they should be considered as candidates for immunization with bacterial capsular polysaccharides. Satisfactory antibody levels, as measured by immunoassay, were reported in splenectomized subjects who received pneumococcal or meningococcal vaccine, provided they were not receiving cytotoxic or lymph node irradiation therapy.[298–300] However, even following vaccination, serum opsonic activity of asplenic hosts can still be deficient.[294,301] Although pneumococcal vaccine is protective in sickle cell patients, it has not yet been proved of benefit in splenectomized subjects.[299] Thus vaccination with capsular antigens does not remove the need for continued surveillance of splenectomized or asplenic subjects for possible sepsis with organisms included in the vaccine preparations. A decrease in infection incidence has been noted in sickle cell patients treated prophylactically with daily oral penicillin.[302]

Mixed Cellular and Humoral Deficiency Secondary to Disease or Therapy

Patients with generalized lymphomas may have both impaired cellular as well as humoral immunity.[273,275] Lymphopenia may occur in severely burned patients, leading to similar impairments.[303] Other disorders that can affect both limbs of the immune response in the absence of disease treatment are quite rare. One such disease is the disorder known as intestinal lymphangiectasia. Small lymphocytes, the majority of which are T cells, are lost in the gastrointestinal tract through dilated lymphatic channels. Patients with these disorders become markedly lymphopenic and can suffer from the same infections as patients with primary combined immunodeficiency.[304]

The majority of patients with secondary impairments in both humoral and cellular immunity are receiving cytotoxic, irradiation, or corticosteroid therapy.[274,275,305–307] By reducing the lymphocyte mass and by providing particular effectiveness against rapidly proliferating cells, cytotoxic agents can markedly impair the immune response. This is especially true when the host is faced with newer antigens for which a rapid proliferative response is called. Secondary responses are less affected by cytotoxic treatment both with respect to cellular and humoral immune components. Whereas patients receiving cytotoxic therapy may experience a reduction in the levels of circulating immunoglobulins, frank hypogammaglobulinemia is rarely seen, and established antibodies remain.[305,307]

Corticosteroid therapy exerts its major immunosuppressive effects against the T-lymphocyte population and against macrophages.[308,309] T-cell "traffic" is markedly disrupted by glucocorticoids.[310] Monocyte traffic, including egress from the circulation, is similarly disrupted, potentially creating a second level of impairment in tissue macrophage–lymphocyte interactions. Macrophage and lymphocyte production of immunoregulatory cytokines may be markedly diminished.[311,312] Glucocorticoid therapy can also reduce polymorphonuclear inflammatory responses; however, because this population is rapidly repleted, the effects are of short duration.[309] The consequences are most evident if glucocorticoid doses exceed 0.3 mg/kg/day/dose of prednisone or its equivalent.[313] A marked increase in susceptibility to a wide variety of infections is experienced within several weeks of steroid therapy if the dosages are in excess of 1 mg/kg/day and is the major cause of infection in patients undergoing renal transplantation[314] or treatment for lupus.[315]

Infection with HIV, the causative agent of AIDS, is associated with aberrant immunoglobulin production.[316] Patients most notably demonstrate polyclonal gammopathy, but specific antibody responses to new antigens are impaired.[317,318] In some patients, this results in an increased frequency of pneumonias caused by encapsulated bacteria.[319] For a more detailed discussion of these phenomena see Chapter 108.

Evaluation and Treatment of Disorders of Humoral Immunity

A summary of common practices used to evaluate and treat disorders of humoral immunity is given in Table 6, and a brief description follows. Chronic, unusually severe, or recurrent infections with bacteria and viruses can be caused by deficiencies in immunoglobulin, complement, or phagocyte-mediated immunity. Abnormal T-cell function is more commonly associated with fungal, protozoan, or viral illnesses. Certain nonimmunologic abnormalities, such as ciliary dyskinesis syndrome and cystic fibrosis, can additionally result in infectious complications. Therefore the measurement of serum immunoglobulin levels should not occur in isolation but must be part of a coordinated diagnostic strategy in the evaluation of suspected immunodeficiencies.[205]

Diagnosis

Information on immunoglobulin synthesis and antibody formation can be derived from a number of readily available studies. Serum protein electrophoresis can be used to screen for grossly hypogammaglobulinemic conditions and for the presence of paraproteins[188]; however, important selective immunoglobulin deficiencies can be missed. Instead, the separate amounts of IgM, IgG, and IgA can be quantitated directly by radial diffusion assay, immunoelectrophoresis, or automated laser nephelometry,[188] and these tests should be used to diagnose Ig class deficiencies. IgG subclasses (IgG_1, IgG_2, IgG_3, and IgG_4) and IgE must be measured using very sensitive enzyme-linked immunosorbent assays (ELISA) or radioimmunoassays that utilize isotype-specific monoclonal antibody reagents.[255] Because normal values for immunoglobulin concentrations vary with age, adjusted reference values must be used. Specific antibody formation against previously experienced antigens can be evaluated by measurements of A and B isohemagglutinins (IgM) or by application of a Schick test in an immunized patient (IgG). Primary responses to new antigens such as keyhole limpet hemocyanin can be evaluated, but this is an investigative procedure. Lymphocyte numbers can be estimated or quantitated by total lymphocyte counts and by enumeration of the circulating B and T cells using fluorescent monoclonal antibodies or other markers as described.[320] Measurement of in vitro responses of B cells to mitogens by immunoglobulin production is a research tool available in a number of centers, as is the quantitation of helper and suppressor T lymphocytes and their functions.[320] In some cases, a rectal or intestinal biopsy will allow further classification of immunodeficiency by providing lymphatic tissue for histologic study. When these tests are coupled with assays of complement, phagocyte, and T-lymphocyte function, a complete picture of the host defense system can be assembled.

REFERENCES

1. Natvig JB, Kunkel HG. Immunoglobulins: classes, subclasses, genetic variants and idiotypes. Adv Immunol. 1973;16:1–59.
2. Porter, RR. Structural studies of immunoglobulins. Science. 1973;180: 713–6.
3. Spiegelberg HL. Biological activities of immunoglobulins of different classes and subclasses. Adv Immunol. 1974;19:259–94.
4. Goodman JW. Immunoglobulins I: Structure and function. In Stites DP, Stobo JD, Wells JV, eds. Basic and Clinical Immunology. ed. 6th Los Altos, CA: Appleton & Lange; 1987:27–36.
5. Fu SM. Occurrence of IgM and IgD on human lymphocytes. J Exp Med. 1974;139:451–6.
6. Koshland ME. The coming of age of the immunoglobulin J chain. Annu Rev Immunol. 1985;3:425–53.
7. Underdown BJ, Schiff MJ. Immunoglobulin A: strategic defense initiative at the mucosal surface. Annu Rev Immunol. 1986;4:389–417.
8. Waldmann TA, Strober W. Metabolism of immunoglobulins. Prog Allergy. 1969;13:1–27.
9. Waldmann TE. The metabolism of IgE: studies in normal individuals and in a patient with IgE myeloma. J Immunol. 1976;117:1139–44.
10. Moller G, ed. Immunoglobulin D: structure, synthesis, membrane representation and function. Immunol Rev. 1977;37:1–62.
11. Yoffey YM, Courtice FC, eds. Lymphatics, Lymph and the Lymphomyeloid Complex. New York: Academic Press; 1970.
12. Virella G, Nunes MAS, Tamagini G. Placental transfer of IgG subclasses. Clin Exp Immunol. 1972;10:475–9.
13. Conley ME, Delacroix DL. Intravascular and mucosal immunoglobulin A: two separate but related systems of immune defense? Ann Intern Med. 1987;106:892–9.
14. Reynolds HY. Immunoglobulin G and its function in the human respiratory tract. Mayo Clin Proc. 1988;63:161–74.
15. Goodman JW. Antigenic determinants and antibody combining sites. In Sela M, ed. The Antigens. vol. 3. New York: Academic Press; 1975;127.
16. Isenman DE, Dorrington KJ, Painter RH. The structure and function of immunoglobulin domains: II. The importance of interchain disulfide bonds and the possible role of molecular flexibility in the interaction between immunoglobulin G and complement. J Immunol. 1975;114:1726–31.
17. Finkelman, FD, Vitetta ES. Role of surface immunoglobulin in B lymphocyte activation. Fed Proc. 1984;43:2624–32.
18. Bruggemann M, Williams GT, Bindon CI, et al. Comparison of the effector functions of human immunoglobulins using a matched set of chimeric antibodies. J Exp Med. 1987;166:1351–61.
19. Morgan EL, Weigle WO. Biological activities residing in the Fc region of immunoglobulin. Adv Immunol. 1987;40:61–134.
20. Anderson CL, Loon JR. Human leukocyte IgG Fc receptors. Immunol Today. 1986;7:264–6.
21. Shen L, Guyre PM, Fanger MW. Polymorphonuclear leukocyte function triggered through the high affinity Fc receptor for monomeric IgG. J Immunol. 1987;139:534–8.
22. Willis HE, Browder B, Feister AJ, et al. Monoclonal antibody to human IgG Fc receptors: cross-linking of receptors induces lysosomal enzyme release and superoxide generation by neutrophils. J Immunol. 1988;140:234–9.
23. Ryan JL, Henkart PA. Fc receptor mediated inhibition of murine B lymphocyte activation. J Exp Med. 1976;144:768–75.
24. Clarkson SB, Ory PA. Developmentally regulated IgG Fc receptors on cultured human monocytes. J Exp Med. 1988;167:408–17.
25. Lanier LL, Phillips JH. Evidence for three types of human cytotoxic lymphocytes. Immunol Today. 1986;7:132–4.
26. Ferreri NR, Howland WC, Spiegelberg HL. Release of leukotrienes C_4 and B_4 and prostaglandin E_2 from human monocytes stimulated with aggregated IgG, IgA, and IgE. J Immunol. 1986;136:4188–92.
27. Metzger H, Alcaraz G, Hohman R, et al. The receptor with high affinity for immunoglobulin E. Annu Rev Immunol. 1986;4:419–70.
28. Bonnefoy JY, Aubry JP, Peronne C, et al. Production and characterization of a monoclonal antibody specific for the human lymphocyte low affinity receptor for IgE: CD 23 is a low affinity receptor for IgE. J Immunol 1987;138:2970–8.
29. Spiegelberg HL, Boltz-Nitulescu G, Plummer JM, et al. Characterization of the IgE Fc receptors on monocytes and macrophages. Fed Proc. 1983;42:124–8.
30. Butterworth AE, David JR, Franks D, et al. Antibody-dependent eosinophil mediated damage to 51 Cr labeled schistosomula by *Schistosoma mansoni*: damage by purified eosinophils. J Exp Med. 1977;145:136–50.
31. Densen P, Mahmoud AAF, Sullivan J, et al. Demonstration of eosinophil degranulation on the surface of opsonized schistosomules by phase-contrast cinemicrography. Infect Immun. 1978;22:282–5.
32. Joseph M, Capron A, Ameisen JC, et al. The receptor for IgE on blood platelets. Eur J Immunol. 1986;16:306–12.
33. Joseph M, Auriault C, Capron A, et al. A new function for platelets: IgE-dependent killing of schistosomes. Nature. 1983;303:810–12.
34. Ishizaka K. Twenty years with IgE: from the identification of IgE to regulatory factors for the IgE response. J Immunol. 1985;135:i–x.
35. Lum LG, Muchmore AV, Keren D, et al. A receptor for IgA on human T lymphocytes. J Immunol. 1979;122:65–71.
36. Daeron M, Yodoi J, Neauport-Sautes C, et al. Receptors for immunoglobulin isotypes (FcR) on murine T cells. Eur J Immunol. 1985;15:662–7.
37. Kiyono H, Mosteller-Barnum IM, Pitts AM, et al. Isotype-specific immunoregulation: IgA-binding factors produced by Fc receptor-positive T cell hybridomas regulate IgA responses. J Exp Med. 1985;161:731–47.
38. Moretta L, Webb SR, Grossi CE, et al. Functional analysis of two human T cell subpopulations: help and suppression of B cell responses by T cells bearing receptors for IgM or IgG. J Exp Med. 1977;146:184–200.
39. Moretta L, Mingari MC, Moretta A, et al. Human lymphocyte surface markers. Semin Hematol. 1982;19:273–84.
40. Fanger MW, Goldstone SN, Shen L. Cytofluorographic analysis of receptors for IgA on human polymorphonuclear cells and monocytes and the correlation of receptor expression with phagocytosis. Mol Immunol. 1983;20:1019–27.
41. Maliszewski CR, Shen L, Fanger MW. The expression of receptors for IgA on human monocytes and calcitrol-treated HL-60 cells. J Immunol. 1985;135:3878–81.
42. Weisbart RH, Kacena A, Schuh A, et al. GM-CSF induces human neutrophil IgA-mediated phagocytosis by an IgA Fc receptor activation mechanism. Nature. 1988;332:647–8.
43. Edwards MS, Nicholson-Weller A, Baker CJ, et al. The role of specific antibody in alternative complement pathway-mediated opsonophagocytosis of type III, group B streptococcus. J Exp Med. 1980;151:1275–87.
44. Winkelstein JA, Shin HS. The role of immunoglobulin in the interaction of pneumococci and the properdin pathway: evidence for its specificity and lack of requirement for the Fc portion of the molecule. J Immunol. 1974;112:1635–42.
45. Wright AE, Douglas SR. An experimental investigation of the role of the body fluids in connection with phagocytosis. Proc R Soc Lond. 1903;72:357.
46. Proctor RA. Fibronectin: an enhancer of phagocyte function. Rev Infect Dis. 1987;9:S412–9.
47. Kilpatrick JM, Volanakis JE. Opsonic properties of C-reactive protein. Simulation by phorbol myristate acetate enables human neutrophils to phagocytize C-reactive protein-coated cells. J Immunol. 1985;134:3364–70.
48. Horowitz J, Volanakis JE, Brites DE. Blood clearance of *Streptococcus pneumoniae* by C-reactive protein. J Immunol. 1987;138:2598–603.
49. Horowitz MA. Phagocytosis of microrganisms. Rev Infect Dis. 1982;4:104–18.
50. Griffin FM, Blanco C, Silverstein SC. Characterization of the macrophage receptor for complement and demonstration of its functional independence from the receptor for the Fc portion of immunoglobulin G. J Exp Med. 1975;141:1269–77.
51. Mantovani B. Different roles of IgG and complement receptors in phagocytosis by polymorphonuclear leukocytes. J Immunol. 1975;115:15–7.
52. Guckian JC, Christensen WD, Fine DP. Evidence for quantitative variability of bacterial opsonic requirements. Infect Immun. 1978;19:822.
53. Jasin HE. Human heat labile opsonins: evidence for their mediation via the alternate pathway of complement activation. J Immunol. 1972;109:26.
54. Peterson PK, Verhoef J, Sabath LD, et al. Effect of protein A on staphylococcal opsonization. Infect Immun. 1977;15:760–4.
55. Williams RC, Quie PG. Opsonic activity of agammaglobulinemic human sera. J Immunol. 1971;106:51–5.
56. Giebink GS, Verhoef J, Peterson PK, et al. Opsonic requirements for phagocytosis of *Streptococcus pneumoniae* types VI, XVIII, XXIII, and XXV. Infect Immun. 1977;18:291–7.

57. Verhoef J, Peterson PK, Kim Y, et al. Opsonic requirements for staphylococcal phagocytosis: heterogeneity among strains. Immunology. 1977;33:191–7.
58. Baker CJ, Edwards MS, Webb BJ, et al. Antibody-independent classical pathway-mediated opsonophagocytosis of type 1a, group B streptococcus. J Clin Invest. 1982;69:394–404.
59. Leist-Welsh P, Bjornson AB. Immunoglobulin-independent utilization of the classical complement pathway in opsonophagocytosis of *Escherichia coli* by human peripheral leukocytes. J Immunol. 1982;128:2643–51.
60. Stjernstrom I, Magnusson KE, Stendahl O, et al. Liability to hydrophobic and charge interaction of smooth *Salmonella typhimurium* 395 MS sensitized with anti-MS immunoglobulin G and complement. Infect Immun. 1977; 18:261–72.
61. Van Oss CJ, Gillman CF. Phagocytosis as a surface phenomenon. II. Contact angles and phagocytosis of encapsulated bacteria before and after opsonization by specific antiserum and complement. J Reticuloendothel Soc. 1972;12:497–502.
62. Stendahl O, Tagesson C, Edebo L. Influence of hyperimmune immunoglobulin G on the physicochemical properties of the surface of *Salmonella typhimurium* 395 MS in relation to interaction with phagocytic cells. Infect Immun. 1974;10:316–9.
63. Absolom CJ, Van Oss CJ, Zingg W, et al. Phagocytosis as a surface phenomenon: opsonization by a specific absorption of IgG as a function of bacterial hydrophobicity. J Reticuloendothel Soc. 1982;31:59–64.
64. Tagesson C, Magnusson KE, Stendahl O. Physicochemical consequences of opsonization. Perturbation of liposomal membranes by *Salmonella ty phimurium* 395 MS opsonized with IgG antibodies. J Immunol. 1977; 119:609–13.
65. Ofeck I, Sharon N. Lectinophagocytosis: a molecular mechanism of recognition between cell surface sugars and lectins in the phagocytosis of bacteria. Infect Immun. 1988;56:539–47.
66. Quie PG, Messner RP, Williams RK. Phagocytosis in subacute bacterial endocarditis: localization of the primary opsonic site to Fc fragment. J Exp Med. 1968;128:553–70.
67. Shigeoka AO, Hall RT, Hemming VG, et al. Role of antibody and complement in opsonization of group B streptococci. Infect Immun. 1978;21:34.
68. Griffis JM. Epidemic meningococcal disease: synthesis of a hypothetical immunoepidemiologic model. Rev Infect Dis. 1982;4:159–79.
69. Johnston RB Jr, Klemperer MR, Alper CA, et al. The enhancement of bacterial phagocytosis by serum: the role of complement components and two cofactors. J Exp Med. 1969;129:1275–90.
70. Young LS. Human immunity to *Pseudomonas aeruginosa*. II. Relationship between heat stable opsonins and type-specific lipopolysaccharides. J Infect Dis. 1972;126:277–87.
71. Anderson P, Johnston RB Jr. Human serum activities against *Hemophilus influenzae*, type B. J Clin Invest. 1972;51:31–8.
72. Hemming VG, Hall RT, Rhodes PG. Assessment of group B streptococcal opsonins in human and rabbit serum by neutrophil chemiluminescence. J Clin Invest. 1976;58:1379–87.
73. Fischetti VA, Gottschlich EC, Siviglia G, et al. Streptococcal M protein: an antiphagocytic molecule assembled on the cell wall. J Infect Dis. 1977; 136:S222–33.
74. Peterson PK, Wilkinson BJ, Kim Y, et al. The key role of peptidoglycan in the opsonization of *Staphylococcus aureus*. J Clin Invest. 1978;61:597–609.
75. Schwartz JS. Pneumococcal vaccine: clinical efficacy and effectiveness. Ann Intern Med. 1982;96:208–20.
76. Baker CJ, Kasper DL. Group B streptococcal vaccines. Rev Infect Dis. 1985;7:458–67.
77. Hill JC. Summary of a workshop on *Haemophilius influenzae* type B vaccines. J Infect Dis. 1983;148:167–75.
78. van Furth R, Leijh PCJ, Klein F. Correlation between opsonic activity for various microorganisms and composition of gammaglobulin preparations for intravenous use. J Infect Dis. 1984;149:511–7.
79. Hill HR, Bathras JM. Protective and opsonic activities of a native, pH 4.25 intravenous immunoglobulin G preparation against common bacterial pathogens. Rev Infect Dis. 1986;8:S396–400.
80. Cunningham-Rundles C, Siegal FP, Smithwick EM, et al. Efficacy of intravenous immunoglobulin in primary immunodeficiency disease. Ann Intern Med. 1984;101:435–9.
81. Pennington JE, Pier GB, Sadoff JC, et al. Active and passive immunization strategies for *Pseudomonas aeruginosa* pneumonia. Rev Infect Dis. 1986;8:S426–33.
82. Allison AC. On the role of mononuclear phagocytes in immunity against viruses. Prog Med Virol. 1974;18:15–7.
83. Sissons JGP, Oldstone MBA. Killing of virus infected cells. The role of antiviral and complement in limiting virus infection. J Infect Dis. 1980;142:442–8.
84. Lehrer RI, Cline MJ. Interaction of *Candida albicans* with human leukocytes and serum. J Bacteriol. 1969;98:996.
85. Diamond RD, Root RK, Bennett JE. Factors influencing killing of *Cryptococcus neoformans* by human leukocytes in vitro. J Infect Dis. 1972;125:367–76.
86. Davies SF, Clifford DP, Hoidal JR, et al. Opsonic requirements for the uptake of *Cryptococcus neoformans* by human polymorphonuclear leukocytes and monocytes. J Infect Dis. 1982;145:870–4.
87. Roantree RJ, Rantz LA. A study of the relationship of the normal bactericidal activity of human serum to bacterial infection. J Clin Invest. 1960;39:72–81.
88. Frank MM, Joiner K, Hammer C. The function of antibody and complement in the lysis of bacteria. Rev Infect Dis. 1987;9:S537–45.
89. Li IW, Mudd S. The heat labile serum factor associated with intracellular killing of *Staphylococcus aureus*. J Immunol. 1965;94:852–62.
90. Wilson LA, Spitznagel JK. Molecular and structural damage to *Escherichia coli* produced by antibody, complement and lysozyme systems. J Bacteriol. 1969;96:1339–42.
91. Pappenheimer AM, Gill DM. Diphtheria. Science. 1973;182:353–8.
92. Pappenheimer AM Jr. The Schick test 1913–1958. Int Arch Allergy Appl Immunol. 1958;12:35–7.
93. Morrison DC. Endotoxins and disease mechanisms. Annu Rev Med. 1987;38:417–32.
94. McCabe WR, Bruins SC, Cralven DE, et al. Cross reactive antigens: their potential for immunization induced immunity to gram negative bacteria. J Infect Dis. 1977;136:S161–76.
95. Braude AI, Ziegler EJ, Douglas H, et al. Antibody to cell wall glycolipid of gram negative bacteria: induction of immunity to bacteremia and endotoxemia. J Infect Dis. 1977;136:S167–73.
96. Ziegler EJ, McCutchan JA, Fierer J, et al. Treatment of gram-negative bacteremia and shock with human antiserum to a mutant *Escherichia coli*. N Engl J Med. 1982;307:1225–30.
97. McCabe WR, Kreger BE, Johns M. Type specific and cross-reactive antibodies in gram negative bacteremia. N Engl J Med. 1972;287:261–7.
98. Baumgartner JD, Glauser MP, McCutchan JA, et al. Prevention of gram-negative shock and death in surgical patients by antibody to endotoxin core glycolipid. Lancet. 1985;2:59–63.
99. Teng NNH, Kaplan HS, Hebert JM, et al. Protection against gram-negative bacteremia and endotoxemia with human monoclonal IgM antibodies. Proc Natl Acad Sci USA. 1985;82:1790–4.
100. Proctor RA. Role of antibody in the prevention and pathogenesis of endotoxin and gram-negative septic shock. In: RA Proctor, ed. Handbook of Endotoxin. Vol 4. New York: Elsevier Science Publishers; 1986:161–84.
101. Beachey EH. Bacterial adherence: adhesion-receptor interactions mediating the attachment of bacteria to mucosal surfaces. J Infect Dis. 1981;143:325–45.
102. Beachey EH, Ofek I: Epithelial cell binding of group A streptococci by lipoteichoic acid on fimbriae denuded of M protein. J Exp Med. 1976;143:759–71.
103. Densen P, Mandell GL. Gonococcal interactions with polymorphonuclear neutrophils. Importance of the phagosome for bactericidal activity. J Clin Invest. 1978;62:1161–71.
104. Levine, MM. Escherichia coli that cause diarrhea: Enterotoxigenic, enteropathogenic, enteroinvasive, enterohemorrhagic and enteroadherent. J Infect Dis. 1987;155:377–88.
105. O'Hanley P, Low D, Romero I, et al. Gal-Gal binding and hemolysin phenotypes and genotypes associated with uropathogenic escherichia coli. N Engl J Med. 1985;313:414–20.
106. Abraham SN, Beachey EH. Host defenses against adhesion of bacteria to mucosal surfaces. In: Gallin JI, Fauci AS, eds. Advances in Host Defense Mechanisms. Vol. 4, New York: Raven Press; 1985:63–88.
107. Williams RC, Gibbons RJ. Inhibition of bacterial adherence by secretory immunoglobulin A: Mechanism of antigen disposal. Science. 1972;177: 697–9.
108. Tramont EC. Inhibition of adherence of *Neisseria gonorrhoeae* by human genital secretions. J Clin Invest. 1977;59:117–24.
109. Kilian M, Mesteoky J, Russell MW. Defense mechanisms involving Fc-dependent functions of immunoglobulin A and their subversion by bacterial immunoglobulin A proteases. Microbiol Rev. 1988;52:296–303.
110. Dimmock NJ. Mechanisms of neutralization of animal viruses. J Gen Virol. 1984;65:1015–22.
111. Daniels CA. Neutralization of sensitized virus by purified components of complement. Proc Natl Acad Sci USA. 1970;65:528–35.
112. Nemerow GR, Jensen FC, Cooper NR. Neutralization of Epstein-Barr virus by nonimmune human serum. J Clin Invest. 1982;70:1081–91.
113. Beebe DP, Schrieber RD, Cooper NR. Neutralization of influenza virus by normal human sera: mechanisms involving antibody and complement. J Immunol. 1983;130:1317–27.
114. Svehag S. Formation and dissociation of virus-antibody complexes with special reference to the neutralization process. Prog Med Virol. 1968;10:1–11.
115. Sissons JGP, Oldstone MBA. Killing of virus infected cells by cytotoxic lymphocytes. J Infect Dis. 1980;142:114–9.
116. Shore SL, Melewicz FM, Gordon DS. The mononculear cell in human blood which mediates antibody-dependent cellular cytotoxicity to virus-infected target cells. I. Identification of the population of effector cells. J Immunol. 1977;118:558–66.
117. Kohl SS, Starr SE, Oleske JM, et al. Human monocyte-macrophage-mediated antibody-dependent cytotoxicity to herpes simplex virus-infected cells. J Immunol. 1977;118:729–35.
118. Clark RA, Klebanoff SJ. Studies on the mechanism of antibody-dependent polymorphonuclear leukocyte-mediated cytotoxicity. J Immunol. 1977; 119:1413–8.
119. Tschopp J, Masson D, Stanley KK. Structural/functional similarity between proteins involved in complement- and cytotoxic T-lymphocyte-mediated cytolysis. Nature. 1986;322:831–4.
120. Podack ER. Molecular mechanisms of cytolysis by complement and by cytolytic lymphocytes. J Cell Biochem. 1986;30:133–70.

121. Ochs HD, Ament ME, Davis ID. Giardiasis with malabsorption in X-linked agammaglobulinemia. N Engl J Med. 1972;287:341–2.
122. Burke BA, Good RA. *Pneumocystis carinii* infection. Medicine. 1973;52:23.
123. Olgilvie BM. Immunity to parasites (helminths and arthropods). Prog Immunol. 1974;2:127–37.
124. Hsu SYL, Hsu HF, Isacson P, et al. In vitro schistomulicidal effect of immune serum and eosinophils, neutrophils and lymphocytes. J Reticuloendothel Soc. 1977;21:153–9.
125. Sher A, Butterworth AE, Colley DG, et al. Immune responses during human schistosomiasis mansoni. II. Occurrence of eosinophil-dependent cytotoxic antibodies in relation to intensity and duration of infection. Am J Trop Med Hyg. 1977;26:909–15.
126. Ottesen EA, Stanley AM, Gelfand JA, et al. Immunoglobulin and complement receptors on human eosinophils and their role in cellular adherence to schistosomules. Am J Trop Med Hyg. 1977;26:135–41.
127. Vadas MA, Butterworth AE, Sherry B, et al. Interactions between human eosinophils and schistosomula of *Schistosoma mansoni*. I. Stable and irreversible antibody-dependent adherence. J Immunol. 1980;124:1441–8.
128. Capron A, Dessaint JP, Capron M. Specific IgE antibodies in immune adherence of normal macrophages to *Schistosoma mansoni* schistosomules. Nature. 1975;253:474–5.
129. Rothwell TLW, Dineen JK, Love RJ. The role of pharmacologically active amines in resistance to *Trichostrongulus colubriformis* in the guinea pig. Immunology. 1971;21:925–32.
130. Murray M, Jarrett WFH, Jennings FW. Mast cells and macromolecular leak in intestinal immunological reactions. Immunology. 1971;21:17–21.
131. Tonegawa S. Somatic generation of antibody diversity. Nature. 1983; 302:575–81.
132. Milstein C. From antibody structure to immunological diversification of immune response. Science. 1986;231:1261–8.
133. Korsmeyer SJ, Waldmann TA. Immunoglobulins II: Gene organization and assembly. In: Stites DP, Stobo JD, Wells JV, eds. Los Altos, CA: Appleton & Lange; 1987.
134. Marrack P, Kappler J. The T cell receptor. Science. 1987;238:1073–9.
135. Williams AF. A year in the life of the immunoglobulin superfamily. Immunol Today. 1987;8:298–302.
136. Yuan D, Gilliam AC, Tucker PW. Regulation of expression of immunoglobulins M and D in murine B cells. Fed Proc. 1985;44:2652–9.
137. McCune M, Fu SM, Kunkel HG, et al. Biogenesis of membrane-bound and secreted immunoglobulins: two primary translation products of the human chain, differentially N-glycosylated to four discrete forms *in vivo* and *in vitro*. Proc Natl Acad Sci USA. 1981;78:5127–31.
138. Griffith GM, Berek C, Kaartinen M, et al. Somatic mutation and the maturation of immune response to 2-phenyl oxazolone. Nature. 1984;312: 271–5.
139. Siekevitz M, Kocks C, Rajewsky K, et al. Analysis of somatic mutation and class switching in naive and memory B cells generating adaptive primary and secondary responses. Cell. 1987;48:757–70.
140. Fu SM, Kunkel HG. Membrane immunoglobulin of B lymphocytes. J Exp Med. 1974;140:895–903.
141. Raff MC, Feldmann M, DePetris S. Monospecificity of B lymphocytes. J Exp Med. 1973;137:1024–30.
142. Cooper MD. B lymphocytes: normal development and function. N Engl J Med. 1987;317:1452–6.
143. Cooper MD, Kearney J, Scher I. B lymphocytes. In: Paul WE, ed. Fundamental Immunology. New York: Raven Press; 1984:43–55.
144. Stobo JD. Lymphocytes. In: Stites DP, Stobo JD, Wells JV, eds. Basic and Clinical Immunology. 6th ed. Los Altos, CA: Appleton & Lane; 1987.
145. Royer HD, Reinherz EL. T lymphocytes: ontogeny, function, and relevance to clinical disorders. N Engl J Med. 1987;317:1136–42.
146. Haynes BF. Human T lymphocyte antigens as defined by monoclonal antibodies. Immunol Rev. 1981;57:127–58.
147. Reinherz EL, Schlossman SF. Regulation of the immune response: inducer and suppressor T-lymphocyte subsets in human beings. N Engl J Med. 1980;303:370–4.
148. Lynch RG. Immunoglobulin-specific suppressor T cells. Adv Immunol. 1987;40:135–51.
149. Shevach EM. Macrophages and other accessory cells. In: Paul WE, eds. Fundamental Immunology. New York: Raven Press; 1984.
150. Unanue ER, Allen PM. The basis for the immunoregulatory role of macrophages and other accessory cells. Science. 236:551–7.
151. Shackleford AA, Kaufman JF, Korman AJ, et al. HLA-DR antigens: structure, separation of subpopulations, gene cloning and function. Immunol Rev. 1982;66:133–52.
152. Dinarello CA. Interleukin-1 and the pathogenesis of the acute-phase response. N Engl J Med. 311:1413–8.
153. O'Garra A, Umland S, DeFrance T, et al. B-cell factors are pleiotropic. Immunol Today. 1988;9:45–54.
154. Kishimoto T. B-cell stimulatory factors (BSFs): molecular structure, biological function, and regulation of expression. J Clin Immunol. 1987;7:343–55.
155. Chestnut RW, Grey HM. Antigen presentation by B cells and its significance in T-B interactions. Adv Immunol. 1986;39:51–95.
156. Hunt P, Robertson D, Weiss D, et al. A single bone marrow-derived stromal cell type supports the in vitro growth of early lymphoid and myeloid cells. Cell. 1987;48:997–1007.
157. Ross GP, Polley MJ, Rabellino EM, et al. Two different complement receptors on human lymphocytes. J Exp Med. 1973;138:798–818.
158. Fingeroth JD, Weiss JJ, Tedder TF, et al. Epstein-Barr virus receptor of human B lymphocytes is the C3d receptor CR2. Proc Natl Acad Sci USA. 1984;81:4510–4.
159. Melchers F, Erdei A, Schulz T. Growth control of activated, synchronized murine B cells by the C3d fragment of human complement. Nature. 1985;317:264–7.
160. Casali P, Burastero E, Nakamura M, et al. Human lymphocytes making rheumatoid factor and antibody to ssDNA belong to Leu-1 + B-cell subset. Science. 1987;236:77–80.
161. DeFranco AL. Molecular aspects of B-lymphocyte activation. Annu Rev Cell Biol. 1987;3:143–78.
162. Maruyama S, Kubagawa H, Cooper MD. Activation of human B cells and inhibition of their terminal differentiation by monoclonal anti-antibodies. J Immunol. 1985;135:192–6.
163. Mingari MC, Gerosa F, Carra G, et al. Human interleukin-2 promotes proliferation of activated B cells via surface receptors similar to those of activated T cells. Nature. 1984;312:641–3.
164. Park LS, Friend D, Sassenfeld HM. Characterization of the human B cell stimulatory factor 1 receptor. J Exp Med. 1987;166:476–88.
165. Taga T, Kawanishi Y, Hardy RR, et al. Receptors for B cell stimulatory factor 2: quantification, specificity, distribution, and regulation of their expression. J Exp Med. 1987;166:967–81.
166. Feldmann M, Basten A, Phil D. The relationship between antigenic structure and the requirement for thymus-derived cells in the immune response. J Exp Med. 1971;134:103–19.
167. Yount WJ, Dorner MM, Kunkel HG, et al. Studies on human antibodies: selective variations in subgroup composition and genetic markers. J Exp Med. 1968;127:633–46.
168. Riesen WF, Skvaril F, Braun DG. Natural infection of man with group A streptococci. Levels; Restriction in class, subclass, and type; and clonal appearance of polysaccharide group-specific antibodies. Scand J Immunol. 1976;5:383–90.
169. Makela O, Mattila P, Rautonen N, et al. Isotype concentrations of human antibodies to *Haemophilus influenzae* type b polysaccharide (Hib) in young adults immunized with the polysaccharide as such or conjugated to a protein (diphtheria) toxoid. J Immunol. 1987;139:1999–2004.
170. Abbas AK. A reassessment of the mechanisms of antigen-specific T-cell dependent B-cell activation. Immunol Today. 1988;9:89–91.
171. Jones B. Cooperation between T and B cells. A minimal model. Immunol Rev. 1987;99:5–18.
172. Sanders VM, Snyder JM, Uhr JW, et al. Characterization of the physical interaction between antigen-specific B and T cells. J Immunol. 1986; 137:2395–404.
173. Fischer A, Durandy A, Sterkers G. Role of the LFA-1 molecule in cellular interactions required for antibody production in humans. J Immunol. 1986;136:3198–203.
174. Mitchison NA. The carrier effect in the secondary response to hapten-carrier conjugates. II. Cellular cooperation. Eur J Immunol. 1971;1:18–26.
175. DeFranco AL, Gold MR, Jakway JP. B-lymphocyte signal transduction in response to anti-immunoglobulin and bacterial lipopolysaccharide. Immunol Rev. 1987;95:161–76.
176. Coffman RL, Ohara J, Bond MW, et al. B cell stimulatory factor-1 enhances the IgE response of lipopolysaccharide-activated B cells. J Immunol. 1986;136:4538–41.
177. Finkelman FD, Katona IM, Urban JF, et al. Suppression of *in vivo* polyclonal IgE responses by monoclonal antibody to the lymphokine B-cell stimulatory factor 1. Proc Natl Acad Sci USA. 1986;83:9675–8.
178. Snapper CM, Paul WE. Interferon-γ and B cell stimulatory factor-1 reciprocally regulate Ig isotype production. Science. 1987;236:944–7.
179. Coffman RL, Shrader B, Carty J, et al. A mouse T cell product that preferentially enhances IgA production. I. Biologic characterization. J Immunol. 1987;139:3685–90.
180. Harriman GR, Strober W. Commentary: Interleukin 5, a mucosal lymphokine? J Immunol. 1987;139:3553–5.
181. Murray PD, McKenzie DT, Swain SL, et al. Interleukin 5 and interleukin 4 produced by Peyer's patch T cells selectively enhance immunoglobulin A expression. J Immunol. 1987;139:2669–74.
182. Siskind GW. Immunologic tolerance. In: Paul WE, ed. Fundamental Immunology. New York: Raven Press; 1984:537–58.
183. Schaper HW, Pierre CW, Aune TM. Identification and initial characterization of concanavalin A- and interferon-induced human suppressor factors: evidence for a human equivalent of murine soluble immune response suppressor (SIRS). J Immunol. 1984;132:2429–34.
184. Burdette S, Schwartz RS. Current concepts: immunology. Idiotypes and idiotypic networks. N Engl J Med. 1987;317:219–24.
185. McNamara MK, Ward RE, Kohler H. Monoclonal idiotype vaccine against *Streptococcus pneumoniae* infection. Science. 1984;226:1325–6.
186. Kennedy RC, Melnick SL, Preesman GR. Antibody to hepatitis B virus induced by injecting antibodies to the idiotype. Science. 1984;223:930–1.
187. McIntosh K. Diagnostic virology. In: Fields BN, et al., eds. Virology 1985. New York: Raven Press; 1985:309–22.
188. Ritzmann SE. Pathology of Immunoglobulins: Diagnostic and Clinical Aspects. New York: Alan R. Liss; 1982:1–10.
189. Bach A. Immunologic manifestations. In: Sande MA, Kaye D, Root RK, eds. Endocarditis. New York: Churchill Livingstone; 1984:33–58.

190. Phair JP, Clarke J. Immunology of infective endocarditis. Prog Cardiovasc Dis. 1979;22:137–44.
191. Turner KS, Feddema L, Quinn EH. Nonspecific potentiation of IgE by parasitic infections in man. Int Arch Allergy Appl Immunol. 1979;58:232–6.
192. Rosen A, Gergely P, Jondal M, et al. Polyclonal Ig production after Epstein-Barr virus infection of human lymphocytes *in vitro*. Nature. 1977;267:52–5.
193. Theofilopoulos AN, Dixon FJ. The biology and detection of immune complexes. Adv Immunol. 1979;28:89–220.
194. Hoiby N, Doring G, Schiotz. The role of immune complexes in the pathogenesis of bacterial infections. Annu Rev Microbiol. 1986;40:29–53.
195. Arnend WP, Joslin FG, Massoni RJ. Effects of immune complexes on production by human monocytes of interleukin 1 or an interleukin 1 inhibitor. J Immunol. 1985;134:3868–75.
196. Couser WG. Mechanisms of glomerular injury in immune-complex disease. Kidney Int. 1985;28:569–83.
197. Gocke DJ. Extrahepatic manifestations of viral hepatitis. Am J Med Sci. 1975;270:49–60.
198. Carson DA, Chen PP, Fox RI, et al. Rheumatoid factor and immune networks. Annu Rev Immunol. 1987;5:109–26.
199. Coulie PG, Van Snick J. Rheumatoid factor (RF) production during anamnestic immune responses in the mouse. III. Activation of RF precursor cells is induced by their interaction with immune complexes and carrier-specific helper T cells. J Exp Med. 1985;161:88–97.
200. Radoux V, Chen PP, Sorge JA, et al. A conserved human germline V gene directly encodes rheumatoid factor light chains. J Exp Med. 1986;164:2119–24.
201. Clarkson AB, Mellow GH. Rheumatoid factor-like immunoglobulin M protects previously uninfected rat pups and dams from *Trypanosoma lewisi*. Science. 1981;214:186–8.
202. Levo Y, Gorevic PD, Kassal HJ, et al. Association between hepatitis B virus and essential mixed cryoglobulinemia. N Engl J Med. 1977;296:1501–3.
203. Oldstone MBA, Molecular mimicry and autoimmune disease. Cell. 1987;50:819–20.
204. Dale JB, Beachey EH. Multiple, heart-cross-reactive epitopes of streptococcal M proteins. J Exp Med. 1985;161:113–23.
205. Schwimmbeck PL, Yu DTY, Oldstone MBA. Autoantibodies to HLA B27 in the sera of HLA B27 patients with ankylosing spondylitis and Reiter's syndrome: Molecular mimicry with *Klebsiella pneumoniae* as potential mechanism of autoimmune disease. J Exp Med. 1987;166:173–81.
206. Srinvasappa J, Saegusa J, Prabhakar BS, et al. Molecular mimicry: frequency of reactivity of monoclonal antiviral antibodies with normal tissues. J Virol. 1986;57:397–401.
207. WHO Scientific Group on Immunodeficiency. Primary immunodeficiency diseases: report of a world health organization scientific group. Clin Immunol Immunopathol. 1986;40:166–96.
208. Rosen FS, Cooper MD, Wedgwood RJP. Medical progress: the primary immunodeficiencies. N Engl J Med. 1984;311:235–42, 300–10.
209. Ammann AJ. Immunodeficiency Diseases. In: Stites DP, Stobo JD, Wells JV, eds. Basic and Clinical Immunology. 6th ed. 1987:317–55.
210. Hermans PE, Diaz-Buxo JA, Stobo JD. Idiopathic late onset immunoglobulin deficiency. Clinical observations in 50 patients. Am J Med. 1976;61:221–32.
211. Davis LE, Bodian D, Price D, et al. Chronic progressive poliomyelitis secondary to vaccination of an immunodeficient child. N Engl J. Med. 1977; 297:241–5.
212. Wilfert CM, Buckley RH, Mohanakumar T, et al. Persistent and fatal central nervous system echo virus infections in patients with agammaglobulinemia. N Engl J Med. 1977;296:1485–9.
213. Saulsbury FT, Winkelstein JA, Yolken RH. Chronic rotavirus infection in immunodeficiency. Pediatrics. 1980;97:61–5.
214. Ament ME, Ochs HD, Davis SD. Structure and function of the gastrointestinal tract in primary immunodeficiency syndromes. Medicine. 1973; 52:227–48.
215. Bruton OC. Agammaglobulinemia. Pediatrics. 1952;9:722–30.
216. Fearon ER, Winkelstein JA, Civin CI, et al. Carrier detection in X-linked agammaglobulinemia by analysis of X-chromosome inactivation. N Engl J Med. 1987;316:427–31.
217. Schwaber J, Molgaard H, Orkin SH, et al. Early pre-B cells from normal and X-linked agammaglobulinaemia produce C without an attached V region. Nature. 1983;304:355–7.
218. Gail-Pezcalskak Lim JD, Good RA. B lymphocytes in primary and secondary deficiencies of humoral immunity. Birth Defects. 1975;11:33.
219. Lederman HM, Winkelstein JA. X-linked agammaglobulinemia: an analysis of 96 patients. Medicine. 1985;64:145–56.
220. Crennan JM, Van Scoy RE, McKenna CH, et al. Echovirus polymyositis in patients with hypogammaglobulinemia: failure of high-dose intravenous gammaglobulin therapy and review of the literature. Am J Med. 1986;81:35–42.
221. McKinney RE, Katz SL, Wilfert CM. Chronic enteroviral meningoencephalitis in agammaglobulinemic patients. Rev Infect Dis. 1987;9:334–56.
222. Roifman CM, Rao CP, Lederman HM, et al. Increased susceptibility to mycoplasma infection in patients with hypogammaglobulinemia. Am J Med. 1986;80:590–4.
223. Taylor-Robinson D, Furr PM, Webster AD. *Ureaplasma urealyticum* in the immunocompromised host. Pediatr Infect Dis 1986;5:236–8.
224. Reinherz EL, Cooper MD, Schlossman SF, et al. Abnormalities of T cell maturation and regulation in human beings with immunodeficiency disorders. J Clin Invest. 1981;68:699–705.
225. Fleisher TA, White RM, Broder S, et al. X-linked hypogammaglobulinemia and isolated growth hormone deficiency. N Engl J Med. 1980;302:1492–34.
226. Stiehm RE, Ashida E, Kim KS, et al. Intravenous immunoglobulins as therapeutic agents. Ann Intern Med. 1987;107:367–82.
227. Wedgwood RJ. Intravenous immunoglobulin. Clin Immunol Immunopathol. 1986;40:147–50.
228. Roifman CM, Levison H, Gelfand EW. High-dose versus low-dose intravenous immunoglobulin in hypogammaglobulinaemia and chronic lung disease. Lancet. 1987;I:1075–7.
229. Lederman HM, Roifman CH, Lari S, et al. Corticosteroids for prevention of adverse reactions to intravenous immune serum globulin infusions in hypogammaglobulinemic patients. Am J Med. 1986;81:443–7.
230. Tiller TL, Buckley RH. Transient hypogammaglobulinemia of infancy: review of the literature, clinical and immunologic features of 11 new cases, and long-term follow-up. J Pedatr. 1978;92:347–53.
231. Wilson CB, Remington JS. Effects of monocytes from human neonates on lymphocyte transformation. Clin Exp Immunol. 1979;36:511–6.
232. Ferguson AC, Cheung SSC. Modulation of immunoglobulin M and G synthesis by monocytes and T lymphocytes in the newborn infant. J Pediatr. 1981;98:385–95.
233. Siegel RL, Issekutz T, Schwaber J, et al. Deficiency of T helper cells in transient hypogammaglobulinemia of infancy. N Engl J Med. 1981;305:1307–13.
234. Rodriquez MA, Bankhurst AD, Cueppens JL, et al. Characterization of the suppressor activity in human cord blood lymphocytes. J Clin Invest. 1981;68:1577–85.
235. Good RA, Zak SJ, Condie RM, et al. Clinical investigation of patients with agammaglobulinemia and hypogammaglobulinemia. Pediatr Clin North Am. 1960;7:397–416.
236. Buckley RH. Humoral immunodeficiency. Clin Immunol Immunopathol. 1986;40:13–24.
237. Geha RS, Schneeberger E, Merter E, et al. Heterogeneity of "acquired" or common variable agammaglobulinemia. N Engl J Med. 1974;291:1–6.
238. Waldmann TA, Durm M, Broder S, et al. Role of suppressor T cells in pathogenesis of common variable hypogammaglobulinaemia. Lancet. 1974;2:609.
239. Reinharz EL, Geha R, Wohl ME, et al. Immunodeficiency associated with loss of T4+ inducer-T cell function. N Engl J Med. 1981;304:811–6.
240. White WB, Ballow M. Modulation of suppressor-cell activity by cimetidine in patients with common variable hypogammaglobulinemia. N Engl J Med. 1985;312:198–202.
241. Stiehm ER, Fudenberg HH. Clinical and immunologic features of dysgammaglobulinemia type I. Am J Med. 1966;40:805–17.
242. Mayer L, Kwan SP, Thompson C, et al. Evidence for a defect in "switch" T cells in patients with immunodeficiency and hyperimmunoglobulinemia M. N Engl J Med. 1986;314:409–13.
243. Burks AW, Steele RW. Selective IgA deficiency. Ann Allergy. 1986;57:3–8.
244. Vanthiel DH, Smith WI Jr., Rabin BS, et al. A syndrome of immunoglobulin A deficiency, diabetes mellitus, malabsorption, a common HLA haplotype. Immunologic and genetic studies of forty-three family members. Ann Intern Med. 1977;86:10–4.
245. Ammann AJ, Hong R. Selective IgA deficiency: presentation of 30 cases and a review of the literature. Medicine. 1971;50:223–36.
246. Walker WA, Isselbacher KJ, Block KJ. Intestinal uptake of macromolecules: effect of oral immunization. Science. 1972;177:608–10.
247. Oxelius VA, Laurell AB, Lindquist B, et al. IgG subclasses in selective IgA deficiency. Importance of IgG_2-IgA deficiency. N Engl J Med. 1981; 304:1476–7.
248. Bjorkander J, Bake B, Oxelius VA, et al. Impaired lung function in patients with IgA deficiency and low levels of IgG2 or IgG3. N Engl J Med. 1985;313:720–4.
249. Migane N, Oliviero S, DeLange G, et al. Multiple-gene deletions within the human immunoglobulin heavy chain cluster. Proc Natl Acad Sci USA. 1984;81:5811–5.
250. Carbonara AO, Demarchi M. Genetics and techniques: Ig isotypes deficiency caused by gene deletions. Monogr Allergy. 1986;20:13–7.
251. Burks AW, Sampson HA, Buckley RH. Anaphylactic reactions after gammaglobulin administration in patients with hypogammaglobulinemia: detection of IgE antibodies to IgA. N Engl J Med. 1986;314:560–3.
252. Hobbs JR, Milner RDG, Watt PJ. Gamma-M deficiency predisposing to meningoccal septicemia. Br Med J. 1967;2:583–5.
253. Schur PH, Borel H, Gelfand EW, et al. Selective gamma-G globulin deficiencies in patients with recurrent pyogenic infections. N Engl J Med. 1970;283:631–4.
254. Ochs HD, Wedgwood RJ. IgG subclass deficiencies. Annu Rev Med. 1987; 38:325–40.
255. Umetsu DT, Ambrosino DM, Quinti I, et al. Recurrent sinopulmonary infection and impaired antibody response to bacterial capsular polysaccharide antigen in children with selective IgG-subclass deficiency. N Engl J Med. 1985;313:1247–51.
256. Pahwa RN, Pahwa SG, Good RA. T-lymphocyte differentiation in severe combined immunodeficiency: defects of stem cells. J Clin Invest. 1979; 64:1632–41.

257. Good RA, Bach FH. Bone marrow and thymus transplants: cellular engineering to correct primary immunodeficiency. Clin Immunobiol. 1974;2:63.
258. Hirschhorn R. Inherited enzyme deficiencies and immunodeficiency: adenosine deaminase (ADA) and purine nucleoside phosphorylase (PNP) deficiencies. Clin Immunol Immunopathol. 1986;40:157–65.
259. Polmar SH, Stem RC, Schwartz AL, et al. Enzyme replacement therapy for adenosine deaminase deficiency and severe combined immunodeficiency. N Engl J Med. 1976;295:1337–43.
260. Gatti RA, Allen HD, Meuwissen HJ, et al. Immunological reconstitution of sex-linked lymphopenic immunological deficiency. Lancet. 1968;2:1366–9.
261. Stoop JW, Zegers BJ, Hendrix GF, et al. Purine nucleoside phosphorylase deficiency associated with selective cellular immune deficiency. N Engl J Med. 1977;296:651–5.
262. Lawlor GJ Jr, Amman AJ, Wright WC Jr. The syndrome of cellular immunodeficiency with immunoglobulins. J Pediatr. 1974;84:183–7.
263. Remold-O'Donnell E, Davis AE, Kenney D, et al. Purification and chemical composition of gpL115, the human lymphocyte surface sialoglycoprotein that is defective in Wiskott-Aldrich syndrome. J Biol Chem. 1986;261:7526–30.
264. Cooper MD, Chase HP, Lowman JT, et al. Wiskott-Aldrich syndrome: an immunologic disease involving the afferent limb of immunity. Am J Med. 1968;44:499–506.
265. Blaese RM, Strober W, Brown RS, et al. Wiskott-Aldrich syndrome. Lancet. 1968;1:1056–7.
266. Parkman R, Rappeport J, Geha R, et al. Correction of the Wiskott-Aldrich syndrome by bone-marrow transplantation. N Engl J Med. 1978;298:291–8.
267. Biggar WD, Good RA. Immunodeficiency in ataxia-telangiectasia. Birth Defects. 1975;11:271–7.
268. Berkel AI. Studies of IgG subclasses in ataxia-telangiectasia patients. Monogr Allergy. 1986;20:100–5.
269. Davis MM, Gatti RA, Sparkes RS. Neoplasia and chromosomal breakage in ataxia-telangiectasia: a 2-14 translocation. In: Gatti RA, Swift M, eds. Ataxia-Telangiectasia: Genetics, Neuropathology, and Immunology of a Degenerative Disease of Childhood. New York: Alan R Liss; 1985:197–203.
270. McKinnon PJ. Ataxia-telangiectasia: an inherited disorder of ionizing-radiation sensitivity in man. Hum Genet. 1987;75:197–207.
271. Oxelius VA, Berkel AI, Hanson LA. IgG2 deficiency in ataxia-telangiectasia. N Engl J Med. 1982;306:515–7.
272. Donabedian H, Gallin JI. The hyperimmunoglobulin E recurrent infection (Job's) syndrome. A review of the NIH experience and the literature. Medicine. 1983;62:195–212.
273. Levine AS, Graw RG Jr, Young RC. Management of infections in patients with leukemia and lymphoma: current concepts and experimental approaches. Semin Hematol. 1972;9:141–26.
274. Miller DG. Patterns of immunologic deficiency in lymphomas and leukemias. Ann Intern Med. 1972;57:703–6.
275. Weitzman SA, Aisenberg AC, Siber GR, et al. Impaired humoral immunity in treated Hodgkin's disease. N Engl J Med. 1977;297:245–8.
275a. Cooperative group for the study of immunoglobulin in chronic lymphocytic leukemia. Intravenous immunoglobulin for the prevention of infection in chronic lymphocytic leukemia. N Engl J Med. 1988;319:902–7.
276. Louie S, Schwartz RS. Immunodeficiency and the pathogenesis of lymphoma and leukemia. Semin Hematol. 1978;15:117–28.
277. Bergsagel DE. Lymphoreticular disorders—malignant proliferative response and/or abnormal immunoglobulin synthesis—plasma cell dyscrasias. In Williams WJ, et al, eds. Hematology. 2nd ed. New York: McGraw-Hill; 1977 :1087.
278. Paglieroni T, MacKenzie MR. Studies on the pathogenesis of an immune defect in multiple myeloma. J Clin Invest. 1977;59:1120–33.
279. Glenchur H, Zinneman HH, Hall WH. A review of fifty-one cases of multiple myeloma: emphasis on pneumonia and other infections as complications. Arch Intern Med. 1959;103:173–9.
280. Myers BR, Hirshman SZ, Azelrod JA. Current patterns of infection in multiple myeloma. Am J Med. 1972;52:87–97.
281. Salmon SE, Samal BA, Hayes D, et al. Role of gammaglobulin for immunoprophylaxis in multiple myelona. N Engl J Med. 1968;277:1336–40.
282. Bjornson AB, Altemeier WA, Bjornson HS. Changes in humoral components of host defense following burn trauma. Ann Surg. 1977;186:88–96.
283. Wilfert CM, Katz SL. Etiology of bacterial sepsis in nephrotic children, 1963–1967. Pediatrics. 1968;42:840–59.
284. Lockwood CM. Immunological functions of the spleen. Clin Haematol. 1983;12:449–65.
285. Bohnsack JF, Brown EJ. The role of the spleen in resistance to infection. Annu Rev Med. 1986;37:49–59.
286. Rosner F, Zarrabi MH, Benach JL, et al. Babesiosis in splenectomized adults: review of 22 reported cases. Am J Med. 1984;76:696–702.
287. Brown EJ, Hosea SW, Frank MM. The role of complement in the localization of pneumococci in the splanchnic reticuloendothelial system during experimental bacteremia. J Immunol. 1981;126:2230–6.
288. Likhite VV. Immunological impairment and susceptibility to infection after splenectomy. JAMA. 1976;236:1376.
289. Martone WJ, Zuehl RW, Minson GE. Postsplenectomy sepsis with DF-2: report of a case with isolation of the organism from the patient's dog. Ann Intern Med. 1980;93:457–8.
290. Eraklis AJ, Kevy SV, Diamond LK, et al. Hazard of overwhelming infection after splenectomy in childhood. N Engl J Med. 1967;276:1225–9.
291. Chilcote RR, Baehner RL, Hammond D, et al. Septicemia and meningitis in children splenectomized for Hodgkin's disease. N Engl J Med. 1976; 295:802.
292. Bisno AL, Gopol V. Fulminant pneumococcal infection in "normal" asplenic hosts. Arch Intern Med. 1977;137:1526–32.
293. Pearson HA, Spencer RP, Cornelius EA. Functional asplenia in sickle-cell anemia. N Engl J Med. 1969;281:923–7.
294. Bjornson AB, Lobel JS. Direct evidence that decreased serum opsonization of *Streptococcus pneumoniae* via the alternative complement pathway in sickle cell disease is related to antibody deficiency. J Clin Invest. 1987;79:388–98.
295. Spirer Z, Zakuth V, Diamant S, et al. Decreased tuftsin concentrations in patients who have undergone splenectomy. Br Med J. 1977;2:1574–6.
296. Brown EJ, Hosea SW, Frank MM. The role of the spleen in experimental pneumococcal bacteremia. J Clin Invest. 1981;67:975–82.
297. Hosea SE, Brown EJ, Hamburger MI, et al. Opsonic requirements for intravascular clearance after splenectomy. N Engl J Med. 1981;304–245.
298. Siber GR, Weitzman SA, Aisenberg CA, et al. Impaired antibody response to pneumococcal vaccine after treatment for Hodgkin's disease. N Engl J Med. 1978;299:442–8.
299. Amman AJ, Addiego J, Wara DW, et al. Polyvalent pneumococcal-polysaccharide immunization of patients with sickle-cell anemia and patients with splenectomy. N Engl J Med. 1977;297:897–900.
300. Ruben FL, Hankins WA, Zeigler Z, et al. Antibody responses to meningococcal polysaccharide vaccine in adults without a spleen. Am J Med. 1984;76:115–21.
301. Giebink GS, Foker JE, Kim Y, et al. Serum antibody and opsonic responses to vaccination with pneumococcal polysaccharide in normal and splenectomized children. J Infect Dis. 1980;141:404–12.
302. Gaston MH, Verter JI, Woods G, et al. Prophylaxis with oral penicillin in children with sickle cell anemia: a randomized trial. N Engl J Med. 1986;314:1593–9.
303. Alexander JW. Immunologic considerations and the role of vaccination in burn injury. In Polk HC, Stone HH, eds. Contemporary Burn Management. Boston: Little, Brown; 1971:265.
304. Strober W, Wochner RD, Carbone PP, et al. Intestinal lymphangiectasia: a protein-losing enteropathy with hypogammaglobulinemia, lymphocytopenia, and impaired homograft rejection. J Clin Invest. 1967;46:1643–56.
305. Heppner GH, Calabresi P. Selective suppression of humoral immunity by antineoplastic drugs. Annu Rev Pharmacol Toxicol. 1976;16:367.
306. Stewart CC, Perez CA. Effect of irradiation on immune responses. Radiology. 1976;118:201–11.
307. Order SE. The effects of therapeutic irradiation on lymphocytes and immunity. Cancer. 1977;39:737–45.
308. Webb DR, Winkelstein A. Immunosuppression, immunopotentiation, and antiinflammatory drugs. In Stites DP, Stobo JD, Wells JV, eds. Basic and Clinical Immunology. 4th ed. Los Altos, CA: Appleton & Lange, 1982:277.
309. Fauci AS, Dale DC, Balow JE. Glucocorticosteroid therapy: mechanisms of action and clinical considerations. Ann Intern Med. 1976;84:304–15.
310. Haynes BF, Fauci AS. The differential effect of in vivo hydrocortisone on the kinetics of subpopulations of human peripheral blood thymus-derived lymphocytes. J Clin Invest. 1978;61:703–10.
311. Arya SK, Wong-Staal F, Gallo RC. Dexamethasone-mediated inhibition of human T cell growth factor and interferon messenger RNA. J Immunol. 1984;133:273–6.
312. Snyder DS, Unanue ER. Corticosteroids inhibit murine macrophage Ia expression and interleukin 1 production. J Immunol. 1982;129:1803–5.
313. Dale DC, Fauci AS, Wolff SM. Alternate day prednisone: leukocyte kinetics and susceptibility to infections. N Engl J Med. 1974;291:1154–8.
314. Anderson RJ, Schafer LA, Olin DB, et al. Infectious risk factors in the immunosuppressed host. Am J Med. 1973;54:453–62.
315. Staples PJ, Gerding DN, Decker JL, et al. Incidence of infection in systemic lupus erythematosus. Arthritis Rheum. 1974;17:1–11.
316. Lane HC, Masur H, Edgar LC, et al. Abnormalities of B-cell activation and immunoregulation in patients with the acquired immunodeficiency syndrome. N Engl J Med. 1983;309:453–8.
317. Ammann AJ, Schiffman G, Abrams D, et al. B-cell immunodeficiency in acquired immune deficiency syndrome. JAMA. 1984;251:1447–9.
318. Pahwa SG, Quilop MTJ, Lange M. Defective B-lymphocyte function in homosexual men in relation to the acquired immunodeficiency syndrome. Ann Intern Med. 1984;101:757–63.
319. Polsky B, Gold JWM, Whimbey E, et al. Bacterial pneumonia in patients with acquired immunodeficiency syndrome. Ann Intern Med. 1986;104:38–41.
320. Buckley RH. Advances in the diagnosis and treatment of primary immunodeficiency diseases. Arch Intern Med. 1986;146:377–84.
321. Waldmann TA, Korsmeyer SJ, Bakhshi A, et al. Molecular genetic analysis of human lymphoid neoplasms. Immunoglobulin genes and the c-myc oncogene. Ann Intern Med. 1985;102:497–510.
322. Wells JV. Metabolism of immunoglobulins. In: Fudenberg HH, et al., eds. Basic and Clinical Immunology. 2nd ed. Los Altos, CA: Lange; 1978:237.
323. Stites DP, Stobo JD, Wells JV, eds. Basic and Clinical Immunology. 6th ed. Los Altos, CA: Appleton & Lange; 1987.
324. Waldmann TA, Korsmeyer SJ, Bakhshi A, et al. Molecular genetic analysis of human lymphoid neoplasms. Ann Intern Med. 1985;102:497–510.

6. COMPLEMENT

PETER DENSEN

Functional activity attributable to the complement system was first described in the period between 1888 and 1894.[1] These experiments demonstrated that fresh serum contained a heat-labile bactericidal factor termed *alexin*. Subsequently it was shown that a heat-stable factor present in convalescent serum also contributed to bactericidal activity. At the turn of the century Paul Erlich employed the term *complement* to describe the heat-labile factor and *amboceptor* (antibody) to describe the heat-stable factor. The early part of the nineteenth century saw the demonstration that complement consisted of more than one component. However, it was not until 1941 that Louis Pillemer was able to separate functionally distinct components of the classical pathway from various serum fractions. In the early 1950s Pillemer and coworkers also described and characterized an antibody-independent mechanism for activating complement that they termed the *properdin pathway*.[1–3] However, the protein purification techniques then available were unable to provide complement components of sufficient purity to convince others of the existence of this pathway. The 1960s and 1970s saw the development of a mathematical model capable of describing the sequential activation of complement as well as new techniques for the purification of the individual complement components. The latter development led to the rediscovery of Pillemer's work, and the characterization of these proteins and the mechanisms controlling the activity of this pathway. With the 1980's has come the recognition that the complement system consists not only of plasma proteins capable of being deposited upon the surface of invading microbes but also of membrane proteins that protect host cells from the detrimental effects of complement activation.

At the present time the complement system is known to consist of 19 plasma and at least 9 membrane proteins (Table 1). Activation of the system results in the sequential triggering of the various proteins and in this regard exhibits many similarities to the clotting cascade. The beneficial effects of complement activation for the host include the development of an inflammatory response and the elimination of microbial pathogens and immune complexes.

The antibody and complement systems are grouped together because of their historical and functional association as well as because they both occur as soluble proteins in serum.[4] However, a number of important differences distinguish the two systems. Antibody-mediated events are characterized by a high degree of specificity dictated by a given antibody for a given antigenic epitope. Consequently, after initial exposure to antigen there is a significant delay while protective antibody is synthesized to influence the course of the disease. In contrast, the complement system is activated by a wide variety of chemically diverse substances even in the absence of antibody. Consequently, the multiplicity of its physiologic effects is felt early in the course of infection. In many instances antibody and complement are synergistic in providing effective host defense. The presence of specific antibody leads to more rapid and efficient complement activation and serves to direct complement deposition to appropriate sites on the surface of invading pathogens. Opsonization of infectious agents with both antibody and complement leads to more efficient ingestion and killing of these microbes than does opsonization with either substance alone. Similarly, the presence of receptors on lymphocytes for immunoglobulin and complement suggest a cooperative role for these substances in both the affector and effector pathways of the immune response. "In such a way a highly specific response mediated by the tertiary structure of an antibody molecule can be coupled with the more general cellular or humoral responses of the phagocytic and complement system to eradicate attacking organisms."[4]

COMPLEMENT SYNTHESIS, CATABOLISM, AND DISTRIBUTION

Studies employing human hepatic cells in culture have demonstrated that most of the complement components can be synthesized by the liver.[5,6] Moreover, examination of complement component polymorphisms in patients before and after orthotopic liver transplantation has shown that hepatic synthesis accounts for at least 90 percent of the quantity of these components in plasma.[7] The normal concentration of many individual complement components may fluctuate widely in a given individual over time. In part this fluctuation reflects the fact that many components are acute-phase reactants, and their synthesis can be modulated by a variety of immune modulators. These substances, including interleukin-1β (IL-1β), tumor necrosis and dexamethasone, can increase hepatic synthesis of these components two- to fivefold.[8,9]

Complement synthesis has also been demonstrated in a variety of other cells, most notably monocytes and macrophages.[10] These cells synthesize C1q, C4, C2, factors D and B, C3, and C5.[6] Synthesis varies with the site of isolation of the cell. For example, bronchoalveolar fluid, breast milk, and monocyte-derived macrophages differ with respect to the proportion of the cells secreting C2, average rate of C2 production per cell, and the amount of C2-specific RNA.[11] Complement synthesis by monocytes can be modulated by γ-interferon and the lipid A component of endotoxin.[12,13] The exact mechanism by which complement synthesis is enhanced has not been delineated in most cases but appears to occur at a pretranslational level.[13] Other sites of complement component synthesis that have been demonstrated on an experimental basis include intestinal and uroepithelial cells and fibroblasts.[6]

Synthesis of the early components of both activating pathways of complement by mononuclear phagocyte cells is believed to be an important aspect of complement-mediated host defense in tissues. In vitro studies have demonstrated that these cells can synthesize sufficient amounts of these components to promote opsonization, ingestion, and killing of bacteria or other target cells with which they have been coincubated.[14]

A detailed examination of the metabolic fate of all complement components has not been carried out. However, studies have demonstrated fractional catabolic rates for C3, C4, C5, and factor B that range from 1 to 2 percent per hour, thus indicating that they are among the most rapidly metabolized of all plasma proteins. Catabolic rates of C3 and C4 are independent of serum levels, whereas their synthetic rates correlate with serum levels, which indicates that in healthy people the rate of synthesis is the major determinant of plasma concentration.[15]

In healthy individuals the vast majority of complement is found in blood. Concentrations of complement proteins in normal mucosal secretions are approximately 5–10 percent of serum levels and in normal spinal fluid even lower, perhaps 1 percent or less of serum levels. In the presence of local infection or inflammation complement levels in mucosal secretions and in cerebrospinal fluid increase, most likely as a result of alterations in vascular permeability barriers as well as by enhanced synthesis and secretion of these components by local mononuclear cells.

Serum complement activity is reduced in preterm infants in proportion to the magnitude of their immaturity.[16] In contrast, complement levels in healthy term infants range from 60 to 100 percent of those in healthy adults. Despite these nearly normal levels, defective complement activation via either the classical or alternative pathway has been noted in as many as 40 percent of such infants.[17–19]

TABLE 1. Complement Components Present in Serum

Component	*Approximate Serum Concentration (μg/ml)*	*Molecular Weight*	*Chain Structure*[a]	*Number of Genetic Loci*	*Chromosomal Assignment*[b]
Classical Pathway					
C1q	70	410,000	(A, B, C) × 6	3 (A, B, C)	1p
C1r	34	170,000	Dimer of 2 identical chains	1	12p
C1s	31	85,000	2 identical chains	1	12p
C4	600	206,000	β-α-γ	2 (C4A, C4B)	6p
C2	25	117,000	1 chain	1	6p
Alternative pathway					
D	1	24,000	1 chain	1	ND
C3	1300	195,000	β-α	1	19q
B	200	95,000	1 chain	1	6p
Membrane attack complex					
C5	80	180,000	β-α	1	9q
C6	60	128,000	1 chain	1	ND
C7	55	120,000	1 chain	1	ND
C8	65	150,000	3 nonidentical chains α---γ, β	3 (α, β, γ)	1p (γ-ND)
C9	60	79,000	1 chain	1	ND
Control proteins					
Positive regulation					
Properdin	25	220,000	Cyclic polymers of a single 57 kD chain	1	Xp
Negative regulation					
C1 INH	200	105,000	1 chain	1	11q
C4 BP	250	550,000	7 identical chains	1	1q
Factor H	500	150,000	1 chain	1	1q
Factor I	34	90,000	β-γ	1	4
Anaphylatoxin inactivator (carboxypeptidase B)	35	280,000	Dimer of 2 nonidentical chains (H, L) × 2	ND	ND
S protein (vitronectin)	500	80,000	1 chain	1	ND

[a] For multichain components parentheses are used to indicate subunit structure; commas indicate noncovalent linkage of chains arising from separate genes; solid lines indicate covalent linkage of chains arising from post-translational cleavage of a proenzyme molecule, chains being listed in order beginning at the amino terminus of the proenzyme molecular; dashed lines indicate covalent linkage of chains arising from separate genes.

[b] p indicates the short arm and q the long arm of the chromosome.

Abbreviations: ND: not determined; C1-INH: C1 inhibitor.

COMPLEMENT ACTIVATION

Generation of the Classical Pathway C3 Convertase

Activation of the classical pathway occurs most commonly as the result of an immunologic reaction between antibody and antigen (Fig. 1). Of the various isotypes only IgM and certain subclasses of IgG ($3 > 1 > 2$) bind C1 and initiate complement activation.[20,21] C1 in serum is a trimolecular complex containing one molecule of C1q and two molecules each of the C1r and C1s subunits. C1q is the subunit responsible for binding to antibody. The C1q molecule consists of a central core with six radiating pods that terminate in globular heads. The globular heads contain the antibody binding site.[21,22]

The mechanism by which the interaction of antibody with antigen facilitates C1q binding and complement activation differs between the two antibody isotypes. In solution or under conditions of antigen excess IgM exists as a planar pentameric structure and displays a weak C1q binding site in the CH3 or CH4 region of each monomeric IgM subunit. Binding of IgM to several antigen molecules on the same particle causes IgM to assume a "staple" configuration. This change results in the appearance of at least two additional C1q binding sites and the firm association of C1q with IgM. In contrast IgG possesses two C1q binding sites in the CH2 domain of its Fc fragment, but functionally effective C1q binding requires that two IgG molecules be cross linked via the globular heads on C1q. This requirement dictates that thousands of IgG molecules be bound to a target particle to ensure sufficient proximity for doublet formation. At a functional level this requirement means that complement activation by IgG is less efficient than that by IgM since the latter requires only that a single molecule be bound in the correct configuration.[21,22]

C1 binding by antibody results in a change in the structural configuration of the C1q molecule such that the C1r and C1s tetramer contained within the cagelike structure formed by the radiating pods of C1q becomes autocatalytically active. This structural alteration may involve the release of C1 inhibitor which binds reversibly to proenzyme C1. C1r and C1s are structurally related molecules consisting of a head bearing the serine esterase enzymatic site and a tail bearing the binding site. The subunits are aligned linearly such that the central portion of the tetramer is formed by two C1r subunits linked through their catalytic domains. Each C1r molecule is joined to a C1s molecule via the binding site in the tail region of the respective subunits. This linear arrangement allows the tetramer to assume a figure eight configuration such that all four catalytic domains are in close proximity. In this configuration each C1r molecule is believed to activate the other C1r molecule, which in turn then activates C1s.[21,23,24]

Expression of enzymatic activity by C1r and C1s represents the initial activation and amplification step in the classical pathway. Thus many molecules of substrate are cleaved by a given enzyme complex, which results in the fixation of subsequent components in the complement cascade to the surface of the target particle in close proximity to the antibody binding site. Hence antibody serves not only to activate complement in a kinetically efficient manner but also to direct complement deposition to specific sites on the target surface.

Activated C1s cleaves a 9 kD fragment, C4a, from the amino terminus of the α-chain of C4. This results in the exposure of an internal thiolester bond linking the SH group of a cysteine residue with the terminal COOH group of glutamic acid. This bond is subject to nucleophilic attack by hydroxyl or amino groups, which leads to the formation of covalent ester or amide linkages.[20,21,25] Through this reaction and the analogous one involving C3 (Fig. 2), the complement system acquires a chemically stable association with the target surface. Of interest with regard to the formation of these covalent bonds is that due to

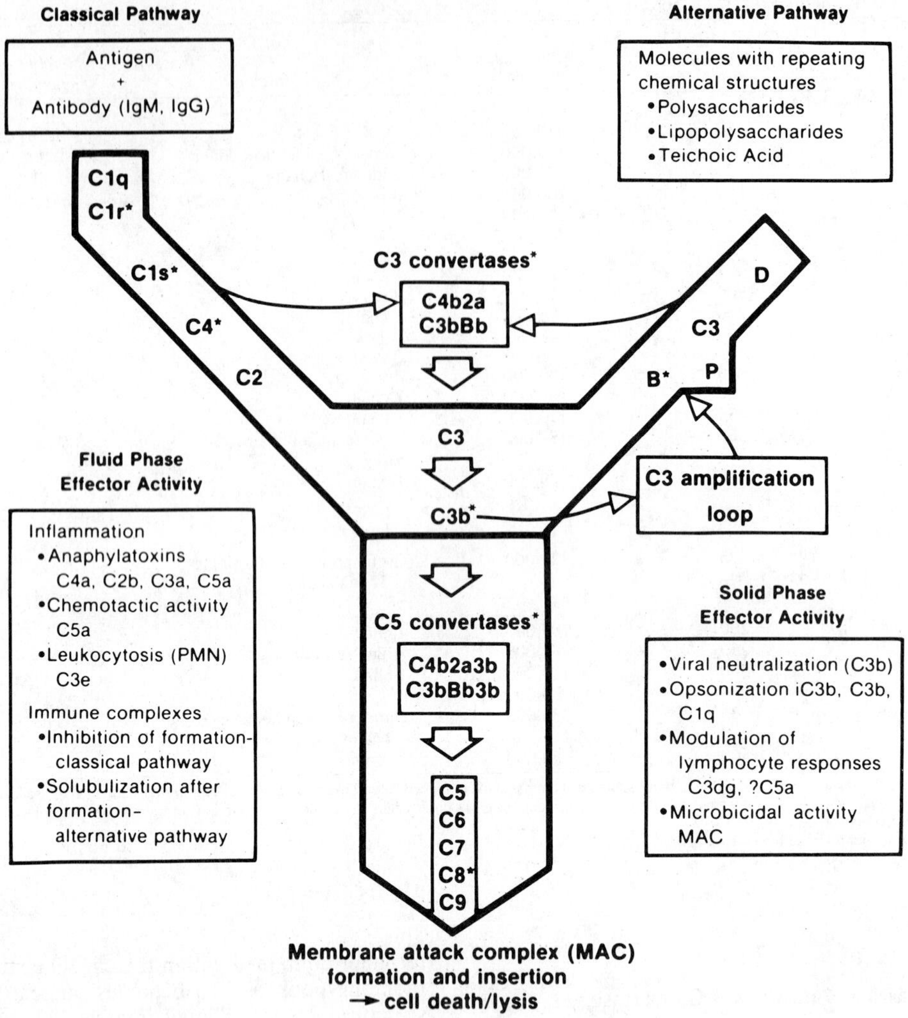

FIG. 1. The complement cascade. Within each pathway the components are arranged in order of their activation and aligned opposite their functional and structural analogue in the opposite pathway. Asterisks (*) indicate sites of downregulation of complement activity (see Table 2).

gene duplication there are two slightly different C4 genes, C4A and C4B. The product of the C4A gene preferentially forms amide bonds with target surfaces and is hemolytically less active than is the product of the C4B gene, which preferentially forms ester bonds.[27–29] Consequently, C4A binds more effectively to proteins, for example, antigen–antibody complexes, than does C4B.[28,30,31] The molecular basis for this difference in binding efficiency appears to be the presence of an aspartic acid residue in the C4A molecule and a histidine residue in the C4B molecule at a site distant from the thiolester. Although distant from the thiolester in the primary structure of C4, the tertiary configuration of the molecule probably brings these charged amino acids into close proximity with the thiolester such that they influence the nucleophilic attack of the thiolester bond by amino or hydroxyl groups on the target surface. The difference in reactivity of the C4A and C4B molecules may play a role in determining the clinical picture observed in patients with inherited deficiencies of these respective genes.[32]

Activated C1s also cleaves C2 to produce a small fragment, C2b, which is released into the environment, and a larger fragment, C2a, which binds to C4b on the surface of the target particle. This complex, C4b2a, is the classical pathway C3 convertase (Fig. 1). It is inherently labile, but after its dissociation C4b can bind fresh C2a derived from further cleavage of C2 by C1s.[20,21]

Generation of the Alternative-Pathway C3 Convertase

Activation of complement by the alternative pathway displays several unique features. First, antibody is not required, although it can facilitate the activation process. Second, activation proceeds both in the fluid phase as well as on cell surfaces. Fluid-phase activation occurs continuously at a low rate that is controlled by regulator proteins in plasma. Spillover from the fluid phase results in complement deposition on cells of the host as well as intruding microorganisms. Thus host cells must possess a mechanism to limit the effects of complement fixation (i.e., they are "nonactivators"), whereas intruding cells must provide a surface that allows complement activation to proceed further (i.e., they are "activators").[20,33,34] Third, a component of the activation process, C3b, is also a product of the reaction, thereby generating a positive-feedback system that amplifies the activation process. Consequently, C3b deposition resulting from C3 cleavage by either the alternative- or the classical-pathway C3 convertase can initiate the alternative-pathway amplification loop (Fig. 1).[20,33,34] The time required until amplification occurs makes complement activation via the alternative pathway three to five times kinetically less efficient than via the classical pathway on the same target.[35] This delay in activation is characteristic for a given target and differs among different target particles.[33,34] Fourth, in contrast to the classical pathway in which antibody directs covalent C4b binding in clus-

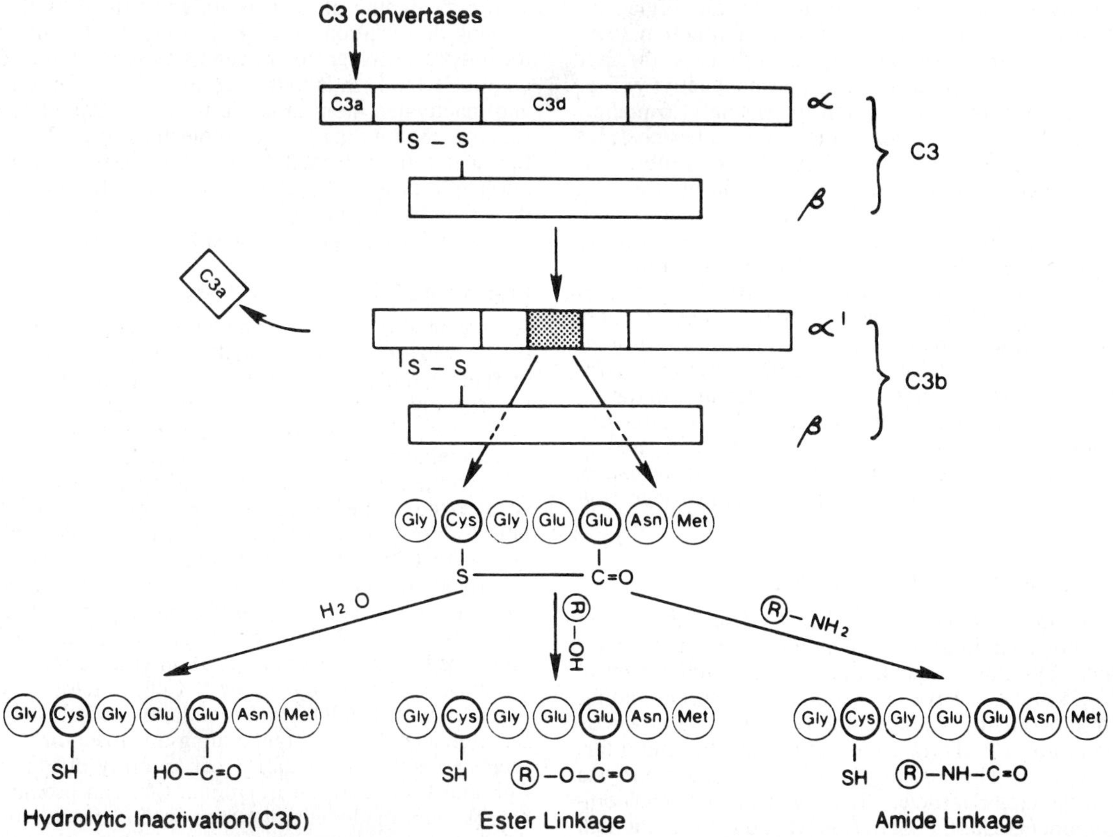

FIG. 2. C3 activation and fate of the internal thiolester bond. During activation C3a is released from the amino terminus of the α-chain of C3. The exposed internal thiolester bond becomes accessible to nucleophilic attack and can react with water or available hydroxyl or amine groups on cell surfaces. Analogous reactions occur with C4. Together these reactions involving C3 and C4 are responsible for covalently linking complement deposition to the cell surface. (From Gordon et al.,[26] with permission.)

ters about the antibody binding site, covalent C3b binding mediated by the alternative pathway occurs randomly over the surface of the target particle.[33,34] The random nature of this process contributes in part to the delay in complement activation via this pathway.

C3 is the critical reactant of the alternative pathway. It is structurally and functionally analogous to C4 (Fig. 1) and contains the same internal thiolester bond within its α-chain. This internal thiolester bond undergoes spontaneous low-rate hydrolysis to form C3(H_2O) as shown in Figure 2. For a brief moment before its inactivation by the control proteins factors H and I, C3(H_2O) can form a complex with factor B. Once bound to C3, factor B can be cleaved by factor D to yield C3 (H_2O) Bb—the fluid-phase C3 convertase. C3(H_2O)Bb reacts with intact C3 to cleave a 9 kD peptide fragment, C3a, from the amino terminus of the α-chain.[33,34] Analogous to the situation with C4, this process results in the exposure of the internal thiolester in the α-chain. The resulting metastable C3b can form covalent ester or amide linkages with appropriate chemical constituents on the surface of nearby cells. Surface-bound C3b can bind additional factor B, which in turn can be cleaved by factor D to produce C3bBb. This complex is the alternative-pathway C3 convertase, which is capable of cleaving additional C3, thereby initiating the amplification phase of the alternative pathway. Like its classical-pathway analogue, this convertase is inherently labile and has a half-life of approximately 90 seconds. Properdin binding to C3bBb stabilizes the complex and prolongs its half-life by 5- to 10-fold,[36,37] thereby providing reaction conditions sufficient for further C3 cleavage and signaling the initiation of the amplification phase of alternative-pathway activation.

From these considerations it is apparent that any substance that stabilizes the alternative-pathway convertase will also promote C3 consumption. This situation arises in patients who develop autoantibodies to C3bBb that stabilize the convertase.[38] In addition, cobra venom contains a C3b-like factor that forms an extremely stable complex with factor B that functions as a C3 convertase except that it is resistant to the action of the control proteins. Thus, the addition of cobra venom factor to serum leads to the dramatic consumption of C3.[33,39–41] Consequently, infusion of this factor can be used in experimental animals to delineate the role of the complement cascade in host defense or other disease processes.

Although antibody is not required for activation of the alternative pathway, it acts synergistically with properdin to facilitate the activation process.[42,43] Facilitation is dependent upon the Fab portion of the antibody molecule rather than the Fc fragment responsible for classical-pathway activation.[43–47] Not all antibodies can enhance activation, for example, guinea pig IgG1 but not IgG2 can augment alternative-pathway activation.[48] The molecular basis for facilitation is uncertain but probably requires carbohydrate moieties present on IgG.[49] Antibody deposited on target surfaces can itself become a potential binding site for the covalent linkage of C3.[44] Moreover, the alternative-pathway C3 convertase, C3bBb that is formed on IgG is relatively resistant to the action of the regulatory proteins.[50,51] This property may contribute to the ability of antibody to facilitate alternative-pathway activation.

C3—The Linchpin of the Complement System

The critical importance of C3 in the complement cascade is evident from its position at the convergence of the classical and alternative pathways, its role in activating and amplifying alternative-pathway activation, the multitude of functional activities associated with its various cleavage products, the fact that it is a major point of regulation of complement activity (Fig. 1), and the fact that its concentration in plasma (1.6 mg/ml) exceeds by 2 to 10-fold the concentration of all other complement components (Table 1).[52] The α-chain of C3b is subject to proteolytic cleavage by factor I to yield iC3b and by less well defined proteases to C3dg and C3d. Each of these progressively smaller C3 fragments remains linked to the cell surface via the original covalent bond. Each of these C3 cleavage products (C3b, iC3b, C3dg, and C3d) can react with specific receptors on phagocytic and lymphocytic cells, but only C3b perpetuates complement activation. C3b binding to the C3 convertases generates new complexes, C4bC2aC3b and C3bBbC3b, the C5 convertases, which are responsible for cleaving C5 and initiating assembly of the membrane attack complex (MAC). Enzymes present in neutrophil granules can proteolytically inactivate C3. Cleavage products have been detected in areas of pus formation such as empyema and may contribute to the impaired ingestion of bacteria in abscesses.[53,54]

Assembly of the Membrane Attack Complex

C5 is the structural hemologue of C4 and C3 except that its α-chain does not contain an internal thiolester bond. Instead, the amino acids cysteine and glutamine, which form the internal thiolester in C4 and C3, have been replaced by serine and alanine.[55,56] Analogous to C4 and C3, activation of C5 proceeds via cleavage of an 11.2 kD fragment, C5a, from the amino terminus of its α-chain. The resulting C5b binds noncovalently to the surface of the target particle.[57] The remaining terminal complement components C6, C7, C8β, C8α-γ, and C9 share a high level of structural organization at both the DNA and protein levels.[58–60] Unlike the early components of the classical and alternative pathways these proteins lack enzymatic activity but as a group are characterized by their amphipathic properties. They circulate in plasma in a hydrophilic form but undergo hydrophobic transformation upon binding to the nascent MAC.[57] Assembly of the MAC begins when C5b binds to hydrophobic sites on the cell surface and expresses a metastable binding site for C6. After C6 binding, C7 also binds to C5b, which results in the formation of a stable trimolecular complex, C5b67.[57] Subsequently, C8 binds to C5b via a site on its β-chain.[61,62] In the final step, C8 initiates polymerization of C9 through a binding site on C8α-γ.[63] A current model of this process suggests that the function of C5b-8 is to create a discontinuity in the membrane lipid bilayer, thereby establishing an environment for the stepwise unfolding, insertion, and polymerization of monomeric C9.[64] In its completely assembled state the MAC consists of a single molecule each of C5b-C8 and multiple (1–18) molecules of C9.[57]

Fully inserted and polymerized C9 has a tubular shape and the properties of an integral membrane protein.[57,64] It is responsible for the characteristic electron microscopic appearance of the membrane holes that appear during effective complement activation. The inner aspect of this tubular structural is hydrophilic and allows the passage of water and ions, whereas the outer surface of the structure is hydrophobic and causes varying degrees of membrane disorganization during insertion.[57,64] Both of these effects are thought to contribute to the microbicidal and cytolytic properties of the MAC. A functionally and structurally related protein called perforin has been isolated from the granules of natural killer (NK) cells. Translocation of this protein from NK cells to the membrane of target cells occurs during the cytolytic process.[58,65–67]

REGULATION OF COMPLEMENT ACTIVATION

Regulation of C1 Activation

As described earlier, C1 esterase inhibitor (C1-INH) binds reversibly to pro-C1, thereby preventing its spontaneous activation.[22] Binding of C1q to antibody subverts this control by causing dissociation of C1-INH from pro-C1 and allowing autocatalytic cleavage to proceed. At some point after C1 activation C1-INH binds to the serine esterase sites on C1r and C1s and inactivates their catalytic function. Complete inactivation requires the binding of four molecules of C1-INH per C1rC1s tetramer (one per catalytic site). In contrast to its reversible binding to pro-C1, C1-INH binding to C1r and C1s is irreversible, thereby preventing cleavage of C4 and controlling the initial amplification step of classical-pathway activation.[22,68]

Regulation of the C3 Convertases

As indicated in Figure 1 the classical- and alternative-pathway C3 convertases are functionally analogous molecules. Control of their activity occurs by three basic mechanisms and uses functionally identical or shared regulator proteins (Table 2).[20,33,34,38] First, both of the convertases are inherently labile and undergo spontaneous decay with the loss of C2a or Bb from the complex. Second, the rate of spontaneous decay can be accelerated by the binding of C4 binding protein (C4bp) or factor H to C4b or C3b, respectively. These regulatory proteins compete with C2a and Bb for binding sites on C4b and C3b, respectively, thereby inhibiting new convertase formation and enhancing the rate of dissociation of the already formed convertases. Third, functionally active C3b and C4b remaining on the cell surface after dissociation of the convertases are proteolytically cleaved by factor I. C4bp, factor H, complement receptor type 1 (CR1), and membrane cofactor protein (MCP) function as cofactors in mediating this reaction.[20,33,34,38,69] Proteolysis results in the display of an array of covalently bound C4b and C3b cleavage fragments that can promote additional complement-mediated functions when present on the appropriate target particle.

C4bp and factor H are soluble molecules that exert their regulatory influence over both fluid-phase and surface-bound C3 convertases.[20,33,69,70] Functionally analogous molecules are present in the membrane of host cells. These proteins include the C3b receptor (CR1), MCP (or GP45-70), and decay accelerating factor (DAF).[71] CR1 is present primarily on peripheral blood cells and facilitates the clearance of immune complexes. MCP and DAF enjoy a wider tissue distribution and play a major role in the inactivation of C3b deposited on host cells during complement activation.[69,70] Thus they serve to distinguish self from nonself with respect to the deleterious effects of complement activation.[70] Like C4bp and factor H all three proteins function to inhibit the assembly and accelerate the decay of the C3 convertases, but unlike the soluble regulator proteins, the membrane-bound proteins do not exhibit pathway specificity.[69,70] Of the membrane-bound proteins, DAF exhibits specificity for C3b and C4b only when these molecules are bound to the same cell on which the DAF is located (intrinsic activity), whereas CR1 and MCP exhibit extrinsic activity. Although the soluble regulator proteins C4bp and factor H contribute to the regulation of cell-bound C3 convertases, their principal role is to control the formation and activity of these convertases in the fluid phase, whereas the membrane-bound regulatory proteins primarily regulate cell-bound C3b and C4b.[69,70] The multiplicity of proteins involved and the existence of both fluid-phase and membrane-bound regulatory proteins all with activity specific for the C3 convertases serve to emphasize the critical importance of the convertases in amplifying complement activation.

Recently the assembly and insertion of the MAC has been shown to inhibit C3 convertase formation and to accelerate the decay of the alternative-pathway convertase. Feedback inhibition of this sort may serve to protect the host from the detrimental affects of continued complement activation.[72,73]

The Basis for Discriminating between Host and Microbial Cell Surfaces

The capacity of C4 and C3 to form covalent bonds with reactive groups on cell surfaces, thereby establishing the nidus for C3

TABLE 2. Plasma and Membrane Proteins That Regulate or Mediate Complement Activity

Location / *Protein*	*Specificity*	*Function*
Plasma		
C1-INH	C1r, C1s	Binds to and removes C1r and C1s from C1 complex
C4bp	C4b	Inhibits assembly and accelerates decay of C4b2a Cofactor for C4b cleavage by factor I
Factor H	C3b	Inhibits assembly and accelerates decay of C3bBb Cofactor for C3b cleavage by factor I
Factor I	C4b, C3b	Proteolytic inactivation of C4b and C3b
S protein	C5b-7	Binds fluid-phase C5b-7; prevents attachment of SC5b-7, C5b-9 to membranes
Carboxypeptidase N	C4a, C3a, C5a	Inactivates these anaphylatoxins by removal of C terminal arginine
Cell Membranes		
CR1	C3b, C4b, iC3b	Inhibit assembly and accelerate decay of C3 convertases
MCP	C3b, C4b	Cofactor for cleavage of C4b/C3b by factor I
DAF	C4b2a, C3bBb	
CR1	C3b, C4b, iC3b	Binds immune complexes to erythrocytes; phagocytosis
CR2	C3d, C3dg, iC3b, C3b	Phagocytosis Modulates B-cell responses Epstein-Barr virus receptor
CR3	iC3b	Phagocytosis
CR4 (p150, 95)	C3dg, C3d	Unknown
HRF	C8 in C5b-8	? Binds to C8 Inhibits polymerization of C9
C3a/C4a receptor	C3a, C4a	Vasodilation
C5a receptor	C5a, C5a des-arg	Chemotaxis
C1qR	C1q	Phagocytosis

convertase formation, is inherently incapable of distinguishing between host and microbial cells. Consequently, in order for the beneficial effects of complement activation to be expressed as an effective host defense mechanism additional factors must allow the discrimination between self and nonself[76]: inhibiting activation of complement amplification on host cells ("nonactivators") yet permitting amplification on the surface of microbial organisms ("activators"). One element of this discriminatory process is the presence of the complement regulatory proteins in the membranes of host cells but not on the cells of microbial organisms.[70] The other important determinant of complement activation is the chemical composition of the cell surface. Moreover, since covalent bond formation is nondiscriminatory, the basis for discrimination must lie in the capacity for chemical differences to affect the outcome of the competition between factor B and factor H for the binding site on C3b, which in turn determines C3 convertase formation or decay and whether or not a particular cell surface will activate the alternative pathway. For example, C3b bound to the surface of a nonactivating particle binds factor H with about a 100-fold greater affinity than C3b bound to an activator particle. Consequently, factor B binding and subsequent amplification of complement activation is favored on the latter particle.[20,33,34,38]

Chemical constituents that influence the competition between factor B and factor H for C3b include sialic acid and sulfated acid mucopolysaccharides (e.g., heparin sulfate). These chemical molecules are present on most human cells and enhance the affinity of factor H for C3b, thereby contributing to the nonactivator status of host cells.[74–76] From the standpoint of infectious diseases it is interesting that sialic acid is a prominent chemical constituent of the capsular polysaccharides present on type 3 group B streptococci, K1 *Escherichia coli*, and group B and C meningococci.[38] Consequently, the capsules of these organisms are nonactivators of the alternative pathway and, being a constituent of host cells, constitute a poor stimulus for antibody production. In this context it is noteworthy that K1 *E. coli*, group B streptococci, and group B meningococci are prominent causes of neonatal and infant sepsis and meningitis. Moreover, the frequent absence in these individuals of specific antibody to activate the classic pathway coupled with bacterial sialic acid–mediated inhibition of alternative-pathway activity may provide the ideal clinical setting for infection with these organisms.

Chemical constituents other than sialic acid must also affect the outcome of the competition between factors B and H for C3b. For example, sheep and human erythrocytes contain an extensive amount of sialic acid on their surface and are normally nonactivators of the alternative pathway.[74,77] Enzymatic removal of sialic acid from these cells converts sheep but not human erythrocytes into activating particles. Moreover, the chemical introduction of lipopolysaccharide molecules capable of activating the alternative pathway into the membrane of sheep erythrocytes converts them from a nonactivating to an activating particle despite the presence of sialic acid.[77]

In summary, the C3 convertases represent the major site of both complement amplification and regulation. The membranes of host cells contain both unique proteins that act specifically to downregulate the C3 convertases and other chemical constituents that enhance the affinity of fluid-phase factor H for surface-bound C3b and promote its regulatory activity. In contrast, most microbial surfaces lack specific factors capable of downregulating complement activation and possess a chemical composition that decreases the affinity of factor H for cell-bound C3b. Thus, factor B binding to C3b and alternative-pathway activation and amplification are favored on microbial surfaces. The composition of the cell surface also influences the efficiency of complement activation by the classic pathway. The mechanism of this modulation is less clearly understood but appears to occur at the level of cellbound C4b.[78]

Regulation of the Membrane Attack Complex

Control of the assembly of the MAC is exerted at two levels. First, S protein in plasma binds to lipophilic sites on the fluid-phase trimolecular C5b-7 complex. This interaction inhibits the binding of C5b-7 to membranes and prevents the assembly of the MAC on innocent bystander cells of the host.[57] Second, homologous restriction protein (HRP) present on many types of peripheral blood cells binds C8 and prevents C9 polymerization.[79–81] This protein was discovered as a result of the observation that appropriately sensitized erythrocytes from a given species were lysed less well when the complement source, in particular the C8 and C9, was derived from the same species rather than from another species.[82]

Nucleated eukaryotic cells are quite resistant to complement-mediated cytolysis even in the face of a nonhomologous complement source. Resistance is associated with the capacity of the cell to maintain high synthetic rates of membrane lipids and the ability to shed MAC from the cell surface.[83–85] Insertion of the MAC in eukaryotic cell membranes is accompanied by a rapid influx of calcium and stimulation of arachidonic acid metabolism.[86–90] These events may contribute to host cell injury in certain disease states.[86]

COMPLEMENT RECEPTORS

During the 1980's, an increasing number of membrane receptors have been recognized for the products of complement activation.[91–93] These receptors have been described primarily on peripheral blood cells including erythrocytes, neutrophils, monocytes, B and T lymphocytes, and platelets. They fall into two broad categories: those that bind complement components deposited on cell surfaces such that the component serves as a bifunctional ligand linking the target cell to the receptor and those that bind diffusable complement fragments released during activation of the complement cascade. The latter are responsible for many of the manifestations of the inflammatory response.

The former category of receptor includes C1qR, CR1, CR2, CR3, and CR4. Little is known about C1qR other than that it is present on phagocytic cells and that binding results from the interaction of the receptor with the central collagenlike core of the molecule. Recent evidence suggests that interaction of C1q with its receptor on granulocytes may mediate particle ingestion and stimulate a respiratory burst in these cells (see Chapter 7).[91,92]

Receptors for the cleavage products of C3 and C4 (CR1, CR2, CR3, and CR4) have been studied more extensively. Despite recognizing closely related ligands each of these receptors is structurally distinct and exhibits a unique pattern of distribution on peripheral blood cells.[93,94] A portion of these receptors is linked to the cellular cytoskeleton, an association that is probably important in the transduction of the binding signal into a cellular response.[95]

CR1, the C3b receptor, is present on erythrocytes, neutrophils, monocytes, B lymphocytes, subpopulations of T lymphocytes, follicular dendritic cells, and glomerular podocytes. It also recognizes C4b and iC3b but with less affinity than for C3b. This receptor mediates immune complex binding and clearance and ingestion of particles bearing C3b and presumably modulates certain immune lymphocyte responses.[91,93,94]

CR3, the iC3b receptor, is the major complement receptor mediating phagocytosis by phagocytic cells.[91,93,94] It is a heterodimer and has recently been shown to be a member of the integrin family[96] It recognizes a three–amino acid sequence, arg-gly-asp, present on C3[97] and other ligands important in adhesion.[98] In addition to recognizing iC3b it plays an important role in the adherence-related functions of neutrophils and is covered more extensively in Chapter 7.

CR4 is the C3dg receptor. It is present on phagocytic cells and appears to be synonomous with p150,95.[99] More CR4 is present on culture-derived macrophages than on freshly isolated monocytes. CR2, the C3d receptor, is present on B lymphocytes and follicular dendritic cells. Its stimulation appears to modulate antibody production by these lymphocytes. It also serves as the Epstein-Barr virus receptor, and its stimulation during viral entry may contribute to the polyclonal gammopathy observed early in the course of infectious mononucleosis.[100,101]

Receptors for complement-derived mediators of the inflammatory response including C4a, C3a, and C5a have also been described. Of these the C5a receptor has been best studied. It is present on neutrophils and monocytes, and its pertubation causes directed migration (chemotaxis) of these cells in the direction of increasing C5a concentration. Experimental evidence suggests the presence of receptors for C3a on guinea pig ileum, vascular endothelium, and mast cells.[102]

FAMILIES OF COMPLEMENT PROTEINS

The preceding material and the representation of the complement cascade presented in Figure 1 emphasize features shared by both pathways with respect to their activation and regulation. It is apparent from these similarities that a number of complement components belong to several different protein families. These include the serine protease family (C1r, C1s, C2, factor D, factor B, and factor I); multichained disulfide-linked molecules with homology to an ancestral protein that contain an internal thiolester bond (C4, C3, and C5); proteins that are the products of class 3 major histocompatibility complex (MHC) genes located on chromosome 6 (C2, factor B, C4A, and C4B); proteins that bind C3 and C4 fragments that belong to a closely clustered supergene family located on the long arm of chromosome 1 (C4bp, factor H, DAF, MCP, CR1, and CR2); and proteins sharing homology with the low-density lipoprotein (LDL) receptor (C9, C8α, C8β, C7, and probably C6). These families also include a number of noncomplement homologues.[103]

Of these families current interest has focused on those components that are the products of the class 3 MHC genes, the regulatory protein supergene family on chromosome 1, and the proteins with homology to the LDL receptor. Class 3 MHC genes are located between the class 1 and class 2 loci on the short arm of chromosome 6 (Fig. 3).[104] The genetic material in this region is of particular interest because it appears to have undergone two duplication events resulting on the one hand in the structurally and functionally related proteins C2 and factor B and on the other hand the C4 and 21-hydroxylase A and B variants.[103–105] The gene for tumor necrosis factor/cachectin has also been localized to this region of chromosome 6.[106] Recombinant events in this region of the chromosome tend to be suppressed, thereby leading to the usual inheritance of the entire region intact from each parent.[107] The polymorphic variants of the complement components encoded by these genes in a given individual are referred to as complotypes.[108] The association of specific complotypes with specific products of the class 1 and 2 MHC genes probably contributes to the association of specific complotypes with certain disease states (e.g., systemic lupus erythematosus [SLE])[109]

Proteins encoded by the complement regulatory protein loci on the long arm of chromosome 1 share a common organization with each other, with other proteins capable of binding to C3 and C4 (e.g., C2 and factor B), and with some complement and noncomplement proteins that do not bind these two components.[110,111] All of these proteins contain tandem repeats of approximately 60 amino acids that share a consensus sequence. Each of these 60 amino acid repeats are encoded within separate exons, and the number of repeats varies from as few as 2 and 3 in C1r and C2/factor B, respectively, to as many as 20 in factor H, although CR1 may contain up to 36 repeats. The functional significance of these repeating structures, particularly with respect to their C3 and C4 binding properties, remains to be delineated.[111]

The LDL receptor-related complement proteins are cysteine-rich molecules. Each molecule contains an even number of cysteine residues that are clustered at the amino and carboxy terminal portions of the protein and participate in disulfide bond formation. Those clustered at the amino terminus of the molecule share homology with epidermal growth factor, while those at the carboxy terminus share homology with the LDL receptor. The large number of disulfide bonds in these molecules is thought to convey a tertiary structure that facilitates the hydrophilic–hydrophobic transition that occurs upon their inter-

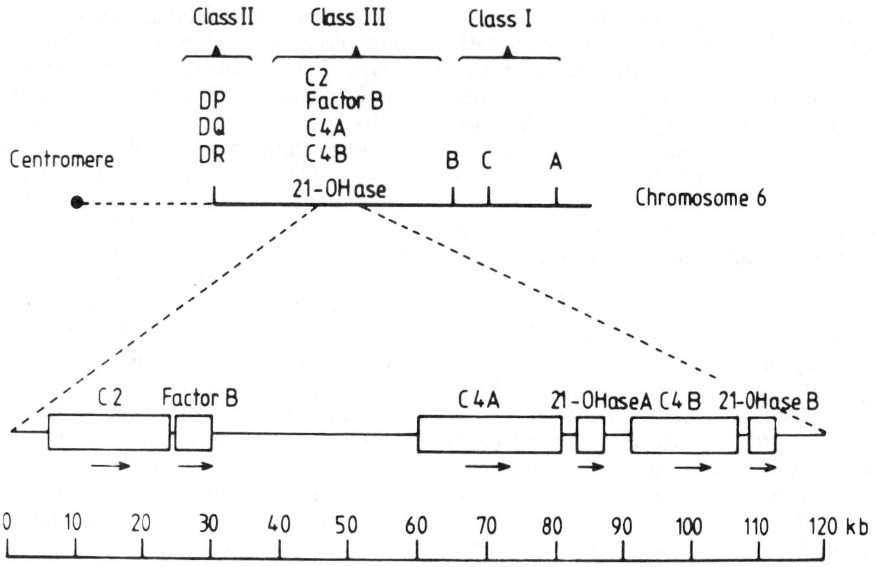

FIG. 3. Organization of the human MHC genes on chromosome 6. The proximity of the class 3 genes to one another and to the class 2 and 1 genes is apparent. C2 and factor B are tightly linked and probably represent duplication of the phylogenetically older factor B gene. Genetic duplication is also apparent in the paired arrangement of the C4 and 21-hydroxylase genes. (From Campbell,[104] with permission.)

action with lipid membranes during the assembly of the MAC.[58,59,102]

COMPLEMENT-MEDIATED FUNCTIONS

Complement plays a major role in initiating the inflammatory response, clearing immune complexes, modulating immunoglobulin production, opsonizing microbial pathogens, and killing certain gram-negative bacteria (Fig. 1). Small, diffusable peptide fragments released from C4, C3, C5, and probably C2 during their activation help mediate the inflammatory response.[102] Collectively C4a, C3a, and C5a are referred to as anaphylatoxins, and together they stimulate histamine release from mast cells (C3a), promote vascular dilation (C3a, C4a), increase endothelial permeability (C3a), and stimulate neutrophil responses (C5a, e.g., adhesiveness, chemotaxis, degranulation, and oxidative burst; see Chapter 7). Each of these structurally related anaphylatoxins contains an arginine residue at its carboxy terminus. Removal of this terminal amino acid by carboxypeptidase B in serum abrogates their functional activity by preventing their interaction with specific receptors.[102] However, in the case of C5a des-arg (the inactivated form of C5a), chemotactic activity is restored by association with a cochemotaxin present in serum[112] that has recently been identified as a vitamin D binding protein.[113,114] The chemotactic activity of this complex can be inhibited by free Bb, a situation that occurs in the sera of some patients with SLE.[115]

The incorporation of complement in immune complexes enhances their clearance and helps to minimize their potential for causing tissue damage.[116,117] This process includes the inhibition of immune complex precipitation from solution, the solubilization of immune complexes, and the clearance of C3b-bearing immune complexes via the CR1 receptor. Under conditions of antibody excess or antibody–antigen equivalence the attachment of both antigen binding sites on a single antibody to epitopes on a single antigen and the binding of multiple antibody molecules to a given molecule of antigen provide an opportunity for antibody–antibody interactions via their Fc fragments, a condition that leads to immune complex precipitation.[117] C1q binding inhibits these Fc–Fc interactions and leads to complement activation with covalent binding of C3b to the immune complex. Subsequent recruitment of the alternative pathway via the C3b amplification loop promotes further C3b deposition within the immune complex lattice, thereby reducing the forces holding the lattice together and causing separation (solubilization) of smaller complexes from the lattice network. Thus the classic pathway functions to inhibit immune complex precipitation, whereas the alternative pathway promotes solubilization of the immune complex.[116,117]

Small immune complexes bearing C3b are bound to cells bearing C3b receptors (CR1). The number of these receptors per cell varies from a low of 950 for erythrocytes to a high of 57,000 for neutrophils.[118] However, since red cells outnumber white cells by a thousandfold, 95 percent of the total CR1 receptors in the peripheral circulation are located on red cells. Consequently, immune complexes bearing C3b are 500–1000 times more likely of being removed from the circulation via red cells than white cells.[118] These complexes are removed from the red cell during passage through the liver by an as yet undefined mechanism.[119]

Most evidence implicates C3 as the major complement-derived stimulus involved in modulating immune responses. These studies suggest that C3 or its fragments may enhance or inhibit both T- and B-cell-mediated immune responses, the observed effect perhaps depending upon the concentration of the relevant C3 fragment.[120,121] This evidence includes the observation that the trapping of aggregated human IgG within splenic germinal centers is dependent upon the presence of C3[122] and the demonstration that lymphocytes, particularly B cells, possess receptors (CR2) with ligand specificity for C3dg and C3d.[100] In addition, impaired antibody responses have been demonstrated after primary immunization with a T-cell-dependent antigen, bacteriophage ϕX174, in C2-, C4-, and C3-deficient guinea pigs[123,124] as well as in a limited number of patients with analogous deficiencies.[125] Moreover, dogs with inherited C3 deficiency or animals rendered C3 deficient by the infusion of cobra venom factor were also unable to respond normally to ϕX174.[124,124a] Immune responsiveness in deficient animals could be restored by repletion of the complement system with the missing component or by increasing the dose of antigen during primary immunization.[123] In addition to the impaired response to primary antigenic exposure, complement-deficient animals exhibit an abnormal anamestic response and fail to demonstrate isotype switching after secondary antigenic presentation.[124] Impaired antibody responses in C3-deficient dogs were also observed after primary and secondary immunization with a T-cell independent antigen. In contrast to the results with T-cell dependent antigens, the impaired response to T-cell independent antigens could not be overcome by increasing the dose of antigen or changing the route of administration.[124a] These results clearly demonstrate a critical role for C3 in the generation of a normal humoral immune response.

Finally, a small fragment, C3e, derived from the α-chain of C3 promotes the development of leukocytosis. This observation may account for the failure of some C3-deficient patients to develop leukocytosis in response to infection.[20]

Cell-bound fragments of C3, particularly C3b and iC3b, serve as bifunctional ligands linking target particles with cells bearing receptors for these fragments. In the case of bacteria, opsonization with C3b or iC3b, especially in conjunction with IgG, promotes ingestion of the organism and triggers the microbicidal mechanisms of phagocytic cells (see Chapter 7). Ingestion is more efficient when the organism is opsonized with iC3b than with C3b.[26,126]

The complete activation of the complement cascade with the assembly of the MAC and its effective insertion into cell membranes results in the death and eventual lysis of the cell. Death and lysis are independent events, and in the case of prokaryotes some evidence suggests that a metabolic response of the organism is required before the lethal effects of the MAC can be expressed.[127] For some organisms the assembly of the MAC through C8 is sufficient to kill the organism[128]; however, in all cases the incorporation of C9 accelerates this process. Complement-mediated virucidal activity has also been well described and frequently requires deposition of only the early components of the classic pathway.[129]

MICROBIAL INTERACTIONS WITH THE COMPLEMENT SYSTEM

A common theme encountered in the pathogenesis of many infectious agents is the evolution of strategies to neutralize or elude normal host defense mechanisms. An example of this principle and one of the first to suggest an important role of the bactericidal capacity of complement in host defense was the demonstration by Roantree and Rance that gram-negative bacteria isolated from the blood of infected patients were almost always resistant to serum (complement)-mediated killing.[130] In contrast, two-thirds of the gram-negative bacteria isolated from mucosal surfaces could be killed by normal serum. This finding has been confirmed many times in relationship to other invasive bacterial infections, although different organisms employ a variety of molecular strategies to achieve this end.

Resistance to the bactericidal effect of complement is influenced by the structural organization and chemical composition of the outer membrane, the capacity of the organism to activate the alternative pathway, and the presence of bactericidal antibody. Virtually all gram-positive organisms and fungi are resistant to complement-mediated killing, not because they fail to activate complement, but because a thick outer membrane prevents access of the MAC to their inner membrane.[131]

Gram-negative bacilli, for example, *Salmonella*, owe their serum resistance to the long 0-antigen side chains on their lipopolysaccharides. These chains lead to complement activation at sites distant from the outer membrane and hinder access of C5b-9 complexes to it.[132] The failure of these complexes to localize to hydrophobic domains in the bacterial outer membrane results in their shedding and the survival of the organism.[133]

Gram-negative bacteria possessing truncated lipopolysaccharide molecules, for example, *Haemophilus influenzae*, meningococci, and gonococci, are not innately resistant to the bactericidal effects of the complement system but require antibody for effective sensitization and complement deposition. Thus, the absence of bactericidal antibody renders these organisms serum resistant and contributes to the greater frequency of *H. influenzae* and meningococcal disease during the first several years of life. Gonococci isolated from individuals with disseminated gonococcal infection are resistant to the bactericidal activity of normal human serum, whereas those isolated from individuals with symptomatic local genital disease are serum sensitive.[134] The MAC is assembled on the surface of both types of gonococci but fails to insert properly in the outer membrane of the resistant isolates.[135,136] However, insertion and killing occur normally in the presence of IgG antilipooligosaccharide antibody found in the convalescent serum of some individuals with this infection.[137,138] These findings emphasize the importance of both the composition of the outer membrane of gram-negative bacteria in determining sensitivity to complement-mediated killing and the importance to the host of specific antibody in overcoming the resistance of these organisms to killing.[139]

Other strains of serum-resistant gonococci appear to owe their serum resistance to the presence in some sera of an IgG specific for protein 3 in the gonococcal outer membrane.[140,141] This antibody competes with bactericidal antibody for binding sites on the surface of the organism, thereby blocking its bactericidal effect. Although the blocking antibody promotes complement deposition on the organism, it apparently does so at sites that do not lead to the killing of the organism.[142] Blocking antibody also appears to account for the resistance of meningococci to killing by the serum of many adults who acquire this infection.[143,144] In contrast to the situation with gonococci, this antibody is a non-complement-fixing IgA that competes with killing antibody for bactericidal sites on the capsular polysaccharide.[144–146]

The importance of the interaction of antibody with different antigenic structures in determining the effectiveness of complement in promoting host defense mechanisms is further emphasized by the observation that both antipneumococcal cell wall antibody and antipneumococcal capsular antibody promote the efficient deposition of C3b on the pneumococcal surface. However, only C3b deposited on the surface of the pneumococcal capsule is opsonically effective. These results imply that the pneumococcal capsule interferes with the interaction of cell wall–bound C3b with receptors on phagocytic cells.[147]

Protozoan parasites, which undergo dramatic metamorphosis from insect to human infective forms, provide a striking testimony to the importance of serum resistance. For example epimastigotes, the insect infective form of *Trypanosoma cruzi*, are efficiently killed in nonimmune normal human serum as a consequence of complement activation via the alternative pathway. In contrast, trypomastigotes, the human infective form of *T. cruzi*, are not killed under identical circumstances.[148] The basis for this difference is the capacity of trypomastigotes but not epimastigotes to *N*- glycosylate a 72 kD surface protein[149] that serves as the C3b acceptor site on both forms of *T. cruzi*.[148] Although C3b is deposited on both organisms, the presence of the glycosylated 72 kD protein on the invasive trypomastigotes reduces the affinity of C3b for factor B, thereby promoting its cleavage to iC3b.[150] Consequently, amplification of the alternative pathway, MAC formation, and killing occurs only on the serum-sensitive epimastigotes containing the unglycosylated 72 kD protein.

Although serum resistance is an important virulence factor for many organisms, this property by itself cannot account for the difference in virulence among various smooth gram-negative bacilli, all of which have outer membranes containing long-chain lipopolysaccharide molecules. This issue has been addressed in experiments correlating virulence with lipopolysaccharide composition and complement activation by three *Salmonella typhimurium* transductants and recombinants.[151] These organisms share identical outer membrane protein patterns but possess lipopolysaccharide side chains that differ in their chemical structure. The relative in vivo virulence of these three isolates was inversely proportional to their ability to activate complement via the alternative pathway. The rates and extent of C3 consumption and C3b deposition on the surface of these bacteria paralleled one another, the greatest consumption and deposition occurring on the least virulent strain.[152–154] Subsequent studies demonstrated that the magnitude of C3b binding was a function of the fine structure of the lipopolysaccharide O antigen and that while this structure affected C3 binding it had no effect on the subsequent cleavage and breakdown of the bound C3b. The effect of O antigen structure was expressed at the level of alternative-pathway amplification rather than degradation as shown by a greater affinity of factor B for C3b on the surface of the least virulent as compared with the most virulent strains, whereas the affinity of factor H for C3b was the same on all strains.[155,156]

The chemical composition of other structures on the bacterial surface also affects complement activation. Thus, K-1 *E. coli*, type 3 group B streptococci, and group B meningococci that possess sialylated capsular polysaccharides are poor activators of the alternative pathway[157,158] due to the higher affinity of C3b for factor H than for factor B in this setting.[38,74–76] Studies of alternative-pathway activation by pneumococci have demonstrated an effect of the chemical composition of the capsule on both the extent and the degradation of C3b. An interesting observation of these studies is an apparent inverse relationship between the degree of C3b degradation on a given capsular polysaccharide and the ability of that capsular polysaccharide to elicit an immune response when administered as part of the polyvalent pneumococcal vaccine.[159]

In addition to the capacity of the microbial surface to modulate the activity of bound C3, some organisms possess glycoproteins that bind C3 noncovalently. These proteins are antigenically similar to C3 receptors on human cells as shown by their ability to bind monoclonal, receptor-specific antibodies.[160–162] In the case of herpes simplex viruses expression of a complement binding protein (glycoprotein C) is associated with resistance to neutralization by complement.[163] In the case of *Candida albicans* the presence of these surface proteins is associated with resistance to phagocytosis.[164]

COMPLEMENT DEFICIENCY STATES

Frequency

Complement deficiency states may be either acquired or inherited. Acquired deficiency states can occur acutely, as part of an abrupt insult such as infection, or in conjunction with more chronic diseases such as rheumatologic or autoimmune processes. The frequency of inherited complement deficiencies in the general population is about 0.03 percent. Since these states are rare, the utility of screening tests is greatest in populations that contain the clinical correlates of abnormal complement inheritance, that is, persons with rheumatologic diseases and/or recurrent bacterial infections.[165] In one such study, a single individual with a homozygous complement deficiency was detected among 545 patients with rheumatologic diseases.[166] This frequency (0.2 percent) is approximately 10-fold greater than that in the general population. In addition, 19 individuals with a definite, probable, or possible heterozygous C2 deficiency state were detected among the 545 rheumatologic patients as compared with only 6 possible heterozygotes among 509 individuals without these diseases. Thus, this study provides clear support for the association of complement deficiency states with certain rheumatologic disorders, in particular, SLE.[166]

Reports of an association between systemic meningococcal and gonococcal infections and an inherited deficiency of C5, C6, C7, or C8[165,167] have led to several studies of the frequency of these deficiencies among patients with these infections. Such studies have uncovered as few as 0 of 47 (<2 percent) to as many as 3 of 20 (15 percent) individuals presenting with a first episode of documented meningococcal disease.[168–171] The wide range in frequency is probably related to the age of the patients in the studies, the relatively small number of patients studied, and a disproportionate genetic influence in relatively insular populations.[165] The best estimate of the frequency of inherited complement deficiency states among patients with endemic neisserial disease is about 5–10 percent, although the likelihood of a complement deficiency increases dramatically (31 percent) among patients who have had more than one episode of meningococcal infection.[172]

Classical-Pathway Deficiencies

The association of immune disorders, in particular SLE, with complement deficiency states is most evident in individuals lacking C1, C4, C2, or C3 (Table 3). The clinical presentation of SLE in individuals with a deficiency of one of these components differs from that in the general population in that males are commonly affected, renal disease is less severe, antinuclear antibody titers are low or absent, and there is an increased prevalence of Ro antibodies.[173–175]

In contrast to the relationship with infection in which an association is apparent only in homozygous deficient individuals, an increased frequency of collagen vascular diseases is apparent in individuals with either homozygous or heterozygous deficiency. The basis for this phenomenon has not been precisely delineated, although impaired immune complex handling and the tight genetic linkage of the C2 and C4 loci with the class I and II MHC genes appear to contribute to the association.[176] Of these variables, impaired immune complex clearance probably exerts a greater impact since the association is apparent for all four of these complement proteins whereas only C4 and C2 are MHC linked (see Fig. 3). The role of the early components of the classical pathway in inhibiting immune complex precipitation has been confirmed in the sera from patients with these deficiencies.[177,178] Moreover, abnormal humoral immune system regulation and the presence of autoantibodies, including rheumatoid factors, have been demonstrated in C2- and C4-deficient guinea pigs.[179]

Consequent to the linkage disequilibrium with other MHC loci, the C2 and C4 null genes occur predominantly as part of distinct extended haplotypes. For C2 deficiency, this haplotype is DR2;C2Q0;BfS;C4A-4;C4B-2;B18;A25,[180] and for C4 deficiency it is DR3;C2C;BfS;C4AQ0;C4B-1;B8.[181] Multivariate analysis of DR and C4 gene types has confirmed an independent contribution of the C4AQ0 and the DR2 antigens to the development of SLE. The C4B null gene (C4Q0) was not associated with SLE.[182] The chemical preference of the internal thiolester in C4A to form amide bonds during complement activation and to react with immune complexes may account for the contribution of the C4A null gene to the development of SLE.[28,30,31]

A preliminary report suggests that C4B deficiency may occur with increased frequency among children with bacterial meningitis. This report is particularly intriguing given the preference of C4B to form covalent ester bonds during complement activation and the abundance of available hydroxyl groups on the surface of the bacterial pathogens usually responsible for meningitis.[183]

The low frequency of infection (20 percent) in individuals with a deficiency of C1, C4, or C2 as compared with other component deficiencies (Table 3) is attributed to the presence of an intact alternative pathway in these patients. When present, bacterial infection is usually caused by encapsulated bacteria, especially *Streptococcus pneumoniae*, and may be recurrent. The most common sites of infection are the sinopulmonary tree, meninges, and blood.[165]

The molecular basis fo C4A deficiency involves gene deletion.[181] In contrast, the C2 gene appears intact in individuals with C2 deficiency and data suggest that this deficiency may be due to a defect in transcription.[184] The existence of two separate C4 genes dictates that complete C4 deficiency, that is, the

TABLE 3. Complement Deficiency States

Component	Number of Reported Patients	Mode of Inheritance	Functional Defect	Disease Associations
Classical pathway				
C1qrs	29	ACD	Impaired IC handling	CVD, 48%
C4	20	ACD	Delayed C′ activation	Infection (encaps bact), 22%
C2	90	ACD	Impaired immune response	Both, 18% Healthy, 12%
Alternative pathway				
D	2	ACD	Impaired C′ activation	Infection (meningococcal), 74%
P	41	XL	In absence of specific antibody	Healthy, 26%
Junction of classical and alternative pathways				
C3	14	ACD	Impaired IC handling opson/phag; granulocytosis, CTX, immune response, and absent SBA	CVD, 79% Recurrent infection (encaps bact), 71%
Terminal components				
C5	17	ACD	Impaired CTX; absent SBA	Infection (*Neisseria*—primarily meningococcal), 69% CVD, 4%
C6	64	ACD	Absent SBA	Both, 1%
C7	47	ACD		Healthy, 25%
C8	55	ACD		
C9	12	ACD	Impaired SBA	Healthy, 92% Infection, 8%
Plasma proteins regulating C′ activation				
C1-INH	Many	AD acq	Uncontrolled generation of an inflammatory mediator upon C′ act	Hereditary angioedema
H	5	ACD	Uncontrolled AP act → low C3[a]	CVD, 40% CVD + infection (encaps bact), 40% Healthy, 20%
I	9	ACD	Uncontrolled AP act → low C3[a]	Infection (encaps bact), 100%
Membrane proteins regulating C′ activation				
DAF HRF	Many	acq	Impaired regulation of C3b and C8 deposited on host RBC, PMN platelets → cell lysis	Paroxysmal nocturnal hemoglobinuria
CR3	>20	ACD	Impaired PMN adhesive functions i.e., margination, CTX, iC3b-mediated opson/phag	Infection (*S. aureus, Pseudomonas* sp.), 100%
Autoantibodies				
C3 nephritic factors	>59	acq	Stabilizes AP C3 convertase → low C3[a]	MPGN, 41%; PLD, 25%; infection (encaps bact), 16% MPGN + PLD, 10%; PLD + infection, 5%; MPGN + PLD + infection, 3%; MPGN + infection, 2%
C4 nephritic factor	4	acq	Stabilizes CP C3 convertase → low C3[a]	Glomerulonephritis, 50% CVD, 50%

Abbreviations: ACD: autosomal codominant; XL: X-linked; AD: autosomal dominant; acq: acquired; IC: immune complex; C′: complement; act: activation; opson/phag: opsonophagocytosis; CTX: chemotaxis; SBA: serum bactericidal activity; AP: alternative pathway; RBC: red blood cells; PMN: polymorphonuclear neutrophils; CVD: collagen vascular disease; encaps bact: encapsulated bacteria; MPGN: membrane proliferative glomerulonephritis; PLD: partial lymphodystrophy.
[a] See Table 3, Section III.
(Data updated to June 1988 from Ross et al.[165])

absence of the products of all four C4 genetic loci, is extremely rare. Conversely, the heterozygous C4 deficiency state is very common and occurs in approximately 25 percent of the general population.[185]

ALTERNATIVE-PATHWAY DEFICIENCIES

Inherited deficiencies of the components of the alternative pathway appear to be less common than those of other complement proteins, and to date, no individuals with homozygous factor B deficiency have been identified (Table 3). In the presence of specific antibody, individuals with alternative-pathway defects can activate the classic pathway normally, but the absence of antibody, coupled with the defect in alternative-pathway activation, leads to a profound defect in complement activation and serum bactericidal activity. Consequently, infection in such individuals might be expected to have dire consequences, a prediction borne out in properdin-deficient individuals (Table 4).

Properdin deficiency is unique because it is an X-linked trait. Three-quarters of properdin-deficient individuals experience infections, most of which are caused by *Neisseria meningitidis*. These infections are frequently characterized by a fulminant course and high mortality rate. Consequently, recurrent infections are uncommon.[186,187] Three properdin-deficient variants have been described: type 1 is characterized by extremely low properdin levels (<0.1 μg/ml) and absent properdin function.[186,187] The serum from individuals with type 2 deficiency contains low levels (~2 μg/ml) of antigenically detectable and functionally altered properdin. Properdin from these individuals has a normal monomeric molecular weight, but oligomer formation and size are altered. Functionally these molecules do not support alternative-pathway activation in the fluid phase but do on target particles, albeit at a slow rate.[188] Type 3 de-

TABLE 4. Comparison of Meningococcal Disease In Normal, Late Complement Component, and Properdin-Deficient Individuals

Characteristic	*Normal*	*LCCD*[a]	*Properdin Deficient*[b]
Number of homozygotes	—	195	41
Number with meningococcal disease	—	124	14–26
Frequency of infection (%)	.0072	64	34–63
Male:female ratio	1.3:1	2.8:1	14:0–25:1
Median age (yr)—first episode	3	17	14–11.5
Recurrence rate (%)	0.34	46.2	0(<2.4)
Relapse rate (%)	0.6	4.7–5.8	0(<2.4)
Mortality/100 episodes (%)	19	1.6–2.7[c]	43–65
Infecting serogroup			
# of isolates	3184	48	11
% B	50.2	20.8	27.3
% Y	4.4	41.7	27.3

[a] Late complement component deficient.
[b] Where a range is given, the first number (e.g., 14) refers to documented cases of meningococcal infection, and the second number (e.g., 26) refers to documented plus probable and possible cases of meningococcal disease.
[c] Larger estimate includes two deaths in individuals with unconfirmed LCCD. The corresponding mortality rate per 100 patients is 2.4–4.0 percent.

ficiency is characterized by normal amounts of antigenically detectable properdin (~25 μg/ml) but absent function.[189]

C3 Deficiency

C3 deficiency is uncommon (see Table 3). As expected from its position and function as the linchpin of the complement cascade, almost all individuals with this defect are seriously ill.[165] Approximately three-quarters develop SLE or a related rheumatologic syndrome. Moreover, the inability to use either the classic or alternative pathway results in a multitude of severe defects in host defense, including impairments in opsonization, immune response, neutrophil chemotaxis, and the ability to generate serum bactericidal activity. Consequently, severe and recurrent pneumococcal, *H. influenzae*, and meningococcal infections involving the sinopulmonary tree, meninges, and blood stream are common, occurring in about 70 percent of such patients.[165]

A comparable clinical picture is observed in individuals with an inherited deficiency of either factor H or factor I and in individuals who develop autoantibody to C3 (C3 nephritic factor).[165] The similar clinical picture results from uncontrolled alternative-pathway activation and the resultant low levels of C3 (less than 10 percent) in serum. Recurrent infection and collagen vascular disorders occur less commonly in individuals with C3 nephritic factor, presumably due to the somewhat higher levels of C3 in these patients. Patients with autoantibody to C3 have an increased incidence of membranoproliferative glomerulonephritis and/or partial lipodystrophy (see Table 3), although the basis for these associations has not been elucidated.[190,191]

Late Complement Component Deficiencies

With the exception of C9, individuals with a deficiency of one of the terminal complement components exhibit a striking susceptibility to systemic neisserial infection, especially meningococcal disease.[33,165] The basis for this association is the inability to express complement-dependent serum bactericidal activity. Support for this conclusion stems from the observation that the serum from C9-deficient individuals can kill meningococci, albeit at a slower rate than is normal, a finding that is consistent with the fact that C9 is not absolutely required for complement-mediated lysis of red cells and presumably accounts for the relative lack of meningococcal infection in these individuals.[128]

Complement-dependent opsonization is unimpaired in late complement component–deficient sera.[192] Nevertheless, phagocytic cells in the tissues and reticuloendothelial system do not seem to prevent neisserial infection in these patients. The reason for this apparent failure seems to be that the serum from unvaccinated and previously uninfected late component–deficient patients as well as healthy individuals contains inadequate amounts of specific IgG anticapsular antibodies. As a result C3 is not deposited on the capsule of these organisms, thereby leading to impaired opsonization as discussed earlier.[147] Bactericidal activity in healthy individuals is mediated primarily by antibodies directed at subcapsular antigens on meningococci. The level of these antibodies in healthy individuals and late complement component–deficient patients who have not experienced previous meningococcal infection are comparable.[193] Thus, the complement deficiency and resulting absence of serum bactericidal activity account for the susceptibility of these patients to meningococcal disease, but the associated lack of anticapsular antibody contributes to this susceptibility by impairing effective elimination of this organism by phagocytes. Conversely, stimulation of an anticapsular antibody response via vaccination may help to protect these individuals by recruiting the phagocytic arm of host defense.[194]

Meningococcal Infection in Complement Deficiency States

Meningococcal disease is the most common infection experienced by complement-deficient individuals (see Table 3).[165] The clinical pattern of the disease is different in complement-deficient and healthy individuals (Table 4). In particular, meningococcal disease in properdin-deficient individuals occurs in males and the first episode of infection usually occurs during the teenage years.[187] The clinical course is frequently fulminant, and there is an associated high mortality,[186,187] presumably as a consequence of low levels of specific outer membrane and anticapsular antibodies, which leads to an impaired capacity to use the classical pathway to opsonize bacteria and develop serum bactericidal activity. The severity of the disease in these individuals contrasts with that in individuals with late complement component deficiencies, presumably because the former are unable to effectively recruit any C3-dependent host defense mechanisms whereas the latter can express some of these activities.

A striking finding in individuals with late complement component deficiencies is the low mortality of meningococcal disease in these individuals as compared with healthy people.[165,171,195] This observation suggests that exuberant complement activation, which occurs frequently in meningococcal disease,[169] may contribute to mortality in healthy individuals and that this contribution is dependent in part upon assembly of an intact MAC. The first occurrence of meningococcal disease at an older age in complement-deficient individuals as compared with healthy people has not been fully explained. Group Y meningococcal disease is relatively more common among complement-deficient than among healthy individuals. The basis for the altered distribution of meningococcal serogroups appears to stem in part from the fact that group Y organisms are more serum sensitive but exhibit a more stringent requirement for elimination by phagocytic cells than do group B strains.[193] However, the absence of complement-dependent bactericidal activity in individuals with late complement component deficiencies does not automatically provide access to the blood stream by the multitude of serum-sensitive organisms present on mucosal membranes.[196] This observation suggests that the serum-sensitive organisms normally present on mucosal surfaces lack factors in addition to serum resistance determinants (e.g., tissue invasion determinants) that contribute to the pathogenesis of infection.

Other Complement Deficiency States

Hereditary Angioedema–C1 Inhibitor Deficiency. Individuals lacking C1-INH present with a distinctive noninfectious, nonrheumatologic clinical picture historically referred to as hereditary angioneurotic edema (HANE or HAE).[197] The hereditary form of this disease was recognized over 100 years ago, whereas an acquired variant has been identified as a distinct entity only within the last 25 years. The genetic form of the disease is inherited as an autosomal dominant trait and exhibits two variants. Type 1 HAE is more common and accounts for 75–85 percent of cases and is characterized by the presence of low (5–30 percent) or normal plasma levels of normally functioning C1-INH protein. In contrast, type 2 HAE is characterized by the presence of normal to elevated levels of antigenic C1-INH that is functionally abnormal.[68,197–199] The acquired forms of this disorder occur considerably less commonly, and two variants are recognized. One, occurring in association with B-lymphocyte disorders, is due to a reaction of circulating anti-idiotype antibodies, with the monoclonal immunoglobulin expressed on the surface of the abnormal B cells.[200] The resulting immune complex leads to C1-INH consumption and secondarily to the clinical picture of angioedema. The second type derives from the presence of autoantibody to the C1-INH. In this situation, angioedema develops as a consequence of inhibition of C1-INH activity.[201]

Since the hereditary form of this disorder is inherited as an autosomal dominant trait, the serum from all of these individuals contains some normally functioning C1-INH.[68] In contrast, individuals with the acquired variants have markedly reduced or absent functional C1-INH activity in their serum. As a consequence of this basic difference, the serum from individuals with the hereditary form of this disorder contains normal amounts of C1 and C1q but reduced levels of C4 and C2, whereas the serum from individuals with the acquired variants contains strikingly reduced amounts of C1, C1q, C4, and C2.[68,197–199]

The health of individuals with this disorder is punctuated by attacks of nonpitting, nonpruritic, and nonpainful edema of the extremities, face, or larynx. Angioedema of the larynx is the most severe complication of the disorder and is a common cause of death in these individuals. The gastrointestional tract may also be affected, and such attacks present as episodes of acute, crampy abdominal pain frequently associated with nausea, vomiting, and occasionally diarrhea. In the inherited form of the disorder, attacks generally begin in childhood, increase in frequency and worsen in severity during adolescence, increase during menstruation, are markedly reduced during pregnancy, and diminish gradually in the fifth and sixth decades of life. A typical attack lasts 2–3 days. Impeded androgens increase the biosynthesis of c1-INH in vitro and have been employed successfully to treat individuals with the hereditary form of the disease.[68,197]

Although C1-INH is the only recognized inhibitor of C1 esterase activity, it also participates in regulating the plasma kinin system and some of the enzymes in the coagulation and fibrinolytic cascades.[68,197] Plasma from these patients exhibits an impaired ability to inactivate kallikrein, and it has been suggested that this impairment is responsible for the manifestations of HAE. However, subcutaneous injection of bradykinin produces pain and swelling, and intravenous infusion induces hypotension, none of which are characteristic of HAE.[68] In contrast, intradermal injection of activated C1s leads to nonpainful, nonpruritic swelling in both humans and guinea pigs. This response does not occur if activated C1 is injected into C2-deficient individuals or guinea pigs, but it was observed upon injection into a C3-deficient patient.[202] Consequently, these data favor the hypothesis that the clinical manifestations of this disorder are due to the release of an anaphylatoxic-like peptide from the C2b fragment of the C2 molecule. It is also possible that symptoms result from the interaction of several factors from these cascade systems.[68]

Studies employing a cDNA probe to examine Southern digests of DNA from families with type 1 HAE[203] and studies of mutant C1-INH molecules from unrelated families with type 2 HAE[204] have shown that the genetic basis for both types of this disorder is an alteration in the structural gene for C1-INH. These studies also make it clear that the molecular basis for this alteration frequently differs among unrelated families.[204]

Paroxysmal Nocturnal Hemoglobinuria. Another syndrome in which the function of complement regulatory proteins is deranged is paroxysmal nocturnal hemoglobinuria (PNH).[205,206] The basic problem in such individuals is an increased susceptibility of their red blood cells to hemolysis. The disease is uncommon but usually presents in young adults during the third to fifth decades. Occasionally it may be observed in association with drug-induced aplastic anemia, but in most instances there is no apparent inciting event. Classically, individuals present with bouts of hemolysis that are worse at night and last for several days to weeks. The precipitating events responsible for these bouts of hemolysis are usually inapparent, although they are occasionally associated with infection. The basis for the increased hemolysis at nighttime is not clear but may relate to a lower pH in the small vessels of the peripheral venous circulation. Although this is the classic picture of the disease, the more common presentation, occurring in about half of the patients, is one of chronic hemolysis. Patients may have back pain, crampy abdominal pain, and headaches. Some of these individuals are prone to venous thrombosis, especially after surgery, while others may have slightly more frequent infections. Thrombocytopenia and/or leukopenia develop in most individuals at some point during their illness.[205,206]

The peripheral blood of individuals with PNH contains varying proportions of three populations of red blood cells. PNH type 1 cells are normal, whereas type 2 and type 3 PNH cells exhibit a 3- to 6- and 15- to 25-fold increase in sensitivity to complement-mediated lysis, respectively. The severity of the clinical picture correlates best with the proportion of type 3 cells present in the peripheral circulation.[207]

Identification of surface proteins that downregulate the effect of C3b deposited on host cells led to the discovery that types 2 and 3 PNH cells lack one of these proteins, decay-accelerating factor (DAF).[208–210] Moreover, if normal erythrocytes are treated with antibody to DAF, they behave like PNH type 2 cells, and if DAF is inserted in the membrane of type 2 cells, they behave like normal (type 1) cells. However, insertion of DAF into the membrane of PNH type 3 cells, while circumventing increased C3b uptake, has no effect on their increased susceptibility to complement-mediated lysis.[211] Thus although both PNH type 2 and 3 cells lack DAF, the greatly increased sensitivity to complement-mediated lysis, which is the physiologic basis[207,211] for the clinical manifestations of the disorder, is determined by another factor. This factor appears to be the absence of a second complement-regulatory protein, homologous restriction protein (HRP or C8 binding protein), from PNH type 3 cells.[212] Thus, the latter cells are missing two important membrane proteins that protect host cells from complement-mediated damage. Other studies have demonstrated that these cells are missing or have reduced amounts of additional surface proteins including acetycholinesterase, alkaline phosphatase, and lymphocyte function-associated antigen 3 (LFA-3).[207,211,213] Some of these molecules are missing from the surface of platelets and neutrophils isolated from patients with PNH,[209,214] a finding that may help to explain the increased susceptibility of these individuals to episodes of venous thrombosis and infection.

The fact that these molecules are present in normal amounts on human cells, for example, endothelial cells, that are not bone marrow derived supports the origin of this disorder as a clonal abnormality within bone marrow precursor cells. Recently it has been established that the surface molecules that are absent or present in reduced amounts on PNH cells are unique in that they are bound to the membrane through a carboxy terminal glycolipid linkage.[215] Thus, although the physiologic basis for the clinical symptomatology observed in this disorder is the absence of the complement-regulatory proteins from PNH cells, the molecular basis for the absence of these proteins is probably an abnormality in the metabolic pathway by which these surface proteins become anchored to the cell membrane through glycolipid linkages[216] or to a basic defect in the membrane lipids themselves, which secondarily affects this process.

Miscellaneous Deficiency States. Additional deficiency states related to the complement system include the neutrophil iC3b (CR3) receptor deficiency[217] (see Chapter 7), the deficiency of a C5a inhibitor molecule in familial Mediterranean fever,[218,219] and a deficiency of anaphylatoxin inactivator (carboxypeptidase B).[220]

COMPLEMENT IN DISEASE STATES

Complement activation has been demonstrated in a wide variety of diseases, which suggests that products of this activation may play a role in the development of symptoms or in the outcome of these disorders. Evidence supporting this suggestion includes the fact that the extent of complement activation parallels disease activity, that complement deposition can be demonstrated at the site of tissue injury, the finding of altered complement metabolism in various disease states, and the demonstration that complement activation modulates the course of disease in animal models of these disorders. In this context, the role of complement has been most extensively studied in infectious diseases, rheumatologic conditions, renal diseases, and hemolytic states. The recent demonstration of the MAC in ischemic myocardium,[221–225] renal tissue in various immune and nonimmunologic renal diseases,[226–233] the skin of individuals with immunologically mediated dermatitis,[234] the cerebrospinal fluid of individuals with central nervous system lupus erythematosus,[235] and the serum and peripheral nerves of individuals with Guillain-Barré syndrome as well as other demyelinating diseases[236–238] implicates this complex in tissue damage in these disorders.

Infectious Diseases

Complement activation probably occurs during most infections but can be particularly impressive in diseases like dengue fever, bacterial endocarditis, and bacteremia in which the organisms or their products react with antibodies to form circulating immune complexes and initiate complement consumption. Complement consumption is particularly striking in meningococcal disease and other forms of gram-negative bacteremia. Complement activation via the alternative pathway has been well documented in gram-negative sepsis, with the greatest degree of activation occurring in patients with shock.[239] Whether complement activation contributes to shock or is a consequence of the development of shock itself has been a matter of debate. Circulating C5a has been associated with the development of the acute respiratory distress syndrome in humans[240,241] and in a monkey model of gram-negative shock.[242] In the latter, mortality could be prevented and morbidity attenuated by the administration of antibody to C5a.[243] The observation that individuals with inherited C5, C6, C7, or C8 deficiency have a 6000-fold greater frequency of meningococcal disease, but 10-fold less mortality than do persons with a normal complement system (see Table 4) suggests that the ability to assemble the MAC may increase mortality.[165] The increase in mortality may relate to the release of endotoxin, which occurs upon insertion of the MAC in the outer membrane of gram-negative bacteria. Endotoxin release under such circumstances may contribute to the development of shock via its role as a potent stimulus for tumor necrosis factor synthesis[243,244] and by the continued activation of both complement pathways.

Complement, in conjunction with the organs of the reticuloendothelial system, plays a critical role in the removal of encapsulated bacteria from the blood stream.[245] Delineation of the contribution of these variables to the clearance process has been accomplished in an animal model of pneumococcal bacteremia and has demonstrated that the more virulent the organism, the greater the role of the spleen in performing this clearance function.[246,247] Complement depletion of the animals led to a significant decrease in the number of pneumococci needed to kill 50 percent of the animals, thus demonstrating an important role for complement in the clearance function. In addition, clearance of pneumococci was similar in healthy and C4-deficient animals, thus indicating that complement activation and fixation to the bacteria via the alternative pathway was particularly relevant in this process. Last, the presence of immune antibody shifted the burden of clearance from the spleen to the liver, but this effect was absolutely dependent upon a functional alternative complement pathway.[248]

An increased susceptibility to infection is observed both in individuals undergoing splenectomy as well as in individuals with intact but nonfunctioning spleens, for example, patients with sickle cell anemia.[249,250] The incidence of infection varies from a low of approximately 1 percent in individuals undergoing incidental splenectomy to a high of approximately 25 percent in individuals undergoing splenectomy as treatment for thalassemia.[250] The mortality rate in these individuals varies between 40 and 80 percent depending on the underlying condition prompting splenectomy. A wide variety of organisms have been reported to cause overwhelming sepsis in splenectomized individuals, but the pneumococcus accounts for 50–70 percent of such infections, with the bulk of the remainder being accounted for by the meningococcus, *H. influenzae*, and to a lesser extent *E. coli*.[250] The typical presentation of such individuals is that of septic shock, disseminated intravascular coagulopathy, and the adult respiratory distress syndrome occurring in the absence of a primary site of infection.[251]

Rheumatologic Disorders

Substantial clinical and experimental evidence links complement deficiency syndromes and complement activation to a variety of rheumatologic diseases, most notably SLE.[252] Additional support for this relationship is the finding that pharmacologic agents, for example, hydralazine and isoniazid, associated with the drug-induced form of SLE inactivate C4 by nucleophilic attack on its internal thiolester and formation of amide bonds.[253] Evidence that complement activation may be associated with the manifestations of the disease and tissue injury includes the demonstration of C3 and immune complex deposition at the dermal–epidermal junction in the cutaneous lesions from patients with both SLE and discoid lupus erthyematosus. Similar immunohistochemical alterations have been demonstrated in biopsy specimens of healthy skin from the same individuals. However, the recent finding of MACs in areas of affected but not unaffected skin from these individuals strengthens the hypothesis that complement activation may partly mediate tissue injury in these disorders.[235]

In addition to these effects in the tissues, the sera from about 40 percent of patients with SLE contain an inhibitor of C5a-derived chemotactic activity.[254–256] Its presence correlates with disease activity and the resultant chemotactic defect with the enhanced susceptibility of these patients to infection. The inhibitor has been identified as the Bb fragment of factor B, and it exerts its effect by blocking the interaction of C5a des-arg with its cochemotaxin in serum.[115] The presence of free Bb in the serum of these individuals reflects alternative-pathway activation and substantiates the utility of complement component quantitation in assessing disease activity.

Incorporation of C3 into immune complexes promotes their binding to C3b receptors (CR1) on erythrocytes, and the number of these receptors is reduced in individuals with disorders like SLE that are characterized by circulating immune complexes.[253,257] The degree of CR1 reduction correlates well with disease activity and the extent of complement activation. These and other data indicate that erythrocyte CR1 is removed along with immune complexes during passage through the liver and spleen. The decrease in CR1 coupled with the inability of circulating red cells to resynthesize them further exacerbates the defect in immune complex clearance, thereby promoting their deposition in the tissues, with resultant damage to the host.

Renal Disorders

Complement deposition in renal disease associated with immune disorders is related to the deposition of immune complexes within the kidney,[226–229,231–233] whereas complement deposition in the absence of immune complexes is postulated to occur by activation of the alternative pathway.[230] Recently, a rat model of chronic tubulointerstitial disease has been used to investigate the mode of complement deposition and its role in producing injury.[230] In the diseased rats, the loss of renal mass and function was correlated with increased ammonia production and systemic acidosis. Under these conditions, peritubular deposition of C3 and the MAC was readily demonstrated. However, deposition of these components and evidence of tubulointerstitial inflammation were markedly decreased in diseased animals treated with sodium bicarbonate. These and other results suggest that ammonia attacks the C3 internal thiolester to form amidated C3. Amidated C3 serves to activate the alternative complement pathway in the fluid phase, leads to C3 and C5b-9 deposition in the tissue, and elicits an inflammatory response and tissue injury.[230,258] The resulting intrarenal complement depletion may also contribute to the development of chronic bacterial pyelonephritis.[259]

Local ammonia production may also play a role in complement deposition in ischemic tissue. The mechanism of ammonia formation in such tissues involves the release of adenosine from affected cells and its deamination to ammonia by the adenosine deamidase present in circulating erthyrocytes.[260,261]

The use of C6-sufficient and -deficient rabbits and the infusion of C8-deficient serum into rats has clearly demonstrated that the development of proteinuria in membranous glomerulonephritis is dependent upon the assembly and deposition of a complete MAC on the glomerular epithelial cells.[228,232] A substantial portion of this injury results from MAC-mediated stimulation of prostaglandin and thromboxane synthesis since the proteinuria could be inhibited by treatment with indomethacin, an inhibitor of cyclo-oxygenase.[262]

Many patients with chronic renal disease ultimately require hemodialysis. Exposure of plasma to first-use filter membranes during dialysis results in complement activation.[263] Anaphylatoxins released during this process, for example, C5a, have been associated in a concentration-dependent and temporal fashion with the onset of respiratory distress in some dialysis patients.[241,263,264] This association is believed to relate in part to C5a-dependent neutrophil aggregation and stimulation and the formation of microemboli and their deposition in the lung[241] (see Chapter 7).

EVALUATION AND TREATMENT OF COMPLEMENT DISORDERS

Evaluation

Evaluation of the complement system is indicated when the diagnosis of a complement deficiency state is being considered or when specific measures of complement proteins are being used to assess disease activity or response to therapy. As pointed out earlier, several clinical clues should lead the clinician to suspect a complement deficiency state.[165] Foremost among these is a medical or family history of recurrent systemic infection caused by encapsulated bacteria, especially meningococci. A family history of fulminant meningococcal disease occurring in males in skipped generations should suggest the possibility of X-linked properdin deficiency. Meningococcal disease occurring in individuals over 10 years of age, especially when caused by non-group B meningococci, warrants evaluation of the complement system since 5–10 percent of these individuals will have a complement deficiency state, even in the absence of recurrent disease. Likewise, a history of SLE in family members or the occurrence of atypical features of SLE should also suggest the need to evaluate the complement system. Specific syndromes including partial lipodystrophy, angioedema, and PNH are other indications for the specific measurement of complement function or related activities.

Since any of a number of specific complement deficiencies can produce one of the typical clinical syndromes associated with these disorders, it is important to use a test that measures the function of the entire complement cascade during the initial evaluation of such patients. The most common of these tests is the CH_{50}, which measures the function of the classical and terminal complement pathways. When defects in the alternative pathway are being considered, an analogous test evaluating alternative-pathway function should be requested. Many hospital laboratories do not perform the latter test, so it may be necessary to contact a research or commercial laboratory with specific expertise in this area. A negative or extremely low result in either of these two assays warrants further diagnostic evaluation. The combined results of the tests of classical- and alternative-pathway function should suggest which additional tests need to be performed. If both the classical- and alternative-pathway CH_{50} values are extremely low, the defect must lie in one of the components shared by both pathways, i.e., C3 through C9 (see Fig. 1). If the alternative pathway is normal but the classical pathway is not, the deficient component must be either C1, C2, or C4. Conversely, a normal classical but defective alternative pathway suggests a defect in factors D or B, or properdin. The diagnosis of these specific defects can frequently be accomplished by using immunochemical methods to demonstrate an absence of the relevant antigen. However, several complement deficiency states involve absent function in the presence of normal amounts of antigenic protein; thus confirmation of the diagnosis of a specific component deficiency should be documented by using functional assays for the protein under consideration. Such assays usually require the expertise of a complement laboratory.

Treatment

There are two aspects of the treatment of complement deficiency states: replacement of the missing protein and prevention of infection. Although advances in our knowledge of the molecular basis for the various complement deficiency states may provide an alternative means of therapy in the future, replacement of a deficient component at the present time generally requires the infusion of fresh frozen plasma. This approach has been successfully employed in therapy for acute attacks of angioedema[68,197] and in restoring C3 levels toward normal in individuals with C3 deficiency. This approach suffers from several drawbacks. First, the half-life of most complement proteins in vivo is short,[15] although a notable exception occurs in patients with low C3 levels secondary to factor I deficiency. In these patients, replacement therapy restores factor I activity, thereby markedly reducing the accelerated breakdown of C3 that is observed in this disorder.[265] Second, replacement of a genetically absent protein may stimulate the production of antibody to the missing component, thereby limiting the value of subsequent therapy. This consideration is of limited concern in individuals with autosomally inherited disorders such as hereditary angioedema whose serum contains some normal protein or in individuals with other complement deficiency disorders characterized by the presence of antigenically normal amounts of a dysfunctional protein. Third, the relative infrequency of infection in most of these individuals must be balanced against the potential risk of acquiring non-A, non-B hepatitis or human immunodeficiency virus (HIV) infection during plasma infusion, especially since alternative modes of therapy are available. Whether the acute infusion of fresh frozen plasma might be beneficial in the treatment of life-threatening infections,[266] especially in properdin-deficient patients, remains an untested possibility. The use of impeded androgens to enhance the in vivo biosynthesis of C1-INH provides a long-term alternative approach to the replacement of this protein.[68,197,267]

Prevention of infection in complement-deficient patients is best achieved through vaccination. Deficient individuals should be vaccinated with the tetravalent meningococcal, polyvalent pneumococcal, and *Haemophilus influenzae* capsular polysaccharide vaccines. Successful vaccination leads to the production of anticapsular antibodies that promote utilization of the classical pathway in individuals with an alternative-pathway defect and facilitate alternative-pathway utilization in individuals lacking one of the classical-pathway components.[42,187] In such individuals, these antibodies may promote bactericidal activity as well as microbial elimination by enhancing opsonophagocytosis. Although anticapsular antibody cannot enhance serum bactericidal activity in individuals with a deficiency of one of the terminal complement proteins, it should promote opsonization and killing of these organisms by phagocytic cells.[193] In view of experimental evidence indicating a suboptimal response to protein and polysaccharide antigens in C1-, C2-, C4-, and C3-deficient humans and animals, documentation of the patient's response to vaccination with these antigens seems prudent.

Anecdotal evidence suggests that prophylactic antibiotics may have use in the rare complement-deficient patient who experiences several episodes of systemic infection over a short period of time.[268] However, the use of this approach is unlikely to be successful in preventing infections for prolonged periods. A potentially more important use of appropriate antibiotics is to eliminate the carrier state in complement-deficient individuals receiving treatment for systemic infections caused by meningococci or *Haemophilus influenzae*.

REFERENCES

1. Ross GD. Introduction and history of complement research. In: Ross GD, ed. Immunobiology of the Complement System. Orlando, FL: Academic Press; 1986:1–20.
2. Ratnoff WD. A war with the molecules: Louis Pillemer and the history of properdin. Perspect Biol Med. 1980;23:638–57.
3. Lepow IH. Louis Pillemer, properdin, and scientific controversy. J Immunol. 1980;125:471–8.
4. Root RK, Ryan JL. Humoral immunity and complement. In: Mandell GL, Douglas RG Jr, Bennett JE, eds. Principles and Practice of Infectious Diseases. 2nd ed. New York: Churchill Livingstone; 1985:31–56.
5. Morris KM, Aden DP, Knowles BB, et al. Complement biosynthesis by the human hepatoma-derived cell line HepG2. J Clin Invest. 1982;70:906–13.
6. Perlmutter DH, Colten HR. Molecular immunobiology of complement biosynthesis: A model of single-cell control of effector–inhibitor balance. Annu Rev Immunol. 1986;4:231–51.
7. Alper CA, Raum D, Awdeh ZL, et al. Studies of hepatic synthesis in vivo of plasma proteins, including orosomucoid, transferrin, α_1-antitrypsin, C8, and factor B. Clin Immunol Immunopathol. 1980;16:84–9.
8. Mier JW, Dinarello CA, Atkins MB, et al. Regulation of hepatic acute phase protein synthesis by products of interleukin 2 (IL 2)-stimulated human peripheral blood mononuclear cells. J Immunol. 1987;139:1268–72.
9. Baumann H, Richards C, Gauldie J. Interaction among hepatocyte-stimulating factors, interleukin 1, and glucocorticoids for regulation of acute phase plasma proteins in human hepatoma (HepG2) cells. J Immunol. 1987;139:4122–8.
10. Beatty DW, Davis AE III, Cole FS, et al. Biosynthesis of complement by human monocytes. Clin Immunol Immunopathol. 1981;18:334–43.
11. Cole FS, Auerbach HS, Goldberger G, et al. Tissue-specific pretranslational regulation of complement production in human mononuclear phagocytes. J Immunol. 1985;134:2610–6.
12. Strunk RC, Cole FS, Perlmutter DH, et al. γ-Interferon increases expression of class III complement genes C2 and factor B in human monocytes and in murine fibroblasts transfected with human C2 and factor B genes. J Biol. Chem. 1985;260:15280–5.
13. Strunk RC, Whitehead AS, Cole FS. Pretranslational regulation of the synthesis of the third component of complement in human mononuclear phagocytes by the lipid A portion of lipopolysaccharide. J Clin Invest. 1985;76:985–90.
14. Hetland G, Eskeland T. Formation of the functional alternative pathway of complement by human monocytes in vitro as demonstrated by phagocytosis of agarose beads. Scand J Immunol. 1986;23:301–8.
15. Ruddy S, Carpenter CB, Chin KW, et al. Human complement metabolism: An analysis of 144 studies. Medicine (Baltimore). 1975;54:165–78.
16. Notarangelo LD, Chirico G, Chaira A, et al. Activity of classical and alternative pathways of complement in preterm and small for gestational age infants. Pediatr Res. 1984;18:281–5.
17. Johnston RB Jr, Altenburger KM, Atkinson AW Jr, et al. Complement in the newborn infant. Pediatrics. 1979;64(Pt 2, Suppl):781–6.
18. Mills EL, Björksten B, Quie PG. Deficient alternative complement pathway activity in newborn sera. Pediatr Res. 1979;13:1341–4.
19. Edwards MS, Buffone GJ, Fuselier PA, et al. Deficient classical complement pathway activity in newborn sera. Pediatr Res. 1983;17:685–8.
20. Fearon DT. Complement. J Allergy Clin Immunol. 1983;71:520–9.
21. Lachmann PJ, Hughes-Jones NC. Initiation of complement activation. Springer Semin Immunopathol. 1984;7:143–62.
22. Cooper NR. The classical complement pathway: Activation and regulation of the first complement component. Adv Immunol. 1985;37:151–216.
23. Arlaud GJ, Colomb MG, Gagnon J. A functional model of the human C1 complex. Immunol Today. 1987;8:106–11.
24. Schumaker VN, Zavodszky, P, Poon RH. Activation of the first component of complement. Annu Rev Immunol. 1987;5:21–42.
25. Müller-Eberhard HJ. Molecular organization and function of the complement system. Annu Rev Biochem. 1988;57:321–47.
26. Gordon DL, Hostetter MK. Complement and host defense against microorganisms. *Pathology*. 1986,18:365–75.
27. Isenman DE, Young JR. The molecular basis for the difference in immune hemolysis activity of the Chido and Rodgers isotypes of human complement component C4. J Immunol. 1984;132:3019–27.
28. Law SKA, Dodds AW, Porter RR. A comparison of the properties of two classes, C4A and C4B, of the human complement component C4. EMBO J. 1984;3:1819–23.
29. Dodds AW, Law SK, Porter RR. The origin of the very variable haemolytic activities of the common human complement component C4 allotypes including C4-A6. EMBO J. 1985;4:2239–44.
30. Schifferli JA, Steiger G, Paccaud J-P, et al. Difference in the biological properties of the two forms of the fourth component of human complement (C4). Clin Exp Immunol. 1986;63:473–7.
31. Schifferli JA, Hauptmann G, Paccaud J-P. Complement-mediated adherence of immune complexes to human erythrocytes. FEBS Lett. 1987;213:415–8.
32. Naama JK, Niven IP, Zoma A, et al. Complement, antigen–antibody complexes and immune complex disease. J Clin Lab Immunol. 1985;17:59–67.
33. Pangburn MK, Müller-Eberhard HJ. The alternative pathway of complement. Springer Semin Immunopathol. 1984;7:163–92.
34. Pangburn MK. The alternative pathway. In: Ross GD, ed. Immunobiology of the Complement System. Orlando, FL: Academic Press; 1986:45–62.
35. Densen P, McRill C, Ross SC. The contribution of the alternative and classical complement pathways to gonococcal killing and C3 fixation. In: Poolman JT, Zanen HC, Meyer TF, et al, eds. Gonococci and Meningococci. Dordrecht: Kluwer Academic Publishers; 1988:693–7.
36. Fearon DT, Austen KF. Properdin: Initiation of alternative complement pathway. Immunology. 1975;72:3220–4.
37. Fearon DT, Austen KF. Properdin: Binding to C3b and stabilization of the C3b-dependent C3 convertase. J Exp Med. 1975;142:856–63.
38. Fearon DT, Austen KF. The alternative pathway of complement—a system for host resistance to microbial infection. N Engl J Med. 1980;303:259–63.
39. Hunsicker LG, Ruddy S, Austen KF. Alternate complement pathway: Factors involved in cobra venom factor (CoVF) activation of the third component of complement (C3). J Immunol. 1973;110:128–38.
40. Müller-Eberhard HJ, Schreiber. Molecular biology and chemistry of the alternative pathway of complement. Adv Immunol. 1980;29:1–53.
41. Vogel C-W, Smith CA, Müller-Eberhard HJ. Cobra venom factor: Structural homology with the third component of human complement. J Immunol. 1984;133:3235–41.
42. Söderström C, Braconier JH, Danielsson D, et al. Bactericidal activity for *Neisseria meningitidis* in properdin-deficient sera. J Infect Dis. 1987;156:107–12.
43. Schenkein HA, Ruddy S. The role of immunoglobulins in alternative complement pathway activation by zymosan. II. The effect of IgG on the kinetics of the alternative pathway. J Immunol. 1981;126:11–5.
44. Ratnoff WD, Fearon DT, Austen KF. The role of antibody in the activation of the alternative complement pathway. Springer Semin Immunopathol. 1983;6:361–71.

45. Winkelstein JA, Shin HS. The role of immunoglobulin in the interaction of pneumococi and the properdin pathway: Evidence for its specificity and lack of requirement for the Fc portion of the molecule. J Immunol. 1974;112:1635–42.
46. Nelson B, Ruddy S. Enhancing role of IgG in lysis of rabbit erythrocytes by the alternative pathway of human complement. J Immunol. 1979;122:1994–9.
47. Schenkein HA, Ruddy S. The role of immunoglobulins in alternative complement pathway activation by zymosan. I. Human IgG with specificity for zymosan enhances alternative pathway activation by zymosan. J Immunol. 1981;126:7–10.
48. Nicholson-Weller A, Daha MR, Austen KF. Different functions for specific guinea pig IgG1 and IgG2 in the lysis of sheep erythrocytes by C4-deficient guinea pig serum. J Immunol. 1981;126:1800–4.
49. Capel PJA, Groeneboer O, Grosveld G, et al. The binding of activated C3 to polysaccharides and immunoglobulins. J Immunol. 1978;121:2566–72.
50. Fries LF, Gaither TA, Hammer CH, et al. C3b covalently bound to IgG demonstrates a reduced rate of inactivation by factors H and I. J Exp Med. 1984;160:1640–55.
51. Joiner KA, Fries LF, Schmetz MA, et al. IgG bearing covalently bound C3b has enhanced bactericidal activity for *Escherichia coli* 0111. J Exp Med. 1985;162:877–89.
52. Lambris JD, Müller-Eberhard HJ. The multifunctional role of C3: Structural analysis of its interactions with physiological ligands. Mol Immunol. 1986;23:1237–42.
53. Suter S, Nydegger UE, Roux L, et al. Cleavage of C3 by neutral proteases from granulocytes in pleural empyema. J Infect Dis. 1981;144:499–508.
54. Manthei U, Strunk RC, Giclas PC. Acute local inflammation alters synthesis, distribution, and catabolism of the third component of complement in rabbits. J Clin Invest. 1984;74:424–3.
55. Wetsel RA, Lemons RS, Le Beau MM, et al. Molecular analysis of human complement component C5: Localization of the structural gene to chromosome 9. Biochemistry. 1988;27:1474–82.
56. Lundwall AB, Wetsel RA, Kristensen T, et al. Isolation and sequence analysis of a cDNA clone encoding the fifth complement component. J Biol Chem. 1985;260:2108–12.
57. Müller-Eberhard HJ. The membrane attack complex of complement. Annu Rev Immunol. 1986;4:503–28.
58. Stanley K, Luzio P. A family of killer proteins. Nature. 1988;334:475–6.
59. Tschopp J, Mollnes T-E. Antigenic crossreactivity of the α subunit of complement component C8 with the cysteine-rich domain shared by complement component C9 and low density lipoprotein receptor. Proc Natl Acad Sci USA. 1986;83:4223–7.
60. Haefliger J-A, Tschopp J, Nardelli D, et al. Complementary DNA cloning of complement C8β and its sequence homology to C9. Biochemistry. 1987;26:3551–6.
61. Monahan JB, Sodetz JM. Binding of the eighth component of human complement to the soluble cytolytic complex is mediated by its β subunit. J Biol Chem. 1980;255:10579–82.
62. Stewart JL, Kolb WP, Sodetz JM. Evidence that C5b recognizes and mediates C8 incorporation into the cytolytic complex of complement. J Immunol. 1987;139:1960–4.
63. Stewart JL, Sodetz JM. Analysis of the specific association of the eighth and ninth components of human complement: Identification of a direct role for the α subunit of C8. Biochemistry 1985;24:4598–602.
64. Stanley KK, Page M, Campbell AK, et al. A mechanism for the insertion of complement component C9 into target membranes. Mol Immunol. 1986;23:451–8.
65. Podack ER. The molecular mechanism of lymphocyte-mediated tumor cell lysis. Immunol Today. 1985;6:21–7.
66. Tschopp J, Masson D, Stanley KK. Structural/functional similarity between proteins involved in complement- and cytotoxic T-lymphocyte-mediated cytolysis. Nature 1986;322:831–4.
67. Shinkai Y, Takio K, Okumura K. Homology of perforin to the ninth component of complement (C9). Nature. 1988;334:525–7.
68. Davis AE III. C1 inhibitor and hereditary angioneurotic edema. Annu Rev Immunol 1988;6:595–628.
69. Holers VM, Cole JL, Lublin DM, et al. Human C3b- and C4b-regulatory proteins: A new multi-gene family. Immunol Today. 1985;6:188–92.
70. Atkinson JP, Farries T. Separation of self from non-self in the complement system. Immunol Today. 1987;8:212–5.
71. Nicholson-Weller A, Burge J, Fearon DT, et al. Isolation of a human erythrocyte membrane glycoprotein with decay-accelerating activity for C3 convertases of the complement system. J Immunol. 1982;129:184–9.
72. Bhakdi S, Maillet F, Muhly M, et al. The cytolytic C5b-9 complement complex: Feedback inhibition of complement activation. Proc Natl Acad Sci USA. 1988;85:1912–6.
73. Densen P, McRill CM, Ross SC. Assembly of the membrane attack complex promotes decay of the alternative pathway C3 convertase on *Neisseria gonorrhoeae*. J Immunol. 1988;141:3902–9.
74. Fearon DT, Austen KF. Activation of the alternative complement pathway with rabbit erythrocytes by circumvention of the regulatory action of endogenous control proteins. J Exp Med 1977;146:22–33.
75. Fearon DT. Regulation by membrane sialic acid of β1H-dependent decay-dissociation of amplification C3 convertase of the alternative complement pathway. Proc Natl Acad Sci USA. 1978;75:1971–5.
76. Kazatchkine MD, Fearon DT, Austen KF. Human alternative complement pathway: membrane-associated sialic acid regulates the competition between B and β1H for cell-bound C3b. J Immunol 1979;122:75–81.
77. Pangburn MK, Morrison DC, Schreiber RD, et al. Activation of the alternative complement pathway: Recognition of surface structures on activators by bound C3b. J Immunol. 1980;124:977–82.
78. Brown EJ, Ramsey J, Hammer CH, et al. Surface modulation of classical pathway activation: C2 and C3 convertase formation and regulation on sheep, guinea pig, and human erythrocytes. J Immunol. 1983;131:403–8.
79. Schönermark S, Rauterberg EW, Shin ML, et al. Homologous species restriction in lysis of human erythrocytes: A membrane-derived protein with C8-binding capacity functions as an inhibitor. J Immunol. 1986;136:1772–6.
80. Shin ML, Hänsch G, Hu VW, et al. Membrane factors responsible for homologous species restriction of complement-mediated lysis: Evidence for a factor other than DAF operating at the stage of C8 and C9. J Immunol. 1986;136:1777–82.
81. Zalman LS, Wood LM, Müller-Eberhard HJ. Isolation of a human erythrocyte membrane protein capable of inhibiting expression of homologous complement transmembrane channels. Proc. Natl Acad Sci USA. 1986;83:6975–9.
82. Hänsch GM, Hammer CH, Vanguri P, et al. Homologous species restriction in lysis of erythrocytes by terminal complement proteins. Proc Natl Acad Sci USA. 1981;78:5118–21.
83. Carney DF, Koski CL, Shin ML. Elimination of terminal complement intermediates from the plasma membrane of nucleated cells: The rate of disappearance differs for cells carrying C5b-7 or C5b-8 or a mixture of C5b-8 with a limited number of C5b-9. J Immunol 1985;134:1804–9.
84. Ramm LE, Whitlow MB, Koski CL, et al. Elimination of complement channels from the plasma membranes of U937, a nucleated mammalian cell line: Temperature dependence of the elimination rate. J Immunol. 1983;131:1411–5.
85. Schlager SI, Ohanian SH, Borsos T. Correlations between the ability of tumor cells to resist humoral immune attack and their ability to synthesize lipid. J Immunol. 1978;120:463–71.
86. Campbell AK, Luzio JP. Intracellular free calcium as a pathogen in cell damage initiated by the immune system. Experientia. 1981;37:1110–2.
87. Imagawa DK, Osifchin NE, Paznekas WA, et al. Consequences of cell membrane attack by complement: Release of arachidonate and formation of inflammatory derivatives. Proc Natl Acad Sci USA. 1983;80:6647–51.
88. Betz M, Hansch GM. Release of arachidonic acid: A new function of the late complement components. Immunobiology. 1984;166:473–83.
89. Hänsch GM, Seitz M, Martinotti G, et al. Macrophages release arachidonic acid, prostaglandin E_2, and thromboxane in response to late complement components. J Immunol. 1984;133:2145–50.
90. Suttorp N, Seeger W, Zinsky S, et al. Complement complex C5b-8 induces PGI_2 formation in cultured endothelial cells. Am J Physiol. 1987;253:13–32.
91. Fearon DT, Wong WW. Complement ligand-receptor interactions that mediate biological responses. Annu Rev Immunol. 1983;1:243–71.
92. Gresham HD, Volanakis JE. Structure and function of human complement receptors: 1985. Year Immunol. 1986;2:177–86.
93. Ross GD, Medof ME. Membrane complement receptors specific for bound fragments of C3. Adv Immunol. 1985;37:217–67.
94. Wilson JG, Andriopoulos NA, Fearon DT. CR1 and the cell membrane proteins that bind C3 and C4. A basic and clinical review. Immunol Res. 1987;6:192–209.
95. Jack RM, Ezzell RM, Hartwig J, et al. Differential interaction of the C3b/C4b receptor and MHC class I with the cytoskeleton of human neutrophils. J Immunol. 1986;137:3996–4003.
96. Hynes RO. Integrins: A family of cell surface receptors. Cell 1987;48:549–54.
97. Wright SD, Reddy A, Jong MTC, et al. C3bi receptor (complement receptor type 3) recognizes a region of complement protein C3 containing the sequence Arg-Gly-Asp. Proc Natl Acad Sci USA. 1987;84:1965–68.
98. Ruoslahti E, Pierschbacher MD. Arg-Gly-Asp: A versatile cell recognition signal. Cell. 1986;44:517–8.
99. Myones BL, Dalzell JG, Hogg N, et al. Neutrophil and monocyte cell surface p150,95 has iC3b-receptor (CR4) activity resembling CR3. J Clin Invest. 1988;81:640–51.
100. Cooper NR, Moore MD, Nemerow GR. Immunobiology of CR2, the B lymphocyte receptor for Epstein-Barr virus and the C3d complement fragment. Annu Rev Immunol. 1988;6:85–113.
101. Fingeroth JD, Weis JJ, Tedder TF, et al. Epstein-Barr virus receptor of human B lymphocytes is the C3d receptor CR2. Proc Natl Acad Sci USA. 1984;81:4510–4.
102. Hugli TE. Biological activities of fragments derived from human complement components. Prog Immunol. 1983:419–26.
103. Perlmutter DH, Colten HR. Complement molecular genetics. In: Gallin JI, Goldstein IM, Snyderman R, eds. Inflammation: Basic Principles and Clinical Correlates. New York: Raven Press; 1988:75–88.
104. Campbell RD. The molecular genetics and polymorphism of C2 and Factor B. Br Med Bull. 1987;43:37–49.
105. Campbell RD, Law SKA, Reid KBM et al. Structure, organization, and regulation of the complement genes. Annu Rev Immunol. 1988;6:161–95.
106. Spies T, Morton CC, Nedospasov SA, et al. Genes for the tumor necrosis factors α and β are linked to the human major histocompatibility complex. Proc Natl Acad Sci USA. 1986;83:8699–702.
107. Awdeh ZL, Raum D, Yunis EJ, et al. Extended HLA/complement allele

haplotypes: Evidence for T/t-like complex in man. Proc Natl Acad Sci USA. 1983;80:259–63.
108. Alper CA, Raum D, Karp S, et al. Serum complement 'supergenes' of the major histocompatibility complex in man (complotypes). Vox Sang. 1983;45:62–7.
109. Porter RR. Complement polymorphism, the major histocompatibility complex and associated diseases: A speculation. Mol Biol Med. 1983;1:161–68.
110. Kristensen T, D'Eustachio P, Ogata RT, et al. The superfamily of C3b/C4b-binding proteins. Fed Proc. 1987;46:2463–9
111. Reid KBM, Bentley DR, Campbell RD, et al. Complement system proteins which interact with C3b or C4b. A superfamily of structurally related proteins. Immunol Today. 1986;7:230–4.
112. Perez HD, Chenoweth DE, Goldstein IM. Attachment of human C5a des Arg to its cochemotaxin is required for maximum expression of chemotactic activity. J Clin Invest. 1986;78:1589–95.
113. Perez HD, Kelly E, Chenoweth D, et al. Identification of the C5a des Arg cochemotaxin. Homology with vitamin D-binding protein (group-specific component globulin). J Clin Invest. 1988;82:360–3.
114. Kew RR, Webster RO. Ge-globulin (vitamin D-binding protein) enhances the neutrophil chemotactic activity of C5a and C5a des Arg. J Clin Invest. 1988;82:364–9.
115. Perez HD, Hooper C, Volanakis J, et al. Specific inhibitor of complement (C5)-derived chemotactic activity in systemic lupus erythematosus related antigenically to the Bb fragment of human factor B. J Immunol. 1987;139:484–9.
116. Miller GW, Nusenzweig V. A new complement function: Solubilization of antigen–antibody aggregates. Proc Natl Acad Sci USA. 1975;72:418–22.
117. Schifferli JA, Ng YC, Peters DK. The role of complement and its receptor in the elimination of immune complexes. N Engl J Med. 1986;315:488–95.
118. Siegel I, Liu TL, Gleicher N. The red-cell immune system. Lancet. 1981;2:556–9.
119. Cornacoff JB, Hebert LA, Smead WL, et al. Primate erythrocyte-immune complex-clearing mechanism. J Clin Invest. 1983;71:236–47.
120. Weiler JM, Ballas ZK, Needleman BW, et al. Complement fragments suppress lymphocyte immune responses. Immunol Today. 1982;3:238–43.
121. Laham MN, Caldwell JR, Panush RS. Modulation of lymphocyte proliferative responses to mitogens and antigens by complement components C1, C4 and C2. J Clin Lab Immunol. 1982;9:39–47.
122. Papamichail M, Gutierrez C, Embling P, et al. Complement dependence of localisation of aggregated IgG in germinal centres. Scand J Immunol. 1975;4:343–7.
123. Ochs HD, Wedgwood RJ, Frank MM, et al. The role of complement in the induction of antibody responses. Clin Exp Immunol. 1983;53:208–16.
124. Böttger EC, Bitter-Suermann D. Complement and the regulation of humoral immune responses. Immunol Today. 1987;8:261–4.
124a. O'Neil KM, Ochs HD, Heller SR, et al. Role of C3 in humoral immunity defective antibody production in C3-deficient dogs. J Immunol. 1988;140:1939–45.
125. Ochs HD, Wedgwood RJ, Heller SR, et al. Complement, membrane glycoproteins, and complement receptors: Their role in regulation of the immune response. Clin Immunol Immunopathol. 1986;40:94–104.
126. Hostetter MK, Krueger RA, Schmeling DJ. The biochemistry of opsonization: Central role of the reactive thiolester of the third component of complement. J Infect Dis. 1984;150:653–61.
127. Taylor PW. Bactericidal and bacteriolytic activity of serum against gram-negative bacteria. Microbiol Rev. 1983;47:46–83.
128. Harriman GR, Esser AF, Podack ER, et al. The role of C9 in complement-mediated killing of *Neisseria*. J Immunol. 1981;127:2386–90.
129. Cooper NR, Nemerow GR. Complement-dependent mechanisms of virus neutralization. In: Ross GD, ed. Immunobiology of the Complement System. Orlando, FL: Academic Press; 1986:139–62.
130. Roantree RJ, Rantz LA. A study of the relationship of the normal bactericidal activity of human serum to bacterial infection. J Clin Invest. 1960;39:72–81.
131. Brown EJ. Interaction of gram-positive microorganisms with complement. Curr Top Microbiol Immunol. 1985;121:159–87.
132. Joiner KA, Grossman N, Schmetz M, et al. C3 binds preferentially to long-chain lipopolysaccharide during alternative pathway activation by *Salmonella montevideo*. J Immunol. 1986;136:710–5.
133. Brown EJ, Joiner KA, Frank MM. The role of complement in host resistance to bacteria. Springer Semin Immunopathol. 1983;6:349–60.
134. Schoolnik GK, Buchanan TM, Holmes KK. Gonococci causing disseminated gonococcal infection are resistant to the bactericidal action of normal human sera. J Clin Invest. 1976;58:1163–73.
135. Joiner KA, Warren KA, Brown EJ, et al. Studies on the mechanism of bacterial resistance to complement-mediated killing. IV. C5b-9 forms high molecular weight complexes with bacterial outer membrane constituents on serum-resistant but not on serum-sensitive *Neisseria gonorrhoeae*. J Immunol. 1983;131:1443–51.
136. Harriman GR, Podack ER, Braude AI, et al. Activation of complement by serum-resistant *Neisseria gonorrhoeae*. J Exp Med. 1982;156:1235–49.
137. Rice PA, Kasper DL. Characterization of gonococcal antigens responsible for induction of bactericidal antibody in disseminated infection. J Clin Invest. 1977;60:1149–58.
138. Densen P, Gulati S, Rice PA. Specificity of antibodies against *Neisseria gonorrhoeae* that stimulate neutrophil chemotaxis. Role of antibodies directed against lipooligosaccharides. J Clin Invest. 1987;80:78–87.
139. Frank MM, Joiner K, Hammer C. The function of antibody and complement in the lysis of bacteria. Rev Infect Dis. 1987;9(Suppl5):537–45.
140. Rice PA, Kasper KL. Characterization of serum resistance of *Neisseria gonorrhoeae* that disseminate. Roles of blocking antibody and gonococcal outer membrane proteins. J Clin Invest. 1982;70:157–67.
141. Rice PA, Vayo HE, Tam MR, et al. Immunoglobulin G antibodies directed against protein III block killing of serum-resistant *Neisseria gonorrhoeae* by immune serum. J Exp Med. 1986;164:1735–48.
142. Joiner KA, Scales R, Warren KA, et al. Mechanism of action of blocking immunoglobulin G for *Neisseria gonorrhoeae*. J Clin Invest. 1985;76:1765–72.
143. Griffiss MJ, Bertram MA. Immunoepidemiology of meningococcal disease in military recruits. II. Blocking of serum bactericidal activity by circulating IgA early in the course of invasive disease. J Infect Dis. 1977;136:733–9.
144. Griffiss JM. Epidemic meningococcal disease: Synthesis of a hypothetical immunoepidemiologic model. Rev Infect Dis. 1982;4:159–72.
145. Griffiss JM, Goroff DK. IgA blocks IgM and IgG-initiated immune lysis by separate molecular mechanisms. J Immunol. 1983;130:2882–5.
146. Griffiss JM. Bactericidal activity of meningococcal antisera. Blocking by IgA of lytic antibody in human convalescent sera. J Immunol. 1975;114:1779–84.
147. Brown EJ, Joiner KA, Cole RM, et al. Localization of complement component 3 on *Streptococcus pneumoniae*: Anti-capsular antibody causes complement deposition on the pneumococcal capsule. Infect Immun. 1983;39:403–9.
148. Joiner K, Hieny S, Kirchhoff LV, et al. gp72, the 72 kilodalton glycoprotein, is the membrane acceptor site for C3 on *Trypanosoma cruzi* epimastigotes. J Exp Med. 1985;161:1196–212.
149. Sher A, Hieny S, Joiner K. Evasion of the alternative complement pathway by metacyclic trypomastigotes of *Trypanosoma cruzi*: Dependence on the developmentally regulated synthesis of surface protein and N-linked carbohydrate. J Immunol. 1986;137:2961–7.
150. Joiner K, Sher A, Gaither T, et al. Evasion of alternative complement pathway by *Trypanosoma cruzi* results from inefficient binding of Factor B. Proc Natl Acad Sci USA. 1986;83:6593–7.
151. Leive LL, Jimenez-Lucho VE. Lipopolysaccharide O-antigen structure controls alternative pathway activation of complement: Effects on phagocytosis and virulence of *Salmonella*. In: Leive L, ed. Microbiology. Washington, DC: American Society for Microbiology; 1986:14–7.
152. Liang-Takasaki C-J, Mäkelä PH, Leive L. Phagocytosis of bacteria by macrophages: Changing the carbohydrate of lipopolysaccharide alters interaction with complement and macrophages. J Immunol. 1982;128:1229–35.
153. Liang-Takasaki C-J, Saxén H, Mäkelä PH, et al. Complement activation by polysaccharide of lipopolysaccharide: An important virulence determinant of *Salmonella*. Infect Immun. 1983;41:563–9.
154. Grossman N, Leive L. Complement activation via the alternative pathway by purified *Salmonella* lipopolysaccharide is affected by its structure but not its O-antigen length. J Immunol. 1984;132:376–85.
155. Grossman N, Joiner KA, Frank MM, et al. C3b binding, but not its breakdown, is affected by the structure of the O-antigen polysaccharide in lipopolysaccharide from *Salmonella*. J Immunol. 1986;136:2208–15.
156. Jimenez-Lucho VE, Joiner KA, Foulds J, et al. C3b generation is affected by the structure of the O-antigen polysaccharide in lipopolysaccharide from *Samonella*. J Immunol. 1987;139:1253–9.
157. Jarvis GA, Vedros NA. Sialic acid of group B *Neisseria meningitidis* regulates alternative complement pathway activation. Infect Immun. 1987;55:174–80.
158. Edwards MS, Kasper DL, Jennings HJ, et al. Capsular sialic acid prevents activation of the alternative complement pathway by type III, group B streptococci. J Immunol. 1982;128:1278–83.
159. Hostetter MK. Serotypic variations among virulent pneumococci in deposition and degradation of covalently bound C3b: Implications for phagocytosis and antibody production. J Infect Dis. 1986;153:682–93.
160. Friedman HM, Cohen GH, Eisenberg RJ, et al. Glycoprotein C of herpes simplex virus 1 acts as a receptor for the C3b complement component on infected cells. Nature. 1984;309:633–5.
161. Friedman HM, Glorioso JC, Cohen GH, et al. Binding of complement component C3b to glycoprotein gC of herpes simplex virus type 1: Mapping of gC-binding sites and demonstration of conserved C3b binding in low-passage clinical isolates. J Virol. 1986;60:470–5.
162. Edwards JE Jr, Gaither TA, O'Shea JJ, et al. Expression of specific binding sites on candida with functional and antigenic characteristics of human complement receptors. J Immunol. 1986;137:3577–83.
163. McNearney TA, Odell C, Holers VM, et al. Herpes simplex virus glycoproteins gC-1 and gC-2 bind to the third component of complement and provide protection against complement-mediated neutralization of viral infectivity. J Exp Med. 1987;166:1525–35.
164. Gilmore BJ, Retsinas EM, Lorenz JS, et al. An iC3b receptor on *Candida albicans*: Structure, function, and correlates for pathogenicity. J Infect Dis. 1988;157:38–46.
165. Ross SC, Densen P. Complement deficiency states and infection: Epidemiology, pathogenesis and consequences of neisserial and other infections in an immune deficiency. Medicine (Baltimore). 1984;63:243–73.
166. Glass D, Raum D, Gibson D, et al. Inherited deficiency of the second component of complement. J Clin Invest. 1976;58:853–61.
167. Cornacoff JB, Hebert LA, Smead WL, et al. Primate erythrocyte-immune complex-clearing mechanism. J Clin Invest 1983;71:236–47.

168. Ellison RT III, Kohler PF, Curd JG, et al. Prevalence of congenital or acquired complement deficiency in patients with sporadic meningococcal disease. N Engl J Med. 1983;308:913–6.
169. Beatty DW, Rynder CR, Hesse HDV. Complement abnormalities during an epidemic of group B meningococcal infection in children. Clin Exp Immunol. 1985;64:465–70.
170. Møller M, Rasmussen J, Brandslund I, et al. Screening for complement deficiencies in unselected patients with meningitis. Clin Exp Immunol. 1987;68:437–45.
171. Zimran A, Rudensky B, Kramer MR, et al. Hereditary complement deficiency in survivors of meningococcal disease: High prevalence of C7/C8 deficiency in sephardic (Moroccan) Jews. Q J Med. 1987;63:349–58.
172. Merino J, Rodriguez-Valverde V, Lamelas JA, et al. Prevalence of deficits of complement components in patients with recurrent meningococcal infections. J Infect Dis. 1983;148:331.
173. Agnello v. Complement deficiency states. Medicine (Baltimore). 1978;57:1–23.
174. Agnello V. Lupus diseases associated with hereditary and acquired deficiencies of complement. Springer Semin Immunopathol. 1986;9:161–78.
175. Provost TT, Arnett FC, Reichlin M. Homozygous C2 deficiency, lupus erythematosus, and anti-Ro (SSA) antibodies. Arthritis Rheum. 1983;26:1279–82.
176. Davis AE III. The efficiency of complement activation in MHC-linked diseases. Immunol Today. 1983;4:250–2.
177. Schifferli JA, Peters DK. Complement, the immune-complex lattice, and the pathophysiology of complement-deficiency syndromes. Lancet. 1983;2:957–9.
178. Schifferli JA, Steiger G, Hauptmann G, et al. Formation of soluble immune complexes by complement in sera of patients with various hypocomplementemic states. J Clin Invest. 1985;76:2127–33.
179. Böttger EC, Hoffmann T, Hadding U, et al. Guinea pigs with inherited deficiencies of complement components C2 or C4 have characteristics of immune complex disease. J Clin Invest. 1986;78:689–95.
180. Awdeh ZL, Raum DD, Glass D, et al. Complement-human histocompatibility antigen haplotypes in C2 deficiency. J Clin Invest. 1981;67:581–3.
181. Kemp ME, Atkinson JP, Skanes VM, et al. Deletion of C4A genes in patients with systemic lupus erythematosus. Arthritis Rheum. 1987;30:1015–22.
182. Howard PF, Hochberg MC, Bias WB, et al. Relationship between C4 null genes, HLA-D region antigens, and genetic susceptibility to systemic lupus erythematosus in Caucasian and Black Americans. Am J Med. 1986;81:187–93.
183. Rowe PC, McLean RH, Wood RA, et al. Association of C4B deficiency with bacterial meningitis (Abstract). Pediatr Res. 1988;23:360.
184. Cole FS, Whitehead AS, Auerbach HS, et al. The molecular basis for genetic deficiency of the second component of human complement. N Engl J Med. 1985;313:11–6.
185. Hauptmann G, Goetz J, Uring-Lambert B, et al. Component deficiencies. 2. The fourth component. Progr Allergy. 1986;39:232–49.
186. Sjöholm, AG, Braconier J-H, Söderström C. Properdin deficiency in a family with fulminant meningococcal infections. Clin Exp Immunol. 1982;50:291–7.
187. Densen P, Weiler JM, Griffiss JM, et al. Familial properdin deficiency and fatal meningococcemia. Correction of the bactericidal defect by vaccination. N Engl J Med. 1987;316:922–6.
188. Sjöholm, AG, Söderström, C. Nilsson L-A. A second variant of properdin deficiency: The detection of properdin at low concentration in affected males. Complement. 1988;5:130–40.
189. Sjöholm AG, Kuijper EJ, Tijssen CC, et al. Dysfunctional properdin in a Dutch family with meningococcal disease. N Engl J Med. 1988;319:33–7.
190. Sissons JGP, West RJ, Fallow J, et al. The complement abnormalities of lipodystrophy. N Engl J Med. 1976;294:461–5.
191. Ipp MM, Minta JO, Gelfand EW. Disorders of the complement system in lipodystrophy. Clin Immunol Immunopathol. 1977;7:281–7.
192. Nicholson A, Lepow IH. Host defense against *Neisseria meningitidis* requires a complement-dependent bactericidal activity. Science. 1979;205:298–9.
193. Densen P. Interaction of complement with *Neisseria meningitidis* and *Neisseria gonorrhoeae*. Clin Microbiol Rev. 1989;2:(April, in press).
194. Ross SC, Rosenthal PJ, Berberich HM, et al. Killing of *Neisseria meningitidis* by human neutrophils: Implications for normal and complement-deficient individuals. J Infect Dis. 1987;155:1266–75.
195. Orren A, Potter PC, Cooper RC, et al. Deficiency of the sixth component of complement and susceptibility to *Neisseria meningitidis* infections: Studies in 10 families and five isolated cases. Immunology. 1987;62:249–53.
196. Ross SC, Berberich HM, Densen P. Natural serum bactericidal activity against *Neisseria meningitidis* isolates from disseminated infections in normal and complement-deficient hosts. J Infect Dis. 1985;152:1332–5.
197. Frank MM, Gelfand JA, Atkinson JP. Hereditary angioedema: The clinical syndrome and its management. Ann Intern Med. 1976;84:580–93.
198. Frank MM. C1 esterase inhibitor: Clinical clues to the pathophysiology of angioedema. J Allergy Clin Immunol. 1986;78:848–50.
199. Frank MM. The C1 esterase inhibitor and hereditary angioedema. J Clin Immunol. 1982;2:65–8.
200. Geha RS, Quinti I, Austen KF, et al. Acquired C1-inhibitor deficiency associated with antiidiotypic antibody to monoclonal immunoglobulins. N Engl J Med. 1985;312:534–40.
201. Alsenz J, Bork K, Loos M. Autoantibody-mediated acquired deficiency of C1 inhibitor. N Engl J Med. 1987;316:1360–6.
202. Strang CJ, Auerbach HS, Rosen FS. C1s-induced vascular permeability in C2-deficient guinea pigs. J Immunol. 1986;137:631–5.
203. Stoppa-Lyonnet D, Tosi M, Laurent J, et al. Altered C1 inhibitor genes in type I hereditary angioedema. N Engl J Med. 1987;317:1–6.
204. Donaldson VH, Harrison RA, Rosen FS. Variability in purified dysfunctional C1-inhibitor proteins from patients with hereditary angioneurotic edema. Functional and analytical gel studies. J Clin Invest. 1985;75:124–32.
205. Rosse WF. Paroxysmal nocturnal hemoglobinuria. In: Williams WJ, Beutler E, Erslev AJ, Rundles RW, eds. Hematology. New York: McGraw-Hill; 1972;460–74.
206. Rosse WF, Parker CJ. Paroxysmal nocturnal haemoglobinuria. Clin Haematol. 1985;14:105–25.
207. Rosse WF. The control of complement activation by the blood cells in paroxysmal nocturnal hemoglobinuria. Blood. 1986;67:268–9.
208. Nicholson-Weller A, March JP, Rosenfeld SI, et al. Affected erythrocytes of patients with paroxysmal nocturnal hemoglobinuria are deficient in the complement regulatory protein, decay accelerating factor. Proc Natl Acad Sci USA. 1983;80:5066–70.
209. Nicholson-Weller A, Spicer DB, Austen KF. Deficiency of the complement regulatory protein, "decay-accelerating factor," on membranes of granulocytes, monocytes, and platelets in paroxysmal nocturnal hemoglobinuria. N Engl J Med. 312:1091–7.
210. Pangburn MK, Schreiber RD, Müller-Eberhard HJ. Deficiency of an erythrocyte membrane protein with complement regulatory activity in paroxysmal nocturnal hemoglobinuria. Proc Natl Acad Sci USA. 1983;80:5430–4.
211. Medof ME, Gottlieb A, Kinoshita T, et al. Relationship between decay accelerating factor deficiency, diminished acetylcholinesterase activity, and defective terminal complement pathway restriction in paroxysmal nocturnal hemoglobinuria erythrocytes. J Clin Invest. 1987;80:165–74.
212. Hänsch GM, Schönermark S, Roelcke D. Paroxysmal nocturnal hemoglobinuria type III. Lack of an erythrocyte membrane protein restricting the lysis of C5b-9. J Clin Invest. 1987;80:7–12.
213. Selvaraj P, Dustin ML, Silber R, et al. Deficiency of lymphocyte function-associated antigen 3 (LFA-3) in paroxysmal nocturnal hemoglobinuria. Functional correlates and evidence for a phosphatidylinositol membrane anchor. J Exp Med. 1987;166:1011–25.
214. Kinoshita T, Medof ME, Silber R, et al. Distribution of decay-accelerating factor in the peripheral blood of normal individuals and patients with paroxysmal nocturnal hemoglobinuria. J Exp Med. 1985;162:75–92.
215. Medof ME, Walter EI, Roberts WL, et al. Decay accelerating factor of complement is anchored to cells by a C-terminal glycolipid. Biochemistry. 1986;25:6740–7.
216. Low MG. Biochemistry of the glycosyl-phosphatidylinositol membrane protein anchors. Biochem J. 1987;244:1–13.
217. Anderson DC, Schmalsteig FC, Finegold MJ. The severe and moderate phenotypes of heritable Mac-1, LFA-1 deficiency: Their quantitative definition and relation to leukocyte dysfunction and clinical features. J Infect Dis. 1985;152:668–89.
218. Matzner Y, Brzezinski A. C5a-inhibitor deficiency in peritoneal fluids from patients with familial Mediterranean fever. N Engl J Med. 1984;311:287–90.
219. Schwabe AD, Lehman TJA. C5a-inhibitor deficiency—a role in familial Mediterranean fever? N Engl J Med. 1984;311:325–6.
220. Mathews KP. Anaphylatoxin inactivator. In: Rother K, Rother U, eds. Hereditary and Acquired Complement Deficiencies in Animals and Man. Basel: S Karger AG; 1986:344–51.
221. Schafer H, Mathey D, Bhakdi HF. Deposition of the terminal C5b-9 complement complex in infarcted areas of human myocardium. J Immunol. 1986;137:1945–9.
222. Rus HG, Niculescu F, Vlaicu R. Presence of C5b-9 complement complex and S-protein in human myocardial areas with necrosis and sclerosis. Immunol Lett. 1987;16:15–20.
223. Rus HG, Niculescu F, Constantinescu E, et al. Immunoelectron-microscopic localization of the terminal C5b-9 complement complex in human atherosclerotic fibrous plaque. Atherosclerosis. 1986;61:35–42.
224. Maroko PR, Carpenter CB, Chiariello M, et al. Reduction by cobra venom factor of myocardial necrosis after coronary artery occlusion. J Clin Invest. 1978;61:661–70.
225. Pinckard RN, O'Rourke RA, Crawford MH, et al. Complement localization and mediation of ischemic injury in baboon myocardium. J Clin Invest. 1980;66:1050–6.
226. Biesecker G, Katz S, Koffler D. Renal localization of the membrane attack complex in systemic lupus erythematosus nephritis. J Exp Med. 1981;151:1790–1.
227. Falk RJ, Dalmasso AP, Kim Y, et al. Neoantigen of the polymerized ninth component of complement. Characterization of a monoclonal antibody and immunohistochemical localization in renal disease. J Clin Invest. 1983;72:560–73.
228. Groggel GC, Adler S, Rennke HG, et al. Role of the terminal complement pathway in experimental membranous nephropathy in the rabbit. J Clin Invest. 1983;72:1948–57.
229. Adler S, Baker PJ, Pritzl P, et al. Detection of terminal complement components in experimental immune glomerular injury. Kidney Int. 1984;26:830–7.
230. Nath KA, Hostetter MK, Hostetter TH. Pathophysiology of chronic tubulo-

interstitial disease in rats. Interactions of dietary acid load, ammonia, and complement component C3. J Clin Invest. 1985;76:667–75.
231. Cybulsky AV, Rennke HG, Feintzeig ID, et al. Complement-induced glomerular epithelial cell injury. Role of the membrane attack complex in rat membranous nephropathy. J Clin Invest. 1986;77:1096–1107.
232. Cybulsky AV, Quigg RJ, Salant DJ. The membrane attack complex in complement-mediated glomerular epithelial cell injury: Formation and stability of C5b-9 and C5b-7 in rat membranous nephropathy. J Immunol. 1986;137:1511–6.
233. Rus HG, Niculescu F, Nanulescu M, et al. Immunohistochemical detection of the terminal C5b-9 complement complex in children with glomerular diseases. Clin Exp Immunol. 1986;65:66–72.
234. Biesecker G, Lavin L, Ziskind M, et al. Cutaneous localization of the membrane attack complex in discoid and systemic lupus erythematosus. N Engl J Med. 1982;306:264–70.
235. Sanders ME, Alexander EL, Koski CL, et al. Detection of activated terminal complement (C5b-9) in cerebrospinal fluid from patients with central nervous system involvement of primary Sjögren's syndrome or systemic lupus erythematosus. J Immunol. 1987;138:2095–9.
236. Koski CL, Sanders ME, Swoveland PT, et al. Activation of terminal components of complement in patients with Guillain-Barré syndrome and other demyelinating neuropathies. J Clin Invest. 1987;80:1492–7.
237. Cammer W, Brosnan CF, Basile C, et al. Complement potentiates the degradation of myelin proteins by plasmin: Implications for a mechanism of inflammatory demyelination. Brain Res. 1986;364:91–101.
238. Mollnes TE, Vandvik B, Lea T, et al. Intrathecal complement activation in neurological diseases evaluated by analysis of the terminal complement complex. J Neurol Sci. 1987;78:17–28.
239. Fearon DT, Ruddy S, Schur PH, et al. Activation of the properdin pathway of complement in patients with gram-negative bacteremia. N Engl J Med. 1975;292:937–40.
240. Weaver LJ, Craddock PR, Jacob HS. Association of complement activation and elevated plasma-C5a with adult respiratory distress syndrome. Pathophysiological relevance and possible prognostic value. Lancet. 1980;1:947–9.
241. Jacob HS, Craddock PR, Hammerschmidt DE, et al. Complement-induced granulocyte aggregation. An unsuspected mechanism of disease. N Engl J Med. 1980;302:789–94.
242. Stevens JH, O'Hanley P, Shapiro JM, et al. Effects of anti-C5a antibodies on the adult respiratory distress syndrome in septic primates. J Clin Invest 1986;77:1812–6.
243. Beutler B, Cerami A. The endogenous mediator of endotoxic shock. Clin Res. 1987;35:192–7.
244. Beutler B, Milsark IW, Cerami AC. Passive immunization against cachectin/tumor necrosis factor protects mice from lethal effect of endotoxin. Science. 1985;229:869–71.
245. Hosea SW, Brown EJ, Frank MM. The critical role of complement in experimental pneumococcal sepsis. J Infect Dis. 1980;142:903–9.
246. Brown EJ, Hosea SW, Frank MM. The role of the spleen in experimental pneumococcal bacteremia. J Clin Invest. 1981;67:975–82.
247. Bohnsack JF, Brown EJ. The role of the spleen in resistance to infection. Annu Rev Med. 1986;37:49–59.
248. Brown EJ, Hosea SW, Frank MM. The role of antibody and complement in the reticuloendothelial clearance of pneumococci from the bloodstream. Rev Infect Dis. 1983;5(Suppl):797–805.
249. Singer DB. Postsplenectomy sepsis. Perspect Pediatr Pathol. 1973;1:285–311.
250. Winkelstein JA, Drachman RH. Deficiency of pneumococcal serum opsonizing activity in sickle-cell disease. N Engl J Med. 1968;279:459–66.
251. Bisno AL, Freeman JC. The syndrome of asplenia, pneumococcal sepsis, and disseminated intravascular coagulation. Ann Intern Med. 1970;72:389–93.
252. Atkinson JP. Complement activation and complement receptors in systemic lupus erythematosus. Springer Semin Immunopathol. 1986;9:179–94.
253. Sim E, Gill EW, Sim RB. Drugs that induce systemic lupus erythematosus inhibit complement component C4. Lancet 1984;2:422–4.
254. Clark RA, Kimball HR, Decker JL. Neutrophil chemotaxis in systemic lupus erythematosus. Ann Rheum Dis. 1974;33:167–172.
255. Perez HD, Lipton M, Goldstein IM. A specific inhibitor of complement (C5)-derived chemotactic activity in serum from patients with systemic lupus erythematosus. J Clin Invest. 1978;62:29–38.
256. Perez HD, Goldstein IM. Polymorphonuclear leukocyte chemotaxis in systemic lupus erythematosus. J Rheumatol. 1987;14:53–8.
257. Ross GD, Yount WJ, Walport MJ, et al. Disease-associated loss of erythrocyte complement receptors (CR1, C3b receptors) in patients with systemic lupus erythematosus and other diseases involving autoantibodies and/or complement activation. J Immunol. 1985;135:2005–14.
258. Gordon DL, Krueger RA, Quie PG, et al. Amidation of C3 at the thiolester site: Stimulation of chemiluminescence and phagocytosis by a new inflammatory mediator. J Immunol. 1985;134:3339–45.
259. Beeson PB, Rowley D. The anticomplementary effect of kidney tissue. Its association with ammonia production. J Exp Med. 1959;110:685–98.
260. Hostetter MK, Gordon DL. Biochemistry of C3 and related thiolester proteins in infection and inflammation. Rev Infect Dis. 1987;9:97–109.
261. Rubio R, Berne RM, Katori M. Release of adenosine in reactive hyperemia of the dog. Am J Physiol. 1969;216:56–62.
262. Cybulsky AV, Lieberthal W, Quigg RJ, et al. A role for thromboxane in complement-mediated glomerular injury. Am J Pathol. 1987;128:45–51.
263. Hakim RM, Breillatt J, Lazarus MJ, et al. Complement activation and hypersensitivity reactions to dialysis membranes. N Engl J Med. 1984;311:878–82.
264. Craddock PR. Complement and granulocyte activation and deactivation during hemodialysis. In: Lysaght MJ, Gurland JG, eds. Plasma Separation and Plasma Fractionation. Basel: S Karger AG; 1983;14–21.
265. Barrett DJ, Boyle MDP. Restoration of complement function in vivo by plasma infusion in factor I (C3b inactivator) deficiency. J Pediatr. 1984;104:76–81.
266. Rao CP, Minta JO, Laski B, et al. Inherited C8β subunit deficiency in a patient with recurrent meningococcal infections: In vivo functional kinetic analysis of C8. Clin Exp Immunol. 1985;60:183–90.
267. Pitts JS, Donaldson VH, Forristal J, et al. Remissions induced in hereditary angioneurotic edema with an attenuated androgen (danazol): Correlation between concentrations of C1-inhibitor and the fourth and second components of complement. J Lab Clin Med. 1978;92:501–7.
268. Densen P, Brown EJ, O'Neill GJ. Inherited deficiency of C8 in a patient with recurrent meningococcal infections: Further evidence for a dysfunctional C8 molecule and nonlinkage to the HLA system. J Clin Immunol. 1983;3:90–9.

7. GRANULOCYTIC PHAGOCYTES

PETER DENSEN
GERALD L. MANDELL

Granulocytes are the most numerous leukocytes in the peripheral circulation. The granulocytic cell series consists of basophils, eosinophils, and neutrophils. These cells share in common a multilobed nucleus, the presence of numerous membrane-bound, characteristically staining cytoplasmic granules, as well as a primary site of action in the tissues. Functionally, however, their differences are greater than are their similarities.

White cells were first recognized in blood in the 1760s by William Hewson in England. A century later, Elya Metchnikoff reported his observations on phagocytosis and formulated his theory of cellular immunity. In 1903–1904, Wright and Douglas demonstrated the importance of serum factors in phagocytosis and coined the term *opsonins* for these factors. Their work provided the impetus for the experimental resolution of the conflict between the theories of cellular and humoral immunity.[1,2] The past 20 years have seen the progressive understanding of neutrophil function in biochemical terms. Central to this understanding has been the clinical recognition of qualitative defects in neutrophil function and the experimental elucidation of the basis for these defects.

NEUTROPHILS

Development

Neutrophils are derived from pluripotential stem cells located in the bone marrow. Granulocyte development and maturation in the bone marrow occurs in two phases, a mitotic phase and a nonmitotic phase. Each phase lasts approximately 1 week. During the mitotic phase, cells mature sequentially from myeloblasts into promyelocytes and myelocytes.[3] Maturation is associated with the appearance of the characteristic granules in the cytoplasm of neutrophils, basophils, and eosinophils. The nonmitotic phase of development includes metamyelocytes, band (or immature) neutrophils, and mature neutrophils.

Morphologic development is accompanied by changes in the physical properties of the cell, the appearance of specific cell surface antigens[4–6] and maturation of cell function.[7] Thus, IgG Fc receptors appear as the cells develop into promyelocytes;

phagocytic ingestion in the early myelocyte stage; complement receptors in the late myelocyte and metamyelocyte stage; oxygen-independent microbicidal activity in the early metamyelocyte stage; oxidative activity and oxygen-dependent microbicidal activity at the metamyelocyte stage; and increased adhesiveness, cell motility, and chemotactic responses in the late metamyelocyte–band stage.[7,8] Morphologically mature neutrophils in the bone marrow exhibit lower stimulated oxidative responses than do mature neutrophils in the peripheral circulation.[8] A reduction in net surface charge, due primarily to the loss of sialic acid, occurs during maturation and has been implicated in the release of cells from the bone marrow.[9,10]

Morphologic and Structural Characteristics

Neutrophils contain two major granule populations, primary or azurophil granules and specific or secondary granules.[11] Careful studies using differential centrifugation, electron microscopy, and biochemical markers have suggested the existence of additional types or subtypes of granules.[12–16] In particular, a gelatinase-containing tertiary granule has been described that is morphologically similar to specific granules but degranulates upon very mild stimulation.[15] The possible role that the tertiary granules play in neutrophil priming requires further delineation.

The characteristics of the two major granule types are summarized in Table 1. Primary granules appear first, stain blue, and are subject to reduction in number during mitosis. Specific granules arise during the nonmitotic stage of cell development and thus do not undergo numerical reduction. Consequently in the mature neutrophil, specific granules outnumber primary granules 2–3:1.[3,11] Primary granules are true lysosomes since they contain acid hydrolases in addition to neutral proteases, myeloperoxidase, cationic proteins, lysozyme and acid mucopolysaccharide. Specific granules contain lactoferrin, lysozyme, vitamin B_{12} binding protein, and cytochrome b, and their membranes serve as a source of receptors. In general, the contents of the primary granule have a lower pH optimum than do those of the specific granule.

During maturation, the nucleus becomes segmented and cytoskeletal elements—microfilaments and microtubules—appear in the cytoplasm. A meshwork of microfilaments makes up the clear cortical veil that surrounds the cell and forms the lamellipodium of an advancing cell (Fig. 1). These structures are polymers of actin, a protein representing 5–10 percent of the total cellular protein. Actin, together with a number of other interacting proteins, constitutes the contractile machinery of the cell that generates locomotion.[17–19] Actin monomers (G-actin), in the presence of actin binding protein, polymerize to form cross-linked actin filaments (F-actin). Regulation of the length of the filaments and the degree of cross-linking provide for the physicochemical fluctuation of actin between the gel and sol states. Filament length is controlled by several different proteins. Profilin serves to sequester G-actin and may provide a mechanism for rapid transport of actin to sites of polymerization. Acumentin, by initiating multiple sites of filament formation (nucleation) and preferentially inhibiting actin monomer exchange from the "slow growing" end of elongating filaments, maintains actin in short filaments. Gelsolin, a calcium-modulated protein that initiates filament nucleation, binds to the "fast growing" end of the filaments and can split preformed actin filaments. In the presence of ATP, myosin repetitively dissociates and binds to cross-linked actin. Myosin binding changes the cross-linking angle between actin filaments from 90 to 45 degrees, which results in movement of the filaments. Thus myosin serves to harness the changes in the physicochemical state of actin to give directionality to cell movement. Changes in calcium concentration that occur with membrane perturbation, directly and in concert with calmodulin, exert control over the contractile process by regulating myosin kinase and gelsolin. As a result, intracellular calcium gradients provide for an increase in polymerized actin in regions of high calcium concentrations.[17–19]

Actin filaments are associated with the cytoskeleton or with the plasma membrane via membrane skeletal proteins.[20] Stimulation of the cell with chemotactic factors causes an abrupt increase in the amount of actin associated with the cytoskeleton[21] and a shift in microfilament organization from a parallel strand to a crosshatched meshwork most evident at the leading edge of the directionally polarized cell.[22]

Microtubules are large, hollow structures composed of dimers of tubulin. In contrast to the role of microfilaments in directed locomotion and changes in cell shape, microtubules appear necessary for the initial orientation of the cell in a chemotactic gradient as well as the spatial organization of structures within the cell during locomotion. They also may be involved in degranulation and in the regulation of cell surface microviscosity during phagocytosis.[23–26]

Mature neutrophils (Figs. 1 and 2) are characterized by a paucity of ribosomal material and mitochondria, which reflects the relative lack of synthetic processes in these cells. Glycogen granules fill the cytoplasm and serve as a source of energy for neutrophil function.

Receptors with specificity for a number of humoral sub-

TABLE 1. Characteristics of Neutrophil Granules

Characteristics	*Primary (Azurophil)*	*Specific (Secondary)*
Contents	Acid hydrolases	Lactoferrin
	β-glucuronidase	Lysozyme
	α-Mannosidase	Vitamin B_{12} binding protein
	Arylsulfatase	
	5′-Nucleotidase	Collagenase (?)
	Acid protease (cathepsin)	Monocyte chemotactic factor
	Neutral proteases	C3 and C5 cleaving proteases
	Cathepsin G	Membrane bound receptors
	Elastase	CR-3
	Collagenase (?)	C5a
	Myeloperoxidase	FMLP
	Cationic proteins	Laminin
	Lysozyme	Membrane-bound components of NADPH oxidase system
	Acid mucopolysaccharide	Cytochrome b_{558}
pH optimum	5.5–6.5	7.0–7.5
Degranulation	Degranulation delayed >50% Into Phagosome	Degranulates first >90% Exocytosis
Function	Microbial killing Digestion	Inflammatory process

Abbreviation: FMLF: formylmethyl-leucyl-phenylalanine.

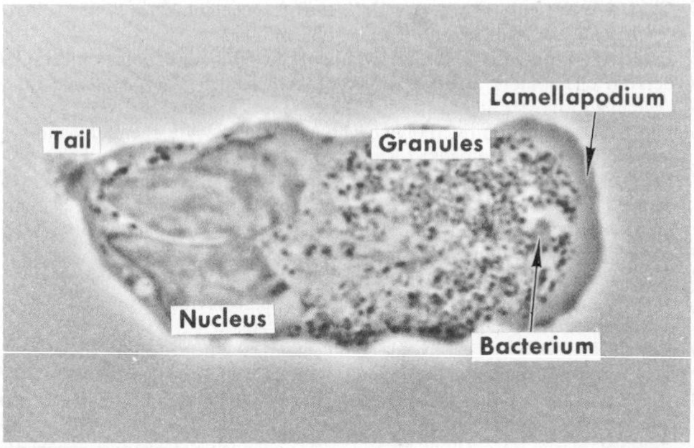

FIG. 1. Phase-contrast photomicrograph of a human neutrophil.

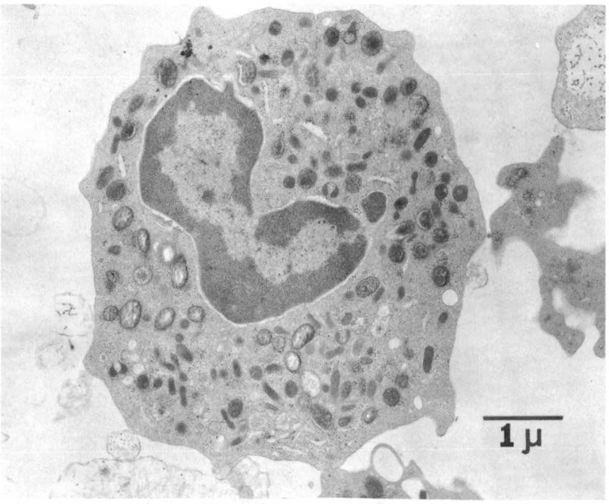

FIG. 2. Electron micrograph of a human neutrophil. Note the granules (large oval structures), glycogen particles (small dark particles), but few other visible organelles.

stances, including IgG, IgA, C3b, iC3b, and several chemotactic factors,[27–31] have been identified and characterized both functionally and structurally. These receptors are homogeneously distributed over the surface of the resting cell. Upon polarization of the cell in response to a chemotactic stimulus, receptors for IgG and concanavalin A undergo an asymmetric clustering at the front of the cell. It is now clear that the distribution of receptors with different ligand specificity can be independently regulated even though stimulation via these receptors may result in similar functional effects.[32–34] Moreover, the various neutrophil functional responses exhibit differential requirements for receptor occupancy. Thus, maximal degranulation requires brief receptor occupancy whereas sustained oxidative responses are dependent upon continuous ligand binding to the receptor.[35]

Neutrophil Kinetics

The daily production of mature neutrophils (PMNs) is on the order of 10^{11} cells. This granulocyte reserve contains up to 10 times the normal daily neutrophil requirement. During acute infection or other inflammatory stresses, neutrophils are mobilized from the marrow reservoir. In the face of a continuing stimulus this reserve may be depleted, thus necessitating additional means for increasing delivery to meet demands. Increased stem cell input, increased mitoses during the mitotic stage of development, use of a store of cells whose maturation had been inhibited (so-called hiatal cells), and shortening of the maturation time within the marrow may all occur.[36] Multiplication and differentiation of stem cells is stimulated by a family of proteins called colony-stimulating factors. These factors are produced by peripheral blood monocytes, tissue macrophages, and stimulated lymphocytes and exhibit a hierarchy with respect to the type(s) of myeloid cells that they stimulate.[36,37] Different proteins induce growth and differentiation, and the interaction of these factors determines the balance between immature and mature cells.[37] Lithium carbonate, a drug used primarily for the treatment of manic-depressive disorders, accelerates neutrophil production by stimulating clonal proliferation. This effect leads to an increase in the total circulating neutrophil mass without a reduction in the delivery of cells to sites of inflammation.[38,39]

Intravascular neutrophils are present in a circulating pool and a marginating pool. The circulating pool contains about 22×10^7 cells/kg and the marginating pool (which can be released with exercise or epinephrine) about 17×10^7 cells/kg. In contrast, more than 1000×10^7 PMNs and PMN percursors/kg are found in the marrow. The half-life of intravascular neutrophils is 6–8 hours. Mature neutrophils leave the body via the gut, respiratory secretions, and urine, and senescent cells may be engulfed by other phagocytic cells in the tissues. Estimates of extravascular survival range from 7 hours to 4 days.

In addition to infection, granulocytosis can be produced by a number of pharmacologic and physiologic stimuli. Most of these situations do not involve an increase in cell production but rather cause granulocytosis by altering the distribution of cells in the various granulocyte pools. Thus, the acute administration of corticosteroids and endotoxin induces the release of cells from a marrow granulocyte reserve, which is analogous to the redistribution observed during acute inflammatory processes. Chronic steroid administration, however, inhibits granulocyte egress from the circulation. Exercise, stress, epinephrine, alcohol, and hypoxia all produce granulocytosis by mobilizing marginating granulocytes. Steroids, aspirin, and alcohol also decrease granulocyte adherence.

Delivery to the Inflammatory Site

The circulating and marginating pools are heterogeneous, being composed of a large subpopulation (80 percent) of neutrophils with IgG rosetting properties and a smaller population lacking this characteristic.[40] It is not clear whether this heterogeneity represents different cellular subsets or is due to maturational differences within a single cell line. The functional significance of neutrophil heterogeneity is uncertain, but differences in the distribution of these cells may contribute to the development of "impaired" neutrophil function in certain disease states.[41] In contrast to circulating granulocytes, tissue neutrophils are homogeneous, greater than 96 percent being capable of IgG rosette formation.[40] Tissue neutrophils contain fewer lysosomal granules but up to 10-fold greater amounts of glycogen than their circulating counterparts have.[42] Anaerobic glycolysis of these glycogen stores provides the energy for neutrophil locomotion.

Although neutrophils within the marginating pool stick to vascular endothelium, they are not truly adherent; rather, they tumble slowly along the vessel wall. After, a local insult these neutrophils become firmly adherent to the side of the vessel wall closest to the injury. Plasma factors,[43] neutrophil and endothelial cell products, and surface glycoproteins on neutrophils and endothelial cells all combine to modulate neutrophil adherence to the endothelium.[44] Inflammatory mediators and chemotactic factors stimulate the limited release of specific granules and probably tertiary granules from neutrophils in the local circulation. The consequences of this degranulation include decreased surface charge, increased neutrophil adhesiveness, and an increase in a number of membrane receptors. The functional result of these changes is a cell that has been primed to a state of enhanced responsiveness.[45–48] Increased expression of the laminin receptor coupled with the release of granule enzymes may facilitate limited digestion of laminin, an endothelial matrix protein, thereby facilitating diapedesis and entry of the neutrophil into the tissues.[44] Several neutrophil surface glycoproteins promote neutrophil-dependent adherence to endothelial cells. These include an 80–100 kD protein, also found on monocytes, eosinophils, and lymphocytes,[49] and the CDw18 glycoproteins (Mo1, MAC-1/LFA-1, GP150,95) that are variably present on granulocytes, monocytes, macrophages, T lymphocytes, and large granular lymphocytes.[50] Mo1 is synonymous with the complement receptor for iC3b, CR3. The CDw18 proteins are heterodimers composed of a common 95 kD β-chain and unique 150–180 kD α-chains. The β-chain exhibits a high degree of structural homology with other cellular adhesion proteins belonging to the integrin family of cell surface receptors.[51,52] Many of these receptors recognize the tripeptide amino acid sequence arg-gly-asp.[53] A 90–110 kD glycoprotein having a broad tissue distribution and termed intercellular adhesion molecule (ICAM-1) facilitates neutrophil adherence to endothelial cells. Surface expression of this molecule is up regulated by interleukin-1 (IL-1)), tumor necrosis factor (TNF), and interferon-γ (IFN-γ).[54] Thus neutrophil adherence to endothelial cells is promoted by glycoproteins present on the surface of both cells.[55]

Neutrophils can arrive at an inflammatory site either by increasing their overall random movement (chemokinesis) or by following a concentration gradient of inflammatory substances in a directional manner (chemotaxis). Most substances that stimulate directed movement on the part of the neutrophil also stimulate an increase in overall motility.[56]

Directed movement of neutrophils requires cell polarization and the orderly making and breaking of cell–substrate contact. There is no evidence that neutrophils can swim, and progress appears to be made either by gliding along a surface with caudad displacement of dorsal folds or cycles of partial release of the lamellipodium from the substrate with anterior advance followed by lamellipodial reassociation with the substrate.[57]

Chemotactic factors fall into two categories: (1) chemotaxins, which act directly to stimulate chemotaxis, and (2) chemotaxigens, which induce the formation of chemotaxins. Bacterial factors may fall into either category. The tripeptide formylmethionyl-leucyl-phenylalanine (FMLP) is directly chemotactic for neutrophils at concentrations as low as 10^{-11} M. Since bacteria and mitochondria initiate protein synthesis with formylmethionine at the N-terminus, it has been suggested that bacterial or mitochondrial proteins released during cell death are responsible for stimulating neutrophil chemotaxis.[58]

The interaction of bacteria or their products with complement generates the chemotactic factor C5a. This fragment is converted rapidly to C5a des arg, which has little inherent chemotactic activity but combines with an anionic polypeptide cochemotaxin via sialic acid residues to form the bulk of chemotactic activity present in activated normal serum.[59,60] Biologically active lipids generated from arachidonic acid are potent mediators of a variety of inflammatory reactions. Products of arachidonic acid metabolism, particularly the hydroxyeicosatetranoic acids (HETEs) and leukotriene B_4 (LTB_4) are potent mediators of the inflammatory response. These substances influence a number of neutrophil functions including chemokinesis, chemotaxis, granule release, and iC3b receptor expression.[61] Substances released during neutrophil degranulation can, either by direct action or via cleavage of C5a from C5, attract other cells to the site of bacterial invasion.[62]

Chemotactic factor concentration differences as little as 0.1–

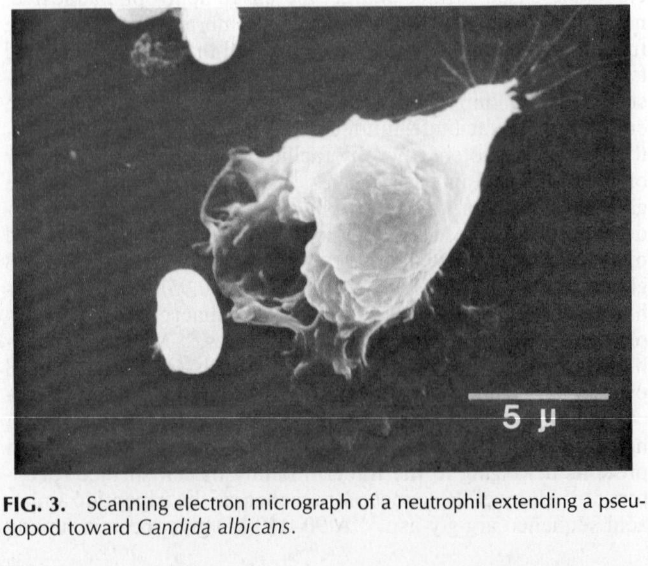

FIG. 3. Scanning electron micrograph of a neutrophil extending a pseudopod toward *Candida albicans*.

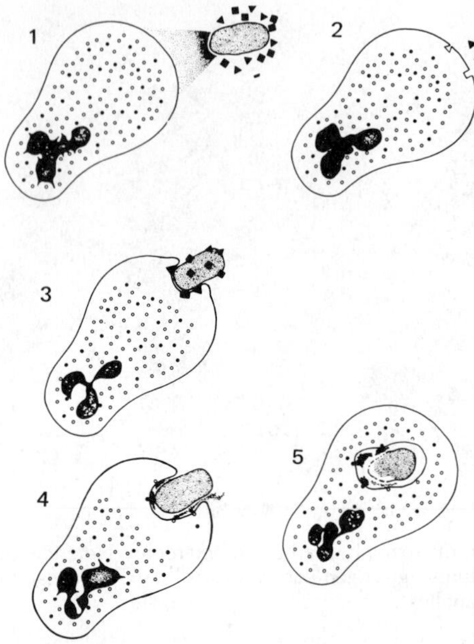

FIG. 4. (1) A neutrophil approaching a bacterium is guided by a concentration gradient of chemotactic factors emanating from the microbe. (2) Antibody and complement attaching to the surface of the bacterium to opsonize the organism. (3) Ingestion taking place by sequential binding of receptors on the neutrophil to opsonins on the bacterium. (4) Early degranulation. Specific granules (open circles) are discharging before the phagocytic vacuole is closed, and thus much of the granule contents are found outside of the cell—"regurgitation during feeding." (5) Later degranulation and destruction of ingested bacteria. Primary granules fire into the closed phagosome. This, in conjunction with an oxidative burst of activity, results in bactericidal activity.

1.0 percent across the neutrophil are sufficient to produce cellular orientation and directed movement (Figs. 3 and 4). The mechanism by which transduction of chemotactic factor binding to specific receptors produces a chemotactic response is unclear, but calcium fluxes and transmethylation of phospholipids appear essential.[24] Fusion of granule and cell membranes during limited degranulation increases the number of chemotactic receptors.[46] As the cell moves in an increasing chemotactic gradient, these receptors become occupied and are rapidly internalized. The resultant decrease in receptor number and perhaps a decrease in affinity of the remaining receptors may control chemotactic responsiveness.[63] Occupied receptors are internalized, stripped of ligand, and recycled to the cell surface.[64,65] Recycling is facilitated by sialic acid on membrane glycoproteins.[65] The oxidative and degranulation responses induced in the neutrophil by increasing concentrations of mediators (Fig. 4) promote the inactivation of unbound chemotactic mediators.[61,66,67] In addition, lysozyme release dampens both the chemotactic and oxidative responsiveness of the cell.[68] In concert, this multitude of effects serves to attract and keep the neutrophil at the site of bacterial invasion.

Phagocytosis

Phagocytosis is a two-step process involving attachment and engulfment of the phagocytic particle. Ingestion but not attachment is an active process requiring energy from anaerobic glycolysis. Optimal ingestion requires the presence of calcium and magnesium ions. Some microorganisms and inert particles may be ingested by neutrophils in the absence of serum factors, but most bacteria must be coated with opsonins (humoral substances that enhance microbial ingestion) for attachment to and ingestion by neutrophils to occur.

Specific IgG and complement are the major opsonic factors promoting recognition and ingestion of microorganisms by neutrophils. Antibody promotes phagocytic uptake by neutralization of antiphagocytic molecules on the bacterial surface, e.g., capsular polysaccharide; physically linking the organism to the neutrophils; efficiently activating the classical pathway of complement and promoting deposition of opsonic fragments of C3 on the bacterial surface; and by activating the neutrophil ingestion mechanism through interaction of IgG with its receptor in the neutrophil membrane (Fig. 4). Activation of complement via either the alternative or classical pathways leads to C3b and iC3b deposition on the microbial surface (Chapter 6). In addition C1q deposition enhances Fc receptor-dependent ingestion.[69]

Receptors for IgG (FcγRI-III), but not other immunoglobulins, and for C3b (CR-1) and iC3b (CR-3) are present in the neutrophil membrane.[27,28,70] These receptors are biochemically, topographically, and functionally distinct. Recent evidence suggests that FcγRs mediate phagocytosis via calcium-dependent pathways whereas CR-1 and 3 use calcium-independent pathways.[71] FcγRII and -III are low to moderate affinity receptors normally present on the cell surface, whereas the high-affinity FcγRI is found on the surface of IFN-γ-stimulated neutrophils.[70] Intracellular pools of Fc receptors have not been identified. In contrast, such pools have been described for both CR-1 and CR-3, the latter clearly being associated with the specific granules.[72,73] These receptor pools are rapidly mobilized to the surface after stimulation of the cell by a variety of inflammatory mediators.[73] It is likely that C3 receptors enjoy only low-level expression on circulating neutrophils and that differences in resting expression levels are attributable to the presence of miniscule amounts of mediators (e.g., endotoxin) in the isolation procedures used during neutrophil purification.

In contrast to upregulation, which occurs primarily through an increase in receptor numbers, downregulation of receptor-mediated processes occurs principally via diminished receptor function. Receptor oxidation as a consequence of the normal stimulation of the neutrophil oxidative burst contributes to decreased receptor function. Consequently, neutrophil receptor half-life and function are enhanced in individuals with either impaired oxidase activity (e.g., chronic granulomatous disease) or in whom the generation of certain oxidative reactants is depressed (e.g., myeloperoxidase deficiency).[74,75] The balance between these regulating events is probably an important modulating factor in the inflammatory response and in limiting tissue damage.

Both IgG and C3 binding increase the rate of phagocytosis of appropriately sensitized erythrocytes, but in the unprimed cell only interactions via the Fc receptor initiate microfilament polymerization and ingestion of this target.[76–78] However, complement deposition alone is sufficient to promote ingestion of a number of bacteria, a finding that emphasizes the heterogeneity among opsonic requirements for different particles. In most cases phagocytosis is most efficient when organisms are coated with both IgG and C3, thereby allowing cooperative interaction of the two types of receptors. In fact, recent data suggest that a subpopulation of CR3 and Fc receptors are physically associated within the membrane.[79]

Ingestion is the result of the sequential interaction between opsonic ligands distributed homogeneously over the particle surface and their receptors on the phagocyte membrane. The sequential interaction of these opsonic ligands with their receptors in the phagocytic membrane initiates polymerization of actin microfilaments in the cytoplasm underlying the site of a particle attachment and results in the circumferential flow of the cell membrane about the opsonized particle and its enclosure within a phagosome (Figs. 4 and 5).[18,80,81]

In addition to acting as ligands between the phagocytic particle and the phagocyte, complement and specific immunoglobulin alter the surface characteristics of the phagocytic particle. The surface of bacteria, which has antiphagocytic properties, is hydrophilic relative to the surface of the neutrophil. Upon opsonization the surface of these bacteria becomes relatively more hydrophobic than that of the neutrophil, and they are readily engulfed. Alterations in surface properties may also promote ingestion by reducing charge repulsion between the particle and the phagocyte.[82] Different bacterial species, as well as mutants within the same species, may vary in their opsonic requirements for optimal phagocytosis.

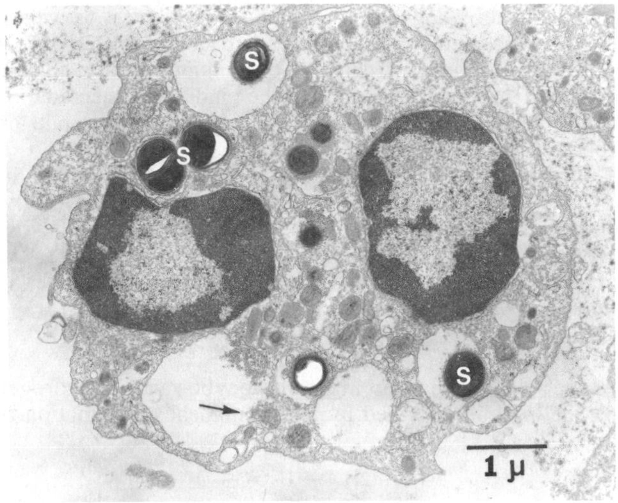

FIG. 5. Electron micrograph of a neutrophil that has ingested *Staphylococcus aureus* (S). Bacteria are in phagocytic vacuoles formed by invagination of external cell membrane. Degranulation into a phagocytic vacuole can be seen at the lower left (arrow).

Increased attention has been paid to the important role that nonspecific factors play in the phagocytic process, especially in soft tissues where the functional impact of the neutrophil is most critical. Chief among these factors are fibronectin and laminin, proteins that constitute part of the extracellular matrix secreted by endothelial cells. These proteins contain the arg-gly-asp amino acid recognition sequence through which they bind to specific but separate membrane receptors.[53] Since the different receptors recognize the same binding sequence, specificity must be conferred by other aspects of the structure of these matrix proteins.[53] In the fluid phase or by themselves these proteins fail to promote ingestion of target particles. However, when neutrophils adherent to surfaces coated with these proteins are stimulated with a variety of chemotactic factors, their capacity to ingest either IgG- or C3-coated particles, in particular, the latter, is substantially enhanced. This effect requires neutrophil adherence to the matrix protein but not the interaction of the matrix protein with the target particles or an increase in FcγR or C3 receptor number. Hence these proteins are not opsonins. Rather, they enhance phagocytosis primarily by promoting the conversion of C3 receptors from a binding to an ingesting function. Thus chemotactic mediators and extracellular matrix proteins cooperate to prepare neutrophils for their primary phagocytic function as they migrate from the circulation to sites of infection.[83,84]

Postphagocytic Events

The term *postphagocytic events* refers to the burst of metabolic activity and the discharge of granule contents that occurs during and after phagocytosis. These events are initiated by the attachment of opsonized microbes to the cell membrane as well as by an array of soluble mediators such as C5a, LTB_4, and platelet activating factor.

The metabolic or respiratory burst is a series of enzymatic

reactions used by stimulated phagocytes to convert oxygen to various active metabolites critical for bactericidal activity. A number of other events including chemiluminescence, iodination of protein, lipid turnover, and the binding and degradation of some hormones are increased during phagocytosis but are secondary to the reduction of oxygen.

The basic series of reactions of the respiratory burst results in (1) oxygen consumption, (2) superoxide production, (3) hydrogen peroxide production, and (4) stimulation of the hexose monophosphate shunt. Oxygen is consumed and reduced to the superoxide anion radical $O_2^{\cdot}$ by the one electron transfer to oxygen from the reduced pyridine nucleotide NADPH:

$$2O_2 + NADPH \rightarrow 2O_2^{\cdot} + H^+ + NADP^+$$

At the acidic pH present in the phagocytic vacuole, hydrogen peroxide is rapidly formed by the spontaneous dismutation of superoxide.

$$2O_2^{\cdot} + 2H^+ \rightarrow H_2O_2 + O_2$$

Detoxification of superoxide and hydrogen peroxide as they diffuse into the surrounding cytoplasm is accomplished by cellular antioxidant systems. At neutral pH, superoxide dismutase catalyzes the above reaction to eliminate superoxide, whereas hydrogen peroxide is destroyed by the glutathione peroxide system.

$$H_2O_2 + 2GSH \rightarrow 2H_2O + GSSG$$

Reduced glutathione (GSH) is regenerated by glutathione (GSSG) reductase.

$$GSSG + 2NADPH \rightarrow 2GSH + 2NADP^+$$

Thus, NADPH serves a critical role both in the primary reduction of oxygen as well as in the protection of the cell from toxic metabolites of oxygen.[85]

The hexose monophosphate shunt, a series of reactions oxidizing glucose to a five-carbon sugar and carbon dioxide, serves to regenerate NADPH. In resting neutrophils only 1–2 percent of glucose metabolism occurs via the hexose monophosphate shunt, but during phagocytosis glucose use via this pathway increases 15- to 30-fold.[86]

The NADPH oxidase lies dormant in resting neutrophils. Stimulation of the cell is followed by a 30–60 second lag during which the dormant enzyme is activated, thereby resulting in the characteristic burst of respiratory activity. In its active state the oxidase is associated with the plasma membrane. Current evidence supports the view that the oxidase is a multicomponent electron transport system. A component on the cytoplasmic face of the cell membrane[87] catalyzes the oxidation of NADPH generated by the hexose monophosphate shunt and initiates the flow of electrons through the membrane via other components to environmental oxygen as the terminal electron acceptor.[88–90] Superoxide is the product of this terminal reduction of oxygen. Evidence supporting a role for a flavoprotein, quinones, cytosolic factors, and cytochrome b_{-558} (previously termed cytochrome b_{-245}) has been generated from several laboratories.[91–95] However, the identity of the individual components in the putative transport chain is a matter of a debate.[89,90] Evidence supporting the participation of a flavoprotein, cytosolic factors, and cytochrome b_{-558} in a multicomponent oxidase system derives from studies of the chronic granulomatous diseases (CGD). Neutrophils from patients with these disorders lack oxidase activity, and this phenotype has been associated with the absence of each of the three aforementioned components.[96–99]

The organization of the components of the oxidase within the membrane requires further delineation. However, it is clear that the NADPH binding site lies on the inner face of the cytoplasmic membrane.[87] Studies using an NADPH analog in chemical cross-linking experiments have identified a 65-kD NADPH membrane binding protein in guinea pig neutrophils.[100] The relationship of this protein to the reported components of the oxidase system is uncertain. The outer face of the plasma membrane must contain the component responsible for the direct transfer of electrons to oxygen. The low midpoint potential of cytochrome b_{-558} argues for its role in this function and thus as the terminal constituent of the transport chain.[89,90] Recent work indicates that the human cytochrome is a 120–135 kD protein composed of two tightly associated polypeptide chains, α (22 kD) and β (91 kD).[101] The α-chain is encoded on chromosome 16 and probably bears the cytochrome heme binding site, whereas the heavily glycosylated β-chain is encoded by an X-linked gene.[102–105]

A major question concerns the mechanism of oxidase activation after stimulation of the cell. Activation appears to involve multiple steps and several pathways since multiple substances, each with a characteristic lag time, can initiate the burst and patients have been identified whose granulocytes respond with a burst to some but not all stimuli.[85,106] Transient depolarization of the cell membrane occurs within 5 to 10 seconds of stimulation, precedes the earliest detectable changes in oxygen metabolism, and seems to be a necessary although insufficient condition for activation.[107,108] The demonstration that 70–90 percent of the cytochrome b_{-558} activity is located in the specific granules[88,109,110] implies that degranulation with translocation of the cytochrome from the granule to the cell membrane may be involved in the assembly and activation of the oxidase system.[109] However, the oxidative burst can occur in the apparent absence of degranulation,[111,112] and certain substances can reversibly activate the oxidase system.[113,114] Hence degranulation alone is not the sole determinant of oxidase activation. In addition not all investigators have found cytochrome b_{-558} associated with specific granules.[115,116]

Evidence is accumulating that suggests that there is more than one pathway for activating the oxidase system.[89,117,118] This conclusion is based on the observations that different stimuli exhibit markedly disparate kinetics for activation[118] and that a comparison of a number of parameters (e.g., phosphoinositide turnover, calcium fluctuations, inhibition by pertussis toxin and protein kinase C dependency) for each of the different stimuli yields a pattern that cannot be accounted for by a simple, stepwise activation pathway.[89] A protein kinase C dependent pathway clearly involves receptors, phosphoinositide metabolism, G proteins and calcium.[117,119] A second pathway used by arachidonic acid and sodium dodecyl sulfate (SDS) is protein kinase C independent.[117] It has been suggested that these latter two stimuli may activate the oxidase by virtue of their detergent properties or by producing changes in membrane fluidity in the vicinity of the oxidase.[120,121] Inactivation of the oxidase may occur by a poorly characterized desensitization mechanism[122] or by myeloperoxidase-dependent oxidation of critical determinants of oxidase activity.[123]

Degranulation, the other major postphagocytic event, is also initiated before completion of ingestion. Ninety percent of the contents released from specific granules during phagocytosis can be found outside the cell. These substances function optimally at the pH encountered extracellularly. Thus specific granules appear to function principally as secretory granules. In contrast, greater than 50 percent of the contents released from primary granules during phagocytosis can be recovered from the phagosome.[124] These enzymes function best at the low pH (6.0–6.5) found in phagosomes. Consequently, the contents of the primary granule appear to function principally in microbial killing and digestion.

Recent evidence links degranulation to calcium fluxes and depolarization of the neutrophil membrane.[125,126] Changes in the intracellular levels of cyclic nucleotides also influence degranulation, perhaps by modulating microtubule assembly, but these changes are unlikely to account directly for granule release induced by stimulation of the cell.[127,128] Inhibition of microtubule assembly by colchicine interferes with degranulation;

however, microtubule assembly does not induce granule release in the absence of surface adherence.[129] Hence, microtubule assembly is necessary but not sufficient for degranulation. Microtubules are believed to promote granule movement toward the phagosome, but microfilaments probably are also involved in the degranulation process.[130] Fusion of the cytoplasmic granules with the phagosome results in the melding of the two membranes, an increase in the size of the phagocytic vacuole, activation of membrane-bound enzymes, and discharge of granule contents into the phagosome.

The extracellular release of the constituents of neutrophil granules occurs by two different routes.[131] The first, known as "regurgitation during feeding," occurs by virtue of granule discharge into the nascent phagosome before closure of the phagosome around the phagocytic particle. Exocytosis may also involve the direct fusion of lysosomes with the external cell membrane and subsequent extracellular extrusion of granule contents. This process is called "reverse endocytosis" or "frustrated phagocytosis." Granule extrusion occurs over a large area of membrane surface and may involve greater quantities of enzyme release than with the regurgitation route.

Signal Transduction

The major neutrophil functions depicted in Figure 4 (chemotaxis, phagocytosis, degranulation, and the oxidative burst) are initiated by the interaction of mediators with specific receptors in the cell membrane. The transduction of a given signal into a specific response has elements unique to the stimulus as well as aspects shared with other stimuli.[132] For example, chemotactic stimuli promote directed cell movement but may also stimulate degranulation or the oxidative burst.

As with other cells a major transduction pathway involves the phosphoinositide–protein kinase C (PKC) system,[133–135] but as discussed above, PKC-independent, calcium-dependent pathways also exist. The basic components of the phosphoinositide pathway include a receptor that communicates via G protein(s) with membrane-bound phospholipase C. Agonist binding to the receptor promotes phosphatidyl-4,5-biphosphate (IP_2) cleavage by phospholipase C, which results in the release of diacylglycerol (DAG) and inositol triphosphate (IP_3), the latter of which can be further converted to IP_4. IP_3 and IP_4 mediate increases in free intracellular calcium by respectively stimulating its release from unique intracellular compartments called calcisomes and by promoting its influx from the cell exterior.[136,137] The increase in intracellular calcium is greatest at the region of stimulation, for example, at the leading edge of the cell during chemotaxis or periphagosomally during phagocytosis, as might be anticipated from the role of calcium in actin polymerization and the importance of microfilaments in cell movement and ingestion.[138]

Free intracellular calcium also acts in conjunction with DAG to promote translocation of PKC from the cytosol to the cell membrane where it functions to phosphorylate critical proteins, thereby regulating the activity of these molecules. Current research is directed at establishing the identity of the phosphorylated molecules in order to delineate their function. That this approach is likely to yield important insights is attested to by the recent demonstration of an association between one form of CGD and failure to phosphorylate a 44–48 kD membrane protein.[139–141] Phorbol myristate acetate, an agent commonly used to activate a variety of neutrophil responses, substitutes for DAG in the phosphoinositide pathway, thereby bypassing the steps between the receptor and PKC activation.[133,134] Pertussis toxin, another commonly used reagent, binds to certain G proteins, thereby inhibiting neutrophil responses.[142]

Priming of Neutrophil Responses

Recently obtained data have emphasized that concentrations of mediators sufficiently low enough not to stimulate neutrophils directly nevertheless prepare the cell for an enhanced response to a second unrelated stimulus.[143,144] This phenomenon is referred to as priming and is likely to be important in vivo since it appears to be cell specific. That is, bacterial infection primes neutrophils, whereas parasitic infection or allergic responses prime eosinophils.[145] A broad array of inflammatory mediators including chemotactic factors, endotoxin, cytokines, and certain lipids can prime the neutrophil, and the primed state exists with respect to each of the major aspects of neutrophil function (Fig. 4). This state of enhanced responsiveness persists for an extended period of time (>20 minutes) relative to the response elicited by direct stimulation of the cell.[122,143] Presentation of the same agonist in both the priming and stimulating steps results in decreased cellular responses indicating the existence of chemical pathways for desensitization in addition to those for priming.[122] The chemical basis for these different pathways is uncertain. Current evidence suggests that, in contrast to directly stimulated responses, primed responses are independent of PKC activation and translocation.[145] Changes in the physicochemical properties of the lipid bilayer have been invoked as the physiologic basis for this phenomenon.[145]

Microbicidal Mechanisms

The postphagocytic events described above are designed to deliver the products of degranulation and the respiratory burst to the phagocytic vacuole. The phagosome plays an important role in this process because it provides a closed space in which an ingested microbe is exposed to high concentrations of toxic substances and the exposure of the phagocyte and other cells to these metabolites is minimized (Fig. 5).[146]

Oxygen-dependent bactericidal mechanisms can be divided into myeloperoxidase-dependent and -independent reactions.[147] The essential requirements for the myeloperoxidase-mediated bactericidal mechanisms as first described by Klebanoff are myeloperoxidase, released from the primary granule; hydrogen peroxide, generated by the respiratory burst; and a halide ion. In addition, the low pH present in the phagocytic vacuole enhances myeloperoxidase activity. Hydrogen peroxide by itself has bactericidal properties, but in the presence of myeloperoxidase the potency of this system for bacteria is enhanced 50-fold. The halide used in the myeloperoxidase–hydrogen peroxide reaction also has an effect on the bactericidal potency in decreasing order of efficacy—ioide, bromide, and chloride. However, on the basis of concentration, chloride appears to be the physiologic cofactor for this reaction in the cell.[147]

Hypochlorous acid, formed by the neutrophil when chloride is the relevant halide, is a potent oxidizing and microbicidal agent.[147] The microbicidal activity of this system probably results from halogenation or oxidation of critical iron-rich catalytic components of the electron transport chain within the microbial membrane. Oxidation of these molecules leads to the release of free iron, which can then participate in the formation of the highly reactive hydroxyl radical.[148–151] In addition to these well-defined effects, the myeloperoxidase-hydrogen peroxide-halide system promotes the formation of singlet oxygen, decarboxylation of amino acids to form toxic aldehydes, and the generation of chloramines.[152,153] These effects probably contribute to neutrophil microbicidal activity.[147,154,155]

Metabolites of oxygen for which a role in neutrophil bactericidal activity has been suggested include hydrogen peroxide, superoxide, singlet oxygen, and hydroxyl radical. The fact that catalase, which destroys hydrogen peroxide, protects bacteria from the bactericidal effects of neutrophils[156] and that the bactericidal activity of myeloperoxidase-deficient neutrophils remains high are strong pieces of evidence supporting a direct germicidal effect of hydrogen peroxide. Superoxide, by itself, is thought to play little role in the killing of microorganisms. This conclusion is based on the demonstration that bacteria incubated in a cell-free, superoxide-generating system survive normally. However, under appropriate conditions superoxide can react with other products of oxygen to generate hydroxyl radical and singlet oxygen. The bactericidal effect of these oxygen-derived free radicals may be due to the initiation of a chain of oxidizing events in the bacterial cell wall.[147,154,155] Hydroxyl radical is a potent bactericidal agent that can be formed by the direct reaction of superoxide with hydrogen peroxide. This reaction occurs too slowly to be of biologic importance, but it can be catalyzed by ferric salts.[157,158] Recent studies support this scenario since hydroxyl radical formation by stimulated neutrophils occurred only in the presence of free iron.[159] Thus the formation of this highly reactive species in vivo is probably determined by the availability of free iron in the environment or its release from oxidatively injured organisms.[158] The demonstration that neutrophils emit light during the metabolic burst and the fact that the relaxation of oxygen from an excited singlet state to the ground state produces light led to the suggestion that neutrophil chemiluminescence was due to singlet oxygen. Both superoxide- and myeloperoxidase-dependent reactions have been implicated in the formation of singlet oxygen. Myeloperoxidase-dependent reactions are clearly an important source of chemiluminsecence, but available evidence at present suggests that chemiluminescence is not directly related to singlet oxygen.[154]

The presence of oxygen-independent microbicidal mechanisms in neutrophils is clearly demonstrated by the ability of these cells to kill some organisms under anaerobic conditions.[160] Substances contributing to oxygen-independent microbicidal activity include acid, lactoferrin, lysozyme, and cationic proteins. In human neutrophils, the pH in the phagosome decreases to about 6.0.[161] Although pneumococci are readily killed by the effect of acid alone, most bacteria are little affected by the acid environment. The main effect of the low pH in the phagocytic vacuole appears to be enhancement of the activity of the granule enzymes important in the killing and digestion of ingested microorganisms.

Lactoferrin is an iron-binding protein found in secretions bathing mucosal membranes as well as in neutrophils.[162] Its presence in the specific granules of neutrophils suggests that the primary site of its action lies extracellularly. Lactoferrin's bacteriostatic effect is related to its ability to deprive bacteria of the iron required for growth, and this effect is eliminated by saturation of both iron binding sites.[162] Lactoferrin plays a role in the alteration of the physicochemical properties of the neutrophil membrane that occurs during degranulation,[163] the modulation of hydroxyl radical production,[158] the regulation of granulopoiesis,[164] and the modulation of complement function.[165]

Lysozyme is found mainly in the specific granules but is also present in the primary granules. This enzyme hydrolyzes the glycoside bond between *N*-acetylmuramic acid and *N*-acetylglucosamine, a component of the peptidoglycan in bacterial cell walls. The bactericidal properties of lysozyme are due to this reaction. However, in most bacteria, peptide substitutions on the *N*-acetylmuramic acid residue make this bond inaccessible to lysozyme. The bacteriolytic properties of lysozyme are correspondingly limited. The action of lysozyme is enhanced by the presence of other substances, for example, complement, which damages the bacterial cell wall, thereby allowing access of lysozyme to its site of action.[147]

A number of highly cationic proteins have been isolated from neutrophil primary granules.[166–168] The reaction of these proteins with acidic groups on the bacterial surface is associated with inhibition of bacterial growth. Some of these proteins preferentially inhibit specific bacterial species.[169] These proteins include a 37 kD cation antimicrobial protein, the activity of which is favored by the intraphagosomal acid pH[166,170,172]; a 59 kD "bactericidal permeability increasing" protein, the activity of which resides in a 25 kD amino terminal fragment[167,172]; and a family of small (3–4 kD) cysteine- and arginine-rich peptides dubbed "defensins".[168,173] The former two proteins are active only against gram-negative bacteria and are more active against strains with a rough (incomplete) rather than a smooth (complete) lipopolysaccharide. Their exact mode of action is incompletely understood but involves temperature-independent binding to the organism via ionic interactions followed by temperature-dependent insertion into the outer membrane via hydrophobic interactions.[166,167,174] These events result in increased permeability of the bacterial outer membrane which in turn is associated with death of the organism. In contrast, the defensins exhibit antimicrobial activity against both gram-negative and gram-positive organisms as well as fungi and viruses.[168,173] The structure of these peptides is highly conserved among different and within the same animal species.[168,175] The mode of action of these peptides may relate more to their detergent-like properties than their cationic nature.[168] Intracellular killing of bacteria may also be enhanced by antibody and complement independently of the role of these ligands in opsonization and triggering the respiratory burst.[176,177]

Microbial Defenses against Phagocytes

In general, microbes involved in the pathogenesis of acute infections must remain extracellular if they are to produce an infection, whereas chronic infections are typically produced by organisms whose pathogenic potential necessitates an intracellular environment, usually in monocytes or macrophages. Both types of microbes possess virulence factors that enable them to persist in their respective locations. Bacteria may elude neutrophils by failing to stimulate chemotaxis or by circumventing attachment or ingestion. Organisms that inhibit degranulation or the oxidative burst may survive inside neutrophils or monocytes and generally cause chronic infections (Table 2).[178]

Tissue Injury—The Dark Side of Neutrophil Function

Ordinarily, degranulation and the oxidative burst are restricted to the points of contact between an opsonized organism and the developing phagolyosome.[179,180] Downregulation of receptor-mediated events during continuous exposure to homologous stimuli (desensitization)[122] and during exposure to products of the oxidative burst,[75] oxidative inactivation of inflammatory mediators[66,181] and the oxidase itself,[74,123] and the release of lactoferrin to bind environmental iron in a form in which it is not available to catalyze hydroxyl radical formation[158,182,183] further limit neutrophil activation and confine the toxic effects of oxygen-dependent and -independent microbicidal systems to the vicinity of the organism. However, the toxic potential of these microbicidal systems can be unleashed and cause damage to host tissues in diseases associated with autoantibody formation, immune complex deposition, the intravascular release of excessive quantities of inflammatory mediators, or chronic low-grade inflammation. Thus various granule proteins and products of the neutrophil oxidative burst have been implicated in the pathogenesis of immune- and non-immune-mediated arthropathies and nephropathies as well as pulmonary and cardiac injury.[184,185]

Inflammatory cytokines such as tumor necrosis factor and interleukin-1 activate neutrophils and may contribute to tissue damage.

The intravascular activation of complement and generation of circulating C5a that can occur during the initiation of hemodialysis, cardiopulmonary bypass, or septic shock has been shown to stimulate neutrophil aggregation, oxidative activity, and degranulation. Aggregation of neutrophils leads to the formation of microemboli that lodge in the lung and accounts for the neutropenia observed in these situations. The release of toxic products of oxygen metabolism, coupled with the discharge of granule contents from aggregated neutrophils in the pulmonary circulation, leads to endothelial damage and has been implicated in the development of the adult respiratory dis-

TABLE 2. Tactics of Microorganisms against Strategies of Phagocytic Cells and the Microbes That Use Them

Function of Phagocyte Inhibited								*Tactic of Microbe*	
						Microbial Activity by Resistance to			
Recognition	*Chemotaxis*	*Attachment and Ingestion*	*Ingestion (Despite Attachment)*	*Oxidative Burst*	*Degranulation*	*Oxidative Attack*	*Granule Substance*	*Escape from Phagosome*	*Leukotoxicity*
Schistosome	*Salmonella typhi*	*Streptococcus pneumoniae*	*N. gonorrhoeae*	*S. typhi*	*M. tuberculosis*	*S. aureus*	*Salmonella typhimurium*	*M. bovis*	*S. pneumoniae*
	Neisseria meningitidis	*Streptococcus pyogenes*	*Mycoplasma*	*Brucella abortus*	*Mycobacterium microti*	*Listeria monocytogenes*	*Salmonella minnesota*	*Rickettsia tsutsugamushi*	*S. pyogenes*
	Neisseria gonorrhoeae	*N. gonorrhoeae*	Influenza virus	Newcastle disease virus	*Mycobacterium bovis*	*E. coli*	*Mycobacterium leprae*	Vaccinia virus	*S. aureus*
	Pseudomonas aeruginosa	*N. meningitidis*		Vaccinia virus	*Toxoplasma gondii*	*Sarcina lutea*	*Mycobacterium lepraemurium*	Reovirus	*P. aeruginosa*
	Serratia species	*Klebsiella pneumoniae*		Herpes simplex virus	*L. pneumophila*	*B. abortus*	*M. tuberculosis*		*Entamoeba histolytica*
	Mycobacterium tuberculosis	*S. aureus*		Reovirus					
	Staphylococcus aureus	*Haemophilus influenzae*		*B. pertussis*					
	Capnocytophaga[a]	*E. coli*		*Legionella micdadei*					
	Escherichia coli	*Yersinia pectis*							
	Vibrio cholera	*Bacillus anthracis*							
	Bordetella pertussis	*Campylobacter fetus*							
		Cryptococcus neoformans							
		P. aeruginosa							
		Pasteurella multocida							
		Bacteroides fragilis							
		B. pertussis							

[a] Known also as *Bacteroides ochraceus.*

tress syndrome both in vitro and in vivo.[186–189] However, the occurrence of the adult respiratory distress syndrome in neutropenic patients indicates that factors other than intravascular neutrophil aggregates also contribute to the development of this syndrome.[190] Substantial evidence implicates neutrophil products in the development of pulmonary emphysema. In this scenario neutrophils infiltrate the lung and are activated consequent to inflammation-provoking substances in cigarette smoke. Cigarette smoke and products of activated neutrophils inactivate α_1-antitrypsin, the major inhibitor of neutrophil elastase. Neutrophil elastase released during cellular stimulation then promotes proteolytic destruction of the lung architecture.[191–194]

Defects in Neutrophil Function

Defects in neutrophil function can result from decreased numbers of mature neutrophils or abnormalities in chemotaxis, ingestion, or bactericidal mechanisms.[195,196] Table 3 summarizes these defects. Infections resulting from quantitative or qualitative defects in neutrophil function share in common a tendency to be prolonged, to respond slowly to antibiotics, and to be recurrent. Staphylococci, gram-negative organisms, and fungi are the usual organisms responsible for these infections. Patients with defective opsonic activity suffer from infections due to encapsulated bacteria.

Qualitative defects may be intrinsic or extrinsic to the neutrophil. In general, the intrinsic defects of qualitative neutrophil function are more severe than are the extrinsic defects. Chemotactic defects are frequently expressed as cutaneous infections with associated adenitis. Unlike quantitative defects or defects in phagocytosis or intracellular killing, they rarely result in bacteremia or metastatic spread of infection. This is probably due to the fact that, although neutrophil accumulation is delayed, phagocytosis and bactericidal activity frequently proceed normally once neutrophils encounter the microorganism.

TABLE 3. Defects in Neutrophil Function

- Neutropenia
  - Acquired
    - Drug induced
    - Autoimmune
    - Cancer related
  - Hereditary
    - Infantile genetic agranulocytosis
    - Familial neutropenia
    - Cyclic neutropenia
- Qualitative defects
  - Adhesion defects
    - Leukocyte adhesion deficiency
  - Chemotactic defects
    - Humoral
      - Complement deficiency
      - Inhibitors
      - Immune complexes
      - Hyperimmunoglobulinemia E (Job's) syndrome
    - Cellular
      - Chédiak-Higashi syndrome
      - Hypophosphatemia
      - Lazy leukocyte syndrome
  - Opsonic defects
    - Complement deficiency
    - Antibody deficiency
  - Defects in intracellular killing
    - Abnormal respiratory burst
      - Chronic granulomatous disease
      - G6PD deficiency
    - Granule abnormalities
      - Myeloperoxidase deficiency
      - Specific granule deficiency
      - Chédiak-Higashi syndrome

Abbreviation: G6PD: glucose-6-phosphate dehydrogenase.

NEUTROPENIA

The most common granulocyte defect encountered is the absolute reduction of circulating neutrophils. The lower limit of normal for circulating neutrophils is 1500–2000/mm^3. The risk of acquiring an infection increases progressively with both the duration and the magnitude of the granulocytopenia below 1500 cells/mm^3. Below 500 neutrophils/mm^3, there is a dramatic increase in the incidence of infection.[197]

The acquired neutropenias are most often related to drug therapy and may be a predictable result of therapy or an idiosyncratic reaction. The former are frequently encountered during chemotherapy for various neoplastic and immunologic disorders. Neutropenia as a result of an idiosyncratic drug reaction is observed with phenothiazines, sulfonamides, penicillins, cephalosporins, and vancomycin. Chloramphenicol can cause both a predictable and an idiosyncratic neutropenia. The latter is uncommon but is frequently fatal. Increased granulocyte destruction may occur as a result of splenic sequestration. Splenic sequestration of neutrophils may be immunologically mediated by antibody[198,199] or secondary to any of the causes of hypersplenism. Splenectomy may be beneficial in restoring neutrophil counts toward normal.

Hereditary neutropenias are observed either as solitary defects or in association with other defects, for example, orotic aciduria. The neutropenia may be severe as in infantile genetic agranulocytosis, moderate as in familial (benign) neutropenia, or cyclic. Infantile genetic agranulocytosis is an autosomal recessive disorder characterized by granulocyte maturation arrest and severe infection with death in infancy. Some hereditary neutropenias are accompanied by an apparent compensatory monocytosis. Cyclic neutropenia is a rare autosomal dominant defect of myelopoiesis that is characterized by the periodic disappearance of neutrophils and other blood elements from the circulation. Early granulocyte precursors are present in the marrow during the neutropenia, which suggests a transient maturation arrest. The duration of neutropenia ranges from 5 to 8 days, followed by a 2- to 5-week period with normal numbers of circulating neutrophils. In a given patient, the periodic oscillations are constant. During the neutropenic state, the patients suffer from aphthous stomatitis, fever, malaise, and cutaneous infections. The disease is usually recognized during childhood, and there is no amelioration with age. Alternate-day predinosolone (25 mg qod) therapy attenuates the oscillation in neutrophil maturation.[200]

LEUKOCYTE ADHESION (Mo-1,Mac-1,LFA-1) DEFICIENCY SYNDROME

The development of monoclonal antibodies to neutrophil antigens and the use of these reagents to probe the cell surface in patients with neutrophil defects has led to the recognition of a new category of neutrophil dysfunction.[50] Previously the defect in these patients had been variously ascribed to actin, chemotactic, or phagocytic dysfunction.[201–205] It is now appreciated that the basic abnormality involves surface glycoproteins that mediate the adherence-related functions of the cell. Thus neutrophil adhesion, chemotaxis, and phagocytosis are all impaired in these patients.

The disorder is inherited in an autosomal recessive manner, and there is frequently a history of consanguinity. Severe and moderate phenotypes are recognized. Patients with this syndrome typically present with prolonged and/or recurrent staphylococcal and *Pseudomonas* infections beginning in infancy, often in the perinatal period. Patients with the severe phenotype often have delayed separation of the umbilical cord and may develop omphalitis. Infections involving the soft tissues, mucosal surfaces, and the intestinal tract are common. Cutaneous infections frequently become necrotic. Initially they may resemble ecthyma gangrenosum, whereas later they may assume a pyoderma gangrenosum appearance. Individuals surviving infancy universally develop acute gingivitis with eruption of primary dentition. The ginivitis persists and results in progressive gingival hypertrophy and alveolar bone loss. Individuals expressing the severe phenotype may also exhibit poor wound healing. Although survival into adulthood is well described, particularly in patients with the moderate phenotype, 41 percent of affected individuals die before the age of 2 years.[50,206]

A hallmark of the disease is a markedly and persistently elevated peripheral white blood cell count. Cell counts typically range from 2 to 20 times normal and remain elevated even in the absence of infection, probably due to impaired cellular margination and egress from the vascular tree. Evaluation of neutrophil function demonstrates impaired adherence to artificial substrates, impaired chemotaxis in vivo and in vitro, and an impaired respiratory burst in response to the ingestion of particles coated with iC3b but not IgG.[50,195,196] Affected neutrophils exhibit an above- or below-normal burst in oxidative metabolism after stimulation with soluble stimuli, depending on which stimulus is used and the nature of the association between its receptor and the cytoskeleton.[207]

The basis for this syndrome is the absence of a family of surface glycoproteins on the neutrophils from affected individuals. These proteins are important molecular determinants of adhesion-related functions and include the iC3b receptor (CR3, Mo-1, or Mac-1), lymphocyte function-associated antigen 1 (LFA-1), and p150,95. The proteins are α,β-heterodimers sharing identical β-chains but possessing distinct α-chains. The β-chain and each α-chain are the products of separate genes located on chromosomes 21 and 16, respectively. All three proteins are normally present on granulocytes and monocytes, whereas only LFA-1 is present on lymphocytes.

Leukocytes from individuals with the severe phenotypic expression of this disorder have less than 0.3 percent of the normal quantity of all three proteins on their surface, whereas moderately affected individuals express levels 2.5–6 percent of that in healthy people.[206] In affected individuals the surface expression of both the α- and β-chains is abnormal. However the α- but not the β-chain can be found in normal amounts within the cell. This finding indicates that the basis for the syndrome lies in the synthesis of the β-chain and that assembly of the α,β-heterodimer is required for transport of the α-chain to the cell surface.[208] Molecular analysis of the abnormal β-gene from a number of patients with this disorder has demonstrated a spectrum of mutations in the β-gene that range from the failure to produce mRNA in some individuals with the severe disease phenotype, to the production of an abnormally sized precursor β-protein, and to no readily apparent defect in some patients with either disease phenotype.[209]

CHEMOTACTIC DEFECTS

Extrinsic Abnormalities

Neutrophil chemotactic defects due to factors extrinsic to the cell may be secondary to abnormalities involving the complement cascade. These include genetic deficiencies (C3, C5), as well as decreased synthesis (cirrhosis, kwashiorkor, premature infants), hypercatabolism, and increased loss (severe burns) of serum proteins. Some investigators have noted a depression in neutrophil chemotactic responses in patients with diabetes mellitus that is independent of serum osmolality. The defect is mild and is most readily demonstrated in juvenile-onset diabetics. Chemotactic responsiveness of diabetic neutrophils can be restored in vitro by incubation with insulin.[210–212]

Chemotactic inhibitors may express their effect directly or indirectly by neutralizing the chemotactic effect of complement. Polymeric IgA is cytophilic for neutrophils and can markedly depress chemotaxis.[213] Defective chemotaxis has been described in a number of diseases characterized by circulating immune complexes. These include rheumatoid arthritis, systemic lupus erythematosus, and subacute bacterial endocarditis. Neutrophils exposed to immune complexes have high rates of oxidative metabolism and granule release in the resting state as well as an abnormal response to chemotactic stimuli. The sera from about 40 percent of patients with systemic lupus erythematosus contain an inhibitor that is specific for C5-derived chemotactic activity. This inhibitory factor does not interfere with the expression of other C5-mediated functions. Its presence correlates with disease activity and the resultant chemotactic defect with the enhanced susceptibility of these patients to infection.[214,215] The inhibitor has been identified as the Bb fragment of complement factor B, and it exerts its effect by inhibiting the interaction of C5a des arg with cochemotaxin in serum.[216,217]

A chemotactic defect has been described in patients with juvenile periodontitis, a familial disorder characterized by periodontitis occurring in the absence of severe dental disease. Serum from some of these patients contains an inhibitor of chemotaxis, and the resultant defect in chemotaxis has been postulated to play a role in the pathogenesis of this disease.[218,219] In addition, neutrophils from some of these patients bear fewer chemotactic receptors as compared with cells from unaffected individuals.[220] Of particular note in this regard is the report of an acquired neutrophil chemotactic defect in two adults with gingival infection due to *Capnocytophaga* (Bacteroides ochraceus). Eradication of infection resulted in a return to normal of neutrophil function. Sonicates of *Capnocytophaga* and filtrates of broth in which the organism had been grown inhibited the chemotactic response of normal neutrophils. These findings suggest that the chemotactic defect associated with some forms of periodontal disease may be due to the presence of bacterial products in the circulation.[221]

Chemotactic inhibitors whose mode of action appears to be the inactivation of chemotactic substances have been described in Hodgkin's disease, sarcoidosis, leprosy, and cirrhosis. These inhibitors are usually present in low concentration in normal serum and affect chemotaxis only when present in high concentrations.[212] Recurrent skin infections and abnormal neutrophil chemotaxis have also been associated with an IgG antineutrophil antibody.[222]

A number of pharmacologic agents including alcohol, steroids, tetracyclines, and amphotericin B inhibit chemotaxis in vitro. Alcohol may exert its effect by elevating cyclic AMP levels. The inhibitory effect of tetracyclines may be related to their ability to chelate calcium.

Intrinsic Abnormalities

Chédiak-Higashi Syndrome. The Chédiak-Higashi syndrome is a rare autosomal recessive trait involving a generalized dysfunction of granule-containing cells. Giant granules have been found in melanocytes, Schwann cells, renal tubular cells, thyroid cells, and all types of leukocytes (Fig. 6). These abnormal granules account for many of the physical findings including partial oculocutaneous albinism, rotatory nystagmus, peripheral neuropathy (both sensory and motor), and recurrent infection. In neutrophils, they are formed during cell maturation by fusion of the two granule types.[223] Laboratory abnormalities include anemia, leukopenia, thrombocytopenia, and evidence of intramedullary destruction of all blood elements with an associated elevation in serum lysozyme levels and deficiencies in iron and folate concentrations. Abnormal natural killer (NK) cell function has also been reported.[224] In a number of patients with the Chédiak-Higashi syndrome, the disease undergoes a transformation to an accelerated phase. This phase is characterized by hepatosplenomegaly, lymphadenopathy, and lymphocytic organ infiltration. Unexplained febrile episodes occur, and patients frequently die of infection or less commonly of hemorrhage at an early age.[225]

Neutrophils from patients with the Chédiak-Higashi syndrome exhibit a defective chemotactic response, but ingestion occurs normally.[226] Many bacteria, including both catalase-positive and catalase-negative species, exhibit prolonged survival within these neutrophils. Bacterial killing rates are most abnormal during the first 20 minutes of contact in vitro but approach normal levels at 2 hours. The faulty release of the large neutrophil granules is associated with the delayed appearance of myeloperoxidase within phagocytic vacuoles. The metabolic burst is normal.[227] The intracellular killing defect thus appears primarily due to delayed delivery of granule enzymes to the phagosome.

The biochemical abnormality underlying the neutrophil dysfunction in the Chédiak-Higashi syndrome is unknown. Abnormal function of a diverse number of cell types suggests that the defect involves some basic aspect of cell function. The bulk of current evidence suggests that the defect involves the microtubule apparatus: cell ultrastructure studies confirm a decreased number of centriole-associated microtubules in some patients; membrane fluidity is enhanced and has been suggested as a possible explanation for the abnormal fusion of the azurophil and specific granules; the level of tyrosylated tubulin is abnormally high; and pharmacologic agents, such as ascorbic acid, that affect microtubule assembly may improve cell function in occasional patients. In addition, agents that decrease the cyclic AMP/GMP ratio have been reported to improve neutrophil function. Many of these agents also affect microtubule assembly, and changes in cyclic nucleotide metabolism now appear to be a consequence of these alterations.[210,228–230]

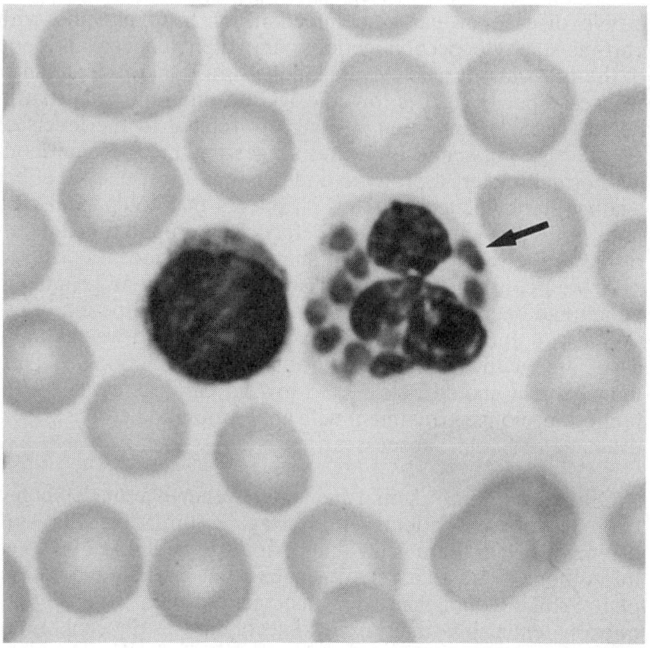

FIG. 6. Neutrophil and lymphocyte from a patient with Chédiak-Higashi syndrome. Note the large abnormal granules (arrow).

Hyperimmunoglobulinemia E with Impaired Chemotaxis (Job's Syndrome). Job's syndrome, as originally described, is an affliction of fair-skinned, red-haired females that is characterized by eczema, recurrent "cold" staphylococcal skin abscesses, sinusitis, and otitis media.[231,232] However, the disorder occurs in blacks and males as well. Many of the patients have coarse facial features and a broad nasal bridge. In addition to cutaneous staphylococcal infection, recurrent pneumonia and mucocutaneous candidiasis are common. Patients may have mild eosinophilia, and although variable, the neutrophils of most patients exhibit a chemotactic abnormality. The chemotactic defect appears to correlate best with the severity of the eczema, and patients have been reported in whom a chemotactic defect could be demonstrated only during relapses of their dermatitis.[211] Mononuclear cells from these patients but not from individuals either with or without atopy spontaneously produce a factor that inhibits the chemotactic responses of normal neutrophils and monocytes.[233] All patients have markedly elevated (>10 times normal) serum levels of IgE due to a decreased fractional catabolic rate of this immunoglobulin.[234] Antistaphylococcal and anti-*Candida* IgE antibodies have been demonstrated in the serum from patients with Job's syndrome but not from healthy people, from patients with hyperimmunoglobulinemia E due to atopic disease or parasitic infection, or from patients with chronic staphylococcal infections. Antistaphylococcal antibody of the IgM class is also elevated in the sera from these patients, whereas specific IgA is low and IgG no different from that in healthy people. Infection is inversely related to the levels of specific IgE, IgA, and IgM, thus suggesting that these antibodies normally exert a protective rather than a permissive effect against staphylococci.[235] Thus it appears that Job's syndrome does not represent an intrinsic defect of neutrophil function but rather is the result of aberrant immune regulation.

A well-controlled clinical trial established that levamisol, which had been reported to improve neutrophil function in patients with Job's syndrome, failed to reduce and was actually associated with an increase in the number of infections.[236] Thus management should be directed toward early detection of infection, prolonged treatment with antibiotics, and early surgical drainage of "cold" abscesses.[232]

Other Disorders. A mild and variable chemotactic defect has been described in patients with Kartagener (immotile cilia) syndrome in which there is an abnormality in the linkage between microtubules and cilia.[210] An acquired but reversible defect in neutrophil function has been documented with severe hypophosphatemia (less than 1 mg/dl) secondary to phosphate-free hyperalimentation. The defect in these cells is thought to be due to an inability to generate ATP from anaerobic glycolysis.[237]

Abnormal Phagocytosis

Defective opsonization occurs with inherited or acquired deficiencies of the early complement components (especially C3) or immunoglobulin. Similar derangements accompany the paraproteinemias as well as a number of other neoplastic and nonneoplastic disorders characterized by hypoglobulinemia and/or hypocomplementemia. Anatomic or functional asplenia results in a deficiency of opsonic factors for a number of encapsulated bacteria. Splenectomy also results in a deficiency in tuftsin, a tetrapeptide synthesized in the spleen and reported to facilitate ingestion of staphylococci.[238] Patients with opsonic disorders frequently have recurrent infections with encapsulated bacteria, particularly pneumococci and *Haemophilus influenzae*. Infection with these organisms in the splenectomized person can present as a fulminant bacteremia or meningitis accompanied by disseminated intravascular coagulation.[239]

Defects in Intracellular Killing

Abnormal Respiratory Burst. CHRONIC GRANULOMATOUS DISEASES OF CHILDHOOD. The chronic granulomatous diseases of childhood (CGDs) are a group of disorders characterized by recurrent infections attributable to defects in neutrophil oxygen-dependent microbicidal activity. The classic form of this disease is an X-linked recessive disorder, but a clinically indistinguishable variant affecting females as well as males exhibits an autosomal mode of inheritance. The relative frequency of these two forms of the disease is uncertain. The disease usually presents early in childhood, 78 percent of affected individuals manifesting recurrent and often prolonged infection during the first year of life. Although an infectious agent is not isolated during the majority of most febrile episodes,[240] the microbiology of this disorder is distinctive for the paucity of infections caused by the encapsulated or catalase-negative organisms (e.g., *S. pneumoniae*) that ordinarily predominate in this age group. Rather, *Staphylococcus aureus* is the causative agent in 52 percent of the infections with an identifiable etiology. Other primary infecting agents include *Salmonella, Pseudomonas aeruginosa, Serratia marcescens, Nocardia asteroides,* and *Aspergillus*. Although *S. aureus* is the pathogen most commonly isolated from infected sites, gram-negative bacteria account for 73 percent of all bacteremic episodes and for 80 percent of fatal septicemias.[241] Pyogenic dermatitis, suppurative adenitis, recurrent pneumonia with abscess formation, stomatitis, enteritis, and colitis are common. Intestinal obstruction secondary to inflammatory masses, especially in the perirectal area, has been reported. A third of the patients have deep-seated abscesses in the liver or perihepatic region. Obstructive uropathy and xanthogranulomatous pyelonephritis also occur. Osteomyelitis is common and is noteworthy for its relatively frequent causation by *Serratia marcescens* and involvement of the metacarpal and metatarsal bones.[242] Physical findings commonly include dermatitis, adenopathy, hepatosplenomegaly, and "failure to thrive." Routine laboratory studies show leukocytosis, anemia of chronic disease, and hyperglobulinemia. Pathologic examination of affected tissues reveals noncaseating granulomas. Although recurrent infection with death by an average age of 3.7 years was the rule in 1955–1965, the average life expectancy in the period 1975–1982 was 9.5 years. The disorder has been diagnosed in adults presenting with "idiopathic" pulmonary fibrosis. These patients frequently have a history of recurrent infections in childhood, but infections seem to occur less frequently during adulthood. Thus, the increased life expectancy in this disease probably reflects both an improvement in medical management and the recognition of milder forms of the disease.[85,106,243]

Female carriers of X-linked CGD have both normal and abnormally functioning neutrophils. Most of these women display no undue susceptibility to infection, although an association with discoid lupus erythematosus has been noted in several reports.[97,244,245] The greater frequency of infection that occurs in some carriers correlates with an increase in the population of defective neutrophils. This increase appears due to the chance inactivation of a disproportionate number of normal X chromosomes as predicted by the Lyon hypothesis.[246]

The defect in CGD is an inability of neutrophils, other granulocytes, and monocytes to display the respiratory burst during phagocytosis. All oxidative events associated with the burst (oxygen consumption, chemiluminescence, production of toxic oxygen species, hexose monophosphate shunt activity, and microbial halogenation) are absent in CGD neutrophils. These cells also fail to undergo membrane depolarization during phagocytosis. Chemotaxis, phagocytosis, and degranulation are normal. Infections caused by catalase-negative organisms are uncommon because hydrogen peroxide produced by these bacteria effectively circumvents the biochemical lesion and reacts with myeloperoxidase and a halide in the phagosome to regenerate microbicidal activity.

Recognition of the complexity of the oxidase system coupled with the identification of patients with CGD due to different biochemical defects has led to the classification of these disorders on the basis of whether they involve oxidase activation pathways or the oxidase system itself (Table 4).[85,89,106] Disorders involving the activation pathways may be due to a defect in signal recognition or transduction. The defect is usually inapparent upon stimulation of the cell with soluble agents but becomes evident when a phagocytic particle is used as the stimulus. This contrasts with disorders involving the oxidase system itself in which neither particulate nor soluble stimuli activate the respiratory burst. Neutrophils from patients with the leukocyte adhesion deficiency syndrome lack CR3 and do not respond to iC3b-coated particles but exhibit a normal oxidative burst upon stimulation with phorbol myristate acetate (PMA). Thus they are representative of the former category of CGD.[201–205] This type of defect emphasizes the importance of using more than one type of stimulus when considering the diagnosis of CGD.

Defects involving the oxidase itself are subclassified as to whether oxidase activity is impaired or totally absent (Table 4). The former category is represented by a clinically mild variant of X-linked CGD described in two unrelated males whose neutrophils exhibited normal membrane depolarization and a nor-

TABLE 4. Classification of the Chronic Granulomatous Diseases

Type of Defect in the Oxidase System	*Relative Frequency*[a] *(%)*	*Inheritance*	*Oxidase Response to Stimuli*		*Cytochrome* b_{-558}		*Flavo-protein*	*Cytosolic Factor*	*Physphorylation of 48 kD Membrane Protein*
			Particulate	*Soluble*					
Impaired activation									
LAD syndrome	<3.3	AR	abs/imp	nl/super nl	nl		nl	nl	depends on stimulus
Abnormal oxidase activity									
Impaired activity	<3.3–18	XL	imp	imp	"abs"–low		nl	nl	imp
Absent activity									
Cytochrome b_{-558} absent					Chain				
					α	β			
a	23–64	XL	abs	abs	abs	abs[b]	nl	nl	imp
b	<3.3–3.3	AR	abs	abs	ND[c]	ND	nl	nl	ND
c	13–18	XL	abs	abs	abs	abs	low	nl	ND
Cytochrome b_{-558} present	18–60								abs
a		AR	abs	abs	nl	nl	nl	47 kD prot—abs 65 kD prot—nl	ND
b		AR	abs	abs	nl	nl	nl	47 kD prot—nl 65 kD prot—abs	ND

[a] Among individuals with the CGD syndrome.[98,247]
[b] The primary defect involes the β-chain encoded by a gene on the X chromosome.
[c] The primary defect probably involves the α-chain encoded by a gene on chromosome 16.
Abbreviations: LAD: leukocyte adhesion deficiency; AR: autosomal recessive; XL: X-linked; abs: absent; imp: impaired; nl: normal; ND: not determined.

mal lag time between stimulation and onset of the respiratory burst. However, the magnitude of the burst was substantially reduced. A reduced affinity of the oxidase system for NADPH was felt to account for this defect.[248,249] An unexplained finding in these two patients has been the associated absence of the b cytochrome.[249]

CGD due to the total absence of neutrophil oxidase activity is inherited in either an X-linked or autosomal manner. That different biochemical lesions underlie these two genetic variants of CGD was originally most clearly demonstrated in a cooperative European study of 27 CGD patients and their families. The b cytochrome was absent from the neutrophils of patients with X-linked CGD and present in half-normal amounts in female carriers of this form of the disease. In contrast, neutrophils from patients with the autosomal recessive form of the disease contained normal quantities of an apparently normal b cytochrome.[97] Subsequently it was shown that oxidase activity could be restored by cross-hybridization of monocytes from patients with different inherited forms of CGD.[250] These studies demonstrated that at least three separate biochemical defects could result in absent oxidase activity.[251] As detailed above, substantial evidence supports a role for cytochrome b_{-558}, a flavoprotein, and cytosolic factors as constituents of the oxidase system. Cytochrome b_{-558} is an α,β-heterodimer consisting of a 22 kD α-chain that contains the heme group responsible for the cytochrome spectral signal and a 91 kD β-chain. These chains appear to be tightly but noncovalently associated in the intact cytochrome.[101,103,104] The α-chain is encoded by a gene on chromosome 16 and the β-chain by an X-linked gene.[102] Neutrophils from patients with X-linked CGD are missing both the α- and the β-chains of the cytochrome as determined by both immunoprecipitation studies and detection of the cytochrome spectral signal.[101,252] The absence of the 22 kD product of a gene on chromosome 16 in X-linked CGD suggests that the 91 kD β-chain, which is the product of the X-linked gene, may be required for cellular processing of the α-chain.[101] Recently four patients with autosomal CGD due to cytochrome b_{-558} deficiency have been identified on the basis of an absent spectral signal for the cytochrome.[247,251] Neither of these reports examined neutrophil membranes for the presence of the α- or the β-chain of the cytochrome. On the basis of the chromosomal location of the genes for the respective polypeptide chains one might speculate that this form of CGD may be due to an abnormality involving the α-gene on chromosome 16 and that the β-chain might be present in these neutrophils. Finally, some patients with X-linked cytochrome b deficiency have an associated flavoprotein deficiency (Table 4).[91,98,247]

Cytochrome b_{-558} and flavoprotein levels are normal in most patients with autosomal recessive CGD.[247] These patients may have a clinically milder form of the disease,[99,106,253] although this is not supported by all studies.[98] Neutrophils from these patients are missing either a 47 kD or 65 kD cytosolic factor that must be translocated to the cell membrane in order to activate the oxidase system.[99,254–256] This type of CGD is associated with the failure of these neutrophils or their cytosol to phosphorylate an uncharacterized 48 kD membrane protein(s)[139,254]; however, the factor does not appear to be protein kinase C since the activity of this enzyme is normal in neutrophils from some of these patients.[254] Although further characterization is obviously required, it is of interest that the molecular size of the 65 kD protein is consistent with that described for the NADPH membrane binding protein in guinea pigs.[100] There is evidence supporting a defect in the phosphorylation of a 48 kD membrane protein in X-linked CGD as well.[257] On the other hand, some investigators have failed to detect such an abnormality in any form of CGD.[258] Thus the role of phosphorylation in the activation of the oxidase system requires further delineation.

The diagnosis of CGD is readily made by using the nitroblue tetrazolium dye (NBT) test.[259] This test depends on the ability of normal neutrophils to reduce the yellow dye, nitroblue tetrazolium, to blue formazan. NBT reduction by neutrophils is primarily dependent on the production of superoxide; therefore, the NBT test is negative in CGD. A properly performed, negative NBT test with appropriate controls is very strong evidence for the diagnosis of CGD. It should be confirmed by the demonstration of normal phagocytosis and a marked reduction in the parameters of the metabolic burst. In order to detect abnormalities in the activation mechanism, both soluble and particulate stimuli should be used in tests of oxidative function.

GLUCOSE-6-PHOSPHATE DEHYDROGENASE DEFICIENCY. Although erythrocyte and leukocyte glucose-6-phosphate dehydrogenase (G6PD) are products of the same gene, the common form of G6PD deficiency that presents as a hemolytic anemia in blacks is not associated with neutrophil dysfunction. This discrepancy is explained by the fact that this deficiency is due to an unstable enzyme, the activity of which diminishes over a period of time that exceeds the life expectancy of the neutrophil. Neutrophil dysfunction does occur in rare cases of G6PD deficiency in whites missing or having less than 5 percent of the normal levels of G6PD. The basis for neutrophil dysfunction in this disorder is that in the absence of G6PD glucose cannot be metabolized via the hexose monophosphate shunt. As a consequence, NADPH, used by the oxidase, cannot be regenerated from NADP. Aside from the presence of a hemolytic anemia, the clinical, laboratory, and genetic (X-linked) presentation is very similar to CGD. The NBT test is negative or low, as are other parameters of the respiratory burst. The failure of methylene blue to stimulate hexose monophosphate shunt activity and low levels of G6PD distinguish this defect from CGD.[85,260]

Granule Abnormalities. MYELOPEROXIDASE DEFICIENCY. Once thought to be a rare disorder, neutrophil myeloperoxidase (MPO) deficiency is now recognized as the most common of all neutrophil functional disorders, with a frequency of 1 per 2000–4000 people for whom leukocyte counts are performed. This discrepancy is accounted for by the fact that the overwhelming majority of such individuals are healthy and that detection of this condition has been greatly facilitated by the widespread use of flow cytometry techniques that use peroxidase staining for leukocyte differential counts.[261] Eosinophil peroxidase is not affected in this disorder. An autosomal recessive manner of inheritance has been reported, but the heterogeneous expression of the defect has led to the suggestion that inheritance may be under polygenic control. Of all the patients recognized with this disorder, only six have had serious infections. Systemic candidiasis occurred in four of these patients, three of whom had diabetes mellitus. This association suggests that diabetics with serious fungal infection should be screened for MPO deficiency and, conversely, that MPO-deficient individuals receiving broad-spectrum antibiotics may be at increased risk for fungal superinfection.[262]

Since the cell is devoid of MPO-dependent but not other oxidative killing mechanisms, there is delayed but not absent intracellular killing in MPO-deficient neutrophils. Delayed killing is more pronounced for fungi than for bacteria,[263] which suggests an explanation for the clinical findings in this disorder. Chemotaxis, phagocytosis, and degranulation are normal, but the respiratory burst is enhanced. The supranormal oxidative metabolism may be due to absent MPO-dependent inactivation of the oxidase system[123] and may help explain the lack of clinical expression of this defect in most patients.

Normal MPO is the product of a single gene on chromosome 17.[264] Post-translational cleavage of a glycosylated (89 kD) primary gene product results in a mature molecule containing heavy α (59 kD) and light β (13.5 kD) chains.[262,265,266] The current structural model suggests that the chain content of mature MPO is $\alpha_2\beta_2$, but this is a matter of some debate.[262,267] Granule extracts from normal neutrophils contain an 80–90 kD MPO-related peptide in addition to the mature α- and β-chains, whereas similar extracts from completely deficient MPO neutrophils contain only the 80–90 kD peptide.[265] This finding strongly suggests that MPO deficiency is due to a defect in the post-translational modification of the 89 kD precursor protein. Restriction endonuclease DNA mapping and analysis of MPO-specific mRNA obtained from the bone marrow of deficient individuals indicates that a number of heterogeneous molecular defects are responsible for the phenotypic deficit in processing.[262] MPO deficiency has also been recognized as an acquired defect accompanying some myeloproliferative disorders, particularly acute myelogenous leukemia (AML). In the leukemic but not the preleukemic state this deficiency is associated with an increased risk of infection.[262] This finding coupled with analogous observations in the inherited form of the disorder indicates that the occurrence of MPO deficiency by itself does not alter the host's susceptibility to infection but in conjunction with an additional insult (e.g., diabetes mellitus, AML) may tip the balance in favor of infection.

SPECIFIC GRANULE DEFICIENCY. The absence of specific granules has been recognized in five patients with recurrent infection.[268] The peripheral white blood cell count in such individuals is normal when they are uninfected, and the diagnosis is established by the apparent absence of intracellular granules on routine Wright stain (primary granules do not take up Wright stain). Close examination reveals a bilobed nuclear morphology with nuclear blocks and clefts. Specific granule contents (e.g., lactoferrin, vitamin B_{12}-binding protein) are absent, as is membrane alkaline phosphatase.[164,268,269] This finding coupled with the presence of apparently empty granule vesicles in one of these patients and the abnormal nuclear morphology suggests that the defect may be a more general disorder involving membrane assembly rather than a defect unique to specific granules.[268]

Specific granules are a rich source of substances that modulate the inflammatory response, and their membranes contain receptors for a number of opsonic ligands and inflammatory mediators. Hence it is not surprising that in vitro upregulation of these receptors is impaired and that there are associated impairments in chemotaxis, phagocytosis, and oxidase activity with certain stimuli. Of particular note, however, is the demonstration of an in vivo chemotactic defect for both neutrophils and monocytes from patients with this disorder, whereas only neutrophils exhibit a chemotactic defect in vitro. This finding supports a role for defective chemotaxis in the genesis of infection in these patients and further suggests that a constitutent of specific granules may normally modulate monocyte infiltration to sites of inflammation.[268] Neutrophils from severely burned patients and from neonates share some of the characteristics of specific granule-deficient cells.[268]

Therapy for Neutrophil Defects

Antimicrobial Therapy. The recurrent and severe infections that occur in many patients with abnormal neutrophil function has made the administration of prophylactic antibiotics common despite concerns about colonization and infection with resistant microorganisms. The low prevalence of these disorders has made controlled trials of prophylactic antibiotics nearly impossible, although one study evaluating cloxacillin prophylaxis in the Chédiak-Higashi syndrome did not show any benefit.[270] The administration of lipid-soluble antibiotics such as rifampin and trimethoprim-sulfamethoxazole that penetrate phagocytic cells[271,272] has been advocated for patients with impaired neutrophil bactericidal activity. In this regard, the broad antimicrobial spectrum of trimethoprim-sulfamethoxazole against both gram-positive and gram-negative bacteria, coupled with its penetration and concentration within neutrophils probably explains its apparent effectiveness in reducing infections in patients with CGD.[273,274] Prophylactic antibiotic therapy in patients with CGD has been associated with an increase in the infection-free interval from 9.6 to 40 months.[240] The effect of antibiotics on the intracellular killing mechanisms has received attention with the demonstration that staphylococci exposed to sublethal concentrations of cell wall-active antibiotics for a short time were more readily killed by neutrophils than were staphylococci grown in the absence of antibiotics. Improved killing was due to an enhancement in nonoxidative bactericidal mechanisms and was both organism and antibiotic specific.[275,276] The significance of these findings for patient management is unknown.

Cytokine Therapy. Incubation of IFN-γ with granulocytic cells from patients with CGD enhances superoxide production, restores killing of *S. aureus* and increases cytochrome b_{-558} content. In total, cells from 15 of 18 patients with cytochrome b positive (primarily autosomal) CGD but only 7 of 21 individuals with cytochrome b negative (primarily X-linked) CGD responded to IFN-γ. In vitro testing appeared predictive of a response in vivo in five patients who received subcutaneous injections of recombinant human IFN-γ. Moreover in vivo responses persisted for 3 to 5 weeks following cessation of therapy.[277,277a,277b] Clinical trials evaluating drug toxicity and efficacy in ameliorating the infectious consequences of this disease are currently in progress.

Granulocyte Transfusion. Granylocyte transfusions have been used therapeutically in febrile granulocytopenic patients. To achieve a theoretic blood neutrophil count of 1000 cells/mm^3 after transfusion, approximately 1×10^{10} neutrophils (all the neutrophils in 2–3 liters of blood) are required for the average adult per day. However, many patients will show no significant rise in the peripheral white cell count after transfusion of this number of cells.[278] Two basic methods of procurement have been devised—centrifugation and filtration leukopheresis. The former method uses differences in density among blood cells to achieve separation. Filtration uses the ability of neutrophils to adhere to nylon wool to achieve separation from other cells. Cells obtained by both procedures are functional both in vitro and in vivo, but those obtained by filtration leukopheresis exhibit cytoplasmic vacuolization and surface distortion as well as a loss of granule contents and reduced bactericidal capacity.[278,279] In addition, up to 75 percent of the recipients of cells obtained by leukopheresis will have transfusion reactions, predominantly fever and chills, as compared with 15 percent of the recipients of cells obtained by centrifugation.[280] Despite these differences, administration of cells obtained by either method to granulocytopenic patients with infection has been beneficial in some but not all controlled trials.[281,282] Granulocytopenic patients with proven bacterial infection who received daily granulocyte transfusions for the duration of their infection survived longer than did infected nontransfused control patients. Both groups received therapy appropriate for their infection.[280,283] Leukocyte transfusions have also been therapeutically successful when administered to a limited number of patients with neutrophil bactericidal defects and progressive infection. By using a positive NBT test as a marker, delivery to and persistence of transfused normal leukocytes at the site of infection has been documented in a patient with CGD.[284]

Although leukocyte transfusions may be lifesaving in certain infected granulocytopenic patients, associated complications have limited their routine use in these febrile patients. These complications include (1) transfusion-associated cytomegalovirus infection; (2) allosensitization to HLA antigens; (3) difficulties in locating adequate numbers of suitable donors; (4) risks to the donor; (5) extreme cost of the procedure; and (6) an increased incidence of acute pulmonary reactions when transfusions are given in conjunction with amphotericin B.[285–287] This latter complication is a major concern since one accepted indication for the use of leukocyte transfusions is the treatment of unrelenting fungal infection in the neutropenic host. This reaction most commonly occurs when amphotericin B treatment is initiated simultaneously with or after transfusion. It is characterized by the acute onset of respiratory decompensation, pulmonary infiltrates, and intra-alveolar hemorrhage.[287] A potentially serious complication of red cell or white cell transfusions in patients with CGD is related to the Kell-related antigen, K_X. This antigen is present on the surface of red and

TABLE 5. Evaluation of Neutrophil Function

White blood cell count and differential count
Migration to site[295]
Chemotaxis[296]
Phagocytosis and bactericidal activity[297]
Postphagocytic activity
Oxygen consumption[298]
Hexose monophosphate shunt[299]
Iodination[300]
NBT reduction[259,301]
Degranulation[302]
Chemiluminescence[303]

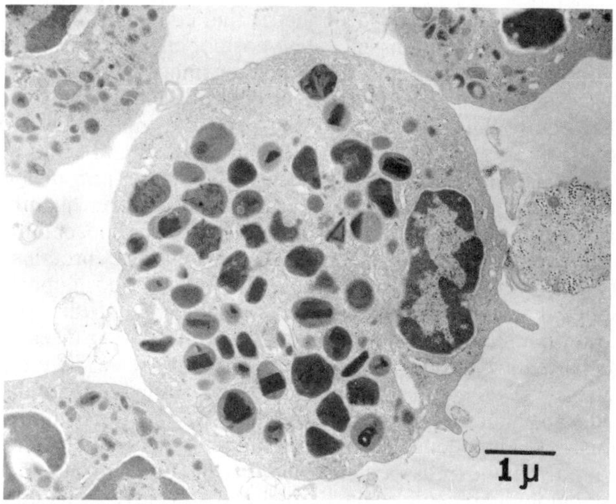

FIG. 7. Electron micrograph of a human eosinophil. Note the prominent granules with crystalloid cores.

white cells from healthy people and patients with autosomally transmitted CGD. K_X is absent from the neutrophils of most patients with the X-linked form of the disease due to the close linkage of the CGD and X_k genes on the X chromosone.[288–290] Failure to recognize this antigenic abnormality can result in severe transfusion reactions.[291] As a consequence of these complicating aspects, leukocyte transfusion seems best reserved for the patient with severe granulocytopenia or functionally defective neutrophils who has a serious bacterial or fungal infection that has not responded to appropriate antimicrobial therapy.

Bone Marrow Transplantation. Several patients, one with leukocyte adhesion deficiency[201] and three with CGD,[292–294] have undergone successful bone marrow engraftment and clinical improvement. Two of the latter patients ultimately rejected their transplant but continued to enjoy clinical improvement.[292,294] This result illustrates the difficulty in the meaningful evaluation of this procedure in these types of patients. Moreover, given the increased infection-free interval and survival observed with the use of prophylactic antibiotics in CGD,[240] it seems reasonable to reserve such aggressive therapy for unusual situations.

Evaluating Phagocyte Function

The single most important test in the evaluation of possible abnormalities of neutrophil function is a white blood cell count with a differential count. Serum immunoglobulin and complement levels should be determined. An NBT test, requiring only a drop or two of blood, is simple and can be performed quickly. Further evaluation depends on the results of these simple screening tests (Table 5).[294]

EOSINOPHILS

Eosinophils are primarily tissue-based granulocytes, the ratio of tissue to blood eosinophils being 100 to 1 in humans.[304] Eosinophils differentiate from stem cells in the bone marrow over the course of 5 to 6 days.[305] Maturation is accompanied by the development of cytoplasmic granules and surface receptors for complement and IgG.[304] The number of these receptors is upregulated during specific stimulation of the eosinophil. There are at least two types of granules present in the cytoplasm of eosinophils. The larger, more numerous eosinophil granules contain an electron-dense crystalloid core (Fig. 7) composed of major basic protein. The crystalloid core is surrounded by a less dense, regularly arranged matrix that contains a number of highly cationic proteins including eosinophil cationic protein, eosinophil-derived neurotoxin, and eosinophil myeloperoxidase. This peroxidase is antigenically and genetically distinct from neutrophil myeloperoxidase. A second, smaller and more homogenous granule containing arylsulfatase B and acid phosphatase is also present in the cytoplasm.[306] Other enzymes and nonenzymatic proteins isolated in relatively greater quantities from eosinophils than from neutrophils include phospholipase D, lysophospholipase, histaminase, and cationic proteins.[304] Oxidative metabolism in resting and stimulated eosinophils is higher than that of neutrophils; the significance of this observation is unknown but may relate to the underlying disease in the patients with hypersinophilia from whom the cells were obtained.[307] Two populations of eosinophils, normodense and hypodense, have been recognized on the basis of their different densities. Hypodense cells are eosinophils that have been activated. They express a greater number of complement and immunoglobulin receptors, have a higher resting level of oxidative metabolism, and predominate in the blood and tissues of individuals with eosinophilia.[306] The half-life of eosinophils in blood is 2 hours.[304] After leaving the circulation, eosinophils are found along with IgE-bearing mast cells and basophils subjacent to the skin and mucosal lining of the respiratory and gastrointestinal tracts.[304,308] The development of eosinophilia[309,310] is dependent in part on a specific cytokine released from sensitized T lymphocytes. An eosinophilopoietin has also been isolated and characterized.[311] These factors produce eosinophilia by increasing eosinophil release from the bone marrow and spleen, shortening the marrow maturation time, and increasing eosinophil production. Eosinophil colony-stimulating factor both stimulates the differentiation of eosinophil precursors and promotes activation of mature eosinophils in the circulation.[306] Certain products of complement activation are chemotactic for eosinophils as they are for neutrophils. Substances specifically chemotactic for eosinophils are released in substantial quantities during immediate hypersensitivity reactions. These substances include eosinophil chemotactic factor of anaphylaxis (ECF-A), histamine, lymphokines, and lipoxygenase metabolites of arachidonic acid, particularly the hydroxyeicosatetranoic acids.[61,304]

Substantial evidence supports a role for eosinophils in immunity to helminthic parasites,[312–314] for modulation of type I hypersensitivity reactions, [304,315] and for the production of tissue damage in certain disease states.[304,306,308,315–317] Although eosinophils can phagocytose bacteria in vitro, they are less efficient in this regard than are neutrophils[307] and probably do not play a role in host defense against bacteria.[316] In contrast, they are a major effector of immunity to helminthic infections as demonstrated by the greater worm burden and tissue damage in animals whose eosinophils have been eliminated by treatment with antieosinophil serum.[314] This conclusion is buttressed by the presence of eosinophils on and around degenerating parasites in vivo and by the ability of eosinophils to kill these organisms in vitro. Killing is also antibody and complement dependent,[312,313] but the transfer of passive immunity requires the presence of eosinophils in the recipient.[314]

Killing of parasites is related to exocytosis of eosinophil granule contents onto the parasite surface while it is in close opposition to the eosinophils.[318,319] The eosinophil peroxidase, hydrogen peroxide, halide oxidation, system plays a minor role in anthelminthic activity.[304,306,308,316] Rather, the cationic granule proteins are responsible for the bulk of this activity. These proteins appear to have different sites of action as inferred from different morphologic alterations in the parasite surface and internal tissues that are observed upon incubation of the organism with purified preparations of the various proteins. Synergistic activity among proteins with different loci of action may occur. On a molar basis eosinophil cationic protein exerts a more potent anthelminthic effect than does major basic protein, but the greater quantity of the latter in the eosinophil makes its contribution more significant.[306] The effect of these proteins is also specific for different stages in the life cycle of the parasite.[306,320]

Recognition that eosinophil granules contain a number of substances capable of inactivating the chemical mediators of anaphylaxis has led to the suggestion that the eosinophil may modulate the severity of type I hypersensitivity reactions.[304,306,317] In this scenario, stimulation of basophils and mast cells by the interaction of surface IgE with specific antigen results in the release of substances important in type I hypersensitivity reactions. These include vasoactive amines, slow-reacting substance of anaphylaxis (leukotrienes C, D, and E), platelet activating factor (PAF), and ECF-A. Histamine and ECF-A attract eosinophils to the site of antigen reaction with basophils and mast cells. ECF-A can also stimulate eosinophil degranulation, as can immune complexes that the eosinophil phagocytizes. Histaminase secreted by the eosinophil may inactivate local histamine, and further histamine secretion by basophils may be inhibited by a substance present in eosinophils. Arylsulfatase and phospholipase present in the smaller eosinophil granules are capable of inactivating leukotrienes C, D, and E and PAF. Thus, eosinophils may modulate immediate hypersensitivity reactions by inhibiting the release of mediators of the type I reaction as well as by destroying mediators that have already been released.[304,315]

The association of eosinophilia of several weeks' duration with the development of endocardial lesions and the isolation of an eosinophil-derived neurotoxin capable of reproducing the neurologic picture observed in patients with cerebrospinal fluid eosinophilia strongly supports a role for the eosinophil in the pathogenesis of tissue injury in certain disorders.[306] Most prominent among these disorders is bronchial asthma. Here substantial evidence indicates that eosinophil major basic protein (MBP) is an important mediator of tissue injury. This evidence can be summarized as follows. (1) Nanomolar concentrations of MBP but not other cationic proteins cause exfoliation of epithelial cells and impaired ciliary function in tracheal ring explants. (2) Immunofluorescent staining of bronchial epithelium in autopsy specimens from patients dying of asthma reveals extensive deposition of MBP in the peribronchial areas and overlying regions of bronchial epithelial denuclation. These findings were not observed in autopsy material obtained from patients whose death was related to other pulmonary diseases. The importance of epithelial denudation lies in the resultant enhanced responsiveness of the underlying bronchial smooth muscle to contractile agonists including leukotriene C_4 produced by eosinophils. (3) Increased quantities of MBP are detectable in the bronchial washings from patients with asthma but not other pulmonary disorders.[306]

BASOPHILS

Basophils are tissue-based granulocytes related to mast cells. Although capable of phagocytosis, they perform this function poorly. Basophil granules are rich in heparin and vasoactive amines, particularly histamine. Basophils circulate with IgE bound to their membrane; recognition of antigen by this cytophilic immunoglobulin results in the external secretion of the contents of the granules. While the pharmacologic actions and importance of these vasoactive amines are well recognized, their physiologic role and the role of the basophils in secreting them is less well understood.[321] Although basophils do not appear to have a primary role in dealing with infection, recent evidence suggests that they may play a role in immunity to ticks.[322]

REFERENCES

1. Silverstein AM. Cellular versus humoral immunity: Determinants and consequences of an epic 19th century battle. Cell Immunol. 1979;48:208.

2. Hirsch JG. Host resistance to infectious diseases—a centennial. Adv Host Defense Mech. 1982;1:1.
3. Bainton DF. Differentiation of human neutrophilic granulocytes: Normal and abnormal. Prog Clin Biol Res. 1977;13:1.
4. Cotter TG, Spears P, Henson PJ. A monoclonal antibody inhibiting human neutrophil chemotaxis and degranulation. J Immunol. 1981;127:1355.
5. Cotter TG, Keeling PG, Henson PM. A monoclonal antibody–inhibiting FMLP-induced chemotaxis of human neutrophils. J Immunol. 1981;127:2241.
6. Nauseef WM, Root RK, Newman SL, et al. Inhibition of zymosan activation of human neutrophil oxidative metabolism by a mouse monoclonal antibody. Blood. 1983;62:635.
7. Glasser L, Fiederlein RL. Functional differentiation of normal human neutrophils. Blood. 1987;69:937–44.
8. Zakhireh B, Root RK. Development of oxidase activity by human bone marrow granulocytes. Blood. 1979;54:429.
9. Lichtman MA, Weed RI. Alteration of the cell periphery during granulocyte maturation: Relationship to cell function. Blood. 1972;39:301.
10. Lichtman MA, Chamberlain JK, Weed RI, et al. The regulation of the release of granulocytes from normal marrow. Prog Clin Biol Res. 1977;13:53.
11. Bainton DF, Farquhar MG. Origin of granules in polymorphonuclear leukocytes. J Cell Biol. 1966;28:277.
12. Bretz U, Baggiolini M. Biochemical and morphological characterization of azurophil and specific granules of human neutrophilic polymorphonuclear leukocytes. J Cell Biol. 1974;63:251.
13. Spitznagel JK, Dalldorf FG, Leffell MS, et al. Character of azurophil and specific granules purified from human polymorphonuclear leukocytes. Lab Invest. 1974;30:774.
14. West BC, Rosenthal AS, Gelb NA, et al. Separation and characterization of human neutrophil granules. Am J Pathol. 1974;77:41.
15. Dewald B, Bretz U, Baggiolini M. Release of gelatinase from a novel secretory compartment of human neutrophils. J Clin Invest. 1982;70:518–25.
16. Brederoo P, van der Meulen J, Mommaas-Kienhuis AM. Development of the granule population in neutrophil granulocytes from human bone marrow. Cell Tissue Res. 1983;234:469–96.
17. Weeds A. Actin-binding proteins—regulators of cell architecture and motility. Nature. 1982;296:811.
18. Southwick FS, Stossel TP. Contractile proteins in leukocyte function. Semin Hematol. 1983;20:305.
19. Stossel TP, Hartwig JH, Yin HL, et al. The motor of leukocytes. Fed Proc. 1984;43:2760–3.
20. Stevenson KB, Nauseef WM, Clark RA. Fodrin and band 4.1 in a plasma membrane–associated fraction of human neutrophils. Submitted for publication.
21. White JR, Naccache PH, Sha'afi RI. Stimulation by chemotactic factor of actin association with the cytoskeleton in rabbit neutrophils. J Biol Chem. 1983;258:14041–7.
22. Ryder MI, Weinreb RN, Niederman R. The organization of actin filaments in human polymorphonuclear leukocytes. Anat Rec. 1984;209:7–20.
23. Berlin RD, Fera JP. Changes in membrane microviscosity associated with phagocytosis: Effects of colchicine. Proc Natl Acad Sci USA. 1977;74:1072.
24. Snyderman R, Goetzl EJ. Molecular and cellular mechanisms of leukocyte chemotaxis. Science. 1981;213:830.
25. Bucher NLR. Microtubules. N Engl J Med. 1972;287:195.
26. Malfunctioning microtubules (Editorial). Lancet. 1978;1:697.
27. Messner RP, Jelinek J. Receptors for human gamma-globulin on human neutrophils. J Clin Invest. 1970;49:2165.
28. Spiegelberg NL, Lawrence DA, Henson P. Cytophilic properties of IgA to human neutrophils. Adv Exp Biol Med. 1974;45:67.
29. Lay WH, Nussenzweig V. Receptors for complement on leukocytes. J Exp Med. 1968;129:991.
30. Williams LT, Snyderman R, Pike MC, et al. Specific receptor sites for chemotactic peptides on human polymorphonuclear leukocytes. Proc Natl Acad Sci USA. 1977;74:1204.
31. Chenoweth DE, Hugli TE. Demonstration of specific C5a receptor on intact human polymorphonuclear leukocytes. Proc Natl Acad Sci USA. 1978;75:3943.
32. Walter RJ, Berlin RD, Oliver JM. Asymmetric Fc receptor distribution on human PMN oriented in a chemotactic gradient. Nature. 1980;286:724.
33. Weinbaum DL, Sullivan JA, Mandell GL. Receptors for concanavalin A cluster at the front of polarized neutrophils. Nature. 1980;286:725.
34. Bender JG, Van Epps DE, Chenoweth DE. Independent regulation of human neutrophil chemotactic receptors after activation. J Immunol. 1987;139:3028–33.
35. Korchak HM, Wildenfeld C, Rich AM, et al. Stimulus response coupling in the human neutrophil. J Biol Chem. 1984;259:7439–45.
36. Walker RI, Willemze R. Neutrophil kinetics and the regulation of granulopoiesis. Rev Infect Dis. 1980;2:282–92.
37. Sachs L. The molecular control of blood cell development. Science. 1987;238:1374–9.
38. Rothstein G, Clarkson DR, Larsen W, et al. Effect of lithium on neutrophil mass and production. N Engl J Med 1978;298:178.
39. Barr RD, Koekebakker M, Brown EA, et al. Putative role for lithium in human hematopoiesis. J Lab Clin Med. 1987;109:159–63.
40. Klempner MS, Gallin JI. Separation and functional characterization of human neutrophil subpopulations. Blood. 1978;51:659.
41. Gallin JI. Human neutrophil heterogeneity exists, but is it meaningful? Blood. 1984;63:977–83.
42. Robinson JM, Karnovsky ML, Karnovsky MJ. Glycogen accumulation in polymorphonuclear leukocytes, and other intracellular alterations that occur during inflammation. J Cell Biol. 1982;95:933.
43. Lentnek AL, Schreiber AD, MacGregor RR: Induction of augmented granulocyte adherence by inflammation. J Clin Invest. 1976;47:1098.
44. Harlan JM. Leukocyte-endothelial interactions. Blood. 1985;65:513–25.
45. Gallin JI. Degranulating stimuli decrease the negative surface charge and increase the adhesiveness of human neutrophils. J Clin Invest. 1980;65:298.
46. Fletcher MP, Gallin JI. Degranulating stimuli increase the availability of human neutrophils for the chemoattractant f-met-leu-phe. J Immunol. 1980;124:1585.
47. Bockenstedt KL, Goetzl EJ. Constituents of human neutrophils that mediate enhanced adherence to surfaces. J Clin Invest. 1980;65:1372.
48. Zimmerli W, Seligmann B, Gallin JI. Exudation primes human and guinea pig neutrophils for subsequent responsiveness to the chemotactic peptide *N*-formylmethionylleucylphenylalanine and increases complement component C3bi receptor expression. J Clin Invest 1986;77:925–33.
49. Lewinsohn DM, Bargatze RF, Butcher EC. Leukocyte–endothelial cell recognition: Evidence of a common molecular mechanism shared by neutrophils, lymphocytes, and other leukocytes. J Immunol. 1987;138:4313–21.
50. Anderson DC, Springer TA. Leukocyte adhesion deficiency: An inherited defect in the Mac-1, LFA-1, and p169,95 glycoproteins. Annu Rev Med. 1987;38:1975–94.
51. Kishimoto TK, O'Connor K, Lee A, et al. Cloning of β subunit of the leukocyte adhesion proteins: Homology to an extracellular matrix receptor defines a novel supergene family. Cell. 1987;48:681–90.
52. Hynes RO. Integrins. A family of cell surface receptors. Cell. 1987;48:549–54.
53. Ruoslahti E, Pierschbacher MD. Arg-Gly-Asp: A versatile cell recognition signal. Cell. 1986;44:517–8.
54. Dustin ML, Rothlein R, Bhan AK, et al. Induction of IL 1 and interferon-γ: Tissue distribution, biochemistry, and function of a natural adherence molecule (ICAM-1). J Immunol. 1986;137:245–54.
55. Zimmerman GA, McIntyre TM. Neutrophil adherence to human endothelium in vitro occurs by CDw18 (Mol, MAC-1/LFA-1/GP 150,95) glycoprotein-dependent and -independent mechanisms. J Clin Invest. 1988;81:531–7.
56. Zigmond SH. Chemotaxis by polymorphonuclear leukocytes. J Cell Biol. 1978;77:269.
57. Sullivan JA, Mandell GL. Motility of human polymorphonuclear neutrophils. J Reticuloendothel Soc. 1983;3:31.
58. Schiffmann E, Corcoran BA, Wahl SM. Formylmethionyl peptides as chemoattractants for leukocytes. Proc Natl Acad Sci USA. 1975;72:1059.
59. Perez HD, Goldstein IM, Webster RO, et al. Enhancement of the chemotactic activity of human C5a des arg by an anionic polypeptide ("cochemotaxin") in normal serum and plasma. J Immunol. 1981;126:800.
60. Perez HD, Chenoweth DE, Goldstein IM. Attachment of human C5a des Arg to its cochemotaxin is required for maximum expression of chemotactic activity. J Clin Invest. 1986;78:1589–95.
61. Goetzl EJ. Mediators of immediate hypersensitivity derived from arachidonic acid. N Engl J Med. 1980;303:822.
62. Wright DG, Gallin JI. A functional differentiation of human neutrophil granules: Generation of C5a by a specific (secondary) granule product and inactivation of C5a by azurophil (primary) granule products. J Immunol. 1977;119:1068.
63. Donabedian H, Gallin JI. Deactivation of human neutrophil chemotaxis by chemoattractants: Effect on receptors for the chemotactic factor f-met-leu-phe. J Immunol. 1981;127:839.
64. Jesaitis AJ, Naemura JR, Painter RG, et al. The fate of an *N*-formylated chemotactic peptide in stimulated human granulocytes. J Biol Chem. 1983;258:1968–77.
65. Perez HD, Elfman F, Lobo E. Removal of human polymorphonuclear leukocyte surface sialic acid inhibits reexpression (or recycling) of formyl peptide receptors. J Immunol. 1987;139:1978–84.
66. Clark RA. Chemotactic factors trigger their own oxidative inactivation by human neutrophils. J Immunol. 1982;129:2725.
67. Lee CW, Lewis RA, Corey EJ, et al. Oxidative inactivation of leukotriene C4 by stimulated human polymorphonuclear leukocytes. Proc Natl Acad Sci USA. 1982;79:4166.
68. Gordon LI, Douglas SD, Kay NE, et al. Modulation of neutrophil function by lysozyme. J Clin Invest. 1979;64:226.
69. Bobak DA, Gaither TA, Frank MM, et al. Modulation of FcR function by complement: Subcomponent C1q enhances the phagocytosis of IgG-opsonized targets by human monocytes and culture-derived macrophages. J Immunol. 1987;138:1150–56.
70. Petroni KC, Shen L, Guyre PM. Modulation of human polymorphonuclear leukocyte IgG Fc receptors and Fc receptor-mediated functions by IFN-γ and glucocorticoids. J Immunol. 1988;140:3467–72.
71. Lew DP, Andersson T, Hed J, et al. Ca^{2+}-dependent and Ca^{2+}-independent phagocytosis in human neutrophils. Nature. 1985;315:509–11.
72. Berger M, O'Shea J, Cross AS, et al. Human neutrophils increase expression of C3bi as well as C3b receptors upon activation. J Clin Invest. 1984;74:1566–71.
73. O'Shea JJ, Brown EJ, Seligmann BE, et al. Evidence for distinct intracellular

pools of receptors for C3b and C3bi in human neutrophils. J Immunol. 1985;134:2580–7.
74. Stendahl O, Coble B-I, Dahlgren C, et al. Myeloperoxidase modulates the phagocytic activity of polymorphonuclear neutrophil leukocytes. Studies with cells from a myeloperoxidase-deficient patient. J Clin Invest. 1984;73:366–73.
75. Gaither TA, Medley SR, Gallin JI, et al. Studies of phagocytosis in chronic granulomatous disease. Inflammation. 1987;11:211–27.
76. Lawrence WD, Packman CH, Rowe JM, et al. Attachment of particle bound IgG and complement to human neutrophils. Blood. 1981;58:772.
77. Stossel TP. Phagocytosis recognition and ingestion. Semin Hematol. 1975;12:83.
78. Newman S, Johnston RB Jr. Role of binding through C3b and IgG in polymorphonuclear neutrophil function: Studies with trypsin generated C3b. J Immunol. 1979;123:1839.
79. Brown EJ, Bohnsack JF, Gresham HD. Mechanism of inhibition of immunoglobulin G-mediated phagocytosis by monoclonal antibodies that recognize the Mac-1 antigen. J Clin Invest. 1988;81:365–75.
80. Griffin FM, Griffin JH, Leider JE, et al. Studies on the mechanism of phagocytosis. I. Requirements for circumferential attachment of particle bound ligands to specific receptors on the macrophage plasma membrane. J Exp Med. 1975;142:1263.
81. Griffin FM, Griffin JA, Silverstein SC. Studies on the mechanism of phagocytosis. II. The interaction of macrophages with anti-immunoglobulin IgG-coated bone marrow derived lymphocytes. J Exp Med. 1976;144:788.
82. van Oss CJ. Phagocytosis as a surface phenomenon. Annu Rev Microbiol. 1978;32:19.
83. Wright SD, Griffin FM. Activation of phagocytic cells' C3 receptors for phagocytosis. J Leukocyte Biol. 1985;38:327–39.
84. Brown EJ. The role of extracellular matrix proteins in the control of phagocytosis. J Leukocyte Biol. 1986;39:579–91.
85. Babior GL, Crowley CA. Chronic granulomatous disease and other disorders of killing by phagocytes. In: Steinbury JB, Wyngaarden JB, Frederickson DS, et al, eds. The Metabolic Basis of Inherited Disease. 5th ed. New York: McGraw-Hill; 1983:1969.
86. Eggleston LV, Krebs AA. Regulation of the pentose phosphate cycle. Biochem J. 1974;138:424.
87. Babior BM, Rosin RE, McMurrich BJ, et al. Arrangement of the respiratory burst oxidase in the plasma membrane of the neutrophil. J Clin Invest. 1981;67:1724.
88. Borregaard N, Tauber AI. Subcellular localization of the human neutrophil NADPH oxidase. J Biol Chem. 1984;259:47–52.
89. Rossi F. The $O_2^{\cdot}$-forming NADPH oxidase of the pahgocytes: Nature, mechanisms of activation and function. Biochim Biophys Acta. 1986;853:65–89.
90. Bellavite P. The superoxide-forming enzymatic system of phagocytes. Free Radic Biol Med. 1988;4:225–261.
91. Cross AR, Jones OTG, Garcia R, et al. The association of the FAD with the cytochrome b_{-245} of human neutrophils. Biochem J. 1982;208:759.
92. Gabig TG, Schervish EW, Santinga JT. Functional relationship of the cytochrome b to the superoxide-generating oxidase of human neutrophils. J Biol Chem. 1982;257:4114–9.
93. McPhail LC, Shirley PS, Clayton CC, et al. Activation of the respiratory burst enzyme from human neutrophils in a cell-free system. J Clin Invest. 1985;75:1735–9.
94. Curnutte JT. Activation of human neutrophil nicotinamide adenine dinucleotide phosphate, reduced (triphosphopyridine nucleotide, reduced) oxidase by arachidonic acid in a cell-free system. J Clin Invest. 1985;75:1740–43.
95. Clark RA, Leidal KG, Pearson DW, et al. NADPH oxidase of human neutrophils. J Biol Chem. 1987;262:4065–74.
96. Segal AW, Jones OTG, Webster D, et al. Absence of a newly described cytochrome b from neutrophils of patients with chronic granulomatous disease. Lancet. 1978;2:446–9.
97. Segal AW, Cross AR, Garcia RD, et al. Absence of cytochrome b_{-245} in chronic granulomatous disease: A multicenter European evaluation of its incidence and relevance. N Engl J Med. 1983;308:245.
98. Ohno Y, Buescher ES, Roberts R, et al. Reevaluation of cytochrome b and flavin adenine dinucleotide in neutrophils from patients with chronic granulomatous disease and description of a family with probable autosomal recessive inheritance of cytochrome b deficiency. Blood. 1986;67:1132–8.
99. Curnutte JT, Berkow RL, Roberts RL, et al. Chronic granulomatous disease due to a defect in the cytosolic factor required for nicotinamide adenine dinucleotide phosphate oxidase activation. J Clin Invest. 1988;81:606–10.
100. Umei T, Takeshige K, Minakami S. NADPH binding component of neutrophil superoxide-generating oxidase. J Biol Chem. 1984;261:5229–32.
101. Parkos CA, Allen RA, Cochrane CG, et al. Purified cytochrome b from human granulocyte plasma membrane is comprised of two polypeptides with relative molecular weights of 91,000 and 22,000. J Clin Invest. 1987;80:732–42.
102. Royer-Pokora B, Kunkel LM, Monaco AP, et al. Cloning the gene for an inherited human disorder—chronic granulomatous disease—on the basis of its chromosomal location. Nature. 1986;322:32–8.
103. Dinauer MC, Orkin SH, Brown R, et al. The glycoprotein encoded by the X-linked chronic granulomatous disease locus is a component of the neutrophil cytochrome b complex. Nature. 1987;327:717–20.
104. Teahan C, Rowe P, Parker P, et al. The X-linked chronic granulomatous disease gene codes for the β-chain of cytochrome b_{-245}. Nature. 1987;327:720–1.
105. Harper AM, Chaplin MF, Segal AW. Cytochrome b_{-245} from human neutrophils is a glycoprotein. Biochem J. 1985;227:783–8.
106. Tauber AI, Borregaard N, Simons ER, et al. Phagocyte oxidase deficiency syndrome (PODS): A revised nosology of chronic granulomatous disease and related acquired disorders. Medicine (Baltimore). 1983;62:286–309.
107. Whitin JC, Chapman CE, Simons ER, et al. Correlation between membrane potential changes and superoxide production in human granulocytes stimulated by phorbol myristate acetate. J Biol Chem. 1980;255:1874.
108. Seligmann BE, Gallin JI. Use of lipophilic probes of membrane potential to assess human neutrophil activation. J Clin Invest. 1980;66:493.
109. Borregaard N, Heiple JM, Simons ER, et al. Subcellular localization of the b-cytochrome component of the human neutrophil microbicidal oxidase: Translocation during activation. J Cell Biol. 1983;97:52.
110. Ohno Y, Seligmann BE, Gallin JI. Cytochrome b translocation to human neutrophil plasma membranes and superoxide release. J Biol Chem. 1985;260:2409–14.
111. Goldstein IM, Kaplan HB, Radin A, et al. Independent effects of IgG and complement upon human PMN leukocyte function. J Immunol. 1976;177:1282.
112. Henson PM, Oades ZG. Stimulation of human neutrophils by soluble and insoluble immunoglobulin aggregates. J Clin Invest. 1975;56:1053.
113. Curnutte JT, Babior BM, Karnovsky ML. Fluoride-mediated activation of the respiratory burst in human neutrophils. A reversible process. J Clin Invest. 1979;63:637.
114. Badwey J, Curnutte JT, Karnovsky ML. *Cis*-polyunsaturated fatty acids induce high levels of superoxide production by human neutrophils. J Biol Chem. 1981;256:12640.
115. Mollinedo F, Schneider DL. Subcellular localization of cytochrome b and ubiquinone in a tertiary granule of resting human neutrophils and evidence for a proton pump ATPase. J Biol Chem. 1984;259:7143–50.
116. Yamaguchi T, Kaneda M, Kakinuma K. Is cytochrome b_{-558} translocated into the plasma membrane from granules during the activation of neutrophils? J Biochem. 1986;99:953–9.
117. Tauber AI. Protein kinase C and the activation of the human neutrophil NADPH-oxidase. Blood. 1987;69:711–20.
118. McPhail LC, Snyderman R. Activation of the respiratory burst enzyme in human polymorphonuclear leukocytes by chemoattractants and other soluble stimuli. J Clin Invest. 1983;72:192–200.
119. Clark RA, Volpp BD, Leidal KG, et al. NADPH oxidase in subcellular fractions of human neutrophils: Evidence for a guanine and adenine nucleotide-dependent activation event (Abstract). Clin Res. 1987;35:655.
120. Badwey JA, Curnutte JT, Robinson JM, et al. Effect of free fatty acids on release of superoxide and on change of shape by human neutrophils. Reversibility by albumin. J Biol Chem. 1984;259:7870.
121. Bromberg Y, Pick E. Activation of NADPH-dependent superoxide production in a cell-free system by sodium dodecyl sulfate. J Biol Chem. 1985;260:13539.
122. McPhail LC, Clayton CC, Snyderman R. The NADPH oxidase of human polymorphonuclear leukocytes. J Biol Chem. 1984;259:5768–75.
123. Jandl RC, Andre-Schwartz J, Borges-Dubois L, et al. Termination of the respiratory burst in human neutrophils. J Clin Invest. 1978;61:1176.
124. Leffell MS, Spitznagel JK. Fate of human lactoferrin and myeloperoxidase in phagocytizing human neutrophils: Effects of immunoglobulin G subclasses and immune complexes coated on latex beads. Infect Immun. 1975;12:813.
125. Naccache PH, Showell HJ, Becker EL, et al. Changes in ionic movements across rabbit polymorphonuclear leukocyte membranes during lysosomal enzyme release. J Cell Biol. 1977;75:665.
126. Korchak HM, Weissmann G. Changes in membrane potential of human granulocytes antecede the metabolic responses to surface stimulation. Proc Natl Acad Sci USA. 1978;75:3818.
127. Weissmann G, Smolen JE, Korchak HM. Release of inflammatory mediators from stimulated neutrophils. N Engl J Med. 1980;303:27.
128. Wright DG. The neutrophil as a secretory organ of host defense. Adv Host Defense Mech. 1982;1:75.
129. Goldstein IM, Hoffstein ST, Weissmann G. Influence of divalent cations upon complement-mediated enzyme release from human PMN leukocytes. J Immunol. 1975;115:665.
130. Moore PL, Bank HL, Brissie NT, et al. Association of microfilament bundles with lysosomes in PMN leukocytes. J Cell Biol. 1976;71:659.
131. Goldstein IM. Polymorphonuclear leukocyte lysosomes and immune tissue injury. Prog Allergy. 1976;20:301.
132. Becker EL. Leukocyte stimulation: Receptor, membrane, and metabolic events. Fed Proc. 1986;7:2148–50.
133. Bell RM. Protein kinase C activation by diacylglycerol second messengers. Cell. 1986;45:631–2.
134. Marx JL. Polyphospoinositide research updated. Science. 1987;235:974–6.
135. Casey PJ, Gilman AG. G protein involvement in receptor-effector coupling. J Biol Chem. 1988;263:2577–80.
136. Krause K-H, Lew PD. Subcellular distribution of Ca^{2+} pumping sites in human neutrophils. J Clin Invest. 1987;80:107–16.
137. Volpe P, Krause K-H, Hashimoto S, et al. "Calciosome," a cytoplasmic organelle: The inositol 1,4,5-trisphosphate–sensitive Ca^{2+} store of nonmuscle cells? Proc Natl Acad Sci USA. 1988;85:1091–5.
138. Sawyer DW, Sullivan JA, Mandell GL. Intracellular free calcium localization in neutrophils during phagocytosis. Science. 1985;230:663–6.

139. Segal AW, Heyworth PG, Cockcroft S, et al. Stimulated neutrophils from patients with autosomal recessive chronic granulomatous disease fail to phosphorylate a M_r-44,000 protein. Nature 1985;316:547–9.
140. Hayakawa T, Suzuki K, Suzuki S, et al. A possible role for protein phosphorylation in the activation of the respiratory burst in human neutrophils. J Biol Chem. 1986;261:9109–15.
141. Caldwell SE, McCall CE, Hendricks CL, et al. Coregulation of NADPH oxidase activation and phosphorylation of a 48-kD protein(s) by a cytosolic factor defective in autosomal recessive chronic granulomatous disease. J Clin Invest. 1988;81:1485–96.
142. Becker EL, Kermode JC, Naccache PH, et al. Pertussis toxin as a probe of neutrophil activation. Fed Proc. 1986;45:2151–5.
143. Van Epps DE, Garcia ML. Enhancement of neutrophil function as a result of prior exposure to chemotactic factor. J Clin Invest. 1980;66:167–75.
144. Bender JG, McPhail LC, Van Epps DE. Exposure of human neutrophils to chemotactic factors potentiates activation of the respiratory burst enzyme. J Immunol. 1983;130:2316–23.
145. Bass DA, Gerard C, Olbrantz P, et al. Priming of the respiratory burst of neutrophils by diacylglycerol. J Biol Chem. 1987;262:6643–9.
146. Densen P, Mandell GL. Gonococcal interactions with polymorphonuclear neutrophils. Importance of the phagosome for bactericidal activity. J Clin Invest. 1978;62:1161.
147. Klebanoff SJ. Antimicrobial mechanisms in neutrophilic PMN leukocytes. Semin Hematol. 1975;12:117.
148. Rosen H, Klebanoff SJ. Oxidation of *Escherichia coli* iron centers by the myeloperoxidase-mediated microbicidal system. J Biol Chem. 1982;257:13731–5.
149. Rosen H, Klebanoff SJ. Oxidation of microbial iron-sulfur centers by the myeloperoxidase-H_2O_2-halide antimicrobial system. Infect Immun. 1985;47:613–8.
150. Rosen H, Rakita RM, Waltersdorph AM, et al. Myeloperoxidase-mediated damage to the succinate oxidase system of *Escherichia coli.* J Biol Chem. 1987;262:15004–10.
151. Repine JE, Fox RB, Berger EM. Hydrogen peroxide kills *Staphylococcus aureus* by reacting with staphylococcal iron to form hydroxyl radical. J Biol Chem. 1981;256:7094–6.
152. Thomas EL, Jefferson MM, Grisham MB. Myeloperoxidase-catalyzed incorporation of amines into proteins: Role of hypochlorous acid and dichloramines. Biochemistry. 1982;24:6299–6308.
153. Grisham MB, Jefferson MM, Melton DF, et al. Chlorination of endogenous amines by isolated neutrophils. J Biol Chem. 1984;259:10404–13.
154. Klebanoff SJ. Oxygen-dependent cytotoxic mechanisms of phagocytes. Adv Host Defense Mech. 1982;1:111.
155. Babior BM. Oxygen-dependent microbial killing by phagocytes. N Engl J Med. 1978;298:659, 721.
156. Mandell GL. Catalase, superoxide dismutase, and virulence of *S. aureus*. J Clin Invest. 1975;55:561.
157. Klebanoff SJ. The iron-H_2O_2-iodide cytotoxic system. J Exp Med. 1982;156:1262–7.
158. Cohen MS, Britigan BE, Hassett DJ, et al. Phagocytes, O_2 reduction, and hydroxyl radical. Rev Infect Dis. 1988;10:1088.
159. Britigan BE, Rosen GM, Chai Y, et al. Do human neutrophils make hydroxyl radical? J Biol Chem. 1986;261:4426–31.
160. Mandell GL. Bactericidal activity of aerobic and anaerobic polymorphonuclear neutrophils. Infect Immun. 1974;9:337.
161. Mandell GL. Intraphagosomal pH of human polymorphonuclear neutrophils. Proc Soc Exp Biol Med. 1970;134:447.
162. Oram JD, Reiter B. Inhibition of bacteria by lactoferrin and other iron-chelating agents. Biochim Biophys Acta. 1968;170:351.
163. Boxer LA, Coates TD, Haak RA, et al. Lactoferrin deficiency associated with altered granulocyte function. N Engl J Med. 1982;387:404.
164. Broxmeyer HE, Smithyman A, Eger RR, et al. Identification of lactoferrin as the granulocyte-derived inhibitor of colony-stimulating activity production. J Exp Med. 1978;148:1052.
165. Kijlstra A, Jeurissen HM. Modulation of classical C3 convertase of complement by tear lactoferrin. Immunology. 1982;47:263.
166. Sptiznagel JK, Shafer WM. Neutrophil killing of bacteria by oxygen-independent mechanisms: A historical summary. Rev Infect Dis 1985;7:398.
167. Elsbach P, Weiss J. Oxygen-independent bactericidal systems of polymorphonuclear leukocytes. In: Weissmann G, ed. Advances in Inflammation Research. v. 2. New York: Raven Press; 1981:95.
168. Ganz T, Selsted ME, Lehrer RI. Antimicrobial activity of phagocyte granule proteins. Semin Respir Infect 1986;1:107.
169. Zeya AT, Spitznagel JK. Arginine-rich proteins of PMN leukocyte lysosomes. J Exp Med. 1968;127:927.
170. Shafer WM, Martin LE, Spitznagel JK. Cationic antimicrobial proteins isolated from human neutrophil granulocytes in the presence of diisopropyl flurophosphate. Infect Immun. 1984;45:29.
171. Shafer WM, Martin LE, Spitznagel JK. Late intraphagosomal hydrogen ion concentration favors the in vitro antimicrobial capacity of a 37-kilodalton cationic granule protein of human neutrophil granulocytes. Infect Immun. 1986;53:651.
172. Ooi CE, Weiss J, Elsbach P, et al. A 25-kD NH_2-terminal fragment carries all the antibacterial activities of the human neutrophil 60-kD bactericidal/permeability-increasing protein. J Biol Chem. 1987;262:14891.
173. Ganz T, Selsted ME, Szklarek D, et al. Defensins. Natural peptide antibiotics of human neutrophils. J Clin Invest. 1985;76:1427.
174. Weiss J, Victor M, Elsbach P. Role of charge and hydrophobic interactions in the action of the bactericidal/permeability-increasing protein of neutrophils on gram-negative bacteria. J Clin Invest. 1983;71:540.
175. Selsted ME, Harwig SSL, Ganz T, et al. Primary structures of three human neutrophil defensins. J Clin Invest. 1985;76:1436.
176. Leijh PCJ, van den Barselaar MTh, van Zwet TL, et al. Requirement of extracellular complement and immunoglobulin for intracellular killing of microorganisms by human monocytes. J Clin Invest. 1979;63:772.
177. Tedesco F, Rottini G, Patriarca P. Modulating effect of the late acting components of the complement system on the bactericidal activity of human polymorphonuclear leukocytes on *E. coli* 0111:34. J Immunol. 1981;127:1910.
178. Densen P, Mandell GL. Phagocyte strategy vs. microbial tactics. Rev Infect Dis. 1980;2:817.
179. Bellavite P, Serra MC, Davoli A, et al. Selective enrichment of NADPH oxidase activity in phagosomes from guinea pig polymorphonuclear leukocytes. Inflammation. 1982;6:21.
180. Ohno YI, Hirai KI, Kanoh T, et al. Subcellular localization of H_2O_2 production in human neutrophils stimulated with particles and an effect of cytochalasin-B on the cells. Blood. 1982;60:253.
181. Clark RA. Extracellular effects of the myeloperoxidase-hydrogen peroxide-halide system. In: Weissmann G, ed. v. 5. Advances in Inflammation Research. New York: Raven Press; 1983;107.
182. Britigan BE, Rosen GM, Thompson BY, et al. Stimulated human neutrophils limit iron-catalyzed hydroxyl radical formation as detected by spin-trapping techniques. J Biol Chem. 1986;261:17026.
183. Britigan BE, Hassett DJ, Rosen GM, et al. Neutrophil degranulation inhibits potential hydroxyl radical formation: Differential impact of myeloperoxidase and lactoferrin release on hydroxyl radical production by iron supplemented neutrophils assessed by spin trapping techniques. Submitted for publication.
184. Henson PM, Johnston RB Jr. Tissue injury in inflammation. J Clin Invest. 1987;79:669.
185. Cross CE, Halliwell B, Borish ET, et al. Oxygen radicals and human disease. Ann Intern Med. 1987;107:526.
186. Jacob HS, Craddock PR, Hammerschmidt DE, et al. Complement induced granulocyte aggregation. An unsuspected mechanism of disease. N Engl J Med. 1980;302:789.
187. Zimmerman G, Renzetti AD, Hill HR. Functional and metabolic activity of granulocytes from patients with adult respiratory distress syndrome. Evidence for activated neutrophils in the pulmonary circulation. Am Rev Respir Dis. 1983;127:290.
188. Hammerschmidt DE. Activation of the complement system and of granulocytes in lung injury: The adult respiratory distress syndrome. In: Weissmann G, ed. Advances in Inflammation Research v. 5. New York: Raven Press; 1983:147.
189. Smedley LA, Tonnesen MG, Sandhaus RA, et al. Neutrophil-mediated injury to endothelial cells: Enhancement by endotoxin and essential role of neutrophil elastase. J Clin Invest. 1968;77:1233.
190. Ognibene FP, Martin SE, Parker MM, et al. Adult respiratory distress syndrome in patients with severe neutropenia. N Engl J Med. 1986;315:547.
191. Janoff A. Elastase in tissue injury. Annu Rev Med. 1985;36:207.
192. Wewers MD, Gadek JE. The protease theory of emphysema. Ann Intern Med. 1987;107:761.
193. Carrell RW. α_1-Antitrypsin: Molecular pathology, leukocytes and tissue damage. J Clin Invest. 1986;78:1427.
194. Desrochers PE, Weiss SJ. Proteolytic inactivation of alpha-1-proteinase inhibitor by a neutrophil metalloproteinase. J Clin Invest. 1988;81:1646.
195. Rotrosen D, Gallin JI. Disorders of phagocyte function. Annu Rev Immunol. 1987;5:127.
196. Malech HL, Gallin JI. Neutrophils in human diseases. N Engl J Med. 1987;317:687.
197. Bodey GP, Buckley M, Sathe YS, et al. Quantitative relationships between circulating leukocytes and infection in patients with acute leukemia. Ann Intern Med. 1966;64:328.
198. Cines DB, Passero F, DuPont GM, et al. Granulocyte-associated IgG in neutropenic disorders. Blood. 1982;59:124.
199. Wright DG. Autoimmune leukopenia. In Lichtenstein LM, Fauci AS, eds: Current Therapy in Allergy and Immunology. Toronto: BC Decker; 1983:277.
200. Wright DG, Fauci AS, Dale DC, et al. Correction of human cyclic neutropenia with prednisolone. N Engl J Med. 1978;298:295.
201. Boxer LA, Hedley-Whyte T, Stossel TP: Neutrophil actin dysfunction and abnormal neutrophil behavior. N Engl J Med. 1974;291:1093.
202. Crowley CA, Curnutte JT, Rosin RE, et al. An inherited abnormality of neutrophil adhesion. N Engl J Med. 1980;302:1163.
203. Arnaout MA, Pitt J, Cohen HJ, et al. Deficiency of a granulocyte-membrane glycoprotein (gp-150) in a boy with recurrent bacterial infections. N Engl J Med. 1982;306:693.
204. Weening RS, Roos D, Weemoes CMR, et al. Defective imitation of the metabolic stimulation in phagocytizing granulocytes: A new congenital defect. J Lab Clin Med. 1976;88:757.
205. Harvath L, Andersen BR. Defective initiation of oxidative metabolism in polymorphonuclear leukocytes. N Engl J Med. 1979;300:1130.
206. Anderson DC, Schmalsteig FC, Finegold MJ, et al. The severe and moderate phenotypes of heritable Mac-1, LFA-1 deficiency: Their quantitative definition and relation to leukocyte dysfunction and clinical features. J Infect Dis. 1985;152:668.

207. Nauseef WM, de Alarcon P, Bale JF, et al. Aberrant activation and regulation of the oxidative burst in neutrophils with Mol glycoprotein deficiency. J Immunol. 1986;137:636.
208. Springer TA, Thompson WS, Miller LJ, et al. Inherited deficiency of the Mac-1, LFA-1, p150,95 glycoprotein family and its molecular basis. J Exp Med. 1984;160:1901.
209. Kishimoto TK, Hollander N, Roberts TM, et al. Heterogeneous mutations in the β subunit common to the LFA-1, Mac-1, and p150,95 glycoproteins cause leukocyte adhesion deficiency. Cell. 1987;50:193.
210. Gallin JI. Abnormal phagocyte chemotaxis: Pathophysiology, clinical manifestations, and management of patients. Rev Infect Dis. 1981;3:1196.
211. Quie PG, Cates KL. Clinical conditions associated with defective PMN leukocyte chemotaxis. Am J Pathol. 1977;88:711.
212. Ward PA. Leukotaxis and leukotactic disorders. Am J Pathol. 1974;77:520.
213. Van Epps DE, Williams RC. Suppression of leukocyte chemotaxis by human IgA myeloma components. J Exp Med. 1976;144:1227.
214. Clark RA, Kimball HR, Decker JL. Neutrophil chemotaxis in systemic lupus erythematosus. Ann Rheum Dis. 1974;33:167.
215. Perez HD, Lipton M, Goldstein IM. A specific inhibitor of complemennt (C5)-derived chemotactic activity in serum from patients with systemic lupus erythematosus. J Clin Invest. 1978;62:29.
216. Perez HD, Hooper C, Volanakis J, et al. Specific inhibitor of complement derived chemotactic activity in systemic lupus erythematosus related antigenically to the Bb fragment of human factor B. J Immunol. 1987;139:484.
217. Perez HD, Goldstein IM. Polymorphonuclear leukocyte chemotaxis in systemic lupus erythematosus. J Rheumatol. 1987;14:53.
218. Cianciola LJ, Genco RJ, Patters MR, et al. Defective polymorphonuclear leukocyte function in a human periodontal disease. Nature. 1977;265:445.
219. Clark RA, Page RC, Wilde G. Defective neutrophil chemotaxis in juvenile periodontis. Infect Immun. 1977;18:694.
220. Van Dyke TE. Role of the neutrophil in oral disease: Receptor deficiency in leukocytes from patients with juvenile periodontitis. Rev Infect Dis. 1985;7:419.
221. Shurin SB, Socransky SS, Sweeney E, et al. A neutrophil disorder induced by capnocytophaga; a dental micro-organism. N Engl J Med. 1979;301:849.
222. Kramer N, Perez HD, Goldstein IM. An immunoglobulin (IgG) inhibitor of polymorphonuclear leukocyte motility in a patient with recurrent infection. N Engl J Med. 1980;303:1253.
223. Rausch PG, Pryzwansky KB, Spitznagel JK. Immunochemical characterization of Chédiak-Higashi neutrophils. N Engl J Med. 1978;298:693.
224. Haliotis T, Roder J, Klein M, et al. Chédiak-Higashi gene in humans. I. Impairment of natural killer function. J Exp Med. 1980;151:1039.
225. Blume RS, Wolff SM. The Chédiak-Higashi syndrome: Studies in four patients and a review of the literature. Medicine (Baltimore). 1972;51:247.
226. Clark RA, Kimball HR. Defective granulocyte chemotaxis in the Chédiak-Higashi syndrome. J Clin Invest. 1971;50:2645.
227. Root RK, Rosenthal AS, Balestra DJ. Abnormal bactericidal, metabolic, and lysosomal functions of Chédiak-Higashi syndrome leukocytes. J Clin Invest. 1972;51:649.
228. Oliver JM. Cell biology of leukocyte abnormalities—membrane and cytoskeletal functions in normal and defective cells. Am J Pathol. 1978;93:219.
229. Baehner RL, Boxer LA. Disorders of polymorphonuclear leukocyte function related to alterations in the integrated reactions of cytoplasmic constituents with the plasma membrane. Semin Hematol. 1979;16:148.
230. Pryzwansky KB, Schliwa M, Boxer LA. Microtubule organization of unstimulated and stimulated adherent human neutrophils in Chédiak-Higashi syndrome. Blood. 1985;66:1398.
231. Davis SD, Schaller J, Wedgwood RJ. Job's syndrome. Recurrent "cold" staphylococcal abscesses. Lancet. 1966;1:1013.
232. Donabedian H, Gallin JI. The hyperimmunoglobulin E recurrent-infection (Job's) syndrome. Medicine (Baltimore). 1983;62:195.
233. Donabedian H, Gallin JI. Mononuclear cells from patients with the hyperimmunoglobulinemia E recurrent infection syndrome produce an inhibitor of leukocyte chemotaxis. J Clin Invest. 1982;69:1155.
234. Dreskin SC, Goldsmith PK, Strober W, et al. Metabolism of immunoglobulin E in patients with markedly elevated serum immunoglobulin E levels. J Clin Invest. 1987;79:1764.
235. Dreskin SC, Goldsmith PK, Gallin JI. Immunoglobulins in the hyperimmunoglobulin E and recurrent infection (Job's) syndrome. J Clin Invest. 1985;75:26.
236. Donabedian H, Alling DW, Gallin JI. Levamisole is inferior to placebo in the hyperimmunoglobulin E recurrent-infection (Job's) syndrome. N Engl J Med. 1982;307:290.
237. Craddock PR, Yawata P, Van Santen L, et al. Acquired phagocyte dysfunction. A complication of the hypophosphatemia of parenteral hyperalimentation. N Engl J Med. 1974;290:1403.
238. Najjar VA, Constantopoulos A. A new phagocytosis stimulating tetrapeptide hormone, tuftsin and its role in disease. J Reticuloendothel Soc. 1972;12:197.
239. Bisno AL, Freeman JC. The syndrome of asplenia, pneumococcal sepsis, and disseminated intravascular coagulation. Ann Intern Med. 1970;72:389.
240. Gallin JI, Buescher ES, Seligmann BE, et al. Recent advances in chronic granulomatous disease. Ann Intern Med. 1983;99:657–74.
241. Lazarus GM, Neu HM. Agents responsible for infection in chronic granulomatous disease of childhood. J Pediatr. 1975;86:415.
242. Johnston RB Jr, Newman SL. Chronic granulomatous disease. Pediatr Clin North Am 1977;24:365.
243. Dilworth JA, Mandell GL. Adults with chronic granulomatous disease of childhood. Am J Med. 1977;63:233.
244. Schaller J. Illness resembling lupus erythematosus in mothers of boys with chronic granulomatous disease. Ann Intern Med. 1972;76:747.
245. Kragballe K, Borregaard N, Brandrup F, et al. Relation of monocyte and neutrophil oxidative metabolism to skin and oral lesions in carriers of chronic granulomatous disease. Clin Exp Immunol. 1981;43:390.
246. Johnston RB Jr. Unusual forms of an uncommon disease (chronic granulomatous disease). J Pediatr. 1976;88:172.
247. Bohler M-C, Seger RA, Mouy R, et al. A study of 25 patients with chronic granulomatous disease: A new classification by correlating respiratory burst, cytochrome b, and flavoprotein. J Clin Immunol. 1986;6:136.
248. Lew PD, Southwick FS, Stossel TP, et al. A variant of chronic granulomatous disease: Deficient oxidative metabolism due to a low-affinity NADPH oxidase. N Engl J Med. 1981;305:1329.
249. Seger RA, Tiefenauer L, Matsunaga T, et al. Chronic granulomatous disease due to granulocytes with abnormal NADPH oxidase activity and deficient cytochrome b. Blood. 1983;61:423.
250. Hamers MN, de Boer M, Meerhof LJ, et al. Complementation in monocyte hybrids revealing genetic heterogeneity in chronic granulomatous disease. Nature. 1984;307:553–5.
251. Weening RS, Corbeel L, De Boer M, et al. Cytochrome b deficiency in an autosomal form of chronic granulomatous disease. J Clin Invest. 1985;75:915–20.
252. Segal AW. Absence of both cytochrome b_{-245} subunits from neutrophils in X-linked chronic granulomatous disease. Nature. 1987;326:88.
253. Weenings RS, Adriaansz LH, Weemaes CMR, et al. Clinical differences in chronic granulomatous disease in patients with cytochrome b-negative or cytochrome b-positive neutrophils. J Pediatr. 1985;107:102.
254. Caldwell SE, McCall CE, Hendricks CL. Coregulation of NADPH oxidase activation and phosphorylation of a 48-kD protein(s) by a cytosolic factor defective in autosomal recessive chronic granulomatous disease. J Clin Invest. 1988;81:1485.
255. Curnutte JT, Kuver R, Scott PJ. Activation of neutrophil NADPH oxidase in a cell-free system. Partial purification of components and characterization of the activation process. J Biol Chem. 1987;262:5563.
256. Gabig TG, English D, Akard LP, et al. Regulation of neutrophil NADPH oxidase activation in a cell free system by guanine nucleotides and fluoride: Evidence for participation of a pertussis and cholera toxin–insensitive G protein. J Biol Chem. 1987;262:1685.
257. Hayakawa T, Suzuki K, Suzuki S, et al. A possible role for protein phosphorylation in the activation of the respiratory burst in human neutrophils. Evidence from studies with cell from patients with chronic granulomatous disease. J Biol Chem. 1986;261:9109.
258. Ishii E, Juta K, Fujita I, et al. Protein phosphorylation of neutrophils from normal children and patients with chronic granulomatous disease. Eur J Pediatr. 1986;145:22.
259. Ochs HD, Igo RP. The NBT slide test: A simple screening method for detecting chronic granulomatous disease and female carriers. J Pediatr. 1973;83:77.
260. Cooper MR, DeChatelet LR, McCall CE, et al. Complete deficiency of leukocyte glucose-6-phosphate dehydrogenase with defective bactericidal activity. J Clin Invest. 1972;51:769.
261. Parry MF, Root RK, Metcalf JA, et al. Myeloperoxidase deficiency. Prevalance and clinical significance. Ann Intern Med. 1981;95:293.
262. Nauseef WM. Myeloperoxidase deficiency. Hematol Oncol Clinics North Am. 1988;2:135.
263. Lehrer RJ, Cline MJ. Leukocyte myeloperoxidase deficiency and disseminated candidiasis: The role of myeloperoxidase in resistance to candida infection. J Clin Invest. 1969;48:1478.
264. van Tuinen P, Johnson KR, Ledbetter S, et al. Localization of myeloperoxidase to the long arm of human chromosome 17: Relationship to the 15:17 translocation of acute promyelocytic leukemia. Oncogene. 1987;1:319.
265. Nauseef WM, Root RK, Malech HL. Biochemical and immunologic analysis of hereditary myeloperoxidase deficiency. J Clin Invest. 1983;71:1297.
266. Koeffler HP, Ranyard J, Pertcheck M. Myeloperoxidase: Its structure and expression during myeloid differentiation. Blood. 1985;65:484.
267. Nauseef WM, Malech HL. Analysis of the peptide subunits of human neutrophil myeloperoxidase. Blood. 1986;67:1504.
268. Gallin JI. Neutrophil specific granule deficiency. Annu Rev Med. 1985; 36:263.
269. Gallin JI, Fletcher MP, Seligmann BE, et al. Human neutrophil-specific granule deficiency: A model to assess the role of neutrophil-specific granules in the evolution of the inflammatory response. Blood. 1982;59:1317.
270. Wolff SM, Dale DC, Clark RA, et al. The Chédiak-Higashi syndrome: Studies of host defenses. Ann Intern Med. 1972;76:293.
271. Ezer G, Soothill JF. Intracellular bactericidal effects of rifampicin in both normal and chronic granulomatous disease polymorphs. Arch Dis Child. 1974;49:463.
272. Mandell GL: Interaction of intraleukocytic bacteria and antibiotics. J Clin Invest. 1973;52:1673.
273. Johnston R, Wilfert CM, Buckley RH, et al. Enhanced bactericidal activity of phagocytes from patients with chronic granulomatous disease in the presence of sulphisoxazole. Lancet. 1975;1:824.
274. Gmümder RK, Seger RA. Chronic granulomatous disease: Mode of action of sulfamethoxazole/trimethoprim. Pediatr Res. 1981;15:1533.

275. Root RK, Isturiz R, Molavi A, et al. Interactions between antibiotics and human neutrophils in the killing of staphylococci. J Clin Invest. 1981;67:247.
276. Yourtee EL, Root RK. Antibiotic-neutrophil interactions in microbial killing. Adv Host Defense Mech. 1982;1:187.
277. Ezekowitz RAB, Orkin SH, Newburger PE. Recombinant interferon gamma augments phagocyte superoxide production and X-chronic granulomatous disease gene expression in X-linked variant chronic granulomatous disease. J Clin Invest. 1987;80:1009.
277a. Sechler JMG, Malech HL, White CJ, et al. Recombinant human interferon-gamma reconstitutes defective phagocyte function in patients with chronic granulomatous disease of childhood. Proc Natl Acad Sci USA. 1988; 85:4874–8.
277b. Ezekowitz RAB, Dinauer MC, Jaffe HS, et al. Partial correction of the phagocyte defect in patients with X-linked chronic granulomatous disease by subcutaneous interferon gamma. N Engl J Med. 1988;319:146.
278. Herzig GP, Graw RG. Granulocyte transfusion for bacterial infections. Prog Hematol. 1975;9:207.
279. Klock JC, Bainton DF. Degranulation and abnormal bactericidal function of granulocytes procured by reversible adhesion to nylon wool. Blood. 1976;48:149.
280. Herzig RH, Herzig GP, Grano RG, et al. Successful granulocyte transfusion therapy for gram-negative septicemia. N Engl J Med. 1977;296:701.
281. Strauss RG, Connett JE, Gale RP, et al: A controlled trial of prophylactic granulocyte transfusions during initial induction chemotherapy for acute myelogenous leukemia. N Engl J Med. 1981;305:597.
282. Winston DJ, Winston GH, Gale RP: Therapeutic granulocyte transfusions for documented infections. Ann Intern Med. 1982;97:509.
283. Alavi JB, Root RK, Djerassi I, et al. A randomized clinical trial of granulocyte transfusions for infections in acute leukemia. N Engl J Med. 1977;296:706.
284. Buescher ES, Gallin JI. Leukocyte transfusion in chronic granulomatous disease. N Engl J Med. 1982;307:800.
285. Young LS. Prophylactic granulocytes in the neutropenic host. Ann Intern Med. 1982;96:240.
286. Rosenshein MS, Farewell VT, Price TH, et al. The cost effectiveness of therapeutic and prophylactic leukocyte transfusion. N Engl J Med. 1980;302:1058.
287. Wright DG, Robichaud KJ, Pizzo PA, et al. Lethal pulmonary reactions associated with the combined use of amphotericin B and leukocyte transfusions. N Engl J Med. 1981;304:1185.
288. Marsh WL, Oyen R, Nichols ME. K_X antigen, the McLeod phenotype, and chronic granulomatous disease: Further studies. Vox Sang. 1976;31:356.
289. Densen P, Wilkinson-Kroovand S, Mandell GL, et al. K_X: Its relationship to chronic granulomatous disease and genetic linkage with Xg. Blood. 1981;58:34.
290. Frey D, Machler M, Seger R, et al. Gene deletion in a patient with chronic granulomatous disease and McLeod syndrome: Fine mapping of the Xk gene locus. Blood. 1988;71:252.
291. Giblett ER, Klebanoff SJ, Pincus SH, et al. Kell phenotypes in chronic granulomatous disease: A potential transfusion hazard. Lancet. 1971;1:1235.
292. Westminster Hospitals Bone Marrow Transplant Team. Bone marrow transplant from an unrelated donor for chronic granulomatous disease. Lancet, 1977;1:210.
293. Kamani N, August CS, Douglas SD, et al. Bone marrow transplantation in chronic granulomatous disease. J Pediatr. 1984;105:42.
294. van der Meer JWM, van den Broek PJ. Present status of the management of patients with defective phagocyte function. Rev Infect Dis. 1984;6:107.
295. Rebuck JW, Crowley JH. A method of studying leukocyte functions in vivo. Ann NY Acad Sci. 1955;59:757.
296. Nelson RB, Quie PG, Simmons RL. Chemotaxis under agarose: A new and simple method for measuring chemotaxis and spontaneous migration of human polymorphonuclear leukocytes and monocytes. J Immunol. 1975;155:1650.
297. Mandell GL, Hook EW. Leukocyte function in chronic granulomatous disease of childhood. Studies on a 17 year old boy. Am J Med. 1969;47:473.
298. Holmes B, Page A, Good R. Studies of the metabolic activity of leukocytes from patients with genetic abnormality of phagocytic function. J Clin Invest. 1967;46:1422.
299. Root RK, Rosenthal AS, Balestra DJ. Abnormal bactericidal metabolic and lysosomal functions of Chédiak-Higashi syndrome leukocyte. J Clin Invest. 1972;51:649.
300. Klebanoff SJ, Clark RA. Iodination of human polymorphonuclear leukocytes: A re-evaluation. J Lab Clin Med. 1977;89:675.
301. Baehner RL, Nathan DG. Quantitative nitroblue tetrazolium dye test in chronic granulomatous disease. N Engl J Med. 1968;278:971.
302. Stossel TP, Root RK, Vaughan M. Phagocytosis in chronic granulomatous disease and the Chédiak-Higashi syndrome. N Engl J Med. 1972;286:120.
303. Allen RC, Loose LD. Phagocytic activation of a luminol-dependent chemiluminescence in rabbit alveolar and peritoneal macrophages. Biochem Biophys Res Commun. 1976;69:245.
304. Weller PF, Goetzl EJ. The human eosinophil. Roles in host defense and tissue injury. Am J Pathol. 1980;100:790.
305. Spry CJE. Mechanisms of eosinophilia. V. Kinetics of normal and accelerated eosinopoiesis. Cell Tissue Kinet. 1971;4:351.
306. Gleich GJ, Adolphson CR. The eosinophilic leukocyte: Structure and function. Adv Immunol. 1986;39:177.
307. Mickenberg ID, Root RK, Wolff SM. Bactericidal and metabolic properties of human eosinophils. Blood. 1972;39:67.
308. Ackerman SJ, Durack DT, Gleich GJ. Eosinophil effector mechanisms in health and disease. Adv Host Defense Mech. 1982;1:269.
309. Basten A, Boyer MH, Beeson PB. Mechanisms of eosinophilia. I. Factors affecting the eosinophil response of rats to *Trichinella spiralis*. J Exp Med. 1970;131:1271.
310. Basten A, Beeson PB. Mechanisms of eosinophilia. II. Role of the lymphocyte. J Exp Med. 1970;131:1288.
311. Mahmoud AAF, Stone MK, Kellermeyer RW. Eosinophilopoietin. A circulating low molecular weight peptide-like substance which stimulates the production of eosinophils in mice. J Clin Invest. 1977;60:675.
312. Butterworth AE, Sturrock RV, Houba V, et al. Eosinophils as mediators of antibody dependent damage to schistosomula. Nature. 1975;257:727.
313. David JR, Vadas MA, Butterworth AE, et al. Enhanced helminthotoxic capacity of eosinophils from patient with eosinophilia. N Engl J Med. 1980;303:1147.
314. Mahmoud AAF, Warren KS, Peters PA. A role for the eosinophil in acquired resistance to *Schistosoma mansoni* infection as determined by antieosinophil serum. J Exp Med. 1975;142:805.
315. Goetzl EJ, Wasserman SI, Austen KF. Eosinophil polymorphonuclear leukocyte function in immediate hypersensitivity. Arch Pathol. 1975;99:1.
316. Bass DA. Eosinophil behavior during host defense reactions. Adv Host Defense Mech. 1982;1:211.
317. Butterworth AE, David JR. Eosinophil function. N Engl J Med. 1981; 304:154.
318. McLaren DJ, MacKenzie CD, Ramalho-Pinto FJ. Ultrastructural observations on the in vitro interaction between rat eosinophils and some parasitic helminths (*Schistosoma mansoni, Trichinella spiralis* and *Nippostrongylus brasiliensis*). Clin Exp Immunol. 1977;30:105.
319. Densen P, Mahmoud AAF, Sullivan J, et al. Demonstration of eosinophil degranulation on the surface of opsonized schistosomules by phase-contrast cinemicrography. Infect Immun. 1978;22:282.
320. Grove DI, Mahmoud AAF, Warren KS. Eosinophils and resistance to *Trichinella spiralis*. J Exp Med. 1977;145:755.
321. Dvorak HF, Dvorak AM. Basophilic leucocytes: Structure, function and role in disease. Clin Haematol. 1975;4:651.
322. Brown SJ, Galli SJ, Gleich GJ, et al. Ablation of immunity to *Ambylomna americanum* by antibasophil serum. Cooperation between basophils and eosinophils in expression of immunity to ectoparasites (tubo) in guinea pigs. J Immunol. 1982;129:790–796.

BIBLIOGRAPHY

Klebanoff SJ, Clark RA: The Neutrophil. Function and Clinical Disorders. Amsterdam: North Holland; 1978.

8. THE CELLULAR IMMUNE SYSTEM AND ITS ROLE IN HOST DEFENSE

CHRISTOPHER B. WILSON

TERMS

Cell Types

Dendritic cell. Bone-marrow-derived, adherent cell that is nonphagocytic, expresses class II HLA (Ia) molecules, and lacks Fc receptors for IgG and receptors for the third component of complement. It is antigenically and morphologically distinct from macrophages, occupies different areas of the spleen from macrophages, and is a potent accessory cell in antigen-specific T-cell proliferation. It stimulates syngeneic and allogeneic mixed lymphocyte reactions and induces specific cytotoxic T cells and cells that mediate delayed-type hypersensitivity (DTH).

Macrophage. Bone-marrow-derived tissue phagocyte that begins as a monocyte progenitor cell in bone marrow. Has class II HLA (Ia) molecules and receptors for IgG (Fc receptors) and for the third component of complement on its surface. Presents antigens to lymphocytes and inhibits or kills microorganisms.

Monocyte. Circulating bone-marrow-derived phagocyte that begins as a monocyte progenitor cell in bone marrow and differentiates into macrophage in tissue.

Mononuclear phagocytes. Monocytes, tissue macrophages, and macrophage-like cells (e.g., microglia).

Natural killer (NK) cell. Large granular lymphocyte with distinct surface antigens. It is cytotoxic to tumor cells, certain virus-infected cells, and certain protozoa.

Null cell. Lymphocyte that lacks surface markers of B or T lymphocytes.

T cell. Thymus-derived lymphocyte that bears a receptor (T-cell antigen receptor, TCR) that recognizes and triggers a response to a specific antigen in the context of host HLA molecules.

T4 cell. T cell that expresses the surface CD4 molecule and recognizes antigen in the context of class II HLA molecules; these cells are commonly called helper T cells but are functionally heterogeneous (see text).

T8 cell. T cell that expresses the surface CD8 molecule and recognizes antigen in the context of class I HLA molecules; these cells are commonly called cytotoxic cells and include cells that inhibit (suppress) B- and T-cell responses.

Genetic Restriction of Cell-Mediated Immunity

Cell-mediated immunity (CMI). Immunity conferred by T lymphocytes and effected by lymphocytes and macrophages.

Major histocompatibility complex (MHC). Cluster of gene loci that encodes class I and class II determinants that provide context for antigen recognition by T lymphocytes.

Class I HLA determinants. Glycoprotein antigens that are encoded by the A, B, and C regions of the MHC of humans, are integral membrane proteins, and restrict interactions of T8 cells.

Class II HLA determinants. Glycoprotein antigens that are encoded by the D region of the MHC of humans, are integral membrane proteins, and restrict interactions of T4 cells.

Haplotype. Constellation of alleles in a particular MHC (i.e., groups of genes that are adjacent and therefore inherited together).

HLA-A, HLA-B, HLA-C. MHC loci encoding class I histocompatibility determinants in humans.

HLA-D. MHC loci encoding class II histocompatibility determinants in humans.

Human leukocyte antigen (HLA) region. MHC region of humans.

I region associated (a) molecule. Product of the Ir gene (D region in humans), which is the I region in mice.

Miscellaneous Terms

Cytokine/lymphokines. Hormone-like or neurotransmitter-like proteins or glycoproteins, secreted by lymphocytes or macrophages, that act as molecular signals for communication between cells of the immune system and as mediators of the systemic response to infection/inflammation.

Epitope. Unique antigenic structure.

T-cell antigen receptor (TCR). Dimeric molecule that contains a unique receptor for antigen and a variable portion of the MHC.

CELL-MEDIATED IMMUNITY

CMI collectively refers to those aspects of the immune response in which T lymphocytes and mononuclear phagocytes induce, regulate, or mediate host response(s), either directly or indirectly, by their effects on other aspects of the immune system. Although CMI is generally thought to play a primary role in protecting against microbes that replicate within host cells (intracellular pathogens),[1–4] including those outlined in Table 1, it has become increasingly apparent that CMI plays a pivotal role in regulating all aspects of the immune system. Central to this role is the critical importance of helper T cells (CD4 antigen-positive cells, hereafter referred to as *T4 cells* or *T4 lymphocytes*) in the induction of specific immune responses[5]; this is clearly illustrated by the devastating effect that selective ablation of functional T4 cells has on all aspects of immunity in acquired immunodeficiency syndrome (AIDS).[6] Thus, although not part of the classic cellular immune system, the optimal function of B lymphocytes, which are the source of specific humoral immunity, and to a lesser degree of granulocytes, which function to ingest and kill antibody-coated microbes, is dependent on intact T4 lymphocyte function.

Historically, CMI was recognized by the delayed-type hypersensitivity (DTH) response, in which, approximately 2 days after intradermal injection of antigen, erythema and induration are detected. This correlates with an influx of lymphocytes and macrophages into the site and can be passively transferred with T lymphocytes but not with serum. Resistance to certain intracellular pathogens can be transferred in a similar fashion.[1–3] Recently, with the rapid increase in knowledge made possible by advances in cell culture, cell cloning, monoclonal antibody techniques, and molecular and structural biologic techniques, our understanding of the cellular immune system and its effects on all aspects of the host response has increased markedly. These discoveries have served to illustrate the complexity of this system. Accordingly, current knowledge, as summarized in this chapter, is necessarily an incomplete and simplistic overview of an elegant system that functions in concert with other aspects of immunity to protect us from the complex microbial environment in which we live. Both T lymphocytes and mononuclear phagocytes function in the inductive and effector phases of the immune response. This chapter discusses these functions separately after describing the origin and differentiation of these cell types and the molecular basis for specific antigen recognition.

T LYMPHOCYTES

T lymphocytes both mediate specific immune functions and modulate those of other cells in the immune system, thereby regulating most aspects of specific immune recognition. These cells recognize antigen via a cell surface receptor for specific antigen, which is structurally similar to immunoglobulin.[7] When activated by antigen in an appropriate context, T cells are stimulated to replicate and/or to mediate one of three principal functions: helping, by stimulating the immune responses of other cells; suppression, by inhibiting the immune response of other cells; and cytotoxicity, by direct killing of target cells. The helper functions are mediated primarily by a subset of T-cell helpers that express the CD4 (T4) surface antigen, whereas the suppressor and cytotoxic functions are mediated primarily by cells expressing the CD8 (T8) surface antigen.[5] However, recent data indicate that the functions of these subsets in part overlap.[8,9] The CD4 molecule is expressed on cells that recognize antigen associated with human leukocyte antigen (HLA) class II molecules; T4 cells can act as helper cells for B-cell responses, as cells that induce other T cells to suppress immune responses and, less commonly, as cytotoxic cells. The CD8 molecule is expressed on cells that respond to antigens (such as viruses) in association with HLA class I antigens and can act as cytotoxic or suppressor cells.

T-Cell Receptors

Structure. Unlike immunoglobulin, the antigen receptor for B cells, the T-cell antigen receptor (TCR) requires simultaneous recognition of antigen with self-major histocompatibility com-

TABLE 1. Pathogens Against Which Cell-Mediated Immunity Contributes to Host Defense in Humans or Experimental Animals

Intracellular					*Extracellular*			
Bacteria	*Viruses*	*Fungi*	*Protozoa*	*Other*	*Bacteria*	*Fungi*	*Protozoa*	*Helminths*
Brucella spp. *Erysipelothrix rhusiopathiae* *Francisella tularenis* *Listeria monocytogenes*[a] *Legionella pneumophila*[a] Mycobacteria, including *M. tuberculosis*[a] *M. leprae*[a] *M. avium intracellulare* *Nocardia asteroides* *Pseudomonas pseudomallei* *Pseudomonas mallei* *Salmonella* spp.[a] *Yersinia* spp.	Cytomegalovirus Herpes simplex Varicella-zoster Epstein-Barr Rubeola (measles) Vaccinia	*Blastomyces dermatidis*[a] *Candida* spp. *Coccidioides immitis*[a] *Cryptococcus neoformans*[a] *Histoplasma capsulatum*[a] *Paracoccidoides brasiliensis*[a]	*Leishmania*[a] *Toxoplasma gondii*[a] *Trypanosoma cruzi*[a]	*Chlamydia*[a] *Rickettsia*[a] *Treponema pallidum*	*Pseudomonas aeruginosa* *Bacteroides fragilis*	*Aspergillus* *Zygomycetes*	*Plasmodia*[a] *Giardia* *Entamoeba histolytica*[a]	*Schistosoma* spp.[a] *Strongyloides stercorales* *Trichinella spiralis*

[a] Organisms susceptible to the IFN-γ-activated monocyte/macrophage in vitro.
(Adapted from Murray,[4] with permission.)

plex (self-MHC).[10] Like immunoglobulin, the TCR is a heterodimer (reviewed in Refs. 7 and 11). Most T cells (more than 95 percent in healthy people) express a heterodimer composed of an α- and a β-chain[7,11,12]; the remainder express a receptor composed of a γ- and a δ-chain.[11,13] TCR chains are synthesized independently from separate genes and then associate to form the TCR molecule (Fig. 1). Both chains have a variable and a constant region. The β- and δ-chain variable regions are derived, like immunoglobulin heavy chains, by sequential rearrangement of diversity (D), joining (J), and variable (V) gene segments to form a contiguous VDJ gene segment; this rearrangement of germ line genomic DNA occurs during thymic development only in cells of the T-cell lineage. The derived variable region and the adjacent constant (C) region, which includes the transmembrane (TM) and cytoplasmic (CY) domains, is then transcribed to form the β- or the δ-chain messenger RNA. The α- and δ-chains are formed by a similar mechanism, although to date no α- or δ-chain D regions have been found, suggesting that these chains, like immunoglobulin light chains, are derived from VJC segments only. Rearrangement of TCR genes appears to be mediated by an enzyme(s) similar or identical to that mediating immunoglubulin gene rearrangement.[14] The mechanisms determining whether a cell will rearrange its immunoglobulin genes and become a B cell, or its TCR genes and become a T cell, is not known. It is also not known with certainty what determines which TCR gene will be rearranged to form a functional receptor.

Gene transfer studies using the α, β TCR indicate that these two chains are sufficient to dictate specific recognition of antigen and HLA[15,16]; this recognition process is discussed more fully below. Specific recognition is thought to be mediated by three hypervariable regions that, because they determine complementary interaction with antigen-HLA, are known as *complementarity-determining regions* (CDR 1, 2, and 3), as shown in Figure 1 for the TCR α-chain. The CDR regions appear to be closely approximated spatially to form the recognition site.[11]

TCR genes are expressed on the surface of T cells in an obligatory fashion with a complex of molecules, the CD3 (T3) complex, that appears to consist of five chains: δ, γ, ϵ, and either two ζ-chains or a ζ plus an η-chain.[17] The CD3 complex appears to act as the signal transduction mechanism whereby antigen binding to the TCR activates T cells.

TCR Diversity. A variety of mechanisms are used to generate the diversity in the nucleotide and the resultant polypeptide sequence of TCR genes sufficient to allow recognition of the variety of antigens to which we are exposed. These include the use of different V, D, and J segments and imprecise joining together of these segments to form the variable region of the TCR. A great deal more information is known about the mouse compared to humans regarding the organization of the genes and the diversity in the V gene segments (Table 2). In the mouse there are estimated to be about 100 Vα and about 25 Vβ gene segments. There are about 50 Jα gene segments and a single Cα. There are two Cβ gene segments, each preceded by one Dβ and six Jβ gene segments. All potential recombinations appear to be possible. The number of γ-chain variable segments appears to be more limited, with three Jγ and Cγ pairs. The TCR δ-locus is located within the TCR α-locus, and certain V segments may be shared. As in the γ-chain, the number of δ-chain V genes appears to be limited. Estimates of potential diversity in humans, although not identical, are similar.[18] As in immunoglobulin, the phenomenon of allelic exclusion appears to be operative, so that a given cell expresses only one αβ or γδ heterodimer.

Additional diversity in the TCR is provided by imprecise joining together of V, D, and J segments so that addition or deletion of nucleotides occurs, producing N-region diversity; this is probably mediated by terminal transferase.[7] However, in contrast to B cells, somatic hypermutation appears either not to occur or to be infrequent in TCR V regions. Nevertheless, the estimated diversity of TCR genes is greater than that of immunoglobulin genes[11] because of greater N-region diversity. This is particularly true for the γδ TCR, which compensates for its more limited V-region repertoire by increased junctional diversity.

Both T4 (helper) cells and T8 (suppressor/cytotoxic) cells can use the same V-region gene segments.[19–21] This suggests that specificity and HLA class I or class II restriction are not determined by the V-region segment alone. Specificity appears to be determined by both the α- and β-chains; specificity is affected both by the germ line gene segments used and by junctional diversity and nucleotide addition or deletion during rearrangement.[15,22,23] A working hypothesis for the mechanism of TCR recognition has recently been published.[11]

Role of Accessory Molecules, Including CD4 and CD8, in T-Cell Recognition

Mature T cells express on their surface accessory molecules that function to enhance T-cell recognition of other cells. The

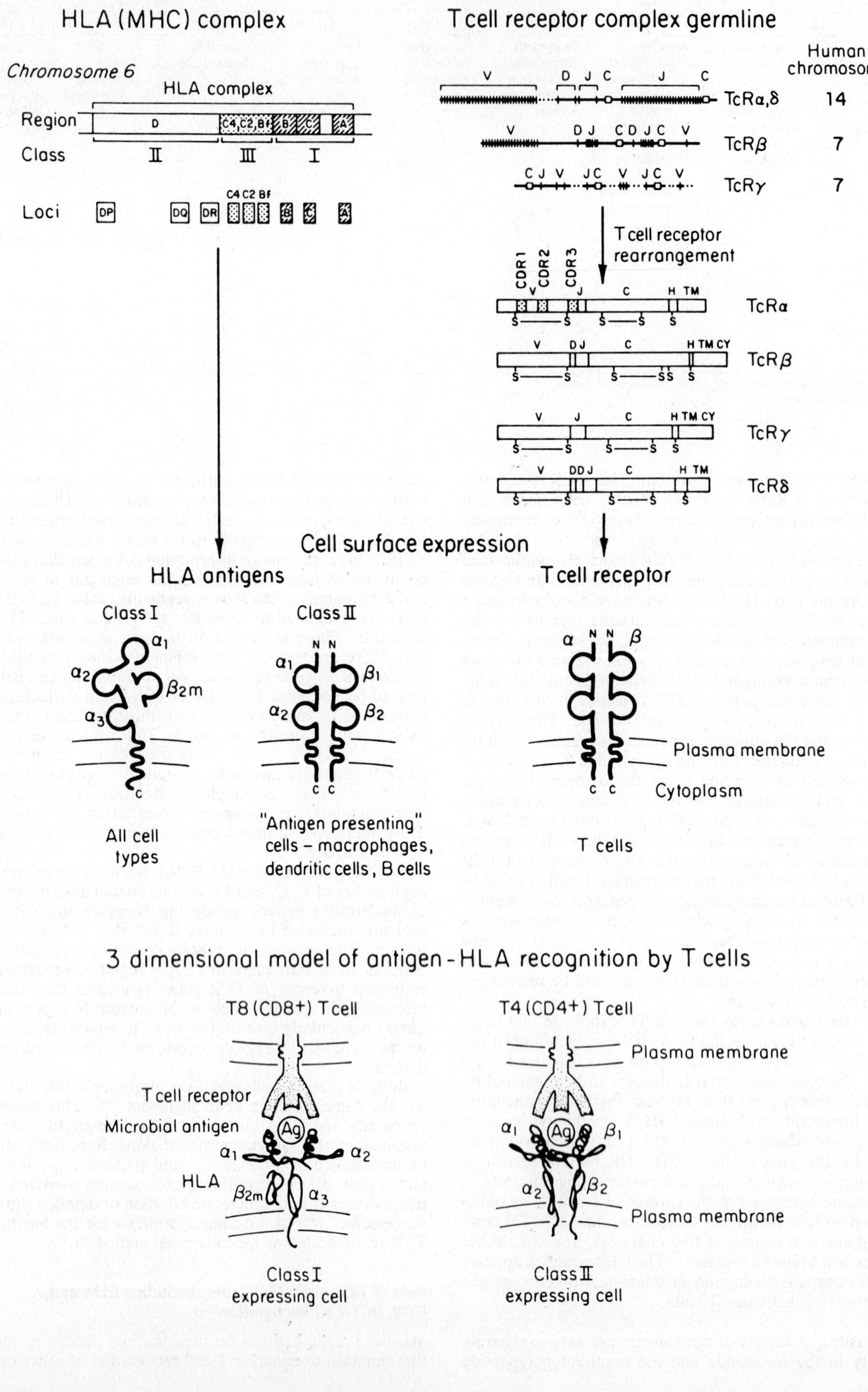
HLA (MHC) complex
Chromosome 6
HLA complex
Region
D
C4,C2,Bf
B
C
A
Class
II
III
I
Loci
DP
DQ
DR
C4 C2 Bf
T cell receptor complex germline
Human chromosome
V
D J C
J
C
TcRα,δ
14
V
D J
C D J C
V
TcRβ
7
C J V
J C
V
J C
V
TcRγ
7
T cell receptor rearrangement
CDR1
CDR2
CDR3
V
J
C
H TM
TcRα
V
D J
C
H TM CY
TcRβ
V
J
C
H TM CY
TcRγ
V
DD J
C
H TM
TcRδ
Cell surface expression
HLA antigens
Class I
α1
α2
β2m
α3
C
All cell types
Class II
N N
α1
β1
α2
β2
C C
"Antigen presenting" cells – macrophages, dendritic cells, B cells
T cell receptor
α
N N
β
Plasma membrane
C C
Cytoplasm
T cells
3 dimensional model of antigen-HLA recognition by T cells
T8 (CD8+) T cell
T cell receptor
Microbial antigen
Ag
α1
α2
HLA
β2m
α3
Class I expressing cell
T4 (CD4+) T cell
Plasma membrane
α1
Ag
β1
α2
β2
Plasma membrane
Class II expressing cell

TABLE 2. Sequence Diversity in T-Cell Receptor and Immunoglobulin Genes in the Mouse

	IG[a]		*TCR I*		*TCR II*	
	H	κ	α	β	γ	δ
Variable segments	250–1000[b]	250	100	25	7	10
Diversity segments	10	0	0	2	0	2
D's read in all frames	Rarely	—	—	Often	—	Often
N-region addition	V–D, D–J	None	V–J	V–D, D–J	V–J	V–D1, D1–2, D1–J
Joining segments	4	4	50	12	3	2
Variable region combinations	62,500–250,000		2500		70	
Junctional combinations	$\sim 10^{11}$		$\sim 10^{15}$		$\sim 10^{18}$	

[a] Immunoglobulin heavy chain.
[b] Number of gene segments.
(From Davis and Bjorkman,[11] with permission.)

CD4 and CD8 molecules are expressed in a mutually exclusive manner on T4 and T8 T cells, respectively. The CD4 and CD8 molecules have structural homology to the immunoglobulin gene superfamily[24–26] but are not variable, as are TCR and HLA molecules. They are believed to act, in part, as a stabilizing ligand for T-cell binding to HLA class II (CD4) or class I (CD8) molecules.[8] This is believed to be mediated by binding of these molecules to nonpolymorphic (nonvariable) regions of the HLA molecule.[16,27] Such interactions may be particularly important in stabilizing binding of T cells to antigen–HLA when the TCR does not have a high affinity for the particular antigen–HLA complex. The importance of these accessory molecules was illustrated in gene transfer experiments in which it was necessary to transfer both the TCR α- and β-chains and the CD8 molecule in order to achieve functional interaction of T cells with an antigen–MHC class I expressing target cell.[16,27] These and other studies have illustrated that the CD4 and CD8 molecules are most closely associated with recognition of antigen in the context of class II and class I MHC molecules, respectively, rather than as determinants of specific types of helper (CD4) or cytotoxic/suppressor (CD8) T-cell function.

The CD2 (sheep erythrocyte receptor) may also facilitate T-cell activation. Recent studies have identified the LFA-3 molecule as its natural ligand.[28] Both have recently been cloned.[29–31] CD2–LFA-3 interaction also may play a role in thymocyte differentiation and selection, an accessory role in T-cell activation, and a primary role in activation of NK cells as discussed below.[31–33] Other T-cell surface molecules,[34–36] particularly the LFA-1 molecule,[37–39] may play ancillary roles in T-cell function by their effects on interaction with other cells, on activation, and on migration.

Derivation of T Cells from Thymocytes

T cells are originally derived from bone marrow precursors (prothymocytes) that migrate to and mature in the thymus. The mass of the thymus relative to body mass is greatest in late fetal life and infancy. The relatively large size of this organ appears to reflect the need for rapid expansion of the T-cell pool at this age. The stages of thymocyte differentiation and the mechanisms leading to differentiation remain to be clearly defined. Much of the work has been performed in the mouse,[39,40] but more recent studies in humans reveal a similar pattern of differentiation.[5,41,42]

Putative pathways of differentiation in the postnatal thymus are schematically depicted in Figure 2. This scheme is a modification of stages originally proposed for humans based on cell surface marker data[5] that has been modified to incorporate recent information from murine studies[39,40] and studies of T-cell receptor gene expression. This represents a working hypothesis rather than established fact.

Prothymocyte precursors are derived from the bone marrow.[41,42] Such cells, as well as all thymocytes and T cells, can be detected by expression of the CD7 surface antigen.[42] In the thymus, cells initially acquire T10 (type 1). Thereafter, CD2 and subsequently a series of different antigens are acquired. The precise precursor–product relationship of cells from type 2 to mature T cell has not been defined. Models in humans[5] and mice[40] in which cells mature sequentially from type 1 to mature T cells seem not to explain fully the heterogeneity recently described in thymocytes. Similarly, the view that immature cells first enter the thymic cortex, mature, and migrate to the medulla, from which they exit, may be overly simplistic.[39,40,43] This complexity is best exemplified by recent findings regarding two aspects of thymocyte development: the TCR and homing receptors. Conventionally, type 1 and type 2 thymocytes, which do not express either CD4 or CD8 (double-negative cells), were thought to be the most immature thymocytes. Support for this belief comes from observations in the mouse. In irradiated mice, transplanted double-negative cells give rise to all other thymocyte populations.[39] If thymus from day 13 or day 14 fetal mice (gestation = 20 days) is cultured in vitro for 7 days, the phenotype of the cells changes from 100 percent double-negative cells to include all types of thymocytes in a proportion similar to that of the mature thymus.[44,45] That mature T cells (CD3+ and either CD4 or CD8+) may also derive from double-positive cells (CD4+, CD8+) under certain conditions is sug-

FIG. 1. Representation of the genetic organization of the HLA and TCR complex, TCR rearrangement, HLA and TCR expression, and TCR recognition of the antigen–HLA complex. In humans, the HLA complex is on chromosome 6; the class I (A, B, and C) antigen locus is separated from the class II (DR, DQ, DP) locus by genes for certain complement components (also called *class III genes*) and for the cytokines, TNF, and lymphotoxin (not shown). Surface expression of class I HLA antigens is ubiquitous (with rare exceptions; see text), whereas class II HLA antigens are restricted in their expression to antigen-presenting cells, primarily macrophages, dendritic cells, and B cells (see text).

The TCR genes are on chromosome 14 (α, δ) or 7 β, γ). The Vα and Vδ gene segments are adjacent to each other on chromosome 14. The Dδ, Jδ, and Cδ gene segments lie between the Vα and Vδ segments and the Jα and Cα segments; the β and γ regions on chromosome 7 do not overlap. In the upper portion of the figure, the germ line configuration of the TCR genes is shown; this is the configuration found in non-T cells. The specific chromosomal relationships are shown for the mouse but are similar in humans. The TCR genes are rearranged in T cells during thymic development in a way that juxtaposes the VDJC (β, δ) or VJC (α, γ) gene segments, usually by deletion of the intervening germ line segments. Following productive rearrangement, a TCR, shown here as an αβ heterodimer, is expressed on the T-cell surface. A model of T-cell recognition of antigen in the context of HLA molecules is shown schematically, based on that proposed by Davis and Bjorkman.[11] It is proposed that the CDR3 region of the TCR is that portion that contacts antigen, and the CDR1 and CDR2 regions contact HLA. Not shown are the T cell accessory molecules CD8 and CD4, which are believed to stabilize the bicellular complex by binding to nonvariable regions of class I and class II HLA molecules, respectively.

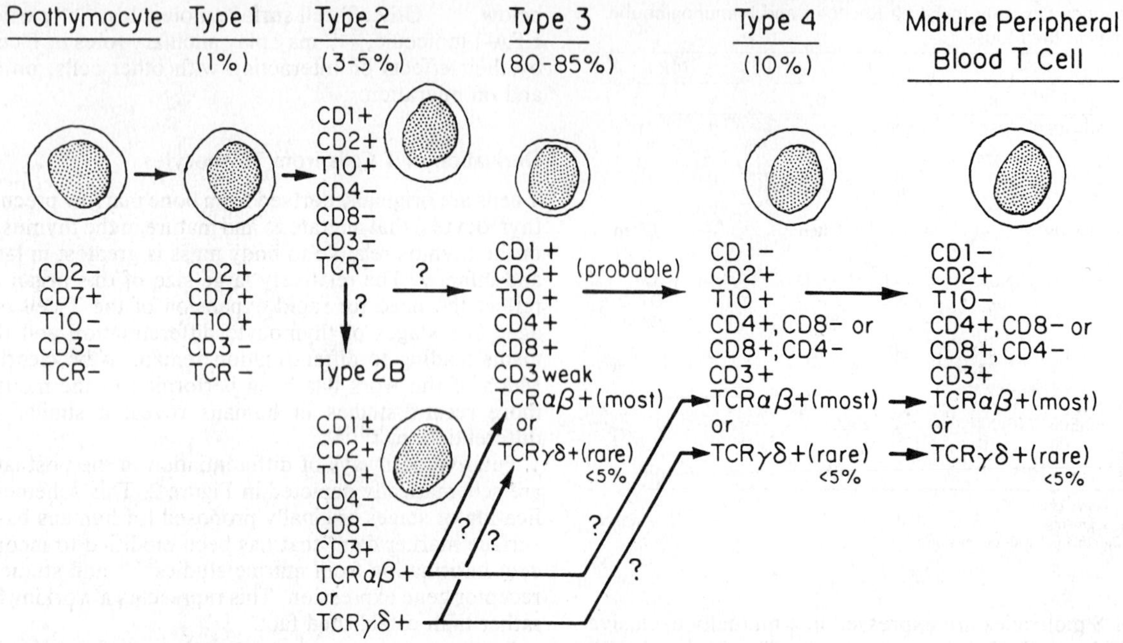

FIG. 2. Putative stages of thymocyte differentiation in postnatal humans. Types of thymocytes are defined by their expression of certain surface antigens. The T cell receptor (TCR), usually composed of an αβ heterodimer or, less commonly, of a γδ heterodimer, is expressed in association with the CD3 surface antigens. Pathways of maturation are indicated by arrows. (?)-uncertain.

gested by in vitro studies.[46] However, in the murine thymus, most double-positive thymocytes die[39,40] and do not differentiate into more mature cells. Thus, it is unclear whether type 4 cells are derived from type 3 or type 2 cells or both. The mechanism determining which thymocytes differentiate into T cells and which die is unknown. Failure to productively rearrange TCR genes and to express cell surface TCR or expression may lead to thymocyte death, but other selection mechanisms also appear to determine which cells survive and mature. One such mechanism is the "education" of cells by self-MHC molecules. Mice that are treated as neonates with antibodies to class I or class II MHC do not develop normal numbers of T8 or T4 cells, respectively; they are accordingly deficient in helper or cytotoxic T-cell function, respectively.[47] Thus, MHC molecules appear to be important in the development of type 4 thymocytes and mature T cells. In addition to this "positive" selection, thymocytes strongly reactive with self-MHC molecules are deleted during thymic maturation.

Recent studies also indicate that type 2 cells are not a single population. Rather, they include a CD3-negative subset, which is the most immature, and two CD3-positive subsets; each of the CD3-positive subsets appears to represent a separate pathway of T-cell development. One of the CD3-positive, CD4- and CD8-negative thymocytes express the uncommon type of TCR composed of the Tγ chain in association with the newly described protein Tδ.[48–52] Even as mature cells, most of these δT lymphocytes with the γδ TCR do not express either the CD4 or the CD8 accessory molecule; a few express the CD8 molecule.[52] The other CD3-positive, CD4- and CD8-negative thymocyte subset expresses the common α-β TCR; these are precursors of most (about 97 percent) mature T cells—those that express the α-β TCR and either the CD4 or the CD8 accessory molecule. The cells expressing the γδ TCR constitute about 3 percent of the circulating T cells.[52,53] The function of the γδ TCR-bearing T cells compared to the α-β TCR-bearing T cells is not clear. Such cells are markedly increased in number in nude mice and in certain patients with primary immunodeficiency.[48]

During fetal development, prothymocytes are first detected in the thymus at 8 weeks in the human[42] and at 14 days in the mouse.[39,40] At this stage, the phenotype of most thymocytes is immature.[42] Data on the sequential appearance of thymocyte types is more complete in the mouse than in the human. There is sequential rearrangement of γ and then β TCR genes, and subsequent expression of their mRNA followed by that of α. At this stage the α-β TCR can first be detected on the surface of thymocytes,[54] and surface expression of CD4 and CD8 is first revealed. The percentage of cells gradually changes to reach values similar to those of adults by about 7 days of postnatal age in the mouse[55] and probably by 12–16 weeks of gestation in humans.[42]

During thymic development in the fetus, T cells that recognize self-antigens appear to be deleted. This has been convincingly shown in mice. Two groups demonstrated the selective loss during thymic maturation of thymocytes bearing a specific TCR variable region gene in inbred mice of one genetic type of histocompatibility antigen but not in those with a different genetic type.[56–59] Although other mechanisms of tolerance to self-antigens are possible, these results suggest that deletion of T cells expressing strongly self-reactive receptors is likely to be the major mechanism.

MONONUCLEAR PHAGOCYTES AND DENDRITIC CELLS

Origin and Differentiation

The mononuclear phagocyte system includes bone marrow precursors, circulating monocytes, and macrophages. In the adult, the promonocyte is the first recognizable marrow precursor cell, although it presumably is derived from a myeloid stem cell precursor. Promonocytes are actively dividing cells that mature into nonreplicating monocytes. Under steady-state conditions, monocytes are released from the marrow within 24 hours and circulate in the blood for 1–3 days before moving to the tissues.[60] Their growth and maturation in the marrow are regulated by specific colony-stimulating factors, as discussed in the section on cytokines.

Once they have left the blood, monocytes do not recirculate but differentiate into macrophages, which are present in all tissues. The estimated life span of macrophages in the tissues is 4–12 weeks. Under steady-state conditions, more than 95 percent of mononuclear phagocytes are mature tissue macrophages and less than 2 percent are monocytes.[60,61] Data from bone marrow transplants indicate that tissue macrophages are ultimately derived from blood monocyte precursors[62]; however, tissue macrophages appear capable of limited replication and self-renewal.[62,63]

Differentiation of monocytes into macrophages is associated with some common maturational changes and others that are unique to the tissue in which they are located. For example, all monocytes lose granule myeloperoxidase as they differentiate into tissue macrophages.[64] Monocytes and peritoneal macrophages rely primarily on anaerobic glycolysis, whereas alveolar (lung) macrophages use aerobic cytochrome oxidation as well.[62] The function of macrophages is readily modulated by lymphokines and they are capable of fusing to form multinucleated giant cells.[60] Thus, unlike granulocytes, mononuclear phagocytes are relatively long-lived cells capable of limited self-renewal and of morphologic and functional modulation, depending on local conditions.

Dendritic cells are also derived from bone marrow precursors.[64] They represent a very small fraction of blood mononuclear cells (less than 1 percent). Like monocytes and macrophages, they express class II MHC molecules and are highly efficient antigen-presenting cells. However, they are phenotypically distinct since they have a dendritic morphology and do not have surface receptors for IgG (Fc receptors) or for the third component of complement. They are found in lymphoid tissue in association with T-lymphocyte-rich areas. Compared to mononuclear phagocytes, less is known regarding their progenitor cells in the bone marrow and their life span in the tissues.

Langerhans cells are related to but phenotypically distinct from macrophages and dendritic cells. They express class II MHC antigens and are efficient antigen-presenting cells.[65] Like macrophages, they express Fc receptors for IgG and receptors for the third component of complement, but they also express the CD1 and S100 antigens not found on other antigen-presenting cells.[66,67] Langerhans cells are abundant in skin, and similar cells are found in the thymus and lymph nodes. They are the normal counterpart of the malignant cells found in histiocytosis X.[66–68]

THE MAJOR HISTOCOMPATIBILITY COMPLEX MOLECULES RESTRICT AND DETERMINE THE CAPACITY FOR THE IMMUNE RESPONSE TO ANTIGENS

Nature of Major Histocompatibility Complex Genes and Molecules

The major histocompatibility complex (MHC) is a cluster of genetic loci, located in humans on the short arm of chromosome 6, that encode genetically polymorphic cell membrane molecules involved in antigen binding and T-cell recognition; these molecules are known in humans as *human leukocyte antigens* (HLAs). These molecules were discovered when investigators studying the rejection of organ transplants in inbred strains of mice found that the capacity to discriminate self from non-self mapped to the MHC. Subsequently, studies by McDevitt and Benacerraf revealed that the capacity to develop an immune response to simple exogenous antigens mapped to a region within the MHC locus, which they named the immune response (Ir) gene locus.[69] Subsequent studies revealed that the Ir locus was identical to the MHC region containing class II MHC molecules.

The MHC locus encodes two structurally distinct types of polymorphic molecules, referred to as *class I* and *class II molecules*.[70–72] As shown in Figure 1, each class contains several individual antigens. The class I molecules in humans are denoted HLA-A, -B, and -C, and the class II molecules are denoted HLA-DR, -DQ, and -DP. The genes for class I and class II molecules are in separate clusters on chromosome 6 and are separated by genes for complement factor C2, C4, and B, and by genes for the lymphokines, tumor necrosis factor α and β. Additional HLA genetic elements are also present, but those studied to date appear not to be functional genes. Each chromosome contains a complete set of these molecules. Accordingly, two alleles each of HLA-A, -B, and -C, and HLA-DR, -DP, and -DQ, are simultaneously present on the cells of each individual. The number of alleles for each HLA molecule varies: at least 50 B but only about 10 C and intermediate numbers of A alleles are known; the number of D region alleles is less well known, but DR appears to be the most diverse. The diversity provided by two alleles of each HLA antigen is sufficient to permit immune recognition by most individuals of the entire array of microbes and antigens that they encounter.

Structure. Structurally, each HLA molecule is a heterodimer, that is, is composed of two different molecules (Fig. 1). Class I molecules are composed of a polymorphic α-chain 45 kD in size that is an integral membrane protein; it is associated on the cell surface with a smaller (12 kD) invariant molecule, β_2-microglobulin by a noncovalent interaction that appears to stabilize the α-chain structure. Class II molecules are composed of an α- (about 30 kD) and a β- (about 26 kD) chain, both of which are polymorphic and are integral membrane proteins. The genes for the α- and β-chains of class II molecules are adjacent to each other on chromosome 6 and are inherited as a paired set.

Both class I and class II molecules contain paired regions that resemble immunoglobulin.[26] Such regions are about 100 amino acids in length and are folded into regions with sheet-like (β-pleated sheets) domains by intramolecular disulfide bonds. The importance of this structure has recently been demonstrated by x-ray crystallographic analysis of the HLA-A2 molecule, the first MHC molecule for which precise structural data are known. These studies showed that the β-pleated sheets of the α_1 and α_2 domains of the molecule, which are exposed on its surface, form an antigen-binding platform within a groove formed by other parts of the molecule.[73] Molecular modeling predicts a similar structure for class II molecules in which the platform is formed by the α_1 and β_1 domains[74] (Fig. 1).

Distribution and Regulation of Expression. In general, class I molecules are expressed by most nucleated cells. However, certain tissues express few or no class I antigens; these include the villous trophoblast, central nervous system neurons, corneal endothelium, and most endocrine cells, including pancreatic β-cells. Expression of class II molecules is much more restricted. B cells express these molecules in a relatively invariant manner; antigen-presenting macrophages, dendritic cells, and Langerhans cells also ordinarily express class II molecules, but expression on cells from different tissues varies in intensity and in which of the three classes (DR, DP, and DQ) are expressed.[75–77] Class II antigen expression is commonly less intense on tissue macrophages than on blood monocytes.[75]

The intensity of HLA antigen expression is an important determinant of the intensity of T-cell recognition and response; this is particularly important for class II antigen expression. Accordingly, the intensity of class II expression can be modulated reciprocally. Interferon-γ (IFN-γ) increases expression on macrophages and dendritic antigen-presenting cells[75,77,78] and can induce expression on cells that ordinarily are class II negative, such as endothelial, epithelial, and endocrine cells. This allows such cells to function as antigen-presenting cells at times of need but to be class II negative normally. Aberrant expression of class II molecules by such cells may be undesirable by leading to autoimmune injury, as seen in models of insulin-dependent diabetes.[79] Class II expression on B cells is not increased by IFN-γ but by another lymphokine, interleukin-4 (see section on lymphokines). Class I expression is increased by IFN-γ, but unlike class II molecules, class I expression is also increased by IFN-α, IFN-β, and tumor necrosis factor (see section on lymphokines). Class II expression is under reciprocal negative control by bacterial lipopolysaccharides, prostaglandins, and glucocorticoids. This system of regulatory controls, particularly for class II molecules, underscores their importance in immune response control.

Interaction of MHC Molecules with T-Cell Subsets

The cell and tissue distribution of class I compared to class II HLA molecules appears to be functionally related to their interaction with T-cell subsets. As noted above, class I and class II molecules restrict antigen recognition by T8 and T4 cells, respectively. T8 cells function primarily as cytotoxic T cells that recognize and destroy virus-infected cells, allogeneic grafts, or tumor cells. Since these target cells may include nucleated cells of all types, it is important that all or most nucleated cells express class I molecules, which they do.

In contrast, T4 cells are critical regulators of the function of other cell types, such as B cells and cytotoxic T cells—both enhancing the response (helper function) or inhibiting the response (suppressor inducer function).[80–83] By limiting class II HLA expression to a few cell types that are present at sites of potential microbial entry or entrapment (skin, lymphoid tissue, and spleen),[64,84–86] the amplitude and location of T4 compared to T8 cell stimulation may be more finely controlled; the ability of the lymphokines IFN-γ and interleukin-4 to induce or increase expression provides a mechanism for increasing the capacity of class II-dependent antigen- presentation at times of need.

Once induced to express class II MHC molecules, cells such as endothelial cells and fibroblasts can also present antigen to helper T cells.[84] Data derived from experiments in which class II MHC genes were expressed in fibroblasts by recombinant DNA techniques or peptide antigens were presented on artificial membranes containing class II suggest that MHC class II expression may be the only absolute requirement for a cell to function in antigen presentation to T4 cells.[10,84,87]

ROLE OF MACROPHAGES AND OTHER ANTIGEN-PRESENTING CELLS IN THE INDUCTIVE PHASE OF THE SPECIFIC IMMUNE RESPONSE

Antigen

Recognition of antigen by T cells differs fundamentally from recognition of antigen by B cells.[10,86,88–90] In most cases, B cells recognize intact antigens, frequently the confirmational determinants provided by the secondary and tertiary structures of the molecule. In contrast, T-cell recognition appears to depend on the primary amino acid sequence, and a relatively small number (about 10–20) of sequential amino acids are recognized in association with a specific MHC molecule.

Antigen Presentation to T4 (Helper) Cells. T4 cells that regulate all immune responses and are necessary for the induction of a primary response to antigen recognize the primary amino acid sequence only in association with class II HLA molecules.[10,86,87,91,92] Therefore, necessary requirements for induction of a primary T-cell response are that antigen-presenting cells both alter complex antigens so that the specific primary sequence is accessible and express class II MHC molecules on their surface. Optimal presentation of most antigens appears to require three important functional components: antigen processing, class II antigen expression, and cytokine (e.g., interleukins-1 and -6) production.[86]

Antigen processing appears most often to involve partial proteolysis or denaturation of an antigen.[88] This appears to take place in acidic endosomes within antigen-presenting cells[90] following endocytosis of microbes or other complex antigens. Such processing appears to be required for most globular proteins. Nonglobular hydrophilic proteins may not require such processing in all cases, as the recognized amino acids may be exposed and not cryptic, as in globular proteins. The efficiency of antigen uptake and subsequent processing by macrophages, Langerhans cells, and B cells may be facilitated by surface receptors for IgG (Fc receptors) and for derivatives of the third component of complement. These opsonic receptors facilitate phagocytosis of microbes or other particulate antigens. Such receptors are absent from other antigen-presenting cells.

The function of processing is to create peptides that will bind to MHC molecules and in so doing display a conformation that is recognized (i.e., that will bind to a specific T-cell antigen receptor).[86,89] Experiments with synthetic peptides derived from the sequences of known antigens, such as viral proteins of influenza and human immunodeficiency virus (HIV), suggest that 10–20 sequential amino acids are sufficient for both binding to MHC and recognition by T cells.[89,92,93]

Binding of processed antigen to class II MHC molecules is thought to occur in most cases intracellularly; then the antigen bound to the class II molecule is transported to the cell surface.[86,89] Such intracellular binding may be required because processed antigen binds to MHC with relatively low affinity (about 10^{-3} to 10^{-6} M), and both binding and release of antigen from MHC occur slowly over hours.[84,94] Thus, on the cell surface, MHC molecules probably have antigen bound at all times, limiting the access of newly processed antigens to newly synthesized or recycled MHC molecules within the cell.

Antigen Presentation to T8 Cytotoxic Cells. Antigens recognized in the context of class I MHC molecules are commonly derived from proteins synthesized within the cell on which they are presented. This is true for viral proteins[94–96] and for proteins of the MHC that are recognized as foreign in an allogeneic host.[97] However, recent studies indicate that the viral antigens recognized by cytotoxic T cells, including those of influenza[96,98] and HIV-1,[99] are often internal viral proteins rather than or in addition to those on the viral envelope or host cell plasma membrane.[95,98] These results suggest that viral or MHC antigens, newly synthesized within the cell but most likely in an incomplete or proteolytically processed form, may associate within the cell with host cell MHC class I molecules. MHC class I antigen complex would then be transported to the cell surface. In this manner, both internal and external viral antigens may be targets for recognition and destruction by cytotoxic T cells. This fact has obvious implications for viral vaccine strategies, since internal viral antigens may be suitable candidates in diseases such as influenza and HIV, in which surface antigens vary considerably among strains.[96,98,99]

MHC Molecular Polymorphism Regulates Responsiveness to Different Antigens

Early studies showed that helper T cells sensitized by immunization in vivo responded to a specific antigen only in the presence of autologous macrophages or macrophages bearing class II MHC molecules of the same allele (haplotypes). The T-cell response was said to be restricted by a specific MHC molecule. Molecular analyses indicate that a single amino acid substitution either in the MHC molecule or in the recognized portion of the antigen molecule is sufficient to alter recognition by T cells.[10,77,86,89,93] Structural analysis of the MHC molecules[73,74,100] and molecular manipulation of antigens[88,91] suggest that this restriction is mediated by variation in the binding affinity of MHC alleles for specific antigenic peptides. This variability is such that a given region of a processed complex antigen may bind strongly, weakly, or not at all; antigens that do not bind cannot be presented by that MHC molecule.

Antigen is predicted to bind in an antigen-binding groove at the exterior surface of the MHC molecule.[73,74] Further, many of the antigenic peptide sequences recognized by T cells are predicted to exist in an amphipathic α-helical conformation[89,92] such that one side of the antigen molecule binds to the MHC molecule and the opposite side binds to the T cell receptor. This is shown schematically in Figure 1. This model illustrates the basic nature of MHC restriction: the structure of the MHC molecule dictates which portions of an antigen will bind in the antigen-binding groove and, once bound, which portion and side of the antigen will be available for recognition by the T-cell receptor.

The Basis for T-Cell Recognition of the Antigen–MHC Complex

As noted, the potential diversity of T-cell receptors (about 10^{15}–10^{18} different possible receptors) is similar to the potential diversity of immunoglobulin.[11] However, unlike immunoglobulin, the diversity within the T-cell receptor genes is more heavily concentrated in the junctional regions, which are the location of the third complementarity determining region (CDR3) and is much more limited in the variable regions, the location of CDR1 and CDR2. Specific recognition of the MHC–antigen complex is mediated entirely by the two-chain T-cell receptor molecule. The recent evidence that antigen binds in a groove in the MHC molecule and other molecular modeling data suggested to Davis and Bjorkman[11] that the highly variable CDR3 region might bind to antigen as it lies within the groove and that the less variable CDR1 and CDR2 regions might contact the MHC molecule on the sides of the groove (Fig. 1). This model is appealing since it would explain the concentration of variability in the CDR3 region of the receptor. Compatible with this model are recent data indicating that for a series of T-cell clones recognizing a specific antigen, the CDR3 regions have been highly conserved.[23] Further experimental data are needed to determine the general applicability of this model.

There is a high degree of specificity present in this system: a specific antigenic peptide–MHC molecule complex is recognized by a given T cell. Although each T cell recognizes only a short peptide region of a larger molecule, each molecule may have many regions capable of binding to one or another of the host's MHC alleles. The T-cell receptor repertoire contains sufficient diversity that in most cases any complex microbial antigen will contain several peptide regions that bind to one or both MHC molecules of an individual and are recognized by T cells with the appropriate receptor. However, as noted above, inbred rodents with certain MHC class II alleles will not respond to a specific antigen; they lack an immune response gene (MHC class II allele) necessary for that response. Such occurrences are likely to be uncommon in highly outbred human populations. However, the association of specific diseases, most commonly autoimmune diseases, with specific HLA alleles in humans suggests that such differences may also account in part for increased susceptibility to certain infectious pathogens in humans.

T-Cell Activation and Proliferation

Binding of the TCR to antigen–MHC triggers a series of intracellular events that ultimately lead to lymphokine production and replication or, in the case of cytolytic T cells, trigger the cytolytic mechanism. Collectively, this process is referred to as *T-cell activation*.[101,102] Transduction of the signal from the T-cell receptor appears to be mediated by the CD3 (T3) complex.[17,101] There follows a series of associated biochemical events, critical among which appear to be an increase in intracellular free calcium concentration[103] and translocation of protein kinase C from cytosol to plasma membrane, whereby the T cell is activated.[104] Together these two events act, through as yet poorly characterized intracellular pathways, to induce transcription of a series of genes, among which are those for interleukin-2, the interleukin-2 receptor, and other lymphokines.[101,102] As described below ("The Role of Cytokines in T-Cell Proliferation"), binding of interleukin-2 to its receptor appears to be the critical event driving T cells to proliferate.

Both the increase in intracellular calcium and the activation of protein kinase C follow the activation of a cell membrane-associated phospholipase C, which releases inositol phosphates and diacylglycerol from membrane phospholipids. Inositol phosphates trigger the intracellular increase in calcium; diacylglycerol and calcium act together to activate membrane-associated protein kinase C.[101,102] This pathway is a common mechanism of intracellular signaling in many cell types. Although these pathways were deduced initially from studies in which stimuli other than the antigen–MHC complex were used to activate T cells, studies in which antigen was used have yielded similar results.[105,106]

The CD4 and CD8 molecules appear to play an accessory role in T-cell activation. Their major role may be to enhance adhesion between the T cell and the antigen-presenting cell or target cell by binding to nonpolymorphic regions of class II or class I MHC molecules, respectively. However, recent data suggest that they may modulate signaling through the T-cell receptor, enhancing the signal in the presence of antigen–MHC, inhibiting the signal in the absence of MHC molecules.[9,37,107–109] The CD2 surface molecule (the sheep erythrocyte receptor) also appears to function as an accessory signal for T-cell activation[32,33,37] and may be important in activation of NK cells.[110]

LYMPHOKINES AND CYTOKINES

Definitions and Overview

Lymphokines are proteins (or glycoproteins) secreted by lymphocytes that act as molecular signals for communication between cells of the immune system and as systemic mediators of the host's response to infection; as such, their function is analogous to that of neurotransmitters and hormones, respectively. It is now clear that other cell types, particularly mononuclear phagocytes, release and/or respond to such substances. In recognition of this, *cytokines*, a more general term that includes lymphokines, monokines (cytokines produced by mononuclear phagocytes), and other such mediators, is now in common use. The two terms are often used interchangeably.

Cytokines were originally detected in experimental systems that defined them by a specific biologic effect. An example is T-cell growth factor, now called *interleukin-2*. Biologic assays were used to monitor purification procedures for this molecule, which was found to be a glycoprotein of about 15 kD.[111] Modern molecular biologic techniques have resulted in the molecular cloning of this lymphokine and subsequently of many others. Once recombinant materials were made available, it became apparent that in most cases more than one lymphokine can mediate a biologic effect previously ascribed to a specific molecule. An example is the ability of interleukin-4 to act as a T-cell growth factor.[112,113] Conversely, many biologic effects originally thought to be mediated by different molecules were subsequently found to be the properties of one. For example, a molecule causing hemorrhagic necrosis of tumors, tumor necrosis factor (TNF), was found to be identical to a molecule causing wasting in rabbits with trypanosomiasis, cachectin.[114,115] Thus, definitions based solely on biologic effects can be misleading. Until it is cloned and molecularly characterized, a cytokine is generally referred to as a *factor* and is named according to its biologic effect(s), recognizing that this may or may not represent a single molecule. Once the amino acid sequence of the human form has been determined, it may be assigned an interleukin (IL) number.[116] However, some lymphokines, including the interferons, TNF, and msot of the colony-stimulating factors, have retained their original names even though cloned and molecularly characterized. For purposes of clarity and because many of the important lymphokines originally described as factors have been cloned in the past few years, this chapter focuses on those that have been molecularly defined. The reader should recognize that this necessarily oversimplifies the true complexity of the system; many factors that are not molecularly characterized and not fully discussed are likely to play a role in the processes that will be discussed.

Cytokines Act to Amplify or Attenuate Immune Responses

Cytokines bind to specific receptors on the surface of cells. In most cases, each cytokine has a unique receptor to which only it will bind with high affinity. However, there are at present two examples of related cytokines that exhibit minimal molecular homology but bind to a common receptor and appear to mediate similar biologic effects. IL-1 biologic activity is mediated by two molecules, IL-1α and IL-1β,[117,118] which are 26 percent homologous at the amino acid level but bind to a common receptor with similar affinities.[119,120] Similarly, TNF/cachectin biologic activity is mediated by two molecules, TNF-α and TNF-β (also called *lymphotoxin*), which are 30 percent homologous at the amino acid level.[121,122] TNF-α and -β bind to a common receptor. Although many of the biologic activities of TNF are also common to IL-1, the receptors for TNF are distinct from those for IL-1 and are not shared with other cytokines. Many cytokine receptors are present in low numbers (less than 500) and increase minimally on stimulated cells, suggesting that few molecules are required to mediate the biologic effect. An exception to this is the high-affinity receptor for IL-2, which is absent on resting T cells but present in moderately high numbers (more than 1000/cell) on activated T cells.[111] Up- and down-regulation of receptor numbers are two mechanisms by which the response to cytokines may be modulated. The molecular mechanism by which the cytokines alter cell function after binding is not well characterized, although receptor internalization after binding is a common feature often required for action.

The actions of cytokines are not antigen specific. However, their effects in many cases serve to transduce antigen-specific signals. Such is the case for the T-cell-derived lymphokines, since their production is stimulated by specific antigen in the context of HLA antigens. Also, in certain cases, their actions are restricted to cells that have first been primed to respond by specific antigen stimulation. Examples are IL-2, which stimulates proliferation of T cells primed to express high-affinity IL-2 receptors by antigen stimulation,[111] and B cells, which respond to IL-5 and IL-6 after antigen-triggered activation.[123] However, in many cases, cytokines act not only on antigen-triggered T and B cells but also on a wide variety of other cell types to amplify specific or nonspecific immune responses or to mediate more general host responses. In addition, many cytokines are produced by NK cells, mononuclear phagocytes, and certain nonimmune system cells in response to infections or inflammatory stimuli of a nonspecific nature. Thus, cytokines serve as transducing or modulating signals in the immune system, mediating both antigen-specific and non-antigen-specific effects.

Table 3 lists the principal cytokines that have been molecularly characterized and describes their basic characteristics, the major cell sources and stimuli triggering their secretion, and their major biologic effects. It should be emphasized that the effects listed are representative of those currently described that appear to be of biologic importance. In many cases, specific receptors for these molecules are much more widely distributed on cells than are the known biologic effects. Thus, it is to be anticipated that additional effects of importance will be discovered with time. The biochemistry, sources, production, and actions of TNF-α,[114,115,123] IL-1,[116,125] IL-2,[111] IL-4, IL-5, IL-6,[123,126,127] the interferons,[4,128–130] and the colony-stimulating factors (CSF), including IL-3,[131–133] have recently been reviewed. Progress in this field has been rapid. I will focus on a general overview of cytokines, including regulation of their production and their role in specific immune pathways relevant to host defense. New findings not available when the cited reviews were prepared have been included where informative.

General Biochemical Properties of Cytokines

Cytokines are not stored preformed within cells. Their production requires new protein and in most cases new mRNA synthesis. As expected from their role as humoral mediators of cellular immunity, they are encoded as propeptides, and with the exception of IL-1 (discussed below) and perhaps TNF-α,[134] they have an NH_2-terminal sequence dictating their transport to the Golgi apparatus, where they are glycosylated (for those that are glycoproteins) and promptly secreted. At this time the signal peptide sequence is removed to yield the mature protein of a lower molecular mass. Each cytokine is encoded by a unique mRNA and those described to date are encoded by a single gene. Monocyte CSF (M-CSF) is actually two different proteins, which are encoded by a single gene and derived by alternate mRNA processing.

Specific Cytokines Produced by Mononuclear Phagocytes and Mechanisms Regulating Their Production

Monocytes and macrophages are important sources of IL-1, IL-6, IFN-α, TNF-α, GM-CSF, G-CSF and M-CSF. Studies performed primarily in vitro indicate that each of these cytokines is also produced by other human cells types; human endothelial and fibroblasts are probably important sources of CSFs,[132,133,135] IL-1,[117,125] and IL-6[127]; B lymphocytes of IL-1,[117,125,136] T lymphocytes of TNF-α[137–139] and probably of IL-6[127,139]; and NK cells of TNF-α.[138] IFN-β, which is a molecule related to IFN-α with similar biologic activity, is produced by fibroblasts and epithelial cells. Other cell types may produce one or more of these cytokines; this may be of physiologic importance in specific anatomic sites. Most cytokines produced by mononuclear phagocytes have potent and diverse systemic effects in addition to their effects on immune function.

In general, appropriate stimulation of mononuclear phagocytes induces synthesis of specific cytokine mRNAs and proteins, followed rapidly by cytokine secretion. In addition, as illustrated by TNF-α, unstimulated monocytes and macrophages isolated from humans[140] and mice[141] appear to contain small amounts of mRNA for TNF-α but produce little or no detectable TNF-α protein until stimulated; stimulation induces increased TNF-α mRNA synthesis and enhances translation of preexisting and newly synthesized TNF-α mRNA. Low-level expression of mRNA in the absence of stimulation has been seen with other macrophage cytokines, including IL-1α and IL-1β,[117] IL-6,[127] M-CSF, and G-CSF in vitro (135, unpubl. obs.); it is not known if this actually occurs in vivo or is an artifact of the procedures used to isolate or culture the cells. Preexisting mRNA may allow more rapid production of cytokine protein by mononuclear phagocytes in response to infectious or inflammatory stimuli in vivo than would be possible if all protein was derived from newly synthesized mRNA.

A common set of stimuli lead to the production of cytokines by mononuclear phagocytes. Bacteria and their products, such as lipopolysaccharide and toxic shock syndrome toxin,[142] are potent inducers of TNF-α,[140,141] IL-1,[117,125,143] IL-6,[144,145] IFN-α/β,[128,146] and M-CSF, G-CSF, and GM-CSF[132,133,135] production by mononuclear phagocytes. Viruses and polynucleotides also induce IFN-α/β[146–148] and perhaps IL-1.[117] An interesting and important property of these cytokines is the capacity to induce or enhance their own or each other's production. Thus, TNF-α and IL-1 directly induce production of IL-1,[143,149–152] TNF-α,[143] IL-6,[144,145] GM-CSF, G-CSF, and M-CSF[132,133,135,153] by human mononuclear phagocytes, endothelial cells, and fibroblasts. Similar results have been observed in many cases with experimental animals in vivo.[149,154] In addition to directly stimulating cytokine production, cytokines can enhance production induced by other stimuli. GM-CSF and INF-γ enhance production of TNF-α and IL-1[140,155] and of M-CSF and G-CSF.[156,157] Activated complement components and immune complexes also stimulate cytokine production by human mononuclear phagocytes.[158]

Under most conditions, stimulation of macrophages induces the coordinate release of each of these cytokines. Although teleologically appealing, examples of selective cytokine production by macrophages are limited. IFN-α/β are in part differentially regulated from other cytokines, since their production is efficiently induced by certain stimuli (viruses) that do not induce or only weakly induce the other macrophage-derived cytokines. Differentially diminished IL-1 relative to TNF production and secretion has also been described. Human monocytes infected with *Leishmania donovani* or cultured under resting conditions have impaired IL-1 but not TNF-α production.[140,159,160] IFN-γ enhances TNF-α production under all conditions[140] and reverses the block in IL-1 production induced by *Leishmania*.[160] There is no clear evidence for subsets of blood monocytes that produce only one or a few cytokines and not others. Differential regulation of cytokine production in tissue macrophages resulting from differences in local conditions is suggested by the studies with cultured monocytes but has not been directly determined.

Stimulation of macrophage cytokine production by microbial products with amplification by other cytokines may be important for a rapid response to minimal microbial invasion but also has the potential for overproduction in response to maximal microbial challenge; this may contribute to some of the deleterious host responses to infection discussed below. However, the host also has pathways for down-regulating production, and for limiting systemic release of these mediators, while focusing their production at the site(s) of infection.

One mechanism for focusing the effects of the cytokines would be to limit their production to the local site. This is accomplished in part by the positive feedback system described above. Resting tissue macrophages appear to have a more limited capacity to release TNF-α, and particularly IL-1, than do inflammatory macrophages and monocytes.[140] The higher capacity of inflammatory macrophages may relate in part to their more recent derivation from monocytes and to their exposure to high local concentrations of microbial products, chemotactic complement components, and cytokines. The end result is that the greatest production will be by macrophages at inflammatory sites. In addition, only part of the IL-1 produced is secreted; the remainder is cell-associated, at least in part, as an integral plasma membrane protein.[161] This is possible because both IL-1α and IL-1β lack a signal peptide sequence directing secretion.[118,125] The pathways by which IL-1α and IL-1β are processed from precursor forms of about 31 kD to their secreted low molecular weight forms (about 17.5 kD) and how they reach the cell membrane or are secreted is unclear.[125,162] However this occurs, the effects of IL-1 are thereby focused, allowing it to act locally to enhance T-cell activation in response to antigen while minimizing systemic effects. We have found that cultured human monocytes as a model of resting macrophages secrete a much smaller fraction of total IL-1 produced than do circulating blood monocytes[140]; results with tissue macrophages were intermediate between those of fresh and cultured monocytes. Thus, in the absence of an influx of large numbers of inflammatory macrophages, IL-1 may be highly focused at local sites of infection. Consistent with this is the finding that alveolar macrophages from people with inflammatory processes secrete greater amounts of IL-1 in response to stimulation than do macrophages from healthy people.[163] Similar to IL-1, a small fraction of TNF-α may be initially expressed as an integral membrane protein.[134]

Cytokines also induce the production of compounds that down-regulate their own production. Both TNF-α and IL-1 induce production of prostaglandins, particularly PGE_2, which down-regulates their production.[114,124,125] PGE_2 also inhibits certain effects of IL-1, such as T-cell activation.[164] IL-1 appears to be unique in its ability to enhance production of certain pituitary hormones, including ACTH and α-melanocyte stimulating hormone.[117,125,165–167] ACTH, by enhancing glucocorticoid production, can negatively regulate production of itself, TNF, and other cytokines, including the CSFs, interferons, and IL-2 to IL-6. In addition to inhibiting cytokine production, glucocorticoids and α-melanocyte stimulating hormone inhibit the effects of IL-1 on many cell types. Other substances may act as endogenous negative regulators of cytokine production and effects, but their precise role in vivo remains to be determined.[168–170] The effects of excessive TNF and IL-1 production are also attenuated by their ability to down-regulate their own receptors.

The relative role that each of these processes plays in vivo in attenuating the potential adverse systemic effects of overproduction of TNF, IL-1, and other macrophage-derived cytokines remains to be determined.

Lymphokines Produced by T Cells and Mechanisms Regulating Their Production

With the exception of certain tumors, T lymphocytes are the sole source of IL-2, -3, and -5 and lymphotoxin (TNF-β), and are the major source of IFN-γ; along with macrophages and NK cells, they produce TNF-α; they are the major source of IL-4, which is also produced by mast cells.[126] Unlike macrophages, which produce and secrete cytokines in response to a number of stimuli, T cells secrete lymphokines in response to activation by antigen in the context of HLA. The molecular events that transduce these signals and mediate the initial events in T-cell activation have been discussed above. Following activation, the genes encoding these lymphokines are transcribed within a few hours, followed rapidly by their production and prompt secretion. Production continues to increase over the first 24–72 hours after stimulation, depending on the conditions, and then declines.

Activation of a mixed population of T lymphocytes and antigen-presenting cells, such as blood, tonsillar, or splenic mononuclear cells, usually leads to coordinate production of each of these lymphokines, although the rate and time to maximal production of each vary slightly. This reflects the aggregate production of lymphokines by all cells in the population. However, evidence suggests that the production of individual lymphokines may be regulated, in part, differentially.

T4 cells of humans and mice produce each of these lymphokines[171–175]; However, the capacity to secrete specific lymphokines may be restricted to subsets of T4 cells. Initially, data derived from murine T-cell clones in vitro indicated that certain ones (known as *TH1 clones*) produced IL-2, IFN-γ, TNF-α, TNF-β (lymphotoxin), and GM-CSF, whereas others (known as *TH2 clones*) produced IL-4 and IL-5; both produced IL-3.[173–175] Interestingly, evidence (discussed below) suggests that this selective lymphokine production may have functional significance in that the lymphokines produced by TH2 cells enhance production of antibody isotypes that sensitize mast cells and eosinophils (IgG1 and IgE in the mouse) and stimulate mar-

TABLE 3. Properties of Lymphokines and Cytokines

Name	Physicochemical Characteristics (Human)	Principal Cell Sources	Stimuli Inducing Release	Major Biologic Effects
Interleukin-1 (Lymphocyte-activating factor, endogenous pyrogen hemopoietin 1)	Two proteins: α and β, both Mr ~17.5 kD; α more acidic than β	Many cell types; mononuclear phagocytes are a major source	Bacteria and their products (e.g., endotoxin), antigens, other cytokines (e.g., TNF)	Induces catabolic state, fever, acute phase protein synthesis, and ACTH release; is a cofactor for T-cell activation, B-cell proliferation, and bone marrow stem cell proliferation; induces PMN release from bone marrow; enhances or induces TNF, IL-1, IFN and CSF production; increases endothelial adherence and procoagulant properties
Interleukin-2 (T-cell growth factor)	Glycoprotein Mr ~15 kD	T cells	Antigen–MHC	Major mediator of T-cell proliferation; promotes production of other T-cell lymphokines; enhances cytotoxic T-cell production and differentiation; enhances NK function; cofactor for B-cell proliferation and immunoglobulin secretion
Interleukin-4 (B-cell stimulating factor, B-cell growth factor I)	Glycoprotein ~20 kD	T cells	Antigen–MHC	Promotes proliferation of B cells; induces IgE isotype synthesis; enhances cytotoxic T-cell production and differentiation; enhances B-cell surface HLA class II and IgE receptors; enhances mast cell production; cofactor with other colony stimulating factors in the mouse
Interleukin-5 (B-cell growth factor II, T-cell replacing factor)	Glycoprotein ~18 kD (circulates as a homodimer)	T cells	Antigen–MHC	Induces IgA and IgM isotype synthesis; enhances eosinophil production and function; unclear whether it promotes proliferation of B cells and immunoglobulin secretion in humans
Interleukin-6 (B-cell stimulating factor 2, interferon-β-2, B-cell differentiation factor)	Glycoprotein 21–29 kD	Mononuclear phagocytes; fibroblasts; T cells; certain tumors	Low-level constitutive, increased by viruses, bacteria and their products, IL-1, TNF, IFN, PDGF	Induces immunoglobulin production in activated B cells; little or no interferon activity; induces fever, acute phase protein synthesis, and ACTH release
Interferon-α	Family of peptides 8–20 kD	Mononuclear phagocytes; lymphocytes	Bacteria and their products, viruses, double stranded RNA, other	Interferes with viral replication; decreases cell replication; increases class I MHC expression;

Interferon-β	Glycoprotein 23 kD	Fibroblasts; epithelial cells	cytokines	increases NK cell function; induces fever
Interferon-γ	Glycoprotein 20–25 kD	T cells; NK cells	Antigen–MHC; NK targets	Same as α and β; also increases class II MHC expression, enhances macrophage functions, enhances IgG subtype production
Tumor necrosis factors (TNF) α (cachectin)	Peptide 17 kD	Mononuclear phagocytes; T cells; NK cells	Bacteria and their products, other cytokines, (e.g., IL-1, CSFs, IFN-γ) Antigen–MHC; NK targets	Induces catabolic state, fever, acute phase protein synthesis; major mediator of septic shock; has direct antiviral and antitumor activity; increases endothelial cell adherence and procoagulant properties; enhances B-cell proliferation and immunoglobulin production; enhances PMN adherence and cidal activity (α > β); increases class I MHC expression; enhances or induces TNF, IL-1, IFN and colony stimulating factor production (α > β); inhibits bone marrow cell proliferation
β (lymphotoxin)	Glycoprotein 25 kD	T cells	Antigen–MHC	
Interleukin-3 (multi-CSF)	Glycoprotein 14–28 kD	T cells	Antigen–MHC	Promotes proliferation of pluripotent marrow stem cells
GM-CSF (granulocyte-macrophage-CSF)	Glycoprotein 14–35 kD	T cells; endothelial cells; mononuclear phagocytes; fibroblasts	Antigen–MHC; bacterial products, other cytokines (e.g., TNF, IL-1, IFN-γ)	Promotes proliferation of neutrophil, macrophage, and eosinophil precursors; enhances neutrophil, eosinophil, and macrophage function
M-CSF (macrophage CSF, CSF-1)	Glycoprotein, two forms: 35–45 kD and 20–25 kD (one gene); both circulate as homodimers	Mononuclear phagocytes; fibroblasts; endothelial cells	Constitutive production, increased in response to bacterial products, other cytokines	Promotes proliferation of monocytes; enhances macrophage function
G-CSF (granulocyte CSF)	Glycoprotein 19 kD	Mononuclear phagocytes; epithelial cells; fibroblasts	Low-level constitutive production increased in response to bacterial products, other cytokines	Promotes proliferation of granulocytes; enhances granulocyte function

row production of eosinophils and mast cells.[126,171–176] In contrast, TH1 cells produce INF-γ, which preferentially enhances production of a complement-fixing antibody isotype (IgG2a in the mouse), thought to be important in antiviral and antibacterial defense.[126,177] There is no direct evidence to date that selective lymphokine production is a property of T cells that have not been passaged and cloned in vitro. However, in the rat, a subset of T4 cells that expresses the surface marker OX22 produces IL-2 but does not support immunoglobulin production by B cells, whereas the subset lacking OX22 does not produce IL-2 but does support immunoglobulin synthesis.[178] The situation in the human may be somewhat different. An antigen analogous to OX22, CD45R (detected by the monoclonal antibody 2H4), is absent on T4 cells that support immunoglobulin production and is present on those that do not.[83] We have recently found that IL-4 production is restricted to a small subpopulation (about 5 percent) of human T4 cells; although IL-4-producing cells are almost all CD45R negative, only 6–8 percent of CD45R-negative T4 cells produce IL-4.[172] In contrast, about 30–50 percent CD45R-positive or -negative T4 cells produce IL-2 and IFN-γ. Initial data with cloned human T4 cells also suggest that there is more overlap in production of lymphokines than in the mouse clones. A single T4 cell clone produced IL-4, IL-5 and GM-CSF, but not IL-2, IL-3, and IFN-γ, whereas all other clones produced IL-2, IL-4, and IFN-γ.[171] Nevertheless, these data indicate that production of specific lymphokines by T cells may be regulated, in part, by differences in the capacity of an individual T cell to produce specific lymphokines.

There is a more clear distinction in the capacity for lymphokine production between T4 and T8 cells than within subsets of T4 cells. Although both T4 and T8 cells produce IL-2 and IFN-γ when stimulated with nonspecific mitogens or in response to allogeneic cells,[179,180] production of IL-2 in response to antigens appears to be restricted primarily to T4 cells. Production of other lymphokines by T8 cells in response to antigens but not nonspecific mitogens appears to be almost completely dependent on IL-2 production by T4 cells.[181–183] These findings highlight the critical importance of T4 (helper) cells in lymphokine production, as in T-cell proliferation (see below), and provide an explanation for the devastating effects that result from ablation of this T-cell subset in AIDS. In addition, to the requirement for IL-2, other cytokines may enhance lymphokine production. IL-1 acts to increase production of IL-2, particularly when antigen or antigen-presenting cells are limiting,[116,184,185] and thereby indirectly augments production of other lymphokines. In addition, IFN-γ and TNF-α and -β augment the production of each other.[116,137,186]

Differential regulation of lymphokine production may also be determined, in part, by differences in the way antigen is presented. For example, antigen-presenting cells that have had surface molecules altered by chemical agents have altered antigen-presenting properties such that they induce little or no IL-2 production, whereas IFN-γ, IL-3, and IL2-R are normally induced.[187] Other evidence suggests that the state of T-cell activation or T-cell surface molecules, which could bind to and be affected differently by altered antigen-presenting cells, may act to regulate in part which lymphokines, are produced.[188] How these changes lead to selective induction of certain lymphokines is unclear, although altered production of putative second mediators, such as arachidonic acid metabolites for IFN-γ production,[189] has been proposed.

Since T cells produce IL-2, which augments production of other T-cell-derived lymphokines, there is a potential for overproduction. Important regulatory mechanisms act to attenuate the response. First, IL-2 does not stimulate its own production.[111] In addition, with mouse T-cell clones, the capacity of IL-2 to enhance lymphokine production is maximum within the first 24–48 hours after T cells have been activated by antigen stimulation and is virtually absent 7 days later.[188,190] Reciprocally, exposure of T cells to high concentrations of IL-2 impairs their activation through the antigen receptor.[191] In addition, activated T cells (192, 193) produce transforming growth factor-β early after activation.[192,193] This factor inhibits IL-2-induced T-cell proliferation and inhibits preferentially IFN-γ production, with less inhibition of TNF-α and TNF-β (lymphotoxin) production. In addition, monocytes that are exposed to IFN-γ produce PGE_2 and 1,25 dihydroxy vitamin D_3 (calcitriol), which inhibit IL-2 and IFN-γ production and the T-cell response to IL-2.[164,194,195] Thus, like the production of cytokines by macrophages, both positive and negative regulatory signals act to modulate the strength and duration of T-cell lymphokine production.

Cytokine Production by NK Cells and B Cells

The repertoire of lymphokines that NK and B cells produce is more limited. Binding to target cells induces NK cells to secret TNF-α but apparently not TNF-β.[138,196] However, unlike T cells, most mitogens are poor inducers of TNF-α production by NK cells.[138] IL-2 and inflammatory stimuli induce NK cells to produce IFNγ.[130,197] B cells and NK cells may release low levels of IL-1 constitutively.[136] It is likely that these cells also release additional cytokines, since tumor cell lines of these lineages have been reported to secrete such lymphokines as IL-6,[123] lymphotoxin,[121] and GM-CSF.[198]

IMPORTANT IMMUNOLOGIC RESPONSE PATHWAYS ARE REGULATED BY CYTOKINES

To provide a conceptual framework for understanding the function of cytokines in the immune response, several examples of cytokine-regulated responses are discussed below. These discussions are necessarily oversimplified. Additional complexity due to the interaction of cell types and cytokines that are not shown, or are still not cloned or molecularly characterized, is likely. The role of cytokines in modifying effector cell function is discussed in the section on these cells.

Fever, the Systemic Acute Phase Response to Infection and Septic Shock

The role of cytokines in the pathogenesis of fever has recently been reviewed (see Chapter 39).[154] Fever is associated with an elevation of the normal temperature set point for an individual; although the mean body temperature is increased, the normal diurnal fluctuation of temperature is not altered. Fever may play a beneficial role in host resistance to infection both by inhibiting the growth of certain microorganisms directly and by enhancing certain aspects of host immune responses.[199,200] The elevation of temperature is mediated primarily by endogenous pyrogens. Studies to define the pyrogenic molecules have, by necessity, been done largely in experimental animals. TNF-α and TNF-β and IL-1α and IL-1β are directly pyrogenic in rabbits. They appear to act directly on vascular endothelial cells in the hypothalamic area to cause local production of PGE_2, which then acts on cells within the anterior hypothalamus to cause fever. The antipyretics, such as aspirin and acetaminophen, act by blocking the production of PGE_2 in the brain. In addition to inducing fever directly, TNF stimulates IL-1 production, accounting for the biphasic fever observed in animals administered TNF. The major mediators of bacterial lipopolysaccharide-induced fever appear to be TNF and IL-1; lipopolysaccharide also acts directly on the hypothalamus to induce fever, accounting for the biphasic fever in response to this substance. Other cytokines, including interferons and IL-6, cause fever in experimental animals,[154,201] although they are less potent, and in the case of IFN-γ perhaps act indirectly by inducing TNF or IL-1 release. The pyrogenic effects of TNF and the interferons have been demonstrated in humans.[154]

The *acute phase reaction* is a term describing collectively a range of metabolic changes occurring in response to infection and inflammation (see Chapter 4). Striking effects include those on hepatic protein synthesis, lipid metabolism, and tissue catabolism. TNF, IL-1, and IL-6 all play a role in altering hepatic protein synthesis. Albumin synthesis is decreased and, concomitantly, synthesis of complement components C3 and factor B, metallothionein, serum amyloid A, α_1-antitrypsin, haptoglobin, fibrinogen, C-reactive protein, and others is increased in human hepatoma cell lines in vitro or in experimental animals in vivo.[117,125,201–205] Both TNF and IL-1 also inhibit lipoprotein lipase production, thereby causing lipemia, which is characteristic of certain chronic infections, including experimental trypanosomiasis.[114,115,117,205] The role of TNF-α in cachexia related to infection or malignancy has been postulated based on its effects on food intake and catabolism; this has been directly demonstrated in experimental transgenic mice bearing tumors continually secreting TNF-α in which progressive anorexia and wasting occurred.[206] It is likely that IL-1 also contributes to the wasting seen in chronic inflammatory conditions.[117]

A striking effect of TNF, which is augmented by IL-1, is its ability to produce profound vascular effects. Both increase the adhesive properties of endothelial cells, due in part to increased synthesis of cell adhesion molecules.[207] TNF increases the adhesiveness of circulating granulocytes, due in part to increased surface expression of the leukocyte cell adhesion molecules (LCAM) of the Mac-1, LFA-1 family.[208,209] Endothelial cell procoagulant activity and platelet activating factor production are also increased by TNF and IL-1.[210,211] These and additional effects likely act to induce granulocyte adhesion, capillary leakage, vessel thrombosis, and hemorrhagic necrosis at local sites of administration in experimental animals.[114,115,125] Systemic administration of TNF to rodents produces a syndrome resembling septic shock and disseminated intravascular coagulation; this is characterized by hemorrhagic necrosis, particularly in the gastrointestinal tract, hypotension, hypoglycemia, and lactic acidosis terminating in death.[212–214] IL-1,[117] IFN-γ,[215] and lipopolysaccharide enhance these toxic effects of TNF. The most convincing evidence for a role for TNF in the pathogenesis of septic shock comes from studies in baboons with experimentally induced *Echerichia coli* bacteremia. In such animals treated with antibody to TNF-α 2 hours before infection, death associated with hypotension, and cardiopulmonary and renal failure were completely prevented, whereas they were observed in 100 percent of controls.[213] Circulating TNF-α concentrations were markedly elevated in controls and were not detectable in the treated animals. It is likely that the effects of TNF-α are mediated, at least in part, indirectly. Data support an important role for cyclooxygenase products in TNF-α-induced septic shock in rats; in this model, PGE_2 concentrations in plasma are markedly increased; this increase and the rapidly fatal course are largely blocked in animals that are pretreated with the cyclooxygenase inhibitors indomethacin or ibuprofen.[216] Other mediators, such as lipoxygenase products of arachidonic acid, platelet activating factor, and kinins, are likely to be involved.

Hematopoiesis

Hematopoietic cells are derived from pluripotent stem cells in the bone marrow. The growth and differentiation of hematopoietic cells are under the control of specific cytokines[132,133,135] (Fig. 3). IL-1α,[217,218] IL-6,[219] and IL-3[220] stimulate proliferation of early pluripotent stem cells; IL-3 and GM-CSF stimulate proliferation of cells capable of forming granulocytes, erythrocytes, macrophages, and megakaryocytes[132,133]; GM-CSF stimulates granulocyte and macrophage precursors to proliferate[221]; M-CSF and G-CSF stimulate proliferation of their respective committed precursors[222–224]; IL-5 stimulates eosinophil production.[176] TNF and interferons may act as negative feedback signals to impede marrow cell growth. Note that the factors acting on the most mature precursors of phagocytes (M-CSF and G-CSF) are rapidly produced by macrophages and other nonhematopoietic cells in response to microbial or inflammatory stimuli. This may be important in allowing rapid mobilization of marrow reserves in response to infection. In contrast, the T-cell-derived products act either to augment production of cells at earlier stages of differentiation (IL-3 and GM-CSF) or to stimulate production of eosinophils (IL-5).

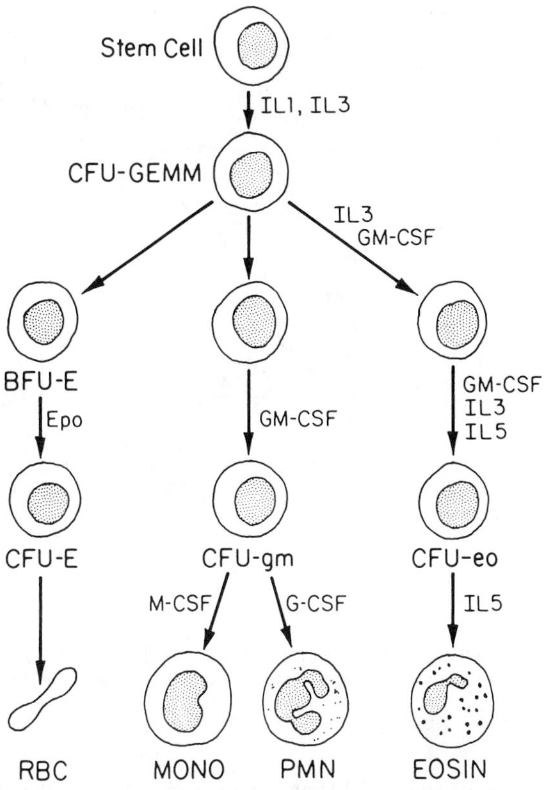

FIG. 3. The role of lymphokines in marrow growth and differentiation. IL, interleukin; CSF, colony-stimulating factor; G, granulocyte; M, monocyte/macrophage.

The Role of Cytokines in T-Cell Proliferation

As discussed above, T cells are activated by antigen in the context of HLA antigens on macrophages or other antigen-presenting cells to produce cytokines, most importantly IL-2, and to express IL-2 receptors on their plasma membrane (Fig. 4). Cognate interaction of T cells with antigen associated with MHC on the antigen-presenting macrophages induces IL-1 production by the macrophages[162,225]; this may be mediated by a direct cell contact mechanism and perhaps also by an as yet undefined soluble factor(s) that T cells release in response to this interaction. IL-1 appears to be most important in enhancing T-cell activation when antigen is limiting.[162] It acts both to increase IL-2 and high-affinity IL-2 receptor expression by T cells. However, IL-1 cannot completely replace antigen-presenting cells in most experimental systems even if a direct signal to the T cell is delivered by a monoclonal antibody that activates the T-cell receptor complex; this indicates that antigen-presenting cells facilitate T-cell activation at multiple levels.

T-cell proliferation appears to be closely regulated by the amount of free IL-2 and by the number and affinity of IL-2 receptors.[112] Since T4 (helper) cells appear to be the primary source of IL-2 produced in response to antigen stimulation, it follows that they are critical to one component of this process—the amount of free IL-2. High-affinity IL-2 receptors are expressed in response to stimulation both by T4 and by T8 (cytotoxic) T cells. High-affinity receptors are composed of two

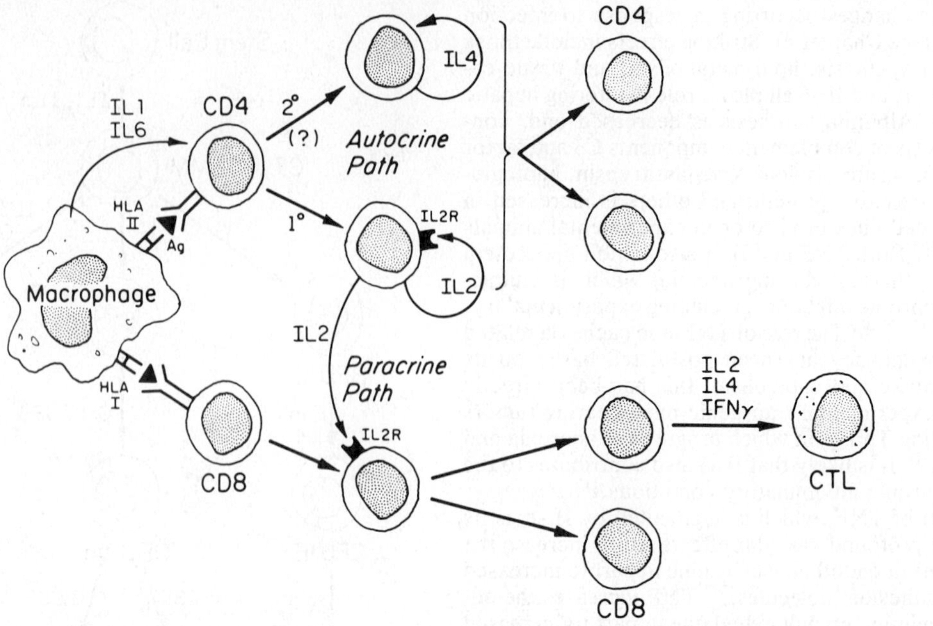

FIG. 4. The role of lymphokines in T-cell proliferation and differentiation. IL: interleukin; IFN-γ: interferon-γ: IL-2R, interleukin-2 receptor; CD4 and CD8: T4 (helper) and T8 (cytotoxic) T cells, respectively; CTL: cytotoxic T lymphocyte.

chains: one of about 55 kD and another of about 70–75 kD.[236–238] Little if any of either chain is present on resting T cells.[229] In the absence of the other, either chain can bind IL-2—the 55 kD chain rapidly but with low affinity and the 70 kD chain slowly and with medium affinity.[230,231] Together they form a receptor with high affinity, which binds IL-2 rapidly but releases it slowly. Current data suggest that the 70 kD chain is critical for induction of IL-2 driven proliferation.[231] Such a receptor permits maximal expression of high-affinity receptors when desirable, shortly after antigen-triggered T-cell activation, that are down-regulated within a few days unless T cells are restimulated by antigen. Thus, when recently triggered by antigen, all T cells express high-affinity receptors and can be driven to proliferate by IL-2. Conversely, the response to IL-2 is limited to cells recently activated by antigen, thereby preventing nonspecific proliferation of T cells not activated by antigen and excessive, sustained proliferation of antigen-activated T cells. This process of negative control is likely to be even more complex, since for a period late after antigen activation, T cells may become refractory to IL-2-driven proliferation even though they still express high-affinity IL-2 receptors; likewise, T cells recently stimulated by high concentrations of IL-2 may be temporarily refractory to antigen-induced activation.[191] The mechanism by which this refractoriness is mediated is not yet clear, but it may be due to a block in signal transduction.

Recent data indicate that there may be alternative pathways by which T-cell proliferation may be driven. IL-4 may augment or replace the need for IL-2 in T-cell proliferation.[112,113] A role for IL-6 has also been suggested.[232] However, it is likely that IL-2 is the major lymphokine required for T-cell proliferation under most conditions. The role of cytokines in differentiation of cytotoxic T cells is discussed in the section on "Cytotoxic T Cells."

Role of Cytokines in B-Cell Activation and Differentiation into Antibody-Secreting Cells

B cells are activated by specific antigens through surface immunoglobulin that acts as an antigen receptor. Once activated, they replicate and then differentiate into immunoglobulin-secreting B cells, and subsequently into memory B cells or plasma cells. This process is controlled by T cells, macrophages, and cytokines from these cells, as shown in Figure 5 (reviewed in Ref. 233). This appears to be a sequential process involving first antigen-induced activation and then DNA synthesis and proliferation, followed by differentiation into immunoglobulin-secreting cells. The requirements for activation vary with the nature of the antigen. Many of the steps were first deduced in the murine system; the relative requirement for T-cell help has been less well studied in humans. It is clear that the actions of specific lymphokines in this process may differ somewhat between the two species; this may reflect species differences or differences in the source of cells and culture conditions used in the in vitro studies. The data shown for the lymphokines are those derived from studies with human cells. The studies on T-cell-independent vs. T-cell-dependent responses are largely extrapolated from those in the mouse; available human data are consistent with these distinctions but require confirmation.

The activation step may be fully T cell independent or dependent on T cells to provide lymphokines (partially T cell independent, type II), or dependent on direct cognate T cell–B cell interaction[234]; cognate T cell–B cell interaction requires that processed antigen be presented in association with class II MHC antigens on B cells to T cells that bind antigen through their antigen receptor. It is unclear if naturally occurring, fully T-cell-independent (type I) antigens exist in humans, although lipopolysaccharide may be an example; in the mouse such antigens are usually large, multivalent, synthetic molecules. Partially T-cell-independent (type II) antigens are oligovalent antigens with repetitive sites, such as the polysaccharide antigens of encapsulated bacteria. Other antigens, including most proteins, are T cell dependent. The activation step triggered by antigen is often mimicked in studies in vitro by antibody to B cell surface IgM or by staphylococcal protein A. These stimuli, like soluble antigen, provide the first signals in B-cell activation, and full activation is facilitated by IL-4. In T-cell-dependent activation, murine studies suggest that cognate T cell–B cell interaction appears to provide one signal independent of IL-4[235,236]; however, IL-4 appears to provide an additional signal and may regulate this process both positively and negatively.[237,238]

Once activated, B cells become responsive to the prolifera-

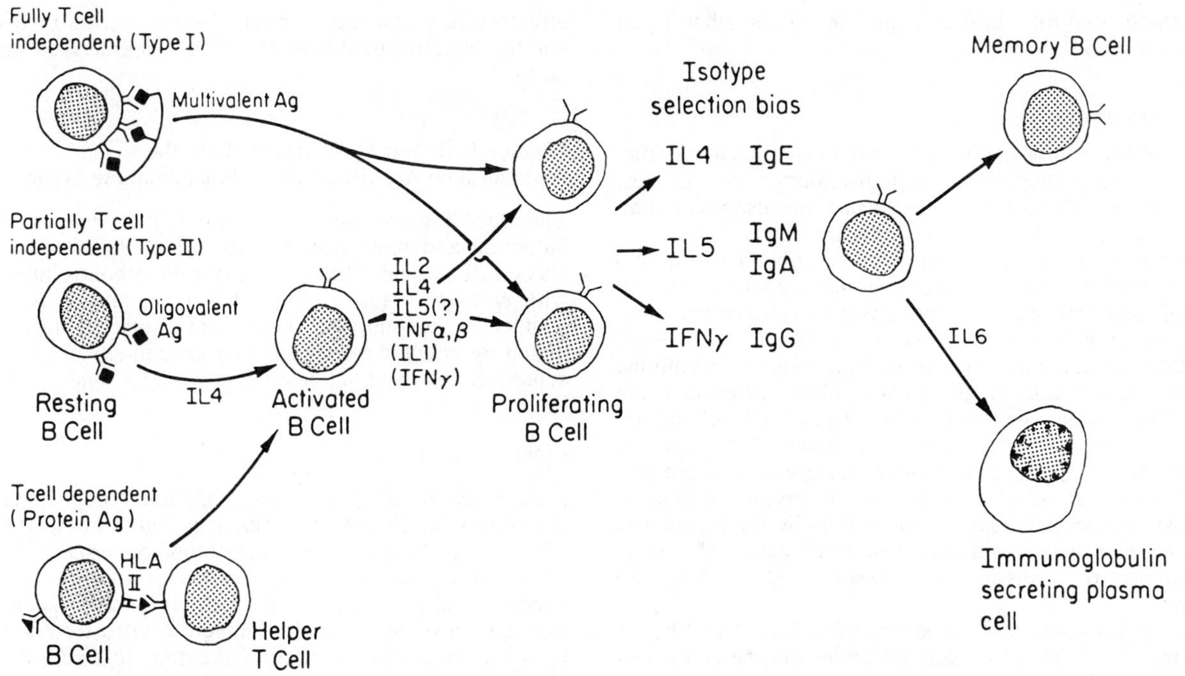

FIG. 5. The role of lymphokines in B-cell growth and differentiation. IL: interleukin; TNF: tumor necrosis factor; IFN-γ: interferon-γ; Ig: immunoglobulin.

tive effects of several lymphokines. In humans, IL-2,[239–242] IL-4,[243,244] and TNF-α[245] and -β[246] appear able to serve as independent signals for proliferation of activated B cells. The effects of one are frequently augmented by those of the others or by the effects of IL-1[233,247] and IFN-γ,[248] which act as cofactors for B-cell proliferation. IL-5, which is a major mediator of B-cell proliferation in the mouse, has not yet been shown to have such activity in the human[233]; conversely, TNF-α and -β have not been shown to drive murine B-cell proliferation, and IFN-γ inhibits this proliferation. After proliferation, B cells either become quiescent memory B cells or differentiate into antibody-secreting plasma cells. IL-6 appears to enhance differentiation into plasma cells and supports the growth of antibody-secreting cells.[249,250] Other lymphokines, such as IFN-γ and IL-2, may also act together to increase the secretion of immunoglobulin.[239]

Lymphokines also influence and may in part determine the class of immunoglobulin secreted. This has most clearly been shown for IL-4, which appears to stimulate a switch from IgM to IgE production in the mouse and in the human.[171,233] In contrast, this switch is antagonized by IFN-γ, which preferentially increases production of IgG in the human[171,233]; in the mouse, IFN-γ increases production of IgG2a, a complement-fixing IgG subclass implicated in antiviral and perhaps antibacterial defenses.[126] IL-5 enhances IgM and IgA production in both species.[176,233,251] There is clearly greater complexity in the system. For example, IL-4 also appears to be important in the B-cell response to polysaccharide antigens such as those of encapsulated bacteria[252]; antibodies to such organisms are commonly of the IgG2 and IgG4 subclasses in humans. Further, with T-cell-dependent antigens, IL-4 may enhance IgM secretion while inhibiting production of all IgG subclasses. These latter effects of IL-4 have been described in the mouse but have not yet been studied in the human.

THE IMMUNOREGULATORY FUNCTION OF T CELLS AND MACROPHAGES

T-cell functions have commonly been divided into three categories: helper, suppressor, or cytotoxic function. The first two roles are immunoregulatory and the final is a direct effector role. These functions correlate in part with surface expression of the CD4 (T4 helper) and CD8 (T8 suppressor/cytotoxic) surface molecules.

T-Cell Help

Traditionally, help is defined as the ability of certain T cells to enhance immunoglobulin synthesis by B cells.[253–256] This capacity appears to be restricted to T4 cells, hence their designation as helper T cells. As discussed above, T4 cells are heterogeneous in that B-cell help is mediated by some but not all T4 cells.[83,173] This heterogeneity has been discerned by assays in which B-cell help is provided only by those cells defined as helper-inducer T cells, which express surface antigens detected by the monoclonal antibodies 4B4 and UCHL1[83]; similarly, heterogeneity has been found in the production by T4 cell clones of specific lymphokines known to regulate B-cell growth and differentiation.[171–175] B-cell help may be both antigen specific and antigen nonspecific. Both types of help appear to be provided by helper-inducer T cells: the antigen-specific help appears to require direct "cognate" interaction through concomitant binding of T cells and B cells to different components of the same complex antigen; the nonspecific help is mediated by release of certain lymphokines. Lymphokines also appear to play a role in antigen-specific help, as discussed more fully in the section on role of lymphokines in B-cell help.

A broader definition of T-cell help includes the role of T4 cells in differentiation of T8 cells[257–259] or macrophages into more competent antigen-presenting or effector cells. It is likely that these effects are mediated primarily by lymphokines. Thus, heterogeneity in the production of certain lymphokines may be one reason why T-cell help for B cells, cytotoxic T cells, and macrophages is not directly correlated. A characteristic of cells in the helper-inducer subset of T4 cells (as defined by the surface antigens detected by monoclonal antibodies 4B4 and UCHL1) is their capacity to respond to soluble antigen. In the absence of these cells, other T4 and T8 cells do not respond to specific antigens, leading to the suggestion that "memory," recognition of antigens to which the individual has previously been exposed, is restricted to these cells.[83] This observation may explain the pivotal role these cells play in helping other T and B cells to respond.

T-Cell Suppression

The proper function of the immune system is efficient destruction of microbial pathogens with minimal injury to host tissues. Accordingly, T cells also attenuate the immune response to balance the potential risks of excessive tissue injury.

Although suppressor T cells are well described from in vivo and in vitro studies, there is no area of immunology more controversial than that regarding the existence, characterization, and specificity of these cells.[260] Suppressor T cells are thought to regulate the immune response by inhibiting the promoting effects of helper T cells on growth and differentiation of T and B cells. These effects were initially defined in bulk cell culture studies in vitro[260] or in adoptive transfer studies of experimental infections, including those due to mycobacteria, fungi, and protozoa.[261] However, it was not possible to produce clones or lines of antigen-induced suppressor T cells by the techniques used to develop helper and cytotoxic T-cell clones,[260] calling the existence of a distinct suppressor T-cell lineage into question.

Initial studies suggested that suppression is mediated by T8 cells, which are known to recognize antigen in the context of class I MHC antigens and to include most functionally cytotoxic T cells. Recent studies propose a complex network whereby a subset of soluble, antigen-responsive T4 cells induce a subset of T8 cells to inhibit the response of the CD4 helper T cells in an antigen-specific fashion; it is suggested that the specificity derives from recognition of the TCR on the helper T cell as antigen by the TCR of the T8 suppressor cells.[260,262] Further complexity may be provided by a network of contrasuppressor cells that block the suppressive effect of the T8 cells on the antigen-specific helper T cells.[263] The requirement for both T4 and T8 cells for suppression induction/mediation may explain the differences in requirements for these subsets to inhibit responses in different animal models of infection (e.g., suppression of resistance to *Leishmania* by T4 cells in BALB-c mice).[264] There is some evidence that antigen-induced enhancement of response occurs with optimum doses of antigen and that attenuation (suppression) occurs with much lower or higher doses of antigen.[260]

The molecular mechanism responsible for antigen-specific suppression is as yet uncharacterized. Direct cell-to-cell interaction is thought to be one mechanism of suppression.[260] Soluble antigen-specific suppressor factors have also been described,[265] but as yet none have been molecularly characterized or cloned convincingly. It is also unclear whether the mechanisms mediating antigen-specific suppression of helper T-cell function and of B-cell growth and differentiation are the same; certain evidence suggests that they are not.[257–260]

Non-antigen-specific suppression of T-cell and B-cell responses by soluble T-cell-derived products has also been described. One well-characterized factor is transforming growth factor-β.[266,267] Other factors that are not yet molecularly characterized are likely to function as attenuators of the immune response. One such factor is a product of T cells that is inactive until modified by oxygen metabolites apparently derived from macrophages.[268] This factor may play a role in attenuating responses in human infection and may be overproduced in AIDS[269]; it is suggested that its effects can be overcome by lymphokine growth factors.[270]

Suppressive Macrophage–Lymphocyte Interactions. The effect of macrophages on lymphocyte responses is dependent on the macrophage-to-lymphocyte ratio in vitro. Low ratios appear to enhance lymphocyte responses, whereas high ratios suppress them. Activated macrophages have an increased capacity to both enhance and suppress lymphocyte responses.[12] Inhibitory effects may be mediated in part by production of PGE_2[164,271] and by oxidative modification of the T-cell-derived suppressor factor.

Effector Cells and Cytokines Mediate the Antimicrobial Activity of the Cellular Immune System

The preceding discussion has focused on the role of CMI in the induction and regulation of host defenses. In addition, CMI plays a direct and often a primary role in controlling infection with pathogens, many of which survive and replicate within host cells. Immunity to these intracellular pathogens is mediated by effector cells, including antigen-specific cytotoxic T cells, NK cells and activated macrophages, and cytokines.

Cytotoxic T Cells

Most cytotoxic T cells express CD8 and recognize antigen in the context of class I MHC antigens found on nearly all cells of the body. As isolated from the blood or tissues, T8 cells are not capable of cytolysis. However, after antigen injection into experimental animals, T8 cells with cytolytic capacity can be isolated. Restimulation with antigen in vitro further enhances cytotoxicity; primary induction of cytotoxic T cells can also be affected in vitro by antigen stimulation. Under most conditions, T4 cells are required for differentiation of T8 cells into cytotoxic cells; this reflects the need for IL-2 for this process in vitro and in vivo[272–274] (Fig. 4). However, IL-2 alone is not sufficient.[272,273] Other factors that appear to play a role as indicated by studies in the human and the mouse, include IL-4,[275–277] produced by a subset of helper T cells,[171,172] IFN-γ,[130,272] and perhaps IL-6.[278] As noted for T-cell proliferation, the ability of these lymphokines to trigger differentiation of T8 cells into cytotoxic cells may be regulated in part by their expression of receptors for the respective lymphokines. As noted, expression of IL-2 receptors is tightly regulated by antigen-induced activation in a time-dependent fashion. However, receptors for IL-4, IFN-γ, and probably IL-6 appear to be constitutively expressed,[279] although they increase in number with activation. Thus, the effects of these cytokines may not be as tightly regulated, indicating the critical role of IL-2 and its receptor in the regulation of this differentiative process as well.

The biochemical processes accounting for the differentiated state of cytotoxic T cells and the mechanisms by which lymphokines mediate this process are only partly understood. Cytotoxic T cells differentiated in vitro have cytoplasmic granules that contain a protein termed *perforin*, which polymerizes to form pores in the membranes of target cells and organisms; these pores resemble those produced by terminal complement components.[280,281] These molecules have been best defined in murine cells but also appear to be present in human cytotoxic T cells.[281,282] Differentiated cytotoxic T cells also contain a family of serine esterases in their granules.[283] Development of cytotoxic function in mouse T cells in vitro correlates with the acquisition of granules containing pore-forming activity but not with serine esterase activity,[284] suggesting that the esterases may not have a direct cytotoxic role. Differentiated cytotoxic T cells may also secrete TNF-α, lymphotoxin (TNF-β), and molecules with activity related to but apparently distinct from those of TNF-α and TNF-β.[285] The precise role that each plays in the cytotoxic function of these cells is not clear. In addition, cytotoxic T cells raised entirely in vivo appear to lack the pore-forming protein but are cytotoxic nevertheless, indicating that other mechanisms are sufficient, if not solely responsible, for cytotoxic activity.[286] Data are not available to determine which properties of differentiated cytotoxic T cells are induced by specific lymphokines. Both IL-2 and IL-4 act, at least in part, by increasing the number of cytotoxic T cells generated in response to antigen stimulation.[285–287]

NK Cells

Natural killer (NK) cells constitute 10–15 percent of blood lymphocytes in adult humans. They are nonadherent, nonphagocytic cells and morphologically are large, granular lymphocytes. They express some surface antigens common to T cells, monocytes, and granulocytes; specifically, most express surface CD2 (the sheep erythrocyte receptor found on all T cells), OKM1, a marker found on monocytes, and CD16 (Leull), a receptor for IgG-Fc found only on NK cells and granulocytes.[287–289] CD16 can be used to define the NK cells in a mixed mononuclear cell population, as can a second antigen, NKH1.[287,288] Only a small portion of NK cells express CD3 and TCR[289–291]; some of these are CD3 cells expressing the unique γδ receptor.[48,52] Other evidence indicating that most NK cells are not T cells includes their lack of T-cell receptor gene rearrangement and messenger RNA expression,[289–291] the presence of normal or increased numbers of NK cells and NK cell precursors in mice that lack mature T and B cells,[290] and differential modulation of T cell and NK cell cytotoxicity.[292]

NK cells were originally defined by their ability to lyse target cells in a manner not restricted by HLA antigens and not requiring presensitization.[293] Recent data suggest that absent or abnormal cell surface HLA antigens, as occur on certain tumor cells and virus-infected cells, are associated with susceptibility to lysis by NK cells; cells expressing abundant, normal HLA antigens are not lysed.[294,295] The molecules that mediate binding of NK cells to targets have not been fully defined, although the leukocyte cell adhesion molecule (LCAM) family plays a role.[296] The CD2 molecule may also be important in NK cell binding and activation.[110]

Studies in experimental animals support a role for these cells in controlling resistance to tumors and viruses,[293] including cytomegalovirus[297] and herpes simplex virus,[298] in vivo. They may also play a role in resistance to other infectious agents, including *Toxoplasma*.[299] The cytolytic mechanisms of NK cells appear to be similar if not identical to those of cytotoxic T cells. IFN-α, -β, or -γ and IL-2 augment NK activity.[130,300–302]

In addition to their cytolytic function, NK cells produce certain lymphokines, as noted above; replicate in response to IL-2, augment cytolytic T-cell responses, inhibit T- and B-cell growth and differentiation, and inhibit hematopoietic cell growth and maturation.[292,303,304] However, their precise functions in vivo have not been fully defined.

NK cells also mediate, in part, antibody-dependent cell-mediated cytotoxicity (ADCC).[293] Cells to which IgG antibodies are bound are lysed. This process is more efficient than antibody-independent NK lysis, presumably because of the increased binding of effector cells to the target. Other cell types, including granulocytes and monocytes, may mediate antibody-dependent cytolysis. Human NK cytotoxicity is most commonly measured against a K562 erythroleukemia cell target. NK and ADCC have also been assessed using cells infected with herpes simplex virus or cytomegaloviruses. In these studies, the cells mediating the cytolytic activity against virus-infected targets appear to be NK cells.[298,305–307]

Monocytes and Activated Macrophages

Properties and Functions of Resting Macrophages as Effector Cells. Resting macrophages play an important role in clearing small numbers of microbes that gain access to tissues and in removing damaged or affected cells and extracellular tissue matrix. Accordingly, these cells contain surface receptors for IgG-Fc, for the derivatives of the third component of complement (C3), and for cell surface carbohydrates (e.g., mannose and frucose) and glycoproteins.[308] These receptors allow marcophages to internalize macromolecules and larger particles that exist in the extracellular environment by pinocytosis and phagocytosis. Pinocytosis consists of the incorporation of small amounts of extracellular material by invagination of a portion of cell membrane and the formation of a cytoplasmic vesicle 1–2 μm in size. Phagocytosis involves larger particles and is greatly enhanced when the particle to be phagocytosed is coated with antibody and/or complement, thereby allowing binding by Fc or C3b receptors on the macrophage surface. The process of phagocytosis involves binding of a particle to macrophage membrane receptors, circumferential enclosure of a particle by a portion of the cell membrane, internalization with formation of a phagosome, fusion of the phagosome with a lysosome, and subsequent digestion. Mechanisms by which macrophages inhibit or kill and degrade phagocytosed organisms include the actions of toxic oxygen metabolites and lysosomal enzymes (e.g., lysozyme). There is some evidence that deprivation of nutrients needed for growth of the organisms, but without which the host cell can survive, might also be involved in some cases.[4,309] Whether killing and/or degradation of phagocytosed organisms is effective depends at least in part on the characteristics of the organisms, the mononuclear phagocytes' innate functional capabilities, the receptor involved in attachment and uptake of the organism, whether the phagocytosing macrophage is activated, and the susceptibility of the particle to the host's microbicidal or digestive mechanisms. Because the macrophage's microbicidal mechanisms may also injure host tissues, it is important that tissue macrophages be limited in the potency of these toxic microbicidal mechanisms. Conversely, resting tissue macrophages are rich in components needed for tissue remodeling, including a wide variety of proteases.

Macrophage Activation and the Role of IFN-γ. At times of infectious challenge, the macrophage adapts. This process, whereby antimicrobial activity is increased at times of need, is known as *macrophage activation*. It was first described by Mackaness and colleagues in the 1960s[310] and has recently been reviewed by others[4,124,308,311]; it is a lymphokine-dependent process central to cellular immunity. The lymphokine dependence of this process was initially suggested by in vivo studies with experimental animals, which indicated that resistance to infection with intracellular pathogens, such as *Mycobacteria, Listeria*, and *Toxoplasma*, could be adoptively transferred by T lymphocytes and did not develop in T-cell-deficient nude mice. Macrophages were also required for resistance. Dissection of this process in vitro indicated that antigen-stimulated T cells secrete lymphokines that alter the macrophage so that it is primed to a state of enhanced microbicidal activity.[4,311,312] Subsequent exposure to microbes or to microbial products, particularly lipopolysaccharide, may either trigger microbial killing directly or provide a second stimulus that fully activates macrophages to lyse tumors or other targets such as virus-infected cells.

It is now apparent that the principal lymphokine that activates macrophages is IFN-γ[313–316] (reviewed in Ref. 4). Macrophages activated by IFN-γ have increased activity against a wide variety of microbes, as indicated in Table 1. The extent to which activated macrophages can kill or inhibit the growth of these organisms varies; for example, activated human macrophages are microbicidal for *Toxoplasma gondii* and *Leshmania donovani*, inhibit but do not kill *Chlamydia psittaci*, and have minimal activity against *Mycobacteria* in vitro. Two types of studies in experimental animals support a role for IFN-γ in resistance to intracellular pathogens. In the first type of study, IFN-γ, when given before or immediately after experimental infection, produced varying degrees of protection against *Listeria*,[317] *T. gondii*,[318] *Mycobacterium intracellulare* or *M. tuberculosis*,[319,320] *L. donovani*,[321] *Salmonella typhimurium*,[322] and *Franciscella tularesis*.[323] In the second type of study, animals treated with antibodies that neutralize IFN-γ had more severe infection with *Listeria*,[324] *L. donovani*,[325] *T. gondii*,[326] and *Rickettsia conarii*.[327] It should be noted that treatment with IFN-γ did not usually protect completely, nor did anti-IFN-γ antibody completely ablate resistance, suggesting IFN-γ-independent mechanisms of resistance. It is also likely that effects of IFN-γ other than macrophage activation, including enhancement of antigen presentation, T-cell help, and cytotoxic T-cell activity, and effects on the survival of pathogens in cells other than macrophages, play an important role.

Although IFN-γ appears to be the lymphokine that induces the broadest range of macrophage antimicrobial activity, other lymphokines activate macrophage activity against a more restricted range of pathogens. TNF enhances macrophage activity against *Trypanosoma cruzi*[328] and *M. avium-intracellulare*,[329] and GM-CSF enhances macrophage activity against *T. cruzi*[330] and *Leshmania tropica* or *L. donovani*.[331,332] In contrast, to date only IFN-γ has been shown to activate macrophage anti-*Toxoplasma* activity.[316]

Characteristics of Activated Macrophages. The properties and functions of mononuclear phagocytes and the effects of macrophage activation on them are shown in Table 4.[308] It is evident that activation is associated with a wide variety of changes that enhance the capacity of these cells to migrate to sites of infection, phagocytose particles coated with IgG or C3 more efficiently, and release increased amounts of potentially microbicidal oxygen metabolites, proteases, and cytokines. The role of enhanced release of oxygen metabolites in the microbicidal activity of activated macrophages has been well characterized (reviewed in Ref. 4). Oxygen-independent mechanisms have been less well characterized but include the degradation of tryptophan, which contributes to activity against *T. gondii* and *C. psittaci* in human cells,[309,333,334] limiting iron availability, which contributes to activity against *Legionella*[335] and arginine catabolism,[336] which contributes to anticryptococcal activity. It is likely that the tissue source, state of activation, and varying susceptibility of given pathogens to different antimicrobial mechanisms determine the relative importance of individual mechanisms in a particular circumstance.

ROLE OF CMI IN DEFENSE AGAINST SPECIFIC TYPES OF INFECTIOUS PATHOGENS

In general, cellular immunity is important in resistance to those infectious pathogens that replicate intracellularly, either in an obligate or a facultative manner. Mechanisms of resistance to intracellular viral pathogens differ somewhat from those to nonviral intracellular pathogens. Accordingly, these will be discussed separately, as will the role of cellular immunity in resistance to certain extracellular pathogens. This section uses representative examples of pathogens in each class to illustrate general concepts. Important differences will be noted, but it should be recognized that this overview is by nature simplistic, and more details are provided in the chapters discussing specific pathogens. Potential approaches for future trials of immunologic intervention are discussed.

TABLE 4. Major Functions of Mononuclear Phagocytes and Their Modification by the Process of Activation[a]

Microbicidal activity (↑)
Tumoricidal activity (↑)
Chemotaxis (↑)
Phagocytosis (varies with particle)
Pinocytosis (↑)
Glucose transport and metabolism (↑)
Microbicidal oxygen-metabolite production (↑)
Antigen presentation (↑)
Secretion
Lysozyme (NC)
Prostaglandins, leukotrienes (↓)
Apolipoprotein E and lipoprotein lipase (↓)
Elastase (↓)
Complement components (↑ or NC)
Acid hydrolases (↑)
Collagenase (↑)
Plasminogen activator (↑)
Cytolytic proteinase (↑)
Arginase (↑)
Fibronectin (↑)
Interleukin-1 (↑ when stimulated)
Tumor necrosis factor-cachectin (↑ when stimulated)
Interferon-α and -β (↑)
Angiogenesis factor (↑)
Colony stimulating factors (↑ when stimulated)

[a] ↑ Indicates that the activity or constituent is increased in activated macrophages, ↓ indicates that it is decreased, and NC indicates no change. This list is based primarily on studies with macrophages from animals and humans infected with intracellular parasites; in some cases, the findings have been confirmed by the addition of IFN-γ in vitro.
(Adapted from Johnston,[308] with permission.)

Nonviral Pathogens—Intracellular

In addition to viruses, certain organisms, facultative and obligate intracellular pathogens, respectively, are capable of or are restricted to replication within cells. Of those noted in Table 1, the intracellular protozoa, *Chlamydia* and *Rickettsia*, are obligate intracellular pathogens, and the remaining organisms are facultative intracellular pathogens. Unlike pyogenic bacteria, for which phagocytosis usually represents death, phagocytosis may represent entry into a comfortable home for these organisms.

Overview of Defense Mechanisms. Animal studies indicate that control of infection with these nonviral organisms is mediated primarily by T lymphocytes, monocytes, and macrophages. The critical role of macrophages has been established in animal studies in which depletion of macrophages increased susceptibility to *Listeria*.[1] The critical role of T lymphocytes is indicated by the marked susceptibility of athymic animals[1] and by passive transfer of resistance with T lymphocytes.[337] Similarly, the important role of T lymphocytes in protecting humans from *Toxoplasma* is suggested by the marked increase in the incidence of severe infection in patients with AIDS,[338] who have a deficiency in helper T4 cells.

In the first days of infection, the rate at which monocytes are recruited to the site of infection and the microbicidal activity of these cells appear to be important in controlling *Listeria* and *Toxoplasma* infection in animals. These findings correlate with the greater microbicidal activity of human monocytes compared with macrophages against *Toxoplasma* and *Listeria*.

Subsequently, resolution of active infection and development of protective immunity in animals depend on appropriate interaction between macrophages and T lymphocytes. On the basis of studies initially performed in animal cells but since reproduced with human cells in vitro, it is thought that this interaction, which is both antigen and host specific, leads to the production of macrophage- and T-cell-derived cytokines. After ingestion and killing by local macrophages, organisms are degraded by these cells. Microbial antigens are then displayed on the macrophage surface in association with class II (HLA-DR) major histocompatibility epitopes. Macrophages stimulated by phagocytosis or by microbial products release IL-1. In the presence of IL-1 and microbial antigen displayed on class II MHC-bearing macrophages, antigen-specific T4 cells are recruited to the site of infection, where they secrete IL-2. Interleukin-2 binds to IL-2 receptors on these and other antigen-activated T lymphocytes, both of the T4 and T8 phenotypes, and stimulates these cells to divide, to release more IL-2, and to release factors that recruit and focus monocytes and macrophages to the site of infection, and enhance monocyte and macrophage microbicidal activity. Interferon-γ appears to be the most important factor mediating these effects on macrophages. In mice, resistance correlates directly with the amount of IFN-γ produced during infection, IFN-γ is protective, and antibody to IFN-γ markedly impairs resistance to *Listeria, Leishmania*, and *Toxoplasma*.[324–326] In addition, depletion of T4 cells in mice causes reactivation of central nervous system toxoplasmosis, illustrating the central role of these cells, as suggested by the frequency and severity of this infection in patients with AIDS.[339]

In contrast to the production by T cells of chemotactic factors and IFN-γ, which are host cell and pathogen specific, monocyte recruitment and macrophage activation are nonspecific.[1] Once recruited to the site of infection and activated, macrophages have increased activity against a wide range of microbes. The basis for the enhanced activity of activated macrophages appears to be multifactorial; both increased generation of microbicidal oxygen metabolites and oxygen-independent mechanisms appear to contribute (reviewed in Ref. 308).

Roles of Cytokines and Mononuclear Phagocytes. Recent studies in patients with leprosy appear to illustrate the importance of these processes. Leprosy is a disease in which the clinical features vary between two polar forms. Patients with the tuberculoid form have a strong cellular immune response, few lesions, and very small numbers of *Mycobacterium leprae*, whereas patients with the lepromatous form have a selective absence of cellular immunity and a high body burden of *M. leprae*.[340] Antibody offers no apparent protection, since patients with lepromatous disease have higher titers than those with tuberculoid disease. Because the disease has major cutaneous manifestations, it has been possible to assess the cellular immune response in vivo as well as in vitro.[341–343] In vitro T cells from tuberculoid but not lepromatous patients fail to produce IL-2 or IFN-γ in response to *M. leprae* antigen, whereas T cells from patients with both types produce these lymphokines in response to other antigens and mitogens.[344,345] In contrast to lesions from tuberculoid patients, biopsied lesions from lepromatous patients have many *M. leprae*. In addition, compared to tuberculoid lesions, in lepromatous lesions the expression of class II MHC antigen on overlying keratinocytes and the number of class II MHC-bearing macrophages and T cells is low. Fewer of the T cells are of the T4 phenotype, and of these, most do not express the 4B4+ phenotype, characteristic of memory T cells with the helper-inducer phenotype, but rather express the CD45R+ phenotype, characteristic of suppressor-inducer cells. Accordingly, fewer T cells in lepromatous lesions are producing IL-2. Addition of IL-2 to T cells from lepromatous patients in vitro allows these cells to proliferate and secrete IFN-γ in response to *M. leprae* antigen.[345] Injection of IFN-γ but not placebo into lepromatous lesions leads to an enhanced mononuclear infiltrate, increased expression of class II MHC on keratinocytes, and a variable decrease in the number of *M. leprae*.

In addition to IFN-γ and IL-2, other cytokines and blood monocytes are likely to be important in the control of nonviral intracellular pathogens. This is suggested by the inability of IFN-γ alone to induce macrophages from mice to be fully activated to kill *Listeria monocytogenes* or *S. typhimurium*, even though these cells are active against *T. gondii*.[346,347] These results are compatible with other data indicating the importance of macrophages derived from newly recruited monocytes rather than from resident macrophages in resistance to *Listeria*.[1] Monocytes have greater antimicrobial activity than resting tissue macrophages against many intracellular pathogens, including *Toxoplasma*[348] and *Leishmania*.[349] Recent data suggest that the CSFs, produced early in the response of mice that resist *Listeria* but later in more susceptible mice, may be important in stimulating the production of monocytes and enhancing their activity[350,351]; production of these CSFs was dependent on T4 cells. As noted in the section on activated macrophages, GM-CSF and TNF-α may contribute to resistance against certain organisms by enhancing macrophage function; in contrast, M-CSF does not appear to enhance activity against *L. tropica* or *T. gondii*.[352]

It is unclear in most cases why certain lymphokines enhance macrophage activity against one pathogen but not another. This may relate in part to differences in the still incompletely characterized effects of specific lymphokines on molecular events associated with macrophage activity. In addition, the nonviral obligate and facultative intracellular pathogens appear to use a wide variety of strategies to survive within the cell.[353,354] For example, *T. gondii* evades killing by several mechanisms: it is relatively resistant to reactive oxygen metabolites,[355] and it does not effectively trigger production of reactive oxygen metabolites (respiratory burst) or phagolysosome fusion in resting macrophages.[348,356] *Leishmania donovani* promastigotes, but not the intracellular amastigotes, are easily killed by oxygen metabolites[4]; promastigotes, but not amastigotes, trigger a respiratory burst in resting macrophages. Both forms are resistant to killing by lysosomes that fuse with phagosomes in which they reside. *Trypanosoma cruzi* evades oxygen metabolites and lysosomal enzymes by escaping from the phagocytic vacuole to reside within the cytoplasm. Other intracellular pathogens, including *Listeria, Legionella, Mycobacteria*, fungi, *Rickettsia*, and *Chlamydia*, use one or more of these strategies to survive within macrophages and other cells. In addition, each pathogen appears to have particular metabolic requirements that are supplied by the host cell and that, in most cases, are still uncharacterized. These differences among pathogens in the mechanisms for establishing intracellular parasitism are likely to provide different targets for attack and thereby dictate which mechanisms must be affected by a lymphokine(s) for it to activate macrophages to kill that organism.

The broad range of pathogens susceptible to IFN-γ-activated macrophages are indicated by an asterisk in Table 1. This broad activity of IFN-γ may relate in part to its much greater capacity, compared to that of other lymphokines, to increase the macrophage production of reactive oxygen metabolites and to uniquely enhance an apparent variety of oxygen-independent mechanisms.[4] Interferon-γ induces expression of a multitude of new proteins in murine and human macrophages[357] and other cell types, some of which are unique and some of which are induced by other lymphokines, including TNF. Further study of these proteins should help elucidate the molecular basis of IFN-γ-induced macrophage activation.

Role of Other Cell Types in Resistance. Activated macrophages may not be sufficient to control infection completely. This may occur either because the pathogen is capable of invading host cells other than macrophages and granulocytes or because activated macrophages are not sufficiently microbicidal. Infection of cells other than macrophages and granulocytes is the rule for infection with *Toxoplasma, Chlamydia*, and *Rickettsia* but may also occur to a limited extent in infections with other nonviral intracellular pathogens. An example is infection of Schwann cells in tuberculoid leprosy.

One mechanism by which infection is controlled in nonmacrophage cells may be the induction of microbistatic or microbicidal activity in fibroblasts and in endothelial, epithelial, and parenchymal cells by IFN-γ (reviewed in Ref. 4). This has been demonstrated for *Toxoplasma, Chlamydia*, and *Rickettsia*.

An alternative control mechanism may be the lysis of infected cells or extracellular organisms by T cells and NK cells. Kaufmann has demonstrated that murine macrophages infected with *L. monocytogenes, M. tuberculosis*, and *M. leprae* are recognized by specific T-cell clones both of the T4 and T8 phenotypes and that both can lyse infected macrophages in an antigen- and MHC-restricted manner.[353] *Nocardia asteroides* also appears to be sensitive to killing by cytotoxic T cells.[358] NK cells may play a role in resistance to *Cryptococcus neoformans, Leishmania, Plasmodium bergheii*, and *T. cruzi* in experimental animals (reviewed in Ref. 359). They may act to lyse extracellular organisms directly, such as *T. cruzi* and *T. gondii*[299,359] or to lyse infected cells, particularly in the presence of antibody. This process may be beneficial to the host if liberated organisms are then killed by another mechanism; however, cytotoxic T-cell activity could lead to pathologic tissue damage. The potential role of NK cells is not well established.

The Role of Antibody. Lymphokine-dependent cellular immunity appears to be the sole mechanism for resistance of animals to *Listeria* and *M. tuberculosis*. Antibody appears to play no role.[310] Based on studies with animals and with human cells in vitro, antibody may play a limited role in protection against other intracellular bacterial pathogens, including *Salmonella* and *Legionella*,[360–362] although this is an area of controversy.

Antibody does contribute to protection against protozoa, including *Toxoplasma*, in experimental animals. Mice that cannot mount an antibody response are slightly more susceptible to late death from *Toxoplasma* than are normal mice. Antibody and complement lyse extracellular *Toxoplasma*, and antibody-coated *Toxoplasma* organisms are killed by resting mouse and human macrophages.[363] Antibody alone provides minimal protection in adult and newborn mice, but antibody enhances protection by activated macrophages.[364] T-lymphocyte-deficient mice are much more susceptible than are antibody-deficient animals and are not protected by antibody.

Leishmania donovani promastigotes are lysed by naturally occurring antibody and complement, but the intracellular amastigote forms are resistant.[349] However, antibody may contribute to protection against amastigotes by inhibiting uptake of amastigotes into resting macrophages in which they replicate.[365] Antibodies also inhibit motility and nucleic acid synthesis by *T. cruzi*.

Nonviral Pathogens—Extracellular Helminths and Bacteria

CMI appears to play an important role in resistance to certain extracellular protozoa and helminths (Table 1).

Of the protozoa, the mechanisms of immunity to *Plasmodia* are the best characterized. Sterile immunity to the sporozoite form (the form passed from the mosquito to the host) of the rodent parasites *P. berghei* and *P. yoelii* requires antibody and T8 but not T4 cells[366–368]; antibody alone or T cells alone may be sufficient to prevent infection with a very small inoculum. T8 cells may act in part by cytotoxic mechanisms and in part by lymphokine production. Interferon-γ appears to play an important role in this process, since antibody to IFN-γ blocks protection in immunized mice and in mice passively protected by antibody and immune T cells.[368] Interferon-γ acts in part by causing destruction of exo-erythrocytic forms within hepatic parenchymal cells. Interferon-γ also activates human and murine macrophages to kill erythrocytic forms of *Plasmodia*.[369] TNF-α has antiplasmodial activity and is detectable in the serum of infected humans.[370] However, data in mice infected with *P. berghei* suggest that overproduction of TNF-α may be an important cause of fatal cerebral malaria by causing cerebrovascular accumulation of macrophages containing phagocytosed, parasitized erythrocytes.[371] Anti-TNF-α antibody protects against cerebral malaria without increasing parasitemia. This illustrates the delicate balance needed in the CMI response to provide protection without excessive tissue injury.

CMI appears to be important in conferring protection but may also contribute to tissue damage in response to helminths. In patients with more intense infections with *Schistosoma mansoni*, killing of schistosomula by monocytes and lymphocytes and the response to schistosome antigens are depressed compared to those with less intense infection[372]; however, it is not known whether this is a cause or an effect of more severe infection. Interferon-γ-activated macrophages have antischistosomal activity,[4] and TNF, released in greater amounts by activated macrophages, enhances eosinophil killing of *S. mansoni* larvae in vitro.[373] In addition to CMI, eosinophils, neutrophils, and IgE antibodies contribute to resistance to schistosomes.[372] Since IgE and eosinophil production is controlled by the T4-cell-derived lymphokines IL-4 and -5, respectively (see above), it is likely that these cells play an important role in resistance to schistosomiasis, as they do in mice infected with *Nippostrongylus brasiliensis* and *Trichinella spiralis*[374]; in these infections, IgE, eosinophils, and immune lymphocytes cause worm expulsion from the intestine of infected rodents.[374–378] An important component of the immune response to schistosomiasis is downmodulation of hepatic CMI. This attenuates the granulomatous response to schistosome larvae that develops in the liver, which may lead to cirrhosis. In mice, attenuation of the granulomatous response appears to correlate with decreased IFN-γ and IL-2 production by T cells. This is mediated by antigen- and MHC-specific T8 (suppressor) cells in *S. mansoni* infection, and by this mechanism and antibody-induced suppression in *S. japonicum* infection.[375]

Recent studies indicate that T cells may also participate directly in defenses against certain pyogenic bacteria. For example, T cells regulate the development of abscesses induced by *Bacteroides fragilis* in mice[379,380]; similar to the studies with schistosome-induced hepatic granulomas, T cells act both to induce abscess formation in naive mice and to inhibit abscess formation in immune mice. In addition, in a murine model, specific immune T8 cells protect against intraperitoneal infection with *Pseudomonas aeruginosa*.[381] Immune T cells alone are protective in the absence of antibody and in granulocytopenic mice.[381–383] The T cells appear to act by secreting a still uncharacterized lymphokine with bactericidal activity. Induction of the lymphokine is antigen specific, but it is protective against a variety of bacteria. In other murine models, lymphokines, including IL-1[384] and IL-2,[385] increase resistance to pyogenic bacterial infections. However, the mechanism by which resistance is increased is unknown.

Viruses

The immune response to certain viral infections, particularly those in which viral transmission occurs by cell-to-cell contact rather than by release of virus into the extracellular environment, appears to be cell mediated. For a particular virus, an individual function or combination of functions of sensitized T lymphocytes may be important; these functions may include (*1*) mobilization and activation of macrophages, (*2*) direct cytotoxicity against virus-infected cells, and (*3*) release of interferon (Table 5). Because they are the most common severe viral infections in patients with cellular immune dysfunction, including neonates and the aged, transplant recipients and individuals with AIDS, infections with the herpes viruses provide

TABLE 5. Mechanisms of Host Defense Against Viruses

		Target	
	Mechanism	*Extracellular Virus*	*Infected Cells*
Humoral			
Antibody	Neutralize	+	−
	ADCC	−	+
Interferon	Inhibit viral replication	−	+
Cellular			
Monocytes/ macrophages	Ingest and clear virus	+	−
	Inhibit viral replication	−	+
	Lyse infected cells ADCC NK cytotoxicity	−	+
Lymphocytes			
NK cells	Lyse infected cells ADCC NKC	−	+
T lymphocytes	Specific cell-mediated cytotoxicity	−	+

Abbreviations: ADCC: antibody-dependent cell-mediated cytotoxicity; NK: natural killer cell.

models for the role of CMI in viral defenses and have recently been reviewed.[386]

Antibody can neutralize extracellular virus or sensitize virus-infected cells to lysis by complement (IgG and IgM) or by effector cels (IgG only).[387] In animal models, T cells appear to be important in herpes simplex virus (HSV) and cytomegalovirus (CMV) infection because depletion of complement does not alter the protective effect of antibody,[388] whereas depletion of T cells by irradiation or by antithymocyte serum does.[389]

Intracellular viral replication may be prevented by noncytotoxic mechanisms and by mechanisms that lyse infected cells. The best-characterized noncytotoxic mechanism is interferon-mediated inhibition of viral replication. Interferon is produced by macrophages, fibroblasts, and nonimmune lymphocytes in response to viral challenge (IFN-α and -β) and by specifically sensitized lymphocytes in response to antigen (IFN-γ)[390]. IFN-β and -γ are highly species specific, whereas IFN-α has some activity in cells from other species.

Ingestion of HSV by human monocytes (and perhaps polymorphonuclear leukocytes, PMNs) is associated with abortive infection, thus effectively clearing extracellular virus.[391] Unlike the monocytes from which they are derived, macrophages may support viral replication. Mouse macrophages can inhibit viral replication within other cells by a noninterferon, noncytotoxic mechanism[392]; human cells have not been studied. Mouse and human lymphocytes and monocytes (and perhaps PMNs) can lyse HSV- and CMV-infected cells in the presence of specific antibody by ADCC.[387] Although less efficient, cell-mediated lysis of virus-infected cells also occurs in the absence of specific antibody by NK cytotoxicity,[393,394] thought to be important in controlling early infection in mice before specific immunity develops.[387] NK cells are the major effector cell of ADCC and NK cytotoxicity in mice and humans; macrophages may also mediate cytotoxicity. Cells from nonimmune humans are as effective[394] or almost as effective in ADCC and NK cytotoxicity as cells from immune individuals.[393] Both ADCC and NK cytotoxicity are augmented by interferon.

Nude mice, which lack T lymphocytes, are more resistant than controls to early overwhelming infection; this is thought to result from high NK cytotoxicity. However, nude mice commonly die late in the infectious process, when specific T-cell-mediated cellular cytotoxicity, which they lack, normally develops.[387]

The relative roles of these processes in protection are not established in humans. Neither humans with isolated T lymphocyte deficiency (DiGeorge syndrome) nor those with isolated immunoglobulin or complement deficiency develop disseminated primary HSV infection.[387] In contrast, primary infection is severe in patients with combined immunodeficiency.[387,395]

In adults, Merigan and coworkers[396] have shown that increased HSV-specific induction of IFN-γ in vivo and in vitro correlates with a longer interval to recurrence of HSV infection; the IFN-γ appeared to be produced primarily by T4 cells. In contrast, IFN-α production did not correlate with time to next recurrence. Human neonates develop severe and often fatal HSV infection, whereas in adults primary HSV infection is much less severe. We have recently found that neonates with HSV infection compared to adults with primary HSV infection have markedly delayed and diminished production of IFN-γ in response to HSV.[397] They also produce less TNF in response to HSV. TNF and IFN-γ-synergistically inhibit HSV replication and lyse HSV-infected cells in vitro.[398] At the time of primary infection nearly all neonates have detectable HSV antibody, whereas antibody is absent in the adults with primary infection.[397] These data suggest a more important role for T-cell-dependent lymphokine production than for antibody in resistance to primary and recurrent HSV infection. The importance of cellular and humoral immunity is also suggested by studies in mice.[399,400]

Overall, based on animal and human data, the following may be hypothesized for HSV infection. High-titer antibody may prevent infection with a low inoculum. With a higher inoculum or in the absence of antibody, infection develops. NK cytotoxicity (and if passively derived antibody is present, as in some neonates, ADCC) may limit the initial spread of infection. Eradication of acute infection and establishment and maintenance of latency may depend on or at least be markedly facilitated by specific cytotoxic T lymphocytes and T-cell-dependent lymphokine production. Further basic and clinical studies are needed to determine the validity of these hypotheses.

Similar mechanisms appear operative in CMV infection.[401,402] Specific HLA-restricted, cytotoxic T lymphocytes have been more strongly implicated in the control of severe CMV[401] than HSV infection, and antibody appears to have a limited role in resistance to CMV infection.[401] Resistance to Epstein-Barr virus (EBV) also appears to be mediated principally by CMI. T8 cells act to restrict EBV-induced polyclonal B cell proliferation.[386] Attenuation of T-cell defenses by cyclosporine in transplant patients is associated with EBV-induced polyclonal B-cell proliferation, which is reversible on discontinuation of the drug. An X-linked defect, apparently in the CMI response to EBV infection, is seen in the X-linked lymphoproliferative syndrome.[403] The precise mechanisms that are aberrant in this syndrome are not known; it appears that some patients have an excessive CMI response associated with fatal infectious mononucleosis or hypogammaglobulinemia and that others have an inadequate CMI response associated with B-cell lymphoma. Impaired production of immune interferon has been proposed as a mechanism in one patient with this syndrome and B-cell lymphoma.[404] Impaired T-cell control of EBV replication may also contribute to EBV-associated complications in AIDS.[405]

In addition to the herpes group viruses, CMI has been shown to play an important role in influenza virus infection. Development of virus-specific, HLA-restricted, cytotoxic T cells appears to be important for resistance.[406,407] Specific antigenic epitopes of influenza recognized by cytotoxic T cells have been extensively studied as models,[408] and results indicate that both internal viral antigens, such as nucleoproteins, as well as surface antigens are recognized.[95,96]

Defense mechanisms acting against HIV infection are reviewed in Chapter 107. They include T8 cells that suppress HIV replication in T4 cells[409] or lyse infected T4 cells[99,410] and perhaps contribute to helper T-cell depletion. Recent studies indicate that IFN-γ, production of which is impaired in those with progressive AIDS, inhibits HIV replication.[411] With IFN-γ, TNF synergistically inhibits HIV replication in T cells.[411] GM-CSF synergistically inhibits HIV infection in the monocytic cell line U937 but increases HIV infection in U1, which is derived from U937.[412]

Cell-mediated cytotoxicity may contribute to tissue damage when directed against critical host cells, as in AIDS. This is an established mechanism for tissue injury in lymphocytic choriomeningitis infection[413] and may play a role in rabies.[414]

PROSPECTS FOR IMMUNOLOGIC INTERVENTION

Cytokines, including purified IL-2 and IFN-γ, TNF, and CSFs, are now available in large quantities through recombinant DNA methods, and clinical trials have been initiated.

Interferon-γ

Interferon-γ has been used in treatment trials of patients with cancer, leprosy, chronic granulomatous disease, and AIDS (reviewed in Ref. 4). In patients with cancer or leprosy who received doses ranging from 10 to 1000 units/M^2, circulating monocytes produced increased amounts of potentially microbicidal oxygen metabolites when stimulated[415–417] and had increased activity against allogeneic tumor cells in vitro.[418] Variable decreases in the number of *M. leprae* organisms were seen in patients receiving intralesional IFN-γ.[340] Blood monocytes from patients with AIDS receiving intermittent IFN-γ intravenously had increased activity against *T. gondii* and *L. donovani*[419] and enhanced NK-cell[420] and T-cell function.[421,422]

However, patients with AIDS have not been fully protected from opportunistic infections by IFN-γ, since cryptococcal meningitis and *Pneumocystis* pneumonia have developed in the first week of therapy[419,421] or during low-dose therapy,[421] and IFN-γ did not affect established CMV infection.[419] The failure of IFN-γ to protect may be due in part to the short interval between initiation of treatment and infection, failure to focus delivery at the site of infection, or lack of activity of IFN-γ or IFN-γ-activated effector cells against *Pneumocystis* and CMV.[4]

The effects of IFN-γ on immune functions does not correlate clearly with the dosage or the dosage interval.[4] This is particularly true in patients with chronic granulomatous disease (CGD). Although these patients suffer from frequent pyogenic infections, infections with intracellular pathogens, such as *Mycobacteria* and *Nocardia*, may also be problematic. Administration of IFN-γ often results in increased microbicidal activity of phagocytes from CGD patients that lasts for 2 or more weeks suggesting actions in addition to direct effects on mature macrophages.[423,423a,423b]

Toxicity of IFN-γ includes fever, fatigue, myalgias, and headaches at dosages greater than 10 μg/m^2 and appears to be dose limiting at dosages of 500 μg/m^2 or greater. Granulocytopenia also develops, as do other transient laboratory abnormalities.

Interleukin-2

Because it enhances T-cell growth and cytotoxic T-cell function, IL-2 is an attractive candidate for immune intervention. Administration of IL-2 to experimental animals has increased resistance to viral, bacterial, and protozoan pathogens. However, therapeutic trials in humans, including AIDS patients, have not yet shown convincing evidence of efficacy. Some increase in the number of lymphocytes in lymph nodes proximal to the site of administration was seen in a child with immunodeficiency, possibly due to Nezeloff syndrome or to AIDS, who had received a bone marrow transplant that did not engraft; the child died of overwhelming infections 5 days after IL-2 therapy was initiated.[424] In the same series, another patient with AIDS had improvement in CMV retinitis while receiving IL-2 but *Salmonella* sepsis subsequently developed. Although no toxicity was seen in this study, which used relatively low dosages of purified IL-2, toxicity has been a significant problem in cancer patients receiving high dosages in conjunction with LAK cells (up to 100,000 units/kg every 8 hours). Severe fluid retention associated with capillary leakage appears to be dose limiting; fever and neuropsychiatric effects have also been problems.[425,426] However, if LAK cells are omitted, toxicity of IL-2 appears to be greatly reduced (C. Henney, personal communication.

More promising is the potential use of the IL-2 gene in recombinant vaccines.[427,428] This strategy involves the incorporation of the IL-2 gene in a vaccinia virus recombinant. Such vaccines result in the localized production of IL-2 only at sites of viral replication; local control of viral replication then stops IL-2 production, thereby focusing its effects both locally and temporally. In T-cell-deficient nude mice given vaccinia virus progressive disease resulted. However, in these mice the infection completely resolved with vaccinia virus recombinants containing the IL-2 gene. In one study, influenza virus hemagglutinin or nucleoprotein genes were included in the recombinant vaccinia virus vectors[427]; in studies also containing the IL-2 gene, antibody production was increased under conditions in which the response to vaccines without the IL-2 gene was often suboptimal. The precise mechanisms by which IL-2 acted are not yet known. However, these results suggest potential sechanisms by which lymphokine therapy can be directed to enhance a specific desired response and limit its undesirable systemic effects.

Colony-Stimulating Factors

The CSFs have been used in clinical trials in patients with AIDS, cancer, and bone marrow transplants. Experience with GM-CSF suggests that it is well tolerated at dosages that increase circulating monocyte and neutrophil counts.[429,430] Whether delivery of monocytes to sites of infection increases resistance to infection with intracellular pathogens remains to be determined. Interleukin-1-α acts early in the hematopoietic pathway to increase production. This may account for its radioprotective effect in experimental animals[217] and may suggest a potential role in limiting the duration and severity of myelosuppression in individuals receiving radiotherapy. However, there is concern about the potential for causing recrudescence of hematologic malignancies by the use of exogenous CSFs to limit therapy-induced cytopenias. Accordingly, trials in patients treated for solid tumors are receiving greater initial attention.

Other Cytokines

TNF-α has been used initially in trials for the treatment of cancer. Toxicity has been problematic and the response minimal. Because of its synergistic activity with IFN-γ, an initial trial of these agents is being undertaken in AIDS patients. Low doses of TNF-α have reduced infection in mice with experimental malaria.[431]

Future studies will need to determine the optimal means for giving cytokines. It may be possible to partially target delivery to sites of infection by administering them in an appropriate vehicle, as in vaccinia virus—IL-2 recombinants. Another example may be the use of lymphokines targeted to the reticuloendothelial system or to the lung. Further, antimicrobial chemotherapy is currently used for many intracellular infections with varying degrees of success. Synergistic effects have been observed in vitro with IFN-γ and antimicrobials.[4] It will be important to determine the potential for synergistic or antagonistic interaction between immunologic and antimicrobial therapy in vivo. It is also likely that combined use of IFN-γ and other cytokines, such as IL-2 or CSFs, may be advantageous.

Noncytokine Immunopotentiators

Use of other nonspecific immunoenhancers has been attempted, but to date success has been limited and has often been overshadowed by toxicity. *Corynebacterium parvum* (killed) and Calmette-Guerin bacillus (BCG) (live or various extracts) are immunologic adjuvants and appear to stimulate both the afferent and efferent limbs of CMI. Although *C. parvum* has been used extensively for immunotherapy in cancer patients, its use for infections in humans has been limited. In one study it had no effect on the chronic carriage of hepatitis B surface antigen. Similarly, transfer factor, an uncharacterized crude extract of peripheral blood leukocytes, was suggested to be useful in certain patients with congenital immunodeficiency,[432] in the treatment of varicella zoster in children with cancer,[433] and in certain other infections with intracellular infections. However, its use has never been properly studied in multicenter controlled trials and in the absence of molecular characterization it is primarily of historical interest. Similarly, studies to date with levamisole and other chemical immune potentiators and with thymic hormones have been limited and have not provided clear evidence of benefit.

Immunoattenuation

In certain disease states, an excessive immune response results in tissue damage and attenuation rather than enhancement is desirable. An example is septic shock (see Chapter 59). Cytokines, particularly TNF-α, appear to be major mediators. In experimental animals, either early administration of corticosteroids, which blocks production of TNF, IL-1, and other cytokines, or specific antibody to TNF-α prevents the development of fatal septic shock. Unfortunately, delay in administration of these treatments until after the disease is established is less successful and may account for the failure of corticosteroids to clearly benefit humans. Whether agents with specific activities, like antibodies to cytokines, or a combination of agents would be more effective must be determined in clinical trials. The use of reagents more specific than corticosteroids offers the potential for relatively selective inhibition of undesirable responses with retention of those critical to resistance. Examples include immunotoxins in which lymphokines or specific monoclonal antibodies may be fused to a toxin. By so doing, the toxin can be targeted to cells expressing specific lymphokine receptors or surface molecules recognized by the antibodies.

Immunoattenuating therapy may be more beneficial in patients with less rapidly progressive diseases. For example, corticosteroids appear to be beneficial in decreasing the severity of lung dysfunction in AIDS patients with *Pneumocystis* pneumonia[434] or lymphoid interstitial pneumonitis.[435]

DEFECTS IN THE FUNCTION OF CMI

The thorough review of this topic by McLeod et al.[311] in the previous edition of this book has been updated and material on the physiologic "immunodeficiency" of infancy and the aged has been added.

Physiologically Diminished CMI in Infants and the Aged

The human fetus and the neonate are unduly susceptible to severe infection with multiple pathogens, including those against which CMI is the major mechanism of host defense. These include *Toxoplasma, Listeria, Treponema pallidum*, and the herpes group viruses. The rate of disease progression in neonates with HIV infection is also more rapid than in older individuals, with a median survival time for infants with AIDS of 6.5 months.[436]

Deficiencies in the cytokine-dependent interaction between T lymphocytes and macrophages have been demonstrated with human neonatal cells in vitro (reviewed in Ref. 437). Interleukin-1 production by monocytes from most newborn infants is normal,[140] and although the density of HLA-DR on neonatal monocytes is somewhat less than on adult monocytes, they support a normal proliferative response of T lymphocytes to microbial antigens. The proliferative response of neonatal T cells to nonspecific mitogens and of T cells from most infants with congenital *Toxoplasma* infections to *Toxoplasma* antigen is normal. However, the response to *Toxoplasma* antigen is less consistent in infants younger than 2 months, and in infants with other congenital or neonatal infections, the proliferative response to specific antigens is often absent or diminished. In contrast, production of the major macrophage activation factor, IFN-γ, by T cells from neonates at birth and in the first weeks of life is markedly decreased.[438] This immaturity of lymphokine production is relatively selective, since production of other T-cell- and macrophage-derived cytokines is similar or only slightly less than by adult cells, with the exception of IL-4.[439]

Human neonatal monocytes migrate somewhat less well than adult monocytes; both efficiently ingest and kill *Toxoplasma*.[356] Macrophages derived from neonatal monocytes and fetal macrophages from the placenta can be activated in vitro by macrophage activiation factor produced by adult lymphocytes or by recombinant or purified IFN-γ.[356] Once activated, these cells are as effective at killing or inhibiting the replication of *Toxoplasma* as are adult cells.[356] These studies suggest that defects in delivery and activation of macrophages at sites of infection may contribute to the susceptibility of the fetus and neonate to infection with nonviral intracellular pathogens.

Antiviral cellular defenses are also immature in the neonate. Although production of IFN-α and -β by human neonatal cells is normal,[440] production of IFN-γ is markedly decreased. Further, IFN-α less consistently inhibits viral replication[441] and enhances cytotoxic activity in human neonatal cells compared with adult cells.[394] In mice, development of interferon soon after challenge is important in conferring protection from large inocula[442] and is delayed in neonates[443]; such data are not available in humans.

Some studies suggest that monocytes[444] and alveolar macrophages from human newborn infants[445] may not clear extracellular virus, as adult cells do. The validity of these results is uncertain, either because the cell preparations contained both monocytes and lymphocytes[444] or because alveolar macrophages from only three patients were studied at the time of death.[445] We have found no consistent difference in this function between adult and neonatal monocytes and macrophages.[446]

More consistent defects have been found in the ability of neonatal human lymphocytes and monocytes to lyse HSV-infected cells. In the extensive studies by Ching and Lopez[447] and by Kohl et al.,[394] neonatal cells had clearly less NK cytotoxicity than did adult cells; ADCC was less severely decreased. However, the total number and percentage of NK cells in neonatal blood are similar to those in adult blood.[448] The relevance of these observations is suggested by studies in newborn mice, which have deficient NK and ADCC cytotoxicity. Newborn mice are protected against lethal HSV infection by either antibody, acyclovir, or interferon in combination with lymphocytes or monocytes from human adults but not from human neonates.[298] The development of specific cytotoxic T cells has not been documented in human neonates; however, lymphocyte proliferation and production of IFN-γ and TNF in response to HSV is delayed in neonates compaed to adults with primary HSV infection.[397]

In summary, the failure of neonates to control HSV may be related in part to decreased production of or reduced response to interferon or to decreased activity of nonimmune and immune cellular cytotoxic mechanisms. In addition, infection with HSV occurs more often in infants born to mothers with primary rather than secondary infection; the lack of passively acquired antibody in such infants is a possible but unproved susceptibility factor. Similarly, infection with *Toxoplasma* and intracellular bacterial pathogens, such as *Listeria*, may be more severe because of the decreased generation of lymphokines and interleukins, which attract macrophages to the site of infection and enable them to kill these organisms. Much of the data on neonatal immunity are based on in vitro and animal studies and summarize current information in a rapidly changing field rather than stating established fact. The data suggest that immature CMI may contribute to the neonate's susceptibility. The precise age at which most of the immune functions discussed reach maturity is unknown. However, the risk of severe infection with these pathogens appears to wane by 2–3 months of age. Although this may partly reflect decreased exposure, it is possible that immune functions that are mature by this age are those most critical for protection.

Aged individuals also have diminished CMI responses in vitro and delayed hypersensitivity skin test responses in vivo.[449] The major consistent change appears to be a decline in proliferative responses to antigens and certain mitogens; this appears to reflect diminished production of and response to IL-2.[450] There is an associated decrease in cytotoxic T-cell generation.[451] Altered T-cell-mediated immunoregulation may contribute to the increased incidence of autoantibodies and to the enhanced susceptibility to viral and nonviral intracellular pathogens seen in the aged.[451]

CMI is also decreased physiologically during pregnancy in response to antigens and less consistently to mitogens. This is associated with an apparent increase in susceptibility to infections, including those due to varicella-zoster virus, *C. immitis*, and *M. leprae*.[452]

Congenital Disorders

A number of congenital disorders of CMI and their associated laboratory abnormalities are listed in Table 6. DiGeorge syndrome, a classic example of a congenital disease with defective CMI, results when the third and part of the fourth pharyngeal pouch fail to develop during embryogenesis. This results in the absence of the thymus and parathyroid glands. Severe hypocalcemia and tetany secondary to hypoparathyroidism occur in the neonatal period and are early clues to the diagnosis. Absence of the thymus gland prevents differentiation of T-lymphocyte precursors into T lymphocytes; lack of T lymphocytes prevents expression of a normal cellular immune response. Children with this disorder are lymphopenic, and thymic-dependent areas of their lymph nodes show depletion of lymphocytes. Their lymphocytes do not undergo transformation when exposed to either mitogen or antigen or when placed in mixed lymphocyte culture. A common feature of this and other disorders affecting T-cell function is defective production of lymphokines, including IFN-γ.[4] DTH skin reactivity to antigens, including streptokinase-streptodornase and candidin, is absent, and they cannot be sensitized with dinitrochlorobenzene. The CMI defects in these patients are associated with increased susceptibility to life-threatening infections by pathogens against which CMI is important, including herpes simplex virus, varicella-zoster virus, *Candida albicans*, and *Pneumocystis carinii*. Other congenital diseases that affect CMI are associated with variable defects in resistance to intracellular pathogens (Table 7). One important clinical corollary in the management of patients suspected or known to have disorders of CMI is the danger associated with their receiving live vaccines such as BCG, vaccinia, measles, rubella, and mumps. The attenuated organisms in these vaccines may disseminate, with fatal consequences in patients with defects in CMI.

Abnormalities of regulatory T cells and T-cell maturation have recently been identified as the possible mechanisms of the immunodeficiency in the common-variable forms of combined immunodeficiency syndrome, DiGeorge syndrome, and acquired agammaglobulinemia.[453] In one study,[453] several disorders of T-cell differentiation occurred in patients with combined immunodeficiency. One subtype of combined immunodeficiency was associated with failure to develop lymphocytes that expressed any thymus-specific antigens; another subtype was associated with failure to differentiate beyond the early prothymocyte–thymocyte stage; a third subtype was associated with failure to differentiate beyond a late thymocyte stage. In contrast, patients with thymic aplasia (DiGeorge syndrome) had a diminished but detectable population of mature T cells. Imbalances in immunoregulatory T cells with a relative excess of suppressor cells were found in approximately half of a group of patients with spontaneously occurring acquired agammaglobulinemia. In one of the latter group, there was an activated suppressor T-cell population that expressed Ia antigens. Another had no inducer (T4) cells. Patients with X-linked agammaglobulinema frequently had an abnormal ratio of inducer to suppressor cells, as well as an absence of circulating surface immunoglobulin-bearing cells. Common variable immunodeficiency is heterogeneous with defects in both cellular and humoral immunity; humoral immune defects may result from B-cell abnormalities or abnormalities in the production of regulatory T-cell lymphokines. Low lytic efficiency of mature NK cells[454] has recently been identified as another facet of immune dysfunction in Chédiak-Higashi syndrome, and defects of secretion of IFN-γ and NK cell activities have been identified in patients with recurrent and unusually severe viral and bacterial infections.[403]

Certain immune deficiency diseases have been associated with a deficiency of particular cellular enzymes. For example, severe combined immunodeficiency disease has been associated with a lack of the enzyme adenosine deaminase. In a patient with severe combined immunodeficiency disease and lack of adenosine deaminase, replacement therapy for the enzyme, using frozen irradiated human red blood cells as a source of adenosine deaminase, restored humoral immunity and CMI.[455] Other examples of defective T-lymphocyte function associated with enzyme deficiencies occurred in patients who lacked purine nucleoside phosphorylase and had abnormal CMI[456] and occurred in two siblings with an autosomally recessive error of pyrimidine metabolism, hereditary orotic aciduria, who had cellular immunodeficiency.[457] A less severe defect in CMI is seen in Down syndrome.[458]

Patients with Chédiak-Higashi syndrome,[454] LCAM deficiency,[459] and chronic granulomatous disease[460] suffer most from severe infection with extracellular bacterial pathogens. However, cytotoxic lymphocyte function is also abnormal in the former two disorders and may explain their greater susceptibility to viral pathogens. Intracellular bacterial pathogens including *Nocardia*, Mycobacteria and *Legionella* also cause serious infections in these patients.[461,469]

Acquired Disorders

Infections. Among the causes of defective CMI that are acquired after birth is infection itself.[462] These infections known to depress DTH skin tests and in vitro lymphocyte transformation to either mitogens or antigens are listed in Table 7; these include infectious mononucleosis and influenza; bacterial infections including tuberculosis, leprosy, bacterial pneumonia, and syphilis; and fungal infections including coccidioidomycosis. Although most studies of the suppression of CMI that occurs during infection have demonstrated defects in response to DTH skin tests and in lymphocyte transformation, data have accumulated that also reveal the presence of acquired defects in monocyte and macrophage function. Suppression of in vitro chemotaxis has been described in monocytes from patients acutely infected with influenza virus. This defect persists for approximately 3 weeks.[463] Suppression of phagocytosis by macrophages from animals infected with viruses is well described.[464] Thus, both lymphocyte and macrophage function may be abnormal during and after acute infections. It is unclear in most cases whether suppression of these in vivo and in vitro correlates of CMI by a given infection results in an increased susceptibility to other organisms or even to the original infecting organism.

Viral infection can inhibit CMI either directly, by infecting lymphocytes and macrophages and thereby altering their function, or indirectly, by altering immune regulatory mechanisms (reviewed in Ref. 465). AIDS is an example of the first mechanism and is discussed fully in Chapter 107. Another example in which viral infection of lymphocytes may be important is measles. Measles virus does this in part by reducing DTH and the response of lymphocytes to mitogens and antigens, as well as by suppression of the number of circulating T lymphocytes by noncytolytic infection, transforming lymphocytes and thereby suppressing lymphocyte transformation and proliferation.[465] Ratios of circulating T-lymphocyte subsets remain normal in measles.[466] The possible clinical relevance of abnormalities in tests of CMI during measles infection is controversial.

Viruses, including influenza, respiratory syncytial virus, and CMV, may inhibit the accessory functions of macrophages for T-cell responses in vitro[465,467–469]; however, results in vivo do

TABLE 6. Congenital Disorders of Cell-Mediated Immunity

	Di George Syndrome[a]	*Nezelof Syndrome*[b]	*Cartilage Hair Hypoplasia*	*Chronic Mucocutaneous Candidiasis*	*Wiskott-Aldrich Syndrome*[c]	*Ataxia Telangiectasia*[d]	*Severe Combined Immunodeficiency Disease (SCID)*	*Adenosine Deaminase Deficiency*[e]	*Purine Nucleoside Phosphorylase Deficiency*[f]	*Chédiak-Higashi Syndrome*[g]	*LCAM Deficiency*[h]	*Chronic Granulomatous Disease of Childhood*[i]
Increased incidence or severity of infections due to												
intracellular bacteria		Yes					Yes	Yes	Yes	Yes	Yes	Yes
Viruses	Yes	Yes	Yes		Yes	Yes	Yes	Yes	Yes	Yes	Yes	
Fungi	Yes	Yes		Yes			Yes	Yes				Yes
Protozoa	Yes	Yes			Yes		Yes	Yes				
Lymphopenia	Yes	Yes	Yes	Variable	Variable	Variable	Yes	Yes	Yes	Yes		
Absent delayed-type hypersensitivity	Yes	Yes	Variable	Variable	Variable	Variable	Yes	Yes	Yes			
Absent lymphocyte transformation to:												
Phytohemagglutinin	Yes	Yes	Variable	Variable	Variable	Variable	Yes	Yes	Yes			
Antigen	Yes	Yes	Yes (Varicella)	Variable	Variable	Variable	Yes	Yes	Yes			

[a] Thymic hypoplasia. Other features include congenital cardiac defects and hypocalcemia.
[b] Autosomal recessive lymphopenia.
[c] Immunodeficiency with thrombocytopenia. Other features include X-linked thrombocytopenia and death in childhood.
[d] Other features include cerebellar ataxia (infancy), cutaneous telangiectasia, sinopulmonary infections, lymphomas, carcinomas, maldevelopment of thymus, ovarian agenesis, increased α-fetoprotein, susceptibility to radiation-induced chromosomal damage.
[e] Other features include symptoms in the first 6 months of life, death in the first year of life, bony abnormalities (cupping of the ribs at the costochondral junctions, abnormal metaphyses, short extremities). Causes one-third of autosoma recessive severe combined immunodeficiency disease. Prenatal diagnosis with amniotic fluid cells. Treatment is bone marrow transplantation or transfusion of normal erythrocytes
[f] Appears normal at birth, but progressive depletion of T lymphocytes occurs between first and second years of life with recurrent infections. Autoimmune hemolytic anemia. It is a rare autosomal recessive trait.
[g] Autosomal inheritance; giant lysosomal granules in leukocytes, melanocytes, Schwann cells, and possibly other tissues; partial oculocutaneous albinism and a lymphoma-like phase with widespread mononuclear cell infiltration. Ascorbic acid, which increases cGMP, is reported to improve a chemotactic defect. There is also defective NK cell function.
[h] Leukocyte cell adhesion molecule deficiency; LCAM are three different molecules composed of a variable α and a common β subunit; the most common defect is autosomal recessive β-chain deficiency, causing deficiency of all three molecules.
[i] More commonly X-linked recessive but also autosomal recessive inheritance, generalized lymphadenopathy, frequent hepatosplenomegaly with granulomas. Inability of monocytes and PMNs to generate superoxide and hydrogen peroxide. Common X-linked form is due to absence of b cytochrome heavy chain.

TABLE 7. Some Infections and Vaccines That May Be Associated with Depressed Delayed-Type Hypersensitivity or CMI

Viral	Bacterial
Human immunodeficiency viruses	Tuberculosis
Measles (and vaccine)	Leprosy
Mumps	Syphilis
Chickenpox	Streptococcal infection
Influenza	Brucellosis
Infectious mononucleosis	Bacterial pneumonia
Yellow fever	Typhoid fever
Rubella vaccine	Other
Measles-mumps-rubella vaccine	Schistosomiasis
Chronic hepatitis B	Toxoplasmosis
Cytomegalovirus infection	Malaria
Fungal	Filiariasis
Coccidioidomycosis	Leishmaniasis
Histoplasmosis	
Blastomycosis	

not always parallel those in vitro, as indicated by the failure of influenza infection to impair induction of the DTH skin test response.[470] Viruses, including influenza virus, may also impair human monocyte migration, phagocytosis, and microbicidal activity[471]; however, the microbicidal activity of human alveolar macrophages is not impaired.[472] Thus, caution is advisable in extrapolation of these variable results to human disease.

Diminished CMI also occurs in patients with infectious mononucleosis due to EBV.[386,403] This virus infects B lymphocytes, which have a specific receptor for the virus, the type 2 complement receptor. Infected B lymphocytes are polyclonally activated to secrete immunoglobulin and are immortalized in vitro; this may account for the development of heterophilic antibodies and autoantibodies in this infection. In vivo cytotoxic/suppressor T8 cells increase in number and act to inhibit infected B cells but may also inhibit other T-cell responses.

In two forms of the X-linked lymphoproliferative syndrome,[403] an accentuation of the T8 response appears to result in fatal infectious mononucleosis or hypogammaglobulinemia. In patients with acute CMV mononucleosis, there are decreased numbers of helper T4 lymphocytes and increased numbers of cytotoxic/suppressor T8 lymphocytes in conjunction with depressed concanavalin A responsiveness, all of which return to normal in convalescence.[473] Parasitic disease as a cause of immunosuppression has recently been reviewed.[474] Immunodepression and alteration of T-cell subsets occur during some *Toxoplasma* infections in humans[475] and in some animal models. A novel mechanism of immunosuppression in malaria is the appearance of cold reactive lymphocytotoxic antibodies.[476]

Malignancies. Malignancies may adversely affect both humoral and cellular immunity (e.g., Hodgkin's disease[477–479]). In patients with Hodgkin's disease, there is lymphopenia, low NK cell activity, depressed DTH, decreased ability to be sensitized to dinitrochlorobenzene, and diminished in vitro lymphocyte transformation to antigens and mitogens and in mixed lymphocyte culture. Depressed lymphocyte function due to Hodgkin's disease has been attributed variously to serum factors,[477] to an adherent mononuclear cell population,[478] to a prostaglandin-producing adherent suppressor cell, and to suppressor T lymphocytes.[479] Lymphocyte responsiveness has been restored by incubating T lymphocytes in fetal calf serum and levamisole, demonstrating that the alteration of T lymphocytes is reversible. Another in vitro correlate of CMI, production of chemotactic factor, is normal in Hodgkin's disease even when responsiveness to mitogens is abnormal. High levels of a naturally occurring chemotactic factor inactivator have been detected in the sera of patients with Hodgkin's disease, which may result in a generalized defect in the ability to mobilize inflammatory cells in these patients. The abnormalities in CMI described above are associated with an increased susceptibility of patients with Hodgkin's disease to a variety of intracellular pathogens.

Although defects in cellular immunity have been clearly established in patients with Hodgkin's disease and certain other lymphomas, they are less well described in other malignancies, and results of testing CMI in many such patients have been reported to be normal. Some patients with advanced neoplasms (e.g., those with squamous cell carcinoma of the head and neck, intracranial tumors, and melanoma) have depressed DTH and/or mitogen-stimulated lymphocyte transformation. In some reports that describe cancer patients, washing lymphocytes has improved lymphocyte responsiveness, suggesting the presence of an elutable inhibitor factor. In addition, monocyte function has been reported to be suppressed in patients with malignancy. In animal models and/or in vitro, tumor cells and/or their products have been reported to block accumulation of macrophages in vivo, inhibit development of macrophage activation, reduce release of lytic substances from macrophages or inhibit injurious effects of these mediators once they have been released, and suppress macrophage anti-microbial activity against *Leishmania* and *Toxoplasma* in conjunction with suppression of oxidative mechanisms.[480]

Pharmacologic Agents and Radiation. CYTOTOXIC AGENTS, CORTICOSTEROIDS, AND RADIATION. Cytotoxic drugs and corticosteroids may have profound effects on CMI.[481–483] Two chemotherapeutic drugs that are highly immunosuppressive, cyclophosphamide and methotrexate, differ both qualitatively and quantitatively in their effects on the immune system and will be used here as examples. Cyclophosphamide is a cycle-specific agent that is toxic to cells in either proliferating or resting stages but has a preferential effect on proliferating cells. Cyclophosphamide inhibits T-lymphocyte proliferation and production of many lymphokines and depletes the intermitotic circulating T-lymphocyte pool, thereby decreasing the number of previously committed lymphocytes as well as those available for sensitization.

Methotrexate is a phase-specific drug that acts primarily on dividing cells. If the drug is administered for 7 days after an animal is exposed to a new antigen, suppression of DTH and antigen-specific lymphocyte transformation occurs; if it is administered before or after the 7-day induction period, no effect on CMI function is seen. Therefore, methotrexate usually will not affect the CMI response to an antigen when sensitization has already been established.

Administration of corticosteroids results in lymphopenia and the shrinkage of organs of the reticuloendothelial system in certain animals. However, there are large differences among different species of animals with regard to susceptibility of the immune system to corticosteroids; the principal effect of administration of the drug in humans is to cause transient lymphopenia by redistribution of lymphocytes.[481] Corticosteroids decrease expression of DTH. The production of most cytokines by lymphocytes and mononuclear phagocytes is inhibited.[484] The effects of cytokines on target cells also may be blocked[485]; however, this varies since corticosteroids do not block IFN-γ-induced activity of human macrophages against *Listeria* but do block IFN-γ-induced activity against *Nocardia* and *Salmonella*. Target cells may be protected from direct cytotoxicity by T lymphocytes without directly affecting the T lymphocytes themselves. Corticosteroids cause monocytopenia, decreased clearance of particulate material, and decreased bactericidal and fungicidal activity of monocytes in vitro.

In animals, increased susceptibility to infection, as well as increased risk of reactivation of latent infections, can result from administration of corticosteroids.[482] Although this is also true in humans, the incidence of infection depends largely on the underlying disease for which the corticosteroids are being administered.

Cytotoxic agents and corticosteroids are frequently administered in combination, and it is the total effect of all the drugs in this combination that dictates the degree and nature of immunosuppression. Studies with combinations of these drugs in the treatment of malignancy in humans show that immunosuppression occurs during therapy but that immunologic competence may return after therapy. In some cases (e.g., patients who have received combined-modality therapy for Hodgkin's disease and who have depressed responses to vaccines many years after completion of therapy), either the underlying diseases or the therapy continues to cause depressed immune function. Continuous therapy has longer, more profound effects than intermittent therapy.[483]

As would be expected from the above, when immunosuppressive agents are given before or simultaneously with experimental infections, CMI fails to develop and mortality frequently increases. Numerous experimental infections produced by intracellular pathogens are exacerbated by immunosuppressive agents. In humans, there is evidence of increased susceptibility to infection with the use of cytotoxic drugs. Transplant recipients who receive immunosuppressive drugs to prevent tissue rejection have a striking susceptibility to opportunistic infections, although the incidence of such infections has decreased with the change to a less immunosuppressive regimen that includes cyclosporin A (see below under "Other Pharmacologic Agents"[486]). In children with acute lymphocytic leukemia, the incidence of *P. carinii* pneumonia increases when the number of cytotoxic agents used to combat the leukemia is increased. In addition, in patients with herpes zoster and stage 3 or 4 lymphoma, a randomized trial revealed that treatment with cytosine arabinoside increased the time for resolution of zoster lesions. The antiviral effects of the drug were apparently less important than its immunosuppressive effect.

Radiation therapy also predisposes the patient to infections by affecting proliferating and nonproliferating lymphoid cell populations and consequently depressing CMI. In animals, suppression of established DTH and interference with initial sensitization of lymphocytes occur as a result of irradiation. The combination of radiation and drugs such as cortisone and nitrogen mustard more frequently resulted in relapse of latent infection with *Toxoplasma* in hamsters than radiation or drugs alone.[482] Extrapolation of these findings to humans is difficult because of the differences in the doses of radiation given to humans and to experimental animals and because of the deficiencies in CMI secondary to the underlying disease process in humans for which the radiation is being administered.

ANTIMICROBIAL AGENTS. Certain antimicrobial agents are associated with abnormalities of CMI.[487,488] The meaning, clinical relevance, and significance of the changes observed are not yet clear. Results have been conflicting, and few controlled clinical studies have been carried out to determine the effect of antibiotics on the immune response in humans. There is a need for better understanding of the influence of antibiotics on the immune response. This is especially important for patients who receive antibiotic therapy for prolonged periods and for immunosuppressed patients.

OTHER PHARMACOLOGIC AGENTS. Cyclosporin A is used to suppress allograft rejection and alters helper T cells, effector T cells, and NK cells.[489] It is a fungal metabolite of *Trichoderma polysporum* and is a cyclic polypeptide containing 11 amino acids. It is an effective immunosuppressant with low myelotoxicity and has been used successfully as the primary drug to suppress the rejection of transplants of nonmatched cadaver kidneys, as well as heart, lung, bone marrow, and liver transplants. It prevents the response of T lymphocytes to alloantigens and certain mitogens. The synthesis of IL-2, the expression of receptors for IL-2 on the cell membrane, and the response to IL-2 are inhibited by cyclosporin A. These effects appear to reflect inhibition of calcium-dependent T-cell activation pathways.[490] Interferon -γ and IL-3 but not GM-CSF production is also inhibited.[491] Allograft recipients treated with cyclosporin A rather than with the more cytotoxic regimens used formerly have less pronounced immunodepression and a reduced incidence of opportunistic infections.[486] It is of interest that cyclosporin A also has antimicrobial effects against malaria, schistosomes, and *Toxoplasma*. Whether this has any effect on the patterns of opportunistic infections that allograft recipients acquire remains to be determined.

Other Disorders. In addition to those factors discussed above, leukocytosis, anemia, and fever depress DTH skin responses. Autoantibodies may alter CMI (e.g., a patient with acquired agammaglobulinemia had an autoantibody to T4 cells and subsequently to T8 cells). Uremia,[492] diabetes mellitus,[493] surgery and anesthesia,[494] sarcoidosis,[495] cystic fibrosis,[496] and prolonged but not brief zinc deficiency[497] have also been reported to be associated with depressed CMI. Anergy, zinc deficiency, and decreased nucleoside phosphorylase activity have been found in patients with sickle cell anemia.[498]

Nutritional status has a profound effect on immune function.[499–501] Chronic protein-calorie malnutrition exerts a suppressive effect on functions of T lymphocytes (e.g., DTH reactions, lymphocyte proliferative responses to mitogens and antigens, and T-cell-dependent antibody responses are all decreased by protein-calorie malnutrition) and to a lesser extent on macrophage function. Depressed T-lymphocyte function has also been documented in deficiencies of trace elements such as copper (as well as zinc; see above) and certain vitamins, such as thiamine and folate. Replacement of deficient nutritional components results in restoration of immune function.

An increasing body of data indicates that the nervous and immune systems interact. As described above, immune cytokines act on the central nervous system to induce fever, sleep, and changes in alertness. Reciprocally, neural transmitters released in response to stress may alter CMI. Norepinephrine and epinephrine block induction by IFN-γ of mouse macrophage activity against herpes simplex virus-infected cells, an effect apparently mediated by increased intracellular cyclic AMP.[502] Cyclic AMP negatively regulates many aspects of CMI, including IL-2 production[503]; thus, adrenergic agents may have more general down-modulating effects on CMI. Deficiency of prolactin, secretion of which is induced by stress and other neuroactive compounds, appears to impair CMI and resistance to the intracellular pathogen *L. monocytogenes* in mice[504]; a major mechanism appears to be impaired IFN-γ production and as a consequence, impaired macrophage activation. Certain opioid peptides enhance IFN-γ production by human mononuclear cells.[505] Another example of neuroregulation of the immune response is the stimulation by IL-1 of adrenocorticotrophic hormone (ACTH) and glucocorticoid release,[166,167] which act to inhibit IL-1 production.[506]

Patients with autoimmune disorders have variable deficiencies of CMI. Interferon-γ production by the cells of patients with systemic lupus erythematosus, rheumatoid arthritis and connective tissue disease, and psoriasis is diminished.[4] CMI in these patients may be further impaired by treatment.

Certain types of infections (e.g., with cytomegalovirus or fungi) appear to occur most frequently at identifiable intervals following bone marrow transplantation, which in part reflects immunosuppressive therapy and in part the development of a graft vs. host (GvH) reaction. In the first phase of GvH disease, recognition of allogeneic MHC antigens activates a potent suppressive signal that rapidly abrogates immunity. The number of helper T4 cells decreases, and the number of regulatory macrophages increases.[507] Acutely, there is a lack of suppressor T-cell activity that leads to increased levels of serum IgE. In the second phase, macrophage production of PGE_2 increases, and later this terminates. In the third phase there is destruction of thymic medullary epithelium, disruption of T-cell maturation, functional defects in B-cell maturation, neutrophil development, chemotaxis, formation of autoantibodies, and more frequently, development of neoplasia (e.g., B-cell lymphomas and mammary carcinomas[507]).

TABLE 8. Evaluation of the Capacity for Immune Response[a]

History
- Increased frequency and severity of infections
- Abnormal responses to live vaccines (e.g., vaccinia)
- Frequent infections with less common pathogens (e.g., fungi)
- Recurrent diarrhea
- Family history of increased susceptibility to infection
- Sexual preference
- Intravenous drug abuse
- Blood product transfusions

Physical examination
- Signs of chronic infection
- Absence of lymphoid tissue
- Signs associated with specific immunodeficiency disorders (see Chapter 9)

Laboratory

I. Preliminary screen[a]
  - A. Complete blood cell count with differential smear
  - B. Quantitative immunoglobulin levels

II. Readily available studies
  - A. B-cell function
    1. Natural or commonly acquired antibodies: isohemagglutinins, "febrile" agglutinins, antibodies to common viruses (rubella, rubeola, influenza), and toxins (diphtheria, tetanus)
    2. Response to immunization (typhoid, polio, diphtheria-tetanus vaccines)
    3. Determination of total B cells by immunofluorescence
  - B. T-cell function
    1. Skin tests (PPD, *Candidin, Trichophyton*, streptokinase-streptodornase), tetanus toxoid (1:100 dilution)
    2. Chest x-ray film (thymus shadow in infants, thymoma in adults)
    3. T-cell subsets CD4, CD8 by immunofluorescence
  - C. Complement
    1. C3
    2. CH_{50} (total hemolytic complement)
  - D. Phagocyte function
    1. Reduction of nitroblue tetrazolium
    2. Inflammatory skin window (Rebuck)
    3. LCAM expression by immunofluorescence
    4. Class II HLA expression on monocytes
  - E. Infectious agents causing immunodeficiency
    1. Antibodies to HIV-1, HIV-2, Epstein-Barr virus (isolation of virus also at reference laboratories)

III. In-depth investigation
  - A. B cell
    1. Pre-B-cell examination in bone marrow samples
    2. B-lymphocyte membrane markers: IgM, IgD, IgG, IgA; receptors for aggregated IgG (Fc receptor), C3; antigens detected by anti-B antibodies
    3. Induction of B-lymphocyte differentiation in vitro stimulated by pokeweed mitogen, Epstein-Barr virus, or other polyclonal B-cell activators
    4. Kinetics and immunoglobulin class of antibody produced in response to specific primary and secondary immunization
    5. Measurement of IgG subclasses and κ:λ ratio
    6. Histologic and immunofluorescent examination of biopsy specimens (intestinal mucosa, lymph node, bone marrow)
  - B. T cell
    1. Surface markers for T-helper subsets: 4B4, 2H4
    2. In vitro correlates of delayed hypersensitivity
       - a. Proliferative response to mitogens; phytohemagglutinin, ConA, specific antigens (purified protein derivative, *Candida*, tetanus); allogeneic cells (one-way mixed lymphocyte response)
       - b. Quantification of lymphokines (interferon, IL-2, etc.) or lymphokine mRNA
       - c. Induction of killer cells by stimulation with allogeneic lymphocytes
    3. Measurement of thymus hormones
    4. Assays for T-cell helper function using supernatants of antigen-activated T cells or T cells plus pokeweed mitogen or antigens to trigger B-lymphocyte differentiation
    5. Skin graft rejection
  - C. Phagocytes and complement
    1. Chemotactic response in vitro
    2. Bactericidal function
    3. Classic and alternative pathway complement components
  - D. Natural killer cells
    1. Enumeration with monoclonal antibodies
    2. Functional assay using appropriate target cells
  - E. Miscellaneous
    1. Lymphocytotoxic antibodies
    2. Measurement of adenosine deaminase and purine nucleoside phosphorylase enzyme activities

[a] Analyses of complement, B, T, and phagocytic cells are included because of interrelated syndromes.

(Adapted from Cooper and Lawton,[508] with permission.)

Evaluation of the Patient with Suspected Deficiency of CMI

Immunodeficiency syndromes—congenital, spontaneously acquired, or iatrogenic—are characterized by unusual susceptibility to infection. Autoimmune disease and lymphoreticular malignancies sometimes occur. The types of infection often provide an early clue to the immunologic defect. T-cell deficiency is almost always accompanied by some abnormality of antibody responses. Since many antibody responses require T-cell help, this may explain in part why patients with primary T-cell defects also develop overwhelming infection with bacterial species against which antibody plays a major role in resistance. An outline of important considerations in the evaluation of patients with suspected defects in CMI is presented in Table 8.[508] It is important to obtain a careful history and to perform a thorough physical examination, as these may indicate whether the antibody–complement–phagocyte system or CMI is defective. A normal response to smallpox vaccination or contact dermatitis due to poison ivy suggests intact cellular immunity. Lymphopenia, absence of palpable lymph nodes or diffuse lymphoid hyperplasia, and signs of specific infections are relevant.

Since at least 80 percent of the population have been sensitized to one of the following—*Candida, Trichophyton*, streptokinase-streptodornase, or purified protein derivative (PPD)—using these antigens for skin tests to elicit DTH is useful in evaluation of CMI. A positive skin test indicates prior sensitization of helper T cells to antigens of the organism. Absence of skin reactivity to these antigen indicates either a defect in CMI, failure to properly inject the antigen intradermally, or a defect in the ability of the patient to develop a nonspecific inflammatory skin response. (The last defect can be tested by placing irritating substances such as benzalkonium chloride on the skin.) For skin testing, an initial evaluation should be made at 2–6 hours after injection of the antigen for immediate hypersensitivity reactions that are not due to CMI and may result in false-positive readings 24–48 hours later.

Basic in vitro tests of CMI are becoming more widely available since the onset of the AIDS epidemic. These include determination of T-cell subsets (T4 and T8), B-cell and NK-cell number, expression of class II HLA antigens, and proliferative responses to mitogens. Tests commonly performed by research or reference laboratories for in-depth investigation are also indicated in Table 8. In certain conditions associated with defects in CMI, there may be a negative correlation between the DTH response in vivo and results of in vitro correlates of DTH (e.g., in mucocutaneous candidiasis, the candidin skin test may be negative in a patient whose lymphocytes transform to candidin antigen in vitro).

ACKNOWLEDGMENT

This chapter was supported in part by grants from the National Institutes of Health.

REFERENCES

1. Hahn H, Kaufmann SHE. The role of cell-mediated immunity in bacterial infections. Rev Infect Dis. 1981;3:1221–50.
2. Blanden RV. Mechanisms of recovery from a generalized viral infection: Mouse-pox-I. The effects of anti-thymocyte serum. J Exp Med. 1970; 132:1035–50.
3. Ruskin J, McIntosh J, Remington JS. Studies on the mechanisms of resistance to phylogenetically diverse intracellular organisms. J Immunol. 1969;103:252–9.
4. Murray HW. Interferon-gamma, the activated macrophage, and the host defense against microbial challenge. Ann Intern Med. 1988;108:595–608.
5. Royer HD, Reinherz EL. T lymphocytes: Ontogeny, function, and relevance to clinical disorders. N Engl J Med. 1987;317:1136–42.
6. Fauci AS. The human immunodeficiency virus: Infectivity and mechanisms of pathogenesis. Science. 1988;239:617.
7. Kronenberg M, Siu G, Hood LE, et al. The molecular genetics of the T-cell

antigen receptor and T-cell antigen recognition. Ann Rev Immunol. 1986;4:529–91.
8. Swain SL. T-cell subsets and the recognition of MHC class. Immunol Rev. 1983;74:129.
9. Fleischer B, Schrezenmeier H, Wagner H. Function of the CD4 and CD8 molecules on human cytotoxic T lymphocytes: Regulation of T cell triggering. J Immunol. 1986;136:1625–8.
10. Schwartz RH. T-lymphocyte recognition of antigen in association with gene products of the major histocompatibility complex. Ann Rev Immunol. 1985;3:237–61.
11. Davis MM, Bjorkman PJ. T cell antigen receptor genes and T cell recognition. Nature. 1988;334:395–402.
12. Fitch FW. T-cell clones and T-cell receptors. Microbiol Rev. 1986;50:50–69.
13. Elliott JF, Rock EP, Patten PA, et al. The adult T-cell receptor δ-chain is diverse and distinct from that of fetal thymocytes. Nature. 1988;331:627–31.
14. Yancopoulous GD, Blackwell TK, Heikyung S, et al. Introduced T cell receptor variable region gene segments recombine in pre-B cells: Evidence that T and B cells use a common recombinase. Cell. 1986;44:251–9.
15. Dembic Z, Haas W, Weiss S, et al. Transfer of specificity by murine alpha and beta T-cell receptor genes. Nature. 1986;320:232–8.
16. Gabert J, Langlet C, Zamoyska R, et al. Reconstitution of MHC Class I specificity by transfer of the T cell receptor and Lyt-2 genes. Cell. 1987;50:545–54.
17. Clevers H, Alarcon B, Wileman T, et al. The T cell receptor/CD3 complex: A dynamic protein ensemble. Ann Rev. Immunol. 1988;6:629–62.
18. Wilson RK, Lai E, Concannon P, et al. Structure, organization and polymorphism of murine and human T-cell receptor alpha and beta chain gene families. Immunol Rev. 1988;101:149–72.
19. Gefter M, Marrack P. Development and modification of the lymphocyte repertoire. Nature. 1986;321:116–8.
20. Garman RD, Ko JL, Vulpe CD, et al. T-cell receptor variable region gene usage in T-cell populations. Proc Natl Acad Sci USA. 1986;83:3987–91.
21. Rupp F, Acha-Obeo H, Hengartner H, et al. Identical Vβ T-cell receptor genes used in alloreactive cytotoxic and antigen plus I-A specific helper T cells. Nature. 1985;315:425–7.
22. Epplen JT, Bartels F, Becker A, et al. Change in antigen specificity of cytotoxic T lymphocytes is associated with the rearrangement and expression of a T-cell receptor beta-chain gene. Proc Natl Acad Sci USA. 1986;83:4441–5.
23. Hedrick SM, Engel I, McElligott DL, et al. Selection of amino acid sequences in the beta chain of the T cell antigen receptor. Science. 1988;239:1541–4.
24. Maddon MJ, Littman DR, Godfrey M, et al. The isolation and nucleotide sequence of a cDNA encoding the T cell surface protein T4: A new member of the immunoglobulin gene family. Cell. 1985;42:93–104.
25. Littman DR, Thomas Y, Maddon PJ, et al. The isolation and sequence of the gene encoding T8: A molecule defining functional classes of T lymphocytes. Cell. 1985;40:237–46.
26. William AF, Barclay AN. The immunoglbulin superfamily—domains for cell surface recognition. Ann Rev Immunol. 1988;6:381–405.
27. Gay D, Maddon P, Sekaly R, et al. Functional interaction between human T-cell protein CD4 and the major histocompatibility complex HLA-DR antigen. Nature. 1987;328:626–9.
28. Shaw S, Ginther GE. The lymphocyte function-associated antigen (LFA)-1 and CD2/LFA-3 pathways of antigen-independent human T cell adhesion. J Immunol. 1987;139:1037–45.
29. Peterson A, Seed B. Monoclonal antibody and ligand binding sites of the T cell erythrocyte receptor (CD2). Nature. 1987;329:842–6.
30. Sewell WA, Brown MH, Dunne J. Molecular cloning of the human T-lymphocyte surface CD2 (T11) antigen. Proc Natl Acad Sci USA. 1986;83:8718–22.
31. Wallner BP, Frey AZ, Tizard R, et al. Primary structure of lymphocyte function-associated antigen 3 (LFA-3). The ligand of the T lymphocyte CD2 glycoprotein. J Exp Med. 1987;166:923–32.
32. Yang SY, Chouaib S, Dupont B. A common pathway for T lymphocyte activation involving both the CD3-Ti complex and CD2 sheep erythrocyte receptor determinants. J Immunol. 1986;137:1097–1100.
33. Fox DA, Scholossman SF, Reinherz EL. Regulation of the alternative pathway of T cell activation by anti-T3 monoclonal antibody. J Immunol. 1986;136:1945–50.
34. June CH, Rabinovitch PS, Ledbetter JA. CD5 antibodies increase intracellular ionized calcium concentration in T cells. J Immunol. 1987;138:2782–92.
35. Martin PJ, Ledbetter JA, Morishita Y, et al. A 44 kilodalton cell surface homodimer regulates interleukin 2 production by activated human T lymphocytes. J Immunol. 1986;136:3282–7.
36. Springer TA, Teplow DB, Dreyer WJ. Sequence homology of the LFA-1 and Mac-1 leukocyte adhesion glycoproteins and unexpected relation to leukocyte interferon. Nature. 1985;314:540–2.
37. Bierer BE, Mentzer SJ, Greenstein JL, et al. Year Immunol. 1986:39–59.
38. Blanchard D, van Els C, Borst J, et al. The role of the T cell receptor, CD8, and LFA-1 in different stages of the cytolytic reaction mediated by alloreactive T lymphocyte clones. J Immunol. 1987;138:2417–21.
39. Fowlkes BJ, Mathieson BJ. Intrathymic differentiation: Thymocyte heterogeneity and the characterization of early T-cell precursors. Surv Immunol Res. 1985;4:96–109.
40. Rothenberg E, Lugo JP. Differentiation and cell division in the mammalian thymus. Dev Biol. 1985;112:1–17.
41. Haynes BF. The human thymic microenvironment. Adv Immunol. 1984; 36:87–142.
42. Lobach DF, Hensley LL, Ho W, et al. Human T cell antigen expression during the early stages of fetal thymic maturation. J Immunol. 1985;135:1752–9.
43. Gallatin M, St. John TP, Siegelman M. Lymphocyte homing receptors. Cell. 1986;44:673–80.
44. Kisielow P, Leiserson W, von Boehmer H. Differentiation of thymocytes in fetal organ culture: Analysis of phenotypic changes accompanying the appearance of cytolytic and interleukin 2-producing cells. J Immunol. 1984;133:1117–23.
45. Kingston R, Jenkinson EJ, Owen JJT. A single stem cell can recolonize an embryonic thymus, producing phenotypically distinct T-cell populations. Nature. 1985;317:811–3.
46. Blue ML, Daley JF, Levine H, et al. Class II major histocompatibility complex molecules regulate the development of the $T4^{+}T8^{-}$ inducer phenotype of cultured human thymocytes. Proc Natl Acad Sci USA. 1985;82:8178–82.
47. Marusic-Galesic S, Stephany DA, Longo DL, et al. Development of $CD4^{-}CD8^{+}$ cytotoxic T cells requires interactions with class I MHC determinants. Nature. 1988;333:180–3.
48. Brenner MB, McLean J, Scheft H, et al. Two forms of the T-cell receptor gamma protein found on peripheral blood cytotoxic T lymphocytes. Nature. 1987;325:6898.
49. Brenner MB, McLean J, Dialynas DP, et al. Identification of a putative second T-cell receptor. Nature. 1986;322:145–9.
50. Bank I, DePinho RA, Brenner MB, et al. A functional T3 molecule associated with a novel heterodimer on the surface of immature human thymocytes. Nature. 1986;322:179–81.
51. Weiss A, Newton M, Crommie D. Expression of T3 in association with a molecule distinct from the T-cell antigen receptor heterodimer. Proc Natl Acad Sci USA. 1986;83:6998–7002.
52. Borst J, van Dongen JJM, Bolhuis RLH, et al. Distinct molecular forms of human T cell receptor γ/δ detected on viable T cells by a monoclonal antibody. J Exp Med. 1988;167:1625–44.
53. Lanier LL, Ruitenberg JJ, Phillips JH. Human $CD3^{+}$ T lymphocytes that express neither CD4 nor CD8 antigens. J Exp Med. 1986;164:339–44.
54. Roehm N, Herron L, Cambier J. The major histocompatibility complex-restricted antigen receptor on T cells: Distribution on thymus and peripheral T cells. Cell. 1984;38:577–84.
55. Lugo JP, Krishnan SN, Sailor RD, et al. Early precursor thymocytes can produce interleukin 2 upon stimulation with calcium ionophore and phorbol ester. Proc Natl Acad Sci USA. 1986;83:1862–6.
56. Kappler JW, Roehm N, Marrack P. T cell tolerance by clonal elimination in the thymus. Cell. 1987;49:273–80.
57. MacDonald HR, Schneider R, Lees RK, et al. T-cell receptor Vβ use predicts reactivity and tolerance to Mls^{a}-encoded antigens. Nature. 1988;332:40–45.
58. Kappler JW, Staerz U, White J, et al. Self-tolerance eliminates T cells specific for Mls-modified products of the major histocompatibility complex. Nature. 1988;332:35–40.
59. Robertson M. Tolerance, restriction and the Mls enigma. Nature. 1988;332:18–9.
60. Hocking WG, Golde DW. The pulmonary–alveolar macrophage. N Engl J Med. 1979;301:580–646.
61. Bitterman PB, Saltzman LE, Adelberg S, et al. Alveolar macrophage replication. One mechanism for the expansion of the mononuclear phagocyte population in the chronically inflamed lung. J Clin Invest. 1984;74:460–9.
62. Nichols BA, Bainton DF, Farquhar MG. Differentiation of monocytes. J Cell Biol. 1984;50:498–515.
63. Keleman E, Janossa M. Macrophages are the first differentiated blood cells formed in human embryonic liver. Exp Hematol. 1980;8:996–1000.
64. Brooks CF, Moore M. Differential MHC class II expression on human peripheral blood monocytes and dendritic cells. Immunology. 1988;63:303–11.
65. Wolff K, Stingl G. The Langerhans cell. J Invest Dermatol. 1983;80:17s–21s.
66. Braathen LR, Bjercke S, Thorsby E. The antigen-presenting function of human Langerhans cells. Immunobiology. 1984;168:301–12.
67. Jaffe R. Pathology of histiocytosis X. Perspect Pediatr Pathol. 1987;9:4–47.
68. Favara BE, McCarthy RC, Mierau GW. Histiocytosis X. Hum Pathol. 1983;14:663–76.
69. McDevitt HO. Regulation of the immune response by the major histocompatibility system. N Engl J Med. 1980;303:1514.
70. Srivastava R, Duceman BW, Biro PA, et al. Molecular organization of the class I genes of human major histocompatibility complex. Immunol Rev. 1985;84:93–120.
71. Bell JI, Denny DW, McDevitt HO. Structure and polymorphism of murine and human class II major histocompatibility antigens. Immunol Rev. 1985;84:52–70.
72. Lee JS, Cohen EB, Hume CR, et al. Organization, polymorphism, and regulation of class II genes of the major histocompatibility complex. Year Immunol. 1986;2:205–21.
73. Bjorkman PJ, Saper MA, Samraoui B, et al. The foreign antigen binding site and T cell recognition regions of class I histocompatibility antigens. Nature. 1987;329:512.

74. Brown JH, Jardetzky T, Saper MA, et al. A hypothetical model of the foreign antigen binding site of class II histocompatibility molecules. Nature. 1988;332:845–50.
75. Glover DM, Brownstein D, Burchett SK, et al. Expression of HLA class II antigens and secretion of interleukin 1 by monocytes and macrophages from adults and neonates. Immunology. 1987;61:195–201.
76. Eckels DD, Lake P, Lamb JR, et al. SB-restricted presentation of influenza and herpes simplex virus antigens to human T-lymphocyte clones. Nature. 1983;301:716–8.
77. Brown MA, Glimcher LA, Nielsen EA, et al. T-cell recognition of Ia molecules selectively altered by a single amino acid substitution. Science 1986;231:255–8.
78. Lyons CR, Ball EJ, Toews GB, et al. Inability of human alveolar macrophages to stimulate resting T cells correlates with decreased antigen-specific T cell macrophage binding. J Immunol. 1986;137:1173–80.
79. Sarvetnick N, Liggitt D, Pitts SL, et al. Insulin-dependent diabetes mellitus induced in transgenic mice by ectopic expression of class II MHC and interferon-gamma. Cell. 1988;52:773–82.
80. Morimoto C, Letvin NL, Distaso JA, et al. The isolation and characterization of the human suppressor inducer T cell subset. J Immunol. 1985;134:1508–15.
81. Morimoto C, Letvin NL, Rudd CE, et al. The role of the 2H4 molecule in the generation of suppressor function in Con A-activated T cells. J Immunol. 1986;137:3247–53.
82. Morimoto C, Letvin NL, Boyd AW, et al. The isolation and characterization of the human helper inducer T cell subset. J Immunol. 1985;134:3762–9.
83. Rudd CE, Morimoto C, Wong LL, et al. The subdivision of the T4 (CD4) subset on the basis of the differential expression of L-C/T200 antigens. J Exp Med. 1987;166:1758–73.
84. Grey HM, Chesnut R. Antigen processing and presentation to T cells. Immunol Today. 1985;6:101–6.
85. Chesnut RW, Grey HM. Antigen presentation by B cells and its significance in T–B interactions. Adv Immunol. 1986;236:3951–94.
86. Unanue ER, Allen PM. The basis for the immunoregulatory role of macrophages and other accessory cells. Science. 1987;236:551–7.
87. Fox BS, Quill H, Carlson L, et al. Quantitative analysis of the T cell response to antigen and planar membranes containing purified Ia molecules. J Immunol. 1987;138:3367–74.
88. Allen PM. Antigen processing at the molecular level. Immunol Today. 1987;8:270–3.
89. Rothbard JB, Taylor WR. A sequence pattern common to T cell epitopes. EMBO J. 1988;7:93–100.
90. Cresswell P. Antigen recognition by T lymphocytes. Immunol Today. 1987;8:67–9.
91. Buus S, Sette A, Colon SM, et al. The relation between major histocompatibility complex (MHC) restriction and the capacity of Ia to bind immunogenic peptides. Science. 1987;235:1353–8.
92. Berzofsky JA. Structural features of protein antigenic sites recognized by helper T cells: What makes a site immunodominant? Year Immunol. 1986;2:28–38.
93. Rothbard JB, Lechler RI, Hoiwland, K, et al. Structural model of HLA-DR1 restricted T cell antigen recognition. Cell. 1988;52:515–23.
94. Buus S, Sette A, Colon SM, et al. Isolation and characterization of antigen–Ia complexes involved in T cell recognition. Cell. 1986;47:1071–7.
95. Rouse BT, Norley S, Martin S. Antiviral cytotoxic T lymphocyte induction and vaccination. Rev Infect Dis. 1988;10:16–33.
96. Yewdell JW, Bennink JR, Hosaka Y. Cells process exogenous proteins for recognition by cytotoxic T lymphocytes. Science. 1988;239:637–40.
97. Maryanski JL, Pala P, Corradin G, et al. H-2-restricted cytolytic T cells specific for HLA can recognize a synthetic HLA peptide. Nature. 1986;324:578–9.
98. Wraith DC. The recognition of influenza A virus-infected cells by cytotoxic T lymphocytes. Immunol Today. 1987;8:239–45
99. Walker BD, Flexner C, Paradis TJ. HIV-1 reverse transcriptase is a target for cytotoxic T lymphocytes in infected individuals. Science. 1988;240:64–6.
100. Bjorkamn PJ, Sasper MA, Samraoui B, et al. Structure of the human class I histocompatibility antigen, HLA-A2. Nature. 1987;329:506–16.
101. Weiss A, Imboden J, Hardy K, et al. The role of the T3/antigen receptor complex in T-cell activation. Ann Rev Immunol. 1986;4:593–619.
102. MacDonald HR. T-cell activation. Ann Rev Cell Biol. 1986;2:231–53.
103. Imboden JB, Weiss A, Stobo JD. The antigen receptor on a human T cell line initiates activation by increasing cytoplasmic free calcium. J Immunol. 1985;134:663–5.
104. Manger B, Weiss A, Imboden J, et al. The role of protein kinase C in transmembrane signaling by the T cell antigen–receptor complex. J Immunol. 1987;139:2755–60.
105. Utsunomiya N, Tsuboi M, Nakanishi M. Early transmembrane events in alloimmune cytotoxic T-lymphocyte activation as revealed by stopped-flow fluorometry. Proc Natl Acad Sci USA. 1986;83:1877–80.
106. Nisbet-Brown E, Cheung RK, Lee JWW, et al. Antigen-dependent increase in cytosolic free calcium in specific human T-lymphocyte clones. Nature. 1985;316:545–7.
107. Rosoff PM, Burakoff SJ, Greenstein JL. The role of the L3T4 molecule in mitogen- and antigen-activated signal transduction. Cell. 1987;49:845–53.
108. Takada S, Engleman EG. Evidence for an association between CD8 molecules and the T cell receptor complex on cytotoxic T cells. J Immunol. 1987;139:3231–5.
109. Leo O, Foo M, Henkart PA, et al. Role of accessory molecules in signal transduction of cytolytic T lymphocyte by anti-T cell receptor and anti-Ly-6.2C monoclonal antibodies. J Immunol. 1987;139:3556–63.
110. Siliciano RF, Pratt JC, Schmidt RE, et al. Activation of cytolytic T lymphocyte and natural killer cell function through the T11 sheep erythrocyte binding protein. Nature 1985;317:428–30.
111. Smith KA. Interleukin 2. Ann Rev Immunol. 1984;2:319–33.
112. Hu-Li J, Shevach EM, Mizuguchi J, et al. B cell stimulatory factor I (interleukin 4) is a potent costimulant for normal resting T lymphocytes. J Exp Med. 1987;165:157–72.
113. Spits H, Yssel H, Takebe Y, et al. Recombinant interleukin 4 promotes the growth of human T cells. J Immunol. 1987;139:1142–7.
114. Beutler B, Cerami A. Cachectin and tumour necrosis factor as two sides of the same biological coin. Nature. 1986;320:584–8.
115. Beutler B, Cerami A. Cachectin: More than a tumor necrosis factor. N Engl J Med. 1987;316:379–85.
116. Dinarello CA, Mier JW. Lymphokines. N Engl J Med. 1987;317:940–5.
117. Dinarello CA. Biology of interleukin 1. FASEB J. 1988;2:108–15.
118. March CJ, Mosley B, Larsen A, et al. Cloning, sequence and expression of two distinct human interleukin-1 complementary DNAs. Nature. 1985; 315:641–7.
119. Bird TA, Saklatvala J. Identification of a common class of high affinity receptors for both types of porcine interleukin-1 on connective tissue cells. Nature. 1986;324:263–6.
120. Dower SK, Kronheim SR, Hopp TP, et al. The cell surface receptors for interleukin-1α and interleukin-β are identical. Nature. 1986;324:266–8.
121. Gray PW, Aggarwal BB, Benton CV, et al. Cloning and expression of cDNA for human lymphotoxin, a lymphokine and tumour necrosis activity. Nature. 1984;312:721–4.
122. Pennica D, Nedwin GE, Hayflick JS, et al. Human tumour necrosis factor: Precursor structure, expression and homology to lymphotoxin. Nature. 1984;312:724–9.
123. Kishimoto T. B-cell stimulatory factors (BSFs): Molecular structure, biological function, and regulation of expression. J Clin Immunol. 1987;7:343–55.
124. Nathan CF. Secretory products of macrophages. J Clin Invest. 1987;79:319–26.
125. Dinarello CA. Interleukin-1: Amino acid sequences, multiple biological activities and comparison with tumor necrosis factor (cachectin). Year Immunol. 1986;2:68–89.
126. Paul WE. Interleukin 4 B cell stimulatory factor 1: One lymphokine, many functions. FASEB J. 1987;1:456–61.
127. Sehgal PB, May LT, Tamm I, et al. Human β^2 interferon and B-cell differentiation factor BSF-2 are identical. Science. 1987;235:731–2.
128. Epstein LB. The comparative biology of immune and classical interferons, in: Cohen S, Pich E, Oppenheim JJ, eds. Biology of the Lymphokines. New York: Academic Press, 1979:443–514.
129. Gray PW, Leung DW, Pennica D, et al. Expression of human immune interferon cDNA in *E. coli* and monkey cells. Nature. 1982;295:503–8.
130. Trinchieri G, Perussia B. Immune interferon: A pleiotropic lymphokine with multiple effects. Immunol Today. 1985;6:131–35
131. Metcalf D. The granulocyte–macrophage colony-stimulating factors. Science. 1985;229:16–22.
132. Sieff CA. Hematopoietic growth factors. J Clin Invest. 1987;79:1549–57.
133. Clark SC, Kamen R. The human hematopoietic colony-stimulating factors. Science. 1987;236:1229–37.
134. Kriegler M, Perez C, DeFay K, et al. A novel form of TNF/cachectin is a cell surface cytotoxic transmembrane protein: Ramifications for the complex physiology of TNF. Cell. 1988;53:45–53.
135. Kaushansky K, Lin N, Adamson JW. Interleukin 1 stimulates fibroblasts to synthesize granulocyte–macrophage and granulocyte colony-stimulating factors. J Clin Invest. 1988;81:92–7.
136. Pistoia V, Cozzolino F, Rubartelli A, et al. In vitro production of interleukin 1 by normal and malignant human B lymphocytes. J Immunol. 1986; 136:1688–92.
137. Nedwin GE, Svedersky LP, Bringman TS, et al. Effect of interleukin 2, interferon-γ and mitogens on the production of tumor necrosis factors α and β. J Immunol. 1985;135:2492–7.
138. Cuturi MC, Murphy M, Costa-Giomi MP, et al. Independent regulation of tumor necrosis factor and lymphotoxin production by human peripheral blood lymphocytes. J Exp Med. 1987;165:1581–94.
139. Hirano T, Yasukawa K, Harada YH, et al. Complementary DNA for a novel human interleukin (BSF-2) that induces B lymphocytes to produce immunoglobulin. Nature. 1986;324:73–6.
140. Burchett SK, Weaver WM, Westall JA, et al. Regulation of tumor necrosis factor/cachectin and interleukin 1 secretion in human mononuclear phagocytes. J Immunol. 1988;140:3473–7.
141. Beutler B, Krochin N, Milsark IW, et al. Control of cachectin (tumor necrosis factor) synthesis: Mechanisms of endotoxin resistance. Science. 1986;232:977–80.
142. Ikejima T, Dinarello CA, Gill DM, et al. Induction of human interleukin-1 by a product of *Staphylococcus aureua* associated with toxic shock syndrome. J Clin Invest. 1984;73:1312–20.
143. Philip RM, Epstein LB. Tumour necrosis factor as immunomodulator and

mediator of monocyte cytotoxicity induced by itself, γ-interferon and interleukin-1. Nature. 1986;323:86–9.
144. Van Damme J, Opdenakker G, Simpson RJ, et al. Identification of the human 26-kD protein, interferon β^2 (IFN-β^2), as a B cell hybridoma/plasmacytoma growth factor induced by interleukin 1 and tumor necrosis factor. J Exp Med. 1987;165:914–9.
145. Tosato G, Seamon KB, Goldman ND, et al. Monocyte-derived human B-cell growth factor identified as interferon-β^2 (BSF-2, IL-6). Science. 1987; 239:502–4.
146. Abb J, Abb H, Deinhardt F. Phenotype of human α-interferon producing leucocytes identified by monoclonal antibodies. Clin Exp Immunol. 1983;52:179–84.
147. Bell DM, Roberts NJ Jr, Hall CB. Different antiviral spectra of human macrophage interferon activities. Nature. 1983;305:319–21.
148. Stevenson HC, Dekaban GA, Miller PJ, et al. Analysis of human blood monocyte activation at the level of gene expression. J Exp Med. 1985;161:503–13.
149. Dinarello CA, Cannon JG, Wolff SM, et al. Tumor necrosis factor (cachectin) is an endogenous pyrogen and induces production of interleukin 1. J Exp Med. 1986;163:1433–50.
150. Broudy VC, Harlan JM, Adamson JW. Disparate effects of tumor necrosis factor-α cachectin and tumor necrosis factor-β lymphotoxin on hematopoietic growth factor production and neutrophil adhesion molecule expression by cultured human endothelial cells. J Immunol. 1987;136:4298–4302.
151. Locksley RM, Heinzel FP, Shepard HM, et al. Tumor necrosis factors α and β differ in their capacities to generate interleukin 1 release from human endothelial cells. J Immunol. 1987;139:1891–5.
152. Kurt-Jones EA, Fiers W, Pober JS. Membrane interleukin 1 induction on human endothelial cells and dermal fibroblasts. J Immunol. 1987;139:2317–24.
153. Munker R, Gasson J, Ogawa M, et al. Recombinant human TNF induces production of granulocyte–monocyte colony-stimulating factor. Nature. 1986;323:79–82.
154. Dinarello CA, Cannon JG, Wolff SM. New concepts on the pathogenesis of fever. Rev Infect Dis. 1988;10:168–89.
155. Cannistra SA, Rambaldi A, Spriggs DR, et al. Human granulocyte–macrophage colony-stimulating factor induces expression of the tumor necrosis factor gene by the U937 cell line and by normal human monocytes. J Clin Invest. 1987;79:1720–8.
156. Herrmann F, Cannistra SA, Griffin JD. T cell–monocyte interactions in the production of humoral factors regulating human granulopoiesis in vitro. J Immunol. 1986;136:2856–61.
157. Horiguchi J, Warren MK, Kufe D. Expression of the macrophage-specific colony-stimulating factor in human monocytes treated with granulocyte–macrophage colony-stimulating factor. Blood. 1987;69:1259–62.
158. Okusawa S, Dinarello CA, Yancey KB, et al. C5a induction of human interleukin 1. J Immunol. 1987;139:2635–40.
159. Crawford GD, Wyler DJ, Dinarello CA. Parasite–monocyte interactions in human leishmaniasis: Production of interleukin-1 in vitro. J Infect Dis 1985;152:315–22.
160. Reiner NE, Behm EA, Ng W, et al. Human monocytes treated with recombinant interferon gamma become responsive to *Leishmania donovani* for the production of interleukin 1 and tumor necrosis factor alpha. Clin Res. 1988;36:468A.
161. Kurt-Jones EA, Virgin HW IV, Unanua ER. In vivo and in vitro expression of macrophage membrane interleukin 1 in response to soluble and particulate stimuli. J Immunol. 1986;137:10–14.
162. Mizel SB. Interleukin 1 and T-cell activation. Immunol Today. 1987;8:330–1.
163. Eden E, Turino GM, Interleukin 1 secretion from huma alveolar macrophages in lung disease. J Clin Immunol. 1986;6:326–33.
164. Goodwin JS, Ceuppens JL, Gualde N. Control of the immune response in humans by prostaglandins. Adv Inflamm Res. 1984;7:79–92.
165. Bernton EW, Beach JE, Holaday JW, et al. Release of multiple hormones by a direct action of interleukin-1 on pituitary cells. Science. 1987;238:519–21.
166. Besedovsky H, del Rey A, Sorkin E, et al. Immunoregulatory feedback between interleukin-1 and glucocorticoid hormones. Science. 1986;233:652–3.
167. Woloski BMRNJ, Smith EM, Meyer WJ III, et al. Corticotropin-releasing activity of monokines. Science. 1985;230:1035–7.
168. Roberts NJ Jr, Prill AH, Mann TN. Interleukin 1 and interleukin 1 inhibitor production by human macrophages exposed to influenza virus or respiratory syncytial virus. J Exp Med. 1986;163:511–9.
169. Fujiwara H, Ellner JJ. Spontaneous production of a suppressor factor by the human macrophage-like cell line U937: I. Suppression of interleukin 1, interleukin 2, and mitogen-induced blastogenesis in mouse thymocytes. J Immunol. 1986;136:181–5.
170. Pennica D, Kohr WJ, Kuang W-J, et al. Identification of human uromodulin as the Tamm-Horsfall urinary glycoprotein. Science. 1987;236:83–8.
171. Jabara HH, Ackerman SJ, Vercelli D, et al. Induction of IgE synthesis and eosinophil differentiation by supernatants of an IL-4, IL-5 producing human helper T cell clone. J Immunol. 1988;140:4211–16.
172. Lewis DB, Prickett K, Larsen A, et al. Restricted production of interleukin-4 by activated T cells. Proc Natl Acad Sci USA. 1988;85:9743–47.
173. Mosmann TR, Cherwinski H, Bond MW, et al. Two types of murine helper T cell clone. I. Definition according to profiles of lymphokine activities and secreted proteins. J Immunol. 1986;136:2348.
174. Cherwinski HM, Schumacher JH, Brown KD, et al. Two types of mouse helper T cell clone. III. Further differences in lymphokine synthesis between Th1 and Th2 clones revealed by RNA hybridization, functionally monospecific bioassays, and monoclonal antibodies. J Exp Med. 1987;166:1229–44.
175. Kurt-Jones EA, Hamberg S, Ohara J, et al. Heterogeneity of helper/inducer T lymphcoytes. I. Lymphokine production and lymphokine responsiveness. J Exp Med. 1987;166:1774–87.
176. Yokota T, Coffman TL, Hagiwara H, et al. Isolation and characterization of lymphokine cDNA clones encoding mouse and human IgA-enhancing factor and eosinophil colony-stimulating factor activities: Relationship to interleukin 5. Proc Natl Acad Sci USA. 1987;84:7388–92.
177. Snapper CM, Paul WE. Interferon-γ and B cell stimulatory factor-1 reciprocally regulate Ig isotype production. Science. 1987;236:944–7.
178. Arthur RP, Mason D. T cells that help B cell responses to soluble antigen are distinguishable from those producing interleukin 2 on mitogenic or allogeneic stimulation. J Exp Med. 1986;163:774–6.
179. Luger TA, Smolen JS, Chused TM, et al. Human lymphocytes with either the OKT4 and OKT8 phenotype produce interleukin 2 in culture. J Clin Invest. 1982;70:470–3.
180. Mizuochi T, Ono S, Malek TR, et al. Characterization of two distinct primary T cell populations that secrete interleukin 2 upon recognition of class I or class II major histocompatibility antigens. J Exp Med. 1986;163:603–19.
181. Kasahara T, Hooks JJ, Dougherty SF, et al. Interleukin-2-mediated immune interferon (IFN-γ) production by human T cells and T cell subsets. J Immunol. 1983;130:1784–9.
182. Vilcek J, Henriksen-Destefano D, Siegal D, et al. Regulation of IFN-γ induction in human peripheral blood cells by exogenous and endogenously produced interleukin 2. J Immunol. 1985;135:1851–6.
183. Kelly CD, Welte K, Murray HW. Antigen-induced human interferon-γ production. Differential dependence on interleukin 2 and its receptor. J Immunol. 1987;139:2325–8.
184. Smith KA, Lachman LB, Oppenheim JJ, et al. The functional relationship of the interleukins. J Exp Med. 1980;151:1551–6.
185. Hagiwara H, Huang H-JS, Arai N, et al. Interleukin 1 modulates messenger RNA levels of lymphokines and of other molecules associated with T cells activation in the T cell lymphoma LBRM33-1A5. J Immunol. 1987;138:2514–9.
186. Scheurich P, Thoma B, Ucer U, et al. Immunoregulatory activity of recombinant human tumor necrosis factor (TNF)-α: Induction of TNF receptors on human T cells and TNF-α-mediated enhancement of T cell responses. J Immunol. 1987;138:1786–90.
187. Jenkins MK, Pardoll DM, Mizuguchi J, et al. Molecular events in the induction of a nonresponsive state in interleukin 2-producing helper T-lymphocyte clones. Proc Natl Acad Sci USA. 1987;84:5409–13.
188. Heckford SE, Gelmann EP, Agnor CL, et al. Distinct signals are required for proliferation and lymphokine gene expression in murine T cell clones. J Immunol. 1986;137:3652–63.
189. Rola-Pleszczynski M. Immunoregulation by leukotrienes and other lipoxygenase metabolites. Immunol Today. 1985;6:302–7.
190. Harris DT, Kozumbo WJ, Cerutti P, et al. Molecular mechanisms involved in T cell activation. I. Evidence for independent signal-transducing pathways in lymphokine production vs proliferation in cloned cytotoxic T lymphocytes. J Immunol. 1987;138:600–5.
191. Otten G, Herold KC, Fitch FW. Interleukin 2 inhibits antigen-stimulated lymphokine synthesis in helper T cells by inhibiting calcium-dependent signalling. J Immunol. 1987;139:1348–53.
192. Derynck R, Harrett JA, Chen EY, et al. Human transforming growth factor-β-complementary DNA sequence and expression in normal and transformed cells. Nature. 1985;316:701–5.
193. Kehrl JH, Wakefield LM, Roberts AB, et al. Production of transforming growth factor β by human T lymphocytes and its potential role in the regulation of T cell growth. J Exp Med. 1986;163:1037–50.
194. Wolf M, Falk W, Mannel D, et al. Inhibition of interleukin 2 production by prostaglandin E_2^- is not absolute but depends on the strength of the stimulating signal. Cell Immunol. 1985;90:190–5.
195. Rigby WFC. The immunobiology of vitamin D. Immunol Today. 1988;9:54–6.
196. Peters PM, Ortaldo JR, Shalaby R, et al. Natural killer-sensitive targets stimulate production of TNF-α but not TNF-β (lymphotoxin) by highly purified human peripheral blood large granular lymphocytes. J Immunol. 1986;137:2592–8.
197. Munakata T, Semba U, Shibuya Y, et al. Induction of interferon-γ production by human natural killer cells stimulated by hydrogen peroxide. J Immunol. 1985;134:2449–51.
198. Bickel M, Amstad P, Tsuda H, et al. Induction of granulocyte–macrophage colony-stimulating factor by lipopolysaccharide and anti-immunoglobulin M-stimulated murine B cell lines. J Immunol. 1987;139:2984–8.
199. Mackowiak PA. Direct effects of hyperthermia on pathogenic microorganisms: Teleologic implications with regard to fever. Rev Infect Dis. 1981;3:508–20.
200. Roberts NJ Jr. Temperature and host defense. Microbiol Rev. 1979;43:241–59.
201. Marx JL. Orphan interferon finds a new home. Science. 1988;239:25–6.
202. Perlmutter DH, Goldberger G, Dinarello CA, et al. Regulation of class III

major histocompatibility complex gene products by interleukin-1. Science. 1986;232:850–2.
203. Perlmutter DH, Dinarello CA, Punsal PI, et al. Cachectin/tumor necrosis regulates hepatic acute-phase gene expression. J Clin Invest. 1986;78:1349–54.
204. Baumann H, Richards C, Gauldie J. Interaction among hepatocyte-stimulating factors, interleukin 1, and glucocorticoids for regulation of acute phase plasma proteins in human hepatoma (HepG2) cells. J Immunol. 1987;139:4122–8.
205. Beutler BA, Cerami A. Recombinant interleukin 1 suppresses lipoprotein lipase activity in 3T3-L1 cells. J Immunol. 1985;135:3969–71.
206. Oliff A, Defeo-Jones D, Boyer M, et al. Tumors secreting human TNF/cachectin induce cachexia in mice. Cell. 1987;50:555–63.
207. Dustin ML, Rothlein R, Bhan AK, et al. Induction by IL 1 and interferon-γ: Tissue distribution, biochemistry, and function of a natural adherence molecule (ICAM-1). J Immunol. 1986;137:245–54.
208. Gamble JR, Harlan JM, Klebanoff SJ, et al. Stimulation of the adherence of neutrophils to umbilical vein endothelium by human recombinant tumor necrosis factor. Proc Natl Acad Sci USA. 1985;82:8667–71.
209. Pohlman TH, Stanness KA, Beatty PG, et al. An endothelial cell surface factor(s) induced in vitro by lipopolysaccharide, interleukin 1 and tumor necrosis factor-α increases neutrophil adherence by a CDw18-dependent mechanism. J Immunol. 1986;136:4548–53.
210. Nawroth PP, Stern DM. Modulation of endothelial cell hemostatic properties by tumor necrosis factor. J Exp Med. 1986;163:740–5.
211. Bevilacqua MP, Pober JS, Majeau GR, et al. Recombinant tumor necrosis factor induces procoagulant activity in cultured human vascular endothelium: Characterization and comparison with the actions of interleukin 1. Proc Natl Acad Sci USA. 1986;83:4533–7.
212. Tracey KJ, Beutler B, Lowry SF, et al. Shock and tissue injury induced by recombinant human cachectin. Science. 1986;234:470–4.
213. Tracey KJ, Fong Y, Hesse DG, et al. Anti-cachectin/TNF monoclonal antibodies prevent septic shock during lethal bacteraemia. Nature. 1987;330:662–4.
214. Rothstein JL, Schreiber H. Synergy between tumor necrosis factor and bacterial products causes hemorrhagic necrosis and lethal shock in normal mice. Proc Natl Acad Sci USA. 1988;85:607–11.
215. Billiau A. Not just cachectin involved in toxic shock. Nature. 1988;331:665.
216. Kettelhut IC, Fiers W, Goldberg AL. The toxic effects of tumor necrosis factor in vivo and their prevention by cyclooxygenase inhibitors. Proc Natl Acad Sci USA. 1987;84:4273–7.
217. Neta R, Oppenheim JJ, Douches SD. Interdependence of the radioprotective effects of human recombinant interleukin 1α, tumor necrosis factor α, granulocyte colony-stimulating factor, and murine recombinant granulocyte–macrophage colony-stimulating factor. J Immunol. 1988;140:108–11.
218. Mochizuki DY, Eisenman JR, Conlon PJ, et al. Interleukin 1 regulates hematopoietic activity, a role previously ascribed to hemopoietin 1. Proc Natl Acad Sci USA. 1987;84:5267–71.
219. Ikebuchi K, Wong GG, Clark SC, et al. Interleukin 6 enhancement of interleukin 3-dependent proliferation of multipotential hemopoietic progenitors. Proc Natl Acad Sci USA. 1987;84:9035–9.
220. Yang Y-C, Ciarletta AB, Temple PA, et al. Human IL-3 (Multi-CSF): Identification by expression cloning of a novel hematopoietic growth factor related to murine IL-3, Cell. 1986;47:3–10.
221. Vadhan-Raj S, Keating M, LeMaistre A, et al. Effects of recombinant human granulocyte–macrophage colony-stimulating factor in patients with myelodysplastic syndromes. N Engl J Med. 1987;317:1545–52.
222. Caracciolo D, Shirsat N, Wong GG, et al. Recombinant human macrophage colony-stimulating factor (M-CSF) requires subliminal concentrations of granulocyte–macrophage (GM) CSF for optimal subliminal concentrations of granulocyte–macrophage (GM) CSF for optimal stimulation of human macrophage colony formation in vitro. J Exp Med. 1987;166:1851–60.
223. Welte K, Bonilla MA, Gillio AP, et al. Recombinant human granulocyte colony-stimulating factor. J Exp Med. 1987;165:941–8.
224. Souza LM, Boone TC, Gabrilove J, et al. Recombinant human granulocyte colony-stimulating factor: Effects on normal and leukemic myeloid cells. Science. 1986;232:61–5.
225. Weaver CT, Unanue ER. T cell induction of membrane IL 1 on macrophages. J Immunol. 1986;137:3868–73.
226. Leonard WJ, Depper JM, Crabtree GR, et al. Molecular cloning and expression of cDNAs for the human interleukin-2 receptor. Nature. 1984;311:626–31.
227. Sharon M, Klausner RD, Cullen BR, et al. Novel interleukin-2 receptor subunit detected by cross-linking under high-affinity conditions. Science. 1986;234:859–63.
228. Teshigawara K, Wang H-M, Kato K, et al. Interleukin 2 high-affinity receptor expression requires two distinct binding proteins. J Exp Med. 1987;165:223–38.
229. Tsudo M, Kozak RW, Goldman CK, et al. Demonstration of a non-Tac peptide that binds interleukin 2: A potential participant in a multichain interleukin 2 receptor complex. Proc Natl Acad Sci USA. 1986;83:9693–8.
230. Lowenthal JW, Greene WC. Contrasting interleukin 2 binding properties of the α (p55) and β (p70) protein subunits of the human high-affinity interleukin 2 receptor. J Exp Med. 1987;166:1156–61.
231. Wang H-M, Smith KA. The interleukin 2 receptor. J Exp Med. 1987;166:1055–69.
232. Lotz M, Jirik F, Kabouridis P, et al. B cell stimulating factor 2/interleukin 6 is a costimulant for human thymocytes and T lymphocytes. J Exp Med. 1988;167:1253–8.
233. O'Garra A, Umland Sh, De France T, et al. "B-cell factors" are pleiotropic. Immunol Today. 1988;9:45–54.
234. Stein P, Dubois P, Greenblatt D, et al. Induction of antigen-specific proliferation in affinity-purified small B lymphocytes: Requirement for BSF-1 by type 2 but not type 1 thymus-independent antigens. J Immunol. 1986;136:2080–9.
235. Krusemeier M, Snow EC. Induction of lymphokine responsiveness of hapten-specific B lymphocytes promoted through an antigen-mediated T helper lymphocyte interaction. J Immunol. 1988;140:367–75.
236. Brian AA. Stimulation of B-cell proliferation by membrane-associated molecules from activated T cells. Proc Natl Acad Sci USA. 1988;85:564–8.
237. Asano Y, Nakayam T, Kubo M, et al. Analysis of two distinct B cell activation pathways mediated by a monoclonal T helper cell. II. T helper cell secretion of interleukin 4 selectively inhibits antigen-specific B cell activation by cognate, but not noncognate, interactions with T cells. J Immunol. 1988;140:419–26.
238. Sanders VM, Fernandez-Botran R, Uhr JW, et al. Interleukin 4 enhances the ability of antigen-specific B cells to form conjugates with T cells. J Immunol. 1987;139:2349–54.
239. Bich-Thuy L, Fauci AS. Recombinant interleukin 2 and gamma-interferon act synergistically on distinct steps of in vitro terminal human B cell maturation. J Clin Invest. 1986;77:1173–9.
240. Jelinek DF, Lipsky PE. Comparative activation requirements of human peripheral blood, spleen, and lymph node B cells. J Immunol. 1987;139:1005–13.
241. Pike BL, Raubitschek A, Nossal GJV. Human interleukin 2 can promote the growth and differentiation of single hapten-specific B cells in the presence of specific antigen. Proc Natl Acad Sci USA. 1984;81:7917–21.
242. Mingari MC, Gerosa F, Carra G, et al. Human interleukin-2 promotes proliferation of activated B cells via surface receptors similar to those of activated T cells. Nature. 1984;312:641–3.
243. Defrance T, Vanbervliet B, Aubry J-P, et al. B cell growth-promoting activity of recombinant human interleukin 4. J Immunol. 1987;139:1135–41.
244. Yokota T, Otsuka T, Mosmann T, et al. Isolation and characterization of a human interleukin cDNA clone, homologous to mouse B-cell stimulatory factor 1, that expresses B-cell- and T-cell-stimulating activities. Proc Natl Acad Sci USA. 1986;83:5894–8.
245. Kehrl JH, Miller A, Fauci AS. Effect of tumor necrosis factor α on mitogen-activated human B cells. J Exp Med. 1987;166:786–91.
246. Kehrl JH, Alvarez-Mon M, Delsing GA, et al. Lymphotoxin is an important T cell-derived growth factor for human B cells. Science. 1987;238:1144–6.
247. Pike BL, Nossal GJB. Interleukin 1 can act as a B-cell growth and differentiation factor. Proc Natl Acad Sci USA. 1985;82:8153–7.
248. Defrance T, Aubry J-P, Vanbervliet B, et al. Human interferon-γ acts as a B cell growth factor in the anti-IgM antibody co-stimulatory assay but has no direct B cell differentiation activity. J Immunol. 1986;137:3861–7.
249. Kawano M, Hirano T, Matsuda T, et al. Autocrine generation and requirement of BSF-2/IL-6 for human multiple myelomas. Nature. 1988;332:83–5.
250. Poupart P, Vandenabeele P, Cayphas S, et al. B cell growth modulating and differentiating activity of recombinant human 26-kd protein (BSF-2, HuIFN-β^2, HPGF). EMBO J. 1987;6:1219–24.
251. Azuma C, Tanabe T, Konishi M, et al. Cloning of cDNA for human T-cell replacing factor (interleukin-5) and comparison with the murine homologue. Nucleic Acid Res. 1986;14:9149–58.
252. Stein P, Dubois P, Greenblatt D, et al. Induction of antigen-specific proliferation in affinity-purified small B lymphocytes: Requirement for BSF-1 by type 2 but not type 1 thymus-independent antigens. J Immunol. 1986;136:2080–9.
253. Reinherz EL, Schlossmann SF. Regulation of the immune response: Inducer and suppressor T lymphocyte subsets in man. N Engl J Med. 1980;303:370.
254. Reinherz EL, Kung PC, Goldstein G, et al. A monoclonal antibody reactive with the human cytotoxic/suppressor T cell subset previously defined by heteroantiserum termed TH^2. J Immunol. 1980;124:1301.
255. Thomas Y, Sosman J, Irigoyen O, et al. Functional analysis of human T cell subsets defined by monoclonal antibodies. I. Collaborative T–T interactions in the immunoregulation of B cell differentiation. J Immunol. 1980;125:2402.
256. Ledbetter J, Evans RL, Lipinski M, et al. Evolutionary conservation of surface molecules that distinguish T lymphocyte inducer and cytotoxic/suppressor subpopulations in mouse and man. J Exp Med. 1981;153:310.
257. Damle NK, Childs AL, Doyle LV. Immunoregulatory T lymphocytes in man: Soluble antigen-specific suppressor inducer T lymphocytes are derived from the CD4 CD45R p80 subpopulation. J Immunol. 1987;139:1501–8.
258. Takeuchi T, Rudd CE, Schlossman SF, et al. Induction of suppression following autologous mixed lymphocyte reaction; role of a novel 2H4 antigen. Eur J Immunol. 1987;17:97–103.
259. Morimoto C, Letvin NL, Distaso JA, et al. The cellular basis for the induction of antigen-specific T8 suppressor cells. Eur J Immunol. 1986;16:198–204.
260. Damle NK. Suppressor T lymphocytes in man. Year Immunol. 1986;2:60–7.
261. Ellner JJ. Suppressor cells of man. Clin Immunol Dev. 1981;1:119–41.
262. Damle NK, Childs AL, Doyle LV. Immunoregulatory T lymphocytes in man. Soluble antigen-specific suppressor-inducer T lymphocytes are derived from the CD4 CD45R p80 subpopulation. J Immunol. 1987;139:1501–8.

263. Green DR, Flood PM, Gershon RK. Immunoregulatory T-cell pathways. Ann Rev Immunol. 1983;1:439–64.
264. Sathish M, Bhutani LK, Sharma AK, et al. Monocyte-derived soluble suppressor factor(s) in patients with lepromatous leprosy. Infect Immun. 1983;42:890–9.
265. Kapp JA, Pierce CW, Sorensen CM. Antigen-specific suppressor T-cell factors. Hosp Pract. 1984;19-8:85–98.
266. Espevik T, Figari IS, Shalaby MR, et al. Inhibition of cytokine production by cyclosporin A and transforming growth factor β. J Exp Med. 1987; 166:571–6.
267. Lee G, Ellingsworth LR, Gillis S, et al. β Transforming growth factors are potential regulators of B lymphopoiesis. J Exp Med. 1987;166:1290–9.
268. Schnaper HW, Pierce CW, Aune TM. Identification and initial characterization of concanavalin A- and interferon-induced human suppressor factors: Evidence for a human equivalent of murine soluble immune response suppressor (SIRS). J Immunol. 1984;132:2429–35.
269. Laurence J, Mayer L. Immunoregulatory lymphokines of T hybridomas from AIDS patients: Constitutive and inducible suppressor factors. Science. 1984;225:66–9.
270. Aune TM. Inhibition of soluble immune response suppressor activity by growth factors. Proc Natl Acad Sci USA. 1985;82:6260–4.
271. Chouaib S, Chatenoud L, Klatzmann D, et al. The mechanisms of inhibition of human IL2 production. II. PGE_2 induction of suppressor T lymphocytes. J Immunol. 1984;132:1851–7.
272. Gromo G, Geller RL, Inverardi L, et al. Signal requirements in the stepwise functional maturation of cytotoxic T lymphocytes. Nature. 1987;327:424–6.
273. Gately MK, Wilson DE, Wong HL. Synergy between recombinant interleukin 2 (rIL 2) and IL 2-depleted lymphokine-containing supernatants in facilitating allogeneic human cytolytic T lymphocyte responses in vitro. J Immunol. 1986;136:1274–82.
274. Hefeneider SH, Conlon PJ, Henney CS, et al. In vivo interleukin 2 administration augments the generation of alloreactive cytolytic T lymphocytes and resident natural killer cells. J Immunol. 1983;130:222–7.
275. Widmer MB, Grabstein KH. Regulation of cytolytic T-lymphocyte generation by B-cell stimulatory factor. Nature. 1987;326:795–8.
276. Widmer MB, Acres RB, Sassenfeld HM, et al. Regulation of cytolytic cell populations from human peripheral blood by B cell stimulatory factor 1 (interleukin 4). J Exp Med. 1987;166:1447–55.
277. Pfeifer JD, McKenzie DT, Swain SL, et al. B cell stimulatory factor 1 (interleukin 4) is sufficient for the proliferation and differentiation of lectin-stimulated cytolytic T lymphocyte precursors. J Exp Med. 1987;166:1464–70.
278. Takai Y, Wong GG, Clark SC, et al. B cell stimulatory factor-2 is involved in the differentiation of cytotoxic T lymphocytes. J Immunol. 1988;140:508–12.
279. Park LS, Friend D, Sassenfeld HM, et al. Characterization of the human B cell stimulatory factor 1 receptor. J Exp Med. 1987;166:476–88.
280. Podack ER. Molecular mechanisms of cytolysis by complement and by cytolytic lymphocytes. J Cell Biochem. 1986;30:133–70.
281. Young JDE, Hengartner H, Podack ER, et al. Purification and characterization of a cytolytic pore-forming protein from granules of cloned lymphocytes with natural killer activity. Cell. 1986;44:849–59.
282. Martin DE, Zalman LS, Jung G, et al. Induction of synthesis of the cytolytic C9 (ninth component of complement)-related protein in human peripheral mononuclear cells by monoclonal antibody OKT3 or interleukin 2: Correlation with cytotoxicity and lymphocyte phenotype. Proc Natl Acad Sci USA. 1987;84:2946–50.
283. Masson D, Tschopp J. A family of serine esterases in lytic granules of cytolytic T lymphocytes. Cell. 1987;49:679–85.
284. Garcia-Sanz JA, Plaetinck G, Velotti F, et al. Perforin is present only in normal activated Lyt2 T lymphocytes and not in L3T4 cells, but the serine protease granzyme A is made by both subsets. EMBO J. 1987;6:933–8.
285. Young JD-E, Liu C-C. How do cytotoxic T lymphocytes avoid self-lysis? Immunol Today. 1988;9:14–15.
286. Dennert G, Anderson CG, Prochazka G. High activity of *N*-benzyloxycarbonyl-L-lysine thiobenzyl ester serine esterase and cytolytic perforin in cloned cell lines is not demonstrable in in vivo-induced cytotoxic effector cells. Proc Natl Acad Sci USA. 1987;84:5004–8.
287. Lanier LL, Le AM, Civin CI, et al. The relationship of CD16 (LEU-11) and LEU-19 (NKH-1) antigen expression on human peripheral blood NK cells and cytotoxic T lymphocytes. J Immunol. 1986;136:4480–6.
288. Lanier LL, Kipps TJ, Phillips JH. Functional properties of a unique subset of cytotoxic CD3 lymphocytes that express Fc receptors for IgG (CD16/LEU-11 antigen). J Exp Med. 1985;162:2089–2106.
289. Lanier LL, Cwirla S, Federspiel N, et al. Human natural killer cells isolated from peripheral blood do not rearrange T cell antigen receptor β chain genes. J Exp Med. 1986;163:209–14.
290. Hackett J, Bosma GC, Bosma MJ, et al. Transplantable progenitors of natural killer cells are distinct from those of T and B lymphocytes. Proc Natl Acad Sci USA. 1986;83:3427–31.
291. Ritz J, Campen TJ, Schmidt RE. Analysis of T-cell receptor gene rearrangement and expression in human natural killer clones. Science. 1985;228:1540–3.
292. Bensussen A, Tourveille B, Chen LI, et al. Phorbol ester induces a differential effect on the effector function of human allospecific cytotoxic T lymphcyte and natural killer clones. Immunology 1985;66:42–6.
293. Herberman RB, Ortaldo JR. Natural killer cells: Their role in defenses against disease. Science. 1981;214:24–30.
294. Bellan AH, Quilet A, Marchiol C, et al. Natural killer susceptibility of human cells may be regulated by genes in the HLA region on chromosome 6. Proc Natl Acad Sci USA. 1986;83:5688–92.
295. Stern P, Gidlund M, Orn A, et al. Natural killer cells mediate lysis of embryonal carcinoma cells lacking MHC. Nature. 1980;285:341–2.
296. Springer TA, Anderson DC. The importance of the Mac-1, LFA-1, glycoprotein family in monocyte and granulocyte adherence, chemotaxis, and migration into inflammatory sites: Insights from an experiment of nature. Ciba Found Symp. 1986;118:102–26.
297. Bukowski JF, Warner JR, Dennert G, et al. Adoptive transfer studies demonstrating the antiviral effect of natural killer cells in vivo. J Exp Med. 1985;161:40–52.
298. Kohl S. Herpes simplex virus immunology: Problems, progress and promises. J Infect Dis. 1985;152:435–40.
299. Hauser WE, Tsai V. Acute toxoplasma infection of mice induces spleen NK cells that are cytotoxic for *T. gondii* in vitro. J Immunol. 1986;136:313–9.
300. Seki H, Ueno Y, Taga K, et al. Mode of in vitro augmentation of natural killer cell activity by recombinant human interleukin 2: A comparative study of $LEU\text{-}11^+$ and $LEU\text{-}11^-$ cell populations in cord blood and adult peripheral blood. J Immunol. 1985;135:2351–6.
301. Herberman RB, Ortaldo JR, Mantovani A, et al. Effect of human recombinant interferon on cytotoxic activity of natural killer (NK) cells and monocytes. Cell Immunol. 1982;67:160–7.
302. Targan S, Stebbing N. In vitro interactions of purified cloned human interferons on NK cells: Enhanced activation. J Immunol. 1982;129:934–5.
303. Shah PD, Gilbertson SM, Rowley DA. Dendritic cells that have interacted with antigen are targets for natural killer cells. J Exp Med. 1985;162:625–36.
304. Callewaert DM. Purification and characterization of NK cells. In: Herberman R, ed. Mechanisms of Cytotoxicity by NK Cells. New York: Academic Press, 1985:17–28.
305. Starr SE, Garrabrant T. Natural killing of cytomegalovirus-infected fibroblasts by human mononuclear leucocytes. Clin Exp Immunol. 1981;46:484–92.
306. Lopez CC. Natural killing of herpes simplex virus type 1-infected target cells: normal human responses and influence of antiviral antibody. Infect Immun. 1979;26:49.
307. Kohl S, Shaban SS, Starr SE, et al. Human neonatal and maternal monocyte–macrophage and lymphocyte-mediated antibody-dependent cytotoxicity to cells infected with herpes simplex. J Pediatr. 1978;93:206–10.
308. Johnston RB Jr. Monocytes and macrophages. N Engl J Med. 1988;318:747–52.
309. Pfefferkorn ER. Interferon-γ blocks the growth of *Toxoplasma gondii* in human fibroblasts by inducing the host cells to degrade tryptophan. Proc Natl Acad Sci USA. 1984;81:908–12.
310. Mackaness GB. The immunological basis of acquired cellular immunity. J Exp Med. 1964;120:105–20.
311. McLeod RE, Wing J, Remington JS. Lymphocytes and macrophages in cell-mediated immunity. In: Mandell GL, Douglas RG Jr, Bennett JE, eds. Principles and Practice of Infectious Diseases. 2nd ed. New York: Churchill Livingstone; 1985:72–93.
312. Hamilton TA, Adams DO. Molecular mechanisms of signal transduction in macrophages. Immunol Today. 1987;8:151–8.
313. Murray HW, Rubin BY, Rothermel CD. Killing of intracellular *Leishmania donovani* by lymphokine-stimulated human mononuclear phagocytes. J Clin Invest. 1983;72:1506–10.
314. Wilson CB, Haas JE. Cellular defenses against *Toxoplasma gondii* in newborns. J Clin Invest. 1984;73:1606–16.
315. Wilson CB, Westall J. Activation of neonatal and adult human macrophages by alpha, beta, and gamma interferons. Infect Immun. 1985;49:351–6.
316. Nathan CF, Prendergast TJ, Wiebe ME, et al. Activation of human macrophages. Comparison of other cytokines with interferon-γ. J Exp Med. 1984;160:600–5.
317. Roberts WK, Vasil A. Evidence for the identity of murine gamma interferon and macrophage activating factor. J Interferon Res. 1982;2:519–32.
318. Edwards CK III, Hedegaard HB, Zlotnik A, et al. Chronic infection due to *Mycobacterium intracellulare* in mice: Association with macrophage release of prostaglandin E_2 and reversal by injection of indomethacin, muramyl dipeptide, or interferon-gamma. J Immunol. 1986;136:1820–7.
319. McCabe RE, Luft BJ, Remington JS. Effect of murine interferon-γ on murine toxoplasmosis. J Infect Dis. 1984;150:961–2.
320. Khor M, Lowrie DB, Coates AR, et al. Recombinant interferon-gamma and chemotherapy with isoniazid and rifampicin in experimental murine tuberculosis. Br J Exp Pathol. 1986;67:587–96.
321. Murray HW, Stern JJ, Welte K, et al. Experimental visceral leishmaniasis: Production of interleukin 2 and interferon-γ, tissue immune reaction, and response to treatment with interleukin 2 and interferon-γ. J Immunol. 1987;138:2290–7.
322. Gould CL, Sonnenfeld G. Effect of treatment with interferon-gamma and concanavalin A on the course of infection of mice with *Salmonella typhimurium* strain LT-2. J Interferon Res. 1987;7:255–60.
323. Anthony LSD, Ghadirian E, Kongshavn PAL. Effect of gamma-interferon treatment on the resistance of mice to experimental tularemia (Abstract). J Leukocyte Biol. 1987;42:415.
324. Buchmeier NA, Schreiber RD. Requirement of endogenous interferon-

gamma production for resolution of *Listeria monocytogenes* infection. Proc Natl Acad Sci USA. 1985;82:7404–8.
325. Squires KE, Schreiber RD, McElrath MJ, et al. Role of endogenous interferon-γ in murine visceral leishmaniasis (Abstract). Clin Res. 1987;35:492.
326. Suzuki Y, Orellana MA, Schreiber RD, et al. Interferon-γ: The major mediator of resistance against *Toxoplasma gondii*. Science. 1988;240:516–8.
327. Li H, Jerrells TR, Spitalny GL, et al. Gamma interferon as a crucial host defense against *Rickettsia conorii* in vivo. Infect Immun. 1987;55:1252–5.
328. De Titto E, Catterall JR, Remington JS. Activity of recombinant tumor necrosis factor on *Toxoplasma gondii* and *Trypanosoma cruzi*. J Immunol. 1986;1342–5.
329. Bermudez LEM, Young LS. Tumor necrosis factor, alone or in combination with IL-2, but not IFN-γ, is associated with macrophage killing of *Mycobacterium avium* complex. J Immunol. 1988;140:3006–13.
330. Reed SG, Nathan CF, Pihl DL, et al. Recombinant granulocyte/macrophage colony-stimulating factor activates macrophages to inhibit *Trypanosoma cruzi* and release hydrogen peroxide. J Exp Med. 1987;166:1734–46.
331. Handman E, Burgess AW. Stimulation by granulocyte–macrophage colony-stimulating factor of *Leishmania tropica* killing by macrophages. J Immunol. 1979;22:1134–7.
332. Weiser WY, Van Niel A, Clark SC, et al. Recombinant human granulocyte/macrophage colony-stimulating factor activates intracellular killing of *Leishmania donovani* by human monocyte-derived macrophages. J Exp Med. 1987;166:1436–46.
333. Byrne GI, Lehmann LK, Landry GJ. Induction of tryptophan catabolism is the mechanism for gamma-interferon-mediated inhibition of intracellular *Chlamydia psittaci* replication in T24 cells. Infect Immun. 1986;53:347–51.
334. Niesel DW, Hess CB, Cho YJ, et al. Natural and recombinant interferons inhibit epithelial cell invasion by *Shigella* spp. Infect Immun. 1986;52:828–33.
335. Byrd TF, Horwitz MA. Intracellular multiplication of *Legionella pneumophila* in human monocytes is iron-dependent and the capacity of activated monocytes to inhibit intracellular multiplication is reversed by iron-transferrin (Abstract). Clin Res. 1987;35:613.
336. Granger DL, Hibbs JB Jr, Perfect JR, et al. Specific amino acid requirement for the microbistatic activity of murine macrophages. J Clin Invest. 1988;81:1129–36.
337. Frenkel JK. Adoptive immunity of intracellular infection. J Immunol. 1966;98:1309–19.
338. Luft BJ, Brooks RG, Conley FK, et al. Toxoplasmic encephalitis in patients with acquired immune deficiency syndrome. JAMA. 1984;252:913–7.
339. Vollmer TL, Waldor MK, Steinman L, et al. Depletion of T-4 lymphocytes with monoclonal antibody reactivates toxoplasmosis in the central nervous system: A model of superinfection in AIDS. J Immunol. 1987;138:3737–41.
340. Sansonetti P, Lagrange PH. The immunology of leprosy: Speculations on the leprosy spectrum. Rev Infect Dis. 1981;3:422–69.
341. Nathan CF, Kaplan G, Levis W, et al. Local and systemic effects of intradermal recombinant interferon-γ in patients with lepromatous leprosy. N Engl J Med. 1986;315:6–15.
342. Modlin RL, Hofman RM, Horwitz DA, et al. In situ identification of cells in human leprosy granulomas with monoclonal antibodies to interleukin 2 and its receptor. J Immunol. 1984;132:3085–90.
343. Modlin RL, Melancon-Kaplan J, Young SMM, et al. Learning from lesions: Patterns of tissue inflammation in leprosy. Proc Natl Acad Sci USA. 1988;85:1213–7.
344. Haregewoin A, Godal T, Mustafa AS, et al. T-cell conditioned media reverse T-cell unresponsiveness in lepromatous leprosy. Nature. 1983;303:342–4.
345. Nogueira N, Kaplan G, Levy E, et al. Defective γ interferon production in leprosy. J Exp Med. 1983;158:2165–70.
346. van Dissel JT, Stikkelbroeck JM, van den Barselaar MT, et al. Divergent changes in antimicrobial activity after immunologic activation of mouse peritoneal macrophages. J Immunol. 1987;139:1665–72.
347. van Dissel JT, Stikkelbroeck JM, Michel BC, et al. Inability of recombinant interferon-γ to activate the antibacterial activity of mouse peritoneal macrophages against *Listeria monocytogenes* and *Salmonella typhimurium*. J Immunol. 1987;139:1673–8.
348. Wilson CB, Tsai V, Remington JS. Failure to trigger the oxidative metabolic burst by normal macrophages. J Exp Med. 1980;151:328–46.
349. Pearson RD, Wheeler DA, Harrison LH, et al. The immunobiology of *Leishmania*. Rev Infect Dis. 1983;5:907–27.
350. Cheers C, Haigh AM, Kelso A, et al. Production of colony-stimulating factors (CSFs) during infection: Separate determinations of macrophage-, granulocyte-, granulocyte-macrophage-, and multi-CSFs. Infect Immun. 1988;56:247–51.
351. Magee DM, Wing EJ. Antigen-specific production of colony-stimulating factors by *Listeria monocytogenes*-immune, L3T4-positive cells. J Infect Dis. 1988;157:941–9.
352. Wing EJ, Ampel NM, Waheed A, et al. Macrophage colony-stimulating factor (M-CSF) enhances the capacity of murine macrophages to secrete oxygen reduction products. J Immunol. 1985;135:2052–6.
353. Kaufmann SHE. Possible role of helper and cytolytic T lymphocytes in antibacterial defense: Conclusions based on a murine model of listeriosis. Rev Infect Dis. 1987;9(S5):S650–9.
354. Moulder JW. Comparative biology of intracellular parasitism. Microbiol Rev. 1985;49:298–337.
355. Murray HW. How protozoa evade intracellular killing. Ann Intern Med. 1983;98:1016–8.
356. Wilson CB, Haas JE. Cellular defenses against *Toxoplasma gondii* in newborns. J Clin Invest. 1984;73:1606–16.
357. MacKay RJ, Russell SW. Protein changes associated with stages of activation of mouse macrophages for tumor cell killing. J Immunol. 1986;137:1392–8.
358. Deem RL, Doughty FA, Beaman BL. Immunologically specific direct T lymphocyte-mediated killing of *Nocardia asteroides*. J Immunol. 1983;130:2401–6.
359. Albright JW, Munger WE, Henkart PA, et al. The toxicity of rat large granular lymphocyte tumor cells and and their cytoplasmic for rodent and African trypanosomes. J Immunol. 1988;140:2774–8.
360. Eisenstein TK, Tamada R, Meissler J, et al. Vaccination against *Legionella pneumophila*: Serum antibody correlates with protection induced by heat-killed or acetone-killed cells against intraperitoneal but not aerosol infection in guinea pigs. Infect Immun. 1984;45:685–91.
361. Eisenstein TK, Killar LM, Sultzer BM. Immunity to infection with *Salmonella typhimurium*: Mouse-strain differences in vaccine- and serum-mediated protection. J Infect Dis. 1984;150:425–35.
362. Horwitz MA, Silverstein SC. Interaction of the Legionnaires' disease bacterium (*Legionella pneumophila*) with human phagocytes. II. Antibody promotes binding of *L. pneumophila* to monocytes but does not inhibit intracellular multiplication. J Exp Med. 1981;153:398–406.
363. Frenkel JK, Taylor DW. Toxoplasmosis in immunoglobulin M-suppressed mice. Infect Immun. 1982;38:360.
364. Eisenhauer P, Mack DG, McLeod R. Prevention of peroral and congenital acquisition of *Toxoplasma gondii* by antibody and activated macrophages. Infect Immun. 1988;56:83–7.
365. Change K-P. Antibody-mediated inhibition of phagocytosis in *Leishmania donovani*–human phagocyte interactions *in vitro*. Am J Trop Med Hyg. 1981;30(2):334–9.
366. Weiss WR, Sedegah M, Beaudoin RL, et al. CD8 T cells (cytotoxic/suppressors) are required for protection in mice immunized with malaria sporozoites. Proc Natl Acad Sci USA. 1988;85:573–6.
367. Cox FEG. Which way for malaria? Nature. 1988;331:486–7.
368. Schofield L, Villaquiran J, Ferreira A, et al. γ-Interferon, CD8 T cells and antibodies required for immunity to malaria sporozoites. Nature. 1987;330:664.
369. Ockenhouse CF, Schulman S, Shea HL. Induction of crisis forms in the human malaria parasite *Plasmodium falciparum* by γ-interferon-activated, monocyte-derived macrophages. J Immunol. 1984;133:1601–8.
370. Scuderi P, Lam KS, Ryan KJ, et al. Raised serum levels of tumour necrosis factor in parasitic infections. Lancet. 1986;1:1364–5.
371. Grau GE, Fajardo LF, Piguet P-F, et al. Tumor necrosis factor (cachectin) as an essential mediator in murine cerebral malaria. Science. 1987;237:1210–2.
372. Ellner JJ. Immunology of human schistosomiasis. Clin Immunol Newsletter. 1983;4:108–17.
373. Silberstein DS, David JR. Tumor necrosis factor enhances eosinophil toxicity to *Schistosoma mansoni* larvae. Proc Natl Acad Sci USA. 1986; 83:1055–9.
374. Katona IM, Urban JF Jr, Finkelman FD. The role of L3T4 and Lyt-2 cells in the IgE response and immunity to *Nippostrongylus brasiliensis*. J Immunol. 1988;140:3206–11.
375. Stavitsky AB. Immune regulation in *Schistosoma japonica*. Immunol Today. 1987;8:228–32.
376. Ogilvie BM, Love RJ. Cooperation between antibodies and cells in immunity to a nematode parasite. Transplant Rev. 1974;19:147.
377. Wakelin D, Wilson MM. Transfer of immunity to *Trichinella spiralis* in the mouse with mesenteric lymph node cells. Time of appearance of effective cells in donors and expression of immunity in recipients. Parasitology. 1977;74:215.
378. Wing EJ, Remington JS. A role for activated macrophages in resistance against *Trichinella spiralis*. Infect Immun. 1978;21:398.
379. Shapiro ME, Kasper DL, Zaleznik DF, et al. Cellular control of abscess formation: Role of T cells in the regulation of abscesses formed in response to *Bacteroides fragilis*. J Immunol. 1986;137:341–6.
380. Onderdonk AB, Markham RB, Zeleznik DF, et al. Evidence for T cell-dependent immunity to *Bacteroides fragilis* in an intraabdominal abscess model. J Clin Invest. 1982;69:9–16.
381. Powderly WG, Schreiber JR, Pier GB, et al. T cells recognizing polysaccharide-specific B cells function as contrasuppressor cells in the generation of T cell immunity to *Pseudomonas aeruginosa*. J Immunol. 1988;140:2746–52.
382. Markham RB, Powderly WG. Exposure of mice to live *Pseudomonas aeruginosa* generates protective cell-mediated immunity in the absence of an antibody response. J Immunol. 1988;140:2039–45.
383. Powderly WG, Pier GB, Markham RB. T lymphocyte-mediated protection against *Pseudomonas aeruginosa* infection in granulocytopenic mice. J Clin Invest. 1986;78:375–80.
384. Ozaki Y, Ohashi T, Minami A, et al. Enhanced resistance of mice to bacterial infection induced by recombinant human interleukin-α. Infect Immun. 1987;55:1436–1450.
385. Iizawa Y, Nishi T, Kondo M, et al. Effect of recombinant human interleukin-2 on the course of experimental chronic respiratory tract infection caused by *Klebsiella pneumoniae* in mice. Infect Immun. 1988;56:45–50.
386. Finberg R, Hom R. The role of T cell immunity in infection with the herpes group viruses. Year Immunol. 1986;2:267–78.

387. Shore SL, Feorino PM. Immunology of primary herpes virus infections in human. In: Nahmias AJ, Dowdle WR, Schinazi RF, eds. The Human Herpes Viruses. New York: Elsevier, 1981;267–8.
388. Oakes JE, Lausch RN. Role of Fc fragments in antibody-mediated recovery from ocular and subcutaneous herpes simplex virus infection. Infect Immun. 1981;33:109.
389. Oakes JE, Davis WB, Taylor JA, et al. Lymphocyte reactivity contributes to protection conferred by specific antibody passively transferred to herpes simplex virus-infected mice. Infect Immun. 1980;29:642.
390. Epstein LB. The comparative biology of immune and classical interferons. In: Cohen S, Pich E, Oppenheim JJ, eds. Biology of the Lymphokines. New York: Academic Press, 1979;443–514.
391. Daniels CA: Kleinerman ES, Snyderman R: Abortive and productive infections of human mononuclear phagocytes by type I herpes simplex virus. Am J Pathol. 1978;91:119.
392. Morahan PS, Morse SS, McGeorge MB. Macrophage extrinsic activity during herpes simplex virus infection. J Gen Virol. 1980;46:291.
393. Ching C, Lopez C. Natural killing of herpes simplex virus type 1-infected target cells: normal human responses and influence of antiviral antibody. Infect Immun. 1979;26:49.
394. Kohl S, Frazier JJ, Greenberg SB, et al. Interferon induction of natural killer cytotoxicity in human neonates. J Pediatr. 1981;98:379–84.
395. St. Geme JW, Prince JT, Burke BA, et al. Impaired cellular resistance to herpes-simplex virus in Wiskott-Aldrich syndrome. N Engl J Med. 1965; 273:229.
396. Torseth JW, Merigan TC. Significance of local γ interferon in recurrent herpes simplex infection. J Infect Dis. 1986;153:979–84.
397. Burchett SK, Mohan K, Corey L, et al. Delayed production of interferon-gamma (IFNγ) and tumor necrosis factor (TNFα) by mononuclear cells (MC) of herpes simplex virus (HSV) infected neonates (NB). Pediatr Res. 1987;21:309A.
398. Wong GHW, Goeddel DV. Tumour necrosis factors α and β inhibit virus replication and synergize with interferons. Nature. 1986;323:819–22.
399. Hayashi Y, Wada T, Mori R. Protection of newborn mice against herpes simplex virus infection by prenatal and postnatal transmission of antibody. J Gen Virol. 1983;64:1007.
400. Kohl S, Loo LS. The relative role of transplacental and mild immune transfer in protection against lethal neonatal herpes simplex virus infection in mice. J Infect Dis. 1984;149:38.
401. Quinnan GV, Kirmani N, Rook AH, et al. Cytotoxic T cells in cytomegalovirus infection. N Engl J Med. 1982;307:7–12.
402. Winston DJ, Ho WG, Lin CH, et al. Intravenous immune globulin for prevention of cytomegalovirus infection and interstitial pneumonia after bone marrow transplantation. Ann Intern Med. 1987;106:12–18.
403. Grierson H, Purtilo DT. Epstein-Barr virus infections in males with the X-linked lymphoproliferative syndrome. Ann Intern Med. 1987;106:538–45.
404. Virelizier J-L, Lenoir G, Griscelli C. Persistent Epstein-Barr virus infection in a child with hypergammaglobulinemia and immunoblastic proliferation associated with a selective defect in immune interferon secretion. Lancet. 1978;2:231–4.
405. Birx DL, Redfield RR, Tosato G. Defective regulation of Epstein-Barr virus infection in patients with acquired immunodeficiency syndrome (AIDS) or AIDS-related disorders. N Engl J Med. 1986;314:874–9.
406. Ennis FA, Yi-Hua Q, Riley D, et al. HLA-restricted virus-specific cytotoxic T-lymphocyte responses to live and inactivated influenza vaccines. Lancet. 1981;2:88–91.
407. McMichael AJ, Gotch FM, Noble GR, et al. Cytotoxic T-cell immunity to influenza. N Engl J Med. 1983;309:13–7.
408. Ennis FA, Martin J, Verbonitz MW, et al. Specificity studies on cytotoxic thymus-derived lymphocytes reactive with influenza virus-infected cells: Evidence for dual recognition of H-2 and viral hemagglutinin antigens. Proc Natl Acad Sci USA. 1977;74:3006–10.
409. Walker CM, Moody DJ, Stites, DP, et al. CD8 lymphocytes can control HIV infection in vitro by suppressing virus replication. Science. 1986;234:1563–6.
410. Walker BD, Chakrabarti S, Moss B, et al. HIV-specific cytotoxic T lymphocytes in seropositive individuals. Nature. 1987;328:345–8.
411. Wong GHW, Krowka FJ, Stites DP, et al. In vitro anti-human immunodeficiency virus activities of tumor necrosis factor-α and interferon-γ. J Immunol. 1988;140:120–4.
412. Folks TM, Justement J, Kinter A, et al. Cytokine-induced expression of HIV-1 in a chronically infected promonocyte cell line. Science. 1987; 238:800–2.
413. Oldstone MBA, Tishon A, Buchmeier MJ. Virus-induced alterations in homeostasis and differentiated functions of infected cells in vivo. Science. 1982;218:1125–9.
414. Hemachudha T, Phanuphak P, Sriwanthana B, et al. Immunologic study of human encephalitic and paralytic rabies. Am J Med. 1988;84:563–77.
415. Nathan CF, Kaplan G, Levis WR, et al. Local and systemic effects of intradermal recombinant interferon-γ in patients with lepromtous leprosy. N Engl J Med. 1986;315:6–15.
416. Nathan CF, Horowitz CR, de la Harpe, et al. Administration of recombinant interferon-γ to cancer patients enhances monocyte secretion of hydrogen peroxide. Proc Natl Acad Sci USA. 1985;82:8686–90.
417. Maluish AE, Urba WJ, Gordon K, et al. Determination of an optimal biological response modifying dose of interferon gamma in melanoma patients (Abstract). In: Abstracts of the Proceedings of the American Society of Chemotherapy and Oncology. V. 6. Chicago: American Society of Chemotherapy and Oncology, 1987:251.
418. Kleinerman ES, Kurzrock R, Wyatt D, et al. Activation or suppression of the tumoricidal properties of monocytes from cancer patients following treatment with human recombinant γ-interferon. Cancer Res. 1986;46:5401–5.
419. Murray HW, Scavuzzo D, Jacobs JL, et al. In vitro and in vivo activation of human mononuclear phagocytes by gamma interferon: Studies with normal and AIDS monocytes. J Immunol. 1987;138:2457–62.
420. Lane HC, Sherwin SA, Masur H, et al. A phase I trial of recombinant immune (γ) interferon in patients with the acquired immunodeficiency syndrome (Abstract). Clin Res. 1985;33:408.
421. Parkin JM, Eales LJ, Moshtael O, et al. A preliminary report of the use of interferon-gamma in patients with the acquired immune deficiency syndrome. In: Staquet MJ, Hemmer R, Baert AE, eds. Clinical Aspects of AIDS and AIDS-Related Complex. Oxford: Oxford University Press, 1986:167–74.
422. Murray HW, Roberts RB. Interferon-γ and interleukin 2 treatment in AIDS: Clinical toxicity and T lymphocyte effects (Abstract). Clin Res. 1987;35:610.
423. Ezekowitz RAB, Orkin SH, Newburger PE. Recombinant interferon gamma augments phagocyte superoxide production and XO chronic granulomatous disease gene expression in X-linked variant chronic granulomatous disease. J Clin Invest. 1987;80:1009–16.
423a Ezekowitz RAB, Newburger PE. New perspectives in chronic granulomatous disease. J Clin Immunol. 1988;8:419–425
423b Sechler JMG, Malech HL, White CJ, Gallin JI. Recombinant human interferon-γ reconstitutes defective phagocyte function in patients with chronic granulomatous disease of childhood. Proc Natl Acad Sci USA. 1988;85:4874–78.
424. Welte K, Mertelsmann T. Human interleukin 2: Biochemistry, physiology, and possible pathogenetic role in immunodeficiency syndromes. Cancer Invest. 1985;3:35–49.
425. Rosenberg SA, Lotze MT, Muul LM, et al. Observations on the systemic administration of autologous lymphokine activated killer cells and recombinant interleukin-2 to patients with metastatic cancer. N Engl J Med. 1985;313:1485–92.
426. Denicoff KD, Rubinow DR, Papa MZ, et al. The neuropsychiatric effects of treatment with interleukin-2 and lymphokine-activated killer cells. Ann Intern Med. 1987;107:293–300.
427. Flexner C, Hugin A, Moss B. Prevention of vaccinia virus infection in immunodeficient mice by vector-directed IL-2 expression. Nature. 1987; 330:259–62.
428. Ramshaw IA, Andrew ME, Phillips SM, et al. Recovery of immunodeficient mice from a vaccinia virus/IL-2 recombinant infection. Nature. 1987; 329:545–6.
429. Groopman JE, Mitsuyasu RT, DeLeo MJ, et al. Effect of recombinant human granulocyte–macrophage colony-stimulating factor on myelopoiesis in the acquired immunodeficiency syndrome. N Engl J Med. 1987;317:593–8.
430. Brandt SJ, Peters WP, Atwater SK, et al. Effect of recombinant human granulocyte–macrophage colony-stimulating factor on hematopoietic reconstitution after high-dose chemotherapy and autologous bone marrow transplantation. N Engl J Med. 1988;318:869–76.
431. Cerami A, Beutler B. The role of cachectin/TNF in endotoxic shock and cachexia. Immunol Today. 1988;9:28–31.
432. Balow M, Hyman LR. Combination immunotherapy in chronic mucocutaneous candidiasis; synergism between transfer factor and fetal thymus tissue. Clin Immunol Immunopathol. 1977;8:504.
433. Steele RW, Myers MG, Vincent MM. Transfer factor for the prevention of varicella-zoster infection in childhood leukemia. N Engl J Med. 1980;1303–355.
434. MacFadden DK, Hyland RH, Inouye T, et al. Corticosteroids as adjunctive therapy in treatment of *Pneumocystis carinii* pneumonia in patients with acquired immunodeficiency syndrome. Lancet. 1987;1:1477–9.
435. Scott GB. Management of HIV infection in children. In: Schimazi RF, Nahmias AJ, eds. AIDS in Children Adolescents, and Heterosexual Adults. Amsterdam: Elsevier; 1988:264–70.
436. Rogers MF, Thomas PA, Starcher ET, et al. Acquired immunodeficiency syndrome in children: Report of the Centers for Disease Control national surveillance, 1982 to 1985. Pediatrics. 1987;79:1008–14.
437. Wilson CB. Developmental Immunology and Role of Host Defenses in Neonatal Susceptibility. Philadelphia: WB Saunders Co; in press.
438. Wilson CB, Westall J, Johnston L, et al. Decreased production of interferon-gamma by human neonatal cells. J Clin Invest. 1986;77:860–7.
439. Lewis DB, Wilson CB. Molecular basis for decreased interleukin-4 (IL4) and interferon-gamma (IFNγ) production by neonatal T cells. Pediatr Res. 1988;23:356A.
440. Handzel ZT, Levin S, Dolphin Z, et al. Immune competence of newborn lymphocytes. Pediatrics. 1980;65:491.
441. Thorley-Lawson DA. The transformation of adult but not newborn human lymphocytes by Epstein-Barr virus and phytohemagglutinin is inhibited by interferon: The early suppression by T cells of Epstein-Barr infection is mediated by interferon. J Immunol. 1981;1126:829–33.
442. Zawatzky R, DeMaeyer E, Kirchner H. The role of interferon in the resistance of C57BL/6 mice to various doses of herpes simplex virus type 1. J Infect Dis. 1982;146:405–10.
443. Pedersen EB, Haahr S, Mogensen SC. X-linked resistance of mice to high doses of herpes simplex virus type 2 correlates with early interferon production. Infect Immun. 1983;142:740–6.

444. Trofatter KF, Daniels CA, Williams RJ, et al. Growth of type 2 herpes simplex virus in newborn and adult mononuclear leukocytes. Intervirology. 1979;11:117–25.
445. Mintz L, Drew WL, Hoo R, et al. Age-dependent resistance of human alveolar macrophages to herpes simplex virus. Infect Immun. 1980;28:417.
446. Cottman GW, Westall J, Corey L, et al. Replication of HSV2 in mononuclear phagocytes from newborns and adults. Clin Res. 1984;32:108A.
447. Ching C, Lopez C. Natural killing of herpes simplex virus type 1-infected target cells: normal human responses and influence of antiviral antibody. Infect Immun. 1979;26:49–56.
448. Perussia B, Starr S, Abraham S, et al. Human natural killer cells analyzed by B73.1, a monoclonal antibody blocking Fc receptor functions. J Immunol. 1983;130:2133–41.
449. Joris F, Girard JP. Immune response in aged and young subjects following administration of large doses of tuberculin. Int Arch Allergy Appl Immunol. 1975;48:584.
450. Gillis S, Kozak R, Durante M, et al. Decreased production of and response to T cell growth factor by lymphocytes from aged humans. J Clin Invest. 1981;67:937–42.
451. Gardner ID. The effect of aging on susceptibility to infection. Rev Infect Dis. 1980;2:801–10.
452. Brunham RC, Martin DH, Hubbard TW, et al. Depression of the lymphocyte transformation response to microbial antigens and to phytohemagglutinin during pregnancy. J Clin Invest. 1983;72:1629–38.
453. Reinherz EL, Cooper MD, Schlossman SF, et al. Abnormalities of T cell maturation and regulation in human beings with immunodeficiency disorders. J Clin Invest. 1981;68:699.
454. Brahmi Z. Nature of natural killer cell hyporesponsiveness in the Chediak-Higashi syndrome. In: Human Immunology. V. 6. New York: Elsevier; 1983:45.
455. Polmar SH, Stern RC, Schwartz AL, et al. Enzyme replacement therapy for adenosine deaminase deficiency and severe combined immunodeficiency. N Engl J Med. 1976;295:1337.
456. Stoop JW, Zegers BJM, Hendricks GFM, et al. Purine nucleoside deficiency associated with selective cellular immunodeficiency. N Engl J Med. 1977;296:651.
457. Girot R, Hamet M, Perignon JL, et al. Cellular immune deficiency in two siblings with hereditary orotic aciduria. N Engl J Med. 1983;308:700.
458. Lockitch G, Singh VK, Putterman ML, et al. Age-related changes in humoral and cell-mediated immunity in Down syndrome children living at home. Pediatr Res. 1987;22:536–40.
459. Anderson DC, Schmalsteig FC, Finegold MJ, et al. The severe and moderate phenotypes of heritable Mac-1, LFA-1 deficiency: Their quantitative definition and relation to leukocyte dysfunction and clinical features. J Infect Dis. 1985;152:668–89.
460. Gallin JI, Buescher S, Seligmann BE, et al. Recent advances in chronic granulomatous disease. Ann Intern Med. 1983;99:657–74.
461. Peerless AG, Liebhaber M, Anderson S, et al. Legionella pneumonia in chronic granulomatous disease. J Pediatr. 1985;106:783–5.
462. Mackowiak PA. Microbial synergism in human infections. N Engl J Med. 1978;298:21.
463. Pike MC, Daniels CA, Sydnerman R. Influenza-induced depression of monocyte chemotaxis: Reversal by levamisole. Cell Immunol. 1977;32:234–40.
464. Warshauer D, Goldstein E, Akers T, et al. Effect of influenza viral infection on the ingestion and killing of bacteria by alveolar macrophages. Am Rev Respir Dis. 1977;115:269–77.
465. Rouse BT, Horohov DW. Immunosuppression in viral infections. Rev Infect Dis. 1986;8:850–73.
466. Arneborn P, Biberfeld G. T-lymphocyte subpopulations in relation to immunosuppression in measles and varicella. Infect Immun. 1983;39:29–37.
467. Roberts NJ. Different effects of influenza virus, respiratory syncytial virus, and Sendai virus on huuman lymphocytes and macrophages. Infect Immun. 1982;35:1142–6.
468. Roberts NJ, Diamond ME, Douglas RG, et al. Mitogen responses and interferon production after exposure of human macrophages to infections and inactivated influenza viruses. J Med Virol. 1980;5:17–23.
469. Roberts NJ, Prill AH, Mann TN. Interleukin 1 and interleukin 1 inhibitor production by human macrophages exposed to influenza virus or respiratory syncytial virus. J Exp Med. 1986;163:511–9.
470. Cate TR, Couch RB. Lack of effect of influenza virus infection on induction and expression of delayed hypersensitivity. J Infect Dis. 1981;144:280.
471. Gardner ID, Lawton JWM. Depressed human monocyte function after influenza infection in vitro. J Reticuloendothel Soc 1982;32:443–48.
472. Nugent KM, Pesanti EL. Effect of influenza infection on the phagocytic and bactericidal activities of pulmonary macrophages. Infect Immun. 1979; 26:651–7.
473. Carney WP, Rubin RH, Hoffman RA, et al. Analysis of T lymphocyte subsets in cytomegalovirus mononucleosis. J Immunol. 1981;126:2114.
474. Nussenzweig RS. Parasitic disease as a cause of immunosuppression. N Engl J Med. 1982;306:423–4.
475. Luft BJ, Kansas G, Engleman EG, et al. Functional and quantitative alterations in T lymphocyte subpopulations in acute toxoplasmosis. J Infect Dis. 1984;150:761–7.
476. Gibreath MJ, Pavanand K, Macdermott RP, et al. Characterization of cold reactive lymphocytotoxic antibodies in malaria. Clin Exp Immunol. 1983; 51:232.
477. Gaines JD, Gilmer MA, Remington JS. Deficiency of lymphocyte antigen recognition in Hodgkin's disease. In: International Symposium on Hodgkin's Disease. National Cancer Institute Monograph 36. 1973:117.
478. Twomey JJ, Laughter AH, Farrow S, et al. Hodgkin's disease: An immunodepleting and immunosuppressive disorders. J Clin Invest. 1975;56:467.
479. Engleman EJ, Benike CJ, Hoppe RT, et al. Autologous mixed lymphocyte reaction in patients with Hodgkin's disease. J Clin Invest. 1980;66:149.
480. Szuro-Sudol A, Murray HW, Nathan CF. Suppression of macrophage antimicrobial activity by a tumor cell product. J Immunol. 1983;131:384.
481. Fauci AS, Dale DC, Balow JE. Glucocorticosteroid therapy: Mechanisms of action and clinical considerations (NIH conference). Ann Intern Med. 1976;84:304.
482. Frenkel JK, Nelson BM, Arias-Stella J. Immunosuppression and toxoplasmic encephalitis, clinical experimental aspects. Hum Pathol. 1975;6:97.
483. Bodey GP, Hersh EM, Valdivieso M, et al. Effects of cytotoxic and immunosupressive agents on the immune system. Postgrad Med. 1975;58:67.
484. Lew W, Oppenheim JJ, Matsushima K. Analysis of the suppression of IL-1α and Il-1β production in human peripheral blood mononuclear adherent cells by a glucocorticoid hormone. J Immunol. 1988;140:1895–1902.
485. Schaffner A, Schaffner T. Glucocorticoid-induced impairment of macrophage antimicrobial activity: Mechanisms and dependence on the stage of activation. Rev Infect Dis. 1987;9:S620–9.
486. Preiksatitis JK, Rosno G, Grumet C, et al. Infections due to herpesviruses in cardiac transplant recipients: Role of the donor heart and immunosuppressive therapy. J Infect Dis. 1983;147:974.
487. Wilson CB, Jacobs RF, Smith AL. Cellular antibiotic pharmacology. Semin Perinatol. 1982;6:205–13.
488. Hauser WE, Remington JS. Effects of antibiotics on the immune response. Am J Med. 1982;72:711–6.
489. Britton S, Palacios R. Cyclosporin A: Usefulness, risks and mechanism of action. Immunol Rev. 1982;65:5.
490. Manger B, Hardy KJ, Weiss A, et al. Differential effect of cyclosporin A on activation signaling in human T cell lines. J Clin Invest. 1986;77:1501–6.
491. Bickel M, Tsuda H, Amstad P, et al. Differential regulation of colony-stimulating factors and interleukin 2 production by cyclosporin A. Proc Natl Acad Sci USA. 1987;84:3274–7.
492. Alevy YG, Hutcheson P, Mueller KR, et al. Suppressor alveolar macrophages in experimentally induced uremia. J Reticuloendothel Soc. 1983; 33:11.
493. MacCuish AC, Urbaniak SJ, Campbell CJ, et al. Phytohemagglutinin transformation and a circulating lymphocyte subpopulation in insulin-dependent diabetic patients. Diabetes. 1974;23:708.
494. Vose BM, Mondgil GC. Postoperative depression of antibody dependent lymphocyte cytotoxicity following minor surgery and anesthesia. Immunology. 1976;30:123.
495. Kataria YP, Sagne AL, LoBuglio AR, et al. In vitro observations on sarcoid lymphocytes and their correlation with cutaneous anergy and clinical severity of disease. Am Rev Respir Dis. 1973;108:767.
496. Lieberman J, Kaneshiro W. Abnormal response of cultured lymphocytes to phytohemagglutinin and autologous serum in cystic fibrosis. Am Rev Respir Dis. 1977;116:1047.
497. Sugarman B. Zinc and infection. Rev Infect Dis. 1983;5:137.
498. Ballester OF, Prasad AS. Anergy, zinc deficiency, and decreased nucleoside phosphorylase activity in patients with sickle cell anemia. Ann Intern Med. 1983;98:180.
499. Chandra RK. Nutrition, immunity and infection: Present knowledge and future directions. Lancet. 1983;1:688–91.
500. Keusch GT, Scrimshaw NS. Selective primary health care strategies for control for disease in the developing world. XXIII. Control of infection to reduce the prevalence of infantile and childhood malnutrition. Rev Infect Dis. 1986;8:273–87.
501. Beisei WR, Edelman R, Nauss K, et al. Single-nutrient effects on immunologic functions. JAMA. 1981;1:53–8.
502. Koff WC, Dunegan MA. Neuroendocrine hormones suppress macrophage-mediated lysis of herpes simplex virus-infected cells. J Immunol. 1986;136:705–9.
503. Mary D, Aussel C, Ferrua B, et al. Regulation of interleukin 2 synthesis by cAMP in human T cells. J Immunol. 1987;4:1179–84.
504. Bernton EW, Meltzer MS, Holaday JW. Suppression of macrophage activation and T-lymphocyte function in hypoprolactinemic mice. Science. 1988;239:401–4.
505. Brown SL, VanEpps DE. Opioid peptides modulate production of interferon-γ by human mononuclear cells. Cell Immunol. 1986;103:1926.
506. Kern JA, Lamb RJ, Reed JC, et al. Dexamethasone inhibition of interleukin-1 beta production by human monocytes. J Clin Invest. 1988;81:237–44.
507. Seemayer TA, Gartner JG, Lapp WA. The graft versus host reaction. Hum Pathol. 1983;14:3.
508. Cooper MD, Lawton AR. Immune deficiency diseases. In: Braunwald E, Isselbacher KJ, Petersdorf RG, et al, eds. Harrison's Principles of Internal Medicine. 11th ed. New York: McGraw-Hill; 1987:1385–92.

9. EVALUATION OF THE PATIENT WITH SUSPECTED IMMUNODEFICIENCY

DANIEL ROTROSEN
JOHN I. GALLIN

Pediatricians, internists, and infectious disease specialists are occasionally involved in the diagnostic evaluation of the patient with suspected immunodeficiency. With the exception of the acquired immunodeficiency syndrome (AIDS), the well-characterized immunodeficiency syndromes are, for the most part, exceedingly uncommon. As a result, physicians generally lack the clinical experience to readily recognize these disorders or proceed toward a diagnosis in an orderly, stepwise fashion. Our experience at a referral center specializing in phagocytic cell disorders suggests that simple, inexpensive, and widely available tests are underused in the initial evaluation of patients with suspected defects in host defense mechanisms. Furthermore, many texts describe a bewildering array of specialized procedures to assess immune function, but their diagnostic utility is limited, and specific guidelines for their application are neither available nor uniformly accepted. As a result, the correct diagnosis may be unduly delayed and patients subjected to repetitive, costly, and inappropriate testing.

With the exception of transplantation of immunocompetent tissue in severe combined immunodeficiency, curative therapy is not available for any of the primary immunodeficiency disorders, and adequate replacement or immunomodulatory treatments remain remote possibilities in all but a few. Nonetheless, a diligent attempt at specific diagnosis still seems warranted in all cases of suspected immunodeficiency. Early diagnosis is critical in treatable forms of severe immunodeficiency to prevent life-threatening infections and morbid complications. In several instances the underlying defects are now understood at a biochemical level, and genes encoding missing or defective proteins have been cloned. Recognition of heterozygote carriers is important for early (in some cases, antenatal) diagnosis and essential for sound genetic counseling. The rare immunodeficiency diseases are rightly viewed as "experiments in nature," and further advances will certainly depend on continued identification of individuals with these disorders. Finally, as in other areas of medicine, earlier diagnosis of affected individuals is likely to result in lesser morbidity and mortality, even without the advent of specific therapies.

GOALS IN THE INITIAL EVALUATION OF PATIENTS WITH SUSPECTED IMMUNODEFICIENCY

Clinical evaluation of patients with recurrent or unusual infections should be grounded on the realization that nearly all of the primary immunodeficiencies are uncommon. Appropriate goals in the initial screening of such patients include the following: (*1*) recognition of clinical features truly indicative of an abnormal frequency or severity of infection and differentiation of these from the range of normal, (*2*) early identification of features suggestive of defects in nonspecific host defense mechanisms (integrity of normal mucocutaneous barriers or clearance mechanisms, for example) that may direct the immediate evaluation away from the immune system, and (*3*) recognition of clinical features suggestive of defects within a particular limb of immune defenses. In addition, a realistic goal in the initial laboratory evaluation of such patients is to expeditiously gather data sufficient to profile immune function despite the fact that neither a precise classification nor specific therapy may be an immediate possibility. These aims should take into account the likelihood that thorough evaluation, accurate diagnosis, and management of patients with unusual, poorly characterized, or clinically severe primary immunodeficiencies are often possible only in specialized research facilities.

INITIAL CLINICAL SCREENING

Despite thorough evaluation the vast majority of patients in whom an immunodeficiency is suspected on the basis of a history of chronic or recurrent infection will not have a clearly defined disorder. A detailed history is always indicated to determine the frequency and severity of infections, sites and organ systems involved, etiologic agents, and age at onset. As a rule, severe congenital immunodeficiencies present with life-threatening infection within the first year of life. In most congenital immunodeficiencies, a convincing history of recurrent or unusual infection dates to early childhood, although in some disorders patients with clinically less severe "variants" may not be recognized until adolescence. Primary immunodeficiency with clinical onset in adulthood occurs (e.g., common variable hypogammaglobulinemia and hypogammaglobulinemia with thymoma) but is the exception.

It is important to appreciate that normal school-age children may have 6–12 respiratory infections per year.[1] Attack rates decline with age and reach adult rates of two to four infections per year by adolescence.[1,2] Furthermore, common colds, nonnecrotizing pharyngitis, and tonsillitis are rarely if ever serious problems in individuals with well-characterized immunodeficiencies. Recurrent skin infections due to gram-positive cocci, without a history of extracutaneous infection, are rarely indicative of immunodeficiency. Likewise, recurrent urinary tract and biliary tree infections suggest obstructive lesions and are unlikely to be due to defects in immune defense mechanisms. Factitious illness may warrant consideration in adults with recurrent infection.

A thorough family history is essential to document consanguinity, to identify risk factors for vertical transmission of AIDS, and to identify relatives with recurrent infections, connective tissue disorders, malignancies, and early demise. Laboratory evaluation of family members may be necessary to assess modes of inheritance and to provide a data base for appropriate genetic counseling.

The clinical presentation may be indicative of deficiencies within a particular limb of host defense. The guidelines in Table 1 and the following discussion are generally useful in directing the emphasis to a given system and in suggesting common disorders of nonimmune defenses that should be excluded. However, due to the complex interdependencies embodied in the immune response there may be considerable overlap in the clinical features of disorders arising from pathophysiologically discrete but functionally interrelated defects in host defenses. For this reason, a complete and encompassing algorithm for the evaluation of patients with suspected immunodeficiency is probably neither possible nor advisable.

Recurrent sinopulmonary infections, meningitis, and bacteremia due to encapsulated organisms suggest deficiencies of complement or antibody and certain types of phagocytic cell dysfunction. In the absence of pneumonia, chronic otitis media, or systemic infection, recurrent sinusitis alone is rarely indicative of immunodeficiency because it occurs so frequently in normal individuals. In such patients anatomic abnormalities of the sinuses and allergic disorders should be considered potential contributing factors. Bronchial obstruction, underlying cystic and cavitary diseases, and disorders of bronchopulmonary clearance such as cystic fibrosis and immotile cilia syndrome should be considered in patients with recurrent pneumonia. Recurrent pneumonia in the same pulmonary lobe suggests an anatomic abnormality as opposed to immunodeficiency.

Recurrent staphylococcal skin infection associated with subcutaneous extension or deep-organ infection suggests phago-

TABLE 1. Common Clinical Syndromes Associated with Immune Deficiency

	Common Clinical Syndromes
B lymphocytes	Sinopulmonary infection due to encapsulated bacteria, chronic otitis media Giardiasis Repeated episodes of common viral illnesses[3] Chronic enteroviral encephalitis[4–7]
Complement	Sinopulmonary infection due to encapsulated bacteria, chronic otitis Neisserial bacteremia and meningitis Autoimmune syndromes, glomerulonephritis
Phagocytic cells	
CR3 deficiency	Delayed separation of the umbilical stump, patent urachus Leukocytosis, necrotizing infections without pus, periodontitis, pneumonitis, perianal abscesses
Chronic granulomatous disease	Infection due to catalase-positive bacteria (e.g., staphylococci, (Enterobacteriaceae), *Nocardia, Candida, Aspergillus* Cellulitis, suppurative lymphadenitis, draining sinuses, osteomyelitis, visceral and brain abscesses, periodontitis Recurrent granulomas
Chédiak-Higashi syndrome Neutrophil-specific granule deficieny	Moderate neutropenia Skin and deep-organ bacterial infection (no particular class of organisms) Periodontitis Oculocutaneous albinism and neuropathy (CHS only)
Myeloperoxidase deficiency	No significant increased susceptibility to infection (perhaps fungal infection in association with immunocompromising systemic illness, e.g., diabetes mellitus)
T lymphocytes	Disseminated infection due to intracellular pathogens, protozoans, opportunistic fungi, normally benign DNA viruses Protracted diarrhea, eczema, endocrinopathy Graft-vs.-host disease after transfusions Malignancies

cytic cell dysfunction. Children with clinically significant phagocytic cell defects generally have moderate to severe periodontal disease, a finding usually lacking in individuals with recurrent skin infections but without phagocyte dysfunction.[8] Most patients with recurrent infection limited to the skin do not have a significant or well-characterized immunodeficiency. In such patients other predisposing factors should be sought. These include chronic nasal carriage of staphylococci phage identical to those in the lesions, needle use, draining sinuses, apocrine gland obstruction, foreign bodies, and chronic excoriating or bullous skin disorders.

Disseminated infection with intracellular pathogens, protozoans, opportunistic fungi, or ordinarily benign viruses strongly suggests defective cell-mediated immunity. Hypocalcemia in the newborn (in DiGeorge syndrome) or intrauterine graft-vs.-host disease (scaling erythroderma and total alopecia) are useful early signs of severe T-cell deficiency. Children with primary disorders of cell-mediated immunity may have failure to thrive, wasting, diarrhea, severe eczema, chronic mucocutaneous candidiasis, a high incidence of malignancies, and early demise.[5–7] This clinical presentation is so striking that confusion with infectious illnesses in immunocompetent individuals is usually not an issue.

CLINICAL AND LABORATORY ASSESSMENT OF B-CELL FUNCTION

Specific humoral immunodeficiency syndromes are considered in detail in Chapters 5 and 6. Antibody deficiencies are the most common and constitute approximately one-half of patients with primary immunodeficiencies.

With rare exceptions, deficiency of humoral immunity is accompanied by decreased levels of one or more classes of serum immunoglobulin. The widely available techniques to measure immunoglobulins use commercially available and well-standardized, immunoglobulin class-specific antisera. Most clinical laboratories quantitate immunoglobulins by radial diffusion or nephelometrically by determination of changes in light scattering that occur in dilute solutions of immunoglobulin on mixing with class-specific antisera. Nephelometry may yield spurious results in the presence of circulating immune complexes, but for most clinical purposes the techniques are essentially equivalent.[9,10] IgE is measured by radioimmunoassay. While immunoelectrophoresis allows detection of three immunoglobulin classes, it is not quantitative and is not a satisfactory technique for the measurement of immunoglobulins. Because serum immunoglobulin concentrations vary among normal individuals and with age, difficulties arise in defining the lower limits of normal. Reasonable estimates for low normal values in adults are 40 mg/dl for IgM, 500 mg/dl for IgG, and 50 mg/dl for IgA; serum immunoglobulins are detectable in the primary hypogammaglobulinemic and agammaglobulinemic disorders but are below the 95 percent confidence limits for age- and race-matched controls. Corresponding normal values in prepubertal children are ≈30–80 percent of adult levels and increase with age.[3,10–12] In protein-losing states with depression of immunoglobulins, IgM levels usually remain normal or are only slightly diminished. Simultaneous determination of serum albumin and transferrin levels may be helpful in identifying these conditions.

A major goal of screening for antibody deficiency is the identification of the subset of patients in whom replacement therapy will be helpful. In all such situations the benefits of therapy (i.e., provision of protective antibody) need to be weighed against the potential risks (suppression of endogenous antibody formation and induction of anti-IgG allotype antibodies). As a general rule, patients with B-cell disorders in which replacement therapy is indicated do not have IgG or IgM antibodies. Knowledge of the IgA concentration is also of pivotal help in guiding initial evaluation because a normal serum IgA content excludes not only isolated IgA deficiency but all of the permanent types of agammaglobulinemia since IgA is low or absent in those conditions as well.[4,6]

Humoral immunodeficiency may exist in the presence of normal or near-normal concentrations of most or all five immunoglobulin classes, as demonstrated by patients with the Wiskott-Aldrich syndrome.[5,6,13] In the presence of borderline immunoglobulin concentrations or if the suspicion of antibody deficiency is strong, humoral immunity should be assessed by responses to "natural" antigens to which the population is commonly exposed or after active immunization. Active immunization should be considered as a diagnostic maneuver only with the following caveats: (*1*) live vaccines (Calmette-Guérin bacillus [BCG], poliomyelitis, measles, rubella, mumps, and smallpox) should never be given when primary or severe secondary immunodeficiency is suspected, (*2*) polysaccharide antigens are ineffective in infants less than 1 year old, (*3*) the capacity to make antibody to T-cell-independent polysaccharide antigens is acquired late in infancy and results in predominantly IgM responses associated with little immunologic memory, and (*4*) immunization of infants (as opposed to adults) with protein antigens results primarily in the production of IgM antibodies with a relatively slow progression to an IgG response.[5,14–16]

Nearly all hospital blood banks can measure isohemagglutinins. These are predominantly IgM antibodies (normally detectable in infants by 6 months of age) against bacterial polysaccharides cross-reactive with type A and B red blood cells. Most hospital laboratories can also measure anti-streptolysin O and febrile agglutinins. Antibody against typhoid H and O antigens can be measured before and after immunization with typhoid vaccine. Production of diphtheria toxin-specific IgG can be demonstrated by the Schick test, and most state and local health department laboratories can titer antibodies to common viral agents, diphtheria/tetanus toxoid, *Escherichia coli*, and pneumococcal polysaccharides. Except in previously unimmunized children, antigen challenge assesses the capacity for secondary (recall) responses. If results are normal, the patient is unlikely to have a clinically significant deficit in antibody production. The primary response can be assessed on an investigational basis by using keyhole limpet hemocyanin, or bacteriophage φX174.[7,17] The use of bacteriophage φX174 demonstrates the capacity for isotype switch (T cell dependent) and allows quantitation of antigen clearance and an assessment of primary and secondary responses. Based on these responses, identification of those who will benefit from IgG replacement is possible. A presumptive diagnosis of B-cell deficiency can be made in the neonate since healthy subjects clear bacteriophage φX174 immediately whereas abnormal subjects show phage persistence for more than 1 week.[17]

IgA deficiency may occur in association with isolated deficits in specific IgG subclasses. In these cases, specific subclass determinations may be necessary to demonstrate the deficiency. Unfortunately, antisera suitable for subclass determinations are neither widely available nor well standardized. An effort by the World Health Organization is likely to improve this situation in the near future.[7] It is important to assess the severity of the deficiency in such individuals by measuring the recall response to a panel of antigens. Because safe replacement therapy (i.e., subclass-specific IgG) is not available, failure to identify patients with deficits in specific IgG subclasses but without severe antibody deficiency is of limited clinical impact.

Measuring levels of antigen-specific antibody may be useful in particular settings. For example, high titers of *Staphylococcus aureus*- and *Candida*-specific IgE or low titers of *S. aureus*-specific IgA may be useful in distinguishing patients with hyperimmunoglobulin E (Job) syndrome from those with atopy, chronic eczema, and elevated IgE levels.[18]

Circulating B cells can be quantitated by immunofluorescence; the information obtained may be useful in classification but is usually not critical to an initial assessment of the level of immunodeficiency. In an investigational setting, mitogen-driven B-cell proliferation has been useful in characterizing B-cell defects and T-''helper'' and -''suppressor'' function in humoral immunodeficiency, but is not generally useful in initial screening.

TABLE 2. Delayed Cutaneous Hypersensitivity Testing (DCH)

Agent	*Dilution*[a]	*Comments*
Tuberculin	2 IU Tween-stabilized PPD	If negative, repeat with 50 IU
Candida[b]	1:100	If no reaction, repeat with 1:10 dilution
Trichophyton[b]	1:30	
Mumps[c]	Undiluted	Read at 6–8 hr for early Arthus reaction (antibody mediated) Read at 48 hr for DCH
Tetanus/diphtheria toxoids[d]	1:100	Ascertain immunization status, repeat DCH testing after active immunization if initially negative
Keyhole limpet hemocyanin[a]	100 ug	DCH testing 2 wk after subcutaneous immuniztion with 2.5 mg KLH

[a] All skin tests intradermal injection of 0.1 ml of antigen diluted in Hollister-Stier–buffered saline.
[b] Hollister-Stier Laboratories.
[c] Mumps skin test, Eli Lilly & Company. Immunization with live viral vaccines is contraindicated in all patients with severe combined or cell-mediated immunodeficiency.
[d] Pediatric diphtheria and tetanus toxoid, Wyeth Laboratories.
[e] Sigma Chemical Company or Calbiochem-Behring, not currently licensed by FDA for use in humans.
(Data from Rosen et al.[7] and deShazo et al.[9])

TABLE 3. In Vitro Lymphocyte Proliferation

Stimulus	*Interpretation*
Mitogens	
Phytohemagglutinin Concanavalin A Anti-thymocyte globulin	Nonspecific stimulation of both helper and suppressor subsets, predominantly T-cell mitogens in humans; response indicates that some of the normal populations are present.
Pokeweed	Stimulates T cells for B-cell help required for immunoglobulin synthesis and secretion.
Staphylococcus aureus (Cowan I strain)	Direct stimulation of B-cell proliferation and polyclonal activation.
Allogenic lymphocytes	Proliferative stimulus to T-helper cells resulting in generation of specific cytotoxic cells against the stimulating histocompatibility antigens. Response may be normal even in the presence of severe T-cell immunodeficiency.
Antigens	Response requires genetically restricted antigen-presenting cell. Most stringent test of immunologic competence and correlates better with state of health than do other tests.

CLINICAL AND LABORATORY EVALUATION OF CELL-MEDIATED IMMUNITY

Cell-mediated and combined immunodeficiency syndromes are considered in detail in Chapter 8. Cellular deficiencies constitute ≈40 percent of patients with primary immunodeficiencies. Of these, approximately three-quarters have associated antibody deficiencies.

Delayed cutaneous hypersensitivity (DCH) testing represents the most informative and cost-effective approach in the initial evaluation of cell-mediated immunity. All skin tests are by intradermal injection of 0.1 ml of antigen and should be read at 48–72 hours for maximum induration. A positive skin test response, defined as induration greater than 5 mm at 48–72 hours, indicates intact cell-mediated immunity. Erythema is not an indication of DCH. To demonstrate defective cell-mediated immunity several antigens must be used; widely available and commonly used preparations are shown in Table 2. Response to sensitization with dinitrochlorobenzene is no longer recommended because it is mutagenic and causes necrosis.[7] An assessment of response after primary sensitization can be made after immunization with keyhole limpet hemocyanin (KLH), but this is an investigational procedure, and KLH preparations are not currently licensed by the Food and Drug Administration (FDA) for use in humans.

Tuberculin reactivity should be ascertained early in all patients with suspected immunodeficiency to identify those who would benefit from chemoprophylaxis.

For practical purposes, normal DCH responses to a panel of test antigens excludes significant cellular immunodeficiency. With rare exceptions in vitro evaluation of T-cell or macrophage function in such patients is not indicated. Selective anergy to specific pathogens appears to play a role (albeit poorly defined) in the impaired immune response in chronic mucocutaneous candidiasis and lepromatous leprosy,[6,7,19] but with rare exceptions defective cell-mediated immunity is not likely to be a significant factor underlying infection in individuals with otherwise normal DCH responses.

DCH testing is of limited value in infants because of inadequate natural sensitization and because they are uniformly anergic during the first few weeks of life regardless of antigen exposure. However, the total lymphocyte count of peripheral blood is normally ≥1200/mm^3, regardless of age. In infants and patients with absent or borderline DCH, further assessment of cell-mediated immunity generally requires T-cell profiling and in vitro functional testing (Table 3). These tests have been useful in elucidating the basic mechanisms of disease and in classification but are not usually essential for the diagnosis of primary immunodeficiency. In vitro functional responses are influenced by steroid administration; viral, bacterial, and fungal infection; or recent vaccination.[3,6,9] In vitro functional studies should be obtained only after consultation with specialists who have reviewed the clinical aspects of the case and who are familiar with the techniques, limitations, and interpretation of such studies. Recent experience in AIDS suggests that changes in the number of CD4+ ("helper") T cells may be a clinically useful predictor of the relative risk of opportunistic infection, but guidelines for periodic T-lymphocyte profiling, based on controlled studies, are not available in AIDS or in other immunodeficiencies. Limited data suggest that determination of the CD4+/CD8+ cell ratio may be helpful in distinguishing certain primary immunodeficiencies from AIDS, particularly in pediatric patients.[20]

The chest radiograph or tomography may be useful in identifying adults with thymoma. In children the thymic shadow (retrosternal lucency) is more easily appreciated on the lateral chest projection than on the frontal view. However, the absence of a thymic shadow on the chest radiograph is of limited predictive value due to rapid involution in normal infants during a stressful illness.[21] Thymic biopsy and lymph node biopsy may be highly informative in infants with signs of severe immunodeficiency but should be performed by experienced surgeons only after careful consideration of diagnostic alternatives. Biopsy should be performed on rapidly enlarging lymph nodes in any patient with immunodeficiency to exclude infection, malignancy, or lymphoreticular hyperplasia. For standardization, lymph node biopsy should be performed 5–7 days after local antigenic challenge with diphtheria/tetanus toxoids and morphologic assessment based on the published criteria of the World Health Organization.[21]

In particular situations additional studies may be diagnostic of specific immunodeficiency disorders. Erythrocyte adenosine deaminase (ADA) levels should be determined in all infants with the clinical features of severe combined immunodeficiency to exclude ADA deficiency as the underlying biochemical lesion. Early diagnosis and treatment are essential in this instance to prevent significant morbidity. Likewise, purine nucleoside phosphorylase (PNP) levels should be determined in all infants with T-cell deficiency or features of Diamond-Blackfan aplastic anemia.[7,22] Other immunodeficiency disorders that are both treatable and associated with specific and easily demonstrated biochemical lesions include transcobalamine II deficiency and acrodermatitis enteropathica (associated with a deficiency of serum zinc). Serum α-fetoprotein (AFP) levels are helpful in distinguishing ataxia teleangiectasia (AFP levels elevated in ≥95 percent) from other neurologic disorders.[7]

Endocrinopathy associated with disorders of impaired cell-mediated immunity (e.g., chronic mucocutaneous candidiasis) may precede or follow clinically apparent immunodeficiency. In addition, endocrine dysfunction in this setting is progressive, thus necessitating careful observation for treatable endocrine dysfunction in patients with immunodeficiency and vice versa.[23]

The role of a number of cytokines and inflammatory mediators in normal immune function is being increasingly recognized.[24–31] Some of these factors have been characterized at the molecular level and their specific receptors on immunocompetent cells identified. Very likely, immunodeficiency disorders due to a lack (or overproduction) of these factors or their corresponding receptors will eventually be recognized. However, outside of specific investigational settings there are presently no indications for measurement of such factors in serum or tissues.

CLINICAL AND LABORATORY EVALUATION OF PATIENTS WITH SUSPECTED COMPLEMENT DEFICIENCY

The synthesis and function of the components of the complement system are described in detail in Chapter 6 and in recent reviews.[32,33] Complement components do not cross the placenta. Total hemolytic complement (CH_{50}) determinations and the levels of most components in term infants correspond to ≈60–80 percent of normal adult levels; levels of C8 and C9 are lower and correspond to ≈10 percent of normal adult levels.[34]

With the exception of properdin, which is X-linked, complement proteins are encoded by genes inherited in an autosomal codominant fashion.[33,35] Congenital deficiency is the consequence of inheritance of a null allele, which codes for nonsynthesis of the protein.[33] In part due to the prevalence of null alleles, the normal range of complement proteins is broad, usually ±50 percent of the normal mean.[34] Since diminished levels but not the absence of complement proteins are adequate for normal host defense mechanisms, complement deficiency syndromes (with the exception of properdin deficiency) are characterized phenotypically by an apparent autosomal recessive pattern of inheritance. In general, absence of the early components is primarily but not strictly associated with autoimmune disease, thus reflecting the overlapping role of the alternative pathway in protection against bacterial infection. In contrast, deficiencies of late components or alternative-pathway factors generally present with a strikingly increased suseptibility to infection accompanied by less prominent autoimmune manifestations.[33,36] Due to the pivotal role C3 plays in both complement activation pathways and the opsonic and pro-inflammatory properties of C3 fragments, C3 deficiency has among the most severe consequences of all the complement deficiency disorders. All homozygous C3-deficient individuals described to date have experienced serious complications including recurrent infection or autoimmune disorders.[33] Individual complement component deficiencies associated with an increased risk of infection are discussed in detail in Chapter 6.

A CH_{50} determination should be the initial step in the laboratory evaluation of all patients with a suspected complement deficiency. Appropriate sample handling is important. Blood should be allowed to clot at room temperature (cold activation of complement may occur at 0°C), centrifuged at 4°C, and serum frozen in aliquots at −70°C. Deficiencies of classical pathway components profound enough to account for infectious complications are easily detected by the CH_{50} assay, but the test is relatively insensitive to even moderate depression of individual components. The CH_{50} value will be 0 or extremely low in the absence of classical pathway or terminal components.[33] If the CH_{50} value is low, levels of individual components should be measured. In homozygous complement component deficiencies, the deficient component will be essentially absent on either antigenic or functional testing. Heterozygotes usually exhibit below-normal levels on careful antigenic or functional testing for the component in question.[33,34] Ideally, the initial investigation of individual components should be based on the clinical presentation and known gene frequencies. Individual components can be assayed by radial immunodiffusion or nephelometry using commercially available antibodies. Assays for C3 and C4 are widely available; antigenic assays for other components and functional titration of individual components are reliable and sensitive tests but are largely confined to reference laboratories. In contrast to the role of structural variants in C1 inhibitor deficiency (hereditary angioedema), reports of immune impairment due to dysfunctional structural variants are exceedingly rare.[33,35]

Routine CH_{50} determinations do not assess alternative-pathway components. Commercial kits for the assay of factor B and properdin are available, but determinations of these and other alternative pathway components are usually done by specialized facilities.

Simultaneous depression of more than a single complement component argues strongly against a hereditary deficiency and is more consistent with consumptive disorders or diminished complement synthesis.

PHAGOCYTIC CELL DYSFUNCTION

Nearly all of the clinically significant and well-characterized defects in phagocytic cell defenses can be identified by widely available and easily performed screening tests. Specific syndromes and appropriate screening procedures are discussed in the following sections.

Neutrophil Kinetics and Neutropenia

Neutropenia is the most commonly encountered defect in phagocytic cell host defenses. The normal range of peripheral blood neutrophil counts is from 1500 to 8000/mm^3 but can be as low as 1000/mm^3 in healthy black individuals.[37–40] The increased risk of bacterial and fungal infection in patients with profound neutropenia secondary to cytotoxic chemotherapy dramatically underscores the central role that phagocytes play in host defense. A moderate neutropenia commonly accompanies clinically significant T-cell deficiency; the underlying mechanisms are poorly understood. Detailed approaches for the evaluation of causes of neutropenia are provided elsewhere.[38]

A severe neutropenia of the newborn occurs as a result of maternal antibody response to neutrophil-specific antigens. This is a self-limited process resolving over several weeks as maternal antibodies are cleared. However, the risk of infection is significant during the neutropenic period. Similar neutrophil-specific antibodies may occur in autoimmune neutropenia as a primary disorder or in association with other immune disorders such as systemic lupus erythematosus.

A complete blood count and white blood cell differential will identify all patients with neutropenia; sequential testing (3 days per week over an 8- to 12-week period) may be necessary to demonstrate cycling and to document the periodicity and duration of neutropenia. Normal neutrophil counts vary among individuals but remain relatively constant in a particular individual followed over a period of several years. Idiopathic acute neutropenia (particularly in the elderly or debilitated) should prompt a work-up for sepsis, even when other signs of infection are lacking. Bone marrow aspiration and biopsy for histology and culture are essential parts of the work-up of neutropenia but may be delayed in some cases of acute neutropenia where a presumptive cause is obvious and recovery likely.

Screening for autoimmune disease is indicated in all neonates and in patients with chronic neutropenia; the evaluation should include lymphocyte profiling with assessment of natural killer cell number. Anti-neutrophil antibodies should be sought by fluorescence-activated cell sorting using patient serum directed against autologous and normal donor cells and by induction of leukoagglutination in normal neutrophils.[41,42]

Bone marrow biopsy is the most direct and informative procedure to assess myeloid maturation and marrow reserves. Kinetic studies (challenge with endotoxin, steroids, or epinephrine) have been used to evaluate marrow reserves and the size of the marginated pool but require close monitoring by experienced physicians.[37–40] Clinical experience with kinetic studies is limited (relative to bone marrow biopsy), and interpretation of abnormal results can be problematic. Nonetheless, used in an investigational setting these tests have been critical to a current understanding of neutrophil kinetics and will likely be important in evaluating the physiologic response to newly described inflammatory mediators and cytokines.

Chronic Granulomatous Disease

Since the initial descriptions of chronic granulomatous disease (CGD) (see Chapter 7) more than 30 years ago well over 300 cases have been reported.[43–45] This is a rare disorder with a frequency of 1:500,000 to 1:1,000,000. Nonetheless, the disease has engendered tremendous interest as a prototype for abnormalities of phagocyte oxidative metabolism, and elucidation of the underlying defects has been critical to an understanding of the activation, structure, and function of the respiratory burst oxidase. Recent studies indicate that CGD represents a genetically heterogenous group of disorders potentially affecting the entire cascade of events leading to the production of toxic oxygen metabolites.[46,47]

Patients with the "classic" form of CGD develop serious infections due to catalase-positive microorganisms. The onset of serious infections is usually within the first year of life. Common infectious syndromes include pneumonia and lung abscesses, skin and soft tissue infections, lymphadenopathy and suppurative lymphadenitis, visceral abscesses, and osteomyelitis, usually involving the small bones of the hands and feet. Septicemia, meningitis, and brain abscesses are less common. Although severe, infection in CGD may follow a rather indolent course characterized only by malaise, low-grade fever, and a mild leukocytosis, but the erythrocyte sedimentation rate is nearly always elevated during infection. There may be incomplete resolution of the inflammatory process (even after infection has been eliminated) that leads to granuloma formation. The resulting granulomatous lesions occasionally cause esophageal, antral, or genitourinary tract obstruction. "Variant" clinical forms of the disease have been recognized including presentation in adolescence or young adulthood; such patients usually have a history of infection since childhood, although typically less severe than in the "classic" form of the disease.[43–45]

Staphylococcus aureus and gram-negative bacilli account for most infections in CGD, but infection due to *Aspergillus, Candida*, and *Nocardia* is not uncommon. Organisms that produce H_2O_2 but are catalase-negative (e.g., streptococci, pneumococci, and lactobacilli) are not major pathogens in CGD; the persistence of H_2O_2 within the phagosome in concert with host cell myeloperoxidase may result in bactericidal activity against these organisms. Alternatively, oxygen-independent microbicidal mechanisms may be sufficient in CGD to kill certain pathogens. In preliminary studies subcutaneous interferon-γ treatment partially corrected the defects in superoxide production and bactericidal activity in neutrophils obtained from some CGD patients and, in vitro, improved function of their cultured monocytes.[48,49] A multicenter cooperative trial of interferon-γ in CGD has been started.

CGD is X chromosome linked in ≈65 percent of cases and autosomal recessively inherited in ≈35 percent of cases. A kindred with probable autosomal dominant inheritance has been described.[44] As a group, patients with autosomal recessive inheritance may have a less severe clinical course than those with X-linked inheritance, but in the individual patient severity of infectious episodes does not reliably predict the mode of inheritance.

Essentially all patients with CGD can be identified on screening by the nitroblue tetrazolium (NBT) dye reduction test.[43–45] Positive tests (no reduction of NBT by neutrophils) should be confirmed by quantitative determination of superoxide production and an assessment of respiratory burst kinetics. Female carriers can be identified by the NBT slide test with the caveat that certain affected individuals (because of chance inactivation of the normal or defective X chromosome) may display an apparently normal or CGD phenotype. A severe deficiency of glucose-6-phosphate dehydrogenase (G6PD) has been reported to result in the phenotypic expression of CGD. These reports predated current concepts of the molecular and genetic heterogeneity of CGD, and in retrospect, it is thought that such patients probably had autosomal recessive CGD. The clinical features in such cases were attributed to impaired activity of the hexose-monophosphate shunt, which normally furnishes reducing equivalents (NADPH) required for oxidase activity. However, NADPH oxidase activity is normal in G6PD deficiency, and such patients would be readily distinguished from those with classic CGD by the history of severe hemolytic anemia, by quantitation of G6PD, and by a failure to stimulate hexose-monophosphate shunt activity with methylene blue. As recent advances have demonstrated, a more complete understanding of the respiratory burst oxidase and elucidation of the underlying genetic and biochemical defects in CGD will depend on continued identification and investigation of patients with unique lesions.

iC3b Receptor (CR3) Deficiency

The adherence of neutrophils to opsonized particles, endothelial cells, and plastic and glass surfaces is mediated in part by a family of cell surface glycoproteins that includes complement receptor type 3 (CR3), lymphocyte function-associated antigen 1 (LFA-1), and p150,95 (see Chapter 7). Neutrophil CR3 deficiency is associated with abnormalities of adherence-related functions including aggregation, margination, chemotaxis, spreading, and phagocytosis of opsonized particles.[50–52] The clinical features include a history of delayed separation of the umbilical stump and patent urachus (sometimes requiring surgical excision and closure), poor wound healing, and the absence of pus formation in a setting of recurrent bacterial and fungal infections. Focal or spreading skin and subcutaneous infections, otitis, mucositis, gingivitis, and periodontitis are common; systemic and deep-seated infections including meningitis, pneumonitis, and perianal abscess formation occur less frequently. The intravascular marginated pool of neutrophils is absent or markedly diminished in CR3 deficiency, and patients have a persistent neutrophilia even in the absence of infection and a striking leukocytosis (up to $\approx 150{,}000/mm^3$) in its presence. Impaired T-cell cytotoxicity and abnormal B-cell function are also seen.[50,51]

A patient from one kindred who was initially shown to have a disorder of neutrophil actin polymerization was later found to be deficient in CR3 as well.[53,54] Neutrophils deficient in CR3 demonstrate a prolonged respiratory burst[55] and fail to adapt normally to repetitive stimulation with formylpeptide chemoattractants.[56] These observations suggest that the CR3 family of adherence-related glycoproteins may additionally be involved in the modulation of cytoskeletal assembly and receptor processing.

Patients with CR3 deficiency are easily recognized by immunofluorescence microscopy or fluorescence-activated cell sorter analysis using commercially available antibodies to CR3 epitopes.[50,51] Since patients may have moderate or profound deficits in CR3 expression, these tests should be performed by laboratories familiar with their interpretation. In the absence of immediate access to such facilities, presumptive evidence supporting the diagnosis can be obtained by the failure of neutrophils to stick and spread normally on glass or a failure to aggregate, despite shape change, upon stimulation with formylpeptide chemoattractants.[57]

Neutrophil-Specific Granule Deficiency

The first granules to appear during neutrophil maturation are the primary or azurophil granules, which account for about one-third of all granules in the mature cell. Azurophil granules are lysosome-like and contain acid hydrolases and a diverse group of degradative enzymes as well as distinct antimicrobial cationic proteins, the defensins, and bactericidal/permeability increasing factor.[58,59] Azurophil granules function primarily in the intracellular milieu (in the phagolysosomal vacuole) where they are involved in the killing and degradation of microorganisms and ultimately in the inactivation of the inflammatory response.

Neutrophil secondary granules appear at approximately the metamyelocyte stage of maturation and have been designated "specific" by virtue of their unique contents, lactoferrin and vitamin B_{12} binding protein.[60] Lactoferrin facilitates the production of hydroxyl radicals and chelates the iron necessary for microbial growth. In addition, specific granules contain lysozyme and collagenase, components of azurophil granules.[61] Recent evidence supports the existence of a population of gelatinase-containing tertiary granules that undergoes exocytosis in response to mild stimuli.[62,63] Neutrophils also contain an intracellular reservoir of various proteins (including receptors for iC3b, laminin, formylpeptide chemoattractants, signal-transducing G-proteins, cytochrome b_{558}, plasminogen activator, and alkaline phosphatase) whose translocation to the cell surface may be important in chemotaxis, activation of microbicidal pathways, and regulation of the inflammatory response.[64–69] Specific granules have been considered the intracellular reservoir for some of these proteins, but other, as yet poorly characterized intracellular membrane vescicles may also be involved.

The importance of neutrophil-specific granules in host defenses is dramatized by the congenital syndrome of specific granule deficiency.[60] This is an exceedingly rare disorder characterized by diminished inflammatory responses and severe bacterial infections of skin and deep tissues without predisposition to a particular class of organisms. Cell motility to all stimuli is strikingly diminished in congenital specific granule deficiency. Decreasing bactericidal activity and a failure to generate chemoattractants and inflammatory mediators from plasma probably also contribute to the increased susceptibility to infection.[60,61]

There is evidence for heterogeneity in the genesis of this disorder since neutrophils from one patient described appear to contain "empty" secondary granules, whereas neutrophils from other patients lack the granule-limiting membrane in addition to granule contents.[70] Azurophil granules from patients with specific granule deficiency are of lighter than normal density, and neutrophils from the few patients studied lack gelatinase and defensins, normally components of tertiary and azurophil granules, respectively.[71] The defect appears to be limited to cells of myeloid lineage since lactoferrin is found in normal amounts in parotid and nasolacrimal secretions in patients with neutrophil-specific granule deficiency.[71] Lactoferrin mRNA is totally absent or greatly diminished in bone marrow cultures of patients with specific granule deficiency, which suggests that the disorder involves regulatory defects in the transcription of specific mRNAs normally produced at a particular stage of myelogenesis.[71]

Neutrophil secondary granules but not primary granules are visualized by Wright staining of peripheral blood. Hence, patients with specific granule deficiency can be recognized because their neutrophils appear devoid of granules on Wright stain but stain normally with peroxidase. Nuclei are bilobed, and the nuclear membrane may be distorted by blebs, clefts, and pockets.[60] The absence of neutrophil-specific granules should be confirmed by a quantitative determination of vitamin B_{12} binding protein (by radioisotope binding) and lactoferrin (by enzyme-linked immunoassay or immunoblot analysis using commercially available antibodies).

Chédiak-Higashi Syndrome

The Chédiak-Higashi syndrome (CHS) is a rare disorder characterized by autosomal recessive inheritance, recurrent infections, moderate neutropenia, characteristic giant lysosomes in many tissues, partial occulocutaneous albinism, and central and peripheral neuropathy. In most patients the disease eventually enters an accelerated phase characterized by extensive non-neoplastic lymphoid infiltration, pancytopenia, serious infection, and progressive peripheral neuropathy.[72,73] In CHS, neutrophils are deficient in elastase (a normal component of azurophil granules that may be important in the degradation of endothelial basement membrane and neutrophil diapedesis[74]) and the giant neutrophil lysosomes contain other constituents normally segregated between azurophil and specific granules.[73] In addition, in vitro abnormalities of cell deformability and microtubule assembly, impaired chemotaxis, and phagolysosomal fusion probably contribute to the increased susceptibility to infection in vivo.

In the appropriate clinical setting examination of the peripheral blood smear is sufficient to identify all patients with CHS. The giant blue-gray lysosomes in granulocytes can be confused with Döhle or May-Hegglin bodies, but in the absence of the characteristic clinical features of CHS the latter abnormalities will be easily distinguished. Moreover, in CHS, giant lysosomes are found within lymphocytes and erythrocytes, whereas Döhle bodies are limited to neutrophils and May-Hegglin bodies to cells of granulocytic lineage.[75]

Myeloperoxidase Deficiency

In the presence of halide, myeloperoxidase (MPO) catalyzes the conversion of H_2O_2 to hypochlorous acid.[46,47] The MPO-halide-H_2O_2 system can damage microorganisms by incorporation of halide into the cell wall, but other mechanisms probably account for the microbicidal potency of the system. In addition to hypochlorous acid, other toxic moieties are ultimately produced including chlorine and potent long-lived *N*-chloro oxidants.[76] MPO is an iron-containing heme protein that is responsible for the peroxidase activity of azurophil granules and for the greenish color of these granules and of pus. Hereditary MPO deficiency is a relatively common disorder occurring as a total (≈1:4000) or a partial (≈1:2000) absence of MPO in neutrophils and monocytes.[77] The MPO gene is on chromosome 17.[78] A full-length cDNA probe has been cloned and used to show that the endonuclease cleavage pattern of genomic DNA from individuals deficient in MPO differs from that of normal individuals in the region of the MPO gene.[78] Native MPO consists of large and small peptide subunits. The relationship between subunits and the location of the heme binding regions have not been fully established. Since myeloid cells from individuals with a complete deficiency of MPO produce normal-sized mRNA for MPO but do not contain mature MPO peptides, hereditary MPO deficiency may represent a genetic defect that affects post-translational processing of an abnormal precursor protein.[79]

In complete MPO deficiency the respiratory burst is prolonged, which supports the concept that MPO plays a role in inactivation of the inflammatory response.[80–82] Otherwise healthy individuals with a complete deficiency of MPO are not at an increased risk of infection, but deep fungal infections have been noted infrequently in poorly controlled diabetics with MPO deficiency. Better identification of MPO-deficient individuals would have little impact on clinical practice since optimal management depends only on careful control of any underlying immunosuppressive diseases. MPO deficiency is easily recognized by peroxidase stains.

Localized Juvenile Periodontitis

Moderate to severe gingivitis, periodontitis, and mucositis are frequent findings in patients with significant neutropenia or phagocytic cell dysfunction. In most cases intraoral infection is associated with recurrent infection at other sites. In contrast, localized juvenile periodontitis (LJP) is a disease of adolescents that is characterized by severe alveolar bone loss limited primarily to the first molars and incisors.[8] Patients are not predisposed to extraoral infection. Patients with LJP have a moderate but reproducible impairment of chemotaxis stimulated by formylpeptides and C5a; neutrophil adherence in LJP is normal. Defective chemotaxis in LJP persists after aggressive local therapy (in distinction to the chemotactic defect described in patients with intraoral *Capnocytophaga* infection[83]) and has been demonstrated in siblings of index patients before the development of clinical disease.[8] Limited data suggest that chemoattractant receptor numbers and affinities are normal in LJP but that receptor processing may be impaired.[84,85] It is unclear whether the latter abnormalities are causally related to the chemotactic defect in LJP or reflect a more fundamental abnormality in membrane processing.

TABLE 4. Secondary Immunodeficiency

Clinical Setting	*Observed Functional Deficiencies*
Infection	
Acute viral infection	Lymphopenia, decreased circulating T cells, depressed CD4/CD8 ratio in some, abnormal monocyte function with influenza and herpes simplex
HIV infection	Lymphopenia, decreased circulating T cells, depressed CD4/CD8 ratio
Tuberculosis, leprosy	Decreased DCH
Malignancy	
Hodgkin's disease	Decreased DCH, impaired antibody response to certain antigens, treatment and splenectomy may contribute to deficits
Leukemia	Variable immunoglobulin levels
Myeloma	Impaired antibody response, decreased immunoglobulins and/or complement
Solid tumors	Impaired monocyte chemotaxis
Autoimmune disorders	
SLE	Decreased DCH, decreased T cells, immunoglobulins usually increased, may be associated with complement deficiency
Rheumatoid arthritis	Decreased DCH, immunoglobulins usually increased, normal response to antigens, abnormal neutrophil chemotaxis
Protein-losing states	Decreased immunoglobulins, complement, and DCH
Immunosuppressive therapy	
Corticosteroids	Transient T-cell sequestration, decreased immunoglobulin synthesis, decreased neutrophil adherence and degranulation
Cytotoxic agents Radiation	Variable decrease in T-cell, B-cell, and granulocyte numbers and function
Anti-thymocyte globulin	Decreased T-cell numbers and function, B-cell function variably impaired
Cyclosporine	Decreased T-cell function and T-cell-dependent B-cell function
Dilantin, penicillamine	IgA deficiency, hypogammaglobulinemia
Miscellaneous	
Sickle cell disease Splenectomy	Decreased antibody response, opsonization
Thermal injury Neonates	Decreased neutrophil chemotaxis and degranulation
Diabetes	Decreased neutrophil chemotaxis and phagocytosis
Aging	Decreased antibody response to certain antigens, decreased DCH

Abbreviations: HIV: human immunodeficiency virus; DCH: delayed cutaneous hypersensitivity; SLE, systemic lupus erythematosus.

ADDITIONAL STUDIES OF PHAGOCYTE FUNCTION

Assays of neutrophil or monocyte chemotaxis, phagocytosis, and microbicidal activity, although frequently recommended in evaluation of patients with suspected immunodeficiency, are of limited value in screening. In an investigational setting such studies have been critical to the current understanding of leukocyte physiology. However, these assays are poorly standardized for clinical testing, are technically demanding, and are subject to considerable biologic variability, even in experienced hands. Unless in vitro function is profoundly impaired, the extent to which the demonstrated abnormalities contribute to impaired host defenses in vivo is usually unclear. Moreover, in and of themselves, the demonstrated abnormalities are not diagnostic of any of the well-characterized disorders of phagocyte function. Migration of leukocytes into Rebuck skin windows or skin blisters is occasionally informative but not essential for diagnosis. These procedures establish a potential portal of entry for microbes and may be hazardous in immunodeficient patients. The foregoing notwithstanding, several poorly understood syndromes of phagocyte dysfunction (e.g., lazy leukocyte syndrome, Papillon-Lefevre syndrome, icthyosis, mannosidosis, Down syndrome) lack specific biochemical markers and were initially characterized on the basis of clinical features accompanied by in vitro deficits in chemotaxis, phagocytosis, or killing.[86,87] These appear to be exceedingly rare conditions and, for practical purposes, may be largely of historic interest. Were such patients studied within a contemporary technical and conceptual framework, other diagnoses would, in some instances, probably be apparent.

CLINICAL ASSESSMENT OF IMMUNOCOMPETENCE IN PATIENTS WITH SYSTEMIC ILLNESS

Aging, systemic illness, and the use of immunosuppressive agents may be accompanied by a decline in immunocompetence (Table 4). In some instances the particular limb or component of the immune system that is involved has been identified. Beyond simple screening (complete blood count and differential, DCH testing, and possibly an assessment of immunoglobulins) there is no advantage to routine immunologic testing. Recognition of the increased risk of infection and attention to immunization status are important. Assays of immune function may provide critical insights into the natural history and basic mechanisms of disease but do not aid in the care of the individual patient.

REFERENCES

1. Dingle JH, Badger GF, Jordan WS Jr. Illness in the Home: Study of 25,000 Illnesses in a Group of Cleveland Families. Cleveland: Western Reserve University Press; 1964:1.
2. Gwaltney JM Jr, Hendley JO, Simon G, et al. Rhinovirus infections in an industrial population. I. The occurrence of illness. N Engl J Med. 1966;275:1261.
3. Cooper MD, Lawton AR III. Immune deficiency diseases. In: Braunwald E, Isselbacher KJ, Petersdorf RG, et al., eds. Harrison's Principles of Internal Medicine. 11th ed. New York: McGraw-Hill; 1987:1385.
4. Buckley RH. Humoral immunodeficiency. Clin Immunol Immunopathol. 1986;40:13.
5. Rosen FS, Cooper MD, Wedgwood, RJP. The primary immunodeficiencies. N Engl J Med. 1984;311:235, 300.
6. Buckley RH: Immunodeficiency diseases. JAMA. 1987;258:2841.
7. Rosen FS, Wedgwood RJ, Eibl M, et al. Primary immunodeficiency diseases: Report of a World Health Organization Scientific Group. Clin Immunol Immunopathol. 1986;40:166.
8. Van Dyke TE, Levine MJ, Genco RJ. Neutrophil function and oral disease. J Oral Pathol. 1985;14:95.
9. deShazo RD, Lopez M, Salvaggio JE. Use and interpretation of diagnostic immunologic laboratory tests. JAMA. 1987;258:3011.
10. Check IJ, Piper M. Quantitation of immunoglobulins. In: Rose NR, Friedman H, Fahey JL, eds. Manual of Clinical Laboratory Immunology. 3rd ed. Washington DC: American Society for Microbiology 1986:138.
11. Stiehm ER, Fudenberg HH. Serum levels of immune globulins in health and disease: A survey. Pediatrics. 1966;37:715.
12. Stiehm ER. Immunodeficiency—general considerations. In: Stiehm ER, Fulginetti VA, eds. Immunologic Disorders in Infants and Children. Philadelphia: WB Saunders; 1980.
13. Nahn MH, Blaese RM, Crain MJ, et al. Patients with Wiskott-Aldrich syndrome have normal IgG2 levels. J Immunol. 1986;137:3484.
14. Claman HN. The biology of the immune response. JAMA. 1987;258:2835.
15. Wall R, Kuehl M. Biosynthesis and regulation of immunoglobulins. Annu Rev Immunol. 1983;1:393.
16. Gathings WE, Kubagawa H, Cooper MD. A distinctive pattern of B-cell immaturity in perinatal humans. Immunol Rev. 1981;57:107.
17. Wedgwood RJ, Ochs HD, Davis SD. The recognition and classification of immunodeficiency diseases with bacteriophage ϕX174. I: Bergsma D, Good RA, Finstad J, eds. Immunodeficiency in Man and Animals. Sunderland, MA: Sinauer Associates; 1975:331.
18. Dreskin SC, Goldsmith PK, Gallin JI. Immunoglobulins in the hyperimmunoglobulin E and recurrent infection (Job's) syndrome. J Clin Invest. 1985;75:26.
19. Nathan CF, Kaplan G, Levis WR, et al. Local and systemic effects of intradermal recombinant interferon-γ in patients with lepromatous leprosy. N Engl J Med. 1986;315:6.
20. Buckley RH. Advances in the diagnosis and treatment of immunodeficiency diseases. Arch Intern Med. 1986;146:377.
21. Hong R. Immunodeficiency. In: Rose NR, Friedman H, Fahey JL, eds. Manual of Clinical Laboratory Immunology. 3rd ed. Washington DC: American Society for Microbiology. 1986:702.
22. Hirschorn R. Inherited enzyme deficiencies and immunodeficiency: Adenosine deaminase (ADA) and purine nucleoside phosphorylase (PNP) deficiencies. Clin Immunol Immunopathol. 1986;40:157.
23. Ammann AJ. Immunodeficiency diseases. In: Stites DP, Stobo JD, Wells JV, eds. Basic & Clinical Immunology. 6th ed. Norwalk, CT: Appleton & Lange; 1987:317.
24. Dinarello CA, Mier JW. Current concepts: Lymphokines. N Engl J Med. 1987;317:940.
25. Johnston RB Jr. Current concepts—immunology: Monocytes and macrophages. N Engl J Med. 1988;318:747.
26. Beutler B, Cerami A. Cachectin and tumor necrosis as two sides of the same biological coin. Nature. 1986;320:584.
27. Adams DO, Hamilton TA. The cell biology of macrophage activation. Annu Rev Immunol. 1984;2:283.
28. Metcalf D. The granulocyte-macrophage colony stimulating factors. Science. 1985;229:16.
29. Walz A, Peveri P, Aschauer W, et al. Purification and amino acid sequencing of NAF, a novel neutrophil-activating factor produced by monocytes. Biochem Biophys Res Commun. 1987;149:755.
30. Yoshimura T, Matsushima K, Oppenheim JJ, et al. Neutrophil chemotactic factor produced by lipopolysaccharide (LPS)-stimulated human blood mononuclear leukocytes: Partial characterization and separation from interleukin 1 (IL 1). J Immunol. 1987;139:788.
31. Murray HW. Interferon-gamma, the activated macrophage, and host defense against microbial challenge. Ann Intern Med. 1988;108:595.
32. Joiner KA, Brown EJ, Frank MM. Complement and bacteria: Chemistry and biology in host defense. Annu Rev Immunol. 1984;2:461.
33. Fries LF, Frank MM. Complement and related proteins: Inherited deficiencies. In: Gallin JI, Goldstein IM, Snyderman R, eds. Inflammation: Basic Principles and Clinical Correlates. New York: Raven Press; 1988:89.
34. Ruddy S. Complement. In: Rose NR, Friedman H, Fahey JL, eds. Manual of Clinical Laboratory Immunology. 3rd ed. Washington DC: American Society for Microbiology. 1986:175.
35. Sjìholm AG, Kuijper EJ, Tijssen CC, et al. Dysfunctional properdin in a Dutch Family with meningococcal disease. N Engl J Med. 1988;319:33.
36. Ross SC, Densen P. Complement deficiency states and infection: Epidemiology, pathogenesis and consequences of neisserial and other infections in an immune deficiency. Medicine (Baltimore). 1984;63:243.
37. Cartwright GE, Athens JW, Wintrobe MM. The kinetics of neutrophilic cells. Blood. 1964;24:780.
38. Finch SC. Granulocytopenia. In: Williams WJ, Beutler E, Erslev AJ, et al., eds. Hematology. 2nd ed. New York: McGraw-Hill; 1977:717.
39. Dancey JT, Deubelbeiss KA, Harker LA, et al. Neutrophil kinetics in man. J Clin Invest. 1976;58:705.
40. Joyce RA, Boggs DR, Hasiba U, et al. Marginal neutrophil pool size in normal subjects and neutropenic patients as measured by epinephrine infusion. J Lab Clin Med. 1976;88:614.
41. Minchinton RM, McGrath KM. Alloimmune neonatal neutropenia—a neglected diagnosis? Med J Aust. 1987;147:139.
42. Ducos R, Madyastha PR, Warrier RP, et al. Neutrophil agglutinins in idiopathic chronic neutropenia of early childhood. Am J Dis Child. 1986;140:65.
43. Gallin JI, Fauci AS, eds. Advances in Host Defense Mechanisms. v. 3. In: Chronic Granulomatous Disease. New York: Raven Press; 1982:262.
44. Gallin JI, Buescher ES, Seligmann BE, et al. Recent advances in chronic granulomatous disease. Ann Intern Med. 1983;99:657.
45. Tauber AI, Borregaard N, Simons E, et al. Chronic granulomatous disease; a syndrome of phagocyte oxidase deficiencies. Medicine (Baltimore). 1983;62:286.
46. Klebanoff SJ. Oxygen metabolism and the toxic properties of phagocytes. Ann Intern Med. 1980;93:480.
47. Babior BM. The respiratory burst of phagocytes. J Clin Invest. 1984;73:599.
48. Ezekowitz RAB, Orkin SH, Newburger PE. Recombinant interferon gamma augments phagocyte superoxide production and X-chronic granulomatous disease gene expression in X-linked variant chronic granulomatous disease. J Clin Invest. 1987;80:1009.
49. Sechler JMG, Malech HL, White CJ, et al. Recombinant interferon-γ reconstitutes defective phagocyte function in patients with chronic granulomatous disease of childhood. Proc Natl Acad Sci USA. 1988;85:4874.

50. Anderson DC, Schmalstieg FC, Finegold MJ, et al. The severe and moderate phenotypes of heritable Mac-1, LFA-1, p150,95 deficiency: Their qualitative definition and relation to leukocyte dysfunction and clinical features. J Infect Dis. 1985;152:668.
51. Anderson DC, Springer TA. Leukocyte adhesion deficiency: An inherited defect in the Mac-1, LFA-1, and p150,95 glycoproteins. Annu Rev Med. 1987;38:175.
52. Harlan JM, Killen PD, Senecal FM, et al. The role of neutrophil membrane glycoprotein GP-150 in neutrophil adherence to endothelium in vitro. Blood. 1985;66:167.
53. Boxer LA, Hedley-Whyte ET, Stossel TP. Neutrophil actin dysfunction and abnormal neutrophil behavior. N Engl J Med. 1974;291:1093.
54. Southwick FS, Holbrook T, Howard T, et al. Neutrophil actin dysfunction is associated with a deficiency of Mol (Abstract). Clin Res. 1986;34:533.
55. Nauseef WM, DeAlarcon P, Bale JF, et al. Aberrant activation and regulation of the oxidative burst in neutrophils with Mol glycoprotein deficiency. J Immunol. 1986;137:636–42.
56. Seligmann B, Gallin JI. Neutrophils from a CR3 (C3bi) receptor deficient patient exhibit low ED-50 values for fmet-leu-phe stimulated responses and do not exhibit affinity adaption (Abstract). Clin Res. 1986;34:679.
57. Rotrosen D, Gallin JI. Disorders of phagocyte function. Annu Rev Immunol. 1987;5:127.
58. Weiss J, Victor M, Elsbach P. Role of charge and hydrophobic interactions in the action of the bactericidal/permeability increasing protein of neutrophils on gram-negative bacteria. J Clin Invest. 1981;71:540.
59. Ganz T, Selsted ME, Szklarek D, et al. Defensins: Natural peptide antibiotics of human neutrophils. J Clin Invest. 1985;76:1427.
60. Gallin JI. Neutrophil specific granule deficiency. Annu Rev Med. 1985;36:263.
61. Wright DG, Gallin JI. A functional differentiation of human neutrophil granules: Generation of C5a by a specific (secondary) granule product and inactivation of C5a by azurophil (primary) granule products. J Immunol. 1977;119:1068.
62. DeWald B, Bretz U, Baggiolini M. Release of gelatinase from a novel secretory compartment of human neutrophils. J Clin Invest. 1982;70:518.
63. Yoon PS, Boxer LA, Mayo LA, et al. Human neutrophil laminin receptors: Activation-dependent receptor expression. J Immunol. 1987;138:259.
64. Borregaard N, Heiple JM, Simons ER, et al. Subcellular localization of the b-cytochrome component of the human neutrophil microbicidal oxidase: Translocation during activation. J Cell Biol. 1983;97:52.
65. Borregaard N, Miller LJ, Springer TA. Chemoattractant-regulated mobilization of a novel intracellular compartment in human neutrophils. Science. 1987;237:1204.
66. Fletcher MP, Gallin JI. Human neutrophils contain an intracellular pool of putative receptors for the chemoattractant N-formyl-methionyl-leucyl-phenylalanine. Blood. 1983;62:792.
67. Heiple JM, Ossowski L. Human neutrophil plasminogen activator is localized in specific granules and is translocated to the cell surface by exocytosis. J Exp Med. 1986;164:826.
68. Ohno Y, Seligmann BE, Gallin JI. Cytochrome b translocation to human neutrophil plasma membranes and superoxide release. J Biol Chem. 1985;260:2409.
69. Rotrosen D, Gallin JI, Spiegel AM, et al. Subcellular localization of Giα in human neutrophils. J Biol Chem. 1988;263:10958.
70. Parmley RT, Tzeng DY, Baehner RL, et al. Abnormal distribution of complex carbohydrates in neutrophils of a patient with lactoferrin deficiency. Blood. 1983;62:538.
71. Lomax KJ, Gallin JI, Rotrosen D, et al. A selective defect in myeloid cell lactoferrin gene expression in neutrophil specific granule deficiency. J Clin Invest. 1989;83:514–519.
72. Blume RS, Wolff SM. The Chédiak-Higashi syndrome: Studies in four patients and a review of the literature. Medicine (Baltimore). 1972;51:247.
73. Klebanoff SJ, Clark RA. Chédiak-Higashi syndrome. In: The Neutrophil: Function and Clinical Disorders. Amsterdam: Elsevier Biomedical; 1978.
74. Smedly LA, Tonnesen MG, Sandhaus RA, et al. Neutrophil mediated injury to endothelial cells: Enhancement by endotoxin and essential role of neutrophil elastase. J Clin Invest. 1986;77:1233.
75. Wintrobe MM, Lee RG, Bithell TC, et al. eds. Clinical Hematology. 7th ed. Philadelphia: Lee & Febriger; 1975:221.
76. Test ST, Lampert MB, Ossanna PJ, et al. Generation of nitrogen-chlorine oxidants by human phagocytes. J Clin Invest. 1984;74:1341.
77. Parry MF, Root RK, Metcalf JA. Myeloperoxidase deficiency. Prevalence and clinical significance. Ann Intern Med. 1981;95:293.
78. Weil SC, Rosner GL, Reid MS, et al. cDNA cloning of human myeloperoxidase: Decrease in myeloperoxidase in RNA upon induction of HL-60 cells. Proc Natl Acad Sci USA. 1987;84:2057.
79. Nauseef WM. Myeloperoxidase biosynthesis by a human promyelocytic leukemia cell line: Insight into myeloperoxidase deficiency. Blood. 1986;67:865.
80. Clark RA, Klebanoff SJ. Chemotactic factor inactivation by the myeloperoxidase-hydrogen peroxide-halide system. J Clin Invest. 1979;64:913.
81. Henderson WR, Klebanoff SJ. Leukotriene production and inactivation by normal, chronic granulomatous disease and myeloperoxidase-deficient neutrophils. J Biol Chem. 1983;258:13522.
82. Clark RA, Borregaard N. Neutrophils autoinactivate secretory products by myeloperoxidase-catalyzed oxidation. Blood. 1985;65:375.
83. Shurin SB, Socransky SS, Sweeney E, et al. A neutrophil disorder induced by capnocytophaga, a dental micro-organism. N Engl J Med. 1979;301:849.
84. Van Dyke TE, Levine MJ, Tabak LA, et al. Reduced chemotactic peptide binding in juvenile periodontitis: A model for neutrophil function. Biochem Biophys Res Commun. 1981;100:1278.
85. Van Dyke TE. Role of the neutrophil in oral disease: Receptor deficiency in leukocytes from patients with juvenile periodontitis. Rev Infect Dis. 1985;7:419.
86. Gallin JI. Abnormalities of phagocyte chemotaxis: Pathophysiology, clinical manifestations, and management of patients. Rev Infect Dis. 1981;3:1196.
87. Elmostehy MR. Papillon-Lefevre syndrome. Precocious periodontosis with epidermal lesions: Review of literature and presentation of five cases. Egypt Dent J. 1976;22:49.

SECTION C. EPIDEMIOLOGY OF INFECTIOUS DISEASE

10. PRINCIPLES AND METHODS

PHILIP S. BRACHMAN

Epidemiology is the evaluation of the determinants, occurrence, distribution, and control of health and disease in a defined population. The word *epidemiology* is derived from the Greek (*epi*, upon; *demos*, people; *logy*, study); it is the study of anything that happens to people.

The science of epidemiology can be applied to the study of any disease or condition, acute or chronic, infectious or noninfectious, communicable or noncommunicable, and to the study of health as well. It is a science of rates, in which, for example, the numerator is the number of cases of a disease that occur in a given period of time and the denominator is the total population at risk, that is, exposed to the etiologic agent.

Epidemiologists should be working colleagues of clinicians. A clinician who sees an individual patient may not relate that patient's condition to the community in which he or she lives. The insularity of the clinician may inhibit definition of a common disease problem occurring among a group of people and thus delay or inhibit the institution of appropriate control and prevention measures. Multiple cases of a single disease entity may appear simultaneously in a population who have had a common exposure to the etiologic agent. If the individual cases diagnosed by different physicians are not reported, no association among the cases can be made. If, however, the individual cases are reported and can be investigated as a group in an *epidemiologic investigation*, the epidemic has a better chance of being characterized, the cases related, and control measures instituted.

Once the outbreak has been identified and the diagnosis confirmed, other cases that are not diagnosable with certainty by themselves may become diagnosable by their similarities with the cases initially identified as epidemic cases. This development of *consensus diagnosis* has obvious benefits for the individual patient as well as allowing a better characterization of the epidemic.

Evaluation of a single case of an infectious disease may not identify the method of transmission since diseases can be transmitted by various routes; however, if multiple cases have occurred and each is investigated, analysis of the combined data may identify the route of transmission.

Additionally, evaluation of multiple cases of the same disease may identify predisposing host factors; with this information, cases may be prevented by removing or protecting people at risk against the predisposing factor.

The epidemiologic investigation provides the opportunity of collating information from cases temporally related into a coherent narrative, examination of which should describe the cause, transmission, and host factors that may suggest an intervention point leading to control and prevention. Without an epidemiologic investigation, cases may continue to occur until the disease has run its natural course and/or there are no susceptibles left in the population.

A parallel may be drawn between the professional activities of the private practitioner or clinician and the practitioner of epidemiology. The private practitioner's initial contact with the situation is through an individual patient, whereas the epidemiologist usually becomes involved because of a collection of cases. The clinician obtains the patient's history, conducts a physical examination, and orders laboratory tests, all of which are necessary in investigating the illness of an individual patient. The epidemiologist is also interested in the history, physical examination, and results of laboratory tests, but he or she collects these data for all the patients involved in the outbreak. The private practitioner considers the results of the examination of one patient, makes a diagnosis, and prescribes appropriate therapy for that person. The epidemiologist analyzes available data from the community of patients and others at risk, makes a prediction as to additional cases, and then prescribes intervention measures for the involved population. The private practitioner is concerned with the prognosis for the patient, whereas the epidemiologist is concerned with the trend of the disease in the community.

It should be apparent that the clinician and the epidemiologist are dependent on each other. The epidemiologist is dependent on the clinician to make the diagnosis and to report the case; the accumulation of individual reports of cases allows the epidemiologist to practice his or her profession. The clinician is dependent on the epidemiologist to investigate a collection of cases of a similar nature and to prescribe the proper control and prevention measures. However, these two professionals should not be isolated within their own specialties. The clinician should know something about epidemiology, just as the epidemiologist should be knowledgeable about clinical medicine. At the same time they need to recognize their own limitations and to consult freely with one another. In this way they both may practice their professions to the advantage of the community in controlling and preventing disease.

The epidemiologist can serve as a connection between the clinicians and their patients, the community, and all the patients ultimately involved in the specific disease problem. It should be apparent that epidemiologic investigations should be beneficial to the patient and to the physician, as well as to the community. In addition to reducing the incidence of disease, there should be financial savings to all involved in the health care system and, ultimately, better use of health resources.

DEFINITIONS

Infection means the presence and replication of microorganisms in the tissues of a host. The host response to infection is highly variable, depending on the interrelationship of many host and agent factors, and ranges from subclinical or inapparent infection to disease. *Disease* is the clinical expression of infection and indicates that not only are microorganisms present and replicating but they also are disrupting the host to the extent that signs and symptoms are being produced. Disease may vary from mild to severe with the most severe form leading to death.

A *subclinical infection* indicates a reaction between the agent and the host limited to an immune response that can only be diagnosed by serologic means with demonstration of either a single high titer or a fourfold rise in titer to the infecting agent.

Colonization indicates the presence of an organism without clinical or subclinical disease. However, the organism is replicating in or on the tissues of the host and can be identified by culture in the laboratory. *Contamination* refers to the presence of microorganisms on a body surface without tissue invasion or reaction or to their presence on the surface of inanimate objects.

A *carrier* is a person who is colonized with an organism but shows no evidence of disease, although disease may have been present earlier. The organisms can be recovered by culture. Carriage may be transient, that is, the organism is carried for a short period of time, intermittent (sporadic), or long term (chronic). The factors that influence the length of carriage are not well defined but may represent partial immunity or be a result of partial therapy directed against the organism. Recovery from clinical disease may result in short-term carriage (*Shigella*) or occasionally in chronic carriage (*Salmonella typhi*).

Dissemination of microorganisms can occur from either a person who is infected or has disease.[1] Usually dissemination is greatest during the latter part of the incubation period, just before the infection becomes clinically apparent. Once disease is evident, dissemination usually decreases, sometimes rather dramatically. However, with some diseases, dissemination may be a serious problem during the clinical phase and until treatment is initiated. A person with disease will arouse suspicion of dissemination, and appropriate precautions can be taken. However, the silent disseminator, that is, the infected person without overt evidence of disease, causes the greatest concern because dissemination can be demonstrated only by special shedding studies or if secondary cases of infection can be proved to have resulted from contact with this person.[2] Dissemination from a carrier may be enhanced by infection or disease with a second microorganism, by development of another (noninfectious) disease, or as a result of unknown causes.[3]

A carrier not disseminating is not necessarily dangerous, and special precautions may be unwarranted. A judgment as to therapy, isolation, or other special actions directed against a carrier should reflect proven dissemination and not just carriage. Special culture surveys to define carriage may lead to an inappropriate decision if there is no evidence of dissemination from the carrier.

Multiple cases of a disease can occur infrequently, at irregular or regular intervals, or at an increased frequency. *Sporadic occurrence* refers to the occasional cases of disease at irregular intervals. *Endemic frequency* refers to a low-level frequency of disease at moderately regular intervals. *Hyperendemic* refers to a gradual increase in the occurrence of a disease beyond the endemic level but not currently at epidemic proportions. The *epidemic occurrence* of disease refers to the sudden increase in incidence of the disease above the expected incidence. *Pandemic disease* is epidemic disease that has spread among continents. For example, the current occurrence of cholera in Africa, Asia, and southern Europe reflects the seventh pandemic of cholera that began in the Celebes Islands in the Pacific.

Disease prevalence refers to the number of cases of the disease that are active at a particular point in time (point prevalence) or that occur over a defined period of time (period prevalence). *Disease incidence* is a rate that reflects the number of new cases of the disease in a defined time period within a specific population.

TECHNIQUES OF EPIDEMIOLOGIC PRACTICE

Three basic epidemiologic techniques—descriptive, analytic, and experimental—are used individually or collectively to investigate an epidemic.

Descriptive Epidemiology

The descriptive technique is most frequently applied initially. If the problem is not solved or if additional questions arise as a result of the initial analysis of the data, then the analytic or the experimental method or both may be applied to the problem.

In descriptive epidemiology, all pertinent data are collected and described according to time, place, and person. In describing time, there are four trends that need to be considered—secular, periodic, seasonal, and acute. The secular trend refers to the long-term variation in the occurrence of the disease; the time interval is years. For example, the secular trend of tetanus shows a gradual but steady decrease in incidence from 1954 to 1987 (Fig. 1).[4] In general, the secular trend is influenced by the overall immunity level of the population and by nonspecific factors, such as socioeconomic, nutritional, and hygienic status.

Periodic trends are the temporary variations in the occurrence of the disease that disrupt the secular trend of the disease. Periodic trends will occur over a time frame of several months to several years. An example is the periodic increase in the incidence of influenza A every 2–3 years, which reflects antigenic drifts in the predominant strain as well as changes in the immunity level of the population.[5] Another example is periodic change in death rates associated with influenza that reflect changes in circulating influenza viruses as well as changes in immunity in the population (Fig. 2).

Seasonal trends are the variations based on climatic factors that directly or indirectly influence disease transmission. Thus, food-borne diseases are more likely to occur in warm months because of the favorable temperature conditions for microorganisms to multiply to disease-producing levels in unrefrigerated foods (Fig. 3).

The acute trend describes the sudden rise in the incidence (rate) of a disease. This trend is referred to as an *epidemic*. The graphic portrayal of these data is called an epidemic curve, which commonly is an analysis of the time of onset (abscissa or horizontal axis) plotted against the number of cases (ordinate or vertical axis).

The time scale for analyzing epidemiologic data varies from minutes for diseases with short incubation periods, such as chemical gastroenteritis, to years for diseases with extremely long incubation periods, such as leprosy. Analysis of these data may allow a judgment to be made as to the mode of transmission.

Frequently the epidemiologist becomes involved in the investigation after the peak of the epidemic has occurred, and the epidemiologic analysis is mainly retrospective; however, if cases are continuing to occur, knowing something about the epidemiology of the disease, including the method of transmission and the shape of its epidemic curve, may allow predictions to be made about the occurrence of additional cases and institution of appropriate controls.

Description of epidemiologic data by place refers to the geographic area in which the contact between the susceptible host and the etiologic agent occurred. This may be a home, public building, or restaurant; a water distribution district; a sanitary district; a political subdivision such as a city, county, region, and so on. The place in which the actual contact between the organism and the person took place may be different from the place in which the vehicle of infection became contaminated. This differentiation may be important with regard to instituting control and prevention measures. For example, a food item contaminated in a delicatessen may have been taken home and then eaten, which would result in the home being the site in which the vehicle of infection came into contact with the susceptible host(s). However, the primary effort toward prevention of additional cases would involve identifying the delicatessen as the site in which the food became contaminated and in which control efforts need to be directed. Place in which exposure to the organism occurred becomes of even greater importance when long-distance travel is considered. Exposure to an infectious agent can occur in one country with the onset of symptoms days

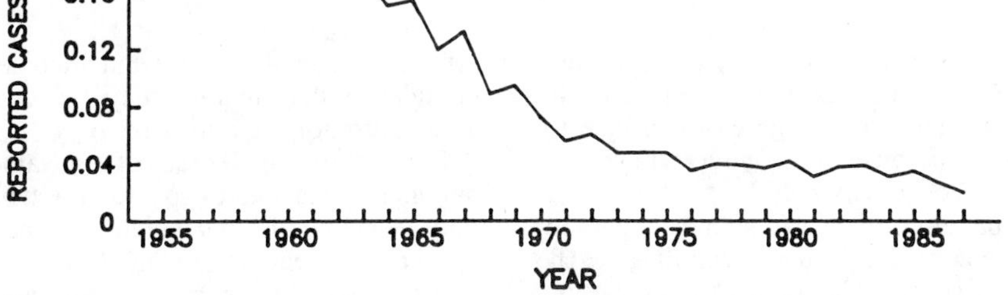

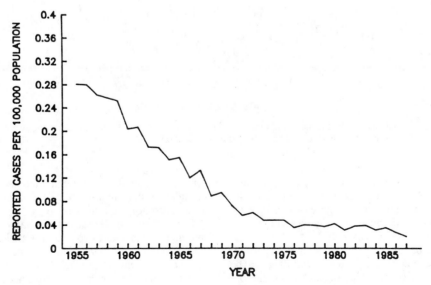

FIG. 1. Reported tetanus cases by year: United States, 1954–1987. (Courtesy of Centers for Disease Control, Epidemiology Program Office, Division of Surveillance and Epidemiologic Studies, Atlanta, GA.)

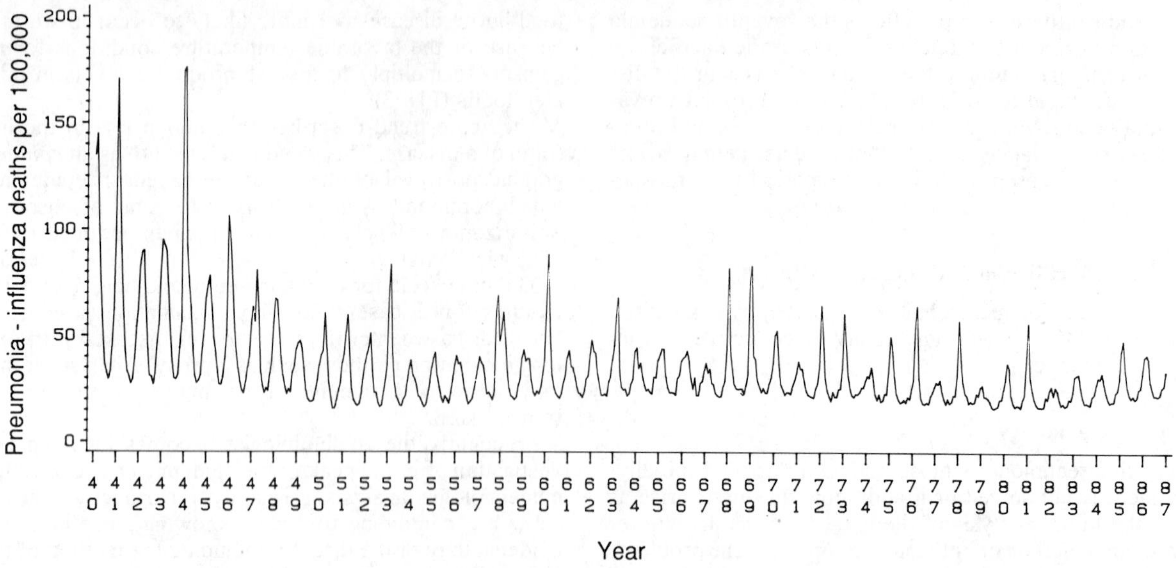

FIG. 2. Pneumonia-influenza death rates by month in the United States, 1940–1987. Monthly rates; annual base. (Courtesy of Centers for Disease Control, Biometrics Activity and Epidemiology Office, Division of Viral Diseases, Atlanta, GA.)

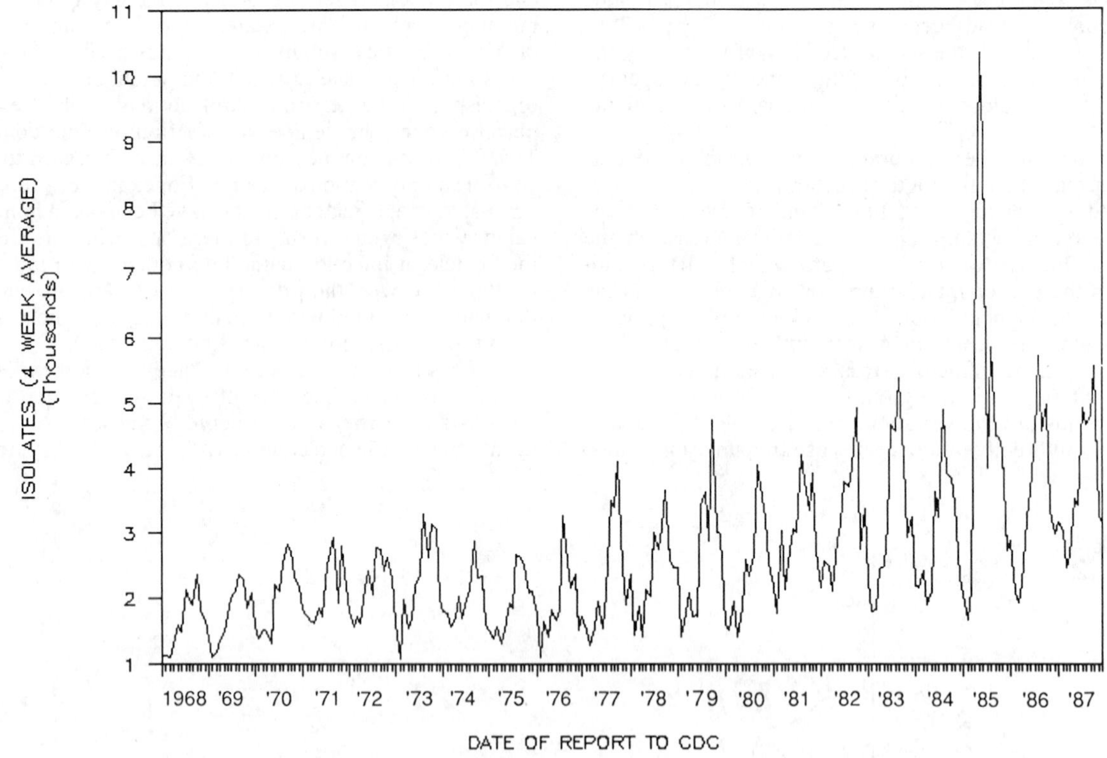

FIG. 3. Reported isolations of salmonellae from humans in the United States, 1968–1987. (Courtesy of Centers for Disease Control, Enteric Diseases Branch, Division of Bacterial Diseases, Atlanta, GA).

later when the traveler is thousands of miles away. The identification of a common-source outbreak may be seriously delayed by the inability to accumulate enough cases to identify the common site of exposure because of the movement of people after exposure to the infective material.

The third component of descriptive epidemiology, person, refers to organizing the epidemiologic data according to the characteristics of the involved people; these include factors such as age, sex, individual susceptibility, race, religion, socioeconomic status, occupation, and social history. These factors collected individually, but analyzed collectively, may show cumulative data important to the overall epidemiologic characterization of the outbreak.

For example, if all cases of a certain disease occurred in boys and men, a place of exposure or a vehicle of infection common only to men and boys would be considered. If all the patients were of one religion, a similar judgment would be made.

A number of years ago an outbreak of gastroenteritis due to *Salmonella new brunswick*, a rare serotype, involving people in eight states occurred.[6] Age-specific attack rates clearly indicated that the cases had primarily occurred in infants; there were three times as many cases in this age group as would be expected. This suggested that the vehicle of infection was something common to infants, commercially distributed over a wide area. These clues led to the identification of the vehicle as a particular batch of powdered skim milk distributed under a variety of brand names but that originated from one processing factory. The source of infection was identified, intervention measures were introduced, and the epidemic was terminated.

The accurate description of the epidemiologic data by personal characteristics may reveal important clues that help to answer the questions of why the epidemic occurred and how to control it and to prevent further spread.

Analytic Epidemiology

The second epidemiologic technique is analytic epidemiology, which is used to investigate the relationships between cause and effect and to evaluate risk factors and disease.[7,8] There are two basic analytic epidemiologic methods—the case-control study and the cohort study. In the case-control method, the investigation starts with an effect and attempts to identify the cause that resulted in that effect. This is conceptually referred to as a *retrospective study*, going back in time to determine what events occurred that resulted in the specific effect. In this type of study, new records are not created; the investigation involves a review of existing records. A critical part of this investigation is the selection of the control group (or comparison group, which is a more accurate term); it is absolutely necessary to avoid having overt or covert bias enter into the selection process. The purpose of a comparison group is to allow comparison with the group to whom the effect occurred to identify quantifiable difference(s) between the two groups that should explain why the effect developed. The comparison group is selected so that it resembles the case group as closely as possible, except that the former group does not have the effect. Thus, if the comparison group is carefully matched to the case group except for the presence of the effect, the reason the case group developed the disease, but the comparison group did not, should become apparent. Case-control studies are used in acute- as well as chronic-disease investigations.

An example of a case-control study is the investigation of an outbreak of gastroenteritis among people at a picnic. It may be difficult or impossible by obtaining food histories only from those ill to identify the common vehicle that transmitted the infection; no one food item may stand out as the contaminated item. Selecting a comparison group of picnickers who selected their meals from the same menu, ate at the same time, were generally of the same age, lived in the same area of town, but were not ill, and obtaining their food histories for the same period of time, should reveal data that incriminate a certain food as the vehicle of infection. That is, those who are ill should have a statistically higher consumption rate of the suspected food than the comparison group.

The second analytic method is the cohort study, which is conceptually referred to as a prospective study. In this method, a population exposed to a specific presumed cause is followed to identify resulting effects. In this type of investigation new records are created. Again, we select a comparison group of people who are similar to the exposed cohort except that they do not have contact with the cause being investigated. Both groups are followed to note the effect of the supposed cause. The comparison group should remain free of the effect. For example, a hospital is experiencing an increase in septicemia and suspects that the cause may be related to use of a certain lot of intravenous fluids. The study cohort is made up of those who receive the suspect fluids; the comparison group should be patients who match them in age, sex, underlying diagnosis, location within the hospital, and other therapeutic procedures but who do not receive the suspect intravenous fluid. If the suspect intravenous fluid is actually contaminated, then some of the group who receive it should develop septicemia, whereas people in the comparison group should not, though some could develop septicemia due to other causes; however, the rates should be statistically significantly different. The difference in attack rates for septicemia between the two groups should be attributable to having received the contaminated fluids.

The case-control study has the advantages over the prospective cohort study of being easier and quicker to conduct and less expensive. One potential difficulty is in selecting an appropriate comparison group without allowing bias to develop in the selection process. Another problem is asking people questions about previous activities, which is fraught with the dangers of poor memory. Another potential problem is inadvertently including subclinical cases among the controls.

The prospective cohort study does not depend on the memory of people and makes it possible to obtain the necessary epidemiologic data as it occurs—not retrospectively. We do have to be careful that there is no bias in selecting the comparison group and in determining the diagnosis. Another problem is the possible need to follow the two groups for a long time. If the incubation period is long, there is the need to follow the participants for an equal or longer period of time. Some of the participants may leave the study, reducing the number of people in the study. Additionally, because of the time involved and the chance of negative findings, the cohort study is usually more expensive to conduct.

Another type of cohort study is a retrospective cohort study in which the effect (disease) occurs and a study is conducted to show whether there is a relationship between the effect and a specific cause. A population exposed to the suspected cause is identified; a comparison group is selected, matching for various factors except that the comparison group lacks exposure to the suspected cause; and the incidence of the effect is calculated. This method of study uses existing records to establish the history of exposure to the cause and then measures the effect of that exposure. Conceptually, this is a cohort study, but temporally, it is a retrospective study.

An additional study method is the cross-sectional study which examines the relationships between cause and effect in a defined population at a specific point in time. This study describes prevalence relationships and allows a direct measurement of the variables.

Experimental Epidemiology

The third epidemiologic technique, the experimental method, involves stating a hypothesis, developing an experimental model that allows for manipulation of one or several factors, and then noting the resultant effect. In this method, the hypothesis is tested. An example is the evaluation of a drug in the treatment of a certain disease. Patients with the disease are selected randomly and divided into two groups; one group is treated with the drug, and the other group is given a placebo. The resultant difference(s) between the two groups is attributed to the drug itself. Animals may be used in experimental epidemiology; if this technique is used on humans, careful consideration must be given to the ethics of the experiment as concerns real or potential danger to the human subjects.

EPIDEMIC INVESTIGATIONS

The objectives of investigating an outbreak of disease are to identify the problem, to ascertain its cause and the method of transmission, and to define the extent of involvement in terms of time, place, and person. The ultimate purpose of the investigation is to determine the appropriate measures necessary to control the outbreak and to prevent similar outbreaks from occurring.

The following paragraphs describe various elements of an epidemic investigation that form the skeleton for investigating the outbreak. There is no rigid rule that an investigation must be investigated in a particular order; it may be appropriate to change the sequence of the elements to meet certain exigencies of the investigation or of the ongoing occurrence of the disease itself. The actual elements may be telescoped or expanded. Additionally, it is important to consider whether control measures can be instituted before completion of the epidemic investigation to prevent the occurrence of additional cases.

An epidemic is an increase in the incidence of a disease above the expected incidence in a specific geographic area within a defined time period. The background occurrence (endemicity) of the disease in the population must be known in order for a judgment to be made as to whether the increased incidence is an epidemic or only normal variation. For example, an increase in the number of *Salmonella* isolates in August in a community may represent the normal increase for that time of year and not an unusual event.

An investigation may be carried out by the physician whose patients are involved, or the local or state health department may be notified and may provide support. Initially, an epidemiologist may be the only resource necessary; however, depending on the complexities of the outbreak, additional personnel may be needed, including nurses, veterinarians, sanitarians, environmental engineers, industrial hygienists, interviewers, statisticians, and laboratorians.

The first element in the investigation is to establish the existence of an epidemic. The initial and possibly other reporting sources should be consulted. This may involve contacting a physician, a health officer, patients, and relatives of patients; examining laboratory reports; reviewing hospital records; and checking absenteeism in industries or schools. This initial effort may be carried out very quickly.

The second element is to verify the diagnosis by obtaining clinical histories, examining patients, and obtaining appropriate specimens for laboratory study. A case definition needs to be developed; it should be broad enough to include all cases that may be important to the overall investigation. In setting a case definition it is important to remember the variability of host responses and that some cases may have been modified by reason of treatment or partial immunity. It is important for the epidemiologist to see "cases" and to discuss the diagnosis with the attending physician(s). It may be that some "noncases" should also be seen to refine the case definition. It might be appropriate to establish a classification system for cases under the headings of definite, probable, and suspected. In reviewing the laboratory data, it must be remembered that the laboratory results may not always be correct because of inadequacies in collection of the laboratory specimens, improper labeling, or improper handling or processing in the laboratory.

The next element is to do a rough case count to get an idea of the magnitude of the problem. Much time should not be spent on individual case data. These data should then be oriented according to time, place, and person (descriptive epidemiology). Time refers to determining the incubation period and graphing the epidemic curve. The shape of the curve may suggest the method of transmission and allow a prediction to be made about the course of the epidemic. As for place, plotting a spot map of the location of cases (where infection occurred) may provide important clues about the reservoir, the source, and the method of transmission. The data should also be oriented according to personal characteristics, that is, age, sex, occupation, socioeconomic status, and so on. It may be possible to make some preliminary judgments not only about the disease but also about intervention points for the institution of control measures that should perhaps be implemented at this time. In spite of implementation of any control measures, it is important to complete the epidemic investigation, not only to develop further information on the outbreak but also to evaluate the effectiveness of the implemented control measures.

The next element is to identify the population at risk, that is, the population exposed to the infectious agent, so attack rates can be calculated. The population may be determined by geographic area, such as those exposed to a specific water distribution area or those who work in a certain building. However, the exposed population may be more diffuse and difficult to identify, such as people who ate in a certain restaurant or who had contact with a certain commercially distributed food. It may be necessary to conduct a survey to determine the population at risk.

At this stage, a tentative hypothesis should be proposed by considering the data developed on the source and the reservoir of the agent, the mode of transmission, and the relevant host factors. Preferably the tentative hypothesis should be one that involves a single explanation for the outbreak. The hypothesis should allow for the best fit of all the data developed up to this point.

The next element is to plan and to conduct more systematic or specific investigations, including surveys, laboratory analyses, environmental examinations, and analytic epidemiologic studies. It may be necessary to reexamine patients or to seek out additional patients who may have been missed. The case definition may need to be narrowed, or cases that were previously listed as probable or suspected may now need to be included. The development of a comparison group may be important. New data should be combined with the previously analyzed data and reanalyzed. The analysis may involve hand tabulation of the data, use of McBee cards, or use of a computer. It may be appropriate to subject the analyzed data to statistical testing. The specific tests used will depend on various factors including the interrelationships between these factors and the quantity and complexity of the data.

The results of this analysis should confirm or challenge the tentative hypothesis. The hypothesis may be further tested by instituting specific control measures, which if successful, would result in a reduction of the number of cases. Knowledge of the past history of the disease in the population is necessary to know whether the change in the occurrence of cases was due to chance or was related to the control measures. If the hypothesis is correct, then it should be possible to predict the duration of the outbreak.

In testing the hypothesis it is important that the hypothesis be compatible with all the known facts. If this is not the case, the areas of incompatibility should be carefully reanalyzed to see whether an error was made in the analyses, whether some facts were missing, or whether some facts were wrong.

The local public health officials should be kept informed as to the progress of the investigation. A report of the investigation and recommended control measures should be prepared and distributed. At the appropriate time, the state and federal public health officials should be made aware of the epidemic and be provided with a copy of the report. Releasing publicity for general consumption may be a positive factor and should be considered.

Preventive measures should be considered, and an appropriate program should be planned and instituted. There may be need for a special surveillance program to evaluate the effectiveness of the recommended control measures. Education and training programs may be considered for selected groups of people.

SURVEILLANCE

General Aspects

Surveillance is a dynamic activity that includes gathering information on the occurrence of disease in a defined population, collating and analyzing these data, and summarizing the publishable findings.[9] If no action resulted from surveillance activities, it would be purely an archival function. Surveillance should be closely tied to control and prevention actions. Surveillance should either stimulate appropriate action or be used to evaluate actions already instituted.

The person responsible for reporting the occurrence of a reportable disease is the health care provider, usually a physician, who sees the patient and makes the diagnosis. The actual reporter, however, may be a representative of the physician, such as an assistant or secretary, a nurse, or hospital personnel. The list of reportable diseases varies from state to state and is modified at intervals. All physicians are required to report the occurrence of the three quarantinable diseases (cholera, plague, and yellow fever), and state health officials have agreed to collect and to report to federal officials cases of certain other communicable diseases. Additionally, depending on the need for additional data in some states, other communicable diseases may be reportable by individual state law.

A question often asked is why the private practitioner should report the occurrence of diseases, since filing a report takes time, and the physician frequently does not reap any noticeable benefits from participating in a surveillance program. An active surveillance program should provide physicians the opportunity to see the relationships of their cases to the occurrence of that disease in the community and should allow them to be more effective providers of health care. They should be interested in knowing whether their patient represents a single case of that disease or whether there are other cases that have occurred or are occurring.

Active surveillance may provide important information about therapy. For example, several years ago there was an epidemic of bacillary dysentery due to *Shigella dysenteriae* 1 in Mexico.[10] Some U.S. travelers became infected in Mexico and then returned to the United States, where clinical disease developed. This particular strain of *Shigella* had an unusual antibiotic resistance pattern (resistant to penicillin, tetracycline, chloramphenicol, and sulfonamide). Since the disease was under surveillance, cases had been reported, and since the organism had been studied in a laboratory, it was possible to recommend specific chemotherapy (ampicillin) when the diagnosis was first suspect. Thus it was not necessary to withhold specific therapy until the patient's organism had been isolated and its antibiogram had been determined.

Surveillance may provide information suggesting the need for institution of specific control and prevention measures, such as vaccination and prophylactic antibiotics. If surveillance reveals an increase in the occurrence of meningococcal meningitis, vaccination of highly susceptible groups of people with type-specific vaccine may clearly be indicated to prevent the occurrence of additional cases. Surveillance of hepatitis B may reveal an increasing incidence, which when investigated may identify a common source. Accordingly, those that have had contact with the common source within a prescribed period of time may be offered prophylactic immune serum or hepatitis B vaccine.

Current surveillance information may show the ineffectiveness of past or present disease control measures against the occurrence of a disease. Analysis of measles surveillance data, for example, has indicated that vaccination at less than 1 year of age did not, because of the presence of maternal antibody, provide all recipients with long-lasting immunity. Thus surveillance had identified a group of children who had been considered to be immune and who needed to be revaccinated.

Reporting may also make it possible to recognize epidemiologically related cases of a disease that without being reported to a central office would be considered sporadic cases. If this association is not recognized, the epidemic could continue smoldering and spreading. A number of years ago, an outbreak of staphylococcal skin infections developed in a newborn nursery, but the infants were being discharged before the infections became clinically apparent. Different pediatricians were seeing the infants, and it was not until two cases were reported by two pediatricians that the extensive outbreak was uncovered.

Surveillance data can be useful to health departments in their use of resources, including personnel, equipment, and money that should lead not only to increased efficiency but also to better control of the diseases under surveillance.

Collection of Data

There are 10 basic sources of surveillance information, some or all of which will be useful in describing a specific disease.[11]

The first element and the one most commonly used is morbidity data. Morbidity data are generated from case reports from health practitioners who report the occurrence of disease by various methods. These data, the backbone of any surveillance program, are dependent on the diagnosis being made by the health practitioner. Reporting methods vary. The traditional method has been the use of a simple card or form that a physician fills out and sends to the local or state health department. Other methods include reporting by telephone using a toll-free number. To encourage reporting, if the telephone report is being made at other than normal working hours, a recording device can be used to transcribe the data; if more information is desired, the physician can be called back.

Another method of obtaining morbidity data is the use of sentinel-physician reporting; a random selection of physicians from among those who are more likely to see infectious diseases (pediatricians, internists, family practice physicians, infectious disease specialists) are contacted and asked to report regularly the occurrence of reportable diseases.

These methods are passive methods: the reporter is asked to report cases when they occur. Active surveillance can be instituted by regularly contacting the reporters, usually by telephone, and asking if they have seen cases of specific diseases. This method may be very useful when attempting to develop information concerning the occurrence of a new disease or during an epidemic of a disease.

The second source of surveillance information is mortality data. Validity is dependent on the accuracy and completeness of the listing of the cause of death on death certificates. An example of the usefulness of this method is the collection of mortality data by the Centers for Disease Control (CDC) from 121 cities throughout the United States as part of the influenza surveillance program.[12] Knowing that excess mortality in the winter is usually due to influenza has made these data very useful in portraying the occurrence of epidemic influenza.

The third method of collecting surveillance data is case investigation. The occurrence of certain diseases, such as poliomyelitis, botulism, and plague, will always be investigated. The specific case investigation may uncover other cases of the same disease that would not have been diagnosed without the case investigation.

The fourth method of developing surveillance data is reporting of epidemics. Not all epidemics will be investigated, possibly because it is felt that nothing new will be gained from a particular investigation or because the health department does not have enough personnel available. During the influenza season, after the initial cases have been confirmed and laboratory specimens collected, it is quite possible that epidemics will be recorded but will not be investigated further unless some unusual feature occurs. Even without a specific investigation, the report of the epidemic will add important data to the surveillance program.

Another method of obtaining surveillance data is from an epidemic investigation. The initial report will indicate the occurrence of a certain number of cases; however, field investigation may result in a significant increase in the case count. In 1965, an outbreak of gastroenteritis due to *Salmonella typhimurium* occurred in Riverside, California.[13] Less than 1000 cases were or would have been reported had there been no further investigation. Because of the need to identify the source of infection, a field investigation was conducted, which included a community survey. As a result of the survey, more than 16,000 cases of gastroenteritis due to *S. typhimurium* were projected to have occurred. Since the majority of acute disease epidemics are not investigated, this method of obtaining surveillance data is undoubtedly underused.

The sixth method of gathering surveillance information is that of reviewing laboratory reports. For some diseases the laboratory identification of the etiologic agent is necessary if the disease is to be diagnosed at all or with any degree of accuracy. For example, it is difficult if not impossible to be specific as to the cause of gastroenteritis without laboratory assistance. An example of a successful surveillance program based on laboratory identification of the etiologic agent is that of salmonellosis. Not only is identification of the genus important but serotype identification of salmonella may show a cluster of cases due to the same serotype; identification of a rare serotype may trigger a specific field investigation. Laboratory identification of the antigenic makeup of influenza viruses is the only way that specific information concerning the occurrence and/or spread of specific types can be documented. These data are of significant value in deciding the formulation and subsequent use of influenza vaccines. The laboratory may also play a valuable part by characterizing the antibiotic sensitivity of organisms.

The seventh method of obtaining surveillance information is that of conducting population surveys to determine who has had a certain illness and to delineate characteristics that are key to the development of an illness.[14] Not all people in the community need actually be questioned; a statistically valid sample can be identified and questioned. If the survey group was properly selected, analysis of the data should produce data that are applicable to the entire population.

The eighth method for consideration is animal and vector disease occurrence data, which may be obtained from surveys of the appropriate populations, from observation of the occurrence of the disease in these populations, or from knowledge of carriage of the infectious agent among animals or vectors. In general, the surveillance of zoonotic diseases is enhanced by maintaining knowledge of the status of the disease in its host animals or insect vectors. For example, reports of tularemia would be investigated if cases of animal tularemia were not being reported from the area.

The ninth method of surveillance is that of noting the usage of certain biologics. For example, by noting requests for specific antitoxin, botulism surveillance is maintained.

The tenth method of surveillance is the use of demographic data that portrays the characteristics of a population. Demographic data may be useful in evaluating surveillance data and in projecting the anticipated occurrence of a disease in the population.

Another source of information that may provide surveillance data is local publicity. As reporters are frequently interested in the occurrence of disease, information from newspapers, radio, or television stations may provide the initial clue to the occurrence of a disease that may not have been reported.

Not all these methods of surveillance will be used to maintain surveillance for any one disease. Most frequently morbidity reporting is the main method used, supported by laboratory reports. The methods used will vary according to the type of surveillance data desired, the use to which it will be put, the sensitivity and specificity desired, and the available resources. Additional methods may be incorporated depending on the occurrence or on the anticipated occurrence of the disease.

The sensitivity and specificity of the surveillance system varies according to the disease, the method of reporting—including the reporting official, the circumstances of disease occurrence, and other nonpredictable factors. In disease of low frequency, such as poliomyelitis, plague, and anthrax, sensitivity is probably quite high, with close to 100 percent of the actual cases being reported. Diseases that occur with a high frequency, such as hepatitis, rubella, and salmonellosis, have a low reporting sensitivity. For example, only approximately 1 percent of the cases of salmonellosis are cultured and subsequently reported, and approximately 10 percent of cases of viral hepatitis are reported. The development of surveillance information is basically to show the linear trends of occurrence of disease. If the surveillance techniques remain fairly consistent, then the data will be adequate for comparison with previously collected data, for defining health problems, and for developing and evaluating control and prevention techniques. However, if there is a significant change in the surveillance technique, then there is need to be concerned about comparing data that may have been developed after the change occurred. For example, when *Shigella* surveillance was initiated in the United States, one-third of the states entered the program. Over the next several years, the other states joined, and there was a significant increase in the number of *Shigella* organisms identified in laboratories and reported to the surveillance system. Without knowing something about the expanding surveillance program throughout the country, we would have interpreted the surveillance data as showing a significant increase in shigellosis in the United States.

ANALYSIS OF DATA

The data, having been collected, must be collated and analyzed for those characteristics of the disease for which the surveillance program was initiated. The data should not be analyzed to any greater extent than they will be used. Depending on the complexities of the data and of the analyses, the statistical treatment of the data may be by hand or by computer. The data should be analyzed at intervals that allow development of relevant and timely information. If surveillance data are collected at weekly intervals, these data must be analyzed weekly. Frequency of analysis should be dictated by the use of the data.

Once the data have been analyzed, a report discussing those data and their analyses should be prepared. Additionally, the reports can provide comparisons with similarly collected data from previous years, discuss control and prevention measures, recount interesting aspects of the disease, and summarize outbreak investigations. The reports should be distributed to people who assisted in obtaining the data, as well as to those who need to see the results of surveillance activities in reference to their roles in control and prevention. Reports may be distributed at weekly or less frequent intervals. The CDC prepares a weekly surveillance report (*Morbidity and Mortality Weekly Report*) that summarizes the data reported weekly by the states and contains surveillance summaries, reports of current field investigations, international summaries, and quarantine-regulation information. Additionallly, the annual summary of these data compares the current year with others. The CDC also prepares quarterly and special surveillance reports at varying intervals for approximately 25 diseases.

Special surveillance programs may be established to meet the need for specific information over a limited period of time. For example, during the fall and winter, when influenza is prevalent, school and factory absenteeism is reported in selected areas. Routine reporting of excess mortality and review of laboratory isolates continues, but the additional data are useful in portraying the epidemic occurrence of influenza. Special surveillance programs may be developed for diseases that become of specific importance to public health such as legionnaires' disease, toxic shock syndrome, Reye syndrome, and acquired immunodeficiency syndrome (AIDS).

International surveillance through the World Health Organization is maintained on the three quarantinable diseases (cholera, plague, and yellow fever) and other diseases such as influenza and salmonellosis.

REFERENCES

1. Williams REO. Airborne staphylococci in the surgical ward. J Hyg (Camb). 1967;65:207.
2. Noble WZ. Dispersal and acquisition of microorganisms. In: Brachman PS, Eickhoff TC, eds. Proceedings of the International Conference on Nosocomial Infections. Chicago: American Hospital Association; 1971:193.
3. Eichenwald HF, Kotsevalov O, Fasso LA. The "cloud baby": an example of bacterial-viral interaction. Am J Dis Child. 1960;100:161.
4. Centers for Disease Control. Epidemiology Program Office, Division of Surveillance & Epidemiologic Studies.
5. Dowdle WR, Coleman MT, Gregg MB. Natural history of influenza type A in the United States, 1957–1972. Prog Med Virol. 1974;17:91.
6. Collins RN, Treger MD, Goldsby JB, et al. Interstate outbreak of *Salmonella new brunswick* infection traced to powdered milk. JAMA. 1968;203:838.
7. Fox JP, Hall CE, Elveback LR. Epidemiology: Man and Disease. New York: Macmillan; 1970:6.
8. MacMahon B, Pugh TF. Epidemiology Principles and Methods. Boston: Little Brown; 1970:41.
9. Thacker SB, Choi K, Brachman PS. The surveillance of infectious diseases. JAMA. 1983;249:1181.
10. Weissman JB, Marton KI, Lewis JN, et al. Impact in the United States of the Shiga dysentery pandemic of Central America and Mexico: a review of surveillance data through 1972. J Infect Dis. 1974;129:218.
11. World Health Organization. The surveillance of communicable diseases. WHO Chron. 1968;22:439.
12. Serfling RE. Methods for current statistical analysis of excess pneumonia-influenza deaths. Public Health Rep. 1963;78:494.
13. A waterborne epidemic of salmonellosis in Riverside, California, 1965, epidemiologic aspects, a collaborative report. Am J Epidemiol. 1971;93:33.
14. Serfling RE, Sherman IL. Attribute Sampling Methods, Publication No. 1230, US Department of Health, Education and Welfare, Public Health Service, 1965.

11. TRANSMISSION AND PRINCIPLES OF CONTROL

PHILIP S. BRACHMAN

Infectious disease results from the interaction between an infectious agent and a susceptible host. If the agent already resides in the host (endogenous infection), disease may develop due to changes in the relationship between the agent and the host. If the agent is transported from an external source to the host (exogenous infection) and if the balance between agent and host favors the agent, disease develops. The relationships among the agent, transmission, and the host may be considered the chain of infection.

There are four exogenous routes by which microorganisms are transmitted from the source to the host: contact, common vehicle, air, and vector. The environment plays an all-encompassing role, impacting on the agent, the route of transmission, and the host. Control and prevention of infections depend on defining the interaction of these factors. The most effective, practical, and appropriate means of interrupting the development of infection can then be identified and implemented. The relationships of these interrelating factors (chain of infection) will be discussed in this chapter.

AGENT

The agent, the first link in the chain of infection, is any microorganism—bacterium, virus, fungus, parasite, rickettsia or *Chlamydia*. The pathogenicity of an agent describes its ability to cause disease. An organism with high pathogenicity is the smallpox virus. There is no known human carrier state for this agent; once infected with the virus, the host will develop disease. Thus its presence in a human is always associated with disease. An organism of low pathogenicity is *Staphylococcus epidermidis*, an organism associated with a high colonization rate but not frequently associated with significant disease. Pathogenicity may be further described by noting the organism's virulence and invasiveness. Virulence may be described according to epidemiologic factors of morbidity, mortality, and communicability and by clinical factors, noting the severity of the disease.

In considering all organisms, there is a spectrum of virulence from low to high. Some organisms are described as avirulent; however, avirulence is a relative term, dependent on agent, host, and possibly other factors. An organism considered to be avirulent when in contact with a normally healthy person may cause disease in a highly susceptible person. For example, years ago *Serratia marcescens* organisms were used for air tracer studies because they were thought to be avirulent and their cultural characteristics made them distinctively identifiable. However, disease has been found to result from infection with *S. marcescens,* primarily in people with increased susceptibility to infectious agents.

Invasiveness is the ability of the agent to enter and to move through tissue. Some organisms move with relative ease, whereas others are likely to remain at the point of first tissue contact. For example, *Vibrio cholerae* organisms are not invasive but remain localized on the intestinal mucosa and produce toxin that on reacting with tissues results in the production of signs and symptoms. On the other hand, *Shigella* organisms are highly invasive and, when they locate on the mucosal surface of the intestine, will invade the submucosal tissue, become established, and cause disease.

Other agent factors to be considered in evaluating the role of the agent in causing infection are the infective dose, physical characteristics, organism specificity, antigenic variations of the organism, elaboration of enzymes and toxins, and genetic factors such as resistance transfer plasmids.

The infective dose, that is, the number of organisms necessary to cause an infection, vary according to the route and conditions of transmission and according to host susceptibility. The influence of transmission on the infective dose is exemplified by the susceptibility of enteric organisms to gastric acidity. For example, if the organisms are freely exposed to the gastric contents, a higher oral infective dose will be necessary than if they are transported through the stomach in milk, which will protect them from the acidity of the gastric contents.[1]

Physical characteristics of agents may influence the occurrence of disease. Some agents such as *Bacillus anthracis* can survive in soil for years, whereas most viruses generally do not survive for long within the inanimate environment.

Agent specificity refers to host preference as shown by some agents. For example, *Salmonella typhi* is host-specific for humans, whereas *Salmonella dublin* has a predilection for cattle. The smallpox virus was found only in humans. *Clostridium botulinum* types A, B, E, and F are associated with human disease, whereas types C and D are associated with disease in birds and mammals.

Within one species there may be antigenic variations that reflect differences in the pathogenicity of that organism. For example, among pneumococci there are 83 different serotypes (U.S. typing system); however, 80 percent of the cases of pneumococcal pneumonia are associated with only 14 types.

Other organisms may show antigenic variations over time. Influenza A virus shows minor antigenic drifts every 2–3 years and major changes or shifts every 7–10 years (A/Japan/305/57 H2N2, 1958–1959, A/Hong Kong/68 H3N2, 1968–1969, and so on).[2] These variations are reflected in changes in the occurrence of influenza A, which are further influenced by the immunity level of the population, which will vary according to the past experiences with that particular virus strain and with the use of influenza vaccines.

Some organisms elaborate enzymes that challenge the defense mechanisms of the host; other organisms produce toxins that damage the host's tissues. Resistance transfer plasmids may have a direct influence on antibiotic resistance and thus have an influence on the pathogenicity of bacterial organisms.

It is important to differentiate between the *reservoir* and the *source* of an organism if control measures are to be effectively directed against the organism. The reservoir is the location in which the organism is normally found, that is, where it becomes established, metabolizes, and multiplies. The source is the location from which the organism is immediately transmitted to the host either directly or indirectly through a vehicle (see below). The reservoir of *C. botulinum* is in the environment, specifically, in soil; the source of *C. botulinum* organisms for human infection is usually improperly processed food contaminated by soil. The reservoir and source may have the same location, such as a nasal carrier of *Staphylococcus aureus* who is disseminating organisms. However, if they have different locations, eradication of the organism at its source may not prevent further spread of infection, since the reservoir may remain and be capable of reinfecting the previous source or establishing new sources.

The presence of an organism depicts a potential for transmission, but the important event is the actual dissemination of the agent. Dissemination is influenced by various factors, including the number of organisms present, physical activity, stress, environmental factors, and the presence of another infection.

The period of infectivity refers to the time during which the source (usually refers to a human source) is infectious or is disseminating organisms. This is usually during the incubation period and the first days of the clinical period of disease as seen in hepatitis A and measles. A patient with influenza is usually only infectious during the clinical period. Some patients may remain infectious during the convalescent period, such as in shigellosis.

The portals of exit of organisms are most likely the respiratory, gastrointestinal, and genitourinary tracts. Additionally, the skin and wounds and blood can be the portals of exit.

TRANSMISSION

Transmission is the second link in the chain of infection, and there are four main routes of infection: contact, common vehicle, airborne, and vector-borne. Identification of the route by which microorganisms are transmitted from the source to the host may allow for specific control measures that are designed to interrupt transmission.

The contact route implies contact between the source and the host; that contact is by direct contact, indirect contact, or droplets. Direct contact means that the source and the host come in physical contact, allowing for direct transfer of microorganisms; this route is frequently called person-to-person. For example, a physician with a staphylococcal furuncle on a finger may directly infect a patient while performing a physical examination.

Indirect contact refers to the transmission of microorganisms from the source to the host via passive transfer—usually on an inanimate object. An example would be a common shaving brush that has become contaminated with *Pseudomonas* organisms and serves to transfer the organisms from an initial human source to the host.[3]

Droplet-spread organisms are those particles usually larger than 5 μm whose route of transmission is through the air, but only for very short distances. Because of their relatively large size, they rapidly settle out because they cannot travel in the air further than approximately 1 m. Transfer of microorganisms by droplets occurs because of the close proximity of the source and the host; droplets are usually produced by talking or sneezing. Measles and streptococcal infection are examples of droplet-spread diseases. When many people are exposed to a single source of droplets, attack rates will show a gradation from high for those closest to the source to low for those furthest away. For example, in a study of streptococcal transmission in an army barracks, where transmission was by the droplet route, susceptible soldiers whose beds were located nearest the source had the highest rates of acquiring streptococci.[4]

In common-vehicle spread, a single inanimate vehicle serves to transmit the infectious agent to multiple hosts. The vehicle may be actively involved in transmission by means of multiplication of the agent in the vehicle (direct), such as *Clostridium perfringens* in gravy, or may be passively involved (indirect) and only serve as a means by which the agent is transmitted to hosts, such as hepatitis A virus in food. The most frequently involved common vehicles are food and water; however, lots or batches of blood, blood products, intravenous fluids, and drugs may be prepared from a single contaminated source and serve as a "common vehicle," resulting in multiple infections.

In airborne transmission, the etiologic agent is truly airborne in its transmission from the source to the host. The airborne infected particles are either contained in droplet nuclei or dust and travel over 1 m in the air from the disseminating source to the host. Droplet nuclei are small particles—less than 5 μm in diameter—that represent the residua resulting from evaporation of larger particles (droplets). Dust represents material that settles out from the air and becomes resuspended by physical forces. Skin squames may also serve as airborne vehicles of infectious agents. The distance airborne particles are carried in the air depends on the force with which the particles are propelled into the air. In some outbreaks of airborne disease, the infective particles were carried several miles from the source to the susceptible hosts.

Humans, animals, and inanimate objects can be sources of airborne agents. When humans and animals are the source, the agent can be propelled by coughing and sneezing into the air from the respiratory tract. Tuberculosis is an example of an airborne spread disease from a human source. Usually the organisms become airborne by coughing. In one case, tubercule bacilli became airborne from a singer whose lesion was on a vocal chord, and he only disseminated when he sang. An example of human disease resulting from the airborne spread of the agent from an animal is psittacosis among bird owners, the source of the agent being psittacine birds.

An example of an inanimate source of airborne particles is an outbreak of Q fever, in which equipment in a rendering plant in which contaminated animal products were being processed produced aerosols containing *Coxsiella burnetii* that were being carried up to 10 miles downwind by the prevailing winds and resulted in 75 cases of disease.[5]

Insects are the source of vector-borne agents, and vector-borne transmission includes external and internal transmission. In external or mechanical transmission, the agent is carried on the body of the insect vector. Carriage is passive, with no change in the organism during transmission. Flies carrying *Salmonella* or *Shigella* organisms on their appendages from a fecal source to food would be an example of external carriage. In internal transmission, the etiologic agent is carried within the insect vector, and there is either harborage or a biologic transmission phase. In harborage transmission, the organism is ingested by the insect but undergoes no changes within the vector while being carried. An example of harborage transmission is carriage of *Yersinia pestis* within a flea during the transmission of plague. The organisms are picked up by the flea while it is feeding on a "source" and carried in the flea gut until deposited on the skin of a host, but they undergo no changes while in the flea.

Biologic transmission indicates that the etiologic agent goes through physiologic changes in the vector, such as in malaria, in which there is maturation of the agent within the mosquito. In investigating vector-borne disease in which there is a true biologic transmission phase, it is important to consider the incubation period of the etiologic agent within the vector, which is known as the extrinsic incubation period, as distinct from the intrinsic incubation period, which is the incubation period within the susceptible host after transmission has occurred.

Usually the route of transmission is predictable; however, some microorganisms may be transmitted by one of several different routes. For example, staphylococci are usually transmitted by direct (person-to-person) contact; however, they can also be transported by the airborne route. Salmonellae are usually transported by means of a common vehicle, but they can also be transported by direct contact and by the airborne route; they also have been reported to be transmitted by vectors (external). Malaria parasites are most frequently transmitted by vectors, but they have also been transmitted in transfused contaminated blood. Knowledge of the most likely route of transmission can be important in rapidly controlling the occurrence of additional cases if it is not possible to conduct definitive studies to define all the circumstances of the epidemic.

HOST

The host is the last link in the chain of infection. The site of entrance of the agent may be the skin, mucous membranes, respiratory tract, urinary tract, or gastrointestinal tract. Some organisms, such as *Leptospira,* are able to penetrate the intact skin, whereas other organisms can only enter the skin through breaks in the integrity of the skin. Microorganisms may also be introduced through the skin by the parenteral route such as by means of contaminated blood (hepatitis B virus) or intravenous fluids (gram-negative organisms or yeasts). Insect vectors may inject organisms through the skin (malaria).

Organisms may be deposited on the mucous membranes by movement through the air (adenovirus 8) or by contact with inanimate objects, such as instruments or medications. Organisms inhaled into the lungs will be deposited at various levels of the pulmonary tree in relation to their size. The larger particles may not reach the bronchi but impinge on the nasal cilia and travel no further; the majority of the smaller particles (less than 5 μm in diameter) will reach the terminal alveoli where they may be deposited and cause disease or be carried across the aveolar membranes in macrophages and may either be deposited in local lymph nodes or spread systemically throughout the body.

Organisms may also enter the host via the urinary tract during the process of catheterization or instrumentation or may travel retrogressively through a urinary catheter. Organisms may be ingested with contaminated food or water or through contamination of an instrument introduced into the gastrointestinal tract.

Infection may also be transmitted via the transplacental route such as rubella viruses and *Toxoplasma* parasites.[6] Transplantation may also result in the introduction of organisms into the body, such as a kidney contaminated with cytomegalovirus or a heart valve contaminated with *S. epidermidis* organisms.

Microorganisms may colonize one site without any evidence of disease, but the same organism located in another site may cause symptomatic disease. For example, *S. aureus* may colonize the external nares without any evidence of disease, but the same organism located beneath the skin may result in a skin infection.

The host defense mechanisms may be categorized as either nonspecific or specific (see Section B for a more complete discussion of host defense mechanisms). Nonspecific mechanisms include the skin, body secretions such as tears, mucus, and saliva, and nasal cilia. Inflammation is another nonspecific action the body uses to mobilize defense mechanisms against microorganisms. Nonspecific defense mechanisms are also influenced by age, sex, genetic factors, nutrition, and behavioral patterns.

Specific defense mechanisms include natural and artificial im munity. Natural immunity follows the natural occurrence of disease, such as measles, rubella, and poliomyelitis. Natural immunity usually has a long duration, at times for the life of the host, and can be demonstrated by specific serologic studies. It may also be demonstrated by noting the lack of the occurrence of disease in a population previously naturally exposed to the agent. For example, people exposed to the HlNl influenza viruses that circulated throughout the world from late 1946 to early 1957 now show relative immunity to the new prevalent strain A/USSR/7/77(HlNl), which is antigenetically related to the prior HlNl virus.[7]

Artificial immunity is either active or passive. Active artificial immunity results from vaccination using killed vaccines (typhoid fever or pertussis), attenuated vaccines (Calmette-Guérin/bacillus—BCG or poliomyelitis), or toxoids (diphtheria, tetanus). Passive immunity is associated with the use of immunoglobulins, antitoxins, or material antibody in newborn infants.

A more complete discussion of immunization will be found in Chapter 296.

The spectrum of host response to infection depends on agent and host factors and varies from subclinical, or inapparent infection, to severe disease with the most severe involvement being death. Subclinical infection can be determined by serologic means. Also, a carrier state may develop. If a host has partial immunity that may develop following imperfect immunization or incomplete therapy and if infection develops, it may result in modified or atypical disease. Also, prophylactic or therapeutic treatment after exposure to an infectious agent may result in an atypical clinical expression of the disease.

ROLE OF THE ENVIRONMENT

Infection develops within the milieu of the environment, and thus any of the determinants involved in the occurrence of an infection may be influenced by environmental factors such as heat, cold, moisture, radiation, air pressure, movement and velocity of the air, and presence of chemicals, gases, and toxins. The influence may promote the development of infection or it may inhibit, limit, or prevent the development of infection.

Environmental factors in effect at the agent's reservoir, such as temperature, humidity, and nutrients, may be beneficial or inhibitory to the growth and multiplication of the agent. The movement of the agent from the source to the susceptible host may be influenced by air velocity, humidity, radiation, and temperature. The host may also be influenced by environmental factors, such as low humidity, which may increase the permeability of mucous membranes to infectious agents.

Environmental studies should be conducted to define the precise role of the environment so control efforts can be directed specifically if indicated and not randomly at the appropriate environmental factor. In hospitals, for example, it is not unusual to find an extremely complex—but random—environmental control program in operation; such programs are more expensive and less effective than programs directed at preventing specific infections. Not only do catchall programs cost more but they may also lead to a false sense of security.

Some hospitals have relied heavily on routine environmental culturing in their efforts to prevent nosocomial infections. They have set unsubstantiated standards for recovery of microorganisms from these environmental specimens and have predicted that when recovery does exceed the standard, disease will result unless special decontamination efforts are instituted. Generally, however, setting such standards is not based on factual data. Another example of the overemphasis on the environment was the promotion of full-room ultraviolet irradiation in operating theaters as a technique to prevent the development of postoperative infections.[8] Full-room irradiation does reduce the number of airborne bacteria, but a double-blind study conducted by the National Research Council indicated that there was no difference in the overall rate of postoperative wound infections. There was a difference in the postoperative wound infection rate for operations with the highest risk of developing postoperative wound infections ("dirty wounds"—such as those where the bowel was transected), but it did not show any statistically valid effect for the rest of the operations, and thus there was no justification for using full-room irradiation for all operative procedures.

There are some appropriate standards, such as the number of coliform organisms in water, which are acceptable as standards for human use. Some routine environmental cultures can be meaningful, such as regular bacteriologic checks of autoclaves and/or hospital-prepared infant formula. Some environmental cultures may be useful in training programs to demonstrate the potential role of the inanimate environment in causing disease.

The environment can play an important role in the development of infections, but before strenuous nonspecific control efforts aimed at influencing environmental factors are instituted, appropriate studies must be conducted to demonstrate the specific role that the environmental factors play in the development of infections. Only after these studies have been completed should measures be adopted aimed at influencing the environmental factors. The environmental emphasis should be in concert with knowledge of the specific role of the environment in particular disease outbreak situations.

CONTROL

Since the development of infections is multifactorial, designing control measures is complex. We have to consider available resources, cost effectiveness, time constraints, adverse effects or complications of the proposed control measures, and effect on prevention of future cases (or epidemics). Control activities may reflect compromises among competing measures. For the most appropriate, effective, and acceptable decision, all the interrelated parameters related to the occurrence of the particular infection (or epidemic) need to be identified. Only then can an intelligent decision be made. Basically, control measures should be directed against the part of the infection cycle most susceptible to such actions. However, other considerations, such as cost and availability of personnel may indicate otherwise.

Control efforts may best be directed toward controlling or eradicating the agent at its reservoir or source. If the reservoir or source is human, then therapy or isolation techniques may be the best method of preventing the spread of infection.[9] If the reservoir or source is an inanimate object, then it may be controlled by either decontamination procedures or by using disposable materials.

If the route of transmission seems to be the best area for approaching control, then the specific type of transmission needs to be identified, for methods of control will vary depending on the route. If the disease is spread by the contact route, then control measures need to be directed toward people or inanimate objects associated with transmission. Personal factors may reflect the need for education or antibiotic therapy. If an inanimate object is involved, improved disinfection or sterilization methods may be necessary. If there is a common-vehicle-spread disease, then the vehicle must be decontaminated by better processing, sterilization, and improved training of humans to prevent contamination from occurring. If airborne infection is involved, effective filtering of the contaminated air or other treatment of the air needs to be instituted. If the disease is spread by vector, the vector must be controlled by spraying or other techniques.

If the best way to control infection is to increase the resistance of the host, then the primary defense mechanisms may need to be strengthened. It may be necessary to improve secondary host defenses by vaccination, either actively or passively.

Thus control must be directed toward the part of the pathway of infection that is most susceptible to the development of infection.

One of the most important areas of control is education, not only for new employees but ongoing, continuing education for all employees. All need to be reminded of old techniques and taught new techniques. Changing human behavioral patterns by education can be a very effective way to reduce the risk of infection.

REFERENCES

1. Hornick RB, Greisman SE, Woodward TE, et al. Typhoid fever: pathogenesis and immunologic control. N Engl J Med. 1970;283:686.
2. Dowdle WR, Coleman MT, Gregg MB. Natural history of influenza type A in the United States, 1957–1972. Prog Med Virol. 1974;17:91.
3. Ayliffe CAJ, Lowbury EJL, Hamilton JG, et al. Hospital infection with *Pseudonomas aeruginosa* in neurosurgery. Lancet. 1965;1:365.
4. Rammelkamp CH Jr, Mortimer EA Jr, Wolinsky E. Transmission of streptococcal and staphylococcal infections. Ann Intern Med. 1964;60:753.
5. Wellock CE. Epidemiology of Q-fever in the urban East Bay area. California Health. 1960;18:73.
6. Benenson AS, ed. Control of Communicable Diseases in Man. 13th ed. Washington, DC: APHA; 1980:296, 356.
7. Gregg MB, Hinman AR, Craven RB. The Russian flu: its history and implications for this year's influenza season. JAMA. 1978;240:2260.
8. Postoperative Wound Infections. The influence of ultraviolet irradiation of the operating room and of various other factors. Report of an ad hoc committee. Ann Surg. 1964;Suppl, August.
9. CDC Guidelines for Isolation Precautions in Hospitals. US Department of Health and Human Services, Public Health Service, Centers for Disease Control; 1983:81.

12. PRINCIPLES OF CHEMOPROPHYLAXIS AND IMMUNOPROPHYLAXIS

PHILIP S. BRACHMAN

CHEMOPROPHYLAXIS

Chemoprophylaxis is the treatment with a drug before, during, or shortly after exposure to an infectious agent or agents in an attempt to prevent the development of infection due to that agent. Chemoprophylaxis may be specific, that is, directed against a specific microorganism—usually an exogenous organism such as *Neisseria meningitidis*—or it may be nonspecific—when more than one organism, any one of which may cause an infection, may be present. These organisms are usually endogenous (or autogenous). An example of nonspecific prophylaxis is the preoperative use of antibiotics to prevent postoperative wound infections.

The greatest possibility for success occurs when chemoprophylaxis is directed against a specific organism with known antibiotic sensitivities. When nonspecific chemoprophylaxis is directed against various organisms, usually the host's nonspecific defense mechanisms have been compromised. If the antibiotic sensitivities of the organisms vary, then the choice of the prophylactic drug is a difficult one. If prophylaxis directed against two or more organisms is not effective against all of them, one or several of the surviving species may multiply to fill the niche vacated by the eradicated organism. This may lead to the development of disease due to the replacement organism.

Other potential problems related to specific or nonspecific prophylaxis are that the prolonged use of a chemoprophylactic agent may lead to the development of hypersensitivity to that agent or to the development of resistant strains for which the specific prophylaxis is no longer effective. Other considerations include the expense of prophylaxis and the development of adverse reactions, such as hepatitis following exposure to isonicotinic acid hydrazide (INH).

When to start, how much to give, which to give, and how long to continue prophylactic therapy depend on the microorganism or microorganisms involved, the period during which it or they may be infectious to the patient, the mode of transmission, and the period during which the patient is susceptible to infection. The patient's susceptibility will reflect the defense mechanisms. These may be normal, but due to a high degree of pathogenicity of the organism, the development of disease is a definite possibility. However, the host's defenses may be compromised as a result of hereditary factors, disease, malnutrition, or therapy, making possible an infection with an organism of low pathogenicity, such as *Staphylococcus epidermidis*. Prophylaxis is often started before potential exposure to the infectious agent, such as preoperatively, but it may be given during exposure, such as chloroquine during travel in a malarious area, or after exposure, such as after contact with a person with gonorrhea.

A potential problem in making a decision about prophylaxis may be in determining the degree of contact the person actually had with the microorganism. The decision to initiate prophylactic therapy is at times made on the basis of an emotional response to the potential pathogenicity of the organism and not on the basis of the actual degree of contact with the organism. When considering chemoprophylaxis, a judgment should be made as to whether the benefits outweigh the possible adverse effects.

Specific Chemoprophylaxis

Specific chemoprophylaxis has been shown to be effective in cholera,[1] gonorrhea (Chapter 190)[2] *Haemophilus influenza* (Chapter 201),[3] influenza (Chapter 142),[4] leprosy (Chapter 230),[5] malaria (Chapter 251),[6] meningococcal infections (Chapter 189),[7] rheumatic fever (Chapter 177), syphilis (Chapter 213),[8,9] and tuberculosis (Chapter 229).[10]

Chemoprophylaxis has also been shown to be effective in preventing certain nosocomial infections. For example, it may be very effective in preventing wound infections after clean-contaminated surgical procedures and has shown effectiveness following some clean surgical procedures. This subject is reviewed in detail by Eickhoff.[11] Prophylactic doxycycline has been reported to be effective in preventing travelers' diarrhea in some areas.[12] However, there is concern over the extrapolation of these results to other areas; the prophylactic use of antibiotics for travelers' diarrhea should be approached with caution.

There are also some infections for which chemoprophylaxis is used, but its effectiveness in preventing infections has not been proven. One example is in contacts of pneumonic plague among whom the use of tetracycline has been recommended.

IMMUNOPROPHYLAXIS

Immunoprophylaxis is the use of vaccines, toxoids, and immune serum to protect otherwise susceptible people against specific diseases. (A more detailed discussion of specific immunoprophylaxis will be found in Chapter 296.) Occurrence of the natural disease usually results in the production of protective antibody against that disease; this usually persists for years and possibly for the life of the person. If one lacks natural antibody against a disease, then active or passive immunoprophylaxis may help provide immunologic protection. In active immunoprophylaxis the body's immune system is stimulated to develop antibody against the antigen. The antigen can be live, or inactivated (killed), or a toxoid. An antibody so produced varies in the duration of effectiveness from months, as in the case of some cholera vaccines, to years, as in the case of diphtheria or tetanus toxoid. With certain vaccines, especially the killed vaccines and toxoids, booster inoculations are necessary to maintain protection. In passive immunoprophylaxis, antibody formed in another host, animal or human, is given to a susceptible person and provides protection for the life (relatively short) of the passively infused antibodies. An example of this is immunoglobulin used against hepatitis A.

Control of current and prevention of future epidemics of some infectious diseases may result from increasing the immunity level (herd immunity) of groups of susceptible people by means of community vaccination programs. These are especially important today in populations in which there may be significant numbers of people susceptible to diseases of relatively high prevalence, such as measles and rubella. In diseases of low prevalence, such as diphtheria and poliomyelitis, there may be small pockets of susceptible people who should be vaccinated to prevent focal epidemics from occurring. Vaccination campaigns supported by public health authorities, medical societies, and other groups have been successful in raising immunity levels and in preventing serious large epidemics of these diseases. However, many of these diseases occur at a frequency that clearly indicates a need to continue to stimulate health care providers to promote routine vaccination actively for their patients as a part of good preventive care. Some of the newer vaccines have been used to control outbreaks of disease in selected populations, such as the outbreak of meningococcal disease in Brazil[13] and in other populations[14] and outbreaks of pneumococcal disease in military recruits.[15]

Active or passive immunization may afford only partial protection, which means that subsequent exposure to the specific etiologic agent may result in the disease or in a modified clinical form of the disease. In some cases the modified or atypical clinical manifestations may be as severe or more severe than the natural disease. For example, this has been seen in some people initially vaccinated with live measles vaccine in combination with measles immune serum globulin who subsequently were exposed to naturally occurring measles virus.

Active Immunoprophylaxis

Recommendations for the use of an active immunizing agent depend on the potential for exposure to that pathogen. The vaccine should be administered far enough in advance of exposure for protective antibody to develop; antibody responses usually take 7–21 days. There are some diseases for which the vaccine should be given as part of a regular "childhood vaccination" program (diphtheria, pertussis, tetanus, poliomyelitis, measles, rubella, mumps; in some countries Calmette-Guérin bacillus [BCG] is considered part of the regular vaccination program).[16] Other vaccines such as cholera, plague, typhoid fever, and yellow fever, should be given as necessary, depending on exposure potential related to travel. At times residence may necessitate recommendations for certain vaccines because of the prevalence of certain diseases in the area such as plague and yellow fever. Professional activity may dictate the need for vaccination programs. In a laboratory in which pathogenic organisms are handled, vaccines against them, if they exist, should be routinely used for the personnel or for those people who may have contact with this laboratory or with the specific agents. These diseases include anthrax, cholera, hepatitis B, plague, rabies, Rocky Mountain spotted fever, typhoid fever, typhus, and yellow fever. Additionally, anthrax vaccination is indicated for people who are exposed to certain imported raw animal materials, and rabies vaccine should be given to people whose occupations may bring them into contact with possibly rabid animals, either domestic or wild.

Some vaccines should be used in selected populations, depending on the disease occurrence and on the population characteristics. Influenza vaccine should be considered for use on an annual basis for those people with chronic debilitating conditions such as pulmonary disease, cardiovascular disease, and metabolic diseases.[17] Additionally, elderly people should be routinely given the current vaccine. Consideration should be given to vaccinating people, such as policemen, firemen, hospital personnel, and utility repair personnel, who provide essential community services. Meningococcal vaccine should be considered in areas of population groups in which the disease is of moderate prevalence, such as in some military recruit populations[18] or in some families with a risk of secondary cases.[19] In some elderly populations, pneumococcal vaccines are recommended as a regular immunization program.[20] In some hospitals, some vaccines are recommended or mandated for employees who work in specific high-risk areas. These include hepatitis B, measles, and rubella vaccines.[21] In some countries, BCG vaccine is recommended for children due to the prevalence of active disease among the population.[16] In addition to some professional groups in hospitals, there are other high-risk groups for which hepatitis B vaccine is recommended.[22]

Passive Immunoprophylaxis

Passive immunoprophylaxis is recommended in circumstances in which a susceptible person is exposed to an infectious agent and there is inadequate time to allow for immunization and antibody formation or there is no appropriate vaccine with which to immunize that person actively. In these instances there should be documentation of the actual exposure before use of the passive immunizing agent. It may be necessary to use epidemiologic evidence to decide whether the passive immunizing agent should be used. For example, when rabies exposure stems from animal contact and the animal is not available for diagnostic studies, a judgment has to be made as to the likelihood of that animal being rabid. In circumstances in which a definite judgment cannot be made, it is usually best to err on the side of providing therapy.

The diseases for which passive immunoprophylaxis should be considered are botulism, diphtheria, viral hepatitis, measles, rabies, tetanus, and varicella-zoster.

It is recommended that a serum sample be taken before the patient is given the passive immunizing agent so diagnostic or therapeutic studies can be conducted if appropriate.

Maternal antibodies are forms of passive immunization that are important in certain situations. For example, in some countries the passive transfer of maternal tetanus antibody is of prophylactic importance in preventing neonatal tetanus. The presence and relative persistence of maternal antibody will influence the effectiveness of active vaccination, which has to be considered in planning the regular vaccination schedule for newborns. This has been of particular importance in scheduling use of measles vaccine.

REFERENCES

1. McCormick WM, Chowdhury AM, Hahangir N, et al. Tetracycline prophylaxis in families of cholera patients. Bull WHO. 1968;38:787.
2. Centers for Disease Control. Sexually Transmitted Diseases Treatment Guidelines—1982. MMWR. 1982;31(Suppl):375.
3. Centers for Disease Control. Prevention of secondary cases of *Haemophilus influenzae* type b disease. MWWR. 1982;31:672.
4. Jackson GG, Stanley ED. Prevention and control of influenza by chemoprophylaxis and chemotherapy. JAMA. 1976;235:2739.
5. Noorden SK. Chemoprophylaxis in leprosy. Lepr India. 1969;41:247.
6. Centers for Disease Control. Prevention of malaria in travelers. MMWR. 1982;31(Suppl):3s.
7. Meningococcal Disease Surveillance Group. Analysis of endemic meningococcal disease by serogroup and evaluation of chemoprophylaxis. J Infect Dis. 1976;134:201.
8. Centers for Disease Control. Sexually Transmitted Diseases Treatment Guidelines—1982. MMWR. 1982;31(Suppl):50s.
9. Elliott WC. Treatment of primary syphilis. J Am Venereal Dis. 1976;3:128.
10. American Thoracic Society/Centers for Disease Control. Treatment of tuberculosis and other mycobacterial diseases. Am Rev Respir Dis. 1983;127:793.
11. Eickhoff TC. Antibiotics and nosocomial infections. In: Bennett JV, Brachman PS, eds. Hospital Infections. Boston: Little, Brown; 1979:195–221.
12. Sack DA, Kaminsky DC, Sack RB, et al. Prophylactic doxycycline for travelers' diarrhea. N Engl J Med. 1978;298:758.
13. Meningococcal meningitis vaccine: Brazil. Bull Pan Am Health Organ. 1976;10:20.
14. Makela PH, Kayhty H, Weckstrom P, et al. Effect of group-A meningococcal vaccine in army recruits in Finland. Lancet. 1975;1:883.
15. MacLeod CM, Hodges RG, Heidelberger M, et al. Prevention of pneumococcal pneumonia by immunization with specific capsular polysaccharides. J Exp Med. 1945;82:445.
16. American Thoracic Society/Centers for Disease Control. Treatment of tuberculosis and other mycobacterial diseases. Am Rev Respir Dis. 1983;127:795.
17. Centers for Disease Control. Influenza vaccines. MMWR. 1983;32:333.
18. Centers for Disease Control. Meningococcal polysaccharides vaccines. Recommendations of the Public Health Service Advisory Committee on Immunization Practices. MMWR. 1978;27:327.
19. Greenwood BM, Hassan-King M, Whittle HC. Prevention of secondary cases of meningococcal disease in household contacts by vaccination. Br Med J. 1978;1:1317.
20. Centers for Disease Control. Pneumococcal polysaccharide vaccine. Recommendation of the Public Health Service Advisory Committee on Immunization Practices. MMWR. 1981;30:410.
21. CDC Guideline for Infection Control in Hospital Personnel. US Dept Health and Human Services, Public Health Service, Centers for Disease Control; 1983:17–8.
22. Centers for Disease Control. Inactivated hepatitis B viral vaccine. Recommendations of the Immunizations Practice Advisory Committee (APIC). MMWR. 1982;31:317–27.

SECTION D. THE CLINICIAN AND THE MICROBIOLOGY LABORATORY

13. BACTERIA, FUNGI, AND PARASITES

JOHN A. WASHINGTON II

The purpose of the microbiology laboratory is to isolate and identify microorganisms that cause disease and to determine their susceptibility to antimicrobial agents that assist in their eradication. There is, however, no other area of the clinical laboratory in which specimen sources and types are so diverse, in which specimen selection and collection are so important, and in which close communication with the clinician is so vital.

SPECIMEN COLLECTION AND PROCESSING

There are several general guidelines on selection and collection of the specimen that bear emphasis. First of all, the specimen selected should be representative of the disease process. Material swabbed from the orifice of a sinus tract is, for example, more apt to yield harmless saprophytic microorganisms present on the skin than would material obtained by curettage or biopsy of the base of the tract. Second, an adequate quantity of material should be obtained for complete examination. All too frequently, a small or even invisible amount of material is obtained with a swab, which makes it nearly impossible for the laboratory to make appropriate smears and adequate cultures. Characteristically, chronic lesions contain few organisms. These may be missed readily in smears, cultures, and histopathologic sections. Third, scrupulous attention must be given to avoiding contamination of the specimen by the many varieties of organisms indigenous to the skin and mucous membranes (Table 1), culture of which may often be more confusing and misleading than helpful. Sterile equipment and aseptic technique should be used for collecting specimens, particularly those from normally sterile sites. Fourth, material should be forwarded promptly to the laboratory. Fastidious organisms may not survive prolonged storage or may be overgrown by less fastidious organisms before cultures can be made. Last, specimens should be obtained before antimicrobial agents have been administered.

Other factors may impair the laboratory's ability to establish the cause of an infectious disease. First, sampling difficulties may preclude obtaining a specimen representative of the disease process. Second, it may be impossible to obtain a specimen that is not contaminated with flora indigenous to the site of infection. Third, patients with serious underlying diseases often become colonized with gram-negative bacilli, so their indigenous flora contains potentially pathogenic bacteria not ordinarily encountered on healthy human body surfaces. A somewhat different problem in the compromised host is that infections may be caused by organisms ordinarily considered to be indigenous on healthy human body surfaces; therefore, the more attention given to collecting the specimen, the greater the level of confidence we can place on the results of its culture. Fourth, technical errors of various types can interfere with the recovery of organisms causing disease. Examples include patients to whom antimicrobials were being administered at the time of specimen collection, the application of topical anesthetics to infected sites before specimen collection, the use of saline or another irrigating solution containing a preservative to collect the specimen, improper transport or storage of specimens, and the inappropriate selection of culture media.

A final limitation on the laboratory's ability to determine the cause of an infectious disease relates to the laboratory's capability of recovering a rare, unusual, or fastidious organism. It is unreasonable to expect equal capabilities from all microbiology laboratories, and varying extents or levels of capability have been recognized in bacteriology, mycobacteriology, mycology, virology, and parasitology by national laboratory accreditation agencies. Thus, a laboratory offering level I service in mycobacteriology, for example, develops a proficiency in the collection of adequate clinical specimens and in their prompt transport to a more specialized laboratory. With existing and anticipated regulations requiring inspection, proficiency testing, and accreditation, we may anticipate that an increased number of clinical laboratories will establish extents and levels of performance and refer materials or cultures to be examined for rare, fastidious, or otherwise unusual organisms to specialized laboratories. Although it is essential for laboratories to recognize their own limitations, it also behooves the clinician to be aware of these limitations and to recommend referral of material or cultures to specialized laboratories when a diagnosis is suspected that cannot be established by the laboratory facilities at hand. It is essential that diagnostic specimens sent to reference laboratories be shipped according to minimum packaging requirements specified by federal regulation.[1]

Hospital procedure guides should contain reasonably precise guidelines for the collection and transport of specimens from various sites (Table 2). There are numerous kinds of devices and containers available for this purpose. Swabs of every description and composition are available. Many commercially manufactured swab tubes contain a transport medium that is designed to preserve a variety of organisms and to prevent the multiplication of rapidly growing organisms. The swab, however, should be limited in its use to collecting material from the skin and mucous membranes, principally because the amount of material that can be collected with it is limited and is often negligible in practice. It should never be submitted in lieu of curettings, biopsy material, pus, or fluid or tissue removed surgically. All too frequently, biopsy specimens or excised materials are placed in their entirety into formalin for histopatho-

TABLE 1. Microorganisms Encountered on Healthy Human Body Surfaces

Organism	*Skin*	*Conjunctiva*	*Upper Respiratory Tract*	*Mouth*	*Intestine*	*External Genitalia*	*Anterior Urethra*	*Vagina*
Bacteria								
Actinomyces			+	+	±			
Bacteroides			+	++	++	+	+	+
Bifidobacteria				+	++			
Clostridia	±			±	++		±	±
Corynebacteria	++	+	+	+	+	+	+	+
Enterobacteriaceae	±		±	±	++	+	+	±
Fusobacteria			+	++	+	+	+	±
Haemophilus		±	++	+				
Lactobacilli				+	+		±	++
Mycoplasmas			+	+			+	+
Neisseriae		±	++	+			+	±
Propionibacteria	++		+	±	±		±	
Staphylococci	++	+	+	+	±	++	+	+
Streptococci								
Enterococcal			±	+	+	+	+	+
Pyogenic			±	±				±
Viridans group	±	±	+	++	+	+	+	+
Spirochetes				+	+			
Cocci, anaerobic								
Gram-positive	+		+	++	++	+	±	+
Gram-negative			+	++	+		±	+
Fungi								
Aspergillus	±	+		+				
Candida	±	+	+	++	+			+
Cryptococcus	±			±				
Penicillium	+	+		+				
Rhodotorula	±	+		+				
Torulopsis	±			+	±			±

Symbols: ±: irregular; +: common; ++: prominent.

TABLE 2. Guidelines for Microbiologic Specimen Collection and Transport

Specimen	Container or Transport Device	Volume (ml)	Other Considerations
Respiratory tract			
Nasopharynx	Flexible wire calcium alginate tipped swab or no. 8 French 16" suction catheter in sterile jar	NA	Used to detect carrier states of *Streptococcus pyogenes*, *Neisseria meningitidis*, *Corynebacterium diphtheriae*, and *Bordetella pertussis*. Aspirates are useful in the diagnosis of pertussis.
Sinus aspirate	Anaerobic transport vial	NA	
Tympanocentesis	Anaerobic transport vial	NA	
Oral cavity	Swab	NA	
Throat	Swab	NA	Swab tonsils, tonsillar areas, posterior pharynx, and areas of inflammation, exudation, ulceration, or capsule formation. Notify laboratory when diphtheria, pertussis, or gonococcal pharyngitis is suspected clinically.
Tracheal aspirate	Sterile, screw-capped tube or jar	NA	Specimen unsuitable for anaerobic culture.
Bronchial washings	Sterile, screw-capped tube or jar	NA	Specimen unsuitable for anaerobic culture unless obtained with double-lumen, distally occluded catheter.
Transtracheal apirate	Anaerobic transport vial	3–5	
Sputum			
Bacteria	Sterile, screw-capped jar	NA	Collect fresh specimen resulting from deep cough. Instruct patient not to expectorate saliva or postnasal discharge into container. Specimen unsuitable for anaerobic culture.
Mycobacteria	Sterile, screw-capped jar	5–10	Collect three early morning, fresh specimens resulting from deep cough or induced by heated aerosol of 10% glycerin and 15% NaCl. Send to laboratory promptly or store under refrigeration. DO NOT COLLECT 24-HOUR SPECIMENS.
Fungi	Sterile, screw-capped jar	3–5	
Lung abscess, empyema fluid	Anaerobic transport vial	NA	
Urinary tract			
Clean-voided midstream urine or urine obtained by catheterization or cystoscopy for	Sterile, screw-capped tube or jar		Send to laboratory promptly or store under refrigeration. DO NOT COLLECT 24-HOUR SPECIMENS. Specimen unsuitable for anaerobic cultures.
Bacteria		1–10	
Mycobacteria		>20	
Fungi		>20	
Suprapubic aspirate	Anaerobic transport vial	(As above)	Only valid means of establishing diagnosis of anaerobic bacteriuria.
Voided urine for parasites	Clean, screw-capped container	24-hour collection	Primarily collected to detect eggs of *Schistosoma haematobium*, trophozoites of *Trichomonas vaginalis* in the male, and microfilariae of *Onchocerca volvulus*.
Blood			
Cultures for			
Bacteria	Blood culture bottles containing broth or lysis–centrifugation tube	20–30 from adults, 1–3 from infants and children	Collect three separate blood samples during a 24-hour period; intervals between cultures are determined by urgency of clinical situation. More than three cultures per 24 hours are rarely necessary.
Brucellae and fungi	Lysis–centrifugation tube or biphasic blood culture bottle	(As for bacteria)	(As for bacteria)
Leptospires	Sterile, heparinized tube	1	(As for bacteria)
Examination for			
Borreliae	Peripheral smear	NA	Examine wet mount by darkfield microscopy or smear stained with aniline dyes
Malaria	Thick and thin films on clean glass slide	NA	
Filaria, Trypanosomes	Sterile tube containing anticoagulant (citrate, oxalate, heparin)	5	Wet mount of drop of blood or concentrated hemolyzed blood preferable to stained thick and thin films.
Fluids			
Exudates, transudates, drainage, pus	Anaerobic transport vial	1–5	
Abdomen, chest	Anaerobic transport vial	1–5 for bacteria, >10 for mycobacteria or fungi	
Synovial	Anaerobic transport vial	1–5 for bacteria, >10 for mycobacteria or fungi	Inoculate modifed Thayer-Martin medium in cases of suspected gonococcal arthritis.
Cerebrospinal	Sterile, screw-capped tube	1–2 for bacteria, >2 for mycobacteria or fungi	Send to laboratory immediately.

(Continued)

logic examination, and the microbiology laboratory receives one swab for a variety of smears and cultures.

Because of the frequency with which anaerobic bacteria play a role in causing infectious diseases, fluids or pus from the brain, thoracic and abdominal cavities, transtracheal and suprapubic aspirations, the pelvis, and the musculoskeletal system should be placed into a transport vial or tube in which anaerobes can survive for several hours. Alternatively, the syringe used to aspirate such materials may be used for their transport to the laboratory, provided the transport time is short. Anaerobe transport vials or tubes are available commercially, or they may be prepared in the laboratory. These contain gaseous mixtures of hydrogen, nitrogen, and carbon dioxide or deoxygenated carbon dioxide alone. Vials should contain a transport medium

TABLE 2. *(Continued)*

Specimen	*Container or Transport Device*	*Volume (ml)*	*Other Considerations*
Catheters			
Intravascular	Sterile, screw-capped tube; Culterette (with swab removed)	NA	Disinfect skin entry site, remove catheter, clip off end into tube.
Suction, drainage	Sterile, screw-capped tube	NA	
Skin and soft tissues			
Cultures	Swab	NA	
	Anaerobic transport vial	NA	
Scrapings for dermatophytes	Sterile Petri dish	NA	
Gastrointestinal tract			
Stool culture or examination for			
Bacteria	Sterile, screw-capped jar Transport medium swab	NA	Freshly collected specimen mandatory; transport medium less desirable. Request cultures for vibrios when suspected clinically.
Fungi	Sterile, screw-capped tube		Refrigerate if storage time exceeds 1 hour.
Ova and parasites	Stool carton sealed in plastic bag PVA preservative	NA	Collect saline purged stools on 3 consecutive days.
Anal swab for pinworm	Sterile plastic swab in tube (SWUBE)	NA	Swab perianal area, preferably on arising in morning and before bathing or defecation.
Sexually transmitted diseases			
Neisseria gonorrhoeae	Swab; modified Thayer-Martin medium (Transgrow, JEMBEC)	NA	Women Cervix—moisten speculum with water; insert swab into cervical canal. Anal canal—insert swab approximately 1 in. to sample anal crypts. Urethral or vaginal—culture if cervix not accessible. Men Urethral—obtain material for smear and culture with swab or a sterile bacteriologic loop, which is used to inoculate medium directly and for preparing smears of exudates from men.
Gardnerella vaginalis	Swab	NA	
Haemophilus ducreyi	Swab	NA	
Treponema pallidum	Serous exudate on clean glass slide or in capillary pipet	NA	Abrade lesion with clean dry sponge. Examine preparation by darkfield microscopy *immediately*.
Chlamydia trachomatis	Sucrose-phosphate solution (2 SP)	NA	Extract urethral or cervical material on swab in solution and refrigerate during storage.
Ureaplasma urealyticum	(As for *Chlamydia*)	(As for *Chlamydia*)	(As for *Chlamydia*)
Candida albicans	Swab	NA	
Trichmonas vaginalis	Swab	NA	
Genitourinary tract excluding sexually transmitted diseases			
Cervical, vaginal discharge	Swab	NA	Specimen unsuitable for anaerobic culture.
Culdocentesis fluid	Anaerobic transport vial	NA	
Abscess			
Pelvic, tubal, ovarian	Anaerobic transport vial	NA	
Prostatic secretion	Sterile, screw-capped bottle	NA	
Eye			
Corneal lesion or scraping	Material should be inoculated directly onto appropriate media and applied directly to clean microscope slides for staining and microscopic examination.		
Conjunctiva examination for			
Bacteria, fungi	Swab		
Neisseria gonorrhoeae	Modified Thayer-Martin medium (Transgrow, JEMBEC)	NA	Inoculate swab directly onto medium.
Chlamydia trachomatis	Sucrose-phosphate solution (2 SP)	NA	Extract material on swab in solution and refrigerate during storage.
Tissue	Sterile, screw-capped bottle	Representative samples	Specimen must be of sufficient size to ensure recovery of small numbers of organisms.

Abbreviations: NA: not applicable; PVA: polyvinyl alcohol.

with an indicator, for example, resazurin, which in its colorless state shows that the interior of the vial is anaerobic at the time a specimen is introduced. Anaerobic swab devices are also commercially available; however, their use is inadvisable because of the limited amount of material generally collected on swabs. Specimen containers should be sterile; they should not contain nonviable but stainable organisms that may provide misleading results.

Protection of Laboratory Workers from Infectious Diseases

Although microbiology laboratory workers are trained to practice aseptic technique and to handle specimens and cultures as being potentially infectious, the advent of infections due to human immune deficiency virus (HIV) and of the practice of universal precautions for preventing infection due to HIV, hepatitis B virus (HBV), and other blood-borne pathogens has led to changes in safety practices in clinical laboratories.

Under universal precautions, blood and body fluids are considered potentially infectious for HIV, HBV, and other blood-borne pathogens. Treating all such specimens as potentially infectious eliminates the need for warning labels on specimen containers. Specimens to which universal precautions should apply are blood and the following fluids: cerebrospinal, synovial, pleural, bronchial (including bronchoalveolar lavage), pericardial, peritoneal, and amniotic as well as vaginal secretions and semen. Universal precautions do not apply to upper respiratory secretions, sputum, urine, and feces unless they contain visible blood.

Specimens should be placed into sturdy, leak-proof containers, and care should be taken not to contaminate the external surface of containers during collection and handling of specimens. Specimen containers should routinely be checked to ensure they are leak-proof before any bulk purchase agreement with manufacturers. When contamination of the external surface of a specimen container is likely, the primary container should be placed into a secondary container such as a plastic sealable bag. In such cases, the specimen requisition should be affixed to the outside of the secondary container.

Laboratory workers should use appropriate barrier protection when handling specimens. In most instances, wearing gloves and a laboratory gown or coat is sufficient; however, the use of masks and protective eyewear or face shields and wearing aprons may be necessary if there is a high degree of likelihood that splashing may occur. Gloves should be removed if they become visibly contaminated with blood or if punctured or torn and the hands washed immediately.

Laboratory-specific precautions also include the use of mechanical pipetting devices (no mouth pipetting); restricted use of needles and syringes; prohibition of eating, drinking, or smoking in the laboratory; and biosafety level 2 practices, including the use of a class I or II biologic safety cabinet when there is a high probability of producing infectious droplets (e.g., homogenization of tissue, vigorous mixing, blending, sonicating), decontamination of work surfaces on a daily basis or after a spill of blood or a body fluid, the use of biohazard disposal techniques, handwashing after completing work and before leaving the laboratory, and the use of laboratory coats and gowns, which should be removed before leaving the laboratory.

More specific guidelines for the protection of laboratory workers are available from the National Committee for Clinical Laboratory Standards (NCCLS, Villanova, PA), the Centers for Disease Control (Atlanta, GA), and for laboratories performing HIV testing, the Division of Safety at the National Institutes of health (Bethesda, MD).

SPECIFIC GUIDELINES FOR SPECIMEN COLLECTION AND PROCESSING

Respiratory Tract

Many types of specimens originate from the respiratory tract. The means of their collection and transport are outlined in Table 2, whereas the procedures recommended for their microscopic examination and culture are listed in Table 3.

Nasopharynx. Cultures of the nose are occasionally made to detect carriers of *Staphylococcus aureus;* however, the results of such cultures are seldom of any epidemiologic value and are not indicated except when serious focal outbreaks of nosocomially acquired staphylococcal infections occur. The results of cultures of the nose have been shown by Evans et al.[2]

TABLE 3. Recommended Procedures for the Isolation and Identification of Respiratory Tract Pathogens

		Microscopic Examination					
Source	*Organism Sought or Disease Suspected*	*Gram Stain*	*FA*[a]	*Acid-Fast*	*KOH*	*Toluidine Blue*	*Methenamine Silver*
Nasopharynx	*Streptococcus pyogenes*		+				
	Neisseria meningitidis						
	Corynebacterium diphtheriae						
	Bordetella pertussis		+				
Paranasal sinus (aspirate)	Sinusitis	+					
Ear (aspirate)	Otitis media	+					
Mouth	Acute necrotizing ulcerative gingivitis (Vincent's)	+					
	Thrush				+		
Throat	*S. pyogenes*		+				
	N. gonorrhoeae						
	C. diphtheriae						
	Mycoplasma pneumoniae						
Sputum	Bacteria	+					
	Legionella		+				
	Mycobacteria			+			
	Nocardia			+[c]			
	Fungi				+		
	Mycoplasma						
Tracheal aspirate	Pneumonitis	+					
Transtracheal aspirate	Pneumonitis, abscess	+				±	
Bronchial washings, lavage, aspirate	Bacteria	+					
	Legionella						
	Mycobacteria			+			
	Nocardia			+[c]			
	Fungi				+		+
	Pneumocystis carinii					+	+
Pleural fluid	Empyema						
	Nonsurgical	+		+			
	Surgical	+					
Lung tissue		+	+	+	+	+	+

Abbreviations: BA: Blood agar; CBA: chocolate blood agar; EMB: eosin–methylene blue (MacConkey's is an acceptable alternative); CNA: colistin–nalidixic acid BA; BCYE: buffered yeast extract medium; BMPA: BCYE with antibiotics; L-J: Lowenstein-Jensen agar; 7H11: Middlebrook 7H11 agar; BHI: brain–heart infusion agar with and without antibiotics; Sab: Sabouraud agar.

[a] Immunofluorescence with specific labeled conjugates can be performed directly with smears prepared from specimens indicated, although *S. pyogenes* is best detected in smears prepared from centrifuged sediment of a 2–4 hour broth culture of the swab.

[b] Anaerobic media: thioglycolate supplemented with vitamin K and hemin; BA with vitamin K and hemin; BA with gentamicin and vancomycin; phenylethyl alcohol agar (PEA).

[c] Modified acid-fast stain.

to correlate poorly with those of sinus aspirates and are, therefore, of little value in establishing the microbial etiology of sinusitis. Since aerobic, anaerobic, and facultatively anaerobic bacteria as well as fungi and viruses have been shown to cause sinusitis,[2] it is necessary to take appropriate precautions with sinus aspirates to ensure the recovery of such a variety of organisms. There is similarly little value in making cultures of the nose to establish the microbial cause of otitis media.[3] Although seldom necessary in acute cases because of the rather predictable findings of *Haemophilus influenzae, Streptococcus pneumoniae,* and *Streptococcus pyogenes,* tympanocentesis is probably warranted in cases with chronic otitis media due to this condition's variable bacteriologic etiology.

Cultures of the nasopharynx may be used to detect carriers of *S. pyogenes* (i.e., group A streptococci), *Neisseria meningitidis, Corynebacterium diphtheriae,* and *Bordetella pertussis.* Some have advocated their use in determining the cause of pneumonia in infants and children; however, nasotracheal aspiration is likely to provide material that is more representative of the disease process. Nasopharyngeal suction, as described by Auger,[4] is preferred for establishing the bacteriologic diagnosis of pertussis. A no. 8 French 16 in. suction catheter with a safety valve is satisfactory in most cases. It is important to remember that cultures for *N. meningitidis, C. diphtheriae,* and *B. pertussis* must be requested specifically since these organisms either will not grow or will fail to be recognized on conventional bacteriologic media. Pertussis may be accurately and rapidly diagnosed by staining a smear of nasopharyngeal aspirate with anti-*B. pertussis* fluorescein-labeled conjugate.

Oral Cavity. Cultures of the oral cavity are seldom helpful because of the millions of microorganisms normally resident in it (Table 1). Direct examination of potassium hydroxide (KOH) preparations may, however, be helpful in confirming the diagnosis of oral thrush, and a Gram or methylene blue-stained smear may be helpful in the diagnosis of acute necrotizing ulcerative gingivitis (Vincent's angina or fusospirochetal disease).

Throat. Most cultures of the throat are made to diagnose streptococcal pharyngitis since its clinical presentation is highly variable and is often indistinguishable from that of viral pharyngitis. Moreover, it is not at all uncommon for there to be concurrent viral and group A streptococcal infections of the throat. Sampling errors in swabbing the throat are frequent, and the patient's interests are best served by vigorous rather than gentle application of the swab to the posterior portion of the pharynx, tonsillar areas, and areas of ulceration, exudation, and membrane formation. Gram-stained smears are of little use or reliability since streptococci of all kinds occur normally and in

Media												
BA	*CBA*	*EMB*	*CNA*	*BCYE, BMPA*	*Anaerobic*[b]	*Loeffler, Tellurite*	*Thayer-Martin*	*Charcoal or Bordet-Gengou*	*L-J, 7H11*	*BHI or Sab*	*Mycoplasma*	*Comments and Other Procedures*
+												
							+					
						+						
								+				
+	+				+							
+	+				+							
										+		
+												Antigen test
							+					
						+						
											+	Serology
+	+	+										
				+								Serology
									+			PPD
+									+	+		
										+		
											+	Serology
+	+	+	+									
+	+	+	+		+							
+	+		+									
									+			PPD
									+	+		
										+		
+	+		+		+				+	+		
+	+	+	+									
+	+	+	+	+					+	+	+	Selection of tests based on clinical and histopathologic findings

large numbers in the mouth and there is little that is distinctive about the microscopic appearance of group A streptococci.

A large number of rapid group A streptococcal antigen detection kits are commercially available for direct testing of throat swabs. Although these tests are highly specific, their sensitivity ranges from 45 to 100 percent, depending on the population studied, culture method used for comparison purposes, and the criteria (i.e., number of colonies) used to define a positive culture. Since the sensitivity of antigen detection kits is directly correlated with the number of group A streptococci present in the specimen, kit sensitivity is lowest with specimens yielding few colonies of group A streptococci in cultures. Manufacturers have tended to discount false-negative kit test results under these circumstances as clinically unimportant; however, since the seroconversion (antistreptolysin O [ASO] and/or anti-DNase B) rate in children with both positive antigen test and culture results is virtually identical to that in children with negative antigen test results and positive cultures,[5] the number of group A streptococci in the specimen often reflect sampling variation and are seldom helpful in distinguishing between infection and colonization or the carrier state. Thus, although antigen tests have a high positive predictive value (100 percent), their negative predictive value may be substantially lower. Antigen tests may, therefore, not be acceptable as a culture substitute, particularly in areas in which there has been a resurgence of acute rheumatic fever. Although it has been shown that the treatment rate is markedly higher for cases detected by antigen tests than for those detected by culture,[6] it is likely that inappropriate treatment rates are also markedly higher when a screening test is known to have a sensitivity of only 45 percent.

In expert hands, a Loeffler's alkaline methylene blue smear of material collected from the margin of a membrane may suggest the diagnosis of diphtheria; however, such expertise is rare in the United States today, and culture remains the principal means of establishing this diagnosis.

It must also be remembered that acute pharyngitis may be caused by *Neisseria gonorrhoeae,* which will not grow on media usually used for throat cultures. If gonococcal pharyngitis is suspected on clinical or epidemiologic grounds, the laboratory should be notified accordingly; however, it is preferable to inoculate modified Thayer-Martin medium directly at the time the swab is taken.

Sputum. The microbiologic examination of sputum is fraught with numerous problems. The patient is usually poorly instructed as to the type of specimen required; supervision is generally lacking during specimen collection; and the specimen often remains on the patient's night table for hours before being delivered to the laboratory, during which time it becomes overgrown with bacteria normally present in saliva. Ideally, patients should be instructed to rinse out their mouths with water and to provide only material resulting from a deep cough. Several attempts may be necessary before a suitable specimen of sputum is obtained. The specimen should then be transported to the laboratory promptly. If bacterial infection is suspected clinically, examination under low power (×100) of a Gram-stained smear of a carefully selected aliquot of the specimen, as described by Chodosh,[7] is a rapid means of determining its suitability for culture (Fig. 1). The presence of many squamous epithelial cells (>25 per low-power field[lpf]) indicates that the specimen consists substantially of saliva and contains an abundance of oropharyngeal microflora.[8,9] It is advisable not to culture this specimen but to try to collect another one. If few squamous epithelial cells (<25/lpf) are present, the smear should be examined carefully under oil immersion (×1000) to determine whether bacteria morphologically typical of certain species (e.g., pneumococci, staphylococci) are present and the specimen should be cultured. In cases of suspected pneumococcal pneumonia it may be helpful to examine a wet mount of sputum that has been mixed with pneumococcal antiserum for evidence of the quellung reaction. In cases of suspected legionellosis, a smear of sputum should be examined by immunofluorescence or genetic probe, and cultures should be made on buffered charcoal yeast extract medium containing antibiotics (BMPA medium). The most important consideration, however, in the laboratory diagnosis of pneumococcal and other bacterial pneumonias is the attention given to proper specimen collection.[10]

Although the degree of oropharyngeal contamination is not as critical in sputum specimens submitted for mycobacterial or fungal examination, every effort should still be made to collect material resulting from a deep cough and to minimize the specimen's contamination since the overgrowth by aerobic and facultatively anaerobic bacteria of mycobacterial and fungal cultures may severely limit the laboratory's ability to recover these pathogens. Twenty-four-hour specimens should not be collected for mycobacterial or fungal cultures. In some cases collection of sputum induced by a heated aqueous aerosol of 10% glycerin and 15% sodium chloride is useful for recovering mycobacteria and fungi. Specimens that cannot be processed within 1 or 2 hours after collection should be refrigerated during their storage and transport; failure to do so may result in a decreased yield of mycobacteria or fungi.

In suspected mycobacterial or fungal disease, appropriately prepared smears should be examined. A fluorochrome stain provides the most rapid means of examining a smear for mycobacteria, while phase-contrast microscopy of a KOH preparation represents the best means of looking for fungi (Fig. 2). It is important to remember that *Nocardia,* which may be seen in Gram-stained smears or KOH preparations (Fig. 3) of respiratory tract specimens, may not be seen in carbol fuchsin (Ziehl-Neelsen or Kinyoun) acid-fast stained smears unless decolorized with 0.5–1% sulfuric acid.

Mycoplasma pneumoniae may be isolated on special media from sputum or from throat swabs from patients with pneumonia due to this organism. Because the growth and isolation of *M. pneumoniae* can be quite slow, it is suggested that serodiagnosis also be attempted by testing acute and convalescent sera for a fourfold or greater increase in complement fixing or immunofluorescent antibody activity.

Transtracheal Aspirate. A transtracheal aspirate (TTA) provides a means of bypassing the upper respiratory tract and obtaining lower respiratory secretions that are suitable for culture of aerobic and anaerobic bacteria as well as mycobacteria and some fungi other than *Candida.*[11] The procedure does require technical expertise and should be reserved for situations in which other less invasive procedures have provided inconclusive results.

Bronchoscopy. Bronchoscopy is a relatively safe technique that provides secretions directly from bronchial drainage sites of infection. Examination of bronchoscopy specimens should be considered in two categories: (*1*) studies to detect microorganisms (e.g., *Legionella, Mycobacterium, Pneumocystis carinii*) that pose no problem in interpretation even in the presence of upper respiratory contamination and (*2*) studies for bacteria that may comprise upper respiratory flora but in which differentiation between upper and lower respiratory origin is necessary.[12] Bronchoscopy, including washings, biopsy, or lavage procedures, is suitable for the first category of examination, whereas bronchoscopy with a double-lumen catheter and a distal occluding plug is useful in the second category, particularly when accompanied by quantitative cultures for aerobic and anaerobic bacteria.[12]

Pleural Fluid. Pleural or empyema fluid is of particular value in the diagnosis of anaerobic pleuropulmonary infections and legionnaires' disease. In such cases, a Gram-stained smear can be very helpful, although it is necessary to prolong the period

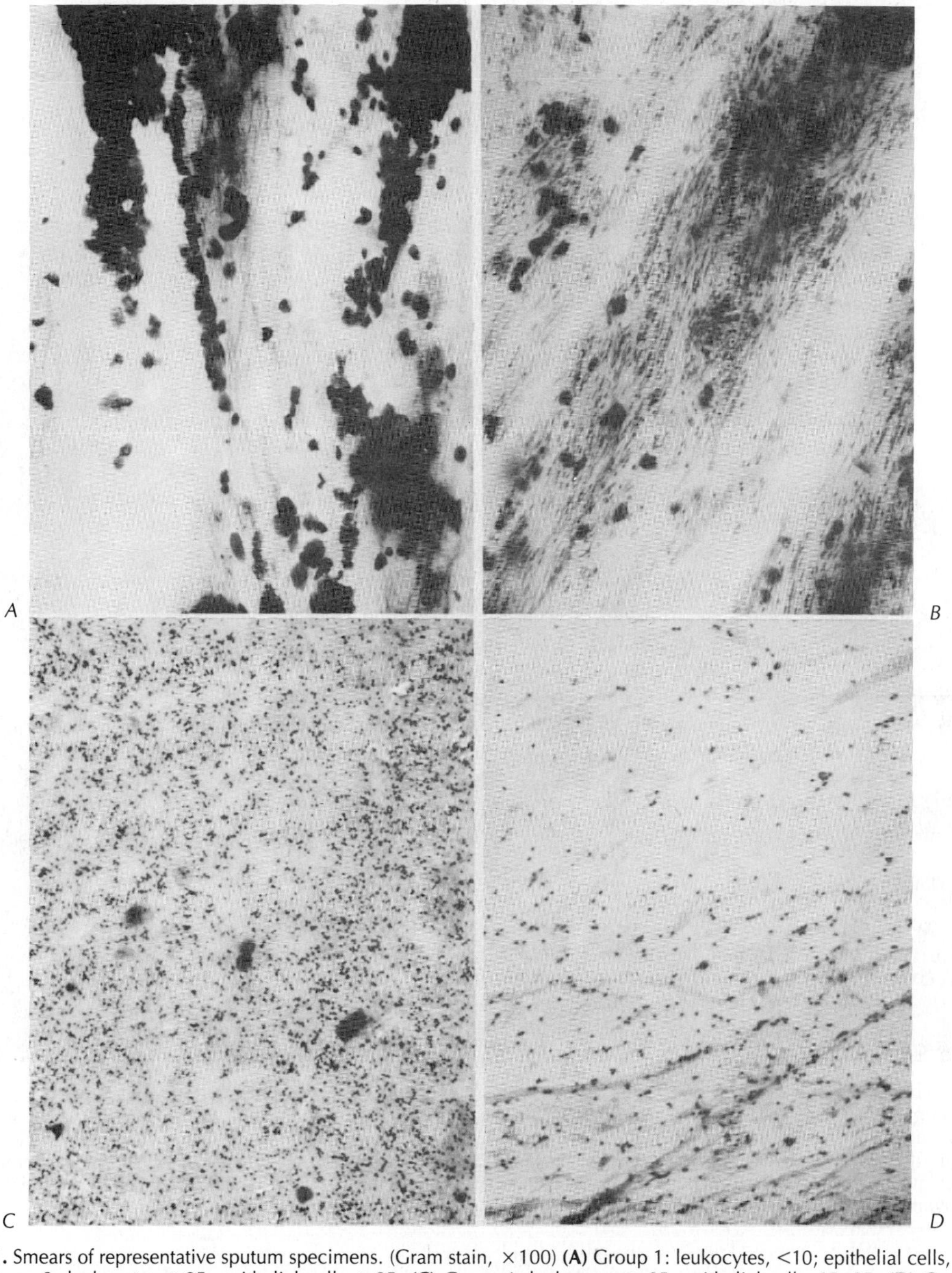

FIG. 1. Smears of representative sputum specimens. (Gram stain, ×100) **(A)** Group 1: leukocytes, <10; epithelial cells, >25. **(B)** Group 3: leukocytes, >25; epithelial cells, >25. **(C)** Group 4: leukocytes, >25; epithelial cells, 10–25. **(D)** Group 5: leukocytes, >25; epithelial cells, <10. (From Murray et al.,[8] with permission.)

of counterstaining with safranin for several minutes to detect *Legionella*. A more specific approach to the diagnosis of this disease is by direct immunofluorescent staining of a smear of pleural fluid. Obviously, pleural or empyema fluid can be examined and cultured for other etiologic agents of pulmonary disease.

Lung Tissue. Obtained at substantial cost and some risk to the patient, lung tissue specimens warrant special attention by all concerned.[12] The microbiologist needs to know the suspected clinical diagnosis and what the histopathologic studies show. It should be stressed that few organisms may be present in a chronic inflammatory lesion and that an adequate quantity of the lesion should be submitted for examination and cultures. Impression smears of tissue are especially useful in the diagnosis of *Pneumocystis carinii* infections and legionnaires' disease. Although *P. carinii* is readily seen in Gomori methenamine silver-stained smears, smears stained with toluidine blue 0 can be easily and rapidly prepared and examined in the microbiology laboratory.[13] Impression smears for *Legionella* are fixed with 10% formalin for 10 minutes and are stained with specific fluorescein-labeled conjugate.

Gram stain, an acid-fast stain, and Gomori methenamine silver stain are satisfactory for screening tissue sections for microorganisms.[12] Dieterle silver-impregnation stain will demonstrate *Legionella* in paraffinized tissue sections.[12]

Tissue for culture is finely minced with sterile scissors and is then ground in a tissue grinder or with a small amount of sterile abrasive (alundum) in a sterile mortar with a pestle. A 10–20 percent suspension is prepared with nutrient broth and is used to inoculate cultures. Alternatively, tissue may be ma-

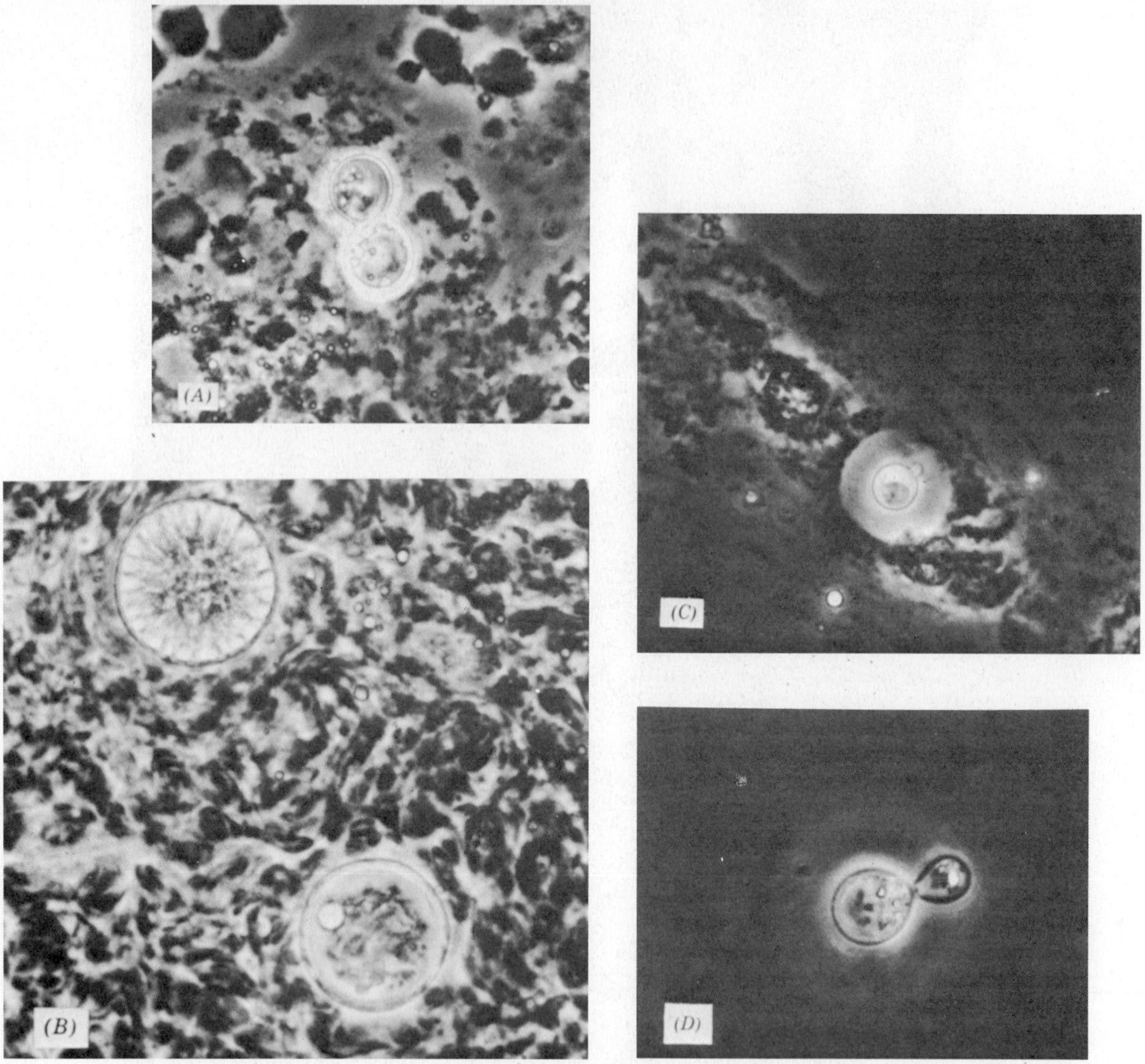

FIG. 2. Phase-contrast microscopy of clinical specimens. (×2000) **(A)** *Blastomyces dermatitidis* in sputum. The characteristic yeast form has a budding cell attached by a broad base. Also note the "double contoured" appearance of the cell wall. **(B)** *Coccidioides immitis* in sputum. Large thick-walled spherules with few endospores are scattered within the interior of the spherule (lower) or cleavage furrows developing along the periphery to form endospores (upper). **(C)** *Cryptococcus neoformans* in sputum. Spherical yeast is surrounded by a large capsule with a small bud arising from the parent cell. **(D)** *C. neoformans* in sputum. An encapsulated yeast form has a budding cell attached by a narrow base. (*Figure continues*)

cerated in a stomaching device and the extract used for microbiologic examination. Such suspensions are saved, most conveniently in a sterile 60 ml dropper bottle, until after the tissue sections and special stains have been reviewed in case additional cultures are indicated.

Urinary Tract

Clean-voided midstream urine is preferred for bacterial, mycobacterial, and fungal cultures. Twenty-four-hour collections are suitable only for parasitologic study (Table 2). Catheterization is not recommended for obtaining urine unless the procedure fulfills a diagnostic or therapeutic purpose. Suprapubic aspiration is recommended for establishing the diagnosis of bacteriuria in infants and small children, for determining the significance of borderline counts of bacteria in repeated clean-voided midstream specimens, and for determining the presence of anaerobic bacteriuria.

Because the distal urethra of both men and women is normally colonized with large numbers of aerobic, facultatively anaerobic, and anaerobic bacteria, the diagnosis of clinically significant bacteriuria in a clean-voided, midstream specimen requires quantitative smears and cultures. A Gram stain of a drop (allow to dry without spreading) of well-mixed urine will not only provide a means of determining the adequacy of its collection but also will provide the diagnosis of significant bacteriuria (≥100,000 cfu/ml) when at least two bacteria per oil immersion (×1000) field are found. The correlation of the results of this test in expert hands with those of quantitative cultures should be at least 90 percent. Essential to the validity of these results is proper specimen collection and transport to the laboratory. Unless refrigerated during storage and transport, no urine arriving in the laboratory more than 2 hours after its collection should be cultured. The presence of many squamous epithelial cells on microscopic examination of the urine is indicative of poor technique in its collection, and another specimen should be requested.

Quantitation of bacteriuria in cultures can be most conveniently accomplished by streaking a measured volume (e.g., 0.01

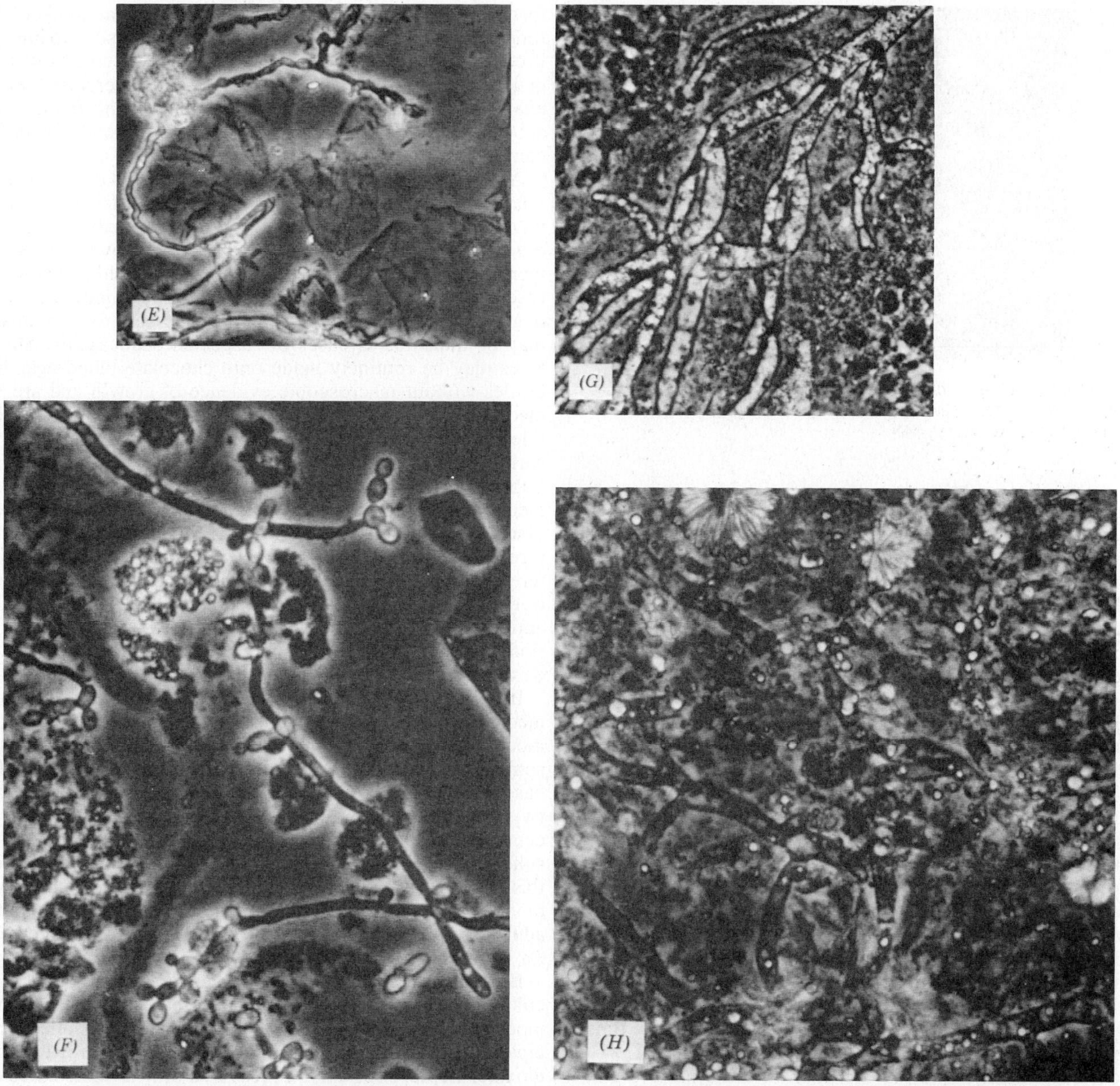

FIG. 2 (*Continued*). **(E)** Dermatophyte in a skin scraping. Septate hyphae intertwine among squamous cells. **(F)** *Candida albicans* in urine. Hyphae and budding yeasts appear among epithelial cells. **(G)** *Mucor* sp. in pus from a skin lesion. The large, branching, ribbonlike aseptate hyphae are indicative of a zygomycete. **(H)** *Aspergillus fumigatus* in sputum. The septate hyphae show dichotomous branching. (Courtesy of Dr. Glenn D. Roberts, Rochester, MN.)

or 0.001 ml) of well-mixed urine onto the surface of culture media with a calibrated milk dilution platinum loop. A general-purpose medium (e.g., blood agar) and a gram-negative differential medium (e.g., eosin–methylene blue [EMB] or MacConkey) should be used. Broth cultures of clean-voided urine are meaningless and should not be made since the growth of even a few bacteria of urethral origin will render the broth turbid and will provide misleading results. Precision in reporting the number of colonies isolated on solid media is unnecessary, and the results can be reported as approximate colony counts (e.g., $<10^3$, 10^4–10^5, $>10^5$ cfu/ml). Provided the specimen has been properly collected, colony counts of $\geq 10^4$/ml are usually significant; however, as few as 100 cfu/ml may be significant in women with the acute dysuric syndrome.

Commercially available screening tests for significant bacteriuria include bioluminescence, miniaturized culture systems, dipstick method for nitrite and leukocyte esterase (Chemstrip L-N) and staining of bacteria and leukocytes on filter paper (Bac-T-Screen, Filtra Check-UTI). Regardless of the principle involved in the test, sensitivity is maximal with at least 10^5 cfu/ml, although it may vary with the populations of patients studied. The sensitivity of the L-N test may be enhanced by using the additional tests for blood and protein that are available on the Chemstrip 9.[14]

Despite the fact that cultures of the urine for other microorganisms (e.g., brucellae, leptospires, mycobacteria, fungi, mycoplasmas, and viruses) entail selective processes for their isolation, the same requirements for careful specimen collection and transport apply because selective procedures are not uniformly successful in eliminating any bacterial contamination that may be present and that may overgrow cultures or otherwise interfere with the isolation of these other microorganisms. Decontamination and selective isolation procedures for these other organisms are described in detail elsewhere.[15]

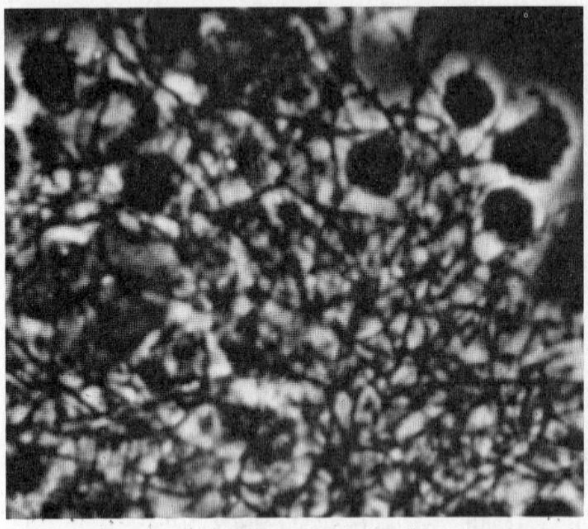

FIG. 3. Phase-contrast microscopy of sputum containing *Nocardia asteroides* shows slender, branching filaments. (×2000) (Courtesy of Dr. Glenn D. Roberts, Rochester, MN.)

Septicemia

The successful isolation of microorganisms from blood requires an understanding of the intermittency and low order of magnitude of most bacteremias, the great variety of organisms capable of causing septicemia, and a broad range of microbiologic considerations involved in the isolation of microorganisms from blood. Each of these factors is reviewed in detail elsewhere.[16,17] There are two major variables that warrant emphasis here: timing of blood collections and the volume of blood collected for culture. Most bacteremias are intermittent, so blood collections for culture should be made intermittently during a 24-hour period. Studies have shown that the sensitivity of two to three separately collected blood cultures within a 24-hour period in establishing the cause of clinically significant bacteremias is nearly 100 percent and that the sensitivity of a single blood culture within this same time period is approximately 80 to 90 percent. The bacteremia associated with subacute bacterial endocarditis is usually continuous, so only two cultures will yield the etiologic agent in nearly all cases. It is apparent, therefore, that two and preferably three separate blood cultures should be collected within a 24-hour period and that it is seldom necessary to perform more than three blood cultures within this same time period.

Most bacteremias, with the exception of those occurring in infants, are of a very low order of magnitude; therefore, an adequate volume of blood should be collected for each set of cultures. It is suggested that 20 ml be obtained from adults and that 1–3 ml be obtained from infants and small children. It is important to consider the volume of blood cultured and the number of blood cultures obtained as independent variables; therefore, we should avoid the obvious temptation to use one venipuncture to obtain an unusually large volume of blood that is then inoculated into several sets of cultures. Although the rate of recovery of bacteria from blood is directly related to the volume of blood cultured, the yield from several separate sets of blood cultures is related, in turn, to the usual intermittency of bacteremia. Both factors, therefore, must be kept in mind when making blood cultures.

The proposed venipuncture site requires careful disinfection since bacteria normally resident in the skin include species that frequently are associated with infections of implanted prosthetic material. Their isolation from blood cultures can cause considerable confusion unless the skin has been carefully prepared for venipuncture with a suitable antiseptic agent and multiple sets of blood cultures have been inoculated with blood obtained from separate venipunctures.

Proper selection of blood culture bottles, although important, is difficult because of differences among manufacturers in their formulations of media, use of additives, and methods of bottling. Published evaluations of media are impossible to interpret if comparisons were made sequentially or if cultures were inoculated with different volumes of blood. Other variables, for example, atmosphere of incubation, timing, and frequency of subcultures, require careful scrutiny before broad conclusions can be drawn.

As a general rule, blood should be inoculated on a 10 percent vol/vol basis into two vacuum bottles, one of which remains unvented (relatively anaerobic) during incubation while the other is vented transiently to permit the growth of pseudomonads and yeasts. Cultures should be examined daily for macroscopic, infrared spectrophotometric, or radiometric evidence of growth for a minimum of 1 week; longer periods of incubation may be indicated in cases of suspected endocarditis. Subcultures may be routinely made onto chocolate blood agar from bottles without macroscopic evidence of growth and are best made between 6 and 24 hours after the initial inoculation. Routine subcultures of anaerobic bottles are not useful. With the early subculture, routine Gram-stained smears are unnecessary. Subcultures of bottles yielding growth should be made onto media suitable for the growth of aerobic, facultatively anaerobic, and anaerobic bacteria and for the differentiation of mixtures of different species of bacteria since polymicrobial bacteremia occurs in nearly 10 percent of the cases. Turbid broth or colonies from bottles yielding growth may be used for direct antimicrobial susceptibility testing after a short incubation period and adjustment of the inoculum size to that used in standardized methodology.

In cases of suspected meningococcemia or gonococcemia, media without sodium polyanetholesulfonate (SPS) should be inoculated because of this polyanion's inhibitory effects on some strains of pathogenic neisseriae. Otherwise, SPS, which has antiphagocytic, anticomplement, and anticoagulant activity, should be incorporated at concentrations of 0.025–0.05 percent into all blood culture media. The use of sodium amylosulfate (SAS) in lieu of SPS appears to be contraindicated at this time. The value of penicillinase in media inoculated with blood from patients receiving penicillins is uncertain, but its addition is probably advisable provided it is tested concurrently for its sterility.

Brucellae are most likely to be recovered from blood that is cultured early in the course of the disease and that has been inoculated into a bottle containing biphasic (Castaneda principle) soybean-casein digest medium and 10 percent carbon dioxide. Leptospires can be recovered only in some cases during the first week of illness and from essentially none thereafter. Cultures should be made by inoculating a few drops of fresh or anticoagulated blood into each of several tubes containing a leptospiral semisolid culture medium such as Fletcher's. Cultures should be incubated at 30°C for 2 or 3 weeks and should be examined with darkfield or immunofluorescent microscopy twice weekly. Direct darkfield microscopic examination of blood or blood cultures should be interpreted very cautiously because of the formation of motile "pseudospirochetes" from blood components.

In cases in which fungal sepsis is suspected, blood should be inoculated into bottles that contain biphasic brain–heart infusion (BHI) medium and that are vented and incubated at 30°C for 1 month. Most yeasts will grow in media in conventional blood culture bottles provided these bottles are vented if under vacuum; however, the growth of yeasts in vented vacuum bottles is significantly slower than in bottles containing biphasic media.

Techniques that lyse blood cells and concentrate the residue by filtration or centrifugation for culture have generally proved more sensitive methods than those of conventional broth culture in detecting bacteria and fungi present in blood. A lysis–centrifugation device is available commercially (Isolator, DuPont) and has generally been found to increase and accelerate the detection of bacteria and, particularly, fungi in blood.[17] Disadvantages of this system include the need for processing specimens within several hours of blood collection, increased yield of presumed contaminants (primarily *Staphylococcus epidermidis*), and decreased yield of *S. pneumoniae*, nutritionally deficient streptococci, *Listeria monocytogenes*, and anaerobic bacteria. For these reasons, it is advisable for the system to be used in conjunction with a suitable vacuum blood culture bottle.

Intra-abdominal Infections

According to Finegold,[18] the incidence of infections involving anaerobic bacteria in this site generally is 86 percent. Anaerobes are involved in pyogenic abscesses of the liver in 50–100 percent of the cases and in at least 90 percent of tuboovarian and pelvic abscesses. Appropriate measures must, therefore, be taken to ensure the survival of anaerobes during the specimen's transport to the laboratory. Fluid or pus should be aspirated into a syringe, and air bubbles expelled, and the syringe transported directly to the laboratory, or its contents should be injected into an anaerobic vial or tube for transport to the laboratory. Swabs are generally not suitable for this purpose.

Granulomatous lesions of the liver, spleen, or lymph nodes should be cultured for mycobacteria, brucellae, and fungi as well as for aerobic and facultatively anaerobic bacteria. Complete microbiologic examination of material removed surgically is essential in patients undergoing abdominal exploration for fever of unexplained origin (Table 4). Because the distribution of organisms in tissue may not be uniform, generous portions of tissue should be removed for histologic and microbiologic examination.

Amebic abscesses of the liver are rarely confused histologically with pyogenic abscesses and are mainly composed of necrotic granular and eosinophilic material with considerable nuclear debris and few or no cells. The amebae are usually found near the capsule and not in the central necrotic material. Microscopic examination of the pus may be facilitated by its enzymatic digestion with streptodornase and the preparation of wet mounts from centrifuged sediment. Indirect hemagglutination titers are usually elevated in sera from patients with extraintestinal amebiasis.

Central Nervous System Infections

The cerebrospinal fluid (CSF) from a patient suspected of having meningitis demands immediate attention from the microbiologist. This urgency is dictated by the lethality of acute bacterial meningitis if untreated, its morbidity if inadequately treated, and its curability if treated early with appropriate antimicrobial agents. The prompt detection, isolation, and identification of the etiologic agent and determination of its antimicrobial susceptibility play a crucial role in the management of meningitis.

Cerebrospinal fluid must be collected aseptically, both to prevent the inadvertent introduction of organisms into the central nervous system and to avoid contamination with organisms indigenous to the skin or other body surfaces, culture of which may delay or confuse the diagnosis. Aspirations of cerebrospinal fluid shunts must be made very carefully since bacteria associated with infections of such shunts frequently belong to species that are ordinarily indigenous to the skin. Careful preparation of the skin must be carried out with a suitable antiseptic such as tincture of iodine or an iodophor; aqueous benzalkonium chloride should be avoided for skin antisepsis.

Specimen containers in lumbar puncture trays, whether prepared in-house or commercially, should be randomly tested by the microbiology laboratory for sterility, absence of stainable but nonviable bacteria, and effectiveness of closure to prevent leakage during transport. Many hospitals now use pneumatic tube systems to transport medically urgent specimens to the laboratory, and it is not uncommon for leakage from certain kinds of tubes to occur under these conditions. Cerebrospinal fluid should not be stored or refrigerated, and it should be transported to the laboratory for examination as rapidly as possible.

Although the number of bacteria per milliliter of cerebrospinal fluid in cases with meningitis usually exceeds 10^5 cfu, numbers significantly below this level do occur.[19] Moreover, if present, the numbers of mycobacteria and fungi in cerebrospinal fluid are often few. It is, therefore, important for a sufficient volume (Table 2) of fluid to be sent to the laboratory to ensure its proper examination. Additional fluid is, of course, required for cell counts and biochemical analyses. Ideally, fluid for microbiologic studies should be placed in separate containers from that needed for other studies to expedite processing and to minimize contamination.

Fluid should be examined microscopically in the laboratory (Table 5). Procedures to be followed for the laboratory diagnosis of viral meningitis and encephalitis are described elsewhere (Chapter 14). Centrifuged sediment is generally examined microscopically; however, it is important to realize that some bacteria usually require a force of at least 10,000 $\times g$ for 10 minutes to sediment and that 60 minutes may be required to accomplish the same purpose with the conventional bench-top laboratory centrifuge, which develops a maximum force of only 1000 $\times g$. In most cases, the presence of inflammatory cells will hasten the sedimentation process; however, there may only be a few polymorphonuclear leukocytes in the cerebrospinal fluid early in the course of acute bacterial meningitis. Published reports of the sensitivity of the Gram-stained smear of cerebrospinal fluid sediment from patients with acute bacterial meningitis vary but approximate 70 percent. For this reason as well as because of possible misinterpretation of findings in the smear, other methods of bacterial detection in cerebrospinal fluid have been developed, the most rapid and specific of which are immunologic.

Counterimmunoelectrophoresis (CIE), latex particle agglutination (LPA), and coagglutination (CoA) tests have been positive upon initial evaluation of cerebrospinal fluid in 82 (range, 68–94), 95 (range, 78–100), and 94 (range, 83–100) percent, respectively, of patients with *Haemophilus influenzae* meningitis.[20] The corresponding figures for CIE, LPA, and CoA in meningococcal meningitis are 60 (range, 17–100), 78 (range, 20–100), and 39 (range, 33–50) percent, respectively, and for pneu-

TABLE 4. Recommended Procedures for Examination and Culture of Intra-abdominal Fluids and Tissue

		Culture Media[a]								
Type of Lesion	*Microscopic Examination*	*BA*	*CBA*	*EMB*	*CNA*	*Thayer-Martin*	*Anaerobic*	*L-J, 7H11*	*BHI or Sab*	*Brucella*[b]
Pyogenic										
Abdominal	Gram stain	X	X	X	X		X			
Pelvic	Gram stain	X	X	X	X	X	X			
Granulomatous	Acid-fast and methenamine silver							X	X	X

[a] Abbreviations as in Table 3.
[b] Brucella media: blood–heart infusion agar, W medium.[15]

TABLE 5. Microbiologic Examination of Cerebrospinal Fluid

	Detection Procedures		
Suspected Cause	Essential	Supplemental	Media
Bacterial	Gram-stained smear	Quellung reaction, immunofluorescence, counterimmunoelectrophoresis, coagglutination, latex agglutination, and limulus lysate assay	BA, CBA, Thiogly/S, MHB/S
Leptospiral	Darkfield microscopy	Macroscopic agglutination for antibody in serum	Fletcher's semisolid medium or albumin fatty acid broth (Ellinghausen)
Mycobacterial	Acid-fast stained smear		L-J, 7H11
Fungal	India ink wet mount	Latex agglutination for cryptococcal antigen in CSF, complement fixation for coccidioidal antibody in CSF	BHI,[a] Sab
Amebae	Phase-contrast microscopy	Cocultivation on plain agar with *E. coli*	1.5% agar in distilled water

Abbreviations: Thiogly/S: thioglycollate medium supplemented with rabbit serum; MHB/S: Mueller-Hinton broth with supplement C; others as in Table 3.
[a] BHI without cycloheximide should be included.

mococcal meningitis are 67 (range, 20–100), 67 (range, 50–100), and 82 (range, 60–100) percent, respectively.[20] The sensitivity of CIE, LPA, and CoA is much less in cases in which the Gram-stained smear of cerebrospinal fluid was negative than in those in which the smear was positive.[20] False-positive immunologic test results (i.e., positive for antigen and a negative culture) on cerebrospinal fluid are uncommon. Whether such false-positive results actually represent false-negative cultures, technical errors, cross-reactions, or in the case of tests of urine in which false-positives occur more frequently, antigenuria in asymptomatic carriers or recently immunized children remains uncertain.[20,21]

The major question regarding rapid antigen tests of cerebrospinal fluid is how the information they provide is used clinically. In one study of this question, appropriate therapy for *H. influenzae* type b meningitis was initiated before the results of latex particle agglutination were known, and in no case did the results of the test alter therapy.[21] Granoff et al. concluded that physicians believed that the risks of error in the test were not acceptable in the management of an infection that is potentially fatal without appropriate antimicrobial therapy and that culture results rather than antigen test results were being used for management decisions.[21] Antigen tests of cerebrospinal fluid may be helpful in partially treated patients and when cerebrospinal fluid indices do not distinguish between bacterial and nonbacterial meningitis.

A high level of sensitivity in the diagnosis of meningitis due to *N. meningitidis, H. influenzae,* and other gram-negative bacteria can be obtained with the limulus lysate test, in which a lysate prepared from amebocytes of the horseshoe crab, *Limulus polyphemus,* undergoes gelation when exposed to endotoxin. A positive response to a limulus lysate test is obviously nonspecific and, therefore, provides less information than do the more specific immunologic tests.

In suspected fungal meningitis, an India ink wet mount preparation of cerebrospinal fluid sediment should be examined carefully for the presence of encapsulated, budding yeasts resembling cryptococci (Chapter 241). Care must be taken not to confuse red blood cells, white blood cells, or starch granules with the characteristically encapsulated cryptococci. The sensitivity of this procedure, however, is only approximately 50 percent; therefore, it is important to supplement it with a latex agglutination test for cryptococcal antigen. Properly controlled, the sensitivity of this test approximates that of culture. Wet mount preparations are not usually useful in establishing the diagnosis of coccidioidal meningitis. Cultures should be made, and most patients develop complement-fixing antibodies to *Coccidioides* in their spinal fluid.

Darkfield microscopy of cerebrospinal fluid may be helpful in establishing the diagnosis of leptospirosis; however, the presence of leptospires in cerebrospinal fluid closely parallels that in blood. Darkfield examinations and cultures should therefore be made during the first week of illness.

The motile amebae (*Naegleria, Hartmannella-Acanthamoeba* group) may be seen with phase microscopy. They may be cultured on plain agar by placing a drop of cerebrospinal fluid onto a loopful of *E. coli* spread in a 1 cm^2 area in the center of the plate.

Brain abscesses contain anaerobic bacteria in nearly 90 percent of cases.[18] Often their presence is suggested in Gram-stained smears made directly with pus from the abscess. Appropriate precautions must be taken to ensure the survival of anaerobes during the specimen's transport to the laboratory, and anaerobic cultures should be prepared.

Media to be inoculated with cerebrospinal fluid are listed in Table 5 according to the etiologic agent suspected. It is important to concentrate the specimen before its inoculation either by centrifugation or by membrane filtration. In the latter case, fluid is forced through a 0.45 μm disposable membrane filter device (e.g., Swinnex, Millipore Corporation), and the filter is cultured by placing it "upstream" side down on the agar surface. After 24–48 hours of incubation, the filter is moved to determine whether colonies may have arisen at its site of application.

Musculoskeletal Infections

Most musculoskeletal infections are due to bacteria (aerobic, facultatively anaerobic, anaerobic, and mycobacterial) and less frequently to fungi. Microorganisms are usually recovered from previously unopened and undrained abscesses, provided the pus has been properly collected and transported to the laboratory. "Sterile" pus is usually due to carelessness on the part of the person collecting the specimen or to the ineptness of the laboratory personnel examining it. In chronic lesions the number of organisms is often small, so an adequate quantity of specimen should be obtained. Swabs are usually unsatisfactory for this purpose, and material should be collected with a sterile syringe and needle. If necessary, irrigation of the lesion with bacteriostat-free saline or Ringer lactate solution is satisfactory. Sinus tracts often originate in bone or lymph nodes, and their microbial cause is seldom elucidated by swabbing the tract's orifice.[22] The orifice should be cleansed with an antiseptic, and curettings should be taken of the tract as close to its base as possible. A biopsy specimen is preferable. Cultures of swabs of ulcers may also be misleading, and it is suggested that curetting or biopsy specimens be taken from the base or undermined edge of such lesions. Cultures of previously opened abscesses usually yield a great variety of microorganisms, identification of which taxes the technologist and defies rational antimicrobial therapy. Again, a carefully collected specimen does much to minimize confusion.

Wounds, both traumatic and nosocomial in origin, are increasingly found to be infected with gram-negative bacilli and anaerobic bacteria. Media appropriate for the isolation and identification of these bacteria should be used for cultures of wound material (see Table 4 for suitable bacteriologic media). Quantitative bacteriology of biopsy specimens from acute and chronic wounds has been shown to provide valuable prognostic information on the risk of sepsis at the time of closure.[23] In addition, quantitative bacteriology of biopsy specimens of burn wounds has been found to reflect infection more accurately than have surface culture techniques.[24] As a general rule, the risk of wound sepsis increases significantly if there are more than 10^5 cfu/g of tissue, whereas wounds with fewer than 10^5 cfu/g have little risk of developing sepsis when closed primarily.[23] Gram-stained smears of biopsy material may be made to provide quantitative results within 30 minutes after receipt of the specimen in the laboratory.[23]

Post-traumatic mycobacterial infections are often due to the *Mycobacterium fortuitum-chelonae* complex and to *Mycobacterium marinum*.[25] Sources of the former group of mycobacteria have included soil, lower animals, dirty skin, foreign bodies, contaminated needles or syringes, and contaminated injectable material, whereas those of *M. marinum* have included tropical fish aquariums, swimming pools, and tributaries. When granulomas are suspected of being due to *M. marinum,* the laboratory should be notified so cultures are incubated at 25°–30°C; *M. marinum* grows slowly if at all at 37°C. Colonies of *M. marinum* require 2 weeks or longer to develop, whereas those of the *M. fortuitum-chelonae* complex will usually appear within 7 days of incubation. Mycobacterial infections of the bones and joints may also be due to several species including *M. tuberculosis, M. bovis,* and *M. kansasii.*[25] Their growth requires at least 2 weeks.

The significance of mycobacteria other than tubercle bacilli that are isolated from the musculoskeletal system and wounds must be interpreted cautiously because of their occurrence in nature as well as in clinically asymptomatic humans, especially in superficial lesions. Their significance is increased if isolated from an abscess or closed lesion, when present in large numbers, and if isolated in repeated cultures. Acid-fast bacteria may not be seen in as many as half of the tissues from which tubercle bacilli are isolated, so acid-fast stains are helpful only when positive.

Osseous lesions may occur in disseminated forms of brucellosis, cryptococcosis, coccidioidomycosis, blastomycosis, and sporotrichosis. The presence of granulomas in frozen sections of bone should therefore prompt a request for cultures for mycobacteria, brucellae, and fungi (see Table 4 for suitable media).

Acute-Onset Diarrhea

Acute-onset diarrhea may be caused by a variety of bacterial, parasitic, and viral agents. Included among bacterial etiologic agents are *Bacillus cereus, Campylobacter jejuni, Clostridium difficile, Clostridium perfringens,* enterotoxigenic and enteroinvasive *E. coli,* salmonellae, shigellae, *Vibrio cholerae* and halophilic vibrios, and *Yersinia enterocolitica*. Among parasitic agents, those most frequently encountered in the United States are *Giardia lamblia* and *Entamoeba histolytica;* however, cryptosporidiosis has become a serious problem in patients with the acquired immunodeficiency syndrome (AIDS). Viral causes of acute-onset diarrhea are rotavirus, Norwalk and similar agents, calicivirus, and adenovirus. With certain exceptions, serotypes of *E. coli,* which were formerly described as "enteropathogenic," have been shown not to be pathogenic and should therefore no longer be routinely identified in stool cultures. Identification of enterotoxigenicity in *B. cereus* or *E. coli* and of cytotoxicity in *C. difficile* requires inoculation of tissue culture cell lines, whereas identification of enteroinvasive *E. coli* requires animal inoculation. Alternative methods for detecting *C. difficile* toxin have included counterimmunoelectrophoresis, which generally lacks sensitivity (41–100 percent) and specificity (78–95 percent), enzyme immunoassay, which has variable sensitivity (56–100 percent) but appears to be highly specific (98–100 percent), and a commercially available latex agglutination that is relatively specific (92–98 percent) and moderately sensitive (80–91 percent) but appears to react with a protein that is not associated with either toxin A or toxin B.[26,27] Although the latex agglutination test is simple and rapid to perform, its use should probably be limited to laboratories that are unable to perform a cytotoxin assay. Although culture for *C. difficile* is the most sensitive test for antibiotic-associated gastroenteritis, isolation of the organism is a nonspecific finding; therefore, testing is usually limited to toxin detection.

DNA hybridization appears to be a highly sensitive and specific approach to the detection of enterotoxigenic *E. coli;* however, reagents for this purpose are as yet not commercially available.

To examine stool for the more conventional pathogenic bacteria, the laboratory should receive a freshly passed stool or freshly collected rectal swab. It may be helpful in distinguishing between diarrhea due to invasive and toxigenic bacteria to examine a fleck of mucus or stool mixed with Loeffler methylene blue stain for the presence of leukocytes.[28] The specimen should then be inoculated onto blood agar, a gram-negative differential medium (EMB or MacConkey agar), a selective medium for *Salmonella* and *Shigella* (xylose-lysine-deoxycholate [XLD] or Hektoen enteric [HE] agar), and enrichment broth (gram-negative [GN] or selenite), and selective media for *C. jejuni* and, when specifically requested, *Y. enterocolitica*. Should infection with vibrios be suspected on the basis of recent travel in an endemic area (*V. cholerae*) or recent ingestion of raw seafood or shellfish (*Vibrio parahaemolyticus*), the laboratory should be so notified so that thiosulfate-citrate-bile salts (TCBS) agar can also be inoculated. *Bacillus cereus* food poisoning has been only infrequently recognized in the United States but becomes manifested either by upper gastrointestinal tract symptoms, similar to those seen in staphylococcal food poisoning, or by lower intestinal tract symptoms, similar to those seen in clostridial food poisoning. Diagnosis of the former syndrome can only be established by the isolation of large numbers of *B. cereus* in incriminated food; however, diagnosis of the latter syndrome is limited to isolation of the organism from stool and determining whether it is enterotoxigenic.

In suspected parasitic infections, loose watery stools should be promptly submitted to the laboratory since protozoan trophozoites may degenerate rapidly, especially at room or incubation temperatures. If the stools are formed, it is preferable to obtain a saline-purged stool on each of 3 consecutive days after having the patient ingest 15 ml of magnesium sulfate (Epsom salt) early in the day. Specimens that are mailed or in which delivery is delayed should be placed in 10% formalin or polyvinyl alcohol (PVA) fixative in a small, plastic, screw-capped container. For brief periods of storage ($\leq$2 hours), refrigeration is advisable. A negative report based on examination of a single specimen is unreliable. Specimens are examined grossly for the presence of proglottids or adult worms and for areas of blood or mucus that should be examined microscopically in direct and concentrated wet mounts and in permanently stained smears. Concentration procedures by formalin-ether sedimentation or zinc sulfate flotation techniques increase the likelihood of detection of protozoan cysts and helminthic eggs and larvae. Trichrome and iron hematoxylin are commonly used for preparing permanent stains.

Norwalk-like agents are important causes of epidemic gastroenteritis but require special immune electron microscopy or radioimmunoassay techniques for their detection (see Chapter 14). Rotavirus causes a syndrome characterized by diarrhea, fever, and vomiting but may also be shed asymptomatically; thus, detection of rotavirus in feces may have little utility in distinguishing between those who are infected (as evidenced by antibody titer rise) and those who are carriers.[29,30] Nonetheless, detection of rotavirus has epidemiologic utility since viral shedding is the major means of transmission of the virus. The major diagnostic tests available commercially for detection of rotavirus in feces are enzyme immunoassay and latex agglutination. Latex agglutination is comparable to enzyme immunoassay in the acute phase of rotaviral infection since large amounts of antigen are excreted during the first days of illness; however, latex agglutination has less sensitivity than does enzyme immunoassay later in the course of disease or in the detection of asymptomatic carriers.[31]

Despite the many advances that have been made in determining the etiology of diarrheal disease, the diagnostic capabilities of the clinical laboratory remain limited to cultures for *Salmonella, Shigella, Campylobacter, Yersinia,* and *Vibrio;* examination for ova and parasites; and detection of *C. difficile* toxin and rotavirus antigen. Detection of enterotoxigenic, enteroinvasive, enterohemorrhagic, and enteropathogenic strains of *E. coli,* Norwalk-like agents, caliciviruses, astroviruses, and adenoviruses await further technologic developments.

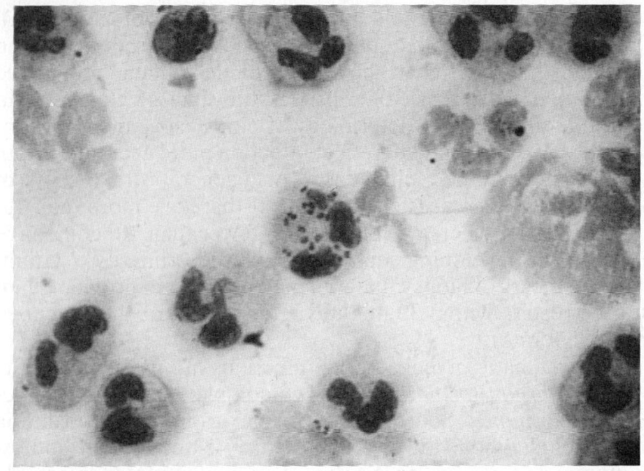

FIG. 4. Intracellular diplococci in a smear of urethral exudate from a male with gonorrhea. (Gram stain, ×1000) (From Washington,[33] with permission.)

Genital Infections

Changing social mores, AIDS, and other poorly definable factors have resulted in significant increases in the incidence of sexually transmitted diseases. At the same time, technical developments in the isolation of anaerobic bacteria and *Chlamydia* have increased our understanding of the cause of these diseases. The laboratory must therefore be prepared to handle a variety of specimens and process them appropriately according to the disease suspected clinically.

Syphilis. Although usually diagnosed serologically, syphilis can in its primary and secondary stages be diagnosed by darkfield or direct fluorescent antibody microscopic examination of serous exudate from infectious lesions. Lesions should be abraded with a dry sponge to provoke exudation; however, it is important to minimize bleeding since the presence of red cells will make the examination more difficult. The exudate is applied directly to a clean coverslip that is inverted on a glass slide. The edges of the coverslip can be sealed to minimize evaporation since *Treponema pallidum* is very sensitive to desiccation. The slide should, at any rate, be examined as soon as possible. Spirochetes of *T. pallidum* are motile, 6–15 μm in length, and have 5–20 rigid and regular spirals. Because of the normal presence of nonpathogenic treponemes in the mouth, darkfield microscopic examinations of material from this source should not be performed.

Serologic tests for syphilis are divided into nontreponemal tests, including the Venereal Disease Research Laboratory (VDRL) test, and treponemal tests, including the fluorescent treponemal antibody absorption (FTA-ABS) test and microhemagglutination tests such as MHA-TP. The sensitivity of the VDRL test is high in secondary syphilis and early latent syphilis and less sensitive in primary syphilis. Its specificity is high (99.5–100 percent) in healthy persons but reduced (75–85 percent) in sick persons.[32] The VDRL test is the preferred test for screening asymptomatic persons and, when positive, should be confirmed by a hemagglutination test. The VDRL should then be followed at 3, 6, and 12 months to determine the adequacy of treatment.[32] Although the CSF-VDRL test is a highly specific indicator of neurosyphilis, it is positive in only 22–69 percent of patients with active neurosyphilis.[32] Because of its lack of specificity, the CSF-FTA-ABS is not recommended for use in this country.[32]

Gonorrhea. The diagnosis of gonorrhea in men can be established presumptively by the findings of gram-negative intracellular diplococci in stained smears of urethral discharge (Fig. 4). Gram-stained smears of cervical drainage lack sensitivity and specificity,[34] and it is probably advisable for laboratories other than those in sexually transmitted disease clinics not to make them at all. Nonpathogenic neisseriae, anaerobic cocci, overdecolorized gram-positive cocci, and short forms of gram-negative bacilli that may normally be found in the vagina and may appear to be within or adherent to leukocytes render interpretation of Gram-stained smears of this area especially difficult and are subject to potentially serious error. To confirm the diagnosis in men and to establish it in women, it is necessary to make cultures for *N. gonorrhoeae*. The sites and types of examination recommended for various gonococcal syndromes are shown in Table 6. In the absence of a urethral discharge, which may sometimes be obtained by "milking" the urethra, material should be obtained either by inserting a thin calcium alginate swab or small-diameter, smooth bacteriologic loop into the urethra. Cervical material should be obtained by direct visualization with the aid of a speculum. In all women and in homosexual men suspected of having gonorrhea it is also recommended that the anal crypts be swabbed for culture since this may be the only site from which gonococci may be recovered. In cases of suspected gonococcal pharyngitis, the posterior portion of the pharynx and tonsillar areas should be vigorously swabbed as for any throat culture. In cases of suspected gonococcemia, blood should be inoculated into media without SPS, as has already been described (see "Septicemia").

Specimens from sites normally inhabited by fungi or other bacteria should be inoculated promptly onto selective media such as modified Thayer-Martin medium (MTM) containing vancomycin (3 μg/ml), colistin (7.5 μg/ml), and nystatin (12.5 units/ml) or, preferably, anisomycin (10 μg/ml). The addition of trimethoprim (5 μg/ml) to MTM is desirable to prevent swarming by *Proteus*. Concurrent inoculation of chocolate blood agar without antibiotics is also recommended to allow growth of vancomycin-susceptible gonococci, another cause of false-positive smears. Incubation in an atmosphere of at least 70 percent humidity and 3–7 percent carbon dioxide should be done as quickly as possible. Gonococci are sensitive to drying and wide fluctuations in temperature.

Several devices are available commercially that permit the physician to inoculate MTM directly with clinical material. The necessary carbon dioxide is either already provided in the device by its manufacturer (e.g., Transgrow) or by placing a carbon dioxide–generating effervescent tablet in a chamber at the time the MTM is inoculated (e.g., JEMBEC). Such devices may then be transported to a laboratory for examination; however, it is important that they be incubated at 35°C overnight before mailing, and failure to do so will significantly decrease recovery of *N. gonorrhoeae*.

An enzyme immunoassay (EIA) for the detection of gonococcal antigen is commercially available and has been found to

TABLE 6. Recommended Specimens for Laboratory Evaluation of Specific Sexually Transmitted Disease Syndromes

	Urethral		*Cervical*		*First-Voided Urine*		*Rectal*	*Pharyngeal*	*Orogastric Aspirate*		*Serous or Synovial Exudate*		*Abscess Pus*		*Conjunctival*		*Biopsy*		*Blood Culture*
Syndrome	*S*	*C*	*S*	*C*	*S*	*C*	*C*	*C*	*S*	*C*	*S*	*C*	*S*	*C*	*S*	*C*	*S*	*C*	*C*
Men																			
Acute urethritis	R	±			±	±													
Chronic urethritis	R	R			±	±													
Suspected gonorrhea in homosexuals without urethritis	±	R					R	R											
Women																			
Acute symptomatic GU gonorrhea	±	R	R	R	±	±	R	±											
Asymptomatic suspected GU gonorrhea (e.g., contact)	–	±	–	R	±	±	R	±											
Bartholin's abscess	±	R	±	R			±						R[a]	R[a]					
Pelvic inflammatory disease	R	R	R	R			R				R[a]	R[a]					R[a]	R[a]	
Both sexes																			
Pharyngitis	R	R	R	R				R											
Suspected neonatal sepsis							±		R	R									R
Neonatal conjunctivitis															R	R			
Disseminated gonococcal infection	R	R	R	R							R[a]	R[a]	R[a]	R[a]			R[a]	R[a]	R
Men																			
Heterosexual	–	R																	
Homosexual	–	R					R												
Women	–	±	–	R															

Abbreviations: S: Gram-stained smear; R: routine examinations; C: culture; ±: optional examinations; GU: genitourinary.
[a] If sites are believed to be infected
(From Kellogg et al., [34] with permission.)

be as sensitive as Gram-stained smears of male urethral specimens and more sensitive than are Gram-stained smears of cervical specimens for the detection of *N. gonorrhoeae*. Compared with culture of endocervical specimens, the sensitivity of EIA has varied between 75 and 100 percent, whereas specificity has varied between 95 and 99 percent. False-positives in endocervical specimens have been troublesome and appear to be due to cross-reactive gram-negative bacteria. Whether EIA can serve as a culture substitute depends upon multiple factors, including the prevalence of gonorrhea in the population being examined, the incidence of antibiotic resistance of isolates from cultures, laboratory resources, turnaround time, and cost. A small false-positive rate may be acceptable in a high-prevalence population seen in a sexually transmitted disease clinic but may be unacceptable in a low-prevalence private practice setting. The turnaround time of the EIA is 4 hours but may be considerably longer if tests are batched to reduce the per-test cost. Even on a batched basis, however, cost of the EIA exceeds that of Gram-stained smear and culture. Finally, if screening for *N. gonorrhoeae* is by EIA only, this obviously precludes determining β-lactamase activity or the susceptibility of gonococci to other antimicrobial agents.

Chlamydia. Infection due to *Chlamydia trachomatis* is most accurately detected by culture (see Chapter 14). Specimens should be collected by rubbing a swab vigorously over the suspected site of infection. In collecting specimens from the cervix it is especially important to remove excess discharge and to rub the swab vigorously along the walls of the endocervical canal. Failure to do so will substantially reduce the detection of *C. trachomatis*, especially when sought in smears stained with the fluorescent antibody technique. Specimens that cannot be cultured immediately should be stored in sucrose-phosphate (2 SP) transport medium at 5°C for up to 72 hours or at −70°C if for longer than 72 hours.[35] Cultures are made by inoculating with centrifugation aliquots of 2 SP onto cycloheximide-treated McCoy cells, incubating for 48 to 72 hours, and then staining the cells with the fluorescent antibody technique or iodine to detect inclusions.[35]

Tests for detecting chlamydial antigen in specimens include enzyme immunoassay (EIA) and direct fluorescent antibody staining (DFA). Although their specificities are generally ≥95 percent, their sensitivities vary from nearly 70 to 100 percent,[36,37] depending upon the quality of the specimen and the skill of the person performing the DFA. EIA is easier to perform than DFA is, but the DFA provides the faster turnaround time and is less expensive to perform than is EIA, regardless of batching. Although culture is less expensive than either antigen detection test, many laboratories do not have tissue culture capabilities. Since the specificity of antigen tests is not 100 percent, only a culture performed in a competent laboratory should be used in evaluating chlamydial infection in sexually abused children.[38]

Mycoplasma. The role of the genital mycoplasmas in producting urethritis and pelvic inflammatory disease remains unclear, although there are circumstantial data implicating *Ureaplasma urealyticum* (T-strain mycoplasmas) in nongonococcal urethritis. Swabs transported in 2 SP are suitable for culture of genital mycoplasmas; however, the results of cultures should be interpreted cautiously because of the frequency of isolation of mycoplasmas from genital sources.

Gardnerella vaginalis. The role of *Gardnerella vaginalis* in causing bacterial vaginosis remains uncertain since it is found in the vaginal flora of many asymptomatic women and since the entity of bacterial vaginosis appears to be associated with the isolation of *G. vaginalis,* anaerobic curved rods, and anaerobic gram-negative bacilli. Amsel et al.[39] have proposed three of the four following criteria adequate for a diagnosis of bacterial vaginosis: (*1*) vaginal pH greater than 4.5; (*2*) thin, homogeneous, milklike discharge; (*3*) release of fishy amine odor on addition of a drop of KOH (10% solution) to a drop of vaginal discharge; and/or (*4*) the presence microscopically of clue cells in a saline wet mount of the vaginal discharge. Culture is not currently recommended for diagnostic purposes.

Pelvic Inflammatory Disease. The cause of pelvic inflammatory disease is difficult to determine and varies according to the population of patients studied, the types of specimens examined, and the investigator bias as to the types of microorganisms being studied. Pelvic inflammatory disease may be classified as gonococcal and nongonococcal or as sexually transmitted and nonsexually transmitted.[40] The major causes of the sexually transmitted disease are *Neisseria gonorrhoeae* and *Chlamydia trachomatis*. The possible roles of *Mycoplasma hominis* and *Ureaplasma urealyticum* remain controversial.[40] The major causes of nonsexually transmitted pelvic inflammatory disease are aerobic and anaerobic bacteria, often in mixed culture.[40] Diagnosis of gonococcal disease is facilitated by the isolation of *N. gonorrhoeae* from the endocervix, while the preferred method of diagnosis of disease due to aerobic and anaerobic bacteria is by aspiration with a needle and syringe or surgical incision and drainage or excision.[18] Anaerobic cultures should be routinely performed with such specimens as well as with material obtained by culdocentesis. Cultures of material aspirated from the uterine cavity should be limited to those obtained with a double-lumen, distally occluded catheter, which will minimize contamination of the specimen by normal vaginal and cervical flora.

Both *Chlamydia trachomatis* and genital tract mycoplasmas have been implicated as causes of acute salpingitis after their recovery from material obtained by laparoscopy.[41] Cultures of endocervical or tubal material for *C. trachomatis* are therefore of value in elucidating the cause of salpingitis. The interpretation of endocervical cultures yielding mycoplasmas, however, remains problematic because of the frequency of isolation of this group of organisms from asymptomatic women.

Ocular Infections

The difficulties of determining the cause of conjunctivitis on the basis of Gram-stained smears and bacteriologic cultures have been emphasized by Leibowitz et al.[42] who found a poor correlation between the initial clinical impression and the results of microbiologic studies and between the findings in Gram-stained smears and in cultures. Although bacteriologic studies of conjunctivitis are useful primarily in gonococcal conjunctivitis, microbiologic studies for chlamydiae and viruses (e.g., adenovirus, herpesvirus) are often warranted. Although Giemsa stains demonstrate chlamydiae in a very high percentage of neonates with inclusion blennorrhea, they are considerably less sensitive than are tissue culture in detecting chlamydiae in adults with follicular conjunctivitis due to *C. trachomatis*. Direct fluorescent antibody-stained smears are highly sensitive in either case.

Corneal ulcers require careful laboratory studies as described elsewhere by Jones et al.[43] and by François and Rysselaere.[44] The microbiologist should ensure that the following materials are available to the ophthalmologist for these studies: sterile swabs, spatula, clean glass microscopic slides and coverslips, proparacaine hydrochloride (Ophthaine, 0.5%), alcohol lamp, and media suitable for cultivation of bacteria, mycobacteria, and fungi. The swabs are used for obtaining conjunctival and lid cultures. Corneal scrapings are taken with the aid of a slit lamp and are spread gently over a small area of each slide and medium to be examined. Multiple areas of the ulcer should be sampled. One slide each should be stained by the Gram and Giemsa methods. Scrapings on a third slide are examined under a coverslip in a potassium hydroxide preparation. If indicated, the remaining slides may be stained with a fluorochrome or carbol fuchsin technique for mycobacteria and by a silver impregnation method for fungi.

Intraocular infections, including those related to surgery, may be due to a variety of microorganisms. Material obtained by ocular paracentesis requires scrupulous attention with appropriate smears and cultures for bacteria (including anaerobic), mycobacteria, fungi, and viruses.

IDENTIFICATION OF ORGANISMS

The laboratory can provide preliminary or definitive identification of etiologic agents based on: (*1*) microscopic examination of specimens, of growth occurring in cultures of those specimens, or of indirect evidence of growth in tissue culture (e.g., cytopathic effects); (*2*) immunologic techniques that detect microbial antigens or antibodies in body fluids or in cultures of those fluids; (*3*) DNA probes to detect microorganisms or genetically encoded characteristics of microorganisms in specimens or cultures; and (*4*) growth or biochemical characteristics of organisms isolated in cultures.

Microscopy

Unstained. Wet mount preparations of specimens can be examined with an ordinary light microscope for evidence of fungi or parasites. The substage condenser should be raised and lowered during examination to achieve optimal illumination and contrast. Practical applications include direct examination for fungi or sputum and other body fluids, transtracheal and bronchial aspirates, skin and hair scrapings, and urinary sediments mixed with 10% potassium hydroxide on a clean glass microscopic slide. A coverslip is placed over the mixture, and the slide is gently heated by passing it through a flame. Wet mounts are also used for examining fecal material for the presence of protozoan trophozoites and helminth larvae. Contrast can be increased in examining cerebrospinal fluid for cryptococci by mixing centrifuged sediment with India ink. Contrast can also be enhanced with phase microscopy (Figs. 2 and 3) or with darkfield microscopy, the latter being the procedure of choice for the detection of spirochetes in skin lesions in early cases of syphilis or in the cerebrospinal fluid or urine in early cases of leptospirosis.

Wet mounts of urinary sediment, with or without methylene blue, will provide reliable evidence of the presence of significant bacteriuria when at least 20 bacteria per high dry objective field (×430) are seen. Capsular swelling (quellung reaction) of pneumococci occurs in wet mounts of cerebrospinal fluid or sputum when polyvalent or type-specific antibody is added to the specimen.

In each of these cases microscopy can provide rapid and definitive identification of an etiologic agent in a specimen, assuming, of course, that organisms display typical morphologic characteristics. All these procedures are limited by the occurrence of small or rare numbers of organisms in the specimen, by the findings of artifacts that may resemble organisms, and by the presence of atypical forms of organisms that are not readily identifiable. Training and experience are required to prevent over- or underinterpretation of findings.

Stained. Innumerable stains have been described for the examination of specimens or organisms. Only those in frequent use will be described here, and the interested reader is referred to standard references for details about reagents and procedures for other stains.

ACID-FAST STAINS

A. Kinyoun carbol fuchsin

Reagents

1. Carbol fuchsin

Basic fuchsin	4 g
Phenol, melted	8 ml
Ethyl alcohol, 95%	20 ml
Distilled water	68 ml

Mix the phenol and alcohol in 50 ml of water in a flask or bottle; add the dye, shake, and allow to stand overnight at room temperature. Add the rest of the water, and filter through coarse paper. Store in the bottle.

2. Decolorizer*

HCl, concentrated	12 ml
Ethyl alcohol, 95%	388 ml

3. Counterstain

Methylene blue	4 g
Water	400 ml

Procedure

1. Air-dry the smears on new, clean glass microscope slides, and heat fix by passing through a flame.
2. Cover the slides with strips of coarse filter paper and flood with carbol fuchsin for 5 minutes.
3. Remove the filter paper and rinse the slide with tap water.
4. Decolorize until thick portions of the smear are clear.
5. Rinse the slide with tap water.
6. Flood the slide with counterstain for 1 minute.
7. Rinse the slide with tap water, drain, and blot dry.

B. Auramine-rhodamine (fluorochrome)

Reagents

1. Auramine-rhodamine

Auramine O (C.I. 41000)	1.5 g
Rhodamine B (C.I. 45170)	0.75 g
Glycerol	75 ml
Phenol, melted	10 ml
Distilled water	50 ml

Dissolve the phenol in water, add dyes, and mix. Add glycerol in 25 ml water and mix with a magnetic stirrer or shake periodically for several hours. Filter through glass wool. Store in the bottle.

2. Decolorizer*

HCl, concentrated	2.5 ml
Ethyl alcohol, 70%	500 ml

3. Counterstain

Potassium permanganate	5 g
Distilled water	1000 ml

* One percent sulfuric acid is used as a decolorizer for acid-fast stains of *Nocardia*.

Procedure

1. Air-dry the smears on new, clean glass microscope slide and heat-fix by passing through a flame.
2. Flood the slide with auramine-rhodamine for 15 minutes.
3. Rinse the slide with distilled water.
4. Flood the slide with decolorizer for 2 minutes.
5. Rinse the slide with distilled water.
6. Flood the slide with counterstain for 2 minutes.
7. Rinse the slide with tap water, drain, and blot dry.

The sensitivity and specificity of the carbol fuchsin and fluorochrome stains are approximately equal. However, because carbol fuchsin stains must be examined with the ×100 oil immersion objective and fluorochrome stains are examined with a ×25 objective, the latter is a far more rapid and efficient method of screening smears. Moreover, the fluorochrome stain may be more sensitive in some observer's hands because of the greater contrast it provides.

GIEMSA STAIN FOR MALARIA AND OTHER ORGANISMS

Reagents

1. Stock Giemsa stain solution (commercially available)
2. Methyl alcohol, absolute
3. Phosphate buffer, M/15, pH 7.0

Working solution is prepared by mixing 15 ml of stock solution in 35 ml phosphate buffer. Filter if necessary.

Procedure

1. Puncture the skin with a sterile, disposable lancet.
2. Apply a drop of blood to surface of a clean (with alcohol or acetone) glass microscope slide.
3. Stir the drop of blood vigorously in a circular motion with the corner of another glass slide so as to cover a surface approximately 1.5 cm in diameter. A proper thick film should be thin enough for newsprint to be read through it.
4. Prepare a thin film as for a conventional hematologic smear.
5. Allow the films to dry gently.
6. Fix the thin film with methyl alcohol (3 minutes). Do not fix the thick film, and if both films are on the same slide, protect the thick film from the alcohol or its fumes.
7. Place the slides into a Coplin jar containing working Giemsa solution for a minimum of 30 minutes.
8. Remove the slides, and rinse in phosphate buffer.
9. Drain the slides, and allow to air-dry.
10. Examine with low power (×100) for microfilariae and with high power (×430) and oil immersion (×1000) for blood and tissue protozoa.

Smears should be prepared whenever malaria is suspected; however, the optimal time is midway between attacks, and the least favorable time is during or immediately after an episode of fever. Care must be taken to differentiate malaria forms from normal blood components (e.g., platelets).

GRAM STAIN

Reagents

1. Crystal violet solution

Crystal violet, 90% dye content	10 g
Methyl alcohol, absolute	500 ml

2. Iodine solution

Iodine crystals	6 g
Potassium iodide	12 g
Distilled water	1800 ml

3. Decolorizer†

Acetone	400 ml
Ethyl alcohol, 95%	1200 ml

4. Counterstain

Safranin, 99% dye content	10 g
Distilled water	1000 ml

Procedure

1. Air-dry smears of clean glass microscope slides and heat-fix by passing through a flame.
2. Flood the slide with crystal violet solution for at least 10 seconds.
3. Rinse the slide with tap water.
4. Flood the slide with iodine solution for at least 10 seconds.
5. Rinse the slide with tap water.
6. Decolorize until no more blue color comes off thin portions of the smear, and rinse immediately with tap water.
7. Flood the slide with counterstain for 10 seconds.
8. Rinse the slide with tap water, drain, and blot dry.

This stain should be used routinely by the bacteriology laboratory in examining material from normally sterile body fluids, abscesses, wounds, sputum, and tissue. The finding of at least two bacteria per oil immersion field (×1000) in well-mixed properly collected and stored urine represents significant bacteriuria (≥70,000 cfu/ml). Although the finding of gram-positive or gram-negative bacteria is not specific, it is often possible to surmise on the basis of the patient's clinical presentation and source of the material examined what the organisms seen in the smear are likely to be. Those inexperienced with the Gram stain technique are most apt to have difficulty with the decolorization step and to over- or underdecolorize. Artifacts such as deposited crystal violet may be misinterpreted as being cocci or bacilli.

PNEUMOCYSTIS CARINII STAIN

A. Toluidine blue[13,45]

Reagents

1. Sulfation reagent

Glacial acetic acid	45 ml
Sulfuric acid, concentrated	15 ml

Pour glacial acetic acid into a Coplin jar that has been placed in a plastic tub containing cool tap water (≥10°C). Add 15 ml concentrated sulfuric acid slowly and mix with a glass rod. Seal the jar with petroleum jelly, and store at room temperature. The reagent should be replaced after 1 week's use.

2. Toluidine blue

Toluidine blue 0	0.3 g
Hydrochloric acid	2 ml
Ethyl alcohol	140 ml
Distilled water	60 ml

Mix the dye in water, and then add acid and finally alcohol. Store at room temperature. The reagent should be replaced after 1 year's use.

Procedure

1. Air-dry the smear and touch preparations on clean glass microscope slides for 30 minutes.
2. Place the slides in sulfation reagent for 10 minutes.
3. Rinse the slides gently with tap water for 5 minutes.
4. Stain the slides in toluidine blue for 3 minutes.
5. Decolorize by dipping once into 95% ethyl alcohol and once into absolute alcohol, each for approximately 10 seconds.
6. Dip in and out of Xyless (Columbia Diagnostics, Inc., Springfield, VA) twice each for approximately 10 seconds, and allow to evaporate.
7. Mount in a suitable mounting medium (e.g., Permount) with a coverslip.

Pneumocystis carinii cysts stain lavender. In contrast with yeasts, which also are stained by toluidine blue, cysts of *P. carinii* do not bud. Nevertheless, a diagnosis of *P. carinii* infection should not be made when specimens contain yeast cells unless at least one cluster of *P. carinii* cysts in seen.[12]

Other stains for *P. carinii* include Giemsa, which demonstrates the internal contents of the cyst and the trophozoite forms but which requires considerable experience on the part of the microscopist for accurate interpretation, and the Gomori methenamine silver (GMS), which provides the most reliable detection of cysts in touch preparations and tissue section. Although GMS staining is usually performed in histopathology laboratories, a simple and reliable rapid method is available that can be readily performed in the clinical laboratory.[46]

TISSUE SECTION STAINS. Hematoxylin and eosin (H&E) is a useful stain for screening tissue to determine whether a lesion is malignant or inflammatory and, if so, whether it is granulomatous or suppurative. Bacteria may be stained by various modifications of the Brown and Brenn Gram stain as well as by the Dieterle stain. The fluorochrome procedure can be used to examine tissue homogenate for mycobacteria; however, the sensitivity of this procedure is less than 50 percent as compared with culture of tissue from non-AIDS patients. Gomori methenamine silver stain is used to detect and characterize actinomycetes, fungi, and *Pneumocystis carinii.* Direct fluorescent antibody stain is the most specific method for detecting *Legionella pneumophila* in tissue sections.

INTESTINAL PARASITE STAINS. Wet preparations can be made by mixing a small quantity of feces on a glass microscope slide with a drop or two of freshly mixed 0.1% eosin in saline. A coverslip is placed over the mixture, which is then examined under low power (×100). The eosin is nontoxic for protozoa and worms and provides a contrasting reddish background for the normally pale green parasites. Concentration procedures are recommended to enhance the detection of cysts, eggs, and larvae. The zinc sulfate centrifugal flotation and the acid–ether centrifugal sedimentation methods are those most widely used in the United States. There are also a variety of permanent staining techniques, of which Heidenhain's iron hematoxylin and the Wheatley trichrome stains are widely used. Concentration methods and stains are described in detail in a number of standard references in parasitology. Care must be exercised in the examination of smears to avoid over- and underinterpretation. Unless skilled examiners are available, it is strongly recommended that the specimen be mixed in 10% formalin or polyvinyl alcohol (PVA) fixative for shipment to a reference laboratory. Laboratories engaging in parasitologic work should have photographs and other illustrated material available. (An excellent three-volume *Atlas of Diagnostic Medical Parasitology* may be obtained from the American Society of Clinical Pathologists.)

Care should be taken not to examine specimens from patients who have had recent cleansing or barium enemas, antidiarrheal compounds, antiparasitic medications, laxatives, or antibiotics. These compounds or procedures will either interfere with the visualization of parasites in stool or cause their disappearance at the time stool is collected for examination.

† Ninety-five percent alcohol may be used instead of acetone-alcohol to reduce the risk of overdecolorization.

LOEFFLER'S METHYLENE BLUE STAIN

Reagents

Methylene blue, certified	0.3 g
Potassium hydroxide, 10% solution	0.1 ml
Ethyl alcohol, 95%	30 ml
Distilled water	100 ml

Dissolve methylene blue with alcohol with a mortar and pestle and transfer to a flask. Add potassium hydroxide to water, wash the mortar, and pour the washings with the remainder of the water into the flask. Filter the mixture through paper 24 hours later.

Procedure

A small fleck of mucus or liquid stool is placed on a clean glass microscope slide and mixed thoroughly with the stain. A coverslip is applied, and after 2 or 3 minutes, the slide is examined under high power (×430) for leukocytes.[28]

Immunoassays and DNA Probe Hybridization Techniques

New technologies that provide rapid detection or identification of specified microorganisms or specific characteristics of microorganisms (e.g., *E. coli* enterotoxins) are exciting developments that are likely to substantially alter the practice of medical microbiology. As new immunoassays and DNA probes are developed, however, certain critical issues need to be addressed before these technologies can be implemented in the clinical laboratory. These issues include the sensitivity, specificity, predictive values, and confidence intervals of the new test in relation to an accepted reference method. The confidence interval allows one to assess the relative precision of the different point estimates provided by an investigator evaluating the test or the manufacturer selling the product.[47] With the appropriate statistical data, it is then possible to assess the clinical value of the test and to decide whether to implement the test in the laboratory. It is important to determine whether the test will be used for screening purposes or for confirming or ruling out a diagnosis. In the former instance a sensitive test is desirable, while in the latter instance a specific test is desirable. A highly sensitive test should be used when knowledge of the disease present is highly important in the management of the patient, while a highly specific test should be used if no confirmatory test is available or there would be serious adverse consequences from a false-positive result. These issues must be addressed whether the test is used to detect a particular microorganism that is either difficult or easy to culture and when there is any question about whether an immunoassay or DNA probe might serve as a culture substitute. For example, DNA probes for *E. coli* enterotoxins appear to be highly specific and to be as, if not more, sensitive than are traditional methods involving culture isolation of colonies of *E. coli* that are then tested for toxinogenicity in either tissue culture or animals. DNA hybridization allows the processing of a large number of specimens on a batch basis in a much shorter period of time than do traditional methods; therefore, a DNA probe for *E. coli* enterotoxin has the attributes of high sensitivity, high specificity, and cost-effectiveness required for its implementation in laboratories investigating diarrheal disease. In contrast, the commercially available *Legionella* probe, although highly specific, has a sensitivity of 60–80 percent and can therefore only be used as a screening test, with culture and/or serology serving as confirmatory tests. Thus, the *Legionella* probe must be compared with the *Legionella* direct immunofluorescent antibody (DFA) test for screening purposes. The sensitivity of both tests is 60–80 percent, while the specificities of the probe and the monoclonal DFA for *L. pneumophila* are >99 percent (specificity of the polyclonal DFA may be ≥97 percent).[48] Since the procedure for the probe requires less technical expertise than that for DFA, the probe may be the preferred screening test, provided the batch size allows for complete utilization of the test kit and the frequency of testing allows for complete utilization of the radiolabeled reagents within the product's short shelf life. If neither of these conditions is met, the per-test cost of the probe is substantially higher than for DFA. In other words, DFA is the most cost-effective procedure for the laboratory processing an average of two to four specimens a day, provided the technical expertise in immunofluorescence microscopy is available in the laboratory. The same considerations arise when comparing DFA and enzyme immunoassay to screen for *Chlamydia trachomatis*.

Replacement of isotopically labeled probes with nonisotopically labeled probes should eventually reduce equipment and reagent expense. Ultimately, however, the use of probes and immunoassays as culture substitutes will depend on improved sensitivity and specificity, simplification of specimen processing, and automation of procedures. As long as these techniques remain culture supplements (vs. substitutes), they represent added costs that may be difficult to implement unless a clear-cut clinical benefit can be demonstrated from their use.

Other Immunologic Techniques

Direct Immunofluorescence. Direct immunofluorescence technique involves the attachment of antigen or antibody labeled with fluorescein isothiocyanate (FITC) to its antibody or antigen, respectively, and detection of the labeled product with fluorescence microscopy. Practical applications of direct staining include the identification of *S. pyogenes* (group A) in throat swabs or cultures; *B. pertussis* in nasopharyngeal swabs, aspirates, or cultures; *H. influenzae, L. monocytogenes, N. meningitidis, S. agalactiae* (group B), and *S. pneumoniae* in cerebrospinal fluid; *T. pallidum* in lesions of early syphilis; *Brucella, Francisella tularensis,* and *Yersinia pestis* in clinical specimens; *Legionella* in lung tissue; colonies of *N. gonorrhoeae* in cultures of genital sources; and *C. trachomatis* in ocular, nasopharyngeal, and genital specimens.

Direct immunofluorescence is a rapid and sensitive method of staining organisms in specimens or cultures. Fluorescent antibody procedures for screening clinical material and cultures for fungi have been described by Kaufman and Reiss at the Centers for Disease Control[49]; however, labeled reagents are not yet available from commercial sources. The accuracy of immunofluorescence depends on many factors, including technical expertise, properly functioning equipment, the sensitivity of the reagents and their specificity, and the source of the specimen being examined. Immunofluorescence is not necessarily a substitute for culture since it does not yield a viable organism for antimicrobial susceptibility testing or other specific studies. Nonetheless, it can provide rapid detection and often at least presumptive identification of many microorganisms, and it has become an indispensable tool for many laboratories.

Reagents for some specific antigen–antibody reactions are only available in larger nongovernmental reference laboratories and in state or federal public health facilities. Specimens or cultures that are mailed to such laboratories must be shipped in accordance with federal packaging requirements.[1]

Agglutination. Agglutination tests to identify etiologic agents in specimens are limited in number. The most important one in use today is the latex agglutination test for *Cryptococcus neoformans* antigen in cerebrospinal fluid and serum. The sensitivity of this test exceeds that of the India ink preparation for examination of cerebrospinal fluid. Specificity of the cryptococcal latex agglutination test may be reduced by the presence of rheumatoid factor or other interfering proteins; however, treatment of the specimen with a protease (pronase) will eliminate false-positive results due to interfering proteins.[49a]

As discussed earlier, latex and coagglutination may be useful in the diagnosis of bacterial meningitis of partially treated children or in those children in whom the inflammatory response and various biochemical indices in the cerebrospinal fluid do not clearly distinguish between bacterial and viral meningitis.

Latex agglutination, coagglutination, the quellung reaction and counterimmunoelectrophoresis have been used to detect pneumococcal antigen in sputum from patients with suspected pneumococcal pneumonia. The sensitivity of each of these tests relative to documented pneumococcal pneumonia is approximately 80 percent and is therefore higher than that of a Gram-stained smear (approximately 50 percent) in which a positive result is defined by a predominance of lancet-shaped diplococci in each of several oil immersion fields (×1000). Specificities of the antigen tests may, however, be only about 70 percent since false-positive results occur, particularly in patients with chronic bronchitis and pneumococci in their sputum. Latex agglutination tests for group A streptococci are widely available commercially. Although highly specific, these tests are only relatively sensitive, so antigen-negative tests should be backed up by cultures, particularly in areas in which there is a high prevalence of acute rheumatic fever or in which there has been a resurgence of acute rheumatic fever.

Latex agglutination has also been used to detect *Candida* antigenemia; however, differences in study populations and criteria for defining invasive candidiasis have made interpretation of published evaluations difficult. Although fairly specific, antigen tests, including a commercially available product, appear to be relatively insensitive, even if patients with candidemias unrelated to intravascular devices are included in the invasive category of disease. The transient nature of antigenemia and its detection relatively late in the course of disease appear to limit the test's utility in the differentiation between invasive and noninvasive candidiasis.[50,51]

Growth or Biochemical Characteristics

The presence of growth can usually be readily recognized by the development of colonies on solid media and colonies or turbidity in liquid media; however, the rate of growth is a function of the original inoculum size and the group of organisms involved. Most pathogenic bacteria, for example, require only a few hours to produce visible growth, whereas it may take many weeks for colonies of mycobacteria to become evident. It is important for the clinician to know what are reasonable reporting times for various kinds of cultures (Table 7). It is equally important for the laboratory to establish a system for reporting important preliminary results by telephone and in writing.

TABLE 7. Reporting Times for Various Microbiologic Procedures

Procedure	Time
Microscopic	
Acid-fast	4–6 hr
Gram stain	½ hr
India ink	1 hr
Toluidine blue (*Pneumocystis*)	1 hr
Direct fluorescent antibody (*Legionella, Chlamydia trachomatis*)	1 hr
Culture	
Actinomyces	10 days
Anaerobic bacteria	2–14 days
Brucella	21 days
Other bacteria	2–7 days
Leptospires	30 days
Mycobacteria	8 wk
Chlamydia	2–3 days
Mycoplasma	30 days
Fungi	4–6 wk
Viruses	2–14 days

The initial identity of an organism may be suggested by the source of the material cultured, its pattern of growth on nutrient and selective media, its colonial morphology on the various media inoculated, its hemolytic or fermentative properties, and its microscopic appearance. This process requires careful training and experience and provides information that is essential for all further procedures required to identify the organism. The experienced microbiologist can often provide a reasonably accurate preliminary identification of an organism at this point.

Bacteria. Most clinically important bacteria grow under both aerobic and anaerobic conditions and are called facultatively anaerobic. Some, such as *Pseudomonas aeruginosa,* are strict aerobes. For practical purposes, anaerobic bacteria are those that grow only in an atmosphere of reduced oxygen tension and do not grow on solid media in an atmosphere with 10% CO_2 in air.[18] The term *microaerophilic* has no standard meaning but is commonly applied to bacteria preferring an incubation atmosphere of 10% CO_2 in air to aerobic or anaerobic atmospheres of incubation. General schemes for differentiating the major groups of gram-positive and gram-negative bacteria are shown in Figures 5 and 6.

AEROBIC AND FACULTATIVELY ANAEROBIC BACTERIA. *Gram-Positive Cocci.* The gram-positive cocci usually grow satisfactorily on blood agar and are inhibited in their growth on gram-negative differential media such as EMB and MacConkey agar. Staphylococci possess catalase that produces oxygen bubbles when a drop of hydrogen peroxide (H_2O_2) is placed on a colony on a glass microscope slide or on a medium without red blood cells; streptococci are catalase-negative. Staphylococci may or may not exhibit hemolytic properties. Streptococci may display β-hemolytic (complete), α-hemolytic (partial), or nonhemolytic (called γ) properties on blood agar. This method of classifying streptococci is complicated by other schema that place them into pyogenes, viridans, and enterococcal groups based on their biologic properties and into serologic (Lancefield) groups based on group-specific carbohydrate precipitin patterns. Although many β-hemolytic strains are pyogenic and belong to a specific Lancefield group, Lancefield's group D includes β- and nonhemolytic strains. Both α- and nonhemolytic strains (other than those belonging to group D) are frequently classified as viridans streptococci.

More recent changes in streptococcal taxonomy include the reclassification of what were formerly salt-tolerant group D streptococci into the genus *Enterococcus,* including the species *E. faecalis, E. faecium,* and *E. durans,* and the reclassification, by some workers, of "*S. milleri,*" *S. intermedius, S. constellatus,* and minute or small colony-forming β-hemolytic streptococci that are nongroupable or possess the group A, C, F, or G antigens into the species *S. anginosus.* (see Chapter 182).

Most clinical laboratories perform the coagulase test directly with catalase-positive cocci resembling staphylococci and report *Staphylococcus aureus* or coagulase-negative *Staphylococcus* accordingly. Although *S. epidermidis* constitutes the predominant coagulase-negative staphylococcal species of clinical importance, *S. saprophyticus* is an important cause of the acute dysuric syndrome. Other coagulase-negative species of *Staphylococcus* are infrequently pathogenic. The novobiocin test for presumptive identification of *S. saprophyticus* can be limited to urinary isolates of coagulase-negative staphylococci from young female outpatients in the sexually active age group. Otherwise, speciation of coagulase-negative staphylococci is seldom indicated.

Bile solubility may be performed by observing lysis of colonies of streptococci when a solution of 10% deoxycholate is applied to the agar surface. Pneumococci are also inhibited by low concentrations of ethyl hydrocuprein hydrochloride or optochin. Presumptive identification of group A streptococci can be made on the basis of their inhibition by low concentrations

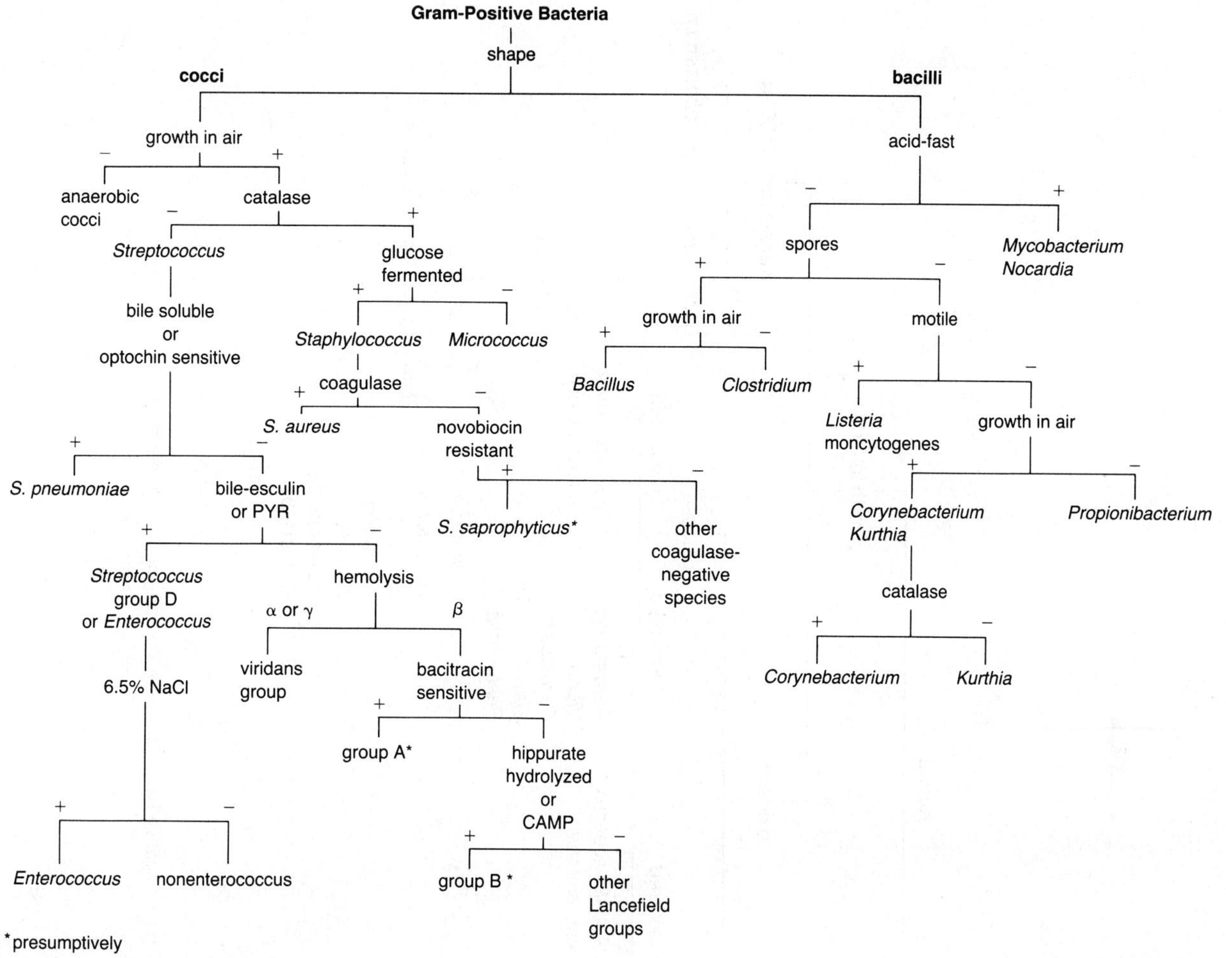

FIG. 5. Schematic outline for the identification of gram-positive bacteria. (From Washington,[15] with permission.)

of bacitracin contained in a paper disk that is applied to the surface of agar to which the organism has been subcultured. Although it is rare for a group A *Streptococcus* to be resistant to bacitracin, between 5 and 10 percent of nongroup A β-hemolytic streptococci (generally belonging to groups B, C, and G) are inhibited. Group B β-hemolytic streptococci can be identified on the basis of their ability to hydrolyze hippurate. Group D streptococci tolerate 40% bile and hydrolyze esculin; those growing in the presence of 6.5% sodium chloride or hydrolyzing L-pyrrolidonyl-β-naphthalamide (PYR) represent enterococcal species. Viridans streptococci represent a group of at least nine species, including *S. pneumoniae*. Most so-called microaerophilic strains belong to these species. In practice, however, it is sufficient to call them viridans streptococci.

Immunofluorescence, latex agglutination, or coagglutination can be used for the rapid identification of group A and group B β-hemolytic streptococci. Lancefield grouping is otherwise performed by capillary precipitin techniques. Typing of group A streptococci, based on their M proteins, may be useful for epidemiologic purposes.

Gram-Negative Cocci. Presumptive identification of the pathogenic neisseriae is based on the growth of gram-negative cocci on modified Thayer-Martin medium and a positive oxidase reaction. Definitive identification and differentiation of *N. gonorrhoeae* and *N. meningitidis* require carbohydrate utilization tests. Immunofluorescence can be used to identify colonies of *N. gonorrhoeae;* however, anti-*N. meningitidis* fluorescein-labeled conjugates tend to cross-react with *N. gonorrhoeae*. Another species, *Neisseria lactamica,* also grows on Thayer-Martin agar and closely resembles *N. meningitidis* in its carbohydrate utilization properties; however, it utilizes lactose, which *N. meningitidis* does not. *Neisseria lactamica* is rarely pathogenic. *Branhamella* (or *Moraxella*) *catarrhalis* has assumed increasing importance in otitis media and as an opportunistic lower respiratory pathogen; it frequently produces β-lactamase.

Gram-Negative Bacilli. The identification of gram-negative bacilli is complex and is based on the interpretation of numerous biochemical tests. The number of tests required for speciation of the various groups in Figure 6 depends on technical expertise, interest, economics, epidemiologic necessity, and clinical relevance. Commercially prepared devices containing multiple tests for identifying the Enterobacteriaceae have become widely used and have generally proved to be convenient and accurate. In most kits individual test results are reduced to profile or code numbers. It should be emphasized that the reproducibility of these numbers reflects the reproducibility of individual test reactions and that some of these reactions are sufficiently variable to render unreliable the use of the numbers ("biotypes") for epidemiologic purposes. Devices are also available for the identification of nonfermenters; however, the identification of these organisms remains rather complex, and the tests provided in the devices often need to be supplemented with other tests to obtain a definitive identification.

There are, in addition, gram-negative bacilli that require enriched media and, in many cases, added carbon dioxide during incubation for their growth. Included in this group are *Campylobacter, Haemophilus, Cardiobacterium, Actinobacillus, Bordetella, Brucella,* and *Francisella.*

Species of *Haemophilus* of clinical importance are *H. influ-*

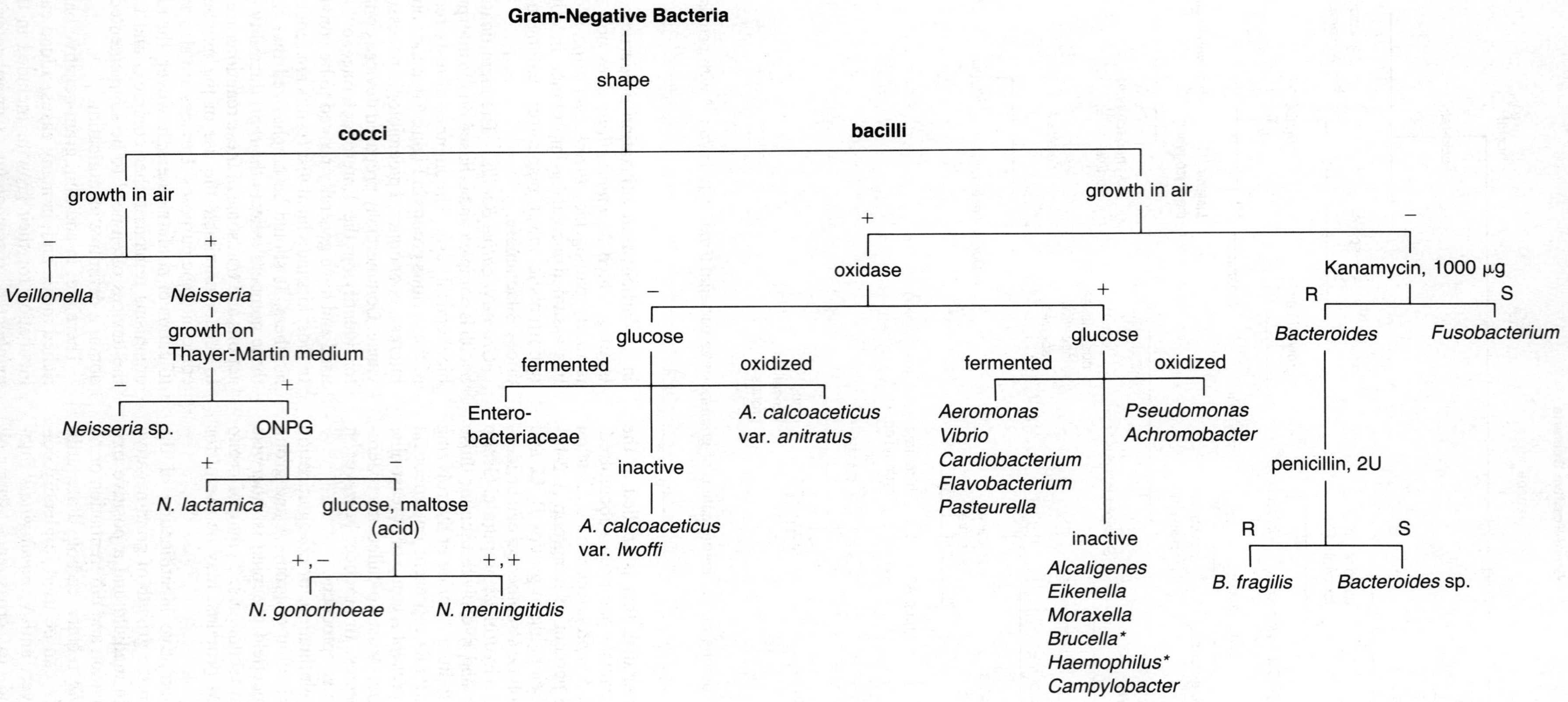

*Carbohydrate utilization not important for differentiation or speciation and can only be demonstrated in special media.

FIG. 6. Schematic outline for the identification of gram-negative bacteria. (From Washington,[17] with permission.)

enzae, H. parainfluenzae, H. aphrophilus, H. paraphrophilus, and *H. ducreyi.* Although *H. influenzae* is readily identifiable on the basis of its colonial morphology, characteristic odor, oxidase activity, requirements for hemin (X factor) and nicotinamide adenine dinucleotide (V factor), and antigenic characteristics, the other species are not and require a more complex series of tests for their differentiation. These species are being recognized increasingly, along with *Actinobacillus, Cardiobacterium,* and *Eikenella,* for their role in causing endocarditis. The identification of *Brucella* and *Francisella* can be expedited with direct immunofluorescent staining.

Gram-Positive Bacilli. Gram-positive bacilli are either sporulating or nonsporulating. The most commonly isolated nonsporulating bacilli are the corynebacteria ("diphtheroids") that normally inhabit the skin but may cause infections of implanted prosthetic material, a possibility that is strongly suggested by their repeated isolation from normally sterile fluids or sites. When isolated from blood or cerebrospinal fluid, it is important to distinguish corynebacteria, which produce catalase and are usually not motile, from another nonsporulating gram-positive bacillus, *L. monocytogenes,* which is motile at room temperature and may cause meningitis in newborn infants and in immunosuppressed hosts.

The isolation of *C. diphtheriae,* a nonsporulating rod, or *Bacillus anthracis,* a large sporulating rod, requires that the laboratory be notified so appropriate media are inoculated and toxigenicity tests performed. Otherwise, these organisms, if isolated, are apt to be discarded as contaminants.

ANAEROBIC BACTERIA. Most infections occurring in proximity to a mucosal surface, particularly those in the abdomen and the pelvis, are due to a combination of facultatively anaerobic (e.g., *E. coli* and *Enterococcus*) and anaerobic bacteria, including *Bacteroides* species, fusobacteria, anaerobic cocci, clostridia, and nonsporulating gram-positive bacilli. The presence of anaerobic bacteria is often suspected on the basis of their pleomorphism in Gram-stained smears of appropriately collected specimens and is subsequently confirmed in cultures on selective and nonselective media. Since cultures are often mixed and since definitive identification of anaerobic bacteria is time-consuming and expensive, the extent of identification provided must first reflect clinical need and then laboratory resources. When several different groups of anaerobic bacteria are present in a culture, it may be sufficient to characterize them superficially according to their Gram-stained morphology and to determine whether any anaerobic gram-negative bacilli that may be present produce β-lactamase. Although not necessarily predictive of β-lactam activity, a positive β-lactamase test (nitrocefin) finding is generally indicative of the presence of the *Bacteroides fragilis* group in the culture. In the case of perirectal lesions and sacral decubiti, it may be sufficient to report the presence of mixed fecal flora. Definitive identification may be reserved for isolates in pure culture and those from blood, brain abscesses, and other critical areas and may be carried out with one of several commercially available rapid identification kits.

Because of continuing debate about the relevance of in vitro susceptibility test results to clinical response, the variability of results provided by the different methods that are available for susceptibility testing of anaerobic bacteria, disagreement over break points for defining susceptibility, and the relatively slow turnaround time for isolating and performing susceptibility test of individual isolates of anaerobic bacteria, testing should be limited to those isolates from brain abscesses, bone and joint infections, infections of implanted prosthetic materials or devices, endocarditis, and persistent or recurrent bacteremia. Otherwise, susceptibility testing should be done to monitor susceptibility patterns on a regional or local basis and to evaluate the activity of new antimicrobial agents.

Mycobacteria. The extent to which laboratories should engage in mycobacterial isolation and identification should reflect the number of specimens received, the frequency of isolation of mycobacteria, technical expertise, availability of suitable facilities to process cultures and identify mycobacteria safely, and accessibility to suitable reference laboratories. Limits of mycobacteriologic services have been suggested by the College of American Pathologists and the American Thoracic Society. These suggested limits range from no services or services limited to acid-fast smears on site with transmittal of specimens to a reference laboratory, the isolation and identification of *M. tuberculosis,* and preliminary grouping of other species on site to isolation, identification, and drug susceptibility testing of isolates on site.

Identification of mycobacteria is based on microscopy, optimal temperature for growth, colonial morphology and pigmentation, growth in liquid medium, cord formation, niacin production, and other tests described elsewhere.[52]

The isolation after 2 or more weeks of incubation of slowly growing, nonpigmented, and rough colonies is strongly suggestive of *M. tuberculosis,* confirmation of which is obtained with a positive niacin test result. Calmette-Guérin bacillus (BCG) mutants of *M. bovis* have been isolated from patients receiving immunotherapy for cancer and are distinguishable from *M. tuberculosis* in that they are inhibited by thiophene-2-carboxylic acid hydrazide (TCH). *Mycobacterium kansasii,* which causes lesions resembling tuberculosis, grows slowly (2–3 weeks) and produces raised, rough, colorless, or buff-colored colonies that become yellow when exposed to light (photochromogenic). Similar characteristics are displayed by *M. marinum,* which, however, grows best at 30°C and is usually isolated from superficial lesions. Also photochromogenic at 25°C is *Mycobacterium szulgai,* which produces lesions resembling tuberculosis; this organism grows slowly and produces pale yellow colonies (scotochromogenic) whether exposed to light or not when incubated at 37°C. *Mycobacterium scrofulaceum* is a slowly growing (1–3 weeks) scotochromogen that is widely distributed in nature and may cause cervical adenitis in children.

Mycobacterium xenopi is a slowly growing (3–4 weeks) organism that grows best at 42°–45°C, is found in water, and has been associated with pulmonary lesions. It resembles *Mycobacterium intracellulare,* which is closely related to *M. avium,* hence the term *M. avium-intracellulare* complex ("Battey bacillus"). Although members of the *M. avium-intracellular* complex are highly resistant to most antimicrobial agents, *M. xenopi* is not.

Mycobacterium fortuitum is a rapidly growing (1–3 days) soil mycobacterium that is closely related to *Mycobacterium chelonae* and for which the term *M. fortuitum-chelonae* has been proposed. Rarely the cause of pulmonary disease, this group of organisms has caused wound infections, postinjection abscesses, and contamination of porcine valves used for heart valve replacement in humans.

Mycobacterium ulcerans grows slowly (3–4 weeks) at 30°C but not at 37°C, is nonphotochromogenic, and produces chronic skin ulcers ("Buruli ulcer") on the extremities of patients living in the tropics. *Mycobacterium leprae* causes leprosy in humans but cannot be cultured on artificial media. It is identified in tissue sections and smears by the arrangement of acid-fast bacilli in intracellular bundles called "globi." Bacilli may be abundant in lepromatous leprosy but are rare in tuberculoid lesions.

Fungi. The diagnosis of fungal infection can often be made by mixing a portion of the specimen with a drop of 10% potassium hydroxide on a clean glass microscope slide, applying a coverslip, gently flaming the slide, and examining the material microscopically (Fig. 2). Fungal cultures most often yield yeasts, the most frequently isolated species of which is *Candida albicans,* followed by *Torulopsis glabrata, C. tropicalis, C. parapsilosis, C. krusei,* and *Saccharomyces.* The interpretation of these results is complicated by the normal occurrence of these yeasts in the oropharynx, gastrointestinal tract, and vagina.

However we decide to identify isolates from these sources, a minimal requirement is that all clinical laboratories should be able to isolate and identify *Cryptococcus neoformans* and *C. albicans* from normally sterile body fluids and tissues. Yeasts isolated from these sources should be screened for urease production. The production of urease should strongly suggest *C. neoformans,* the identification of which should be confirmed with carbohydrate and nitrate assimilation tests or Niger seed agar.[15] *Candida albicans* is identified by inoculating a colony into 0.5 ml of normal human serum, incubating the test at 37°C for 3 hours, and examining the suspension microscopically for germ tube formation. Carbohydrate assimilation and fermentation tests may be used to identify other species of *Candida.*[15]

The identification of the filamentous fungi is more complex and time-consuming. Their colonial morphology is seldom characteristic and is highly medium dependent. Rates of growth vary widely. *Coccidioides immitis* colonies may appear after only a day's incubation, whereas colonies of *Blastomyces dermatitidis* and *Histoplasma capsulatum* may take as long as a month to appear. Definitive identification is based therefore on microscopic examination of the hyphae and the arrangement and appearance of the spores. Demonstration of the saprobic and parasitic forms of the dimorphic fungi is usually required. In some cases animals, most often mice, must be inoculated to convert the dimorphic fungi to the parasitic or yeast form. Recognition of the morphology characteristic of the various species requires experience, and it is suggested that photographs and other illustrative material be used as reference material with which to compare the morphology of isolates. An excellent six-volume *Atlas of Clinical Mycology* may be obtained for this purpose from the American Society of Clinical Pathologists.

DETECTION OF ANTIBODIES

Cultures of certain bacteria, fungi, parasites, and viruses may be unavailable because the methodology remains undeveloped (e.g., *T. pallidum,* hepatitis and Epstein-Barr viruses), is unsafe (e.g., rickettsiae), or is impractical for all but a few research and reference laboratories. Moreover, cultures may be negative because of prior antimicrobial therapy or because of the chronic state of the disease. Under these circumstances, the detection of nonspecific (Table 8) or specific antibodies may be of considerable diagnostic and epidemiologic use. Antibody response to infection is, however, quite variable, so serologic tests may vary considerably in sensitivity and specificity. An elevated single antibody titer usually does not permit a distinction to be made between active and past infection, and the absence of a measurable antibody titer may reflect a lack of immunogenicity of the etiologic agent, the use of an inappropriate test for detecting the antibody, or insufficient time from the onset of infection for an antibody response to have occurred. For these reasons, test selection and timing of the collection of specimens are essential to the proper use and interpretation of serologic tests. As a general rule, therefore, tests should be performed concurrently with a specimen taken during the acute phase of the disease and a specimen (convalescent) taken 1 or more weeks thereafter. A fourfold or greater rise in antibody titer usually provides unequivocal evidence of recent infection. Serologic testing is for this reason often of confirmatory or epidemiologic value.

Antibodies may be detected by agglutination, immunodiffusion, immunofluorescence, immunoassay, and many other techniques. No single technique is universally applicable for measuring antibody responses to all microorganisms. Techniques are selected on the basis of their sensitivity, specificity, ease and speed of performance, and cost-effectiveness.

The commonly available bacterial antibody tests are described in Table 9. Antibodies to the 0 antigens of *Proteus vulgaris* (Table 8), *Brucella, Francisella,* and *Salmonella* have commonly been included in a "febrile agglutinin" test battery, which, either because of the infrequency of the diseases involved or the lack of specificity of the tests involved, has very limited use and the individual components of which should be selectively ordered when clinically indicated. Moreover, certain tests within the battery should be replaced by more specific tests (e.g., rickettsial group-specific complement fixation or immunofluorescent antibody for *P. vulgaris* agglutinins [Weil-Felix test]) or eliminated (*Salmonella* agglutinins [Widal test]).

The commonly available fungal serologic tests are described in Table 10. Those pertinent to virology are discussed elsewhere (Chapter 14).

DETERMINATIONS OF ANTIMICROBIAL ACTIVITY

Susceptibility Tests

General indications for performing susceptibility tests are (*1*) the isolation of organisms with unpredictable susceptibility to antimicrobial agents (e.g., staphylococci, Enterobacteriaceae, and pseudomonads) and (*2*) the isolation of organisms of clinical significance (e.g., isolates from normally sterile sources, wounds and abscesses, and urine if present in significant numbers). Susceptibility tests are usually performed with organisms that grow rapidly and well on artificial media, so variables such as inoculum size, medium, atmosphere and duration of incubation, and interpretative criteria can be standardized. Standards, therefore, have been established for testing the rapidly growing aerobic and facultatively anaerobic bacteria.[54,55] Standards are under development for testing anaerobic bacteria, mycobacteria and fungi, although procedures have been described in the literature for testing these organisms.

Susceptibility testing of anaerobic bacteria should be limited to isolates from more serious or persistent infections (e.g., bacteremia); brain abscess; and bone, joint, or intraocular infections. Periodic testing of large numbers of anaerobes should be carried out by large reference laboratories to determine whether any alterations in susceptibility have occurred.

TABLE 8. Nonspecific Antibody Tests

Disease	*Test*	*Antigen or Hapten*	*Comments*
Infectious mononucleosis	Heterophile agglutination	Sheep erythrocytes	Test is negative in about 10% of cases
Inflammation disorder, acute infection	C-reactive protein	C-reactive protein	Nonspecific indicator of active tissue-damaging process
Mycoplasma pneumoniae	Cold agglutinins	Human O erythrocytes	Titers rise in only about 50% of cases and may rise in cases with hemolytic anemias and liver disease
Rickettsial diseases	Weil-Felix	O antigen of *Proteus vulgaris* OX 2, OX 19, and OX K	Nonspecific; questionable reliability unless more than fourfold rise in titer occurs
Syphilis	Nontreponemal (VDRL, RPR, ART)	Cardiolipin	If reactive, test should be confirmed with specific treponemal antigen test

Abbreviations: RPR: rapid plasma reagin; ART: automated reagin test.

TABLE 9. Commonly Available Bacterial Serologic Tests

Disease	*Antigen(s)*	*Test(s)*	*Interpretation*
Brucellosis	*Brucella abortus*	Agglutination	Titers of more than 1:80 are suggestive of past infection, whereas titers of more than 1:160 are highly suggestive of active infection. Titers of less than 1:80 occur occasionally in cases of active infection. Cross-reactions occur in patients with *Francisella, Yersinia,* or *Vibrio* infections or immunizations.
Tularemia	*Francisella tularensis*	Agglutination	Titers of 1:40 or more are indicative of past infection; titers usually rise to more than 1:160 during active infection. Minor cross-reactions occur in patients with *Brucella* infection or immunization.
Legionellosis	*Legionella pneumophila* and other species	Immunofluorescence	Fourfold titer rise to 1:128 is indicative of recent infection. Titers of 1:256 or more may occur in asymptomatic population.
Leptospirosis	Multiple *Leptospira* serovars	Agglutination	Titers of 1:100 or more are indicative of recent or past infection.
Rickettsioses	Group specific	Immunofluorescence	Fourfold titer rise, single titer of 1:128 or more, or any IgM titer is indicative of infection.
		Complement fixation	Fourfold titer rise is significant; however, CF test is less sensitive and specific than is the immunofluorescent antibody test.
Salmonellosis	O and H antigens of *Salmonella typhi* and *S. enteritidis,* bioser *paratyphi* A–C	Agglutination (Widal)	Elevated titers may represent a cross-reaction from past infection with group A, C, or nontyphoidal D *Salmonella* or result from past immunization with typhoid–paratyphoid vaccine. Early antibiotic therapy may prevent a titer rise. *Salmonella* agglutinins are the least accurate of any diagnostic test for typhoid–paratyphoid fever.
Streptococcal infection (group A)	Streptolysin O DNase B	Neutralization (ASO) Neutralization (anti-DNase B)	Approximately 45% of children with pharyngitis and positive throat cultures for group A streptococci have a fourfold rise in ASO and/or anti-DNase B titers. Approximately 10% of such children will have a fourfold rise in ASO but not in anti-DNase B titer or vice versa. ASO titers usually do not rise in cases of streptococcal pyoderma.
	"Extracellular products"	Agglutination (streptozyme)	Sensitivity is equivalent to but the specificity is less than either ASO or anti-DNase B. False-positives may be due to non-group A β-hemolytic streptococci.
Syphilis	*Treponema pallidum*	Immunofluorescence (FTA-ABS) Hemagglutination (MHA-TP)	These tests are used to confirm positive nontreponemal or reagin test.
Psittacosis	*Chlamydia trachomatis* (LGV-1)	Immunofluorescence (Micro-IF)	Fourfold titer rise (IgG) or presence of IgM antibody is indicative of recent chlamydial infection. LGV-1 antigen cannot distinguish between infection by *C. trachomatis* and *C. psittaci.*
Other chlamydial	*Chlamydia trachomatis* (LGV-1)	Immunofluorescence (Micro-IF)	There is a high incidence of seroreactors among venereal disease populations. IgM antibody (>1:32) and IgG antibody (≥1:2000) titers occur in patients with active lymphogranuloma venereum. IgM antibody titers of 1:128 or more occur in infants with *C. trachomatis* pneumonitis.
Mycoplasmal	*Mycoplasma pneumoniae*	Complement fixation	Fourfold titer rise is indicative of recent infection. High titers may persist for more than 1 year.

Mycobacteria usually do not require susceptibility testing when isolated from previously untreated patients; however, susceptibility testing is probably indicated for mycobacteria isolated from previously treated patients who have relapsed after a course of chemotherapy, from patients whose sputum smears continue to show acid-fast bacilli after 2–3 months of treatment or whose cultures are persistently positive after 5 or 6 months of treatment, and from patients who acquired their disease outside the United States or from possible contacts with drug-resistant tuberculosis. Because they are often resistant to the commonly recommended antimycobacterial agents, clinically significant mycobacteria other than *M. tuberculosis* probably should be tested. Susceptibility testing of mycobacteria is based on the principle that when more than 1 percent of tubercle bacilli are drug resistant in vitro therapy with that agent is not likely to be effective. Inocula of mycobacteria are therefore adjusted so that colony-forming units can be enumerated, and the percentage or proportion surviving in the presence of various agents is calculated.[52] Direct drug susceptibility studies of specimens may be performed if the initial smear demonstrates that sufficient numbers of acid-fast bacilli are present. Radiometric procedures are suitable alternatives for testing *M. tuberculosis*.[52] Agents to be tested against mycobacteria include the primary antituberculous drugs, isoniazid, streptomycin, rifampin, and ethambutol. The secondary drugs include ethionamide, kanamycin, capreomycin, cycloserine, pyrazinamide, and para-aminosalicylic acid and are usually only given in cases with infections due to mycobacteria that are resistant to the primary drugs. As has already been discussed, susceptibility testing of mycobacteria should be limited to laboratories expert in this area.

The indications for performing susceptibility tests of fungi are quite limited, probably reflecting the small number of antifungal agents available, the limited number of people expert in their administration, and the technical difficulties involved in testing yeasts and, especially, filamentous fungi reproducibly. Amphotericin B has a broad range of activity in vitro against fungi, including the yeasts, dimorphic fungi, and strictly filamentous

TABLE 10. Commonly Available Fungal Serologic Tests

Infection	*Antigen(s)*	*Test(s)*	*Interpretation*
Aspergillosis	*Aspergillus fumigatus* *Aspergillus niger* *Aspergillus flavus*	Immunodiffusion	One or more precipitin bands is suggestive of active infection. Precipitin bands have been shown to correlate with complement fixation titers—the greater the number of bands, the higher the titer. Preciptins can be found in 95% of the fungus ball cases and 50% of the allergic bronchopulmonary cases. They are sometimes positive in invasive infection, depending on the immunologic status of the patient.
Blastomycosis	*Blastomyces dermatitidis* Yeast form	Complement fixation	Titers of 1:8 to 1:16 are highly suggestive of active infection; titers of 1:32 or greater are indicative. Cross-reactions occur in patients having coccidioidomycosis or histoplasmosis; however, titers are usually lower. A decreasing titer is indicative of regression. Most patients (75%) having blastomycosis have negative test findings.
	Yeast culture filtrate	Immunodiffusion	An A precipitin band may occur in as many as 80% of proven cases of blastomycosis.
Candidiasis	*Candida albicans*	Immunodiffusion, CIE	The test is difficult to interpret because precipitins are found in 20–30% of the normal population, and reports in the literature are conflicting. Clinical correlation must exist for the test to be useful.
Coccidioidomycosis	Coccidioidin	Complement fixation	Titers of 1:2 to 1:4 have been seen in active infection. Low titers should be followed by repeat testing at 2–3 wk intervals. Titers of greater than 1:16 are usually indicative of active infection. Cross-reactions occur in patients having histoplasmosis, and false-negative results occur in patients with solitary pulmonary lesions. Titer parallels the severity of infection.
	Coccidioidin	Immunodiffusion	Results correlate with complement fixation test and can be used as a screening test—should be confirmed by performing complement fixation test. A concentration (8- to 10-fold) of specimen enhances antibody detection.
	Coccidioidin	Latex agglutination	Precipitins occur during first 3 wk of infection and are diagnostic but not prognostic—useful as a screening test for precipitins in early infection. False-positive tests are frequent when diluted serum or cerebrospinal fluid specimens are used.
Cryptococcosis	No antigen—latex particles coated with hyperimmune anticryptococcal globulin	Latex agglutination for cryptococcal antigen	The presence of cryptococcal polysaccharide in body fluids is indicative of cryptococcosis. Rheumatoid factor presents false-positive reactions, and an RA test must be performed as a control. A decrease in antigen titer indicates regression. Positive tests (in CSF) have been seen in 95% of cryptococcal meningitis cases and 30% of nonmeningitis cases. Serum is less frequently positive than CSF. Disseminated infections usually present positive results in serum. The test may be performed by using serum and CSF, and is more sensitive than the India ink preparation.
Histoplasmosis	Histoplasmin and yeast form of *Histoplasma capsulatum*	Complement fixation	Titers of 1:8 to 1:16 are highly suspicious of infection; however, titers of 1:32 or greater are usually indicative of active infection. Cross-reactions occur in patients having aspergillosis, blastomycosis, and coccidioidomycosis, but titers are usually lower. Several follow-up serum samples should be tested—drawn at 2–3 week intervals. Rising titers indicate progressive infection, and decreasing titers indicate regression. Some disseminated infections are nonreactive to the complement fixation test. Recent skin tests in persons who have had prior exposure to *H. capsulatum* will cause an elevation in the complement fixation titer. This occurs in 17–20% of persons tested. The yeast antigen gives positive reactions in 75–80% of cases, and the histoplasmin gives positive reactions in 10–15% of cases. In 10% of cases both are positive simultaneously.
	Histoplasmin	Immunodiffusion	H and M bands appearing simultaneously are indicative of active infection. M band may appear alone and can indicate early infection or chronic infection. Also the M band may appear after a recent skin test. The H band appears later than the M band does and disappears earlier, and its disappearance may indicate regression of the infection.
	Histoplasmin	Latex agglutination	The test is unreliable. Many false-positive and negative test results may be observed. Any positive test result should be confirmed by the complement fixation test.
Sporotrichosis	Yeast of *Sporothrix schenckii*	Agglutination	Titers of 1:80 or greater are usually indicative of active infection. Some cutaneous infections present negative test findings; however, extracutaneous infections present positive test results.

(From Koneman et al.,[53] with permission.)

fungi; therefore, determination of its antifungal activity is rarely indicated in clinical practice. Although most clinically significant yeasts are initially susceptible to flucytosine, resistance is acquired during therapy in a substantial number of cases. For this reason, the drug is seldom administered alone, and it is usually used in conjunction with amphotericin B, with which it acts synergistically unless the organism is resistant to it. It is therefore probably important to determine the susceptibility to flucytosine of yeasts isolated from serious infections so that its use with amphotericin B can be considered. A standard method has not been agreed on; however, the choice of medium is important since some media are inhibitory to flucytosine. Most authors seem to agree on the use of yeast nitrogen base (YNB) for this purpose. The activity of ketoconazole is also highly medium dependent. Be that as it may, it seems reasonable to suggest that susceptibility testing of fungi be limited to those centers with expertise in antifungal chemotherapy.

Because of the specialized nature of antimycobacterial and antifungal susceptibility testing, the remainder of this discussion will be limited to antibacterial susceptibility tests.

Selection of Antimicrobial Agents

Agents selected for susceptibility testing should be confined to those that are clinically useful and relevant to the kind of bacterium isolated as well as to its source. Closely related analogues with activity in vitro that do not differ significantly from that of the parent or an established compound should not be tested routinely. Suggested guidelines for selecting agents to be tested are listed in Table 11. Additions to and perhaps deletions from this list can be anticipated as new agents are introduced and older ones become infrequently used. Close coordination between the laboratory and the hospital formulary committee is of utmost importance for the final selection of antimicrobial agents to be tested. Sulfonamides, except in combination with trimethoprim, are not included in this list because their principal use is in the treatment of uncomplicated lower urinary tract infections that are usually due to susceptible strains of *E. coli,* the most accurate susceptibility test of which is their eradication within the first 48–72 hours of therapy. Oxacillin or nafcillin is preferable to methicillin because of its greater stability in disks or solution. Resistance of staphylococci to the penicillinase-resistant penicillins often requires the addition of NaCl (2% in broth, 4% in agar) to Mueller-Hinton medium and incubation at temperatures not exceeding 35°C. Cephalosporins, imipenem, and some β-lactam/β-lactamase inhibitor combinations may appear to be active against methicillin-resistant staphylococci in vitro; however, there is clinical evidence that these compounds are not effective in treating serious infections due to methicillin-resistant staphylococci. Thus, staphylococci that are resistant in vitro to oxacillin, nafcillin, or methicillin should be considered resistant to other β-lactams and reported as such. Because of this characteristic, cephalosporins are not tested in some laboratories against staphylococci, and all oxacillin-, nafcillin-, or methicillin-susceptible staphylococci are considered to be susceptible to cephalosporins.

Of the currently available aminoglycosides, only three—gentamicin, tobramycin, and amikacin—generally appear in hospital formularies. Testing of any one or all of these should depend on which one or ones are in the formulary, which might, in turn, reflect the local prevalence of resistance to gentamicin or tobramycin and local bias regarding the relative toxicity of each aminoglycoside. Since resistance of enterococci to the synergistic activity of penicillin or ampicillin plus streptomycin or gentamicin can be predicted from their resistance to 2000 μg streptomycin/ml or 500 μg gentamicin/ml, it is suggested that susceptibility testing of enterococci from blood, tissue, and normally sterile body fluid cultures be tested at these high concentrations of streptomycin and gentamicin. Netilmicin may be tested if local resistance patterns to other aminoglycosides indicate that netilmicin may be useful.

The most complex issue facing formulary committees and microbiologists is the proliferation of expanded-spectrum β-lactams. Selection of a few from among the many for the hospital formulary and for laboratory testing requires familiarity with their similarities and dissimilarities in vitro and in vivo and a substantial amount of commitment and fortitude. Aztreonam and all third-generation cephalosporins available to date are equally active in vitro against the Enterobacteriaceae; therefore, aztreonam, cefotaxime, ceftazidime, ceftizoxime, ceftriaxone, or moxalactam could be selected for testing. Although cefotaxime, ceftriaxone, or moxalactam could be selected for testing against *Pseudomonas,* aztreonam has somewhat greater activity, and cefoperazone and ceftazidime have substantially greater activity than do other third-generation cephalosporins, and it would be advisable to test either cefoperazone or ceftazidime against *Pseudomonas.* Whether to test aztreonam against *Pseudomonas* in this instance might reflect its position in the formulary, and it might simply not be relevant to test cefotaxime, ceftriaxone, or moxalactam against *Pseudomonas.* Although neither aztreonam nor all third-generation cephalosporins are listed as primary antibiotics in Table 11, there are probably few settings in which one or more of these compounds are not included in the formulary and are not being tested. The situation with the *Pseudomonas*-active penicillins is complicated by some similarities and dissimilarities in their activity in vitro, their usual administration with an aminoglycoside, and the general lack of much clinical data, even among febrile granulocytopenic patients, that demonstrate statistically significant differences among them. Thus, selection of the one for the formulary and for testing should probably not be based solely on in vitro activity and could be based on competitive bidding.

Resistance among microorganisms such as *Haemophilus influenzae, Neisseria gonorrhoeae,* and *Streptococcus pneumoniae* that were previously considered to be uniformly susceptible to penicillins and some other commonly recommended alternatives has created a need for determining their susceptibility on a more routine basis. Initially, it was sufficient to test isolates of *H. influenzae* and *N. gonorrhoeae* to detect plasmid-mediated β-lactamases; however, chromosomally mediated resistance to penicillins, which is not related to β-lactamase production and is, therefore, not detectable by β-lactamase testing, has occurred in both species so that susceptibility testing of β-lactamase–negative isolates to penicillins is becoming necessary. Moreover, resistance of *H. influenzae* to cefuroxime and chloramphenicol and of *N. gonorrhoeae* to tetracycline and spectinomycin has been reported, so additional testing may be indicated in certain instances. Although susceptibility testing of *H. influenzae* by diffusion or dilution methods is reasonably well standardized and readily accomplished in most clinical laboratories, the same is not true of susceptibility testing of *N. gonorrhoeae* in which lot-to-lot differences in GC medium base produce highly variable results. Although isolates of pneumococci with penicillin minimal inhibitory concentrations (MICs) between 0.12 and 1.0 have been recognized for many years, strains with penicillin MICs of ≥2 μg/ml have only been recognized in recent years, initially in South Africa but subsequently in other parts of the world including the United States. Since pneumococci with MICs of 0.12–1.0 μg/ml may not respond to penicillin therapy in cases of meningitis and since infections due to penicillin-resistant pneumococci fail to repond to therapy with penicillin and antibiotics other than vanco-

TABLE 11. Guidelines for Selection of Antibacterial Agents for Susceptibility Testing

Agent	*Staphylococci*	*Enterococci*	*Nonenterococcal Streptococci*	*Pseudomonads*	*Enterobacteriaceae*
Amikacin				P	P
Ampicillin	S	P			P
Ampicillin/sulbactam (or amoxicillin/clavulanate)	S				S
Azlocillin (or mezlocillin, carbenicillin, piperacillin or ticarcillin)				P	
Aztreonam				S	S
Cefamandole (or cefonicid or cefuroxime)					S
Cefotaxime (or cefoperazone, ceftazidime, ceftizoxime, ceftriaxone, or moxalactam)					P
Cefoxitin (or cefotetan)					S
Ceftazidime (or cefoperazone)				P	
Cephalothin	P[a]		P		P[b]
Chloramphenicol	S			S	S
Ciprofloxacin	S			S	S
Clindamycin	P		P		
Erythromycin	P	U	P		
Gentamicin (or tobramycin)	S	S[c]		P	P
Imipenem				S	S
Mezlocillin (or piperacillin or ticarcillin)					P
Netilmicin				S	S
Oxacillin (or methicillin or nafcillin)	P[b]				
Penicillin G	P		P		
Tetracycline	S				S, U
Ticarcillin/clavulanate					S
Trimethoprim/sulfamethoxazole	S			S[d]	P
Vancomycin	P	S			
Cinoxacin (or nalidixic acid)					U
Nitrofurantoin	U	U	U		U
Norfloxacin	U	U	U	U	U
Trimethoprim	U				U

Abbreviations: P: primary agents to be tested routinely; S: secondary agents to be tested under special circumstances such as in institutions harboring endemic or epidemic resistance to one or more of the primary agents, for therapy for patients allergic to a primary agent, or as an epidemiologic aid; U: urinary tract–specific agent to be tested against urinary isolates only.

[a] Oxacillin (or methicillin- or nafcillin)-resistant staphylococci should be considered resistant to cephalosporins, penicillins (including combinations with β-lactamase inhibitors), and imipenem.

[b] Although cephalothin can be used to predict the in vitro activity of other first-generation cephalosporins, cefazolin should not be used for the same purpose because cefazolin is more active than are other first-generation cephalosporins vs. *E. coli*.

[c] Gentamicin should be tested at concentration of 500 or 2000 μg/ml to detect high-level resistant strains that are not synergistically affected by the combination of a penicillin and gentamicin.

[d] Applies only to species other than *P. aeruginosa*.

(Data from National Committee for Clinical Laboratory Standards.[54,55])

mycin, it is imperative for the laboratory to test clinically significant isolates of pneumococci against penicillin.

Methods

Dilution. The principle of dilution tests is to determine the lowest or minimal concentration of antimicrobial agent that is required to inhibit the growth of a microorganism. The MIC is usually expressed in micrograms per milliliter, although SI units may be used in the future. Approved standards describing the methods to be used for dilution testing have been published by the National Committee for Clinical Laboratory Standards.[55] Dilution tests may be performed in agar or in broth, the latter of which can be readily adapted to microdilution, which is currently in widespread use in clinical and research laboratories. Dilution tests are often preferred because they are incorrectly perceived as being more accurate than disk diffusion tests are and because laboratory personnel incorrectly assume that MICs are preferred by clinicians. In fact, dilution and diffusion tests are directly correlated, and most clinicians other than those with subspecialty interest in infectious diseases require interpretation of MICs. Thus, the indications for dilution testing are (*1*) investigations of new antimicrobial agents, (*2*) testing of microorganisms that grow slowly or have special growth requirements, (*3*) determination of precise susceptibility when the preferred therapy is with a relatively nontoxic but not highly active β-lactam, and (*4*) as an alternative to disk diffusion testing when inocula replica plating is deemed cost-effective. Replicate inoculation of a single microorganism into microwells containing biochemical substrates for microbial identification and antimicrobial agents for susceptibility testing is a common feature of many commercially available devices today.

Discrepancies between dilution methods in broth and in agar are largely limited to tests of aminoglycosides against *Pseudomonas aeruginosa*. Tests in Mueller-Hinton broth that has been supplemented with Ca^{2+} and Mg^{2+} at concentrations of 50 and 25 mg/liter, respectively, appear to provide an unacceptably high false-resistance rate relative to results obtained with a reference lot of Mueller-Hinton agar when aminoglycosides are tested against *P. aeruginosa*. As a consequence, the recommended concentrations of Ca^{2+} and Mg^{2+} will be reduced so as to bring the results of testing with agar and broth into agreement.[55]

Interpretative guidelines for translating MIC results into susceptible, moderately susceptible, intermediate, or resistant categories have been published by the National Committee for Clinical Laboratory Standards.[55] As a rule, these interpretative criteria should be made available in laboratory reports of MICs.

With appropriate modifications of media and the duration and atmosphere of incubation, dilution procedures may be adapted for use with slow-growing or fastidious microorganisms.

The greatest day-to-day variability in MICs is due to variations in inoculum size. The recommended inoculum is approximately 5×10^5 cfu/ml,[55] and it is not sufficient to rely on a manufacturer's directions for attaining this inoculum size, particularly when performing microdilution methods. It is incumbent on each user of a susceptibility testing device to establish procedures through quantitative studies that ensure a final inoculum of approximately 5×10^5 cfu/ml. Attainment of this inoculum is critical to the accurate detection of penicillin- and methicillin-resistant staphylococci as well as of mutants of Enterobacteriaceae and *P. aeruginosa* that are selectively derepressed for the chromosomal class I β-lactamase and that are resistant to expanded-spectrum β-lactam antibiotics. Conversely, preparation of the inoculum of *Haemophilus influenzae* by visual comparison with the recommended McFarland standard is likely to yield an inoculum exceeding 1×10^6 cfu/ml and result in false resistance to expanded-spectrum cephalosporins.

Disk Diffusion. The principle of the disk diffusion technique is that the diameter of a zone of inhibition about an antimicrobial-impreganated paper disk relates approximately linearly to the antimicrobial's $\log_2$ MIC. Zone diameters are interpreted as signifying susceptibility, intermediate susceptibility, or resistance to each antimicrobial agent tested according to published criteria. Obviously, these criteria retain their validity only as long as standard procedures are followed.[54] It should be equally obvious that the interpretative criteria apply only to organisms that grow rapidly on Mueller-Hinton agar, with or without whole or chocolatized blood, when incubated at 35°C for 16–18 hours in room air, that is, staphylococci, Enterobacteriaceae, and pseudomonads. The disk diffusion test may also be used reliably to determine whether *H. influenzae* is susceptible to ampicillin. No disk diffusion method is uniformly reliable for determining the susceptibility of anaerobic bacteria.

Disk Elution. Elution of antimicrobial agents into liquid or solid media occurs rapidly and completely. The concept has been applied to automated rapid susceptibility testing using procedures including the Organon Teknika Autobac and the Abbott MS-2 as well as to the testing of anaerobic bacteria.

Quality Control. All susceptibility tests must undergo frequent performance controls to ensure accurate and reproducible results. Methods for quality control of disk diffusion methods are described elsewhere[54] and involve the testing on weekly basis of *S. aureus* (ATCC 25923), *E. coli* (ATCC 25922), and *P. aeruginosa* (ATCC 27853), for which acceptable zone diameter control limits have been established. Control of dilution tests is performed with *S. aureus* (ATCC 29213), *S. faecalis* (ATCC 29212), *E. coli* (ATCC 25922), and *P. aeruginosa* (ATCC 27853).[55] *E. coli* (ATCC 35218) should be included when testing β-lactam/β-lactamase inhibitor combinations.

Bactericidal Tests

Broth. The principle of this test is to determine the lowest or minimal concentration of antimicrobial agent that kills ≥99.9 percent of the inoculum used for the test. The minimal bactericidal concentration (MBC) or minimal lethal concentration (MLC) is obtained by subculturing measured aliquots from broth in tubes containing no visible growth (inhibitory phase) to antimicrobial-free media. Although the inhibitory phase of this test has been standardized, the volume of the aliquot subcultured, the subculture medium, the subculture method (pour vs. streak plates), and the duration of incubation have not. There are consequently numerous technical variations of this test in the literature. Most investigators agree on the need to quantify the original inoculum to determine the lowest concentration of antimicrobial agent that destroys at least 99.9 percent of it. Recommended procedures for performing bactericidal tests have been described by Pearson et al.[56] and in a proposed guideline published by the National Committee for Clinical Laboratory Standards.[57] Critical components of the methodology include an inoculum of at least 5×10^5 cfu/ml and a subculture volume of 0.01 ml to allow accurate estimation of ≥99.9 percent killing.[56,57]

There are very few indications for bactericidal testing. Although the MBC is an accepted parameter in the evaluation of a new antimicrobial agent, its clinical value is debatable, especially since the test is so method dependent and interpretation of the results is not well defined. A related issue is that of tolerance, about which much has been written but about which there are substantial definitional problems.[58,59] Among the technical problems involved are (*1*) the fact that stationary-phase cultures result in diminished killing rates, (*2*) bacteria may escape exposure to the antibiotic by adhering to the side of the tube above the meniscus, (*3*) sufficient antibiotic may be transferred in subcultures to inhibit surviving organisms, and (*4*) the rate of bactericidal activity may vary according to duration of incubation, medium content, and pH.[58,59] For all of these reasons it appears that the most reliable method for determining tolerance, defined as a reduced rate of killing, is by timed killing curve studies in which an exponential phase of growth of the organism is adjusted to provide an inoculum of approximately 5×10^5 cfu/ml that is exposed to a concentration of the antibiotic that is eight times its MIC and the number of survivors after 4 to 6 hours of incubation is compared with those at 2-hour or 0 time.[59] Determination of the number of persisters can be made by quantitative subculture after 24 hours of incubation.[59]

Combination Studies. Studies of combinations of antimicrobial agents are performed when there is multiple resistance to antimicrobials singly, when there are contraindications to the use of preferred antimicrobials, when therapeutic failure has occurred with a current antimicrobial regimen, and when the potential for toxicity exists during a prolonged therapeutic regimen.

There are two major approaches to performing combination studies.[60]

METHODS WITH SOLID MEDIUM. Antimicrobials can be combined in a single disk to determine whether their activity is greater (or less) than that of either agent singly. A frequently used example of this approach is the cotrimoxazole (trimethoprim-sulfamethoxazole) disk. The synergistic interaction of this combination can be seen if its components are tested separately by placing disks containing each proximately on the seeded agar surface. A modification of this technique is to place two filter paper strips, each containing a different antimicrobial, at right angles to one another on the seeded agar surface. Bacteriostatic synergism is indicated by inhibition of growth within the angle formed by the two strips. Bactericidal interactions between two antimicrobial agents may be determined by the cellophane transfer technique wherein a cellophane tambour inoculated on the inside with the test organism is applied to an agar surface into which antimicrobials have prediffused from filter paper

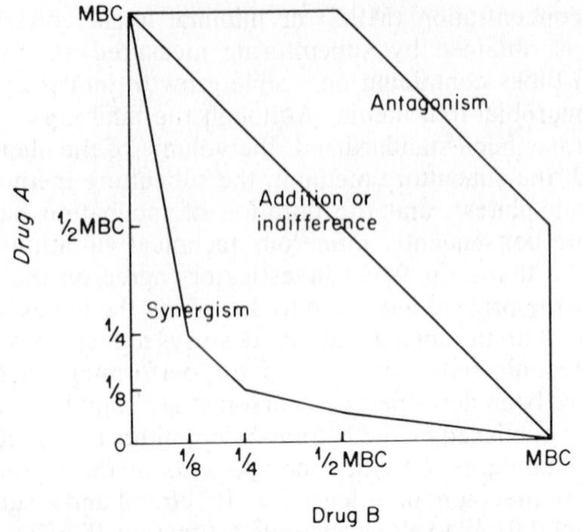

FIG. 7. Isobologram depicting three possible interactions between two antimicrobial agents when tested in combination by the two-dimensional ("checkerboard") technique. (From Washington,[15] with permission.)

strips placed at right angles.[60] The antimicrobials and nutrients from the agar diffuse through the cellophane. After overnight incubation, the tambour is removed from the agar surface, transferred to an antimicrobial-free medium, and incubated for an additional 24 hours. Synergism is indicated when growth is absent within the area formerly encompassed by the angle formed by the two antimicrobial-containing strips.

METHODS WITH LIQUID MEDIUM. There are two techniques for combination studies in liquid medium.[60] In the two-dimensional ("checkerboard") method serial, twofold dilutions of two agents, alone and in combination, are inoculated with the test organism. After incubation for 16–18 hours, those tubes containing broth without visible growth are subcultured, as for the MBC, to antimicrobial-free media. The results are then depicted according to isobologram criteria as demonstrating synergy, antagonism, or indifference (Fig. 7). In the timed killing curve two or more fixed concentrations of two or more antimicrobials, singly and in combination, are inoculated with the test organism and subcultured quantitatively over time to compare the rate of killing by the combinations with that of either antimicrobial by itself[61] (Fig. 8).

Synergism is usually defined by the significantly greater activity of the combination than would be expected from the sum of the separate effects of the antimicrobials being tested.[60] In the checkerboard method, synergism is defined when the fractional inhibitory concentration (FIC) or fractional bactericidal concentration (FBC) index is ≤ 0.5, whereas in killing curve studies synergy is defined as a $\geq 2 \log_{10}$ cfu/ml decrease between the combination and its most active component after 24 hours of incubation, assuming that at least one of the antimicrobials in the combination does not produce inhibitory or killing activity by itself. Antagonism is defined in the checkerboard method by an FIC or FBC index of >4.0 and in the killing curve method by $\leq 2 \log_{10}$ decrease in killing by the combination at 24 hours as compared with the most active antimicrobial by itself. Between synergy and antagonism are additive and indifferent effects.[60]

In either test it is important to standardize the inoculum. In the case of the checkerboard method, all of the variables discussed previously in determining MBCs apply. In killing curve studies, it is important to define the lower threshold of sensitivity of the detectable number of colony-forming units per milliliter and to limit the effects of antimicrobial carryover either by inactivating one or both antimicrobials in the subculture or serially diluting subcultures to the point at which each antimicrobial is present only in subinhibitory concentrations.

Although the interpretative results of both the checkerboard and timed killing curve methods often agree, differences do occur, often reflecting differences between methods in inoculum size and growth phase as well as in sampling times.[62] Because of the extremely laborious nature of these methods and because of difficulties in applying the results in clinical practice, their use should probably be restricted to investigational studies.

Serum Bactericidal Test. The dilution of serum that is inhibitory or bactericidal to an organism isolated from a patient receiving antimicrobial therapy has been used for years as an indirect method of monitoring the antimicrobial dosage. First described by Schlichter et al.[63] as a test of the serum's bacteriostatic activity at the anticipated trough level of antibiotics, the test has undergone innumerable modifications as regards the timing of blood collection, inoculum size, serum diluent, subculture volume and medium, and end points. Proposed guidelines for performing the test have been published by the National Committee for Clinical Laboratory Standards[64]; however, the interpretative guidelines provided are limited by sev-

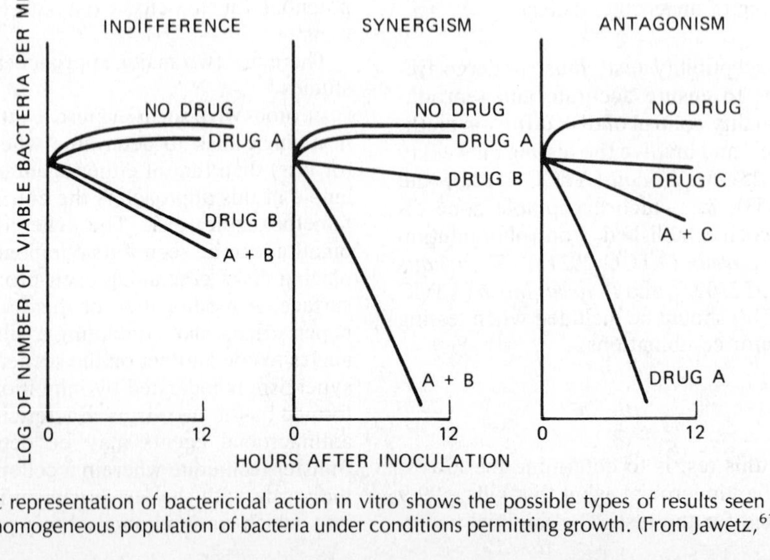

FIG. 8. Schematic representation of bactericidal action in vitro shows the possible types of results seen when one drug or two drugs act on a homogeneous population of bacteria under conditions permitting growth. (From Jawetz,[61] with permission.)

eral factors. First, exclusive of infections associated with implanted prosthetic materials, most cases of endocarditis and osteomyelitis are successfully treated with currently recommended antibiotic regimens, so the correlation between treatment failure and any range of titers is based on a very small sample. Accordingly although the predictive value of a titer, for example, ≥1:16, for cure may be high, that for failure with a lesser titer is not, particularly when confidence limits are applied to any published predictive values for failure related to titers below 1:16. Second, although the serum bactericidal test is considered an indirect assay of antimicrobial activity in vitro, the test is subject to all of the methodological variables that have been described for the MBC. Third, there is an inherent risk in promoting a particular minimal acceptable titer in that efforts to increase a low titer might result in an inappropriate increase in the dosage of a potentially toxic antibiotic. In conclusion, although the determination of serum bactericidal titers may provide another piece of information about the antimicrobial properties in vivo of a new investigational antimicrobial agent, there are few clinical indications for their use.

Assays

Assays of antimicrobial concentrations in serum should be made when there is dysfunction of excretory or metabolic organs or systems, when there is an in vivo response that is inconsistent with in vitro susceptibility test results, when there is variability in the pharmacokinetics of an antimicrobial agent, and when potentially toxic antimicrobial agents are being administered. Assays are particularly useful when therapeutic concentrations of an agent approximate its potentially toxic concentrations. For example, therapeutic concentrations of gentamicin are in the range of 4–6 μg/ml, whereas potentially toxic concentrations are 12 μg/ml or greater. Assays in this case assist in adjusting the antibiotic dosage to achieve therapeutic concentrations in serum and, at the same time, provide a means of monitoring the dosage to ensure that potentially toxic levels are not being attained. Although many formulas have been published to assist in adjusting antibiotic dosage, changing renal status often renders these calculations invalid, and assays should be made to monitor antimicrobial therapy.

There are many methods for performing antimicrobial assays, the details of which are described in several excellent books devoted to the subject.[15,65–69] The methods most frequently used in clinical laboratories are microbiologic assay or bioassay, radioenzymatic assay (REA), radioimmunoassay (RIA), chromatography, and nonisotopic immunoassays (e.g., fluorescence polarization).

Bioassay. Bioassays compare the response of a highly susceptible test organism to known concentrations of an antimicrobial with the response of the same organism under identical test conditions to an unknown concentration of the same antimicrobial. Bioassays may be made by serial dilution methods (Table 12); however, since the reproducibility of such methods is ±1 $\log_2$ dilutions, their accuracy is generally not suitable for

TABLE 12. Sample Protocol for Broth Dilution Assay Method

	Tube Number							
Series	*1*	*2*	*3*	*4*	*5*	*6*	*7*	*8*
First								
Antimicrobial (μg/ml)	4	2	1	0.5	0.25	0.12	0.06	0.03
Second								
Serum (reciprocal titer)	4	8	16	32	64	128	256	512

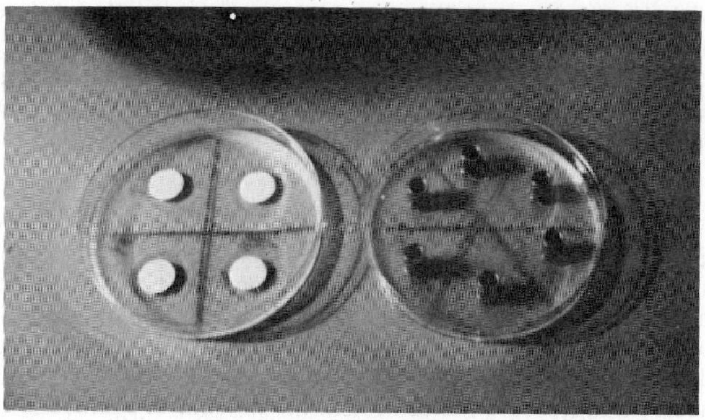

FIG. 9. Agar diffusion assays using stainless steel cylinders (right) and paper disks (left) to contain the standards and samples to be tested.

assays of agents with narrow toxic:therapeutic ratios. In the example shown (Table 12), the antimicrobial to be assayed is serially diluted, as is the patient's serum containing an unknown concentration of the antimicrobial. Both series of tubes are inoculated with a standardized suspension of the test organism. Should the organism be inhibited after overnight incubation by 0.12 μg/ml of the antibiotic and by a 1:16 dilution of the patient's serum, the concentration of the antibiotic in the patient's serum would be 1.9 μg/ml (16 × 0.12).

Many bioassays are performed by the diffusion method, which is more accurate and reproducible than is the dilution method because response is measured as a zone of inhibition and therefore as a progression of antimicrobial activity in agar. In the diffusion assay a standard curve is constructed from the inhibitory zone diameters produced by standards with varying concentrations of antimicrobial. The zone diameter of inhibition produced by an unknown sample is extrapolated from the standard curve to a concentration (μg/ml). Standards and unknown materials to be assayed are placed into a cylinder or onto a paper disk applied to the seeded agar surface (Fig. 9). Alternatively, samples can be placed into wells punched out of the seeded agar. By increasing the inoculum size, it is often possible to shorten the incubation time of the bioassay. Most aminoglycosides, for example, can be assayed within a 4-hour period.

Fluids to be assayed often contain more than one antimicrobial agent. In the bioassay this problem is circumvented by selecting a test organism that is very susceptible to the agent to be assayed and resistant to other agents, by inactivating interfering antimicrobials, or by diluting the fluid to eliminate detectable activity of any agents present in low concentrations to assay one that is present in high concentrations. In practice, the first two approaches are commonly used. Organisms with the desired susceptibility patterns can be obtained from reference laboratories or can be selected from isolates encountered in the laboratory. These organisms should be tested at regular intervals to ensure that they have retained their original susceptibility patterns. Penicillins and cephalosporins can be inactivated with β-lactamases, whereas aminoglycosides can be inactivated with calcium hydroxide or sodium polyanetholsulfonate.

It is essential for physicians ordering assays to provide the laboratory with information on the dosage and time interval since the last dose of the antimicrobial to be assayed as well as what other antimicrobials are being administered concurrently. Failure to do so may not only delay completion of the assay but can also lead to spurious results.

Radioenzymatic Assay. In the REA a radiolabeled functional group, for example, ^{14}C-adenosine triphosphate (ATP), that serves as the source of an adenyl or acetyl group is transferred enzymatically to an aminoglycoside. The adenylylated or acetylated aminoglycoside is strongly cationic and binds to phosphocellulose paper; therefore, phosphocellulose-bound radioactivity measures the amount of aminoglycoside present. The procedure is rapid, accurate, and reproducible but requires access to a liquid scintillation spectrometer.

Radioimmunoassay. The RIA depends on the noncovalent binding of an antigen, the antimicrobial agent, by a specific antibody. If the amount of antibody is limited and kept constant, the percentage of antigen bound will be inversely related to the total amount of antigen present in the standard or sample. This distribution is determined by adding a small amount of radiolabeled antigen as a tracer so that the amount of radioactivity in the bound fraction can be counted and expressed as a percentage of total counts.

The RIA is rapid, accurate, and reproducible. As with the REA, access to a liquid scintillation spectrometer is required. The RIA is expensive to perform unless large numbers of specimens can be tested in batches. Neither the REA nor the RIA are particularly well suited for handling single specimens on demand, as often occurs in hospital practice. Alternatives to assays requiring radioisotopes and scintillation spectrometry are highly desirable.

Chromatography. Chromatographic assays are very sensitive, rapid, and specific and lend themselves readily to handling single specimens on demand. In contrast to REA and RIA, chromatography usually requires only a single internal standard that is run with each specimen. The two types of chromatography that have been developed to the point of practicality for antimicrobial assays are gas–liquid (GLC) and high-pressure liquid (HPLC) chromatography, the latter of which does not require volatility of the antimicrobial or derivatization and is, therefore, simpler and more rapid. Antimicrobial agents that may be assayed by GLC include clindamycin, chloramphenicol, thiamphenicol, sulfonamides, flucytosine, miconazole, griseofulvin, and metronidazole. HPLC methodology exists for assay of most antibacterial, antimycobacterial, antifungal, and antiparasitic agents.

Nonisotopic Immunoassays. Nonisotopic immunoassays differ from radioimmunoassays in that the drug is labeled with a fluorophore or enzyme instead of a radionuclide. Because of the greater stability of nonisotopic labels, the lack of potential exposure to radioactive materials, and the more moderate equipment costs, nonisotopic immunoassays have replaced radioimmunoassays for measuring aminoglycoside and vancomycin levels.[69]

Chemical Tests for β-Lactamase

The determination of production of β-lactamase by staphylococci, *H. influenzae,* and *N. gonorrhoeae* is of considerable clinical value in the treatment of diseases caused by these organisms. There are both rapid acidimetric and iodometric methods, as well as a rapid chromogenic cephalosporin test, available for this purpose. These can be used with isolated colonies of bacteria and provide results within a few minutes.

REFERENCES

1. Huffaker RH, ed. Collection, Handling and Shipment of Microbiological Specimens. Atlanta: US Department of Health, Education, and Welfare. Public Health Service. Centers for Disease Control. DHEW Publication No. CDC 75-8263; 1974.
2. Evans FO, Sydnor JB, Moore WEC, et al. Sinusitis of the maxillary antrum. N Engl J Med. 1975;293:735–9.
3. Schwartz R, Rodriguez WJ, Mann R, et al. The nasopharyngeal culture in acute otitis media: A reappraisal of its usefulness. JAMA. 1979;241:2170–3.
4. Auger WJ. An original method of obtaining sputum from infants and children with reference to the incidence of pneumococci in the nasopharynx. J Pediatr. 1939;15:640–5.
5. Gerber MA. Rapid diagnosis of group A beta-hemolytic streptococcal pharyngitis. Use of antigen detection tests. Diagn Microbiol Infect Dis. 1986;4(Suppl):5–15.
6. Lieu TA, Fleisher GR, Schwartz JS. Clinical performance and effect on treatment rates of latex agglutination testing for streptococcal pharyngitis in an emergency department. Pediatr Infect Dis. 1986;5:655–9.
7. Chodosh S. Examination of sputum cells. N Engl J Med. 1970;282:854–7.
8. Murray PR, Washington JA II. Microscopic and bacteriologic analysis of sputum. Mayo Clin Proc. 1975;50:339–44.
9. Geckler RW, Gremillion DH, McAllister CK, et al. Microscopic and bacteriological comparison of paired sputa and transtracheal aspirates. J Clin Microbiol. 1977;6:396–9.
10. Thorsteinsson SB, Musher DM, Fagan T. The diagnostic value of sputum culture in acute pneumonia. JAMA. 1975;233:894–5.
11. Bartlett JG, Rosenblatt JE, Finegold SM. Percutaneous transtracheal aspiration in the diagnosis of anaerobic pulmonary infection. Ann Intern Med. 1973;79:535–40.
12. Bartlett JG, Ryan KJ, Smith TF, et al. Cumitech 7A. In: Washington JA II, ed. Laboratory Diagnosis of Lower Respiratory Tract Infections. Washington: American Society for Microbiology; 1987.
13. Chalvardjian AM, Grawe LA: A new procedure for the identification of *Pneumocystis carinii* cysts in tissue sections and smears. J Clin Pathol. 1963;16:383–4.
14. Jones RN. Contemporary perspectives on clinical laboratory diagnosis of urinary tract infections: Two protocols that function in a cost-containment outpatient medical practice. In: Smith JW, ed. The Role of Clinical Microbiology in Cost-Effective Health Care. Skokie, IL: College of American Pathologists; 1985:427–36.
15. Washington JA II (ed): Laboratory Procedures in Clinical Microbiology, 2nd ed. New York: Springer-Verlag; 1985.
16. Reller LB, Murray PR, MacLowry JD. Cumitech 1A. In: Washington JA II, ed. Blood Cultures II. Washington: American Society for Microbiology; 1982.
17. Washington JA II. Blood cultures: Issues and controversies. Rev Infect Dis. 1986;8:792–802.
18. Finegold SM: Anaerobic bacteria in Human Disease. New York: Academic Press; 1977.
19. Feldman WE. Concentrations of bacteria in cerebrospinal fluid of patients with bacterial meningitis. J Pediatr. 1976;88:549–52.
20. Wilson CB, Smith AL. Rapid tests for the diagnosis of bacterial meningitis. In: Remington JS, Swartz MN, eds. Current clinical topics in infectious diseases 7. New York: McGraw Hill; 1986:134–56.
21. Granoff DM, Murphy TV, Ingram DL, et al. Use of rapidly generated results in patient management. Diagn Microbiol Infect Dis. 1986;4(Suppl):157–66.
22. Mackowiak PA, Jones SR, Smith JW. Diagnostic value of sinus-tract cultures in chronic osteomyelitis. JAMA. 1978;239:2772–5.
23. Krizek TJ, Robson MC: Evolution of quantitative bacteriology in wound management. Am J Surg. 1975;130:579–84.
24. Loebel EC, Marvin JA, Heck EL, et al. The method of quantitative burn-wound biopsy cultures and its routine use in the care of the burned patient. Am J Clin Pathol. 1974;61:20–4.
25. Woods GL, Washington JA II. Mycobacteria other than *Mycobacterium tuberculosis:* Review of microbiologic and clinical aspects. Rev Infect Dis 1987;9:275–94.
26. Ryan RW. Considerations in the laboratory diagnosis of antibiotic-associated gastroenteritis. Diagn Microbiol Infect Dis. 1986;4(Suppl):79–86.
27. Lyerly DM, Ball DW, Toth J, et al. Characterization of cross-reactive proteins detected by Culturette brand rapid latex test for *Clostridium difficile.* J Clin Microbiol. 1988;26:397–400.
28. Harris JC, DuPont HL, Hornick RB: Fecal leukocytes in diarrheal illness. Ann Intern Med. 1972;76:697–703.
29. Champsaur H, Questiaux E, Prevot J, et al. Rotavirus carriage, asymptomatic infection, and disease in the first two years of life. I. Virus shedding. J Infect Dis. 1984;149:667–74.
30. Champsaur H, Henry-Amar M, Goldszmidt D, et al. Rotavirus carriage, asymptomatic infection, and disease in the first two years of life. II. Serological response. J Infect Dis. 1984;149:675–82.
31. Yolken RH, Miotti P, Viscidi R. Immunoassays for the diagnosis and study of viral gastroenteritis. Pediatr Infect Dis. 1986;5(Suppl):46–52.
32. Hart G. Syphilis tests in diagnostic and therapeutic decision making. Ann Intern Med. 1986;104:368–76.
33. Washington JA II. What can you reasonably ask and expect of the microbiology laboratory? Med Times. 1977;105:20–7.
34. Kellogg DS, Holmes KK, Hill GA: Cumitech 4. In: Marcus S, Sherris JC, eds. Laboratory Diagnosis of Gonorrhea. Washington: American Society for Microbiology; 1976.
35. Clyde WA Jr, Kenny GE, Schachter J. Cumitech 19. In: Drew L, ed. Laboratory Diagnosis of Chlamydial and Mycoplasmal Infection. Washington: American Society for Microbiology; 1984.
36. Chernesky MA, Mahony JB, Castriciano S, et al. Detection of *Chlamydia trachomatis* antigens by enzyme immunoassay and immunofluorescence in

genital specimens from symptomatic and asymptomatic men and women. J Infect Dis. 1986;154:141–8.
37. Tilton RC, Judson FN, Barnes RC, et al. Multicenter comparative evaluation of two microscopic methods and culture for detection of *Chlamydia trachomatis* in patient specimens. J Clin Microbiol. 1988;26:167–70.
38. Hammerschlag MR, Rettig PJ, Shields ME. False positive results with the use of chlamydial antigen detection tests in the evaluation of suspected sexual absue in children. Pediatr Infect Dis. 1988;7:11–14.
39. Amsel R, Totten PA, Spiegel CA, et al. Nonspecific vaginitis: Diagnostic criteria and microbial and epidemiologic associations. Am J Med. 1983;74:14–22.
40. Burnakis TG, Hildebrandt NB. Pelvic inflammatory disease: A review with emphasis on antimicrobial therapy. Rev Infect Dis. 1986;8:86–116.
41. Mardh P-A. An overview of infectious agents of salpingitis, their biology, and recent advances in methods of detection. Am J Obstet Gynecol. 1980;138:933–51.
42. Leibowitz HM, Pratt MV, Flagstad IJ, et al. Human conjunctivitis. I. Diagnostic evaluation. Arch Ophthalmol. 1976;94:1747–9.
43. Jones DB, Liesegang TJ, Robinson NM. Cumitech 13. In: Washington JA II, ed. Laboratory Diagnosis of Ocular Infections. Washington: American Society for Microbiology; 1981.
44. François J, Rysselaere M: Oculomycoses. Springfield, IL, Charles C Thomas; 1972.
45. Gosey LL, Howard RM, Witebsky FG, et al. Advantages of a modified toluidine blue O stain and bronchoalveolar lavage for the diagnosis of *Pneumocystis carinii* pneumonia. J Clin Microbiol. 1985;22:803–7.
46. Shimono LH, Hartman B. A simple and reliable rapid methenamine silver stain for *Pneumocystis carinii* and fungi. Arch Pathol Lab Med. 1986;110:855–6.
47. Braitman LE. Confidence intervals extract clinically useful information from data. Ann Intern Med. 1988;108:296–8.
48. Edelstein PH. The laboratory diagnosis of legionnaires' disease. Semin Respir Infect 1987;2:235–41.
49. Kaufman L, Reiss E. Serodiagnosis of fungal diseases. In: Rose NR, Friedman H, Fahey JL, eds. Manual of Clinical Immunology. 3rd ed. Washington: American Society for Microbiology; 1986;446–66.
49a. Stockman L, Roberts GD. Specificity of latex test for cryptococcal antigen: A rapid, simple method for eliminating interference factors. J Clin Microbiol. 1982;16:965–7.
50. Bailey JW, Sada E, Brass C, et al. Diagnosis of systemic candidiasis by latex agglutination for serum antigen. J Clin Microbiol. 1985;21:749–52.
51. Kahn FW, Jones JM. Latex agglutination for detection of *Candida* antigens in sera of patients with invasive candidiasis. J Infect Dis. 1986;153:579–85.
52. Sommers HM, Good RC. *Mycobacterium*. In Lennette EH, Balows A, Hausler WJ Jr, et al., eds. Manual of Clinical Microbiology. 4th ed. Washington: American Society for Microbiology; 1985;216–48.
53. Koneman EW, Roberts GD. Clinical and laboratory diagnosis of mycotic disease. In: Henry JB, ed. Clinical Diagnosis and Management by Laboratory Methods. 16th ed. Philadelphia: WB Saunders; 1979:1276–7.
54. National Committee for Clinical Laboratory Standards. Performance Standards for Antimicrobial Disk Susceptibility Tests. Tentative Standard NCCLS Publication M2T4. Villanova, PA: NCCLS; 1988.
55. National Committee for Clinical Laboratory Standards. Methods for Dilution Antimicrobial Susceptibility Tests for Bacteria That Grow Aerobically. Tentative Standard NCCLS Publication M7-T2. Villanova, PA: NCCLS; 1988.
56. Pearson RD, Steigbigel RT, Davis HT, et al. Method for reliable determination of minimal lethal concentrations. Antimicrob Agents Chemother. 1980;18:699–708.
57. National Committee for Clinical Laboratory Standards. Methods for Determining Bactericidal Activity of Antimicrobial Agents. Proposed Guideline. NCCLS Document M26-P. Villanova, PA: NCCLS; 1987.
58. Handwerger S, Tomasz A. Antibiotic tolerance among clinical isolates of bacteria. Rev Infect Dis. 1985;7:368–86.
59. Sherris JC. Problems in in vitro determination of antibiotic tolerance in clinical isolates. Antimicrob Agents Chemother. 1986;30:633–7.
60. Krogstad DJ, Moellering RC Jr. Antimicrobial combinations. In Lorian V, ed. Antibiotics in Laboratory Medicine. 2nd ed. Baltimore: Williams & Wilkins; 1986;537–95.
61. Jawetz E. Combined antibiotic action. Some definitions and correlations between laboratory and clinical results. Antimicrob Agents Chemother. 1967:203–9.
62. Bayer AS, Morrison JO. Disparity between timed-kill and checkerboard methods for determination of in vitro bactericidal interactions of vancomycin plus rifampin versus methicillin-susceptible and -resistant *Staphylococcus aureus*. Antimicrob Agents Chemother. 1984;26:220–3.
63. Schlichter JG, Maclean H, Milzer A. Effective penicillin therapy in subacute bacterial endocarditis and other chronic infections. Am J Med Sci. 1949;217:600–8.
64. National Committee for Clinical Laboratory Standards. Methodology on the Serum Bactericidal Test. Proposed Guideline. NCCLS Document M21-P. Villanova, PA: NCCLS; 1987.
65. Grove DC, Randall WA: Assay Methods of Antibiotics: A Laboratory Manual (Anitibiotics Monograph 2). New York: Medical Encyclopedia; 1955.
66. Kavanagh F, ed. Analytical Microbiology. New York: Academic Press; 1963.
67. Kavanagh F, ed. Analytical Microbiology. v. 2. New York: Academic Press; 1972.
68. Hash JH, ed. Antibiotics. Methods in Enzymology. V. 43. New York: Academic Press; 1975.
69. Edberg SC. The measurement of antibiotics in human body fluids: Techniques and significance. In Lorian V, ed. Antibiotics in Laboratory Medicine. 2nd ed. Baltimore: Williams & Wilkins; 1986;381–476.

14. VIRUSES, RICKETTSIAE, CHLAMYDIAE, AND MYCOPLASMAS

MARILYN A. MENEGUS
R. GORDON DOUGLAS, JR.

VIRUSES

As a result of discovery of the viral etiology of a number of diseases and of the increasing interest in antiviral chemotherapy, a number of hospitals and health care facilities now have active viral diagnostic laboratories. Currently, the major emphasis is placed on isolation of viruses and on serologic tests.[1–6] Serologic tests suffer from the requirement for convalescent serum, usually obtained 10 or more days after the acute serum specimen, thus providing diagnoses in retrospect. Viral isolation techniques, on the other hand, are expensive and relatively slow because of the dependence on the rate of replication of virus in cell cultures. Today, techniques such as electron microscopy (EM), immunofluorescence (IFA), radioimmunoassay (RIA), enzyme-linked immunosorbent assay (ELISA), and nucleic acid hybridization (NAH) are being adapted to detect viruses in clinical specimens.[7–11] Using these techniques, results can be obtained rapidly, often on the day the specimen is submitted. The isolation of viruses in cell culture systems, however, remains the most widely available system; it is sensitive and highly specific and is the "gold standard" against which all new techniques must be measured. The relative efficiency with which the common human viruses can be isolated in cell culture systems is shown in Table 1. Appropriate choice of specimen and proper collection and transportation of such specimens to the laboratory are essential to viral diagnosis. Communication between laboratory personnel and clinicians is critical to ensuring that these processes are carried out properly.

General Principles

The first step in making a viral diagnosis is to decide the following: (*1*) Are viral studies warranted for this patient at this time? (*2*) If so, what specimens should be collected? (*3*) How should specimens be cared for until they reach the laboratory?

Since virus shedding may be of short duration, it is important to collect specimens early in illness. Virus is excreted or shed at its highest titer at this time, and quantities generally diminish as illness progresses. Thus, sampling late in the course of an illness may result in false-negative reports. Because nosocomial viral infections are reasonably common,[12] special care should be taken to collect specimens from the hospitalized patient as close to the time of admission as possible. The dilemma of whether a positive virus isolation should be attributed to the illness that required admission or to a nosocomially acquired infection is thus avoided.

Choosing the type of specimen to be collected is also important in viral diagnosis. In contrast to bacteriologic diagnosis, fluid specimens rather than swabs are inoculated onto cell mon-

TABLE 1. Relative Efficacy of the Viral Diagnostic Laboratory in the Isolation of Human Viral Pathogens

Viruses commonly and easily isolated by routine cell culture technique
Adenoviruses
Coxsackieviruses
type A (few types)
type B
Echoviruses
Herpes simplex virus types 1 and 2
Influenza viruses types A and B
Polioviruses
Vaccinia virus
Reovirus
Viruses more difficult to isolate by virtue of viral instability or requirement of specialized culture conditions
Cytomegalovirus
Measles virus
Mumps virus
Parainfluenzaviruses
Respiratory syncytial virus
Rhinovirus
Rubella virus
Varicella-zoster virus
Viruses best isolated in animal systems
Bunyaviruses
Coxsackievirus type A (most types)
Lymphocytic choriomeningitis virus
Orbivirus
Rabies virus
Togaviruses
Viruses that are only isolated by specialized laboratories
Coronavirus (some types)
Epstein-Barr virus
Coronavirus (most)
Virus of progressive multifocal leukoencephalopathy
Virus of subacute sclerosing panancephalitis
Hepatitis A
Rotavirus
Human immunodeficiency viruses
Viruses that cannot be isolated
Hepatitis B
Molluscum contagiosum
Human papillomavirus
Paravaccinia
Parvovirus
Norwalk-like viruses

olayers. Thus, if swab specimens are collected, the secretions and cells that adhere to the cotton or Dacron swab are eluted by vigorously agitating the swab in a fluid-transport medium, usually contained in a tube or a vial. On the other hand, specimens that are fluid by nature, such as urine or cerebrospinal fluid, are satisfactory as obtained from the patient. Solid specimens or those containing mucus such as sputum are processed by homogenizing in a glass tissue grinder in the presence of transport medium followed by centrifugation to obtain a fluid specimen.

Gross contamination of specimens with bacteria or fungi may result in the growth of the contaminating microorganisms in cell culture with destruction of the cell monolayers. To help minimize contamination, grossly contaminated specimens are usually centrifuged to remove bacteria, fungi, and cell debris before inoculation of cell cultures. In addition, both transport media and cell culture media usually contain broad-spectrum antibiotics for this purpose. A frequently used combination is penicillin, gentamicin, and amphotericin B.

Many viral transport media have been devised. Although they may differ from laboratory to laboratory, the basic elements are similar. One of the most widely used is veal infusion broth, although Hanks' or Earle's balanced salt solutions are satisfactory.[13] In either case, the medium is supplemented with antibiotics as indicated above, and a protein such as gelatin or albumin is added to stabilize virus and to preserve viral infectivity. Transport media should be stored in a refrigerator or freezer to maintain the antibiotic potency. Phenol red is often used as a pH indicator, giving viral transport media its characteristic pink color. Since viral transport media contain several potential allergens, instruments or swabs should not be immersed in transport media before obtaining specimens from patients. It should also be noted that the antibiotics generally contained in viral transport media make specimens placed in it unsuitable for the isolation of most other infectious agents, such as fungi, bacteria, mycoplasmas, and chlamydiae. Thus, it is often necessary to obtain more than one specimen from a single site if multiorganism etiology is suspected.

Many viruses are thermolabile, and a large decrease in the amount of virus in a specimen may occur even after storage for only a few minutes at room temperature. Optimally, specimens for virus isolation should be taken to the laboratory immediately after collection, because the delays in transportation often encountered in busy hospitals explain some of the inability to make a viral diagnosis. Either a special system that provides rapid transportation for specimens for viral diagnosis must be devised or, as is more often practical, specimens should be placed in wet ice (0°C) as soon as they are collected and until they arrive in the laboratory. If delay in delivery is unavoidable and will not exceed 24 hours, the specimens should be refrigerated (4°C); if delay will exceed 24 hours, the specimens should be frozen, preferably at −70°C. It should be remembered, however, that freezing and thawing reduces the infectivity of many viruses; thus, the yield is less frequent from specimens exposed to a freeze–thaw cycle. Repeated freezing and thawing should definitely be avoided.

Specimens

Respiratory Tract. Specimens from the respiratory tract are commonly collected for virus isolation procedures and include throat swabs and washings, nasopharyngeal swabs and washings, and sputum. Throat and nasal swabs must be placed in transport medium after collection. Such swabs when well collected are saturated with approximately 0.1–0.15 ml of secretions. In contrast, washings contain larger quantities of secretions, up to 1.0 ml and are superior for that reason for isolation of many viruses. Swab specimens may be preferred by patients because of familiarity with the technique; however, it should be noted that a vigorously applied swab may be more uncomfortable than a washing technique.

Some viruses, for example, rhinoviruses and respiratory syncytial virus, are best isolated from nasopharyngeal washings. On the other hand, a throat swab is the specimen of choice for the isolation of others, for example, adenoviruses and enteroviruses, probably because these viruses replicate to a greater extent in the pharynx than in the nose.[14,15] Unfortunately, the optimal specimen is not always easily obtained. An uncooperative patient or the lack of equipment often makes nasal washings or sputum difficult to obtain. Also, due to the multiple etiology of respiratory tract syndromes, the optimum specimen is not always easy to establish.[16] Probably the best compromise is a vigorously obtained nasopharyngeal swab specimen and a throat swab specimen that are then combined in a single container of transport medium. Fortunately, unlike the parallel situation in bacteriology and mycology, specimens from the upper respiratory tract can be quite useful in the diagnosis of lower respiratory infections. Isolation of a virus from the upper respiratory tract generally indicates recent infection, since shedding of most viruses from this site usually ceases 10–14 days after onset of illness. Subclinical infections occur, but shedding ceases after several days in these cases as well.[15,17–20] The only virus that can properly be called "normal flora" of the upper respiratory tract is herpes simplex virus in that it may be recovered from 5 percent of normal adults.[21]

Nasal swab specimens are collected by inserting a dry swab into the nares until resistance is met at the level of the turbinates, then swabbing the entire surface of the cavity at that level, and repeating the process on the other side. Throat swab specimens are best obtained with direct visualization and, without a tongue blade if possible, swabbing first one, then the other tonsil or tonsillar crypt, and finally the posterior pharyngeal wall with a dry swab. Gagging or coughing frequently ensues. Nasal washings are performed by instilling 5 ml of sterile saline (not containing antibiotics) into each nostril with the head hyperextended and the subject told not to swallow, then tilting the head forward, allowing the fluid to run out of the nares into a sterile container. Saline washes are then placed in an equal volume of viral transport media.[22,23]

Tissue. Virtually any type of tissue can be tested for the presence of viruses. The standard method of processing tissue consists of making a 10 percent suspension of tissue in cell culture medium, homogenizing it in a glass tissue grinder, sedimenting larger debris by centrifugation, and then testing the supernatant fluid for presence of viruses.[1,3,5,6] Whenever possible, at least 1 g of tissue should be sent to the laboratory, either hand-carried by the physician immediately or transported in a sterile container on wet ice. If tissues from several organs are sent for examination, each should be taken with a separate set of instruments and should be put into individual sterile containers. Large specimens can be transported intact, but if only a small amount of tissue can be obtained, care should be taken to keep it from drying out before it reaches the laboratory. This can be done by placing the specimen in a sterile Petri dish on a gauze wetted with saline or directly into a vial of transport medium. In some instances viruses are more easily isolated by outgrowth of the tissue itself (see "Cocultivation" and "Organ Culture" below). This special procedure is available in few institutions, and the laboratory should be contacted in advance.

Cerebrospinal Fluid (CSF). The diagnosis of viral meningitis or encephalitis is presumptive until virus is isolated from a central nervous system (CNS) source. Because of its diagnostic value, therefore, CSF should always be sent for viral culture in suspected cases of CNS infection. Controversy exists among virologists over the frequency of recovery of virus from the CSF. Some have reported poor rates of isolation,[17] while others detected virus in CSF more frequently.[24–26] The rate of isolation varies with the etiologic agent. Mumps virus, for example, is relatively easy to recover from CSF, and in one series was isolated in up to 77 percent of the cases examined.[27] On the other hand, herpes simplex virus, poliovirus, and many togaviruses are isolated only rarely from the CSF.[28–30] A major impediment to successful isolation frequently encountered by the laboratory is the small amount of CSF submitted. At least 1 ml is required for adequate testing. Since CSF is usually a bacteriologically sterile fluid, the specimen is generally tested unprocessed.

Feces. Fecal specimens for virus isolation have been recommended in a number of clinical situations, but, in fact, they are useful in very few. The viruses most commonly associated with viral gastroenteritis (rotavirus and Norwalk-like agents) cannot be isolated by conventional cultural methods.[31,32] Because virus is shed in stools for a long time after the onset of illness and after oropharyngeal excretion has ceased, fecal specimens have been said to be useful for the diagnosis of enteroviral aseptic meningitis, encephalitis, and pericarditis, and adenoviral pneumonia.[1,4,6] It is just this prolonged shedding, however, that minimizes the diagnostic value of the stool specimen isolate. For example, as many as 15–20 percent of well children sampled in the summertime, when enteroviruses are prevalent, may be found to be shedding these viruses in their stools.[29,33] Although generally not useful for diagnosis in the individual patient, stools and sewage have been used for surveillance of enteroviral activity in the community.[34] Either bulk stool or an anal swab specimen in viral transport medium can be sent for culture. In the former case, stool is homogenized in transport medium and centrifuged by the laboratory before inoculation of cell culture. Anal swabs are obtained by inserting a dry cotton or Dacron swab several centimeters in the anal canal, twirling it, and then eluting the absorbed material in transport medium. Like stool specimens, anal swab specimens are centrifuged before inoculation of cell cultures.

Vesicular Fluid and Lesion Swabs. The virus most commonly isolated from vesicular fluids and swabs of skin lesions is herpes simplex. It is easily isolated from such specimens taken in the early stages of the illness. Even later, when scabs have already formed, removal of the scab and vigorous rubbing of the vesicle base with a swab will occasionally lead to recovery of virus. Although not a common diagnostic problem, vaccinia virus is also readily isolated from swab specimens. On the other hand, coxsackieviruses, echoviruses, and varicella-zoster virus are generally more difficult to recover from such lesions, but recovery can be accomplished if proper technique is used. If infection with one of these agents is suspected, obtaining vesicular fluid rather than a swab specimen is recommended. Fluid should be obtained by puncturing the intact vesicle with a sterile needle, expressing the fluid through the puncture hole, and then drawing it up with a syringe or capillary pipette. The advantage of using a capillary pipette is that the amount of fluid obtained can be easily visualized. Even if the amount obtained may be too little to see when collected with a syringe, washing of the needle and syringe several times, by moving the plunger back and forth with the needle immersed in transport medium, will remove the fluid trapped in the needle. Although collection of vesicular fluid in transport medium is adequate for those viruses that are more difficult to isolate, direct inoculation into cell cultures is ideal and should be arranged with the laboratory if at all possible.

Eye. The most common causes of viral conjunctivitis are adenovirus and herpes simplex virus infections. Varicella-zoster, vaccinia, cytomegalovirus, and enterovirus 70 have also been isolated from ocular specimens. Conjunctival swabs or corneal scrapings may be used for isolation of viruses from the eye. Studies suggest that corneal scraping is superior for the isolation of herpes simplex virus, but these studies have not been extended to include other viruses.

Conjunctival swab specimens should be collected by placing a dry sterile swab in the lower medial conjunctival sac so as to occlude the nasolacrimal duct and waiting until the swab is saturated or nearly saturated with fluid. The swab is then placed in viral transport medium. Corneal scrapings should be obtained by an ophthalmologist or other experienced person with a sterile spatula, which is then washed off in viral transport medium. It should be remembered that viral transport media generally contain antibiotics and foreign protein and should not be introduced into the eye during the process of specimen collection.

Urine. Urine is commonly used only for the isolation of cytomegalovirus. It can be useful, as well, for isolation of mumps virus because urinary excretion often continues for weeks after oral excretion has ceased. Enteroviruses, adenoviruses, and herpes simplex have also been isolated from urine specimens, but generally these isolates represent contamination from fecal or genital sources. Adenovirus, however, has been cultured from the urine of patients with acute hemorrhagic cystitis and is thought to be etiologically related to this syndrome.

Clean-voided urine samples, collected in conventional containers, are satisfactory for virus isolation. Like other specimens, urine should be kept at 4°C until it can be delivered to the laboratory, but unlike other specimens, it should not be frozen, even if delivery is delayed.

Blood. Blood cultures are not commonly used in the diagnosis of virus infections, but recent studies suggest they may be quite useful, particularly in young children with enterovirus infection and in the immunocompromised host.[35–37] Buffy coat preparations, separated subpopulations of leukocytes, and serum have all been successfully used to demonstrate viremia in patients with a number of different virus infections. Depending on the virus sought, either serum or anticoagulated whole blood should be submitted to the laboratory for culture.

Other Specimens. Occasionally other specimens such as pleural fluid, semen, cervical secretions, and urethral secretions are submitted for viral culture. If sufficient fluid can be obtained, that fluid is a satisfactory specimen; if not, a swab can be used to absorb secretions and then can be immersed in transport medium.

Isolation and Identification. Viruses require living cells to support their replication. Several methods of using living cells for viral isolation are available: cell cultures, embryonated hen's eggs, and experimental animals. Cell culture is by far the most widely used technique.

Cell Cultures. Cell cultures, often inappropriately called tissue cultures, are initiated by dissociating tissue with proteolytic enzymes and chelating agents, generally trypsin and ethylenediamine-tetraacetic acid (EDTA), into a suspension of single cells. The dissociating agents are removed by centrifugation, and the cells are resuspended in cell culture medium that is basically a balanced salt solution containing glucose, vitamins, amino acids, antibacterial and antifungal agents, sodium bicarbonate as a buffer, and phenol red as a pH indicator. The suspended cells are placed in culture vessels, which for most diagnostic laboratories, consist of 130 × 15 mm screw cap tubes. The cells settle on and attach to the surface of the vessel and replicate, eventually forming a single layer (monolayer) of firmly adherent cells.

Cell cultures are divided into three general classes:

1. *Primary cultures*. These consist of cells derived directly from tissue (e.g., kidney, lung). They generally contain a mixed cell population of epithelial cells, fibroblasts, and trapped leukocytes.
2. *Semicontinuous cell cultures*. These are obtained by "splitting" (dissociating and dividing) or subculturing of primary cultures; epithelial cells and trapped leukocytes do not survive, so generally these cell populations consist of fibroblasts that are diploid and undergo a finite number of subpassages.
3. *Continuous cell cultures*. These are derived from malignant tissue that is generally epithelial in origin. They grow rapidly, are heteroploid, and can be subpassaged indefinitely.

Cell cultures can be prepared in the diagnostic laboratory or can be purchased from commercial sources. Most virus laboratories have available a primary monkey (rhesus, African green, or cynomolgus) kidney cell culture, a semicontinuous cell line such as WI-38 human embryonic lung fibroblast or human foreskin fibroblast, and one or more continuous cell lines such as KB human nasopharyngeal carcinoma, HeLa human cervical carcinoma. Hep-2 human epidermoid laryngeal carcinoma, or Madin–Darby canine kidney (MDCK). In addition, many also use primary human embryonic kidney cells. Each type of cell culture has its own spectrum of viral sensitivity, just as different bacteriologic media have differing selective and restrictive properties for growth of bacteria (Table 2).

Specimen Inoculation and Viral Effects. Based on clinical history, the clinician, in consultation with the virologist, decides which viruses may be responsible for the patient's illness (Table 3) and then selects and collects the appropriate specimen(s), as indicated in Table 4. The virologist selects for inoculation a combination of cell cultures with the appropriate sensitivity range (Table 2), and the cell cultures are inoculated with the fluid specimen. Viruses contained in the specimen are then free to attach to and to penetrate the cells and begin their replicative cycle. Depending on the viruses sought, the cultures are incubated for 7–21 days at either 33°C or 36°C. The cells are examined daily or every other day at a total magnification of 40×–100× using a conventional light microscope.

The presence of viral replication in cell cultures is tradition-

TABLE 2. Optimal System for Primary Isolation of Human Viral Pathogens

Virus Family	*Virus Type*	*Suckling Mouse*	*Embryonated Egg*	*Primary Monkey Kidney*	*Primary Human Embryonic Kidney*	*Semicontinuous Human Diploid*	*Continuous Human Heteroploid*
Picornaviridae	Rhinovirus		0	+	±	++	0 to ++
	Polioviruses 1–3	0	0	++	++	++	++
	Coxsackievirus A1–24	++	0	0 to ++[a]	0 to ++[a]	0 to ++[a]	0 to ++[a]
	Coxsackievirus B1–6	++	0	++	++	±	++
	Echovirus 1–32	0 to ++	0	++	+	++ ±	0
Orthomyxoviridae	Influenza A, B, C	0	++	0 to ++	±	±	0
Paramyxoviridae	Parainfluenza 1,2,3,4	0	0	++	+	+	±
	Respirtory syncytial	0	0	+	+	++	++
	Measles	0	0	+	++	0	±
	Mumps	0	++	++	++	+	0
Adenoviridae	Adenovirus types 1–34	0	0	± to +	++	+	+
Herpesviridae	Herpes simplex	0	++	0 to ++	++	++	0 to ++
	Varicella-zoster	0	0	0	+	++	0
	Cytomegalovirus	0	0	0	0	++	0
Togaviridae	Rubella virus	0	0	+	+	0	0
	Eastern equine encephalitis	++	0	±		0	±
	Western equine encephalitis	++	0	+		0	+
	St. Louis encephalitis	++	0	0		0	+
Bunyaviridae	California encephalitis virus	++	0	0		0	+
Reoviridae	Rotavirus	0	0	0	0	0	0
	Colorado tick fever	+	0	0	0	0	0
Poxviridae	Vaccinia	+	++	++	++	++	++
Arenaviridae	Lymphocytic choriomeningitis	++	++	++	++	++	++

Key: 0: not suitable for isolation; ±: some strains may be recovered; +: many strains may be recovered; ++: most strains will be recovered.
[a] Coxsackievirus A-7, A-9, and A-16 strains grow well in cell culture.

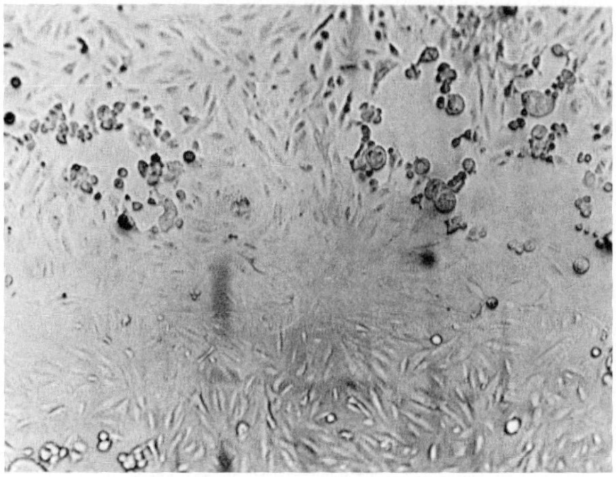

FIG. 1. Human embryonic kidney cell culture infected with herpes simplex. The focal rounding seen is the typical CPE of this virus. This photograph was taken 24 hours after inoculation of the cell culture with a specimen obtained from an ulcerative penile lesion.

ally detected in three ways: (*1*) by the observation of cytopathic effect (CPE), (*2*) by hemadsorption, and (*3*) by the use of interference. In addition, more recently, EM, immunoassays, and NAH (described in detail later in this chapter) have been applied to cell cultures to detect the presence of virus.

Cytopathic Effect. Cytopathic effect, generally a prelude to cell death, is an observable change that occurs in cells as a result of viral replication. Among the changes that occur are rounding, ballooning, syncytial formation, and clustering. The CPE of herpes simplex virus is illustrated in Figure 1. Because cells are examined live and unstained, if a suspected area of CPE is observed, the culture can be further incubated and reexamined for progression of the effect. The nature of the CPE, is rapidity of development, and the cell types in which it occurs all aid the virologist in identifying the putative virus. Some viruses exhibit such characteristic patterns of CPE that definitive identification can be based on CPE alone. For example, herpes simplex virus can often be identified on this basis.[38] Others, however, such as adenoviruses and picornaviruses, produce a CPE characteristic of the virus family, and serologic methods, which can take several weeks to complete, must be used for specific identification of virus type.[1–3,5,6] The tendency, especially among hospital-based laboratories, is to issue a preliminary report when definite CPE is observed, followed by a final report when serotyping is completed.

Hemadsorption. As well as examining cell cultures for the development of CPE at staggered intervals during the incubation period, a suspension of red blood cells (usually guinea pig) is added to selected cultures. Several viruses during their replicative cycle alter the cell membrane in such a way that red blood cells adhere firmly to it. When this phenomenon, called *hemadsorption*, is observed, the virologist issues a preliminary report stating that a hemadsorbing virus has been isolated. Specific serologic typing is then carried out, and a final report is issued. The commonly encountered hemadsorbing viruses include influenza virus types A and B, parainfluenza virus types 1, 2, and 3, and mumps virus.

Interference. Some viruses produce no CPE and cause no hemadorption in cell culture. Cells infected with these viruses, although they appear normal, are resistant to superinfection with certain other cytopathic viruses. This phenomenon, known as *interference,* is used by the diagnostic laboratory primarily for the detection of rubella virus. When interference is found, a preliminary report that an interfering virus has been isolated is issued; following serologic typing, a final report is sent.

Isolation of viruses in cell cultures can be achieved far more rapidly than is commonly appreciated. Table 5 summarizes some of our recent experience with the more frequently isolated virus types. As can be seen, a positive report can often be issued within several days of receipt of specimen.

Embryonated Hen's Eggs. Before the advent of cell cultures, embryonated hen's eggs were widely used for virus isolation. Because cell cultures provide a broader range of sensitivity (Table 2) and are easier to maintain, most laboratories have abandoned eggs in lieu of cell cultures. Even in the case of influenza virus, where embryonated hen's eggs were thought to be the optimal system for isolation, equivalent or superior rates of virus isolation from clinical specimens with A/H1N1 and A/H3N2 and B strains have been achieved using rhesus monkey kidney, cynomolgus monkey kidney, or MDCK cells.[39] There are three main routes of egg inoculation for virus isolation: (*1*) the allantoic cavity, (*2*) the amniotic cavity, and (*3*) the chorioallantoic membrane. Virus replication is recognized by the development of pocks on the chorioallantoic membrane,

TABLE 3. Viruses Associated with Different Categories of Disease

	Associated Virus	
Disease Category	*Common*	*Less Common*
Respiratory tract		
Upper respiratory infection (including common cold and pharyngitis)	Rhinoviruses	Coronaviruses
	Parainfluenza 1–3	Influenza C
	Influenza A, B	Parainfluenza 4
	Herpes simplex	Echoviruses[b]
	Adenoviruses[a]	Coxsackieviruses[b]
	Echoviruses[a]	Adenoviruses[b]
	Coxsackieviruses[a]	
	Epstein-Barr virus	
	Respiratory syncytial	
Croup	Influenza A, B	Measles
	Respiratory syncytial	Adenovirus[a]
	Parainfluenza 1–3	
Bronchiolitis	Respiratory syncytial	Influenza A
	Parainfluenza 1–3	
Pneumonia (adults)	Influenza A	Adenovirus
		Herpes simplex[c]
		Varicella-zoster[c]
		Cytomegalovirus[c]
Pneumonia (children)	Respiratory syncytial	Measles
	Parainfluenza 1–3	Varicella-zoster
	Influenza A	Adenovirus

(Continued)

TABLE 3. (Continued)

Disease Category	Associated Virus: Common	Associated Virus: Less Common
Central nervous system		
Aseptic meningitis	Mumps Coxsackievirus B1–5 Coxsackievirus A9 Echovirus 4, 6, 9, 11, 14, 18, 30, 31	Human immunodeficiency virus Other enteroviruses Herpes simplex 2 (adults) Lymphocytic choriomeningitis Varicella-zoster Many other viruses
Paralysis	Polio 1–3	Enterovirus 71 Coxsackievirus A7 Many other enteroviruses (rarely)
Encephalitis and encephalopathy	Human immunodeficiency virus Alphaviruses, Flaviviruses, Bunyaviruses (formerly arboviruses) Herpes simplex 1 Enterovirus 71 Mumps	Rabies Herpes virus B Enteroviruses (rarely) Polyomaviruses (BK and JC)[c]
Genitourinary tract		
Vulvovaginitis, cervicitis	Herpes simplex 2	Herpes simplex 1 Cytomegalovirus (?)[d]
Penile and vulvar lesions	Herpes simplex 2 Molluscum contagiosum Warts	Herpes simplex 1
Acute hemorrhagic cystitis	Adenovirus 11	Adenovirus 2, 21
Glomerulonephritis		Hepatitis B
Ocular		
Conjunctivitis	Adenovirus 3, 4, 7, 8, 19 Herpes simplex Varicella-zoster Enterovirus 70 Measles	Vaccinia Dengue Newcastle disease virus
Subacute opticoneuropathy	New herpetovirus (?)[d]	
Gastrointestinal tract		
Gastroenteritis	Rotavirus Norwalk-like viruses Adenoviruses	Enteroviruses (?)[d]
Hepatitis	Hepatitis A Hepatitis B Delta hepatitis virus Epstein-Barr virus Cytomegalovirus[c]	Herpes simplex[c] Arenaviruses Togaviruses (e.g., yellow fever)
Skin		
Maculopapular rash	Measles Rubella Parvovirus Echoviruses[a] Coxsackievirus[a]	Adenovirus Epstein-Barr virus Cytomegalovirus
Vesicular rash	Varicella-zoster Herpes simplex Coxsackievirus A16 Enterovirus 71	Vaccinia Coxsackieviruses A and B[a] Echovirus[a]
Hemorrhagic rash	Alphavirus, Bunyavirus, Flaviviruses[a] (formerly arboviruses)	
Localized lesions	Herpes simplex Warts Molluscum contagiosum Varicella-zoster virus	Cowpox Milker's nodule ORF
Neonatal		
Teratogenic effects	Rubella Cytomegalovirus	Others (?)[d]
Disseminated disease	Coxsackievirus B1–5 Echoviruses[a] Hepatitis B Parvovirus Cytomegalovirus	Varicella Herpes simplex Adenovirus
Lower respiratory disease	Respiratory syncytial Influenza	Adenovirus Measles Parainfluenza 1–3
Enteritis	Rotavirus	
Other		
Arthritis	Rubella Parvovirus Hepatitis B	
Myositis	Togaviruses Influenza B	Coxsackieviruses
Carditis	Coxsackievirus B	Other enteroviruses
Parotitis, pancreatitis, and orchitis	Mumps	Coxsackieviruses

[a] Several serotypes.
[b] Many serotypes.
[c] Particularly in the "compromised host."
[d] (?) Association questioned.

TABLE 4. Clinical Specimen(s) to Be Obtained for Viral Diagnosis

Disease Category	*Specimens that Should Be Taken Routinely*	*Specimens Also of Value*[a]	*Comment*
Respiratory tract	Nasal wash *or* throat wash *or* nasal/throat swab *or* sputum	Bronchial brush *or* wash, bronchoalveolar lavage transtracheal aspirate, lung biopsy	Urine if cytomegalovirus is suspected
Central nervous system			
Aseptic meningitis	Cerebrospinal fluid, throat swab, rectal swab	Urine (for mumps virus)	Adults should be examined for genital lesions (see genitourinary tract); whole blood should be obtained in cases of suspected toga and bunya viral meningitis
Encephalitis	Cerebrospinal fluid, throat swab, rectal swab	Brain biopsy, whole blood	
Genitourinary tract			
Vaginitis and cervicitis	Cervicovaginal swab		
Penile and vulvar lesions	Lesion swab		
Acute hemorrhagic cystitis	Urine	Throat swab, rectal swab *or* stool	
Ocular			
Conjunctivitis	Conjunctival swab *or* corneal scraping	Throat swab	
Gastrointestinal			
Gastroenteritis	Stool[b]		Most viruses associated with these syndromes not diagnosed by conventional isolation techniques; antigen detection and serologic techniques currently most useful for diagnosis
Hepatitis	Serum	Urine (for cytomegalovirus)	
Skin			
Maculopapular rash	Throat swab	Rectal swab *or* stool, urine	
Vesicular rash	Vesicular fluid	Throat swab, rectal swab *or* stool	
Hemorrhagic rash	Whole blood		
Localized lesions	Vesicular fluid *or* lesion swab		
Neonatal disease			
Teratogenic effects	Nasal/throat swab and urine		Virus isolation techniques generally more useful than serodiagnostic procedures for the diagnosis of neonatal disease
Disseminated disease	Cerebrospinal fluid, nasal/throat swab, urine, blood		
Lower respiratory disease	Stool *or* rectal swab, nasal/throat swab, urine		
Other			
Arthritis	Nasal/throat swab		
Myositis	Nasal/throat swab, rectal swab *or* stool		
Carditis	Throat swab, rectal swab *or* stool		
Parotitis, pancreatitis and orchitis	Throat swab, urine	Stool *or* rectal swab	

[a] Autopsy tissues may often be useful in cases of death thought to be associated with viral infection. The value of serodiagnostic procedures varies widely based on the agent sought. Always consider serodiagnositc procedures.
[b] If electronmicroscopy or other rapid diagnostic techniques are available.

by the development of hemagglutinins in the allantoic and amniotic fluid, and by death of the embryo.

Laboratory Animals. Laboratory animals, especially infant mice, were also widely used for virus isolation before the advent of cell cultures. Although they, too, have been largely supplanted by cell cultures, there are a number of viruses that are best isolated in laboratory animals, among them, many members of the Togaviridae and Bunyaviridae families, most of the 24 types of coxsackievirus A, and several members of the Arenaviridae family. Inoculated animals are observed for specific signs of disease or death. For some viruses, hemagglutinins can be extracted from infected tissues for serotyping. Others, once isolated in laboratory animals, can be adapted to growth in cell cultures and then serotyped. A few viruses remain, however, that can be serotyped only by using laboratory animals as the indicator system, an expensive and laborious procedure.

Cocultivation. Cocultivation consists of the incorporation of cells from a diagnostic tissue specimen into an already established cell culture. The established culture serves to support and maintain the viability of the cells under investigation and sometimes as an indicator for viral replication. This technique gained prominence after its successful use for the detection of SV40 virus in experimental tumors in animals and of measles virus in brain tissue of patients with subacute sclerosing panencephalitis.[40] It is now widely used by research laboratories attempting to demonstrate latent virus infection. Although most viral diagnostic laboratories do not routinely perform cocultivation techniques, some have the capabilities and attempt cocultivation on special request.

Organ Culture. Certain viruses (e.g., coronaviruses and rotaviruses), although they do not replicate in conventional cell monolayers, do replicate in tissue whose normal architecture has been preserved; such cultures are called *organ cultures*. Organ culture is accomplished by placing small fragments of organs (e.g., tracheal rings, intestinal rings) intact into cell culture medium. Specimens are then inoculated into the cell culture medium. Loss of ciliary function, histopathologic changes, electron microscopy, and serologic tests have all been used as measures of viral replication in organ culture. This technique is generally available only in specialized research laboratories.

Organ culture has also been used to reveal latent virus. The best known example of this is the demonstration of herpes simplex virus in sensory ganglia.[41] The ganglia are removed and placed intact in cell culture medium. Virus replication is assessed by removing aliquots of the medium in which the ganglion is being maintained and inoculating the aliquots onto indicator cultures.

TABLE 5. Rate of Development of Reportable Cytopathic Effect for Different Viruses[a]

Virus or Virus Group	*No. of Isolates Examined*	*Earliest Day of Positivity*	*Day ≥50% Cultures Positive*	*Day ≥90% Cultures Positive*
Adenoviruses	30	1	5	13
Cytomegalovirus	60	2	7	13
Enteroviruses (echovirus, coxsackievirus, poliovirus)	80	1	3	6
Herpes simplex virus	100	1	2	4
Influenza virus	80	1	3	5
Parainfluenza virus	30	3	7	14
Respiratory syncytial virus	40	3	7	14
Rhinovirus	20	2	6	14
Varicella-zoster virus	40	3	5	10

[a] Based on readings made daily for the first 7 days and every fourth day thereafter.

Practical Application of Virus Culture

Although more widely available than in the past, viral diagnostic laboratories are still not often present in hospitals. When they are, the frequency with which they are used generally increases rather rapidly, indicating that they can produce important diagnostic information. For example, at the Strong Memorial Hospital and Monroe County Department of Health Viral Diagnostic Laboratory in Rochester, New York, the number of specimens submitted for virus isolation has increased from 354 specimens in 1970 to approximately 6800 specimens in 1983. This laboratory serves as the only viral diagnostic facility serving a community of 750,000 people with 2500 hospital beds.

The frequency of isolation and spectrum of viruses isolated from clinical specimens in a current hospital diagnostic facility are illustrated in Table 6. In this laboratory, primary cynomolgus monkey kidney, primary human embryonic kidney, and human embryonic fibroblast cell cultures are used routinely. Hep-2 cells are added in the winter months, primarily for the detection of respiratory syncytial virus. The isolation rate achieved is affected by both the season and the type of specimen submitted. A broad spectrum of viruses can be obtained especially from specimens from the respiratory tract. Diagnostic laboratories differ significantly in their ability to isolate certain viruses, depending on experience and on the spectrum of cell cultures used. If a particular agent that is more difficult to isolate (Table 1) is being sought, the laboratory should be consulted about its experience with the agent.

Other Methods for Detection of Virus and Viral Components

Electron Microscopy. Many investigators recommend EM as a tool for rapid diagnosis. One advantage is that EM is more frequently found in hospitals than in the viral diagnostic laboratory. Using EM, viruses have been demonstrated by the direct negative-staining technique in a wide variety of specimens including spinal fluid, urine, tissue, stools, nasal secretions, and throat swabs.[42–47] A diagnosis can often be made within hours of receiving the specimen. Direct EM, however, has its limitations. It requires expensive equipment, highly trained technicians, and is only applicable to specimens in which a high density of intact virus (10^6 virions/ml of specimen or greater) are present. The sensitivity of direct EM can be increased by application of several techniques including ultracentrifugation, agar gel diffusion, and immune electron microscopy.[43,44,46] Immune EM can also be used for virus identification. Unfortunately, each of these methods is time-consuming and therefore cannot be used routinely.

Specimens for EM examination may also be embedded and sectioned, but because this technique is also quite time-consuming, only carefully selected specimens should be submitted. Cold gluteraldehyde is the most widely recommended fixative, but the herpesviruses, the viruses of progressive multifocal leucoencephalopathy (PML) and subacute sclerosing panencephalitis (SSPE), and adenoviruses, among others, have been successfuly demonstrated in formalin-fixed and even paraffin-embedded tissue. Figure 2 illustrates adenovirus particles in a lung specimen that had been formalin-fixed before EM study. Although tissue architecture is sometimes lost in suboptimally fixed specimens, viral morphologic characteristics are generally well preserved.

A valuable contribution of the EM to viral diagnosis has been the detection of viruses that are difficult or even impossible to culture by conventional methods. Examples include hepatitis A virus, a number of viruses associated with gastroenteritis including rotaviruses and Norwalk-like agents, the viruses of PML and SSPE, and wart virus.

Immunofluorescence. Detection of viral antigen in clinical specimens by immunofluorescence (FA) can be used to demonstrate infection with a number of viruses including respiratory syncytial virus, influenza viruses, parainfluenza virus, mumps virus, measles virus, rabies virus, herpesviruses, variola virus,, adenoviruses, rubella virus, and some togaviruses.[11,48] Both direct and indirect methods are used. In the direct test, specific antiserum is tagged with the fluorescein label. In the indirect test, an unlabeled, virus-specific antiserum is allowed to react with antigen, and fluorescein-labeled antibody to the specific antiviral antiserum is then added.

The great advantage of FA is speed; often results are available within a few hours of specimen collection. In practice, FA is

TABLE 6. Types of Virus Isolated from Clinical Specimens over a 1-Year Period (1980) by the Strong Memorial Hospital—Monroe County Health Department Virus Laboratory

Type of Specimen Submitted	*Number Submitted*	*Percentage Yielding Virus*	*Number and Type of Viruses Isolated*
Genital culture	1,149	27.8	304 Herpes simplex 15 Cytomegalovirus
Eye culture	76	9.2	5 Herpes simplex 2 Adenovirus
Urine and saliva	365	9.0	26 Cytomegalovirus 4 Enterovirus 2 Herpes simplex 1 Adenovirus
Fecal	630	12.9	55 Enterovirus 19 Adenovirus 4 Herpes simplex 2 Reovirus 1 Cytomegalovirus (22 Poliovirus)[a]
CSF	362	7.2	25 Enterovirus 1 Herpes simplex
Lesion culture and vesicular fluid (extragenital)	338	42.3	126 Herpes simplex 15 Varicella-zoster 2 Enterovirus
Respiratory tract culture	1,324	24.3	71 Influenza B 61 Enterovirus 44 Herpes simplex 39 Rhinovirus 28 Parainfluenza virus 27 Respiratory syncytial virus 24 Adenovirus 17 Cytomegalovirus 11 Influenza A (6 Poliovirus)[a]
Tissues and effusions	172	6.4	8 Herpes simplex 2 Cytomegalovirus 1 Enterovirus

[a] Presumed to be vaccine strain, not included in calculating percentage of specimens yielding virus.

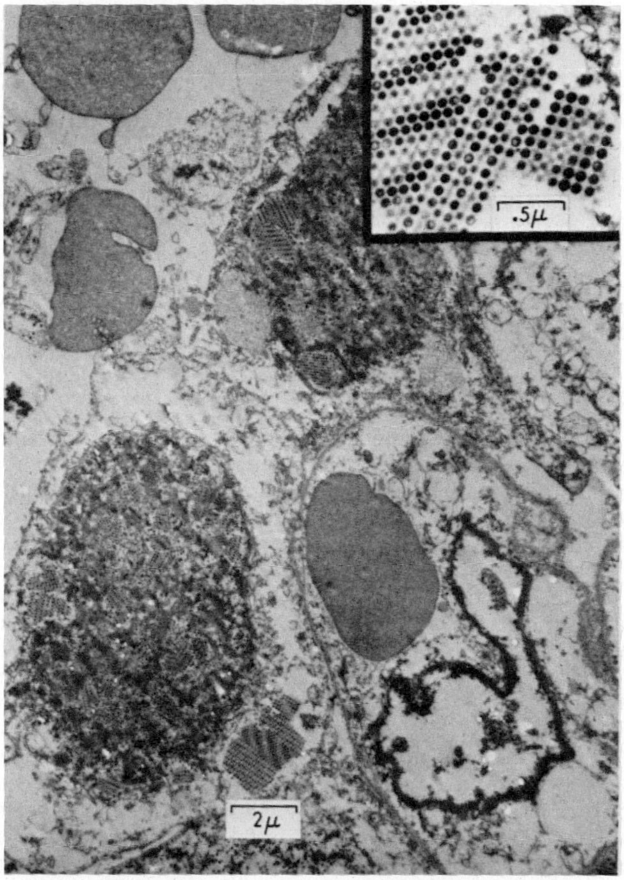

FIG. 2. Crystaline arrays of adenovirus particles seen in the lung of an infant with fatal adenovirus pneumonia. Although the tissue was fixed in formalin before preparation for electron microscopy, viral structure is well preserved.

very successful in the hands of experienced personnel, however, it does have some serious drawbacks. FA requires highly trained and experienced personnel to interpret the results. Although specific and sensitive when tested against virus grown in cell culture, there are problems of nonspecific absorption to leukocytes, mucus, and other materials in clinical specimens that make interpretation of results an "art." Finally, FA is dependent on collection of adequate numbers of intact infected cells rather than extracellular fluids containing viruses. This necessitates specialized specimen collecting and processing techniques, time-consuming for both the laboratory and those obtaining the specimens.

Immunohistochemical Assay. A modification of immunofluorescent staining using indicator antibody conjugated with an enzyme rather than a fluorescent tag has been developed.[49] After addition of the enzyme-labeled antibody, the appropriate substrate is added, and, if positive, a fixed color reaction develops that can be read with an ordinary light microscope. The advantages of this technique are that it does not require a fluorescent microscope and that fixed slides can be permanently mounted and kept indefinitely.

Radioimmunoassay. The first widespread application of RIA for the diagnosis of viral infections was for the detection of HBsAg. A number of RIA formats have been described, but the one most frequently used for antigen detection is the indirect solid-phase RIA.[50] The indirect solid-phase RIA uses the "sandwich" principle, in which test samples are added to plastic tubes or beads coated with a "capture" antibody directed against the antigen being sought. After a suitable incubation period, the sample is removed, and the tubes or beads are washed. Antibody to the antigen in question labeled with radioisotope (generally ^{125}I) is then added. Following a second incubation and washing step, the tubes or beads are counted in a gamma counter. The counts are compared with counts given by known negative specimens to establish a cut-off point for distinguishing negative from positive specimens.

The major advantage of RIA is its high degree of sensitivity. RIA never gained widespread acceptance by routine diagnostic laboratories for other than HBsAg detection. Lack of standardized commercially available reagents, high equipment costs, and instability of reagents are major contributing factors to the limited use of RIA in routine diagnosis. RIA has for the most part been replaced by ELISA for routine diagnostic purposes.

Enzyme-Linked Immunosorbent Assay. A relatively new technique, ELISA is similar in principle to the solid-phase RIA and is now widely used for the detection of both antibody and antigen in clinical specimens.[51,52] It makes use of enzyme-labeled rather than radioactively labeled reagents. Commonly used enzymes include peroxidase and alkaline phosphatase. Enzyme activity is easily assayed by color change, obviating the need for expensive radioactive counting equipment. Reagents are stable and relatively easy to standardize. Commercial ELISA kits are already available for the detection of several viruses including hepatitis B, rotavirus, and respiratory syncytial virus. The use of monoclonal antibodies has improved the sensitivity and specificity of current methods and led to the more widespread use of ELISA as a diagnostic tool.[53]

Nucleic Acid Technology

In recent years, nucleic acid techniques have been used to address a variety of problems in clinical microbiology. Although many methods remain research tools, a number are already in use in clinical laboratories. The general principles of such tests and their applications are summarized below.

Restriction Endonuclease Analysis. Restriction endonucleases are enzymes that recognize defined DNA nucleotide sequences and cleave viral nucleic acid at specific sites. Once cleaved, the fragmented viral genome can be separated on gels based on the fragment size. When identical patterns result, regardless of the number of enzymes used, the viruses under analysis are considered identical. Identity is more certain if it is established with a number of enzymes with different specificities.[54] Restriction enzyme analysis has been used to establish epidemiologic links among cases of viral infection[55] and to resolve questions surrounding the reactivation of latent infection and reinfection.[56]

Nucleic Acid Hybridization. Through the advances that have been made in recent years in the field of molecular biology, it is now possible to demonstrate viral nucleic acid as well as viral antigen in clinical specimens. The technique used, NAH, makes use of labeled, single-stranded DNA or RNA probes (specific viral nucleic acid sequences) for virus detection. The probe is applied to the clinical specimen, and hybridization takes place if a complementary strand of viral nucleic acid is present. A variety of hybridization techniques, including filter, Southern blot, Northern blot, and in situ hybridization are now in common use, and each exploits the technology in a slightly different way.[9]

Many viruses, including herpes simplex virus,[57] cytomegalovirus,[58] rotavirus,[59] papillomavirus,[60] and human immunodeficiency virus (HIV)[61] have been detected in clinical specimens by NAH techniques and at least one commercial NAH assay has already been approved for diagnostic use by the Food and Drug Administration. Like antigen detection methods, NAH is particularly useful for the diagnosis of viruses that cannot be readily grown in cell culture. Unfortunately, while NAH appears to be slightly more specific than antigen detection for the demonstration of viruses in clinical specimens, its sensitivity in most cases is comparable to antigen detection methods and significantly less than that of cell culture. The recent development of biotinylated (nonradioactive) probes has made NAH much more practical for use in the routine diagnostic laboratory.[62,63]

Polymerase Chain Reaction. PCR, first described in 1985, is a novel method for the *in vitro* amplification of specific DNA sequences.[64–66] In 1986 a modification of the technique (the thermolabile DNA polymerase initially used was replaced by the thermostable DNA polymerase *Taq*) greatly simplified the procedure and permitted automation of the reaction.[67] Now, within a few hours, a single viral DNA sequence in a clinical specimen can be amplified to over a million copies. The procedure involves repeated cycles of heat denaturation of the targeted DNA, annealing of the primers to their complementary sequences, and extension of the annealed primers with a DNA polymerase. The specificity of PCR is based on the selection of the viral oligonucleotide sequences used to prime the reaction. Once amplified, the product DNA can be detected and characterized by a variety of methods, including NAH and endonuclease restriction analysis.

The extraordinary sensitivity of PCR is also the basis for one of its limitations. Since even a single DNA sequence is amplified a million times during one reaction, contamination of the sample being examined even with minute amounts of DNA will create false-positive reactions. For this reason scrupulous care must be taken to avoid the introduction of extraneous DNA into the sample being examined.

Despite its very recent discovery, PCR has already been used to detect HIV-1,[68] HTLV-1,[69] and cytomegalovirus[70] in fresh clinical specimens. Concurrent infection with HIV-1 and HIV-2 has also been demonstrated.[71] In addition, PCR has also been used to detect human papillomavirus (HPV) DNA in thin sections of formalin-fixed, paraffin-embedded material, underscoring the power and flexibility of the technique.[72] Within the next few years, PCR will undoubtedly assume a prominent place in the clinical virology laboratory.

Virus Serology

In years past, serology was the primary laboratory means used to diagnose viral infections.[2] However, with the shift from remote diagnostic facilities to hospital-based laboratories, greater emphasis is now being placed on testing methods such as culture, EM, and antigen detection, which can provide results in time to influence patient management. Although serologic results are for the most part retrospective, there are still clinical situations in which they can be quite helpful.

General Considerations. A large number of tests and test formats are available.[1,3,5,6] The criteria used for interpreting results depend not only on the test used but also on the virus substrate. The best approach for detecting antibody to specific viruses should be sought in the chapters in Part III.

Clotted blood is the preferred specimens for all serologic tests. Whole blood can be refrigerated for several days; however, if a longer delay in sending the specimen to the laboratory is anticipated, the blood should be centrifuged and the serum should be frozen at $-20°C$. Anticoagulants should be avoided because they are incompatible with many serologic tests. CSF specimens can also be tested for virus-specific antibody, but, with the exception of measles titers in patients with subacute sclerosing panencephalitis, there is very little basis for interpreting the results. Any efforts to draw conclusions based on CSF antibody titers should take into account the integrity of the blood-brain barrier.[73]

Virus serology is often the preferred diagnostic method for viruses that are difficult to isolate in cell culture (Table 1). In addition, it may be a useful alternative to culture if optimal conditions of storage and transport of isolation specimens are not available.

Even in instances in which virus isolation in cell culture is more desirable, serology can contribute to a more accurate diagnosis by establishing the significance of an isolate. Some viruses such as cytomegalovirus and enterovirus can be shed for prolonged periods, and a rise in antibody titer strengthens the etiologic association with disease.

Virus serology can be used to diagnose acute infection and to determine immune status.

Diagnosis of Acute Infection. The serodiagnosis of viral infections is best accomplished by demonstrating a significant rise in antibody titer between sera collected during the acute phase of the patient's illness and convalescence. The acute serum should be collected as early as possible, and the convalescent specimen should be obtained 2–3 weeks later. The examiner risks missing a titer rise if sera are more closely spaced and may have difficulty determining when the infection occurred if the sera are taken too far apart. Test-to-test variation is common. Therefore, paired sera must be tested in parallel in the same test run. Results cannot be interpreted reliably unless this is done.

Traditional serologic tests (e.g., complement fixation) employ serial twofold dilutions of serum, and titers are expressed as the reciprocal of the highest serum dilution that produces a positive reaction. For such tests, a fourfold rise in titer is considered diagnostic. However, many of the newer serologic tests (e.g., ELISA) measure antibody concentration using a linear scale. The criteria for interpreting such tests are not yet standardized; therefore most laboratories provide an interpretation with the numerical test results.

In some cases, serodiagnosis can be accomplished by testing a single acute-phase serum. Virus-specific IgM appears early during primary infection, persists for a short time, and then declines to undetectable levels. Therefore, demonstration of specific IgM correlates well with primary infection. Many assay systems have been decribed for this purpose.[74–77] However, a number of factors limits the reliable interpretation of results.[75,77,78] Caution in the interpretation of results should always be exercised when using specific IgM tests as a diagnostic tool.

Immune Status Testing. In a number of clinical situations, knowing the immune status of a patient for a particular virus is important. Immunization with rubella vaccine is advised for all women of childbearing age with negative antibody titers unless, of course, they are pregnant. The cytomegalovirus antibody status of both donor and recipient is an important consideration in transplantation and blood transfusion in neonates.[79,80] Varicella-zoster immune status results are used to establish if exposed immunocompromised patients require passive immunization and to guide institution of infection control precautions.[81] Finally, the enormous consequences associated with a positive test for HIV have made the examination of sera for antibody to this virus the single most important test of immune status performed in the clinical laboratory. Sophisticated and extremely accurate protocols for determining the immune status of individuals to HIV are now in routine use throughout the world.[82]

The ideal antibody status test should be highly sensitive and highly specific; however, selecting for sensitivity sometimes compromises specificity and vice versa. The selection of the test that provides the appropriate balance between the two should be based on which is more undesirable from a clinical standpoint—a false-negative or a false-positive result.

RICKETTSIAE

Rickettsial diseases can be diagnosed serologically and by isolation of the organism. Because isolation is both hazardous to laboratory personnel and expensive, serodiagnostic methods are preferred. Isolation of rickettsiae is generally confined to reference laboratories and specialized research laboratories.

Although rickettsiae can be propaged in embryonated hen's eggs and some cell cultures, inoculation of adult male guinea pigs or adult white mice is the method of choice for the isolation of all known species of rickettsiae, save for *R. quintana,* which can be cultivated on artificial medium. Several animals per specimen are inoculated and observed daily for 14 days for signs of illness. On the second or third day of illness, one animal is sacrificed, a postmortem examination is performed, and smears are made for microscopic examination. *Rickettsia mooseri* and the members of the spotted fever group evoke scrotal edema and erythema in the guinea pig that may be useful in preliminary identification. Generally, however, postmortem examination reveals only mild peritonitis. Smears are made by touching the serosal surface of the spleen, the parietal peritoneum, and in the guinea pig, the tunica vaginalis to glass slides. The slides are stained either with analine dyes (Macchiavello or Giemsa stains) or with fluorescent antibody reagents. The organisms are found intracytoplasmically in serosal cells. Several passages in animals are often required before organisms can be detected with certainty. Inoculated animals are examined for evidence of seroresponse as well as for the presence of organisms.

Definitive identification of isolates can be established by complement-fixation and agglutination tests with specific antigens, in some cases by type-specific fluorescent antibody tests, and by toxin neutralization and cross-protection tests in mice.

A rickettsemia is associated with the early febrile period of all rickettsial infections in humans. For isolation attempts, 20–30 ml of clotted blood should be taken at this time. It is important that the blood be drawn before treatment with antibiotics. The serum and clot should be separated as soon as possible. The clot should be "snap" frozen in either a dry ice-alcohol bath or liquid nitrogen. Since loss of viability occurs at higher temperatures, storage at −70°C is recommended. The serum can be stored at 4–20°C for serodiagnosis. Tissue specimens should be taken aseptically and also "snap" frozen and stored at −70°C. Because of the unique epidemiology of rickettsial disease, information on the patient's travel history and possible exposure to vectors can aid the laboratory significantly.[83]

Immunofluorescence of skin specimens in cases of Rocky Mountain spotted fever may be positive as early as the third or fourth day of illness, and if the reagents are available, the diagnosis may be established in a few hours.[84]

CHLAMYDIAE

The increased emphasis on chlamydiae as etiologic agents of nongonococcal urethritis, cervicitis, and pelvic inflammatory disease in adults and of conjunctivitis and pneumonia in children as well as their well-recognized association with psittacosis and lymphogranuloma venereum has resulted in the widespread availability of diagnostic services for this class of organisms.[85] Although culture is still accepted as the most sensitive and specific technique for the laboratory diagnosis of chlamydia infections, immunodetection methods (direct fluorescent antibody [DFA] and ELISA) have supplanted the use of culture in many laboratories because such tests are in general more rapid, easier to perform, and less costly than culture.

A variety of cell cultures and methods can be used for the cultivation of chlamydiae.[85,86] The most commonly employed protocol includes inoculation of the clinical specimen into cyclohexamide-treated McCoy cells, centrifugation of the inoculum into the cell monolayer, and incubation of the culture for 2–3 days. Following the incubation period, chlamydiae are detected by examining the cell monolayer for cytoplasmic inclusions stained with either iodine, Giemsa, or immunofluorescent stains. The sensitivity of cell culture varies somewhat from laboratory to laboratory depending on the methods used, but, as with most other culture methods, the specificity is usually equal or close to 100 percent. Although cell culture is the most sensitive diagnostic test available, there is ample evidence that its sensitivity is not 100 percent. Therefore, a negative culture result does not reliably exclude infection.[85]

Many immunodiagnostic kits and reagents are now commercially available for the direct detection of clinical specimens of chlamydia antigens. Most use either a DFA or an ELISA format. For the DFA tests fluorescein-conjugated antibodies specific for *C. trachomatis* are used to stain smears prepared from the clinical specimen. The smears are then examined for elementary bodies (rather than inclusions) by a microscopist. The quality of the results obtained with DFA tests depends a great deal on the interpretative skills of the microscopist. ELISA tests for the direct detection of chlamydiae in clinical specimens are available in a variety of configurations for use in the clinical laboratory. In addition, very simple ELISA tests (similar in format to those described to detect rotavirus), which take only minutes to perform, have recently been approved by the Food and Drug Administration and are now being actively marketed for use in the office setting.[87] ELISA methods have the advantage of being far less subject to interpreter variation than DFA tests. Many studies of DFA and ELISA for the detection of *C. trachomatis* have been published, and most conclude that the sensitivity and specificity of the two methods are essentially equal and range from 70 to 95 percent and from 90 to 100 percent, respectively, relative to cell culture.[88–93]

MYCOPLASMAS

Mycoplasma and *Ureaplasma* species comprise the two genera of the family Mycoplasmataceae. Although many mycoplasma species have been isolated from humans, only three—*Mycoplasma pneumoniae, Ureaplasma urealyticum,* and *Mycoplasma hominis*—have been associated with disease.

Mycoplasma pneumoniae is well established as a cause of upper and lower respiratory tract disease, but the role played by *U. urealyticum* and *M. hominis* as human pathogens remains poorly defined. *Ureaplasma urealyticum* and *M. hominis* are frequently found in specimens obtained from the respiratory and genital tract both in the presence and absence of disease. In addition, *U. urealyticum* and *M. hominis* have been recovered from the blood of women with postpartum fever, from the lower respiratory tract, blood, and CSF of newborn infants, and from postoperative wound infections.[94–99]

Unlike most other organisms discussed in this chapter, mycoplasmas can be grown on artificial media. However, they are significantly more fastitidious than most bacteria, and the media used for their isolation must be supplemented with horse serum and yeast extract to assure growth. In addition, antibiotics and inhibitors must be added to the medium to prevent overgrowth by bacteria and fungi.

Unfortunately, no single medium can be used for the recovery of all mycoplasmas because of their heterogeneous growth requirements. The medium most frequently used for the recovery of *M. pneumoniae* is the diphasic medium (an agar layer covered by broth), SP-4.[100] Specimens are inoculated into the broth phase, and growth is indicated by a change in the pH of the fluid phase. The presence of *M. pneumoniae* is then confirmed by subculture of the broth phase to an agar plate and the observation of colonies with a typical morphology. Recovery of the organism usually takes 8–15 days. *Ureaplasma urealyticum* and *M. hominis* are less fastidious than *M. pneumoniae*. Consequently, they can be recovered on a variety of different media.[101,102] One, A-7, has been found useful for the recovery of both organisms and is presently the medium most widely used by clinical laboratories.[102] However, some investigators still prefer the use of two media to prevent overgrowth of *U. urealyticum* by *M. hominis*. *Ureaplasma urealyticum* and *M. hominis* are easily distinguished by their unique colonial morphology; they usually take 2–3 days to grow.

Mycoplasmas produce small characteristic colonies on agar, which are barely visible to the naked eye and are best seen using 40× –100× magnification. The organisms do not stain well with ordinary bacterial stains but can be stained with specialized mycoplasma stains (Dienes and Romanovksy).

Although definitive identification of *Mycoplasma* species is established by serologic methods, *M. pneumoniae* can be tentatively identified by its ability (*1*) to grow in the presence of methylene blue under aerobic conditions, (*2*) to rapidly hemolyze guinea pig erythrocytes, and (*3*) to adsorb guinea pig erythrocytes. The serologic methods used for definitive identification of mycoplasmal isolates include growth inhibition (the most widely used), immunofluorescence, and metabolic inhibition.

Recently, NAH technology has been applied to the detection of *M. pneumoniae* in clinical specimens with some success.[103] The major advantage offered by this technique is the speed with which the diagnosis can be made.

Specimens for *Mycoplasma* isolation are best collected in veal infusion broth containing no antibiotics, in contrast to the transport medium used for viral isolation procedures. If the broth is kept cold during transport to the laboratory, growth of bacteria is minimized, and the specimen may be used for the isolation of viruses and other organisms. If, however, there is a risk that specimens will remain at room temperature for prolonged periods, thallium acetate and/or penicillin should be added to the medium to prevent bacterial overgrowth. For best results specimens should be tested soon after they are obtained; if this cannot be done, they should be frozen and stored at −70°C until such tests can be performed.

REFERENCES

1. Grist NR, Ross CA, Bell EJ, et al. Diagnostic Methods in Clinical Virology. 2nd ed. Oxford: Blackwell; 1974.
2. Herrmann EC Jr. The tragedy of viral diagnosis. Postgrad Med. 1970;46:545.
3. Hsuing GD. Diagnostic Virology: An Illustrated Handbook. 3rd ed. New Haven: Yale University Press; 1982.
4. Timbury M. Notes on Medical Virology. 7th ed. Edinburgh: Churchill Livingstone; 1983.
5. Lennette EH. Manual of Clinical Microbiology. 4th ed. Washington, DC: American Society for Microbiology; 1985.
6. Lennette EH, Schmidt NJ. Diagnostic Procedures for Viral and Rickettsial Infections. 5th ed. New York: American Public Health Association; 1979.
7. World Health Organization. Rapid laboratory techniques for the diagnosis of virus infections. WHO Tech Rep Ser. 1981;661.
8. Atanasiu P, Avrameas S, Beale J, et al. Progress in the rapid diagnosis of viral infections: A memorandum. Bull WHO. 1978;56:241–4.
9. Zwadyk P Jr, Cooksey RC. Nucleic acid probes in clinical microbiology. Clin Lab Sci. 1987;25:71.
10. McIntosh K, Wilfert C, Chernesky M, et al. Summary of a workshop on new and useful methods in viral diagnosis. J Infect Dis. 1980;142:793–802.
11. Gardner PS. Rapid viral diagnosis. J Gen Virol. 1977;36:1–28.
12. Douglas RG Jr, Betts RF, Hruska JF, et al. Epidemiology of nosocomial viral infections. In: Weinstein L, ed. Seminars in Infectious Disease. New York: Stratton Intercontinental; 1979.
13. Baxter BD, Couch RB, Greenberg SB, et al. Maintenance of viability and comparison of identification methods for influenza and other respiratory viruses of humans. J Clin Microbiol. 1977;6:19–22.
14. Jackson GG, Muldoon RL. Viruses Causing Common Respiratory Infections in Man. New York: University of Chicago Press; 1975.
15. Wenner HA, Behbehani AM. Echoviruses. In: Gard S, Hallaner C, Meyer KF, eds. Virology Monographs 1. New York: Springer-Verlag; 1968.
16. Report of a WHO Scientific Group. Respiratory viruses. WHO Tech Rep Ser. 1969;408.
17. Herrmann EC Jr, Herrmann JA. Laboratory diagnosis of viral disease. In: Drew WL, ed. Viral Infections. Philadelphia: FA Davis; 1976:23–45.
18. Douglas RG Jr, Cate TR, Gerone PJ, et al. Quantitative rhinovirus shedding patterns in volunteers. Am Rev Respir Dis. 1966;94:159–67.
19. Knight V, Kasel JA. Influenza. In: Knight V, ed. Viral and Mycoplasmal Infections of the Respiratory Tract. Philadelphia: Lea & Febiger; 1973:87–123.
20. Hall CB, Douglas RG Jr, Geiman JM. Quantitative shedding patterns of respiratory syncytial virus in infants. J Infect Dis. 1975;132:151–6.
21. Douglas RG Jr, Couch RB. A prospective study of chronic herpes simplex virus infection and recurrent herpes labialis in humans. J Immunol. 1970;104:289–95.
22. Cate TR, Couch RB, Johnson KM. Studies with rhinoviruses in volunteers: production of illness, effect of naturally acquired antibody and determination of a protective effect not associated with serum antibody. J Clin Invest. 1964;43:56–67.
23. Hall CB, Douglas RG Jr. Clinically useful method for the isolation of respiratory syncytialvirus. J Infect Dis. 1975;131:1–5.
24. Haynes RE, Cramblett HG, Kronfol HJ. Echovirus 9 meningoencephalitis in infants and children. JAMA. 1969;208:1657–60.
25. Chonmaitree T, Menegus MA, Powell KR. The clinical relevance of "CSF viral culture." JAMA. 1982;247:1843–47.
26. Lake AM, Lauer BA, Clark JC, et al. Enterovirus infections in neonates. J Pediatr. 1976;89:787–91.
27. Wolontis S, Bjorvatn B. Mumps meningoencephalitis in Stockholm, November 1964–July 1971. Scand J Infect Dis. 1973;5:261–71.
28. Johnson RT, Olson LC, Buescher EL. Herpes simplex infections of the nervous system: problems in laboratory diagnosis. Arch Neurol. 1968;18:260–4.
29. Melnick JL. Enteroviruses. In: Evans AS, ed. Viral Infections of Humans. New York: Plenum; 1982;187–251.
30. Downs WB. Arboviruses. In: Evans AS, ed. Viral Infections of Humans. New York: Plenum; 1982;95–126.
31. Cukor G, Blacklow NR. Human viral gastroenteritis. Microbiol Rev. 1984;48:157–79.
32. Madeley CR. Viruses and diarrhoea: problems of proving causation. In: de la Maza LM, Peterson EM, eds. Medical Virology II. New York: Elsevier Biomedical; 1983;81–109.
33. Kepfer PD, Hable KA, Smith TF. Viral isolation rates during summer from children with acute upper respiratory tract disease and healthy children. Am J Clin Pathol. 1974;61:1–5.
34. Lund E, Hedström C-E, Strannegord O. A comparison between virus isolations from sewage and from fecal specimens from patients. Am J Epidemiol. 1966;84:282–66.
35. Prather SL, Jenista JA, Menegus MA. The isolation of nonpolio enteroviruses from serum. Diagn Microbiol Infect Dis. 1984;2:353–7.
36. Murray DL, Zonana J, Seidel JS, et al. Relative importance of bacteremia and viremia in the course of acute fevers of unknown origin in outpatient children. Pediatrics. 1981;68:157–60.
37. Howell CL, Miller MJ, Martin WJ. Comparison of rates of virus isolation from leukocyte subpopulations separated from blood by conventional and Ficoll-Paque/macrodex methods. J Clin Microbiol. 1979;10:533–7.
38. Herrmann EC Jr. Experiences in the laboratory diagnosis of herpes simplex, varicella-zoster, and vaccinia virus infections in routine medical practice. Mayo Clin Proc. 1967;42:744–53.
39. Frank AL, Couch RB, Griffis CA, et al. Comparison of different tissue cultures for isolation and quantitation of influenza and parainfluenza viruses. J Clin Microbiol. 1979;10:32–6.
40. Horta-Barbosa L, Fuccilo DA, Sever JL, et al. Subacute sclerosing panencephalitis: isolation of measles virus from a brain biopsy. Nature. 1969;221:974.
41. Stevens JG, Cook ML. Latent herpes simplex virus in the spinal ganglia of mice. Science. 1971;173:843–5.
42. Chernesky MA. The role of electronmicroscopy in diagnostic virology. In: Lennette D, Specter S, Thompson K, eds. Diagnosis of Viral Infections: The Role of the Clinical Laboratory. Baltimore: University Park Press; 1979;125–42.
43. Doane FW, Anderson N. Electron and immune electron microscopic procedures for diagnosis of viral infections. In: Kurstak E, Kurstak C, eds. Comparative Diagnosis of Viral Diseases. New York: Academic Press; 1977:2:505–39.
44. Hsuing GD, Fong CKY, August MJ. The use of electronmicroscopy for the diagnosis of virus infections: an overview. In: Melnick JL, ed. Progress in Medical Virology. Basal: S Karger; 1979:25:133–59.
45. Almeida JD. Practical aspects of diagnostic electron microscopy. Yale J Biol Med. 1980;53:5–25.
46. Field AM. Diagnostic virology using electron microscopic technique. In: Lauffer MA, Maramorosch K, Bang FB, et al., eds. Advances in Virus Research. New York: Academic Press; 1982:7:1–69.
47. Yunis EJ, Hashida Y, Haas J. The role of electronmicroscopy in the identification of viruses in human disease. In: Sommers SC, Rosen PP, eds. Pathology Annual. New York: Appleton-Century-Crofts; 1977:311–30.
48. Gardner PS, McQuillin J. Rapid Virus Diagnosis. London: Butterworths; 1974.
49. Nakane PK. Recent progress in the perioxidase-labeled antibody method. In: Hijmans W, Schaeffer M, eds. Fifth International Conference on Immunofluorescence and Related Staining Techniques. Ann NY Acad Sci. 1975;254:203–11.
50. Halonen P, Meurman O. Radioimmunoassay in diagnostic virology. In: Howard CR, ed. New Developments in Practical Virology. New York: Alan R Liss, Inc; 1982;83–124.

51. Voller A, Bidwell DE, Bartlett A. ELISA techniques in virology. In: Howard CR, ed. New Developments in Practical Virology. New York: Alan R Liss; 1982;59–81.
52. Avrameas S. Enzyme immunoassays and related techniques: Development and limitations. In: Bachman PA, ed. Current Topics in Microbiology and Immunology: New Developments in Diagnostic Virology. Berlin: Springer-Verlag; 1983;93–9.
53. Yolken RH. Use of monoclonal antibodies for viral diagnosis. In: Bachman PA, ed. Current Topics in Microbiology and Immunology: New Developments in Diagnostic Virology. Berlin: Springer-Verlag; 1983;177–95.
54. Wilhelm JM. Introduction to methods or characterization of viruses and viral macromolecules. In: Belshe RB, ed. Textbook of Human Virology. Littleton, MA: PSG Publishing Co; 1984;29–48.
55. Buchman TG, Roizman B, Adams G, et al. Restriction endonuclease fingerprinting of herpes simplex virus DNA: a novel epidemiological tool applied to a nosocomial outbreak. J Infect Dis. 1978;138:488–98.
56. Yow MD, Lakeman AD, Stagno S, et al. Use of restriction enzymes to investigate the source of a primary cytomegalovirus infection in a pediatric nurse. Pediatrics. 1982;70:713–6.
57. Redfield DC, Richman DD, Albinil S, et al. Detection of herpes simplex virus in clinical specimens by DNA hybridization. Diagn Microbiol Infect Dis. 1983;1:117–28.
58. Chou S, Merrigan TC. Rapid detection and quantitation of human cytomegalovirus in urine through DNA hybridization. N Engl J Med. 1983;308:921–5.
59. Flores J, Goeggeman E, Purcell RH, et al. A dot hybridization assay for detection of rotavirus. Lancet. 1983;1:55–7.
60. Lörincz AT. Detection of human papillomavirus infection by nucleic acid hybridization. In: Reid R, ed. Obstetrics and Gynecology Clinics of North America. Philadelphia: WB Saunders; 1987;14:451–69.
61. Pezzella M, Pezzella F, Galli C, et al. In situ hybridization of human immunodeficiency virus (HTLV-III) in cryostat sections of lymph nodes of lymphadenopathy syndrome patients. J Med Virol. 1987;22:135–42.
62. Langer PR, Waldrop AA, Ward DC. Enzymatic synthesis of biotin-labeled polynucleotides. Novel nucleic acid affinity probes. Proc Natl Acad Sci USA. 1981;78:6633–7.
63. Leary JJ, Brigati DJ, Ward DC. Rapid and sensitive colorimetric method for visualizing biotin-labeled DNA probes hybridized to DNA or RNA immobilized on nitrocellulose: bioblots. Proc Natl Acad Sci USA. 1983;80:4045–9.
64. Marx JL. Multiplying genes by leaps and bounds. Science. 1988;240:1408.
65. Erlich HA, Gelfand DH, Saiki RK. Specific DNA amplification. Nature. 1988;331:461–2.
66. Schochetman G, Ou CY, Jones W. Polymerase chain reaction. J Infect Dis. 1988;158:1154–7.
67. Saiki RK, Gelfand DH, Stoffel S, et al. Primer-directed enzymatic amplification of DNA with a thermostable DNA polymerase. Science. 1988;239:487–91.
68. Ou CY, Kwok S, Mitchell SW, et al. DNA amplification for direct detection of HIV-1 in DNA of peripheral blood mononuclear cells. Science. 1988;239:295–7.
69. Kwok S, Ehrlich G, Poiesz B, et al. Enzymatic amplification of HTLV-1 viral sequences from peripheral blood mononuclear cells and infected tissues. Blood. 1988;72:1117–23.
70. Demmler GJ, Buffone GJ, Schimbor CM, et al. Detection of cytomegalovirus in the urine of newborns by using polymerase chain reaction amplification. J Infect Dis. 1988;1177–84.
71. Rayfield M, DeCock K, Heyward W, et al. Mixed human immunodeficiency virus (HIV) infection of an individual: demonstration of both HIV type 1 and type 2 proviral sequences by using polymerase chain reaction. J Infect Dis. 1988;158:1170–6.
72. Shibata DK, Arnheim N, Martin WJ. Detection of human papilloma virus in paraffin-embedded tissue using the polymerase chain reaction. J Exp Med. 1988;167:225–30.
73. Eickhoff K, Heipertz R. Discrimination of elevated immunoglobulin concentrations in CSF due to inflammatory reaction of the central nervous system and blood-brain-barrier dysfunction. ACTA Neurol Scand. 1977;56:475–82.
74. Ziegler DW. Determination of IgM antibodies in diagnostic virology. In: Lennette D, Specter S, Thompson D, eds. Diagnosis of Viral Infections: The Role of the Clinical Laboratory. Baltimore: University Park Press; 1979:63–73.
75. Schmidt NJ. Application of class-specific antibody assays to viral serodiagnosis. Clin Immunol Newsl. 1980;1:1–3.
76. Handsher R, Fogel A. Modified staphylococcal absorption method used for detecting rubella-specific immunoglobulin M antibodies during a rubella epidemic. J Clin Microbiol. 1977;5:588–92.
77. Herrmann, KL. Problems associated with immunoglobulin M detection in the diagnosis of acute viral infections. In: Schlessinger D, ed. Microbiology. Washington, DC: American Society for Microbiology; 1981;280–9.
78. Salonen EM, Vaheri A, Suni J, et al. Rheumatoid factor in acute viral infections: interference with determination of IgM, IgG, and IgA antibodies in an enzyme immunoassay. J Infect Dis. 1980;142:250–5.
79. Stagno S, Pass RF, Reynolds DW, et al. Comparative study of diagnostic procedures for congenital cytomegalovirus infection. Pediatrics. 1980;65:251–7.
80. Yeager AS, Grumet FC, Hafleigh EB, et al. Prevention of transfusion acquired cytomegalovirus infection in new born infants. J Pediatr. 1981;98:281–7.
81. Grandien M, Appelgren P, Espmark A, et al. Determination of varicella immunity by the indirect immunofluorescence test in urgent clinical situations. Scand J Infect Dis. 1976;8:65–9.
82. Hausler WJ Jr. Report of the third consensus conference on HIV testing sponsored by the association of state and terratorial public health laboratory directors. Infect Control Hosp Epidemiol. 1988;9:345–9.
83. Elisberg BL, Bozeman FM. Rickettsiae. In: Lennette EH, Schmidt NJ, eds. Diagnostic Procedures for Viral and Rickettsial Infections. 5th ed. New York: American Public Health Association; 1979;1061–108.
84. Woodward TE, Pederson CE Jr, Oster CN, et al. Prompt confirmation of Rocky Mountain spotted fever: identification of rickettsiae in skin tissues. J Infect Dis. 1976;134:297–305.
85. Batteiger BE, Jones RB. Chlamydial infections. Infect Dis Clin North Am. 1987;1:55–81.
86. Clyde WA Jr, Kenny GE, Schacter J. Laboratory diagnosis of chlamydial and mycoplasmal infections. In: Drew WL, ed. Cumitech 19. Washington, DC: American Society for Microbiology; 1984;1–5.
87. Chernesky M, Castriciano S, Mahony J, et al. Ability of Testpack Rotavirus enzyme immunoassay to diagnose rotavirus gastroenteritis. J Clin Microbiol. 1988;26:2459–61.
88. Chernesky MA, Mahony JB, Castrciano S, et al. Detection of *Chlamydia trachomatis* antigens by enzyme immunoassay and immunofluoresence in genital specimens from symptomatic and asymptomatic men and women. J Infect Dis. 1986;154:141–8.
89. Lipkin ES, Moncada JV, Shafer MA et al. Comparison of monoclonal antibody staining and culture in diagnosing cervical chlamydial infection. J Clin Microbiol. 1986;23:114–7.
90. Tilton RC, Judson FN, Barnes BC, et al. Multicenter comparative of two rapid microscopic methods and culture for detection of *Chlamydia trachomatis* in patient specimens. J Clin Microbiol. 1988;26:167–9.
91. Forbes BA, Bartholomoa N, McMillan J, et al. Evaluation of a monoclonal antibody test to detect chlamydia in cervical and urethral specimens. J Clin Microbiol. 1986;23:1136–7.
92. Quinn TC, Warfield P, Kappus E, et al. Screening for *Chlamydia trachomatis* infection in an inner city population: a comparison of diagnostic methods. J Infect Dis. 1984;152:419–23.
93. Stamm WE, Tam M, Koester M, et al. Diagnosis of *Chlamydia trachomatis* infections by direct immunofluoresence staining of genital secretions: a multi-center trial. Ann Intern Med. 1984;101:638–41.
94. Moller BR. The role of mycoplasmas in the upper genital tract of women. Sex Transm Dis. 1983;10:281–4.
95. Mufson MA. *Mycoplasma hominis*: a review of its role as a respiratory tract pathogen of humans. Sex Transm Dis. 1983;10:335–40.
96. Taylor-Robinson D, McCormack WM. Medical progress: the genital mycoplasmas. N Engl J Med. 1980;302:1003–10,1063–7.
97. Cassell GH, Cole BC. Mycoplasmas as agents of human disease. N Engl J Med. 1981;304:80–9.
98. Murray HW, Masur H, Senterfit LB, et al. The protean manifestations of *Mycoplasma pneumoniae* infection in adults. Am J Med. 1975;58:229–42.
99. Kenny GE. Mycoplasmas: In: Lennette EH, Balows A, Hausler WJ Jr, Shadomy HJ, eds. Manual of Clinical Microbiology. Washington, DC: American Society for Microbiology; 1985;407–11.
100. Tulley JG, Rose DL, Witcomb RF, et al. Enhanced isolation of *Mycoplasma pneumoniae* from throat washings with a newly modified culture medium. J Infect Dis. 1979;139:478–82.
101. Phillips LE, Goodrich KH, Turner RM, et al. The isolation of *Mycoplasma* species and *Ureaplasma urealyticum* from obstetrical and gynecological patients by using commercially available medium formulations. J Clin Microbiol. 1986;24:377–9.
102. Yajko DM, Balston E, Wood D, et al. Evaluation of PPLO, A7B, E, and NYC agar media for the isolation of *Ureaplasma urealyticum* and *Mycoplasma* species from the genital tract. J Clin Microbiol. 1984;19:73–6.
103. Dular R, Kajioka R, and Kasatiya S. Comparison of Gen-Probe commercial kit and culture technique for the diagnosis of *Mycoplasma pneumoniae* infection. J Clin Microbiol. 1988;26:1068–9.

SECTION E. ANTI-INFECTIVE THERAPY

15. PRINCIPLES OF ANTI-INFECTIVE THERAPY

ROBERT C. MOELLERING, JR.

Although the discovery of effective agents to prevent and treat infection caused by bacteria and other pathogenic microorganisms is one of the most important developments of modern medicine, the use of such agents has not been limited to the present era. Substances with anti-infective potential have been applied medically for thousands of years. Indeed, more than 2500 years ago the Chinese were aware of the therapeutic properties of moldy soybean curd applied to carbuncles, boils, and other infections,[1] and the ancient Greek physicians, including Hypocrates, routinely used substances with antimicrobial activity including wine, myrrh, and inorganic salts in their treatment of wounds.[2] Until the discovery of the microbiologic basis of infections in the nineteenth century, however, the therapy for infections remained strictly empirical. Heavy metals such as arsenic and bismuth were found to be useful against a number of infections including syphilis in the early 1900s; but the modern era of chemotherapy did not really begin until the discovery and initial clinical use of the sulfonamides in 1936.[1] This was followed in the 1940s by the discovery of the therapeutic value of penicillin and streptomycin, and by 1950 the "golden age" of antimicrobial chemotherapy was well underway.

It is the result of the relatively recent work in this area since 1936 that forms the basis for this and each of the succeeding chapters on anti-infective therapy. The major emphasis in this chapter is on antibacterial agents because there are more data available on these drugs. However, many of the principles to be discussed can also be applied to the use of antifungal, antiviral, and to some extent, antiparasitic drugs.

CHOICE OF THE PROPER ANTIMICROBIAL AGENT

In choosing the appropriate antimicrobial agent for therapy for a given infection, a number of important factors must be considered. First, the identity of the infecting organism must be known, or at the very least, it must be possible to arrive at a reasonable statistical guess as to its identity on the basis of clinical information. Second, we must have as accurate information as possible about the antimicrobial susceptibility (or potential susceptibility) of the infecting organism. Finally, a series of so-called host factors must be taken into consideration to arrive at the optimal choice of antimicrobial agent. Each of these items will be considered in this section.

Identification of the Infecting Organism

Several methods for the rapid identification of pathogenic bacteria in clinical specimens are available. A Gram stain preparation is perhaps the simplest, least expensive, and most useful of all the "rapid methods" of identification of bacterial (and some fungal) pathogens. This technique can be used to identify the presence and morphologic features of microorganisms in body fluids that are normally sterile (cerebrospinal fluid, pleural fluid, synovial fluid, peritoneal fluid, urine). On occasion, Gram staining of a buffy coat preparation of blood will reveal phagocytosed organisms in the polymorphonuclear leukocytes of patients with bacteremia or fungemia. Similar preparations of sputum will also be helpful in revealing the nature of the infecting organism in patients with bacterial bronchitis or pneumonia. Gram stain of a stool specimen may also produce useful information. In patients with staphylococcal enterocolitis, the Gram stain reveals sheets of gram-positive cocci replacing the normal stool flora. The presence of polymorphonuclear leukocytes in the stool also provides a helpful clue to the cause of certain cases of diarrhea. Polymorphonuclear leukocytes are not found in normal stools. When present, they suggest the possibility of a bacterial gastroenteritis such as shigellosis, salmonellosis, or campylobacteriosis, or invasive *Escherichia coli* gastroenteritis. Polymorphonuclear leukocytes are not found in the stools of patients with viral gastroenteritis, food poisoning, cholera, and diarrhea due to noninvasive toxigenic *E. coli*.[3] *Campylobacter* may be identified in the stools of patients by its characteristic gull-wing appearance on smears of stool.[4]

Immunologic methods for antigen detection (such as enzyme-linked immunoabsorbent assay [ELISA] or latex agglutination) may also provide clues for the rapid identification of the infecting pathogens. Final and definitive identification of pathogenic organisms usually requires cultural techniques. It is thus imperative that appropriate specimens be obtained for culture before beginning antimicrobial therapy. Once anti-infective therapy has been started, cultures often are rendered sterile, even though viable organisms remain in the host.

In most cases, it may be impossible to determine the exact nature of the infecting organisms before the institution of antimicrobial therapy. In these cases the use of bacteriologic statistics may be particularly helpful.[5,6] The term *bacteriologic statistics* refers to the application of knowledge of the organisms most likely to cause infection in a given clinical setting. For example, a person with normal host defense mechanisms who develops cellulitis of the arm after a minor abrasion most likely has an infection due to *Staphylococcus aureus* or group A streptococci, and antimicrobial therapy should be tailored accordingly, even though there is no material available for examination with Gram stain. Similarly, a young child with acute otitis media almost certainly has an infection due to either a virus or to one of four major bacterial pathogens: *Haemophilus influenzae, Streptococcus pneumoniae, Branhamella catarrhalis,* or a group A streptococcus.

Determination of Antimicrobial Susceptibility of Infecting Organisms

Since different organisms vary in their susceptibility to antimicrobial agents, it is imperative that we have some means for determining the antimicrobial susceptibility of the actual (or presumed) infecting organism(s). If the pathogen is isolated from a culture, it can be subjected to direct susceptibility testing as described in Chapter 13. A number of methods for determining antimicrobial susceptibility are available. The commonly used disk-diffusion method is simple to perform and is relatively inexpensive, but it provides at best only semiquantitative or qualitative data about the susceptibility of a given organism to a given agent. It is not useful for slow-growing or fastidious organisms and has not been standardized for anaerobes. Nonetheless, if the test is carefully done, it provides data that are clinically useful. Quantitative data are provided by methods that incorporate serial dilutions of antimicrobials in agar-containing or broth culture media. The lowest concentration of the antimicrobial agent that prevents visible growth after an 18- to 24-hour incubation period is known as the minimal inhibitory concentration (MIC). The minimal bacterial concentration (MBC) or minimal lethal concentration (MLC) may be determined in broth dilution tests by subculturing the containers that show no growth onto antibiotic-free agar-containing media. The lowest concentration of antimicrobial that totally suppresses growth on antibiotic-free media (or results in a 99.9 percent or greater decline in colony count) after overnight incubation is known as the MBC (or MLC). The aforementioned techniques are based on an 18- to 24-hour incubation period. A variety of "rapid methods" are now available as well.[7] These are based on a determination of changes in bacterial growth rates caused by antimicrobial agents and can provide susceptibility in 4 to 8 hours.

Susceptibility testing is particularly important for certain organisms such as *S. aureus* and the various facultative and aerobic gram-negative bacilli. The widespread clinical and agricultural use of antibiotics since the 1930s and 1940s has resulted in the emergence of many strains of bacteria resistant to one or more antimicrobial agents.[8] In most cases in which adequate studies have been done, it appears that the role of antimicrobial agents is to exert selective pressure that results in the emergence of resistant organisms. In some cases the organisms are naturally resistant to the antibiotic used. Examples of this include gram-positive organisms such as staphylococci and streptococci, which are naturally resistant to the polymyxins. Many gram-negative bacilli are naturally resistant to penicillin G, erythromycin, and clindamycin. In other cases the resistant bacterial strains have acquired R factors or plasmids that enable them to resist antimicrobial inhibition. These plasmids may provide the organisms with the ability to synthesize enzymes that modify or inactivate the antimicrobial agent; they may result in changes in the bacterial cell's ability to accumulate the antimicrobial agent or may permit the cell to produce metabolic enzymes resistant to inhibition by the antimicrobial agent.[8] Examples of each of these mechanisms of resistance are well known. Most strains of *S. aureus* that are resistant to penicillin contain plasmids that enable them to produce an extracellular β-lactamase that hydrolyzes and inactivates penicillin G.[8] Many gram-negative bacilli that are resistant to aminoglycosidic aminocyclitol antibiotics such as streptomycin, kanamycin, tobramycin, gentamicin, and amikacin contain plasmids that code for the production of periplasmic enzymes that catalyze a modification of the aminoglycosidic aminocyclitols by phosphorylation, acetylation, or adenylylation.[8] R-factor–mediated tetracycline resistance in both gram-negative bacilli and *S. aureus* involves an inducible decrease in the uptake of tetracycline, although the actual mechanism for this decreased uptake is not yet understood.[8] *Escherichia coli* organisms resistant to trimethoprim have been found to contain R factors that enable them to synthesize a new dihydrofolate reductase (the enzyme specifically inhibited by trimethoprim) that is 10,000 times less susceptible to the in vitro effects of trimethoprim than is the host bacteria's own chromosomal enzyme.[8]

The aforementioned developments provide the rationale for performing tests of antimicrobial susceptibility whenever there is reasonable doubt about the susceptibility of a given organism. There are certain cases in which routine susceptibility testing need not be done, but they make up an ever-diminishing list. All group A streptococci remain susceptible to the penicillins and cephalosporins; meningococci likewise are universally susceptible to chloramphenicol; virtually all anaerobes except *Bacteroides* species are susceptible to penicillin G. Thus, testing these organisms against the agents listed need not be routinely carried out at the present time. Even a statement such as this is fraught with a certain amount of danger. The discoveries of penicillin-resistant meningococci and pneumococci in South Africa, the emergence of penicillin-resistant gonococci in Asia and Africa, the rapid spread of ampicillin-resistant (and even chloramphenicol-resistant) strains of *H. influenzae* in the United States and Europe and the proliferation of vancomycin-resistant enterococci and staphylococci make us realize that, in time, strains of virtually any organism may be found that are resistant to antimicrobial agents that previously had been effective against them.[9]

It is important to consider geographic differences in patterns of susceptibility of organisms when choosing antimicrobial agents. In many cases, there may be variations in susceptibility patterns between hospitals and the community or among hospitals themselves. The emergence of gram-negative bacilli that are resistant to gentamicin is a good example of this. Most of the aminoglycoside-resistant organisms are found in hospitals, whereas most isolates from nonhospitalized patients remain susceptible to gentamicin.[8,10] The possibility of significant geographic variations in antimicrobial susceptibility must be remembered as we examine Table 1, which is a compendium of antimicrobial agents of choice for various commonly encountered infectious agents. The data in this table are based on material accumulated primarily in the United States and are similar in many aspects to data published periodically in the *Medical Letter on Drugs and Therapeutics*.[11]

Host Factors

It is obviously important to determine the identity and antimicrobial susceptibility of the organism(s) causing a given infection. However, optimal therapy is impossible unless we also consider a number of host factors that may influence the efficacy and toxicity of antimicrobial agents.[12]

History of Previous Adverse Reactions to Antimicrobial Agents. Simply obtaining an adequate history of previous adverse reactions to drugs may prevent the inadvertent administration of an antimicrobial agent to which the patient is allergic. A failure to do so can have serious (and sometimes fatal) consequences.

Age. The age of the patient is a major factor to consider in the choice of antimicrobial agents. Gastric acidity varies with age. The pH of gastric secretions is higher in young children and does not reach adult levels of acidity until approximately the age of 3 years. At the other end of the age spectrum, there is also a decline in gastric acidity such that gastric achlorhydria is found in 5.3 percent of people 20–29 years of age, in 16 percent of those 40–49, and in 35.4 percent of those over 60.[12] The absorption of a number of antimicrobials via the oral route depends on their acid stability and the pH of gastric secretions. Penicillin G is an excellent example of this phenomenon. The oral absorption of penicillin G is markedly reduced by gastric acid. However, in young children and in older achlorhydric patients, the absorption of the drug is markedly enhanced. As a result, various orally administered penicillins will produce high serum levels in young children and in elderly patients who have achlorhydria. It makes no sense to give such a patient the more expensive acid-resistant forms of penicillin such as phenoxymethyl penicillin (penicillin V) since these drugs will not be absorbed any better than the less expensive penicillin G. The absorption of other orally administered β-lactam antibiotics is probably also enhanced in achlorhydric patients; however, evidence is convincing only in the case of the penicillins.[13] Gastric acidity does not always have a negative influence on the absorption of antimicrobials. Drugs that are weak acids such as ketoconazole may be better absorbed at a low pH. Thus, absorption of ketoconazole is impaired by the administration of antacids, cimetidine, or even food.[14]

Renal function, likewise, varies with age. It is relatively diminished in premature and newborn children and reaches "adult levels" between 2 and 12 months of age.[12] Thus the serum half-lives of drugs that are primarily excreted by the kidneys may be considerably increased in neonates. As a result, doses of antimicrobial agents such as penicillin G and its various

TABLE 1. Antimicrobial Agents of Choice

Organism	*Antimicrobial of Choice*	*Alternative Agents*
Gram-positive cocci		
Staphylococcus aureus		
Non-penicillinase producing	Penicillin	A cephalosporin,[a] vancomycin, clindamycin, imipenem, erythromycin
Penicillinase producing	A penicillinase-resistant penicillin[b]	A cephalosporin,[a] vancomycin, clindamycin, imipenem, erythromycin
β-Streptococci (groups A, B, C, and G)	Penicillin	A cephalosporin,[a] erythromycin, vancomycin
α-Streptococci (*Streptococcus viridans*)	Penicillin	A cephalosporin,[a] vancomycin, erythromycin
Streptococcus bovis	Penicillin	A cephalosporin,[a] vancomycin, erythromycin
Enterococci		
Endocarditis or other serious infection	Penicillin (or ampicillin) plus gentamicin or streptomycin	Vancomycin plus gentamicin or streptomycin
Uncomplicated urinary tract infection	Ampicillin or amoxicillin	Nitrofurantoin, erythromycin
Streptococcus pneumoniae	Penicillin	A cephalosporin,[a] erythromycin, chloramphenicol, vancomycin
Gram-negative cocci		
Neisseria meningitidis	Penicillin	Chloramphenicol, cefuroxime, ceftriaxone, cefotaxime, moxalactam, a sulfonamide
Neisseria gonorrhoeae		
Non-β-lactamase producing	Penicillin	Spectinomycin, ampicillin, amoxicillin, cefoxitin, ceftriaxone, cefuroxime, cefotaxime, trimethoprim-sulfamethoxazole, ciprofloxacin
β-Lactamase producing	Ceftriaxone	Cefoxitin, cefuroxime, amoxicillin clavulanate, spectinomycin, chloramphenicol, cefotaxime, trimethoprim-sulfamethoxazole, ciprofloxacin
Gram-negative bacilli		
Acinetobacter sp. (*Mima, Herellea*)	Imipenem	Tobramycin or kanamycin (± carbenicillin), sulfisoxazole, trimethoprim-sulfamethoxazole, ticarcillin, mezlocillin, piperacillin, doxycycline
Brucella sp.	Tetracycline (± streptomycin)	Chloramphenicol (± streptomycin)
Campylobacter jejuni	Erythromyycin	Ciprofloxacin[c,f], tetracycline, chloramphenicol, gentamicin
Enterobacter sp.	Gentamicin or tobramycin	Carbenicillin, ticarcillin, mezlocillin, piperacillin, netilmicin, amikacin, third-generation cephalosporin,[d] cefoperazone, tetracycline, chloramphenicol, imipenem, trimethoprim-sulfamethoxazole, ciprofloxacin
Escherichia coli		
Uncomplicated urinary tract infection	Ampicillin, amoxicillin, or trimethoprim-sulfamethoxazole	A cephalosporin,[a] a tetracycline, trimethoprim, sulfisoxazole
Systemic infection	Ampicillin or amoxicillin (for serious infections, third-generation cephalosporin[d], cefoperazone)	A cephalosporin,[a] carbenicillin, mezlocillin, piperacillin, gentamicin, tobramycin, kanamycin, amikacin, netilmicin, ciprofloxacin, imipenem, aztreonam
Francisella tularensis	Streptomycin	Tetracycline, chloramphenicol
Haemophilus influenzae		
Meningitis	Chloramphenicol, third-generation cephalosporin[d]	Ampicillin (if β-lactamase–negative), cefuroxime
Other infections	Ampicillin or amoxicillin[e]	Trimethoprim-sulfmethoxazole, cefuroxime cefaclor, cefamandole, sulfisoxazole, amoxicillin clavulanate, ciprofloxacin
Klebsiella pneumonia	A cephalosporin[a] (for serious infections, third-generation cepholosporin[d])	Imipenem, aztreonam, trimetheprim-sulfamethoxazole, cefuroxime, cefamandole, amikacin, netilmicin, gentamicin, tobramycin, ciprofloxacin, chloramphenicol, tetracycline
Legionella sp.	Erythromycin	Rifampin plus erythromycin, trimethoprim-sulfamethoxazole
Proteus mirabilis	Ampicillin	Gentamicin or tobramycin, a cephalosporin,[a] imipenem, aztreonam, ticarcillin, mezlocillin, piperacillin
Other *Proteus* sp. (*P. rettgeri, M. morganii, P. vulgaris*	Gentamicin or tobramycin	Third-generation cephalosporin,[d] carbenicillin, ticarcillin, mezlocillin, piperacillin, amikacin, kanancycin, netilmicin, imipenem, aztreonam, trimethoprim-sulfamethoxazole, chloramphenicol, ciprofloxacin
Providencia sp.	Gentamicin or tobramycin	Third-generation cephalosporin,[d] amikacin, kanamcycin, netilmicin, carbenicillin, ticarcillin, mezlocillin, piperacillin, imipenem, aztreonam, trimethoprim-sulfamethoxazole, chloramphenicol, ciprofloxacin
Pseudomonas aeruginosa	Tobramycin or gentamicin plus ticarcillin, carbenicillin, azlocillin, mezlocillin, or piperacillin	Amikacin, netilmicin, imipenem, aztreonam, ceftazidime, ciprofloxacin
Salmonella sp.	Chloramphenicol	Ampicillin or amoxicillin, trimethoprim-sulfamethoxazole,[f] ciprofloxacin

(Continued)

TABLE 1. (Continued)

Organism	*Antimicrobial of Choice*	*Alternative Agents*
Serratia marcescens	Gemtamicin or amikacin	Third-generation cephalosporin,[d] carbenicillin, ticarcillin, mezlocillin, piperacillin, imipenem, aztreonam, tobramycin, netilmicin, chloramphenicol
Shigella sp.	Trimethoprim-sulfamethoxazole	Ciprofloxacin, ampicillin, chloramphenicol, nalidixic acid
Yersinia pestis	Streptomycin	Tetracycline, chloramphenicol, gentamicin
Anaerobes		
Anaerobic streptococci	Penicillin	Clindamycin, erythromycin, chloramphenicol, a cephalosporin,[a] tetracycline
Bacteroides sp.		
Oropharyngeal stains	Penicillin	Clindamycin, tetracycline, chloramphenicol metronidazole, cefoxitin, cefotetan
Gastrointestinal strains	Clindamycin or metronidazole	Chloramphenicol, cefoxitin, cefotetan, moxalactam, carbenicillin, ticarcillin, piperacillin, mezlocillin, imipenam, ticarcillin clavulanate, ampicillin-sulbactam
Clostridium sp.	Penicillin	Chloramphenicol, clindamycin, metronidazole

[a] The term *cephalosporin* refers to the first-generation cephalosporins cephalothin, cefazolin, cephapirin, cephradine, cephalexin, cefaclor, and cefadroxil.
[b] Methicillin, nafcillin, oxacillin, or dicloxacillin.
[c] For adults.
[d] The term *third-generation cephalosporin* refers to ceftriaxone, cefotaxime, ceftizoxime, ceftazidime, and moxalactam.
[e] For strains that do not produce β-lactamase.
[f] Not approved for this indication by the U.S. Food and Drug Administration.

semisynthetic derivatives as well as the aminoglycosides must be altered in neonates.

Aging results in the decline of a number of physiologic processes, including renal function.[13] It is especially important to realize that creatinine clearance may be significantly reduced in elderly patients even though they have normal blood urea nitrogen (BUN) or serum creatinine concentrations. In view of this, high doses of the penicillins or cephalosporins must be given with caution to elderly patients to prevent the development of excessively high serum levels that may produce severe neurotoxic reactions such as myoclonus, seizures, and coma.[12,13] It is likewise possible that other adverse reactions to the penicillins such as reversible neutropenia may be dose related and may occur with increased frequency when high doses of such drugs are given to elderly patients with physiologic renal impairment.[13] This, however, has not been proved. Impaired renal excretion of the aminoglycoside antibiotics may result in elevated serum concentrations, which in turn may be associated with an increasing incidence of ototoxicity in elderly patients.[15]

In addition to the toxicity that may result from impaired renal excretion in neonates and elderly patients, other adverse effects of antimicrobial agents may also be age related.[14,16] Hepatic function in the neonate is underdeveloped by adult standards. This can result in difficulties if such patients are administered drugs that are normally excreted or inactivated by the liver. Chloramphenicol is inactivated by conjugation to the glucuronide form in the liver. However, in the neonate, hepatic levels of glucuronyl transferase are relatively insufficient. Thus when neonates are given large doses of chloramphenicol, high serum levels of unconjugated chloramphenicol result. Such high concentrations of unconjugated chloramphenicol are toxic and can result in shock, cardiovascular collapse, and death (the so-called gray syndrome).[12,17] For this reason, chloramphenicol should be avoided if possible in the neonate. If it is necessary to use the drug, however, it may be safely administered if given in a dosage that has been reduced appropriately for the patient's age.[17,18]

The sulfonamides compete with bilirubin for binding sites on serum albumin. When given to neonates, they produce increased serum levels of unbound bilirubin that predispose the child to kernicterus.[17,18] For this reason, these agents should not be administered to neonates. Hyperbilirubinemia per se may be associated with the administration of novobiocin to neonates.[17] This is due to the ability of this drug to inhibit hepatic glucuronyl transferase, which in turn diminishes the ability of the liver to conjugate and excrete bilirubin. Hence, novobiocin should be avoided in newborn infants.

The tetracyclines are avidly bound to developing bone and tooth structures. As they bind to developing teeth, tetracyclines may cause a number of adverse effects ranging from purplish to brownish discoloration of the teeth to actual enamel hypoplasia.[12,17] The tetracyclines readily cross the placenta.[19] Thus, when administered during the latter half of pregnancy or from birth to the age of 6 months, they may cause these effects on the deciduous teeth of the infant. From the age of 6 months to 6–8 years, similar damage to the permanent teeth may occur. In view of this, tetracycline should be avoided, if possible, in young children.

The quinolone antimicrobials including the newer agents such as ciprofloxacin, norfloxacin, ofloxacin, pefloxacin, and others have been shown to cause cartilage damage and arthropathy in young animals. As a result, they are not recommended for use in prepubertal children.[20]

Adverse effects due to a number of antimicrobial agents have been noted to occur with increased incidence in the elderly.[13] In some cases (and perhaps in all if adequately studied), this relationship may be shown to be due to specific disease states or to impairment of physiologic processes associated with aging as noted earlier. However, in certain cases no specific factors other than age can be identified. The hepatotoxicity associated with isoniazid administration is a good example of this. A small percentage of patients receiving isoniazid develop toxic hepatitis that may be fatal if not recognized in time.[21] Liver damage from isoniazid almost never occurs in patients under 20 years of age. In patients 20–34 years of age, the incidence of isoniazid hepatotoxicity is 0.3 percent and rises steadily with age to reach 2.3 percent in patients 50 years of age or more. Because of this, it is currently recommended that routine prophylactic use of isoniazid for patients discovered to have positive tuberculin test reactions be limited to people under the age of 35.[22]

Nephrotoxic reactions to certain antimicrobial agents likewise appear to be more frequent or to occur with lower doses of drugs among the elderly. This has been demonstrated to occur with cephaloridine[23] and colistin[12,24] and may be true for other nephrotoxic antimicrobials as well.

Finally, hypersensitivity reactions to antimicrobial agents also appear to be more common in elderly than in younger patients.[12] This appears to be due to the fact that older patients are more likely to have been previously exposed and, thus, sensitized to these agents. In addition, prior exposure to drugs such as the aminoglycosidic aminocyclitols, which produce irreversible cochlear damage, can result in cumulative toxicity on repeat exposure.[13]

Genetic or Metabolic Abnormalities. The presence of genetic or metabolic abnormalities may also have a significant effect on the use or toxicity of a given antimicrobial agent. The rate at which isoniazid is conjugated and biologically inactivated by acetylation in the liver is genetically determined.[12] Rapid acetylators are more commonly found among Oriental populations, whereas 45–65 percent of U.S. and North European populations are slow acetylators. Several studies have suggested that polyneuritis is seen more frequently as a complication of isoniazid therapy in slow than in rapid acetylators.[12] It was once thought that hepatotoxicity due to isoniazid is related to the conversion of isoniazid to acetylhydrazine and other related hepatoxic derivatives and is more common among rapid acetylators,[25] but this does not appear to be true.

A number of antimicrobial agents have been shown to be capable of provoking hemolysis in patients with glucose-6-phosphate dehydrogenase (G6PD) deficiency, including the sulfonamides, nitrofurantoin, furazolidone, diaminodiphenylsulfone, and chloramphenicol.[12] Sulfonamides may likewise cause hemolytic reactions in the presence of certain hemoglobinopathies, including hemoglobin Zurich and hemoglobin H.[12]

The presence of metabolic disorders such as diabetes mellitus may also pose problems in antimicrobial therapy. Certain agents such as the sulfonamides (especially the long-acting types) and chloramphenicol can potentiate the hypoglycemic activity of sulfonylurea hypoglycemic agents such as tolbutamide and chlorpropamide.[13] In the case of the sulfonamides, this action may be related to their structural similarity to the sulfonylurea drugs. Chloramphenicol inhibits microsomal enzyme activity in the liver, and this impairs the metabolism of the sulfonylurea hypoglycemic agents. The dextrose load infused with intravenous antibiotics dissolved in dextrose-containing vehicles may be sufficient to produce hyperglycemia and glucosuria in diabetic patients. Another kind of ''glucosuria'' can occur in patients receiving antimicrobial agents. The cephalosporins, chloramphenicol, isoniazid, nalidixic acid, nitrofurantoin, penicillin, streptomycin, sulfanilimide, and the tetracyclines can all cause false-positive test results when urine sugar levels are determined by a method (such as the Benedict test or Clinitest) that measures reducing substances in the urine.[23] Tests that are specific for glucose (i.e., that use glucose oxidase) such as Dextrostix or Labstix are not affected by antimicrobial agents.

The absorption of intramuscularly administered antibiotics may be impaired in diabetic patients. Diabetics with bacterial endocarditis who failed to respond to intramuscular penicillin have been described.[12] Administration of the same dose of penicillin by the intravenous route, however, resulted in bacterial eradication.[12] Because of the potential impaired absorption of intramuscularly administered antimicrobial agents, it is probably prudent to initiate therapy by the intravenous route when using drugs such as the aminoglycosides to treat diabetic patients with gram-negative bacteremia (especially if accompanied by hypotension) or other serious infections.

The concomitant administration of chloramphenicol has been noted to delay the reticulocyte response to vitamin B_{12} or iron therapy in patients with pernicious anemia or iron deficiency anemia.[12] As noted previously, patients with pernicious anemia and gastric achlorhydria may exhibit enhanced serum levels of antimicrobials such as penicillin G when given by the oral route.

Rifampin may increase the hepatic metabolism and therefore decrease the effect of oral anticoagulants, oral contraceptives, and barbiturates. See Rizack and Hilman[27] for a comprehensive list of drug interactions.

Pregnancy. Patients who are pregnant and nursing mothers also pose certain problems in the selection of appropriate antimicrobial agents. All antimicrobial agents cross the placenta in varying degrees.[28,29] Thus, the use of such agents in pregnant women provides direct exposure of the fetus to the adverse effects of the drug. Although there are few solid data on the teratogenic potential of most antimicrobial agents in humans, experience suggests that certain drugs such as the penicillins (with the possible exception of ticarcillin[30]), the cephalosporins, and erythromycin are unlikely to be teratogenic and are safe for pregnant women to use.[17,28,29] Metronidazole and ticarcillin have been shown to be teratogenic in rodents and thus should be avoided in pregnancy.[30,31] The teratogenic potential of many other drugs in humans, including rifampin and trimethoprim, is simply unknown.

A number of antimicrobials have been shown to be deleterious in pregnancy. Tetracycline heads the list. The possible adverse effects of this drug on fetal dentition have already been noted. In addition, pregnant women receiving tetracycline are particularly vulnerable to certain toxic effects including acute fatty necrosis of the liver, pancreatitis, and probably renal damage,[12] The liver damage may be severe and can result in death. When administered to patients with impaired renal function, these effects may be magnified, particularly if the agent is one of the tetracyclines that is primarily excreted by the kidneys. These adverse effects are dose related and may be more frequent after intravenous administration. Although it has been suggested that tetracyclines may be given to pregnant women by the oral route in doses of 1 g or less per 24 hours, it is probably safer to avoid these agents entirely in pregnancy.[12,17]

The aminoglycosidic aminocyclitol antibiotics cross the placenta. So far fetal toxicity has been reported only for streptomycin when used to treat tuberculosis in pregnant women. Even in that setting, the toxicity has been mild, detectable only by formal vestibular testing or by an audiogram.[32] Psychomotor retardation, myoclonus, and convulsions have been reported in a small uncontrolled series of children whose mothers received isoniazid for tuberculosis during pregnancy.[33] This observation has not been confirmed to date.

Another aspect of drug therapy in pregnancy has recently been examined. It has been found that serum levels after a given dose of ampicillin are lower in pregnant than in nonpregnant women.[34] This is related to more rapid clearance of the drug and to a greater volume of distribution (probably due to increased plasma volume) in pregnancy. Thus, higher doses of ampicillin are required to achieve therapeutic blood levels in pregnancy. It is likely that these observations will also apply to other antimicrobial agents, but data on this are not presently available.

Virtually all antimicrobial agents appear in measurable concentrations in breast milk when administered in therapeutic doses to nursing women.[35] The amount of drug excreted into breast milk depends on its degree of ionization, its molecular weight, and its solubility in fat and water. Under usual circumstances, the concentrations of antibiotics found in breast milk are quite low. However, even these small amounts may cause significant adverse reactions in the nursing infant. Nalidixic acid and the sulfonamides in breast milk have been shown to cause hemolysis in infants with G6PD deficiency. Sulfonamides in breast milk may be dangerous to premature babies because even small doses of ingested sulfonamides may produce increased levels of unbound bilirubin by displacing bilirubin from its albumin binding sites. As noted previously, this predisposes the child to kernicterus.[35] The possibility that antimicrobial agents in breast milk can sensitize newborn children is a theoretic one, but it has not been convincingly demonstrated. Although tetracycline is excreted in breast milk, it is unlikely to produce damage to the nursing child's bones or teeth because the calcium in the milk forms an insoluble chelate with tetracyclines, which is not absorbable by the oral route.[35]

Renal and Hepatic Function. The ability of the patient to metabolize or excrete antimicrobial agents is one of the most important host factors to consider, especially when high serum or tissue concentrations of the administered drugs are potentially toxic. From a practical point of view, this means that one must carefully assess the patient's renal and hepatic function since these organs serve as the major (and in most cases the *only*) routes of excretion and/or inactivation of antimicrobials. Renal excretion is the most important route of elimination for most antimicrobial agents.[36–41] Table 2 lists those drugs that must be used with particular care in patients with decreased renal function. Doses for these drugs may be found in the chapters dealing with the individual agents and in Chapter 38. In general those agents that require no dosage change in impaired renal function are excreted effectively by extrarenal routes (usually the hepatobiliary system) in patients with renal failure. Their use in normal doses does not result in the appearance of toxic serum levels in this situation, although the urine levels of a number of these agents such as doxycycline and chloramphenicol may be significantly diminished.

Toxic serum levels of the remaining agents may develop if they are used without dosage modification in patients with impaired renal function. Excessive serum levels of penicillin G, carbenicillin, or imipenem may be associated with neuromuscular hyperexcitability, myoclonus, seizures, or coma.[12] Excessive serum levels of semisynthetic penicillins such as carbenicillin and ticarcillin or of cephalothin or moxalactam may cause hemostatic defects in patients with impaired renal failure because of interference with platelet function.[42,43] Elevated serum levels of aminoglycosidic aminocyclitol antibiotics or vancomycin may result in eighth nerve damage.[15,41] Neurotoxic reactions including respiratory arrest and death may occur in patients with excessive serum levels of certain aminoglycosidic aminocyclitols or the polymyxins.[12,24] Bone marrow suppression may occur in patients with renal failure who receive inappropriately high doses of 5-fluorocytosin.[44] In all the above situations, the possibility of toxic reactions can be significantly lessened or eliminated if the doses of the antimicrobial agents are appropriately reduced in the presence of renal insufficiency.

The tetracyclines (except doxycycline and possibly minocycline) are contraindicated in patients with impaired renal function because the elevated serum levels that result may produce a significant worsening of the uremic state due to their antianabolic effect. Moreover, they may cause enhanced hepatotoxicity in this situation.[12] Cephaloridine and the long-acting sulfonamides should be avoided in this situation because they are potentially nephrotoxic.

Certain antimicrobial agents, including erythromycin, chloramphenicol, lincomycin, and clindamycin, should be used with caution in patients with impaired hepatic function.[45] These drugs are primarily excreted or detoxified in the liver. Bone marrow suppression due to chloramphenicol is much more likely to occur in patients with impaired hepatic function; because of this, it has been suggested that the dose of chloramphenicol be cut at least in half in patients with cirrhosis and other severe liver disease.[46] The serum half-life of clindamycin is increased in patients with severe liver disease; because of this, the dose should be decreased in this situation. The tetracyclines may produce elevations in serum transaminase levels in patients recovering from viral hepatitis.[12] They should be avoided or used with extreme caution in patients with underlying liver disease. The serum half-lives of both rifampin and isoniazid are prolonged in patients with cirrhosis.[47] Other drugs that should be used with caution or for which serum levels should be monitored in patients with severe liver disease include metronidazole, ketoconazole, miconazole, nitrofurantoin, fusidic acid, and pyrazinamide.[45] Hepatobiliary disease influences antimicrobic therapy in still another way. The biliary concentrations of many antimicrobial agents, including ampicillin and nafcillin, that are normally excreted in high concentration in the bile may be significantly reduced in patients with liver disease or biliary obstruction.[12]

TABLE 2. Antimicrobial Use in Patients with Varying Degrees of Impaired Renal Function

Antimicrobial agents requiring no dosage change regardless of renal function
Erythromycin, clindamycin, chloramphenicol, doxycycline, cefoperazone, oxacillin, cloxacillin, dicloxacillin, nafcillin, rifampin, amphotericin B,[a] cefaclor, ceftriaxone, metronidazole
Antimicrobial agents requiring dosage change only with severe renal failure
Penicillin G, amoxicillin, ampicillin, methicillin, cephalothin, cephalexin, cefamandole, cefoxitin, cefotaxime, ceftizoxime, piperacillin, isoniazid, ethambutol, trimethoprim-sulfamethoxazole, cefotetan, ceftazidime, cefuroxime, cefonicid, mezlocillin, nalidixic acid, ciprofloxacin, norfloxacin
Antimicrobial agents requiring dosage change with impaired renal function
Carbenicillin, ticarcillin, cefazolin, moxalactan, streptomycin, kanamycin, gentamicin, tobramycin, amikacin, netilmicin, polymxyin B, colistin, vancomycin, flucytosine, imipenem
Antimicrobial agents contraindicated in renal failure
Tetracyclines (except doxycycline and possibly minocycline), nitrofurantoin, cephaloridine, long-acting sulfonamides, methenamine, para-aminosalicyclic acid

[a] Even though amphotericin B is excreted primarily by nonrenal means, this drug must be used with caution in patients with impaired renal function because of its nephrotoxicity.

Site of Infection. Of all the host factors to be considered in the choice of an antimicrobial agent, none is more important than the site of infection. The locus of the infectious process determines not only the choice of the agent but also its dose and the route by which it should be administered. For antimicrobial therapy to be effective, an adequate concentration of the drug must be delivered to the site of infection. In most cases, this means that the local concentration of the antimicrobial agent should at least equal the MIC of the infecting organism. Concentrations representing multiples of the MIC are generally felt more likely to be efficacious, but in many cases such local concentrations may be difficult or impossible to achieve. A failure to achieve local concentrations of antibiotics higher than the MIC of the infecting organism may not always be disastrous, however, because there is evidence that subinhibitory concentrations of drugs may produce antimicrobial effects that aid the host defenses against infections. It has been clearly demonstrated that subinhibitory concentrations of antibiotics can alter bacterial morphology,[48] adherence properties,[49] and opsonic requirements[50]; can enhance phagocytosis[51]; and can even aid intracellular killing of bacteria by polymorphonuclear leukocytes.[52] This may explain the clinical observation that, on occasion, doses of antimicrobials that produce seemingly inadequate serum levels may still result in clinical cure. In spite of such observations, most infectious disease clinicians feel that optimal therapy requires concentrations of antimicrobials that are above the MIC.

Serum concentrations of antimicrobial agents are relatively easy to determine and therefore are often used as a guide in the therapy. However, except in cases of bacteremia, antimicrobial efficacy is more likely determined by the tissue concentration than by blood level, as noted earlier. Moreover, there are some agents such as spiromycin and certain macrolides that are effective in vivo despite an inability to achieve serum levels above the MICs of certain organisms. This may be explained by the ability to achieve intracellular and tissue concentrations that far exceed those obtained in serum.[53] Binding to serum proteins may affect both the tissue distribution and the activity of antimicrobial agents in the blood. Although much careful investigation has been done on protein binding, the precise clinical significance of this phenomenon remains to be determined. For example, it has been shown that only the unbound form of a given antimicrobial agent is active in vitro (and presumably also in vivo) against infecting organisms.[54] However, since protein binding is rapidly reversible,[55] the activity of even highly protein-bound agents may not be absolutely limited by protein binding. The penetration of antimicrobial agents into interstitial fluid and lymph is related to protein binding since only the free form of the agent is able to pass through the capillary wall.[54] Penetration of antibiotics into fibrin clots (which may be analogous to the penetration of the drugs to reach the site of infection in patients with bacterial endocarditis) is likewise related to the amount of unbound antibiotic in the surrounding fluid.[56] Nevertheless, it is often difficult to correlate therapeutic outcome with in vitro susceptibility and protein binding unless several variables are carefully controlled.[51,58] The reason for this is simply that it is the concentration of antibiotic at the site of infection that is the major determinant in the successful therapy. Such concentrations are often difficult to assess because they are the result of a complex interaction between local factors that may bind, inactivate, or enhance the activity of a given antimicrobial agent. The ability of an antibiotic to pass through membranes by nonionic diffusion is related to its lipid solubility. Thus, lipid-soluble agents such as chloramphenicol, rifampin, trimethoprim, and isoniazid are all more adept at penetrating membranes than are the more highly ionized compounds.[54] These agents rapidly cross the blood-brain barrier and produce better cerebrospinal fluid levels than do more highly ionized compounds such as the aminoglycosidic aminocyclitols. Except in neonates, none of the aminoglycosides produces effective cerebrospinal fluid levels when given parenterally. To be effective for the treatment of meningitis, they must be given via the intrathecal or intraventricular route in adults.[59] This is an excellent example of the importance of the site of infection in determining the most efficacious antimicrobial therapy. For the treatment of bacterial meningitis in adults, we either must choose agents such as chloramphenicol or the third-generation cephalosporins (e.g., cefotaxime, ceftriaxone, or ceftazidime) that cross the blood-brain barrier reasonably well, or we must use high concentrations of parenteral doses of drugs such as penicillin G, ampicillin, or nafcillin that penetrate into the cerebrospinal fluid only with difficulty. Agents such as the aminoglycosidic aminocyclitols and first-generation cephalosporins that produce inadequate cerebrospinal fluid levels even after high-dose parenteral therapy must be administered directly into the cerebrospinal fluid or must be avoided entirely.

The vegetations of bacterial endocarditis, bones, and devitalized tissue represent examples of other areas in which the penetration of antimicrobial agents to the site of infection may be borderline or inadequate. Because of this, high-dose and prolonged parenteral therapy is usually required for the effective treatment of bacterial endocarditis and osteomyelitis. In some cases, we may take advantage of the physiologic handling of antimicrobials to achieve therapeutic success. Agents that are excreted by the liver and are concentrated in the bile such as ampicillin or doxycycline may be more effective in treating cholangitis than are agents such as the first-generation cephalosporins or aminoglycosidic aminocyclitols that are not greatly concentrated in bile. The new fluoroquinolones may owe some of their effectiveness in the treatment of osteomyelitis to their ability to achieve superior concentrations in bone.[60]

Even the achievement of "therapeutic concentrations" of antimicrobial agents at the site of infection may not be sufficient for cure. The reason for this is that a number of local factors may influence the activity of antimicrobial agents. These, too, must be considered in designing an appropriate therapeutic regimen. Aminoglycosidic aminocyclitols and the polymyxins are bound to and inactivated by purulent material.[61] This is one of many reasons why surgical drainage is imperative when treating abscesses with agents such as these. Interestingly, carbenicillin does not lose activity in pus.[61] Although carbenicillin (and other penicillins) may be more active in purulent material, clinical experience strongly suggests that appropriate drainage procedures greatly enhance the efficacy of these agents as well. Although penicillin G, like carbenicillin, is not inactivated by purulent material per se,[54] recent studies suggest that the presence of β-lactamase–producing organisms such as *Bacteroides fragilis* in abscesses may result in local inactivation of penicillin G and other β-lactam antibiotics.[62]

Pencillins and tetracyclines are also bound by hemoglobin and thus may be less effective in the presence of significant hematoma formation.[54] In vitro *Pseudomonas aeruginosa* is protected from the action of the aminoglycosidic aminocyclitols and polymyxins by high concentrations of calcium or magnesium in the culture medium.[63] The clinical significance of this observation, if any, remains to be determined. Local decreases in oxygen tension such as occur in abscesses and intraperitoneal infections may also have an effect on the activity of certain antimicrobial agents. The aminoglycosidic aminocyclitols, for example, are inactive against anaerobes and may also be less effective against facultative organisms under anaerobic conditions because oxygen is required for the transport of these agents into the bacterial cell.[64]

Local alterations in pH such as occur in abscesses and especially in the urine may have an important effect on the activity of a number of antimicrobial agents. Methenamine, nitrofurantoin, novobiocin, and chlortetracycline are more active at an acid pH, whereas alkalinization enhances the activity of erythromycin, lincomycin, clindamycin, and the aminoglycosidic aminocyclitol antibiotics. Indeed, the aminoglycosidic aminocyclitols show a marked loss of activity at a low pH. These observations have been used in treating patients with urinary tract infections, a situation in which the local pH can be altered by the addition of acidifying or alkalinizing agents.[65,66]

The presence of foreign bodies also has a profound effect on the activity of antimicrobial agents. Thus, it is often necessary to remove the foreign material to cure an infection in the vicinity of a prosthetic heart valve or joint implant.[67] The mechanism by which foreign bodies potentiate infection is not clear, but they probably cause localized impairment of host defense mechanisms.[68] In addition, the foreign body often serves as a nidus on which organisms can adhere and produce extracellular substances such as glycocalyx or slime that may interfere with phagocytosis and impair the penetration of antibiotics to the underlying organisms.[69] It has also been demonstrated that antimicrobial agents themselves may cause alterations in host defenses. Clinically achievable concentrations of many different agents have been shown to have adverse effects on leukocyte chemotaxis, lymphocyte transformation, monocyte transformation, delayed hypersensitivity, antibody production, phagocytosis, and the microbicidal action of polymorphonuclear leukocytes.[70–76] It is not clear, however, whether any of these effects (largely demonstrated by in vitro studies) are of clinical significance.[76] Nonetheless, the possibility that antimicrobial agents can cause immunosuppression exists, and this fact should discourage the indiscriminate use of antibiotics, especially in patients who are already immunosuppressed because of their underlying disease or because of their concomitant drug therapy.[74]

ANTIMICROBIAL COMBINATIONS

Most infections in humans can be treated with a single antimicrobial agent, but there are clear-cut (as well as borderline) indications for the use of combinations (usually two) of antimicrobials. Because combinations may provide more broad-spectrum coverage than single agents can, the physician is often tempted to use combinations for the sense of security they provide, even in situations in which they are not indicated. Such inappropriate use of antimicrobial combinations may have significantly deleterious effects. In this section we will examine indications for the use of combinations and the potential disadvantages of this approach to therapy.

In Vitro Results of Combination Therapy

When two antimicrobial agents are combined, they may have one of three types of activity against a given organism in vitro: (*1*) an additive effect (sometimes called an indifferent effect), (*2*) synergism, and (*3*) antagonism.[77] Two drugs are said to be additive when the activity of the drugs in combination is equal to the sum (or a partial sum) of their independent activities when studied separately. The combined effect of a synergistic pair of antimicrobials is greater than the sum of their independent activities when measured separately. If two drugs are antagonistic, the activity of the combination is less than the sum of their independent effects when measured alone. These concepts are illustrated by "time-kill curves" in Figure 1. The various methods used to determine the in vitro effects of antibiotic combinations are beyond the scope of this chapter but have been reviewed in detail.[78]

Indications for the Clinical Use of Antimicrobial Combinations

Five reasons have been advanced to justify the use of antimicrobial combinations. The first three of these are discussed in detail in other chapters and, therefore, will be given only brief mention here.

Prevention of the Emergence of Resistant Organisms. Although the use of antimicrobial agents to prevent the emergence of resistant organisms would seem to be a major indication for the use of such therapy, combination therapy has been clearly documented as effective in preventing resistance only during the treatment of tuberculosis (see Chapters 32 and 229). There is somewhat less epidemiologic evidence in support of this concept as it applies to the use of rifampin for the treatment of nonmycobacterial infections, but it nonetheless appears that one of the major benefits of using rifampin in combination with a second agent for treating staphylococcal infections, for example, is that the combination prevents the rapid emergence of resistance to rifampin, which is evident when this drug is used alone.[80,81]

Polymicrobial Infections. In most infections, even those due to more than one organism, a single effective agent can be found. For example, cellulitis due to *S. aureus* and group A streptococci can be treated with a penicillinase-resistant penicillin alone. However, there are certain types of infections due to such a broad variety of organisms that more than one antimicrobial agent may be required to provide adequate coverage. Examples of such infections include intraperitoneal and pelvic infections due to mixed bowel flora and certain brain abscesses (see Chapters 60, 70, and 96).

Initial Therapy. In neutropenic patients or other patients with presumed infection in whom the nature of the infection is not clear, it may be reasonable to begin broad-spectrum coverage, usually with two agents such as ticarcillin plus gentamicin or tobramycin while awaiting the results of cultures. In this setting, it is often possible to discontinue treatment with one of the agents or to switch to an alternate single drug after the results of cultures are available (see Chapter 29). The development of new drugs with broad spectra of activity makes it possible to use a single agent for most cases of initial therapy, but it would be premature to advocate a general application of this concept at present.

Decreased Toxicity. Many of the drugs used in therapy for infections are potentially toxic (e.g., aminoglycosidic aminocyclitols). Therefore, a major goal of combination therapy has been to reduce the amount of drug required for treatment and, thus, to reduce dose-related toxicity. Unfortunately, at present there are no data from clinical trials that establish beyond doubt that combination therapy with different agents permits a reduction of the drug dose sufficient to reduce dose-related toxicity. There is evidence that the use of a mixture of similar agents (e.g., triple sulfonamides) can reduce the incidence of a dose-related complication: crystalluria with stone formation.[82] The explanation for this effect is that the solubility of each component (sulfadiazine, sulfamerazine, sulfamethazine) in urine is independent of the others, although their antibacterial activity is cumulative.

Synergism. The use of synergistic combinations of antimicrobial agents to treat infections due to resistant or relatively resistant organisms represents one of the most appealing ways to use these agents. There are numerous examples of in vitro synergism, but thus far synergistic antimicrobial combinations have proved more effective than are single agents in only a limited number of clinical settings.[79,83]

Perhaps the best known application of synergistic combinations of antimicrobial agents is for the treatment of enterococcal endocarditis. Treatment of this disease with penicillin alone results in an unacceptable relapse rate because enterococci are relatively resistant to penicillin.[84] Indeed, penicillin alone seems to act as a bacteriostatic and not a bactericidal agent.[85] The addition of an aminoglycoside such as streptomycin or gentamicin results in both in vitro and in vivo synergism and yields clinical cure rates comparable to those achieved for endocarditis caused by less resistant streptococci.[84,85] Penicillin enhances the uptake of aminoglycosides by enterococci; the result of this interaction is the synergistic killing of the organisms.[86] In recent years some enterococci have been found to be resistant to penicillin-streptomycin, penicillin-kanamycin, and penicillin-amikacin synergism due to high-level resistance (MIC > 2000 μg/ml) to streptomycin and/or to kanamycin.[87] Strains may resist synergism if they are ribosomally resistant to streptomycin[88] or if they contain plasmid-mediated enzymes

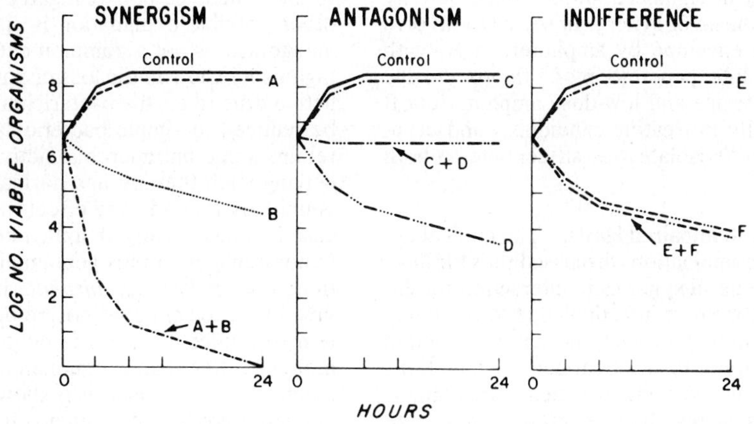

FIG. 1. Antibacterial effects of antibiotic combinations. *Left* (A and B): synergism; *center* (C and D): antagonism; *right* (E and F): indifference (additive). (From Moellering,[79] with permission.)

that inactivate streptomycin, kanamycin, or amikacin.[89] The prevalence of enterococci with high-level resistance to gentamicin appears to be increasing rapidly.[91] Moreover, the use of penicillin-gentamicin therapy in such patients may result in a failure to eradicate the infecting organisms.[92] Therefore it is important to test for high-level resistance to streptomycin and gentamicin before embarking on a therapeutic regimen for enterococcal endocarditis or meningitis.

Penicillin-streptomycin combinations are also synergistic against viridans streptococci and have been used for the treatment of endocarditis due to these organisms.[83] However, viridans streptococci are usually very susceptible to penicillin, and penicillin alone has been used successfully for treatment of this kind of endocarditis.[93,94]

A similar type of synergism occurs when semisynthetic penicillinase-resistant penicillins such as nafcillin or oxacillin are combined with gentamicin against *S. aureus*.[95] So far there are no data to document that the use of combination therapy for *S. aureus* infections in humans has any advantage over therapy with a penicillin or cephalosporin alone.[96]

Combinations of carbenicillin, ticarcillin, mezlocillin, azlocillin, or piperacillin with gentamicin, tobramycin, or amikacin exhibit synergism against many strains of *P. aeruginosa*.[97,98] The mechanism of synergism in this setting is similar to that described for enterococci (i.e., enhanced uptake of the aminoglycoside in the presence of the antipseudomonal penicillin). Studies with experimental animals convincingly demonstrate the superiority of such combinations for the treatment of serious *Pseudomonas* infections.[99] Although the information available from limited human trials to date is also consistent with enhanced activity of these combinations for *Pseudomonas* infections, this form of therapy has not been subjected to definitive controlled study.[78]

Synergism occurs by a different mechanism when sulfonamides are combined with trimethoprim. In this case, the two agents are synergistic because they act to inhibit sequential steps in the microbial pathway of folic acid metabolism.[100] As a result, combinations of sulfonamides with trimethoprim are often useful for the treatment of infections due to organisms that may be resistant to sulfonamides alone. A fixed combination of sulfamethoxazole and trimethoprim is available for clinical use and has been shown effective for the treatment and prevention of chronic urinary tract infections, even when due to sulfonamide-resistant organisms.[101] The combination has also been shown to be useful for the treatment of typhoid fever and shigellosis caused by organisms resistant to ampicillin and/or chloramphenicol, for the treatment of infections due to ampicillin-resistant *H. influenzae* and for therapy for a wide variety of other infections as well.[78,102–104]

Combinations of amphotericin B with a number of other agents including 5-fluorocytosine, rifampin, and tetracycline have been shown to result in enhanced antimicrobial activity against fungi.[105] The mechanism of synergism seems to involve damage to the fungal cell envelope by amphotericin B, with resultant enhanced intracellular penetration of 5-fluorocytosine and other agents.[105] Flucytosine and low-dose amphotericin B have been used successfully in treating candidiasis and cryptococcosis when the patient's isolate was susceptible to both drugs.[106,107]

Synergism and Infections in Impaired Hosts. The clinical applications of antimicrobial combinations discussed thus far have all represented attempts to use a synergistic interaction for enhanced efficacy in the treatment of infections due to relatively resistant organisms. Another use of such therapy is to obtain enhanced antimicrobial activity in the treatment of infections due to susceptible organisms occurring in patients with abnormalities of host defense systems. Several groups have conducted randomized trials of various combinations of two agents chosen from among carbenicillin, ticarcillin, piperacillin, the cephalosporins, gentamicin, tobramycin, and amikacin for the treatment of severe infections in patients with impaired host defense mechanisms. Both Lau et al.[108] and Klastersky et al.[109] have demonstrated improved survival rates in such patients treated with combinations that were synergistic against the infecting organisms as compared with patients receiving nonsynergistic combinations. These studies add strong support to the concept that synergistic combinations of antimicrobials may be an important determinant of success in the treatment of serious infections, especially when due to gram-negative organisms in patients with impaired host defenses. However, there is no absolute proof that synergistic combinations are more effective in this setting than are single agents that have a sufficiently broad spectrum and that produce sufficiently high serum bactericidal titers against the infecting organisms.[110]

Disadvantages of the Inappropriate Use of Antimicrobial Combinations

Whereas the clinical use of synergistic combinations of antimicrobial agents may have beneficial results as noted above, the inappropriate use of antimicrobial combinations may have important adverse effects, three of which will be discussed below.

Antagonism. The medical literature contains a large number of reports of in vitro antagonism between antimicrobial agents.[79,83] In view of this, it is surprising that there are only a few well-documented clinical examples of antagonism. Perhaps the most impressive is the study of Lepper and Dowling, who demonstrated conclusively in 1951 that penicillin is more effective than is the combination of penicillin with chlortetracycline for the treatment of pneumococcal meningitis.[111] The fatality among patients treated with penicillin alone was 21 percent, whereas that among patients treated with penicillin plus chlortetracycline was 79 percent. A study of childhood meningitis has also demonstrated the superiority of single-drug therapy. Mathies et al. treated a group of children suffering from bacterial meningitis with either ampicillin alone or a combination of ampicillin, chloramphenicol, and streptomycin.[112] The mortality among 140 children treated with ampicillin alone was 4.3 percent, whereas the mortality among 124 children receiving the antibiotic combination was 10.5 percent, a difference that reached statistical significance. There are several other reports of the influence of antagonism on the treatment of urinary tract infections and streptococcal pharyngitis, but none are particularly impressive.[79] Considering the extensive clinical use of antimicrobial combinations and especially in view of the large number of reports of in vitro antagonism, it is surprising that there are so few reports of in vivo antagonism. This may be due in part to the paucity of well-controlled studies in this area or to the reluctance of investigators to report adverse results. Another possible explanation is simply that clinically significant antagonism is not a common event. In most cases, in vitro antagonism results in the loss or partial loss of activity of the most active drug (e.g., the bactericidal activity of such an agent may be reduced to simple bacteriostasis), but the combination still retains some antimicrobial activity. As long as the patient receiving such therapy has normal host defense mechanisms, it is unlikely that adverse effects will be seen. This has been the case in studies using an antagonistic combination of antibiotics (chloramphenicol plus gentamicin) to treat experimental infections due to *Proteus mirabilis* in mice.[113] In healthy mice, in vivo antagonism could not be demonstrated, but after irradiation to render the animals neutropenic, gentamicin alone was more effective than gentamicin plus chloramphenicol was. This combination has also been shown to be antagonistic in experimentally produced meningitis due to *P. mirabilis* in rabbits.[114] Thus, it seems that clinically important antagonism is most likely to be manifested in patients with generalized impairment of host defense mechanisms (such as seen in leukemia, cancer patients who are neutropenic, etc.) or in patients with infections such as meningitis or endocarditis where localized host defenses may be inadequate.

The observation of in vivo antagonism in the treatment of bacterial meningitis raises some questions about the recommendations of the use of ampicillin plus chloramphenicol in the initial treatment of childhood meningitis (see Chapter 66) because of the emergence of ampicillin-resistant strains of *H. influenzae*.[8] Combinations of penicillin plus chloramphenicol have been shown to exhibit in vitro antagonism against pneumococci and other organisms.[83] However, this antagonism takes the form of lessened bactericidal activity of penicillin in the presence of chloramphenicol. Since chloramphenicol alone is quite active against the organisms likely to cause childhood meningitis. (*H. influenzae, S. pneumoniae, Neisseria meningitidis*) and since there is no evidence that penicillin or ampicillin antagonizes the activity of chloramphenicol, it seems unlikely that the current recommendations for pediatric meningitis will result in in vivo antagonism when used to treat meningitis due to the organisms listed above.[83]

Studies documenting the effectiveness of some of the newer cephalosporins such as cefuroxime and ceftriazone[115,116] for childhood meningitis may ultimately make it unnecessary to continue to use combination therapy in this setting.

There has been a recent upsurge of interest in the use of the newer broad-spectrum β-lactams in combination with each other to obtain broad-spectrum coverage without exposing the patient to the possible toxicity of an agent such as chloramphenicol or an aminoglycosidic aminocyclitol.[117] For the most part, this seems reasonable. However, there is in vitro and in vivo evidence that some β-lactam–β-lactam combinations may be antagonistic against certain organisms such as *Enterobacter, Serratia,* or *Pseudomonas*. This antagonism seems to be the result of the induction or derepression inactivation of the second.[118] The exact clinical significance of this phenomenon is not presently clear, but it must be kept in mind when one considers the clinical use of such combinations.

Most of the examples of in vitro antagonism are the result of interactions of the antimicrobial agents as they react at a subcellular level on a given microorganism. However, another type of antagonism should also be included in this discussion. This may result from the direct interaction of drugs before they reach the microorganism. If chloramphenicol and erythromycin are inadvertently mixed together in the same parenteral infusion solution, they form insoluble precipitates and hence lose activity. In recent years, it has become clear that the mixing of penicillins (especially carbenicillin or ticarcillin) with aminoglycosides results in the inactivation of the aminoglycoside.[119] Because the reaction occurs slowly, this is usually not a problem in vivo, provided the drugs are given by separate routes of administration. However, in uremic patients in whom the serum half-life of aminoglycosides is greatly prolonged, in vivo inactivation can occur.[120] The clinical significance of this observation, however, has not yet been elucidated.

Cost. With the possible exception of penicillin G and certain of the tetracyclines and sulfonamides, antimicrobials are expensive drugs. Thus the inappropriate use of antimicrobial combinations (when a single agent would be adequate) can add greatly to the cost of the patient's illness. This important consideration is discussed in greater detail in Chapter 37.

Adverse Effects. It has been estimated that approximately 5 percent of the patients receiving a given antibiotic in the hospital will experience some sort of adverse reaction.[14,121] Obviously the possibility of such adverse reactions (including hypersensitivity reactions and direct toxic effects) is increased without any enhanced therapeutic benefit when one inappropriately uses combinations of antimicrobial agents. Moreover, when an adverse reaction occurs in a patient receiving more than one drug, it is often difficult to be certain of the agent that caused the reaction. This may mean that treatment with several or all drugs must be stopped. If combination drug therapy is to be used in such a patient, each drug must be tested carefully before use to make certain that it was not the cause of the original adverse reaction. This is time-consuming and expensive and may needlessly deprive the patient of the benefits of a useful agent.

CHOICE OF APPROPRIATE ROUTE OF ADMINISTRATION OF ANTIMICROBIAL AGENTS AND EVALUATION OF EFFICACY

Route of Administration

Once the physician has determined the most appropriate drug or drugs with which to treat a given infection, he must decide which route of administration to use to obtain maximum benefits from the therapy. In most cases this is a choice between oral and parenteral routes. In general, the oral route of administration is chosen for those infections that are mild and can be treated on an outpatient basis. Not all antibiotics can be administered in this way. Drugs such as vancomycin, the polymyxins, the aminoglycosidic aminocyclitols, and amphotericin B are absorbed so poorly from the gastrointestinal tract that they cannot be administered orally to treat systemic infections. When drugs are administered by the oral route, the physician must ascertain that the patient will reliably take them as ordered. The absorption of certain agents such as penicillin G is markedly impaired if taken with meals, whereas the absorption of acid-stable penicillins such as penicillin V is not affected by food or gastric acidity. The concomitant administration of antacids or iron-containing preparations may severely impair the absorption of tetracycline since this drug forms insoluble chelates in the presence of Mg^{2+}, Ca^{2+}, or Fe^{2+} ions. Antacids and histamine antagonists may also interfere with the absorption of the fluoroquinolones such as ciprofloxacin and norfloxacin.[122] More detailed information on the oral absorption of antimicrobial agents may be found in the chapters on the individual drugs.

The parenteral route of administration is used for agents that are inefficiently absorbed from the gastrointestinal tract and for the treatment of patients with serious infections in whom high serum concentrations of antimicrobial agents are required. The aminoglycosidic aminocyclitols and polymyxins may be given by intramuscular injection and are well tolerated when given this way. For most infections, adequate serum concentrations are achieved after the intramuscular administration of these drugs. However, in life-threatening infections, especially in the presence of shock (or in diabetic patients as discussed earlier), intravenous administration is preferred. Intravenous administration allows large doses of drugs to be given with a minimum of discomfort to the patient when high serum concentrations are required for the effective treatment of disease processes such as meningitis, endocarditis, and osteomyelitis. Whether intravenously administered drugs should be given by continuous infusion or by intermittent bolus infusion remains a matter of controversy. The former method has the advantage of simplicity; because pulses containing very high concentrations of drugs are avoided, it may result in less venous irritation and phlebitis. Studies in animal models suggest that the concentration of drugs such as penicillins and cephalosporins in fibrin clots is related to the peak serum levels achieved. Thus, greater concentrations of drugs are achieved in the clots in the face of intermittent bolus therapy.[123] It has been suggested that this data may be applicable to therapy for infective endocarditis and other infections in which high tissue concentrations of antibiotics are required. Convincing clinical proof of this concept, however, does not exist.

As discussed earlier, the intrathecal or intraventricular route of administration may be necessary for the treatment of meningeal infections with drugs such as the aminoglycosidic aminocyclitols, polymyxins, bacitracin, and possibly vancomycin, all of which cross the blood-brain barrier with considerable difficulty. The parenteral administration of antimicrobial agents results in adequate concentrations in pleural, peritoneal, pericardial, and synovial fluids. Thus, direct instillation of antibiotics into these areas is not necessary.

Monitoring the Response of the Patient to Antimicrobial Therapy

Although several laboratory tests are available to assist in the monitoring of antimicrobial therapy, clinical assessment remains the most important method for determining the efficacy of treatment. It is not uncommon to see patients fail to respond in the face of laboratory studies that suggest adequate therapy and vice versa. The reasons for this may usually be found among the many host factors that affect therapy as described earlier.

Nonetheless, the measurement of serum concentrations of antimicrobial agents and a determination of serum bactericidal titers are often of considerable use. The details concerning these tests are given in Chapter 13 and will not be repeated here. The major value of the direct determination of serum concentrations of antimicrobial agents is to avoid toxicity from excessive levels of agents such as the aminoglycosidic aminocyclitols and vancomycin, especially in patients with impaired renal or hepatic function. These tests are also useful for determining inadequate serum levels due to insufficient dosing or unusually rapid clearance.

Another method used to monitor the effectiveness of antimicrobial therapy is the serum bactericidal titer (sometimes called the serum antimicrobial dilution titer). This test was originally described by Schlichter and MacLean as a guide for effective therapy for subacute bacterial endocarditis.[126] Subsequently this test has been used to monitor therapy in patients with infective endocarditis, osteomyelitis, septic arthritis, empyema, and bacteremia.[109,127] In this test, serial dilutions of the patient's serum are incubated with an inoculum of the infecting organism; after incubation, the highest dilution that inhibits and/or kills the organism is determined. Most investigators feel that a serum bactericidal titer of at least 1:8 can be correlated with a successful therapeutic outcome.[109,126,128,130] A more recent multicenter study has suggested that peak and trough titers of at least 1:64 and 1:32, respectively, are good predictors of a successful therapeutic outcome in patients with infective endocarditis.[129] However, a lack of standardization and a lack of consistency in specifying the point (peak, trough, or midpoint serum levels) at which the test should be done have hindered attempts at more widespread application and evaluation of this test.[131–134]

CONCLUSION

Optimal use of antimicrobial agents demands consideration of a large number of important factors that may influence the choice of an appropriate agent and that determine the most effective dose and route of administration of a drug. A number of these factors have been outlined in this chapter. In the final analysis, sound clinical judgment remains the most important determinant of a successful outcome.

REFERENCES

1. Weinstein L. General considerations. In: Goodman LS, Gilman A, eds. The Pharmacological Basis of Therapeutics. New York. Macmillan; 1970:1154.
2. Majno G. The Healing Hand: Man and Wound in the Ancient World. Cambridge, MA: Harvard University Press; 1975:154,215.
3. Harris JC, Dupont HL, Hornick RB. Fecal leukocytes in diarrheal illness. Ann Intern Med. 1972;76:697.
4. Ho D, Ault MJ, Ault MA, et al. *Campylobacter* enteritis. Early diagnosis with Gram's stain. Arch Intern Med. 1982;142:1858.
5. Weinstein L. Common sense (clinical judgment) in the diagnosis and antibiotic therapy of etiologically undefined infections. Pediatr Clin North Am. 1968;15:141.
6. Moellering RC Jr. A rational approach to the choice of antimicrobial agents in bacterial infections. In: Seminar on Gram-Negative Infections. St Louis: 1974:5.
7. Thornsberry C. Automated procedures for antimicrobial susceptibility tests. In: Lennette EH, Balows A, Hausler WJ Jr, et al., eds. Manual of Clinical Microbiology. Washington DC: American Society for Microbiology; 1985:1015.
8. Murray BE, Moellering RC Jr. Patterns and mechanisms of antibiotic resistance. Med Clin North Am. 1978;62:899.
9. Puoff KL. Gram-positive vancomycin-resistant clinical isolates. Clin Microbiol Newsletter. 1989;11:1.
10. Moellering RC Jr, Kunz LJ, Poitras JW, et al. Microbiologic basis for the rational use of antibiotics. South Med J. 1977;70(Suppl):8.
11. Abramowicz M, ed. The choice of antimicrobial drugs. Med Lett. 1988;30:33.
12. Weinstein L, Dalton AC. Host determinants of response to antimicrobial agents. N Engl J Med. 1968;279:467.
13. Moellering RC Jr. Factors influencing the clinical use of antimicrobial agents in elderly patients. Geriatrics. 1978;33:83.
14. Mannisto PT, Mantyla R, Nykanen S, et al. Impairing effect of food on ketoconazole absorption. Antimicrob Agents Chemother. 1982;21:730.
15. Jackson GG, Arcieri G. Ototoxicity of gentamicin in man: A survey and controlled analysis of clinical experience in the United States. J Infect Dis. 1969;119:432.
16. Calderwood S, Moellering RC Jr. Common adverse effects of antibacterial agents on major organ systems. Surg Clin North Am. 1980;60:65.
17. Moellering RC Jr. Antimicrobial agents in pregnancy and the postpartum period. Clin Obstet Gynecol. 1989;22:277.
18. McCracken GH Jr. Pharmacologic basis for antimicrobial therapy in newborn infants. Am J Dis Child. 1974;128:407.
19. Kline AH, Blattner RJ, Lunin M. Transplacental effect of tetracyclines on teeth. JAMA. 1964;118:178.
20. Hoyer D, Walfson J. Adverse effects of quinolone antibiotics. In: Hooper D, Wolfson J, eds. Quinolone Antimicrobial Agents. Washington DC: American Society for Microbiology; 1989:249–271.
21. Garibaldi RA, Drusin RE, Ferebee SH, et al. Isoniazid-associated hepatitis. Am Rev Respir Dis. 1972;106:357.
22. Anonymous. Preventive therapy of tuberculous infection. MMWR. 1975;24:71.
23. Foord RD. Cephaloridine, cephalothin and the kidney. J Antimicrob Chemother. 1975;1(Suppl):119.
24. Koch-Weser J, Sidel VW, Federman EB, et al. Adverse effects of sodium colistimethate. Ann Intern Med. 1970;72:857.
25. Van Scoy RE. Antituberculous agents. Mayo Clin Proc. 1977;52:694.
26. Young DS, Thomas DW, Friedman RB, et al. Effects of drugs on clinical laboratory tests. Clin Chem. 1972;18:1041.
27. Rizack MA, Hilman CDM. The Medical Letter Handbook of Drug Interactions. New Rochelle, NY: The Medical Letter; 1983.
28. Sabath LD. Antibiotics in obstetric practice. In: Charles D, Finland M, eds. Obstetric and Perinatal Infections. Philadelphia: Lea & Febiger; 1973:563.
29. Monif GRG. Infectious Diseases in Obstetrics and Gynecology. Hagerstown, MD: Harper & Row; 1974:18.
30. Anonymous. Ticarcillin. Med Lett. 1977;19:17.
31. Anonymous. Is Flagyl dangerous? Med Lett. 1975;17:53.
32. Conway N, Birt BD. Streptomycin in pregnancy: Effect in foetal ear. Br Med J. 1965:2:260.
33. Monnet P, Kalb JC, Pujol M. Toxic influence of isoniazid on fetus. Lyon Med. 1967;218:431.
34. Philipson A. Pharmakokinetics of ampicillin during pregnancy. J Infect Dis. 1977;136:370.
35. Vorherr H. Drug excretion in breast milk. Postgrad Med. 1974;56:97.
36. Reeves DS. The effect of renal failure on the pharmacokinetics of antibiotics. J Antimicrob Chemother. 1988;21:5.
37. Jackson EA, McLeod DC. Pharmacokinetics and dosing of antimicrobial agents in renal impairment, part i. Am J Hosp Pharm. 1974;31:36.
38. Jackson EA, McLeod DC. Pharmacokinetics and dosing of antimicrobial agents in renal impairment, part ii. Am J Hosp Pharm. 1974;31:137.
39. Cheigh J. Drug administration in renal failure. Am J Med. 1977;62:555.
40. Bennett WM, Singer I, Coggins CJ. A guide to drug therapy in renal failure. JAMA. 1974;230:1544.
41. Appel GB, Neu HC. The nephrotoxicity of antimicrobial agents. N Engl J Med. 1977;296:663,722.
42. Natelson EA, Brown CH III, Bradshaw MW, et al. Influence of cephalosporin antibiotics on blood coagulation and platelet function. Antimicrob Agents Chemother. 1976;9:91.
43. Neu HC. Adverse effects of new cephalosporins. Ann Intern Med. 1983;98:415.
44. Kaufman CA, Frame PT. Bone marrow toxicity associated with 5-fluorocytosine therapy. Antimicrob Agents Chemother. 1977;11:244.
45. Davey PG. Pharmacokinetics in liver disease. J Antimicrob Chemother. 1988;21:1.
46. Suhrland LG, Weisberger AS. Choramphenicol toxicity in liver and renal disease. Arch Intern Med. 1963;112:747.

47. Pessayre D, Allemand H, Benhamou J-P. Effets des maladies du foie et des voies biliaires sur le métabolisme des médicaments. Nouv Presse Med. 1977;35:3209.
48. Lorian V, Atkinson B. Killing of oxacillin-exposed staphylococci in human polymorphonuclear leukocytes. Antimicrob Agents Chemother. 1980;18:807.
49. Ofek IE, Beachey H, Eisenstein BI, et al. Suppression of bacterial adherence by subminimal inhibitory concentration of β-lactam and aminoglycoside antibiotics. Rev Infect Dis. 1979;1:832.
50. Gemmell CG, Peterson PK, Schmeling DJ, et al. Potentiation of opsonization and phagocytosis of *Streptococcus pyogenes* following growth in the presence of clindamycin. J Clin Invest. 1981;67:1249.
51. Friedman HH, Warren GH. Enhanced susceptibility of penicillin-resistant staphylococci to phagocytosis after in vitro incubation with low dose of nafcillin. Proc Soc Exp Biol Med. 1974;146:707.
52. Elliott GR, Peterson PK, Verbrugh HA, et al. Influence of subinhibitory concentrations of penicillin, cephalothin, and clindamycin on *Staphyloccus aureus* growth in human phagocytic cells. Antimicrob Agents Chemother. 1982;22:781.
53. Smith CR. The spiramycin paradox. J Antimicrob Chemother. 1988;22(Suppl B):141.
54. Craig WA, Kunin CM. Significance of serum protein and tissue binding of antimicrobial agents. Annu Rev Med. 1976;27:287.
55. Peterson LR, Gerding DN. Interaction of cephalosporins with human and canine serum proteins. J Infect Dis. 1978;137:452.
56. Barza M, Samuelson T, Weinstein L. Penetration of antibiotics into fibrin loci in vivo. II. Comparison of nine antibiotics: Effect of dose and degree of protein binding. J Infect Dis. 1974;129:66.
57. Kunst MW, Mattie H. Cefazolin and cephradine. Relationship between antibacterial activity in vitro and in mice experimentally infected with *Escherichia coli*. J Infect Dis. 1978;137:391.
58. Merrikin DJ, Briant J, Rolinson GN. Effect of protein binding on antibiotic activity in vivo. J Antimicrob Chemother. 1983;11:233.
59. Kaiser AB, McGee ZA. Aminoglycoside therapy of gram-negative bacillary meningitis. N Engl J Med. 1975;293:1215.
60. Waldvogel FW. Treatment of osteomyelitis and septic arthritis with quinolone antimicrobial agents. In: Hooper D, Wolfson J, eds. Quinolone antimicrobial Agents. Washington DC: American Society for Microbiology; 1989:177–86.
61. Bryant RE, Howard D. Interaction of purulent material with antibiotics used to treat *Pseudomonas* infections. Antimicrob Agents Chemother. 1974;6:702.
62. O'Keefe JP, Tally FP, Barza M, et al. Inactivation of penicillin G during experimental infection with *Bacteroides fragilis*. J Infect Dis. 1978;137:437.
63. Zimelis VM, Jackson GG. Activity of aminoglycoside antibiotics against *Pseudomonas aeruginosa*. Specificity and site of calcium and magnesium antagonism. J Infect Dis. 1973;127:663.
64. Bryan LE, Van Den Elzen HM. Streptomycin accumulation in susceptible and resistant strains of *Escherichia coli* and *Pseudomonas aeruginosa*. Antimicrob Agents Chemother. 1976;9:928.
65. Zinner SH, Sabath LD, Casey JI, et al. Erythromycin and alkalinization of the urine in the treatment of urinary tract infections due to gram-negative bacilli. Lancet. 1971;1:1267.
66. Sabath LD, Gerstein DA, Leaf CD, et al. Increasing the usefulness of antibiotics: Treatment of infections caused by gram-negative bacilli. Clin Pharmacol Ther. 1970;11:161.
67. Karchmer AW, Dismukes WE, Buckley MJ, et al. Late prosthetic valve endocarditis. Am J Med. 1978;64:99.
68. Zimmerli W, Waldvogel FA, Vaudaux P, et al. Pathogenesis of foreign body infection: Description and characteristics of an animal model. J Infect Dis. 1982;146:487.
69. Dickinson GM, Bisno AL. Infections associated with indwelling medical devices. Antimicrob Agents Chemother. In press.
70. Forsgren A, Schmeling D, Quie PG. Effect of tetracycline on the phagocytic function of human leukocytes. J Infect Dis. 1974;130:412.
71. Seklecki MM, Quintiliani R, Maderazo EG. Aminoglycoside antibiotics moderately impair granulocyte function. Antimicrob Agents Chemother. 1978;13:552.
72. Chaperon EA, Sanders WE Jr. Suppression of lymphoctye responses by cephalosporins. Infect Immun. 1978;19:378.
73. Mandell LA. Effects of antimicrobial and antineoplastic drugs on the phagocytic and microbicidal function of the polymorphonuclear leukocyte. Rev Infect Dis. 1982;4:683.
74. Hauser WE, Remington JS. Effect of antibiotics on the immune response. Am J Med. 1982;72:711.
75. Manzella JP, Clark JK. Effects of moxalactam and cefuroxime on mitogen-stimulated human mononuclear leukocytes. Antimicrob Agents Chemother. 1983;23:360.
76. Daschner FD. Antibiotics and host defense with special reference to phagocytosis by human polymorphonuclear leukocyte function in vivo. Antimicrob Agents Chemother. 1985;27:712.
77. Jawetz E. Combined antibiotic action: Some definitions and correlations between laboratory and clinical results. Antimicrob Agents Chemother. 1967,1968;203.
78. Krogstad DJ, Moellering RC Jr. Antimicrobial combinations. In: Lorian V, ed. Antibiotics in Laboratory Medicine. 2nd ed. Baltimore: Williams & Wilkins; 1986:537–95.
79. Moellering RC Jr. Use and abuse of antibiotic combinations. RI Med J. 1972;55:341.
80. VanderAuwera P, Meunier-Carpentier F, Klastersky J. Clinical study of combination therapy with oxacillin and rifampin for staphylococcal infections. Rev Infect Dis. 1983;5(Suppl 3):515.
81. Karchmer AW, Archer GL, Dimukes WE. Rifampin treatment of prosthetic valve endocarditis due to *Staphylococcus epidermidis*. Rev Infect Dis. 1983;5(Suppl 3):543.
82. Lehr D. Inhibition of drug precipitation in the urinary tract by the use of sulfonamide mixtures. I. Sulfathiazole-sulfadiazine mixture. Proc Soc Exp Biol Med. 1945;58:11.
83. Rahal JJ Jr. Antibiotic combinations: The clinical relevance of synergy and antagonism. Medicine (Baltimore). 1978;57:179.
84. Mandell GL, Kaye D, Levison ME, et al. Enterococcal endocarditis. An analysis of 38 patients observed at the New York Hospital–Cornell Medical Center. Arch Intern Med. 1970;125:258.
85. Moellering RC Jr, Wennersten C, Weinberg AN. Studies on antibiotic synergism against enterococci: I. Bacteriologic studies. J Lab Clin Med. 1971;77:821.
86. Moellering RC Jr, Weinberg AN. Studies on antibiotic synergism against enterococci: II. Effect of various antibiotics on the uptake of ^{14}C-labelled streptomycin by enterococci. J Clin Invest. 1971;50:2580.
87. Moellering RC Jr, Wennersten CBG, Medrek T, et al. Prevalence of high-level resistance ot aminoglycosides in clinical isolates of enterococci. Antimicrob Agents Chemother. 1970, 1971;335.
88. Zimmermann RA, Moellering RC Jr, Weinberg AN. Mechanism of resistance to antibiotic synergism in enterococci. J Bacteriol. 1971;105:873.
89. Krogstad DJ, Korfhagen TR, Moellering RC Jr, et al. Aminoglycoside-inactivating enzymes: An explanation for resistance to penicillin-aminoglycoside synergism in enterococci. J Clin Invest. 1978;62:480.
90. Mederski-Samoraj BD, Murray BE. High-level resistance to gentamicin in clinical isolates of enterococci. J Infect Dis. 1983;147:751.
91. Moellering RC Jr. The enterococcus: High-level resistance to gentamicin and production of beta-lactamase. Clin Microbiol Newsletter. 1988;10:129.
92. Fernandez-Guerrero ML, Barros C, Tudela JLR, et al. Aortic endocarditis caused by gentamicin-resistant *Enterococcus*. Eur J Clin Microbiol. 1988;7:525.
93. Wolfe JC, Johnson WD Jr. Penicillin-sensitive streptococcal endocarditis. Ann Intern Med. 1974;81:178.
94. Karchmer AW, Moellering RC Jr, Maki D, et al. Single antibiotic therapy of streptococcal endocarditis. JAMA. 1979;241:1801.
95. Watanakunakorn C, Glotzbecker C. Enhancement of the effects of antistaphylococcal antibiotics by aminoglycosides. Antimicrob Agents Chemother. 1974;6:802.
96. Korzeniowski O, Sande MA. The National Collaborative Endocarditis Study Group: Combination antimicrobial therapy for *Staphylococcus aureus* endocarditis in patients addicted to parenteral drugs and in nonaddicts. Ann Intern Med. 1982;97:496.
97. Smith CB, Dans PE, Wilfert JN, et al. Use of gentamicin in combination with other antibiotics. J Infect Dis. 1969;119:370.
98. Eliopoulos GM, Moellering RC Jr. Azlocillin, mezlocillin and piperacillin: New broad-spectrum penicillins. Ann Intern Med. 1982;97:755.
99. Adriole VT. Antibiotic synergy in experimental infection with *Pseudomonas:* II. The effect of carbenicillin, cephalothin or cephanone combined with tobramycin or gentamicin. J Infect Dis. 1974;129:124.
100. Then R. Synergism between trimethoprim and sulfonamides. Science. 1977;197:1301.
101. Harding GKM, Ronald AR. A controlled study of antimicrobial prophylaxis of recurrent urinary tract infections in women. N Engl J Med. 1974;291:597.
102. Gilman RN, Terminel M, Levine MM, et al. Comparison of trimethoprim-sulfamethoxazole and amoxicillin in therapy of chloramphenicol-resistant and chloramphenicol-sensitive typhoid fever. J Infect Dis. 1975;132:630.
103. Chang MJ, Dunkle LM, Van Reken D, et al. Trimethoprim-sulfamethoxazole compared to ampicillin in the treatment of shigellosis. Pediatrics. 1977;59:726.
104. Quintiliani R, Levite RE, Nightingale CH. Potential role of trimethoprim-sulfamethoxazole in the treatment of serious hospital-acquired infections. Rev Infect Dis. 9(Suppl 2):S160, 1987;9(Suppl 2):160.
105. Kwan CN, Medoff G, Kobayashi G, et al. Potentiation of the anti-fungal effects of antibiotics by amphotericin B. Antimicrob Agents Chemother. 1972;2:61.
106. Titsworth E, Grunberg E. Chemotherapeutic activity of 5-fluorocytosine and amphotericin B against *Candida albicans* in mice. Antimicrob Agents Chemother. 1973;4:306.
107. Bennett J, Dismukes W, Duma R, et al. A comparison of amphotericin B alone with amphotericin B plus flucytosine in the treatment of cryptoccal meningitis. N Engl J Med. 1979;301:126.
108. Lau WK, Young LS, Block RE, et al. Comparative efficacy and toxicity of amikacin/carbenicillin versus gentamicin/carbenicillin in leukopenic patients. Am J Med. 1977;62:959.
109. Klastersky J, Hensgens C, Meunier-Carpentier F. Comparative effectiveness of combinations of amikacin with penicillin G and amikacin with carbenicillin in gram-negative septicemia: Double-blind clinical trial. J Infect Dis. 1976;134(Suppl):433.
110. Moellering RC Jr. Monotherapy with expanded-spectrum cephalosporins for empiric treatment of serious infections diseases. In Hoepelman IM, Moell-

ering RC Jr, eds. New Directions in Cephalosporin Therapy: The Expanded Spectrum Cephalosporins. Winchester, UK: Theracom; 1988:49.
111. Lepper MH, Dowling HF. Treatment of pneumococcic meningitis with penicillin compared with penicillin plus aureomycin. Arch Intern Med. 1951;88:489.
112. Mathies AW Jr, Leedom JM, Ivier D, et al. Antibiotic antagonism in bacterial meningitis. Antimicrob Agents Chemother. 1967;7:218.
113. Sande MA, Overton JW. In vivo antagonism between gentamicin and chloramphenicol in neutropenic mice. J Infect Dis. 1973;128:247.
114. Strausbaugh LJ, Sande MA. Factors influencing the therapy of experimental *Proteus mirabilis* meningitis in rabbits. J Infect Dis. 1978;137:251.
115. Swedish Study Group: Cefuroxime versus ampicillin and chloramphenicol for the treatment of bacterial meningitis. Lancet. 1982;1:295.
116. Del Rio MDL, Chrane D, Shelton S, et al. Ceftriaxone versus ampicillin and chloramphenicol for treatment of bacterial meningitis in children. Lancet. 1983;1:1241.
117. Moellering RC Jr. Rationale for the use of antibiotic combinations. Am J Med. 1983;75(2A):4.
118. Sanders CC. Novel resistance selected by the new expanded spectrum cephalosporins: A concern. J Infect Dis. 1983;147:585.
119. McLaughlin JE, Reeves DS. Clinical and laboratory evidence for inactivation of gentamicin by carbenicillin. Lancet. 1971;1:261.
120. Riff LJ, Jackson GG. Laboratory and clinical conditions for gentamicin inactivation by carbenicillin. Arch Intern Med. 1972;130:887.
121. Seidl LG, Thornton GF, Smith SW, et al. Studies on epidemiology of adverse drug reactions. III. Reactions in patients on general medical service. Bull Johns Hopkins Hosp. 1966;119:299.
122. Drusano GL. Pharmacokinetics of quinolone antimicrobial agents. In: Hooper D, Wolfson J, eds. Quinolone Antimicrobial Agents. Washington DC: American Society for Microbiology; 1989:71–105.
123. Barza M, Brusch J, Bergeron M, et al. Penetration of antibiotics into fibrin loci in vivo. III. Intermittent versus continuous infusion and the effect of probenicid. J Infect Dis. 1974;129:73.
124. Nelson JD. Antibiotic concentrations in septic joint effusions. N Engl J Med. 1971;284:349.
125. Gerding DN, Hall WH. The penetration of antibiotics into peritoneal fluid. Bull NY Acad Med. 1975;51:1016.
126. Schlichter JG, MacLean H. A method of determining the effective therapeutic level in the treatment of subacute bacterial endocarditis with penicillin. Am Heart J. 1947;34:209.
127. Reller LB, Stratton CW. Serum dilution test for bactericidal activity. II. Standardization and correlation with antimicrobial assays and susceptibility tests. J Infect Dis. 1977;136:196.
128. Carrizosa J, Kaye D. Antibiotic concentrations in serum, serum bactericidal activity, and results of therapy of streptococcal endocarditis in rabbits. Antimicrob Agents Chemother. 1977;12:479.
129. Weinstein MP, Stratton CW, Ackley A, et al. Multicenter collaborative evaluation of a standardized serum bactericidal test as a prognostic indicator in infective endocarditis. Am J Med 1985;78:262.
130. Levy J, Klastersky J. Serum bactericidal test: A review with emphasis on its role in the evaluation of antibiotic combination. In: Klastersky J, Staquet MJ, eds. Combination Antibiotic Therapy in the Compromised Host. New York: Raven Press; 1982:43.
131. Pien FD, Vosti KL. Variation in performance of the serum bactericidal test. Antimicrob Agents Chemother. 1974;6:330.
132. Stratton CW, Reller LB. Serum dilution test for bactericidal activity. I. Selection of a physiologic diluent. J Infect Dis. 1977;136:187.
133. Mellors JW, Colman DL, Andriole VT. Value of the serum bactericidal test in management of patients with bacterial endocarditis. Eur J Clin Microbiol. 1986;5:67.
134. Reller LB. The serum bactericidal test. Rev Infect Dis. 1986;8:803.

16. MECHANISMS OF ANTIBIOTIC RESISTANCE

KENNETH H. MAYER
STEVEN M. OPAL
ANTONE A. MEDEIROS

MOLECULAR GENETICS OF ANTIBIOTIC RESISTANCE

Genetic variability is essential in order for microbial evolution to occur. Antimicrobial agents exert strong selective pressures upon bacterial populations and favor those organisms that are capable of resisting them.[1,2] Genetic variability may occur by a variety of mechanisms. Point mutation may occur at a nucleotide base pair, a process referred to as microevolutionary change. Point mutations may alter the target site of an antimicrobial agent, thereby interfering with its activity.

A second level of genomic variability in bacteria is referred to as a macroevolutionary change and results in whole-scale rearrangements of large segments of DNA as a single event. Such rearrangements may include inversions, duplications, insertions, deletions, or transpositions of large sequences of DNA from one location of the bacterial chromosome to another. These whole-scale rearrangements of large segments of the bacterial chromosome are frequently created by specialized genetic elements known as transposons, or insertion sequences that have the capacity to move independently of the rest of the bacterial chromosome.[2]

A third level of genetic variability in bacteria is created by the acquisition of foreign DNA carried by plasmids, bacteriophages, or transposable genetic elements. Inheritance of these extrachromosomal elements further contributes to the organism's ability to cope with selection pressures imposed by antimicrobial agents.[3] These mechanisms endow bacteria with the seemingly unlimited capacity to develop resistance to any antimicrobial agent. Once an antibiotic resistance gene evolves, this resistance determinant may spread to other bacteria by transformation, transduction, conjugation, or transposition. Favored clones of bacteria may then proliferate in the flora of patients exposed to antibiotics.

Plasmids

Extrachromosomal elements were present in bacteria before the advent of antibiotics.[4] However, the introduction of antibiotics into clinical medicine over the past five decades has created selection pressures that favored the dissemination of antibiotic resistance genes via mobile genetic elements, i.e., plasmids and transposons. Rapid increases in the spread of antibiotic resistance within species and between species is often correlated with the dissemination of resistance (R). Plasmids are particularly well adapted to serve as agents of genetic evolution and resistance gene dissemination.[5] Plasmids are extrachromosomal genetic elements that are made of circular double-stranded DNA molecules that range in size from less than 10 to greater than 400 kilobase pairs and are extremely common in bacteria.[6] While multiple copies of a specific plasmid and/or multiple different plasmids may be found in a single bacterial cell, closely related plasmids often cannot coexist in the same cell. This observation has led to a classification scheme of plasmids that is based upon incompatibility groups.[7]

Plasmids may determine a wide range of functions besides antibiotic resistance, including virulence and metabolic capacities. Plasmids are autonomous, self-reproducing genetic elements that require an origin of replication and a region of the plasmid that is essential for its stable maintenance in host bacteria.[7] Conjugative plasmids require additional genes that can initiate self-transfer.[8]

The transfer of plasmid DNA between bacterial species is a complex process, and thus conjugative plasmids tend to be larger than nonconjugative plasmids. Some small plasmids may be able to use the conjugation apparatus of a coresident conjugative plasmid. Many plasmid-encoded functions enable bacterial strains to persist in the environment by resisting noxious agents. Compounds such as hexachlorophene are used as topical bacteriostatic agents, and plasmid-mediated resistance to these agents has increased significantly in recent years.[9]

Plasmids may be involved in the dissemination of antibiotic resistance in several ways (Fig. 1). A single clone of a specific organism may become resistant by mutation or by the inheritance of a resistance plasmid. The resultant resistant organism may have genes that are particularly well adapted to a specific niche and thus be able to disseminate widely. The single clone

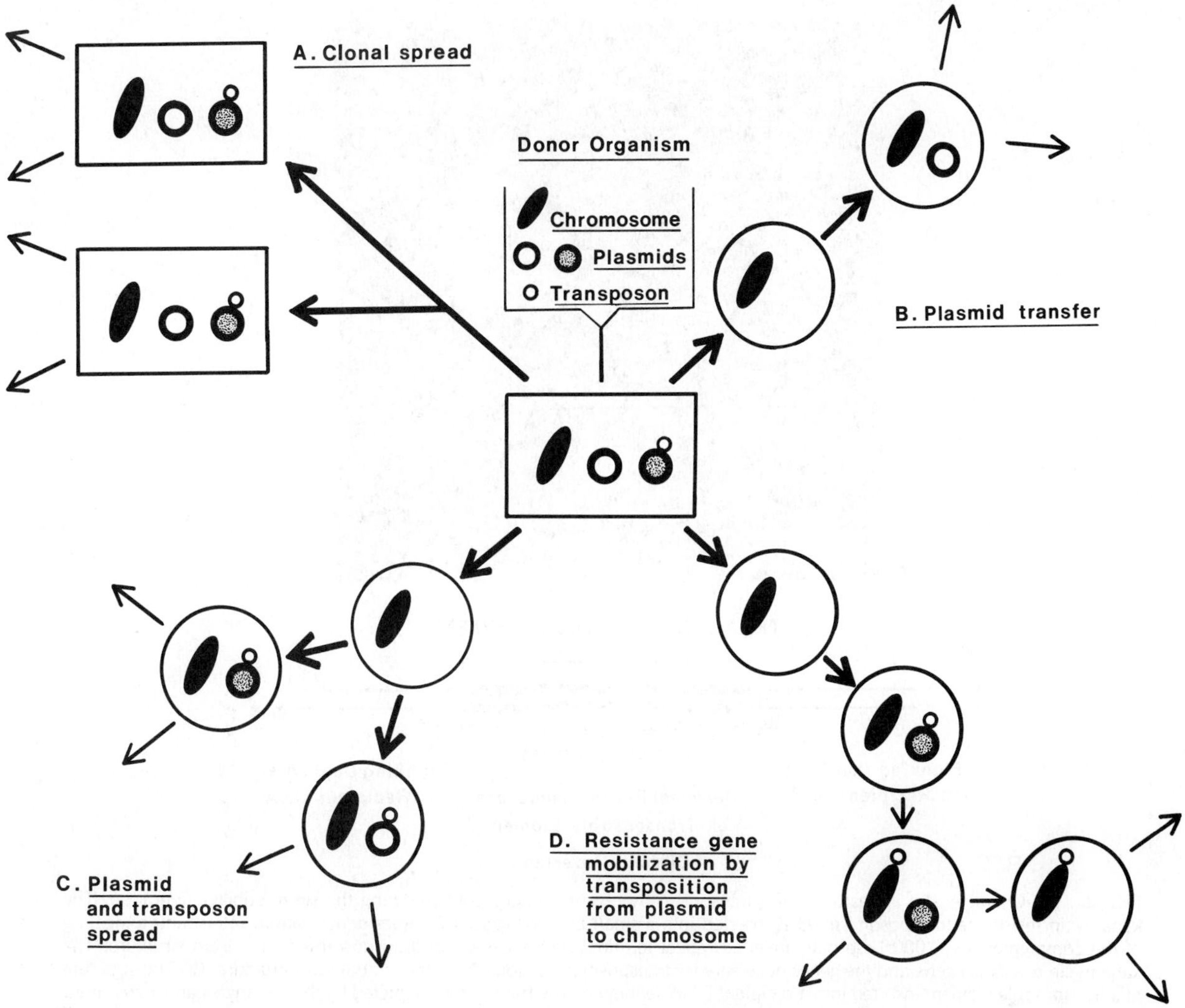

FIG. 1. Examples of the molecular spread of antibiotic resistance. The donor organism has a chromosome, two plasmids, and a transposon. If it is well adapted to a particular niche, it may remain stable in the environment and continue to replicate itself and thus disseminate through clonal spread **(A)**. If the organism comes into close physical contact with another bacterium that may not possess extrachromosomal DNA, attachment between the two cells from different bacterial species may allow for the introduction of one of the plasmids by conjugation **(B)**. The donor organism may be able to spread resistance genes through several mechanisms including the spread of transposons as well as plasmids **(C)**. Transposons may be able to hop between plasmids **(C)**, or they may be able to allow for the mobilization of resistance genes by being transferred on a conjugative plasmid into new bacterial species and then hop from the plasmid to the chromosome **(D)**. Some transposons may subsequently become integrated into the host chromosome and be spread as a stable genetic element in the chromosome without any subsequent transfer via plasmid DNA.

may be responsible for multiple outbreaks of antibiotic resistance. Conjugative plasmids may be transferred from one species to another and result in new outbreaks of antibiotic-resistant organisms.[10] Transposons create the potential for even wider dissemination of antibiotic resistance genes.[11]

Transposable Genetic Elements

Transposons can translocate from one area of the bacterial chromosome to another or between the chromosome and plasmid or bacteriophage DNA. Transposable genetic elements possess a specialized system of recombination that is independent of the generalized recombination system that classically permits recombination of largely homologous sequences of DNA by crossover events (the recA system of bacteria). The recA-independent recombination system of transposable elements usually occurs in a random fashion between nonhomologous sequences of DNA and results in whole-scale modifications of large sequences of DNA as a single event (Fig. 2).[1,3]

There are two types of transposable genetic elements, referred to as transposons and insertion sequences, that have similar characteristics. Transposons (Tn) differ from insertion sequences in that they mediate a recognizable phenotypic characteristic such as an antibiotic resistance marker. Either element can translocate as an independent unit. Transposons and insertion sequences are incapable of autonomous self-replication and therefore must exist on a replicon such as the chromosome, bacteriophage, or plasmid in order to be replicated and maintained in a bacterial population. Recently, a new class of transposable elements has been described that have the capability to move from the chromosome of one bacterium to another without being part of a plasmid or bacteriophage. These elements are referred to as "conjugative" transposons and have been found in aerobic and anaerobic gram-positive organisms.[12,13]

Transposition usually results in localized replication of the transposable element from the original donor sequence of DNA as well as the insertion of a copy of the transposable element

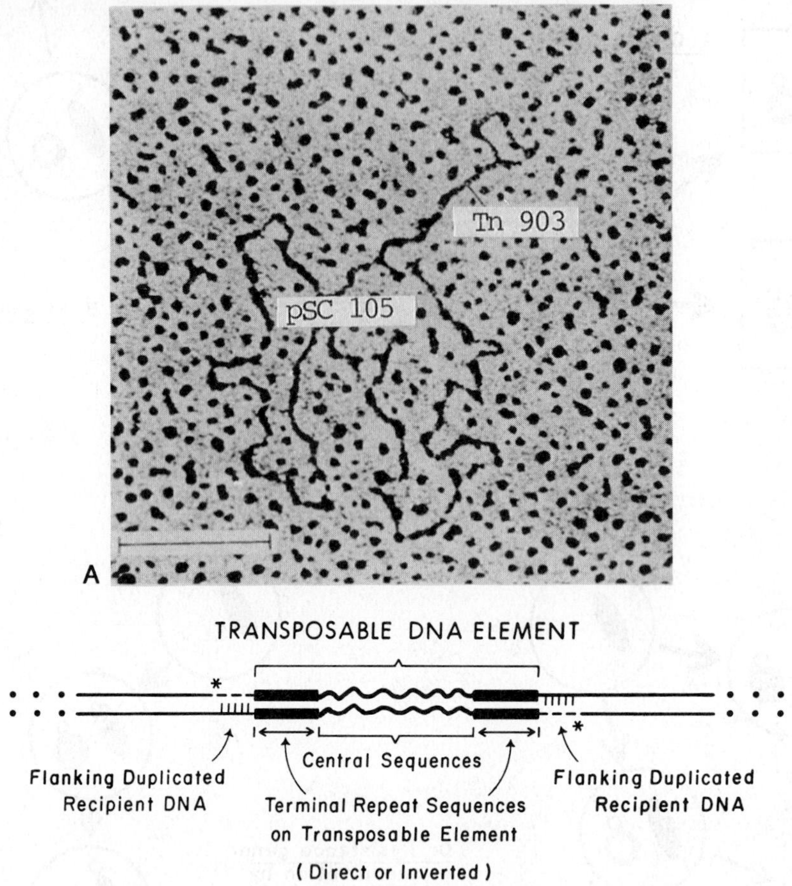

FIG. 2. **(A)** Characteristic appearance of a transposon by electron microscopy showing the stem-loop configuration. The kanamycin resistance transposon Tn903 is inserted into a small plasmid (pSC105). After denaturation, intrastrand annealing of the complementary, 1000 base pair, inverted repeat terminal sequences of the transposon form the stem structure. The kanamycin resistance gene and the genes necessary for transposition are located in the central loop structure. **(B)** The structure of a transposable element inserted into a recipient DNA sequence. The transposon (depicted by the rectangles and wavy lines) consists of a central sequence containing the phenotypic marker gene(s) (antibiotic resistance gene) and the "transposase" genes. The terminal repeat sequences of the transposon flank the central sequences on both sides. Insertion of the transposon results in single-strand, staggered cuts in the recipient DNA (marked by asterisks). Subsequent gap-filling DNA synthesis and ligation results in duplication of a short sequence of recipient DNA at either end of the transposon. (From Kopecko,[1] with permission.)

into the recipient sequence of DNA (replicative transposition).[1–3] Transposition is a continuous and ongoing process in bacterial populations. A recent example of this phenomenon is the spread of a tetracycline resistance transposon among *Neisseria gonorrhoeae, Mycoplasma hominis,* and *Ureaplasma urealyticum.*[14,15] Transposons are also essential in the evolution of R plasmids that contain multiple antibiotic resistance determinants.[11] Single transposons may encode multiple antibiotic resistance determinants within their inverted repeat termini as well.[3]

MECHANISMS OF ANTIBIOTIC RESISTANCE

At least seven distinctive mechanisms of antibiotic resistance have been described in bacteria (Table 1).

Enzymatic Inhibition

β-Lactamases. Resistance to β-lactam antibiotics is due mainly to the production of β-lactamases, enzymes that inactivate these antibiotics by splitting the amide bond of the β-lactam ring. Numerous β-lactamases exist, encoded either by chromosomal genes or by transferable genes located on plasmids or transposons.[17]

Three evolutionarily distinct classes of β-lactamases have been defined on the basis of amino acid and nucleotide sequence studies. Class A β-lactamases have molecular weights around 29,000, possess a serine residue at their active site, and preferentially hydrolyze penicillins. An example is the TEM-1 β-lactamase widely prevalent in gram-negative bacilli. Class B β-lactamase is a metalloenzyme with a molecular weight of 23,000 that attacks cephalosporins preferentially. Class C includes the chromosomally determined β-lactamase of *Escherichia coli,* which shares extensive sequence homology with chromosomally mediated β-lactamases of *Shigella* and *Klebsiella* species. These enzymes are large proteins with molecular weights about 39,000 and also have serine at their active site but share no homology with the class A β-lactamases.[18]

GRAM-POSITIVE BACTERIA. Among the gram-positive bacteria staphylococci are the major pathogens that produce β-lactamase. Staphylococcal β-lactamases preferentially hydrolyze penicillins. Most are inducible and are excreted extracellularly.[17] The genes that determine staphylococcal β-lactamases are usually carried on small plasmids that can be transferred from cell to cell by transduction. Larger plasmids encoding β-lactamase and other resistances also exist and can transfer by conjugation, not only between strains of *Staphylococcus aureus* but also between *S. aureus* and *Staphylococcus epidermidis.*[19]

TABLE 1. Major Mechanisms of Antibiotic Resistance

	Type of Antibiotic											
Resistance Mechanism	*β-Lactams*	*Aminoglycosides*	*Chloramphenicol*	*Macrolides*	*Lincosamides*	*Sulfonamides*	*Trimethoprim*	*Tetracyclines*	*Quinolones*	*Vancomycin*[a]	*Rifampin*	*Polymyxin*
1. Enzymatic inhibition	B	B	P	P	—	—	—	—	—	—	—	—
2. Membrane impermeability	C	C	P	—	—	C	C	B	—	C	—	C
3. Alteration in intracellular target site	—	C	C	B	B	—	—	B	—	—	—	C
4. Alteration in target enzyme	B	—	—	—	—	B	B	—	C	—	C	—
5. Overproduction of target enzyme	—	—	—	—	—	C	C	—	—	—	—	—
6. Auxotrophs that bypass inhibited steps	—	—	—	—	—	B	B	—	—	—	—	—
7. Active pumping out of substrate	—	—	—	—	—	—	—	B	—	—	—	—

[a] Plasmid-mediated vancomycin resistance has been described, but its mechanism has not yet been characterized.[16]
Abbreviations: P: plasmid mediated; C: chromosomally mediated; B: both; —: not yet described.

The streptococci also produce β-lactamase; an *Enterococcus faecalis* strain produces a plasmid-determined β-lactamase that appears to be of staphylococcal origin.[20]

GRAM-NEGATIVE BACTERIA. Gram-negative bacteria produce a much greater variety of β-lactamases than do gram-positive bacteria. This diversity has led to several classification schemes. Over 30 different plasmid-determined β-lactamases have been discovered.[21] All are produced constitutively and can be grouped into three broad classes: (*1*) those that hydrolyze benzylpenicillin and cephaloridine at similar rates (broad-spectrum enzymes), (*2*) those that hydrolyze oxacillin and related penicillins rapidly (oxacillinases), and (*3*) those that break down carbenicillin readily (carbenicillinases). The properties of the plasmid-determined β-lactamases are summarized in Table 2.

ANAEROBIC BACTERIA. The resistance of anaerobic bacteria to β-lactam antibiotics also involves the production of β-lactamases. The β-lactamases of fusobacteria and clostridia are principally penicillinases. Those produced by *Bacteroides fragilis* are predominantly cephalosporinases, some of which have been found to hydrolyze cefoxitin and imipenem and may be transferable.[22,23]

DISTRIBUTION IN CLINICAL ISOLATES. The existence of β-lactamase genes on plasmids and transposons ensures that a β-lactamase originally confined to one group of bacteria sooner or later may appear in other groups. The widespread use of antibiotics fosters selection of the resistant organisms, which rise in prevalence locally and then spread worldwide. A prime example of this process occurred with the TEM-1 β-lactamase, which has spread from the Enterobacteriaceae to *Haemophilus influenzae*[24] and *N. gonorrhoeae*.[25] Clinical isolates may produce two and even three plasmid-determined β-lactamases. In nearly all cases TEM-1 is one of the β-lactamases produced. A large number of strains from South America and the Far East have had novel and/or multiple plasmid β-lactamases.[19]

The success of the pharmaceutical industry in developing new β-lactams resistant to hydrolysis by β-lactamases led to the introduction into clinical use of the third-generation cephalosporins around 1978 in Europe and 1981 in the United States. These antibiotics were very resistant to hydrolysis by the known plasmid-determined β-lactamases. Then in 1983 in Germany, isolates of *Klebsiella pneumoniae* and then other Enterobacteriaceae were discovered that produced a plasmid-determined β-lactamase that hydrolyzed cefotaxime as well as other newer cephalosporins. This new β-lactamase, called SHV-2, derived from a mutation in the well-known SHV-1 β-lactamase commonly found in *Klebsiella*. The mutation resulted in an enhanced affinity of the SHV-1 β-lactamase for cefotaxime.[26] More recently, cefotaxime-resistant strains of *K. pneumoniae* producing a novel plasmid-encoded, TEM-like, cefotaxime-hydrolyzing β-lactamase, designated CTX-1, have been recovered from several French hospitals.[27] Also, three novel plasmid-encoded β-lactamases that hydrolyze ceftazidime and aztreonam have appeared in clinical isolates from France and Germany.[28,29] On the basis of DNA hybridization studies these new β-lactamases appear to be derivatives of the TEM-2 β-lactamase.[30] Thus, in response to new selection pressures engendered by the frequent use of third-generation cephalosporins, mutations have occurred among the well-established plasmid-determined β-lactamases, which has resulted in the dissemination of novel transferable β-lactamases with an expanded spectrum of activity.

β-LACTAMASES DETERMINED BY CHROMOSOMAL GENES. Virtually all gram-negative bacteria produce some chromosomally determined β-lactamase. Furthermore, the types of β-lactamase produced are often specific for species and sometimes for subspecies. β-Lactamase activity is frequently very low, particularly in ampicillin-susceptible isolates, but may increase due to induction or to alterations in the number of β-lactamase genes on the chromosome; also, mutation of genes that regulate induction may lead to constitutive hyperproduction of inducible β-lactamases.[31] Most of the chromosomally determined β-lactamases preferentially hydrolyze cephalosporins, including many of the third-generation agents that are resistant to hydrolysis by the plasmid-determined β-lactamases (Table 3).[31a]

Chromosomally determined β-lactamases nearly always differ in their biochemical properties from the plasmid-determined enzymes. The exception is a chromosomal β-lactamase found in many isolates of *K. pneumoniae* that is indistinguishable from the SHV-1 β-lactamase. It may be that the SHV-1 β-lactamase gene evolved as a chromosomal gene in *Klebsiella* and was later incorporated into a plasmid.[32] As yet no such ancestral chromosomal gene has been found for the much more common TEM-1 β-lactamase or for any of the other plasmid-determined β-lactamases.

CONTRIBUTION OF β-LACTAMASES TO β-LACTAM ANTIBIOTIC RESISTANCE. The level of antibiotic resistance mediated by a particular β-lactamase in a population of bacteria is determined by several variables. The efficiency of the β-lactamase in hydrolyzing an antibiotic depends on both its rate of hydrolysis (V_{max}) and its affinity for the antibiotic (K_m). Other variables are the amount of β-lactamase produced by the bacterial cell, the susceptibility of the target protein (penicillin binding protein [PBP]) to the antibiotic, and the rate of diffusion of the antibiotic into the periplasm of the cell.

Within the bacterial cell, β-lactamases contribute to antibiotic resistance in several ways. The simplest model is that of penicillinase-producing staphylococci in which the bacteria, upon exposure to penicillin, begin to produce β-lactamase, which they excrete extracellularly. Two events then take place concurrently: (*1*) penicillin lyses bacteria, and (*2*) β-lactamase hydrolyzes penicillin. If viable bacterial cells remain after the level

TABLE 2. Properties of Plasmid-Determined β-Lactamases

β-Lactamase	*pI*	*Prevalence*	*Host Bacteria*	*Specific Features*
Broad Spectrum				
HMS-1	5.2	Rare	Enterobacteriaceae	
TEM-1	5.4	Very common	Enterobacteriaceae *P. aeruginosa* *H. influenzae* *N. gonorrhoeae* *Vibrio cholerae*	Most common type in nearly all bacterial species
TLE-1	5.55	Rare	*E. coli*	Closely related to TEM-1
TEM-2	5.6	Common	Enterobacteriaceae	Differs from TEM-1 by 1 amino acid
LCR-1	5.85	Rare	*P. aeruginosa*	
NPS-1	6.5	Rare	*P. aeruginosa*	Cefsulodin induces conformational change
TLE-2	6.5	Rare	*K. pneumoniae*	High affinity for cefsulodin and cefotetan
LXA-1	6.7	Uncommon	Enterobacteriaceae	Very low affinity for benzylpenicillin confers low-level β-lactam resistance
OHIO-1	7.0	Uncommon	Enterobacteriaceae	Only found in isolates from Ohio
SHV-1	7.6	Common	Enterobacteriaceae	Often encoded by chromosomal genes in *K. pneumoniae*
ROB-1	8.1	Uncommon	*H. influenzae* *H. pleuropneumoniae* *P. multocida*	Found in both human and animal isolates
Oxacillinase				
Unnamed (Gn11499)	6.9	Rare	*B. fragilis*	
OXA-3	7.1	Uncommon	Enterobacteriaceae *P. aeruginosa*	
OXA-1	7.4	Common	Enterobacteriaceae *P. aeruginosa*	Second most common type in *E. coli*
OXA-4	7.45	Rare	Enterobacteriaceae	Closely related to OXA-1
OXA-5	7.62	Rare	*P. aeruginosa*	
OXA-7	7.65	Rare	*E. coli*	
OXA-6	7.68	Rare	*P. aeruginosa*	
OXA-2	7.7	Common	Enterobacteriaceae *P. aeruginosa*	Second most common type in salmonellae
Carbenicillinase				
CARB-4	4.3	Rare	*P. aeruginosa*	Confers resistance to cefsulodin
SAR-1	4.9	Rare	*V. cholerae*	
PSE-4 (CARB-1)	5.3	Uncommon	*P. aeruginosa* Enterobacteriaceae	
BRO-1	5.6	Common	*Branhamella* *Moraxella*	Confers resistance to ampicillin and cefaclor
PSE-1 (CARB-2)	5.7	Common	*P. aeruginosa* Enterobacteriaceae	Most common type in *P. aeruginosa*
CARB-3	5.75	Rare	*P. aeruginosa*	
AER-1	5.9	Rare	*A. hydrophila*	
Unnamed (N-3)	6.0 (5.73)	Rare	*P. mirabilis*	Similar to PSE-1
PSE-2	6.1	Uncommon	*P. aeruginosa* Enterobacteriaceae	Hydrolyzes oxacillin rapidly
PSE-3	6.9	Uncommon	*P. aeruginosa* Enterobacteriaceae	
Unnamed (N-29)	6.9 (6.93)	Rare	*P. mirabilis*	
Cephalosporinase				
CEP-1	8.0	Rare	*P. mirabilis*	
CEP-2	8.1	Rare	*Achromobacter*	
Cefotaximase				
RHH-1	5.5	Rare	Enterobacteriaceae	
CAZ-1	5.55	Common (France)	Enterobacteriaceae	Derivative of TEM-2
CAZ	5.85	Uncommon (Germany)	Enterobacteriaceae	Derivative of TEM-2
CTX-1	6.3	Common (France)	Enterobacteriaceae	Derivative of TEM-2
SHV-2	7.6	Uncommon but widespread (Germany, France, Greece, Chile, China)	Enterobacteriaceae	Derivative of SHV-1

TABLE 3. Classification of Chromosomal β-Lactamases

Broad-spectrum cephalosporinases—hydrolyze benzylpenicillin, ampicillin, and carbenicillin as well as cephalosporins
P. vulgaris
K. pneumoniae
K. oxytoca
K. aerogenes K-1
Typical cephalosporinases—little or no activity against penicillins
Constitutive
E. coli
B. fragilis
Inducible
E. aerogenes
E. cloacae
P. rettgeri
P. aeruginosa
A. anitratus
S. marcescens

(Data from Sawai.[31a])

of penicillin has fallen below the minimal inhibitory concentration, regrowth of bacteria occurs.[18]

Another model is exemplified by gram-negative bacilli, which (*1*) produce a β-lactamase that remains trapped in the periplasmic space and (*2*) have no barrier to antibiotic penetration. An example is *H. influenzae* strains that produce the TEM-1 β-lactamase.[33] In both this model and the first one discussed, a marked inoculum effect occurs in that the minimal inhibitory concentration (MIC) for a large inoculum (10^6 organisms/ml) may be 1000-fold greater than with a small inoculum (10^2 organisms/ml). The low level of resistance of single cells has made it possible for ampicillin to cure some infections caused by β-lactamase-producing strains of *H. influenzae* when the inoculum of infecting bacteria was low.

Another model is exemplified by ampicillin resistance of *E. coli* strains that produce the TEM-1 β-lactamase. These bacteria have a barrier to the entry of β-lactam molecules (the outer membrane), and they produce a β-lactamase that remains localized to the periplasmic space. In this model, the kinetics are more complicated. The enzyme is strategically situated between the barrier to antibiotic penetration (outer membrane) and the antibiotic targets (penicillin binding proteins on the cytoplasmic membrane). In this position the enzyme can sequentially destroy antibiotic molecules as they make their way through the barrier in a manner analogous to a sharpshooter with abundant ammunition who aims at targets passing through a single entry point. As a consequence, high levels of resistance occur with single bacterial cells, unlike the previous example.[18]

Variations on this model may occur when the amount of β-lactamase produced increases with exposure to a β-lactam (induction) as occurs in *Enterobacter* and *Pseudomonas* species. High levels of β-lactamase are produced only after a period of exposure to the inducing antibiotic, and hence resistance may be expressed late. When *Enterobacter* strains are exposed to two β-lactam antibiotics, one of which is a potent inducer (e.g., cefamandole), antagonism between the two antibiotics may result.[34]

Aminoglycoside Resistance-Modifying Enzymes. Among aerobic bacteria, aminoglycoside resistance is most commonly due to modifying enzymes that are coded by genes on plasmids or the chromosome.[35] Several of the aminoglycoside-modifying enzymes have been shown to be carried on transposons.[11]

More than two dozen aminoglycoside-modifying enzymes that have been identified are capable of three general reactions: *N*-acetylation, *O*-nucleotidylation, and *O*-phosphorylation. For each of these general reactions there are several different enzymes that attack a specific amino or hydroxyl group. The nomenclature for these enzymes lists the molecular site where the modification occurs after the type of enzymatic activity. For example an aminoglycoside acetyltransferase (AAC) that acts at the 3′ site is designated AAC(3′)[36] (Table 4). However, there may be more than one enzyme that will catalyze the same reaction, and thus roman numerals may be necessary (e.g., AAC(3′)-IV).

Enzymatic aminoglycoside resistance is achieved by modification of the antibiotic in the process of transport across the cytoplasmic membrane.[35] Resistance to a particular aminoglycoside is a function of two different rates, that of drug uptake vs. that of drug inactivation. An important factor in determining the level of resistance is the affinity of the modifying enzyme for the antibiotic. If an enzyme has a high affinity for the specific aminoglycoside, then drug inactivation can occur at very low concentrations.

The differences in the worldwide distribution of aminoglycoside-modifying enzymes may partially be a function of antibiotic selection pressures and have had profound implications on the choice of antibiotics used at specific centers.[37] APH(3′) and APH(3″) are widely distributed among gram-positive and gram-negative species worldwide and thus have led to decreased utilization of kanamycin and streptomycin. The ANT(2″) gene has been associated with multiple nosocomial outbreaks over the past decade across the United States.AAC(6′)-I gene has been found to be more prevalent in East Asia.[38] The AAC(3) group of enzymes have been responsible for outbreaks of antibiotic resistance in South America, Western Europe, and the United States. Although each outbreak of aminoglycoside-resistant Enterobacteriaceae in the United States has its own pattern, the most typical manner of spread has been the appearance of a plasmid-carrying aminoglycoside-resistant strain of *K. pneumoniae,* usually carrying the ANT(2″) gene, with subsequent dissemination to other strains of the species and further spread later to other species and genera of Enterobacteriaceae.[39] A recent global survey detected an increased prevalence of amikacin-resistant isolates from hospitals in the United States and Western Europe,[39a] reflecting ongoing changes in the deployment of different aminoglycoside-modifying enzymes among gram-negative bacilli.

Chloramphenicol Acetyltransferase. Resistance to chloramphenicol in gram-positive and gram-negative organisms is primarily mediated by an inactivating enzyme known as chloramphenicol acetyltransferase. This is an intracellular enzyme that inactivates the drug by 3-*O*-acetylation[40] and is encoded by plasmid-borne or chromosomal genes. Despite homology at the active site of this enzyme, there is considerable diversity between chloramphenicol acetyltransferase enzymes isolated from gram-positive and gram-negative organisms.[41]

Erythromycin Esterase. While resistance to erythromycin and other macrolides is generally the result of an alteration in the ribosomal target site, an additional mechanism of resistance

TABLE 4. Examples of Where Common Aminoglycoside-Modifying Enzymes Are Found

Enzymes	*Usual Antibiotics Modified*	*Common Genera*
Phosphorylation		
APH(2″)	K, T, G	SA, SR
APH(3′)-I	K	E, PS, SA, SR
APH(3′)-III	K, + A	E, PS, SA, SR
Acetylation		
AAC(2′)	G	PR
AAC(3)-I	± T, G	E, PS
AAC(3)-III, IV, or -V	K, T, G	E, PS
AAC(6′)	K, T, ± A	E, PS, SA
Adenylation		
ANT(2″)	K, T, G	E, PS
ANT(4′)	K, T, A	SA

Abbreviations: K: kanamycin; T: tobramycin; G: gentamicin; A: amikacin; E: Enterobacteriaceae; SA: staphylococci; SR: streptococci; PS: pseudomonads; PR: providencia/proteus.

that is based upon enzymatic destruction has recently been characterized. An enzyme known as erythromycin esterase has been isolated from *E. coli* that hydrolyzes the lactone ring of the antibiotic, thereby resulting in its inactivation.[42] This is a plasmid-mediated resistance determinant that is constitutively produced and results in high-level resistance to erythromycin (MIC > 2000 μg/ml).[43] This resistance determinant may limit the utility of oral erythromycin in reducing the aerobic gram-negative flora of the intestinal tract before gastrointestinal surgical procedures.

Alterations in Bacterial Membranes

Outer Membrane Permeability. It was recognized early in the history of antibiotic development that penicillin was effective against gram-positive bacteria but not against gram-negative bacteria.[44] This difference in susceptibility to penicillin is due in large part to the outer membrane, a lipid bilayer that acts as a barrier to the penetration of antibiotics into the cell.[45] Situated outside the peptidoglycan cell wall of gram-negative bacteria, this outer membrane is absent in gram-positive bacteria. The outer portion of this lipid bilayer is composed principally of lipopolysaccharide made up of tightly bound hydrocarbon molecules that impede the entry of hydrophobic antibiotics such as nafcillin or erythromycin.[46,47] Agents that disrupt the integrity of the lipopolysaccharide layer such as polymyxin or mutations that lead to the production of defective lipopolysaccharide result in increased permeability of hydrophobic antibiotics.[48]

The passage of hydrophilic antibiotics through this outer membrane is facilitated by the presence of porins, proteins that are arranged so as to form water-filled diffusion channels through which antibiotics may traverse.[49] Bacteria usually produce a large number of porins; approximately 10^5 porin molecules are present in a single cell of *E. coli*. Bacteria are able to regulate the relative number of different porins in response to the osmolarity of the surrounding media. Thus, in hyperosmolar media *E. coli* may repress production of the larger porins (OmpF) while continuing to express smaller ones (OmpC).[50]

The rate of diffusion of antibiotics through this outer membrane is a function not only of the number and properties of the porin channels but also of the physicochemical characteristics of the antibiotic. Generally, the larger the antibiotic molecule, the more negative the charges, and the greater the degree of hydrophobicity, the less likely it is to penetrate through the outer membrane.[45,51] Small, hydrophilic molecules with a zwitterionic charge such as imipenem are highly permeable. Conversely, larger highly charged molecules such as carbenicillin are much less permeable.

Mutations resulting in the loss of specific porins can occur in clinical isolates and determine increased resistance to β-lactam antibiotics. For example, a strain of *Salmonella typhimurium* obtained from a perirenal abscess became resistant to various cephalosporins during therapy with cephalexin.[52] The parent strain produced both OmpF and OmpC proteins, but the mutant produced only OmpF. The mutant was resistant to β-lactam antibiotics only when tested in media of high osmolarity, comparable to that in the patient's tissues. Under these conditions the production of the OmpF protein was repressed completely, leaving the microorganism devoid of either species of porin and impermeable to the cephalosporins. Resistance to aminoglycosides and carbapenems that emerges during therapy has also been associated with a lack of production of outer membrane proteins, probably by mechanisms other than diffusion through porins.[53,54]

Resistance to nalidixic acid and other quinolones may also be associated with alterations of outer membrane proteins.[55] Plasmid-mediated chloramphenicol resistance due to decreased permeability has been demonstrated in *E. coli*.[56] The mechanism by which plasmid-mediated vancomycin and teicoplanin resistance in *Enterococcus faecium* occurs has not yet been elucidated but may be related to outer membrane impermeability.[16]

Inner Membrane Permeability. The rate of entry of aminoglycoside molecules into bacterial cells is a function of their binding to a usually nonsaturable anionic transporter whereupon they retain their positive charge and are subsequently "pulled" across the cytoplasmic membrane by the internal negative charge of the cell.[57] This process requires energy and a threshold minimal level of internal negative charge of the cell that has to be present before significant transport occurs ("proton motive force").[58] The level of the internal charge that is required may depend on the actual aminoglycoside concentration at a given time. The energy generation or the proton motive force that is required for substrate transport into the cell may be altered in mutants resistant to aminoglycosides.

These aminoglycoside-resistant isolates with altered proton motive force occur rarely but develop in the course of long-term aminoglycoside therapy.[59] These isolates usually have a "small-colony" phenotype due to their reduced rate of growth. They may be unstable and revert back to a sensitive phenotype in the absence of selective amingolycoside pressure. The clinical significance of these isolates is not clear. They may retain some virulence[60] and may cause fatal bacteremia rarely.[61] Because oxidative metabolism is essential for aminoglycoside uptake, *Pseudomonas* mutants deficient in specific cytochrome action as well as cell growth and development have been found.[57] Resistant mutants with defective electron transport systems have been described in *E. coli, S. aureus,* and *Salmonella* species. Facultative organisms grown anaerobically are resistant to aminoglycosides because of a marked reduction of the uptake of the antibiotic.[35]

Promotion of Antibiotic Efflux

The major mechanism of resistance to tetracycline found in enteric gram-negative organisms results from the decreased accumulation of tetracycline. This reduced uptake is an energy-dependent process that is related to the generation of an inner membrane protein produced by the tetracycline resistance determinant. The primary mechanism for decreased accumulation of tetracycline is due mainly to active efflux of the antibiotic across the cell membrane.[62,63] Decreased uptake of tetracycline from the extracellular environment also accounts for decreased accumulation of tetracycline inside resistant cells. These resistance determinants may be found on the chromosome or plasmids and are frequently found on transposable genetic elements. Tetracycline resistance genes are generally inducible by subinhibitory concentrations of tetracycline. An active efflux system for the removal of fluoroquinolones has recently been demonstrated in *E. coli*.[64] This system may represent a potential mechanism for resistance to the newer quinolone antimicrobial agents.

Alteration in Ribosomal Target Sites

Resistance to a wide variety of antimicrobial agents including tetracyclines, macrolides, lincosamides, and the aminoglycosides may result from an alteration in ribosomal binding sites. Failure of the antibiotic to bind to its target site(s) on the ribosome disrupts its ability to inhibit protein synthesis and cell growth. For the macrolides (such as erythromycin) and lincosamides (such as clindamycin), this is the principal mechanism of resistance among gram-positive organisms.[65] Resistance occurs as the result of a methylase enzyme that dimethylates adenine residues on the 23S ribosomal RNA of the 50S subunit of the prokaryotic ribosome, thereby disrupting the binding of macrolides and lincosamides to the ribosome. There are four classes of this resistance determinant that may be located on plasmids or the bacterial chromosome.[66] Tetracycline resistance may also occur by a mechanism that interferes with the ability of tetracycline to bind to the ribosome. The ubiquitous *tetM* resistance gene protects the ribosome from tetracycline action. The precise mechanism of action of this resistance gene is unclear at present.[67] The *tetM* determinant is widely dispersed in gram-positive organisms[67] in addition to *Mycoplasma,*[68] *Ureaplasma,*[15] *Campylobacter,*[69] and *Neisseria* spp.[14]

Resistance to aminoglycosides may also be mediated at the ribosomal level. Mutations of the S12 protein of the 30S subunit has been shown to interfere with binding streptomycin to the ribosome. Ribosomal resistance to streptomycin may be a significant cause of streptomycin resistance among enterococcal isolates.[70] Ribosomal resistance to the 2-deoxystreptamine aminoglycosides (gentamicin, tobramycin, amikacin) appears to be uncommon and may require multiple mutations in that these aminoglycosides appear to bind to several sites on the 30S and 50S subunits of the prokaryotic ribosome. Ribosomal resistance is often associated with decreased intracellular accumulation of the drug.[71]

Alteration in Target Enzymes

β-Lactams. β-Lactam antibiotics inhibit bacteria by binding covalently to penicillin binding proteins (PBPs) in the cytoplasmic membrane. These target proteins catalyze the synthesis of the peptidoglycan that forms the cell wall of bacteria.[72] Alterations in PBPs can lead to β-lactam antibiotic resistance.[73]

In gram-positive bacteria, resistance to β-lactam antibiotics may be associated either with a decrease in the affinity of the PBP for the antibiotic[74] or with a change in the amount of PBP produced by the bacterium.[75] Multiple mechanisms appear to be present in some clinical isolates. For example, penicillin-resistant strains of *Streptococcus pneumoniae* isolated in South Africa have shown several changes in their PBPs, i.e., decreased affinity of some PBPs, loss of others, and appearance of PBPs not present in the more susceptible cells.[76] In *S. aureus*[77–79] and *Enterococcus faecium*[79,80] additional PBPs may be inducible, i.e., their production is stimulated by exposure of the microorganism to the β-lactam antibiotic. These inducible PBPs have a lower affinity for β-lactam antibiotics, which makes them less susceptible to inhibition by low concentrations of drug. Changes in the types of PBPs observed in susceptible and resistant strains have also been seen with a viridans streptococcal species, *S. mitis*.[81]

Factors that regulate the induction of PBPs are poorly understood. The induction of a low-affinity PBP in methicillin-resistant *S. aureus* (MRSA) occurs to a larger extent when the microorganisms are grown at 32°C rather than at 37°C, conditions known to favor the expression of methicillin resistance.[82] There is evidence that the production of this inducible PBP is under the control of plasmid-borne genes that regulate staphylococcal penicillinase production. The structural gene that determines the low-affinity PBP of MRSA shares extensive sequence homology with a PBP of *E. coli,* and the genes that regulate the production of the low-affinity PBP have considerable sequence homology with the genes that regulate the production of staphylococcal penicillinase.[83] Thus, the production of this low-affinity penicillin-binding protein in MRSA may be mediated by a fusion of genes scavenged from *E. coli* and *S. aureus*.

The PBPs of chromosomally mediated, penicillin-resistant strains of *N. gonorrhoeae* have shown reduced penicillin binding of some of their PBPs.[84] Mutations leading to a loss of outer membrane proteins may also be associated with acquisition of penicillin resistance in non-penicillinase-producing strains of *N. gonorrhoeae,* thus suggesting that altered permeability may also contribute to the resistance.[85] Permeability changes and a decreased affinity of PBPs are mechanisms jointly found in clinical isolates of *P. aeruginosa*[86] and non beta-lactamase producing strains of *H. influenzae* as well.[87] Thus, multiple mutations may be necessary in order to effect this type of resistance.

Sulfonamides and Trimethoprim. Sulfonamides compete with para-aminobenzoic acid to bind the enzyme dihydropteroate synthetase, thereby halting the generation of pteridines and nucleic acids. Sulfonamide resistance may be mediated by the production of a dihydropteroate synthetase that is resistant to binding by sulfonamides.[88] The high prevalence of resistance to sulfonamides among gram-negative bacteria may be attributed to the spread of R plasmids that contain genes that elaborate resistant enzymes. The most common mechanism of transferable trimethoprim resistance occurs in a similar fashion, by making a drug-resistant dihydrofolate reductase (DHFR).[89] Trimethoprim-resistant DHFRs have been found on the chromosome, and multiple forms have been found to be plasmid mediated.[90]

Quinolones. DNA gyrase is necessary for the supercoiling of chromosomal DNA in bacteria in order to have efficient cell division.[91] This enzyme consists of two A subunits encoded by the *gyr* A gene and two B subunits encoded by the *gyr* B gene. Although spontaneous mutations in the *gyr* A locus have resulted in resistance to multiple fluoroquinolones, B-subunit alterations may also affect resistance to these drugs. Mutations in a variety of chromosomal loci have been described that result in altered DNA gyrases that are resistant to nalidixic acid and the newer fluoroquinolones in Enterobacteriaceae and *P. aeruginosa*.[92,93]

Bypass of Antibiotic Inhibition

Another mechanism for acquiring resistance to specific antibiotics is by the development of auxotrophs, which have growth factor requirements different from those of the wild strain. These mutants require substrates that normally are synthesized by the target enzymes, and thus if the substrates are present in the environment, the organisms are able to grow despite inhibition of the synthetic enzyme. For example, bacteria that lose the enzyme thymidilate synthetase are "thymine dependent" and cannot synthesize thymidilate in the usual way. They therefore require exogenous supplies of thymidine to synthesize thymidilate via salvage pathways and are thus highly resistant to trimethoprim.[94]

CONTROL OF ANTIBIOTIC RESISTANCE

Although the emergence of antibiotic-resistant bacteria has generally been correlated with the rise and fall of specific antibiotic use in clinical practice, the chain of causality is not always clear-cut.[95] Bacterial strains contain complex aggregations of genes that may be linked together. Thus the use of one antibiotic may select for the emergence of resistance to another. Although the development of antibiotic resistance may be inevitable, the rate at which it develops may be diminished by the rational use of antibiotics.[96]

The wider accessibility of minicomputers as well as the ability to track antibiotic resistance genes with molecular techniques has enhanced the ability to track the spread of antibiotic resistance. With the appropriate computerized surveillance, a hospital laboratory may be able to rapidly detect the emergence of a new type of resistance or the presence of a new microbial strain within a specific unit or patient population. Techniques such as restriction endonuclease digestion analyses of bacterial plasmids and chromosomes and genetic probes of resistance genes make it possible to confirm the presence of new genes in the environment. This information may then be correlated with the phenotypic measures determined by the clinical microbiology surveillance system.[97] Utilization of molecular techniques greatly augments routine surveillance (Fig. 3) since large data

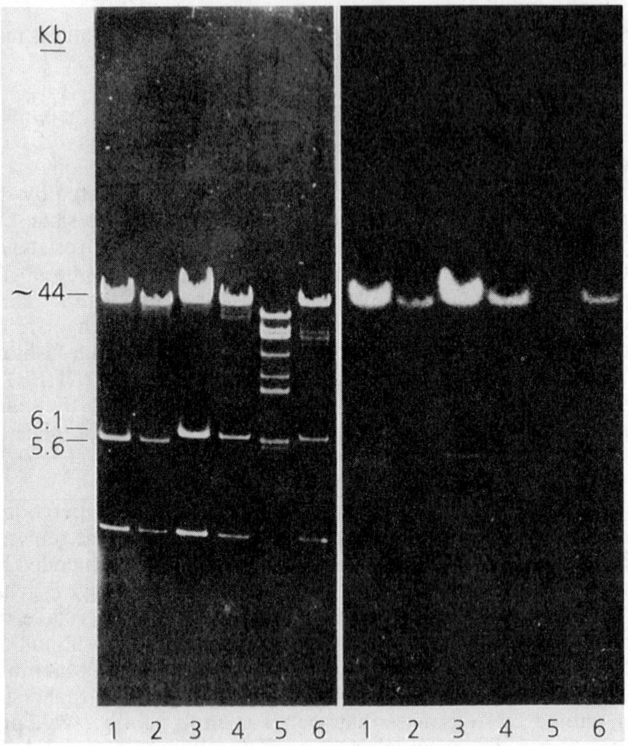

FIG. 3. **(A)** Agarose gel of *Eco*RI-digested plasmids derived from four isolates that contain a nosocomial trimethoprim resistance plasmid (known as pBWH10) from a Boston hospital (lanes 1–4). Another nosocomial plasmid from the same hospital that does not contain trimethoprim resistance genes (lane 5), and one in which both the trimethoprim-resistant and -sensitive plasmids are present in the same isolate (lane 6). **(B)** In order to show that the "fingerprints" from the trimethoprim-resistant plasmids in lanes 1–4 and 6 contain the same gene, DNA–DNA hybridization of the same six plasmids was performed by using a type II DHFR probe. The probe and the restriction endonuclease analyses helped to pinpoint the location and genetic homology of this trimethoprim resistance gene. (From Mayer et al.,[98] with permission.)

sets may obscure subtle changes ("miniepidemics") that may be more amenable to the institution of stringent infection control measures.

Study of the genetics of antibiotic resistance, particularly the awareness of the great mobility of plasmids and transposons, leads one to the conclusion that ultimately each antibiotic used may inexorably alter its microenvironment and create selective advantages for resistant organisms. Since prokaryotic organisms all contribute to a common "gene pool," favorable genes mediating antibiotic resistance may disseminate among bacterial populations. In less than a decade, newly used inexpensive drugs such as trimethoprim have gone from being highly effective in the treatment of dysentery in developing countries to becoming unusable in several of these areas.[99] Rational antibiotic usage policies would suggest the curtailment of the unnecessary use of antibiotics in situations such as animal husbandry, although the causal link between the use of antibiotics for animal growth promotion and their augmentation of the resistance in human pathogens has been disputed.[100] New drug discoveries have allowed us to be one step ahead of the bacterial pathogens. Nonetheless, the rapid evolution of resistance has limited the duration of the effectiveness of specific agents against certain pathogens. The best hope for the future is the development of greater understanding of how antimicrobial resistance spreads and the implementation of effective infection control strategies. Newer antimicrobial agents have had a substantial impact in decreasing human morbidity and mortality over the past half century. It behooves us to expand our surveillance of antibiotic resistance determinants and to exercise caution in dispensing antibiotics in order to maximize their continued efficacy.

REFERENCES

1. Kopecko D. Specialized genetic recombination systems in bacteria: Their involvement in gene expression and evolution. Prog Mol Subcell Biol. 1980;7:135–243.
2. Kopecko DJ. Involvement of specialized recombination in the evolution and expression of bacterial genes. In: Stuttgart C, Rozel KR, eds. Plasmids and Transposons. New York: Academic Press; 1980:165–206.
3. Lupski JR. Molecular mechanisms for transposition of drug-resistance genes and other movable genetic elements. Rev Infect Dis. 1987;9:357–68.
4. Datta N. Plasmids as organisms. In: Helinski DR, Cohen SN, Clevwell DB, et al., eds. *Plasmids in Bacteria.* New York: Plenum Press; 1985:383–95.
5. O'Brien T, del Pilar Pla M, Mayer KH, et al. Intercontinental spread of a new antibiotic resistance gene on an epidemic plasmid. Science. 1985; 230:87–8.
6. Timmis KN, Gonzalez-Carrero MI, Sekizaki T, et al. Biological activities specified by antibiotic resistance plasmids. J Antimicrob Chemother. 1986;18:1–12.
7. Nordstrom K. Replication, incompatibility and partition. In: Helinski DR, Cohen SN, Clewell DB, et al., eds. Plasmids in Bacteria. New York: Plenum Press; 1985:119–23.
8. Thompson R. R plasmid transfer. J Antimicrob Chemother. 1986;18:13–23.
9. Foster TJ. Plasmid-determined resistance to antimicrobial drugs and toxic metal ions in bacteria. Microbiol Rev. 1983;43:361–409.
10. Mayer KH, Hopkins JD, Gilleece ES, et al. Molecular evolution, species distribution and clinical consequences of an endemic aminoglycoside resistance plasmid. Antimicrob Agents Chemother. 1986;29:628–33.
11. Rubens CE, McNeill WF, Farrar WE Jr. Evolution of multiple-antibiotic-resistance plasmids mediated by transposable plasmid deoxyribonucleic acid sequences. J Bacteriol. 1979;140:713–9.
12. Franke AE, Clewell DB. Evidence for a chromosome-borne resistance transposon (Tn916) in *Streptococcus faecalis* that is capable of "conjugal" transfer in the absence of a conjugative plasmid. J Bacteriol. 1981;145:494–502.
13. Solh NE, Allignet J, Bismuth R, et al. Conjugative transfer of staphylococcal antibiotic resistance markers in the absence of detectable plasmid DNA. Antimicrob Agents Chemother. 1986;30:161–69.
14. Morse SA, Johnson SR, Biddle JW, et al. High-level tetracycline resistance in *Neisseria gonorrhoeae* is the result of acquisition of streptococcal *tetM* determinant. Antimicrob Agents Chemother. 1986;30:664–70.
15. Roberts MC, Kenny GE. Dissemination of the *tetM* tetracycline resistance determinant to *Ureaplasma urealyticum.* Antimicrob Agents Chemother. 1986;29:350–52.
16. Leclеq R, Derlot E, Duval J, et al. Plasmid-mediated resistance to vancomycin and teicoplanin in *Enterococcus faecium.* N Engl J Med. 1988;319:157–61.
17. Medeiros AA. Beta-lactamases. Br Med Bull. 1984;40:18–27.
18. Sykes RB, Matthew M. The beta-lactamases of gram-negative bacteria and their role in resistance to beta-lactam antibiotics. J Antimicrob Chemother. 1976;2:115–57.
19. McDonnell RW, Sweendy HM, Cohen S. Conjugational transfer of gentamicin resistance plasmids intra- and interspecifically in *Staphylococcus aureus* and *Staphylococcus epidermidis.* Antimicrob Agents Chemother. 1983;23:151–60.
20. Murray BE, Mederski-Samoraj B, Foster SK, et al. In-vitro studies of plasmid-mediated penicillinase from *Streptococcus faecalis* suggest a staphylococcal origin. J Clin Invest. 1986;77:289–93.
21. Medeiros AA. Plasmid-determined beta-lactamases. Microbial resistance to drugs. In: Bryan LE, ed. Handbook of Experimental Pharmacology. Berlin: Springer-Verlag. 1989:102–27.
22. Cuchural GJ Jr, Tally FP, Storey JR, et al. Transfer of beta-lactamase-associated cefoxitin resistance in *Bacteroides fragilis.* Antimicrob Agents Chemother. 1986;29:918–20.
23. Cuchural GJ Jr, Mulamy MH, Tally FP. Beta-lactamase-mediated imipenem resistance in *Bacteroides fragilis.* Antimicrob Agents Chemother. 1986; 30:645–48.
24. Medeiros AA, O'Brien TF. Ampicillin-resistant *Haemophilus influenzae* type B possessing a TEM-type beta-lactamase but little permeability barrier to ampicillin, Lancet. 1975;1:716.
25. Elwell LP, Roberts M, Mayer LW, et al. Plasmid-mediated beta-lactamase production in *Neisseria gonorrhoeae.* Antimicrob Agents Chemother. 1977;11:528–33.
26. Kliebe C, Nies BA, Meyer JF, et al. Evolution of plasmid-coded resistance to broad-spectrum cephalosporins. Antimicrob Agents Chemother. 1985; 28:302–7.
27. Brun-Buisson C, Legrand P, Philippon A, et al. Transferable enzymatic resistance to third-generation cephalosporins during nosocomial outbreak of multiresistant *Klebsiella pneumoniae.* Lancet. 1987;302–6.
28. Bauernfeind A, Horl G. Novel R-factor borne beta-lactamase of *Escherichia coli* conferring resistance to cephalosporins. Infection. 1987;15:257–9.
29. Sirot J, Labia R, Thabaut A. *Klebsiella pneumoniae* strains more resistant to ceftazidime than to other third-generation cephalosporins (Abstract). J Antimicrob Chemother. 1987;20:611–2.

30. Goussard S, Sougakoff W, Gerbaud G, et al. CTX-1, a wide-substrate-range enzyme, is a derivative of a TEM beta-lactamase (Abstract). Proceedings of the 27th Interscience Conference on Antimicrobial Agents and Chemotherapy. New York: American Society for Microbiology; 1987.
31. Jaurin B, Grundstrom T, Edlund T, et al. The *E. coli* beta-lactamase attenuator mediates growth rate–dependent regulation. Nature. 1981;290:221–5.
31a. Sawai T, Kanno M, Tsukamoto K. Characterization of eight beta-lactamases of gram-negative bacteria J. Bacteriol. 1982;152:567–71.
32. Nugent ME, Hedges RW. The nature of the genetic determinant for the SHV-1 beta-lactamase. Mol Gen Genet. 1979;175:239–43.
33. Moxon ER, Medeiros AA, O'Brien TF. Beta-lactamase effect on ampicillin treatment of *Haemophilus influenzae* B bacteremia and meningitis in infant rats. Antimicrob Agents Chemother. 1977;12:461–4.
34. Sanders CC, Sanders WE, Goering RV. In vitro antagonism of beta-lactam antibiotics by cefoxitin. Antimicrob Agents Chemother. 1982;21:968–75.
35. Bryan LE. Aminoglycoside resistance. In: Bryan LE, ed. Antimicrobial Drug Resistance. Orlando, FL: Academic Press; 1984:241–77.
36. Davies J, Smith DI. Plasmid-determined resistance to antimicrobial agents. Annu Rev Biochem. 1978;32:469.
37. Mayer KH. Review of epidemic aminoglycoside resistance worldwide. Am J Med. 1986;80(Suppl 6B):56–64.
38. Shimizu K, Kumada T, Hsieh W, et al. Comparison of aminoglycoside resistance patterns in Japan, Formosa, and Korea, Chile, and the United States. Antimicrob Agents Chemother. 1985;28:282–8.
39. John JF Jr, Twitty JA. Plasmids as epidemiologic markers in nosocomial gram-negative bacilli: Experience at a university and review of the literature. Rev Infect Dis. 1986;8:693–704.
39a. Hare RS, Shaw KJ, Miller GH, et al. The activity of isepamicin (ISM) against amikacin resistant gram-negative bacteria from the USA, Europe, Argentina, and Japan (Abstract). Proceedings of the 28th Interscience Conference on Antimicrobial Agents and Chemotherapy. Los Angeles: American Society for Microbiology. 1988:Abstract 1495;376.
40. Gaffney DF, Foster TJ, Shaw WV. Chloramphenicol acetyl transferases determined by R-plasmids from gram (−) bacteria. J Gen Microbiol. 1978;109:351–8.
41. Davies J. General mechanisms of antimicrobial resistance. Rev Infect Dis. 1979;1:23–7.
42. Barthelemy P, Autissier D, Gerbaud G, et al. Enzymatic hydrolysis of erythromycin by a strain of *Escherichia coli*: A new mechanism of resistance. J Antibiot. 1984;37:1692–6.
43. Andremont A, Gerbaud G, Courvalin P. Plasmid-mediated high-level resistance to erythromycin in *Escherichia coli*. Antimicrob Agents Chemother. 1986;29:515–8.
44. Fleming A. On the antibacterial action of cultures of a *Penicillium,* with special reference to their use in the isolation of *B. influenzae*. Br J Exp Pathol. 1929;10:226–36.
45. Nikaido H. Role of permeability barriers in resistance to beta-lactam antibiotics. Pharmacol Ther. 1985;27:197–231.
46. Labischinski H, Barnickel G, Bradaczek H, et al. High state of order of isolated bacterial lipopolysaccharide and its possible contribution to the permeation barrier property of the outermembrane. J Bacteriol. 1985;162:9–20.
47. Takeuchi Y, Nikaido H. Physical interaction between lipid A and phospholipids: A study with spin-labeled phospholipids. Rev Infect Dis. 1984;6:488–92.
48. Vaara M. Polymyxin B nonapeptide complexes with lipopolysaccharide (Letter). FEMS Microbiol. 1983;18:117–21.
49. Nikaido H, Vaara M. Molecular basis of the permeability of outer membrane permeability. Microbiol Rev. 1985;49:1–32.
50. Hasegawa Y, Yamada H, Mizushima S. Interactions of outer membrane proteins 0-8 and 0-9 with peptidoglycan sacculus of *Escherichia coli* K-12. J Biochem. 1976;80:1401–9.
51. Yoshimura F, Nikaido H. Diffusion of beta-lactam antibiotics through the porin channels of *Escherichia coli* K-12. Antimicrob Agents Chemother. 1985;27:84–92.
52. Medeiros AA, O'Brien TF, Rosenberg EY, et al. Loss of OmpC porin in a strain of *Salmonella typhimurium* causes increased resistance to cephalosporins during therapy. J Infect Dis. 1987;156:751–7.
53. Goldstein FW, Gutmann L, Williamson R, et al. In vivo and in vitro emergence of simultaneous resistance to both beta-lactam and aminoglycoside antibiotics in a strain of *Serratia marcescens* (Abstract). Ann Microbiol (Paris). 1983;134:329–37.
54. Quinn JP, Dudek EJ, DiVincenzo CA, et al. Emergence of resistance to imipenem during therapy for *Pseudomonas aeruginosa* infections. J Infect Dis. 1986;154:289–94.
55. Sanders CC, Sanders WE Jr, Goering RV, et al. Selection of multiple antibiotic resistance by quinolones, beta-lactams, and aminoglycosides with special reference to cross-resistance between unrelated drug classes. Antimicrobial Agents Chemother. 1984;26:797–801.
56. Gaffney DF, Cundiffe E, Foster TJ. Chloramphenicol resistance that does not involve chloramphenicol acetyltransferase encoded by plasmids from gram (−) bacteria. J Gen Microbiol. 1981;125:113–121.
57. Bryan LE, Kwan S. Roles of ribosomal binding membrane potential and electron transport in bacterial uptake of streptomycin and gentamicin. Antimicrob Agents Chemother. 1983;23:835–45.
58. Mates SM, Esenberg ES, Mandel LF, et al. Membrane potential and gentamicin uptake in *Staphylococcus aureus*. Proc Natl Acad Sci USA. 1982;79:6693–7.
59. Rusthoven JJ, Davies A, Lerner SA. Clinical isolation and characterization of aminoglycoside-resistant small colony variants of *Enterobacter aerogenes*. Am J Med. 1979;67:702–6.
60. Musher DN, Baughan RE, Merrell GL. Selection of small-colony variants of Enterobacteriaceae by *in vitro* exposure to aminoglycosides: Pathogenicity for experimental animals. J Infect Dis. 1979;140:209–14.
61. Funada H, Hattori K, Kosaki N. Catalase-negative *Escherichia coli* isolated from the blood. J Clin Microbiol. 1978;7:474–8.
62. McMurry L, Petrucci RE, Levy SB. Active efflux of tetracycline encoded by four genetically different tetracycline resistance determinants in *Escherichia coli*. Proc Natl Acad Sci USA. 1980;71:3974–7.
63. McMurry LM, Park BH, Burdette V, et al. Energy-dependent efflux mediated by Class L (*tetL*) tetracycline resistance determinant from streptococci. Antimicrob Agents Chemother. 1987;31:1648–50.
64. Cohen SP, Hooper DC, Wolfson JS, et al. Endogenous active efflux of norfloxacin in susceptible *Escherichia coli*. Antimicrob Agents Chemother. 1988;32:1187–90.
65. Engel HWB, Soedirman N, Rost JA, et al. Transferability of macrolide, lincomycin, and streptogramin resistances between group A, B, and D streptococci, *Streptococcus pneumoniae,* and *Staphylococcus aureus*. J Bacteriol. 1980;142:407–13.
66. Weisblum B. Inducible resistance to macrolides, lincosamides and streptogramin type B antibiotics: The resistance phenotype, its biological diversity, and structural elements that regulate expression—a review. J Antimicrob Chemother. 1985;16(Suppl A):63–90.
67. Burdette V. Streptoccal tetracycline resistance mediated at the level of protein synthesis. J Bacteriol. 1986;165:564–9.
68. Roberts MC, Koutsy LA, Holmes KK, et al. Tetracycline-resistant *Mycoplasma hominis* strains contain streptococcal *tetM* sequences. Antimicrob Agents Chemother. 1985;28:141–3.
69. Taylor DE, Kiratsuka K, Ray H, et al. Characterization and expression of a cloned tetracycline resistance determinant from *Campylobacter jejuni* plasmid pUA466. J Bacteriol. 1987;169:2984–9.
70. Eliopoulos GM, Farber BF, Murray BE, et al. Ribosomal resistance of clinical enterococcal isolates to streptomycin. Antimicrob Agents Chemother. 1984;25:398–9.
71. Ahmad MH, Rechenmacher A, Boch A. Interaction between aminoglycoside uptake and ribosomal resistance mutations. Antimicrob Agents Chemother. 1980;18:798–806.
72. Waxman DJ, Strominger JL. Penicillin-binding proteins and the mechanism of action of beta-lactam antibiotics. Annu Rev Biochem 1983;52:825–69.
73. Malouin F, Bryan LE. Modification of penicillin-binding proteins as mechanisms of beta-lactam resistance. Antimicrob Agents Chemother. 1986;30: 1–5.
74. Williamson R. Resistance of *Clostridium perfringens* to beta-lactam antibiotics mediated by a decreased affinity of a single essential penicillin-binding protein. J Gen Microbiol. 1983;129:2339–42.
75. Giles AF, Reynolds PE. *Bacillus megaterium* resistance to cloxacillin accompanied by a compensatory change in penicillin binding proteins. Nature. 1979;280:167–8.
76. Hakenbeck R, Tarpay M, Tomasz A. Multiple changes of penicillin-binding proteins in penicillin-resistant clinical isolates of *Streptococcus pneumoniae*. Antimicrob Agents Chemother. 1980;17:364–71.
77. Hartman BJ, Tomasz A. Low-affinity penicillin-binding protein associated with beta-lactam resistance in *Staphylococcus aureus*. J Bacteriol. 1984;158:513–6.
78. Ubukata K, Yamashita N, Konno M. Occurrence of a beta-lactam-inducible penicillin-binding protein in methicillin-resistant staphylococci. Antimicrob Agents Chemother. 1985;27:851–7.
79. Fontana R. Penicillin-binding proteins and the intrinsic resistance to beta-lactams in gram positive cocci. J Antimicrob Chemother. 1985;16:412–6.
80. Fontana R, Grossato A, Rossi L, et al. Transition from resistance to hypersusceptibility to beta-lactam antibiotics associated with loss of low-affinity penicillin-binding protein in a *Streptococcus faecium* mutant highly resistant to penicillin. Antimicrob Agents Chemother. 1985;28:678–83.
81. Farber BF, GM Eliopoulos, Ward JI, et al. Multiply resistant viridans streptococci: Susceptibility to beta-lactam antibiotics and comparison of penicillin-binding protein patterns. Antimicrob Agents Chemother. 1983;24:702–5.
82. Sabath LD. Chemical and physical factors influencing methicillin resistance of *Staphylococcus aureus* and *Staphylococcus epidermidis*. J Antimicrob Chemother. 1977;3(Suppl C):47–51.
83. Song MD, Wachi M, Doi M, et al. Evolution of an inducible penicillin target protein in methicillin-resistant *Staphylococcus aureus* by gene fusion. FEBS Lett. 1987;226:167–71.
84. Dougherty TJ, Koller AE, Tomasz A. Penicillin binding proteins of penicillin-susceptible and intrinsically resistant *Neisseria gonorrhoeae*. Antimicrob Agents Chemother. 1980;18:730–7.
85. Faruki H, Kohmescher RN, McKinney WP, et al. A community based outbreak of infection with penicillin-resistant *Neisseria gonorrhoeae* not producing penicillinase (chromosomally mediated resistance). N Engl J Med. 1985;313:607–11.
86. Mirelman D, Nuchamowitz Y, Rubinstein E. Insensitivity of peptidoglycan biosynthetic reactions to beta-lactam antibiotics in a clinical isolate of *Pseudomonas aeruginosa*. Antimicrob Agents Chemother. 1981;19:687–95.
87. Parr TR, Bryan LE. Mechanism of resistance of an ampicillin-resistant beta-

lactamase-negative clinical isolate of *Haemophilus influenzae* type b to beta-lactam antibiotics. Antimicrob Agents Chemother. 1984;25:747–53.
88. Hamilton-Miller JMT. Resistance to antibacterial agents acting on antifolate metabolism. In: Bryan LE, ed. Antimicrobial Drug Resistance. Orlando, FL: Academic Press; 1984:173–88.
89. Huovinen P. Trimethoprim resistance. Antimicrob Agents Chemother. 1987;31:1451–6.
90. Steen R, Skold O. Plasmid-borne or chromosomally mediated resistance by Tn7 is the most common response to ubiquitous use of trimethoprim. Antimicrob Agents Chemother. 1985;27:933–7.
91. Wolfson JS, Hooper DC. The fluoroquinolones: Structures, mechanisms of action and resistance, and spectra of activity in vitro. Antimicrob Agents Chemother. 1985;28:581–6.
92. Hane MW, Wood TH. *Escherichia coli* K-12 mutants resistant to nalidixic acid: Genetic mapping and dominance studies. J Bacteriol. 1969;99:238–41.
93. Robillard NJ, Scarpa AL. Genetic and physiological characterization of ciprofloxacin resistance in *Pseudomonas aeruginosa* PAO. Antimicrob Agents Chemother. 1988;32:535–9.
94. Maskell R, Okubagejo OA, Payne RH. Human infections with thymine-requiring bacteria. J Med Microbiol. 1978;11:33–42.
95. McGowan JE. Antimicrobial resistance in hospital organisms and its relation to antimicrobial use. Rev Infect Dis. 1983;5:1033–48.
96. Levy SB. Resistance to the tetracyclines. In: Bryan LE, ed. Antimicrobial Drug Resistance. Orlando, FL: Academic Press; 1984:192–234.
97. Mayer KH, Hopkins JD, Gilleece ES, et al. Computer-assisted correlations between antibiotypes of clinical isolates and the endonuclease restriction fragment of types of their plasmids. In: Mitsuhasi S, Rosival L, Krcmery V, eds. Transferrable Antibiotic Resistance: Plasmids and Gene Manipulation. Prague and Heidelberg: Czechoslovak Press and Springer-Verlag; 1984:163–9.
98. Mayer KH, Fling ME, Hopkins JD, et al: Trimethoprim resistance in multiple genera of Enterobacteriaceae at a U.S. hospital: Spread of type II dihydrofolate reductase gene by a single plasmid. J Infect Dis. 1985;151:783–89.
99. Murray BE, Alvarado T, Kim K-H. Increasing resistance to trimethoprim-sulfamethoxazole among isolates of *Escherichia coli* in developing countries. J Infect Dis. 1985;152:1107–13.
100. Holmberg SD, Solomon SL, Blake PA. Health and economic impacts of antimicrobial resistance. Rev Infect Dis. 1987;6:1065–78.

17. PHARMACOKINETICS OF ANTIMICROBIAL AGENTS

PAUL S. LIETMAN

The pharmacokinetics of antimicrobial agents should be considered in terms of the time-dependent interactions with both microorganisms and humans.

The time-dependent interactions of antimicrobial agents with microorganisms are important to the effectiveness of the drug.[1] This effectiveness is influenced by both the kinetics of microbial growth and the drug concentration in the environment of the microbe. Usually, the drug concentration in the environment of the microbe changes over time, with peaks and troughs that roughly parallel the plasma levels when intermittent doses are administered. Although much is unknown about the interplay between microbial growth kinetics and constantly changing drug concentrations in the microbial environment, some generalizations can be made. Penicillin G (and probably other penicillins, β-lactams, and inhibitors of cell wall synthesis) can inhibit bacterial cell growth and can produce cell lysis even though the concentration of antibiotic drops quite low during some of each dosing interval if the target organism is *Staphylococcus* sp., *Streptococcus pyogenes,* or *Streptococcus pneumoniae.*[2] With these organisms and drugs, the physician does not need to keep the level of these antibiotics above the minimum bacteriostatic concentration (MIC) throughout all of each dosing interval. Although there is insufficient evidence about any other drugs and these organisms, it can be assumed that the level of drug in the environment of these bacteria should be maintained above the MIC throughout each dosing interval. The MIC should be considered as the lowest concentration, which, if constantly maintained adjacent to the bacterium, will prevent bacterial growth. β-Lactam antibiotics behave quite differently with gram-negative bacilli, and there is mounting evidence that bacterial regrowth begins as soon as the concentration of drug falls below the MIC.[2,3] In these situations, the β-lactam level should be maintained above the MIC throughout each dosing interval. Aminoglycoside antibiotics also appear to be dependent on the bacterial species being treated. When aminoglycosides interact with *Pseudomonas aeruginosa,* there is a significant lag between the time the bacteria begin to regrow and the time the antibiotic concentration falls below the MIC.[2] With *Escherichia coli,* however, and probably other Enterobacteriaceae as well, bacterial regrowth commences very quickly after the adjacent antibiotic concentration falls below the MIC.[2] Since data exist for only a very few combinations of antimicrobial agents and microbes, the physician is often forced to act without the benefit of adequate information. Thus, a dosing regimen that would maintain the drug level above the MIC throughout each entire dosing interval would be the conservative approach.

The time-dependent interactions of antimicrobial agents with humans are important to both effectiveness and toxicity. The interactions of drugs and microorganisms depend on attaining antibiotic concentrations immediately adjacent to bacteria, and consequently these levels depend on human drug interactions including absorption, distribution, metabolism, and excretion. In addition, the plasma and tissue concentrations of drugs may correlate with dose-related toxicities. The time-dependent interactions with humans can also be used to construct dosing regimens.

Although the precise description of the pharmacokinetics of any drug can be exceedingly complex, the clinician can benefit considerably from approximations that are reasonably accurate and yet comprehensible. The goal of this chapter is to provide a foundation of pharmacokinetics of chemotherapeutic agents that is useful in the construction of therapeutic regimens and in the modification of these regimens for individualization of antimicrobial therapy. More extensive discussions of pharmacokinetics can be found in several excellent books.[4–6]

VOLUME OF DISTRIBUTION (V_D)

The volume of distribution (V_D) of a drug is defined as that volume in which the total amount of drug in the body (A) would have to be uniformly distributed in order to give the observed plasma concentration (C_P).

$$V_D = \frac{A}{C_P} \quad (1)$$

Thus if 140 mg of gentamicin were given to a 70 kg patient and the plasma concentration was found to be 8 μg/ml (= 8 mg/liter), then the volume of distribution would be (140 mg) ÷ (8 mg/liter) = 17.5 liters.

The volume of distribution is often expressed in terms of the body weight, liters/kg. If expressed as liters/kg, then the actual V_D is obtained simply by multiplying the volume of distribution per kg by the body weight.

By rearranging Equation 1, the dose (or amount) necessary to produce any desired plasma concentration can be calculated with a drug whose volume of distribution is known or the plasma concentration that can be expected with any chosen dose. Thus, if the goal is to produce a plasma gentamicin concentration of 10 μg/ml (= 10 mg/liter) in a 70 kg man and the V_D is known to be 0.25 liter/kg, then the dose must = $(V_D)(C_P)$ = (0.25 liter/kg)(70 kg)(10 mg/liter) = 175 mg.

The volume of distribution need not and usually does not correspond to any actual anatomic or physiologic space. It is simply a mathematical tool.

Most antimicrobial agents have volumes of distribution of

between 0.15 liter/kg and 0.40 liter/kg. However, a few have larger volumes of distribution. For example, flucytosine, isoniazid, and erythromycin have volumes of distribution of 0.6 liter/kg to 0.7 liter/kg while chloramphenicol, doxycycline, nafcillin, and tetracycline have volumes of distribution of about 1 liter/kg. A few antimicrobial agents have volumes of distribution that exceed the body weight. Trimethoprim, ethambutol, and rifampin have volumes of distribution of 1.6 liters/kg to 1.8 liters/kg, and amphotericin B has a V_D of 4 liters/kg.

The important clinical use of the V_D is that it provides an initial or loading dose that promptly provides a therapeutic plasma concentration. The V_D is also useful, as is described below, in calculating subsequent or maintenance doses to achieve therapeutic and yet safe plasma concentrations.

HALF-LIFE ($T_{\frac{1}{2}}$)

The half-life of a drug is defined as the time required for the plasma concentration to fall to one-half its former value as it is being eliminated from the body.

It is usually assumed that the half-life associated with a drug is the half-life of the predominant phase of drug elimination, that absorption of the drug is completed, and that the distribution of the drug throughout the entire volume of distribution has been completed. It is also assumed that the fall in the plasma concentration parallels the fall in the total amount of drug in the body.

The half-life of a drug remains constant over time if there has been no change in the processes of drug elimination. During each half-life, 50 percent of the total amount of drug in the body is eliminated, and the plasma concentration falls by 50 percent. Generally, a constant percentage (or fraction) of drug is eliminated from the body in any constant period of time.

The half-lives of antimicrobial agents vary considerably. All of the currently marketed β-lactam antibiotics except ceftriaxone have very short half-lives (usually <1.5 hours). The aminoglycosides have somewhat longer half-lives (2–3 hours). Ceftriaxone, chloramphenicol, flucytosine, sulfisoxazole, and vancomycin have half-lives of 3–6 hours. Sulfamethoxazole, tetracycline, and trimethoprim have half-lives of 6–12 hours. Doxycycline has a relatively long half-life of 20 hours.

The usually quoted half-life of a drug is applicable as a generalization to young adults without renal or hepatic dysfunction. Clinically significant prolongation of a drug's half-life often accompanies renal dysfunction and occasionally occurs with hepatic dysfunction. The half-life may also be influenced by age with prolongations of the half-life in the newborn and the elderly and with shortened half-lives in young children when compared with young adult values. Other drugs administered concomitantly can also alter a drug's half-life as, for example, probenecid prolongs the half-life of many β-lactam antibiotics.

The half-life data are used to calculate continuing (or maintenance) doses of a drug and provide important information about oscillations of plasma concentrations of a drug given intermittently and repetitively.

REPETITIVE DOSING: THE PLATEAU PRINCIPLE

With repetitive dosing of a drug at regular intervals, the maximal or peak plasma concentrations and the minimal or trough plasma concentrations rise to a steady state or plateau, and after such a plateau is reached, the peak and trough plasma concentrations remain constant if the dose remains constant and if there is no change in the rate of drug elimination. The attainment of a plateau is also applicable to continuous dosing at a constant rate where the plasma concentrations climb until a plateau is reached and then remain constant.

The rate at which the plateau is attained is a function exclusively of the half-life of drug elimination and is independent of the rate of drug administration. Thus, giving twice as much drug per dose or per unit of time ultimately provides a higher plasma concentration at the plateau but the plateau is still reached at the same time. A useful concept is that the plateau is reached after four half-lives. Actually, after one half-life the peak and trough or mean plasma concentrations are about 50 percent, after three half-lives 88 percent, and after four half-lives 94 percent of the ultimate plateau levels. Similarly, when a dosage change is made or when a drug is discontinued, the new plateau is reached after about four half-lives.

The plateau principle is especially important in antimicrobial chemotherapy where the physician often wishes to provide therapeutic levels of the antimicrobial agent very promptly and where waiting four half-lives to achieve a desired level may be disastrous. In such situations an initial, or loading dose, of the drug should be given in order to achieve quickly the desired therapeutic level of the antimicrobial agent. As mentioned above, the loading dose is determined exclusively by the volume of distribution and not by the half-life.

Clearly, the plateau principle has greater clinical significance when a half-life is several hours or longer than when the half-life is an hour or less. As a generalization in antimicrobial chemotherapy, a loading dose should be considered whenever the half-life of the chosen drug in the patient is estimated to be longer than 3 hours and whenever a delay of 12 hours or longer to achieve a therapeutic level is unacceptable. A loading dose should also be considered whenever the half-life of the chosen drug is estimated to be prolonged beyond 3 hours by renal or hepatic dysfunction.

It is often useful to estimate the peak and trough plasma concentrations that can be expected with a chosen dose and dosing interval. This can be easily calculated if the volume of distribution and half-life are known. At steady state the minimal plasma concentrations (C_{min}) or trough levels are related to the V_D, $T_{\frac{1}{2}}$ and dose (D) by the following equation where n equals the dosing interval expressed in half-lives.

$$C_{min} = \frac{D}{(V_D)(2^n - 1)} \qquad (2)$$

Thus, if a 6 g dose of carbenicillin (V_D = 0.18 liter/kg; $T_{\frac{1}{2}}$ = 1.0 hour) is given every 6 hours (i.e., every six half-lives; n = 6) to an 80 kg man, the minimal of trough plasma concentration can be anticipated to be (6000 mg) ÷ (0.18 liter/kg)(80 kg)(2^6 − 1) = 6.6 mg/liter = 6.6 μg/ml.

The relationship between the maximal plasma concentrations (C_{max}) or peak levels and the minimal plasma concentrations (C_{min}) or trough levels is given by Equation 3 where n is again the dosing interval expressed in half-lives.

$$\frac{C_{max}}{C_{min}} = 2^n \qquad (3)$$

Thus, to continue with the example of carbenicillin given above, the drug was to be given every six half-lives and the ratio of C_{max} to C_{min} = 2^6 or 64. Thus, the peak plasma levels at steady state will be 64 times the trough levels of (64)(6.6 μg/ml) = 422 μg/ml. The oscillations during every dosing interval of 6 hours at steady state will be from a peak of 422 μg/ml to a trough of 6.6 μg/ml.

It may be desirable to give an antimicrobial agent by continuous intravenous infusion rather than intermittently. In such a case a plateau can be reached in about four half-lives as with intermittent dosing but there will be no peaks and troughs but only a plasma concentration at steady state (C_{ss}). The plasma concentration can also be easily estimated from a fourth simple equation.

$$C_{ss} = \frac{\text{Dose per half-life}}{(0.693)(V_D)} \qquad (4)$$

Thus, to extend the example of carbenicillin cited above, assume that the same total daily dose (i.e., 24 g) is given by continuous intravenous infusion without a loading dose. The dose per half-life is then 1 g/hr, and the plasma concentration at steady state will be 1000 mg ÷ (0.693)(V_D) = 1000 mg ÷ (0.693)(0.18 liter/kg)(80 kg) = 100 mg/liter = 100 μg/ml.

By rearranging Equations 3 or 4, it is easy to solve for the dose that needs to be given to achieve any desired plasma concentration or alternatively the dosing interval that can provide any desired oscillation from peak to trough level.

DOSE-RELATED KINETICS

Most antimicrobial agents behave pharmacokinetically in a manner that can be described with reasonable accuracy by the above four equations. However, Equations 2, 3, and 4 all used the half-life, and we have stated that the half-life in constant over time. This constancy of the half-life is dependent on there being no process of elimination (renal, hepatic, or other) that is saturable at the concentrations of drug realized. If, however, the concentration of drug begins to exceed that which can be removed from the body, then the drug is said to exhibit dose-related kinetics. With dose-related kinetics, it is as if the half-life of the drug were not constant. Although it is theoretically possible to exceed the renal secretory mechanism or the renal reabsorption mechanism, this is rarely, if ever, seen in clinical practice. The hepatic drug metabolizing capacity is, however, occasionally exceeded, in which case the drug may exhibit dose-related kinetics. A specific example is chloramphenicol where at high plasma concentrations the half-life is prolonged. This is especially pertinent to the newborn or the patient with hepatic disease.

ALTERATIONS OF DOSE WITH RENAL OR LIVER DISEASE

In general, antibiotics are eliminated from the body either into the gut after secretion into the bile or into the urine. In either case, the drug may be eliminated unchanged or may be metabolized, usually by the liver, before excretion. Thus, liver disease can impair drug elimination either as a result of impaired drug metabolism or impaired drug secretion into the bile. Kidney disease can impair drug elimination as a result of impaired glomerular filtration or, occasionally, impaired tubular secretion. The extent to which renal or hepatic processes are rate-limiting is quite variable for different drugs and is pivotal in the construction of a dosing regimen in the presence of reduced renal or hepatic function. In the presence of liver disease, the elimination of a few antimicrobial agents is slowed, that is, the half-life is prolonged. There are, however, no clear and useful correlations between any test of liver structure or function and the rate of drug elimination from the body. Thus, in a patient with known liver disease, the examiner cannot predict how the half-life of any drug will be affected, and the patient must be monitored, either clinically or with plasma drug levels, in order to be provided with safe and effective dosing.

In the presence of renal disease the elimination of many antimicrobial agents is slowed and the half-life prolonged. The prolongation of the half-life can often be estimated, however, and rational dosing adjustments can be calculated.

REFERENCES

1. Drusano GL. Role of pharmacokinetics in the outcome of infections. Antimicrob Agents Chemother. 1988;32:289.
2. Bundtzen RW, Gerber AU, Cohn DL, et al. Postantibiotic suppression of bacterial growth. Rev Infect Dis. 1981;3:28.
3. Rolinson GN. Plasma concentrations of penicillin in relation to the antibacterial effect. In Davies DS, Pritchard BNC, eds. Biological Effects of Drugs in Relation to Their Plasma Concentrations. Baltimore: University Park Press; 1973:183.
4. Gladtke E, von Hattingberg HM. Pharmacokinetics: An Introduction. New York: Springer-Verlag; 1979.
5. Rowland M, Tozer TN. Clinical Pharmacokinetics: Concepts and Applications. Philadelphia: Lea & Febiger; 1980.
6. Tedrell T, Dedrick RL, Condliffe PG. Pharmacology and Pharmacokinetics. New York: Plenum Press; 1974.

18. PENICILLINS

HAROLD C. NEU

Penicillin was isolated from *Penicillium notatum* by Fleming in 1929. The fortuitous isolation of this compound did not bear fruit until the work of Florey, Chain, and associates in 1941 made possible the commercial production of penicillin G. In 1928 Fleming found that the mold *Penicillium* produced a substance, which he named penicillin, that inhibited the growth of *Staphylococcus aureus*.[1] Fleming was not successful in attempts to obtain significant amounts of the agent and let the matter rest while he continued his work on lysozyme. In 1939 Florey at the Sir William Dunn School of Pathology began to work out the isolation, structure, and properties of the compound. In 1940 his group showed that penicillin protected mice experimentally infected with streptococci, and by 1941 they had produced enough penicillin to treat a few patients, the first of whom was a British policeman infected with both staphylococci and streptococci. As a result of the war, production of penicillin was undertaken in the United States. Initial clinical trials at Yale and the Mayo Clinic were so successful that the U.S. Army began to use the material to treat streptococcal, gonococcal, and treponemal infections. As fermentation techniques improved, production of large amounts of pure drug became possible, and by the end of the 1940s penicillin G was available for general use in the United States.

Initial production of penicillin was from *P. notatum*, but it was discovered that greater yields could be achieved from *Penicillium chrysogenum* and from growing the organism in different media. It was soon apparent that the growth medium affected the type of natural penicillin produced. Although a number of penicillins were found, for example, F, X, N, K, none of these were superior to the benzylpenicillin that was designated as penicillin G.

CHEMISTRY

The basic structure of the majority of commercially available penicillins is a nucleus that consists of three components—a thiazolidine ring, the β-lactam ring, and a side chain (Fig. 1). The side chain determines in large part the antibacterial spectrum and pharmacologic properties of a particular penicillin. The penicillin nucleus is a condensation of alanine and β-dimethylcysteine. Penicillins currently in use are dextrorotatory and usually exist as salts combined with alkaline earth metals such as sodium or potassium. The β-lactam nucleus is essential for antibacterial activity. Although biosynthesis of penicillin has been achieved, it has not proved to be a useful technique, and fermentation remains the method of production of penicillin G.

The appearance of β-lactamase-producing organisms, particularly of *S. aureus*, prompted studies to develop compounds with resistance to hydrolysis by β-lactamases and also to find agents that had increased activity over that of penicillin G against gram-negative species. In 1959 Batchelor et al.[2] isolated the penicillin nucleus 6-amino-penicillanic acid from a precursor-depleted fermentation of *P. chrysogenum*. This made possible the production and testing of numerous semisynthetic penicillins, the first of which was methicillin, active against β-lactamase-producing *S. aureus*; followed by ampicillin, active

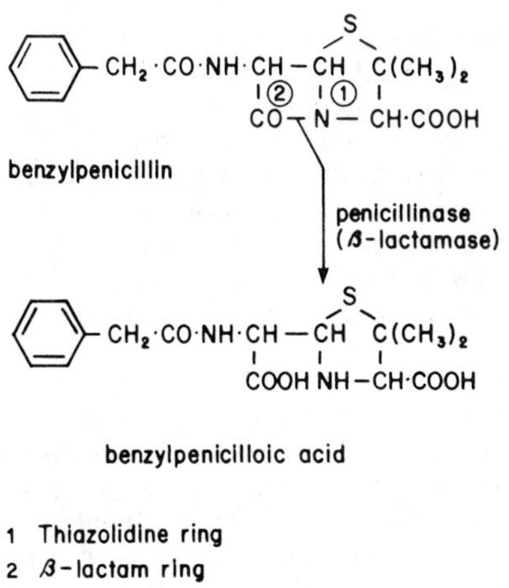

FIG. 1. Structure of penicillin and site of β-lactamase attack.

against selected gram-negative bacilli; and in 1957 by carbenicillin, which had activity against *Pseudomonas aeruginosa*. The past few years have seen the development of a score of agents with different pharmacologic and antimicrobial properties, which will be discussed subsequently in this chapter.

MECHANISM OF ACTION

We do not know precisely how penicillins kill bacterial cells. Study of the action of penicillins has elucidated many aspects of bacterial physiology, but recent advances suggest that the concept that penicillin inhibited the last step in cell wall synthesis is a simplistic one. The cell wall of bacteria is assembled in a series of enzymatic steps that involve at least 30 enzymes.

Bacterial Cell Walls

The cell walls of both gram-positive and gram-negative bacteria are held in a rigid manner protecting against osmotic rupture by the peptidoglycan, also called murein sacculus.[3,4] The cell wall of gram-positive bacteria is a large, 50–100 molecular layer, whereas the peptidoglycan component of gram-negative bacteria is only 1 or 2 molecules thick.

There is an outer lipopolysaccharide layer on top of the peptidoglycan in gram-negative species such as Enterobacteriaceae and the pseudomonads, which is absent in gram-positive species.

All peptidoglycans are long polysaccharide chains in which *N*-acetylglucosamine (NAG) and *N*-acetylmuramic (NAM) acid alternate in a linear form. These long chains are cross-linked by short peptides linked in amide linkage to the D-alanyl group of the *N*-acetylmuramic acid. In gram-negative species the 6-amino group of diaminopimelic acid is linked to the carboxy-alanine terminus of another chain.[4] Interestingly, cross-linking is less common in *Escherichia coli* (25 percent), compared with the 90 percent cross-linking in *S. aureus*.[5]

Peptidoglycan synthesis has been divided into three stages. The first is the synthesis of the nucleotide precursors with uridine diphosphate (UDP) by cytoplasmic enzymes to make UDP-*N*-acetylmuramyl-LAra-Disglu-LX-DAla-Dala and UDP-*N*-acetylglucosamine. The "X" in gram-negative species is diaminopimelic acid. The next step is the translocation of the NAM-pentapeptide and NAG across the cytoplasmic membrane by a lipid-soluble carrier, which is a C_{55} isoprenyl alcohol phosphate. Transglycosylation into peptidoglycan polymer occurs at this stage. The final reaction is the incorporation of new peptidoglycan into the existing peptidoglycan. In this final reaction a free amino group on the third amino acid of the NAM-pentapeptide of one strand displaces the terminal D-alanine from a pentapeptide of a second strand in a transpeptidation reaction. This final step was the step thought to be the sole penicillin-sensitive reaction, but we now realize that the other earlier steps also can be inhibited.

It has been shown that penicillin can inhibit transpeptidation without altering transglycosylation of the disaccharide units. There appear to be distinct transpeptidases that provide for anchoring of new peptidoglycan to old, that cross-link special structures, and that make the cell wall septum. Although there are other penicillin-susceptible reactions, such as the effects on carboxypeptidase, these reactions do not seem to be critical in gram-negative species. The most telling argument that penicillin inactivates transpeptidases was the stereo chemistry modeling of Strominger's group,[6] which supports an acylenzyme intermediate because of the structural similarity of penicillin and the acyl-D-alanyl-D-alanine.

Penicillin-Binding Proteins

In 1972 Suginaka and Blumberg and Strominger detected penicillin-binding proteins (PBPs). Subsequently Spratt's studies[7,8] of the PBPs in *E. coli* provided the biggest advance in our understanding of the effect of β-lactams on cell walls. Since then the PBPs of almost all species have been studied.

The PBPs of a given organism are numbered in order of decreasing molecular weight, for example, PBP-1 weighs about 120,000 and PBP-6 weighs 40,000. The particular number of a PBP will not readily relate from one species to another, and the PBP numbering system of gram-positive bacteria bears no relation to the PBP numbering of gram-negative bacteria. The PBPs probably account for only 1 percent of the membrane protein.

The PBPs vary greatly in the amount present. In *E. coli* and *P. aeruginosa*, high molecular weight PBPs, that is, 1, 2, 3, are in low amounts compared with PBPs 5 and 6, which account for 78 percent of the PBPs in *E. coli*. The PBPs also vary greatly in their affinity for certain β-lactams. In general, the affinity of a β-lactam to a particular PBP has been expressed as the concentration of antibiotic needed to reduce the ^{14}C-penicillin G binding to that PBP. The PBPs bind β-lactams covalently. It is believed that penicillins bind to PBPs through the carbonyl as a penicilloyl moiety and the binding of penicilloyl moiety is to a serine residue in the PBP via a bimolecular reaction.

Since the 1940s it has been known that low concentrations of penicillins cause filamentation of *E. coli*, whereas at high concentrations lysis occurs. It seems most likely that binding of a β-lactam to PBP-1Bs, or its substitute enzyme PBP-1A, results in rapid cell lysis and that this PBP is the most important protein for cell elongation.[8]

The role of PBP-2 in cell shape of bacteria was delineated by the availability of amdinocillin (mecillinam). *Escherichia coli* in the presence of amdinocillin form osmotically stable large round forms.[9] After several hours in the presence of amdinocillin, these bacteria lyse. It is probable that PBP-2 catalyzes a specific topologically restricted transpeptidase or carboxypeptidase reaction during a particular part of the cell cycle of division.

The third major PBP is PBP-3, which is important in cell division of *E. coli* and other enterobacteriaceae and pseudomonads. The PBP-3 is activated upon completion of DNA replication and subsequently catalyzes a carboxypeptidase reaction needed for the special peptidoglycan synthesis that ensues when cells divide.[10] The other low molecular weight PBPs have been thought to lack importance in the killing events associated with β-lactam binding to the proteins since mutants lacking PBP-4, -5, -6 have been isolated and grow well.[11]

The PBPs that are important in gram-positive organisms are PBPs-1, -2, and -4, since their antibiotic susceptibility closely resembles the effect of the agents on whole organisms.[12] In general, low molecular PBP-5, the carboxypeptidases, are not killing targets. Analysis of the lack of activity of β-lactams such as amdinocillin or aztreonam against gram-positive species and anaerobes shows that these agents fail to bind to PBPs of gram-positive species and anaerobes.[13]

The high activity of penicillins such as penicillin G against staphylococci can be correlated with binding to essential PBPs in these agents. Alteration of PBPs in gram-positive species has been correlated with resistance of *Streptococcus pneumoniae*, *S. aureus*, coagulase-negative staphylococci, and *Enterococcus faecium* to penicillin.

"Unleashing" of bacterial autolysins by β-lactam antibiotics may be responsible for cell death in certain species.

BACTERIAL RESISTANCE

Since there are many components involved in cell wall synthesis, variation in the composition of the wall components among bacteria accounts for some of the differences in susceptibility of individual bacterial strains to a particular penicillin. The differential binding of specific penicillins to target sites also accounts for differences in activity of different penicillins against a single organism or species. Mutation in a gene that specifies a binding site may lead to resistance to a penicillin, but this has been uncommon since most penicillins attack more than one of the peptidoglycan targets, and a coordinated mutation in a number of genes is an unlikely event. Resistant organisms with altered penicillin-binding proteins have been shown to produce an altered peptidoglycan structure.[14]

Some organisms are resistant to penicillins because the penicillin fails to reach its receptor site. Failure of a penicillin to reach its target is unlikely to be a mechanism of resistance in gram-positive species since the peptidoglycan layer lies outside the bacterial membrane,[15] but in gram-negative bacteria, two membranes compose the cell envelope, and the peptidoglycan lies inside the outer membrane. Thus in gram-negative bacteria a penicillin must pass through the outer membrane to reach its target site. Formerly it was supposed that lipophilicity of a molecule determined its activity. We now know that the protein layers on the outer surface of the bacterial membrane are held together by protein molecules that pass through the structure from one surface to the other. It is probable that penicillins that conform to the structural and charge properties of these stability proteins pass through to their receptor sites, whereas those β-lactam antibiotics that are structurally "different" do not enter the envelope and hence fail to reach a receptor site. Changes in structural protein components of the outer membrane due to mutations yield organisms more or less susceptible to penicillins. It is uncommon for naturally occurring resistant bacterial strains to owe their resistance to an alteration in membrane properties that prevents the particular penicillin from reaching its target.

The most important mechanism of bacterial resistance to penicillins is enzymatic hydrolysis of the β-lactam bond by β-lactamases with loss of antibiotic activity of the molecule.[16] A classification of β-lactamases is shown in Figure 2. The enzymes are classified on the basis of affinity for specific β-lactam compounds and amino acid composition. In gram-positive bacteria such as staphylococci, β-lactamase production is plasmid-mediated. The enzyme is both inducible and is an exoenzyme, that is, it is liberated into the surrounding medium in which it carries out its protective role by destroying the penicillins in the environment before they reach the cell surface. This mechanism of production of an exoenzyme is a protective one for bacteria such as staphylococci since they produce a large amount of enzyme with a very high affinity for penicillins.

On the other hand, β-lactamases of gram-negative bacteria are located in the periplasmic space that lies between the inner and outer membranes of gram-negative bacteria. Thus the enzymes are strategically located to protect the β-lactam target. Gram-negative β-lactamases may be either chromosomally or plasmid-mediated, constitutive or inducible enzymes, with an affinity for penicillins or for cephalosporins or both types of compounds. It is probable that all gram-negative species contain small amounts of a β-lactamase. The activity of the β-lactamase stable compounds, methicillin, and the isoxazolyl penicillins against staphylococci, is due to their β-lactamase stability. Differences in β-lactamase stability also account for some of the differences in activity of different penicillins against gram-negative bacteria. For example, carbenicillin is destroyed at a much slower rate than is ampicillin by *Enterobacter cloacae* or *Morganella morganii*.

Increased β-lactamase stability may decrease overall antibacterial activity since addition of bulky side chains that prevent β-lactamase hydrolysis also interfere with passage of the molecule across the outer membrane of gram-negative bacteria.[17] In general, increased activity of penicillins against β-lactamase-producing gram-negative bacteria is not associated with stability against β-lactamase hydrolysis but with affinity to penicillin receptor proteins and with increased entry into the bacterial cell. The one exception is temocillin, which contains a methoxy group on the β-lactam ring. Plasmid β-lactamases have markedly increased in number in the past decade, and some of the recent enzymes will destroy many cephalosporins as well as penicillins.

One final mechanism of resistance to penicillins seen in some gram-positive species is that of tolerance. This has been reported primarily for *S. aureus* and *S. pneumoniae*. Bacterial loss of viability, that is, cell death, is the result of secondary responses to inhibition of cell wall assembly. In some organisms the lytic effect of β-lactam antibiotics can be eliminated by inactivation of peptidoglycan hydrolyases (autolysins). For example, in pneumococci, lipoteichoic acids inhibit amidases. These acids are secreted into the surrounding milieu when penicillins are present. Suppression of autolytic activity protects the bacterium from the lytic effect of cell wall inhibition by penicillin. Thus an isolate that lacks autolysins will be inhibited but not killed by penicillin, that is, it is tolerant. At certain pHs the cellular autolysins are inactive and the bacteria although inhibited are not killed. The relevance of these observations to clinical situations is unclear.

CLASSIFICATION

Penicillins can be conveniently divided into classes on the basis of antibacterial activity (Table 1). Great overlaps do exist among the groups, but differences within a group usually are of a pharmacologic nature, although one compound in a group may be more active than another.

The susceptibility patterns of various species of microorganisms are given in Tables 2, 3, and 4. Gram-positive bacteria inhibited by natural penicillins in general are more susceptible to these penicillins than to semisynthetic penicillins.[18–23] Penicillin V (used orally) can be substituted for penicillin G, except against gram-negative species since it is less active than penicillin G against *Neisseria* and *Haemophilus*. Semisynthetic penicillinase-resistant penicillins are the drugs of choice only for penicillin-resistant *S. aureus* and *Staphylococcus epidermidis*, even though they will inhibit streptococci at concentrations below that needed to inhibit staphylococci.[19,20] Carboxypenicillins such as carbenicillin and ticarcillin are less active than the ureidopenicillins against streptococcal and *Haemophilus* species. The susceptible gram-negative organisms that are members of the Enterobacteriaceae or *Pseudomonas* vary from hospital to hospital and from community to community. Most of the anaerobic gram-positive bacteria are susceptible to all the penicillins. Gram-negative anaerobic bacteria are susceptible to most penicillins with the exception of isolates of *Bacteroides fragilis*, which are inhibited by high levels of penicillin G or the semisynthetic anti-*Pseudomonas* agents—azlocillin, carbenicillin, mezlocillin, piperacillin, and ticarcillin.[22] *Fusobacterium varium* often are resistant to all penicillins.

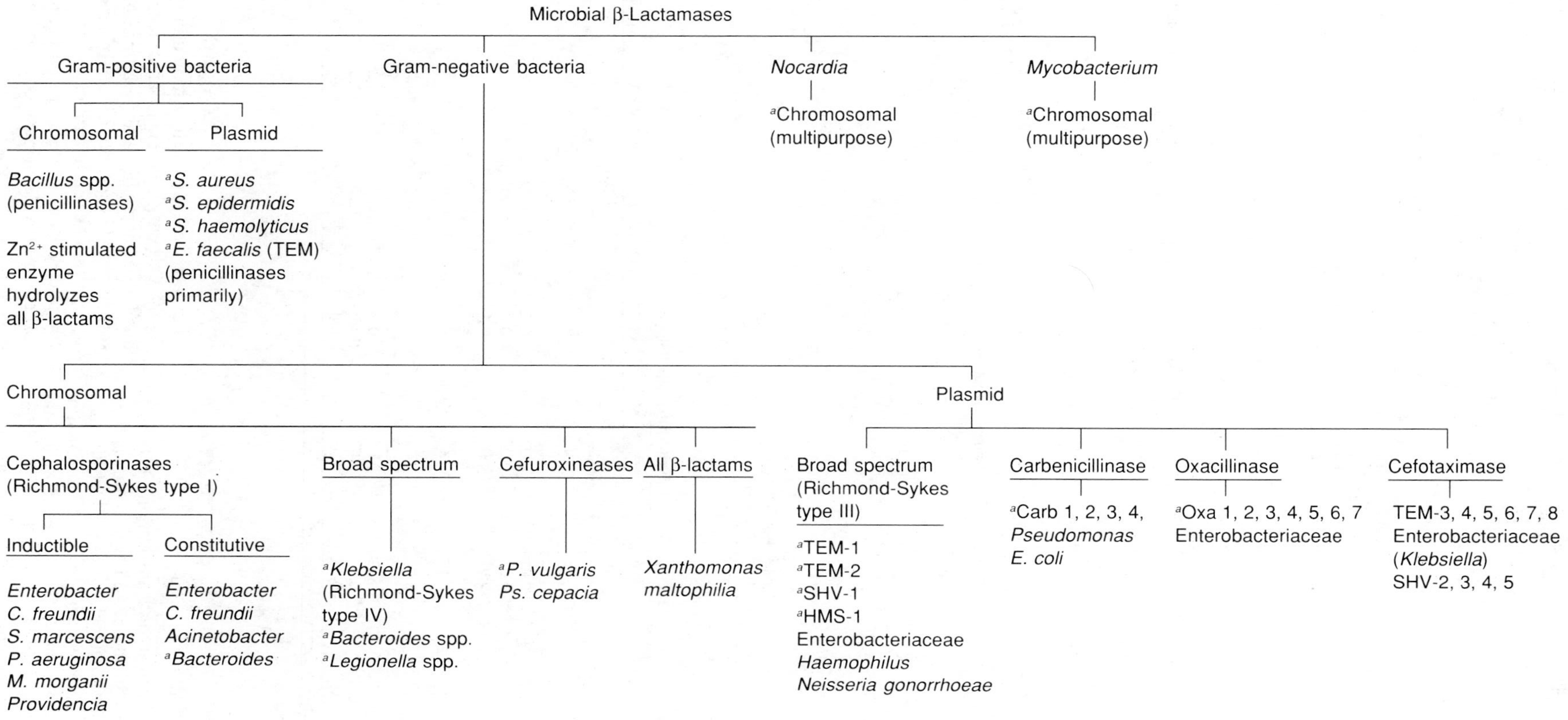

[a] Inhibited by clavulanate, sulbactam, and tazobactam

FIG. 2. Diagrammatic representation of β-lactamases.

TABLE 1. Classification of Penicillins

	Routes of Use	*Trade Names*
Natural penicillins		
Penicillin G	PO	Pfizerpen, Pentids, Kesso-Pen
	IM	Procaine—Wycillin, Duracillin, Crysticillin
	IM	Benzathine—Permapen, Bicillin
Penicillin G potassium or sodium	IV	
Penicillin V	PO	Ledercillin, Compocillin, Betapen, V-cillin, Veetids, Uticillin, S-K penicillin, Robicillin, Pen-Vee, Penapar
Phenethicillin	PO	Broxil, Syncillin, Maxipen, Pensig
Penicillinase-resistant penicillins		
Methicillin	IM, IV	Staphcillin, Celbenin
Nafcillin	IM, IV	Unipen
Isoxazolyl penicillins		
Cloxacillin	PO	Tegopen
Dicloxacillin	PO	Veracillin, Pathocil, Dynapen
Flucloxacillin	PO	
Oxacillin	PO, IM, IV	Prostaphlin, Bactocill
Aminopenicillins		
Ampicillin	IM, IV	Alpen, Amcil, Pen A/N, Omipen, Totacillin, Supen, S-K ampicillin, Principen, Probampcin, Polycillin, Pensyn, Penbritin
Amoxicillin	PO	Amoxil, Larotid, Polymox
Bacampicillin	PO	Spectrobid
Cyclacillin	PO	Cyclapen
Epicillin	PO	
Hetacillin	PO	Versapen
Pivampicillin	PO	
Anti-Pseudomonas penicillins		
Azlocillin	IM, IV	Azlin
Carbenicillin	IM, IV	Pyopen, Geopen
Indanylcarbenicillin	PO	Geocillin
Ticarcillin	IM, IV	Ticar
Extended-spectrum penicillins		
Mezlocillin	IM, IV	Mezlin
Piperacillin	IM, IV	Pipral, Pipracil
Amidino penicillins		
Amdinocillin	IM, IV	
Pivamdinocillin	PO	
Stable against gram-negative β-lactamases		
Temocillin	IM IV	

TABLE 2. Usual Minimal Inhibitory Concentrations (MIC) of Penicillins Against Cocci

	Mean Minimum Inhibitory Concentration (μg/ml)							
	Penicillin G	*Penicillin V*	*Ampicillin, Amoxicillin*	*Methicillin*	*Oxacillin, Cloxacillin Dicloxacillin*	*Nafcillin*	*Carbenicillin, Ticarcillin*	*Azlocillin Mezlocillin, Piperacillin*
Streptococcus pneumoniae	0.01[a]	0.02[a]	0.02[a]	0.1[a]	0.04	0.02	0.4	0.02
Streptococcus pyogenes	0.005	0.01	0.02	0.2	0.04	0.02	0.2	0.02
Streptococcus agalactiae	0.005	0.01	0.02	0.2	0.06	0.02	0.2	0.15
Viridans streptococci	0.01	0.01	0.05	0.1	0.1	0.06	0.2	0.12
Enterococcus faecalis	3.0	6.0	1.5[c]	>25	>25	>25	50	1.5
Peptostreptococcus	0.2	0.5	0.2	2.0	0.6	0.5	0.4	0.8
Staphylococcus aureus								
Penase-negative	0.02	0.02	0.05	1.0	0.3	0.25	1.2	0.8
Penase-positive	>25	>25	>25	2.0	0.4	0.25	25	25
Staphylococcus epidermidis	0.02[b]	0.02[b]	0.05[b]	0.8[b]	0.2[b]	0.2[b]	0.8[b]	1.6[b]
Neisseria gonorrhoeae[d]	0.01[b]	0.1	0.03[b]	12.0	12.0	12.0	0.3[b]	0.05[b]
Neisseria meningitidis	0.05	0.25	0.05	6.0	6.0	6.0	0.1	0.05

[a] Rare isolates resistant to penicillins have been found MIC >5 μg/ml.
[b] Many isolates resistant.
[c] Amoxicillin has a mean MIC of 0.4.
[d] Can range from 0.005 to 100.

PHARMACOLOGIC PROPERTIES

Penicillins differ markedly in their oral absorption (Table 5). Penicillin G is not stable to acid and has a half-life of less than 20 minutes at pH 2. In contrast, at pH 4 it has a half-life of 1 hour. The other penicillins, which are acid-labile, are methicillin and all the anti-*Pseudomonas* penicillins. However, acid stability is not a guarantee of oral absorption, and there are major differences in oral absorption of compounds within a group. Penicillin V is well absorbed even when ingested with food, and the greatest absorption of penicillin V is with the potassium salt.[24] The semisynthetic penicillins, with the exception of nafcillin, are well absorbed. Ampicillin is only partially absorbed, 30–60 percent,[19] whereas amoxicillin and the "proampicillins"—bacampicillin and pivampicillin—are almost totally absorbed.[23,25] The pivaloyl ester of amdinocillin is absorbed orally. Although carbenicillin is not absorbed, esters of the compound such as indanyl carbenicillin are adequately absorbed to provide urinary concentration to treat urinary tract infections.[26]

The majority of penicillins are absorbed so they yield peak levels 1–2 hours after ingestion. When ingested with food, absorption is delayed to yield peak serum levels 2–3 hours after

TABLE 3. Activity of Penicillins Against Selected Bacilli and Anaerobic Organisms

	Mean Minimum Inhibitory Level (μg/ml)				
Organism	*Penicillin G*	*Ampicillin, Amoxicillin*[a]	*Oxacillin*[b]	*Carbenicillin, Ticarcillin*[a]	*Azlocillin, Mezlocillin, Piperacillin*[a]
Clostridium perfringens	0.5	0.05	0.5	0.5	0.05
Corynebacterium diphtheriae	0.1	0.02	0.1	0.1	1.0
Listeria monocytogenes	0.5	0.5	4.0	4	0.5
Haemophilus influenzae[c]	0.8	0.5	25	0.5	0.1
Bacteroides melaninogenicus	0.5	0.5	25	0.5	0.2
Fusobacterium nucleatum	0.5	0.1	>100	0.5	0.5
Bacteroides fragilis	32	32	>500	64	32

[a] Minor differences do occur.
[b] Oxacillin is used as representative of isoxazoyl penicillins.
[c] β-lactamase-producing strains occur and are resistant to the penicillins.

TABLE 4. Activity of Penicillins Against Enterobacteriaceae and *Pseudomonas*

	Mean Minimum Inhibitory Levels (μg/ml)						
	Penicillin G	*Ampicillin, Amoxicillin*	*Oxacillin*[a]	*Carbenicillin, Ticarcillin*	*Azlocillin,*[d] *Mezlocillin, Piperacillin*	*Amdinocillin*	*Temocillin*
Escherichia coli[b]	100	3	>1000	6	8	0.5	10
Proteus mirabilis	50	3	>1000	1.5	1	25	5
Klebsiella spp.	>400	200	>1000	>400	16	1.5	10
Enterobacter spp.	>500	>500	>1000	50	16	1.5	10
Citrobacter diversus	>500	>100	>1000	12	8	1.5	2.5
Citrobacter freundii	>500	50	>1000	12	32	1.5	2.5
Serratia	>500	>500	>1000	100	32	100	25
Salmonella[b]	10	1.5	>1000	3	4	1	5
Shigella[b]	20	1.5	>1000	3	8	1	5
Proteus vulgaris	>500	>500	>1000	12	16	100	2.5
Providencia	>500	>500	>1000	12	8	100	2.5
Morganella	>500	200	>1000	25	8	8	2.5
Pseudomonas, other	>500	>500	>500	100	>100	>100	<100
Acinetobacter	>500	250	>1000	25	32	400	>100
Pseudomonas aeruginosa	>500	>500	>1000	50[c]	16[a]	100	>100

[a] Used as representative antistaphylococcal penicillin.
[b] Amoxicillin is twofold more active against *Salmonella* and twofold less active against *Shigella*. Strains containing the TEM plasmid β-lactamase are resistant except to temocillin.
[c] Ticarcillin two- to fourfold more active.
[d] Some isolates, particularly *Klebsiella*, are resistant to azlocillin but susceptible to mezlocillin and piperacillin.
[e] Mezlocillin is less active than azlocillin or piperacillin.

ingestion, and peak levels are lower, except for the pivaloyl esters and amoxicillin.

Repository forms of penicillin G are available. These are procaine penicillin G and benzathine penicillin G. These are absorbed more slowly from intramuscular sites than are the crystalline salts. Procaine or lidocaine can also be used as a diluent for intramuscular injection of anti-*Pseudomonas* penicillins, but the half-life of these drugs is not prolonged by this maneuver.

Penicillins are bound to protein in varying degrees from 17 percent for the aminopenicillins to 97 percent for dicloxacillin (Table 5). The major protein to which they bind is albumin.[19] Only an unbound (free) drug exerts antibacterial activity, since the bound drug cannot reach a receptor site within the bacteria. However, protein binding is a reversible process, and it is possible for bound penicillin to be released and to kill bacteria in tissue or in the blood stream. Penicillins are metabolized to a minor degree.[27] However, differences in metabolism explain the differences in half-lives in the presence of renal failure. The major mechanism by which they are removed from the body is by excretion as intact molecules via the kidney.[28] Biliary excretion of penicillins does occur, but it probably is important only for nafcillin and the anti-*Pseudomonas* penicillins.[29]

The mechanism of excretion of penicillins is via renal tubular cells. Penicillins are rapidly excreted into urine, and hence they have a short half-life, ranging from less than 30 minutes for penicillin to 72 minutes for carbenicillin. The one exception is temocillin, which has a half-life of 4 hours in healthy people.[30] The ability of the renal tubular cells to excrete penicillin varies with the agents, but up to 4 g/hr of penicillin G can be excreted. This excretion can be blocked by probenecid, which prolongs the serum half-life of all the penicillins.[31] Probenecid also competes for binding sites on albumin; hence, there is more free drug in the presence of probenecid. Renal excretion of all penicillins by the newborn is markedly less than in older children since tubular function is not fully developed. Hence, the dosage programs for penicillins must be modified when given to newborns or low birth weight infants.

Reduction in renal function is an important consideration in the administration of certain penicillins, namely, carbenicillin, ticarcillin, and temocillin. If the creatinine clearance is greater than 10 ml/min, it is necessary to make only minor adjustments in the dosage of other penicillins. In the presence of anuria, reduction in total daily dose of the natural penicillins, of many of the penicillinase-resistant penicillins, and of the aminopenicillins is necessary[32] (Table 6).

Peritoneal dialysis removes variable amounts of the penicillins. In general, after peritoneal dialysis only the dosage programs of carbenicillin and ticarcillin need to be adjusted. After hemodialysis it is necessary to replace the dialyzed penicillin G, ampicillin, amoxicillin, carbenicillin, ticarcillin, azlocillin, mezlocillin, piperacillin, and temocillin, but not nafcillin or the isoxazolyl penicillins.[32]

Penicillins are well distributed to most areas of the body such as lung, liver, kidney, muscle, bone, and placenta. The levels

TABLE 5. Pharmacokinetic Properties of Penicillins

					Serum Level[a]		Serum $T_{\frac{1}{2}}$ (hr)[b]			
Antibiotic	*Oral Adsorption (%)*	*Food Decreases Adsorption*	*Protein Binding (%)*	*Percentage of Dose Metabolized (%)*	*Total Drug (μg/ml)*	*Free Drug (μg/ml)*	*Normal (C_{cr} > 90 ml/min)*	*Renal Failure (C_{cr} < 10 ml/min)*	*Liver Impairment Increases ($T_{\frac{1}{2}}$)*	*Na^+ Content[d] (mEq/g)*
Penicillin G	20	Yes	55	20	2	0.9	0.5	10	+	2.7
Penicillin V	60	No	80	55	4	0.8	1	4		
Methicillin	Nil		35	10			0.5	4		3.1
Oxacillin	30	Yes	93	45	6	0.4	0.5	1		
Cloxacillin	50	Yes	94	20	10	0.6	0.5	1	++	
Dicloxacillin	50	Yes	97	10	15	0.45	0.5	1.5	++	
Nafcillin	Erratic	Yes	87				0.5	1.5	+++	
Ampicillin[c]	40	Yes	17	10	3.5	2.9	1	8	++	3.4
Amoxicillin	75	No	17	10	7.5	6.2	1	8	+	
Carbenicillin	Nil		50	2			1.1	15	++, 18–20 hr	4.7
Indanyl carbenicillin	30	No	50		15	7.5	1.1	15	++	
Ticarcillin	Nil		50	15			1.2	15	++, 18–20 hr	4.7
Amdinocillin	Nil		20				0.8	4	+	
Pivamdinocillin	50	No	20		3		1	4	+	
Mezlocillin	Nil		50				1.1	4	++	1.8
Piperacillin	Nil		50				1.3	4	++	1.8
Azlocillin	Nil		20				0.8	4	++	2.2
Temocillin	Nil		85	10			4	17	++	

[a] After 500 mg dose taken fasting.
[b] Values have been rounded of to approximate values.
[c] Proampicillins (bacampicillin, pivampicillin) are absorbed twice as well as ampicillin and food does not decrease absorption, but other properties are those of the parent ampicillin. Bacampicillin would give a serum level of 9 μg/ml after 500 mg.
[d] Na^+ content based on IV preparations.

TABLE 6. Antibiotic Dosage Change in Renal Disease and after Dialysis

	Dosage Change in Renal Failure[a]		
Agent	*Creatinine Clearance (30–50 ml/min)*	*Creatinine Clearance (<10 ml/min)*	*Dosage after Hemodialysis*
Penicillin G	NC	1.6×10^6 units/6 hr	Yes (1.6×10^6 units)
Penicillin V	NC	250 mg/6 hr	Yes (250 mg)
Methicillin	NC	2 g/8 hr	Slight (2 g)
Oxacillin	NC	NC	Slight (as in uremia)
Cloxacillin	NC	NC	Slight (as in uremia)
Dicloxacillin	NC	NC	Slight (as in uremia)
Nafcillin	NC	NC	Slight (as in uremia)
Ampicillin[c]	NC	0.5–1 g/8 hr	Yes (500 mg)
Amoxicillin	NC	500 mg/12 hr	Yes (250 mg)
Carbenicillin[b]	3 g/4 hr	2 g/8 hr	Yes (2 g)
Ticarcillin[b]	2 g/4 hr	2 g/12 hr	Yes (2 g)
Indanyl carbenicillin	NC	Avoid	
Azlocillin	NC	3 g/8–12 hr	Yes (2 g)
Mezlocillin	NC	3 g/8–12 hr	Yes (2 g)
Piperacillin	NC	3 g/8–12 hr	Yes (2 g)
Temocillin	1 g/24 hr	1 g/48 hr	Yes (1 g)
Amdinocillin	NC	1 g/8 hr	Yes (1 g)

[a] Refers to maximum dose used.
[b] Only carbenicillin and ticarcillin need adjustment of dosage after peritoneal dialysis.
[c] Dosage adjustments of "pivampicillins" should be the same as those of amoxicillin.
Abbreviations: NC: no change.

of penicillins in abscesses, middle ear, and pleural, peritoneal, and synovial fluids are sufficient in the presence of inflammation to inhibit most susceptible bacteria.[33–37] Most penicillins are relatively insoluble in lipid and so do not penetrate cells, including polymorphonuclear cells. Distribution of all the penicillins to eye, brain, cerebrospinal fluid, or prostate is nil in the absence of inflammation.[38] Inflammation alters normal barriers, permitting entry of penicillins, but more importantly it interferes with the anion pump that removes penicillins from areas such as cerebrospinal fluid. Low protein-bound penicillins reach levels in fetal serum equivalent to levels in maternal serum 30–60 minutes after injection. In contrast, the highly protein-bound semisynthetic penicillins achieve low concentrations in both amniotic fluid and fetal serum.[39]

Urinary concentrations of all penicillins are high, even in the presence of moderately reduced renal function, but in people with creatinine clearances below 10 ml/min the urinary levels may not exceed those in the blood. Cortical and medullary concentrations of penicillins during normal hydration and in hydropenia exceed serum levels.[40]

Most penicillins are actively secreted into the bile, yielding biliary concentrations well in excess of those in serum. The levels of penicillin G, ampicillin, and amoxicillin are at least 10 times those in the serum, and the levels of nafcillin and mezlocillin are as high as 100 times the simultaneous serum level. In the presence of common duct obstruction, the levels of all penicillins in bile are markedly reduced. Since the biliary transport system is a saturable one, at very high serum levels the biliary levels are not significantly increased over those obtained at lower serum levels.

UNTOWARD REACTIONS

The major adverse effects of the penicillins are hypersensitivity reactions, which range in severity from rash to immediate anaphylaxis (Table 7)[41,42] (see Chapter 21). Penicillins are capable of acting as haptens to combine with proteins contaminating the solution or with human protein after the penicillin has been administered to humans. The most important antigenic component of penicillins is the penicolloyl determinant, which is produced through opening of the β-lactam ring, thereby allowing amide linkage to body proteins (Fig. 3). Penicillanic acid and derivatives of penicillanic acid are produced when reconstituted penicillins break down in solution due to acidity or temperature elevation. The penicillolyl and penicillanic derivatives are the major determinants of penicillin allergy. Minor determinants of allergy are benzyl penicillin itself or sodium benzyl penicilloate, which can act either as sensitizing agents or on their own elicit an allergic reaction.[41,42] Both major and minor determinants may be involved in anaphylactic reactions, as well as in urticarial reactions. These reactions are mediated by IgE antibody. Minor determinants are the major cause of anaphylactic reactions. When a person has been sensitized by the hapten–carrier complex, he or she can have a reaction to penicillin alone or to penicillin that has formed dimers or polymers in

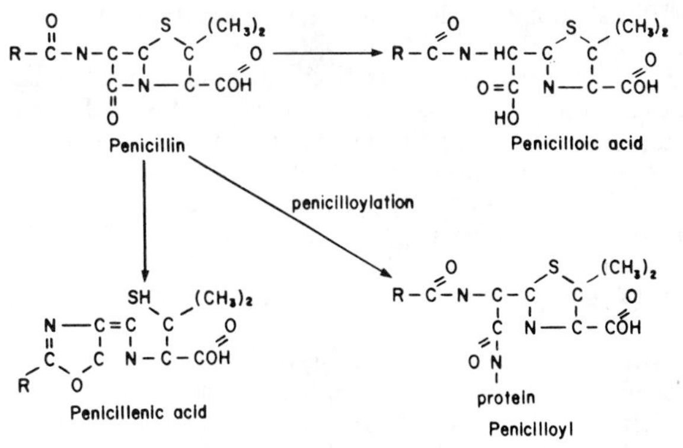

FIG. 3. Mechanisms for formation of antigens from penicillins.

solution. Anaphylactic reactions to penicillins are uncommon, occurring in only 0.2 percent of 10,000 courses of treatment, with 0.001 percent out of 100,000 cases resulting in fatality.[43] People with atopic dermatitis or allergic rhinitis appear not to be at increased risk of a penicillin reaction.[44]

Serum sickness does occur with penicillins, but it is very uncommon today. It probably is due to IgG antibodies to the benzyl penicilloyl hapten. The illness is characterized by fever, urticaria, joint pains, and angioneurotic edema. Exfoliative dermatitis and Stevens-Johnson syndrome are rare forms of allergic reactions to penicillins. The morbilliform eruptions that develop after penicillin therapy probably are due to IgM antibody to the benzyl penicilloyl hapten and to the minor determinants. In many patients these rashes will disappear, even if the penicillin is continued, due to the production of IgG blocking antibody. There is a risk, however, that the rash could progress to generalized desquamation. If an allergic reaction does occur, epinephrine given intramuscularly or intravenously will usually abort the reaction. Antihistamines and corticosteroids have not been shown to be of benefit.

Another allergic reaction to penicillins is that of allergic vasculitis with development of cutaneous and visceral lesions similar to that found with periarteritis nodosa. This reaction is extremely rare.

Hematologic toxicity is rare, although neutropenia has been encountered with the use of all types of penicillins, particularly when large doses are used.[45] The mechanism of the neutropenia is unknown, and white blood cell counts return to normal rapidly if the offending agent is discontinued. Sometimes a lower dose of drug can be used without production of neutropenia. Coombs-positive hemolytic anemia occurs rarely.[46] All penicillins at high concentrations, but particularly carbenicillin and ticarcillin, bind to the adenosine diphosphate receptor site in platelets, preventing normal platelet aggregation. A clinically significant bleeding disorder occurs relatively infrequently.[47]

Renal toxicity from penicillins has varied from allergic angiitis to interstitial nephritis.[48,49] Interstitial nephritis has occurred most commonly with the use of methicillin, but it has been seen with all penicillins. The clinical syndrome is one of fever, macular rash, eosinophilia, proteinuria, eosinophiluria, and hematuria. Initially the reaction is one of nonoliguric renal failure with a decrease in creatinine clearance and a rise in serum urea nitrogen and serum creatinine concentrations. This reaction can progress to anuria and renal failure. Biopsy specimens of the kidney show an interstitial infiltrate of mononuclear and eosinophilic cells with tubular damage but no glomerular lesions. Discontinuation of the penicillin will result in the return of renal function to normal in the majority of situations.[50]

Administration of massive doses of any penicillin, but most often carbenicillin and ticarcillin, may result in hypokalemia due to the large dose of nonreabsorbable anion presented to the

TABLE 7. Adverse Reactions to Penicillins

Type of Reaction	Frequency (%)	Occurs Most Frequently with[a]
Allergic		
IgE antibody	0.004–0.4	Penicillin G
Anaphylaxis		
Early urticaria (<72 hr)		
Cytotoxic antibody	Rare	Penicillin G
Hemolytic anemia		
Ag-Ab complex disease	Rare	Penicillin G
Serum sickness		
Delayed hypersensitivity	4–8	Ampicillin
Contact dermatitis		
Idiopathic	4–8	Ampicillin
Skin rash		
Fever		
Late onset urticaria		
Gastrointestinal	2–5	
Diarrhea	2–5	Ampicillin
Enterocolitis	<1	Ampicillin
Hematologic		
Hemolytic anemia	Rare	Penicillin G
Neutropenia	1–4	Penicillin G Oxacillin Piperacillin
Platelet dysfunction	3	Carbenicillin
Hepatic		
Elevated SGOT level	1–4	Oxacillin Nafcillin Carbenicillin
Electrolyte disturbance		
Sodium overload	Variable	Carbenicillin
Hypokalemia	Variable	Carbenicillin
Hyperkalemia—acute	Rare	Penicillin G
Neurologic		
Seizures	Rare	Penicillin G
Bizarre sensations		Procaine Penicillin
Renal		
Interstitial nephritis	1–2	Methicillin
Hemorrhagic cystitis	Rare	Methicillin

[a] All the reactions can occur with any of the penicillins.

distal renal tubules, which alters [H^+] excretion and secondarily results in K^+ loss.[48]

Central nervous system toxicity in the form of myoclonic seizures can follow administration of massive doses of penicillin G, ampicillin, carbenicillin, or methicillin. If there is reduced renal function, the drugs accumulate, and this toxicity is more likely.[51] Direct instillation of small doses of methicillin, oxacillin, or nafcillin into the ventricles at the time of surgery for placement of atrioventricular shunts has not resulted in seizures. Direct application of penicillin to the cortex will provoke seizure activity.

Gastrointestinal disturbances have followed the use of any of the oral forms but have been most pronounced with ampicillin. Enterocolitis due to *Clostridium difficile* has followed the use of all of the penicillins (see Chapter 83). All the penicillins used at high doses for prolonged periods will abolish normal bacterial flora with resulting colonization with resistant gram-negative bacilli and/or with fungi such as *Candida*. Abnormalities in hepatic function tests such as elevation of the alkaline phosphatase and serum glutamic oxaloacetic (SGOT) levels have been reported most often after the use of oxacillin and carbenicillin.[45,52] The pathogenesis of the hepatic reaction is unknown. Major hepatic injury is very uncommon, and liver enzymes return to normal values within a few days of stopping therapy.

CLINICAL USE

Table 8 lists some uses of penicillins. Penicillin G remains the primary agent for treatment of *Streptococcus pyogenes* and *S. pneumoniae* infections (regardless of the site). None of the newer penicillins or agents in other classes has been shown to be more effective. *Streptococcus pneumoniae* resistant to penicillin have been isolated in South Africa and the United States, but these are rarely encountered. In the United States *S. pneumoniae* of relative resistance to penicillin, minimum inhibitory concentration (MIC) values of 0.1–1 μg/ml, have been seen. Much higher doses of penicillin are required to kill these organisms. Nearly all *Neisseria meningitidis* strains are susceptible to penicillin G. *Neisseria gonorrhoeae* vary in susceptibility to penicillin G. Strains can be resistant due to β-lactamase production, to altered PBPs, or to membrane changes (see Chapter 16). Penicillin G is the drug of choice for treponemal infection in all its forms. Puerperal infections due to anaerobic streptococci or group B streptococci (*Streptococcus agalactiae*), as well as genital clostridial infections, are treated with penicillin G. Infections produced by anaerobic mouth flora including gram-positive and gram-negative cocci and the *Actinomyces* can be treated with penicillin G, although *Bacteroides melaninogenicus* producing a β-lactamase and resistant to penicillin are being encountered.

PROPHYLACTIC USE

Penicillins have been used in a number of situations for prevention of infection. Oral administration of 200,000 units of penicillin G or penicillin V every 12 hours has resulted in a significant reduction in recurrences of rheumatic fever. Because of the problems with compliance with oral therapy, intramuscular injections of 1.2 or 2.4 million units of benzathine penicillin given once each month have also been used with excellent results.

Outbreaks of streptococcal infection due to *S. pyogenes* have been aborted by the use of oral penicillin G or V given twice a day for 5 days, by single injections of procaine penicillin daily, or by administration of benzathine penicillin.

One of the most important prophylactic uses of penicillin is for prevention of bacterial endocarditis (see Chapter 63).

Antistaphylococcal penicillins may be used prophylactically at the time of implantation of an artificial joint or heart valve. These agents should be given just before the surgery, during the procedure, and in the immediate postoperative period. There are no studies that delineate the best penicillin agent for such procedures, and many physicians prefer to use a cephalosporin (see Chapter 285).

Ampicillin or amoxicillin has been administered orally to asplenic children or to children with agammaglobulinemia to prevent infections caused by *H. influenzae* and *S. pneumoniae*.

Penicillin prophylaxis has not been of benefit in prevention of meningococcal infection, bacterial infection after viral respiratory infection, or pneumonia after coma, shock, or congestive heart failure.

PROPERTIES OF INDIVIDUAL PENICILLINS

Dosages of penicillins are given in Tables 9 and 10.

Natural Penicillins

Penicillin G. Penicillin G or benzylpenicillin G (Fig. 4) is available in oral, parenteral, and respository salts. Oral salts are either the sodium or potassium forms, which are available as suspensions for pediatric use or as tablets in doses of 50,000 to 1 million units (200,00 units equals 125 mg). Penicillin G should be used orally only if it is taken 1 hour before or 2 hours after a meal to prevent its destruction by gastric acid. There is little reason to use oral penicillin G for acute infection at the present time, and penicillin V should be the oral preparation used.

Crystalline penicillin G in aqueous solution has been used intramuscularly, subcutaneously, intravenously, and intrathecally. It is available either as the potassium or sodium salt. The sodium salt is much more expensive than the potassium salt, and it rarely needs to be used since the amount of potassium present in 6 million units, an amount a patient with reduced renal function would receive, is less than 10 mEq. Given intramuscularly as an aqueous solution, penicillin G is very rapidly cleared from the body, and it is preferable to use a repository form. It is available as sterile dry powder in ampules or vials containing 200,000–20 million units per vial. Each million units of penicillin G contains 1.7 mEq of sodium or potassium.

Repository penicillins provide tissue depots from which the drug is absorbed over hours in the case of procaine penicillin or over days in the case of benzathine penicillin. Repository penicillins are only for intramuscular use and cannot be used intravenously or subcutaneously or to irrigate wounds. Procaine penicillin is a mixture of equal molar parts of procaine and penicillin. Thus 300,000 units contains 120 mg of procaine. Use of this suspension delays the peak of activity but provides serum and tissues levels for at least 12 hours. Doubling the dose of procaine penicillin given at a single injection site does not double the serum level. To increase the peak level it is necessary to use two body sites as was done in the treatment of gonorrhea, for example, with 2.4 million units of procaine penicillin given in each buttock. Marketed procaine penicillin preparations are of two types: One is an aqueous solution of the crystalline salt, and the other contains 2% aluminum monosterate as a dispensing agent. The preparations are marketed in cartridges and vials in doses of 300,000, 500,000, and 600,000 units in 1–4 ml and as 2.4 million units/4 ml.

Benzathine penicillin is a repository form of penicillin, which is a combination of 1 mole of penicillin and 2 moles of an ammonium base. It is available for intramuscular injection in 10 ml vials containing 300,000 units/ml and as prefilled syringes containing 600,000 units/ml in 1-, 2-, and 4 ml sizes. It provides detectable serum levels for 15–30 days depending on the size of the dose. Concentrations of penicillin G in the spinal fluid after use of benzathine penicillin probably are inadequate to treat treponemal infections of the nervous system.

TABLE 8. Antimicrobial Spectrum of Penicillins[a]

Organisms	*Penicillin of Choice*	*Alternate Acceptable Penicillin*	*Frequency of Resistance to Penicillins (%)*
Gram-positive cocci			
Streptpcoccus pneumoniae	G	V	Uncommon
Streptococcus pyogenes (A)	G	V	None
Streptococcus agalactiae (B)	G	Ampicillin	None
Viridans streptococci	G		None
Streptococcus bovis (D)	G		None
Enterococcus faecalis	Ampicillin	Mezlocillin	Rare, <1
Staphylococcus aureus (nonpenicillinase)	G	Penase-resistant	80
Staphylococcus aureus (penicillinase)	Penase-resistant		100
Staphylococcus aureus (methicillin-resistant)	None	None	100
Staphylococcus epidermidis	Penase-resistant		80
Staphylococcus epidermidis (methicillin-resistant)	None	None	100
Gram-negative cocci			
Neisseria meningitidis	G	Ampicillin	Very rare
Neisseria gonorrhoeae	G	Ampicillin	1–40
Gram-positive bacilli			
Bacillus anthracis	G		None
Corynebacterium diphtheriae	G		None
Listeria monocytogenes	Ampicillin	G	None
Anaerobic species			
Peptostreptoccoccus	G	Ampicillin	None
Actinomyces israeli	G	V	None
Bacteroides melaninogenicus	G	C, T	10
Fusobacterium	G	Ampicillin	1–10
Bacteroides fragilis	M, PA		75
Clostridium	G	Ampicillin	<1
Gram-negative bacilli			
Haemophilus	Ampicillin	G	5–30
Escherichia coli	Ampicillin		30
Proteus mirabilis	Ampicillin	G	<5
Salmonella typhi	Ampicillin		20
Salmonella, other sp.	Ampicillin		20
Klebsiella	None		95
Enterobacter spp.	M, P, T, C		70
Citrobacter freundii	M, P, T		80
Proteus, indole-positive	M, P, T, C		20
Serratia	M, P, T, C		90
Pseudomonas aeruginosa	A, P, T		20–30
Pseudomonas, other	None		95
Acinetobacter	T	A, G, P	50
Providencia	M, P, TC		20–30
Xanothomonas	None		95
Other organisms infrequently encountered			
Erysipelothrix	G	Ampicillin	None
Pasturella multocida	G		Rare, <1
Streptobacillus moniliformis	G		None
Spirillum minus	G		None
Fucospirochetes	G	Ampicillin	None
Treponema pallidum	G		None

[a] In each case it is assumed that a route of administration would be used that would achieve levels in serum and tissue to eradicate the organism. If there is no entry in the alternate column, it means that an antibiotic in another class would be a more appropriate choice. Amoxicillin can be used in place of ampicillin in all situations except with *Shigella*.
Abbreviations: A: azlocillin; C: carbenicillan; M: mezlocillin, P: piperacillin; T: ticarcillin.

Penicillin V. Phenoxymethyl penicillin (Fig. 4) is available only for oral use as sodium or potassium salts in suspension or tablets in doses of 125, 250, and 500 mg. The potassium salt produces higher blood levels than the other salts. Serum levels are from two to five times those obtained with penicillin G. Absorbed penicillin V is handled in the body similarly to penicillin G. Penicillin V can be substituted for penicillin G in most situations in which it is reasonable to treat an infection by the oral route. However, penicillin V is less active than penicillin G against *Haemophilus, Neisseria*, and enteric organisms. Blood levels after 500 mg given to an adult are equivalent to the levels achieved with 600,000 units of procaine penicillin given intramuscularly. The usual dosage for children is 25–50 mg/kg/day and for adults, 1–4 g/day. The interval between dosages is 6–8 hours.

Phenethicillin. This phenoxyethyl analogue of penicillin G (Fig. 4) has microbiologic properties similar to penicillin G. It is acid-stable and better absorbed from the gastrointestinal tract. Blood levels are high, but food delays its absorption. It is available only as the potassium salt in the form of 125 and 250 mg tablets and an oral suspension of 125 mg in 5 ml. Once absorbed it is handled in the body the same way as is penicillin G.

Penicillanse-Resistant Penicillins (Fig. 5)

Methicillin. Methicillin (2,6-dimethoxyphenylpenicillin) is a penicillin resistant to staphylococcal β-lactamase.[36] Its activity against staphylococci is low, with most strains inhibited by 2–3 μg/ml. Methicillin-resistant *S. aureus* are resistant not because of β-lactamase activity but by virtue of altered penicillin-binding proteins. These organisms have become a serious problem in some parts of the United States. Methicillin inhibits *S. pyogenes* and *S. pneumoniae* at levels of 0.2 μg/ml, but it has no activity against *Enterococcus fecalis* and gram-negative bacilli. Methicillin is acid-unstable and must be given parenterally. Absorption after an intramuscular injection is rapid, as is excretion, with peak levels after 1 g of 17 μg/ml but subinhibitory levels by 4 hours. Methicillin is less protein bound than the

TABLE 9. Dosage of Penicillins

Compound	*Oral*	*Intramuscular*	*Intravenous*
Penicillin G			25,000–500,000 units/kg/day, 6 doses
Procaine		300,000–600,000 units every 12 hr	
Benzathine		1.2–2.4 mega units every 15–20 days	
Pencillin V	Infant: 50 mg/kg/day, 3 doses 125–500, 4 doses		
Ampicillin[a]	25–200 mg/kg/day, 4 doses	100–200 mg/kg/day, 4 doses	100–400 mg/kg/day, 6 doses
Amoxicillin	25–50 mg/kg/day, 3 doses		
Methicillin Oxacillin Nafcillin		100 mg/kg/day, 4 doses	100–300 mg/kg/day, 6 doses
Cloxacillin	25–100 mg/kg/day, 4 doses		
Dicloxacillin	12–25 mg/kg/day, 4 doses		
Carbenicillin		50–100 mg/kg/day, 4 doses	50–500 mg/kg/day, 6 doses
Ticarcillin		50–100 mg/kg/day, 4 doses	50–300 mg/kg/day, 6 doses
Indanylcarbenicillin	50–65 mg/kg/day, 4 doses		
Azlocillin		50–100 mg/kg/day, 4 doses	200–300 mg/kg/day, 4 doses
Mezlocillin		50–100 mg/kg/day, 4 doses	200–300 mg/kg/day, 4 doses
Piperacillin		50–100 mg/kg/day, 4 doses	200–300 mg/kg/day, 4 doses

[a] Proampicillins are given at the same dose as amoxicillin.

TABLE 10. Dosage of Antibiotics in Newborn Infants

	Infants Less than 1 Week Old		*Infants 1 Week–1 Month Old*	
Compound	*Dose (per kg/day)*	*Interval between Doses (in hours)*	*Dose (per kg day)*	*Interval between Doses (in hours)*
Penicillin G	50,000–100,000 units	12	100,000 units	8
Ampicillin	100 mg	12	200 mg	6
Oxacillin	100 mg	12	200 mg	6
Methicillin	100 mg	12	300 mg	6
Nafcillin	100 mg	12	200 mg	6
Carbenicillin	250 mg	8	400 mg	6
Ticarcillin	150 mg	8	300 mg	6
Mezlocillin	75 mg	12	300 mg	6
Azlocillin	75–100 mg	12	300 mg	6

other antistaphylococcal penicillins, and although its intrinsic activity is less than the other antistaphylococcal penicillins, it is as active in the presence of serum as are the more intrinsically active oxacillin and nafcillin. Methicillin is available as a sodium salt, but since it is unstable in acidic media, it is used as a buffered solution. It is packaged as 1, 4, and 6 g vials and can be diluted with sodium chloride or dextrose in water. When diluted, buffered solutions are stable at room temperature for 8 hours. It is preferable to administer the drug every 4 hours if

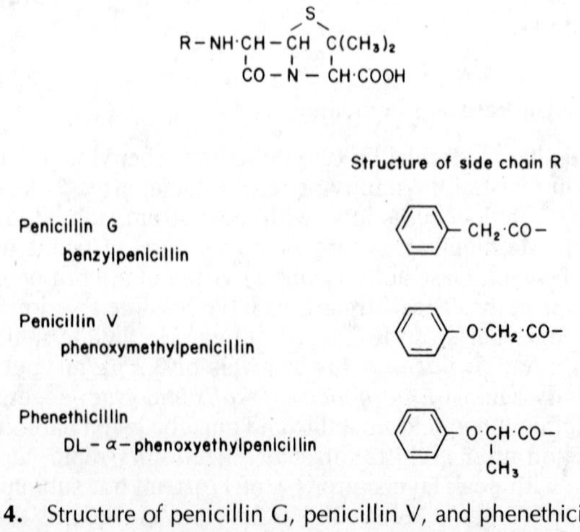

FIG. 4. Structure of penicillin G, penicillin V, and phenethicillin.

used intravenously. Methicillin should be used only for the treatment of penicillin G-resistant staphylococcal infections. Toxicity is that seen with any penicillin, although interstitial nephritis may be more common. The usual dosage is 4–12 g/day for adults and 200–300 mg/kg/day for children given in 4 or 6 doses.

Nafcillin. Nafcillin (2-ethoxy-1-naphthylpenicillin) has more intrinsic activity than methicillin against both staphylococci and streptococci but is not active against gram-negative bacteria. Nafcillin is highly protein bound, and in the presence of serum its activity is similar to methicillin. Although nafcillin is absorbed when taken by mouth, absorption is erratic whether the drug is taken fasting or with food, and hence serum levels are low.[36] Levels after intramuscular injection are low, and the preferred route of administration is intravenously. The antibiotic is primarily excreted by the liver and to a lesser extent by the kidney. Serum levels are elevated and the half-life is prolonged by probenecid. Although available as capsules (250 mg) and a suspension, one of the other agents in this class would be preferred for oral use. Sterile vials of 500 mg/1, 2, or 4 g of the sodium salt can be reconstituted in most solutions and are stable for up to 4 hours at room temperature. The usual dosage of nafcillin is 4–9 g/day, depending on the severity of the infection, and 100–200 mg/kg/day for children.

Isoxazolyl Penicillins. All these agents are stable to staphylococcal β-lactamase and inhibit both penicillin-sensitive and penicillin-resistant staphylococci at mean concentrations of 0.2–0.4 μg/ml. Methicillin-resistant *S. aureus* is resistant to

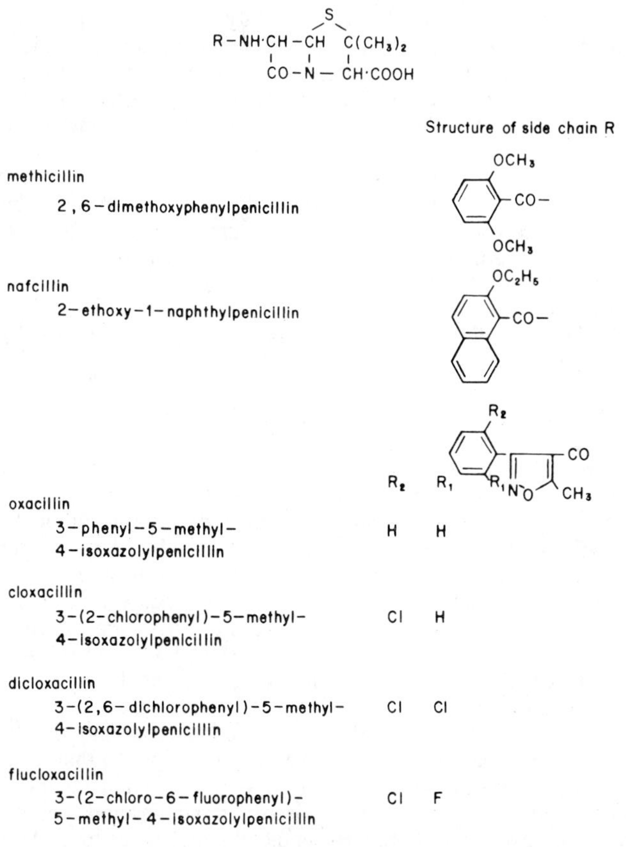

FIG. 5. Antistaphylococcal penicillins.

these penicillins. Recently an increasing number of *S. epidermidis* isolates resistant to these penicillins has been found as the cause of serious infections. The mechanism of resistance is altered PBPs. Isoxazolyl penicillins inhibit streptococci and pneumococci but are virtually inactive against gram-negative bacilli. All are absorbed after oral administration, but absorption is adversely affected by food. There are differences in serum levels among the drugs after oral ingestion, with the serum level of cloxacillin twice that of oxacillin and the levels of dicloxacillin and flucloxacillin twice that of cloxacillin; all the drugs are highly bound to serum proteins; oxacillin, cloxacillin, and flucloxacillin are equally bound, but dicloxacillin is bound to a greater extent. Thus, actual free serum concentrations of the drugs are greatest for flucloxacillin followed by cloxacillin and dicloxacillin as equals and oxacillin the least (Table 5). After intravenous infusion of 1 g over 15 minutes, peak serum levels are 70–100 μg/ml, with levels of 25 μg/ml at 1 hour and less than 1 μg/ml at 6 hours. The isoxazolyl penicillins undergo some metabolism but are excreted primarily by the kidney with slight biliary excretion. Oxacillin undergoes more rapid degradation in the body than does cloxacillin or dicloxacillin.

OXACILLIN. Oxacillin is available as a sodium salt for oral use in 250 and 500 mg capsules and as a powder for suspension at 250 mg/5 ml. It should be taken 1–2 hours before meals. The daily dosage for adults is 1–4 g taken in four parts. The dosage for children is 50–100 mg/kg/day taken in four parts. Oxacillin sodium for injection may be given intramuscularly or intravenously. It is available in 500 mg and 1, 2, or 4 g vials and is stable in most saline and dextrose solutions for 6 hours at room temperature. Adult dosage is 2–12 g/day and for children, 100–300 mg/kg/day given every 4–6 hours.

CLOXACILLIN. Cloxacillin sodium is available in the United States only as an oral solution (125 mg/5 ml), or capsules of 250 and 500 mg. Dosage for children is 50–100 mg/kg/day given as four equal doses. Dosage for adults is 1–4 g/day given as four equal doses. In Europe cloxacillin is available as a parenteral for intramuscular or intravenous administration in 250 mg vials. It yields serum levels similar to those achieved with oxacillin.

DICLOXACILLIN. Dicloxacillin sodium is available as a suspension (62.5 mg/5 ml) and as capsules of 125 and 250 mg. The dosage for children less than 40 kg is 25 mg/kg/day given as four doses. Some authorities recommend doses as above for cloxacillin. For adults, a dosage of 250 mg–1 g every 6 hours can be given, depending on the severity of the infection.

FLUCLOXACILLIN. Flucloxacillin sodium is not available in the United States. It is available in Europe in the form of suspension and capsules similar to the forms of cloxacillin, 250 mg capsules, and for parenteral use in 250 mg vials.

Aminopenicillins (Fig. 6)

The antibacterial activity of all these penicillins is similar.[53] They are not stable to β-lactamases of either gram-positive or gram-negative bacteria. The aminopenicillins are only slightly less active than penicillin G against *S. pyogenes, S. pneumoniae*, and *S. agalactiae*. They are more active against *E. fecalis*. Activity of the compounds against clostridial species, *Actinomyces*, corynebacteria, and *N. meningitidis* is equal to that of penicillin G. They are more active than penicillin G against *Listeria monocytogenes*. Sensitivity of *N. gonorrhoeae* (see Chapter 190) varies from highly sensitive to completely resistant strains that bear a plasmid-mediating production of a β-lactamase. *Haemophilus influenzae* (both typeable and nontypeable strains) and *Haemophilus parainfluenzae* are usually susceptible, except for the isolates that produce β-lactamases (see Chapter 201). Although many domiciliary *E. coli* are sensitive to aminopenicillins, plasmid resistance is common in hospital isolates. *Shigella sonnei*, many salmonellae, including many *Salmonella typhi*, are resistant because of β-lactamases. Most *Klebsiella, Serratia, Acinetobacter*, indole-positive *Proteus, Pseudomonas*, and *B. fragilis* are resistant to the penicillins of this class.

Ampicillin. Ampicillin is moderately well absorbed after oral administration, but peak levels are delayed and lowered if it is ingested with food. Peak blood levels of 3 μg/ml occur 1–2 hours after ingestion of 0.5 g. Peak blood levels occur later in diabetic patients with neurologic disease and in patients with renal failure. Drug can be detected in the serum for 4–6 hours. After intramuscular injection of 0.5 g peak levels of 10 μg are achieved in 1 hour and persist for 4 hours. Probenecid increases the height of peak levels and prolongs the period in which the drug can be detected in serum. Ampicillin is well distributed to body compartments and achieves therapeutic concentrations in cerebrospinal fluid (CSF) and in pleural, joint, and peritoneal fluids

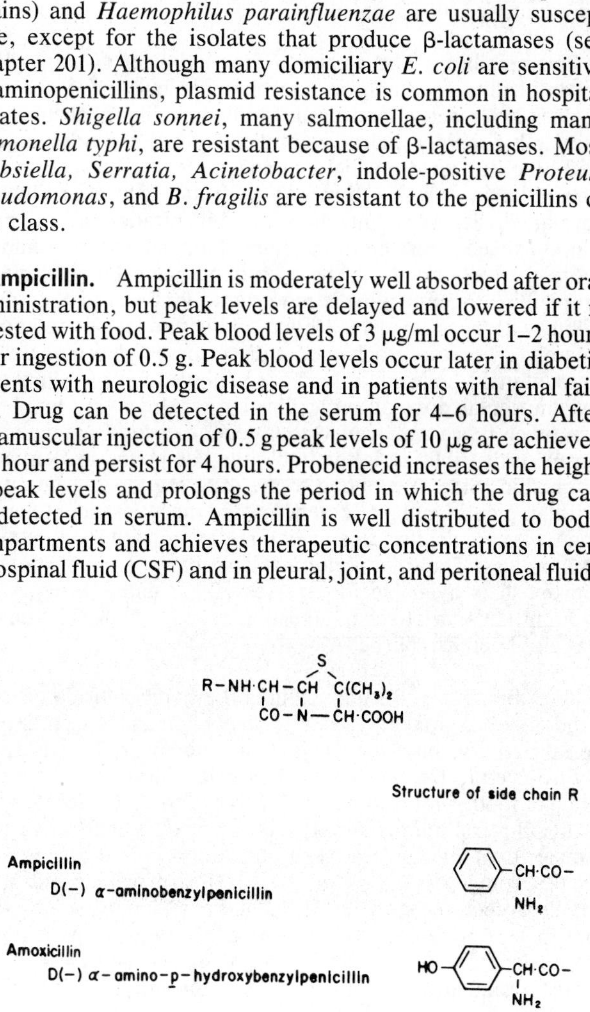

FIG. 6. Aminopenicillins.

in the presence of inflammation after parenteral administration. Urinary levels are high even in the presence of markedly reduced renal function. Peritoneal dialysis is ineffective in removing the drug, but hemodialysis removes approximately 40 percent in a 6 hour period.

Ampicillin is available for oral use as the sodium salt or as the trihydrate in capsules of 125, 250, and 500 mg, as a suspension of 125 and 250 mg/5 ml, as drops of 100 mg/ml, and as 125 mg chewable tablets. It is also prepared as a suspension, which contains 3.5 g of ampicillin trihydrate and 1 g of probenecid. It is available as ampicillin trihydrate in 2.5 g vials only for intramuscular use. As a sodium salt in vials of 0.125, 0.5, 2, and 4 g it can be used either intramuscularly or intravenously. It is stable in sodium chloride for 8 hours at concentrations up to 30 mg/ml, but for intravenous use at concentrations greater than 2 mg/ml it is stable at room temperature for less than 4 hours and hence would preferably be administered by "piggy back" within 0.5–1 hour. Dosage varies with the age of the patients, the status of renal function, and the severity of the disease. For children above 1 month of age the oral dosage is 50–100 mg/kg/day in four doses; the intramuscular or intravenous dosage is 100–400 mg/kg/day in four or six doses. For adults the oral dosage is 2–4 g/day given in a dose every 6 hours. For severe infection the parenteral dosage is 6–12 g/day given in divided doses every 4 hours. See Chapter 20 for a discussion of ampicillin–sulbactam.

Hetacillin. This is a condensation product of ampicillin and acetone that is rapidly hydrolyzed to ampicillin either as it crosses the gastrointestinal mucosa or in the serum.[54] It offers no advantage over ampicillin.

Pivampicillin. The pivaloyloxymethyl ester of ampicillin—pivampicillin—is stable in aqueous acid but undergoes rapid hydrolysis in serum and tissue.[55] Pivampicillin is absorbed intact and is rapidly hydrolyzed by nonspecific esterases in cells and blood to yield pivalic acid and the hydroxyl methyl ester of ampicillin, which are rapidly hydrolyzed to ampicillin and formaldehyde. At no time does the concentration of ester in the blood exceed 2 percent of the ampicillin, and within 15 minutes more than 99 percent of the compound has been converted to ampicillin. Pivampicillin is more rapidly absorbed than ampicillin, with peak levels at 1 hour, and serum levels are approximately twice those achieved with a comparable oral dose of ampicillin and are equal to those achieved with a comparable intramuscular dose of ampicillin. Urinary recovery and levels are twice those achieved with the same dose of ampicillin. In terms of distribution in the body, the compound is identical to ampicillin. Side effects due to the drug are those encountered with ampicillin, although there may be more gastric intolerance than with ampicillin, especially if not taken with food, but diarrhea is less. The drug is not available in the United States. In Europe it is available in capsules of 178 and 358 mg, which contain 125 and 250 mg of ampicillin. An advantage for the drug has not been established.

Bacampicillin. Bacampicillin is the hydrochloride of the 1-ethoxycarboxyloxyethyl ester of ampicillin. It has no antibacterial activity, but when it is adminsitered orally it is totally hydrolyzed to free ampicillin. It is better absorbed in the presence of food, with peak serum levels occurring earlier than with ampicillin and approximately from one and a half to two times greater than that achieved with an equimolar dose of ampicillin. Peak serum levels of 9 μg/ml follow a dose of 500 mg, and serum levels exceed those of ampicillin and amoxicillin for 2.5 hours, but thereafter serum levels of ampicillin from bacampicillin are equivalent to those of amoxicillin.[25] Clinical studies have shown efficacy similar to that of ampicillin.[56] Bacampicillin is available as an oral suspension containing 125 mg per 5 ml as 400 mg tablets, which is the equivalent of 280 mg of ampicillin.

Talampicillin. This is the phthalidyl ester of ampicillin. It has no antibacterial activity but is hydrolyzed to free ampicillin as it is absorbed. It produces serum levels earlier and three times those achieved with equimolar doses of ampicillin. It is not available in the United States. It has no merit over ampicillin.

Epicillin. Epicillin is a compound in which the benzene ring has been replaced by a 1,4-cyclohexadienyl ring. It has a bacterial spectrum similar to ampicillin. It is acid-stable and has oral absorption, serum binding, excretion, and tissue distribution similar to ampicillin. It has been effective in treatment of a variety of infections. It is not available in the United States. It has no value over ampicillin.

Cyclacillin. Cyclacillin, 6-(1-aminocyclohexande carboxyamido) penicillanic acid, is an acid-stable aminopenicillin with antibacterial activity similar to ampicillin. It is the most rapidly absorbed aminopenicillin, with levels of 10–18 μg/ml 30 minutes after ingestion of 500 mg—levels four times that of ampicillin. However, it is extremely rapidly cleared, and levels at 2 hours are less than those achieved with a comparable dose of ampicillin. Probenecid causes appreciably less delay in excretion than with other penicillins. It has no merit over ampicillin.

Amoxicillin. Amoxicillin differs from ampicillin only in the presence of a hydroxyl group in the para position of the benzene side chain. It has in vitro activity similar to ampicillin. It is significantly better absorbed when given by mouth than is ampicillin.[23] Peak blood levels are from two to two and a half times those achieved with a similar dose of ampicillin, and food does not decrease absorption. Oral amoxicillin produces blood levels similar to those produced by intramuscularly administered sodium ampicillin or ampicillin trihydrate. Urinary excretion of amoxicillin is greater than that of ampicillin. Tissue distribution is similar to that of ampicillin. Clinical studies with amoxicillin have been extensive, and it has been used in the treatment of otitis media, bronchitis, pneumonia, typhoid, gonorrhea, and urinary tract infections.[57] It has been used as a single 3 g dose for therapy for bacterial cystitis in women.[59] It is not useful as treatment of shigellosis. Side effects of amoxicillin are similar to those seen with ampicillin, although diarrhea may be less common than with ampicillin. It is available as the trihydrate in suspensions of 125 and 250 mg/5 ml, as drops of 50 mg/ml, and as capsules of 250 and 500 mg. Usual dosage for children is 20–40 mg/kg/day given in three doses every 8 hours, and for adults the dosage is 250 mg every 8 hours, although it has been used in doses up to 1 g every 4 hours. It has been useful in pediatric infections, except for shigellosis, and may be preferred to ampicillin. In adult infections its use would depend on cost factors and tolerance. See Chapter 20 for a discussion of amoxicillin–clavulanate.

Carboxy Penicillins (Fig. 7)

Carbenicillin. Carbenicillin was the first penicillin with activity against *P. aeruginosa* and certain indole-positive *Proteus* species that were not susceptible to other penicillins or to the cephalosporins.[37] It is destroyed by β-lactamases of both gram-positive and gram-negative organisms, but it is more stable against hydrolysis by the β-lactamases of species such as *Pseudomonas, Enterobacter, Morganella*, and *Proteus-Providencia*, which function primarily as cephalosprorinases. Carbenicillin is less active than ampicillin against *S. pyogenes, S. pneumoniae*, and *E. fecalis*. It is less active than the ureidopenicillins against streptococcal species and *Listeria*. Its activity against *Haemophilus, N. gonorrhoeae*, and *N. meningitidis* is similar to ampicillin. It has gram-negative activity similar to ampicillin against *E. coli, Proteus mirabilis, Salmonella* species, and *Shigella* species, but it is inactive against *Klebsiella*.

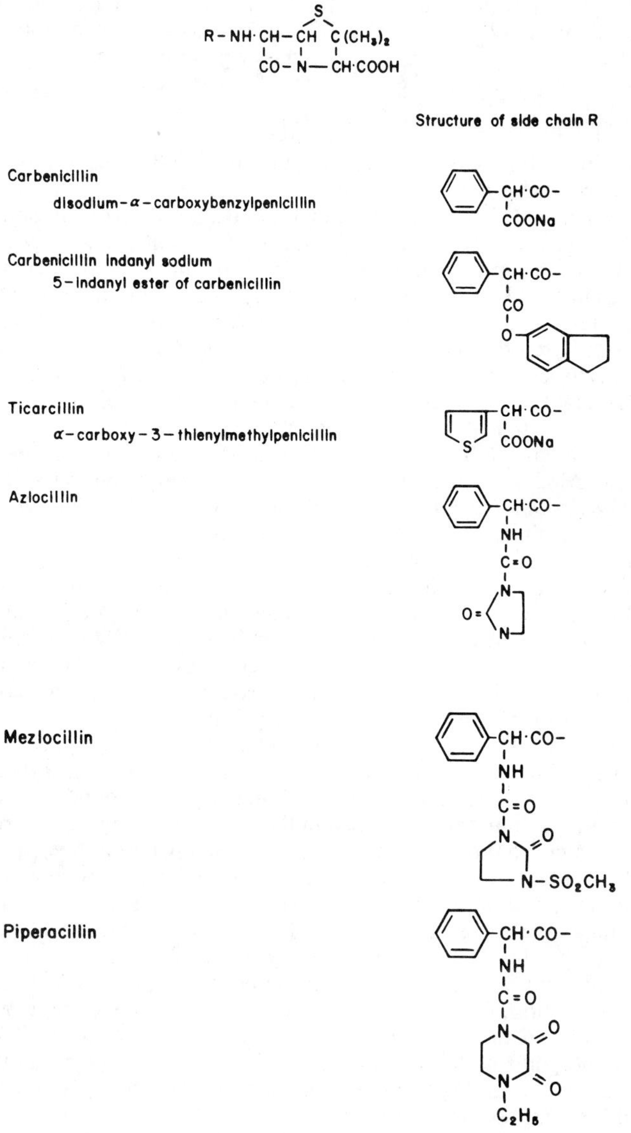

FIG. 7. Penicillins active against gram-negative bacteria.

It inhibits some *Enterobacter* and *Serratia* strains and many *B. fragilis*, although high concentrations are required. Carbenicillin acts synergistically with amikacin, gentamicin, and tobramycin to inhibit *P. aeruginosa*. Carbenicillin is not absorbed by mouth but can be given by intramuscular or intravenous administration. After an intramuscular dose of 1 g, peak serum levels of 20 μg/ml are reached in 1 hour, but the drug is not detectable at 4 hours. These levels are not adequate for treatment of tissue *Pseudomonas* infections, but levels of 2000–4000 μg/ml are achieved in the urine, and, therefore, it could be used by this route for urinary infections. Serum levels of 150–200 μg/ml will be maintained when it is given at dosages of 70–100 mg/kg over 1–2 hours. Carbenicillin is excreted by renal tubules, but since less is converted to penicilloic acid, its half-life (72 minutes) is longer than that of penicillin G, and it accumulates in the presence of renal failure.[37,60] Greater accumulation occurs if there is combined hepatic and renal dysfunction. Hemodialysis reduces plasma concentrations. Probenecid delays renal excretion and increases serum concentrations. Tissue distribution is simlar to ampicillin, but concentrations in the cerebrospinal fluid are not adequate for *Pseudomonas*. Side effects due to carbenicillin are similar to those seen with penicillins, but since it is a disodium salt and each gram contains 4.7 mEq of sodium, when administered at doses of 30–40 g/day congestive failure may occur. Carbenicillin causes more hypokalemia than other penicillins due to the load of nonreabsorbable anion in the distal tubule. Carbenicillin binds to the adenosine 5′-diphosphate (ADP) receptor site on platelets and prevents normal contraction; hence, bleeding occurs on occasion in the presence of high serum levels such as may occur in renal failure.

Carbenicillin is available as the disodium salt in vials of 1, 2, 5, and 10 g. It should never be mixed or administered in the same solution with aminoglycosides, since it complexes with these drugs and the activity of both compounds is inhibited. Intravenous dosages of 400–600 mg/kg/day given over 1–2 hours every 4 hours are used for treatment of systemic *Pseudomonas* infections. In the presence of markedly decreased renal function (creatinine clearance less than 10 ml/min) 2 g every 8 hours will provide adequate levels without toxicity. It should be replaced by one of the following agents.

Ticarcillin. The antibacterial spectrum of ticarcillin is identical to that of carbenicillin, except that it is from two to four times more active against *P. aeruginosa*.[61] The pharmacokinetics of ticarcillin and carbenicillin are virtually identical, as are side effects.[62] Ticarcillin can be used at dosages of 200–300 mg/kg/day. It is available in 1, 3, and 6 g vials. The advantage of ticarcillin over carbenicillin is that it inhibits some *Pseudomonas* that could be achieved with safety.[63] Another advantage is a reduced dose of ticarcillin (with the same therapeutic efficacy) resulting in less platelet dysfunction and less hypokalemia. See Chapter 20 for a discussion of ticarcillin-clavulanate.

Oral Antipseudomonas Penicillins

Indanyl Carbenicillin. Indanyl carbenicillin (carindacillin) is an α-carboxy ester of carbenicillin. It has no intrinsic activity of its own, but as a sodium ester it is highly acid-stable and relatively well absorbed from the gastrointestinal tract. Ingestion with food may actually enhance absorption. The ester is immediately hydrolyzed to free carbenicillin, and only trace amounts of ester are found in serum or urine. Peak serum levels after 1 g taken orally are 10 μg at 1–2 hours. Urine levels are 300–1000 μg/ml with 30 percent of a dose recovered in the first 6 hours. The compound does not provide adequate serum or tissue levels for systemic infections, and it is useful only for the treatment of urinary tract infections. In the presence of decreased renal function, urine levels are lower and may be inadequate to treat *Pseudomonas* infections. Side effects are those of all the penicillins, but gastrointestinal irritation has been a problem in some people. It is available as 500 mg capsules (containing 382 mg of carbenicillin). The usual dosage is 1 g every 6 hours for adults. Quinolones should replace this agent for treatment of urinary tract infections and prostatitis.

Carfecillin. Carfecillin is the phenyl ester of carbenicillin. It is also well absorbed and rapidly hydrolyzed to yield carbenicillin. Serum levels are similar to those of the indanyl ester. It is useful only to treat urinary infections due to *Pseudomonas*. It has been better tolerated due to a less bitter taste. It is not available in the United States.

Ureidopenicillins

Azlocillin. Azlocillin is an acylureido penicillin that is 8–16 times more active than carbenicillin against *P. aeruginosa* and is less active against indole-positive *Proteus* species. It has the same activity as ampicillin against streptococcal species.[64] It is destroyed by β-lactamases of both gram-positive and gram-negative bacteria. It is not orally absorbed and must be given by the intravenous route to provide adequate serum levels to treat

Pseudomonas infection. The half-life is approximately 50 minutes, and administration of 4 g yields peak levels of 285 μg/ml.

Azlocillin shows nonlinear pharmacokinetics. The peak serum concentrations and the area under the drug curve are not proportional; that is, a 4 or 5 g dose produces serum levels that are greater than four or five times the 1 g dose.[65] The drug thus could be administered in larger doses at intervals of 6 hours rather than the 4 hour intervals used for carbenicillin. Azlocillin also does not accumulate in renal failure to the same degree as do carbenicillin and ticarcillin since its half-life rises only to 4 hours with creatinine clearances below 7 ml/min.[66–68] Azlocillin enters the cerebrospinal fluid in the presence of meningeal inflammation, but levels are only 10 percent of the serum level. Azlocillin also causes less increase in bleeding time than does carbenicillin since it apparently has less affinity for the ADP receptor site. Azlocillin is used primarily to treat *Pseudomonas* infections. It has proved to be a useful drug in a variety of clinical situations.[67] It is available as 1, 2, 3, and 4 g vials, which contain 2.17 mEq sodium per gram of drug.

Mezlocillin. Mezlocillin is an acylureido penicillin similar in antibacterial spectrum to carbenicillin and ticarcillin but with some significant differences.[64] It is more active in vitro against *E. faecalis* than either of the above-mentioned agents. It inhibits about 75 percent of *Klebsiella* species at a concentration of 25 μg/ml, whereas less than 5 percent would be inhibited by 100 μg/ml of carbenicillin.[69] It is also more active than carbenicillin or ticarcillin against *H. influenzae* and is more active than carbenicillin against *B. fragilis*. It is, however, not more stable to β-lactamase hydrolysis than is carbenicillin; hence its greater intrinsic activity is due to other factors such as greater affinity for penicillin-binding proteins and better entry into the bacterial periplasmic space. It acts synergistically against gram-negative bacteria when combined with aminoglycosides. The drug must be given parenterally. Its pharmacokinetics are different from carbenicillin since, like azlocillin and piperacillin, it shows dose-related nonlinear kinetics. Peak serum levels, half-life, and area under the time curve are greater with larger doses. Administration of 4 g produces peak levels of 300 μg/ml.[70] Its half-life increases only to 4 hours in patients in renal failure. Mezlocillin is the least likely of the broad-spectrum penicillins to alter bleeding times. Clinical studies in the United States and Europe have shown that it is effective therapy for respiratory, urinary, gynecologic, and surgical infections.[67,71–76] It causes less increase in bleeding time than does carbenicillin. Usual doses have been 12–18 g/day for adults. It is available as 1, 2, 3, and 5 g vials, which contain 1.85 mEq of sodium per gram.

Piperacillin. Piperacillin is an acylureido penicillin derivative that is similar in activity to ampicillin against gram-positive species.[77] It has excellent activity against streptococcal species and against *Neisseria* and *Haemophilus* and many Enterobacteriaceae. It also has excellent activity against both cocci and bacilli anaerobic species. It inhibits 60 percent of *Pseudomonas* species at 3 μg/ml and 90 percent at 12 μg/ml.[77,78] It is hydrolyzed by plasmid-mediated β-lactamases of gram-positive and gram-negative bacteria. Its acts synergistically against *Pseudomonas* and against some of the Enterobacteriaceae when combined with aminoglycosides.[77] The human pharmacology of piperacillin is similar to that of azlocillin and mezlocillin.[79–82] Administration of 4 g by the intravenous route produces peak serum levels of 300 μg/ml. It shows kinetics that are dose-dependent. It accumulates in renal failure to a lesser degree than does carbenicillin, and its half-life is only 4 hours in renal failure.[83] It is removed by hemodialysis. Piperacillin has shown adverse reactions similar to those of the other penicillins noted earlier. After prolonged administration at high doses neutropenia has been reported. Alteration of bleeding time and hypokalemia occur but less frequently than with carbenicillin. Clinical studies have shown that it is a useful agent in treatment of a variety of infections.[67,84–90] It is administered in daily doses to adults of 12–18 g. It is available in vials of 2, 3, and 4 g, which contain 1.85 mEq of sodium per gram of drug.

Amdinopenicillanic Acid Derivatives

Amdinocillin, formerly called mecillinam, is a 6-β-acylaminopenicillanic acid. It has unusual antibacterial properties for a penicillin.[91,92] It has poor antigram-positive activity. In situations in which 0.01 μg/ml of penicillin G inhibits *S. pyogenes*, 6 μg/ml of amdinocillin are needed to inhibit streptococci. It does not bind to the penicillin-binding proteins of gram-positive species. It has poor activity against *Haemophilus* and *Neisseria*. However, it is extremely active against *E. coli*, inhibiting many β-lactamase-containing strains even though it is hydrolyzed by the plasmid-mediated β-lactamases. The reason for its activity is that it binds only to PBP-2 in Enterobacteriaceae, and this protein is critical in cell wall production in these species. Amdinocillin is active against many ampicillin-resistant *Shigella* and *Salmonella* species. In contrast to ampicillin, it is active against many *Klebsiella, Enterobacter*, and *Citrobacter* species. It has variable activity against *Proteus*, both *P. mirabilis* and the indole-positive *Proteus*, and it fails to inhibit *Pseudomonas* and anaerobic species such as *B. fragilis* and *Clostridium*. Amdinocillin acts synergistically with other penicillins such as ampicillin or carbenicillin and also with cephalosporins.[92] It does not act synergistically with aminoglycosides nor is its activity inhibited by chloramphenicol.

Amdinocillin is not acid-stable and cannot be used orally except in the form of a pivaloyl ester. This ester is well absorbed and immediately hydrolyzed, yielding free compound in the serum. Serum levels of pivamdinocillin after ingestion are equivalent to those obtained with pivampicillin (see above), and absorption is improved in the presence of food. Amdinocillin administered parenterally as a sodium salt yields serum levels comparable to those achieved with equimolar doses of ampicillin.[93,94] The compound is renally excreted similarly to ampicillin and is distributed within the body in the same manner as ampicillin. Clinical studies have shown the compound to be effective in the treatment of infections caused by susceptible microorganisms.[95,96] It is available in Europe as the pivaloyl ester for oral use and as the sodium salt for parenteral administration.

6-Methoxy Penicillin Derivatives

Temocillin is a 6-α-methoxy derivative of ticarcillin. The presence of the methoxy group on the β-lactam ring renders the compound extremely resistant to hydrolysis by both plasmid and chromosomally mediated β-lactamases. However, there has been a marked loss in activity against gram-positive species and *Pseudomonas*.[97,98] Temocillin inhibits the majority of *E. coli, Klebsiella, Enterobacter* species, *Proteus, Serratia*, and *Citrobacter* species at 10 μg/ml or less. *Haemophilus* and *Branhamella* are inhibited by less than 1 μg/ml. *Bacteroides* species are resistant. Temocillin is not hydrolyzed by the common chromosomal and plasmid β-lactamases. It is not destroyed by the cefotaxine–ceftazidime-destroying β-lactamases. Although it does not inhibit *Pseudomonas*, this is due to failure to cross the outer cell wall.

Peak serum concentrations of temocillin after 500 mg and 1 g are administered by the intramuscular route average 50 and 70 μg/ml, respectively.[30,99] Serum half-life of temocillin after intramuscular administration ranges from 4 to 6 hours. After bolus intravenous administration of temocillin peak serum concentrations have been 75 μg/ml for 500 mg and 170 μg/ml for 1 g. Serum half-life after intravenous administration averages 4½ hours. Urinary recovery of temocillin is 70–80 percent, with urine concentrations of 100–500 μg/ml for 12 hours after a 500 mg intramuscular injection. Temocillin accumulates in the presence of renal failure with serum half-life reaching 15–20 hours.[30] It is partially removed by hemodialysis but not by peritoneal dialysis. Temocillin has been used in Europe to treat urinary infections and tissue infections due to gram-negative bacilli.[100–102] It is not available in the United States.

REFERENCES

1. Fleming A. On the antibacterial action of cultures of a penicillium, with special reference to their use in the isolation of *B. influenzae*. Br J Exp Pathol. 1929;10:226.
2. Batchelor FR, Doyle FP, Naylor JHC, et al. Synthesis of penicillin: 6-aminopenicillanic acid in penicillin fermentations. Nature. 1959;183:257.
3. Tipper DJ, Wright A. The structure and biosynthesis of bacterial cell walls. In: Sokatch JR, Ornstein LA, eds. The Bacteria. v. 7. New York: Academic Press; 1979:291.
4. Strominger JL. Penicillin-sensitive enzymatic reactions in bacterial cell wall synthesis. Harvey Lect. 1970;64:179.
5. Mirelman D. Biosynthesis and assembly of cell wall peptidoglycan. In: Inouye M, ed. Bacterial Outer Membranes. New York: John Wiley & Sons; 1980:166.
6. Waxman DL, Yocum RR, Stominger JL. Penicillins and cephalosporins are active site-directed acylating agents: evidence in support of the substrate analogue hypothesis. Philos Trans R Soc Lond [Biol]. 1980;289:257.
7. Spratt BG. Distinct penicillin binding proteins involved in the division, elongation and shape of *Escherichia coli*, K 12. Proc Natl Acad Sci USA. 1975;72:2999.
8. Spratt BG. Biochemical and genetical approaches to the mechanism of action of penicillin. Philos Trans R Soc Lond (Biol). 1980;289:273.
9. Tamaki S, Nakajima S, Matsuhashi M. Thermosensitive mutation in *Escherichia coli* simultaneously causing defects in penicillin-binding protein 1 Bs and in enzyme activity for peptidoglycan synthesis in vivo. Proc Natl Acad Sci USA. 1977;74:5472.
10. Spratt BG, Bowler LB, Edelman A, et al. Membrane topology of PBPs 7B and 3 of *E. coli* and the production of water-soluble forms of high molecular weight PBPs. In: Shockman GD, ed. Antibiotic Inhibition of Bacterial Cell Surface Assembly and Function. Washington, DC: American Society for Microbiology; 1988:292–300.
11. Suzuki H, Nishimuka Y, Hirota Y. On the process of cellular division in *Escherichia coli*: a series of mutants of *E. coli* altered in penicillin-binding proteins. Proc Natl Acad Sci USA. 1978;75:664.
12. Yocum RR, Waxman DW, Strominger JL. The mechanism of action of penicillin. J Biol Chem. 1980;255:3977.
13. Georgopapadakou NH, Liu FY. Binding of β-lactam antibiotics to penicillin-binding proteins of *Staphylococcus aureus* and *Streptococcus faecalis* in relation to antibacterial activity. Antimicrob Agents Chemother. 1980;18:834.
14. Garcia-Bustos JF, Chait BT, Tomasz A. Altered peptidoglycan structure in a pneumococcal transformant resistant to penicillin. J Bacteriol. 1989; 170:2143–7.
15. Tomaz A. Penicillin tolerance and the control of the murein hydrolases. In: Salton M, Shockman GD, eds. Beta-lactam Antibiotics. New York: Academic Press; 1980:227–47.
16. Sykes RB, Matthew M. The β-lactamases of gram-negative bacteria and their role in resistance to β-lactam antibiotics. J Antimicrob Agents Chemother. 1976;2:115.
17. Neu HC. β-Lactam antibiotics: structural relationships affecting in vitro activity and pharmacologic properties. Rev Infect Dis. 1986;8(Suppl 3):237–59.
18. Barber M, Waterworth PM. Antibacterial activity of the penicillins. Br Med J. 1962;1:1159.
19. Rolinson GN, Sutherland R. Semisynthetic penicillins. Adv Pharmacol Chemother. 1973;11:152.
20. Marcy SM, Klein JO. The isoxazolyl penicillins: oxacillin, cloxacillin and dicloxacillin. Med Clin North Am. 1970;54:1127.
21. Finland M, Garner C, Wolcox C, et al. Susceptibility of pneumococci and *Haemophilus influenzae* to antibacterial agents. Antimicrob Agents Chemother. 1976;9:274.
22. Sutter VL, Finegold SM. Susceptibility of anaerobic bacteria to 23 antimicrobial agents. Antimicrob Agents Chemother. 1976;10:736.
23. Neu HC. Antimicrobial activity and human pharmacology of amoxicillin. J Infect Dis. 1974;129 (Suppl):123.
24. McCarthy CG, Finland M. Absorption and excretion of four penicillins: penicillin G, penicillin V, phenethicillin and phenylmercaptomethyl penicillin. N Engl J Med. 1960;263:315.
25. Neu HC. The pharmacokinetics of bacampicillin. Rev Infect Dis. 1981;3:110.
26. Butler K, English AR, Briggs B, et al. Indanyl carbenicillin: chemistry and laboratory studies with a new semisynthetic penicillin. J Infect Dis. 1973;127(Suppl):97.
27. Cole M, Kening MD, Hewitt VA. Metabolism of penicillins to penicilloic acidosis and 6-aminopenicillanic acid in man and its significance in assessing penicillin absorption. Antimicrob Agents Chemother. 1973;3:463.
28. Eagle H, Newman E. Renal clearance of penicillin F, G, K, and X in rabbits and man. J Clin Invest. 1947;26:903.
29. Acocella G, Mattiussi R, Nichols FB, et al. Biliary excretion of antibiotics in man. Gut. 1968;9:536.
30. Bodaert J, Daneels R, Schurgers M, et al. The pharmacokinetics of temocillin in patients with normal and impaired renal function. J Antimicrob Chemother. 1983;11:349.
31. Gilbaldi M, Swartz MA. Apparent effect of probenecid on the distribution of penicillins in man. Clin Pharmacol Ther. 1968;9:345.
32. Appel GB, Neu HC. Infections and antibiotic usage in patients with renal diseases. In: Martinez-Maldonado M, ed. Handbook of Renal Therpeutics. New York: Plenum; 1983:227.
33. Parker RH, Schmid FR. Antibacterial activity of synovial fluid during therapy of septic arthritis. Arthritis Rheum. 1971;14:96.
34. Barza M, Weinstein L. Penetration of antibiotics into fibrin loci in vivo. I. Comparison of penetration of ampicillin into fibrin clots, abscesses and interstitial fluid. J Infect Dis. 1974;129:59.
35. Pancoast SJ, Neu HC. Antibiotic levels in human bone and synovial fluid. Orthopedics Rev. 1980;9:49.
36. Neu HC. Antistaphylococcal penicillins. Med Clin North Am. 1982; 66:51.
37. Neu HC. Carbenicillin and ticarcillin. Med Clin North Am. 1982;66:61.
38. Fishman RA. Blood-brain and CSF barriers to penicillin and related organic acids. Arch Neurol. 1966;15:13.
39. Depp R, Kind AC, Kirby WMM, et al. Transplacental passage of methicillin and dicloxacillin into the fetus and amniotic fluid. Am J Obstet Gynecol. 1970;197:1054.
40. Whelton A, Carter GG, Bryant HH, et al. Carbenicillin concentrations in normal and diseased kidneys. A therapeutic consideration. Ann Intern Med. 1973;78:659.
41. Levine BB, Redmond AP, Feller MF, et al. Penicillin allergy and the heterogeneous immune response of man to benzylpenicillin. J Clin Invest. 1966;45:1895.
42. Saxon A. Immediate hypersensitivity reactions to β-lactam antibiotics. Rev Infect Dis. 1983;5(Suppl 2):368.
43. Idsoe O, Gothe T, Wilcox RR, et al. Nature and extent of penicillin side reactions with particular reference to fatalities from anaphylactic shock. Bull WHO. 1968;38:159.
44. Green GR, Rosenblum A. Report of the penicillin study group, American Academy of Allergy. J Allergy Clin Immunol. 1971;48:331.
45. Parry MF, Neu HC. The safety and tolerance of mezlocillin. J Antimicrob Chemother. 1982;9(Suppl A):273.
46. Kerr RO, Cardamone J, Dalmasso AP, et al. Two mechanisms of erthrocyte destruction in penicillin-induced hemolytic anemia. N Engl J Med. 1972;287:1322.
47. Brown CH, Natelson EA, Bradshaw W, et al. The hemostatic defect produced by carbenicillin. N Engl J Med. 1974;291:265.
48. Appel GB, Neu HC. The nephrotoxicity of antimicrobial agents. N Engl J Med. 1977;296:63.
49. Appel GB, Neu HC. Acute interstitial nephritis induced by β-lactam antibiotics. In: Fillastre JP, ed. Nephrotoxicity-ototoxicity of Drugs. Rouen: Inserum Publ de l'Université de Rouen; 1981:195.
50. Baldwin DS, Levine BB, McCluskey RT, et al. Renal failure and interstitial nephritis due to penicillin and methicillin. N Engl J Med. 1968;279:1245.
51. Bloomer HA, Barton LJ, Maddock RJ Jr. Penicillin-induced encephalopathy in uremic patients. JAMA. 1967;200:121.
52. Wilson FM, Belamavic J, Lauter CB, et al. Anicteric carbenicillin hepatitis. Eight episodes in four patients. JAMA. 1967;232:818.
53. New HC. Aminopenicillins: clinical pharmacology and use in disease states. Int J Clin Pharmacol Biopharm. 1975;11:132.
54. Tuano SD, Johnson LD, Brodie JL, et al. Comparative blood levels of hetacillin, ampicillin and penicillin G. N Engl J Med. 1966;275:635.
55. Daehne W von, Godfredsen WO, Rotrott K, et al. Pivampicillin, a new orally active ampicillin ester. Antimicrob Agents Chemother. 1971;10:431.
56. Scheife RT, Neu HC. Bacampicillin hydrochloride: chemistry, pharmacology and clinical use. Pharmacotherapy. 1982;2:313.
57. Prince AS, Neu HC. New penicillins and their use in pediatrics. Pediatr Clin North Am. 1983;30:3.
58. McCracken GH Jr. Selection of antimicrobial agents for treatment of acute otitis media with effusion. Pediatr Infect Dis J. 1987;6:985–8.
59. Fang LST, Tolokoff-Rubin NE, Rubin RH. Efficacy of single-dose and conventional amoxicillin therapy in urinary tract infection localized by antibody-coated bacteria technique. N Engl J Med. 1978;298:413.
60. Hoffman TA, Cestero R, Bullock WE. Pharmacodynamics of carbenicillin in patients with hepatic and renal failure. Ann Intern Med. 1970;73:173.
61. Fuchs PC, Thornsberry C, Barry AL, et al. Ticarcillin: a collaborative in vitro comparison with carbenicillin against 9,000 clinical bacterial isolates. Am J Med Sci. 1977;274:255.
62. Neu HC, Garvey GG. Comparative in vitro activity and clinical pharmacology of ticarcillin and carbenicillin. Antimicrob Agents Chemother. 1975;8:457.
63. Parry MF, Neu HC. Ticarcillin for treatment of serious infections with gram-negative bacteria. J Infect Dis. 1976;134:476.
64. Fu KP, Neu HC. Azlocillin and mezlocillin: new ureido penicillins. Antimicrob Agents Chemother. 1978;13:930.
65. Bergen T. Review of the pharmacokinetics and dose dependency of azlocillin in normal subjects and patients with renal insufficiency. J Antimicrob Agents. 1983;11(Suppl B):101.
66. Whelton A, Stout RL, Delgado FA. Azlocillin kinetics during extracorporeal haemodialysis and peritoneal dialysis. J Antimicrob Chemother. 1983;11(Suppl B):89.

67. Drusano GL, Schimpff SC, Hewitt WL. The acylampicillins: mezlocillin, piperacillin, and azlocillin. Rev Infect Dis. 1984;6:13–32.
68. Lowenbraun S, Fox N, Cunitz D. Azlocillin, cephalothin and tobramycin therapy in solid tumor patients with chemotherapy-induced leukopenia. Cancer. 1987;60:14–7.
69. Parry MF, Folta D. The in vitro activity of mezlocillin against community hospital isolates in comparison to other penicillins and cephalosporins. J Antimicrob Chemother. 1983;11(Suppl C):97.
70. Meyers BR, Mendelson MH, Srulevitch-Chin E, et al. Pharmacokinetic properties of mezlocillin in ambulatory elderly subjects. J Clin Pharmacol. 1987;27:678–81.
71. Pancoast SJ, Jahre JA, Neu HC. Mezlocillin in the therapy of serious infections. Am J Med. 1979;67:747.
72. Issell BF, Bodey GP. Mezlocillin for treatment of infections in cancer patients. Antimicrob Agents Chemother. 1980;17:1008.
73. Melikian V, Wise R, Allum WH, et al. Mezlocillin and gentamicin in the treatment of infections in seriously ill and immunosuppressed patients. J Antimicrob Chemother. 1981;7:657.
74. Ramirez-Ronda CH, Gotierrez J, Bermudez RH. Comparative effectiveness, safety and tolerance of mezlocillin and ticarcillin: a prospective randomized trial. J Antimicrob Chemother. 1982;9 (Suppl A):125.
75. Faro S, Phillips LE, Baker JL, et al. Comparative efficacy and safety of mezlocillin, cefoxitin, and clindamycin plus gentamicin in post-partum endometritis. Obstet Gynecol. 1987;69:760–6.
76. Alvarez RD, Kilgore LC, Huddlestone JF. A comparison of mezlocillin versus clindamycin/gentamicin for the treatment of post-caesarean endomyometritis. Am J Obst Gynecol. 1988;158:425–9.
77. Fu KP, Neu HC. Piperacillin, a new penicillin active against many bacteria resistant to other penicillins. Antimicrob Agents Chemother. 1978;13:358.
78. Verbist L. Comparison of the activities of the new ureido-penicillins—piperacillin, mezlocillin, azlocillin and Bay K4999—against gram-negative organisms. Antimicrob Agents Chemother. 1979;16:115.
79. Bergen T. Overview of acylureidopenicillin pharmacokinetics. Scand J Infect Dis. 1981;29:33.
80. Tjandramaga TB, Mollie A, Verbesselt R, et al. Piperacillin pharmacokinetics after intravenous and intramuscular administration. Antimicrob Agents Chemother. 1978;14:829.
81. Martens MG, Faro S, Feldman S, et al. Pharmacokinetics of the acylureidopenicillins piperacillin and mezlocillin in the post-partum patient. Antimicrob Agents Chemother. 1987;31:2015–7.
82. Brattstrom C, Malmborg AS, Tyden G. Penetration of clindamycin, cefoxitin, and piperacillin into pancreatic juice in man. Surgery. 1988;103:563–7.
83. Francke EL, Appel GB, Neu HC. Pharmacokinetics of intravenous piperacillin in patients undergoing chronic hemodialysis. Antimicrob Agents Chemother. 1979;16:788.
84. Winston DJ, Murphy W, Young LS, et al. Piperacillin therapy for serious bacterial infections. Am J Med. 1980;69:255.
85. Wade JC, Schimpff SC, Newman KA, et al. Piperacillin or ticarcillin plus amikacin: a double blind prospective comparison of empiric antibiotic therapy for febrile granulocytopenic cancer patients. Am J Med. 1981;71:983.
86. Pancoast SJ, Prince AS, Francke EL, et al. Clinical evaluation of piperacillin for therapy of infection. Arch Intern Med. 1981;141:1447.
87. Prince AS, Neu HC. Use of piperacillin, a semisynthetic penicillin, in the therapy of acute exacerbations of pulmonary disease in patients with cystic fibrosis. J Pediatr. 1980;97:148.
88. Hemsell DL, Hemsell PG, Heard MC. Piperacillin and a combination of clindamycin and gentamicin for the treatment of hospital and community-acquired acute pelvic infections including pelvic abscess. Surg Gynecol Obstet. 1987;165:223–9.
89. Menichetti F, Del Favero A, Guerciolini R, et al. Empiric antimicrobial therapy in febrile granulocytopenic patients. Randomized prospective comparison of amikacin plus piperacillin with or without parenteral trimethoprim/sulfamethoxazole. Infection. 1986;14:61–267.
90. Holmes B, Richard DM, Brodgen RN, et al. Piperacillin: a review of its antibacterial activity, pharmacokinetic properties, and their therapeutic use. Drugs. 1984;28:375–425.
91. Neu HC. Mecillinam, a novel penicillanic acid derivative with unusual activity against gram-negative bacteria. Antimicrob Agents Chemother. 1976;9:793.
92. Neu HC. Mecillinam: an amdinocillin which acts synergistically with other β-lactam compounds. J Antimicrob Cheother. 1977;3(Suppl B):43.
93. Neu HC, Srinivasan S, Francke EL, et al. Pharmacokinetics of amdinocillin and pivamdinocillin in normal volunteers. Am J Med. 1983;75(Suppl 2A):60.
94. Moukhtar I, Nawishy S, Sabbour M. Pharmacokinetics of mecillinam after a single intravenous dose in patients with impaired renal function. Int J Clin Pharmacol Res. 1987;7:59–62.
95. Demos CH, Green E. Review of clinical experience with amdinocillin monotherapy and comparative studies. Am J Med. 1983;75(Suppl 2A):72.
96. King JW, Beam TR Jr, Neu HC, et al. Systemic infections treated with amdinocillin in combination with other beta-lactam antibiotics. Am J Med. 1983;75(Suppl 2A):90.
97. Jules K, Neu HC. Antibacterial activity and β-lactamase stability of temocillin. Antimicrob Agents Chemother. 1982;22:453.
98. Gobernado M, Conton E. Comparative in vitro activity of temocillin. Drugs. 1985;29(Suppl 5):24–31.
99. Hampel B, Feike M, Koeppe P, et al. Pharmacokinetics of temocillin in volunteers. Drugs. 1985;29(Suppl 5):99–102.
100. Kosmidis J. The treatment of complicated and uncomplicated urinary tract infections with temocillin. Drugs. 1985;29(Suppl 5):172–4.
101. VanLanduyt HW, Lambert A, vanCouter A, et al. Temocillin in the treatment of gram-negative septicemia. Drugs. 1985;29(Suppl 5):182–5.
102. Lindsay G, Beattie AD, Taylor EW. Temocillin in the treatment of serious gram-negative infections. Drugs. 1985;29(Suppl 5):191–3.

19. CEPHALOSPORINS

GERALD R. DONOWITZ
GERALD L. MANDELL

Most of the new antibiotics introduced for clinical use in recent years are cephalosporins. These agents are now the most prescribed of all antimicrobials and account for a large segment of the health care budget. It all started in 1945 when Professor Giuseppe Brotzu began searching for antibiotic-producing microorganisms. He hypothesized that the process of self-purification of water might be due in part to substances produced by certain organisms inhibiting other microbes. He isolated a fungus, *Cephalosporium acremonium*, from seawater near a sewage outlet in Kaglara, Sardinia, and found that this organism inhibited the growth of a variety of gram-positive and gram-negative bacteria. Broth cultures produced a filtrate that showed some antibacterial effect on infections in animals and later in patients.

Professor Brotzu sent a culture of his organism to Oxford in 1948, and attempts were made by several workers, led by Professor Edward P. Abraham, to isolate the active antibacterial factors. Several different antibiotic fractions were isolated from these broth cultures. These included cephalosporin C, which is the parent substance from which the first cephalosporins for clinical use were derived. In addition to its fairly broad range of antimicrobial activity, it had the interesting features of being relatively acid stable and resistant to penicillinase.[1]

CLASSIFICATION

Cephalosporins may be classified by their chemical structure, major differences in clinical pharmacology, β-lactamase resis-

TABLE 1. Selected Cephalosporins Listed by Generation

Generic Name	*Proprietary Name*
First generation	
Cefazolin	Ancef, Kefzol
Cephalothin	Keflin, Seffin
Cephapirin	Cefadyl
Cefadroxil	Duricef
Cephalexin	Keflex
Cephradine	Anspor, Velasef
Second generation	
Cefamandole	Mandol
Cefoxitin	Mefoxin
Cefuroxime	Zinacef, Kefurox
Cefotetan	Cefotan
Cefonicid	Monocid
Cefaclor	Ceclor
Cefuroxime axetil	Ceftin
Third generation	
Cefotaxime	Claforan
Ceftizoxime	Cefizox
Ceftriaxone	Rocephin
Moxalactam	Moxam
Ceftazidime	Fortaz, Taxidime, Tazicef
Cefoperazone	Cefobid
Cefpirome	—
Cefpiramide	—
Cefixime	Suprax

tance, or antibacterial spectrum. The well-accepted "generations scheme" is a somewhat arbitrary but useful way to classify these agents (Table 1). *Generations* are based on antimicrobial activity and not on the time of introduction of the agents.

CHEMISTRY

The three active fermentation products of *Cephalosporium* were identified as cephalosporin C, cephalosporin N, and cephalosporin P. Cephalosporin N is actually a penicillin, with an aminocarboxybutyl side chain. Cephalosporin P is a steroid with a very narrow range of antibacterial activity. Cephalosporin C is the major product, and it is the basis for the new cephalosporins. Cephalosporin C resembles a penicillin since it has a β-lactam structure, but the five-member thiazolidine ring characteristic of the penicillins is replaced by a six-member dihydrothiazine ring (Fig. 1). Previous experience has shown that the potency of penicillins was improved by substitution of different groups at the 6-acylamino function adjacent to the β-lactam ring. Attempts were made to cleave the side chain off enzymatically, but these failed. Acid treatment, however, did hydrolyze cephalosporin C to 7-aminocephalosporanic acid (7-ACA) (Fig. 2). This compound has been subsequently modified with different side chains to create a whole family of cephalosporin antibiotics. In general, modifications at position 7 of the 7-aminocephalosporanic acid nucleus are associated with alteration in antibacterial activity, and substitutions at position 3 of the dihydrothiazine ring are associated with changes in the pharmacokinetics and the metabolic parameters of the drug (Fig. 3).[2,3] Hepatic metabolism occurs at the 3-acetoxymethyl position. There has been an association made with certain adverse side effects such as disulfuram-like (Antabuse) reactions, and the potential for bleeding associated with the methylthiotetrazole group at position 3 of the dihydrothiazoladine ring.[4] Molecules with a methoxy group in position 7 of the 7-aminocephalosporanic acid nucleus are called cephamycins.

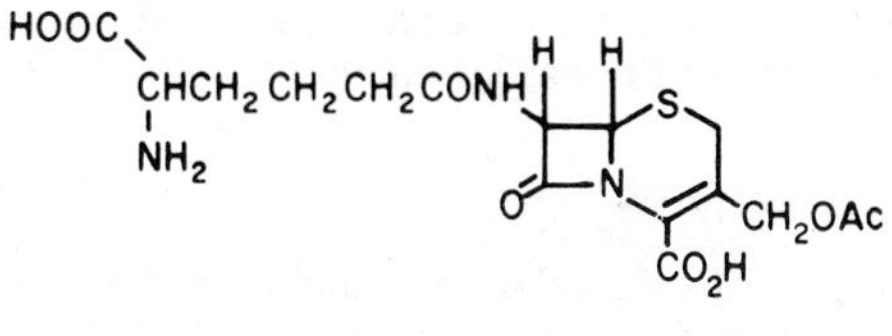

FIG. 1. Structure of cephalosporin C.

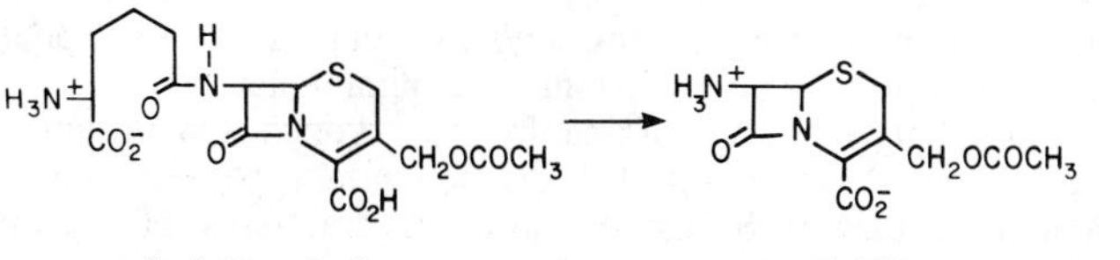

FIG. 2. Preparation of 7-aminocephalosporanic acid (7-ACA) from cephalosporin C.

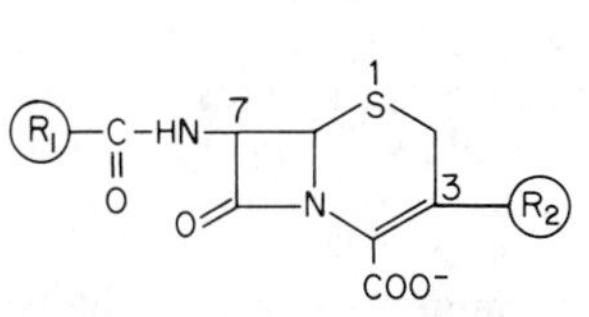

FIG. 3. Basic structure of a cephalosporin.

MECHANISM OF ACTION

The mechanism of action of the β-lactam antibiotics could be explained with confidence and precision a decade ago. It was thought that all β-lactam antibiotics had the same mechanism of action and that this was related to interference with cell wall structure. A brilliant series of experiments by a number of investigators identified the particular step in the cross-linking of the peptidoglycan polymer that was interfered with by the β-lactam antibiotics.[5] It was thought that these weak or defective cell walls then allowed for growth of bizarre bacterial forms with subsequent lysis and death of bacterial cells.

It became clear that this explanation of the mechanism of action of the β-lactam antibiotics was oversimplified and failed to explain various observations of drug–bacteria interactions. First, antibiotic-induced lysis of bacteria appeared to be an enzymatic process rather than a process resulting from a weakened bacterial cell wall.[6] It also became clear that multiple targets for β-lactam molecules existed within bacteria and differed from each other biochemically and functionally.[7,8] Furthermore, different agents produced greatly different effects on bacteria. Some β-lactam antibiotics produced lytic effects such as those seen with cephalothin acting on *Staphylococcus aureus*. Other agents, such as cephalexin, produced long filamentous forms when they interacted with *Escherichia coli*, while yet other agents such as amdinocillin produced round, osmotically fragile forms.

At present, our understanding of the specific mechanisms involved in the antibacterial activity of β-lactam antibiotics, including the cephalosporins, remains incomplete. However, several basic elements have been established. These agents act by binding to and inactivating specific targets located on the inner aspect of the bacterial cell membrane.[7,8] These targets, or penicillin-binding proteins (PBPs), are enzymes, including transpeptidases, carboxypeptidases, and endopeptidases, that are important for the biosynthesis of the peptidoglycan component of the bacterial cell wall. β-Lactam antibiotics have different binding affinities to the various PBPs. The effect of an antibiotic on a bacterium is, in part, dependent on which PBP or combination of PBPs are bound and inactivated.[9–11] Some PBPs (PBP1A, -1BS, -2, and -3) are of critical importance, and their inactivation leads to cell death. Other PBPs (PBP4, -5, and -6) are not essential for bacterial survival, and their inhibition causes nonlethal changes.[12,13] Actual lysis of a bacterium by a β-lactam appears to involve inhibition of protein synthesis and the loss from the cell of an inhibitor of an enzyme that functions as an autolysin. Bacterial cells containing the autolysins are often lysed by the activity of the β-lactam antibiotics. Bacterial cells not containing the autolysin may develop bizarre forms, and their growth may be only inhibited.[14,15] Thus the β-lactam exhibits a bacteriostatic effect rather than a bactericidal effect. This phenomenon has been called tolerance.

Some of the newer concepts of the mechanism of action of the β-lactam antibiotics may be of clinical importance. In the past it was thought that there would be no reason to combine β-lactam antibiotics, since it was thought that they all worked in an identical fashion and thus true synergism would not be seen. However, since these agents may bind to different proteins in the bacterial cell, it may be feasible to use two β-lactam antibiotics together to achieve a synergistic effect.[16]

MECHANISM OF BACTERIAL RESISTANCE TO THE CEPHALOSPORINS

The antibacterial activity of cephalosporins is dependent on their ability to penetrate the bacterial cell wall, resist inactivation by bacterial enzymes known as β-lactamases, and bind to and inactivate penicillin-binding proteins. Bacterial resistance may develop at each of these steps. The peptidoglycan structure of the cell wall of gram-positive organisms offers little resistance to the entry of antibiotic molecules. In contrast, the outer cell wall of gram-negative organisms, consisting of lipids, proteins, and polysaccharides, represents a formidable barrier to entry of many molecules, including cephalosporins.[17] Passage of these agents through the cell wall occurs through channels lined by proteins called porins. Porin channels allow selective movement of molecules through the bacterial cell wall based on size, change, and hydrophilic properties.[18] This selective permeability of the cell wall may be an inherent property of a bacterium but may also result from changes caused by exposure to antibiotics. Difficulty in penetration may by itself offer a means of resistance for bacteria like *Pseudomonas aeruginosa* and *Enterobacter cloacae*. This mechanism may also interact synergistically with other bacterial mechanisms of resistance.[19]

Decreased binding affinity of penicillin-binding proteins for antibiotics is another mechanism of bacterial resistance and is the reason that cephalosporins are ineffective against methicillin-resistant *S. aureus*. Exposure of these organisms to β-lactam antibiotics stimulates the production of a novel PBP termed PBP2′ or PBP2a, which has a markedly lowered binding affinity for cephalosporins as well as penicillinase-resistant penicillins.[20,21] The most important bacterial mechanism of resistance to the cephalosporins is the production of β-lactamases.[22–25] These enzymes are present in virtually all gram-negative and gram-positive bacteria and hydrolyze the cyclic amide bond of the β-lactam ring, rendering it inactive. Among gram-positive organisms, the staphylococcal β-lactamses are the most significant and are released into the surrounding media. While the penicillins are highly susceptible to these enzymes, most cephalosporins, with the exception of cephaloridine, are poorly hydrolyzed. Gram-negative bacilli produce a variety of β-lactamses that may be encoded chromosomally or extrachromosomally via plasmids or transposons. Although gram-negative organisms seem to produce less β-lactamase, the location of their β-lactamases in the periplasmic space makes the enzymes more effective in destroying cephalosporins as they attempt to reach their target on the inner membrane.[22]

The cephalosporins have variable susceptibility to β-lactamase. Cephaloridine is the most sensitive to both gram-positive and gram-negative β-lactamases, and thus more antibiotic is hydrolyzed by the enzyme. Cefazolin is more susceptible to hydrolysis by β-lactamases from *S. aureus* than is cephalothin.[26] Cefoxitin, cefuroxime, and the third-generation cephalosporins are the most resistant to hydrolysis by the β-lactamases produced by gram-negative organisms.[27] However, the correlation between antimicrobial activity and β-lactamase resistance is not linear. Some bacterial strains that fail to hydrolyze the antibiotics are nevertheless resistant. Conversely, some bacteria with β-lactamases that can destroy cephalosporins are susceptible to the cephalosporins.[28]

Although most of the third-generation cephalosporins are relatively resistant to hydrolysis by bacterial β-lactamases, there are increasing reports of development of resistance to the third-generation cephalosporins by *Enterobacter, Serratia, Citrobacter*, and *Pseudomonas* species.[27] Sanders and Sanders[29] have suggested that the derepression of chromosomally mediated β-lactamases in these organisms has resulted in the production of large amounts of enzyme that have a high affinity for the antibiotics although they slowly hydrolyze them. They propose that the complex of a β-lactamase and a cephalosporin prevents binding to penicillin-binding proteins, thereby leading to antibiotic resistance.[30,31] That the binding of a drug rather than its hydrolysis can be a major factor in the development of resistance is still debated.[32]

It is important to remember that cephalosporins do not have reliable activity or effectiveness against penicillin-resistant *Streptococcus pneumoniae*, methicillin-resistant *S. aureus*, methicillin-resistant *Staphylococcus epidermidis, Enterococcus faecalis, Listeria monocytogenes, Legionella pneumophila, Legionella micdadei, Clostridium difficile, Xanthomonas maltophila, Pseudomonas putida, Campylobacter jejuni*, and, of course, *Candida albicans*.

PHARMACOLOGY

The pharmacologic features of selected cephalosporins are shown in Table 2.[33–48] Six of the agents may be absorbed orally and include the first-generation agents cephradine, cephalexin, and cefadroxil, the second-generation agents cefaclor and cefuroxime axetil, and the third-generation agent cefixime. The remaining drugs must be given parenterally. Cephalothin and cephapirin are painful when given intramuscularly and are therefore restricted to intravenous use. The rest of the agents may be administered intramuscularly and intravenously.

Peak serum levels for most of these agents are similar for a given dose and route of administration. Serum levels about 100 μg/ml can be expected for parenteral doses of 2 g.

Several cephalosporins penetrate into cerebrospinal fluid in sufficient amounts to be useful for treating meningitis. These include cefuroxime, moxalactam, cefotaxime, ceftriaxone, and ceftazidime.

Cephalosporins are found in high concentrations across the placenta and in synovial[49] and pericardial fluid. Penetration into the aqueous humor of the eye after systemic administration is relatively good for third-generation cephalosporins, but vitreous penetration is poor. There is some evidence that therapeutic levels for eye infections due to gram-positive and certain gram-negative organisms can be achieved after systemic administration. Bile levels are usually high, with those after cefoperazone administration being the highest.

Most cephalosporins are excreted primarily via the kidneys. Probenecid slows their renal excretion and may be used to increase serum levels. These agents require dosage adjustments in patients with renal failure. Two cephalosporins with different means of elimination are cefoperazone and ceftriaxone, which are eliminated primarily in the liver. Neither of these agents requires dosage adjustments in renal failure.

Agents with the acetyl group at the R2 position, including cephalothin, cephapirin, and cefotaxime (Figs. 4 and 5) undergo in vivo metabolism to the desacetyl forms, which have less biologic activity than the parent compounds.

ADVERSE REACTIONS

The cephalosporins are relatively safe drugs. Thrombophlebitis occurs with intravenous administration of all the cephalosporins. There are no conclusive data indicating significant differences.[50,51]

Hypersensitivity reactions related to the cephalosporins are the most common systemic side effects.[52] Unlike the penicillins, where metabolites of the bicyclic core structure are the major allergenic determinents, the acyl side chains of the cephalosporins appear to be important determinants as well.[53–56]

Immediate reactions of anaphylaxis, bronchospasm, and urticaria have been reported. More commonly, patients develop maculopapular rash, usually after several days of therapy. These patients may or may not have fever and eosinophilia. Fever and lymphadenopathy have been associated with cephalosporin administration without other manifestations of allergic phenomena.[57]

The specific haptens involved in producing allergic responses to cephalosporins are unknown. It is therefore difficult to assess the degree of cross-reactivity of cephalosporins with each other. Limited evidence suggests that cross-reactivity is less than that noted with the penicillins.[58] There is no data to suggest that immune-mediated allergic reactions are more common with one cephalosporin versus any other.

Of major clinical importance is the incidence of cross-reacting allergic responses occurring in penicillin-allergic patients who

TABLE 2. Pharmacologic Properties of the Cephalosporine

Generic Name	*Adult Dose for Serious Infection*[a]	*Peak Serum Concentration*[b] *(μg/ml)*	*Half-Life (hr)*	*Cerebrospinal Fluid Concentration (μg/ml)*	*Route of Excretion*
First generation					
Cefazolin	1g q8h	80 (1)	1.5	NA	Renal
Cephalothin	1g q4h	30 (1)	0.6	NA	Renal
Cefadroxil	0.5g q12h PO	16 (1)	1.2	NA	Renal
Cephalexin	0.5–1g q6h PO	18 (1)	0.75	NA	Renal
Cephradine	0.5g q6h PO	(18) (1)	0.7	NA	Renal
Second generation					
Cefamandole	1g 4q–6h	150 (2)	0.8	NA	Renal
Cefonicid	1–2g q24h	260 (2)	4.5	NA	Renal
Cefotetan	2–3g q12h	230 (2)	3.5	NA	Renal
Cefoxitin	2g q6–8h	150 (2)	0.8	NA	Renal
Cefuroxime	1.5g q8h	100 (1.5)	1.3	7	Renal
Cefaclor	0.25–0.5g q8h PO	13 (0.5)	0.8	NA	Renal
Cefuroxime axetil	0.25–0.5g q12h PO	8–9 (0.5)	1.3	NA	Renal
Third generation					
Cefixime	0.4g q24h PO	3.9 (0.4)	3.0	Data not available	Renal (15–20%); other?
Cefotaxime	2g q6–8h	130 (2)	1.0	44	Renal
Ceftizoxime	2g q8–12h	130 (2)	1.7	29	Renal
Ceftriaxone	1–2g q12h	250 (2)	8.0	10	Renal (50%); hepatic (40%)
Moxalactam	1–2g q8h	200 (2)	2.2	65	Renal
Third-generation cephlasporins with anti-Pseudomonas activity					
Cefoperazone	2g q8–12	250 (2)	2.0	8	Hepatic (70%); renal (25%)
Cefpiramide[c]	1–4g q12–24h	166 (1)	4.4	Data not available	Biliary (80%); renal (20%)
Cefpirome[c]	1–2g q12h	100 (1)	2.0	Data not available	Renal
Ceftazidime	2g q8h	160 (2)	1.8	40	Renal

[a] All doses are parenteral unless otherwise stated.
[b] Level after noted gram amount (in parentheses) of drug is given intravenously or, where noted in column 2, orally. Peak serum concentrations reported in the literature vary, depending on the time over which drug is given and time of serum sampling. Represented values are noted.
[c] Not yet available.
Abbreviations: NA: not clinically applicable.

receive a cephalosporin. Unfortunately, definitive data on this point is lacking. Early series indicated that the incidence of allergic reactions to cephalosporins was higher in patients with a history of penicillin allergy (5–16 percent) than in patients with no history of penicillin allergy (1–2.5 percent).[59,60] Flaws in these studies make evaluation difficult. Since only 15–40 percent of patients with a history of penicillin allergy will have positive skin tests,[61,62] many patients listed as penicillin-allergic were probably not. In addition, not all reactions described as allergic were shown to be immune-mediated. Adverse drug reactions in general are three times more common in patients with a penicillin allergy even when the drugs used are immunologically dissimilar to penicillin.[63] The increased incidence of reactions to cephalosporins in these studies may therefore have been due in part to this predisposition, rather than true allergic cross-reactivity.[64]

Cephalosporins have been given to patients in whom penicillin allergy was documented with skin testing including penicilloyl polylysine.[64–66] While the numbers of patients have been small, only one of ninety-nine (1 percent) developed a clinically significant reaction. Since IgE antibodies diminish over time, fewer allergic reactions to cephalosporins may occur in patients whose allergic reactions to penicillin were in the distant past.[67] Until the specific haptens involved in cephalosporin allergy have been identified and until testing for cephalosporin allergy is standardized, all that can be said definitively is that allergic reactions to cephalosporins do occur in penicillin-allergic patients, the incidence appears to be low, and mechanisms for the accurate prediction of allergic cross-reactions are not available.

Use of cephalosporins in penicillin-allergic patients should be guided by the severity of the allergy to penicillin, the availability of effective noncephalosporin treatment regimens, and clinical judgment. In most instances, a non-β-lactam agent should be used in patients with a definite history of severe penicillin or cephalosporin allergy. If possible, a history of penicillin allergy should be documented by skin testing with penicilloyl polylysine and a minor determinant mixture (See Chapter 21). Patients having no immediate reaction to either test probably can be given a cephalosporin safely. Practices differ when one of the tests is positive. There are insufficient data to make a reliable decision. Some experts do not recommend use of a cephalosporin under these circumstances (see Chapter 21). We feel that if a patient is skin test-positive to penicillin but has no history of anaphalaxis or other significant IgE-mediated reaction to penicillin, cephalosporins may be used with caution *if* no other suitable regimen is available. Where skin test positivity to penicillin is associated with a recent history of a severe IgE-mediated response, alternative, noncephalosporin regimens should be sought.

A positive Coombs reaction appears frequently in patients receiving large doses of cephalosporin drugs. Hemolysis is not usually associated with this phenomenon, although it has been reported. Rare cases of bone marrow depression characterized by granulocytopenia have been reported.

The cephalosporins have been implicated as potentially nephrotoxic agents, although they are not nearly as toxic to the kidney as are the aminoglycosides or the polymyxins.[68] Renal tubular necrosis has been described with cephaloridine in doses greater than 4 g/day. Other cephalosporins are much less toxic and, in recommended doses, rarely produce significant renal toxicity when used by themselves. High doses of cephalothin have produced acute tubular necrosis in certain cases, and usual doses (8–12 g/day) have been nephrotoxic in patients with preexisting renal disease[69] There is fairly good evidence that the combination of cephalothin plus gentamicin or tobramycin is synergistically nephrotoxic.[70] Interstitial nephritis, identical to that occurring during therapy with semisynthetic penicillins, may result from cephalosporin therapy. This is especially marked in patients over 60 years of age. Diarrhea has been reported with cephalosporin administration and may be more frequent with cefoperazone, perhaps because of its greater biliary excretion. Alcohol intolerance (a disulfuram-like reaction) has been noted with cefamandole, moxalactam, and cefotetan.

Ceftriaxone has recently been associated with the formation of biliary sludge in the gallbladder, which may lead to signs and symptoms of cholecystitis. This phenomenon appears to be unusual and is reversible once the drug is discontinued.[71–73] Ceftriaxone competes with bilirubin for albumin binding sites,

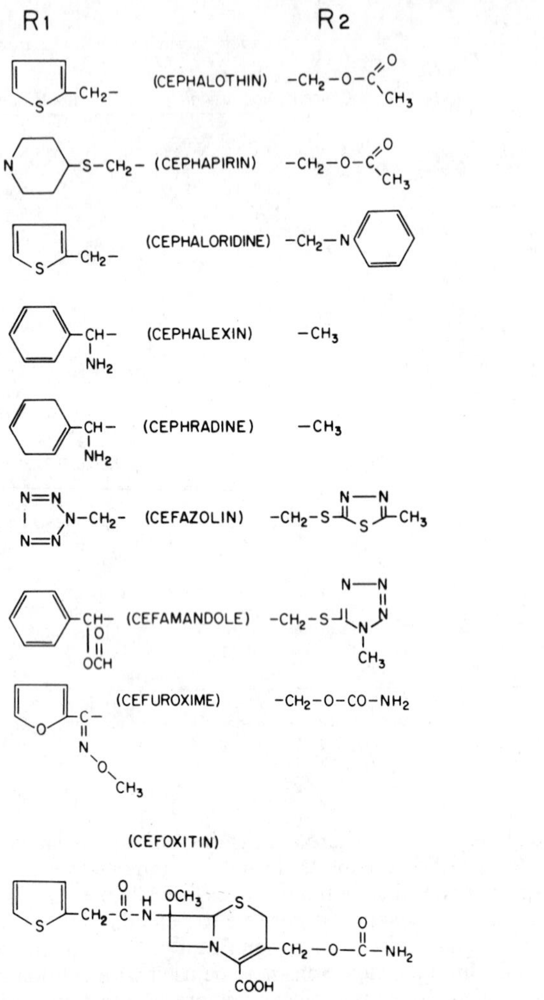

FIG. 4. Structures of selected first- and second-generation cephalosporins (see Fig. 3).

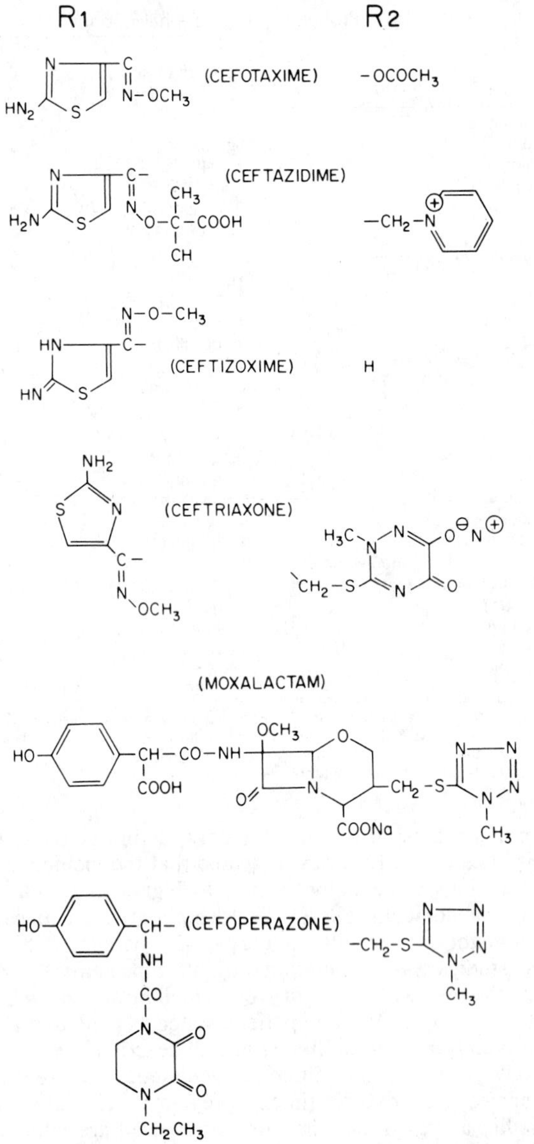

FIG. 5. Structures of selected third-generation cephalosporins (see Fig. 3).

which in neonates could theoretically be a factor in the development of bilirubin encephalopathy.[74,75] Its use in the neonate has therefore been discouraged.

Bleeding due to hypoprothrombinemia, platelet aggregation abnormalities, and thrombocytopenia have been associated with cephalosporin use.[76–78] The cause of hypoprothrombinemia is due to several factors. Inhibition of vitamin K synthesis by suppression of gut flora may occur with any of these agents.[79] The methylthiotetrazole side chain in cefamandole, cefotetan, moxalactam, and cefoperazone may inhibit the conversion of clotting factors II, VII, IX, and X to their active form and may also inhibit the formation of active vitamin K from its inactive precursor.[80–83] Use of these agents has been associated with abnormal coagulation parameters in 20–60 percent of patients.[84,85] Consequently vitamin K prophylaxis has been recommended when these agents are used in nutritionally deprived or otherwise seriously ill patients. Platelet aggregation abnormalities have been seen only with moxalactam among the cephalosporins.[86,87] This agent, more than any other of the cephalosporins, has been associated with significant bleeding[76] and for this reason has been removed from many formularies.

MODIFICATION OF DOSE WITH RENAL INSUFFICIENCY

The cephalosporins, although largely excreted by the kidney, require only moderate dose reduction in patients with renal insufficiency (see Chapter 38).

FIRST-GENERATION CEPHALOSPORINS

First-generation cephalosporins are the most active cephalosporins against gram-positive cocci, including *S. aureus* and streptococci[88] (Table 3). Two important exceptions to this are methicillin-resistant staphylococci and penicillin-resistant *S. pneumoniae*, which are not usually sensitive.[89] First-generation agents have moderate activity against a limited number of aerobic gram-negative bacilli, including *E. coli, Klebsiella pneumoniae*, and indole-negative *Proteus*.[90,91] Both parenteral and oral preparations of first-generation agents are available.

Cephalothin (Keflin) is not well absorbed orally and is available only in parenteral form. Because of pain on intramuscular injection, it is rarely administered via that route. After intravenous use, cephalothin has a large volume of distribution, indicating wide dispersal throughout body tissues and fluids. Cephalothin has a short half-life (30–40 minutes) and is actively metabolized in addition to being excreted. From 20 to 30 percent of cephalothin is excreted as the desacetyl metabolite. Unmetabolized active cephalothin does not appreciably enter the cerebrospinal fluid, and thus this drug and other first-generation

TABLE 3. In Vitro Activities of Selected Cephalosporins[a]

	S. aureus	*S. epidermidis*	*S. pyogenes*	*H. influenzae*	*E. coli*	*K. pneumoniae*	*S. marcesens*	*P. aeruginosa*	*B. fragilis*
First generation									
Cefazolin	1.0	0.8	0.1	10	5.0	6.0	>100	>100	>100
Cephalothin	1.0	0.5	0.1	10	5.0	32	>100	>100	>100
Second generation									
Cefamandole	1.0	2.0	0.06	1.0	4.0	8.0	>100	>100	>100
Cefoxitin	3.0	12.5	0.7	6.0	8.0	5.0	>100	>100	16
Cefuroxime	2.0	1.0	0.06	2.0	4.0	4.0	>100	>100	>100
Cefotetan	8.0	32	2.0	1.6	0.5	0.5	16	>100	16
Third generation									
Cefotaxime	2.0	8.0	0.03	0.03	0.25	0.25	2.0	>32	64
Ceftizoxime	3.0	2.5	0.03	0.01	0.13	0.25	2.0	>32	32
Moxalactam	8.0	32	2.0	0.1	0.25	0.25	4.0	64	16
Ceftriaxone	4.0	16	0.03	0.1	0.1	0.1	4.0	>32	>64
Third generation with good anti-*Pseudomonas* activity									
Cefoperazone	4.0	8.0	0.12	0.06	2.0	4.0	16	32	>64
Ceftazidime	16.0	32	0.25	0.1	0.5	0.5	1	4	>64
Cefpirome	1.0	2.0	0.1	0.03	0.06	0.03	0.12	16	32
Cefpiramide	8.0	8.0	0.25	0.25	32	32	>128	16	>256

[a] Minimum inhibitory concentration (μg/ml) for 90 percent of strains (MIC_{90}).
Values are approximations and are derived from Refs. 46, 88, 90–92, 94, 95, 105, 113, 117, 143, 147, 149, 150, 153, 154, 164, 165, 167.

cephalosporins should not be used for the treatment of meningitis. Since cephalothin is the cephalosporin most impervious to attack by staphylococcal β-lactamase, some authorities consider it to be the cephalosporin of choice in severe staphylococcal infections such as endocarditis.

Cefazolin (Ancef and Kefzol) has a spectrum of activity similar to that of cephalothin. However, cefazolin is more active against *E. coli* and *Klebsiella* species.[92] Cefazolin is somewhat more sensitive to staphylococcal penicillinase than is cephalothin.[93,94] Serum levels of cefazolin are higher after intramuscular and intravenous injections than are levels of cephalothin due in part to a smaller volume of distribution. The half-life is also appreciably longer, being 1.8 hours as compared with 0.5 hour for cephalothin.[95] The renal clearance of cefazolin is lower than that of cephalothin. This is probably related to the fact that cefazolin is excreted by glomerular filtration, whereas cephalothin is also excreted by the kidney tubule. Cefazolin is highly (about 80 percent) protein-bound. Cefazolin is relatively well tolerated after intramuscular or intravenous injections. It is the usually preferred first-generation cephalosporin since it can be administered less frequently.[96]

Cephradine (Anspor—oral, Velosef—oral and parenteral) is similar in structure to cephalexin, and its in vitro activity is almost identical. Cephradine is unmetabolized and after rapid oral absorption is excreted unchanged in the urine. Cephradine can be administered intramuscularly or intravenously. When administered by mouth the clinical pharmacology of cephradine is very much like that of cephalexin. Because cephradine is so well absorbed, the serum levels after an oral or intramuscular dose are nearly equivalent (about 10–18 μg/ml after 0.5 g orally or intramuscularly). The peak serum level for the oral dose is actually higher, but the area under the curve for both routes of administration is equivalent.[97]

Cephapirin (Cefadyl) is very similar to cephalothin. Like cephalothin, it is painful after intramuscular injection. Also like cephalothin, it is metabolized as the desacetyl derivative, which is about half as active as the parent compound. The half-life and excretion pattern of cephapirin are like that of cephalothin.[98]

Cefadroxil monohydrate (Duricef, Ultracef) is the parahydroxy analogue of cephalexin. Serum and urine concentrations of cefadroxil are somewhat more sustained than those noted with cephalexin. The drug may be used once or twice a day for treatment of urinary tract infections. In vitro activity is similar to that of cephalexin.[99]

Cephalexin (Keflex) is a cephalosporin for oral use that has the same antibacterial spectrum as other first-generation cephalosporins. It is less active, however, against penicillinase-producing staphylococci. Oral cephalexin therapy (0.5 g) results in peak serum levels of 16 μg/ml, which are adequate for the inhibition of many cephalosporin-sensitive gram-positive and gram-negative pathogens. The drug is unmetabolized, and more than 90 percent is excreted in the urine.[100]

Clinical Uses

The first-generation cephalosporins most commonly in use are the parenteral agents cefazolin and cephalothin and the oral agent cephalexin. Because of their activity against gram-positive cocci, they are useful alternatives to penicillin for therapy of a variety of infections due to staphylococci and nonenterococcal streptococci. The first-generation cephalosporins are the agents of choice for prophylaxis of most surgical procedures including orthopaedic and cardiovascular operations.[101–104] Because cefazolin has a longer half-life than cephalothin, it is the preferred agent in this regard. For procedures in which anaerobic infections are likely (colorectal surgery, appendectomies), agents with better anaerobic coverage such as cefoxitin or cefotetan are suggested. The first-generation agents can be used to treat a variety of infections caused by susceptible aerobic gram-negative bacilli, but the activity of these drugs against gram-negative rods is inconsistent and their empiric use is not suggested.

SECOND-GENERATION CEPHALOSPORINS

As a group, the second-generation cephalosporins are more potent than first-generation cephalosporins against *E. coli, Klebsiella* sp., and indole-negative *Proteus* (Table 3). Individual members of the second generation extend the spectrum of activity of first-generation agents to include strains of *Haemophilus influenzae*, *Enterobacter* sp., *Serratia* sp., indole-positive *Proteus*, anaerobes, *Neisseria meningitidis*, and *Neisseria gonorrhoeae*. None of the agents has activity against *Pseudomonas* sp.[44,105,106]

Specific Agents

Cefamandole (Mandol) is more active than the first-generation cephalosporins against certain species of gram-negative organisms. This is especially evident for *H. influenzae*,[107] *Enterobacter* sp., indole-positive *Proteus* sp., *E. coli*, and *Klebsiella* sp.[108] Its activity against β-lactamase-producing, ampicillin-resistant *H. influenzae* is inconsistent, and heavy bacterial inocula show decreased susceptibility. Most gram-positive cocci are susceptible to cefamandole.

Cefoxitin (Mefoxin) is a cefamycin produced by *Streptomyces lactamdurans*. It is highly resistant to β-lactamases produced by gram-negative rods.[109] This antibiotic is more active than cephalothin against certain gram-negative organisms, including *E. coli, Klebsiella*, indole-positive and -negative *Proteus*, and *Serratia* sp. It is less active than cefamandole against *Enterobacter* sp. and many strains of *H. influenzae*. It is also less active than both cefamandole and the older cephalosporins against gram-positive bacteria. Cefoxitin is more active than other first-, second-, and most third-generation agents against anaerobes, especially *Bacteroides fragilis*. Cefoxitin's special role seems to be for treatment of certain mixed anaerobic–aerobic infections.[110–112]

Cefuroxime (Zinacef, Kefurox) is similar to cefamandole in structure and antibacterial activity.[113] It is relatively more resistant to β-lactamases than is cefamandole, including those produced by ampicillin-resistant *H. influenzae*. Its serum half-life is longer (1.5 vs. 0.5 hours), and the drug may be given every 8 hours. Cefuroxime is the only second-generation cephalosporin with consistent penetration into cerebrospinal fluid.

Cefuroxime axetil (Ceftin) is the 1-acetoxyethyl ester of cefuroxime. Taken orally, cefuroxime axetil is hydrolyzed to cefuroxime after absorption.[114–116] Bioavailability varies between 30 and 50 percent and is increased after food ingestion. Mean peak serum levels occur 1.5–2.5 hours after a 500 mg dose. The half-life is 1.2 hours, but adequate serum levels persist long enough to allow for twice a day dosing.

Cefotetan (Cefotan) is a cephamycin that has characteristics of both second- and third-generation agents.[117,118] Its activity against gram-positive cocci and *B. fragilis* is similar to that of cefoxitin. It is less active than cefoxitin against other *Bacteroides* species.[119] Its activity against aerobic gram-negative bacilli is superior to that of cefoxitin and most other second-generation agents. Its half-life is 3.3 hours, and it may be used with twice daily dosing.

Cefaclor (Ceclor) is a cephalosporin for oral administration. The serum levels after an oral dose are about 50 percent of those achieved after equivalent oral doses of cephalexin. However, cefaclor is more active against gram-negative bacilli. This may be especially important for *H. influenzae, E. coli*, and *Proteus mirabilis*, although some β-lactamase-producing strains of *H. influenzae* may be resistant.[120]

Ceforanide (Precef) is similar in structure and antimicrobial activity to cefamandole. However, it is less active against strains of *H. influenzae*. Peak plasma concentrations after 1 g given intramuscularly are approximately 65 μg/ml. Ninety percent of a dose is excreted unchanged in the urine, and the half-life is approximately 3 hours. The drug has been effective when administered every 12 hours.[121]

Cefonicid (Monicid) has similar in vitro activity to cefamandole. The plasma half-life of the drug is about 4½ hours, and one dose a day has been effective for certain infections caused by susceptible organisms.[122]

Clinical Uses

Cefuroxime, because of its activity against *S. pneumoniae, S. aureus*, and *H. influenzae*, including ampicillin-resistant strains, has been used widely as therapy for community-acquired pneumonia when a specific pathogen is not suggested by sputum examination.[123,124] Cefamandole's relative lack of efficacy against some strains of ampicillin-resistant *H. influenzae* makes it a less attractive alternative in this situation.[125] Cefuroxime has been used to treat meningitis caused by *H. influenzae, S. pneumoniae*, and *N. meningitidis*, but since third-generation agents have greater activity and better penetration into the cerebrospinal fluid, these agents are usually preferred.[126–128]

Cefuroxime axetil has been used to treat a variety of mild-to-moderate infections including skin and soft tissue infections, urinary tract infections, pneumonia, bronchitis, otitis media, and uncomplicated gonococcal urethritis.[129,130] In most but not all of these cases, cefuroxime has proved at least as effective as other oral agents including cefaclor and amoxicillin with and without clavulanic acid. Failure to cure cases of purulent bronchitis and recurrent urinary tract infections has been reported, and its utility in more serious infections remains to be proved.[131,132]

Cefoxitin has been used successfully to treat mixed aerobic–anaerobic infections. It has often been used with an aminoglycoside to maximize coverage of aerobic gram-negative bacilli. Intra-abdominal infections, pelvic infections, nosocomial aspiration pneumonia, and foot infections in the diabetic have all been successfully treated.[133,134] Because of its anaerobic activity cefoxitin has been suggested as the agent of choice for prophylaxis of colorectal surgery, appendectomies, and procedures in which anaerobic infections are likely.[135] Cefoxitin has been used as effective therapy for gonorrhea including disease caused by penicillin-resistant strains.[136,137] Cefotetan has been suggested as a replacement for cefoxitin because of its similar spectrum of activity against anaerobes and its longer half-life. It has proven to be as effective as cefoxitin for prophylaxis in pelvic and abdominal surgery and is as effective as either cefoxitin or moxalactam for therapy of obstetric and gynecologic infections and intra-abdominal infections.[138–141]

THIRD-GENERATION CEPHALOSPORINS

The third-generation cephalosporins have the broadest spectrum and most potent activity of all cephalosporins against gram-negative bacilli[44,46] (Table 3). They are resistant to many of the β-lactamases produced by gram-negative bacteria and retain their activity against organisms resistant to first- and second-generation agents, aminoglycosides, and extended spectrum penicillins. Their activity against gram-positive cocci adds nothing to that of first- and second-generation agents. Activity against anaerobes is agent-dependent but is usually no better than that provided by cefoxitin. The third-generation agents may be divided into two groups, based on their activity against *P. aeruginosa*. Cefotaxime, ceftizoxime, ceftriaxone, moxalactam, and the oral agent cefixime have poor anti-*Pseudomonas* activity. (Moxalactam is an oxa-β-lactam and not a true cephalosporin since it has an oxygen molecule instead of a sulphur molecule at the C_1 position of the dihydrothiazine ring [see Fig. 5]. It is usually placed in this group due to similar antimicrobial activity and pharmacologic properties.) Ceftazidime, cefoperazone, and the investigational agents cefpirome and cefpiramide are third-generation agents with activity against *P. aeruginosa*.

Specific Agents

Cefotaxime (Claforan) was the first of the third-generation cephalosporins to become available in the United States and is the agent with which there has been the greatest experience. Cefotaxime is highly resistant to bacterial β-lactamases and has good activity against gram-positive organisms, with the exception of enterococci and *Listeria monocytogenes*, and to gram-negative aerobic organisms, with the exception of all strains of *Pseudomonas*.[142,143] Ninety to one hundred percent of strains of *E. coli, Klebsiella*, indole-positive and -negative *Proteus, H. influenzae, N. meningitidis*, and *N. gonorrhoeae* are inhibited. *Enterobacter cloacae* and strains of *Acinetobacter* show moderate susceptibility to the drug. The majority of strains of *P. aeruginosa* are resistant. While peptococci and peptostreptococci are usually susceptible to cefotaxime, many strains of anaerobes are resistant. Cefotaxime penetrates reliably into cerebrospinal fluid.[144]

Moxalactam (Moxam) has a unique structure (designated

oxa-β-lactam), which is created by the substitution of an oxygen for the sulfur atom in the six-membered ring of the cephem nucleus (see Fig. 5). Moxalactam has the broad antimicrobial activity characteristic of the third-generation cephalosporins.[145] In comparison with cefotaxime, it is less active against gram-positive organisms including streptococci and staphylococci. It is somewhat less active against *H. influenzae* and has very similar activity against most of the Enterobacteraceae. It is slightly more active against *Pseudomonas* and appreciably more active against *B. fragilis* than is cefotaxime. Clinically significant bleeding has been reported with moxalactam administration and for this reason we no longer recommend it for clinical use.[146]

Ceftizoxime (Cefizox) has in vitro activity similar to that of cefotaxime, with more activity against strains of *Serratia marcescens* and *Bacteroides*.[147] Like cefotaxime, ceftizoxime penetrates well into the cerebrospinal fluid.[148] Its half-life is slightly longer than that of cefotaxime, allowing it to be dosed at 8 hour intervals.

Ceftriaxone (Rocephin) has a spectrum of activity that mirrors that of cefotaxime and ceftizoxime.[149,150] It is the most potent agent against both *N. meningitidis* and *N. gonorrhoeae*, with an MIC_{90} of 0.025 μg/liter. Like cefotaxime and ceftizoxime, reliable cerebrospinal fluid levels can be attained. The truly outstanding feature of ceftriaxone is its half-life of 8 hours, significantly longer than any other cephalosporin. This has allowed serious infections to be treated with once a day, or twice a day dosing.

Cefixime (Suprax) is the first oral third-generation cephalosporin. Its spectrum of activity against aerobic gram-negative rods is similar to that of ceftizoxime and superior to those of cephalexin, cefaclor, and cefuraxime axetil—the other oral cephalosporins.[151,152] Its activity against nonenterococcal streptococci is similar to that of other oral cephalosporins, but its activity against *S. aureus* is inferior. Clinical experience is limited.

Specific Agents with Anti-Pseudomonas Activity

Cefoperazone (Cefobid) is less active than cefotaxime against gram-positive cocci and the majority of aerobic gram-negative rods.[46,153–156] Cefoperazone does, however, have activity against *P. aeruginosa*, with greater than 50 percent of strains susceptible to ≤16 μg/ml. Activity against anaerobes is not different from that of cefotaxime and is inferior to that of cefoxitin. Cefoperazone's half-life of 2 hours allows for twice a day dosing for selected situations, although severe infections should be treated with shorter dosing intervals. Serum levels are among the highest for all cephalosporins, and its biliary levels are greater than any other currently available third-generation agent.[157] Penetration into the cerebrospinal fluid is poor and mitigates against its use in meningitis. As with other agents containing a methylthiotetrazole side chain at the C_3 position, cefoperazone causes a disulfiram-like reaction in patients ingesting alcohol. Bleeding abnormalities due to hypoprothrombinemia have been reported,[158–161] and prophylactic vitamin K has been recommended when the drug is used in seriously ill or malnourished patients.

Ceftazidime (Fortaz, Taxidime, Tazicef) is the most active third-generation cephalosporin against *P. aeruginosa*.[46,162] Approximately 90 percent of strains will be inhibited by 4 μg/ml. Ceftazidime's activity against other gram-negative bacilli is comparable to that of cefotaxime. Ceftazidime is the least active third-generation agent against *S. aureus* and has little activity against anaerobes. Peak serum levels are comparable to that of other third-generation agents. Penetration into cerebrospinal fluid is adequate to treat meningitis.[163]

Cefpiramide is a new third-generation agent with activity against *P. aeruginosa* that is comparable to that of cefoperazone.[164,165] In general, it is less active than many of the other third-generation agents against other gram-negative organisms. This agent has consistent activity against gram-positive cocci and is unique in that it has activity against *Enterococcus* sp.

Cefpirome is a new cephalosporin with an extremely wide spectrum of activity.[166–168] Its activity against gram-positive cocci is similar to that of first- and second-generation agents but includes *Enterococcus* sp. The activity of cefpirome against most anaerobes and aerobic gram-negative bacteria is comparable to that of cefotaxime and is better than cefotaxime for strains of *Enterobacter, Acinetobacter*, and *Serratia*. It possesses activity against *Pseudomonas* comparable to that of cefoperazone but is inferior to that of ceftazidime.

Clinical Uses

The major use of the third-generation cephalosporins is in the therapy of serious aerobic gram-negative infections. The third-generation agents should not be used for most community-acquired infections. Multiply-resistant organisms are unusual in this circumstance, and agents with a narrower spectrum of activity and equal efficacy are available.

Cefotaxime, ceftriaxone, and ceftazidime have been successfully used to treat meningitis caused by *H. influenzae, S. pneumoniae*, and *N. meningitidis*. In children, these drugs appear to be as effective as the standard combination regimens of ampicillin and chloramphenicol or ampicillin and gentamicin.[144,169–176] Delayed sterilization of cerebrospinal fluid has been noted in small numbers of patients treated with ceftriaxone and, at the very least, suggests that close scrutiny of patients treated for meningitis is needed.[177] Ceftizoxime has also proved effective for meningitis, although experience with this drug remains limited.[148]

Third-generation cephalosporins, especially cefotaxime and ceftazidime, are the drugs of choice for the therapy of meningitis in adults caused by aerobic gram-negative bacilli.[144,169,170,172] Success rates of 80–90 percent have been reported with disease caused by *E. coli, Klebsiella pneumoniae*, and *Serratia* sp. Lower response rates have been noted with *Enterobacter* and *Salmonella*. This is in marked contrast to the 60–80 percent mortality noted in cases treated before the development of these agents.[178] Because of its excellent penetration into the cerebrospinal fluid and excellent activity against *Pseudomonas*, ceftazidime has been used to treat *P. aeruginosa* meningitis with responses rates of approximately 80 percent.[172,179]

The third-generation agents are extremely useful for therapy of nocosomial infections, especially those caused by multiply-resistant gram-negative organisms, where aminoglycosides and extended spectrum penicillins may be of limited use. Pneumonias, bacteremias, urinary tract infections, intra-abdominal infections, and skin and soft tissues have all been treated with success rates of over 80–90 percent.[180–192] It remains unclear whether these agents should be used in conjunction with other β-lactam antibiotics or aminoglycosides for maximum efficacy. There is no convincing data to indicate clinical superiority of any specific third-generation agent in the therapy of a given disease.

Because of its extended half-life ceftriaxone may be used to treat a variety of severe infections with once daily or twice daily dosing; it has been used successfully and with demonstrated cost savings for outpatient therapy of skin and soft-tissue infections and urinary tract infections.[193–195] Because of its potent activity against penicillin-sensitive and -resistant strains of *N. gonorrhoeae*, ceftriaxone has become the agent of choice for treating uncomplicated urethral, anorectal, and pharyngeal gonorrhoeae.[196,197] Limited data suggest that ceftriaxone may be effective in eradicating oropharyngeal carriage of *N. meningitidis*.[198] Ceftriaxone is effective therapy for Lyme disease.

Cefoperazone and ceftazadime have been used in patients when *P. aeruginosa* infections are suspected. When used as monotherapy in neutropenic patients, cefoperazone has led to resonse rates lower than those usually seen with antibiotic combinations.[199,200] Combination regimens of cefoperazone plus mezlocillin and cefoperazone plus aminoglycoside have proved as efficacious as other combination regimens.[201,202] Ceftazadime has been used as monotherapy or as modified monotherapy (used with an aminoglycoside for 3 days and then continued as monotherapy thereafter) in patients with fever and neutropenia.[203,204] The findings suggest that ceftazidime alone is adequate for the majority of infections, but its use with an aminoglycoside may be more effective in documented gram-negative rod bacteremia.

REFERENCES

1. Abraham EP, Loder PB. Cephalosporin C. In: Flynn EH, ed. Cephalosporins and Penicillins. New York: Academic Press; 1972:2.
2. Huber FM, Chauvette RR, Jackson BG. Preparative methods for 7-aminocephalosporanic acid and 6-aminopenicillanic acid. In: Flynn EH, ed. Cephalosporins and Penicillins. New York: Academic Press; 1972:27.
3. Neu HC. Structure-activity relations of new beta-lactam compounds and in vitro activity against common bacteria. Rev Infect Dis. 1983;5(Suppl):S319–37.
4. Neu HC. The new beta-lactamase-stable cephalosporins. Ann Intern Med. 1982;97:408–17.
5. Strominger JL. How penicillin kills bacteria: a short history. In: Schlessinger D, ed. Microbiology—1977. Washington, DC: ASM Publications; 1977:177.
6. Tomasz A, Albino A, Zanatle E. Multiple antibiotic resistance in a bacterium with suppressed autolytic system. Nature. 1970;227:138–40.
7. Tomasz A. The mechanism of the irreversible antimicrobial effects of penicillins: how the beta-lactam antibiotics kill and lyse bacteria. Annu Rev Microbiol. 1979;33:113–37.
8. Blumberg PM, Strominger JL. Interaction of penicillin with the bacterial cell: penicillin-binding proteins and penicillin-sensitive enzymes. Bacteriol Rev. 1974;38:291–335.
9. Spratt BG. Proerties of the penicillin-binding proteins of *Escherichia coli* K 12. Eur J Biochem. 1977;72:341–52.
10. Neu HC. Penicillin-binding proteins and role of amdinocillin in causing bacterial cell death. Am J Med. 1983;75:(Suppl 2A):9–20.
11. Matsuhashi S, Kamiryo T, Blumberg PM, et al. Mechanism of action and development of resistance to a new amidino penicillin. J Bacteriol. 1974;117:578–87.
12. Waxman DJ, Strominger JL. Penicillin-binding proteins and the mechanism of action of β-lactam antibiotics. Annu Rev Biochem. 1983;52:825–69.
13. Tomasz A. Penicillin-binding proteins and the antibacterial effectiveness of β-lactam antibiotics. Rev Infect Dis. 1986;8(Suppl 3):S260–78.
14. Tomasz A, Waks S. Enzyme replacement in a bacterium: phenotypic correction by the experimental introduction of the wild type enzyme into a live enzyme defective mutant pneumococcus. Biochem Biophys Res Commun. 1975;65:1311–9.
15. Tomasz A, Holtje SV. Murein hydrolases and the lytic and killing action of penicillin. In: Schlessinger D, ed. Microbiology—1977. Washington, DC: American Society for Microbiology; 1977:209–15.
16. Tomasz A. Penicillin-binding proteins in bacteria. Ann Intern Med. 1982;96:502–4.
17. Nikaido H, Nakae T. The outer membrane of gram-negative bacteria. Adv Microb Physiol. 1979;20:163–250.
18. Nikaido H, Rosenberg EY, Foulds J. Porin channels in *Escherichia coli*: studies with β-lactams in intact cells. J Bacteriol. 1983;153:232–40.
19. Sawai T, Yamaguchi A, Hiruma R. Effect of interaction between outer membrane permeability and β-lactamase production on resistance to β-lactam agents in gram-negative bacteria. Rev Infect Dis. 1988;10:761–4.
20. Hartman BJ, Tomasz A. Low affinity penicillin binding protein associated with β-lactam resistance in *Staphylococcus aureus*. J Bacteriol. 1984;158:513–6.
21. Utsui Y, Yokota T. Role of an altered penicillin-binding protein in methicillin and cephem-resistant *Staphylococcus aureus*. Antimicrob Agents Chemother. 1985;28:397–403.
22. Richmond MH, Sykes RB. The beta-lactamases of gram-negative bacteria and their possible physiological role. Adv Microb Physiol. 1973;9:31–88.
23. Sykes RM, Matthew M. The β-lactamases of gram-negative bacteria and their role in resistance to β-lactam antibiotics. J Antimicrob Chemother. 1976;2:115–57.
24. Novick RP, Richmond MH. Nature and interactions of the genetic elements governing penicillinase synthesis in *Staphylococcus aureus*. J Bacteriol. 1965;90:467–80.
25. Dyke KGH. β-lactamases of *Staphylococcus aureus*. In: Hamilton-Miller JMT, Smith JT, eds. Beta-Lactamases. New York: Academic Press; 1979:291–310.
26. Farrar WE Jr, O'Dell NM. Comparative beta-lactamase resistance and antistaphylococcal activities of parenterally and orally administered cephalosporins. J Infect Dis. 1978;137:490–3.
27. Sykes RB, Bush K. Interaction of new cephalosporins with beta-lactamases and beta lactamase-producing gram-negative bacilli. Rev Infect Dis. 1983;5(Suppl 5):S356–67.
28. Farrar WE, Krause JM. Relationship between beta-lactamase activity and resistance of *Enterobacter* to cephalothin. Infect Immun. 1970;2:610–6.
29. Sanders CC, Sanders WE. Emergence of resistance during therapy with the newer beta-lactam antibiotics: role inducible beta-lactamases and implications for the future. Rev Infect Dis. 1983;5:639–48.
30. Sanders CC. Inducible β-lactamases and non-hydrolytic resistance mechanisms. J Antimicrob Chemother. 1984;13:1–3.
31. Sanders CC, Sanders WE Jr. Trapping and hydrolysis are not mutually exclusive mechanisms for β-lactamase-mediated resistance (Letter). J Antimicrob Chemother. 1986;17:121–2.
32. Charnas RL, Then RL. Mechanism of inhibition of chromosomal β-lactamases by third-generation cephalosporins. Rev Infect Dis. 1988;10:752–60.
33. Brumfitt W, Kosmidis J, Hamilton-Miller JMT, et al. Cefoxitin and cephalothin: antimicrobial activity, human pharmacokinetics, and toxicology. Antimicrob Agents Chemother. 1974;6:290–9.
34. Tauber MG, Hackbarth CJ, Scott KG, et al. New cephalosporins cefotaxime, cefpirizole, BMY 289142, and HR 810 in experimental pneumococcal meningitis in rabbits. Antimicrob Agents Chemother. 1985;27:340–2.
35. Bodian M, Molerczyk V, Collins JD, et al. Safety, tolerance and pharmacokinetics of 2.0 g of cefpirome (HR810) after single and multiple dosing. Chemotheray 1988;34:367–73.
36. Nakagawa K, Koyama M, Matsui H, et al. Pharmacokinetics of cefpiramide (SM-1652) in humans. Antimicrob Agents Chemother. 1984;25:221–5.
37. Barza M, Srikumaran M, Berger S, et al. Comparative pharmacokinetics of cefamandole, cephapirin and cephalothin in healthy subjects and effect of repeated dosing. Antimicrob Agents Chemother. 1976;10:421–5.
38. Pitkin D, Dubb J, Altor P, et al. Kinetics and renal handling of cefonicid. Clin Pharmacol Ther. 1981;30:587–93.
39. Malerczyk V, Maab L, Verho M, et al. Single and multiple dose pharmacokinetics of intravenous cefpirome (HR810), a novel cephalosporin derivative. Infection 1987;15:211–4.
40. Maab L, Malerczyk V, Verho M. Pharmacokinetics of cefpirome (HR810), a new cephalosporin deriative administered intramuscularly and intravenously to healthy volunteers. Infection. 1987;15:207–10.
41. Yates RA, Adam HK, Donnelly RJ, et al. Pharmacokinetics and tolerance of single intravenous doses of cefotetan disodium in male Caucasian volunteers. J Antimicrob Chemother. 1983;11(Suppl A):185–91.
42. Sommers DK, Van Wyk M, Williams PEO et al. Pharmacokinetics and tolerance of cefuroxime axetil in volunteers during repeated dosing. Antimicrob Agents Chemother. 1987;25:374–7.
43. Jones RN, Antimicrobial activity, spectrum and pharmacokinetics of old and new orally administered cephems. Antimicrob Newsletter. 1988;5:1–7.
44. Thompson RL, Wright AJ. Cephalosporin antibiotics. Mayo Clin Proc. 1983;58:79–87.
45. Fried JS, Hinthrom DR. The cephalosporins. DM. 1985;31:1–60.
46. Donowitz GR, Mandell GL. Beta-lactam antibiotics. N Engl J Med. 1988;318(2 Pt 2):490–500.
47. Fong IW, Ralph ED, Engelking FR, et al. Clinical pharmacology of cefamandole as compared with cephalothin. Antimicrob Agents Chemother. 1976;9:65–9.
48. Neu HC. Comparison of the pharmacokinetics of cefamandole and other cephalosporin compounds. J Infect Dis. 1978;137(Suppl):S80–7.
49. Nelson JD. Antibiotic concentration in spectic joint effusion. N Engl J Med. 1971;284:349.
50. Berger S, Ernest E, Barza M. Comparative incidence of phlebitis due to buffered cephalothin, cephapirin and cefamandole. Antimicrob Agents Chemother. 1976;9:575–9.
51. Carrizosa J, Levison ME, Kaye D. Double-blind controlled comparison of phlebitis produced by cephapirin and cephalothin. Antimicrob Agents Chemother. 1973;3:306–7.
52. Petz LD. Immunologic cross-reactivity between penicillins and cephalosporins: a review. J Infect Dis. 1978;137(Suppl):S74–9.
53. Petersen BH, Graham J. Immunologic cross-reactivity of cephalosporin and penicillin. J Lab Clin Med. 1974;833:860–70.
54. Iwata M, Tokiwa H, Matuhasi T. Detection and characterization of polymers in cephalothin by passive cutaneous anaphylaxis in mice. Int Arch Allergy Appl Immunol. 1983;70:132–7.
55. Batchelor FR, Dewdney JM, Weston RD, et al. The immunogenicity of cephalosporin derivatives and their cross-reaction with penicillin. Immunology 1966;10:21–33.
56. Hamilton-Miller JMT, Abraham EP. Specificities of haemagglutinating antibodies evolved by members of the cephalosporin C family and benzyl penicillin. Biochem J. 1971;123:183–90.
57. Sanders WE, Johnson JE, Taggart JG. Adverse reactions to cephalothin and cephapirin. N Engl J Med. 1974;290:424.
58. Scholond JF, Tennenbaum JL, Cerilliu GJ. Anaphylaxis to cephalothin in a patient allergic to penicillin. JAMA. 1968;206:130–2.
59. Thoburn R, Johnson JE, Cliff LE. Studies on the epidemiology of adverse drug reactions. JAMA. 1966;198:345–8.
60. Petz LD. Immunologic reactions of humans to cephalosporins. Postgrad Med J. 1971; Feb[Suppl]64–9.
61. Sullivan TJ, Wedner HJ, Shatz GS, et al. Skin testing to detect penicillin allergy. J Allergy Clin Immunol. 1981;68:171–80.
62. Sogn DD. Prevention of allergic reactions to penicillin. J Allergy Clin Immunol. 1986;78:1051–2.
63. Smith JW, Johnson JE, Cliff LE. Studies on the epidemiology of adverse

drug reactions. II. An evaluation of penicillin allergy. N Engl J Med. 1966;274:998–1002.
64. Saxon A, Beall GN, Rohn AS, et al. Immediate hypersensitivity reaction to beta-lactam antibiotics. Ann Intern Med. 1987;107:204–15.
65. Solley GO, Cleich GJ, Van Dellen RG. Penicillin allergy-clinical experience with a battery of skin-test reagents. J Allergy Clin Immunol. 1982;69:238–44.
66. Saxon A. Immediate hypersensitivity reactions to beta-lactam antibiotics. Rev Infect Dis. 1983;5:S368–78.
67. Finke SR, Grieco MH, Connel JT, et al. Results of comparative skin tests with penicilloyl-polylysine and penicillin in patients with penicillin allergy. Am J Med. 1965;38:71–82.
68. Barza M. The nephrotoxicity of cephalosporins: an overview. J Infect Dis. 1978;137(Suppl):S60–S73.
69. Pasternack DP, Stephen BG. Reversible nephrotoxicity associated with cephalothin therapy. Arch Intern Med. 1975;135:599–602.
70. Wade JC, Petty BG, Conrad G, et al. Cephalothin plus an aminoglycside is more nephrotoxic than methicillin plus an aminoglycoside. Lancet. 1978;2:604–6.
71. Jacobs RF. Ceftriaxone-associated cholecystitis. Pediatr Infect Dis J. 1988;7:434–6.
72. Schaad UB, Tschappeler H, Lentze MJ. Transient formation of precipitations in the gallbladder associated with ceftriaxone therapy. Pediatr Infect Dis J. 1986;5:708–10.
73. Schaad UB, Gianella-Borradori A, Sutter S. Ceftriaxone versus cefuroxime for bacterial meningitis in infants and children. 27th Interscience Conference on Antimicrobial Agents and Chemotherapy. 1987;#789:234.
74. Finke S, Karp W, Robertson A. Ceftriaxone effect in bilirubin-albumin binding. Pediatrics 1987;80:873–5.
75. Gulian JM, Dalmasso C, Pontier F, et al. Displacement effect of ceftriaxone on bilirubin bound to human serum albumin. Chemotherapy 1986;32:399–403.
76. Sattler FR, Weitekamp MR, Ballard JO. Potential for bleeding with the new beta-lactam antibiotics. Ann Intern Med. 1986;105:924–31.
77. Nichols RL, Wikler MA, McDevitt JT, et al. Coagulopathy associated with extended-spectrum cephalosporins in patients with serious infections. Antimicrob Agents Chemother. 1987;31:231–5.
78. Bank NU, Kammer RB. Hematologic complications associated with beta-lactam antibiotics. Rev Infect Dis. 1983;5(Suppl 2):S380–93.
79. Conly JM, Ramotar K, Chubb H, et al. Hypoprothrombinemia in febrile, neutropenic patients with cancer: association with antimicrobial suppression of intestinal microflora. J Infect Dis. 1984;150:202–12.
80. Lipsky JJ, Lewis JC, Novick WJ Jr. Production of hypoprothrombinemia by moxalactam and 1-methyl-5-thiotetrazole in rats. Antimicrob Agents Chemother. 1984;25:380–1.
81. Bechtold H, Andrassy K, Jahnchen E, et al. Evidence for impaired hepatic vitamin K_1 metabolism in patients treated with N-methyl-thiotetrazole cephalosporins. Thromb Haemost. 1984;51:358–61.
82. Barza M, Furie B, Brown AE, et al. Defects in vitamin K-dependent carboxylation associated with moxalactam treatment. J Infect Dis. 1986;153:1166–9.
83. Agnelli G, Del Favero A, Parise P, et al. Cephalosporin-induced hypoprothrombinemia: is the N-methylthiotetrazole side chain the culprit? Antimicrob Agents Chemother. 1986;29:1108–9.
84. Sattler FR, Colao DJ, Caputo GM, et al. Cefoperazone for empiric therapy in patients with impaired renal function. Am J Med. 1986;81:229–36.
85. Baxter JG, Marble DA, Whitfield LR, et al. Clinical risk factors for prolonged PT/PTT in abdominal sepsis patients treated with moxalactam or tobramycin plus clindamycin. Ann Surg. 1985;201:96–102.
86. Meyers BR. Comparative toxicities of third-generation cephalosporins. Am J Med. 1985;79(Suppl 2A):96–103.
87. Weitekamp MR, Caputo GM, Al-Mondhiry HA, et al. The effect of latamoxef, cefotaxime, and cefoperazone on platelet function and coagulation in normal volunteers. J Antimicrob Chemother. 1985;16:95–101.
88. Moellering RC Jr, Swartz MN. The newer cephalosporins. N Engl J Med. 1976;294:24–8.
89. Hartman B, Tomasz A. Altered penicillin-binding proteins in methicillin-resistant strains of *Staphylococcus aureus*. Antimicrob Agents Chemother. 1981;19:726–35.
90. Chang TW, Weinstein L. In vitro biological activity of cephalothin. J Bacteriol. 1963;85:1022.
91. Klein JO, Eickhoff TC, Tilles JG, et al. Cephalothin: activity in vitro, absorption and excretion in normal subjects and clinical observations in 40 patients. Am J Med Sci. 1964;248:640.
92. Sabath LD, Wilcox C, Garner C, et al. In vitro activity of cefazolin against recent clinical bacterial isolates. J Infect Dis. 1973;128(Suppl):S320–6.
93. Regamey C, Libke RD, Engelking ER, et al. Inactivation of cefazolin, cephaloridine, and cephalothin by methicillin-sensitive and methicillin-resistant strains of *Staphylococcus aureus*. J Infect Dis. 1975;131:291–4.
94. Fong IW, Engelking ER, Kirby WMM. Relative inactivation by *Staphylococcus aureus* of eight cephalosporin antibiotics. Antimicrob Agents Chemother. 1976;9:939–44.
95. Bergeron MG, Brusch JL, Barza M, et al. Bactericidal activity and pharmacology of cefazolin. Antimicrob Agents Chemother. 1973;4:396–401.
96. Quintiliani R, Nightingale CH. Cefazolin: diagnosis and treatment. Ann Intern Med. 1978;89:650–6.
97. Neiss E. Cephradine: summary of preclinical studies and clinical pharmacology. J Irish Med Assoc. 1973;66(Suppl):1–12.
98. Renzini G, Ravagnan G, Oliva B. In vitro and in vivo microbiological evaluation of cephapirin, a new antibiotic. Chemotherapy. 1975;21:289.
99. Hartstein AI, Patrick KE, Jones SR, et al. Comparison of pharmacological and antimicrobial properties of cefadroxil and cephalexin. Antimicrob Agents Chemother. 1977;12:93–7.
100. Meyers BR, Kaplan K, Weinstein L. Cephalexin microbiological effects and pharmacologic parameters in man. Clin Pharmacol Ther. 1969;10:810.
101. Cartwright PS, Pittaway DE, Jones HW III, et al. The use of prophylactic antibiotics in obstetrics and gynecology: a review. Obstet Gynecol Surv. 1984;39:537–4.
102. DiPiro JT, Bowden TA Jr, Hooks VH III. Prophylactic parenteral cephalosporins in surgery: are the newer agents better? JAMA. 1984;252:3277–9.
103. Gilbert DN. Current status of antibiotic prophylaxis in surgical patients. Bull NY Acad Med. 1984;60:340–57.
104. Norden CW. A critical review of antibiotic prophylaxis in orthopedic surgery. Rev Infect Dis. 1983;5:928–32.
105. Sanders CV, Greenberg RN, Marier RL. Cefamandole and cefoxitin. Ann Intern Med. 1985;103:70–8.
106. Fraser DG. Drug therapy reviews: antimicrobial spectrum, pharmacology and therapeutic use of cefamandole and cefoxitin. Am J Hosp Pharm. 1979;36:1503–8.
107. Delgado DG, Crau CJ, Cobbs CG, et al. Clinical and laboratory evaluation of cefamandole in the therapy of *Haemophilus* sp. Bronchopulmonary infections. Antimicrob Agents Chemother. 1979;15:807–12.
108. Meyers BR, Hirschman SZ. Antibacterial activity of cefamandole in vitro. J Infect Dis. 1978;137(Suppl):S25–31.
109. Kass EH, Evans DA. Future prospects and past problems in antimicrobial therapy: the role of cefoxitin. Rev Infect Dis. 1979;1:1.
110. Chow AW, Bednorz D. Comparative in vitro activity of newer cephalosporins against anaerobic bacteria. Anttimicrob Agents Chemother. 1978;14:668–71.
111. Sutter VL, Finegold SM. Susceptibility of anaerobic bacteria to carbenicillin, cefoxitin, and related drugs. J Infect Dis. 1975;131:417–22.
112. Bach VT, Roy I, Thadepalli H. Susceptibility of anaerobic bacteria to cefoxitin and related compounds. Antimicrob Agents Chemother. 1977;11:912–3.
113. Smith BR, LeFrock JL. Cefuroxime: antimicrobial activity, pharmacology, and clinical efficacy. Ther Drug Monit. 1983;5:149–60.
114. Williams PEO, Harding SM. The absolute bioavailability of oral cefuroxime axetil in male and female volunteers after fasting and after food. J Antimicrob Chemother. 1984;13:191–6.
115. Harding SM, Williams PEO, Ayrton J. Pharmacology of cefuroxime as the 1-acetoxyethyl ester in volunteers. Antimicrob Agents Chemother. 1984;25:78–82.
116. Sommers D, Van Wyk M, Williams PEO, Harding SM. Pharmacokinetics and tolerance of cefuroxime axetil in volunteers during repeated dosing. Antimicrob Agents Chemother. 1984;25:344–7.
117. Morel C, Vergnaud M, Langeard MM, et al. Cefotetan: comparative study in vitro against 266 gram-negative clinical isolates. J Antimicrob Chemother. 1983;11(Suppl A):31–6.
118. Ruckdeschel G. Activity in vitro of cefotetan against nonsporing anaerobes: a comparative study. J Antimicrob Chemother. 1983;11(Suppl A):117–24.
119. Wexler HM, Finegold SM. In vitro activity of cefotetan compared with that of other antimicrobial agents against anaerobic bacteria. Antimicrob Agents Chemother. 1988;32:601–4.
120. Silver MS, Counts GW, Zeleznik D, et al. Comparison of in vitro antibacterial activity of three oral cephalosporins: cefaclor, cephalexin, and cephradine. Antimicrob Agents Chemother. 1977;12:591–6.
121. Barriere SL, Mills J. Ceforanide: antibacterial activity, pharmacology, and clinical efficacy. Pharmacotherapy. 1982;2:322–7.
122. Gremillion DH, Winn RE, Vandenbout E. Clinical trial of cefonicid for treatment of skin infections. Antimicrob Agents Chemother. 1983;23:944–6.
123. Pines A, Raafat HH, Khorasani M, et al. Cefuroxime and ampicillin compared in a double-blind study in the treatment of lower respiratory tract infections. Chemotherapy. 1981;27:459–65.
124. Mehtar S, Parr JH, Morgan DJR. A comparison of cefuroxime and cotrimoxazole in severe respiratory tract infections. J Antimicrob Chemother. 1982;9:479–84.
125. Bergeron MG, Claveau S, Simard P. Limited in vitro activity of cefamandole against 100 beta-lactamase and non-beta-lactamase producing *H. influenzae* strains: Comparison of moxalactam, chloramphonical and ampicillin. Antimicrob Agents Chemother. 1981;19:101–5.
126. Swedish Study Group, Cefuroxime versus ampicillin and chloramphonical for the treatment of bacterial meningitis. Lancet. 1982;1:295–9.
127. Pfenninger J, Schaad UB, Lutschg J, et al. Cefuroxime in bacterial meningitis. Arch Dis Child. 1982;57:539–45.
128. Sirinavin S, Chiemchanya S, Visudhipan P, et al. Cefuroxime treatment of bacterial meningitis in infants and children. Antimicrob Agents Chemother. 1984;25:273–5.
129. Schleupner CJ, Anthony WC, Tan J, et al. Blinded comparison of cefuroxime to cefaclor for lower respiration tract infections. Arch Intern Med. 1988;148:343–8.
130. Reichman RC, Nolte FS, Wolinsky SM, et al. Single dose cefuroxime axetil for treatment of uncomplicated gonorrhea: a controlled trial. Sex Transm Dis. 1985;12:184–7.

131. Davies BL, Maesen FDV, Teengs JP. Cefuroxime axetil in acute purulent exacerbations of chronic bronchitis infections. 1987;15:253–6.
132. Brumfitt W, Hamilton-Miller JMT, Smith GW. Comparative trial of cefuroxime axetil in recurrent urinary tract infections, illustrating the importance of 6-week follow-up. Antimicrob Agents Chemother. 1987;31:1442–3.
133. Lefrock JL, Blais F, Schell RD, et al. Cefoxitin in the treatment of diabetic patients with lower extremity infections. Infect Surg. 1983;2:361–74.
134. Drusano GL, Warren W, Saah AJ, et al. A prospective randomized controlled trial of cefoxitin versus clindamycin-aminoglycoside in mixed anaerobic-aerobic infections. Surg Gynecol Obstet. 1982;154:715–20.
135. Antimicrobial prophylaxis in surgery. Med Lett. 1987;29(Issue 750):91.
136. Rice RJ, Thompson SE. Treatment of uncomplicated infections due to *Neisseria gonorrhoeae*: a review of clinical efficacy and in vitro susceptibility studies from 1982 through 1985. JAMA. 1986;255:1739–46.
137. Sanchez PL, Wingall FS, Zajdowicz TR, et al. One gram of cefoxitin cures uncomplicated gonococcal urethritis caused by penicillinase-producing *Neisseria gonorrhoeae* (PPNG). Sex Transm Dis. 1973;10:135–7.
138. Orr JW, Varner RE, Kilgore LC, et al. Cefotetan versus cefoxitin as prophylaxis in hysterectomy. Am J Obstet Gynecol. 1986;154:960–3.
139. McGregor JA, French JI, Makowski E.Single dose cefotetan versus multidose cefoxitin for prophylaxis in cesarean section in high risk patients. Am J Obstet Gynecol. 1986;154:955–60.
140. Wilson SE, Boswick JA, Duma RJ, et al. Cephalosporin therapy in intraabdominal infections: a multicenter randomized, comparative study of cefotetan, moxalactam and cefoxitin. Am J Surg. 1988;155(Suppl 5A):61–6.
141. Sweet R, Gall SA, Gobbs RS, et al. Multicenter clinical trial comparing cefotetan with moxalactam or cefoxitin as therapy for obstetric and gynecologic infections. Am J Surg. 1988;155(Suppl 5A):56–60.
142. Richmond MH. β-Lactamase stability of cefotaxime. J Antimicrob Chemother. 1980;6(Suppl A):13–7.
143. Schrinner E, Limbert M, Penasse L, et al. Antibacterial activity of cefotaxime and other newer cephalosporins (in vitro and in vivo). J Antimicrob Chemother. 1980;6(Suppl A):25–30.
144. Mullaney DT, John JF. Cefotaxime therapy: evaluation of its effects on bacterial meningitis, CSF drug levels, and bactericidal activity. Arch Intern Med. 1983;143:1705–8.
145. Moellering RC, Young LS. Moxalactam international symposium. Rev Infect Dis. 1982;4:S489–90.
146. Weitekamp MR, Aber RC. Prolonged bleeding times and bleeding diathesis associated with moxalactam administration. JAMA. 1983;249:69
147. Fu KP, Neu HC. Antibacterial activity of ceftizoxime, a β-lactamase stable cephalosporin. Antimicrob Agents Chemother. 1980;17:583–90.
148. Overturf GD, Cable DC, Forthal DN, et al. Treatment of bacterial meningitis with ceftizoxime. Antimicrob Agents Chemother. 1984;25:158–61.
149. Cleeland R, Squires E. Antimicrobial activity of ceftriaxone, a review. Am J Med. 1984;77:3–11.
150. Neu HC, Meropol NJ, Fu KP. Antibacterial activity of ceftriaxone (Ro 13-9904) a β-lactamase stable cephalosporin. Antimicrob Agents Chemother. 1981;19:414–23.
151. Neu HC, Chin NX, Labthavikul P. Comparative in vitro activity and β-lactamase stability of FR 17027, a new orally active cephalosporin. Antimicrob Agents Chemother. 1984;26:174–80.
152. Jones RN. Antimicrobial activity spectrum and pharmacokinetics of old and new orally administered cephens. Antimicrob Newslett. 1988;5:1–8.
153. Neu HC. The new beta-lactamase stable cephalosporins. Ann Intern Med. 1982;97:408–19.
154. Fass RJ. Comparative in vitro activities of third generation cephalosporins. Arch Intern Med. 1983;143:1743–5.
155. Trabulsi LR, Almada NP, Marqus LRM. Inhibitory concentrations of cefoperazone, cefazolin, cefamandole, cephaloridine and cefoxitin for 300 gram-negative clinical isolates. Clin Ther. 1980;3:145–8.
156. Brogden RN, Carmine A, Heel RC, et al. Cefoperazone, a review of its in vitro antimicrobial activity, pharmacological properties and therapeutic efficacy. Drugs. 1981;22:423–60.
157. Kemmerich B, Lode H, Borner K, et al. Biliary excretion and pharmacokinetics of cefoperazone in humans. J Antimicrob Chemother. 1983;12:27–37.
158. Sattler FN, Weitekamp MR, Ballard JO. Potential for bleeding with the new beta-lactam antibiotics. Ann Intern Med. 1986;105:924–30.
159. Shenkenberg TD, Mackowiak PA, Smith JW. Coagulopathy and hemorrhage associated with cefoperazone therapy in a patient with renal failure. South Med J. 1985;78:488–9.
160. Osborne JC. Hypoprothrombinemia and bleeding due to cefoperazone. Ann Intern Med. 1985;102:721–2.
161. Sattler FR, Colao DJ, Caputo GM, et al. Cefoperazone for empiric therapy in patients with impaired renal function. Am J Med. 1986;81:229–36.
162. Neu HC, Labthavikul P. Antibacterial activity and beta-lactamase stability of ceftazidime, an aminothiazolyl cephalosporin potentially active against *Pseudomonas aeruginosa*. Antimicrob Agents Chemother. 1982;21:11–8.
163. Modai J, Vittecoq D, DeCazes JM, et al. Penetration of ceftazidime into cerebral spinal fluid of patients with bacterial meningitis. Antimicrob Agents Chemother. 1983;24:126–8.
164. Pfaller MA, Niles AC, Murray PR. In vitro antibacterial activity of cefpiramide. Antimicrob Agents Chemother. 1984;25:368–72.
165. Fukasawa M, Noguchi H, Okuda T, et al. In vitro antibacterial activity of SM-1652 a new broad-spectrum cephalosporin with anti-pseudomonal activity. Antimicrob Agents Chemother. 1983;3:195–200.
166. Jones RN, Thornsberry C, Barry AL. In vitro evaluation of HR810, a new wide-spectrum aminothiazolyl—methoxyimino cephalosporin. Antimicrob Agents Chemother. 1984;25:710–8.
167. Jones RN, Gerlach EH. Antimicrobial activity of HR810 against 419 strict anaerobic bacteria. Antimicrob Agents Chemother. 1985;27:413–5.
168. Bauernfeind A. Susceptibility of gram positive aerobic cocci to the new cephalosporin HR810. Eur J Clin Microbiol. 1988;2:354–5.
169. Lecour H, Seara A, Miranda AM, et al. Treatment of 160 cases of acute bacterial meningitis with cefotaxime. J Antimicrob Chemother. 1984;14(Suppl B):195–202.
170. Belohradsky BH, Geiss D, Marget W, et al. Intravenous cefotaxime in children with bacterial meningitis. Lancet. 1980;i:61–3.
171. Rodriquez WJ, Khan WN, Gold B, et al. Ceftazidime in the treatment of meningitis in infants and children over one month of age. Am J Med. 1985;79(Suppl 2A):52–5.
172. Norrby SR. Role of cephalosporins in the treatment of bacterial meningitis in adults: overview with special emphasis on ceftazidime. Am J Med. 1985;(Suppl 2A):56–61.
173. Jacobs RF, Wells TG, Steele RW, et al. A prospective randomized comparison of cefotaxime vs ampicillin and chloramphenicol for bacterial meningitis in children. J Pediatr. 1985;107:129–33.
174. Barson WJ, Miller MA, Brady MT, et al. Prospective comparative trial of ceftriaxone vs conventional therapy for treatment of bacterial meningitis in children. Pediatr Infect Dis. 1986;4:362–8.
175. Congeni BL. Comparison of ceftriaxone and traditional therapy of bacterial meningitis. Antimicrob Agents Chemother. 1984;25:40–4.
176. Bryan JP, Rocha H, da Silva HR, et al. Comarison of ceftriaxone and ampicillin plus chloramphenicol for therapy of acute bacterial meningitis. Antimicrob Agents Chemother. 1985;28:361–8.
177. Jacobs RF, Wright MW, Deskin RL, et al. Delayed sterilization of *Haemophilus influenzae* type B meningitis with twice-daily ceftriaxone. JAMA. 1988;259:392–4.
178. Cherubin CE, Marr JS, Sierra MF, et al. *Listeria* and gram-negative bacillary meningitis in New York City 1972–1979: frequent causes of meningitis in adults. Am J Med. 1981;71:199–209.
179. Fong IW, Tompkins KB. Review of *Pseudomonas aeruginosa* meningitis with special emphasis on treatment with ceftazidime. Rev Infect Dis. 1985;7:604–12.
180. Francke EL, Neu HC. Use of cefotaxime, a β-lactamase stable cephalosporin in the therapy of serious infections, including those due to multiresistant organisms. Am J Med. 1981;71:435–42.
181. Young JPW, Husson JM, Bruch K, et al. The evaluation of efficacy and safety of cefotaxime: a review of 2500 cases. J Antimicrob Chemother. 1980;6(Suppl A):293–300.
182. Daikos GK, Kosmidis J, Giamarellou H, et al. Evaluation of cefotaxime in a hospital with high antibiotic resistance rates. J Antimicrob Chemother. 1980;6(Suppl A):255–61.
183. Scully BE, Neu HC. The use of ceftizoxime in the treatment of critically ill patients infected with multiply antibiotic resistant bacteria. J Antimicrob Chemother. 1982;10(Suppl C):141–50.
184. Johnson ES, Smith LG. Ceftrizoxime in moderate-to-severe infections. J Antimicrob Chemother. 1982;10(Suppl C):151–7.
185. Baumgartner J-D, Glauser MP. Single daily dose treatment of severe refractory infections with ceftriaxone: cost savings and possible parenteral outpatient treatment. Arch Intern Med 1983;143:1868–73.
186. Eron LJ, Park CH, Goldenberg RI, et al. Ceftriaxone therapy of serious bacterial infections. J Antimicrob Chemother. 1983;12:65–78.
187. Cohen MS, Washton HE, Barranco SF. Multicenter clinical trial of cefoperazone sodium in the United States. Am J Med. 1984;77(Suppl 1B):35–41.
188. Warren JW, Miller EH Jr, Fitzpatrick B, et al. A randomized, controlled in trial of cefoperazone vs cefamandole-tobramycin in the treatment of putative, severe infections with gram-negative bacilli. Rev Infect Dis. 1983;5(Suppl 1):S173–80.
189. Mangi RJ, Greco T, Ryan J, et al. Cefoperazone versus combination antibiotic therapy of hospital acquired pneumonia. Am J Med. 1988;84:68–74.
190. Bergeron MG, Mendelson J, Harding GK, et al. Cefoperazone compared with ampicillin plus tobromycin for severe biliary tract infections. Antimicrob Agents Chemother. 1988;32:1231–6.
191. Scully BE, Neu HC. Clinical efficacy of ceftazidime: treatment of serious infection due to multiresistant pseudomonas and other gram negative bacteria. Arch Intern Med. 1984;144:57–62.
192. Young LS. Ceftazidime in the treatment of nosocomial sepsis. Am J Med. 1985;79(Suppl 2A):89–95.
193. Bradsher RW JR, Snow RM. Ceftriaxone treatment of skin and soft tissue infections in a once daily regimen. Am J Med. 1984;77(Suppl 4C):63–7.
194. Eron LJ, Park CH, Hixon DL, et al. Ceftriaxone therapy of bone and soft tissue infections in hospital and outpatient settings. Antimicrob Agents Chemother. 1983;23:731–7.
195. Poretz DM, Woolard D, Eron LJ, et al. Outpatient use of ceftriaxone: a cost-benefit analysis. Am J Med. 1984;77(Suppl 4C):77–83.
196. Judson FN, Ehret JM, Handsfield HH. Comparative study of ceftriaxone and spectinomycin for treatment of uncomplicated gonorrhoea in men. Lancet. 1983;2:67–70.
197. Collier AC, Judson FN, Murphy VL, et al. Comparative study of ceftriaxone and spectinomycin in the treatment of uncomplicated gonorrhea in women. Am J Med. 1984;77(Suppl 4C):68–72.
198. Schwartz B, Al-Ruwais A, A'ashi J, et al. Comparative efficacy of ceftriax-

one and rifampian in eradicating pharyngeal carriage of group A *Neisseria meningitidis*. Lancet. 1988;1:1239–45.
199. Bolivar R, Fainstein V, Elting L, et al. Cefoperazone for the treatment of nfections in patients with cancer. Rev Infect Dis. 1983;5(Suppl 1):S181–7.
200. Piccart M, Klastersky J, Meunier F, et al. Single-drug versus combination empirical therapy for gram-negative bacillary infections in febrile cancer patients with and without granulocytopenia. Antimicrob Agents Chemother. 1984;26:870–5.
201. Gucalp R, Lia S, McKitrick JC, et al. Cefoperaxone plus tobramycin versus ticarcillin plus tobramycin in febrile granulocytopenic cancer patients. Am J Med. 1988;85(Suppl 1A):31–3.
202. Winston DJ, Ho WG, Bruckner DA, et al. Controlled trials of double beta-lactam therapy with cefoperazone plus piperacillin in febrile granulocytopenic patients. Am J Med. 1988;85(Suppl 1A):21–30.
203. Pizzo PA, Hathorn JW, Hiemenz J, et al. A randomized trial comparing ceftazidime alone with combination antibiotic therapy in cancer patients with fever and neutropenia. N Engl J Med. 1986;315:552–8.
204. EORTC International Antimicrobial Therapy Cooperative Group. Ceftazidime combined with a short or long course of amikacin for empirical therapy of gram-negative bacteremia in cancer patients with granulocytopenia. N Engl J Med. 1987;317:1692–8.

20. OTHER β-LACTAM ANTIBIOTICS

HAROLD C. NEU

Several antimicrobial agents belonging to the β-lactam class of antibiotics have been developed in recent years. Since these agents differ widely in their antibacterial and pharmacologic properties, they will be discussed as separate entities.

CARBAPENEMS

Imipenem is the prototype drug of this class of compounds. In the early 1970s scientists in Spain discovered a new *Streptomyces* species called *Streptomyces cattleya*, which produced a carbapenem compound that was subsequently named thienamycin.[1]

Chemistry

Figure 1 shows the chemical structure of the stable *N*-formimidoyl derivative of thienamycin. The presence of an azetidiome group caused thienamycin to undergo aminolysis of the β-lactam ring through reaction of the amino group of one molecule with another. *N*-formimidoyl thienamycin is called imipenem.

Carbapenems possess novel stereochemical features that differentiate them from penicillins and cephalosporins. They are in an S transconfiguration, and the endocyclic sulfur is replaced by a methylene group, with the sulfur adjacent to the bicyclic ring system.

Antibacterial Activity

Imipenem has excellent in vitro activity against aerobic gram-positve species such as the hemolytic streptococci of the Lancefield classifications A, B, C, and G, with minimal inhibitory values (MICs) of 0.2 μg/ml or less (Table 1).[2,3] *Streptococcus*

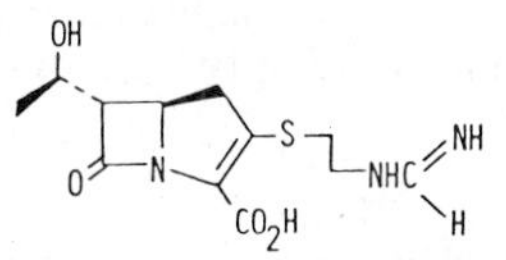

FIG. 1. Imipenem (*N*-formimidoyl thienamycin).

TABLE 1. Activity of Imipenem against Aerobic and Anaerobic Bacteria

Organism	*MIC_{90} (μg/ml)*
Staphylococcus aureus[a]	0.1
S. epidermidis[a]	0.2
Streptococcus pyogenes	0.1
S. agalactiae	0.1
Viridans streptococci	0.1
S. pneumoniae	0.01
S. bovis	0.1
Enterococcus faecalis	0.8
Haemophilus influenzae	0.1
Neisseria gonorrhoeae	0.1
N. meningitidis	0.02
Listeria monocytogenes	0.02
Klebsiella pneumoniae[a]	0.4
Enterobacter cloacae[a]	1.6
E. aerogenes[a]	0.2
E. agglomerans[a]	0.4
E. hafnia[a]	0.4
Escherichia coli[a]	0.4
Klebsiella oxytoca[a]	0.2
Arizona hinshawii[a]	0.1
Aeromonas hydrophila[a]	0.1
Citrobacter freundii	1.6
C. diversus[a]	0.2
Serratia marcescens[a]	6.3
Proteus mirabilis	1.6
Morganella morganii[a]	1.6
Proteus rettgeri[a]	1.6
P. vulgaris[a]	0.6
Providencia stuart[a]	1.6
Salmonella	0.1
Shigella	0.2
Acinetobacter	0.8
Pseudomonas aeruginosa[a]	12.5
P. maltophilia	>50
P. cepacia	>50
Bacteroides fragilis	1
Bacteroides bivius	0.03
Bacteroides melaninogenicus	0.12
Bacteroides disiens	0.03
Bacteroides thetaiotamicron	1
Bacteroides vulgatus, B. ovatus	1
Fusobacterium nucleatum	0.25
Fusobacterium species	0.5
Veillonella species	1
Clostridium difficile	16
Clostridium perfringens	1
Clostridium species	2
Peptostreptococci	0.12
Peptococci	0.12
Propionibacterium species	0.01
Eikenella corrodens	0.25
Campylobacter fetus	0.12

[a] Both β-lactamase- and non-β-lactamase-containing strains.

pneumoniae organisms are inhibited by less than 0.1 μg/ml, and *S. pneumoniae* strains resistant to by penicillin (MIC values >4 μg/ml) are inhibited by 1 μg/ml or less. *Enterococcus faecalis* organisms are inhibited by less than 1.5 μg/ml, but there is a discrepancy between inhibitory and bactericidal levels just as exists for ampicillin and vancomycin, and *Enterococcus faecium* strains resistant to ampicillin are resistant to imipenem. *Staphylococcus aureus* and *Staphylococcus epidermidis* are inhibited by less than 0.2 and 1.5 μg/ml, respectively. Methicillin-resistant staphylococci are resistant and have MICs of ≥16 μg/ml. *Listeria* and *Bacillus* sp. are also inhibited by less than 1 μg/ml.[4]

Most of the Enterobacteriaceae are inhibited by concentrations of imipenem less than or equal to 1 μg/ml. Some *Proteus* strains have MIC values of 2–4 μg/ml. *Haemophilus infuenzae* and *Neisseria gonorrhoeae*, including their β-lactamase–producing isolates, are inhibited by less than 0.5 μg/ml.

Pseudomonas aeruginosa, including strains resistant to penicillins such as piperacillin and to cephalosporins such as ceftazidime and cefsulodin, are inhibited by 1–6 μg/ml.[5] Some *Pseudomonas cepacia* strains are inhibited by imipenem, but

Pseudomonas maltophilia is resistant. Most *Acinetobacter* organisms are inhibited by less than 1 μg/ml.

Imipenem inhibits most anaerobic species, including *Bacteroides fragilis* and some isolates resistant to moxalactam and cefoxitin, at concentrations of less than 0.5 μg/ml.[6,7] Most *Clostridium* sp. are inhibited by 1 μg/ml or less, with the exception of *Clostridium difficile*, which requires 6–8 μg/ml. *Fusobacterium, Actinomyces, Campylobacter*, and *Yersinia* are inhibited by imipenem, and many *Nocardia asteroides* strains are inhibited by 1 μg/ml. It also inhibits *Mycobacterium-avium* and some *Legionella* spp.

Mechanism of Action

Imipenem binds to penicillin-binding protein 2 (PBP-2) of gram-negative aerobic bacteria and to critical PBPs in *S. aureus* and streptococci. Unlike the situation with amdinocillin, imipenem causes rapid death of bacteria, and there is no major discrepancy between inhibitory and bactericidal activity. Imipenem shows a marked postantibiotic effect on both gram-positive and gram-negative bacteria.

Imipenem is not hydrolyzed by most β-lactamases, penicillinases, cephalosporinases, plasmid or chromosomally mediated, of *S. aureus, Escherichia coli, Enterobacter cloacae, Citrobacter freundii, Proteus rettgeri, Serratia marcescens, Proteus vulgaris, Klebsiella oxytoca, P. aeruginosa, P. cepacia* and *B. fragilis*. It is hydrolyzed by a *P. maltophilia* β-lactamase, some *Bacillus*, and *Bacteroides* enzymes.

Pharmacology

Imipenem cannot be absorbed after oral ingestion due to its instability in gastric acid. Although initial studies of imipenem after iv infusion showed high serum levels, urinary recovery was only 6–38 percent of an administered dose. Extrarenal metabolism is minimal but renal peptidase, dehydropeptidase-1, which hydrolyzes L-L and L-D dipeptides, is located on the brush border of the proximal renal tubules. After imipenem is removed from the circulation by glomerular filtration and secretion, it is hydrolyzed. Metabolites of imipenem in the absence of cilastatin are nephrotoxic.

Imipenem in the circulation is not destroyed and is widely distributed to various body compartments.[8,9] There is minimal biliary secretion of imipenem, and there is minimal change in bowel flora. In the absence of meningeal inflammation only minor amounts of imipenem enter the cerebrospinal fluid (CSF). In the presence of meningeal inflammation CSF levels of 1–5 μg/ml have been recorded. Imipenem has a high affinity for brain cells.

To overcome the problem of the destruction of imipenem in urine, a dehydropeptidase inhibitor was synthesized. This molecule, called cilastatin, is administered in equal amounts to imipenem. Cilastatin has no antibacterial activity, nor does it alter the antibacterial activity of imipenem. Cilastatin does not affect zinc metalloenzyme peptidases or angiotensin-converting enzymes.

After 20–30 minutes of infusion of 250 mg imipenem plus 250 mg cilastatin, mean peak serum levels of imipenem are 13 μg/ml. After 500 mg, mean peak serum levels are 33 μg/ml; 1000 mg produces a peak concentration of 52 μg/ml[10,11]; the half-life of imipenem is 1 hour in healthy people. The serum half-life increases to 4 hours with a fall in creatinine clearance in patients whose creatinine clearance is less than 10 ml/min. The half-life of cilastatin increases to a much greater extent than does that of imipenem and reaches 16 hours in anuria.[12] Imipenem is removed from the body by hemodialysis. Cilastatin is also removed by dialysis less completely. With dialysis the half-life of imipenem is 2.5 hours, and for cilastatin it is 3.8 hours.

In the presence of cilastatin, urinary recovery of imipenem is 70 percent, with a 25–29 percent recovery of the metabolites. Fecal elimination of imipenem is less than 1 percent.[13]

Adverse Reactions. Imipenem has generally been well tolerated.[14] It causes minimal phlebitis when used iv. It can cause immediate hypersensitivity,[15] and cross-reactions with penicillins have occurred. No major adverse effects such as diarrhea, pseudomembranous colitis, coagulation abnormalities, nephrotoxicity, or hepatotoxicity have been reported. Rapid infusion of imipenem has produced nausea and emesis in about 1 percent of patients. About 2–4 percent of imipenem-treated patients will have from a one- to two-fold elevation of serum glutamic-oxaloacetic transaminase and/or serum glutamic-pyruvic transaminase (SGOT, SGPT) values. Leukopenia has occurred, but infrequently. No drug interactions have been reported. The most serious toxicity is seizure, which occurs infrequently but most often in patients with underlying central nervous system pathology and in individuals with decreased renal function in whom dose adjustment has not been made.

Clinical Use. Animal infection studies have demonstrated the utility of imipenem in therapy for staphylococcal endocarditis (but not enterococcal endocarditis where high relapse rates were noted),[16,17] bacteremia due to *P. aeruginosa* in neutropenic rats,[18] and pyelonephritis in rats.

These observations have been extended to humans where imipenem has been found to be useful in the treatment of bone and soft tissue infections,[19,20] obstetric and gynecologic infections,[21] complicated urinary tract infections,[22] intra-abdominal sepsis,[23] pneumonia,[24] and endocarditis due to *S. aureus*.[25] In addition, imipenem has been found to be effective as a single agent in the treatment of febrile neutropenic patients, although the number of patients treated to date has been small.[26]

Since imipenem is not active against *Chlamydia trachomatis* a tetracycline would also have to be administered for the treatment of pelvic inflammatory disease. Imipenem has activity against *Nocardia asteroides* in vitro and in a murine model of cerebral infection.[27] Clinical experience is limited.[28]

In cystic fibrosis patients receiving imipenem as a single agent for the treatment of pulmonary exacerbations, a significant number of *P. aeruginosa* isolates resistant to imipenem have been encountered.[29] In addition, the treatment of pneumonia due to *P. aeruginosa* in non-cystic fibosis patients with imipenem as a single agent has had a disappointingly low success rate.[30] These observations suggest that imipenem not be used alone in therapy for serious pseudomonal infections, particularly those involving the respiratory tract.

The use of imipenem is most appropriate in the treatment of infections due to cephalosporin-resistant *Enterobacteriaceae*, particularly those due to *Citrobacter freundii* and *Enterobacter* spp.; as empirical therapy in the treatment of serious infections in patients previously treated with multiple antibiotics because the likelihood of encountering organisms resistant to more conventional β-lactams is high; possibly as a single agent in the treatment of febrile, neutropenic patient, although this is not clearly established at present; and in the treatment of polymicrobial infections where otherwise multiple-drug regimens of higher cost and potentially more adverse side effects would be necessary.

Based on their pharmacokinetic profiles, imipenem/cilastatin can be administered safely on an q6h or q8h basis to patients with normal renal function. Based on the available MIC data and the knowledge that a 500 mg infusion of imipenem results in a peak serum concentration of about 35 μg/ml, most infections can be treated with a regimen of 500 mg every 6 hours.

In Europe imipenem is available in a different formulation that permits im administration twice a day.

MONOBACTAMS

The development of new methods by Sykes and his colleagues[31] to screen large numbers of organisms for the production of β-lactam antibiotics showed that a number of bacteria, particularly *Gluconobacter* and *Acinetobacter*, produced monocyclic β-lactam antibiotics with antibacterial activity. From *Chromobacterium violaceum* a monocyclic compound was isolated and the structure confirmed. This compound was subsequently modified to yield a highly active therapeutic agent, aztreonam.

AZTREONAM

Chemistry

Aztreonam is a monocyclic β-lactam (Fig. 2) in which there is a sulfate group affixed to the nitrogen at position 1, an acyl side chain at position 3 that consists of an aminothiazolyl nucleus and an iminocarboxypropyl group, and a methyl group at position 4 of the ring.

Mechanism of Action

Aztreonam has no appreciable antibacterial activity against gram-positive or anaerobic bacteria. This is because it does not bind to penicillin-binding proteins in these species. Aztreonam binds primarily to PBP-3 in Enterobacteriaceae, *Pseudomonas*, and other gram-negative aerobic organisms. It produces long filamentous structures that are not viable. Aztreonam readily passes through the outer wall of gram-negative species, and it is not hydrolyzed by most plasmid and chromosomal β-lactamases but is hydrolyzed by some *K. oxytoca* and *P. cepacia* and the cefotaxime-hydrolyzing plasmid enzymes.

Antibacterial Activity

Aztreonam inhibits most Enterobacteriaceae at concentrations below 0.5 μg/ml (Table 2); some *P. aeruginosa*. *E. cloacae*, and *C. freundii* strains are resistant. Most *P. aeruginosa* organisms are inhibited by less than 16 μg/ml. Most *C. cepacia* and *P. maltophilia* are resistant, as are many *Aceintobacter* sp.; *Haemophilus* and *Neisseria*, including β-lactamase–producing isolates, are inhibited by less than 0.2 μg/ml. *Yersinia* and *Aeromonas* are inhibited by less than 0.5 μg/ml. In general, the antibacterial activity is minimally affected by inoculum size except for *P. aeruginosa*, and there is no major difference between MIC and minimum bactericidal concentration (MBC) values.[32,34] Aztreonam acts synergistically with aminoglycosides against *P. aeruginosa* and some *Enterobacteriaceae*. It also acts synergistically with amdinocillin against *Enterobacteriaceae*.

Bacterial Resistance. *Enterobacteriaceae* and *P. aeruginosa* can be resistant due to a failure to cross the outer cell wall, destruction by β-lactamases i.e., *P. maltophilia*, CTX-1, and related enzymes, and a failure to bind to PBPs.

Adverse Reactions

No new major adverse reactions to aztreonam have been reported.[35] Skin rashes have occurred. Neither anaphylaxis nor rashes have followed its use in patients with positive skin test reactions to penicillins (see Chapter 21). About 2–4 percent of

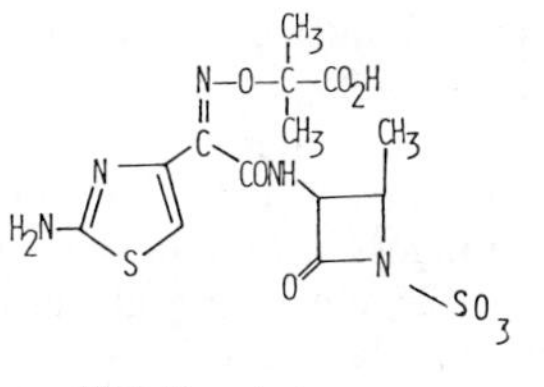

FIG. 2. Aztreonam.

TABLE 2. In Vitro Activity of Aztreonam

Organism	MIC90 (μg/ml)
Escherichia coli	0.25
Klebsiella pneumoniae	1
K. oxytoca	1
Enterobacter cloacae	16
E. aerogenes	8
E. agglomerans	1
Citrobacter freundii	8
C. diversus	0.25
Serratia marcescens	4
Proteus mirabilis	0.01
P. vulgaris	0.12
P. rettgeri	0.12
Morganella morganii	0.25
Providencia	0.025
Salmonella enteritidis	0.25
Shigella	0.12
Arizona hinshawii	0.12
Aeromonas hydrophila	0.12
A. shigelloides	0.12
Yersinia enterocolitica	2
Pasteurella multocida	0.12
Salmonella typhi	0.12
Haemophilus influenzae	0.12
Neisseria gonorrhoeae	0.25
N. meningitidis	0.025
Pseudomonas aeruginosa	16
P. maltophilia	>128
Pseudomonas, other (*P. cepacia, P. diminuta, P. stutzeri, P. fluorescens*)	>128
S. pyogenes	16
S. pneumoniae	16
Enterococci	>128
Clostridium	>128
Bacteroides sp.	>128

patients will have increases in serum transaminase values two times above normal when receiving aztreonam. No hematologic, gastrointestinal, nephrotoxic, or neurotoxic reactions have been noted with this agent.

Pharmacokinetics

Aztreonam is not absorbed from the gastrointestinal tract. It is rapidly and completely absorbed after im administration, with peak serum concentrations attained within 1 hour.[37–40] A 500 mg im aztreonam dose produces serum concentrations of 21–27 μg/ml at 1 hour, 3.8–5.9 μg/ml at 6 hours, 1.5–3.3 μg/ml at 8 hours, and 0.1–1.7 μg/ml at 12 hours. A 1 g im dose yields peaks of 3.5 μg/ml at 8 hours and 0.7 μg/ml at 12 hours.[40] Aztreonam serum concentrations 1 hour after an im dose are the same as after an iv dose.

After iv infusion of a single 0.5, 1, or 2 g dose of aztreonam in healthy adults over a period of 30 minutes, peak serum concentrations of the drug immediately after completion of the infusion average 55–65, 90–160, or 200–255 μg/ml, respectively.[40] After repeated dosing the drug does not accumulate. In healthy adults receiving 1 or 2 g doses of aztreonam im or iv every 8 hours, steady-state trough serum concentrations of the drug average 1–1.8 and 2.5–3.8 μg/ml, respectively.[37]

Aztreonam is widely distributed into body tissues and fluids.[37] Therapeutic levels are present in adipose tissue, bone, gallbladder, liver, lungs, kidney, heart, intestinal tissue, and prostatic tissue. It is also present in saliva, sputum, bronchial secretions, bile, and pericardial, pleural, peritoneal, and synovial fluids.

Azteonam enters the CSF after iv administration, with CSF concentrations at 1 and 4 hours after a 2 g dose of 2 and 3.2 μg/ml, respectively.[41] In neonates and children 3 months to 2 years of age with bacterial meningitis who received a 30 mg/kg dose of aztreonam by iv injection over a period of 3 minutes, CSF aztreonam concentrations ranged from 2.1 to 20.8 μg/ml at 0.8 to 4.3 hours after the dose.[42]

Aztreonam concentrations in peritoneal fluid are approximately equal to concurrent serum concentrations of the drug,[37] and concentrations 1 hour after a 2 g dose average 300 μg/ml in common duct bile and 100 μg/ml in gallbladder bile. At serum concentrations of 1–100 μg/ml aztreonam is 45–60 percent bound to serum proteins in patients with normal serum albumin levels, but in patients with impaired renal function and decreased serum albumin concentrations, aztreonam is 22–40 percent bound.[37] Aztreonam is primarily removed from the body by renal mechanisms of both glomerular filtration and tubular secretion. No active metabolites have been found in serum or urine. In adults with normal renal and hepatic function, the distribution half-life of aztreonam averages 0.2–0.7 hours, and the elimination half-life averages 1.3–2.2 hours.

The half-life of aztreonam averages 1.7 hours in children 2 months to 12 years of age.[42] In neonates 7 days old, the half-life of aztreonam averages 5.5–9.9 hours in neonates weighing less than 2.5 kg.[42]

Serum concentrations of aztreonam are higher and the serum half-life prolonged in patients with renal impairment.[43,44] In adults with renal impairment, the half-life of aztreonam averages 3.5, 5.6, 7.8, and 8.5 hours in adults with creatinine clearances of 30–80, 10–30, ≤10, and 2 ml/min, respectively. The half-life of aztreonam is only slightly prolonged in patients with hepatic impairment.

Aztreonam is excreted as unchanged drug by both glomeruler filtration and tubular secretion, with approximately 58–74 percent of the dose excreted unchanged and 1–7 percent as open ring metabolites.[37] In adults with normal renal function, urinary concentrations of aztreonam after a single 0.5 or 1 g iv dose average 250–330 and 710–720 μg/ml, respectively 4–6 hours after the dose.[40]

Aztreonam and its renal metabolite are removed by hemodialysis.[43,44] The amount of the drug removed depends on the type of coil used and the dialysis flow rate. The serum half-life of aztreonam averages 2.7 hours during hemodialysis and 6–8 hours between dialysis sessions. A 4-hour period of hemodialysis removes 25–50 percent of a dose. Aztreonam is removed to a lesser extent by peritoneal dialysis. With a 6-hour dwell time, about 10 percent of a single 1 g iv dose of aztreonam is removed.[45]

Clinical Use

Aztreonam has been used for the treatment of a variety of infections such as urinary tract infections (including pyelonephritis and cystitis), lower respiratory tract infections including pneumonia and bronchitis, septicemia, skin and skin structure infections including those associated with postoperative wounds or ulcers and burns, intra-abdominal infection including peritonitis, and gynecologic infections including endometritis and pelvic cellulitis due to gram-negative aerobic bacteria.[35,46–55]

Because aztreonam has a spectrum of activity limited to aerobic gram-negative bacteria, the drug should not be used singly for empirical therapy in seriously ill patients if there is any possibility that the infection may be caused by gram-positive aerobic bacteria or if a mixed aerobic–anaerobic bacterial infection is suspected, an anti-infective agent effective against the suspected organism(s) should be used concomitantly. Aztreonam has been used safely and effectively in conjunction with clindamycin, erythromycin, metronidazole, penicillins, and vancomycin.

β-LACTAMASE INHIBITORS

Clavulanate

Clavulanate (Fig. 3) is a β-lactamase inhibitor. This compound was found in cultures of *Streptomyces clavuligerus*. It showed only a low level of antibacterial action, but when the compound was combined with penicillin G, inhibition of a *Klebsiella* isolate normally resistant to penicillin was noted. Clavulanate has subsequently been shown to inhibit β-lactamases from a number of clinically important gram-positive and gram-negative organisms.[56,57]

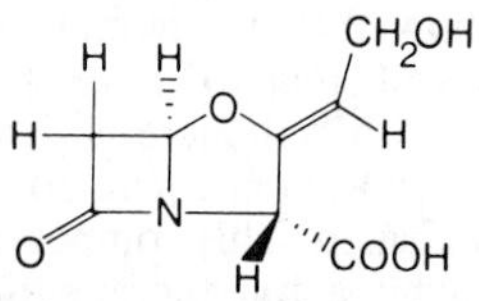

FIG. 3. Clavulanate.

Mechanism of Action. β-Lactamases account for the major form of resistance to penicillins and cephalosporins. These enzymes hydrolyze the cyclic amide bond in β-lactam–containing molecules. When the β-lactam ring is hydrolyzed, an inactive penicilloate is produced, or in the case of cephalosporins because of the unsaturated bond between carbons 3 and 4, both rings decompose to smaller fragments.

β-Lactamases of gram-positive species are exoenzymes, and in *S. aureus* the enzyme is plasmid mediated and inducible. Generally endemic hospital *S. aureus* produces large amounts of β-lactamase. The β-lactamases of gram-negative bacteria, aerobic and anaerobic, are situated in the periplasmic space and are either of chromosomal or plasmid origin. Richmond and Sykes developed a classification for gram-negative β-lactamases that lists them as I–V.[58] The most important chromosomal β-lactamases, most of which fall into class I, are present in *Acinetobacter, Citrobacter, Enterobacter, Proteus, Pseudomonas*, and *Serratia*. These are inducible enzymes and are not inhibited by clavulanate except at very high concentrations, which are only possible in test tube conditions. β-Lactamases are produced constitutively by some *Enterobacter, E. coli*, and *Shigella*. These are not inhibited by clavulanate. Conversely, β-lactamases of *Legionella* and *Bacteroides* are inhibited by clavulanate. Other important chromosomally mediated β-lactamases are the class IV enzymes produced by *Klebsiella*. These are also inhibited by clavulanate.[59–62]

Plasmid-mediated β-lactamases are of a number of types. The most common is TEM-1, so-called for the initials of the original patient from whom the *E. coli* β-lactamase–containing isolate was derived. There are also TEM-2; oxacillin-hydrolyzing enzymes; OXA-1, -2, and -3; sulfhydro-inhibited enzymes SHV-1 and HMS; and finally PSE-1, PSE-2, PSE-3, and PSE-4, originally felt to be enzymes found only in *Pseudomonas* but now found occasionally in *E. coli*. All of these plasmid enzymes are inhibited by clavulanate (Table 3), as are the new cefotaxime-ceftazidime hydrolyzing enzymes TEM-3, -4, -5, -6, -7, and -8 and SHV-2, -3, -4, and -5. Concentrations needed to inhibit bacteria are shown in Table 4.

Since clavulanate inhibits β-lactamases, it has been shown to act synergistically with amoxicillin, ampicillin, piperacillin, mezlocillin, and cefoperazone, all of which can be destroyed by *Staphylococcus, Klebsiella*, or plasmid-mediated β-lactamases.

The mode of inhibition of a β-lactamase by clavulanate is characteristic of the particular enzyme studied.[60] Although competitive inhibition is seen, clavulanate primarily acts as a suicide inhibitor that, after forming an acyl enzyme intermediate with the enzyme, causes destruction of the enzyme.

Pharmacology. Clavulanate is moderately well absorbed from the gastrointestinal tract, with peak serum levels occurring 40–120 minutes after ingestion. Mean peak serum levels for 62.5 mg are 1 μg/ml; for 125 mg, 4 μg/ml; and for 250 mg, 6 μg/ml.[63,64] Combining clavulanate with amoxicillin does not significantly alter the pharmacologic parameters of either drug.

TABLE 3. Inhibition of β-Lactamases by β-Lactam inhibitors

β-Lactamases	Name	Organisms	Inhibited by Clavulanate-Sulbactam
Plasmid		*S. aureus*	Yes
Plasmid	TEM-1	*E. coli* *Haemophilus* *N. gonorrhoeae* *Salmonella* *Shigella*	Yes
Plasmid	TEM-2	*E. coli*	Yes
Plasmid	TEM-3 to -8	*Klebsiella*	Yes
Plasmid	SHV-1	*Klebsiella*	Yes
Plasmid	SHV-2 to -5	Enterobacteriaceae	Yes
Plasmid	OXA-1, 2, 3	*E. coli*	Variable
Plasmid	PSE-1, 2, 3	*Pseudomonas*	Variable
Chromosomal	Type 1a[a]	*Enterobacter* *Morganella* *Citrobacter* *Serratia*	No
Chromosomal	Type Id[a]	*Pseudomonas*	No
Chromosomal	Type IV, K1[a]	*Klebsiella*	Yes
Chromosomal		*Bacteroides*	Yes
Chromosomal		*Legionella*	Yes
Chromosomal		*Branhamella*	Yes

[a] Richmond-Sykes classification.[58]

The pharmacokinetics of orally administered clavulanate in children in terms of peak serum levels and plasma half-lives of the drug are similar to those in adults.[65,66]

The absorption of clavulanate in the adult is unaffected by the simultaneous administration of food, milk, or aluminum hydroxide–containing antacids. After iv infusion of calvulanate combined either with amoxicillin or ticarcillin, the drug is rapidly distributed. Peak serum concentration are approximately 11 μg/ml after a 200 mg iv dose, with drug detectable to levels of 0.2 μg/ml at 6 hours.[67,68] Peak serum concentrations of clavulanate in children receiving 5 mg/kg have been 19 μg/ml with less than 1 μg/ml present at 3 hours.[66]

The serum half-life of clavulanate is slightly less than that of amoxicillin, 0.76–1.4 hours. No accumulation of clavulanate occurs until creatinine clearances fall below 10 ml/min.[69] Dose adjustment usually is made by adjustment for amoxicillin or ticarcillin. Clavulanate has been shown to be degraded in vivo in animals, with metabolites being excreted via lung, feces, and urine and only 20–60 percent appearing unchanged in urine 6 hours after an oral dose. After a dose of 125 mg of clavulanate urine levels are 115–508 μg/ml for 0–2 hours and 45–74 μg/ml for 4–6 hours.[69]

Concentrations less than 1 μg/ml of clavulanate are achieved in sputum after the oral administration of amoxicillin-clavulanate, but pleural fluid levels are 46–91 percent of peak serum levels. There is rapid penetration of clavulanate into peritoneal fluid, with mean peritoneal fluid levels of clavulanate 66 percent of serum levels.[67,70] After 200 mg of clavulanate, peritoneal fluid levels fall below 5 μg/ml after about 0.5 hours and below 1 μg/ml after about 3 hours. Clavulanate does not penetrate noninflamed meninges, but after large iv doses in patients with meningitis, CSF levels of clavulanate have been in the range of 1 μg/ml. Clavulanate produces therapeutic levels in bile, middle ear fluid, and tonsil tissue.[70]

Clavulanate crosses the placenta and may be found in the cord blood of newborns and in the amniotic fluid, but no clavulanate can be detected in breast milk.

Adverse Reactions. No new or major adverse reactions to the use of clavulanate combined with amoxicillin or of clavulanate combined with ticarcillin have been reported. The incidence of skin reactions has been similar to that of penicillin used alone. Diarrhea has followed the use of 250 mg clavulanate given three times daily, and some nausea has occurred with this dose program. Parenteral amoxicillin-clavulanate and ticarcillin-clavulanate have not caused undue diarrhea.

Amoxicillin-Clavulanate

Amoxicillin-clavulanate (Augmentin) has been used in a number of different clinical settings. The combination has proved useful as therapy for acute otitis media in children that is caused by β-lactamase–producing *Haemophilus influenzae* and *Branhamella catarrhalis*.[71] It has also been used to treat sinusitis and, rarely, pharyngitis in individuals where large tonsillar tissue contains β-lactamase–producing *Bacteroides melaninogenicus*.[71] Amoxicillin-clavulanate has proved useful in lower respiratory tract infections such as exacerbations of bacterial bronchitis or pneumonitis due to β-lactamase–producing bacteria. It has proved particularly useful to treat bite wounds of human or animal origin. Skin structure infections due to streptococci and staphylococci have responded to amoxicillin-clavulanate with results comparable to oral antistaphylococcal agents and oral cephalosporins.[72] Amoxicillin-clavulanate has been used to treat diabetic foot infections since it has activity against staphylococci, anaerobes, and aerobic gram-negative bacteria.

Amoxicillin-clavulanate is available as a parenteral agent in many countries and has been used to treat gynecologic infections and intra-abdominal infections.

Ticarcillin-Clavulanate

Ticarcillin-clavulanate has been used as treatment of community- and hospital-acquired pneumonia, particularly where there has been aspiration of oral secretions and aerobic gram-negative bacilli.[73] Intra-abdominal infections and gynecologic infections have been treated successfully, as have skin structure infections and osteomyelitis.[74,75] When ticarcillin-clavulanate has been used to treat febrile neutropenic patients, it has been necessary to combine it with an aminoglycoside. The usual doses are either 3.1 or 3.2 g administered every 4 or 6 hours.

TABLE 4. Activity of Augmentin against Amoxicillin-Resistant Organisms

Organism	Amoxicillin	Augmentin[a]
Staphylococcus aureus	256	1.0
Staphylococcus epidermidis	256	2.0
Staphylococcus aureus (MRSA)	256	16.0
Haemophilus influenzae	64	0.5
Branhamella catarrhalis	16	0.25
Neisseria gonorrhoeae	128	1.0
Escherichia coli	>256	8.0
Klebsiella pneumoniae	128	4.0
Proteus mirabilis	>256	4.0
Proteus vulgaris	>256	2.0
Bacteroides fragilis	32	0.5
Enterobacter, Citrobacter, Serratia sp. and *Pseudomonas aeruginosa*	>128	>128

[a] Contains amoxicillin and clavulanate in a 2:1 ratio.

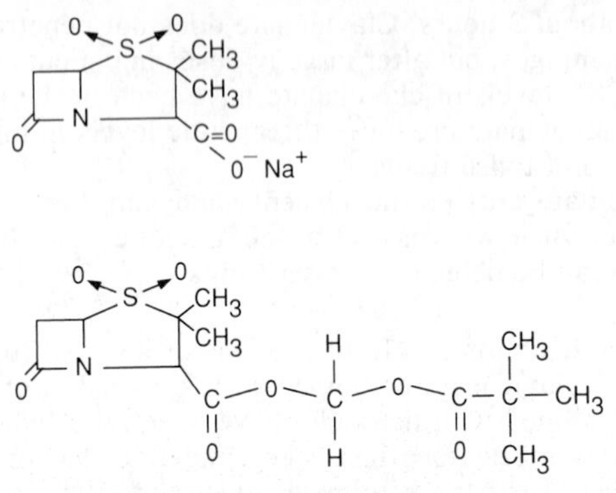

FIG. 4. Sulbactam and sulbactam oral ester (lower).

Sulbactam

Sulbactam (Fig. 4) is a 6-desaminopenicillin sulfone that resembles clavulanate structurally by a lack of substitution at carbon 6 of the β-lactam ring and by the presence of an activated center at carbon 5. Sulbactam has weak antibacterial activity against most gram-positive cocci, Enterobacteriaceae, and *Pseudomonas* but has reasonable activity against *Neisseria* sp., *Bacteroides* sp., and some *Acinetobacter* sp.[76–78]

Sulbactam acts similarly to clavulanate as a suicide inhibitor of certain plasmid- and chromosomally mediated β-lactamases. It does not inhibit β-lactamases of the Richmond-Sykes type Ia classification. These are chromosomally mediated β-lactamases of *Enterobacter, Citrobacter freundii*, and the indole-positive *Proteus-Providencia* organisms. Like clavulanate, it inhibits the β-lactamases of *Staphylococcus aureus*, Enterobacteriaceae with TEM-1 to -8 and SHV-1 to -5, *Klebsiella, Bacteroides, Branhmaella, Legionella*, and *Mycobacterium*. It does not inhibit the *Pseudomonas maltophilia* β-lactamase.

Sulbactam does not induce β-lactamases, nor does it select for derepressed β-lactamase–producing bacteria.

Sulbactam penetrates some bacteria less well than does clavulanate, particularly some *Klebsiella* species, but like clavulanate, it is a suicide inhibitor.

Sulbactam acts synergistically with penicillins and cephalosporins that are degraded by β-lactamases. In the presence of 8 μg/ml of sulbactam and 16 μg/ml of ampicillin, most staphylococci, *Klebsiella, Haemophilus, E. coli*, and *Bacteroides* sp. that would normally be resistant to ampicillin are inhibited.[77,78]

Pharmacology. Sulbactam has pharmacokinetics in humans similar to ampicillin.[79,80] Peak serum levels after 250 mg are 6.4 μg/ml, with 1.1 μg/ml at 4 hours.[79] Peak serum levels after im injections of 0.250 and 0.5 g are 7 and 13 μg/ml, respectively, with a serum half-life of 1.1–1.3 hours. After the iv infusion of 0.5 g, peak serum levels of 30 μg/ml are achieved, and after 1 g, 68 μg/ml are achieved. The serum half-life is 1 hours. Sulbactam is excreted by the kidney and has a urinary recovery of 70–80 percent of a dose. Biliary excretion is minimal, and metabolism is <25 percent. Concentrations of sulbactam in interstitial fluid and peritoneal secretions are comparable to levels in serum. Penetration of sulbactam into inflamed meninges is low, with levels of 0.1–10 μg/ml found in the CSF after a 1 g infusion. Excretion is blocked by probenecid. The half-life does not increase down to creatinine clearances of 30 ml/min. With clearances between 15 and 30, the half-life is 5.1 hours; with clearances of 5–15, the half-life is 9.2 hours, and the half-life of anuric patients is 20 hours. It can be removed by hemodialysis.

Adverse Reactions. The clinical studies of the combination of sulbactam plus ampicillin have reported no major hematologic, renal, hepatic, or central nervous system reactions.[81–83] Diarrhea has not been a major problem after iv use. Skin reactions are similar to those found for ampicillin, and there is occasional elevation of transaminase levels.

Clinical Use. Sulbactam-ampicillin in the United States is available only as a parenteral agent where it is used primarily intravenously. It has been used in treatment of mixed bacterial infections such as intra-abdominal infections, obstetric and gynecologic infections, and soft tissue and bone infections.[84,85] It has been used to treat meningitis in infants and children and to treat epiglottitis and selected other pediatric infections.[86,87] However, the pediatric experience is limited, and it would seem that third-generation cephalosporins would be preferred in such infections.

REFERENCES

1. Kahan JS, Kahan FM, Goegleman R, et al. Thienamycin, a new beta-lactam antibiotic. 1. Discovery, isolation and physical properties. J Antibiot. 1979;32:1–12.
2. Neu HC, Labthavikul P. Comparative in vitro activity of *N*-formimidoyl thienamycin against gram-positive and gram-negative aerobic and anaerobic species and its beta-lactamase stability. Antimicrob Agents Chemother. 1982;21:180–7.
3. Wise R, Andrews JM, Patel N. *N*-formimidoyl thienamycin a novel beta-lactam: An in vitro comparison with other beta-lactam antibiotics. J Antmicrob Chemother. 1981;7:521–9.
4. Jones RN. Review of the in vitro spectrum of activity of imipenem. Am J Med. 1985;78:22–32.
5. Prince AS, Neu HC. Activities of new beta-lactam antibiotics against isolates of *Pseudomonas aeruginosa* from patients with cystic fibrosis. Antimicrob Agents Chemother. 1981;20:545–6.
6. Brown JE, Del Benes VE, Collins CD. In vitro activity of *N*-formimidoyl thienamycin, moxalactam and other new beta-lactam agents against *Bacteroides fragilis*: Contribution of beta-lactamase to resistance. Antimicrob Agents Chemother. 1981;19:248–52.
7. Kesado T, Hashizume T, Ashi Y, et al. Susceptibilities of anaerobic bacteria to *N*-formimidoyl thienamycin (MK0787) and to other antibiotics. Antimicrob Agents Chemother. 1982;21:1016–22.
8. Norrby SR, Alestig K, Björngard B, et al. Urinary recovery of *N*-formimidoyl thienamycin (MK0787) as affected by coadminstration of *N*-formimidoyl thienamycin dehydropeptidase inhibitors. Antimicrob Agents Chemother. 1983;23:300–7.
9. Norrby SR, Alestig K, Ferber F, et al. Pharmacokinetics and tolerance of *N*-formimidoyl thienamycin (MK0787) in humans. Antimicrob Agents Chemother. 1983;23:293–9.
10. Drusano GL, Standiford HC, Ruslamante C, et al. Multiple dose kinetics of imipenem/cilastatin. Antimicrob Agents Chemother. 1984;26:715–21.
11. Drusano GL, Standiford HC. Pharmacokinetic profile of imipenem/cilastatin in normal volunteers. Am J Med. 1985;78:47–53.
12. Berman SJ, Sugihara JG, Nakumara JM, et al. Multiple dose study of imipenem/cilastatin in patients with end-stage renal disease undergoing long-term hemodialysis. Am J Med. 1985;78:105–8.
13. Norrby SR, Rogers JD, Ferber F, et al. Disposition of radio labeled imipenem and cilastatin in normal human volunteers. Antimicrob Agents Chemother. 1985;26:707–14.
14. Calandra GB, Ricci FM, Wang C, et al. Safety and tolerance comparison of imipenem-cilastatin to cephalothin and cefazolin. J Antimicrob Chemother. 1983;12(Suppl D):125–31.
15. Sadon A, Gilden BN, Rohr AS, et al. Immediate hypersensitivity reactions to beta-lactam antibiotics. Ann Intern Med. 1987;127:204–15.
16. Baumgardner JD, Galuser MP. Comparative imipenem treatment of *Staphylococcus aureus* endocarditis in the rat. J Antimicrob Chemother. 1983;12(Suppl D):79–87.
17. Scheld WM, Keely J. Imipenem therapy of experimental *Staphylococcus aureus* and *Streptococcus faecalis* endocarditis. J Antimicrob Chemother. 1983;12(Suppl D):69–78.
18. Johnson DE, Calia IM, Snyder MJ, et al. Imipenem therapy of *Pseudomonas aeruginosa* bacteremia in neutropenic rats. J Antimicrob Chemother. 1983;12(Suppl D):89–96.
19. MacGregor RR, Gentry LO. Imipenem/cilastatin in the treatment of osteomyelitis. Am J Med. 1985;78:92–5.
20. Marier RL. Role of impenem in the treatment of soft tissue infections. Am J Med. 1985;78:132–6.
21. Berkeley AS, Freedman K, Hirsch J, et al. Imipenem/cilastatin in the treatment of obstetric and gynecologic infections. Am J Med. 1985;78:71–6.

22. Cox CE, Corrado ML. Safety and efficacy of imipenem/cilastatin in treatment of complicated urinary tract infections. Am J Med. 1985;78:84–91.
23. Kager L, Nord CE. Imipenem/cilastatin in the treatment of intraabdominal infections: A review of worldwide experience. Rev Infect Dis. 1985;7(Suppl 3):518–21.
24. Salata RA, Gebhart RC, Palmer DL, et al. Pneumonia treated with imipenem/cilastatin. Am J Med. 1985;78:96–101.
25. Dickson G, Rodriguez K, Arcey S, et al. Efficacy of imipenem/cilastatin in endocarditis. Am J Med. 1985;78:109–18.
26. Bodey GP, Alvarez ME, Jones PG, et al. Imipenem/cilastatin as initial therapy for febrile cancer patients. Antimicrob Agents Chemother. 1986;30:211–4.
27. Gombert ME, Aulicino TM, duBouchet L, et al. Therapy of experimental cerebral nocardiosis with imipenum, amikacin, trimethoprim-sulfamethoxazole, and minocycline. Antimicrob Agents Chemother. 1986;30:270–3.
28. Ertl G, Schall K, Kochsiek K. Nocardial endocarditis of an aortic valve prosthesis. Br Heart J. 1987;57:384–6.
29. Krilov LR, Blumer JL, Stern RC, et al. Imipenem/cilastatin in acute pulmonary exacerbations of cystic fibrosis. Rev Infect Dis. 1985;7(Suppl 3):482–9.
30. Acar JF. Therapy for lower respiratory tract infections with imipenem/cilastatin: A review of worldwide experience. Rev Infect Dis. 1985;7:S513–7.
31. Sykes RB, Cimarausti CM, Bonner DP, et al. Monocyclic beta-lactam antibiotics produced by bacteria. Nature. 1981;291:489–91.
32. Neu HC, Labthavikul P. Antibacterial activity of a monocyclic beta-lactam SQ 26,776. J Antimicrob Chemother. 1981;9(Suppl E):111–2.
33. Barry AL, Thornsberry C, Jones RN, et al. Aztreonam: Antibacterial activity, beta-lactamase stability, and interpretive standards and quality control guidelines for disk-diffusion susceptibility tests. Rev Infect Dis. 1985;7(Suppl 4):594–604.
34. Sykes RB, Bonner DP, Bush K, et al. Aztreonam (SQ 26,776), a synthetic monobactam specifically active against aerobic gram-negative bacteria. Antimicrob Agents Chemother. 1982;21:85–92.
35. Henry SA, Bendush CB. Aztreonam: Worldwide overview of the treatment of patients with gram-negative infections. Am J Med. 1985;78(Suppl 2A):57–64.
36. Swabb EA, Sugerman AA, Stern M. Oral bioavailability of the monobactam aztreonam (SQ 26,776) in healthy subjects. Antimicrob Agents Chemother. 1983;23:548–550.
37. Swabb EA. Review of the clinical pharmacology of the monobactam antibiotic aztreonam. Am J Med. 1985;78(Suppl 2A):11–8.
38. Jones PG, Bodey GP, Swabb EA, et al. Clinical pharmacokinetics of aztreonam in cancer patients. Antimicrob Agents Chemother. 1984;26:455–61.
39. Janicke DM, Cafarell RF, Parker SW, et al. Pharmacokinetics of aztreonam in patients with gram-negative infections. Antimicrob Agents Chemother. 1985;27:16–20.
40. Scully BE, Swabb EA, Neu HC. Pharmacology of aztreonam after intravenous infusion. Antimicrob Agents Chemother. 1983;24:18–22.
41. Duma RJ, Berry AJ, Smith SM, et al. Penetration of aztreonam into cerebrospinal fluid of patients with and without inflammed meninges. Antimicrob Agents Chemother. 1984;26:730–3.
42. Stutman HR, Marks MI, Swabb EA. Single-dose pharmacokinetics of aztreonam in pediatric patients. Antimicrob Agents Chemother. 1984;26:196–9.
43. Fillastre JP, Leroy A, Baudoin C, et al. Pharmacokinetics of aztreonam in patients with chronic renal failure. Clin Pharmacokinet. 1985;10:91–100.
44. Mihindu JC, Scheld WM, Bolton ND, et al. Pharmacokinetics of aztreonam in patients with various degrees of renal dysfunction. Antimicrob Agents Chemother. 1983;24:252–61.
45. Gerig JS, Bolton ND, Swabb EA, et al. Effect of hemodialysis and peritoneal dialysis on aztreonam pharmacokinetics. Kidney Int. 1984;26:308–18.
46. Daikos GK. Clinical experience with aztreonam in four Mediterranean countries. Rev Infect Dis. 1985;7(Suppl 4):831–9.
47. Giamarellou H, Galanakis N, Douzinas E, et al. Evaluation of aztreonam in difficult-to-treat infections with prolonged post-treatment follow-up. Antimicrob Agents Chemother. 1984;26:245–9.
48. Gibbs RS, Blanco JD, Bernstein S. Role of aerobic gram-negative bacilli in endometritis after cesarean section. Rev Infect Dis. 1985;7(Suppl E):690–5.
49. Rodriguez JR, Ramirez-Ronda CH. Efficacy and safety of aztreonam versus tobramycin for aerobic gram-negative bacilli lower respiratory tract infections. Am J Med. 1985;78(Suppl 2A):42–3.
50. Romero-Vivas J, Rodriguez-Creixems M, Bouza E, et al. Evaluation of aztreonam in the treatment of severe bacterial infections. Antimicrob Agents Chemother. 1985;28:222–6.
51. Scully BE, Henry SA. Clinical experience with aztreonam in the treatment of gram-negative bacteremia. Rev Infect Dis. 1985;7(Suppl 4):789–93.
52. Scully BE, Neu HC. Use of aztreonam in the treatment of serious infections due to multiresistant gram-negative organisms, including *Pseudomonas aeruginosa*. Am J Med. 1985;78:251–61.
53. Scully BE, Ores CN, Prince AS, et al. Treatment of lower respiratory tract infections due to *Pseudomonas aeruginosa* in patients with cystic fibrosis. Rev Infect Dis. 1985;7(Suppl):669–74.
54. Simons WJ, Lee TJ. Aztreonam in the treatment of bone and joint infections caused by gram-negative bacilli. Rev Infect Dis. 1985;7(Suppl 4):783–8.
55. Gudiol F, Pallares R, Ariza X, et al. Comparative clinical evaluation of aztreonam versus aminoglycosides in gram-negative septicaemia. J Antimicrob Chemother. 1986;17:661–71.
56. Reading C, Cole M. Clavulanic acid: A beta-lactamase inhibiting beta-lactam from *Streptomyces clavuligerus*. Antimicrob Agents Chemother. 1977;11:852–7.
57. Neu HC, Fu KP. Clavulanic acid: A beta-lactamase–inhibiting beta-lactamase. Antimicrob Agents Chemother. 1978;14:650–5.
58. Richmond MM, Sykes RB. The beta-lactamases of gram-negative bacteria and their possible physiological role. Adv Microb Physiol. 1973;9:31–88.
59. Neu HC. The contribution of beta-lactamases to bacterial resistance and mechanisms to inhibit beta-lactamases. Am J Med. 1986;79(Suppl 5B):2–12.
60. Neu HC. The role of beta-lactamase inhibitors in chemotherapy. In: Tipper PJ, ed. Antibiotic Inhibitors of Bacterial Cell Wall Biosynthesis. Oxford: Pergamon Press; 1987:241–58.
61. Neu HC. Penicillin-binding proteins and beta-lactamases: Their effects on the use of cephalosporins and other new beta-lactams. In: Remington JS, Swartz MN, eds. Current Clinical Topics in Infectious Diseases. New York: McGraw-Hill; 1987:37–83.
62. Bush K: Recent developments in beta-lactamase research and their implications for the future. Rev Infect Dis. 1988;10:681–90.
63. Munch P, Luthy R, Blaser J, et al. Human pharmacokinetics and CSF penetration of clavulanic acid. J Antimicrob Chemother. 1981;8:29–37.
64. Adam D, Visser I, Koeppe P. Pharmacokinetics of amoxicillin and clavulanic acid administered alone and in combination. Antimicrob Agents Chemother. 1982;22:353–7.
65. Nelson JD, Kusmiesz H, Shelton S. Pharmacokinetics of potassium clavulanate in combination with amoxicillin in pediatric patients. Antimicrob Agents Chemother. 1982;21:681–2.
66. Schaad UB, Casey PA, Copper DL. Single-dose pharmacokinetics of intravenous clavulanic acid with amoxicillin in pediatric patients. Antimicrob Agents Chemother. 1983;23:252–5.
67. Bennett S, Wise R, Weston D, et al. Pharmacokinetics and tissue penetration of ticarcillin combined with clavulanic acid. Antimicrob Agents Chemother. 1983;23:831–4.
68. Scully BE, Chin NX, Neu HC. Pharmacology of ticarcillin combined with clavulanic acid in humans. Am J Med. 1985;79(Suppl 5B):39–43.
69. Jackson D, Cockburn A, Cooper DL, et al. Clinical pharmacology and safety evaluation of Timentin. Am J Med. 1985;79(Suppl 5B):44–55.
70. Walsted RA, Hellum KB, Thurmann-Nielson E, et al. Pharmacokinetics and tissue penetration of Timentin: A simultaneous study of serum, urine, lymph, suction blister, and subcutaneous treatment fluid. J Antimicrob Chemother. 1986;17(Suppl C):71–80.
71. Kaleida PH, Bluestone DC, Rockette HE, et al. Amoxicillin-clavulanate potassium compared with cefaclor for acute otitis media in infants and children. Pediatr Infect Dis. 1987;6:265–71.
72. Neu HC, ed. Progress and perspectives on beta-lactamase inhibition: a review of Augmentin. Postgrad Med. 1984;3–295.
73. Neu HC, ed. Beta-lactamase inhibition: Therapeutic advances. Am J Med. 1985;79(Suppl 5B):1–196.
74. Gentry LO, Macko V, Lind R, et al. Ticarcillin plus clavulanic acid (Timentin) therapy for osteomyelitis. Am J Med. 1985;79(Suppl 5B):116–21.
75. Leigh DA, Phillips I, Wise R, eds. Timentin-ticarcillin plus clavulanic acid, a laboratory and clinical perspective. J Antimicrob Chemother. 1986;17(Suppl C):1–244.
76. Aswapokee N, Neu HC. A sulfone, beta-lactam compound which acts as a beta-lactamase inhibitor. J Antibiot. 1978;31:1238–43.
77. Retsema VA, English AR, Girard AR. CP-45,899 in combination with penicillin or ampicillin against penicillin-resistant staphylococci. Antimicrob Agents Chemother. 1980;17:615–22.
78. Jones RN. In vitro evaluation of aminopenicillin–beta-lactamase inhibitor combinations. Drugs. 1988;36(Suppl 7):17–26.
79. Foulds G, Stankewich JP, Marshall DC, et al. Pharmacokinetics of sulbactam in humans. Antimicrob Agents Chemother. 1983;23:692–9.
80. Hampel B, Lode H, Bruchnor G, et al. Comparative pharmacokinetics of sulbactam/ampicillin and clavulanic acid/amoxicillin in human volunteers. Drugs. 1988;35(Suppl 7):29–33.
81. Guneren MF. Clinical experience with intramuscular sulbactam/ampicillin in the out-patient treatment of various infections: A multicenter trial. Drugs. 1988;35(Suppl 7):57–68.
82. Dajani AS. Sulbactam/ampicillin in pediatric infections. Drugs. 1988;35(Suppl 7):35–8.
83. Kass EH, Lode H, eds. Enzyme-mediated resistance to beta-lactam antibiotics: A symposium on sulbactam/ampicillin. Rev Infect Dis. 1986;8(Suppl 5):465–650.
84. Reinhardt JF, Johnston L, Ruane P, et al. A randomized, double-blind comparison of sulbactam/ampicillin and clindamycin for the treatment of aerobic and aerobic-anaerobic infections. Rev Infect Dis. 1986;8(Suppl 5):569–75.
85. Hemsell DL, Heard MC, Hemsell PG, et al. Sulbactam/ampicillin versus cefoxitin for uncomplicated and complicated acute pelvic inflammatory disease. Drugs. 1988;35(Suppl 7):39–42.
86. Rodriguez WJ, Kahn WN, Puig N, et al. Sulbactam/ampicillin vs. chloramphenicol/ampicillin for the treatment of meningitis in infants and children. Rev Infect Dis. 1986;8(Suppl 5):620–9.
87. Wald E, Reilly JS, Bluestone CD, et al. Sulbactam/ampicillin in the treatment of acute epiglottis in children. Rev Infect Dis. 1986;8(Suppl 5):617–9.

21. β-LACTAM ALLERGY

MICHAEL E. WEISS
N. FRANKLIN ADKINSON

After the clinical introduction of penicillin in the mid-1940s, it soon became clear that its principal toxicity was allergic in origin. The first reported case of anaphylaxis due to penicillin was in 1946,[1] and the first reported death was in 1949.[2] Subsequently, a broad spectrum of allergic reactions to β-lactam antibiotics have been recognized. Allergic reactions occur in 0.7–4 percent of penicillin treatment courses.[3]

REACTIONS

Gell and Coombs have classified four types of immunopathologic reactions,[4] all of which have been seen with penicillin (Table 1).

Type I—Immediate Hypersensitivity

These reactions result from the interaction of penicillin haptenic determinants with preformed penicillin-specific IgE antibodies that are bound to tissue mast cells and/or circulating basophils via high-affinity IgE receptors. Cross-linking of two or more IgE receptors by penicillin antigens leads to the release of both preformed (histamine, proteases, and chemotactic factors) and newly generated (prostaglandins, leukotrienes, and platelet activating factor) mediators from cell membrane phospholipids.[5] Release of these mediators can lead to urticaria, laryngeal edema, and bronchospasm with or without cardiovascular collapse. Anaphylactic reactions occur in 0.004–0.015 percent of penicillin treatment courses.[6] Fatality from penicillin anaphylaxis occurs about once in every 50,000–100,000 treatment courses.[6] β-Adrenergic antagonists apparently increase the risk of a fatal outcome from anaphylaxis by rendering treatment more difficult.[7] IgE-mediated reactions may be the most important allergic reaction to β-lactam drugs clinically, because of the risk of life-threatening anaphylaxis.

Type II—Cytotoxic Antibodies (Usually IgG and/or IgM)

Penicillin determinants can become chemically bound to circulating blood cells (or renal interstitial cells), leading to their accelerated destruction via IgG or IgM antibodies and complement. Long-term, high-dose penicillin treatment is usually required for this form of immunopathology. Interstitial nephritis, seen most frequently with methicillin, may also be caused by a type II mechanism.

Type III—Immune Complexes

Penicillin-specific IgG or IgM antibodies form circulating complexes with penicillin haptenized to serum proteins, largely albumin. These circulating complexes can fix complement and then lodge in tissue sites, causing serum sickness and possibly drug fever. Immune complex reactions typically appear 7–14 days after the initiation of high-dose β-lactam therapy; the syndrome sometimes appears after termination of therapy.

Type IV—Cell-mediated Hypersensitivity

Contact dermatitis from penicillin involves drug-sensitized, thymus-derived lymphocytes. The high rate of penicillin contact dermatitis (5–10 percent) in the 1940s led to the discontinuation of its use as a topical antibiotic. Contact dermatitis is still occasionally seen in individuals who are occupationally exposed to penicillins, particularly those involved in antibiotic manufacturing and packaging.[6,8]

Idiopathic Reactions

Some reactions to β-lactam antibiotics have an obscure pathogenesis. Among these are the very common maculopapular rash that appears late in the treatment course in 2–3 percent of penicillin treatments. Ampicillin-induced rashes occur with much greater frequency (5.2–9.5 percent of treatment courses in uncomplicated cases).[9–11] When ampicillin is given during infections with Epstein-Barr virus or cytomegalovirus, or to patients with acute lymphocytic leukemia, a much higher incidence of rash (69–100 percent) occurs.[12] The participation of immune mechanisms in the origin of the measles-like (non-urticarial) rash is unclear. Exfoliative dermatitis and the Stevens-Johnson syndrome also have obscure immunologic origins. Pseudoanaphylactic reactions have been observed after im or inadvertent iv injection of procaine penicillin. These reactions are probably due to a combination of toxic and embolic phenomena from procaine.[13]

Levine proposed a classification of adverse reactions to penicillin according to their time of onset[14] (Table 2). Immediate reactions occur within the first hour after penicillin administration, and they are almost always IgE-mediated (anaphylaxis and urticaria). Accelerated reactions occur 1–72 hours after initial treatment with penicillin; they most commonly involve urticaria. Late reactions begin more than 72 hours after the onset of penicillin therapy. Anaphylaxis does not occur later in the course of continuous β-lactam therapy; maculopapular erup-

TABLE 1. Classification of Immunopathologic Reactions to Penicillin

Type[a] of reaction	Description	Primary Effector Mechanism(s): Antibody	Cells	Other	Clinical Reactions
I	Anaphylactic (reaginic) hypersensitivity	IgE	Basophils, mast cells		Anaphylaxis, urticaria
II	Cytotoxic or cytolytic damage	IgG IgM	Any cell with isoantigen	C′, RES	Coombs + hemolytic anemia; drug-induced nephritis
III	Immune complex disease	Soluble immune complexes (Ag-Ab)	None directly	C′	Serum sickness; drug fever
IV	"Delayed" or cell-mediated hypersensitivity	None known	Sensitized T lymphocytes		Contact dermatitis
V	Idiopathic	IgM(?) ? ? ?	? ? ? ?	? ? ? ?	Maculopapular eruptions Eosinophilia Stevens-Johnson syndrome Exfoliative dermatitis

[a] According to the scheme of Gell and Coombs.[4]
Abbreviations: C′: complement; RES: reticuloendothelial system; Ag-Ab: antigen-antibody; (?): immunopathologic mechanism in doubt.

TABLE 2. Classification of Allergic Reactions to Penicillin

Reaction Type	Onset	Spectrum of Clinical Reactions
Immediate	0–1 hr	Anaphylaxis Hypotension Laryngeal edema Urticarial/angioedema Wheezing
Accelerated	1–72 hr	Urticaria/angioedema Laryngeal edema Wheezing
Late	>72 hr	Morbilliform rash Interstitial nephritis Hemolytic anemia Neutropenia Thrombocytopenia Serum Sickness Drug fever Stevens-Johnson syndrome Exfoliative dermatitis

(Adapted from Levine,[14] with permission.)

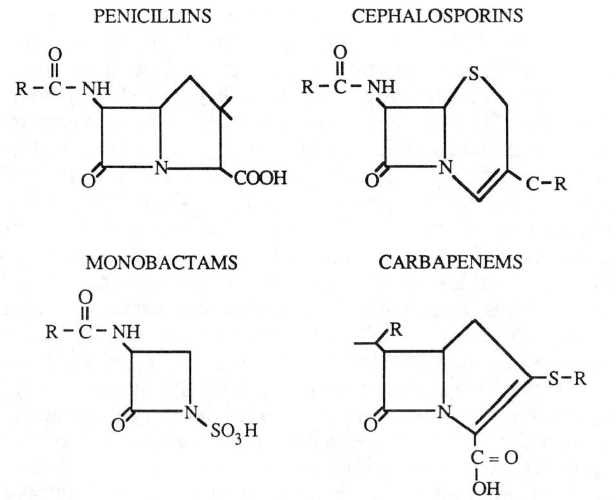

FIG. 1. Structure of the four classes of β-lactam antibiotics in use today. All contain the four-membered β-lactam ring.

tions are most common, but types II–IV reactions also occur in this time frame.

IMMUNOCHEMISTRY

Penicillins consist of a β-lactam ring, on which antimicrobial activity depends, and a five-membered thiazolidine ring (Fig. 1). Penicillin (MW 356) is a low molecular weight chemical and as such must first covalently combine with tissue macromolecules (presumably proteins) to produce multivalent hapten-protein complexes, which are required both for the induction of an immune response and the elicitation of an allergic reaction.[15]

Levine and Parker showed that the β-lactam ring spontaneously opens under physiologic conditions forming the penicilloyl group.[16] This penicilloyl group has been designated the *major determinant* because about 95 percent of the penicillin molecules that irreversibly combine with protein form penicilloyl groups (Fig. 2).[14] Recent evidence suggests that penicillin haptenization is facilitated by dializable serum molecules.[16a] This reaction occurs with the prototype benzylpenicillin and virtually all semisynthetic penicillins. Multiple penicilloyl determinants have been synthetically coupled to a weakly immunogenic polylysine carrier molecule to form penicilloyl-polylysine (PPL), which has been successfully used as a skin test reagent for the detection of penicilloyl IgE antibody.[17]

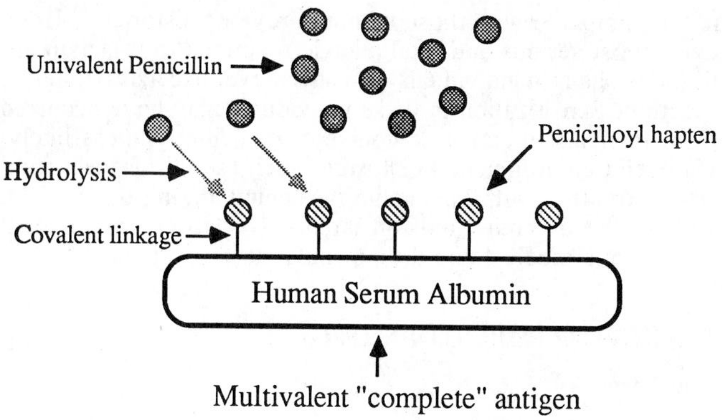

FIG. 2. Formation of penicilloyl-protein conjugates.

Benzylpenicillin can also be degraded by other metabolic pathways to form additional antigenic determinants.[18] These derivatives are formed in small quantities and stimulate a variable immune response; hence they have been termed the *minor determinants*. Because some of the determinants are labile and cannot be readily synthesized in multivalent form, skin testing for minor determinant specificities is usually accomplished using a mixture of benzylpenicillin, its alkaline hydrolysis product (benzylpenicilloate), and its acid hydrolysis product (benzylpenilloate), collectively called the *minor determinant mixture* (MDM). Therefore, for penicillin and other β-lactams, IgE antibodies can be produced against a number of haptenic derivatives labeled the major and minor determinants.

Anaphylactic reactions to penicillin are usually mediated by IgE antibodies directed against minor determinants, although some anaphylactic reactions have occurred in patients with only penicilloyl-specific IgE antibodies.[14,18,19] Accelerated and late urticarial reactions are generally mediated by penicilloyl-specific IgE antibody (major determinant).[14]

RISK FACTORS FOR IgE-DEPENDENT PENICILLIN REACTIONS

It is generally agreed, despite sparse evidence, that penicillin reactions occur less frequently in both children and the elderly than in nonelderly adults.[20,21] Although the frequency of anaphylactic reactions may be less in the elderly, fatal outcomes are more common due to compromised cardiopulmonary reserve.

Serial measurements in patients who mounted an immune response to penicillin showed that the half-life of penicilloyl-specific IgE antibody ranged from as short as 10 days to an indeterminantly long interval (more than 1,000 days).[22] An individual whose penicillin-specific IgE antibody response persists is at greater cumulative risk for allergic reactions to penicillin than one whose IgE antibody quickly disappears. Recent evidence suggests that as a group, patients allergic to penicillin dehaptenate penicillin determinants from albumin more slowly than non-penicillin-allergic subjects.[23]

A history of atopy does not seem to be an independent risk factor for the development of penicillin allergy,[20,22] although atopic individuals may be predisposed to fatal reactions to penicillin should anaphylaxis occur.[6]

Parenteral administration of penicillin produces more allergic reactions than orally administered penicillin.[24] Recent evidence suggests that this may be more related to dose than route of administration. When higher oral doses are given, as in the treatment of gonorrhea, the incidence of allergic reactions is no different from that of im procaine penicillin at a comparable dose.[25]

Individuals with a history of a prior penicillin reaction have a four- to sixfold increased risk of subsequent reactions to penicillin compared with those without previous histories.[20] However, most serious and fatal allergic reactions to β-lactam antibiotics occur in individuals who have never had a prior allergic reaction. Sensitization in these individuals may have occurred from their last therapeutic course of penicillin or (less likely) via occult environmental exposures such as milk or meat from cows treated with penicillin,[26] penicillin in other food sources,[2,27] or breast milk in infants,[21] or from occupational exposure in medical and drug manufacturing personnel.[8]

TESTING FOR PENICILLIN ALLERGY

Skin Tests

The most useful single piece of information in assessing an individual's potential for an immediate IgE-mediated reaction is his skin test response to major (PPL) and minor (MDM) penicillin determinants. When therapeutic doses of penicillin are given to patients with histories of penicillin allergy but with negative skin tests to PPL and MDM, IgE-mediated reactions occur very rarely and are almost always mild and self-limited. About 1 percent of skin test-negative patients will develop accelerated urticarial reactions, and approximately 3 percent will develop other mild reactions.[28] Penicillin anaphylaxis has not been reported in skin test-negative patients. Therefore negative skin tests indicate that β-lactam antibiotics may be safely given.

A limited number of skin test-positive patients have been treated with therapeutic doses of penicillin. The risk of an acute immediate or accelerated allergic reaction ranges from about 10 percent in history-negative subjects to 50–70 percent in history-positive subjects (Fig. 3).[28] The risk appears, with limited experience, to be somewhat higher when patients have positive skin tests to minor determinant reagents.[29] Therefore, if skin tests are positive, an equally effective, non-cross reacting antibiotic should be substituted when available. Since semisynthetic penicillins contain the same nucleus as penicillin G, and since the nuclear conformation determines the major antigenic specificity, skin testing with reagents derived from semisynthetic penicillins is generally not necessary.[30]

Skin testing to penicillin preferably should be done immediately before its intended use and repeated before each course of β-lactam therapy in patients with a history of an IgE-dependent reaction. Patients with a history of exfoliative dermatitis or Stevens-Johnson or Lyell syndromes, reactions that constitute nearly absolute contraindications for penicillin administration, should not be evaluated by skin testing. Skin tests have no predictive value in non-IgE-mediated reactions, such as serum sickness, hemolytic anemia, drug fever, interstitial nephritis, contact dermatitis, exfoliative dermatitis, or maculopapular exanthems.

In numerous studies in which both PPL and minor determinant skin tests were performed, only 7–35 percent of patients who gave histories of penicillin allergy were skin test-positive to either reagent,[28] although one study found a positive rate of 63 percent.[31] In general, with increasing time from the allergic reaction to penicillin, the prevalence of positive skin tests to penicillin determinants decreases, although some patients have penicillin-specific IgE antibody indefinitely.[31,32] Therefore skin tests in patients who gave a history of penicillin allergy confirm that 65–93 percent can safely be given a β-lactam antibiotic. With negative histories of penicillin allergy, the rate of positive skin tests is about 2 percent (Fig. 3).[33]

Ideally, all patients should be skin tested before receiving β-lactam drugs, but a systematic study of routine skin testing in history-negative patients from a sexually transmitted disease clinic indicated that such testing is probably not cost-effective.[33] Therefore we believe skin testing should be restricted to patients with a history of prior penicillin allergy for whom a β-lactam antibiotic is presently the indicated drug of choice.

A scratch or puncture (epicutaneous) test should be performed first. If there is no induration (or systemic symptoms) after 15 minutes, duplicate intradermal injections are placed, raising 3–4-mm blebs. Testing should be done with PPL, MDM, a positive control (histamine phosphate, 100 μg/ml), and a negative diluent control. The diameter of induration at 15–20 minutes is read; if it is greater than 5 mm, the test is considered positive.[34] Antihistamines, tricyclic antidepressants, and adrenergic drugs, all of which may inhibit skin test results, should be discontinued at least 24 hours prior to skin testing. Antihistamines with long half-lives (hydroxyzine, terfenadine, astemazole, etc.) may attenuate skin test results up to a week, or longer after discontinuation. Unfortunately, a minor determinant mixture is not commercially available in the United States at present. A minor determinant mixture can be prepared as described previously,[34] or benzylpenicillin can be used as the sole minor determinant reagent.

Presently only PPL (PRE-PEN; Kremers-Urban) at a concentration of 6×10^{-5} M (re: penicilloyl) is commercially available in the United States for use as a skin test reagent. Use of PPL alone would miss between 10 and 25 percent of all positive

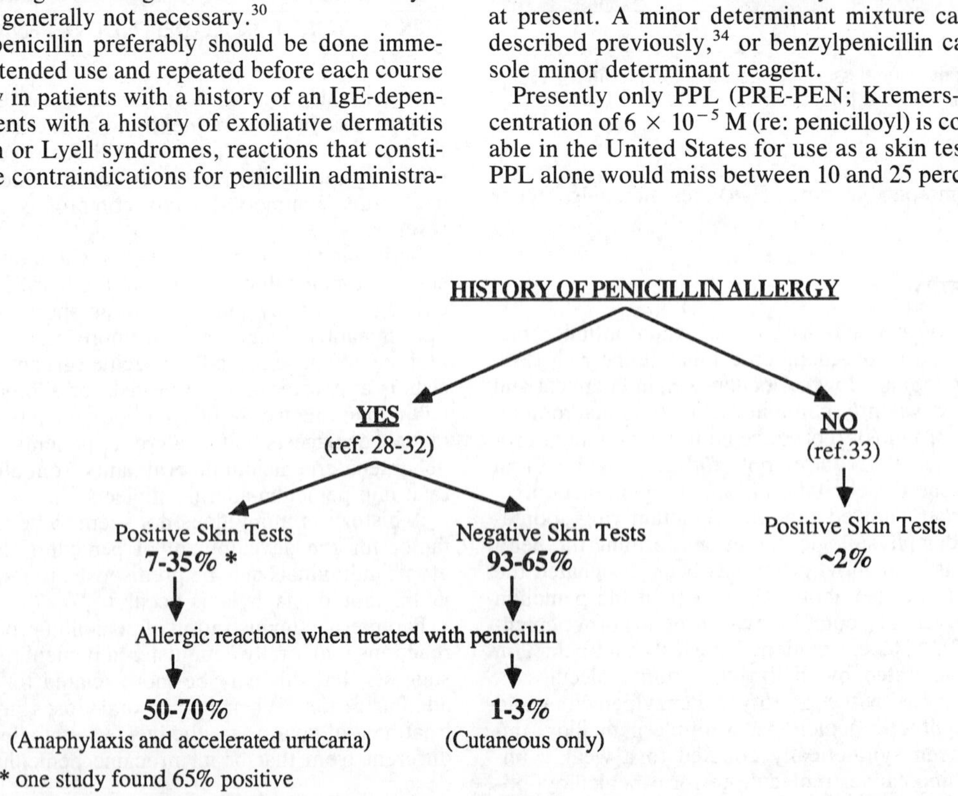

FIG. 3. Prevalence of positive and negative skin tests, and subsequent allergic reactions in patients treated with penicillin (based on studies using both penicilloyl-polylysine and minor determinant mixture as skin test reagents).

skin test reactions.[3,31] If one uses benzylpenicillin diluted to a concentration of 10,000 units/ml (10^{-2} M) as the sole minor determinant reagent, about 5–10 percent of skin test-reactive patients will be missed.[3,31] However, some of those missed may be at risk for serious, anaphylactic reactions.[35] Nevertheless, this is a reasonable alternative to MDM for use in patients *without* impressive histories of IgE-mediated reactions. Unfortunately, the lack of general access to a licensed minor determinant reagent has hindered the general application of penicillin skin testing for risk assessment.

When properly performed with due consideration for preliminary scratch tests and appropriate dilutions, skin testing with penicillin reagents can almost always be safely accomplished. Systemic reactions accompany about 1 percent of positive skin tests[36]; these are usually mild but can be serious. Therefore skin tests should be done in the presence of a physician and with immediate access to medications and equipment needed to treat anaphylaxis.

Other Tests

Solid-phase immunoassays such as the radioallergosorbent test (RAST) have been developed to detect serum IgE antibodies directed against the penicilloyl determinant. At present there is no in vitro RAST for minor determinant antibodies.[34] The penicilloyl-specific RAST is positive in 60–95 percent of patients with a positive skin test to PPL. Because it is more time-consuming, more expensive, less sensitive for detection of the major determinant IgE than skin testing, and unavailable for minor determinant detection, the RAST and other in vitro analogs have limited clinical utility.

MONITORING PATIENTS TREATED WITH β-LACTAM ANTIBIOTICS

Traditionally, outpatients treated with parenteral β-lactam antibiotics have been observed for 30 minutes following treatment. As most anaphylactic reactions to β-lactam antibiotics occur within 30 minutes of dosing,[6] this is a reasonable observation period. We have shown that a high-dose oral treatment (e.g., ampicillin 3.5 g with probenecid) is as likely to cause allergic reactions as comparable doses of parenteral procaine penicillin.[25] Therefore it is suggested that patients treated with high-dose oral β-lactam antibiotics be observed for 30 minutes also. More worrisome patients, such as those with histories of acute allergic reactions to penicillin in whom skin testing has not been done, should be observed for longer periods if they must receive β-lactams without skin testing. For such patients treated orally or parenterally as outpatients, 2 hours is a reasonable period for observation. For hospitalized patients considered at risk, the first intravenous dose may be infused slowly over a 1–2-hour period, sacrificing the initial peak antibiotic level, to observe for signs of an allergic reaction.

TABLE 3. Oral Desensitization Protocol

Step[a]	*Phenoxymethyl Penicillin (units/ml)*	*Amount (ml)*	*Dose (units)*	*Cumulative Dosage (units)*
1	1,000	0.1	100	100
2	1,000	0.2	200	300
3	1,000	0.4	400	700
4	1,000	0.8	800	1,500
5	1,000	1.6	1,600	3,100
6	1,000	3.2	3,200	6,300
7	1,000	6.4	6,400	12,700
8	10,000	1.2	12,000	24,700
9	10,000	2.4	24,000	48,700
10	10,000	4.8	48,000	96,700
11	80,000	1.0	80,000	176,700
12	80,000	2.0	160,000	336,700
13	80,000	4.0	320,000	656,700
14	80,000	8.0	640,000	1,296,700
Observe patient for 30 minutes				
Change to benzylpenicillin G iv				
15	500,000	0.25	125,000	
16	500,000	0.50	250,000	
17	500,000	1.00	500,000	
18	500,000	2.25	1,125,000	

[a] Interval between steps, 15 min.
(Adapted from Sullivan,[36] with permission.)

TABLE 4. Parenteral Desensitization Protocol: Typical Schedule

Injection No.	*Benzylpenicillin Concentration (units/ml)*	*Vol. and Route (cc)[a]*
1[b]	100	0.1 id
2	↓	0.2 sc
3	↓	0.4 sc
4	↓	0.8 sc
5[b]	1,000	0.1 id
6	↓	0.3 sc
7	↓	0.6 sc
8[b]	10,000	0.1 id
9	↓	0.2 sc
10	↓	0.4 sc
11	↓	0.8 sc
12[b]	100,000	0.1 id
13	↓	0.3 sc
14	↓	0.6 sc
15[b]	1,000,000	0.1 id
16	↓	0.2 sc
17	↓	0.2 im
18	↓	0.4 im
19	Continuous iv infusion (1,,000,000 units/hr)	

[a] Administer progressive doses at intervals of not less than 20 minutes
[b] Observe and record skin wheal and flare response to intradermal dose.
Abbreviations: id: intradermal; sc: subcutaneous; im: intramuscular; iv: intravenous.

PENICILLIN DESENSITIZATION

Effective, non-cross reacting alternative antibiotics to penicillin are usually available for patients with positive penicillin skin tests. If alternative drugs fail, induce unacceptable side effects, or are clearly less effective, then the administration of a penicillin using a desensitization protocol may be justified. Infections in which this may be considered include subacute bacterial endocarditis due to enterococci, brain abscess, bacterial meningitis, overwhelming infections with staphylococci or *Pseudomonas* organisms such as osteomyelitis or sepsis, *Listeria* infections, neurosyphilis, or syphilis during pregnancy. Use of a desensitization protocol for penicillin skin test-positive patients markedly reduces the risk of anaphylaxis.

Acute penicillin desensitization should only be performed in an intensive care setting. Any remedial risk factor should be corrected. All β-adrenergic antagonists such as propranolol or even timolol ophthalmic drops should be discontinued. Asthmatic patients should be under optimal control. An intravenous line should be established, baseline electrocardiogram (ECG) and spirometry should be performed, and continuous ECG monitoring should be instituted. Premedication with antihistamines or steroids is not recommended, as these drugs have not proven effective in suppressing severe reactions but may mask early signs of reactivity that would otherwise result in a modification of the protocol.[37,38]

Protocols have been developed for penicillin desensitization using both the oral and parenteral route[24,39] (Tables 3 and 4). As of 1987 there were 93 reported cases of oral desensitization, 74 of which were done by Sullivan and his collaborators.[40] Of these 74 patients, 32 percent experienced a transient allergic reaction either during desensitization (one-third) or during penicillin treatment after desensitization (two-thirds). These reactions were usually mild and self-limited in nature. Only one

IgE-mediated reaction (wheezing and bronchospasm) required discontinuation of the procedure before desensitization could be completed.[41] It has been argued that oral desensitization may be safer than parenteral desensitization,[39] but most patients can also be safely desensitized by the parenteral route.[42]

During desensitization any dose that causes mild systemic reactions such as pruritus, fleeting urticaria, rhinitis, or mild wheezing should be repeated until the patient tolerates the dose without systemic symptoms or signs. More serious reactions such as hypotension, laryngeal edema, or asthma require appropriate treatment, and if desensitization is continued, the dose should be decreased by at least 10-fold and withheld until the patient is stable.[39]

Once desensitized, the patient's treatment with penicillin must not lapse or the risk of an allergic reaction increases. If the patient requires a β-lactam antibiotic in the future and still remains skin test-positive to penicillin reagents, desensitization would be required again.

Several patients have been maintained on long-term, low-dose penicillin therapy (usually bid-tid) to sustain a chronic state of desensitization. Such individuals usually require chronic desensitization because of continuous occupationally related exposures to β-lactam drugs.[43,44]

ALLERGY TO OTHER β-LACTAM ANTIBIOTICS

Cephalosporins

Like penicillin, cephalosporins possess a β-lactam ring, but the five-member thiazolidine ring is replaced by the six-member dihydrothiazine ring (Fig. 1). Shortly after the cephalosporins came into clinical use, allergic reactions including anaphylaxis were reported, and the question of cross-reactivity between cephalosporins and penicillins was raised.[45] Complicating matters, the early cephalosporin antibiotics were contaminated with trace amounts of penicillin,[46] potentially leading to overestimates of the degree of cross-reactivity. Nevertheless, studies in both animals and man have clearly demonstrated cross-reactivity between penicillins and the cephalosporins using immuno- and bioassays to evaluate IgG, IgM, and IgE antibodies.[47–49]

When patients with positive skin tests to any penicillin reagents are skin tested with native cephalosporins (relevant degradation products are unknown), approximately 50 percent are positive,[31,50] but some of these studies used concentrations of cephalosporins above 1 mg/ml, which tends to give irritative, false-positive reactions in the skin. Very few cephalosporin skin test-positive individuals have been challenged with cephalosporins to allow estimation of the predictive value of a positive skin test. Small numbers of penicillin skin test-positive patients have been treated with cephalosporin antibiotics without allergic reactions.[51,52] Primary cephalosporin allergy in non-penicillin-allergic patients has been reported, but the exact incidence is not clear.[53,54]

The incidence of clinically relevant cross-reactivity between the penicillins and the cephalosporins is probably small, but rare cases of life-threatening anaphylactic cross-reactivity have occurred. There is no proven test to predict cephalosporin hypersensitivity. Patients with positive skin tests to any penicillin reagents probably should not receive cephalosporin antibiotics unless alternative drugs are clearly less desirable. If cephalosporin drugs are to be used, they should be administered with caution using a modified desensitization protocol.

Monobactams

The monobactams are a new group of β-lactam antibiotics that contain a monocyclic ring structure rather than the bicyclic structure of the penicillins and cephalosporins (Fig. 2). In animal studies, aztreonam, a monobactam prototype, showed negligible cross-reactivity with either benzylpenicillin or cephalothin.[55] Skin tests with aztreonam determinants analogous to the major and minor penicillin determinants were undertaken in patients with positive skin tests to penicillin; these tests also failed to demonstrate appreciable cross-reactivity between penicillin and aztreonam.[56] Out of 72 penicillin-allergic patients, 4 showed weak skin test responses to one or more aztreonam reagents.[56,57] In a subsequent trial, 20 patients with positive penicillin skin tests were treated with therapeutic doses of aztreonam, and none had IgE-mediated reactions.[57] Taken together, these data suggest weak cross-reactivity between aztreonam and other β-lactam antibiotics and indicate that aztreonam may be safely administered to most if not all penicillin-allergic subjects. Preliminary studies also suggest that the immunogenicity of aztreonam appears to be lower than penicillins and cephalosporins.[55]

Carbapenems

Another new class of β-lactam antibiotics are the carbapenems, of which imipenem is the prototype. Like penicillin, this class of β-lactams has a bicyclic nucleus containing a β-lactam ring and an adjacent five-membered ring (Fig. 1). Recent studies showed that 9 of 20 penicillin skin test-positive patients had positive skin reactions to analogous imipenem determinants, suggesting appreciable cross-reactivity and indicating the prudence of withholding carbapenems from penicillin skin test-positive patients.[58]

REFERENCES

1. Gorevic PD. Drug-induced autoimmune disease. In: Kaplan A, ed. Allergy. New York: Churchill Livingston; 1985:480.
2. Schwartz HJ, Sher TH. Anaphylaxis to penicillin in a frozen dinner. Ann Allergy. 1984;52:342–3.
3. Parker CW. Drug therapy (first of three parts). N Engl J Med. 1975;292:511.
4. Gell PGH, Coombs RRA. Classification of allergic reactions responsible for clinical hypersensitivity and disease. In: Gell PGH, Coombs RRA, Hachmann PJ, eds. Clinical Aspects of Immunology. Oxford: Blackwell Scientific Publications; 1975:761–82.
5. Plaut M, Lichtenstein LM. Cellular and chemical basis of the allergic inflammatory response. In: Middleton E Jr, Reed CE, Ellis EF, eds. Allergy: Principles and Practice. St. Louis: CV Mosby; 1983:119–46.
6. Idsoe O, Guthe T, Willcox RR, et al. Nature and extent of penicillin side-reactions, with particular reference to fatalities from anaphylactic shock. Bull World Health Org. 1968;38:159–88.
7. Jacobs RL, Geoffrey WR Jr, Fournier DC, et al. Potentiated anaphylaxis in patients with drug-induced beta-adrenergic blockade. J Allergy Clin Immunol. 1981;68:125–7.
8. Shmunes E, Taylor JS, Petz LD, et al. Immunologic reactions in penicillin factory workers. Ann Allergy. 1976;36:313.
9. Levine B. Skin rashes with penicillin therapy: current management. N Engl J Med. 1972;286:42.
10. Shapiro S, Siskin V, Slone D, et al. Drug rash with ampicillin and other penicillins. Lancet. 1969; 2:7628.
11. Arndt KA, Jick H. Rates of cutaneous reactions to drugs. A report from the Boston Collaborative Drug Surveillance Program. JAMA. 1976;235:918–22.
12. Kerns DL, Shira JE, Go S, et al. Ampicillin rash in children. Relationship to penicillin allergy and infectious mononucleosis. Am J Dis Child. 1973;125:187.
13. Galpin JE, Chow AW, Yoshikawa TT, et al. "Pseudoanaphylactic" reactions from inadvertent infusion of procaine penicillin G. Ann Intern Med. 1974;81:358.
14. Levine BB. Immunologic mechanisms of penicillin allergy. A haptenic model system for the study of allergic diseases of man. N Engl J Med. 1987;275:1115.
15. Eisen HN. Hypersensitivity to simple chemicals. In: Lawrence HS, ed. Cellular and Humoral Aspects of the Hypersensitive States. New York: PB Hoeber, 1959.
16. Levine BB. Immunochemical mechanisms involved in penicillin hypersensitivity in experimental animals and in human beings. Fed Proc. 1965;24:45.

16a. Lee M, Sullivan T. Facilitated haptenation of human proteins by penicillin (Abstract). J Allergy Clin Immunol. 1989;83:255.

17. Parker CW. The immunochemical basis for penicillin allergy. Postgrad Med J. 1964;40:141–55.
18. Levine BB, Redmond AP. Minor haptenic determinant-specific reagins of penicillin hypersensitivity in man. Int Arch Allergy. 1969;35:445–55.
19. Levine BB, Redmond AP, Fellner MJ, et al. Penicillin allergy and the heterogeneous immune responses of man to benzylpenicillin. J Clin Invest. 1966;45:1895.

20. Sogn DD. Prevention of allergic reactions to penicillin. J Allergy Clin Immunol. 1987;78:1051.
21. Sogn DD. Penicillin allergy. J Allergy Clin Immunol. 1984;74:589.
22. Adkinson NF Jr. Risk factors for drug allergy. J Allergy Clin Immunol. 1984;74:567–72.
23. Sullivan TJ. Dehaptenation of albumin substituted with benzylpenicillin G determinants (Abstract). J Allergy Clin Immunol. 1988;81:222.
24. Sullivan TJ, Yecies LD, Shatz GS, et al. Desensitization of patients allergic to penicillin using orally administered beta-lactam antibiotics. J Allergy Clin Immunol. 1982;69:275–82.
25. Adkinson NF Jr, Wheeler B. Risk factors for IgE-dependent reactions to penicillin. In: Kerr JW, Ganderton MA, eds. XI International Congress of Allergology and Clinical Immunology. London: Macmillan; 1983;55–9.
26. Wicher K, Reisman RE, Arbesman CE. Allergic reaction to penicillin present in milk. JAMA. 1969;208:143–5.
27. Wicher K, Reisman RE. Anaphylactic reaction to penicillin (or penicillin-like substance) in a soft drink. J Allergy Clin Immunol. 1980;66:155–7.
28. Weiss ME, Adkinson NF Jr. Immediate hypersensitivity reactions to penicillin and related antibiotics. Clin Allergy. 1988;18:515–40.
29. Levine BB, Zolov DM. Prediction of penicillin allergy by immunological tests. J Allergy. 1969;43:231.
30. Warrington RJ, Simons FER, Ho HW, et al. Diagnosis of penicillin allergy by skin testing: the Manitoba experience. CMA J. 1978;11:787.
31. Sullivan TJ, Wedner HJ, Shatz GS, et al. Skin testing to detect penicillin allergy. J Allergy Clin Immunol. 1981;68:171–80.
32. Chandra RK, Joglekar SA, Tomas E. Penicillin allergy: antipenicillin IgE antibodies and immediate hypersensitivity skin reactions employing major and minor determinants of penicillin. Arch Dis Child. 1980;55:857–60.
33. Adkinson NF Jr, Spence M, Wheeler B. Randomized clinical trial of routine penicillin skin testing (Abstract). J Allergy Clin Immunol. 1984;73:163.
34. Adkinson NF Jr. Tests for immunological drug reactions. In: Rose NF, Friedman H, eds. Manual of Clinical Immunology. Washington, DC: American Society for Microbiology; 1986:692–7.
35. Gorevic PD, Levine BB. Desensitization of anaphylactic hypersensitivity specific for the penicilloate minor determinant of penicillin and carbenicillin. J Allergy Clin Immunol. 1981;68:267–72.
36. Sullivan TJ. Penicillin allergy. In: Lichtenstein LM, Fauci A, eds. Current Therapy in Allergy. Philadelphia: BC Decker, 1985:57.
37. Mathews KP, Hemphill FM, Lovell RG, et al. A controlled study on the use of parenteral and oral antihistamines in preventing penicillin reactions. J Allergy. 1956;27:1.
38. Sciple GW, Knox JM, Montgomery CH. Incidence of penicillin reactions after an antihistaminic simultaneously administered parenterally. N Engl J Med. 1959;261:1123.
39. Adkinson NF Jr. Penicillin allergy. In: Lichtenstein LM, Fauci A, eds. Current Therapy in Allergy, Immunology and Rheumatology. Ontario, Canada: BS Decker; 1983:57–62.
40. Stark BJ, Earl HS, Gross GN, et al. Acute and chronic desensitization of penicillin-allergic patients using oral penicillin. J Allergy Clin Immunol. 1987;79:523–32.
41. Earl HS, Sullivan TJ. Acute desensitization of a patient with cystic fibrosis allergic to both beta-lactam and aminoglycoside antibiotics. J Allergy Clin Immunol. 1987;79:477–83.
42. Graybill JR, Sande MA, Reinarz JA, et al. Controlled penicillin anaphylaxis leading to desensitization. South Med J. 1974;67:62–4.
43. Naclerio R, Mizrahi EA, Adkinson NF Jr. Immunologic observations during desensitization and maintenance of clinical tolerance to penicillin. J Allergy Clin Immunol. 1983;71:294–301.
44. O'Driscoll BJ. Desensitization of nurses allergic to penicillin. Br Med J. 1955;2:473.
45. Grieco MH. Cross-allergenicity of the penicillins and the cephalosporins. Arch Intern Med. 1967;119:141.
46. Pedersen-Bjergaard J. Cephalothin in the treatment of penicillin sensitive patients. Acta Allergol. 1967;XXII:299–306.
47. Petz L. Immunologic cross-reactivity between penicillins and cephalosporins: A review. J Infect Dis. 1978;137:S74.
48. Shibata K, Atsumi T, Itorivchi Y, et al. Immunological cross-reactivities of cephalothin and its related compounds with benzylpenicillin (penicillin G). Nature. 1966;212:491.
49. Abraham GN, Petz LD, Fudenberg HH. Immunohaematological cross-allergenicity between penicillin and cephalothin in humans. Clin Exp Immunol. 1968;3:343–57.
50. Assem ESK, Vickers MR. Tests for penicillin allergy in man. II. The immunological cross-reaction between penicillins and cephalosporins. Immunology 1964;27:255.
51. Saxon A. Immediate hypersensitivity reactions to beta-lactam antibiotics. Rev Infect Dis. 1983;5:S368.
52. Solley GO, Gleich GJ, Van Dellen RG. Penicillin allergy: clinical experience with a battery of skin-test reagents. J Allergy Clin Immunol. 1982;69:238–44.
53. Abraham GN, Petz LD, Fudenberg HH. Cephalothin hypersensitivity associated with anti-cephalothin antibodies. Int Arch Allergy. 1968;34:65–74.
54. Ong R, Sullivan T. Detection and characterization of human IgE to cephalosporin determinants (Abstract). J Allergy Clin Immunol 1988;81:222.
55. Adkinson NF Jr, Swabb EA, Sugerman AA. Immunology of the monobactam aztreonam. Antimicrob Agents Chemother. 1984;25:93–7.
56. Saxon A, Hassner A, Swabb EA, et al. Lack of cross-reactivity between aztreonam, a monobactam antibiotic, and penicillin in penicillin-allergic subjects. J Infect Dis. 1984;149:16–22.
57. Adkinson NF Jr, Wheeler B, Swabb EA. Clinical tolerance of themonobactam aztreonam in penicillin allergic subjects (Abstract WS-26-4). Presented at the 14th International Congress of Chemotherapy, June 23–28, 1985, Kyoto, Japan.
58. Saxon A, Beall GN, Rohr AS, et al. Immediate hypersensitivity reactions to beta-lactam antibiotics. Ann Intern Med. 1987;107:204–215.

22. AMINOGLYCOSIDES AND SPECTINOMYCIN: AMINOCYCLITOLS

PAUL S. LIETMAN

Since the introduction of streptomycin in the mid-1940s, one or another of the aminoglycosides has been a mainstay in our therapeutic armamentarium. Their bactericidal activity against aerobic gram-negative bacilli, their coverage of *Pseudomonas* species, and their antitubercular activity are their three most acclaimed attributes. However, their dose-related toxicity is a major consideration, limiting their dosage and making them prime targets for competition by other, and presumably safer, classes of antibiotics. Nevertheless, they continue to be widely used in serious infections.

HISTORY

Waksman and colleagues derived streptomycin from *Streptomyces griseus* in 1943. This drug was used for tuberculosis but resistance rapidly emerged when used alone. In 1949 neomycin was isolated from *Streptomyces fradiae*. The agent proved to be too toxic for systemic administration. Kanamycin was isolated by Japanese investigators in 1957 and became the dominant aminoglycoside until its replacement by newer agents, including gentamicin, tobramycin, netilmicin, and amikacin. [Fig. 1]

STRUCTURES

The family of aminoglycoside antibiotics is defined by the presence of two or more aminosugars linked by glycosidic bonds to an aminocyclitol ring.[1–3] The six-member aminocyclitol ring is either streptidine (as in streptomycin) or 2-deoxystreptamine (as in neomycin, kanamycin, gentamicin, tobramycin, amikacin, and netilmicin). Spectinomycin is often included as a member of the family, although it contains no aminosugar and no glycosidic bond. Since spectinomycin does contain an aminocyclitol ring, as do the aminoglycosides, a general term that includes both aminoglycosides and spectinomycin is *aminocyclitol antibiotics*. However, the term *aminoglycoside* is sanctioned by common usage.

Streptomycin, neomycin, kanamycin, and tobramycin have each been isolated from a different species of *Streptomyces*, whereas the gentamicins and netilmicin have been isolated from *Micromonospora* species. The spelling of gentamicin and netilmicin with -micin rather than -mycin denotes this difference in origin. The two newest aminoglycosides, amikacin and netilmicin, are semisynthetic aminoglycosides since they are both artificial derivatives of naturally occurring aminoglycosides. Amikacin is the 1-*N*-hydroxyaminobutyric acid derivative of kanamycin A, and netilmicin is the 1-*N*-ethyl derivative of si-

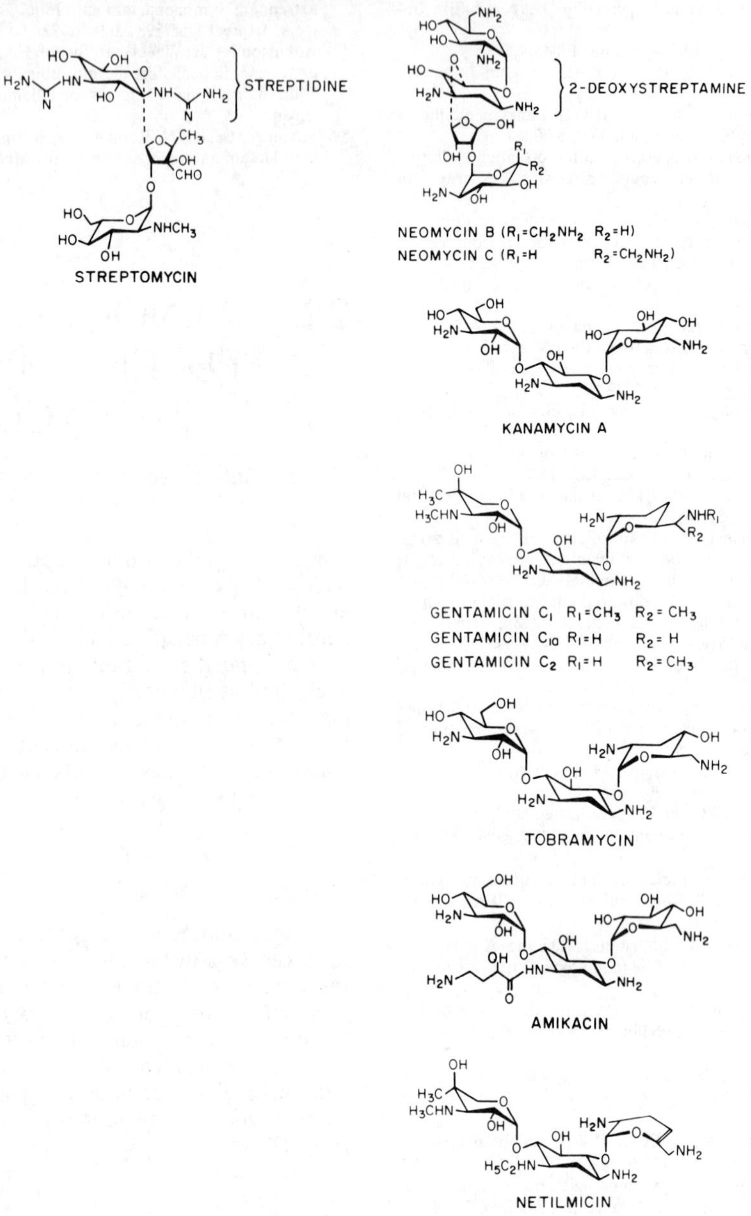

FIG. 1. Structures of aminoglycosides.

somicin, a naturally occurring aminoglycoside derived from a *Micromonospora* species.[4]

The structure–activity relationships of the aminoglycosides are incompletely understood, but the importance of the several hydroxyl and amino groups attached to the various rings is established by the loss of antibacterial activity when these groups are modified, either by synthetic chemists or by numerous bacterial enzymes.[4,5] Numerous intriguing similarities between aminoglycosides and polyamines such as spermine and spermidine suggest that aminoglycosides might be viewed as unusual polyamines with respect to their interactions with both bacteria and humans.

The groups of aminoglycosides differ from one another in the nature of the aminosugars that are linked to the central aminocyclitol ring. Structures of the aminoglycosides currently marketed in the United States are shown in Figure 1.

Although most of the aminoglycosides are unique chemical entities, gentamicin consists of a mixture of roughly equal amounts of three individual components, gentamicin C_1, C_{1a}, and C_2, and neomycin consists of roughly equal amounts of neomycin B and neomycin C. The inherent difficulties in separating the closely related gentamicins and neomycins have accounted for the inclusion of two or three components in the commercial formulations of each.

INTERACTIONS WITH MICROBES

Mechanism of Action

The precise biochemical mechanism of action of the aminoglycosides remains enigmatic in spite of an enormous amount of sophisticated attention. The difficulty lies in an inability to correlate the known biochemical effects of aminoglycosides with their lethal action. Aminoglycosides clearly inhibit bacterial protein synthesis, and this effect appears to be a necessary component of the lethal event. However, inhibition of bacterial protein synthesis is not a sufficient explanation for aminoglycoside lethality, and a second target for aminoglycoside effect appears to be necessary. The second target has remained elusive.[6–10]

Aminoglycosides inhibit protein synthesis after interacting

with one or more ribosomal binding sites. The interactions appear to be specifically localized to the interface between the smaller ribosomal subunit and the larger ribosomal subunit, an area that includes individual proteins of the smaller ribosomal unit (S3, S4, S5, and S12), as well as at least one protein of the larger ribosomal subunit (L6).[10–14] Streptomycin binds specifically, rapidly, tightly, and reversibly in a 1:1 stoichiometric ratio with the smaller 30s ribosomal subunit.[15,16] The binding of streptomycin is dependent on the S12 protein, although the actual binding is not to this protein but to an adjacent area in the vicinity of S3 and S5.[17,18] The other aminoglycosides that have been studied (including neomycin, kanamycin, gentamicin, and tobramycin) appear to bind to multiple ribosomal binding sites on both the larger and smaller ribosomal subunits and fail to compete with streptomycin binding to the smaller subunit.[15] Thus the exact site of aminoglycoside binding may differ among the aminoglycosides, and there appear to be at least two different types of ribosomal binding, one unique to streptomycin and one shared by other aminoglycosides.

The consequences of the interactions of aminoglycosides with ribosomes are numerous.[7,8] The two best documented consequences are the inhibition of protein synthesis and an infidelity in correctly reading the genetic code.

Streptomycin prevents the maintenance of polysomal function by stimulating polysome breakdown to monosomes, thereby precluding effective peptide bond formation and chain elongation.[19] These "streptomycin monosomes" dissociate into ribosomal subunits more slowly than do normally released monosomes.[20] Furthermore, "streptomycin monosomes" may be considered as abortive initiation complexes, since effective initiation cannot occur.[20–22] The effects of the deoxystreptamine-containing aminoglycosides on protein synthesis are less well understood. In general, there is less of an effect of these aminoglycosides on protein synthesis and more of an effect on the fidelity of reading the genetic code.[10]

The effects of aminoglycosides on the correct reading of the genetic code have also received considerable attention. The localization of interactions to the area of the interface between the smaller ribosomal subunit and the larger ribosomal subunit appears quite relevant to the fidelity with which the genetic code is read. This area is believed to consist of messenger RNA (mRNA) binding sites and aminoacyl transfer RNA (tRNA) acceptor sites. The faithful translation of the RNA depends on the error-free interaction between ribosomes, RNA, and the anticodon associated with each incoming aminoacyl tRNA.[10–13] The identification of ribosomal protein L6 as a protein involved with the fidelity of codon–anticodon recognition and its function in terms of determining aminoglycoside sensitivity or resistance suggests an important role for this protein in the process of aminoglycoside-induced misreading of the genetic code.[12] As a result of faulty codon–anticodon recognition, "fraudulent" proteins and proteins of abnormal length are synthesized in the presence of aminoglycosides. These effects of aminoglycosides are less prominent with streptomycin and more prominent with deoxystreptamine-containing members of the family.

Unfortunately, the relationship between either of the two prominent ribosomal effects of aminoglycosides and aminoglycoside lethality remains inconclusive.[7,8,10] Other antibacterial agents inhibit protein synthesis at least as effectively as do the aminoglycosides and yet fail to cause a lethal event, that is, produce only bacteriostasis. Thus the inhibition of protein synthesis appears insufficient to explain the bactericidal effect of aminoglycosides. Similarly, the production of "fraudulent" proteins correlates imperfectly with lethality. Based on the inadequacy of either of these two ribosomal effects to explain lethality, other targets for aminoglycoside action must be considered. Hancock has recently provided a thoughtful review of the issues involved in identifying the second target for aminoglycoside lethality.[7] Its nature, however, remains speculative.[8,10]

Although the precise biochemical events leading to aminoglycoside lethality remain to be divined, it is clear that an essential element in the process leading to lethality is the transport of aminoglycosides from the external milieu across the cell membrane and into the interior of the bacterium.[6,7,11,23,24] Aminoglycoside transport by bacteria results in the accumulation of aminoglycosides inside bacterial cells to concentrations far in excess of the external concentration. Ineffective transport precludes aminoglycoside lethality.

The transport process is energy-dependent, and the energetics of transport depend on an electrochemical gradient of protons (designated Δu_{H+}) that is generated by proton extrusion during respiration or adenosine 5′-triphosphate (ATP) hydrolysis.[9,23,25,26] The electrochemical gradient of protons is composed of both an electrical potential (designated $\Delta\Psi$) and a chemical component (designated ΔpH), which represents the difference in proton concentrations across a membrane. The transport of aminoglycosides is well correlated with the electrical potential ($\Delta\Psi$), and the effects of several situations in which aminoglycoside transport is impaired can be rationalized by considering this component of the electrochemical gradient of protons.[25,26] For example, anaerobiasis is associated with a low magnitude of $\Delta\Psi$ and impaired aminoglycoside transport, a low external pH is associated with a diminution of $\Delta\Psi$ and impaired aminoglycoside transport, an increase in the osmolarity of the environment is associated with a lower $\Delta\Psi$ and less aminoglycoside transport, and bacterial mutants that are unable to maintain a proton gradient are unable to generate a $\Delta\Psi$ or transport aminoglycosides. In each of these situations in which the electrical potential ($\Delta\Psi$) is diminished, aminoglycoside transport is impaired, and relative aminoglycoside resistance is seen.

The transport of aminoglycosides also appears to involve a transporter molecule to which the aminoglycosides bind during their internalization. Although the nature of this putative carrier molecule has not been defined, it seems likely that both divalent calcium or magnesium and polyvalent polyamines bind to the same carrier.[6,7,24,27] This competition could explain the fact that high external concentrations of calcium, magnesium, or polyamines prevent aminoglycoside transport. The interactions with calcium and magnesium are particularly relevant to the creation of appropriate and consistent media for the in vitro assessment of minimum inhibitory or minimum bacteriocidal concentrations (MIC or MBC) of aminoglycosides.

Aminoglycoside transport is also blocked by low and clinically relevant concentrations of chloramphenicol.[24,28] Thus, in the presence of chloramphenicol, the aminoglycosides will be ineffective, at least in those organisms sensitive to chloramphenicol. Whether or not the same phenomenon exists in bacteria resistant to chloramphenicol is unknown.

Mechanisms of Resistance

The usefulness of aminoglycosides depends on their selective toxicity to bacteria as opposed to eucaryotic (including human) cells. This selective toxicity to bacterial cells or, conversely, this selective resistance of eucaryotic cells is due to the inability of the cells of most human organs to transport aminoglycosides and to the failure of aminoglycosides to interact with eucaryotic cytosoline ribosomes.[10] Although mitochondrial ribosomes are sensitive to aminoglycosides, mitochondria cannot transport aminoglycosides, and mitochondrial protein synthesis is probably unaffected in vivo, even in the few tissues (such as the proximal renal tubule and cochlea) that can internalize aminoglycosides.

Bacterial resistance to aminoglycosides can occur by at least three different mechanisms: ribosomal resistance, ineffective transport, or enzymologic modification of the aminoglycoside.[29–31]

Ribosomal resistance to streptomycin is dependent on one specific aberrant protein (S12) in the smaller ribosomal subunit. A mutation in S12 leads to loss of ribosomal binding of streptomycin and to very high levels of resistance in a single mutational event.[17] At a clinical level, this type of streptomycin resistance is very uncommon in gram-negative bacilli. Ribosomal resistance can also exist for the deoxystreptamine group of aminoglycosides. In contrast to the ribosomal resistance to streptomycin, however, this resistance requires multiple mutational events before high-level resistance is seen, suggesting that more than one site must be altered.[12–14] This type of ribosomal resistance is also exceedingly uncommon clinically.

Resistance due to ineffective transport appears to be uncommon in most geographic areas, although a few centers have reported that this is the most common mechanism for aminoglycoside resistance. Genetic defects associated with ineffective transport can be localized to any of numerous proteins that have in common an involvement in bacterial electron transport or adenosine triphosphatase (ATPase) activity.[6,7,9] An inability to maintain the requisite electrical potential appears to be pivotal to each of the known mutants. It is fortunate that this mechanism for aminoglycoside resistance is uncommon, since these transport mutants are defective in the transport of all aminoglycosides.

The most common mechanism for aminoglycoside resistance involves the conjugation of the aminoglycoside with one of three groups, an acetyl group, an adenyl group, or a phosphoryl group, thereby rendering the aminoglycoside inactive.[29–32] The conjugation, in each case, is catalyzed by an enzyme produced in the bacterial cell from information contained in an extrachromasomal plasmid. Plasmid-mediated resistance is particularly worrisome because the responsible plasmids can infect other gram-negative bacteria, even of different species, and because information for multiple-resistance mechanisms involving other antibacterial classes can be simultaneously introduced into bacterial cells. A very large number of individual enzymes has been identified, each of which catalyzes the addition of one of the above groups onto a specific site on one or more than one aminoglycoside. The overlapping substrate specificities of the individual inactivating enzymes leads to a bewildering array of possibilities for cross-resistance to several aminoglycosides.[29–32] For example, an enzyme capable of acetylating an aminoglycoside at the 6′ position (i.e., the 6 position of one of the aminosugar rings adjacent to the deoxystreptamine ring) can inactivate neomycin, kanamycin, tobramycin, amikacin, and netilmicin but not streptomycin or gentamicin. An enzyme capable of phosphorylating the 3′ position, however, can inactivate only neomycin and kanamycin. To complicate the picture even further, isoenzymes have been identified for many of the specific enzymatic functions. Thus there may be several unique isoenzymes, each capable of catalyzing the addition of an acetyl group to the 6 prime position of an aminoglycoside but each possessing different substrate specificity so that one might inactivate kanamycin where as another might inactivate tobramycin. Thus an incredible multiplicity of possibilities exists for cross-resistance to multiple aminoglycosides.

The prevalence of individual aminoglycoside-inactivating enzymes varies widely with respect to both place and time. Thus, whereas 2″-adenyltransferase, 3-acetyltransferase, and 6′-acetyltransferase are predominant in that order in the United States, 6′-acetyltransferase is most common in Japan, and 3-acetyltransferase is most common in Chile.[31] Further geographic variability exists between hospitals in any one country, state, or city and even between wards in one hospital. The reasons for this variability have remained an enigma. A simple relationship to patterns of aminoglycoside usage does not exist. This may be explicable in part by the overlapping of aminoglycoside resistance generated by each of the inactivating enzymes. Thus the prevalence of resistance to amikacin might be expected to be lessened by the infrequent use of amikacin and the consequent diminished genetic pressure for the emergence of amikacin-inactivating enzymes. This may well be partially negated by the continued use of other aminoglycosides that can also be inactivated by the same enzymes that are capable of inactivating amikacin. For example, the continued use of kanamycin, tobramycin, or netilmicin should provide genetic pressure for the emergence of 6′-acetylating enzyme; the continued use of kanamycin or tobramycin should provide pressure for the emergence of a 4′-adenylating enzyme; and the continued use of any of the available deoxystreptamine-containing aminoglycosides should provide pressure for the emergence of a 2″-phosphorylating enzyme.

At a clinical level, several conclusions are justified by the current information on aminoglycoside resistance.

First, we cannot predict the precise enzymologic mechanism responsible for aminoglycoside resistance in an individual patient. Although resistance patterns may be known for a particular time and place, these patterns can be helpful only in the selection of an initial aminoglycoside to be used before the determination of the specific sensitivity of the individual patient's pathogen.

Second, it is seldom feasible to determine the precise enzymologic mechanism responsible for aminoglycoside resistance, and we must rely on more general tests of sensitivity and resistance such as the MIC or MBC.

Third, it may be futile to reserve an individual aminoglycoside for future use in hopes of delaying the emergence of resistance, since the continued use of other aminoglycosides that are inactivated by the same enzyme may provide sufficient genetic pressure for the emergence of the enzyme that can inactivate the reserved drug.

Sepectrum of In Vitro Activity

The spectrum of in vitro activity of the aminoglycosides includes primarily aerobic and facultative gram-negative bacilli and *Staphylococcus aureus*. A representative summary of MICs at which 75 or 100 percent of the strains of various bacteria are sensitive in one laboratory is shown in Table 1.[33] Some hospitals have more aminoglycoside resistance than that shown in the table. In general, aminoglycosides are not often used for known staphylococcal infections since a number of alternative antibiotics has considerably more data backing clinical efficacy. Aminoglycosides are considered excellent choices for serious infections caused by aerobic or facultative gram-negative bacilli and especially those caused by *Pseudomonas aeruginosa*. For these latter infections, in spite of some in vitro differences in MICs, there is no clinical evidence to substantiate an advantage for anyone of the aminoglycosides in treating an infection due to a susceptible organism. Thus, although the percentage of resistant strains in a given locale may dictate the most rational initial aminoglycoside to be used, equivalent effectiveness should be expected from any of this group in treating a patient with a sensitive organism. Nevertheless, differences in in vitro activity do exist with respect to some bacteria. Streptomycin has the greatest in vitro activity against *Mycobacterium tuberculosis*, is considered the drug of choice for *Francisella tularensis* and *Yersinia pestis*, and is often used in brucellosis.[34] Streptomycin is seldom used for aerobic or facultative gram-negative bacillary infections due to the frequency of resistance.[34] Kanamycin is limited in its spectrum, compared with the other 2-deoxystreptamine-containing aminoglycosides, because of the common resistance of *P. aeruginosa*.[34] Kanamycin is also inactivated by a large number of the plasmid-mediated enzymes, and consequently kanamycin resistance among other gram-negative bacilli is prevalent in many locales. Gentamicin and tobramycin share very similar in vitro profiles, although gentamicin is somewhat more potent in vitro against *Serratia* species and tobramycin somewhat more potent against *P. aeruginosa*.[33] However, these minor differences in in vitro potencies

TABLE 1. In Vitro Susceptibility of Various Bacteria to Five Aminoglycosides[a]

	Kanamycin		Gentamicin		Tobramycin		Amikacin		Netilmicin	
Organism (No.)	*75%*	*100%*	*75%*	*100%*	*75%*	*100%*	*75%*	*100%*	*75%*	*100%*
Staphylococcus aureus (25)	1.6	3.1	≤0.2	0.8	≤0.2	6.2	1.6	3.1	0.4	0.8
Enterococci (20)	12.5	>50	3.1	6.2	6.2	12.5	25	50	3.1	6.2
Neisseria gonorrhoeae (20)	12.5	25	6.2	12.5	6.2	12.5	25	50	6.2	12.5
Escherichia coli (40)	12.5	>50	1.6	6.2	3.1	12.5	6.2	12.5	1.6	6.2
Klebsiella sp. (20)	3.1	>50	0.4	1.6	0.4	1.6	1.6	6.2	0.4	0.8
Enterobacter sp. (40)	3.1	>50	0.8	1.6	1.6	6.2	1.6	6.2	0.4	6.2
Citrobacter sp. (15)	12.5	25	1.6	6.2	1.6	1.6	3.1	6.2	0.8	3.1
Serratia sp. (15)	3.1	6.2	1.6	1.6	3.1	6.2	3.1	6.2	1.6	3.2
Proteus mirabilis (20)	3.1	25	1.6	3.1	1.6	3.1	6.2	12.5	1.6	3.1
Morganella morganii (29)	3.1	6.2	0.8	0.8	0.8	1.6	3.1	6.2	0.8	1.6
Proteus vulgaris (6)	6.2	6.2	1.6	1.6	1.6	3.1	3.1	6.2	0.8	0.8
Providencia rettgeri (6)	3.1	3.1	3.1	6.2	3.1	6.2	1.6	1.6	12.5	12.5
Providencia stuartii (8)	1.6	3.1	3.1	6.2	3.1	12.5	3.1	3.1	3.1	12.5
Pseudomonas aeruginosa (40)	ND	ND	0.8	3.1	≤0.2	1.6	0.8	12.5	0.8	6.2

[a] MIC (μg/ml) for percent of strains indicated.
(Data from Sanders et al.[33])

have not been demonstrated to correlate with greater in vivo effectiveness. Since gentamicin and tobramycin are both susceptible to the same enzymologic modifications (save for a few uncommon enzymes that can inactivate gentamicin and not tobramycin), the percentage of resistant strains to these two aminoglycosides is also quite similar.[33] Amikacin has a clear advantage over gentamicin or tobramycin as a result of its resistance to many of the common plasmid-mediated enzymes. Consequently, the percentage of strains susceptible to amikacin is significantly greater for amikacin compared with gentamicin or tobramycin.[33] The in vitro potency of amikacin with respect to many of the gram-negative bacilli is less than that of gentamicin or tobramycin, but the dose that is allowed by its lesser toxicity (i.e., three to four times the dose of gentamicin or tobramycin) compensates for this lesser potency. Again, there is no clinical evidence to suggest lesser or greater effectiveness against sensitive bacteria. Netilmicin shares the spectrum of gentamicin and tobramycin in general. However, netilmicin is resistant to aminoglycoside-adenylating enzymes and as a result some *Escherichia coli*, *Klebsiella*, *Enterobacter*, and *Citrobacter* isolates that are resistant to gentamicin remain sensitive to netilmicin.[32] Gentamicin-resistant *Serratia*, *Proteus*, *Providencia*, and *Pseudomonas* strains are, however, usually also netilmicin-resistant.[35]

In vitro sensitivity and resistance to aminoglycosides is usually determined as a minimum inhibitory concentration. Since the minimum bacteriocidal concentration is nearly always close to the MIC, there is no advantage associated with this more cumbersome technique. The MIC is most frequently assessed by a disk diffusion method but may be more accurately quantified by either agar dilution or broth dilution methods.[34] For the disk diffusion method, standards have been set for the aminoglycoside content of the individual disks, zone diameters, and agar composition.[36] Standardization of agar diffusion and broth dilution methods is also important, since several variables in the media can significantly influence the MIC, especially pH and cation concentration.[37] These variables affect the MIC determinations primarily by affecting transport of the aminoglycosides into the bacteria. An acid pH of the media will provide erroneously high MICs, whereas an alkaline pH will give an erroneously low MIC. The pH of the agar or broth should be kept at pH 7.3–7.5. High concentrations of cations, especially calcium, magnesium, and sodium, yield erroneously high MICs, especially with *P. aeruginosa*.[37] Standardization of the calcium salt concentration at about 50 μg/ml and the magnesium salt concentration at about 25 μg/ml has been proposed.[37] The number of bacteria used should also be standardized, although the "inoculum effect" is far less important with aminoglycosides than with β-lactams.[34] The relative lack of inoculum effect is attributable to the failure of aminoglycoside-inactivating enzymes to be released into the medium. Thus the concentration of aminoglycoside in the medium will remain nearly constant, even with large inocula of resistant bacteria.

Time Course of Antibacterial Effects

Each of the routine methods of determining an MIC provides a constant concentration of antibiotic adjacent to the bacterium for the entire period of incubation. Thus the MIC should be interpreted as the lowest concentration that inhibits bacterial growth *if constantly adjacent to the bacterium*.

Recent interest has focused on more sophisticated systems to assess both the in vitro effects and the in vivo effects in laboratory animals of changing concentrations of antibiotics over time.[38–55] Although these systems are not feasible for the routine definition of sensitivity and resistance to antibiotics, they contribute significantly to an understanding of the complex interrelationships between the pharmacokinetics of the antibiotic and the kinetics of bacterial growth. In these systems, with continuously changing aminoglycoside concentrations adjacent to continuously growing bacteria, there is evidence of a significant "postantibiotic effect" by aminoglycosides on *P. aeruginosa*. There is also a suggestion that a lesser, but potentially significant, "postantibiotic effect" is exerted by aminoglycosides on *E. coli* and *Klebsiella pneumoniae*.[50–52] The presence of such a "postantibiotic effect" would support the possible feasibility of longer dosing intervals (12 or even 24 hours) for aminoglycosides in man. While preliminary human studies have been compatible with both the safety and the effectiveness of a 24-hourly dosing regimen, larger clinical trials are needed to ascertain the true comparative value of such regimens compared with the existing standard regimen using an 8-hourly dosing regimen.[49]

Synergism

Aminoglycosides frequently exhibit synergism with other antibiotics. Especially noteworthy is the synergism usually found in enterococcal species between penicillin or vancomycin and the aminoglycosides.[56] The mechanism of this synergism involves the enhancement of aminoglycoside uptake into cells whose wall has been damaged by the cell wall inhibitor.[57] Numerous other synergistic combinations involving an aminoglycoside also exist.

INTERACTIONS WITH HUMANS

Pharmacokinetics

The pharmacokinetics of all of the aminoglycosides are quite similar. Subtle differences among individual members of the family may have importance with respect to the pathophysiology of their toxicities, but these minor differences are unimportant with respect to rational dosing.

Absorption. The extent of absorption of oral aminoglycosides is unpredictable but always low.[58–62] Consequently, aminoglycosides are generally considered nonabsorbable antibiotics and are occasionally used to alter the gut flora. In the presence of impaired elimination, however, even a small amount of absorbed aminoglycoside may accumulate to toxic levels.[63–66]

Absorption after intramuscular aminoglycoside administration is both complete and rapid, with maximal plasma levels achieved between 30 and 90 minutes.[67–68] Impaired tissue perfusion, as in shock, delays the absorption of intramuscular aminoglycosides.

Intravenous aminoglycoside administration is frequently used in patients with serious infections, and the dose is completely delivered to the vascular space. When the intravenous infusion lasts for 20–30 minutes, the plasma levels are similar to those achieved by intramuscular administration.

Topical aminoglycosides generally either are not absorbed or only minimally absorbed. Exceptions include patients with extensive epidermal loss due to burns or epidermolysis and patients with open wounds in which significant absorption can occur.[69,70]

Intraperitoneal or intrapleural aminoglycosides are rapidly absorbed, quickly providing plasma levels that are dependent on the concentration of drug instilled into the peritoneal or pleural fluid.[71,72] Administration of large amounts of aminoglycosides can result in very high plasma levels and toxicity.

Bladder irrigation is not associated with significant aminoglycoside absorption,[73] intratracheal or aerosolized aminoglycosides are poorly absorbed,[74,75] and intrathecal or intraventricular aminoglycosides produce negligible plasma levels.[76]

Distribution. Aminoglycosides are freely distributed in the vascular space and are relatively freely distributed in the interstitial spaces of most tissues. Although the mean aminoglycoside concentration in interstitial fluids approximates the mean plasma concentration at steady state with repetitive dosing, the peak concentrations are lower, the oscillations between peak and trough concentrations are less, and the rate of elimination is lower from interstitial fluids.[77]

Because of their size and polycationic charge, aminoglycosides cross biologic membranes that lack transport mechanisms very poorly. This accounts for their low intracellular concentrations in nearly all human tissues. An exception is the proximal renal tubular cell, which appears to have a unique transport mechanism and can concentrate aminoglycosides to levels far in excess of plasma or interstitial fluid levels.[78]

Aminoglycosides enter bronchial secretions poorly, attaining mean levels approximately 20 percent of mean plasma levels.[79] Intermittent administration produces higher peak levels in bronchial secretions than does continuous infusion, but areas under the concentration versus time curves as similar.[79,80] Neither mode of delivery produces high aminoglycoside levels in bronchial secretions, however, and the direct intratracheal administration of aminoglycosides to patients with serious gram-negative pneumonitis has been advocated on the basis of higher levels in bronchial secretions and greater clinical effectiveness.[80]

Intravenous or intramuscular administration of aminoglycosides to adults produces very low aminoglycoside levels in the cerebrospinal fluid.[76,81,82] In newborns cerebrospinal fluid levels are higher relative to plasma levels.[83] Intrathecal administration in the lumbar area produces high lumbar cerebrospinal fluid levels but poor intraventricular levels, whereas intraventricular administration produces high levels in both ventricular fluid and lumbar cerebrospinal fluid.[81] Based on these findings, intraventricular aminoglycoside administration has been proposed for gram-negative bacillary meningitis in adults.[81,82] In the newborn, intraventricular aminoglycoside administration has been shown to be no more effective and possibly more toxic than intravenous administration alone.[83]

Aminoglycoside distribution in the eye has been studied after repetitive intramuscular or continuous intravenous dosing in the rabbit. The cornea and aqueous fluids attain levels approximating serum levels, whereas entry into vitreous fluid is slow, and mean vitreous levels are only about 40 percent of serum levels over a 12-hour period.[84] Subconjunctival injection produces high aqueous fluid levels of aminoglycosides in humans.[85] However, neither systemic nor subconjunctival aminoglycoside administration in single doses produces reliable levels in the vitreous humor of humans, and intravitreal injection has been advocated in the treatment of endophthalmitis.[86]

Aminoglycosides enter the synovial fluid rather easily and achieve levels only modestly less than simultaneously measured plasma levels.[87–91]

Aminoglycosides penetrate into prostatic fluid poorly, and levels are low compared with plasma levels.[92]

Aminoglycosides do not enter saliva.[93]

The biliary concentrations of aminoglycosides are significantly less than the plasma levels.[94,95]

Urinary concentrations of aminoglycosides reach levels about 25–100 times peak plasma aminoglycoside concentrations within an hour after dosing and remain well above therapeutic levels for several days after even a single dose.[96–99] After termination of a multiple dosing regimen, urinary aminoglycoside concentrations remain above therapeutic levels for many days, with a terminal half-life of about 48–200 hours.[97–100]

Metabolism. Aminoglycosides are not metabolized by humans.

Excretion. Aminoglycosides are eliminated entirely as unchanged drugs and almost entirely from the kidneys. Less than 1 percent of a parenterally administered dose appears in the feces and none in saliva.[101,102]

Aminoglycosides are filtered by the glomerulus. Although they are negligibly protein bound, their filtration is not completely free, since their polycationic nature appears to impede filtration through the glomerular capillary wall.[103] After entering the luminal fluid of the proximal renal tubule, a small but toxicologically important portion of the total filtered aminoglycoside is reabsorbed exclusively into the proximal renal tubular cells.[78,104,105] This reabsorption appears to involve binding of the aminoglycosides to negatively charged phospholipids in the renal tubular brush border membranes, with subsequent internalization by pinocytosis.[106–110] There is no conclusive evidence for secretion of aminoglycosides into the urine. Quantitatively, most of the filtered aminoglycoside is excreted into the urine.

Overall Pharmacokinetics

The overall pharmacokinetics of aminoglycosides can be quite accurately described as a composite of contributions from absorption and three phases of elimination.[111,112] Since absorption is predictably complete and rapid after either intramuscular or intermittent intravenous administration, it is the three phases of elimination that deserve emphasis.

The three phases of aminoglycoside elimination can be considered to be related to three connected compartments in the commonly used model of the pharmacokinetic behavior of drugs or simply as mathematical components of a triexponential equation that has been found to fit the experimentally derived decay curve of plasma aminoglycoside levels versus time. Although neither of the above approaches allows the designation of anatomic or physiologic spaces for the compartments or for the components of the equation, it is clearly of practical value to consider the disposition of aminoglycosides in physiologic terms. The first (or alpha or distributive) phase of aminoglycoside elimination is made up predominantly of the process of drug distribution from the vascular space to some extravascular space. Since aminoglycosides enter most cells poorly, the extravascular space may be considered to be similar to the extracellular fluid volume. The time course of this phase can be described as having a half-life of about 15–30 minutes.[111–113] Measurement of plasma aminoglycoside levels after the end of this phase provides levels that approach the levels in interstitial fluid and avoids the rapidly changing plasma levels that occur earlier. For this reason it has been suggested that "peak" aminoglycoside levels should be drawn 30 minutes to 1 hour after the end of an intravenous infusion.[114]

The second (or beta) phase of aminoglycoside elimination involves the excretion of the drug from the plasma and simultaneously from most of the extravascular space. The time course of this beta phase is determined nearly exclusively by the glomular filtration rate, and it is this phase that is most important in terms of clinical dosing. It is also this phase that is altered by a number of clinically important factors, as discussed below. In the young healthy adult with normal renal function, this phase can be reasonably described by a small number of pharmacokinetic parameters. The volume of distribution is about 25–30 percent of body weight,[115–117] the half-life is 1.5–3.5 hours,[115–118] and the plasma clearance is about 1 ml/min/kg.[119] Each of these pharmacokinetic parameters can be altered, however, by a number of clinically important conditions, and rational dosing of the aminoglycosides must take cognizance of these alterations, which are described below.

The third (or gamma) phase of aminoglycoside elimination involves the prolonged and slow excretion of the drug from the plasma and simultaneously from a relatively small portion of an extravascular space either through the plasma space or directly into the urine. This portion of the extravascular space has been termed a *deep compartment* to distinguish it from the portion of the extravascular space that readily equilibrates with the vascular space. It has also been considered to represent primarily the kidneys, since aminoglycosides accumulate in kidney parenchymal tissue and leave very slowly. The importance of this third phase of aminoglycoside elimination has been clearly demonstrated in terms of rigorously describing the overall pharmacokinetics of aminoglycoside elimination.[111,120–122] However, the importance of this phase in terms of rational aminoglycoside dosing remains unclear. The third phase can be described in pharmacokinetic terms as having a large volume of distribution (the volume of distribution at steady state) of 45–100 percent of the body weight, a very long half-life of 35–200 hours, and a clearance of about 1 ml/min/kg.[100,101,109–111] The influence of various clinical conditions on the pharmacokinetics of the third phase has not been defined, although individual aminoglycosides appear to vary with respect to their volumes of distribution at steady state.[111,112,120–122]

Alterations with Age. The pharmacokinetics of aminoglycosides in both children and the elderly differ significantly from those in young healthy adults. The differences are attributable to known differences in glomerular function in newborns, children, and the elderly and are seen primarily as deviations during the second phase of elimination.

In the newborn the volume of distribution is considerably larger as a percentage of body weight (34–78 percent), and the half-life of the second phase is significantly prolonged (3–14 hours). Both the volume of distribution and the half-life of the second phase are inversely correlated with either gestational age or postnatal age.[123–131]

After the newborn period, infants and children have volumes of distribution that are close to those of young adults and half-lives that are shorter (.4–3 hours) than those of young adults.[123,131–141]

In the elderly the volumes of distribution are similar to those of young adults, but the half-lives are considerably longer due to decreased glomerular function with age.[142] Since the diminution in glomerular function in the elderly is not necessarily reflected in a higher serum creatinine (Cr) (due to a decrease in creatinine production in the elderly), it is important to use a calculated creatinine clearance (C_{cr}) in order to estimate the half-life or clearance of an aminoglycoside in the elderly.[143] The equation of Cockcroft and Gault is as follows:

$$C_{cr}(\text{ml/min}) = \frac{(140 - \text{age}) \times \text{weight}}{\text{Cr} \times 72}$$

The modification by Spyker and Guerrant is

$$C_{cr}(\text{ml/min}) = \frac{(140 - \text{age}) \times (1.03 - 0.053 \times \text{Cr})}{\text{Cr}}$$

The nomogram of Siersbaek-Nielson et al. is useful in calculating the creatinine clearance.[143–145] In the above equations weight is in kilograms, creatinine in milligrams per deciliter, and age in years.

Alterations with Disease States. Kidney disease with glomerular dysfunction is the most common disease state associated with altered aminoglycoside pharmacokinetics. The clearance of an aminoglycoside is linearly related to the clearance of creatinine since aminoglycosides are nearly entirely eliminated renally and their elimination rate is highly dependent on the glomerular filtration rate. A useful estimation of aminoglycoside clearance[146] is given by the following equation:

$$\text{Aminoglycoside clearance} = (C_{cr})\,(0.6) + 10$$

Since the creatinine clearance, as a measure of glomerular filtration rate, can also be calculated reasonably accurately using the equation of Cockcroft and Gault (given above), we can easily estimate the clearance of an aminoglycoside in a patient with renal disease. The volume of distribution as a percent of body weight of an aminoglycoside may be increased in patients with marked renal dysfunction.[146–148] The half-life, which is a function of the ratio of the volume of distribution to clearance, is prolonged in patients with renal disease and may in fact be somewhat longer than would be predicted on the basis of the creatinine clearance alone due to the somewhat larger volume of distribution.

In obese patients, the volume of distribution of aminoglycosides as a fraction of the total body weight is about 75 percent of that seen in nonobese patients, or about 20 percent of total body weight. The rates of elimination and half-lives, however, are similar in obese and nonobese patients.[149,150]

Conversely, in protein–calorie malnutrition (marasmus), the volume of distribution of aminoglycosides as a fraction of the total body weight is about 120 percent of that seen in well-nourished patients.[151]

Fever appears to alter aminoglycoside pharmacokinetics. Lower plasma aminoglycoside levels are found in febrile patients.[152]

In severe burns the glomerular filtration rate and consequently the rate of elimination of aminoglycosides may be markedly enhanced.[153,154]

Alterations with Other Drugs. The aminoglycosides can be inactivated by many of the β-lactam antibiotics in vitro and to a lesser extent in vivo. The inactivation occurs because a covalent bond is formed between the carboxyl group of a broken β-lactam ring and an amino group on the aminoglycoside. The reaction occurs at high molar ratios of β-lactam to aminoglycoside and is thus especially important when carbenicillin or ticarcillin is used with an aminoglycoside, since large doses of these β-lactams provide the requisite high molar ratios. Since 1 mol of β-lactam is inactivated at the same time that 1 mol of aminoglycoside is being inactivated, theoretically there should be a loss of both activities. The disproportionate number of β-lactam molecules, however, is not significantly diminished by having lost a few molecules through these interactions. The reaction occurs more readily in a protein-free setting, and therefore the reaction is more relevant to the situation in an intravenous bottle containing both drugs than to the patient containing both drugs. The rapid elimination of most β-lactams also tends to minimize the ability of the β-lactam to inactivate the aminoglycoside, since the required molar ratios of the two antibiotics exist for only a brief period in patients with normal renal function. The shortening of the half-life of the aminoglycoside in patients with renal failure may be clinically significant.

DOSING

Extensive pharmacokinetic data on aminoglycosides permit the construction of dosage regimens that will achieve and maintain plasma aminoglycoside levels within practically any desired range. Numerous dosage regimens have been proposed, and extensive and rigorous clinical trials have been conducted with a few of the proposed regimens. However, studies comparing one regimen with another with respect to both effectiveness and safety are virtually nonexistent. A dosage regimen that has been used extensively and rigorously and that has been carefully assessed with respect to both effectiveness and toxicity is presented as one approach.[114,155] Although other regimens may be equally or even more effective and equally or even less toxic, there is currently no comparative information to verify such differences.

Initiation of therapy should involve the administration of a loading dose of aminoglycoside in order to achieve therapeutic aminoglycoside plasma levels quickly. This principle is especially relevant when elimination of the aminoglycoside is delayed, since in such situations it will take many hours to achieve a plateau level unless a loading dose is given. The loading dose will be determined exclusively by the volume of distribution of the aminoglycoside and the desired maximum plasma aminoglycoside level. Considerable evidence suggests that a reasonable goal in terms of the maximum plasma aminoglycoside level is between 5 and 10 μg/ml for gentamicin, tobramycin, and netilmicin and between 20 and 40 μg/ml for kanamycin and amikacin.[156–162] Based on an average volume of distribution of 25 percent of the body weight, a loading dose of 1.5–2 mg/kg for gentamicin, tobramycin, or netilmicin or 7.5–8 mg/kg for kanamycin or amikacin will provide plasma levels of 6–8 and 30–32 μg/ml, respectively.

Several aspects of the loading dose deserve emphasis. First, the loading dose should be the same whether or not there is reason to believe that elimination will be impaired. Thus, no matter what the degree of renal dysfunction, the same loading dose should be given. Second, in calculating a loading dose, we should aim at the maximal plasma level desired, since some drug will be eliminated before the first maintenance dose and we would not choose to provide suboptimal levels during the critical initiation of aminoglycoside therapy. Third, the loading dose should be given intravenously over 20–30 minutes or intramuscularly rather than as a rapid intravenous bolus in order to minimize the risk of transient neuromuscular paralysis.

The next step is to calculate a maintenance dosage regimen, including the size of individual doses and the dosing intervals. In adult patients with normal renal function, a dose of 1.5–2 mg/kg of gentamicin, tobramycin, or netilmicin given every 8 hours or 7.5–8 mg/kg of kanamycin or amikacin given every 12 hours will provide levels that oscillate between peaks of about 8 or 32 μg/ml, respectively, and troughs of about 1 or 4 μg/ml, respectively.

In patients with diminished renal glomerular function, the total daily dose of aminoglycosides must be reduced. A convenient method of calculating the appropriate daily dose of an aminoglycoside in the presence of renal glomerular dysfunction is to multiply the usual daily dose for a patient with normal renal function by the ratio of the clearance of the drug in renal insufficiency to the clearance of the drug with normal renal function. Since the clearance of aminoglycosides is linearly related to the endogenous creatinine clearance, the ratio of the patient's creatinine clearance to normal creatinine clearance will closely approximate the ratio of aminoglycoside clearances. Thus, if the calculated creatinine clearance, taking into account the patient's age, sex, weight, and serum creatinine, is 40 ml/min/1.73 m^2, the appropriate ratio is (40 ml/min/1.73 m^2)/(100 ml/min/1.73 m^2) = 0.4, and the total daily aminoglycoside dose should be 0.4 times or 40 percent of the usual daily aminoglycoside dose. Instead of 4.5–6 mg/kg/day, the reduced dose should be 1.8–2.4 mg/kg/day.

Having derived a reduced daily maintenance dose, there are two commonly advocated methods of giving the reduced dose. One can either reduce the individual dose given at the usual dosage interval or give the usual individual dose at less frequent intervals. There is currently no evidence to support one method over the other.

It must be emphasized that any calculation of dosage reduction will be approximate and should only be used to provide an estimate of the appropriate maintenance dose. As soon as convenient (usually within 24–48 hours), plasma aminoglycoside levels should be measured and the maintenance doses adjusted to provide selected plasma levels. Plasma levels of 5–10 μg/ml 30 minutes to 1 hour after the end of an intravenous infusion over 20–30 minutes or after an intramuscular injection of gentamicin, tobramycin, or netilmicin have been associated with effectiveness and acceptibly low toxicity as have plasma levels of 20–40 μg/ml for amikacin (and presumably kanamycin).[114,155]

TOXICITY

All aminoglycosides share three principal toxicities, although there are quantitative differences among individual aminoglycosides for each of the three. The principal toxicities are neuromuscular paralysis, ototoxicity, and nephrotoxicity. Although the detailed mechanisms involved in these toxicities remain to be defined, an intriguing thread that appears to run through each involves the interactions of the polycationic aminoglycosides, polyamines, calcium, and magnesium with the polyanionic phosphatidylinositol, phosphatidylinositol diphosphate, and phosphatidylinositol triphosphate.

Neuromuscular Paralysis

The aminoglycosides are all capable of producing clinically significant neuromuscular paralysis. Although this phenomenon is rare, it is potentially quite serious.

The mechanism responsible for aminoglycoside-induced neuromuscular paralysis appears to involve both an inhibition of the presynaptic release of acetylcholine and a blockade of the postsynaptic receptor sites for acetylcholine. The presynaptic site of inhibition is dependent on the ability of an aminoglycoside to inhibit the internalization of calcium into the presynaptic region of the neuronal axon, thus preventing an event that necessarily precedes the release of acetylcholine.[163] This presynaptic effect is manifest more by neomycin or tobramycin than by streptomycin and is prevented or reversed by the provision of additional local calcium.[150–152] The postsynaptic site of blockade involves an effect on the postsynaptic receptor for acetylcholine such that the response to acetylcholine is blunted. The postsynaptic effect is produced more potently by streptomycin or netilmicin than by neomycin.[164,165]

The neuromuscular paralysis associated with aminoglycosides is enhanced by the presence of curare-like drugs, succinylcholine, and magnesium, by the simultaneous presence of botulin toxin in patients with botulism, and in patients with myasthenia gravis.[166–171]

The neuromuscular paralysis of aminoglycosides is clearly associated with the presence of very high concentrations of drug at the neuromuscular junctions. Sufficiently high concentrations are achieved only by the very rapid intravenous administration of a bolus of aminoglycoside or as a result of absorption of the drug from the pleural or peritoneal space after instillation of a highly concentrated solution.

The neuromuscular paralysis of aminoglycosides can be prevented by administering intravenous doses over 20–30 minutes, by the intramuscular administration of the drugs, and by the instillation of less concentrated solutions into the pleural or peritoneal spaces.

Once manifest, the neuromuscular paralysis of aminoglycosides can be treated by the prompt administration of calcium. Neostigmine has also been advocated, but neostigmine may be less rational if it is the presynaptic release of acetylcholine that is inhibited by aminoglycosides.

Aminoglycosides are capable of inhibiting both myocardial and vascular smooth muscle contractility in experimental situations, but the clinical relevance is uncertain.[172–174]

Ototoxicity

All aminoglycosides are capable of causing ototoxicity. Although individual aminoglycosides preferentially reduce either auditory toxicity or vestibular toxicity in experimental animals, all aminoglycosides are capable of producing both in humans. Although relatively uncommon, ototoxicity is especially worrisome because of its frequent irreversibility, its occurrence even after discontinuation of the drug, and its cumulative nature with repeated courses of the drug.[175]

The mechanism of auditory toxicity of aminoglycosides involves the selective destruction of the outer hair cells of the organ of Corti, especially those located in the basal turn.[175–178] Subsequently, retrograde degeneration of the auditory nerve occurs.[179] Inner hair cells and cells of the stria vascularis are affected with more extensive damage. The vestibular system is affected primarily by damage to type I hair cells of the summit of the ampullar cristae.[180] Neither cochlear nor ampullar cells can regenerate once they have been destroyed, thus accounting for irreversibility.

The cellular damage may be related to the concentrations of aminoglycosides in the perilymph and endolymph that bathe the relevant cells. Aminoglycosides enter and leave the perilymph slowly, compared with their pharmacokinetics in plasma.[181] Endolymph levels rise and disappear even more slowly.[181] Thus cells bathed by these fluids may be exposed to aminoglycosides for prolonged periods of time even after discontinuation of the drug.

The biochemical events associated with aminoglycoside ototoxicity appear to be biphasic, with an immediate effect that is reversible by calcium and a subsequent irreversible event that may involve binding of the aminoglycoside by phosphatidylinositol biphosphate.[182,183] An inhibition of a sodium–potassium ATPase has also been found.[184] This inhibition might lead to alterations in endolymph or perilymph ion gradients with subsequent effects on the integrity of cochlear cells.

The incidence of aminoglycoside-induced auditory and vestibular toxicity in humans is quite low if clinically detectable hearing loss or vestibular dysfunction is required, but it is clearly higher if more sensitive measures of auditory or vestibular function, such as audiometry or electronystagmography, are used. Large prospective comparative clinical trials of aminoglycosides, usually using rigorous dosing regimens, have delineated relative incidents of aminoglycoside ototoxicity and have also contributed significantly to an understanding of the clinical course of the ototoxicity and risk factors involved with the development of ototoxicity.

Clinically detectable toxicity has been reported to occur in 3–5 percent of patients receiving gentamicin, tobramycin, or amikacin in whom audiometric testing could be performed.[185,186] In other extensive clinical trials of gentamicin, tobramycin, and amikacin, only 3 patients with clinically detectable hearing loss were seen out of a total of 674 patients receiving an aminoglycoside. Thus another estimate of the incidence of clinically detectable hearing loss is less than 0.5 percent of those receiving an aminoglycoside.[114,155]

Using audiometric testing, the incidence of auditory toxicity in patients receiving gentamicin, tobramycin, or amikacin has not been shown to differ significantly when individual aminoglycosides are directly compared.[114,155,185,186] Netilmicin, however, has been shown to produce auditory toxicity less frequently than tobramycin in one multicenter study.[187]

Vestibular dysfunction has been reported as clinically significant in 0.4 percent of patients receiving gentamicin, tobramycin, or amikacin[185,186] and present by electronystagmography in 4 percent of patients receiving gentamicin and 6 percent of patients receiving amikacin.[172] In a prospective but unblinded study tobramycin produced vestibular dysfunction significantly less frequently than did gentamicin.[186]

Auditory toxicity associated with aminoglycosides is seen clinically as hearing loss. Although tinnitus and a feeling of fullness in the ears have been said to precede hearing loss, these are clearly unreliable premonitors of auditory toxicity since they often occur without subsequent hearing loss and hearing loss often occurs without these symptoms. The hearing loss is usually bilateral, although unilateral hearing loss has been reported and usually involves the loss of high-tone hearing before the loss of low-tone hearing. The occurrence and severity of the hearing loss are related to the dose and duration of aminoglycoside therapy.[187,188] There is, however, a somewhat less clear relationship between plasma aminoglycoside levels and auditory toxicity. In prospective clinical trials in which aminoglycoside levels have been carefully monitored and adjusted, there has been no correlation of auditory toxicity and plasma aminoglycoside levels within the narrow range of levels seen. However, if plasma aminoglycoside levels are not carefully adjusted, high plasma levels would surely be associated with greater auditory toxicity. Transient aminoglycoside levels above the usual limits of 10 μg/ml for gentamicin, tobramycin, and netilmicin or 40 μg/ml for amikacin (and presumably kanamycin) are unlikely to be ototoxic.

Even when plasma aminoglycoside levels are carefully monitored, some patients will suffer hearing loss by audiometry and even clinical hearing loss. Risk factors for the development of auditory toxicity include the duration of aminoglycoside use, the presence of bacteremia, fever, liver dysfunction, and the ratio of serum urea nitrogen to serum creatinine as a measure of hypovolemia.[189]

Another important risk factor for auditory aminoglycoside toxicity is the concurrent use of ethacyrnic acid.[190–192] Fortunately, furosemide at clinically used doses and with proper attention to hydration does not appear to be associated with enhanced aminoglycoside auditory toxicity.[192]

Several other potential risk factors that have been identified in experimental animals but that have not yet been proven in humans include noise and age, with increased susceptibility in the very young and the elderly.[193–196]

It should be emphasized that auditory toxicity is cumulative. Thus, with repeated aminoglycoside courses, hearing loss may become detectable as a result of cumulative damage even during a carefully monitored course of therapy.[186–189] This is surely related to the inability of damaged or destroyed cochlear hair cells to regenerate.

Vestibular dysfunction is manifest clinically by nausea, vomiting, vertigo, dizziness, and an unsteady gait with nystagmus. These symptoms and signs are difficult to evaluate in ill patients. More sophisticated laboratory tests are too cumbersome for use in most ill patients.[188]

As with auditory toxicity, vestibular toxicity is dose-related, duration-related, and probably related to plasma levels outside the therapeutic range. However, because of the difficulties of evaluating vestibular function, it has been less well defined than has been auditory toxicity.

Nephrotoxicity

All aminoglycosides are capable of causing nephrotoxicity, although individual differences exist among members of the family with respect to nephrotoxic potential.

The mechanisms involved in aminoglycoside nephrotoxicity include the rapid transport, extensive accumulation, and avid retention of aminoglycosides for prolonged periods of time. In addition, the aminoglycosides are assumed to produce biochemical effects on proximal tubular metabolism that lead to pathophysiologic effects linking proximal tubular damage to diminished glomerular function.

The transport of aminoglycosides is primarily across the luminal brush border of the proximal renal tubular cells and involves an initial binding of the positively charged aminoglycoside to the negatively charged phosphatidylinositol within the membrane.[104,106,107,110] Internalization is believed to occur by pinocytosis into vesicles that eventually coalesce with lysosomes whose highly negative interior effectively traps the aminoglycoside.[105,197] The extensive accumulation of aminoglycosides is confined to the renal cortex, where concentrations 5–50-fold higher than plasma concentrations are found.[198] Within the renal cortex the aminoglycosides are further localized exclusively to the proximal renal tubular cells.[78,105]

It remains unclear whether the proximal tubular cell damage that is characteristic of the aminoglycosides is attributable to lysosomal or extralysosomal effects. Lysosomes may be a primary site of aminoglycoside toxicity or may be salvage organelles responsible for keeping the intracellular aminoglycoside in a nontoxic site. Morphologically, aminoglycosides cause an accumulation of multilamellar structures within lysosomes called myeloid bodies.[197,199,200] Biochemically, aminoglycosides inhibit lysosomal phospholipases A_1, A_2, and C_1 and are also associated with a loss of sphingomyelinase activity.[201,202] Extralysosomal effects of aminoglycosides include both structural and functional effects on mitochondria,[203–205] the inhibition of a sodium–potassium adenosine triphosphatase localized on the basolateral portion of the plasma membrane,[206] and the inhibition of a cytosolic phosphatidylinositol specific phospholipase C.[207] The inhibition of this cytosolic phospholipase may be particularly important since this enzyme may be responsible for an early and pivotal step in the biosynthesis of prostaglandins and prostacyclin. Such an effect might be quite relevant to the reduction of glomerular filtration that is produced by the aminoglycosides subsequent to proximal tubular damage, since an inhibition of the production of vasodilatory prostaglandins would allow the unopposed vasoconstrictor action of angiotensin II, leading to arteriolar vasoconstriction and a decrease in glomerular filtration.[208] Structural and functional alterations of glomeruli have also been identified and may be directly related to aminoglycosides or secondary to effects on prostaglandin or angiotensin systems.[209–212]

Clinical nephrotoxicity, as defined by a reduced glomerular filtration rate (GFR), occurs in between 5 and 25 percent of aminoglycoside recipients.[114,155] The earliest manifestation of an effect of aminoglycosides on the kidney is an increase in the urinary excretion of several renal tubular enzymes, including alanine aminopeptidase, B-D-glucosaminidase, and alkaline phosphatase.[213] In addition, the reabsorption of β_2-microglobulin is competitively inhibited, and its excretion is enhanced.[214] These early indicators of renal effects are too sensitive and too nonspecific to be of clinical value, since every patient receiving an aminoglycoside will exhibit these effects.[213] It appears to be more useful to define aminoglycoside nephrotoxicity in terms of a reduction in GFR as reflected by a rise in serum creatinine, and the serum creatinine is an adequate and convenient parameter to follow when monitoring for aminoglycoside nephrotoxicity.

The onset of glomerular dysfunction usually occurs several days after the initiation of therapy, although a more rapid onset is possible. The glomerular dysfunction in humans increases in severity over a few days, although in experimental animals a cyclic phenomenon of damage and repair occurs even with continuing administration of the aminoglycoside.[215] Whether the same phenomenon occurs in humans remains unknown.

The extent of human kidney damage associated with aminoglycosides is most often mild, occasionally moderate, and rarely severe.[216] It appears that severe nephrotoxicity does not occur if the aminoglycoside dosage is carefully adjusted for changing glomerular function.

The degree of reversibility of renal dysfunction associated with aminoglycosides is remarkable, since the potential of the proximal renal tubule for regeneration is extensive and no or very little irreversible damage is associated with aminoglycosides. The type of renal dysfunction is nonoliguric.

Although individual functions served by the proximal renal tubule such as glucose reabsorption or amino acid reabsorption have been abnormal in experimental animals, these individual proximal tubular functions are usually remarkably well preserved in humans. A syndrome of hypokalemia, hypocalcemia, and hypomagnesemia has been reported in a very few patients.[217–221]

Considerable attention has centered on risk factors in an effort to identify patients who are likely to develop renal dysfunction while receiving an aminoglycoside. Risk factors include older age, female sex, concomitant liver disease, and concomitant hypotension at the onset of aminoglycoside therapy.[222–224] Concomitant cephalothin administration has been reported to be associated with an increased incidence of renal dysfunction.[225] Other nephrotoxic drugs including *cis*-platinum, amphotericin B, and cyclosporin also contribute to the renal dysfunction associated with aminoglycosides.

In addition, different aminoglycosides possess differing degrees of inherent nephrotoxic potential. Of the currently available aminoglycosides, gentamicin is more nephrotoxic than tobramycin.[155] Amikacin is also less nephrotoxic than gentamicin on a weight basis in animals. At a clinical level, however, higher doses of amikacin are allowed because of this lesser nephrotoxicity, and at least some of the difference may be abolished. Netilmicin is also less nephrotoxic than gentamicin in animal studies, but the evidence in humans is currently unconvincing.

Since aminoglycoside nephrotoxicity is usually mild and reversible, we should not err on the side of undertreatment as a result of excessive fear of this adverse effect.

INDIVIDUAL DRUGS

Streptomycin

Streptomycin is available as streptomycin sulfate for intramuscular administration in vials either premixed or to be reconstituted to concentrations of 400 or 500 mg/ml.

Streptomycin is primarily considered as an antituberculous drug with good activity against both *M. tuberculosis* and *Mycobacterium bovis* and less activity against atypical mycobacteria. Streptomycin is also considered the drug of choice for *F. tubarensis* (tularemia) and *Y. pestis* (plague) and is often used for infections caused by *Brucella*. In addition, streptomycin is frequently used, in combination with penicillin or vancomycin, for infections caused by *Enterococcus* (*Streptococcus*) *faecalis* or *Streptococcus viridans*, especially endocarditis, and in prophylactic regimens designed to prevent endocarditis. Enterococcal resistance to streptomycin in some areas, however, may preclude the use of streptomycin and favor gentamicin.[46]

The dosage of streptomycin for tuberculosis is generally 1

g/day followed in a few weeks by 1 g three times a week. For tularemia an accepted dosage is 2 g/day in divided doses (12 hourly), for plague 2 g/day in divided doses (12 hourly), and for brucellosis 1 g/day in divided doses (12 hourly) along with tetracycline. For the treatment of enterococcal endocarditis a recommended dosage regimen is 1 g/day in divided doses (12 hourly) for 4–6 weeks. Enterococci may be highly resistant to streptomycin, and gentamicin is usually recommended for treatment of endocarditis caused by streptomycin-resistant organisms. For the prevention of endocarditis, a recommended dosage regimen of streptomycin is 1 g given ½–1 hour before dental or surgical intervention and for genitourinary or gastrointestinal surgery an additional 1 g at 12 hours and again at 24 hours postoperatively.

As with other aminoglycosides, the dosage should be reduced in the elderly, in newborns, and in patients with diminished glomerular function.

Neomycin

Neomycin is available as neomycin sulfate for oral administration in tablets containing 500 mg each. In addition, neomycin sulfate is available either alone or in combination with other agents in numerous ophthalmologic, otic, and dermatologic formulations for topical application.

For preoperative suppression of intestinal bacteria a dosage regimen of 6 g/day (divided four hourly) for 2–3 days has been recommended. In hepatic coma a dosage regimen of 4–12 g/day (divided four or six hourly) has been recommended. It is imperative to recognize that a small percentage of the oral dose of neomycin will be absorbed and that this may provide toxic systemic levels in a patient with renal dysfunction.

Kanamycin

Kanamycin is available as kanamycin sulfate in both parenteral and oral formulations. For parenteral use kanamycin sulfate is available at concentrations of 250, 333, or 37.5 mg/ml. All parenteral formulations contain sodium bisulfite as a preservative. For oral use kanamycin sulfate is available in capsules of 500 mg each.

The place of kanamycin for treatment of systemic infections is debatable. Its widespread usage during the 1960s was sharply curtailed in the 1970s as a result of the relatively common emergence of resistance in common gram-negative bacillary organisms in conjunction with the usual resistance of *Pseudomonas* species. With its disuse, however, the level of resistance has decreased in many areas, and it has again enjoyed some increase in use in infections unlikely to be associated with *Pseudomonas* species. In general, however, its place has been taken by gentamicin, tobramycin, and amikacin.

The dosage of kanamycin (either intramuscularly or intravenously) for systemic infections has been 15 mg/kg/day in divided doses (usually 12 hourly) with a maximal dose of 1.5 g/day. If given intravenously, the dose should be administered over at least 30 minutes.

The parenteral formulation of kanamycin sulfate may be diluted with sterile distilled water to provide solutions for intraperitoneal instillation or for the irrigation of abscess cavities, pleural or peritoneal spaces, the bladder, or wounds. Although concentrations of 25 mg/ml for intraperitoneal instillation and 2.5 mg/ml for irrigating solutions have been recommended, it is important to recognize that absorption can occur, especially from the peritoneum, pleura, or open wounds, and that very large daily systemic doses can be achieved inadvertently with these concentrated solutions. It would seem more prudent to use solutions of 25 μg/ml since this is the peak level achieved in plasma with systemic dosing and since this level is unlikely to produce toxicity in the absence of renal dysfunction.

The oral dose of kanamycin for the suppression of intestinal bacteria preoperatively or in hepatic coma is 8–12 g/day in divided doses (four or six hourly). As with neomycin, some kanamycin will be absorbed, and toxic systemic levels may result in patients with renal dysfunction.

As with all aminoglycosides, the systemic dosing of kanamycin must be adjusted for renal glomerular dysfunction, including that seen in the elderly and the newborn.

Gentamicin

Gentamicin is available as gentamicin sulfate for parenteral and topical use. For parenteral use gentamicin sulfate is available in concentrations of 2 mg/ml (without methyl and propylparabens, ethylenediaminetetraacetic acid (EDTA), and sodium bisulfite as preservatives) for intrathecal or intraventricular use, 10 mg/ml (pediatric), 40 mg/ml (intravenous or intramuscular), or 1 mg/ml (intravenous piggyback without preservative) in various sized vials, prefilled syringes, or piggyback units.

Gentamicin sulfate is also available in several topical formulations for ophthalmologic or dermatologic use.

Gentamicin remains a mainstay in the treatment of gram-negative bacillary infections, in part because of its relatively low cost after the expiration of its patent.

Gentamicin dosing is discussed above.

Tobramycin

Tobramycin is available as tobramycin sulfate for parenteral or topical use. For parenteral use tobramycin sulfate is available in concentrations of 10 mg/ml (pediatric) and 40 mg/ml (intravenous or intramuscular) in vials or prefilled syringes. Each of these formulations contains phenol, EDTA, and sodium bisulfite as preservatives. In addition, a powder for injection is available, which can be reconstituted with sterile water to a concentration of 40 mg/ml. This formulation contains no preservatives and may be a more reasonable choice for intrathecal or intraventricular injections.

Tobramycin sulfate is also available as ophthalmic drops containing 3 mg/mg.

Tobramycin is widely used in the treatment of gram-negative bacillary infections. At a clinical level there is no evidence for its superiority or inferiority when compared with gentamicin, amikacin, or netilmicin with respect to effectiveness in infections caused by susceptible organisms. Its in vitro activity is somewhat greater than gentamicin for *P. aeruginosa* and somewhat less for *Serratia*, but this has not led to demonstrable differences in clinical effectiveness. A few organisms are resistant to gentamicin and yet sensitive to tobramycin, but the resistance profiles of the two are highly similar. Tobramycin is somewhat less nephrotoxic than gentamicin and may be somewhat less ototoxic as well, but the lesser ototoxicity that exists in animals has been supported only with respect to vestibular dysfunction in humans.

Tobramycin dosing is discussed above and is identical to gentamicin dosing.

Amikacin

Amikacin is available as amikacin sulfate for parenteral use in solutions containing 50 or 250 mg/ml. Only one formulation of amikacin sulfate contains no preservatives (sodium bisulfite and sulfuric acid), and this is probably the preferred formulation for intrathecal or intraventricular use.

Amikacin is widely used in the treatment of gram-negative bacillary infections. At a clinical level there is no evidence for its superiority or inferiority when compared with gentamicin, tobramycin, or netilmicin with respect to effectiveness in infections caused by susceptible organisms. Although its in vitro potency is somewhat less, or a weight basis, than that of gentamicin, tobramycin, or netilmicin, the larger dosages used compensate for this lesser potency. A clear advantage of amikacin lies in its resistance profile. Many of the aminoglycoside-inactivating enzymes that inactivate other aminoglycosides cannot inactivate amikacin, and consequently many organisms that are resistant to gentamicin, tobramycin, or netilmicin remain sensitive to amikacin. Thus amikacin has clear-cut advantages in treating infections caused by organisms known to be resistant to other aminoglycosides and in nosocomial infections in which the likelihood of resistant organisms is increased. The use of amikacin in other and more general settings currently presents a dilemma for the clinician. On the one hand, the restriction of amikacin usage is often believed to be wise in order to delay the emergence of resistance to this valuable drug. On the other hand, there is no evidence that the restriction of amikacin usage will delay the emergence of resistance, and there is a theoretical reason that resistance may not be delayed. This is based on the fact that each of the relatively few aminoglycoside-inactivating enzymes that can inactivate amikacin can also inactivate other aminoglycosides. Thus the continued use of other aminoglycosides may provide ecologic pressure for the development of those enzymes capable of inactivating amikacin even though amikacin use is restricted.

With respect to toxicity, amikacin is probably less nephrotoxic and less ototoxic than gentamicin on a weight basis. However, since larger doses of amikacin are used, the differences on a weight basis may be at least partially lost. On a clinical level there have been no direct prospective and blinded comparisons between amikacin and either tobramycin or netilmicin with respect to toxicity. Therefore, the precise placement of amikacin with respect to its relative toxicity remains unclear.

Netilmicin

Netilmicin is available as netilmicin sulfate for parenteral use, in formulations containing 10 mg/ml (neonatal; with sodium metabisulfite and sodium sulfite as preservatives), 25 mg/ml (pediatric; with methyl and propyl parabens, EDTA, sodium metabisulfite, and sodium sulfite as preservatives) and 100 mg/ml (with benzyl alcohol, EDTA, sodium metabisulfite, and sodium sulfite as preservatives) in vials or prefilled syringes.

Netilmicin has only recently been marketed, and its place in therapy is yet to be established. Its clinical effectiveness is probably similar to gentamicin, tobramycin, and amikacin. In vitro its resistance profile resembles gentamicin and tobramycin, with only a few strains of bacteria being resistant to gentamicin or tobramycin and sensitive to netilmicin. From a toxicologic point of view, netilmicin is less nephrotoxic than gentamicin in experimental animals, but this has not been confirmed in humans. Subclinical auditory toxicity, as detected by audiometry, is less with netilmicin than with tobramycin.[187] Clinically detectable auditory toxicity is very rare with any of the commonly used aminoglycosides if dosing is appropriately controlled.

Spectinomycin

Spectinomycin is isolated from *Streptomyces spectabilis* and is classified as an aminocyclitol antibiotic but is not an aminoglycoside since it contains neither an aminosugar nor a glycosidic bond (Fig. 2).[226,227]

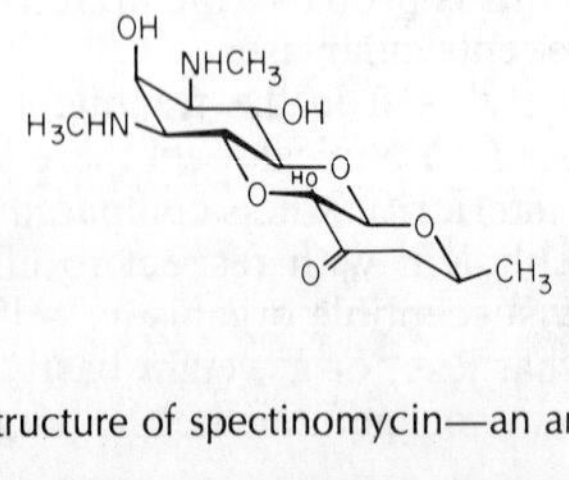

FIG. 2. Structure of spectinomycin—an aminocyclitol.

The site of action of spectinomycin may be similar to the aminoglycosides since spectinomycin binds to the smaller (30s) ribosomal subunits, and protein synthesis is inhibited.[228] However, misreading of the genetic code does not occur, and a membrane effect does appear to exist by electron microscopy.[229]

Resistance to spectinomycin is rarely seen in *Neisseria gonorrhoea*, and there is no cross-resistance with penicillins.[226]

Although the spectrum of activity of spectinomycin is broader, spectinomycin is used only as an agent for infections caused by *N. gonorrhoea*. Significantly, it is not effective against *Treponema pallidum* or *Chlamydia trachomatis*, but it may be somewhat effective against *Ureaplasma urealyticum* and *Gardnerella vaginalis*.[226,227,230]

Spectinomycin is rapidly and completely absorbed after intramuscular administration.[231] Its volume of distribution is about 0.33 liter/kg and its half-life about 1 hour.[216] It is not metabolized and is excreted completely into the urine as unchanged drug. Spectinomycin does not enter saliva and is not predictably effective in eliminating pharyngeal *Neisseria*.[212]

Toxicologically, spectinomycin differs considerably from the aminoglycosides in that it is neither ototoxic nor nephrotoxic, and, in fact, few side effects exist with the usual dosing of the drug. Urticaria, chills, fever, dizziness, nausea, and insomnia have been reported.

Therapeutically, spectinomycin is clearly highly effective in the treatment of uncomplicated gonorrhea and disseminated gonococcal infection. It is unpredictable in the treatment of pharyngeal gonorrhea. Spectinomycin is the drug of choice in the treatment of penicillinase-producing gonococcal infections and in the treatment of patients who fail to respond to treatment.

Spectinomycin is available as spectinomycin hydrochloride in a powder form that is reconstituted with 0.9% benzyl alcohol as a diluent to a concentration of 400 mg/ml. It can be given only intramuscularly.

For uncomplicated gonorrheal infections 2 g as a single intramuscular dose is recommended. For disseminated gonococcal infections the recommended dose is 4 g/day in divided doses (12 hourly) for 3 days.

REFERENCES

1. Rinehart KL. Comparative chemistry of the aminoglycoside and aminocyclitol antibiotics. J Infect Dis. 1969;119:345.
2. Daniels PJL: Antibiotics (aminoglycosides). In: Grayson M, ed. Kirk-Othmer: Encyclopedia of Chemical Technology. v. 5. 3rd ed. New York: John Wiley Sons; 1978:819.
3. Hooper IR. The naturally occurring aminoglycoside antibiotics. In: Umezawa H, Hooper IR, eds. Aminoglycoside Antibiotics. New York: Springer-Verlag; 1982:1.
4. Umezawa S, Tsuchiya T. Total synthesis and chemical modification of the aminoglycoside antibiotics. In: Umezawa H, Hooper IR, eds. Aminoglycoside Antibiotics. New York: Springer-Verlag; 1982:37.
5. Price KE, Godfrey JC, Kawaguchi H. Effect of structural modifications on the biological properties of aminoglycoside antibiotics containing 2-deoxystreptamine. Adv Appl Microbiol. 1974;18:191.
6. Hancock REW. Aminoglycoside uptake and mode of action: with special reference to streptomycin and gentamicin. I. Antagonists and mutants. J Antimicrob Chemother. 1981;8:249.
7. Hancock REW. Aminoglycoside uptake and mode of action: with special reference to streptomycin and gentamicin. II. Effects of aminoglycosides on cells. J Antimicrob Chemother. 1981;8:429.
8. Davis BD. The lethal action of aminoglycosides. J Antimicrob Chemother. 1988;22:1.
9. Nichols WW. On the mechanism of translocation of dihydrostreptomycin across the bacterial cytoplasmic membrane. Biochim Biophys Acta. 1987;895:11.
10. Pestka S. Inhibitors of protein synthesis. In: Weissback H, Pestka S, eds. Molecular Mechanisms of Protein Synthesis. New York: Academic Press; 1977:467.
11. Stoffler G, Wittmann HG. Primary structure and three-dimensional arrangement of proteins within the *Escherichia coli* ribosome. In: Weissbach H, Pestka S, eds. Molecular Mechanisms of Protein Synthesis. New York: Academic Press; 1977:117.
12. Hummel H, Piepersberg W, Bock A. 30s subunit mutations relieving restriction of ribosomal misreading caused by L6 mutations. Mol Gen Genet. 1980;179:147.
13. Kuhberger R, Piepersberg W, Petzet A, et al. Alteration of ribosomal protein

L6 in gentamicin-resistant strains of *Escherichia coli*. Effects on fidelity of protein synthesis. Biochemistry. 1979;18:187.
14. Tai P-C, Davis BD. Triphasic concentration effects of gentamicin on activity and misreading in protein synthesis. Biochemistry. 1979;18:193.
15. Chang FN, Flaks JG. Binding of dihydrostreptomycin to *Escherichia coli* ribosomes: characteristics and equilibrium of the reaction. Antimicrob Agents Chemother. 1972;2:294.
16. Chang FN, Flaks JG. Binding of dihydrostreptomycin to *Escherichia coli* ribosomes: kinetics of the reaction. Antimicrob Agents Chemother. 1972;2:308.
17. Ozaki M, Mizushima S, Nomura M. Identification and functional characterization of the protein controlled by the streptomycin-resistant locus in *E. coli*. Nature. 1969;222:333.
18. Schreiner G, Nierhaus KH. Protein involved in the binding of dihydrostreptomycin to ribosomes of *Escherichia coli*. J Mol Biol. 1973;81:71.
19. Wallace BJ, David BD. Cyclic blockade of initiation sites by streptomycin-damaged ribosomes in *Escherichia coli*: an explanation for dominance of sensitivity. J Mol Biol. 1973;75:377.
20. Wallace BJ, Tai P-C, Davis BD. Effect of streptomycin on the response of *Escherichia coli* ribosomes to the dissociation factor. J Mol Biol. 1973;75:391.
21. Luzzatto L, Apirion D, Schlessinger D. Mechanism of action of streptomycin in *E. coli*: Interruption of the ribosome cycle of the initiation of protein synthesis. Proc Natl Acad Sci USA. 1968;60:873.
22. Luzzatto L, Apirion D, Schlessinger D. Polyribosome depletion and blockage of the ribosome cycle by streptomycin in *Escherichia coli*. J Mol Biol. 1969;42:315.
23. Bryan LE, van den Elzen HM. Effects of membrane-energy mutations and cations on streptomycin and gentamicin accumulation by bacteria: a model for entry of streptomycin and gentamicin in susceptible and resistant bacteria. Antimicrob Agents Chemother. 1977;12:163.
24. Mak L, Lietman PS. Aminoglycoside transport by bacteria. In: Fillastre J-P, ed. Nephrotoxicité et Ototoxicité Medicamenteuses. Rouen: Editions INSERM; 1981:55.
25. Damper PD, Epstein W. Role of the membrane potential in bacterial resistance to aminglycoside antibiotics. Antimicrob Agents Chemother. 1981;20:803.
26. Mates SM, Patel L, Kaback HR, et al. Membrane potential in anaerobically growing *Staphylococcus aureus* and its relationship to gentamicin uptake. Antimicrob Agents Chemother. 1983;23:526.
27. Holtje J-V. Regulation of polamine and streptomycin transport during stringent and relaxed control in *Escherichia coli*. J Bacteriol. 1979;137:661.
28. Hurwitz C, Rosano CL. Chloramphenicol-sensitive and -insensitive phases of the lethal action of streptomycin. J Bacteriol. 1962;83:1202.
29. Bryan LE. General mechanisms of resistance to antibiotics. J Antimicrob Chemother. 1988;22(Suppl A):1.
30. Mitsuhashi S, Kawabe H. Aminoglycoside antibiotic resistance in bacteria. In: Whelton A, New HC, eds. The Aminoglycosides. New York: Marcel Dekker; 1983:97.
31. Davies JE. Resistance to aminoglycosides: mechanism and frequency. Rev Infect Dis. 1983;5(Suppl):3261.
32. Kabins SA, Nathan C, Cohen S. *In vitro* comparison of netilmicin, a semisynthetic derivative of sisomicin, and four other aminoglycoside antibiotics. Antimicrob Agents Chemother. 1976;10:139.
33. Sanders CC, Sanders WE, Jr, Goering RV. *In vitro* studies with Sch 21420 and Sch 22591: activity in comparison with six other aminoglycosides and synergy with penicillin against enterococci. Antimicrob Agents Chemother. 1978;14:178.
34. Moellering RC Jr. Clinical microbiology and the *in vitro* activity of aminoglycosides. In: Whelton A, Neu HC, eds. The Aminoglycosides: Microbiology, Clinical Use, and Toxicology. New York: Marcel Dekker; 1982:65.
35. Fu K, Neu HC. *In vitro* study of netilmicin compared with other aminoglycosides. Antimicrob Agents Chemother. 1976;10:526.
36. National Committee for Clinical Laboratory Standards. Performance standards for antimicrobial disc susceptibility tests. Approved Standard: ASM-2, Villanova, PA, 1979.
37. Thornsberry C, Gavan TL, Gerlach EH, et al. New developments in antimicrobial agent susceptibility testing. In: Sherris JC, ed. Cumitech 6. Washington, DC: American Society of Microbiology; 1977:1.
38. McDonald PJ, Craig WA, Konin CM. Persistent effect of antibiotics on *Staphylococcus aureus* after exposure for limited periods of time. J Infect Dis. 1977;135:217.
39. Grasso S, Meinardi G, DeCarneri J, et al. New *in vitro* model to study the effect of antibiotic concentration and rate of elimination on antibacterial activity. Antimicrob Agents Chemother. 1978;13:570.
40. Al-Asadi MJS, Greenwood D, O'Grady F. *In vitro* model simulating the form of exposure of bacteria to antimicrobial drugs encountered in infection. Antimicrob Agents Chemother. 1979;16:77.
41. Murakawa T, Sakamoto H, Hinrose T, et al. New *in vitro* model for evaluating bactericidal efficacy of antibiotics. Antimicrob Agents Chemother. 1980;18:77.
42. Bergan T, Carlsen IB, Fuglesang JE. An *in vitro* model for monitoring bacterial responses to antibiotic agents under simulated *in vivo* conditions. Infection. 1980;8(Suppl 1):S96.
43. Longstreth JA. Interaction of aminoglycoside pharmacokinetics and bacterial population kinetics in a chemostat. PhD dissertation. Johns Hopkins University, 1982.
44. Hammond BJ, Kogot M, Lightbown JW. Analogue computer studies of the growth characteristics of *Escherichia coli* following dihydrostreptomycin treatment. J Gen Microbiol. 1967;48:189.
45. Kogot M, Lightbown JW, Isaacson P. Effects of dihydrostreptomycin treatment on the growth of *Escherichia coli* after removal of extracellular antibiotic. J Gen Microbiol. 1965;39:165.
46. Bundtzen RW, Gerber AU, Cohn DL, et al. Postantibiotic suppression of bacterial growth. Rev Infect Dis. 1981;3:28.
47. Gerber AU, Wippraechtiger P, Stettler U, et al. Constant infusions versus intermittent doses of gentamicin against Pseudomonas *in vitro*. J Infect Dis. 1982;145:554.
48. Gerber AU, Craig WA, Brugger H-P, et al. Impact of dosing intervals on activity of gentamicin and ticarcillin against *Pseudomonas aeruginosa* in granulocytopenic mice. J Infect Dis. 1983;147:910.
49. Powell SH, Thompson WL, Luthe MA, et al. Once-daily versus continuous aminoglycoside dosing: efficacy and toxicity in animal and clinical studies of gentamicin, netilmicin and tobramycin. J Infect Dis. 1983;147:918.
50. Vogelman BS, Craig WA. Postantibiotic effects. J Antimicrob Chemother. 1985;15(Suppl A):37.
51. Blaser J, Stone BB, Zinner SH. Efficacy of intermittent versus continuous administration of netilmicin in a two-compartment *in vitro* model. Antimicrob Agents Chemother. 1985;27:343.
52. Craig WA, Vogelman B. The postantibiotic effect. Ann Intern Med. 1987;106:900.
53. Vogelman B, Gudmundsson S, Turnidge J, et al. *In vivo* postantibiotic effect in a thigh infection in neutropenic mice. J Infect Dis. 1988;157:287.
54. Isaksson B, Nilsson L, Maller R, et al. Postantibiotic effect of aminoglycosides on Gram-negative bacteria evaluated by a new method. J Antimicrob Chemother. 1988;22:23.
55. Wood CA, Norton DR, Kohlhepp SJ, et al. The influence of tobramycin dosage regimens on nephrotoxicity, ototoxicity and antibacterial efficacy in a rat model of subcutaneous abscess. J Infect Dis. 1988;158:13.
56. Klastersky J, Cappel R, Danpau D. Clinical significance of *in vitro* synergism between antibiotics in gram-negative infections. Antimicrob Agents Chemother. 1972;2:470.
57. Moellering RC Jr, Wennerstein C, Weinberg AN. Studies on antibiotic synergism against enterococci: I. Bacteriologic studies. J Lab Clin Med. 1971;77:821.
58. Kunin CM, Chalmers TC, Leevy CM. Absorption of orally administered neomycin and kanamycin. N Engl J Med. 1960;262:380.
59. Last PM, Sherlock S. Systemic absorption of orally administered neomycin in liver disease. N Engl J Med. 1960;262:385.
60. Kunin CM. Absorption, distribution, excretion and fate of kanamycin. Ann NY Acad Sci. 1966;132:811.
61. Breen KF, Bryant RE, Levinson JD, et al. Neomycin absorption in man. Ann Intern Med. 1972;76:211.
62. Mitch WE, Lietman PS, Walser M. Effects of oral neomycin and kanamycin in chronic uremic patients. I. Urea metabolism. Kidney Int. 1977;11:116.
63. King JT. Severe deafness in an infant following oral administration of neomycin. J Med Assoc Ga. 1962;51:530.
64. Ruben RJ, Daly JF. Neomycin ototoxicity and nephrotoxicity. Laryngoscope. 1968;78:1734.
65. Kalbian VV. Deafness following oral use of neomycin. South Med J. 1972;65:499.
66. Ward KM, Rounthwaite FJ. Neomycin ototoxicity. Ann Otol. 1978;87:211.
67. Doluisio JT, Dittert LW, LaPiana JC. Pharmacokinetics of kanamycin following intramuscular administration. J Pharmacokinet Biopharm. 1973;1:253.
68. Barza M, Lauermann M. Why monitor serum levels of gentamicin. Clin Pharmacokinet. 1978;3:202.
69. Little PJ, Lynn KL. Neomycin toxicity. NZ Med J. 1975;81:445.
70. Bamford MFM, Jones LF. Deafness and biochemical imbalance after burns treatment with topical antibiotics in young children. Arch Dis Child. 1978;53:326.
71. Somani P, Shapiro RS, Stockard H, et al. Unidirectional absorption of gentamicin from the peritoneum during continuous ambulatory peritoneal dialysis. Clin Pharmacol Ther. 1982;32:113.
72. DePaepe M, Lameire N, Belpaire F, et al. Peritoneal pharmacokinetics of gentamicin in man. Clin Nephrol. 1983;19:107.
73. Chamberlain G, Needham P. The absorption of antibiotics from the bladder. J Urol. 1976;116:172.
74. Lifschitz MI, Denning CR. Safety of kanamycin aerosol. Clin Pharmacol Ther. 1971;12:91.
75. Odio W, VanLeier E, Klastersky J. Concentrations of gentamicin in bronchial secretions after intramuscular and endotracheal administration. J Clin Pharmacol. 1975;15:518.
76. Rahal JJ Jr, Hyams PJ, Simberkoff MS, et al. Combined intrathecal and intramuscular gentamicin for gram-negative meningitis. N Engl J Med. 1974;290:1394.
77. Van Etta LL, Kravitz GR, Russ TE, et al. Effect of method of administration on extravascular penetration of four antibiotics. Antimicrob Agents Chemother. 1982;21:873.
78. Kuhar MJ, Mak LL, Lietman PS. Localization of ^{3}H-gentamicin in the proximal renal tubule of the mouse. Antimicrob Agents Chemother. 1979;15:131.
79. Thys JP, Klastersky J, Mombelli G. Peak or sustained antibiotic levels for optimal tissue penetration. J Antimicrob Chemother. 1981;8(Suppl C):29.
80. Klastersky J, Meunier-Carpentier F, Kahan-Coppens L, et al. Endotra-

cheally administered antibiotics for gram negative bronchopneumonia. Chest. 1979;75:586.
81. Kaiser AB, McGee ZA. Aminoglycoside therapy of gram-negative bacillary meningitis. N Engl J Med. 1975;293:1215.
82. Wirt TC, McGee ZA, Oldfield EH, et al. Intraventricular administration of amikacin for complicated gram-negative meningitis and ventriculitis. J Neurosurg. 1979;50:95.
83. McCracken GH Jr, Mize S, Threlkeld N. Intraventricular gentamicin therapy in gram-negative bacillary meningitis of infancy. Lancet. 1980;i:787.
84. Barza M, Kane A, Baum J. Comparison of the effects of continuous and intermittent systemic administration on the penetration of gentamicin into infected rabbit eyes. J Infect Dis. 1983;147:144.
85. Gorden TB, Cunningham RD. Tobramycin levels in aqueous humor after subconjunctival injection in humans. Am J Ophthalmol. 1982;93:107.
86. Rubenstein E, Goldfarb J, Keren G, et al. The penetration of gentamicin into the vitreous humor in man. Invest Ophthalmol Vis Sci. 1983;24:637.
87. Marsh DC Jr, Matthew EB, Perselin RA. Transport of gentamicin into synovial fluid. JAMA. 1974;228:607.
88. Dee TH, Koein F. Gentamicin and tobramycin penetration into synovial fluid. Antimicrob Agents Chemother. 1977;12:548.
89. Chow A, Hecht R, Witners R. Gentamicin and carbenicillin penetration into the septic joint. N Engl J Med. 1971;285:178.
90. Baciocco EA, Iles RI. Ampicillin and kanamycin concentration in joint fluid. Clin Pharmacol Ther. 1971;12:858.
91. Schurman DJ, Wheeler R. Bone and joint gram-negative infection and amikacin treatment. Am J Med. 1977;62(Suppl):160.
92. Alftan O, Renkonen OV, Sironen A. Concentration of gentamicin in serum, urine and urogenital tissue in man. Acta Pathol Microbiol Scand [B]. 1973;81(Suppl 241):92.
93. Mahmod S, Al-Hakiem MHH, Landon J, et al. Aminoglycoside antibiotics do not appear in saliva. Clin Chem. 1983;29:988.
94. Pitt HA, Roberts RB, Johnson WD Jr. Gentamicin levels in the human biliary tract. J Infect Dis. 1973;127:299.
95. Mendelson J, Portnoy J, Sigman H. Pharmacology of gentamicin in the biliary tract of humans. Antimicrob Agents Chemother. 1973;4:538.
96. Wood MJ, Farrell W. Comparison of urinary excretion of tobramycin and gentamicin in adults. J Infect Dis. 1976;134(Suppl):S133.
97. Kahlmeter G, Kamme C. Prolonged excretion of gentamicin in a patient with unimpaired renal function. Lancet. 1975;i:286.
98. Kahlmeter G, Jonsson S, Kamme C. Multiple-compartment pharmacokinetics of tobramycin. J Antimicrob Chemother. 1978;4(Suppl A):5.
99. Kahlmeter G. Netilmicin: clinical pharmacokinetics and aspects on dosage schedules. An overview. Scand J Infect Dis. 1980;23:74.
100. Laskin OL, Longstreth JA, Smith CR, et al. Netilmicin and gentamicin multidose kinetics in normal subjects. Clin Pharmacol Ther. 1983;34:644.
101. Wilson TW, Mahon WA, Inaba T, et al. Elimination of tritiated gentamicin in normal human subjects and in patients with severely impaired renal function. Clin Pharmacol Ther. 1973;14:815.
102. Kahlmeter G. Gentamicin and tobramycin: clinical pharmacokinetics and nephrotoxicity: aspects on assay techniques. Thesis, Department of Medical Microbiology, University of Lund, Sweden, 1979.
103. Pastoriza-Munoz E, Timmerman D, Feldman S, et al. Ultrafiltration of gentamicin and netilmicin *in vivo*. J Pharmacol Exp Ther. 1982;220:604.
104. Collier VU, Lietman PS, Mitch WE. Evidence for luminal uptake of gentamicin in perfused rat kidney. J Pharmacol Exp Ther. 1979;210:247.
105. Silverblatt FJ, Kuehn C. Autoradiography of gentamicin uptake by the rat proximal tubular cell. Kidney Int. 1979;15:335.
106. Lipsky JJ, Cheng L, Saktor B, et al. Gentamicin uptake by renal tubule brush border membrane vesicles. J Pharmacol Exp Ther. 1980;215:390.
107. Sastrasinh M, Knauss TC, Weinberg JM, et al. Identification of the aminoglycoside binding site in rat renal brush border membranes. J Pharmacol Exp Ther. 1982;222:350.
108. Senekjian HO, Knight TF, Weinman EJ. Micropuncture study of the handling of gentamicin by the rat kidney. Kidney Int. 1981;19:416.
109. Pastoriza-Munoz E, Bowman RL, Kaloyanides GJ. Renal tubular transport of gentamicin in the rat. Kidney Int. 1979;16:440.
110. Frommer JP, Senekjian HO, Babino H, et al. Intratubular microinjection study of gentamicin transport in the rat. Mineral Electrolyte Metab. 1983;9:108.
111. Wenk M, Spring P, Vozeh S, et al. Multicompartment pharmacokinetics of netilmicin. Eur J Clin Pharmacol. 1979;16:331.
112. Laskin OL, Longstreth JA, Smith CR, et al. Netilmicin and gentamicin multidose kinetics in normal subjects. Clin Pharmacol Ther. 1983;34:644.
113. Lanao JM, Dominguez-Gil A, Tobernero JM, et al. Pharmacokinetics of amikacin (BB-K8) in patients with normal or impaired renal function. Int J Clin Pharmacol Biopharm. 1979;17:171.
114. Smith CR, Baughman KL, Edwards CQ, et al. Controlled comparison of amikacin and gentamicin. N Engl J Med. 1977;296:349.
115. Gyselynck A-M, Forrey A, Cutler R. Pharmacokinetics of gentamicin: distribution and plasma and renal clearance. J Infect Dis. 1971;124(Suppl):S70.
116. Plantier J, Forrey AW, O'Neill MA, et al: Pharmacokinetics of amikacin in patients with normal or impaired renal function: radioenzymatic acetylation assay. J Infect Dis. 1976;134(Suppl):S323.
117. Barza M, Brown RB, Shen D, et al. Predictability of blood levels of gentamicin in man. J Infect Dis. 1975;132:165.
118. Clarke JT, Libke RD, Regamey C, et al. Comparative pharmacokinetics of amikacin and kanamycin. Clin Pharmacol Ther. 1974;15:610.
119. Walker JM, Wise R, Mitchard M. The pharmacokinetics of amikacin and gentamicin in volunteers: a comparison of individual differences. J Antimicrob Chemother. 1979;5:95.
120. Kahlmeter G, Jonsson S, Kamme C. Multiple-compartment pharmacokinetics of tobramycin. J Antimicrob Chemother. 1978;4(Suppl A):5.
121. Kahlmeter G. Gentamicin and Tobramycin: Clinical Pharmacokinetics and Nephrotoxicity: Aspects on Assay Techniques. Lund; Berlings; 1979.
122. Adelman M, Evans E, Schentag JJ. Two-compartment comparison of gentamicin and tobramycin in normal volunteers. Antimicrob Agents Chemother. 1982;22:800.
123. Assael BM, Cavanna G, Jusko WJ, et al. Multiexponential elimination of gentamicin. A kinetic study during development. Dev Pharmacol Ther. 1980;1:171.
124. Driessen OMJ, Sorgedrager N, Michel MF, et al. Pharmacokinetic aspects of therapy with ampicillin and kanamycin in new-born infants. Eur J Clin Pharmacol. 1978;13:449.
125. Haughey DB, Hilligoss DM, Grassi A, et al. Two compartment gentamicin pharmacokinetics in premature neonates. A comparison to adults with decreased glomerular filtration rate. J Pediatr. 1980;96:325.
126. Herngren L, Boreaus LO, Jalling B, et al. Pharmacokinetic aspects of streptomycin treatment of neonatal septicemia. Scand J Infect Dis. 1977;9:301.
127. Howard JB, McCracken GH. Reappraisal of kanamycin usage in neonates. J Pediatr. 1975;86:949.
128. Howard JB, McCracken GH, Trujillo H, et al. Amikacin in newborn infants: comparative pharmacology with kanamycin and clinical efficacy in 45 neonates with bacterial diseases. Antimicrob Agents Chemother. 1976;10:205.
129. McCracken GH Jr, Gay Jones L. Gentamicin in the neonatal period. Am J Dis Child. 1970;120:524.
130. McCracken GH Jr, Nelson JD. Antimicrobial Therapy for Newborns: Practical Application of Pharmacology to Clinical Use. New York: Grune & Stratton; 1977.
131. Yoshioka H, Takimoto M, Matsudi I, et al. Dosage schedule of gentamicin for chronic renal insufficiency in children. Arch Dis Child. 1978;53:334.
132. Echeverria P, Siber GR, Paisley J, et al. Age dependent dose response to gentamicin. J Pediatr. 1975;87:805.
133. Evans WE, Feldman S, Barker LF, et al. Use of gentamicin serum levels to individualize therapy in children. J Pediatr. 1978;93:133.
134. Evans WE, Huntley Taylor R, Feldman S, et al. A model for dosing gentamicin in children and adolescents that adjusts for tissue accumulation with continuous dosing. Clin Pharmacokinet. 1980;5:295.
135. Hoecker JL, Pickering LK, Swaney J, et al. Clinical pharmacology of tobramycin in children. J Infect Dis. 1978;137:592.
136. Karetzis DA, Sinaniotis CA, Papadatos CJ, et al. Pharmacokinetics of amikacin in infants and preschool children. Acta Paediatr Scand. 1979;68:419.
137. Kramer WG, Cleary T, Frankel LS, et al. Multiple-dose amikacin kinetics in pediatric oncology patients. Clin Pharmacol Ther. 1979;26:635.
138. Marks MI, Vose A, Hammerberg S, et al. Clinico-pharmacological studies of sisomicin in ill children. Antimicrob Agents Chemother. 1978;13:753.
139. McCracken GH Jr. Clinical pharmacology of gentamicin in infants 2 to 24 months of age. Am J Dis Child. 1972;124:884.
140. Siber GR, Echeverria P, Smith AL, et al. Pharmacokinetics of gentamicin in children and adults. J Infect Dis. 1975;132:637.
141. Vogelstein B, Kowarski AA, Lietman PS. The pharmacokinetics of amikacin in children. J Pediatr. 1977;91:333.
142. Wellilng PG, Baumueller A, Lau CC, et al. Netilmicin pharmacokinetics after single intravenous doses to elderly male patients. Antimicrob Agents Chemother. 1977;12:328.
143. Spyker DA, Guerrant RL. Dosage nomograms for aminoglycoside antibiotics. Hosp Formulary. 1981;16:132.
144. Cockcroft DW, Gault MH. Prediction of creatinine clearance from serum creatinine. Nephron. 1976;16:31.
145. Siersbaek-Nielsen K, Molholm-Hansen J, Kampmann J. Rapid evaluation of creatinine clearance. Lancet. 1971;i:1133.
146. Plantier J, Forrey AW, O'Neill MA, et al. Pharmacokinetics of amikacin in patients with normal or impaired renal function: radioenzymatic acetylation assay. J Infect Dis. 1976;134(Suppl):5323.
147. Gyscelynck A-M, Forrey A, Cutler R. Pharmacokinetics of gentamicin: distribution and plasma and renal clearance. J Infect Dis. 1971;124(Suppl):570.
148. Lanao JM, Dominguez-Gil A, Tabernero JM, et al. Pharmacokinetics of amikacin (BB-K8) in patients with normal or impaired renal function. Int J Clin Pharmacol Biopharm. 1979;17:171.
149. Schwartz SN, Pazin GJ, Lyon JA, et al. A controlled investigation of the pharmacokinetics of gentamicin and tobramycin in obese subjects. J Infect Dis. 1978;138:499.
150. Blouin RA, Mann HJ, Griffen WO Jr, et al. Tobramycin pharmacokinetics in morbidly obese patients. Clin Pharmacol Ther. 1979;26:508.
151. Bravo ME, Arancibia A, Jarpa S, et al. Pharmacokinetics of gentamicin in malnourished infants. Eur J Clin Pharmacol. 1982;21:499.
152. Pennington JE, Dale DC, Reynolds HY, et al. Gentamicin sulfate pharmacokinetics: lower levels of gentamicin in blood during fever. J Infect Dis. 1975;132:270.
153. Sawchuk RJ, Zaske DE. Pharmacokinetics of dosing regimens which utilize multiple intravenous infusions: gentamicin in burn patients. J Pharmacokinet Biopharm. 1976;4:183.
154. Loirat P, Rohan J, Baillet A, et al. Increased glomerular filtration rate in patients with major burns and its effect on the pharmacokinetics of tobramycin. N Engl J Med. 1978;299:915.

155. Smith CR, Lipsky JJ, Laskin OL, et al. Double-blind comparison of the nephrotoxicity and auditory toxicity of gentamicin and tobramycin. N Engl J Med. 1980;302:106.
156. Noone P, Parsons TMC, Pattison JR, et al. Experience in monitoring gentamicin therapy during treatment of series gram-negative sepsis. Br Med J. 1974;1:477.
157. Tally FP, Louie TJ, Weinstein WM, et al. Amikacin therapy for severe gram-negative sepsis. Ann Intern Med. 1975;83:484.
158. Anderson ET, Young LS, Hewitt WL. Simultaneous antibiotic levels in "breakthrough" gram-negative and bacteremia. Am J Med. 1976;61:493.
159. Klastersky J, Meunier-Carpentier F, Prevase J. Significance of antimicrobial synergism for the outcome of gram-negative sepsis. Am J Med Sci. 1977;273:157.
160. Moore RD, Smith CR, Lietman PS. The association of aminoglycoside plasma levels with mortality in patients with gram-negative bacteremia. J Infect Dis. 1984;149:443.
161. Moore RD, Smith CR, Lietman PS. Association of aminoglycoside plasma levels with therapeutic outcome in gram-negative pneumonia. Am J Med. 1984;77:657.
162. Moore RD, Lietman PS, Smith CR. Clinical response to aminoglycoside therapy: importance of the ratio of peak concentration to minimal inhibitory concentration. J Infect Dis. 1987;155:93.
163. Wright JM, Collier B. The effects of neomycin upon transmitter release and action. J Pharmacol Exp Ther. 1977;200:576.
164. Lee C, DeSilva JC. Acute and subchronic neuromuscular blocking characteristics of streptomycin: a comparison with neomycin. Br J Anaesth. 1979;51:431.
165. Caputy AJ, Kim YI, Sanders DB. The neuromuscular blocking effects of therapeutic concentrations of various antibiotics on normal rat skeletal muscle: a quantitative comparison. J Pharmacol Exp Ther. 1981;217:369.
166. Chinyanga HM, Stoyka WW. The effect of colymycin M, gentamycin and kanamycin on depression of neuromuscular transmission induced by pancuronium bromide. Can Anaesth Soc J. 1974;21:569.
167. L'Hommedieu CS, Huber PA, Rasch DK. Potentiation of magnesium-induced neuromuscular weakness by gentamicin. Crit Care Med. 1983;11:55.
168. L'Hommedieu C, Stough R, Brown L, et al. Potentiation of neuromuscular weakness in infant botulism by aminoglycosides. J Pediatr. 1979;95:1065.
169. Hokkanen E. The aggravating effect of some antibiotics on the neuromuscular blockade in myasthenia gravis. Acta Neurol Scand. 1964;40:346.
170. Sanders DB, Kim YI, Howard JF, et al. Intercostal muscle biopsy studies in myasthenia gravis: clinical correlations and the direct effects of drugs and myasthenic serum. Ann NY Acad Sci. 1981;377:544.
171. Pittinger CB, Adamson R. Antibiotic blockade of neuromuscular function. Annu Rev Pharmacol. 1972;12:169.
172. Adams HR. Direct myocardial depressant effects of gentamicin. Eur J Pharmacol. 1975;30:272.
173. Descotes J, Evreux JC. Cardiac depressant effects of some recent aminoglycoside antibiotics. J Antimicrob Chemother. 1981;7:197.
174. Adams HR, Goodman FR, Wass GB. Alteration of contractile function and calcium ion movements in vascular smooth muscle by gentamicin and other aminoglycoside antibiotics. Antimicrob Agents Chemother. 1974;5:640.
175. Lerner SA, Matz GJ, Hawkins JE, eds. Aminoglycoside Ototoxicity. Boston: Little, Brown and Company; 1981.
176. Brummett RE, Meikle MM, Vernon JA. Ototoxicity of tobramycin in guinea pigs. Arch Otolaryngol. 1971;94:59.
177. Theopold HM. Comparative surface studies of ototoxic effects of various aminoglycoside antibiotics on the organ of Corti in the guinea pig. Acta Otolaryngol. 1977;84:57.
178. Johnson L-G, Hawkins JE Jr, Kinesley TC, et al. Aminoglycoside-induced cochlear pathology in man. Acta Otolaryngol [Suppl] (Stockh). 1981;383:1.
179. Koitchev K, Guilhaume A, Cazals Y, et al. Spiral ganglion changes after massive aminoglycoside treatment in the guinea pig. Acta Otolaryngol (Stockh). 1982;94:431.
180. Igarashi M. Vestibular ototoxicity in primates. Audiology. 1973;12:337.
181. Tran Ba Hay P, Muelemans A, Wassef M, et al. Gentamicin persistence in rat endolymph and perilymph after a two-day constant infusion. Antimicrob Agents Chemother. 1983;23:344.
182. Takada A, Sachacht J. Calcium antagonism and reversibility of gentamicin-induced loss of cochlear microphonics in the guinea pig. Hear Res. 1982;8:179.
183. Schacht J. Biochemistry of neomycin ototoxicity. J Acoust Soc Am. 1978;59:940.
184. Iinuma T, Mizukoshi O, Daly JF. Possible effects of various ototoxic drugs upon the ATP-hydrolyzing system in the stria vascularis and spiral ligament of the guinea pig. Laryngoscope. 1967;77:159.
185. Matz GJ, Lerner SA. Prospective studies of aminoglycoside ototoxicity in adults. In: Lerner SA, Matz GJ, Hawkins JE, eds. Aminoglycoside Ototoxicity. Boston: Little Brown and Company; 1981:327.
186. Fee WE Jr. Aminoglycoside ototoxicity in the human. Laryngoscope. 1980;90(Suppl 24):1.
187. Lerner AM, Reyes MP, Cone LA, et al. Randomized, controlled trial of the comparative efficacy, auditory toxicity, and nephrotoxicity of tobramycin and netilmicin. Lancet. 1983;i:1123.
188. Bendush CL. Ototoxicity: clinical considerations and comparative information. In: Whelton A, Neu HC, eds. The Aminoglycosides. New York: Marcel Dekker; 1982:453.
189. Moore RD, Smith CR, Lietman PS. Risk factors for the development of auditory toxicity in patients receiving aminoglycosides. J Infect Dis. 1984;149:23.
190. Mathog RH, Klein WJ, Jr. Ototoxicity of ethacrynic acid and aminoglycoside antibiotics in uremia. N Engl J Med. 1969;280:1223.
191. Brummett RE, Brown RT, Himes DL. Quantitative relationships of the ototoxic interaction of kanamycin and ethacrynic acid. Arch Otolaryngol. 1979;105:240.
192. Smith CR, Lietman PS. Effect of furosemide on aminoglycoside-induced nephrotoxicity and auditory toxicity in humans. Antimicrob Agents Chemother. 1983;23:133.
193. Dodson HC, Bannister LH, Dovek EE. The effects of combined gentamicin and white noise on the spiral organ of young guinea pigs. Acta Otolaryngol (Stockh). 1982;94:193.
194. Ryan AF, Bone RC. Non-simultaneous interaction of exposure to noise and kanamycin intoxication in the chinchilla. Am J Otolaryngol. 1982;3:264.
195. Henry KR, Chole RA, McGinn MD, et al. Increased ototoxicity in both young and old mice. Arch Otolaryngol. 1981;107:92.
196. Dumas G, Charachon R. Ototoxicity of kanamycin in developing guinea pigs: an electrophysiological study. Acta Otolaryngol (Stockh). 1982;94:203.
197. Silverblatt F. Pathogenesis of nephrotoxicity of cephalosporins and aminoglycosides. A review of current concepts. Rev Infect Dis. 1982;4(Suppl):S360.
198. Edwards CQ, Smith CR, Baughman KL, et al. Concentrations of gentamicin and amikacin in human kidneys. Antimicrob Agents Chemother. 1976;9:925.
199. Luft FC, Yun MN, Walker PD, et al. Gentamicin gradient patterns and morphological changes in human kidneys. Nephron. 1977;18:167.
200. Houghton DC, Campbell-Boswell MV, Bennett WM, et al. Myeloid bodies in the renal tubules of humans: relationship to gentamicin therapy. Clin Nephrol. 1978;10:140.
201. Aubert-Tulkens G, Van Hoof F, Tulkens P. Gentamicin-induced lysosomal phospholipidosis in cultured rat fibroblasts. Quantitative ultrastructural and biochemical study. Lab Invest. 1979;40:481.
202. Carlier MB, Laurent G, Claes PJ, et al. Inhibition of lysosomal phospholipases by aminoglycoside antibiotics: *in vitro* comparative studies. Antimicrob Agents Chemother. 1983;23:440.
203. Bennett WM, Gilbert DN, Houghton D, et al. Gentamicin nephrotoxicity: morphologic and pharmacologic features. West J Med. 1977;126:65.
204. Wellwood JM, Simpson PM, Tighe JR, et al. Evidence of gentamicin nephrotoxicity in patients with renal allographs. Br Med J. 1975;3:278.
205. Simmons CF, Bogusky RT, Humes HD. Inhibitory effects of gentamicin on renal mitochondrial oxidative phosphorylation. J Pharmacol Exp Ther. 1980;214:709.
206. Lipsky JJ, Lietman PS. Neomycin inhibition of adenosine triphosphatase: evidence for a neomycin-phospholipid interaction. Antimicrob Agents Chemother. 1980;18:532.
207. Lipsky JJ, Lietman PS. Aminoglycoside inhibition of a renal phophatidylinositol phospholipase C. J Pharmacol Exp Ther. 1981;220:287.
208. McNeil JS, Jackson B, Nelson L, et al. The role of prostaglandins in gentamicin-induced nephrotoxicity in the dog. Nephron. 1983;33:202.
209. Baylis C, Rennke HR, Brenner BM. Mechanism of the defect in glomerular ultrafiltration associated with aminoglycoside administration. Kidney Int. 1977;12:344.
210. Cojocel C, Hook JB. Differential effect of aminoglycoside treatment on glomerular filtration and renal reabsorption of lysozyme in rats. Toxicity. 1981;22:261.
211. Luft FC, Aronoff GR, Evan AP, et al. The effect of aminoglycosides on glomerular endothelium: a comparative study. Res Commun Chem Pathol Pharmacol. 1981;34:89.
212. Cojocel C, Dociu N, Maita K, et al. Effects of aminoglycosides on glomerular permeability, tubular reabsorption, and intracellular catabolism of the cation low-molecular-weight protein lysozyme. Toxicol Appl Pharmacol. 1983;68:96.
213. Carlier B, Ninane G. Effects of aminoglycosides on enzymuria and beta 2 microglobulinuria. Acta Clin Belg. 1982;37:23.
214. Walenkamp GHIM, Vree TB, Guelen PJM, et al. Interaction between the renal excretion rates of beta-2-microglobulin and gentamicin in man. Clin Chim Acta. 1983;127:229.
215. Elliott WC, Houghton DC, Gilbert DN, et al. Gentamicin nephrotoxicity: 1. Degree and permanence of acquired insensitivity. J Lab Clin Med. 1982;100:501.
216. Lietman PS, Smith CR. Aminoglycoside nephrotoxicity in humans. J Infect Dis. 1983;5(Suppl 2):S284.
217. Holmes AM, Hesling CM, Wilson TM. Drug-induced secondary hyperaldosteronism in patients with pulmonary tuberculosis. Q J Med. 1970;39:299.
218. Bar RS, Wilson HE, Mazzaferri EL. Hypomagnesemic hypocalcemia secondary to renal magnesium wasting: a possible consequence of high-dose gentamicin therapy. Ann Intern Med. 1975;82:646.
219. Roediger WEW, Ludwin D, Hinder RA. Hypocalcaemic response to streptomycin in malignant hypercalcaemia. Postgrad Med J. 1975;51:399.
220. Keating MJ, Seth MR, Bodey GP, et al. Hypocalcemia with hypoparathyroidism and renal tubular dysfunction associated with aminoglycoside therapy. Cancer. 1977;39:1410.
221. Patel R, Savage A. Symptomatic hypomagnesemia associated with gentamicin therapy. Nephron. 1979;23:50.
222. Moore RD, Smith CR, Lipsky JJ, et al. Risk factors for renal dysfunction in patients treated with aminoglycosides. Ann Intern Med. 1984;100:352.

223. Moore RD, Smith CR, Lietman PS. Increased risk of renal dysfunction due to interaction of liver disease and aminoglycosides. Am J Med. 1986;80:1093.
224. Lietman PS. Liver disease, aminoglycoside antibiotics, and renal dysfunction. Hepatology. 1988;8:966.
225. Wade JC, Petty BG, Conrad G, et al. Cephalothin plus an aminoglycoside is more nephrotoxic than methicillin plus an aminoglycoside. Lancet. 1978;ii:604.
226. Davies J, Anderson P, Davis BD. Inhibition of protein synthesis by spectinomycin. Science. 1965;149:1096.
227. Ward ME. The bactericidal action of spectinomycin on *Neisseria gonorrhoeae*. J Antimicrob Chemother. 1977;3:323.
228. Holloway WJ. Spectinomycin. Med Clin North Am. 1982;66:169.
229. McCormack WM, Finland M. Spectinomycin. Ann Intern Med. 1976;84:712.
230. Virtanen S. Sensitivity of *Haemophilus vaginalis* (*Corynebacterium vaginale*) to oleandomycin and spectinomycin. Pathol Microbiol. 1975;42:36.
231. Wagner JG, Novak E, Leslie LG. Absorption, distribution and elimination of spectinomycin dihydrochloride in man. Int J Clin Pharmacol Biopharm. 1967;14:261.

23. TETRACYCLINES AND CHLORAMPHENICOL

HAROLD C. STANDIFORD

THE TETRACYCLINES

All the tetracyclines are primarily bacteriostatic at therapeutic concentrations and have a broad spectrum that includes gram-positive, gram-negative, aerobic, and anaerobic bacteria, spirochetes, mycoplasmas, rickettsia, chlamydiae, and some protozoa. The analogues can be divided into three groups based on differences in their pharmacology: (*1*) the short-acting compounds chlortetracycline, oxytetracycline, and tetracycline; (*2*) an intermediate group consisting of demeclocycline and methacycline; and (*3*) the more recently discovered, longer-acting compounds doxycycline and minocycline.

Structure, Derivation, Nomenclature, and Brand Names

Unlike the fortuitous discovery of penicillin by Flemming, the first tetracycline, chlortetracycline, was discovered by screening organisms obtained from the soil for their antimicrobial properties. Benjamin M. Duggar, a meticulous mycologist in his 70s, noted unusual antimicrobial activity from organisms that formed a golden yellow colony.[1] He designated the organism *Streptomyces aureofaciens* (L. *aurum*, golden) and named the product aureomycin. Oxytetracycline was derived from *Streptomyces rimosus* in 1950, and tetracycline was produced by the catalytic dehalogenation of chlortetracyline in 1953. The two long-acting compounds were derived semisynthetically: doxycycline in 1966 and minocycline in 1967. The generic names of the analogues are determined by the substitutions on the basic structure of tetracycline, which consists of a hydronaphthacene nucleus containing four fused rings (Fig. 1). The compounds currently available in the United States and their major brand names, doses, and costs are listed in Table 1. Of these, tetracycline HCl and doxycycline have emerged as the most useful clinically. Chlortetracycline (aureomycin), the first member of the family, is no longer available except for topical use.

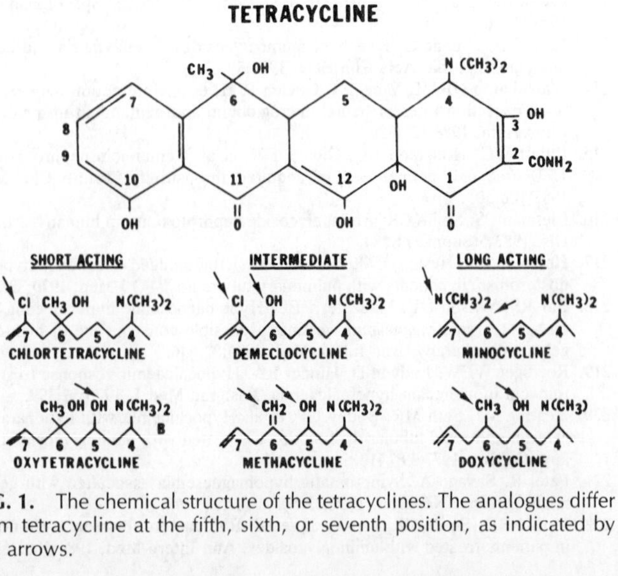

FIG. 1. The chemical structure of the tetracyclines. The analogues differ from tetracycline at the fifth, sixth, or seventh position, as indicated by the arrows.

TABLE 1. The Names, Preparations, Usual Adult Oral Dose, and Costs for the Tetracyclines Currently Available in the United States

Generic Name (Major Brand Name[a])	*Oral Preparations*	*Usual Adult Oral Dose*	*Cost for 10 Days[f]*
Short acting[b]			
Oxytetracycline (Terramycin, Pfizer)	Capsules: 125, 250 mg	500 mg q6h	45.00
Tetracyclone HCl[c] (Achromycin V, Lederle)	Capsules: 100, 250, 500 mg	500 mg q6h	7.50[g]
	Syrup: 125 mg/5 ml		5.75
Intermediate			
Methacycline (Rondomycin, Wallace)	Capsules: 150, 300 mg	300 mg q12h	31.50
Demeclocycline HCl (Declomycine, Lederle)	Capsules: 150 mg Tablets: 150, 300 mg	300 mg q12h	71.90
Long Acting[d]			
Doxycycline (Vibramycin, Pfizer)	Capsules (hyclate): 50, 100 mg	200 mg (or 100 q12h for first day), then 100 mg q24h[e]	25.60
	Syrup (calcium): 50 mg/5 ml Suspension (monohydrate): 25 mg/5 ml		5.65[g]
Minocycline (Minocin, Lederle)	Capsules and tablets: 50, 100 mg Suspension: 50 mg/5 ml	200 mg, then 100 mg q12h	35.65

[a] Many other brands are available for some of the analogues.
[b] The short-acting tetracyclines are also available for intravenous administration at usual doses of 500 mg every 6–12 hours not to exceed 2 g daily. However, most prefer doxycycline for this route of administration. Preparations combined with a local anesthetic agent can be given intramuscularly, but these are not recommended.
[c] Tetracycline is also available as a tetracycline phosphate complex (Tetrex, Bristol) intended to enhance absorption, but its superiority has not been established.
[d] The longer-acting agents can be given intravenously in the same doses that are recommended for oral therapy. Doxycycline is available at 100 or 200 mg per vial and minocycline at 100 mg per vial.
[e] The treatment schedules for sexually transmitted diseases use 100 mg twice daily.
[f] The costs (in dollars) are those for a 10-day adult treatment regimen when the antibiotics are purchased by the patient at a community pharmacy. (Courtesy of Robert Plummer, Dell's Pharmacy, Aberdeen, MD.)
[g] Cost for the generic form.

Mechanism of Action

The tetracyclines enter bacteria by an initial rapid phase driven by the proton-motive force followed by a slower accumulation over a period of hours that is energy dependent.[2] Once within the cell, they reversibly bind primarily to the 30S ribosomal subunit at a position that blocks the binding of the aminoacyl-tRNA to the accepter site on the mRNA–ribosome complex.[3] This prevents the addition of new amino acids into the growing peptide chain. The tetracyclines also inhibit protein synthesis in mammalian cells but do not accumulate within these cells by an active process.[4] This may partially explain the difference in the degree of protein inhibition produced in the host and in the microorganism.

In Vitro Activity

The antimicrobial spectra of all the tetracyclines are almost identical. Some differences, however, in the degree of activity against these organisms do exist among the analogues. In general, the lipophilic congeners are more active than are those that are more hydrophilic. It follows, therefore, that minocycline is the most active of the analogues, closely followed by doxycycline. The minimum inhibitory concentration (MIC) of the more hydrophilic congeners oxytetracycline and tetracycline are two- to fourfold higher against many bacteria and are the least-active analogues. Despite these differences, for cost reasons, it is recommended that tetracycline be used in the clinical microbiology laboratory to evaluate susceptibility for all the analogues.[5] Minimum inhibitory concentrations of tetracycline and doxycycline for many aerobic bacteria are given in Table 2. For the activity of the other analogues, the reader is referred to the extensive work from the laboratory of Finland et al.[7–9]

Although many of the aerobic and facultative anaerobic organisms are within the spectrum of the tetracyclines, more effective agents are available for the treatment of infections caused by most of these bacteria. The pneumonococci and many *Haemophilus influenzae* can be inhibited by concentrations of tetracyclines achieved in the serum, and this provides a rationale for their use in sinusitis and acute exacerbations of chronic bronchitis.[13] Gonococci and meningococci are extremely susceptible; unfortunately, gonococci resistant to penicillin G also tend to be resistant to tetracycline and are becoming more common.[6,14] Most *Escherichia coli* acquired outside the hospital setting can be inhibited by concentrations achieved in the serum or urine. Tetracyclines, therefore, are useful agents for the treatment of acute, uncomplicated, urinary tract infections. *Pseudomonas pseudomallei* organisms are generally sensitive, and this has therapeutic importance, as does the high degree of susceptibility of *Brucella* sp.[10,15] *Vibrio cholerae, vulnificus*, and other vibrios are generally susceptible, and the tetracyclines are important for therapy for diseases caused by this group of organisms.[16] Although *Campylobacter* sp. are generally susceptible, a high percentage of resistant isolates has been noted in some countries.[11,17,18] Therefore, it is not the drug of choice for infections caused by these bacteria. *Shigella* organisms have become increasingly resistant to these agents.[12] *Mycobacterium marinum* is susceptible and appears to respond clinically.[19]

The tetracyclines have activity against many anaerobic organisms[20] (Table 3). Their activity against *Actinomyces* is particularly relevant clinically. Doxycycline is more active against *Bacteroides fragilis* than tetracycline is, but clindamycin or metronidazole are the preferred agents for infections caused by this organism. The activity of the tetracyclines against anaerobic bacteria, however, may be partially responsible for the effectiveness of the neomycin–tetracycline combination and doxycycline alone as oral presurgical bowel preparations.[21,22] Many pathogenic spirochetes are susceptible including *Borrelia burgdorferi*, the agent of Lyme disease.[23] Other organisms generally inhibited by this group of antibiotics include rickettsia, chlamydiae, mycoplasmas, and to a limited degree protzoa (malariae and *Entamoeba histotytica).*[24]

Bacteria develop resistance to the tetracyclines predominantly by preventing the accumulation of tetracycline within the cell. This is accomplished by decreasing the influx transport system and/or increasing the ability of the cell to export the antibiotic. Rarely if ever are the tetracyclines inactivated bio-

TABLE 2. Minimum Inhibitory Concentration of Tetracycline and Doxycycline for Common Aerobic and Facultative Anaerobic Bacteria[a]

Organism	*Number of Strains*	*Antibiotic*	*Cumulative Percentage Inhibited by Indicated Concentrations (μg/ml)* 0.4	0.8	1.6	3.1	6.3	12.5	25
Gram-positive									
S. aureus	56	Tetracycline	0	2	20	65	67	67	67
		Doxycycline	2	25	63	65	68	80	87
S. pyogenes[b]	63	Tetracycline	10	50	80	87	90	92	98
		Doxycycline	56	90	90	95	95	98	100
S. pneumoniae[c]	35	Tetracycline	70	96	96	100			
		Doxycycline	100						
Streptococcus (group B)	12	Tetracycline	0	0	50	50	50	50	75
		Doxycycline	0	50	50	50	50	58	100
Streptococcus (group D)	36	Tetracycline	0	0	0	0	10	15	15
		Doxycycline	0	0	0	0	10	18	22
Gram-negative[d]									
N. gonorrhoeae[e]	25	Tetracycline	5	60	85	88	100		
		Doxycycline	60	75	80	92	100		
N. meningitidis[f]	10	Tetracycline	0	50		100			
		Doxycycline	0		50		100		
H. influenzae	15	Tetracycline	0	0	0	33	87	100	
		Doxycycline	0	0	60	93	100		
E. coli	48	Tetracycline	0	0	0	5	35	60	65
		Doxycycline	0	0	0	5	35	60	70
K. pneumoniae	17	Tetracycline	0	0	0	0	5	30	40
		Doxycycline	0	0	0	0	12	35	40
Enterobacter sp.	10	Tetracycline	0	10	30	50	70	80	90
		Doxycycline	0	0	0	0	10	30	60
Pseudomonas pseudomallei	10	Tetracycline	0	0	60	100			
Campylobacter	172	Tetracycline	44	62	74	81	84	85	88
jejuni	107	Doxycycline	68	74	79	80	86	98	100
Shigella sp.	213	Tetracycline	0	10	12	50	50	55	62

[a] Organisms should be considered susceptible if the MICs are 4 μg/ml or less. A moderate susceptibility range of up to 8 μg/ml may be useful for the treatment of urinary tract infections.[5]
[b] More recent series indicate that 20–40 percent of *S. pyogenes* have become resistant to the tetracyclines.
[c] Tetracycline-resistant *S. pneumoniae* strains are more common in some areas.
[d] *Proteus mirabilis*, indole-positive *Proteus* sp., and *P. aeruginosa* are generally resistant to 25 μg/ml.
[e] Many individual cases and clusters of tetracycline-resistant *Neisseria gonorrhoeae* have been reported.[6]
[f] The medium inhibitory concentration of minocycline for meningococci is 1.6 μg/ml (range, 0.8–1.6 μg/ml).
(Data from refs. 7–12.)

TABLE 3. Minimum Inhibitory Concentrations of Tetracycline and Doxycycline for Common Anaerobic Bacteria[a]

Organism	Number of Strains	Antibiotic	Cumulative Percentage Susceptible to Indicated Concentration (μg/ml) 0.5	1.0	2.0	4.0	8.0	16.0	32.0
Gram-positive									
Peptococcus and *Gaffkya*	59	Tetracycline	25	29	36	36	37	61	92
		Doxycycline	28	35	40	70	93	98	100
Peptostreptococcus	29	Tetracycline	38	41	48	52	72	86	97
		Doxycycline	45	45	66	79	97	100	
Streptococci, anaerobic and microaerophilic	10	Tetracycline	50	60	70	90	90	90	100
		Doxycycline	70	90	90	90	100		
Eubacterium	17	Tetracycline	24	59	65	65	77	82	94
		Doxycycline	59	65	77	82	88	100	
Propioni bacterium	12	Tetracycline	58	75	83	83	83	83	100
		Doxycycline	75	83	83	92	92	92	100
Clostridium perfringens	9	Tetracycline	22	22	56	67	67	78	78
		Doxycycline	67	67	67	78	89	100	
Other clostridia	33	Tetracycline	36	46	49	52	61	67	76
		Doxycycline	49	52	61	68	82	97	97
Actinomyces	16	Tetracycline	56	69	94	94	94	100	
		Doxycycline	63	69	94	100			
Gram-negative									
Gram-negative cocci	26	Tetracycline	54	69	73	73	73	85	92
		Doxycycline	58	69	73	81	96	100	
Fusobacterium	34	Tetracycline	94	97	97	97	97	100	
		Doxycycline	94	94	94	94	100		
Bacteroides fragilis	76	Tetracycline	25	40	40	42	46	68	63
		Doxycycline	41	42	50	75	88	97	100
Bacteroides melaninogenicus	67	Tetracycline	75	76	79	87	94	96	99
		Doxycycline	75	78	90	96	97	99	99
Other *Bacteroides*, *Selenomonas*	72	Tetracycline	33	35	43	50	60	75	93
		Doxycycline	40	43	53	68	79	85	96

[a] An organism with a MIC of 4 μg/ml or less should be considered susceptible.
(Modified from Sutter et al.,[20] with permission.)

logically or altered chemically by resistant bacteria.[25–28] Resistance to one tetracycline usually implies resistance to all, although there are marked differences in the degree of resistance among species. The resistance among bacteria can be mediated by transferable resistance plasmids, a mechanism particularly important for *Shigella*. The tetracyclines have been widely used in feeds to promote growth in animals. This may be a major factor in providing selective antibiotic pressure for the spread of plasmid-mediated resistance to these and other antibiotics.[29–31]

Pharmacology

Serum levels achieved by usual oral doses in adults are seen in Figure 2. Absorption occurs primarily in the proximal small bowel and produces peak serum concentrations 1–3 hours after administration. The commonly used 500 mg therapeutic dose of tetracycline gives a serum level of 4 μg/ml, highest of all the short-acting analogues.[32] Doxycycline and minocycline (200 mg) achieve serum levels of about 2.5 μg/ml, slightly higher than levels attained by the larger therapeutic doses of the intermediate agents.[33–37]

After the intravenous administration of 500 mg, serum levels of the short-acting agents (not shown) are approximately 8 μg/ml at 30 minutes and decrease to 2–3 μg/ml by 5 hours.[38] Intravenous injection of the usual 200 mg loading dose of the long-acting agents doxycycline and minocycline produces serum levels of approximately 4 μg/ml at 30 minutes. Once tissue distribution occurs for the long-acting analogues, levels are almost identical to concentrations achieved orally.[33,39] Thrombophlebitis is a frequent complication of the intravenous preparations. Intramuscular preparations are available for the short-acting compounds but are not recommended because of the severe pain produced on injection, even when they are mixed with local anesthetics.

Some of the pharmacokinetic properties of the tetracyclines are compared in Table 4. The high levels obtained orally with tetracycline as compared with other short-acting agents are due primarily to better absorption from the gastrointestinal tract. The long-acting analogues doxycycline and minocycline are absorbed almost completely; thus, high serum levels are achieved with relatively small doses.[33,34] The tetracyclines can be differentiated into three groups on the basis of their different half-lives. Doxycycline has the longest of all and allows therapeutic levels to be maintained with a single daily dose.[33] The 8-hour half-life of tetracycline[38] suggests that the dosage interval could

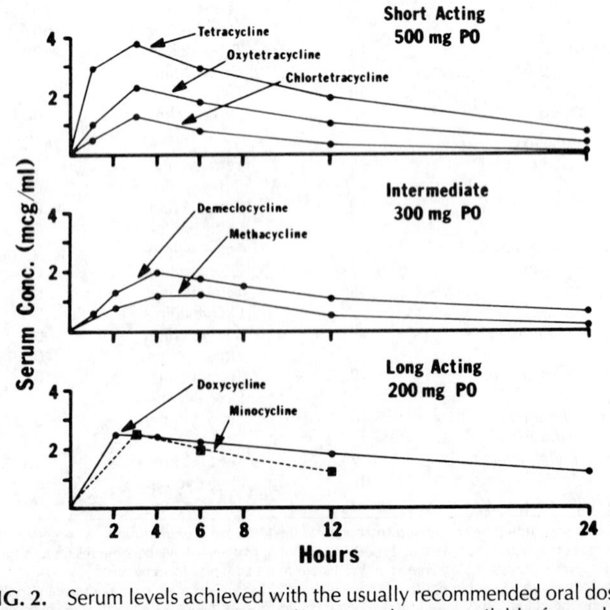

FIG. 2. Serum levels achieved with the usually recommended oral doses of the tetracyclines. Chlortetracycline is no longer available for oral or parenteral administration. (Data from refs. 32–36.)

TABLE 4. Pharmacokinetic Features of the Tetracyclines[a]

Antibiotic	*GI Absorption (%)*	*Half-Life (hr)*	*Renal Clearance*[b] *(ml/min/1.73 m²)*	*Urinary Recovery (%)*	*Apparent Volume of Distribution*[b] *(Liters)*	*Protein Binding*[c] *(%)*
Short acting						
Chlortetracycline	30	6	32	18	100	47
Oxytetracycline	58	9	99	70	128	35
Tetracycline	77	8	74	60	108	65
Intermediate						
Demeclocycline	66	12	35	39	121	91
Methacycline	58	14	31	60	79	90
Long acting						
Doxycycline	93	18	20	42	50	93
Minocycline	95	16	9	6	60	76

[a] The pharmacokinetic values vary considerably from laboratory to laboratory. These values were selected in most instances because comparative data were available from reliable investigators.
[b] After single-dose intravenous administration.
[c] Ultrafiltration technique.
(Data from refs. 33–35 and 38–41.)

be 8 hours for this antibiotic when it is used to treat minor infections. The half-lives of the compounds are determined mainly by the rate of excretion by the kidneys. Chlortetracycline is an exception: it has a short half-life despite a slow rate of clearance as a result of the marked instability of the compound in vitro as well as in vivo.[38] With the possible exception of chlortetracycline and minocycline, adequate therapeutic concentrations of all the tetracyclines are achieved in the urine for treatment of urinary tract infections caused by sensitive organisms. The degree of protein binding of the analogues is variable, depending on the methods used for the determination, but it tends to be greater for the intermediate and long-acting compounds.[39–41] This may be one of the factors that determines their slow rate of renal excretion. The apparent volume of distribution for most of the tetracyclines is greater than that of extracellular body water, thus indicating sequestration in tissues, presumably the liver.[38] Minocycline and doxycycline have the smallest volume of distribution, another factor that tends to enhance their serum levels.[39]

Tissue Distribution. The tetracyclines can be found in small amounts in many tissues and fluids, including the lung, liver, kidney, brain, sputum, and mucosal fluid. For tetracycline, the levels in the cerebral spinal fluid are approximately 10–26 percent of the serum levels,[42,43] whereas concentrations in synovial fluid and the maxillary sinus mucosa approach serum levels.[44,45] All the tetracyclines are concentrated in unobstructed bile and produce levels in this fluid 5–20 times those obtained in the serum. It has been suggested that lipid solubility is a primary determinant for the diffusion in many tissues. Minocycline, followed by doxycycline, is more lipophilic at a physiologic pH than are the other drugs. This may explain why minocycline reaches sufficient concentrations in saliva and tears to eradicate the meningococcal carrier state whereas the other tetracyclines do not.[46,47] The tetracyclines cross the placenta, accumulate in fetal bone and teeth, and therefore, should not be given during pregnancy.[48] Because they are excreted in breast milk, caution is advised in the postpartum period.

Renal and Hepatic Insufficiency. The tetracyclines should not be used in patients with renal failure. Doxycycline, the only exception, is excreted in the gastrointestinal tract under these circumstances. Neither the half-life nor the therapeutic dose of this antibiotic varies with alterations in renal function.[49] The tetracyclines are slowly removed by hemodialysis but not effectively by peritoneal dialysis. Hepatic disease is not known to cause elevated serum levels of the tetracyclines. However, they should be used very cautiously in such situations because they have been noted to cause hepatic toxicity.

Assay

The tetracyclines generally are measured by bioassay using *Bacillis cereus* as the test organism.[50] A spectrofluorometric assay is available for some of the analogues,[51] but monitoring of serum levels during therapy is rarely indicated.

Toxicity

Skin and Allergy. Hypersensitivity reactions including anaphylaxis, urticuria, periorbital edema, fixed drug eruptions, and morbilliform rashes occur with tetracyclines but are not common.[52–54] When a patient is allergic to one analogue, he should be considered to be allergic to all. Photosensitivity reactions consisting of a red rash on areas exposed to sunlight that is frequently associated with onycholysis are most common in patients receiving demeclocycline but occur with all analogues.[55,56] They appear to be a toxic rather than an allergic reaction. Prolonged administration of minocycline has been noted rarely to cause nail, skin, and scleral pigmentation, which is usually reversible, as well as an asymptomatic black pigmentation of the thyroid.[57,58]

Teeth and Bones. A gray-brown to yellow discoloration of the teeth has been noted in 80 percent of the children taking tetracyclines in some communities.[59] This side effect is permanent and may be associated with hypoplasia of the enamel[55,60] and depression of skeletal growth in premature infants.[61] The darkening effect of tetracyclines on permanent teeth appears to be related to the total dose of the antibiotic administered. In a retrospective study, cosmetically noticeable, but mild darkening of the permanent teeth occurred in 3 of 14 children receiving five courses of tetracycline, whereas 4 of 6 children receiving eight courses had moderate darkening of the enamel.[62] Primary teeth generally show more darkening than do the larger, thicker, and more opaque permanent teeth. Since there is some variability in staining with similar tetracycline exposure, it is prudent not to administer these agents to pregnant women and to children up to the age of 8 years, the period when tooth enamel is being formed. For this reason, the Food and Drug Administration (FDA) has withdrawn from the market the concentrated liquid dosage forms (drops) specifically intended for pediatric use.[63] It is not unreasonable, however, to administer a single course of tetracycline therapy to young children for specifically defined indications where the alternative regime may produce more severe toxicity. Thus, the tetracyclines are indicated for children suspected of having Rocky Mountain spotted fever who can tolerate oral medications. Doxycycline binds less with calcium than do other tetracyclines and may cause dental changes less frequently in children.[64]

Gastrointestinal. The tetracyclines are irritative substances and frequently produce gastrointestinal symptoms after oral administration. Esophageal ulcerations that are manifested as retrosternal pain exacerbated by swallowing have been clearly documented after tetracycline and doxycycline administration. In most cases, the patients were taking the capsules with little or no fluid just before going to bed. A word of caution to the patient is indicated in order to prevent this toxicity. The complication may also occur in patients with esophageal obstruction or motility disorders.[65,66] Nausea, vomiting, and epigastric distress are dose related and limit the dose of most the analogues. The administration of food with doxycycline, minocycline, or oxytetracycline may ameliorate some of these symptoms, but food seriously decreases the absorption of the other tetracyclines. Diarrhea is most often associated with analogues that are poorly absorbed and appears to be related to alterations in the enteric flora. Doxycycline produces less of an effect on bowel flora than does tetracycline.[67] The diarrhea usually subsides when treatment with the antibiotic is stopped, but prolonged symptoms due to pseudomembranous colitis have been reported.[68] Tetracycline also has been noted, rarely, to cause pancreatitis with or without overt liver disease.[69]

Liver. The hepatoxicity of the tetracyclines, first described in patients receiving intravenous chlortetracycline but now described with other analogues, appears pathologically as a fine droplet fatty metamorphosis and results in a high mortality.[70,71] The administration of less than 2 g/day intravenously is not associated with liver dysfunction or injury except in pregnant women, who are particularly at risk,[72] and in patients with an excessive serum level due to renal failure.[73]

Renal Function. The tetracyclines aggravate pre-exisitng renal failure by inhibiting protein synthesis, which increases the azotemia from amino acid metabolism.[74] Nephrogenic diabetes insipidus is produced by demeclocycline, a side effect that has been used therapeutically to reverse chronic inappropriate antidiuretic hormone secretion[75]; renal failure has complicated its use for this purpose in patients with cirrhosis.[76] Outdated tetracycline has produced a reversible Fanconi-like syndrome with renal tubular acidosis, but tetracycline formulations producing this syndrome have been modified. It is unlikely that this complication will recur.[49]

Nervous and Sensory Systems. Vertigo is a side effect unique to minocycline. Symptoms of light-headedness, loss of balance, dizziness, and tinnitus usually begin on the second and third days of therapy and have been noted more frequently in women (70 percent) than in men (28 percent). The symptoms are reversible within several days after discontinuation of therapy with the antibiotic, but this side effect has seriously limited the use of minocycline.[77] Benign intracranial hypertension (pseudotumor cerebri) has been described in infants and adults with many of the analogues.[78,79]

Superinfection. Colonization by tetracycline-resistant organisms is a frequent occurrence during tetracycline therapy and is generally of little clinical significance. Rarely, a fulminating diarrhea resulting from staphylococcal enteritis may occur after oral or parenteral therapy.[80,81] More often and less serious, oral or vaginal monaliasis complicates treatment, a complication that may require specific therapy.

Significant Drug Interactions

Food adversely affects the absorption of tetracycline, chlortetracycline, methacycline, and demeclocycline. All the tetracyclines form complexes with divalent or tivalent cations. Therefore, absorption is markedly decreased when these drugs are administered simultaneously with calcium, magnesium, and aluminum in antacids, milk, or iron and iron-containing tonics.[82] Sodium bicarbonate also has an adverse effect on absorption and should not be administered simultaneously.[83] Cimetidine has been shown to decrease the absorption of tetracycline, but this is unlikely to be significant in the clinical situation.[84] Carbamazepine (Tegretol), diphenylhydantoin, and barbiturates decrease the normal half-life of doxycycline to almost one-half by increasing the hepatic metabolism of the antibiotic.[85,86] Chronic ethanol ingestion has also resulted in a shorter half-life of doxycycline but not tetracycline, presumably also through induction of hepatic microsomal enzymes.[87] Methyoxyflurane anesthesia may cause nephrotoxicity when administered with tetracyclines.[88] It has been suggested that this adverse interaction occurs with the newer, less nephrotoxic fluorinated anesthetic agents as well.[89] The use of these antibiotics concurrently with diuretics produces an elevated blood urea nitrogen (BUN) level, although th exact mechanism has not been determined.[90] It has been reported that women receiving oral contraceptives have become pregnant while receiving tetracycline. This may be caused by the reduction in bacterial hydrolysis of conjugated estrogen in the intestine.[91,92]

Indications

The tetracyclines are the drugs of choice or effective alternative therapy for a wide variety of infections (Table 5). Their role in the therapy for many of the sexually transmitted diseases, including infections caused by the gonococci and chlamydiae, and for the treatment of the syndromes of acute pelvic inflammatory disease, nonspecific urethritis, and sexually transmitted epididymo-orchitis in young adults is particularly noteworthy.[93] The reader is referred to the specific chapter for details. They have no role in the treatment of viral or fungal diseases. Tetracycline, the least expensive of the analogues, is sometimes preferred for oral administration. Doxycycline, however, ap-

TABLE 5. Major Therapeutic Indications for the Tetracyclines[a]

Therapy of Choice	*Effective Therapy*
Brucellosis (with streptomycin in seriously ill patients	Acne, severe
Chlamydial infections	Actinomycosis
Ornithosis	Anthrax
Trachoma	*Campylobacter fetus, jejuni*
Urethral, endocervical, or rectal infections in adults	Chronic bronchitis (acute exacerbations)
Cholera	Glanders (*Pseudomonas mallei*)
Lymphogranuloma venereum	Gonococcal infections (resistance is a problem)
Epididymitis, acute (sexually transmitted form)	*Pasteurella multocida*
Granuloma inguinale	Prostatitis
Leptospirosis	Rat-bite fever (*Spirillum minus, Streptococcus moniliformis*)
Lyme disease (early stages)	Syphilis
Melioidosis (with chloramphenicol in seriously ill patients)	Tularemia
Mycobacterium marinum (minocycline)	Vincent's infection
Mycoplasma pneumoniae (some prefer erythromycin)	Whipple's disease
Pelvic inflammatory disease (acute, in combination with other antibiotics)	Yaws, nasopalatal
Relapsing fever (*Borrelia recurrentis*)	*Yersinia enterocolitica*
Rickettsial infections (some prefer chloramphenicol for severe infections)	*Effective Alternative Prophylaxis*
Rocky Mountain spotted fever	Oral bowel preparation for intestinal surgery (tetracycline in combination with neomycin or doxycycline alone)
Typhus fever	Meningococcal disease (only minocycline)
Q fever	Traveler's diarrhea (doxycycline)
Rickettsial pox	
Ehrlichiosis	
Urethritis, nonspecific	
Urethral syndrome (dysuria-frequency syndrome)	
Vibrio vulnificus	

[a] Unless otherwise specified, tetracycline hydrochloride is the preferred analogue for oral administration.

pears equally effective and is preferred by most when intravenous administration is required.

CHLORAMPHENICOL

Soon after chloramphenicol was released in the United States in 1949, reports linked this highly effective agent with aplastic anemia, and it quickly fell into disfavor. The increased awareness of the pathogenicity of anaerobic organisms and the development of ampicillin-resistant *H. influenzae* accounted for an increase in the use of the compound. However, the availability of other agents for anaerobic infections has reduced the need for chloramphenicol for this indication, and its use for ampicillin-resistant *H. influenzae* is currently being challenged by the newer cephalosporins. Chloramphenicol remains a useful antibiotic, but only for well-defined indications in seriously ill patients.

Structure, Derivation, Brand Names, and Preparations

Like the early tetracyclines, chloramphenicol was discovered by screening organisms for their antimicrobial activity. Isolated independently by Burkholder from a mulched field near Caracas, Venezuela,[94] and by workers at the University of Illinois from compost,[95] the organism producing the active compound was named *Streptomyces venezuelae*.[96] The structure of chloramphenicol is shown in Figure 3. It was the first antibiotic whose chemical synthesis was economically and technically practical for large-scale production.[97] Preparations currently available and the usual doses are given in Table 6.

Thiamphenical, not available in the United States, is an analogue in which the *p*-nitro group on the benzene ring is replaced by a methylsulfonyl group. Its spectrum of activity is similar to chloramphenicol, but it has not been reported to cause aplastic anemia.

Mechanism of Action

Chloramphenicol appears to enter the cell by an energy-dependent process.[98] Once within the cell it inhibits protein synthesis. This is accomplished by reversibly binding to the larger 50S subunit of the 70S ribosome at a locus that prevents the attachment of the amino acid-containing end of the aminoacyl-tRNA to its binding region. Without this attachment, the association of the amino acid substrate with peptidyl transferase does not occur, and peptide bond formation is prevented.[2] This block in protein synthesis produces a static effect against most sensitive microorganisms. However, in vitro evidence indicates that chloramphenicol is bactericidal against some meningeal pathogens such as *H. influenzae, Streptococcus pneumoniae*, and *Neisseria meningitidis* but not group B streptococci or enteric gram-negative bacilli at concentrations that can be achieved therapeutically.[99–101] Although mammalian cells contain primarily 80S ribosomes that are unaffected by chloramphenicol, the mitochondria do contain 70S particles. The effect of chloramphenicol on these has been suggested as a cause for the dose-related bone marrow suppression of the compound but not the idiosyncratic aplastic anemia.[102]

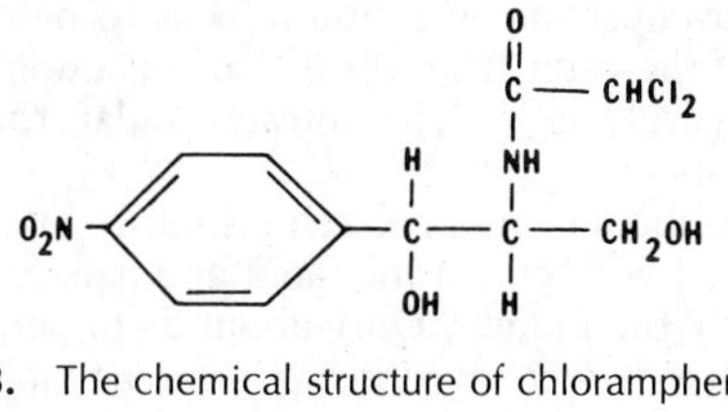

FIG. 3. The chemical structure of chloramphenicol.

TABLE 6. Systemic Chloramphenicol Preparations Currently Available in the United States[a]

Preparation	How Supplied	Usual Dose
Oral		
Capsules		
Chloromycetin (Parke-Davis)	250 mg	25 mg/kg/day for neonates less than 1 wk old; 25 mg/kg q12h for infants 1–4 wk; 50 mg/kg/day in 6-hr intervals for older children and adults; 100 mg/kg/day for older children and adults with meningitis
Mychel (Rachelle)	250 mg	
Suspension		
Chloromycetin Palmitate (Parke-Davis)	150 mg/5 ml	Same as above
Parenteral (intravenous)		
Chloromycetin Sodium Succinate (Parke-Davis)	1 g (powder)	Same as above

[a] Other pharmaceutical companies also make chloramphenicol.

In Vitro Activity

Chloramphenicol is extremely active against a variety of organisms, including bacteria, spirochetes, richettsia, chlamydiae, and mycoplasmas. The MICs required for bacteria are listed in Table 7. Most of the gram-positive and gram-negative aerobic bacteria are inhibited by concentrations easily achieved in the serum of patients, but more active or less toxic therapeutic agents are available for most of these pathogens.[8–10,20,97,103–107] Salmonellae icluding *Salmonella typhi* are generally susceptible.[105] In the United States, resistant strains occasionally occur,[109] but imported strains may be highly resistant. The three most common organisms causing meningitis in childhood (*H. influenzae, S. pneumoniae*, and *N. meningitidis*) are highly susceptible,[9,110,111] although rare resistant strains of each species have been reported. The overall rate of *H. influenzae* resistance among clinical strains in the United States is approximately 0.6 percent.[112] Indeed, strains of *H. influenzae* that cause clinical infections and are resistant to both chloramphenicol and ampicillin have been isolated in several parts of the world.[113–115] These resistant isolates are rare in the United States but rather frequent in Spain.[116–118] Chloramphenicol is one of the most active antibiotics against anaerobic bacteria including *B. fragilis*, but clindamycin, metronidazole, and imipenem have become more important clinically to treat infections caused by these bacteria.[20,108,119,120]

Bacteria develop resistance to chloramphenicol by becoming impermeable to the drug or by producing an enzyme, acetyltransferase, that acetylates the antibiotic to an inactive diacetyl derivative.[121,122] This latter mechanism has been R factor–mediated and has been responsible for widespread epidemics of chloramphenicol-resistant typhoid fever and *Shigella* dysentery in Central and South America, Vietnam, and other countries.[123–126] It has been suggested that the unrestricted over-the-counter sale of chloramphenicol in the countries involved may be an important factor that provides antibiotic pressure for the development of these resistant strains.[125,126] In the United States, chloramphenicol resistance in *Salmonella* has been traced to the use of chloramphenicol on dairy farms.[31]

Pharmacology

Chloramphenicol serum levels achieved by different routes of administration and with different product forms are listed in Figure 4. Chloramphenicol in the encapsulated form is well absorbed from the gastrointestinal tract and results in peak serum levels of 12 μg/ml of active antibiotic after a 1 g dose.[127,128] Since

TABLE 7. Activity of Chloramphenicol against Bacteria[a]

Bacteria	Number of Strains	Cumulative Percentage Inhibited at Indicated Concentration (μg/ml)						
		0.4	*0.8*	*1.6*	*3.1*	*6.3*	*12.5*	*25*
Aerobic bacteria								
Gram-positive								
S. aureus	291	0	0	0	5	55	95	96
S. aureus (methicillin-resistant)	22	0	0	0	0	20	20	20
S. pyogenes	303	0	0	20	92	99	100	
Streptococci, group B	146	0	0	0	85	99	100	
S. viridans	193	0	0	0	60	90	100	
Streptococci, group D	382	0	0	0	0	0	12	48
S. pneumoniae	78				50	100		
Gram-negative								
H. influenzae	17			50	100			
N. meningitidis	7		50		100			
N. gonorrhoeae	106	5	52	97	100			
E. coli	71	0	0	5	30	75	95	95
K. pneumoniae	35	0	0	6	70	75	75	75
Enterobacter	10	0	0	0	10	20	50	80
Serratia marcescens	111	0	0	0	0	5	33	60
P. mirabilis	209	0	0	0	20	60	90	95
Proteus (indole-positive)	32	0	0	0	10	40	50	65
Salmonella typhosa	81	0	0	0	50	95	100	
S. paratyphi A	31				28	97	97	97
Shigella sp.	44		20	30	75	90	90	95
Vibrio cholera	64					84		89
Brucella sp.	25	0	0	28	92	100		
P. aeruginosa	11	0	0	0	0	0	0	0
P. pseudomallei	10	0	0	0	0	50	100	
Bordetella pertussis	31	20	45	85	97	99		
Anaerobic bacteria								
Gram-positive								
Peptococcus sp.	145	8	25	67	97	98	98	99
Peptostreptococcus sp.	72	11	37	63	96	100		
Propionibacterium acnes	16	12	31	94	100			
Eubacterium lentum	14	14	14	28	71	100		
Clostridium perfringens	34	0	0	15	100			
Clostridium sp.	17	12	12	53	88	100		
Gram-negative								
Veillonella sp.	13	23	46	85	100			
B. fragilis	195	0	1	2	23	98	100	
B. melaninogenicus	29	14	31	93	96	100		
Fusobacterium fusiforme	18	39	44	56	89	100		

[a] The National Committee for Clinical Laboratory Standards suggests that 4 μg/ml or less be considered susceptible when testing *H. influenzae* and 12 μg/ml or less be considered susceptible when testing other organisms.[5]
(Data from refs. 8–10, 12, 20, 97, and 103–108.)

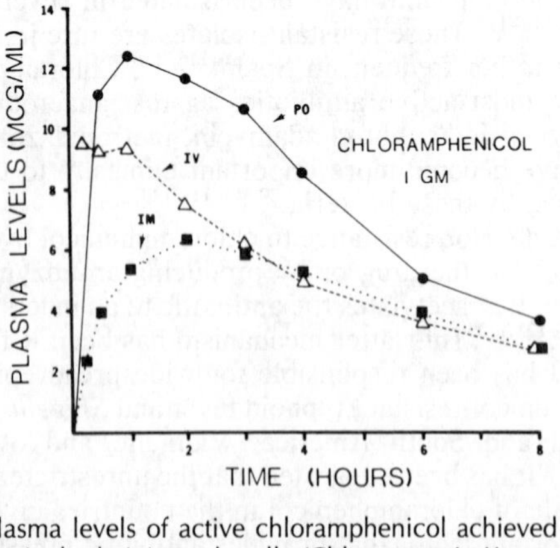

FIG. 4. Plasma levels of active chloramphenicol achieved with 1 g of chloramphenicol administered orally (Chloromycetin Kapseals) and with chloramphenicol sodium succcinate intravenously (iv) and intramuscularly (im). (Modified from Glazko,[127] with permission.)

it is a very bitter substance, aqueous solutions may not be accepted by children. A tasteless suspension in the form of chloramphenicol palmitate is available. This preparation must be hydrolized in the intestine to produce active chloramphenicol. Although earlier formulations sometimes produced erratic serum levels, the bioavailability of chloramphenicol palmitate in the current formulation is the same as in the capsules and is effective for children with *H. influenzae* meningitis (A. J. Glazko, Warner-Lambert/Parke-Davis Pharmaceutical Research Division, Ann Arbor, Michigan, personal communication).[129,130]

The intravenous preparation of the drug is the soluble but inactive chloramphenicol succinate ester that is rapidly hydrolized within the body to biologically active chloramphenicol.[131] This preparation produces active chloramphenicol levels in the serum that are 70 percent of those obtained after oral administration due to incomplete hydrolysis.[127] Intramuscular injection is well tolerated and in most studies produces peak serum levels and areas under the serum level curve similar to intravenous administration.[132–136] One study in adults, however, showed peak concentrations of only one-half to two-thirds of those obtained by the intravenous route, and this was associated with a delayed therapeutic response and increased relapse rate of typhoid fever.[137] Since 30 percent of the unhydrolyzed inactive succinate ester is found in the urine regardless of which parenteral route is used, the lower serum levels produced by intramuscular injection appear to be due to delayed absorption of the ester from the site of injection rather than to decreased hydrolysis.[127] The intramuscular route should be used cautiously.

Chloramphenicol is metabolized primarily by the liver where it is conjugated with glucuronic acid and is excreted in this inactive form by the kidney. Only about 5–10 percent of the administered dose is recovered in the urine as biologically active chloramphenicol. Nevertheless, in the absence of renal disease, concentrations of 150–200 μg/ml of active drug are achieved, which is sufficient to treat urinary tract infections if necessary. Urinary concentrations are markedly diminished, however, in patients with renal failure.[138]

The increased use of chloramphenicol in children has led to a better understanding of the pharmacokinetics. It is clear that there is a wide variation in the metabolism and excretion in that age group. Dosage requirements may vary threefold in children of the same age, with even greater variation noted in newborn and young infants. Because they metabolize the antibiotic at a slow rate, the initial dose for newborns less than 1 week old should be 25 mg/kg every 24 hours and for infants from 1–4 weeks old, 25 mg/kg every 12 hours instead of the usual 50 mg/kg/day divided into 6-hour dosing intervals for older children and adults. However, the wide variation makes monitoring serum levels imperative.[136,139,140]

Chloramphenicol has a half-life in adults of 4.1 hours after single intravenous injections, is not highly bound to protein (25–50 percent), and has an apparent volume of distribution of 100 liters.[97,127,141] The antibiotic diffuses well into many tissues and body fluids. Kramer et al.[142] have shown levels in the brain to be 36 μg/ml, whereas corresponding serum levels were 4 μg/ml. These high levels may reflect the antibiotic's high degree of lipid solubility in conjunction with low protein binding and small molecular size.[143] Levels in the cerebral spinal fluid even without inflamed meninges are generally 30–50 percent of serum concentrations, much higher than those of most other antibiotics.[97] Therapeutic levels are obtained in pleural, ascitic, and synovial fluids.[97,144] In the aqueous humor levels are approximately 50 percent of those in the serum,[145] but studies in rabbits and humans suggest that topical administration may be more efficient in providing high aqueous concentrations.[146,147] Subconjuctival injections are not satisfactory.[148] The antibiotic crosses the placenta to the fetal circulation but produces negligible amounts in the amniotic fluid.Only small amounts of active chloramphenicol are recovered in the bile (0.14 percent of a 1 g dose).[97]

Renal and Hepatic Insufficiency. The half-life of biologically active chloramphenicol in patients with renal disease differs only slightly from healthy subjects, whereas its metabolites increase markedly. The dose, however, should not be modified if therapeutic levels of the active drug are to be maintained. Fortunately, the metabolites do not appear to be as toxic as the active compound. Neither peritoneal nor hemodialysis alters serum levels sufficiently to require dose alterations.[141,149]

Patients with hepatic failure, as evidenced by jaundice or ascites, conjugate chloramphenicol at a slower rate. Serum levels of active chloramphenicol increase to levels capable of bone marrow suppression.[150] The regimen suggested for adults with hepatic insufficiency is an initial 1 g loading dose followed by 500 mg every 6 hours. The course of therapy should be limited where possible to 10–14 days.

Assay

Because of the narrow therapeutic-to-toxic ratio, it is important to monitor serum levels of this antibiotic, particularly in newborn and premature infants, in patients with hepatic disease, and in those patients taking interacting drugs. There are a number of very effective assays that can be used, including bioassays, radioenzymatic assays, competitive enzyme-linked immunoassays, and high-performance chromotography.[151–158] Serum levels in most cases should be maintained between 10 and 30 μg/ml.

Toxicity

Hematologic. The most important toxic effects of chloramphenicol occur in the bone marrow. The effects can be divided into two types. The first is a reversible bone marrow depression due to a direct pharmacologic effect of the antibiotic as a result of inhibition of mitochondrial protein synthesis. It is manifested by reticulocytopenia, anemia, leukopenia, thrombocytopenia, or any combination thereof. There is an increase in serum iron in association with a reduced uptake of radioactive iron by the red blood cells, thus indicating diminished hemoglobin synthesis. The bone marrow reveals vacuolization of the erythyroid and myeloid precursors, but these changes are not specific for chloramphenicol. This type of toxicity is extremely common, occurs during the course of therapy, and is dose related.[159] It is more likely to occur in patients receiving 4 g or more per day or in patients in whom serum levels are above 25 μg/ml, a level that may occur in patients with severe liver disease who are receiving usual doses. It is reversible when treatment with the antibiotic is discontinued.[160]

The second type of toxicity is a rare but generally fatal "idiosyncratic" response that is most frequently manifested as aplastic anemia.[161] Indeed, chloramphenicol is the most common cause of this syndrome. According to the best epidemiologic studies in the United States, aplastic anemia occurs once in 24,500–40,800 patients who receive the antibiotic, a risk about 13 times greater than that for aplastic anemia in the general population.[162] The aplastic anemia most commonly occurs weeks to months after completion of therapy and is not necessarily dose related. It appears that this toxic effect is caused by a mechanism different from the direct bone marrow suppression previously described. Although the pathogenesis of this idiosyncratic response is not known, there have been several observations and theories that deserve comment. This type of toxicity has occurred in identical twins, which suggests a genetic predisposition.[163] Morley et al.[164] have observed that mice given chloramphenicol after treatment with busulfan had a progressive decrease in the number of pluripotential stem cells whereas control mice did not. Since most of the animals had entirely normal hemograms before receiving chloramphenicol, they suggest that the aplastic anemia might result in patients with unrecognized pre-existing residual marrow damage either genetic or acquired. In 1967 Holt observed that the aplastic anemia occurred only after oral administration of the antibiotic.[165] He postulates that the fatal reaction may be caused by the absorption of toxic products produced by enzymatic degradation of chloramphenicol, perhaps as a result of specific types of bacteria colonizing the gut of affected people. Supporting this hypothesis, Jimenez and colleagues have shown that one of chloramphenicol's metabolites, dehydrochloramphenicol, is 10- to 20-fold more cytotoxic than chloramphenicol is yet only one-third as effective in inhibiting protein synthesis, thus suggesting that this metabolite and perhaps others may play a significant role in this toxicity.[166] However, a number of cases of aplastic anemia from parenteral chloramphenicol and after the administration of eye drops have also been reported. Although the number of cases reported is greater after oral therapy, the parenteral form of the antibiotic should also be considered to be potentially toxic.[167–169] It has been speculated that the nitrobenzene moiety of chloramphenicol may be the culprit responsible for the aplastic anemia. Thiamphenicol, an analogue of chloramphenicol that is currently used in Europe and Japan, has the nitro group on the benzene ring replaced by methysulfone. This analogue produces the reversible bone marrow suppression as readily as chloramphenicol does but has not been associated with the aplastic anemia.[170] Although most cases of aplastic anemia from chloramphenicol become apparent after the completion of therapy, it should be emphasized that 22 percent of the cases occur concurrently with antibiotic administration.[161,169] Whether some of these episodes can be prevented by checking the blood counts of patients is not known. Until the pathogenesis of the toxicity is clearly understood, it is recommended that a complete blood count be obtained on a twice-a-week basis on all patients receiving chloramphenicol. If the white blood cell count decreases below 2500/mm^3, it is desirable to discontinue treatment with the antibiotic if the clinical condition allows. It should be recognized, however, that low numbers of white blood cells may occur in illnesses for which chloramphenicol is used such as typhoid fever.

Also of concern are the reports of childhood leukemia after the use of chloramphenicol. Although these cases generally follow the aplastic anemia, a recent population-based case control interview study of 309 childhood leukemia cases and 618 age- and sex-matched controls showed a significant dose-response relation between chloramphenicol and the risk of both acute lymphocytic and nonlymphocytic leukemia, particularly after treatment for greater than 10 days in children without prior aplastic anemia. Until this is more clearly defined, it seems prudent to change therapy as quickly as possible to alternate agents when organisms prove susceptible to other equally effective and less toxic antibiotics.[171]

Chloramphenicol may also produce a hemolytic anemia in patients with the Mediterranean form of glucose-6-phosphate dehydrogenase (G6PD) deficiency. This apparently does not occur with the milder A type G6PD deficiency, which is the most common form in blacks.[172]

Gray Baby Syndrome. The gray baby syndrome of neonates is characterized by abdominal distension, vomiting, flaccidity, cynosis, circulatory collapse, and death. The side effect results from a diminished ability of neonates to conjugate chloramphenicol and to excrete the active form in the urine.[173] If chloramphenicol is necessary in premature infants and neonates, the dose should be reduced to 25 mg/kg/day, and the antibiotic levels should be monitored. This syndrome has also been recognized in toddlers and after accidental overdoses in adults.[174,175] It is generally associated with serum concentrations of chloramphenicol of greater than 50 μg/ml and may present with unexplained metabolic acidosis.[176] Large-volume exchange transfusions or charcoal hemoperfusion has been used to accelerate drug removal.[177,178]

Optic Neuritis. Optic neuritis resulting in decreased visual acuity has been described in patients receiving prolonged chloramphenicol therapy.[179] The symptoms are generally reversible, but a loss of vision has occurred. Other neurologic sequelae such as peripheral neuritis, headache, depression, opthalmoplegia, and mental confusion have also been described.

Other Types. Hypersensitivity reactions including rashes and drug fevers and anaphylaxis are rare. Herxheimer-like responses during therapy for syphilis, brucellosis, and typhoid fever have been observed. Symptoms involving the gastrointestinal tract, including nausea, vomiting and diarrhea, glossitis, and stomatitis, occur but have not been a major problem. Bleeding due to decreased vitamin K synthesis has resulted from prolonged administration.

Significant Drug Interactions

Chloramphenicol prolongs the half-life of tolbutamide, chlorpropamide, phenytoin, cyclophosphamide, and warfarin (Coumadin), apparently by inhibiting hepatic microsomal enzymes.[180–183] Severe toxicity and death have occurred. Phenytoin, rifampin, and phenobarbital have been observed to decrease the serum concentration and increase the total body clearance of chloramphenicol, perhaps by inducing hepatic microsomal enzymes. Serum concentrations should be monitored when these drugs are administered concurrently.[184,185] The physician should be on the alert for toxicity from other agents that are metabolized by the liver when administering this agent and should monitor serum levels when these drugs are administered concurrently. Chloramphenicol may delay the response of anemias to iron, folic acid, and vitamin B_{12}.[186]

TABLE 8. Indications for Chloramphenicol

Indication	*Usual Adult Dose*	*Comment*
Therapy of choice		
Brain abscess	100 mg/kg/day	Used with a penicillin; some prefer penicillin plus metronidazole for this indication
Typhoid fever and invasive salmonellosis	50 mg/kg/day	Strains in some areas may be chloramphenicol resistant; not used for gastroenteritis or carrier state
Effective alternative therapy		
Bacterial meningitis *H. influenzae* *S. pneumoniae* *N. meningitidis*	100 mg/kg/day	For penicillin-allergic patients; can be used for empirical therapy when these pathogens are suspected; also used for *S. pneumoniae* relatively resistant to penicillin
Rickettsial infections Rocky Mountain spotted fever Typhus (murine) Scrub typhus Tick bite fever Q fever	50 mg/kg/day	Preferred drug when patients require parenteral therapy, in pregnancy, and in young children
Melioidosis, acute	50 mg/kg/day	Used with tetracycline

Chloramphenicol is primarily a bacteriostatic agent and will antagonize in vitro the bactericidal activity of the penicillins, cephalosporins, and aminoglycoside antibiotics. This has doubtful clinical significance in most instances. However, care should be exercised in the use of such combinations for infections that require bactericidal activity for efficacy such as for infections in the granulocytopenic host or in the treatment of endocarditis.[187] In the treatment of meningitis, the bacteriostatic activity of chloramphenicol against group B streptococci and its in vitro antagonism with ampicillin against this organism are of concern and should be considered in selecting therapy when this organism is likely to be a pathogen.[101]

Indications

The clinical indications for the use of chloramphenicol are listed in Table 8. In most cases, these indications are clearly defined. Many experts feel that the third-generation cephalosporins have superseded chloramphenicol for the treatment of bacterial meningitis in infants and children. The antibiotic is still used for the treatment of meningitis in the penicillin-allergic patients, for meningitis cases by relatively penicillin-resistant pneumococci, and as an oral alternative where the use of parenteral therapy is impossible.[188–190] Occasionally, the antibiotic is useful when the differential diagnosis includes both meningococcemia and Rocky Mountain spotted fever, diseases that may be difficult to distinguish on clinical characteristics. It also may be useful in the place of a nephrotoxic agent for the treatment of severe infections due to sensitive organisms in patients with decreased renal function.

Chloramphenicol is a valuable antimicrobial agent. Like many other agents, it is toxic and can cause death. When the rare clinical indications are present, however, the antibiotic should not be avoided because of its possible toxicity.

REFERENCES

1. Finland M. Twenty-fifth anniversary of the discovery of Aureomycin: The place of the tetracyclines in antimicrobial therapy. Clin Pharmacol Ther. 1974;15:3.
2. Pratt WB, Fekety R. The Antimicrobial Drugs. New York: Oxford University Press; 1986:205–8.
3. Craven GR, Gavin R, Fanning T. The transfer RNA binding site of the 30

s ribosome and the site of tetracycline inhibition. Symp Quant Biol. 1969;34:129.
4. Beard HS, Armentrout SA, Weisberger. Inhibition of mammalian protein synthesis by antibiotics. Pharmacol Rev. 1969;21:213.
5. National Committee for Clinical Laboratory Standards. Methods for dilution antimicrobial susceptibility tests for bacteria that grow aerobically: Approved standard. NCCLS Publication M7-A. Villanova, PA: NCCLS; 1985.
6. Centers for Disease Control. Antibiotic-resistant strains of *Neisseria gonorrhoeae*. MMWR. 1987;36(Suppl 55)1–18.
7. Steigbigel NH, Reed CR, Finland M. Susceptibility of common pathogenic bacteria to seven tetracycline antibiotics in vitro. Am J Med Sci. 1968;255:179.
8. Finland M. Changing patterns of susceptibility of common bacterial pathogens to antimicrobial agents. Ann Intern Med. 1972;76:1009.
9. Sabath LD, Stumpf LL, Wallace SJ, et al. Susceptibility of *Diplococcus pneumoniae, Haemophilus influenzae*, and *Neisseria meningitidis* to 23 antibiotics. Antimicrob Agents Chemother. 1970, 1971;53.
10. Eickhoff TC, Bennett JV, Hayes PS, et al. *Pseudomonas pseudomallei* susceptibility to chemotherapeutic agents. J Infect Dis. 1970;121:95.
11. Karmali MA, DeGrandis S, Fleming PC. Antimicrobial susceptibility of *Campylobacter jejuni* with special reference to resistance patterns of Canadian isolates. Antimicrob Agents Chemother. 1981;19:593.
12. Gordon RC, Thompson TR, Carlson W, et al. Antimicrobial resistance of shigellae isolated in Michigan. JAMA. 1975;231:1159.
13. Neu HC. A symposium on the tetracyclines: A major appraisal. Introduction. Bull NY Acad Med. 1978;54:141.
14. Sparling PF. Antibiotic resistance in *Neisseria gonorrhoeae*. Med Clin North Am. 1972;56:1133.
15. Farrell ID, Hinchliffe PM, Robertson L. Susceptibility of *Brucella* spp. to tetracycline and its analogues. J Clin Pathol. 1976;29:1097.
16. Morris J Glenn Jr, Black RE. Chloera and other vibrioses in the United States, N Engl J Med. 1985;312:343–50.
17. Chow AW, Patten V, Dominick B. Susceptibility of *Campylobacter fetus* to twenty-two antimicrobial agents. Antimicrob Agents Chemother. 1978;13:416.
18. Michel J, Rogol M, Dickman D. Susceptibility of clinical isolates of *Campylobacter jejuni* to sixteen antimicrobial agents. Antimicrob Agents Chemother. 1983;23:796.
19. Wallace RJ, Wiss K. Susceptibility of *Mycobacterium marinum* to tetracyclines and aminoglycosides. Antimicrob Agents Chemother. 1981;20:610.
20. Sutter VL, Finegold SM. Susceptibility of anaerobic bacteria to 23 antimicrobial agents. Antimicrob Agents Chemother. 1976;10:736.
21. Washington JA, Dearing WH, Judd ES, et al. Effect of preoperative antibiotic regimen on development of infection after intestinal surgery: Prospective, randomized, double-blind study. Ann Surg. 1974;180:567.
22. Hojer H, Wetterfors J. Systemic prophylaxis with doxycycline in surgery of the colon and rectum. Ann Surg. 1978;187:362.
23. Johnson SE, Klein GP, Schmid GP, et al. Susceptibility of the Lyme disease spirochete to seven antimicrobial agents. Yale J Biol Med. 1984;57:549–53.
24. Pang LW, Limsomwong N, Boudreau EF, et al. Doxycycline prophylaxis for *falciparum malaria*: Lancet. 1987;1:1161–4.
25. Benveniste R, Davies J. Mechanisms of antibiotic resistance in bacteria. Annu Rev Biochem. 1973;42:471.
26. Sompolinsky D, Zemira S. Plasmid-determined resistance to tetracycline. Microbios. 1981;30:109.
27. Park BH, Hendricks M, Malamy MH, et al. Cryptic tetracycline resistance determinant (class F) isolated from *Bacteroides fragilis* mediates resistance in *Escherichia coli* by actively reducing tetracycline accumulation. Antimicrob Agents Chemother. 1987;31:1739–43.
28. Roberts MC, Kenny GE, Tet M. Tetracycline resistance determinants in *Ureaplasma urealyticum*. Antimicrob Agents Chemother. 1986:29:350–2.
29. Rapoport MI, Calia FM. The use of antibiotics in animal feeds. JAMA. 1974;229:1212.
30. VanLeeuwen WJ, VanEmbden J, Guinee PAM, et al. Decrease in drug resistance in *Salmonella* in the Netherlands. Antimicrob Agents Chemother. 1979;16:237.
31. Spika JS, Waterman SH, Soo Hoo GW, et al. Chloramphenicol-resistant *Salmonella newport* traced through hamburger to dairy farms. N Engl J Med. 1987;316:565–70.
32. Finland M, Garrod LP. Demethylchlortetracycline. Br Med J. 1960;2:959.
33. Fabre J, Milek E, Kalfopoulos P, et al. The kinetics of tetracyclines in man: Digestive absorption and serum concentrations. In: Doxycycline (Vibramycin): A Compendium of Clinical Evaluation. New York: Pfizer Laboratories; 1973:13.
34. Lederle Laboratories. Minocin: Minocycline. Pearl River, NY: Lederle Laboratories; 1975.
35. Rosenblatt JE, Barrett JE, Brodie JL, et al. Comparison of in vitro activity and clinical pharmacology of doxycycline with other tetracyclines. Antimicrob Agents Chemother. 1966, 1967;134.
36. Kirby WMM, Roberts CE, Burdick RE. Comparison of two new tetracyclines with tetracycline and demethylchlortetracycline. Antimicrob Agents Chemother. 1961,1962;286.
37. Fabre J, Pitton JS, Junz JP, et al. Distribution and excretion of doxycycline in man. Chemotherapia. 1966;11:73.
38. Kunin CM, Dornbush AC, Finland M. Distribution and excretion of four tetracycline analogues in normal young men. J Clin Invest. 1959;38:1950.
39. MacDonald H, Kelley RG, Allen ES, et al. Pharmacokinetic studies on minocycline in man. Clin Pharmacol Ther. 1973;14:852.
40. Kunin CM. Comparative serum binding distribution and excretion of tetracycline and a new analogue methacycline. Proc Soc Exp Biol Med. 1962;110:311.
41. Bennett JV, Mickewait JS, Barrett JE, et al. Comparative serum binding of four tetracyclines under simulated in vivo conditions. Antimicrob Agents Chemother. 1965, 1966;180.
42. Wood WS, Kipnis GR. The concentrations of tetracycline, chlortetracycline and oxytetracycline in the cerebrospinal fluid after intravenous administration. In: Antibiotics Annual, 1953–1954. New York: Medical Encyclopedia; 1953:98.
43. Yim CW, Flynn NM, Fitzgerald FT. Penetration of oral doxycycline into the cerebrospinal fluid of patients with latent or neurosyphilis. Antimicrob Agents Chemother. 1985;28:347.
44. Parker RH, Schmid F. Antimicrobial activity of synovial fluid during therapy of septic arthritis. Arthritis Rheum. 1971;14:96.
45. Lundberg C, Malmburg A, Ivemark BI. Antibiotic concentrations in relation to structural changes in maxillary sinus mucosa folowing intramuscular or peroral treatment. Scand J Infect Dis. 1974;6:187.
46. Fabre J, Milek E, Kalopoulos P, et al. The kinetics of tetracyclines in man II. Excretion, penetration in normal and inflammatory tissues, behavior in renal insufficiency and hemodialysis. In: Doxycycline (Vibramycin): A Compendium of Clinical Evaluations. New York: Pfizer Laboratories; 1973:19.
47. Hoeprich PD, Warshauer DM. Entry of four tetracyclines into saliva and tears. Antimicrob Agents Chemother. 1974;5:330.
48. LeBlanc AL, Perry JE. Transfer of tetracycline across the human placenta. Tex Rep Biol Med. 1967;25:541.
49. Whelton A. Tetracyclines in renal insufficiency: Resolution of a therapeutic dilemma. Bull NY Acad Med. 1978;54:223.
50. Bennett JV, Brodie JL, Benner EJ, et al. Simplified accurate method for antibiotic assay of clinical specimens. Appl Microbiol. 1966;14:170.
51. Kohn KW. Determination of tetracyclines by extraction of fluorescent complexes: Application to biological materials. Anal Chem. 1961;33:862.
52. Csonka GW, Rosedale N, Walkden L. Balanitis due to fixed drug eruption associated with tetracycline therapy. Br J Vener Dis. 1970;47:42.
53. Fellner MJ, Baer RL. Anaphylactic reaction to tetracycline in a penicillin-allergic patient: Immunologic studies. JAMA. 1965;192:997.
54. Furey WW, Tan C. Anaphylactic shock due to oral demethylchlortetracycline. Ann Intern Med. 1969;70:357.
55. Carey BW. Photodynamic response of a new tetracycline. JAMA. 1960;172:1196.
56. Frost P, Weinstein GD, Gomez EC. Phototoxic potential of minocycline and doxycycline. Arch Dermatol. 1972;105:681.
57. Angeloni VL, Salasche SJ, Ortiz R. Nail, skin and scleral pigmentation induced by minocycline. Cutis. 1987;40:229–33.
58. Atwood HD, Dennet X. A black thyroid and minocycline treatment. Br Med J. 1976;2:1109.
59. Brearley LJ, Storey E. Tetracycline-induced tooth changes: Part 2. Prevalence, localization and nature of staining in extracted deciduous teeth. Med J Aust. 1968;2:714.
60. Witkop CJ, Wolf RO. Hypoplasia and intrinsic staining of enamel following tetracycline therapy. JAMA. 1963;185:1008.
61. Cohan S, Bevelander G, Tiamsic T. Growth inhibition of prematures receiving tetracycline. Am J Dis Child. 1963;105:453.
62. Grossman ER, Walcheck A, Freedman H. Tetracycline and permanent teeth: The relationship between doses and tooth color. Pediatrics. 1971;47:567.
63. Department of Health Education and Welfare. Tetracycline pediatric drops to be withdrawn from the market. FDA Drug Bull. 1978;8:23.
64. Forti G, Benincori C. Doxycycline and the teeth. Lancet. 1969;1:782.
65. Schneider R. Doxycycline esophageal ulcers. Am J Dig Dis. 1977;22:805.
66. Winckler K. Tetracycline ulcers of the oesophagus: Endoscopy, histology, and reoentgenology in two cases, and review of the literature. Endoscopy. 1981;13:225.
67. Hinton NA. The effect of oral tetracycline HCl and doxycycline on the intestinal flora. Curr Ther Res. 1970;12:341.
68. Gorbach SL, Bartlett JG. Anaerobic infections. N Engl J Med. 1974;290:1289.
69. Elmore MF, Rogge JD. Tetracycline induced pancreatitis. Gastroenterology. 1981;81:1134.
70. Lepper MH, Wolfe CK, Zimmerman HJ, et al. Effect of large doses of Aureomycin on human liver. Arch Intern Med. 1951;88:271.
71. Schultz JC, Adamson JS Jr, Workman WW, et al. Fatal liver disease after intravenous administration of tetracycline in high doses. N Engl J Med. 1963;269:999.
72. Whalley PJ, Adams RH, Combes B. Tetracycline toxicity in pregnancy: Liver and pancreatic dysfunction. JAMA. 1964;189:357.
73. Damjanov I, Arnold R, Faour M. Tetracycline toxicity in a non-pregnant woman. JAMA. 1968;204:934.
74. Shils ME. Renal disease and the metabolic effects of tetracycline. Ann Intern Med. 1963;58:389.
75. Forrest JN, Cox M, Hong C, et al. Superiority of demeclocycline over lithium in the treatment of chronic syndrome of inappropriate secretion of antidiuretic hormone. N Engl J Med. 1978;298:173.
76. Carrilho F, Bosch J, Arroyo V, et al. Renal failure associated with demeclocycline in cirrhosis. Ann Intern Med. 1977;87:195.

77. Fanning WL, Gump DW, Sofferman RA. Side effects of minocycline: A double blind study. Antimicrob Agents Chemother. 1977;11:712.
78. Koch-Weser J, Gilmore EB. Benign intracranial hypertension in an adult after tetracycline therapy. JAMA. 1967;200:345.
79. Walters BNJ, Gubbay SS. Tetracycline and benign intracranial hypertension: Report of five cases. Br Med J. 1981;282:19.
80. Jackson GG, Haight TH, Kass EH, et al. Tetramycin therapy of pneumonia: Clinical and bacteriologic studies in 91 cases. Ann Intern Med. 1951;35:1175.
81. Lundsgaard-Hansen P, Senn A, Roos B, et al. Staphylococcal enteritis: Report of six cases with two fatalities after intravenous administration of *N*-(pyrrolidinomethyl) tetracycline. JAMA. 1960;173:1008.
82. Neuvonen PJ, Gothoni G, Hackman R, et al. Interference of iron with the absorption of tetracyclines in man. Br Med J. 1970;4:532.
83. Bar WH, Adir J, Garrettson L. Decrease of tetracycline in man by sodium bicarbonate. Clin Pharmacol Ther. 1971;12:779.
84. Fisher P, House F, Inns P, et al. Effect of cimetidine on the absorption of orally administered tetracycline. Br J Clin Pharmacol. 1980;9:153.
85. Neuvonen PJ, Pentitila O. Interaction between doxycycline and barbiturates. Br Med J. 1974;1:535.
86. Pentitla O, Neuvonen PJ, Lehtovaara R. Interaction between doxcycline and some antiepileptic drugs. Br Med J. 1974;2:470.
87. Neuvonen PJ, Penttila O, Roos M. Effect of long-term alcohol consumption on the half-life of tetracycline and doxycycline in man. Int J Clin Pharmacol. 1976;14:303.
88. Kuzucu EY. Methoxyflurane, tetracycline and renal failure. JAMA. 1970;211:1162.
89. Semel JD. Renal failure and multiple organ toxicity associated with tetracycline operative prophylaxis. Infect Surg. 1988;June:405–8.
90. Boston collaborative drug surveillance program. Tetracycline and drug-attributed rises in blood urea nitrogen. JAMA. 1972;220:377.
91. Bacon JF, Chenfield GM. Pregnancy attributable to interaction between tetracycline and oral contraceptives. Br Med J. 1980;280:293.
92. Hansen PD. Drug Interactions. 5th ed. Philadelphia: Lea & Febiger; 1985:239.
93. U.S. Department of Health and Human Services. 1985 STD treatment guidelines. MMWR. 1985;34(Suppl 4):81–6.
94. Ehrlich J, Bartz QR, Smith RM, et al. Chloromycetin, a new antibiotic from a soil actinomycete. Science. 1947;106:417.
95. Carter HE, Gottliebb D, Anderson HW. Comments and communications. Science. 107;113:947.
96. Ehrlich J, Gottlieb D, Burkholder PR, et al. *Streptomyces venezuelae*, N. sp., the source of Chloromycetin. J Bacteriol. 1948;56:467.
97. Woodward TE, Wisseman CL. Chloromycetin (Chloramphenicol). New York: Medical Encyclopedia; 1958.
98. Abdel-Sayed S. Transport of chloramphenicol into sensitive strains of *Escherichia coli* and *Pseudomonas aeruginosa*. J Antimicrob Chemother. 1987;19:7–20.
99. Turk DC. A comparison of chloramphenicol and ampicillin as bactericidal agents for *Haemophilus influenzae* type B. J Med Microbiol. 1977;10:127.
100. Rahal JJ, Simberkoff MS. Bactericidal and bacteriostatic action of chloramphenicol against meningeal pathogens. Antimicrob Agents Chemother. 1979;16:13.
101. Weeks JL, Mason EO Jr, Baker CJ. Antagonism of ampicillin and chloramphenicol for meningeal isolates of group B streptococci. Antimicrob Agents Chemother. 1981;20:281.
102. Roodyn DB, Wilkie D. The Biogenesis of Mitochondria. London: Methuen; 1968.
103. McGowan JE, Garner C, Wilcox C, et al. Antibiotic susceptibility of gram negative bacilli isolated from blood cultures: Results of tests with 35 agents and strains from 169 patients at Boston City Hospital during 1972. Am J Med. 1974;57:225.
104. Yow EM, Spink WW. Experimental studies on the action of streptomycin, Aureomycin and Chloromycetin on *Brucella*. J Clin Invest. 1949;28:871.
105. Robertson RP, Wahab MFA, Raasch FO. Evaluation of chloramphenicol and ampicillin in *Salmonella* enteric fever. N Engl J Med. 1968;278:171.
106. Rubinstein E, Shainberg B. In vitro activity of cinoxacin, ampicillin, and chloramphenicol against *Shigella* and non-typhoid *Salmonella*. Antimicrob Agents Chemother. 1977;11:577.
107. Wells EB, Chang SM, Jackson GG, et al. Antibiotic spectrum of *Hemophilus pertussis*. J Pediatr. 1950;36:752.
108. Martin WJ, Gardner M, Washington JA II. In vitro antimicrobial susceptibility of anaerobic bacteria isolated from clinical specimens. Antimicrob Agents Chemother. 1972;1:148.
109. Cherubin CE, Neu HC, Rahal JJ, et al. Emergence of resistance to chloramphenicol in *Salmonella*. J Infect Dis. 1977;135:807.
110. Long SS, Phillips SE. Chloramphenicol-resistant *Hemophilus influenzae*. J Pediatr. 1976;90:1030.
111. Mathies AW Jr. Penicillins in the treatment of bacterial meningitis. *J R Coll Physicians Lond*. 1972;6:139.
112. Doern GV, Jorgensen JH, Thornsberry C, et al. Prevalance of antimicrobial resistance among clinical isolates of *Haemophilus influenzae*: A collaborative study. Diagn Microbiol Infect Dis. 1986;4:95–107.
113. MacMahon P, Sills J, Hall E, et al. *Haemophilus influenzae* type b resistant to both chloramphenicol and ampicillin in Britain. Br Med J. 1982;24:1229.
114. Bergeron MC, Claveau S, Simard P. Limited in vitro activity of cefamandole against 100 beta-lactamase and non–beta-lactamase-producing *Haemophilus influenzae* strains: Comparison of moxalactam, chloramphenicol and ampicillin. Antimicrob Agents Chemother. 1981;19:101.
115. Kenny JF, Isburg CD, Michaels RH. Meningitis due to *Haemophilus influenzae* type b resistant to both ampicillin and chloramphenicol. Pediatrics. 1980;66:14.
116. Campos J, Garcia-Tornel S, San Feliu I. Susceptibility studies of multiply resistant *Haemophilus influenzae* isolated from pediatric patients and contacts. Antimicrob Agents Chemother. 1984;25:706.
117. Centers for Disease Control. Ampicillin and chloramphenicol resistance in systemic *Haemophilus influenzae* disease. MMWR. 1984;33:35.
118. Williams JD, Mossdeen F. Antibiotic resistance in *Haemophilus influenzae*; epidemiology, mechanisms, and therapeutic possibilities. Rev Infect Dis. 1986;8(Suppl 5):555–61.
119. Cuchural GJ Jr, Talley FP, Jacobus NV, et al. Susceptibility of the *Bacteroides fragilis* group in the United States: Analysis by site of isolation. Antimicrob Agents Chemother. 1988;32:717–22.
120. Finegold SM, Wexler HM. Therapeutic implications of bacteriologic findings in mixed aerobic-anaerobic infections. Antimicrob Agents Chemother. 1988;32:611–6.
121. Okamoto S, Mizuno D. Mechanism of chloramphenicol and tetracycline resistance in *Escherichia coli*. J Gen Microbiol. 1964;35:125.
122. Okamoto S, Suzuki Y. Chloramphenicol-, dihydrostreptomycin-, and kanamycin-inactivating enzymes from multiple drug-resistant *Escherichia coli* carrying episome "R." Nature. 1965;208:1301.
123. Gangarosa EJ, Bennett JV, Wyatt C, et al. An epidemic-associated episome? J Infect Dis. 1972;126:215.
124. Butler T, Linh NN, Arnold K, et al. Chloramphenicol-resistant typhoid fever in Vietnam associated with R-factor. Lancet. 1973;2:983.
125. Editorial: Drug resistance in salmonellas. Lancet. 1982;1:1391.
126. Anderson ES, Smith HR. Chloramphenicol resistance in the typhoid bacillus. Br Med J. 1972;3:329.
127. Glazko AJ, Dill WA, Kinkel AW, et al. Absorption and excretion of parenteral doses of chloramphenicol sodium succinate in comparison with peroral doses of chloramphenicol (Abstract). Clin Pharmacol Ther. 1977;21:104.
128. Bartelloni PJ, Calia FM, Minchew BH, et al. Absorption and excretion of two chloramphenicol products in humans after oral administration. Am J Med Sci. 1969;258:203.
129. Pickering LK, Hoecker JL, Kramer WG, et al. Clinical pharmacology of two chloramphenicol preparations in children: Sodium succinate (IV) and palmitate (oral) esters. J Pediatr. 1980;96:757.
130. Tuomen EI, Powell KR, Marks MI, et al. Oral chloramphenicol in the treatment of *Haemophilus influzenae* meningitis. J Pediatr. 1981;99:968.
131. McCrumb FR, Snyder MJ, Hicken WJ. The use of chloramphenicol acid succinate in the treatment of acute infections. In: Antibiotics Annual, 1957–1958. New York: Medical Encyclopedia; 1958:837.
132. Ross S, Puig JR, Zarembra EA. Chloramphenicol acid succinate (sodium salt); some preliminary clinical and laboratory observations in infants and children. In Antibiotics Annual, 1957–1958. New York: Medical Encyclopedia; 1958:803–19.
133. McCrumb FR Jr, Snyder MJ, Hicken WJ. The use of chloramphenicol acid succinate in the treatment of acute infections. In Antibiotics Annual, 1957–1958. New York: Medical Encyclopedia; 1958:837.
134. Ciocatto E, Marchiaro G. Chloramphenicol in resuscitation and cardiac surgery. Postgrad Med J. 1967;43(Suppl):90–3.
135. Shann F, Linnenmann V, MacKenzie A, et al. Absorption of chloramphenicol sodium succinate after intramuscular administration in children. N Engl J Med. 1985;313:410–4.
136. Smith AL, Weber A. Pharmacology of chloramphenicol. Pediatr Clin North Am. 1983;30:209–36.
137. DuPont HL, Hornick RB, Weiss CF, et al. Evaluation of chloramphenicol acid succinate therapy of induced typhoid fever and Rocky Mountain spotted fever. N Engl J Med. 1970;282:53.
138. Lindberg AA, Nilsson LH, Bucht H, et al. Concentration of chloramphenicol in the urine and blood in relation to renal function. Br Med J. 1966;2:724.
139. Kauffman RE, Miceti JN, Strebel L, et al. Pharmacokinetics of chloramphenicol and chloramphenicol succinate in infants and children. J Pediatr. 1981;98:315.
140. Kauffman RE, Thirumoorthi MC, Buckley JA, et al. Relative bioavailability of intravenous chloramphenicol succinate and oral chloramphenicol palmitate in infants and children. J Pediatr. 1981;99:363.
141. Kunin CM. A guide to use of antibiotics in patients with renal disease. Ann Intern Med. 1967;67:151.
142. Kramer PW, Griffith RS, Campbell RL, et al. Antibiotic penetration of the brain: A comparative study. J Neurosurg. 1969;31:295.
143. Braude AI: Antimicrobial Drug Therapy. Philadelphia: WB Saunders; 1976:82.
144. Rapp GF, Griffith RS, Hebble WM. The permeability of traumatically inflamed synovial membrane to commonly used antibiotics. J Bone Joint Surg [Am]. 1966;48:1534.
145. Abraham RK, Burnett HH. Tetracycline and chloramphenicol studies on rabbit and human eyes. Arch Ophthalmol. 1955;54:641.
146. Beasley H, Boltralik JJ, Baldwin HA. Chloramphenicol in aqueous humor after topical application. Arch Ophthalmol. 1975;93:184.
147. George FJ, Hanna C. Ocular penetration of chloramphenicol. Arch Ophthalmol. 1977;95:879.
148. McPherson SD Jr, Presley GD, Crawford JR. Aqueous humor assays of subconjunctival antibiotics. Am J Ophthalmol. 1968;66:430.

149. Kunin CM, Glazko AJ, Finland M. Persistence of antibiotics in blood of patients with acute renal failure. II. Chloramphenicol and its metabolic products in the blood of patients with severe renal disease or hepatic cirrhosis. J Clin Invest. 1959;38:1498.
150. Suhrland LG, Weisberger AS. Chloramphenicol toxicity in liver and renal disease. Arch Intern Med. 1963;112:161.
151. Louie TJ, Tally FP, Bartlett JG, et al. Rapid microbiological assay for chloramphenicol and tetracyclines. Antimicrob Agents Chemother. 1976;9:874.
152. Jorgensen JH, Alexander GA. Rapid bioassay for chloramphenicol in the presence of other antibiotics. Am J Clin Pathol. 1981;76:474.
153. Lietman PS, White TJ, Shaw WV. Chloramphenicol: An enzymological microassay. Antimicrob Agents Chemother. 1976;10:347.
154. Smith AL, Smith DH. Improved enzymatic analysis of chloramphenicol. Clin Chem. 1978;24:1452.
155. Aravind MK, Miceli JN, Kauffman RE, et al. Simultaneous measurements of chloramphenicol and chloramphenicol succinate in body fluids utilizing HPLC. J Chromatogr. 1980;221:176.
156. Nahata MC, Powell DA. Simultaneous determination of chloramphenicol and its succinate ester by high-performance liquid chromatography. J Chromatogr. 1981;223:247.
157. Cambell GS, Mageau RP, Schwab B, et al. Detection and quantitation of chloramphenicol by competitive enzyme-linked immunoassay. Antimicrob Agents Chemother. 1984;25:205–11.
158. Abou-Khalil S, Abou-Khalil WH, Masoud AM, et al. High-performance liquid chromatographic determination of chloramphenicol and four analogues usingg reductive and oxidative electrochemical and ultraviolet detection. J Chromatogr. 1987;417:111–9.
159. Yunis AA. Chloramphenicol-induced bone marrow suppression. Semin Hematol. 1973;10:225.
160. Scott JL, Finegold SM, Belkin GA, et al. A controlled double-blind study of the hematologic toxicity of chloramphenicol. N Engl J Med. 1965;272:1137.
161. Best WR. Chloramphenicol-associated blood dyscrasias. A review of cases submitted to the American Medical Association Registry. JAMA. 1967;201:181.
162. Wallerstein RO, Condit PK, Kasper CK, et al. Statewide study of chloramphenicol therapy and fatal aplastic anemia. JAMA. 1969;208:2045.
163. Nagao T, Mauer AM. Concordance for drug-induced aplastic anemia in identical twins. N Engl J Med. 1969;281:7.
164. Morley A, Trainor K, Remes J. Residual marrow damage: Possible explanation for idiosyncrasy to chloramphenicol. Br J Haematol. 1976;32:525.
165. Holt R. The bacterial degradation of chloramphenicol. Lancet. 1967;1:1259.
166. Jimenez JJ, Arimura GK, Abou-Khalil WH, et al. Chloramphenicol-induced bone marrow injury: Possible role of bacterial metabolites of chloramphenicol. Blood. 1987;70:1180–5.
167. Polin HB, Plaut ME. Chloramphenicol. NY State J Med. 1977;77:378.
168. Plaut ME, Best WR. Aplastic anemia after parenteral chloramphenicol: Warning renewal (Letter). N Engl J Med. 1982;306:1486.
169. Daum RS, Cohen DL, Smith AL. Fatal aplastic anemia following apparent "dose-related" chloramphenicol toxicity. J Pediatr. 1979;94:403.
170. Keiser G. Introduction: Symposium on thiamphenicol. Postgrad Med J. 1974;50(Suppl 5):13.
171. Shu XO, Linet MS, Gao RN, et al. Chloramphenicol use and childhood leukaemia in Shanghai. Lancet. 1987;2:934–7.
172. Beutler E. Glucose 6-phosphate dehydrogenase deficiency. In: Williams WJ, Beutler E, Erslev AJ, et al., eds. Hematology. New York: McGraw-Hill; 1977:466.
173. Burns LE, Hodgman JE, Cass AB. Fatal circulatory collapse in premature infants receiving chloramphenicol. N Engl J Med. 1959;261:1318.
174. Craft AW, Brocklebank JT, Hey EN, et al. The "grey toddler": Chloramphenicol toxicity. Arch Dis Child. 1974;49:235.
175. Thompson WL, Anderson SE, Lipsky JJ, et al. Overdoses of chloramphenicol. JAMA. 1975;234:149.
176. Evans LS, Kleiman MB. Acidosis as a presenting feature of chloramphenicol toxicity. J Pediatr. 1986;108:475–7.
177. Stevens DC, Kleinman MB, Lietman PS, ett al. Exchange transfusion in acute chloramphenicol toxicity. J Pediatr. 1981;99:651.
178. Freundlick M, Cynamon H, Tamer A, et al. Management of chloramphenicol intoxication in infancy by charcoal hemoperfusion. J Pediatr. 1983;103:485.
179. Chloramphenicol blindness (Editorial). Br Med J. 1965;1:1511.
180. Christensen LK, Skovsted L. Inhibition of drug metabolism by chloramphenicol. Lancet. 1969;2:1397.
181. Petitpierre B, Fabre J. Chlorpropamide and chloramphenicol. Lancet. 1970;1:789.
182. Rose JQ, Choi HK, Schentag JJ. Intoxication caused by interaction of chloramphenicol and phenytoin. JAMA. 1977;237:2630.
183. Faber OK, Mouridsen HT, Skovsted L, et al. The effect of chloramphenicol and sulphaphenazole on the biotransformation of cyclophosphamide in man. Br J Clin Pharmacol. 1975;2:281.
184. Powell DA, Nahata MC, Durrell DC, et al. Interactions among chloramphenicol, phenytoin and phenobarbital in a pediatric patient. J Pediatr. 1981;98:1001.
185. Prober CG. Effect of rifampin on chloramphenicol levels. N Engl J Med. 1985;312:788–9.
186. JiJi RM, Gangarosa EJ, de la Macorra F. Chloramphenicol and its sulfamoyl analogue. Report of reversible erythropoietic toxicity in healthy volunteers. Arch Intern Med. 1963;11:70.
187. Sande MA, Overton JW. In vivo antagonism between gentamicin and chloramphenicol in neutropenic mice. J Infect Dis. 1973;128:247.
188. del Rio M, Chrane D, Shelton S, et al. Cefriaxone versus ampicillin and chloramphenicol for treatment of bacterial meningitis in children. Lancet. 1983;1:1241–4.
189. Odio CM, Faingezicht I, Salas JL, et al. Cefotaxime versus conventional therapy for the treatment of bacterial meningitis of infants and children. Pediatr Infect Dis. 1986;5:402.
190. McCracken GH, Nelson JD, Kaplan SL, et al. Consensus report: Antimicrobial therapy for bacterial meningitis in infants and children. Pediatr Infect Dis J. 1987;6:501–5.

24. RIFAMYCINS

BARRY M. FARR
GERALD L. MANDELL

Rifampin is a semisynthetic derivative of rifamycin B, a macrocyclic antibiotic compound produced by the mold *Streptomyces mediterranei*. First isolated from fermentation culture of a soil isolate in 1957, rifamycins were named for a then current French movie, *Le Riffi*.[1] Rifampin, which is the 3-4-methylpiperazinyl-iminomethyl derivative of rifamycin SV, is more soluble and active in vitro than is its parent compound[2] (Fig. 1). Rifampin is a zwitterion (inner salt) that is soluble in acidic aqueous solution, is even more soluble in organic solvents, and displays remarkable diffusion through lipids.[3]

MECHANISM OF ACTION

The rifamycins exert a bactericidal effect by inhibition of DNA-dependent RNA polymerase at the β-subunit, which prevents chain initiation but not elongation.[4] Mammalian mitochondrial RNA synthesis is not impaired at clinically achievable concentrations.

PHARMACOLOGY

Rifampin is available in the United States as a capsule of orange-red powder that is almost completely absorbed from the gastrointestinal tract to yield peak plasma concentrations of approximately 7–10 μg/ml (range, 4–32) within 1–4 hours after ingestion of 600 mg in adults or 10 mg/kg of body weight in children. Higher doses such as 1200 mg in adults result in a similar, more-than-proportional increase in the peak (≥30 μg/ml) serum concentration because such doses exceed the biliary Tm for excretion of rifampin.[5] The area under the curve (AUC) shows a similar, more-than-proportional increase after saturation of the biliary Tm. For this reason, a single daily dose of 1200 mg results in higher AUC values for rifampin than does divided doses totaling 1200 mg.

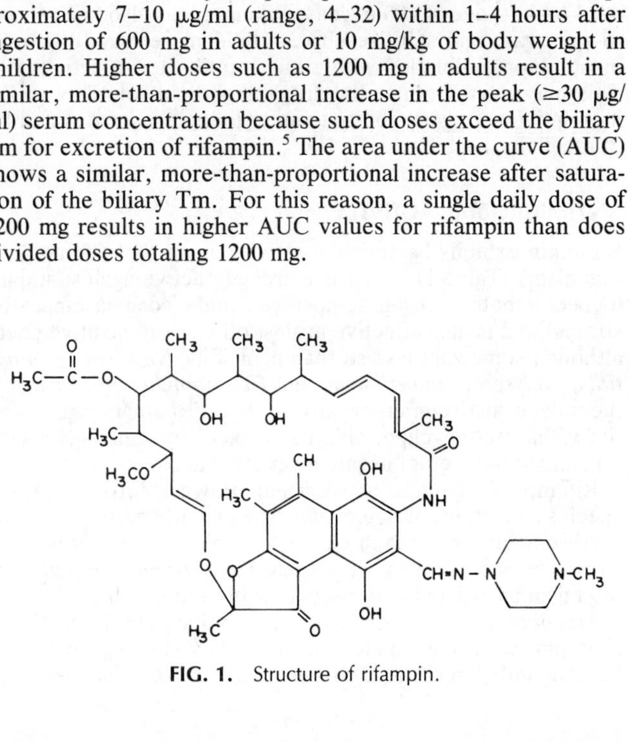

FIG. 1. Structure of rifampin.

The recommended dosage is usually 10 to 20 mg/kg (600 mg maximum) in a single daily administration. A 1% weight/volume oral suspension containing 10 mg/ml may be prepared by mixing the contents of four 300 mg capsules with 120 ml of any of several commercially available syrups according to the directions in the package insert or the *Physician's Desk Reference*.[6] Dosage adjustment is unnecessary in renal failure, but rifampin should be avoided or used with caution (perhaps at a lower dosage) in patients with hepatic dysfunction. Food with a high fat concentration interferes with absorption by lowering and delaying peak blood levels.[7] Para-aminosalicylic acid also interferes with absorption.

The drug is 80 percent protein bound in serum and distributes into a volume calculated to be 160 percent of body weight. Plasma clearance is through hepatic uptake, deacetylation to an active metabolite, and biliary excretion. Deacetylation diminishes reabsorption and increases fecal excretion, but there is significant enterohepatic circulation. The half-life is initially 2–5 hours, but it decreases by 40 percent during the first 2 weeks of therapy due to enhanced biliary excretion. Slow acetylators of isoniazid have an accelerated clearance of rifampin. From 6 to 30 percent of a dose is excreted in the urine. Probenecid does not consistently affect rifampin serum levels. Renal excretion is reduced in the elderly, but serum levels remain similar to those in young adults because of hepatic clearance.[8] Pharmacokinetics in pediatric patients are similar to those in adults.[9] An intravenous preparation commercially available in several countries but not yet licensed in the United States yields higher peak concentrations of about 27 μg/ml but otherwise similar pharmocokinetics.[10] An investigational parenteral formulation is available from Merrell Dow Laboratories in the United States.

Rifampin penetrates well into almost all body tissues. It achieves concentrations in lung, liver, bile, cholecystic wall, and urine that exceed peak blood levels.[11] Peak concentrations average 300–350 μg/ml in urine.[5] The concentration in tears is similar to that in serum, and salivary concentrations are about 20 percent of those in serum. It achieves therapeutic levels in pleural exudate, sputum,[5] ascites, cavity fluid, milk, urinary bladder wall, skin blister fluid,[12] and soft tissues. It penetrates bone, with higher levels being reached in the presence of osteomyelitis.[11] Levels in cerebrospinal fluid (CSF) of 0–0.5 μg/ml have been achieved in healthy people, and higher levels (up to 1.3 μg/ml) have been observed during meningitis after a standard oral dosage of 600 mg/day. Rifampin has also been shown to penetrate and sterilize abscess fluid more readily than do most other antibiotics with similar antibacterial activity.[13,14] This may relate both to the drug's high lipid solubility and to its relatively unusual ability to enter living phagocytes and kill intracellular bacteria.[3,12,15]

ANTIMICROBIAL ACTIVITY

Rifampin exhibits bactericidal activity against a wide range of organisms (Table 1).[16,17] It is extremely active against staphylococci (both coagulase-positive and coagulase-negative strains) and is also effective against other gram-positive cocci, although somewhat less so than penicillin. *Neisseria meningitidis, Neisseria gonorrhoeae*, and *Haemophilus influenzae* are the most sensitive gram-negative species. Rifampin has less activity than tetracycline, chloramphenicol, or aminoglycosides do against most gram-negative aerobic bacilli.

Rifampin is the most active agent known against the various species and strains of *Legionella*, being clearly more active than erythromycin, the drug of choice for legionellosis.[17] It is as active as vancomycin in vitro against *Clostridium difficile*, the organism associated with pseudomembranous colitis.

Mycobacterium tuberculosis has remained quite sensitive to rifampin, with most epidemiologic surveys finding less than 1 percent initial resistance to the drug.[18,19] *Mycobacterium ulcerans* is equally sensitive. A spiropiperidyl rifamycin called rifabutin (ansamycin) has remarkable in vitro activity against many mycobacteria including the *Mycobacterium avium-intracellulare* complex and *Mycobacterium fortuitum*.[20]

TABLE 1. Susceptibility of Various Bacteria to Rifampin

	MICs (μg/ml)		
Species (n)	Range (Mode)	MIC_{50}	MIC_{90}
Gram-positive bacteria			
Staphylococcus aureus (26)	0.008–0.015 (0.015)	0.015	0.015
Staphylococcus epidermidis (25)	0.004–0.015 (0.015)	0.015	0.015
Group A streptococci (25)	0.03–0.12 (0.12)	0.12	0.12
Group B streptococci (25)	0.25–1 (1)	1.0	1.0
Streptococcus pneumoniae (28)	0.06–32 (0.06)	0.12	4.0
Viridans group			
Streptococci (34)	0.03–8 (0.06)	0.06	0.12
Enterococcus faecalis (16)	1.0–8 (2)	2.0	8.0
Haemophilus influenzae (26)	0.5–64 (1)	1.0	1.0
Neisseria gonorrhoeae (29)	0.06–2 (0.25)	0.25	0.5
Neisseria meningitidis (26)	0.015–1 (0.03)	0.03	0.5
Listeria monocytogenes (40)	≤0.12–0.25 (≤0.12)	≤0.12	0.25
Mycobacterium fortuitum (18)	16.0–>64 (>64)	>64	>64
Mycobacterium chelonae (15)	>64 (>64)	>64	>64
Gram-negative bacteria			
Escherichia coli (15)	8–16 (8)	8	16
Klebsiella pneumoniae (14)	16–32 (32)	32	32
Enterobacter agglomerans (14)	8–64 (32)	32	64
Enterobacter cloacae (13)	16–64 (32)	64	64
Enterobacter aerogenes (15)	16–64 (32)	32	64
Citrobacter freundii (4)	32 (32)	32	32
Citrobacter diversus (4)	32 (32)	32	32
Proteus mirabilis (15)	4–8 (4)	4	8
Proteus vulgaris (17)	8–32 (32)	16	32
Morganella morganii (15)	8–32 (32)	16	32
Providencia rettgeri (15)	8–64 (8, 16)	16	32
Providencia stuartii (15)	4–16 (8)	8	16
Serratia marcescens (15)	32–64 (64)	64	64
Acinetobacter species (15)	4–16 (8)	8	8
Pseudomonas aeruginosa (17)	32–>64 (32)	32	64
Pseudomonas species (12)	4–>64 (8)	8	32

Abbreviation: MIC: minimal inhibitory concentration.
(From Thornsberry et al.,[17] with permission.)

The rifamycins possess antiviral and possible antitumor activity, which have not proved clinically useful at usual therapeutic levels. Rifampin is among the most active agents against *Chlamydia*, including *Chlamydia trachomatis* (lymphogranuloma venereum [LGV] and non-LGV strains) and *Chlamydia psittaci*.[21] *Ureaplasma urealyticum* and *Treponema pallidum* are usually resistant. Rifampin has shown synergy with amphotericin B in vitro and in animal models of infection with fungal species such as *Histoplasma capsulatum* and *Aspergillus* species.[22]

Bacteria rapidly develop resistance to rifampin in vitro or in vivo due to mutations altering the β-subunit of the DNA-dependent RNA polymerase. These mutations may occur at many different sites in the RNA polymerase and lead to various degrees of resistance to rifampin.[23] Approximately 1 out of every 10^{10} tubercule bacilli is a resistant mutant. A recent national survey found the incidence of rifampin resistance among previously untreated tuberculous patients to be 0.6 percent as compared with 3.3 percent of patients previously treated for tuberculosis. The rates of isoniazid resistance in this same survey were much higher, 5.3 and 19.3 percent for untreated and previously treated patients, respectively.[19]

The mutation rate to rifampin resistance among other bacteria is higher than that for *M. tuberculosis* (e.g., *Staphylococcus aureus*, 10^{-7}; *Streptococcus* spp., 10^{-7}; *H. influenzae* type B, 10^{-7}; meningococcus, 10^{-7}; and *Escherichia coli*, 10^{-8}).[16,24] Except for short-term meningitis prophylaxis, rifampin should not be used alone because of this rapid development of resistance during monotherapy.

ADVERSE EFFECTS

Short-term meningitis prophylaxis with rifampin has been associated with mild, reversible symptoms in 20–25 percent of recipients as compared with about 10 percent of placebo recipients.[25,26] The symptoms reported most frequently have been dizziness, drowsiness, abdominal pain, diarrhea, nausea, vomiting, headache, visual change, pruritus, and rash. Each of these symptoms usually occurs in less than 5–10 percent of recipients.[26] An orange-red discoloration of urine and permanent staining of soft contact lenses may also occur with such brief regimens.

Chronic daily therapy is associated with a mild, usually self-limited maculopapular rash in up to 5 percent of patients, gastrointestinal complaints in 1–2 percent of patients, asymptomatic elevation of serum enzyme levels in up to 14 percent of adult patients, and overt hepatitis in fewer than 1 percent of patients.[16] More severe rashes such as exfoliative dermatitis and toxic epidermal necrolysis have been rarely reported as being associated with rifampin.[27,28] Of 430 children treated with rifampin and isoniazid for tuberculosis, 14 (3.3 percent) were reported to have hepatotoxic reactions in a recent national survey.[29] In a study of rifampin (15 mg/kg/day) and higher-dose isoniazid (15–20 mg/kg/day) therapy for children with severe tuberculosis, 36 of 44 developed an elevation of hepatic enzyme levels during therapy, and 1 child died of hepatitis.[30] Acute renal failure has been reported during daily therapy and has occasionally required dialysis.[31] The renal failure has been related to a variety of different mechanisms including interstitial nephritis, glomerulonephritis, and massive hemolysis.[32,33] Light-chain proteinuria has been reported to occur in a majority of patients receiving rifampin without apparent ill effect, but in the setting of dehydration these proteins may contribute to development of a cast nephropathy and acute renal failure on this basis.[34,35]

Intermittent administration (less than twice per week) and high individual dosages (greater than or equal to 1200 mg) have been associated with an increased incidence of side effects. A flulike syndrome with fever, chills, and myalgias may develop in up to 20 percent of patients after several months of intermittent therapy and correlates with the presence of anti-rifampin antibodies.[36] These patients may develop eosinophilia, interstitial nephritis, acute tubular necrosis, thrombocytopenia, hemolytic anemia, and even shock.[37] Acute massive hemolysis is rarely associated with such flulike reactions after intermittent therapy, in which case nausea, vomiting, flank pain, and brown turbid urine may be observed; most patients with massive hemolysis develop acute renal failure.[38]

Various effects of rifampin on the central nervous system have been reported, including rare cases of organic brain syndrome. Pseudomembranous colitis has been observed in animal models after rifampin administration to animals colonized with a rifampin-resistant strain of *C. difficile*. One patient has also been reported with pseudomembranous colitis that developed with a rifampin-resistant *C. difficile* during rifampin therapy. This appears to be a very rare side effect with only a few reports of such an association despite widespread chronic use of rifampin in antituberculous chemotherapy.[39] Pancreatitis has been reported in rare cases. Patients have survived overdoses of up to 12 g, turning "lobster red" for several days; facial or periorbital edema, pruritus of the head, and vomiting each occur in a majority of cases of the "red man syndrome" after an overdose.[40]

Rifampin causes an increase in serum bile acid levels and may cause slight elevations of serum bilirubin concentrations that return to normal during the first week of therapy in the absence of hepatitis. Rifampin causes a reduction in 25-hydroxycholecalciferol levels without changing the levels of 1,25-dihydroxycholecalciferol or parathyroid hormone, and osteomalacia has been mentioned as a possible side effect with long-term treatment. It causes increased deiodination and biliary clearance of thyroxine and lowers the serum concentration of thryoxine. The serum concentration of triiodothyronine remains normal.

Immunosuppression has been an alleged side effect of rifampin therapy. Contradictory studies have found diminished or normal antibody responses to various antigens such as sheep red blood cells, pneumococcal vaccine, and tetanus toxoid. Some workers have suggested blunted cell-mediated immunity with a diminished response to phytohemagglutinin in vitro, whereas others have shown no change in response to phytohemagglutinin, concanavalin A, pokeweed mitogen, or purified protein derivative (PPD). Skin tests with PPD have not been consistently altered by rifampin therapy, and no ill effect from this possible immunosuppression in the form of opportunistic infection or an inability to heal tuberculosis has been reported.[41]

Rifampin readily crosses the placenta and has caused teratogenic effects in rodents treated with high doses; such effects have not been observed in humans, except in patients with severe tuberculosis, but rifampin should only be used for severe tuberculous infections during pregnancy.[42]

DRUG INTERACTIONS

Rifampin competitively inhibits the hepatic uptake of several compounds such as cholecystografin and sulfobromophthalein. The addition of isoniazid to rifampin increases the risk of hepatitis slightly, but the combination is usually safe in the absence of prior liver disease.[43] Rifampin is one of the most potent inducing agents for hepatic microsomal enzymes[44] and leads to a decreased half-life for a number of compounds including prednisone, norethisterone, digitoxin, quinidine, ketoconazole, and the sulfonylureas (Table 2).[45–49] These effects have been reported to cause decreased efficacy of oral contraceptive agents, relapse of arrhythmias during quinidine therapy, decompensation of heart failure during digoxin or digitoxin therapy, and exacerbation of diabetes during oral hypoglycemic therapy. Rifampin also reduces the efficacy of warfarin by causing a reduction in prothrombin time in patients anticoagulated with this drug. Patients receiving glucocorticoid therapy for Addison's disease or asthma have relapsed, and transplant patients receiving cyclosporine therapy have developed acute rejection when given rifampin. Hypothyroid patients receiving replacement L-thyroxine may require an increased dosage.[48]

THERAPEUTIC USES

Mycobacterial Infections

The unique pharmacology and bactericidal activity of rifampin have revolutionized chemotherapy for pulmonary tuberculosis, with rifampin-containing treatment courses of 6–9 months yielding cure rates equal to those achieved with 18 months of regimens without rifampin.[50] The regimen of choice for uncomplicated pulmonary or extrapulmonary tuberculosis is now 6 months of daily rifampin (15 mg/kg/day; maximum, 600 mg) and isoniazid (10 mg/kg/day; maximum, 300 mg), with daily pyrazinamide being added for the first 2 months. Additional regimens include isoniazid and rifampin daily for 9 months or twice-weekly, supervised adminstration of isoniazid and rifampin for 9 months in noncompliant patients.[51] It should be emphasized that rifampin monotherapy is contraindicated in mycobacterial

TABLE 2. Medications for Which the Half-Life Is Reduced through Enhancement of Hepatic Metabolism by Rifampin

Barbituates	Ketoconazole
Chloramphenicol	Metaprolol
Cimetidine	Methadone
Clofibrate	Phenytoin
Contraceptives, oral	Propranolol
Cyclosporine	Sulfonylureas
Dapsone	Theophylline
Digitoxin	Thyroxine
Digoxin	Verapamil
Estrogens	Warfarin

disease, as illustrated by one study in which 5 out of 11 tuberculous patients developed rifampin-resistant isolates within 3 months when receiving rifampin alone.[52] The American Thoracic Society has recommended the use of rifampin alone or in conjunction with isoniazid or ethambutol as prophylactic therapy for infected contacts of persons with known isoniazid-resistant tuberculosis. Data regarding the efficacy of such prophylaxis are not available, however, and one failure of rifampin monoprophylaxis in such an instance has been reported in an alcoholic with questionable compliance.[53]

Rifampin-containing regimens have proved useful in therapy for *M. avium-intracellulare*,[54,55] *Mycobacterium kansasii*,[56] *Mycobacterium xenopi*,[57] *Mycobacterium marinum*,[58] and Calmette-Guérin bacillus (BCG) infections.[59,60]

Rifampin kills *Mycobacterium leprae* faster than do the sulfones. If used in patients with lepromatous leprosy, however, it should be combined with dapsone to prevent the development of resistance. Monthly rifampin doses may be added to daily dapsone therapy without producing the flulike side effects frequently seen with intermittent rifampin administration.[61,62]

Meningitis Prophylaxis

Rifampin has been approved by the Food and Drug Administration (FDA) as prophylaxis for close contacts of patients with meningococcal meningitis at a daily dose of 10 mg/kg (600 mg maximum) for 4 days. The Centers for Disease Control (CDC) recommends 600 mg every 12 hours for 2 days for adults and 10 mg/kg every 12 hours for 2 days for children. Rifampin has been shown to eradicate meningococci from the nasopharynx in approximately 90 percent of carriers.[63–66] Sulfadiazine was formerly recommended for meningococcal prophylaxis, but up to 70 percent of recent meningococcal isolates are resistant to sulfa. Minocycline is also an effective prophylactic agent, but it is associated with a higher incidence of side effects, especially vestibular symptoms.[67] Recent studies have suggested the efficacy of oral ciprofloxacin (4–10 doses) and also of a single intramuscular injection of ceftriaxone (250 mg for adults, 125 mg for children less than 15 years old).[68,69]

Epidemiologic studies of *H. influenzae* type B meningitis have shown a high incidence of secondary disease among preschool contacts.[70] Secondary disease attack rates for this group have been approximately one percent, which yields a relative risk approximately 600 times that of the general population.[71] Rifampin at a single daily dose of 20 mg/kg (up to a maximum dose of 600 mg) for 4 days has been shown to eradicate *H. influenzae* from the nasopharynx in over 90 percent of carriers and to significantly reduce the risk of secondary infection.[25] It has been recommended that families with young children exposed to another member of the household with invasive *H. influenzae* type B disease (e.g., meningitis, epiglottitis, or pneumonia) take rifampin prophylaxis.[71–73] The age below which child household contacts and their families should receive prophylaxis has been debated. All agree that prophylaxis should be given when there are children younger than two years, and some recommend prophylaxis when there are children under 4 years (see Chapter 200).[71,73] Pregnant family members should not take rifampin prophylaxis. Day care center staff (excluding pregnant women) and day care classmates of a child with such disease have also been advised to take rifampin prophylaxis if any of the exposed classmates are younger than 2 years old. Some authorities recommend prophylaxis after a single case in a day care center, while others have advocated instituting prophylaxis only if a second case occurs within 60 days.[73,74] Failure to provide simultaneous rifampin prophylaxis to all day care center contacts including those who have received *Haemophilus* b polysaccharide vaccine has been associated with persistent colonization of children in the center and subsequent cases of disease.[75] The prophylaxis should be given as rapidly as possible after identification of the index case to provide maximal benefit since a majority of secondary cases appear to occur in the week after the onset of the index case. Index cases with invasive *H. influenzae* disease should also be given the same rifampin regimen before hospital discharge because of the 1 percent rate of recurrent systemic disease in index cases after therapy and also the risk of exposing other children to the organism.[76] Attempts to eradicate nasopharyngeal carriage with other drugs active against *H. influenzae*, including ampicillin and trimethoprim-sulfamethoxazole, have been less successful; data regarding the efficacy of quinolones and third-generation cephalosporins for this indication are not yet available.

Endocarditis

The use of rifampin in the treatment of staphylococcal endocarditis remains an unsettled and controversial issue.[77] Rifampin was shown to be superior to therapy with vancomycin, gentamicin, or β-lactams in an experimental model of *S. epidermidis* endocarditis in rabbits.[78] In another rabbit model of *S. epidermidis* endocarditis, rifampin plus teicoplanin proved more effective therapy than either agent alone.[79] A retrospective series of 75 cases of prosthetic valve endocarditis due to *S. epidermidis*, the most common cause of prosthetic valve endocarditis, suggested a trend toward higher survival ($p = .10$) in patients receiving rifampin (900–1200 mg/day) or an aminoglycoside plus vancomycin as opposed to vancomycin alone.[80] The only randomized trial of rifampin therapy in endocarditis compared patients with prosthetic valve endocarditis due to methicillin-resistant *S. epidermidis* who were treated with vancomycin (30 mg/kg/day) and rifampin (300 mg q8h) or with vancomycin and rifampin (same doses) plus gentamicin (3 mg/kg/day). The cure rate was 77 percent with the two-drug regimen and 85 percent with the three-drug regimen. Rifampin resistance developed in six patients receiving the two-drug regimen as compared with none receiving the three-drug regimen.[81] A separate study identified three patients in whom rifampin resistance developed during therapy for prosthetic valve *S. epidermidis* endocarditis with rifampin plus vancomycin.[82]

Several patients with endocarditis due to *S. aureus* have been reported to respond only after the addition of rifampin to nafcillin or vancomycin.[16,83,84] Rifampin therapy for experimental endocarditis due to *S. aureus* in rabbits has been examined by Sande et al.[13,85] In one study, the combination of rifampin with penicillin was antagonistic in vitro against a strain of *S. aureus*, and there was a trend toward slower sterilization of vegetations with the rifampin combination than with penicillin alone. Sterilization of renal abscesses, however, occurred faster in the group receiving the rifampin combination than in the group receiving penicillin alone despite in vitro antagonism. It was suggested that this was due to rifampin's unique ability to penetrate and sterilize abscess fluid and living polymorphonuclear neutrophil (PMN) leukocytes.

In a subsequent study using the same animal model and a methicillin-sensitive strain of *S. aureus* it was found that rifampin plus cloxacillin was additive or synergistic in four of five different regimens studied; the only regimen showing antagonism combined a high dose of cloxacillin (100 mg/kg) with a low dose of rifampin (2 mg/kg).[85] Sande and associates have concluded that rational treatment of staphylococcal endocarditis might involve initial therapy with a β-lactam or vancomycin alone or in combination with an aminoglycoside, which should result in rapid elimination of organisms from vegetations. He suggests the addition of rifampin for cases in which myocardial or metastastic abscesses are detected, while emphasizing the necessity of surgical drainage of abscesses.[86] Adding rifampin after several days of effective therapy with nafcillin or vancomycin plus gentamicin might be less likely to result in the development of rifampin resistance because the titer of organisms exposed to rifampin should then be lower.

The problem of methicillin-resistant *S. aureus* (MRSA) endocarditis has been studied in a rabbit model by Bayer et al., who found that a combination of rifampin (20 mg/kg/day) plus vancomycin (30 mg/kg/day) was significantly more effective than was either drug alone in eliminating organisms from the valve and curing the animal. Rifampin resistance developed in 2 of 4 animals that were sacrificed after treatment with rifampin alone but was not found in any of the 21 animals given the combination.[87] One retrospective study of treatment of MRSA endocarditis in drug addicts did not demonstrate a higher cure rate for rifampin-containing regimens than for vancomycin alone, but such studies are likely to be biased with only the more severely ill patients receiving rifampin. Randomized trials are needed to accurately assess the efficacy of rifampin for endocarditis due to MRSA.

The problem of rifampin resistance developing during therapy for endocarditis that has been noted with methicillin-resistant *S. epidermidis* has also been observed with MRSA during treatment with rifampin and vancomycin.[88,89] Acar and colleagues reported that two of three patients with *S. aureus* endocarditis who had failed therapy with another regimen developed rifampin resistance when rifampin was added to either vancomycin or pristinamycin.[84] It has been suggested by the results of one study that, although rifampin resistance may develop in the presence of a β-lactam such as nafcillin in vitro, the rate of developing such resistance is lower with this combination than with rifampin alone; by contrast, this study found that vancomycin did not suppress the emergence of rifampin resistance when incubated with rifampin in vitro.[90] The results of other studies, however, have suggested that incubation of vancomycin with rifampin in vitro can suppress the emergence of rifampin resistance.[91,92]

The efficacy of rifampin in *S. aureus* endocarditis will have to be proved by randomized controlled trials. In the meantime, it would appear reasonable to consider using rifampin in cases with renal, myocardial, splenic, or cerebral abscess formation or because of failure of conventional therapy. If rifampin were to be added, an optimal regimen would probably include at least two other drugs such as gentamicin and either nafcillin or vancomycin to minimize the probability of developing rifampin resistance during therapy.

The value of serum bactericidal titers and of in vitro synergy studies of antibiotic combinations including rifampin are of unclear value. Serum bactericidal titers have not been clearly demonstrated to predict the clinical outcome in patients with endocarditis,[93] and in vitro studies of rifampin and vancomycin or nafcillin with large batteries of staphylococcal isolates have produced inconsistent results in different laboratories, with most studies finding indifference for a majority of isolates.[94–101] Synergy studies performed with the same strain of *S. aureus* and the same concentrations of antibiotics have yielded directly contradictory results using checkerboard and time-kill methods.[94,97,102] Faster sterilization of renal abscesses has been shown in one animal model when a combination of rifampin and penicillin was administered despite in vitro evidence of antagonism.[13]

One theme that has emerged from several synergy studies is that lower ratios of the concentration of rifampin to the concentration of oxacillin appear to be less bactericidal in vitro. Since highest peak concentrations and AUC values are achieved by administering a single large daily dose of rifampin (e.g., ≥600 mg for an adult),[5] this approach may be more effective than smaller divided doses would be.

Rifampin (300 mg po bid) has also been recommended in combination with vancomycin and gentamicin for the treatment of endocarditis due to *Corynebacterium* spp.[103] One case of endocarditis due to psittacosis was refractory to several other antibiotics but subsequently responsive to rifampin.[104]

Tolerant Staphylococci

Staphylococci with an antibiotic minimal bactericidal concentration (MBC) much greater than the minimal inhibitory concentration (MIC) (MBC equal to or greater than 32 × MIC) are said to be tolerant to the antibiotic in question. Tolerance to nafcillin and/or vancomycin has been described in several cases of persistent staphylococcal infection. The addition of rifampin has led to improved serum bactericidal levels and the successful treatment of such infections in several cases.[105,106] No randomized trials of such therapy for this indication are available.

Staphylococcal Carriage and Furunculosis

Rifampin has been shown to reduce the rate of staphylococcal nasal colonization markedly,[107–109] whereas systemic penicillinase-resistant penicillins or intranasal gentamicin cream has not eradicated nasal carriage.[110] Mandell and Sande (unpublished data) have used cloxacillin plus rifampin to eradicate nasal carriage and interrupt the course of recurrent furunculosis. Methicillin-resistant staphylococcal nasal carriage in nosocomial epidemics has been successfully eradicated by using a combination of rifampin plus either vancomycin or trimethoprim-sulfamethoxazole.[110–113]

Methicillin-Resistant Staphylococcal Infection

Methicillin-resistant infections should be treated with vancomycin, to which they are uniformly sensitive. There are no data to support the routine addition of rifampin to vancomycin, but if there is inadequate response to vancomycin alone, then the addition of gentamicin, rifampin, or both should be considered. The development of rifampin resistance has been reported during therapy for MRSA infections with vancomycin plus rifampin,[84,89] and the addition of gentamicin to the regimen may help prevent the development of rifampin resistance.[81]

Streptococcal Carriage

Chronic pharyngeal carriage of *Streptococcus pyogenes* in children has sometimes resulted in multiple courses of antibiotic therapy for apparent streptococcal pharyngitis with each new cold because of continuing positive cultures after completion of each course of therapy, and even in tonsillectomy. Eradication of carriage is not usually medically indicated for chronic carriers, but when carriage eradication is desired, rifampin, 10 mg po bid for 4 days, plus benzathine penicillin has been shown to eradicate *S. pyogenes* in 93 percent of cases.[114] Such therapy for the eradication of *S. pyogenes* has been tried in patients with psoriasis, with apparent benefit to their skin disease.[115]

Group B streptococci are the leading cause of sepsis and meningitis in neonates, and efforts to eradicate colonization are now being studied. A recent study of treatment of experimentally exposed infant rats showed that rifampin plus penicillin eradicated group B streptococci for 80 percent of the animals, a significantly higher rate than for either drug alone.[116] Clinical data are not available.

Osteomyelitis and Septic Arthritis

Experimental animal data suggest that rifampin combined with another antistaphylococcal drug such as nafcillin or vancomycin provides better results than does single drug therapy for chronic staphylococcal osteomyelitis, even when the drug combination is antagonistic in vitro.[117] Controlled trials are necessary to confirm these data in human infection, however. The only randomized trial evaluating a rifampin-containing regimen in chronic staphylococcal osteomyelitis was halted after the enrollment of 18 patients: there was a trend toward a higher rate of favorable response in the group receiving rifampin and nafcillin (8 of 10) as compared with the group receiving nafcillin alone (4 of 8). The difference was not statistically significant ($p = .2$), but the statistical power was only 40 percent for detecting significance in the 30 percent higher rate of response that was observed because of the small sample size.[118]

Rifampin is not part of the usual regimen for staphylococcal arthritis, but it has been added with success in occasional patients initially refractory to nafcillin alone[119]; however, rifampin resistance has developed in one patient due to MRSA treated with vancomycin and rifampin.[90]

Legionella

Both *L. pneumophila* and *L. micdadei* are sensitive to rifampin. It has been suggested that rifampin be added to erythromycin for patients with legionnaires' disease when the illness does not respond to erythromycin alone, but data from randomized trials are lacking.

Brucellosis

Rifampin has been shown to be superior to tetracycline in therapy for experimental brucellosis in rodents, and there have been several case reports of successful therapy for human infections. In one uncontrolled study, relapses occurred after rifampin monotherapy, thus suggesting the need for combination therapy if rifampin is used.[120] A randomized trial comparing tetracycline (or doxycycline) regimens containing either rifampin or streptomycin found that all patients responded to both regimens but a significantly higher proportion of the rifampin recipients relapsed (39 percent) as compared with streptomycin recipients (7 percent).[121] Rifampin resistance has also developed during such therapy and has been documented during clinical relapse. Several studies of rifampin and doxycycline therapy for patients with neurobrucellosis have suggested a high rate of efficacy, with relapse rates between 0 and 10 percent.[122]

Infection Occurring in Patients with Chronic Granulomatous Disease of Childhood

Rifampin has been shown to kill living intracellular staphylococci in neutrophils from healthy people and from patients with chronic granulomatous disease.[123] One patient with an axillary staphylococcal abscess responded dramatically to the addition of rifampin after months of unsuccessful therapy with vancomycin, nafcillin, and gentamicin.[124]

Infected Cerebrospinal Fluid Shunts and Vascular Grafts

Cerebrospinal fluid shunt infections have responded to the addition of rifampin in several cases after an initial failure with multiple-drug therapy excluding rifampin.[125–127] Data from controlled trials are lacking.

Therapy with rifampin plus clinadamycin for aortic Dacron grafts experimentally infected with *S. aureus* was found to cure the infection in seven of seven dogs as compared with five of seven dogs cured with cefazolin therapy.[128] Data from clinical trials are not available.

Cutaneous Leishmaniasis

When a patient with *Leishmania mexicana amazonensis* refractory to previous antileishmanial therapy was treated with rifampin and isoniazid for intercurrent mycobacterial infection, the cutaneous leishmaniasis improved.[129] Several uncontrolled series have suggested that rifampin may be efficacious for this disease,[130] but controlled trials are still needed.[131]

Urinary Tract Infections

A number of studies have been conducted that show the efficacy of rifampin in the treatment of urinary tract infections. Rifampin resistance has arisen with monotherapy, but combination therapy with trimethoprim has resulted in cure rates that are comparable to those of trimethoprim-sulfamethoxazole.[132] Rifampin combined with trimethoprim has been used with success in eradicating persistent, relapsing infections of the kidney or prostate.[132] Rifampin combinations are not the drug of choice for infections of the urinary tract but may be considered when conventional therapy fails.

Urethritis

Although not a first-line drug for gonococcal urethritis, rifampin (900 mg) plus erythromycin (1 g) as a single oral dose has been shown to cure 95 percent of patients with gonorrhea, with equivalent efficacy against penicillinase-producing *Neisseria gonorrhoeae* (PPNG) strains.[133,134] Despite excellent activity against chlamydia in vitro, a single dose of rifampin in combination with erythromycin showed poor efficacy in the treatment of chlamydial urethritis.[134]

Chancroid

Rifampin has good activity against *Haemophilus ducreyi*, the causative agent of chancroid, and has been shown effective in treatment,[135] but intramuscular ceftriaxone and oral erythromycin are the treatments of choice.[136]

Infections Due to Multiply Resistant Pseudomonas aeruginosa

Most isolates of *Pseudomonas aeruginosa* are relatively resistant to rifampin, with MICs ranging from 32 to 64 μg/ml. Occasional isolates of *P. aeruginosa*, however, are also resistant to available β-lactams, aminoglycosides, or both. In vitro data have suggested synergy of ticarcillin, tobramycin, and rifampin against such resistant strains,[137] and case reports of patients refractory to conventional therapy who responded dramatically after the addition of rifampin to their regimen suggest that rifampin may be of value in combination therapy for such infections.[138] Rifampin combined with imipenem has also shown in vitro syngery against *P. aeruginosa* and *Enterobacter* spp. and an additive effect against *Serratia marcescens*; in vitro synergy was also shown for the combination of rifampin, imipenem, and ciprofloxacin against each of these three species.[139] Data from clinical trials are needed on the use of rifampin in such combination therapy.

Anaerobic Infections

Data from experimental animal models suggest that rifampin is as effective as metronidazole in the prevention of abscess formation and eradication of *Bacteriodes fragilis* after intraperitoneal injection of the organism. Clinical data are not available.[140,141]

Rifampin is highly active against *C. difficile* and has been used in combination with vancomycin to successfully interrupt relapsing pseudomembranous colitis in one series.[142]

Meningitis

Rifampin has been used successfully in the therapy for several cases of meningitis refractory to other available antibiotics. *Flavobacterium meningosepticum* is a rare cause of meningitis and occurs primarily in neonates but sometimes in adults after surgery as well. Most strains are susceptible to trimethoprim-sulfamethoxazole, imipenem, vancomycin, and rifampin. Rifampin has been used successfully as part of combination therapy with one or more of these other agents in curing such patients.[131,143] Randomized trials of such therapy are not available.

Rifampin was also added to the regimen of a patient with *H. influenzae* meningitis who had not responded clinically to therapy with chloramphenicol or subsequently with ampicillin and trimethoprim-sulfamethoxazole. The patient responded dramatically after the addition of rifampin.[144]

Rifapentine

Rifapentine is a new cyclopentyl rifamycin with antibacterial[145,146] and antimycobacterial[147,148] activity similar to that of rifampin but has a longer half-life of approximately 14 to 18 hours in animals (rat, mouse, and rabbit).[149] Sixty-five percent of an oral dose of 10 mg/kg is absorbed by such animals; its hepatic metabolism, biliary excretion, and wide distribution throughout body tissues are each similar to that of rifampin, as is its marked induction of hepatic microsomal oxidase activity.[150] This drug appears to be several times more active against *M. tuberculosis* and *M. leprae* than rifampin is, and its longer half-life may facilitate therapy by allowing less frequent administration. Data from clinical trials are not yet available.

Rifabutin

Rifabutin (ansamycin, LM 427) is a semisynthetic spiropiperidyl derivative of rifamycin S that shows good activity against most species of mycobacteria including all rifampin-sensitive *M. tuberculosis* strains and about one-third of rifampin-resistant strains; strains highly resistant to rifampin are usually resistant to rifabutin. Rifabutin shows better activity against the *M. avium-intracellulere* complex (MAC) of organisms than do other rifamycins; it inhibits 81 percent of MAC strains at a concentration of 1.0 mg/ml as compared with only 6 percent being inhibited by rifampin at this concentration.[151]

Rifabutin is absorbed from the gastrointestinal tract with a peak level of 0.49 mg/ml about 4 hours after ingestion of 300 mg in an adult. The serum half-life is 16 hours, and protein binding is 20 percent. The drug is taken up by all tissues and especially concentrated in the lungs, where levels may be 10-fold higher than in serum. Both hepatic and renal clearance occur as with other rifamycins, and although animal models suggest less of an effect on hepatic microsomal enzyme activity than rifampin has, several reports have suggested that rifabutin may increase corticosteroid metabolism in patients. The rates and types of side effects from rifabutin appear to be comparable to rifampin from initial reports, but better quantification of these reactions is needed from controlled clinical trials.[151]

Rifabutin has been used in open trials for the treatment of MAC disease in patients with acquired immunodeficiency syndrome (AIDS) without dramatic benefit,[152,153] but it may prove more useful in the treatment of pulmonary MAC disease in non-AIDS patients because of higher concentrations in lung tissue and a better immune system.

Randomized clinical trials of rifabutin therapy for patients with newly diagnosed pulmonary tuberculosis, MAC pulmonary disease, and drug-resistant tuberculosis are needed.

REFERENCES

1. Sensi P. History of the development of rifampin. Rev Infect Dis. 1983;5(Suppl):402.
2. Sensi P, Maggi N, Furesz S, et al. Chemical modifications and biological properties of rifamycins. Antimicrob Agents Chemother. 1966;6:699.
3. Mandell GL. Interaction of intraleukocytic bacteria and antibiotics. J Clin Invest. 1973;52:1673.
4. Wehrli W, Knusel F, Schmid K, et al. Interaction of rifamycin with bacterial RNA polymerase. Proc Natl Acad Sci USA. 1968;61:667.
5. Acocella G. Pharmacokinetics and metabolism of rifampin in humans. Rev Infect Dis. 1983;5(Suppl):428.
6. Krukenberg CC, Mischler PG, Massad EN, et al. Stability of 1% rifampin suspensions prepared in five syrups. Am J Hosp Pharm. 1986;43:2225–8.
7. Purohit SD, Gupta ML, Gupta PR. Dietary constituents and rifampicin absorption. Tubercle. 1987;68:151.
8. Advenier C, Gobert C, Houin G, et al. Pharmacokinetic studies of rifampicin in the elderly. Ther Drug Monit. 1983;5:61–5.
9. Koup JR, Williams-Warren J, Viswanathan CT, et al. Pharmacokinetics of rifampin in children II. Oral bioavailability. Ther Drug Monit. 1986;8:17–22.
10. Koup JR, Williams-Warren J, Weber A, et al. Pharmacokinetics of rifampin in children I. Multiple dose intravenous infusion. Ther Drug Monit. 1986;8:11–6.
11. Furesz S. Chemical and biological properties of rifampicin. Antibiot Chemother. 1970;16:316.
12. Solberg CO, Halstensen A, Digranes A, et al. Penetration of antibiotics into human leukocytes and dermal suction blisters. Rev Infect Dis. 5:S468, 1983.
13. Sande MA, Johnson ML. Antimicrobial therapy of experimental endocarditis caused by *Staphylococcus aureus*. J Infect Dis. 1975;131:367.
14. Mandell GL, Vest TK. Killing of intraleukocytic *Staphylococcus aureus* by refampin: In vitro and in vivo studies. J Infect Dis. 1972;125:486.
15. Mandell GL. The antimicrobial activity of rifampin: Emphasis on the relation to phagocytes. Rev Infect Dis. 1983;5(Suppl):463.
16. Farr B, Mandell GL. Rifampin. Med Clin North Am. 1982;66:157.
17. Thornsberry C, Hill BC, Swenson JM, et al. Rifampin: Spectrum of antibacterial activity. Rev Infect Dis. 1983;5(Suppl):412.
18. Collins CH, Yates MD. Low incidence of rifampin resistant tubercle bacilli. Thorax. 1982;37:526.
19. Cauthen GM, Kilburn JO, Kelly GD, et al. Resistance to anti-tuberculosis drugs in patients with and without prior treatment: Survey of 31 state and large city laboratories, 1982–1986. Am Rev Respir Dis. 1988;137:260.
20. Woodley CL, Kilburn JO. In vitro susceptibility of *Mycobacterium avium* complex and *Mycobacterium tuberculosis* strains to a spiro-piperidyl rifamycin. Am Rev Respir Dis. 1982;126:586.
21. Schachter J. Rifampin in chalmydial infections. Rev Infec Dis. 1983;5(Suppl):562.
22. Medoff G. Antifungal action of rifampin. Rev Infect Dis. 1983;5(Suppl):614.
23. Wehrli W. Rifampin: Mechanisms of action and resistance. Rev Infec Dis. 1983;5(Suppl):407.
24. Yogev R, Melick C, Glogowski W. In vitro development of rifampin resistance in clinical isolates of *Haemophilus* influenzae type B. Antimicrob Agents Chemother. 1982;21:387.
25. Band JD, Fraser DW, Ajello G, et al. Prevention of *Hemophilus* influenzae type b disease. JAMA. 1984;251:2381–6.
26. Band JD, Fraser DW. Adverse effects of two rifampicin dosage regimens for the prevention of meningococcal infection. Lancet. 1984;1:101.
27. Goldin HM, Schweitzer WJ, Bronson DM. Rifampin and exfoliative dermatitis. Ann Intern Med. 1987;107:789.
28. Okano M, Kitano Y, Igarashi T. Toxic epidermal necrolysis due to rifampicin. J Am Acad Dermatol. 1987;17:303.
29. O'Brien RJ, Long MW, Cross FS, et al. Hepatotoxicity from isoniazid and rifampin among children treated for tuberculosis. Pediatrics. 1983; 72:491–9.
30. Tsagaropoulou-Stinga H, Mataki-Emmanouilidou T, Karida-Kavalioti S, et al. Hepatotoxic reactions in children with severe tuberculosis treated with isoniazid-rifampin. Pediatr Infect Dis. 1985;4:270–3.
31. Qunibi WY, Godwin J, Eknoyan G. Toxic nephropathy during continuous rifampin therapy. South Med J. 1980;73:791.
32. Grosset J, Leventis S. Adverse effects of rifampin. Rev Infect Dis. 1983;5(Suppl):440.
33. Murray AN, Cassidy MJD, Templecamp C. Rapidly progressive glomerulonephritis associated with rifampicin therapy for pulmonary tuberculosis. Nephron. 1987;46:373.
34. Soffer O, Nassar VH, Campbell WG Jr. Light chain cast nephropathy and acute renal failure associated with rifampin therapy. Am J Med. 1987;82:1052.
35. Winter RJD, Banks RA, Collins CMP, et al. Rifampicin induced light chain proteinuria and renal failure. Thorax. 1984;39:952.
36. Poole G, Stradling P, Worlledge S. Potentially serious side-effects of high dose twice weekly rifampicin. Postgrad Med J. 1971;47:742–7.
37. Girling DJ, Hitze HL. Adverse reactions to rifampicin. Bull WHO. 1979;57:45.
38. Tahan SR, Diamond JR, Blank JM, et al. Aute hemolysis and renal failure with rifampicin-dependent antibodies after discontinuous administration. Transfusion. 1985;25:124–7.
39. Fekety R, O'Connor R, Silva J. Rifampin and pseudomembranous colitis. Rev Infect Dis. 1983;5(Suppl):524–7.
40. Bolan G, Laurie RE, Broome CV. Red man syndrome: Inadvertent administration of an excessive dose of rifampin to children in a day-care center. Pediatrics. 77:633, 1986.
41. Humber DP, Nsanzumuhire H, Aluoch HA, et al. Controlled double-blind study of the effect of rifampin on humoral and cellular immune responses in patients with pulmonary tuberculosis and in tuberculosis contacts. Am Rev Respir Dis. 1980;122:425.
42. Snider DE Jr, Layde PM, Johnson MW, et al. Treatment of tuberculosis during pregnancy. Am Rev Respir Dis. 1980;122:65.
43. Mandell GL, Sande MA. Drugs used in the chemotherapy of tuberculosis and leprosy. In: Goodman AG, Goodman LS, Gilman A, eds. The Pharmacological Basis of Therapeutics. 6th ed. New York: Macmillan; 1980:1203–6.
44. Ohnhaus EE, Kirchhof B, Peheim E. Effect of enzyme induction on plasma lipids using antipyrine, phenobarbital, and rifampicin. Clin Pharmacol Ther. 1979;25:591.

45. Twum-Barima Y, Carruthers SG. Quinidine-rifampin interaction. N Engl J Med. 1981;304:1466.
46. Brass C, Galgiani JN, Blaschke TF, et al. Disposition of ketoconazole, an oral antifungal, in humans. Antimicrob Agents Chemother. 1982;21:151.
47. Baciewicz AM, Self TH, Bekemeyer WB. Update on rifampin drug interactions. Arch Intern Med. 1987;147:565.
48. Baciewicz AM, Self TH. Rifampin drug interactions. Arch Intern Med. 1984;144:1667–71.
49. Isley WL. Effect of rifampin therapy on thyroid function tests in a hypothyroid patient on replacement L-thyroxine. Ann Intern Med. 1987;107:517.
50. British Thoracic Association: A controlled trial of six months chemotherapy in pulmonary tuberculosis. Second report: Results during the 24 months after the end of chemotherapy. Am Rev Respir Dis. 1982;126:460.
51. Anonymous. Drugs for tuberculosis. Med Lett 1988;30:43.
52. Baronti A, Lukinovich N. A pilot trial of rifampicin in tuberculosis. Tubercle. 1968;49:180.
53. Livengood JR, Sigler TG, Foster LR, et al. Isoniazid resistant tuberculosis: A community outbreak and report of a rifampin prophylaxis failure. JAMA. 1985;253:2847–9.
54. Hunter AM, Campbell IA, Jenkins PA, et al. Treatment of pulmonary infections caused by mycobacteria of the *Mycobacterium avium-intracellulare* complex. Thorax. 1981;36:326.
55. Baron EJ, Young LS. Amikacin, ethambutol, and rifampin for treatment of disseminated *Mycobacterium avium-intracellulare* infections in patients with acquired immune deficiency syndrome. Diagn Microbiol Infect Dis. 1986;5:215–20.
56. Ahn CH, Lowell JR, Ahn SS, et al. Chemotherapy for pulmonary disease due to *Mycobcterium kansasii*: Efficacies of some individual drugs. Rev Infect Dis. 1981;3:1028.
57. Bogaerts Y, Elinck W, van Renterghem D, et al. Pulmonary disease due to *Mycobacterium xenopi*: Report of two cases. Eur J Respir Dis. 1982;63:298.
58. Donta ST, Smith PW, Levitz RE, et al. Therapy of *Mycobacterium marinum* infections. Arch Intern Med. 1986;146:902–4.
59. Kallenius G, Moller E, Ringden O, et al. The first infant to survive a generalized BCG infection. Acta Paediatr Scand. 1982;71:161.
60. Izumi AK, Matsunaga J. BCG vaccine-induced lupus vulgaris. Arch Dermatol. 1982;118:171.
61. Yawalkar SJ, McDougall AC, Longuillon J, et al. Once monthly rifampicin plus daily dapsone in initial treatment of lepromatous leprosy. Lancet. 1982;1:1119.
62. Bullock WE. Rifampin in the treatment of leprosy. Rev Infect Dis. 1983;5(Suppl):606–13.
63. Deal WB, Sanders E. Efficacy of rifampin in treatment of meningococcal carriers. N Engl J Med. 1969;281:641–5.
64. Devine LF, Rhode SL, Pierce WE. Rifampin: Effect of two-day treatment on the meningococcal carrier state and the relationship to the levels of drug in sera and saliva. Am J Med Sci. 1971;261:79–83.
65. Weidmer CE, Dunkel TB, Pettyjohn FS, et al. Effectiveness of rifampin in eradicating the meningococcal carrier state in a relatively closed population: Emergence of resistant strains. J Infect Dis. 1971;124:172–8.
66. Beaty HN. Rifampin and minocycline in meningococcal disease. Rev Infect Dis. 1983;5(Suppl):451–8.
67. Jacobson JA, Daniel B. Vestibular reactions associated with minocycline. Antimicrob Agents Chemother. 1975;8:453–6.
68. Schwartz B, Al-Ruwais A, A'Ashi J, et al. Comparative efficacy of ceftriaxone and rifampicin in eradicating pharyngeal carriage of group A *Neisseria meningitidis*. Lancet. 1988;1:1239–42.
69. Pugsley MP, Dworzack DL, Horowitz EA, et al. Efficacy of ciprofloxacin in the treatment of nasopharyngeal carriers of *Neisseria meningitidis*. J Infect Dis. 1987;156:211–3.
70. Broome CV, Mortimer EA, Katz SL, et al. Use of chemoprophylaxis to prevent the spread of *Hemophilus enfluenzae* B in day-care facilities. N Engl J Med. 1987;316:1226–8.
71. Anonymons. Update: Prevention of *Haemophilus influenzae* type b disease. MMWR. 1986;35:170–80.
72. Respiratory and Special Pathogens Epidemiology Branch (CDC): Prevention of secondary cases of *Haemophilus influenzae* type B disease. MMWR. 1982;31:672.
73. Brunnel PA, Bass JW, Daum RS, et al. Revision of recommendation for use of rifampin prophylaxis of contacts of patients with *Haemophilus influenzae* infection. Pediatrics. 1984;74:301–2.
74. Dashefsky B, Wald E, Li K. Management of contacts of children in day care with invasive *Haemophilus influenzae* type b disease. Pediatrics. 1986;78:939–40.
75. Wilde J, Adler SP. Molecular epidemiology of *Haemophilus influenzae* type B: failure of rifampin prophylaxis in a day care center. Pediatr Infect Dis. 1986;5:505–8.
76. Cates KL, Krause PJ, Murphy TV, et al. Second episodes of *Haemophilus influenzae* type b disease following rifampin prophylaxis of the index patients. Pediatr Infect Dis J. 1987;6:512–5.
77. Sande MA. The use of rifampin in treatment of nontuberculous infections. Rev Infect Dis. 1983;5(Suppl):399.
78. Vazquez GJ, Archer GL. Antibiotic thrapy of experimental *Staphylococcus epidermidis* endocarditis. Antimicrob Agents Chemother. 1980;17:280–5.
79. Tuazon CU, Washburn D. Teicoplanin and rifampicin singly and in combination in the treatment of experimental *Staphylococcus epidermidis* endocarditis in the rabbit model. J Antimicrob Chemother. 1987;20:233–7.
80. Karchmer AW, Archer GL, Dismukes WE. *Staphylococcus epidermis* causing prosthetic valve endocarditis: Microbiological and clinical observations as guides to therapy. Ann Intern Med. 1983;48:447.
81. Karchmer AW, Archer GA. Methicillin-resistant *Staphylococcus epidermidis* (SE) prosthetic valve (PV) endocarditis (E): A therapeutic trial (Abstract 476). Program and Abstracts of the Twenty-fourth Interscience Conference on Antimicrobial Agents and Chemotherapy. October 8–10, 1984.
82. Chamovitz B, Bryant RE, Gilbert D, et al. Prosthetic valve endocarditis caused by *Staphylococcus epidermidis*. JAMA. 1985;253:2867–8.
83. Swanberg L, Tuazon CU. Rifampin in the treatment of serious staphylococcal infections. Am J Med Sci. 1984;287:49–54.
84. Acar JF, Goldstein FW, Duval J. Use of rifampin for the treatment of serious staphylococcal and gram-negative bacillary infections. Rev Infect Dis. 1983;5(Suppl):502–6.
85. Zak O, Scheld M, Sande M. Rifampin in experimental endocarditis due to *Staphylococcus aureus* in rabbits. Rev Infect Dis. 1983;5(Suppl):481–90.
86. Kapusnik JE, Parenti F, Sande M. The use of rifampicin in staphyloccal infections—a review. J Antimicrob Chemother. 1984;13:61–6.
87. Bayer AS, Lam K. Efficacy of vancomycin plus rifampin in experimental aortic-valve endocarditis due to methicillin-resistant *Staphylloccus aureus*: In vitro–in vivo correlations. J Infect Dis. 1985;151:157–65.
88. Eng RHK, Smith SM, Tillem M, et al. Rifampin resistance. Development during the therapy of methicillin-resistant *Staphylococcus aureus* infection. Arch Intern Med. 1985;145:146–8.
89. Simon GL, Smith RH, Sande MA. Emergence of rifampin-resistant strains of *Staphylococcus aureus* during combination therapy with vancomycin and rifampin: A report of two cases. Rev Infect Dis. 1983;5(Suppl):507–8.
90. Eng RHK, Smith SM, Buccini FJ, et al. Differences in ability of cell-wall antibiotics to suppress emergence of rifampicin resistance in *Staphylococcus aureus*. J Antimicrob Chemother. 1985;15:201–7.
91. Hackbarth CJ, Chambers HF, Sande MA. Serum bactericidal activity of rifampin in combination with other antimicrobial agents against *Staphylococcus aureus*. Antimicrob Agents Chemother. 1986;29:611–3.
92. Foldes M, Munro R, Sorrell TC, et al. In-vitro effects of vancomycin, rifampicin, and fusidic acid, alone and in combination, against methicillin-resistant *Staphylococcus aureus*. J Antimicrob Chemother. 1983;11:21–6.
93. Coleman DL, Horwitz RI, Andriole VT. Association between serum inhibitory and bactericidal concentrations and therapeutic outcome in bacterial endocarditis. Am J Med. 1982;73:260–7.
94. Traczewski MM, Goldmann DA, Murphy P. In vitro activity of rifampin in combination with oxacillin against *Staphylococcus aureus*. Antimicrob Agents Chemother. 1983;23:571.
95. Watanakunakorn C, Guerriero JC. Interaction between vancomycin and rifampin against *Staphylococcus aureus*. Antimicrob Agents Chemother. 1981;19:1089.
96. Walsh TJ, Auger F, Tatem BA, et al. Novobiocin and rifampicin in combination against methicillin-resistant *Staphylococcus aureus*: An in-vitro comparison with vancomycin plus rifampicin. J Antimicrob Chemother. 1986;17:75–82.
97. Varaldo PE, Debbia E, Schito GC. In vitro activity of teichomycin and vancomycin alone and in combination with rifampin. Antimicrob Agents Chemother. 1983;23:402–6.
98. Zinner SH, Lagast H, Klastersky J. Antistaphylococcal activity of rifampin with other antibiotics. J Infect Dis. 1981;144:365–71.
99. Van der Auwera P, Klastersky J. In vitro study of the combination of rifampin with oxacillin against *Staphylococcus aureus*. Rev Infect Dis. 1983;5(Suppl):509–14.
100. Van der Auwera P, Klastersky J. Bactericidal activity and killing rate of serum in volunteers receiving teicoplanin alone or in combination with oral or intravenous rifampin. Antimicrob Agents Chemother. 1987;31:1002–5.
101. Ho JL, Klempner MS. In vitro evaluation of clindamycin in combination with oxacillin rifampin or vancomycin against *Staphylococcus aureus*. Diagn Microbiol Infect Dis. 1986;4:133.
102. Bayer AS, Morrison JO. Disparity between timed-kill and checkerboard methods for determination of in vitro bactericidal interactions of vancomycin plus rifampin versus methicillin-susceptible and resistant *Staphylococcus aureus*. Antimicrob Agents Chemother. 1984;26:220–3.
103. Sande MA, Scheld WM. Combination antibiotic therapy of bacterial endocarditis. Ann Intern Med. 1980;92:390.
104. Jariwalla AG, Davies BH, White J. Infective endocarditis complicating psittacosis: Response to rifampicin. Br Med J. 1980;280:155.
105. Faville RJ, Zaske DE, Kaplan EL, et al. *Staphylococcus aureus* endocarditis: Combined therapy with vancomycin and rifampin. JAMA. 1978;240:1963.
106. Simmons NA. Synergy and rifampicin. J Antimicrob Chemother. 1977;3:109.
107. Wheat LJ, Kohler RB, White AL, et al. Effect of rifampin on nasal carriers of coagulase-positive staphylococci. J Infect Dis. 1981;144:177.
108. Wheat LJ, Kohler RB, Luft FC, et al. Long term studies of the effect of rifampin on nasal carriage of coagulase-positive staphylococci. Rev Infect Dis. 1983;5(Suppl):459–62.
109. McNally TP, Lewis MR, Brown DR. Effect of rifampin and bacitracin on nasal carriers of *Staphylococcus aureus*. Antimicrob Agents Chemother. 1984;25:422–6.
110. Locksley RM, Cohen ML, Quinn TC, et al. Multiply antibiotic-resistant *Staphylococcus aureus*: Introduction, transmission, and evolution of nosocomial infection. Ann Intern Med. 1982;97:317.
111. Ward TT, Winn RE, Hartstein AI, et al. Observations relating to an inter-

hospital outbreak of methicillin resistant *Staphylococcus aureus*: Role of anticrobial therapy in infection control. Infect Control. 1981;2:453.
112. Ellison H, Judson FN, Peterson LC, et al. Oral rifampin trimethoprim-sulfamethoxazole therapy in symptomatic carriers of methicillin-resistant *Staphylococcus aureus* infections. West J Med. 1984;140:735–40.
113. Pearson JW, Christiansen KJ, Annear DI, et al. Control of methicillin-resistant *Staphylococcus aureus* (MRSA) in an Australian metropolitan teaching hospital complex. Med J Aust. 1985;142:103–8.
114. Tanz RR, Shulman ST, Barthel MJ, et al. Penicillin plus rifampin eradicates pharyngeal carriage of group A streptococci. J Pediatr. 1985;106:876–80.
115. Rosenberg EW, Noah PW, Zanolli MD, et al. Use of rifampin with penicillin and erythromycin in the treatment of psoriasis. J Am Acad Dermatol. 1986;14:761–4.
116. Millard DD, Shulman ST, Yogev R. Rifampin and penicillin for the elimination of group B streptococci in nasally colonized infant rats. Pediatr Res. 1985;19:1183–6.
117. Norden CW, Shaffer M. Treatment of experimental chronic osteomyelitis due to *Staphylococcus aureus* with vancomycin and rifampin. J Infect Dis. 1983;147:352.
118. Norden CW, Bryant R, Palmer D, et al. Chronic osteomyelitis caused by *Staphylococcus aureus*: Controlled clinical trial of nafcillin therapy and nafcillin-rifampin therapy. South Med J. 1986;79:947–51.
119. Beam TR. Sequestration of *Staphylococcus aureus* at an inaccessible focus. Lancet. 1979;2:227.
120. LLoren-Terol J, Busquets RM. Brucellosis treated with rifampicin. Arch Dis Child. 1980;55:486.
121. Ariza J, Gudiol F, Pallares R, et al. Comparative trial of rifampin-doxycycline versus tetracycline-streptomycin in the therapy of human brucellosis. Antimicrob Agents Chemother. 1985;28:548–51.
122. Perez MAH, Rodriguez BA, Garcia AF, et al. Treatment of nervous system brucellosis with rifampin and doxcycline (Letter). Neurology. 1986;36:1408–9.
123. Ezer G, Soothill JF. Intracellular bactericidal effect of rifampicin in both normal and chronic granulomatous disease polymorphs. Arch Dis Child. 1974;49:463.
124. Lorber B. Rifampin in chronic granulomatous disease. N Engl J Med. 1980;303:111.
125. Archer G. Tenenbaum JM, Haywood HB. Rifampin therapy of *S. epidermidis*: Use in infections from indwelling artificial devices. JAMA. 1978;240:751.
126. Bolton WK, Sande MA, Normansell DE, et al. Ventriculojugular shunt nephritis with *Corynebacterium bovis*. Am J Med. 1975;59:417.
127. Ring JC, Cates KL, Belani KK, et al. Rifampin for CSF shunt infections caused by coagulase-negative staphylococci. J Pediatr. 1979;95:317.
128. Wakefield TW, Schaberg DR, Pierson CL, et al. Treatment of established prosthetic vascular graft infection with antibiotics preferentially concentrated in leukocytes. Surgery. 1987;102:8–14.
129. Peters W, Shaw JJ, Lainson R, et al. Potentiating action of rifampicin and isoniazid against *Leishmania mexicana amazonensis*. Lancet. 1981;1:1122.
130. Even-Paz Z, Weinrauch L, Livshin R, et al. Rifampicin treatment of cutaneous leishmaniasis. Int J Dermatol. 1982;21:110.
131. Conti R, Parenti F. Rifampin therapy for brucellosis, *Flavobacterium meningitis*, and cutaneous leishmaniasis. Rev Infect Dis. 1983;5(Suppl):600–5.
132. Brumfitt W, Dixson S, Hamilton-Miller JMT. Use of rifampin for the treatment of urinary tract infections. Rev Infect Dis. 1983;5(Suppl):573–82.
133. Desudchit P, Nunthapisud P, Rukjutitum S, et al. Rifampicin-erythromycin combination for the treatment of gonococcal urethritis in men. Southeast Asian J Trop Med Public Health. 1984;15:360–3.
134. Oriel JD, Ridway GL, Goldmeir D, et al. Treatment of gonococcal urethritis in men with a rifampicin-erythromycin combination. Sex Transm Dis. 1982;9:208–11.
135. Plummer FA, Nsanze H, D'Costa LJ, et al. Short-course and single-dose antimicrobial therapy for chancroid in Kenya: Studies with rifampin alone and in combination with trimethoprim. Rev Infect Dis. 1983;5(Suppl):565–72.
136. Treatment of sexually transmitted diseases. Med Lett. 1988;30:5–10.
137. Zuravleff JJ, Yu VL, Yee RB. Ticarcillin-tobramycin-rifampin: In vitro synergy of the triplet combination against *Pseudomonas aeruginosa*. J Lab Clin Med. 1983;101:896–902.
138. Yu VL, Zuravleff JJ, Peacock JE, et al. Addition of rifampin to carboxypenicillin-aminoglycoside combination for the treatment of *Pseudomonas aerugionosa* infection: Clinical experience with four patients. Antimicrob Agents Chemother. 1984;26:575–7.
139. Chin NX, Heu HC. Synergy of imipenen, a novel carbapenem, and rifampin and ciprofloxacin against *Pseudomonas aeruginosa*, *Serratis marcescens* and *Enterobacter* species. Chemotherapy. 1987;33:183–8.
140. Fu KP, Lasinski ER, Zoganas HC, et al. Therapeutic efficacy and pharmacokinetic properties of rifampicin in a *Bacteroides fragilis* intra-abdominal abscess. J Antimicrob Chemother. 1984;14:633–40.
141. Fu KP, Lasinski ER, Zoganas HC, et al. Efficacy of rifampicin in experimental *Bacteroides fragilis* and *Pseudomonas aeruginosa* mixed infections. J Antimicrob Chemother. 1985;15:579–85.
142. Buggy BP, Fekety R, Silva J Jr. Therapy of relapsing *Clostridium difficile*-associtaed diarrhea and colitis with the combination of vancomycin and rifampin. J Clin Gastroenterol. 1987;9:155–9.
143. Hirsh BE, Wong B, Kiehn TE, et al. A case of *Flavobacterium meningoseptícum* bacteremia in an adult with acute leukemia. Use of rifampin to clear persistent infection. Diagn Microbiol Infect Dis. 1986;4:65–9.
144. Lewis MA, Priestley BL. Addition of rifampicin in persistent *Haemophilus influenzae* type B meningitis. 1986;292:448–9.
145. Varaldo PE, Debbia E, Schito GC. In vitro activities of rifapentine and rifampin, alone and in combination with six other antibiotics, against methicillin-susceptible and methicillin-resistant staphylococci of different species. Antimicrob Agents Chemother. 1985;27:615–8.
146. Korvic J, Yu VL, Sharp JA. Interaction of rifampicin or rifapentine with other agents against *Pseudomonas aerugionosa*. J Antimicrob Chemother. 1987;19:847–8.
147. Dickinson JM, Mitchison DA. In vitro properties of rifapentine (MDL473) relevant to its use in intermittent chemotherapy of tuberculosis. Tubercle. 1987;68:113–8.
148. Bermudez LEM, Wu M, Young LS. Intracellular killing of *Mycobacterium avium* complex by rifapentine and liposome-encapsulated amikacin. J Infect Dis. 1987;156:510–3.
149. Assandri A, Ratti B, Cristina T. Pharmacokinetics of rifapentine, a new long lasting rifamycin, in the rat, the mouse and the rabbit. J Antibiot (Tokyo). 1984;37:1066–73.
150. Durand DV, Hampden C, Boobis AR, et al. Induction of mixed function oxidase activity in man by rifapentine (MDL473), a long-acting rifamycin derivative. Br J Clin Pharmacol. 1986;21:1–7.
151. O'Brien RJ, Lyle MA, Snider DE. Rifabutin (ansamycin LM 427): A new rifamycin-S derivative for the treatment of mycobacterial diseases. Rev Infect Dis. 1987;9:519–30.
152. Hawkins CC, Gold JWM, Whimbey E, et al. *Mycobacterium avium* complex infections in patients with the acquired immunodeficiency syndrome. Ann Intern Med. 1986;105:184–8.
153. Masur H, Tuazon C, Gill V, et al. Effect of combined clofazimine and ansamycin therapy on *Mycobacterium avium–Mycobacterium intracellulare* bacteremia in patients with AIDS. J Infect Dis. 1987;155:126–29.

25. METRONIDAZOLE

SYDNEY M. FINEGOLD
GLENN E. MATHISEN

DESCRIPTION

Metronidazole was introduced in 1959 for the treatment of *Trichomonas vaginalis* infections. It is now known to be effective against most infections involving anaerobic bacteria and against certain other parasitic infections. Metronidazole diffuses well into all tissues including the central nervous system. It is well tolerated and has the best bactericidal activity of all drugs active against anaerobic bacteria.

Metronidazole is a nitroimidazole drug with the chemical formula 1-(2-hydroxyethyl)-2-methyl-5-nitroimidazole. It has a low molecular weight, 171.

SPECTRUM OF ACTIVITY, RESISTANCE

Table 1 from Sutter[1] summarizes the activity of metronidazole against 793 strains of anaerobic and microaerophilic bacteria. Note that virtually all of the organisms tested were inhibited by 16 μg/ml or less except for one-third of gram-positive nonspore-forming bacilli and 7 percent of *Capnocytophaga* sp. Metabolites are found in serum and urine, and Sutter found that the hydroxy metabolite of metronidazole was slightly less active than was the parent compound against many anaerobes but had equivalent or better activity against some. The acid metabolite has poor activity against anaerobes. In general, studies by other workers have given comparable results in terms of the in vitro activity of metronidazole. Wüst[2] found that seven strains of *Propionibacterium acnes* required 100 μg/ml for inhibition. Werner et al.[3] also noted that the hydroxy metabolite of metronidazole was roughly comparable in activity to the parent compound. We found that only about 25 percent of the strains of *Actinomyces* and *Arachnia* are susceptible to metronidazole at achievable levels. In a recent study, Rosenblatt and Edson[4]

TABLE 1. Activity of Metronidazole against Anaerobic and Microaerophilic Bacteria

Bacteria	No. Strains	Cumulative Percentage Susceptible to Indicated Concentration (μg/ml) 4	8	16	32
Bacteroides fragilis[a]	161	90	99	100	—
B. melaninogenicus[b]	60	98	100	—	—
Other bacteroides and *Selenomonas* sp.	154	95	98	100	—
Fusobacterium sp.	65	100	—	—	—
Anaerobic gram-negative cocci	24	92	96	100	—
Anaerobic gram-positive cocci	124	98	—	—	—
Clostridium perfringens	18	94	100	—	—
Other *Clostridium* sp.	73	97	99	—	100
Gram-positive nonsporulating bacilli	87	57	60	62	66
Capnocytophaga sp.	27	52	70	93	—

[a] Includes all species of the *B. fragilis* group.
[b] Includes *B. melaninogenicus* and *B. asaccharolyticus* ssp.
(From Sutter,[1] with permission.)

noted somewhat less activity against anaerobic gram-positive cocci (a minimum inhibitory concentration for 70 percent of strains [MIC_{70}] of 6.25 and MIC_{90} of >25 μg/ml). *Propionibacterium acnes* was highly resistant. The study by Chow et al.[5] found significantly more resistance among anaerobes to metronidazole than was indicated by the studies previously cited.

Also sensitive to metronidazole are *Treponema pallidum,* oral spirochetes, *Campylobacter fetus,* and *Gardnerella vaginalis*. In certain animal models, *Escherichia coli* may be inhibited by metronidazole when it is present together in a mixture with *Bacteroides fragilis*. However, in another animal model[6] there was no activity against *E. coli*. We have noted decreased counts of *E. coli* initially present together with anaerobes in the bypassed loop of patients with ileal bypass for obesity who were treated with metronidazole for "bypass enteropathy."

Resistance to metronidazole develops rarely. Resistant strains identified include one strain each of *Bacteroides fragilis, Bacteroides distasonis,* what was originally described as *Bacteroides melaninogenicus* ss *melaninogenicus* and *Bacteroides bivius*. Phillips et al.[7] note that they have seen occasional marginally resistant isolates of *B. bivius, Bacteroides ureolyticus,* and perhaps *B. melaninogenicus*. Tally et al.[8] studied a metronidazole-resistant strain of *B. fragilis*. They found that the uptake of metronidazole by cells was slower than in a sensitive strain. Also, the rate of reduction of metronidazole was four times less than with a sensitive control strain, possibly due to decreased nitroreductase activity. Although rare, case reports suggest that resistant organisms may develop in patients receiving therapy, and this could lead to a clinical relapse of infection.[9,10] *Trichomonas vaginalis* may become resistant to metronidazole, and several case reports have described recalcitrant vaginal trichomoniasis secondary to resistant strains.[11–13]

MODE OF ACTION

Mechanism of Action

It is convenient to think of the action as occurring in four successive steps[14]: (*1*) entry of the drug into the bacterial cell, (*2*) reductive activation, (*3*) toxic effect of the reduced intermediate product(s), and (*4*) release of inactive end products. A key feature is reduction of the nitro group of the drug; the drug acts as a preferential electron acceptor, being reduced by low–redox potential electron transport proteins (ferredoxin-like and flavodoxin-like). Reduction of the drug decreases the intracellular concentration of unchanged drug, thus maintaining a gradient that drives the uptake and generates compounds that are toxic to the cell. The toxicity is due to short-lived intermediate compounds or free radicals that produce damage by interaction with DNA and possibly other macromolecules. The cytotoxic intermediates decompose into nontoxic and inactive end products, including acetamide and 2-hydroxethyl oxamic acid.

Metabolic Products

As noted before, the hydroxy derivation of metronidazole has significant antianaerobic activity; it is more active than metronidazole is on *G. vaginalis*. The acid derivative of metronidazole has relatively little activity, less than one-tenth as much as metronidazole against *B. fragilis* and *Trichomonas*.[14] The drug is also conjugated; the glucuronide has no activity on *Trichomonas* and is not taken up.[14]

Bactericidal Activity

Metronidazole is a potent bactericidal agent. It typically kills organisms at the same concentration or within one twofold dilution of that required for inhibition.[15] Under reduced conditions, metronidazole has a rapid onset of bactericidal activity. Killing rates are not affected by inoculum size, nutritional requirements, or growth rate.[16,17]

Bartlett et al.[18] found metronidazole to be the most effective drug in a *B. fragilis* subcutaneous abscess model in mice even when treatment was delayed for 8–120 hours after challenge.

PHARMACOLOGY

When given orally, metronidazole is absorbed rapidly and almost completely. Serum levels are similar during the elimination phase after equivalent doses by the intravenous and oral routes. Blood levels are proportional to the administered dose. The standard intravenous dosage regimen that has been used in the United States consists of a loading dose of 15 mg/kg of body weight followed by 7.5 mg/kg every 6 hours. This results in peak and trough steady-state plasma levels averaging 25 μg/ml and 18 μg/ml, respectively. There is very little protein binding of metronidazole. The half-life is 8 hours. Absorption of metronidazole is not affected by ingestion of food, but peak levels may be markedly delayed. Metronidazole is absorbed after vaginal administration, but peak serum levels (mean, 1.2 μg/ml) and bioavailability (20 percent) are lower than by oral or intravenous administration.[19] Absorption after rectal administration is quite good, although peak serum levels occur approximately 3 hours after insertion. Metronidazole is rapidly transferred across the placenta; peak serum levels in the fetus are equivalent to maternal levels after intravenous administration to pregnant women.[20]

There is a large apparent volume of distribution of metronidazole that is equivalent to about 80 percent of body weight; it reaches all tissues and fluids. Therapeutic levels are achieved in amniotic fluid, the unobstructed biliary tract, alveolar bone, cerebrospinal fluid and brain abscess contents, cord blood, pleural empyema fluid, hepatic abscesses, middle ear discharge, middle ear mucosa, breast milk, pelvic tissues (concentrations attained in the myometrium and fallopian tubes are nearly the same as concomitant serum levels), saliva, seminal fluid, and vaginal secretions. Levels achieved in the aqueous humor were between one-third and one-half those attained in the serum.[21]

During metabolization of metronidazole, five major products are formed. The most important one is the hydroxy derivative. In addition, there is an acid metabolite, acetylmetronidazole, metronidazole glucuronide, and the glucuronide conjugate of hydroxy metronidazole. A sulfate conjugate may also be found on occasion. Metronidazole and its metabolites are eliminated primarily in the urine (60–80 percent of the dose). From 6 to 15 percent is excreted in the feces.

The elimination half-life of metronidazole in patients with no renal function is the same as in healthy people. However, the hydroxy metabolite may accumulate in patients with absent renal function, and although dosage adjustment is usually not considered necessary in the absence of hepatic disease, consideration might be given to dosage adjustment in patients initially receiving large doses. Metronidazole and its metabolites are rapidly removed by hemodialysis; the elimination half-life of metronidazole is reduced to 2.6 hours. Dose reduction is generally not necessary in patients undergoing chronic ambulatory peritoneal dialysis.[22] In patients with impaired hepatic function, even without concomitant renal function impairment, the plasma clearance of metronidazole is delayed. Although data are limited, pharmacokinetic studies in patients with significant liver disease suggest that doses should be reduced by at least 50 percent in this patient population.[23,24]

ADMINISTRATION AND DOSAGE

Table 2 gives dosage recommendations and routes of administration for the major indications for metronidazole therapy. The intravenous route is recommended initially for seriously ill patients. Since oral therapy gives blood levels comparable to those achieved by the intravenous route, we may switch when conditions warrant.

As noted, the standard regimen in the United States for intravenous administration has been a loading dose of 15 mg/kg of body weight followed by a maintenance schedule of 7.5 mg/kg every 6 hours. Clearly, the half-life of the drug would warrant administration at longer intervals such as every 8 or even every 12 hours. The manufacturer recommends that intravenous infusions be administered over a period of 1 hour. However, a number of foreign investigators have administered the drug in as little as 20 minutes without any apparent adverse effects. The maximum daily dose recommended is 4 g.

After reconstitution, metronidazole hydrochloride should be diluted with intravenous fluid to a concentration not exceeding 8 mg/ml and should be neutralized to pH 6.0–7.0 with sodium bicarbonate before administration. There is also a metronidazole intravenous solution (Flagyl IV RTU), a ready-to-use isotonic solution that does not require dilution or buffering before infusion.

The duration of therapy will vary according to the entity being treated. Certain recommendations are made in Table 2. For serious infections, however, we may often need to treat the patient for 2–4 weeks or longer.

Comments regarding dosage in patients with impaired renal and/or hepatic function have been noted in the earlier section on pharmacology.

ADVERSE REACTIONS, PRECAUTIONS

In general, metronidazole is well tolerated. The more commonly encountered major and minor adverse reactions are listed in Table 3. There may also be furring of the tongue, glossitis, stomatitis, dry mouth, headache, fever, dizziness, syncope, and occasionally overgrowth of *Candida* in the oral cavity or vagina. Thrombophlebitis has been reported with intravenous infusion but is seldom seen now with proper buffering of the preparation. Gastrointestinal side effects include nausea, epigastric distress, anorexia, and less commonly, vomiting or diarrhea. Although pseudomembranous colitis has been reported rarely with metronidazole therapy, the drug has proved effective therapeutically for this condition and is comparable to vancomycin in effectiveness. The most serious adverse effects are those involving the central nervous system. These are rare unless large doses and/or prolonged therapy is used. If abnormal neurologic symptoms are observed, treatment with the drug must be discontinued immediately. Metronidazole should be used with caution in people with a history of seizures or other central nervous system disorders. The peripheral neuropathy may take a considerable period of time to resolve.

There has been concern about mutagenicity in the Ames *Salmonella* mutant system and carcinogenicity of metronidazole. Reduction of the nitro group of the compound is necessary for both antibacterial activity and mutagenic activity. Mutagenic activity has been detected in the urine of patients receiving 750 mg/day of metronidazole. When a mutant *Salmonella* that did not possess nitroreductase was used in the mutagenic testing system, metronidazole could not be demonstrated to be a mutagen. Thus, the drug itself is not mutagenic, but rather it is one or more reduction products of it. Some protozoa, bacteria (including facultative anaerobes), and fungi possess nitroreductase activity. Eukaryotic tissues have very little nitroreductase activity. It has been suggested that during metronidazole therapy some reduction products of the drug might escape from the bacterial cells and serve as mutagens to the host's mammalian tissue. However, these active derivatives are very short-lived and either promptly bind to macromolecules within the bacterial cell or are promptly reduced to compounds that are not mutagenic or carcinogenic. The drug has been studied specifically for mutagenic potential in eukaryotic test systems (human lymphocytes in vitro and lymphocytes of patients receiving metronidazole therapy). No chromosomal aberrations or sister chromatid exchanges could be detected in vitro with metronidazole or its metabolites in concentrations of 1000–10,000 μg/ml. No lymphocyte abnormalities were noted in patients receiving a short course of metronidazole therapy.[25,26] Metronidazole has shown tumorigenic activity in several studies in mice involving lifetime (or almost lifetime) oral administration. Female rats given metronidazole over long periods (sometimes for life) had a significant increase in neoplasms, especially mammary tumors, as compared with controls. Interestingly, in one study drug-fed rats lived longer than did controls. Two lifetime studies in hamsters were negative (see Finegold[27]). It should be noted that acetamide has been found in the urine of patients

TABLE 2. Major Indications for Metronidazole: Administration and Dosage

Indication	*Route of Administration*	*Dosage*
Susceptible anaerobic infections	iv	Loading dose of 15 mg/kg, then 7.5 mg/kg q6h
	po	1–2 g/day in 2–4 doses q6–12h
Nonspecific vaginitis	po	500 mg bid for 7 days
Trichomonas vaginitis	po	250 mg tid for 7 days *or* 5000 mg bid for 5 days *or* 2 g in single dose
Amebiasis (intestinal or extraintestinal)	iv or po	750 mg tid for 10 days
Giardiasis	po	250 mg bid or tid for 5–7 days *or* 2 g/day for 3 days

TABLE 3. Adverse Effects Related to Metronidazole Therapy

- Major adverse reactions (rare)
  - Seizures, encephalopathy
  - Cerebellar dysfunction, ataxia
  - Peripheral neuropathy
  - Disulfiram reaction with alcohol
  - Potentiation of effects of warfarin
  - Pseudomembranous colitis
  - Pancreatitis
- Minor adverse reactions
  - Minor gastrointestinal disturbances
  - Reversible neutropenia
  - Metallic taste
  - Dark or red-brown urine
  - Maculopapular rash, urticaria
  - Urethral, vaginal burning
  - Gynecomastia

receiving metronidazole and prolonged feeding of high doses of this compound to rats has produced hepatocarcinomas.[28] A study in rats[29] using the dimethylhydrazine (DMH) model for colon neoplasia noted that the addition of metronidazole on a long-term basis had an apparent cocarcinogenic effect. As Condon notes in the discussion of this paper, the DMH tumor model is relatively specific and may not readily be extrapolated to humans.[29] Indeed, in another study looking at bile salt–induced colorectal cancer in rats, metronidazole administration appeared to reduce the carcinogenic effect of sodium deoxycholate.[30]

Long-term follow-up of a cohort of 771 women who received metronidazole therapy for the treatment of vaginal trichomoniasis during the 1960s has not shown an increased incidence of malignancy.[31] It should be recognized that these patients received relatively low doses of the drug for brief periods of time (7–10 days). A recent report raises the possibility of carcinogenicity in three patients with Crohn's disease who had received prolonged therapy with metronidazole[32]; these observations remain anecdotal, and further studies are clearly needed. Although metronidazole appears to be safe, the long-term effects of high-dose prolonged therapy are not completely known, and such usage should be avoided if other alternatives are available.

Metronidazole crosses the placental barrier, and concerns have been raised about possible teratogenic effects in light of the evidence for mutagenicity in bacterial systems. To date, there has been little evidence for this in animal models, although one study has raised the possibility of fetal "genotoxicity" in pregnant golden Syrian hamsters fed high doses of metronidazole.[33] Studies in pregnant women who had received metronidazole during pregnancy for the treatment of vaginal trichomoniasis have not shown an increased incidence of stillbirths, small-for-age infants, premature infants, or teratogenicity.[34] Although there is one paper that raises the possibility of a metronidazole-induced teratogenic effect,[35] again, this may well be a coincidence and is not supported by other human or animal studies; nevertheless, the use of metronidazole during pregnancy should be reserved for situations in which it is clearly needed. Metronidazole during the first trimester should be avoided.

Because metronidazole is excreted into breast milk, nursing should be discontinued during and for 2 days after therapy with metronidazole.

Drug Interactions, Interference with Laboratory Tests

In patients ingesting alcohol, metronidazole may cause reactions similar to those produced by disulfiram. Patients should be advised not to drink alcohol when taking this drug. Metronidazole inhibits the metabolism of warfarin and other oral coumarin-type anticoagulants. Therefore, if concomitant use must be carried out, the dosage of the anticoagulant should be reduced to maintain the desired prothrombin time.

Metronidazole interferes with certain chemical analyses for the serum enzyme glutamic oxaloacetic transaminase, which results in falsely low or negative values.

EFFECT ON NORMAL FECAL FLORA

In subjects who have a healthy gastrointestinal tract and are not receiving other drugs, metronidazole has very little effect on the fecal flora.[36] This is thought to be due to the drug being rapidly reduced by the bowel flora under the usual anaerobic conditions in the colon. Why this would not have an impact on the organisms carrying out the reduction, as it does in the course of treating infections, is not at all clear. In patients on high-dosage regimens, in patients with diarrhea, and in patients receiving certain other antimicrobial agents concurrently, there may be a significant impact of metronidazole on the fecal flora. For example, when oral neomycin or kanamycin (active primary against nonanaerobes) is given with metronidazole, there is a significant impact on both the anaerobic and aerobic flora. Thus, it has been feasible to use metronidazole for therapy in certain conditions such as ileal bypass enteropathy and for preoperative "bowel preparation" along with an oral aminoglycoside.

CLINICAL USES

Parasitic Infections

Metronidazole has been used successfully for therapy for *Trichomonas* vaginitis for many years. It is also an effective agent for therapy of amebic liver abscess and has been used with generally good results in intestinal amebiasis. The drug is also effective against giardiasis, being at least as active as quinacrine for this purpose.

Some workers have felt that metronidazole has been effective in *Balantidium coli* infection and in infection due to *Dracunculus medinensis,* but these indications are certainly not well established. Metronidazole has been used in the treatment of cutaneous leishmaniasis, although it appears to be less effective than are other available agents.[37]

Anaerobic Infections

As is suggested by the spectrum of activity of metronidazole, this drug is useful for the vast majority of anaerobic infections. Certainly actinomycosis is one notable exception, and infections with *P. acnes,* which are quite rare, would be another. There is one other setting in which metronidazole may represent less than optimum therapy—anaerobic infections of the lower respiratory tract. Data from Sanders et al.[38] show a relatively high rate of suboptimal response. Most treatment failures had mixed infections with aerobic bacteria as well as anaerobes. The addition of penicillin G or ampicillin for mixed infections involving streptococci, pneumococci, or *Haemophilus influenzae* or the addition of erythromycin in the case of a penicillin-allergic patient would likely provide an excellent regimen. In the case of aspiration pneumonia involving aerobic and/or facultative gram-negative bacilli and/or *Staphylococcus aureus,* other appropriate therapy to cover these agents would be needed along with metronidazole. Many anaerobic infections are mixed with aerobic or facultative bacteria, of course, and particularly in sicker patients, therapy aimed at both categories of organisms is desirable.

The excellent distribution of metronidazole throughout the body, including the central nervous system, and the impressive bactericidal activity of this compound, even against organisms that are not actively multiplying, make it an excellent choice for a number of serious infections, including brain abscess and other central nervous system infections involving anaerobes, endocarditis due to anaerobic bacteria, and perhaps, any anaerobic infection of serious nature in patients who are immunocompromised.

The *B. fragilis* group of organisms is the one most commonly encountered in anaerobic infections overall. Until recently, there were only three drugs that were consistently active against this group—metronidazole, chloramphenicol, and clindamycin. Recently, a number of centers have been encountering varying degrees of resistance of the *B. fragilis* group to clindamycin. Thus, metronidazole may become an even more important part of our armamentarium for the management of anaerobic infections. It should be noted, however, that in intra-abdominal infections, in which *B. fragilis* is almost always involved, comparative studies[16] failed to show any significant difference among metronidazole, clindamycin, chloramphenicol, ticarcillin, or cefoxitin; most of these were used together with an aminoglycoside.

The resistance of a number of clostridia other than *Clostrid-*

ium perfringens to cefoxitin and clindamycin again suggests that metronidazole might have an advantage in selected intra-abdominal and obstetric and gynecologic infections. However, there are no specific data to back up this point.

Metronidazole has been useful against other types of anaerobic infections including bacteremia, infections of bones and joints, soft tissue infections, oral and dental infections, and head and neck infections. Metronidazole has also provided good results in the therapy for nonspecific vaginitis, a condition in which various anaerobes, *G. vaginalis,* or both may be important.[39] As noted elsewhere, it has been effective in the management of pseudomembranous colitis due to *Clostridium difficile*. Limited studies have shown that fecal levels of metronidazole (up to 1,212 μg/g dry weight and 24.2 μg/g wet weight feces) may be attained by using either an oral or parenteral route in patients with active colitis.[40,41] The parenteral route may be especially useful in patients who have *C. difficile*–induced toxic megacolon and are unable to take oral medications. A recent clinical study suggests that metronidazole may be more effective than penicillin is for antimicrobial therapy for tetanus.[42] Metronidazole is not a suitable alternative to penicillin for syphilis.

Other Therapeutic Uses

Metronidazole has been used experimentally in very high doses as a hypoxic cell sensitizer in radiotherapy for malignancy.

Metronidazole has been useful in a number of types of bowel bacterial overgrowth syndromes such as complications of jejunoileal bypass for obesity[43] and dysfunction of the continent ileostomy,[44] and for the prevention of intrahepatic cholestasis associated with total parenteral nutrition.[45] Although not everyone agrees, it appears that metronidazole has had a beneficial effect in Crohn's disease by producing a lessening of diarrhea (in patients with colonic involvement) and promoting the healing of perianal lesions and erythema nodosum.[46] The prolonged use of the drug, however, may result in a significant incidence of metronidazole-induced peripheral neuropathy,[47] and concerns have been raised about possible carcinogenic effects of the drug.[32]

Metronidazole is said to be beneficial in the treatment of acne rosacea whether used orally or topically.[48]

An intriguing report[49] notes striking decreases in serum cholesterol and triglyceride levels in patients receiving metronidazole for other indications. Only short courses of therapy were used. There is no information as to the mechanism of this effect.

Prophylactic Use

Several groups have carried out prospective controlled studies of metronidazole, alone or in combination with other agents, for prophylaxis in patients undergoing elective colonic surgery, gynecologic surgery, or emergency appendectomy. In the case of appendectomy, a perforated appendix is an indication for therapy rather than prophylaxis, and in uncomplicated appendicitis, the frequency of postoperative infection is quite low. In general, however, in these studies metronidazole has appeared to be as effective as other effective prophylactic agents. It should be kept in mind, however, that the prophylactic use of metronidazole is not an approved indication for the drug in the United States at present. Finally, it should be appreciated that not all of the prophylactic trials have found metronidazole effective. Metronidazole was not effective prophylactically in one study of hysterectomy[50] and in one study of appendectomy for nonperforated appendicitis.[51]

REFERENCES

1. Sutter VL. In vitro susceptibility of anaerobic and microaerophilic bacteria to metronidazole and its hydroxy metabolite. In: Finegold SM, George WL, Rolfe RD, eds. Proceedings of the First United States Metronidazole Conference. Tarpon Springs, FL, February 1982. New York: Biomedical Information Corp; 1982:61.
2. Wüst J. Susceptibility of anaerobic bacteria to metronidazole, ornidazole, and tinidazole and routine susceptibility testing by standardized methods. Antimicrob Agents Chemother. 1977;11:631.
3. Werner H, Schädler G, Krasemann C. In vitro activity of azlocillin, metronidazole and its hydroxy metabolite against anaerobes. Arzneimittelforsch Drug Res. 1983;33:574.
4. Rosenblatt JE, Edson RS. Metronidazole. Mayo Clin Proc. 1983;58:154.
5. Chow AW, Bednorz D, Guze LB. Susceptibility of obligate anaerobes to metronidazole: An extended study of 1,054 clinical isolates. In: Finegold SM, McFadzean JA, Roe FJC, eds. Metronidazole. Proceedings of the International Metronidazole Conference, Montreal, May 1976. Princeton, NJ: Excerpta Medica; 1977:286.
6. Reznikov M, McDonald PJ. Effect of metronidazole on *Escherichia coli* in the presence of *Bacteroides fragilis:* An investigation in mice. Chemotherapy. 1983;29:225.
7. Phillips I, Warren C, Taylor E, et al. The antimicrobial susceptibility of anaerobic bacteria in a London teaching hospital. J Antimicrob Chemother. 1981;8:17.
8. Tally FP, Snydman DR, Shimell MJ, et al. Mechanisms of antimicrobial resistance of *Bacteroides fragilis*. In: Phillips I, Collier J, eds. Metronidazole. Proceedings of the Second International Symposium on Anaerobic Infections, Geneva, April 1979. London: The Royal Society of Medicine and Academic Press, New York: Grune & Stratton, 1979:19.
9. Ingham HR, Eaton S, Venables CW, et al. *Bacteroides fragilis* resistant to metronidazole after long-term therapy. Lancet. 1978;1:214.
10. Sprott MS, Ingham HR, Hickman JE, et al. Metronidazole-resistant anaerobes. Lancet. 1983;1:1220.
11. Krajden S, Lossick JG, Wilk E, et al. Persistent *Trichomonas vaginalis* infection due to a metronidazole-resistant strain. Can Med Assoc J. 1986;134:1373–4.
12. Müller M, Meingassner JG, Miller WA, et al. Three metronidazole-resistant strains of *Trichomonas vaginalis* from the United States. Am J Obstet Gynecol. 1980;138:808–12.
13. Dombrowski MP, Sokol RJ, Bronsteen RA. Intravenous therapy of metronidazole-resistant *Trichomonas vaginalis*. Obstet Gynecol. 1987;69:524–5.
14. Müller M. Mode of action of metronidazole on anaerobic bacteria and protozoa. In: Rhône-Poulenc Pharma Inc, Montreal. Proceedings of the North American Metronidazole Symposium on Anaerobic Infections, Scottsdale, AZ, October 1981. Surgery. 1983;93:165.
15. Nastro LJ, Finegold SM. Bactericidal activity of five antimicrobial agents against *Bacteroides fragilis*. J Infect Dis. 1972;126:104.
16. Tally FP, Sullivan CE. Metronidazole: In vitro activity, pharmacology and efficacy in anaerobic bacterial infections. Pharmacotherapy. 1981;1:28.
17. Corrodi P, Busch DF, Sutter VL, et al. Factors affecting the in vitro antibacterial activity of metronidazole In: Finegold SM, McFadzean JA, Roe FJC, eds. Metronidazole. Proceedings of the International Metronidazole Conference, Montreal, May 1976. Princeton, NJ: Excerpta Medica; 1977:299.
18. Bartlett JG, Dezfulian M, Joiner K. Relative efficacy and critical interval of antimicrobial agents in experimental infections involving *Bacteroides fragilis*. Arch Surg. 1983;118:181.
19. Fredricsson B, Hagström B, Nord C-E, et al. Systemic concentrations of metronidazole and its main metabolites after intravenous, oral and vaginal administration. Gynecol Obstet Invest. 1987;24:200–7.
20. Visser AA, Hundt HKL. The pharmacokinetics of a single intravenous dose of metronidazole in pregnant patients. J Antimicrob Chemother. 1984;13:279–83.
21. Mattila J, Nerdrum K, Rouhiainen H, et al. Penetration of metronidazole and tinidazole into the aqueous humor in man. Chemotherapy. 1983;29:188.
22. Guay DR, Meatherall RC, Baxter H, et al. Pharmacokinetics of metronidazole in patients undergoing continuous ambulatory peritoneal dialysis. Antimicrob Agents Chemother. 1984;25:306–10.
23. Lau AH, Evans R, Chang C-W, et al. Pharmacokinetics of metronidazole in patients with alcoholic liver disease. Antimicrob Agents Chemother. 1987;31:1662–4.
24. Loft S, Sonne J, Dossing M, et al. Metronidazole pharmacokinetics in patients with hepatic encephalopathy. Scand J Gastroenterol. 1987;22:117–23.
25. Lambert B, Lindblad A, Lindsten J, et al. Genotoxic effects of metronidazole in human lymphocytes in vitro and in vivo. In: Phillips I, Collier J, eds. Metronidazole. Proceedings of the Second International Symposium on Anaerobic Infections, Geneva, April 1979. London: The Royal Society of Medicine and Academic Press; New York: Grune & Stratton; 1979:229.
26. Hartley-Asp B. Chromosomal studies on human lymphocytes exposed to metronidazole in vivo and in vitro. In: Phillips I, Collier J, eds: Metronidazole. Proceedings of the Second International Symposium on Anaerobic Infections, Geneva, April 1979. London: The Royal Society of Medicine and Academic Press; New York: Grune & Stratton; 1979:237.
27. Finegold SM. Metronidazole. Ann Intern Med. 1980;93:585.
28. Koch RL, Chrystal EJT, Beaulieu BB, et al. Acetamide—a metabolite of metronidazole formed by the intestinal flora. Biochem Pharmacol. 1979;28:3611.
29. Sloan DA, Fleiszer DM, Richards GK, et al. Increased incidence of experimental colon cancer associated with long-term metronidazole therapy. Am J Surg. 1983;145:66.
30. Rainey JB, Maeda M, Williams C, et al. The cocarcinogenic effect of intra-

rectal deoxycholate in rats is reduced by oral metronidazole. Br J Cancer. 1984;49:631–6.
31. Beard CM, Noller KL, O'Fallon WM, et al. Cancer after exposure to metronidazole. Mayo Clin Proc. 1988;63:147–53.
32. Krause JR, Ayuyang HQ, Ellis LD. Occurrence of three cases of carcinoma in individuals with Crohn's disease treated with metronidazole. Am J Gastroenterol. 1985;80:978–82.
33. Garry VF, Nelson RL. Host-mediated transformation: Metronidazole. Mutat Res. 1987;190:289–95.
34. Robbie MO, Sweet RL. Metronidazole use in obstetrics and gynecology: A review. Am J Obstet Gynecol. 1983;145:865–81.
35. Cantú JM, Garcia-Cruz D. Midline facial defect as a teratogenic effect of metronidazole. March Dimes Birth Defect Fdn 1982;18:85–8.
36. Lewis RP, Wideman P, Sutter VL, et al. The effect of metronidazole on human fecal flora. In. Finegold SM, McFadzean JA, Roe FJC, eds. Metronidazole. Proceedings of the International Metronidazole Conference, Montreal, May 1976. Princeton, NJ: Excerpta Medica; 1977:307.
37. Chong H. Oriental sore. A look at trends in and approaches to the treatment of leishmaniasis. Int J Dermatol. 1986;25:615–23.
38. Sanders CV, Hanna BJ, Lewis AC, et al. The use of metronidazole in the treatment of anaerobic pleuropulmonary infections. In: Phillips I, Collier J, eds. Metronidazole. Proceedings of the Second International Symposium on Anaerobic Infections, Geneva, April 1979. London: The Royal Society of Medicine and Academic Press; New York: Grune & Stratton, 1979:83.
39. Swedberg J, Steiner JF, Deiss F, et al. Comparison of single-dose vs one-week course of metronidazole for symptomatic bacterial vaginosis. JAMA. 1985;254:1046–9.
40. Kleinfeld DI, Sharpe RJ, Donta ST. Parenteral therapy for antibiotic-associated pseudomembranous colitis. J Infect Dis. 1988;157:389.
41. Bolton RP, Culshaw MA. Faecal metronidazole concentrations during oral and intravenous therapy for antibiotic associated colitis due to *Clostridium difficile*. Gut. 1986;27:1169–72.
42. Ahmadsyah I, Salim A. Treatment of tetanus: An open study to compare the efficacy of procaine penicillin and metronidazole. Br Med J. 1985;291:648–50.
43. Drenick EJ. Extraintestinal complications of jejunoileal bypass for obesity. In: Finegold SM, George WL, Rolfe RD, eds. Proceedings of the First United States Metronidazole Conference, Tarpon Springs, FL, February 1982. New York: Biomedical Information Corp; 1982:371.
44. Kelly DG, Phillips SF, Kelly KA, et al. Dysfunction of the continent ileostomy: Clinical features and bacteriology. Gut. 1983;24:193.
45. Capron J-P, Herve M-A, Gineston J-L, et al. Metronidazole in prevention of cholestasis associated with total parenteral nutrition. Lancet. 1983;1:446.
46. Gilat T. Metronidazole in Crohn's disease (Editorial). Gastroenterology. 1982;83:702.
47. Duffy LF, Daum F, Fisher SE, et al. Peripheral neuropathy in Crohn's disease patients treated with metronidazole. Gastroenterology. 1985;88:681–4.
48. Nielsen PG. Metronidazole treatment in rosacea. Int J Dermatol. 1988;27:1–5.
49. Davis JL, Schultz TA, Mosley CA. Metronidazole lowers serum lipids. Ann Intern Med. 1983;99:43.
50. Vincelette J, Finkelstein F, Aoki FY, et al. Double-blind trial of perioperative intravenous metronidazole prophylaxis for abdominal and vaginal hysterectomy. In: Rhône-Poulenc Pharma Inc, Montreal. Proceedings of the North American Metronidazole Symposium on Anaerobic Infections, Scottsdale, AZ, October 1981. Surgery. 1983;93:185.
51. Keiser TA, MacKenzie RL, Feld R, et al. Prophylactic metronidazole in appendectomy: A double-blind controlled trial. In: Rhône-Poulenc Pharma Inc, Montreal. Proceedings of the North American Metronidazole Symposium on Anaerobic Infections, Scottsdale, AZ, October 1981. Surgery. 1983;93:201.

BIBLIOGRAPHY

Finegold SM, McFadzean JA, Roe FJC, eds. Metronidazole. Proceedings of the International Metronidazole Conference, Montreal, May 1976. Princeton, NJ: Excerpta Medica; 1977.
Finegold SM. Metronidazole. Ann Intern Med. 1980;93:585.
Finegold SM, George WL, Rolfe RD, eds. Proceedings of the First United States Metronidazole Conference, Tarpon Springs, FL, February 1982. New York: Biomedical Information Corp; 1982.
Kucers A, Bennett N McK, Kemp RJ, eds. Metronidazole. In: The Use of Antibiotics. Philadelphia: JB Lippincott; 1987.
May & Baker, Ltd. "Flagyl" (Metronidazole) in Anaerobic Infections. Essex, England: May & Baker, Ltd; 1979.
Phillips I, Collier J, eds. Metronidazole. Proceedings of the Second International Symposium on Anaerobic Infections, Geneva, April 1979. London: The Royal Society of Medicine and Academic Press; New York: Grune & Stratton 1979.
Rhône-Poulenc Pharma Inc., Montreal. Proceedings of the North American Metronidazole Symposium on Anaerobic Infections, Scottsdale, AZ, October 1981. Surgery. 1983;93:123.
Rosenblatt JE, Edson RS. Metronidazole. Mayo Clin Proc. 1987;62:1013–17.
Stranz MH, Bradley WE. Metronidazole (Flagyl IV, Searle). Drug Intell Clin Pharm. 1981;15:838.

26. ERYTHROMYCIN, LINCOMYCIN, AND CLINDAMYCIN

NEAL H. STEIGBIGEL

Erythromycin and the lincosamide antibiotics, lincomycin and clindamycin, are chemically unrelated but possess similar biologic properties in terms of mechanisms of action and resistance, antimicrobial activity, and clinical pharmacology. Erythromycin, currently the most important of the macrolide antibiotics, has a few primary indications in therapy and is often useful as an alternative to penicillin G. It is one of the safest antibiotics in clinical use. Clindamycin has been restricted in use by its potential gastrointestinal toxicity but remains particularly important in the treatment of certain anaerobic infections. Lincomycin is now mainly of historic interest.

ERYTHROMYCIN

Derivation, Chemistry, and Preparations

Erythromycin was derived in 1952 from a strain of *Streptomyces erythreus* obtained from soil from the Philippines. The structure (Fig. 1) consists of a 14-membered macrocyclic lactone ring, therefore the class name *macrolide*, attached to two sugar moities. Erythromycin base is poorly soluble in water, has a pK of 8.8, is rapidly inactivated by gastric acid, and is often inconsistently absorbed after oral administration. Pharmaceutical preparations for oral use have been made with an aim to diminish destruction by gastric acid and to promote better absorption. Six preparations for oral use are available: enteric-coated tablets (Ilotycin, E-mycin, Ery-Tab, Robimycin, and generics), enteric-coated pellets in capsules (Eryc), and "film"-coated (Filmtab, Abbott) tablets of the base; stearate salt (formed in association with the amino group on desosamine) and available as film-coated tablets (Erythrocin, Bristamycin, other brand names, and generics); ethylsuccinate ester (formed with the hydroxyl group on desosamine), available in tablet, chewable, and liquid forms (Erythrocin, Eryped, EES, Pediamycin); and lauryl sulfate salt of the propionyl ester (the estolate), available in tablet, capsule, or liquid forms (Ilosone). There are two water-soluble salts of erythromycin prepared for intravenous use, erythromycin gluceptate (Ilotycin gluceptate) and erythromycin lactobionate (Erythrocin lactobionate). The drug is not given intramuscularly because of pain on injection. Erythromycin base is also available in 1.5 and 2 percent topical solutions, gels, and creams for treatment of acne vulgaris and in an ophthalmic ointment for treatment of bacterial conjunc-

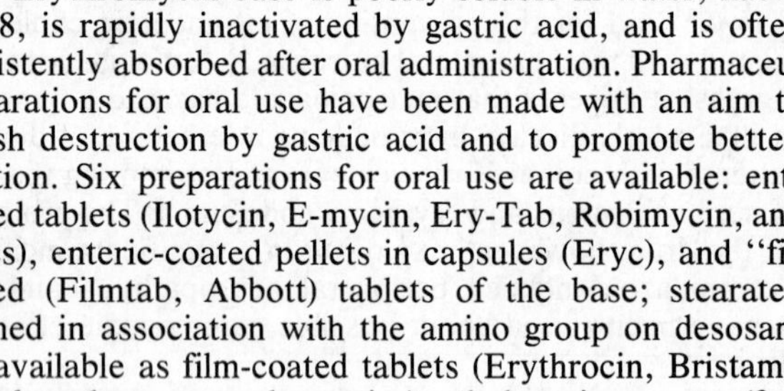

FIG. 1. Erythromycin base.

tivitis and prevention of neonatal gonococcal and chlamydial conjunctivitis.

Mechanisms of Action

Erythromycin inhibits RNA-dependent protein synthesis at the step of chain elongation in susceptible prokaryotic organisms. A single molecule of the antibiotic reversibly binds to the 50S ribosomal subunit, resulting in blockage of the transpeptidation and/or translocation reactions.[1–3] In some bacteria erythromycin interferes with the ribosomal binding of other macrolides, lincomycin, and chloramphenicol, suggesting common or overlapping binding sites for these antibiotics.

Antimicrobial Activity and Mechanisms of Resistance

The antimicrobial activity of erythromycin is broad in spectrum, being exhibited against gram-positive and gram-negative bacteria, including actinomycetes and mycobacteria, as well as against treponemes, mycoplasmas, *Chlamydia*, and rickettsia. Depending on the drug concentration, bacterial species, phase of growth, and density of the inoculum, erythromycin may be primarily bacteriostatic or bactericidal. Bacterial killing is favored by higher antibiotic concentrations, lower bacterial density, and rapid growth.[4] The activity of erythromycin, which is a weak base, increases markedly with increasing pH over the range 5.5–8.5, for both gram-positive and gram-negative bacteria,[5,6] possibly reflecting increased entry into the bacterial cell of the un-ionized drug that is more plentiful at the higher pH.

The in vitro susceptibilities of potential pathogens to erythromycin are listed in Table 1.[7–13] Erythromycin shows high activity against pneumococci and group A streptococci, although occasional resistant clinical isolates have been encountered, especially from patient populations recently exposed to erythromycin or lincomycin.[14,15] Of 200 strains of *Streptococcus pneumoniae* isolated from patients with pneumococcal disease in a survey conducted in Spain, 5 were found to be highly resistant to erythromycin and clindamycin.[16] In a study in Japan, 60 percent of strains of group A streptococci isolated from infected children were highly resistant to erythromycin and lincomycin.[17] Almost all of these resistant strains were of type 12, and erythromcyin had been widely used to treat respiratory infections in Japan in the several years before the study. A survey of 474 group A streptococcal strains isolated from patients in Oklahoma in 1980 indicated that 5 percent had minimal inhibitory concentrations (MIC) to erythromycin by microtiter broth dilution ≥ 1 μg/ml.[18] The emergence of resistance to erythromycin encountered in clinical isolates of these organisms from patient populations treated with this antibiotic is consistent with in vitro studies with pneumococci and streptococci subcultured sequentially in the presence of erythromycin, demonstrating the selection of erythromycin resistance and often cross-resistance to other macrolides and lincomycin. Similar in vitro results are obtained with staphylococci.[19] Although resistance to erythromycin by *Staphylococcus aureus* may be selected by its use in hospitals,[20] most clinical isolates are presently sensitive, to this agent. However, there is always a potential for the emergence, during treatment in an individual patient, of erythromycin resistance by *S. aureus*.[7,19,21,22] These strains may demonstrate the emergence of one-step high-level resistance to erythromycin alone or may show cross-resistance to other macrolides and to lincomycin and clindamycin. In addition, staphylococci isolated from patients treated with erythromycin may exhibit a phenomenon called *dissociated resistance* by Garrod.[23] Only a small proportion of the population of such staphylococcal isolates exhibit resistance when grown in large concentrations of erythromycin; however, in the presence of lower concentrations of erythromycin almost the entire population demonstrates resistance to erythromycin, to other macrolides, and to the lincosamide antibiotics. In the absence of erythromycin these organisms appear sensitive to these antibiotics.

TABLE 1. In Vitro Susceptibilities to Erythromycin

Organism	Minimum Inhibitory Concentration (μg/ml) Range	Median
S. pneumoniae	0.001–0.2[a]	0.05
S. pyogenes	0.005–0.2[a]	0.04
S. "viridans"	0.02–3.1[a]	0.06
Enterococcus	0.1–>100	1.5
S. aureus	0.005–>100	0.4
S. epidermidis	0.2–>100	0.6
C. diphtheriae	0.006–3.1[a]	0.02
C. perfringens	0.1–6[a]	0.8
L. monocytogenes	0.1–0.3	0.2
B. pertussis	0.02–1.6	0.3
N. gonorrhoeae	0.005–0.4[a]	0.1
N. meningitidis	0.1–1.6	0.4
H. influenzae	0.1–6	3.1
C. jejuni	0.05–>50	0.2
B. fragilis	0.1–>100	≤0.25
L. pneumophila	0.06–0.5	0.1
M. pneumoniae	0.001–0.02	0.005
C. trachomatis	0.1–0.5	0.1
B. catarrhalis	0.03–0.125	0.07

[a] Occasional clinical isolates are more resistant.

The majority of strains of the "viridans" group of streptococci, *Listeria monocytogenes*, and *Corynebacterium diphtheriae* show appreciable susceptibility to erthromycin. Many strains of *Clostridium perfringens* may be only moderately sensitive.[24] Appreciable in vitro activity has been demonstrated against *Actinomyces israelii*, *Mycobacterium scrofulaceum*, and *Mycobacterium kansasii*,[25] and against *Nocardia asteroides* when combined with ampicillin.[26]

With gram-negative bacteria, erythromycin displays consistent and useful activity against *Neisseria meningitidis*, *Neisseria gonorrhoeae*, and *Bordetella pertussis*[8] and somewhat lower activity against *Haemophilus influenzae*.[27] High bacteriostatic and bactericidal activity is demonstrated against over 90 percent of strains of *Campylobacter jejuni*.[10] Erythromycin has activity against some species of gram-negative anaerobes, but *Bacteroides fragilis* strains are usually resistant.[28] The Enterobacteriaceae are usually resistant, except as the pH rises to 8.5.[6]

The extensive spectrum of activity of erythromycin is also demonstrated by its clinically useful activity against such diverse organisms as *Treponema pallidium*, *Legionella pneumophila*,[9] *Mycoplasma pneumoniae*, *Ureaplasma urealyticum*, some strains of *Rickettsia*, and *Chlamydia trachomatis*. Erythromycin is about 50 times more potent against *M. pneumoniae* than tetracycline.[29] Erythromycin-resistant variants of *M. pneumoniae* have been isolated in the laboratory and from a patient.[30]

Resistance to erythromycin may be the result of the following: (*1*) Decreased permeability of the cell envelope to the drug is exhibited by the Enterobacteriaceae; cell-free systems and protoplasts of these organisms are susceptible to the drug.[31,32] Plasmid-mediated erythromycin resistance in *S. epidermidis* due to decreased permeability to the drug has also been described.[33] (*2*) Alteration in a single 50S ribosomal protein of the receptor site confers resistance to erythromycin and often to other macrolides, lincomycin, and clindamycin; in some but not all strains this is associated with a decreased binding affinity for erythromycin.[2] This one-step high-level resistance is the result of chromosomal mutation, has been demonstrated in some strains of *Bacillus subtilis*, *Streptococcus pyogenes*, and *Escherichia coli* and probably occurs in *S. aureus*. (*3*) Alteration in the 23S ribosomal RNA of the 50S ribosomal subunit by methylation of adenine.[34–37] This is associated with resistance to erythromycin and often to other macrolides (M), lincocasamides (L, lincomycin and clindamycin), and streptogramin type B (S_B); this pattern of resistance is referred to as the MLS_B

phenotype. The resistance is due to decreased binding of the antibiotics to their targets on the ribosome and is usually mediated by a plasmid. It can be exhibited by strains of *S. aureus*, streptococci (including *S. pneumoniae*), *C. diphtheriae*, *B. fragilis*, *C. perfringens*, *Listeria* species, and *Legionella* species.[38] This phenomenon may be constitutive or inducible by subinhibitory concentrations of erythromycin that bring about induction of the methylating enzyme. The inducible mechanism seems to explain the phenomenon of dissociated resistance already described. Several determinants of MLS_B resistance have been defined,[39,40] including the erm A, erm B, and erm C genes, which occupy plasmids in *S. aureus*. The nucleotide sequence of erm A has been determined.[41] *(4)* Inactivation of erythromycin by enzymatic hydrolysis brought about by strains of Enterobacteriaceae with high-level resistance has been demonstrated.[42] These organisms possess an erythromycin esterase encoded by a plasmid-mediated determinant.[43]

Clinical Pharmacology

The peak serum levels obtained after single doses of various erythromycin preparations are given in Table 2.[7,8,28,44,45] Erythromycin base is subject to destruction by gastric acid, and preparations of the base have been made with an acid-resistant coating to delay drug dissolution until it reaches the small bowel. The esters and ester salts of erythromycin are more acid stabile, form a stable suspension in water, and are tasteless. These characteristics are used in the liquid suspensions for children. Erythromycin base (absorbed intact), stearate (absorbed as the base), and ethylsuccinate (absorbed both as the intact ester and as the free base after hydrolysis in the intestine) are usually absorbed more completely in the fasting state, although one study demonstrated increased absorption of a stearate preparation when taken with a meal.[45] After absorption, about 45 percent of the ethylsuccinate preparation is present in the serum as the inactive ester and about 55 percent as the active base. Average serum levels achieved under fasting conditions with these preparations are similar; however, results with the base may be erratic. Erythromycin base has become available in a capsule containing enteric-coated granules; this preparation is promoted as giving more uniform absorption,[46,48] but some enteric-coated tablets may provide similar blood levels.[47] The absorption of the estolate is not affected by food, and the resulting peak serum level consists of both free base (20–30 percent) (active form) and estolate (70–80 percent) (much less active); the level of base thus achieved is similar to that achieved by the other oral preparations taken in comparable doses in the fasting state. The clinical significance of the much less active esterified form of the drug that is present in serum in appreciable concentration is controversial. It would seem that in treatment of infections of only moderate severity by organisms highly sensitive to erythromycin (*S. pneumoniae*, *S. pyogenes*, *M. pneumoniae*), differences in therapeutic results using the various oral preparations will be insignificant. Limited clinical comparisons confirm that suspicion.[49] However, in the treatment of group A streptococcal pharyngitis in children, substantially higher rates of bacteriologic eradication and lower rates of gastrointestinal side effects have been reported with the estolate preparation in comparison with the ethylsuccinate formulation.[50] Intravenous preparations of erythromycin achieve appreciably higher serum levels and should be used to treat serious infections requiring erythromycin.

TABLE 2. Serum Levels of Erythromycin in Adults

			Peak Serum Level	
Preparation	*Dose (mg)*	*Route*	*Hours After Dose*	*μg/ml*
Base	250	Oral	4	0.3–1.0[a]
	500			0.3–1.9
Stearate	250 (fasting)	Oral	3	0.2–1.3
	500 (fasting)		3	0.4–1.8
	500 (after food)		3	0.1–0.4[b]
Ethylsuccinate	500	Oral	0.5–2.5	1.5[c] (0.6[d])
Estolate	250	Oral	2–4	1.4–1.7
	500		3.5–4	4.2[c] (1.1[d])
Lactobionate	200	Intravenous	Immediately	3–4
	500		1	9.9
Gluceptate	250	Intravenous	Immediately	3.5–10.7
	1000		1	9.9

[a] Somewhat higher levels reported with some enteric-coated preparations after repeated doses.[46,47]
[b] One study demonstrated higher levels (to 2.8 μg/ml) with dose taken during a meal.[45]
[c] Total drug (inactive ester and free base).
[d] Free base.

Erythromycin is distributed through total body water.[51] Values given for protein binding vary from 40 to 90 percent; however, the significance of such binding is speculative.[52] The drug persists in tissues longer than in the blood. The ratios of tissue or body fluid concentrations to simultaneous serum concentrations (usually at peak) are for aqueous humor, 0.3; ascites, 0.4; bile, 28; middle ear exudate in otitis media, 0.3–0.7; pleural fluid, 0.7; prostatic fluid, 0.4; cerebrospinal fluid without meningitis, 0–0.02, with meningitis, 0.05–0.1; infected maxillary paranasal sinus, 0.4–0.8; tonsil, 0.3. Concentrations achieved in the middle ear in otitis media are adequate to treat pneumococcal and group A streptococcal infections but are not adequate to eradicate consistently *H. influenzae*.[53,54] High concentrations of erythromycin are achieved in alveolar macrophages[55] and polymorphonuclear leukocytes[56] compared to those in extracellular fluid.

There are very limited data on concentrations of erythromycin achieved in the cerebrospinal fluid of patients with meningitis, which suggest that large parenteral doses may be effective against meningeal infection by highly susceptible organisms such as *S. pneumoniae*.[57] Limited data from patients with septic arthritis suggest poor penetration of synovial fluid. Erythromycin is transferred across the placenta; fetal serum concentrations are about 2 percent of those in maternal serum, but higher concentrations accumulate in fetal tissue and amniotic fluid.[58] The drug is excreted in breast milk.

Up to 4.5 percent of an oral dose and 15 percent of a parenteral dose of erythromycin are recoverable in the urine.[7,8] Urine concentrations after oral doses are often high, but quite variable. Erythromycin is concentrated by the liver and excreted into the bile in high concentrations; however, only about 1.5 percent of the dose of the base and 0.2 percent of the ester can be recovered in bile in the first 8 hours, and some of this is reabsorbed from the intestine.[59] The higher serum levels achieved by the estolate have been attributed to both better absorption and lower biliary excretion. After an oral dose, large concentrations of the antibiotic are found in feces, probably representing ingested drug that was never absorbed as well as some that was excreted in bile. A large proportion of absorbed drug cannot be accounted for by urinary or biliary excretion or by tissue binding and may be inactivated in the liver by demethylation.[60]

The normal serum half-life of erythromycin is 1.4 hours, and appreciable serum levels are maintained for 6 hours. In anuric patients, the half-life is only prolonged to about 5 hours, and dosage reduction in patients with renal failure is generally therefore not necessary.[61] Erythromycin is not removed by peritoneal dialysis or hemodialysis.

ADVERSE REACTIONS

Erythromycin is one of the safest antibiotics in clinical use. Untoward reactions except for pseudomembranous colitis are not life threatening and, with the exception of the irritative reactions, are rare.

1. Irritative reactions are as follows:

a. Dose-related abdominal cramps, nausea, vomiting, and diarrhea occur more commonly in children and young adults than in older individuals and may be associated with intravenous as well as oral administration. These side effects appear to be due to a gastrointestinal motility-stimulating effect of the 14-membered ring macrolides.[62,63]
b. Thrombophlebitis with intravenous use can be decreased by appropriate dilution of the dose in at least 250 ml of solution and by avoiding rapid bolus infusions (infuse over about 45–60 minutes).

2. Allergic reactions include skin rash, fever, and eosinophilia.
3. Cholestatic hepatitis occurs rarely[64] and almost always with the estolate preparation and chiefly in adults.[65] The syndrome typically begins after 10 days of therapy, but more rapidly in those previously treated, and consists of nausea, vomiting, and abdominal pain followed by jaundice, fever, and abnormal liver function tests consistent with cholestatic hepatitis. These findings are sometimes accompanied by rash, leukocytosis, and eosinophilia. The abnormalities generally clear within days to a few weeks after stopping the drug but may return rapidly on rechallenge. The syndrome appears to represent a hypersensitivity reaction to the specific structure of the estolate compound.[66] However, hepatocyte toxicity induced by the drug or its metabolites, as well as allergy to altered hepatocyte components, may be contributory.[67] Milder forms of the syndrome occur with the estolate and may be more common in pregnant women.[68] It must be distinguished from false-positive serum glutamic-oxaloacetic transaminase (SGOT) elevations that occur in patients taking the estolate.[69] The latter may be found when SGOT is determined by colorimetric procedures rather than by an enzymatic method and seems to result from an interfering substance present in the blood in association with estolate administration. Reversible hepatotoxicity has occurred with the stearate salt and the ethylsuccinate ester of erythromycin.[70,71]
4. Transient hearing loss has been reported very rarely in association with the use of large intravenous doses of erythromycin lactobionate or large doses of oral erythromycin.[72,73] This may occur more commonly in elderly patients with renal insufficiency.[74–76]
5. Hypertrophic pyloric stenosis developed in five infants during administration of erythromycin estolate.[77]
6. Superinfection, especially of the gastrointestinal tract or vagina, with *Candida* species or gram-negative bacilli may occur, as with other antibiotics.
7. Psudomembranous colitis caused by overgrowth of toxin-producing *Clostridium difficile* occurs rarely with the use of erythromycin.[78,79]

Drug Interactions

Incompatibility during administration between intravenous preparations of erythromycin and other drugs has been reported; the latter include vitamin B complex and vitamin C, cephalothin, tetracycline, chloramphenicol, colistin, heparin, metraminol, and diphenylhydantoin. Erythromycin may produce interactions with other drugs by interfering with their hepatic metabolism through the cytochrome P-450 enzyme system.[80] When oral theophylline and oral erythromycin are used concurrently, increased blood levels of theophylline and potential theophylline toxicity may result.[81] By the same mechanism, erythromycin can increase the anticoagulant effect of warfarin[82] and interfere with the metabolism of methylprednisolone,[83] carbamazapine,[84] and cyclosporine,[85] sometimes leading to toxicity with the latter two drugs. Erythromycin can increase the bioavailability of digoxin by interfering with its inactivation by gut flora.[80] Erythromycin may inhibit the assay organism used in some determinations of serum folic acid. Sequential use of erythromycin and clindamycin should be avoided when possible because of the potential for the development of cross or "dissociated" resistance.

Uses of Erythromycin

Erythromycin has a few indications for use as the drug of choice and a larger number of important applications as an alternative drug to penicillin G (Table 3).[86] When used in adults by the oral route, preparations other than the estolate are generally preferable because they have less risk of cholestatic hepatitis. Absorption, particularly with the enteric-coated base, stearate, or ethylsuccinate preparations taken in the fasting state or before meals, is usually adequate. The estolate preparation should be particularly avoided during pregnancy, when hepatotoxicity may be more common.[68] When higher serum levels are needed in more severe infections requiring erythromycin therapy, the drug should be given intravenously.

Treatment of *M. pneumoniae* infection with erythromycin, as with tetracycline, shortens the clinical course of the infection; radiologic clearing of pulmonary lesions occurs earlier with erythromycin.[87] Clinical experience and studies in vitro and in guinea pigs suggest that erythromycin is the most active available agent in treating pneumonia caused by L. pneumophila or *L. micdadei*.[9,88,89] Erythromycin treatment of patients with gastroenteritis caused by *C. jejuni* hastens the eradication of the organism from the feces, but it does not appear to alter the clinical course of uncomplicated infection when therapy begins 4 days or more after the onset of symptoms.[90] However, earlier treatment of young children with acute dysentery associated with *C. jejuni* has recently been shown to shorten the course of diarrhea and fecal excretion of the organism.[91] Nevertheless, in an institutional setting in Thailand where *C. jejuni* strains were frequently resistant to erythromycin in vitro, early treatment of infants with diarrhea due to this organism was not beneficial.[92] Treatment of infants with erythromycin for pneumonia due to *C. trachomatis* appears to speed recovery and eradication of the shedding of organisms.[93] Erythromycin is preferable to tetracycline in treating chlamydial pelvic infection during pregnancy.[86] Erythromycin base given orally together with neomycin on the day before colorectal surgery and combined with vigorous purgation is about as effective as parenteral cephalosporin administration just before surgery in decreasing the incidence of septic complications.[94] However, in the presence of bowel obstruction or when there is need for emergency surgery, the parenteral antibiotic regimen should be used.[86] The results of treating syphilis with erythromycin during pregnancy must be considered uncertain at best; fetal syphilis may not be eradicated, and therefore convincing evidence of potentially dangerous penicillin allergy should be obtained before this type of therapy is used.[95] When erythromycin is used to treat syphilis in pregnancy, the infant should be treated with penicillin at birth. Erythromycin may occasionally be useful in treating urinary tract infections due to gram-negative bacilli that might otherwise require the use of more toxic agents.[96] Urine pH must generally be raised to 8.0 or above to achieve effective activity at urinary concentrations against the gram-negative bacilli. Erythromycin may be used as an alternative antibiotic in the treatment of anthrax and in infections by *B. catarrhalis, E. corrodens,* and *L. monocytogenes*. Erythromycin is not consistently effective in treatment of infections due to *H. influenzae*,[53,54] and in vitro studies suggest resistance by some strains of *C. perfringens*.[24] In view of the availability of more effective alternative drugs, erythromycin should not be used alone in the treatment of deep-seated staphylococcal infections because of the potential for the emergence of resistant strains during therapy.[19,21,22] Experimental studies and limited clinical data suggest that erythromycin combined with a penicillin may demonstrate synergy[21,97] against S. aureus; further studies are needed to exploit the potential in therapy.

TABLE 3. Major Uses of Erythromycin

Indication	*Doses of Erythromycin for Adults*	*Alternative Drug*
Infection in which erythromycin is the drug of first choice		
M. pneumoniae infections	0.5 g tid-qid po[a]	Tetracycline
Legionella pneumonia	0.5–1.0 g qid po[a]	Rifampin + erythromycin
Diphtheria[b]	Carrier state: 500 mg qid po for 10 days	Penicillin G
	Disease:[a] followed by oral for 10 days	Penicillin G
Pertussis	0.5 g qid po	Ampicillin
Chl. trachomatis pneumonia or conjunctivitis	10 mg/kg qid po[a]	Trimethoprim-sulfamethoxazole
Chlamydial pelvic infection in pregnancy	0.5–1.0 g qid po[a,c]	Sulfisoxazole
C. jejuni gastroenteritis	250 mg qid po	Ciprofloxacin
Prevention of infection after colorectal surgery	1 g po each of neomycin and erythromycin base at 1, 2, and 11 P.M. on the day before surgery combined with vigorous purgation over the 2 days before surgery	Parenteral cephalosporin
Infections in which erythromycin is an important alternative drug		*Drug of first choice*
Groups A, C, C, G streptococcal infection	250–500 mg qid po[a,d]	Penicillin G
S. pneumoniae infection	250–500 mg qid po[a]	Penicillin G
Rheumatic fever prophylaxis	250 mg bid po	Penicillin G
Prevention of bacterial endocarditis (in dental procedures)	1.0 g po 2 hr before procedure, then 500 mg 6 hr later	Penicillin V
Lymphogranuloma venereum	500 mg qid po for 21 days	Tetracycline
Chancroid	500 mg qid po for 7 days	Ceftriaxone
Nongonococcal urethritis	500 mg qid po for 7 days	Tetracycline
Syphilis 1°, 2°, latent (<1 yr) in pregnancy	500 mg qid po for 15 days[e]	Penicillin G
latent (>1 yr) in pregnancy	500 mg qid po for 30 days[e]	Penicillin G
Bronchopulmonary anaerobic infections	0.5 gm qid po	Penicillin G; clindamycin
Acne vulgaris	250 mg qid po or topical preparation	Tetracycline po and a number of topical drugs
Urinary tract infection	500 mg qid po[f]	Many agents

[a] Intravenous therapy (2–4 g/day) should be used in serious illness or when oral therapy is not possible or reliable.
[b] Antitoxin is essential primary therapy for disease.
[c] Severe pelvic inflammatory disease is often polymicrobial in origin; treatment of such cases should include other agents more active against likely facultative and anaerobic enteric bacteria and/or *N. gonorrhoeae*.
[d] Treatment should be continued for 10 days for Group A.
[e] Effectiveness uncertain. Careful follow-up needed when used in pregnancy. Infants should be treated with penicillin at birth.
[f] Urine pH must be raised to greater than 8 with sodium bicarbonate.

Other Macrolides

Trioleandomycin, an ester of the 14-membered ring macrolide oleandomycin, has no advantages over erythromycin and may occasionally cause cholestatic hepatitis. Spiramycin, a 16-membered ring macrolide, has been reported to have some effectiveness in the treatment of diarrhea due to cryptosporidium[98] and in toxoplasmosis,[99] but confirmation of its effectiveness is needed.

Several investigational macrolides are of current interest. Clarithromycin (A-56268) (TE-031) (Abbott Laboratories) is a 6-0-methyl derivative of erythromycin with in vitro antibacterial activity equal to or slightly greater than that of erythromycin.[100] Roxithromycin (RU-28965) (Roussel) is an ether oxime derivative of erythromycin with somewhat less in vitro antibacterial activity than erythromycin, but with a longer half-life, which may allow twice daily oral dosing.[100,101] Azithromycin (CP 62,993) (Pfizer Laboratories) is a 15-membered ring macrolide differing from erythromycin by having a methyl-substituted nitrogen in the macrolide ring. Compared to erythromycin, it is somewhat less active in vitro against gram-positive bacteria, substantially more active against *H. influenzae*, and generally somewhat more active against *B. catarrahalis*, *N. gonorrhoeae*, and *Campylobacter* species.[100,102] Azithromycin also shows promising activity against *T. gondii* in mouse protection studies involving both intraperitoneal and intracerebral infections.[103] It shows more stability to gastric acid, a longer half-life, and increased concentrations in tissues compared to erythromycin.[104]

LINCOMYCIN AND CLINDAMYCIN

Derivation, Chemistry, and Preparations

Lincomycin was isolated in 1962 from an organism, *Streptomyces lincolnensis*, obtained from soil near Lincoln, Nebraska. Its biologic properties are similar to those of erythromycin, but it is chemically unrelated, consisting of an amino acid linked to an amino sugar (Fig. 2). Chemical modification provided clindamycin (7-chloro-7-deoxy-lincomycin) (Fig. 2) with increased antibacterial potency and absorption after oral administration.[105] Since there are no therapeutic advantages for lincomycin over clindamycin, the discussion will concentrate on the latter, although both are still marketed as pharmaceuticals. Both are weak bases that are readily water soluble when provided as salts.

Lincomycin (Lincocin) is available as the hydrochloride salt in 250- and 500-mg capsules and syrup for oral administration and in solution (300 mg/ml) for parenteral use. Clindamycin (Cleocin) is prepared as the hydrochloride salt of the base in 75- and 150-mg capsules and of the palmitate ester for pediatric suspension. It is supplied as the phosphate ester for intramuscular or intravenous use (150 mg/ml). It is also available in a topical solution for the treatment of acne vulgaris.

Mechanisms of Action

The lincosamide antibiotics have, in susceptible organisms, the same or overlapping 50S ribosomal binding sites as those for the macrolides and chloramphenicol, and they may compete with these drugs for binding.[2,3] Protein synthesis is inhibited primarily in early chain elongation by interference with the transpeptidation reaction.[1,3]

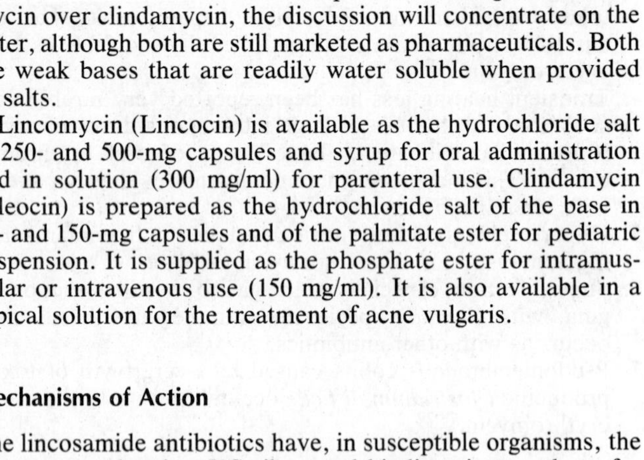

FIG. 2. The lincosamide antibiotics; lincomycin, R = OH; clindamycin, R = Cl.

Antimicrobial Activity and Mechanisms of Resistance

In vitro susceptibilities to clindamycin are given in Table 4.[7,12,105,106] Clindamycin is more potent than lincomycin but similar in degree of activity to erythromycin against staphylococci, pneumococci, *S. pyogenes*, and streptococci of the "viridans" group. However, while erythromycin demonstrates at least moderate activity against the enterococcus, *H. influenzae*, and *N. meningitidis*, clindamycin is generally inactive against these organisms at clinically achievable concentrations. In contrast, clindamycin shows significantly greater activity than erythromycin against most clinically significant anaerobic bacteria, particularly *B. fragilis*[107,108] and some erythromycin-resistant strains of *S. aureus*.[109] Clindamycin is one of the most active antibiotics available against *B. fragilis*. In a survey of nine hospitals in the United States that provided 750 strains of the *B. fragilis* group in 1981, 6 percent of isolates were resistant to clindamycin (MIC > 4 μg/ml by an agar dilution method); this represented 0–13 percent of strains in individual institutions.[12] In a similar survey by the same group involving eight centers and 678 isolates of the *B. fragilis* group collected in 1984 and 1985, 5 percent were resistant to clindamycin, representing 0–10 percent of the strains in individual institutions.[106] Of the species belonging to the *B. fragilis* group, clindamycin resistance was found in 5 percent of *B. fragilis*, 10 percent of *Bacteroides thetaiotaomicron*, 15 percent of *B. vulgatus*, 6 percent of *B. distasonis*, and 7 percent of *B. ovatus*.[106] Resistance to clindamycin by anaerobes also includes 10–20 percent of clostridial species other than *C. perfringens*, about 10 percent of peptococci, and most *Fusobacterium varium* strains.[107,108] All the Enterobacteriaceae are resistant to clindamycin.

There have been occasional reports of clinical isolates of lincosamide-resistant *S. pneumoniae*,[15,16] *S. pyogenes*,[14,17] and "viridans" group streptococci; these strains are usually also resistant to erythromycin. In most hospitals at present, the majority of isolates of *S. aureus* are sensitive to lincomycin or clindamycin[108]; however, resistance occurs in 15–20 percent of strains.[110] Lincomycin resistance has been reported in 20 percent of methicillin-resistant strains[111] and in 50 percent of erythromycin-resistant strains[112] of *S. aureus*. Cross resistance of *S. aureus* between lincomycin and clindamycin is complete. The minimal inhibitory concentrations of clindamycin and erythromycin in vitro are generally similar for *S. aureus* strains that are sensitive to both agents; however, resistance can be selected in vitro by serial subculture in the presence of subinhibitory concentrations of either, and it occurs slowly for clindamycin and more rapidly for erythromycin.[109,113] In contrast, strains that are sensitive to clindamycin and resistant to erythromycin can be rapidly selected for clindamycin resistance by serial subculture on clindamycin. Consistent with these in vitro observations, the emergence of clindamycin-resistant *S. aureus* has been noted in clindamycin-treated patients, in particular when the organisms had demonstrated erythromycin resistance at the onset of treatment.[109] Clindamycin resistance, often crossing to erythromycin, has also emerged from treated patients infected with *S. aureus* that were initially sensitive to erythromycin.[114] Resistance of the "dissociated" type may also emerge during treatment of patients.[113]

The antibacterial activity of lincomycin and clindamycin has been shown, in limited in vitro studies, to be bactericidal for *S. pneumoniae, S. pyogenes*, and *S. aureus*. Its killing activity is similar to that of erythromycin and therefore probably varies with the concentration, bacterial species, and inoculum. It is more slowly bactericidal for *S. aureus* than are the penicillins[115] and is inconsistently bactericidal for *B. fragilis*.[116]

Mechanisms of resistance to the lincosamide antibiotics include the following: (*1*) Alteration in a single 50S ribosomal protein of the receptor site confers resistance to erythromycin and often to the lincosamides[2]; this mechanism has already been discussed for erythromycin. (*2*) Alteration in the 23S ribosomal RNA of the 50S ribosomal subunit by methylation of adenine[34–37] has also been discussed. It is usually plasmid mediated and provides the MLS_B type of resistance, which includes that exhibited by some strains of *S. aureus* and *B. fragilis* to clindamycin.[39] (*3*) Inactivation of lincomycin and clindamycin by a few isolates of staphylococci, including *S. aureus*, which possess a 4-lincosamide 0-nucleotidyltransferase that catalyzes the nucleotidylation of the hydroxyl group in position 4 of the antibiotics.[117] This adenylation of the lincosamides is associated with high-level resistance to lincomycin, but clindamycin resistance may not be detected by routine methods. The adenylation of clindamycin is associated with impaired bactericidal activity and decreased activity at high inoculum levels. The nucleotide sequences of the plasmid-mediated genes, lin A and lin A′, which encode for the inactivating enzymes, have been determined.

TABLE 4. In Vitro Susceptibilities to Clindamycin

	Minimum Inhibitory Concentration (μg/ml)	
Organism	*Range*	*Median*
S. pneumoniae	0.002–0.04[a]	0.01
S. pyogenes	0.02–0.1[a]	0.04
S. viridans	0.005–0.04[a]	0.02
Enterococcus	12.5–>100	100
S. aureus	0.04–>100	0.1
S. epidermidis	0.1–>100	0.1
C. perfringens	<0.1–8	0.8
N. gonorrhoeae	0.01–6.3	3.1
N. meningitidis	6.3–25	12.5
H. influenzae	0.4–50	12.5
B. fragilis group	<0.125–>256	0.25
B. melaninogenicus	≤0.1–1	≤0.1
Fusobacterium spp.	≤0.5[a]	≤0.5
Peptococcus spp.	≤0.1–>100	≤0.5
Peptostreptococcus spp.	≤0.1–0.8	≤0.5
M. pneumoniae	1.6–3.1	3.1

[a] Occasional clinical isolates are more resistant.

Clinical Pharmacology

Peak serum levels achieved after oral administration of clindamycin occur earlier and are at least twice as high as those of lincomycin. Absorption of clindamycin is about 90 percent and is slightly delayed, but not decreased, by ingestion of food, whereas that of lincomycin is markedly decreased.[105] Mean peak serum concentrations of clindamycin in adults after single oral doses of 150 and 300 mg occur at 1 hour and are 2.5 and 3.6 μg/ml, respectively; at 6 hours they are 0.7 and 1.1 μg/ml, respectively. The esters, clindamycin palmitate in suspension for oral use and clindamycin phosphate for parenteral use, are absorbed as the inactive ester and rapidly hydrolyzed in the blood to the active base. After intramuscular administration, which causes little pain, mean peak serum levels are reached in 3 hours and are about 6 μg/ml after a 300-mg dose and 9 μg/ml after a 600-mg dose; at 12 hours they are 0.7 and 0.9 μg/ml, respectively.[118] In adult healthy volunteers, immediately following 20–45-minute intravenous infusions of 600, 900, or 1200 mg of clindamycin phosphate, serum levels of base are 10, 11, and 14 μg/ml, respectively. Higher levels after intravenous infusion have been reported in infected patients under treatment.[119] Dose regimens of intravenous clindamycin using 900 mg every 8 hours or 600 mg every 6 hours are considered acceptable.[120]

Limited studies have demonstrated good penetration of most tissues by the lincosamides excepting clinically insignificant entry of clindamycin into the cerebrospinal fluid, even with meningitis.[7,121] The concentration in bone in relationship to serum levels is particularly high.[122] Clindamycin administered to pregnant women readily passes the placental barrier and enters fetal blood and tissues.[58] Clindamycin is actively transported into polymorphonuclear leukocytes and macrophages[123] and is present in relatively high concentrations, compared to peak serum levels, in experimental abscesses.[124]

The normal half-life of clindamycin is 2.4 hours. Most of the absorbed drug is metabolized, probably by the liver, to products with variable antibacterial activity, including *N*-demethyl-clindamycin (more active than the parent compound) and clindamycin sulfoxide (less active), which have been detected in bile and urine but not in serum.[118] High bioactivity is found in bile, mostly as the *N*-demethyl metabolite; this represents a minor route of excretion and accounts for the activity assayed in feces after parenteral administration.[118,125] Clindamycin activity in feces persists for at least 5 days after 48 hours of parenteral administration and is associated with a major reduction in the population of sensitive bacteria in the colon lasting for up to 14 days.[126] Clindamycin concentration in bile is markedly diminished or absent when the common bile duct is obstructed.[127] High clindamycin bioactivity, also mostly in the *N*-demethyl form, is found in the urine and persists for up to 4 days after a single dose, suggesting slow release from tissues.[118] Accurate data on the proportion of absorbed clindamycin that is excreted in the urine are not available because of the variable activity of the metabolites and their unknown proportions in urine.

The half-life of clindamycin is increased from 2.4 to about 6 hours in patients with severe renal failure, and peak blood levels after parenteral administration are about twice those in healthy people.[128] If modified at all, parenteral doses should be halved in such patients. Some prolongation of clindamycin activity in serum is noted in patients with severe liver disease.[129] Appreciable dose modification should be made when there is concomitant severe renal and hepatic disease in the same patient. Neither hemodialysis nor peritoneal dialysis removes significant amounts of clindamycin.

Adverse Reactions

1. Allergic reactions include a variety of rashes, fever, and rare cases of erythema multiforme and anaphylaxis.
2. Diarrhea occurs in up to 20 percent of patients and is more common with oral administration. However, the major toxicity of lincomycin and clindamycin that now appreciably limits their use is the occurrence of pseudomembranous colitis caused by a toxin secreted by *C. difficile* that overgrows in the presence of these antibiotics.[130–132] This has been reported in 0.01–10 percent of clindamycin-treated patients.[108,133] The syndrome may occur in association with administration of other antibiotics but does so less frequently; it is not related to the dose and may occur after oral or parenteral therapy. The variable incidence of colitis in different reports has been ascribed to different diagnostic methods and the variable epidemiology of *C. difficile*.[108,133] It may begin during or as long as several weeks after a course of lincomycin or clindamycin therapy and is characterized by diarrhea, sometimes bloody, with fever and cramps and the appearance of yellow-white plaques on the colonic mucosa, seen by proctoscopy. The toxin of *C. difficile* can be detected in the stool of nearly all patients with antibiotic-associated pseudomembranous colitis and in about 20 percent of patients with antibiotic-associated diarrhea by a cytotoxicity assay using tissue culture cells.[79,132] The cytotoxic effect can be prevented by neutralization of the toxin in the stool extract with *Clostridium sordelli* antitoxin. The syndrome can be protracted and may end fatally. Prompt cessation of the antibiotic is essential. Use of antiperistaltic drugs should be avoided since they may worsen the condition. Vancomycin given by mouth in doses of 125–500 mg qid is the drug of choice for treatment of this type of pseudomembranous colitis, although oral bacitracin and oral metronidazole may be effective as well.[134,135] Relapse after treatment may occur.
3. Hepatotoxicity: Minor reversible elevation of transaminase levels, unassociated with other evidence of liver abnormality, has been commonly observed in patients receiving clindamycin, especially by the parenteral route. Some of these may have been false-positive reactions associated with colorimetric rather than specific enzymatic measurements.[105] However, rare cases of frank hepatotoxicity, including jaundice associated with hepatocellular damage, have been observed.[136]
4. Isolated cases of reversible neutropenia, thrombocytopenia, and agranulocytosis associated with lincomycin or clindamycin therapy have been reported; their relationship to the antibiotic administration was uncertain.
5. Occasional reports of hypotension, ECG changes, and rarely cardiopulmonary arrest have been reported when large intravenous doses of lincomycin were given rapidly. This has not been reported with clindamycin.
6. Local irritative reactions are rare with these drugs. Intramuscular and intravenous administration is generally well tolerated.

Drug Interactions

Clindamycin may block neuromuscular transmission and may enhance the action of other blocking agents.[137] Clindamycin phosphate in solution is physically incompatible with ampicillin, diphenylhydantoin, barbiturates, aminophylline, calcium gluconate, and magnesium sulfate.

Uses of Clindamycin

The higher activity and absorption properties of clindamycin, along with no greater potential for toxicity, compared with lincomycin, favors the former in all indications for use of these antibiotics. The lincosamides have been used in a variety of infections, often with good effect; however, the appreciation of the potential for serious or even fatal toxicity with pseudomembranous colitis and the availability of safer alternative antibiotics should now generally limit the use of clindamycin to a few indications[86]:

1. Infections that are outside of the central nervous system and are likely to involve *B. fragilis* or other penicillin-resistant anaerobic bacteria. These particularly involve polymicrobial intra-abdominal or gynecologic pelvic infections.[108] Clindamycin is likely to be beneficial where there is spillage of fecal flora associated with tissue damage, as in cases involving bowel damage or perforation. In these situations, studies of experimental animal models and patients with infection suggest that clindamycin decreases the likelihood of abscess formation involving fecal organisms, especially *B. fragilis*.[138,139] In these conditions, clindamycin is administered together with an aminoglycoside, because additional activity is required against Enterobacteriaceae. The beneficial effect of clindamycin in preventing or ameliorating morbidity from fecal abscess formation or other infections appears to be superior to that of penicillin, cephalothin, or aminoglycosides.[138,140] However, in comparative trials of therapy for intra-abdominal or pelvic sepsis, clindamycin, cefoxitin, metronidazole, imipenem, and chloramphenicol have shown similar effectiveness.[108,141] In addition, given its excellent in vitro activity against the *B. fragilis* group,[106] regimens including ticarcillin-clavulanic acid can be expected to give similar clinical results.

Clindamycin may offer no advantage over penicillin G in the treatment of anaerobic bronchopulmonary infections,[142] except that it serves as an alternative in patients allergic to penicillin. However, in a prospective randomized study of 39 patients with community-acquired putrid lung abscess, clindamycin was more effective than penicillin in terms of the time until eradication of fever and fetid sputum and the "overall response" to treatment.[143] The study involved small numbers of patients and had some flaws in the analysis;[144] however, the superiority of clindamycin for some patients was demonstrated and may relate to observations that 15–25 percent of anaerobic pulmonary infections involve β-lactamase-producing strains of *B. fragilis*, *B. melaninogenicus, B. ruminicola,* and *B. ureolyticus,* which are resistant to penicillin.[108,144] Clindamycin may therefore be preferable for the treatment of this condition, particularly in seriously ill patients or in those who have responded poorly to penicillin.

2. Clindamycin is useful as an alternative to penicillin in treatment of *C. perfringens* infections.
3. Clindamycin may sometimes be useful as an alternative to a penicillin in the treatment of staphylococcal infections. However, its more limited bactericidal rate for staphylococci compared with that of the penicillins, and particularly the real potential for the emergence of clindamycin-resistant strains in treated patients, are disadvantages. The latter problem, noted especially but not only with erythromycin-resistant strains, appreciably limits its effectiveness in the therapy of deep-seated staphylococcal infections, particularly endocarditis.[114,122] Vancomycin or the cephalosporins are usually better alternatives to the penicillins for the latter. Although high concentrations of clindamycin are achieved in bone, an advantage of clindamycin for the treatment of osteomyelitis in patients has not been established.
4. The topical solution of clindamycin may be used to treat acne vulgaris.[145] However, it should be noted that pseudomembranous colitis associated with the use of topical clindamycin has been reported.[146]
5. Clindamycin has been reported to have some success in treating experimental animals and small numbers of patients with toxoplasmosis of the central nervous system.[147,148] These studies require confirmation in controlled clinical trials.
6. Clindamycin has been reported to be effective in the treatment of falciparum malaria,[149] but its relative place in the treatment of this infection compared to that of other regimens has not been established. It has also been reported to be useful in the treatment of babesiosis[86,150]; it is suggested that clindamycin be used together with quinine for such treatment.[86]
7. Several studies have suggested that the coexistence of β-lactamase-producing *S. aureus* or *Bacteroides* species and group A streptococci may be associated with the failure of penicillin to eradicate the latter, resulting in recurrent tonsillitis. These studies suggest lower recurrence rates when clindamycin is used.[151] Most recurrences of streptococcal pharyngitis are reinfections rather than relapses, and widespread use of clindamycin for this common problem will likely lead to a substantial number of cases of pseudomembranous colitis,[152] as well as selection for clindamycin-resistant strains of group A streptococci.

Doses of clindamycin, for adults depend on the site, severity of the infection, and condition of the patient. Oral doses are usually 150–300 mg every 6 hours and parenteral doses, given every 6–12 hours, usually total 600–2700 mg/day, occasionally higher.

REFERENCES

1. Pestka S. Inhibitors of protein synthesis. In: Weissbach H, Pestka S, eds. Molecular Mechanisms of Protein Biosynthesis. New York: Academic Press; 1977:467.
2. Oleinick NL. The erythromycins. In Corcoran JW, Hahn FE, eds. Mechanism of Action of Antimicrobial and Antitumor Agents. New York: Springer-Verlag; 1975:396.
3. Franklin TJ, Snow GA. Biochemistry of Antimicrobial Action. 3rd ed. London: Chapman and Hall; 1981:128.
4. Haight TH, Finland M. Observations on mode of action of erythromycin. Proc Soc Exp Biol Med. 1952;81:188–93.
5. Haight TH, Finland M. The antibacterial action of erythromycin. Proc Soc Exp Biol Med. 1952;81:175–83.
6. Sabath LD, Gerstein DA, Loder PB, et al. Excretion of erythromycin and its enhanced activity in urine against gram-negative bacilli with alkalinization. J Lab Clin Med. 1968;72:916–23.
7. Garrod LP, Lambert HP, O'Grady F. Antibiotic and Chemotherapy. 5th ed. Edinburgh: Churchill Livingstone; 1981:183.
8. Washington JA II, Wilson WR. Erythromycin: A microbial and clinical perspective after 30 years of clinical use. I. Mayo Clin Proc. 1984;60:189–203; II. 1985;60:271–8.
9. Edelstein PM, Meyer RD. Susceptibility of *Legionella pneumophila* to twenty antimicrobial agents. Antimicrob Agents Chemother. 1980;18:403–8.
10. Vanhoff R, Gordts B, Dierickx R, et al. Bacteriostatic and bactericidal activities of 24 antimicrobial agents against *Campylobacter fetus* subsp. jejuni. Antimicrob Agents Chemother. 1980;18:118–21.
11. Kuo C, Wang S, Grayston T. Antimicrobial activity of several antibiotics and a sulfonamide against *Chlamydia trachomitis* organisms in cell culture. Antimicrob Agents Chemother. 1977;12:80–3.
12. Tally FP, Cuchural GJ, Jacobus NV, et al. Susceptibility of the *Bacteroides fragilis* group in the United States in 1981. Antimicrob Agents Chemother. 1983;23:536–40.
13. Ahmad F, McLeod DT, Croughan MJ, et al. Antimicrobial susceptibility of *Branhamella catarrhalis* isolates from bronchopulmonary infections. Antimicrob Agents Chemother. 1984;26:424–5.
14. Sanders E, Foster MT, Scott D. Group A beta-haemolytic streptococci resistant to erythromycin and lincomycin. N Engl J Med. 1968;278:538–40.
15. Dixon JM: Pneumococcus resistant to erythromycin and lincomycin. Lancet. 1967;1:573.
16. Linares J, Garau J, Dominiquez C, et al. Antibiotic resistance and serotypes of *Streptococcus pneumoniae* from patients with community acquired pneumococcal disease. Antimicrob Agents Chemother. 1983;23:545–7.
17. Maruyama S, Yoshioka H, Fujita K, et al. Sensitivity of group A streptococci to antibiotics. Am J Dis Child. 1979;133:1143–5.
18. Istre GR, Welch DF, Marks MI, et al. Susceptibility of group A beta-hemolytic *Streptococcus* isolates to penicillin and erythromycin. Antimicrob Agents Chemother. 1981;20:244–6.
19. Haight TH, Finland M. Resistance of bacteria to erythromycin. Proc Soc Exp Biol Med. 1952;81:183–8.
20. Lepper MH, Dowling HF, Jackson GG, et al. Effect of antibiotic usage in the hospital on the incidence of antibiotic-resistant strains among personnel carrying staphylococci. J Lab Clin Med. 1953;42:832.
21. Griffith RS, Black HR. Erythromycin. Med Clin North Am. 1970;54:1199–215.
22. Haight TH, Finland M. Laboratory and clinical studies on erythromycin. N Engl J Med. 1952;247:227–32.
23. Garrod LP. The erythromycin group of antibiotics. Br Med J. 1957;2:57–63.
24. Sapico FL, Kwok Y, Sutter V, et al. Standardized antimicrobial disc susceptibility testing of anaerobic bacteria: In vitro susceptibility of *Clostridium perfringens* to nine antibiotics. Antimicrob Agents Chemother. 1972;2:320–5.
25. Molavi A, Weinstein L. In vitro activity of erythromycin against atypical mycobacteria. J Infect Dis. 1971;123:216–9.
26. Finland M, Bach MC, Garner C, et al. Synergistic action of ampicillin against *Nocardia asteroides*: Effect of time of incubation. Antimicrob Agents Chemother. 1974;5:344–53.
27. Fernandes PB, Hardy D, Bailer R, et al. Susceptibility testing of macrolide antibiotics against *Hemophilus influenzae* and correlation of in vitro results with in vivo efficacy in a mouse septicemia model. Antimicrob Agents Chemother. 1987;31:1243–50.
28. Kucers A. Chloramphenicol, erythromycin, vancomycin, tetracyclines. Lancet. 1982;ii:425–9.
29. Jao RL, Finland M. Susceptibility of *Mycoplasma pneumoniae* to 21 antibiotics in vitro. Am J Med Sci. 1967;253:639–50.
30. Niitu Y, Hasegawa S, Kubota H. In vitro development of resistance to erythromycin, other macrolide antibiotics, and lincomycin in *Mycoplasma pneumoniae*. Antimicrob Agents Chemother. 1974;5:513–9.
31. Mao JC-H, Putterman M. Accumulation in gram-positive and gram-negative bacteria as a mechanism of resistance to erythromycin. J Bacteriol. 1968;95:1111–7.
32. Taubeneck U. Susceptibility of *Proteus mirabilis* and its stable L-forms to erythromycin and other macrolides. Nature. 1962;196:195–6.
33. Lampson BC, von David W, Parisi JT. Novel mechanism for plasmid-mediated erythromycin resistance by pNE24 from *Staphylococcus epidermidis*. Antimicrob Agents Chemother. 1986;30:653–8.
34. Weisblum B, Siddhikol C, Lai CJ, et al. Erythromycin inducible resistance in *Staphylococcus aureus*: Requirements for induction. J Bacteriol. 1971;106:835–47.
35. Lai CJ, Weisblum B, Fahnestock SR, et al. Alteration of 23S ribosomal RNA and erythromycin-induced resistance to lincomycin and spiramycin in *Staphylococcus aureus*. J Mol Biol. 1973;74:67–72.
36. Fujisawa Y, Weisblum B. A family of *r*-determinants in *Streptomyces* spp. that specifies inducible resistance to macrolide, lincosamide, and streptogramin type B antibiotics. J Bacteriol. 1981;146:621–31.
37. Lai CJ, Weisblum B. Altered methylation of ribosomal RNA in an erythromycin-resistant strain of *Staphylococcus aureus*. Proc Natl Acad Sci USA. 1971;68:856–60.

38. Dowling JN, McDevitt DA, Pasculle WA. Isolation and preliminary characterization of erythromycin-resistant variants of *Legionella micdadei* and *Legionella pneumophila*. Antimicrob Agents Chemother. 1985;27:272–4.
39. Courvalin P, Ounissi H, Arthur M. Multiplicity of macrolide–lincosamide–streptogramin antibiotic resistance determinants. J Antimicrob Chemother. 1985;16(Suppl A):91–100.
40. Weisblum B. Inducible resistance to macrolides, lincosamides and streptogramin type B antibiotics: The resistance phenotype, its bacteriological diversity and structural elements that regulate expression. A review. J Antimicrob Chemother. 16(Suppl A):726–30.
41. Murphy E. Nucleotide sequence of erm A, a macrolide–lincosamide–streptogramin B determinant in *Staphylococcus aureus*. J Bacteriol. 1985;162(2):633–40.
42. Barthelemy P, Autissier D, Gerbaud G, et al. Enzymatic hydrolysis of erythromycin by a strain of *Escherichia coli*. J Antibiot. 1984;37:1692–6.
43. Ounissi H, Courvalin P. Nucleotide sequence of the gene ere A encoding the erythromycin esterase in *Escherichia coli*. Gene. 1985;35:271–8.
44. Bechtol LD, Stephens VC, Pugh CT, et al. Erythromycin esters: Comparative in-vivo hydrolysis and bioavailability. Curr Ther Res. 1976;20:610–22.
45. Malmborg A. Effect of food on absorption of erythromycin. A study of two derivatives, the stearate and the base. J Antimicrob Chemother. 1979;5:591–9.
46. McDonald PJ, Mather LE, Story MJ. Studies on absorption of a newly developed enteric-coated erythromycin base. J Clin Pharmacol. 1977;17:601–6.
47. DiSanto AR, Chodos DJ. Influence of study design in assessing food effects on absorption of erythromycin base and erythromycin stearate. Antimicrob Agents Chemother. 1981;20:190–6.
48. Yakatan GJ, Rasmussen CE, Feis PJ et al. Bioinequivalence of erythromycin ethylsuccinate and enteric-coated erythromycin pellets following multiple oral doses. J Clin Pharmacol. 1985;25:36–42.
49. Janicki RS, Garnham JC, Worland MC, et al. Comparison of erythromycin ethylsuccinate, stearate and estolate treatments of group A streptococcus infections of the upper respiratory tract. Clin Pediatr (Phila). 1975;14:1098–1107.
50. Ginsburg CM, McCracken GH Jr, Crow SD, et al. Erythromycin therapy for group A streptococcal pharyngitis. Results of a comparative study of the estolate and ethylsuccinate formulation. Am J Dis Child. 1984;138:536–9.
51. Osono T, Umezawa H. Pharmacokinetics of macrolides, lincosamides and streptogramins. J Antimicrob Chemother. 1985;16(Suppl A):151–66.
52. Welling PG. The esters of erythromycin. J Antimicrob Chemother. 1979;5:633–4.
53. Bass JW, Steele RW, Wiebe RA, et al. Erythromycin concentrations in middle ear exudates. Pediatrics. 1971;48:417–22.
54. Howard JE, Nelson JD, Clahsen J, et al. Otitis media of infancy and early childhood. Am J Dis Child. 1976;130:965–70.
55. Hand WL, Corwin RW, Steinberg TH, et al. Uptake of antibiotics by human alveolar macrophages. Am Rev Respir Dis. 1984;129(6):933–7.
56. Miller MF, Martin JR, Johnson P, et al. Erythromycin uptake and accumulation by human polymorphonuclear leukocytes and efficacy of erythromycin in killing ingested *Legionella pneumophila*. J Infect Dis. 1984;149(5):714–8.
57. Romansky MJ, Nasou JP, Davis DS, et al. The treatment of 171 patients with erythromycin, including 132 with bacterial pneumonia. Antibiotics Annual. New York: Medical Encyclopedia; 1956, 1955–1956:48.
58. Phillipson A, Sabath LD, Charles D. Transplacental passage of erythromycin and clindamycin. N Engl J Med. 1973;288:1219–21.
59. Hammond JB, Griffith RS. Factors affecting the absorption and biliary excretion of erythromycin and two of its derivatives in humans. Clin Pharmacol Ther. 1961;2:308–12.
60. Mao JC-H, Tardrew PL. Demethylation of erythromycin by rabbit tissues in vitro. Biochem Pharmacol. 1965;14:1049–58.
61. Kunin CM. A guide to use of antibiotics in patients with renal disease. Ann Intern Med. 1967;67:151–8.
62. Itoh Z, Suzuki T, Nakaya M, et al. Gastrointestinal motor-stimulating activity of macrolide antibiotics and analysis of their side effects on the canine gut. Antimicrob Agents Chemother. 1984;26:863–9.
63. Itoh Z, Suzuki T, Nakaya M, et al. Structure–activity relation among macrolide antibiotics in initiation of interdigestive migrating contractions in the canine gastrointestinal tract. Am J Physiol. 1985;11:G320–5.
64. Inman WHW, Rawson NSB. Erythromycin estolate and jaundice. Br Med J. 1983;286:1954–5.
65. Braun P. Hepatotoxicity of erythromycin. J Infect Dis. 1969;119:300–6.
66. Tolman KG, Sannella JJ, Freston JW. Chemical structure of erythromycin and hepatotoxicity. Ann Intern Med. 1974;81:58–60.
67. Pessayre D, Larrey D, Funck-Brentano C, et al. Drug interactions and hepatitis produced by some macrolide antibiotics. J Antimicrob Chemother. 1985;16(Suppl A):181–94.
68. McCormack WM, George H, Donner A, et al. Hepatotoxicity of erythromycin estolate during pregnancy. Antimicrob Agents Chemother. 1977;12:630–5.
69. Sabath LD, Gerstein DA, Finland M. Serum glutamic oxalacetic transaminase: False elevation during administration of erythromycin. N Engl J Med. 1968;279:1137–9.
70. Sullivan D, Csuka ME, Blanchard B. Erythromycin ethylsuccinate hepatotoxicity. JAMA. 1980;243:1074.
71. Auckenthaler RW, Zwahlen A, Waldvogel FA. Macrolides. In: Peterson, PK, Verhoef J, eds. The Antimicrobial Agents Annual. v. 2. Amsterdam: Elsevier; 1987:120.
72. Karmody CS, Weinstein L. Reversible sensorineural hearing loss with intravenous erythromycin lactobionate. Ann Oral Rhinol Laryngol. 1977;86:9–11.
73. Eckman MR, Johnson T, Riess R. Partial deafness after erythromycin (Letter). N Engl J Med. 1975;292:649.
74. Mery JP, Kanfer A. Ototoxicity of erythromycin in patients with renal insufficiency (Letter). N Engl J Med. 1979;301:944.
75. Taylor R, Schofield IS, Ramos JM, et al. Ototoxicity of erythromycin in peritoneal dialysis patients (Letter). Lancet. 1981;2:935–6.
76. Haydon RC, Thaelin JW, Davis WE. Erythromycin ototoxicity: Analysis and conclusions based on 22 case reports. Otolaryngol Head Neck Surg. 1984;92:678–84.
77. Filippo JA. Infantile hypertrophic pyloric stenosis related to ingestions of erythromycin estolate: A report of five cases. J Pediatr Surg. 1976;11:177–80.
78. Gantz NM, Zawacki JK, Dickerson J, et al. Pseudomembranous colitis associated with erythromycin. Ann Intern Med. 1979;91:866–7.
79. Bartlett JG. Antimicrobial agents implicated in *Clostridium difficile* toxin-associated diarrhea or colitis. Johns Hopkins Med J. 1981;149:6–9.
80. Ludden TM. Pharmacokinetic interactions of the macrolide antibiotics. Clin Pharmacokinet. 1985;10:63–79.
81. Reisz G, Pingleton SK, Melethil S, et al. The effect of erythromycin on theophylline pharmacokinetics in chronic bronchitis. Ann Rev Respir Dis. 1983;127:581–4.
82. Bachmann K, Schwartz JI, Forney R Jr, et al. The effect of erythromycin on the desposition kinetics of warfarin. Pharmacology. 1984;28:171–6.
83. LaForce CF, Szefler SJ, Miller ME, et al. Inhibition of methylprednisolone elimination in the presence of erythromycin therapy. J Allergy Clin Immunol. 1983;72:34–9.
84. Wong YY, Lundden TD, Bell RD. Effect of erythromycin on carbamazepine kinetics. Clin Pharmacol Ther. 1983;33:460–4.
85. Martell R, Heinrichs D, Stiller CR, et al. The effects of erythromycin in patients treated with cyclosporine. Ann Intern Med. 1986;104:660–1.
86. Handbook of Antimicrobial Therapy. The Medical Letter on Drugs and Therapeutics. New Rochelle, NY: Medical Letter; 1988.
87. Rasch JR, Mogabgab WJ. Therapeutic effect of erythromycin on *Mycoplasma pneumoniae* pneumonia. Antimicrob Agents Chemother. 1965;5:693–9.
88. Kirby BD, Synder KM, Myer RD, et al. Legionnaires' disease: Report of sixty-five nosocomially acquired cases and review of the literature. Medicine. 1980;59:188–205.
89. Muder RF, Yu VL, Zuravleff MS. Pneumonia due to the Pittsburgh pneumonia agent: New clinical perspective with a review of the literature. Medicine. 1983;62:120–8.
90. Anders BJ, Lauer BA, Paisley JW, et al. Double-blind placebo controlled trial of erythromycin for treatment of *Campylobacter* enteritis. Lancet. 1982;1:131–2.
91. Salazar-Lindo E, Sack B, Chea-Woo E, et al. Early treatment with erythromycin of *Campylobacter jejuni*-associated dysentery in children. J Pediatr. 1986;109:355–60.
92. Taylor DN, Blaser MJ, Escheverria P. Erythromycin-resistant *Campylobacter* infections in Thailand. Antimicrob Agents Chemother. 1987;31:438–42.
93. Beem MD, Saxon E, Tipple MA. Treatment of chlamydial pneumonia of infancy. Pediatrics. 1979;63:198–203.
94. Clarke JS, Condon RE, Fenton LJ, et al. Preoperative oral antibiotics reduce septic complications of colon operations: Results of prospective randomized, double-blind clinical study. Ann Surg. 1977;186:251–9.
95. Fenton LJ, Light IJ. Congenital syphilis after maternal treatment with erythromycin. Obstet Gynecol. 1976;47:492–4.
96. Zinner SK, Sabath LD, Casey JI, et al. Erythromycin and alkalinization of the urine in treatment of urinary tract infections due to gram-negative bacilli. Lancet. 1971;1:1267–8.
97. Steigbigel RT, Greenman RL, Remington JS. Antibiotic combinations in the treatment of experimental *Staphylococcus aureus* infection. J Infect Dis. 1975;131:245–51.
98. Soave R. Cryptosporidiosis and isosporiasis in patients with AIDS. Infectious Dis Clin North Am. 1988;2:485–92.
99. Chang HR, Pechere J-C. In vitro effects of four macrolides (roxithromycin, spiramycin, azithromycin [CP-62,993], and A-56268) on *Toxoplasma gondii*. Antimicrob Agents Chemother. 1988;32:524–9.
100. Barry AL, Jones RN, Thornsberry C. In vitro activities of azithromycin (CP 62,993), clarithromycin (A-56268; TE-031), erythromycin, roxithromycin, and clindamycin. Antimicrob Agents Chemother. 1988;32:752–4.
101. Puri SK, Lassman HB. Roxithromycin: A pharmacokinetic review of a macrolide. J Antimicrob Chemother. 1987;20(Suppl B):89–100.
102. Retsema J, Girard A, Schelkly W, et al. Spectrum and mode of action of azithromycin (CP62,993), a new 15-membered ring macrolide with improved potency against gram-negative organisms. Antimicrob Agents Chemother. 1987;31:1939–47.
103. Araujo FG, Guptill DR, Remington JS. Azithromycin, a macrolide with potent activity against *Toxoplasma gondii*. Antimicrob Agents Chemother. 1988;32:755–7.
104. Girard AE, Girard D, English AR, et al. Pharmacokinetic and in vivo studies with azithromycin (CP 62,993), a new macrolide with an extended half-life

and excellent tissue distribution. Antimicrob Agents Chemother. 1987;31:1948–54.
105. McGehee RF Jr, Smith CB, Wilcox C, et al. Comparative studies of antibacterial activity in vitro and absorption and excretion of lincomycin and clindamycin. Am J Med Sci. 1968;256:279–92.
106. Cuchural GJ Jr, Tally FP, Jacobus NV, et al. Susceptibility of the *Bacteroides fragilis* group in the United States: Analysis by site of isolation. Antimicrob Agents Chemother. 1988;32:717–22.
107. Sutter VL: In vitro susceptibility of anaerobes: Comparison of clindamycin and other antimicrobial agents. J Infect Dis. 1977;135(Suppl):S7–12.
108. Bartlett JG. Anti-anaerobic antibacterial agents. Lancet. 1982;2:478–81.
109. McGehee RF, Barrett FF, Finland M. Resistance of *Staphylococcus aureus* to lincomycin, clindamycin and erythromycin. Antimicrob Agents Chemother. 1969;1968:392–7.
110. Nunnery AW, Riley HD. Clinical and laboratory studies of lincomycin in children. Antimicrob Agents Chemother–1964;1965:142–6.
111. Barrett FF, McGehee RF Jr, Finland M. Methicillin resistance *Staphylococcus aureus* at Boston City Hospital. N Engl J Med. 1968;279:441–8.
112. Desmyter J, Reybrouck G. Lincomycin sensitivity of erythromycin-resistant staphylococci. Chemotherapia. 1964;9:183–9.
113. Duncan IBR. Development of lincomycin resistance by staphylococci. Antimicrob Agents Chemother–1967. 1968:723–9.
114. Watanakunakorn C. Clindamycin therapy of *Staphylococcus aureus* endocarditis. Clinical relapse and development of resistance to clindamycin, lincomycin and erythromycin. Am J Med. 1976;60:419–25.
115. Sande MA, Johnson ML. Antimicrobial therapy of experimental endocarditis caused by *Staphylococcus aureus*. J Infect Dis. 1975;131:367–75.
116. Nastro LJ, Finegold SM. Bactericidal activity of five antimicrobial agents against *Bacteroides fragilis*. J Infect Dis. 1972;126:104–7.
117. Leclercq R, Brisson-Noel A, Duval J, et al. Phenotypic expression and genetic heterogeneity of lincosamide inactivation in *Staphylococcus* spp. Antimicrob Agents Chemother. 1987;31:1887–91.
118. DeHaan RM, Metzler CM, Schellenberg D, et al. Pharmacokinetic studies of clindamycin phosphate. J Clin Pharmacol. 1973;13:190–209.
119. Fass RJ, Salow S. Clindamycin: Clinical and laboratory evaluations of parenteral therapy. Am J Med Sci. 1972;263:369–82.
120. Townsend RJ, Baker RP. Pharmacokinetic comparison of three clindamycin phosphate dosing schedules. Drug Intell Clin Pharmacol. 1987;21:279–81.
121. Panzer JD, Brown DC, Epstein WL, et al. Clindamycin levels in various body tissues and fluids. J Clin Pharmacol. 1972;12:259–62.
122. Nicholas P, Meyers BR, Levy RN. Concentrations of clindamycin in human bone. Antimicrob Agents Chemother. 1975;8:220–1.
123. Prokesch RC, Hand WL. Antibiotic entry into human polymorphonuclear leukocytes. Antimicrob Agents Chemother. 1982;23:373–80.
124. Joiner KA, Lowe BR, Dzink JL, et al. Antibiotic levels in infected and sterile subcutaneous abscesses in mice. J Infect Dis. 1981;143(3):487–94.
125. McCall CE, Steigbigel NH, Finland M. Lincomycin: Activity in vitro and absorption and excretion in normal young men. Am J Med Sci. 1967;254:144–55.
126. Kager L, Liljeqvist L, Malmborg AS, et al. Effect of clindamycin prophylaxis on the colonic microflora in patients undergoing colorectal surgery. Antimicrob Agents Chemother. 1981;20:736–40.
127. Brown RB, Martyak SN, Barza M, et al. Penetration of clindamycin phosphate into the abnormal human biliary tract. Ann Intern Med. 1976;84:168–70.
128. Joshi A, Stein R. Altered serum clearance of intravenously administered clindamycin phosphate in patients with uremia. J Clin Pharmacol. 1974;14:140–4.
129. Williams DN, Crossley K, Hoffman C, et al. Parenteral clindamycin phosphate: Pharmacology with normal and abnormal liver function and effect on nasal staphylococci. Antimicrob Agents Chemother. 1975;7:153–8.
130. Rifkin GD, Fekety FR, Silva J Jr, et al. Antibiotic-induced colitis: Implication of a toxin neutralized by *Clostridium sordellii* antitoxin. Lancet. 1977;11:1103–6.
131. Bartlett JG, Chang TW, Gurwith M, et al. Antibiotic-associated pseudomembranous colitis due to toxin-producing clostridia. N Engl J Med. 1978;298:531–4.
132. Bartlett JG. Antibiotic-associated pseudomembranous colitis. Rev Infect Dis. 1979;1:530–9.
133. Tedesco FJ. Clindamycin and colitis: A review. J Infect Dis. 1977; 135(Suppl):S95–8.
134. George WL, Rolfe RD, Finegold SM. Treatment and prevention of antimicrobial agent-induced colitis and diarrhea. Gastroenterology. 1980;79:366–72.
135. Bartlett JG. Treatment of *Clostridium difficile* colitis. Gastroenterology. 1985;89:1192–5.
136. Elmore M, Rissing JP, Rink L, et al. Clindamycin-associated hepatotoxicity. Am J Med. 1974;57:627–30.
137. Fogdall RP, Miller RD. Prolongation of a pancuronium-induced neuromuscular blockade by clindamycin. Anesthesiology. 1974;41:407–8.
138. Thadepalli H, Gorbach SL, Broido PW, et al. Abdominal trauma, anaerobes, and antibiotics. Surg Gynecol Obstet. 1973;137:270–6.
139. Weinstein WM, Onderdonk AB, Bartlett JG, et al. Antimicrobial therapy of experimental intra-abdominal sepsis. J Infect Dis. 1975;132:282–6.
140. diZerega G, Yonekura L, Roy S, et al. A comparison of clindamycin–gentamicin and penicillin–gentamicin in the treatment of post-cesarean section endometritis. Am J Obstet Gynecol. 1979;134:238–42.
141. Solomkin JS, Fant WK, Rivera JD, et al. Randomized trial of imipenem/cilastatin versus gentamicin and clindamycin in mixed flora infections. Am J Med. 1985;78:85–91.
142. Bartlett JG, Gorbach SL. Treatment of aspiration pneumonia and primary lung abscess: penicillin G vs. clindamycin. JAMA. 1975;234:935–7.
143. Levison ME, Mangura CT, Lorber B, et al. Clindamycin compared with penicillin for the treatment of anaerobic lung abscess. Ann Intern Med. 1983;98:466–71.
144. Bartlett JG, Gorbach SL. Penicillin or clindamycin for primary lung abscess? (Editorial). Ann Intern Med. 1983;98:546–8.
145. Leyden JJ, Shalita AR, Saatjian GD, et al. Erythromycin 2% gel in comparison with clindamycin phosphate 1% solution in acne vulgaris. Am J Am Acad Dermatol. 1987;16:822–7.
146. Parry MF, Rha CK. Pseudomembranous colitis caused by topical clindamycin phosphate. Arch Dermatol. 1986;122:583–4.
147. Hofflin JM, Remington JS. Clindamycin in a murine model of toxoplasmic encephalitis. Antimicrob Agents Chemother. 1987;31:492–6.
148. Israelski DM, Remington JS. Toxoplasmic encephalitis in patients with AIDS. Infect Dis Clin North Am. 1988;2:429–45.
149. el Wakeel ES, Homeida MM, Ali HM, et al. Clindamycin in the treatment of falciparum malaria in Sudan. Am J Trop Med Hyg. 1985;34:1065–8.
150. Wittner M, Rowin KS, Tanowitz HB, et al. Successful chemotherapy of transfusion babesiosis. Ann Intern Med. 1982;96:601–4.
151. Brook I, Hirokawa R. Treatment of patients with a history of recurrent tonsillitis due to group A beta-hemolytic streptococci. A prospective randomized study comparing penicillin, erythromycin and clindamycin. Clin Pediatr. 1985;24:331–6.
152. Hermans P. Lincosamides. In Peterson PK, Verhoef J, eds. The Antimicrobial Agents Annual. v. 2. Amsterdam: Elsevier; 1987:114.

27. VANCOMYCIN AND TEICOPLANIN

ROBERT FEKETY

VANCOMYCIN

Structure

Vancomycin is a complex soluble glycopolypeptide that has a molecular weight of approximately 1450 daltons. While similar to two new glycopeptide antimicrobials, teichomycin and daptomycin (LY 146032), it is unrelated to all other antibiotics. When vancomycin was first introduced, commercial preparations contained as much as 30 percent of another substance of unknown nature that probably contributed to its side effects.[1,2] Current preparations are more pure and appear to be less toxic than the early preparations were.

Derivation and Nomenclature

Vancomycin (Vancocin from Lilly and Vancoled from Lederle) is a narrow-spectrum bactericidal antibiotic obtained from *Streptomyces orientales*. Introduced in 1956 because of its effectiveness against penicillin-resistant staphylococci, it was relegated because of its toxicity to the role of alternate therapy when methicillin became available. With spread of methicillin-resistant staphylococci in the United States in recent years, vancomycin underwent a marked increase in frequency of use and popularity, and it is now the drug of choice for treating infections with this organism. It is also the drug of choice for oral treatment of patients with severe antibiotic-associated colitis caused by *Clostridium difficile*.

Mechanism of Action

Vancomycin inhibits synthesis and assembly of the second stage of cell wall peptidoglycan polymers by complexing with the D-alanyl-D-alanine precursor. In addition, it injures protoplasts by altering the permeability of their cytoplasmic membrane and also impairs RNA synthesis. The multiple mechanisms of its action may contribute to the observed low frequency of the development of resistance. Rapidly and tightly bound to organisms, vancomycin exerts a bactericidal effect without a lag period, but only on multiplying organisms.

Antimicrobial Activity

Both *Staphylococcus aureus* and *Staphylococcus epidermidis* are susceptible to vancomycin. Marked resistance has not been observed. Concentrations of 1–5 μg/ml or less are almost invariably inhibitory, even with isolates resistant to methicillin, and most organisms are killed at about the same concentrations. A small proportion of strains require 10–20 μg/ml for inhibition, and about 20 percent of organisms are deficient in autolysins and relatively tolerant to the bactericidal action of vancomycin.[3,4] Slime biofilms on plastic foreign bodies also may be responsible for the persistence of staphylococci, particularly *S. epidermidis,* and treatment failures.[5] Recently, a coagulase-negative staphylococcus, speciated as *Staphylococcus haemolyticus,* was shown to be relatively resistant to vancomycin (minimum inhibitory and bactericidal concentrations [MIC, MBC] increased fourfold to 8 and 12 μg/ml, and the MBC with heavy inocula was as high as 32 μg/ml) and associated with the failure of treatment until a foreign body was removed. These organisms were also resistant to teicoplanin but were killed at low concentrations of daptomycin.[6] *Streptococcus pygoenes,* group B streptococci, corynebacteria JK, *Streptococcus pneumoniae,* and *Clostridium difficile* are highly susceptible. *Listeria monocytogenes* is usually susceptible. Anaerobic or microaerophilic streptococci, clostridia including *Clostridium perfringens, Bacillus anthracis, Actinomyces,* lactobacilli, diphtheroids, *C. diphtheriae,* corynebacteria CDC-D2, and *Neisseria gonorrheae* are usually susceptible.[7,8] Nutritionally variant streptococci may be killed by vancomycin alone.[9] Viridans streptococci, *Streptococcus agalactiae, Streptococcus bovis,* and *Enterococcus faecalis* (formerly *S. faecalis*) isolates are usually inhibited at concentrations attainable in serum, but few if any *Enterococcus* isolates are killed at concentrations less than 100 μg/ml.[4] A synergistic bactericidal effect is shown by 40–70 percent of *Enterococcus* isolates when vancomycin is combined with streptomycin, and the combinatin of vancomycin plus gentamicin is almost always bactericidal at attainable concentrations[10,11] unless so-called high-level gentamicin-resistant isolates are implicated.[12] Recently, vancomycin-resistant isolates of *Enterococcus faecalis, Enterococcus faecium,*[13] *Enterococcus gallinarum,*[14] and *Leukonostoc* species (which may be misidentified as streptococci)[15] have been detected. The mechanism of resistance is unknown. There is no cross-resistance between vancomycin and other unrelated antibiotics, and significant resistance rarely if ever develops during therapy. Cross-resistance with teicoplanin or daptomycin occurs but is variable. Antibacterial activity varies little between pH 6.5 and 8. Some *Neisseria gonorrhoeae* isolates are susceptible enough to be missed on cultures when vancomycin-containing selective media (Thayer-Martin) are used. *Flavobacterium meningosepticum* is susceptible at attainable concentrations (between 16 and 25 μg/ml), but other gram-negative bacilli, mycobacteria, fungi, and *Bacteroides* are not susceptible.

Pharmacology

Administration. After being dissolved in sterile water, vancomycin should be given intravenously in 100–250 ml of 5% dextrose or 0.9% NaCl over a period of at least 30–60 minutes.[1] It can also be given by continuous intravenous drip, but intermittent infusion is preferred. Rapid or bolus administration is dangerous, especially if 1 g doses are used, because it causes histamine release by basophiles and mast cells,[16] which can cause flushing (the "red-neck syndrome"), anaphylactoid reactions and even cardiac arrest.[9] Antihistamines may help prevent this. Hydrocortisone (20 mg) can be added to the infusion to reduce side effects, but this mixture may precipitate at high concentrations. Heparin and vancomycin also can precipitate at high concentrations, so they should not be infused simultaneously through the same intravenous line.[17] Because of pain on injection, no satisfactory intramuscular preparation is available. Vancomycin is absorbed poorly from the gastrointestinal tract, even when the colon is inflamed, and it is used orally for the treatment of enterocolitis[1,18–20] and for the prevention of infection in cancer patients.[21]

Distribution, Excretion, and Protein Binding. Vancomycin is eliminated from the body almost exclusively by glomerular filtration. Within 24 hours 80–90 percent of an administered dose appears in the urine. A small amount may be eliminated via the liver and biliary tract. The half-life of vancomycin in serum is 6–8 hours in persons with normal renal function. In anuria, it may be prolonged to about 9 days, and it may be detected in serum for as long as 21 days after a single 1 g dose.[22,23] From 10 to 55 percent is protein bound in serum; this is believed to have a negligible effect on clinical results.

Concentrations in Body Fluids and Tissue. Serum levels 1–2 hours after the intravenous administration of a 500 mg dose to adults range from 6 to 10 μg/ml, with an average of 8 μg/ml after repeated dosing. Peak levels of up to 50 μg/ml may be seen. When 1 g is given slowly intravenously, peak and trough levels of 20–50 μg/ml and 5–10 μg/ml, respectively, can be achieved; these are considered desirable and appropriate concentrations. Urinary concentrations range from 100 to 300 μg/ml. When vancomycin (0.5 g q6h) is given orally, levels of 1000–9000 μg/ml are found in stool, but only trace amounts are ordinarily found in serum[7,8,19]; levels as high as therapeutic levels have been found occasionally in the serum of anuric patients given the drug orally to treat colitis.[24] When 125 mg is given orally, stool concentrations have ranged from 100 to 800 μg/ml. When vancomycin is given intravenously, levels of up to 100 μg/ml may be found in stools of some patients, but the drug is undetectable in the stools of most patients.[8] Vancomycin is not found in the cerebrospinal fluid (CSF) of persons without meningitis, but bactericidal levels have been found in the CSF of most but not all patients with meningitis (<1–7 μg/ml). Small supplemental amounts (3–5 mg) may be given intrathecally in meningitis if there is no response after 48 hours of intravenous therapy.[25] A larger intrathecal dose may be needed for less susceptible organisms such as flavobacteria. Vancomycin is irritating when injected into serous or synovial cavities, and peritonitis has been reported after direct instillation.[26] Adequate concentrations are reached in pleural, pericardial, synovial, and ascitic fluids after intravenous administration, and low levels are found in bile.[7]

Since the kidney is the only significant organ of elimination of vancomycin, high and potentially toxic serum levels can be attained in patients with renal insufficiency unless the dosage is reduced appropriately.[21,23,27] It is recommended that a loading dose of 15 mg/kg may be given to all adults, regardless of renal function. To achieve a mean therapeutic concentration of 20 μg/ml in the serum of adults with renal impairment, a simple formula can be used to estimate maintenance dosage: the daily parenteral dose of vancomycin in milligrams is 150 plus 15 times the creatinine clearance in milliliters per minute.[27] Another strategy is to give 1 g every 36 hours when the serum creatinine concentration is 1.5–5 mg/100 ml and 1 g every 10–14 days when it is greater than 5 mg/100 ml. As little as 1 g may yield effective serum concentrations for 7–14 days in anuric patients.[23] There is a nomogram[28] that may be more accurate than the aforementioned simple rules for dosing patients with renal failure. In difficult situations, serum concentrations should be monitored whichever method is used to estimate the dosage. It is designed to provide steady-state concentrations of 15 μg/ml[28] and is probably the most accurate dosing method.[29] Hemodialysis does not remove significant amounts of vancomycin, but peritoneal dialysis can.[21,23,26] Hemofiltration may be very efficient at removing it and useful in managing overdosage in patients with renal failure.[30] Serum levels should be monitored at frequent, regular intervals in dialyzed, uremic, or seriously ill patients to ascertain that safe, yet adequate concentrations are present. Cardiopulmonary bypass is associated with a fall in serum levels because of dilution.[31] A preoperative dose of 15 mg/kg is needed before bypass surgery, and 10 mg/kg should be given after bypass surgery if renal function is normal. Pediatric dosing is discussed in the later section on major uses and doses.

Toxicity and Adverse Reactions

With the purified preparations now available, adverse reactions seem to be much less frequent than when vancomycin was first introduced. The most frequent side effects consist of fever, chills, and phlebitis at the site of the infusion. These are less frequent if the drug is infused slowly in a large volume of fluid. Tingling and flushing of the face, neck, and thorax (the "red-neck syndrome") are frequently experienced, especially if 1 g doses are given [32] and if the drug is infused very rapidly[33]; this is related to histamine release, not to allergic hypersensitivity. Shock has occurred after rapid intravenous infusion of the drug, especially during surgery. Reversible leukopenia or eosinophilia sometimes develop.[34] Maculopapular or diffuse erythomatous rashes, presumably on a hypersensitivity basis, occur in 4–5 percent of patients and may persist for weeks despite discontinuation of vancomycin treatment in patients with marked renal failure. They may respond to steroid or antihistamine therapy. Lacrimation has been reported.[16] One case of antibiotic-induced *C. difficile* colitis has been reported after the intravenous use of vancomycin.[35]

An important adverse reaction to vancomycin is neurotoxicity, which is manifested by auditory nerve damage and hearing loss. This is infrequent if serum concentrations are maintained below 30 μg/ml and is more common with concentrations of 80 μg/ml or more. Tinnitus and high-tone hearing loss are frequently an antecendent to deafness. Hearing occasionally improves when treatment with the drug is discontinued but usually continues to deteriorate and is permanent.[36,37] Nephrotoxicity was relatively common with early impure preparations of vancomycin, especially when given in high doses; it is usually transient or reversible. With appropriate doses selected by monitoring renal function and serum concentrations, nephrotoxicity is now uncommon.[37–39] Though vancomycin is no longer appreciably nephrotoxic, high doses given by the parenteral route should be avoided, and serum levels should be carefully monitored when other nephrotoxic drugs are being given. The risk of nephrotoxicity appears to be enhanced even with safe levels when drugs such as aminoglycosides or ethacrynic acid are given concomitantly.

Drug Interactions

Vancomycin is incompatible with many drugs in intravenous solutions, especially chloramphenicol, adrenal corticosteroids, and methicillin. Heparin (at very high concentrations) may inactivate vancomycin in intravenous solutions and be responsible for persistent bacteremia.[17] Vancomycin is not stable enough for use with certain implantable pumps.[40]

Major Uses and Doses

The usual intravenous dose of vancomycin for adults with normal renal function is 1 g every 12 hours (15 mg/kg) or 500 mg (6.5–8 mg/kg) every 6 hours. In severely ill patients with normal renal function such as those with meningitis, 1 g may be given every 8 hours for 2 or 3 days until the infection is under control. Morbidly obese patients with severe infections may require high doses, which should be based upon total body weight, creatinine clearance, and monitoring serum levels.[41] Various dosage regimens have been proposed for pediatric usage. For newborn infants, 15 mg/kg should be given slowly intravenously every 12 hours during the first week of life or every 8 hours in those 8–30 days of age; 10 mg/kg every 6 hours is recommended for older infants and children and 15 mg/kg every 6 hours for infants and children with staphylococcal central nervous system infections. Monitoring serum levels is desirable, especially in preterm infants.[42] A continuous drip can be used.[43,44] An oral dose of 125–500 mg four times per day has been used to treat adults with *Clostridium difficile* colitis (R. Fekety, J. Silva, C. Kauffman, et al., unpublished observations). In infants and children with *Clostridium difficile* colitis, an oral dose of 500 mg/1.73 m^2 every 6 hours has been recommended.[45] Oral therapy is much more reliable than intravenous therapy is for the treatment of *Clostridium difficile* colitis.

The intravenous dosage must be reduced in patients with renal impairment and monitored to achieve peak serum concentrations no higher than 30–40 μg/ml and troughs ranging from 5 to 10 μg/ml; if a continuous infusion is used, a steady-state concentration of 15 μg/ml seems desirable.[25,26,35,46] Recent evidence indicates that impaired liver function may also delay the elimination of vancomycin and require a dosage modification.[47]

Vancomycin should be used primarily for serious infections. Intravenous vancomycin is the therapy of choice for serious staphylococcal infections in patients with methicillin-, oxacillin-, nafcillin-, or cephalothin-resistant organisms or in patients who cannot be given these primary drugs.[7,38,48–52]

All strains of methicillin-resistant staphylococci have been susceptible to low concentrations of vancomycin, but rare isolates show clinically significant tolerance to its bactericidal action.[4,48,51,53] When treatment of serious infections with vancomycin given alone has failed, the addition of gentamicin, rifampin, or trimethoprim-sulfamethoxazole may be tried. Since antagonism may occur rarely with some of these combinations of antimicrobials,[48] these combinations should not be routine, and serum bacteriostatic and bactericidal levels ideally should be monitored as a guide to therapy when they are used. When vancomycin is used for adults in conjunction with an aminoglycoside, its dosage should rarely exceed 0.5 g every 8 hours.[38] However, methicillin-resistant *S. epidermidis* endocarditis involving a prosthetic valve is best treated with the usual doses of vancomycin for 4 weeks in combination with rifampin plus the addition of an aminoglycoside for the first 2 weeks only.[52]

Vancomycin has a very rapid and potent bactericidal effect, and were it not for its potential toxicity, it might be the preferred drug for treating all serious staphylococcal infections. Survival rates of 60–75 percent have been achieved with vancomycin in patients with staphylococcal endocarditis or bacteremia.[1,7] Survival in patients aged 70 years or older is about 50 percent. The usual duration of therapy is 4–6 weeks. Success rates of 75 percent or greater have been reported in patients with pneumonia, parotitis, or meningitis.

While vancomycin penetrates into the central nervous system in most ill patients in amounts adequate to treat meningitis and shunt infections, this is not always the case,[25] and removal of foreign bodies or supplemental intraventricular or intrathecal instillation of vancomycin may be required in patients with a poor response.[53–55] Cerebrospinal fluid concentrations need not be greater than about 25 μg/ml, so intrathecal doses of 3 mg are usually adequate.

Vancomycin is the treatment of choice in patients with *E. faecalis* (enterococcal) endocarditis who are allergic to penicillin. In this setting it is best given along with an aminoglycoside since vancomycin alone is not dependably bactericidal against these streptotocci.[10,11,56,57] Since bactericidal synergism between gentamicin and vancomycin has been demonstrated with most enterococci (until recently),[12,58] gentamicin is preferable to streptomycin, which is not synergistic with as many as 40 percent of these organisms. Laboratory studies of synergism with the patient's organism or Schlicter tests on their serum may be helpful in determining the best regimen during the course of treatment. A vancomycin dose of 0.5 g every 8 hours iv plus streptomycin, 0.5 g every 12 hours im, or gentamicin, 60–80 mg (1 mg/kg) every 8 hours iv for 1 month, is recommended for adults with normal renal function. More vigorous or prolonged therapy may be needed for complicated cases, as when a prosthetic valve is infected. Patients should be monitored closely for signs of ototoxicity or nephrotoxicity, and drug dosages should be carefully adjusted in renal failure. Viridans streptococcal or *S. bovis* endocarditis may be treated with vancomycin alone if the MBC for the isolate is no more than 10 μg/ml; otherwise it should be combined with streptomycin or another aminoglycoside.[7,38]

Other serious infections with resistant organisms that have been responsive to vancomycin include *Corynebacterium* endocarditis in patients with prosthetic valves and *Flavobacterium meningosepticum* meningitis.[7,25,54]

Vancomycin has been considered the drug of choice for treating acute staphylococcal pseudomembranous enterocolitis, which is now a rare disease. In two series of cases, 67 of 72 patients were cured (93 percent).[18,59] It was usually given orally, 500 mg diluted in water every 6 hours for adults.

Although metronidazole is less expensive and also effective,[61] orally administered vancomycin is considered the drug of choice by most investigators for treating *seriously* ill patients with antibiotic-associated *Clostridium difficile* (pseudomembranous) colitis. This organism is always susceptible to vancomycin, and treatment failures are very rare unless treatment is delayed.[18,19,62,63] Dosages of either 125 or 500 mg four times daily have been effective and the lower and less expensive dose seems as good as the larger one.[63a] Vancomycin is very useful in treating relapses of colitis cause by *C. difficile*.[62] Preferably, vancomycin should be given orally to treat colitis since the drug is needed to inhibit toxin production in the lumen of the bowel and not for inhibition of the organism in tissues.[62] Intravenous vancomycin is not as reliable since adequate concentrations may not be achieved within the lumen when it is given in this way. In patients with ileus, vancomycin should be given orally or by nasogastric tube in 500 mg doses every 6 hours, and both vancomycin (in full parenteral doses) plus metronidazole should be given intravenously. Even though little vancomycin will be absorbed from the intestinal tract, serum levels should be monitored to prevent toxicity when it is used by both routes. When nasogastric tubes are needed for administering vancomycin, they can be clamped for 30–60 minutes after administration. When patients have ileus, the drug has been given by enema or via an ileostomy or colostomy.

Staphylococcal peritonitis occurring during peritoneal dialysis can be treated with intravenous vancomycin alone. The administration of 1 g intravenously will yield peritoneal fluid concentrations greater than 5 μg/ml for a week or more in this setting.[26,42] Others have noted that peritoneal dialysis may remove vancomycin from the blood and have recommended instilling vancomycin into the peritoneal cavity at a concentration of 25 μg/ml in addition to parenteral vancomycin to ensure good levels in peritoneal fluid.[63] In fact, it may be possible to treat staphylococcal peritonitis in chronic peritoneal dialysis patients solely by the intraperitoneal administration of vancomycin at a concentration of 50 μg/ml in the dialysate.[63,64] However, vancomycin given intraperitoneally with some preparations can be irritating[65]; furthermore, organisms protected by a biofilm on the catheter may be clinically tolerant and responsible for a relapse.[5] The addition of rifampin to vancomycin to treat refractory staphylococcal peritonitis in chronic dialysis can be curative.[66]

According to an American Heart Association Advisory Committee,[67,68] vancomycin is useful in the prevention of bacterial endocarditis in patients who are allergic to penicillin and undergoing dental or respiratory tract procedures.[67] The mechanism of prevention may be either by the bactericidal action of vancomycin or by interference with the ability of the organism to adhere to the endocardium. One gram is given slowly intravenously over a period of 60 minutes before the procedure; no repeat dose is necessary. For genitourinary or gastrointestinal surgery or instrumentation, vancomycin can be given as above plus gentamicin, 1.5 mg/kg; these may be repeated once 8–12 hours later.[67] Vancomycin can be used prophylactically for the placement of prosthetic valves, with an initial intravenous dose of 15 mg/ml given over a period of 1 hour just before surgery, followed by 10 mg/kg immediately after bypass surgery (if renal function is normal),[31] and 1.7 mg/kg gentamicin before surgery and 8 hours later. The efficacy of this regimen has not been proved, but it is designed to prevent *S. aureus, S. epidermidis,* and coliform infections of the prosthesis and sternum. Vancomycin is often included in empirical therapy for febrile neutropenic patients, but unless there is good evidence to suggest a staphylococcal infection, its use probably should not be routine.[69]

Vancomycin has been used in prophylactic oral nonabsorbable antibiotic regimens designed to prevent endogenous infections in patients with cancer or leukemia.[21] Such patients seem to experience a lower rate of *C. difficile* colitis complicating their chemotherapy. Otherwise, these regimens are probably of no value unless protective environments and leukocyte transfusions are available and used.

Vancomycin has been used prophylactically in order to prevent staphylococcal infections in patients receiving chronic dialysis, but this has resulted in the emergence of vancomycin-resistant enterococci and serious enterococcal infections.[14]

It is obvious that there has been a resurgence of the use of vancomycin in the last 2 decades. Many new indications for its use have been established, and much new information has been accumulated. An excellent review of newer knowledge about vancomycin has been published.[70]

TEICOPLANIN

Teicoplanin (formerly named teichomycin A) is a new glycopeptide antibiotic derived from the fermentation products of *Actinoplanes teichomyceticus*.[71] While it is widely used in Europe for the treatment of gram-positive infections, it is still investigational in the United States. Teicoplanin is a complex of six analogues having the same linear heptapeptide base and an aglycone containing aromatic amino acids with D-mannose and *N*-acetyl-D-glycosamine as sugars, with a molecular weight ranging from 1562 to 1891. Teicoplanin is chemically similar to vancomycin and ristocetin but with important differences responsible for the unique physical and chemical properties of the complex.[72] It has greater lipophilicity than vancomycin does, which results in excellent tissue penetration. Other consequences are a long elimination half-life, slow release from tissues, and water solubility at physiologic pH. It has few if any inactive metabolites.[73]

Mechanism of Action and Pharmacokinetics

Teicoplanin has an antibacterial spectrum and mechanism of action similar to that of vancomycin. It is bactericidal, although tolerance has been observed to its bactericidal action. The development of resistance during treatment has not been reported. It impairs cell wall synthesis by inhibiting polymerization of peptidoglycan, but at different sites from those inhibited by β-lactams.[74,75] It does this by forming a complex with the terminal D-alanyl-D-alanine precursor, which fits into a "pocket" in the teicoplanin molecule.[76] It has an elimination half-life of 40–70 hours after intravenous administration, a disappearance curve that fits both a two- and a three-compartment model, and a volume of distribution of 0.5–0.8 liter/kg.[77,78] Protein binding is as high as 90 percent,[76] which may account for its slow renal clearance. Because of its long half-life, it can be given intramuscularly or intravenously once per day.[79] It has usually been given in a daily intravenous dose of 2–3 mg/kg after a loading dose of 6 mg/kg (400 mg).[80] When single intravenous injections of 3 or 6 mg/kg were given rapidly (over a period of 5 minutes) to healthy volunteers, peak plasma concentrations of 53 and 112 μg/ml were observed, and concentrations of 2.1 and 4.2 μg/ml were observed at 24 hours. Similar concentrations were seen after intramuscular dosing with 3 mg/kg. When 3 mg/kg was administered to volunteers at a constant rate over a period of 30 minutes, peak concentrations were about 22 μg/ml. After six intramuscular doses of 200 mg (3 mg/kg) over a 5-day period, mean peak levels of 12.1 μg/ml were reached. Trough levels were 5.4–7.3 μg/ml,[78] and the calculated elimination half-life was about 99 hours. Urinary concentrations ranged from 16 to 156 μg/ml from day 1 through day 7. About 80 percent of the drug was eliminated in urine.[79] Teicoplanin was not significantly absorbed from the intestinal tracts of human volunteers.[73] In patients with renal impairment, serum concentrations are related to creatinine clearance, which can be used for adjusting the dosage.[80] Teicoplanin is well tolerated by children. A dose of 10 mg/kg/day has been recommended for children and 6 mg/kg/day for neonates.[81]

ANTIBACTERIAL ACTIVITY

Teicoplanin has excellent bactericidal activity against gram-positive organisms, including *S. pneumoniae, S. pyogenes,* other streptococci, *Enterococcus faecalis, S. aureus* (both penicillinase-producing and methicillin-resistant organisms), *S. epidermidis, Clostridium* species, corynebacteria JK, *Propionibacterium acnes,* and *Listeria monocytogenes.*[82–84] Inhibitory concentrations range from 0.025 to 3.1 μg/ml. Some strains of *S. epidermidis* and *S. haemolyticus* are relatively resistant to teicoplanin but susceptible to vancomycin.[85,86] Against many susceptible organisms, teicoplanin is two to four times as active as vancomycin. Teicoplanin was the most active antimicrobial agent against *E. faecalis,* but like vancomycin, it is rarely bactericidal for this species. Teicoplanin is more active than vancomycin is against *Clostridium difficile,* but it is even more highly bound by cholestyramine.[87] It is not active against gram-negative organisms, mycobacteria, or fungi. Teicoplanin does not give rise to stably resistant mutants in vitro, and it shows no cross-resistance with nonglycopeptide antibiotics. Like vancomycin, teicoplanin can be synergistic with rifampin or aminoglycosides against staphylococci, enterococci, other streptococci, and *Listeria.*[88–92]

Toxicity

Teicoplanin produces only mild pain at the site of injection. After slow intravenous infusion, it has not caused thrombophlebitis[93] or adverse effects on platelet function or coagulation.[94] Studies with 100 human volunteers showed no untoward effects at doses of up to 7.5 mg/kg. When used by rapid intravenous infusion in 310 hospitalized infected patients with infections, significant adverse effects were uncommon (2 percent), and no patient developed flushing or the "red-man syndrome."[95] However, ototoxicity has been reported.[95–97]

Clinical Uses

Teicoplanin is similiar to vancomycin, with the advantage of less frequent dosing and, because of its greater potency and therapeutic ratio, the potential for less nephrotoxicity and ototoxicity. It may be useful for patients who have had neutropenic or allergic reactions to vancomycin.[98]

Clinical cures were seen in 96 percent of 88 patients treated with 200–400 mg teicoplanin once daily for coagulase-negative staphylococcal infections[99,100] and in 79–91 percent of 1781 patients with various gram-positive infections.[97,99] These included methicillin-resistant *S. aureus* (MRSA) infections, pneumonia, endocarditis, septicemia, and joint infections. Some of these patients developed ototoxicity or nephrotoxicity, but many of them had also received an aminoglycoside.[97]

When patients with serious staphylococcal infections were treated with doses of 200 mg/day, only 44 percent were cured.[101] Treatment failure was related to the presence of foreign bodies and poor tissue concentrations. The high degree of protein binding of teicoplanin may have been an important factor in these low-doses treatment failures. Doses of 400 mg/day or more will probably be needed for the successful treatment of severe infections. When used once daily for prophylaxis in cardiac surgery, teicoplanin was associated with higher than expected numbers of sternal wound and urinary tract infections.[102] Other potential indications include shunt infections and treatment of gram-positive peritonitis in chronic dialysis patients.[103,104]

REFERENCES

1. Alexander MR. Review of vancomycin after 15 years of use. Drug Intell Clin Pharm. 1974;8:520.
2. Perkins HR, Nieto M. The chemical basis for the action of the vancomycin group of antibiotics. Ann NY Acad Sci. 1974;235:348.
3. Gopal V, Bisno AL, Silverblatt FJ. Failure of vancomycin treatment in *Staphylococcus aureus* endocarditis. In vivo and in vitro observations. JAMA. 1976;236:1604.
4. Sabath L, Wheeler N, Laverdiere M, et al: A new type of penicillin resistance in *Staphylococcus aureus.* Lancet 1977;1:443.
5. Evans RC, Holmes CJ. Effect of vancomycin hydrochloride on *staphylococcus epidermidis* biofilm associated with silicone elostomen. Antimicrob Agents Chemother. 1987;31:889–94.
6. Schwalke RS, Stapleton JT, Gilligan PH. Emergence of vancomycin resistance in coagulase-negative staphylococci. N Engl J Med. 1987;316:927–31.
7. Geraci JE. Vancomycin. Mayo Clin Proc 1977;52:631.
8. Geraci JE, Heilman FR, Nichols DR, et al. Some laboratory and clinical experiences with a new antibiotic, vancomycin. Proc Staff Meet Mayo Clin. 1956;31:564.
9. Reimer LG. Measurement of serum bactericidal activity and use of vancomycin for treatment of nutritionally variant streptococcal bacteremia. Diagn Microbiol Infect Dis. 1987;6:319–22.
10. Watanakunakorn C, Bakie C. Synergism of vancomycin-gentamicin and vancomycin-streptomycin against enterococci. Antimicrob Agents Chemother. 1973;4:120.
11. Harwick HJ, Kalmanson GM, Guze LB: In vitro activity of ampicillin or vancomycin combined with gentamicin or streptomycin against enterococci. Antimicrob Agents Chemother. 1973;4:383.
12. Mederski-Samoraj BD, Murray BE. High level resistance to enterococci in clinical isolates of staphylococci. J Infect Dis. 1983;147:751–7.
13. Uttley AC, Collins CH, Naidoo J, et al. Vancomycin-resistant enterococci. Lancet 1988;1:57–8.
14. Kaplan AH, Gilligan PH, Facklam RR. Recovery of resistant enterococci during vancomycin prophylaxis. J Clin Microbiol. 1988;26:1216–8.
15. Rubin LG, Velozzi E, Shapiro J, et al. Infection with vancomycin-resistant "streptococci", due to *Leuconostoc* species. J Infect Dis. 1988;157:216.
16. Polk RE, Healy DP, Schwartz LB, et al. Vancomycin and the red-man syndrome: Pharmacodynamics of histamine release. J Infect Dis. 1988;157:502–7.
17. Barg NL, Fekety R, Supena R: Persistant staphylococcal bacteremia in an intravenous drug abuser. Antimicrob Agents Chemother. 1986;29:209–11.
18. Khan MY, Hall WH: Staphylococcal enterocolitis-treatment with oral vancomycin. Ann Intern Med. 1966;65:1.
19. Tedesco F, Markham R, Gurwith M, et al. Oral vancomycin for antibiotic-associated pseudomembranous colitis. Lancet 1978;2:226–8.
20. Silva J, Batts DH, Fekety R, et al. Treatment of *Clostridium difficile* colitis and diarrhea with vancomycin. Am J Med. 1981;71:815–22.
21. Bodey G: Oral antibiotic prophylaxis in protected environment units: Effect of nonabsorbable and absorbable antibiotics on the fecal flora. Antimicrob Agents Chemother. 1972;1:343.
22. Lindholm DD, Murray JS. Persistance of vancomycin in the blood during renal failure and its treatment by hemodialysis. N Engl J Med. 1966;274:1047.
23. Eykyn S, Phillip I, Evans J: Vancomycin for staphylococcal shunt infections in patients on regular hemodialysis. Br Med J. 1970;3:80.
24. Spitzer PC, Eliopoulos GM. Systemic absorption of enteral vancomycin in a patient with pseudomembranous colitis. Ann Intern Med. 1984;100:533–4.
25. Hawley HB, Gump DW. Vancomycin therapy of bacterial meningitis. Am J Dis Child. 1973;126:261.
26. Ayus JC, Enkas JF, Tong TG, et al. Peritoneal clearance and total body elimination of vancomycin during chronic intermittent peritoneal dialysis. Clin Nephrol. 1979;11:129–32.
27. Nielsen HE, Hansen JE, Korsager B, et al. Renal excretion of vancomycin in kidney disease. Acta Med Scand. 1975;197:261.
28. Moellering RC, Krogstad DJ, Greenblatt DJ. Vancomycin therapy in patients with impaired renal function. A nomogram for dosage. Ann Intern Med. 1981;94:343–6.
29. Matzke G, Kovarik JM, Rybak MJ, et al. Evaluation of the vancomycin clearance: Creatinine-clearance relationship for predicting vancomycin dosage. Clinical Pharm 1985;4:311–5.
30. Matzke GR, O'Connell MB, Collins AJ, et al. Disposition of vancomycin during hemofiltration. Clin Pharmacol Ther. 1986;40:425–30.

31. Austin TW, Leake J, Coles JC, et al. Vancomycin blood levels during cardiac surgery. Card J Surg 1981;24:423–5.
32. Healy DP, Polk RE, Garson ML, et al. Comparison of steady-state pharmacokinetics of two dosage regimens of vancomycin in normal volunteers. Antimicrob Agents Chemother. 1987;31:393–7.
33. Newfield P, Roizen MF. Hazards of rapid administration of vancomycin. Ann Intern Med. 1979;91:581.
34. Mordenti J, Ries C, Brooks GF, et al. Vancomycin-induced neutropenia complicating bone marrow recovery in a patient with leukemia. Case report and a review of the literature. Am J Med. 1986;30:333–5.
35. Miller SN, Ringler RP. Vancomycin-induced pseudomembranous colitis. J Clin Gastroenterol. 1987;9:114–5.
36. Traber PG, Levine DP. Vancomycin ototoxicity in a patient with normal renal function. Ann Intern Med. 1981;95:458–60.
37. McHenry MC, Gavan TL. Vancomycin. Pediatr Clin North Am 1983;30:31–47.
38. Geraci JE, Hermans PE. Vancomycin. Mayo Clin Proc. 1983;58:88–91.
39. Appel GB, Neu HC. The nephrotoxicity of antimicrobial agents. N Engl J Med. 1977;296:722.
40. Greenberg RN, Saud AMK, Kennedy DJ, et al: Instability of vancomycin in Infusaid drug pump model 100. Antimicrob Agents Chemother. 1987;31:610–1.
41. Blovin RA, Bauer LA, Miller DD, et al. Vancomycin pharmacokinetics in normal and morbidity obese subjects. Antimicrob Agents Chemother. 1982;21:575–80.
42. Nagvi SH, Kennan WJ, Reichley RM, et al: Vancomycin pharmcokinetics in small, seriously ill infants. Am J Dis Child. 1986;140:107–10.
43. Riley HD. Vancomycin and novobiocin. Med Clin North Am 1970;54:1277.
44. Schaad CVB, McCracken GH, Nelson JD. Clinical pharmacology and efficacy of vancomycin in pediatric patients. J Pediatr. 1980;96:119–26.
45. Batts DH, Martin D, Holmes R, et al. Treatment of antibiotic-associated *Clostridium difficile* diarrhea with oral vancomycin. J Pediatr. 1980;97:151–53.
46. Rotschafer JC, Crossley K, Zaski DE, et al. Pharmacokinetics of vancomycin. Observations in 28 patients and dosage recommendations. Antimicrob Agents Chemother. 1982;22:391–94.
47. Brown N, Ho DHW, Fong KL, et al. Effects of hepatic function on vancomycin clinical pharmacology. Antimicrob Agents Chemother. 1983;23:603–9.
48. Watanakunakorn C. Treatment of infections due to methicillin-resistant *Staphylococcus aureus*. Ann Intern Med. 1982;97:376–8.
49. Myers JP, Linnemann CC. Bacteremia due to methicillin-resistant *Staphylococcus aureus*. J Infect Dis. 1982;4:532–6.
50. Sorrell TC, Packham DR, Shanker S, et al. Vancomycin therapy for methicillin-resistant *Staphylococcus aureus*. Ann Intern Med. 1982;97:344–50.
51. Levine DP, Cushing R, Jim J, et al. Community-acquired methicillin-resistant *Staphylococcus aureus* endocarditis in the Detroit Medical Center. Ann Intern Med. 1982;330–8.
52. Karchmer AW, Archer GL, Dismukes WE. *Staphylococcus epidermidis* causing prosthetic-valve endocarditis. Microbiologic and clinical observations as guides to therapy. Ann Intern Med. 1983;98:447–55.
53. Sutherlan GE, Palitang EG, Marr JJ, et al. Sterilization of Ommaya reservoir by instillation of vancomycin. Am J Med. 1981;71:1068–70.
54. Gump DW. Vancomycin for treatment of bacterial meningitis. Rev Infect Dis. 1981;3(Suppl):289–92.
55. Swayne RS, Rampling A, Newsom SWB. Intraventricular vancomycin for treatment of shunt-associated ventriculitis. J Antimicrob Chemother. 1987;19:249–53.
56. Westenfelder GO, Paterson PY, Reisberg BE, et al. Vancomycin–streptomycin synergism in enterococcal endocarditis. JAMA. 1973;223:37.
57. Harwick HJ, Kalmanson GM, Guze LB. Pyelonephritis. XVII. Comparison of combinations of vancomycin, ampicillin, streptomycin, and gentamicin in the treatment of enterococcal infection in the rat. J Infect Dis. 1974;129:358.
58. Zervos MJ, Kauffman CA, Therasse PM, et al. Nosocomial infection by gentamicin-resistant *Streptococcus faecalis*. Ann Intern Med. 1987;106:687–91.
59. Esposito AL, Gleckman RA: Vancomycin, a second look. JAMA. 1977;238:1756.
60. Teasley DG, Gerding DN, Olson MM, et al. Prospective randomised trial of metronidazole versus vancomycin for *Clostridium difficile*–associated diarrhea and colitis. Lancet 1983;2:1043–6.
61. Fekety R, Silva J, Armstrong J, et al. Treatment of antibiotic-associated enterocolitis with vancomycin. Rev Infect Dis. 1981;3(Suppl):273–81.
62. Tedesco FJ. Treatment of recurrent antibiotic-associated pseudomembranous colitis. Am J Gastroenterol. 1982;77:220–1.
63. Nielsen HE, Sorensen I, Hansen HE. Peritoneal transport of vancomycin during peritoneal dialysis. Nephron. 1979;24:274–7.
63a. Fekety R, Silva J, Kauffman C, et al. Treatment of antibiotic-associated *Clostridium difficile* colitis with oral vancomycin: Comparison of two dosage regimens. Am J Med. 1989;86:15–19.
64. Morse GD, Farolino DF, Apicella MA, et al. Comparative study of intraperitoneal and intravenous vancomycin pharmcokinetics during continuous ambulatory peritoneal dialysis. Antimicrob Agents Chemother. 1987;31:173–7.
65. Piraino B, Bernardini J, Johnston J, et al. Chemical peritonitis due to intraperitoneal vancomycin. Peritoneal Dialysis Bull. 1987;7(Suppl):59.
66. Buggy BP, Schaberg DR, Swartz RD. Intraleukocytic sequestration as a cause of persistent *Staphylococcus aureus* peritonitis in continuous ambulatory peritoneal dialysis. Am J Med. 1984;76:1035–40.
67. Kaye D. Prophylaxis for infective endocarditis: An update. Ann Intern Med. 1986;104:419–23.
68. Kaplan EL, Anthony BF, Bisno A, et al. Prevention of bacterial endocarditis (abstract). Circulation. 1977;56:139–43.
69. Rubin M, Hathorn JW, Marshall D, et al. Gram-positive infections and the use of vancomycin in 550 episodes of fever and neutropenia. Ann Intern Med. 1988;108:30–35.
70. Wise RI, Kory M, ed. Reassessments of vancomycin—a potentially useful antibiotic. Rev Infect Dis. 1981;3(Suppl):199–300.
71. Williams AH, Gruneberg RN. Teicoplanin. J Antimicrob Chemother. 1984;14:441–8.
72. Parenti F. Structure and mechanism of action of teicoplanin. J Hosp Infect. 1986;7(Suppl A):79–83.
73. Neville LD, Baillod R, Grady D, et al. Teicoplanin in patients with chronic renal failure on dialysis: Microbiological and pharmakokinetic aspects. Int J Clin Pharm Res. 1987;7:485–90.
74. Somma S, Gastaldo L. Mechanism of action of teichomycin A_2, a new antibiotic. In: Current Chemotherapy and Immunotherapy, Proceedings of the 12th International Congress of Chemotherapy, Florence, Italy, July 1981:19–24. Project Report, Clinical Investigator Brochure, Merrell Dow Research Institute, Cincinnati, June 1984.
75. Greenwood D. Microbiological properties of teicoplanin. J Antimicrob Agents Chemother. 1988;21(Suppl A):1–13.
76. Parenti F. Glycopeptide antibiotics. J Clin Pharmacol. 1988;28:136–40.
77. McNulty CAM, Garden GMF, Wise R, et al: The pharmacokinetics and tissue penetration of teicoplanin. J Antimicrob Chemother. 1985;16:743–9.
78. Verbist L, Tjandramaga B, Hendrickx B, et al. In vitro activity and human pharmacokinetics of teicoplanin. Antimicrob Agents Chemother. 1984;12:119–28.
79. Buniva G, DelFavero A, Bernareggi A, et al. Pharmacokinetics of ^{14}C-teicoplanin in healthy volunteers. J Antimicrob Chemother. 1988;21(Suppl A):23–8.
80. Bonati M, Traina GL, Rosiva R, et al. Pharmacokinetics of a single intravenous dose of teicoplanin in subjects with various degrees of renal impairment. Antimicrob Agents Chemother. 1988;21(Suppl A):29–37.
81. Tarral E, Jehl F, Tarral A, et al. Pharmacokinetics of teicoplanin in children. J Antimicrob Chemother. 1988;21(Suppl A):47–51.
82. Domart Y, Pierre C, Clair B, et al. Pharmacokinetics of teicoplanin in critically ill patients with various degrees of renal impairment. Antimicrob Agents Chemother. 1987;31:1600–4.
83. Bauernfeind A: Teichomycin and AM-715 activity on staphylococci enterococci in comparison to other antibiotic agents (abstract). In: Proceedings of the 21st Interscience Conference on Antimicrobiol Agents and Chemotherapy. Chicago: American Society for Microbiology; November 1981.
84. Jadeja L, Fainstein V, LeBlanc B, et al. Comparative in vitro activities of teichomycin and other antibiotics against JK diphtheroids. Antimicrob Agents Chemother. 1983;24:145–6.
85. Greenwood D. Microbiological properties of teicoplanin. J Antimicrob Chemother. 1988;21(Suppl A):1–3.
86. Felmingham D, Solomonides K, O'Hare MD, et al. The effect of medium and inoculum on the activity of vancomycin and teicoplanin against coagulase-negative staphylococci. Antimicrob Agents Chemother. 1987;10:609–19.
87. Pantosti A, Luzzi I, Cardine R, et al. Comparison of the in vitro activities of teicoplanin and vancomycin against *Clostridium difficile* and their interactions with cholestyramine. Antimicro Agents Chemother. 1985;28:847–8.
88. Van der Auwera P, Klastersky J. Bactericidal activity and killing rate of serum in volunteers receiving vancomycin or teicoplanin with and without amikacin given intravenously. J Antimicrob Chemother. 1987;19:623–35.
89. Van der Auwera P, Joly P. Comparative in-vitro activities of teicoplanin, vancomycin, coumermycin and ciprofloxacin, alone and in combination with rifampicin or LM427, against *Staphylococcus aureus*. J Antimicrob Chemother. 1987;19:313–20.
90. Watanakunakorn C. In-vitro activity of teicoplanin alone and in combination with rifampicin, gentamicin or tobramycin against coagulase-negative staphylococci. J Antimicrob Chemother. 1987;19:439–43.
91. Tuazon CU, Washburn D. Teicoplanin and rifampicin singly and in combination in the treatment of experimental *Staphylococcus epidermidis* endocarditis in the rabbit model. J Antimicrob Chemother. 1987;20:233–7.
92. Shanson DC, Todayon M. Activity of teicoplanin compared with vancomycin alone, and combined with gentamicin, against penicillin tolerant viridans streptococci and enterococci causing endocarditis. J Hosp Infect. 1986;7(Suppl A):65–72.
93. Williams AH, Gruneberg RN, Webster A, et al. Teicoplanin in the treatment of infection caused by gram-positive organisms. J Hosp Infect. 1986;7(Suppl A):101–3.
94. Agnelli G, Longetti M, Guerciolini R, et al. Effects of the new glycopeptide antibiotic teicoplanin on platelet function and blood coagulation. Antimicrob Agents Chemother. 1987;31:1609–12.
95. Stille W, Sietzen W, Dieterich HA, et al. Clinical efficacy and safety of teicoplanin. J. Antimicrob. Chemother. 1988;21(Suppl A):69–79.
96. Maher ER, Hollman A, Gruneberg RN. Teicoplanin-induced ototoxicity in Down's Syndrome. Lancet. 1986;1:613.
97. Drabu YJ, Walsh B, Blakemore PH, et al. Teicoplanin in infections caused by methicillin-resistant staphylococci. J Antimicrob Chemother. 1988;21(Suppl A):89–92.

98. Schlemmer B, Falkman H, Boudjadja A, et al. Teicoplanin for patients allergic to vancomycin. N Engl J Med. 1988;318:1127–8.
99. Lewis P, Garaud JJ, Parenti F. A multicentre open clinical trial of teicoplanin in infections caused by gram-positive bacteria. J Antimicrob Chemother. 1988;21(Suppl A):61–7.
100. Harding I, Garaud JJ. Teicoplanin in the treatment of infections caused by coagulase-negative staphylococci. J Antimicrob Chemother. 1988;21(Suppl A):93–103.
101. Galanakis N, Giamarellou H, Vlachogiannis N, et al: Poor efficacy of teicoplanin in treatment of deep-seated staphylococcal infections. Eur J Clin Microbiol Infect Dis. 1988;7:130–4.
102. Wilson APR, Treasure T, Gruneberg RN, et al. Antibiotic prophylaxis in cardiac surgery: A prospective comparison of two dosage regimens of teicoplanin with combination of flucloxacillin and tobramycin. J Antimicrob Chemother. 1988;21:213–33.
103. Neville LO, Baillod RA, Brumfitt W, et al. Efficacy and safety of teicoplanin in gram-positive peritonitis in patients on peritoneal dialysis. J Antimicrob Chemother. 1988;21(Suppl A):123–31.
104. Bowley JA, Pickering SJ, Scantlebury AJ, et al. Intraperitoneal teicoplanin in the treatment of peritonitis associated with continuous ambulatory peritoneal dialysis. J Antimicrob Chemother. 1988;21(Suppl A):133–9.

28. POLYMYXINS

ROBERT FEKETY

STRUCTURE

Polymyxin A, B, C, D, and E are related cyclic basic polypeptides characterized by poor diffusibility, a molecular weight of about 1100, an antimicrobial spectrum limited to gram-negative aerobes, and significant toxicity. All but polymyxin B and E are too toxic for therapeutic use in humans.[1] Colistin is identical to polymyxin E; it differs from polymyxin B in only 1 of its 10 amino acids.[2]

DERIVATION AND NOMENCLATURE

Polymyxins are derived from *Bacillus polymyxa*. Polymyxin B sulfate was introduced for clinical use in 1947. It is marketed in units that are only 65–75 percent pure; 1 unit of polymyxin B sulfate is equivalent to 0.1 μg of pure polymyxin base. Colistin (polymyxin E, Coly-Mycin) was introduced clinically in 1961 as the methanesulfonate (colistimethate) derivative. Its advatage is that it is less painful than polymyxin B sulfate is after intramuscular injection.[3] Methanesulfonation of the free amino groups of polymyxins has a (temporarily) detrimental effect on their antibacterial action; colistimethate is essentially inactive until hydrolyzed within the body to the colistin base.[4] Thus, colistimethate may be thought of as a repository form of intramuscular polymyxin.

MECHANISM OF ACTION

The polymyxins act like cationic detergents or surfactants. They disrupt the osmotic integrity of the cell membrane by interacting with its phospholipids and increasing cellular permeability. This effect allows vital intracellular constituents such as nucleic acids and proteins to leak out, with subsequent death of the cell. The polymyxins are bactericidal and kill resting cells without necessarily lysing them. Susceptibility may be related to the phospholipid content of the cell wall–membrane complex.[3] Resistant organisms have cell walls that prevent access of the drug to the membrane. Calcium reduces the antibacterial action of polymyxins by interfering with their attachment to the membrane. Interestingly, polymyxins may also interfere with some of the actions of bacterial endotoxins, but this effect is inhibited by calcium and is of uncertain clinical significance.

ANTIMICROBIAL ACTIVITY

Polymyxin B and colistin (polymyxin E) have identical antibacterial spectra and show complete cross-resistance.[1,3,5] On a weight basis, polymyxin B sulfate is slightly more active and toxic than colistin sulfate is and is much more active than colistin methanesulfonate is.[6] The polymyxins are almost exclusively active against gram-negative bacilli. Their primary clinical usefulness is for *Pseudomonas* infections. *Pseudomonas aeruginosa* isolates are almost always inhibited by concentrations lower than 8 μg/ml. *Escherichia coli, Klebsiella pneumoniae, Enterobacter, Salmonella, Shigella, Vibrio, Haemophilus, Pasteurella, Bordetella,* and the other *Pseudomonas* species are usually susceptible. *Proteus, Providencia, Serratia,* and *Neisseria* isolates are usually resistant, as are gram-positive organisms and obligate anaerobes.[1,5] There is no cross-resistance with other antibiotics, and resistance rarely develops during therapy. Polymyxins have some slight activity against various fungi, but this has had no clinical significance. Rifampin combined with polymyxin B may be synergistic against multiply resistant *Serratia* isolates. Synergism against *Pseudomonas* has been demonstrated in vitro between polymyxins and tetracycline, chloramphenicol, carbenicillin, and trimethoprim/sulfamethoxazole, but the clinical significance of this enhancement for the most part is not known.[1,3,6] The combination of polymyxin and trimethoprim/sulfamethoxazole has been useful in severe *Pseudomonas cepacia* or *maltophilia* infections.

PHARMACOLOGY: ADMINISTRATION AND ABSORPTION

The polymyxins are not absorbed when given orally. They are intended primarily for parenteral use. Polymyxin B sulfate is the only derivative of polymyxin B that is available for treatment. It can be given intravenously, intramuscularly, intrathecally, orally, topically, endobronchially, or by aerosol. Polymyxins are quite painful when given intramuscularly, and the pain may persist for several hours. However, when the drugs are given intravenously, local adverse effects are minimal. Colistin is available as the sulfate for oral use and as the sodium salt of the colistimethate derivative for parenteral use. Colistimethate is less painful than polymyxin B is on intramuscular injection. Colistimethate can be given by slow intravenous infusion, but even when given slowly its intravenous use may result in inadequate serum and tissue antibacterial activity if colistimethate is eliminated from the body by the kidneys before hydrolysis to the active base can take place.[4] (A bioassay of colistimethate in serum after intravenous or intramuscular administration encounters a related problem in that unhydrolyzed drug may become hydrolyzed and therefore may become more active during the assay.)

When a total daily dose of parenteral polymyxin B of 2.5 mg (25,000 units)/kg is infused in 300–500 ml of 5% dextrose in water (D_5W), peak serum concentrations of approximately 5 μg/ml are obtained. Ninety-five percent of *P. aeruginosa* isolates are susceptible to this concentration. These organisms are also susceptible at the serum levels of 5–8 μg/ml that are achieved with intramuscular colistin (2.5–5.0 mg/kg/day). By virtue of the renal excretion of colistimethate, urinary concentrations of 10–160 μg/ml are achieved with it. The serum half-life of colistin is 2–4.5 hours and that of polymyxin B, 6–7 hours. With an intramuscular injection, there may be a delay of several hours before effective urinary levels are achieved with both drugs, but colistimethate, being less bound to kidney tissues, is excreted more rapidly than is polymyxin B.[4] These drugs may be found in the urine for 2–3 days after treatment has been discontinued. Polymyxins do not pass into the cerebrospinal fluid well, even in the presence of inflammation, and in the treatment of meningitis they must be given intrathecally.[3] Nor do they pass readily into pleural, synovial, or brain tissues. Furthermore, they may combine with tissue cell membranes and the constituents of exudates (such as polyphosphates), which may explain why the polymyxins seem to be relatively ineffective in infections of the pleura, synovium, or brain.[3] Polymyxins cross the placental barrier, and concentrations of 1 μg/ml may be found in the fetus.

The excretion of the polymyxins is mostly via the kidneys. They are excreted primarily by glomerular filtration; there is no tubular secretion or reabsorption. Renal insufficiency results in decreased renal excretion of polymyxins, increased serum levels, and a greater likelihood of toxicity. The half-life in serum of polymyxin B or E in anuric patients is 48–72 hours. Doses must be reduced appropriately and renal function monitored carefully to avoid toxicity (Table 1). Urinary concentrations are reduced in the presence of renal failure.[5] Hemodialysis has no appreciable effect on serum concentrations, but peritoneal dialysis removes small amounts (1 mg/hr), and it may be useful in an overdosage.[7]

While orally administered polymyxins are poorly absorbed from the intact gastrointestinal tract of adults, they may be absorbed from the gastrointestinal tract of premature or newborn infants, and their oral use is thus hazardous and contraindicated in this population.[5] After being administered orally, polymyxins are not found in the tissues of the bowel wall in significant amounts, which may account for their ineffectiveness in the treatment of shigellosis.

Polymyxin is often used topically, usually in concentrations of 0.1% polymyxin (1 mg/ml or 1 mg/g), in combination with other antibiotics such as bacitracin or neomycin for the treatment of skin, mucous membrane, eye, and ear infections. Polymyxins are poorly absorbed from these surfaces. Polymyxin B is sometimes used for irrigation of various sites of infection. This can be dangerous since polymyxin B is absorbed well from serous cavities such as the peritoneum and the resultant high serum concentrations may result in the induction of apnea.

The protein binding of polymyxins has not been studied extensively but may be as high as 75 percent. These drugs lose much of their antibacterial activity in the presence of serum.[1]

TOXICITY AND ADVERSE REACTIONS

The two most important side effects of polymyxins are neurotoxicity and nephrotoxicity. Allergic reactions (including fever and skin rashes) are rare after polymyxin administration, but they are histamine releasers, and some patients have developed urticaria or shock after the rapid intravenous infusion of polymyxins. Pain at the site of injection is common. This can be reduced by mixing with a local anesthetic. For example, 50 mg polymyxin B may be mixed with 2 ml of 2% procaine in saline; colistimethate formerly was supplied mixed with dibucaine. When a serum concentration of 1–2 μg/ml or more of polymyxins is achieved, most patients will experience circumoral or stocking-glove paresthesias, sometimes with flushing, dizziness, vertigo, ataxia, slurred speech, drowsiness, or confusion. These are less frequent with lower doses, in children, and when injections are given no more frequently than every 8 hours. These neurotoxic side effects disappear soon after therapy with the drugs has been discontinued. Polymyxins also have a curare-like action on striated muscles and block neuromuscular transmission. High serum concentrations may result in apnea, which can be treated with intravenous calcium chloride.

Dose-related nephrotoxicity is the most important side effect of polymyxins. In general, the more antibacterially active derivative, polymyxin B, is more toxic than colistin is. At therapeutically equivalent doses, they are frequently and equally nephrotoxic,[3,6] and renal function should be carefully monitored during therapy. Renal toxicity probably follows attachment of the antibiotics to the membrane of the renal convoluted tubular epithelium. This may be accentuated or potentiated by aminoglycosides or other nephrotoxic drugs, which should therefore be avoided. At appropriate therapeutic dosages, approximately 20 percent of patients experience nephrotoxicity manifested by a rising serum creatinine level and an abnormal urinary sediment, and 1–2 percent develop acute tubular necrosis. Nitrogen retention, probably related to a reduction in the glomerular filtration rate, frequently increases for a week or so after treatment with these drugs has been discontinued but is usually reversible.[8] Anuria and tubular necrosis with serious renal failure are particularly common in patients who have received excessive doses or in whom the drug therapy is continued in usual doses in the face of impaired renal function. In renal failure, polymyxins should be used only with great care and in reduced doses (Table 1).[3,5,8,9] Patients receiving no more than 2.2 mg/kg daily usually tolerate polymyxin B well even for long periods.

Little diarrhea or disturbance of the gastrointestinal flora results when these drugs are used. Dyspnea may occur after the use of polymyxin by aerosol, and respiratory arrest has been reported.

MAJOR USES AND DOSES

The polymyxins are used infrequently parenterally and almost exclusively for serious, life-threatening *Pseudomonas* or gram-negative bacillary infections caused by organisms resistant to other drugs or in patients with these infections who are intolerant or allergic to the preferred drugs. The usual dose of polymyxin B for adults with normal renal function is 1.5–2.5 mg (15,000–25,000 units)/kg/day given by continuous intravenous infusion. The intramuscular dosage is 2.5–3.0 mg/kg/day given at 4- or 6-hour intervals. Septic infants may receive up to 40,000–45,000 units/kg/day. Adults with normal renal function may be given 2.5–5.0 mg/kg colistimethate/day in two or three divided doses (iv or im). Polymyxin B is preferred to colistimethate for intravenous use since it does not require hydrolysis for activation.[5]

Polymyxins are second-line or alternate drugs since they are relatively ineffective in patients with bacteremia and involvement of deep tissues, and they are especially ineffective in compromised hosts with granulocytopenia.[10] Endocarditis usually cannot be cured with the polymyxins without the aid of surgery or other drugs. When bacteremia is associated with a removable or treatable focus, these drugs may be useful. Best results have been obtained with urinary tract infections or septicemias arising from the urinary tract.[3,7]

The rare patient with meningitis requiring polymyxins should be treated intrathecally. The usual intrathecal dose of polymyxin B is 5–10 mg/day in adults; in children younger than 2 years of age, a dose of 2 mg/day is used. Amounts greater than 10 mg (100,000 units) should never be used intrathecally for meningitis alone. It is believed that nothing is gained by adding intravenous therapy when patients are treated intrathecally. Daily intrathecal therapy should be given for 3–5 days and then every other day for 3 weeks or for 2 weeks after cultures are negative and the cerebrospinal fluid (CSF) glucose level is normal.

Urinary tract infections can be treated with relatively low and

TABLE 1. Reduction in Polymyxin Dosage to Avoid Drug-Induced Renal Injury

	Parenteral Dose (mg/kg Body Weight) When Creatinine Clearance Is			
Drug	*Normal, or ≥80% of Normal*	*80–≥30% of Normal*	*<30% of Normal*	*With Anuria*
Polymyxin B, sulfate	2.5–3.0 mg/day	1st day, 2.5 mg; daily thereafter at 1.0–1.5 mg	1st day, 2.5 mg; every 2–3 days thereafter, 1.0–1.5 mg	1st day, 2.5 mg; every 5–7 days thereafter, 1.0 mg
Colistimethate (polymyxin E)	3.0–5.0 mg/day	1st day, 3.0 mg; daily thereafter at 1.5–2.5 mg	1st day, 3.0 mg; every 2–3 days thereafter, 1.5–2.5 mg	1st day, 2.5 mg; every 5–7 days thereafter, 1.5 mg

well-tolerated doses of intramuscular colistimethate (2.5 mg/kg/day in divided dosage for 7–10 days). Results are better with acute than with chronic urinary infections, in which relapses are frequent within a few months.

Some investigators believe that the prevention of urinary tract infections in patients requiring indwelling (Foley) catheters for periods up to 2 weeks may be achieved by using triple-lumen catheters and continuous irrigation of the bladder with a solution of neomycin (40 mg/liter) and polymyxin B (20 mg/liter). Usually, no more than 1 liter of irrigant is used per day unless urine flow rates are very high.[11]

Aerosolized polymyxins have been used in the treatment of respiratory infections due to *Pseudomonas* in patients with cystic fibrosis or bronchiectasis and in the prevention of *Pseudomonas* infections in respiratory intensive care units during periods of high risk.[12] Usually, the solution contains 2–10 mg/ml, and 2 ml is aerosolized six to eight times per day. Ultimately, the development of resistant organisms has limited the efficacy of this measure; to delay this, intermittent use of the regimens has been tried. Polymyxin has been combined with neomycin and amphotericin B, other nonabsorbed antimicrobials, via the oral route for infection prophylaxis and selective decontamination of the digestive tract in patients with acute leukemia.[13] The oropharynx and stools of most patients became free of gram-negative bacilli within 1 week.

In creams, sprays, and solutions containing 0.5–3 mg/ml, polymyxins are useful in the prevention and treatment of skin infections and in the treatment of external otitis or corneal ulcers. When administered topically, it is often combined with neomycin and bacitracin. Subconjunctival injection of up to 100,000 units polymyxin B per day may be used in the treatment of *Pseudomonas* infections of the cornea and conjunctivae. A total dose of 200 mg/day should not be exceeded.

Polymyxins may be useful when administered orally to small children with localized gastroenteritis due to enteropathogenic *E. coli*, but they are relatively useless in patients with *Salmonella* or invasive *Shigella* enteritis. An oral dose of colistin sulfate of 15–20 mg/kg/day in three divided doses for 5–20 days has been used with *E. coli* outbreaks, but 3–5 mg/kg/day is the usual oral dose. These drugs should not be used orally in neonates and premature infants.

When polymyxins are combined with sulfamethoxazole and trimethoprim, they are often synergistic and can be useful in the treatment of serious infections with multiply drug-resistant *Serratia* and *Pseudomonas cepacia, P. maltophilia*, or *P. aeruginosa* isolates.[14–16] A combination of polymyxin B and rifampin has also been used successfully in seriously ill patients with drug-resistant nosocomial *Serratia* infections.[17]

REFERENCES

1. Jawetz E. Polymyxin, colistin and bacitracin. Pediatr Clin North Am. 1961;8:1057.
2. Wilkinson S. Identity of colistin and polymyxin E. Lancet. 1963;1:922.
3. Goodwin NJ. Colistin and sodium colistimethate. Med Clin North Am. 1970;54:1267.
4. Barnett M, Bushby SRM, Wilkinson S. Sodium sulphomethyl derivatives of polymyxins. Br J Pharmacol. 1964;23:552.
5. Hoeprich PD. The polymyxins. Med Clin North Am. 1970;54:1257.
6. Nord NM, Hoeprich PD. Polymyxin B and colistin. A critical comparison. N Engl J Med. 1964;270:1030.
7. Goodwin N, Friedman E. The effects of renal impairment, peritoneal dialysis, and hemodialysis on serum sodium colistimethate levels. Ann Intern Med. 1968;68:984.
8. Fekety FR, Norman PS, Cluff LE. The treatment of gram-negative bacillary infections. The toxicity and efficacy of large doses in forty-eight patients. Ann Intern Med. 1962;57:214.
9. Appel GB, Neu HC. The nephrotoxicity of antimicrobial agents. N Engl J Med. 1977;296:663.
10. Whitecar JP, Luna M, Bodey GP. *Pseudomonas* bacteremia in patients with malignant disease. Am J Med Sci. 1970;260:216.
11. Marten CM, Bookrajian EN. Bacteriuria prevention after indwelling urinary catheterization. Arch Intern Med. 1962;110:703.
12. Feeley TW, duMoulin GC, Hedley-Whyte J, et al. Aerosol polymyxin and pneumonia in seriously ill patients. N Engl J Med. 1975;293:471.
13. van der Waaij D, Gaus W, Krieger D, et al. Bacteriological data on a prospective multicenter study of the effect of two different regimens for selective decontamination in patients with acute leukemia. Infection. 1986;14:268–74.
14. Thomas FE, Leonard JM, Alford RH. Sulfamethoxazole-trimethoprim polymyxin therapy of serious multiply drug-resistant *Serratia* infections. Antimicrob Agents Chemother. 1976;9:201.
15. Rosenblatt JE, Stewart PR. Combined activity of sulfamethoxazole, trimethoprim, and polymyxin B against gram-negative bacilli. Antimicrob Agents Chemother. 1974;6:84.
16. Nord C, Wadstrom T, Wretlind B. Synergistic effects of combinations of sulfamethoxazole, trimethoprim and colistin against *Pseudomonas maltophilia* and *P. cepacia*. Antimicrob Agents Chemother. 1974;6:521.
17. Ostenson RC, Fields BT, Nolan CM. Polymyxin B and rifampin: New regimen for multiresistant *Serratia marcescens* infections. Antimicrob Agents Chemother. 1977;12:655.

29. SULFONAMIDES AND TRIMETHOPRIM

STEPHEN H. ZINNER
KENNETH H. MAYER

The modern era of antimicrobial chemotherapy began in 1932 with the first reports by Gerhard Domagk of the protective activity of prontosil against murine streptococcal infections. This drug was an outgrowth of the German dye industry and had been commercially available since the early twentieth century. Prontosil (sulfachrysoidine) exerted its antibacterial activity due to the release in vivo of para-aminobenzenesulfonamide (sulfanilamide). This agent was the first antibacterial used in the United States, in an unsuccessful attempt, in July, 1935, to treat a 10-year-old girl late in the course of meningitis and sepsis due to *Haemophilus influenzae*.[1] During the late 1930s, the basic sulfanilamide compound was modified to remove unpleasant side effects while expanding its spectrum of activity. More recent modifications have resulted in compounds of specific usefulness, for example, in urinary infections (those compounds that are highly soluble), or those nonabsorbable sulfonamides that act only within the gastrointestinal tract.

Trimethoprim is a 2,4-diamino-pyrimidine and, as such, inhibits the enzyme dihydrofolate reductase, resulting in interference in folic acid and subsequent pyrimidine synthesis in the bacterial cell. Trimethoprim is one of several such compounds synthesized and studied by Hitchings and coworkers in the 1950s and 1960s. The use of trimethoprim as a potentiator of sulfonamide activity was introduced by Bushby and Hitchings in 1968.[2] In the subsequent decade the combination of trimethoprim-sulfamethoxazole has been introduced clinically and has found a place in the chemotherapy of many infectious diseases. These agents, available in a fixed drug combination, show true antibacterial synergism against a wide variety of organisms.

SULFONAMIDES

Structure

The clinically useful sulfonamides are derived from sulfanilamide (para-aminobenzenesulfonamide) that is similar in structure to para-aminobenzoic acid (PABA), a factor required by bacteria for folic acid synthesis (Fig. 1).

A free amino group at the 4 position is associated with enhanced activity. Increased activity due to increased PABA inhibition is associated with substitutions at the sulfonyl radical (SO_2)—attached to the 1 carbon, as seen with sulfadiazine, sulfisoxazole, and sulfamethoxazole, all of which are more active than the parent compound, sulfanilamide. The nature of these substitutions determines other pharmacologic properties of the drug such as absorption, solubility, and gastrointestinal

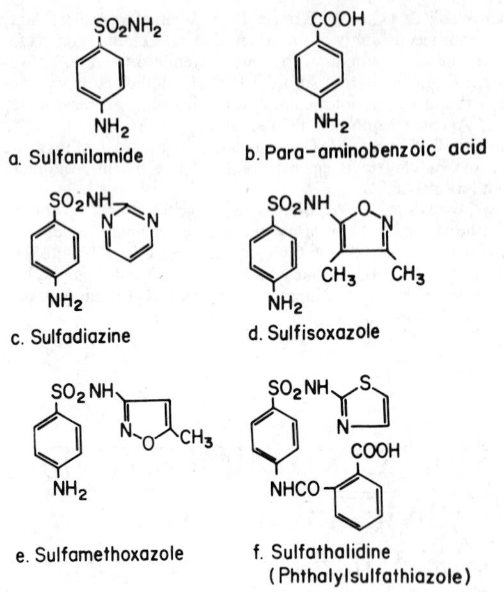

FIG. 1. Structural formulas of selected sulfonamides.

tolerance. Substitutions at the 4-amino group result in decreased absorption from the gastrointestinal tract (e.g., phthalylsulfathiazole).

Derivation and Nomenclature

Since the introduction of sulfonamides into clinical medicine, dozens of compounds have been used. However, relatively few survive today, and they can be classified as (*1*) short- or medium-acting sulfonamides, (*2*) long-acting sulfonamides, (*3*) sulfonamides limited to the gastrointestinal tract, and (*4*) topical sulfonamides.

Short- or Medium-Acting Sulfonamides. Sulfisoxazole *United States Pharmacopeia* (USP) (sulphafurazole *British Pharmacopeia*–BP, 3,4-dimethyl-5-sulfanilamidoisoxazole, Gantrisin, SK-Soxazole) is a highly soluble drug especially useful in urinary tract infections. Sulfamethoxazole USP (5-methyl-3-sulfanilamidoisoxazole; Gantanol) is somewhat less soluble than sulfisoxazole and yields higher blood levels. It is the sulfonamide presently most frequently combined with trimethoprim. Sulfadiazine USP (2-sulfanilamidopyridine) is highly active, attains high blood and cerebrospinal fluid levels, and is associated with low protein binding and lower solubility than the above drugs. Sulfamethizole USP (2-sulfanilamide-5-methyl-1:3:4-thiazole; Microsul, Thiosulfil) is used for urinary tract infections. Sulfadimidine and sulfacarbamide are available in the United Kingdom.

Short-acting sulfonamides are also available in several combinations. Sulfisoxazole, sulfamethoxazole, and sulfamethizole are each combined with phenazopyridine, a urinary analgesic, as Azo Gantrisin, Azo Gantanol, Microsul-A, Sul-Azo, and Thiosulfil-A Forte. Phenazopyridine is also present with sulfamethazole and sulfadiazine in Suladyne. Sulfamethizole is also combined with tetracycline and phenazopyridine in Urobiotic and Azotrex, but these two preparations have been classified by the Food and Drug Administration (FDA) as lacking evidence of effectiveness as a fixed drug combination.

Long-Acting Sulfonamides. Sulfamethoxypyridazine (3-sulfanilamido-6-methoxy-pyridazine) and sulfameter [4-amino-*N*-(5-methoxy-2-pyrimidinyl)] benzene-sulfonamide are no longer available for single daily dose therapy, as they were associated with hypersensitivity reactions such as Stevens-Johnson syndrome. Neither sulfadimethoxine (Madribon) nor any other long-acting sulfonamides other than sulfadoxine are currently available in the United States.

Sulfadoxine, originally known as sulformethoxine [*N*′-(5,6-dimethoxy-4-pyrimidyl) sulfanilamide] is a very long-acting sulfonamide that, combined with pyrimethamine, is available as Fansidar. Sulfadoxine has a half-life of 100–230 hours and reaches a peak serum level of 51–76 μg/ml 2.5–6 hours after an oral dose of 500 mg. Fansidar is active in the treatment and prophylaxis of malaria due to chloroquine-resistant *Plasmodium falciparum*.[3] Due to the unknown teratogenic potential of pyrimethamine, Fansidar should not be recommended for prophylaxis of pregnant women, and its use has been associated with Stevens-Johnson syndrome. Also, some strains of *P. falciparum* from Southeast Asia and South America may be resistant.

Sulfonamides Limited to the Gastrointestinal Tract. Sulfaguanidine (*N*′amidinosulfanilamide), sulfasuxidine (2-(para-succinylsulfanilamido)-thiazole, succinylsulfathiazole), and sulfathalidine [2(para-phthalyl-sulfanilamido)-thiazole] are relatively poorly absorbed from the gastrointestinal tract. They have been used in the past to suppress the susceptible bowel flora before surgery.

Salicylazosulfapyridine (sulfasalazine, Azulfidine) is a sulfonamide derivative used in the treatment of ulcerative colitis. This drug is absorbed in its parent form as sulfapyridine, and significant blood levels of this compound are measurable.

Topical Sulfonamides. Mafenide acetate (para-aminomethylbenzene sulfonamide, Sulfamylon cream) is available for use in the topical therapy of burns. However, its use has been limited by metabolic acidosis due to carbonic anhydrase inhibition. Silver sulfadiazine has fewer side effects and is used extensively for burns.[4] Here the sulfonamide acts primarily as a vehicle for release of silver ions that exert an antibacterial effect. Recent reports of outbreaks of silver-resistant infections in burn units may ultimately limit its usefulness.[5,6] Various combinations of other sulfonamides are available as vaginal creams or suppositories (e.g., Sultrin vaginal cream and tablets, AVC cream and suppositories, Sulfamel, Vagitrol).

There are a variety of ophthalmic ointments and solutions of sulfacetamide sodium USP (a highly soluble sulfonamide) available for use in treating conjunctivitis due to susceptible bacteria and as adjunctive therapy of trachoma (e.g., Bleph, Cetamide, Isoph, Sulamyd).

Mechanisms of Action

Although a wide variety of chemical modifications of the sulfonamides has been synthesized, all basically share the same mechanism of action. The sulfonamides are bacteriostatic in that they inhibit bacterial growth via interference with microbial folic acid synthesis. More specifically, sulfonamides inhibit competitively the incorporation of PABA into tetrahydropteroic acid,[7–9] and they in turn may be incorporated into dihydropteroate.[10] Sulfonamides may have a higher affinity for the microbial enzyme tetrahydropteroic acid synthetase than the natural substrate PABA. Richmond[11] has suggested that sulfonamides may act on bacterial repressor genes or by feedback inhibition to decrease formation of new enzyme. The ultimate result of decreased folic acid synthesis is a decrease in bacterial nucleotides, with subsequent inhibition of bacterial growth.

Antimicrobial Activity In Vitro

Sulfonamides exhibit in vitro inhibitory activity against a broad spectrum of gram-positive and gram-negative bacteria as well as *Actinomyces*, *Chlamydia*, *Plasmodia*, and *Toxoplasma* (Table 1). The in vitro antimicrobial sensitivity of sulfonamides

TABLE 1. In Vitro Activity of Sulfonamides Against Representative Organisms[a]

	Range of MIC[b] (μg/ml)
Gram-positive	
Staphylococcus aureus	8–64
Streptococcus pneumoniae	4–128
Streptococcus pyogenes	0.5–16
Enterococcus faecalis	25–250
Corynebacterium diphtheriae	25–75
Listeria monocytogenes	3–75
Bacillus anthracis	12–100
Gram-negative	
Escherichia coli	4–64
Klebsiella spp.	8–128
Proteus mirabilis	8–128
Serratia marcescens	25–>1000
Salmonella sp.	16–128
Shigella sp.	2–32
Haemophilus influenzae	1–16
Neisseria gonorrhoeae	4–32
Neisseria meningitidis	0.25–>10
Pseudomonas aeruginosa	>100–200
Other	
Chlamydia trachomatis	0.1
Nocardia asteroides	2–16

[a] The acquisition of plasmids may increase MICs.
[b] Minimum Inhibitory Concentration. Range is expressed for a variety of sulfonamide compounds.
(Data from Garrod et al.,[27] Bushby,[28] and Bach et al.[23])

is strongly influenced by the size of the inoculum and the composition of the test media. High concentrations of PABA and thymidine inhibit sulfonamide activity.

Antimicrobial Resistance. Resistance to sulfonamides is widespread and may be found in more than 20 percent of community and nosocomial strains of bacteria, including staphylococci, Enterobacteriaceae, *Neisseria meningitidis*, and *Pseudomonas* sp.[12]

Organisms may develop resistance or partial resistance by mutation, resulting in either microbial overproduction of PABA[13] or a structural change in dihydropteroate synthetase, an enzyme that has lowered affinity for sulfonamide.[14] The former mechanism has been implicated in resistant strains of *Neisseria gonorrhoeae* and *Staphylococcus aureus*,[13,15] and the latter has been found in strains of *Escherichia coli*.[16] Resistance also may be mediated by plasmids, episomal-resistance transfer factors (R factors) that may code for the production of drug-resistant enzymes, such as dihydropteroate synthetase,[17] or may result in decreased bacterial cell permeability to sulfonamides.[18] R-factor transfer can occur in the gastrointestinal tract as well as in vitro and has been seen especially with Enterobacteriaceae.[19] More than one resistance mechanism may be operating simultaneously.[20]

Plasmid-mediated sulfonamide resistance has greatly increased in recent years, often in conjunction with trimethoprim resistance. More than one-fourth of the uropathogens and one-half of the clinical *Shigella* isolates studied in Sweden,[21,22] England,[12,23] and the United States[24] were sulfonamide-resistant. *Salmonella* resistance to sulfonamides has also increased in the United States,[25] often in conjunction with resistance to other antibiotic classes. The increase in sulfonamide-resistant *Haemophilus ducreyi* in Asia and Africa has been associated with a plasmid related to those found in Enterobacteriaceae.[26]

Pharmacology

Routes of Administration. Sulfonamides are usually administered orally, although sulfadiazine and sulfisoxazole are available for use as intravenous or subcutaneous preparations. These latter forms are used rarely, if at all. Sulfacetamide is available as ophthalmic preparations, and silver sulfadiazine and mafenide acetate are applied topically in burn patients and are associated with significant absorption of sulfonamide percutaneously. Vaginal preparations are available for topical application.

Absorption. Most of the short- and medium-acting sulfonamides are absorbed rapidly and almost completely in the unionized state from the small intestine and stomach. Compounds with *N*-1 substitutions are absorbed poorly, as are more acidic compounds (e.g., phthalylsulfathiazole, Fig. 1f). Long-acting sulfonamides also are absorbed rapidly but have a much slower excretion rate. Topical sulfonamides are absorbed and may result in detectable blood levels.

Distribution. The sulfonamides generally are well distributed throughout the body, entering the cerebrospinal fluid and synovial, pleural, and peritoneal fluids with concentrations approaching 80 percent of serum levels. Blood and tissue levels are related to the degree of protein binding (Table 2) and lipid solubility. Sulfonamides administered in pregnancy readily cross the placenta and are present in the fetal blood and amniotic fluid.[31]

Excretion. Acetylation and glucuronidation occur in the liver, and free and metabolized drug appears in the urine. Glomerular filtration is probably a route of excretion, although partial reabsorption and active tubular secretion also are involved, especially at low creatinine clearance rates. Urinary excretion is more rapid for those sulfonamides with low pKa values (e.g., sulfamethizole, sulfisoxazole), and alkalinization of the urine increases excretion by this route. Plasma half-lives vary widely and are related inversely to lipid solubility and directly to pKa but are not clearly related to the degree of protein binding.[30] Small amounts of sulfonamides are found in bile, human milk, prostatic secretions, saliva, and tears.

Protein Binding and Blood or Tissue Levels. Sulfonamides are bound variably and not irreversibly to plasma albumin, and the bound drug is inactive (Table 2). Levels obtainable in cerebrospinal and other body fluids are inversely related to the degree of protein binding. The amount of free drug in plasma is directly related to pKa.[30]

Use in Renal Insufficiency. Sulfonamides can be used in renal failure, but therapeutic serum levels will persist longer because of reduced excretion, and the dosage must be reduced and the interval between doses extended proportional to the degree of renal impairment. Protein binding of sulfonamides is decreased in severe renal insufficiency.[32] The *N*-4 acetylated metabolite of sulfonamides may accumulate in patients with renal failure, especially during prolonged therapy. This derivative loses its antibacterial effect but still may have toxic properties. Plasma levels of sulfonamide should be measured every 3 days, and peak concentrations of sulfamethoxazole should be less than 120 μg/ml.

TABLE 2. Levels in Blood, Cerebrospinal Fluid, Plasma Half-life, and Protein Binding of Some Sulfonamides

Drug	Peak Blood Level[a] (μg/ml)	Serum Level in CSF (%)	Plasma Half-life (hours)	Protein Binding (%)
Sulfadiazine	30–60	40–80	17	45
Sulfisoxazole	40–50	30–50	5–6	92
Sulfamethoxazole	80–100	25–30	11	70
Sulfadoxine	50–75	20–30	100–230	80–98

[a] Approximate free sulfonamide level after a 2 g oral dose.
(Data from Anand[30] and Garrod et al.[27])

Toxicity and Adverse Reactions

Sulfonamides may cause nausea, vomiting, diarrhea, rash, fever, headache, depression, jaundice, hepatic necrosis, and a serum sicknesslike syndrome. Earlier, less soluble compounds (sulfadiazine, sulfathiazole) used in excessively high doses were associated with crystalluria and tubular deposits of sulfonamide crystals. These complications could be minimized by the maintenance of high urine flow and alkalinization of the urine. This complication usually is not seen with modern soluble sulfonamides. Tubular necrosis, interstitial nephritis, or necrotizing angiitis may be associated rarely with sulfonamide sensitivity.

More serious adverse reactions due to sulfonamides may include acute hemolytic anemia (sometimes related to a deficiency in erythrocyte glucose-6-phosphate dehydrogenase—G6PD), aplastic anemia, agranulocytosis, thrombocytopenia, and leukopenia. A recent study showed that G6PD-deficient patients who received trimethoprim-sulfamethoxazole did not have hemolytic reactions during therapy.[33]

Sulfonamides should not be administered during the last month of pregnancy because they compete for bilirubin-binding sites on plasma albumin and may increase fetal blood levels of unconjugated bilirubin, increasing the risk of kernicterus. Also, because of the immature fetal acetyl transferase system, blood levels of free sulfonamide may be increased, further adversely affecting the risk of kernicterus.[30]

Finally, significant hypersensitivity reactions may occur due to sulfonamides administered via any route. The most important of these include erythema nodosum, erythema multiforme (including Stevens-Johnson syndrome), drug eruption, vasculitis similar to periarteritis nodosa, and anaphylaxis. Long-acting sulfonamides have been associated with fatal hypersensitivity reactions, especially in children, and this severely limits their use. Locally applied sulfonamides (e.g., to skin) may be associated with any of these adverse reactions.

Drug Interactions

Sulfonamides may displace from albumin-binding sites drugs such as warfarin, thus increasing the effective activity of the displaced drug. Anticoagulant dosage therefore should be reduced during sulfonamide therapy. Sulfonamides also displace methotrexate from its bound protein, thereby increasing methotrexate toxicity. An increased hypoglycemic effect of chlorpropamide and tolbutamide may occur during sulfonamide therapy, possibly due to the same mechanism or to structural similarities. Sulfonamides may potentiate the action of some thiazide diuretics, phenytoin, and uricosuric agents. Conversely, sulfonamides themselves may be displaced from binding sites by indomethacin, phenylbutazone, salicylates, probenecid, and sulfinpyrazone, resulting in increased sulfonamide activity.

The activity of sulfonamides may be decreased by procaine and other local anesthetics derived from PABA. Methenamine compounds should not be used with sulfonamides because of the formation of insoluble urinary precipitates. Intravenous solutions of sulfonamides are physically incompatible with chloramphenicol, aminoglycosides, lincomycin, methicillin, tetracyclines, vancomycin, norepinephrine, insulin, procaine, Ringer lactate solution, and others. Sulfonamides may decrease protein-bound iodine and ^{131}I uptake and may produce false-positive Benedict tests for urine glucose and false-positive sulfosalicylic acid tests for urine proteins.[34–36]

Major Clinical Use

Sulfonamides are primarily used in the treatment of acute urinary tract infections, but increasing resistance has diminished their effectiveness. Most first episodes of infection in the unobstructed urinary tract will be due to *E. coli* that are often sensitive to sulfonamides. Sulfisoxazole is administered orally in a usual dosage of 1 g qid. Since the infecting organism of any urinary tract infection may or may not be sensitive to sulfonamides, the choice of therapy should be based on appropriate sensitivity tests (see Chapter 58).

Sulfonamides are also quite effective in the therapy of infections due to *Nocardia asteroides*. Therapy must include 4–6 g or more daily after a loading dose of 4 g and should be continued for 4–6 months or longer if necessary (see Chapter 94). Sulfonamides may be useful in combination with other antimycobacterial drugs for the management of infections due to rifampin-resistant *Mycobacterium kansasii*.[37]

Sulfonamides are effective in the prophylaxis of patients against recurrent attacks of rheumatic fever associated with group A β-hemolytic streptococcal infections, but they are not effective for therapy for established streptococcal pharyngitis. Sulfonamide prophylaxis of close contacts of patients with meningitis due to *N. meningitidis* is effective if the infecting organism is known to be sulfonamide-sensitive (adult dose for sulfadiazine is 1 g q12h for 2 days). Sulfonamides have been used to treat toxoplasmosis and *P. falciparum* malaria (with pyrimethamine), meliodosis, dermatitis herpetiformis, lymphogranuloma venereum, and chancroid; topical and systemic therapy is effective for trachoma and inclusion conjunctivitis (usually with topical tetracycline). Nongonococcal urethritis due to *Chlamydia*, but not *Ureaplasma urealyticum*, responds well to sulfonamide therapy (see Chapter 94). Sulfasalazine is used in the treatment of inflammatory bowel diseases and has had some success in patients with rheumatoid arthritis and other inflammatory conditions.[38,39] Currently, sulfonamides are used frequently in combination with trimethoprim (see below).

TRIMETHOPRIM

Structure and Derivation

Trimethoprim is a 2,4-diamino-5-(3′,4′,5′-trimethoxybenzyl) pyrimidine (Fig. 2). This drug was synthesized by Hitchings and coworkers as a dihydrofolate reductase inhibitor thought to potentiate the activity of sulfonamides by sequential inhibition of folic acid synthesis.[2] In the United States, trimethoprim is now available as a single agent as well as in combination with sulfamethoxazole (see below). Trimethoprim does have antibacterial activity of its own, and its pharmacology will be reviewed.

Mechanism of Action

Trimethoprim owes its activity to powerful inhibition of bacterial dihydrofolate reductase, which is the enzyme step after the step in folic acid synthesis blocked by sulfonamides. Trimethoprim is 50,000–100,000 times more active against bacterial dihydrofolate reductase than against the human enzyme. Trimethoprim interferes with the conversion of dihydrofolate to tetrahydrofolate, the precursor of folinic acid and ultimately purine and DNA synthesis (Fig. 3). The sequential blockage of the same biosynthetic pathway by sulfonamides and trimethoprim results in a high degree of synergistic activity against a wide spectrum of microorganisms. Humans do not synthesize

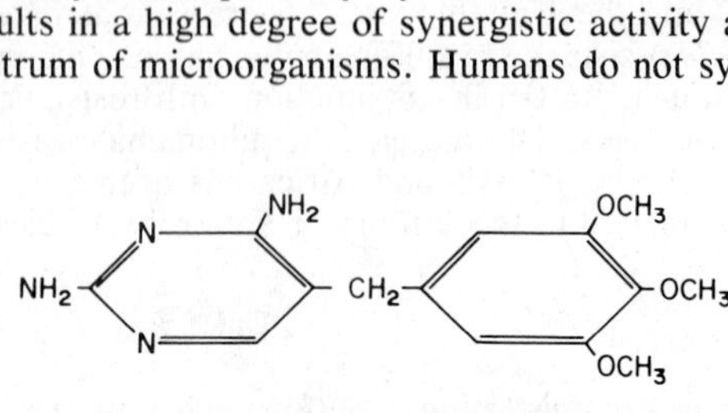

TRIMETHOPRIM
(2,4-diamino-5-(3′,4′,5′-trimethoxybenzyl)pyrimidine)

FIG. 2. Chemical structure of trimethoprim.

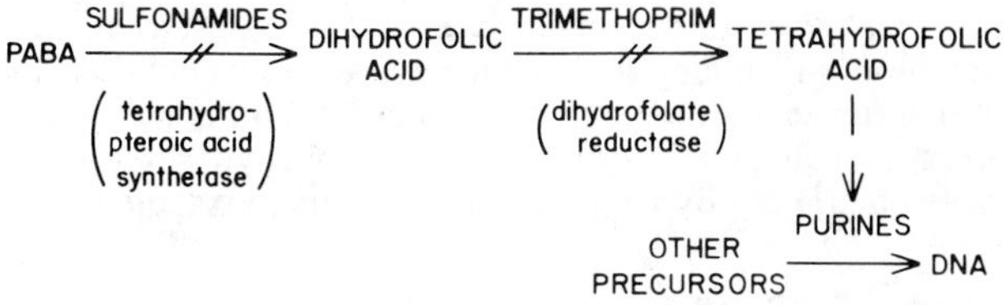

FIG. 3. Action of sulfonamides and trimethoprim on the metabolic pathway of bacterial folic acid synthesis.

folic acid but require it in their diet, and therefore human purine synthesis is not affected significantly by the enzyme inhibition by trimethoprim.[40,41]

Antimicrobial Activity

Trimethoprim is quite active in vitro against many gram-positive cocci and most gram-negative rods except for *Pseudomonas aeruginosa* and *Bacteroides* sp. (Table 3). *Treponema pallidum*, *Mycobacterium tuberculosis*, *Mycoplasma* sp., and most anaerobes are resistant. Thymidine will inhibit the in vitro activity of trimethoprim, but the addition of thymidine phosphorylase or 5 percent lysed horse blood to Mueller-Hinton or other sensitivity media removes this inhibition. The minimum inhibitory concentration (MIC) will vary considerably with the media used.[46]

Potentiation of the action of trimethoprim is seen in combination with sulfamethoxazole (see below and Table 3). Antibacterial synergism has been demonstrated in vitro for trimethoprim and polymyxins[47] and for trimethoprim and aminoglycosides against some gram-negative bacilli.[48] The combination of trimethoprim–sulfamethoxazole is active in vitro against many isolates of tested *S. aureus*.[49] *Streptococcus pyogenes, Streptococcus pneumoniae, E. coli, Proteus mirabilis, Shigella* sp., *Salmonella* sp., *Pseudomonas cepacia, Pseudomonas pseudomallei, Yersinia enterocolitica*, and *N. gonorrhoeae*.[50]

Variable bactericidal effects have been noted when enterococci are tested against trimethoprim–sulfamethoxazole.[45,45a] The susceptibility of Enterobacteriaceae may vary greatly between locations and within the same location from year to year, due to the spread of trimethoprim-resistant plasmids and transposons.[50] Almost all strains of *P. aeruginosa* are resistant in vitro to trimethoprim–sulfamethoxazole.[49]

Trimethoprim combined with sulfamethoxazole or dapsone has been effective in the treatment of *Pneumocystis carinii* pneumonia in immunocompromised patients (see below). *Listeria monocytogenes*,[51] *Branhamella catarrhalis*,[52] and atypical mycobacteria[53] have been shown to be susceptible to the combination of trimethoprim and sulfamethoxazole.

The optimal ratio for in vitro synergism of trimethoprim–sulfamethoxazole in combination is 1:20, but this ratio does not always obtain in vivo. The synergism seen with trimethoprim–sulfamethoxazole depends somewhat on the sensitivity of the organism to each drug. In one study[54] over 95 percent of organisms sensitive to both drugs showed synergism, whereas 60 percent of sulfamethoxazole-resistant strains and 45 percent of trimethoprim-resistant strains showed synergism.

Resistance to Trimethoprim. Bacteria may develop trimethoprim resistance by frequent passage in media containing the drug. Clinical resistance has increased. In one hospital in France[50] trimethoprim-resistant Enterobacteriaceae (MIC ≥ 4 μg/ml) increased from 18 to 25 percent of isolates. A decrease in the ratio of strains resistant to both sulfamethoxazole and trimethoprim compared with stains resistant only to trimethoprim may reflect an increase in independent trimethoprim resistance, and this might be a useful monitoring parameter in hospitals.[55]

TABLE 3. In Vitro Activity of Trimethoprim Against Representative Organisms

Organism	*MIC[a] Alone (μg/ml)*	*MIC with Sulfamethoxazole (μg/ml, 1:20)[b]*
Gram-positive		
Staphylococcus aureus	0.15–2	0.04–1.6
S. epidermidis	0.02	—
Streptococcus pneumoniae	0.004–5	0.05–1.5
S. pyogenes	0.02–1	0.015–0.4
Enterococcus faecalis	0.15–0.5	0.015–0.4[b]
Corynebacterium diphtheriae	0.15–0.5	0.05–0.15
Listeria monocytogenes	0.05–1.5	0.015–0.15
Clostridium perfringens	2–50	—
Propionibacterium acnes	0.07	—
Gram-negative		
Escherichia coli	0.01–>5	0.005–>5
Klebsiella sp.	0.15–5	0.05–3.1
Proteus mirabilis	0.15–1.5	0.05–0.15
Serratia marcescens	0.8–50	0.4–50
Salmonella sp.	0.01–0.4	0.05–0.15
Shigella sp.	0.04–0.8	0.02–0.5
Citrobacter freundii	0.2	—
Vibrio cholera	0.2	—
Haemophilus influenzae	0.1–12.5	0.04–50
Neisseria gonorrhoeae	0.2–128	0.15–3.1
N. meningitidis	3.1–50	0.01–1.6
Pseudomonas aeruginosa	50–1000	3.1–100
P. cepacia	1–2	—
P. maltophilia	>32	>32
Bacteroides fragilis	≥4.0	—
Other		
Nocardia asteroides	3–100	1.5
Chlamydia trachomatis	20	—

[a] MIC vanes with the method, inoculum size, and media used. Acquisition of residence plasmids may increase MIC's.
[b] MBC may be much higher.[45]
(Data from refs. 27–29 and 42–44.)

Trimethoprim resistance may be due to changes in cell permeability, loss of bacterial drug-binding capacity, and overproduction of or alterations in dihydrofolate reductase. However, the clinically most important mechanism is due to plasmid-mediated dihydrofolate reductases that are resistant to trimethoprim.[56–58]

Eleven distinctive dihydrofolate reductases have been described in recent years in Enterobacteriaceae, *P. aeruginosa*, or *S. aureus*.[58,59] They are frequently plasmid-mediated[50,58,59a] and may be disseminated by highly mobile transposons (such as Tn7) with wide host species' ranges.[60] Outbreaks due to trimethoprim-resistant conjugative plasmids have been noted in Europe,[58–62] East Asia,[63,64] South America,[65] and the United States.[65,66] Increases in endemic trimethoprim resistance, particularly among Enterobacteriaceae, have been especially marked in developing countries.[67] With more than one-third of the *E. coli* and *Salmonella* resistant to trimethoprim in several South American and Asian nations, the use of this low-cost agent for the treatment of urinary tract infections and serious enteric infections is imperiled.

Permeability changes may occur in the bacterial cell and result in resistance to both trimethoprim and sulfonamides. Thymine requiring auxotrophs may also account for clinically significant resistance to both drugs. These mutants lack thymidylate synthetase and are probably less virulent than are sensitive strains.[68,69]

Pharmacology

Routes of Administration. Trimethoprim is available as 100 mg tablets for oral use. Trimethoprim is absorbed readily and almost completely from the gastrointestinal tract. Peak serum levels after taking 100 mg appear 1–4 hours after ingestion and approach 1 μg/ml. The coadministration of sulfamethoxazole does not affect the rate of absorption or serum levels of trimethoprim.

Trimethoprim is also available in fixed combination with sulfamethoxazole in a ratio of 1:5 for oral use (trimethoprim, 80 mg; sulfamethoxazole, 400 mg; Bactrim, Septra); double-strength and quarter-strength pediatric tablets are available, as is an oral suspension containing 40 mg trimethoprim and 200 mg sulfamethoxazole per 5 ml. Intravenous trimethoprim (16 mg/ml) plus sulfamethoxazole (80 mg/ml) is available. When administered intravenously, 10 ml or 160 mg trimethoprim (with 800 mg sulfamethoxazole) produces a peak serum trimethoprim concentration of 3.4 μg/ml in 1 hour. After repeated doses, the peak trimethoprim concentration may approach 9 μg/ml.[70] Similar peak levels may be reached with oral therapy, but at 2–4 hours after taking the dose.[71,72]

Distribution. Trimethoprim is widely distributed in tissues and may appear in kidney, lung, and sputum in higher concentrations than in plasma, as well as in bile, saliva, human breast milk, and seminal fluid.[73] Trimethoprim is also found in prostatic fluid at two to three times the serum concentration, but lower levels may be present in patients with chronic prostatitis.[74,75] Cerebrospinal fluid levels are about 40 percent of serum levels.

Metabolism and Excretion. Approximately 60–80 percent of an administered dose of trimethoprim is excreted in the urine via tubular secretion within 24 hours. The remainder of the drug is excreted by the kidney in one of four oxide- or hydroxyl-derivatives. The urinary metabolites are bacteriologically inactive.[70] Trimethoprim is also excreted in the bile. The serum half-life ranges from 9 to 11 hours in healthy subjects and is prolonged in patients with renal insufficiency. Unlike sulfamethoxazole, the excretion rate of trimethoprim is increased with acidification of the urine, and serum protein binding (65–70 percent) does not decrease significantly with increasing degrees of uremia.[32] Urine concentrations in healthy subjects (60–1000 μg/ml) are usually in excess of the MIC of most urinary pathogens.[32] Trimethoprim–sulfamethoxazole can be given in the usual doses to patients with creatinine clearances of 30 ml/min or greater. One-half the usual daily dose can be given to patients with creatinine clearances of 15–30 ml/min, but trimethoprim-sulfamethoxazole is not recommended for use in patients with clearances less than 15 ml/min.[32,76,77] Both trimethoprim and nonacetylated sulfamethoxazole are removed by hemodialysis.[32] Patients needing chronic peritoneal dialysis can receive the equivalent of one double-strength trimethoprim–sulfamethoxazole tablet every 48 hours.

Toxicity and Side Effects

The toxic and undesired effects of trimethoprim–sulfamethoxazole include all those discussed above for sulfonamides. Nausea, vomiting, diarrhea, anorexia, and hypersensitivity reactions are the most frequent.[78,79] Rash has been noted frequently in patients with the acquired immunodeficiency syndrome (AIDS).[80–82] In 2 patients with AIDS, transient pulmonary infiltrates and hypotension developed following reexposure to trimethoprim–sulfamethoxazole.[83] In addition, impaired folate utilization may be seen in humans with prolonged administration. This is usually manifest as a megaloblastic marrow, with hypersegmented polymorphonuclear leukocytes. Also leukopenia, thrombocytopenia, and granulocytopenia may be seen. The administration of folinic acid usually prevents or treats effectively the antifolate effects of trimethoprim, and the latter drug's antibacterial efficacy is not impaired except possibly against enterococci. Pseudomembranous colitis has been described with trimethoprim–sulfamethoxazole but is uncommon.[84] Renal dysfunction may occur in patients with pre-existing renal disease, but this is reversible with dose reduction.[85] Trimethoprim–sulfamethoxazole may cause an increase in measured serum creatinine.[86] Drug-induced hepatitis has been reported infrequently.[81] Active levels of phenytoin may be increased markedly by trimethoprim–sulfamethoxazole.[87]

Trimethoprim Plus Other Antimicrobial Agents

Other sulfonamides, such as sulfamoxole, sulfadiazine, sulfadimidine, and sulfametrol, have been combined with trimethoprim, but more clinical studies are needed to recommend their use over the currently used combination.[88–90] Trimethoprim–sulfadiazine was reported to be less likely to accumulate in the kidneys of elderly patients with impaired renal function than trimethoprim–sulfamethoxazole.[89] Combinations of trimethoprim with other agents such as rifampin[91–93] polymyxin,[47] amikacin,[94] and metronidazole[95] have been suggested or used. Extensive clinical experience with these combinations is lacking. Recent reports suggest that trimethoprim–dapsone is more efficacious for the treatment of *P. carinii* pneumonia than dapsone alone.[80,96,97]

Clinical Use

Urinary Tract Infections. Trimethoprim–sulfamethoxazole is useful in the treatment of recurrent or chronic urinary tract infections due to sensitive organisms. Many Enterobacteriaceae are sensitive to the combined action of these drugs. The combination is also effective in acute pyelonephritis and cystitis (see Chapter 58), although either antibiotic alone could be appropriate for susceptible isolates.

Because trimethoprim accumulates in prostatic secretions, trimethoprim–sulfamethoxazole is often effective in bacterial prostatitis,[75] as well as in orchitis and epididymitis due to susceptible bacteria.

The usual dosage in an adult for the treatment of acute prostate or urinary infection is two tablets every 12 hours or one double-strength tablet every 12 hours. The pediatric dose for urinary tract infection is 150–185 mg/m^2 for trimethoprim and 750–925 mg/m^2 for sulfamethoxazole daily in two divided doses. Single-dose therapy with one or two double-strength tablets may be effective in women with uncomplicated lower urinary tract infection.[98,99] However, in patients with chronic tissue invasive urinary infections, longer-term therapy of up to 6 weeks might be required.[100]

Trimethoprim–sulfamethoxazole has been shown to be useful in the long-term suppressive therapy of adults and children with chronic or recurrent urinary infections, and extremely low doses (one-half to one tablet at bedtime or every other night) are effective.[101,102] Trimethoprim is thought to achieve effective concentrations in the vaginal secretions, and it is believed by some that it exerts its protective effect on reducing the number of recurrent infections in this manner despite the fact that trimethoprim–sulfamethoxazole-resistant organisms may be present in the vaginal and stool flora.[103] Trimethoprim alone is effective therapy for uncomplicated and recurrent urinary infections in women. Usual doses are 100–200 mg bid,[103–105] and nightly doses of 100 mg may be effective suppressive therapy.[105,106] Trimethoprim alone has been felt by some to be preferable to the combination of trimethoprim–sulfamethoxazole for acute urinary tract infections and possibly other infections as well.[107,108] However, trimethoprim-resistant organisms might increase with extended use.

Respiratory Tract Infections. Trimethoprim–sulfamethoxazole is effective in the treatment of acute bronchitis and pneumonitis due to sensitive organisms, although it is not the treatment of choice for any single organism. Trimethoprim–sulfamethoxazole may be as effective as tetracyclines in the reduction of acute exacerbations in patients with chronic bronchitis,[108–110] but full doses should be used. Although not usually considered for use in seriously ill patients with pneumonia, intravenously administered trimethoprim–sulfamethoxazole may be effective in patients with infections due to susceptible gram-negative bacteria.[111]

Consistent with its antibacterial spectrum, trimethoprim–sulfamethoxazole may be as effective as ampicillin for the treatment of sinusitis and otitis media,[112] and ampicillin-resistant strains of *H. influenzae* and *Branhamella catarrhalis* might be susceptible.[52]

Gastrointestinal Infections. Although antibiotics per se prolong the carrier state in acute gastroenteritis due to *Salmonella* sp., trimethoprim–sulfamethoxazole may be effective in eliminating chronic *Salmonella* carriage including carriers of *Salmonella typhi*, especially in patients over 2 years of age. Typhoid fever also may be treated successfully with this combination, although the development of resistant strains has been increasingly reported.[50,67] Trimethoprim–sulfamethoxazole is effective in shigellosis,[113] especially due to ampicillin-resistant strains; however, susceptibility testing is necessary given reports of plasmid-mediated outbreaks of resistant organisms.[114] Intravenous administration may be necessary for patients with some of these infections. Trimethoprim–sulfamethoxazole also may be effective in the treatment of diarrhea due to enteropathogenic *E. coli* and in the treatment and prophylaxis of traveler's diarrhea[115–117] if the prevalence of resistant strains in the area to be visited is low. The combination may be a useful adjunct to fluids in the treatment of cholera[118]; however, plasmid-mediated trimethoprim resistance has been reported in East Asia.[119]

Sexually Transmitted Diseases. Trimethoprim–sulfamethoxazole may be effective in the treatment of uncomplicated gonorrhea when used in several dosage regimens (e.g., 2 tabs po bid for 5 days, 4 tabs bid for 2 days, and a single dose of 8 tabs).[120–122] For pharyngeal gonorrhea, especially that due to penicillinase producing *N. gonorrhoeae*. 9 tablets/day for 5 days has been recommended.[123] However, almost half of the *N. gonorrhoeae* that were chromosomally resistant to penicillin in one study were resistant to trimethoprim–sulfamethoxazole as well.[124] Nongonococcal urethritis due to *Chlamydia trachomatis* may be treatable with the combination, but its activity is due to the sulfonamide.[125] The combination is also effective therapy for chancroid and lymphogranuloma venereum. It is ineffective for syphilis. Trimethoprim plus sulfametrole has been successful as a single-dose regimen for chancroid.[90]

Other Infections. Trimethoprim–sulfamethoxazole is useful against brucellosis (long-term therapy for 6 weeks),[126] biliary tract infections, acute and chronic osteomyelitis,[127,128] periodontal infection,[129] mycetoma due to paracoccidioidomycosis and other fungi,[130] and nocardiosis.[131,132] Individual cases of successful response to combination therapy have been described for melioidosis,[133] *P. cepacia* bacteremia,[134] Whipple's disease,[135] and Wegener's granulomatosis.[135a]

Intravenous trimethoprim–sulfamethoxazole has been useful in treating gram-negative rod bacteremia and staphylococcal bacteremia and endocarditis, although other agents may be preferred.[95,136,137,137a] Trimethoprim–sulfamethoxazole plus extended spectrum β-lactams and/or aminoglycosides provide effective broad-spectrum antimicrobial coverage in the management of febrile neutropenic patients.[138,139] Meningitis due to susceptible organisms may be successfully treated,[139a] but other agents are usually preferred. The combination may be effective in meningitis due to *Listeria monocytogenes*.[51]

Trimethoprim plus sulfalene and trimethoprim–sulfamethoxazole have been used in the treatment of susceptible *P. falciparum* infections, although these combinations are not very active against multiple-resistant strains. In vitro efficacy has been suggested for *Toxoplasma gondii*[140] and *M. kansasii*, *Mycobacterium marinum*, and *Mycobacterium scrofulaceum*, and some clinical successes have been reported.[37,53,141]

PNEUMOCYSTIS CARINII INFECTIONS. Trimethoprim–sulfamethoxazole has been highly efficacious in the treatment of *P. carinii* pneumonia in immunocompromised patients with and without AIDS[80,81,142,143] (see Chapters 110 and 256). The usual daily dose is trimethoprim 20 mg/kg/day; sulfamethoxazole 100 mg/kg/day in up to four divided doses iv, or two to three doses orally. Patients with AIDS frequently respond to therapy but have a higher incidence of toxic reactions, particularly neutropenia and rash.[81] Although the toxicities are different, the efficacy and drug reactions associated with systemic pentamidine are comparable.[144] The recommended duration of therapy is 21 days. Trimethoprim–sulfamethoxazole has been successfully used for the chemoprophylaxis of *P. carinii* pneumonia.[81,145,146]

PROPHYLACTIC THERAPY OF NEUTROPENIC PATIENTS. Several studies have presented evidence of a striking reduction in gram-negative rod bacteremia in neutropenic patients treated prophylactically with trimethoprim–sulfamethoxazole (2 tabs bid or more until stools were free of Enterobacteriaceae) compared with untreated control neutropenic patients.[147–149] Other studies have not universally shown benefit in preventing bacteremia in neutropenic patients with acute myelocytic leukemia.[150] Trimethoprim–sulfamethoxazole may prolong recovery from induction chemotherapy-induced neutropenia, as has been reported in some but not all studies.[151,152]

Trimethoprim Use in Pregnancy. The teratogenicity of trimethoprim in humans is not clearly defined, but this drug is not recommended for use in pregnancy at this time. It is, however, well tolerated in pediatric populations.[153]

REFERENCES

1. Carithers HA. The first use of an antibiotic in America. Am J Dis Child. 1974;128:207–11.
2. Bushby SRM, Hitchings GH. Trimethoprim, a sulphonamide potentiator. Br J Pharmacol Chemother. 1968;33:72–90.
3. Pearson RD, Hewlett EL. Use of pyrimethamine–sulfadoxine (Fansidar) in prophylaxis against chloroquine-resistant *Plasmodium falciparum* and *Pneumocystis carinii*. Ann Intern Med. 1987;106:714–8.
4. Ballin JC. Evaluation of a new topical agent for burn therapy. Silver sulfadiazine (Silvadene). JAMA. 1974;230:1184–5.
5. Mayer KH, Hopkins JD, Gilleece ES, et al. Molecular evolution, species distribution, and clinical consequences of an endemic aminoglycoside resistance plasmid. Antimicrob Agents Chemother. 1986;29:628–33.
6. McHugh G, Moellering RC Jr, Hopkins CC, et al. *Salmonella typhimurium* resistant to silver nitrate, chloramphenicol and ampicillin: a new threat in burn units? Lancet. 1975;1:235–40.
7. Woods DD. Relation of p-aminobenzoic acid to mechanism of action of sulphamilamide. Br J Exp Pathol. 1940;21:74–90.
8. Fildes P. Rational approach to research in chemotherapy. Lancet. 1940;1:955–7.
9. Miller AK, Bruno P, Berglund RM. The effect of sulfathiazol on the in vitro synthesis of certain vitamins by *Escherichia coli*. J Bacteriol. 1947;54:9.
10. Brown GH. The biosynthesis of pteridines. Adv Enzymol. 1971;35:35–77.
11. Richmond MH. Structural analogy and chemical reactivity in the action of antibacterial compounds, In: Biochemical Studies of Antimicrobial Drugs. Proceedings of the Sixteenth Symposium of the Society of General Microbiology. London: Cambridge University Press; 1966:301.
12. Hamilton-Miller JMJ. Mechanisms and distribution of bacterial resistance to diaminopyrimidines and sulphonamides. J Antimicrob Chemother. 1979;5(Suppl B):61–73.
13. Landy M, Larkun NW, Oswald EJ, et al. Increased synthesis of p-aminobenzoic acid associated with the development of resistance in *Staph aureus*. Science. 1943;97:265–67.
14. Wolf B, Hotchkiss RD. Genetically modified folic acid synthesising enzymes in pneumococcus. Biochemistry. 1940;2:145–50.
15. Landy M, Gerstung RB. p-Aminobenzoic acid synthesis by *Neisseria gonorrhoeae* in relation to clinical and cultural sulfonamide resistance. J Bacteriol. 1944;47:448.
16. Swedberg G, Castensson S, Sköld O. Characterization of mutationally altered dihydropteroate synthase and its ability to form a sulfonamide-containing dihydrofolate analog. J Bacteriol. 1979;137:129–36.
17. Sköld O: R-factor mediated resistance to sulfonamides by a plasmid-borne, drug resistant dihydropteroate synthase. Antimicrob Agents Chemother. 1976;9:49–54.

18. Kabins SA, Panse MV, Cohen S. Role of R-factor and bacterial host in sulfonamide resistance mediated by R-factor in *Escherichia coli*. J Infect Dis. 1971;123:158–68.
19. Watanabe T. Infective heredity of multiple drug resistance in bacteria. Bacteriol Rev. 1963;27:87–115.
20. Then RL. Mechanisms of resistance to trimethoprim, the sulfonamides and trimethoprim–sulfamethoxazole. Rev Infect Dis. 1982;4:261–9.
21. Burman LG. Apparent absence of transferable resistance to nalidixic acid in pathogenic gram-negative bacteria. J Antimicrob Chemother. 1977;3:509–14.
22. Hansson HB, Walder M, Juhlin I. Susceptibility of shigellae to mecillinam, nalidixic acid, trimethoprim, and five other antimicrobial agents. Antimicrob Agents Chemother. 1981;19:271–4.
23. Davies JR, Farrant WN, Uttley AHC. Antibiotic resistance of *Shigella sonnei*. Lancet. 1970;2:1157–60.
24. Gordon RC, Thompson TR, Carlson W, et al. Antimicrobial resistance of shigellae isolated in Michigan. JAMA. 1975;231:1159–64.
25. Ryder RW, Blake PA, Murlin AC, et al. Increase in antibiotic resistance among isolates of salmonella in the United States, 1967–1975. J Infect Dis. 1980;142:485–91.
26. Albritton WL, Brunton JL, Slaney L, Maclean I. Plasmid-mediated sulfonamide resistance in *Haemophilus ducreyi*. Antimicrob Agents Chemother. 1982;21:159–66.
27. Garrod LP, Lambert HP, O'Grady F. Antibiotic and Chemotherapy. 4th ed. Edinburgh and London: Churchill Livingstone; 1973.
28. Bushby SRM. Trimethoprim–sulfamethoxazole: in vitro microbiologic aspects. J Infect Dis. 1973;128:S442–62.
29. Bach MC, Finland M, Gold W, et al. Susceptibility of recently isolated pathogenic bacteria to trimethoprim and sulfamethoxazole separately and combined. J Infect Dis. 1973;128:S508–33.
30. Anand N. Sulfonamides and sulfones, In: Corcoran JW, Hahn FE, eds. Antibiotics III: Mechanism of Action of Antimicrobial and Antitumor Agents. Berlin: Springer-Verlag; 1975:668.
31. Sparr RA, Pritchard JA. Maternal and newborn distribution and excretion of sulfamethoxypyridazine (Kynex). Obstet Gynecol. 1958;12:131–4.
32. Craig WA, Kunin CM. Trimethoprim–sulfamethoxazole: pharmacodynamic effects of urinary pH and impaired renal function. Ann Intern Med. 1973;78:491–7.
33. Markowitz N, Saravolatz LD. Use of trimethoprim–sulfamethoxazole in a glucose-6-phosphate dehydrogenase-deficient population. Rev Infect Dis. 1987;9:S218–25.
34. Dunea G, Freedman P. Proteinuria. JAMA. 1968;203:973–84.
35. Hansten PD. Drug Interactions. 2nd ed. Philadelphia: Lea & Febiger; 1973.
36. Griffin JP, D'Arcy PF. A Manual of Adverse Drug Interactions. Bristol: John Wright and Sons; 1975:63.
37. Ahn CH, Wallace RJ Jr, Steel LC, et al. Sulfonamide-containing regimens for disease caused by rifampin-resistant *Mycobacterium kansasii*. Am Rev Respir Dis. 1987;135:10–6.
38. Peppercorn MA. Sulfasalazine: pharmacology, clinical use, toxicity, and related new drug development. Ann Intern Med. 1984;3:377–84.
39. Pullar T, Hunter JA, Capell HA. Sulphasalazine in rheumatoid arthritis: a double-blind comparison of sulphasalazine with placebo and sodium aurothiomalate. Br Med J. 1983;287:1102–6.
40. Burchall JJ. Trimethoprim and pyrimethamine, In: Corcoran JW, Hahn FE, eds. Antibiotics III: Mechanism of Antimicrobial and Antitumor Agents. Berlin: Springer-Verlag; 1975:304.
41. Hitchings GT. The biochemical basis for the antimicrobial activity of septrin. In: Bernstein LS, Salter AJ, eds. Trimethoprim/Sulphamethoxazole in Bacterial Infections. Edinburgh and London: Churchill Livingstone, 1973:7–16.
42. Phillips I, Warren C. Activity of sulfamethoxazole and trimethoprim against *Bacteroides fragilis*. Antimicrob Agents Chemother. 1976;9:736–40.
43. Trehane JD, Day J, Yeo CK, et al. Susceptibility of chlamydiae to chemotherapeutic agents. In Hobsen D, Holmes KK, eds. Nongonococcal Urethritis and Related Infections. Washington, DC: Am Soc Microbiology; 1977:214–22.
44. Moody MR, Young VM. In vitro susceptibility of *Pseudomonas cepacia* and *Pseudomonas maltophilia* to trimethoprin and trimethoprim–sulfamethoxazole. Antimicrob Agents Chemother. 1975;7:836–9.
45. Najjar A, Murray BE. Failure to demonstrate a consistent in vitro bactericidal effect of trimethoprim sulfamethoxazole against enterococci. Antimicrob Agents Chemother. 1987;31:808–10.
45a. Goodhart GL. In vivo versus in vitro susceptibility of enterococcus to trimethoprim-sulfamethoxazole. JAMA. 1984;252:2748–9.
46. Dornbusch K, Moore WB. The effects of different media on the response of bacteria to sulphonamides and trimethoprim using the disc-diffusion method and regression line analysis, In: Bernstein LS, Salter AJ, eds. Trimethoprim/Sulphamethoxazole in Bacterial Infections. Edinburgh and London: Churchill Livingstone; 1973:39–51.
47. Simmons NA. Colistin, sulphamethoxazole and trimethoprim in synergy against gram-negative bacilli. J Clin Pathol. 1970;23:757–64.
48. Parsley TL, Provonchee RB, Glicksman C, et al. Synergistic activity of trimethoprim and amikacin against gram-negative bacilli. Antimicrob Agents Chemother. 1977;12:349–54.
49. Bushby SRM. Sensitivity patterns and use of a combined disc of trimethoprim–sulphamethoxazole, In: Bernstein LS, Salter AJ, eds. Trimethoprim/Sulphamethoxazole in Bacterial Infections. Edinburgh and London: Churchill Livingstone; 1973:31–8.
50. Goldstein FW, Papadopoulou B, Acar JF. The changing of trimethoprim resistance in Paris, with a review of worldwide experience. Rev Infect Dis. 1986;8:725–37.
51. Armstrong RW, Slater B. *Listeria monocytogenes* meningitis treated with trimethoprim–sulfamethoxazole. Pediatr Infect Dis J. 1986;5:712–3.
52. Riley TV, Degiovanni C, Hoyne GF. Susceptibility of *Branhamella catarrhalis* to sulphamethoxazole and trimethoprim. J Antimicrob Chemother. 1987;19:39–43.
53. Wallace RJ Jr, Swanson JM, Silcox VA, et al. Treatment of nonpulmonary infections due to *Mycobacterium fortuitum* and *Mycobacterium chelonei* based on in vitro susceptibility. J Infect Dis. 1985;152:500–14.
54. Bohni E. Vergleichende bakteriologishe untersuchungen mit der Kombination Trimethoprim Sulfamethoxazole in vitro and in vivo. Chemotherapy. 1969;14(Suppl):1–21.
55. O'Brien TF, Acar JF, Altmann G, et al. Laboratory surveillance of synergy between and resistance to trimethoprim and sulfonamides. Rev Infect Dis. 1982;4:351–7.
56. Richards HN, Datta N, Sojka NJ, et al. Trimethoprim resistance plasmids and transposons in Salmonella. Lancet. 1978;2:1194–5.
57. Burchall JJ, Pelwell L, Fling ME. Molecular mechanisms of resistance to trimethoprim. Rev Infect Dis. 1982;4:246–54.
58. Houvinen P. Trimethoprim resistance. Antimicrob Agents Chemother. 1987;31:1451–6.
59. Goldstein FW, Labigne-Roussel A, Gerbaud G, et al. Transferable plasmid-mediated antibiotic resistance in *Acinetobacter*. Plasmid. 1983;10:138–47.
59a. Sundstrom L, Vinayagamoorthy T, Skold O. Novel type of plasmid-borne resistance to trimethoprim. Antimicrob Agents Chemother. 1987;31:60–6.
60. Steen R, Sköld O. Plasmid-borne or chromosomally mediated resistance by Tn7 is the most common response to ubiquitous use of trimethoprim. Antimicrob Agents Chemother. 1985;27:933–7.
61. Fleming MP, Datta N, Grüneberg RN. Trimethoprim resistance determined by R factors. Br Med J. 1972;1:726–8.
62. Saroglou G, Parakevopoulou P, Paniara O, Kontomichalou P. Trimethoprim resistance plasmids from Enterobacteriaceae isolated in Greece. In: Mitsuhashi S, Rosival L, Krcméry V, eds. Antibiotic Resistance. Berlin: Springer-Verlag; 1980:267–71.
63. Agarwal KC, Panhotra BR, Mahanta J, et al. Typhoid fever due to chloramphenicol resistant *Salmonella typhi* associated with R-plasmid. Indian J Med Res. 1981;73:484–8.
64. Goldstein FW, Chumpitaz JC, Guevara JM, et al. Plasmid-mediated resistance to multiple antibiotics in *Salmonella typhi*. J Infect Dis. 1986;153:261–6.
65. O'Brien TF, Hopkins JD, Gilleece ES, et al. Molecular epidemiology of antibiotic resistance in *Salmonella* from animals and human beings in the United States. N Engl J Med. 1982;307:1–6.
66. Mayer KH, Fling ME, Hopkins JD, et al. Trimethoprim resistance in multiple genera of Enterobacteriaceae at a U.S. hospital: spread of the type II dihydrofolate reductase gene by a single plasmid. J Infect Dis. 1985;5:783–9.
67. Murray BE, Alvarado T, Kim K-H, et al. Increasing resistance to trimethoprim–sulfamethoxazole among isolates of *Escherichia coli* in developing countries. J Infect Dis. 1985;152:1107–3.
68. Smith HW, Tucker JF. The virulence of trimethoprim resistant thymine-requiring strains of *Salmonella*. J Hyg (Lond). 1976;76:97–108.
69. Maskell R, Okubadejo OA, Payne RH, et al. Human infections with thymine-requiring bacteria. J Med Microbiol. 1978;11:33–45.
70. Grose WE, Bodey GP, Loo TL. Clinical pharmacology of intravenously administered trimethoprim–sulfamethoxazole. Antimicrob Agents Chemother. 1979;15:447–51.
71. Bach MC, Gold O, Finland M. Absorption and urinary excretion of trimethoprim, sulfamethoxazole, and trimethoprim–sulfamethoxazole: results with single doses in normal young adults and preliminary observations during therapy with trimethoprim–sulfamethoxazole. J Infect Dis. 1973;128:S584–98.
72. Kaplan SA, Weinfeld RE, Abruzzo CW, et al. Pharmacokinetic profile of trimethoprim–sulfamethoxazole in man. J Infect Dis. 1973;128:S547–55.
73. Pater RB, Welling PG. Clinical pharmacokinetics of co-trimoxazole (trimethoprim/sulfamethoxazole). Clin Pharmacokinet. 1980;5:405–23.
74. Winningham DG, Nemoy NJ, Stamey TA. Diffusion of antibiotics from plasma into prostatic fluid. Nature. 1968;219:139–43.
75. Meares EM Jr. Prostatitis: Review of pharmacokinetics and therapy. Rev Infect Dis. 1982;4:475–83.
76. Welling PG, Craig WA, Amidon GL, et al. Pharmacokinetics of trimethoprim and sulfamethoxazole in normal subjects and in patients with renal failure. J Infect Dis. 1973;128(Suppl):556–66.
77. Salter AJ. Trimethoprin sulfamethoxazole: an assessment of more than 12 years of use. Rev Infect Dis. 1982;4:196–236.
78. Jick H. Adverse reactions to trimethoprim–sulfamethoxazole in hospitalized patients. Rev Infect Dis. 1982;4:426–8.
79. Lawson DH, Paice BJ. Adverse reactions to trimethoprim–sulfamethoxazole. Rev Infect Dis. 1982;4:429–33.
80. Masur H, Kovacs JA. Treatment and prophylaxis of *Pneumocystis carinii* pneumonia. In: Moellering RC Jr, ed. Infectious Disease Clinics of North America (Medical Management of AIDS). Philadelphia: WB Saunders; 1988:419–28.
81. Wofsy CB. Use of trimethoprim–sulfamethoxazole in the treatment of *Pneumocystis carinii* pneumonitis in patients with acquired immunodeficiency syndrome. Rev Infect Dis. 1987;9:S184–91.

82. Gordin FM, Simon GL, Wofsy CB, et al. Adverse reactions to trimethoprim–sulfamethoxazole in patients with acquired immunodeficiency syndrome. Ann Intern Med. 1984;100:495–9.
83. Silvestri RC, Jensen WA, Zibrak JD, et al. Pulmonary infiltrates and hypoxemia in patients with the acquired immunodeficiency syndrome re-exposed to trimethoprim–sulfamethoxazole. Am Rev Respir Dis. 1987;136:1003–4.
84. Cameron A, Thomas M. Pseudomembranous colitis and co-trimoxazole. Br Med J. 1977;1:1321.
85. Bailey RR, Little PJ. Deterioration in renal function in association with co-trimoxazole therapy. Med J Aust. 1976;1:914–6.
86. Trollfors B, Wahl, Alestig K. Co-trimoxazole, creatinine and renal function. J Infect. 1980;2:221.
87. Hansen JM, Kampmann JP, Sierbaek-Nielsenk, et al. The effect of different sulfonamides on phenytoin metabolism in man. Acta Med Scand [Suppl] 1979;624:106–10.
88. Bernstein LS. Combination of trimethoprim with sulfonamides other than sulfamethoxazole. Rev Infect Dis. 1982;4:411–8.
89. Bergan T, Allgulander S, Fellner H. Pharmacokinetics of co-trimazine (sulphadiazine plus trimethoprim) in geriatric patients. Chemotherapy. 1986;32:478–85.
90. Dylewski J, D'Costa LJ, Nsanze H, et al. Single dose therapy with trimethoprim—sulfametrole for chancroid in females. Sex Transm Dis. 1986;13:166–8.
91. Brumfitt W, Hamilton-Miller JMT. Rifamprim (rifampicin plus trimethoprim): pharmacokinetics and effects on the normal flora of man. Biopharm Drug Dispos. 1981;2:157–66.
92. Kerry DW, Hamilton-Miller JMT, Brumfitt W. Trimethoprim and rifampicin: in vitro activities separately and in combination. J Antimicrob Chemother. 1975;1:417–27.
93. Alvarez S, DeMaria A Jr, Kulkarni R, et al. Interactions of rifampin and trimethoprim in vitro. Rev Infect Dis. 1982;4:390–401.
94. Zinner SH, Lagast H, Kasry A, et al. Synergism of trimethoprim combined with aminoglycosides in vitro and in serum of volunteers. Eur J Clin Microbiol. 1982;1:144–8.
95. Salter AJ. Trimethoprim–sulfamethoxazole in treatment of severe infections. Rev Infect Dis. 1982;4:338–50.
96. Leoung GS, Mills J, Hopewell PC, et al. Dapsone–trimethoprim for *Pneumocystis carinii* pneumonia in acquired immunodeficiency syndrome. Ann Intern Med. 1986;105:48–54.
97. Mills J, Leoung G, Medina I, et al. Dapsone is ineffective therapy for *Pneumocystis* pneumonia in patients with AIDS (Abstract). Clin Res. 1986;34:101A.
98. Tolkoff-Rubin NE, Weber D, Fang LST, et al. Single dose therapy with trimethoprim–sulfamethoxazole for urinary tract infection in women. Rev Infect Dis. 1982;4:444–8.
99. Counts GW, Stamm WE, McKevitt M, et al. Treatment of cystitis in women with a single dose of trimethoprim–sulfamethoxazole. Rev Infect Dis. 1982;4:484–90.
100. Gleckman R, Crowley M, Natsios GA. Treatment of recurrent invasive urinary-tract infections of men. N Engl J Med. 1979;301:878–80.
101. Harding GKM, Ronald AR, Nicolle LE, et al. Long-term antimicrobial prophylaxis for recurrent urinary tract infection in women. Rev Infect Dis. 1982;4:438–43.
102. Stamey TA. Recurrent urinary tract infections in female patients: an overview of management and treatment. Rev Infect Dis. 1987;9:S195–208.
103. Brumfitt W, Pursell R. Double-blind trial to compare ampicillin, cephalexin, co-trimoxazole and trimethoprim in treatment of urinary infection. Br Med J. 1972;2:673–6.
104. Kasanen A, Toivanen P, Sourander L, et al. Trimethoprim in the treatment of long-term control of urinary tract infection. Scand J Infect Dis. 1974;6:91–6.
105. Iravani A, Richard GA, Baer H. Treatment of uncomplicated urinary tract infection with trimethoprim versus sulfisoxazole with special reference to antibody-coated bacteria and faecal flora. Antimicrob Agents Chemother. 1981;19:842–50.
106. Stamm WE, Counts GW, Wagner KR, et al. Antimicrobial prophylaxis or recurrent urinary tract infections. Ann Intern Med. 1980;92:770–5.
107. Reeves D. Sulphonamides and trimethoprim. Lancet. 1982;2:370–3.
108. Amyes SGB, Doherty CJ, Wonnacott S. Trimethoprim and co-trimoxazole: a comparison of the use in respiratory tract infections. Scand J Infect Dis. 1986;18:561–6.
109. Pandy GJ. Trimethoprim/sulphamethoxazole and doxycycline in acute exacerbations of chronic bronchitis in general practice: a comparative study. Med J Aust. 1979;1:264–6.
110. Pines A. Trimethoprim–sulfamethoxazole in the treatment and prevention of purulent exacerbations of chronic bronchitis. J Infect Dis. 1973;128:S706–9.
111. Schmidt U, Sen P, Kapila R, et al. Clinical evaluation of intravenous trimethoprim sulfamethoxazole for serious infections. Rev Infect Dis. 1982;4:332–7.
112. Shurin PA, Pelton SI, Donner A, et al. Trimethoprim–sulfamethoxazole compared with ampicillin in the treatment of acute otitis media. J Pediatr. 1980;96:1081–87.
113. Nelson JD, Kusmiesz H, Shelton S. Oral or intravenous trimethoprim–sulfamethoxazole therapy for shigellosis. Rev Infect Dis. 1982;4:546–50.
114. Bannatyne RM, Toma S, Cheung R, et al. Resistance to trimethoprim and other antibiotics in Ontario shigellae (Letter). Lancet. 1980;1:425–6.
115. Thoren A, Wolde-Mariam I, Stintzing G, et al. Antibiotics in the treatment of gastroenteritis caused by enteropathogenic *Escherichia coli*. J Infect Dis. 1980;141:27–31.
116. DuPont HL, Evans DG, Rios N, et al. Prevention of travelers' diarrhea with trimethoprim–sulfamethoxazole. Rev Infect Dis. 1982;4:533–9.
117. DuPont HL, Reves RR, Galindo E, et al. Treatment of travelers' diarrhea with trimethoprim-/sulfamethoxazole and with trimethoprim alone. N Engl J Med. 1982;307:841–4.
118. Francis TI, Lewis EA, Oyediran ABOO, et al. Effect of chemotherapy on the duration of diarrhoea, and on vibrio excretion by cholera patients. J Trop Med Hyg. 1971;74:172–6.
119. Threlfall EJ, Rowe B, Huq I. Plasmid-encoded multiple antibiotic resistance in *Vibrio cholerae* El Tor from Bangladesh (Letter). Lancet. 1980;1:1247–8.
120. Svindland HB. Treatment of gonorrhoea with sulphamethoxazole–trimethoprim. Lack of effect on concomitant syphilis. Br J Vener Dis. 1973;49:50–3.
121. Lawrence A, Phillips E, Nicol C. Various regimens of trimethoprim–sulfamethoxazole in the treatment of gonorrhea. J Infect Dis. 1973;128(Suppl):S673–8.
122. Rahim G. Single dose treatment of gonorrhoea with cotrimoxazole. A report on 1,223 cases. Br J Vener Dis. 1975;51:179–82.
123. Centers for Disease Control. 1985 STD treatment guidelines. MMWR [Suppl]. 1985;34:4S.
124. Centers for Disease Control. Chromosomally mediated resistant *Neisseria gonorrhoeae*—United States. MMWR. 1984;33:408–10.
125. Hammerschlag MR. Activity of trimethoprim–sulfamethoxazole against *Chlamydia trachomatis* in vitro. Rev Infect Dis. 1982;4:500–5.
126. Daikos GK, Papapolyzos N, Marketos N, et al. Trimethoprim–sulfamethoxazole in brucellosis. J Infect Dis. 1973;128(Suppl):S731–3.
127. Bajpai J, Chaturvedi Sn, Khanuja SPS. Chemotherapy of acute bone and joint infections. Int Surg. 1977;62:172–4.
128. Millard FJC. Trimethoprim/sulphamethoxazole in the treatment of chronic osteomyelitis. In Bernstein LS, Salter AJ, eds. Trimethoprim–Sulphamethoxazole in Bacterial Infections. Edinburgh: Churchill Livingstone; 1973:195–9.
129. Lakshmanan CDS. Comparative evaluation of cotrimoxazole and demeclocycline in periodontal bacterial infection (Abstract 128). J Dent Res. 1976;55(Special issue D):D137.
130. Mahgoub ES. Medical management of mycetoma. Bull WHO. 1976;54:303.
131. Welsh O, Sauceda E, Gonzalez J, et al. Amikacin alone and in combination with trimethoprim–sulfamethoxazole in the treatment of actinomycotic mycetoma. J Am Acad Dermatol. 1987;17:443–8.
132. Wallace RJ, Septimus EJ, Williams JH, et al. Use of trimethoprim–sulfamethoxazole for the treatment of infections due to *Nocardia*. Rev Infec Dis. 1982;4:315–25.
133. Morrison IM. Chronic melioidosis. Proc R Soc Med. 1970;63:239–49.
134. Neu HC, Garvey GJ, Bleach MP. Successful treatment of *Pseudomonas cepacia* endocarditis in a heroin addict with trimethoprim sulfamethoxazole. J Infect Dis. 1973;128(Suppl):768–70.
135. Viteri AL, Greene JF Jr, Chandler JB Jr. Whipple's disease, successful response to sulfamethoxazole–trimethoprim. Am J Gastroenterol. 1981;75:309–14.
135a. Deremee RA, McDonald TJ, Weiland LH. Wegener's granulomatosis: observations on treatment with antimicrobial agents. Mayo Clin Proc. 1985;60:27–32.
136. Geddes AM, Ball AP, Farrell ID. Co-trimoxazole for the treatment of serious infections. J Antimicrob Chemother. 1979;5(Suppl B):221–30.
137. Quintiliani R, Levitz RE, Nightingale CH. Potential role of trimethoprim–sulfamethoxazole in the treatment of serious hospital-acquired infections. Rev Infect Dis. 1987;9:S160–5.
137a. Sattler FR, Remington JS. Intravenous sulfamethoxazole and trimethoprim for serious gram-negative bacillary infection. Arch Intern Med. 1983; 143:1709–12.
138. Menichetti F, Del Favero A, Guerciolini R, et al. Empiric antimicrobial therapy in febrile granulocytopenic patients. Randomized prospective comparison of amikacin plus piperacillin with and without parenteral trimethoprim sulphamethoxazole. Infection. 1986;14:261–7.
139. Young LS, Hindler J. Use of trimethoprim–sulfamethoxazole singly and in combination with other antibiotics in immunocompromised patients. Rev Infect Dis. 1987;9:S177–81.
139a. Levitz RE, Quintilliani R. Trimethoprim-sulfamethoxazole for bacterial meningitis. Ann Int Med. 1984;100:881–90.
140. Israelski DM, Remington JS. Toxoplasmic encephalitis in patients with AIDS. In: Moellering RC Jr, ed. Infectious Disease Clinics of North America (Medical Management of AIDS). Philadelphia: WB Saunders; 1988:429–45.
141. Wallace RJ, Wissk, Bushby MB, et al. In vitro activity of trimethoprim and sulfamethoxazole against nontuberculosis mycobacteria. Rev Infect Dis. 1982;4:326–31.
142. Sattler RF, Remington JS. Intravenous trimethoprim–sulfamethoxazole therapy for *Pneumocystis carinii* pneumonia. Am J Med. 1981;70:1215–21.
143. Young LS. Trimethoprim–sulfamethoxazole in the treatment of adults with pneumonia due to *Pseumocystis carinii*. Rev Infect Dis. 1982;4:608–13.
144. Wharton JM, Coleman DL, Wofsy CB, et al. Trimethoprim-sulfamethoxa-

zole or pentamidine for *Pneumocystis carinii* pneumonia in the acquired immunodeficiency syndrome, Ann Int Med. 1986;105:37–44.
145. Hughes WT, Smith BL. Intermitten chemoprophylaxis for *Pneumocystis carinii* pneumonia. Antimicrob Agents Chemother. 1983;24:300–5.
146. Fischl MA, Dickinson GM. Trimethoprim–sulfamethoxazole prophylaxis of *Pneumocystis carinii* pneumonia in acquired immunodeficiency syndrome (Abstract 436). In: Program and Abstracts of the 25th Interscience Conference on Antimicrobial Agents and Chemotherapy. Washington, DC: American Society for Microbiology; 1985:230.
147. Gurwith M, Brunton J, Lank B, et al. A prospective controlled investigation of prophylactic trimethoprim/sulfamethoxazole in hospitalized granulocytopenic patients. Am J Med. 1979;66:248–56.
148. Kauffman CA, Liepman MA, Bergman AG, et al. Trimethoprin/sulfamethoxazole prophylaxis in neutropenic patients: reduction of infections and effect on bacterial and fungal flora. Am J Med. 1983;74:599–607.
149. Gualtieri RJ, Donowitz GR, Kaiser DC, et al. Double-blind randomized study of prophylactic trimethoprim/sulfamethoxazole in granulocytopenic patients with hematologic malignancies. Am J Med. 1983;74:934–40.
150. EORTC International Antimicrobial Therapy Project Group. Trimethoprim–sulfamethoxazole in the prevention of infection in neutropenic patients. J Infect Dis. 1984;150:372–9.
151. Wade JC, Schimpff SC, Hargadon MT, et al. A comparison of trimethoprim–sulfamethoxazole plus nystatin with gentamicin plus nystatin in the prevention of infections in acute leukemia. N Engl J Med. 1981;304:1057–62.
152. Wade JC, de Jongh CA, Newman KA, et al. Selective antimicrobial modulation as prophylaxis against infection during granulocytopenia: trimethoprim–sulfamethoxazole vs. nalidixic acid. J Infect Dis. 1983;147:624–34.
153. Overturf GD. Use of trimethoprim–sulfamethoxazole in pediatric infections: relative merits of intravenous administration. Rev Infect Dis. 1987;9:S168–73.

30. QUINOLONES

VINCENT T. ANDRIOLE

Most of the new antimicrobial agents that either have been or will be introduced for clinical use in the near future are the newer 4-quinolone antibacterial agents, particularly the 6-fluorinated piperazinyl quinolones. Nalidixic acid, described by Lescher and colleagues in 1962,[1] was the first in this series of agents. Oxolinic acid and cinoxacin were introduced in the 1970s. Shortly thereafter the development of the newer quinolones progressed rapidly and was spearheaded by the introduction of a fluorine at the 6 position in the basic nucleus. This procedure enhanced and broadened the antibacterial activity of these agents and led to the development of newer 4-quinolones with antibacterial activities 1000 times that of nalidixic acid.[2] The newer quinolones have an extremely broad antibacterial spectrum, unique mechanism of action, good absorption from the gastrointestinal tract after oral administration, excellent tissue distribution, and low incidence of adverse reactions.[3]

CHEMISTRY AND CLASSIFICATION

All of the compounds in the quinolone class of antibacterial agents are structurally similar. Yet, there are some differences in the basic nucleus so that they can be divided into four general groups, i.e., naphthyridines, cinnolines, pyrido-pyrimidines, and quinolones (Fig. 1). The addition of an oxygen at the 4 position in the basic nucleus of each of these groups produces a common skeleton, 4-oxo-1,4-dihydroquinolone, more commonly called *4-quinolone*.[2] The naphthyridines (nalidixic acid and enoxacin) have an additional nitrogen in the 8 position and are 8-aza-4-quinolones. The cinnolines (cinoxacin), with an additional nitrogen in the 2 position, are 2-aza-4-quinolones. The pyrido-pyrimidines (pipemidic and piromidic acids), with additional nitrogens in the 6 and 8 positions, are 6,8-diaza-4-quinolones (Fig. 2). All of the other agents (oxolinic acid, norfloxacin, ciprofloxacin, ofloxacin, pefloxacin, amifloxacin, fleroxacin, flumequine, lomefloxacin, temafloxacin, difloxacin, acrosoxacin [rosoxacin], piroxacin, and irloxacin [pirfloxacin]) are classified simply as 4-quinolones (Fig. 3).[2,3] Numerous additional compounds have been synthesized and are undergoing development.[3]

Structural features common to the 4-quinolones include a carboxyl group at the 3 position and a piperazine ring (except flumequine and oxolinic acid) at the 7 position of the quinolone nucleus. The introduction of a fluorine at the 6 position and substitutions at the 1 and 8 positions of the quinolone or naphthyridine nucleus and the para position of the piperazine ring are responsible for differences in the in vitro activity and pharmacologic properties of these compounds (Figs. 2 and 3).[4]

Nalidixic acid (1-ethyl-7-methyl-1, 8-naphthyridine-4-one-3-carboxylic acid) is one of a series of 1,8-naphthyridine derivatives first described by Lesher and colleagues in 1962.[1] This compound is only slightly soluble in water but is readily soluble in dilute alkali and is stable in urine. Nalidixic acid is marketed as Neggram (Winthrop, 1964). Oxolinic acid (5-ethyl-5,8-dihydro-8-oxo-1,3-dioxolo-[4,5-g]-quinolone-7-carboxylic acid), a quinolone derivative, is a crystalline substance that is a weak organic acid.[5–7] Oxolinic acid is marketed by Utibid (Warner-Lambert, 1975). Cinoxacin [1-ethyl-1,4-dihydro-4-oxo (1,3)dioxolo(4,5-g)cinnoline-3-carboxylic acid] is similar to nalidixic acid.[8] It is a yellow-white crystalline solid with a pKa of 4.7, which is insoluble in water and poorly lipid soluble but is soluble in alkaline solution. Cinoxacin is marketed as Cinobac (Dista/Lilly, 1981). Norfloxacin [1-ethyl-6-fluoro-1,4-dihydro-4-oxo-7-(1-piperazinyl)-3-quinolone carboxylic acid (AM 715 or MK-0366) is similar to nalidixic acid.[9,10] It is a yellow-white crystalline solid only slightly soluble in water. Norfloxacin is marketed as Noroxin (Merck). Ciprofloxacin [1-cyclopropyl-6-fluoro-1,4-dihydro-4-oxo-7-(1-piperazinyl)-3-quinolone carboxylic acid hydrochloride] (Bay 09867) is also a new quinolone derivative similar in structure to nalidixic acid.[11] It is a light yellow crystalline substance slightly soluble in water. Ciprofloxacin is marketed as Cipro (Miles/Bayer). Additional new antibacterial agents that are currently under development and that will most likely be marketed in the near future include enoxacin [1-ethyl-6-fluoro-1,4-dihydro-4-oxo-7-(1-piperazinyl)-1,8-naphthyridine-3-carboxylic acid] (Warner-Lambert); ofloxacin [9-fluoro-2,3-dihydro-3-methyl-10-(4-methyl-1-piperazinyl)-7-oxo-7H-pyrido-[1,2,3,de][1,4]-benzoxacine-6-carboxylic acid] (Ortho); fleroxacin [6,8-difluoro-1-(2-fluoro-ethyl)-1,4-dihydro-7-(4-methyl-1-piperazinyl)-4-oxo-3-quinolone carboxylic acid] (Roche); lomefloxacin [1-ethyl-6-8-difluoro-1,4-dihydro-7-(3-methyl-1-piperazinyl)-4-oxo-3-quinolone carboxylic acid] (Searle); and pefloxacin [1-ethyl-6-fluoro-1,4-dihydro-7-(4-methyl-1-piperazinyl)-4-oxo-3-quinolone carboxylic acid] (Bellon/Dianippon).[3]

Also, acrosoxacin (rosoxacin) [1-ethyl-1,4-dihydro-4-oxo-7-(4-pyridyl)3-quinolone carboxylic acid] (Sterling), amifloxacin [6-fluoro-1,4-dihydro-1-methylamino-7-(4-methyl-1-piperazinyl)-4-oxo-3-quinolone carboxylic acid] (Sterling), flumequine [9-fluoro-6,7-dihydro-5-methyl-1-ozo-1H,5H-benzo-(ij)-2-quinolicine carboxylic acid] (Riker), difloxacin [6-fluoro-1(4-fluoro-phenyl -1,4-dihydro-7- (4-methyl-1-piperazinyl) -4-oxo-3-quinolone carboxylic acid] (Abbott), irloxacin (pirfloxacin) [1-ethyl-6-fluoro-1,4-dihydro-4-oxo-7- (1-pyrrolyl) -3-quinolone carboxylic acid] (Esteve), piroxacin [1-ethyl-1,4-dihydro-4-oxo-7-(1-pyrrolyl)-3-quinolone carboxylic acid] (Esteve), and temafloxacin [6-fluoro-1-(2,4-difluoro-phenyl)-1,4-dihydro-7-(4-methyl-1-piperazinyl)-4-oxo-3-quinolone carboxylic acid] (Abbott) along with a number of other compounds are also new antibacterial quinolones currently under development.[3,4]

MECHANISM OF ACTION

Early studies have shown that nalidixic acid rapidly inhibits DNA synthesis in susceptible bacterial cells, although not in mammalian cells, whereas protein and RNA synthesis continue.[12,13] Inhibition of DNA synthesis by nalidixic acid has

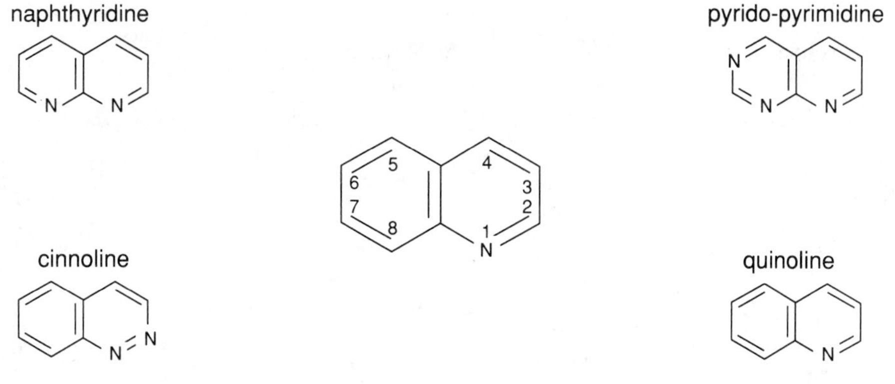

FIG. 1. Chemical structure of the four general groups of the 4-quinolones and its system of ring numbering. (Modified from Smith et al.,[2] with permission.)

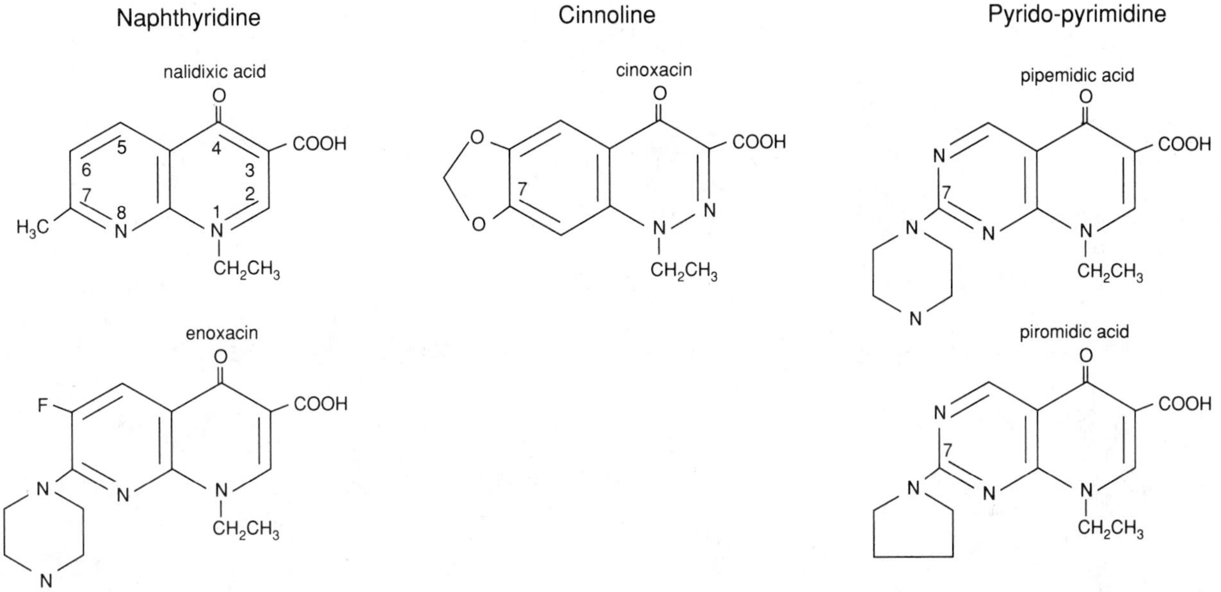

FIG. 2. Structures of naphthyridine, cinnoline, and pyrido-pyrimidine derivatives. (Modified from Smith et al.,[2] with permission.)

been shown to be reversible since bacterial cells exposed to the drug will resume growth when placed in drug-free media.[14] Nalidixic acid does not bind to purified DNA,[15] although recent work suggests that some quinolones may bind to DNA. Nalidixic acid does affect replication at a stage beyond the production of deoxynucleoside triphosphates and inhibits synthesis taking place on the double-stranded DNA template.[16] Recent studies indicate that the bactericidal activity of nalidixic acid as well as 4-quinolones is reduced significantly if RNA or protein synthesis is inhibited.[17] Although all 4-quinolones are bactericidal, these drugs exhibit a single most-bactericidal concentration, so greater or lesser concentrations result in less bacterial death.[2,13] This paradoxical effect of decreased killing at higher concentrations is most likely a dose-dependent inhibition of RNA synthesis.[2,13,14]

Other studies indicate that the mechanism of action of nalidixic acid is by inhibition of DNA topoisomerases (gyrases), of which four subunits (two A monomers and two B monomers) have been defined.[18,19] The topoisomerases, which have been found in every organism examined, are required to supercoil strands of bacterial DNA into the bacterial cell.[20,21] Each chromosomal domain is transiently nicked during supercoiling, which results in single-stranded DNA. When supercoiling is completed, the single-stranded DNA state is abolished by an enzyme that seals the nicked DNA. The sealing action of this enzyme is inhibited specifically by nalidixic acid.[2,13] The same enzyme, identified by Gellert et al.[22] and termed DNA gyrase or topoisomerase II (nicking–closing enzyme), nicks double-stranded chromosomal DNA, introduces supercoils, and seals the nicked DNA.[2,3,22–24] The A subunits are thought to introduce the nicks, the B subunits are thought to cause supercoiling, and then the A subunits seal the nick they produced initially.[2,24] Some of the newer 4-quinolones may act slightly differently from nalidixic acid, which prevents the A subunits from sealing the nicks in chromosomal DNA. The newer 4-quinolones may affect both the A and B subunits of DNA gyrase since mutations that affect the B subunit change the bacterial sensitivity to the 4-quinolones.[2,17,25,26] The identification of DNA gyrase has led to the development of new quinolone compounds that may have increased activity against DNA gyrase.

ANTIMICROBIAL ACTIVITY

Nalidixic acid has greater antimicrobial activity against gram-negative rods than against gram-positive bacteria (Table 1). It is active against most enterobacteriaceae. Approximately 99 percent of the strains of *Escherichia coli*, 98 percent of *Proteus mirabilis*, 75–97 percent of other *Proteus* sp., 92 percent of

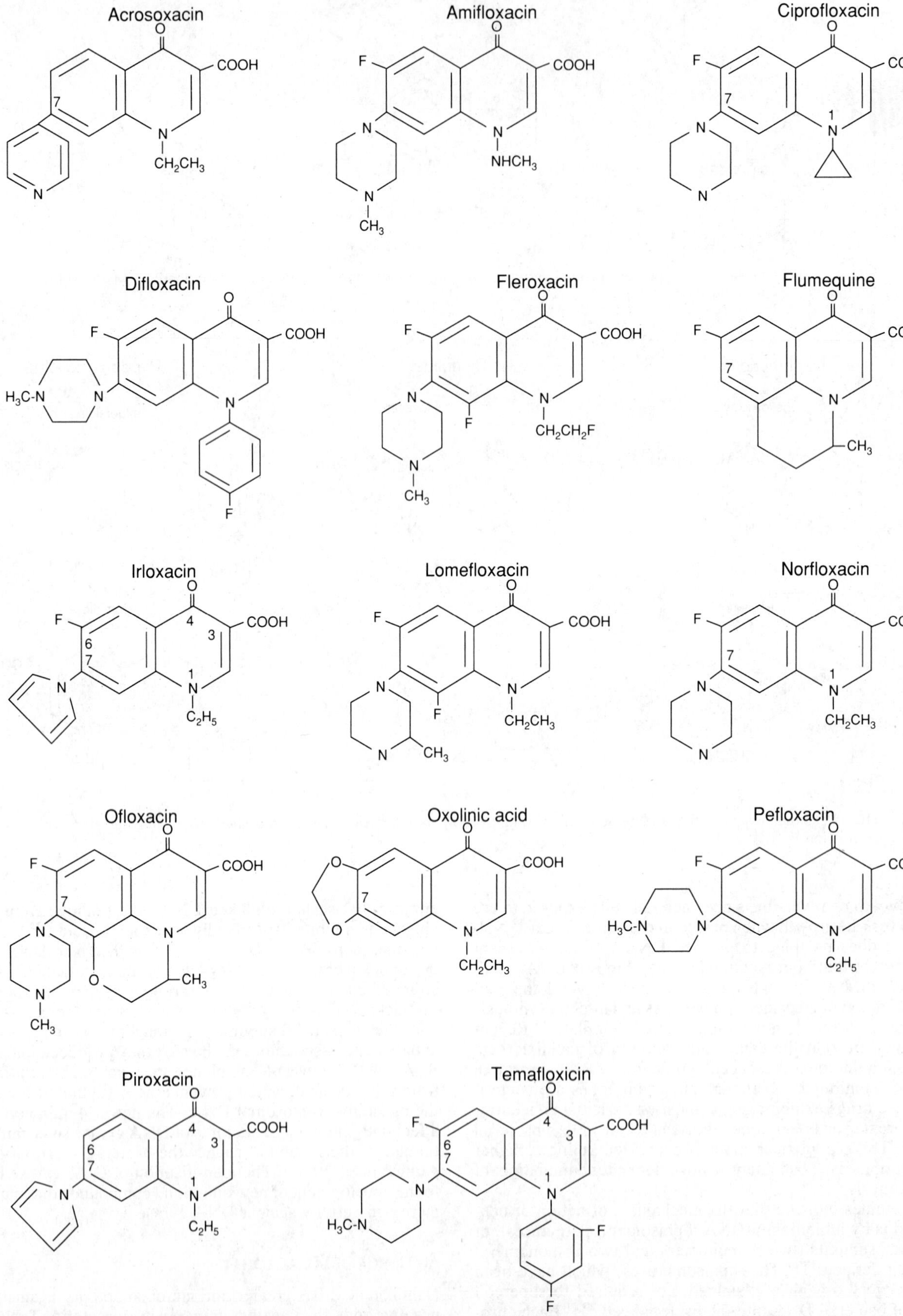

FIG. 3. Chemical structure of the 4-quinolones that are derivatives of the quinoline nucleus.

TABLE 1. In Vitro Activity of Selected 4-Quinolones

Organism	*Nalidixic Acid*	*Ciprofloxacin*	*Enoxacin*	*Norfloxacin*	*Ofloxacin*	*Perfloxacin*
Gram-negative aerobes						
E. coli	8 (4–128)[a]	0.03 (0.015–0.06)	0.5 (0.25–1)	0.125 (0.06–0.5)	0.125 (0.06–0.25)	0.125 (0.125–0.25)
K. pneumoniae	8 (1–128)	0.125 (0.06–0.25)	0.5	0.25 (0.125–1)	0.25	0.5
Enterobacter sp.	32 (4–128)	0.125 (0.03–0.5)	0.5 (0.25–4)	0.5 (0.125–2)	0.5 (0.125–1)	0.5 (0.25–1)
Citrobacter sp.	8 (4–>100)	0.03 (0.03–0.06)	0.5	0.25 (0.125–0.5)	0.5	0.5
S. marcescens	>128 (16–>256)	1 (0.25–2)	2 (0.5–4)	1 (0.5–8)	1 (0.25–2)	1 (0.25–2)
Shigella sp.	4	0.03 (0.015–0.06)	0.125	0.06 (0.03–0.125)	0.125 (0.06–0.125)	0.125
Salmonella sp.	8 (4–8)	0.015 (≤0.015–0.03)	0.25 (0.125–0.25)	0.125 (0.06–0.125)	0.125 (0.06–0.125)	0.125 (0.06–0.25)
P. mirabilis	16 (4–32)	0.06 (0.03–0.125)	0.5 (0.25–1)	0.25 (0.125–0.5)	0.25 (0.25–0.5)	0.5 (0.25–1)
Proteus sp. (indole-positive)	8 (4–16)	0.06	0.25 (0.25–0.5)	0.125 (0.06–0.125)	0.25	0.25
M. morganii	8 (2–8)	0.015 (0.015–0.03)	0.25 (0.25–0.5)	0.125 (0.03–0.25)	0.125 (0.125–0.25)	0.25 (0.25–0.5)
P. aeuruginosa	≥128	0.5 (0.25–1)	4 (2–8)	2 (0.06–8)	4 (2–4)	4 (2–8)
H. influenzae	1 (1–2)	0.015 (0.015–0.03)	0.125 (0.06–0.25)	0.06 (0.03–0.125)	0.03 (0.03–0.06)	0.06 (0.03–0.06)
L. pneumophila	NA	(0.03–0.125)	NA	(0.125–0.5)	NA	NA
N. gonorrhoeae	1 (1–2)	≤0.015	0.03 (0.015–0.06)	0.06 (0.015–0.125)	0.03 (0.015–0.06)	0.06 (0.03–0.06)
N. meningitidis	2	0.004	0.06	0.03	0.015	0.03
Gram-negative anaerobes						
B. fragilis	128 (64–256)	8 (4–32)	32 (16–128)	64 (16–>128)	4 (4–8)	16 (8–16)
Bacteroides sp.	256	16 (16–32)	32 (32–64)	128 (128–256)	NA	NA
Gram-positive aerobes						
S. aureus (MS)	≥128 (32–>128)	0.5 (0.25–1)	2 (1–4)	2 (1–4)	0.5 (0.25–1)	0.5 (0.125–1)
S. aureus (MR)	>64 (32–128)	0.5 (0.5–1)	2	2	0.5 (0.25–0.5)	1 (0.5–1)
S. epidermidis	>64 (64–128)	0.25 (0.125–0.5)	1	2 (1–4)	0.5 (0.25–1)	1 (0.5–2)
S. pneumoniae	≥128 (64–≥256)	1 (0.5–2)	16	16 (4–16)	2 (1–2)	8 (8–16)
S. pyogenes	≥128	1 (0.5–2)	8 (8–16)	16 (8–32)	4	8
S. agalactiae	>128 (>128–512)	1 (0.5–2)	16 (16–32)	16 (8–32)	2 (1–4)	16
Enterococcus	>128 (64–>128)	2 (0.5–2)	8 (8–16)	8 (4–32)	2 (2–4)	4
Gram-positive anaerobes						
Peptococcus	256	2	8	8	4	NA
Peptostreptococcus	≥64	1 (0.5–8)	8	4 (2–4)	2	NA
Clostridium sp.	≥256	16 (8–32)	32 (32–64)	64 (32–128)	16 (8–16)	NA

Abbreviations: NA: not available; MS: methicillin sensitive; MR: methicillin resistant.
[a] Values are means of the minimum 90 percent inhibitory concentration in micrograms per milliliter.
(From Norris et al.,[27] with permission.)

Klebsiella and *Enterobacter* spp., and 80 percent of other coliform bacteria are sensitive to the drug at concentrations that are easily achieved in the urine, that is, 16 μg/ml or lower.[1,28] Some strains of *Salmonella* and *Shigella* are also sensitive, and *Brucella* sp. may be sensitive. *Pseudomonas* sp. and *Serratia* sp. are resistant. Resistance of sensitive gram-negative bacteria to the drug can be induced in vitro by serial passage of these bacteria in increasing concentrations of nalidixic acid.[29] Resistance may also be acquired during treatment of bacteriuria, so repeat urine culture and sensitivity testing are of practical clinical importance.[30] Gram-positive bacteria including *Staphylococcus aureus*, *Streptococcus pneumoniae*, and *Enterococcus faecalis* are resistant to nalidixic acid.[1,18]

The antibacterial spectrum of activity of oxolinic acid is similar to nalidixic acid. It is primarily active against gram-negative bacteria with the exception of *Pseudomonas* sp. Oxolinic acid is significantly more active than nalidixic acid is in vitro and is two to four times more active in vivo.[5,31] Oxolinic acid inhibits 95 percent of the strains of *E. coli*, 92 percent of *P. mirabilis*, 89 percent of other *Proteus* sp., 91 percent of other coliform bacteria, and 64 percent of *Klebsiella–Enterobacter* isolates at concentrations of 1.56 μg/ml or less.[32] Although *Klebsiella–Enterobacter* isolates are less susceptible, 93 percent are inhibited by 6.25 μg/ml, an amount of oxolinic acid easily achieved in urine.[32] *Neisseria gonorrhoeae* and *Neisseria meningitidis* are also inhibited at concentrations of 0.01–0.19 μg/ml of the drug.[5] Except for *S. aureus* strains that are inhibited at concentrations of 6.25 μg/ml, oxolinic acid has no significant activity against other gram-positive bacteria or fungi.[5] Sensitive gram-negative bacteria can acquire resistance to oxolinic acid in a stepwise manner in vitro similar to that observed with nalidixic acid. Cross-resistance between these two agents has been demonstrated, that is, oxolinic acid–resistant strains are also resistant to nalidixic acid and vice versa. Also, resistance is not reversed in vitro even after 10–12 consecutive passages in drug-free media.[6] As with nalidixic acid, resistance to oxolinic acid may also be acquired during treatment of patients with bacteriuria, so follow-up urine culture and sensitivity testing are clinically important.[33]

The antibacterial spectrum of activity of cinoxacin, although similar to that of nalidixic acid, is greater against some bacterial species[8,34] but is less than that of oxolinic acid.[35] Cinoxacin is active against most strains of gram-negative bacteria that cause urinary tract infections at concentrations that are readily attained in the urine. Cinoxacin inhibits more than 90 percent of *E. coli* strains at a concentration of 16 μg/ml. It is active against all *Proteus* sp. and most strains of *Klebsiella*, *Enterobacter*, *Citrobacter*, *Providencia*, and *Serratia* spp. Cinoxacin also demonstrates in vitro activity against *Salmonella*, *Shigella*, *Alcaligenes*, *Acinetobacter*, *Moraxella*, and *Haemophilus* spp. as well as against *Clostridium perfringens*, *Clostridium tetani*, *N. meningitidis*, and *Pseudomonas pseudomallei*. Cinoxacin has negligible activity against *Pseudomonas aeruginosa* and gram-positive cocci such as *S. aureus*, *Staphylococcus saprophyticus*, *Streptococcus* sp., and enterococci.[8,34–36] Cross resistance among bacterial isolates develops among cinoxacin, nalidixic acid, and oxolinic acid.[35,37] Resistance to cinoxacin of organisms that are usually susceptible can be induced in vitro and is mediated presumably via chromosomes since there is no evidence that resistance is transferred as an extrachromosomal plasmid.[38]

Norfloxacin is 100 times more active than nalidixic acid is, with a spectrum that includes enterococci and staphylococci as well as *Pseudomonas*.[9] Norfloxacin is active against most strains of gram-negative and gram-positive bacteria that cause urinary tract infections at concentrations that are readily attained in the urine. Norfloxacin inhibits more than 90 percent of strains of *E. coli* at a concentration of 0.2 μg/ml, *Klebsiella* species at 0.4 μg/ml; *Salmonella* and *Shigella* species at 0.1 μg/ml; *Citrobacter* species at 0.4 μg/ml; *Enterobacter cloacae* at 0.2 μg/ml; *Enterobacter aerogenes* at 0.4 μg/ml; *Enterobacter agglomerans* at 0.2 μg/ml; *Proteus mirabilis* at 0.1 μg/ml; *Mor-*

ganella species at 0.2 μg/ml; *Proteus vulgaris* at 0.8 μg/ml; *Proteus rettgeri* at 0.3 μg/ml; *Providencia* species at 1.6 μg/ml; *Pseudomonas aeruginosa*, including gentamicin-resistant strains, at 0.8 μg/ml; *Pseudomonas maltophilia* at 3.1 μg/ml; *Serratia marcescens* at 3.1 μg/ml; *Acinetobacter calcoaceticus* at 8 μg/ml; and *Yersinia*, *Arizona*, *Aeromonas*, and *Campylobacter* at concentrations below 1 μg/ml. Norfloxacin is also active against *Haemophilus influenzae* at concentrations of 0.12 μg/ml; *Neisseria gonorrhoeae*, regardless of β-lactamase activity, at 0.016 μg/ml; and *Branhamella catarrhalis* at 0.25 μg/ml. Norfloxacin is somewhat less active against gram-positive species, with 90 percent of strains of *Staphylococcus aureus* inhibited at concentrations of 2 μg/ml, methicillin-resistant strains of *S. aureus* at 4.0 μg/ml, *S. saprophyticus* at 4 μg/ml, *S. epidermidis* at 1 μg/ml, *Streptococcus pyogenes* at 4–6 μg/ml, *Streptococcus agalactiae* at 8 μg/ml, *Enterococcus faecalis* at 12.5 μg/ml, *Streptococcus pneumoniae* at 16 μg/ml, and *Listeria* species at 3.1 μg/ml. Members of the *Bacteroides fragilis* group of anaerobes are relatively resistant to norfloxacin since they are inhibited at concentrations of 8–128 μg/ml, as are most other anaerobes. Norfloxacin has some activity against *Gardnerella vaginalis*, inhibiting 90 percent of isolates at 16–32 μg/ml, and *Ureaplasma urealyticum* at concentrations of 8 μg/ml.[10,31,39–43]

Ciprofloxacin, although similar in antibacterial activity, is even more potent than norfloxacin is. Ciprofloxacin is active against most strains of gram-negative and gram-positive bacteria that cause infections at concentrations that are easily attained in most tissues and body fluids. Ciprofloxacin inhibits more than 90 percent of strains of *E. coli* at a concentration of 0.06 μg/ml, *Klebsiella* species at 0.25 μg/ml, *Salmonella* and *Shigella* species at 0.015 and 0.008 μg/ml respectively, *Citrobacter diversus* at 0.03 μg/ml, *Citrobacter freundii* at 0.125 μg/ml, *Enterobacter cloacae* at 0.03 μg/ml, *Enterobacter aerogenes* at 0.06 μg/ml, *Proteus mirabilis* at 0.06 μg/ml, *Proteus vulgaris* at 0.06 μg/ml, *Morganella morganii* at 0.016 μg/ml, *Providencia stuartii* at 0.5 μg/ml, *Pseudomonas aeruginosa* at 0.25 μg/ml, *Pseudomonas maltophilia* at 4 μg/ml, *Pseudomonas cepacia* at 8 μg/ml, *Serratia marcescens* at 0.13 μg/ml, *Acinetobacter calcoaceticus* at 0.5 μg/ml, *Yersinia enterocolitica* at 0.06 μg/ml, *Campylobacter jejuni* at 0.12 μg/ml, *Aeromonas hydrophilia* at 0.008 μg/ml, and *Pasteurella multocida* at 0.016 μg/ml. Ciprofloxacin is also active against *H. influenzae* at concentrations of 0.015 μg/ml, *Branhamella catarrhalis* at 0.03 μg/ml, *Gardnerella vaginalis* at 1 μg/ml, and *Neisseria gonorrhoeae*, regardless of β-lactamase activity, at 0.004 μg/ml. In contrast to norfloxacin, ciprofloxacin is more active against *Bacteroides fragilis*, with 90 percent of strains inhibited at concentrations of 4 μg/ml, *Bacteroides melaninogenicus/oralis* group at 4 μg/ml, *Bacteroides urealyticus* at 0.06 μg/ml, *Fusobacteria* sp. at 4 μg/ml, *Mobiluncus* sp. at 1 μg/ml, and *Peptococcus* sp. at 2 μg/ml, *Peptostreptococcus* sp. at 2 μg/ml, and *Clostridia* sp. at 16 μg/ml. Similarly, ciprofloxacin is more active than norfloxacin is against gram-positive bacteria, with 90 percent of strains of *Staphylococcus aureus*, including methicillin-resistant strains, inhibited at concentrations of 0.5 μg/ml; *Staphylococcus epidermis* at 0.25 μg/ml; *Streptococcus pyogenes* at 1 μg/ml; *Streptococcus agalactiae* at 1 μg/ml; *Enterococcus faecalis* at 2 μg/ml; *Streptococcus pneumoniae* at 2 μg/ml; viridans streptococci at 2 μg/ml; *Legionella pneumophila* at 0.03–0.125 μg/ml; *Mycobacterium tuberculosis* at 0.25–1 μg/ml (atypical mycobacteria are less susceptible); and *Listeria monocytogenes* at 1 μg/ml. Compared with norfloxacin, ciprofloxacin has increased activity against all bacterial species studied. Ciprofloxacin has excellent activity against *Chlamydia trachomatis* and inhibits 90 percent of isolates at 1 μg/ml.[11,27,31,44–48]

The antibacterial activity of the newer 4-quinolones under development (listed before) are similar to that of ciprofloxacin, which, with few exceptions, is the most potent of the newer 4-quinolones.[31]

MECHANISMS OF BACTERIAL RESISTANCE

The selection in vitro of bacterial variants with reduced susceptibility to the quinolones has occurred after serial exposure of bacteria to subinhibitory drug concentrations.[27,31] These variants with reduced quinolones susceptibility have been obtained from gram-negative and gram-positive organisms. The resulting strains may exhibit cross-resistance to other quinolones. The mechanism of resistance usually involves either (1) mutations in the gene coding for DNA gyrase so that there is reduced quinolone affinity for the A subunit or (2) mutations that change the outer membrane porins.[27,31,45–51] Relative resistance to antibiotics unrelated to the quinolones has been observed when reduced susceptibility to the quinolones is caused by reduced outer membrane porin F activity.[31,52]

The exact mechanism for the development of bacterial resistance to the quinolones has not been determined. However, recent work suggests that the quinolones are unable to bind to DNA gyrase subunit A if serine, in the 83 position of subunit A, is replaced by tryptophan (L.M. Fisher, personal communication).

Since quinolones interfere with DNA gyrase activity, which is necessary for plasmid replication, plasmid-mediated quinolone resistance was not expected to occur. In fact, quinolones were expected to promote a loss of plasmids and inhibit the transfer of R-factor–mediated resistance.[27,53] However, recent reports suggest that plasmid-mediated resistance may be possible, although rare.[31,54,55]

PHARMACOLOGY

Nalidixic acid is administered by the oral route and is well absorbed (96 percent) from the gastrointestinal tract.[56] It is rapidly metabolized in the liver to hydroxynalidixic acid, which is biologically active, and to antibacterially inactive monoglucuronide conjugates, both of which, along with the parent compound, are rapidly excreted by the kidney into the urine. The biologically active drug in the plasma consists of the hydroxylated metabolite (one-third) and the parent compound (two-thirds), which are 63 and 93 percent, respectively, bound to plasma proteins.[57] Plasma levels of 20–50 μg/ml may be attained 2 hours after a single oral dose of 1 g of the drug.[58] The drug does not accumulate in tissues even after prolonged administration, and the kidney is the only organ in which tissue concentrations may exceed plasma levels.[56] Nalidixic acid does not diffuse into prostatic fluid.[59] It will appear in human milk of lactating mothers and therefore may be harmful to the newborn.[60] Excretion is almost completely via the kidney into the urine. About 85 percent of the drug in the urine is in the conjugated inactive form. Most of the remainder is present as biologically active hydroxynalidixic acid, which is 16 times more active than is the parent compound and is primarily responsible for the therapeutic effect of this drug in the treatment of urinary tract infection.[57] Urine concentrations of the active drug after a 0.5–1.0 g single oral dose in adults range from 25 to 250 μg/ml and remain between 100 and 500 μg/ml with a 1 g oral dose administered every 6 hours.[29,58] Bactericidal levels of the drug are also attained in the urine of patients with moderate or advanced renal failure.[58] The antibacterially active component of the drug does not accumulate in the serum of azotemic patients during continuous therapy[58] as do the inactive monoglucuronides that may also contribute to toxicity.[61] Although increased toxicity has not been observed in patients with advanced renal failure who were given the usual doses of nalidixic acid, the drug should be used cautiously in these patients as well as in patients with liver disease since conjugation of the drug may be impaired in this latter group.

Oxolinic acid is also administered orally, after which active and inactive metabolites are excreted in the urine and eliminated in the feces. Plasma levels of oxolinic acid after oral administration are low to borderline with respect to antimicrobic activity against susceptible bacteria. An effective bactericidal concentration for most susceptible microorganisms is achieved in the urine within 4 hours and is sustained for 12 hours after the recommended oral dose. The concentration of oxolinic acid attained in 24-hour urine collections after an oral dose of 2 g/day averaged 38 μg/ml with a range of 16–64 μg/ml.[62] Although oxolinic acid given to patients with moderate or advanced renal failure did not further impair or damage the kidney or interfere with the drug's renal excretion, it should be used cautiously in patients with severely impaired renal function. Since oxolinic acid is excreted in human milk, it is contraindicated in nursing mothers.

Cinoxacin is also administered orally and is rapidly and almost completely absorbed from the gastrointestinal tract. Peak plasma levels usually occur in 2–3 hours and are in the range of <4–14.8 and 2.8–28 μg/ml after an oral dose of 250 and 500 mg, respectively. Approximately 70 percent of cinoxacin is bound to plasma proteins. It has a serum half-life of approximately 1 hour, which may increase threefold in patients with creatinine clearance of less than 30 ml/min/1.73 m^2. Although concomitant ingestion of food delays the absorption of cinoxacin and causes a 30 percent reduction in mean peak plasma levels, overall recovery of the drug in urine is not affected significantly. Peak urine concentrations (88–925 μg/ml) occur within 4–6 hours and are decreased in patients with impaired renal function. Cinoxacin concentrations in human prostatic tissue range from 0.6 to 6.3 μg/g, whereas concentrations in renal tissue exceed those in serum.[63] Approximately 60 percent of an orally administered dose is excreted into the urine unchanged in patients with normal renal function, and 40 percent is metabolized by the liver. Cinoxacin is metabolized to at least four microbiologically inactive metabolites that represent approximately 30–40 percent of the ingested dose.[64] The renal clearance of cinoxacin exceeds the glomerular filtration rate, and probenecid inhibits cinoxacin excretion by the kidney. Thus, this drug is excreted by both glomerular filtration and tubular secretion.[65] Changes in urinary pH do not influence cinoxacin excretion significantly. It is not known whether cinoxacin is excreted into human milk. Because other drugs in this class are excreted into human milk and because of the potential for serious adverse reactions from cinoxacin in nursing infants, the drug should not be used in nursing women.

Norfloxacin is also administered orally and is readily absorbed from the gastrointestinal tract. Peak plasma levels usually occur 1–2 hours after each dose and are in the range of 0.75, 1.58, 2.41, 3.15, and 3.87 μg/ml for doses of 200, 400, 800, 1200, and 1600 mg, respectively. The half-life of norfloxacin is 3–4.5 hours for all doses studied. Concentrations in urine peak at 1–2 hours after administration. Mean peak values for increasing doses of norfloxacin (200, 400, 800, 1200, and 1600 mg) are 200, 478, 697, 992, and 1045 μg/ml, respectively. Renal clearances approximate 285 ml/min. Approximately 30 percent of each dose is excreted into urine as unmetabolized norfloxacin, with lesser quantities of glucuronide conjugate and six active metabolites with modifications in the piperazine ring being excreted.[27,66–68] Crystals of norfloxacin are occasionally observed during microscopic examination of freshly voided urine collected after the 1200 and 1600 mg doses. However, crystalluria is not encountered at lower doses.[66] Concentrations of norfloxacin in human milk are below the bioassay detection limits.[67]

Ciprofloxacin is also administered orally and is rapidly absorbed from the gastrointestinal tract. Peak plasma levels usually occur in 1–1.5 hours and are approximately 2–3 μg/ml after an oral dose of 500 mg. Approximately 35 percent of ciprofloxacin is bound to plasma proteins. It has a serum half-life 3–4.5 hours. Peak urine concentrations occur within 4 hours. Approximately 20 percent of the administered dose can be recovered as active drug in the urine during the first 4 hours, with a total of 30–60 percent by 24 hours. Renal clearance of ciprofloxacin is 4.9 ml/min/kg or 267 ml/min.[67,68] Approximately 10 percent of ciprofloxacin is excreted into the urine in the form of four different metabolites.[67] Approximately 15 percent of ciprofloxacin is recoverable in feces (10 percent as ciprofloxacin, 5 percent as metabolites); less than 1 percent appears in bile. Ciprofloxacin is the most thoroughly studied quinolone in all respects. Its extravascular penetration into tissues and other body compartments is better than or comparable to other newer quinolones.[67] For example, ciprofloxacin penetrates blister fluid well, with 57 percent of the serum concentration recoverable. Also, the concentration of ciprofloxacin in blister fluid exceeds that in serum about 3 hours after administration.[69] It is not known whether ciprofloxacin is excreted into human milk. A parenteral preparation of ciprofloxacin is also available and is currently under investigation.

The pharmacokinetic properties of some of the newer quinolones are summarized in Table 2. The newer quinolones in general exhibit linear pharmacokinetics. Peak serum concentrations occur 1–3 hours after oral administration. Food delays absorption so that serum peaks appear later and are moderately lower.[67] Absorption is also reduced by concomitant administration of magnesium or aluminum hydroxide antacids, by H-2 blockers (ranitidine), and by other drugs that decrease peristalsis or delay the gastric emptying time.[27,67] None of the newer quinolones is extensively bound (only up to 30 percent) to serum proteins. Their long serum half-life allows twice-daily or once-daily dosing. The newer quinolones undergo renal and hepatic metabolism. Renal elimination is by glomerular filtration and active tubular secretion, which is blocked by probenicid (except fleroxacin). Urinary recovery of the newer quinolones after oral administration ranges from 70 to 85 percent for lomefloxacin and ofloxacin to 5 to 15 percent for pefloxacin and difloxacin,[70] with 62 percent for enoxacin, 50–60 percent for fleroxacin, 31 percent for ciprofloxacin, and 27 percent for norfloxacin.[3,27,67,70] The antibacterial activity of the quinolones is reduced at lower urinary pH values (pH 5.5–6.0 vs. pH 7.4).[3] Hepatic metabolism includes conjugation with glucuronic acid as well as carboxylation, hydroxylation, and demethylation.[71] Pefloxacin and difloxacin undergo extensive hepatic metabolism, followed by enoxacin and, to a lesser degree, norfloxacin, ciprofloxacin, and fleroxacin. Lomefloxacin and ofloxacin undergo the least hepatic metabolism. Biliary concentrations of the quinolones (ciprofloxacin, enoxacin, ofloxacin, and pefloxacin) are two to 8 times the simultaneous serum concentrations.[67]

The quinolones penetrate well into body fluids and into cells and tissues by passive diffusion across capillary membranes. Those quinolones with a longer half-life have smaller penetration ratios.[67] Also, ciprofloxacin and norfloxacin have high intracellular concentrations inside human neutrophils, whereas pefloxacin penetrates poorly into alveolar macrophages and neutrophils.[67] The tissue penetration of some of the newer quinolones is summarized in Table 3.

Intravenous preparations of some of the newer four-quinolones are undergoing clinical investigation. The intravenous preparation of ciprofloxacin will probably be approved and released for clinical use before the parenteral preparations of other newer quinolones; it is prepared as the 0.1 percent excess lactate salt.[71a] The pharmacology of intravenously administered ciprofloxacin has been studied with doses ranging from 25 to 200 mg, though most studies have used either 100 or 200 mg administered by bolus injection. These dose-ranging studies demonstrate a linear increase in the area under the concentration-time curve, and produce a half-life of approximately 4 hours.[71b] Peak serum concentrations of 3.80 ± 0.62 μg/ml are achieved with intravenous infusions of 200 mg. Although renal clearance accounts for two-thirds of the total serum clearance, approximately 75 percent is recovered in the urine as parent compound plus metabolites.[71b] Intravenous ciprofloxacin is excreted into bile unchanged and 14 percent is recovered in feces.

TABLE 2. Pharmacokinetic Properties of Selected Newer Quinolones

Drug	Dose (mg)	C_{max} (mg/L)	Half-life (hr)	Protein Binding (%)	Bioavailability (%)	VD (liters)	Urinary Excretion (%)	
							Unchanged	Metabolites
Ciprofloxacin	500	2–3	3–4.5	35	85	250	30–60	10
Norfloxacin	400	1.5	3–4.5	15	80	225	20–40	20
Ofloxacin	400	3.5–5.0	5–6	8–30	85–95	100	70–90	5–10
Enoxacin	400	2–3	4–6	43	90	190	50–55	15
Pefloxacin	400	4–5	10–11	25	90	110	5–15	55
Fleroxacin	400	4–6	10	23	96	100	60–70	10
Lomefloxacin	400	3	8	NA	NA	190	70	10
Difloxacin	400	4–5	26	42	NA	140	10	20

Abbreviations: C_{max}: peak serum concentration; VD: volume of distribution; NA: data not available.

TABLE 3. Penetration of Selected Quinolones into Body Fluids and Tissues

Fluid/Tissue	Ciprofloxacin	Norfloxacin	Ofloxacin	Enoxacin	Pefloxacin	Fleroxacin
Blister fluid	++++	++++	++++	++++	+++	++++
Saliva	++	++	+++	+++	+++	+++
Bronchial secretions	++	—	+++	++++	++++	—
Pleural fluid	+++	—	—	—	—	—
Nasal secretions	+++	+++	++++	++++	+++	++++
Tears	++	++	+++	++	+++	+++
Sweat	+	+	++	++	++	++
Cerebrospinal fluid	+	—	++	—	+++	—
Prostatic fluid	+++	++	++++	++	—	++
Ejaculate	+++++	—	++++	++++	—	++++
Lung	++++	—	++++	+++++	++++	—
Kidney	+++++	+++++	+++++	++++	—	—
Bone	++++	—	++	++	++	—
Skin	++++	—	—	++++	—	—
Muscle	++++	—	—	++++	—	—
Fat	++++	—	—	+++	—	—

Abbreviations: +: area under the curve (AUC) ratios or concentration ratios <0.1; ++: AUC ratios or concentration ratios 0.1–0.5; +++: AUC ratios or concentration ratios 0.5–1; ++++: AUC ratios or concentration ratios 1–4; +++++: AUC ratios or concentration ratios >4 of tissue or fluid vs. serum.
(Modified from Sörgel et al.,[68] with permission.)

Also, renal impairment reduces the serum clearance of ciprofloxacin, with a doubling of the half-life in anephric patients; thus, the dose should be reduced by 50 percent in patients with creatinine clearances of 20 to 30 ml/min/1.73m^2.[71b]

DOSAGE ADJUSTMENTS IN RENAL OR HEPATIC INSUFFICIENCY

Dosage adjustments in patients with renal insufficiency (creatinine clearance below 80 ml/min) are recommended for ofloxacin and lomefloxacin since they undergo minimal hepatic metabolism and are excreted predominantly unchanged in the urine.[70] Adjustments in the dose of enoxacin, fleroxacin, and pefloxacin may be necessary in patients with moderate renal insufficiency; this also holds for norfloxacin and ciprofloxacin but only when creatinine clearance is severely impaired.[3,48,67]

Dosage adjustments in patients with hepatic disease may be required for pefloxacin, difloxacin, and possibly enoxacin,[67,70,71] whereas norfloxacin and ciprofloxacin may accumulate only in patients with severe hepatic failure.[27,67]

TOXICITY AND ADVERSE REACTIONS

Oral nalidixic acid is usually well tolerated, although a number of adverse reactions have been reported. Gastrointestinal side effects include nausea, vomiting, diarrhea, and abdominal pain. Dermatologic reactions include pruritus, nonspecific rashes, and urticaria associated with eosinophilia as well as photosensitivity reactions involving skin surfaces exposed to sunlight that are most commonly manifested as a sunburn and rarely as a bullous eruption.[72–74] Patients receiving the drug should be cautioned to avoid excessive exposure to direct sunlight. Ophthalmologic side effects include blurred vision, diplopia, photophobia, abnormal accommodation, and changes in color perception, all of which disappear with cessation of therapy. Central nervous system reactions include headaches, drowsiness, asthenia, giddiness, vertigo, syncope, sensory changes, grand mal seizures, and acute reversible toxic psychosis[75–77] as well as pseudotumor cerebri with intracranial hypertension, papilledema, and bulging fontanelles in infants and young children,[78–81] which reverses after the cessation of therapy. Also, convulsions, hyperglycemia, and glycosuria without abnormal serum ketone levels has been reported in one patient who took an overdose of nalidixic acid.[82] Therefore, the drug should not be given to patients with convulsive disorders, pre-existing mental instability, parkinsonism, or cerebral vascular insufficiency, nor to infants or pregnant women in the first trimester, and it probably should not be used in children.

Nalidixic acid has rarely been associated with blood dyscrasias and hemolytic anemia that sometimes is associated with glucose-6-phosphate dehydrogenase (G6PD)-deficient red blood cells.[60,83] The drug has also rarely been associated with cholestatic jaundice and possibly may precipitate acute respiratory failure in patients with impaired respiratory function.[84]

Oxolinic acid has been associated frequently with excitative central nervous system responses, which include restlessness, insomnia, nervousness, dizziness, headache, and nausea.[56] This potential is increased in elderly patients and is more common with oxolinic acid than with nalidixic acid. Less frequent reactions include abdominal pain, vomiting, anorexia, diarrhea, constipation, pruritus, and weakness. Abnormal liver function test results and reduced leukocyte counts have also been observed. Rare reactions include photophobia, palpitations, swelling of extremities, reduction in hematocrit or hemoglobin values, eosinophilia, urticaria, rash, soreness of mouth and gums, and metallic taste. A seizure occurred in one patient with known epilepsy, and hallucinations and hysteria occurred in one patient who received a larger dose than was recommended. All reactions are reversible with cessation of treatment.

Oral cinoxacin is well tolerated, and adverse reactions occur infrequently (4.4 percent) and are reversible.[65] Gastrointestinal reactions are the most common side effects, and nausea is the most frequent (3 percent of patients), followed by vomiting, anorexia, abdominal cramps, and diarrhea. The frequency of adverse central nervous system reactions is less than 1 percent. These consist of headache, dizziness, insomnia, paresthesias, perineal burning, photophobia, and tinnitus. Hypersensitivity reactions (less than 3 percent) include urticaria, morbilliform rash, pruritus, and edema. Abnormal liver (serum glutamic-oxaloacetic transaminase [SGOT], serum glutamic-pyruvic transaminase [SGPT], and alkaline phosphatase) and renal (blood urea nitrogen [BUN] and serum creatinine) function values have been observed in fewer than 1 percent of patients who have received cinoxacin. This drug should be used with caution in patients with a history of liver disease. Also, the use of cinoxacin in prepubertal children and during pregnancy is not recommended.

The newer fluoroquinolones norfloxacin, ciprofloxacin, ofloxacin, enoxacin, and pefloxacin have similar toxicities and incidences of adverse reactions.[85] Compared with other antimicrobial agents, the newer quinolones can be considered relatively safe agents. Even so, adverse effects have been observed during clinical trials with these agents. Gastrointestinal side effects are the most frequent (0.8–6.8 percent of patients) and include nausea, vomiting, dyspepsia, epigastric/abdominal pain, anorexia, diarrhea, flatulence, and dry mouth.[85] Antibiotic-associated colitis has been seen but only very rarely.[86]

Central nervous system side effects are the next most commonly observed adverse reactions (0.9–1.8 percent of patients) and can be divided into mild reactions and severe neurotoxic side effects that require interruption of therapy. Mild reactions include headache, dizziness, tiredness, insomnia, faintness, agitation, listlessness, restlessness, abnormal vision, and bad dreams. Severe reactions are rare (<0.5 percent) and include hallucinations, depressions, psychotic reactions and grand mal convulsions. In general, these side effects occur after only a few days of treatment and stop when therapy is discontinued.[85,86] The exact mechanism of central nervous system toxicity associated with quinolone therapy has not been defined. Although the quinolones do inhibit the receptor binding of γ-aminobutyric acid (GABA), which is an inhibitory neurotransmitter, the concentrations required for inhibition are higher than can probably be attained clinically.[87,88]

Skin and allergic reactions are the third most commonly observed side effects (0.6–2.4 percent of patients) and include erythema, urticaria, rash, pruritus, and photosensitivity reactions of skin surfaces exposed to sunlight.[85,86] Very rare cases of hypotension, tachycardia, nephrotoxicity (elevations in serum creatinine levels), thrombocytopenia, leukopenia, anemia, and transient elevations in liver enzyme concentrations have been observed.[85,86] Animal toxicology has described testicular toxicity, ocular damage (including subcapsular cataracts, retinal changes, and altered visual acuity), as well as arthropathy, gait abnormalities, and articular cartilage lesions in weight-bearing joints in juvenile animals.[85] Although the significance of these findings in human adults is unclear, there is concern about the effect of the newer quinolones in children and adolescents. Thus, the newer quinolones have not been approved for use in pediatric patients in the United States.

DRUG INTERACTIONS

Nalidixic acid–glucuronide conjugates may produce a false-positive reaction for urine glucose when tested with Benedict solution such as Clinitest, but not with glucose oxidase test strips such as Clinistix. Diabetic patients treated with this drug should be so alerted. Nitrofurantoin interferes with the therapeutic action of nalidixic acid.

The safety of the concomitant use of oxolinic acid and other central nervous system stimulants has not been established. Also, oxolinic acid may enhance the effects of the oral anticoagulants bishydroxycoumarin and warfarin by displacing these drugs from serum albumin binding sites. Nitrofurantoin also interferes with the therapeutic action of oxolinic acid.[89]

Some of the newer quinolones increase significantly the peak and trough serum concentrations of theophylline in patients receiving theophylline therapy. Increases in theophylline plasma concentrations are very significant with enoxacin (111 percent) and, to a much lesser extent, with ciprofloxacin (23 percent), pefloxacin (20 percent), and ofloxacin (12 percent).[90–92] The 4-oxo metabolite of the piperazine ring in these quinolones is thought to compete with theophylline for liver enzymes and interfere with theophylline clearance.[91] Thus, the dose of theophylline probably should be halved in patients also receiving enoxacin, whereas no routine reduction in the theophylline dose is recommended for ciprofloxacin, ofloxacin or pefloxacin. However, monitoring theophylline levels is recommended in patients also receiving one of these quinolones.

Some of the newer quinolones also interfere with the clearance of caffeine. Enoxacin increases the plasma concentration of caffeine by 41 percent and reduces the clearance by 78 percent. Ciprofloxacin increases the half-life of caffeine only modestly (15 percent), and ofloxacin does so only minimally.[93,94]

CLINICAL USES

The newer quinolones have proved to be effective therapies for infection of the urinary tract, respiratory tree, gastrointestinal tract, skin, soft tissue, and bone and for sexually transmitted bacterial diseases.

Urinary Tract Infections

Nalidixic acid, oxolinic acid, cinoxacin, norfloxacin, and ciprofloxacin have established roles in treating urinary tract infections. Nalidixic acid (*adults*: 1 g qid for 1–2 weeks, thereafter 0.5 g qid if needed; *children*: 55 mg/kg/day in four divided doses for 1–2 weeks, thereafter 33 mg/kg/day if needed), oxolinic acid (*adults*: 750 mg bid for 2 weeks; *children*: not recommended), and cinoxacin (*adults*: 250 mg qid 500 mg bid for 1–2 weeks; *children*: not recommended) have been used in acute and recurrent uncomplicated urinary infections due to susceptible organisms. Nalidixic acid has also been used as long-term therapy for frequently recurrent bacteriuria, in adults, and in children with bacteriuria associated with urinary tract abnormalities. [29,95] The follow-up cure rate was disappointingly similar to that observed with other agents, and resistance to nalidixic acid commonly emerged during treatment.[29] In contrast, the rapid emergence of resistant organisms during acute and long-term treatment with cinoxacin has not been observed. The efficacy of cinoxacin prophylaxis for frequently recurrent urinary infections is less clear.[96,97] Nalidixic acid, oxolonic acid, and cinoxacin should not be used in patients with renal carbuncles or perinephric abscesses.

The newer quinolones are also at least as effective as other well established agents for the treatment of *uncomplicated* urinary infections.[3] Single doses of norfloxacin (800 mg), ciprofloxacin (100 or 250 mg), and ofloxacin (200 mg) are highly effective in women with simple cystitis caused by enterobacteriacae but may be less effective against *Staphylococcus saprophyticus*.[3,98] Also, 3–10 days of therapy with norfloxacin, ciprofloxacin, ofloxacin, or enoxacin resulted in excellent bacteriologic cure rates in uncomplicated urinary infections.[3,27,98]

Norfloxacin, ciprofloxacin, ofloxacin, and enoxacin, given for 5–10 days to patients with nosocomial or *complicated* urinary infections, resulted in higher cure rates than did amoxicillin, amoxicillin plus clavulanic acid, trimethoprim-sulfamethoxazole, or parenteral antibiotic therapy.[3,27,98]

The newer quinolones ciprofloxacin (1000 mg/day), ofloxacin

(300–600 mg/day), pefloxacin (800 mg/day), and norfloxacin (800 mg/day), given to patients with either acute or chronic *prostatitis* for 28 (range, 5–84) days, cured 63–92 percent of patients.[3,99–102]

Respiratory Tract Infections

Ciprofloxacin, ofloxacin, enoxacin, and pefloxacin, given for 10 (range, 7–15) days to patients with purulent bronchitis, acute exacerbations of chronic bronchitis, or pneumonia, resulted in clinical cure or improvement (76–91 percent) and bacteriologic cure (68–83 percent) in most patients. However, bacteriologic persistence, relapse, or treatment failure occurred in 49 percent of patients with *Pseudomonas aeruginosa* infections, in 39 percent with *Streptococcus pneumoniae* infections, and in 33 percent with *Staphylococcus aureus* infections.[3,103] Although the newer quinolones are effective for the treatment of bronchitis, they should not be used to treat either community-acquired or aspiration pneumonia because of their reduced activity against *S. pneumoniae* and against those microaerophilic and anaerobic bacteria associated with aspiration pneumonia. In contrast, the newer quinolones may have value for the treatment of hospital-acquired pneumonia caused by aerobic gram-negative bacteria.[3,27] Also, ciprofloxacin (750 mg twice daily) has proved to be a useful alternative to conventional parenteral therapy for cystic fibrosis patients with acute exacerbations of their pulmonary infections, although resistant organisms may emerge.[3,104,1005] Ciprofloxacin may have value also for treating malignant external otitis caused by *Pseudomonas aeruginosa*, which currently requires parenteral combination therapy.

The newer quinolones should not be used for acute sinusitis because of the possible presence of pneumococci and anaerobic streptococci. However, these agents may be useful in specific cases of chronic sinusitis when aerobic gram-negative bacteria susceptible to the newer quinolones are responsible. These agents should not be used for otitis media since they are currently not recommended for use in pediatric patients. Of importance, norfloxacin has not been approved for and should not be used for any type of respiratory tract infection.

Gastrointestinal Infections

The bacterial pathogens causing diarrheal disease, including toxigenic *E. coli*, *Salmonella*, *Shigella*, *Campylobacter* and *Vibrio spp.*, are highly susceptible to the newer quinolones, which also provide high drug concentrations in the lumen of the gut and the mucosa. These factors contribute to the eradication of these pathogens from the intestine within 48 hours of initiating therapy.[106–108] Ciprofloxacin (500 mg bid for 5 days) and norfloxacin (400 mg bid for 5 days) have been studied extensively in patients with either acute bacterial diarrhea or acute traveller's diarrhea. Both of these agents have a greater than 90 percent cure rate and are comparable to trimethoprim-sulfamethoxazole.[3,106–108] Although these newer agents are effective in treating bacterial and traveller's diarrhea, they should not be used as prophylactic agents to prevent acute traveller's diarrhea because this disease responds promptly to treatment once symptoms develop and because of the concern that resistance may develop more rapidly with the indiscriminate use of the newer quinolones. These agents should probably be reserved and used as an alternative for persons with a history of trimethoprim-sulfamethoxazole hypersensitivity or for persons in areas where resistance to trimethoprim-sulfamethoxazole is common.[3,109] Ciprofloxacin, 500 mg twice daily for 2–15 (mean, 13) days, and ofloxacin, 200 mg twice daily for 6–30 days, given to patients with typhoid fever cured all patients; none relapsed or became a chronic carrier.[3] Preliminary reports suggest that ciprofloxacin, 500–750 mg twice daily for 4 weeks, eliminated the chronic *Salmonella* carrier state in 86 percent of patients treated and followed for 10–12 months.[3]

Although the newer quinolones inhibit *Campylobacter pylori*, which has been associated with antral gastritis, these agents have not been effective in the treatment of *C. pylori*–associated gastritis.[3,110] Also, some relapses have been reported in patients with *Brucella* infections who have been treated with the newer quinolones.[3]

Skin and Soft Tissue Infections

Oral therapy with some of the newer quinolones, i.e., ciprofloxacin, ofloxacin, and enoxacin, appear to be as effective as alternative parenteral agents in treating a variety of skin and skin structure infections.[3,27] Patients with bacterial infections of the skin and soft tissue, including patients with cellulitis, subcutaneous abscesses, wound infections, and infected ulcers, generally in diabetic patients, have been treated successfully with the newer oral quinolones, primarily ciprofloxacin.[3,111–114] Most patients received 750 mg ciprofloxacin orally twice daily for 14 days, with clinical cure or improvement observed in 95 percent of patients. Bacteriologic cure rates were lower in patients infected with gram-positive organisms than were observed for infections caused by gram-negative aerobic bacteria.[3,112] Also, therapy failed in 25 percent of anaerobic infections. Ciprofloxacin, 750 mg orally twice daily for 7–28 days, eradicated colonization with methicillin-resistant *Staphylococcus aureus* (MRSA) in 79 percent of evaluable patients.[115] Although ciprofloxacin has the potential to eradicate MRSA colonization, there is the potential for the development of increased resistance to this and other newer quinolones.[3]

Osteomyelitis

Current experience with the newer oral quinolones as monotherapy for osteomyelitis, particularly when caused by gram-negative aerobic pathogens, is very encouraging. Most patients with osteomyelitis who have been treated with one of the newer quinolones received ciprofloxacin orally in a dose of 750 mg twice daily. The mean duration of therapy was 8 weeks (range, 4 days to 6 months). Patients with either acute or chronic osteomyelitis either in native bone or complicating a foreign body were treated. Clinical cure or improvement occurred in approximately 80 percent of patients with adequate follow-up of at least 6 months to more than 1 year. Treatment failures occurred in 15 percent, and a few patients developed recurrence of their infection. The infecting organism developed resistance to the newer quinolone used in therapy in only a small number (0.5 percent) of patients, primarily those with *Pseudomonas aeruginosa* infections.[3,116] Thus, ciprofloxacin has an established efficacy in the treatment of osteomyelitis and should facilitate home therapy for many patients with osteomyelitis.

Sexually Transmitted Diseases

Ciprofloxacin, ofloxacin, difloxacin, amifloxacin, lomefloxacin, norfloxacin, fleroxacin, pefloxacin, and enoxacin are extremely active in vitro against *Neisseria gonorrhoeae*, including penicillinase-producing strains (PPNG), and ciprofloxacin is especially active against *Haemophilus ducreyi*.[3,31] *Chlamydia trachomatis* isolates are susceptible to ciprofloxacin, ofloxacin, and difloxacin but are resistant to enoxacin and norfloxacin.[117,118] *Gardnerella vaginalis* isolates are relatively resistant to these agents, as are *Ureaplasma urealyticum*, although ciprofloxacin is active against the latter about 50 percent of the time.[3,119] Thus, the newer quinolones, on the basis of their in vitro activity, have been used to treat a variety of sexually transmitted diseases.

Gonococcal Infections

In uncomplicated gonococcal infections in both men and women, single oral doses of either 500, 250, or 100 mg of ciprofloxacin, 660, 400, or 200 mg of enoxacin, 400 mg of pefloxacin, 800, 600, 400, or 200 mg of ofloxacin, or 800 mg of norfloxacin cured 95–100 percent of patients, including patients infected with PPNG. Thus, the lowest effective oral single dose of the newer quinolones has been 100 mg of ciprofloxacin, which has cured almost 100 percent of patients with urethral as well as rectal gonorrhea and is probably effective for pharyngeal gonococcal infections. However, there is little experience with these newer agents in the treatment of *disseminated gonococcal* infections.[3]

Chlamydia Urethritis, Postgonococcal Urethritis, Nongonococcal Urethritis

None of the current quinolones is effective as single-dose therapy for *C. trachomatis* urethritis, nor are they able to prevent postgonoccal urethritis (PGU) when used as single-dose therapy in gonococcal infections. Ciprofloxacin, however, in a dose of 750 mg orally twice daily for 4 days eradicated *C. trachomatis* in 60 percent of co-infected patients and reduced the incidence of PGU from 35 percent to 12.8 percent.[3,120] Currently, ciprofloxacin in a dose of 500 mg three times daily and ofloxacin in a dose of 100 mg three times daily for 14 days have cured most patients with nongonococcal urethritis (NGU) caused by *C. trachomatis*, whereas norfloxacin is not effective.[3,120] However, the newer quinolones are less effective than is doxycycline in NGU patients with chlamydial infections alone.[120] Thus, further studies are needed to accurately define the efficacy of the newer quinolones in NGU.

Chancroid

Patients with chancroid and *H. ducreyi* infections have responded successfully to either a 500 mg oral single dose (95 percent cure rate) of ciprofloxacin or 500 mg twice daily for 3 days (100 percent cure rate). Currently the 3-day, six-dose ciprofloxacin regimen, which cured all patients with chancroid, is preferred.[3,121]

Nonspecific Vaginitis

Ciprofloxacin in an oral dose of 500 mg twice daily for 7 days given to women with nonspecific vaginitis caused by *Corynebacterium* spp., *Bacteroides* spp., and *Gardnerella vaginalis* produced clinical and bacteriologic cures in 73 percent of patients. Clinical improvement without bacteriologic eradication occurred in an additional 18 percent, and 9 percent failed to respond,[3,122] Vaginal colonization with *Candida albicans* occurred in 32 percent of these patients, but without clinical signs or symptoms of yeast infection.[3]

Other Infections

Immunocompromised Host. Ciprofloxacin and norfloxacin have been used successfully as *prophylactic* agents in granulocytopenic patients.[3,124–128] Prophylaxis was begun 1–2 days before the initiation of cytotoxic therapy and continued until the granulocyte count rose above 500 cells/mm^3. Ciprofloxacin prevented whereas norfloxacin reduced but did not prevent colonization by gram-negative bacilli, nor did norfloxacin influence the incidence of gram-positive bacteremia.[124] Clinical experience with the newer quinolones in the *treatment* of severe infections in immunocompromised patients is very preliminary.[3,128] Limited experience with ciprofloxacin, ofloxacin, and pefloxacin suggest a potential role for these agents in immunocompromised patients, but further trials are needed to establish their value.

Central Nervous System Infections. Ciprofloxacin, ofloxacin, and pefloxacin do penetrate into cerebrospinal fluid and brain tissue.[3,68,129,130] However, clinical experience with the newer quinolones as therapeutic agents for central nervous system bacterial infections is only anecdotal.[3] These agents should not be used empirically for central nervous system infections but should be reserved for special cases caused by multiantibiotic-resistant aerobic gram-negative bacteria. Of note, in *meningococcal carriers* oral ciprofloxacin in a dose of either 500 mg twice daily for 5 days or 250 mg twice daily for 2 days eradicated the meningococci in 100 and 96 percent, respectively, of nasopharyngeal carriers.[131,132]

The newer quinolones, particularly ciprofloxacin and ofloxacin, inhibit *M. tuberculosis* and *M. avium-intracellulare* and may be useful in drug-resistant mycobacterial infections with these organisms, but clinical studies are needed to define their effectiveness.[3]

REFERENCES

1. Lesher GY, Froelich EJ, Gruett MD, et al. 1,8-naphthyridine derivatives. A new class of chemotherapeutic agents. J Med Pharmacol Chem. 1962; 5:1063.
2. Smith JT, Lewin CS. Chemistry and mechanisms of action of the quinolone antibacterials. In: Andriole VT, ed. The Quinolones. London: Academic Press; 1988;23–81.
3. Andriole VT. Clinical overview of the newer 4-quinolone antibacterial agents. In: Andriole VT, ed. The Quinolones. London: Academic Press; 1988;155–200.
4. Crumplin G. Aspects of chemistry in the development of 4-quinolone antibacterial agents. Rev Infect Dis. 1988;1(Suppl):2–9.
5. Turner FJ, Ringel SM, Martin JF, et al. Oxolinic acid, a new synthetic antimicrobial agent. I. In vitro and in vivo activity. Antimicrob Agents Chemother. 1967;475.
6. Ringel SM, Turner FJ, Lindo FL, et al. Oxolinic acid, a new synthetic antimicrobial agent. II. Bactericidal rate and resistance development. Antimicrob Agents Chemother. 1967;480.
7. Ringel SM, Turner FJ, Roemer S, et al. Oxolonic acid, a new synthetic antimicrobial agent. III. Concentrations in serum, urine, and renal tissue. Antimicrob Agents Chemother. 1967;486.
8. Wick WE, Preston DS, White WA, et al. Compound 64716, a new synthetic antibacterial agent. Antimicrob Agents Chemother. 1973;4:415.
9. Ito A, Hirai K, Inoue M, et al. In vitro antibacterial activity of AM 175, a new nalidixic acid analog. Antimicrob Agents Chemother. 1980;17:103.
10. Downs JT, Andriole VT, Ryan JL. In vitro activity of MK 0366 against clinical urinary pathogens including gentamicin-resistant *Pseudomonas aeruginosa*. Antimicrob Agents Chemother. 1982;21:670.
11. Wise R, Andrew JM, Edwards LJ. In vitro activity of Bay 09867, a new quinolone derivative, compared with those of other antimicrobial agents. Antimicrob Agents Chemother. 1983;23:559.
12. Goss WA, Deitz WH, Cook TM. Mechanism of action of nalidixic acid on *Escherichia coli*. II. Inhibition of deoxyribonucleic acid synthesis. J Bacteriol. 1965;89:1068.
13. Crumplin GC, Smith JT. Nalidixic acid: An antibacterial paradox. Antimicrob Agents Chemother. 1975;8:251–61.
14. Deitz WH, Cook TM, Goss WA. Mechanism of action of nalidixic acid on *Escherichia coli*. III. Conditions required for lethality. J Bacteriol. 1966; 91:768.
15. Bourguignon GJ, Levitt M, Sternglanz R. Studies on the mechanism of action of nalidixic acid. Antimicrob Agents Chemother. 1973;4:479.
16. Pratt WB. The urinary tract antiseptics. In: Pratt WB, ed. Chemotherapy of Infection. New York: Oxford University Press; 1977:215.
17. Smith JT. Awakening the slumbering potential of the 4-quinolone antibacterials. Pharmacol J. 1984;233:299–305.
18. Higgens NP, Peebles CL, Sugino A, et al. Purification of subunits of *Escherichia coli*. DNA gyrase and reconstitution of enzymic activity. Proc Natl Acad Sci USA. 1978;75:1773–7.
19. Pedrini A. Nalidixic acid. In: Hahn FE, ed. Antibiotics. v. 5. Berlin: Springer-Verlag. 1979:154.
20. Wang JC. Interactions between DNAs and enzymes. The effect of superhelical turns. J Mol Biol. 1974;87:797–816.
21. Wang JC. DNA topoisomerases. Annu Rev Biochem. 1985;54:665–7.
22. Gellert M, Mizuuchi K, O'Dea MH, et al. DNA gyrase. An enzyme that introduces superhelical turns into DNA. Proc Natl Acad Sci USA. 1976;73:3872–6.
23. Sugino A, Peebles CL, Krenzer KN, et al. Mechanism of action of nalidixic acid. Purification of *E. coli* Nal A gene production and its relationship to DNA gyrase and a novel nicking–closing enzyme. Proc Natl Acad Sci USA. 1977;74:4767.
24. Gellert M, Mizuuchi K, O'Dea MH, et al. Nalidixic acid resistance. A second genetic character involved in DNA gyrase activity. Proc Natl Acad Sci USA. 1977;74:4772–6.
25. Inoue S, Ohue T, Yamagishi J, et al. Mode of incomplete cross-resistance among pipemidic, piromidic, and nalidixic acids. Antimicrob Agents Chemother. 1978;14:240–5.

26. Yamagishi J, Yoshida H, Yamayoshi M, et al. Nalidixic acid–resistant mutations of the gyr B gene of *Escherichia coli*. Mol Gen Genet. 1986;204:367–73.
27. Norris S, Mandell GL. The quinolones: History and overview. In: Andriole VT, ed. The Quinolones. London: Academic Press; 1988:1–22.
28. Barlow AM. Nalidixic acid in infections of urinary tract. Br Med J. 1963;2:1308.
29. Buchbinder M, Webb JC, Anderson LV, et al. Laboratory studies and clinical pharmacology of nalidixic acid (WIN 18,320). Antimicrob Agents Chemother. 1962;308.
30. Ronald AR, Turck M, Petersdorf RG. A critical evaluation of nalidixic acid in urinary tract infections. N Engl J Med. 1966;275:1081.
31. Phillips I, King A, Shannon K. In vitro properties of the quinolones. In: Andriole VT, ed. The Quinolones. London: Academic Press; 1988:83–117.
32. Cox CE. Oxolinic acid therapy of recurrent urinary tract infections. Del Med J. 1970;42:327.
33. D'Alessio DJ, Olexy VM, Jackson GG. Oxolinic acid treatment of urinary tract infections. Antimicrob Agents Chemother. 1967;490.
34. Mardh PA, Colleen S, Andersson KE. Studies in cinoxacin. I. In vitro activity of cinoxacin as compared to nalidixic acid, against urinary tract pathogens. J Antimicrob Chemother. 1977;3:411.
35. Gordon RG, Stevens LI, Edmiston CE, et al. Comparative in vitro studies of cinoxacin, nalidixic acid, and oxolinic acid. Antimicrob Agents Chemother. 1976;10:918.
36. Jones RN, Fuchs PC. In vitro antimicrobial activity of cinoxacin against 2,968 clinical bacterial isolates. Antimicrob Agents Chemother. 1976;10:146.
37. Goss WA, Deitz WH, Cook TM. Mechanism of action of nalidixic acid on *Escherichia coli*. II. Inhibition of deoxyribonucleic acid synthesis. J Bacteriol. 1965;89:1068.
38. Ott JL, Gordee RS. Inhibition of R-factor transfer by cinoxacin. Current chemotherapy. In: Proceedings of the 10th International Congress on Chemother. Washington, DC: American Society for Microbiology; 1978:688.
39. King A, Warren C, Shannon K, et al. In vitro antibacterial activity of norfloxacin (MK 0366). Antimicrob Agents Chemother. 1982;21:604.
40. Neu HC, Labthavikul P. In vitro activity of norfloxacin, a quinolone-carboxylic acid, compared with that of beta-lactams, aminoglycosides, and trimethoprim. Antimicrob Agents Chemother. 1982;22:23.
41. Norrby SR, Jonsson M. Antibacterial activity of Norfloxacin. Antimicrob Agents Chemother. 1983;23:15.
42. Corrado ML, Cherubin CE, Shulman M. The comparative activity of norfloxacin with other antimicrobial agents against gram-positive and gram-negative bacteria. J Antimicrob Chemother. 1983;11:369.
43. Gadebusch HH, Shungu DL, Weinberg E, et al. Comparison of the antibacterial activity of norfloxacin (MK 0366, AM 715), a new organic acid, with that of other orally absorbed chemotherapeutic agents. Infection. 1982;10:41.
44. Bauernfeind A, Petermuller C. In vitro activity of ciprofloxacin, norfloxacin and nalidixic acid. Eur J Clin Microbiol. 1983;2:111.
45. Muytjens HL, van der Ros–van de Repe J, van Veldhuizen G. Comparative activities of ciprofloxacin (Bay 09867), norfloxacin, pipemidic acid, and nalidixic acid. Antimicrob Agents Chemother. 1983;24:302.
46. Fass RJ. In vitro activity of ciprofloxacin (Bay 09867). Antimicrob Agents Chemother. 1983;24:568.
47. Heessen FWA, Muytjens HL. In vitro activities of ciprofloxacin, norfloxacin, pipemidic acid, cinoxacin, and nalidixic acid against *Chylamydia trachomatis*. Antimicrob Agents Chemother. 1984;25:123.
48. Wolfson JS, Hooper DC. The fluoroquinolones: Structure, mechanisms of action and resistance, and spectra of activity in vitro. Antimicrob Agents Chemother. 1985;28:581–6.
49. Olsson-Lilejequist B, Gezelius L, Svensson SB. Selection of multiple antibiotic resistance by norfloxacin and nalidixic acid in *Klebsiella* and *Enterobacter* (Abstract 106). In: Proceedings of the 25th Interscience Conference on Antimicrobial Agents and Chemotherapy, Minneapolis. Washington, DC: American Society for Microbiology; 1985.
50. Hirai K, Aoyama H, Suzue S, et al. Isolation and characterization of norfloxacin-resistant mutants *Escherichia coli* K-12. Antimicrob Agents Chemother. 1986;30:248–53.
51. Hiraei K, Suzue S, Irikura T, et al. Mutations producing resistance to norfloxacin in *Pseudomonas aeruginosa*. Antimicrob Agents Chemother. 1987;31:582–6.
52. Sanders CC, Sanders WE, Goering RV, et al. Selection of multiple antibiotic resistance by quinolones, beta-lactams, and aminoglycosides with special reference to cross-resistance between unrelated drug classes. Antimicrob Agents Chemother. 1984;26:797–801.
53. Hirai K, Irikura T, Iyobe S, et al. Inhibition of conjugal transfer of R-plasmids by norfloxacin in *Pseudomonas aeruginosa*. Chemotherapy. 1984;32:471–6.
54. Crumplin GC. Plasmid-mediated resistance to nalidixic acid and new 4-quinolones? Lancet. 1987;2:854–5.
55. Munshi MH, Sack DA, Haider K, et al. Plasmid-mediated resistance to nalidixic acid in *Shigella dysenteriae* type I. Lancet. 1987;2:419–21.
56. McChesney EW, Froelich EJ, Lesher GY, et al. Absorption, excretion and metabolism of a new antibacterial agent, nalidixic acid. Toxicol Appl Pharmacol. 1964;6:292.
57. Portmann GA, McChesney EW, Stander H, et al. Pharmacokinetic model for nalidixic acid in man. II. Parameters for absorption, metabolism and elimination. J Pharm Sci. 1966;55:72.
58. Stamey TA, Nemoy NJ, Higgins M. The clinical use of nalidixic acid. A review of some observations. Invest Urol. 1969;6:582.
59. Stamey TA, Meares EM, Winningham DG. Chronic bacterial prostatitis and the diffusion of drugs into prostatic fluid. J Urol. 1970;103:187.
60. Belton EM, Jones RV. Haemolytic anaemia due to nalidixic acid. Lancet. 1965;2:691.
61. Adam WR, Dawborn JK. Plasma levels and urinary excretion of nalidixic acid in patients with renal failure. Aust NZ J Med. 1971;1:126.
62. Atlas E, Clark H, Silverblatt F, et al. Nalidixic acid and oxolinic acid in the treatment of chronic bacteriuria. Ann Intern Med. 1969;70:713.
63. Burt RAP, Morgan T, Payne JP, et al. Cinoxacin concentrations in plasma, urine, and prostatic tissue after oral administration to man. Br J Urol. 1977;49:147.
64. Black HR, Israel KS, Wolen RL, et al. Pharmacology of cinoxacin in humans. Antimicrob Agents Chemother. 1979;15:165.
65. Scavone JM, Gleckman RA, Fraser DG. Cinoxacin: Mechanism of action, spectrum of activity, pharmacokinetics, adverse reactions, and therapeutic indications. Pharmacotherapy. 1982;2:266.
66. Swanson BN, Boppana VK, Vlasses PH, et al. Norfloxacin disposition after sequentially increasing oral doses. Antimicrob Agents Chemother. 1983; 23:284.
67. Bergan T. Pharmacokinetics of fluorinated quinolones. In: Andriole VT, ed. The Quinolones. London: Academic Press; 1988:119–54.
68. Sörgel F, Jaehde U, Naber K, et al. Pharmacokinetic disposition of quinolones in human body fluids and tissues. Clin Pharmacokinet. In press.
69. Crump B, Wise R, Dent J. Pharmacokinetics and tissue penetration of ciprofloxacin. Antimicrob Agents Chemother. 1983;24:784.
70. Lode H, Hoffken G, Olschewski P, et al. Pharmacokinetics of ofloxacin after parenteral and oral administration. Antimicrob Agents Chemother. 1987;31:1338–42.
71. White LO. Metabolism of 4-quinolones. Quinolones Bull. 1987;3:1–4.
71a. Bergan T, Thorsteinsson SB, Solberg R, et al. Pharmacokinetics of ciprofloxacin: intravenous and increasing oral doses. Am J Med. 1987;82(Suppl 4A):97–102.
71b. Drusano GL. An overview of the pharmacology of intravenously administered ciprofloxacin. Am J Med. 1987;82(Suppl 4A):339–345.
72. Zelickson AS. Phototoxic reaction with nalidixic acid. JAMA. 1964; 190:556.
73. Burry JN, Crosby RWL. A case of phototoxicity to nalidixic acid. Med J Aust. 1966;2:698.
74. Mathew TH. Nalidixic acid. Med J Aust. 1966;2:243.
75. Cahal DA. Reactions to nalidixic acid. Br Med J. 1965;2:590.
76. Finegold SM, Miller LG, Posnick D, et al. Nalidixic acid: Clinical and laboratory studies. Antimicrob Agents Chemother. 1966;189.
77. Kremer L, Walton M, Wardle EN. Nalidixic acid and intracranial hypertension. Br Med J. 1967;4:488.
78. Boreus LO, Sundstrom B. Intracranial hypertension in a child during treatment with nalidixic acid. Br Med J. 1967;2:744.
79. Fisher OD. Nalidixic acid and intracranial hypertension. Br Med J. 1967;3:370.
80. Cohen DN. Intracranial hypertension and papilledema associated with nalidixic acid therapy. Am J Ophthalmol. 1973;76:680.
81. Rao KG. Pseudotumor cerebri associated with nalidixic acid. Urology. 1974;4:204.
82. Islam MA, Sreedharan T. Convulsions, hyperglycaemia, and glycosuria from overdose of nalidixic acid. JAMA. 1965;192:1100.
83. Mandal BK, Stevenson J. Haemolytic crisis produced by nalidixic acid. Lancet. 1970;1:614.
84. Today's drugs. Nalidixic acid. Br Med J. 1967;1:741.
85. Stahlmann R, Lode H. Safety overview: Toxicity, adverse effects and drug interactions. In: Andriole VT, ed. The Quinolones. London: Academic Press; 1988:201–33.
86. Adam D, Andrassy K, Christ W, et al. [Arbeitsgemeinschaft "Arzneimittelsicherheit" der Paul-Ehrlich-Gesellschaft fur Chemotherapie]. Vertraglichkeit der Gyrase-Hemmer. Munch Med Wochenschr. 1987;129:45–46.
87. Hori S, Shimada J, Saito A, et al. Effect of new quinolones on gamma-aminobutyric acid receptor binding (Abstract 396). In: Proceedings of the 25th Interscience Conference on Antimicrobial Agents and Chemotherapy, Minneapolis. Washington, DC: American Society for Microbiology; 1985.
88. Hori S, Shimada J, Saito A, et al. Inhibitory effect of quinolones on gamma-aminobutyric acid receptor binding. Structure activity relationship (Abstract 438). In: Proceedings of the 26th Interscience Conference on Antimicrobial Agents and Chemotherapy, New Orleans. Washington, DC: American Society for Microbiology; 1986.
89. Westwood GPC, Hooper WL. Antagonism of oxolinic acid by nitrofurantoin. Lancet. 1975;1:460.
90. Wijnands WJA, van Herwaarden CLA, Vree TB. Enoxacin raises plasma theophylline concentrations (Letter). Lancet. 1984;2:108–9.
91. Wijnands WJA, Vree TB, van Herwaarden CLA. The influence of quinolone derivatives on theophylline clearance. Br J Clin Pharmacol. 1986;22:677–83.
92. Gregoire SL, Grasela ThH Jr, Freer JP, et al. Inhibition of theophylline effects. Antimicrob Agents Chemother. 1987;31:375–378.
93. Staib AH, Harder S, Mieke S, et al. Gyrase-inhibitors impair caffeine elimination in man. Methods Find Exp Clin Pharmacol. 1987;9:193–8.
94. Stille W, Harder S, Mieke S, et al. Decrease of caffeine elimination in man

during co-administration of 4 quinolones. J Antimicrob Chemother. 1987;20:729–734.
95. Kneebone GM. A clinical appraisal of nalidixic acid in urinary tract infections in childhood. Med J Aust. 1965;2:947.
96. Landes RR. Long term dose cinoxacin therapy for the prevention of recurrent urinary tract infections. J Urol. 1980;123:47.
97. Schaeffer AJ, Jones JM, Flynn SS. Prophylactic efficacy of cinoxacin in recurrent urinary tract infection: Biologic effects on the vaginal and fecal flora. J Urol. 1982;127:1118.
98. Malinverni R, Glauser MP. Comparative studies of fluoroquinolones in the treatment of urinary tract infections. Rev Infect Dis. 1988;10(Suppl):153–63.
99. Bologna M, Vaggi L, Flammini D, et al. Norfloxacin in prostatitis: Correlation between HPLC tissue concentrations and clinical results. Drugs Exp Clin Res. 1985;11:95–100.
100. Suzuki K, Tamai H, Naide Y, et al. Laboratory and clinical study of ofloxacin in the treatment of bacterial prostatitis. Hinyokika Kijo. 1984;30:1505–18.
101. Weidner W, Schiefer HG, Dalhoff A. Treatment of chronic bacterial prostatitis with ciprofloxacin. Am J Med. 1987;82(Suppl):280–3.
102. Remy G, Rouger C, Chavanet P, et al. Use of ofloxacin for prostatitis. Rev Infect Dis. 1988;10(Suppl):173–4.
103. Thys JP. Quinolones in the treatment of bronchopulmonary infections. Rev Infect Dis. 1988;10(Suppl):212–7.
104. Bosso JA, Black PG, Matsen JM. Ciprofloxacin versus tobramycin plus azlocillin in pulmonary exacerbations in adult patients with cystic fibrosis. Am J Med. 1987;82(Suppl):180–4.
105. Scully BE, Nakatomi M, Ores C, et al. Ciprofloxacin therapy in cystic fibrosis. Am J Med. 1987;(Suppl):196–201.
106. DuPont HL, Ericsson CD, Robinson A, et al. Current problems in antimicrobial therapy for bacterial enteric infection. Am J Med. 1987;82:324–8.
107. Pichler HET, Diridl G, Stockler K, et al. Clinical efficacy of ciprofloxacin compared with placebo in bacterial diarrhea. Am J Med. 1987;82:329–32.
108. DuPont HL, Corrado ML, Sabbaj J. Use of norfloxacin in the treatment of acute diarrheal disease. Am J Med. 1987;82(Suppl):79–83.
109. Ericsson CD, Johnson PC, DuPont HL, et al. Ciprofloxacin or trimethoprim-sulfamethoxazole as initial therapy for traveler's diarrhea. Ann Intern Med. 1987;106:216–20.
110. Glupczynski Y, Labbe M, Burette A, et al. Treatment failure of ofloxacin in *Campylobacter pylori* infection. Lancet. 1987;2:1096.
111. Fass RJ. Treatment of skin and soft tissue infections with oral ciprofloxacin. J Antimicrob Chemother. 1986;18(Suppl):153–7.
112. Eron LJ. Therapy of skin and skin structure infections with ciprofloxacin. Am J Med. 1987;82(Suppl):244–6.
113. Valainis GT, Pankey GA,, Katner HP, et al. Ciprofloxacin in the treatment of bacterial skin infections. Am J Med. 1987;82(Suppl):230–2.
114. Self PL, Zeluff BA, Sollo D, et al. Use of ciprofloxacin in the treatment of serious skin and skin structure infections. Am J Med. 1987;82(Suppl):239–41.
115. Mulligan ME, Ruane RJ, Johnston L, et al. Ciprofloxacin for eradication of methicillin-resistant *Staphylococcus aureus* colonization. Am J Med. 1987;82(Suppl):215–9.
116. Andriole VT. Treatment of osteomyelitis with quinolones. Quinolones Bull. 1987;3:15–7.
117. Schachter J, Moncada J. In vitro activity of ciprofloxacin against *Chlamydia trachomatis*. Am J Med. 1987;82 (Suppl):42–3.
118. Hartinger A, Hartmut B, Korting HC. In vitro activity of ciprofloxacin and ofloxacin against clinical isolates of *Chylamdia trachomatis*. Rev Infect Dis. 1988;10(Suppl):151–2.
119. Krausse R, Ullmann U. In-vitro-Aktivitat von Enoxazin Ciprofloxacin und Tetracyclin gegenuber *Mycoplasma hominis* und *Ureaplasma urealyticum*. Z Antimikrob Antineoplast Chemother. 1984;2:83–8.
120. Fong IW. Treatment of chlamydial urethritis with ofloxacin or ciprofloxacin. Quinolones Bull. 1986;2:10–1.
121. Naamara W, Plummer FA, Greenblatt RM, et al. Treatment of chancroid with ciprofloxacin. Am J Med. 1987;82(Suppl):317–20.
122. Carmona O, Hernandez-Gonzalez, Kobelt R. Ciprofloxacin in the treatment of nonspecific vaginitis. Am J Med. 1987;82(Suppl):321–3.
123. Neu HC. The quinolones: Prospects. In: Andriole VT, ed. The Quinolones. London: Academic Press; 1988:235–54.
124. Winston DJ, Ho WG, Champlin RE, et al. Norfloxacin for prevention of bacterial infections in granulocytopenic patients. Am J Med. 1987; 82(Suppl):40–6.
125. Winston DJ, Ho WG, Nakao SL, et al. Norfloxacin versus vancomycin/polymyxin for prevention of infections in granulocytopenic patients. Am J Med. 1986;80:884–90.
126. Karp JE, Merz WG, Hendricksen C, et al. Oral norfloxacin for prevention of gram-negative bacterial infections in patients with acute leukemia and granulocytopenia. Ann Intern Med. 1987;106:1–6.
127. Dekker AW, Rozenberg-Arska M, Verhoef J. Infection prophylaxis in acute leukemia: A comparison of ciprofloxacin with trimethoprim-sulfamethoxazole and colistin. Ann Intern Med. 1987;106:7–12.
128. Webster A, Gaya H. Quinolones in the treatment of serious infections. Rev Infect Dis. 1988;10(Suppl):225–33.
129. Norrby SR. 4-Quinolones in the treatment of infections of the central nervous system. Rev Infect Dis. 1988;10(Suppl):253–5.
130. Wolff M, Regnier B, Daldoss C, et al. Penetration of pefloxacin into cerebrospinal fluid of patients with meningitis. Antimicrob Agents Chemother. 1984;26:289–91.
131. Renkonen OV, Sivonen A, Visakorpi R. Effect of ciprofloxacin on carrier rate of *Neisseria meningitidis* in army recruits in Finland. Antimicrob Agents Chemother. 1987;31:962–3.
132. Pugsley MP, Dworzack DL, Horowitz EA, et al. Efficacy of ciprofloxacin on the treatment of nasopharyngeal carriers of *Neisseria meningitidis*. J Infect Dis. 1987;156:211–3.

31. URINARY TRACT AGENTS: NITROFURANTOIN AND METHENAMINE

VINCENT T. ANDRIOLE

Several antibacterial drugs are concentrated primarily in the urinary tract, that is, in the renal tubules with back diffusion into the renal parenchyma, and/or in the urine of the renal pelves and bladder. Since effective plasma concentrations are not obtained with safe doses of these agents, they cannot be used to treat patients with systemic infections and should only be used to treat patients with infections of the urinary tract. For this reason these drugs (nitrofurantoin and methenamine) are known as urinary tract antiseptics.

NITROFURANTOIN

Nitrofurantoin, *O*-(5-nitrofurfurylideneamino)-hydantoin, is one of a series of synthetic nitrofuran compounds that belong to a class of organic substances characterized by a heterocyclic ring consisting of four carbon atoms and one oxygen atom. (Fig. 1). This compound has been available for clinical use in a microcrystalline form since 1953 and is marketed as Furadantin (Eaton). Since nitrofurantoin is of limited solubility in water, a macrocrystalline form of the drug was prepared in 1967 and is marketed as Macrodantin (Eaton).

Mechanism of Action

The precise mechanism of action of nitrofurantoin is not known, although there is evidence that the drug inhibits a variety of enzyme systems in bacteria.[1] Nitrofurans can also enter mammalian cells and have been shown to affect several enzymes in these cells, the most notable of which is to arrest spermatogenesis in animals.[2] Also, at high local concentrations nitrofurantoin immobilizes human sperm.[3]

Antimicrobial Activity

Nitrofurantoin is active against a wide spectrum of gram-positive and gram-negative bacteria and particularly against many strains of the common urinary tract pathogens (Table 1).

Bacterial species with a minimum inhibitory concentration (MIC) of 32 μg/ml or less of nitrofurantoin are considered sensitive since this concentration of the drug can easily be achieved

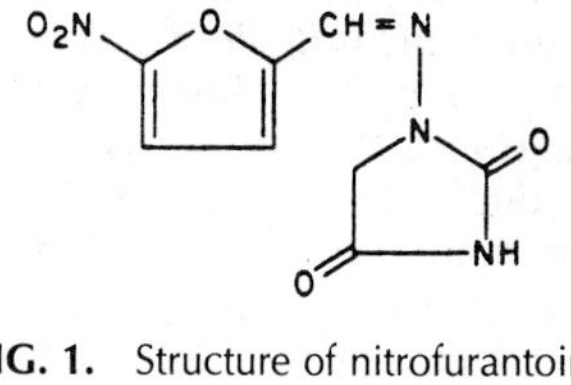

FIG. 1. Structure of nitrofurantoin.

TABLE 1. Nitrofurantoin Antibacterial Spectrum In Vitro

Gram-positive organisms	Gram-negative organisms
Bacillus subtilis	*Enterobacter aerogenes*
Corynebacterium sp. (diphtheroids)	*Alcaligenes faecalis*
Staphylococcus aureus	*Escherichia coli*
Enterococcus faecalis	*Klebsiella pneumoniae*
	Proteus mirabilis
	Proteus morganii
	Proteus rettgeri
	Proteus vulgaris
	Pseudomonas aeruginosa

in the urine with usual therapeutic doses. *Escherichia coli* is very sensitive (96 percent) to nitrofurantoin at this concentration, as are other coliform bacteria (68 percent), whereas *Enterobacter* and *Klebsiella* spp. are less susceptible (36 percent).[4] Most *Proteus* sp. (92 percent) are moderately resistant, and *P. aeruginosa* is almost always resistant.[4] The usual MIC of nitrofurantoin for *E. coli* is 16 μg/ml, whereas *Enterobacter* and *Klebsiella* spp. may require 100 μg/ml and *P. mirabilis*, 200 μg/ml.[4] The drug is also active against staphylococci and enterococci, and the MICs are lower, 4.0 μg/ml for *S. aureus* and 25.0 μg/ml for *Enterococcus faecalis*.[1] Salmonellae, shigellae, and *Neisseria* sp. are also susceptible to nitrofurantoin, as are *S. pyogenes*, *S. pneumoniae*, and *Corynebacterium* spp. including *C. diphtheriae*, but their susceptibility to the drug is of little practical importance.[1] In contrast to nalidixic and oxolonic acid, microorganisms sensitive to nitrofurantoin do not readily become resistant to this drug.

Pharmacology

Nitrofurantoin is usually administered orally and is rapidly and completely absorbed from the gastrointestinal tract. The drug crosses the blood-brain and the placental barrier. Only very low levels of antibacterial activity are attained in serum after usual oral doses of the drug, and nitrofurantoin does not accumulate in the serum of patients with normal renal function when given continuously in recommended doses. Also, therapeutically active concentrations of the drug are not attained in most body tissues. The serum half-life is about 20 minutes in patients with normal renal function because about two-thirds of the drug is rapidly metabolized in tissues, with inactivation apparently occurring in all body tissues, although the liver may play a major role.[5] One-third of the drug is rapidly excreted into the urine by both glomerular filtration and tubular secretion, with significant reabsorption when the urine is acid.[5] Nitrofurantoin acts as a weak acid, so in an aciid urine more of the drug is in the undissociated form, and more of the drug is reabsorbed, with less appearing in the urine. In an alkaline urine, more of the drug is in the dissociated or ionized form, little of the drug is reabsorbed, and more appears in the urine,[6] but the antibacterial efficacy is decreased.[7] Therefore, the urine should not be alkalinized. Nitrofurantoin has been shown to diffuse into the interstitial tissue of the renal medulla[8] and to be present in higher concentrations in the lymphatics draining the medulla than in serum.[9] Since one-third of an orally administered dose of the drug is excreted unchanged (i.e., in a therapeutically active form) into the urine,[5] an average dose of nitrofurantoin yields a urine concentration of approximately 200 (range, 50–250) μg/ml in patients with normal renal function. (Nitrofurantoin may color the urine brown.) However, recovery of the drug from the urine is linearly related to creatinine clearance, so the concentration of the drug in the urine of uremic patients may be insufficient to inhibit common urinary tract pathogens when the glomerular filtration rate is less than 30 ml/min.[10] Furthermore, nitrofurantoin accumulates in the serum of patients with creatinine clearances of less than 60 ml/min,[10] and blood levels may range between 5 and 6.5 μg/ml in severe uremia,[11] which increases the danger of systemic toxicity developing, particularly peripheral neuropathy.[12] Although nitrofurantoin is removed by hemodialysis, it is contraindicated in patients with significant renal impairment as well as in newborn and premature infants, who may also develop toxic blood levels.

The macrocrystalline form of nitrofurantoin (Macrodantin) was introduced to delay absorption from the gastrointestinal tract. Since nitrofurantoin is of limited solubility in water, an increase in size of the drug particles might significantly retard it solution rate in and consequently its absorption from the alimentary tract. Delaying the drug's entrance into body fluids was hoped to lower its peak serum concentration and decrease the incidence and severity of nausea and vomiting without significantly affecting its concentration in the urinary tract.[13] Studies on humans have shown that, although the urinary excretion of the macrocrystals is prolonged, there is no difference between macrocrystals and fine particles in the percentage of dose recovered from the urine. The macrocrystalline form results in maximum urinary concentrations of about 150 μg/ml after a dose of 100 mg and is probably associated with a lower incidence of side effects and better patient tolerance than the microcrystalline form is.[14] The mechanism of action, antimicrobic activity, and pharmacology of the macrocrystalline form is otherwise similar to conventional microcrystalline nitrofurantoin.

Toxicity and Adverse Reactions

Gastrointestinal irritation is the most common side effect of nitrofurantoin therapy, particularly anorexia, nausea, and vomiting, which may be controlled by a reduction in dosage or by the concomitant administration of food or milk, although sometimes it is severe enough to require discontinuation of treatment with the drug. Diarrhea and abdominal pain occur less frequently. Gastrointestinal intolerance appears to occur less frequently in patients receiving nitrofurantoin macrocrystals than in those receiving microcrystalline tablets.[14] The crystalline and macrocrystalline forms are therapeutically equivalent.

Hypersensitivity reactions occur occasionally and may involve the skin, lungs, blood, and liver. Also chills, drug fever, arthralgia, a lupus erythematosis syndrome, and anaphylaxis have been observed.

Dermatologic allergic manifestations include maculopapular, erythematous, or eczematous rashes, urticaria, angioneurotic edema, and pruritus and usually subside when treatment of the drug is stopped.[1] Pulmonary reactions include asthmatic attacks in patients with a history of asthma as well as acute, subacute, or chronic reactions. Acute pneumonitis is commonly manifested by the sudden onset of fever, chills, cough, dyspnea, chest pain, pulmonary infiltration with consolidation or pleural effusion seen on x-ray films, and eosinophilia.[15] This syndrome is more common in elderly patients, and the symptoms usually occur within the first week of treatment but may become evident within hours or days or in some cases after a prolonged period after starting nitrofurantoin therapy. This pneumonitis is probably immunologically mediated and is rapidly reversible with cessation of therapy. Corticosteroid treatment may be beneficial and necessary in severe cases.[16] The syndrome rapidly recurs after rechallenge with the drug,[17] and there is some evidence that cell-mediated immunity is implicated in this type of nitrofurantoin sensitivity.[18] In *subacute* pneumonitis the symptoms are more insidious, fever and eosinophilia are observed less often, and recovery may be slower. *Chronic* pulmonary reactions are rare and usually occur in patients receiving continuous therapy for 6 months or more. An insidious onset of malaise, dyspnea on exertion, cough, altered pulmonary function, and roentgenographic and histologic findings of interstitial fibrosis with or without interstitial pneumonitis are common.[19,20] Fever is rarely prominent. This syndrome may also have an immunologic basis. In some cases improvement occurs with cessation of nitrofurantoin and institution of steroid therapy. However, the severity of this reaction and the degree of resolution appear to be related to the amount of time therapy is continued after the onset of clinical signs and symptoms. Permanently impaired pulmonary function may occur even after treatment with the drug is discontinued, especially when the syndrome is not recognized early.

Hematologic reactions include leukopenia, granulocytopenia, eosinophilia, megaloblastic anemia, and hemolytic anemia. Megaloblastic anemia is rare and appears to be due to folic acid deficiency, particularly when repeated courses of the drug are used.[21] Nitrofurantoin can precipitate an acute hemolytic anemia in patients with glucose-6-phosphate dehydrogenase–deficient red blood cells, which is found in 10 percent of blacks and a small percentage of Mediterranean and Near-Eastern ethnic groups. Also the drug should not be given to infants with immature red cell enzyme systems.

Hepatotoxic reactions are very rare and include cholestatic jaundice with prodromal fever, rash, and eosinophilia[22] and hepatocellular damage.[23]

Neurologic reactions include headache, drowsiness, dizziness, nystagmus, which is readily reversible, and peripheral polyneuropathy. This peripheral neuritis is an ascending sensorimotor neuropathy, which may be progressive if treatment with the drug is continued and is one of the most serious side effects of nitrofurantoin therapy.[24] Although it occurs more commonly in patients with renal failure,[12] it also occurs in patients with normal blood urea nitrogen levels and low creatinine clearances[25] as well as in patients, especially the elderly, with normal renal function who receive prolonged courses of nitrofurantoin. The mechanism is unknown,[26] but demyelination and degeneration of both sensory and motor nerves occur. Treatment with the drug should be stopped at the earliest signs of neuritis such as paresthesias.

Transient alopecia may occur. Also, a 17-month-old infant who received nitrofurantoin for 68 days developed permanent yellow discoloration of those teeth that erupted during therapy.[21]

Drug Interactions

Nitrofurantoin antagonizes the action of nalidixic and oxolinic acids.[28]

METHENAMINE

Methenamine (hexamethylenetetramine, hexamethyleneamine, hexamine) is a tertiary amine and has the properties of a monoacidic base in its salt formation and can be combined with an unlimited number of organic and inorganic compounds. It is a colorless, odorless compound that is readily soluble in water and forms weakly basic solutions of pH 8.0–8.5. Its chemical structure is shown in Figure 2.

Methenamine was introduced by Nicolaier in 1895 for the treatment of urinary infections[29] and is available, as the pure base, in 0.5 g tablets as methenamine, *National Formulary* (NF) (Lilly). Methenamine has also been combined with mandelic acid, apparently because of Rosenheim's observations in 1935[30] that mandelic acid is excreted in the urine unchanged and, when given in large doses, renders the urine bactericidal. The combination of methenamine and mandelic acid is marketed as methenamine mandelate under the trade name Mandelamine (Warner-Chilcott). Methenamine has also been combined with hippuric acid to form the salt methenamine hippurate, and this combination is marketed as Hiprex (Merrell-National) and Urex (Riker).

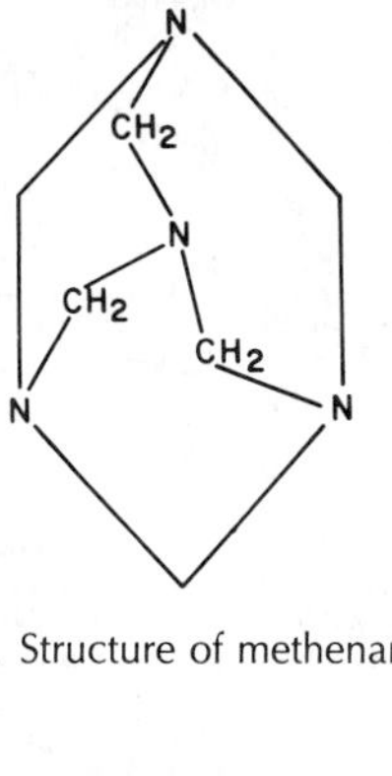

FIG. 2. Structure of methenamine.

Mechanism of Action

Methenamine itself is not bactericidal, nor, regardless of concentration, is it antibacterial in alkaline solutions. Its mechanism of action is due to its hydrolysis, at an acid pH, to ammonia and formaldehyde according to the following reaction:

$$N_4(CH_2)_6 + 6H_2O + 4H^+ \rightleftarrows 4NH_4^+ + 6HCHO$$

Formaldehyde is the active degradation product of methenamine[29] and can only be liberated from methenamine at a pH below 7.0,[31] for example, 6% is yielded at pH 6 and 20% at pH 5. Only two body fluids, gastric juice and urine, are capable of releasing formaldehyde from methenamine.[31–34] Although methenamine has no antimicrobial activity in the presence of alkaline fluids, formaldehyde is equally bactericidal at acid and alkaline pHs.[33] Nevertheless, the degradation of methenamine to formaldehyde is entirely dependent on two factors: proper acidification of the urine and time for hydrolysis of methenamine to occur. Furthermore, the ultimate antibacterial effect of methenamine, that is, through the generation of formaldehyde, is also dependent on the concentration of methenamine in the urine as well as on the urine pH and the time the drug remains in the urine.[35,36] Specifically, at an average urinary methenamine concentration of 0.75 mg/ml and in a quite acid urine (pH 5.0–5.5), at least 1 hour is needed to generate approximately 25 μg/ml of free formaldehyde, 2 hours more reliably produces bactericidal levels of free formaldehyde, and 3 hours is required to reach 90 percent of the final equilibrium.[36] Low concentrations of methenamine in the urine are inadequate to generate bactericidal levels of free formaldehyde regardless of urine pH and time.[36]

Since the proper function of methenamine is dependent on an acid urine, various poorly metabolized acids have been used to acidify the urine putatively during therapy with methenamine. The acids most commonly used are mandelic acid, hippuric acid, ascorbic acid, and acid-producing foods such as cranberry juice. Also, a low pH alone is bacteriostatic, so acidification could possibly serve a double function. Furthermore, mandelic acid and hippuric acid are bacteriostatic in vitro aside from their effect on pH. These organic acids inhibit the metabolism of bacteria by means of their un-ionized molecules.[37] For these reasons, these acids are widely thought to contribute to the lowering of urinary pH as well as to producing an antibacterial effect in urine, which, if true, would be an advantage. However, it is important to emphasize that to achieve this effect, that is, bacteriostasis, in urine it is necessary to administer these acids (mandelic, hippuric, ascorbic, and cranberry juice) in prohibitively large doses, otherwise the urine is not rendered inhibitory. Equally important is that the prepared combinations of the methenamine salts of organic acids, methenamine mandelate and hippurate, when given as currently recommended, contain only a fraction of the dosage of the organic acid (mandelic or hippuric) that is required to either exert an antibacterial effect in the urine or to influence the pH of the urine. Unfortunately, there is little evidence that the acid forms (mandelic or hippuric) of the methenamine salt contribute in any way to the antibacterial activity of methenamine.[38] Fortunately, in most circumstances normal urine, in the absence of diuresis, is sufficiently acid to liberate free formaldehyde from methenamine.[39]

Antimicrobial Activity

Methenamine, through the liberation of free formaldehyde into the urine, is active against all gram-positive and gram-negative bacteria and also against fungi. Almost all bacteria are susceptible to free formaldehyde at about the same concentration, that is, 20 μg/ml.[38] However, urinary tract infections due to urea-splitting organisms such as *Proteus* sp. may not respond to methenamine because it is difficult to acidify the urine in the presence of these infections and free formaldehyde is not liberated. Significant resistance cannot be induced in vitro[40] and is not a problem with methenamine because bacteria and fungi do not become resistant to formaldehyde.

Pharmacology

Methenamine, methenamine mandelate, and hippurate are rapidly absorbed from the gastrointestinal tract, but 10–30 percent is hydrolyzed by the gastric juice in the stomach unless the drug is protected by enteric coating. Because of the ammonia produced, methenamine is contraindicated in patients with hepatic insufficiency. Antimicrobial activity is not achieved in the blood since methenamine does not liberate formaldehyde in serum and mandelic or hippuric acid serum levels are too low to produce any antibacterial effect. Methenamine diffuses widely into body fluids since it is distributed through total body water including that of red blood cells; cerebrospinal, synovial, and pericardial fluids; and both aqueous and vitreous humors of the eye.[31] Only methenamine, not formaldehyde, is present in these body fluids since almost no formaldehyde is generated at physiologic pH, so there is no antibacterial activity in tissues, body fluids, or blood. Methenamine is rapidly excreted into urine. Its clearance from the blood is considerably less than its glomerular filtration rate,[41] and its half-life in blood is quite long. Also, in the presence of an optimally acid urine, only 2–20 percent of the methenamine present is converted to free formaldehyde. Over 90 percent of an administered dose will be excreted into the urine within 24 hours. Although some antibacterial activity may be demonstrated within half an hour, adequate antibacterial activity through the generation of sufficient formaldehyde does not occur, even in a properly acid urine (pH 5.0–5.5), until at least 1 hour and more likely 2 hours after the administration of methenamine. This antibacterial activity is not found in urine from the renal pelvis or ureter but only in bladder urine because the transit time down the renal tubules, calyces, and pelvis into the bladder is too short to allow the generation of significant amounts of formaldehyde.[32,38,42] Exceptions may occur in extremely dehydrated patients with highly acid urine or in those with some degree of obstructive renal residual urine. The antibacterial activity in bladder urine may be maintained for at least 6 hours or until the patient voids, after which hydrolysis of new methenamine will have to occur to render newly formed urine bactericidal.[38] It is probably best not to force fluids on a patient receiving methenamine because a diuretic urine may be more alkaline and diuresis may reduce the concentration of free formaldehyde to a noninhibitory (<20 μg/ml) level. Except for urine, so little methenamine decomposes in body fluids and tissues that it is virtually nontoxic systemically, and renal insufficiency is no contraindication to methenamine alone. Also, since the acidifying ability of the renal tubules functions in azotemia, these patients can convert methenamine to formaldehyde. However, the acid salts are contraindicated, and methenamine mandelate may precipitate crystalluria.

Toxicity

Methenamine is usually well tolerated, as are both the methenamine salts mandelate and hippurate, but some patients develop gastrointestinal side effects such as gastric distress, nausea, vomiting, and diarrhea. Some patients complain of bladder irritation, with dysuria, frequency, albuminuria, and hematuria, particularly with high doses or prolonged administration. Various rashes may also occur. The methenamine salts should be avoided in patients with gout because these drugs may precipitate urate crystals in the urine.

Drug Interactions

Methenamine combines with sulfamethizole and possibly other sulfonamides in the urine, which results in mutual antagonism.

MAJOR USES AND DOSAGE

In addition to the general uses and doses described in Table 2, these urinary tract agents have also been used as prophylactic and suppressive agents in patients with recurrent urinary tract infections as well as in catheterized patients with bacteriuria and in chronically infected patients with neurogenic bladders subjected to long-term indwelling catheter drainage. Nitrofurantoin has also been used for long-term suppressive therapy, particularly during pregnancy and in children with persistent or frequently recurrent bacteriuria, with reasonably good results.[43–45] Bacterial resistance was not a problem with nitrofurantoin. Methenamine has also been used successfully as prophylactic therapy in men with recurrent bacteriuria[46] as well as in patients with recurrent bacteriuria caused by multiply antibiotic-resistant gram-negative bacilli or by yeasts because these pathogens are susceptible to formaldehyde.[7,41,47,48] In addition, it has been successfully used as a prophylactic agent in otherwise healthy girls and women who have recurring urinary tract infection in the absence of structural abnormalities of the urinary tract,[47,49] although it does not appear to be as effective as trimethoprim sulfamethoxazole administered once daily in these patients.[49] In short, nitrofurantoin, methenamine, or trimethoprim-sulfamethoxazole appear to be the reasonable

TABLE 2. Urinary Tract Agents

Agent	Dosage	Use
Nitrofurantoin	Adults: 50 or 100 mg qid for 1–2 wk Children: 1.25–1.75 mg/kg qid for 1–2 wk	Acute and recurrent uncomplicated urinary tract infections due to susceptible organisms or long-term suppressive therapy for frequently recurrent bacteriuria (single dose of 50–100 mg in adults or 1 mg/kg bid in children). Do not use in patients with renal insufficiency, renal carbuncle, perinephric abscess, or in infants.
Methenamine	Adults: 0.5–2 g (usually 1 g) qid or bid Children: 15 mg/kg qid	Chronic suppressive treatment of urinary tract infections when urine pH is 5.5 or less. Not a primary drug for acute urinary tract infections.
Methenamine mandelate	Adults: 1 g qid Children: 15 mg/kg qid	Chronic suppressive treatment of urinary tract infections when urine pH is 5.5 or less. Not a primary drug for acute urinary tract infections.[a]
Methenamine hippurate	Adults: 1 g bid Children age 6–12 yr: 0.5–1 g bid	Chronic suppressive treatment of urinary tract infections when urine pH is 5.5 or less. Not a primary drug for acute urinary tract infections.[a]

[a] One gram of methenamine mandelate or hippuric acid contains only 480 mg of methenamine and 520 mg of mandelic or hippuric acid. These combinations contain an amount of acid that is unlikely to contribute significant antibacterial activity to the urine. Also, there is little evidence that these acid forms contribute to the antibacterial activity of methenamine.

agents for the prophylaxis of frequently recurrent urinary tract infections.

Methenamine has also been used regularly to treat patients with chronic bacteriuria in the presence of indwelling bladder catheters or patients who are receiving intermittent bladder catheterization as well as patients with neurogenic bladders with indwelling catheters. There is little evidence that methenamine, when given as methenamine mandelate or hippurate, prevents the acquisition of or eradicates bacteriuria in patients with suprapubic or indwelling Foley catheters.[50,51] This is understandable since the mechanism of action of methenamine requires the generation of formaldehyde, which takes a minimum of 1 hour to be made in sufficient antibacterial concentrations. It is unlikely that urine remains in the bladder long enough for this reaction to occur in patients with constant bladder drainage. On the other hand, methenamine could potentially be effective in patients with neurogenic bladders who are receiving intermittent catheterization since urine would remain in the bladder for sufficient periods of time. However, recent observations indicate that methenamine, when given as the mandelic acid salt methenamine mandelate, was ineffective as either a suppressive or prophylactic agent in patients undergoing intermittent catheterization.[51] It is important to emphasize that the methenamine used in all these studies was combined with mandelic or hippuric acid as methenamine mandelate or hippurate. The actual amount of methenamine in these combinations is less than half of the total dose administered, which may have provided inadequate urine concentrations of methenamine for the generation of sufficient formaldehyde.

In summary, the urinary tract agents discussed in this chapter seem to be effective in treating acute, uncomplicated symptomatic bacteriuria of the lower urinary tract. Nitrofurantoin is effective in treating upper tract infection and frequent bacteriuria as well as a long-term suppressive agent in children and pregnant women. Methenamine, used properly, is also effective in women with uncomplicated recurrent bacteriuria, including those that are multiply antibiotic resistant, and as a prophylactic agent in men with recurrent infection. There is little convincing evidence that methenamine combined with mandelic or hippuric acid has any advantage over the use of methenamine alone. In fact, there is a strong possibility that, when these salts are used in the doses currently recommended, insufficient methenamine is delivered to the urine to generate adequate concentrations of formaldehyde.

REFERENCES

1. Kucers A, Bennett NM. Nitrofurans. In: Kucers A, Bennett NM, eds. The Use of Antibiotics. Philadelphia: JB Lippincott; 1979:749.
2. Paul HE, Paul MF. The nitrofurans—chemotherapeutic properties. In: Schnitzer RJ, Hawking F, eds. Experimental Chemotherapy. New York; Academic Press; 1966:521.
3. Albert PS, Mininberg DJ, Davis JE. Nitrofurans: Sperm-immobilizing agents. Their tissue toxicity and clinical application. Urology. 1974;4:307.
4. Turck M, Ronald AR, Petersdorf RG. Susceptibility of Enterobacteriaceae to nitrofurantoin correlated with eradication of bacteriuria. Antimicrob Agents Chemother. 1966;446.
5. Reckendorf HK, Castringius RG, Spingler HK. Comparative pharmacodynamics, urinary excretion, and half-life determinations of nitrofurantoin sodium. Antimicrob Agents Chemother. 1962:531, 1963.
6. Andriole VT. Factors affecting antibiotic concentrations in urine and kidney tissue. In: Proceedings of the Fourth International Congress on Nephrology Stockholm. Basel: S. Karger; 1969:338.
7. Pratt WB. The urinary tract antiseptics. In: Pratt WB, ed. Chemotherapy of Infection. New York: Oxford University Press; 1977:215.
8. Currie GA, Little PJ, McDonald SJ. The localization of cephaloridine and nitrofurantoin in the kidney. Nephron. 1966;3:282.
9. Katz YJ, Cockett ATK, Moore RS. Renal lymph and antibacterial levels in the treatment of pyelonephritis. Life Sci. 1964;3:1249.
10. Sachs J, Greer T, Noell P, et al. Effect of renal function on urinary recovery of orally administered nitrofurantoin. N Engl J Med. 1968;278:1032.
11. Loughridge L. Peripheral neuropathy due to nitrofurantoin. Lancet. 1962; 2:1133.
12. Felts JH, Hayes DM, Gergen JA, et al. Neural, hematologic and bacteriologic effects of nitrofurantoin in renal insufficiency. Am J Med. 1971;51:331.
13. Hailey FJ, Glascock HW. Gastrointestinal tolerance to a new macrocrystalline form of nitrofurantoin: A collaborative study. Curr Ther Res. 1967;9:600.
14. Kalowski S, Radford N, Kincaid-Smith P. Crystalline and macrocrystalline nitrofurantoin in the treatment of urinary tract infection. N Engl J Med. 1974;290:385.
15. Dawson RB. Pulmonary reactions to nitrofurantoin. N Engl J Med. 1966; 274:522.
16. Morgan LK. Nitrofurantoin pulmonary hypersensitivity. Med J Aust. 1970; 2:136.
17. Murray MJ, Kronenberg R. Pulmonary reactions simulating cardiac pulmonary edema caused by nitrofurantoin. N Engl J Med. 1965;273:1185.
18. Pearsall HR, Ewalt J, Tsoi MS, et al. Nitrofurantoin lung sensitivity: Report of a case with prolonged nitrofurantoin lymphocyte sensitivity and interaction of methenamine-stimulated lymphocytes with alveolar cells. J Lab Clin Med. 1974;83:728.
19. Rosenow EC, DeRemee RA, Dines DE. Chronic nitrofurantoin pulmonary reaction: Report of five cases. N Engl J Med. 1968;279:1258.
20. Holmberg L, Boman G, Bottiger LE, et al. Adverse reactions to nitrofurantoin. Analysis of 921 reports. Am J Med. 1980;69:733.
21. Bass BH: Megaloblastic anaemia due to nitrofurantoin. Lancet. 963;1:530.
22. Ernaelsteen D, Williams R. Jaundice due to nitrofurantoin. Gastroenterology. 1961;41:590.
23. Bhagwat AG, Warren RE. Hepatic reaction to nitrofurantoin. Lancet. 1969; 2:1369.
24. Ellis FG. Acute polyneuritis aftter nitrofurantoin therapy. Lancet. 1962; 2:1136.
25. Craven RS. Furadantin neuropathy. Aust NZ J Med. 1971;1:246.
26. Toole JF, Parrish ML. Nitrofurantoin polyneuropathy. Neurology (NY). 1973;23:554.
27. Ball JS, Ferguson AW. Permanent discoloration of primary definition by nitrofurantoin. Br Med J. 1962;2:1103.
28. Westwood GPC, Hooper WL. Antagonism of oxolonic acid by nitrofurantoin. Lancet. 1975;1:460.
29. Nicolaier A. Ueber die therapeutische verwendung des Urotropin (Hexamethylente tramin). Dtsch Med Wochenschr. 1895;21:541.
30. Rosenheim ML. Mandelic acid in the treatment of urinary infections. Lancet. 1935;1:1032.
31. Hanzlik PJ, Collins AB. Hexamethylenamine: The liberation of formaldehyde and the antiseptic efficiency under different chemical and biological conditions. Arch Intern Med. 1913;12:578.
32. Levy LH, Strauss A. A clinical and bacteriological study of hexamethylenamin as a urinary antiseptic. Arch Intern Med. 1914;14:730.
33. Shohl AT, Deming CL. Hexamethylenamin: Its quantitative factors in therapy. J Urol 1920;4:419.
34. De Eds F. Fate of hexamethylenamin in the body and its bearing on systemic antisepsis. Arch Intern Med. 1924;34:511.
35. Heathcote RSA. Hexamine as an urinary antiseptic. 1. Its rate of hydrolysis at different hydrogen ion concentrations. II. Its antiseptic power against various bacteria in urine. Br J Urol. 1935;7:9.
36. Jackson J, Stamey TA. The Riker method for determining formaldehyde in the presence of methenamine. Invest Urol. 1971;9:124.
37. Draskoczy P, Weiner N. Effect of organic acids on oxidative metabolism of *Escherichia coli*. Fed Proc. 1960;19:140.
38. Stamey TA. General and specific principles of therapy. In: Stamey TA, ed. Urinary Infections. Baltimore: Williams & Wilkins; 1972:253.
39. Elliot JS, Sharpe RF, Lewis L. Urinary pH. J Urol. 1959;81:339.
40. Duca CJ, Scudi JV. Some antibacterial properties of Mandelamine (methenamine mandelate). Proc Soc Exp Biol Med. 1947;66:123.
41. Scudi JV, Reinhard JF. Absorption, distribution and renal excretion of mandelamine (methenamine mandelate). J. Lab Clin Med. 1948;33:1304.
42. Hinman F. An experimental study of the antiseptic value in the urine of the internal use of hexamethylenamin. JAMA. 1913;61:1601.
43. Marshall M, Johnson SH. Use of nitrofurantoin in chronic and recurrent urinary tract infections in children. JAMA 1959;169:919.
44. Normand ICS, Smellie JM. Prolonged maintenance chemotherapy in the management of urinary infection in childhood. Br Med J. 1965;1:1023.
45. Brumfitt W, Smith GW, Hamilton-Miller JMT, et al. A clinical comparison between macrodantin and trimethoprim for prophylaxis in women with recurrent urinary infection. J Antimicrob Agents Chemother. 1985;16:111–120
46. Freeman RB, Smith WM, Richardson JA, et al. Long-term therapy for chronic bacteriuria in men: U.S. Public Health Service cooperative study. Ann Intern Med. 1975;83:133.
47. Holland NH, West CD. Prevention of recurrent urinary tract infections in girls. Am J Dis Child. 1963;105:560.
48. Brumfitt W, Hamilton-Miller JMT, Gargon RA, et al. Long-term prophylaxis of urinary infections in woman: Comparative trial of trimethoprim, methenamine hippurate, and topical povidone-iodine. J Urol. 1983;130:1110–4.
49. Harding GK, Roland AR. A controlled study of antimicrobial prophylaxis of recurrent urinary infection in women. N Engl J Med. 1974;291:597.
50. Gerstein AR, Okun R, Gonick HC, et al. The prolonged use of methenamine hippurate in the treatment of chronic urinary tract infections. J. Urol. 1968;100:767.
51. Vainrub B, Musher DM. Lack of effect of methenamine in suppression of, or prophylaxis against, chronic urinary infection. Antimicrob Agents Chemother. 1977;12:625.

32. ANTIMYCOBACTERIAL AGENTS

ROBERT H. ALFORD

Drugs for mycobacterial infections will be categorized under three headings: those primarily for *Mycobacterium tuberculosis,* drugs for "atypical" mycobacterial infections, and agents principally for the treatment of leprosy. Traditionally, antimicrobials for tuberculosis have been classified further as "first-line drugs" having superior efficacy with acceptable toxicity and "second-line" drugs either having less efficacy, greater toxicity, or both.[1–4]

Antituberculous drugs vary according to bactericidal function and site of action in tuberculous lesions.[4] All of the first-line agents are bactericidal except for ethambutol. The bactericidal action of pyrazinamide (PZA) against actively metabolizing tubercle bacilli was overlooked initially because infections in PZA-treated animals relapsed due to metabolically inactive organisms ("persisters") that regrew.

In site of action, drugs may exert their effects against mycobacteria either within cavities, intracellularly, or intermittently replicating in closed caseous lesions: (*1*) four agents have activity against the large, actively dividing extracellular populations in cavities—isoniazid (INH), rifampin, streptomycin, and ethambutol. Pyrazinamide is inactive at the neutral or slightly alkaline pH encountered in such areas. (*2*)Against intracellular mycobacteria, isoniazid, rifampin, and pyrazinamide are active, whereas streptomycin, other aminoglycosides, and capreomycin lose their activity at acidic pH. (*3*) Slowly replicating organisms in caseous lesions are killed only by rifampin and, somewhat less readily, by INH. Thus, the combination of INH and rifampin is bactericidal for all three populations in tuberculous lesions. (*4*) A fourth population of dormant organisms may be particularly difficult to eradicate. These principles are especially important in designing "short-course" chemotherapy and for resistant or relapsing infections.[4,5]

FIRST-LINE ANTITUBERCULOSIS DRUGS

Isoniazid

Derivation and Structure. Isoniazid, isonicotinic acid hydrazide (INH), a synthetic agent, was demonstrated in 1952 to be effective in the treatment of human tuberculosis.[6] Its structure is indicated in Figure 1.

Mechanism of Action. Isoniazid, bactericidal against growing *Mycobacterium tuberculosis* in vitro, is static against "resting" organisms. It acts primarily by inhibition of the synthesis of mycolic acid,[3] an important component of mycobacterial cell walls. Against certain "atypical" mycobacteria, INH in higher concentration also affects energy-requiring metabolic pathways.[7]

Antimicrobial Activity. Against *M. tuberculosis,* 0.025–0.05 μg/ml of INH is inhibitory. Isoniazid can kill intracellular organisms provided they are replicating. Tubercle bacilli become resistant to INH administered alone. Initially susceptible isolates will become INH-resistant in 71 percent of cases treated for 3 months with INH alone.[6] Resistance results from selection under the antimicrobic pressure of less susceptible variants of *M. tuberculosis* that initially number 1 in 10^6 bacilli among untreated mycobacterial populations. Surviving bacilli exhibit decreased INH uptake. Large populations like the 10^9–10^{10} bacilli in open pulmonary cavities are especially likely to contain significant numbers of resistant mycobacteria that subsequently overgrow and lead to secondary resistance. Emergence of resistance depends on the type and duration of prior therapy.[8] Significant primary resistance to INH in untreated cases occurs in approximately 6 percent of isolates in the United States and should be anticipated, particularly in immigrants from regions having high levels of endemic drug resistance. Primary resistance has been documented in 43 percent of Korean isolates of *M. tuberculosis.*[9]

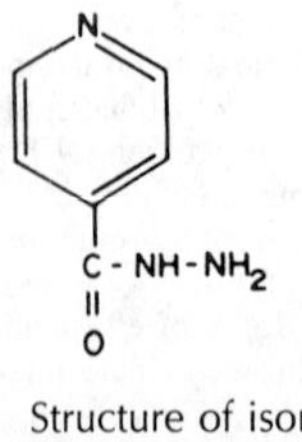

FIG. 1. Structure of isoniazid.

Pharmacology. Isoniazid, well absorbed orally or intramuscularly, is subsequently distributed throughout the body including the cerebrospinal fluid. CSF levels are usually about 20 percent of plasma levels but in the presence of meningeal inflammation may equal plasma concentrations.

Metabolism of INH is initially by liver *N*-acetyl transferase. Its rate of acetylation is determined genetically, with slow acetylation inherited as an autosomal recessive trait[3] that varies from 5 percent in Canadian eskimos to 83 percent in Egyptians; 10–15 percent of Orientals are slow acetylators, as are 58 percent of American whites.[3] Six hours after a 4 mg/kg oral dose, slow acetylators have INH serum levels of >0.8 μg/ml and rapid acetylators, <0.2 μg/ml.[1] The striking bimodal distribution of serum half-lives caused by acetylation status is depicted in Figure 2. Acetylator status does not affect outcome with daily therapy because plasma levels are well above inhibitory concentrations. However, weekly intermittent therapy may be adversely affected, with rapid acetylators faring less well. Primarily excreted as metabolically altered drug in the urine, some unaltered INH appears there as well. Dosage modification in hepatic or renal failure is not usually necessary, but in the presence of severe hepatic insufficiency, a reduction in dosage by one-half is recommended, and with significant renal failure, a dosage reduction to 150–200 mg/day is recommended for slow acetylators.[10] Table 1 indicates antituberculous drugs requiring dosage modification in hepatic or renal failure.

Adverse Reactions. Isoniazid has infrequent major toxicities that include hepatitis. Approximately 15 percent of INH recipients will have some elevation in serum glutamic-oxaloacetic transaminase (SGOT) levels that resolves with continued therapy. Although fatal INH hepatitis had been clearly documented by 1970,[11] early reports infrequently recognized it. Documen-

TABLE 1. Dosage Modification Requirement for Antituberculous Drugs Used in Hepatic or Renal Failure

Antimicrobial	*Hepatic Failure*	*Renal Failure*
Ethionamide	Yes	No
Isoniazid	Yes	Minor
Pyrazinamide	Yes	Yes[a]
Rifampin	Yes	No
Thiacetazone	Yes	Minor
Amikacin	No	Yes
Capreomycin	No	Yes
Cycloserine	No	Yes
Ethambutol	No	Yes
Kanamycin	No	Yes
Para-aminosalicylic acid	No	Yes
Streptomycin	No	Yes
Viomycin	No	Yes

[a] Accumulation of toxic metabolites.

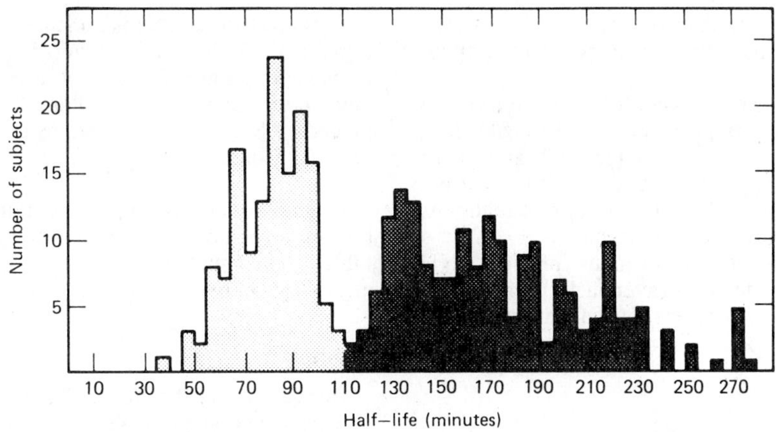

FIG. 2. Bimodal distribution of isoniazid half-lives as related to acetylation status. Patients received 5 mg/kg intravenously. Light bars indicate rapid acetylators and dark bars, slow acetylators. (From Pratt,[3] with permission.)

tation of the incidence of major INH hepatotoxicity awaited a large prophylactic trial reported in 1972 in which 19 of 2321 recipients developed serious hepatitis and 2 died.[12] Hepatotoxicity occurs at any time but is most likely to occur 4–8 weeks after the onset of treatment. Isoniazid hepatotoxicity is clearly correlated with age, as is indicated in Table 2, presumably due to the diminished capacity for repair of INH hepatocellular damage in the elderly. Hepatotoxicity is also more likely to occur in alcoholics with pre-existing liver damage.[12,14] Hepatocellular damage is usually evident histologically, while toxic cholestasis is infrequent. Chronic infection caused by hepatitis B is not a contraindication to the prophylactic use of INH.[15] Isoniazid hepatotoxicity was initially thought to reflect acetylator status, with increased risk for toxicity in rapid acetylators because of an acetylhydrazine metabolite. Subsequent studies have demonstrated that INH hydrolase induced by rifampin apparently increased the production of hepatotoxic hydrazine in *slow* acetylators treated daily with INH and rifampin.[16] Monitoring of concentrations of hepatic enzymes in plasma is generally unnecessary except in the elderly. Patients should be advised to discontinue INH therapy at the onset of symptoms consistent with beginning hepatitis.

Appreciation of the frequency of INH hepatotoxicity has not significantly limited therapeutic indications but has had a major impact on "chemoprophylactic" usage. No longer is "routine" INH chemoprophylaxis of adult purified protein derivative (PPD) skin test converters recommended, with special caution indicated in people over the age of 35.[13]

Neurotoxicity. Peripheral neuropathy occurs in 17 percent of those receiving 6 mg/kg/day of INH but less frequently with a conventional dosage. Neuropathy is especially likely in people with poor nutrition or underlying neuropathy resulting from alcoholism, diabetes, or uremia and is more frequent in slow acetylators who have higher serum levels of unaltered drug. Increased pyridoxine excretion is caused by INH administration. Pyridoxine replacement does not affect INH antimicrobial action[3] but does ameliorate the neuropathy.

TABLE 2. Age-Related Incidence of Isoniazid Hepatotoxicity

Age (yr)	*Serious Hepatotoxicity (% Patients)*
<20	"Rare"
20–34	0.3
35–49	1.2
50>	2.3

(From Centers for Disease Control.[13])

Central nervous system (CNS) INH toxicity may cause aberrations ranging from memory loss to psychosis or seizures. Particular caution should be exercised when administering INH to people with convulsive disorders. Optic neuropathy has been reported. Toxic CNS reactions are not related directly to pyridoxine deficiency for certain but have responded to its administration.[1]

Hypersensitivity Reactions. Fever that may be sustained or "spiking," skin eruptions, or hematologic abnormalities may occur. A substantial number of INH recipients develop positive antinuclear antibody (ANA) reactions, and some will manifest an INH-induced lupuslike syndrome that is usually reversible upon discontinuation of treatment with the drug.

Other Reactions. Arthritic disorders associated with INH administration have included Dupuytren's contracture and the "shoulder–hand" syndrome. Pellagra may occur in malnourished recipients of INH.[1,3] Pyridoxine deficiency–related anemia can occur.

Significant Drug Interactions. Phenytoin (Dilantin) toxicity is potentiated by INH. Mental changes, nystagmus, and ataxic gait can result, especially in slow acetylators in whom high INH levels inhibit phenytoin metabolism. Combined INH and rifampin therapy predisposes to elevation of serum hepatic enzyme levels in up to 29 percent of recipients of that combination. Plasma INH levels are increased by concurrent para-aminosalicylic acid (PAS) because of interference with acetylation.

Usage. Isoniazid is indicated for all forms of tuberculosis. In 1952, pulmonary disease was found to respond favorably to INH.[6] Tuberculous meningitis was almost always fatal before the advent of chemotherapy. Isoniazid-containing regimens yielded 83 percent survival rates as compared with 45 percent with streptomycin plus PAS.[17] Survival in miliary disease reached 77 percent with INH as compared with 22 percent with streptomycin plus PAS.[18] Therapeutic regimens include one or more companion drugs to discourage emergence of INH-resistant bacilli. Indications for INH include preventive therapy or "chemoprophylaxis" of selected PPD skin test converters.

Availability and Dosage. Isoniazid is available as INH, Nydrazid, Hyzyd, and Niconyl, for example. Dosage forms include 100 and 300 mg tablets, syrup containing 10 mg/ml, and a 100 mg/ml solution for parenteral injection. The usual dosage is 5–10 mg/kg/day (preferably 300 mg as a single daily dose), with the lower dosage range used routinely in adults for most therapy or "prophylaxis." Higher dosage schedules may be used for serious infections and for infants and children. Divided doses result in plasma concentrations below recommended therapeutic levels.

Intermittent therapy such as twice-weekly high-dose INH (15 mg/kg orally) combined with streptomycin (25–30 mg/kg im), ethambutol (50 mg/kg po), low-dose rifampin (600 mg po), or pyrazinamide is being used more frequently after an initial period of daily drug administration.[19] Such intermittent regimens are less expensive and encourage compliance.

Although not recommended for intravenous infusion, INH for injection has been administered intravenously[10] and can be given in this way cautiously when other routes of administration are contraindicated.

Ethambutol

Derivation and Structure. Ethambutol was discovered in 1961 among synthetic compounds being screened for antituberculous activity. Its structure is indicated in Figure 3.

Mechanism of Action. Ethambutol is tuberculostatic. Its precise mechanism of action is not known, although it is probably an antimetabolite affecting RNA synthesis.

Pharmacology. Ethambutol administered orally is 75–80 percent absorbed and yields peak plasma levels of 5 μg/ml after a dose of 25 mg/kg. It is distributed throughout the body, including the CSF. Although little ethambutol crosses normal meninges, levels 10–50 percent of those in serum appear in CSF with meningeal inflammation. After conversion of approximately 15 percent of absorbed ethambutol to inactive metabolites, 80 percent of the parent and metabolized drug is excreted in the urine. Thus, it becomes necessary to modify the dosage in significant renal failure.

Antimicrobial Activity. Ethambutol is bacteriostatic in vitro and also within macrophages[20] at concentrations of approximately 1 μg/ml against most strains of *M. tuberculosis,* even those that are INH-resistant. Resistance of a stepwise nature occurs when ethambutol is administered without companion drugs. Primary resistance has been reported only occasionally, and cross-resistance with other antimycobacterial drugs is unusual. Thus, ethambutol's principal role is as a "companion" drug to retard emergence of resistance.

Adverse Reactions. The major toxicity of ethambutol is neuropathic. Peripheral neuropathy may occur, but more common is the retrobulbar neuritis that is reported regularly with a dosage of 50 mg/kg/day. Characteristically, impairment of visual acuity or color vision develops, and there may be constriction of visual fields. More likely in association with high-dose or prolonged ethambutol administration, retrobulbar neuritis is usually reversible. Blindness has occurred in the elderly with as little as 15 mg/kg/day. Consequently, patients receiving ethambutol should be instructed to report optic symptoms, and visual acuity and color perception should be tested every 4–6 weeks. Gastrointestinal intolerance is infrequent. Hyperuricemia occurs secondary to decreased urinary uric acid excretion. Infrequent hypersensitivity reactions include dermatitis, arthralgias, and fever.

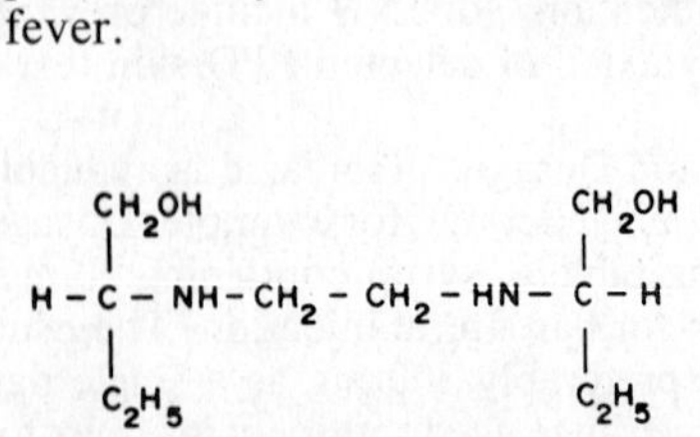

FIG. 3. Structure of ethambutol.

Usage. Ethambutol is indicated for infections due to *M. tuberculosis*. With combined therapy, resistance develops slowly. Because of its greater activity, lower incidence of side effects, and better record of compliance, ethambutol has largely replaced PAS in the United States as a bacteriostatic companion drug for isoniazid.

Availability and Dosage. Ethambutol is available as ethambutol hydrochloride (Myambutol) supplied in 100 and 400 mg tablets. The usual dosage is 15–25 mg/kg/day initially, followed after 60 days by 15 mg/kg/day as a single daily dose.

Rifampin

Derivation and Structure. Rifampin (termed rifampicin in the United Kingdom) is a semisynthetic derivative of a complex macrocyclic antibiotic, rifamycin B, produced by *Streptomyces mediterranei*. In 1967, it was introduced for clinical trials against mycobacterial infections. Its complex macrocyclic structure is indicated in Figure 4.

Mechanism of Action. Rifampin inhibits mycobacterial DNA-dependent RNA polymerase. Human RNA polymerase is insensitive to rifampin's action. It is bactericidal against *M. tuberculosis* at 0.005–0.2 μg/ml. Rifampin's lipid solubility enhances intracellular penetration.

Unlike any other combination, rifampin and INH have consistently sterilized tissue in experimental murine tuberculosis.

Pharmacology. Rifampin is well absorbed orally and yields peak levels of 7–8 μg/ml after 600 mg po. It is widely distributed throughout the body, including cerebrospinal fluid. CSF levels have ranged from undetectable to 0.5 μg/ml in healthy people and reach 50 percent of the plasma concentration with meningeal irritation. Rifampin is deacetylated to an active form that undergoes biliary excretion and enterohepatic recirculation. Due to autoinduction of rifampin's metabolizing enzymes (cytochrome P-450–coupled), biliary excretion increases with continued therapy. Excretion is primarily into the gastrointestinal tract, with lesser excretion in the urine. Both serum concentrations and urinary excretion increase in the presence of hepatic failure.[21] Probenecid causes decreased excretion by blocking hepatic uptake. In liver failure, some dosage reduction is indicated, but a full dosage can be administered in renal failure.

Antimicrobial Activity. Rifampin is active against *M. tuberculosis* to a degree comparable with INH. It affects intracellular, slowly replicating bacilli in caseous foci or intracavitary organisms as noted previously. In vitro, rapid, one-step resistance emerges with a low frequency, which precludes rifampin's use alone. Low-frequency resistance has been reported among clinical isolates of *M. tuberculosis*.[22]

Hepatotoxicity. Adverse reactions are rather frequent with

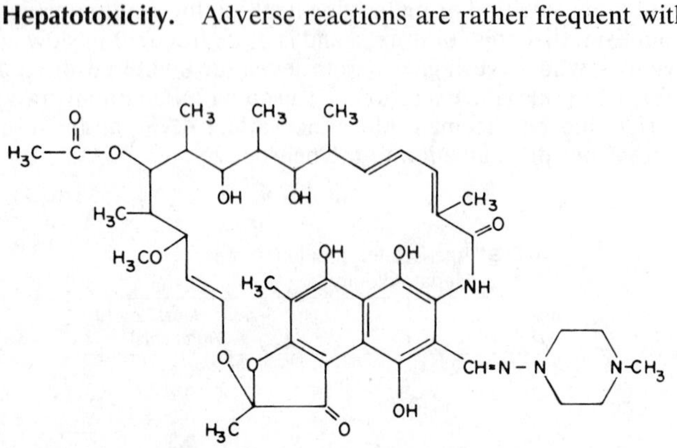

FIG. 4. Structure of rifampin.

rifampin, but only 6 of 372 patients taking the drug for 20 weeks had to discontinue therapy because of adverse effects.[23] The major adverse effect is hepatotoxicity, which has caused 16 deaths in 500,000 rifampin recipients.[1]

Minimal abnormalities in liver function test findings are common in people receiving rifampin and usually resolve even with continuation of the drug. Characteristically, elevations of bilirubin and alkaline phosphatase levels are noted, whereas elevations of hepatocellular enzymes such as SGOT can result from rifampin, INH, or both. Rifampin-induced toxic liver changes occur earlier and produce a patchier cellular abnormality with less marked periportal inflammation than does the hepatitis caused by INH.[24] Alcoholics with pre-existing liver damage appear to be especially prone to serious rifampin-induced liver toxicity. Concomitant INH appears to increase the risk of rifampin-related hepatotoxicity. It has been suggested that rifampin not be given to alcoholics with underlying liver damage "unless other drug combinations are contraindicated."[24] Such advice is hard to follow since alcoholism also predisposes to INH hepatitis and because alternatives such as PZA, PAS, and ethionamide also may be hepatotoxic. Children appear to be at an increased risk of serious rifampin-associated hepatotoxicity, perhaps in part because of relatively higher doses. Jaundice has been frequent (27 percent) in children with tuberculous meningitis who were receiving rifampin in combination regimens but could have been potentiated by phenytoin or other seizure medications.[25]

Effects on Immune Parameters. The effects of rifampin on humoral and cell-mediated immunity appear to be extensive but are of uncertain significance. Light-chain proteinuria occurs in 85 percent of those receiving rifampin.[26] It inhibits blastic transformation of phytohemagglutinin-stimulated lymphocytes and interferes with cutaneous reactivity to intradermal tuberculin.[27]

Hypersensitivity Reactions. Flushing, fever, pruritus without a rash, urticaria, eosinophilia, hemolysis, and renal failure due to interstitial nephritis[28] may occur after rifampin administration. A systemic flulike syndrome, at times associated with thrombocytopenia, appears to have an immunologic basis and has been described most often with intermittent high-dose rifampin. However, regimens employing 600 mg of rifampin twice weekly have recently produced the flulike syndrome very infrequently.[29]

Other Side Effects. The widespread systemic distribution of rifampin is reflected in the orange color appearing in urine, feces, saliva, sputum, pleural fluid, tears, soft contact lenses, sweat, semen, and CSF of people receiving the drug. Patients should be appropriately forewarned. With overdosage, a "red-man" syndrome caused from drug discoloration has occurred. Infrequently, gastrointestinal intolerance may result.

Significant Drug Interactions. By potentiating hepatic microsomal cytochrome P-450–related enzymatic reactions, rifampin induces increased hepatic excretion of a number of drugs and other compounds metabolized by the liver. A list of many of this expanding number of substances is given in Table 3. Several of these interactions appear clinically significant.[30,31] In this manner, it causes decreased activity of the coumarin-type anticoagulants that persists 5–7 days after rifampin therapy is discontinued. Menstrual irregularities and decreased efficacy of oral contraceptives have been reported due to potentiation of steroid hormone metabolism. On the other hand, competition for excretion with contrast materials used in cholecystography may result in a failure to visualize the gallbladder. Rifampin crosses the placenta readily and is not approved for use in pregnancy. There is interference with gastrointestinal absorption of rifampin by PAS. Probenecid administration causes increased plasma rifampin concentrations.

TABLE 3. Compounds Having Rifampin-Induced Reduction in Plasma Levels[a]

Barbiturates	Ketoconazole
Bile acids	Methadone
Chloramphenicol	Metoprolol
Clofibrate	Phenytoin
Cyclosporine	Prednisone—glucocorticoids
Digoxin	Propranolol
Digitoxin	Sulfonylureas
Estrogens	Theophylline
Itraconazole	Verapamil

[a] Reviewed in Baciewicz et al.[30]

Usage. Rifampin's efficacy is indicated in pulmonary tuberculosis by sputum conversion 2 weeks earlier with rifampin than with non-rifampin-containing regimens.[23] Because of rifampin's potent antimycobacterial action, combination regimens with it have yielded gratifying results in short-duration therapy and in retreatment of drug-resistant tuberculosis. Rifampin in combination with INH has been recommended for extrapulmonary tuberculous infections including tuberculous meningitis.

Availability and Dosage. Rifampin is available in the United States as Rifadin and Rimactane, supplied as 300 mg capsules. The usual dose is 600 mg once daily for adults and 10–20 mg/kg/day for children (not to exceed 600 mg/day). Twice weekly 1200 and 900 mg dosage regimens have largely been abandoned due to unacceptably high numbers of toxic reactions. A 600 mg twice-weekly regimen has been generally well tolerated. Rifampin capsules can be opened and the drug suspended in simple or flavored sugar syrup for pediatric administration. The suspension can be refrigerated for up to 2 weeks.

Rifabutin

Several other spiropiperidyl rifamycins have a high degree of activity against mycobacteria including *M. tuberculosis, M. avium-intracellulare* complex, and *M. fortuitum.*[32] Rifabutin (ansamycin, LM-427), a derivative of rifamycin-S is more active in vitro and effective in experimental murine tuberculosis than is rifampin, even against some rifampin-resistant strains.[33–35] Characterized by a long half-life (16 hours) in humans and marked tissue tropism producing tissue concentrations 5- to 10-fold greater than in plasma, rifabutin in animals is no more toxic than is rifampin. Clinical investigations are underway to define rifabutin's role in the treatment of tuberculosis and *M. avium-intracellulare* infections.

Streptomycin

Derivation and Structure. Streptomycin, an aminoglycoside antimicrobic introduced in the 1940s, was the first drug to reduce tuberculosis mortality. Its structure, mechanism of action, and pharmacology are given in Chapter 22. Briefly, the drug is administered intramuscularly and yields serum levels of 25–30 μg/ml after a 1 g injection. It is practically excluded from the CNS. Streptomycin's toxicities are similar to other aminoglycoside antibiotics but has less nephrotoxicity and greater vestibular toxicity than do most aminoglycosides.

Antimicrobial Activity. In vitro, streptomycin is bactericidal for *M. tuberculosis,* but in animals it can be only suppressive and is inactive against intracellular tubercle bacilli. Concentrations of 0.4–10 μg/ml are inhibitory. Rapid emergence of resistance has long been recognized as a hazard of single-drug therapy with streptomycin. Approximately 1 bacterium in 10^6 is primarily resistant to streptomycin. Such high concentrations of tubercle bacilli most often reside in cavitary pulmonary lesions. Primarily occurring cross-resistance to streptomycin is found most often among patient populations having a high incidence of INH resistance. Among other aminoglycosides, amikacin and dibukacin appear to possess superior activity to streptomycin against *M. tuberculosis*.[36] However, familiarity, low toxicity, and reasonable price cause streptomycin to remain the aminoglycoside of choice for tuberculosis.

Usage. Streptomycin is indicated in multiple-drug therapy for tuberculosis. Caution must be exercised with a prolonged dosage of greater than 1 g/day and with administration to the elderly or persons with impaired renal function. Care must also be taken if streptomycin is used in combination with other nephrotoxic or ototoxic antibiotics.

Availability and Dosage. Streptomycin sulfate for injection is provided in 0.5 g/ml single-injection vials and mulidose vials. The customary dose in adults ranges from 2 g daily to 1 g twice weekly (most often 500 mg to 1 g daily). Higher dosage schedules are indicated for initial short-term (2–4 weeks) therapy, with subsequent reduction to 1 g/day or less. Children should receive 20–40 mg/kg/day in two divided doses q12h.

Pyrazinamide

Derivation. Pyrazinamide (PZA) is a synthetic analog of nicotinamide that has been elevated to first-line usage for "short-course" therapy regimens because of its bactericidal action[4] plus acceptable toxicity at relatively low doses. Its structure is indicated in Figure 5

Mechanism of Action. Pyrazinamide is bactericidal for the tubercle bacillus at 12.5 μg/ml. Its maximal activity in vitro is at an acid pH, like that existing intracellularly in tuberculous lesions. Its precise action is unknown. Despite good activity at an acid pH in vitro and inhibitory concentrations within mononuclear cells,[20] PZA is barely active in macrophages pretreated with the drug, which leaves unanswered the mechanism of its apparently selective intracellular action.[37] Resistance evolves rapidly when PZA is used alone. Metabolically inactive tubercle bacilli are resistant to PZA, thus rendering it inappropriate for long-term therapy.[4] Primary resistance is less than 1 percent.

Pharmacology. Well absorbed orally, PZA is widely distributed throughout the body in concentrations exceeding inhibitory levels for the tubercle bacillus. Peak plasma concentrations are approximately 50 μg/ml. A half-life of 12–24 hours lends itself to once-daily dosing. Pyrazinamide crosses inflamed meninges. It is metabolized by the liver, and its metabolic products, including principally pyrazinoic acid, are excreted mainly in the urine, so it is best avoided in renal failure.

Toxicity. Hepatotoxicity occurring in up to 15 percent of people receiving pyrazinamide in initial trials long ago discouraged its use. Early trials of PZA employed dosages of 40–50 mg/kg/day for prolonged periods. Currently recommended regimens of 20–35 mg/kg/day appear to be much safer.[38,39] Patients with pre-existing liver disease probably should not receive the drug; symptoms and hepatic function tests should be monitored in those receiving PZA. Other side effects include urate retention in 56 percent of PZA recipients.[39] Photosensitivity and rash have been reported.

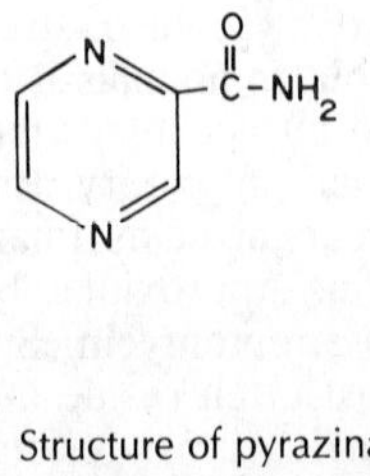

FIG. 5. Structure of pyrazinamide.

Usage. Because of a fear of hepatotoxicity, PZA has been reserved in the United States for the treatment of patients with drug-resistant infections. In other nations, it has played a role in initial therapy, particularly in areas of high primary resistance. Low in price, it can be administered once weekly, thus favoring its usage in developing nations. Now PZA is receiving attention worldwide as a component of multidrug short-course chemotherapy.[4,29,39]

Availability and Dosage. Pyrazinamide is available in 500 mg tablets. The usual dose is 20–35 mg/kg/day orally in two to four spaced doses equivalent to 1.5–2.0 g daily. Apparently it has been well tolerated in a twice-weekly dosage of 50 mg/kg, not to exceed 3 g/day, for short-course regimens. It has even been administered in a 90 mg/kg dose once weekly with little overt hepatotoxicity.

SECOND-LINE ANTITUBERCULOUS DRUGS

Para-aminosalicylic Acid

This synthetic compound, supplied as a sodium or calcium salt or resin, inhibits the growth of mycobacteria by impairment of folate synthesis. Para-aminosalicylic acid is incompletely absorbed orally. A 4 g oral dose yields plasma concentrations of 7–8 μg/ml. Eighty-five percent of absorbed PAS is excreted in the urine in the form of various degradation products.

Toxicity. Chief among side effects of PAS is gastrointestinal intolerance, which may be severe and thus often causes poor patient compliance with treatment regimens. Para-aminosalicylic acid can cause a reversible drug-induced lupus-like syndrome or can produce lymphoid hyperplasia. Recipients can develop a mononucleosis-like syndrome with fever, rash, lymphadenopathy, hepatosplenomegaly, and occasionally toxic hepatitis. Hypersensitivity to PAS is frequent, occurring in 5–10 percent. Further, it seems to cross-sensitize to streptomycin and INH in patients who are receiving multidrug regimens. Readministration of any of the components in a combination regimen after PAS hypersensitivity may subsequently result in reaction to the companion drug. Increased toxicity of INH in association with para-aminosalicylate may result from PAS inhibition of INH acetylation.

Usage. Para-aminosalicylic acid was once included in standard combination therapy for *M. tuberculosis*. In the United States, it has, to a large extent, been supplanted by ethambutol. Due to its low cost, PAS retains a place in multidrug therapy in developing countries but is becoming less favored because of poor compliance.

Availability and Dosage. Para-aminosalicylic acid is provided as acid salts (Pamisyl), as a sodium-potassium-free ascorbate (Pascorbic), and as a resin (Resipas). Dosage forms include 500 mg tablets and 4 g resin packets. The customary dose is 10–12 g/day in three to four divided doses for adults (6–8 g/day of the sodium-potassium–free ascorbate) and, in children, 200–300 mg/kg/day in divided doses.

Cycloserine

Derivation. Initially produced by fermentation, cycloserine is now synthesized. By virtue of inhibition of cell wall synthesis, cycloserine possesses antimicrobial activity against a broad range of prokaryotic microorganisms including mycobacteria. Five to 20 μg/ml inhibits *M. tuberculosis*.

Pharmacology. Cycloserine is readily absorbed orally, with peak serum levels of 20–50 μg/ml. Widely distributed among tissues, no blood-brain barrier exists to cycloserine.[1] Approximately two-thirds of the drug is excreted unchanged in urine, and the remainder is metabolized to inactive forms.

Side Effects. Peripheral neuropathy or CNS dysfunction can be caused by cycloserine. Behavioral alterations or seizures can result. In patients with latent seizures, treatment with the drug is contraindicated.

Usage. Cycloserine is one of several agents to choose from for retreatment or treatment of primarily resistant *M. tuberculosis*.

Availability and Dosage. Cycloserine is provided as Seromycin in 250 mg capsules. The usual dose is 500–1000 mg/day in two divided doses, with 500 mg daily used most frequently.

Ethionamide

Derivation. Ethionamide, a derivative of isonicotinic acid, was synthesized in 1956. It is tuberculostatic at 0.6–2.5 μg/ml against susceptible strains.

Pharmacology. Ethionamide is absorbed well orally and yields peak plasma concentrations of 20 μg/ml. It is widely distributed and penetrates both normal and inflamed meninges to yield CSF concentrations approximately the same as in serum. The drug is metabolized by the liver, with metabolites excreted mainly in the urine. Ethionamide interferes with INH acetylation.

Side Effects. Most people taking ethionamide will experience gastrointestinal irritation with nausea and, frequently, vomiting. Various neurologic disorders can be caused by ethionamide, including peripheral neuropathy or psychiatric disturbances that may require discontinuation of therapy with the drug and reportedly are alleviated by pyridoxine and nicotinamide. Reversible hepatotoxicity, heralded by increasing SGOT values, may occur in approximately 5 percent of ethionamide recipients. Hypersensitivity-type rash or poor diabetic control are infrequent complications.

Usage. Ethionamide is among the choices of agents for treatment of primarily or secondarily resistant tuberculosis.

Availability and Dosage. Ethionamide is available as Trecator-SC in 250 mg tablets. The usual initial dosage is 250 mg twice daily (or as a single dose on retiring) and is increased by 125 mg/day until 1 g/day is reached. Commonly, 500–750 mg becomes the maximum dose because of gastrointestinal intolerance.

Kanamycin, Viomycin, Capreomycin, Amikacin

These agents are considered as a group because all must be administered by intramuscular injection, have similar pharmacokinetics and toxicities, and are excreted by the kidneys. The first three have been employed principally as alternative agents in retreatment regimens for resistant tuberculosis. These agents have additive ototoxicity and nephrotoxicity and should not be given, as a rule, in combination with each other, streptomycin, or another aminoglycoside.

Kanamycin. Kanamycin is an aminoglycoside antibiotic described in Chapter 19 to which some resistant tubercle bacilli are susceptible. Except for lower price, kanamycin has no advantages over amikacin as an alternative in treatment schedules. (See "Amikacin.")

AVAILABILITY AND DOSAGE. Kanamycin sulfate is supplied as Kantrex, 0.5 g/2 ml, 1 g/3 ml, or 75 mg/2 ml (pediatric dose form), for intramuscular injection. The usual dose is 15 mg/kg/day, which for practical purposes is 1 g/day in most adults.

Viomycin. Viomycin is a complex basic polypeptide antibiotic for injection.[2] Certain resistant *M. tuberculosis* strains are susceptible. Cross-resistance to viomycin and capreomycin occurs regularly and is seen less consistently between viomycin and kanamycin.[40] Susceptible strains of *M. tuberculosis* are inhibited by 1–10 μg/ml.

AVAILABILITY AND DOSAGE. Viomycin sulfate for injection is supplied as Viocin in 1 and 5 g vials. The usual dosage is 2 g twice weekly, administered as 1 g every 12 hours on the days of injection. One to 2 g daily has been used for periods of not longer than 1 to 2 weeks.

Capreomycin. Capreomycin is a polypeptide antibiotic produced by *Streptomyces capreolus*. Susceptible *M. tuberculosis* strains are susceptible to 1–50 μg/ml (usually 10 μg/ml), depending on the culture medium. Average peak serum concentrations of 30 μg/ml are achieved. Cross-resistance occurs chiefly between capreomycin and viomycin but also between capreomycin and kanamycin. According to some authorities, capreomycin is less toxic than viomycin is and especially less toxic than is kanamycin.[40] Capreomycin may be employed in the retreatment of resistant tuberculosis as one component of a multiple-drug regimen.

AVAILABILITY AND DOSAGE. Capreomycin sulfate is supplied as Capastat. The dosage is 1 g intramuscularly daily for 2–4 months and is reduced to 1 g two to three times weekly thereafter.

Amikacin. In vitro and in animal trials amikacin is among the most active if not the most active aminoglycoside against *M. tuberculosis*.[36] It has not been used extensively in human tuberculosis. Due to expense and toxicity, it should not supplant streptomycin as the first-line aminoglycoside for the initial treatment of susceptible tuberculosis. Except for cost it probably would replace its congener kanamycin since both have similar pharmacokinetics and toxicities. In renal failure, amikacin might be chosen because assays for it are more generally available.

USAGE. Amikacin appears to have merit as an alternative drug for the retreatment of resistant *M. tuberculosis* infections.

Amithiozone

Amithiozone (thiacetazone), a thiosemicarbazole, is quite active against most strains of *M. tuberculosis*. Susceptible strains are inhibited by 1 μg/ml.[1,2] Peak serum concentrations are 1–2 μg/ml. Resistance to amithiozone readily develops with single-drug therapy and necessitates combination regimens. Toxicity (gastrointestinal irritation and marrow suppression) has precluded use of this agent in Europe and the United States. (The drug is unavailable in the United States.) Gastrointestinal toxicity is comparable to that of PAS. Additionally, hepatic damage has occurred, usually in patients receiving INH concomitantly. Apparently there is a lower incidence of untoward effects in African populations. Consequently, because of its low price, amithiozone has been used as a "first-line" drug particularly in East African developing nations.[2] Amithiozone (Panthrone, Tibione) is administered orally in a dose of 150 mg/day or 450 mg twice weekly.

β-Lactams

Most mycobacteria produce β-lactamases, and several β-lactamase–resistant β-lactam antibiotics or combinations with β-lactamase inhibitors such as clavulanic acid are active in vitro against *M. tuberculosis*[41] and various atypical mycobacteria. The activity of β-lactam agents on intracellular mycobacterial replication is greatly diminished. Ceforanide, active in vitro in the macrophage model in concentrations as high as 50 μg/ml is unable to retard the tubercle bacillus.[20] Similarly, cefotaxime, ceftizoxime, or cefoperazone lack intracellular activity against *M. avium-intracellulare* strains that were susceptible in vitro.[42] However, cefoxitin has proved efficacious in susceptible *M. fortuitum* infections,[43] which gives hope that stable β-lactams sufficiently active against problem mycobacteria may be forthcoming.

DRUGS FOR THE TREATMENT OF ATYPICAL MYCOBACTERIAL INFECTIONS

"Atypical" (i.e., nontuberculous) mycobacteria vary greatly in susceptibility to antimicrobics. Some are susceptible to agents used principally for the treatment of tuberculosis; other atypicals respond to various antibiotics used more commonly for treating pyogenic bacterial infections; and still others, especially among the *M. avium-intracellulare* group, are frequently broadly resistant. Mycobacteria of the *M. avium-intracellulare* complex often contain plasmids that contribute to their broad antimicrobial resistance.[44] Choosing appropriate therapy for atypicals is further confounded because methodology for susceptibility testing varies. Standardization of atypical mycobacterial identification and susceptibility testing methods is in progress.[45] Rational chemotherapy for atypical mycobacterial infections that is based on susceptibility results has become feasible.[46] Regardless of therapy with combinations of drugs active in vitro against *M. avium-intracellulare,* outcomes in the acquired immunodeficiency syndrome (AIDS) are poor.[47]

ANTITUBERCULOUS DRUGS USED FOR THE TREATMENT OF ATYPICAL MYCOBACTERIA

Isoniazid

Agents used principally for the treatment of *M. tuberculosis* were evaluated years ago for activity against "atypical" mycobacteria.[48] Isoniazid inhibits nearly 40 percent of the strains of *M. kansasii* at a concentration of 1–5 μg/ml, as contrasted with only 10–30 percent of *M. avium-intracellulare* strains that are inhibited by that concentration. Some authorities include INH in multidrug regimens for the treatment of many atypical mycobacterial infections even in the face of in vitro INH resistance. Because of borderline susceptibilities of most atypical mycobacteria, doses of INH up to 10–15 mg/kg/day have been used with accompanying increased toxicity.

Rifampin, Rifabutin

Rifampin is used for the treatment of many atypical mycobacterial infections. In vitro, 93–100 percent of *M. kansasii* strains are inhibited by 0.25–1 μg/ml, and virtually all *M. marinum* are susceptible.[49,50] About one-half of *M. scrofulaceum* or *M. avium-intracellulare* strains are inhibited in vitro by 4–16 μg/ml of rifampin. The *M. fortuitum* complex is universally resistant to rifampin, although *M. ulcerans* bacilli are generally susceptible. The response of *M. marinum* infections to rifampin has been particularly encouraging. Synergy of rifampin and other agents is often demonstrable in vitro. Its role as a single agent is discouraged to prevent the emergence of resistance. Rifabutin (ansamycin, LM-427) is inhibitory against all strains of *M. avium-intracellulare* in a concentration of <2 μg/ml.[33–35] It is concentrated severalfold in tissue and apparently has no greater toxicity than rifampin. Controlled clinical trials are underway.

Aminoglycosides

Aminoglycosides have been extensively used for the treatment of atypical mycobacterial infections. Of *M. kansasii* strains, 86 percent are streptomycin susceptible, as are 93 percent of *M. scrofulaceum*. Forty-four percent of strains of *M. avium-intracellulare* have been streptomycin sensitive. The *M. fortuitum* complex is generally resistant, whereas *M. ulcerans* strains demonstrate universal susceptibility to streptomycin in vitro.[51] Despite in vitro susceptibility, streptomycin has not been effective in *M. ulcerans* infections, probably because of inactivity against bacilli located intracellularly, and indeed, surgical excision of Buruli ulcers remains the only effective treatment. Kanamycin is not active in vitro against most *M. kansasii* strains, whereas most *M. scrofulaceum* isolates are kanamycin susceptible, and *M. avium-intracellulare* and *M. fortuitum* are not predictably kanamycin sensitive.

Amikacin and dibekacin,[52] congeners of kanamycin, appear to have greater activity against atypical mycobacteria than the parent compound does. Many atypicals are susceptible to 12.5 μg/ml of amikacin.[36] However, marked variability exists between mycobacteria in susceptibility to amikacin. Virtually all *M. marinum* strains are susceptible to 3 μg/ml of amikacin,[50] but only 50 percent of the *M. fortuitum* group are susceptible to 12.5 μg/ml,[53] whereas other aminoglycosides are even less active.[54] Susceptibility of *M. avium-intracellulare* varies.

Ethambutol, ethionamide, and cycloserine possess variable activity against *M. avium-intracellulare* and have been employed in combination for infections caused by that group. Capreomycin frequently is the only antituberculous drug showing activity against *M. fortuitum*.

MISCELLANEOUS ANTIMICROBIALS FOR THE TREATMENT OF ATYPICAL MYCOBACTERIA

Erythromycin

Nearly all strains of *M. kansasii* and *M. scrofulaceum* and some of those of *M. avium-intracellulare* are susceptible to concentrations of erythromycin that can be achieved in plasma by conventional therapy.[55] Erythromycin has been effective in susceptible *M. chelonae* infections.[43]

Tetracyclines

Some strains included in the *M. fortuitum-chelonae* complex are tetracycline susceptible. Although extensive in vitro testing has not been performed, encouraging clinical results have occurred with tetracyclines, especially minocycline (Minocin) in *M. marinum* infections.[49]

Sulfonamides

Sulfamethoxazole is active against *M. fortuitum*. Localized infections have been cured with sulfamethoxazole alone or in combination with trimethoprim.[43]

M. marinum infections have responded to therapy with trimethoprim-sulfa, but most strains are resistant to concentrations in vitro.[50]

Clofazimine

Discussed more fully under antileprosy drugs, clofazimine (Lamprene) has shown promising in vitro activity against *M. avium-intracellulare*. Most strains tested are inhibited by 1.6–2.0 μg/ml.[32,56] However, trials of clofazimine in combination therapy against *M. avium-intracellulare* in persons having AIDS yielded disappointing results.[48]

Other Antimicrobics

Active chemotherapeutic agents for serious *M. fortuitum* and *M. avium-intracellulare* infections are greatly needed. Cefoxitin (Mefoxin), cefmetazole, and imipenem-cilastatin (Primaxin), apparently because of resistance to *M. fortuitum* β-lactamase, are active in vitro against approximately 80 percent of *M. fortuitum* strains at achievable plasma concentrations.[57] Ciprofloxacin (Cipro) is active against most *M. avium-intracellulare* strains in vitro and consequently deserves further study.[58]

A summary of in vitro susceptibility data of atypical mycobacteria is supplied in Table 4. The table serves as a guide only. It is a compilation of data from a number of laboratories, some using nonstandard methodology or testing a small number of strains. Furthermore, in vitro susceptibility of atypical mycobacteria to an antimicrobial agent fails to guarantee therapeutic efficacy. The earlier cited failure of clofazimine in *M. avium-intracellulare* infections and of streptomycin against *M. ulcerans* indicates the limitations of extrapolating in vitro data to clinical experience. As a rule, good therapeutic outcomes are more likely when agents are used to which atypical mycobacteria are susceptible in vitro, and poor outcomes can be anticipated when there is in vitro resistance. Especially for more resistant atypical mycobacterial infections like those caused by *M. avium-intracellulare* or the *M. fortuitum* complex, well-designed clinical trials with active antimicrobials are needed. Readily available analyses of plasma levels of the antimycobacterial agents are also needed to assess the efficacy and toxicity of drug regimens. The polypharmacy of atypical mycobacterial infections without confirmatory susceptibility testing and plasma concentrations continues to foster unnecessary toxicity and expense.

DRUGS FOR THE TREATMENT OF LEPROSY

Background

The special parasite–host relationship of *Mycobacterium leprae* (Hansen's bacillus), which is characterized by persistence of the organism in tissue for years, has mandated prolonged chemotherapy to prevent relapses. Thus bacillary persistance has long been the major consideration in designing therapy for leprosy (Hansen's disease). Now the second factor is resistance.

Chemotherapy for leprosy for years has consisted, for practical purposes, of dapsone alone. This produced gratifying clinical results and was affordable. Because of monotherapy, however, resistance of leprosy bacilli, both secondary and now primary, has emerged as a worldwide concern[63] and has led to the long overdue use of multidrug therapeutic regimens for leprosy.[64]

Dapsone and Other Sulfones

Derivation and Structure. Diaminodiphenyl sulfone (dapsone, DDS), a synthetic compound, was demonstrated to be effective against rat leprosy in 1941 and soon thereafter was used successfully in human trials. Its structure is indicated in Figure 6.

Mechanism of Action. Sulfones are bacteriostatic presumably by the same mechanism by which sulfonamides interfere with folate synthesis.

Antimicrobial Activity. By mouse footpad inoculation, as little as 0.003 μg/ml of dapsone inhibits *Mycobacterium leprae*.[65] Dapsone appears "weakly bactericidal" for most leprosy bacilli. It has been estimated that 99.9 percent of bacillary populations are killed after 3–4 months of therapy with dapsone.[64] However, despite initial susceptibility, "persister" bacilli apparently exist for years. Secondary dapsone resistance is evident, principally in lepromatous (multibacillary) patients in whom resistance has emerged 5–24 years after commencing therapy.[66] The incidence of secondary resistance varies widely between geographic regions and occurs in up to 19 percent of cases. Fully resistant *M. leprae* should be suspected when patients supervised on 100 mg dapsone daily relapse during treatment.[63] Apparently because of the spread of infection from secondarily resistant cases, primary dapsone resistance is now encountered as frequently as is secondary resistance. Partial (usual) to fully developed (infrequent) primary dapsone resistance varies in frequency, depending on geographic area.

Pharmacology. Oral dapsone is well absorbed. Distributed throughout body fluids, tissue levels are approximately 2 μg/ml. The serum half-life of dapsone is 21–44 hours, with some drug retention for up to 3 weeks. Dapsone is acetylated, with 70–80 percent being excreted as metabolites in the urine. The dosage thus should be reduced in significant renal failure.

Side Effects and Adverse Reactions. Dapsone, an oxidant drug, can produce minor hemolysis in patients receiving 200–300 mg/day. Insignificant hemolysis occurs at doses under 100 mg/day in healthy people or at doses of 50 mg/day or less in people with glucose-6-phosphate dehydrogenase (G6PD) deficiency. Methemaglobinemia is common. Gastrointestinal intolerance occurs and is manifested by anorexia with occasional

TABLE 4. Antimicrobials for "Atypical" Mycobacteria: Likelihood of In Vitro Susceptibilities Being within Range of Achievable Serum Concentrations

Category	Runyon Group	Mycobacterial Species	Likelihood of Susceptibility to Antimicrobial[a]
Photochromogens	I	*M. kansasii*	Erythromycin (4+), rifampin (4+), streptomycin (4+), ethionamide (4+), amikacin (3+), cycloserine (3+), ethambutol (3+), viomycin (3+), INH (2+)
		M. marinum	Rifampin (4+), amikacin (4+), kanamycin (4+), minocycline (3+)
Scotochromogens	II	*M. scrofulaceum*	Amikacin (4+), erythromycin (4+), kanamycin (4+), streptomycin (4+), rifampin (3+), ethionamide (2+), INH (1+)
Nonchromogens	III	*M. avium-intracellulare*	Amikacin (4+), rifabutin (4+), clofazimine (3+), ethionamide (2+), rifampin (2+), streptomycin (2+), cycloserine (2+), kanamycin (1+), INH (1+), ethambutol (1+), viomycin (1+), erythromycin (1+)
Rapid growers	IV	*M. fortuitum*	Cefoxitin (4+), cefmetazole (3+), imipenem-cilastatin (3+), amikacin (3+), minocycline (2+), capreomycin (2+), kanamycin (2+), ethionamide (1+), gentamicin (1+), viomycin (1+)
		M. chelonae ssp. *chelonae*	Amikacin (3+), kanamycin (3+), erythromycin (2+)
		M. chelonae ssp. *abscessus*	Cefoxitin (4+), amikacin (3+), kanamycin (3+), erythromycin (2+)
Other		*M. ulcerans*	Rifampin (4+), streptomycin (4+), clofazimine (2+)

[a] Compilation of data from published sources ranked according to the percentage of tested strains that were found susceptible to achievable serum concentrations of the antimicrobials: 81–100% = (4+), 61–80% = (3+), 41–60% = 2+, 21–40% = (1+).
(Data from references 32, 34–37, 42–44, 47–51, 52–62.)

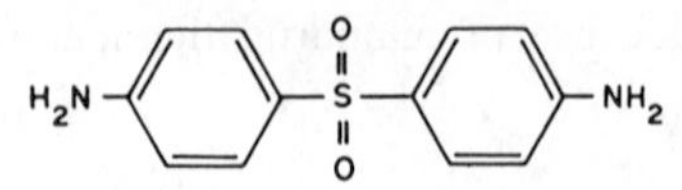

FIG. 6. Structure of dapsone.

nausea and vomiting. Hematuria, fever, pruritus, and skin rashes can occur.

Reactions encountered with dapsone or other sulfones may be difficult to extricate from the reactions that occur because of the disease itself.[67] A *sulfone syndrome* has been reported 5–6 weeks after initiation of therapy and is characterized by fever, jaundice, dermatitis, and lymphadenopathy—a picture somewhat like infectious mononucleosis.[68] Its likelihood is diminished by a gradual increase in dapsone doses until a full therapeutic dosage is attained. Also, during dapsone administration, erythema nodosum leprosum (ENL, type 2) reactions commonly become manifested in persons with multibacillary disease. In borderline or intermediate cases, reactional states (lepra, type 1, upgrade or downgrade) may be accentuated by dapsone therapy.[67] Although apparently infrequent, hypersensitivity reactions to dapsone may thus be difficult to recognize due to the complexity of the illness.

Usage. Dapsone continues to be the basic therapeutic agent for *M. leprae* infections, often as a component of multidrug programs.

Availability and Dosage. Dapsone is available as Alvosulfon tablets of 25 or 100 mg. To avoid untoward reactions, it is begun in a dose of one 25 mg tablet per week with a gradual increase by one tablet per week or so until a full therapeutic dose is reached—usually 100 mg/day. An appropriately reduced dosage is given to children.

Acedapsone

Derivation. Acedapsone (4,4′-diacetyldiaminodiphenylsulfone) is a long-acting repository derivative of dapsone.

Pharmacology. Slow absorption of acedapsone occurs from injection sites, with peak concentrations occurring between 22 and 35 days later. The parent compound has little activity against *M. leprae* but is converted into active dapsone. Its half-life is 46 days and 43 days for the derived dapsone.[69] Because of its long half-life, injections only five times yearly have been used. A 300 mg im dose maintained dapsone levels in volunteers above the inhibitory concentration for *M. leprae,* which was measured in mice for approximately 100 days.

Usage. This repository drug has been employed in *M. leprae* infections with promising results. Microbiologic and clinical responses are somewhat slower than with daily dapsone, which raises the concern that resistance may become a problem. Long-term studies with acedapsone by injection five times yearly have yielded encouraging results indicated by the fact that 91 percent of patients improved or "healed" after 6 years.[70] Acedapsone shows promise, especially in areas where other routes of therapy are not feasible. Trials incorporating widely spaced doses of rifampin plus acedapsone are in progress with the hope of reducing the burden of *M. leprae* more rapidly, thus lessening the likelihood of acedapsone—dapsone resistance.

Sulfoxone

Less well absorbed and more expensive, the disubstituted sulfone sulfoxone is sometimes better tolerated by the gastrointestinal tract than is dapsone. It is formulated in 165 mg enteric-coated tablets with a usual daily dose of 330 mg.[1]

Rifampin

Mechanism of Action and Resistance. The mechanism of action of rifampin against *M. leprae* is presumed to be by inhibition of DNA-dependent RNA polymerase, which produces a relatively rapid bactericidal effect. The inhibitory concentration of rifampin for human strains of *M. leprae* tested in mice is 0.3 μg/ml. A tabulation of the relative activity of antileprosy drugs in clearing tissue of viable bacilli is shown in Table 5.

Usage. Clinical trials of rifampin have indicated that rifampin differs by several orders of magnitude in its initial effectiveness as compared with other antileprosy drugs. Demonstration by skin biopsy that a single dose of 1500 mg of rifampin can reduce the viability of leprosy bacilli to undetectable levels by 3–5 days is truly remarkable. However, limitations of biopsy evaluations are inherent since the method can only account for a decrease to about 10^8 total leprosy bacilli.[71] Prolonged therapy for multibacillary lepromatous disease with 600 mg of rifampin daily has failed to eradicate large bacterial populations. Evidently, in leprosy as in other infections rifampin as a solitary therapeutic agent promotes bacterial resistance. Despite generally satisfactory clinical results with rifampin alone, relapses have occurred.[64]

Although it causes a rapid decrease in *M. leprae* populations, rifampin should be used with another, preferably two, companion drugs, including dapsone for multibacillary disease. The high cost of rifampin has discouraged its use in economically deprived areas. However, once-monthly therapy with 600–1200 mg of rifampin in combination-drug regimens has produced satisfactory clinical responses without adverse reactions.[64,72] Lepra and ENL reactions with rifampin have been comparable or less severe than with sulfones.

Rifabutin (ansamycin) and rifapentine, two investigational substituted rifamycins, have activity against *M. leprae*. In mice, these compounds are even more active than rifampin,[73] which raises interest in human therapeutic trials.

Clofazimine (B-663)

Derivation and Structure. The structure of clofazimine, a phenazine dye, is indicated in Figure 7.

Mechanism of Action and Antimicrobial Activity. Clofazimine's precise mechanism of action is not known. Highly lipophilic and binding to mycobacterial DNA, clofazimine is weakly bactericidal against *M. leprae*. Its action may relate to iron chelation with resulting production of nascent oxygen radicals intracellularly.[74] The inhibitory concentration of clofazimine in mouse tissue is between 0.1 and 1 mg/kg.[75] A delay of some 50 days ensues before tissue antimicrobic activity can be demonstrated in humans.

TABLE 5. Efficacy of Antileprosy Agents in Rendering Tissue Free of Bacilli[a]

Antimicrobial	Adult Human Dosage	Time until Tissue Negative by Mouse Footpad Assay (Days): Range	Median
Rifampin	1500 mg once	<3–<5	<3
Rifampin	600 mg/day	3–<14	<7
Dapsone	50 mg/day[a]	21–>134	61
Clofazimine	200 mg/day[b]	94–138	113
Acedapsone	225 mg/q 75 days	44–>306	214

[a] Dosage raised to 50 mg/day over a period of 4 weeks.
[b] Dosage decreased to 100 mg/day in some patients having excessive skin pigmentation.
(Modified from Shepard et al.,[71] with permission.)

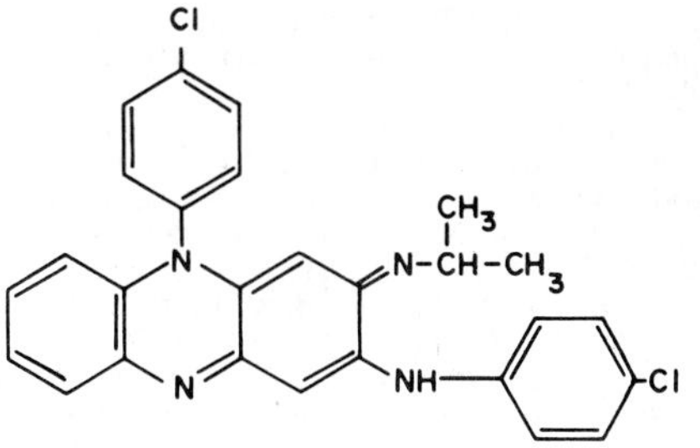

FIG. 7. Structure of clofazimine.

Pharmacology. Clofazimine's pharmacokinetics are complex. Absorption is quite variable, with 9–74 percent of an administered dose appearing in feces. The route of administration is oral and results in plasma concentrations of 0.4–3 μg/ml with a half-life of approximately 70 days. Clofazimine is widely distributed through reticuloendothelial tissues, especially in the liver, spleen, lung, adrenals, adipose tissue, and skin lesions. Red-orange crystals of clofazimine can be observed microscopically in phagocytic reticuloendothelial cells. Precise concentrations in tissues can only be estimated because of the very uneven distribution of the drug. It is largely unmetabolized and subsequently excreted slowly, with less than 1 percent of a dose appearing in urine. Biliary excretion appears to be the major route of disposition of clofazimine. Excretion also occurs in breast milk. A dosage of 100 mg/day has been calculated to eventually result in total accumulation of at least 10 g of drug in human tissue.[75]

Adverse Reactions. Gastrointestinal intolerance may occur. Skin pigmentation is the major side effect from drug accumulation and results in red-brown to almost black skin discoloration in susceptible people. Other side effects are negligible.

Usage. Clofazimine is expensive. Its principal role has been as therapy for sulfone-resistant infections and for people who are sulfone intolerant, usually because of severe sulfone-associated ENL or lepra reactions. These reactions occur much less frequently with clofazimine than with dapsone,[76] possibly promoted by the anti-inflammatory properties of clofazimine.

Availability and Dosage. Clofazimine is available as Lamprene in 100 mg capsules. For monotherapy, its dose has ranged from 300 mg monthly to 600 mg daily and has usually been 100–300 mg/day. The administration of clofazimine alone once weekly or less frequently has resulted in diminished efficacy.[76] In combination therapeutic regimens for multibacillary disease, the recommended dosage has been either 300 mg monthly or 50–100 mg daily.

ADDITIONAL DRUGS FOR THE TREATMENT OF MULTIBACILLARY LEPROSY

Amithiozone (Thiacetazone)

Derivation, structure, pharmacokinetics, untoward reactions, and dosage of this thiosemicarbazone are described under second-line drugs for tuberculosis.

Usage. Amithiozone's efficacy is greater in tuberculoid than in lepromatous (multibacillary) disease. The drug can be administered when sulfones cannot be tolerated. Considerable cross-resistance occurs with sulfones. Amithiozone is not available in the United States.

Long-Acting Sulfonamides

Hypersensitivity reactions including erythema multiforme (Stevens-Johnson syndrome) can result from long-acting sulfonamides. Used with varying degrees of success for the treatment of leprosy, they have no particular advantage over sulfones, share cross-resistance with them, and consequently have been supplanted by the sulfones.

Ethionamide and Prothionamide

Ethionamide has been described under second-line agents for tuberculosis. It and its congener prothionamide possess similar pharmacokinetics and dosing and provide alternatives to clofazimine in multidrug regimens for multibacillary disease, principally in people who are unable to tolerate or who will not accept clofazimine due to skin pigmentation. Ethionamide and prothionamide are apparently weakly bactericidal for *M. leprae*. Both drugs are available as 125 or 250 mg tablets. The dosage with either is 375–500 mg daily.[64] Both agents are expensive, cause a considerable degree of gastrointestinal intolerance, and rarely cause drug-induced hepatitis.

CHEMOTHERAPY-ASSOCIATED REACTIONS IN LEPROSY

Febrile reactions in people with leprosy can be treated with acetylsalicylic acid (aspirin) in conventional dosages. Chloroquine phosphate (Aralen, Avloclor, Resochin) in a dose of 250–500 mg of diphosphate daily has been used in some centers for treatment-associated reactions. Methylprednisolone, 60 mg daily initially, followed by tapering of the dosage, has been reasonably efficacious.[77] Thalidomide in an initial dosage of 400 mg daily has been used to lessen therapy-associated reactions. Thalidomide therapy should not be abruptly discontinued due to exacerbations of reactions. Consequently, a gradually tapering dosage and even maintenance with 50 mg/day has been recommended.[78] Because of teratogenic potential, thalidomide should never be administered to pregnant women or those of childbearing age. Patients who manifest puzzling severe reactions are best managed by a specialist.[67]

REFERENCES

1. Mandell GL, Sande MA. Drugs used in the chemotherapy of tuberculosis and leprosy. In: Gilman AS, Goodman LS, Rall TW, et al., eds. The Pharmacological Basis of Therapeutics. ed. 7. New York: MacMillan Publishing Co, 1985:199–1218.
2. Kucers A, Bennett NM. Drugs Mainly for Tuberculosis. Part III. In: *The Use of Antibiotics*. 4th ed. Philadelphia: JB Lippincott, 1987:1351–437.
3. Pratt WB. Chemotherapy of tuberculosis. In: Chemotherapy of Infection. New York: Oxford University Press; 1977:231–62.
4. Stead WW, Dutt AK. Chemotherapy for tuberculosis today. Am Rev Respir Dis. 1982;125(suppl 3):94–101.
5. National ACCP Consensus Conference on Tuberculosis. Standard therapy for tuberculosis 1985. Chest. 1985;87(suppl 2):117–24.
6. Tuberculosis Chemotherapy Trials Committee. Interim report to the Medical Research Council; the treatment of pulmonary tuberculosis with isoniazid. Br Med J. 1952;2:735–46.
7. Herman, RP, Weber MM. site of action of isoniazid on the electron transport chain and its relationship to nicotinamide adenine dinucleotide regulation in *Mycobacterium phlei*. Antimicrob Agents Chemother. 1980;17:450–4.
8. Costello HD, Caras GJ, Snider DE. Drug resistance among previously treated tuberculosis patients: A brief report. Am Rev Respir Dis. 1980;121:313–6.
9. Carpenter JL, Covelli HD, Avant ME, et al. Drug resistant *Mycobacterium tuberculosis* in Korean isolates. Am Rev Respir Dis. 1982;126:1092–5.
10. Bowersox DW, Winterbauer RH, Steward GL, et al. Isoniazid doses in patients with renal failure. N Engl J Med. 1973;289:84–7.
11. Grossman LA, Kaplan HJ, Brittingham TE. Jaundice and death from isoniazid. J Tenn Med Assoc. 1970;63:23–8.
12. Kopanoff DE, Snider DE, Caras GJ. Isoniazid-related hepatitis. Am Rev Respir Dis. 1978;117:991–1001.
13. Centers for Disease Control. National Consensus Conference on Tuberculosis. Preventive treatment of tuberculosis. Chest. 1985;87(suppl 2):128–32.
14. Gronhagen-Riska C, Hellstrom PE, Froseth B. Predisposing factors in hepatitis induced by isoniazid-rifampin treatment of tuberculosis. Am Rev Respir Dis. 1978;118:461–6.

15. McGlynn KA, Lustabader ED, Sharrar, RG, et al. Isoniazid prophylaxis in hepatitis B carriers. Am Rev Respir Dis. 1986;134:666–8.
16. Gangadharam PRJ. Isoniazid, rifampin, and hepatotoxicity. Am Rev Respir Dis. 1986;133:963–5.
17. Falk A. US Veterans Administration–Armed Forces cooperative study on the chemotherapy of tuberculosis. XIII. Tuberculous meningitis in adults with special reference to survival, neurologic residuals, and work status. Am Rev Respir Dis. 1965;91:823–31.
18. Falk A. US Veterans Administration–Armed Forces cooperative study on the chemotherapy of tuberculosis. XII. Results of treatment in miliary tuberculosis: A followup study of 570 adult patients. Am Rev Respir Dis. 1965;91:6–12.
19. American Thoracic Society. Intermittent therapy for adults with tuberculosis. Am Rev Respir Dis. 1974;110:374–6.
20. Crowle AJ. Studies of antituberculosis chemotherapy with an in vitro model of human tuberculosis. Semin Respir Infect. 1986;1:262–4.
21. Acocella G, Bonollo M, Garimoldi M, et al. Kinetics of rifampicin and isoniazid administered alone and in combination to normal subjects and patients with liver disease. Gut. 1972;13:47–53.
22. Stottmeier KD. Emergence of rifampin-resistant *Mycobacterium tuberculosis* in Massachusetts. J Infect Dis. 1976;133:88–90.
23. Newman R, Doster BE, Murray FJ, et al. Rifampin in initial treatment of pulmonary tuberculosis. A US Public Health Service tuberculosis therapy trial. Am Rev Respir Dis. 1974;109:216–32.
24. Thompson JE. The effect of rifampicin on liver morphology in tuberculous alcoholics. Aust NZ J Med. 1976;6:111–6.
25. Rahajoe NN, Rahajoe N, Boediman I, et al. The treatment of tuberculous meningitis in children with a combination of isoniazid, rifampicin, and streptomycin—preliminary report. Tubercle. 1979;60:245–50.
26. Braber CD, Jebaily J, Galphin RL, et al. Light chain proteinuria and humoral immunocompetence in tuberculosis patients treated with rifampin. Am Rev Respir Dis. 1973;107:713–7.
27. Grassi GG, Pozzi E. Effect of rifampin on delayed hypersensitivity reactions. J Infect Dis. 1972;126:542–4.
28. Flynn CT, Rainford DJ, Hope E. Acute renal failure and rifampin: Danger of unsuspected intermittent dosage. Br Med J. 1974;2:482.
29. Dutt AK, Stead WW. Present chemotherapy for tuberculosis. J Infect Dis. 1982;146:698–704.
30. Baciewicz AM, Self TH, Bekemeyer WB. Update on rifampin drug interactions. Arch Intern Med. 1987;147:565–8.
31. Langhof E, Madsen S. Rapid metabolism of cyclosporin and prednisone in kidney transplant patient receiving tuberculostatic treatment. Lancet. 1983;2:1031.
32. Greene JB, Sidhu GS, Lewin S, et al. *Mycobacterium avium intracellulare:* A cause of disseminated life-threatening infection in homosexuals and drug abusers. Ann Intern Med. 1982;97:539–46.
33. Heifets LB, Iseman MD, Lindholm-Levy PJ, et al. Determination of ansamycin MICs for *Mycobacterium avium* complex in liquid medium by radiometric and conventional methods. Antimicrob Agents Chemother. 1985;28:570–5.
34. Masur H, Tuazon C, Gill V, et al. Effect of combined clofazimine and ansamycin therapy on *Mycobacterium avium–Mycobacterium intracellulare* bacteremia in patients with AIDS. J Infect Dis. 1987;155:127–9.
35. O'Brien RJ, Lyle MA, Snider DE Jr. Rifabutin (ansamycin LM 427): A new rifamycin-S derivative for the treatment of mycobacterial diseases. Rev Infect Dis. 1987;9:519–30.
36. Sanders WE Jr, Cacciatore R, Valdez J, et al. Activity of amikacin against mycobacteria in vitro and in experimental infections with *M. tuberculosis*. Am Rev Respir Dis. 1976;113(suppl 4):59.
37. Nalin R, Potar M, David HL. Pyrazinamide is not effective against intracellularly growing *Mycobacterium tuberculosis*. Antimicrob Agents Chemother. 1987;31:287.
38. Girling DJ. The hepatic toxicity of antituberculous regiments containing isoniazid, rifampicin, and pyrazinamide. Tubercle. 1978;59:13–32.
39. Zierski M, Bek E. Side effects of drug regimens used in short-course chemotherapy for pulmonary tuberculosis. A controlled clinical study. Tubercle. 1980;61:41–9.
40. McClatchy JK, Kanes W, Davidson PT, et al. Cross-resistance in *M. tuberculosis* to kenamycin, capreomycin, and viomycin. Tubercle. 1977;58:29–34.
41. Cynamon MH, Palmer GS. In vitro activity of amoxicillin in combination with clavulanic acid against *Mycobacterium tuberculosis*. Antimicrob Agents Chemother 1983;24:429–31.
42. Nozawa RT, Kato H, Yokota T, et al. Susceptibility of intra- and extracellular *Mycobacterium avium-intracellulare* to cephem antibiotics. Antimicrob Agents Chemother. 1985;27:132–134.
43. Wallace RJ Jr, Swenson JM, Silcox VA, et al. Treatment of nonpulmonary infections due to *Mycobacterium fortuitum* and *Mycobacterium chelonei* on the basis of in vitro susceptibilities. J Infect Dis. 1985;152:500–14.
44. Crawford JT, Bates JH. Isolation of plasmids from mycobacteria. Infect Immun. 1979;24:979–81.
45. Sommers HM, McClatchy JK. Laboratory diagnoses of the mycobacterioses. Cumitech 16. In: Morello JA, ed. Cumulative Techniques and Procedures in Microbiology. Washington, DC: American Society for Microbiology; 1983.
46. Irwin RS, Pratter MR, Corwin RW, et al. Pulmonary infection with *Mycobacterium chelonei:* Successful treatment with one drug based on disk diffusion susceptibility data. J Infect Dis. 1981;145:772.
47. Hawkins CC, Gold JWM, Whimbey E, et al. *Mycobacterium avium* complex infections in patients with the acquired immunodeficiency syndrome. Ann Intern Med. 1986;105:184–8.
48. Hobby GL, Redmond WB, Runyon EH, et al. A study on pulmonary disease associated with mycobacteria other than *Mycobacterium tuberculosis:* Identification and characterization of the mycobacteria. XVIII. A report of the Veterans Administration–Armed Forces cooperative study. Am Rev Respir Dis. 1967;95:954–71.
49. Rynearson TK, Shronts JS, Wolinsky E. Rifampin: In vitro effect on atypical mycobacteria. Am Rev Respir Dis. 1971;104:272–74.
50. Sanders WJ, Wolinsky E. In vitro susceptibility of *Mycobacterium marinum* to eight antimicrobial agents. Antimicrob Agents Chemother. 1980;18:529–31.
51. Leach RH, Fenner F. Studies on *Mycobacterium ulcerans* and *Mycobacterium balnei*. III. Growth in semisynthetic culture media of Dubos and drug sensitivity in vitro and in vivo. Aust J Exp Biol Med Sci. 1954;32:835–52.
52. Nozawa RT, Kato H, Yokota T. Intra- and extracellular susceptibility of *Mycobacterium avium-intracellulare* complex to aminoglycoside antibiotics. Antimicrob Agents Chemother. 1984;26:841–4.
53. Sanders WE Jr, Hartwig EC, Schneider NJ, et al. Susceptibility of organisms in the *Mycobacterium fortuitum* complex to antituberculous and other antimicrobial agents. Antimicrob Agents Chemother. 1977;12:295–7.
54. Clegg HW, Foster MT, Sanders WE Jr, et al. Infection due to organisms of the *Mycobacterium fortuitum* complex after augmentation mammoplasty: Clinical and epidemiologic features. J Infect Dis. 1983;147:427–33.
55. Molavi A, Weinstein L. In vitro activity of erythromycin against atypical mycobacteria. J Infect Dis. 1971;123:216–9.
56. Gangadharam PRJ, Candler ER. Activity of some antileprosy compounds against *Mycobacterium intracellulare* in vitro. Am Rev Respir Dis. 1977;115:705–8.
57. Cynamon MH, Palmer GS. In vitro susceptibility of *Mycobacterium fortuitum* to *N*-formidoyl thienamycin and several cephamycins. Antimicrob Agents Chemother. 1982;22:1079–81.
58. Swenson JM, Thornsberry C, Silcox VA. Rapidly growing mycobacteria: Testing of susceptibility to 34 antimicrobial agents by broth microdilution. Antimicrob Agents Chemother. 1982;22:186–92.
59. Loria PR. Minocycline hydrochloride treatment for atypical acid-fast infection. Arch Dermatol. 1976;112:517–9.
60. Donta ST, Smith PW, Levitz RE, et al. Therapy of *Mycobacterium marinum* infections. Use of tetracyclines vs rifampin. Arch Intern Med. 1986;146:902–4.
61. Yajdo DM, Nassos PS, Hadley WK. Therapeutic implication of inhibition versus killing of *Mycobacterium avium* complex by antimicrobial agents. Antimicrob Agents Chemother. 1987;31:117–20.
62. Brown TH. The rapidly growing mycobacteria—*Mycobacterium fortuitum* and *Mycobacterium chelonei*. Infect Control. 1985;6:283–7.
63. US Public Health Service Centers for Disease Control. Increase in prevalence of leprosy caused by dapsone-resistant *Mycobacterium leprae*. MMWR. 1982;30:637–8.
64. WHO Study Group. Chemotherapy of Leprosy for Control Programmes. Geneva: World Health Organization; 1982.
65. Levy L, Peters JH. Susceptibility of *Mycobacterium leprae* to dapsone as a determinant of patient response to acedapsone. Antimicrob Agents Chemother. 1976;9:102–12.
66. Pearson JMH, Rees RJW, Waters MFR. Sulphone resistance in leprosy. A review of one hundred proven clinical cases. Lancet. 1975;2:69–72.
67. Case records of the Massachusetts General Hospital. Weekly clinicopathological exercises. Case 49-1985. Erythema nodosum leprosum reaction in patient with lepromatous leprosy. N Engl J Med. 1985;313:1464–72.
68. Adverse reactions to dapsone (editorial). Lancet. 1981;2:184–5.
69. Peters JH, Murray JF, Gordon GR, et al. Acedapsone treatment of leprosy patients: Response versus drug disposition. Am J Trop Med Hyg. 1977;26:127–36.
70. Russell DA, Shepard CC, McRae DH, et al. Acedapsone (DADDS) treatment of leprosy patients in the Karimui of Papua New Guinea: Status at six years. Am J Trop Med Hyg. 1975;24:485–95.
71. Shepard CC, Levy L, Fasal P. Further experience with the rapid bactericidal effect of rifampin on *Mycobacterium leprae*. Am J Trop Med Hyg. 1974;23:1120–4.
72. Yawalkar SJ, Languillon J, Hajra SK, et al. Once-monthly rifampicin plus dapsone in initial treatment of lepromatous leprosy. Lancet. 1982;1:1199–202.
73. Pattyn SR. Rifabutin and rifapentime compared with rifampin against *Mycobacterium leprae* in mice. Antimicrob Agents Chemother. 1987;31:134.
74. Niwa Y, Sakance T, Miyachi Y, et al. Oxygen metabolism in phagocytes of leprotic patients: Enhanced endogenous superoxide dismutase activity and hydroxyl radical generation by clofazimine. J Clin Microbiol. 1984;20:837–42.
75. Levy L. Pharmacologic studies of clofazimine. Am J Trop Med Hyg. 1974;23:1097–109.
76. US Leprosy Panel. Spaced clofazimine therapy of lepromatous leprosy. Am J Trop Med Hyg. 1976;25:437–44.
77. Grove DI, Warren KS, Mahmoud AAF. Algorithms in the diagnosis and management of exotic diseases. XV. Leprosy. 1976;134:205–10.
78. Convit J, Browne SG, Languillon J, et al. Therapy of leprosy. Bull WHO. 1970;42:667–72.

33. ANTIFUNGAL AGENTS

JOHN E. BENNETT

The broad array of topical agents already available and the gratifying number of systemic agents now entering clinical trial have necessitated that this chapter be limited to major drugs either now on the market or likely to be marketed in the near future.

TOPICAL AGENTS

Topical Agents for Cutaneous Use

Use of topical agents is confined to infections of the epidermis, hair, nails, and cornea. This form of application is not effective in deeper cutaneous infections, such as sporotrichosis, blastomycosis, or chromomycosis. The choice between treating superficial infections with a topical or systemic agent depends on the fungus and on the site and extent of the lesion. For example, topical therapy is rarely used for ringworm of the scalp, nails, or extensive *Trichophyton rubrum* lesions of the trunk. The efficacy of topical agents in ringworm of the beard or in chronic noninflammatory sole and palm lesions also tends to be poor. Among the topical agents, the choice of formulation is important. Creams or solutions are preferred for fissured or inflamed intertriginous areas such as on the toe webs, groin, or scrotum. Use of powder, whether administered by a shake container or aerosol, is confined to mild lesions in those same areas or to preventive therapy in patients with repeated relapses of tinea pedis. Sprays are not recommended for the face. None of the preparations for cutaneous use should be applied to the vagina or eye. Secondary bacterial infection requires ancillary measures. Despite some antibacterial effect of the imidazoles in vitro, none of the antifungals included here have useful antibacterial activity.

The plethora of agents used for topical application necessitates that older agents with limited indications, such as iodine, sulfur, and gentian violet, not be discussed. Undecylenic acid and its salts, while widely used in nonprescription formulations, has too little efficacy to warrant further comment. While a list of nonprescription drugs would also include tolnaftate and miconazole, other agents can be expected to be added. Changes are also frequent as to which formulations of antifungal agents are marketed in combination with corticosteroids or antibacterial agents.

Details of the treatment of cutaneous mycoses are beyond the scope of this chapter, except to note that the agents listed below are generally applied twice daily and do not differ substantially in the duration of therapy necessary for cure.

Salicylic and Benzoic Acids (Whitfield's ointment). Salicylic acid is widely used in topical preparations as a keratolytic agent, often combined with other agents. The ointment marketed for nonprescription use in ringworm usually contains 3% salicylic acid and 6% benzoic acid. Although Whitfield's ointment can be used in mild tinea pedis, occlusive effects of the ointment and mild irritation of the salicylic acid make the undiluted preparation inappropriate for inflamed or macerated toe webs or scrotal infections. Except for its low cost, there is little to recommend the use of Whitfield's ointment in ringworm.

The most commonly used topical preparations for cutaneous use are given in Table 1. *Ciclopirox olamine* (Loprox), *haloprigin* (Halotex), and *naftifine* (Naftin) creams are all active against both ringworm, tinea versicolor, and candidiasis. *Tolnaftate* (Tinactin, Aftate, Zeasorb-AF) is active against ringworm and tinea versicolor but not against candidiasis.

TABLE 1. Topical Antifungals for Cutaneous Application

	Preparations Available in the United States			
Agent	Cream	Solution	Ointment	Powder
Polyenes				
Nystatin	X		X	X
Amphotericin	X		X	
Imidazoles and triazoles				
Clotrimazole	X	X	X	
Econazole	X			
Ketoconazole	X			
Miconazole	X			
Other agents				
Ciclopirox	X			
Haloprigin	X	X		
Naftifine	X			
Tolnaftate	X	X		X

Polyenes. A large number of macrolide polyene antibiotics are known and have broad-spectrum antifungal activity in vitro.[1] Topically, they are useful only against *Candida*, not ringworm. The hypertrophic skin lesions of chronic mucocutaneous candidiasis do not respond to these antibiotics, although macerated or intertriginous lesions typically respond well. These polyenes are derived by biosynthesis from aerobic actinomycetes, are poorly soluble in water, and share a common mechanism of action. The antifungal activity depends upon binding to the cytoplasmic membrane sterols such as ergosterol and thereby increasing membrane permeability.[2] Other pharmacologic properties are discussed later. Only *nystatin* and *amphotericin B* are readily available for topical use in the United States. *Natamycin* (pimaricin, Natacyn) is available from the manufacturer (Alcon) as a 5% suspension for ophthalmic use in fungal keratitis.

Imidazoles. These synthetic compounds and the triazoles, a closely related class, remain the object of active drug development. Lists of these agents rapidly become outdated. A current list of compounds marketed in the United States and their commercial names includes *clotrimazole* (Lotrimin, Mycelex), *econazole* nitrate (Spectazole), and *ketoconazole* (Nizoral). *Bifonazole* and *tioconazole*, both imidazoles, and *terconazole*, a triazole, have been effective in clinical trials, and some are available overseas. Others are available only for vaginal use, as will be discussed later. The structural formulas of the most commonly used agents are included in Figure 1. These compounds all share the same mechanism of action and the same indications for use. As will be discussed later in this chapter, in systemic use the compounds differ in solubility, human metabolism, and side effects. The imidazoles and triazoles inhibit fungal cytochrome P-450-dependent 14-α-demethylase, blocking the conversion of lanosterol and other 14-methylsterols to ergosterol.[3] The abnormal sterols interfere with membrane permeability. At the high concentrations that might be achieved topically, these agents directly damage the cytoplasmic membrane. The antifungal spectrum is extremely broad in vitro but fungistatic. Clinical efficacy has been demonstrated in ringworm of the body, foot, hand, and perineum, as well as in cutaneous candidiasis and tinea versicolor.[4]

Topical Agents for Vaginal Use

Vulvovaginal candidiasis is a common disease that can cause substantial chronic discomfort. Except for ineffective nostrums, all the agents are available by prescription only. Both tablets and creams are marketed for once-a-day use, preferably at bedtime to facilitate retention. If candidiasis has extended onto the vulva or perineum, creams that can be applied topically as well as vaginally may have an advantage over tablets. Cream dispensers are designed to administer 5 g per use. The differences between creams and vaginal troches are less important

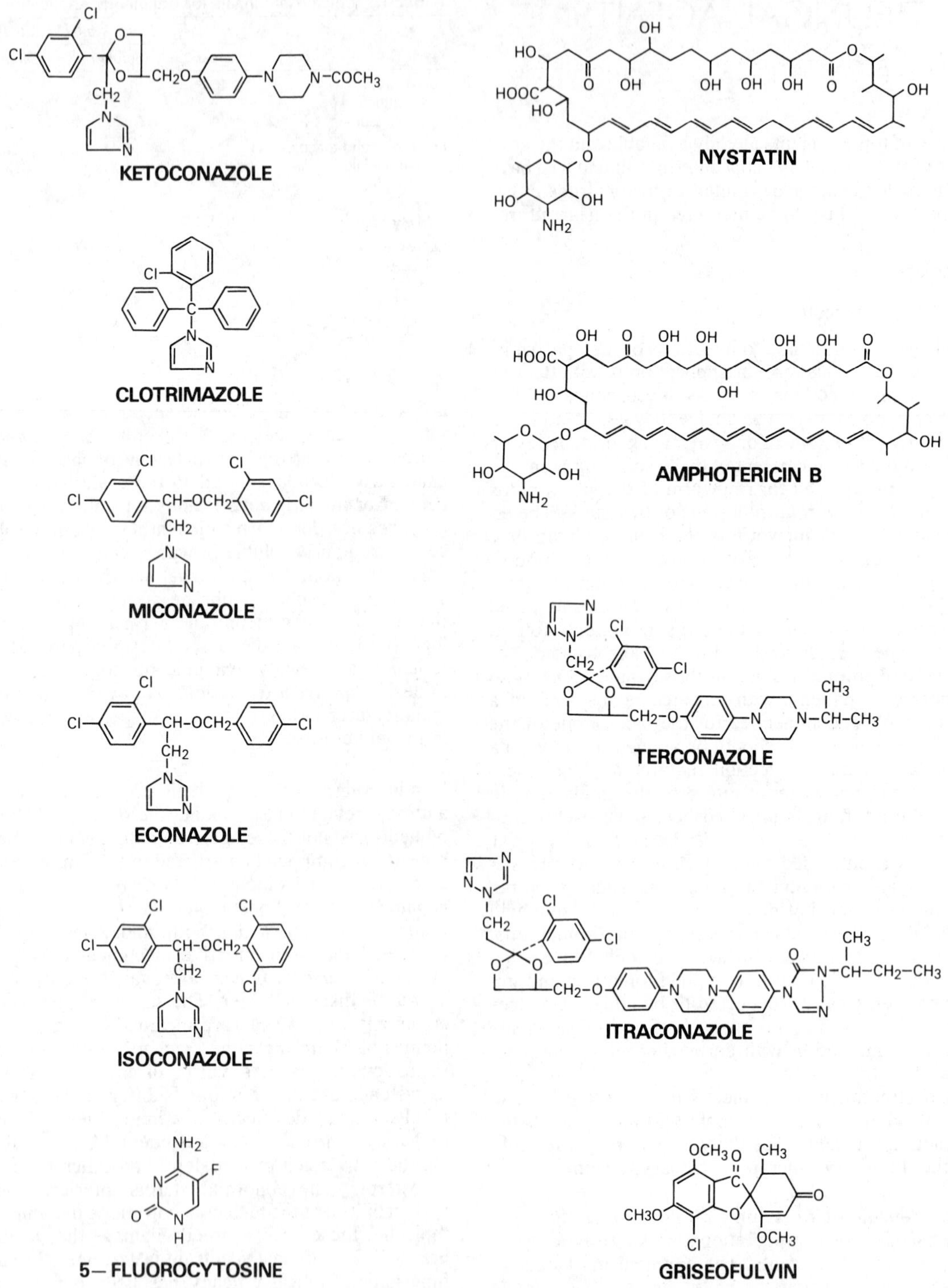

FIG. 1. Structures of the major antifungal agents.

than correct insertion deep in the vagina. Some preparations have a patient package insert with a clear set of instructions. The duration of therapy is longer for polyene troches than for the imidazoles, leading to increasing use of the latter class. The duration of therapy for the imidazoles, as stated in the literature or in the package insert, seems more dependent on the design of the original clinical studies than on the efficacy of the product. Most of the studies of imidazoles have shown short-term efficacy of roughly 80–90 percent if high-risk patients are excluded, such as patients relapsing from recent treatment.[5–8] Data on late relapse after treatment with these drug are hard to find, although relapse is acknowledged to be common. Ingestion of nystatin tablets to decrease the fecal *Candida* concentration has been recommended to aid treatment and prevent relapse of vulvovaginal candidiasis, but the evidence of efficacy remains unconvincing. Although a fecal reservoir for relapse appears likely, the reduction in fecal colony counts by oral nystatin is small. Even the massive doses of oral nystatin used in laminar flow units usually have not eradicated *Candida* from the feces.

Adverse effects of vaginal therapy are few. Allergy to any

one imidazole probably precludes the use of other imidazoles, Local irritation or burning, rarely a serious problem, does vary among preparations. Some systemic absorption, generally less than 10 percent of the dose, has been documented for many of the vaginal imidazoles and may be a general phenomenon. This is of theoretical interest in that it might cause birth defects during the first trimester of pregnancy or alter the metabolism of other medications taken by the patient. However, none of these consequences has been observed. Systemic absorption of vaginal polyenes probably does not occur. A list of agents currently available for vaginal use is given in Table 2. Compounds available in Canada, such as *econazole* (Ecostatin), or only overseas, such as isoconazole, are not listed. *Butoconazole* (Femstat), *miconazole* (Monistat 3 and Monistat 7), and econazole are formulated as the nitrate for vaginal use. The triazole *terconazole* (Terazol 3 and Terazol 7) and *clotrimazole* (Gyne-Lotrimin and Mycelex-G) are marketed as the base, not as a salt. Trade names differ in Canada.

ORAL THERAPY FOR SUPERFICIAL MYCOSES

Agents for the Treatment of Oral Candidiasis (Thrush)

Nystatin (Mycostatin, Nilstat, and generic), named for New York State, is produced by *Streptomyces noursei*. The drug is available as an oral suspension of 100,000 units/ml. Adults should swish 5–10 ml around in the mouth three times a day. Swallowing the suspension rather than expectorating it may help to treat subclinical esophageal candidiasis in immunosuppressed patients. Nystatin suspension is not absorbed from the gastrointestinal tract and, except for its bitter taste, is remarkably free from adverse effects. Vaginal tablets of nystatin can be held in the mouth and used as troches, but these are bitter and not designed for this use. A better alternative is the use of *clotrimazole* troches. These pleasant-tasting 10-mg tablets are effective in oral thrush when used five times a day.[9] Each tablet should not be chewed but kept in the mouth until it dissolves. Although some absorption occurs after the drug is swallowed, no adverse effects or systemic efficacy occurs. Oral ketoconazole, 200–400 mg/day, is also effective in oral candidiasis and may the drug of choice when concomitant esophagitis is present.[10–12] Unfortunately, none of the above regimens is very effective for oral or esophageal candidiasis in severely neutropenic patients. Intravenous amphotericin B may be necessary in such patients.

Oral Therapy of Superficial Cutaneous Infections

Systemic therapy of ringworm of the scalp, beard, and nails of the hand is preferred to topical therapy. Chronic noninflammatory ringworm of the soles and palms, as well as extensive ringworm of the trunk or groin, may also require systemic therapy. The preferred drug for these indications is griseofulvin because of its efficacy and low incidence of adverse effects. Although ketoconazole can be used for griseofulvin-resistant ringworm, the chance of serious side effects indicates that readily remedial causes of griseofulvin failures should be sought: erratic drug ingestion, too low a dose, and incorrect diagnosis. Candidiasis of the nail or skin, particularly of the groin, can resemble ringworm closely and does not respond to griseofulvin. None of the currently available topical or systemic agents is very effective against ringworm of the toenail. White superficial onychomycosis, while rare, is more responsive to griseofulvin. In young adult women who are concerned about the cosmetic problem, a 12- to 18-month course of griseofulvin may be worth a trial. Duration of therapy depends on the rate of nail growth, which may be slower than normal.

TABLE 2. Topical Agents for Vaginal Candidiasis

Agent	Formulation[a]	Days of Therapy
Polyene		
Nystatin (generic, Korostatin, Mycostatin, Nilstat)	100,000 unit tablet	14
Imidazole/Triazole		
Butoconazole (Femstat)	2% cream	3[b] 6[c]
Clotrimazole (Gyne-Lotrimin, Mycelex-G)	100-mg tablet	7 for 1 tablet/day 3 for 2 tablets/day[b]
	500-mg tablet	1
	1% cream	7–14
Miconazole (Monistat)	100-mg suppository	7
	200-mg suppository	3
	2% cream	7
Terconazole (Terazol)	0.4% cream	7
	80-mg suppository	3

[a] All formulations are designed to be used once a day, preferably at bedtime. The creams are dispensed in 5 gs per use, irrespective of concentration. Tablets are for vaginal use.
[b] Recommendation for nonpregnant women.
[c] Recommendation for pregnant women.

Griseofulvin. This agent, derived from a species of *Penicillium*, is active against ringworm but not against *Candida* or tinea versicolor. It is poorly active topically but reaches the skin and hair after ingestion. Absorption is favored by reducing the particle size and perhaps by ingestion with a fatty meal. A microcrystalline form (generic, Fulvicin-U/F, Grifulvin V and Grisactin) is available as 125-, 250-, and 500-mg tablets, plus a pediatric suspension of 125 mg/5 ml. The ultramicrocrystalline form (Fulvicin-P/G, Gris-PEG, and Grisactin Ultra) comes in 125-, 165-, 250-, and 330-mg tablets. The two forms have comparable efficacy. Griseofulvin is metabolized in the liver with a serum half life of 24–36 hours. Blood levels can be depressed by phenobarbital therapy and may require increasing the griseofulvin dose. Conversely, metabolism of warfarin anticoagulants is increased by griseofulvin. Adverse reactions to griseofulvin are uncommon. Headache may be observed early in therapy but usually disappears with continued use. Allergic reactions can occur, apparently unrelated to penicillin allergy. Hepatotoxic reactions have been observed in patients with acute intermittent porphyria. A variety of other side effects have also been observed, but a causal relationship is much less clear. Safety during pregnancy has not been established.

The usual daily dose is 500, 750, or 1000 mg daily for the microcrystalline drug, with children receiving 10 mg/kg. The 500 mg/day dose is reserved for mild infections and small adults. A dose of 330 mg daily is recommended for the ultramicrocrystalline form. Either preparation can be given once daily at the end of a meal, but dividing the dose into twice daily administration may help maintain therapeutic levels in the epidermis and is recommended for refractory infections.

Ketoconazole. The pharmacologic properties of this synthetic agent will be discussed later. Of relevance here is that the drug readily reaches the skin surface from the blood, most prominently by the way of apocrine sweat. Ketoconazole has definite activity against ringworm, chronic mucocutaneous candidiasis, and tinea versicolor.[13] At least in part because ketoconazole is reserved for griseofulvin failures, the efficacy of ketoconazole may not be striking. Certainly, the poor efficacy and potential toxicity of ketoconazole contraindicate its use in onychomycosis. In contrast, ketoconazole is the drug of choice for patients with chronic mucocutaneous candidiasis.[10] For tinea versicolor, topical therapy with selenium sufide shampoo or one of the many other agents is preferred. However, oral ketoconazole can be a very effective and useful drug for patients with extensive relapsing tinea versicolor.

Terbinafine. This oral agent, an allylamine structurally related to naftifine, has been evaluated in Europe for treatment of ringworm. In early short-term studies, the agent appeared to be comparable to griseofulvin. Evidence that the drug and its metabolites accumulate substantially during long-term administration may limit its use in onychomycosis.

Systemic Therapy of Candida Vulvovaginitis

Ketoconazole. The efficacy of oral ketoconazole in *Candida* vulvovaginitis is comparable to that of the topical imidazoles and triazoles. Ketoconazole is given as 400 mg/day for 5 days. However, the drug is contraindicated during pregnancy because of its potential teratogenicity and during breast-feeding because of its secretion into breast milk. Hepatotoxic and other adverse reactions also overweigh the convenience of oral administration and the possibility of use during menstruation. Perhaps for the woman with smear-positive chronic relapsing vaginal candidiasis, prophylactic courses could be considered, as recommended by Sobel.[14]

TREATMENT OF DEEP MYCOSIS

Oral iodides are useful only in cutaneous sporotrichosis and possibly in *Basidiobolus* infections, and therefore will not be included here. The of hydroxystilbamidine in blastomycosis has been eclipsed by better drugs and is also omitted.

Amphotericin B

Structure and Mechanism of Action. Amphotericin B is produced by *Streptomyces nodosus*. The major mechanism of antifungal effect appears to be combination of the drug with ergosterol, fungisterol, or similar sterols in the fungal cytoplasmic membrane, altering membrane permeability.[2] Drug-resistant strains in usually susceptible species remain a rarity. Other proposed mechanisms of chemotherapeutic effect include oxidative damage[15] and immunomodulation. Although the seven conjugated double bonds (Fig. 1) are essential for activity, alteration of the carboxyl primary amino group or the internal lactam linkage has also decreased activity. The negligible aqueous solubility of this drug at neutral pH has led to several formulations for intravenous use.

Desoxycholate Formulation. The commercially available intravenous formulation is a colloidal complex of amphotericin B, 50 mg, and desoxycholate, 41 mg, together with 25.2 mg sodium phosphate buffer. When the desoxycholate-amphotericin B powder is dissolved in 5% dextrose in water, a clear yellow colloidal solution results. Although low ionic strength additives such as hydrocortisone or heparin may be added, the solution becomes cloudy due to aggregation of the colloid if sodium or potassium salts are added to the bottle. The likelihood that cloudy solutions give lower blood levels has led to the recommendation that cloudy solutions be discarded. The colloidal solution is stable at room temperature under normal illumination for the usual infusion intervals. The older recommendation that infusion bottles be covered with foil to protect them from light has been convincingly demonstrated to be wrong.[16] Infusion bottles can also be stored for 24–48 hours under refrigeration before use. Another incorrect assertion has been that hydrocortisone added to the bottle inactivates amphotericin B. An important precaution is that 0.22-μm filters should not be placed in the infusion line because some drug may be removed. Filters with 0.45-μm-diameter pores do not remove drug.

Other Formulations. Alternative solutions to the problem of intravenous infusion have been proposed because of the toxicity of the desoxycholate complex. Esterification of the carboxyl group and N-acylation result in water-soluble micellar preparations but have reduced antifungal activity. Various salts of the methyl ester were given to animals and a small group of patients and seemed to cause less nephrotoxicity. Leukoencephalopathy with this derivative has halted further clinical studies.[17] None of the N-acyl derivatives have reached clinical trial.

Currently, interest has centered on liposomal encapsulated preparations of amphotericin B. In these preparations amphotericin B is intercalated into the phospholipid bilayer membrane, rather than included in the enclosed aqueous phase. Two entirely different formulations have reached early clinical trial. One preparation is 5 mol% amphotericin B in a 7:3 mixture of dimyristoylphosphatidylcholine:dimyristoylphosphatidyl glycerol (DMPC:DMPG). This preparation is quite heterogeneous in size and shape on scanning electron microscopy, containing both sheets and multilamellar spherical liposomes, the former containing more amphotericin B than the latter. The size of the sheets and spheres ranges from roughly 0.5 to 6 μm,[18] which is considerably larger than the micelles of the desoxycholate complex. Although little data on toxicity and pharmacology have been reported, more than 30 patients have received doses of 1 mg/kg or more, apparently with little toxicity. Blood levels with comparable preparations have been too low to be measured readily at these doses. The majority of the drug appears to be cleared by macrophages in the lung, liver, and spleen. Chemotherapeutic activity in experimental murine infections was not lost, although larger doses were necessary for an effect equivalent to that of the desoxycholate complex. Future clinical studies are planned with 30 mol% amphotericin B in the same phospholipid, a formulation that provides only sheets and ribbons, not spherical particles.[19] A different approach to liposomal amphotericin B has been to create unilamellar liposomes less than 0.2 μm in diameter. The two unilamellar preparations given to humans thus far both used a fatty acid with a longer chain length than DMPC:DMPG (i.e., stearic acid rather than myristic acid) and differed in net charge and the presence of cholesterol. Pharmacologic studies on one of these preparations have found blood levels at least as high as with the desoxycholate complex, but with much less toxicity.[20] No data on the efficacy of the unilamellar preparations in humans have been reported to date, although efficacy in experimental murine candidiasis and cryptococcosis has been reported.

Pharmacology. Concentrations of amphotericin B in biologic fluids have usually been measured by bioassay,[21] but high-pressure liquid chromatography,[22] ^{86}Rb release,[23] and radiometric respirometry[24] have been described. Despite the proliferation of methods, routine determination of amphotericin B serum, urine, or cerebrospinal fluid concentrations has no definite clinical value. Nonetheless, amphotericin B assays have revealed some remarkable pharmacologic properties of this drug. When colloidal amphotericin B is admixed in serum, desoxycholate separates from amphotericin B,[25] and more than 95 percent of the latter binds to serum proteins,[26] principally to β-lipoprotein.[27] Presumably the drug is bound to the cholesterol carried on this protein. The majority of the drug leaves the circulation promptly, perhaps bound to cholesterol-containing cytoplasmic membranes. Amphotericin B is stored in the liver and other organs; the drug appears to reenter the circulation slowly.[28] Most of the drug is degraded in situ with only a small percentage being excreted in urine[21,28] or bile.[29] Blood levels are uninfluenced by hepatic or renal failure.[26,29] Hemodialysis does not alter blood levels, except for an occasional patient with lipemic plasma who may be losing drug by adherence to the dialysis membrane.[26] Concentrations of amphotericin B in fluids from inflamed areas, such as pleura, peritoneum, joint, vitreous humor,[30] and aqueous humor, are roughly two-thirds of the trough serum level. Cord blood from one infant contained an amphotericin B concentration of 0.37 μg/ml, half the simultaneous maternal trough blood level. Amphotericin B penetrates poorly into either normal or inflamed meninges, vitreous humor, or normal amniotic fluid. Urine concentrations are similar to serum concentrations. Peak serum concentrations with conventional intravenous doses are roughly 0.5–2.0 μg/ml but fall rapidly initially to slowly approach a plateau of roughly 0.2–0.5 μg/ml.[21,31,32]

Clinical Use. Toxicity of intravenous amphotericin B is formidable, but nearly all patients can complete a conventional course of therapy. Therapy is best begun with a small test dose, such as 1 mg in adults, to assess the patient's febrile response. This dose can be given in 20 ml of 5% dextrose over 10–20 minutes. The patient's temperature, pulse and respiration rates, and blood pressure are recorded every 30 minutes for 4 hours.

Acute reactions due to amphotericin B follow a distinctive time course. The onset, often associated with a rigor, begins about 30–90 minutes after the start of the infusion and rarely lasts for more than 2–4 hours. Hypoxemia and hypotension or hypertension may occur during the rigor. These reactions are less marked in patients who are already receiving therapeutic doses of adrenal corticosteroids or who are given hydrocortisone, 25–50 mg, with amphotericin B. Giving hydrocortisone by intravenous bolus before amphotericin B may be preferable to administering the two drugs together when reactions occur early in the infusion, before much hydrocortisone has been received. Infants and young children also seem less prone to acute reactions. Intravenous meperidine has been advocated to ameliorate a rigor once it has begun, but the rigor usually lasts for only 15–45 minutes. Meperidine given when the rigor is about to end anyway makes little sense. Acetaminophen premedication may be used to replace hydrocortisone when reactions are mild. The rapidity of the dose escalation during initiation of therapy depends upon the severity of the acute reactions, the patient's ability to tolerate the reaction, and the rate of progression of the mycosis.

A patient with a rapidly progressing infection, with good cardiopulmonary status, and with a mild reaction to the test dose can for the next dose be given amphotericin B, 0.3 mg/kg, with hydrocortisone hemisuccinate, approximately 0.7 mg/kg. Patients already receiving supraphysiologic doses of adrenal corticosteroids receive little or no benefit from additional steroid in the infusion. A smaller second dose is appropriate for fragile patients with marked reactions to the test dose. Therapy for indolent mycoses may also be initiated slowly and without the addition of hydrocortisone. Tolerance to the febrile reactions develops with time, allowing diminution and eventual discontinuance of the hydrocortisone. The amphotericin B dose is advanced progressively to about 0.5 mg/kg/day by the third to fifth day in patients with prior normal renal function. This dose is maintained or advanced slowly to 0.6 mg/kg/day or, at most, 0.7 mg/kg/day while biweekly determinations of blood creatinine, hematocrit, potassium, and bicarbonate levels are observed. Each infusion is given over 2–3 hours in 500 ml of 5% dextrose in water. I prefer to add heparin, 1000 units, to this infusion, although there is no proof that this decreases phlebitis.

Azotemia is a normal concomitant of amphotericin B therapy.[33] The azotemia reaches a plateau during therapy at a level commensurate with the daily dose. Other nephrotoxic drugs, including cyclosporine,[34] increase azotemia. Salt repletion can improve renal function in the sodium-depleted patient.[35,36] A therapeutic course of amphotericin B is usually followed by a permanent reduction in glomerular filtration rate. This reduction is unrelated to the azotemia during therapy but is correlated with the total dose.[33] Dosage reduction during therapy to keep the serum creatinine level below 3.5 mg/dl is recommended only to help keep nausea and vomiting from causing dehydration and cachexia. Adequate oral intake of high-potassium foods, such as certain fruits and meat, can help prevent hypokalemia.

During an average course of therapy, the patient's serum creatinine level rises to 2.0–3.0 mg/dl, cyllindruria occurs, the hematocrit falls to 20–30 percent and, in one-fourth of the patients, hypokalemia necessitates oral potassium supplements. Weight loss of 15 lb is common. Renal tubular acidosis may occur but rarely requires treatment.[37] Headache and phlebitis are common. Rare side effects include thrombocytopenia, mild leukopenia, anaphylaxis, and burning sensations on the soles of the feet. Neither rash nor hepatotoxicity has been clearly documented. Side effects disappear in the first 3 months after therapy. The slow disappearance of side effects perhaps reflects the slow catabolism of the drug, which can be found in serum and urine up to 6 weeks after a course of therapy.[21,31] Several pregnant patients have received intravenous amphotericin B during the second or third trimester without fetal damage. However, safety in pregnancy is not clearly established.

Mechanisms for the toxic reactions are not fully understood. Amphotericin B-induced cell permeability probably accounts for the loss of intracellular potassium into the blood and excreted with the urine. Ventricular tachycardia in experimental animals given rapid injections of 5 mg/kg may also result from membrane damage. Renal damage morphologically is primarily injury to both proximal and distal tubular cells.[38] Glomerular damage is subtle or absent. Conceivably, nephrotoxicity in humans results from renal vascular constriction, such as occurs in dogs.[39] Anemia is normocytic, normochromic, and accompanied by a normal-appearing bone marrow. Erythrocyte survival is normal.[40] The serum erythropoietin level is abnormally low for the degree of anemia.[41] Acute respiratory deterioration was thought to have occurred in one institution when amphotericin B was given during or right after leukocyte transfusion.[42] Aggregation of leukocytes by amphotericin B[43] with trapping in the lung has been proposed. The rarity of this phenomenon has raised consideration of a third factor, perhaps bacterial endotoxin, necessary to create the syndrome. Febrile reactions to amphotericin B are usual and may be mediated by an entirely different process than renal toxicity. In vitro, the drug causes release of interleukin-1 and tumor necrosis factor from human peripheral blood monocytes.[44] Both mediators can cause fever.

Administration of amphotericin B on alternate days rather than daily does not reduce nephrotoxicity if the alternate-day dose is doubled. The number of venipunctures is decreased, and ambulation is facilitated by an alternate-day double-dose schedule, but more febrile reactions may be encountered. The therapeutic effects of both regimens are indistinguishable. Adequate hydration and salt replacement remain the best measures to minimize azotemia.

Mycoses with a useful response to amphotericin B include blastomycosis, candidiasis, histoplasmosis, cryptococcosis, paracoccidioidomycosis, coccidioidomycosis, aspergillosis, mucormycosis, and extracutaneous sporotrichosis. Doses range from 0.4 to 0.6 mg/kg/day, depending on the mycosis. Lower doses (−0.3 mg/kg) have been used largely in situations in which spontaneous recovery is a good possibility, such as esophagitis due to *Candida*. The duration of therapy in systemic mycoses is 6–12 weeks in most patients. Esophagitis due to *Candida* is often treated for only 5–7 days.

Localized injections of amphotericin B may be useful. Sporotrichosis or coccidioidomycosis of joints may benefit by intraarticular injections of 5–15 mg, depending on joint size. Intrathecal amphotericin B is essential in coccidioidal meningitis. After test doses of 0.05 and 0.1 mg, doses of 0.2–0.5 mg are given from one to three times per week into the lumbar, cisternal, or ventricular cerebrospinal fluid. Hydrocortisone, 5–15 mg, in the injection helps to decrease the resulting fever, headache, and nausea. Lumbar injections may cause temporary radicular pain and loss of motor function in the legs, rectum, and bladder.[45] Use of 10% glucose as a diluent and positioning the patient during injection to permit hyperbaric flow toward the brain may decrease local myelopathy.[46] Injections into the lateral cerebral ventricle through a subcutaneous siliconized rubber reservoir are useful, but the complication rate is high.[47] Bladder irrigations with amphotericin B, 50 μg/ml, in distilled water have been used in *Candida*-induced cystitis.[48] Corneal baths with 1 mg/ml are irritating but beneficial in keratomycosis.

Amphotericin B in Combination with Other Drugs

Under certain conditions, the antifungal activity of amphotericin B can be enhanced with flucytosine, rifampin, or tetracycline. Use of the amphotericin B–flucytosine combination will be discussed in the section dealing with the latter drug. Rifampin, which is not antifungal when used alone, decreases the in vitro concentration of amphotericin B necessary to inhibit the growth of *Candida*,[49] *Histoplasma*,[50] *Cryptococcus*,[51] and *Aspergillus* spp.[52] The amount of reduction is roughly from twofold to fourfold. In experimental mouse infections with *Histoplasma*,[53] *Blastomyces*,[53] and *Aspergillus*,[54] but not *Coccidioides*[55] or *Candida*,[56] rifampin therapy resulted in a significant decrease in the dose of amphotericin B necessary to prolong life. Perhaps significant is the fact that the combination did not result in a therapeutic effect superior to that obtainable with optimum doses of amphotericin B alone. This would suggest an amphotericin-B-sparing rather than amphotericin-B-enhancing effect. Anecdotal clinical experiences with this combination have revealed neither a noticeable improvement in therapeutic efficacy nor a definite synergistic toxicity.

Tetracycline provided an amphotericin-B-sparing effect in experimental murine coccidioidomycosis.[57] In vitro, minocycline decreased the concentration of amphotericin B necessary to inhibit many strains of *Candida* and *Cryptococcus*.[58] This combination has attracted little clinical attention thus far because of all the potential toxic interactions between tetracyclines and amphotericin B.

Combinations of amphotericin B with antitumor agents have received clinical trial based on favorable experience in experimental animals.[59]

Amphotericin B combined with ketoconazole has not appeared particularly promising in vitro or in vivo. The effect in vitro is very method dependent.[60] Under some conditions, antagonism can be demonstrated.[61] In experimentally infected mice, the effect of the combination in candidiasis,[62] histoplasmosis,[63] and cryptococcosis[62,63] was not superior to that of the better single drug.

FLUCYTOSINE

Flucytosine (5-fluorocytosine [5-FC], Ancobon) is the fluorine analogue of a normal body constituent, cytosine (Fig. 1). The drug was synthesized as a potential antitumor agent, but that property was lacking. Routine screening discovered the antifungal effect, which became the sole use of this drug.[64] Flucytosine is a white powder, moderately soluble in water, very stable on dry storage, and marketed as 250- and 500-mg capsules. Absorption from the gastrointestinal tract is rapid and complete. Approximately 90 percent is excreted unchanged in the urine. Protein binding is barely measurable.[26] Cerebrospinal fluid concentrations approximate 74 percent of simultaneous serum concentrations. The drug is readily cleared by hemodialysis.[26,65] Peritoneal dialysis also removes flucytosine from the body.

The half-life of the drug in the serum of patients with normal renal function is 3–5 hours.[66] Abnormal hepatic function has no influence, but decreased renal function can prolong the half-life to beyond 24 hours.

Mechanism of flucytosine's antifungal action appears to be by deamination to 5-fluorouracil (5-FU) and then conversion through several steps to 5-fluorodeoxyuridylic acid monophosphate, a noncompetitive inhibitor of thymidylate synthetase.[67] This interferes with DNA synthesis. Additional mechanisms of action may also be operative.[68]

Flucytosine is usually given as 150 mg/kg/day in four divided doses. Patients with a serum creatinine level of 1.7 mg/dl or greater usually require dose reduction. As an approximation, the total daily dose should be reduced to 75 mg/kg, with a creatinine clearance of 26–50 ml/min, and to 37 mg/kg when the creatinine clearance is 13–25 ml/min.[69] Ideally, the blood level should be measured in azotemic patients 2 hours after the last dose and immediately before the next dose. These values should range between 50 and 100 μg/ml. Patients receiving hemodialysis may be given a single postdialysis dose of 37.5 mg/kg. Further doses are adjusted by blood level. Reliable biologic,[70] enzymatic,[71] and physical[72] methods are available to assay flucytosine, even in the presence of amphotericin B.

Flucytosine given alone to patients with normal renal, hematologic, and gastrointestinal function is associated with very infrequent adverse effects. These include rash, diarrhea, and, in about 5 percent, hepatic dysfunction. In the presence of azotemia or concomitant amphotericin B, leukopenia, thrombocytopenia, and enterocolitis may appear and can be fatal. These complications seem to be far more frequent among patients whose flucytosine blood levels exceed 100–125 μg/ml.[69] Patients receiving flucytosine should have their leukocyte count and platelet count determined twice a week. Serum alkaline phosphatase and transaminase levels should be followed weekly. Appearance of loose stools or dull abdominal pain should prompt withholding of the drug to evaluate the progression of symptoms. Patients with bone marrow and gastrointestinal toxicity from flucytosine often tolerate the drug at reduced dosages. Patients with rash or hepatotoxicity have not been rechallenged. Flucytosine is teratogenic for rats and is contraindicated in pregnancy.

Conversion of flucytosine to 5-FU within the human body occurs in sufficient degree to be a possible explanation for toxicity to bone marrow and gastrointestinal tract.[73] It is possible that secretion of the drug into the colon occurs, where flucytosine becomes deaminated by intestinal bacteria and is reabsorbed as 5-FU.[74]

Flucytosine has a beneficial effect in cryptococcosis, candidiasis, and chromomycosis. It is not the drug of choice for any infection except chromomycosis because the clinical efficacy in the first two mycoses is inferior to that of amphotericin B and because secondary drug resistance is common in all three infections. Although the frequency and clinical significance of primary drug resistance are debatable, drug resistance arising during therapy is usually profound and accompanied by clinical deterioration. Mechanisms for the drug resistance may include loss of deaminase and decreased permeability to the drug. This problem has been significant enough to cause flucytosine to be used largely in combination with amphotericin B.

Flucytosine in Combination with Amphotericin B

Flucytosine and amphotericin B are at least additive in their effects in vitro and in mice experimentally infected with doubly sensitive isolates of *Candida* and *Cryptococcus*.[75,76] Results with *Aspergillus* are contradictory.[52,63] In animals, the combination has never been better than an optimum dose of amphotericin B alone. Flucytosine permitted a lower dose of amphotericin B to be used to gain the same therapeutic effect, and amphotericin B prevented the emergence of secondary drug resistance. These same advantages have been confirmed in two large multicenter studies of cryptococal meningitis.[77,78] Experience with candidiasis remains limited, but the combination has been recommended in *Candida* meningitis[79] and arthritis.

Physicians not familiar with the combination are more likely to encounter serious toxicity than with amphotericin B alone. This is particularly true in patients with rapidly changing azotemia or poor bone marrow reserve. Leukopenia and diarrhea are common and difficult to manage in patients with the acquired immunodeficiency syndrome (AIDS). Oral flucytosine may not be reliably ingested by patients who are confused or vomiting. Intravenous flucytosine has to be obtained directly from the manufacturer but is used at the same dose as the capsule formulation. There is no less diarrhea or leukopenia with intravenous administration.

Combination regimens with amphotericin B doses in excess of 0.3 mg/kg/day or 0.6 mg/kg every other day cause sufficient azotemia to make the safe administration of flucytosine difficult. The amphotericin-B-sparing function of flucytosine in this setting is lost. At present, there are no clear indications for adding flucytosine to amphotericin B regimens containing these higher doses.

Flucytosine resistance has occurred, albeit uncommonly, during combination therapy. Use of the combination in such patients incurs the risk of toxicity without evidence that flucytosine adds to the therapeutic effect. Whenever flucytosine is used to treat a patient who has received that drug before, the isolate should be tested for susceptibility. In most laboratories, a minimum inhibitory concentration (MIC) of 15 μg/ml or less is considered sensitive.

IMIDAZOLES

The imidazole ring (Fig. 1) confers antifungal activity upon a variety of synthetic organic compounds. Unlike the 5-nitroimidazoles such as metronidazole, activity against bacteria and protozoa, although measurable, has not been clinically significant. Most of the imidazoles reaching clinical trials have had similar in vitro activity, encompassing a broad range of superficial and deep pathogens.[13,80] Determination of activity in vitro has shown a marked dependence of the result upon inoculum size, pH, culture medium, and incubation time.[80,81] There are no widely accepted methods for measuring in vitro activity, and no firm indications for performing such tests can be offered. Secondary drug resistance has been encountered but is extremely rare.[82]

N-substitution of imidazoles has created a family of drugs called *triazoles* that have the same antifungal spectrum and mechanism of action as imidazoles but less effect upon human sterol metabolism. Both imidazoles and triazoles inhibit 14-α-demethylation of lanosterol in fungi by binding to one of the cytochrome P-450 (cyt. P-450) enzymes.[3] This leads to accumulation of 14-α-methylsterols and reduced concentrations of ergosterol, a sterol essential for a normal fungal cytoplasmic membrane. Inhibition of cyt. P-450 also decreases the synthesis of testosterone and cortisol in mammals. By studying cyt. P-450 inhibition in vitro, new drugs can be selected that are more active in inhibiting fungal ergosterol synthesis and less active in mammalian sterol synthesis. For example, in vitro study of itraconazole found that 14-α-demethylation of lanosterol in *Candida albicans* was inhibited at 100-fold lower concentrations than those required to inhibit mammalian sterol synthesis.[3] It is not surprising, then, that the newer triazoles, such as itraconazole and fluconazole, have not caused decreased cortisol and testosterone levels in patients, as was seen with ketoconazole.

Many of the newer triazoles have properties that may allow them to replace ketoconazole—not only less hormonal inhibition but also fewer drug interactions, a parenteral formulation, better distribution into body fluids, less gastrointestinal distress, and less hepatotoxicity. N-substitution of the imidazole ring is thought to confer greater metabolic stability on the triazoles and to offer the potential for slower elimination. Both itraconazole and fluconazole have longer serum half-lives than ketoconazole.

Ketoconazole

This synthetic agent differs from its closely related congener, miconazole, in its solubility at pH less than 3. Solubility in acidic aqueous solutions is conferred in large part by the basic piperazine ring.

The pharmacology of ketoconazole has been reviewed.[13,83] The drug is metabolized in the liver and excreted as inactive drug in the bile and, to a small extent, in the urine. Very little biologically active drug appears in urine. Serum protein binding exceeds 90 percent. The drug is not removed significantly by hemodialysis or peritoneal dialysis. Decreased renal or hepatic function does not alter plasma drug levels. Based on studies of oral ingestion by volunteers, the initial half-life is approximately 2 hours, with a β-phase half-life of about 9 hours commencing 8–12 hours after ingestion.

Oral absorption of ketoconazole varies among different individuals. Serious gastrointestinal disease, such as the graft-versus-host reaction,[84] may lead to low blood levels. H_2-receptor blocking agents, such as ranitidine, famotidine, or cimetidine, should not be given to patients taking ketoconazole because blood levels of the latter drug are drastically reduced. Although oral ingestion of hydrochloric acid along with ketoconazole has been said to reverse this effect in volunteers, acid administration would be contraindicated in patients requiring H_2-blocking agents. Citric acid does not seem acidic enough to overcome the effect of H_2-blocking agents.[83] Antacids can be given to patients taking ketoconazole but should be separated in time. Rifampin causes a substantial lowering of ketoconazole blood levels, probably by accelerating metabolism. Isoniazid possibly has the same effect. Occasional patients have had elevated phenytoin or oral anticoagulant levels while taking ketoconazole. Cyclosporine blood levels should be monitored during ketoconazole therapy because these levels sometimes increase, causing nephrotoxicity.[85] Penetration into the cerebrospinal fluid is very poor, even in the presence of inflammation.[86] Low concentrations are found in vaginal secretions,[87] saliva, and breast milk.

Ketconazole is presently available only as scored 200-mg tablets. Used as two tablets daily (400 mg), the drug is effective in nonmeningeal histoplasmosis and blastomycosis of the non-immunosuppressed host.[88] Therapy is continued for 6–12 months. Improvement may require 2–4 weeks to be evident. Although the dose can be advanced to 600 or 800 mg daily in patients not responding to therapy, there is more evidence of increased toxicity than increased efficacy.[86,88] Both disseminated and chronic pulmonary histoplasmosis respond to ketoconazole therapy. Histoplasmosis in AIDS responds too poorly to risk the use of this drug for acute therapy, although long-term ketoconazole has been used to prevent relapse after amphotericin B treatment.[89] Paracoccidioidomycosis responds well to ketoconazole.[90] Disseminated nonmeningeal coccidioidomycosis may be partially and temporarily controlled by ketoconazole.[91] Among patients with disseminated coccidioidomycosis who respond well, relapse is usual if the drug is stopped. With all these mycoses, patients with grave, rapidly progressing infection should receive amphotericin B. The slow therapeutic response and variable absorption of ketoconazole make it a poor choice in such patients. If the mycosis involves the meninges, ketoconazole is too ineffective to warrant trial.

Ketoconazole is of no value in cryptococcosis. There is no evidence that it accelerates the normal resolution of pulmonary lesions or prevents spread to the central nervous system. Patients who have been treated with amphotericin B for cryptococcal meningitis have relapsed while taking ketoconazole. The response is also negligible in chromomycosis and extracutaneous sporotrichosis. Although the response in cutaneous sporotrichosis also tends to be poor, a dose of 400 mg/day may be tried in patients with allergic reactions to iodide, the drug of choice. As will be mentioned later, itraconazole may be a better choice. Ketoconazole has been used in Old World leishmaniasis and was useful in *Leishmania major* but not in *L. tropica or L. aethiopica* infections (see Chapter 252). Studies on New World leishmaniasis are still inconclusive but not encouraging.

Aspergillosis does not respond to ketoconazole. Additionally, there is concern, based upon experience with mice, that subsequent use of amphotericin B may be antagonized.[92] The agents of mucormycosis have all been resistant to imidazoles and triazoles in vitro, discouraging clinical use for that indication.

The most frequent toxic effects of ketoconazole are anorexia, nausea, and vomiting. These reactions occurred in 17 percent of 71 patients taking 400 mg/day and in 29 percent of those receiving 800 mg/day.[88] Gastrointestinal distress is most common when the drug is first begun and can be partially controlled by taking the tablets with food. Dividing doses above 400 mg/day has not been recommended because hormonal suppression is prolonged. Ketoconazole causes a dose-dependent depression of serum testosterone and adrenocorticotropic hormone (ACTH)-stimulated cortisol response.[93,94] While this effect is quite modest at the recommended dose of 400 mg/day, doses of 800–1,200 mg/day cause a profound enough effect to have prompted trials in the treatment of ACTH-secreting tumors and prostatic cancer. Hypertension has been seen in a few of these high-dose patients in association with increased deoxycorticosterone, corticosterone, and 11-deoxycortisol levels. Gynecomastia, impotence, decreased libido, oligospermia, and azospermia in men and menstrual irregularities in women may also be seen during prolonged therapy.[88,93] Allergic rash has been seen in 10 percent of patients.[88] Pruritus occurs with equal frequency, sometimes associated with a complaint of dry skin. Perhaps the most grave complication of ketoconazole therapy is hepatitis.[95] Fortunately, this complication is quite rare, estimated to appear in 1 in 15,000 exposed individuals. Asymptomatic slight elevation of transaminases is not rare and is generally transient. This event is distinguished from the potentially lethal hepatitis by the presence of symptoms and the progressive course. Ketoconazole hepatitis begins as anorexia, malaise, nausea, and vomiting. Abnormalities of either or both serum transaminase and alkaline phosphatase become increasingly profound, soon accompanied by jaundice. Eighty percent of cases occur within the first 3 months, but the onset can occur at any time. Progression can be surprisingly swift. Patients should be instructed to discontinue ketoconazole if they experience the above symptoms and told to call their physician. If hepatotoxicity is suspected, serum transaminase and alkaline phosphatase should be measured within a day or two of discontinuing therapy. Symptomatic patients with abnormal liver function should not be rechallenged with ketoconazole. Of course, if serum chemistries are normal, the drug can be reinstituted. Some authorities have recommended that liver function be measured periodically.[95] This procedure does not protect the patient who has a rapid onset of hepatitis in the interval between tests but does require that all patients with abnormalities be contacted in order to inquire about symptoms and arrange for repeat testing.

Itraconazole

Despite its marked structural similarity to ketoconazole, itraconazole differs in several respects. Peak blood levels are lower than with ketoconazole, but tissue levels are higher. Antifungal activity is better in both susceptibility testing and in in vitro systems measuring the inhibition of *C. albicans* cyt. P-450.[3] Ingesting this lipophilic drug with meals substantially enhances absorption. With 200 mg once daily taken with breakfast, peak blood levels by day 15 were 1.07 μg/ml, as measured by high-pressure liquid chromatography.[96] Elimination from serum is triexponential, making calculations of half-life somewhat variable, being reported as roughly 20–36 hours.[96] Itraconazole is extensively metabolized in the liver, but neither renal dysfunction, hemodialysis, nor continuous peritoneal dialysis alters metabolism.[97] About 99 percent of serum itraconazole is protein bound. Drug concentrations are negligible in the urine and cerebrospinal fluid. At the doses used to date, there has been no effect on serum testosterone or ACTH-stimulated cortisol concentrations. Rifampin can reduce itraconazole levels. Interactions with H_2-receptor blocking agents, oral anticoagulants, and phenytoin have not yet been studied. The ability of itraconazole to elevate blood levels of cyclosporine has been reported in some patients[98,99] but not in others.[100] Dose-related nausea has been the most common adverse effect. Headache, hypertension, or edema has been noted in a few patients, but the relationship to itraconazole is not firmly established. Early indications are that hepatotoxicity is less common than with ketoconazole.

Conclusions about clinical utility are based upon the reactions of only small numbers of patients but suggest that primary indications for itraconazole will be the same as those for ketoconazole (i.e., coccidioidomycosis, paracoccidioidomycosis, blastomycosis, histoplasmosis, mucocutaneous candidiasis, and refractory cases of tinea versicolor or tinea corporis).[101–103] Itraconazole is given only by the oral route. The dose in systemic mycoses has been 200–400 mg/day, or half the dose of ketoconazole. A few reports of responses in cutaneous sporotrichosis[104] and invasive aspergillosis[105] have encouraged further study of these mycoses and may be evidence of an expanded spectrum of activity.

Fluconazole

This low molecular weight, fluorine-substituted bis-triazole has pharmacologic properties that differ strikingly from those of ketoconazole and itraconazole. The drug is water soluble, essentially completely absorbed from the gastrointestinal tract, administered by oral or intravenous routes, excreted unchanged in the urine, only 11 percent bound to serum proteins, and distributed throughout the body.[106,107] Penetration into cerebrospinal fluid is excellent, cerebrospinal fluid levels being about 70 percent of serum levels. The elimination half-life from serum is about 25 hours.[106,108] There does not appear to be any inhibition of testosterone[109] or cortisol synthesis at the doses used so far. Little is known about drug interactions. Oral absorption is not dependent upon gastric acid, as with ketoconazole. A major issue yet to be resolved is the necessity of obtaining blood levels when fluconazole is administered to azotemic patients. Although the drug clearly accumulates in azotemic patients, no dose-related toxicity has yet been reported. Nomograms for adjusting the dose in azotemic patients are available, but determination of blood levels is preferred.

Efficacy has been reported so far in oral thrush of AIDS patients,[110] in denture stomatitis,[111] and in one patient with *Candida* endocarditis.[112] Of greater interest are the anecdotes about responses in cryptococcal meningitis.[113–115] Some patients with cryptococcal meningitis, mostly AIDS patients, have clearly improved during fluconazole therapy. A multicenter study is in progress to determine whether the drug, given orally, can decrease the incidence of relapse in AIDS patients whose cryptococcal meningitis has been treated with amphotericin B.

REFERENCES

1. Hamilton-Miller JMT. Chemistry and biology of the polyene macrolide antibiotics. Bacteriol Rev. 1973;37:166.
2. Kerridge D, Whelan WL. The polyene macrolide antibiotics and 5-fluorocytosine: Molecular actions and interactions. In: Trinci APJ, Riley JF, eds. Mode of Action of Antifungal Agents. London: British Mycological Society; 1984:343–75.
3. Vandem Bossche H, Bellens D, Cools W, et al. Cytochrome P-450: Target for itraconazole. Drug Dev Res. 1986;8:287–98.
4. Fromtling RA. Imidazoles as medically important antifungal agents: An overview. Drugs Today. 1984;20:325–49.
5. Stern GE, Gurwith D, Mummaw N, et al. Single dose tioconazole compared with 3-day clotrimazole treatment in vulvovaginal candidiasis. Antimicrob Agents Chemother. 1986;29:969–71.
6. Gabriel G, Thin RNT. Clotrimazole and econazole in the treatment of vaginal candidosis. Br J Vener Dis. 1983;59:56–8.
7. Svendsen E, Lie S, Gunderson TH, et al. Comparative evaluation of miconazole, clotrimazole and nystatin in the treatment of *Candida* vulvo-vaginitis. Curr Ther Res. 1978;23:666.

8. Franklin R. Seven day clotrimazole therapy for vulvovaginal candidiasis. South Med J. 1978;71:141.
9. Shechtman LB, Funaro L, Robin T, et al. Clotrimazole treatment of oral candidiasis in patients with neoplastic disease. Am J Med. 1984;76:91.
10. Horsbaugh CR, Kirkpatrick CH. Long-term therapy of chronic mucocutaneous candidiasis with ketoconazole: Experience with twenty-one patients. Am J Med. 1983;74:23.
11. Fazio RA, Wickremesinghe PC, Arsure EL. Ketoconazole treatment of *Candida* esophagitis; a prospective study of 12 cases. Am J Gastroenterol. 1983;78:261.
12. Hughes WT, Bartley DL, Patterson GG, et al. Ketoconazole and candidiasis: A controlled study. J Infect Dis. 1983;147:1060.
13. Heel RC, Brogden RN, Carmine A, et al. Ketoconazole: A review of its therapeutic efficacy in superficial and systemic fungal infections. Drugs. 1982;23:1.
14. Sobel JD. Recurrent vulvovaginal candidiasis. A prospective study of the efficacy of maintenance ketoconazole therapy. N Engl J Med. 1986;315:1455–8.
15. Sokol-Anderson ML, Brajtburg, Medoff G. Amphotericin B-induced oxidative damage and killing of *Candida albicans*. J Infect Dis. 1986;154:76–83.
16. Block ER, Bennett JE. Stability of amphotericin B in the infusion bottle. Antimicrob Agents Chemother. 1973;4:648.
17. Ellis WG, Sobel RA, Nielsen SL. Leukoencephalopathy in patients treated with amphotericin B methyl ester. J Infect Dis. 1982;146:125.
18. Lopez-Berestein G, Fainstein V, Hopfer R, et al. Liposomal amphotericin B for the treatment of systemic fungal infections in patients with cancer: A preliminary study. J Infect Dis. 1985;151:704–10.
19. Janoff AS, Boni LT, Popescu MC, et al. Unusual lipid structures selectively reduce the toxicity of amphotericin B. Proc Natl Acad Sci USA. 1988;85:6122–6.
20. Sculier JP, Coune A, Meunier F, et al. Pilot study of amphotericin B entrapped in sonicated liposomes in cancer patients with fungal infections. Eur J Cancer Clin Oncol. 1988;24:527–38.
21. Bindschadler DD, Bennett JE. A pharmacologic guide to the clinical use of amphotericin B. J Infect Dis. 1969;120:427.
22. Mayhew JW, Fiore C, Murray T, et al. An internally standardized assay for amphotericin B in tissues and plasma. J Chromatog. 1983;274:271.
23. Cosgrove RF, Fairbrother JE. Bioassay method for polyene antibiotics based on the measurement of rubidium efflux from rubidium-loaded yeast cells. Antimicrob Agents Chemother. 1977;11:31.
24. Merz WG, Fay D, Thumar B, et al. Susceptibility testing of filamentous fungi to amphotericin B by a rapid radiometric method. J Clin Microbiol. 1984;19:54.
25. Jagdis FA, Monji N, Lawrence RM, et al. Distribution of radiolabeled amphotercin B methyl ester and amphotericin B in nonhuman primates. Sixteenth Interscience Conference of Antimicrobial Agents and Chemotherapy. Washington, DC: American Society of Microbiology; 1976:abstract 305.
26. Block ER, Bennett JE, Livoti LG, et al. Flucytosine and amphotericin B: Hemodialysis effects on the plasma concentration and clearance. Ann Intern Med. 1974;80:613.
27. Bennett JE. Amphotericin B binding to serum betalipoprotein. In Iwata K, ed. Recent Advances in Medical and Veterinary Mycology. Tokyo: University of Tokyo Press; 1977:107.
28. Atkinson AJ, Bennett JE. Amphotericin B pharmacokinetics in humans. Antimicrob Agents Chemother. 1978;13:271.
29. Craven PC, Ludden TM, Drutz DJ, et al. Excretion pathways of amphotericin B. J Infect Dis. 1979;140:329.
30. Fisher JF, Taylor AT, Clark J, et al. Penetration of amphotericin B into the human eye. J Infect Dis. 1983;147:164.
31. Christiansen KJ, Bernard EM, Gold JWM, et al. Distribution and activity of amphotericin B in humans. J Infect Dis. 1985;152:1037–43.
32. Starke JR, Mason EO, Kramer WG, et al. Pharmacokinetics of amphotericin B in infants and children. J Infect Dis. 1987;155:766–74.
33. Butler WT, Bennett JE, Alling DW, et al. Nephrotoxicity of amphotericin B. Early and late effects in 81 patients. Ann Intern Med. 1964;61:175.
34. Kennedy MS, Deeg HJ, Siegel M, et al. Acute renal toxicity with combined use of amphotericin B and cyclosporine after marrow transplantation. Transplantation. 1982;35:211.
35. Heidemann HT, Gerkens JF, Spickard WA, et al. Amphotericin B nephrotoxicity in humans decreased by salt repletion. Am J Med. 1983;75:475.
36. Branch RA. Prevention of amphotericin B-induced renal impairment. Arch Intern Med. 1988;148:2389–94.
37. McCurdy DK, Frederic M, Elkinton JR. Renal acidosis due to amphotericin B. N Engl J Med. 1968;278:124.
38. Utz JP, Bennett JE, Brandriss MW, et al. Amphotericin B toxicity. Ann Intern Med. 1964;61:334.
39. Gerkens JF, Heidemann HT, Jackson EK, et al. Effect of aminophylline on amphotericin B nephrotoxicity in the dog. J Pharmacol Exp Ther. 1983;224:609.
40. Brandriss M, Wolff S, Moores R, et al. Anemia induced by amphotericin B. JAMA. 1964;189:663.
41. MacGregor RR, Bennett JE, Erslev AJ. Erythropoietin concentration in amphotericin B-induced anemia. Antimicrob Agents Chemother. 1978;14:270.
42. Wright DG, Robichaud KJ, Pizzo PA, et al. Lethal pulmonary reactions associated with the combined use of amphotericin B and leukocyte transfusions. N Engl J Med. 1981;304:1185.
43. Boxer LA, Ingraham LM, Allen J, et al. Amphotericin-B promotes leukocyte aggregation of nylon-wool-fiber-treated polymorphonuclear leukocytes. Blood. 1981;58:518.
44. Gelfand JA, Kimball K, Burke JF, et al. Amphotericin B treatment of human mononuclear cells in vitro results in secretion of tumor necrosis factor and interleukin-1. Clin Res. 1988;36:456A.
45. Carnevale NT, Galgiani JN, Stevens DA, et al. Amphotericin B-induced myelopathy. Arch Intern Med. 1980;140:1189.
46. Alazraki NP, Fierer J, Halpern SE, et al. Use of a hyperbaric solution for administration of intrathecal amphotericin B. N Engl J Med. 1974;290:641.
47. Diamond RD, Bennett JE. A subcutaneous reservoir for intrathecal therapy of fungal meningitis. N Engl J Med. 1973;288:186.
48. Wise GJ, Wainstein S, Goldberg P, et al. *Candida* cystitis. Management by continuous bladder irrigation with amphotericin B. JAMA. 1973;224:1636.
49. Edwards JE, Morrison J, Henderson DK, et al. Combined effect of amphotericin B and rifampin on *Candida* species. Antimicrob Agents Chemother. 1980;17:484.
50. Kobayashi GS, Medoff G, Schlessinger D, et al. Amphotericin B potentiation of rifampicin as an antifungal agent against the yeast phase of *Histoplasma capsulatum*. Science. 1972;177:709.
51. Fujita NK, Edwards JE: Combined in vitro effect of amphotericin B and rifampin on *Cryptoccus neoformans*. Antimicrob Agents Chemother. 1981;19:196.
52. Kitahara M, Seth UK, Medoff G, et al. Activity of amphotericin B, 5-fluorocytosine and rifampin against six clinical isolates of *Aspergillus*. Antimicrob Agents Chemother. 1976;9:915.
53. Kitahara M, Kobayashi GS, Medoff G. Enhanced efficacy of amphotericin B and rifampicin in treatment of murine histoplasmosis and blastomycosis. J Infect Dis. 1976;133:663.
54. Arroyo J, Medoff G, Kobayashi GS. Therapy of murine aspergillosis with amphotericin B in combination with rafampin or 5-fluorocytosine. Antimicrob Agents Chemother. 1977;11:21.
55. Huppert M, Pappagianis D, Sun SH, et al. Effect of amphotericin B and rifampin against *Coccidioides immitis* in vitro and in vivo. Antimicrob Agents Chemother. 1976;9:406.
56. Graybill JR, Ahrens J. Interaction of rifampin with other antifungal agents in experimental murine candidiasis. Rev Infect Dis. 1983;5:S620.
57. Huppert M, Sun SH, Vukovich KR. Combined amphotericin B-tetracycline therapy for experimental coccidioidomycosis. Antimicrob Agents Chemother. 1974;5:473.
58. Lew M, Beckett KM, Levin MJ. Combined activity of minocycline and amphotericin B in vitro against medically important yeasts. Antimicrob Agents Chemother. 1978;14:465.
59. Presant CA, Klahr C, Santala R. Amphotericin B induction of sensitivity to adriamycin, 1,3-*bis* (2-chloroethyl)-1-nitrosourea (BCNU) plus cyclophosphamide in human neoplasia. Ann Intern Med. 1977;86:47.
60. Brajtburg J, Kobayashi D, Medoff G, et al. Antifungal action of amphotericin B in combination with other polyene or imidazole antibiotics. J Infect Dis. 1982;146:138.
61. Sud IJ, Feingold DS. Effect of ketoconazole on the fungicidal action of amphotericin B in *Candida albicans*. Antimicrob Agents Chemother. 1983;23:185.
62. Graybill JR, Williams DM, Cutsem EV, et al: Combination therapy of experimental histoplasmosis and cryptococcosis with amphotericin B and ketoconazole. Rev Infect Dis. 1980;2:551.
63. Polak A, Scholer HJ, Wall M. Combination therapy of experimental candidiasis and aspergillosis in mice. Chemotherapy. 1982;28:461.
64. Bennett JE: Flucytosine. Ann Intern Med. 1977;86:319.
65. Ittel TH, Legler UF, Polak A, et al. 5-Fluorocytosine kinetics in patients with acute renal failure undergoing continuous hemofiltration. Chemotherapy. 1987;33:77–84.
66. Cutler RE, Balir AD, Kelly MR. Flucytosine kinetics in subjects with normal renal function. Clin Pharmacol Ther. 1978;24:333.
67. Diasio RB, Bennett JE, Myers CE: Mode of action of 5-fluorocytosine. Biochem Pharmacol. 1978;27:703.
68. Oliver SO, Williamson DH. The molecular events involved in the induction of petite yeast mutants by fluorinated pyrimidines. Mol Gen Genet. 1976;146:253.
69. Stamm AM, Diasio RB, Dismukes WE, et al. Toxicity of amphotericin B plus flucytosine in 194 patients with cryptococcal meningitis. Am J Med. 1987;83:236–42.
70. Kaspar RL, Drutz DJ. Rapid, simple bioassay for 5-Fluorocytosine in the presence of amphotericin B. Antimicrob Agents Chemother. 1975;7:462.
71. Huang CM, Kroll MH, Ruddel M, et al. An enzymatic method for 5-fluorocytosine. Clin Chem. 1988;34:59–62.
72. Harding SA, Johnson GF, Solomon HM. Gas chromatographic determination of 5-fluorocytosine in human serum. Clin Chem. 1976;22:772.
73. Diasio RB, Lakings DE, Bennett JE. Evidence for conversion of 5-fluorocytosine to 5-fluorouracil in humans. Possible factor in 5-fluorocytosine clinical toxicity. Antimicrob Agents Chemother. 1978;14:903.
74. Harris BE, Manning BW, Federle TW, et al. Conversion of 5-fluorocytosine to 5-fluorouracil by human intestinal microflora. Antimicrob Agents Chemother. 1986;29:44–8.
75. Medoff G, Comfort M, Kobayashi GS. Synergistic action of amphotericin

B and 5-fluorocytosine against yeast-like organisms. Proc Soc Exp Biol Med. 1971;138:571.
76. Polak A. Synergism of polyene antibiotics with 5-fluorocytosine. Chemotherapy. 1978;24:2.
77. Dismukes WE, Cloud GC, Gallis HA, et al. Treatment of cryptococcal meningitis with combination amphotericin B and flucytosine for four as compared with six weeks. N Engl J Med. 1987;317:334–41.
79. Smego RA, Perfect JR, Durack DT. Combined therapy with amphotericin B and 5-fluorocytosine for *Candida* meningitis. Rev Infect Dis. 1984;6:791–801.
80. Custem JV. The antifungal activity of ketoconazole. Am J Med. 1983;74(Suppl):9.
81. Galgiani JN. Antifungal susceptibility tests. Antimicrob Agents Chemother. 1987;31:1867–70.
82. Ryley JF, Wilson RG, Barrett-Bee KJ. Azole resistance in *Candida albicans*. Sabouraudia. 1984;22:53.
83. Daneshmend TK, Warnock DW. Clinical pharmacokinetics of ketoconazole. Clin Pharmacokinet. 1988;14:13–34.
84. Van HV, Piens MA, Archimbaud E, et al. Serum levels of ketoconazole in bone marrow transplanted patients. Nouv Rev Fr Hematol. 1983;25:241–4.
85. Schroeder TJ, Melvin DB, Clardy CW, et al. Use of cyclosporine and ketoconazole without nephrotoxicity in two heart transplant recipients. J Heart Transplant. 1987;6:84–9.
86. Sugar AM, Alsip SG, Galgiani JN, et al. Pharmacology and toxicity of high-dose ketoconazole. Antimicrob Agents Chemother. 1987;31:1874–8.
87. Nusch W, Plempel M. Microbiological determination of bay N 7133 and ketoconazole after oral application in cervical and vaginal smears of patients. Mykosen. 1983;26:12.
88. NIAID Mycoses Study Group. Treatment of blastomycosis and histoplasmosis with ketoconazole. Results of a prospective randomized clinical trial. Ann Intern Med. 1985;103:861–72.
89. Johnson PC, Khardori N, Najjar AF, et al. Progressive disseminated histoplasmosis in patients with acquired immunodeficiency syndrome. Am J Med. 1988;85:152–8.
90. Restrepo A, Gomez I, Cano LE, et al. Post-therapy status of paracoccidioidomycosis treated with ketoconazole. Am J Med. 1983;74:53.
91. Galgiani JN, Stevens DA, Graybill JR, et al. Ketoconazole therapy of progressive coccidioidomycosis. Comparison of 400 and 800 mg doses and observations at higher doses. Am J Med. 1988;84:603–10.
92. Schaffner A, Frick PG. The effect of ketoconazole on amphotericin B in a model of disseminated aspergillosis. J Infect Dis. 1985;151:902–10.
93. Pont A, Graybill JR, Craven PC, et al. High-dose ketoconazole therapy and adrenal and testicular function in humans. Arch Intern Med. 1984;144:2150–3.
94. De Coster R, Caers R, Haelterman C, et al. Effect of a single administration of ketoconazole on total and physiologically free plasma testosterone and 17-beta-oestradiol levels in healthy male volunteers. Eur J Clin Pharmacol. 1985;29:489–93.
95. Lewis JH, Zimmerman HJ, Benson GD, et al. Hepatic injury associated with ketoconazole therapy. Gastroenterology. 1984;86:503–13.
96. Hardin TC, Graybill JR, Fetchick R, et al. Pharmacokinetics of itraconazole following oral administration to normal volunteers. Antimicrob Agents Chemother. 1988;32:1310–13.
97. Boelaert J, Schurgers M, Matthys E, et al. Itraconazole pharmacokinetics in patients with renal dysfunction. Antimicrob Agents Chemother. 1988;32:1595–7.
98. Kwan JTC, Foxall PJD, Davidson DGC, et al. Interaction of cyclosporin and itraconazole. Lancet. 1987;2:282.
99. Trenk D, Brett W, Jahnchen E, et al. Time course of cyclosporin/itraconazole interaction. Lancet. 1987;2:1335–6.
100. Novakova I, Donnelly P, de Witte T, et al. Itraconazole and cyclosporin nephrotoxicity. Lancet. 1987;2:920–1.
101. Phillips P, Fetchick R, Weisman I, et al. Tolerance to and efficacy of itraconazole in treatment of systemic mycoses: Preliminary results. Rev Infect Dis. 1987;9(Suppl 1):S87–S93.
102. Lavalle P, Suchil P, de Ovando F, et al. Itraconazole for deep mycoses: Preliminary experience in Mexico. Rev Infect Dis. 1987;9(Suppl 1):S64–S70.
103. Borelli D. A clinical trial of itraconazole in the treatment of deep mycoses and leishmaniasis. Rev Infect Dis. 1987;9(Suppl 1):S57–S63.
104. Restrepo A, Robledo J, Gomez I, et al. Itraconazole therapy in lymphangitic and cutaneous sporotrichosis. Arch Dermatol. 1986;122:413–7.
105. Viviani MA, Tortorano AM, Woenstenborghs R, et al. Experience with itraconazole in deep mycoses in northern Italy. Mykosen. 1987;30:233–44.
106. Dismukes WE. Azole antifungal drugs: Old and new. Ann Intern Med. 1988;109:177–9.
107. Farrow PR, Faulkner JK, Brammer KW. The pharmacokinetics and tissue penetration of fluconazole in man. Rev Infect Dis. In press.
108. Tucker RM, Williams PI, Arathoon EG, et al. Pharmacokinetics of fluconazole in cerebrospinal fluid and serum in human coccidioidal meningitis. Antimicrob Agents Chemother. 1988:32:369–73.
109. Hanger DP, Jevons S, Shaw JTB. Fluconazole and testosterone: In vivo and in vitro studies. Antimicrob Agents Chemother. 1988;32:646–8.
110. Dupont B, Drouhet E. Fluconazole in the management of oropharyngeal candidosis in a predominantly HIV antibody-positive group of patients. J Med Vet Mycol. 1988;26:67–71.
111. Budtz-Jorgensen E, Holmstrup P, Krogh P. Fluconazole in the treatment of *Candida*-associated denture stomatitis. Antimicrob Agents Chemother. 1988;32:1859–63.
112. Isalska BJ, Stanbridge TN. Fluconazole in the treatment of candidal prosthetic valve endocarditis. Br Med J. 1988;297:178–9.
113. Byrne WR, Wajszczuk CP. Cryptococcal meningitis in the acquired immunodeficiency syndrome (AIDS): Successful treatment with fluconazole after failure of amphotericin B. Ann Intern Med. 1988;108:384–5.
114. Stern JJ, Hartman BH, Sharkey P, et al. Oral fluconazole therapy for patients with acquired immunodeficiency syndrome and cryptococcosis: Experience with 22 patients. Am J Med. 1988;85:477–80.
115. Sugar AM, Saunders C. Oral fluconazole as suppressive therapy of disseminated cryptococcosis in patients with acquired immunodeficiency syndrome. Am J Med. 1988;85:481–9.

34. ANTIVIRAL AGENTS

FREDERICK G. HAYDEN
R. GORDON DOUGLAS, JR.

Antiviral drugs with proven therapeutic (Table 1) and prophylactic effectiveness are currently available for a number of common and, in some instances, clinically severe viral infections. In part as a response to acquired immunodeficiency syndrome (AIDS) and its sequelae, the search for new antiviral agents and therapeutic approaches for managing viral diseases has become increasingly intense. Recently licensed agents include zidovudine for human immunodeficiency virus (HIV)-1 infections, aerosolized ribavirin for respiratory syncytial virus (RSV) infections in infants, and intralesional recombinant α-interferon for genital papilloma. Ganciclovir and foscarnet have shown impressive activity against cytomegalovirus (CMV) infections. A number of antiretroviral and antiherpes agents are currently in various stages of development.

MECHANISMS OF ACTION

Chemotherapeutic agents for viral infections can be categorized into three broad groups: agents that directly inactivate intact viruses (virucidal), those that inhibit viral replication at the cellular level (antiviral), and those that augment or modify the host response to infection (immunomodulating). Virucidal agents may cause direct inactivation in a single step, such as with detergents, organic solvents like ether or chloroform, and ultraviolet light, or in multiple steps, as with photodynamic inactivation. However, such agents have not proved clinically useful in the treatment of established mucocutaneous herpes simplex virus (HSV) infections. Treatments that destroy both host tissues and virus simultaneously, such as cryotherapy, cautery, or podophyllin treatment of warts, are useful only in discrete mucocutaneous infections. One potential use of virucidal agents may be in preventing transmission of certain viral infections.

Antivirals

Since viral replication depends primarily on host cell metabolic functions, the challenge has been to identify agents that inhibit virus-specific events such as attachment to the cell, uncoating of the viral genome, or assembly of progeny virions, or that preferentially inhibit virus-directed, as contrasted to host cell-directed, macromolecular synthesis. While many compounds exist that exhibit antiviral activity in vitro, most affect some host cell function and are associated with low therapeutic ratios or unacceptable toxicity in humans.[1]

Currently useful antivirals selectively inhibit specific events in viral replication and, consequently, most have a restricted spectrum of antiviral activity. Similarly, since these agents inhibit ongoing replication at the host cell level, they are not effective in elimination of nonreplicating or latent viruses.

TABLE 1. Viral Infections in Which Antiviral Agents Have Proved Therapeutic Efficacy

Type of Infection	*Antiviral Drug*	*Route of Administration*	*Usual Dosage*
Herpes simplex virus (HSV) encephalitis	Acyclovir[a]	IV	10 mg/kg/8 hr in constant 1 hr infusion for 14–21 days
	Vidarabine	IV	15 mg/kg/day for 14–21 days. Less effective than acyclovir
Neonatal HSV	Acyclovir[a]	IV	10 mg/kg/8 hr in constant 1 hr infusion for 10–14 days
	Vidarabine[a]	IV	30 mg/kg/day for 10–14 days; constant infusion over 12–24 hours
Genital HSV			
Primary	Acyclovir	IV	5 mg/kg/8 hr for 5 days; constant infusion over 1 hr; indicated in severe initial infections
	Acyclovir	Oral	1,000 mg/day in five divided doses for 10 days
	Acyclovir	Topical	4–6 applications/day for 7–14 days; ½ in. ribbon of 5% ointment per 4 square in. applied with gloved finger
Recurrent	Acyclovir	Oral	1,000 mg/day in five divided doses for 5 days; see text regarding long-term suppression
HSV keratoconjunctivitis[b]	Idoxuridine	Topical	One drop of 0.1% solution every 1 hr while awake and every 2 hr at night; instillation of 0.5% ointment 5 times/day
	Vidarabine	Topical	½ in. ribbon of 3% ointment 5 times/day
	Trifluridine	Topical	One drop of 1% solution every 2 hr (up to 9 drops/day)
	Acyclovir[a]	Topical	½ in. ribbon of 3% ophthalmic ointment 5 times/day
Mucocutaneous HSV Immunocompromised host	Acyclovir	IV	250 mg/m²/8 hr for 7–10 days; dosage of 5 mg/kg/8 hr effective in adults
	Acyclovir	PO	2,000–4,000 mg/day in five divided doses for 10 days
	Acyclovir	Topical	Six applications/day for 7 days; ½ in. ribbon of 5% ointment per 4 square in. applied with gloved finger; useful only in limited, non-life-threatening infections
Herpes zoster	Acyclovir[a]	IV	500 mg/m²/8 hr for 7 days[d]; constant infusion over 1 hr; oral route of administration under study
Immunocompromised hosts[c]	Vidarabine[a]	IV	10 mg/kg/day for 5–7 days; constant infusion over 12–24 hr
Normal hosts	Acyclovir[a,e]	PO	4,000 mg/day in five divided doses for 5–7 days
Varicella Immunocompromised hosts	Acyclovir[a]	IV	500 mg/m²/8 hr for 7 days[d]
	Vidarabine[a]	IV	10 mg/kg/day for 5–7 days; constant infusion over 12–24 hr
Cytomegalovirus retinitis[h]	Ganciclovir[a,g]	IV	5.0 mg/kg/12 hr or 2.5 mg/kg/8 hr in 1 hr infusion for 14–21 days; see text regarding long-term suppression
Influenza A virus[f]	Amantadine	Oral	200 mg/day for 5–7 days; 4.4 mg/kg/day in children 1–9 yr to maximum of 150 mg; see text regarding prophylactic administration
	Rimantadine[a]	Oral	200–300 mg/day for 5–7 days; optimal dosage under study
RSV bronchiolitis/pneumonia	Ribavirin	Aerosol	Requires small particle aerosol generator; exposure 18–22 hr/day for 3–5 days at reservoir conc. 20 mg/ml, the delivered dose 0.8–1.8 mg/kg/hr depending on age
HIV-1 disease	Zidovudine	Oral	200 mg every 4 hr; alternative dose schedules under study
Genital papilloma (refractory)	Interferon (rIFN-α2b)	Intralesional	1 × 10⁶ units intralesional injection (0.1 ml) in up to 5 warts three times per week on alternate days for 3 weeks

[a] Not currently approved by the Food and Drug administration for this indication (January, 1989).
[b] Treatment of HSV ocular infections should be supervised by an ophthamologist. Duration of therapy and dosage depends on response.
[c] Antiviral therapy is most effective in localized herpes zoster ≤3 days duration.
[d] Dosage recommendations are those used in studies that showed efficacy in this condition. Acyclovir dosage of 250 mg/m² is approximately 6.2 mg/kg, and 500 mg/m² is approximately 12.4 mg/kg in a 70 kg adult. Dosage of 10 mg/kg/8 hr for 5–10 days recommended for VZV infection by some authorities.
[e] Efficacy established in older adults treated within 1–2 days of rash onset and in ophthalmic zoster.
[f] Efficacy documented only in uncomplicated influenza ≤48 hr duration.
[g] Currently available on compassionate use basis from Syntex Corp., Palo Alto, CA.
[h] See text regarding efficacy of the investigational drug foscarnet.

Drug Resistance

A related problem, which may limit the effectiveness of an antiviral drug, is the development of viral resistance to the inhibitory action of the drug. A well documented laboratory phenomenon for a variety of antiviral agents, in vivo development of drug resistance has been found during use of idoxuridine in HSV keratitis, acyclovir therapy of mucocutaneous HSV infection,[2–7] rimantadine treatment of influenza,[8–10] and recently ganciclovir treatment of CMV disease in AIDS patients.[11]

Host Immune Response

Since antivirals are virustatic or inhibitory in their activity, viral infection may resume when the compound is removed. Intact host immunologic responses remain essential for recovery from virus infections. Immunosuppression due to transplantation, cancer chemotherapy, or AIDS has been associated with high rates of recrudescent or chronic viral infections. Responses to antiviral treatment may be delayed and the risk of selecting drug-resistant viruses higher in such patients. Antivirals that impair host responses to infection, such as cytosine arabinoside in herpes zoster, may actually prolong the course of infection. Even effective antiviral agents, like acyclovir in primary HSV infections, may alter humoral and cellular immune responses, possibly by reducing viral antigen exposure.[12–16] Factors other than inhibition of viral replication alone are important in healing certain viral diseases, particularly mucocutaneous HSV infections, in which it has been possible to demonstrate antiviral effects without clinical benefit.

Combination Chemotherapy

The combined use of antiviral agents with different mechanisms of action has been investigated as a means of increasing antiviral activity, reducing the risk of toxicity, and preventing the development of drug-resistant virus. Combination therapy has been used successfully in experimental infections due to enteroviruses, influenza, HIV, and various herpesviruses.[17–22] Combined treatment with vidarabine and human leukocyte interferon has been reported to be clinically useful in chronic hepatitis B virus infections but is also associated with an increased risk of toxicity.[23,24] Combinations of vidarabine and acyclovir are expected to undergo testing in life-threatening HSV infections,[25] and alternating use of toxic agents, such as zidovudine and dideoxycytidine in AIDS, is being explored.[26]

Immunomodulation

Immunomodulating agents used for treating viral infections include those that supplement deficient host immune responses, such as exogenous antibody in chronic echovirus infection or interferon in herpes zoster of immunocompromised hosts. Intravenous immunoglobulin in combination with ganciclovir has been shown to be effective in CMV pneumonitis in bone marrow recipients.[27,28] Administration of transfer factor from persons recovering from chickenpox was shown to transfer cell-mediated immune (CMI) responses and to protect susceptible leukemic children from varicella, whereas a subsequent study in seropositive bone marrow was negative.[29] Chemical agents that appear to augment CMI responses, such as levamisole or inosiplex, have been used with variable success; all of these agents remain investigational.[29]

Drug Administration

Prophylaxis vs. Therapy. Prophylactic administration, as in amantadine hydrochloride for influenza A virus infection or methisazone in smallpox, is generally more effective than therapeutic administration. Since most antivirals probably serve to protect uninvolved cells and limit the spread of infection, rapid etiologic diagnosis and early administration of antiviral drugs are necessary for therapeutic efficacy.

Clinical and Laboratory Evaluation. Clinical efficacy depends on achieving effective antiviral concentrations at the site of infection, and specifically, adequate intracellular concentrations of an antiviral agent or its active metabolites. Pharmacokinetic studies that define absorption, stability in body fluids, tissue distribution, and metabolic fate of antiviral drugs are important in selecting proper dosage. Unfortunately, no standardized or generally accepted correlations exist between in vitro inhibitory concentrations, achievable blood or body fluid concentrations of antiviral agents, and clinical response.[1,30] Animal models are useful in testing antiviral agents, but may differ from the corresponding human infection in regard to pathogenesis, drug sensitivity of the virus, and drug pharmacology or toxicity.

Topical Administration. Topical application of antivirals to the cornea, skin, mucous membranes, or respiratory tract attempts to provide high concentrations at the site of infection and to avoid the possible toxicity of systemic administration. Topically applied drugs must be able to penetrate such barriers as stratified epithelium or local secretions to reach the site of active viral replication. For example, although beneficial in the treatment of HSV keratitis, topically applied vidarabine and its monophosphate derivative are ineffective in recurrent genital or labial HSV infections, except when applied by iontophoresis.[31,32]

Delivery of antiviral drugs to the respiratory tract in the form of small particle aerosols has been used with some benefit in influenza A, influenza B, and particularly RSV infections,[33–39] and the use of intranasally administered interferon has been shown to be protective in rhinovirus colds.[40]

ANTIVIRALS OF PROVEN EFFECTIVENESS

Acyclovir (Acycloguanosine, ACV, Zovirax)

Spectrum. Acyclovir (9-[2-hydroxyethoxymethyl]guanine) is a guanosine analogue that has an acyclic side chain, instead of the cyclic sugar moiety of natural nucleosides (Fig. 1). Its antiviral activity is limited to herpesviruses, including HSV types 1 and 2, varicella zoster virus (VZV), and Epstein-Barr virus.[41–45] Depending on the type of cell culture, acyclovir concentrations causing 50 percent reduction in plaque formation average 0.02–0.2 μg/ml for type 1 HSV, 0.03–0.5 μ/ml for type 2 HSV, and 0.8–1.2 μg/ml for VZV. Concentrations of approximately 1.6 μg/ml inhibit the replication of Epstein-Barr virus DNA in productively infected cells, but higher concentrations do not affect latent or persistent infection.[44] CMV plaque formation is inhibited by concentrations of 22.7 μg/ml and greater.[45] Acyclovir has shown antiviral activity in various animal models of HSV infection when administered topically, parenterally, or orally and in simian varicella when given systemically.[46–48] In HSV-induced skin infections of mice, early topical application prevents both lesions and the development of latent infection in sensory ganglia.

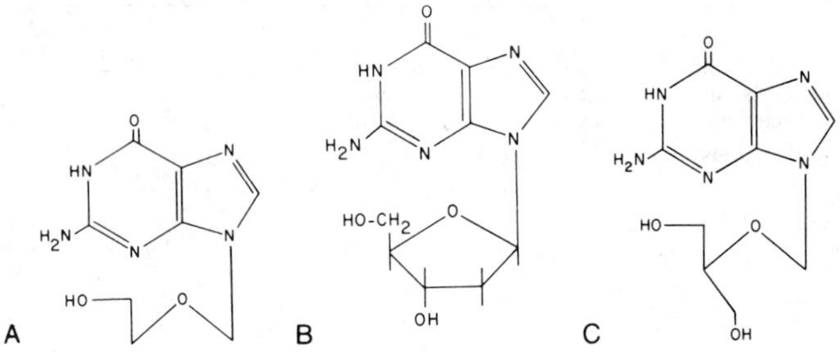

FIG. 1. Chemical structures of acyclovir **(A)**, the nucleoside deoxyguanosine **(B)**, and ganciclovir **(C)**.

Uninfected mammalian cells are generally unaffected by acyclovir concentrations ≤70 μg/ml. Acyclovir (20 μg/ml) does not alter cell-mediated immune responses of human peripheral blood leukocytes (PBL)[49] or affect human granulocyte progenitor cell growth[50] in vitro. Other studies have found that concentrations of 6.4–22.7 μg/ml inhibited the proliferative responses of human PBL to mitogens or herpesvirus antigens.[51,52]

Enhanced antiherpesvirus activity has been reported in combination with different agents[18,21,22] under laboratory conditions, and acyclovir potentiates the in vitro inhibition of HIV-1 by zidovudine.[53]

Mechanism of Action. The antiviral mechanism of action of acyclovir involves inhibition of viral DNA synthesis. It is the prototype of a group of antiviral agents that are activated by thymidine kinase to become inhibitors of viral polymerases.[41,54] Acyclovir uptake and intracellular phosphorylation to the monophosphate derivative are facilitated by HSV-induced thymidine kinase.[54] Cellular enzymes convert the monophosphate to acyclovir triphosphate, which is present in 40- to 100-fold higher concentrations in HSV-infected than in uninfected cells. The triphosphate form selectively inhibits viral DNA polymerase, and to a much smaller extent cellular DNA polymerases, and competes with guanosine triphosphate as a substrate for this enzyme.[55] Acyclovir triphosphate is also incorporated into viral DNA, where it acts as a chain terminator, because of the lack of a 3′-hydroxyl group.[56] Formation of a complex between the terminated DNA template containing acyclovir and the enzyme may lead to irreversible inactivation of the DNA polymerase.[57] The DNA polymerases of various herpesviruses differ in their degree of inhibition by acyclovir triphosphate; the polymerase of Epstein-Barr virus appears to be especially sensitive to its inhibitory action.[58]

Resistance. Alterations in either the viral thymidine kinase (TK) or DNA polymerase can cause acyclovir resistance in vitro.[59,60] Such mutants usually require acyclovir concentrations ≥3 μg/ml for inhibition. Most clinical acyclovir-resistant isolates have been TK-deficient ones recovered from immunocompromised patients receiving multiple courses of therapy. In animal models, acyclovir-resistant mutants with deficient TK activity appear to be less virulent and less likely to cause latent central nervous system (CNS) infection than wild-type strains, but some of these strains cause progressive mucocutaneous disease in highly immunocompromised hosts.[59,61,62] Clinical isolates that are acyclovir-resistant because of an altered TK substrate specificity or because of altered DNA polymerase also have been rarely recovered from treated patients.[59,63] One study found that 40 percent of HSV strains from untreated patients contained acyclovir-resistant virus, accounting for at least one percent of the total virus population.[6,7] Acyclovir-resistant strains of HSV with diminished TK activity have been isolated from immunocompromised patients given intravenous acyclovir for mucocutaneous HSV infections[2–5] and from patients with genital HSV infections before and after therapy.[64] One study of bone marrow transplant patients treated with intravenous acyclovir for recurrent mucocutaneous HSV infections recovered acyclovir-resistant virus in 1 of 52 first-treatment courses and 2 of 22 second courses.[5] Breakthrough isolates recovered during oral suppressive therapy include both resistant and sensitive phenotypes.[65,66] Lack of response to acyclovir associated with the presence of acyclovir-resistant mutants has been a particular problem in AIDS patients with mucocutaneous HSV infections.[11] Although documented,[59] VZV resistance has not yet been recognized as a clinical problem.[67] TK mutants remain sensitive to drugs like vidarabine and phosphonoformate that are not phosphorylated by the viral enzyme,[68] and these agents, particularly foscarnet, may be useful in such patients.

Pharmacology. The bioavailability of oral acyclovir is low (15 to 30 percent) and decreases with increasing doses.[69,70] Peak concentrations of 0.3–0.9 μg/ml occur at about 1.5 hours after 200 mg oral doses taken every 4 hours,[71] and peak levels average 1.8 μg/ml with 800 mg doses.[72] Bioavailability is lower in transplant patients, in whom doses of 400 mg five times daily provide peak levels of 0.7–0.9 μg/ml.[73] A liquid suspension has somewhat lower oral bioavailability; peak plasma concentrations average 1.0 μg/ml in children receiving 600 mg/m^2 doses.[74] An acyclovir prodrug, desciclovir or 6-deoxyacyclovir, is rapidly absorbed and converted to acyclovir by xanthine oxidase and provides blood levels comparable to those following intravenous dosing.[75,76]

Peak and trough plasma concentrations at the end of a 1-hour acyclovir infusion average 9.8 μg/ml and 0.7 μg/ml after 5 mg/kg/8 hr and 20.7 and 2.3 after 10 mg/kg/8 hr, respectively.[69] The volume of distribution corresponds to total body water. Cerebrospinal fluid concentrations are approximately one-half of plasma values.[69] After oral administration, salivary concentrations average 13 percent of simultaneous plasma concentrations, but vaginal secretion concentrations range from 15 to 170 percent of plasma values.[71] Zoster vesicular fluid levels are similar to those in plasma.[75] Aqueous humor levels average 37 percent of concurrent plasma values.[77] Breast milk concentrations average over threefold higher than those in serum.[78] Percutaneous absorption of acyclovir after topical administration appears to be low; plasma concentrations ranging from <0.01 to 0.3 μg/ml have been detected in herpes zoster patients treated topically. In patients with genital HSV infections treated with topical acyclovir, concentrations in genital lesions at 4 to 12 hours after application range widely (0.002–38 μg/ml), and no detectable acyclovir is present in cervicovaginal secretions.[64]

The plasma elimination $T_{1/2}$ of systemic acyclovir averages about 3 hours (range 1.5–6.3 hours) in adults with normal renal function, but is slightly longer (mean 3.8 hours) in neonates and increases to 19.5 hours in anuric patients.[69,79,80] Renal excretion of unmetabolized acyclovir by glomerular filtration and tubular secretion accounts for 60 to 91 percent of an administered dose, while less than 15 percent is excreted as 9-carboxymethoxymethylguanine or minor metabolites.[81,82] By competing for the organic acid secretory pathway, acyclovir may decrease the renal clearance of other drugs eliminated by active renal secretion, such as methothexate.[70] Dosage reductions are indicated in patients with creatinine clearances less than 50 ml/min/1.73 m^2 (see Table 2). Acyclovir is readily hemodialyzable, and 60 percent of the drug in the body will be removed during a 6-hour hemodialysis.[80,83] Peritoneal dialysis is severalfold less efficient in removing acyclovir, so that dosing supplementation is not needed during CAPD. An intravenous dose of 2.5 mg/kg/day has been proposed in CAPD patients.[84]

Toxicity. Acyclovir has shown mutagenic activity in some in vitro assays at high concentrations. No significant immunosuppressive activity, carcinogenicity, or teratogenicity has been noted in animal studies,[85] but safety in the pregnant human has not been established. High doses decrease spermatogenesis and causes testicular atrophy in animals.

Topical acyclovir may cause transient burning when applied to genital lesions, more commonly in first episodes and in female patients.[64] The polyethylene glycol base of topical acyclovir may cause mucosal irritation and is not approved for intravaginal use.

Intravenous acyclovir is generally well tolerated,[86] although inflammation, phlebitis, and rarely vesicular eruption[81] may occur at the injection site following extravasation of the alkaline solution (pH 9–11). Uncommonly reported side effects include rash, diaphoresis, hematuria, hypotention, headache, and nausea.[70] Approximately 1 percent of patients receiving intravenous acyclovir have manifested encephalopathic changes characterized by lethargy, obtundation, tremors, confusion, hallucinations, delerium, seizures, or coma.[86,88–91] Neurotoxicity is associated with renal insufficiency and unexpectedly high serum acyclovir concentrations.[91] Concurrent interferon administration or intrathecal methotrexate may be risk factors. One study found that 4 percent of bone marrow transplant recipients developed one or more neurotoxic symptoms after 2 to 18 days of intravenous acyclovir therapy (750–3,000 mg/m^2/day) for herpesvirus infection.[89] Most had diffuse electroencephalogram (EEG) abnormalities and increased cerebrospinal fluid concentrations of myelin basic protein. Improvement or resolution of symptoms occurred within 1 to 2 weeks after stopping treatment with acyclovir, but two patients developed neurologic symptoms again after reinstitution of therapy.

Reversible renal dysfunction has been observed in approximately 5 percent of patients treated with intravenous acyclovir at a dosage of 5 mg/kg/8 hr. In animals acyclovir can cause a crystalline nephropathy. Acyclovir solubility decreases to 2.5 mg/ml at 37°C, and crystalluria has been described in several adult and pediatric patients.[92,93] Bolus infusion, dehydration, pre-existing renal insufficiency, and high dose appear to be associated risk factors. Obstructive nephropathology related to high intravenous doses may be manifested by nausea, emesis, flank pain, and azotemia in patients without other risk factors.[93]

TABLE 2. Acyclovir Dosage Adjustments Suggested for Patients with Impaired Renal Function

Creatinine Clearance (ml/min/1.73 m^2)	*Standard Dose (%)*	*Dosing Interval (hours)*
>50	100	8
25–50	100	12
10–25	100	24
0–10[a,b,c]	50	24

[a] An alternative in patients with end-stage renal disease is administration of 14 percent of standard dose every 8 hr after loading with 37 percent of the standard dose.[80]
[b] Posthemodialysis administration of 60–100 percent of standard dose.[83]
[c] Oral acyclovir dose adjustments are needed for severe renal insufficiency; suggested dosage is 200 mg every 12 hr at creatinine clearance <10 ml/min/1.73 m^2.
(Recommendations taken from Blum et al.[69] and Lanskin et al.[80])

One study found that one-half of adults receiving 500 mg/m²/dose for treatment of herpes zoster had reversible increases in serum creatinine of at least 25 percent,[94] although a subsequent study at the same dose found renal dysfunction in only 6 percent of acyclovir recipients.[95] Adverse symptoms and renal dysfunction have been related to high acyclovir plasma levels (>25 μg/ml) following intravenous use.[90]

Oral acyclovir has been associated infrequently with nausea, emesis, and headache. During long-term suppression of genital herpes, no effects on sperm motility or morphology have been recognized.[96]

No serious adverse drug interactions have been documented. Probenecid decreases the renal clearance and prolongs the plasma $T_{1/2}$.

Clinical Studies. Extensive clinical testing has established acyclovir as the treatment of choice in many types of HSV and VZV infections (Table 1). Comparative trials with vidarabine have found acyclovir to be superior in regard to efficacy and/or toxicity in HSV encephalitis[97,98] and in varicella[99] or herpes zoster[100] of immunocompromised patients, whereas comparable activity has been found in neonatal HSV infections.[101] Ease of administration has also led many physicians to prefer acyclovir.

A number of placebo-controlled, double-blind clinical trials have demonstrated the therapeutic efficacy of acyclovir in primary genital HSV infections.[102–107] Topical acyclovir is associated with therapeutic and antiviral effects of smaller magnitude than oral or intravenous administration (see Table 3), and does not influence the frequency of new lesion formation after initiation of treatment. Because some patients treated with topical acyclovir develop new lesions and/or increased symptoms after stopping therapy, longer durations of application (10–14 days) have been advocated.[64,105] Topical acyclovir has minimal clinical efficacy in patients with pre-existing HSV antibodies (nonprimary initial infection), such as individuals with a history of orofacial HSV infection, and although associated with an antiviral affect, topical acyclovir offers no significant clinical benefit in recurrent genital HSV infections.[105,108,109]

Intravenous acyclovir has been shown to reduce markedly the duration of viral shedding, time to healing, and duration of symptoms in patients hospitalized with severe primary genital HSV infections.[103] Similarly, in outpatients with initial genital HSV infections, oral acyclovir (200 mg 5 times daily for 10 days) has been associated with significant reductions in virus shedding, symptoms, and time to healing, as well as prevention of new vesicle formation compared with placebo.[103,107] Oral acyclovir has become the best outpatient regimen for initial genital HSV infections at the present time. None of these regimens has been associated with consistent reductions in the risk of recurrent genital lesions. Higher oral doses (400 mg five times daily for 10 days) provides similar benefit in first-episode HSV proctitis.[110] Acyclovir therapy decreases the humoral and cellular immune response to HSV following first-episode genital herpes.[15,16]

TABLE 3. Relative Effectiveness of Different Acyclovir Formulations in Treating First-Episode or Recurrent Genital Herpes Simplex Virus

	Percent Reduction Compared with Placebo		
	Duration of Viral Shedding	*Duration of Pain*	*Duration of Lesions*
First episode			
Intravenous	85	57	57
Oral	80	44	35
Ointment	55	26	29
Recurrent[a]			
Oral	46	12	21
Ointment	45[b]	0	0

[a] Patient-initiated therapy.
[b] Women only; no effect in males.
(Data from refs. 109, 111, and 113.)

Controlled clinical trials have also shown that oral acyclovir is associated with antiviral activity and statistically significant but modest clinical affects (Table 3) in recurrent genital HSV infections.[107,111] One study found that when therapy was initiated by patients during the prodrome or at the first sign of lesions, oral acyclovir was associated with significant but modest reductions in the durations of shedding (mean 2.1 vs. 3.9 days), time to healing (5.7 vs. 7.2 days), and frequency of new lesion formation (7 vs. 22 percent), but no difference in the duration of pain.[111]

In patients with frequently recurring genital herpes, chronic oral acyclovir (400–1,000 mg/day in divided doses) reduces the frequency of recurrences (~90 percent reduction) and protects 65–85 percent of patients from recurrence during a 4-month period.[65,102,112,113] Doses of 400 mg twice daily are well-tolerated and associated with 85 percent reduced frequency of recurrences over 2 years' use.[114] A dose regimen of 200 mg three times daily may be as effective and less costly. Ingestion of 800 mg doses once daily appears efficacious, but weekend only use is unsuccessful.[115,116] Asymptomatic shedding may occur during suppression, and occasional cases of transmission to sexual partners have been documented.[117] Following completion of acyclovir administration, patients generally return to their previous pattern of recurrent infection. Guidelines for this expensive intervention have been published.[102,113] Chronic suppression may be useful in other patients with disabling recurrences of herpes whitlow or HSV-related erythema multiforme.

In recurrent orolabial HSV infections, topical acyclovir reduces the duration of virus shedding in patients treated within hours of symptom onset but is not associated with clinical benefit compared with placebo.[119] Topical application of 5% acyclovir in a cream formulation, not currently available in the United States, has been reported to be therapeutically effective in both recurrent labial and genital HSV infections,[118] which suggests that penetration of intact skin is the crucial factor in effectiveness. Oral acyclovir (200–400 mg five times daily for 5 days) provides modest clinical benefit in recurrent orolabial herpes and cannot be routinely recommended.[119] In patients with a history of sun-induced recurrences, short-term prophylaxis (400 mg twice daily for 1 week) reduces the risk of recurrence by 75 percent in a high-risk setting.[120]

Systemic acyclovir in various regimens has been used successfully for both the prevention and treatment of mucocutaneous HSV infections in immunosuppressed patients.[111–127] Prophylactic intravenous acyclovir (250 mg/m²/8 to 12 hours), begun prior to transplantation and continuing for several weeks, is highly effective in reducing the incidence of HSV disease in seropositive bone marrow transplant recipients,[121,122] but patients may develop mild or asymptomatic HSV infections after acyclovir therapy is discontinued, and no effect on CMV infections is found. Once daily administration is inadequate. In patients who can tolerate oral medications, oral acyclovir (400 mg five times daily for 5 weeks) is also effective in preventing HSV relapses in marrow transplant patients.[73,123] Low doses of oral acyclovir (200 mg/8 hr for 30 days) appear to be effective in renal transplant patients.[124] In marrow transplant patients, long-term oral acyclovir (400 mg three times daily for 6 months) also reduces the risk of herpes zoster.[122] No immunosuppressive effects or adverse effects on marrow engraftment have been found. High-dose intravenous acyclovir (500 mg/m²/8 hr) beginning 5 days before bone marrow transplantation and continuing for 30 days afterwards is associated with delayed CMV excretion, 50 percent lower risk of CMV disease, and significantly improved survival compared with placebo in CMV-seropositive patients.[125] Chronic oral acyclovir (200 mg/6 hr) reduces the frequency of recurrent mucocutaneous HSV infections in immunosuppressed hosts[126] and during intense periods of leukemia chemotherapy.[127]

In therapeutic trials in immunocompromised patients with established mucocutaneous HSV infection, intravenous acyclovir (250 mg/m^2/8 hr for 7 days) shortens the median healing time by 25–65 percent, duration of pain and local symptoms by 30–60 percent, and the period of virus shedding by 60–80 percent when compared with placebo,[113,128] but recurrences are common after cessation of therapy. Oral acyclovir (800 mg five times per day) is also effective in marrow transplant patients.[129] Topical acyclovir theapy for labial or facial HSV infections in immunocompromised patients diminishes the duration of virus shedding and may shorten the time to loss of pain and healing of lesions.[130] However, topical acyclovir should be used only in limited extraoral mucocutaneous HSV infections in such patients.

The clinical usefulness of acyclovir in varicella zoster virus infections is established in immunocompromised patients but less clear in othewise healthy adults and children. In immunocompetent older adults, several studies have found that intravenous acyclovir is associated with significant reductions in the time to healing of skin lesions and the duration of pain during the acute phase of herpes zoster, if administered within 72–96 hours of the onset of symptoms.[94,131] In one study, acyclovir therapy (500 mg/m^2/8 hr for 5 days) significantly shortened the duration of virus shedding (2 vs. 5 days), duration of pain (2 vs. 5 days), duration of new lesion formation (2 vs. 4 days), and time to 50 percent healing (7 vs. 14 days) compared with placebo.[94] Because of the lower acyclovir sensitivity of VZV relative to HSV and acyclovir's low bioavailability, high oral doses are needed in treating VZV infections. Oral acyclovir (600–800 mg five times daily for 7–10 days) reduces acute pain, new lesion formation, and healing time in older adults, if treatment can be initiated within 1–2 days of rash onset.[72,132–135] Lower doses and later initiation of therapy are ineffective. Reductions in ocular complications (keratopathy, stromal keratitis, anterior uveitis) have been reported with oral acyclovir treatment of zoster ophthalmicus, even in patients treated after 72 hours of rash onset.[133] Unfortunately, no consistent effect on the incidence or severity of postherpetic neuralgia has been found with intravenous or oral acyclovir in herpes zoster, although one trial found a lower incidence of chronic pain (4 vs. 17 percent) during the first three months after oral treatment.[132] The combined use of oral prednisolone and acyclovir does not decrease the likelihood of postherpetic neuralgia compared to acyclovir alone.[135a] Patients with ophthalmic zoster and older adults ($\geq$60 years) with zoster of short duration appear to be appropriate candidates for this expensive treatment. Topical application of opthalmic acyclovir is more effective than topical corticosteroids in reducing ocular relapses of zoster ophthalmicus.[136] In varicella of previously healthy adults, intravenous acyclovir was associated with reductions in fever and vesicle duration but not in local symptoms.[137] Anecdotal reports suggest efficacy in varicella pneumonia or encephalitis.[138–140] Studies of oral acyclovir in childhood varicella are in progress.

In immunocompromised patients, intravenous acyclovir (500 mg/m^2/8 hr for 7 days) reduced the frequency of cutaneous dissemination (4 vs. 21 percent) and visceral complications (0 vs. 8 percent) compared with placebo.[95] Similar trends were seen in patients who had disseminated zoster at the time of initiating therapy, but no significant differences were observed in resolution of lesions or pain. One trial in severely compromised patients found that intravenous acyclovir reduced the duration of new lesion formation (3 vs. 6 days), time to complete healing (17 vs. 20 days), and risk of cutaneous dissemination (0 vs. 50 percent) compared with vidarabine,[100] whereas another comparative trial found no differences in efficacy between the drugs.[141] In immunosuppressed children with varicella, intravenous acyclovir (500 mg/m^2/8 hr for 5–7 days) is associated with a lower frequency of visceral complications (0 vs. 45 percent), compared with placebo,[142] and about 1-day reductions in the duration of vesicle formation and time to full crusting.[143] Early relapses of infection may occur following cessation of therapy, and treatment may be ineffective in established visceral disease.[144]

Intravenous acyclovir has been shown to be more effective and less toxic than vidarabine in treating HSV encephalitis.[97,98] The proportion of patients surviving at 6 months is increased from 46 to 50 percent with vidarabine to 81 percent with acyclovir. In neonates, immunosuppressed patients, and rarely in apparently healthy adults, early relapses of encephalitis may follow initial acyclovir therapy,[12–14,145] such that longer courses of treatment may be warranted. Progressive neurologic deterioration in infants has been managed with chronic suppressive oral acyclovir.[13]

Trials of intravenous acyclovir in established CMV infections have shown no consistent clinical benefit, although reductions in viremia and viral titers in the urine have been observed in some patients.[88,146,147] In an uncontrolled study of bone marrow transplant recipients with pneumonia, high-dose acyclovir was associated with possible bone marrow and neurologic toxicity but no clinical benefit.[88]

In infectious mononucleosis of normal hosts, intravenous or oral acyclovir is associated with transient suppression of virus excretion in the saliva and possibly slight reductions in upper respiratory symptoms but no effects on other disease parameters.[148,149] In one case of Epstein-Barr virus-related post-transplant lymphoma, acyclovir therapy appeared to suppress orofacial shedding of virus and induced transient remissions, although the patient ultimately died from a polyclonal B cell lymphoma.[150] Some but not all cases of severe Epstein-Barr virus infections have apparently responded to acyclovir.[150–152] Epstein-Barr virus-related oral hairy leukoplakia responds to oral acyclovir.[153] Acyclovir is ineffective in controlled studies in patients with chronic fatigue syndrome.[154]

Intravenous acyclovir has been reported to inhibit hepatitis B virus replication and enhance the effect of interferon in chronic infection,[155] but intravenous therapy for 4 weeks was of no significant benefit in a controlled trial in chronic hepatitis B patients.[156]

Amantadine (Symmetrel)

Spectrum. Amantadine (1-adamantanamine hydrochloride) is a symmetrical tricyclic amine (Fig. 2) that specifically inhibits the replication of influenza A viruses at low concentrations ($\leq$1.0 μg/ml).[157] By plaque assay, the 50 percent inhibitory concentrations of amantadine range from 0.2 to 0.4 μg/ml for human influenza A viruses including H1N1, H2N2, and H3N2 subtypes.[158,159] Clinical isolates vary in their susceptibility to amantadine,[160] but the significance of such differences is not defined. Higher concentrations (25–50 μg/ml) have variable in vitro inhibitory activity against some influenza B, rubella, paramyxo-, and arenaviruses,[157,161] but these concentrations are too high to be clinically relevant. Such amantadine concentrations may also be cytotoxic and can inhibit lymphocyte transformation responses to mitogen and specific antigens.

Both prophylactic and therapeutic activity has been demonstrated in experimental influenza A virus infection of ani-

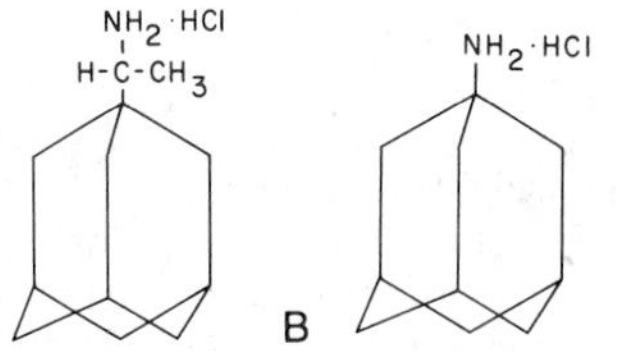

FIG. 2. Chemical structures of **(A)** rimantadine hydrochloride and amantadine hydrochloride **(B)**.

mals.[162] In animals, aerosol delivery of amantadine directly to the respiratory tract has greater efficacy than systemic administration.[19] Amantadine and ribavirin combinations show enhanced antiviral and therapeutic effects in vitro and in experimental murine influenza.[163]

Mechanism of Action. The exact mechanism of action of amantadine is undefined, but it appears to inhibit an early stage in viral replication, possibly uncoating of the viral genome in lysosomes.[157,164–167] Attachment and penetration of influenza virus appear to proceed normally in the presence of amantadine, and no direct effect on virus-associated RNA-dependent RNA polymerase activity has been found. Amantadine is readily concentrated and retained in the lysosomal fraction of mammalian cells, but its antiviral effect is quickly lost upon its removal from surrounding medium.[164] These findings indicate that most of the cell-associated amantadine may not contribute to its anti-influenza action and that amantadine mediating antiviral action may be taken up from the extracellular fluid with the virus.[165] Amantadine-mediated increases in lysosomal pH may inhibit virus-induced membrane fusion events and account for its broad antiviral spectrum at higher concentrations.[157,168] Effects on late replicative steps with impaired assembly of virions has been found for certain avian influenza viruses.[167]

Genetic reassortment studies indicate that amantadine sensitivity is primarily influenced by gene segment 7 coding for the M proteins, although the gene coding for the hemagglutinin may influence the sensitivity of certain strains.[167] Sensitivity of human isolates to low concentrations (1 μg/ml) of amantadine is a property conferred by the M2 protein, which is incorporated into the plasma membranes of influenza A, but not influenza B, virus-infected cells and into the virion.[8,167] Single amino acid changes in a critical transmembrane region of the M2 protein are associated with drug resistance, which indicates that this domain is the prime target of action.

Resistance. Resistance to amantadine is readily achieved in the laboratory by serial passage of influenza A virus strains in the presence of amantadine in vitro or in animals. Such isolates are cross-resistant to rimantadine. When amantadine treatment is given to birds infected with a highly pathogenic avian influenza virus, drug-resistant virus may emerge and cause death in the treated animals.[169] Furthermore, under conditions stimulating natural transmission, contact birds receiving amantadine prophylaxis frequently develop severe disease due to virulent drug-resistant virus after exposure to treated birds.[170] Administration of vaccine and amantadine together, but not vaccine alone, is protective for contact birds. Amantadine-resistant virus generated in the avian influenza model are virulent, genetically stable, and able to compete for infection with wild-type virus, such that transmission of drug-resistant virus may occur after cessaton of amantadine use.[171] Drug-resistant strains have been isolated from untreated patients[160] and recently from pediatric patients treated with rimantadine.[8–10,172] More studies are needed to define the clinical importance of such viruses.

Pharmacology. Amantadine is well absorbed after oral administration of capsule, tablet, or syrup forms.[173–176] The time to peak plasma level averages 2–4 hours but varies widely. Peak plasma concentrations average 0.2–0.4 μg/ml after administration of single 100 mg doses.[174] Steady-state peak plasma concentrations average 0.5–0.8 μg/ml on a 100 mg twice daily regimen in healthy young adults.[173,174] The elderly require only one-half of the weight-adjusted dose needed for young adults to achieve equivalent trough plasma levels of 0.3 μg/ml.[175] In children with cystic fibrosis, mean plasma concentrations were 0.6 μg/ml during long-term ingestion of 6 mg/kg/day, which suggests that such children require relatively large doses. Disproportionate increases in plasma concentrations as a function of dose may explain the high rates of neurotoxicity, including seizures, observed in one study employing 6.6 mg/kg/day doses in mentally handicapped patients.[176] Although some evidence suggests that amantadine is concentrated in pulmonary tissues,[177] nasal secretion and salivary levels of amantadine approximate those found in the serum.[174] Cerebrospinal fluid levels are about one-half of those in plasma, and amantadine is excreted in breast milk. After intermittent small-particle aerosol administration, nasal wash concentrations range from 2 to 19 μg/ml,[33] and the drug readily appears in the urine, indicating rapid absorption.

Amantadine is excreted unmetabolized in the urine through glomerular filtration and probably tubular secretion.[178] The plasma elimination $T_{1/2}$ is about 12–18 hours but ranges widely in apparently healthy young adults. Because of age-related declines in renal function, plasma $T_{1/2}$ increases up to twofold in the elderly,[174] and even more in patients with impaired renal function, in whom plasma concentrations from 1.0 to 5.0 μg/ml have been associated with confusion, delerium, hallucinations, seizures, and other signs of neurotoxicity.[178] In patients with creatinine clearance less than 10 ml/min/1.73 m^2, the $T_{1/2}$ may be as long as 30 days. Dosage guidelines for patients with renal insufficiency are summarized in Table 4. Amantadine is poorly excreted in hemodiaysis patients, and the amount removed by a single dialysis is only a small portion of the total body stores.[178,179] Monitoring of plasma concentrations in such patients is desirable but impractical.

Toxicity. In preclinical testing, amantadine lacked anti-inflammatory, antipyretic, or anticholinergic effects, but clinical observations of dry mouth, pupillary dilation, toxic psychosis, and urinary retention in acute overdose suggest that anticholinergic activity is present in humans.[173] Amantadine demonstrates indirect activity on the adrenergic nervous system by affecting accumulation, release, and reuptake of catecholamines in the central and peripheral nervous systems. The dopamine-enhancing effects of amantadine are probably the basis for its beneficial effects in parkinsonian patients. Ventricular irritability occurs in animals given high doses of intravenous or oral amantadine, and one case of malignant ventricular arrhythmia after amantadine overdose has been described in humans.[180] Amantadine is teratogenic in rodents, and its safety has not been established during pregnancy or lactation.

Orally administered amantadine is generally well tolerated, and no serious renal, hepatic, or hematopoetic toxicity has been documented. Long-term amantadine ingestion has been associated with livido reticularis, peripheral edema, orthostatic hypotension, and in isolated cases congestive heart failure, vision loss, and urinary retention. Patients with pre-existing seizure disorders have been reported to develop an increased frequency of major motor seizures during relatively high-dose amantadine

TABLE 4. Amantadine Dosage Regimens for Prophylaxis and Alterations in Renal Failure

	Suggested Dosage
No renal insufficiency	
Children, 1–9 yr	4.4 mg/kg/day once daily or in divided doses, up to 150 mg/day
Ages 10–64 yr	200 mg once daily or in divided doses
Ages ≥65 yr	100 mg/day
Creatinine clearance (ml/min/1.73 m^2)	
≥80[a]	200 mg once daily or in divided doses
60–80	200 mg/100 mg alternate days
40–60	100 mg daily
30–40	200 mg twice weekly
20–30	100 mg three times a week
10–20	200 mg/100 mg alternating every 7 days

[a] Based on adult dosage of 200 mg per day.
(Data from Horadan et al.[178] and Advisory Committee on Immunization Practices.[195])

ingestion,[181] but amantadine has also been used to treat refractory childhood epilepsy.[182] Psychiatric side effects in parkinsonian patients and psychotic exacerbations in schizophrenic patients have occurred with addition of amantadine.[183]

The most common side effects related to amantadine ingestion are minor gastrointestinal and central nervous system complaints. These include nervousness, lightheadedness, difficulty concentrating, insomnia, and loss of appetite or nausea.[173,184] Amantadine-associated side effects are related to dosage and duration of administration. Although higher doses have been used in the treatment of parkinsonian symptoms, dosages of 300 mg/day are poorly tolerated by healthy working adults and are also associated with significantly decreased performance on psychomotor tests designed to measure sustained attention and problem-solving ability.[185] In contrast, dosages of 200 mg/day has not been associated with consistent changes in psychomotor or academic performance in healthy adults.[185–188] When used for long-term influenza prophylaxis at dosages of 200 mg/day, adverse complaints have occurred in 5–33 percent of subjects and excess withdrawals because of drug side effects in 6–11 percent, relative to placebo.[173,184,188,189] Complaints typically develop within the first week of administration, often resolve despite continued ingestion, and are promptly reversible on discontinuation of the drug. During repeated dosing, trough steady-state plasma concentrations >0.45 μg/ml or peak concentrations >1.0 μg/ml are associated with an increased risk of CNS side effects.[190,191] Serious neurotoxic reactions may be transiently reversed by physostigmine administration.

The potential of CNS adverse effects appears to be increased by concomitant ingestion of antihistamines or anticholinergic drugs. Coadministration with anticholinergics in elderly patients may cause toxic delirum and visual hallucinations including lilliputian (small) and colored human figures. A diuretic combination of triamterene and hydrochlorothiazide was associated with CNS toxicity and a 50 percent increase in plasma amantadine concentration due to decreased renal clearance in one case.[192]

Clinical Studies. The clinical usefulness of amantadine as an antiviral agent is limited to the prevention and treatment of influenza A virus infections.[173,193] Early studies showed that amantadine was ineffective in the prophylaxis of influenza B or experimentally induced measles virus infections. A number of placebo-controlled, blinded studies have documented the prophylactic efficacy of amantadine at a dosage of 200 mg/day against the development of clinical illness in experimentally induced and naturally occurring influenza A virus infections.[173,184] The efficacy of amantadine in preventing illness documented to be secondary to influenza infection has ranged from 50 to over 90 percent, rates comparable to those obtained with inactivated influenza A virus vaccines. Prophylactic efficacy has been demonstrated in preventing nosocomial influenza and possibly in curtailing established nosocomial outbreaks.[181,182] Postexposure prophylaxis in family contacts has been associated with inconsistent protection.[173] Dosages of 100 mg/day have been shown to be protective against influenza A infection in semiclosed populations of teenaged students,[194] and studies to assess the efficacy of nontoxic lower doses are in progress.

Seasonal prophylaxis with amantadine is an alternative in high-risk patients, if the influenza vaccine cannot be administered because of toxicity or allergy, may be ineffective because the epidemic strain differs substantially from the antigens represented in the vaccine, or is unlikely to induce an adequate immune response, as in patients with primary or acquired immunodeficiency.[195] Because of the additive effect of antibody-associated protection and that provided by amantadine, the combined use of preseason vaccine and chemoprophylaxis during an outbreak provides optimal protection for particularly high-risk patients. To prevent the spread of influenza to high-risk patients, amantadine prophylaxis can be used in unimmunized health care workers and household members who have regular contact. Prophylaxis should be begun as soon as influenza is identified in a community or region and should be continued throughout the period of risk (usually 4–8 weeks), since any beneficial effects diminish rapidly after discontinuation of the drug. Alternatively, since amantadine does not interfere with the response to inactivated vaccine, the drug can be started in conjunction with immunization and continued for 2 weeks until protective antibody develops.

A series of controlled trials has demonstrated that amantadine is also an effective therapeutic agent in naturally occurring influenza A virus infection of previously healthy young adults.[173,90,196,197] When begun within 1–2 days of onset of symptoms, a dosage of 200 mg/day has been shown to reduce the duration of fever and systemic complaints by 1–2 days and in some studies to decrease the duration of virus shedding compared with placebo. One study found that amantadine-treated students were able to return to class more rapidly compared with placebo recipients.[196] One study comparing the efficacy of aspirin and amantadine treatment of naturally occurring H1N1 subtype influenza found that aspirin-treated patients defervesced more rapidly but experienced significantly higher rates of drug-related side effects and slower symptomatic improvement than amantadine recipients.[197] Other studies of adults with infection due to H3N2 subtype influenza viruses have found that certain abnormalities of peripheral airway function, but not airway hyperreactivity, resolve more quickly in amantadine-treated patients. However, trials to date have not determined whether amantadine prevents the pulmonary complications of influenza in high-risk patients or whether it is therapeutically useful in patients with established pulmonary complications. Therapeutic efficacy in children has received little study. Intermittent aerosol administration of amantadine has also proven therapeutically active in uncomplicated, naturally occurring influenza.[33] An injectable formulation is currently not available.

Ganciclovir (DHPG, 2′-NDG, BIOLF-62, B759U, Cytovene)

Spectrum. Ganciclovir (9-[1,3-dihydroxy-2-propoxymethyl]guanine) is an acyclic nucleoside analogue of guanine that differs from acyclovir in having an additional hydroxymethyl group on the side chain (Fig. 1). This agent has in vitro activity against all herpesviruses, but its unique characteristic is potent inhibition of CMV replication.[198–203] In plaque reduction assays, strains of HSV-1 and HSV-2 are inhibited by 0.05–0.6 μg/ml ganciclovir, CMV by 0.2–2.8 μg/ml, and VZV by 0.4–10 μ/ml. Thus, 50 percent inhibitory concentrations are similar to acyclovir against HSV and VZV but 10- to 50-fold lower against human CMV strains. Concentrations of 1–5 μg/ml also inhibit Epstein-Barr virus-mediated transformation of cord blood lymphocytes.[198] Systemic ganciclovir is effective at relatively low dosages (5–10 mg/kg/day) in rodent models of CMV[201] and HSV[198,199] infections. Effective doses in HSV encephalitis in mice are lower than those of acyclovir. Topically applied ganciclovir is active in models of HSV keratitis[204] and CMV pneumonia.[205] The combination of ganciclovir and β-interferon is synergistic in simian varicella.[206]

Although high concentrations are needed to inhibit the growth of uninfected cells, the 50 percent inhibitory concentrations for human bone marrow progenitor cells are about 0.6 μg/ml ganciclovir, compared with >25 μg/ml acyclovir.[207] In vitro, significant inhibition of human lymphocyte proliferative responses to mitogen and antigen occurs at 5–10 μg/ml ganciclovir.[208] Immune reactions that require active DNA synthesis may be depressed at therapeutic ganciclovir concentrations.

Mechanism of Action. Ganciclovir is an inhibitor of viral DNA synthesis. Intracellular ganciclovir is phosphorylated to the monophosphate derivative by infection-induced kinases, the viral thymidine kinase during HSV infection, and possibly a cellular deoxyguanosine kinase during CMV infection.[198,201,209,210] Ganciclovir di- and triphosphates are formed through the action of cellular enzymes. At least 10-fold higher concentrations of the triphosphate are present in CMV-infected cells compared with uninfected cells exposed to ganciclovir.[201] Intracellular ganciclovir triphosphate concentrations are also over 10-fold higher than those of acyclovir triphosphate in CMV-infected cells exposed to the drugs under similar conditions, and ganciclovir triphosphate levels decline much more slowly after drug removal.[209,210] These differences may account in part for ganciclovir's greater anti-CMV activity and explain how single daily doses are effective in suppressing human CMV infections.

Ganciclovir triphosphate is a competitive inhibitor of dGPT incorporation into DNA and preferentially inhibits viral rather than host cellular DNA polymerase.[211,212] Incorporation of ganciclovir triphosphate into viral DNA causes a slowing and subsequent cessation of viral DNA chain elongation.[213] Because of the two hydroxyl groups on the acyclic side chain, ganciclovir is incorporated internally into both host cell and viral DNA.[211]

Resistance. Ganciclovir is over 40-fold less active against acyclovir-resistant, thymidine kinase-deficient HSV strains.[198,199] HSV strains resistant to ganciclovir because of DNA polymerase mutation have been demonstrated in the laboratory, although some HSV strains resistant to gancyclovir because of DNA polymerase mutations retain sensitivity to ganciclovir.[212,214] A CMV strain resistant to ganciclovir because of reduced intracellular accumulation of ganciclovir triphosphate has been produced in the laboratory.[215] Ganciclovir-resistant strains of CMV have been uncommonly isolated from immunocompromised patients who remain culture-positive despite receiving the drug.[11,216,217]

Pharmacology. The oral bioavailability of ganciclovir in humans is very low (<5 percent of the administered dose),[218] and, consequently, almost all clinical trials have used intravenous administration. Peak and 6-hour trough plasma levels average 0.7–0.8 μg/ml and 0.2–0.3 μg/ml, respectively, after 20 mg/kg oral doses.[218] Oral doses of 1 gm three times daily are associated with greater bioavailability, perhaps related to gradual absorption, and peak plasma concentrations of 3–4 μg/ml. Prodrugs that are converted to ganciclovir and that have greater oral bioavailability are under development. The peak plasma concentrations at the end of a 1-hour 5 mg/kg or 2.5 mg/kg intravenous infusion average 8–11 μg/ml and 4–6 μg/ml, respectively.[217,219,220] Eight-hour trough concentrations after 2.5 mg/kg are 0.4–0.6 μg/ml. Following intravenous dosing, limited evidence suggests that aqueous and subretinal fluid levels are similar to those in serum and may persist longer.[221,222] Cerebrospinal fluid levels average 24–70 percent and brain tissue 38 percent of those in plasma.[217,220] After intravitreal injection of 200 μg ganciclovir, levels of about 1.2 μg/ml (51 hours) and 0.1 μg/ml (97 hours) have been found.[223]

The plasma elimination $T_{1/2}$ averages 3–4 hours in patients with normal renal function. In patients with mild renal insufficiency (serum creatinine (SCr) 1.4–2.5 mg/dl), plasma elimination $T_{1/2}$ averages 5.3 hours and increases to 9.7 hours in those with moderate (SCr 2.5–4.5) and to 28.5 hours in those with severe renal insufficiency (SCr >4.5).[224] Dose-independent kinetics are observed over the usual dose range, and twice daily administration of 5 mg/kg intravenously does not result in accumulation of ganciclovir in the plasma. Because ganciclovir is eliminated unmetabolized by renal excretion (>90 percent of dose), the clearance of ganciclovir correlates with creatinine (CrCl) clearance, and dose reductions are necessary in patients with renal impairment (CrCl <50 ml/min). A hemodialysis run reduces the plasma levels of ganciclovir by approximately 50 percent.

Toxicity. Ganciclovir is teratogenic in rabbits and is mutagenic in several different systems.[224] Systemic ganciclovir in mice and dogs causes significant toxicity involving the male and female reproductive, hematopoietic, and gastrointestinal systems. Testicular atrophy and bone marrow hypocellularity have been observed in animals at ganciclovir dosages comparable to those used in humans. Ganciclovir has carcinogenic potential in animals.

Evaluation of ganciclovir toxicity in humans has been difficult, because its use is restricted to severely ill patients with various concurrent illnesses and medications. The most common adverse events have been leukopenia, specifically neutropenia (<1,000 cells/mm^3) occurring in 40 percent or more of patients and thrombocytopenia (<50,000 platelets/mm^3) in up to 20 percent.[219,224–231] Neutropenia is most commonly observed during the second week of treatment, but may begin months later, and has been reversible in most patients, although persistent neutropenia complicated by fatal infections has been reported. The risk of neutropenia is higher in AIDS patients and is greatly enhanced by concurrent zidovudine therapy.[232] It may also be higher with tid dosing. Central nervous system side effects ranging in severity from headache to behavioral changes and psychosis to convulsions and coma have been described in 5–15 percent of treated patients. About one-third of patients receiving ganciclovir treatment have had to interrupt or prematurely stop therapy because of bone marrow or CNS toxicity. Frequent monitoring of blood counts for leukopenia is necessary to adjust doses, and treatment should be temporarily discontinued if the absolute neutrophil count falls below 500 cells/mm^3.

Anemia, rash, fever, liver function test abnormalities, azotemia, nausea or vomiting, and eosinophilia have also been reported. Phlebitis at the infusion site may be due to the alkaline pH of the solution. In the event of massive overdosage, hemodialysis and hydration may be effective in reducing plasma ganciclovir levels. Limited studies have found that about one-third of AIDS patients treated with long-term ganciclovir have greater than 50 percent increases in blood follicle-stimulating hormone (FSH), luteinizing hormone (LH), and testosterone values, perhaps related to gonadal toxicity.[231] Oral ganciclovir is associated with nausea.

Clinical Studies. Because of its toxicity, ganciclovir use has been limited to patients with life- or sight-threatening CMV infections. Compassionate use studies began in 1984 in AIDS patients and others with various immunodeficiency states related to transplantation or chemotherapy. The lack of placebo-controlled studies involving significant patient numbers and the use of various treatment regimens have compromised the interpretation of the results. The typical initial or induction treatment dosages have been 7.5–10 mg/kg/day in two or three divided doses given for 10 to 21 days. The largest experience and the clearest clinical responses have been in AIDS patients with CMV retinitis, over 85 percent of whom have improved or stabilized their disease with the initial treatment course.[219,227,232–235] Fundoscopic improvement is usually evident by 10–14 days. Historical controls indicate that over 90 percent of untreated AIDS patients will have progressive retinal disease leading to blindness, whereas retinitis in transplant patients may resolve spontaneously with reduction in immunosuppression. Approximately 90 percent of treated patients have a conversion of urine, blood, and throat cultures to negative or at least a greater than 100-fold reduction in viral titers. The median time to virologic response at these sites ranges from 3 to 8 days. Among AIDS patients who have responded to initial ganciclovir treatment, almost all have relapsed at a median of 2–5 weeks after cessation of therapy.[219,224,227] High doses of ganciclovir (25 to

35 mg/kg/week given once daily on 5 days/week), but not low doses (10–20 mg/kg/week), are effective suppressive therapy and increase the proportion of subjects free of relapse at 120 days from less than 15 percent to nearly 60 percent. Retinal detachments are common during long-term follow-up.[236] Ganciclovir-treated AIDS patients maintained on long-term suppressive therapy appear to have improved survival compared with historical controls.[231] Optimal dose schedules for initial and suppressive therapy have not been established.

Clinical improvement in 65 percent or more of patients and virologic responses have been found in uncontrolled studies of other CMV syndromes in AIDS patients, particularly CMV esophagitis, colitis, wasting syndrome, and possibly pneumonia.[219,226–228] Variable responses have been described in CNS syndromes.[219,229] In bone marrow transplant recipients, virologic responses but no reduction in mortality have been observed in patients with biopsy-proven CMV pneumonia treated with ganciclovir alone[217] or in combination with corticosteroids.[237] The combined use of ganciclovir and anti-CMV immune globulin has been associated with improved survival (43–80 percent) in CMV pneumonia compared with historical controls.[27,28] Uncontrolled studies suggest that renal or heart transplant and other immunosuppressed patients with pneumonia or other CMV syndromes respond to ganciclovir.[230,239,240]

Intravitreal ganciclovir is well tolerated in the rabbit eye[241] and has been used in limited studies for treating CMV retinitis in patients who are unable to tolerate systemic ganciclovir.[223]

Idoxuridine (IDU, IUDR, Stoxil, Herplex, Dendrid)

Idoxuridine (5-iodo-2′-deoxyuridine) is an iodinated thymidine analogue that inhibits the in vitro replication of various DNA viruses, particularly herpesviruses and poxviruses.[242] Plaque production by most clinical isolates of HSV type 1 is inhibited by concentrations of 2–10 μg/ml. Idoxuridine's antiviral mechanism of action is not completely defined, but the phosphorylated derivatives interfere with various enzyme systems, and the triphosphate inhibits viral DNA synthesis and is incorporated into both viral and cellular DNA. Resistance to the antiviral effect of idoxuridine readily develops under laboratory conditions and has occurred in viral isolates recovered from idoxuridine-treated patients with HSV keratitis. In humans, intravenously administered idoxuridine is rapidly metabolized to iodouracil and uracil. Extremely low plasma concentrations of idoxuridine (0.1–0.4 ppm) were detected in about one-half of patients treated topically with 40% idoxuridine in dimethyl sulfoxide. Idoxuridine is teratogenic, mutagenic, and immunosuppressive in certain experimental systems.

Clinical Studies. Parenteral idoxuridine is not useful because of liver function abnormalities and serious bone marrow toxicity.

The therapeutic usefulness of topically applied idoxuridine depends on the site of infection and the vehicle of administration. Idoxuridine in ointment or solution form is ineffective in recurrent herpes labialis, varicella, or localized herpes zoster, whereas frequent application of idoxuridine dissolved in dimethyl sulfoxide (5–40% idoxuridine in 100% DMSO) has been reported to hasten the healing of skin lesions and shorten the duration of pain in localized herpes zoster. Topical application of 30% idoxuridine in DMSO may shorten the duration of viral shedding in recurrent or primary genital HSV infections, but does not reduce the duration of symptoms or healing time.[243] Mild local burning after topical application of DMSO is common, and headache, dizziness, sedation, nausea, and localized and generalized dermatitis have also been reported. DMSO is teratogenic and can cause adverse ocular effects in laboratory animals.

In the United States, idoxuridine is approved by the FDA only for topical treatment of HSV keratitis.[244,245] Controlled trials and extensive clinical experience have indicated greater efficacy in epithelial infections, especially initial episodes, than in stromal infections. Adverse reactions include pain, pruritis, inflammation, or edema involving the eye or lids and rarely allergic reactions.

Ribavirin (Virazole)

The synthetic nucleoside ribavirin (1-beta-D-ribofuranosyl-1,2,4-triazole-3-carboxamide) is a guanosine analogue (Fig. 3), in which both the base and the D-ribose sugar are necessary for antiviral activity.[246] Ribavirin inhibits the in vitro replication of a wide range of RNA and DNA viruses, including myxo-, paramyxo-, arena-, bunya-, RNA tumor, herpes, adeno-, pox-, and retroviruses including HIV-1.[246–250] By plaque assay the ED_{50} concentrations range from 3 to 10 μg/ml for influenza A and B[248] and RSV[241] viruses. Inhibitory concentrations for a particular virus differ markedly in different cell types, and the ability of cells to take up ribavirin and form active metabolites may be important determinants of antiviral activity. Ribavirin is generally not active against viruses with single-stranded RNA genomes that act directly as messenger RNA, such as entero- and rhinoviruses. Relatively high concentrations (30–50 μg/ml) inhibit acute HIV infection of human lymphocytes.[249] Ribavirin antagonizes the anti-HIV-1 effects of zidovudine but enhances the activity of purine dideoxynucleosides.[250]

Low concentrations of ribavirin (2–10 μg/ml) reversibly inhibit macromolecular synthesis and the proliferation of certain rapidly dividing, uninfected mammalian cells.[248] Ribavirin suppresses nucleic acid synthesis in quiescent and mitogen-stimulated human peripheal blood lymphocytes in vitro,[252] but does not adversely affect polymorphonuclear leukocyte functions.[253] Inhibition of mast cell secretory responses occurs after in vitro ribavirin exposure.[254]

Aerosol administration has greater therapeutic activity than the parenteral route in animal models of influenza[19] and RSV infection.[255] Brief aerosol exposures (4 hr/day) employing threefold higher reservoir concentrations are also effective in models of influenza and RSV infection.[256] Parenterally administered ribarivin has antiviral and therapeutic activity in animal models of lassavirus, other arenaviruses, and bunyavirus infections,[251,257–259] but late deaths due to central nervous system infection may occur despite ribavirin therapy.[258] Enhanced therapeutic efficacy occurs in certain animal models when ribavirin is administered in liposomes or in combination with other antivirals or immune modulators.[163,259–261] Parenteral immunoglobulin potentiates the antiviral activity of aerosol ribavirin in the cotton rat model of RSV infection,[261] and increased anti-influenza activity is seen with combinations of ribavirin and amantadine or rimantadine.[163]

Mechanism of Action. The antiviral mechanism of action of ribavirin is not fully defined but relates to alteration of cellular nucleotide pools and of viral messenger RNA formation.[246] Intracellular phosphorylation to the mono-, di-, and triphosphate

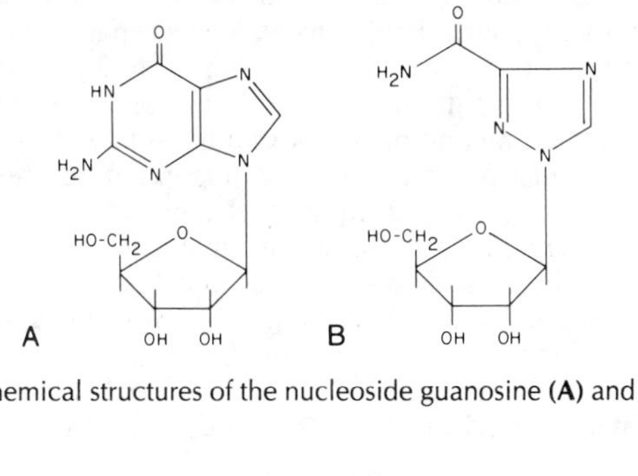

FIG. 3. Chemical structures of the nucleoside guanosine **(A)** and ribavirin **(B)**.

derivatives is mediated by host cell enzymes. In both uninfected and RSV-infected cells, the predominant derivative (>80 percent) is the triphosphate, which is rapidly degraded ($T_{1/2}$ <2 hours) after removal of drug from the surrounding medium.[262] Ribavirin monophosphate competitively inhibits inosine-5'-phosphate dehydrogenase (IMPDH) and interferes with the synthesis of guanosine triphosphate (GTP) and thus nucleic acid synthesis. However, inhibition of this normal cellular enzyme would not fully account for a selective antiviral action, although inhibition of IMPDH and resultant decreased concentrations of competing guanosine could potentiate other antiviral effects. Ribavirin triphosphate has been reported to selectively inhibit influenza virus RNA polymerase activity and to be a competitive inhibitor of the GTP-dependent 5'-capping of viral messenger RNA. Ribavirin triphosphate appears to inhibit the initiation and particularly the elongation of capped mRNA primer fragments by the influenza virus polymerase complex,[263] which in turn causes inhibition of viral protein synthesis.

Ribavirin has biologic activities beyond its antiviral and cytotoxic effects. In rodents, parenteral ribavirin inhibits the serum antibody but not cellular immune responses to inactivated influenza vaccine and diminishes in vivo primary antibody responses and memory cell generation to T-dependent and T-independent antigens.[264] In experimental animals, ribavirin has therapeutic activity against transplantable virus-induced tumors and autoimmune diseases.

Resistance. In contrast to other synthetic antiviral agents, resistance to ribavirin has not been produced under experimental conditions, except for the recent description of ribavirin-resistant sindbis virus mutants.[265] No ribavirin-resistant RSV have been detected during aerosol therapy of children.[36]

Pharmacology. Following oral administration, bioavailability averages 45 percent.[266] Following single oral doses of 600, 1200, or 2400 mg, peak plasma concentrations occur at 1–2 hours and average 1.3, 2.5, and 3.2 μg/ml, respectively. Tenfold higher peak plasma levels occur 0.5 hours after intravenous administration of equivalent doses.[266] Ribavirin accumulates during prolonged oral dosing, such that trough plasma levels average 1.3 and 3.3 μg/ml during the second week of treatment with 200 and 400 mg every 8 hours, respectively.[267] Plasma concentrations average approximately 24 μg/ml and 17 μg/ml after intravenous doses of 1000 and 500 mg, respectively, in Lassa fever patients.[268] During chronic oral administration of 300 mg twice daily cerebrospinal fluid levels average more than two-thirds of those in plasma (1.5–3 μg/ml).[269]

The disposition of ribavirin is complex. The β-phase $T_{1/2}$ is about 2.0 hours, but a prolonged terminal (γ)-phase $T_{1/2}$ of 36 hours occurs after single doses.[266] Ribavirin triphosphate concentrates in erythrocytes (~3 percent of dose), and RBC levels gradually decrease, with an apparent $T_{1/2}$ of about 40 days.[270] With chronic administration and RBC accumulation of ribavirin, the terminal plasma $T_{1/2}$ increases to 1–2 weeks.[267] Renal excretion accounts for approximately one-third of the drug's clearance, but hepatic metabolism is the major route of elimination.

With aerosol administration, plasma levels increase with the duration of exposure. Peak plasma levels range from 0.5 to 2.2 μg/ml after 8 hours exposure and from 0.8 to 3.3 μg/ml after 20 hours in pediatric patients.[268] Respiratory secretion levels often exceed 1000 μg/ml and persist with a half-life of 1.4–2.5 hours. The amount of ribavirin actually deposited in different regions of the respiratory tract during aerosol administration in different pathologic conditions or during mechanical ventilation is not certain. Revised estimates indicate that the delivered dose is twice as high in infants (1.8 mg/kg/hr) as in adults and that various other factors influence dosage.[270]

Toxicity. Ribavirin has been found to have cell-transforming, mutagenic, tumor-promoting, and possibly gonadotoxic activities in preclinical testing. Ribavirin is teratogenic and embryotoxic in small mammals[271] and is consequently contraindicated in pregnancy.

Prolonged administration causes a dose-dependent, macrocytic anemia in animals and humans,[271] and increased reticulocyte counts occur in ribavirin-treated patients after cessation of oral therapy.[272] Systemic ribavirin causes dose-related anemia due to extravascular hemolysis[267] and, at higher doses, suppression of bone marrow release of erythroid elements. Reversible increases of serum bilirubin in up to one-quarter of recipients, serum iron, and uric acid concentrations occur during short-term administration of oral ribavirin.[271,272] Chronic oral therapy is also associated with dose-related gastrointestinal and central nervous system complaints, including headache, lethargy, insomnia, and mood alteration in HIV-infected patients.[267]

Aerosolized ribavirin has been well tolerated except for mild conjunctival irritation and rash, transient wheezing, and occasional reversible deterioration in pulmonary function.[36,39,274] No adverse hematologic effects have been associated with aerosol ribavirin. One study did not find evidence of ribavirin absorption in health care providers working in the environment of aerosol-treated infants,[275] but another detected environmental contamination and ribavirin absorption in one nurse.[275a] When used in conjunction with mechanical ventilation, in-line filters, modified circuitry, and frequent monitoring are required to prevent plugging of ventilator valves and tubing with precipitates of ribavirin.[276–279] The possible effects of such modifications on drug delivery to the lower respiratory tract are undefined.

Clinical Studies. Ribavirin aerosol is approved by the Food and Drug Administration for treatment of RSV bronchiolitis and pneumonia in children.[279] A special aerosol generator utilizing a modified Collison nebulizer is needed to produce particles of proper aerodynamic size to reach the lower respiratory tract (SPAG-2, Viratek Corp). In infants less than 1 year old, the estimated delivered dose is 1.8 mg/kg/hr of aerosol exposure, when the reservoir concentration is 20 mg/ml ribavirin.[270] An initial controlled trial found that aerosolized ribavirin (20 hours exposure/day for 3–6 days) shortened the duration of virus shedding and improved certain clinical measures, including arterial oxygen saturation, in infants hospitalized with RSV pneumonia.[36] Similar studies of infants with RSV disease found that aerosolized ribavirin (12–22 hr/day for 3–5 days) was associated with some reductions in illness severity but not in duration of hospitalization or virus shedding.[37–39,276] More rapid improvements in illness severity and oxygenation have been documented in high-risk subjects with bronchopulmonary dysplasia or congenital heart disease.[38,39] Expert opinion varies about the overall clinical value, indications for use, and optimal length of aerosol ribavirin therapy in RSV infections.[279–282] Trials to date have not determined whether this costly intervention reduces the likelihood of intubation or death, shortens hospitalization time, or provides long-term benefit. Decreased RSV-specific serum neutralizing antibody titers, as well as diminished nasopharyngeal secretion RSV-specific IgE and IgA responses, may occur in ribavirin-treated children compared with placebo,[37,283] but the clinical significance of these findings is uncertain.

Anecdotal reports also suggest efficacy of aerosol ribavirin in severe influenza and parainfluenza virus infection.[284] Ribavirin aerosol treatment for an average of 12–18 hours per day for 3 days was associated with reductions in viral titers, fever, and systemic illness compared with placebo in young adults with uncomplicated influenza A or B virus infection in some but not all studies.[284,285] The relative therapeutic activity of aerosolized ribavirin and oral amantadine or rimantadine in influenza A virus infections and the value of aerosolized or intravenous ribavirin in high-risk groups, such as infants or adults hospitalized with influenza, are undetermined. Oral doses of 1000 mg/day had no clinical or antiviral activity in naturally occurring influenza A virus infection of adults.[272] An oral regimen with loading doses (3.6 mg over 3 hours) may provide clinical benefit in uncomplicated influenza.[286]

In Lassa fever patients at high risk of death because of elevated serum asparate aminotransferase levels or high-titer viremia, intravenous (4 gm/day) or oral ribavirin significantly reduced mortality, especially when therapy was initiated during the first 6 days of illness.[287] High-dose intravenous therapy has also been associated with reduced mortality in Korean hemorrhagic fever[288] and with antiviral effects in Argentine hemorrhagic fever.[289] Uncontrolled studies of chronic oral ribavirin 600 mg/day have found acceptable tolerance and possible antiviral effects in AIDS and ARC patients, but no consistent effects on T4 counts, viral isolation, or serum p24 antigen levels have been documented.[267,290] A placebo-controlled trial reported that ribavirin 800 mg/day reduced the risk of progression from lymphadenopathy syndrome to AIDS.[291] Oral ribavirin has also been reported to provide clinical benefit in measles, acute hepatitis, and mucocutaneous herpes virus infections,[292–294] but confirmation of such observations is needed.

Rimantadine Hydrochloride (Flumadine)

Spectrum. Rimantadine (alpha-methyl-1-adamantane methylamine hydrochloride) is a structural analogue of amantadine (Fig. 2) and shares its antiviral spectrum and mechanism of action. In yield reduction assays, most clinical isolates of influenza A virus are inhibited by ≤ 1 μg/ml, and concentrations of 0.1–0.4 μg/ml inhibit plaque formation by 50 percent or more.[158,159] In ferret tracheal organ culture, rimantadine has comparable antiviral activity to amantadine at four- to eightfold lower concentrations.[295] Concentrations of 10 μg/ml and higher are inhibitory for other enveloped viruses, including parainfluenza, influenza B, rubella, and dengue.[296] Such concentrations are also toxic to ciliated epithelium[295] and inhibitory to lymphocyte blastogenic responses in vitro.

Orally or parenterally administered rimantadine is effective in the prevention and treatment of influenza in various animal models, in which it appears to be more effective than amantadine on a weight basis. Treatment of infected mice limits the extent of virus replication and reduces the risk of transmission to exposed, uninfected animals. In mice, small particle aerosol delivery of rimantadine appears to be associated with greater antiviral and clinical effects than does intraperitoneal administration of comparable doses. Rimantadine exhibits enhanced antiviral activity in combination with ribavirin, interferon, or protease inhibitors.[163,297]

Mechanism of Action. Rimantadine inhibits an early step in the influenza virus replicative cycle, probably viral uncoating at the lysosomal stage.[298,299] Some studies suggest that rimantadine inhibits hemagglutinin-mediated fusion of the viral envelope and lysosomal membrane through increases in lysosomal pH.[300] Such an effect may account for the nonselective inhibitory effect of higher concentrations. However, interference with the removal of M protein from influenza viral ribonucleoproteins has been described,[299] and genetic studies have found that rimantadine's specific effect on human influenza A virus replication at low concentrations relates to gene 7 and its product the M2 protein.[8,167] Single amino acid changes at one of four or five sites in a critical hydrophobic transmembrane region of the M2 protein are associated with drug resistance.

Resistance. Rimantadine-resistant strains of influenza A virus may be readily recovered after passage of the virus in cell culture (frequency 10^{-3}–10^{-4}) or in animals in the presence of the compound.[8,170] Such isolates are cross-resistant to amantadine. In an avian model of influenza, treatment of infected birds is associated with the excretion of rimantadine-resistant virus within several days, and such viruses are capable of infecting and causing severe disease in contact animals receiving rimantadine prophylaxis.[170]

Young children treated with oral rimantadine for established influenza A virus infections may excrete drug-resistant virus by days 4–6 of therapy.[8,9] Transmission of drug-resistant influenza viruses to household contacts receiving rimantadine prophylaxis has also been found in families.[172] The clinical significance of these observations requires further study, but the finding raises questions about the routine use of these drugs in treating pediatric patients, who tend to shed virus longer and in higher titers than adults.

Pharmacology. Rimantadine in tablet form is well but slowly absorbed, and oral absorption does not appear to be decreased by the presence of food.[174,304] A syrup formulation, intended for pediatric use, has oral bioavailability slightly lower than the tablet.[305] The mean time to maximum plasma concentration averages 2–6 hours after administration. With multiple doses of 100 mg twice daily, the steady-state peak and trough plasma concentrations in healthy adults are approximately 0.4–0.5 μg/ml and 0.2–0.4 μg/ml, respectively.[306] In infants receiving doses of 3 mg/kg each day, steady-state peak serum levels range from 0.1 to 0.6 μg/ml.[307] No important age-related changes in plasma levels or pharmacokinetics have been found in healthy elderly adults or in children.[174,308,309] However, steady-state plasma concentrations in elderly nursing home residents receiving 100 mg twice daily averaged over twofold higher (mean, 1.2 μg/ml) than those observed in healthy adults,[303] which indicates the need for dose reductions in such patients. Rimantadine has an exceedingly large volume of distribution, and concentrations in nasal mucus average 50 percent higher than those in plasma.[174,309] Concentration of rimantadine in respiratory secretions could in part account for its efficacy despite lower plasma concentrations than with amantadine.

In contrast to amantadine, rimantadine is extensively metabolized following oral administration. Less than 15 percent of the dose is excreted unchanged in the urine, and approximately 20 percent of the dose is excreted in the urine as hydroxylated metabolites.[174,310] The remaining metabolites have not been fully identified. The plasma elimination $T_{1/2}$ of rimantadine averages 24–36 hours, approximately twofold longer than that of amantadine. In patients with chronic liver disease, without significant hepatocellular dysfunction, no clinically important differences in single-dose pharmacokinetics were found in one study.[311] In hemodialysis patients with severe renal failure, the clearance of rimantadine is decreased by 40 percent, and the elimination $T_{1/2}$ is about 55 percent longer.[310] Guidelines for dose adjustment in less severe renal insufficiency are being developed. Hemodialysis removes only a small amount of rimantadine, so that supplemental doses are not required.[310]

Toxicity. In animals given 5–20 times the recommended human doses, central nervous system (tremors, convulsions) and gastrointestinal side effects, as well as renal glomerular changes at very high doses, are observed during long-term administration. Rimantadine is not mutagenic in vitro and does not appear to cause teratogenic effects in rabbits or rats. However, safety in pregnancy has not been established.

Rimantadine administration is associated with dose-related, reversible side effects qualitatively similar to those observed with amantadine.[173] However, central nervous system side effects are significantly less frequent with rimantadine at dosages of 200 or 300 mg per day.[184,185,196] Rimantadine 300 mg/day is associated with significantly higher rates of gastrointestinal complaints, but not central nervous system or sleep disturbances compared with placebo.[185] Unlike amantadine, it is not associated with alterations of psychomotor test performance at this dosage. Most studies in adults and children have found excess withdrawal rates of less than 5 percent compared with placebo.[301,302] However, conventional 200 mg per day doses are associated with higher plasma levels and side effect rates in elderly nursing home residents.[303] The wider therapeutic margin of rimantadine, relative to amantadine, relates to differences in pharmacokinetics between the drugs.[190] Similar rates of CNS side effects are observed at comparable plasma concentrations. Rimantadine use has been anecdotally associated with exacerbations of seizures.

No clinically important laboratory abnormalities have been described, except for slight (less than threefold) elevations in transaminases in small numbers of subjects, and no serious end organ toxicity of rimantadine is recognized.[302] Drug interactions with rimantadine have not been studied, but patients receiving it concurrently with drugs affecting CNS function (e.g., antihistamines, antidepressants, and minor tranquilizers) should be watched for increased evidence of side effects.

Clinical Studies. Placebo-controlled, double-blind trials have shown that rimantadine is effective in preventing either experimentally induced or naturally occurring influenza virus infection.[173,184,193,312–314] Daily dosages of 200 mg in adults and of 5 mg/kg/day in children[313] have proven effective in preventing illness due to various influenza A subtypes during seasonal prophylaxis. One 6-week field trial comparing equivalent 200 mg/day dosages of rimantadine and amantadine found that the drugs were 85 and 91 percent effective, respectively, in preventing laboratory-documented influenza A illness.[184] In immunized nursing home patients, rimantadine (100 mg bid) had 75 percent efficacy in preventing influenza A illness compared with placebo during a community epidemic.[193] During a 5-week household-based study, rimantadine (5 mg/kg/day) administration to school-aged children decreased the risk of influenza A illness in recipients (100 percent efficacy) and possibly in their family contacts.[313] Studies to determine the minimally effective dose for long-term prophylaxis in healthy and high-risk elderly adults and the utility of postexposure prophylaxis in the family setting are currently in progress.

Therapeutic use of rimantadine is effective in uncomplicated influenza A virus infections, if treatment is begun within 48 hours of illness onset.[173,196,314,315] Oral rimantadine (300 mg/day) has therapeutic effects in uncomplicated, naturally occurring influenza A virus infection comparable to those of amantadine (200 mg/day). One study employing equivalent 100 mg bid dosing found that amantadine-treated patients tended to improve more rapidly than rimantadine-treated patients over the first 24 hours, but that by 48 hours after initiating therapy, both groups had significantly less fever, greater symptomatic improvement, and lower frequencies of virus shedding than placebo-treated patients.[196] Similar therapeutic benefit has been found in elderly influenza patients treated with rimantadine.[314] Because of rimantadine's slow absorption, low initial plasma levels, and long elimination half-life, therapeutic regimens using larger doses (400–600 mg in divided doses) over the first 24 hours of treatment may provide greater antiviral and clinical effects.[315] The possible value of rimantadine in treating acute influenza in high-risk patients to prevent complications and in treating severe influenza in hospitalized patients is currently under study. Aerosolized rimantadine has received limited study.[316]

In children with influenza A/H3N2 subtype infection, rimantadine treatment (6 mg/kg/day, up to 150 mg for those <9 years) for 5 days was associated with lower symptom burden, fever, and viral titers during the first 2 days of treatment compared with acetaminophen administration, but rimantadine-treated children had more prolonged shedding of influenza virus.[8,9] A similar study involving children with milder H1N1 subtype infection found reductions in viral shedding on the first and second days of treatment but no significant clinical benefit of rimantadine compared with acetaminophen.[10] No effects on antibody responses have been found when rimantadine is used for treatment of established influenza, but effects on other host responses to infection have not been critically evaluated. The optimal dose and duration of therapy have not been established in children, and the problem of rapid emergence of drug-resistant virus[8,10] may limit its therapeutic application in this age group.

Trifluridine (5-trifluoromethyl-2′-deoxyuridine, trifluorothymidine, Viroptic)

Trifluridine is a fluorinated pyrimidine nucleoside that has in vitro inhibitory activity against HSV types 1 and 2, cytomegalovirus, vaccinia, and some strains of adenovirus.[242,317] Its antiviral mechanism of action is undefined but involves inhibition of viral DNA synthesis. It also inhibits cellular DNA synthesis at relatively low concentrations. The triphosphate derivative is incorporated into viral, and to a lesser extent cellular DNA, in competition with deoxythymidine triphosphate. Trifluridine is active against thymidine kinase-negative strains of HSV, which indicates that this enzyme is not essential to its action. It also exhibits mutagenic, teratogenic, and antineoplastic activities in experimental systems.

Its use as an antiviral agent is currently limited to topical therapy of ocular HSV infections, in which it is approved by the Food and Drug Administration for treatment of primary keratoconjuctivitis and recurrent epithelial keratitis due to HSV types 1 and 2.[244,245] Topical trifluridine has been found to be more active than idoxuridine, but trials comparing its efficacy with that of topical vidarabine have generally found no significant differences.[318] Topical trifluridine has been effective in some patients who have not responded clinically to idoxuridine or vidarabine. Adverse reactions include discomfort upon instillation, palpebral edema, and, uncommonly, hypersensitivity reactions, irritation, superficial punctate, or epithelial keratopathy.

Vidarabine (ara-A, adenine arabinoside, Vira-A)

Spectrum. Vidarabine (9-beta-D-ribofuranosyladenine) is an analogue of adenine deoxyriboside (Fig. 4), which has in vitro antiviral activity against HSV types 1 and 2, VZV, Epstein-Barr virus, animal herpesviruses, vaccinia and variola viruses, and rhabdo and some RNA tumor viruses. Vidarabine also inhibits the in vitro replication of idoxuridine or acyclovir-resistant HSV strains and acyclovir-resistant VZV strains, but has variable activity against cytomegalovirus.[319–321] Plaque formation by most HSV and VZV strains is completely inhibited by 3.0 μg/ml or less of vidarabine. This concentration does not inhibit mytogen-or antigen-induced lymphocyte blastogenesis or lymphocyte cytotoxicity to herpesvirus-infected target cells in vitro.

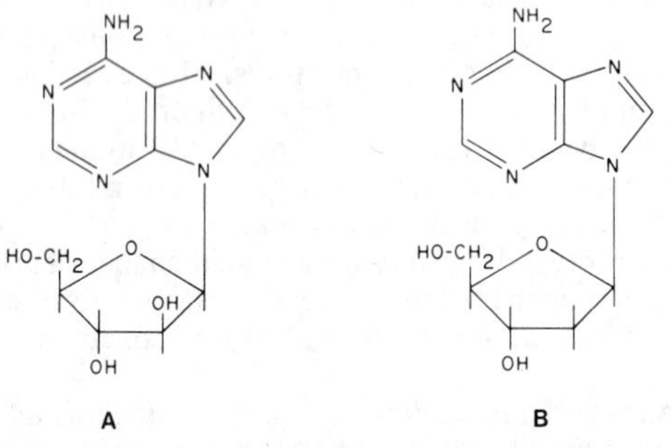

FIG. 4. Chemical structures of vidarabine (**A**) and the nucleoside deoxyadenosine (**B**).

Mechanism of Action. The antiviral mechanisms of vidarabine are not completely understood but it is an inhibitor of HSV DNA synthesis. Vidarabine is phosphorylated by cellular enzymes to the triphosphate derivative, which competitively inhibits HSV, and, to a lesser extent, cellular DNA polymerase activity. Vidarabine triphosphate is incorporated into both cellular and viral DNA, where it may act as a chain terminator for newly synthesized HSV nucleic acid.[322] The principal metabolite in vivo and in cell culture is hypoxanthine arabinoside (ara-Hx), a compound with 30- to 50-fold less antiviral activity than vidarabine.[320] However, ara-Hx appears to enhance the antiviral activity of vidarabine both in vitro and in specimens from patients receiving vidarabine. The carbocyclic analogue of vidarabine (cycladadine) is resistant to the action of adenosine deaminase and retains comparable antiviral activity in vitro and in animal models.[323,324]

Vidarabine triphosphate inhibits other enzyme systems, including ribonucleoside reductase, RNA polyadenylation, and S-adenosylhomocysteine hydrolase, an enzyme involved in transmethylation reactions, both in vitro and in RBC collected from treated patients.[54,325,326] This effect continues for over 1 week following cessation of therapy and may contribute to the antiviral and toxic effects of vidarabine. In mice, vidarabine administration augments humoral immune responses and delayed hypersensitivity reactions and prolongs survival in cryptococcal infection, perhaps mediated through interference with normal suppressor cell function.[327] Changes in the viral DNA polymerase can cause drug resistance, but it is not a recognized clinical problem.

Pharmacology. Following intravenous infusion, vidarabine is rapidly deaminated to ara-Hx by adenosine deaminase.[328] This enzyme is widely distributed through body tissues but in animals is present in relatively low concentrations in blood and brain. Samples for measurement of vidarabine levels need to be collected in the presence of an inhibitor of adenosine deaminase, such as 2-deoxycorformicin, and quickly frozen to prevent in vitro deamination. During a constant 12-hour infusion (10 mg/kg/12 hr), plasma ara-Hx concentrations peak at 3–6 μg/ml, but no or minimal concentrations of vidarabine (0.2–0.4 μg/ml) are detectable in adults by HPLC assay.[328,329] Ara-Hx is present in CSF at concentrations averaging 35 percent of plasma values, although CSF/plasma ratios over 90 percent have been found in infants.[330] Another study found that peak ara-Hx concentrations averaged 3.7 μg/ml in full-term infants and 8.5 μg/ml in preterm infants at a dosage of 15 mg/kg/12 hr[330] indicating that higher weight-adjusted dosages may be required in full-term infants.

The primary route of clearance is renal, and 40–53 percent of the total of the daily dose is recovered in the urine as ara-Hx and 1–3 percent as the parent drug.[228] The serum half-life of ara-Hx is approximately 3.5 hours in adults. Studies with labeled vidarabine have found accumulation of radioactivity in RBC over 5–7 days and lasting up to 3 weeks. In patients with impaired renal function, plasma ara-Hx concentrations rise and may be associated with neurologic or other side effects.[331] A dosage reduction of 25 percent has been recommended for patients with severe renal insufficiency,[331] but guidelines of proven value have not been established. Ara-Hx is readily cleared during hemodialysis (50 percent over 6 hours), so that dosages should be given after dialysis.[331]

Toxicity. Vidarabine has been shown to be mutagenic, teratogenic, and oncogenic in experimental systems, and its use should be restricted to serious infections. During human use, dose-related gastrointestinal toxicity is common with vidarabine and may be manifested by anorexia, nausea, vomiting, diarrhea, and/or weight loss.[328] The principal difficulty encountered during systemic administration of vidarabine relates to its poor solubility (≤0.45 mg/ml) and the consequent infusion of large fluid volumes, often 1.5–2.5 liters at a dosage of 15 mg/kg/day.

At dosages higher than normally used (20 mg/kg/day), vidarabine is associated with megaloblastic bone marrow changes and sometimes with anemia, leukopenia, or thrombocytopenia. Infusion-related thrombophlebitis, weakness, hypokalemia, rash, and the syndrome of inappropriate secretion of antidiuretic hormone (SIADH) have been described, but controlled trials in serious herpes virus infections at dosages of 10–15 mg/kg/day have not documented serious bone marrow, liver, or renal toxicity.

A variety of neurologic side effects have been reported during vidarabine therapy. High dosages, concurrent interferon or possibly allopurinol therapy, acute leukemia and its treatment, and the presence of pre-existing hepatic or renal insufficiency have been predisposing risk factors.[332–335] The reported neurotoxicities include pain syndromes, usually in the extremities and sometimes lasting up to 6 months after cessation of therapy; tremor, often accentuated by intention and at times associated with facial grimacing, myoclonus, ataxia, or dysgraphia; and alterations in behavior or mentation, including disorientation, depression, aphasia, akinetic mutism, agitation, hallucinations, and, rarely, coma or seizures. Electroencephalograms have shown diffuse changes consistent with metabolic encephalopathy in some cases, but may not correlate with clinical manifestations. In several patients, an unusual brain pathology consisting of chromatolysis and neuronal degeneration has been described.[335] Monitoring of ara-Hx concentrations in patients with hepatic or renal insuffiency is desirable, but not available in most laboratories.

Clinical Studies. The most notable successes with vidarabine have been observed in patients with HSV and VZV infections, but acyclovir has replaced it for most indications. The efficacy of vidarabine administered topically in HSV keratoconjunctivitis is well established and is superior to idoxuridine, in that topical vidarabine is effective in patients who cannot receive idoxuridine because of allergy, toxicity, or clinical drug resistance. Vidarabine (15 mg/kg/day for 10 days) increases survival in biopsy-proven HSV encephalitis to 46–61 percent at 6 months, but recent comparative studies have found intravenous acyclovir to be superior in efficacy.[97,98,336] Trials using combinations of acyclovir and vidarabine are planned. Vidarabine treatment reduces the mortality of neonatal HSV infection complicated by visceral dissemination or CNS involvement to 38–40 percent, compared with 74 percent in placebo recipients.[337] A trial comparing the efficacy of acyclovir and vidarabine (30 mg/kg/day) for neonatal infection did not find differences in survival between these treatments.[101] Development of disseminated HSV infection in a neonate has occurred despite vidarabine prophylaxis.[338] Vidarabine (10 mg/kg/day for 7 days) is of limited usefulness in mucocutaneous HSV infections of immunocompromised hosts.[339] Clinically modest reductions in the durations of pain, fever, and shedding of HSV type 1 are observed in vidarabine recipients,[339] but it is an alternative in patients with acyclovir-resistant HSV infections.

In immunocompromised patients with localized herpes zoster of less than 72-hour duration, vidarabine (10 mg/kg/day for 7 days) decreases the frequency of cutaneous dissemination (8 vs. 24 percent), visceral complications (5 vs. 19 percent), time to healing, and total duration of postherpetic neuralgia.[340] A comparative trial with acyclovir in disseminating zoster is in progress. In immunocompromized patients with varicella, vidarabine accelerated the resolution of new vesicle formation and fever and reduced the risk of varicella-related complications.[341] However, a comparative trial in varicella of immunocompromised children was stopped because of neurotoxicity, which occurred in 16 percent of vidarabine recipients.[335]

No therapeutic benefit has been observed in smallpox, despite use of high vidarabine doses (20 mg/kg/day for 7 days), or in patients with advanced progressive multifocal leukoencephalopathy. Uncontrolled studies in patients with congenital CMV infection or the CMV mononucleosis syndrome found transient suppression of virus excretion in the urine during vidarabine therapy. A randomized study of bone marrow transplant recipients found that intermittent administration of low vidarabine doses (5 mg/kg/day) did not reduce the frequency of interstitial pneumonia or CMV isolations. Administration of higher doses (10 mg/kg/day) to renal transplant patients with CMV-associated illness was associated not only with no therapeutic effect compared to placebo, but also with neurologic toxicity in 29 percent of recipients.[334]

In chronic hepatitis B virus infection, vidarabine is associated with reductions in plasma HBV-specific DNA polymerase activity and titers of HBsAg and HBeAg in some patients.[342] The phosphorylated ester of vidarabine, ara-AMP or vidarabine phosphate, is much more water soluble than the parent drug and can be administered intravenously or intramuscularly in chronic hepatitis.[343] The antiviral activity and the pharmacokinetics, metabolism, and toxicities of ara-AMP in man are similar to those of vidarabine.[343–345] Bone marrow toxicity and severe pain syndromes, typically involving lower extremity muscles and sometimes lasting more than 3 months after therapy, have been described in vidarabine phosphate recipients.[345] However, double-blind, placebo-controlled studies found that vidarabine phosphate alone or alternating with human leukocyte interferon does not provide long-term benefit to patients with chronic active or persistent hepatitis B.[346,347] Corticosteroid pretreatment followed by chronic vidarabine or vidarabine phosphate may increase response rates in chronic hepatitis B,[348,349] but steroid withdrawal can be associated with hepatic failure.[350] Vidarabine phosphate conjugated with lactosaminated human serum albumin, which selectively enters hepatocytes, is effective in inhibiting HBV replication at three- to sixfold lower doses than the free phosphate and is well tolerated during short-term administration.[351]

Zidovudine [azidothymidine, AZT, Retrovir]

Spectrum. Zidovudine (3′-azido-3′-deoxythymidine) is a thymidine analog in which the 3′ hydroxyl has been replaced by an azido ($-N_3$) group (Fig. 5). Zidovudine has antiviral activity against HIV-1 and other mammalian retroviruses.[53,352–355] Concentrations of 0.013 μg/ml produce a 50 percent decrease in supernatant reverse transcriptase activity in either HIV-1-infected human T-cell lines or peripheral blood lymphocytes.[352] Depending on the assay method and cell type, zidovudine 0.02–1.3 μg/ml is inhibitory for HIV-1 replication and cytopathology during exogenous infection of various cell types, whereas much higher concentrations are required to block replication in chronically infected cells.[355–361] High concentrations do not inhibit the spread of HIV through giant cell formation in cocultivation studies,[362] and viral replication may proceed in T-cell lines despite the presence of inhibitory concentrations of zidovudine.[363] Zidovudine appears to have minimal phosphorylation and negligible antiviral activity (>20 μg/ml) in human monocyte-derived macrophages, which may serve as a reservoir for HIV replication in vivo.[364] Anti-HIV-1 activity is potentiated by acyclovir, interferon, mismatched double-stranded RNA (ampligen), granulocyte–macrophage colony stimulating factor, and neutralizing antibody, but is antagonized by thymidine or ribavirin in vitro.[53,352,357–360] Zidovudine is inhibitory for HTLV-I,[365] but it appears to be less active against HIV-2.[361] Zidovudine 1.4–2.7 μg/ml is also inhibitory for Epstein-Barr virus replication but not for HSV or VZV. Many Enterobacteriaceae and *Vibrio* strains are inhibited at low concentrations of zidovudine (0.03–1.0 μg/ml), but bacterial resistance to zidovudine develops rapidly.[366] Inhibition of *G. lambia* but not other protozoans has also been described.[367]

Zidovudine concentrations that inhibit the growth of human cell lines are generally >50 μg/ml,[367] although one T-cell line was inhibited by 5 μg/ml. Human myeloid and erythroid progenitor cells are inhibited by low concentrations (0.3–0.6 μg/ml, respectively).[207,368] Uridine partially reverses zidovudine's hematopoietic toxicity for human granulocyte–macrophage progenitor cells without impairing its anti-HIV-1 activity in mononuclear cells.[368] Partial inhibition of mitogen-induced blastogenesis of peripheral blood mononuclear cells is observed at concentrations of ≥2.7 μg/ml.[352]

In animal models of retroviral infection, zidovudine administration after virus exposure can suppress or prevent the development of infection,[353,369,370] which suggests possible usefulness in postexposure prophylaxis. Administration during gestation to pregnant females delays the onset of virus-induced CNS infection in offspring infected in utero in a murine model of retroviral infection.[369]

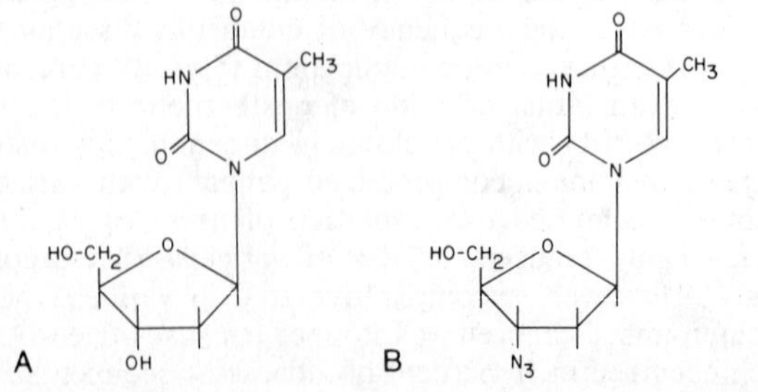

FIG. 5. Chemical structures of the nucleoside thymidine **(A)** and zidovudine **(B)**.

Mechanism of Action. Zidovudine's primary antiviral mechanism of action is inhibition of viral RNA-dependent DNA polymerase (reverse transcriptase).[371–373] Phosphorylation by cellular kinases results in high intracellular levels of the monophosphate, but low levels of the di- and triphosphates.[371] Concentrations of the phosphorylated forms of zidovudine are similar in uninfected and infected cells. Zidovudine triphosphate competitively inhibits the viral reverse transcriptase and is also inhibitory for cellular α-DNA polymerase at 100-fold higher concentrations. Thus, the antiviral selectivity of zidovudine is due to its greater affinity for HIV reverse transcriptase than for human DNA polymerases. In T-lymphocytic cell lines, triphosphate levels peak at 5 hours but then decline during further incubation with zidovudine.[355] The monophosphate is a competitive inhibitor of cellular thymidylate kinase, which leads to reduced intracellular levels of thymidine triphosphate.[371] Because thymidine triphosphate competes for the HIV reverse transcriptase, reduced levels may enhance the inhibition of the enzyme by zidovudine. Reduced levels of normal pyrimidines may also contribute to bone marrow toxicity.[372] The triphosphate is also incorporated into the growing DNA chain by reverse transcriptase. Because the 3′-azido groups prevents the formation of 5′-3′phosphodiester linkages, zidovudine acts as a chain terminator of DNA synthesis.

Resistance. Selection of zidovudine-resistant HIV mutants is difficult in the laboratory. Gene transfer studies employing site-specific mutagenesis have enabled the construction of zidovudine-resistant HIV-1 reverse transcriptases. Recent evidence indicates that zidovudine-resistant HIV strains may be recovered from patients who remain virus-positive on long-term therapy.[373] The frequency and clinical significance of such isolates and their mechanisms of resistance and possible sensitivity to other agents are under study.

Pharmacology. The oral bioavailability of zidovudine is approximately 60–65 percent.[374] Zidovudine is rapidly absorbed from the gastrointestinal tract, with peak serum concentrations occurring at 0.5–1.5 hours, although some patients may have poor or delayed absorption.[375] Following chronic oral administration of 250 mg every 4 hours, the steady-state peak (1.5 hours postdose) and trough plasma concentrations average 0.6–1.0 μg/ml and 0.1–0.2 μg/ml, respectively, although the range of observed concentrations is very broad.[367,375] Mean peak and trough levels of 0.4 to 0.5 and 0.1 μ/ml, respectively, have been found in those receiving 100 mg q4h.[376] Oral doses of 80–120 mg/m^2 give peak plasma concentrations of 1.1–1.4 μg/ml in children. No plasma drug accumulation occurs during prolonged dosing in those with normal renal function. Cerebrospinal fluid concentrations average 24–100 percent of those in plasma, which indicates significant penetration into the central nervous system.[367,374–378] Semen concentrations are 1.3- to 20-fold higher than serum,[375] which suggests sequestration due to the low pH of prostatic secretions. Zidovudine plasma protein binding is only 34–38 percent.

The plasma elimination $T_{1/2}$ is approximately 1 hour (0.8–1.9 hours). Zidovudine is rapidly metabolized to the 5′-glucuronide derivative, (GAZT) which has a similar elimination $T_{1/2}$ but lacks the HIV inhibitory activity of the parent compound. Following oral administration, the urinary recovery of zidovudine and GAZT averages 14 percent and 74 percent, respectively, of the dose. Renal clearance involves both glomerular filtration and tubular secretion. Definitive guidelines for dose adjustments of zidovudine in patients with impaired renal or hepatic function are not available at present. Accumulation of GAZT, but not zidovudine, occurs in renal failure but without obvious toxicity. Concomitant acyclovir does not affect zidovudine pharmacokinetics.[376]

Toxicity. Zidovudine causes transformation of mammalian cells in vitro at ≥0.5 μg/ml and chromosome abnormalities in cultured human lymphocytes at ≥3 μg/ml. In monkeys treated for 3–6 months, dose-related anemia and bone marrow suppression occur. The potential carcinogenicity and teratogenicity of the compound have not been fully studied.

The major toxicities of zidovudine recognized in clinical trials are granulocytopenia and anemia, which occur in up to 45 percent of recipients during relatively short-term administration.[367,379,380] The risk of hematologic toxicities is inversely related to the pretreatment T4 lymphocyte, hemoglobin, and granulocyte values and is directly related to the zidovudine dose and duration of therapy. Patients with more advanced disease or vitamin B_{12} deficiency are also at greater risk of marrow toxicity. The risk of significant granulocytopenia (<750/mm^3) is 19 percent in those with initial T4 counts >100/mm^3 and 51 percent in those with counts ≤100/mm^3.[379] During prolonged treatment the incidence of granulocytopenia remains relatively constant. Anemia associated with erythroid hypoplasia or megaloblastic bone marrow changes may occur as early as 2–4 weeks, but most commonly after the first 6 weeks of therapy,[381] whereas granulocytopenia usually occurs after 6–8 weeks. Macrocytosis is common but does not predict transfusion-requiring anemia. Pancytopenia related to partially reversible bone marrow failure has occurred at 14–17 weeks after starting therapy in up to 5 percent of patients.[382] Careful hematologic monitoring is required. Anemia can be managed by transfusion support, which is required by about 30 percent of patients, whereas zidovudine-induced erythroid hypoplasia, granulocytopenia (≤750/mm^3), or thrombocytopenia may require dose interruption or reduction.

Significantly higher rates of severe headache, nausea, insomnia, and myalgia occur in zidovudine recipients compared with placebo.[379] These symptoms sometimes require dose adjustment or discontinuation but may resolve despite continued zidovudine use. Severe neurotoxicity with seizures, as early as 48 hours after starting therapy,[383,384] Wernicke's encephalopathy, and a polymyositislike syndrome occurring at 6–17 months of therapy have been reported.[385] Late-onset progressive wasting with proximal muscle weakness, reduced exercise tolerance, and myalgia or less commonly acute rhabdomyolisis with muscle tenderness and high CPK levels have been described. After recovery, resumption of zidovudine can cause recurrence. Progressive nail pigmentation may occur in black patients.[386] A variety of other clinical adverse events have been reported in zidovudine-treated patients but at rates similar to those observed in placebo-treated.

Drugs that inhibit glucuronidation and/or renal excretion of zidovudine (e.g., probenicid) may increase the risks of marrow toxicity. Acetaminophen, which may increase plasma levels by inhibiting zidovudine metabolism, has been specifically associated with an increased frequency of leukopenia in one study.[379] Coadministration with drugs that are nephrotoxic or cytotoxic may increase the risk of hematologic toxicity. Concurrent ganciclovir markedly increases the risk of myelosuppression, and interferon of neutropenia and hepatotoxicity. Concomitant dapsone has been associated with severe anemia. Zidovudine therapy may alter plasma diphenylhydantion levels. Several cases of neurotoxicity (lethargy, convulsion) have been described during concomitant use of zidovudine and acyclovir, but subsequent studies have not documented an excessive risk. Acute overdose of zidovudine causes CNS depression but apparently no severe marrow toxicity.[387]

Clinical Studies. An initial 6-week dose escalating study of intravenous and oral zidovudine found that 79 percent of patients showed increased circulating T4 lymphocyte counts and that over 30 percent of anergic patients recovered cutaneous delayed-type hypersensitivity to at least one antigen.[380] In 1986 a randomized, double-blind, placebo-controlled, multicenter trial[378,388] established the efficacy of zidovudine therapy in adult AIDS patients with recently documented *Pneumocystis carini* pneumonia (PCP) and in symptomatic HIV-infected patients, the majority of whom had T4 counts ≤200 cells/mm^3. Treatment (250 mg q4h) over a mean period of 17 weeks was associated with a 91 percent efficacy in reducing mortality at 24 weeks and 56 percent in preventing opportunistic infections acquired after the first 6 weeks of treatment. Significant increases in T4 counts (transient in AIDS patients), return of cutaneous DTH reactivity in 29 percent of patients, weight gain, and stabilization of functional status also occurred. However, over one-third of patients required dose reduction or discontinuation because of hematologic toxicity. After 36 weeks of follow-up, zidovudine treatment was associated with a sixfold decrease in mortality compared with placebo, and the estimated mortality of the zidovudine group followed for 72 weeks was about 30 percent.[388,388a] Those with higher performance status, hemoglobin >12 g/dl, or with treatment initiated <90 days after PCP diagnosis have better prognosis. Concurrent prophylaxis for PCP is associated with much lower mortality during maintenance zidovidine (8 percent vs. 39 percent without prophylaxis at 1 year).[389] Chronic oral zidovudine is also associated with significant decreases in serum HIV p24 core antigen levels as early as 4 weeks.[391] However, zidovudine does not significantly reduce the rate of virus recovery from peripheral blood samples, and treated-patients must be regarded as infections.[388]

The minimally effective dosage of zidovudine for long-term use is currently undefined for different target groups. Dose schedules involving less frequent administration (250 mg or 500 mg q6h or 500 mg q12h) appear to be effective in reducing p24 antigenemia and increasing T4 cell counts in a majority of asymptomatic HIV-infected patients.[391] Studies in small numbers of AIDS or ARC patients found that full-dose zidovudine treatment (200–250 q4h) is associated with 90 percent or greater decreases in circulating p24 antigenemia in those with high antigen levels (>100 pg/ml), but that increases may be observed with lower doses (100 q4h or 250 q8h).[392] The addition of acyclovir to zidovudine does not appear to increase anti-HIV activity or toxicity during short-term use,[376,391] but may reduce

TABLE 5. Selected Antiviral Agents of Investigative Interest

Drug [Ref. No.]	*Mechanism of Action*	*Toxicities*	*Comments/Clinical Use*
Dideoxycytidine (DDC) [407]	Reverse transcriptase inhibition.	Skin rash, stomatitis, arthritis, fever. Dose-related painful peripheral neuropathy after several months.	Oral bioavailability 70–80%. Dose-related reductions in p24 antigenemia. Proposed use is to alternate monthly or weekly with zidovudine.
Dextran sulfate [408]	Blocks attachment of virus to CD4 receptor; inhibits syncytia formation.	Oral use: gastrointestinal upset, possibly CNS effects, abnormal LFT.	Synergistic in vitro with zidovudine. Efficacy and oral bioavailability not established.
Ampligen (mismatched, double-stranded RNA) [409]	Uncertain, interferon-like effects.	Myalgia, fever, chills, hypotension after IV administration.	Antiviral effects in initial clinical tests.
Suramin [409]	Reverse transcriptase inhibition.	Fever, rash, malaise, CNS, bone marrow, proteinuria, abnormal LFT.	No clinical or immune benefit in AIDS/ARC found to date.
Antimoniotungstate (HPA-23) [409]	Reverse transcriptase inhibition.	Thrombocytopenia, renal dysfunction, abnormal LFT.	No clinical or immune benefit in AIDS/ARC found to date.
CD4 receptor protein [410]	Inhibition of attachment/penetration.	Not defined.	Clinical trials with soluble recombinant CD4 molecules in progress. Peptide fragments and conjugates under development.

severe opportunistic infections and mortality to a greater extent than zidovudine alone during chronic administration in AIDS patients.[389]

Uncontrolled studies suggest a beneficial effect on HIV-associated neurologic disease.[377,378,393] Objective improvements in dementia and peripheral neuropathy are apparent within 8 weeks, and up to one-half of patients show sustained neurologic improvement 5–10 months after starting therapy.[378] Recent controlled studies indicate that AIDS patients show significantly improved sustained attention, memory, and visual-motor skills at 8 and 16 weeks of therapy.[390] Continuous intravenous infusion has improved neurodevelopmental abnormalities in encephalopathic children and IQ scores in children without overt encephalopathy.[377] Rebounds in serum and CSF p24 antigen levels and development of acute, self-limited meningoencephalitis have occurred shortly after zidovudine dose reductions.[394] Zidovudine treatment may benefit HIV-associated thrombocytopenia, psoriasis, and lymphocytic interstitial pneumonia.[367,395] The clinical value of zidovudine in pediatric infections, in patients with less severe manifestations of HIV infection (e.g., asymptomatic seropositivity, persistent generalized lymphodenopathy), in postexposure prophylaxis (e.g., needlestick exposure in health care workers), and the efficacy and toxicity of various combination regimens (zidovudine plus interferon, dideoxycitidine, or immunomodulators) are subjects of ongoing controlled clinical trials.

Foscarnet (PFA)

Foscarnet (trisodium phosphonoformate hexahydrate) is a simple inorganic pyrophosphate analogue that inhibits herpesvirus DNA polymerase and retroviral reverse transcriptase. It is active in vitro against most herpes viruses, including cytomegalovirus, hepadna viruses and human immunodeficiency virus. Unlike zidovudine, it also enters macrophages and inhibits HIV in these cells.[396] Resistance due to altered viral DNA polymerase can be generated in the laboratory but has not been observed in clinical isolates.

The drug is nephrotoxic, causing tubular trophy in animals, and other side effects have been noted in humans.[397,398] The drug increases urinary output and fluid intake. It has been associated with malaise, nausea, vomiting, fatigue, and headache. Anemia is common, but granulocytopenia does not occur. Tremor, seizures, irritability, and hallucinosis have been associated with high plasma concentrations. Phlebitis, hypo- and hypercalcemia, hyperphosphatemia, and abnormal transaminase values may also develop. Hypocalcemia may be enhanced by simultaneous administration of pentamidine.

Foscarnet is usually given by the intravenous route, often as a bolus of 20 mg/kg over 30 minutes followed by a continuous infusion of 230 mg/kg/24 h for 2–3 weeks.[399] Alternative dosing regimens to avoid continuous infusions include 60 mg/kg 3 times daily for 2 weeks, followed by a single dose 5 to 7 days per week for maintenance therapy.[400,401] Oral absorption is low. Intermittent infusions of 60 mg/kg/8 hours give peak plasma concentrations averaging 150 μg/ml.[400] The initial plasma T 1/2 averages 3–6 hours. Foscarnet penetrates into the CSF and the eye. Its disposition is complex, and bone deposition accounts for up to 20 percent of the administered dose. The drug is excreted by the kidney, and, because of its nephrotoxicity, the dose must be reduced if serum creatinine levels rise. It is suggested that the infusion be reduced by 20 mg/kg/24 hr for each 20 μmol/liter increase in the serum creatinine above 70 μmol/liter.[399]

Foscarnet has been used primarily to treat cytomegalovirus and HIV infections. In CMV retinitis in patients with AIDS, clinical responses appear to be similar to those observed with ganciclovir.[399,401,402] However, foscarnet has been less well studied. The problem of relapse after discontinuation of foscarnet is similar to that observed with ganciclovir. In a study of patients with AIDS and ARC treated with intravenous foscarnet for 3 weeks, eight patients converted from virus-positive to virus-negative during the study period, and six remained virus-free during 3 months of follow-up.[403] In another study, 15 patients with AIDS were treated for 14 days. No effect on HIV cultures was observed, but p24 antigen disappeared in five of eight patients, only to reappear 4–23 weeks later.[397] Interestingly, CMV culture positivity fell from 46 percent before treatment to 17 percent during treatment, and returned to 37 percent after foscarnet treatment. Other studies have confirmed the effect on p24 antigen.[404]

Foscarnet thus offers a major advantage over ganciclovir for the treatment of CMV infection in persons with AIDS, in that it does not affect granulocyte numbers. However, optimal dose schedules for initial treatment and chronic suppression have not been defined. It also appears to be a useful agent in severe acyclovir-resistant HSV infections.[405] Topical application of 3% foscarnet cream provides marginal clinical benefits in recurrent mucocutaneous HSV infections.[398,406] If the problem of renal toxicity can be overcome, it could become a useful agent.

For information on other antiretroviral agents of investigative interest, see Table 5.

REFERENCES

1. Newton AA. Tissue culture methods for assessing antivirals and their harmful effects. In: Field HJ, ed. Antiviral Agents: the Development and Assessment of Antiviral Chemotherapy. v. 1. Boca Raton, FL: CRC Press; 1988:23–67.
2. Crumpacker CS, Schnipper LE, Marlowe SI, et al. Resistance to antiviral drugs of herpes simplex virus isolated from patients treated with acyclovir. N Engl J Med. 1982;306:343–6.
3. Burns WH, Saral R, Santos GW, et al. Isolation and characterization of

resistant herpes simplex virus after acyclovir therapy. Lancet. 1982;1:421–3.
4. Sibrack CD, Gutman LT, Wilfert CM, et al. Pathogenicity of acyclovir-resistant herpes simplex virus type 1 from an immunodeficient child. J Infect Dis. 1982;146:673–82.
5. Wade JC, McLaren C, Myers JD. Frequency and significance of acyclovir-resistant herpes simplex virus isolated from marrow transplant patients receiving multiple courses of treatment with acyclovir. J Infect Dis. 1983;148:1077–82.
6. Parris DS, Harrington JE. Herpes simplex virus variants resistant to high concentrations of acyclovir exist in clinical isolates. Antimicrob Agents Chemother. 1982;22:71–7.
7. Smith KO, Kennell WL, Poirier RH, et al. In vitro and in vivo resistance of herpes simplex virus to 9-(2-hydroxyethoxymethyl)guanine (acycloguanosine). Antimicrob Agents Chemother. 1980;17:144–50.
8. Belshe RB, Smith MH, Hall CB, et al. Genetic basis of resistance to rimantadine emerging during treatment of influenza virus infection. J Virol. 1988;62:1508–12.
9. Hall CB, Dolin R, Gala CL, et al. Children with influenza A infection: treatment with rimantadine. Pediatrics. 1987;80:275–82.
10. Thompson J, Fleet W, Lawrence E, et al. A comparison of acetaminophen and rimantadine in the treatment of influenza A infection in children. J Med Virol. 1987;249–55.
11. Erice A, Chou S, Biron KK, et al. Progressive disease due to ganciclovir-resistant cytomegalovirus in immunocompromised patients. N Eng J Med. 1989;320:289–93.
12. Yeager AS. Genital herpes simplex infections: effect of asymptomatic shedding and latency on management of infections in pregnant women and neonates. J Invest Dermatol. 1984;83:053s–6s.
13. Gutman LT, Wilfert CM, Eppes S. Herpes simplex virus encephalitis in children: analysis of cerebrospinal fluid and progressive neurodevelopmental deterioration. J Infect Dis. 1986;154:415–21.
14. Brown ZA, Ashley R, Douglas J, et al. Neonatal herpes simplex virus infection: relapse after initial therapy and transmission from a mother with an asymptomatic genital herpes infection and erythema multiforme. Pediatr Infect Dis J. 1987;6:1057–61.
15. Bernstein DI, Lovett MA, Bryson YJ. The effects of acyclovir on antibody response to herpes simplex virus in primary genital infections. J Infect Dis. 1984;150:7–13.
16. Lafferty WE, Brewer LA, Corey L. Alteration of lymphocyte transformation response to herpes simplex virus infection by acyclovir therapy. Antimicrob Agents Chemother. 1984;26:887–91.
17. Hirsch MS. Antiviral drug development for the treatment of human immunodeficiency virus infections. Am J Med. 1988;85(Suppl 2A):182–85.
18. Hall MJ, Duncan IB. Antiviral drugs and interferon combinations. In: Field HJ, ed. Antiviral Agents: The Development and Assessment of Antiviral Chemotherapy. v. 1. Boca Raton, FL: CRC Press; 1988;29–85.
19. Wilson SZ, Knight V, Wyde PR, et al. Amantadine and ribavirin aerosol treatment of influenza A and B infection in mice. Antimicrob Agents Chemother. 1980;17:642–8.
20. Hayden FG, Douglas RG, Jr, Simons R. Enhancement of activity against influenza viruses by combinations of antiviral agents. Antimicrob Agents Chemother. 1980;18:536–41.
21. Stanwick TL, Schinazi RF, Campbell DE, et al. Combined antiviral effect of interferon and acyclovir on herpes simplex virus types 1 and 2. Antimicrob Agents Chemother. 1981;19:672–4.
22. Schinazi RF, Peters J, Williams CC, et al. Effect of combinations of acyclovir with vidarabine or its 5′-monophosphate on herpes simplex viruses in cell culture and in mice. Antimicrob Agents Chemother. 1982;22:499–507.
23. Sacks SL, Scullard GH, Pollard RB, et al. Antiviral treatment of chronic hepatitis B virus infection: pharmacokinetics and side effects of interferon and adenine arabinoside alone and in combination. Antimicrob Agents Chemother. 1982;21:93–100.
24. Smith CI, Kitchen LW, Scullard GH, et al. Vidarabine monophosphate and human leukocyte interferon in chronic hepatitis B infection. JAMA. 1982;247:2261–5.
25. Besser R, Krämer G, Rambow A, et al. Combined therapy with acyclovir and adenosine arabinoside in herpes simplex encephalitis. Eur Neurol. 1987;27:197–200.
26. Yarchoan R, Thomas RV, Allain J-P, et al. Phase I studies of 2′,3′-dideoxycytidine in severe human immunodeficiency virus infection as a single agent and alternating with zidovudine (AZT). Lancet. 1988;1:76–80.
27. Schmidt GM, Forman SJ, Zaia JA, et al. Treatment of cytomegalovirus associated pneumonitis with ganciclovir (DHPG) and immunoglobin following allogeneic bone marrow transplantation: antiviral and therapeutic response. Clin Res. 1988;36:470A.
28. Reed EC, Bowden RA, Dandliker PS, et al. Treatment of cytomegalovirus pneumonia with ganciclovir and intravenous cytomegalovirus immunoglobin in patients with bone marrow transplants. Ann Intern Med. 1988;109:783–8.
29. Steele RW, Charlton RK. Immune modulators as antiviral agents. In: Drew WL, ed. Clinics in Laboratory Medicine. v. 7. Philadelphia: WB Saunders; 1987:911–24.
30. Hayden FG, Laskin OL, Douglas RG Jr. Antiviral agents. In: Lourian V, ed. Antibiotics in Laboratory Medicine, 2nd ed. Baltimore: Williams & Wilkins; 1986:359–80.
31. Hatcher VA, Friedman-Kien AE, Marcus EL, et al. Arabinosyladenine monophosphate in genital herpes: a double-blind, placebo-controlled study. Antiviral Res. 1982;2:283–90.
32. Gangarosa LP, Hill JM, Thompson BL, et al. Iontophoresis of vidarabine monophosphate for herpes orolabialis. J Infect Dis. 1986;154:930–4.
33. Hayden FG, Hall WJ, Douglas RG, Jr. Therapeutic effects of aerosolized amantadine in naturally acquired infection due to influenza A virus. J Infect Dis. 1980;141:535–42.
34. Knight V, Wilson SZ, Quarles JM, et al. Ribavirin small-particle aerosol treatment of influenza. Lancet. 1981;2:945–9.
35. McClung HW, Knight V, Gilbert BE, et al. Ribavirin aerosol treatment of influenza B virus infection. JAMA. 1983;249:2671–4.
36. Hall CB, McBride JT, Walsh EE, et al. Aerosolized ribavirin treatment of infants with respiratory syncytial viral infection. N Engl J Med. 1983;308:1443–47.
37. Taber LH, Knight V, Gilbert BE, et al. Ribavirin aerosol treatment of bronchiolitis associated with respiratory syncytial virus infection in infants. Pediatrics. 1983;72:613–18.
38. Hall CB, McBride JT, Gala CL, et al. Ribavirin treatment of respiratory syncytial infection in infants with underlying cardiopulmonary disease. JAMA. 1985;254:3047–51.
39. Rodriguez WJ, Kim HW, Brandt CD, et al. Aerosolized ribavirin in the treatment of patients with respiratory syncytial virus disease. Pediatr Infect Dis J. 1987;6:159–63.
40. Hayden FG. Intranasal interferons for control of respiratory viral infections. In: Revel M, ed. Clinical Aspects of Interferons. Boston: Kluwer Academic Publishers; 1988;3–16.
41. Dorsky DI, Crumpacker CS. Drugs five years later: acyclovir. Ann Intern Med. 1987;107:859–74.
42. Biron KK, Elion GB. In vitro susceptibility of varicella-zoster virus to acyclovir. Antimicrob Agents Chemother. 1980;18:443–7.
43. Colby BM, Shaw JE, Elion GB, et al. Effect of acyclovir [9-(2-hydroxyethoxymethyl)guanine] on Epstein-Barr virus DNA replication. J Virol. 1980;34:560–8.
44. Lin J-C. Smith MC, Cheng YC, et al. Epstein-Barr virus: inhibition of replication by three new drugs. Science. 1983;221:578–9.
45. Lang DJ, Cheung K-S. Effectiveness of acycloguanosine and trifluorothymidine as inhibitors of cytomegalovirus infection in vitro. Am J Med. 1982;73(Suppl):49–53.
46. Kern ER. Acyclovir treatment of experimental genital herpes simplex virus infections. Am J Med. 1982;73(Suppl):100–8.
47. Collins P, Oliver NM. Acyclovir treatment of cutaneous herpes in guinea pigs and herpes encephalitis in mice. Am J Med. 1982;73(Suppl):96–9.
48. Soike KF, Gerone PJ, Acyclovir in the treatment of simian varicella virus infection of the African green monkey. Am J Med. 1982;73(Suppl):112–7.
49. Steele RW, Marmer DJ, Keeney RE. Comparative in vitro immunotoxicology of acyclovir and other antiviral agents. Infect Immun. 1980;28:957–62.
50. McGuffin RW, Shiota FM, Meyers JD. Lack of toxicity of acyclovir to granulocyte progenitor cells in vitro. Antimicrob Agents Chemother. 1980;10:471–3.
51. Levin MJ, Leary PL, Arbeit RD. Effect of acyclovir on the proliferation of human fibroblasts and peripheral blood mononuclear cells. Antimicrob Agents Chemother. 1980;17:947–53.
52. Wingard JR, Hess AD, Stuart RK, et al. Effect of several antiviral agents on human lymphocyte functions and marrow progenitor cell proliferation. Antimicrob Agents Chemother. 1983;23:593–7.
53. Mitsuya H, Broder S. Strategies for antiviral therapy in AIDS. Nature. 1987;325:773–8.
54. Elion GB. History, mechanism of action, spectrum and selectivity of nucleoside analogs. In: Mills J, Corey L, eds. Antiviral Chemotherapy: New Directions for Clinical Application and Research. New York: Elsevier; 1986;118–37.
55. Derse D, Cheng Y-C, Furman PA, et al. Inhibition of purified human and herpes simplex virus-induced DNA polymerases by 9-(2-hydroxyethoxymethyl)granine triphosphate. J Biol Chem. 1981;256:11447–51.
56. McGuirt PV, Furman PA. Acyclovir inhibition of viral DNA chain elongation in herpes simplex virus-infected cells. Am J Med. 1982;73(Suppl):67–71.
57. Furman PA, St. Clair MH, Spector T. Acyclovir triphosphate is a suicidal inactivator of the herpes simplex virus DNA polymerase. J Biol Chem. 1984;259:9575–9.
58. Pagano JS, Datta AK. Perspectives on interactions of acyclovir with Epstein-Barr and other herpes viruses. Am J Med. 1982;73(Suppl):18–26.
59. Collins P. Viral sensitivity following the introduction of acyclovir. Am J Med. 1988;85(Suppl 2A):129–34.
60. Coen D, Schaffer PA. Two distinct loci confer resistance to acycloguanosine in herpes simplex virus type 1. Am J Med. 1982;73(Suppl):2265–9.
61. Norris SA, Kessler HA, Fife KH. Severe, progressive herpetic whitlow caused by an acyclovir-resistant virus in a patient with AIDS. J Infect Dis. 1988;157:209–10.
62. Erlich KS, Mills J, Chatis P, et al. Acyclovir-resistant herpes simplex virus infections in patients with the acquired immunodeficiency syndrome. N Engl J Med. 1989;320:293–6.
63. Ellis MN, Keller PM, Fyfe JA, et al. Clinical isolate of herpes simplex virus type 2 that induces a thymidine kinase with altered substrate specificity. Antimicrob Agents Chemother. 1987;31:1117–25.
64. Corey L, Holmes KK. Genital herpes simplex virus infections: current concepts in diagnosis, therapy, and prevention. Ann Intern Med. 1983;98:973–83.

65. Straus SE, Takiff HE, Seidlin M, et al. Suppression of frequently recurring genital herpes. N Engl J Med. 1984;310:1545–50.
66. Lehrman SN, Douglas JM, Corey L, et al. Recurrent genital herpes and suppressive oral acyclovir therapy. Ann Intern Med. 1986;104:786–90.
67. Cole NL, Balfour HH Jr. Varicella-zoster virus does not become more resistant to acyclovir during therapy. J Infect Dis. 1986;153:605–8.
68. Larder BA, Darby G. Susceptibility to other antiherpes drugs of pathogenic variants of herpes simplex virus selected for resistance to acyclovir. Antimicrob Agents Chemother. 1986;29:894–9.
69. Blum RM, Liao SHT, de Miranda P. Overview of acyclovir pharmacokinetic disposition in adults and children. Am J Med. 1982;73(Suppl):186–92.
70. Laskin OL. Clinical pharmacokinetics of acyclovir. Clin Pharmocokinet. 1983;8:187–201.
71. Van Dyke RB, Connor JD, Wyborny C, et al. Pharmacokinetics of orally adminsitered acyclovir in patients with herpes progenitalis. Am J Med. 1982;73(Suppl):172–5.
72. McKindrick MW, McGill JI, White JE, et al. Oral acyclovir in acute herpes zoster. Br Med J. 1986;293:1529–32.
73. Wade JC, Newton B, Flournoy N, et al. Oral acyclovir for prevention of herpes simplex virus reactivation after bone marrow transplantation. Ann Intern Med. 1984;100:823–8.
74. Sullender WM, Arvin AM, Diaz PS, et al. Pharmacokinetics of acyclovir suspension in infants and children. Antimicrob Agents Chemother. 1987;31:1722–6.
75. Peterslund NA, Esmann V, Geil JP, et al. Open study of 2-amino-9-(hydroxyethoxymethyl)-9H-purine (desciclovir) in the treatment of herpes zoster. J Antimicrob Chemother. 1987;20:743–51.
76. Petty BG, Whitley RJ, Liao S, et al. Pharmacokinetics and tolerance of desciclovir, a prodrug of acyclovir, in healthy human volunteers. Antimicrob Agents Chemother. 1987;31:1317–22.
77. Hung SO, Patterson A, Rees PJ. Pharmacokinetics of oral acyclovir (Zovirax) in the eye. Br J Ophthamol. 1984;68:192–5.
78. Meyer LJ, de Miranda P, Sheth N, et al. Acyclovir in human breast milk. Am J Obstet Gynecol. 1988;158:586–8.
79. Hintz M, Connor JD, Spector SA, et al. Neonatal acyclovir pharmacokinetics in patients with herpes virus infections. Am J Med. 1982;72(Suppl):210–4.
80. Laskin OL, Longstreth, Whelton A, et al. Effect of renal failure on the pharmacokinetics of acyclovir. Am J Med. 1982;73(Suppl):197–201.
81. DeMiranda P, Good SS, Laskin OL, et al. Disposition of intravenous radioactive acyclovir. Clin Pharmacol Ther. 1981;30:662.
82. De Miranda P, Good SS, Krasny HC, et al. Metabolic fate of radioactive acyclovir in humans. Am J Med. 1982;73(Suppl):215–20.
83. Krasny HC, Liao SHT, de Miranda P, et al. Influence of hemodialysis on acyclovir pharmacokinetics in patients with chronic renal failure. Am J Med. 1982;73(Suppl):202–4.
84. Boelaert J, Schurgers M, Daneels R, et al. Multiple dose pharmacokinetics of intravenous acyclovir in patients on continuous ambulatory peritoneal dialysis. J Antimicrob Chemother. 1987;20:69–76.
85. Quinn RP, Wolberg G, Medzihradsky J, et al. Effect of acyclovir on various murine in vivo and in vitro immunologic assay systems. Am J Med. 1982;73(Suppl):62–6.
86. Keeney RE, Kirk LE, Bridgen D. Acyclovir tolerance in humans. Am J Med. 1982;73(Suppl):176–81.
87. Sylvester RK, Ogden WB, Draxler CA, et al. Vesicular eruption. JAMA. 1986;255:385–6.
88. Wade JC, Hintz M, McGuffin RW, et al. Treatment of cytomegalovirus pneumonia with high-dose acyclovir. Am J Med. 1982;73(Suppl):249–56.
89. Wade JC, Meyers JD. Neurologic symptoms associated with parenteral acyclovir treatment after marrow transplantation. Ann Intern Med. 1983;98:921–5.
90. Bean B, Aeppli D. Adverse effects of high-dose intravenous acyclovir in ambulatory patients with acute herpes zoster. J Infect Dis. 1985;151:362–4.
91. Feldman S, Rodman J, Gregory B. Excessive serum concentrations of acyclovir and neurotoxicity. J Infect Dis. 1988;157:385–8.
92. Potter JL, Krill CE. Acyclovir crystalluria. Pediatr Infect Dis. 1986;5:710–2.
93. Sawyer MH, Webb DE, Balow JE, et al. Acyclovir-induced renal failure: clinical course and histology. Am J Med. 1988;84:1067–71.
94. Bean B, Braun C, Balfour HH Jr. Acyclovir therapy for acute herpes zoster. Lancet. 1982;2:118–21.
95. Balfour HH Jr, Bean B, Laskin OL, et al. Acyclovir halts progression of herpes zoster in immunocompromised patients. N Engl J Med. 1983;308:1448–53.
96. Douglas JM Jr, Davis LG, Remington ML, et al. A double-blind, placebo-controlled trial of chronically administered oral acyclovir on sperm production in men with frequently occurring genital herpes. J Infect Dis. 1988;157:588–93.
97. Whitley RJ, Alford CA, Hirsch MS, et al. Vidarabine versus acyclovir therapy in herpes simplex encephalitis. N Engl J Med. 1986;314:144–9.
98. Sköldenberg B, Alestig K, Burman L, et al. Acyclovir versus vidarabine in herpes simplex encephalitis. Lancet. 1984;2:706–11.
99. Feldman S, Lott L. Varicella in children with cancer: impact of antiviral therapy and prophylaxis. Pediatrics. 1987;80:465–72.
100. Shepp DH, Dandliker PS, Meyers JD. Treatment of varicella-zoster virus infection in severely immunocompromised patients. N Engl J Med. 1986;314:208–12.
101. Whitley RJ, Arvin A, Corey L, et al. Vidarabine versus acyclovir therapy of neonatal herpes simplex virus, HSV, infection (Abstract #986). Pediatr Res. 1986;20:323A.
102. Mertz GJ. Diagnosis and treatment of genital herpes infections. In: Knight V, Gilbert BE, eds. Infectious Disease Clinics of North America, Philadelphia: WB Saunders; 1987;341–66.
103. Corey L, Fife KH, Benedetti JK, et al. Intravenous acyclovir for the treatment of primary genital herpes. Ann Intern Med. 1983;98:914–21.
104. Bryson YJ, Dillon M, Lovett M, et al. Treatment of first episodes of genital herpes simplex virus infection with oral acyclovir. N Engl J Med. 1983;308:916–21.
105. Corey L, Nahmias AJ, Guinan ME, et al. A trial of topical acyclovir in genital herpes simplex virus infections. N Engl J Med. 1982;306:1313–9.
106. Mindel A, Adler MW. Intravenous acyclovir treatment for primary genital herpes. Lancet. 1982;1:697–700.
107. Nilsen AE, Aasen T. Efficacy of oral acyclovir in the treatment of initial and recurrent genital herpes. Lancet. 1982;2:571–3.
108. Reichman RC, Badger GJ, Guinan ME, et al. Topically administered acyclovir in the treatment of recurrent herpes simplex genitalis: a controlled trial. J Infect Dis. 1983;147:336–40.
109. Luby JP, Gnann JW Jr, Alexander WJ, et al. A collaborative study of patient-initiated treatment of recurrent genital herpes with topical acyclovir or placebo. J Infect Dis. 1984;150:1–6.
110. Rompalo AM, Mertz GJ, Davis LG, et al. Oral acyclovir for treatment of first-episode herpes simplex virus proctitis. JAMA. 1988;259:2879–81.
111. Reichman RC, Badger GJ, Mertz GJ, et al. Patient-initiated therapy of recurrent herpes simplex genitalis with orally administered acyclovir. JAMA. 1984;251:2103–07.
112. Douglas JM, Critchlow C, Benedetti J, et al. A double-blind study of oral acyclovir for suppression of recurrences of genital herpes simplex virus infection. N Engl J Med. 1984;310:1551–6.
113. Gold D, Corey L. Acyclovir prophylaxis for herpes simplex virus infections. Antimicrob Agents Chemother. 1987;31:361–7.
114. Mertz GJ, Eron L, Kaufman R, et al. prolonged continuous versus intermittent oral acyclovir treatment in normal adults with frequently recurring genital herpes simplex virus infection. Am J Med. 1988;85(Suppl 2A):14–19.
115. Mostow SR, Mayfield JL, Marr JJ, Drucker JL. Suppression of recurrent genital herpes by single daily dosages of acyclovir. Am J Med. 1988;85(Suppl 2A):30–3.
116. Straus SE, Seidlin M, Takiff HE, et al. Double-blind comparison of weekend and daily regimens of oral acyclovir for suppression of recurrent genital herpes. Antiviral Res. 1986;6:151–9.
117. Rooney JF, Felser JM, Ostrove JM, et al. Acquisition of genital herpes from an asymptomatic sexual partner. N Engl J Med. 1986;314:1561–4.
118. Kinghorn GR, Turner EB, Barton IG, et al. Efficacy of topical acyclovir cream in first and recurrent episodes of genital herpes. Antiviral Res. 1983;3:291–301.
119. Raborn GW, McGaw WT, Grace M, et al. Treatment of herpes labialis with acyclovir: review of three clinical trials. Am J Med. 1988;85(Suppl 2A):39–42.
120. Spruance S, Hamill M, Hoge W, et al. Suppression of herpes simplex labialis at ski resorts with oral acyclovir (Abstract #1182). Programs and Abstracts of the Twenty-sixth International Conference on Antimicrobial Agents and Chemotherapy. 1986:312.
121. Saral R, Burns WH, Laskin OL, et al. Acyclovir prophylaxis of herpes-simplex-virus infections. N Engl J Med. 1981;305:63–7.
122. Lundgren G, Wilczek H, Lonnqvist B, et al. Acyclovir prophylaxis in bone marrow transplant recipients. Scand J Infect Dis. 1985;47:137–44.
123. Gluckman E, Devergie A, Melo R, et al. Prophylaxis of herpes infections after bone marrow transplantation by oral acyclovir. Lancet. 1983;2:706–8.
124. Seale L, Jones CJ, Kathpalia S, et al. Prevention of herpesvirus infections in renal allograft recipients by low-dose oral acyclovir. JAMA. 1985;254:3435–8.
125. Meyers JD, Reed EC, Shepp DH, et al. Acyclovir for prevention of cytomegalovirus infection and disease after allogeneic marrow transplantation. N Engl J Med. 1988;318:70–5.
126. Straus S, Seidlin M, Takiff H, et al. Oral acyclovir to suppress recurrent herpes simplex virus infections in immunodeficient patients. Ann Intern Med. 1984;100:522–24.
127. Saral R, Ambinder RF, Burns WH, et al. Acyclovir prophylaxis against herpes simplex virus infection in patients with leukemia. Ann Intern Med. 1983;99:773–76.
128. Wade JC, Newton B, McLaren C, et al. Intravenous acyclovir to treat mucocutaneous herpes simplex infection after marrow transplantation. Ann Intern Med. 1982;96:265–69.
129. Shepp DH, Newton BA, Dandliker PS, et al. Oral acyclovir therapy for mucocutaneous herpes simplex infections in immunocompromised marrow transplant recipients. Ann Intern Med. 1985;102:783–5.
130. Whitley R, Barton N, Collins E, et al. Mucocutaneous herpes simplex virus infections in immunocompromised patients. Am J Med. 1982;73(Suppl):236–40.
131. Peterslund NA, Ipsen J, Schonheyder H, et al. Acyclovir in herpes zoster. Lancet. 1981;2:827–30.
132. Huff JC, Bean B, Balfour HH Jr, et al. Therapy of herpes zoster with oral acyclovir. Am J Med. 1988;85(Suppl 2A):84–9.
133. Cobo M. Reduction of the ocular complications of herpes zoster ophthalmicus by oral acyclovir. Am J Med. 1988;85(Suppl 2A):90–3.

134. Wassilew SW, Reimlinger S, Nasemann T, Jones D. Oral acyclovir for herpes zoster: a double-blind controlled trial in normal subjects. Br J Dermatol. 1987;117:495–501.
135. Wood MJ, Ogan PH, McKendrick MW, et al. Efficacy of oral acyclovir treatment of acute herpes zoster. Am J Med. 1988;85(Suppl 2A):79–83.
135a. Esmann V, Kroon S, Peterslund NA, et al. Prednisolone does not prevent post-herpetic neuralgia. Lancet. 1987;2:126–9.
136. McGill J, Chapman C. A comparison of topical acyclovir with steroids in the treatment of herpes zoster keratouveitis. Br J Ophthalmol. 1983;67:46–50.
137. Al-Nakib W, Al-Kandari S, El-Khalik DMA, et al. A randomised controlled study of intravenous acyclovir (Zovirax) against placebo in adults with chickenpox. J Infect. 1983;6:49–56.
138. Schlossberg D, Littman M. Varicella pneumonia. Arch Intern Med. 1988;148:1630–2.
139. Boyd K, Walker E. Use of acyclovir to treat chickenpox in pregnancy. Br Med J. 1988;296:393–4.
140. Johns DR, Gress DR. Rapid response to acyclovir in herpes zoster-associated encephalitis. Am J Med. 1987;82:560–2.
141. Vilde JL, Bricaire F, Leport C, et al. Comparative trial of acyclovir and vidarabine in disseminated varicella-zoster virus infections in immunocompromised patients. J Med Virol. 1986;20:127–34.
142. Prober CG, Kirk LE, Keeney RE. Acyclovir therapy of chickenpox in immunosuppressed children—a collaborative study. J Pediatr. 1982;101:622–5.
143. Nyerges G, Meszner Z, Gyarmati E, et al. Acyclovir prevents dissemination of varicella in immunocompromised children. J Infect Dis. 1988;157:309–13.
144. Balfour HH Jr. Intravenous acyclovir therapy for varicella in immunocompromised children. J Pediatr. 1984;104:134–6.
145. VanLandingham KE, Marsteller HB, Ross GW, et al. Relapse of herpes simplex encephalitis after conventional acyclovir therapy. JAMA. 1988;259:1051–3.
146. Balfour HH Jr, Bean B, Mitchell CD, et al. Acyclovir in immunocompromised patients with cytomegalovirus disease. Am J Med. 1982;73(Suppl):241–248.
147. Plotkin SA, Starr SE, Bryan CK. In vitro and in vivo responses of cytomegalovirus to acyclovir. Am J Med. 1982;73(Suppl):257–261.
148. Andersson J, Britton S, Ernberg I, et al. Effect of acyclovir on infectious mononucleosis: a double-blind, placebo-controlled study. J Infect Dis. 1986;153:283–90.
149. Andersson J, Skoldenberg B, Henle W, et al. Acyclovir treatment in infectious mononucleosis: a clinical and virological study. Infection. 1987;15:S14–20.
150. Hanto DW, Frizzera G, Gajl-Peczalska KJ, et al. Epstein-Barr virus-induced B-cell lymphoma after renal transplantation. N Engl J Med. 1982;306:913–8.
151. Sullivan JL, Bryon KS, Brewster FE, et al. Treatment of life-threatening Epstein-Barr virus infections with acyclovir. Am J Med. 1982;73(Suppl):262–6.
152. Schooley RT, Carey RW, Miller G, et al. Chronic Epstein-Barr virus infection associated with fever and interstitial pneumonitis. Ann Intern Med. 1986;104:636–43.
153. Resnick L, Herbst JS, Ablashi DV, et al. Regression of oral hairy leukoplakia after orally administered acyclovir therapy. JAMA. 1988;259:384–8.
154. Straus SE, Dale JK, Tobi M, et al: Acyclovir treatment of the chronic fatigue syndrome: lack of efficacy in a placebo-controlled trial. N Engl J Med. 1988;319:1692–8.
155. Schalm SW, VanBuuren HR, Heytink RA, DeMan RA. Acyclovir enhances the antiviral effect of interferon in chronic hepatitis B. Lancet. 1985;2:358–60.
156. Alexander GJM, Fagan EA, Hegarty JE, Yeo J, Eddleston ALWF, Williams R. Controlled clinical trial of acyclovir in chronic hepatitis B virus infection. J Med Virol. 1987;21:81–7.
157. Couch RB, Six HR. The antiviral spectrum and mechanism of action of amantadine and rimantadine. In: Mills J, Corey L, eds. Antiviral Chemotherapy: New Directions for Clinical Application and Research, New York: Elsevier; 1986;50–57.
158. Hayden FG, Cote KM, Douglas RG, Jr. Plaque inhibition assay for drug susceptibility testing of influenza viruses. Antimicrob Agents Chemother. 1980;17:865–70.
159. Browne MJ, Moss MY, Boyd MR. Comparative activity of amantadine and ribavirin against influenza virus in vitro: possible clinical relevance. Antimicrob Agents Chemother. 1983;23:503–5.
160. Pemberton RM, Jennings R, Potter CW, Oxford JS. Amantadine resistance in clinical influenza A (H3N2) and (H1N1) virus isolates. J Antimicrob Chemother. 1986;18(Suppl B):135–40.
161. Koff WC, Elm JL, Jr., Halstead SB. Inhibition of dengue virus replication by amantadine hydrochloride. Antimicrob Agents Chemother. 1980;18:125–9.
162. Hayden FG. Animal models of influenza virus infection for evaluation of antiviral agents. In: Zak O, Sande MA, eds. Experimental Models in Antiviral Chemotherapy. v. 3. London: Academic Press; 1986;353–71.
163. Hayden FG. Combinations of antiviral agents for treatment of influenza virus infections. J Antimicrob Chemother. 1986;18(Suppl B):177–83.
164. Richman DD, Yazaki P, Hostetler KY. The intracellular distribution and antiviral activity of amantadine. Virology. 1981;112:81–90.
165. Richman DD, Hostetler KY, Yazaki PJ, Clark S. Fate of influenza A virion proteins after entry into subcellular fractions of LLC cells and the effect of amantadine. Virology. 1986;151:200–10.
166. Oxford JS, Galbraith A. Antiviral activity of amantadine: a review of laboratory and clinical data. Pharmacol Ther. 1980;11:181.
167. Hay AJ, Zambon MC, Wolstenholme AJ, Skehel JJ, Smith MH. Molecular basis of resistance of influenza A viruses to amantadine. J Antimicrob Chemother. 1986;18(Suppl B):19–29.
168. Beyer WEP, Ruigrok RWH, van Driel H, Masurel N. Influenza virus strains with a fusion threshold of pH 5.5 or lower are inhibited by amantadine. Arch Virol. 1986;90:173–81.
169. Beard CW, Brugh M, Webster RG. Emergence of amantadine-resistant H5N2 avian influenza virus during a simulated layer flock treatment program. Avian Dis. 1987;31:533–7.
170. Webster RG, Kawaoka Y, Bean WJ, Beard CW, Brugh M. Chemotherapy and vaccination: a possible strategy for the control of highly virulent influenza virus. J Virol. 1985;55:173–6.
171. Bean WJ, Webster RG. Biological properties of amantadine-resistant influenza virus mutants. Antiviral Res. 1988;9:128.
172. Belshe RB, Tomlinson DL, Burk B, Pizzuti D. Occurrence and transmission of amantadine/rimantadine resistant influenza A virus (Abstract). Intersci Conf Antimicrob Agents Chemother. 1988;no. 99:127.
173. Tominack RL, Hayden FG. Rimantadine hydrochloride and amantadine hydrochloride use in influenza A virus infections. In: Moellering RC, Knight V, Gilbert BE, eds: Infectious Disease Clinics of North America. Philadelphia: WB Saunders; 1987;1:459–78.
174. Hayden FG, Minocha A, Spyker DA, Hoffman HE. Comparative single-dose pharmacokinetics of amantadine hydrochloride and rimantadine hydrochloride in young and elderly adults. Antimicrob Agents Chemother. 1985;28:216–21.
175. Aoki FY, Sitar DS. Amantadine kinetics in healthy elderly men: implications for influenza prevention. Clin Pharmacol Ther. 1985;37:137–44.
176. Aoki FY, Sitar DS. Clinical pharmacokinetics of amantadine hydrochloride. Clin Pharmacokinet. 1988;14:35–51.
177. Fishaut M, Mostow S. Amantadine for severe influenza A pneumonia in infancy. Am J Dis Child. 1980;134:321–23.
178. Horadam VW, Sharp JG, Smilack JD, et al. Pharmacokinetics and amantadine hydrochloride in subjects with normal and impaired renal function. Ann Intern Med. 1981;94:454–8.
179. Soung L-S, Ing TS, Daugirdas JT, et al. Amantadine hydrochloride pharmacokinetics in hemodialysis patients. Ann Intern Med. 1980;93:46–9.
180. Sartori M, Pratt CM, Young JB. Malignant cardiac arrhythmia induced by amantadine poisoning. Am J Med. 1984;77:388–91.
181. Atkinson WL, Arden NH, Patriarca PA, Leslie N, Lui K-J, Gohd R. Amantadine prophylaxis during an institutional outbreak of type A (H1N1) influenza. Arch Intern Med. 1986;146:1751–6.
182. Shields WD, Lake JL, Chugani HT. Amantadine in the treatment of refractory epilepsy in childhood: an open trial in 10 patients. Neurology. 1985;35:579–81.
183. Nestelbaum Z, Siris SG, Rifkin A, Klar H, Reardon GT. Exacerbation of schizophrenia associated with amantadine. Am J Psychiatry 1986;143:1170–1.
184. Dolin R, Reichman RC, Madore HP, et al. A controlled trial of amantadine and rimantadine in the prophylaxis of influenza A infection. N Engl J Med. 1982;307:580–4.
185. Hayden FG, Gwaltney JM Jr, Van de Castle RL, et al. Comparative toxicity of amantadine hydrochloride and rimantadine hydrochloride in healthy adults. Antimicrob Agents Chemother. 1981;19:226–33.
186. Millet VM, Dreisbach M, Bryson YJ. Double-blind controlled study of central nervous system side effects of amantadine, rimantadine, and chlorpheniramine. Antimicrob Agents Chemother. 1982;21:1–4.
187. Kantor RJ, Stevens D, Potts DW, et al. Prevention of influenza A/USSR/77 (H1N1): an evaluation of the side effects and efficacy of amantadine in recruits at Fort Sam Houston. Milit Med. May, 1980;312–5.
188. Bryson YJ, Monahan C, Pollack M, et al. A prospective double-blind study of side effects associated with the administration of amantadine for influenza A virus prophylaxis. J Infect Dis. 1980;141:543–47.
189. Pettersson RF, Hellström P-E, Penttinen K, et al. Evaluation of amantadine in the prophylaxis of influenza A (H1N1) virus infection: a controlled field trial among young adults and high-risk patients. J Infect Dis. 1980;142:377–83.
190. Hayden FG, Hoffman HE, Spyker DA. Differences in side effects of amantadine hydrochloride and rimantadine hydrochloride relate to differences in pharmacokinetics. Antimicrob Agents Chemother. 1983;23:458–64.
191. Arden NH, Patriarca PA, Fasano MB, et al. The roles of vaccination and amantadine prophylaxis in controlling an outbreak of influenza A (H3N2) in a nursing home. Arch Intern Med. 1988;148:865–8.
192. Wilson TW, Rajput AH. Amantadine-dyazide interaction. Can Med Assoc J. 1983;129:974–5.
193. World Health Organization. Current status of amantadine and rimantadine as anti-influenza-A agents. Bull WHO. 1985;63:51–56.
194. Payler DK, Purdham PA. Influenza A prophylaxis with amantadine in a boarding school. Lancet. 1984;1:502–4.
195. Advisory Committee on Immunization Practices. Prevention and control of influenza. MMWR. 1988;37:361–73.
196. Van Voris LP, Betts RF, Hayden FG, et al. Successful treatment of naturally occurring influenza A/USSR/77 H1N1. JAMA. 1981;245:1128–31.
197. Younkin SW, Betts RF, Roth FK, et al. Reduction in fever and symptoms

in young adults with influenza A/Brazil/78 H1N1 infection after treatment with aspirin or amantadine. Antimicrob Agents Chemother. 1983;23:577–82.
198. Field AK, Davies ME, DeWitt C, et al. 9-[2-hydroxy-1-(hydroxymethyl)ethoxy]methyl guanine: A selective inhibitor of herpes group virus replication. Proc Natl Acad Sci USA. 1983;80:4139–43.
199. Smee DF, Martin JC, Verheyden JPH, Matthews TR. Antiherpesvirus activity of the acyclic nucleoside 9-(1,3-dihydroxy-2-propoxymethyl)guanine. Antimicrob Agents Chemother. 1983;23:676–82.
200. Mar E-C, Cheng Y-C, Huang E-S. Effect of 9-(1,3-dihydroxy-2-propoxymethyl)guanine on human cytomegalovirus replication in vitro. Antimicrob Agents Chemother. 1983;24:518–21.
201. Freitas VR, Smee DF, Chernow M, Boehme R, Matthews TR. Activity of 9-(1,3-dihydroxy-2-propoxymethyl)guanine compared with that of acyclovir against human, monkey, and rodent cytomegaloviruses. Antimicrob Agents Chemother. 1985;28:240–5.
202. Baba M, Konno K, Shigeta S, deClercq E. Inhibitory effects of selected antiviral compounds on newly isolated clinical varicella-zoster virus strains. Tohoku J Exp Med. 1986;148:275–83.
203. Plotkin SA, Drew WL, Felsenstein D, Hirsch MS. Sensitivity of clinical isolates of human cytomegalovirus to 9-(1,3-dihydroxy-2-propoxymethyl)guanine. J Infect Dis. 1985;152:833–4.
204. Shiota H, Naito T, Mimura Y. Anti-herpes simplex virus (HSV) effect of 9-(1,3-dihydroxy-2-propoxymethyl)guanine (DHPG) in rabbit cornea. Curr Eye Res. 1987;6:241–5.
205. Debs RJ, Montgomery AB, Brunette EN, deBruin M, Stanley JD. Aerososl administration of antiviral agents to treat lung infection due to murine cytomegalovirus. J Infect Dis. 1988;157:327–31.
206. Soike KF, Eppstein DA, Gloff CA, Cantrell C, Chou T-C, Gerone PJ. Effect of 9-(1,3-dihydroxy-2-propoxymethyl)-guanine and recombinant human beta interferon alone and in combination on simian varicella virus infection in monkeys. J Infect Dis. 1987;156:607–14.
207. Sommadossi J-P, Carlisle R. Toxicity of 3′-azido-3′-deoxythymidine and 9-(1,3-dihydroxy-2-propoxymethyl)guanine for normal human hematopoietic progenitor cells in vitro. Antimicrob Agents Chemother. 1987;31: 452–4.
208. Bowden RA, Digel J, Reed EC, Meyers JD. Immunosuppressive effects of ganciclovir on in vitro lymphocyte responses. J Infect Dis. 1987;156:899–903.
209. Biron KK, Stanat SC, Sorrell JB, et al. Metabolic activation of the nucleoside analog 9-[2-hydroxy-1-(hydroxy-methyl)ethoxy]methyl guanine in human diploid fibroblasts infected with human cytomegalovirus. Proc Natl Acad Sci USA. 1985;82:2473–7.
210. Smee DF, Boehme R, Chernow M, Binko B, Mathhews TR. Intracellular metabolism and enzymatic phosphorylation of 9-(1,3-dihydroxy-2-propoxymethyl)guanine and acyclovir in herpes simplex virus-infected and uninfected cells. Biochem Pharmacol. 1985;34:1049–56.
211. Frank KB, Chiou J-F, Cheng Y. Interaction of herpes simplex virus-induced DNA polymerase with 9-(1,3-dihydroxy-2-propoxymethyl)guanine triphosphate. J Biol Chem. 1984;259:1566–9.
212. St Clair MH, Miller WH, Miller RL, Lambe CU, Furman PA. Inhibition of cellular alpha DNA polymerase and herpes simplex virus-induced DNA polymerases by the triphosphate of BW759U. Antimicrob Agents Chemother. 1984;25:191–4.
213. Reid R, Mar E-C, Huang E-S, Topal MD. Insertion and extension of acyclic, dideoxy, and ara nucleotides by herpesviridae, human α and human β polymerases. J Biol Chem. 1988;263:3898–904.
214. Crumpacker CS, Kowalsky PN, Oliver SA, Schnipper LE, Field AK. Resistance of herpes simplex virus to 9-[2-hydroxy-1-(hydroxymethyl)ethoxy]methyl guanine: Physical mapping of drug synergism within the viral DNA polymerase locus. Proc Natl Acad Sci USA. 1984;81:1556–60.
215. Biron KK, Fyfe JA, Stanat SC, et al. A human cytomegalovirus mutant resistant to the nucleoside analog. 9-[(2-hydroxy-1-(hydroxymethyl)ethoxy)methyl]guanine (BW B759U), induces reduced levels of BW B759U-triphosphate. Proc Natl Acad Sci USA. 1986;83:8769–73.
216. Cole NL, Balfour HH Jr. In vitro susceptibility of cytomegalovirus isolates from immunocompromised patients to acyclovir and ganciclovir. Diagn Microbiol Infect Dis. 1987;6:255–61.
217. Shepp DH, Dandliker DH, deMiranda P, et al. Activity of 9-[(2-hydroxy-1-(hydroxymethyl)ethoxymethyl)]guanine in the treatment of cytomegalovirus pneumonia. Ann Intern Med. 1984;103:368–73.
218. Jacobson MA, deMiranda P, Cederberg DM, et al. Human pharmacokinetics and tolerance of oral ganciclovir. Antimicrob Agents Chemother. 1987;31:1251–4.
219. Laskin OL, Cederberg DM, Mills J, Eron LJ, Mildvan D, Spector SA. Canciclovir for the treatment and suppression of serious infections caused by cytomegalovirus. Am J Med. 1987;83:201–7.
220. Fletcher C, Sawchuk R, Chinnock B, deMiranda P, Balfour HH Jr. Human pharmacokinetics of the antiviral drug DHPG. Clin Pharmacol Ther. 1986;40:281–6.
221. Jabs DA, Newman C, deBustros S, Polk F. Treatment of cytomegalovirus retinitis with ganciclovir. Ophthalmology. 1987;94:824–30.
222. Jabs DA, Wingard JR, deBustros S, deMiranda, Saral R. BW B759U for cytomegalovirus retinitis: intraocular drug penetration. Arch Ophthalmol. 1986;104:1436–7.
223. Henry K, Cantrill H, Fletcher C, Chinnock BJ, Balfour HH Jr. Use of intravitreal ganciclovir (dihydroxy propoxy methyl guanine) for cytomegalovirus retinitis in a patient with AIDS. Am J Ophthamol. 1987;103:17–23.
224. Investigator's Monograph. Ganciclovir [9-(1,3-dihydroxy-2-propoxymethyl)guanine]. 5th ed. Palo Alto, CA: Syntex Inc., December, 1987.
225. Collaborative DHPG Treatment Study Group. Treatment of serious cytomegalovirus infections with 9-(1,3-dihydroxy-2-propoxymethyl)guanine in patients with AIDS and other immunodeficiencies. N Engl J Med. 1986;314:801–5.
226. Mills J. 9-(1,3-dihydroxy-2-propoxymethyl)guanine (DHPG) for treatment of cytomegalovirus infections. In: Mills J, Corey L, eds. Antiviral Chemotherapy: New Directions for Clinical Application and Research. New York: Elsevier; 1986:195–203.
227. Jacobson MA, Mills J. Serious cytomegalovirus disease in the acquired immunodeficiency syndrome (AIDS). Ann Intern Med. 1988;108:585–94.
228. Chachoua A, Dieterich D, Krasinski K, et al. 9-(1,3-2-propoxymethyl)guanine (ganciclovir) in the treatment of cytomegalovirus gastrointestinal disease with the acquired immunodeficiency syndrome. Ann Intern Med. 1987;107:133–7.
229. Fiala M, Cone LA, Cohen N, et al. Responses to neurologic complications of AIDS to 3′-azido-3′-deoxythymidine and 9-(1,3-dihydroxy-2-propoxymethyl) guanine. I. Clinical features. Rev Infect Dis. 1988;10:250–6.
230. Erice A, Jordan C, Chace BA, Fletcher C, Chinnock BJ, Balfour HH Jr. Ganciclovir treatment of cytomegalovirus disease in transplant recipients and other immunocompromised hosts. JAMA. 1987;257:3082–7.
231. Kotler DP, Culpepper-Morgan JA, Tierney AR, Klein EB. Treatment of disseminated cytomegalovirus infection with 9-(1,3 dihydroxy-2-propoxymethyl)guanine: evidence of prolonged survival in patients with the acquired immunodeficiency syndrome. AIDS Res. 1986;2:299–308.
232. Jacobson MA, DeMiranda P, Gordon SM, et al. Prolonged pancytopenia due to combined ganciclovir and zidovudine therapy. J Infect Dis. 1988;158:489–90.
233. Henderly DE, Freeman WR, Causey DM, Rao NA. Cytomegalovirus retinitis and response to therapy with ganciclovir. Ophthalmology. 1987;94:425–34.
234. Holland GN, Sidikaro Y, Kreiger AE, et al. Treatment of cytomegalovirus retinopathy with ganciclovir. Ophthalmology. 1987;94:815–23.
235. Orellana J, Teich SA, Friedman AH, Lerebours F, Winterkorn J, Mildvan D. Combined short- and long-term therapy for the treatment of cytomegalovirus retinitis using ganciclovir (BW B759U). Ophthalmology. 1987;94:831–8.
236. Freeman WR, Henderly DE, Wan WL, et al. Prevalence, pathophysiology, and treatment of rhegmatogenous retinal detachment in treated cytomegalovirus retinitis. Am J Ophthalmol. 1987;103:527–36.
237. Reed EC, Dandliker PS, Meyers JD. Treatment of cytomegalovirus pneumonia with 9-[2-hydroxy-1-(hydroxymethyl)ethoxymethyl]guanine and high-dose corticosteroids. Ann Intern Med. 1986;105:214–5.
238. Emanuel D, Cunningham I, Jules-Elysee K, et al. Cytomegalovirus pneumonia after bone marrow transplantation successfully treated with the combination of ganciclovir and high-dose intravenous immune globulin. Ann Intern Med. 1988;109:777–82.
239. Hecht DW, Snydman DR, Crumpacker CS, Werner BG, Heinze-Lacey B, the Boston Renal Transplant CVM Study Group. Ganciclovir for treatment of renal transplant-associated primary cytomegalovirus pneumonia. J Infect Dis. 1988;157:187–90.
240. Keay S, Bissett J, Merigan TC. Ganciclovir treatment of cytomegalovirus infections in iatrogenically immunocompromised patients. J Infect Dis. 1987;156:1016–21.
241. Pulido J, Peyman GA, Lesar T, Vernot J. Intravitreal toxicity to hydroxyacyclovir (BW-B759U), a new antiviral agent. Arch Ophthalmol. 1985;103:840–1.
242. Prusoff WH. Idoxuridine or how it all began. In: DeClercq E, ed. Clinical Use of Antiviral Drugs. Norwell: Martinus Nijhoff; 1988:15–24.
243. Silvestri DL, Corey L, Holmes KK. Ineffectiveness of topcial idoxuridine in dimethyl sulfoxide for therapy of genital herpes. JAMA. 1982;248:953–59.
244. Kaufman HE. The treatment of herpetic eye infections with trifluridine and other antivirals. In: DeClercq E, ed. Clinical Use of Antiviral Drugs. Norwell: Martinus Nijhoff; 1988:25–38.
245. Pavan-Langston DR. Ocular viral diseases. In: Galasso GJ, Merigan TC, Buchanan RA, eds. Antiviral Agents and Viral Diseases of Man. 2nd ed. New York: Raven Press; 1984:207–45.
246. Gilbert BE, Knight V. Minireview: biochemistry and clinical applications of ribavirin. Antimicrob Agents Chemother. 1986;30:201–5.
247. Hruska JF, Bernstein JM, Douglas RG Jr, et al. Effects of ribavirin on respiratory syncytial virus in vitro. Pharmacol Ther. 1980;6:770–75.
248. Browne MJ. Comparative inhibition of influenza and parainfluenza virus replication by ribavirin in MDCK cells. Antimicrob Agents Chemother. 1981;19:712–15.
249. McCormick JB, Mitchell SW, Getchell JP, Hicks DR. Ribavirin suppresses replication of lymphadenopathy-associated virus in cultures of human adult T lymphocytes. Lancet. 1984;2:1367–9.
250. Baba M, Pauwels R, Balzarini J, Herdewijn P, DeClercq E, Desmyter J. Ribavirin antagonizes inhibitory effects of pyrimidine 2′,3′-dideoxynucleosides but enhances inhibitory effects of purine 2′,3′-dideoxynucleosides on replication of human immunodeficiency virus in vitro. Antimicrob Agents Chemother. 1987;31:1613–7.
251. Stephen EL, Jones DE, Peters CJ, et al. Ribavirin treatment of toga-, arena-

and bunyavirus infections in subhuman primates and other laboratory animal species. In: Smith RE, Kirkpatric W, eds. Ribavirin: Broad Spectrum Antiviral Agent. New York: Academic Press; 1980:169.
252. Peavy DL, Koff WC, Hyman DS, et al. Inhibition of lymphocyte proliferative responses by ribavirin. Infect Immun. 1980;29:583–89.
253. Steele RW, Crosby DL, Steele RW, Pilkington NS Jr, Charlton RK. Effects of ribavirin on neutrophil function. Am J Med Sci. 1988;295:503–6.
254. Marquardt DL, Gruber HE, Walker LL. Ribavirin inhibits mast cell mediator release. J Pharmacol Exp Ther. 1987;240:145–9.
255. Hruska JF, Morrow PE, Suffin SC, et al. In vivo inhibition of respiratory syncytial virus by ribavirin. Antimicrob Agents Chemother. 1982;21:125–30.
256. Wyde PR, Wilson SZ, Patrella R, Gilbert BE. Efficacy of high dose-short duration ribavirin aerosol in the treatment of respiratory syncytial virus infected cotton rats and influenza B virus infected mice. Antiviral Res. 1987;7:211–20.
257. Jahrling PB, Hesse RA, Eddy GA, et al. Lassa virus infection of rhesus monkeys: pathogenesis and treatment with ribavirin. J Infect Dis. 1980;141:580–89.
258. Weissenbacher MC, Calello MA, Merani MS, McCormick JB, Rodriguez M. Therapeutic effect of the antiviral agent ribavirin in junin virus infection of primates. J Med Virol. 1986;20:261–7.
259. Kende M, Lupton HW, Rill WL, Levy HB, Canonico PG. Enhanced therapeutic efficacy of poly(ICLC) and ribavirin combinations against Rift Valley Fever virus infection in mice. Antimicrob Agents Chemother. 1987;31:986–90.
260. Gangemi JD, Nachtigal M, Barnhart D, Krech L, Jani P. Therapeutic efficacy of liposome-encapsulated ribavirin and muramyl tripeptide in experimental infection with influenza or herpes simplex virus. J Infect Dis. 1987;155:510–7.
261. Gruber WC, Wilson SZ, Throop BJ, Wyde PR. Immunoglobulin administration and ribavirin therapy: efficacy in respiratory syncytial virus infection of the cotton rat. Pediatr Res. 1987;21:270–4.
262. Smee DF, Mathews TR. Metabolism of ribavirin in respiratory syncytial virus-infected and uninfected cells. Antimicrob Agents Chemother. 1986;30:117–21.
263. Wray SK, Gilbert BE, Knight V. Effect of ribavirin triphosphate on primer generation and elongation during influenza virus transcription in vitro. Antiviral Res. 1985;5:39–48.
264. Peavy DL, Powers CN, Knight V. Inhibition of murine plaque-forming cell responses in vivo by ribavirin. J Immunol. 1981;126:861–64.
265. Scheidel LM, Durbin RK, Stollar V. Sindbis virus mutants resistant to mycophenolic acid and ribavirin. Virology. 1987;158:1–7.
266. Laskin OL, Longstreth JA, Hart CC, et al. Ribavirin disposition in high-risk patients for acquired immunodeficiency syndrome. Clin Pharmacol Ther. 1987;41:546–55.
267. Roberts RB, Laskin OL, Laurence J, et al. Ribavirin pharmacodynamics in high-risk patients for acquired immunodeficiency syndrome. Clin Pharmacol Ther. 1987;42:365–73.
268. Connor JD, Hintz M, Van Dyke R, McCormick JB, McIntosh K. Ribavirin pharmacokinetics in children and adults during therapeutic trials. In: Smith RA, Knight V, Smith JAD, eds. Clinical Applications of Ribavirin. Orlando: Academic Press; 1984:107–23.
269. Crumpacker C, Bubley G, Lucey D, Hussey S, Connor J. Ribavirin enters cerebrospinal fluid. Lancet. 1986;2:45–6.
270. Knight V, Yu CP, Gilbert BE, Divine GW. Estimating the dosage of ribavirin aerosol according to age and other variables. J Infect Dis. 1988;158:443–8.
271. Hillyared IW. The preclinical toxicology and safety of ribavirin. In: Smith RA, Kirkpatric W, eds. Ribavirin: A Broad Spectrum Antiviral Agent. New York: Academic Press; 1980:59.
272. Smith CB, Charette RP, Fox JP, et al. Lack of effect of oral ribavirin in naturally occurring influenza A virus (H1N1) infection. J Infect Dis. 1980;141:548–54.
273. Minkoff DI, Connor DJ. Clinical use of ribavirin and the treatment of herpes zoster in otherwise normal adults. In: Smith RA, Kirkpatric W, eds. Ribavirin: A Broad Spectrum Antiviral Agent. New York: Academic Press; 1980:185–99.
274. Light B, Aoki FY, Serrette C. Tolerance of ribavirin aerosol inhaled by normal volunteers and patients with asthma or chronic obstructive airway disease. In: Smith RA, Knight V, Smith JAD, eds. Clinical Applications of Ribavirin. New York: Academic Press; 1984:97–105.
275. Rodriguez WJ, Dang Bui RH, Connor JD, et al. Environmental exposure of primary care personnel to ribavirin aerosol when supervising treatment of infants with respiratory syncytial virus infections. Antimicrob Agents Chemother. 1987;31:1143–6.
275a. Harrison RJ, Bellows JD. Reproductive risk to health care workers administering ribavirin aerosol (Abstract). Intersci Conf Antimicrob Agents Chemother. 1988;no. 96:126.
276. Conrad DA, Christenson JC, Waner JL, Marks MI. Aerosolized ribavirin treatment of respiratory syncytial virus infection in infants hospitalized during an epidemic. Pediatr Infect Dis J. 1987;6:152–8.
277. Frankel LR, Wilson CW, Demers RR, et al. A technique for the administration of ribavirin to mechanically ventilated infants with severe respiratory syncytial virus infection. Crit Care Med. 1987;15:1051–4.
278. Outwater KM, Meissner C, Peterson MB. Ribavirin administration to infants receiving mechanical ventilation. Am J Dis Child. 1988;142:512–5.
279. Rodriguez WJ, Parrott RH. Ribavirin aerosol treatment of serious respiratory syncytial virus infection in infants. In: Moellering RC, ed. Infectious Disease Clinics of North America, Antiviral Chemotherapy. Philadelphia: WB Saunders; 1987:425–39.
280. American Academy of Pediatrics. Policy statement: ribavirin therapy of respiratory syncytial virus. AAP News. December, 1986.
281. Wald ER, Dashefsky B, Green M. In re ribavirin: a case of premature adjudication? J Pediatr. 1988;1:155–8.
282. McIntosh K. Chemotherapy of respiratory syncytial virus infections. In: Mills J, Corey L, eds. Antiviral Chemotherapy: New Directions for Clinical Application and Research. New York: Elsevier; 1986:83–8.
283. Rosner IK, Welliver RC, Edelson PJ, Geraci-Ciardullo K, Sun M. Effect of ribavirin therapy on respiratory syncytial virus-specific IgE and IgA responses after infection. J Infect Dis. 1987;155:1043–7.
284. Knight V, Gilbert BE. Ribavirin aerosol treatment of influenza. In: Moellering RC, ed. Infectious Disease Clinics of North America, Antiviral Chemotherapy. Philadelphia: WB Saunders; 1987;441–57.
285. Bernstein DI, Reuman PD, Sherwood JR, Young EC, Schiff GM. Ribavirin small-particle-aerosol treatment of influenza B virus infection. Antimicrob Agents Chemother. 1988;32:761–4.
286. Stein DS, Creticos CM, Jackson GG, et al. Oral ribavirin treatment of influenza A and B. Antimicrob Agents Chemother. 1987;31:1285–7.
287. McCormick JB, King IJ, Webb PA, et al. Lassa fever: effective therapy with ribavirin. N Engl J Med. 1986;314:20–6.
288. Canonico PG. Efficacy of ribavirin against viral hemorrhagic fevers and other exotic RNA viral infections. Programs and Abstracts of the International Symposium: Basic and Clinical Approaches to Virus Chemotherapy, June 19–22, 1988, Helsinki, Finland. Final Programme Antivirals 88, p. 68.
289. Enria DA, Briggiler AM, Levis S, Vallejos D, Maiztegui JI, Canonico PG. Preliminary report, tolerance and antiviral effect of ribavirin in patients with Argentine hemorrhagic fever. Antiviral Res. 1987;7:353–9.
290. Crumpacker C, Heagy W, Bubley G, et al. Ribavirin treatment of acquired immunodeficiency syndrome (AIDS) and the acquired-immunodeficiency-syndrome-related complex (ARC). Ann Intern Med. 1987;107:664–74.
291. Mansell PW, Haseltine PN, Roberts RB, Dickinson GM, Leeder JM. Ribavirin delays progression of lymphadenopathy syndrome (LAS) to the acquired immune deficiency syndrome (AIDS) (Abstract). In: Abstracts Volume: III International Conference on AIDS. Washington, DC: National Institutes of Health and the World Health Organization; 1987:58.
292. Palmieri G, Ambrosi G, Ferrano G, Agrati AM, Palazzini E. Clinical and immunological evaluation of oral ribavirin administration in recurrent herpes simplex infections. J Internat Med Res. 1987;15:264–75.
293. Patki SA, Gupta P. Evaluation of ribavirin in the treatment of acute hepatitis. Chemotherapy. 1982;28:298–303.
294. Bierman SM, Kirkpatric W, Fernandez H. Clinical efficacy of ribavirin in the treatment of genital herpes simplex virus infection. Chemotherapy. 1981;27:139–45.
295. Burlington DB, Meiklejohn G, Mostow SR. Anti-influenza A virus activity of amantadine hydrochloride and rimantadine hydrochloride in ferret tracheal ciliated epithelium. Antimicrob Agents Chemother. 1982;21:794–9.
296. Koff WC, Elm JL Jr, Halstead SB. Suppression of dengue virus replication in vitro by rimantadine hydrochloride. Am J Trop Med Hyg. 1981;30:184–9.
297. Zhirnov OP. High protection of animals lethally infected with influenza virus by aprotinin-rimantadine combination. J Med Virol. 1987;21:161–7.
298. Bukrinskaya AG, Vorkunova NK, Kornilayeva GV, Narmanbetova RA, Vorkunova GK. Influenza virus uncoating in infected cells and effect of rimantadine. J Gen Virol. 1982;60:49–59.
299. Bukrinskaya AG, Vorkunova NK, Pushkarskaya NL. Uncoating of a rimantadine-resistant variant of influenza virus in the presence of rimantadine. J Gen Virol. 1982;60:61–6.
300. Donath E, Herrmann A, Coakley WT, Groth T, Egger M, Teager M. The influence of the antiviral drugs amantadine and rimantadine on erythrocyte and platelet membranes and its comparison with that of tetracaine. Biochem Pharmacol. 1987;36:481–7.
301. Levin M. Experience with amantadine and rimantadine in children. J Respir Dis. 1987;8(Suppl 11A):S60–6.
302. Reele SB. Adverse drug experiences during rimantadine trials. J Respir Dis. 1987;8(Suppl 11A):S81–6.
303. Patriarca PA, Kater NA, Kendal AP, Bregman DJ, Smith JD, Sikes RK. Safety of prolonged administration of rimantadine hydrochloride in the prophylaxis of influenza A infections in nursing homes. Antimicrob Agents Chemother. 1984;26:101–3.
304. Wills RJ, Rodriguez LC, Choma N, Oakes M. Influence of a meal on the bioavailability of rimantadine HCl. J Clin Pharmacol. 1987;27:821–3.
305. Wills RJ, Choma N, Buonpane G, Lin A, Keigher N. Relative bioavailability of rimantadine HCl tablet and syrup formulations in healthy subjects. J Pharm Sci. 1987;76:886–8.
306. Wills RJ, Farolino DA, Choma N, Keigher N. Rimantadine pharmacokinetics after single and multiple doses. Antimicrob Agents Chemother. 1987;31:826–8.
307. Nahata MC, Brady MT. Serum concentrations and safety of rimantadine in paediatric patients. Eur J Clin Pharmacol. 1986;30:719–22.
308. Anderson EL, Van Voris LP, Bartram J, Hoffman HE, Belshe RB. Pharmacokinetics of a single dose of rimantadine in young adults and children. Antimicrob Agents Chemother. 1987;31:1140–2.
309. Tominack RL, Wills RJ, Gustavson LE, Hayden FG. Multiple-dose phar-

macokinetics of rimantadine in elderly adults. Antimicrob Agents Chemother. 1988;32:1813–19.
310. Capparelli EV, Stevens RC, Chow MSS, Izard M, Wills RJ. Rimantadine pharmacokinetics in healthy subjects and patients with end stage renal failure. Clin Pharmacol Ther. 1988;43:536–41.
311. Wills RJ, Belshe R, Tomlinsin D, et al. Pharmacokinetics of rimantadine hydrochloride in patients with chronic liver disease. Clin Pharmacol Ther. 1987;42:449–54.
312. Zlydnikov DM, Kubar OI, Kovaleva TP, et al. Study of rimantadine in the USSR: a review of the literature. Rev Infect Dis. 1981;3:408–21.
313. Clover RD, Crawford SA, Abell TD, Ramsey CN Jr, Glezen WP, Couch RB. Effectiveness of rimantadine prophylaxis of children within families. Am J Dis Child. 1986;140:706–9.
314. Betts RF, Treanor JJ, Graman PS, Bentley DW, Dolin R. Antiviral agents to prevent or treat influenza in the elderly. J Respir Dis. 1987;8(Suppl 11A):S56–9.
315. Hayden FG, Monto AS. Oral rimantadine hydrochloride therapy of influenza A virus H3N2 subtype infection in adults. Antimicrob Agents Chemother. 1986;29:339–41.
316. Hayden FG, Zylidnikov DM, Iljenko VI, et al. Comparative therapeutic effect of aerosolized and oral rimantadine HCl in experimental human influenza A virus infection. Antiviral Res. 1982;2:147–53.
317. Spector SA, Tyndall M, Kelly E. Inhibition of human cytomegalovirus by trifluorothymidine. Antimicrob Agents Chemother. 1983;23:113–18.
318. Van Bijsterveld OP, Post H. Trifluorothymidine versus adenine arabinoside in the treatment of herpes simplex keratitis. Br J Ophthalmol. 1980;64:33–6.
319. Field H, McMillan A, Darby G. The sensitivity of acyclovir-resistant mutants of herpes simplex virus to other antiviral drugs. J Infect Dis. 1981;143:281–4.
320. Gephart JF, Lerner AM. Comparison of the effects of arabinosyladenine, arabinosylhypoxanthine, and arabinosyladenine 5′-monophosphate against herpes simplex virus, varicella-zoster virus, and cytomegalovirus with their effects on cellular deoxyribonucleic acid synthesis. Antimicrob Agents Chemother. 1981;19:170–8.
321. Biron KK, Fyfe JA, Noblin JE, et al. Selection and primary characterization of acyclovir-resistant mutants of varicella zoster virus. Am J Med. 1982;73(Suppl):383–6.
322. Pelling JC, Drach JC, Shipman C, Jr. Internucleotide incorporation of arabinosyladenine into herpes simplex virus and mammalian cell dna. Virology. 1981;109:323–35.
323. Shannon WM, Westbrook L, Arrett G, et al. Comparison of the efficacy of vidarabine, its carbocyclic analog (cyclaradine), and cyclaradine-5′-methoxy-acetate in the treatment of herpes simplex type 1 encephalitis in mice. Antimicrob Agents Chemother. 1983;24:538–43.
324. Vince R, Dalarge S, Lee H, et al. Carbocyclic arabinofuranosyladenine (cyclaradine): efficacy against genital herpes in guinea pigs. Science. 1983;221:1405–6.
325. Sacks SL, Merigan TC, Kaminska J, et al. Inactivation of S-adenosylhomocysteine hydrolase during adenine arabinoside therapy. J Clin Invest. 1982;69:226–30.
326. Cantoni GL, Aksamit RR, Kim I-K. Methionine biosynthesis and vidarabine therapy. N Engl J Med. 1982;307:1079.
327. Hinrichs J, Kitz D, Kobayashi G, et al. Immune enhancement in mice by ARA-A. J Immunol. 1983;130:829–33.
328. Whitley R, Alford C, Hess F, et al. Vidarabine: a preliminary review of its pharmacological properties and therapeutic use. Drugs. 1980;20:267–82.
329. Buchanan RA, Kinkel AW, Alford CA Jr, et al. Plasma levels and urinary excretion of vidarabine after repeat dosing. Clin Pharmacol Ther. 1980;27:690–6.
330. Shope TC, Kauffman RE, Bowman D, et al. Pharmacokinetics of vidarabine in infants and children treated for herpes infection. J Infect Dis. 1983;148:721–25.
331. Aronoff GR, Szwed JJ, Nelson RL, et al. Hypoxanthine-arabinoside pharmacokinetics after adenine arabinoside administration to a patient with renal failure. Antimicrob Agents Chemother. 1980;18:212–4.
332. Friedman HM, Grasela T. Adenine arabinoside and allopurinol—possible adverse drug interaction. N Engl J Med. 1981;304:423.
333. Etta LV, Brown J, Mastri A, et al. Fatal vidarabine toxicity in a patient with normal renal function. JAMA. 1981;246:1703–5.
334. Marker SC, Howard RJ, Groth KE, et al. A trial of vidarabine for cytomegalovirus infection in renal transplant patients. Arch Intern Med. 1980;140:1441–4.
335. Feldman S, Robertson PK, Lott L, Thornton D. Neurotoxicity due to adenine arabinoside therapy during varicella-zoster virus infections in immunocompromised children. J Infect Dis. 1986;154:889–93.
336. Whitley RJ, Soong S-J, Hirsch MS, et al. Herpes simplex encephalitis, vidarabine therapy and diagnostic problems. N Engl J Med. 1981;304:313–8.
337. Whitley RJ, Yeager A, Kartus P, et al. Neonatal herpes simplex virus infection: follow-up evaluation of vidarabine therapy. Pediatrics. 1983;72:778–85.
338. Feder HM Jr. Disseminated herpes simplex infection in a neonate during prophylaxis with vidarabine. JAMA. 1988;259:1054–5.
339. Whitley RJ, Spruance S, Hayden F, et al. Vidarabine therapy of mucocutaneous herpes simplex virus infections in the immunocompromised host. J Infect Dis. 1984;149:1–8.
340. Whitley RJ, Soong S-J, Dolin R, et al. Early vidarabine therapy to control the complications of herpes zoster in immunosuppressed patients. N Engl J Med. 1982;307:971–5.
341. Whitley R, Hilty M, Haynes R, et al. Vidarabine therapy of varicella in immunosuppressed patients. J Pediatr. 1982;101:125–31.
342. Bassendine MF, Chadwick RG, Salmeron J, et al. Adenine arabinoside therapy in HBsAg-positive chronic liver disease: a controlled study. Gastroenterology. 1981;80:1016–22.
343. Weller IVD, Bassendine MF, Murray AK, et al. HBsAg-positive chronic liver disease: inhibition of viral replication by highly soluble adenine arabinoside 5′-monophosphate (ARA-AMP). Gastroenterology. 1980;79:1129.
344. Whitley RJ, Tucker BC, Kinkel AW, et al. Pharmacology, tolerance, and antiviral activity of vidarabine monophosphate in humans. Antimicrob Agents Chemother. 1980;18:709–15.
345. Preiksaitis JK, Lank B, Ng PK, et al. Effect of liver disease on pharmacokinetics and toxicity of 9-b-D-arabinofuranosyladenine-5′-phosphate. J Infect Dis. 1981;144:358–64.
346. Garcia G, Smith CI, Weissberg JI, et al. Adenine arabinoside monophosphate (vidarabine phosphate) in combination with human leukocyte interferon in the treatment of chronic hepatitis B. Ann Intern Med. 1987;107:278–85.
347. Hoofnagle JG, Hanson RG, Minuk GY, et al. Randomized controlled trial of adenine arabinoside monophosphate for chronic type B hepatitis. Gastroenterology. 1984;86:150–7.
348. Perrillo RP, Regenstein FG, Bodicky CJ, Campbell CR, Sanders GE, Sunwoo YC. Comparative efficacy of adenine arabinoside 5′ monophosphate and prednisone withdrawal followed by adenine arabinoside 5′ monophosphate in the treatment of chronic active hepatitis type B. Gastroenterology. 1985;88:780–6.
349. Yokosuka O, Omata M, Imazeki F, et al. Combination of short-term prednisolone and adenine arabinoside in the treatment of chronic hepatitis B. Gastroenterology. 1985;89:246–51.
350. Perrillo RP. Severe hepatic failure after ARA-A-prednisolone for chronic type B hepatitis (Reply to letter). Gastroenterology. 1987;274–5.
351. Fiume L, Bonino F, Mattioli A, et al. Inhibition of hepatitis B virus replication by vidarabine monophosphate conjugated with lactosaminated serum albumin. Lancet. 1988;2:13–15.
352. Mitsuya H, Weinhold KJ, Furman PA, et al. 3′-azido-3′-deoxythymidine (BW A509U): an antiviral agent that inhibits the infectivity and cytopathic effect of human T-lymphotropic virus type III/lymphadenopathy-associated virus in vitro. Proc Natl Acad Sci USA. 1985;82:7096–100.
353. Ruprecht RM, O'Brien LG, Rossoni LD, Nusinoff-Lehrman S. Suppression of mouse viraemia and retroviral disease by 3′-azido-3′-deoxythymidine. Nature. 1986;323:467–9.
354. Dahlberg JE, Mitsuya H, Balm SB, Broder S, Aaronson SA. Broad spectrum antiretroviral activity of 2′,3′-dideoxy-nucleosides. Proc Natl Acad Sci USA. 1987;84:2469–73.
355. Balzarini J, Pauwels R, Baba M, et al. The *in vitro* and *in vivo* anti-retrovirus activity, and intracellular metabolism of 3′-azido-2′,3′-dideoxythymidine and 2′,3′-dideoxycytidine are highly dependent on the cell species. Biochem Pharmacol. 1988;37:897–906.
356. Nakashima H, Matsui T, Harada S, et al. Inhibition of replication and cytopathic effect of human T cell lymphotropic virus type III/lymphadenopathy-associated virus by 3′-azido-3′-deoxythymidine in vitro. Antimicrob Agents Chemother. 1986;30:933–7.
357. Hartshorn KL, Vogt MW, Chou T-C, et al. Synergistic inhibition of human immunodeficiency virus in vitro by azidothymidine and recombinant alpha A interferon. Antimicrob Agents Chemother. 1987;31:168–72.
358. Vogt MW, Hartshorn KL, Furman PA, et al. Ribavirin antagonizes the effect of azidothymidine on HIV replication. Science. 1987;235:1276–9.
359. Mitchell WM, Montefiori DC, Robinson WE Jr, Strayer DR, Carter WA. Mismatched double-stranded RNA (ampligen) reduces concentration of zidovudine (azidothymidien) required for in-vitro inhibition of human immunodeficiency virus. Lancet. 1987;1:890–2.
360. Hammer SM, Gillis JM. Synergistic activity of granulocyte-macrophage colony-stimulating factor and 3′-azido-3′-deoxythymidine against human immunodeficiency virus in vitro. Antimicrob Agents Chemother. 1987;31:1046–50.
361. Richman DD. Dideoxynucleosides are less inhibitory in vitro against human immunodeficiency virus type 2 (HIV-2) than against HIV-1. Antimicrob Agents Chemother. 1987;31:1879–81.
362. Nakashima H, Tochikura T, Kobayashi N, Matsuda A, Ueda T, Yamamoto N. Effect of 3′-azido-2′,3′-dideoxythymidine (AZT) and neutralizing antibody on human immunodeficiency virus (HIV)-induced cytopathic effects: implication of giant cell formation for the spread of virus in vivo. Virology. 1987;159:169–73.
363. Smith MS, Brian EL, Pagano JS. Resumption of virus production after human immunodeficiency virus infection of T lymphocytes in the presence of azidothymidine. J Virol. 1987;61:3769–73.
364. Richman DD, Kornbluth RS, Carson DA. Failure of dideoxynucleosides to inhibit human immunodeficiency virus replication in cultured human macrophages. J Exp Med. 1987;166:1144–9.
365. Matsushita S, Mitsuya H, Reitz MS, Broder S. Pharmacological inhibition of in vitro infectivity of human T lymphotropic virus type 1. J Clin Invest. 1987;80:394–400.
366. Elwell LP, Ferone R, Freeman GA, et al. Antibacterial activity and mechanism of action of 3′-azido-3′-deoxythymidine (BW A5509U). Antimicrob Agents Chemother. 1987;31:274–80.

367. Hirsch MS. AIDS commentary—azidothymidine. J Infect Dis. 1988;157:427–31.
368. Sommadossi J-P, Carlisle R, Schinazi RJ, Zhou Z. Uridine reverses the toxicity of 3′-azido-3′-deoxythymidine in normal human granulocyte-macrophage progenitor cells in vitro without impairment of antiretroviral activity. Antimicrob Agents Chemother. 1988;32:997–1001.
369. Sharpe AH, Jaenisch R, Ruprecht RM. Retroviruses and mouse embryos: a rapid model for neurovirulence and transplacental antiviral therapy. Science. 1987;236:1671–4.
370. Tavares L, Roneker C, Johnston K, Nusinoff-Lehrman S, deNoronha F. 3′-azido-3′-deoxythymidine in feline leukemia virus-infected cats: a model for therapy and prophylaxis of AIDS. Cancer Res. 1987;4:3190–4.
371. Furman PA, Fyfe JA, St Clair MH, et al. Phosphorylation of 3′-azido-3′-deoxythymidine and selective interaction of the 5′-triphosphate with human immunodeficiency virus reverse transcriptase. Proc Natl Acad Sci USA. 1986;83:8333–7.
372. Yarchoan R, Broder S. Development of antiretroviral therapy for the acquired immunodeficiency syndrome and related disorders. N Engl J Med. 1987;316:557–64.
373. Larder BA, Darby G, Richman DD. HIV with reduced sensitivity to zidovudine (AZT) isolated during prolonged therapy. Science. 1989;243:1731–4.
374. Klecker RW Jr, Collins JM, Yarchoan R, et al. Plasma and cerebrospinal fluid pharmacokinetics of 3′-azido-3′-deoxythymidine: a novel pyrimidine analog with potential application for the treatment of patients with AIDS and related diseases. Clin Pharmacol Ther. 1987;41:407–12.
375. Henry K, Chinnock BJ, Quinn RP, Fletcher CV, deMiranda P, Balfour JJ Jr. Concurrent zidovudine levels in semen and serum determined by radioimmunoassay in patients with AIDS or AIDS-related complex. JAMA. 1988;259:3023–3026.
376. Surbone A, Yarchoan R, McAtee N, et al. Treatment of the acquired immunodeficiency syndrome (AIDS) and AIDS-related complex with a regimen of 3′-azido-2′,3′-dideoxythymidine (Azidothymidine or Zidovudine) and acyclovir. Ann Intern Med. 1988;108:534–40.
377. Pizzo PA, Eddy J, Falloon J, et al. Effect of continuous intravenous infusion of zidovudine (AZT) in children with symptomatic HIV infection. N Engl J Med. 1988;319:889–96.
378. Yarchoan R, Thomas RV, Grafman J, et al. Long-term administration of 3′-azido-2′,3′-dideoxythymidine to patients with AIDS-related neurological disease. Ann Neurol. 1988;23:S82–7.
379. Richman DD, Fischl MA, Grieco NH, et al. The toxicity of azidothymidine (AZT) in the treatment of patients with AIDS and AIDS-related complex. N Engl J Med. 1987;317:192–7.
380. Yarchoan R, Weinhold KJ, Lyerly HK, et al. Administration of 3′-azido-3′-deoxythymidine, an inhibitor of HTLV-III/LAV replication, to patients with AIDS or AIDS-related complex. Lancet. 1986;1:575–80.
381. Walker RE, Parker RI, Kovacs JA, et al. Anemia and erythropoiesis in patients with the acquired immunodeficiency syndrome (AIDS) and Kaposi sarcoma treated with zidovudine. Ann Intern Med. 1988;108:372–6.
382. Gill PS, Rarick M, Brynes RK, Causey D, Loureiro C, Levine AM. Azidothymidine associated with bone marrow failure in the acquired immunodeficiency syndrome (AIDS). Ann Intern Med. 1987;107:502–5.
383. Hagler DN, Frame PT. Azidothymidine neurotoxicity (Letter). Lancet. 1986;2:1392–3.
384. Davtyan DG, Vinters HV. Wernicke's encephalopathy in AIDS patient treated with zidovudine. Lancet. 1987;1:919–20.
385. Bessen LJ, Greene JB, Louie E, Seitzman P, Weinberg H. Severe polymyositis-like syndrome associated with zidovudine therapy of AIDS and ARC (Letter). N Engl J Med. 1988;318:708.
386. Furth PA, Kazakis AM. Nail pigmentation changes associated with azidothymidine (zidovudine). Ann Intern Med. 1987;107:350.
387. Pickus OB. Overdose of zidovudine. N Engl J Med. 1988;318:1206.
388. Fischl MA, Richman DD, Grieco MH, et al. The efficacy of azidothymidine (AZT) in the treatment of patients with AIDS and AIDS-related complex. N Engl J Med. 1987;317:185–91.
388a. Richman D, Andrews J, and the AZT Collaborative Working Group. Results of continued monitoring of participants in the placebo-controlled trial of zidovudine for serious human immunodeficiency virus infection. Am J Med. 1988;85(Suppl 2A):208–13.
389. Fiddian AP. Clinical experience with anti-HIV agents. Presented at the International Symposium: Basic and Clinical Approaches to Virus Chemotherapy, June 19–22, 1988, Helsinki, Finland. Final Program Antivirals 88, p. 65.
390. Schmitt FA, Bigley JW, McKinnis R, et al. Neuropsychological outcome of zidovudine (AZT) treatment of patients with AIDS and AIDS-related complex. N Engl J Med. 1988;319:1573–8.
391. de Wolf F, Goudsmit J, de Gans J, et al. Effect of zidovudine on serum human immunodeficiency virus antigen levels in symptom-free subjects. Lancet. 1988;1:373–6.
392. Jackson GG, Paul DA, Falk LA, et al. Human immunodeficiency virus (HIV) antigenemic (p24) in the acquired immunodeficiency syndrome (AIDS) and the effect of treatment with zidovudine (AZT). Ann Intern Med. 1988;108:175–80.
393. Dalakas MC, Yarchoan R, Spitzer R, Elder G, Sever JL. Treatment of human immunodeficiency virus-related polyneuropathy with 3′-azido-2′,3′-dideoxythymidine. Ann Neurol. 1988;23:S92–4.
394. Helbert M, Peddle B, Kocsis A, et al. Acute meningo-encephalitis on dose reduction of zidovudine. Lancet. 1988;1:1249–52.
395. Greisman SE, Johnston CA. The effect of azidothymidine on HIV-related thrombocytopenia. N Engl J Med. 1988;318:516–7.
396. Crowe S, Kirihara J, McGrath M, et al. Contrasting antiretroviral efficacy of zidovudine (AZT) and phosphonoformate (PFT) in HIV-infected macrophages. Fourth International Conference on AIDS, Stockholm, 1988, #3132.
397. Gaub J, Pederson C, Poulsen A-G, et al. The effect of focarnet (phosphonoformate) on human immunodeficiency virus isolation, T-cell subsets and lymphocyte function in AIDS patients. AIDS. 1987;1:27–33.
398. Öberg B, Behrnetz S, Eriksson B, et al. Clinical use of foscarnet (phosphonoformate). In: DeClercq E, ed. Clinical Use of Antiviral Drugs. Martinus Nijoff Publishing; 1988;223–40.
399. Walmsley SL, Chew E, Read SE, et al. Treatment of cytomegalovirus retinitis with trisodium phosphonoformate hexahydrate (foscarnet). J Infect Dis. 1988;157:569–572.
400. Jacobson MA, Crowe S, Levy J, et al. Effect of foscarnet therapy on infection with human immunodeficiency virus in patients with AIDS. J Infect Dis. 1988;158:862–5.
401. Singer DRJ, Fallon TJ, Schulenburg WE, et al. Foscarnet for cytomegalovirus retinitis (Letter). Ann Intern Med. 1985;103:962.
402. Bloom JN, Palestine AG. The diagnosis of cytomegalovirus retinitis. Ann Intern Med. 1988;109:963–9.
403. Farthing CF, Dalgleish AG, Clark A, et al. Phosphonoformate (foscarnet): a pilot study in AIDS and AIDS related complex. AIDS. 1987;1:21–25.
404. Bergdahl S, Sonnerborg A, Larsson A, Strannegard O. Declining levels of HIV p24 antigen in serum during treatment with foscarnet (Letter). Lancet. 1988;1:1052.
405. Chatis PA, Miller CH, Schrager LE, et al. Successful treatment with foscarnet of an acyclovir-resistant mucocutaneous infection with herpes simplex virus in a patient with acquired immunodeficiency syndrome. N Engl J Med. 1989;320:297–300.
406. Lawee D, Rosenthal D, Aoki FY, et al. Efficacy and safety of foscarnet for recurrent orolabial herpes: a multicenter randomized double-blind study. CMAJ. 1988;138:329–33.
407. Merigan TC, Skowron G, Bozzette SA, et al. Circulating p24 antigen levels and response to dideoxycytidine in human immunodeficiency virus (HIV) infections: a phase I and II study. Ann Intern Med. 1989;110:189–94.
408. Abrams DI, Kuno S, Wong R, et al. Oral dextran sulfate (UA001) in the treatment of the acquired immunodeficiency syndrome (AIDS) and AIDS-related complex. Ann Intern Med. 1989;110:183–8.
409. Clumeck N, Hermans P. Antiviral drugs other that zidovudine and immunomodulating therapies in human immunodeficiency virus infection. Am J Med. 1988;85(Suppl 2A):165–72.
410. Öberg B. Antiviral therapy. J Acq Imm Def Syn. 1988;1:257–66.

35. INTERFERONS

FREDERICK G. HAYDEN

Since their discovery in 1957 as mediators of the phenomenon of viral interference, that is, inhibition of the growth of one virus by another, interferons (IFNs) have become recognized as potent cytokines that are associated with complex antiviral, immunomodulating, and antiproliferative actions.[1] Interferons can be broadly defined as proteins or glycoproteins that are synthesized by host cells in response to various inducers and that in turn cause biochemical changes leading to a nonselective antiviral state in exposed cells of the same species. Production of IFN requires both de novo RNA and protein synthesis. Inducers include viruses, particularly double-stranded RNA viruses; various organisms capable of intracellular growth; bacterial endotoxins; polyanions; and certain low-molecular-weight organic compounds. Interferon activity is usually measured in terms of antiviral effects in cell culture. Typically, 1 unit of IFN activity is the amount present in a sample dilution that causes a 50 percent reduction in virus replication or expression in certain cell lines and is generally expressed as international units (IU) relative to National Institutes of Health (NIH) or World Health Organization (WHO) reference standards.

Early investigations of the possible clinical usefulness of IFNs were largely dependent on the use of inducers and limited quantities of human leukocyte IFN. Since the early 1980s, the availability of purified IFNs produced by recombinant DNA technology has allowed extensive study of these proteins in viral infections, malignancies, and certain other disorders. Parenteral IFN is currently approved for use in hairy cell leukemia, selected patients with Kaposi sarcoma, and intralesionally in refractory condyloma acuminata.

CLASSIFICATION

Formally designated on the basis of the cell types from which they were derived, three major classes of human IFNs are currently recognized (Table 1). Each type is immunologically distinct and has a fixed pattern of species specificity in addition to differing physiochemical characteristics.[1,3] Interferon-α and -β may be produced by nearly all cells in response to viral infection, whereas IFN-γ is restricted to T lymphocytes responding to mitogens or antigenic stimuli. The principal antiviral interferons, IFN-α and -β, are approximately 30 percent homologous at the amino acid level, whereas IFN-γ shares less than 20 percent homology. Human IFN-α actually comprises a family of over two dozen species that share a high degree of amino acid sequence homology (>50 percent) but have differing in vitro antiproliferative and antiviral effects on human cells. Human leukocyte- or lymphoblastoid-derived IFN preparations contain at least 18 distinct subtypes of IFN-α, as well as small amounts of IFN-β. Recombinant IFNs in clinical testing are over 95 percent pure and have very high specific activities (1 to 4 $\times$ 10^8 IU/mg protein).

Interferon-γ has a different spectrum of antiviral and immunomodulating properties from the other IFNs, with which it shows synergistic antiviral effects in certain test systems.[5,6] Interferon-γ is a potent macrophage-activating factor, and consequently, it is being evaluated in human infections associated with cellular parasites and/or defective macrophage function, including lepromatous leprosy[7] and human immunodeficiency virus (HIV) infection[8] (see Chapter 8). It also activates polymorphonuclear leukocytes (see Chapter 7).

MECHANISMS OF ACTION

Antiviral Effects

A wide range of different RNA and DNA animal viruses are sensitive to the antiviral actions of IFNs, although considerable differences exist for different viruses and assay systems.[4,9] Synergistic antiviral effects have been seen with combinations of IFN-γ and IFN-α or -β. Also, IFNs exhibit additive or synergistic antiviral activity with various synthetic antivirals against herpes, influenza, picorna-, retro-, and arboviruses under laboratory conditions.[6]

Interferons are not directly antiviral but cause biochemical changes in exposed cells that lead to viral resistance. The initial step involves IFN binding to specific cell surface receptors, which are shared between IFN-α and -β, but are different for IFN-γ.[1] The onset of IFN antiviral action is rapid, and alterations in cellular mRNA occur within minutes. Depending on the virus and cell type, IFN's antiviral effects are mediated through the inhibition of viral penetration or uncoating (e.g., papovaviruses), synthesis or methylation of messenger RNA, translation of viral proteins, or viral assembly and release (e.g., retroviruses).[9] For most viruses the principal replicative step inhibited by IFN is viral protein synthesis. After IFN exposure, cells produce a series of proteins, usually including a unique 2′,5′-oligoadenylate synthetase and a protein kinase, either of which can inhibit protein synthesis in the presence of double-stranded RNA. The 2′,5′-oligoadenylate synthetase produces adenylate oligomers that activate a latent cellular endoribonuclease (RNase L) in the presence of double-stranded RNA to cleave both cellular and viral RNAs. The protein kinase selectively phosphorylates two proteins involved in protein synthesis, eukaryotic initiation factor 2 (eIF-2) and a ribosome-associated one called P_1. Interferon may also block mRNA capping by inhibiting transmethylation reactions. Interferon induction of a phosphodiesterase, which cleaves a portion of transfer RNA and thus prevents peptide elongation, also contributes to the inhibition of protein synthesis. However, except possibly for the Mx protein in influenza virus infections, no consistent correlations exist between induction of a particular enzyme or protein and resistance to specific viruses across a range of cell types.[1,4,9] The specific effects important in inhibiting a particular virus are likely to be different for the different groups of viruses. Interferon exposure may also reduce the expression of certain cellular genes, including selected oncogenes and those involved in collagen synthesis.

The assay of IFN in clinical specimens has received study as a means of viral diagnosis.[10] Similarly, elevated levels of 2′,5′-oligoadenylate synthetase activity in peripheral white blood cells have been used for a marker for IFN exposure or endogenous release in different conditions.

TABLE 1. Nomenclature and Classification of Human Interferons

Characteristics	Class α	β	γ
Former designations	Type I, leukocyte	Type I, fibroblast	Type II, immune
No. species	>24	1[a]	1
No. amino acids	165–166	166	143
Apparent MW[b]	16,000–27,000	20,000	15,500–25,000
Disulphide bonds	2	1	0
Glycosylation	Variable[c]	Yes	Yes
Acid stability (pH 2)	Yes[d]	Yes	No
Chromosome coding for IFN[e]	9	9	12

[a] Interferon-β_2 (designated interleukin-6) has negligible antiviral effects and functions primarily as a β-cell differentiation factor (BSF-2). It has minimal sequence homology with classic IFN-β and is encoded by a different chromosome.[2] Its classifiction as an IFN is unsettled.
[b] The molecular weight (MW) range relates to post-translation modifications including the formation of dimers, glycosylation, and protein binding. The MW of nonglycosylated recombinant IFN-$\alpha_2$is approximately 19,500.
[c] Generally not, but several species are glycosylated.
[d] Acid-labile IFN-α occur in certain pathologic states.
[e] The action of IFNs are mediated through chromosome 21, which encodes a glycoprotein receptor for IFN-α and -β. The IFN-γ receptor is encoded on human chromosome 6.
(Data from Zoon[3] and Greenberg.[4])

Non-antiviral Actions

The non-antiviral effects of IFN include inhibiting delayed-type hypersensitivity responses and lymphocyte blastogenesis and prolonging survival of allogeneic grafts, enhancing (low concentration) or suppressing (high concentration) antibody formation, increasing natural killer cell activity and antibody-dependent cellular cytotoxicity, enhancing phagocytic and cytolytic activity of macrophages, inhibiting macrophage migration, increasing the expression of major histocompatibility (MHC) antigens on cell surfaces, inhibiting the growth of intracellular parasites, augmenting IgE-mediated histamine release, increasing the expression of Fc receptors on lymphocytes and accessory cells, interfering with the attachment of hormones and certain toxins to ganglioside receptors on the cell membrane, priming for (low concentration) or inhibiting (high concentration) IFN production; inhibiting the growth of rapidly dividing cells; and enhancing (low concentration) or inhibiting the differentiation (high concentration) of cells.[1,3,5]

Interferon-γ generally has more potent immunoregulatory effects than IFN-α or -β does, particularly with respect to macrophage function, expression of class II MHC antigens, and mediation of local inflammatory responses.[11] Interferon-γ is also approximately 1000-fold more active than IFN-α is in inhibiting the hepatic schizogony of *Plasmodium falciparum* in human hepatocyte cultures[12] (see Chapter 8).

The pleomorphic effects of IFN on immune functions suggests that immunoregulation may be one of its major functions in the host. Complex interactions exist between IFNs and other parts of the immune system. For example, IFN-γ enhances the expression of interleukin-2 (IL-2) receptors on T lymphocytes, and IL-2 appears to modulate IFN-γ production, probably through effects on cellular cyclic guanosine monophosphate (cGMP) levels. The induction of cytotoxic T-lymphocyte responses appears to require both IL-2 and IFN-γ. Interferon-α is both produced by macrophages and can modify macrophage functions by increasing phagocytosis and cytolytic activity. The antiviral action of tumor necrosis factor appears to be mediated by IFN-β.[2]

Role in Viral Infections

Interferons may ameliorate viral infections by exerting antiviral effects and by modifying the immune response to infection. For example, IFN-induced expression of MHC antigens may contribute to the antiviral actions of IFN by enhancing the lytic effects of cytotoxic T lymphocytes. Many observations suggest that IFN titers generally appear at the sites of viral replication at the time of or just after peak titers of virus and before humoral antibody responses. High IFN titers are usually followed by a reduction in virus titer, although persistently elevated IFN titers have been recognized in certain chronic and acute (e.g., hemorrhagic fevers) viral infections. Interferon and its inducers are effective in preventing a variety of viral infections when administered before virus exposure. In animal models, the severity of viral infections is increased by administering antisera to species-specific IFN. In humans, the lack of endogenous IFN responses has been observed in severe viral infections including herpes zoster in immunocompromised hosts, fatal influenza viral pneumonia, chronic hepatitis B virus (HBV) infection, and in HIV infection complicated by opportunistic infections.

In contrast to resolution of viral infection, IFN production may be involved in immunologically mediated tissue damage in various viral diseases.[13] Interferon elaboration has been associated with disease in lymphocytic choriomeningitis virus infection of newborn mice and visna virus infection of sheep. Unusual acid-labile IFN-α has been observed in patients with certain autoimmune disorders and the acquired immunodeficiency syndrome (AIDS), where its presence appears to predict disease progression.[8] In more general terms, IFNs may mediate some of the systemic symptoms associated with viral infections.

HUMAN PHARMACOKINETICS

The pharmacokinetics of IFN are not well characterized. These molecules appear to behave like other small circulating plasma proteins such that after systemic administration low levels of IFN are detected in respiratory secretions, cerebrospinal fluid, eye, and brain.[4] Interferon-α is relatively stable in most body fluids, whereas IFN-β and -γ appear to readily lose activity. However, it is unknown whether measurable IFN levels at a particular site accurately reflect its antiviral or other biologic activities.

Oral administration does not result in detectable serum levels and is not used clinically. After the intramuscular or subcutaneous injection of IFN-α, plasma levels are dose related, peak at 4–8 hours, and return to baseline by 18–36 hours. Accumulation occurs with repetitive dosing. In contrast, intramuscular or subcutaneous injections of IFN-β or -γ results in negligible plasma levels, although increases in peripheral blood leukocyte 2′,5′-oligoadenylate synthetase levels may occur. Peak serum levels average 400–500 units/ml after intramuscular IFN-α doses of approximately 18×10^6 units.

Levels of 2′,5′-oligoadenylate synthetase have been considered to be an index of biologic responsiveness to IFN. After a single intramuscular injection (18×10^6 units of IFN-α), peripheral blood mononuclear cells show increases in their 2′-5′-oligoadenylate synthetase activity beginning at 6 hours and lasting through 4 days and an antiviral state in the same cells starting at 1 hour, peaking at 24 hours, and slowly decreasing to baseline by 6 days after injection.[14] Thus the biologic effects of IFN last days longer than do detectable serum levels. Similarly, after intranasal administration, an antiviral effect lasts at least 18 hours in exposed respiratory mucosa.

After intravenous dosing, both IFN-α and -β are cleared rapidly in a biphasic fashion. Leukocyte and recombinant IFN-α species have an elimination half-life ($T_{1/2}$) of approximately 2 hours in the circulation. The clearance of IFN includes inactivation by various body fluids and metabolism by different organs, primarily the kidney and to some extent the liver, heart and skeletal muscle, and lung. The rate of IFN clearance is less than 2 percent of the glomerular infiltration rate, and negligible biologically active IFN is excreted in the urine.

TOXICITY

Both purified natural and recombinant IFNs are associated with dose-related toxicities that limit their clinical use. With systemic administration, an influenza-like syndrome consisting of fever, chills, headache, myalgia, and occasionally nausea, vomiting, or diarrhea is expected within several hours after initiating doses of 10^4–10^5 units/kg. A systemic dose of approximately 1×10^6 IU/day is generally well tolerated by most patients. Temperatures may range over 40°C, but the fever usually resolves within 12 hours after intramuscular administration.

Up to one-half of patients receiving intralesional therapy for genital warts experience the flulike illness, although symptoms usually decrease during the first week of therapy. The febrile responses are mediated through the production of hypothalamic prostaglandins[15] and can be moderated by pretreatment with various antipyretics.

Major toxicities that limit parenteral therapy are bone marrow suppression with granulocytopenia and thrombocytopenia; neurotoxicity manifested by somnolence, confusion, behavioral disturbance, electroencephalogram (EEG) changes, and rarely seizures[16]; reversible neurasthenia with profound fatigue and anorexia, weight loss, and myalgia during long-term use; and possibly cardiotoxicity with hypotension, arrhythmias, and congestive cardiomyopathy. Leukopenia tends to be most marked by the second week of therapy. Elevations in hepatic enzyme and triglyceride levels are common, and renal insufficiency may occur. Interferon prophylaxis has been associated with severe leukoencephalopathy in bone marrow transplant recipients[17] and with acute steroid-resistant rejection and nephrotic syndrome in kidney transplant recipients. Interferon and its inducers reduce the metabolism of various drugs by the hepatic cytochrome P-450–dependent mixed-function oxidase system and significantly increase plasma half-lives and levels of drugs like theophylline.[18] The development of serum neutralizing antibodies to exogenous IFNs varies with the IFN type, dose, and route of administration but may be associated with a loss of clinical responsiveness.[19,20] Antibodies directed against recombinant IFN-α may or may not cross react with natural IFN-α or other recombinant species, and patients with neutralizing antibodies against recombinant IFN-α subtypes may respond to natural IFN-α.

Local reactions consisting of tenderness and erythema occur after subcutaneous injection. Intranasal administration avoids systemic side effects but is associated with mucosal friability and ulceration and complaints of nasal dryness, stuffiness, and bleeding in up to 50 percent of recipients, depending on the dose and duration of administration.[21] Clinical irritation is preceded by marked histopathologic changes consisting of infiltration by lymphocytic cells in the nasal submucosa.

Interferon is an abortifacient in monkeys at high doses, and its safety during pregnancy is not established.

CLINICAL STUDIES

Extensive clinical testing has been done with various IFN formulations and routes of administration to assess IFN's possible value in the treatment and prevention of viral infections.[4,22] Clinical use of IFNs has been limited by its relative lack of potency, dose-limiting side effects, and the availability of competing antiviral agents. Although various trials have established that IFN is clearly superior to placebo in certain situations (Table 2), convincing clinical benefit has been demonstrated in very few viral diseases. Therapeutic use has generally been limited to the treatment of select chronic viral infections or acute ones associated with the failure of endogenous IFN responses.

Herpes Viruses

Several controlled studies have documented some clinical and virologic efficacy with IFN in the prevention or treatment of herpesvirus infections (Table 2). Although some trials have reported beneficial effects, no consistent reductions in symptoms and lesion duration have been observed with topical or parenteral IFN treatment of recurrent or initial genital herpes.[4,22–25] In such studies, parenteral IFN has been frequently associated with febrile responses and often with reversible neutropenia. The magnitude of the clinical benefit when used for the treatment or suppression of recurrent genital herpes is less than that seen with oral acyclovir.[23] In localized herpes zoster of cancer patients, early treatment with high-dose (approximately 36 × 10^6 units/day for 5–7 days) intramuscular leukocyte-derived IFN reduces progression of the primary dermatome, the risk of cutaneous or visceral dissemination, and the severity of post-herpetic neuralgia.[22] Lower doses or shorter durations of therapy are less effective. A 69 percent lower rate of cutaneous dissemination of localized zoster was found in cancer patients treated with recombinant IFN-α 36 MU/day for 7 days, as compared with placebo, but side effects were common in IFN recipients.[26] Parenteral IFN-α is also effective in reducing the risk of visceral dissemination in varicella of immunocompromised children, but alternative treatments, acyclovir and vidarabine, are available. In cytomegalovirus (CMV) infections, long-term administration reduces the risk of CMV disease in seropositive renal allograft recipients, but systemic IFN is not effective in preventing CMV infection or improving survival in bone marrow recipients when begun after marrow allografting.[17] Interferon is also ineffective in treating established CMV infections.[22]

In superficial herpes simplex virus (HSV) keratitis, the combined administration of topical IFN-α with trifluridine or acyclovir appears to be more effective than single-agent therapy is.[4]

TABLE 2. Viral Infections in which Interferons Have Efficacy

Systemic administration
Chronic hepatitis B
Chronic non-A, non-B hepatitis
Suppression of CMV infections (renal transplantation)
Herpes zoster in immunocompromised hosts
Varicella in immunocompromised hosts
Prevention of orofacial HSV after trigeminal surgery
Condyloma acuminatum
Juvenile laryngeal papillomatosis
Intralesional
Condyloma acuminata, verucca vulgaris
Topical application
Herpes simplex keratoconjunctivitis
Prevention of rhinovirus colds

Hepatitis

Chronic hepatitis B virus (HBV) infections have also shown responsiveness to parenterally administered leukocyte and recombinant IFN-α.[27–29] In addition to acute reductions in serum HBV DNA concentrations and Dane particle markers, interferon administration on a long-term basis (up to 6 months) is associated with the permanent loss of DNA polymerase activity in the serum with or without the loss of hepatitis B surface antigen (HBsAg) in up to one-third of patients. DNA polymerase activity declines to 15–35 percent of pretreatment values within 48 hours of initiating therapy with intramuscular IFN (3–20 × 10^6 units/day). One trial employing 6 months' treatment with lymphoblastoid IFN-α found a 26 percent seroconversion rate to antibody to hepatitis B e antigen (HBeAg) that was associated with a hepatitis-like illness in the third month of therapy and later with clearance of HBsAg.[27] Clearance of serum HBeAg is often associated with symptomatic improvement and normalization of aminotransferase levels. Another study using recombinant IFN-α (2.5–10 × 10^6 units/m^2 intramuscularly three times per week) for 3–6 months found that 70 percent of Chinese patients had undetectable serum HBV DNA levels at the end of therapy but that 47 percent experienced reactivation of HBV infection and only 15 percent had sustained clearance of HBeAg 12 months after the end of therapy.[29] Female patients appear to be more responsive than males are, and Caucasian carriers more responsive than Chinese, most of whom are infected from birth.[29,29a] Concurrent steroid administration or HIV infection are associated with reduced response rates. The combined results of various trials indicate that relatively low doses of parenteral IFN (2.5–5 × 10^6 units/day) are as effective as higher doses in inhibiting HBV replication and are better tolerated, that prolonged administration (2–4 months) is needed to increase the likelihood of a lasting response, but that overall rates of seroconversion from HBeAg to anti-HBe are below 50 percent with single-agent IFN therapy.[27,29a] Optimal dose schedules and possible effects on long-term sequelae remain under study.

Despite evidence indicating short-term enhancement of antiviral effects by combinations of systemic IFN-α with vidarabine, acyclovir, or corticosteroid pretreatment, no dual therapies have yet emerged that provide greater long-term benefit or reductions in toxicity compared with IFN above.[29a,29b] The combination of vidarabine monophosphate and interferons has been disappointing.[30] Suppression of DNA polymerase activity has also been observed with recombinant IFN-β–serine (IFN-β_{ser}) during short-term use, but the addition of IFN-γ to IFN-β_{ser} did not improve responsiveness and may have been associated with additive toxicity in one short-term study.[31] A recent trial found that a 6-week tapered regimen of prednisone followed by 90 days' treatment with subcutaneous recombinant IFN-α (5 × 10^6 IU/day) was associated with clearing of HBV DNA markers and the normalization of aminotransferase values in 50 percent and the disappearance of HBsAg in 22 percent of treated subjects.[32]

Long-term, low-dose IFN-α therapy may be effective in reducing serum aminotransferase levels and improving hepatic histology in some patients with chronic non-A, non-B hepatitis.[33] Sustained biochemical and some hepatic histologic improvements have been observed in some patients with chronic non-A, non-B hepatitis treated with recombinant IFN-α at doses as low as 1 × 10^6 IU three times per week.[33] Controlled trials are in progress.

Papillomavirus

Responses in condylomata acuminata have been observed with various IFN preparations administered topically, intralesionally, and parenterally.[4,34] Intralesional IFN has been demonstrated to be a clinically useful intervention in refractory condylomata acuminata.[34–38] In one trial employing recombinant IFN-α_2 (1 × 10^6 IU per lesion three times weekly for 3 weeks), complete resolution of injected warts occurred in 36 percent of patients by 13 weeks follow-up, but no effects on untreated lesions were observed.[35] In a study of purified leukocyte-derived IFN-α (2.5–5.5 × 10^5 IU/25 mm^2 of lesion twice weekly for 8 weeks), complete responses occurred in 62 percent of patients.[38] Response rates are two- to threefold higher than those observed in placebo recipients, and further complete responses occur with a second course of therapy. No differences in response rates have been found in lymphoblastoid IFN-α, recombinant IFN-α, and fibroblast-derived IFN-β.[37] Responding lesions generally show involution within 4 weeks and maximal decreases at 4–12 weeks after initiating therapy. Intralesional therapy does not benefit uninjected warts and may miss asymptomatic areas of infection, but complete responders appear to have relatively low relapse rates (21–33 percent) during short-term follow-up. Efficacy has been demonstrated in patients previously failing conventional therapies, but responsiveness is poor in HIV-infected patients.[35] Mild to moderate systemic side effects (8–10 percent dropout rate), discomfort at the injection site, and leukopenia (up to 30 percent) are common with intralesional IFN. Thus, intralesional therapy for discreet lesions appears to be effective and reasonably tolerated, although the cost-effectiveness of this intervention relative to ablative therapies like cryosurgery has not been determined.

In extensive disease, intramuscular or subcutaneous administration has been advocated but may be associated with greater toxicity than is observed with intralesional dosing,[34,39,40] Parenteral doses of 1 × 10^6 IU/mm^2/day for 14 days followed by three doses per week for 1 monthe are well tolerated but associated with complete resolution of lesions in a minority of patients.[40a] Intramuscular recombinant IFN-γ is also associated with therapeutic activity in refractory genital papillomavirus infections, including those involving the cervix.[41] Multimodality treatments involving systemic IFN have not yet documented greater response rates than with topical podophyllin or with laser therapy used above.[40a] Interferon use should be currently reserved for patients with recalcitrant disease, those who have repeatedly failed conventional therapy, or those who have such extensive involvement that conventional therapy is impractical.[39] The possible usefulness of IFN in managing human papillomavirus (HPV)-induced cervical dysplasia has not been critically evaluated, but one trial employing an IFN gel was unsuccessful.[42]

Plantar warts appear to be substantially less responsive to intramuscular recombinant IFN-α than are genital warts.[36] Limited evidence suggests that verruca vulgaris may respond to intralesional IFN-α.[43] Responses to intralesional and systemic IFN have also been observed in the rare HPV-related condition of epidermodysplasia verruciformis.[34]

In juvenile laryngeal papillomatosis (JLP), most of the children have some initial decrease in lesions in response to systemic IFN.[4,34] However, HPV DNA persists despite lesion regression such that recurrence rates are high after the cessation of therapy. The long-term response to parenteral IFN-α in recurrent JLP is quite variable.[44] One recent trial employing intramuscular leukocyte-derived IFN, 2 MU/m^2 three times per week for 12 months, found significant reductions in papilloma growth rates during the first 6 months and in the need for urgent surgical procedures but no long-term benefits when compared with laser therapy alone.[45] Adult-onset laryngeal disease appears to be more responsive than that in children. Optimal dose schedules have not been determined in laryngeal papillomatosis, and multicenter controlled trials in conjunction with carbon dioxide laser therapy are in progress.

Respiratory Viruses

Except for adenovirus, IFN has broad-spectrum antiviral activity against respiratory viruses in vitro. In experimentally induced infections in humans, the intranasal administration of leukocyte or recombinant IFN-α has been found to be protective against rhinovirus, coronavirus, and to a lesser extent influenza virus infections.[21] However, during long-term daily use under natural conditions, prophylactic intranasal IFN-α is protective only against rhinovirus colds, and chronic use is limited by the occurrence of local nasal side effects. Studies to date have failed to determine an IFN type and dosage that is both protective against rhinovirus infections and well tolerated during long-term use. When used for postcontact prophylaxis in the family setting, intranasal recombinant IFN-α_2 (5 × 10^6 units once daily for 7 days) is associated with approximately 40 percent reductions in secondary respiratory illnesses and nearly 90 percent protection against rhinovirus colds during the period of use.[46,47] However, protection against other respiratory viral infections has not been observed in such studies, and intranasal IFN-α_2 is therapeutically ineffective in established rhinovirus colds.[48]

Human Immunodeficiency Virus

The interaction of the IFN system with HIV infection is complex, and it is currently difficult to predict the clinical usefulness of exogenous IFNs. Unusual IFN species and IFN inactivators are frequently present in the sera of AIDS patients.[49] Interferons have dose-related inhibitory activity against HIV in T-lymphocyte cultures.[8] High doses of IFN-α induce 10–50 percent response rates in Kaposi sarcoma patients without benefiting concurrent herpesvirus infections or immune function.[8,50] Recent open trials of prolonged IFN-α_2 therapy (up to 36 × 10^6 IU/day) have found that responding KS patients have higher pretreatment T4 lymphocyte counts and may experience T4 count increases, falls in p24 antigen levels, and fewer opportunistic infections compared with nonresponders.[51,52] Initial clinical trials with high doses of IFN-α or -γ have found some antiviral effects but no significant immune reconstitution in patients with advanced AIDS. One controlled study of IFN found no survival benefit in such patients.[53] Studies of lower-dose regimens and combination therapy with other cytokines are in progress. In vitro synergy between IFN and zidovudine, phosphonoformate, or ribavirin has led to clinical testing of drug combinations.

REFERENCES

1. Pestka S, Langer JA, Zoon KC, et al. Interferons and their actions. Annu Rev Biochem. 1987;56:727–77.
2. Reis LFL, Le J, Hirano T, et al. Antiviral action of tumor necrosis factor in human fibroblasts is not mediated by B cell stimulatory factor 2/IFN-beta$_2$, and is inhibited by specific antibodies to IFN-beta. J Immunol. 1988; 140:1566–70.
3. Zoon KC. Human interferons: Structure and function. In: Interferon 9, London: Academic Press; 1987:1–12.
4. Greenberg SB. Human interferon in viral diseases. Infect Dis Clin North Am. 1987;1:383–423.
5. Johnson HM. Interferon-mediated modulation of the immune system. In: Pfeffer LM, ed. Mechanisms of Interferon Actions. v. 2. Boca Raton, FL: CRC Press; 1987:59–77.
6. Hall MJ, Duncan IB. Antiviral drug and interferon combinations. In: Field JH, ed. Antiviral Agents: The Development and Assessment of Antiviral Chemotherapy. v. 2. Boca Raton, FL: CRC Press; 1988:29–84.
7. Nathan CF, Kaplan G, Levis WR, et al. Local and systemic effects of intradermal recombinant interferon-gamma in patients with lepromatous leprosy. N Engl J Med. 1986;315:6–15.
8. Pomerantz RJ, Hirsch MS. Interferon and human immunodeficiency virus infection. In: Interferon 9. London: Academic Press; 1987:113–27.
9. Whitaker-Dowling P, Youngner JS. Antiviral effects of interferon in different virus–host cell systems. In: Pfeffer LM, ed. Mechanisms of Interferon Actions. v. 1. Boca Raton, FL: CRC Press; 1987:83–98.
10. Skidmore SJ, Jarlow MJ. Interferon assay as a viral diagnostic test. J Virol Methods. 1987;16:155–8.
11. Heremans H, Dijkmans R, Sobis H, et al. Regulation by interferons of the local inflammatory response to bacterial lipopolysaccharide. J Immunol. 1987;138:4175–9.
12. Mellouk S, Maheshwari RK, Rhodes-Feuillette A, et al. Inhibitory activity of interferons and interleukin 1 on the development of *Plasmodium falciparum* in human hepatocyte cultures. J Immunol. 1987;139:4192–5.

13. Hooks JJ, Detrick B. The interferon system and disease. In: Pfeffer LM, ed. Mechanisms of Interferon Actions. v. 2. Boca Raton, FL: CRC Press; 1987:113–328.
14. Barouki FM, Witter FR, Griffin DE, et al. Time course of interferon levels, antiviral state, 2′,5′-oligoadenylate synthetase and side effects in healthy men. J Interferon Res. 1987;7:29–39.
15. Dinarello CA, Cannon JG, Wolff SM. New concepts on the pathogenesis of fever. Rev Infect Dis. 1988;10:168–89.
16. McDonald EM, Mann AH, Thomas HC. Interferons as mediators of psychiatric morbidity. Lancet. 1987;2:1175–8.
17. Meyers JD, Flournoy N, Sanders JE, et al. Prophylactic use of human leukocyte interferon after allogeneic marrow transplantation. Ann Intern Med. 1987;107:809–16.
18. Williams SJ, Baird-Lambert JA, Farrell GC. Inhibition of theophylline metabolism by interferon. Lancet. 1987;2:939–41.
19. Steis RG, Smith JW II, Urba WJ, et al. Resistance to recombinant interferon alfa-2a in hairy-cell leukemia associated with neutralizing anti-interferon antibodies. N Engl J Med. 1988;318:1409–13.
20. Spiegel RJ, Spicehandler JR, Jacobs SL, et al. Low incidence of serum neutralizing factors in patients receiving recombinant alfa-2b interferon (Intron A). Am J Med. 1986;80:223–8.
21. Hayden FG. Intranasal interferons for control of the common cold. In: Revel M, ed. Clinical Aspects of Interferon. Boston: Kluwer Academic Publishers; 1988:3–16.
22. Ho M. Interferon for the treatment of infections. Annu Rev Med. 1987;38:51–9.
23. Kuhls TL, Sacher J, Pineda E, et al. Suppression of recurrent genital herpes simplex virus infection with recombinant alfa2 interferon. J Infect Dis. 1986;154:437–42.
24. Pazin GJ, Harger JH, Armstrong JA, et al. Leukocyte interferon for treating first episodes of genital herpes in women. J Infect Dis. 1987;156:891–8.
25. Eron LJ, Toy C, Salsitz B, et al. Therapy of genital herpes with topically applied interferon. Antimicrob Agents Chemother 1987;31:1137–9.
26. Winston DJ, Eron LJ, Ho M, et al. Recombinant interferon alpha-2a for treatment of herpes zoster in immunosuppressed patients with cancer. Am J Med. 1988;85:147–51.
27. Davis GL, Hoofnagle JH. Interferon in viral hepatitis: Role in pathogenesis and treatment. Hepatology. 1986;6:1038–41.
28. Alexander GJM, Fagan EA, Daniels HM, et al. Loss of HBsAg with interferon therapy in chronic hepatitis B virus infection. Lancet. 1987;2:66–9.
29. Lok ASF, Wu P-C, Lai C-L, et al. Long-term follow-up in a randomised controlled trial of recombinant alpha$_2$-interferon in Chinese patients with chronic hepatitis B infection. Lancet. 1988;2:298–302.
29a. Thomas HC. Hepatitis B viral infection. Am J Med. 1988;85(Suppl 2A):135–40.
29b. DeMan RA, Schalm SW, Heijtink RA, et al. Long-term follow-up of antiviral combination therapy in chronic hepatitis B. Am J Med. 1988;85(Suppl 2A):150–54.
30. Garcia G, Smith CI, Weissberg JI, et al. Adenine arabinoside monophosphate (vidarabine phosphate) in combination with human leukocyte interferon in the treatment of chronic hepatitis B. Ann Intern Med. 1987;107:278–85.
31. Bissett J, Eisenberg M, Gregory P, et al. Recombinant fibroblast interferon and immune interferon for treating chronic hepatitis B virus infection: Patients' tolerance and the effect on viral markers. J Infect Dis. 1988;157:1076–80.
32. Perrillo RP, Regenstein FG, Peters MG, et al. Prednisone withdrawal followed by recombinant alpha interferon in the treatment of chronic type B hepatitis. Ann Intern Med. 1988;109:95–100.
33. Hoofnagle JH, Mullen KD, Jones DB, et al. Treatment of chronic non-A, non-B hepatitis with recombinant human alpha interferon. N Engl J Med. 1986;315:1575–8.
34. Weck PK, Brandsma JL, Whisnant JK. Interferons in the treatment of human papillomavirus diseases. Cancer Metastasis Rev. 1986;5:139–65.
35. Eron LJ, Judson F, Tucker S, et al. Interferon therapy for condylomata acuminata. N Engl J Med. 1986;315:1059–64.
36. Vance JC, Bart BJ, Hansen RC, et al. Intralesional recombinant alpha-2 interferon for the treatment of patients with condyloma acuminatum or verruca plantaris. Arch Dermatol. 1986;122:272–7.
37. Reichman RC, Oakes D, Bonnez W, et al. Treatment of condyloma acuminatum with three different interferons administered intralesionally. Ann Intern Med. 1988;108:675–9.
38. Friedman-Kien AE, Eron LJ, Conant M, et al. Natural interferon alfa for treatment of condylomata acuminata. JAMA. 1988;259:533–8.
39. Trofatter KF Jr. Interferon. Obstet Gynecol Clin North Am. 1987;14:569–79.
40. Gall SA, Hughes CE, Mounts P, et al. Efficacy of human lymphoblastoid interferon in the therapy of resistant condyloma acuminata. Obstet Gynecol. 1986;67:643–51.
40a. Weck PK, Buddin DA, Whisnaut JK. Interferons in the treatment of genital papillomavirus infections. Am J Med. 1988;85(Suppl 2A):159–164.
41. Kirby PK, Kiviat N, Beckman A, et al. Tolerance and efficacy of recombinant human interferon gamma in the treatment of refractory genital warts. Am J Med. 1988;85:183–8.
42. Byrne MA, Moller BR, Tayor-Robinson D, et al. The effect of interferon on human papillomaviruses associated with cervical intraepithelial neoplasia. Br J Obstet Gynecol. 1986;93:1136–44.
43. Berman B, Davis-Reed L, Silverstein L, et al. Treatment of verrucae vulgaris with alfa2 interferon. J Infect Dis. 1986;154:328–30.
44. Lusk RP, McCabe BF, Mixon JH. Three-year experience of treating recurrent respiratory papilloma with interferon. Ann Otol Rhinol Laryngol. 1987; 19:158–62.
45. Healy GB, Gelber RD, Trowbridge AL, et al. Treatment of recurrent respiratory papillomatosis with human leukocyte interferon. N Engl J Med. 1988;319:401–7.
46. Hayden FG, Albrecht JK, Kaiser DL, et al. Prevention of natural colds by contact prophylaxis with intranasal alpha2-interferon. N Engl J Med. 1986; 314:71–5.
47. Douglas RB, Moore BW, Miles HB, et al. Prophylactic efficacy of intranasal alpha2-interferon against rhinovirus infections in the family setting. N Engl J Med. 1986;314:65–70.
48. Hayden FG, Kaiser DL, Albrecht JK. Intranasal recombinant alfa-2b interferon treatment of naturally occurring common colds. Antimicrob Agents Chemother. 1988;32:224–30.
49. Ikossi-O'Connor MG, Chadha KC, Lillie MA, et al. Interferon inactivator(s) in patients with AIDS and AIDS-related Kaposi''s sarcoma. Am J Med. 1986;81:783–5.
50. Krown SE. The role of interferon in the therapy of epidemic Kaposi's sarcoma. Semin Oncol. 1987;14:27–33.
51. Lane HC, Feinberg J, Davey V, et al. Anti-retroviral efects of interferon-α in AIDS-associated Kaposi sarcoma. Lancet. 1988;2:1218–1222.
52. DeWit R, Boucher CAB, Veenhof KHN, et al. Clinical and virological effects of high-dose recombinant interferon-α in disseminated AIDS-related Kaposi sarcoma. Lancet. 1988;2:1214–1217.
53. Friedland GH, Landesman SH, Crumpocker CS, et al. A clinical trial of recombinant α-IFN in patients with AIDS. III International Conference on AIDS. Washington DC, June 1987;165.

36. ANTIPARASITIC AGENTS

DAVID E. VAN REKEN
RICHARD D. PEARSON

A comprehensive discussion of antiparasitic chemotherapy must take into account the large number of parasites that can infect humans, the complexity of their life cycles, differences in their metabolism, and the wide array of drugs that have been developed to treat them. Taxonomically, parasites are divided into protozoa and helminths.[1–4] The protozoa often have complex life cycles but are unicellular. Helminths, on the other hand, have highly developed neuromuscular systems, digestive tracts, reproductive organs, and integuments. It is not surprising that most drugs effective against the helminths are not active against protozoa, and vice versa.

The susceptibility of the parasites to chemotherapeutic agents correlates to a high degree with taxonomy and metabolism (Table 1). The parasites can be grouped along these two parameters. The protozoa that inhabit the gastrointestinal lumen and vagina form one group. Although they arise from several taxonomic classes,[1] they share a common microenvironment and in many instances have similar metabolic adaptations. Included in this group are the various amoebae of the superclass Rhizopodia, the luminal flagellates of the class Zoomastigophorea, and *Balantidium coli* of the class Ciliata. The second major group includes members of the phylum Apicomplexa. These protozoa are important causes of morbidity and mortality worldwide. Included are *Plasmodium* spp., which cause malaria, *Babesia* spp., *Toxoplasma gondii, Cryptosporidium* spp., and *Isospora belli*. The latter three "coccidians" have emerged as important pathogens in persons with acquired immunodeficiency syndrome (AIDS). *Pneumocystis carinii*, which has not yet been classified, shares with members of the Apicomplexa the propensity to cause severe disease in the setting of AIDS and susceptibility to certain drugs. The third group of protozoan pathogens include flagellates of the class Zoomastigophorea, family Trypanosomidiae. They are arthropod borne and produce leishmaniasis, Chagas disease, and African sleeping sickness.

The susceptibility of helminths also correlates relatively closely with taxonomy. The helminths can be divided into ne-

TABLE 1. Spectrum of Activity of the Major Antiparasitic Drugs Licensed for Use in the United States, Available in the United States Only from the Manufacturer (*), Available from the CDC Drug Service, Centers for Disease Control (**), or Not Currently Available in the United States (***)

Drug	*Indications*
Amoebae, intestinal and vaginal Flagellates, and *Balantidium coli*	
Metronidazole	*Entamoeba histolytica* (invasive disease) *Entamoeba polecki* *Trichomonas vaginalis* *Blastocystis hominis* *Giardia lamblia* *Balantidium coli* (alternative)
Emetine, dehydroemetine**	*Entamoeba histolytica* (invasive disease)
Iodoquinol	*Entamoeba histolytica* (luminal infection) *Dientamoeba fragilis* *Blastocystis hominis* *Balantidium coli* (alternative)
Diloxanide furoate**	*Entamoeba histolytica* (asymptomatic luminal infection) *Entamoeba polecki* (luminal infection)
Paromomycin	*Entamoeba histolytica* (asymptomatic luminal infection) *Dientamoeba fragilis*
Quinacrine	*Giardia lamblia*
Furazolidone	*Giardia lamblia* (alternative)
Tetracycline	*Balantidium coli* *Dientamoeba fragilis*
Amphotericin B	*Naegleria* spp. (used with miconazole and rifampin)
Apicomplexa and *Pneumocystis carinii*	
Chloroquine	Suppressive prophylaxis and treatment of the asexual erythrocytic phase of *Plasmodium vivax, P. ovale, P. malariae,* and susceptible *P. falciparum.*
Primaquine	Radical cure of the exoerythrocytic hypnozoites of *P. vivax* and *P. ovale.*
Quinine	Treatment of chloroquine-resistant *P. falciparum*; effective against asexual erythrocytic phase of other *Plasmodium* spp.
Quinidine	Treatment of chloroquine-resistant *P. falciparum* when parenteral therapy is required; effective against asexual erythrocytic phase.
Mefloquine***	Prophylaxis and treatment of chloroquine-resistant *P. falciparum*; effective against asexual erythrocytic phase of other *Plasmodium* spp.
Tetracyclines	
Tetracycline	Used with quinine to treat asexual erythrocytic state of chloroquine-resistant *P. falciparum* in Southeast Asia.
Doxycycline	Used alone or with chloroquine for suppressive prophylaxis in Southeast Asia in areas where there is endemic chloroquine-resistant *P. falciparum.*
Dihydrofolate reductase inhibitors and sulfonamides	
Pyrimethamine/short-acting sulfonamides	Used with quinine to treat asexual erythrocytic phase of chloroquine-resistant *P. falciparum* acquired in areas other than Southeast Asia. *Toxoplasma gondii* (when treatment is indicated).
Pyrimethamine-sulfadoxime (Fansidar)	Presumptive treatment of chloroquine-resistant *P. falciparum* in areas where isolates remain sensitive; occasionally used for suppressive prophylaxis of chloroquine-resistant *P. falciparum* in persons at high risk.
Trimethoprim-sulfamethoxazole (cotrimoxazole)	*Pneumocystis carinii* *Isospora belli*
Proguanil***[a]	Used with chloroquine for suppressive prophylaxis in areas of East Africa where there is chloroquine-resistant *Plasmodium falciparum*
Macrolide antibiotics	
Clindamycin	Used with steroids for treatment of ocular *Toxoplasma gondii* in immunocompetent hosts; used with pyrimethamine for *T. gondii* encephalitis in persons with AIDS who cannot tolerate sulfonamides. Used with quinine for treatment of *Babesia* spp.
Spiramycin***[b]	*Toxoplasma gondii* during pregnancy and in the neonate *Cryptosporidium* species (efficacy uncertain)
Pentamidine isethionate	Treatment and prophylaxis of *Pneumocystis carinii* (alternative when given parenterally; aerosolized administration may become prophylaxis of choice in persons with AIDS)
Members of the Family Trypanosomatidae	
Suramin**	*Trypanosoma brucei gambiense* and *Trypanosoma brucei rhodesiense* (hemolymphatic stage)
Melarsoprol B**	*Trypanosoma brucei gambiense* and *Trypanosoma brucei rhodesiense* (late disease with central nervous system involvement)
Eflornithine*	*Trypanosoma brucei gambiense* (both stages; still considered investigational but will likely emerge as the treatment of choice)
Nifurtimox**	*Trypanosoma cruzi*
Benznidazole***	*Trypanosoma cruzi* (alternative)
Stibogluconate sodium**	*Leishmania* spp.
Meglumine antimoniate***	*Leishmania* spp.

(*Continued*)

TABLE 1. *(Continued)*

Drug	*Indications*
Members of the Family Trypanosomatidae *continued*	
Amphotericin B	*Leishmania* spp. (alternative)
Pentamidine isethionate	*Leishmania* spp. (alternative) *Trypanosoma brucei gambiense* (alternative for use in the hemolymphatic stage)
Helminthic diseases: Nematodes (roundworms)	
Benzimidazoles	
Mebendazole	*Ascaris lumbricoides* Hookworm *Trichuris trichiura* *Enterobius vermicularis* *Capillaria philippinensis* *Gnathostoma spinigerum* (surgical removal is an alternative) *Mansonella perstans* *Angiostrongylus cantonensis* *Trichinella spiralis* (recommended by some; used with steroids) Visceral larva migrans (alternative) *Echinococcus granulosus* and *Echinococcus multilocularis* (investigational; for treatment of inoperable lesions)
Albendazole*	*Echinococcus granulosus* and *Echinococcus multilocularis* (investigational; probably the best choice for treatment of inoperable lesions) Intestinal nematodes (alternative; investigational)
Thiabendazole	*Strongyloides stercoralis* Cutaneous larva migrans Visceral larva migrans *Trichostrongylus* spp. *Angiostrongylus costaricensis* (surgical intervention is the alternative) *Dracunculus medinensis* (alternative) *Capillaria philippensis* (alternative) *Trichinella spiralis* (used with steroids; some recommend mebendazole)
Piperazine citrate	*Ascaris lumbricoides* (alternative)
Pyrantel pamoate	*Enterobius vermicularis* *Ascaris lumbricoides* Hookworm *Trichostrongylus* spp. (alternative)
Diethylcarbamazine	*Wuchereria bancrofti* *Brugia malayi* *Mansonella ozzardi* *Loa loa* Tropical eosinophilia Visceral larva migrans *Onchocerca volvulus* (alternative; usually followed by suramin to kill adult worms; ivermectin is now the drug of choice)
Ivermectin*	*Onchocerca volvulus* Broad range of nematodes and blood sucking arthropods (use for these indications is investigational)
Metronidazole	*Dracunculus medinensis*
Helminthic diseases: Trematodes (flukes) and Cestodes (tapeworms)	
Praziquantel	*Schistosoma* spp. *Clonorchis sinensis* *Opisthorchis viverrini* *Paragonimus westermani* *Fasciolopsis buski* *Heterophyes heterophyes* *Metagonimus yokogawai* *Diphyllobothrium latum* (alternative) Taenia solium (adult worm and cysticercosis) *Taenia saginata* (alternative) Dipylidium caninum (alternative) *Hymenolepis nana*
Metrifonate	*Schistosoma haematobium* (alternative)
Oxamniquine	*Schistosoma mansoni* (alternative)
Bithionol	*Fasciola hepatica* *Paragonimus westermani* (alternative)
Niclosamide	*Diphyllobothrium latum* *Taenia saginata* *Taenia solium* *Dipylidium caninum* *Hymenolepis nana* (alternative) *Fasciolopsis buski*

[a] Can be purchased over the counter in London and major cities in East Africa (e.g., Nairobi, Kenya).
[b] Can be used with the approval of the FDA.

matodes (roundworms),[2] which are subdivided into those that live in the lumen of the intestine and those that reside in tissue; trematodes (flukes); and cestodes (tapeworms).[3,4] Chemotherapeutic agents are often active against multiple genera within these groups. Major advances have been made in the treatment of helminthic diseases during the past decade. Specifically, praziquantel has revolutionized the treatment of trematode infections, including schistosomiasis, as well as cerebral cysticercosis, and ivermectin the treatment of onchocerciasis.

The discussion of antiparasitic drugs that follows is arranged according to these groups. The approach is imperfect in that some drugs are active against pathogens in more than one group. This is particularly true for praziquantel, which is active against a broad spectrum of trematodes and cestodes, and two investigational drugs, albendazole, with activity against nematodes and cestodes, and ivermectin, with activity against nematodes and blood-sucking arthropods. Nonetheless, the approach taken provides a logical framework in which to organize the data. Drugs that have broad spectrums of activity are discussed in the context of their primary indications.

The dosage and duration of therapy for specific parasitic diseases are provided in Tables 2–4.[5] Not all of these drugs are available through pharmacies in the United States. Some can be obtained only from the manufacturer (indicated by *). Others have not been licensed in the United States but are available only from the CDC Drug Service (**), Centers for Disease Control, Atlanta, Georgia 30333. Some cannot be obtained in the United States (***), but they are discussed because they are used elsewhere or hold promise for the future.

DRUGS ACTIVE AGAINST LUMINAL PROTOZOA: AMEBAE, INTESTINAL AND VAGINAL FLAGELLATES, AND THE CILIATE BALANTIDIUM COLI

Metronidazole and Other Nitroimidazoles

Metronidazole (Fig. 1), tinidazole,*** and ornidazole*** have selective toxicity against numerous anaerobic and microaerophilic organisms. Only metronidazole, 2-methyl-5-nitroimidazole-1-ethanol, has been licensed in the United States. It is highly effective in the treatment of symptomatic *Entamoeba histolytica*[6,7] and *E. polecki* infections,[8] enteritis due to *Giardia lamblia*,[9,10] and vaginitis due to *Trichomonas vaginalis*.[11,12] It is also considered an alternative drug for the treatment of two other enteric pathogens, *Blastocystis hominis*[13] and *B. coli*.[14] Metronidazole is active against trophozoites of *Entamoeba* species, but it does not invariably eradicate the cysts.[15] A luminally active agent is required for this purpose and to treat asymptomatic cyst passers. Metronidazole has also been advocated as empiric therapy for presumptive protozoal enterocolitis in areas of the world where laboratory facilities are insufficient to provide a specific diagnosis.[16] Finally, metronidazole is recommended for the treatment of the guinea worm, *Dracunculus medinensis*,[17] but its clinical effects are related to a reduction in inflammation rather than to a lethal effect on the worm. The use of metronidazole against anaerobic bacterial pathogens is summarized in Chapter 25.

Metronidazole has Food and Drug Administration (FDA) approval for the treatment of amebiasis and trichomoniasis, but not giardiasis. This does not prevent physicians from using metronidazole for diseases like giardiasis, in which data support its efficacy.[18] The cure rate with the doses of metronidazole recommended for giardiasis (Table 2) is slightly lower than with quinacrine,[9,10,16] but metronidazole is generally better tolerated and many physicians prefer it over quinacrine.

Metronidazole is available as 250- and 500-mg tablets for oral use and in vials with 500 mg lyophilized powder for parenteral administration. When it is administered orally, 90–95 percent is absorbed[19,20]; peak serum levels are reached within 1 hour. It is widely distributed throughout the body and penetrates well into tissues, abscesses, fluid compartments, vaginal secretions, bone, the central nervous system, and breast milk.[21] Only 1–11 percent of the drug is bound to protein. The elimination half-

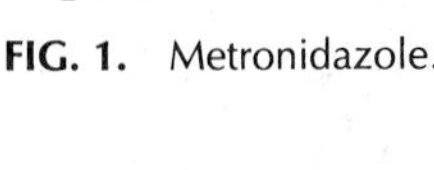

FIG. 1. Metronidazole.

life is 6.2–11.5 hours.[21] Approximately 80 percent of metronidazole and its metabolites are excreted via the kidney. The principal metabolites result from oxidation of side chains and glucuronide formation. Although renal failure prolongs the half-life of these metabolites, the hepatic metabolism is such that the drug dosage need not be modified during renal failure, but it should be adjusted in liver failure. The metabolites are removed by dialysis.

Metronidazole is activated in anaerobic organisms by reduction of the 5-nitro group through a sequence of intermediate steps involving microbial electron transport proteins of low redox potential.[22] This results in a concentration gradient across the membrane of the parasite and permits accumulation of high concentrations of the reduced compound within the cell. Metronidazole acts as an electron sink, depriving the anaerobe of reducing equivalents. Furthermore, the reduced form of metronidazole causes loss of the helical structure of DNA, strand breakage, and impaired template function.[23,24]

Side effects are seldom severe enough to cause discontinuation of the drug. Gastrointestinal side effects include nausea, vomiting, diarrhea, and a metallic aftertaste. They are less common with the low doses (250 mg tid) recommended for giardiasis than with the high doses (750 mg tid) used for amebiasis. Other less frequent side effects include headache, dizziness, rash, urethral burning, vaginal or oral candidiasis, and reversible neutropenia.[25] The urine of some persons may become red or brown due to the presence of metabolites. Metronidazole may potentiate the anticoagulant effects of coumarin.[26] Rarely, patients treated with metronidazole experience sensory neuropathies or central nervous system toxicity with vertigo, ataxia, seizures, or encephalopathy.[27] Pseudomembranous colitis is also rare. Alcohol should be avoided because of the disulfiram (Antabuse)-like effects of metronidazole and the drug–drug interaction that can result in acute psychosis or a confusional state.[28]

The potential role of metronidazole in human carcinogenesis has been the subject of debate. Metronidazole has not been shown to be carcinogenic in humans, but it is mutagenic for certain strains of *Salmonella typhimurium*.[29] Furthermore, human urine contains metabolites that are carcinogenic in rodents.[30] However, 10-year follow-up of patients who received metronidazole for trichomoniasis has revealed no increase in the prevalence of cancer.[31,32]

Tinidazole and ornidazole, two other 5-nitroimidazole derivatives, have amebicidal and trichomonicidal activity similar to that of metronidazole, but fewer side effects.[7,33] A single 2-gr dose of tinidazole has been used successfully to treat giardiasis. Both tinidazole and ornidazole are well absorbed orally, have good tissue penetration, and are widely distributed in the body. Tinidazole and ornidazole have half-lives of 14 and 12–13 hours, respectively.[34] They are excreted primarily in urine, 50 percent of tinidazole and 96 percent of ornidazole in the form of metabolites.[35] These drugs have a favorable side effects profile in comparison to metronidazole. Reported side effects include anorexia, headache, and dizziness.

Emetine and Dehydroemetine**

Emetine, for many years the drug of choice for invasive amebiasis, is a tissue-active amebicide prepared from ipecac, which comes from the root of *Cephaëlis ipecacuanha*. The root is still used as a traditional medicine for the treatment of bloody diarrhea in some rural areas of South and Central America. Emetine and dehydroemetine have appreciable toxicity. They are reserved for persons with extraintestinal amebiasis, usually amebic liver abscesses,[36] who do not respond to metronidazole or for the rare person in whom metronidazole cannot be used. They are often given concomitantly with choroquine, which at high doses is a tissue active amebicide.[37] Iodoquinol or another luminally active agent is necessary to eradicate amebic cysts from the gastrointestinal tract.

TABLE 2. Drugs for Treatment of Parasitic Infections

Infection	*Drug*	*Adult Dosage**	*Pediatric Dosage**
Amebiasis (*Entamoeba histolytica*)			
Asymptomatic			
Drug of choice:	Iodoquinol[1]	650 mg tid × 20d	30–40 mg/kg/d in 3 doses × 20d
Alternatives:	Diloxanide furoate[2]	500 mg tid × 10d	20 mg/kg/d in 3 doses × 10d
	Paromomycin	25–30 mg/kg/d in 3 doses × 7d	25–30 mg/kg/d in 3 doses × 7d
Mild to moderate intestinal disease			
Drugs of choice:	Metronidazole[3,4]	750 mg tid × 10d	35–50 mg/kg/d in 3 doses × 10d
	followed by iodoquinol[1]	650 mg tid × 20d	30–40 mg/kg/d in 3 doses × 20d
Alternative:	Paromomycin	25–30 mg/kg/d in 3 doses × 7d	25–30 mg/kg/d in 3 doses × 7d
Severe intestinal disease			
Drugs of choice:	Metronidazole[3,4]	750 mg tid × 10d	35–50 mg/kg/d in 3 doses × 10d
	followed by iodoquinol[1]	650 mg tid × 20d	30–40 mg/kg/d in 3 doses × 20d
Alternatives:	Dehydroemetine[2,5]	1 to 1.5 mg/kg/d (max. 90 mg/d) im for up to 5d	1 to 1.5 mg/kg/d (max. 90 mg/d) im in 2 doses for up to 5d
	followed by iodoquinol[1]	650 mg tid × 20d	30–40 mg/kg/d in 3 doses × 20d
OR	Emetine[5]	1 mg/kg/d (max. 60 mg/d) im for up to 5d	1 mg/kg/d in 2 doses (max. 60 mg/d) im for up to 5d
	followed by iodoquinol[1]	650 mg tid × 20d	30–40 mg/kg/d in 3 doses × 20d
Hepatic abscess			
Drugs of choice:	Metronidazole[3,4]	750 mg tid × 10d	35–50 mg/kg/d in 3 doses × 10d
	followed by iodoquinol[1]	650 mg tid × 20d	30–40 mg/kg/d in 3 doses × 20d
Alternatives:	Dehydroemetine[2,5]	1 to 1.5 mg/kg/d (max. 90 mg/d) im for up to 5d	1 to 1.5 mg/kg/d (max. 90 mg/d) im in 2 doses for up to 5d
	folllowed by chloroquine phosphate	600 mg base (1 gram)/d × 2d, then 300 mg base (500 mg)/d × 2–3 wks	10 mg base/kg (max. 300 mg base)/d × 2–3 wks
	plus iodoquinol[1]	650 mg tid × 20d	30–40 mg/kg/d in 3 doses × 20d
OR	Emetine[5]	1 mg/kg/d (max. 60 mg/d) im for up to 5d	1 mg/kg/d (max. 60 mg/d) im in 2 doses for up to 5d
	followed by chloroquine phosphate	600 mg base (1 gram)/d × 2d, then 300 mg base (500 mg)/d × 2–3 wks	10 mg base/kg (max. 300 mg base)/d × 2–3 wks
	plus iodoquinol[1]	650 mg tid × 20d	30–40 mg/kg/d in 3 doses × 20d
Amebic meningoencephalitis, primary			
Naegleria spp.			
Drug of choice:	Amphotericin B[6,7]	1 mg/kg/d iv, uncertain duration	1 mg/kg/d iv, uncertain duration
Acanthamoeba spp.			
Drug of choice:	see footnote 8		
Ancylostoma duodenale, see Hookworm			
Angiostrongyliasis			
Angiostrongylus cantonensis			
Drug of choice:	Mebendazole[7,9,10]	100 mg bid × 5d	100 mg bid × 5d for children >2 years
Angiostrongylus costaricensis			
Drug of choice:	Thiabendazole[7,9]	25 mg/kg tid × 3d[11] (max. 3 grams/day)	25 mg/kg tid × 3d[11] (max. 3 grams/day)
OR	surgical intervention		
Anisakiasis (*Anisakis* spp.)			
Treatment of choice:	Surgical removal		
Ascariasis (*Ascaris lumbricoides*, roundworm)			
Drug of choice:	Mebendazole	100 mg bid × 3d	100 mg bid × 3d for children >2 years
OR	Pyrantel pamoate	11 mg/kg once (max. 1 gram)	11 mg/kg once (max. 1 gram)
Alternative:	Piperazine citrate	75 mg/kg (max. 3.5 grams)/d × 2d	75 mg/kg (max. 3.5 grams)/d × 2d
Babesiosis (*Babesia* spp.)			
Drugs of choice:[12]	Clindamycin[7]	1.2 grams bid parenteral or 600 mg tid oral × 7d	20–40 mg/kg/d in 3 doses × 7d
	plus quinine	650 mg tid oral × 7d	25 mg/kg/d in 3 doses × 7d
Balantidiasis (*Balantidium coli*)			
Drug of choice:	Tetracycline[7]	500 mg qid × 10d	10 mg/kg qid × 10d (max. 2 grams/d)
Alternatives:	Iodoquinol[1,7]	650 mg tid × 20d	40 mg/kg/d in 3 doses × 20d
	Metronidazole[3,7]	750 mg tid × 5d	35–50 mg/kg/d in 3 doses × 5d
Blastocystis hominis infection			
Drug of choice:	Iodoquinol[1]	650 mg tid × 20d	30–40 mg/kg/d in 3 doses × 20d
OR	Metronidazole[3,7]	750 mg tid × 10d	35–50 mg/kg/d in 3 doses × 10d
Capillariasis (*Capillaria philippinensis*)			
Drug of choice:	Mebendazole[7]	200 mg bid × 20d	200 mg bid × 20d
Alternative:	Thiabendazole[7]	25 mg/kg/d × 30d	25 mg/kg/d × 30d
Chagas disease, see Trypanosomiasis			
Clonorchis sinensis, see Fluke infection			

(*Continued*)

* The letter d indicates day.
[1] Dosage and duration of administration should not be exceeded because of possibility of causing optic neuritis; maximum dosage is 2 grams/day.
[2] In the USA, this drug is available from the CDC Drug Service, Centers for Disease Control, Atlanta, Georgia 30333; telephone: 404-639-3670 (evenings, weekends, and holidays: 404-639-2888).
[3] Metronidazole is carcinogenic in rodents and mutagenic in bacteria; it should generally not be given to pregnant women, particularly in the first trimester.
[4] Outside the USA, ornidazole and tinidazole are also used.
[5] Dehydroemetine is probably as effective and probably less toxic than emetine. Because of its toxic effects on the heart, patients receiving emetine should have electrocardiographic monitoring and should remain sedentary during therapy.
[6] One patient with a *Naegleria* infection was successfully treated with amphotericin B, micronazole, and rifampin (JS Seidel et al, N Engl J Med, 306:346, 1982).
[7] Considered an investigational drug for this condition by the U.S. Food and Drug Administration.
[8] Experimental infections with *Acanthamoeba* spp. have been reported to respond to sulfadiazine (CG Culbertson, Annu Rev Microbiol, 25:231, 1971). Amebic keratitis due to *Acanthamoeba* sp. has been reported to respond to topical miconazole, propamidine isethionate, and antibiotics (MB Moore et al, Am J Ophthalmol, 100:396, 1985).
[9] Effectiveness documented only in animals.
[10] Analgesics, corticosteroids, and careful removal of CSF at frequent intervals can relieve symptoms. Albendazole and ivermectin have been used successfully in animals.
[11] This dose is likely to be toxic and may have to be decreased.

TABLE 2. *(Continued)*

Infection	*Drug*	*Adult Dosage**	*Pediatric Dosage**
Cryptosporidiosis (*Cryptosporidium* spp.)			
Drug of choice:[13]	Spiramycin	1 gram tid PO × 14d or more	
Cutaneous larva migrans (creeping eruption)			
Drug of choice:	Thiabendazole	25 mg/kg bid (max. 3 grams/d) × 2–5d and/ or topically	25 mg/kg bid (max. 3 grams/d) × 2–5d and/ or topically
Cysticercosis, see Tapeworm infection			
Dientamoeba fragilis infection			
Drug of choice:	Iodoquinol[1]	650 mg tid × 20d	40 mg/kg/d in 3 doses × 20d
OR	Tetracycline[7]	500 mg qid × 10d	10 mg/kg qid × 10d (max. 2 grams/d)
OR	Paromomycin	25–30 mg/kg/d in 3 doses × 7d	25–30 mg/kg/d in 3 doses × 7d
Diphyllobothrium latum, see Tapeworm infection			
Dracunculus medinensis (guinea worm) infection			
Drug of choice:	Metronidazole[3,7]	250 mg tid × 10d	25 mg/kg/d (max. 750 mg/d) in 3 doses × 10d
Alternative:	Thiabendazole[7]	25–37.5 mg/kg bid × 3d[11]	25–37.5 mg/kg bid × 3d[11]
Echinococcus, see Tapeworm infection			
Entamoeba histolytica, see Amebiasis			
Entamoeba polecki infection			
Drugs of choice:	Metronidazole[3,7]	750 mg tid × 10d	35–50 mg/kg/d in 3 doses × 10d
	followed by diloxanide furoate[2]	500 mg tid × 10d	20 mg/kg/d in 3 doses × 10d
Enterobius vermicularis (pinworm) infection			
Drug of choice:	Pyrantel pamoate	A single dose of 11 mg/kg (max. 1 gram); repeat after 2 weeks	A single dose of 11 mg/kg (max. 1 gram); repeat after 2 weeks
OR	Mebendazole	A single dose of 100 mg; repeat after 2 weeks	A single dose of 100 mg for children >2 years; repeat after 2 weeks
Fasciola hepatica, see Fluke infection			
Filariasis			
Wuchereria bancrofti, Brugia (W.) malayi, Mansonella ozzardi, Loa loa			
Drug of choice:[14]	Diethylcarbamazine[15]	Day 1: 50 mg, oral, p.c. Day 2: 50 mg tid Day 3: 100 mg tid Days 4 through 21: 2 mg/kg tid	Day 1: 25–50 mg Day 2: 25–50 mg tid Day 3: 50–100 mg tid Days 4 through 21: 2 mg/kg tid
Mansonella perstans			
Drug of choice:[16]	Mebendazole[7]	100 mg bid × 30d	
Tropical eosinophilia			
Drug of choice:	Diethylcarbamazine	2 mg/kg tid × 7–10d	2 mg/kg tid × 7–10d
Onchocerca volvulus			
Drug of choice:	Ivermectin[7,17]	150 μg/kg PO once, repeated every 6 to 12 months	150 μg/kg PO once
Alternatives:	Diethylcarbamazine[15]	25 mg/d × 3d, then 50 mg/d × 5d, then 100 mg/d × 3d, then 150 mg/d × 12d	0.5 mg/kg tid × 3d (max. 25 mg/d), then 1.0 mg/kg tid × 3–4d (max. 50 mg/d), then 1.5 mg/kg tid × 3–4d (max. 100 mg/d), then 2.0 mg/kg tid × 2–3 wks
	followed by suramin[2,18]	100–200 mg (test dose) iv, then 1 gram iv at weekly intervals × 5 wks	10–20 mg (test dose) iv, then 20 mg/kg iv at weekly intervals × 5 wks
Fluke, hermaphroditic, infection			
Clonorchis sinensis (Chinese liver fluke)			
Drug of choice:	Praziquantel[7]	25 mg/kg tid × 2d	25 mg/kg tid × 2d
Fasciola hepatica (sheep liver fluke)			
Drug of choice:[19]	Bithionol[2]	30–50 mg/kg on alternate days × 10–15 doses	30–50 mg/kg on alternate days × 10–15 doses
Fasciolopsis buski (intestinal fluke)			
Drug of choice:	Praziquantel[7]	25 mg/kg tid × 1d	25 mg/kg tid × 1d
OR	Niclosamide[7]	a single dose of 4 tablets (2 g) chewed thoroughly	11–34 kg: a single dose of 2 tablets (1 g) >34 kg: a single dose of 3 tablets (1.5 g)
Alternative:	Tetrachloroethylene[20]	0.1 ml/kg (max. 5 ml)	0.1 ml/kg (max. 5 ml)
Heterophyes heterophyes (intestinal fluke)			
Drug of choice:	Praziquantel[7]	25 mg/kg tid × 1d	25 mg/kg tid × 1d
Metagonimus yokogawai (intestinal fluke)			
Drug of choice:	Praziquantel[7]	25 mg/kg tid × 1d	25 mg/kg tid × 1d
Opisthorchis viverrini (liver fluke)			
Drug of choice:	Praziquantel[7]	25 mg/kg tid × 1d	25 mg/kg tid × 1d
Paragonimus westermani (lung fluke)			
Drug of choice:	Praziquantel[7]	25 mg/kg tid × 2d	25 mg/kg tid × 2d
Alternative:	Bithionol[2]	30–50 mg/kg on alternate days × 10–15 doses	30–50 mg/kg on alternate days × 10–15 doses

(Continued)

* The letter d indicates day.

[12] Concurrent use of pentamidine and trimethoprim-sulfamethoxazole has been reported to cure an infection with *B. divergens* (D Raoult et al, Ann Intern Med, 107:944, 1987).

[13] Limited clinical results suggest a decrease in diarrhea with therapy. Prospective studies of efficacy are ongoing. Infection is self-limiting in immunocompetent patients.

[14] Several reports indicate that ivermectin may be effective for treatment of *W. bancrofti* (S Diallo et al, Lancet, 1:1030, 1987) and *M. ozzardi* (TB Nutman et al, J Infect Dis, 156:662, 1987).

[15] Diethylcarbamazine should be administered with special caution in heavy infections with *Loa loa* because it can provoke ocular problems or an encephalopathy. Antihistamines or corticosteroids may be required to decrease allergic reactions due to disintegration of microfilariae in treatment of all filarial infections, especially those caused by *Onchocerca* and *Loa loa*. Surgical excision of subcutaneous *Onchocerca* nodules is recommended by some authorities before starting drug therapy.

[16] Ivermectin may also be effective.

TABLE 2. *(Continued)*

Infection	*Drug*	*Adult Dosage**	*Pediatric Dosage**
Giardiasis (*Giardia lamblia*)			
Drug of choice:	Quinacrine HCl	100 mg tid p.c. × 5d	2 mg/kg tid p.c. × 5d (max. 300 mg/d)
Alternatives:	Metronidazole[3,4,7]	250 mg tid × 5d	5 mg/kg tid × 5d
	Furazolidone	100 mg qid × 7–10d	1.25 mg/kg qid × 7–10d
Gnathostomiasis (*Gnathostoma spinigerum*)			
Treatment of choice:	Surgical removal		
OR	Mebendazole[7,21]	200 mg q3h × 6d	
Hookworm infection (*Ancylostoma duodenale, Necator americanus*)			
Drug of choice:[22]	Mebendazole	100 mg bid × 3d	100 mg bid × 3d for children >2 years
OR	Pyrantel pamoate[7]	11 mg/kg (max. 1 gram) × 3d	11 mg/kg (max. 1 gram) × 3d
Hydatid cyst, see Tapeworm infection			
Hymenolepis nana, see Tapeworm infection			
Isosporiasis (*Isospora belli*)			
Drug of choice:	Trimethoprim-sulfamethoxazole[7,23]	160 mg TMP, 800 mg SMX qid × 10d, then bid × 3 wks	
Leishmaniasis			
L. braziliensis, L. mexicana (American cutaneous and mucocutaneous leishmaniasis)			
Drug of choice:[24]	Stibogluconate sodium[2]	20 mg/kg/d (max. 800 mg/d) iv or im × 20d may be repeated or continued until there is a response	20 mg/kg/d im or iv (max. 800 mg/d) × 20d
Alternative:	Amphotericin B[7]	0.25 to 1 mg/kg by slow infusion daily or every 2d for up to 8 wks	0.25 to 1 mg/kg by slow infusion daily or every 2d for up to 8 wks
L. donovani (kala azar, visceral leishmaniasis)			
Drug of choice:	Stibogluconate sodium[2,25]	20 mg/kg/d (max. 800 mg/d) im or iv × 20d (may be repeated)	20 mg/kg/d im or iv (max. 800 mg/d) × 20d
Alternative:	Pentamidine isethionate	2–4 mg/kg/d im for up to 15 doses	2–4 mg/kg/d im for up to 15 doses
L. tropica. L. maior (oriental sore, cutaneous leishmaniasis)			
Drug of choice:	Stibogluconate sodium[2,26]	10 mg/kg/d (max. 600 mg/d) im or iv × 6–10d (may be repeated)	10 mg/kg/d im or iv (max. 600 mg/d) × 6–10d
Alternative:	Topical treatment[27]		
Lice infestation (*Pediculus humanus, capitis, Phthirus pubis*)[28]			
Drug of choice:	1% Permethrin[29]	Topically	Topically
Alternatives:	Pyrethrins with piperonyl butoxide	Topically[30]	Topically[30]
	Lindane	Topically[30]	Topically[30]
Loa loa, see Filariasis			
Malaria, see Tables 3 and 4			
Mites, see Scabies			
Naegleria spp., see Amebic meningoencephalitis, primary			
Necator americanus, see Hookworm infection			
Onchocerca volvulus, see Filariasis			
Opisthorchis viverrini, see Fluke infection			
Paragonimus westermani, see Fluke infection			
Pediculus capitis, humanus, Phthirus pubis, see Lice			
Pinworm, see *Enterobius*			
Pneumocysts carinii pneumonia[31]			
Drug of choice:	Trimethoprim-sulfamethoxazole	TMP 20 mg/kg/d, SMX 100 mg/kg/d oral or iv in 4 doses × 14d	TMP 20 mg/kg/d, SMX 100 mg/kg/d oral or iv in 4 doses × 14d
Alternative:	Pentamidine isethionate	4 mg/kg/d im × 14d	4 mg/kg/d im × 14d
Roundworm, see Ascariasis			
Scabies (*Sarcoptes scabiei*)			
Drug of choice:[32]	Lindane	Topically once	Topically
Alternatives:	Sulfur in petrolatum	Topically	Topically
	10% Crotamiton	Topically	Topically
Schistosomiasis			
S. haematobium			
Drug of choice:	Praziquantel	20 mg/kg tid × 1d	20 mg/kg tid × 1d
S. japonicum			
Drug of choice:	Praziquantel	20 mg/kg tid × 1d	20 mg/kg tid × 1d
S. mansoni			
Drug of choice:	Praziquantel	20 mg/kg tid × 1d	20 mg/kg tid × 1d
Alternative:	Oxamniquine	15 mg/kg once[33]	10 mg/kg bid × 1d[33]

(Continued)

* The letter d indicates day.

17 Ivermectin in a dose of 200 μg/kg has been reported to be as effective as diethylcarbamazine in decreasing the number of microfilaria and causes fewer adverse ophthalmologic reactions (BM Greene et al, N Engl J Med, 313:133, 1985; AT White et al, J Infect Dis, 156:463, 1987). Semiannual to annual prophylaxis appears to be effective in keeping microfilarial counts at low levels.

18 Some Medical Letter consultants use suramin only if ocular microfilariae persist after diethylcarbamazine therapy and nodulectomy.

19 Unlike infections with other flukes, *Fasciola hepatica* infections may not respond to praziquantel. Limited data indicate that albendazole may be effective in this condition.

20 Given on empty stomach. Although approved for human use, it is available currently only as a veterinary product. No alcoholic beverage should be consumed before or for 12 hours after therapy. Keep patient at bedrest for 4 hours after treatment.

21 In felines, ancylol (2, 6, diodo-4-nitrophenol) by subcutaneous injection has been effective against migrating larvae.

22 Albendazole is also effective (RNG Pugh, Ann Trop Med Parasitol, 80:565, 1986).

23 Shorter courses of trimethoprim-sulfamethoxazole may be equally effective. Preliminary studies suggest that a 7–10 day initial course of trimethoprim-sulfamethoxazole may be as effective as a 4.5 week course and that recurrences may be prevented by weekly doses of pyrimethamine-sulfadoxine (R Soave and WD Johnson, Jr, J Infect Dis, 157:225, 1988). In sulfonamide-sensitive patients, such as some patients with AIDS, pyrimethamine 50–75 mg daily has been effective. In immunocompromised patients, it may be necessary to continue therapy indefinitely.

24 Limited data indicate that ketoconazole, 400 to 600 mg daily for 28 days, may be effective for treatment of *L. panamensis* and *L. mexicana* (cutaneous).

TABLE 2. *(Continued)*

Infection	*Drug*	*Adult Dosage**	*Pediatric Dosage**
S. mekongi			
Drug of choice:	Praziquantel	20 mg/kg tid × 1d	20 mg/kg tid × 1d
Sleeping sickness, see Trypanosomiasis			
Strongyloidiasis (*Strongyloides stercoralis*)			
Drug of choice:[34]	Thiabendazole	25 mg/kg bid (max. 3 grams/d) × 2d[35]	25 mg/kg bid (max. 3 grams/d) × 2d[35]
Tapeworm infection, adult or intestinal stage			
Diphyllobothrium latum (fish), *Taenia saginata* (beef), *Taenia solium* (pork),[36] *Dipylidium caninum* (dog)			
Drug of choice:	Niclosamide	A single dose of 4 tablets (2 grams) chewed thoroughly	11–34 kg: a single dose of 2 tablets (1 gram); >34 kg: a single dose of 3 tablets (1.5 grams)
OR	Praziquantel[7]	10–20 mg/kg once	10–20 mg/kg once
Hymenolepsis nana (dwarf tapeworm)			
Drug of choice:	Praziquantel[7]	25 mg/kg once	25 mg/kg once
Alternative:	Niclosamide	A single daily dose of 4 tablets (2 grams) chewed thoroughly, then 2 tablets daily × 6d	11–34 kg: a single dose of 2 tablets (1 gram) × 1d, then 1 tablet (0.5 g)/d × 6d; >34 kg: a single dose of 3 tablets (1.5 grams) × 1d, then 2 tablets (1 gram)/d × 6d
Tapeworm infection, larval or tissue stage			
Echinococcus granulosus			
Drug of choice:	See footnote 37		
Echinococcus multilocularis[38]	See footnote 38		
Cysticercus cellulosae (cysticercosis)			
Drug of choice:[39]	Praziquantel[7]	50 mg/kg/d in 3 divided doses × 14d	50 mg/kg/d in 3 divided doses × 14d
Alternative:	Surgery		
Toxocariasis, see Visceral larva migrans			
Toxoplasmosis (*Toxoplasma gondii*)[40]			
Drugs of choice:	Pyrimethamine[41]	25 mg/d × 3–4 wks	2 mg/kg/d × 3d, then 1 mg/kg/d[42] (max. 25 mg/d) × 4 wks
	plus trisulfapyrimidines	2–6 grams/d × 3–4 wks	100–200 mg/kg/d × 3–4 wks
Alternative:	Spiramycin	2–4 grams/d × 3–4 wks	50–100 mg/kg/d × 3–4 wks
Trichinosis (*Trichinella spiralis*)			
Drugs of choice:	Steroids for severe symptoms		
	plus thiabendazole or mebendazole[43]	25 mg/kg bid × 5d (max. 3 grams/d)	25 mg/kg bid × 5d
Trichomoniasis (*Trichomonas vaginalis*)			
Drug of choice:[44]	Metronidazole[3]	2 grams once or 250 mg tid orally × 7d	15 mg/kg/d orally in 3 doses × 7d
Trichostrongylus infection			
Drug of choice:	Thiabendazole[7]	25 mg/kg bid × 2d (max. 3 grams/d)	25 mg/kg bid × 2d
Alternative:	Pyrantel pamoate[7]	11 mg/kg once (max. 1 gram)	11 mg/kg once (max. 1 gram)
Trichuriasis (*Trichuris trichiura, whipworm*)			
Drug of choice:	Mebendazole	100 mg bid × 3d	100 mg bid × 3d for children >2 yrs
Trypanosomiasis			
T. cruzi (South American trypanosomiasis, Chagas' disease)			
Drug of choice:	Nifurtimox[2]	8–10 mg/kg/d orally in 4 divided doses × 120d	1–10 yrs: 15–20 mg/kg/d in 4 divided doses × 90d; 11–16 yrs: 12.5–15 mg/kg/d in 4 divided doses × 90d
Alternative:	Benznidazole[45]	5–7 mg/kg × 30–120d	

(Continued)

* The letter d indicates day.

[25] For the African form of visceral leishmaniasis, therapy may have to be extended to at least 30 days and may have to be repeated.

[26] Ketoconazole, 400 mg daily for four to eight weeks, has also been reported to be effective (J Viallet et al, Am J Trop Med Hyg, 35:491, 1986).

[27] Application of heat 39° to 42°C directly to the lesion for 20 to 32 hours over a period of 10 to 12 days has been reported to be effective in *L. tropica* (FA Neva et al, Am J Trop Med Hyg, 33:800, 1984).

[28] For infestation of eyelashes with crab lice, use petrolatum.

[29] FDA-approved for head lice only.

[30] Some consultants recommend a second application one week later to kill hatching progeny.

[31] AIDS patients may need longer duration of therapy. For AIDS patients who develop hypersensitivity or resistance to both TMP/SMX and pentamidine, trimetrexate with leucovorin rescue or a combination of dapsone and trimethoprim may be effective. Aerosolized pentamidine has been tried for both treatment and prophylaxis (Medical Letter, 29:103, 1987).

[32] 5% permethrin, not yet marketed in the USA, could prove to be the drug of choice when it becomes available.

[33] In East Africa, the dose should be increased to 30 mg/kg/d, and in Egypt and South Africa, 30 mg/kg/d × 2d. Neuropsychiatric disturbances and seizures have been reported in some patients (H Stokvis et al, Am J Trop Med Hyg, 35:330, 1986).

[34] Albendazole or ivermectin have also been effective.

[35] In disseminated strongyloidiasis, thiabendazole therapy should be continued for at least five days. In immunocompromised patients it may be necessary to continue therapy or use other agents (see footnote 34).

[36] Niclosamide is effective for the treatment of *T. solium* but, since it causes disintegration of segments and release of viable eggs, its use creates a theoretical risk of causing cysticercosis. It should therefore be followed in three or four hours by a purge. Quinacrine is preferred by some clinicians because it expels *T. solium* intact. Others prefer praziquantel, which also kills larvae.

[37] Surgical resection of cysts is the treatment of choice. When surgery is contraindicated, or cysts rupture spontaneously during surgery, mebendazole (experimental for this purpose in the USA) can be tried (JF Wilson and RL Rausch, Ann Trop Med Parasitol, 76:165, 1982; ADM Bryceson et al, Trans R Soc Trop Med Hyg, 76:510, 1982). Albendazole has also been reported to be effective (DL Morris et al, JAMA, 253:2053, 1985). Flubendazole has also been used with some success (E Tellez-Giron et al, Am J Trop Med Hyg, 33:627, 1984). Praziquantel and albendazole will kill protoscolices and may be useful in case of spill during surgery.

[38] Surgical excision is the only reliable means of treatment although recent reports have been encouraging about use of albendazole or mebendazole (JF Wilson et al, Am J Trop Med Hyg, 37:162, 1987; A Davis et al, Bull WHO, 64:383, 1986.)

[39] Corticosteroids should be given for two to three days before and during praziquantel therapy. Praziquantel should not be used for ocular or spinal cord cysticercosis. Albendazole, 15 mg/kg × 30d, which can be repeated, has been used successfully (F Escobedo et al, Arch Intern Med, 147:738, 1987).

[40] In ocular toxoplasmosis, corticosteroids should also be used for anti-inflammatory effect on the eyes.

[41] Pyrimethamine is teratogenic in animals. To prevent hematological toxicity from pyrimethamine, it is advisable to give leucovorin (folinic acid), about 10 mg/day, either by injection or orally. Pyrimethamine alone 50–75 mg daily has been used to treat CNS toxoplasmosis after sulfonamide sensitivity develops. Pyrimethamine 25 mg/d plus clindamycin 1.2 to 2.4 gm/d in divided doses has also been used. In AIDS patients treatment should continue indefinitely.

[42] Every two to three days for infants. Most authorities would treat congenitally infected newborns for about one year.

[43] The efficacy of thiabendazole for trichinosis is not clearly established; it appears to be effective during the intestinal phase but its effect on larvae that have migrated is questionable. In the tissue phase, mebendazole 200–400 mg tid × 3 days, then 400–500 mg tid × 10 days, may be effective. Albendazole may also be effective for this indication.

[44] Sexual partners should be treated simultaneously. Outside the USA, ornidazole and tinidazole have been used for this condition. Metronidazole-resistant strains have been reported; higher doses of metronidazole for longer periods of time are sometimes effective against these strains.

TABLE 2. *(Continued)*

Infection	*Drug*	*Adult Dosage**	*Pediatric Dosage**
T. gambiense, T. rhodesiense (African trypanosomiasis, sleeping sickness)			
Hemolymphatic stage			
Drug of choice:[46]	Suramin[2]	100–200 mg (test dose) iv, then 1 gram iv on days 1, 3, 7, 14, and 21	20 mg/kg on days 1, 3, 7, 14 and 21
Alternative:	Pentamidine isethionate	4 mg/kg/d im × 10d	4 mg/kg/d im × 10d
Late disease with CNS involvement			
Drug of choice:[46]	Melarsoprol[2,47]	2–3.6 mg/kg/d iv × 3 doses; after 1 wk 3.6 mg/kg/d iv × 3 doses; repeat again after 10–21 days	18–25 mg/kg total over 1 mo. Initial dose of 0.36 mg/kg iv, increasing gradually to max. 3.6 mg/kg at intervals of 1–5d for total of 9–10 doses
Alternatives:	Tryparsamide	One injection of 30 mg/kg iv every 5d to total of 12 injections; may be repeated after 1 mo.	Unknown
	plus suramin[2]	One injection of 10 mg/kg iv every 5d to total of 12 injections; may be repeated after 1 mo.	
Visceral larva migrans[48]			
Drug of choice:[49]	Diethylcarbamazine[7]	2 mg/kg tid × 7–10d	2 mg/kg tid × 7–10d
OR	Thiabendazole	25 mg/kg bid × 5d (max. 3 grams/d)	25 mg/kg bid × 5d (max. 3 g/d)
Alternative:	Mebendazole[7]	200–400 mg/d × 5d[50]	
Whipworm, see Trichuriasis			
Wuchereria bancrofti, see Filariasis			

* The letter d indicates day.
[45] Limited data.
[46] In drug-resistant cases of *T. gambiense* infections, elflornithine (difluoromethylornithine, Merrell Dow) has been used successfully; field trials are now underway (H Taelman et al, Am J Med, 82:607, 1987; F Doua et al, Am J Trop Med Hyg 37:525, 1987; J Pepin et al, Lancet, 2:1431, 1987). It is highly effective in both CNS and non-CNS infections with *T. gambiense*.
[47] In frail patients, begin with as little as 18 mg and increase the dose progressively. Pretreatment with suramin has been advocated for debilitated patients.
[48] For severe symptoms or eye involvement, corticosteroids can be used in addition.
[49] Ivermectin and albendazole have been effective in some animal studies.
[50] One report of a cure using 1 gram tid for 21 days has been published (A Bekhti, Ann Intern Med, 100:463, 1984).
(From Ref. 5, with permission.)

Emetine is administered by deep intramuscular injection; oral administration is prevented by severe gastrointestinal irritation. Emetine is well absorbed from muscle and is excreted very slowly.[38] It can be detected in the urine for 1–2 months after completion of treatment. It is distributed to the spleen, kidney, and lung, but the highest concentrations are found in the liver, which enhances its activity in the treatment of amebic liver abscesses.[38] Negligible amounts are detected in the blood. Emetine acts by inhibiting protein synthesis in eukaryotic cells.[38,39]

Emetine is responsible for toxicity in multiple organs. Diarrhea, nausea, and vomiting are frequent. Muscle weakness, aching, tenderness, and stiffness are experienced by the majority of persons who receive a cumulative dose of 1300 mg.[40] The most serious untoward effects are cardiovascular. These include precordial pain, weakness, arrhythmias, hypotension, tachycardia, congestive heart failure, and occasionally death.[41] Electrocardiographic (ECG) changes are characterized by a prolonged Q-T interval, T-wave inversion, and S-T depression. The ECG tends to return to normal 1–2 weeks after cessation of therapy.[42] Emetine has direct toxic effects on skeletal and cardiac muscles.[43] Local toxicity at the site of injection includes muscle pain, tenderness, and stiffness. Less common are urticarial reactions. Persons receiving emetine require hospitalization and careful monitoring for signs of toxicity. Emetine is contraindicated in persons with cardiac and renal disease and is relatively contraindicated in children and pregnant women.

Dehydroemetine has a shorter half-life than emetine, as well as diminished frequency and severity of side effects.[56] It is also less potent then emetine, and higher doses must be used to obtain the desired therapeutic effect.

Iodoquinol

Iodoquinol (diiodohydroxyquin), a halogenated oxyquinoline (5,7-diiodo-8-quinolinol), is a luminally active agent used to eradicate cysts in persons with asymptomatic *E. histolytica* infection or after metronidazole administration in persons with invasive intestinal or extraintestinal disease. Iodoquinol is also recommended for the treatment of *Dientamoeba fragilis* and *B. hominis*, and it is used as an alternative drug for the treatment of *B. coli*.

Iodoquinol is available in 210- and 250-mg tablets. It is poorly absorbed and best tolerated if given with meals. The mechanism of action is not known. Reported side effects include headache, diarrhea, nausea, vomiting and abdominal pain, fever, and itching. Occasionally, the drug is associated with iodine dermatitis (iodine toxicoderma). The high iodine content (63 percent) can interfere with the results of thyroid function tests for months after completion of therapy. Iodoquinol is contraindicated in persons with iodine intolerance.

A related compound, iodochlorhydroxyquin***, which is better absorbed than iodoquinol, gained notoriety as a cause of subacute myelo-optic neuropathy. This syndrome and its relationship to iodochlorhydroxyquin were first described in Japan, where the syndrome occurred in near-epidemic proportions. The discontinuation of iodochlorhydroxyquin led to an almost immediate reduction in the number of cases of subacute myelo-optic neuropathy.[44] Optic nerve damage or inflammation and a peripheral neuropathy may occur with prolonged high doses of iodoquinol as well. The dosage regimen recommended for amebic disease (Table 2) avoids these complications, but the recommended doses and duration of therapy should never be exceeded.[21]

Diloxanide Furoate**

Diloxanide furoate, a substituted acetanilide, 4-(*N*-methyl-2,2-dichloroacetamido)phenyl-2-furoate, is a luminally active agent used for the treatment of asymptomatic *E. histolytica* infection.[45–48] It is also used to eradicate cysts of *E. polecki* after treatment with metronidazole. It is ineffective in the treatment of extraintestinal amebiasis. Diloxanide furoate is hydrolyzed by intestinal esterases releasing diloxanide, the absorbed form of the amebicide. Delayed or reduced absorption of the ester results in higher concentrations in the large intestine and the desired luminal effect.

Diloxanide furoate is formulated in 500-mg tablets. In experimental animals, 60–90 percent of the drug is excreted in the urine within 48 hours.[41] Excretion in the feces accounts for 4–9 percent. Diloxanide is amebicidal at low concentrations, but the mechanism of action is unknown. There are rarely serious side effects at the recommended dosage. The most common untoward effect is flatulence.[48] Mild gastrointestinal complaints may also occur. The low cost of the drug makes it an excellent alternative for the treatment of asymptomtic intestinal amebic infections in developing countries.

Paromomycin

Paromomycin, an aminoglycoside, is a luminally active, poorly absorbed durg that is used for the treatment of asymptomatic intestinal amebiasis.[49,50] It acts directly on amebae and has antibacterial activity in the colon.

Paromomycin is available in 250-mg capsules. Side effects are primarily gastrointestinal and include nausea, vomiting, abdominal cramps, and diarrhea in some patients. Paromomycin, like other aminoglycosides, is potentially ototoxic and nephrotoxic when administered parenterally. Very little is adsorbed from the gastrointestinal tract, but it is contraindicated in persons with renal failure. Paromomycin also has some activity against human tapeworms,[51] but it is rarely used for that purpose.

Quinacrine

Quinacrine (Fig. 2), 3-chloro-7-methoxy-9-(1-methyl-4-diethylaminobutylamino)acridine, a yellow dye with a 4-aminoquinoline radical linked to a benzene ring, is widely used for the treatment of giardiasis.[9,10,52–54] Many experts in the United States consider it the drug of choice for this disease (Table 2). The cure rate in adults is approximately 90 percent,[9] but it may be lower in children.[53] It is the least expensive of the three drugs that are commonly used to treat *G. lamblia*. Quinacrine is also active against adult tapeworms but has largely been replaced by niclosamide, which is less toxic. During World War II, quinacrine was used for malaria prophylaxis and treatment.

Quinacrine is available in 100-mg tablets. It is well absorbed from the gastrointestinal tract and is widely distributed throughout the body. Quinacrine can intercalate into DNA and inhibit nucleic acid synthesis.[55] Whether this relates to its antiparasitic activity is unknown. Quinacrine has strong tissue-binding properties and can be detected in urine for up to 2 months after cessation of therapy.

Data on toxicity were accumulated during the widespread use of quinacrine as an antimalarial.[56] Quinacrine has a bitter, unpleasant taste and can induce nausea and vomiting, especially in children. Other common side effects include headache and dizziness. At high doses, quinacrine can turn the skin and urine yellow. This effect is seen in 4–5 percent of persons treated for giardiasis.[10,57] The sclerae are usually spared. A bright yellow-green fluorescence under Wood's light confirms that the discoloration is due to quinacrine and not bilirubin. The yellow skin discoloration lasts for periods ranging from a few weeks to several months.

Uncommon side effects of quinacrine include skin rashes, fever, and reversible acute, toxic psychosis. The last occurs in 0.1–1.5 percent of persons receiving the drug and usually lasts for 2–4 weeks.[58] The mechanism is unknown. Quinacrine is contraindicated in patients with a history of psychosis. Very rarely, blood dyscrasias have been reported to follow treatment. Quinacrine is also contraindicated in pregnancy, since it readily crosses the placental barrier. Patients with psoriasis occasionally develop extensive exfoliative dermatitis and should not receive the drug.

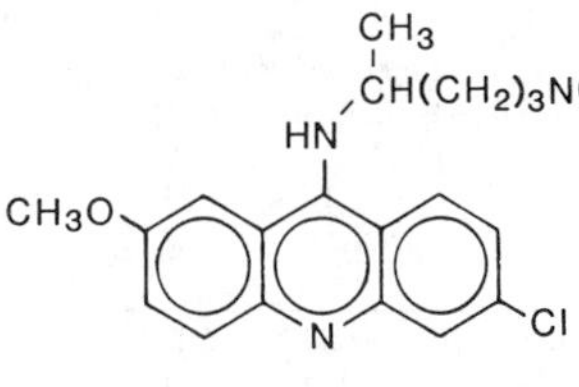

FIG. 2. Quinacrine.

There are two important potential drug interactions with quinacrine. First, like metronidazole, quinacrine has a disulfiram-like effect. Adult patients should be warned not to drink alcohol, and children taking quinacrine should not be given ethanol-containing medications. Second, quinacrine interferes with the metabolism of primaquine and may result in toxic levels of primaquine. The inhibitory effect on primaquine metabolism may last for up to 3 months after the last dose of quinacrine is administered.

Furazolidone

Furazolidone, 3-[(5-Nitro-2furanyl)methylene)-amino]-2-oxazolidinone, is a nitrofuran derivative. Like other nitrofurans, it acts by damaging DNA. It is the only anti-*Giardia* drug available as a liquid, and it is commonly used for the treatment of giardiasis in children.[53,59,60] Furazolidone also has some activity against *I. belli* and a variety of bacteria.[61]

Furazolidone is available as a suspension containing 25 mg/5 ml and 100-mg tablets. It is largely unabsorbed after oral administration.[61] Common side effects include nausea, vomiting, diarrhea, and fever. Some of the metabolites are brown and may discolor the urine. Other rare side effects are hypotension, urticaria, serum sickness, and hypersensitivity reactions. A mild to moderate hemolysis may occur in patients with glucose-6-phosphate dehydrogenase (G6PD) deficiency. As with metronidazole and quinacrine, alcohol should not be ingested because furazolidone has disulfiram-like activity. It is also a monoamine oxidase inhibitor. Furazolidone should not be administered to mothers who are breast-feeding their infants or given to neonates, since hemolytic anemia due to glutathione instability may occur.

DRUGS USED AGAINST MEMBERS OF THE PHYLUM APICOMPLEXA AND PNEUMOCYSTIS CARINII

Members of the phylum Apicomplexa pose substantial risks to people throughout the world. *Plasmodium* spp. continue to cause morbidity and mortality throughout the tropics. Attempts to eradicate malaria by mass residual insecticide spraying have failed, and there has been a resurgence of malaria in some areas.[62] Increasing resistance of *Plasmodium* spp. to prophylactic and therapeutic regimens has further complicated the situation. The four *Plasmodium* spp. that infect humans are responsible for 100–125 million estimated cases of malaria worldwide each year. It is estimated that between 0.7 and 1 million deaths annually in sub-Saharan Africa alone are due to malaria. As of 1984, 56 percent of the world's population lived in areas where malaria is a serious problem.[63]

As travel has increased, so has the exposure of nonimmune hosts to malaria. Every year approximately 1 million Americans travel to tropical or subtropical areas where they are at risk of acquiring malaria. Prophylaxis is effective, but the evolution of drug resistance among *Plasmodium falciparum* continues to pose problems.[64] The erythrocytic stage of malaria is the most sensitive to chemotherapy. The exoerythrocytic stage is difficult to treat, and the sporozoite stage is resistant to all known forms of chemotherapy.

Toxoplasma gondii infects people throughout the world.[65] It is an important cause of birth defects, and it has emerged as the most frequent opportunistic pathogen causing encephalitis in persons with AIDS.[66] *Cryptosporidium* spp. and *I. belli* are other coccidians that have emerged as important pathogens among persons with AIDS. They produce chronic diarrhea with weight loss in that setting. *Cryptosporidium* has increasingly been recognized as a cause of self-limited diarrhea in immunologically normal hosts as well.[67]

Another pathogen, *P. carinii*, which causes pneumonia in over 60 percent of persons with AIDS, has not yet been classified taxonomically.[68,69] Recent evidence suggests that it may be a fungus.[69a] Although not in the phyla Apicomplexa, its chemotherapy will be discussed here, since several drugs active against *P. carinii* are active against organisms within the Apicomplexa.

Aminoquinolines Used for the Prophylaxis and Treatment of Malaria

Chloroquine. Chloroquine (Fig. 3), 7-chloro-4-(4-diethylamino-1-methylbutylamino)-quinoline, the best known of the 4-aminoquinolines, has been the mainstay of antimalarial chemotherapy and prophylaxis (Tables 3 and 4). It is active against the erythrocytic stages of *Plasmodium vivax, Pl. ovale, Pl. malaria*, and, in a decreasing number of regions, *Pl. falciparum*.[62,70] The emergence of resistant strains of *Pl. falciparum* has been increasing steadily over the past 20 years.[71] The majority of strains in East Africa, Southeast Asia, and areas of South America are now chloroquine resistant. Since 1980 chloroquine resistance has become frequent in Central Africa, and reports of chloroquine resistance have come from West Africa.[72,73]

Chloroquine has also been used for the treatment of amebic liver abscess concurrently with emetine and for rheumatoid arthritis and systemic lupus erythematosus (SLE). It was once recommended for persons with *Babesia* infection, but it was found to be ineffective.[74]

Chloroquine phosphate is available as a bitter white medication, which is dispensed in tablets containing 250 or 500 mg (150 and 300-mg base, respectively). Chloroquine is rapidly absorbed after oral ingestion and is slowly excreted. The therapeutic blood concentration is reached within 2 or 3 hours. Chloroquine is widely distributed throughout the body but is relatively concentrated in the liver, spleen, kidneys, and erythrocytes. It is metabolized by alkylation in the liver, but approximately 50 percent of the drug is excreted in the urine. The half-life is 4 days, which allows for once-a-week prophylaxis.[75,76] Approximately 50 percent of chloroquine is protein bound. The renal status of the patient does not affect the amount used for acute malaria, but prophylactic doses need to be reduced for those with reduced renal function.[76]

Chloroquine is concentrated in parasitized erythrocytes 100-fold more than in nonparasitized ones.[77] In erythrocytes with schizonts, the concentration of chloroquine is 600-fold greater than in plasma. Chloroquine is toxic for the asexual erythrocytic stages of *Plasmodium* spp. It has a marked and rapid effect on the hemoglobin-containing digestive vesicles of intraerythrocytic parasites. After therapy, there is fusion of adjacent vesicles, followed by sequestration of the fused vesicles and their malaria pigment into a large autophagic vacuole.[78,79] Chloroquine binds with high affinity to ferriprotoporphyrin IX, which is a product of hemoglobin degradation by the parasite, and to its oxo-dimer. Complexing of chloroquine to this metabolite of hemoglobin may prevent it from being detoxified, and the complex is known to damage membranes. This complex may be responsible for the killing of intraerythrocytic parasites, but the hypothesis has not been proven. At high concentrations, chloroquine also intercalates into DNA, but it is doubtful that this is the mechanism of its antimalarial activity. It can also inhibit ornithine decarboxylase.[80]

Recently, attention has focused on the concentration of chloroquine in the acid-vesicle system of susceptible *Pl. falciparum*.[81,82] It is thought that chloroquine may thus interfere with the endocytosis and proteolysis of hemoglobin and the intracellular targeting of lysosomal enzymes. Resistant parasites transport chloroquine out of intraparasitic compartments more rapidly than susceptible strains and maintain lower chloroquine concentrations in their acid vesicles.[82] There is experimental

TABLE 3. Drugs Used in the Prophylaxis and Presumptive Treatment of Malaria

	Prophylaxis		*Presumptive Treatment for Travelers to Areas of Chloroquine Resistance*	
Drug	*Adult Dose*	*Pediatric Dose*		
Chloroquine phosphate (Aralen[a])	300 mg base (500 mg salt) orally, once/week	5 mg/kg base (8.3 mg/kg salt) orally, once/week, up to maximum adult dose of 300 mg base	Chloroquine is not recommended for the presumptive treatment of malaria acquired in areas of known chloroquine resistance.	
Hydroxychloroquine sulfate (Plaquenil[a])	310 mg base (400 mg salt) orally, once/week	5 mg/kg base (6.5 mg/kg salt) orally, once/week, up to maximum adult dose of 310 mg base	Hydroxychloroquine is not recommended for the presumptive treatment of malaria acquired in areas of known chloroquine resistance.	
Doxycycline	100 mg orally, once/day	>8 years of age: 2 mg/kg of body weight orally, once/day up to adult dose of 100 mg/day	Tetracyclines are not recommended for the presumptive treatment of malaria.	
Proguanil (Paludrine[a])	200 mg orally, once/day, in combination with weekly chloroquine	<2 yrs: 50 mg/day 2–6 yrs: 100 mg/day 7–10 yrs: 150 mg/day >10 yrs: 200 mg/day	Proguanil is not recommended for the presumptive treatment of malaria.	
			Adult Dose	*Pediatric Dose*
Pyrimethamine-sulfadoxine[b] (Fansidar[a])	1 tablet (25 mg pyrimethamine and 500 mg sulfadoxine) orally, once/week	2–11 mos: ⅛ tab/wk 1–3 yrs: ¼ tab/wk 4–8 yrs: ½ tab/wk 9–14 yrs: ¾ tab/wk >14 yrs: 1 tab/wk	3 tablets (75 mg pyrimethamine and 1,500 mg sulfadoxine), orally, as a single dose	2–11 mos: ¼ tab 1–3 yrs: ½ tab 4–8 yrs: 1 tab 9–14 yrs: 2 tabs >14 yrs: 3 tabs as a single dose
Primaquine	15 mg base (26.3 mg salt) orally, once/day for 14 days, or 45 mg base (79 mg salt) orally, once/week for 8 weeks	0.3 mg/kg base (0.5 mg/kg salt) orally, once/day for 14 days, or 0.9 mg/kg base (1.5 mg/kg salt) orally, once/week for 8 weeks	Primaquine is only recommended for use after leaving an endemic area to prevent relapses of *Plasmodium vivax* and *P. ovale*.	

[a] Use of trade names is for identification only and does not imply endorsement by the U.S. Department of Health and Human Services or the Public Health Service.
[b] Not usually recommended for prophylaxis. See text.
(From Centers for Disease Control.[115])

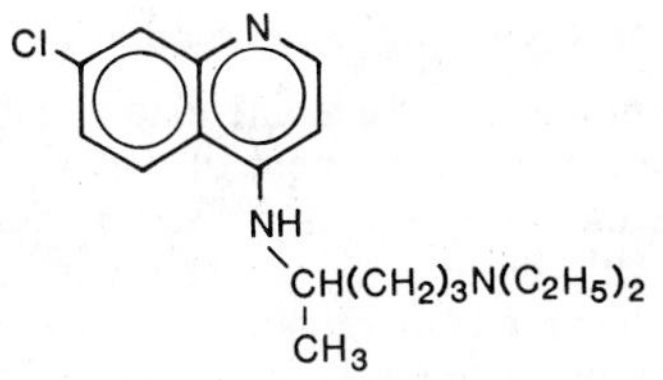

FIG. 3. Chloroquine.

evidence that this can be reversed with calcium channel blockers, raising the theoretical possibility that chloroquine plus an additional agent that blocks the efflux of chloroquine might be effective against chloroquine-resistant strains.[83]

Chloroquine is a relatively safe chemoprophylactic and therapeutic drug when used at the recommended doses for malaria. Oral administration is preferred. Occasional temporary side effects include headache, nausea, vomiting, blurred vision, dizziness, fatigue, and confusion.[70,76] Some Africans experience pruritis, which responds to an antihistamine. Rare side effects include depigmentation of the hair, corneal opacities, weight loss, insomnia, leukopenia, myalgias and exacerbation of psoriasis, and eczema or other exfoliative dermatoses. Extremely rare reactions include blood dyscrasias, toxic psychosis, and photophobia. Permanent retinal damage is rarely associated with malaria prophylaxis and treatment but has occurred with long-term, high-dose therapy given to persons with collagen vascular diseases.[84] Chloroquine is contraindicated in persons with retinal disease, psoriasis, or porphyria.

Chloroquine can also be given by intravenous infusion, but it must be administered slowly and with great caution.[70,85] Respiratory depression, hypotension, cardiovascular collapse, and seizures can follow excessively rapid parenteral administration. These are apparently due to toxic levels of chloroquine in the circulation. Heart block and cardiac arrest are thought to be due to a direct toxic effect on the myocardium at high plasma concentrations. It is recommended that oral administration be substituted for parenteral administration as soon as possible.[70] Deaths from chloroquine toxicity also occur in accidental ingestion by children, in adults who habitually self-medicate, and in those who attempt suicide. The ingestion of 5 g of chloroquine is fatal unless treatment is initiated immediately with mechanical ventilation, diazepam, and epinephrine.[86]

Chloroquine has been implicated in severe cochleovestibular abnormalities in the fetus of a mother taking high doses for the treatment of SLE.[87] There has been no such association between chloroquine administered in antimalarial doses and fetal abnormalities.[76]

Amodiaquine*.** Amodiaquine is another 4-aminoquinolone, which has been used for more than 40 years. Its mechanism of action is thought to be the same as that of chloroquine, although it has activity against some strains of *Pl. falciparum*

TABLE 4. Treatment of Malaria

Drug		*Adult Dosage*	*Pediatric Dosage*
All *Plasmodium* except chloroquine-resisttant *P. falciparum*			
Oral			
Drug of choice:	Chloroquine phosphate[1,2]	600 mg base (1 gram), then 300 mg base (500 mg) 6 hrs later, then 300 mg base (500 mg)/d × 2d	10 mg base/kg (max. 600 mg base), then 5 mg base/kg 6 hrs later, then 5 mg base/kg/d × 2d
Parenteral			
Drug of choice:	Quinine dihydrochloride[3]	600 mg in 300 ml normal saline iv over 2 to 4 hrs; repeat q8h until oral therapy can be started (max. 1800 mg/d)	25 mg/kg/d; give ⅓ of daily dose over 2 to 4 hrs; repeat q8h until oral therapy can be started (max. 1800 mg/d)
OR	Quinidine gluconate[4,5]		
Alternative:	Chloroquine HCl[2]	200 mg base (250 mg) im q6h if oral therapy cannot be started	Not recommended
Chloroquine-resistant *P. falciparum*			
Oral			
Drugs of choice:	Quinine sulfate[6,7]	650 mg tid × 3–7d	25 mg/kg/d in 3 doses × 3d
	plus pyrimethamine	25 mg bid × 3d	<10 kg: 6.25 mg/d × 3d 10–20 kg: 12.5 mg/d × 3d 20–40 kg: 25 mg/d × 3d
	plus sulfadiazine	500 mg qid × 5d	100–200 mg/kg/d in 4 doses × 5d (max. 2 grams/d)
Alternatives:	Quinine sulfate[7,8]	650 mg tid × 7d	25 mg/kg/d in 3 doses × 3d
	plus tetracycline	250 mg qid × 7d	5 mg/kg qid × 7d
Parenteral			
Drug of choice:	Quinine dihydrochloride[3]	same as above	same as above
OR	Quinidine gluconate[4,5]		
Prevention of relapses: *P. vivax and P. ovale* only			
Drug of choice:	Primaquine phosphate[9]	15 mg base (26.3 mg)/d × 14d or 45 mg base (79 mg)/wk × 8 wks	0.3 mg base/kg/d × 14d

[1] If chloroquine phosphate is not available, hydroxychloroquine sulfate is as effective; 400 mg of hydroxychloroquine sulfate is equivalent to 500 mg of chloroquine phosphate.
[2] In *P. falciparum* malaria, if the patient has not shown a response to conventional doses of chloroquine in 48–72 hours, parasitic resistance to this drug should be considered. Intramuscular injection of chloroquine is painful and can cause abscesses.
[3] Available in the USA only from the Centers for Disease Control, telephone 404-488-4046 (nights, weekends, or holidays call 404-639-2888). *P. falciparum* infections from Southeast Asia may require a loading dose of 20 mg/kg (NJ White et al, Am J Trop Med Hyg, 32:1, 1983).
[4] Considered an investigational drug for this condition by the U.S. Food and Drug Administration.
[5] Optimal dosage for treatment of malaria is currently under investigation. For up-to-date information, telephone the Centers for Disease Control (daytime 404-488-4046; nights, weekends, holidays 404-639-2888). ECG monitoring is necessary to detect arrhythmias. Some experts consider quinidine more effective than quinine.
[6] Quinine alone will usually control an attack of resistant *P. falciparum* but, in a substantial number of infections, particularly with strains from Southeast Asia, it fails to prevent recurrence; addition of pyrimethamine and sulfadiazine or tetracycline lowers the rate of recurrence. The duration of quinine sulfate therapy depends on the geographic site.
[7] For treatment of *P. falciparum* infections acquired in Thailand, quinine should be given for seven days instead of three, combined with seven days of tetracycline. Ref. 5 recommends quinine sulfate for 3 days.
[8] Quinine plus tetracycline may be the regimen of choice in areas such as Thailand where resistance to pyrimethamine plus sulfonamides is common.
[9] Primaquine phosphate can cause hemolytic anemia, especially in patients whose red cells are deficient in glucose-6-phosphate dehydrogenase. This deficiency is most common in Blacks, Orientals, and Mediterranean peoples. Patients should be screened for G-6-PD deficiency before treatment. Primaquine should not be used during pregnancy.
(From Ref. 5, with permission.)

resistant to chloroquine. Amodiaquine is not available in the United States. It was briefly recommended for travelers to areas with chloroquine-resistant *Pl. falciparum*, but that recommendation was quickly withdrawn when reports of fatal agranulocytosis appeared in persons taking it as weekly antimalarial prophylaxis.[88,89] Amodiaquine is no longer recommended for malaria prophylaxis or therapy.

Primaquine. Primaquine (Fig. 4) is an 8-aminoquinoline, 8-(4-amino-1-methylbutylamino)-6-methoxyquinoline. It is the only drug available that is effective in eradicating the exoerythrocytic, hypnozoite forms of *Pl. vivax* and *Pl. ovale* in the liver.[90] It has some activity against the asexual blood stages of *Pl. vivax*, but this action is not sufficient to allow it to be used alone for suppressive prophylaxis. The 8-aminoquinolines also have gametocytocidal activity against all four *Plasmodium* spp. that infect humans, but this is not of clinical significance. Primaquine is used after chloroquine to provide a radical cure for persons with acute *Pl. vivax* or *Pl. ovale* malaria or after chloroquine prophylaxis in persons exposed to these forms of malaria.[91] The relapse rate of persons infected with *Pl. vivax* is low after primaquine therapy, except for those with some strains of *Pl. vivax* from the southwestern Pacific, such as the Chesson strain, which requires higher doses given either daily or at weekly intervals.[92,93]

Primaquine phosphate is supplied in tablets containing 26.3 mg of the salt, which is equivalent to 15 mg of the base. It has a bitter taste, and may be crushed and added to sweet liquid or fruit to make it more palatable. The dosage is usually expressed in terms of the base. Primaquine is readily absorbed when taken orally. Plasma concentrations reach a peak at 6 hours and decline to undetectable levels by 24 hours.

Primaquine interferes with the mitochondrial function of *Plasmodium*. It is fully active only after metabolism by the host, but the nature of the active metabolites is not clear. Based on studies with pamoquine***, the first of this series of drugs, the metabolites are thought to affect both the mitochondrial electron transport chain and pyrimidine synthesis.[78]

The major toxicity with primaquine is hemolysis in persons with G6PD deficiency.[94,95] G6PD deficiency is rare in whites, but there are more than 100 million people worldwide with this deficiency (1 percent of males in the Middle East, 5 percent of Chinese males, and 10 percent of black males). Persons from these groups should be tested for G6PD deficiency before primaquine is prescribed. Similarly, the administration of primaquine should be discontinued if darkening of the urine or a fall in hematocrit is noted. For persons with the more mild African form of G6PD deficiency, a dose of 45 mg (base) weekly for 8 weeks has been used.[92] For patients with the more severe Mediterranean variety, 30 mg weekly for 30 weeks has been recommended.[95]

Apart from the potential for hemolysis, primaquine is usually well tolerated.[76] Abdominal cramps, epigastric distress, and nausea occur in some patients. Mild anemia, cyanosis (methemoglobinemia), and leukocytosis are observed in some persons given higher doses. Rare complications include granulocytopenia or agranulocytosis, hypertension, and arrhythmia.

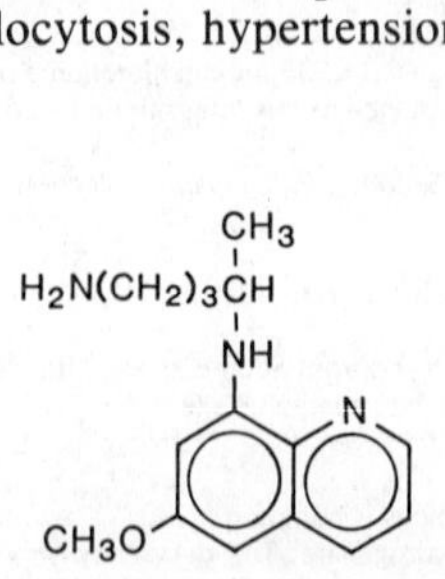

FIG. 4. Primaquine.

Cinchona Alkaloids, Quinine, and Quinidine

Quinine. Quinine (Fig. 5), a cinchona alkaloid, was the first successful agent for the treatment of malaria.[70] It is effective against the asexual blood stages of *Plasmodium* spp. With the introduction of chloroquine, the use of quinine fell dramatically, but with the widespread emergence of chloroquine-resistant *Pl. falciparum*, quinine has once again become widely used.[70] Only in Thailand has progressively decreased sensitivity to quinine been a problem. Quinine acts rapidly against asexual erythrocytic stages of all four *Plasmodium* spp. that infect humans.

Quinine sulfate is supplied as 260- and 325-mg tablets and in capsules of 130, 200, 260, 300, and 325 mg. The tablets have a very bitter taste. Quinine is rapidly absorbed after oral administration and reaches peak levels in 1–3 hours. Peak serum concentrations after a dose of 10 mg/kg are 7–17 μg/ml; side effects can be seen at concentrations above 10 μg/ml.[76] Quinine is formulated for parenteral use as quinine hydrochloride** in 2-ml ampules containing 300 mg/ml. The parenteral preparation is available in the United States only through the Centers for Disease Control. Intravenous quinidine, its dextrostereoisomer, is effective and available in virtually all hospitals, It is usually used instead.

Quinine is metabolized in the liver and excreted in the urine, mainly as metabolites.[96] Only 20 percent of the drug is excreted unchanged.[97] It is not as avidly bound to tissues as chloroquine and has a shorter half-life of 5–15 hours. Monitoring blood levels is recommended for persons with impaired renal or hepatic function, and dose reduction is necessary in severe renal failure.[98]

The exact mechanism of action as an antimalarial is unknown, but quinine, like chloroquine, appears to act at the level of the hemoglobin-containing digestive vesicles of the intraerythrocytic parasite. Quinine is a competitive inhibitor of pigment clumping by chloroquine,[78] and malaria pigment first becomes translucent and then disappears with therapy. Quinine also intercalates into DNA, but this does not appear to be its primary mode of action.

Quinine has the poorest therapeutic-to-toxic ratio of all of the antimalarial drugs.[99] The side effects of quinine are collectively referred to as *cinchonism* and include tinnitis, decreased hearing, headache, dysphoria, nausea, vomiting, and mild visual disturbances.[70,99] These alterations are dose related and reversible. Other less common side effects include skin rashes, including urticaria, angioedema of the face, pruritis, agranulocytosis, and, rarely, massive hemolysis in persons with falciparum malaria (blackwater fever). Quinine can cause respiratory depression in patients with myasthenia gravis. It has a curare-like effect on skeletal muscle and has been useful in the treatment of painful nocturnal leg cramps. Other potential adverse reactions include hypoglycemia in patients with high *Pl. falciparum* parasitemia. This is due to the parasites' consumption of glucose and the release of insulin from the pancreas by quinine.[100] It responds to the administration of intravenous glucose. Quinine causes hemolysis in patients with G6PD deficiency. It can stimulate uterine contractions and may produce abortion if given in high doses. However, quinine has been used

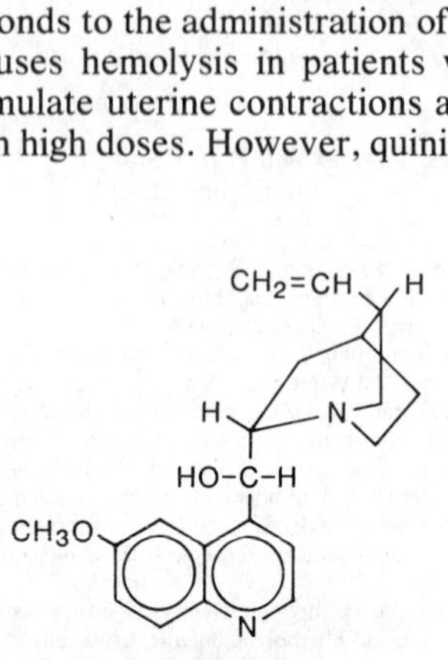

FIG. 5. Quinine.

successfully to treat seriously ill women with malaria in the third trimester of pregnancy.[101] Quinine must be used cautiously by the intravenous route, since rapid intravenous infusion may cause shock due to myocardial depression and peripheral vasodilatation. Overdoses are associated with convulsions, coma, delirium, depressed respiration, circulatory collapse, and death.

Quinidine. Quinidine is the dextrostereoisomer of quinine. It is used in the United States on an investigational basis for the parenteral treatment of chloroquine-resistant falciparum malaria in persons who cannot take oral quinine. A major advantage of parenteral quinidine over parenteral quinine is that quinidine is available in virtually every hospital because of its role in the treatment of cardiac arrhythmias. Quinidine gluconate has been successfully used to treat severe malaria in children and adults unable to take oral medications.[102,103]

Quinidine gluconate is available for intravenous administration. The half-life of quinidine is 12.8 hours. ECG changes including prolonged Q-Tc intervals are common, but life-threatening arrhythmias are rare if proper doses are used. Hypotension may occur if the infusion is too rapid. The rate of infusion, blood pressure, and ECGs of persons receiving intravenous quinidine should be monitored closely.[104]

4-Quinoline-Carbinolamines (Quinoline Methanols): Mefloquine***

Mefloquine (Fig. 6) is a quinolone-methanol derived chemically from quinine. Mefloquine was the result of a search for a new antimalarial drug by researchers at the Walter Reed Army Institute of Research.[70,71] Like quinine and chloroquine, mefloquine is a blood schizontocidal drug and has no effect on exoerythrocytic schizonts or gametocytes.[77] Used as a single dose, it has been effective against all *Plasmodium* spp., including chloroquine-resistant and pyrimethamine-sulfadoxime-resistant isolates of *Pl. falciparum*.[105–108] West African strains of *Pl. falciparum* appear less susceptible to mefloquine in vitro than Southeast Asian strains.[109] A unified effort has been made to restrict its use for treatment and prophylaxis to areas with chloroquine-resistant *Pl. falciparum*. It has not yet been licensed for use in the United States.

Mefloquine is available only for oral administration. Administered in tablet form, it is slowly and incompletely absorbed.[110] Mefloquine is widely distributed in the body, and 99 percent of the drug is protein bound. It has a long half-life in humans, ranging from 6 to 23 days, with a mean of 14 days. It is extensively metabolized and excreted through bile and feces. Mefloquine concentrates on red blood cell membranes and seems to interfere with the food vacuoles of *Plasmodium* in a manner similar to that of quinine.[111] It has been administered as a suspension via a nasogastric tube to unconscious patients with cerebral malaria. Absorption was rapid, with an absorption half-life of 1.5 hours. Plasma mefloquine levels were over 200 ng/ml within 3 hours.[112] While intravenous quinidine is usually the drug of choice for severe malaria in patients who cannot take oral medications, mefloquine through a nasogastic tube is necessary in areas where quinine resistance is encountered (e.g., Thailand).[112] Mefloquine cannot be administered parenterally because it causes intense local irritation.

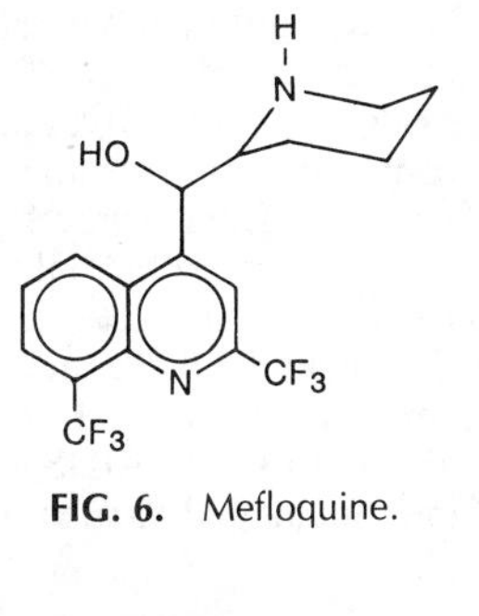

FIG. 6. Mefloquine.

Mefloquine is generally well tolerated. Large amounts can produce nausea and dizziness. Sinus bradycardia has been observed in approximately 7 percent of persons treated with this drug. The heart rate returns to normal within 2 weeks. Patients have been asymptomatic, and ECGs have revealed no sign of myocardial damage.[113] Repeated high doses have caused histologic abnormalities in the retinas of experimental animals.

Tetracycline and Doxycycline

Tetracycline has been used with quinine to treat acute falciparum malaria in areas such as Thailand where *Pl. falciparum* is resistant to pyrimethamine, sulfonamides, and chloroquine and has decreased susceptibility to quinine.[114] Doxycycline, a long-acting tetracycline, has been used prophylactically in these regions. It has not been as thoroughly evaluated as other prophylactic drugs. The Centers for Disease Control recommend the use of daily doxycycline alone[115]; others advise using doxycycline with weekly chloroquine to provide optimal protection against *Pl. vivax*.[5]

Tetracyclines are well absorbed orally. Their pharmacology is discussed in Chapter 23. They inhibit protein synthesis in prokaryotic ribosomes, and it is likely that they affect parasite protein synthesis as well.[78] The most common untoward effects are gastrointestinal. Photosensitivity occurs in approximately 3 percent of recipients and is a potential problem for travelers to the tropics. Candida vaginitis can also complicate tetracycline use. Finally, the tetracyclines are not recommended during pregnancy or for children less than 8 years of age because they are concentrated in bone and teeth and may cause dental staining, hypoplasia of dental enamel, and impaired bone growth in young children.

Artemisinine (Qinghaosu)***

Artemisinine is a sesquiterpene lactone derived from the wormwood plant *Artemisia annua*.[70,77] It has been used as a traditional medication by the Chinese for the treatment of malaria and has activity against chloroquine-resistant *Pl. falciparum* in humans.

The mode of action is poorly understood but appears to be unique to this group of drugs. Artemisinine is thought to act primarily on the integrity of the parasite's membrane. The first biochemical effect, cessation of protein synthesis, is observed within an hour of exposure. Resistance to artemisinine in *Plasmodium yoelii* has been produced in mice.[77] Troublesome was the observation that artemisinine-resistant parasites also displayed marked cross-resistance to chloroquine, quinine, and mefloquine, possibly due to a modification of the membrane composition of the parasite. The use of artemisinine or related compounds for the treatment of chloroquine-resistant falciparum malaria is still investigational.

Dihydrofolate Reductase Inhibitors and Sulfonamides

The diaminopyrimidine dihydrofolate reductase inhibitors, pyrimethamine and trimethoprim, have been used alone or, more commonly, in conjunction with sulfonamides for the prevention and treatment of malaria,[78,116] *I. belli*,[117] *P. carinii* pneumonia,[68,69,118–120] and toxoplasmosis.[121–125] They act at sequential steps in the folic acid cycle. *Plasmodium* spp. and presumably other sensitive parasites carry out pyrimidine synthesis de novo, in which reduced folic acid derivatives are essential cofactors. Unlike mammalian cells, these parasites cannot use preformed pyrimidines obtained through salvage pathways. Pyrimethamine is more active than trimethoprim in inhibiting the dihydrofolate reductases of *Plasmodium* spp. and *T. gondii*.

Conversely, trimethoprim has greater activity against bacteria and has been widely used for the treatment of *P. carinii* and *I. belli*. Both of these drugs can inhibit mammalian dihydrofolate reductase when used at high concentrations. This is more of a problem with pyrimethamine than with trimethoprim. In most instances, a sulfonamide is administered concurrently to inhibit a second step in the folic acid metabolic pathway.

Recent studies indicate that trimetrexate, a low molecular weight, lipid-soluble dihydrofolate reductase inhibitor, is active against *P. carinii*[126] and *T. gondii*.[127] Folinic acid has been used with trimetrexate to minimize its inhibitory effects on bone marrow. Development of new dihydrofolate reductase inhibitors that are preferentially active against protozoal enzymes is now underway.

Pyrimethamine and Short-Acting Sulfonamides. Pyrimethamine (Fig. 7), a 2,4-diaminopyrimidine, has been used on a weekly basis for malaria prophylaxis and with sulfadiazine and quinine for the treatment of chloroquine-resistant *Pl. falciparum*.[5] The usefulness of pyrimethamine with a sulfonamide has been limited by the emergence of resistant *Pl. falciparum* and *Pl. vivax*. Pyrimethamine and sulfadiazine or trisulfapyrimidines are the treatment of choice for toxoplasmosis. The majority of persons who acquire toxoplasmosis have self-limited disease and do not require treatment. In immunocompromised persons, including those with AIDS, toxoplasmic encephalitis is life-threatening. Therapy with high doses of pyrimethamine and sulfonamides is recommended for prolonged periods of time.[121,123] Congenital toxoplasmosis is also treated with pyrimethamine and sulfonamides.[124,125] The optimal treatment for acute toxoplasmosis during pregnancy is uncertain; pyrimethamine is contraindicated, at least for the first trimester, and sulfonamides cannot be used close to the time of delivery because they displace bilirubin from binding sites on albumin. Spiramycin is an alternative, but it is available in the United States only with special approval from the FDA.[128]

Pyrimethamine is well absorbed orally; the half-life is 4–6 days.[129] It is extensively metabolized; less than 3 percent of the drug is excreted unchanged in the urine in 24 hours. Pyrimethamine acts preferentially to inhibit the parasite's dihydrofolate reductase. It mimics dihydrofolate, competing with this metabolite to inhibit the enzyme. Pyrimethamine is approximately 1000-fold more active against the parasite than the host's dihydrofolate reductase.[130]

Pyrimethamine is very well tolerated at a dose of 25 mg/week, which has been used for malaria prophylaxis. Blood dyscrasias, rash, vomiting, seizures, and shock are all rare side effects.[76] Bone marrow suppression with neutropenia, anemia, and thrombocytopenia are seen with the higher doses used for the treatment of toxoplasmosis (25 mg/day). Careful follow-up with complete blood counts is necessary, but concurrent administration of folinic acid usually prevents these complications. Pyrimethamine is teratogenic in animals and is contraindicated during the first 16 weeks of pregnancy.[131,132] It has been used to treat pregnant women with primary toxoplasmosis after this period, but concern remains about its safety. Some experts have argued that there has not been unequivocal documentation of pyrimethamine-associated birth defects at the dose levels used for malaria prophylaxis.[133,134]

Sulfonamides decrease the activity of dihydropteroate synthetase and reduce the binding of *p*-aminobenzoic acid (PABA) to this enzyme in several members of the Apicomplexa. The sulfonamides are described in detail in Chapter 29. They are well absorbed orally. The most common untoward effects are allergic reactions and gastrointestinal complaints. Allergic reactions include fever and rash. Less common are toxic epidermal necrolysis, erythema multiforme, Stevens-Johnson syndrome, hepatitis, pneumonitis, bone marrow depression, and serum sickness.[135]

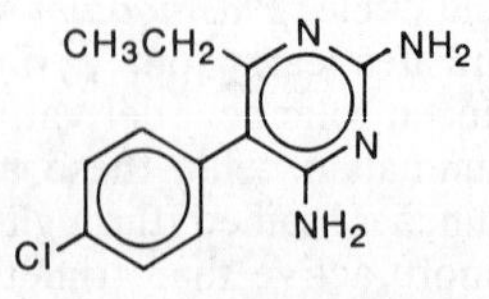

FIG. 7. Pyrimethamine.

Untoward effects are encountered in 60 percent of persons with AIDS treated for toxoplasmic encephalitis[122] with pyrimethamine and a sulfonamide. These effects include fever, skin rashes, bone marrow suppression, and hepatotoxicity. When these effects occur, pyrimethamine or an alternative investigational drug such as trimetrexate or spiramycin has been used as a single agent, but their effectiveness has not been well documented.

Fansidar (Pyrimethamine and Sulfadoxine). Fansidar, which consists of pyrimethamine 25 mg and sulfadoxine 500 mg, was previously recommended as prophylaxis for travelers to areas with chloroquine-resistant *Pl. falciparium*.[116] It is seldom indicated for prophylaxis now because it has been associated with life-threatening allergic reactions. In addition, Fansidar resistance has emerged in many areas. Fansidar has been administered to prevent *P. carinii* pneumonia in patients with AIDS, but the risk of serious untoward allergic reactions has limited its acceptance.[136]

Sulfadoxine, like pyrimethamine, is well absorbed from the gastrointestinal tract. Its half-life is 5–9 days.[129] The severe reactions observed with Fansidar have been attributed to sulfadoxine. Fatalities with prophylactic Fansidar have occurred in 1 in 11,000 to 1 in 26,000 users.[137,138] In 1984, American travelers who took Fansidar as weekly malaria prophylaxis in Kenya were as likely to die from Fansidar toxicity as from malaria. Most of the severe cutaneous reactions, including toxic epidermal necrolysis, erythema multiforme, and the Stevens-Johnson syndrome, have occurred soon after the start of prophylaxis, usually within the first 5 weeks of therapy.[137,138] Other serious but unusual side effects with sulfadoxine include serum sickness, bone marrow suppression, hepatitis, hepatic granuloma, and pneumonitis.[116] No fatal reactions have yet been reported when Fansidar (three tablets in a single dose) has been used for the treatment of chloroquine-resistant falciparum malaria. It is still prescribed as empiric treatment for persons who develop symptoms of malaria abroad and cannot promptly obtain medical evaluation.[5]

Pyrimethamine-Sulfadoxime-Mefloquine (Fansimef).*** The combination of pyrimethamine, sulfadoxine, and mefloquine has been used for the treatment of chloroquine-resistant *Pl. falciparum*.[107,114,139,140] The goal is to reduce the likelihood of developing further resistance. This combination, formulated as Fansimef[140] (pyrimethamine 25 mg, sulfadoxime 500 mg, and mefloquine 250 mg), has also been used prophylactically, but has the potential for the severe allergic cutaneous reactions observed with sulfadoxime.

Trimethoprim-Sulfamethoxazole (Cotrimoxazole). The combination of trimethoprim-sulfamethoxazole, formulated at a ratio of 1:5, is the treatment of choice for *P. carinii*.[68,69,118–120,141] The response rate of patients treated for *P. carinii* pneumonia is 80–85 percent and is comparable to that with pentamidine. It has been postulated that trimethoprim-sulfamethoxazole has a static rather than a microbicidal effect on *P. carinii*.[142] Daily[143] or intermittent[144] prophylactic trimethoprim-sulfamethoxazole has been shown to decrease the incidence of *P. carinii* infection among immunocompromised children and has been proposed for use with patients with AIDS who tolerate the drug. Trimethoprim-sulfamethoxazole has also been used effectively to treat *I. belli* infection in AIDS patients, but relapses are common even after high-dose, prolonged therapy.[117]

Both trimethoprim and sulfamethoxazole are well absorbed when administered orally. Peak blood levels are reached in 1–4 hours. The half-lives are similar: 10–12 hours for trimethoprim and 9–11 hours for sulfamethoxazole.[135] Excretion is through the kidney; renal failure prolongs the half-lives of both drugs. Trimethoprim has greater lipid solubility than sulfamethoxazole, and its apparent volume of distribution is five to six times greater. As a result, the drugs are formulated at a trimethoprim/sulfamethoxazole ratio of 1:5. Single-strength tablets contain 80 mg trimethoprim and 400 mg sulfamethoxazole; double-strength tablets have 160 mg trimethoprim and 800 mg sulfamethoxazole. It is also available in suspension for oral use containing 40 mg trimethoprim and 200 mg sulfamethoxazole per 5 ml for children. For intravenous use, trimethoprim-sulfamethoxazole is available as a solution containing 16 mg trimethoprim and 80 mg sulfamethoxazole per milliliter.

In patients without AIDS, common side effects include gastrointestinal upset (4 percent) and skin reactions (3 percent).[145] Rare adverse reactions include agranulocytosis, aplastic anemia, acute interstitial nephritis, Stevens-Johnson syndrome, jaundice, headaches, depression, and hallucinations.[146] Malnourished individuals on prolonged therapy may require concomitant therapy with folinic acid to prevent megaloblastic anemia. The drug combination is not recommended during pregnancy.[135]

For unknown reasons, patients with AIDS have an unusually high incidence of severe adverse reactions when given trimethoprim-sulfamethoxazole.[69] Approximately 65 percent of AIDS patients experience significant drug-related symptoms, half of which are severe enough to result in discontinuation of therapy.[68,69,147–149] These adverse reactions include neutropenia, fever, and rashes in one-third of these patients and thrombocytopenia, intolerable gastrointestinal effects, and hepatitis in one-tenth.[148,149] Prophylaxis against *P. carinii* is likely to be effective in this group but is often impossible because of the frequency of side effects.

Dapsone and Pyrimethamine or Trimethoprim. Dapsone, a sulfone that has been widely used in the treatment of leprosy, is used outside the United States in combination with pyrimethamine as prophylaxis against malaria. Maloprim, a combination of pyrimethamine 25 mg and dapsone 100 mg, has been used weekly for malaria prophylaxis. More recently, dapsone has been used with trimethoprim for the treatment of *P. carinii* pneumonia[150,151] and for its prevention.[152] When used with trimethoprim for the treatment of nonmoribund AIDS patients with *P. carinii*, the combination appears as effective as and less toxic than trimethoprim-sulfamethoxazole.[150,151]

Like the sulfonamides, dapsone interferes with folic acid metabolism by competitively inhibiting the enzyme dihydropteroate synthetase. Dapsone is available in 25-mg and 500-mg tablets. It is well absorbed after oral administration and is widely distributed in body tissues.[153] About 70–80 percent of the drug is bound to plasma protein. After acetylation and deacetylation, the drug is excreted in the urine as glucuronide or sulfate conjugates. The half-life is variable but averages 25–27 hours.[154] Serious side effects of dapsone include hemolytic anemia, methemoglobinemia, and bone marrow suppression. Very rarely, when maloprim has been used in high doses, the agranulocytosis has been fatal.[155] Uncommon side effects include peripheral neuropathy, anorexia, vomiting, vertigo, blurred vision, tinnitis, fever, headache, pruritis, psychosis, hematuria, and skin rash. Severe skin rashes occur in some AIDS patients given dapsone and trimethoprim; some resolve after the trimethoprim dose is reduced. Trimethoprim is contraindicated in patients with G6PD deficiency or known hypersensitivity to sulfonamides. Complete blood counts should be performed at least weekly on patients receiving dapsone.

Proguanil.*** Proguanil, also known as *chloroquanide*, was the first agent found to inhibit plasmodial dihydrofolate reductase. The elucidation of its mechanism of action led to the synthesis of the diaminopyrimidines, pyrimethamine and trimethoprim.[156] Proguanil has been used for prophylaxis against *Pl. falciparum* and *Pl. vivax*. It acts too slowly to be employed for the treatment of acute malaria. Proguanil is currently used with chloroquine as prophylaxis in travelers to East Africa.[5] It provides protection against chloroquine-resistant strains of *Pl. falciparum* there[157]; chloroquine is administered concurrently because of the potential resistance of *Pl. vivax* to proguanil. The use of proguanil outside of East Africa has been limited by the resistance of *Pl. falciparum*. Proguanil is not available in the United States but can be purchased in Canada, England, and pharmacies in East Africa.

Proguanil is formulated in 100-mg tablets. It is slowly absorbed after oral administration. It reaches peak serum concentrations in 2–4 hours, and the serum levels decline to practically zero by 24 hours.[76] It must be taken daily to provide effective prophylaxis. The concentration of proguanil in erythrocytes is six times that in plasma. Approximately 40–60 percent is excreted in the urine and 10 percent in the feces. It is the metabolite 2,4-diamino-1-*p*-chlorophenyl-1,6-dihydro-6,6-dimethyl-1,3,5-triazine that inhibits parasite dihydrofolate reductase.[76]

Proguanil is thought to be innocuous at the daily dose levels used for malaria prophylaxis. At higher levels, it can produce nausea, vomiting, abdominal pain, and diarrhea. Excessive amounts have been associated with hematuria, proteinuria, and casts in the urine.

Lipid-Soluble Antifolates: Trimetrexate* and Piritrexin***.** Trimetrexate (2,4-diamino 5-methyl-6-[3,4,5-trimethyl-oxyanilino) methyl] quinazoline) is a low molecular weight dihydrofolate reductase inhibitor. It was developed as a myelosuppressive agent but was found to have antiparasitic activity. In preliminary studies, trimetrexate has been effective for the treatment of *P. carinii*[126] and *T. gondii*.[127] It is 1500 times more potent in inhibiting protozoal dihydrofolate reductase than trimethoprim. Trimetrexate is lipid soluble and readily enters host cells as well as protozoa. It has been used effectively with sulfadiazine to treat experimental murine toxoplasmosis.[127] When it was used without a sulfonamide or sulfone to treat *P. carinii* in persons with AIDS, the frequent allergic side effects seen with those compounds were avoided. Folinic acid (leucovorin) was administered concurrently to prevent bone marrow suppression. Adverse effects in patients receiving trimetrexate and leucovorin include leukopenia, rash, elevated aminotransferase levels, and reversible peripheral neuropathy, but they are usually mild. Piritrexin is another lipid-soluble dihydrofolate reductase inhibitor, which in combination with sulfadiazine has been shown to have activity against *T. gondii* in the murine model.[158]

Macrolide Antibiotics Active against Apicomplexa

Clindamycin. Clindamycin, a macrolide antibiotic, has been used along with prednisone for the treatment of ocular toxoplasmosis in immunocompetent patients.[159,160] It has relatively good penetration into the eye and inhibits replication of *T. gondii*. Although the outcome of therapy has been good, there are no prospective studies comparing clindamycin with the combination of pyrimethamine and a sulfonamide. Clindamycin also is of potential use with quinine in the treatment of malaria, and this combination is the treatment of choice for symptomatic human babesiosis.[161]

The pharmacokinetics and untoward effects of clindamycin are discussed in Chapter 26. The major concern is the development of pseudomembranous colitis, a side effect that increases in incidence with age.

Spiramycin* (Available by Special Request from the FDA) and Roxithromycin.*** ** Spiramycin, another macrolide antibiotic, is widely used as an additive in animal feeds. It is active against *T. gondii*, but it has not yet been licensed for use in the United States. Spiramycin has been used to treat primary toxoplasmosis acquired during pregnancy. In a recent study, only 3.7 percent of fetuses became infected in mothers who acquired toxoplasmosis during the first 16 weeks of pregnancy when they received spiramycin.[128] Spiramycin has been reported to be effective in a few persons with AIDS and *Cryptosporidium* infection. Prospective studies of its efficacy are ongoing. Spiramycin is dispensed in 500-mg capsules.

Roxithromycin, an ether oxime derivative of erythromycin, has shown activity against *T. gondii* in mice.[162,163] It acts synergistically with interferon-γ in the murine model of toxoplasmosis.

Pentamidine

Pentamidine isethionate (Fig. 8) is a diamidine that has been used as an alternative drug for the treatment of *P. carinii* pneumonia,[68,69,118,120] the hemolymphatic stage of *Trypanosoma brucei gambiense* infection,[164] and some forms of leishmaniasis.[165–167] Approximately 80–85 percent of patients with *P. carinii* pneumonia respond to intravenously administered pentamidine isethionate, but 50 percent or more suffer ontoward effects with the drug.[68,69,118,120] Parenteral pentamidine is usually reserved for patients who cannot tolerate trimethoprim-sulfamethoxazole. The concurrent use of pentamidine with trimethoprim-sulfamethoxazole has not increased the response rate but may increase the toxicity.[168] Recent studies indicate that aerosolized pentamidine is effective for the prevention of *P. carinii* pneumonia and possibly for its treatment.[169–171b] The effectiveness of therapy is dependent on the nebulization system and the size of the particles.

Pentamidine isethionate is a white powder that is water soluble; each 1.74 mg contains 1 mg of pentamidine base.[172] It is available in 300-mg ampules for intramuscular or intravenous administration. Intramuscular injections are frequently complicated by pain, swelling, and sterile abscesses at the administration site. Pentamidine is now most commonly given intravenously after being diluted in 100–250 ml of 5% dextrose in water. It must be administered slowly over 1–2 hours.[173] Pentamidine is highly tissue bound and excreted slowly over an extended period of time. It does not penetrate the central nervous system.

The mechanism of action has not yet been defined. Pentamidine is known to bind to DNA in a nonintercalative manner.[174] It interacts selectively with trypanosomal kinetoplast DNA, resulting in swelling and loss of structure of the kinetoplast.[175] Pentamidine also inhibits RNA polymerase,[176] ribosomal function,[177] nucleic acid, protein, and phospholipid synthesis,[178] and polyamine synthesis.[179] It can inhibit folic acid synthesis,[180] but this does not appear to be its mode of action. It can also inhibit trypsin and related proteases.[181] At a high concentration, pentamidine impairs oxygen consumption.[182]

The administration of pentamidine isethionate, either by the intravenous or intramuscular routes, is associated with toxicity in 50 percent of persons.[183] Adverse effects include tachycardia, nausea, vomiting, dizziness, rash, facial flushing, breathlessness, and a metallic taste. Severe hypotension may result after an intramuscular injection or after rapid intravenous infusion.[173]

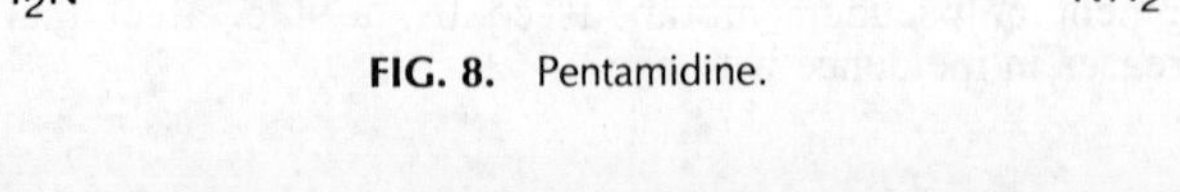

FIG. 8. Pentamidine.

Hypoglycemia has been reported during therapy in 6–9 percent of persons treated in the United States.[183,184] It can be severe and life-threatening, and may even occur after the completion of therapy. It is probably due to a direct toxic effect of pentamidine on pancreatic β cells.[185,186] The hypoglycemia may be followed by the development of insulin-dependent diabetes mellitus. Severe hypoglycemia may be controlled with diazoxide,[187] but it is not known if this will prevent the subsequent development of diabetes mellitus. Reversible renal failure occurs in approximately 25 percent of persons who receive pentamidine.[184] Although severe renal failure has been reported in a few patients, it has been impossible to attribute the renal toxicity solely to pentamidine because of the concurrent administration of other nephrotoxic agents. Other adverse effects of pentamidine include leukopenia and thrombocytopenia, elevated transaminases, fever, hypocalcemia, confusion, hallucinations, and, rarely, cardiac arrhythmias. Rare cases of fatal pancreatitis have been reported in patients with AIDS who received pentamidine.

In preliminary studies, aerosolized pentamidine seems to have been much better tolerated.[170,171] Only a small amount of drug reaches the systemic circulation.[171] Untoward effects include bronchospasm, particularly in patients with a history of asthma or chronic obstructive pulmonary disease, pharyngeal irritation, and a metallic taste. Pretreatment with inhaled bronchodilators may prevent bronchospasm. If subsequent studies confirm the efficacy and safety of inhaled pentamidine, it may replace parenterally administered pentamidine and trimethoprim-sulfamethoxazole for the prevention of *P. carinii* in persons with AIDS.

DRUGS FOR TREATMENT OF TRYPANOSOMATIDAE

Members of the genera *Trypanosoma* and *Leishmania* are important pathogens. *Trypanosoma brucei gambiense* and *Tr. brucei rhodesience* cause African sleeping sickness. The early hemolymphatic stage of disease has traditionally been treated with suramin or pentamidine isethionate.[5] Neither of these compounds reaches therapeutic levels in the central nervous system. Once central nervous system involvement is documented, melarsoprol B, a highly toxic trivalent arsenical, has been the treatment of choice. In recent studies, eflornithine, an inhibitor of ornithine decarboxylase, has been shown to be effective even in patients with far advanced central nervous system involvement with *Tr. brucei gambiense*.[188–190] It has not been associated with serious toxicity. Although still experimental, eflornithine will probably emerge as the treatment of choice for *Tr. brucei gambiense*. The therapeutic situation is worse with *Trypanosoma cruzi*, the cause of Chagas disease in Central and South America.[191] The drug currently available, nifurtimox, is variably effective and frequently associated with sufficiently severe toxicity to necessitate discontinuation of therapy.[191] The alternative, benznidazole, seems to offer no advantage. Efforts continue to identify more effective, less toxic compounds.

The various *Leishmania* spp. produce cutaneous, mucosal, or visceral disease on every continent except Antarctica and Australia. The pentavalent antimonials, stibogluconate sodium, and meglumine antimoniate, are widely used for the treatment of leishmaniasis, but some *Leishmania* spp. (e.g., *Leishmania ethiopica*) and persons with syndromes such as mucosal leishmaniasis or diffuse cutaneous leishmaniasis respond poorly.[192] Pentamidine isethionate[166–168] and amphotericin B serve as alternative drugs. Several new compounds are currently under study.[192]

Suramin**

Suramin is a nonmetallic compound that is used for the treatment of the hemolymphatic stage of African trypanosomiasis.

It has also been used on occasion as chemoprophylaxis against *Tr. brucei gambiense* in persons working in highly endemic regions.[5] Suramin is also active against adult *Onchocerca volvulus*. When used to treat onchocerciasis, it is administered after a course of diethylcarbamazine, which kills microfilariae.

Suramin sodium is a white microcrystalline powder that is readily soluble in water.[193] It is dispensed in 1.0-g vials for parenteral administration. It cannot be given orally. Suramin binds to plasma proteins and persists at low levels in the serum for up to 3 months after infusion. There seems to be negligible metabolism of the drug. Suramin does not penetrate the central nervous system, which limits its usefulness to the hemolymphatic stage of African trypanosomiasis.

Its mechanism of action is uncertain, but at low concentrations suramin is known to inhibit multiple enzymes. It is a polyanion and forms firm complexes with proteins. The antitrypanosomal activity of suramin correlates with its inhibition of glycerol-3-phosphate oxidase and glycerol-3-phosphate dehydrogenase, parasitic enzymes involved in energy metabolism.[194]

Suramin causes a variety of untoward effects.[195] Immediate reactions include nausea, vomiting, shock, loss of consciousness, and occasionally death. Fever and urticaria may also occur. Later reactions, which appear up to 24 hours after administration, include fever, papular rash, exfoliative dermatitis, stomatitis, paresthesias of the palms and soles, photophobia, lacrimation, palpebral edema, and hyperesthesia. These may be followed by renal dysfunction with albuminuria, hematuria, and renal casts. Other reactions include chronic diarrhea and severe prostration. Jaundice, hemolytic anemia, and agranulocytosis are rare. The frequency and severity of side effects are more severe in malnourished hosts.[193] Suramin is relatively contraindicated in persons with pre-existing kidney or liver disease.

In persons treated for onchocerciasis, additional side effects occur, apparently due to the release of worm antigens. These include the formation of abscesses around the adult worms, papular eruptions and desquamation, and aggravation of ocular inflammation.

Melarsoprol**

Melarsoprol, or Mel B, is a trivalent arsenical used for the treatment of central nervous system trypanosomiasis. It is effective in some but not all cases. Melarsoprol is also potentially effective in treatment of the hemolymphatic phase, but it is too toxic to be recommended in that setting.

Melarsoprol is only slightly soluble in water, but it is readily soluble in propylene glycol, in which it is dispensed as a 3.6% weight/volume solution.[193] Melarsoprol is administered intravenously. A small but sufficient amount of the drug penetrates the central nervous system, where it can have a lethal effect on trypanosomes. Arsenicals react avidly with sulfhydryl groups. They thereby interact with a number of proteins and inactivate enzymes. This is the most likely mechanism of action against trypanosomes, as well as the cause of melarsoprol's pronounced toxicity. There is evidence to suggest that melarsoprol acts differentially on parasite pyruvate kinase, which is a terminal glycolytic enzyme.[196] Melarsoprol is oxidized to a nontoxic or less toxic pentavalent metabolite that is excreted.

Melarsoprol is a highly toxic drug.[197] Febrile reactions are common and may be accompanied by hypertension, abdominal pain, vomiting, and arthralgia. Reactive encephalopathy is the most serious side effect and results in death in approximately 6 percent of recipients.[198] It usually appears in the first 3 or 4 days of therapy. The clinical manifestations include headache, dizziness, mental dullness, confusion, and ataxia with progression to obtundation and seizures. Less common untoward effects include hemorrhagic encephalopathy and agranulocytosis. Allergic reactions including rashes may complicate subsequent courses of therapy. On occasion, the appearance of numerous casts in the urine or evidence of hepatotoxicity necessitates a modification of therapy. Severe hemolysis can occur in patients with G6PD deficiency. The gastrointestinal side effects can be reduced by administering the drug slowly to fasting patients. Melarsoprol therapy may precipitate erythema nodosum in patients who have leprosy.

Eflornithine*

Eflornithine (DL-α-difluoromethylornithine) has proven to be highly effective in the treatment of African sleeping sickness due to *Tr. brucei gambiense*, even in patients with advanced central nervous system disease.[188–190] Eflornithine has also been effective in 35–40 percent of patients with *P. carinii* pneumonia refractory to pentamidine and/or trimethoprim-sulfamethoxazole.[199–201]

Eflornithine hydrochloride can be administered intravenously or orally; 80 percent of the drug is excreted unchanged in the urine.[202] Serum levels during administration of 20 g/day by intravenous infusion approach 1200 nmol/ml; oral administration of 5 g every 4 hours produces levels of approximately 500 nmol/ml.[188] The ratio of cerebrospinal fluid to serum concentration ranges from 0.09 to 0.45.[188] The highest cerebrospinal fluid levels have been found in persons with the most severe central nervous system involvement. Eflornithine is an enzyme-activated, irreversible inhibitor of the enzyme ornithine decarboxylase, which is involved in the first step in the polyamine pathway. Polyamines play an essential role in the growth, differentiation, and replication of the trypanosomatids.[202–205]

Eflornithine is well tolerated. Adverse effects are usually mild and reversible. They include anemia, thrombocytopenia, leukopenia, nausea, vomiting, diarrhea, and transient hearing loss. Eflornithine is a much safer drug than either pentamidine, suramin, or melarsoprol, all of which it is likely to replace for the treatment of *Tr. brucei gambiense*. Further studies are needed to document its efficacy and to establish the optimal dose and duration of therapy.

Nifurtimox**

Nifurtimox, 4-[(5-Nitrofurfurylidene)amino]-3-methylthiomorpholine-1,1-dioxide, a nitrofuran, is the most widely used drug for the treatment of acute Chagas disease.[191,206] It can reduce the duration of symptoms of acute disease, and it decreases mortality due to myocarditis and meningoencephalitis. The level and duration of parasitemia are also reduced. However, in the clinical trials done to date, there have been significant numbers of treatment failures. There also seems to be geographic variation in responsiveness. Treatment has been found to be most effective in Argentina and Chile; therapy in Brazil and in some other countries has been less successful. Prolonged therapy for 120 days is recommended,[5] and it is not unusual for a treatment course to be terminated prematurely because of drug toxicity. The effectiveness of nifurtimox in the treatment of patients with the indeterminant phase or chronic Chagas disease has not been documented.

Nifurtimox is formulated as 100-mg tablets. It is well absorbed orally. Biotransformation occurs rapidly, and only low concentrations are found in blood and tissue.[193] Nifurtimox is active against both the trypomastigote and amastigote forms of *T. cruzi*. The trypanocidal action relates to the ability of nifurtimox to form reactive oxygen radicals that are toxic to the parasite.[206]

Toxicity is experienced by 40–70 percent of persons who receive nifurtimox. This is probably due, at least in part, to free radical formation and oxidative damage to host tissues.[207] Most of the symptoms are related to the gastrointestinal tract and the central and peripheral nervous systems.[193] Nifurtimox seems to be better tolerated by children than adults. Nausea, vomiting, abdominal pain, anorexia, and weight loss are common and may require premature termination of therapy. Neurologic sequelae include restlessness, disorientation, insomnia, twitching, paresthesias, polyneuritis, weakness, and stiffness. Convulsions may occur. Rashes, neutropenia, and decreased sperm counts have also been reported. The side effects are usually reversible with discontinuation of the drug, but they frequently pose a therapeutic dilemma given the prolonged course of therapy that is necessary. More effective, less toxic agents are clearly needed for the treatment of Chagas disease.

Benznidazole***

Benznidazole, a nitroimidazole derivative, is another relatively toxic drug that has been used for the treatment of Chagas disease.[191,208] It has not been studied as extensively as nifurtimox, but it seems to be of relatively similar efficacy.[209] Benznidazole is administered orally, usually for several weeks. Therapy is often limited by peripheral neuropathy, rash, or bone marrow suppression. It is not available for use in the United States.

Pentavalent Antimony; Stibogluconate Sodium** and Meglumine Antimoniate***

The leishmaniases are a group of clinical syndromes caused by multiple *Leishmania* spp. The manifestations of infection and the response to chemotherapy depend on the immune responses of the host, as well as the susceptibility of the causative organism to antimicrobial agents. The pentavalent antimonials, stibogluconate sodium and meglumine antimoniate, have been widely used for the treatment of leishmaniasis.[192] The compounds are thought to be of comparable efficacy and toxicity. Stibogluconate is the only pentavalent antimonial available in the United States. It has been the most extensively studied and is used in Africa and India.[210–212] Meglumine antimoniate is used in francophone countries, as well as in Central and South America.

The efficacy of the pentavalent antimonials varies with the leishmanial syndrome and the causative *Leishmania* sp. (see Chapter 252). Good responses are observed in the majority of persons with visceral leishmaniasis. Responses in persons with cutaneous leishmaniasis depend on the causative *Leishmania* sp. Pentamidine isethionate and amphotericin B have been used as alternative drugs when the antimonials fail. Efforts continue to develop new drugs active against the *Leishmania*. spp. Attention has focused on the pyrazolopyrimidines, allopurinol and allopurinol ribonucleoside[213–215]; on ketaconazole,[216] which appears to be effective in the treatment of some forms of New World leishmaniasis; on topical paromomycin with methylbenzethonium chloride for *Leishmania major* infection[217]; and on several other drugs.

Sodium stibogluconate is available in sterile aqueous solution for parenteral administration. It is supplied in 10-ml bottles; each milliliter contains 330 mg of drug, which is equivalent to 100 mg of pentavalent antimony. Meglumine antimoniate is available in 5-ml bottles, with 85 mg of antimony per milliliter. These drugs are prescribed on the basis of their antimony content. They can be administered intramuscularly but are usually given intravenously, either undiluted over a 5-minute period or diluted in 50 ml of 5% dextrose in water or saline and administered over 20 minutes. The antimony concentration in blood is best described by a three-compartment model, with a short initial distribution phase followed by biexponential elimination, primarily through the kidney.[218–220] The mean half-lives for the elimination phases have been reported to be 1.7 and 33 hours after intravenous administration and 2 and 766 hours after the drug is given intramuscularly. The slow terminal elimination phase may be due to conversion of pentavalent to trivalent antimony. The latter may be responsible for the toxicity seen with long-term, high-dose therapy. The mechanism of action is uncertain. Pentavalent antimony is concentrated in cells of reticuloendothelial origin, where the drug is thought to affect parasite metabolism.

The pentavalent antimonials are relatively well tolerated.[192,210,211,219,220] Most of the data on toxicity have come from studies of children or adolescents. Common adverse effects include abdominal pain, nausea, vomiting, malaise, headache, elevated transaminase levels, nephrotoxicity, weakness, myalgias, arthralgias, fever, skin rash, cough, and pneumonitis, but these seldom prevent completion of the treatment course. Dose-related changes are observed in the ECG. The most common are ST-T wave changes and prolonged Q-T intervals. Rarer but more serious effects are atrial and ventricular arrhythmias; sudden death has been associated with high-dose therapy. The use of pentavalent antimonials is relatively contraindicated in patients with myocarditis, hepatitis, and nephritis.

Pyrazolopyrimidines (Allopurinol and Allopurinol Ribonucleoside***)

Allopurinol, allopurinol riboside, and other purine analogues can inhibit the growth of *Leishmania* spp.[213–215] and *Tr. cruzi*.[191,221] The metabolism of purines in the kinetoplastids differs significantly from that in humans. The trypanosomatids rely on salvage pathways to obtain purine analogues, whereas humans synthesize purines de novo. Allopurinol, a pyrazolopyrimidine, inhibits *Leishmania* spp. and *Tr. cruzi* in vitro and in animal models. Allopurinol has been shown to be effective when administered with stibogluconate sodium to persons with visceral leishmaniasis who failed to respond to stibogluconate sodium alone.[215] The usefulness of allopurinol in humans has been limited by its rapid metabolism by xanthine oxidase. Allopurinol ribonucleoside, an inosine analogue, also is active against *Leishmania* spp. and some strains of *Tr. cruzi*. It is not metabolized as rapidly as allopurinol in humans and is currently being evaluated. Some other purine analogues, such as formycin B, are also lethal for these organisms but are too toxic to be used in humans.[221]

Amphotericin B and Ketaconazole

Amphotericin B has been used as an alternative drug in the treatment of visceral and mucocutaneous leishmaniasis.[222,223] The precise mechanism of its antiparasitic activity is uncertain, but it probably affects the parasite's surface membrane. Its use in the treatment of leishmaniasis is limited by its appreciable toxicity, the requirement for intravenous administration, and the prolonged course of therapy. Amphotericin B has also been used with miconazole and rifampin to treat amebic encephalitis due to *Naegleria* spp.[5] The pharmacokinetics and toxicity are detailed in Chapter 33.

Preliminary studies suggest that ketaconazole may be effective for the treatment of cutaneous leishmaniasis due to *Leishmania mexicana*.[216] Prospective, randomized, controlled studies are needed to document its efficacy, since the natural course of infection is self-resolution.

DRUGS FOR TREATMENT OF INTESTINAL NEMATODES (ROUNDWORMS)

The intestinal nematodes remain prevalent in areas of the world where sanitation is poor. As many as 80 percent of rural inhabitants in developing areas may be infected with one or more spp. In the United States, intestinal helminths are most likely to be encountered among immigrants from endemic areas or occasionally in returning travelers who have had intense rural exposure. Transmission of intestinal nematodes continues to occur in some areas of North America.

Mebendazole

Mebendazmole (Fig. 9), a synthetic benzimidazole, methyl 5-benzoylbenzimidazole-2 carbamate, is widely used for treat-

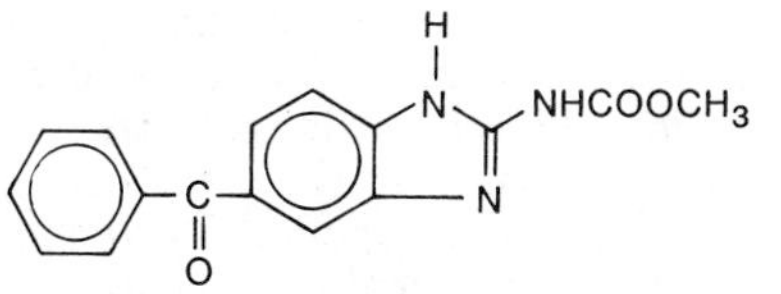

FIG. 9. Mebendazole.

ment of intestinal nematodes.[224] It is highly effective against *Ascaris lumbricoides*,[225] *Necator americanus* and *Ancylostoma duodenale*,[226] and *Trichuris trichiura*[225,227] at doses of 100 mg twice a day for 3 days. It is also effective in persons infected with more than one of these nematodes, which is the norm in impoverished areas.[226] Treatment over several days is often more effective than a single larger dose of mebendazole for these organisms. In contrast, *Enterobius vermicularis* responds to a single dose of 100 mg with a repeat dose given after 2 weeks.[227] The effect of mebendazole on *Strongyloides stercoralis* has been variable[228–231]; thiabendazole remains the drug of choice.[5] Mebendazole has been used at higher doses, 200 mg twice a day for 20 days, for the treatment of *Capillaria philippinensis*, an uncommon cause of chronic malabsorption in Southeast Asia.[224]

Mebendazole has been used at very high doses, 40 mg/kg body weight per day, for prolonged periods of time to treat inoperable cysts of *Echinococcus granulosus* and *E. multilocularis*.[232–235] Although usually not curative, mebendazole prevents progression of the primary lesion and suppresses or prevents metastasis. In general, mebendazole seems to be more effective against *E. multilocularis*. Mebendazole has also been used in the perioperative period to decrease the likelihood of peritoneal implants in case cyst contents are accidentally spilled at surgery.[236,237] Recent studies indicate that anthelmintic metabolites of albendazole attain higher serum and cyst concentrations than those of mebendazole. Albendazole will likely replace mebendazole for the treatment of inoperable echinococcosis.[238–241]

Mebendazole is active against adult *Trichinella spiralis* and appears to have some activity against invading larvae.[242,243] No comparative data are available for humans, but mebendazole has been relatively effective in the treatment of experimental trichinosis in animals and is much less toxic than thiabendazole. Some recommend it for human trichinosis. Mebendazole has activity against two filaria spp., *Loa loa* and *Mansonella perstans*.[244,245] It is considered the drug of choice, 100 mg twice a day for 30 days, for *M. perstans*,[244] against which diethylcarbamazine is not active. Diethylcarbamazine remains the treatment of choice for *L. loa*.

Mebendazole is dispensed in 100-mg tablets. It is only slightly soluble in water and is poorly absorbed from the gastrointestinal tract.[246] This contributes to its low frequency of side effects but limits its usefulness in treating tissue larvae. Up to 10 percent of an orally administered dose of mebendazole is recovered within 48 hours in the urine. Most of the drug excreted by the kidney is the decarboxylated metabolite. Mebendazole selectively blocks glucose uptake by nematodes without affecting blood glucose levels in the host.[246] It selectively blocks microtubule assembly in helminths.[247] Parasite immobilization and death follow, but it can take several days for susceptible nematodes to be cleared from the gastrointestinal tract. Mebendazole also inhibits the development of the ova of hookworms and *Trichuris*.

Side effects are uncommon when mebendazole is used at low doses (100 mg twice a day for 3 days) for the treatment of the common intestinal helminths.[224,246] Transient abdominal pain and diarrhea occur in a small number of persons, usually those with massive parasite burdens. Migration of adult *A. lumbricoides* to the nose or mouth occurs occasionally. Mebendazole produce embryotoxicity and teratogenicity in pregnant rats after a single oral dose of 10 mg/kg; it is therefore contraindicated in pregnant women.[248]

At the high doses (40 mg/kg/day) used for the treatment of inoperable echinococcal cysts, systemic side effects such as alopecia, liver enzyme abnormalities, and transient bone marrow suppression with severe but reversible neutopenia have been observed.[224,249,250] The white blood cell count should be followed closely after initiation of high-dose therapy, since neutropenia is usually observed within the first 30 days.

Albendazole* and Flubendazole***

Neither of these benzimidazole compounds is licensed for use in the United States. Albendazole, methyl (5-(propylthio)-1H-benzimidazol-2-yl) carbamate, has a broad spectrum of activity. It is highly effective when used in a single dose of 400 mg for oral treatment of intestinal helminth infections including *A. lumbricoides, Tri. trichiura*, and the hookworms.[251–255] It is thus ideally suited for mass treatment programs. Albendazole at high doses (10 mg/kg body weight per day for 28 days, followed by a 2-week rest period, then repeated for up to five cycles) appears to be more effective against inoperable echinococcal cysts than mebendazole.[238–240] Albendazole may also be effective in preventing postsurgical recurrence of echinococcal cysts, as demonstrated by animal and, less conclusively, human data.[241] Albendazole has activity against tapeworms in the human intestine, but it is less active than niclosamide.[253] Finally, albendazole (15 mg/kg for 1 month) has recently been shown to be effective in the treatment of a small group of patients with parenchymal neurocysticercosis.[256]

Albendazole is dispensed as 200-mg tablets or as a 2% solution for oral administration. It is not well absorbed. It is metabolized to albendazole sulfoxide in the liver. This metabolite is scolicidal and achieves relatively high levels in serum and within echinococcal cysts. Albendazole is well tolerated when used in single-dose regimens for intestinal helminths. High-dose, prolonged therapy for echinococcal disease has occasionally been complicated by hepatitis and obstructive jaundice.[257] The liver toxicity has reversed after discontinuation of the drug.

Flubendazole is the parafluoro analogue of mebendazole. It has a spectrum of activity against intestinal helminths that is similar to that of mebendazole. Flubendazole is not as well absorbed. Initially, flubendazole was thought to lack teratogenicity, but recent animal studies suggest that it is teratogenic when administered by gavage.[258] Flubendazole has also led to clinical improvement in a small group of persons with neurocysticercosis, but given its poor absorption, it is unlikely to replace praziquantel for the treatment of cysticercosis.[259]

Thiabendazole

Thiabendazole, 2-(4′-thiazolyl)-1H-benzimidazole, is among the most potent anthelmintic drugs,[260] but its use has been limited by the high frequency of untoward effects. Thiabendazole is active against a number of adult nematodes that infect the gastrointestinal tract and against larvae in tissues. It is much better absorbed then mebendazole. The most common indication for thiabendazole is the treatment of *S. stercoralis*[5,261,262] or *S. fuelleborni*[263] infection. It is also used for *Trichostrongylus* infections,[264] cutaneous larvae migrans,[265] visceral larva migrans,[261] and trichinosis.[5,266,267] Some cases of human trichinosis have shown marked clinical improvement with thiabendazole. Anti-inflammatory, antipyretic, and analgesic effects of thiabendazole may have contributed to the clinical response. Studies in animals experimentally infected with *Trich. spiralis* suggested that some but not all larvae are killed by thiabendazole. Although thiabendazole is active against the hookworms, *A. lumbricoides, Ent. vermicularis*, and, to a lesser extent, *Tri. trichiura*,[261] mebendazole in general has higher response rates and is far less toxic.

Thiabendazole is available in 500-mg tablets and as an oral suspension of 500 mg/5 ml. It is rapidly absorbed after oral administration; peak concentrations occur in plasma about 1 hour after treatment.[246] It is recommended that the drug be given with meals. Unfortunately, no parenteral preparation is available, which poses a problem for some patients with disseminated *S. stercoralis* infection. Most of the drug is excreted in urine within 24 hours as 5-hydroxythiabendazole conjugated as the glucuronide or as the sulfate. The precise mechanism of action is not known. Thiabendazole inhibits the fumarate reductase of susceptible helminths, and this may prevent them from eliminating reducing equivalents such as succinic acid.[268–270] Recent studies suggest that thiabendazole, like mebendazole, may interfere with microtubule assembly.[271]

Approximately half of the persons who receive thiabendazole experience one or more side effects. Most frequent are nausea, anorexia, vomiting, and dizziness.[246] Less common are diarrhea, epigastric pain, pruritus, drowsiness, giddiness, and headache. Rare side effects include tinnitus, abnormal sensation in the eyes, numbness, decreased pulse and blood pressure, elevated liver enzymes, and progressive bile duct injury.[246,272] Seizures have been reported in a child with Down syndrome.[273] Transient neutropenia has been observed in some patients. Allergic manifestations such as fever, facial flush, angioneurotic edema, lymphadenopathy, perianal rash, and skin rashes are also observed; some or all of these may be due to the release of parasite antigens or the underlying disease process. Thiabendazole can give urine an asparagus-like odor, and crystalluria has been observed. Because of the central nervous system effects, activities requiring alertness should be avoided during therapy. The drug should be used with caution in persons with hepatic disease or decreased hepatic function. Thiabendazole has been found to be genotoxic in in vitro and in vivo assays,[274] and it is relatively contraindicated in pregnancy.

Pyrantel Pamoate

Pyrantel pamoate is recommended for the treatment of *Ent. vermicularis, A. lumbricoides, N. americanus*, and *Ancylostoma duodenale*.[275,276] It is considered an alternative drug for *Trichostrongylus* infection. It is not active against the whipworm, *Tri. trichura*. Oxantel***, an m-oxyphenol derivative that has not been licensed in the United States, is effective against *Tri. trichura*.

Pyrantel is available as a suspension (250 mg of pyrantel base/5 ml). It is poorly absorbed; less than 15 percent is excreted in the urine as the parent drug or metabolite.[277–279] Pyrantel and its analogues are depolarizing neuromuscular blocking agents. The resulting nicotinic activation results in spastic paralysis of the worm. Pyrantel also inhibits acetylcholinesterases. There is depolarization and increased spike discharge frequency in muscle cells of susceptible nematodes.

Pyrantel pamoate has minimal toxicity at the oral doses used to treat intestinal helminths. Mild, transient gastrointestinal symptoms, headache, drowsiness or insomnia, and dizziness are occasionally encountered. The nitrosated metabolites of pyrantel pamoate are mutagenic in bacteria. Pyrantel pamoate has not been studied in pregnancy, and it is not recommended for pregnant women or children under 1 year of age. Pyrantel and piperazine, which produces hyperpolarization with a reduction in spike wave activity in helminthic muscle cells, appear to be mutually antagonistic and should not be used together.[277–278]

Pyrvinium pamoate***

Pyrvinium pamoate, a cyanide dye, is an alternative drug for the treatment of *Ent. vermicularis*.[280,281] It is still considered an alternative drug for the treatment of pinworm infections, but pyrvinium pamoate has largely been replaced by pyrantel pamoate and mebendazole and is no longer marketed in the United States. Pyrvinium pamoate has some activity against *S. stercoralis*, but thiabendazole is superior. Pyrvinium pamoate has not been effective in the treatment of *Tri. trichura* or *N. americanus*.

Pyrvinium pamoate is a deep red crystalline solid that is insoluble in water.[279] It is available in tablets containing 50 mg of pyrvinium base and as a suspension containing the equivalent of 10 mg of pyrvinium base per milliliter. Its anthelmintic activity is thought to be associated with inhibition of respiration in aerobic organisms and with interference with the absorption of exogenous glucose in intestinal helminths.

Pyrvinium pamoate is generally well tolerated. Side effects, which occur in a minority of recipients, include nausea, vomiting, and abdominal cramping. Emesis has been associated with the suspension. It is recommended that the tablets be swallowed without chewing. Patients should be told that the drug will color stools bright red and that the suspension will stain if spilled. Pyrvinium pamoate is genotoxic in *Saccharomyces cerevisiae*, but little if any of it is absorbed after oral administration, and human and animal studies have not demonstrated mutagenic metabolites in the urine after a single therapeutic dose.[282]

Piperazine

Piperazine citrate is effective in the treatment of *A. lumbricoides*. It has largely been replaced in the United States by mebendazole, which is less toxic, but piperazine is less expensive and is still used in some developing areas. Piperazine also has activity against *Ent. vermicularis*. Piperazine derivatives have a broad range of pharmacologic activity. Some substituted piperazines are central serotonin agonists; others depress monosynaptic spinal cord excitation, block chloride channels, have antioxidant effects, display antiarrhythmic activity, or act as vasodilators. One, diethylcarbamazine, is effective against filariae.

Piperazine salts are available as tablets containing 250 mg and as syrups and suspensions containing 100 per milliliter.[246] Piperazine is well absorbed orally. Some of the drug is metabolized; the remainder is excreted in the urine. Piperazine causes flaccid paralysis of susceptible intestinal helminths. It acts as a low-potency agonist at extrasynaptic γ-aminobutyric acid (GABA) receptors on the bag region of *Ascaris suum*.[283] Activation of these receptors gives rise to an increase in chloride conductance. There is also hyperpolarization and suppression of spontaneous action potentials.[284] Worms are excreted alive, usually without migrating.

Piperazine is generally well tolerated. On occasion, there are gastrointestinal symptoms, transient neurologic side effects, or urticarial reactions. Lethal overdoses are associated with convulsions and respiratory depression. Epileptic activity may be exaggerated, and piperazine is contraindicated in persons with a history of seizures.[285] Neurotoxicity has also been observed in persons with impaired renal function. Visual disturbances, ataxia, and hypotonia occur rarely.[286] The drug has been used during pregnancy without apparent adverse effects, but it has not been thoroughly evaluated in this setting. Although adverse dermatologic reactions are rare, they have been reported in persons sensitized to topical ethylenediamine.[287]

DRUGS FOR TREATMENT OF SYSTEMIC NEMATODES

Diethylcarbamazine*

Diethylcarbamazine (Fig. 10) is a piperazine derivative, *N,N*-diethyl-4-methyl-1-piperazinecarboxamide dihydrogen citrate. It results in the rapid destruction of microfilariae of *Wuchereria*

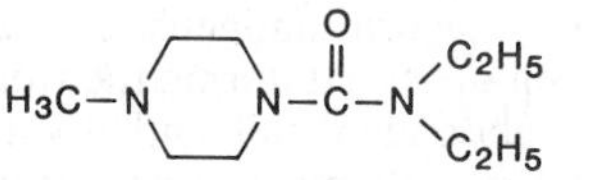

FIG. 10. Diethylcarbamazine.

bancrofti, Brugia malayi, and *B. timori*, the three lymphatic-dwelling filariae infecting humans.[288,289] There is presumptive evidence that it kills the adult worms of these species, and it currently is the drug of choice for each of them. It has been successfully used in community-based mass treatment programs.[290] Diethylcarbamazine is also the treatment of choice for *L. loa*[5,291] and has been recommended for *Mansonella ozzardi*,[5] but the results have been variable.[292,293] It has been used successfully to treat persons with pulmonary infiltrates with eosinophilia in the tropics,[294] presumably because this syndrome is in many instances caused by microfilariae in the lungs. Diethylcarbamazine has also been used as an alternative mode of therapy for visceral larva migrans, with variable success.[295]

Diethylcarbamazine rapidly kills microfilariae of *Onchocerca volvulus* in the skin and eye, but the resulting inflammatory reaction can cause severe damage.[296–298] Prednisone and antihistamines have been administered concomitantly to limit inflammation. Diethylcarbamazine does not affect adult *O. volvulus*, and microfilariae reaccumulate after completion of therapy[299] unless suramin (see above under "Drugs for Treatment of Trypanosomatidae") is administered concurrently to kill adult worms. Ivermectin, which has not yet been licensed in the United States, has emerged as the drug of choice for the treatment of onchocerciasis.

Diethlycarbamazine is available in 50-mg tablets.[246] It is readily absorbed from the gastrointestinal tract. Peak blood levels are reached in 1–2 hours; the serum half-life is approximately 8 hours.[300] The parent compound and its metabolites are cleared through the kidney.[301,302] Diethylcarbamazine is distributed equally throughout all body compartments except adipose tissue, and there is little accumulation even after repeated doses are given. The drug seems to have two types of effects on microfilariae. First, it is associated with a decrease in muscle activity, leading eventually to immobilization of the worm.[303] The piperazine moiety may result in hyperpolarization, resulting in the observed paralysis.[246] Second, the drug appears to alter the surface membranes of microfilariae, resulting in enhanced killing by the host's immune system.[304,305] Diethylcarbamazine has also been shown to enhance the adherence properties of eosinophils and polymorphonuclear leukocytes,[306] and there is evidence to suggest that platelets may mediate the action on microfilariae.[307] Untoward effects include those produced directly by the drug and inflammatory reactions that follow the release of filarial antigens. Common reactions include headache, malaise, weakness, arthralgia, anorexia, nausea, and vomiting. The gastrointestinal effects are usually dose related. Acute psychotic reactions have been reported but are rare.

During treatment of onchocerciasis with diethylcarbamazine, systemic reactions include severe pruritus, edema of the skin, fever, hypotension, heightened eosinophilia, lymphadenopathy, splenomegaly, and proteinuria.[308,309] Ocular complications may result in permanent sequelae and include visual field constriction, optic nerve pallor, chorioretinitis, anterior uveitis, and punctate keratitis.[296–299,308–311] These systemic and ocular reactions are apparently due to the release of filarial antigens and generally correlate with the degree of microfilaremia in the skin and eye. They follow the onset of therapy and may be severe. The acute effects usually last for only 3–7 days. The elicitation of such reactions by even low doses of diethylcarbamazine is the basis for the Mazzotti test,[312] which has been used to diagnose onchocerciasis. Steroids are usually administered to patients with ocular involvement who receive diethlycarbamazine. Ivermectin also is microfilaricidal, but kills slowly and is much less toxic. It has replaced diethylcarbamazine for the treatment of persons with ocular onchocerciasis. In *W. bancrofti* and *B. malayi* infections, localized swellings or nodules may develop along lymphatics, and there may be accompanying lymphadenitis.[309] Transient hydrocele formation or lymphedema may be observed. Encephalopathy has occurred rarely in persons treated for *L. loa*.

Ivermectin*

Ivermectin is the 22,23-dihydro derivative of avermectin B1, a macrocyclic lactone produced by the actinomycete *Streptomyces avermitilis*.[313] It is active at low doses against a broad spectrum of nematodes and blood-sucking arthropod parasites of animals. One of the major recent advances in anthelmintic therapy has been the introduction of ivermectin for treatment of human onchocerciasis.[296–299,313–315] Ivermectin kills microfilariae in the skin as well as in the eye, but the local inflammatory responses are less severe than with diethylcarbamazine. This is particularly important in the eye, where microfilariae disappear slowly after ivermectin therapy. Ivermectin does not kill adult *O. volvulus*, but it does inhibit oviposition. It is active against other filarial pathogens such as *W. bancrofti*.[316] Ivermectin has an extremely broad spectrum of antinematodal activity.[313] It is now widely used in veterinary practice for control and treatment of helminthic and arthropod infestations.

Ivermectin is odorless and colorless, and has been effective when administered as a single oral or parenteral dose. It is concentrated in the liver and adipose tissues. Only a small percentage of the drug is excreted in the urine; the rest is excreted in the stool. Ivermectin acts by blocking signal transmission from interneurons to excitatory motor neurons. GABA is the neurotransmitter that is blocked, but ivermectin does not appear to compete with GABA for binding and does not bind directly to the GABA binding site.[313] In animals, GABA-mediated nerves are present only in the central nervous systems, whereas they are found in peripheral muscle in susceptible invertebrates. Ivermectin is usually well tolerated. The initiation of therapy in persons with onchocerciasis may be complicated by fever, pruritus, headache, and cutaneous edema, but the side effects are less frequent and less severe than those of diethylcarbamazine or suramin.[296–299,313–315] In cattle, 30 times the recommended dose was tolerated without signs of toxicity, but death was reported at 40 times the recommended dose. No teratogenicity has been reported in animals.

DRUGS FOR TREATMENT OF PLATHYHELMINTHS: TREMATODES (FLUKES) AND CESTODES (TAPEWORMS)

Praziquantel

The most important recent addition to the therapeutic armamentarium against helminths has been praziquantel (Fig. 11), 2-(cyclohexylcarbonyl-(1,2,3,6,7,11b)-hexyahydro-4H-pyrazino(2,1-*a*)isoquinoline-4-one), a compound that has a broad spectrum of activity against tematodes and cestodes, is well absorbed orally, is given in several doses in 1 or a few days, and has mild untoward effects.[18,317–320] Praziquantel is highly

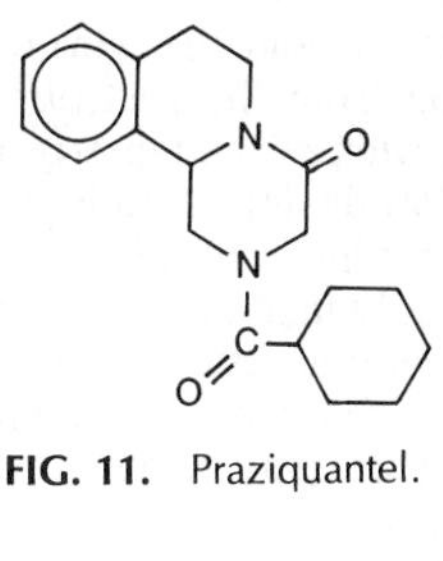

FIG. 11. Praziquantel.

effective against all of the *Schistosoma* spp. that infect humans,[317–330] includin *S. japonicum*, against which there was previously no good form of chemotherapy. It has even been effective in the treatment of *S. japonicum* infection of the central nervous system.[331] Praziquantel is also the drug of choice for the liver flukes *Clonorchis sinensis* and *Opisthorchis viverrini*,[317–320,332–334] the lung flukes *Paragonimus westermani, P. kellicoti*, and other *Paragonimus* spp.[317–320,335–338] and the intestinal flukes *Heterophyes heterophyes, Fasciolopsis buski*, and *Metagonimus yokogawai*.[317–320] Only against the liver fluke, *Fasciola hepatica*, have praziquantel failures been frequent.[339,340]

Praziquantel is also highly active against adult and larval forms of the cestodes.[317–319] Although double-blind, placebo-controlled studies have not been performed, the cumulative experience indicates that praziquantel is the drug of choice for the treatment of neurocysticercosis due to *Taenia solium*.[341–349] It is very effective in the treatment of parenchymal disease. Praziquantel is less effective when there is subarachnoid involvement and is ineffective against cysts in the ventricular system[349] or eye.[350,351] Some prefer praziquantel for the treatment of intestinal *Ta. solium* infestation.[352] It is highly effective against adult *Ta. saginata, Diphyllobothrium latum*, and *D. pacificum*,[352] but niclosamide is equally effective, less expensive, has fewer side effects, and is therefore more widely used against those organisms. In the case of *Hymenolepis nana*, praziquantel may be preferable to niclosamide; praziquantel can be given as a single dose, whereas niclosamide must be given daily for 6 days. Unfortunately, praziquantel is unlikely to be effective in the treatment of human hydatid disease. It is active against adult *Echinococcus* spp. in the canine gastrointestinal tract and damages protoscolices in hydatids, but the germinal layer of the hydatid is not destroyed.[353–357]

Praziquantel is a heterocyclic pyrazino-isoquinoline derivative with an unusually broad range of anthelmintic activity. It is dispensed as 600-mg tablets. The drug is crystalline and nearly colorless.[318,319] It is nearly insoluble in water. A peak serum concentration of 1 μm/ml is reached 1–2 hours after an oral dose of 50 mg/kg body weight is administered. Praziquantel is approximately 80 percent protein bound. There is pronounced first pass metabolism.[358] Approximately 80 percent of praziquantel is excreted in the urine in 4 days; 90 percent of that amount is excreted within the first 24 hours. The remainder is excreted in the feces. The pharmacokinetics of the drug were not significantly altered in one patient undergoing hemodialysis. The concentration of praziquantel in the cerebrospinal fluid is approximately 14–20 percent of the concentration of free plus protein-bound drug in the plasma.[359,360] Plasma levels have been decreased in patients with neurocysticercosis receiving dexamethasone simultaneously.

Praziquantel is rapidly taken up by flukes and tapeworms. It is uniformly distributed in these organisms but is not metabolized. Praziquantel increases the permeability of the flukes' tegument to calcium ions.[361–364] In adult schistosomes, an influx of calcium is followed by tetanic contraction and paralysis of the musculature. The initial effects are very rapid, and intense vacuolation of the tegument is observed.[361] Adult worms are then swept to the liver, where they are attacked by phagocytes. Praziquantel also results in increased exposure of parasite antigens on the surface of adult schistosomes.[365] In the tapeworm *Hymenolepis diminuta*, praziquantel causes calcium release from endogenous stores, and the worm suffers massive contraction.[366] Expulsion from the gastrointestinal tract follows. The tegument of the neck of the tapeworm develops blebs, but the scolex and proglottids appear to be unaffected.

Praziquantel is generally well tolerated.[317–320] Reactions are common, but are usually mild and transient. The most frequent ones are nausea, vomiting, abdominal pain, dizziness, headache, and lassitude. Only rarely is vomiting severe. In some instances, adverse effects may be due to allergic responses that follow the release of worm antigens. For example, urticarial reactions have been observed during the treatment of paragonimiasis.[367] Intense abdominal pain and bloody diarrhea have on occasion occurred in patients heavily infected with *Schistosoma mansoni*.[368–370] Finally, increased intracranial pressure, cerebral edema, and inflammation have been observed during the treatment of neurocysticercosis, and corticosteroids are now used concomitantly in this setting.[371,372] There has been no evidence of mutagenicity or teratogenicity in vitro, but there is an increase in the abortion rate in rats given three times the single human therapeutic dose. Praziquantel is also excreted in breast milk, and it is recommended that women not nurse on the day that praziquantel is given or during the subsequent 72 hours.

Metrifonate***

Metrifonate, an organophosphate that is metabolized in humans to dichlorvos,[373] is an alternative to praziquantel for the treatment of *Schistosoma hematobium*. Metrifonate is less expensive than praziquantel and of comparable efficacy, and it has been used in mass treatment programs.[374,375]

Metrifonate is an organophosphorus inhibitor of acetylcholinesterase.[376] It is well absorbed after oral ingestion.[377] When given to humans, metrifonate causes a decrease of 95 percent in plasma cholinesterase activity within 6 hours of administration. This activity usually returns to normal relatively quickly. Erythrocyte cholinesterase is inhibited to approximately 50 percent of pretreatment values but takes 2 or 2.5 months to return to normal levels.[377] Persons treated with metrifonate should not receive neuromuscular blocking agents or be exposed to insecticides with anticholineserase effects for at least 48 hours. Although the drug is usually well tolerated, mild vertigo, lassitude, nausea, vomiting, and occasionally bronchospasm have been reported. One limitation in large-scale treatment programs is that metrifonate must be given at intervals of 2 weeks, whereas praziquantel is administered in 1 day.

Oxamniquine

Oxamniquine, a tetrahydroquinoline, provides an alternative to praziquantel for the treatment of *S. mansoni* infections.[378–381] It seems to be more effective against strains of *S. mansoni* found in the New World, and it is less expensive than praziquantel. Oxamniquine has been used in mass treatment programs; a large-scale control program based on community therapy has been quite successful in Brazil.[382]

Oxamniquine is dispensed in 250-mg capsules. It is well absorbed orally, and the parent drug and its metabolites are excreted in the urine. It is given as a single dose. Side effects include dizziness, which may occur in 40 percent of the treated population, and drowsiness. Convulsions have occasionally been reported, and oxamniquine should not be used in persons with epilepsy. Orange to red discoloration of the urine has been associated with treatment.

Niridazole***

Niridazole, a nitrothiazole derivative, 1-(5-nitro-2-thiazolyl)-2-imidazolidinone, once widely used for the treatment of schistosomiasis,[383,384] is now seldom if ever indicated. It is far more toxic than praziquantel, metrifonate, and oxamniquine and offers no advantage in efficacy. In addition to schistosomiasis, it is effective in the treatment of dracunculiasis (guinea worm disease), where it acts by reducing swelling and pain and permitting relatively easy extraction of the adult worm.[383]

Niridazole is absorbed orally over several hours and is largely metabolized in the liver.[383] It can cause agitation, confusion, hallucinations, seizures, and electroencephalographic changes, particularly in persons with impaired hepatic function due to hepatosplenic schistosomiasis. It should not be used in persons with hepatic dysfunction or neuropsychiatric disorders.[385] Niridzole can also produce electrocardiographic changes, as well as transitory decreases in fertility. Other side effects include nausea, vomiting, diarrhea, loss of appetite, and headache. Less commonly encountered are insomnia, skin rash, and paresthesis. Niridazole can initiate hemolysis in persons with G6PD deficiency.[386]

Oltipaz***

Oltipaz is a new antischistosomal compound that has been studied in human schistosomiasis. Although it appears to be effective in the treatment of *S. mansoni* infection,[387] it offers no advantage over praziquantel.

Bithionol**

Bithionol is the drug of choice for treatment of *F. hepatica*[5] and is an alternative to praziquantel for the treatment of paragonimiasis.[388] Bithionol is administered orally, usually on alternate days, for 10–15 doses. It has been associated with urticaria, photosensitivity reactions, and gastrointestinal complaints. These allergic reactions may be due, in part or solely, to the release of worm antigens.

Niclosamide

Niclosamide (Fig. 12), *N*-(2′-chloro-4′-nitrophenyl)-5-chlorosalicylamide, given as a single dose, is the drug of choice for *Ta. saginata*, the beef tapeworm, *D. latum*, the fish tapeworm, and *Dipylidium caninum*, the dog tapeworm.[389] It is poorly absorbed, less expensive and less toxic than praziquantel, and highly effective against adult cestodes in he gastrointestinal tract. In the case of *Taenia solium*, treatment with niclosamide is usually followed by a purge to reduce the theoretical risk of autoinfection. Niclosamide results in disintegration of the adult tapeworm. Some physicians prefer to use quinacrine (see above under "Drugs Active Against Luminal Protozoa") for *Ta. solium*, since it causes the expulsion of the adult worm intact. Others prefer praziquantel, which is active against larval as well as adult forms, and might prevent cysticercosis if autoinfection occurred. Niclosamide is as active against *H. nana*, the dwarf tapeworm, as is praziquantel, but a single dose of praziquantel is effective, whereas niclosamide must be administered daily for 6 days.[5]

Niclosamide is very poorly absorbed and nontoxic. It is supplied in 500-mg vanilla-flavored tablets, which should be chewed thoroughly and then washed down with water. The anthelminthic mechanisms of niclosamide are not completely understood. The drug appears to uncouple oxidative phosphorylation in the scolex and proximal segments of the adult tapeworm and to stimulate adenosine triphosphatase activity of mitochondria, resulting in death of the worm and rapid disintegration of the scolex.[390] Niclosamide is remarkably free of toxicity, except for occasional mild gastrointestinal complaints, light-headedness, and, rarely, rash. Information on side effects has been collected in an uncontrolled manner, and it is uncertain whether a placebo group would differ significantly in respect to these symptoms.[391] When expulsion of the worm is delayed, neither the scolex nor the proglottids may be identifiable in the stool.

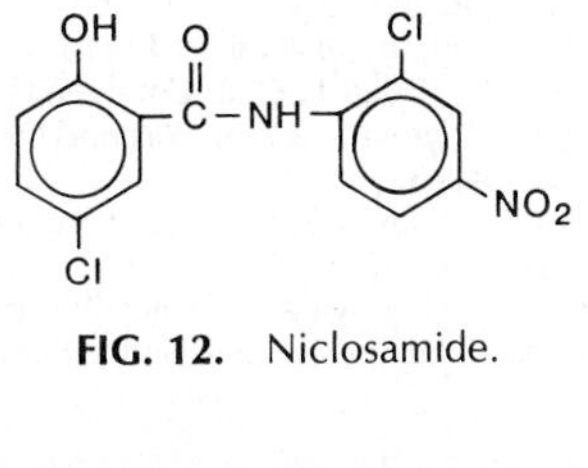

FIG. 12. Niclosamide.

REFERENCES

1. Lee JJ, Hutner SH, Bovee EC. An Illustrated Guide to the Protozoa. Lawrence, Kans.: Society of Protozoologists; 1985.
2. Levine ND. Nematode Parasites of Domestic Animals and of Man. Minneapolis: Burgess; 1968.
3. Burt DRR. Platyhelminthes and Parasitism. An Introduction to Parasitology. New York: American Elsevier; 1970.
4. Erasmus DA. The Biology of Trematodes. New York: Crane, Russak; 1972.
5. Drugs for parasitic infections. Med Lett Drugs Ther. 1988;30:15–22.
6. Powell SJ, Wilmot AJ, Elsdon-Dew R. Further trials of metronidazole in amoebic dysentery and amoebic liver abscess. Ann Trop Med Parasitol. 1967;61:511–4.
7. Welsh JS, Rowsell BJ, Freeman C. Treatment of intestinal amoebiasis and giardiasis: Efficacy of metronidazole and tinidazole compared. Med J Aust. 1978;1:469–71.
8. Salaki JS, Shirey JL, Strickland GT. Successful treatment of symptomatic *Entamoeba polecki* infection. Am J Trop Med Hyg. 1979;28:190–3.
9. Wolfe MS. Giardiasis. N Engl J Med. 1978;298:319–21.
10. Lerman SJ, Walker RA. Treatment of giardiasis. Literature review and recommendations. Clin Pediatr. 1982;21:409–14.
11. Lossick JG. Treatment of *Trichomonas vaginalis* infections. Rev Infect Dis. 1982;4(Suppl):S801–18.
12. Rein MF. Current therapy of vulvovaginitis. Sex Transm Dis. 1981;8:316–20.
13. Wolfe MS. *Blastocystis hominis* infection. In: Strickland GT, ed. Hunter's Tropical Medicine. 6th ed. Philadelphia: Saunders; 1984:513.
14. Walzer PD, Judson FN, Murphy KB, et al. Balantidiasis outbreak in Truk. Am J Trop Med Hyg. 1973;22:33–41.
15. Spillman R, Ayala SC, DeSanchez CE. Double blind test of metronidazole and tinidazole in the treatment of asymptomatic *Entamoeba histolytica* and *Entamoeba hartmanni* carriers. Am J Trop Med Hyg. 1976;25:549–51.
16. Dupont HL, Sullivan PS. Giardiasis: The clinical spectrum, diagnosis and therapy. Pediatr Infect Dis. 1986;5:S131–8.
17. Sharma VP, Rathore HS, Sharma MM. Efficacy of metronidazole in dracunculiasis: A clinical trial. Am J Trop Med Hyg. 1979;28:658–60.
18. Weniger BG, Schantz PM. Praziquantel and refugee health. JAMA. 1984;251:2391–2.
19. Houghton GW, Smith J, Thorpe PS, et al. The pharmacokinetics or oral and intravenous metronidazole in man. J Antimicrob Chemother. 1979;5:621–3.
20. McGilveray IJ, Midha KK, Loo JCK, et al. The bioavailability of commercial metronidazole formulations. Int J Clin Pharmacol. 1978;16:110–5.
21. Norris SM, Ravdin JI. The pharmacology of antiamebic drugs. In: Ravdin JI, ed. Amebiasis: Human Infection by *Entamoeba histolytica*. New York: Wiley; 1988:734–40.
22. Lindmark DG, Müller M. Antitrichomonad action, mutagenicity, and reduction of metronidazole and other nitroimidazoles. Antimicrob Agents Chemother. 1976;10:476–82.
23. Knight RC, Skolimowski IM, Edwards DI. The interaction of reduced metronidazole with DNA. Biochem Pharmacol. 1978;27:2089–93.
24. LaRusso NF, Tomasx M, Müller M, et al. Interaction of metronidazole with nucleic acids in vitro. Mol Pharmacol. 1977;13:872–82.
25. Lefebver Y, Hesseltine HC. The peripheral white blood cells and metronidazole. JAMA. 1965;194:15–8.
26. Kazmier FJ. A significant interaction between metronidazole and warfarin. Mayo Clin Proc. 1976;51:782–4.
27. Kusumi RK, Plouffe JF, Wyatt RH, et al. Central nervous system toxicity associated with metronidazole therapy. Ann Intern Med. 1980;93:59–60.
28. Rothstein E, Clancy DD. Toxicity of disulfiram combined with metronidazole. N Engl J Med. 1969;280:1006–7.
29. Rosenkranz HS, Speck WT. Studies on the significance of the mutagenicity of metronidazole for *Salmonella typhimurium*. In: Finegold SM, ed. Metronidazole, Proceedings of the International Metronidazole Conference, Montreal, Quebec, Canada, May 26–28, 1976. Princeton, N.J.: Excerpta Medica; 1977:119–25.
30. Koch RL, Beaulieu BB Jr, Chrystal EJT, et al. A metronidazole metabolite in human urine and its risk. Science. 1981;211:398–400.
31. Beard CM, Noller KL, O'Fallon WM, et al. Lack of evidence for cancer due to use of metronidazole. N Engl J Med. 1979;301:519–22.
32. Friedman GD, Cancer after metronidazole (Letter). N Engl J Med. 1980;302:519.
33. Bassily S, Farid Z, El-Masry NA, et al. Treatment of intestinal *E. histolytica* and *G. lamblia* with metronidazole, tinidazole and ornidazole: A comparative study. J Trop Med Hyg. 1987;90:9–12.
34. Goldman P. The development of 5-nitroimidazoles for the treatment and prophylaxis of anaerobic bacterial infections. J Antimicrob Chemother. 1982;10(Suppl A):23–33.
35. Rossignol JF, Maisonneuve H, Cho YW. Nitroimidazoles in the treatment of trichomoniasis, giardiasis, and amebiasis. Int J Clin Pharmacol Ther Toxicol. 1984;22:63–72.
36. Powell SJ, Wilmot AJ, MacLeod IN, et al. A comparative trial of dehydroemetine and emetine hydrochloride in identical dosage in amoebic liver abscess. Ann Trop Med Parasitol. 1967;61:26–8.

37. Scragg JN, Powell SJ. Emetine hydrochloride and dehydroemetine combined with chloroquine in the treatment of children with amoebic liver abscess. Arch Dis Child. 1968;43:121–3.
38. Yang WCT, Dubick M. Mechanism of emetine cardiotoxicity. Pharmacol Ther. 1980;10:15–26.
39. Grollman AP. Inhibitors of protein synthesis. V. Effects of emetine on protein and nucleic acid biosynthesis in HELA cells. J Biol Chem. 1968;243:4089–94.
40. Klatskin G, Friedman H. Emetine toxicity in man: Studies on the nature of early toxic manifestations, their relation to the dose level, and their significance in determining safe dosage. Ann Intern Med. 1948;28:892–915.
41. Webster LT Jr. Drugs used in the chemotherapy of protozoal infections: Amebiasis, giardiasis, and trichomoniasis. In: Gilman AG, Goodman LS, Rall TW, et al, eds. The Pharmacological Basis of Therapeutics. 7th ed. New York: Macmillan; 1985:1049–57.
42. Kent L, Kingsland RC. Effects of emetine hydrochloride on the electrocardiogram in man. Am Heart J. 1950;39:576–87.
43. Bradley WG, Fewings JD, Harris JB, et al. Emetine myopathy in the rat. Br J Pharmacol. 1976;57:29–41.
44. Oakley GP Jr. The neurotoxicity of the halogenated hydroxyquinolines. JAMA. 1973;225:395–7.
45. Wolfe MS. The treatment of intestinal protozoal infections. Med Clin North Am. 1982;66:707–20.
46. Krogstad DJ, Spencer HC Jr, Healy GR. Amebiasis. N Engl J Med. 1978;298:262–5.
47. Pehrson P, Bengtsson E. Treatment of non-invasive amoebiasis. A comparison between tinidazole alone and in combination with diloxanide furoate. Trans R Soc Trop Med Hyg. 1983;77:845–6.
48. Wolfe MS. Nondysenteric intestinal amebiasis: Treatment with diloxanide furoate. JAMA. 1973;224:1601–4.
49. Simon M, Shookhoff HB, Terner H, et al. Paromomycin in the treatment of intestinal amebiasis: A short course of therapy. Am J Gastroenterol. 1967;48:504–11.
50. Soderman WA Jr. Amebiasis (clinical seminar). Am J Dig Dis. 1971;16:51–60.
51. Botero D. Paromomycin as effective treatment of *Taenia* infections. Am J Trop Med. 1970;19:234–7.
52. Smith JW, Wolfe MS. Giardiasis. Ann Rev Med. 1980;31:373–83.
53. Craft JC, Murphy T, Nelson JD. Furizolidone and quinacrine. Comparative study of therapy for giardiasis in children. Am J Dis Child. 1981;135:164–6.
54. Bassily S, Farid Z, Mikhail JW, et al. The treatment of *Giardia lamblia* infection with mepacrine, metronidazole and furazolidone. J Trop Med Hyg. 1970;73:15–8.
55. Rollo IM. Miscellaneous drugs used in the treatment of protozoal infections. In: Gilman AG, Goodman LS. Gilman A, eds. The Pharmacological Basis of Therapeutics. 6th ed. New York: Macmillan; 1980:1070–9.
56. Findlay GM. Recent Advances in Chemotherapy. v. II. 3rd ed. London: J & A Churchill; 1951:341–68.
57. Sokol RJ, Lichtenstein PK, Farrell MK. Quinacrine hydrochloride-induced yellow discoloration of the skin in children. Pediatrics. 1982;69:232–3.
58. Lindenmayer JP, Vargas P. Toxic psychosis following use of quinacrine. J Clin Psychiatry. 1981;42:162–4.
59. Wolfe MS. Giardiasis. JAMA. 1975;233:1362–5.
60. Pratt WB, Fekety R. Chemotherapy in protozoal diseases. In: The Antimicrobial Drugs. New York: Oxford University Press; 1986:385–413.
61. Levi GC, de Avila CA, Neto VA. Efficacy of various drugs for treatment of giardiasis. A comparative study. Am J Trop Med Hyg. 1977;26:564–5.
62. Wyler DJ. Malaria—resurgence, resistance, and research. N Engl J Med. 1983;308:875–8, 934–40.
63. Hilton D. Malaria: A new battle plan. Contact. 1987;95:1–5.
64. Lobel HO, Campbell CC, Pappaioanou M, et al. Use of prophylaxis for malaria by American travelers to Africa and Haiti. JAMA. 1987;257:2626–7.
65. Remington JS, Desmonts G. Toxoplasmosis. In: Remington JS, Klein JO, eds. Infectious Diseases of the Fetus and Newborn Infant. 2nd ed. Philadelphia: Saunders; 1983:143–263.
66. Wong B, Gold JWM, Brown AE, et al. Central-nervous-system toxoplasmosis in homosexual men and parenteral drug abusers. Ann Intern Med. 1984;100:36–42.
67. Current WL, Reese NC, Ernst JV, et al. Human cryptosporidiosis in immunocompetent and immunodeficient persons: Studies of an outbreak and experimental transmission. N Engl J Med. 1983;308:1252–7.
68. Kaufman DL. *Pneumocystis carinii* pneumonia. Adv Exp Med Biol. 1986;202:153–69.
69. Kovacs JA, Hiemenz JW, Macher AM, et al. *Pneumocystis carinii* pneumonia: A comparison between patients with the acquired immunodeficiency syndrome and patients with other immunodeficiencies. Ann Intern Med. 1984;100:663–71.
69a. Edman JC, Kovacs JA, Mazur H, et al. Ribosomal RNA sequence shows *Pneumocystis carinii* to be a member of the fungi. Nature. 1988;334:519–22.
70. Krogstad DJ, Herwaldt BL, Schlesinger PH. Antimalarial agents: Specific treatment regimens. Antimicrob Agents Chemother. 1988;32:957–61.
71. Development of mefloquine as an antimalarial drug. *Bull WHO*. 1983;61:169–78.
72. Chloroquine-resistant *Plasmodium falciparum* malaria in West Africa. JAMA. 1987;257:2556–9.
73. LeBras J, Hatin I, Bouree P, et al. Chloroquine-resistant falciparum malaria in Benin. Lancet. 1986;2:1043–4.
74. Miller LH, Neva FA, Gill F. Failure of chloroquine in human babesiosis (*Babesia microti*): Case report and chemotherapeutic trial in hamsters. Ann Intern Med. 1978;88:200–2.
75. Brohult J, Rombo L, Sirleaf V, et al. The concentration of chloroquine in serum during short and long term malaria prophylaxis with standard and "double" dosage in non-immunes: Clinical implications. Ann Trop Med Parasitol. 1979;73:401–5.
76. Webster LT Jr. Drugs used in the chemotherapy of protozoal infections: Malaria. In: Gilman AG, Goodman LS, Rall TW, et al, eds. The Pharmacological Basis of Therapeutics. 7th ed. New York: Macmillan; 1985:1029–48.
77. Andrews P, Haberkorn A, Thomas H. Antiparasitic drugs: Mechanisms of action, pharmacokinetics, and in vitro and in vivo assays of drug activity. In: Lorian V, ed. Antibiotics in Laboratory Medicine. 2nd ed. Baltimore: Williams & Wilkins; 1986;282–345.
78. Warhurst DC. Antimalarial drugs: Mode of action and resistance. J Antimicrob Chemother. 1986;18(Suppl B):51–9.
79. Warhurst DC, Homewood CA, Baffaley VC. The chemotherapy of rodent mlaria. XX. Autophagic vacuole formation in *Plasmodium berghei* in vitro. Ann Trop Med Parasitol. 1974;68:265–81.
80. Konigk E, Putfarken B. Inhibition of ornithine decarboxylase in vitro cultured *Plasmodium falciparum* by chloroquine. Tropenmed Parasitol. 1983;34:1–3.
81. Krogstad DJ, Schlesinger PH. The basis of antimalarial action: Non-weak base effects of chloroquine on acid vesicle pH. *Am J Trop Med Hyg*. 1987;36:213–20.
82. Krogstad DJ, Schlesinger PH. Acid-vesicle function, intracellular pathogens and the action of chloroquine against *Plasmodium falciparum*. N Engl J Med. 1987;317:542–9.
83. Martin SK, Oduola AMJ, Milhous WK. Reversal of chloroquine resistance in *Plasmodium falciparum* by verapamil. Science. 1987;235:899–901.
84. Marks JS. Chloroquine retinopathy: Is there a safe daily dose? Ann Rheum Dis. 1982;41:52–8.
85. White NJ, Watt G, Bergvist Y, et al. Parenteral chloroquine for treating falciparum malaria. J Infect Dis. 1987;155:192–201.
86. Riou B, Barriot P, Rimailho A, et al. Treatment of severe chloroquine poisoning. N Engl J Med. 1988;318:1–6.
87. Hart CW, Naunton RF. The ototoxicity of chloroquine phosphate. Arch Otolaryngol. 1964;80:407–12.
88. Hatton CSR, Peto TEA, Bunch C, et al. Frequency of severe neutropenia associated with amodiaquine prophylaxis against malaria. Lancet. 1986;1:411–4.
89. Cook GC. *Plasmodium falciparum* infection: Problems in prophylaxis and treatment in 1986. Q J Med. 1986;61:1091–115.
90. Saxena AK, Saxena M. Advances in chemotherapy of malaria. Prog Drug Res. 1986;30:221–80.
91. Looareesuwan S, White NJ, Chittamas S, et al. High rate of *Plasmodium vivax* relapse following treatment of falciparum malaria in Thailand. Lancet. 1987;2:1052–5.
92. Alving AS, Johnson CF, Tarlov AR, et al. Mitigation of the haemolytic effect of primaquine and enhancement of its action against exoerythrocytic forms of the Chesson strain of *Plasmodium vivax* by intermittent regimens of drug administration: A preliminary report. Bull WHO. 1960;22:621–31.
93. Clyde DF, McCarthy VC. Radical cure of Chesson strain vivax malaria in man by 7, not 14, days of treatment with primaquine. Am J Trop Med Hyg. 1977;26:562–3.
94. Kellermeyer RW, Tarlov AR, Brewer GJ, et al. Hemolytic effect of therapeutic drugs: Clinical considerations of the primaquine-type hemolysis. JAMA. 1962;180:388–94.
95. Clyde DF. Clinical problems associated with the use of primaquine as a tissue schizontocidal and gametocytocidal drug. Bull WHO. 1981;59:391–5.
96. Brodie BB, Baer JE, Craig LC. Metabolic products of the cinchona alkaloids in human urine. J Biol Chem. 1951;188:567–81.
97. White NJ, Looareesuwan S, Warrell DA, et al. Quinine pharmacokinetics and toxicity in cerebral and uncomplicated falciparum malaria. Am J Med. 1982;73:564–72.
98. Canfield CJ, Miller LH, Bartelloni PJ, et al. Acute renal failure in *Plasmodium falciparum* malaria. Arch Intern Med. 1968;122:199–203.
99. Pratt WB, Fekety R. Chemotherapy of malaria. In: The Antimicrobial Drugs. New York: Oxford University Press; 1986:355–84.
100. White JN, Warrell DA, Chanthavanich P, et al. Severe hypoglycemia and hyperinsulinemia in falciparum malaria. N Engl J Med. 1983;309:61–6.
101. Phillips RE, Looareesunwan S, White NJ, et al. Quinine pharmacokinetics and toxicity in pregnant and lactating women with falciparum malaria. Br J Clin Pharmacol. 1986;21:677–83.
102. Phillips RE, Warrell DA, White NJ, et al. Intravenous quinidine for the treatment of severe falciparum malaria. N Engl J Med. 1985;312:1273–8.
103. Rudnitsky G, Miller KD, Padua T, et al. Continuous-infusion quinidine gluconate for treating children with severe *Plasmodium falciparum* malaria. J Infect Dis. 1987;155:1040–3.
104. Swerdlow CD, Yu JO, Jacobsen E, et al. Safety and efficacy of intravenous quinidine. Am J Med. 1983;75:36–42.
105. Botero D, Restrepo M, Montoya A. Prospective double-blind trial of two different doses of mefloquine plus pyrimethamine-sulfadoxine compared

with pyrimethamine-sulfadoxine alone in the treatment of falciparum malaria. Bull WHO. 1985;63:731–7.
106. De Sousa JM, Sheth UK, Oliveira RMG, et al. An open, randomized, phase III clinical trial of mefloquine and of quinine plus sulfadoxime-pyrimethamine in the treatment of symptomatic falciparum malaria in Brazil. Bull WHO. 1985;63:603–9.
107. Tin F, Hlaing N, Tun T, et al. Falciparum malaria treated with a fixed combination of mefloquine, sulfadoxine and pyrimethamine: A field study in adults in Burma. Bull WHO. 1985;63:727–30.
108. Chongsuphajaisiddhi T, Sabchareon A, Chantavanich P, et al. A phase-III clinical trial of mefloquine in children with chloroquine-resistant falciparum malaria in Thailand. Bull WHO. 1987;65:223–6.
109. Oduola AMJ, Milhous WK, Salako LA, et al. Reduced in-vitro susceptibility to mefloquine in West African isolates of *Plasmodium falciparum*. Lancet. 1987;2:1304–5.
110. Desjardins RW, Pamplin CL III, von Bredow J, et al. Kinetics of a new antimalarial, mefloquine. Clin Pharmacol Ther. 1979;26:372–9.
111. Jacobs GH, Aikawa M, Milhous WK, et al. An ultrastructural study of the effects of mefloquine on malaria parasite. Am J Trop Med Hyg. 1987;36:9–14.
112. Chanthavanich P, Looareesuwan S, White NJ, et al. Intragastic mefloquine is absorbed rapidly in patients with cerebral malaria. Am J Trop Med Hyg. 1985;34:1028–36.
113. Harinasuta T, Bunnag D, Wensdorfer WH. A phase II clinical trial of mefloquine in patients with chloroquine-resistant falciparum malaria in Thailand. Bull WHO. 1983;61:299–305.
114. Meek SR, Doberstyn EB, Gaürzère BA, et al. Treatment of falciparum malaria with quinine and tetracycline or combined mefloquine/sulfadoxine/pyrimethamine on the Thai–Kampuchean border. Am J Trop Med Hyg. 1986;35:246–50.
115. Centers for Diease Control. Recommendations for the prevention of malaria in travelers. MMWR. 1988;37:277–84.
116. Pearson RD, Hewlett EL. Use of pyrimethamine-sulfadoxine (Fansidar) in prophylaxis against chloroquine-resistant *Plasmodium falciparum* and *Pneumocystis carinii*. Ann Intern Med. 1987;106:714–18.
117. DeHovitz JA, Pape JW, Boncy M, et al. Clinical manifestations and therapy of *Isospora belli* infection in patients with the acquired immunodeficiency syndrome. N Engl J Med. 1986;315:87–90.
118. Hughes WT, Feldman S, Chaudhary SC, et al. Comparison of pentamidine isethionate and trimethoprim-sulfamethoxazole in the treatment of *Pneumocystis carinii* pneumonia. J Pediatr. 1978;92:285–91.
119. Young LS. Trimethoprim-sulfamethoxazole in the treatment of adults with pneumonia due to *Pneumocystis carinii*. Rev Infect Dis. 1982;4:608–13.
120. Siegel SE, Wolff LJ, Baehner RL, et al. Treatment of *Pneumocystis carinii* pneumonitis: A comparative trial of sulfamethoxazole-trimethoprim v. pentamidine in pediatric patients with cancer: Report from Childrens Cancer Study Group. Am J Dis Child. 1984;138:1051–4.
121. Luft BJ, Conley F, Remington JS. Outbreak of central-nervous-system toxoplasmosis in Western Europe and North America. Lancet. 1983;1:781–4.
122. Haverkos HW. Assessment of therapy for toxoplasma encephalitis. The TE study group. Am J Med. 1987;82:907–14.
123. Luft BJ, Remington JS. Toxoplasmic encephalitis. J Infect Dis. 1988;157:1–6.
124. Wilson CB, Remington JS. Toxoplasmosis. In: Feigin RD, Cherry JD, eds. Textbook of Pediatric Infectious Diseases. 2nd ed. Philadelphia: Saunders; 1987:2067–78.
125. McCabe R, Remington JS. Toxoplasmosis: The time has come. N Engl J Med. 1988;318:313–5.
126. Allegra CJ, Chabner BA, Tuazon CU, et al. Trimetrexate for the treatment of *Pneumocytis carinii* pneumonia in patients with the acquired immunodeficiency syndrome. N Engl J Med. 1987;317:978–85.
127. Kovacs JA, Allegra CJ, Chabner BA, et al. Potent effect of trimetrexate, a lipid-soluble antifolate, on *Toxoplasma gondii*. J Infect Dis. 1987;155:1027–32.
128. Daffos F, Forestier F, Capella-Pavlovsky M, et al. Prenatal management of 746 pregnancies at risk for congenital toxoplasmosis. N Engl J Med. 1988;318:271–5.
129. Weidekamm E, Plozza-Nottebrock H, Forgo I, et al. Plasma concentrations of pyrimethamine and sulfadoxine and evaluation of pharmacokinetic data by computerized curve fitting. Bull WHO. 1982;60:115–22.
130. Jaffe JJ. Dihydrofolate reductase in parasitic protozoa and helminths. In: Van den Bossche H, ed. Biochemistry of Parasites. London: Academic Press: 1972;219–33.
131. Hayama T, Kokue E. Use of the Goettingen miniature pig for studying pyrimethamine teratogenesis. CRC Crit Rev Toxicol. 1985;14:403–21.
132. Petter C, Bourbon J. Foetal red cell macrocytosis induced by pyrimethamine; its teratogenic role. Experientia. 1975;31:369–70.
133. Pyrimethamine combinations in pregnancy. Lancet. 1983;2:1005–7.
134. Harpey, JP, Darbois Y, LeFèbvre G. Teratogenicity of pyrimethamine (Letter). Lancet. 1983;2:399.
135. Mandell GL, Sande MA. Antimicrobial agents: Sulfonamides, trimethoprim-sulfamethoxazole, and urinary tract antiseptics. In: Gilman AG, Goodman LS, Rall TW, et al, eds. The Pharmacological Basis of Therapeutics. 7th ed. New York: Macmillian; 1985:1095–1114.
136. Navin TR, Miller KD, Satriale RF, et al. Adverse reactions associated with pyrimethamine-sulfadoxine prophylaxis for *Pneumocystis carinii* infections in AIDS (Letter). Lancet. 1985;1:1332.
137. Miller KD, Lobel HO, Satriale RF, et al. Severe cutaneous reactions among American travelers using pyrimethamine-sulfadoxine (Fansidar) for malaria prophylaxis. Am J Trop Med Hyg. 1986;35:451–8.
138. Rombo L, Stenbeck J, Lobel HO, et al. Does chloroquine contribute to the risk of serious adverse reactions to Fansidar? Lancet. 1985;2:1298–9.
139. Karbwang J, Bunnag D, Breckenridge AM, et al. The pharmacokinetics of mefloquine when given alone or in combination with sulphadoxine and pyrimethamine in Thai male and female subjects. Eur J Clin Pharmacol. 1987;32:173–7.
140. De Sousa JM, Sheth UK, Oliveira RMG, et al. A phase I clinical trial of Fansimef (mefloquine plus sulfadoxine-pyrimethamine) in Brazilian male subjects. Bull WHO. 1985;63:611–5.
141. Young LS. Treatment and prevention of *Pneumocystis carinii* infection. In: Young LS, ed. *Pneumocystis carinii* Pneumonia: Pathogenesis, Diagnosis, Treatment. New York: Marcel Dekker; 1984:175–94.
142. Wharton JM, Coleman DL, Wolfsy CB, et al. Trimethoprim-sulfamethoxazole or pentamidine for *Pneumocystis carinii* pneumonia in the acquired immunodeficiency syndrome. Ann Intern Med. 1986;105:37–44.
143. Hughes WT. Five year absence of *Pneumocystis carinii* pneumonitis in a pediatric oncology center. J Infect Dis. 1984;150:305–6.
144. Hughes WT, Rivera GK, Schell MJ, et al. Successful intermittent chemoprophylaxis for *Pneumocystis carinii* pneumonitis. N Engl J Med. 1987;316:1627–32.
145. Jick H. Adverse reactions to trimethoprim-sulfamethoxazole in hospitalized patients. Rev Infect Dis. 1982;4:426–8.
146. Pratt WB, Fekety R. The antimetabolites. In: The Antimicrobical Drugs, New York: Oxford University Press; 1986:229–51.
147. Kaufman DL. *Pneumocystis carinii* pneumonia. Adv Exp Med Biol. 1986;202:153–69.
148. Gordin FM, Simon GL, Wofsy CB, et al. Adverse reactions to trimethoprim-sulfamethoxazole in patients with the acquired immunodeficiency syndrome. Ann Intern Med. 1984;100:495–9.
149. Small CB, Harris CA, Friedland GH, et al. The treatment of *Pneumocystis carinii* pneumonia in the acquired immunodeficiency syndrome. Arch Intern Med. 1985;145:837–40.
150. Leoung GS, Mills J, Hopewell PC, et al. Dapsone-trimethoprim for *Pneumocystis carinii* pneumonia in the acquired immunodeficiency syndrome. Ann Intern Med. 1986;105:45–8.
151. Medina I, Leoung G, Mills J, et al. Oral therapy for *Pneumocystis carinii* pneumonia in AIDS: A randomized double blind trial for trimethoprim-sulfamethoxazole versus dapsone-trimethoprim for first episode (abstract). Third International Conference on AIDS, Washington, D.C., June 1–5, 1987.
152. Metroka CE, Lange R, Braun N, et al. Successful chemoprophylaxis for *Pneumocystis carinii* pneumonia with dapsone in patients with AIDS and ARC (abstract). Third International Conference on AIDS, Washington, D.C., June 1–5, 1987.
153. Mandell GL, Sande MA. Antimicrobial agents: Drugs used in the chemotherapy of tuberculosis and leprosy. In: Gilman AG, Goodman LS, Rall TW, et al, eds. *The Pharmacological Basis of Therapeutics*. 7th ed. New York: Macmillan; 1985:1199–218.
154. Pratt WB, Fekety R. Drugs that act on mycobacteria: Isoniazid, rifampin, ethambutol, and streptomycin; the minor antituberculosis drugs; drugs effective against leprosy. In: Pratt WB, Fekety R, eds. The Antimicrobial Drugs. New York: Oxford University Press; 1986:277–314.
155. Cook GC. Prevention and treatment of malaria. Lancet. 1988:1:32–7.
156. Rollo IM. The mode of action of sulphonamides, Proguanil and pyrimethamine on *Plasmodium gallinaceum*. Br J Pharmacol Chemother. 1955;10:208–14.
157. Fogh S, Schapira A, Bygbjerg IC, et al. Malaria chemoprophylaxis in travellers to East Africa: A comparative prospective study of chloroquine plus proguanil with chloroquine plus sulfadoxine-pyrimethamine. Br Med J. 1988;296:820–2.
158. Araujo FG, Guptill DR, Remington JS. In vivo activity of piritrexin against *Toxoplasma gondii*. J Infect Dis. 1987;156:828–30.
159. Lakhanpal V, Schocket SS, Nirankari VS. Clindamycin in the treatment of toxoplasmic retinochoroiditis. Am J Ophthalmol. 1983;95:605–13.
160. Ferguson JG Jr. Clindamycin therapy for toxoplasmosis. Ann Ophthalmol. 1981;13:95–100.
161. Clindamycin and quinine treatment for *Babesia microti* infections. MMWR. 1983;32;65–6.
162. Chan J, Luft BJ, Activity of roxithromycin (RU28965), a macrolide, against *Toxoplasma gondii* infection in mice. Antimicrob Agents Chemother. 1986;30:323–4.
163. Hofflin JM, Remington JS. In vivo synergism of roxithromycin (RU965) and interferon against *Toxoplasma gondii*. Antimicrob Agents Chemother. 1987;31:346–8.
164. King H, Lourie EM, York W. Studies in chemotherapy XIX: Further report on new trypanocidal substances. Ann Trop Med Parasitol. 1938;32:117–92.
165. Kager PA, Rees PH, Manguyu FM, et al. Clinical, haematological and parasitological response to treatment of visceral leishmaniasis in Kenya: A study of 64 patients. Trop Geogr Med. 1984;36:21–35.
166. Jha TK. Evaluation of diamidine compound (pentamidine isethionate) in the treatment of resistant cases of kala-azar occurring in North Bihar, India. Trans R Soc Trop Med Hyg. 1983;77:167–70.
167. Thakur CP. Epidemiological, clinical and therapeutic features of Bihar kala-azar (including post kala-azar dermal leishmaniasis). Trans R Soc Trop Med Hyg. 1984;78:391–8.

168. Kluge RM, Spaulding DM, Spain AJ. Combination of pentamidine and trimethoprim-sulfamethoxazole in the therapy of *Pneumocystis carinii* pneumonia in rats. Antimicrob Agents Chemother. 1978;13:975–8.
169. Montgomery AB, Debs JR, Luce JM, et al. Aerosolised pentamidine as sole therapy for *Pneumocystis carinii* pneumonia in patients with acquired immunodeficiency syndrome. Lancet. 1987;2:480–3.
170. Conte JE Jr, Hollander H, Golden JA. Inhaled or reduced-dose intravenous pentamidine for *Pneumocystis carinii* pneumonia. Ann Intern Med. 1987;107:495–8.
171. Bernard E, Schmitt H, Pagel L, et al. Safety and effectiveness of aerosol pentamidine for prevention of PCP in patients with AIDS (abstract). 27th Interscience Conference on Antimicrobial Chemotherapy. New York: 1987.
171a. Corkery KJ, Luse JM, Montgomery AB. Aerosolized pentamidine for treatment and prophylaxis of *Pneumocystis carinii* pneumonia: An update. Respiratory Care. 1988;33:676–85.
172. Pearson RD, Hewlett EL. Pentamidine for the treatment of *Pneumocystis carinii* pneumonia and other protozoal diseases. Ann Intern Med. 1985;103:782–6.
173. Navin TR, Fontaine RE. Intravenous versus intramuscular administration of pentamidine (Letter). N Engl J Med. 1984;311:1701–2.
174. Williamson J. Effects of trypanosides on the fine structure of target organisms. Pharmacol Ther. 1979;7:445–512.
175. Croft SL, Brazil RP. Effect of pentamidine isethionate on the ultrastructure and morphology of *Leishmania mexicana amazonensis* in vitro. Ann Trop Med Parasitol. 1982;76:37–43.
176. Waring MJ. The effects of antimicrobial agents on ribonucleic acid polymerase. Mol Pharmacol. 1965;1:1–13.
177. Wallis OC. The effect of pentamidine on ribosomes of the parasitic flagellate *Crithidia* (*Strigomonas*) *oncopelti*. J Protozool. 1966;13:234–9.
178. Gutteridge WE. Some effects of pentamidine di-isethionate on *Crithidia fasciculata*. J Protozool. 1969;16:306–11.
179. Bachrach U, Brem S, Wertman SB, et al. *Leishmania* spp: Effect of inhibitors on growth and on polyamine and macromolecular syntheses. Exp Parasitol. 1979;48:464–70.
180. Waalkes TP, Makulu DR. Pharmcologic aspects of pentamidine. Natl Cancer Inst Monogr. 1976;43:171–7.
181. Geratz JD. Inhibitory effect of aromatic diamidines on trypsin and enterokinase. Experientia. 1969;25:1254–5.
182. Hill GC, Hutner SH. Effect of trypanocidal drugs on terminal respiration of *Crithidia fasciculata*. Exp Parasitol. 1968;22;207–12.
183. Walzer PD, Perl DP, Krogstad DJ, et al. *Pneumocystis carinii* pneumonia in the United States: Epidemiologic, diagnostic, and clinical features. Ann Intern Med. 1974;80:83–93.
184. Western KA, Perera DR, Schultz MG. Pentamidine isethionate in the treatment of *Pneumocystis carinii* pneumonia. Ann Intern Med. 1970;73:695–702.
185. Bouchard P, Sai P, Reach G, et al. Diabetes mellitus following pentamidine-induced hypoglycemia in humans. Diabetes. 1982;31:40–5.
186. Osei K, Falko JM, Nelson KP, et al. Diabetogenic effect of pentamidine: In vitro and in vivo studies in a patient with malignant insulinoma. Am J Med. 1984;77:41–6.
187. Fitzgerald DB, Young IS. Reversal of pentamidine-induced hypoglycemia with oral diazoxide. J Trop Med Hyg. 1984;87:15–9.
188. Taelman H, Schechter PJ, Marcelis L, et al. Difluoromethylornithine, an effective new treatment of Gambian trypanosomiasis. Am J Med. 1987;82:607–14.
189. Di Bari C, Pastore G, Roscigno G, et al. Late-stage African trypanosomiasis and eflornithine (Letter). Ann Intern Med. 1986;105:803–4.
190. Van Nieuwenhove S, Schechter PJ, Declercq J, et al. Treatment of gambiense sleeping sickness in the Sudan with oral DFMO (DL-α-difluoromethylornithine), an inhibitor of ornithine decarbopxylase; first field trial. Trans R Soc Trop Med Hyg. 1985;79:692–8.
191. Marr JJ, Docampo R. Chemotherapy for Chagas' disease: A perspective of current therapy and considerations for future research. Rev Infect Dis. 1986;8:884–903.
192. Pearson RD, Navin TR, Sousa AQ, et al. Leishmaniasis. In: Kass EH, Platt R, eds. Current Therapy in Infectious Diseases. Toronto: BC Decker; 1989, in press.
193. Webster LT Jr. Drugs used in the chemotherapy of protozoal infections: Leishmaniasis, trypanosomiasis and other protozoal infections. In: Gilman AG, Goodman LS, Rall TW, et al, eds. The Pharmacological Basis of Therapeutics. 7th ed. New York: Macmillan; 1985:1058–65.
194. Fairlamb AH, Bowman IB. *Trypanosoma brucei*: Suramin and other trypanocidal compounds: Effects on sn-glycerol-3 phosphate oxidase. Exp Parasitol. 1977;43:353–61.
195. Fuglsang H, Anderson J. Side effects of suramin. In: Research and Control of Onchocerciasis in the Western Hemisphere. Pan American Health Organization, Scientific Publication No 298:54–7.
196. Flynn IW, Bowman IBR. Further studies on the mode of arsenicals on trypanosome pyruvate kinase (Abstract). Trans R Soc Trop Med Hyg. 1969;63:121.
197. Robertson DHH. Chemotherapy of African trypanosomes. Practitioner. 1962;188:80–3.
198. Arrox JOL. Melarsoprol and reactive encephalopathy in *Trypanosoma brucei rhodesiense*. Trans R Soc Trop Med Hyg. 1987;81:192.
199. Golden JA, Sjoerdsma A, Santi DV. *Pneumocystis carinii* pneumonia treated with alpha-difluoromethylornithine. West J Med. 1984;141:613–23.
200. Gilman TM, Paulson YJ, Boylen CT, et al. Eflornithine treatment of *Pneumocystis carinii* pneumonia in AIDS. JAMA. 1986;256:2197–8.
201. McLess BD, Barlow JLR, Kuzma RJ, et al. Studies on successful eflornithine treatment of *Pneumocystis carinii* pneumonia in AIDS patients failing conventional therapy (Abstract). Third International Conference on AIDS, Washington, D.C., June 1–5, 1987.
202. Bacchi CJ. Content, synthesis, and function of polyamines in trypanosomatids: Relationship to chemotherapy. J Protozool. 1981;28:20–7.
203. Sjoerdsma A, Schechter PJ. Chemotherapeutic implications of polyamine biosynthesis inhibition. Clin Pharmacol Ther. 1984;35:287–300.
204. Brener Z. Present status of chemotherapy and chemoprophylaxis of human trypanosomiasis in the Western Hemisphere. Pharmacol Ther. 1979;7:71–90.
205. Haegele KD, Alken RG, Grove J, et al. Kinetics of alpha-difluromethylornithine: An irreversible inhibitor of ornithine decarboxylase. Clin Pharmacol Ther. 1981;30:210–7.
206. Docampo R, Morena SNJ. Free radical metabolites in the mode of action of chemotherapeutic agents and phagocytic cells on *Trypanosoma cruzi*. Rev Infect Dis. 1984;6:223–38.
207. Moreno SNJ, Palmero DJ, de Palmero KE, et al. Stimulation of lipid peroxidation and ultrastructural alternations by nifurtimox in mammalian tissues. Medicina (B Aires). 1980;40:553–9.
208. Apt W, Arribada A, Arab F, et al. Clinical trial of benznidazole and an immunopotentiator against Chagas' disease in Chile (Letter). Trans R Soc Trop Med Hyg. 1986;80:1010.
209. Andrade SG, Magalhaes JB, Pontes AL. Evaluation of chemotherapy with benznidazole and nifurtimox in mice infected with *Trypanosoma cruzi* strains of different types. Bull WHO. 1985;63:721–6.
210. Anabwani GM, Ngira JA, Dimiti G, et al. Comparison of two dosage schedules of sodium stibogluconate in the treatment of visceral leishmaniasis in Kenya. Lancet. 1983;1;210–2.
211. Report of a WHO Expert Committee. The leishmaniases. Geneva: WHO Technical Report Series 701; 1984.
212. Ballou WR, McClain JB, Gordon DM, et al. Safety and efficacy of high-dose sodium stibogluconate therapy of American cutaneous leishmaniasis. Lancet. 1987;2:13–6.
213. Marr JJ, Berens RL. Pyrazolopyrimidine metabolism in the pathogenic trypanosomatides. Mol Biochem Parasitol. 1983;7:339–56.
214. Neal RA, Croft SL, Nelson DJ. Anti-leishmanial effect of allopurinol ribonucleoside and the related compounds, allopurinol, thiopurinol, thiopurinol ribonucleoside, and of formycin B, sinefungin and the lepidine WR 6026. Trans R Soc Trop Med Hyg. 1985;79:122–8.
215. Kager PA, Rees PH, Wellde BT, et al. Allopurinol in the treatment of visceral leishmaniasis. Trans R Soc Trop Med Hyg. 1981;75:556–9.
216. Weinrauch L, Livshin R, El-On J. Cutaneous leishmaniasis: Treatment with ketaconazole. Cutis. 1983;32:288–9, 294.
217. El-On J, Weinrauch L, Livshin R, et al. Topical treatment of recurrent cutaneous leishmaniasis in ointment containing paromomycin and methylbenzethionium chloride. Br Med J. 1985;291:704–5.
218. Chulay JD, Fleckenstein L, Smith DH. Pharmacokinetics of antimony during treatment of visceral leishmaniasis with sodium stibogluconate or meglumine antimoniate. Trans R Soc Trop Med Hyg. 1988;82:69–72.
219. Information material for physicians—Pentostam (sodium antimony gluconate), HHS, PHS, CDC protocol. Provided by the Centers for Disease Control to physicians administering Pentostam in the United States.
220. Berman JD. Chemotherapy for leishmaniasis: Biochemical mechanisms, clinical efficacy, and future strategies. Rev Infect Dis. 1988;10:560–86.
221. Croft SL, Neal RA. The effect of allopurinol ribonucleoside and formycin B on *Trypanosoma cruzi* infections in mice. Trans R Soc Trop Med Hyg. 1985;79:517–8.
222. Sampaio SAP, Godoy JT, Paiva L, et al. The treatment of American (mucocutaneous) leishmaniasis with amphotericin B. Arch Dermatol. 1960;82:627–35.
223. Crofts MAJ. Use of amphotericin B in mucocutaneous leishmaniasis. J Trop Med Hyg. 1976;79:111–3.
224. Keystone JS, Murdoch JK. Mebendazole. Ann Intern Med. 1979;91:582–6.
225. Wolfe MS, Wershing JM. Mebendazole. Treatment of trichuriasis and ascariasis in Bahamian children. JAMA 1974;230:1408–11.
226. Partono F, Purnomo, Tangkilisan A. The use of mebendazole in the treatment of polyparasitism. Southeast Asian J Trop Med Public Health. 1974;5:258–64.
227. Miller MJ, Krupp IM, Little MD, et al. Mebendazole: An effective anthelmintic for trichuriasis and enterobiasis. JAMA. 1974;230:1412–4.
228. Abadi K. Single dose mebendazole therapy for soil-transmitted nematodes. Am J Trop Med Hyg. 1985;34:129–33.
229. Islam N, Chowdhury NA. Mebendazole and pyrantel pamoate as broad-spectrum anthelmintics. Southeast Asian J Trop Med Public Health. 1976;7:81–4.
230. Pelletier LL Jr, Baker CB. Treatment failures following mebendazole therapy for chronic strongyloidiasis. J Infect Dis. 1987;156:532–3.
231. Wilson KH, Kauffman CA. Persistent *Strongyloides stercoralis* in a blind loop of the bowel. Successful treatment with mebendazole. Arch Intern Med. 1983;143:357–8.
232. Witassek F, Bircher J. Chemotherapy of larval echinococcosis with mebendazole: Microsomal liver function and cholestasis as determinants of plasma drug level. Eur J Clin Pharmacol. 1983;25:85–90.
233. Luder J, Witassek F, Weigand K, et al. Treatment of cystic echinococcosis

(*Echinococcus granulosus*) with mebendazole: Assessment of bound and free drug levels in cyst fluid and of parasite vitality in operative specimens. Eur J Clin Pharmacol. 1985;28:279–85.
234. Rudwan MA, Mousa A-RM, Muhtaseb SA. Abdominal hydatid disease: Follow-up of mebendazole therapy by CT and ultrasonography. Int Surg. 1986;71:22–6.
235. Rausch RL, Wilson JF, McMahon BJ, et al. Consequences of continuous mebendazole therapy in alveolar hydatid disease—with a summary of a ten-year clinical trial. Ann Trop Med Parasitol. 1986;80:403–19.
236. Smego DR, Smego RA Jr. Hydatid cyst: Preoperative sterilization with mebendazole. South Med J. 1986;79:900–1.
237. Sayek I, Cakmakci M. The effect of prophylactic mebendazole in experimental peritoneal hydatidosis. Surg Gynecol Obstet. 1986;163:351–3.
238. Wilson JF, Rausch RL, McMahon BJ, et al. Albendazole therapy in alveolar hydatid disease: A report of favorable results in two patients after short-term therapy. Am J Trop Med Hyg. 1987;37:162–8.
239. Mansueto S, Di Rosa S, Farinella E, et al. Albendazole in the treatment of hydatid disease: More than a hope (Letter). Trans R Soc Trop Med Hyg. 1987;81:168.
240. Okelo GBA. Hydatid disease: Research and control in Turkana, III. Albendazole in the treatment of inoperable hydatid disease in Kenya—a report on 12 cases. Trans R Soc Trop Med Hyg. 1986;80:193–5.
241. Morris DL. Pre-operative albendazole therapy for hydatid cyst. Br J Surg. 1987;74:805–6.
242. Levin ML. Treatment of trichinosis with mebendazole. Am J Trop Med Hyg. 1983;32;980–3.
243. Hess JA, Chandrasekar PH, Mortiere M, et al. Comparative efficacy of ketoconazole and mebendazole in experimental trichinosis. *Antimicrob Agents Chemother.* 1986;30:953–4.
244. Van Hoegaerden M, Ivanoff B, Flocard F, et al. The use of mebendazole in the treatment of filariasis due to *Loa loa* and *Mansonella perstans*. Ann Trop Med Parasitol. 1987;81:275–82.
245. Van Hoegaerden M, Flocard F. Mebendazole treatment of loiasis (Letter). Lancet. 1985;1:1278.
246. Webster LT Jr. Drugs used in the chemotherapy of helminthiasis. In: Gilman AG, Goodman LS, Rall TW, et al, eds. The Pharmacologic Basis of Therapeutics. 7th ed. New York: Macmillan; 1985:1009–28.
247. Howells RE, Delves CJ. A simple method for the identification of compounds which inhibit tubulin polymerization in filarial worms. Ann Trop Med Parasitol. 1985;79:507–12.
248. Official Product Monographs, Vermox Tablets. Raritan, NJ: Ortho Pharmaceutical Corp; June 11, 1978 (cited in Ref. 224).
249. Levin MH, Weinstein RA, Axelrod JL, et al. Severe, reversible neutropenia during high-dose mebendazole therapy for echinococcosis. JAMA. 1983;249:2929–31.
250. Fernández-Bañares F, González-Huix F, Xiol X, et al. Marrow aplasia during high dose mebendazole treatment. Am J Trop Med Hyg. 1986;35:350–1.
251. Rossignol JF, Maisonneuve H. Benzimidazoles in the treatment of trichuriasis: A review. Ann Trop Med Parasitol. 1984;78:135–44.
252. Bassily S, El-Masry NA, Trabolsi B, et al. Treatment of ancyclostomiasis and ascariasis with albendazole. Ann Trop Med Parasitol. 1984;78:81–2.
253. Hui-lan Z, Wei-ji C, Rossignol JF, et al. Albendazole in nematode, cestode, trematode and protozoan (giardia) infections. Chin Med J. (Engl.) 1986;99:912–5.
254. Jagota SC. Albendazole, a broad-spectrum anthelmintic, in the treatment of intestinal nematode and cestode infections: A multicenter study in 480 patients. Clin Ther. 1986;8:226–31.
255. Pugh RNH, Teesdale CH, Burnham GM. Albendazole in children with hookworm infection. Ann Trop Med Parasitol. 1986;80:565–7.
256. Escobedo F, Penagos P, Rodriguez J, et al. Albendazole therapy for neurocysticercosis. Arch Intern Med. 1987;147:738–41.
257. Morris DL, Smith PG. Albendazole in hydatid disease—hepatocellular toxicity. Trans R Soc Trop Med Hyg. 1987;81:343–4.
258. Yoshimura H. Teratogenicity of flubendazole in rats. Toxicology. 1987;43:133–8.
259. Téllez-Girón E, Ramos MC, Dufour L, et al. Treatment of neurocysticercosis with flubendazole. Am J Trop Med Hyg. 1984;33:627–31.
260. Brown HD, Matzuk AR, Ilves IR, et al. Antiparasitic drugs. IV. 2-(4′-Thiazolyl)-benzimidazole; a new anthelmintic (Letter). J Am Chem Soc. 1961;83:1764–5.
261. Campbell WC, Cuckler AC. Thiabendazole in the treatment and control of parasitic infections in man. Tex Rep Biol Med. 1969;27 (Suppl 2):665–92.
262. Berk SL, Verghese A, Alvarez S, et al. Clinical and epidemiological features of strongyloidiasis—a prospective study in rural Tennessee. Arch Intern Med. 1987;147:1257–61.
263. Barnish G, Barker J. An intervention study using thiabendazole suspension against *Strongyloides fulleborni*-like infections in Papua, New Guinea. Trans R Soc Trop Med Hyg. 1987;81:60–3.
264. Gordon H McL. Thiabendazole: A highly effective anthelmintic for sheep. Nature. 1961;191:1409–10.
265. Stone OJ. Systemic and topical thiabendazole for creeping eruption. Tex Rep Biol Med. 1969;27(Suppl 2):659–63.
266. Campbell WC, Denham DA. Chemotherapy. In: Campbell WC, ed. *Trichinella* and Trichinosis. New York: Plenum Press; 1983:335–66.
267. Hennekeuser HH, Pabst K, Poeplau W, et al. Thiabendazole for the treatment of trichinosis in humans. Tex Rep Biol Med. 1969;27(Suppl 2):581–96.
268. Criado Fornelio A, Rodriguez Caabeiro F, Jimenez Gonzalez A. The mode of action of some benzimidazole drugs on *Trichinella spiralis*. Parasitology. 1987;95:61–70.
269. Robinson HJ, Silber R, Graessle OE. Thiabendazole: Toxicological, pharmacological and antifungal properties. Tex Rep Biol Med. 1969;27(Suppl 2):537–60.
270. Köhler P, Bachmann R. The effects of the antiparasitic drugs levamisole, thiabendazole, praziquantel, and chloroquine on mitochondrial electron transport in muscle tissue from *Ascaris suum*. Mol Pharmacol. 1978;14:155–63.
271. Watts SDM, Rapson EB, Atkins AM, et al. Inhibition of acetylcholinesterase secretion from *Nippostrongylus brasiliensis* by benzimidazole anthelmintics. Biochem Pharmacol. 1982;31:3035–40.
272. Manivel JC, Bloomer JR, Snover DC. Progressive bile duct injury after thiabendazole administration. Gastroenterology. 1987;93:245–9.
273. Tchao P, Templeton T. Thiabendazole-associated grand mal seizures in a patient with Down syndrome. J Pediatr. 1983;102:317–8.
274. De Pargament MDM, de Vinuesa ML, Larripa I. Mutagenic bioassay of certain pharmacological drugs. I. Thiabendazole (TBZ). Mutat Res. 1987;188:1–6.
275. Austin WC, Courtney W, Danilewicz JC, et al. Pyrantel tartrate, a new anthelmintic effective against infections of domestic animals. Nature. 1966;212:1273–4.
276. Bumbalo TS, Fugazzoto DJ, Wyczalek JV. Treatment of enterobiasis with pyrantel pamoate. Am J Trop Med Hyg. 1969;18:50–2.
277. Aubry ML, Cowell P, Davey MJ, et al. Aspects of the pharmacology of a new anthelminthic: Pyrantel. Br J Pharmacol. 1970;38:332–44.
278. Eyre P. Some pharmacodynamic effects of the nematocides: Methyridine, tetramisole and pyrantel. J Pharm Pharmacol. 1970;22:26–36.
279. Rollo IM. Drugs used in the chemotherapy of helminthiasis. In: Gilman AG, Goodman LS, Gilman A, eds. The Pharmacological Basis of Therapeutics. 6th ed. New York: Macmillan; 1980:1013–37.
280. Royer A. Preliminary report on a new antioxyuritic Poquil. Can Med Assoc J. 1956;74:297.
281. Sawitz WG, Karpinski FE Jr. Treatment of oxyuriasis with pyrrovinyquinium chloride (Poquil). Am J Trop Med Hyg. 1956;5:538–43.
282. Hennig UGG, Galindo-Prince OC, Cortinas da Nava, C, et al. A comparison of the genetic activity of pyrvinium pamoate with that of several other anthelmintic drugs in *Saccharomyces cerevisiae*. Mutat Res. 1987;187:79–89.
283. Martin RJ. γ-Aminobutyric acid- and piperazine-activated single-channel currents from *scaris suum* body muscle. Br J Pharmacol. 1985;84:445–61.
284. Saz HJ, Bueding E. Relationships between anthelmintic effects and biochemical and physiological mechanisms. Pharmacol Rev. 1966;18:871–94.
285. Nickey LN. Possible precipitation of petit mal seizures with piperazine citrate. JAMA. 1966;195:1069–70.
286. Parsons AC. Piperazine neurotoxicity: "Worm wobble." Br Med J. 1971;4:792.
287. Wright S, Harman RRM. Ethylenediamine and piperazine sensitivity. Br Med J. 1983;287:463–4.
288. Ottesen EA. Efficacy of diethylcarbamazine in eradicating infection with lymphatic-dwelling filariae in humans. Rev Infect Dis. 1985;7:341–56.
289. Partono F. Treatment of elephantiasis in a community with timorian filariasis. Trans R Soc Trop Med Hyg. 1985;79:44–6.
290. Kim JS, No BU, Lee WY. Brugian filariasis: 10-year follow-up study on the effectiveness of selective chemotherapy with diethylcarbamazine on Che Ju island, Republic of Korea. Bull WHO. 1987;65:67–75.
291. Hawking F. Chemotherapy of filariasis. Antibiot Chemother. 1980;30:135–62.
292. Montestruc E, Blanche R, Laborde R. Action du 1-diethylcarbamyl 4-methylpiperazine sur *Filaria ozzardi*. Bull Soc Pathol Exot. 1950;43:275–8 (cited in Ref. 293).
293. Bartholomew CF, Nathan MD, Tikasingh ES. The failure of diethylcarbamazine in the treatment of *Mansonella ozzardi* infections. Trans R Soc Trop Med Hyg. 1978;72:423–4.
294. Nesarajah MS. Pulmonary function in tropical eosinophilia before and after treatment with diethylcarbamazine. Thorax. 1975;30:574–7.
295. Wiseman RA, Woodruff AW, Pettitt LE. The treatment of toxocaral infection: Some experimental and clinical observations. Trans R Soc Trop Med Hyg. 1971;65:591–8.
296. Taylor HR. Recent developments in the treatment of onchocerciasis. Bull WHO. 1984;62:509–15.
297. Lariviere M, Vingtain P, Aziz M, et al. Double-blind study of ivermectin and diethylcarbamazine in African onchocerciasis patients with ocular involvement. Lancet. 1985;2:174–7.
298. Diallo S, Aziz MA, Lariviere M, et al. A double-blind comparison of the efficacy and safety of ivermectin and diethylcarbamazine in a placebo controlled study of Senegalese patients with onchocerciasis. Trans R Soc Trop Med Hyg. 1986;80:927–34.
299. Dadzie KY, Bird AC, Awadzi K, et al. Ocular findings in a double-blind study of ivermectin versus diethylcarbamazine versus placebo in the treatment of onchocerciasis. Br. J Ophthalmol. 1987;71:78–85.
300. Hawking F. Chemotherapy of filariasis. In: Schnitzer RJ, Hawking F, eds. Experimental Chemotherapy. v. 1. New York: Academic Press; 1963:893–912.
301. Rée GH, Hall AP, Hutchinson DBA, et al. Plasma levels of diethylcarbamazine in man. Trans R Soc Trop Med Hyg. 1978;71:542–3.
302. Faulkner JK, Smith KJ. Dealkylation and N-oxidation in the metabolism of

1-diethyl-carbamyl-4-methylpiperazine in the rat. Xenobiotica. 1972;2:59–68.
303. Langham ME, Kramer TR. The in vitro effect of diethylcarbamazine on the motility and survival of *Onchocerca volvulus* microfilariae. Tropemed Parasitol. 1980;31:59–66.
304. Hawking F. Diethylcarbamazine and new compounds for the treatment of filariasis. Adv Pharmacol Chemother. 1979;16:129–94.
305. Van den Bossche H. A look at the mode of action of some old and new antifilarial compounds. Ann Soc Belg Med Trop. 1981;16;287–96 (cited in Ref. 264).
306. King CH, Greene BM, Spagnuolo PJ. Diethylcarbamazine citrate, an antifilarial drug, stimulates human granulocyte adherence. Antimicrob Agents Chemother 1983;24:453–6.
307. Cesbron J-V, Capron A, Vargaftig BB, et al. Platelets mediate the action of diethylcarbamazine on microfilariae. Nature. 1987;325:533–6.
308. Greene BM, Taylor HR, Brown EJ, et al. Ocular and systemic complications of diethylcarbamazine therapy for onchocerciasis: Association with circulating immune complexes. J Infect Dis. 1983;147:890–7.
309. Ottesen EA. Description, mechanisms and control of reactions to treatment in the human filariases. Ciba Found Symp. 1987;127:265–83.
310. Rivas-Alcala AR, Greene BM, Taylor HR, et al. Chemotherapy of onchocerciasis: A controlled comparison of mebendazole, levamisole, and diethylcarbamazine. Lancet. 1981;2:485–90.
311. Dominguez-Varquez A, Taylor HR, Greene BM, et al. Comparison of flubendazole and diethylcarbamazine in treatment of onchocerciasis. Lancet. 1983;1:139–43.
312. Francis H, Awadzi K, Ottesen EA. The Mazzotti reaction following treatment of onchocerciasis with diethylcarbamazine: Clinical severity as a function of infection intensity. Am J Trop Med Hyg. 1985;34:529–36.
313. Campbell WC, Fisher MH, Stapley EO, et al. Ivermectin: A potent new antiparasitic agent. Science. 1983;221:823–8.
314. Coulaud JP, Lariviere M, Aziz MA, et al. Ivermectin in onchocerciasis (Letter). Lancet. 1984;2:526–7.
315. Aziz MA, Diallo S, Diop IM, et al. Efficacy and tolerance of ivermectin in human onchocerciasis. Lancet. 1982;2:171–3.
316. Kumaraswami V, Ottesen EA, Vijayasekaran V, et al. Ivermectin for the treatment of *Wuchereria bancrofti* filariasis: Efficacy and adverse reactions. JAMA. 1988;259:3150–3.
317. Mahmoud AAF. Praziquantel for the treatment of helminthic infections. Adv Intern Med. 1987;32:193–206.
318. Pearson RD, Guerrant RL. Praziquantel: A major advance in anthelminthic therapy. Ann Intern Med. 1983;99:195–8.
319. Pearson RD, Wilson ME. Role of praziquantel in the treatment of helminthic diseases. Int Med Specialist. 1986;7:183–204.
320. Wegner DHG. The profile of the trematodicidal compound praziquantel. Arzneim Forsch. 1984;34:1132–6.
321. Davis A, Biles JE, Ulrich A-M. Initial experience with praziquantel in the treatment of human infections due to *Schistosoma haematobium*. Bull WHO. 1979;57:773–9.
322. Katz N, Rocha RS, Chaves A. Preliminary trials with praziquantel in human infections due to *Schistosoma mansoni*. Bull WHO. 1979;57:781–5.
323. Da Silva LC, Sette H Jr, Christo CH, et al. Praziquantel in the treatment of the hepatosplenic form of schistosomiasis mansoni. Arzneim Forsch. 1981;31:601–3.
324. Coutinho A, Domingues ALC, Neves J, et al. Treatment of hepatosplenic schistosomiasis mansoni with praziquantel. Preliminary report on tolerance and efficacy. Arzneim Forsch. 1983;33:787–91.
325. Bassily S, Farid Z, Dunn M, et al. Praziquantel for treatment of schistosomiasis in patients with advanced hepatosplenomegaly. Ann Trop Med Parasitol. 1985;79:629–34.
326. Santos AT, Blas BL, Noseñas JS, et al. Preliminary clinical trials with praziquantel in *Schistosoma japonicum* infections in the Philippines. Bull WHO. 1979;57:793–9.
327. Santos AT, Blas BL, Portillo G, et al. Phase III clinical trials with praziquantel in *S. japonicum* infections in the Philippines. Arzneim Forsch. 1984;34:1221–3.
328. Fu F-Y, Zheng JS, Chen W-Q, et al. Further experience with praziquantel in schistosoma japonicum infections. Chin Med J (Engl). 1984;97:47–52.
329. Nash TE, Hofstetter M, Cheever AW, et al. Treatment of *Schistosoma mekongi* with praziquantel: A double-blind study. Am J Trop Med Hyg. 1982;31:977–82.
330. Keittivuti B, Keittivuti A, O'Rourke T, et al. Treatment of *Schistosoma mekongi* with praziquantel in Cambodian refugees in holding centers in Prachinburi Province, Thailand. Trans R Soc Trop Med Hyg. 1984;78:477–9.
331. Watt G, Adapon B, Long GW, et al. Praziquantel in treatment of cerebral schistosomiasis. Lancet. 1986;2:529–32.
332. Rim H-J, Lyu K-S, Lee J-S, et al. Clinical evaluation of the therapeutic efficacy of praziquantel (Embay 8440) against *Clonorchis sinensis* infection in man. Ann Trop Med Parasitol. 1981;75:27–33.
333. Liu Y-H, Qiu Z-D, Wang X-G, et al. Praziquantel in clonorchiasis sinensis: A further evaluation of 100 cases. Chin Med J (Engl). 1982;95:89–94.
334. Bunnag D, Harinasuta T. Studies on the chemotherapy of human opisthorchiasis in Thailand: I. Clinical trial of praziquantel. Southeast Asian J Trop Med Public Health. 1980;11:528–31.
335. Spitalny KC, Senft AW, Meglio FD, et al. Treatment of pulmonary paragonimiasis with a new broad-spectrum antihelminthic, praziquantel. J Pediatr. 1982;101:144–6.
336. Rim H-J, Chang Y-S. Chemotherapeutic effect of niclofolan and praziquantel in the treatment of paragonimiasis. Korean Univ Med J. 1980;17:113–28.
337. Knobloch J, Paz G, Feldmeier H, et al. Serum antibody levels in human paragonimiasis before and after therapy with praziquantel. Trans R Soc Trop Med Hyg. 1984;78:835–6.
338. Pachucki CT, Levandowski RA, Brown VA, et al. American paragonimiasis treated with praziquantel. N Engl J Med. 1984;311:582–3.
339. Farid Z, Trabolsi B, Boctor F, et al. Unsuccessful use of praziquantel to treat acute fascioliasis in children (Letter). J Infect Dis. 1986;154:920–1.
340. Farag HF, Ragab M, Salem A, et al. A short note on praziquantel in human fascioliasis. J Trop Med Hyg. 1986;89:79–80.
341. Botero D, Castano S. Treatment of cysticercosis with praziquantel in Columbia. Am J Trop Med Hyg. 1982;31:811–21.
342. Gomez JG, Sanchez E, Pardo R. Treatment of cysticercosis with praziquantel (Letter). Arch Neurol. 1984;41:1022.
343. De Ghetaldi LD, Norman RM, Douville AW Jr. Cerebral cysticercosis treated biphasically with dexamethasone and praziquantel. Ann Intern Med. 1983;99:179–81.
344. Biller J, Azar-Kia B, O'Keefe P. Cysticercosis and praziquantel therapy (Letter). Neurology. 1984;34:1621–2.
345. Sotelo J, Torres B, Rubio-Donnadieu F, et al. Praziquantel in the treatment of neurocysticercosis: Long-term follow-up. Neurology. 1985;35:752–5.
346. Robles C, Sedano AM, Vargas-Tentori N, et al. Long-term results of praziquantel therapy in neurocysticercosis. J Neurosurg. 1987;66:359–63.
347. Leblanc R, Knowles KF, Melanson D, et al. Neurocysticercosis: Surgical and medical management with praziquantel. Neurosurgery. 1986;18:419–27.
348. Norman RM, Kapadia C. Cerebral cysticercosis: Treatment with praziquantel. Pediatrics. 1986;78:291–4.
349. Vasconcelos D, Cruz-Segura H, Mateos-Gomez H, et al. Selective indications for the use of praziquantel in the treatment of brain cysticercosis. J Neurol Neurosurg Psychiatry. 1987;50:383–8.
350. Santos R, Chavarria M, Aguirre AE. Failure of medical treatment in two cases of intraocular cysticercosis. Am J Ophthalmol. 1984;97:249–50.
351. Kestelyn P, Taelman H. Effect of praziquantel on intraocular cysticercosis: A case report. Br J Ophthalmol. 1985;69:788–90.
352. Groll E. Praziquantel for cestode infections in man. Acta Trop (Basel). 1980;37:293–6.
353. Gemmell MA, Johnstone PD, Oudemans G. The effect of praziquantel on *Echinococcus granulosus, Taenia hydatigena*, and *Taenia ovis* infections in dog. Res Vet Sci. 1977;23:121–3.
354. Morris DL, Richards KS, Chinnery JB. Protoscolicidal effect of praziquantel—in vitro and electron microscopical studies of *Echinococcus granulosus*. J Antimicrob Chemother. 1986;18:687–91.
355. Heath DD, Lawrence SB. The effect of mebendazole and praziquantel on the cysts of *Echinococcus granulosus, Taenia hydatigena*, and *T. ovis* in sheep. NZ Vet J. 1978;26:11–5.
356. Thomas H, Gonnert R. Zur Wirksamkeit von Praziquantel bei der experimentellen Cysticercose und Hydatidose. Z Parasitenkd. 1978;55:165–79.
357. Marshall I, Edwards GT. The effects of sustained release praziquantel on the survival of protoscolices of *Echinococcus granulosus equinus* in laboratory mice. Ann Trop Med Parasitol. 1982;76:649–51.
358. Leopold G, Ungethum W, Groll E, et al. Clinical pharmacology in normal volunteers of praziquantel, a new drug against schistosomes and cestodes: An example of a complex study covering both tolerance and pharmacokinetics. Eur J Clin Pharmacol. 1978;14:281–91.
359. Andrews P. Pharmakokinetische Tieruntersuchungen mit Droncit unter Verwendurg einer biologischen Prufmethode. Vet Med Nachr. 1976;2:154–6.
360. Thomas H, Andrews P, Mehlhorn H. New results on the effect of praziquantel in experimental cysticercosis. Am J Trop Med Hyg. 1982;31:803–10.
361. Andrews P. Praziquantel: Mechanisms of anti-schistosomal activity. Pharmacol Ther. 1985;29:129–56.
362. Xiao S-H, Friedman PA, Catto BA, et al. Praziquantel-induced vesicle formation in the tegument of male *Schistosoma mansoni* is calcium dependent. J Parasitol. 1984;70:177–9.
363. Gardner DR, Brezden BL. The sites of action of praziquantel in smooth muscle of *Lymnaea stagnalis*. Can J Physiol Pharmacol. 1984;62:282–7.
364. Ruenwongsa P, Hutadilok N, Yuthavong Y. Stimulation of Ca^{2+} uptake in the liver fluke *Opisthorchis viverrini* by praziquantel. Life Sci. 1983;32:2529–34.
365. Harnett W, Kusel JR. Increased exposure of parasite antigens at the surface of adult *Schistosoma mansoni* exposed to praziquantel in vitro. Parasitology. 1986;93:401–5.
366. Prichard RK, Bachmann R, Hutchinson GW, et al. The effect of praziquantel on calcium in *Hymenolepis diminuta*. Mol Biochem Parasitol. 1982;5:297–308.
367. Johnson RJ, Jong EC, Dunning SB, et al. Paragonimiasis: Diagnosis and the use of praziquantel in treatment. Rev Infect Dis. 1985;7:200–6.
368. Polderman AM, Gryseels B, Gerold JL, et al. Side effects of praziquantel in the treatment of *Schistosoma mansoni* in Maniema, Zaire. Trans R Soc Trop Med Hyg. 1984;78:752–4.

369. Farid Z, Wallace CK. Schistosomiasis and praziquantel (Letter). Ann Intern Med. 1983;99:883.
370. Watt G, Baldovino PC, Castro JT, et al. Bloody diarrhoea after praziquantel therapy (Letter). Trans R Soc Trop Med Hyg. 1986;80:345–6.
371. Markwalder K, Hess K, Valavanis A, et al. Cerebral cysticercosis: Treatment with praziquantel. Am J Trop Med Hyg. 1984;33:273–80.
372. Sotelo J, Escobedo F, Rodriguez-Carbajal J, et al. Therapy of parenchymal brain cysticercosis with praziquantel. N Engl J Med. 1984;310:1001–7.
373. Davis A, Bailey DR. Metrifonate in urinary schistosomiasis. Bull WHO. 1969;41:209–24.
374. Omer AHS, Teesdale CH. Metrifonate trial in the treatment of various presentations of *Schistosoma haematobium* and *S. mansoni* infections in the Sudan. Ann Trop Med Parasitol. 1978;72:145–50.
375. Feldmeier H, Doehring E, Daffala AA, et al. Efficacy of metrifonate in urinary schistosomiasis: Comparison of reduction of *Schistosoma haematobium* and *S. mansoni* eggs. Am J Trop Med Hyg. 1982;31:1188–94.
376. Reiner K, Krauthacker B, Simeon V, et al. Mechanism of inhibition in vitro of mammalian acetylcholinesterase and cholinesterase in solutions of 0,0-dimethyl 2,2,2-trichloro-1-hydroxyethyl phosphonate (Trichlorphon). Biochem Pharmacol. 1975;24:717–22.
377. Nordgren I, Bengtsson E, Holmstedt B, et al. Levels of metrifonate and dichlorvos in plasma and erythrocytes during treatment of schistosomiasis with Bilarcil. Acta Pharmacol Toxicol. 1981;49 (Suppl V):79–86.
378. Katz N, Zicker F, Pereira JP. Field trials with oxamniquine in a schistosomiasis mansoni-endemic area. Am J Trop Med Hyg. 1977;26:234–7.
379. Katz N. Chemotherapy of schistosomiasis mansoni. Adv Pharmacol Chemother. 1977;14:1–70.
380. Omer AHS. Oxamniquine for treating *Schistosoma mansoni* infection in Sudan. Br Med J. 1978;2:163–5.
381. Kilpatrick ME, Farid Z, Bassily S, et al. Treatment of schistosomiasis mansoni with oxamniquine—five years' experience. Am J Trop Med Hyg. 1981;30:1219–22.
382. Machado PA. The Brazilian program for schistosomiasis control, 1975–1979. Am J Trop Med Hyg. 1982;31:76–86.
383. Goble FC, ed. The pharmacological and chemotherapeutic properties of niridazole and other antischistosomal compounds. Ann NY Acad Sci. 1969;160:423–946.
384. Farid Z, Bassily S, Lehman JS Jr, et al. A comparative evaluation of the treatment of *Schistosoma mansoni* with niridazole and potassium antimony tartrate. Trans R Soc Trop Med Hyg. 1972;66:119–24.
385. Davidson JC. Neuropsychiatric effects and EEG changes in niridazole therapy. Trans R Soc Trop Med Hyg. 1969;63:579–81.
386. Sonnet J, Doyen A. Effects of niridazole on erythropoiesis of Congolese treated for schistosomiasis and amoebiasis. Ann NY Acad Sci. 1969; 160:786–98.
387. De Carvalho SA, Neto V, Zeitune JM, et al. Avaliaco terapeutica do oltipraz na infeccao humana pelo *S. mansoni*. Rev Inst Med Trop Sao Paulo. 1986;28:271–7.
388. Kim JS. Treatment of *Paragonimus westermani* infections with bithionol. Am J Trop Med Hyg. 1970;19:940–2.
389. Pearson RD, Hewlett EL. Niclosamide therapy for tapeworm infections. Ann Intern Med. 1985;102:550–1.
390. Hecht VG, Gloxhuber C. Experimentelle Untersuchungen mit N-(2'-Chlor-4'-Nitrophenyl)-5-Chlorsalicylamid, einem neuen Bandwurmmittel: 2. Mitteilung: toxikologische Untersuchungen. Arzneim Forsch. 1960;10:884–5.
391. Perera DR, Western KA, Schultz MG. Nicclosamide treatment of cestodiasis: Clinical trials in the United States. Am J Trop Med Hyg. 1970; 19:610–2.

37. PROBLEMS IN ANTIBIOTIC USAGE

CALVIN M. KUNIN

The general problem of appropriate use of drugs has existed for a long time. Osler could assume a position of therapeutic nihilism in the early 1900s since there were few effective agents available to him. The antibiotic era, which began less than 45 years ago, is much more complex. There are a wealth of excellent agents from which to choose, each with its own special benefits and economic, toxic, and ecologic costs. We now have the luxury of debating the value of using antibiotics to prevent complications of relatively simple problems such as the common cold or a sore throat, and we can more readily deal with serious surgical and life-threatening infections.

Soon after antibiotics were introduced, it was recognized that they were being overused and misused. A review of the subject by Jawetz in 1956[1] eloquently stated the problems of the attractiveness of new antibiotics to physicians, exaggerated claims, and the enormous impact of promotion by the drug companies on medical practice. The following year, based on a nationwide study, Welch et al.[2] described the relatively high frequency of severe reactions to antibiotics. In 1959, Finland et al.[3] documented the increasing occurrence of serious bacterial infections since the introduction of antibacterial agents. Reimann and D'Ambola[4] conducted one of the earliest surveys on the appropriate use of antibiotics in 1966 and clearly demonstrated that antibiotics were often used inappropriately. In 1974, Lockwood[5] described the syndrome of compulsive antibiotic prescribing and advocated the formation of an organization called Antibiotics Anonymous to deal with the problem. More recently, the Alliance for Prudent Use of Antibiotics has been formed to monitor the problem worldwide. It is therefore appropriate that a chapter appear in this book on infectious disease to examine the problem and explore potential solutions.

MAGNITUDE OF ANTIMICROBIAL USE IN THE UNITED STATES

Antimicrobial drugs are the second most commonly used class of drugs, second only to cardiovascular agents. According to data from the *U.S. Industrial Outlook,* published by the Department of Commerce, the value of pharmaceutical industry shipments was 27.1 billion dollars in 1986. It is estimated that about 12–15 percent, or about 3–4 billion dollars, was for anti-infective agents. These figures do not include costs of markup or administration of the agents, which could readily double the expenditure. About 45 percent of the expenditure for anti-infective drugs was for outpatient use. The remainder, consisting mostly of the more expensive parenteral agents, was used in hospitals and long-term care facilities. According to the Food and Drug Administration (FDA), 196 million outpatient prescriptions for anti-infective agents were filled in 1984. This accounted for 13.1 percent of all prescriptions. Much of this expenditure is for treatment of conditions such as sinusitis, bronchitis, and respiratory infecions. Since most of these are caused by viruses, much of this expenditure is wasted.[6]

In hospitals, antimicrobial agents are given to 20–40 percent of patients and account for about 25 percent of total drug acquisition costs.[7] We will later show that much of this antimicrobial use is not only unnecessary but also a waste of resources and is potentially harmful to the patient and society.

REASONS FOR CONCERN ABOUT APPROPRIATE USE OF ANTIMICROBIAL AGENTS

Selection of Resistant Bacteria

The development of resistant organisms was recognized by Paul Ehrlich as a potential problem during his early studies of organic arsenicals almost 100 years ago. The overall problem of the emergence of resistant strains is discussed in Chapter 16 and is a persistent theme throughout the sections on antimicrobial chemotherapy. Multiple-drug-resistant organisms derived through the transfer of plasmids or through transduction by bacteriophages have amplified the problem. At first, the focus was on the emergence of resistant bacteria in hospitals, where antimicrobial agents are used most heavily. A causal relationship between antibiotic usage and resistance of organisms in hospitals has been established on the basis of evidence of consistent associations of the emergence of resistant strains with concurrent variations in use in populations over time.[8] More recently, common virulent organisms resistant to previously effective agents have been encountered in office practice as well; this problem is particularly troublesome in developing nations, which can least afford it. This phenomenon has forced physicians to alter their cost/benefit equation and to use expensive and potentially toxic drugs for the treatment of infections due to staphylococci, gonococci, *Haemophilus influenzae, Shigella,* and the pneumococci in focal outbreaks.

Three approaches to the problem of emerging resistant strains are being explored. The simplest and least costly measure is to decrease the selective pressure exerted by antibiotics. Several groups have presented evidence that control of usage will result in reversion of the bacterial population to sensitive organisms.[9,10] A second approach is to develop immunogens that can enhance host resistance to virulent organisms. Development of a polyvalent pneumococcal vaccine is an example of this approach. The major difficulty with the use of vaccines is the complex problems of effective delivery to the target high-risk population and the multiplicity of immunogens needed to deal with an expanding number of microorganisms for which vaccines are being developed. The third and most costly approach is to develop and exploit new antimicrobial agents or alter the chemical structure of older agents to circumvent mechanisms of resistance developed by the microorganisms. This has been the major path taken by the pharmaceutical industry and is most accepted by the medical community.

Rising Costs of Medical Care: Emergence of the "Drugs of Fear"

A new antimicrobial era emerged during the 1970s, the era of the "drugs of fear,"[11] a term that refers to fear on the part of physicians of failing to provide patients with the very best drug for a presumed infection. Although many lives have been saved by these drugs, the underlying conditions that precipitate infection with "difficult hospital bacteria" have not been resolved, and therefore in many cases, the drugs have been used without effect or have simply delayed death. Widespread use of these agents ensures their own phased obsolescence as new resistant organisms emerge, and it also increases the costs of medical care. We can expect costs to increase with only modest improvement in therapeutic efficacy.

Adverse Reactions to Antimicrobial Agents

Untoward toxic effects of antibiotics are well known; they range from death from anaphylaxis or aplastic anemia with penicillin and chloramphenicol, respectively, to severe diarrhea from lincosamides, rash from ampicillin, nephrotoxicity and ototoxicity from the aminoglycosides, and bleeding disorders with some of the new β-lactam antibiotics. Cluff[12] and Seidl et al.[13] reported that approximately 5 percent of the hospitalized patients who are given an antibiotic will experience some adverse reaction to the drug and about 20 percent of patients requiring medical care have a history of adverse reaction(s) to an antibiotic.

EVIDENCE OF INAPPROPRIATE USE OF ANTIMICROBIAL AGENTS

Office Practice

Drug prescribing was examined in a careful epidemiologic study by Stolley et al.[14] They reported that market research data indicated that about 95 percent of physicians will issue one or more prescriptions to a patient whom they diagnose as having the "common cold." Almost 60 percent of these prescriptions are for antibiotics, with the tetracyclines and penicillins being the most popular choices. In their own study in a U.S. community, they found that antibiotics were the most commonly dispensed drugs (15.3 percent of all prescriptions). Another analysis by the same group of investigators[15] showed that prescribing patterns are largely determined by educational experiences. Higher ratings for appropriate drug use and lower frequency of chloramphenicol use in particular were found among more recently trained physicians who had more postgraduate training. Currently amoxicillin, erythromycin, and penicillins are among the 10 most commonly used antibiotics in office practice. Trimethoprim combinations and cephalexin are among the top 30 agents (National Center for Health Statistics advance data, 1987). It is only a matter of time before impact is felt of the use of the orally absorbed quinolones.

We can roughly estimate the magnitude of overuse. Approximately 750 million dollars is spent annually on prescriptions for sinusitis, bronchitis, and respiratory infections. If 60 percent of these prescriptions are for antimicrobial agents,[14] the cost for these drugs is 450 million dollars. Assuming that at least one-half of the prescriptions are inappropriate, about 225 million dollars are wasted each year.

It has been argued that antibiotics should be used more often to treat the bacterial complications of upper respiratory infections,[16] but carefully conducted clinical studies have clearly demonstrated the lack of efficacy with this approach in otherwise healthy adults.[17] It has also been argued that the major reason for the marked decrease in rheumatic fever may be due to the widespread use of antibiotics in office practice, but Stollerman[18] has presented forceful arguments that this is more closely associated with changes in the pathogenetic characteristics of the group A streptococci. There is still considerable disagreement among practitioners of various specialities concerning the proper use of antibiotics to treat respiratory infections.[19] In one study of usage in an emergency room,[20] 31 percent of infections encountered were respiratory. Antibiotic prescribing was appropriate in 78 percent of the cases.

The problem of antibiotics overusage in office practice has been compounded in recent years by the promotion of new high-cost proprietary agents such as oral cephalosporins, new derivatives of ampicillin, and the new quinolones. These agents rarely cure more patients, but do cost more.

Despite the widespread use of new antibiotics in office practice, there are still practitioners who continue to prescribe chloramphenicol, mostly for upper respiratory infections, and tetracycline to children under the age of 8 years, despite repeated recommendations against this practice by the Committee on Drugs of the American Academy of Pediatrics. According to the studies of Ray et al.,[21,22] a small group of physicians located in rural, primary care settings account for most of these inappropriate prescriptions. The most alarming finding is that physicians who recently finished training also take part in these poor practices.

Hospital Practice

There are now numerous studies in representative hospital populations that document that antimicrobial agents are used for unjustifiable reasons or that the wrong drug, dose, or duration of therapy is selected *about half the time* (Table 1). One of the remarkable findings of all these studies is that even though criteria for justified or acceptable usage may differ the results are generally the same.

Virtually all the studies identify the same reasons for overuse and excessive costs of antimicrobial agents in hospitals. These are (*1*) inappropriate use of agents for prophylaxis of surgical infections and (*2*) high cost of parenteral agents, particularly the cephalosporin and aminoglycoside antibiotics, which account for 70 percent of the total antibiotic costs.[7,26,30,31]

In recent years the proportion of costs for cephalosporins has increased because of the introduction of many new expensive agents. They have tended to replace the portion of usage occupied by aminoglycosides. The most representative study of the use of antimicrobial drugs in general hospitals in the United States was conducted by Shapiro et al.[32] They studied 20 short-stay general hospitals in Pennsylvania selected by a stratified random-sampling technique. Approximately 30 percent of the

TABLE 1. Summary of Studies Evaluating Appropriate Use of Antimicrobial Agents in Hospitals

Hospitals	*Investigators*	*No. Patients*	*Findings*
Community (7 hospitals surveyed)	Scheckler and Bennett[23]	2094	62% of patients treated had no evidence of infection
Community	Roberts and Visconti[24]	340	13% rational, 21% questionable, 66% irrational
Pediatric	Gibbs et al.[25]	167	32% rational, 49% questionable, 19% irrational
University	Kunin et al.[11]	500	52% inappropriate[a]
University	Castle et al.[26]	50	64% inappropriate[a]
University	Petrello et al.[27 b]	65	42.6% rational, 48% irrational, 9.3% insufficient data
University	Maki and Schuna[28]	549	41% inappropriate
VA	Jones et al.[29] Before	145	64% inappropriate NS
	After[c]	200	51% inappropriate
Community	Achong et al.[30] Before	219	42%[d] 50%[e] irrational 0.02[f]
	After	240	24%[d] 25%[e] irrational

[a] Judged inappropriate according to criteria in Table 3.
[b] Use of clindamycin only.
[c] Education program in appropriate use of antimicrobial agents.
[d] Surgical service.
[e] Gynecologic service.
[f] Degree of significant difference.

patients received an antimicrobial drug during hospitalization, and about 30 percent received the drugs for prophylaxis in operations or invasive nonsurgical procedures. Despite indications that prophylaxis, when useful at all, is effective only when given concurrently with and for 24–48 hours after an operation, it was usually continued throughout hospitalization. Almost 80 percent of prophylactic antimicrobial agents were administered at least 48 hours after an operation or procedure (Fig. 1). It is apparent that most of the costs were for periods when the drugs would not be helpful to the patient. Similar results were obtained in a survey of 27 hospitals in Minnesota.[33] Savings of 18–50 percent could be achieved by limiting the duration of drug administration. A benefit/cost analysis of antimicrobial prophylaxis in abdominal and vaginal hysterectomy demonstrated that using three doses of cefazolin would markedly reduce costs.[34] The benefits would be eroded by use of newer, more expensive cephalosporins.

Self-Administration

It is quite common to learn from patients that they often treat themselves with drugs prescribed in the past or given to them by friends or relatives. Chretien et al.,[35] in a study of students going to a university health service, have reported that this is a frequent practice, especially for the treatment of respiratory symptoms.

Usage in Other Countries

Misuse of antibiotics is a major problem all over the world. In many Asian and South American countries, potent antibiotics are sold without prescription. A review of antibiotics marketed in Central America[36] revealed that in most countries more than 200 different antibiotic drug products were sold. At least one-third of these were drug combinations of questionable value. Most of the drugs used in the Third World originate from the major Western pharmaceutical companies that promote agents unacceptable in their own countries. Large-scale epidemics of typhoid fever, gonorrhea, and meningococcal meningitis may be traced to resistant strains originating in Third World countries in which antibiotic use is poorly controlled, self-prescribing is common,[37] and physicians often use antibiotics inappropriately.[38] A study in Israel[39] revealed that 30 percent of pharmacy costs could be accounted for by antibiotics (as in the United States), but that Israeli physicians tend to use less expensive agents such as ampicillin more widely than cephalosporins. In the United Kingdom, a study of antibiotic usage for prophylaxis in surgery revealed enormous variation among London teaching hospitals in regard to choice of drug, dose, and timing of administration.[40] In a district general hospital in Londin, ampicillin, cloxacillin, and other penicillins accounted for 61 percent of all antibiotic usage.[41] This is quite different from the United States, in which much more expensive agents are used. Nevertheless, most of the patients were treated without bacteriologic evidence of the infecting agent, and only 7 percent of antibiotics prescribed for surgical prophylaxis fulfilled reasonable criteria for their use. Similar results were obtained in a National Prevalence Survey conducted in 43 hospitals in England.[42] Although oral agents were most commonly used, parenteral agents accounted for 72 percent of the costs.

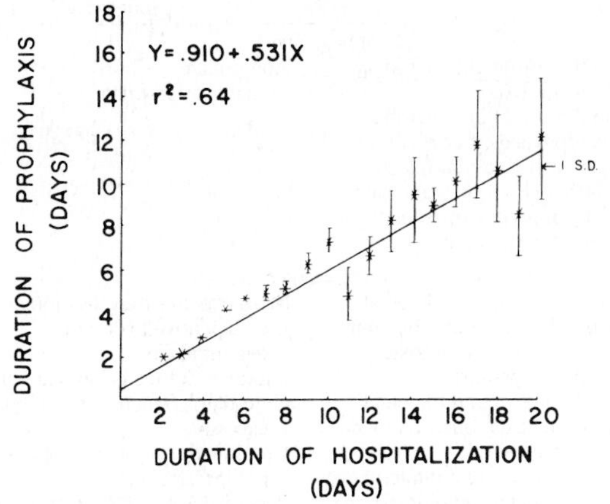

FIG. 1. Duration of antimicrobial prophylaxis in relation to duration of hospitalization. (From Shapiro et al.,[32] with permission.)

Antibiotic Use in Animals

Antibiotics are commonly used in farm animals for growth promotion and for therapeutic and prophylactic purposes. The magnitude of use in the world is highly variable. It is somewhat less in Europe than in the United States and is more sporadic and uncontrolled in Third World countries. The major fear is that plasmid-mediated, multiply resistant strains originating in farm animals will spread to the human population. The issues of control of the use of antibiotics in animals as they relate to human health are complex and controversial. Not all animal pathogens cause disease in humans. For example, staphylococci in cattle, poultry, and dogs are distinct from those that present a problem in humans. In contrast, *Salmonella* and some strains of *Campylobacter* infect humans as well as animals. *Escherichia coli* is a rich source of R plasmids that are potentially transferable in the human gut. Outbreaks of food-borne *Salmonella* infections due to multiply resistant strains may present a major problem, particularly when they produce invasive disease in compromised hosts. In one carefully studied outbreak of infection due to multiple-antibiotic-resistant *Salmonella newport,* the organisms could be traced to meat distributed from beef cattle fed subtherapeutic amounts of antimicrobial agents. Most of the infected patients had been taking penicillin derivatives, before the onset of salmonellosis.[43]

There is very little evidence that the major problem of antibiotic resistance observed in hospitals can be attributed to use in animals, but rather it is the result of excessive use of therapeutic or prophylactic antibiotics in humans. Experts agree, however, that antibiotics important for treating human infections should not be used for animals.[44]

Methods to Define the Problem and Evaluate Appropriate Usage

As awareness of the excessive use of antimicrobial agents increases, demands for accountability will require the development of clear-cut methods to evaluate the problem.

Because of control over the use of medical care services, physicians have a unique fiduciary responsibility to patients and the public. If this is perceived to be misused, the freedom enjoyed by physicians to prescribe whatever drugs they choose will be limited by action of the government or third-party payers. We are beginning to witness this in implementation of diagnostic related groups (DRGs) by Medicare and by the powerful forces in the community that seek to reduce care costs. This also offers an opportunity for implementing programs to improve prescribing as the financial emphasis in hospitals shifts from billing for all goods and services to fixed reimbursement.[45–47] An exciting development in this regard is the enormous cost savings that can be obtained by the use of long-acting parenteral antibiotics in outpatient or home therapy.[48–50] Cost savings are achieved by eliminating the need for prolonged hospital stay and by less frequent dosage intervals. Under these circumstances even the most expensive agents can be used with considerable cost-effectiveness.

Most of the studies reported in the literature use different criteria for appropriateness of use. This makes it difficult to compare data gathered in different institutions. Broad categories of surveillance methods are presented in Table 2 together with a brief list of the advantages and disadvantages of each. The simplest and least expensive method is to obtain gross utilization data from hospital pharmacies. This method can often identify a special problem such as overuse of chloramphenicol or a newly introduced agent. Attention can then be focused on individual services, particularly on patterns of use in a major problem area such as surgical prophylaxis. Drug orders can also be audited in relation to specific indications such as the use of antibiotics for upper respiratory infections. Case reviews can be conducted by using broad judgmental criteria established by specialists in the field. Examples of evaluation categories proposed by Kunin et al.[11] and modified by Jones and his group[29] are presented in Table 3.

An advisory committee on infectious disease to the Veterans Administration (VA) established specific guidelines and audits for antibiotic use to aid individual hospital staffs in conducting their own programs of surveillance.[51] The Infectious Diseases Society of America has developed a set of guidelines for control of the use of antimicrobial agents in hospitals.[52] It is recommended that the guidelines be implemented by a team delegated with this responsibility by the Pharmacy and Therapeutics and Infection Control Committees. The teams consist of a physician knowledgeable in infectious diseases, an infection control practioner, a clinical pharmacist, and a clinical microbiologist. The savings to the hospital in costs and potential reduction of resistant organisms should more than offset the support needed for the team.

Several groups have experimented with methods to evaluate appropriate use of antimicrobial agents in ambulatory practice. Useful data are being gathered by the Kaiser-Permanente group in California and by others. Ray et al.[21,22] have reported that Medicaid data can be used as a surveillance method of individual practitioners. The major advantage is the ability to detect a small group of aberrant physicians who appear to account for most of the inappropriate usage.

CONSTRAINTS OF MEDICAL PRACTICE THAT LEAD TO INAPPROPRIATE USAGE

To solve the problem of inappropriate usage, we must understand the constraints under which physicians work and the pressures that are exerted on them to prescribe drugs. An overall scheme of the elements that motivate the patient to seek help and to comply with the physician and the forces that lead the physician to prescribe drugs are outlined in Figure 2. Each of

TABLE 2. Methods of Surveillance of Antimicrobial Agent Usage in Hospitals

Gross use data based on pharmacy records
Inexpensive; provides secular trends on usage of individual agents and costs; may be used for interhospital comparisons when adjusted for patient hospital days; may identify unusual practices that may lead to more detailed studies

Utilization by services
Inexpensive if pharmacy record system is on unit dose system or can identify shipment to specific wards; will provide data on problems of use by different groups of physicians and may lead to detailed studies of potential problem areas; will refine gross utilization for more appropriate interhospital coomparisons

Survey of routine orders for prophylaxis in surgery
Requires chart review of all cases for specific operations; provides data on actual practices of individual surgeons; permits comparison of practices in different hospitals; identifies unusual practices and can be used for feedback to the surgical service

Survey of orders for specific infectious diseases
Based on discharge diagnosis such as pneumonia, bronchitis, urinary tract infection; provides data on actual practices of individual physicians; permits comparison of practice according to specialty groups and can be used for feedback in education programs

Case review by independent experts
Requires establishment of strict criteria to avoid subjective or varying standards; requires establishment of feedback loops to practicing physicians; may identify specific problems of individual physicians

Guidelines audit
Hospital staffs establish standards of practice and guidelines based on national criteria; audit is used to evaluate compliance with self-imposed standards; enables peer pressure to provide checks and balances; mutes external judgmental evaluations; must be altered as new knowledge of new agents is introduced; may be used for interhospital comparisons

TABLE 3. Suggested Categories for Determining Appropriate Use of Antimicrobial Agents by Peer Review

Categories	
Kunin et al.	*Jones et al.*
Appropriate use	
Agree with the use of antimicrobial therapy/prophylaxis	Appropriate Probably appropriate
Agree with the use of antimicrobial therapy/prophylaxis, but a potentially fatal bacterial infection cannot be ruled out or prophylaxis is probably appropriate; advantages derived remain controversial	
Inappropriate use	
Agree with the use of antimicrobial therapy/prophylaxis, but a different (usually less expensive or toxic) antimicrobial is preferred	More effective drug recommended Less expensive/toxic drug recommended Improper dosage or dosage interval
Agree with the use of antimicrobial therapy/prophylaxis, but a modified dose is recommended	Unjustified, length of treatment excessive Unjustified, use of any antimicrobial not indicated
Disagree with the use of antimicrobial therapy/prophylaxis; administration is unjustified	Records insufficient for categorization

(Data from Kunin et al.[11] and Jones et al.[29])

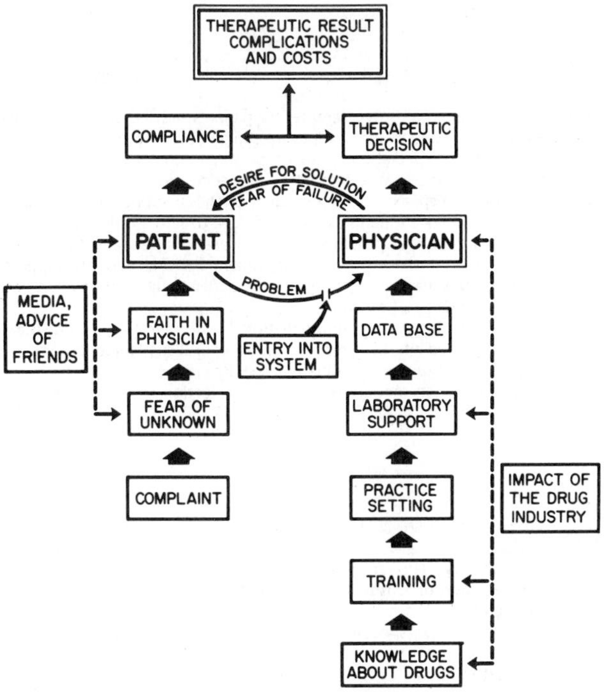

FIG. 2. Outline of the elements and complex interrelationships that influence the patient to use drugs.

the factors leading to misuse of antimicrobial agents is described in Table 4. They begin with the desire of physicians to help their patients and end with the ready solution offered by the pharmaceutical manufacturers to satisfy these needs.

The pharmaceutical manufacturers are keenly aware of the needs of the practicing physician. Dr. Donald Kennedy, a former FDA commissioner, estimated that in 1977 the industry spent $4000 per physician on direct drug advertising. IMS America, Limited, reported that advertising by U.S. drug companies in 1984 cost almost 1.4 billion dollars and was rising at a rate of about 8 percent per year. This does not include funds spent for premarketing evaluation of new drugs by clinical investigators. It is apparent that enormous pressure is exerted on the physician. Not all these funds are spent directly on individual physicians but are often invested in medical education programs. Some of the methods of promotional attack and their objectives are presented in Table 5. We must realize that every step in the medical educational process, beginning with the undergraduate years and upward, is subjected to heavy pharmaceutical promotion, including pressure on academic physicians who tend to set standards of practice.[53]

PROPOSALS FOR IMPROVEMENT OF ANTIBIOTIC USE

Methods to improve the use of antibiotics have been proposed in several editorials and reviews. Most emphasize the need for improved education of physicians in the diagnosis and treatment of infectious diseases. Some institutions have developed effective programs by requiring consultation for high-cost oral cephalosporins,[54] compulsory prospective antibiotic control,[55] antibiotic prescription forms that justify the reason for antibiotic use,[56] or routine surveillance.[57] The efficacy of each of the proposed methods to control the misuse of antibiotics (Table 6) depends on whether they meet the needs of the practicing physician.

The first method is education.[58] Neu and Howrey[59] demonstrated that there were major deficiencies in the physician's knowledge of antibiotic use, and they emphasized the need for further postgraduate education in this field. However, even though continued medical education is expanding in the United States, there is no concrete evidence that it improves actual practice. One study evaluating the effect of education was conducted by Jones et al.[29] The staff at a VA hospital did not show improvement in antibiotic use after an intensive educational program (Table 1). Gilbert and Jackson[60] reported success in improving antibiotic use by targeting their campaign for one drug, gentamicin. Achong et al.[30] reported remarkable success that in large part was attributable to improved use of antibiotics in surgical prophylaxis.

Another method, control of contact between pharmaceutical representatives and staff physicians, is only sporadically successful in a few institutions. The representative is usually visualized as a helpful colleague who provides quick information and favors and is properly obsequious. Entry is aided by advertising gimmicks and gifts, provision of funds for education, guest speakers, and funds for research or fellowship training.

TABLE 4. Factors That Lead to Inappropriate Use of Antimicrobial Agents

Motivation of the physician to give the best treatment	Desire to provide the patient with the very best drug available without regard to outside influences such as cost; fear of failure to provide the patient with the most appropriate drugs; desire to prevent infection before it may occur
Belief that if a small amount of drug will be effective, higher and more prolonged usage might be better	For example, the use of high dose intravenous penicillin for pneumococcal infections rather than equally effective smaller doses of procaine penicillin
Use of multiple antimicrobial agents or broad-spectrum agents to cover unusual organisms	Often appropriate in patients with severe leukopenia, but usually used as a substitute for diagnostic judgment
Inappropriate use of resources of clinical microbiology laboratory	Failure to obtain appropriate cultures; delay in transport of specimens and receiving needed information; poor interpersonal relations with the diagnostic laboratory; lack of explanation of results of tests by the laboratory; resistance of the laboratory to use simple culture methods in wards and clinics; need for consultant for interpretation of stained specimens; availability of rapid tests such as penicillinase production, Quellung reactions, tube dilution sensitivities, serum bactericidal levels; inappropriate sensitivity testing of ineffective agents (e.g., nitrofurantoin for systemic gram-negative infection)
Pressure from the patient to be treated with an antimicrobial agent	Desire to get rid of infection as soon as possible to avoid interference with lifestyle; concern of parents about febrile illness in their child; enhanced expectation for a solution of problems by drugs; fear of the unknown
Cost and availability of radiographic studies and diagnostic tests in relation to ready solution offered by drugs	Depends on practice setting, availability and costs of radiographic studies and diagnostic tests, policy of third-party payors, and distribution of physicians and other health care providers
Adequacy of the physician's knowledge of diagnostic procedures and management of patients with infectious disease	Depends on the extent of exposure to these disciplines in medical school and during postgraduate training; number of years since graduation, medical discipline, continuing education, self-instruction from literature, source(s) of information, experience in caring for patients with simple vs. complicated infectious disease
Malpractice considerations	Have forced physicians to practice defensive medicine by ordering excessive tests and using drugs to solve anticipated problems; explain in part, the overuse of oral cephalosporins in the hope that these new, more expensive, but relatively safe drugs will prevent embarrassment later; the threat of malpractice tends to decrease the usage of more toxic agents such as aminoglycoside antibiotics
Solution provided by pharmaceutical manufacturers	Take advantage of the above concerns and problems by offering often expensive and inappropriate panaceas and using heavy promotion; exploitation of the fear of failure by the physician to help his patient and of the concept that "if it might do some good and probably will do little harm, why not try it?"

TABLE 5. Methods Used by the Pharmaceutical Industry to Influence Physician Prescribing Habits

Group	*Objectives*	*Methods*
Medical students	Develop confidence in industry	Gifts of books, equipment, drugs for family; visits to plant; distribution of learning aids
House staff and fellows	Develop confidence in specific products	Same as for students, plus free samples for patients; advice on products by representatives; support for travel to meetings, throw-away journals
Practicing physicians	Create image of common goal of the physician and industry	Same as above plus special emphasis on personal contact with firm representatives; small medical-related gifts, stationery, forms
Hospital and medical societies	Create general goodwill for entry of representatives of the firm	Support for outside speakers, often product-oriented; support of meetings, entertainment, educational aids films, books—usually product oriented
General media	Raise public expectation for new drugs	News releases timed with development or release of a new agent
Academic physicians	Influence leaders to introduce new drugs to students and physicians	Support of directed studies of new agents; general research support; support for trainees; consultant arrangements, provide teaching aids; travel to national and international meetings
Medical media	Increase awareness of new products; blunt attack of critics	Direct advertising; throw-away journals (totally supported by advertising), published proceedings of symposia on new drugs; planted articles in throw-away news media, *Physicians' Desk Reference*
Diagnostic laboratories	Increase awareness of new agents	Special diagnostic tests that are related to the selection of new drugs

TABLE 6. Methods Used to Control the Use of Antimicrobial Agents in Hospitals

Education programs on the use of antimicrobial agents
- Staff conferences
- Lectures by outside authorities
- Audiovisual programs
- Clinical pharmacist consultants
- Hospital–Pharmacy Committee newsletters
- Independent sources of information (medical letter, AMA drug evaluations)

Control of contact between pharmaceutical representatives and staff physicians
- Registration in the pharmacy
- Visits to staff physicians by appointment only
- Policy concerning entry of salesmen to patient care areas
- Restricted time and place of displays
- Policy on free samples, gifts
- Policy on sponsoring speakers, distribution of literature, and advertising note paper

Hospital formulary
- Restriction of formulary to minimum number of agents needed for most effective therapy
- Elimination of duplicative agents
- Substitution rules for least expensive, most effective agent among a given class of agents
- Generic terminology required for all orders and labels

Diagnostic microbiology laboratory sensitivity tests
- Appropriate selection of sensitivity tests for organism and site
- Use of generic class disks
- Restriction of reports on specialized agents unless specifically requested or indicated
- Print own resort forms with generic terminology

Automatic stop orders for specific high-cost agents

Written justification for high-cost agents
- In cases where alternative, equally effective, less expensive or toxic agents may be used (e.g., oral cephalosporins, new parenteral aminoglycosides, and cephalosporins, lincosamides, chloramphenicol)

Required consultation
- This is to be done after first 3 doses of specific high-cost agents are ordered (e.g., aminoglycosides, parenteral cephalosporins, carbenicillin-ticarcillin, lincosamides)

Controlled agents
- Release of specific agents that may alter the ecology of hospital flora requires approval by infectious disease consultants (e.g., amikacin, carbenicillin-ticarcillin)

Guidelines and audits of antimicrobial usage
- These permit the hospital staff to set standards of use based on local needs and judgments, guided by independent criteria. An audit is based on compliance with these standards but requires a well-structured, authoritative feedback loop.

It is extremely difficult even for the academic physician to restrict these people since the information they bring is often valuable and the companies do develop many excellent antimicrobial agents. However, I believe that contact with drug representatives should be limited and restricted only to providing new information in a physician- and hospital-controlled setting. Some have proposed that "counterdetailing" by clinical pharmacists may help.[61] Schaffner et al.[62] have shown that visits to office-based practitioners by physician counselors was the most effective method to reduce the prescribing of overused antibiotics.

The hospital formulary committee can be extremely useful in examining the claims and need for new agents. It is in this area that the clinical pharmacist may be of greatest help by advising the committee on the relative benefits of adding or deleting agents from the formulary.

In many ways, the diagnostic laboratory also plays a key role in the selection of antimicrobial agents by physicians. So it is exceedingly important that antibiotic sensitivity tests results be reported by generic name and class and be tailored to the best agents according to the organism and site of infection.[63]

Several imaginative methods have been developed to control antibiotic usage. These include automatic "stop" orders for specific high-cost agents, the use of single daily doses of long-acting agents that can also be given intramuscularly,[48–50] prospective monitoring of use, computer surveillance,[64–66] and cost sharing by outpatients.[67] A rational approach described by Quintiliani et al. is to "streamline" the sequence of therapy.[68] A modification of this approach is shown in Table 7. The physician can move rapidly from presumptive therapy in stage I to definitive therapy in stage II by the early use of rapid diagnostic procedures such as examination of wounds and body fluids with Gram stains and specific antibodies.

Written justification for the use of antibiotics on the prescription is an effective method to decrease inappropriate usage. This forces physicians to explain their actions, and the requirement to write even a brief justification tends to blunt unnecessary prescribing. McGowan and Finland[69] have demonstrated that the removal of this requirement has been followed by increased use of these agents.

Required consultations and control of high-cost or toxic agents by experts have been shown to work well in an institution in which there is an active training program in infectious disease and a strong infectious disease group interested in antimicrobial therapy. However, these measures are not applicable at this time to many hospitals in the United States. Nevertheless, the results of these two approaches are instructive. They clearly demonstrate that most antibiotic usage is wasteful and unnecessary. For example, we have been able to reduce overusage markedly by generating an automatic consultation through the hospital pharmacy once the first three doses of an expensive, potentially toxic agent are ordered. This avoids denying the

TABLE 7. Three Typical Stages of Antibiotic Therapy in Hospital-Associated Infections

Stage	*Patient's Condition*	*Diagnosis/Treatment*
Initial	Presumed to have an infectious process	Blood cultures, aspiration of wound or body fluid, gram or other specific stain Specific, established agents may be used effectively
I (days 1–3)	Clinically unstable; uncertain of cause or site of infection	Empirical therapy, β-lactam and aminoglycoside or extended-spectrum β-lactam
II (days 4–6)	Begins to stabilize; causative agent identified	Specific therapy often with single, long-acting, narrow spectrum; parenteral or even oral agent may be used
III (days 7 and beyond)	Clinically stable, completion of therapy	Oral therapy or long-acting parenteral agent administered as outpatient or at home

(Modified from Quintiliani et al.,[68] with permission.)

patient a needed drug but permits early appraisal of the appropriateness of the antibiotic. As the program continues, less consultation is required since physicians soon become aware that their practice will be reviewed with them. Cephalosporin antibiotic use fell dramatically during the period of control. In most cases, a less expensive agent such as penicillin G was used instead, or postsurgical use of a cephalosporin was curtailed. Evaluation of patient records revealed that no patient was denied adequate therapy during the control period. The difference between the use of this class of drugs before and after control measures indicates the amount of this drug unnecessarily prescribed in the hospital.

Since most hospital staffs must function without the aid of experts in antimicrobial therapy, independent guidelines for appropriate use are needed. These guidelines need to be updated continuously. They potentially offer a basis for local discussion of the issues and modifications that best suit the judgment and needs of the practicing physicians. The most critical guidelines are for prophylaxis in surgery and for the use of oral and parenteral cephalosporin antibiotics. It is in these areas that the highest cost and greatest waste occurs. The guidelines are not excessively restrictive since they are based on the best available data from the surgical literature that emphasize short perioperative courses of the most effective agents. This auditing function measures compliance with local standards and provides feedback to the hospital staff who fail to adhere to guidelines accepted by their peers. The report of success in controlling overuse by Achong et al.[30] supports the idea that a well-informed and concerned staff can reduce the inappropriate use of antibiotics.

SUMMATION AND COMMENTARY

This chapter has described the problem of overuse of antibiotics. It is part of a larger problem of overuse of medical care facilities, diagnostic tests, and other drugs. The problem and its solution depend on knowledge of the constraints in medical practice that tend to lead the physician to overprescribe antibiotics. Instruction in infectious disease and antimicrobial therapy has been severely curtailed recently in most medical schools. This error, in my view, must be redressed by greater rather than less formal instruction. The problem, however, extends well beyond the formative years of the physician's education and cannot be solved by a punitive approach to the pharmaceutical industry. The industry simply exploits the constraints of medical practice to sell its products.

The overuse of antibiotics is not simply an economic problem, even though it is easily measured by these standards, nor is it just poor practice because of the heavy price paid for ecologic changes with new, resistant microbial strains. Most importantly, in my view, it reveals how effectively we as physicians use scientific technology to help our patients. The solution to the problem rests on our willingness to use this technology wisely.

REFERENCES

1. Jawetz E. Antimicrobial chemotherapy. Annu Rev Microbiol. 1956;10:85.
2. Welch H, Lewis CN, Weinstein HI, et al. Severe reactions to antibiotics: A nationwide survey. Antibiot Med Chem Ther. 1957;4:800.
3. Finland M, Jones WF, Barnes MW. Occurrence of serious bacterial infections since introduction of antibacterial agents. JAMA. 1959;170:84.
4. Reimann HA, D'Ambola J. The use and cost of antimicrobics in hospitals. Arch Environ Health. 1966;13:631.
5. Lockwood, WR. Antibiotics anonymous. N Engl J Med. 1974;290:465.
6. Simmons HE, Stolley PD. This is medical progress? Trends and consequences of antibiotic use in the United States. JAMA. 1974;227:1023.
7. Craig WA, Sarver KP. Antimicrobial usage in the USA. In: Williams JD, Geddes AM, eds. Chemotherapy, v. 4. New York: Plenum; 1976:293.
8. McGowan JE Jr. Antimicrobial resistance in hospital organisms and its relation to antibiotic use. Rev Infect Dis. 1983;5:1033.
9. Sogaard H, Zimmerman-Nielsen C, Sibioni K. Antibioticresistant gram-negative bacilli in a urological ward for male patients during a 9-year period: Relationship to antibiotic consumption. J Infect Dis. 1974;130:646.
10. Bulger RJ, Sherris JC. Decreased incidence of antibiotic resistance among *Staphylococcus aureus*. A study in a university hospital over a 9-year period. Ann Intern Med. 1968;69:1099.
11. Kunin CM, Tupasi T, Craig WA. Use of antibiotics: A brief exposition of the problem and some tentative solutions. Ann Intern Med. 1973;79:555.
12. Cluff LE. The prescribing habits of physicians. Hosp Pract. 1967;2:100.
13. Seidl LG, Thornder GF, Smith SW, et al. Studies on epidemiology of adverse drug reactions. III. Reactions in patients on general medical service. Bull Johns Hopkins Hosp. 1966;119:299.
14. Stolley PD, Becker MH, McEvilla JB, et al. Drug prescribing and use in an American community. Ann Intern Med. 1972;76:537.
15. Becker MH, Stolley PD, Lasagna L, et al. Differential education concerning therapeutics and resultant physician prescribing patterns. J Med Educ. 1972;47:118.
16. Antibiotics for common colds? (Editorial). Lancet. 1976;1:132.
17. Stott NCH, West RR. Randomized controlled trial of antibiotics in patients with cough and purulent sputum. Lancet. 1976;2:556.
18. Stollerman GH: The relative rheumatogenicity of strains of group A streptococci. Mod Concepts Cardiovasc Dis. 1975;44:35.
19. Greenberg RA, Wagner EH, Wolf SH, et al. Physician opinions on the use of antibiotics in respiratory infections. JAMA. 1978;240:650.
20. Bernstein LR, Barriere SL, Conte JE. Utilization of antibiotics: Analysis of appropriateness of use. Ann Emerg Med. 1982;11:400.
21. Ray WA, Federspiel CF, Schaffner W. Prescribing of chloramphenicol in ambulatory practice. An epidemiologic study among Tennessee Medicaid recipients. Ann Intern Med. 1976;84:266.
22. Ray WA, Federspiel CF, Schaffner W. Prescribing of tetracycline to children less than 8 years old. JAMA. 1977;237:2069.
23. Scheckler WE, Bennett JV. Antibiotic usage in seven community hospitals. JAMA. 1970;213:264.
24. Roberts AW, Visconti JA. The relational and irrational use of systemic antimicrobial drugs. Am J Hosp Pharm. 1972;29:1054.
25. Gibbs CW Jr, Gibson JT, Newton DS. Drug utilization review of actual versus preferred pediatric antibiotic therapy. Am J Hosp Pharm. 1973;30:892.
26. Castle M, Wilfert CM, Cate TR, et al. Antibiotic use at Duke University Medical Center. JAMA. 1977;237:2819.
27. Petrello MA, Linkewich JA, Gluckman SJ, et al. Clindamycin prescribing patterns in a university hospital. Am J Hosp Pharm. 1975;32:1111.
28. Maki DG, Schuna AA. A study of antimicrobial misuse in a university hospital. Am J Med Sci. 1978;275:271.
29. Jones SR, Bratton T, McRee E. The effect of an educational program upon hospital use. Am J Med Sci. 1977;273:79085.
30. Achong MR, Theal HK, Wood J, et al. Changes in hospital antibiotic therapy after a quality-of-use study. Lancet. 1977;2:1118.
31. McGowan JE Jr, Finland M. Effects of minitoring the use of antibiotics: An interhospital comparison. South Med J. 1976;69:193.
32. Shapiro M, Townsend TR, Rosner B, et al. Use of antimicrobial drugs in general hospitals. N Engl J Med. 1979;301:351.
33. Crossley K, Gardner LC. Antimicrobial prophylaxis in surgical patients. JAMA. 1981;245:722.

34. Shapiro M, Schoenbaum SC, Tager IB, et al. Benefit–cost analysis of antimicrobial prophylaxis in abdominal and vaginal hysterectomy. JAMA. 1983;249:1290.
35. Chretien JH, McGarvey M, de Stowlinski A, et al. Abuse of antibiotics, a study of patients attending a university clinic. Arch Intern Med. 1975;135:1063.
36. Gustafsson LL, Wide K. Marketing of obsolete antibiotics in Central America. Lancet. 1981;1:31.
37. Tomson G, Sterky G. Self-prescribing by way of pharmacies in three Asian developing countries. Lancet. 1986;2:620–1.
38. Kunin CM, Lipton HL, Tupasi T, et al. Social, behavior, and practical factors affecting antibiotic use worldwide: Report of task force 4. Rev Infect Dis. 1987;9(Suppl):270.
39. Levy M, Nir I, Superstine E, et al. Antimicrobial therapy in patients hospitalized in a medical ward. A report from the Boston collaborative drug surveillance program. Isr J Med Sci. 1975;11:322.
40. Study group in the use of antimicrobial drugs: Prophylactic antimicrobial drug therapy at five London teaching hospitals. Lancet. 1977;1:1351.
41. Cook D, Salter AJ, Phillips I: Antimicrobial misuse, antibiotic policies and information responses. J Antimicrob Chemother. 1980;6:435.
42. Leigh DA. Antimicrobial usage in forty-three hospitals in England. J Antimicrob Chemother. 1982;9:75.
43. Holmberg SD, Osterholm MT, Senger KA, et al. Drug-resistant *Salmonella* from animal fed antimicrobials. N Engl J Med. 1984;311:617.
44. DuPont HL, Steele JH. Use of antimicrobial agents in animal feeds: Implications for human health. Rev Infect Dis. 1987;9:447.
45. Kunin CM. The responsibility of the infectious disease community for the optimal use of antimicrobial agents. J Infect Dis. 1985;151:388.
46. Gitch DW. New ways of managing under prospective payment and their impact on the principles and practice of infectious diseases. Rev Infect Dis. 1986;8:494.
47. Iannini PB. DRGs and outpatient antibiotics. Infect Control. 1986;7:289.
48. Poretz DM, Eron LJ, Goldenberg RI, et al. Home intravenous antibiotic therapy: A team approach. JAMA. 1982;248:336.
49. Smego RA Jr. Home intravenous antibiotic therapy. Arch Intern Med. 1985;145:1001.
50. Eisenberg JM, Kitz DS. Savings from outpatient antibiotic therapy for osteomyelitis. Economic analysis of a therapeutic strategy. JAMA. 1986;255:1584.
51. Kunin CM. Guidelines and audits for use of antimicrobial agents in hospitals. J Infect Dis. 1977;135:335.
52. Marr JJ, Moffet HL, Kunin CM. Guidelines for improving use of antimicrobial agents in hospitals: A statement of the Infectious Diseases Society of America. J Infect Dis. 1988;157:869.
53. Musher DM. Antibiotics: The medium is the message (Letter). Rev Infect Dis. 1983;5:809.
54. Seligman SJ. Reduction in antibiotic costs by restricting use of an oral cephalosporin. Am J Med. 1981;71:941.
55. Recco RA, Gladstone JL, Friedman SA, et al. Antibiotic control in a municipal hospital. JAMA. 1979;241:2283.
56. Durbin WA, Lapidas B, Goldmann DA. Improved antibiotic usage following introduction of a novel prescription system. JAMA. 1981;246:1796.
57. Feldman L, Lamson M, Gallelli JF, et al. Surveillance of nosocomial infections by antibiotic monitoring. JAMA. 1979;241:2806.
58. Counts GW. Review and control of antimicrobial usage. JAMA. 1977;238:2170.
59. Neu HC, Howrey SP. Testing the physician's knowledge of antibiotic use: Self-assessment and learning via videotape. N Engl J Med. 1975;293:1291.
60. Gilbert DN, Jackson J. Effect of an education program on the proper use of gentamicin in a community hospital (Abstract). Clin Res. 1976;24:112.
61. Hendeles L. Need for "counter-detailing" antibiotics. Am J Hosp Pharm. 1976;33:918.
62. Schaffner W, Ray WA, Federspiel CF, et al: Improving antibiotic prescribing in office practice. A controlled trial of three educational methods. JAMA. 1983;250:1728.
63. Kunin CM. Antibiotic sensitivity tests: How to get the most out of them. Wis Med J. 1971;70:206.
64. Williams RR, Gross PA, Levin JF. Cost containment of the second-generation cephalosporins by prospective monitoring at a community teaching hospital. Arch Intern Med. 1985;145:1978.
65. Evans RS, Larsen RA, Burke JP, et al. Computer surveillance of hospital-acquired infections and antibiotic use. JAMA. 1986;256:1007.
66. Heineman HS, Watt VS. All-inclusive concurrent antibiotic usage review: A way to reduce misuse without formal controls. Infect Control. 1986;7:168.
67. Foxman B, Valdez RB, Lohr KN, et al. The effect of cost sharing on the use of antibiotics in ambulatory care: Results from a population-based randomized controlled trial. J Chronic Dis. 1987;40:429.
68. Quintiliani R, Cooper BW, Briceland LL, et al. Economic impact of streamlining antibiotic administration. Am J Med. 1987;82(Suppl 4A):391.
69. McGowan JE Jr, Finland M. Usage of antibiotics in a general hospital: Effect of requiring justification. J Infect Dis. 1974;130:165.
70. Kunin CM, Efron HY. Audits of antimicrobial guidelines for peer review. JAMA.. 1977;237:1001, 1003, 1134, 1241, 1243, 1366, 1367, 1481, 1482, 1605, 1607, 1723, 1724, 1725, 1859, 1860, 1967, 1968, 1969.

38. TABLES OF ANTIMICROBIAL AGENT PHARMACOLOGY

SANDRA NORRIS
CHARLES H. NIGHTINGALE
GERALD L. MANDELL

The selection of an appropriate dose of an antimicrobial agent is based on information such as the site of infection, the identity and known or presumed antibiotic susceptibility of the infecting organism, dose-related drug toxicity, and the patient's ability to eliminate the drug. This chapter serves as a centralized source of pharmacologic information frequently sought for antimicrobial agents. For more detailed information about specific agents, see the appropriate chapter.

Generic and trade name tables for antimicrobial agents are provided. The antimicrobial "family" classification is also included to help the reader locate specific information in subsequent tables.

DOSING GUIDELINES

Generally, *dosage* selections from the upper end of the dosage range are recommended for severe, life-threatening infections (sepsis, meningitis). The lowest dosages are used for urinary tract infections. A sizable range in dosing *intervals* exists for some antimicrobial agents, with the longer duration between doses appropriate for less severe infections in which a critical threshold level in serum or other site of infection (e.g., central nervous system) is not mandatory or the drug concentrates significantly at the site of infection (urine, bile).

Dosing recommendations for the following drugs result from preliminary, premarketing clinical trials and at the time of publication have not been officially approved by the U.S. Food and Drug Administration: apalcillin, carumonam, cefepime, cefmenoxime, cefotiam, cefpiramide, cefpirome, cefsulodin, clarithromycin, enoxacin, fleroxacin, fluconazole, ganciclovir, itraconazole, lomefloxacin, ofloxacin, pefloxacin, rimantadine, roxithromycin, teicoplanin, temafloxacin, and temocillin. To prevent dosing errors, these recommendations should be checked with recent package inserts or current reference sources.

DOSAGE ADJUSTMENT FOR RENAL IMPAIRMENT

Drug half-life in *adults* with impaired renal function and changes related to dialysis procedures (HD: hemodialysis, PD: peritoneal dialysis) are summarized for the user. An alternative to the elongation of the interval between doses is reduction of the daily dose given at the "usual" dosing interval (Bennett et al.). Antimicrobial serum levels should be determined and patient-specific dosage adjustments made on the basis of these determinations.

Unless otherwise stated, the doses indicated for hemodialysis should supplement "anuric doses." The "usual adult dose" is for parenteral therapy unless designated oral (po).

With the increasing use of chronic ambulatory peritoneal dialysis (CAPD), drug addition to the dialysate solution with direct instillation into the peritoneal cavity is becoming a widely used method of drug delivery. Generally, one adds an amount of drug to dialysate solution to mimic the target serum concentration. For example, add 5 mg gentamicin per liter of dialysate solution for a desired serum level of 5 μg/ml.

BODY FLUID CONCENTRATIONS

In determining the appropriateness of a particular antibiotic for a given site of infection, the ultimate concentration of a drug as compared with the minimum inhibitory concentration for the infecting organism is critical rather than percent penetration as compared with serum. For example, the aminoglycosides are ineffective therapy for meningitis although they penetrate into the cerebrospinal fluid to a higher degree than does penicillin G, which is effective therapy for certain organisms. Percent penetration (relationship between peak concentration in a specific body fluid to serum) is, however, a valuable tool for comparisons among similar agents.

GENERIC-TRADE NAMES

Generic	Trade	Family
Acyclovir	Zovirax	Antiviral agents
Amantadine	Symmetrel	Antiviral agents
Amdinocillin	Coactin	Penicillins
Amikacin	Amikin	Aminoglycosides
Aminosalicylic acid	PAS Para Parasal Rexipas	Antimycobacterial agents Antimycobacterial agents Antimycobacterial agents Antimycobacterial agents
Amoxicillin	Amoxil Larotid Polymox Robamox Trimox	Penicillins Penicillins Penicillins Penicillins Penicillins
Amphotericin B	Fungizone	Antifungal agents
Ampicillin	Ampen Amcill Omnipen Omnipen N PenA Penbritin Pensyn Polycillin Polycillin N Principen Probampacin Supen Totacillin	Penicillins Penicillins Penicillins Penicillins Penicillins Penicillins Penicillins Penicillins Penicillins Penicillins Penicillins Penicillins Penicillins
Ampicillin probenecid	Polycillin-PRB Trojacillin-Plus	Penicillins Penicillins
Ansamycin	—	Antimycobacterial agents
Apalcillin	—	Penicillins
Azlocillin	Azlin	Penicillins
Aztreonam	Azactam	Other β-lactams
Bacampicillin	Spectrobid	Penicillins
Benzathine penicillin	Bicillin Permapen	Penicillins Penicillins
Bithionol	Bitin	Antiparasitic agents
Capreomycin	Capastat	Antimycobacterial agents
Carbenicillin	Geopen Pyopen	Penicillins Penicillins
Carbenicillin indanyl sodium	Geocillin	Penicillins
Cefaclor	Ceclor	Cephalosporins
Cefadroxil	Duricef	Cephalosporins
Cefamandole	Mandol	Cephalosporins
Cefazolin	Ancef Kefzol	Cephalosporins Cephalosporins
Cefmenoxime	Cefmax	Cephalosporins
Cefonicid	Monocid	Cephalosporins
Cefoperazone	Cefobid	Cephalosporins

Generic	Trade	Family
Ceforanide	Precef	Cephalosporins
Cefotaxime	Claforan	Cephalosporins
Cefotetan	Cefotan	Cephalosporins
Cefotiam	—	Cephalosporins
Cefoxitin	Mefoxin	Cephalosporins
Cefsulodin	Cefomonil	Cephalosporins
Ceftazidime	Fortaz Tazicef Tazidime	Cephalosporins
Ceftizoxime	Cefizox	Cephalosporins
Ceftriaxone	Rocephin	Cephalosporins
Cefuroxime	Zinacef	Cephalosporins
Cephalexin	Keflex	Cephalosporins
Cephaloglycine	Kafocin	Cephalosporins
Cephaloridine	Loridine	Cephalosporins
Cephalothin	Keflin	Cephalosporins
Cephapirin	Cefadyl	Cephalosporins
Cephradine	Anspor Velosef	Cephalosporins Cephalosporins
Chloramphenicol	Chloromycetin	Chloramphenicol
Chloroquine	Aralen	Antiparasitic agents
Chlortetracycline	Aureomycin	Tetracyclines
Cinoxacin	Cinobac	Other urinary tract agents
Ciprofloxacin	Cipro	Quinolones
Clavulanate + amoxicillin	Augmentin	β-Lactamase inhibitors
Clavulanate + ticarcillin	Timentin	β-Lactamase inhibitors
Clindamycin	Cleocin	Lincosamides
Clofazimine	Lamprene	Antimycobacterial agents
Clotrimazole	Mycelex Lotrimin	Antifungal agents Antifungal agents
Cloxacillin	Tegopen	Penicillins
Colistimethate	Colymycin M	Polymyxins
Colistin	Colymycin S	Polymyxins
Cotrimoxazole	Bactrim Septra	Sulfonamides + trimethoprim
Cyclacillin	Cyclapen	Penicillins
Cycloserine	Oxamycin Seromycin	Antimycobacterial agents Antimycobacterial agents
Dapsone	Avlosulfon	Antimycobacterial agents
Demeclocycline	Declomycin	Tetracyclines
Dicloxacillin	Dycill Dynapen Pathocil Veracillin	Penicillins Penicillins Penicillins Penicillins
Diethylcarbamazine	Hetrazan	Antiparasitic agents

(*Continued*)

GENERIC-TRADE NAMES *(Continued)*

Generic	*Trade*	*Family*
Diiodohydroxyquin	Panaquin	Antiparasitic agents
Diloxanide furoate	Furamide	Antiparasitic agents
Doxycycline	Doxy II	Tetracyclines
	Doxychel	Tetracyclines
	Vibramycin	Tetracyclines
Emetine	—	Antiparasitic agents
Enoxacin	Comprecin	Quinolones
Erythromycin	E-mycin	Erythromycins
	Erypar	Erythromycins
	Ethril	Erythromycins
	Ilotycin	Erythromycins
	Kesso-mycin	Erythromycins
	Robimycin	Erythromycins
Erythromycin estolate	Ilosone	Erythromycins
Erythromycin ethylsuccinate	E.E.S.	Erythromycins
	Pediamycin	Erythromycins
Erythromycin ethylsuccinate plus sulfisoxazole	Pediazole	
Erythromycin stearate	Bristamycin	Erythromycins
	Erythrocin	Erythromycins
	Pfizer-E	Erythromycins
Ethambutol	Myambutol	Antimycobacterial agents
Ethionamide	Trecator-SC	Antimycobacterial agents
Flucytosine	Ancobon	Antifungal agents
Furazolidone	Furoxone	Antiparasitic agents
Fusidic acid	—	Fusidic acid
Ganciclovir	Cytovene	Antivirals
Gentamicin	Garamycin	Aminoglycosides
Griseofulvin	Fulvicin P-G	Antifungal agents
	Fulvicin U F	Antifungal agents
	Grifulvin V	Antifungal agents
	Gris-PEG	Antifungal agents
	Grisactin	Antifungal agents
Hetacillin	Versapen	Penicillins
	Versapen K	Penicillins
Idoxuridine	Dendrid	Antiviral agents
	Herplex	Antiviral agents
	Stoxil	Antiviral agents
Imipenem + cilastatin	Primaxin	Other β-lactams
Iodoquinol (diiodohydroxyquin)	Yodoxin	Antiparasitic agents
Isoniazid	Hyzyd	Antimycobacterial agents
	INH	Antimycobacterial agents
	Niadox	Antimycobacterial agents
	Niconyl	Antimycobacterial agents
	Nydrazid	Antimycobacterial agents
Itraconazole	Sporanox	Antifungal agents
Kanamycin	Kantrex	Aminoglycosides
Ketoconazole	Nizoral	Antifungal agents
Lincomycin	Lincocin	Lincosamides
Mafenide	Sulfamylon	Sulfonamides + trimethoprim
Mebendazole	Vermox	Antiparasitic agents
Melarsoprol	Arsobal	Antiparasitic agents
	Mel B	Antiparasitic agents
Methacycline	Rondomycin	Tetracyclines
Methenamine hippurate	Hiprex	Other urinary tract agents
	Urex	Other urinary tract agents
Methenamine mandelate	Mandelamine	Other urinary tract agents
Methicillin	Celbenin	Penicillins
	Dimocillin RT	Penicillins
	Staphcillin	Penicillins
Metrifonate	Bilarcil	Antiparasitic agents
Metronidazole	Flagyl	Metronidazole
Mezlocillin	Mezlin	Penicillins
Miconazole	Micatin	Antifungal agents
	Monistat	Antifungal agents
Minocycline	Minocin	Tetracyclines
	Vectrin	Tetracyclines
Moxalactam	Moxam	Cephalosporins

Generic	*Trade*	*Family*
Nafcillin	Nafcil	Penicillins
	Unipen	Penicillins
Nalidixic acid	Cybis	Quinolones
	NegGram	Quinolones
Neomycin	Mycifradin	Aminoglycosides
Netilmicin	Netromycin	Aminoglycosides
Niclosamide	Niclocide	Antiparasitic agents
	Yomesan	Antiparasitic agents
Nifurtimox	Lampit	Antiparasitic agents
Niridazole	Ambilhar	Antiparasitic agents
Nitrofurantoin	Cyantin	Other urinary tract agents
	Furadantin	Other urinary tract agents
	Macrodantin	Other urinary tract agents
	Trantoin	Other urinary tract agents
Norfloxacin	Noraxin	Other urinary tract agents
Novobiocin	Albamycin	—
Nystatin	Mycostatin	Antifungal agents
	Nilstat	Antifungal agents
Oxacillin	Bactocill	Penicillins
	Prostaphlin	Penicillins
	Resistopen	Penicillins
Oxamniquine	Vansil	Antiparasitic agents
Oxolinic acid	Utibid	Quinolones
Oxytetracycline	Terramycin	Tetracyclines
	Uri-Tet	Tetracyclines
Para-aminosalicylic acid, *see* aminosalicylic acid		
Paromomycin	Humatin	Antiparasitic agents
Penicillin G	Pentids	Penicillins
	Pfizerpen	Penicillins
Penicillin G procaine	Crysticillin	Penicillins
	Duracillin AS	Penicillins
	Wycillin	Penicillins
Penicillin G sodium + penicillin G procaine	Duracillin FA	Penicillins
Penicillin G + phenoxymethyl penicillin	Kesso-pen	Penicillins
Penicillin V potassium (phenoxymethyl penicillin)	Betopen VK	Penicillins
	Ledercillin VK	Penicillins
	Penapar VK	Penicillins
	Pen Vee K	Penicillins
	Robicillin VK	Penicillins
	Uticillin VK	Penicillins
	V-Cillin K	Penicillins
	Veetids	Penicillins
Pentamidine	Pentam 300	Antiparasitic agents
	Lomidine	Antiparasitic agents
Phenazopyridine	Azo Gantrisin	—
Phenethicillin	Darcil	Penicillins
	Maxipen	Penicillins
	Synicillin	Penicillins
Piperacillin	Pipracil	Penicillins
Piperazine	Antepar	Antiparasitic agents
Pivmecillinam	Selexid	Penicillins
Pivmecilliam sulfamicillin		Penicillins
Polymyxin B	Aerosporin	Polymyxins
Praziquantel	Biltricide	Antiparasitic agents
Primaquine phosphate	Primaquine	Antiparasitic agents
Pyrantel pamoate	Antiminth	Antiparasitic agents
Pyrazinamide	—	Antimycobacterial agents
Pyrimethamine	Daraprim	Antiparasitic agents
Pyrimethamine-sulfadoxine	Fansidar	Antiparasitic agents
Pyrivinium pamoate	Povan	Antiparasitic agents
Quinacrine	Atabrine	Antiparasitic agents
Quinine sulfate	—	Antiparasitic agents
Ribavirin	Virazole	Antiviral agents

(*Continued*)

GENERIC-TRADE NAMES *(Continued)*

Generic	*Trade*	*Family*
Rifampin	Rifadin Rimactane	Antimycobacterial agents Antimycobacterial agents
Rifampin-isoniazid	Rifamate	Antimycobacterial agents
Rimantadine	Flumadine	Antiviral agents
Silver sulfadiazine	Silvadine	Sulfonamides + trimethoprim
Spectinomycin	Trobicin	Aminoglycosides
Stibogluconate	Pentostam	Antiparasitic agent
Succinylsulfathiazole	Rolsul Sulfasuxidine	Sulfonamides + trimethoprim Sulfonamides + trimethoprim
Sulbactam + ampicillin	Unasyn	β-Lactamase inhibitors
Sulbactam + cefoperazone	—	β-Lactamase inhibitors
Sulfacetamide	Bleph Isopto cetamide Sulamyd sodium	Sulfonamides + trimethoprim Sulfonamides + trimethoprim Sulfonamides + trimethoprim
Sulfachlorpyridazine	Sonilyn	Sulfonamides + trimethoprim
Sulfacytine	Renoquid	Sulfonamides + trimethoprim
Sulfadiazine	Sulfadyne	Sulfonamides + trimethoprim
Sulfadoxine	Fansidar	Sulfonamides + trimethoprim
Sulfamethizole	Thiosulfil Urifon	Sulfonamides + trimethoprim Sulfonamides + trimethoprim Sulfonamides + trimethoprim
Sulfamethoxazole	Gantanol	Sulfonamides + trimethoprim
Sulfasalazine	Azulfidine	Sulfonamides + trimethoprim
Sulfisoxazole	Gantrisin	Sulfonamides + trimethoprim
Sultamicillin	—	β-Lactamase inhibitors
Suramin	Germanin	Antiparasitic agents
Teichomycin	—	—
Temocillin	—	Penicillins
Tetracycline	Achromycin Kesso-tetra Panmycin Polycycline Robitet Steclin Sumycin Tetracyn Tetrex	Tetracyclines Tetracyclines Tetracyclines Tetracyclines Tetracyclines Tetracyclines Tetracyclines Tetracyclines Tetracyclines
Thiabendazole	Mintezol	Antiparasitic agents
Ticarcillin	Ticar	Penicillins
Tobramycin	Nebcin	Aminoglycosides
Tolnaftate	Tinactin	Antifungal agents
Trifluridine	Viroptic	Antiviral agents
Trimethoprim	Proloprim Trimpex	Sulfonamides + trimethoprim Sulfonamides + trimethoprim
Trimethoprim-sulfamethoxazole	Bactrim Septra	Sulfonamides + trimethoprim Sulfonamides + trimethoprim
Trisulfapyrimidines	Terfonyl	Sulfonamides + trimethoprim
Troleandomycin	TAO	—
Vancomycin	Vancocin	Vancomycin
Vidarabine	Vira-A	Antiviral agents
Viomycin	Vinactane Viocin	Antimycobacterial agents Antimycobacterial agents
Zidovudine (AZT)	Retrovir	Antiviral agents

TRADE-GENERIC NAMES

Trade	*Generic*	*Family*
Achromycin	Tetracycline	Tetracyclines
Aerosporin	Polymyxin B	Polymyxins
Albamycin	Novobiocin	—
Ampen	Ampicillin	Penicillins
Ambilhar	Niridazole	Antiparasitic agents
Amcill	Ampicillin	Penicillins
Amikin	Amikacin	Aminoglycosides
Amoxil	Amoxicillin	Penicillins
Ancef	Cefazolin	Cephalosporins
Ancobon	Flucytosine	Antifungal agents
Anspor	Cephradine	Cephalosporins
Antepar	Piperazine citrate	Antiparasitic agents
Antiminth	Pyrantel pamoate	Antiparasitic agents
Apace	Cefotetan	Cephalosporins
Aralen	Chloroquine	Antiparasitic agents
Arsobal	Melarsoprol	Antiparasitic agents
Atabrine	Quinacrine	Antiparasitic agents
Augmentin	Clavulanate + amoxicillin	β-Lactamase inhibitors
Aureomycin	Chlortetracycline	Tetracyclines
Avlosulfon	Dapsone	Antimycobacterial agents
Azactam	Aztreonam	Other β-lactams
Azlin	Azlocillin	Penicillins
Azo Gantrisin	Phenazopyridine	—
Azulfidine	Sulfasalazine	Sulfonamides + trimethoprim
Bactocill	Oxacillin	Penicillins
Bactrim	Trimethoprim-sulfamethoxazole	Sulfonamides + trimethoprim
Betopen VK	Penicillin V potassium	Penicillins
Bicillin	Benzathine penicillin G	Penicillins
Bilarcil	Metrifonate	Antiparasitic agents
Biltricide	Praziquantel	Antiparasitic agents
Bitin	Bithionol	Antiparasitic agents
Bleph	Sulfacetamide	Sulfonamides + trimethoprim
Bristamycin	Erythromycin stearate	Erythromycins
Canesten	Clotrimazole	Antifungal agents
Capastat	Capreomycin	Antimycobacterial agents
Ceclor	Cefaclor	Cephalosporins
Cefadyl	Cephapirin	Cephalosporins
Cefizox	Ceftizoxime	Cephalosporins
Cefmax	Cefmenoxime	Cephalosporins
Cefobid	Cefoperazone	Cephalosporins
Cefomonil	Cefsulodin	Cephalosporins
Celbenin	Methicillin	Penicillins
Chloromycetin	Chloramphenicol	Chloramphenicol
Cinobac	Cinoxacin	Other urinary tract agents
Cipro	Ciprofloxacin	Quinolones
Claforan	Cefotaxime	Cephalosporins
Cleocin	Clindamycin	Lincosamides
Coactin	Amdinocillin	Penicillins
Colymycin M	Colistimethate	Polymyxins
Colymycin S	Colistin	Polymyxins

(Continued)

Trade	Generic	Family
Compresin	Enoxacin	Quinolones
Crysticillin	Penicillin G procaine	Penicillins
Cyantin	Nitrofurantoin	Other urinary tract agents
Cybis	Nalidixic acid	Quinolones
Cyclapen	Cyclacillin	Penicillins
Cytovene	Ganciclovir	Antivirals
Daraprim	Pyrimethamine	Antiparasitic agents
Darcil	Phenethicillin	Penicillins
Declomycin	Demeclocycline	Tetracyclines
Dendrid	Idoxuridine	Antiviral agents
Dimocillin RT	Methicillin	Penicillins
Doxy II	Doxycycline	Tetracyclines
Doxychel	Doxycycline	Tetracyclines
Duracillin AS	Penicillin G procaine	Penicillins
Duracillin FA	Penicillin G sodium + penicillin G procaine	Penicillins
Duricef	Cefadroxil	Cephalosporins
Dycill	Dicloxacillin	Penicillins
Dynapen	Dicloxacillin	Penicillins
E-mycin	Erythromycin	Erythromycins
E.E.S.	Erythromycin ethylsuccinate	Erythromycins
Erypar	Erythromycin	Erythromycins
Erythrocin	Erythromycin stearate	Erythromycins
Ethril	Erythromycin	Erythromycins
Fansidar	Pyrimethamine-sulfadoxine	Antiparasitic agents
Flagyl	Metronidazole	Metronidazole
Flumadine	Rimantadine	Antiviral agents
Fortaz	Ceftazidime	Cephalosporins
Fulvicin P-G	Griseofulvin	Antifungal agents
Fulvicin U-F	Griseofulvin	Antifungal agents
Fungizone	Amphotericin B	Antifungal agents
Furadantin	Nitrofurantoin	Other urinary tract agents
Furamide	Diloxanide furoate	Antiparasitic agents
Furoxone	Furazolidone	Antiparasitic agents
Gantanol	Sulfamethoxazole	Sulfonamides + trimethoprim
Gantrisin	Sulfisoxazole	Sulfonamides + trimethoprim
Garamycin	Gentamicin	Aminoglycosides
Geocillin	Carbenicillin indanyl sodium	Penicillins
Geopen	Carbenicillin	Penicillins
Germanin	Suramin	Antiparasitic agents
Grifulvin V	Griseofulvin	Antifungal agents
Gris-PEG	Griseofulvin	Antifungal agents
Grisactin	Griseofulvin	Antifungal agents
Herplex	Idoxuridine	Antiviral agents
Hetrazan	Diethylcarbamazine	Antiparasitic agents
Hiprex	Methenamine hippurate	Other urinary tract agents
Humatin	Paromomycin	Antiparasitic agents
Hyzyd	Isoniazid	Antimycobacterial agents
Ilosone	Erythromycin estolate	Erythromycins
Ilotycin	Erythromycin	Erythromycins
INH	Isoniazid	Antimycobacterial agents
Isopto cetamide	Sulfacetamide	Sulfonamides + trimethoprim
Kafocin	Cephaloglycine	Cephalosporins
Kantrex	Kanamycin	Aminoglycosides
Keflex	Cephalexin	Cephalosporins
Keflin	Cephalothin	Cephalosporins
Kefzol	Cefazolin	Cephalosporins
Kesso-mycin	Erythromycin	Erythromycins
Kesso-pen	Penicillin G + phenoxymethyl penicillin	Penicillins
Kesso-tetra	Tetracycline	Tetracyclines
Lampit	Nifurtimox	Antiparasitic agents
Lamprene	Clofazimine	Antimycobacterial agents
Larotid	Amoxicillin	Penicillins
Ledercillin VK	Penicillin V potassium	Penicillins
Lincocin	Lincomycin	Lincosamides
Lomidine	Pentamidine	Antiparasitic agents
Loridine	Cephaloridine	Cephalosporins
Lotrimin	Clotrimazole	Antifungal agents
Macrodantin	Nitrofurantoin	Other urinary tract agents
Mandelamine	Methenamine mandelate	Other urinary tract agents
Mandol	Cefamandole	Cephalosporins
Maxipen	Phenethicillin	Penicillins
Mefoxin	Cefoxitin	Cephalosporins
Mel B	Melarsoprol	Antiparasitic agents
Mezlin	Mezlocillin	Penicillins
Micatin	Miconazole	Antifungal agents
Minocin	Minocycline	Tetracyclines
Mintezol	Thiabendazole	Antiparasitic agents
Monocid	Cefonicid	Cephalosporins
Monistat	Miconazole	Antifungal agents
Moxam	Moxalactam	Cephalosporins
Myambutol	Ethambutol	Antimycobacterial agents
Mycifradin	Neomycin	Aminoglycosides
Mycostatin	Nystatin	Antifungal agents
Nafcil	Nafcillin	Penicillins
Nebcin	Tobramycin	Aminoglycosides
NegGram	Nalidixic acid	Quinolones
Netromycin	Netilmicin	Aminoglycosides
Niadox	Isoniazid	Antimycobacterial agents
Niclocide	Niclosamide	Antiparasitic agents
Niconyl	Isoniazid	Antimycobacterial agents
Nilstat	Nystatin	Antifungal agents
Nizoral	Ketoconazole	Antifungal agents
Noraxin	Norfloxacin	Other urinary tract agents
Nydrazid	Isoniazid	Antimycobacterial agents
Omnipen	Ampicillin	Penicillins
Omnipen-N	Ampicillin	Penicillins
Oxamycin	Cycloserine	Antimycobacterial agents
PAS	Aminosalicylic acid	Antimycobacterial agents
Panaquin	Diiodohydroxyquin	Antiparasitic agents
Panmycin	Tetracycline	Tetracyclines
Para	Aminosalicylic acid	Antimycobacterial agents
Parasal	Aminosalicylic acid	Antimycobacterial agents
Pathocil	Dicloxacillin	Penicillins
Pediamycin	Erythromycin ethylsuccinate	Erythromycins
Pediazole	Erythromycin ethylsuccinate plus sulfisoxazole	Erythromycins
Pen Vee K	Penicillin V potassium	Penicillins
PenA	Ampicillin	Penicillins
Penapar VK	Penicillin V potassium	Penicillins
Penbritin	Ampicillin	Penicillins
Pensyn	Ampicillin	Penicillins
Pentam 300	Pentamidine	Antiparasitic agents
Pentids	Penicillin G	Penicillins
Pentostam	Stibogluconate	Antiparasitic agents

(Continued)

Trade	*Generic*	*Family*
Permapen	Benzathine penicillin G	Penicillins
Pfizer-E	Erythromycin stearate	Erythromycins
Pfizerpen	Penicillin G	Penicillins
Pipracil	Piperacillin	Penicillins
Polycillin	Ampicillin	Penicillins
Polycillin-N	Ampicillin	Penicillins
Polycillin-PRB	Ampicillin probenecid	Penicillins
Polycycline	Tetracycline	Tetracyclines
Polymox	Amoxicillin	Penicillins
Povan	Pyrivinium pamoate	Antiparasitic agents
Precef	Ceforanide	Cephalosporins
Primaquine	Primaquine phosphate	Antiparasitic agents
Primaxin	Imipenem + cilastatin	Other β-lactams
Principen	Ampicillin	Penicillins
Probampacin	Ampicillin	Penicillins
Proloprim	Trimethoprim	Sulfonamides + trimethoprim
Prostaphlin	Oxacillin	Penicillins
Pyopen	Carbenicillin	Penicillins
Renoquid	Sulfacytine	Sulfonamides + trimethoprim
Resistopen	Oxacillin	Penicillins
Retrovir	Zidovudine (AZT)	Antiviral agents
Rezipas	Aminosalicylic acid	Antimycobacterial agents
Rifadin	Rifampin	Antimycobacterial agents
Rifamate	Rifampin-isoniazid	Antimycobacterial agents
Rimactane	Rifampin	Antimycobacterial agents
Robamox	Amoxicillin	Penicillins
Robicillin VK	Penicillin V potassium	Penicillins
Robimycin	Erythromycin	Erythromycins
Robitet	Tetracycline	Tetracyclines
Rocephin	Ceftriaxone	Cephalosporins
Rolsul	Succinylsulfathiazole	Sulfonamides + trimethoprim
Rondomycin	Methacycline	Tetracyclines
Selexid	Pivmecillinam	Penicillins
Septra	Trimethoprim-sulfamethoxazole	Sulfonamides + trimethoprim
Seromycin	Cycloserine	Antimycobacterial agents
Silvadine	Silver sulfadiazine	Sulfonamides + trimethoprim
Sonilyn	Sulfachlorpyridazine	Sulfonamides + trimethoprim
Spectrobid	Bacampicillin	Penicillins
Sporanox	Itraconazole	Antifungal agents
Staphcillin	Methicillin	Penicillins
Steclin	Tetracycline	Tetracyclines
Stoxil	Idoxuridine	Antiviral agents
Sulamyd sodium	Sulfacetamide	Sulfonamides + trimethoprim
Sulfadyne	Sulfadiazine	Sulfonamides + trimethoprim
Sulfamylon	Mafenide	Sulfonamides + trimethoprim
Sulfasuxidine	Succinylsulfathiazole	Sulfonamides + trimethoprim
Sumycin	Tetracycline	Tetracyclines
Supen	Ampicillin	Penicillins
Symmetrel	Amantadine	Antiviral agents
Synicillin	Phenethicillin	Penicillins
TAO	Troleandomycin	—
Tazicef	Ceftazidime	Cephalosporins
Tazidime	Ceftazidime	Cephalosporins
Tegopen	Cloxacillin	Penicillins
Terfonyl	Trisulfapyrimidines	Sulfonamides + trimethoprim
Terramycin	Oxytetracycline	Tetracyclines
Tetracyn	Tetracycline	Tetracyclines
Tetrex	Tetracycline	Tetracyclines
Thiosulfil	Sulfamethizole	Sulfonamides + trimethoprim
Ticar	Ticarcillin	Penicillins
Timentin	Clavulanate + ticarcillin	β-Lactamase inhibitors
Tinactin	Tolnaftate	Antifungal agents
Totacillin	Ampicillin	Penicillins
Trantoin	Nitrofurantoin	Other urinary tract agents
Trecator-SC	Ethionamide	Antimycobacterial agents
Trimox	Amoxicillin	Penicillins
Trimpex	Trimethoprim	Sulfonamides + trimethoprim
Trobicin	Spectinomycin	Aminoglycosides
Trojacillin-Plus	Ampicillin probenecid	Penicillins
Unasyn	Ampicillin + Sulbactam	β-Lactamase inhibitors
Unipen	Nafcillin	Penicillins
Urex	Methenamine hippurate	Other urinary tract agents
Uri-tet	Oxytetracycline	Tetracyclines
Urifon	Sulfamethizole	Sulfonamides + trimethoprim
Utibid	Oxolinic acid	Quinolones
Uticillin VK	Penicillin V potassium	Penicillins
V-Cillin K	Penicillin V potassium	Penicillins
Vancocin	Vancomycin	Vancomycin
Vansil	Oxamniquine	Antiparasitic agents
Vectrin	Minocycline	Tetracyclines
Veetids	Penicillin V potassium	Penicillins
Velosef	Cephradine	Cephalosporins
Veracillin	Dicloxacillin	Penicillins
Vermox	Mebendazole	Antiparasitic agents
Versapen	Hetacillin	Penicillins
Versapen-K	Hetacillin	Penicillins
Vibramycin	Doxycycline	Tetracyclines
Vinactane	Viomycin	Antimycobacterial agents
Viocin	Viomycin	Antimycobacterial agents
Vira-A	Vidarabine	Antiviral agents
Virazole	Ribavirin	Antiviral agents
Viroptic	Trifluridine	Antiviral agents
Wycillin	Penicillin G procaine	Penicillins
Yodoxin	Iodoquinol	Antiparasitic agents
Yomesan	Niclosamide	Antiparasitic agents
Zinacef	Cefuroxime	Cephalosporins
Zovirax	Acyclovir	Antiviral agents

ANTIMICROBIAL AGENT PHARMACOLOGY: PENICILLINS

Drug (Oral Absorption, %)	Serum and Urine Concentration for Selected Doses: Dose (g)	Peak Serum (μg/ml)	Peak or Range, Urine (μg/ml)	Dosage Recommendations: Adults, Oral (Dose/Interval)	Adults, Parenteral (Dose/Interval)	Adults, Maximum Daily Dose (g)	Children, Oral (Dose/Interval)	Children, Parenteral (Dose/Interval)	Newborn (Parenteral), Up to 1 wk (Dose/Interval)	Newborn (Parenteral), 1–4 wk (Dose/Interval)
Amdinocillin	10 mg/kg[c]	50	1260		10 mg/kg q4–6h			10 mg/kg q4–6h (not approved)		
Amoxicillin (89)	0.25 po[d] 0.5 po[d]	4.7 (avg) 7.5 (avg)	 600–2000	0.25–0.5 g q8h		3	6.6–13.3 mg/kg q8h		Not recommended	
Ampicillin (50 avg)	0.25 po[d] 0.5 po[d] 1 po[d] 0.5 IV 0.5 IM 1 IV	1.8–2.9 2.5–4 2–6 2.9–7.1 8 40	90 100–700 100–1450 130–610 500–1000	0.5–1 g q6h	1–2 g q4–6h[e]	12	12.5–25 mg/kg q6h	25–50 mg/kg q6h[f]	50–100 mg/kg/day q12h	150–200 mg/kg/day q6–8h
Apalcillin	0.5 IM 1 IV[i,j] 2 IV[j]	28–37 47–58 208	 835							
Azlocillin[k] (minimal)	2 IV[c] 2 IV[j] 3 IV[c] 3 IV[j]	300 165 350 214	2200–8100		2–4 g q4–6h[l]	24		50 mg/kg q4h or 75 mg/kg q6h[m] (not approved)	Not recommended	
Bacampicillin[n] (60–90)	0.4 po 0.8 po	6–8 11–14		0.4–0.8 g q12h		1.6	12.5–25 mg/kg q12h			
Carbenicillin (minimal)	1 IM 2 IM 1 IV 1 g/hr IV 3 IV[c]	15–20 47 45–71 160 278	 2500 1000 4165		5–6.5 g q4–6h[o]	40		25–100 mg/kg q4–6h	200–300 mg/kg/day q8h	400 mg/kg/day q6–8h
Carbenicillin indanyl sodium (30–50)	0.382 po (1 tablet)	6.5	1130	1–2 tablets q6h		3	7.5–12.5 mg/kg q6h			
Cloxacillin (50)	0.5 po	7–14	410–1080	0.5–1 g q6h		4	12.5–25 mg/kg q6h		Not recommended	
Cyclacillin	0.25 po 0.5 po	6–7 11–12		0.25–0.5 g q6h		2	12.5–25 mg/kg q6h		Not recommended	
Dicloxacillin (37–74)	0.5 po	15–18		0.25–0.5 g q6h		4	3.125–6.25 mg/kg q6h		Not recommended	
Hetacillin[p]	0.225 po 0.45 po	1.7–2.1 2.5–2.7		0.225–0.45 g q6h			5.6–11.25 mg/kg q6h			
Methicillin (minimal)	1 IV[c] 1 IM 2 IV[j]	60 18 80			1–2 g q4–6h	12		25–33.3 mg/kg q4–6h	25 mg/kg q8–12h[q]	25 mg/kg q6–8h[r]
Mezlocillin[k] (minimal)	1 IM 2 IV[c] 3 IV[c] 3 IV[j]	15 199 310 263	 >4000		3–4 g q4–6h	24		50 mg/kg q4–6h	150 mg/kg/day q12h	300 mg/kg/day q6h[s]
Nafcillin (10–20 erratic)	0.5 IV[j]	11		0.5–1 g q6h	0.5–1.5 g q4–6h	9	12.5–25 mg/kg q6h	150 mg/kg/day q4–6h	25 mg/kg q12h	25 mg/kg q8h
Oxacillin (33)	0.5 po 0.5 IM	5–6 11	 200–2000	0.5–1 g q6h	0.5–2 g q4–6h	12	12.5–25 mg/kg q6h	37.5–50 mg/kg q6h	50–75 mg/kg/day q8–12h	100–150 mg/kg/day q6–8h
Penicillin G (15–30)	0.25 po 0.5 po 3 IV[j] (4.8 × 10^6 U) 12 g/day IV (19.2 × 10^6 U)[t]	0.6 1.5–2.7 400 16	85	0.5–1 g q6h	1.2–24 × 10^6 U/day q2–12h[u]	24 × 10^6 U	6.25–12.5 mg/kg q6h	100,000–250,000 U/kg/day q2–12h[u]	50,000–150,000 U/kg/day q8–12h	75,000–250,000 U/kg/day q6–8h
Penicillin V (60) (phenoxymethyl penicillin)	0.5 po	3–5		0.25–0.5 g q6h		4	6.25–12.5 mg/kg q6h		Not recommended	
Procaine penicillin G	600,000 U IM	1			0.3–4.8 × 10^6 U/day IM			25,000 U/kg q12–24h		
Penicillin G benzathine	1.2 × 10^6 U IM	0.12 U/ml	20 U/ml		2.4 × 10^6 U IM[w]	2.4 × 10^6 U IM		50,000 U/kg IM	50,000 U/kg IM	50,000 U/kg IM
Piperacillin[k] (minimal)	2 IV[c] 4 IV[j] 4 IV[c]	220 244 412	 1,000–8,500		3–4 g q4–6h	24		50 mg/kg q4–6h (Not approved)		
Ticarcillin (minimal)	1 IM 3 IV 5 IV	35 190 327	2000		3 g q4–6h	24–30		50 mg/kg q4–6h	150–225 mg/kg/day q8–12h[x]	225–300 mg/kg/day q6–8h[x]
Temocillin (minimal)	0.5 IV[c] 1 IV[c] 2 IV[c]	78 160 236	100–500		0.5–1 g q12h					

[a] Penicillins penetrate minimally across uninflamed meninges into the CSF.
[b] Penicillins do not appear in sufficient quantities to treat infections in the infant but do appear in quantities that could lead to allergic sensitization.
[c] IV push (over 2–5 min).
[d] Fasting.
[e] Meningitis should be treated q4h.
[f] Up to 400 mg/kg/day for *Haemophilus influenzae* type b meningitis in children.
[g] Mean concentration.
[h] Candidiasis and diarrhea in infants may result from ampicillin administration to nursing mothers. (*Pharm J.* 1976;217:219.)
[i] Remarkable differences in peak serum levels measured immediately after a 2-minute bolus (1 g: 825 μg/ml) as compared with a 2-hour infusion.
[j] Infusion (over 15–30 minutes).
[k] Dose-dependent pharmacokinetics.
[l] For severe, life-threatening infections: 4 g q4h.

Serum Half-life (hr)				Usual Adult Dose and Interval Adjustment					Dosage for Dialysis						
For Creatinine Clearance (ml/min)		With Dialysis		For Creatinine Clearance (ml/min)					Dose after HD Supplemental to Anuric	Daily Dose during PD	CSF/Serum (%) Inflamed Meninges[a]	Newborn Serum/Maternal Serum (%)	Breast Milk/Maternal Serum[b] (%)	Bile/Serum (%)	Aqueous Humor/Serum (%)
>80	<10	HD	PD	Dose	>80	80–50	50–10	<10 (Anuric)							
0.8–1	3.4–5.6	1.8		10 mg/kg	4 hr	4 hr	6–8 hr	8 hr	10 mg/kg					400	
1	16	2.2–4.5		0.25–0.5 g po	8 hr	8 hr	12 hr	12–24 hr	0.25 g		5–10	100	5		
0.5–1	8–20	2–5	10.9	1–2 g	4–6 hr	6 hr	8 hr	12 hr	0.5 g		8–13[g]	100	11[h]	100–1000	2–8
1.5–2															
1	5	1.5–2.6	Minimal	2–4 g	4–6 hr	4–6 hr	8 hr	12 hr	3 g		13.3[g]				
1	8–20	2–5		0.4–0.8 g po	12 hr	12 hr	12 hr	24 hr				65–75	1.7–3.6	17	
0.5–1	12.5	6	4.2–7.4	5–6.5 g	4–6 hr	6 hr	2–3 g q6–8h	2 g q12h	2 g	2 g q6h	9.4[g]	50–100	0.4	50–75	Up to 3
0.5	0.8	Minimal	Minimal	0.5–1 g po	6 hr	6 hr	6 hr	6 hr							
0.5	3.5			0.25–0.5 g po	6 hr	6 hr	12–24 h	24 h							
0.7	1–2	1.6	Minimal	0.25–0.5 g po	6 hr	6 hr	6 hr	6 hr			Minimal	0–10		5–8	
0.3			0.225–0.45 g po	6 hr											
0.5	4	Minimal	Minimal	1–2 g	4–6 hr	6 hr	8 hr	12 hr	2 g		3–12	50–100		20–50	1–2
1.1[j]	1.6–2.6	1.2–1.4	Minimal	3–4 g	4–6 hr	4–6 hr	6–8 hr	8–12 hr	2–3 g	Anuric dosage	14[g]	100		1000	
0.5	1.2	Minimal	Minimal	0.5–1.5 g	4–6 hr	4–6 hr	4–6 hr	4–6 hr			9–20	10–15		4000	1–2
0.5	2	Minimal	1.4	0.5–2 g	4–6 hr	4–6 hr	4–6 hr	4–6 hr				10–15	≤3.5	20–40	0–20
0.5	7–10	5		1.2–24 × 10^6 U/day	2–12 hr	2–12 hr	2–12 hr	$\frac{1}{3}$–$\frac{1}{2}$ maximum daily dose[v]	0.5 × 10^6 U		2–6	100	6 avg	200–800	
1	4			0.25–0.5 g po	6 hr	6 hr	8 hr	12 hr	0.25 g						
1.3–1.5	2.1–5	1.2–2.4	3.6	3–4 g	4–6 hr	4–6 hr	6–12 hr	12 hr	2 g q8h + 1 g after HD		15.7[g]		1	1000	
1–1.5	13	6	Minimal	3 g	4–6 hr	4–6 hr	2–3 g q6–8h	2 g q12h	3 g	3 g q12h	9.5[g]				
4.5–5	18–27	4.5		0.5–1 g	12 hr	12 hr	12–24 hr	36–48 hr	0.5 g						

[m] Up to 450 mg/kg/day for patients with cystic fibrosis.
[n] 100% of a dose of bacampicillin is metabolized to ampicillin.
[o] 4–8 g/day usually sufficient for urinary tract infections.
[p] The antibiotic activity of hetacillin is provided by its rapid conversion to ampicillin.
[q] For meningitis, 50 mg/kg q8–12h.
[r] For meningitis, 50 mg/kg q6–8h.
[s] For infants weighing less than 2000 g, 75 mg/kg q8h.
[t] By continuous infusion.
[u] The interval between parenteral doses is variable: it can be as frequent as every 2 hours for initial therapy of meningococcemia or as long as 12 hours between IM doses of procaine penicillin G.
[v] Patients on low daily doses usually tolerate full dosage. Upper dosage limit approximation: dose (10^6 U/day) = 3.2 + (CLCR/7). (*Ann Intern Med.* 1975;82:194).
[w] Patients with latent syphilis of more than 1 year's duration should be treated with penicillin G benzathine, 2.4 million units weekly for 4 weeks.
[x] For infants <2000 g: 75 mg/kg q12h for first week and 75 mg/kg q8h for 1–4 weeks old. Those >2000 g: 75 mg/kg q8h for the first week and 100 mg/kg q8h for 1–4 weeks old.

ANTIMICROBIAL AGENT PHARMACOLOGY: CEPHALOSPORINS

Drug (Oral Absorption, %)	Serum and Urine Concentration for Selected Doses: Dose (g)	Peak Serum (μg/ml)	Peak or Range, Urine (μg/ml)	Dosage Recommendations: Adults Oral (Dose/Interval)	Adults Parenteral (Dose/Interval)	Maximum Daily Dose (g)	Children Oral (Dose/Interval)	Children Parenteral (Dose/Interval)	Newborn (Parenteral) Up to 1 wk	Newborn (Parenteral) 1–4 wk
First generation										
Cefadroxil[c] (90–100)	0.25 po 0.5 po 1 po	9 18 28–34	 1200–1800	1–2 g/day q12–24h		2	15 mg/kg q12h			
Cefazolin	0.5 IM 1 IM 1 IV	40 59–68 188	2460 4010		0.5–1.5 g q6–8h	6		8.3–25 mg/kg q6–8h	15–20 mg/kg q12h	15–20 mg/kg q8–12h
Cephalexin[c] (80–100)	0.25 po[f] 0.50 po[f]	8 15–18	 1000–2300	0.25–1 g q6h		4	6.25–25 mg/kg q6h		Not recommended	
Cephalothin	1 IV[g] 1 IM 2 IV[g]	40–60 20 80–100	2500		0.5–2 g q4–6h	12		75–160 mg/kg/day q4–6h	40 mg/kg/day q8–12h	60–80 mg/kg/day q6–8h
Cephapirin	1 IV[j] 2 IV[k] 1 IM	70 129 9.4	2560 1280		0.5–2 g q4–6h	12		10–20 mg/kg q6h		
Cephradine Oral (90–100)	 0.5 po[f] 1 IM	 15–19 10–14	 1000	 0.25–1 g q6–12h		 4	 6.25–12.5 mg/kg q6–12h			
Parenteral	1 IV	60–86	1975		0.5–2 g q6h	8		12.5–25 mg/kg q6h	Not recommended	
Second generation										
Cefaclor[c,d]	0.25 po 0.5 po 1 po	5–7 15 35	600 900	0.25–0.5 g q8h		4	6.6–13.3 mg/kg q8h			
Cefamandole	1 IM 1 IV[g] 2 IV	20–35 90 165	 5000		0.5–2 g q4–6h	12		50–150 mg/kg/day q4–8h		
Cefonicid	7.5 mg/kg IV[k] 0.5 IM 1 IV[g] 1 IV[k]	95–155 40–60 150 221–261	500		0.5–2 g q24h	2				
Cefotetan	0.5 IM 1 IV[k] 2 IV[j]	35 142–180 200	1000 1400–2000 3500–4000		1–2 g q12h	6		20–30 mg/kg q12h		
Cefotiam	1 IV[g] 2 IV[g]	50 135			1–2 g q12h					
Cefoxitin	1 IM 1 IV[g]	20 110–125	450 3000	1–2 g q4–6h or 3 g q6h	12		20–26.6 mg/kg q4–6h			30 mg/kg q8h
Cefuroxime	0.5 IM 1 IM 1 IV[k] 1.5 IV[g]	25 40 100 65	 5000–7000		0.75–1.5 g q8h[m]	9		50–240 mg/kg/day[n] q6–8h	Not recommended	30–50 mg/kg/day q8–12h
Cefuroxime axetil (30–40)	0.25 po 0.5 1	4.1 7.0 13.6		0.125–0.5 g q12h			0.125–0.5 g q12h			
Third generation										
Cefepime	0.5 IV[g]	34								
Cefixime (50)	0.2 po 0.4 po	1.7–1.9 2.7–3.0	52 84	0.4 g/day q12–24h			8 mg/kg/day q12–24h			
Cefmenoxime	1 IV[g] 1 IM 2 IV[g]	40 15 95	1740 3620		0.5–2 g q4–6h	12		10–20 mg/kg q6h	Not recommended	
Cefoperazone	1 IV[j] 2 IV	100–125 200	1600 2000		1–4 g q8h or 0.5–3 g q6h	12 16 by continuous infusion in immunocompromized patient		25–100 mg/kg q12h		
Cefotaxime (desacetyl cefotaxime)	1 IM 1 IV[j] 2 IV[j] 1 IV[k] 2 IV[k]	20 40 80–90 102 9.8	2010		1–2 g q4–12h	12		50–180 mg/kg/day q4–6h	25–50 mg/kg q12h	25–50 mg/kg q8h
Cefpiramide	1IV[k] 2 IV[g]	303 320	1087							
Cefpirome	1 IM 1 IV	28.6 97.1								

Serum Half-life (hr)				Usual Adult Dose and Interval Adjustment					Dosage for Dialysis		CSF/Serum (%) Inflamed Meninges[a]	Newborn Serum/Maternal Serum (%)	Breast Milk/Maternal Serum[b] (%)	Bile/Serum (%)	Aqueous Humor/Serum (%)
For Creatinine Clearance (ml/min)		With Dialysis		For Creatinine Clearance (ml/min)					Dose after HD Supplemental to Anuric	Daily Dose during PD					
>80	<10	HD	PD	Dose	>80	80–50	50–10	<10 (Anuric)							
1.2–1.6[d]	20–25	2.5–3.4		1 g po	12–24 hr	12–24 hr	25–50: q12h 10–25: q24h	36–48 hr	0.5–1 g			50	0.9–1.9	22	
1.5–2	20–70	6.5–9.0	20–46[e]	0.5–1.5 g	6–8 hr	8 hr	0.5–1 g q8–12h	0.5–1 g q24h	0.25–0.5 g		1–4	35–69	3	29–300	<1.7
0.5–1.2	11–20	4.5–6		0.25–1 g po	6 hr	6 hr	500 mg 8–12 hr	250 mg q12–24h	0.25–1 g		Minimal	60	2	216	11
0.5–1	3–18[h]	2.5–3	5.1	0.5–2 g	4–6 hr	6 hr	8 hr	0.5 g q6–8h	Supplemental dose	No supplemental dose[i]	1.2–5.6	16–41	7–26[j]	22–172	4
0.5–1	1.5–2.4	1.8		0.5–2 g	4–6 hr	6 hr	8 hr	12 hr	7.5–15 mg/kg before dialysis			60	7		
0.75–1.5	8–15			1–2 g	6 hr[l]	6 hr	8 h or 250–500 mg q6h	250 mg q12–24 hr	1–2 g	500 mg q6h for CAPD	≤1	9–22	14–20	10–400	5–9
0.5–1	2–3	1.5–2		0.25–0.5 g po	8 hr	8 hr	8 hr (50–100% usual dose)	8 hr (25–33% usual dose)	Repeat dose after HD				2	≥60	1–3
0.5–1	11	6.6	7.2	0.5–2 g	4–6 hr	1–2 g q6h	1–2 g q8h	0.5–1 g q12h	Supplemental dose	No supplemental dose	0.5–20		2.4	300–400	1.5
4.4	50–100	70		0.5–2 g	24 hr	0.5–1.5 g q24h	0.25–1 g q24–48h	0.25–1 g q3–5 days	No extra dose				<1	<10	<1
3–4.6	12–35.1	5.6–7.5	5–9% removed	1–2 g	12 hr	12 hr	24 hr	48 hr	Supplemental dose		0.8–3.6		2.3	1000	
0.7–1		2.4						Reduce the dose by 25%			10	75–130	0–trace	20–25	
0.75–1	10–22	4	Minimal (7.8 with CAPD)	1–3 g	4–6 hr	1–2 g q8h	1–2 g q12h	0.5–1 g q12–24h	1–2 g		<1–77	33–50	up to 3	280	4–7
1–2	15	3.75	5.4–13.6[o]	0.75–1.5 g	8 hr	8 hr	8–12 hr	24 hr	Supplemental dose	No supplemental dose	11–56	20–33	up to 3	35–80	10–14
1.2–1.3															
2															
3.3–4.0	11.1	8.2	14.9 (CAPD)					0.2 g q24h[s]	No supplemental dose						
0.8–1.2	8			0.5–2 g	4–6 hr	6–8 hr	12–24 hr	24h	30–50% maintenance dose		3	30	<25	81–526	2.6–5
1.6–2.6	2.5	2.2		1–4 g	6–8 hr	6–8 hr	6–8 hr	6–8 hr[p]	Schedule the dose after dialysis		1.8–3.1	20–50	Up to 1.5	800–1200	1–6
0.9–1.1	2.5–3.4	1.6	2.9	1–2 g	4–8 hr	4–8 hr	6–12 hr	12 hr	Maintenance dose × 50%		10–25	25[q]	Up to 3–8	59	0.5–4
1.3	10–15	3.16												493	
4.4–5.4	8.3														
2															

ANTIMICROBIAL AGENT PHARMACOLOGY: CEPHALOSPORINS *(Continued)*

Drug (Oral Absorption, %)	Serum and Urine Concentration for Selected Doses: Dose (g)	Peak Serum (μg/ml)	Peak or Range, Urine (μg/ml)	Dosage Recommendations: Adults: Oral (Dose/Interval)	Adults: Parenteral (Dose/Interval)	Adults: Maximum Daily Dose (g)	Children: Oral (Dose/Interval)	Children: Parenteral (Dose/Interval)	Newborn (Parenteral): Up to 1 wk (Dose/Interval)	Newborn (Parenteral): 1–4 wk (Dose/Interval)
Cefsulodin	1 IM 1 IV[g] 2 IV[g]	20 65 140	 1500–3500		1–2 g q6–8h	12		15–25 mg/kg q6h		
Ceftazidime	1 IV[g] 1 IM 2 IV[g]	70–80 38–43 170–180	4000–6000		0.5–2 g q8–12h	6		30–50 mg/kg q8h	60–100 mg/kg/ day q8–12h	60–150 mg/kg/ day q8–12h
Ceftizoxime	0.5 IM 1 IV[g] 2 IV[g]	13.3 60–90 120–130	1120		1–4 g q8–12h	12		50 mg/kg q6–8h		
Ceftriaxone[t]	0.5 IM 1 IV[g] 2 IV[g]	50 150 270	 995 2700		0.5–2 g q12–24h[u]	4[v]		50–100 mg/kg/ day q12–24h[w]	50 mg/kg/day	50–75 mg/kg/day
Moxalactam	0.5 IV[j] 1 IV[g] 2 IV[k] 1 IM	57 60–100 150–200 27	446 2100 4200		0.5–4 g q8–12h[y]	12[y]		50 mg/kg q6–8h[y,z]	50 mg/kg q12h[y,z]	50 mg/kg q8h[y,z]

[a] Cephalosporins penetrate minimally across uninflamed meninges into the CSF.
[b] Cephalosporins do not appear in sufficient systemic quantities via breast milk to treat infections in the infant but could theoretically sensitize the newborn.
[c] Oral.
[d] Dose-dependent pharmacokinetics.
[e] Only two patients studied.
[f] Fasting.
[g] Infusion (over a period of 30 minutes).
[h] Biphasic elimination.
[i] Peritoneal dialysis is reported to diminish the mean peak concentration of cephalothin by 24 percent as well as reducing the subsequent cephalothin levels by as much as 50 percent from baseline. Despite this enhanced elimination during peritoneal dialysis, the cephalothin serum level persisted above 16 μg/ml for 12 hours. (*Am J Med Sci.* 1969;257:116.)
[j] Data from rabbits.
[k] Intravenous push (over a period of 2–5 minutes).
[l] Parenteral doses can be divided q4–6h.
[m] Up to 3 g every 8 hours for meningitis.
[n] Up to 240 mg/kg/day divided every 6–8 hours for meningitis.

ANTIMICROBIAL AGENT PHARMACOLOGY: OTHER β LACTAMS AND β-LACTAMASE INHIBITORS

Drug (Oral Absorption, %)	Serum and Urine Concentration for Selected Doses: Dose (g)	Peak Serum (μg/ml)	Peak or Range, Urine (μg/ml)	Dosage Recommendations: Adults: Oral (Dose/Interval)	Adults: Parenteral (Dose/Interval)	Adults: Maximum Daily Dose (g)	Children: Oral (Dose/Interval)	Children: Parenteral (Dose/Interval)	Newborn (Parenteral): Up to 1 wk (Dose/Interval)	Newborn (Parenteral): 1–4 wk (Dose/Interval)
Other β-lactams										
Aztreonam (minimal)	0.5 IV[a] 0.5 IM 1 IV[a] 1 IM 2 IV[a]	54 22 90 47 205	1400 3000 6500		0.5–2 g q6–12h	8		18.75–37.5 mg/kg q6h (not approved)		
Carumonam	1 2	190 300			0.5–2 g q8h					
Impenem (minimal)	0.25 IV 0.5 IV 1 IV	22 43 68–78	50 100[c] > or = 100		0.5–1 g q6–8h	4		15–25 mg/kg q6h[d]	16.6–33.3 mg/kg q8h (preliminary)	
β-lactamase inhibitors										
Clavulanate (50)	0.125 po 0.25 po 0.2 IV[a]	4 6 13.4	380 680	0.25–0.5 g q8h[e]	3.1 g q4–6h[f]		6.7–13.3 mg/kg q8h[g]			
Sulbactam (60–80)	0.5 IV[l] 1 IV[i] 0.25 po[j] 0.5 po	30 60 3.6 4.4–5.1	 480		1.5–3 g q6–8h[k]	4 g[l]		37.5 mg/kg q6h or 50 mg/kg q8h[k]	75 mg/kg q12h[k]	112.5 mg/kg q8h[k]

[a] IV infusion over 30 minutes.
[b] Animal data.
[c] Urine concentrations are obtained with concomitant administration of dehydropeptidase inhibitor, cilastatin.
[d] For children 3 years of age or less: 25 mg/kg/dose; for children over 3 years: 15 mg/kg/dose to a maximum of 3 g/day.
[e] As Augmentin: 250 mg and 500 mg tablets contain 250 mg and 500 mg, respectively, of amoxicillin and 125 mg and 250 mg, respectively, of clavulanate (2:1 ratio).
[f] As Timentin: 3 g ticarcillin plus 0.1 g clavulanate.

Serum Half-life (hr)				Usual Adult Dose and Interval Adjustment					Dosage for Dialysis		CSF/Serum (%) Inflamed Meninges[a]	Newborn Serum/Maternal Serum (%)	Breast Milk/Maternal Serum[b] (%)	Bile/Serum (%)	Aqueous Humor/Serum (%)
For Creatinine Clearance (ml/min)		With Dialysis			For Creatinine Clearance (ml/min)				Dose after HD Supplemental to Anuric	Daily Dose during PD					
>80	<10	HD	PD	Dose	>80	80–50	50–10	<10 (Anuric)							
1.6–1.9	10–13	2.1–3.3	8.9	0.5–3 g	6 hr	8 hr	0.25–1.5 g q6h or 1 g q12h	0.5 g q12h or 1 g q24h	0.25 g	1 g q18–24h	11		1		16
1.8	16.1–25	2.8	8.7	0.5–2 g	8–12 hr	8–12 hr	1–1.5 g q12–24h	0.5–0.75 g q24–48h	1 g loading 1 g post dialysis	1 g then 0.5 g q24h	21.5		7	33	3–12
1.7	25–36	4–4.9	10.2–12 (CAPD)	1–4 g	8–12 hr	0.5–1.5 g q8h	0.25–1 g q12h	0.25–1 g q24–48h	Give scheduled dose after dialysis	3 g q48h	21–22	28–33	1–6	34–82	3.6–6
8[d]	11.9–15.4	16.1	12.2 (CAPD)	0.5–1 g	12–24 hr	12–24 hr	12–24 hr	12–24 h[x]	No supplemental dose		7–11	18–25	4	Up to 1000	
2.5	5–22	4	16.7	0.5–4 g	8–12 hr	0.5–3 g q8h	0.25–2 g q8h or 0.25–3 g q12h	0.25 g q12h to 1 g q24h	1–2 g	1 g q36–48h or 0.5g q18–24h	4–55[aa]	30–40	2.7	152–224	1–16

[o] The bioavailability of cefuroxime axetil is variable depending on the presence of food in the GI tract. In general, the degree of absorption increases when given with or shortly after food (f = 52%) compared with fasting state (f = 37%).

[p] From manufacturer's data: "When hepatic function is essentially normal, cefoperazone generally does not require adjustment of usual dosages in cases of renal impairment, including end-stage renal failure." Antibiotic serum concentrations are recommended, however, to assess the drug accumulation for patients with renal compromise receiving greater than 4 g/day.

[q] From fetal samples after abortion.

[r] From investigator's brochure: fetal rat data.

[s] Dose for CrCl < 20 ml/min.

[t] Nonlinear kinetics; 35 μg/ml at 12 hours and 15 μg/ml at 24 hours.

[u] For the treatment of uncomplicated gonococcal infections, 0.125 to 0.25 g as a single intramuscular dose is effective.

[v] The maximum recommended daily dose is currently 2 g; however, data for adult meningitis are incomplete.

[w] For gram-negative meningitis in children, the manufacturer recommends initial loading dose of 75 mg/kg.

[x] Serum levels of ceftriaxone should be monitored in patients with severe renal impairment or concomitant renal and hepatic compromise.

[y] Bleeding time should be monitored in patients receiving more than 4 g/day for more than 3 days. Prophylactic vitamin K, 10 mg/wk, should be given to patients treated with moxalactam.

[z] For gram negative meningitis in children, the manufacturer recommends an initial loading dose of 100 mg/kg.

[aa] Data from clinical studies have reported CSF penetration up to 40 percent.

Serum Half-life (hr)				Usual Adult Dose and Interval Adjustment					Dosage for Dialysis		CSF/Serum (%) Inflamed Meninges	Newborn Serum/Maternal Serum (%)	Breast Milk Maternal Serum (%)	Bile/Serum (%)	Aqueous Humor/Serum (%)
For Creatinine Clearance (ml/min)		With Dialysis			For Creatinine Clearance (ml/min)										
>80	<10	HD	PD	Dose	>80	80–50	50–10	<10 (Anuric)	Dose after HD Supplemental to Anuric	Daily Dose during PD					
1.7–2	6–8.7	2.7	3–7.1	0.5–2 g	6–12 hr	8–12 hr	12–24 hr	24–36 hr	15 mg/kg	30 mg/kg q24h	8[b]		Minimal	60–100	5–14
1.3–1.7	11.3			0.5–2 g	8hr	8–12 hr	12–24 hr	0.25–1 g q 24 hr							
1	4	2.5		0.5–1 g	6–8 hr	0.5 g q6–8 h	0.5 g q6–12 h	0.25–0.5 g q24h	2 g/day max and one dose after HD		20–30			Minimal	3
0.7–1.4	3.8	1.2		0.25–0.5 g po 3.1 g[f]	8 hr 4–6 hr	8 hr 4–6 hr	12 hr 2 g q4–8h	12–24 hr 2 g q12h	3.1 g[f]	3.1 g q12h[f]	8.4	100	Minimal	50[h]	
1	20	2.4		1.5–3 g[k]	q6–8h	q6–8h	q8–12h	q24h			2–20	100	Minimal	33	

[g] Based on the amoxicillin component.

[h] Data obtained 1 hour after a dose of oral Augmentin (amoxicillin plus clavulanic acid).

[i] Administered as Unasyn (2:1 ratio of ampicillin and sulbactam) over a period of 15 minutes.

[j] As sultamicillin, a double ester of ampicillin and the β-lactamase inhibitor sulbactam.

[k] As Unasyn: ampicillin plus sulbactam in 2:1 combination; 1 g + 0.5 g and 2 g + 1 g, respectively.

[l] Expressed as the sulbactam component.

ANTIMICROBIAL AGENT PHARMACOLOGY: AMINOGLYCOSIDES

Drug (Oral Absorption, %)	Serum and Urine Concentration for Selected Doses: Dose (g)	Peak Serum (μg/ml)	Peak or Range, Urine (μg/ml)	Dosage Recommendations: Adults, Oral (Dose/Interval)	Adults, Parenteral (Dose/Interval)	Maximum Daily Dose (g)	Children, Oral (Dose/Interval)	Children, Parenteral (Dose/Interval)	Newborn (Parenteral), Up to 1 wk (Dose/Interval)	Newborn (Parenteral), 1–4 wk (Dose/Interval)
Amikacin	5 mg/kg IM 7.5 mg/kg IM 7.5 mg/kg IV	16 21 38	830 700		5 mg/kg q8h or 7.5 mg/kg q12h	1.5 g		5 mg/kg q8h or 7.5 mg/kg q12h	7.5–10 mg/kg q12h	7.5–10 mg/kg q8h
Gentamicin (minimal)	1.25 mg/kg IM	5–7	5–100		1–1.7 mg/kg q8h[f]	5 mg/kg		1–2.5 mg/kg q8h[f]	2.5 mg/kg q12h	2.5 mg/kg q8h
Kanamycin	0.5 g IM	14–29	140–250		5 mg/kg q8h or 7.5 mg/kg q12h	1.5 g	150–250 mg/kg/day q1–6h	5–10 mg/kg q8h	7.5–10 mg/kg q12h	7.5–10 mg/kg q8h
Neomycin (minimal)	4.0 g po[j]	4		6.6 mg/kg q4h ≤3 days[k]		3 g po	12.5–25 mg/kg q6h			
Netilmicin	2 mg/kg IM 2.5 mg/kg IM	6 7.5			1.5–3.25 mg/kg q12h or 1.3–2.2 mg/kg q8h	6.5 mg/kg		1–2.5 mg/kg q8h	2.5 mg/kg q12h	2.5 mg/kg q8h
Spectinomycin	2 g IM 4 g IM	74 199	9000		2 g once[l]	4 g		40 mg/kg once IM	Not recommended	
Streptomycin	0.5 g IM 1 g IM	6–42 25–50	300–400 1000		0.5–1 g q12h	2 g		10–15 mg/kg q12h	Not recommended	
Tobramycin	1 mg/kg IM 2 mg/kg IV	4 3.1–14	75–100 320		1–1.7 mg/kg q8h	5 mg/kg		1–2 mg/kg q8h[f]	2 mg/kg q12h	2 mg/kg q8h

[a] The dosing strategy for aminoglycosides involves the use of ideal (lean) body weight (IBW) for dosage calculation. In obese patients, this approach would result in serum antibiotic concentrations less than expected. Alternative dosing recommendations have been proposed that account for the change in drug distribution volume with obesity:
(1) Lean body weight + 40 percent of the excess weight, defined as total body weight (TBW) minus ideal body weight (IBW). (*J Infec Dis.* 138:499–505, 1978;138:499–505.)
(2) IBW + 58 percent of excess weight (TBW-IBW). (*Clin Pharmacol Ther.* 1979;26:508.)
(3) IBW + 38 percent of excess weight (TBW-IBW). (*Am J Hosp Pharm.* 1980;37:519–22.)

[b] Or calculate the dosage interval in hours as nine times the serum creatinine concentration in mg/100 ml (amikacin, kanamycin) or eight times the serum creatinine concentration in mg/100 ml (gentamicin, netilmicin, tobramycin). Alternatively, refer to nomogram in F.A. Sarubbi, Jr., et al., *Ann Intern Med.* 1978;89:612–18. The simplicity of these predictive methods makes them useful for establishing initial dosing schedules, but serum antimicrobial concentrations should be determined subsequently to ensure therapeutic, nontoxic blood levels.

[c] Mean percentage penetration into CSF of aminoglycoside antibiotics in normal rabbits has been reported to be less than 10 percent.

[d] Aminoglycosides do not penetrate the biliary tree in the presence of obstruction.

ANTIMICROBIAL AGENT PHARMACOLOGY: TETRACYCLINES

Drug (Oral Absorption, %)	Serum and Urine Concentration for Selected Doses: Dose (g)	Peak Serum (μg/ml)	Peak or Range, Urine (μg/ml)	Dosage Recommendations: Adults, Oral (Dose/Interval)	Adults, Parenteral (Dose/Interval)	Maximum Daily Dose (g)	Children, Oral (Dose/Interval)	Children, Parenteral (Dose/Interval)	Newborn (Parenteral), Up to 1 wk (Dose/Interval)	Newborn (Parenteral), 1–4 wk (Dose/Interval)
Chlortetracycline (30)	0.25 po 0.5 po	1.5–2.5 7	320	See tetracycline			See tetracycline		Not recommended	
Demeclocycline (66)	0.3 po	1.5–1.7		0.15 g q6h or 0.3 g q12h		1.2	6.6–13.2 mg/kg/day q6–12h		Not recommended	
Doxycycline (90–100[g])	0.1 po[f] 0.1 IV[g] 0.2 po 0.2 IV[g]	1.8–2.9 2.5 3.7–6.7 4	100–200 200–300	0.1 g q12–24h	0.1 g q12–24h	0.2	2.2 mg/kg q12–24h	2.2 mg/kg q12–24h	Not recommended	
Methacycline (58)	0.15 po 0.3 po	1.3 2.4		0.15 g q6h or 0.3 g q12h		1.2	6.6–13.2 mg/kg/day q6–12h		Not recommended	
Minocycline (95–100[g])	0.2 po 0.2 IV	2–3 4.2–6.6	15[h]	0.2 g once then 0.1 g q12h	0.2 g once then 0.1 g q12h	0.4	4 mg/kg once then 2 mg/kg q12h	4 mg/kg once then 2 mg/kg q12h	Not recommended	
Oxytetracycline (59)	0.25 po 0.5 po	1.3–1.4 4–4.2	300	See tetracycline	0.25–0.5 g q12h	4	See tetracycline	6 mg/kg q12h	Not recommended	
Tetracycline (75[g])	0.25 po 0.5 po 0.5 IV[f]	1.5–2.2 3–4.3 8	300	0.25–0.5 g q6h	0.125–0.5 g q6–12h	2	25–50 mg/kg/day q6–12h	10–20 mg/kg/day q6–12h	Not recommended	

[a] The tetracyclines cause a brown discoloration of the teeth and may retard the growth of bone in the human fetus and children. They are not recommended for use in patients younger than 12 years of age.

[b] Patients in the convalescent stage of poliomyelitis.

[c] Not detected at a dose of 300 mg/day.

[d] Biliary levels determined after an IV injection of 500 mg of the antibiotic.

[e] Serum levels of doxycycline are reduced by 20 percent if given with food, whereas serum levels of tetracycline are reduced up to 50 percent. The oral absorption of minocycline is not significantly impaired by food or milk.

Serum Half-life (hr)				*Usual Adult Dose and Interval Adjustment*					*Dosage for Dialysis*		*CSF/ Serum (%) Inflamed Meninges*	*Newborn Serum/ Maternal Serum (%)*	*Breast Milk Maternal Serum (%)*	*Bile/ Serum (%)*	*Aqueous Humor/ Serum (%)*
For Creatinine Clearance (ml/min)		*With Dialysis*			*For Creatinine Clearance (ml/min)*										
>80	*<10*	*HD*	*PD*	*Dose*	*>80*	*80–50*	*50–10*	*<10 (Anuric)*	*Dose after HD Supplemental to Anuric*	*Daily Dose during PD*					
2–2.5	44–86[e]	3.75–5.6	17.9–29	5–7.5 mg/kg	8–12 hr	12 hr	24–36 hr	36–48 hr	2.5–3.75 mg/kg	3–4 mg/2 liters dialysate removed	15–24	20		30	0–4
2–3	48–72	8–10	5–15[g]	1.5 mg/kg	8 hr	8–12 hr	12–24 hr	24–48 hr	1–1.5 mg/kg	1 mg/2 liters dialysate removed	10–30	30–40		30–60	<8
2.2–3	30–80[h]	4.9	5[f]	5–7.5 mg/kg	8–12 hr	24 hr	24–72 hr	72–96 hr	5 mg/kg	3.75 mg/kg qd	43	50	35	100	
3				6.6 mg/kg po	4 hr										
2.2–2.5	33	5.5		1.3–2.2 mg kg	8 hr	8–12 hr	12–24 hr	24–48 hr	2 mg/kg		21–26				
1.7	18.5–29.3			2 g once[f]											
2–3	100–110			0.5–1 g	12 hr	24 hr	24–72 hr	72–96 hr	5 mg/kg		20	10–40	<25	40–300	
2–2.75	50–70	2.9–10	12–16	1.5 mg/kg	8 hr	8–12 hr	12–24 hr	24–48 hr	1 mg/kg	1 mg/2 liters dialysate removed	14–23	50		10–20	18

[e] Half-life of 86.5 h in anephric patients and 44.3 h in patients with minimal residual kidney function.
[f] For meningitis, aminoglycosides may be administered intraventricularly in single, supplemental daily doses until CSF cultures are negative. (Gentamicin and tobramycin dose: 5–10 mg for adults; 1–2 mg for infants; not recommended for the newborn). Up to 10 mg/kg/day may be administered parenterally for cystic fibrosis.
[g] In the absence of an inflammatory response, peritoneal clearance is diminished, and the half-life is reported as approximately 29 hours. The elimination half-life during CAPD is 36 hours.
[h] The serum half-life of kanamycin in severely uremic patients may be prolonged to 70–80 hours.
[i] As dialysis continues, removal of drug is slower, and the half-life is reportedly prolonged to 48 hours.
[j] Although neomycin is classified as nonabsorbable, some absorption from the GI tract does occur. A review of neomycin-induced deafness has identified ototoxicity as a consequence of all modes of administration—parenteral, aerosol, oral, wound and bowel irrigation, and cutaneous.
[k] The recommended dosage schedule for bowel evacuation; as adjunctive therapy for hepatic coma; 25 mg/kg q6h for 24 hours, then 12.5 mg/kg q6h thereafter.
[l] For disseminated gonoccocal infections, spectinomycin may be administered at 2 g every 12 hours for 3 days.

Serum Half-life (hr)				*Usual Adult Dose and Interval Adjustment*					*Dosage for Dialysis*		*CSF/ Serum (%) Inflamed Meninges*	*Newborn Serum/ Maternal Serum (%)*	*Breast Milk Maternal Serum (%)*	*Bile/ Serum (%)*	*Aqueous Humor/ Serum (%)*
For Creatinine Clearance (ml/min)		*With Dialysis*			*For Creatinine Clearance (ml/min)*										
>80	*<10*	*HD*	*PD*	*Dose*	*>80*	*80–50*	*50–10*	*<10 (Anuric)*	*Dose after HD Supplemental to Anuric*	*Daily Dose during PD*					
5.6	6.8–11	Minimal		0.25–0.5 g po	6 hr	Not recommended					2–6[b]		40	333	
10–16				0.15–0.3 g po	6–12 hr	Not recommended							70[c]	2000[d]	10–30
18.5	19.5–25	18.8		0.1 g po	12–24 hr	12–24 hr	12–24 hr	12–24 hr	No supplemental dose		12–20		30–40	300–2000	10–13
7–15	Up to 44 hr			0.15–0.3 g po	6–12 hr	Not recommended									
11–26	12–30[i]			0.1 g po	12–24 hr	Not recommended						77	8–26	3000	17
9	48–66	24	Minimal	0.25–0.5 g po	6 hr	Not recommended					0–6.7		20–140	400–1000	
8.5	57–108	[j]		0.25–0.5 g po	6 hr	Not recommended					10–25	60–70	25–150	500–1000	9–11

[f] Infused over 60 min.
[g] Infused over 30 min.
[h] Urine concentration of minocycline approximates 5–10 times the serum concentration (lowest of the tetracyclines).
[i] Little accumulation in renal failure but aggravation of uremia reported even with a reduced dosage.
[j] Tetracycline plasma level decreased by 14–27 percent with hemodialysis.

ANTIMICROBIAL AGENT PHARMACOLOGY: ERYTHROMYCIN, LINCOSAMIDES, CHLORAMPHENICOL, AND METRONIDAZOLE

	Serum and Urine Concentration for Selected Doses			*Dosage Recommendations*						
				Adults			*Children*		*Newborn (Parenteral)*	
		Peak Serum	*Peak or Range, Urine*	*Oral*	*Parenteral*	*Maximum Daily Dose*	*Oral*	*Parenteral*	*Up to 1 wk*	*1–4 wk*
Drug (Oral Absorption, %)	*Dose (g)*	*(μg/ml)*		*Dose/Interval*		*(g)*	*Dose/Interval*			
Clarithromycin 14-OH metabolite	0.5 g po	2.4 1.0		0.25–0.5 g q12h			7.5 mg/kg q12h			
Erythromycin (18–45[a])				0.25–0.5 g q6h	0.25–1 g q6h	4	7.5–12.5 mg/kg q6h	3.75–12.5 mg/kg q6h	Not recommended	
base stearate ethyl succinate[d]	0.25 po[b] 0.5 po[b] 0.5 po	0.3–1 0.4–1.9 1.5 (0.6)	13–46[c] 30	0.333 g q8h or 0.25–0.5 g q6–12h 0.4 g q6–12h						
lactobionate	0.5 IV	9.9			0.25–0.5 g IV q6h			30–50 mg/kg/day q6h IM		
gluceptate	1 IV	9.9			0.25–0.5 g IV q6h			30–50 mg/kg/day q6h IM		
estolate	0.5 po	4.2[e]		0.25–0.5 g q6–12h			40 mg/kg/day q6–12h			
Clindamycin (approx. 90[f])	0.15 po 0.3 IM 0.6 IV[g]	1.9–3.9 4.8–6 10	3–4	0.15–0.45 g q6h	0.15–0.9 g q6–8h	8	2–8 mg/kg q6–8h	2.5–10 mg/kg q6h[h]	5 mg/kg q6–8h	
Lincomycin (20–30)	0.6 IV[j] 0.5 po 0.6 IM	19 2.6 9.5	 13–259	0.5 g q6–8h	0.6–1 g q8–12h	8	10–15 mg/kg q6–8h	2.5–5 mg/kg q6h[h]	Not recommended	
Chloramphenicol (75–90)	0.5 po 1 po[u] 1 IV	3–4 11.2–18.4 5–12[l]	70–150[m] 200	12.5–25 mg/kg q6h	12.5–25 mg/kg q6h	4.8	12.5–25 mg/kg q6h	12.5–25 mg/kg q6h	25 mg/kg q24h[n]	25 mg/kg q12–24h[n]
Metronidazole[o] (95[p]) (67–82 rectal[q]) (19 vaginal)	0.25 po 0.5 po 0.5 IV 0.5 rectal suppository 0.5 vaginal	5 10 10[g] 20–25[k] 5.1 1.2–1.8	50–390	7.5 mg/kg q6h[r]	7.5 mg/kg q6h[r]	4	7.5 mg/kg q6h	7.5 mg/kg q6h	15 mg/kg once, then 7.5 mg/kg q12h	15 mg/kg once, then 7.5 mg/kg q8–12h
Roxithromycin (72–85)	0.15 g po 0.3 g po	5.4–7.9 10.4	17.4 37.7	0.15 g q12h or 0.3 g q24h			2.5–5 mg/kg q12h			

[a] The extent of gastrointestinal absorption of erythromycin formulations relates to the chemical structure and its susceptibility to gastric acid, the protective enteric coating, and the concomitant presence of food. (*Am J Hosp Pharm.* 1980;37:1119–205.)
[b] Fasting.
[c] Alkalinization of the urine pH to 8 increases the amount of nonionized drug that remains in the urine and enhances the local antibacterial activity.
[d] Absorption of the ethylsuccinate preparation is enhanced by food. After absorption, 45 percent of the ethylsuccinate preparation is present in serum as the inactive ester and 55 percent as the active base; 1.5 μg/ml total (0.6 μg/ml free base).
[e] Erythromycin estolate total drug concentration with 500 mg dosing is 4.2 μg/ml (ester plus base) or 1.1 μg/ml free base.
[f] Absorption is not decreased by food.
[g] IV infusion (over 30 minutes).
[h] Total daily dose may be divided every 8 hours
[i] Dose modification should be made with coexisting renal and hepatic disease.
[j] IV infusion over 2 h.
[k] Multiple dose (500 mg q8h).

ANTIMICROBIAL AGENT PHARMACOLOGY: POLYMYXINS, VANCOMYCIN, AND FUSIDIC ACID

	Serum and Urine Concentration for Selected Doses			*Dosage Recommendations*						
				Adults			*Children*		*Newborn (Parenteral)*	
		Peak Serum	*Peak or Range, Urine*	*Oral*	*Parenteral*	*Maximum Daily Dose*	*Oral*	*Parenteral*	*Up to 1 wk*	*1–4 wk*
Drug (Oral Absorption, %)	*Dose*	*(μg/ml)*		*Dose/Interal*		*(g)*	*Dose/Interval*			
Colistimethate (minimal)	75 mg IM 150 mg IM 150 mg IV	1–2 6–8 10–13	50 200–270		0.8–1.7 mg/kg q8h	5 mg/kg		1.7–2.3 mg/kg q8h	Not recommended	
Polymyxin B (minimal[d])	50 mg IM 2.5 mg/kg IV (infused in 0.3–0.5 liters)	2–8 5			1.5–2.5 mg/kg/day continuous IV infusion[e]	2.5 mg/kg		up to 4–4.5 mg/kg/day continuous IV infusion[f]	Not recommended	
Vancomycin (minimal)	0.5 g IV 1 g IV 0.125 g q6h po	6–10 20–50 <1[h]	 100–300	0.125–0.5 g q6h	15 mg/kg q12h or 6.5–8 mg/kg q6h[i]	2g	12.5 mg/kg q6h	10 mg/kg q6h[i]	15 mg/kg q12h	15 mg/kg q8h

Serum Half-life (hr): For Creatinine Clearance (ml/min) >80	Serum Half-life (hr): For Creatinine Clearance (ml/min) <10	Serum Half-life (hr): With Dialysis HD	Serum Half-life (hr): With Dialysis PD	Usual Adult Dose and Interval Adjustment: Dose	For Creatinine Clearance (ml/min) >80	80–50	50–10	<10 (Anuric)	Dosage for Dialysis: Dose after HD Supplemental to Anuric	Dosage for Dialysis: Daily Dose during PD	CSF/Serum (%) Inflamed Meninges	Newborn Serum/Maternal Serum (%)	Breast Milk Maternal Serum (%)	Bile/Serum (%)	Aqueous Humor/Serum (%)
6.7	21.6										Minimal		30	7000	
1.4	4–6	No change	No change	0.25–1 g	6 hr	6 hr	6 hr	6 hr	None	No change	6–10	5–25	50	400–2800	25–30
2.4	3.4–6	1.9–6	4.6	0.15–0.9 g	6–8 hr	6–8 hr	6–8 hr	6–8 hr[l]	None	No change	Minimal	6–46	38–50	250–300	
4–6	10–13		10.3–15.4	0.5 g po	6 hr	6 hr	12 hr	24 hr or 25–50% dose	None	No change	1–7	25–36	13	250–400	8–75
1.5–3.5	3.2–4.3	0.8–2.7	3.8	12.5–25 mg/kg	6 hr	6 hr	6 hr	6 hr	Schedule the dose after dialysis	No change	45–99	30–106	51–61	100–200	
6–14[s]	8–15[t]	2.6	5.6–10.9	7.5 mg/kg	6 hr[r]	6 hr	6 hr	6 hr	No change	No change	43–100	97	60–100	100	33–50
8.3–13	16–17.9										Minimal	30–40	0.05		50–200

[l] Intramuscular administration may produce a plasma level of active drug that is but one-half that achieved with a comparable oral dose and is therefore not recommended. The intravenous preparation (succinate ester) produces serum chloramphenicol levels 30–50 percent less than those achieved with a comparable oral dose.
[m] The urine concentration of unmetabolized chloramphenicol is inversely correlated with the renal function. When the creatinine clearance is below 20 ml/min, less than 1 percent of the dose is excreted in the active form as compared with 5–10 precent in patients with normal renal function.
[n] Initial dosage. Subsequent dosage should be based on the determination of serum concentrations (10 to 25 μg/ml, desired). For premature infants throughout the first month of life, the initial dosage is 25 mg/kg/day.
[o] Dosage for anaerobic bacterial infections. The first dose (loading dose) should be 15 mg/kg. The dosage shuld be reduced with severe hepatic disease.
[p] Absorption of metronidazole is not significantly decreased by food.
[q] Rectal absorption is inversely dependent on the dose.
[r] Clinical work with metronidazole completed outside the United States supports the use of an 8-hour dosing interval.
[s] Patients with alcoholic liver disease eliminate metronidazole more slowly, a half-life of 18.3 hours, than do subjects with normal liver function and may therefore require dosage modification to avoid accumulation of metronidazole and its metabolites. (*Antimicrob Agents Chemother.* 1987;31:1662–4.)
[t] The hydroxy metabolite may accumulate in anuric patients.
[u] Multiple dose (1 g q6h).

Serum Half-life (hr): For Creatinine Clearance (ml/min) >80	Serum Half-life (hr): For Creatinine Clearance (ml/min) <10	Serum Half-life (hr): With Dialysis HD	Serum Half-life (hr): With Dialysis PD	Usual Adult Dose and Interval Adjustment: Dose	For Creatinine Clearance (ml/min) >80	80–50	50–10	<10 (Anuric)	Dosage for Dialysis: Dose after HD Supplemental to Anuric	Dosage for Dialysis: Daily Dose during PD	CSF/Serum (%) Inflamed Meninges	Newborn Serum/Maternal Serum (%)	Breast Milk/Maternal Serum (%)	Bile/Serum (%)	Aqueous Humor/Serum (%)
2–3	10–20	1.5	Poor	0.8–1.7 mg/kg	8 hr	2.5 mg/kg on day 1, then 1–1.5 mg/kg q24h	2.5 mg/kg on day 1, then 1–1.5 mg/kg q24–72h	2.5 mg/kg on day 1, then 1–1.5 mg/kg q48–72h[a]	[b]	[c]	Minimal	50	18	Not detectable	25–30
6	48–72			1.5–2.5 mg/kg/day	24 hr	3 mg/kg on day 1, then 1.5–2.5 mg/kg q24h	3 mg/kg on day 1, then 1.5–2.5 mg/kg q24–72h	3 mg/kg on day 1, then 1.5–2.5 mg/kg q48–72h[a]			Minimal[g]			Not detectable	
4–6[k]	240	Negligible effect	18	15 mg/kg q12h or 6.5–8 mg/kg q6h	6–12 hr	See the nomogram, Chapter 27 or *Antimicrob Agents Chemother.* 1984;25:433			No change	[l]	7–21	20[m]	33–66[n]	50	Minimal

Drug (Oral Absorption, %)	Dose	*Serum and Urine Concentration for Selected Doses* Peak Serum (μg/ml)	Peak or Range, Urine (μg/ml)	*Dosage Recommendations* Adults Oral (Dose/Interal)	Adults Parenteral (Dose/Interal)	Maximum Daily Dose (g)	Children Oral (Dose/Interval)	Children Parenteral (Dose/Interval)	Newborn (Parenteral) Up to 1 wk (Dose/Interval)	Newborn (Parenteral) 1–4 wk (Dose/Interval)
Teichoplanin	3 mg/kg IV[q] 6 mg/kg IV[q]	53 112			0.2–0.4 g q24h			10 mg/kg q24h	6 mg/kg q24h (preliminary)	
Fusidic acid	0.5 g po	14–38[o]	<1	0.5–1 g q8h	580 mg q8h IV[p]		6.6–16.6 mg/kg q8h	6.6 mg/kg q8h		

[a] The interval is extended to every 5–7 days for the anuric patient.
[b] The rate of removal of colistimethate by hermodialysis or peritoneal dialysis remains controversial. Studies using a Koiff twin coil dialyzer demonstrate no removal (*N Engl J Med.* 1964;270:394–7; *Ann Intern Med.* 1968;68:984–94.), whereas studies using the Kiil type dialyzer recommend the dose be adjusted so that the patient receives a 2–3 mg/kg dose after dialysis. (*Br Med J.* 1968;1:484–5; *Antimicrob Agents Chemother.* 1964;373–8.)
[c] Small quantities of colistimethate are removed by PD with clearance rates ranging from 5.8–11.3 ml/min. Supplemental doses may be considered on the basis of the duration of dialysis and the need to maintain target serum levels.
[d] The only significant absorption from the gastrointestinal tract has been observed in newborn animals and small infants.
[e] Although not recommended, the IM dosage of polymyxin B for adults is 2.5–3.0 mg/kg/day given in 4–6 divided doses.
[f] Although not recommended, the daily dose may be divided and given by the IM route.
[g] Although rarely used, the daily intrathecal dose of polymyxin B is 5–10 mg for adults and 2 mg for children over 2 years of age. Intrathecal therapy should be administered on a daily basis for the first 3–5 days and then every other day for 3 weeks or for 2 weeks after negative CSF cultures and a normal CSF glucose concentration.

ANTIMICROBIAL AGENT PHARMACOLOGY: SULFONAMIDES AND TRIMETHOPRIM

Drug (Oral Absorption, %)	Dose (%)	*Serum and Urine Concentration for Selected Doses* Peak Serum (μg/ml)	Peak or Range, Urine (μg/ml)	*Dosage Recommendations* Adults Oral (Dose/Interal)	Adults Parenteral (Dose/Interal)	Maximum Daily Dose (g)	Children Oral (Dose/Interval)	Children Parenteral (Dose/Interval)	Newborn (Parenteral) Up to 1 wk (Dose/Interval)	Newborn (Parenteral) 1–4 wk (Dose/Interval)
Trimethoprim-sulfamethoxazole (TMP-SMX) (85–90)	0.16/0.8 po 0.16/0.8 IV[a]	2/40 3.4/47.3	120/300[b]	2 tablets q12h or 1 tablet q6h[c]	4–5 mg/kg q6–12h (as TMP)[c]	4 tablets orally or 1.2 g TMP, 6 g SMX intravenously (usual)	4–5 mg/kg q6–12h (as TMP)[c]	4–5 mg/kg q6–12h (as TMP)[c]	Not recommended[d]	
Trimethoprim (80)	0.32 po 0.1 po	5.5 1	30–160[f]	0.1 g q12h		0.2	2 mg/kg q12h (not approved in children less than 12 years old)			
Sulfonamides (70–90)										
Sulfisoxazole	2 po	40–50 (free)		0.5–1 g q6h[g]	25 mg/kg q6h[g]	8	120–150 mg/kg/day q4–6h	100 mg/kg/day q6–8h[g]	Not recommended	
Sulfamethoxazole	2 po	80–100 (free)		1 g q8–12h[i]		3	25–30 mg/kg q12h[j]		Not recommended	
Sulfamethizole	2 po	60		0.5–1 g q6–8h		6	7.5–11.25 mg/kg q6h		Not recommended	
Sulfacytine	0.25 po	17	420	0.5 g initial dose, then 0.25 g q6h		1	Not recommended		Not recommended	
Sulfadiazine	0.5 po	20–40		2–4 g initial dose, then 0.5–1 g q4–6h	Not recommended	6	120–750 mg/kg/day q4–6h[g]		Not recommended	
Sulfadoxine[l]	2 po	50–75 (free)		1 tablet every wk or 2 tablets every other wk[m]		1.5	By age[n]		Not recommended	
Sulfasalazine (10–15)	2 po	14 sulfasalazine 21 sulfapyridine (total)		0.5–1 g q4–6h		4[o]	30–60 mg/kg/day q4–8h		Not recommended	
Sulfaphenazole	2 po	100–150		2–3 g, then 1 g q12h		2	66 mg/kg, then 33 mg/kg q12h		Not recommended	

[a] Infused over 60 minutes.
[b] The urine concentrations of the drugs depend on the urine flow rate, urine pH, and the time of collection. The approximate urine concentration for trimethoprim is 100 times the plasma concentration; for sulfamethoxazole the level is 5 times the concentration in plasma. Alkalinization of the urine increases the renal excretion of sulfonamides. See footnote f.
[c] Each tablet contains 80 mg trimethoprim and 400 mg sulfamethoxazole. Double-strength tablets are also available and are usually administered at one tablet q12h. The suspension contains 40 mg trimethoprim and 200 mg sulfamethoxazole per 5 ml. Parenteral dosage ranges from 8 to 20 mg/kg/day trimethoprim and 40 to 100 mg/kg/day sulfamethoxazole.
[d] Unsuitable for the newborn because the appropriate dosage requires a ratio of trimethoprim : sulfamethoxazole of 1 : 3 and the only formulation available is a 1 : 5 combination. (*J Pediatr.* 1982;100:647–50.)
[e] Nonacetylated SMX.
[f] Renal clearance of trimethoprim is increased with acidification of the urine.

Serum Half-life (hr)				Usual Adult Dose and Interval Adjustment					Dosage for Dialysis						
For Creatinine Clearance (ml/min)		With Dialysis			For Creatinine Clearance (ml/min)										
>80	<10	HD	PD	Dose	>80	80–50	50–10	<10 (Anuric)	Dose after HD Supplemental to Anuric	Daily Dose during PD	CSF/Serum (%) Inflamed Meninges	Newborn Serum/ Maternal Serum (%)	Breast Milk/ Maternal Serum (%)	Bile/ Serum (%)	Aqueous Humor/ Serum (%)
40–70	125	163		0.4 g	24 hr	0.2 g q24h or 0.4 g q48h	0.2 g q24h or 0.4 g q48h	0.13 g q24 or 0.4 g q72h							
				0.5–1 g po	8 hr	8 hr	8 hr	8 hr							

[h] The stool concentration ranges from 100 to 800 μg/ml.
[i] The incidence of "red-man syndrome" may be decreased by using a 500 mg dose instead of 1 g (*Antimicrob Agents Chemother.* 1987;31:393–7.)
[j] Doses as high as 60 mg/kg/day may be necessary for staphylococcal CNS infections.
[k] The elimination half-life of vancomycin varies with age: 5.9–9.8 hours in newborns, 4.1 hours in older infants, 2.2–3 hours in children.
[l] Conflicting opinion exists with regard to the dosage alteration of vancomycin during PD. The regimen chosen will depend upon the frequency and duration of dialysis as well as the nature of the infection being treated. Serum concentrations should be measured and the dosage regimen adjusted accordingly.
[m] Data from animals (rabbits).
[n] Data from animals (cats).
[o] Accumulation occurs with multiple doses of 0.5 g given every 8 hours; a mean serum level of 71 μg/ml has been reported after 96 hours of therapy.
[p] Diethanolamine fusidate, 580 mg = 500 mg sodium fusidate.
[q] IV infusion over a period of 5 minutes.

Serum Half-life (hr)				Usual Adult Dose and Interval Adjustment					Dosage for Dialysis						
For Creatinine Clearance (ml/min)		With Dialysis			For Creatinine Clearance (ml/min)										
>80	<10	HD	PD	Dose	>80	80–50	50–10	<10 (Anuric)	Dose after HD Supplemental to Anuric	Daily Dose during PD	CSF/Serum (%) Inflamed Meninges	Newborn Serum/ Maternal Serum (%)	Breast Milk/ Maternal Serum (%)	Bile/ Serum (%)	Aqueous Humor/ Serum (%)
11/9	25/27	9.4/11.7[e]		4–5 mg/kg (as TMP)	6–12 hr	12 hr	18 hr	24–48 hr	4–5 mg/kg (as TMP)	0.16/0.8 q48h[f]	30–50/25–30	100/70–90	125/10	100–200/ 40–70	10–45/ 20–30
7.5	14–46	9.4		0.1 g po	12 hr	12 hr	24 hr	24–48 hr			30–50	70–100	100	100	10
											30–80	70–90	10	40–70	20–30
4–6[h]	12			0.5–1 g po	6 hr	6–8 hr	8–12 hr	12–24 hr			30–50				
10–12[k]	22–50			1 g po	8–12 hr						25–30				
2	58			0.5–1 g po	6–8 hr										
4				0.25 g po	6 hr										
10–12	34			0.5–1 g po	4–6 hr						50–80				
150–200				0.5 g po or 1 g po	every wk every other wk										
7.6				0.5–1 g po	4–6 hr										
				1 g po	12 hr										

[g] Administer one-half of the daily dose as the initial dose.
[h] Under normal conditions the half-life of elimination was determined as 6 hours, whereas under alkaline conditions the half-life approached 4 hours.
[i] Administer a 2 g loading dose: 4 regular strength tablets or 2 double-strength tablets.
[j] Administer a 50–60 mg/kg loading dose. The maximum dose for children should not exceed 75 mg/kg/24 h.
[k] Under acidic conditions, the half-life of elimination is slightly longer (11 hours) than under alkaline conditions (9 h).
[l] For malaria prophylaxis. The first dose should be given 1–2 days before departure to an endemic area and the course continued throughout the stay and 4–6 weeks thereafter.
[m] One tablet = 500 mg sulfadoxine and 25 mg pyrimethamine.
[n] Under 4 years: ¼ tablet weekly or ½ tablet every other week; 4–8 years: ½ tablet weekly or 1 tablet every other week; 9–14 years: ¾ tablet weekly or 1½ tablet every other week.
[o] Although doses up to 12 g have been administered, a daily dosage exceeding 4 g is associated with an increased incidence of adverse effects.

ANTIMICROBIAL AGENT PHARMACOLOGY: QUINOLONES AND OTHER URINARY TRACT AGENTS

	Serum and Urine Concentration for Selected Doses			Dosage Recommendations						
				Adults			Children		Newborn (Parenteral)	
		Peak Serum	Peak or Range, Urine	Oral	Parenteral	Maximum Daily Dose	Oral	Parenteral	Up to 1 wk	1–4 wk
Drug (Oral Absorption, %)	Dose	(μg/ml)		Dose/Interal			Dose/Interval			
Quinolones										
Cinoxacin (97)	0.25 po 0.5 po	8 16	400	0.25 g q6h or 0.5 g q12h[a]		1	Not recommended			
Ciprofloxacin (69–85)	0.5 po 0.75 po 0.2 IV[d]	2.9 4 3.8	300–450 550–700	0.25–0.75 g q12h	0.2–0.3 g q12h		Not recommended			
Enoxacin (80–90)	0.4 po 0.6 po 0.2 IV	2.8–3.6 4 1.8	250–300 337	0.4 g q12h	0.4 g q12h		Not recommended			
Fleroxacin (99)	0.4 po 0.1 IV	4.4 2.85	210	0.4 g q12–24h (preliminary)			Not recommended			
Lomefloxacin	0.2 po 0.4 po	2.1 3–4.7	170	0.4 g q12–24h (preliminary)			Not recommended			
Nalidixic acid (96)	1 po	25–35	150–400	1 g q6h[a]		4	Not recommended		Not recommended	
Norfloxacin (30–40)	0.2 po 0.4 po 0.8 po	0.75 1.6 2.4	200 480 700	0.2–0.4 g q12h[a]		0.8				
Ofloxacin (85–90)	0.2 po 0.4 po 0.6 po	2.6 8.6 11	218	0.2–0.4 g q12h			Not recommended			
Oxolinic acid (poor)	0.75 po	0.9–3.6	45–100 avg	0.75 q12h[a]		2	Not recommended		Not recommended	
Pefloxacin (98)	0.4 po 0.4 IV[g]	3.8–5.6 5.8	100–115	0.4 g q12–24h			Not recommended			
Temafloxacin (100)	0.2 po 0.4 po 0.6 po	2 3.7 7		0.2–1.2 g/day q12–24h						
Other urinary tract agents										
Indanyl carbenicillin (30–40)	0.382 po (1 tablet) 1 po	6.5 6–17	1130	1–2 tablets q6h[a]		3	7.5–12.5 mg/kg q6h[a]			
Methenamine mandelate[h] (70[i])	1 po		40 (formaldehyde)	1 g q6h[a]		4	12.5–18.75 mg/kg q6h[a]		Not recommended	
Methenamine hippurate[h] (100)	1	70–100 μmol/liter[k]	1100–1500 (methenamine) approx 50 (formaldehyde)	1 g q12h[a]		4	12.5–25 mg/kg q12h[a]		Not recommended	
Nitrofurantoin (good but variable)	0.1 po	<1	150[j]	0.05–0.1 g q6h[a]		0.4	1.25–1.75 mg/kg q6h[a]		Not recommended	

[a] Used primarily for the treatment of urinary tract infections.
[b] Use during pregnancy not recommended.
[c] Animal pharmacology studies indicate the presence of drug in the milk of lactating rats receiving oral doses of cinoxacin. Human data are currently unavailable.
[d] Infused over a period of 30 minutes.
[e] Ineffective urinary concentrations expected with compromised renal function.
[f] Breast milk percentage extrapolated from data indicating 4 μg/ml breast milk concentration in four patients (*Lancet*. 1965;2:691). Hemolytic anemia has been described in one nursing infant whose mother received nalidixic acid.
[g] Infused over a period of 60 minutes.
[h] Usually coadministered with an acidifying agent to convert the methenamine salts in urine to ammonia and bactericidal formaldehyde (pH < OR = 5.5). Mandelic and hippuric acids are mildly antiseptic and contribute to urine acidification.

ANTIMICROBIAL AGENT PHARMACOLOGY: ANTIMYCOBACTERIAL AGENTS

	Serum and Urine Concentration for Selected Doses			Dosage Recommendations						
				Adults			Children		Newborn (Parenteral)	
		Peak Serum	Peak or Range, Urine	Oral	Parenteral	Maximum Daily Dose	Oral	Parenteral	Up to 1 wk	1–4 wk
Drug (Oral Absorption, %)	Dose	(μg/ml)		Dose/Interal			Dose/Interval			
Ansamycin	0.075–0.3 g	0.2–0.5		0.15–0.3 g/day		0.3 g				
Capreomycin[a] (minimal)	1 g	30	1685		0.75–1 g q24h 15–20 mg/kg/day IM[b]	20 mg/kg/day		15–30 mg/kg/day IM (not approved)		
Clofazimine				0.1 g/day[c]		0.6 g				
Cycloserine (70–90)	0.25 g po 0.5 g po	10	 55–340	0.25–0.5 g q12h		1 g	3.5–5 mg/kg q12h (not approved)			

Serum Half-life (hr)				Usual Adult Dose and Interval Adjustment					Dosage for Dialysis		CSF/ Serum (%) Inflamed Meninges	Newborn Serum/ Maternal Serum (%)	Breast Milk/ Maternal Serum (%)	Bile/ Serum (%)	Aqueous Humor/ Serum (%)
For Creatinine Clearance (ml/min)		With Dialysis			For Creatinine Clearance (ml/min)										
>80	<10	HD	PD	Dose	>80	80–50	50–10	<10 (Anuric)	Dose after HD Supplemental to Anuric	Daily Dose during PD					
1.5	8.4	3–4.4		0.25–0.5 g po	6–12 hr	0.25 g q8h	0.25 g q12–24h	Not recommended				[b]	<100 (18–78)[c]		
3–5	5–10			0.25–0.75	12 hr	12 hr	0.25–0.5 g 12–18 hr	0.25–0.5 g 24 hr	Give dose after dialysis		15–40			500–1000	3–22
5–7	40	9.8									67			900	
9–12	30														
7–8.5	21													700	
1.5	21			1 g po	6 hr	6 hr	6 hr	Not recommended[e]					13[f]	100	
3–4	5–10			0.2–0.4 g po	12 hr	12 hr	12–24 hr	24 hr				Nil	Nil	300–700	
5–8	25–50	10		0.2	12 hr	12 hr	24–48 hr	48 hr	None			60–90	15–75	250	
6–7				0.75 g po	12 hr		Not recommended[e]	Not recommended[e]					Not recommended	200–300	
8–12	11–15										45–60			200–600	
7.7															
0.5–1	12.5			1–2 tablets po	6 hr	6 hr	6 hr	Not recommended[e]							
3–6				1 g po	6 hr	6 hr	Not recommended[e]	Not recommended[e]			[j]			[j]	[j]
4				1 g po	12 hr	12 hr	Not recommended[l]	Not recommended[l]			[j]	50	70–100	[j]	[j]
0.3	1			0.05–0.1 g po	6 hr	6 hr	Not recommended[e,m]	Not recommended[e,m]				100	<25[n]	200–400	

[i] Oral absorption is decreased 30 percent by enteric coating.
[j] Methenamine penetrates a number of body fluids, including bile and cerebrospinal fluid. This penetration proves clinically inconsequential since negligible amounts of formaldehyde are generated at physiologic pH (see Chapter 31).
[k] The serum concentration of methenamine has no clinical significance.
[l] Alkaline conditions reduce tubular reabsorption, which yields higher nitrofurantoin concentrations in urine.
[m] Nitrofurantoin accumulates in the serum of patients with a creatinine clearance <60 ml/min, which leads to systemic toxicity.
[n] Although only small amounts of nitrofurantoin have been detected in breast milk, the drug could cause hemolytic anemia in a glucose-6-phosphate dehydrogenase–deficient infant exposed in this manner.

Serum Half-life (hr)				Usual Adult Dose and Interval Adjustment					Dosage for Dialysis		CSF/ Serum (%) Inflamed Meninges	Newborn Serum/ Maternal Serum (%)	Breast Milk/ Maternal Serum (%)	Bile/ Serum (%)	Aqueous Humor/ Serum (%)
For Creatinine Clearance (ml/min)		With Dialysis		For Creatinine Clearance (ml/min)											
>80	<10	HD	PD	Dose	>80	80–50	50–10	<10 (Anuric)	Dose after HD Supplemental to Anuric	Daily Dose during PD					
				0.15–0.3 g po	24 hr	24 hr	0.15 g q24h	0.075 g q72h							
				0.75–1 g	24 hr									Minimal	
70 days				0.1 g po	24 hr										
				0.25–0.5 g po	12 hr						100	100	72		

ANTIMICROBIAL AGENT PHARMACOLOGY: ANTIMYCOBACTERIAL AGENTS *(Continued)*

	Serum and Urine Concentration for Selected Doses			Dosage Recommendations						
				Adults			Children		Newborn (Parenteral)	
		Peak Serum	Peak or Range, Urine	Oral	Parenteral	Maximum Daily Dose	Oral	Parenteral	Up to 1 wk	1–4 wk
Drug (Oral Absorption, %)	Dose	(μg/ml)		Dose/Interal			Dose/Interval			
Ethambutol (80)	25 mg/kg po	2–5		15 mg/kg/day[d]		15 mg/kg/day[d]	15 mg/kg/day (not approved)			
Ethionamide	1 g po	20		0.25–0.5 g q12h		1 g	5–10 mg/kg q12h (not approved)			
Isoniazid[e]	0.3 g po	7		5 mg/kg/day (0.3 g)[f]	5 mg/kg/day IM	0.6 g	10–20 mg/kg/day q12–24h[g]	10–20 mg/kg/day q12–24h IM		
Para-amino salicylic acid	4 g po (free acid)	75 7–8		3 g q6–8h		12 g	66.6–75 mg/kg q6–8h			
Pyrazinamide	1 g po	45	60	15–30 mg/kg/day[k]		3 g	15–30 mg/kg/day q12–24h			
Rifampin (100)	0.6 g po (fasting)	10[l]	240	0.6 g/24 hr[m]		1.2 g[m]	10–20 mg/kg/day q12–24h			
Streptomycin	1 g IM	25–50	1000		15 mg/kg/day IM[o]	2 g		10–15 mg/kg q12h IM		
Viomycin					1 g q12h twice weekly	2 g				

[a] Pharmacokinetics similar to streptomycin.
[b] The dosage is 1 g IM daily for 2–4 months and is reduced to 1 g two to three times weekly thereafter.
[c] In combination therapeutic regimens, 300 mg monthly to 50–100 mg daily is recommended.
[d] Doses as high as 25 mg/kg/day are occasionally administered during the first 2–3 months of therapy. Intermittent therapy consists of 50 mg/kg/day administered twice weekly.
[e] To minimize the risk of polyneuritis from isoniazid-induced pyridoxine deficiency, pyridoxine (15–50 mg) is often given concurrently.
[f] For noncompliant patients, 15 mg/kg can be given twice weekly under supervision. For prophylaxis, isoniazid is usually given for a year in a daily dose of 300 mg for adults and 10 mg/kg (up to 300 mg maximum for children.
[g] In children with tuberculosis meningitis, some clinicians use 30 mg/kg/day for the first few weeks.
[h] Specific elimination kinetics of isoniazid depend on the acetylator phenotype of the individual; the half-life for rapid acetylators is 0.5–1.5 hours and for slow acetylators, 2–4 hours.

ANTIMICROBIAL AGENT PHARMACOLOGY: ANTIFUNGAL AGENTS

	Serum and Urine Concentration for Selected Doses			Dosage Recommendations						
				Adults			Children		Newborn (Parenteral)	
		Peak Serum	Peak or Range Urine	Oral	Parenteral	Maximum Daily Dose	Oral	Parenteral	Up to 1 wk	1–4 wk
Drug (Oral Absorption, %)	Dose	(μg/ml)		Dose/Interval			Dose/Interval			
Amphotericin (poor)	0.1–1 mg/kg	0.5–5.5	≤5		0.25–1 mg/kg q24h[a]	1 mg/kg[b]		0.25–1 mg/kg q24h[a]	0.1–1 mg/kg/day[a]	0.1–1 mg/kg/day[a]
Fluconazole	0.1 po 0.2 po	4.5–8 10	50	0.2–0.4 g q24h	0.2–0.4 g q24h	0.4 g				
Flucytosine (90)	150 mg/kg/day po	50–80	5800	37.5 mg/kg q6h	37.5 mg/kg q6h	150 mg/kg	37.5 mg/kg q6h		Not recommended	
Giseofulvin (50[d])	1 g po	1–2.8[e]	Minimal	0.5–1 g/day in single or 2–4 doses[d]		2 g	10 mg/kg/day[d]			
Itraconazole	0.2 po	0.6	Not detected	0.2–0.4 g q24h		0.4 g				
Ketoconazole[f]	0.2 g po 0.4 g po	3–4.5 7	Minimal	0.2–0.4 g q24h		0.8 g	5–10 mg/kg/day q12–24h[g]			
Miconazole (25–30)	0.5 g IV[i]	2–9			0.066–1.2 g q8h[j]	3.6 g		6.6–13.3 mg/kg q8h		
Nystatin (minimal)[m]	All doses	Minimal		400,000–600,000 units q6h (4–6 ml)		4×10^4 units	250,000–500,000 units q6h (2.5–5 ml)		100,000 units q6h (0.25 ml) (po)	100,000 units q6h (0.25 ml) (po)

[a] A test dose of 1 mg infused over 15 minutes is often given to assess febrile reactions prior to proceeding to higher doses.
[b] Or up to 1.5 mg/kg every other day.
[c] Data from rabbits.
[d] Dose for conventional microsize griseofulvin. Significant interindividual variation exists with griseofulvin absorption. Bioavailability studies have demonstrated a 150 percent greater absorption of ultramicrosize products (Fulvicin P-G, Gris-PEG). Dosing guidelines for ultramicrosize griseofulvin are 330–660 mg daily for adults and 7.25 mg/kg/day for children (*J Pharmokinet Biopharm.* 1980;8:347–62).
[e] The serum level is increased with a high-fat meal.
[f] Oral absorption is variable and is decreased during simultaneous administration of H_2 antagonists or antacids.

Serum Half-life (hr) For Creatinine Clearance (ml/min) >80	<10	With Dialysis HD	PD	Usual Adult Dose and Interval Adjustment: Dose	For Creatinine Clearance (ml/min) >80	80–50	50–10	<10 (Anuric)	Dosage for Dialysis: Dose after HD Supplemental to Anuric	Daily Dose during PD	CSF/Serum (%) Inflamed Meninges	Newborn Serum/Maternal Serum (%)	Breast Milk/Maternal Serum (%)	Bile/Serum (%)	Aqueous Humor/Serum (%)
4–6	7–32			15 mg/kg/day po	15 mg/kg/day	15 mg/kg/day	7.5 mg/kg/day	5 mg/kg/day	15 mg/kg/day on dialysis day	15 mg/kg/day during PD	25–50	~100			
2–4				0.25–0.5 g po	12 hr						100				
0.5–4[h]	8 (avg)	3.4		5 mg/kg po	24 hr	24 hr	24 hr	24 hr[i]	5 mg/kg	[j]	100	High	100		
1	23			3 g po	6–8 hr						Poor				
9–10				25 mg/kg/day po	6–12 hr						100				
2.5–5[n]	2–5	Minimal	Minimal	0.6 g po	24 hr	24 hr	24 hr	24 hr	No supplemental dose	No supplemental dose	10–30	33	20–60	10,000	
2–3	100–110			15 mg/kg/day	24 hr	24 hr	24–72 hr	72–96 hr	5 mg/kg		20	10–40	<25	40–300	
				1 g	12 hr twice weekly						Poor				

[i] For slow acetylators (at least one-half of white Americans), the daily dose should be reduced to 200 mg.
[j] In cases where peritoneal dialysis has been used for the management of acute isoniazid intoxication, the procedure decreased INH serum concentration by 68% over 24 hours (*N Engl J Med* 269:852–3 1963).
[k] When given intermittently, the adult dosage is 50 mg/kg twice weekly. The daily dosage is divided in two to four equally spaced doses.
[l] An increase in dose results in a disproportionate increase in peak serum concentration: after 300, 600, and 1200 mg doses, the peak serum levels reached 4, 10, and over 30 μg/ml, respectively.
[m] For noncompliant patients, supervised therapy with 600 mg rifampin twice a week can be given. The dose for the prophylaxis of meningococcal meningitis is 600 mg twice daily for 2 days.
[n] The serum half-life increases with the dose: 2.5, 3, and 5 hours after doses of 300, 600, and 900 mg, respectively.
[o] An alternative dosage schedule is 25–30 mg/kg twice weekly.

Serum Half-life (hr) For Creatinine Clearance (ml/min) >80	<10	With Dialysis HD	PD	Usual Adult Dose and Interval Adjustment: Dose	For Creatinine Clearance (ml/min) >80	80–50	50–10	<10 (Anuric)	Dosage for Dialysis: Dose after HD Supplemental to Anuric	Daily Dose during PD	CSF/Serum (%) Inflamed Meninges	Newborn Serum/Maternal Serum (%)	Breast Milk/Maternal Serum (%)	Bile/Serum (%)	Aqueous Humor/Serum (%)
24 or more	24 or more	Minimal		0.25–1 mg/kg IV	24 hr	24 hr	24 hr	24 hr	No change		2–3	50			25
24	48			0.2–0.4 g po	24 hr	24 hr	48 hr	≥72 hr			50–90				64[c]
4–6	30–70	5–6		37.5 mg/kg po	6 hr	6 hr	12–24 hr	15–25 mg/kg q24h or by plasma level of 50–75	20–37.5 mg/kg		70				
20	20			0.5–1 g po	24 hr	24 hr	24 hr	24 hr				80			
18–36	18–36	18–36	18–36	0.2–0.4 g po	24 hr	24 hr	24 hr	24 hr			Not detected				43[c]
6.5–9.6[h]		Minimal	Minimal	0.2–0.4 g po	24 hr	24 hr	24 hr	24 hr			Minimal			Minimal	~10
2.1/24.1[k]	24[l]	Minimal	Minimal	0.066–1.2 g IV	8 hr	8 hr	8 hr	8 hr			Minimal				
				400,000–600,000 units po	6 hr	6 hr	6 hr	6 hr							

[g] Less than 20 kg: 50 mg; 20–40 kg: 100 mg; greater than 40 kg: 200 mg.
[h] Ketoconazole has a dose-dependent elimination with half-lives of 6.5, 8.1, and 9.6 hours after doses of 100, 200, and 400 mg, respectively.
[i] Over a period of 15 minutes.
[j] The manufacturer recommends an initial test dose of 200 mg.
[k] Triphasic half-life with a 0.4-hour absorption half-life and 2.1- and 24-hour elimination half-lives.
[l] Neither renal impairment nor hemodialysis affects elimination, although plasma concentrations are greater in patients with azotemia due to decreased distribution volume.
[m] Dosage for oral candidiasis. Nystatin suspension = 100,000 units/ml.

ANTIMICROBIAL AGENT PHARMACOLOGY: ANTIVIRAL AGENTS

Drug (Oral Absorption, %)	Dose	Serum and Urine Concentration for Selected Doses: Peak Serum (μg/ml)	Peak or Range Urine (μg/ml)	Dosage Recommendations: Adults: Oral (Dose/Interval)	Adults: Parenteral (Dose/Interval)	Maximum Daily Dose	Children: Oral (Dose/Interval)	Children: Parenteral (Dose/Interval)	Newborn (Parenteral): Up to 1 wk (Dose/Interval)	Newborn (Parenteral): 1–4 wk (Dose/Interval)
Acyclovir (15–20)	2.5 mg/kg[a] 5 mg/kg[a] 0.2 po q4h	6.8 9.8 0.3–0.9		0.2–0.8 g q4h (5 doses/day)	5–10 mg/kg q8h[a]	30 mg/kg		5–15 mg/kg q8h	5–15 mg/kg q8h	5–15 mg/kg q8h
Amantadine (85–90)	0.1 po	0.3–0.4		0.1 g q12h or 0.2 g q24h[c]		0.2 g	2.2–4.4 mg/kg q12h[d]			
Ganciclovir (DHPG) (<5%)	2.5 mg/kg	4.8–6.2			2.5–5 mg/kg q8–12h[a]		Aerosol 190 μg/liter at 12.5 liter/min over 12–18 hr/day			
Ribavirin (50)	Aerosol over 20 hr 0.6 po 1.2 po	0.8–3.3 μg/ml 1.3 μg/ml 2.5 μg/ml		0.3–1.2 g q12h[g] (preliminary)						
Rimantadine (>90)	0.1 po	0.44–0.86 μg/ml		0.1–0.15 g q12h[i]			3 mg/kg q12h			
Vidarabine	10–15 mg/kg/day (12 h)	0.2 vidarabine 6–8 arahypoxanthine			10–15 mg/kg/day over 12 h	15 mg/kg		10–15 mg/kg/day over 12 hours	15–30 mg/kg/day over 12 hours	15–30 mg/kg/day over 12 hours
Zidovudine (63–95)	0.1 q4h po	0.4–0.5 μg/ml		0.2 g q4h (around the clock)						

[a] Intravenous infusion over a period of 1 hour.
[b] Data from manufacturer's product information using animals.
[c] Decrease to 0.1 g q24h for patients older than 65 years or with active seizure disorder.
[d] The dose for children 1–9 years old should not exceed 150 mg/day.
[e]

Creatinine Clearance (ml/min · 1.73 meter^2)	Suggested Maintenance Regimen
50	100 mg daily
40	100 mg daily
30	200 mg twice weekly
20	100 mg thrice weekly
10	200 mg/100 mg alternating every 7 days

(From *Ann Intern Med.* 1981;94:454.)

ADVERSE DRUG INTERACTION INVOLVING ANTIMICROBIAL AGENTS

Interacting Drugs	*Adverse Effect*	*Probable Mechanism*
Acyclovir with		
Narcotics	Increased meperidine effect	Decreased renal excretion
Probenecid	Possible increased acyclovir toxicity	Decreased renal excretion
Amantadine with		
Anticholinergics	Hallucinations, confusion, nightmares	Mechanism not established
Aminoglycoside antibiotics with		
Amphotericin B	Nephrotoxocity	Synergism
Bumetanide	Increased ototoxicity	Additive
Cephalosporins	Increased nephrotoxicity	Mechanism not established
Cisplatin	Increased nephrotoxicity	Mechanism not established
Cyclosporine	Increased renal toxicity	Possibly additive or synergism
Digoxin	Probable decreased digoxin effect with oral gentamicin or neomycin	Decreased absorption
Ethacrynic acid	Increased ototoxicity	Additive
Furosemide	Increased ototoxicity and nephrotoxicity	Additive
Magnesium sulfate	Increased neuromuscular blockade	Additive
Methotrexate	Possible increased methotrexate toxicity with kanamycin	Mechanism not established
	Possible decreased methotrexate effect with oral aminoglycosides	Decreased absorption
Miconazole	Possible decreased tobramycin concentration	Mechanism not established
Neuromuscular blocking agents	Neuromuscular blockade	Additive
Nonsteroidal anti-inflammatory drugs	Possible aminoglycoside toxicity in preterm infants with indomethacin given for patent ductus closure	Decreased renal clearance
Penicillins	Decreased aminoglycoside effect with high concentrations of carbenicillin or ticarcillin	Inactivation
Polymyxins	Increased nephrotoxicity; neuromuscular blockade	Additive
Vancomycin	Possible increased nephrotoxicity and ototoxicity	Additive
Aminosalicylic acid (PAS) with		
Probenecid	Increased PAS toxicity	Decreased renal excretion
Rifampin	Rifampin effectiveness may be decreased; separate doses by 8–12 hr	Decreased GI absorption due to excipient bentonite

(*Continued*)

Serum Half-life (hr)				Usual Adult Dose and Interval Adjustment					Dosage for Dialysis						
For Creatinine Clearance (ml/min)		With Dialysis			For Creatinine Clearance (ml/min)										
>80	<10	HD	PD	Dose	>80	80–50	50–10	<10 (Anuric)	Dose after HD Supplemental to Anuric	Daily Dose during PD	CSF/Serum (%) Inflamed Meninges	Newborn Serum/Maternal Serum (%)	Breast Milk/Maternal Serum (%)	Bile/Serum (%)	Aqueous Humor/Serum (%)
2.2–5	20	5.7		5 mg/kg	8 hr	8 hr	12–24 hr	2.5 mg/kg q24h	Give daily dose after HD		50	100[b]	300		37
12–17	Up to 30 days	Minimal		200 mg q24h or 100 mg q12h po	12 hr	100 mg q12–24h	200 mg/day alternate days to alternating q7days[e]		None		50–60				
2–3	29								[f]		24–67				
24–72[h]											67–115				
25–36	44	Minimal effect							None						
1.5	Decreased			10–15 mg/kg/day	10–15 mg/kg/day	10–15 mg/kg/day	10–15 mg/kg/day	7.5–15 mg/kg/day	Give daily dose after HD		35 to >90				
1											50–100				

[f] Hemodialysis reduces the ganciclovir plasma concentration by approximately 50 percent.
[g] Respiratory syncytial virus bronchiolitis/pneumonia requires a small-particle aerosol generator. After exposure 18–22 hours per day for 3–5 days at a reservoir concentration of 20 mg/ml, the delivered dose is 0.8–1.4 mg/kg/hr depending on age.
[h] Ribavirin accumulates in RBCs with chronic administration and prolongs the terminal plasma half-life up to 2 weeks.
[i] A dosage reduction may be necessary in the elderly, whose plasma levels exceed by twofold those observed in healthy, young adults receiving equivalent doses.

ADVERSE DRUG INTERACTION INVOLVING ANTIMICROBIAL AGENTS *(Continued)*

Interacting Drugs	*Adverse Effect*	*Probable Mechanism*
Amphotericin B with		
Aminoglycoside antibiotics	Nephrotoxicity	Synergism
Cyclosporine	Increased renal toxicity	Possible synergism
Digitalis glycosides	Increased digitalis toxicity	Hypokalemia
Neuromuscular blocking agents	Increased neuromuscular blocking effect	Hypokalemia
Cephalosporins with		
Alcohol	Disulfiram-like effect with cefamandole, cefoperazone, and moxalactam	Inhibition of intermediary metabolism of alcohol
Aminoglycoside antibiotics	Increased nephrotoxicity	Mechanism not established
Anticoagulants, oral	Possible increased anticoagulant effect with moxalactam or cefamandole	Mechanism not established
Aspirin	Possible increased bleeding risk with moxalactam	Additive
Ethacrynic acid	Increased nephrotoxicity	Mechanism not established
Furosemide	Increased nephrotoxicity	Mechanism not established
Heparin	Possible increased bleeding risk with moxalactam	Additive
Penicillins	Possible increased cefotaxime toxicity with azlocillin in patients with renal impairment	Decreased excretion
Vancomycin	Increased nephrotoxicity	Additive
Chloramphenicol with		
Acetaminophen	Possible decreased chloramphenicol effect	Increased metabolism
Anticoagulants (oral)	Increased dicumarol effect	Decreased metabolism
Barbiturates	Increased barbiturate effect; decreased chloramphenicol effect	Decreased metabolism Increased metabolism
Cimetidine	Aplastic anemia	Possibly additive or synergism
Etomidate	Prolonged anesthesia	Decreased metabolism
Hypoglycemics, sulfonylurea	Increased hypoglycemic effect	Mechanism not established
Phenytoin	Increased phenytoin toxicity Possible increased chloramphenicol toxicity	Decreased metabolism Mechanism not established
Rifampin	Decreased chloramphenicol effect	Increased metabolism
Clindamycin with		
Neuromuscular blocking agents	Increased neuromuscular blockade	Additive

(Continued)

ADVERSE DRUG INTERACTION INVOLVING ANTIMICROBIAL AGENTS (*Continued*)

Interacting Drugs	*Adverse Effect*	*Probable Mechanism*
Colistimethate, same as polymyxin B		
Cycloserine with		
Alcohol	Increased alcohol effect or convulsions	Mechanism not established
Isoniazid	CNS effects, dizziness, drowsiness	Mechanism not established
Erythromycins with		
Anticoagulant, oral	Hypoprothrombinemia potentiated	Possible decreased metabolism
Carbamazepine	Increased carbamazepine toxicity	Possibly decreased metabolism
Corticosteroids	Increased effect and possible toxicity of methylprednisolone	Decreased excretion
Cyclosporine	Increased cyclosporine toxicity	Probably decreased metabolism
Digoxin	Increased digoxin effect	Decreased gut metabolism and increased absorption
Ergot alkaloids	Increased ergot toxicity	Mechanism not established
Phenytoin	Possible increased or decreased effect	Altered metabolism
Theophyline	Increased theophylline effect and possible toxicity	Decreased metabolism
Fluoroquinolones with		
Antacids	Decreased fluoroquinolone effect with aluminum or magnesium antacids	Decreased absorption
Theophyllines	Possible theophylline toxicity	Decreased metabolism
Griseofulvin with		
Anticoagulants, oral	Decreased anticoagulant effect	Mechanism not established
Contraceptives, oral	Decreased contraceptive effect	Increased metabolism
Hydroxychloroquine with		
Digoxin	Increased digoxin effect	Mechanism not established
Isoniazid with		
Alcohol	Increased incidence of hepatitis	Mechanism not established
	Decreased isoniazid effect in some alcoholic patients	Increased metabolism
Aluminum antacids	Decreased isoniazid effect	Decreased absorption
Anticoagulants, oral	Possible increased anticoagulant effect	Decreased metabolism
Benzodiazepines	Pharmacologic effects of benzodiazepines may be increased; documented with diazepam and triazolam	Decreased metabolism
Carbamazepine	Increased toxicity of both drugs	Altered metabolism
Cycloserine	CNS effects, dizziness, drowsiness	Mechanism not established
Disulfiram	Psychotic episodes, ataxia	Altered dopamine metabolism
Enflurane	Possible nephrotoxicity	Increased metabolism of enflurane caused increased fluoride concentration
Ketoconazole	Decreased ketoconazole effect	Decreased concentration
Phenytoin	Increased phenytoin toxicity	Decreased metabolism
Rifampin	Possible increased isoniazid hepatotoxicity	Possible increased toxic metabolites
Ketoconazole with		
Alcohol	Possible disulfiram-like reaction	Mechanism not established
Antacids	Decreased ketoconazole effect	Decreased absorption
Anticoagulants, oral	Increased anticoagulant effect	Mechanism not established
Corticosteroids	Increased methylprednisolone effect	Decreased metabolism
Cyclosporine	Increased concentration of cyclosporine in blood	Mechanism not established
H_2 antagonists	Possible decreased antifungal effect	Decreased absorption
Isoniazid	Decreased ketoconazole effect	Decreased blood concentrations
Phenytoin	Altered effects of one or both drugs	Altered metabolism
Rifampin	Decreased rifampin and ketoconazole effects	Decreased blood concentrations
Lincomycin with		
Kaolin-pectin	Decreased lincomycin effect	Decreased absorption
Neuromuscular blocking agents	Increased neuromuscular blockade	Additive
Metronidazole with		
Alcohol	Mild disulfiram-like symptoms	Possible inhibition of intermediary metabolism of alcohol
Anticoagulants, oral	Increased anticoagulant effect	Decreased metabolism
Barbiturates	Decreased metronidazole effect with phenobarbital	Probably increased metabolism
Cimetidine	Possible increased metronidazole toxicity	Decreased metabolism
Disulfiram	Organic brain syndrome	Mechanism not established
Lithium	Lithium toxicity	Mechanism not established
Miconazole with		
Aminoglycosides	Possible decreased tobramycin concentration	Mechanism not established
Anticoagulants, oral	Increased anticoagulant effect	Mechanism not established
Hypoglycemics, sulfonylurea	Severe hypoglycemia	Mechanism not established
Phenytoin	Increased phenytoin toxicity	Decreased metabolism
Nalidixic acid with		
Anticoagulants, oral	Increased anticoagulant effect	Displacement from binding sites
Nitrofurantoin with		
Antacids	Possible decreased nitrofurantoin effect	Decreased absorption
Para-aminosalicylic acid, *see* aminosalicylic acid		
Penicillins with		
Allopurinol	Increased incidence of rash with ampicillin	Mechanism not established
Aminoglycosides	Decreased aminoglycoside effect with high concentrations of carbenicillin or ticarcillin	Inactivation
Anticoagulants, oral	Decreased anticoagulant effect with nafcillin and didoxacillin	Increased metabolism
β-Adrenergic blockers	Possible decreased atenolol effect with ampicillin	Decreased absorption
Cephalosporins	Possible increased cefotaxime toxicity with azlocillin in patients with renal impairment	Decreased excretion

(*Continued*)

ADVERSE DRUG INTERACTION INVOLVING ANTIMICROBIAL AGENTS *(Continued)*

Interacting Drugs	*Adverse Effect*	*Probable Mechanism*
Contraceptives, oral	Decreased contraceptive effect with ampicillin or oxacillin	Decreased enterohepatic circulation of estrogen
Lithium	Hypernatremia with ticarcillin	Large sodium load from ticarcillin and decreased renal excretion
Methotrexate	Possible increased methotrexate toxicity	Decreased excretion
Polymyxin B with		
Aminoglycoside antibiotics	Increased nephrotoxicity; increased neuromuscular blockade	Additive
Neuromuscular blocking agents	Increased neuromuscular blockade	Additive
Vancomycin	Increased nephrotoxicity	Additive
Rifampin with		
Aminosalicylic acid	Rifampin effectiveness may be decreased; separate doses by 8–12 h	Decreased GI absorption due to excipient bentonite
Anticoagulants, oral	Decreased anticoagulant effect	Increased metabolism
Barbiturates	Decreased barbiturate effect	Increased metabolism
Benzodiazepines	Possible decreased oral and IV diazepam effect	Increased metabolism
β-Adrenergic blockers	Decreased β-blocker effect	Increased metabolism
Chloramphenicol	Decreased chloramphenicol effect	Increased metabolism
Clofibrate	Pharmacologic effects of clofibrate may be decreased	Increased metabolism–enzyme induction
Contraceptives, oral	Decreased contraceptive effect	Increased metabolism
Corticosteroids	Decreased corticosteroid effect	Increased metabolism
Cyclosporine	Decreased cyclosporine effect	Increased metabolism
Digitalis	Decreased digitoxin and digoxin effect	Increased metabolism
Disopyramide	Decreased disopyramide effect	Probably increased metabolism
Hypoglycemics, sulfonylurea	Decreased hypoglycemic effect	Increased metabolism
Isoniazid	Possible increased hepatotoxicity	Possible increased toxic metabolites
Ketoconazole	Decreased effect of both drugs	Increased metabolism
Methadone	Methadone withdrawal symptoms	Increased metabolism
Mexiletene	Decreased antiarrhythmic effect	Increased metabolism
Phenytoin	Decreased phenytoin effect	Increased metabolism
Progestins	Decreased norethindrone effect	Increased metabolism
Quinidine	Decreased quinidine effect	Increased metabolism
Theophyllines	Decreased theophylline effect	Increased metabolism
Verapamil	Decreased verapamil effect	Increased metabolism
Spectinomycin with		
Lithium	Increased lithium toxicity	Decreased renal excretion
Sulfonamides with		
Anticoagulants, oral	Increased anticoagulant effect	Decreased metabolism and displacement from binding sites
Barbiturates	Increased thiopental effect	Decreased albumin binding
Cyclosporine	Decreased cyclosporine effect with sulfamethazine	Possibly increased metabolism
Digoxin	Possible decreased digoxin effect with sulfasalazine	Decreased digoxin absorption
Hypoglycemics, sulfonylurea	Increased hypoglycemic effect	Mechanism not established
Methotrexate	Possible increased methotrexate toxicity	Decreased renal clearance and displacement from binding
Monoamine oxidase inhibitors	Possible increased phenelzine toxicity with sulfisoxazole	Decreased metabolism
Phenytoin	Increased phenytoin effect, except possibly with sulfisoxazole	Decreased metabolism
Tetracyclines with		
Alcohol	Decreased doxycycline effect in alcoholics	Increased metabolism
Antacids, oral	Decreased oral tetracycline effects	Decreased tetracycline absorption
Anticoagulants, oral	Increased anticoagulant effect	Mechanism not established
Antidepressants, tricyclic	Localized hemosiderosis with amitriptyline and minocycline	Possible synergism
Barbiturates	Decreased doxycycline effect	Increased metabolism
Bismuth subsalicylate	Decreased tetracycline effect	Decreased absorption
Carbamazepine	Decreased doxycycline effect	Increased metabolism
Contraceptives, oral	Decreased contraceptive effect	Possible decreased enterohepatic circulation of estrogen
Digoxin	Increased digoxin effect	Decreased gut metabolism and increased absorption
Iron, oral	Decreased tetracycline effect, but not with doxycycline	Decreased absorption
	Decreased iron effect	Decreased absorption
Lithium	Increased lithium toxicity	Decreased renal excretion
Methotrexate	Possible increased toxicity	Displacement from binding
Molindone	Decreased tetracycline effect	Calcium as an excipient inhibits absorption
Phenformin	Increased lactic acidosis	Possible decreased phenformin excretion
Phenytoin	Decreased doxycycline effect	Increased metabolism
Rifampin	Possible decreased doxycycline effect	Increased metabolism
Theophyllines	Possible theophylline toxicity	Mechanism not established
Zinc sulfate	Decreased tetracycline effect	Decreased absorption
Thiabendazole with		
Theophyllines	Increased theophylline toxicity	Decreased metabolism
Trimethoprim with		
Amiloride	Trimethoprim may potentiate hyponatremia caused by the concomitant use of amiloride with thiazide diuretics	Additive
Azathioprine	Leukopenia	Mechanism not established
Cyclosporine	Increased nephrotoxicity	Synergism
Digoxin	Possible increased digoxin effect	Decreased renal excretion and possibly decreased metabolism
Thiazide diuretics	Trimethoprim may potentiate hyponatremia caused by the concomitant use of amiloride with thiazide diuretics	Additive

(Continued)

ADVERSE DRUG INTERACTION INVOLVING ANTIMICROBIAL AGENTS *(Continued)*

Interacting Drugs	*Adverse Effect*	*Probable Mechanism*
Trimethoprim-sulfamethoxazole with		
Anticoagulants, oral	Increased anticoagulant effect	Decreased metabolism
Antidepressants, tricyclic	Recurrence of depression	Mechanism not established
Lidocaine	Methemoglobinemia	Probably additive
Mercaptopurine	Decreased antileukemic effect	Mechanism not established
Methotrexate	Megaloblastic anemia	Additive inhibition of folate metabolism
Phenytoin	Increased phenytoin toxicity	Probably decreased metabolism
Pimozide	Decreased pimozide effect	Mechanism not established
Vancomycin with		
Aminoglycosides	Possible increased nephrotoxicity and ototoxicity	Possibly additive
Cephalosporins	Increased nephrotoxicity	Additive
Digoxin	Possible decreased digoxin effect	Possibly decreased absorption
Paromomycin	Increased nephrotoxicity	Additive
Polymyxins	Increased nephrotoxicity	Additive
Vidarabine with		
Allopurinol	Increased neurotoxicity	Decreased metabolism
Theophyllines	Increased theophylline effect	Decreased metabolism
Zidovudine with		
Acetaminophen	Granulocytopenia	Mechanism not established
Acyclovir	Neurotoxicity	Mechanism not established

(Data from Rizack et al.)

BIBLIOGRAPHY

Abramowicz M. Handbook of Antimicrobial Therapy. revised ed. New York: Medical Letter; 1986.

Anderson PO. Drugs and breast feeding: A review. Drug Intell Clin Pharm. 1977;11:208–23.

Bennett WM. Update on drugs in renal failure. In Advances in Nephrology. Chicago: Year Book Medical Publishers; 1986.

Bennett WM, Aronoff GR, Morrison G, et al. Drug prescribing in renal failure; dosing guidelines for adults. Am J Kidney Dis. 1983;3:155–93.

Biller JA, Yeager AM. The Harriet Lane Handbook. 9th ed. Chicago: Year Book Medical Publishers; 1981.

Briggs GG, Freeman RK, Yaffe SJ. Drugs in Pregnancy and Lactation. 2nd ed. Baltimore: Williams & Wilkins; 1986.

Keller F, Offerman G, Lode H. Supplementary dose after hemodialysis. Nephron. 1982;30:220–7.

Kucers A, Bennet NM. The Use of Antibiotics. 4th ed. London: William Heinemann; 1987.

Lorian V. Antibiotics in Laboratory Medicine. 2nd ed. Baltimore: Williams & Wilkins; 1986.

Manuel MA, Paton TW, Cornish WR. Drugs and peritoneal dialysis. Peritoneal Dialysis Bull 1983;117–25.

Matsuda SL. Transfer of antibiotics into maternal milk. Biol Res Preg. 1984;5:57–60.

McCracken GH, Nelson JD. Antimicrobial Therapy for Newborns. 2nd ed. New York: Grune & Stratton; 1983.

Nelson JD. 1987–1988 Pocketbook of Pediatric Antimicrobial Therapy. Baltimore: Williams & Wilkins; 1987.

Paton TW, Cornish WR, Manuel MA, et al. Drug therapy in patients undergoing peritoneal dialysis. Clin Pharmacokinet. 1985;10:404–26.

Peterson PK, Matzke G, Keane WF. Current concepts in the management of peritonitis in patients undergoing continuous ambulatory peritoneal dialysis. Rev Infec Dis. 1987;9:604–12.

Platzker ACD, Lew CD, Steward D. Drug administration via breast milk. Hosp Pract. 1980;15:111–22.

Reynolds JE, Prasad AB. Martindale The Extra Pharmacopoeia. 28th ed. London: Pharmaceutical Press; 1982.

Richards ML, Prince RA, Kenaley KA, et al. Antimicrobial penetration into cerebrospinal fluid. Drug Intell Clin Pharm. 1981;15:341–68.

Rizack MA, Hillman CDM: The Medical Letter Handbook of Adverse Drug Interactions. New York: Medical Letter; 1989:5–143.

Rollins DE, Klaassen DC. Biliary excretion of drugs in man. Clin Pharmacokinet. 1979;4:368–79.

Sanford JP. Guide to Antimicrobial Therapy United States of America. J.P. Sanford, M.D., 1988.

Schonfeld H, ed. Pharmacokinetics. Antibiot Chemother. 1978;25:1–320.

Schonfeld H, ed. Pharmacokinetics II. Antibiot Chemother. 1982;31:1–224.

Wilson JT, Brown RD, Cherek DR, et al. Drug excretion in human breast milk: Principles, pharmacokinetics and projected consequences. Clin Pharmacokinet. 1980;5:1–65.

MAJOR CLINICAL SYNDROMES

PART II

SECTION A. FEVER

39. PATHOGENESIS OF FEVER

CHARLES A. DINARELLO
SHELDON M. WOLFF

Fever is an elevation of temperature above the normal daily variation. Infections are most commonly associated with fever, but noninfectious causes such as inflammatory, neoplastic, and immunologically mediated diseases may also have fever as their primary clinical presentation. Fever is best understood at the hypothalamic level. The thermoregulatory center located in the anterior region of the hypothalamus regulates interal temperature at about 37°C (98.6°F) primarily by its ability to balance heat loss from the periphery with heat production from tissues, particularly the liver and muscles. During fever, the balance is adjusted to increase the internal temperature.

Individuals maintain body temperature at about 37°C despite wide variations in environmental temperatures. For some individuals, normal body temperature can be below or above 37°C without constituting a pathologic process. During a 24-hour period, body temperature varies from a low point in the early morning to the highest levels at 4–6 PM. The amplitude of this daily variation, also called the circadian temperature rhythm, is about 0.6°C (1°F), and individuals retain their circadian rhythm throughout life despite intervening bouts of prolonged illness. During fever, the morning low and evening high temperature pattern can still be observed. In the occasional situation in which elevated temperature is really hyperthermia (see below), this rhythm is absent.

Endogenous pyrogens are polypeptides produced by the host in response to infection, injury, inflammation, or antigenic challenge. These polypeptides cause fever by their ability to trigger biochemical changes in the hypothalamus, particularly prostaglandin synthesis. The first endogenous pyrogen described has now been identified as interleukin-1 (IL-1). Recombinant human IL-1s produce fever in experimental animals at doses of 100 ng/kg. Interferons (IFNs), produced as a consequence of viral infection, are also endogenous pyrogens. Recombinant human IFN-α produces chills and fever in humans. Two other endogenous pyrogens are tumor necrosis factor (TNF) and IL-6.

PYROGENS

Pyrogens are substances that cause fever and may be exogenous or endogenous.[1] Exogenous pyrogens are derived from outside the host, and the vast majority of exogenous pyrogens are microbial products, toxins, or the microbes themselves. The best studied of an exogenous pyrogen is the lipopolysaccharide produced by all gram-negative bacteria and commonly called "endotoxin." Endotoxins are large molecules (>300,000 daltons). Another group of bacterial substances that are potent pyrogens are produced by gram-positive organisms. There are the enterotoxins of *Staphylococcus aureus* and the group A streptococcal erythrogenic toxins. A staphylococcal toxin of clinical importance is the toxic shock syndrome toxin associated with strains of *S. aureus* isolated from patients with the toxic shock syndrome. The gram-positive exotoxins are polypeptides in the 20,000–30,000 dalton range. Like the endotoxins from gram-negative bacteria, the toxins produced by staphylococci and streptococci produce fever in experimental animals when injected intravenously in the submicrogram per kilogram range. Of considerable importance is the fact that endotoxin is a highly pyrogenic molecule in humans since 2–3 ng/kg produces fever and generalized symptoms in volunteers.[2]

ENDOGENOUS PYROGENS

In contradistinction to exogenous pyrogens, endogenous pyrogens are polypeptides produced by various host cells, particularly the monocyte/macrophage. They initiate fever by their ability to trigger the hypothalamic thermoregulatory center. Early concepts of the pathogenesis of fever proposed that exogenous pyrogens produced fever by their ability to act directly on the brain. This was later shown to be an unlikely explanation since there was a requirement for an intermediate role for leukocytes. It was subsequently shown that exogenous pyrogens produce fever by first inducing the release of endogenous pyrogens. Endogenous pyrogens then gain entrance to the circulation, either directly or through the lymph, and reach the hypothalamus. There they initiate a cascade of changes in arachidonic acid metabolites, neurotransmitters, and ions that raise the set-point.

It was originally believed that there was a single endogenous pyrogen characterized by its ability to produce fever in rabbits and other experimental animals. After the injection of endogenous pyrogen-containing leukocyte supernatants, there is a rapid rise in body temperature, usually within 5–10 minutes, whereas exogenous pyrogens cause a more delayed onset of fever. In addition, the fever-inducing property of endogenous pyrogens is destroyed by mild heat (70°C), whereas most exogenous pyrogens are more heat resistant.

Initial characterization of human endogenous pyrogen revealed two polypeptides with molecular weights of 14,000–15,000 daltons and two isoelectric points of 6.8 and 5.1. These have been subsequently respectively renamed IL-1β and IL-1α. The two IL-1s have been cloned,[3,4] their entire amino acid sequences are known, and recombinant IL-1s produce typical endogenous pyrogen fever when injected into animals. In rabbits, 50–100 ng/kg induces a peak rise of 0.5–0.8°C within 50 minutes.[1]

Other molecules have been cloned, and the recombinant forms have produced fever when injected into animals or humans. These are tumor necrosis factor (TNF-α),[5] lymphotoxin (TNF-β), IL-6,[6] and IFN-α.[1] Together with IL-1β and IL-1α, these substances can be classified as endogenous pyrogens or as endogenous *pyrogenic cytokines*. The term *cytokine* refers to polypepides produced by a variety of cells that induce biochemical changes in other cells. Each pyrogenic cytokine is a product of a separate gene; elevated plasma levels of some pyrogenic cytokines are found in humans during fever (discussed below).

Interleukin-1, TNF, IL-6, and IFN possess other biologic properties in addition to producing fever (discussed in the section on acute-phase responses). A wide spectrum of exogenous pyrogens induce the synthesis and release of these pyrogenic cytokines. These are listed in Table 1. Most of the exogenous pyrogenic substances can be recognized by their association with febrile diseases. In addition, there are substances produced by the host that cause fever because they stimulate the synthesis and release of the endogenous pyrogenic cytokines. For example, antigen–antibody complexes derived from blood incom-

TABLE 1. Organisms and Substances Inducing Pyrogenic Cytokines[a]

Viruses (influenza, Newcastle disease virus, cytomegalic disease virus)
Bacteria (whole cells, *Staphylococcus epidermidis, Borrelia burgdorferi*)
Peptidoglycans (cell walls of all bacteria)
Muramyl peptides (naturally occurring breakdown products of peptidoglycans)
Endotoxins (lipopolysaccharides of gram-negative bacteria)
Enterotoxins (A, B, C, D from *Staphylococcus aureus*)
Toxic shock syndrome toxin-1 (from toxic shock syndrome-associated *Staphylococcus aureus*)
Erythrogenic toxins (from group A streptococci)
Capsular polysaccharides (from *Cryptococcus neoformans*)
Yeasts (whole cells of *Candida albicans*, other yeasts)
Tuberculin (from mycobacteria in sensitive individuals)
Antigen–antibody complexes (requires the activation of complement)
Complement components (C5a, C3a)
Lymphocyte products (IL-2, interferons-γ^{b})
Polynucleic acids (poly I:C)
Pyrogenic steroids (etiocholanolone, bile salts)
Drugs (via the production of lymphocyte products in sensitized individuals, for example, penicillin)
Pyrogenic cytokines (IL-1, TNF)
Drugs (bleomycin)

[a] Data are derived from both in vitro and in vivo studies.
[b] Interferon-α augments the production of pyrogenic cytokines induced by microbial products.

patibility are pyrogens because they induce the production of IL-1 and TNF.

THE HYPOTHALAMIC CONTROL OF CORE TEMPERATURE

The control of body temperature in humans takes place at the hypothalamic level. Clusters of neurons located in both the preoptic anterior and posterior portions of the hypothalamus receive two kinds of signals: one pathway is from other neurons with connections in the periphery to cold and warm receptors. The other signal is provided by the temperature of the blood bathing the hypothalamic region. These signals are integrated by both "warm" and "cold" neurons whose discharge rate varies with the blood temperature and levels of several neurotransmitters. Together, the area is called the "thermoregulatory center." In health, this center maintains the body temperature of the internal organs between 37° and 38°C. This is the core temperature, and it is best measured in the esophagus close to the great vessels.

Parts of the brain and the liver can have a higher temperature, about 38°C, and the skin is maintained at a lower temperature. The lower temperature of the skin varies with the state of vasoconstriction and the distance to large arteries. Therefore, the axillary temperature tends to be about 1° lower (36°C) than the core temperature is. Oral and rectal temperatures reflect core temperature. Oral readings are probably lower because of mouth breathing, which is particularly important in patients with respiratory infections and rapid breathing. Freshly voided urine temperatures also can reflect the core temperature. In general, with the exception of young children, a correct measurement of the oral temperature is a very good approximation of the true core temperature in most clinical settings.

Using vasoconstriction, vasodilation, sweating, and at times, shivering, the body maintains its temperature in the face of moderate environmental cold or heat. However, these physiologic manipulations cannot overcome severe temperature differences in the environment. Thus the hypothalamic thermoregulatory center also sends signals to the cerebral cortex where behavioral changes such as seeking less severe environmental temperatures, special posturing, or the use of special clothing to help maintain normal body temperature are initiated. The metabolic rate of humans is constantly producing more heat than is necessary to maintain the core body temperature at 37°C; therefore, hypothalamic temperature control is often regulating the amount of heat loss by vasodilation and evaporation. In severe cold, the hypothalamus triggers rapid muscle contractions (shivering) to produce more heat.

Hyperthermia

Despite physiologic and behavioral control of body temperature, excessive heat production or the inability to lose heat may result in elevated core temperatures; this is called hyperthermia. For example, overinsulating clothing can result in elevated core temperatures. Thus, although most patients with elevated body temperatures have fever, there are instances in which an elevated temperature is not fever but hyperthermia.

Hyperthermia is an elevation of the core temperature at a time when the hypothalamic set-point is at normothermic levels. In hyperthermia, elevation of the core temperature occurs because heat loss mechanisms are inhibited or are not adequate. These include heat stroke syndromes in which excessive heat is produced by work or environmental conditions (such as high humidity) that prevent adequate heat loss. Certain metabolic diseases such as hyperthyroidism can result in mild elevations of core temperature. Some pharmacologic agents that interfere with thermoregulation by blocking sweating or vasodilation can also produce an elevation of the core temperature. Once again, these syndromes represent hyperthermia because they take place in the presence of a normal hypothalamic set-point. Hyperthermia characteristically does not respond to antipyretics. Even overinsulation of children can elevate the core temperature, which appears to be fever but is, in fact, hyperthermia.

In some patients the hypothalamic set-point is elevated owing to local trauma, hemorrhage, tumor, or intrinsic hypothalamic malfunction. The term *hypothalamic fever* is sometimes used to describe elevated temperatures caused by abnormal hypothalamic function. However, most patients with hypothalamic damage have *hypo*thermia or do not respond properly to mild environmental temperature changes. In those few patients in whom hypothalamic fever is suspected, a diagnosis depends on demonstrating other abnormal hypothalamic functions such as the production of hypothalamic releasing factors, an abnormal response to cold, and an absence of circadian temperature and hormonal rhythms. Hyperthermia can also occur when certain anesthetics produce a rapid uncoupling of oxidative phosphorylation in susceptible individuals. This is known as malignant hyperthermia[7] and is often fatal. Another form of hyperthermia is seen in patients taking certain neuroleptic drugs.[8]

There is no way to rapidly differentiate fever from hyperthermia. Clinical history usually plays an important role. However, in addition to the clinical history of the patient, there are aspects of some forms of hyperthermia that may alert the clinician; for example, in heat stroke syndromes and in patients taking drugs that block sweating, the skin is very hot but dry. Antipyretics do not reduce the elevated temperature in hyperthermia, whereas there is usually some decrease in body temperature in febrile patients after adequate doses of either aspirin or acetaminophen.

The Febrile Response

Fever is due to an upward shift of the set-point in the hypothalamus to febrile levels. In fever, the hypothalamic set-point is raised, and this triggers the vasomotor center to commence vasoconstriction. Blood is shunted from the periphery, essentially decreasing the usual heat loss and resulting in an increase in blood temperature. For most fevers, this is sufficient to raise body temperatures 2–3°C. Shivering is also triggered at this time in order to increase heat production from the muscles, but shivering is frequently not required if heat conservation mechanisms raise the blood temperature to the required level.

The processes of heat conservation and heat production continue until the temperature of the blood bathing the hypothalamic neurons matches the new setting. At that point, the hypothalamus maintains the new febrile temperature just as it does at normothermic levels. In fact, studies have shown that the mechanisms of heat balance in fever are the same as in the afebrile state, the only difference being that, in fever, the body temperature is maintained at the higher level.

When the hypothalamic set-point is reset downward, the processes of heat loss through vasodilation and sweating are initiated. Behavioral changes are also triggered at this time, and the removal of insulating clothing or bedding takes place.

Persistent fevers are sometimes classified as "intermittent" or "remittent"; intermittent fevers are characterized as daily fever spikes followed by a return to normal body temperature, whereas remittent fevers do not return to normal body temperatures. The biochemical or neurologic basis for these different fever patterns in some infectious diseases remains unknown.

Some hypothalamic substances have been reported to reduce fever; these include various neuropeptides such as somatostatin, arginine vasopressin,[9] and α-melanocyte–stimulating factor.[10] These substances appear to be produced in greater amounts during fever. In animal models, they suppress fever at the hypothalamic level and can be considered to function as intrinsic central antipyretics. For example, arginine vasopressin is thought to prevent fever in pregnant animals immediately before and after birth. In the pre-antibiotic era, fever due to a variety of infectious diseases rarely exceeded 106°F, and there has been speculation that this natural "thermal ceiling" is mediated by these neuropeptides functioning as central antipyretics. It is possible that an absence of the production of these natural antipyretics may account for the failure of some febrile patients to return to baseline body temperature.

Effect of Endogenous Pyrogenic Cytokines on the Hypothalamus

Each endogenous pyrogenic cytokine is a product of a separate gene. Interleukin-1β and IL-1α both recognize the IL-1 receptor, and TNF-α and TNF-β also share a common receptor. Receptors for these pyrogenic cytokines have been observed to be distributed in several areas in the brain, including the hypothalamus. There does not appear to be a particular concentration of cytokine receptors in the hypothalamus, but rather they appear throughout the brain.

During fever, hypothalamic tissue and third cerebral ventricle levels of prostaglandin E_2 (PGE_2) are elevated.[11] The highest concentrations of PGE_2 are near the circumventricular vascular organs (organum vasculosum lamina terminalis), which are networks of enlarged capillaries. Destruction of these organs reduces the ability of pyrogens to produce fever. Experiments have not been able to show, however, that pyrogenic cytokines pass from the circulation into the brain substance. Thus, it appears that endogenous pyrogens interact with the endothelium of these capillaries, which is probably the first step in initiating fever.

The interaction of endogenous pyrogens with the hypothalamic circumventricular vascular organs is poorly understood; however, cultured endothelial cells produce PGE when stimulated with IL-1 or TNF. In addition, these pyrogenic cytokines induce a variety of other changes in endothelial cells including increased adhesion of leukocytes, the release of platelet-activating factor, and the synthesis of plasminogen activator inhibitor.[1,12]

Figure 1 illustrates the key events in the generation of fever. Infections and toxins produced by many microorganisms stimulate the monocyte/macrophage to synthesize and release the various endogenous pyrogenic cytokines. As shown, other cells have the potential to produce these endogenous pyrogens. The pyrogenic cytokines cause fever by their ability to initiate metabolic changes in the hypothalamic thermoregulatory center. Of these, the synthesis of PGE_2 appears to play a critical role. The ability of systemic drugs such as aspirin to inhibit the synthesis of prostaglandins at the hypothalamic level accounts for their antipyretic effect. The elevation in the hypothalamic temperature set-point that is brought about by elevated prostaglandin levels triggers the brain centers controlling heat production and peripheral vascular tone. Neuronal transmission delivers this information to the periphery, and the core temperature begins to rise.

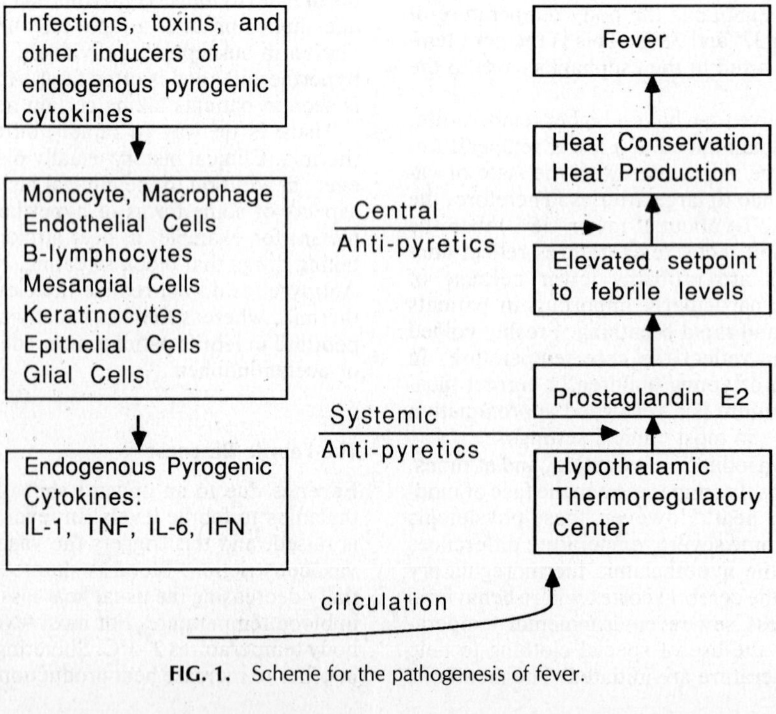

FIG. 1. Scheme for the pathogenesis of fever.

FEVER THERAPY

Throughout history, fever therapy has been used to treat a variety of diseases, both physical and psychological. Sometimes these therapies have been quite successful, for example, the treatment of tertiary syphilis with malarial fever, which brought its inventor a Nobel prize. Most often, however, fever therapies have been replaced with drugs for specific infections. Nevertheless, there is continued interest and investigation into fever therapy. One problem in interpreting the data of such studies is the need to differentiate fever therapy in which a pyrogen or infection induces a fever from what occurs in hyperthermic therapy in which the core temperature is elevated directly by applying heat or preventing its removal. The use of hyperthermia in the treatment of various malignancies is being used today with some success. In these situations, microwave energy is delivered to the patient, and the core temperature can be raised under controlled conditions. Hyperthermia is particularly successful when combined with chemotherapy or radiation. However, hyperthermia treatment should not be equated with fever therapy. In fever therapy, the inducing agent causes a febrile response, but in addition, a variety of pyrogenic and nonpyrogenic cytokines are produced that can affect the host defense.

ANTIPYRETIC THERAPY

There is a continuing debate on whether physicians should recommend reducing the elevated temperature that occurs in a variety of infectious diseases. A decision not to treat the fever may be based on evidence that the elevated temperature may offer the patient a benefit because under some experimental conditions host defense mechanisms are enhanced by an elevated temperature. Is this evidence sufficient to advise patients not to take antipyretics? Unfortunately, there are few human studies, and these do not show a dramatic difference in recovery from viral upper respiratory infections between groups taking or not taking antipyretics. There are, on the other hand, limited animal data and more extensive in vitro data that support the concept that certain host defense functions are enhanced by elevated temperatures. Temperatures of 39°C augment T- and B-cell responses, the generation of cytolytic T cells, B-cell activity, and immunoglobulin synthesis.[13,14] For example, in vitro microbial growth is suppressed at elevated temperatures, and lymphocyte activation and antibody formation are increased. But there are no studies showing that patients not taking antipyretics eliminate their viral infections faster or produce more antibodies. Witholding aspirin from children with viral-like illnesses appears warranted on the basis that this is a risk factor for the development of Reye syndrome. Children with fever, particularly those at risk for a febrile seizure, can be treated with acetaminophen.

An extraordinarily high fever (>41.5°C) is often called hyperpyrexia. Hyperpyrexia can be observed in patients with severe infections, but it most common occurs in patients with central nervous system hemorrhages. Antipyretics reduce the fever but because of the dangerously high temperatures, cooling blankets and water–alcohol bathing are employed to accelerate peripheral heat losses. There are effective means of reducing elevated temperatures, but in the absence of antipyretics that lower the hypothalamic set-point, peripheral cooling can be counterproductive since cold receptors in the skin send signals to the spinal cord and brain for reactive vasoconstriction, thus reducing heat loss mechanisms. Similarly, drugs such as atropine and other muscarinics block sweating and make heat loss more difficult.

Studies in patients receiving controlled hyperthermia treatment for various neoplasms have shown that temperatures as high as 42°C can be tolerated for 4 hours without irreversible organ damage. Nevertheless, fever increases the demand for oxygen and can aggravate pre-existing cardiac or pulmonary insufficiency. For every increase of 1°C over 37°C, there is a 13 percent increase in O_2 consumption. In addition, elevated temperatures can induce mental changes in patients with organic brain disease. Therefore, treatment of fever in some patient groups is recommended.

Children with previous febrile or nonfebrile seizures also should be aggressively treated to reduce fever. However, it is unclear what triggers the febrile seizure since there is no absolute correlation between the temperature elevation and the onset of a febrile seizure in susceptible children.

Antipyretics and the Treatment of Fever

The ability of the pyrogenic cytokines to induce PGE_2 synthesis is an important event in the production of fever. Numerous experiments have shown that the inhibitors of the cyclooxygenase enzyme system are potent antipyretics. There is a direct correlation of the antipyretic potency of various drugs and the inhibition of brain cyclooxygenase.[15] Acetaminophen is a poor cyclooxygenase inhibitor in peripheral tissue and is without noteworthy anti-inflammatory activity; however, in the brain acetaminophen is oxidized, and the oxidized form inhibits cyclooxygenase activity.[16,17] This oxidation explains the potent antipyretic effect of acetaminophen.

Studies have shown that there is no difference between oral aspirin and acetaminophen in reducing fever in humans. Nonsteroidal anti-inflammatory agents (indomethacin, ibuprofen, etc.) are also antipyretics and can be used for this purpose. Chronic high-dose antipyretic therapy such as aspirin or nonsteroidal anti-inflammatory agents used in arthritis does not reduce the normal core body temperature. Thus, there appears to be no role of PGE_2 in normal thermoregulation. There is some evidence in rats that the increase in body temperature that takes place during the day is, in part, due to cytokine release as a result of physical activity and is reducible by antipyretics. However, there are no similar studies in humans, and the evidence suggests that circadian variation in humans is unaffected by antipyretics.

Corticosteroids are also effective antipyretics. However, they act at two levels: (*1*) similar to the cyclooxygenase inhibitors, corticosteroids reduce PGE_2 synthesis by inhibiting the activity of phospholipase A_2, and (*2*) unlike the cyclooxygenase inhibitors, corticosteroids block the transcription of the mRNA for the pyrogenic cytokines. Drugs that interfere with vasoconstriction (phenothiazines, for example) can also act as antipyretics, as can drugs that block muscle contractions. However, these are not true antipyretics because they can also reduce the core temperature independently of hypothalamic control.

MEASUREMENT OF CIRCULATING PYROGENIC CYTOKINES

Radioimmunoassays (RIAs) and enzyme-linked immunosorbent assay (ELISA) kits for each pyrogenic cytokine are available commercially. Because the pyrogenic cytokines are products of blood leukocytes that are affected by the clotting process, the collection of freshly obtained plasma in the presence of protease inhibitors is preferred.[18] Although there are relatively few comprehensive studies on febrile patients, a pattern appears to be emerging: the height of temperature elevation does not correlate with the concentration of the cytokine in the circulation. For example, in human volunteers given an injection of endotoxin, the peak of the fever occurs 4 hours after intravenous injection, but the peak elevation in circulating TNF occurs after 90 minutes.[19] In these same studies, IL-1β concentrations in the plasma increase slowly and reach peak elevation after 180 minutes, whereas maximal IL-6 levels occur at 120 minutes.

In studies of septic patients, there is no correlation between the level of IL-1β and TNF in the same sample. This is supported by evidence showing that the genes for these two cytokines are independently regulated and are on two difference chromosomes. In patients receiving high-dose IL-2 therapy, plasma TNF, IL-1β, and IL-6 concentrations are elevated, but once again, these are not similarly elevated among the patients, and peak plasma levels do not correlate with the peak of the fever. Deficiencies in cytokine production in vitro from blood leukocytes have been described in various disease states.

Despite no overt evidence of fever or illness, some healthy individuals have elevated plasma TNF, IL-1, or IL-6 levels. Studies do show that some of the pyrogenic cytokines are elevated in burns, sepsis, malaria, exacerbations of rheumatoid arthritis,[20] and renal allograft rejection. They are also elevated after strenuous exercise and ovulation.[21]

Pyrogenic cytokines may be present in the circulation but bound to carrier molecules that reduce or prevent interaction with the capillary network in the hypothalamic thermoregulatory center. There is evidence to support this concept since IL-1β requires extraction from plasma proteins such as α_2-macroglobulin before being assayed.[18] The concentration of cytokine-binding proteins appears to increase in chronic diseases and may be due to an increased production of hepatic acute-phase proteins.

Aspirin and nonsteroidal anti-inflammatory agents prevent fever but do not prevent the synthesis and release of pyrogenic cytokines. In fact, the in vitro production of the pyrogenic cytokines from blood leukocytes from human subjects taking oral cyclooxygenase inhibitors is enhanced. Hence, it is possible to measure elevated plasma cytokine levels in individuals who are afebrile because of antipyretic therapy. There are no studies on plasma pyrogenic cytokine levels as a function of diurnal temperature variation; however, preprandial and postprandial levels of IL-1β are within the coefficient of variation.

ACUTE PHASE CHANGES

Infections, trauma, inflammatory processes, and some malignant diseases induce a constellation of host responses that are collectively referred to as the "acute-phase response." This response is associated with characteristic metabolic changes in liver protein synthesis, but on closer examination, changes also occur in several other systems including the hematologic, endocrinologic, neurologic, and immunologic. These changes are called acute because most are observed within hours or days after the onset of infection or injury. The full spectrum of the response includes dramatic increases in the synthesis of several unique hepatic proteins that are not produced in health. One of these, C-reactive protein, is a marker of the acute-phase response and can be used as an indicator of disease. The increased plasma concentrations of acute-phase hepatic proteins, glycoproteins, and globulins are responsible for elevated erythrocyte sedimentation rates. Increases in gluconeogenesis, energy expenditure, and muscle proteolysis occur and contribute to the weight loss. Increased sleep and lethargy are frequent clinical complaints. Thyroid dysfunction can be present, and there is often abnormal glucose tolerance and lipid metabolism. In addition, anemia develops despite adequate stores of iron. This may be due to the suppressive effect of TNF on hematopoiesis. The hypergammaglobulinemia that is often a component of the acute-phase response may be mediated by IL-6. This pyrogenic cytokine induces hepatic acute-phase protein synthesis.[22] and is a potent B-lymphocyte growth and differentiation factor.

Although the most striking changes in the acute-phase response is observed in patients with bacterial infections, burns, or multiple injuries, clinicians also encounter acute-phase changes in patients with occult infections or chronic illnesses such as rheumatoid arthritis, Crohn's disease, and several autoimmune diseases. The presence of acute-phase changes can also serve as an indicator of silent cancers, particularly renal cell carcinoma and Hodgkin's disease. The various components of the response are remarkably consistent despite the considerable variety of pathologic processes that induce it. For example, plasma levels of several acute-phase proteins are elevated after myocardial infarction, a bone fracture, or bacterial pneumonia.

The pyrogenic cytokines IL-1,[23,24] TNF,[25] IL-6,[22] and to a lesser extent, INF-α can induce, in part, many of the acute-phase changes in animals that are observed in humans. Interferon-α is produced primarily during viral infections. Although it shares with IL-1, TNF, and IL-6 the ability to produce fever, sleep, and lethargy, IFN-α does not induce hepatic acute-phase protein synthesis. Thus, elevated erythrocyte sedimentation rates and neutrophilia are not commonly observed during viral infections. Interferon-γ, produced during immunologic reactions such as organ transplant rejection and drug fever, induces some hepatic acute-phase proteins in vitro but, like IFN-α, is a weak inducer of acute-phase changes in the liver. Table 2 compares the multiple biologic effects of the different cytokines involved in acute-phase responses.

The patient with a localized bacterial infection represents an excellent example of the development of the acute-phase response. At the onset of the infection, blood monocytes and tissue macrophages become activated either by phagocytosis of the invading microbe or by exposure to its products or toxins; the process results in the synthesis and release of the pyrogenic cytokines. These mediators enter the circulation and reach the brain where they initiate fever. Although fever is clearly one of the most obvious signs of the acute-phase response, other components of the response can be present without apparent clinical manifestations. One of the most sensitive measures of the acute-phase response is an increase in the number and immaturity of circulating neutrophils. The release of neutrophils is due to the direct action of IL-1 on the bone marrow neutrophil stores. In addition, IL-1 stimulates stem cells to become more responsive to various colony-stimulating factors. In human subjects injected with small doses of endotoxin, marked neutrophilia can be measured in the absence of fever. Serum zinc and iron levels are depressed. Low serum iron levels associated with anemia in the face of adequate iron stores is characteristic of the acute-phase response. A decreased serum iron content probably plays an important role in protecting the host against various bacteria. For example, the reduction in serum iron concentration can suppress the growth rate of several microorganisms and certain tumor cells that have a strict requirement for iron as a growth factor.

Within 8–12 hours after the onset of infection or trauma, the liver increases the synthetic rate of the so-called acute-phase proteins. The response includes increases in protein levels nor-

TABLE 2. Biologic Properties of IL-1, TNF, and IL-6

Biological Property	*IL-1*[a]	*TNF*[b]	*IL-6*
Endogenous pyrogen	+	+	+
Hepatic acute-phase proteins	+	+	+
Decreased albumin synthesis	+	+	+
Fibroblast proliferation	+	+	+
B-lymphocyte activation	+	+	+
T-lymphocyte activation	+	+	+
B-lymphocyte immunoglobulin synthesis	+	+	+
Hematopoietic stem cell activation	+	−	+
Nonspecific resistance to infection	+	+	+
Radioprotection	+	+	−
Endothelial cell activation	+	+	−
Synovial cell stimulation	+	+	−
Bone resorption	+	+	−
Induction of IL-1 and TNF	+	+	−
Induction of IL-6	+	+	−

[a] Data derived from recombinant IL-1β or IL-1α.
[b] Similar data obtained using either TNF-α or TNF-β (lymphotoxin).

mally found in health as well as the appearance of new proteins that serve as markers of a pathologic event.[26] Several normal plasma proteins increase severalfold during the acute-phase response. These include haptoglobin, certain protease inhibitors, complement components, ceruloplasmin, and fibrinogen. However, true acute-phase reactants increase several hundredfold. These include serum amyloid A protein (a precursor of the amyloid fibril in secondary amyloidosis) and C-reactive protein. C-reactive protein was named for its ability to interact with the C-polysaccharide of pneumococci and was the first acute-phase protein described. Albumin and cytochrome synthesis is depressed during acute-phase responses.[26]

Of all the acute-phase proteins, C-reactive protein and serum amyloid A protein are clinically the most important because their presence serves as an indicator of disease. These proteins are structurally related. C-reactive protein is particularly useful as a marker of the hepatic acute-phase protein response and can be measured easily in most clinical laboratories.

Despite the anabolic processes of the liver, the acute-phase response is accompanied by a pronounced catabolism of muscle protein that is associated with a loss of body weight and an overall negative nitrogen balance.[27] Fever increases oxygen and caloric demands, and a negative nitrogen balance can result from the oxidation of amino acids from skeletal muscle, which contributes to wasting. These amino acids are largely used for gluconeogenesis. In addition, there can be demineralization of bone. Although the metabolic demands of elevated temperature contribute to the increased need for energy substrates, the host also requires a large supply of amino acids for the synthesis of new protein at a time when food intake may be severely impaired or appetite reduced. Amino acids are required for immunologic and reparative processes such as the clonal expansion of lymphocytes and the proliferation of fibroblasts. Also, they are needed for the synthesis of hepatic acute-phase proteins, immunoglobulins, and collagen. The mechanism of providing ample amino acids for these cellular functions seems to be well orchestrated during the acute-phase response. The catabolism during infection and inflammation differs from that of starvation. Unlike starvation, in which large amounts of ketones are spilled into the urine, a septic individual excretes protein with small amounts of ketones. Interleukin-1 and TNF inhibit lipoprotein lipase and hence interfere with lipid metabolism.

In addition to the biochemical changes during acute-phase responses, appetite is depressed. In fact, a depressed appetite may play a greater role in the negative nitrogen balance of chronic disease than the mobilization of tissue does. Interleukin-1 and TNF are potent suppressors of appetite in animals.

The presence of certain acute-phase changes in an otherwise healthy individual can alert the physician to hidden disease. Measuring the levels of adrenocorticotropic hormone (ACTH), cortisol, growth hormone, and vasopressin is not particularly useful, although they are elevated during acute-phase responses. Measurement of C-reactive protein can assist the physician in determining the presence of disease in patients with vague, constitutional complaints. C-reactive protein levels are usually less than 100 μg/liter but increase within hours 10- to 1000-fold. In severe bacterial infections, the serum level can rise from undetectable to over 100 mg/liter in 48 hours. The presence of elevated levels of C-reactive protein or serum amyloid A protein, even in the absence of fever or neutrophilia, may indicate occult infection or malignant change. Increases in C-reactive protein and serum amyloid A protein occur in patients of any age and also in immunocompromised patients with opportunistic infections.

Not all inflammatory diseases are associated with elevated C-reactive protein levels. Patients with scleroderma, ulcerative colitis, and lupus erythematosus may not show rises in C-reactive protein levels. A failure to develop hepatic protein changes and the neutrophilia of the acute-phase response seems to be related to the presence of circulating inhibitors of IL-1 and TNF.

The role of acute-phase proteins in host defense and repair is not entirely clear. Studies suggest that the major role of C-reactive protein is to bind serum lipids or opsonize pneumococci, whereas serum amyloid A is thought to be immunosuppressive. Ceruloplasmin scavenges toxic free oxygen radicals that are injurious to many tissues. What is clear, however, is that the production and physical structure of these acute-phase proteins have been conserved through 400 million years of evolution, and therefore they have presumably been useful to the host. This argues that the acute-phase response, like fever, is a positive aspect of the host defense against infection.

REFERENCES

1. Dinarello CA, Cannon JG, Wolff SM. New concepts on the pathogenesis of fever. Rev Infect Dis. 1988;10:168–89.
2. Wolff SM. Biological effects of bacterial endotoxins in man. J Infect Dis. 1973;128(Suppl):733.
3. Auron PE, Webb AC, Rosenwasser LJ, et al. Nucleotide sequence of human monocyte interleukin-1 precursor cDNA. Proc Natl Acad Sci USA. 1984;81:7907.
4. Lomedico PT, Gubler U, Hellmann CP, et al. Cloning and expression of murine interleukin-1 cDNA. Nature. 1984;312:458.
5. Dinarello CA, Cannon JG, Wolff SM, et al. Tumor necrosis factor (cachectin) is an endogenous pyrogen and induces interleukin-1. J Exp Med. 1986;163:1433–50.
6. Helle M, Brakenhoff JP, DeGroot ER, et al. Interleukin-6 is involved in interleukin-1–induced activities. Eur J Immunol. 1988;18:957.
7. Smith RJ. Malignant hyperthermia. Preoperative assessment of the risk factors. Br J Anaesth. 1988;60:317.
8. Allsop P, Twigley AJ. The neuroleptic malignant syndrome. Case report with a review of the literature. Anesthesia. 1987;42:49.
9. Naylor AM, Ruwe WD, Veale WL. Antipyretic action of centrally administered arginine vasopressin but not oxytocin in the cat. Brain Res. 1986;385:156.
10. Lipton JM, Clark WG. Neurotransmitters in temperature control. Annu Rev Physiol. 1986;48:613.
11. Coceani F, Lees J, Bishai I. Further evidence implicating prostaglandin E_2 in the genesis of pyrogen fever. Am J Physiol. 254:R463, 1988;254:463.
12. Dejana E, Breviario F, Erroi A, et al. Modulation of endothelial cell function by different molecular species of interleukin-1. Blood. 1987;69:695–9.
13. Duff GW, Durum SK. Fever and immunoregulation: Hyperthermia, interleukin-1 and 2, and T-cell proliferation. Yale J Biol Med. 1982;55:437.
14. Hanson DF, Murphy PA, Silicano R, et al. The effect of temperature on the activation of thymocytes by interleukin-1 and interleukin-2. J Immunol. 1983;130:216.
15. Flower R, Vane JR. Inhibition of prostaglandin synthetase in brain explains the anti-pyretic activity of paracetamol. Nature. 1972;240:410.
16. Peterson RG. Consequences associated with nonnarcotic analgesics in the fetus and newborn. Fed Proc. 1985;44:2309.
17. Harvison PJ, Egan RW, Gale PH, et al. Acetaminophen and analogs as cosubstrates and inhibitors of prostaglandin H synthetase. Chem Biol Interact. 1988;64:251.
18. Cannon JG, Van der Meer JWM, Kwiatkowski D, et al. Interleukin-1β in human plasma: Optimization of blood collection, plasma extraction and radioimmunoassay. Lymphokine Res. 1988;7:457–67.
19. Michie HR, Manogue KR, Spriggs DR, et al. Detection of circulating tumor necrosis factor after endotoxin administration. N Engl J Med. 1988;318:1481–6.
20. Eastgate JA, Symons JA, Wood NC, et al. Correlation of plasma interleukin-1 levels with disease activity in rheumatoid arthritis. Lancet. 1988;2:706.
21. Cannon JG, Dinarello CA. Increased plasma interleukin-1 activity in women after ovulation. Science. 1985;227:1247–49.
22. Gauldie J, Richards C, Harnish D, et al. Interferon beta-2/B-cell stimulating factor type 2 shares identity with monocyte-derived hepatocyte stimulating factor and regulates the major acute phase protein response in liver cells. Proc Natl Acad Sci USA. 1987;84:7251.
23. Dinarello CA. The biology of interleukin-1. FASEB J. 1988;2:108.
24. Ramadori G, Sipe JD, Dinarello CA, et al. Pretranslational modulation of acute phase hepatic protein synthesis by murine recombinant interleukin-1 and purified human IL-1. J Exp Med. 1985;162:930–42.
25. Perlmutter DH, Dinarello CA, Punsal PI, et al. Cachectin/tumor necrosis factor regulates hepatic acute-phase gene expression. J Clin Invest. 1986;78:1349–54.
26. Pepys MB, Baltz ML. Acute phase proteins with special reference to C-reactive protein and related proteins (pentaxins) and serum amyloid A protein. In: Dixon FJ, Kunkel HG, eds. Advances in Immunology. v. 34. New York: Academic Press; 1983:141–211.
27. Beisel WR. Magnitude of the host nutritional responses to infection. Am J Clin Nutr. 1977;30:1236–47.

40. FEVER OF UNKNOWN ORIGIN

CHARLES A. DINARELLO
SHELDON M. WOLFF

Fever is such a common manifestation of illness that it is not surprising to find accurate descriptions of the febrile patient in early recorded history. There is evidence that the symbol of a flaming brazier was used by the ancient Sumerians to denote fever and that cuneiform inscriptions of the sixth century BC had adapted this symbol into a single ideogram for fever and inflammation.[1] By the time of Hippocrates and later during the Roman Empire, physicians were so well acquainted with the signs and symptoms of febrile diseases that their detailed descriptions of typhoid and malarial fevers can still be used as examples of these protracted fevers. However, only some fevers of prolonged nature can be diagnosed from descriptive histories, and most patients with long-standing fevers require a careful and thorough investigation. Today, the physician charged with the problem of determining the cause of a prolonged fever must consider the spectrum of febrile diseases, which, through the years, has changed under the influence of nutritional, hygienic, and environmental effects. In addition, age, geographic location, and iatrogenic involvement are also important factors that play a role in determining the cause of prolonged fever.

In most patients with fever lasting 1 or 2 weeks, the underlying cause is soon discovered or the patient recovers spontaneously. In the latter case, a protracted viral illness is usually presumed to be the source of the fever. In other patients, however, fever continues for 2 or 3 weeks during which time physical examination, chest x-ray films, blood tests, and routine cultures do not reveal the cause of fever. In these patients a provisional diagnosis of fever of unknown origin (FUO) is made. Some physicians, for the purpose of retrospective studies, have set strict criteria for undiagnosed, febrile illness to be classified as a FUO. In general, a patient may be considered to have a FUO if a cause of the fever cannot be found after 2 to 3 weeks despite thorough physical examination and related laboratory tests. Although a provisional diagnosis of FUO is made after 2 weeks of fever, many patients with FUO have fever for months and some more than a year. In the latter situation, the fever is often present for varying periods of time, disappears, and returns again.

In some studies, FUO has been defined as a daily elevation in oral temperature of 100.2°F (38°C) or higher for 3 weeks without an identified cause. Since the daily rhythm in core temperature varies from individual to individual, we believe that an FUO is best defined when considering the normal temperature rhythm for the patient and the presence of an associated pathologic change. Chronic fatigue syndrome, previously called chronic Epstein-Barr infection, has attracted considerable attention recently; one of the major clinical complaints of this syndrome is recurrent "feverish feelings."[2] Most patients are afebrile, and even those with fever have temperatures generally below 101°F.

There are no shortcuts in determining the cause of a FUO. Only a well-organized systematic approach that is carried out with an awareness of the multiple causes of fever shortens the duration of the investigation. In this regard, reports on patients with FUOs have been helpful, since they call attention to both the varied causes and incidence of long-standing fevers. From these studies several general conclusions can be made. It is best to divide patients into three age groups: under 6 years; 6–14 years; and over 14 years. Patients under 6 years of age have a high incidence of infection, primarily upper respiratory or urinary tract and systemic-viral, while collagen–vascular diseases and inflammatory bowel disease are the most prevalent causes in the 6-to 16-year age group (Table 1). Rheumatic fever as a cause of FUO in American children has decreased in the last 2 decades, although recent reports suggest that the incidence of rheumatic fever in the USA may be rising again. On the other hand, the incidence of tuberculosis as a cause of FUO in children has dropped less sharply.

In adults, infections are also the most common cause of FUO. Using studies made in the antibiotic era only, Table 2 indicates that infection predominates as the most frequently diagnosed source of persistent fever. However, it can be generally stated that as the duration of fever increases, the likelihood of an infectious cause decreases. This statement has been substantiated by studies of patients with FUOs lasting for longer than 1 year in which infections were the third most common cause of the FUO.[12] Following infections, malignancies compose the next most frequent source of FUO in adults. Recent studies on large groups of patients with FUOs have been reported.[13–16] In general, infectious causes of FUO are still as common, but malignancies are increasingly identified as the cause of FUOs. This is not the case, however, in children. Nevertheless, in both adults and children with neoplastic disease as a source of fever, lymphomas and leukemias are the most prevalent. The third most common diagnosis in adult patients with FUO is collagen–vascular disease. The actual incidence of collagen–vascular disease in patients with FUO is possibly higher than is shown in Table 2, since some studies limit this diagnosis to systemic lupus erythematosus, rheumatoid arthritis, and systemic vasculitis. It may be better to classify these diseases as autoimmune rather than collagen–vascular. It is useful then to consider the three major causes of FUO, i.e., infection, malignancy, and autoimmune disease, since more than 70 percent of patients fall into one of these three groups. However, there are many diseases that have been grouped in studies as "miscellaneous," and in adults these include drug fever,[17] erythema multiforme, granulomatous hepatitis, regional enteritis, pulmonary embolism, sarcoidosis, familial Mediterranean fever, Fabry's disease, hypertriglyceridemia, alcoholic hepatitis, and factitious fever.[18–20] In children, miscellaneous causes of FUO have been milk allergy, Behçet syndrome, and heavy metal intoxication. Although fever can be the presenting sign of the initial infection with human immunodeficiency virus (HIV), most FUOs in these patients are due to other infectious agents. Because of the high incidence of unusual infections in HIV-infected patients, any patient from a high-risk group seeking medical attention for an FUO requires a test for the presence of HIV antibodies.

Other important factors in determining the causes of FUO are the type of institution in which the patient is evaluated. A tertiary care facility may see more unusual illness because of the nature of their referral patterns. Inner city hospitals may have much higher incidence of infectious disease since patients may lack proper evaluation or therapy before being seen in the hospital. In the same type of hospital, adult patients may be older and thus more likely to have a malignant neoplasm as a cause of their FUO. Thus, other factors such as economics, race, geography, and so forth may determine the distribution of diagnoses in a given report.

In patients in whom fever persists for longer than 6 months without an identifiable source, the spectrum of diagnoses is different. In these patients a high incidence of granulomatous disease has been seen as well as the adult manifestation of Still's disease.[21] The diagnoses in these patients are shown in Table 3. In all studies, there is a group of patients in whom diagnosis cannot be made after years of fever, and the diagnosis remains FUO. A few of these patients may have abnormal hypothalamic thermoregulation, but in most patients this diagnosis remains speculative. Factitious fevers are consistently reported in studies on FUO, and these include adults and children. Also in-

TABLE 1. Fever of Unknown Origin in Children

References	Dates of Study	No. of Cases	Established Causes (%) Infections	Collagen–Vascular Disease	Neoplasms	Miscellaneous	Undiagnosed
McClung[3]	1959–69	99	29	11	8	19	32
Pizzo, Lovejoy, and Smith[4]	1966–72	100	52	20	6	10	12
Lohr and Hendley[5]	1967–74	54	33	18	13	15	19

TABLE 2. Fever of Unknown Origin in Adults

References	Dates of Study	No. of Cases	Established Causes (%) Infections	Collagen–Vascular Disease	Neoplasms	Miscellaneous	Undiagnosed
Petersdorf and Beeson[6]	1952–57	100	36	13	19	25	7
Sheon and Van Ommen[7]	1959–60	60	21	13	6	20	40
Deal[8]	1970	34	35	15	20	9	20
Frayha and Uwaydah[9]	1967–70	49	43	14	27	6	10
Howard, Hahn, Palmer, and Hardin[10]	1969–76	100	37	19	31	8	5
Larson, Featherstone, and Petersdorf[11]	1970–80	105	30	16	31	10	12

TABLE 3. Prolonged Fever of Unknown Origin[a]

	Percentage of Cases
No fever[b]	27
FUO	19
Miscellaneous	13
Factitious	9
Granulomatous hepatitis	8
Neoplasm	7
Still's disease	6
Infections	6
Colagen–vascular disease	4
Familial Mediterranean fever	3

[a] Evaluation of 347 patients studied from 1961 to 1977 at the National Institutes of Health.[2] Fever was present for more than 1 year in 75 percent of the cases (mean = 4 years).[3]
[b] Includes patients with exaggerated circadian temperature rhythm.

cluded in the diagnosis of a factitious fever are patients who inject themselves with contaminated materials.[22]

Searching for the underlying cause of prolonged fever requires an open mind and a carefully organized approach by the physician. Since most patients who receive a provisional diagnosis of FUO have no obvious source of fever, we recommend an investigation that includes certain clinical tests that can be considered "routine" for these patients. The work-up may be divided into the following categories: (*1*) observation of temperature pattern, (*2*) historical aspects, (*3*) physical examinations, (*4*) laboratory tests, (*5*) noninvasive procedures, and (*6*) invasive procedures.

TEMPERATURE PATTERN

It is important to establish that the patient with a presumptive diagnosis of FUO is, in fact, having fever. There are a few patients who seek medical assistance with a chief complaint of persistent fever and, on closer investigation, do not have fever but rather an exaggerated circadian temperature rhythm. This conclusion can be reached by measuring the daily temperature at approximately 6 AM and 6 PM.[23] In the absence of associated symptoms like sweating, chills, and elevated pulse rate and in the absence of abnormal laboratory, radiologic, or physical findings, these patients can be considered to be normal. In a large series of patients referred to us at the National Institutes of Health with a presumptive diagnosis of FUO for longer than 6 months, 27 percent failed to manifest evidence of ongoing disease during the 2–3 weeks of inpatient observation.[12] In fact, many patients with so-called benign fever of unknown origin probably belong in this category.[24] It is not uncommon for children of overly concerned parents or from troubled families to seek medical work-up for nonexistent fever that they consider "low grade."

Fever patterns have been classified as continuous, remittent, and intermittent; however, observation and characterization of fever patterns have little or no significance in the diagnosis of prolonged fevers. There are two notable exceptions: malaria and cyclic neutropenia. To a lesser extent the fever associated with Hodgkin's disease (Pel-Ebstein) may be helpful in making this diagnosis. The well-synchronized malarial paroxysm can be used to help to make a diagnosis of malaria, although demonstration of the malarial parasite in blood smears is required for diagnostic confirmation. In nonendemic areas, well-synchronized malarial fevers are rarely seen, and this diagnosis is usually suspected on learning of recent travel to malaria-infested areas.[25] Patients with tertian malaria (fever every other day) and quartan malaria (fever on day 1 and day 4 and so forth) can have low-grade fever in between the paroxyms, and most new malarial infections take 1–2 weeks before the paroxyms are synchronized.

The other fever pattern that is most suggestive of a specific diagnosis consists of a 21-day cycle. This fever accompanies cyclic neutropenia in which the peripheral neutrophil count falls to very low levels every 21 days.[26] It is common for these patients to have concurrent ulcers of the mucous membranes.

Other fevers that have been previously considered to be periodic are those of familial Mediterranean fever and Hodgkin's disease. Although such fevers can occur at regular intervals, patients with these diseases do not have a strict periodicity to their fevers like those of malaria or cyclic neutropenia but rather periods of no fevers or irregular fevers.

HISTORICAL ASPECTS

Clues to the diagnosis of certain febrile diseases may be obtained from historical characteristics and symptoms; examples include transient skin rashes in patients with autoimmune and collagen–vascular disease, the injection of medications in patients with drug fever, and hematuria in patients with renal cell carcinoma. Since patients with FUO often have atypical manifestations of their diseases, many symptoms are present only transiently and are not easily recalled during routine questioning. History of other symptoms such as myalgias, malaise, rigors, sweating, and weight loss may be nonspecific in that they are characteristic of elevated body temperature due to a diversity of causes.

Travel and exposure to certain agents or animals is critical information needed to make a diagnosis of several febrile diseases. For example, in the period from 1970 to 1975 there was a threefold increase in the number of civilian cases of malaria imported into the United States.[25] Clearly, knowledge of travel to regions where malaria is indigenous can be key in suspecting this disease. Knowledge of tick bites is often absent in some cases of tick-transmitted diseases, but awareness of the endemic tick-infested areas is valuable even when the patient denies a tick bite. Certain parts of the United States are endemic areas for *Coccidioides, Histoplasma,* and *Blastomyces,* and the diagnosis of disease due to these organisms can be aided by a history of travel to such areas. Occupational hazards are important aspects of an accurate history. For example, exposure to beryllium can lead to a febrile illness, and knowledge of such exposure should expedite the diagnostic work-up of patients with berylliosis.

PHYSICAL EXAMINATION

There is no substitute for a complete physical examination in evaluating a patient with FUO. Furthermore, these patients require repeated physical examinations on a regular basis during investigation into their disease. Such patients may develop skin lesions, fundoscopic changes, organomegaly, and masses late in the course of their disease. All too often patients receive a thorough physical examination at the time of initial medical evaluation for persistent fever, and subsequently the caring physician focuses on laboratory and other diagnostic procedures, never returning to the bedside to repeat the entire physical examination. There are some areas in particular that require almost daily inspection, and these include examination of the skin, eyes, nail beds, lymph nodes, and abdomen, and auscultation of the heart. The rashes of Still's disease are usually faint and fade quickly, the skin lesions of patients with systemic vasculidites who have an FUO may appear late in the disease and in very few numbers. Atypical areas, for example under the scrotal and breast folds, must be inspected for a complete examination of the skin. To make a diagnosis of vasculitis, the involved skin lesion must be located and a biopsy must be done.

Regular inspection of the peripheral lymph nodes is necessary. Many febrile diseases involving the lymph nodes that manifest as FUO may involve only a single node. Illnesses such as Hodgkin's disease, toxoplasmosis, or infectious mononucleosis can manifest atypically with a single node enlargement.[27] Draining lymph nodes of the head and neck, breast, and pelvic regions can be involved in neoplastic and infectious processes in these areas.

The importance of a complete eye examination in patients with FUO cannot be overstated. Because many FUOs manifest with no apparent localizing symptoms and because the eye is often involved in systemic disease, proper examination of the eye is indicated in every patient with prolonged fevers even in the absence of ophthalmalogic symptoms. Examination of the eye can be divided into the orbit, cornea, conjunctiva, uveal tract, and retina. Proptosis due to orbital involvement can be seen in isolated lymphomas of the orbit, retrorbital granulomatous disease such as Wegener's granulomatosis, neurofibromas, and metastatic disease to the orbit.

Band keratopathy can be seen in children with Still's disease and sarcoidosis. Punctate epithelial loss associated with tear deficiency and dry eyes is a striking finding of rheumatoid arthritis and can be an initial sign of lupus erythematosus and other collagen–vascular diseases. Marginal ulceration of the cornea can be observed in arteritides as an early manifestation of these diseases.[28]

Conjunctival lesions can be present in several systemic infections, especially viral and chlamydial infections.[29] Frank conjunctivitis can accompany tuberculosis, syphilis, tularemia, fungal infections (particularly histoplasmosis), cat-scratch fever, erythema multiforme, and erythema nodosum. Petechial hemorrhages associated with bacterial endocarditis are often observed in conjunctival as well as in retinal vessels.

The uveal tract is often involved in granulomatous as well as nongranulomatous diseases. The latter include lupus erythematosus, vasculidites, serum sickness, and other hypersensitivity diseases. Sarcoidosis, toxoplasmosis, syphilis, tuberculosis, and Still's disease can result in significant uveitis. Thus, a slit-lamp examination is desirable in the evaluation of a patient with FUO, even in the absence of ocular complaints. Ophthalmoscopy will reveal diseases that involve the optic nerve, retinal vessels, and choroidal tissues. Many systemic febrile diseases can have retinal as well as uveal manifestations.

LABORATORY TESTS

Cultures, antibody titers, complete blood counts, urine analyses, and direct examination of blood and other body fluids are mandatory procedures used in the evaluation of unexplained fevers. Most patients who are given a presumptive diagnosis of FUO have already had some or many laboratory investigations without revealing a specific cause. Some tests need to be repeated at regular intervals during a work-up of a patient with FUO, and these include serum samples for rising antibody titers and, most importantly, repeated cultures of blood and other body fluids for infectious agents. It should be emphasized that in both adults and children, the most often encountered cause of unexplained fever is infection. The importance of multiple blood cultures (e.g., up to six over a period of time) cannot be overstressed in uncovering many infections, especially endocarditis and osteomyelitis. The failure in diagnosing these and other infections sometimes lies with insufficient numbers of blood cultures and to a lesser extent in the inadequacy of cultures taken during concurrent antibiotic therapy. Polymicrobial sepsis often indicates self-induced infection.[22] Multiple urine cultures are also necessary, particularly in the absence of urinary tract symptoms and pyuria. In children, although urine cultures may be difficult to obtain, these are important. Silent urinary tract infections are common in the pediatric age group. In smaller children, direct bladder needle aspiration should be considered if routine procedures fail to yield adequate samples. Urine cultures are also important for the diagnosis of tuberculosis in children and adults. Other body fluids and tissues that may require multiple cultures include sputum, CSF, stool, and bone marrow. Morning gastric contents can also be cultured for mycobacteria. It is critical to culture tissues such as liver or lymph nodes that are removed during biopsy. Sputa, CSF, bone marrow, liver, and lymph nodes are cultured for aerobic and anaerobic bacteria, mycobacteria, and fungi. Viral cultures and inoculation of material into embryonated chick eggs, mice, and guinea pigs should also be considered. It is sometimes easier to isolate and to identify some infectious agents using animal and yolk sac inoculation. The recognition of the cause of the legionnaires' disease outbreak of 1976 illustrates an example of the usefulness of such procedures.[30]

Direct examination of the blood is necessary to confirm a diagnosis of malaria, trypanosomiasis, and relapsing fever. Thick and thin smears of blood stained with Giemsa or Wright stain require careful examination, particularly in light infections. Demonstration of *Borrelia* may require multiple smears. Wet mounts using phase contrast microscopy are also useful in the detection of spirochetes. Direct examination of spinal fluid sediment with India ink remains a fast and reliable method for detecting cryptococci. In the latter infection, large amounts of spinal fluid and repeated cultures are sometimes needed to make a diagnosis. Direct examination of stool samples is still the preferred method for demonstrating several parasitic infections. Although schistosomiasis and amebic abscess of the liver can both manifest as FUO, the diagnosis is much more likely to be made by means other than stool examination.

Rising antibody titers can be diagnostic in many infectious diseases, and it behooves the clinician who is working up a patient for FUO to obtain serum samples from the patient at regular intervals. It is advisable to freeze and to retain a portion of each sample in the event it is necessary to demonstrate a rising antibody titer to an agent isolated or suspected subsequently. Lyme disease is a good example, although some patients with Lyme disease fail to manifest antibodies to the spirochete. This is particularly true of viral and other infectious agents that are difficult to culture on artificial media.

Each antibody determination has its limitations as to specificity in that there are sometimes more false-positive than false-negative results. In addition, some antibody titers may reveal a recent infection with an organism that is not responsible for the prolonged fever. Newer and more specific immunologic methods are constantly being developed, and it is the responsibility of the physician to be aware of these while considering which immunologic test is most specific in uncovering the underlying cause of an FUO.

Patients with FUO often have elevated serum levels of "acute-phase reactants." These may include fibrinogen, haptoglobin, ceruloplasmin, C-reactive protein, and other α_2-globulins. These are part of the nonspecific changes often measurable and elevated with fever. Other nonspecific changes that accompany fever that are frequently found in patients with FUO include elevations in the erythrocyte sedimentation rate, increased ability of neutrophils to reduce nitroblue tetrazolium, low serum iron and zinc concentrations, and an increased peripheral neutrophil count. To what degree these determinations are useful in working up a patient with FUO depends on the characteristics of certain disease processes. In general, they are nonspecific and are of little value (see chapter 39). However, the erythrocyte sedimentation rate, for example, is usually markedly high in patients with temporal arteritis and Still's disease. It must be pointed out, however, that certain acute changes may be absent in some patients with FUO, and that these changes are by themselves not indicative of a specific diagnosis. Levels of etiocholanolone do not correlate with fever, and this substance plays no role in causing fever.[31]

NONINVASIVE PROCEDURES

The technical advances in diagnostic radiology, radionuclide scanning, and other methods have reduced the need for invasive procedures in evaluating a patient with FUO. These include plain film contrast studies, tomography, selective cinearteriography, radionuclide scans, computerized tomographic scanning, ultrasonography, and magnetic resonance imaging. There are advantages to using each procedure depending on the pathologic process. Some radiologic procedures should be considered "routine" in working up patients with FUO and include chest x-ray films, upper gastrointestinal contrast study with small-bowel follow-through, and barium enema. Chest x-ray films should be repeated periodically, and any radiologic study should be repeated if symptoms arise pertaining to a specific area. There are a large number of pulmonary diseases that cause prolonged fever and, in rare patients, show no demonstrable involvement on chest x-ray films; for example, in sarcoidosis, mycoses, tuberculosis, many of the pneumoconioses, and infiltrative lung disease, chest x-ray films may be normal in the presence of biopsy-proven disease.[32]

Radionuclide scanning procedures using technetium (Tc) 99m sulfur colloid, gallium (Ga) citrate or indium-III are available for the evaluation of many infectious, inflammatory, or neoplastic processes. Success in localizing a process using these radiopharmaceuticals depends on the pathogenic process. ^{67}Ga was initially used to detect bone tumors, but it now has been shown that the radionuclide concentrates in many neoplastic and inflammatory tissues. The mechanism by which ^{67}Ga localizes in inflammatory tissue is thought to be related to the presence of sequestered leukocytes.[33] Whole body gallium citrate (^{67}Ga) scans are often used as a screening procedure in patients with FUO and can localize abscesses, lymphomas, and infectious and other neoplastic processes.[34] However, there are known false-positive and false-negative results with this procedure. Technetium 99m sulfur colloid is also used in scanning and seems to be especially useful in the early diagnosis of osteomyelitis. Radiographic abnormalities develop late in this disease, and scanning techniques are able to localize the disease early, probably because of increased blood flow. To reduce false-positive results, it is advisable to use radionuclide scanning techniques in combination with computed tomography and ultrasonography.[35] Recently, it was reported that indium-111 granulocyte scintigraphy in FUO patients might be useful in diagnosing those with infections.[36]

Computed tomography (CT) scanning is one of the more important noninvasive diagnostic methods available in evaluation of patients with FUO. It appears that CT scanning of the head can detect intracranial lesions early and is superior to angiography for demonstrating cerebral abscesses. CT scanning is also useful in detecting epidural abscesses, retrobulbar masses, and diseases involving the sinus and nasopharynx.[37] Although intracranial tumors, hemorrhages, and hydrocephalus are not common causes of FUO, the usefulness of CT scanning for localizing these processes in the hypothalamus and, in particular, for hypothalamic tumors, has been documented.[38] The efficacy of whole body CT scanning in working up a patient with FUO depends on the extent and location of the disease.[39] For example, CT scanning is effective in delineating intra-abdominal abscesses and retroperitoneal, retrosternal, and mesenteric lymph nodes that may be the causes of FUO. The procedure can also detect defects in the spleen, liver, kidney, adrenals, pancreas, heart, mediastinum, and pelvis, but radionuclide scanning and ultrasonography are also efficacious in demonstrating disease in these organs and regions. For some patients, more than one noninvasive method may be necessary to demonstrate and to confirm abnormalities. Greater use of CT scanning has reduced the need for invasive procedures.[40]

Ultrasonography has been helpful in demonstrating the presence of cardiac abnormalities that may be a cause of fever. Echocardiography can detect valvular vegetations[41] and atrial tumors; it should be included as a "screening" procedure in patients with FUO. Ultrasonography is particularly useful in diagnosing abnormalities in the pancreas, gallbladder, liver, spleen, pelvis, and abdomen.[42–44]

Lymphangiography is a well-established method for demonstrating retroperitoneal, iliac, and periaortic lymph nodes. The involvement of these nodes in patients with lymphomas and Hodgkin's disease that manifest as FUO has been noted in several studies. With the advent of CT scanning, lymphangiography is infrequently used.

SKIN TESTING

With a few exceptions, such as the purified protein derivative (PPD) test for tuberculosis, most skin tests are of limited value in the diagnosis of FUO. Nevertheless, it is important to test for reactivity to tuberculin in patients with FUO. It is necessary at the same time to test for reactivity to other antigens such as mumps, streptodornasestreptokinase, or *Candida*. The lack of sensitivity to these latter antigens often suggests diseases like miliary tuberculosis or Hodgkin's disease. However, patients with FUO, particularly debilitated patients, may have depressed immunologic reactions secondary to nutritional factors.

INVASIVE PROCEDURES

Biopsy of liver and bone marrow should be considered routine in the work-up of FUO if the studies mentioned above are unrevealing. Other biopsy sites may include skin, pleura, lymph nodes, kidney, muscle, nerve, intestine or any tissue that may be involved either on physical examination, scans, or radiographs. Bronchoscopy, peritonoscopy, and other endoscopies are used for both inspection and obtaining tissues and fluids. Proper disposition of the biopsy material requires an organized plan to divide the tissue for maximal information. This is particularly true with needle biopsy material. Bacterial, viral, fungal, and mycobacterial cultures must be done on appropriate tissue. Reports of unusual organisms cultured from the biopsy material of many patients with FUO underscore the importance of this procedure. There is no substitute for a positive culture in uncovering the cause of fever. Microscopic examination also requires advanced organization. Proper staining may be critical to identification of organisms in tissues as well as in certain tissue and intracellular deposits. For example, formalin-fixed tissue should be stained with Brown–Brenn or Brown–Hopps for bacteria, Ziehl–Neelsen for mycobacteria, methenamine silver and periodic acid–Schiff for fungi, and the Dieterle silver-impregnation method for other bacteria and organisms. If possible, a section of the tissue block should always be retained for further sections or stains. Frozen sections can also be used for immunologic procedures. Using anti-IgG, anti-IgM, other anti-immunologlobin and anticomplement sera coupled to fluorescein dyes, these proteins can be identified in certain tissues of patients with autoimmune and collagen–vascular diseases.

With the increasing specificity and safety of noninvasive diagnostic methods, the need for diagnostic laparotomy in patients with FUO has markedly decreased. A diagnostic laparotomy may be indicated in patients with FUO and abdominal pain when the approaches outlined above have failed.[45] Percutaneous liver biopsy is a highly valuable procedure and should be performed on all patients with prolonged FUO.[18,46] Liver biopsy provides tissues for microscopic and microbiologic studies and is safe for most patients. A normal finding on liver biopsy is also helpful in that it is reassuring in those cases in which no diagnosis can be made.[46]

CAUSES OF FEVER OF UNKNOWN ORIGIN

Bacterial Infections

Any bacterial infection can be the source of prolonged fever, especially those that produce little or no obvious inflammation. In these situations localizing symptoms that would indicate the site of infection are missing.

Abscesses. Abscesses are frequently encountered as causes of FUO, and intra-abdominal sites are the most common. Liver and subphrenic abscesses are often seen in patients who have had previous abdominal surgery or in whom intestinal disease had resulted in a small perforation with intestinal leakage. Abdominal abscesses are potential complications in patients undergoing colonoscopy or sigmoidoscopy. Similarly, abdominal abscesses can occur in women following certain gynecologic procedures such as culdoscopy or curetage. Abscesses also can occur following ruptured ovarian cysts. Dental and brain abscesses are less common than an abdominal site as causes of unexplained fever because localizing symptoms are usually present early in the disease; nevertheless, these should be considered as possible causes of a FUO.

Osteomyelitis. Osteomyelitis is a common cause of FUO since symptoms are often masked or are interpreted as nervous or muscular in origin. For example, patients with osteomyelitis of the vertebral bodies or the leg may have symptoms of nerve root compression. Osteomyelitis of the mandible or maxilla can manifest as headache or toothache. Thus, osteomyelitis of any bone can be a cause of FUO because inflammation and pain may occur later in such patients. In this regard, sinusitis can cause prolonged fever without local symptoms except for mild headache.[47]

Subacute Bacterial Endocarditis. Another bacterial source for an FUO in which there may be no localizing symptoms is subacute bacterial endocarditis. This disease is sometimes a cause of FUO because it may not be diagnosed early due to either insufficient or negative blood cultures or to the absence of characteristic physical findings. There have been reports of culture–negative bacterial endocarditis in the past, but modern bacteriologic techniques appear to have reduced this number substantially. Drug addicts and the occasional user of intravenous contaminated materials are at increased risk of developing tricuspid valve infections, which are sometimes abacteremic. Another cause of negative blood cultures in bacterial endocarditis is concomitant antimicrobial therapy, since small doses of antibiotics can render blood cultures negative. For this reason, blood cultures should be repeated several days following cessation of antibiotics. The presence of bacterial endocarditis in the absence of an audible murmur is rare, but some murmurs, particularly in very young and elderly patients, are mistaken as physiologic. In these circumstances, bacterial endocarditis is not considered as a cause of fever, and hence these patients are given a diagnosis of FUO.

Biliary System Infections. Bacterial infections of the biliary system include ascending cholangitis, cholecystitis, frank empyema of the gallbladder, and infection of the pancreatic duct. The organisms gain entrance from the duodenum, and in the majority of cases there is a pre-existing disease like pancreatitis or cholelithiasis. However, patients with bacterial infections of the biliary system who have been diagnosed as having FUO have little or no right upper quandrant discomfort that would indicate the site of infection. Patients with suppurative biliary tract infection had no localizing physical findings or tenderness before laparotomy.[6,48,49] Furthermore, in these patients liver function tests had been normal and hence the diagnosis had been made primarily at laparotomy. Newer methods such as computerized scanning and sonography have lessened the need for such operations in these patients.

Urinary Tract Infections. Urinary tract infections due to bacteria are infrequently encountered as causes of FUO because positive urine cultures make this diagnosis early in a febrile illness. Thus, patients with urinary tract infections that manifest as FUO have negative or intermittently positive urine cultures. Perinephric abscesses may spill bacteria into the urine inconsistently, and some urinary tract infections have such a low titer of bacteria (1000–5000 organisms/ml) that the culture results do not suggest the urinary tract as a source of the fever. In children, particularly in girls with bladder reflux and in boys with posterior urethral valves, urinary tract infections are common causes of FUO. Obtaining urine for culture in small children is difficult, and contaminating organisms are often misleading. Bladder aspiration is indicated in such children with bacteriuria to rule out urinary tract infection as a cause of FUO. When urinary tract infections are a cause of prolonged fever, there usually is absence of symptoms like dysuria, frequency, or lower back pain.

Tuberculosis. *Mycobacterium tuberculosis* is perhaps the single most often cultured organism as a cause of FUO. Although its incidence in producing disease has been markedly reduced, *M. tuberculosis,* nevertheless, continues as a cause of prolonged, unexplained fevers. This is particularly true in patients with certain immunologic deficiency states as well as in those patients with acquired increased susceptibility to infection due to immunosuppressive therapy. There are some patients in whom fever is the only symptom and whose chest x-ray films appear normal. Extrapulmonary tuberculosis is probably the most common manifestation of this infection as a FUO.[50] Miliary tuberculosis including tuberculosis of the spleen, liver, bone, kidney, meninges, peritoneum, and pericardium have all been reported as causes of prolonged fever. Even in cases of overwhelming miliary tuberculosis, the lung fields and other organ sites do not always show signs of involvement until weeks following the onset of fever,[51] and hence diagnosis may be delayed. In addition, the diagnosis of tuberculosis as a cause of fever may not be apparent, since cultures may not become positive before 4–6 weeks. Furthermore, a negative skin test may be due to disseminated disease, and when such is the case, the clinician is often misled by the absence of a positive reaction. Although atypical mycobacteria cause disease, they usually do not manifest as FUO.

Miscellaneous Infections. Intestinal bacterial infections rarely manifest as prolonged fever in the absence of other symptoms. The notable exception to this is salmonellosis, in which fever may be the only abnormality. The causative agent in Whipple's disease (intestinal lipodystrophy) is thought to be bacterial in nature, and this disease has been encountered as a cause of prolonged fever.[48,52] The vast majority of bacterial infections causing prolonged, unexplained fever are confined to specific sites, that is, abscess in organs or infection in certain spaces. There are also a few bacterial infections that may cause prolonged fevers and in which the causative organism is disseminated, residing primarily in the reticuloendothelial and lymphatic systems. These include brucellosis, bartonellosis, and listeriosis. Of these diseases, brucellosis is clearly most frequently encountered as an FUO. Diagnosis rests, as in all bacterial infections, on positive bacterial cultures as well as on the presence of increasing serum antibody titers.

Spirochetal Infections

Relapsing fever. Of the three medically important genera of spirochetes, *Treponema, Leptospira,* and *Borrelia,* only the last is often associated with prolonged fever and is sometimes called "relapsing fever" because the fever characteristically occurs in paroxysms separated by afebrile intervals. Although louse-borne relapsing fever due to infections of *Borrelia recurrentis* occurs worldwide, it is most prevalent in times of war or famine; the tick-borne form of this disease caused by *B. pakeri, B. hermsi,* or *B. turicatae* has been reported in the western and southwestern United States and frequently manifests as a FUO.[53,54] Louse-borne relapsing fever usually occurs in epidemics, and diagnosis is made during the initial febrile episodes. However, tick-borne relapsing fever affects campers and hikers in a sporadic fashion, and patients often are given a provisional diagnosis of FUO until careful direct examination of the blood for the presence of spirochetes or culture in chick embryos suggests the etiology of the infection. The patient may be unaware of a recent tick bite, and during the second or third fever relapse the disease may be overlooked as having an infectious etiology. The initial clinical manifestations of louse-borne relapsing fever can be confused with those caused by tick-borne rickettsiae, but subsequent attacks of relapsing fever may manifest with only fever and no localizing signs.

Leptospirosis. Leptospirosis is a spirochetal infection that can manifest as an FUO, although illness is usually acute and self-limited. During the first phases of leptospirosis, the organisms can be cultured from the blood, but during the second and third phases ("immune phases"), organisms may be absent from body fluids and fever may be the only manifestation. In these cases the cause of prolonged fever may be ascertained by serologic tests.[55]

Rat-Bite Fever. *Spirillum minor,* the spirochete that causes rat-bite fever, cannot be cultured on artificial media, but inoculation of the patient's blood into mice confirms a diagnosis in 10 days to 2 weeks. The history of a rat bite should alert the physician to the diagnostic possibility. Rarely, mouse bites have also been shown to cause the disease. Darkfield microscopy of blood may demonstrate the organism; however, in patients with spirochetal infection who appear to have an FUO, the organism may be absent from body fluids, and diagnosis depends on the presence of specific antibody titers.

Rickettsial Infections In the preantibiotic era, it was not uncommon for typhus to be the cause of undiagnosed fevers. Although rickettsial infections are often associated with high fevers that in untreated cases may last up to 20 days, these diseases are rarely encountered as FUOs today. Clinical manifestations such as the cutaneous exanthem and severe headache, which are present in almost all cases,[56] and the specificity of serologic tests alert physicians to the cause of fever early in the disease.

Chlamydial Infections Psittacosis caused by *Chlamydia psittaci* can occur in the absence of cough and respiratory symptoms and with normal chest x-ray findings. In these situations, fever may be the sole symptom of the disease and splenomegaly the only physical finding. Because fever in psittacosis may be prolonged as long as 3 months, psittacosis has been reported as an infectious cause of FUO in several studies. Isolation of the organism may be difficult in these cases, but diagnosis can be made from a rising titer of complement-fixing antibody. Other chlamydial diseases such as trachoma as well as genital tract infections are usually not associated with fever. Lymphogranuloma venereum, although usually diagnosed without difficulty, may manifest as an FUO.

Viral Infections Viruses can cause prolonged fever in some patients. This is particularly true in children, and the spectrum of infectious causes of FUO in young children includes more viral etiologies than in adults. The proof of a viral agent causing prolonged, unexplained fever rests with two criteria: isolation of the agent and immunologic evidence of infection. Problems arise when the patient does not have a typical immunologic response to the agent and when associated signs and symptoms such as skin rashes and lymphadenopathy are missing or have gone unnoticed. This is particularly true of some viral infections in children. Infectious mononucleosis is perhaps the most commonly encountered viral disease producing prolonged fever without appropriate immunologic response. For example, not all patients develop significant titers of heterophile antibody early in the course of the disease. The disease can thus often be diagnosed by the presence of antibody to Epstein-Barr virus-associated antigens. Rarely, the development of both heterophile and Epstein-Barr virus antibodies is delayed several weeks and diagnosis is difficult. Other viral illnesses associated with FUO include hepatitis, cat-scratch fever, and cytomegalovirus infections.

Fungal Diseases

There is little question that the incidence of fungal diseases, particularly deep mycoses, has increased as a result of the use of antibiotics and immunosuppressive therapy. Many fungal diseases, for example, histoplasmosis, blastomycosis, and coccidiomycosis, manifest primarily as pulmonary infections and are detected early in the disease process. Other fungal diseases, notably cryptococcosis and disseminated histoplasmosis, are less easily detected, and fever may be the major manifestation.

Histoplasmosis involving the reticuloendothelial and lymphatic system may manifest as prolonged, unexplained fever. The clinical manifestations of this form of histoplasmosis are not unlike that of disseminated tuberculosis. Cryptococcal meningitis is often undiagnosed for several weeks and may manifest as an FUO. Headaches and behavioral changes usually lead to an examination of the spinal fluid. With increasing use of antibiotics, particularly in patients being treated with immunosuppressive agents, some of the indigenous fungi, for example, *Candida albicans,* have caused disseminated disease and fever.

Parasitic Disease

Malaria. In endemic areas, malaria is seldom a cause of unexplained fever, but in nonendemic areas, this infection has the potential to go undetected. This may be due to several factors, including the failure of travelers to use prophylactic antimalarials properly, resistant forms, nonsynchronized febrile paroxysms, and the physician's unawareness of travel to endemic areas by the patient. In fact, most reports of malaria as a cause of FUO are due to failure to suspect malaria early in the disease. Blood transfusion as a cause of malarial transmission occurs rarely but increases during periods of war in malarious areas.

Toxoplasmosis. Toxoplasmosis can manifest as FUO and is often discovered in patients with lymph node enlargement during lymph node biopsy. A few patients have minimal lymph node swelling and may have fever as the predominant symptom. Rising antibody titers can detect the disease when it is suspected.

Trypanosomiasis. Trypanosomiasis due to *Trypanosoma rhodesiense* is carried by the tsetse fly vector in East and Central Africa, and visitors to these areas, even for periods as brief as an overnight flight stop, can contract the disease. The disease is rather acute, accompanied by prominent erythematous rash, central nervous system alterations, and high fever. Trypanosomes can be detected in routine blood smears during the disease. *Trypanosoma gambiense* is found in West and Central Africa and produces a more subtle form of onset. Fever begins irregularly and is accompanied by an evanescent rash, splenomegaly, and lymphadenopathy. The disease is less acute than that caused by *T. rhodesiense* and may be present for months as an FUO before blood smears are examined. Visitors to Africa or natives arriving in the United States from endemic areas can have delayed onset of disease.

Other Parasitic Diseases. Leishmaniasis, trichinosis, and amebic liver abscess are parasitic diseases that can have prominent febrile manifestations and, because of their relative infrequency in the United States, may be missed as a cause of unexplained fever.

NEOPLASTIC DISEASES

Unexplained fever is a common manifestation of many malignancies (Table 4). All solid tumors have the potential to cause obstruction and subsequent infection; hence, malignancy and fever may coexist. In these situations, the neoplastic process indirectly causes the fever. However, even in the absence of infection, certain neoplasms are particularly associated with fever, and when these are treated the fever may disappear. In these cases, the neoplasm is thought to be a direct source of the fever.

The mechanism by which a neoplastic process causes fever may be related to its ability either to produce endogenous pyrogens itself or to induce the production of endogenous pyrogens from normal leukocytes. Tissue obtained from patients with Hodgkin's disease, histiocytic lymphomas, and renal cell carcinoma liberate endogenous pyrogens spontaneously in vitro,[57–60] and it is likely that the same process takes place in vivo. In addition to some tumors producing their own endogenous pyrogens, others undergo necrosis as a result of rapid growth, and necrotic debris induces the infiltration of leukocytes in the inflammatory response.[61] Endogenous pyrogens can be the products of inflammatory leukocytes and may be produced in association with tumor necrosis.

TABLE 4. Malignancies Commonly Manifesting as FUO

Hodgkin's disease
Non-Hodgkin's lymphoma
Leukemia (including aleukemia and preleukemia)
Renal cell carcinoma
Hepatoma
Atrial myxomas

Certain neoplasms have a high incidence of manifestation as FUO, and some patients with these malignancies seek medical attention primarily because of recurrent fevers. These neoplasms include lymphoma and other reticuloses, renal cell carcinoma, atrial myxoma, hepatoma, and carcinoma of the intestinal tract. Disseminated carcinomatosis is also a cause of FUO. Nonmalignant neoplasms that are associated with prolonged fever are giant lymph node hyperplasia[62,63] and infantile cortical hyperostosis.[64] It should be pointed out, however, that these benign neoplasms may have an infectious or inflammatory etiology, athough no agent has yet been isolated. Angiomyolipoma is a benign renal tumor that occurs almost exclusively in patients with tuberous sclerosis and can manifest as an FUO.[65]

Lymphomas and Leukemias. Of all the lymphomas, Hodgkin's disease is most commonly associated with recurrent fever, although non-Hodgkin's lymphoma may cause FUO. The likelihood of fever as an initial symptom in Hodgkin's disease increases with the number of lymph nodes involved, and fever is a prominent symptom when disease is present in retroperitoneal nodes. In these latter instances, routine studies to detect a cause of the persistent fever fail, and patients require more specific investigation to uncover the source of fever. Lymphomas that primarily involve the spleen have a high incidence of fever and can manifest along with anorexia, malaise, and weight loss as an FUO.[66] When present, a Pel-Ebstein pattern of fever (3- to 10-day cycles of febrile and afebrile periods) is highly suggestive of Hodgkin's disease.

Acute leukemias may be associated with fever, and sometimes this occurs in the presence of a normal peripheral blood smear, as seen in aleukemic leukemia and preleukemia. In such patients diagnosis is often delayed. Bone marrow aspiration may uncover the aleukemic phase, but in preleukemic forms, fever may persist, and bone marrow aspirates remain nondiagnostic for very long periods.[67] The incidence of fever in the preleukemic form of monocytic leukemia is high and, in general, the number of preleukemias, including myelogenous leukemia, that manifest as FUO varies from 10 to 30 percent in different studies.[67–69]

Renal Cell Carcinoma. Carcinoma of the kidney is often insidious, and many patients do not have hematuria but rather fever as the major symptom.[70] Two large series put the incidence of persistent fever as a manifesting symptom at 11 percent and 12 percent[71] of the cases. There also seems to be a high incidence of a sedimentation rate greater than 100 mm/hr in patients with fever and renal cell carcinoma.[72] In many cases there are no metastases but rather a well-encepsulated neoplasm. Removal of the tumor almost always results in the cessation of fever. Of interest is the fact that investigators have found that the tumor cells synthesize and release endogenous pyrogens spontaneously in vitro, while renal tumor cells taken from patient's who did not have fever did not release endogenous pyrogen.[73]

Tumors of the Liver. There is a greater incidence of metastatic adenocarcinoma to the liver than primary hepatomas, but the latter tumor is often considered as a likely cause of an FUO. Some patients with hepatomas seek medical help because of persistent fever,[74] and several reports of FUO have listed hepatoma as the final diagnosis. Primary or metastatic tumors to the liver that are associated with prolonged fever are not diagnostic problems when accompanied by jaundice or abnormal liver function tests. However, patients with normal liver functions and only fever are admitted to hospitals with the diagnosis of FUO.

Atrial Myxomas. Although myxomas of the atria are very rare neoplasms, they have a high association of fever and manifest as FUO.[75,76] The mechanism of producing fever is not understood but may be related to embolic phenomena or the production of interleukin-6. Murmurs may not be present.

Other Tumors. The list of other tumors that can manifest as FUO is varied. Adenocarcinoma of the large intestine, bronchogenic carcinoma, and adenocarcinoma of the breast particularly when they metastisize can cause a FUO. Children tend to have a different spectrum of neoplasms that manifest as FUO. Acute leukemias are most prevalent in children and can manifest as unexplained fever. Solid tumors in children that may manifest as FUO include neuroblastoma and central nervous system tumors.

Hypersensitivity and Autoimmune Diseases There is a sizable group of diseases that manifest as FUO and that fall into the general categories of hypersensitivity, autoimmune, rheumatic, or collagen–vascular diseases (Table 5). Patients with these diseases may have prolonged, unexplained fever as the prominent symptom of disease, while other clinical manifestations such as cutaneous lesions and joint involvement are either absent or go undetected. Similarly, laboratory tests that would ordinarily alert the physician to the diagnosis are normal. For example, patients with systemic lupus erythematosus (LE) may have fever as a predominant symptom and a negative LE preparation. In several series, 12, 18, and 20 percent of the patients with an unequivocal diagnosis of systemic lupus erythematosus had negative LE preparations.[77,78] Using immunofluorescence, antinuclear antibodies can be found in more than 90 percent of the patients.[78] Fever can be the initial manifestation of the disease in 5 percent of the cases,[78] and such patients are considered to have FUO when they have only fever and no serologic evidence of lupus. Later, additional clinical manifestations may appear such as arthritis, and serologic tests may become positive, which assures a diagnosis of lupus erythematosus.

Patients with various forms of vasculitis can initially have fever as a prominent sign, and cutaneous manifestations may not occur. Biopsy of affected areas, when they appear, confirms the diagnosis. Drug-induced vasculitis is often associated with fever and can manifest as FUO.[79] Drugs that are often associated with hypersensitivity vasculitis include penicillin, sulfonamides, isoniazid, and propylthiouracil, but any drug can cause hypersensitivity vasculitis.

Rheumatoid arthritis can be associated with persistent fever, but in adults, joint involvement usually indicates the proper diagnosis. In children, however, joint involvement may be minimal or absent, and many patients have an FUO. In fact, of all the autoimmune diseases that manifest as FUO in the pediatric age group, juvenile rheumatoid arthritis is undoubtedly the most common.[80,81] Still's disease is the diagnosis given to those children who have primarily systemic manifestations in the absence of arthritis. A complex of high fever, evanescent rash, lymphadenopathy, and splenomegaly with varying degrees of arthralgias and myalgias is typical for Still's disease. Because of its acute onset, it may stimulate other diseases and may pose diagnostic difficulties.

Adults with FUO may also have Still's disease. Onset of the adult form of Still's disease occurs most often between ages 20 and 30, but in some patients onset occurs in childhood and is followed by asymptomatic intervals that may be as long as 10 years. The clinical manifestation in adults is almost identical to that in children. However, adults often have other associated symptoms such as sore throat during febrile episodes.[82] Radiologic evidence of joint changes are often absent in the adult form of Still's disease, and there is no rheumatoid factor present. An elevated white blood cell count with an increase in polymorphonuclear leukocytes and an elevated erythrocyte sedimentation rate are characteristic. The diagnosis of Still's disease as the cause of unexplained fever in adults rests with the presence of its symptom complex in the absence of other diseases.[82,83]

TABLE 5. Hypersensitivity and Autoimmune Diseases Causing FUO

Systemic lupus erythematosus	Polyarteritis nodosa
Still's disease	Erythema multiforme
Polymyalgia rheumatica	Mixed connective tissue disease
Drug fever	Serum sickness
Hypersensitivity vasculitis	Rheumatic fever
Idiopathic vasculitis	

Although rare in the United States, rheumatic fever can manifest as FUO, but in such patients, the classic criteria as established by Jones,[84] are not all present.[15] Although more prevalent in children, acute rheumatic fever in the adult may manifest with less than the full constellation of signs. Rheumatic fever must be differentiated from bacterial endocarditis, rheumatoid arthritis, and systemic lupus erythematosus.

There are also patients in whom a diagnosis of an autoimmune or collagen–vascular disease is almost certain, but its classification is difficult. Although these patients may have fever as the prominent symptom, other symptoms and laboratory data suggest unclassified collagen–vascular disease. Mixed connective tissue disease can manifest as FUO, and in such patients elevated titers of extractable nuclear antigen will confirm the diagnosis. Erythema multiforme with fever may be found in this group of illnesses.

Fever may be the only manifestation of hypersensitivity to drugs, including propriety preparations. Some drugs can cause fever in the absence of an immunologically based hypersensitivity reaction; these include atropine, lyseric acid, some antidepressants, amphotericin B, and bleomycin. The mechanism for atropine and central nervous system-acting drugs causing elevated temperature is through interference with heat regulatory mechanisms, and, as such, the elevated temperature is not fever but rather hyperthermia (see Chapter 39). True drug fever is an immunologically based disease in which, either through previous exposure or recent administration, sensitization takes place to the drug as a foreign antigen. It has been proposed that sensitized T lymphocytes release endogenous pyrogen-inducing substances that cause the fever. Removal of the antigen usually brings about a decrease in the fever within 48 hours.

Fever due to first use of amphotericin B or bleomycin is not due to hypersensitivity reactions but rather to the direct ability of these drugs to stimulate production of endogenous pyrogenic cytokines. In some cases, these drugs, which are given parenterally, may contain endotoxins as contaminants.

In a study published in 1964, cutaneous manifestations were present in a majority of the cases of drug fever.[85] In a large study of 148 episodes of drug fever in 142 patients, cutaneous manifestations were present in only 18 percent of patients, and less than half of these were urticarial in nature.[86]

The most common manifestation of drug fever is seen in the patient being treated with antibiotics and in whom the protracted fever is due to drug hypersensitivity and not to the infection. Withdrawing the drug usually results in disappearance of the fever. For this reason, the patient's history is critical in establishing a diagnosis of drug fever. Some patients suddenly develop fever to common drugs like INH or other agents that have been taken for years without evidence of any hypersensitivity. The variety of agents that have been reported to be the source of FUO is broad. Some agents, however, tend to be particularly associated with fever in the absence of other clinical manifestations and include salicylates, thiouracil, diphenylhydantoin (Dilantin), iodides, isoniazid, methyldopa, and penicillin.

Thyroiditis is usually associated with local pain and fever, and does not manifest as FUO. However, a small number of patients with subacute thyroiditis may be unaware of local tenderness and may have persistent fever. Examination of the thyroid gland reveals local tenderness even when there is limited involvement,[61] and appropriate thyroid function tests and serologic measurements assure the diagnosis.

Granulomatous Diseases

The four major types of granulomatous diseases that produce prolonged, unexplained fevers are: granulomatous hepatitis, sarcoidosis, inflammatory bowel disease, and temporal arteritis. In general, granulomatous disease can go undetected for many months and yet be the cause of high fevers. In fact, in patients with FUO lasting for longer than 1 year, granulomatous causes were more numerous than neoplasms or autoimmune diseases.[12,21] When the patient has a FUO, localizing symptoms are often absent, while diagnosis requires identification of granulomas in biopsy material or radiologic evidence of lesions typical of the process (e.g., Crohn's disease).

Granulomatous Hepatitis. Granulomatous hepatitis of unknown etiology accounts for a large number of cases of prolonged FUO. Granulomas in the liver represent a pathologic response to injury in that they are induced by many infectious diseases. Some of the diseases that are commonly associated with hepatic granulomas include tuberculosis and other mycobacterial infections, histoplasmosis, syphilis, some parasitic diseases, sarcoidosis, and neoplasms.[21,87–89] It is essential to rule out these and other underlying diseases. However, there is a group of patients with FUO and granulomas in the liver in whom no specific underlying process can be found.[88] The disease is usually associated with high fever intermittently present for periods of months to years and occurs most often during the fifth or sixth decade of life. The only laboratory data that suggest granulomatous hepatitis are mildly elevated alkaline phosphatase levels in many patients and elevated serum transaminase determinations in even fewer. However, these may be normal in a small number of patients, and only liver biopsy confirms the diagnosis.

Sarcoidosis. Sarcoidosis is a systemic granulomatous disease that commonly manifests with pulmonary, skin, or lymphoid involvement. However, a small percentage of patients with sarcoidosis have fever, weight loss, and weakness as initial symptoms without localizing signs or symptoms. In fact, some patients with sarcoidosis have a daily temperature elevation greater than 101°F for months, and in these patients granulomas usually can be found in the liver, while the lung fields remain clear. Fever in sarcoidosis is sometimes associated with erythema nodosum.

Inflammatory Bowel Disease. Crohn's disease or granulomatous colitis are granulomatous processes primarily involving the terminal ileum and colon, and nearly one-third of the patients have fever. A small percentage of these patients can have no gastrointestinal symptoms and only high fevers.[21,90–92] This is particularly true of young adults in whom fever can be present for months or years without symptoms referable to the gastrointestinal tract. For this reason, it is important to obtain a detailed small bowel contrast study in patients with FUO. Of all gastrointestinal diseases that cause fever, Crohn's disease is the most likely to be a cause of FUO. Ulcerative colitis, although not a granulomatous disease, rarely manifests as a FUO. There have been reports, however, of patients with high fevers and no intestinal symptoms who later have sigmoidoscopic evidence of this disease.[61,92,93]

Temporal Arteritis. Giant cell arteritis with polymyalgia rheumatica affects patients usually in the sixth and seventh decades of life and may manifest as FUO. The symptom complex includes headache, visual disturbances, and myalgias and arthralgias. It should be pointed out, however, that none of these symptoms need be present for temporal arteritis to cause prolonged fever. Patients with unexplained recurrent fevers and mild headaches or visual disturbance should be considered for temporal artery biopsy, particularly in the sixth and seventh decades of life.[21] Associated laboratory findings are anemia and very high sedimentation rates. Biopsy specimens of the temporal artery reveal granulomas even in cases in which no temporal artery tenderness was demonstrated. In one series, 44 percent of the patients with biopsy-proven temporal arteritis had no tenderness to palpation,[94] and hence it is important to consider this disease in the absence of clinical signs or symptoms in patients with FUO. Takayasu's disease can also manifest as a FUO.[95]

Inherited Disorders

There are at least four inherited diseases that are associated with intermittent fever, sometimes unexplained for years. These are familial Mediterranean fever, which is inherited in about one-half of the patients as an autosomal recessive trait[96]; Fabry's disease or angiokeratoma corporis difusum, an X-linked disorder[97]; hypertriglyceridemia; and a syndrome of deafness, urticaria and progressive amyloidosis that is familial or associated with chromosomal aberration.[98,99]

Familial Mediterranean Fever. Familial Mediterranean fever (FMF) is always associated with unexplained intermittent fever, usually beginning in childhood. Besides fever, FMF has distinct clinical signs and symptoms and laboratory data that, although nonspecific, together suggest this diagnosis in the absence of other disease.[100] These are fever, evidence of serosal inflammation—usually peritoneal or pleural, distinctive skin lesions (painful erythematous swellings), occasional joint pains, and headache. FMF is not periodic but rather a disease characterized by intermittent attacks of fever and serosal pain. In some patients, the attacks may be separated by a number of years, while in others they may occur weekly or more frequently. Spontaneous remissions and recurrence are typical of the disease. Attacks are associated with leukocytosis, elevated sedimentation rate, and elevated levels of several acute phase reactants. Admittedly nonspecific, these usually return to normal following the attacks. Although rarely seen in the United States, amyloidosis is often diagnosed in patients with FMF in the Middle East.

Familial Mediterranean fever is initially diagnosed as FUO because of the misconception that this disease is found only in Sephardic Jews, Armenians, and Arabs. Although there is unquestionably a much higher incidence of this disease in such patients, FMF occurs in patients of other extractions such as western Europeans.[100] The expression of the disease also seems milder in those patients living in the United States in that the skin lesions, joint involvement, and the development of amyloidosis are rarely encountered. Most patients primarily have recurrent bouts of abdominal or chest pain with fever. The fever in FMF may be high during some attacks, and during others, the temperature may be only minimally elevated. After a careful diagnostic work-up in which no evidence of infectious, hypersensitive, or autoimmune disease can be found in patients with symptoms and signs of FMF, this diagnosis can be made. A diagnosis of FMF is usually made after years of recurrent attacks. Prophylactic oral colchicine therapy has been shown to prevent attacks of FMF.[101]

Fabry's Disease. Fabry's disease is an X-linked inborn error of glycosphingolipid metabolism resulting from the deficient activity of a specific alphaglactosidase.[97] There is a systemic accumulation of the glycosphingolipid substrate trihexosyl ceramide, and this results in vascular and renal insufficiency and death in the third or fourth decade. Clinically, the disease is recognized by punctate skin lesions that are most numerous around the genitals and buttocks. Patients have unexplained attacks of fever and pain and also have severe acroparethesias. The recurrent fever can manifest as an FUO, particularly when the characteristic lesions are missed. The enzymatic defect can be detected in plasma, urine, and leukocytes.[97]

Hypertriglyceridemia. Hypertriglyceridemia associated with recurrent fever and abdominal pain can present as FUO, and reduction of saturated fat intake results in the disappearance of the fever and pain.[21] Hyperlipidemia type V may be associated with recurrent bouts of abdominal pain, with evidence of pancreatitis, with elevated amylase levels and may manifest as FUO.

Deafness, Urticaria, and Amyloidosis. The syndrome of deafness, urticaria, and amyloidosis has been described as a heredofamilial disease that is associated with bouts of high-spiking fever and a nonitching urticarial exanthem.[98,99] Progressive deafness is usually present since early childhood, and the febrile episodes begin in adolescence. Amyloidosis with renal failure occurs later. During the second decade of life this syndrome can manifest as FUO.

Central Nervous System Causes of FUO

The term *central* fever has been used to describe fever that is due to pathologic processes in or near the thermoregulatory center of the hypothalamus. There are several diseases that can affect the region of the thermoregulatory center, and these include metastatic tumor, primary CNS tumors, hemorrhage, degenerative diseases, vascular abnormalities, metabolic disorders, and infectious processes. In addition, such lesions more commonly produce endocrine disturbances. It should be pointed out, however, that lesions in or near the hypothalamus that affect thermoregulation are more likely to produce persistent hypothermia rather than hyperthermia. For example, sarcoid granulomas, degenerative processes,[102] tumor invasion,[103] hemorrhage into the third cerebral ventricle,[104] Wernicke's encephalopathy with hypothalamic hemorrhages,[105] and other hypothalamic lesions[106] are most often associated with hypothermia. Nevertheless, a few patients with hypothalamic disturbances may have persistent or intermittently elevated body temperature.[21,106–108] These patients with fever, like the patients with hypothermia, do not have normal mechanisms of thermoregulation and may exhibit poikilothermia.[107] In addition, these patients may lose their daily temperature rhythm.[109] Patients with local infectious processes, like encephalitis, may have an FUO and minimal changes in the CSF.

Children with central nervous system disease are more likely to develop hyperthermia than are adults. Diencephalic seizure disorders, degenerative brain diseases, chronic heavy metal intoxication, and central nervous system tumors, including CNS leukemia, are often associated with fever.[3–5] Nevertheless, hypothalamic lesions or disorders that are thought to be a cause of persistent unexplained fevers are extremely rare.

Factitious Illness

Careful observation of the daily temperature pattern can often lead to a diagnosis of factitious fever, since the circadian temperature rhythm may be absent; in some, the temperature may always be elevated. In addition to abnormal circadian temperature rhythms in patients with factitious fevers, evidence of vasoconstriction, sweating, or increased pulse rate are usually absent despite thermometer readings in excess of 39°C. The use of numbered and electronic thermometers and the simultaneous measurement of urine and body temperature are methods that help in making a diagnosis of factitious fevers.[110,111] Factitious fevers are usually suspected late in the work-up of patients with FUO,[22] but awareness of these methods can alert the attending physician before institution of a costly investigation. Most of these patients have false fevers, and the methods by which they manipulate thermometers is varied and often very ingenious. Others may inject pyrogenic materials or bacteria and induce real fever. Whatever the method used, diagnosis can be difficult, and many patients undergo extensive investigation before the factitious source of their illness is uncovered. There is a high incidence of patients with factitious illness in the health professions, particularly young women.[21] Once the factitious nature of the illness is discovered and the patient is confronted, psychiatric therapy often proves to be very beneficial. In patients with prolonged FUO, usually longer than 6 months, factitious illness accounts for 9 percent of the cases.[12] In addition, there is a higher incidence of association of self-mutilation in those patients with FUO lasting for prolonged periods. Repeated recovery of multiple and unusual organisms from blood and other cultures also suggests factitious illness.

Miscellaneous Causes of FUO

Postoperative fever due to halothane sensitization can persist and can manifest as FUO, although this is usually a self-limited febrile disease.[112] In general, cardiac surgical procedures, particularly those using pump-bypass, are most often followed by prolonged or recurrent fevers that may continue into the second or third postoperative week. In these patients, no infectious cause can be found, although approximately 6 percent have a postpericardiotomy syndrome.[113] The pathogenetic mechanisms proposed for these persistent fevers include exacerbation of pre-existing rheumatic fever, inflammatory response to blood in the pericardial cavity, and autoimmune response to traumatized cardiac tissue.[113] Neurosurgical procedures are also commonly associated with postoperative fever, and this may be related to the presence of blood in the third cerebral ventricle. A low-grade, aseptic meningitis can manifest as persistent fever after the excision of certain tumors from the CNS.[114] Septic thrombophlebitis, particularly of the pelvic veins, and small pulmonary embolization can manifest as FUO.[115] Inflammation resulting from radiation therapy may cause fever.[116] Pheochromocytomas can manifest as FUO years before the tumor is detected.[117] Laennec's cirrhosis is frequently accompanied by fever and is present in over one-third of the patients.[118] Fever due to cirrhosis is moderate but prolonged, and patients with cirrhosis have laboratory and pathologic evidence of active hepatic disease. However, these patients may be diagnosed as FUO only when the evidence of hepatic disease is undetected. The diagnosis of alcoholic hepatitis is frequently made in patients who are admitted to community hospitals with FUOs.

The only true cyclic or periodic cause of fever is cyclic neutropenia, in which the neutrophils are low or absent from the peripheral blood at 21-day intervals.[26] During this time, patients are susceptible to infection. Fever may be prominent during the neutropenic phase, and these patients are considered to have periodic fever before the correct diagnosis is made.

Many patients with the acquired immunodeficiency syndrome (AIDS) initially have an FUO. In the majority, the fever is due to an infection that is often relatively easy to diagnose. Thus, as in all FUO patients, AIDS patients should be evaluated thoroughly, with particular attention to the wide variety of infectious agents that may cause fever.

Exaggerated Circadian Temperature Rhythm

A large number of young children of both sexes, as well as young female adolescents, have been evaluated because of

FUO. These persons have often had a previous acute, self-limited febrile illness of infectious origin. The patient or the family then becomes involved in the frequent monitoring of temperature. Following recovery from this illness, it is noted that the temperature (usually in the early evening) never returns to "normal." These persons seem to have exaggerated daily swings, and their normal evening temperature may be 99–100°F.[109] After a minimal work-up, which is completely normal, we observe such persons and encourage them to not take their temperature unless they are ill. Unfortunately, many of these persons have been subjected to unnecessarily expensive, painful, and often dangerous procedures when, in fact, they are normal. Many years of follow-up have substantiated that these patients were not ill but merely had this exaggerated daily swing in temperature brought to their attention by a routine, self-limited infectious illness.

MANAGEMENT

There are a few general principles in approaching the patient with prolonged fever in whom no underlying source can be determined. A significant number of patients with undiagnosed fevers have good prognoses in that they eventually recover. Another group have intermittent bouts of fever for years but are otherwise well. These groups require no therapy, and mortality in the undiagnosed groups has been found in several studies to be low.[21] Nonspecific therapy for those patients with persistent fever and debilitating nutritional and physiologic imbalances may be instituted with caution. Clinical and laboratory evidence suggest that processes of amino acid oxidation contribute to the negative nitrogen balance of chronic fevers and that this may be partially reversed by cyclooxygenase inhibitors. The approach to empiric therapy in a patient with FUO must first consider whether the risk of the therapy outweighs potential benefit. Thus, there are few, if any indications for empiric antibiotic or cytotoxic chemotherapy. Our approach is to use antipyretics such as acetylsalicylic acid or acetaminophen first. These are given in maximum dosages, and if the patient improves, they are continued for varying periods of time. If these drugs fail, then other prostaglandin synthetase inhibitors such as indomethacin or ibuprofen are tried. If these agents prove ineffective and the patient continues to be ill, then adenal corticosteroid therapy should be considered if the physician is convinced that the underlying cause of the FUO is not infectious. Initially, we give prednisone around the clock and at a reasonable anti-inflammatory dosage (e.g., 10 mg every 6 hours). If improvement occurs and signs of inflammation recede, then we switch the patient to a single daily dose and eventually to alternate-day therapy. The latter is done to minimize undersirable side effects.

It must be emphasized that if the source of the fever defies diagnosis despite a thorough work-up as outlined then, depending on the severity of the illness, reevaluation must be done at reasonable intervals. Most empiric therapy is nonspecific, and the patient may have a relapse after treatment. With such patients or with therapeutic failures, it may be necessary to perform another complete evaluation as often as every 4–6 months, since in rare patients abnormalities may become apparent only after prolonged periods.

REFERENCES

1. Atkins E, Bodel P. Clinical fever: its history, manifestations and pathogenesis. Fed Proc. 1979;38:57.
2. Holmes GP, Kaplan JE, Grant NM, et al. Chronic fatigue syndrome: a working case definition. Ann Intern Med. 1988;108:387–9.
3. McClung HJ. Prolonged fever of unknown origin in children. Am J Dis Child. 1972;124:544.
4. Pizzo PA, Lovejoy FH, Smith DH. Prolonged fever in children: Review of 100 cases. Pediatrics. 1975;55:486.
5. Lohr JA, Hendley JO. Prolonged fever of unknown origin: a record of experiences with 54 childhood patients. Clin Pediatr. 1977;16:768.
6. Petersdorf RG, Beeson PB. Fever of unexplained origin. Medicine. 1961;40:1.
7. Shoen RP, Van Ommen RA. Fever of obscure origin. Am J Med. 1963;34:486.
8. Deal WB. Fever of unknown origin. Postgrad Med. 1971;50:182.
9. Frayha R, Uwaydah M. Fever of unknown origin. Leb Med J. 1973;26:49.
10. Howard P Jr, Hahn HH, Palmer PL, et al. Fever of unknown origin: a prospective study of 100 patients. Tex Med. 1977;73:56.
11. Larson EB, Featherstone HJ, Petersdorf RG. Fever of undetermined origin: diagnosis and follow up of 105 cases, 1970–80. Medicine. 1982;61:269.
12. Aduan R, Fauci A, Dale D, et al. Prolonged fever of unknown origin. Clin Res. 1978;26:558A.
13. Brusch JL, Weinstein L. Fever of unknown origin. Med Clin North Am. 1988;72:1247–61.
14. Petersdorf RG. FUO: how it has changed in 20 years. Hosp Pract. 1985;20:84I–84M, 84P, 84T–84V passim.
15. Barbado FJ, Vazquez JJ, Pena JM, et al. Fever of unknown origin: a survey on 133 patients. J Med. 1984;15:185–92.
16. Kerttula Y, Hirvonen P, Pettersson T. Fever of unknown origin: a follow-up investigation of 34 patients. Scand J Infect Dis. 1983;15:185–7.
17. Young EJ, Feinstein V, Mosher DM. Drug-induced fever: cases seen in the evaluation of unexplained fever in a general hospital population. Rev Infect Dis. 1982;4:69.
18. Jacoby GA, Swartz MN. Fever of undetermined origin. N Engl J Med. 1973;289:1407.
19. Gleckman R, Crowley M, Esposito A. Fever of unknown origin: a view from the community hospital. Am J Med Sci. 1977;274:21.
20. Oppel TW, Bernstein CA. The differential diagnosis of fevers. Med Clin North Am. 1954;38:891.
21. Wolff SM, Fauci AS, Dale DC. Unusual etiologies of fever and their evaluation. Annu Rev Med. 1975;26:277.
22. Aduan R, Fauci A, Dale D, et al. Factitious fever and self-induced infection. Ann Intern Med. 1979;90:230.
23. Dinarello C, Wolff, SM. Pathogenesis of fever in man. N Engl J Med. 1978;298:607.
24. Weinstein L. Clinically benign fever of unknown origin: a personal retrospective. Rev Infect Dis. 1985;7:692–9.
25. Reilly PC, Reilly MC. High-risk travel and malaria. N Engl J Med. 1977;296:1536.
26. Wright DG, Dale DC, Fauci AS, et al. Human cyclic neutropenia: clinical review and long term follow-up of patients. Medicine. 1981;60:1.
27. Krick JA, Remington JA. Toxoplasmosis in the adult—an overview. N Engl J Med. 1978;298:550.
28. Thoft RA. Corneal disease. N Engl J Med. 1978;298:1239.
29. Schacter J. Chlamydial infection. N Engl J Med. 1978;298:428.
30. McDade JE, Shepard CC, Fraser DW, et al. Legionnaires' disease. N Engl J Med. 1977;297:1197.
31. Wolff SM, Kimball HR, Perry S, et al: The biological properties of etiocholanolone. Ann Intern Med. 1967;67:1268.
32. Epler GR, McLoud TC, Graensler EA, et al. Normal chest roentgenograms in chronic diffuse infiltrative lung disease. N. Engl J Med. 1978;298:934.
33. Blain DC, Carroll M, Carr EA, et al. ^{67}Ga citrate for scanning experimental staphylococcal abscesses. J Nucl Med. 1973;14:99.
34. Habibian MR, Staab EV, Matthews HA. Gallium citrate Ga 67 scans in febrile patients. JAMA. 1975;233:1073.
35. McNeil BJ, Sanders R, Alderson PO, et al. A prospective study of computed tomography, ultrasound, and gallium imaging in patients with fever. Radiology. 1981;139:647.
36. Schmidt KG, Rasmussen JW, Sorensen PG, et al. Indium-111 granulocyte scintigraphy in the evaluation of patients with fever of undetermined origin. Scand J Infect Dis. 1987;19:339.
37. Abrams HL, McNeil BJ. Medical implications of computed tomography. N Engl J Med. 1978;298:255.
38. Spiegel AM, DiChiro G, Gordon P, et al. Diagnosis of radiosensitive hypothalamic tumors without craniotomy. Ann Intern Med. 1976;85:290.
39. Abrams HL, McNeil BJ. Medical implications of computed tomography. N Engl J Med. 1978;298:310.
40. Rowland MD, Del Bene VE. Use of body computed tomography to evaluate fever of unknown origin. J Infect Dis. 1987;156:408.
41. Nomeir AM. Bacterial endocarditis: echocardiographic and clinical evaluation during therapy. J Clin Ultrasound. 1976;4:23.
42. DiMagno EP, Malagelada JR, Taylor WF, et al. A prospective comparison of current diagnostic tests for pancreatic cancer. N Engl J Med. 1977;297:737.
43. Ulrich PC, Sanders RC. Ultrasonic characteristics of pelvic inflammatory masses. J Clin Ultrasound. 1976;4:199.
44. Rau J. Ultrasonic or radiologic cholecystography. N Engl J Med. 1977;297:62.
45. Rothman DL, Schwartz SI, Adams JT. Diagnositic laparotomy for fever or abdominal pain of unknown origin. Am J Surg. 1977;133:273.
46. Mitchell DP, Hanes TE, Hoyumpa AM, et al. Fever of unknown origin. Arch Intern Med. 1977;137:1001.
47. Katz P, Fauci AS. *Nocardia asteroides* sinusitis. JAMA. 1977;238:2397.
48. Geraci JE, Weed LA, Nichols DR. Fever of obscure origin. The value of abdominal exploration in diagnosis. JAMA. 1959;169:1302.

49. Fisher HC, White MH Jr. Biliary tract disease in the aged. Arch Surg. 1951;63:536.
50. Fung WO, Ong SC, Lee YS. Splenic tuberculosis presenting as pyrexia of unknown origin. Med J Aust. 1973;1:446.
51. Boettinger LE, Nordenstam HH, Wester PO. Disseminated tuberculosis as a cause of fever of obscure origin. Lancet. 1962;1:19.
52. Maizel H, Ruffin JM, Dobbins WO III. Whipple's disease: a review of 19 patients from one hospital and a review of the literature since 1950. Medicine. 1970;49:175.
53. Smith L. Relapsing fever: a case history. Calif Med. 1969;110:322.
54. Southern PM Jr, Sanford JP. Relapsing fever. Medicine. 1969;48:129.
55. Sundahragiati B, Kasemsuvan P, Harinasuta C, et al. Leptospirosis as a cause of pyrexia of unknown origin in Thailand. Ann Trop Med Parasitol. 1966;60:247.
56. Hattwick MA, O'Brien RJ, Hanson BF. Rocky Mountain spotted fever: epidemiology of an increasing problem. Ann Intern Med. 1976;84:732.
57. Cranston WI, Luff RH, Owen D, et al. Studies on the pathogenesis of fever in renal carcinoma. Clin Sci Mol Med. 1973;45:459.
58. Bodel P. Pyrogen release *in vitro* by lymphoid tissue from patients with Hodgkin's disease. Yale J Biol Med. 1974;47:101.
59. Bodel P. Generalized perturbations in the host physiology caused by localized tumors. Tumors and fever. Ann NY Acad Sci. 1974;230:6.
60. Bodel P. Spontaneous pyrogen production by mouse histiocytic and myelomonocytic tumor cell lines in vitro. J Exp Med. 1978;147:1503.
61. Molavi A, Weinstein L. Persistent perplexing pyrexia: some comments on etiology and diagnosis. Med Clin North Am. 1970;54:379.
62. Lee SL, Rosner F, Rivero I, et al. Refractory anemia with abnormal iron metabolism. N Engl J Med. 1965;272:761.
63. Miller JS, Miller JJ. Benign giant lymph node hyperplasia presenting as fever of unknown origin. J Pediatr. 1975;87:237.
64. Padfield R, Hicken P. Cortical hyperostosis in infants: a radiological study of sixteen patients. Br J Radiol. 1970;43:231.
65. Campbell EW, Brantley R, Harrold M, et al. Angiomyolipoma presenting as fever of unknown origin. Am J Med. 1974;57:843.
66. Ahmann DL, Kiely JM, Harrison EG, et al. Malignant lymphoma of the spleen. Cancer. 1966;19:461.
67. Zanger B, Dorsey HN. Fever: a manifestation of preleukemia. JAMA. 1976;236:1266.
68. Meachan GC, Weisberger AS. Early atypical manifestations of leukemia. Ann Intern Med. 1954;41:780.
69. Kumar S, Bhargava M. Preleukemia acute myelogenous leukemia. Acta Haematol. 1970;43:21.
70. Bowman HS, Martinez E. Fever, anemia and hyperhaptoglobinemia. Ann Intern Med. 1968;68:613.
71. Boettiger LE. Fever of unknown origin: IV. Fever in carcinoma of the kidney. Acta Med Scand. 1957;156:477.
72. Gordon DA. The extra-renal manifestations of hypernephroma. Can Med Assoc J. 1963;88:61.
73. Rawlins MD, Luff RH, Cranston WI. Pyrexia in renal carcinoma. Lancet. 1970;1:1371.
74. Berman C. Primary carcinoma of the liver. In: Greenstein JP, Haddow H (eds). Advances in Cancer Research 5. New York: Academic Press; 1958:67.
75. Goodwin JF, Stanfield CA, Steiner RE. Clinical features of left atrial myxoma. Thorax. 1962;17:91.
76. Petersdorf RG. Fever of unknown origin. Ann Intern Med. 1969;70:864.
77. Rothfield N, Phythin JM, McEwen C, et al. The role of antinuclear reactions in the diagnosis of systemic lupus erythematosus: a study of 53 cases. Arthritis Rheum. 1961;4:223.
78. Estes D, Christian CL. The natural history of systemic lupus erythematosus by prospective analysis. Medicine. 1971;50:85.
79. Fauci AS, Haynes B, Katz P. The spectrum of vasculitis. Ann Intern Med. 1978;89:660.
80. Calabro JJ, Marchesano JM. Fever associated with juvenile rheumatoid arthritis. N Engl J Med. 1967;276:11.
81. Calabro JJ, Marchesano JM. Juvenile rheumatoid arthritis. N Engl J Med. 1967;277:696.
82. Bujak JS, Aptekar RG, Decker JL, et al. Juvenile rheumatoid arthritis presenting in the adult as fever of unknown origin. Medicine. 1973;52:431.
83. Fabricant MS, Chandor SB, Friou GJ. Still's disease in adults. JAMA. 1973;225:273.
84. Jones TD. The diagnosis of rheumatic fever. JAMA. 1944;126:481.
85. Cluff LE, Johnson JE III. Drug fever. Prog Allergy. 1964;8:149.
86. Mackowiak PA. Southwestern Internal Medicine Conference. Drug fever: mechanisms, maxims, and misconceptions. Am J Med Sci. 1987;294:275–86.
87. Wolff SM, Simon HB. Granulomatous hepatitis and prolonged fever of unknown origin. Trans Am Climatol Assoc. 1973;84:149.
88. Simon HB, Wolff SM. Granulomatous hepatitis and prolonged fever of unknown origin: a study of 13 patients. Medicine. 1973;52:1.
89. Fauci AS, Wolff SM. Granulomatous hepatitis. Prog Liver Dis. 1976;5:609.
90. Crohn BB, Yarnis H. Regional Ileitis. 2nd ed. New York: Grune & Stratton; 1958.
91. Lee FI, Davies DM. Crohn's disease presenting as pyrexia of unknown origin. Lancet. 1961;1:1205.
92. Tumen HJ. Fever as a symptom of gastrointestinal disease. Am J Dig Dis. 1964;9:314.
93. Fransen H, Boettiger LE. Fever of more than two weeks' duration. Acta Med Scand. 1966;179:147.
94. Fauchald P, Rygvold O, Oipstese B. Temporal arteritis and polymyalgia rheumatica. Ann Intern Med. 1972;77:845.
95. Roberts WC, MacGregor RR, DeBlanc HJ, et al. The prepulseless phase of pulseless disease, or pulseless disease with pulses. Am J Med. 1969;46:313.
96. Sohar E, Prass M, Heller J, et al. Genetics of familial Mediterranean fever (FMF). Arch Intern Med. 1961;107:529.
97. Desnick RJ, Allen KV, Desnick SJ, et al. Fabry's disease: enzymatic diagnosis of hemizygotes and heterozygotes. J Lab Clin Med. 1973;81:157.
98. Andersen V, Buch NH, Jensen MK, et al. Deafness, urticaria and amyloidosis. Am J Med. 1967;42:449.
99. Muckle TJ, Wells M. Urticaria, deafness and amyloidosis. A new heredofamilial syndrome. Q J Med. 1962;31:325.
100. Wolff SM. Familial Mediterranean fever. In: Wintrobe MM, Isselbacher KJ, Petersdorf RG, et al., eds. Harrison's Principles of Internal Medicine. 11th ed. New York: McGraw-Hill; 1987:1450.
101. Dinarello CA, Wolff SM, Goldfinger SE, et al. Colchicine therapy for familial Mediterranean fever. N Engl J Med. 1974;291:934.
102. Bauer HG. Endocrine and other clinical manifestations of hypothalamic disease: a survey of 60 cases with autopsies. J Clin Endocrinol. 1954;14:13.
103. Fox RH, Davies TW, Marsh FP, et al. Hypothermia in a young man with an anterior hypothalamic lesion. Lancet. 1970;2:185.
104. Hey EN. Thermal regulation in the newborn. Br J Hosp Med. 1972;8:51.
105. Philip G, Smith JF. Hypothermia and Wernicke's encephalopathy. Lancet. 1973;2:122.
106. Johnson RH, Spalding JMK. Disorders of the Autonomic Nervous System. Philadelphia: FA Davis; 1974:153.
107. Wolff SM, Adler RC, Buskirk ER, et al. A syndrome of periodic hypothalamic discharge. Am J Med. 1964;36:956.
108. Simon HB. Extreme pyrexia. JAMA. 1976;236:2419.
109. Dinarello CA, Wolff SM. Molecular basis of fever in humans. Am J Med. 1982;72:799.
110. Kleinman M. Letter to editor. N Engl J Med. 1977;296:886.
111. Murray H, Tuazon C, Guerero IC, et al. Urinary temperature. N Engl J Med. 1977;296:23.
112. Dykes MHM. Unexplained postoperative fever. JAMA. 1971;216:641.
113. Ross DF, Rose MR, Rapaport FT. Febrile responses associated with cardiac surgery. J Thorac Cardiovasc Surg. 1974;67:251.
114. Cantu RC, Moses JM, Kjellberg RN, et al. An unusual cause of aseptic postoperative fever in a neurosurgical patient. Clin Pediatr. 1966;5:747.
115. Dunn LJ, Van Voorhis LW. Enigmatic fever and pelvic thrombophletitis. N Engl J Med. 1967;276:262.
116. Van Herik M. Fever as a complication of radiation therapy for carcinoma of the cervix. Am J Roentgenol Rad Ther Nucl Med. 1965;93:104.
117. Wallberg AV. Operat phaeochromocytoin med lycklig utgang. Nord Med. 1949;41:470.
118. Tisdale WA, Klatskin G. The fever of Laennec's cirrhosis. Yale J Biol Med. 1960;33:94.

41. THE ACUTELY ILL PATIENT WITH FEVER AND RASH

DAVID J. WEBER
WALTER R. GAMMON
MYRON S. COHEN

A recognizable rash can lead to immediate diagnosis and appropriate therapy. Material isolated from involved skin, when properly handled, can confirm a specific diagnosis. Unfortunately, rashes are often quite bewildering. Dermatologists, who are generally more comfortable with evaluation of the skin, are not always available for immediate consultation. Furthermore, not infrequently, dermatologists and infectious disease specialists differ in their approach to the patient with a rash.

In this chapter we will provide a framework emphasizing the following: (*1*) diagnostic approach to patients with fever and rash, (*2*) categories of skin lesions, and (*3*) brief description of the most important febrile illnesses characterized by a rash.

APPROACH TO THE PATIENT

In the initial evaluation of patients with fever and rash three problems are critical. First, whether the patient is well enough to provide further history, or immediate cardiorespiratory support is required. Second, whether the nature of the rash (in the context of presentation) demands institution of isolation precautions. Isolation is required primarily for patients whose illnesses allow airborne spread of the pathogen and includes both viral and bacterial diseases. Hospital isolation guidelines should be employed with urgency. All patients with undiagnosed infectious diseases should be treated with caution by personnel who should avoid intimate contact with secretions and employ universal blood and body fluid precautions.[1] Third, a skin lesion consistent with meningococcal disease (see below) requires emergent antibacterial therapy. Similar urgency may be warranted when lesions suggest bacterial septic shock since appropriate use of antibiotics may improve survival.[2]

The history obtained from the patient should elicit the following information:

1. Drug ingestion within the past 30 days
2. Travel outside of the local area
3. Occupational exposures
4. Sun exposure
5. Immunizations
6. Sexually transmitted disease exposure including risk factors for infection with human immunodeficiency virus (HIV)
7. Immunologic status including chemotherapy, steroid use, hematologic malignancy, and functional or anatomic asplenia
8. Valvular heart disease
9. Prior illnesses including a history of drug and/or antibiotic allergies
10. Exposure to febrile or ill individuals within the recent past
11. Exposure to wild or rural habitats and wild animals
12. Pets and habits

TABLE 1. Systemic Infections with Prominent Cutaneous Manifestations

Organism (Disease)	*Macules, Papules*	*Vesicles, Bullae*	*Petechia, Purpura*
Viruses			
Human immunodeficiency (HIV-1) virus	X		
Echoviruses	X	X	X
Coxsackieviruses	X	X	X
Rubeola (measles)	X		
Atypical measles	X		X
Adenovirus	X		X
Lymphocytic choriomeningitis virus	X		
Dengue virus	X		X
Viral hemorrhagic fevers			X
Rubella (German measles)	X		X
Arboviruses	X		
Colorado tick fever	X		
Yellow fever			X
Varicella-zoster (disseminated)		X	
Herpes simplex (disseminated)		X	
Varicella (Chickenpox)		X	
Vaccinia		X	
Cytomegalovirus	X		
Congenital cytomegalovirus			X
Epstein-Barr virus	X		X
Hepatitis B	X		
Parvovirus (erythema infectiosum)	X		
Bacteria			
Chlamydia psittaci	X		
Mycoplasma pneumoniae	X	X	
Rickettsia			
R. rickettsia (Rocky Mountain spotted fever)	X		X
R. akari (rickettsialpox)	X	X	
R. prowazekii (epidemic/louse-borne typhus)	X		X
R. typhi (endemic/murine typhus)	X		
R. tsutsugamushi (scrub typhus)	X		
Salmonella typhi	X		
Francisella tularensis	X		
Streptobacillus moniliformis (rat-bite fever)	X		X
Treponema pallidum (secondary)	X		
Neisseria gonorrhoeae			X
Neisseria meningitidis			X
Leptospira sp.	X		
Borrelia sp. (relapsing fever)	X		X
Borrelia burgdorfii (Lyme)	X (annular)		
Spirillum minor (rat-bite fever)	X		
Staphylococcal aureus	X		X
Streptococci–Group A (scarlet fever)	X		
Fungi (disseminated)			
Candida sp.	X		
Cryptococcus neoformans	X		
Histoplama capsulatum	X		
Blastomyces dermatitidis	X		
Coccidioidomycosis immitis	X		
Protozoal			
Toxoplasma gondii	X		
Plasmodium falciparum (malaria)			X

(Data from references 5–10.)

The clinician should pay particular attention to the season of the year, which dramatically affects the epidemiology of febrile rashes. Physical examination should focus on the following:

1. Vital signs
2. General appearance
3. Signs of toxicity
4. Presence and location of adenopathy
5. Presence of genital, mucosal, and/or conjunctival lesions
6. Detection of hepatosplenomegaly
7. Arthritis
8. Signs of nuchal rigidity, meningismus, or neurologic dysfunction

Key ingredients in arriving at a correct diagnosis include (*1*) dermatologic classification of the rash[3–5] (Table 1),[5–10] (*2*) distribution of the rash, (*3*) pattern of progression, and (*4*) timing of the development of rash (relative to the onset of illness and fever) (Table 2). Rashes may be classified by histologic or pathophysiologic criteria,[11] which is generally not of immediate benefit to the clinician. It must be emphasized that noninfectious processes often include skin rash and fever and should be considered strongly during the initial evaluation. Drug reactions, which occur with about 1 in 20 courses of drug therapy, should be considered in any patient presenting with a rash.[12]

HOST DEFENSE PROPERTIES OF SKIN

The skin is a relatively inhospitable environment for the growth of most pathogenic microorganisms. The hostility of that environment is mainly attributed to two factors. The relative dryness of most cutaneous surfaces provides an insufficient amount of moisture to support significant growth of pathogens, and colonization with strains of bacteria and yeast (normal resident flora), generally regarded as nonpathogenic, appears to exclude more pathogenic species.[13–15] Resident flora may actually produce metabolites that are inhibitory to the growth of more pathogenic species. Examples include bacterial lipases that liberate from sebum free fatty acids that inhibit various strains of *Streptococcus pyogenes* and antibiotic metabolites derived from *S. epidermidis* that kill strains of *Micrococcus* and *Streptococcus*.[16–18] Eradication of resident flora greatly enhances the survival of *S. aureus* and the subsequent development of infection.[19]

Normal skin is an impenetrable barrier to microorganisms. The barrier to penetration is the outermost layer of skin known as the stratum corneum. The stratum corneum is composed of corneified envelopes of dead keratinocytes joined by a relatively impermeable intercellular substance. Together, the cell envelopes and intercellular substance form a physical barrier approximately 10–15 μm thick.[20] The skin is richly supplied with both endogenous and exogenous cellular and humoral mediators of inflammation that subserve host defense functions.[21]

Epidermis and dermis are home to several cell types that may

TABLE 2. Skin Lesions and Systemic Infections

Lesion	*Common Pathogens*	*Histologic Findings*	*Smears Positive for Pathogens*	*Time of Appearance (After Onset of Illness)*
Symmetric peripheral gangrene, acrocyanosis	Noninfectious or gram-negative bacteria	Bleeding in skin, vascular thrombosis, perivascular infiltration	No	12–36 hr
Multiple purpuric lesions in seriously ill patients	*Neisseria meningitidis, Rickettsia,* other gram-negative bacteria	Vascular thrombosis, perivascular hemorrhage	Yes[a]	12–36 hr[b]
Ecthyma gangrenosum, erythema multiforme, bullous lesions	*Pseudomonas,* other gram-negative bacteria	Veins mainly involved, intima spared, inflammatory reaction	Yes	Several days
Macronodular lesions	*Candida*	Hyphae, mononuclear perivascular reaction	No	Several days
Delayed-onset rash with nonsymmetrical scattered maculopapular or vesicular lesions	*Neisseria gonorrhoeae, N. meningitidis*	Perivascular mononuclear infiltrate, immune complex	Occasionally (few bacteria only)	3–10 days
Polymorphous lesions	*N. meningitidis, N. gonorrhoeae, Salmonella*			
Rose spots	*Salmonella,* various bacteria	Perivascular mononuclear inflammation	No	5–10 days
Toxic erythema	*S. aureus, Streptococcus*	Dilation and perivascular edema	No	At presenation

[a] Except for Rocky Mountain spotted fever, in which biopsy and immunofluorescent staining are important for early diagnosis.
[b] In Rocky Mountain spotted fever, 1–7 days.
(From Kingston et al.,[11] with permission.)

generate soluble factors that initiate and amplify the inflammatory response. Those cells include the keratinocyte, fibroblast, mast cell, Langerhans cell, endothelial cell, and monocyte/macrophage. Recent studies show that keratinocytes are capable of synthesizing a number of proinflammatory and immunostimulatory cytokines (the interleukins IL-1, IL-3, and IL-6; tumor necrosis factor-α; and granulocyte-macrophage colony-stimulating factor), complement proteins and arachidonate metabolites including prostaglandins and leukotrienes.[22,23] The mast cells that reside around dermal vessels can be stimulated by a variety of factors including those derived from microorganisms to make and release promotors of inflammation such as histamine, arachidonate metabolites, proteinases, and factors that can recruit and activate leukocytes.[24] The skin may play an active role in the initiation, development, and expression of specific immune responses to microorganism through a system of skin-associated lymphoid tissues and keratinocytes.[25,26]

PATHOGENESIS OF SKIN RASH

Skin rash with fever can result from a local infectious process due to virtually any class of microbe that has been allowed to penetrate the stratum corneum and multiply locally. However, exanthems are more cogent to this discussion. An exanthem is a cutaneous eruption due to the systemic effects of a microorganism on the skin. An enanthem is an eruption of similar etiology involving the mucus membranes.

Microorganisms produce eruptions by (*1*) multiplication in the skin (e.g., herpesviruses); (*2*) release of toxins that act on skin structures (e.g., scarlet fever, *Pseudomonas aeruginosa*); (*3*) evoking an inflammatory response involving phagocytes and lymphocytes (in this case the microbicidal/tumorcidal metabolism of host defense cells is directed at the skin); and (*4*) via effects on vasculature, including vaso-occlusion and necrosis and/or vasodilation with edema and hyperemia. Obviously, for many eruptions several mechanisms can play a role.

DIFFERENTIAL DIAGNOSIS AND SKIN RASH

There are two ways to approach the investigation of infectious rash, either by the type of lesion visualized or by knowledge of individual pathogens and the rashes they produce. Unfortunately, neither system is inclusive. Accordingly, both approaches are taken in this section.

Characteristics of the Lesion

Morphologic types of skin lesions include macules, papules, plaques, nodules, vesicles, bullae, and pustules. Macules are flat, nonpalpable lesions in the plane of the skin. Papules are small palpable lesions elevated above the plane of the skin. Large papules are referred to as nodules. Vesicles and bullae are small and large blisters, respectively, and pustules are palpable lesions filled with pus. Plaques are large flat lesions that are palpable. In addition to morphology, lesions are characterized by their color and particularly by the presence or absence of hemorrhage. Lesions may be skin colored, hyperpigmented or hypopigmented, or one of several other colors of which redness is the most common. Blanching erythematous lesions are those in which erythema is due to vasodilation, while nonblanching erythemas may be due to extravasation of blood. Purpuric lesions are those in which there is hemorrhage into the skin and may be small, petechial or large, ecchymotic. We have divided our discussion into rashes that are maculopapular (a rash characterized by flat and elevated lesions), nodular, vesiculobullous, erythematous, and purpuric.

Maculopapular Eruptions

Maculopapular eruptions are usually seen in viral illnesses and immune-mediated syndromes. Common viral etiologies include the classic childhood viral diseases such as measles, rubella, erythema infectiosum, and roseola.[27] Other viral agents that often produce a rash are atypical measles, coxsackieviruses, echoviruses, cytomegalovirus, and hepatitis B.[28] Erythema multiforme is considered a special category of maculopapular rash. Erythema infectiosum (fifth disease) is now known to be caused by parvovirus B19. Besides erytherma infectiosum, other disease manifestations of infection with parvovirus B19 include aplastic crisis in patients with sickle cell anemia, arthritis, and, most recently, fetal death and hydrops fetalis. Erythema infectiosum is characterized by a three-stage rash. The initial stage is that of an erythematous, warm but nontender "slapped cheek" facial rash. Simultaneously up to four days later, a variable rash appears on the extremities, which has a morbilliform, confluent, or annular appearance. Later the rash may remit and recur with stress, exercise, sunlight, or bathing. The rash usually disappears within one to two weeks.[27a]

Lesions of erythema multiforme usually begin as round to oval macules and papules that vary in size from less than a centimeter up to 1–2 cm in diameter. Typical lesions have central erythema surrounded by a narrow ring of normal-appearing skin that is in turn surrounded by another thin ring of erythema to form target lesions. The central area may be dark red, blue, or dusky grey in color and may develop into a blister (bullous erythema multiforme). Lesions are typically symmetrically distributed on the trunk and extremities and may show a predilection for knees, elbows, palms, and soles. Mucosal involvement is usually present and painful. The degree of mucosal involvement varies from oral blisters and erosions to a hemorrhagic conjunctivitis and stomatitis. When the latter are present with fever, the term *Stevens-Johnson syndrome* is applied. The distribution, symmetry, tendency to iris formation, and bulla should allow proper identification. Most cases of erythema multiforme are idiopathic. In children and adults infections are a leading etiology, but in adults many cases are idiopathic or due to drug exposure. Infectious diseases linked to erythema multiforme are summarized in Table 3. Atypical rashes suggestive of erythema multiforme may occur in chronic meningococcemia, bacterial endocarditis, secondary syphilis, staphylococcal scalded skin syndrome, Kawasaki disease, toxic shock syndrome, Rocky Mountain spotted fever, collagen vascular disease, and a variety of viral disorders.

Several life-threatening infections may present with blanching erythematous maculopapular lesions before evolving into petechiae. These include meningococcemia, Rocky Mountain spotted fever, and dengue fever. Although rheumatic fever has as one of its diagnostic findings a configurate, migrating erythema known as erythema marginatum, it may also be associated with a maculopapular eruption and subcutaneous nodules. Patients with enteric fever due to *Salmonella* may develop "rose spots," a transient scattering of rose-colored macules over the abdomen.

Secondary syphilis is often accompanied by a rash with highly variable morphology. Lesions may be macular, maculopapular, papulosquamous, or pustular. Occasionally all types of lesions may occur in the same individual.

Nodular Lesions

A nodule is a palpable, solid round or ellipsoidal lesion, usually resulting from disease in the dermis. Nonerythematous nodules may suggest candidal sepsis (see below), but other fungal disease including blastomycosis, histoplasmosis, coccidioidomycosis, sporotrichosis, and histoplasmosis may produce skin nodules. Bacteria such as *Nocardia* and atypical mycobacteria may also cause nodular lesions. Lesions consistent with ecthyma gangrenosum suggest *Pseudomonas* sepsis. A skin biopsy specimen with appropriate stains and cultures will define the diagnosis.

The lesions of erythema nodosum are characterized by tender, erythematous nodules that vary in diameter from less than a centimeter to several centimeters. They are usually multiple and located on the anterior portions of the legs but may be solitary and occur on the upper part of the body. They typically do not suppurate but rarely may do so. The lesions will often develop in crops and usually heal in days to a few weeks without scarring. Infectious agents are a prominant cause of this lesion (Table 4).

TABLE 3. Differential Diagnosis of Erythema Multiforme

Noninfectious
Drugs
X-ray therapy
Infectious
Herpes simplex infections
Epstein-Barr virus
Adenovirus
Coxsackie B5
Vaccinia (smallpox innoculation)
Mycoplasma pneumoniae
Chlamydia (psitticosis, lymphagranuloma venereum)
Cat scratch (?)
Salmonella typhi
Yersinia
Mycobacterium tuberculosis
Histoplasma capsulatum
Coccidioides immitis

TABLE 4. Differential Diagnosis of Erythema Nodosum

Noninfectious
Systemic lupus erythematosus
Sarcoidosis
Ulcerative colitis
Crohn's colitis
Behçet's disease
Drugs
Pregnancy
Infectious
Streptococcal infection
Mycobacterium tuberculosis
Mycobacterium leprae
Chlamydia trachomatus (lymphagranuloma venereum)
Yersinia infection
Histoplasma capsulatum
Blastomyces dermatitidis
Coccidioides immitis

Diffuse Erythema

Diffuse erythema, especially if desquamation or peeling is present, should lead to consideration of scarlet fever, toxic shock syndrome, mucocutaneous lymph node syndrome (Kawasaki disease), staphylococcal scalded skin syndrome, Stevens-Johnson syndrome, and toxic epidermal necrolysis. Desquamation may occur late in all of these syndromes, and its absence early in the disease course should not be considered a reason for excluding any disease process. Most of these disorders can be easily differentiated by the patient's history and appropriate diagnostic tests.

Vesiculobullous Eruptions

A vesicle is a circumscribed, elevated lesion containing free fluid. A vesicular lesion larger than 0.5 cm is termed a bulla. Most vesiculobullous eruptions are immunologic or primarily dermatologic. Infectious diseases to be considered include varicella, disseminated herpes simplex, eczema herpeticum, enteroviruses, and coxsackieviruses (includes A16, the cause of hand, foot, and mouth disease). Tzanck smear of a scraping from a blister may allow determination of a herpes infection, either zoster or varicella. Vesicles can be confused with pustules. A pustule is an elevation of the skin enclosing a purulent exudate. Vesicular lesions may become pustules, but diffuse pustular diseases usually represent a dermatologic illness (e.g., pustular psoriasis) or a cutaneous infection (e.g., pustular *Pseudomonas* lesions after the use of contaminated hot tubs or staphylococcal folliculitis). Pustular skin lesions associated with arthralgias should lead to a consideration of gonoccemia, *Moraxella* bacteremia, chronic meningococcemia, subacute bacterial endocarditis, coxsackie infection, and Behçet syndrome.

Petechial Purpuric Eruptions

Petechiae are lesions less than 3 mm in diameter containing extravascated red blood cells or hemoglobin. Larger lesions are termed ecchymoses. Diffuse petechial lesions should always prompt emergent investigation. In critically ill patients these lesions are often associated with symmetric peripheral gangrene, consumptive coagulopathy, and shock. The most common infectious etiologies include gram-negative organisms, especially *N. meningitidis* and *Rickettsia*. Less commonly *Listeria monocytogenes* or staphylocci may be associated with a similar clinical picture. Asplenic patients are at an increased risk of overwhelming sepsis, which may be accompanied by symmetric peripheral gangrene.[29–36] About half of the infections are due to *S. pneumoniae*.[29,31,36]

Viral illnesses associated with petechial rashes include coxsachie A9, echovirus 9, Epstein-Barr virus, cytomegalovirus, atypical measles and the viral hemorrhagic fevers (see Chapter 142). Children with coxsackievirus and echovirus infections may appear very ill, and differential diagnosis from meningococcemia is difficult.

Rashes are a prominent characteristic of rickettsial disease except for Q fever. Although Rocky Mountain spotted fever is the most common rickettsial disease in the United States, endemic typhus has been noted on the Gulf Coast and epidemic typhus among immigrants and in the mid-Atlantic states. Lesions caused by rickettsiae are usually generalized and symmetric. An eschar (tache noire) characteristically develops at the site of inoculation in the following rickettsial infections: African tick typhus (*R. conorii*), North Asian tick-borne rickettsiosis (*R. siberica*), Queensland tick typhus (*R. australis*), rickettsialpox (*R. akari*), and scrub- or chigger-borne typhus (*R. tsutsugamushi*).

In patients with an appropriate travel history, infection with *P. falciparum* must be considered. Heavy parasitization may lead to severe hemolysis, renal failure, central nervous system findings, and petechiae secondary to thrombocytopenia.

The most important causes of noninfectious petechiae are thrombocytopenia, large and small vessel necrotizing vasculitis, and pigmented purpuric eruptions.

Enanthem

While attempting to classify the exanthem, it is critical that a thorough search (including the mouth, conjunctiva, vagina, rectum, and glans penis) be made for enanthems. In allergic reactions the mucous membranes are frequently involved. Koplick spots, diagnostic of rubeola, are blue-grey spots on red—a grain of sand on the buccal mucosa opposite the end molar. A strawberry tongue suggests Kawasaki disease, toxic shock syndrome, or scarlet fever. Petechiae of the palate are common in scarlet fever, and with infectious mononucleosis petechiae of the hard and soft palate are common. Oral ulcers occur in a variety of immunologic diseases presenting with exanthems and also with coxsackie A16.

PATHOGENS OR INFECTIOUS CONDITIONS STRONGLY ASSOCIATED WITH RASH

Having outlined the general categories by which skin lesions due to infectious agents should be divided, it is worth describing in more detail the spectrum of skin lesions associated with discrete pathogens or pathogenic processes.

Septicemia

Kingston and Mackey have classified the skin lesions associated with septicemia into five pathogenic processes[11] (major infectious etiologies): (*1*) disseminated intravascular coagulation (DIC) and coagulopathy (*Neisseria meningitidis, Streptococcus* sp., enteric gram-negative bacilli); (*2*) direct vascular invasion and occlusion by bacteria and fungi (*N. meningitidis, P. aeruginosa, Candida* sp., *Aspergillus* sp., *Rickettsia* sp.); (*3*) immune vasculitis and immune complex formation (*N. meningitidis, N. gonorrhoeae, Salmonella typhi*); (*4*) emboli from endocarditis (*S. aureus, Streptococcus* sp.); and (*5*) vascular effects of toxins (staphylococcal scalded skin syndrome, toxic shock syndrome, scarlet fever). A variety of bacteria may spread to the skin, generally producing discrete lesions from which bacteria can be isolated or recognized on biopsy.

Cutaneous manifestations of DIC include symmetric peripheral gangrene, purpura fulminans, localized gangrene, acrocyanosis, purpura, ecchymosis, bleeding from wound and venipuncture sites, and subcutaneous hematoma.[11,37] Symmetric peripheral gangrene is defined as ischemic necrosis simultaneously involving the distal portions of two or more extremities without proximal arterial obstruction.[38] Etiologies include cardiogenic shock and other low flow states, disorders that induce severe vasospasm such as ergot poisoning and Raynaud syndrome, disorders that lead to obstruction of small blood vessels such as cold agglutinins or primary polycythemia, snake bites, and infectious agents.[38–40] *Neisseria meningitidis* is the organism most commonly responsible for symmetric peripheral gangrene, but is may occur due to *S. pneumoniae, S. aureus, Streptococcus* sp., *E. coli, Klebsiella* sp., *Proteus* sp., *Aeromonas hydrophila, Aspergillus,* and other gram-negative organisms.[37,39,41] Symmetric peripheral gangrene is preceded by bleeding into the skin, ecchymosis, purpura, and acrocyanosis (a grayish cyanosis that does not blanch on pressure and occurs on the lips, legs, nose, ear lobes, and genitalia). Subsequently the ecchymotic lesions become confluent, blister and necrose, and develop into eschars.[11] The histology reveals a Shwartzman-like reaction in the skin with diffuse and extensive hemorrhages, perivascular cuffing, and intravascular thrombosis. Bacteria are usually absent from smears of the lesions. Shock rather than DIC appears to be the major factor in the pathogenesis of symmetric peripheral gangrene.

The term *purpura fulminans* has been used synonymously with symmetric peripheral gangrene and in a more restricted sense to describe symmetric bleeding into the skin and subsequent necrosis after a benign infection.[11] This latter syndrome is best described in children and usually follows by several days pharyngitis or a viral exanthem.[39,42,43] Common agents include varicella, measles, or streptococci. Histologically, it resembles an Arthus reaction or localized Shwartzman reaction[44] with deposition of antigen–antibody complexes in tissues.

Infections Due to Neisseria Species

N. meningitidis. Purpuric skin lesions have been noted in 80–90 percent of patients with fulminant meningococcemia.[44–46] The lesions characteristically are petechial but may blanch early in the course of infection and resemble a viral exanthem. The petechiae are irregular, small, and often raised with pale centers. Lesions most commonly occur on the extremities and truck but may also be found on the head, palms, soles, and mucous membranes. Symmetric peripheral gangrene may occur, often in association with DIC. Histology reveals diffuse endothelial damage, fibrin thrombi, necrosis of the vessel walls, and perivascular hemorrhage in the involved skin.[46,47] Aspirates of the involved areas frequently will reveal organisms when Gram stained.[45,48] Meningococcal endotoxin is a potent producer of the dermal Shwartzman reaction in mice and probably plays an important role in the frequency of hemorrhagic cutaneous manifestations in meningococcal infections.[49] Skin lesions and bacteremia are rarely seen in patients with meningococcal pneumonia.[50]

Chronic meningococcemia is a rare disease. The classic clinical constellation of symptoms includes intermittent or sustained fevers; recurring maculopapular, nodular, or petechial eruptions; and migratory arthritis or arthralgias with little systemic toxicity.[51,52] Skin lesions were noted to occur in 93 percent of 148 patients.[52] A variety of skin lesions may occur in chronic meningococcemia. The most frequently reported lesions are pale to pink-colored macular and papular lesions, which occur in over 40 percent of cases. Nodular lesions, mostly on the lower extremities, may occur. These lesions may be distinguished from those of erythema nodosum by their tendency to be less painful and lack the bluish border characteristic of erythema nodosum. Petechiae of variable size may occur with vesicular or pustular centers. Small, irregularly round, subcutaneous hemorrhages with a bluish gray center containing pus cells are a distinctive lesion of this syndrome. Ecchymotic areas or hemorrhagic tender nodules that are located deep in the dermis may also occur. Lesions associated with chronic meningococcemia tend to appear in showers in association with the onset of fever. In contrast to the lesions associated with fulminant meningococcemia, the lesions associated with chronic meningococcemia rarely include organisms demonstrable by Gram-stained smear or biopsy.[53]

Neisseria gonorrhoeae. Disseminated gonococcal infection (DGI) follows untreated mucosal infection in about 0.5–3 percent of patients.[54,55] Skin lesions are the most common manifestation of DGI and occur in 50–70 percent of patients.[56] The eruption typically appears during the first day of symptoms and may recur with each bout of fever.[57] The skin lesions associated with DGI begin as tiny red papules or petechiae 1–5 mm in diameter, many of which evolve rapidly through vesicular or pustular stages to develop a grey necrotic center, often on a hemorrhagic base.[57,58] Papules, bullae, pustules, and hemorrhagic lesions may all be present simultaneously. The lesions tend to be scanty but widely distributed. The distal portions of the extremities are most commonly involved, with sparing of the scalp, face, trunk, and oral mucous membranes. Histologic examination will reveal local vasculitis, fibrin deposition, necrosis, and neutrophil infiltration.[59] Gram-stained smears of material from skin lesions infrequently reveal organisms, although most smears are positive for gonococci when examined by immunofluorescence techniques. Circulating immune complexes may play a role in the pathogenesis of DGI-associated skin lesions.[60]

Pseudomonas Infection

Skin lesions have been reported to accompany *P. aeruginosa* sepsis in 13–39 percent of patients.[61–63] The dermatologic manifestations of *P. aeruginosa* sepsis include ecthyma gangrenosum,[62,63–71] subcutaneous nodules,[62,72–76] vesicular lesions,[62] gangrenous cellulitis,[62,63] small papules resembling the rose spots of typhoid fever,[77] and grouped petechiae.[70] Ecthyma gangrenosum, the most characteristic skin lesion caused by *P. aeruginosa,* has generally been reported to occur in 1.3–2.8 percent of septic patients,[61,78,79] but one report noted ecthyma gangrenosum in 28 percent of patients with *Pseudomonas* bacteremia.[63]

Ecthyma gangrenosum lesions begin as a painless round erythematous macule with or without an adherent vesicle that soon becomes indurated and progresses to a hemorrhagic bluish bulla. Later the lesion sloughs to form a gangrenous ulcer with a gray-black eschar and a surrounding erythematous halo. The process evolves rapidly over a period of 12–24 hours. Lesions may be discrete or multiple and are usually found in the groin, axilla, or perianal areas but may occur anywhere on the body. Although most commonly associated with *P. aeruginosa* sepsis, ecthyma gangrenosum has also been reported in sepsis with other pseudomonal species,[80] *A. hydrophila,*[81,82] *Candida* sp.,[83] *Serratia marcescens,*[65] *S. aureus,*[65] *Aspergillus* sp.,[65] and *Mucur* sp.[65] It may also result from vasculitis or malignant infiltration.[84] Rarely ecthyma gangrenosum due to *P. aeruginosa* may occur in the absence of sepsis.[71,85,86]

Histologically ecthyma gangrenosum is characterized by three features: bacterial invasion of the media and adventitia of vein walls deep in the dermis, sparing of the intima and lumen, and minimal inflammation.[67,69,81,84] Bacterial invasion results in marked fibrin exudation and frank hemorrhage, followed by ballooning of the upper dermis with resulting bullous formation. Finally, necrosis of the exudated dermis occurs. Bacteria are readily visible in biopsy samples and can be demonstrated in Gram-stained material scraped from the base of the lesion.[66]

Subcutaneous nodules may result from *P. aeruginosa* bacteremia. Characteristically, the nodules are erythematous and warm and may be either fluctuant or nonfluctuant and either tender or nontender. Despite prolonged antibiotic therapy, these lesions may contain viable bacteria weeks after the blood has been cleared of infection. The absence of fluctuance may be due to either the lack of pus in neutropenic patients and/or the deep location of the abscess. Although therapy may require incision and drainage,[74,75] prolonged therapy with drainage may result in a cure.[72,76]

Subacute Bacterial Endocarditis

Skin lesions have been reported to accompany bacterial endocarditis in 15–50 percent of cases in recent series.[87–90] Skin lesions include Osler nodes, Janeway lesions, and petechiae.

Osler nodes occur in about 5–15 percent of patients with subacute bacterial endocarditis. They are tender, indurated, erythematous nodules with a pale center about 1.0–1.5 mm in diameter.[91,92] Osler nodes most commonly occur on the pads of the fingers or toes but may occur on the thenar and hypothenar eminences and over the arms. Pain may be elicited by palpating the tips of the digits. They tend to occur in crops, are rarely numerous, and tend to be transient. The lesions usually resolve without necrosis or suppuration 1–3 days after antibiotic therapy. Histologically, Osler nodes show microabscesses with microemboli in adjacent arterioles. Osler nodes are most commonly associated with subacute bacterial endocarditis due to infection with streptococci but may occur in endocarditis due to fungi and gram-negative bacilli[92] or in systemic lupus erythematosus, typhoid, and gonococcemia.[11] Osler nodes probably represent microemboli leading to vascular occlusion with localized vasculitis.

Janeway lesions consist of small erythematous macules or less commonly small nodular hemorrhages in the palms and soles. Although they may be seen in subacute bacterial endocarditis, they are more common in acute endocarditis, especially that due to *S. aureus*. Unlike Osler nodes, they are painless. Histologically they show microabscesses with neutrophil infiltration of capillaries.

Petechiae are the most common skin and mucous membrane lesions in endocarditis and occur in about 50 percent of patients. The lesions are small, flat, reddish brown lesions that do not blanch on pressure. Mucous membrane involvement is common. Petechiae frequently occur in small crops. Lesions usually are transient.

Infections Due to Staphylococcus aureus

Staphylococcus aureus is responsible for a variety of infectious syndromes that may produce local or diffuse skin lesions.[93–97] Mechanisms of diffuse skin lesions include (*1*) production of toxins (staphylococcal scalded skin syndrome, toxic shock syndrome), (*2*) as a consequence of shock, and (*3*) due to vascular invasion often in association with endocarditis.

Staphylococcal scalded skin syndrome. *Staphyloccus aureus* belonging to phage group II (types 3A, 3B, 3C, 55, 71) may produce exfoliative toxins. These toxins are capable of causing a clinical spectrum of disease that includes bullous impetigo, a generalized scarlatiniform eruption without exfoliation, and exfoliative disease (staphylococcal scalded skin syndrome [SSSS]).[95,97,98–101] Bullous impetigo, the most limited variant that results from toxin-producing *S. aureus,* is characterized by discrete, flaccid bullae containing clear or cloudy yellow fluid. Lesions are frequently localized to the umbilicus or axillae, and the surrounding skin is normal or mildly erythematous. The bullae rapidly rupture and leave raw, denuded areas that re-epithelialize in 5–7 days. Affected infants are afebrile and lack constitutional signs.

SSSS usually occurs in neonates (Ritter's disease) or young children but may occur in older children or rarely in adults. Most cases in adults occur in association with renal impairment or immunosuppression.[102–104] Unlike bullous impetigo where the staphylococcal infection is in the skin at the site of the lesion, in SSSS the infection is often at a distant site or not on the skin at all. SSSS begins abruptly with a diffuse, blanchable erythema in association with marked skin tenderness, fever, and irritability. Light stroking of the ill-defined bullae will cause rupture and separation of the upper portion of the epidermis (Nikolsky sign). Generalized desquamation usually occurs. Unless secondary infection intervenes, the skin heals within 10–14 days. A skin biopsy (or a frozen section for presumptive diagnosis) may be employed to distinguish between SSSS and toxic epidermal necrolysis (TEN). In SSSS the cleavage plane of the early intraepidermal bulla is just beneath the granular cell layer, whereas in TEN the bulla is subepidermal and is seen at the basement membrane zone. Early distinction between these two diseases is important because the therapy for SSSS includes antistaphylococcal antibiotics whereas in TEN discontinuation of treatment with the offending drug may be lifesaving.

A mild form of SSSS is characterized by a generalized scarlatiniform eruption with exfoliation (staphylococcal scarlet fever). The skin has a sandpaper roughness and Pastia's lines are present, but the strawberry tongue and palatal enanthem of streptococcal scarlet fever are not present.

Toxic shock syndrome. Toxic shock syndrome (TSS) is an acute febrile illness characterized by a generalized erythematous eruption almost certainly due to in vivo production of a toxin at the site of localized, often relatively asymptomatic or unnoticed infection caused by *S. aureus* capable of toxin production.[95] The putative toxin, TSS toxin 1, has been shown to be identical[105] to enterotoxin F[106] and exotoxin C.[107] TSS toxin 1 has been demonstrated to be a potent, nonspecific inducer of IL-1 production; to be a potent, nonspecific T-cell mitogen; and to induce the suppression of a number of immune responses. The exact pathogenesis of TSS is still unclear.[108] Recently, TSS Toxin-1-producing coagulase-negative staphylococci have been linked to TSS.[109] Most cases of TSS have occurred in menstruating females, often in association with tampon use.[110,111] Nonmenstrual TSS has been associated with a variety of infections including postoperative, cutaneous, and burn infections and postpartum complications.[112–114] More recently TSS has been linked to *S. aureus* respiratory infection, often after viral influenza.[115–118]

TSS may vary from a relatively mild disease, often misdiagnosed as a viral syndrome, to a severe life-threatening illness. The most common symptoms include a temperature greater than 40°C, hypotension, and diffuse erythroderma with desquamation 1–2 weeks after the onset of illness. Additional early features include conjunctival, oropharyngeal, and/or vaginal hyperemia; vomiting and diarrhea; and myalgias.[119–122] Most patients have abnormalities in three or more organ systems: (*1*) muscular—rhabdomyolysis; (*2*) central nervous system—toxic encephalopathy; (*3*) renal—azotemia; (*4*) liver—abnormal transaminases; and (*5*) hematologic—thrombocytopenia. The rash of TSS is almost always present within the first 24 hours of illness. Desquamation occurs after 7–10 days, most prominently on the hands and feet. Histologically, the epidermis exhibits cleavage in the basilar layers, which differentiates TSS from SSSS and from viral and drug eruptions.[123]

Staphylococcus aureus septicemia may be associated with erythematous, petechial, or pustular lesions.[124] In addition, lesions associated with endocarditis such as Osler nodes, Janeway lesions, and splinter hemorrhages may occur. Such skin lesions have been reported in 10–64 percent of patients with staphylococcal septicemia.[125] Purpuric lesions may at times be so extensive as to mimic meningococcemia or Rocky Mountain spotted fever.[126–129] Gram-stained smears of the material in these lesions will usually reveal gram-positive cocci.

Rickettsial Infections

Rickettsiae are obligate intracellular parasites whose primary target in humans appears to be the endothelial cell.[130] After parasitization of the endothelial cell, necrosis of the media and intima results in thrombosis, microinfarcts, and extravasation of blood. The end result is increased vascular permeability and vasculitis.

Rash is a hallmark of Rocky Mountain spotted fever,[131–135] the most common rickettsial disease in the United States. Initially, the patient develops a maculopapular rash that may not be appreciated by the patient or the physician. Subsequently, the rash becomes more definite and petechial. Characteristically, the rash appear between the second and sixth days of illness (average, 4 days). However, the rash may be absent in 5–17 percent of patients, and in up to 50 percent it may not appear within the first 3 days of illness.[131,132,134,136,137] Most commonly, the rash begins on the extremities, often around the wrists and ankles, and spreads centripetally to the trunk, with relative sparing of the face. However, the rash may begin on the trunk (10 percent) or have a diffuse onset (10 percent). Characteristically, the rash involves the palms and/or soles in the later stages of infection. Over time, the rash, which begins as maculopapular lesions, may progress to become petechial or ecchymotic. Rarely, the rash may be urticarial or pruritic. Since the mortality of infection may be decreased from 15 to 3 percent[132] with appropriate therapy, antibiotics should never be delayed by the absence of rash.

Candidiasis

The incidence and relative frequency of *Candida* as a nosocomial pathogen appear to be increasing.[138–141] Disseminated candidiasis is frequently fatal and is a major cause of death in immunocompromised patients.[142,143] Predisposing factors are malignancy with cytotoxic therapy, neutropenia, antimicrobial therapy, hyperalimentation, severe burn injuries, very low weight neonates, intravenous catheters, systemic adrenocortical steroids, and gastrointestinal surgery.[142,143]

Disseminated candidiasis may be accompanied by a characteristic macronodular skin rash in up to 13 percent of patients.[143] The lesions are discrete, firm, nontender, subcutaneous raised erythematous areas or nodules.[144–146] Nodules may have a pale center, and some may become hemorrhagic. Often the lesions are diffuse, but they may be localized to a small area. The face is usually spared. Histologically the middle and lower dermis are involved and show vessels distended by fungal pseudohyphae, platelet aggregates, and fibrin. Scant lymphocytic perivenular infiltrate may be present.

The diagnosis of disseminated candidiasis may be established by biopsy and culture of these lesions. However, the diagnosis may be missed unless multiple sections of the subcutaneous tissue are carefully examined.

Chronic mucocutaneous candidiasis results from impaired function of the T-lymphocyte system and may be a manifestation of a variety of cutaneous syndromes.[147]

Many other fungi produce nodular lesions identical to *Candida* and must be considered in the immunocompromised host. In patients with the acquired immunodeficiency syndrome (AIDS), cryptococci may cause umbilicated nodules that look like molluscum contagiosum.

Immunocompromised Patients

The diagnosis of skin lesions in the immunocompromised patient is complex because of the wide range of potential microbial pathogens that may occur in patients with abnormal immune responses.[148,149] Cutaneous lesions of suspected infectious etiology should undergo biopsy. Biopsy samples should be processed by using the most rapid and sensitive methods for detecting microbes both histologically and immunologically, and appropriate stains and cultures should be obtained to optimize the chance for identifying the pathogen. Biopsy samples should be divided into two portions: the first should be sent to histology for evaluation by routine and special stains to detect fungi, mycobacteria, and bacteria. The second portion should be sent to microbiology and cultured for aerobic and anaerobic bacteria, mycobacteria, and fungi. Direct fungal touch preparations and Gram, acid-fast, and modified acid-fast stains should be performed. Viral culture should be considered when herpesviruses are considered.

Human Immunodeficiency Virus

HIV infection commonly results in dermatologic disorders.[150–153] After initial exposure to HIV many patients appear to develop a "seroconversion" disease that is clinically similar to mononucleosis. Manifestations may include transient fevers, myalgias, headache, urticaria, aseptic meningitis and rash.[150,154–161] The rash is maculopapular and usually confined to the trunk.

Kaposi sarcoma in the patient with HIV infection usually begins as multiple reddish to salmon-colored round or oval macules with a halo of surrounding pallor. Lesions are usually multiple, symmetric, and widely distributed over the body, but occasionally only one or a few lesions will develop, usually on the head, neck, or distal parts of the extremities. About 50 percent of patients will develop lesions in the mouth or sites within the gastrointestinal tract. The lesions slowly enlarge and rapidly develop nodularity and a deep red-blue color. Lesions vary in size from a few millimeters to a centimeter in diameter. The lesions are usually asymptomatic and rarely show evidence of necrosis. The diagnosis is made by biopsy.

Well-described primary dermatologic disorders of HIV infection patients include seborrheic dermatitis,[150,151,153,162] ichthyosis,[150,162–164] infectious eczemoid dermatitis,[150,162] yellow nail syndrome,[162] papular eruption,[162] vitiligo,[165] telangiectasias of the anterior portion of the chest,[166] and alopecia.[150,162,167] Several patients with HIV have developed an eosinophilic pustular rash responsive to ultraviolet therapy.[168]

Oral manifestations of HIV infection include oral candidiasis, hairy leukoplakia, herpes infection, and Kaposi sarcoma.[150,169] Oral candidiasis occurs in greater than 50 percent of HIV patients and takes the following forms: (*1*) overt thrush with pseudomembranous patches on the tongue and/or buccal mucosa; (*2*) erythematous, atrophic patches on the hard mucosa; or (*3*) a hypertrophic coating on the dorsum of the tongue.

Cutaneous lesions in HIV-infected persons may be caused by a variety of microorganisms, even when the classic target organs for a particular infectious agent do not include the skin.[170–172] Also, common cutaneous infections may occur in florid or unusual forms in AIDS patients. Herpes zoster occurs with a higher than expected frequency in HIV-infected persons.[150,152,162] Chronic varicella-zoster infection has been reported.[171,173] Severe, chronic herpes simplex lesions have been reported.[162] These ulcers are frequently perianal in homosexual men but may also involve the lips and perioral area. Secondary syphilis may produce a diffuse, erythematous, nonpruritic, maculopapular skin eruption.[174] In patients with AIDS, typical serologic tests (i.e., VDRL and fluorescent treponemal antibody absorption test [FTA-ABS]) for syphilis may be unreliable, and a biopsy of the skin lesion with silver staining to show the spirochetes may be required for diagnosis. Cytomegalovirus,[170] disseminated candidiasis, *C. neoformans*, [170,175] *H. capsulatum*,[170] *C. immitis*,[176] *Acanthamoeba castellani*,[173] and *M. avium-intracellulare* infection[173] may involve the skin. Skin lesions may yield multiple pathogens.[177,178] Recently several groups have reported AIDS patients with papules and nodules histologically identified as epithelioid angiomatosis that may be mistaken for Kaposi sarcoma. A microorganism consistent with the cat-scratch bacillus has been identified in these lesions by use of the Warthin-Starry stain.[179,180]

Drug reactions are common in patients with AIDS. Up to 50 percent of patients treated with trimethoprim-sulfamethoxazole will develop a rash, usually an erythematous, maculopapular rash involving the entire body[181,182] that is commonly associated with fever. Stevens-Johnson syndrome may develop. Rash may also accompany pentamadine therapy[181] or dapsone-trimethoprim.[183]

Dermatologic signs that have been suggested as early evidence of HIV infection include the following: macular exanthematous rash, especially in conjunction with a mononucleosis-like illness; seborreic dermatitis, extensive folliculitis; herpes zoster in young persons; oral candidiasis in patients not recently treated with antibiotics; prolonged herpes eruption; explosive new psoriasis; and oral hairy leukoplakia.

REFERENCES

1. Centers for Disease Control. Recommendations for prevention of HIV transmission in the health-care setting. MMWR. 1987;36(Suppl 2):3–18.
2. Kreger BE, Craven DE, McCabe WR. Gram-negative bacteremia. IV. Reevaluation of clinical features and treatment in 612 patients. Am J Med. 1980;68:344–55.
3. Valman HB. Common rashes. Br Med J. 1981;283:970–1.
4. Fitzpatrick TB, Bernhard JD. The structure of skin lesions and fundamentals of diagnosis. In: Jeffers JD, Scott E, White J, eds. Dermatology in General Medicine. Textbook and Atlas. 3rd ed. New York: McGraw-Hill; 1987:20–49.
5. Lazarus GS, Goldsmith LA, Tharp MD. Diagnosis of skin disease. Philadelphia: FA Davis; 1980
6. Fitzpatrick TB, Johnson RA. Differential diagnosis of rashes in the acutely ill febrile patient and in life-threatening diseases. In: Jeffers JD, Scott E, White J, eds. Dermatology in General Medicine. Textbook and Atlas. 3rd ed. New York: McGraw-Hill; 1987:21–2.
7. Johnson M-L. Dermatologic problems. In: Samily AH, ed. Textbook of Diagnostic Medicine. Philadelphia: Lea & Febiger; 1987:768–89.
8. Corey L, Kirby P. Rash and fever. In: Braunwald E, Isselbacher KJ, Petersdorf RG, et al., eds. Harrison's Principles of Internal Medicine. 11th ed. New York: McGraw-Hill; 1987:240–4.
9. Oblinger MJ, Sande MA. Fever and Rash. In: Stein JH, ed. Internal Medicine. Boston: Little, Brown; 1983:1173–8.
10. Kline PP. Fever and rash. Emerg Decisions. 1988;April:27–37.
11. Kingston ME, Mackey D. Skin clues in the diagnosis of life-threatening infections. Rev Infect Dis. 1986;8:1–11.
12. Swinyer LJ. Drug eruptions in an emergency department setting. Emerg Med Clin North Am. 1985;3:717–35.
13. Fitzpatrick TB, Bernhard JD, Soter NA. Correlation of pathophysiology of skin. In: Jeffers JD, Scott E, White J, eds. Dermatology in General Medicine. Textbook and Atlas. 3rd ed. New York: McGraw-Hill; 1987:69–73.
14. Kligman AM, Leyden JJ, McGinley KJ. Bacteriology. J Invest Dermatol. 1976;67:160–8.
15. Leyden JJ, McGinley KJ, Nordstrom KM, et al. Skin microflora. J Invest Dermatol. 1987;88(Suppl):65–72.
16. Aly R, Maiback HI, Strauss WG, et al. Survival of microorganisms on human skin. J Invest Dermatol. 1972;58:205–10.
17. Selwyn S, Ellis H. Skin bacteria and skin disinfection reconsidered. Br Med J. 1972;1:136–40.
18. Milyani RM, Selwyn S. Quantitative studies on competitive activities of skin bacteria growing on solid media. J Med Microbiol. 1977;11:379–86.
19. Singh G, Marples RR, Kligman AM. Staphylococcus infections in humans. J Invest Dermatol. 1971;57:149–62.
20. Blank IH. The skin as an organ of protection. In: Fitzpatrick TB, Eisen AZ, Wolff K, et al., eds. Dermatology in General Medicine. 3rd ed. New York: McGraw-Hill; 1987:337–42.
21. Ray TL, Wuepper KD. Experimental cutaneous candidiasis in rodents. Arch Dermatol. 1978;114:539–43.
22. Sauder DN, Wong D, McKenzie R, et al. The pluripotent keratinocyte: Molecular characterization of epidermal cytokines (abstract). Clin Res. 1988;36:692.
23. Grabbe J, Rosenback T, Czarnetzki BM. Production of LTB4-like chemotactic arachidonate metabolities from human keratinocytes. J Invest Dermatol. 1985;85:527–30.
24. Siraganian RP. Mast cells and basophils. In: Gallin JI, Goldstein IM, Snyderman R, eds. Inflammation, Basic Principles and Clinical Correlates. New York: Raven Press; 1988:513–42.

25. Streilein JW. Circuits and signals of the skin-associated lymphoid tissues (SALT). J Invest Dermatol. 1985;85(Suppl):10–13.
26. Morhenn VB, Nickoloff BJ, Mansbridge JN. Induction of the synthesis of triton-soluble proteins in human keratinocytes by gamma interferon. J Invest Dermatol. 1985;85(Suppl):27–9.
27. Valman HB. Infectious diseases. Br Med J. 1981;283:1038–9.
27a. Thurn J. Human parvovirus B19: Historical and clinical review. Rev Infect Dis. 1988;10:1005–11.
28. Cohen MS. Relationship between host defense defects and infectious disease. Infect Med. 1986;3:182–88.
29. Baccarani M, Fiacchini M, Galieni P, et al. Meningitis and septicaemia in adults splenectomized for Hodgkin's disease. Scand J Haematol. 1986;36:492–8.
30. Scully RE, Mark EJ, McNeely BU, eds. Case records of the Massachusetts General Hospital. Case 29-1986. N Engl J Med. 1986;315:241–9.
31. Scully RE, Mark EJ, McNelly BU, eds. Case records of the Massachusetts General Hospital. Case 20-1983. N Engl J Med. 1983;308:1212–8.
32. O'Neal BJ, McDonald JC. The risk of sepsis in the asplenic adult. Ann Surg. 1981;194:775–8.
33. Sekikawa T, Shatney CH. Septic sequelae after splenectomy for trauma in adults. Am J Surg. 1983;145:667–73.
34. Zarrabi MH, Rosner F. Serious infections in adults following splenectomy for trauma. Arch Intern Med. 1984;144:1421–4.
35. Green JB, Shackford, SR, Sise MJ, et al. Late septic complications in adults following spenectomy for trauma: A prospective analysis in 144 patients. J Trauma 1986;26:999–1004.
36. Evans D. Postsplenectomy sepsis 10 years or more after operation. J Clin Pathol. 1985;38:309–11.
37. Robboy SJ, Mihm MC, Colman RW, et al. The skin in disseminated intravascular coagulation. Prospective analysis of thirty-six cases. Br J Dermatol. 1973;88:221–9.
38. Goodwin JN, Berne TV. Symmetrical peripheral gangrene. Arch Surg. 1974;108:780–4.
39. Chu DZJ, Blaisdell FW: Purpura fulminans. Am J Surg. 1982;143:356–62.
40. McGouran RCM, Emmerson GA. Symmetrical peripheral gangrene. Br Heart J. 1977;39:569–72.
41. Thisyakorn U, Ningsanond V. Purpura fulminans produced by *Aeromonas hydrophila:* A case report. Southeast Asian J Trop Med. 1985;16:532–3.
42. Dudgeon DL, Kellogg DR, Gilchrist GS, et al. Purpura fulminans. Arch Surg. 1971;103:351–8.
43. Hjort PF, Rapaport SI, Jorgensen L. Purpura fulminans. Report of a case successfully treated with heparin and hydrocortisone. Review of 50 cases from the literature. Scand J Haematol. 1964;1:169–92.
44. Hjort PF, Rapaport SI. The Shwartzman reaction: Pathogenetic mechanisms and clinical manifestations. Annu Rev Med. 1965;16:135–69.
45. Hill WR, Kinney TD. The cutaneous lesions in meningococcemia: A clinical and pathologic study JAMA. 1947;134:513–8.
46. DeVoe IW. The meningococcus and mechanisms of pathogenicity. Microbiol Rev. 1982;46:162–90.
47. Sotto MN, Langer B, Hoshino-Shimizu S, et al. Pathogenesis of cutaneous lesions in acute meningococcemia in humans: Light, immunofluorescent, and electron microscopic studies of skin biopsy specimens. J Infect Dis. 1976;133:506–14.
48. Bernhard WG, Jordan AC. Purpuric lesions in meningococcic infections. 1944;29:273–81.
49. Davis CE, Arnold K. Role of meningococcal endotoxin in meningococcal purpura. J Exp Med. 1974;140:159–71.
50. Koppes GM, Ellenbogen C, Gebhart RJ. Group Y meningococcal disease in United States Air Force recruits. Am J Med. 1977;62:661–6.
51. Leibel RL, Fangman JJ. Chronic meningococcemia in childhood. Am J Dis Child. 1974;127:94–8.
52. Benoit FL. Chronic meningococcemia. Am J Med. 1963;35:103–12.
53. Ognibene AJ, Dito WR. Chronic meningococcemia. Arch Intern Med 1964;114:29–32.
54. Barr J, Danielsson D. Septic gonococcal dermatitis. Br Med J. 1971;1:482–5.
55. Holmes KK, Weisner PJ, Pederson AHB, et al. The gonococcal arthritis–dermatitis syndrome. Ann Intern Med. 1971;75:470–1.
56. Handsfield HH. Disseminated gonococcal infection. Clin Obstet Gynecol. 1975;18:131–42.
57. Abu-Nassar H, Hill N, Fred HL, et al. Cutaneous manifestations of gonococcemia. Arch Intern Med. 1963;112:731–7.
58. Holmes KK, Counts GW, Beaty HN. Disseminated gonococcal infection. Ann Intern Med. 1971;74:979–93.
59. Tronca E, Handsfield HH, Wiesner PJ, et al. Demonstration of *Neisseria gonorrhoeae* with fluorescent antibody in patients with disseminated gonococcal infection. J Infect Dis. 1974;129:583–6.
60. Walker LC, Ahlin TD, Tung KSK, et al. Circulating immune complexes in disseminated gonorrheal infection. Ann Intern Med. 1978;89:28–33.
61. Flick MR, Cluff LE. *Pseudomonas* bacteremia. Am J Med. 1976;60:501–8.
62. Forkner CE, Frei E, Edgcomb JH, et al. *Pseudomonas* septicemia. Am J Med. 1958;25:877–89.
63. Whitecar JP, Luna M, Bodey GP. *Pseudomonas* bacteremia in patients with malignant diseases. Am J Med Sci. 1970;260:216–23.
64. Anderson MG. *Pseudomonas* septicaemia and ecthyma gangrenosum. S Afr Med J. 1979;55:504–9.
65. Bodey GP, Bolivar R, Fainstein V, et al. Infections caused by *Pseudomonas aeruginosa*. Rev Infect Dis. 1983;5:279–313.
66. Curtin JA, Petersdorf RG, Bennett IL. *Pseudomonas* bacteremia: Review of ninety-one cases. Ann Intern Med. 1961;54:1077–107.
67. Dorff GJ, Geimer NF, Rosenthal DR, et al. *Pseudomonas* septicemia. Arch Intern Med. 1971;128:591–5.
68. Fast M, Woerner S, Bowman W, et al. Ecthyma gangrenosum. Can Med Assoc J. 1979;120:332–4.
69. Greene SL, Su WPD, Muller SA. Ecthyma gangrenosum: Report of clinical, histopathologic, and bacteriologic aspects of eight cases. J Am Acad Dermatol. 1984;11:781–7.
70. Hall JH, Callaway JL, Tindall JP, et al. *Pseudomonas aeruginosa* in dermatology. Arch Dermatol. 1968;97:312–24.
71. van den Broek PJ, van der Meer JWM, Kunst MW. The pathogenesis of ecthyma gangrenosum. J Infect. 1979;1:263–7.
72. Bagel J, Grossman ME. Subcutaneous nodules in *Pseudomonas* sepsis. Am J Med. 1986;80:528–9.
73. Llistosella E, Revella A, Moreno A, et al. Panniculitis in *Pseudomonas aeruginosa* septicemia. Acta Derm Venereol (Stockh) 1984;64:447–9.
74. Picou KA, Jarratt MT. Persistent subcutaneous abscesses following *Pseudomonas* sepsis. Arch Dermatol. 1979;115:459–60.
75. Reed RK, Larter WE, Sieber OF, et al. Peripheral nodular lesions in *Pseudomonas* sepsis: The importance of incisions and drainage. J Pediatr. 1976;88:977–9.
76. Schlossberg D. Multiple erythematous nodules as a manifestation of *Pseudomonas aeruginosa* septicemia. Arch Dermatol. 1980;116:446–7.
77. Stanley MM. Bacillus pyocyaneus infections. Am J Med. 1947;9:253–367.
78. Baltch AL, Griffin PE. *Pseudomonas aeruginosa* bacteremia: A clinical study of 75 patients. Am J Med Sci. 1977;274:119–29.
79. Bodey GP, Jadeja L, Elting L. *Pseudomonas* bacteremia. Arch Intern Med. 1985;145:1621–9.
80. Mandell IN, Feiner HD, Price NM, et al. *Pseudomonas cepacia* endocarditis and ecthyma gangrenosum. Arch Dermatol. 1977;113:199–202.
81. Ketover BP, Young LS, Armstrong D. Septicemia due to *Aeromonas hydrophila:* Clinical and immunologic aspects. J Infect Dis. 1973;127:284–90.
82. Shackelford PG, Ratzan SA, Shearer WT. Ecthyma gangrenosum produced by *Aeromonas hydrophilia*. J Pediatr. 1973;83:100–1.
83. Fine JD, Miller JA, Harrist TJ, et al. Cutaneous lesions in disseminated candidiasis mimicking ecthyma gangrenosum. Am J Med 1981;70:1133–5.
84. Musher DM. Cutaneous and soft-tissue manifestations of sepsis due to gram-negative enteric bacilli. Rev Infect Dis. 1980;2:854–66.
85. El Baze P, Ortonne J-P. Ecthyma gangrenosum. J Am Acad Dermatol. 1985;13:299–300.
86. Huminer D, Siegman-Igra Y, Morduchowicz G, et al. Ecthyma gangrenosum without bacteremia. Arch Intern Med. 1987;147:299–310.
87. Von Reyn CF, Levy BS, Arbeit RD, et al. Infective endocarditis: An analysis based on strict case definitions. Ann Intern Med. 1981;94:505–18.
88. Venezio FR, Westenfelder GO, Cook FV, et al. Infective endocarditis in a community hospital. Arch Intern Med. 1982;142:789–92.
89. Terpenning MS, Buggy BP, Kauffman CA. Infective endocarditis: Clinical features in young and elderly patients. Am J Med. 1987;83:626–34.
90. King K, Harkness JL. Infective endocarditis in the 1980s. Part 1. Aetiology and diagnosis. Med J Aust. 1986;144:536–40.
91. Alpert JS, Krous HF, Dalen JE, et al. Pathogenesis of Osler's nodes. Ann Intern Med. 1976;85:471–3.
92. Yee J, McAllister CK. Osler's nodes and the recognition of infective endocarditis: A lesion of diagnostic importance. South Med J. 1987;80:753–7.
93. Harvey D. Staphylococcal infections. J Antimicrob Chemother. 1979;5(suppl. A):21–26.
94. Sheagren JN. *Staphylococcus aureus*. The persistent pathogen (first of two parts). N Engl J Med. 1984;310:1368–73.
95. Sheagren JN. *Staphylococcus aureus*. The persistent pathogen (second of two parts). N Engl J Med. 1984;310:1437–42.
96. Sheagren JN. Staphylococcal infections of the skin and skin structures. Cutis. 1985;361:2–6.
97. Wickboldt LG, Fenske NA. Streptococcal and staphylococcal infections of the skin. Hosp Pract. 1986;21:41–7.
98. Dowsett EG. The staphylococcal scalded skin syndrome. J Hosp Infect. 1984;5:347–54.
99. Elias PM, Fritsch P, Epstein EH. Staphylococcal scalded skin syndrome. Arch Dermatol. 1977;113:207–19.
100. Hebert AA, Esterly NB. Bacterial and candidal cutaneous infections in the neonate. Dermatol Clin. 1986;4:3–21.
101. Melish ME, Glasgow LA. Staphylococcal scalded skin syndrome: The expanded clinical syndrome. J Pediatr. 1971;78:958–67.
102. Borchers SL, Gomez EC, Isseroff RR. Generalized staphylococcal scalded skin syndrome in anephric boy undergoing hemodialysis. Arch Dermatol. 1984;120:912–8.
103. O'Keefe R, Dagg JH, MacKie RM. The staphylococcal scalded skin syndrome in two elderly immunocompromised patients. Br Med J. 1987;295:179–80.
104. Richard M, Mathieu-Serra A. Staphylococcal scalded skin syndrome in a homosexual adult. J Am Acad Dermatol. 1986;15:385–9.
105. Igarashi H, Fujikawa H, Usami H, et al. Purification and characterization of *Staphylococcus aureus* FRI 1169 and 587 toxic shock syndrome exotoxins. Infect Immun. 1984;44:175–81.

106. Bergdoll MS, Crass BA, Reiser RF, et al. A new *Staphylococcus* enterotoxin, enterotoxin F, associated with toxic-shock-syndrome *Staphylococcus aureus* isolates. Lancet. 1981;1:1017–21.
107. Schlievert PM, Shands KN, Dan BB, et al. Identification and characterization of an exotoxin from *Staphylococcus aureus* associated with toxic-shock syndrome. J Infect Dis. 1981;143:509–16.
108. Kass EH. The toxic shock syndrome revisited. Postgrad Med J. 1985;61(Suppl 1):45–48.
109. Crass BA, Bergdoll MS. Involvement of coagulase-negative staphylococci in toxic shock syndrome. J Clin Microbiol 1986;23:43–5.
110. Davis JP, Chesney PJ, Wand PJ, et al. Toxic shock syndrome. Epidemiologic features, recurrence, risk factors, and prevention. N Engl J Med. 1980;303:1429–35.
111. Fisher RF, Goodpasture HC, Peterie JD, et al. Toxic shock syndrome in menstruating women. Ann Intern Med. 1981;94:156–63.
112. Holt PA, Armstrong AM, Norfolk GA, et al. Toxic-shock syndrome due to staphylococcal infection of a burn. Br J Clin Pract. 1987;41:582–83.
113. Reingold AL, Dan BB, Shands KN, et al. Toxic-shock syndrome not associated with menstruation. Lancet. 1982;1:1–4.
114. Reingold AL, Hargrett NT, Dan BB, et al. Nonmenstrual toxic shock syndrome. A review of 130 cases. Ann Intern Med. 1982;96:871–4.
115. Bates I. Characteristic rash associated with staphylococcal pneumonia. Lancet. 1987;2:1026–7.
116. Center for Disease Control. Toxic shock syndrome associated with influenza-Minnesota. MMWR. 1986;35:143–4.
117. Center for Disease Control. Toxic shock syndrome following influenza-Oregon; Update on influenza activity—United States. MMWR. 1987;36:64–5.
118. Wilkins EGL, Ney F, Roberts C, et al. Probable toxic shock syndrome with primary staphylococcal pneumonia. J Infect. 1985;11:231–2.
119. Finch R, Whitby M: Toxic shock syndrome. J R Coll Physicians Lond. 1985;19:219–23.
120. Tofte RW, Williams DN. Clinical and laboratory manifestations of toxic shock syndrome. Ann Intern Med. 1982;96:843–7.
121. Tofte RW, Williams DN. Toxic shock syndrome: Clinical and laboratory features in 15 patients. Ann Intern Med. 1981;94:149–56.
122. Tofte RW, Williams DN. Toxic shock syndrome. Recognition and management of a diverse disease. Postgrad Med. 1983;73:275–88.
123. Todd J, Fishuat M, Kapral F, et al. Toxic-shock syndrome associated with phage-group-1 staphylococci. Lancet. 1978;2:1116–7.
124. Plaut MD. Staphylococcal septicemia and pustular purpura. Arch Dermatol 1969;99:82–5.
125. Musher DM, McKenzie SO. Infections due to *Staphylococcus aureus*. Medicine (Baltimore). 1977;56:383–409.
126. Aach R, Kissane J, eds. A thirty-eight year old woman with overwhelming sepsis. Am J Med. 1972;53:233–41.
127. Murray HW, Tuazon CU, Sheagren JN. Staphylococcal septicemia and disseminated intravascular coagulation. Arch Intern Med. 1977;137:844–47.
128. Milunski MR, Gallis HA, Fulkerson WJ. *Staphylococcus aureus* septicemia mimicking fulminant Rocky Mountain spotted fever. Am J Med. 1987;83:801–3.
129. Rahal JJ, MacMahon E, Weinstein L. Thrombocytopenia and symmetrical peripheral gangrene associated with staphylococcal and streptococcal bacteremia. Ann Intern Med. 1968;69:35–43.
130. Walker DH. Rickettsial disease: An update. In: Majno G, Cotran RS, Kaufman N, eds. Current Topics in Inflammation and Infection. Baltimore: Williams & Wilkins; 1982:188–204.
131. Current trends. Rocky Mountain spotted fever—United States, 1986. MMWR. 1987;36:314–5.
132. Helmick CG, Bernard KW, D'Angelo LJ. Rocky Mountain spotted fever: Clinical, laboratory, and epidemiological features of 262 cases. J Infect Dis. 1984;150:480–8.
133. Hazard GW, Ganz RN, Nevin RW, et al. Rocky Mountain spotted fever in the Eastern United States. N Engl J Med. 1969;280:57–62.
134. Kaplowitz LG, Fischer JJ, Sparling PF. Rocky Mountain spotted fever: A clinical dilemma. In: Remington JS, Swartz MN: Current Clinical Topics in Infectious Diseases. New York: McGraw-Hill; 1981:89–108.
135. Sexton DJ, Burgdorder W. Clinical and epidemiologic features of Rocky Mountain spotted fever in Mississippi, 1933–1973. South Med J. 1975;68:1529–35.
136. Cohen JI, Corson AP, Corey GR. Late appearance of skin rash in Rocky Mountain spotted fever. South Med J. 1983;76:1457–8.
137. Ramsey PG, Press OW. Successful treatment of Rocky Mountain 'spotless' fever. West J Med. 1984;140:94–6.
138. Centers for Disease Control. Nosocomial infection surveillance. MMWR. 1984;35(Suppl):17–29.
139. Drutz DJ, Jarvis WR, de Repentigny L, et al. Severe nosocomial yeast infections. Conversations Infect Control. 1985;6:1–12.
140. Morrison AJ, Freer CV, Searcy MA, et al. Nosocomial bloodstream infections: Secular trends in a statewide surveillance program in Virginia (abstract 452). In: Proceedings of the 25th Interscience Conference on Antimicrobial Agents and Chemotherapy. Minneapolis: American Society for Microbiology, 1985.
141. Weber DJ, Rutala WA. Epidemiology of nosocomial fungal infections. In: McGinnis MR, ed. Current Topics in Medical Mycology. v. 2. New York: Springer Publishing; 1988:305–37.
142. Bodey GP. Fungal infection and fever of unknown origin in neutropenic patients. Am J Med. 1986;80:112–9.
143. Maksymiuk AW, Thongprasert S, Hopfer R, et al. Systemic candidiasis in cancer patients. Am J Med. 1984;77(Suppl):20–7.
144. Bodey GP. Candidiasis in cancer patients. Am J Med. 1984;77(Suppl):13–9.
145. Balandran L, Rothschild H, Pugh N, et al. A cutaneous manifestation of systemic candidiasis. Ann Intern Med. 1973;78:400–3.
146. Jacobs MI, Magid MS, Jarowski CI. Disseminated candidiasis. Arch Dermatol. 1980;116:1277–9.
147. Kirkpatrick CH. Host factors in defense against fungal infections. Am J Med. 1984;77(Suppl):1–12.
148. Dreizen S, McCredie KB, Bodey GP, et al. Unusual mucocutaneous infections. Postgrad Med. 1986;79:287–94.
149. Wolfson JS, Sober AJ. Dermatologic manifestations of infection in the compromised host. In: Rubin RH, Young LS, eds. Clinical Approach to Infection in the Compromised Host. New York: Plenum; 1988:115–30.
150. Valle S. Dermatologic findings related to human immunodeficiency virus infection in high-risk individuals. J Am Acad Dermatol. 1987;17:951–61.
151. Triana AF, Shapiro RS, Polk BF, et al. Mucocutaneous findings in acquired immunodeficiency syndrome/AIDS-related complex patients. J Am Acad Dermatol. 1987;16:888–9.
152. Koslow RA, Phair JP, Friedman HB, et al. Infection with the human immunodeficiency virus: Clinical manifestations and their relationship to immune deficiency. Ann Intern Med. 1987;107:474–80.
153. Matis WL, Triana A, Shapiro R, et al. Dermatologic findings associated with immunodeficiency virus infection. J Am Acad Dermatol. 1987;17:746–51.
154. Calabrese LH, Proffitt MR, Levin KH, et al. Acute infection with the human immunodeficiency virus (HIV) associated with acute brachial neuritis and exanthematous rash. Ann Intern Med. 1987;107:849–51.
155. Denning DW, Amos A, Wall RA. Oral and cutaneous features of acute human immunodeficiency virus infection. Cutis. 1987;40:171–5.
156. Ho DD, Sarngadharan MG, Resnick L, et al. Primary human T-lymphotrophic virus type III infection. Ann Intern Med. 1985;103:880–3.
157. Kessler HA, Blaauw B, Spear J, et al. Diagnosis of human immunodeficiency virus infection in seronegative homosexuals presenting with an acute viral syndrome. JAMA. 1987;258:1196–9.
158. Ruutu P, Suni J, Oksanen K, et al. Primary infection with HIV in a severely immunosuppressed patient with acute leukemia. Scand J Infect Dis. 1987;19:369–72.
159. Valle S-L. Febrile pharyngitis as the primary sign of HIV infection in a cluster of cases linked by sexual contact. Scand J Infect Dis. 1987;19:13–7.
160. Biggs B, Newton-John HF. Acute HTLV-III infection. Med J Aust. 1986;144:545–7.
161. Boyko WJ, Schechter MT, Craib KJP, et al. The Vancouver lymphadenopathy-AIDS study: 7. Clinical and laboratory features of 87 cases of primary HIV infection. Can Med Assoc J. 1987;137:109–13.
162. Goodman DS, Teplitz ED, Wishner A, et al. Prevalence of cutaneous disease in patients with acquired immunodeficiency syndrome (AIDS) or AIDS-related complex. J Am Acad Dermatol. 1987;17:210–20.
163. Brenner S. Acquired ichthyosis in AIDS. Cutis. 1987;39:421–6.
164. Young L, Steinman HK. Acquired ichthyosis in a patient with acquired immunodeficiency syndrome and Kaposi's sarcoma. J Am Acad Dermatol. 1987;16:395–6.
165. Duvic M, Rapini R, Hoots WK, et al. Human immunodeficiency virus–associated vitiligo: Expression of autoimmunity with immunodeficiency? J Am Acad Dermatol. 1987;17:656–62.
166. Fallon R, Abell E, Kingsley L, et al. Telangiectasias of the anterior chest in homosexual man. Ann Intern Med. 1986;105:679–82.
167. Schonwetter RS, Nelson EB: Alopecia areata and the acquired-immunodeficiency-syndrome–related complex. Ann Intern Med. 1986;104:287.
168. Buchness MR, Lim HW, Hatcher VA, et al. Eosinophilic pustular folliculitis in the acquired immunodeficiency syndrome. N Engl J Med. 1988;318:1183–6.
169. Cohen PR, Kurzrock R. Tongue lesions in the acquired immunodeficiency syndrome. Cutis. 1987;40:406–9.
170. Penneys NS, Hicks B. Unusual cutaneous lesions associated with acquired immunodeficiency syndrome. J Am Acad Dermatol. 1985;13:847–52.
171. Kaplan MH, Sadick N, McNutt NS, et al. Dermatologic findings and manifestations of acquired immunodeficiency syndrome (AIDS). J Am Acad Dermatol. 1987;16:485–506.
172. Laurence J. Dermatologic manifestations of HIV infection. Infections in Surgery. 1987;6:488–95.
173. Janier M, Hillion B, Baccard M, et al. Chronic varicella zoster infection in acquired immunodeficiency syndrome. J Am Acad Dermatol. 1988;18:584–5.
174. Hicks CB, Benson PM, Lupton GP, et al. Seronegative secondary syphilis in a patient infected with the human immunodeficiency virus (HIV) with Kaposi sarcoma. Ann Intern Med. 1987;107:492–5.
175. Libow LF, Dobert D, Sibulkin D. Co-existent cutaneous cryptococcosis and Kaposi's sarcoma in a patient with the acquired immunodeficiency syndrome. Cutis. 1988;41:159–64.
176. Pichard JG, Sorotzkin RA, James RE III. Cutaneous manifestations of disseminated coccidioidomycosis in the acquired immunodeficiency syndrome. Cutis. 1987;39:203–5.
177. Gretzula J, Penneys NS. Complex viral and fungal skin lesions of patients with acquired immunodeficiency syndrome. J Am Acad Dermatol. 1987;16:1151–4.
178. Kwan TH, Kaufman HW. Acid-fast bacilli with cytomegalovirus and her-

pesvirus inclusions in the skin of an AIDS patient. Am J Clin Pathol. 1986;85:236–8.
179. Angritt P, Tuur SM, Macher AM, et al. Epithelioid angiomatosis in HIV infection: Neoplasm or cat-scratch disease? Lancet. 1988;1:996.
180. LeBoit PE, Berger TG, Egbert BM, et al. Epitheloid haemangioma-like vascular proliferation in AIDS: Manifestation of cat scratch disease bacillus infection? Lancet 1988;1:960–3.
181. Gordin FM, Simon GL, Wofsy CB, et al. Adverse reactions to trimethoprim-sulfamethoxazole in patients with the acquired immunodeficiency syndrome. Ann Intern Med. 1984;100:495–9.
182. Wofsy CB. Use of trimethoprim-sulfamethoxazole in the treatment of *Pneumocystis carinii* pneumonitis in patients with acquired immunodeficiency syndrome. Rev Infect Dis. 1987;9(Suppl 2):184–94.
183. Leoung GS, Mills J, Hopewell PC, et al. Dapsone-trimethoprim for *Pneumocystis carinii* pneumonia in the acquired immunodeficiency syndrome. Ann Intern Med. 1986;105:45–8.

SECTION B. UPPER RESPIRATORY INFECTIONS

42. THE COMMON COLD

JACK M. GWALTNEY, JR.

While the designation "the common cold" is a time-honored phrase used by both physician and lay persons alike for the identification of acute minor respiratory illness, current scientific knowledge discloses that there is no basis for the concept of a single entity implied by the use of such a term. Instead, "the common cold" is a group of diseases caused, for the most part, by members of five families of viruses. The viruses in these families have distinctive biochemical properties that govern their differing pathogenic and epidemiologic behavior. In addition, the immunotypes of the different viral families have antigenic variations that are of biologic importance to the immune system of their human host. The problem of controlling acute respiratory disease presents a complex challenge that will require specific approaches suitable for the properties of the individual virus groups. Thus the hope for the development of a single "cure for the common cold" is an unrealistic expectation, which has historically led to the diversion of resources into attempts at simplistic and unrealistic solutions.

As a clinical entity, the common cold is a mild, self-limited, catarrhal syndrome that is the leading cause of acute morbidity and of visits to a physician in the United States. It is also a major cause of industrial and school absenteeism.[1] A small proportion of colds is complicated by bacterial infections of the paranasal sinuses and the middle ear, which require antimicrobial therapy.

Based on early observations of their contagious nature, colds have long been thought to be due to infectious agents. It was not until the isolation of a number of new respiratory viruses in tissue culture in the 1950s that the specific etiology of colds was known. The first of these, a parainfluenza virus, was shown to cause acute respiratory disease in 1955.[2] In 1956, the first of the rhinoviruses was isolated from adults with common colds.[3,4] The following year, respiratory syncytial virus was related to acute respiratory illness in infants,[5] and, in 1958, one of the enteroviruses, coxsackievirus A21, was recovered from military recruits with mild respiratory disease.[6] The latest group of common cold viruses to be discovered, the coronaviruses, was first reported in the 1960s.[7,8] Since that time no new cold viruses have been found, although the specific cause of some colds remains unknown. Other respiratory viruses, such as influenza virus and adenovirus, produce the common cold syndrome but are characteristically associated with a more severe illness, which often involves the lower respiratory tract. The discovery of the large number of cold viruses revealed for the first time the complexity of the problem and indicated that it will be a difficult one to control.

ETIOLOGY

The major respiratory viruses causing colds and similar upper respiratory illnesses are found in the myxovirus, paramyxovirus, adenovirus, picornavirus, and coronavirus groups (Table 1).[9–12] Within these groups of viruses are many different antigenic types. The rhinovirus group, which accounts for approximately 30 percent of colds in adults, has 100 antigenically different types. The percentage of colds caused by the coronavirus group and the number of serologic types of this virus have not been fully determined, but it is believed that these viruses are an important cause of colds. The three parainfluenza viruses and the respiratory syncytial virus each account for a proportion of colds on an annual basis. Influenza virus and adenovirus produce a spectrum of illness that overlaps the common cold syndrome. Some of the enteroviruses produce coryza, as do some viruses that usually produce more characteristic findings, such as exanthem. Because mild streptococcal pharyngitis cannot be differentiated from viral pharyngitis on clinical grounds, it also is included as a cause of "colds." The etiology of approximately 35 percent of colds in adults remains unknown. Some undiagnosed illnesses may result from the insensitivity of methods currently used for detecting known viruses, and others may be due to undiscovered agents. Colds in children are caused by the same viruses in roughly the same proportion, but the total number of colds that can be diagnosed in children is significantly lower. In some studies, as high as 70 percent of acute respiratory illnesses in children could not be assigned an etiology.

Colds are a frequent illness because of the large number of different causative viruses and also because reinfections may

TABLE 1. Viruses Associated with the Common Cold

	Antigenic Types	*Percentage of Cases*[a]
Rhinoviruses	100 types and 1 subtype	30–35
Coronavirus	3 or more types	≥10
Parainfluenza virus	4 types	10–15
Respiratory syncytial virus	1 type	
Influenza virus	3 types	
Adenovirus	33 types	
Other viruses (enterovirus, rubeola, rubella, varicella)		5
Presumed undiscovered viruses		30–35
Group A β-hemolytic streptococci[b]		5–10

[a] Estimated percentage of colds annually.
[b] Included because differentiation of streptococcal and viral pharyngitis is not possible by clinical means.

occur with the same virus type. Second infections probably occur with members of all the viral groups; with some, such as coronavirus, reinfections appear to be particularly common. Up to 80 percent of persons infected with coronavirus OC43 have had prior neutralizing antibody to the virus.[13]

SEASONAL INCIDENCE

The respiratory viruses have a worldwide distribution. Annual epidemics of upper respiratory tract disease occur in the colder months in temperate areas and during the rainy season in the tropics. In the United States the respiratory disease season begins in late August to mid-September.[14,15] Respiratory illness rates rise sharply over a few weeks and then remain elevated until spring. During March, April, and May, rates decline to the low summer level.

The events controlling the seasonal variation in attack rates of acute respiratory disease are not well understood. Adding to the complexity of the problem has been the discovery that some of the virus groups have their own seasonal pattern within the overall respiratory disease season. Rhinovirus outbreaks occur in the early fall and in mid- to late-spring,[15] and coronaviruses are most prominent in the winter.[13] Studies with a specific virus, rhinovirus type 15, showed that chilling of volunteers did not increase their susceptibility to infection and illness.[16] Thus the effect of thermal cold per se on the host does not appear to be the explanation for the seasonal outbreaks of colds.

Undoubtedly, among the responsible variables for seasonal fluctuations in colds are the bringing together of children during school periods and the increased crowding indoors of populations during colder months.[17] Also, seasonal changes in relative humidity may be an important variable controlling prevalence of the different virus families because of the effect of differing relative humidities on virus survival. In general, enveloped viruses survive better under conditions of low relative humidity, as found in colder months of the year, while the converse is true for nonenveloped viruses.

ATTACK RATES

During peak months in the respiratory disease season in the United States, adults average six to eight colds per 1000 persons per day.[15] In the summer, rates fall to two to three colds per 1000 per day. Overall, adults in the United States average two to four colds per year and children six to eight.[14,15] In one 10-year study of illness in families, young children in nursery school averaged up to nine colds for the period of September through May! Illness rates decline in older children and reach adult levels in adolescence. Men have slightly more colds than women up to the age of adolescence, but after that the incidence is slightly higher in women, perhaps reflecting their exposure to young children. Adults with children in the home have more colds than those without this exposure.[14,18] Tonsillectomy does not reduce the incidence of colds.[14] Cigarette smokers have the same incidence of colds as nonsmokers, but the severity of their illness is greater.[15,19]

TRANSMISSION

The main reservoir of respiratory viruses is in young children. Spread of colds takes place most commonly in the home[14,18] and school.[20] Children acquire new viral strains from their schoolmates, which they then bring home and pass to other family members. Two- to five-day intervals occur between cases. Secondary attack rates of family members vary, depending on age, position in the family, and prior immunity to the virus. Age and immunity are related risk factors. Young children and mothers have high secondary attack rates as a result of close and prolonged exposure to school children in the family. The secondary attack rate of fathers is relatively low.

The mechanism(s) for the spread of cold viruses has not been well established. Possible means of transmission include (*1*) direct contact with infectious secretions on skin and environmental surfaces, (*2*) large particles of respiratory secretions that are briefly transported in air, (*3*) infectious droplet nuclei suspended in air, and (*4*) combinations of these methods.[21] For some viruses, such as rhinovirus, close physical contact appears necessary for efficient spread. Infectious rhinovirus is produced primarily in the nose and is shed in highest concentrations in nasal secretions. Peak viral titers in nasal mucus occur on the second to fourth day of experimental infection and coincide with the period of maximum communicability.[21] A high proportion of persons with natural and experimental rhinovirus colds have recoverable virus on their hands. With experimental rhinovirus infection, brief hand contact permits ready transfer of virus-contaminated nasal secretions from the hands of infected subjects to the hands of susceptible subjects. When the contaminated fingers of the susceptible subjects are then placed in contact with the nasal and conjunctival mucosa, infection results in a high percentage of cases.[22] In a recent study, which has not been confirmed, treatment of the fingers with a virucidal solution reduced the rate of infection in mothers exposed to other family members with fresh colds.[23] This latter study provides the only direct evidence on the mechanisms of common cold transmission under natural conditions and suggests that a proportion of colds are spread by a hand contamination/self-inoculation route.

Another rhinovirus transmission model has been developed in which virus is reliably transmitted through the air in large- and/or small-particle aerosol.[24] This model demonstrates the feasibility of the aerosol route of spread but does not prove that it occurs under natural conditions. Studies conducted in the field with intervention techniques specific for aerosol transmission are needed to address that question. There is epidemiologic evidence that influenza and adenovirus may spread, at least in part, by small airborne droplets. Thus, all the respiratory viruses may not behave in the same way, and further studies are necessary to determine which route or routes of transmission are important in the natural dissemination of all these viruses.

PATHOGENESIS

Viral invasion of the upper respiratory tract is the basic mechanism in the pathogenesis of colds, but the specific events leading to clinical illness are not well understood. Infection with common cold viruses is characteristically of short duration and self-limited. For example, maximum rhinovirus shedding lasts 3 weeks or less in young adults with experimental colds,[25,26] and coronavirus excretion has been detected for only 1–4 days.[13] Cold viruses are not usually present in asymptomatic persons,[27] although subclinical infections do occur and viral carriage may be somewhat prolonged in children.[28]

Characteristic changes have been described in sloughed columnar epithelial cells in nasal secretions of persons with natural colds of unknown etiology.[29] Cells with persistent ciliary activity have been found in nasal secretions in the first through the third day of illness. Also, some exfoliated cells show degenerative changes characterized by progressive nuclear pyknosis and the formation of apparent inclusion bodies. More recently ciliated epithelial cells containing viral antigen have been found in the nasal mucus of volunteers with experimental rhinovirus colds.[30]

Attempts to demonstrate specific histopathologic changes in nasal biopsy specimens of volunteers with rhinovirus colds[31] or in rhinovirus-infected nasal polyp cultures[32] have not been successful. A subsequent study by light and electron microscopy of nasal biopsy specimens from young adults with natural colds confirmed the absence of destruction of the nasal epithelium.[33] In this study there was a significant increase in the number of neutrophils in the epithelium and in the lamina propria. The number of epithelial mast cells was not increased. The findings with rhinovirus contrast with the destructive changes to the respiratory epithelium that are seen with influenza virus infection.

With rhinovirus colds, the period of maximum viral excretion in nasal secretions coincides with the peak of clinical illness[34] and of appearance of ciliated epithelial cells in nasal mucus.[30] At that time, large quantities of protein, including immunoglobulins, are present in nasal secretions. In addition to any direct destructive effect that the virus may have on the respiratory mucous membrane, it is possible that immunologic mechanisms and chemical mediators may play a role in the pathogenesis of the common cold. In this regard, high concentrations of bradykinin and lysylbradykinin have been measured in nasal secretions of volunteers with experimental rhinovirus colds.[35] Pathogenic mechanisms for the various respiratory viruses are undoubtedly somewhat different.

The self-limited cold virus infection may lead to pathogenic events that affect the resident bacterial flora of the upper respiratory tract and result in secondary bacterial infection. Bacteria become able to invade normally sterile areas such as the sinuses, middle ear, and perhaps the tracheobronchial tree. The variables involved in triggering invasive bacterial infection are unknown but probably include viral damage to the mucociliary cleansing mechanism of the upper respiratory tract. It is currently unknown whether direct viral invasion of the sinus, middle ear, and tracheobronchial tree is necessary for subsequent bacterial infection to occur or whether the viral involvement can remain localized to the nasal and pharyngeal mucous membrane. However, respiratory viruses have been recovered from sinus[36] and middle ear[9] aspirates obtained by direct puncture from patients with acute infections at these sites. Abnormalities in eustachian tube function and middle ear pressures have been consistently observed in volunteers with experimental rhinovirus infection.[37] During colds, increases have also been noted in titers of resident bacterial populations of the upper airways, but the significance of this is unknown.[38,39]

CLINICAL CHARACTERISTICS

The incubation period of the common cold varies somewhat with the different viruses but is usually between 48 and 72 hours. The cardinal symptoms are nasal discharge, nasal obstruction, sneezing, sore or "scratchy" throat, and cough.[14,19] Slight fever may be found, but temperature elevation of more than a degree is distinctly uncommon in the adult. Infants and young children may have more frequent temperature elevation. The early symptoms may be minimal with only mild malaise and nasal complaints. With rhinovirus infection, sneezing, nasal discharge, and nasal obstruction usually begin simultaneously on the first day of illness and rapidly increase to maximum severity by the second or third day. Paralleling the nasal symptoms are sore, dry, or "scratchy" throat. Cough and hoarseness may also begin early in the course of illness and, when present, tend to persist until the end of the first week of symptoms by which time nasal and pharyngeal complaints have usually subsided. Limited information is available suggesting that symptom patterns are similar with coronavirus colds.[13]

The median duration of rhinovirus colds is 1 week, but in approximately one-quarter the illnesses last up to 2 weeks. In cigarette smokers with rhinovirus colds, cough is increased and prolonged. Other complaints include mild burning of the eyes; true conjunctivitis is not seen except in some adenovirus and enterovirus infections. There may also be loss of sense of smell and taste and a feeling of pressure in the ears or sinuses due to obstruction and/or mucosal swelling. The voice may have a nasal quality. Painful maceration of the skin around the nostrils is often bothersome when rhinorrhea has been profuse and persistent.

On physical examination the findings may be few despite the subjective discomfort of the patient. A red nose and a dripping nasal discharge are the characteristic features of the cold sufferer, but many patients have minimal outward manifestations of the infection. The nasal mucous membrane may have a glassy appearance due to the exudation of serum proteins and increased mucus secretions. It is difficult to judge accurately the presence of increased erythema of the mucous membrane of the nose and throat due to normal variations in the color of these structures. Marked pharyngeal erythema and exudate are not seen with rhinovirus and coronavirus infections, but they do occur with pharyngoconjunctival fever of adenovirus infection. Examination of the chest may reveal the presence of rhonchi.

The clinical picture of the common cold is similar in children and adults. However, in young children parainfluenza virus and respiratory syncytial virus infection may lead to viral pneumonia, croup, and bronchiolitis, while in adults these viruses usually cause only colds. In both adults and children the upper airway manifestations of rhinovirus, coronavirus, parainfluenza virus, and respiratory syncytial virus infections are indistinguishable in the individual patient.

DIAGNOSIS

The manifestations of the common cold are so typical that self-diagnosis by the patient is usually correct. Hay fever and vasomotor rhinitis may give similar nasal symptoms, but the recurrent and chronic nature of these diseases is soon recognized by the patient and easily diagnosed by the physician from the patient's history. Diagnosis of the specific virus involved is usually not possible on the basis of clinical observation. Some acute respiratory infections, such as influenza and pharyngoconjunctival fever, when seen in a typical epidemiologic setting, can be recognized without benefit of viral culture or serologic tests. Knowledge of the characteristic seasonal patterns for the different virus groups may also aid in the identification of a particular virus.

The main challenge to the physician is to distinguish the uncomplicated cold from the approximately 0.5 percent of cases with secondary bacterial sinusitis and the 2 percent with otitis media.[14] This is not easy because of the lack of inexpensive and noninvasive diagnostic tests for these infections. A complete examination should be performed on the pharynx, nasal cavity, ears, and sinuses. In the pharynx, marked injection or exudate should raise suspicion of streptococcal or adenovirus infection, Vincent's angina, mononucleosis, or diphtheria. Occasionally, patients have small vesicles on the palate due to coxsackievirus A infections. The presence of nasal polyps is suggestive of an underlying allergic problem. In children, a foreign body may lead to persistent nasal discharge. Examination of the ears is directed at finding changes in the appearance of the tympanum, indicating infection (see Chapter 46). The use of the pneumatic otoscope is helpful in determining if fluid is present behind the ear drum. The sinuses should be examined by transillumination under optimal conditions (see Chapter 47).

Sinus radiography is a sensitive diagnostic test for infection of the sinuses, but the expense of the procedure has prevented its widespread use. The most valuable laboratory test in patients with pharyngeal complaints is rapid antigen detection for group A β-hemolytic streptococci. Many of the respiratory viruses can be isolated in cell culture, although specific virologic diagnosis is not usually available in clinical practice. Rhinoviruses grow in human embryonic lung cells (WI-38), myxo- and paramyxoviruses in primary Rhesus monkey kidney cells, and respiratory syncytial virus in Hep 2 cells. Isolation of coronavirus in cell culture has proved difficult with currently available techniques. The sensitivity of the tests for isolating viruses can vary widely with changes in the sensitivity of the cell cultures.

The serologic diagnosis of influenza, parainfluenza, respiratory syncytial, and adenovirus infection is available in some state health department laboratories. Serum specimens should be obtained in the acute phase of illness and approximately 3 weeks later and tested simultaneously. A fourfold or greater rise in antibody titer is indicative of infection. Serologic diagnosis of rhinovirus infection is not practical because of the many different antigenic types. Rapid techniques using fluorescent antibody or other immunodiagnostic procedures on respiratory secretions may become practical in the future and would be useful if antiviral chemotherapy becomes available.

TREATMENT

Only symptomatic treatment is available for the uncomplicated common cold. Individual measures directed at controlling nasal and pharyngeal complaints and cough are more effective than all-inclusive cold remedies found in tablets and capsules. Direct application to the nasal membrane of vasoconstrictors such as 0.5 or 0.25% phenylephrine or 1% ephedrine drops or sprays are recommended to provide symptomatic relief of nasal obstructions and to promote drainage of nasal secretions. Patients should be instructed to place themselves in a head down position when administering decongestants to achieve penetration of the drug to inaccessible areas of the nasal cavity. An interval of approximately 1 minute should be allowed between three separate applications of drops or spray. Decongestants should be used every 4 hours on a regular basis. Patients should be cautioned on the rebound effect that results if decongestants are used continuously for more than 3 or 4 days. Recently, it has been shown that intranasal application of a topically active parasympatholygic, ipratropium, was effective in reducing nasal secretions.[40]

Sore throat is relieved by warm saline gargles and cough by liquids or cough drops containing dextromethorphan. Cough suppression in the severe case is best achieved with preparations containing codeine. The regular application of an ointment containing a petrolatum base is useful in controlling painful maceration of the nares. Aspirin and bed rest are of value when headache and constitutional symptoms are prominent. The patient should restrict his activities during the height of the illness, at which time he is most contagious to others. Regular handwashing and care to avoid contamination of the environment with nasal secretions may also help to prevent spread.

Antibiotics have no place in the treatment of uncomplicated colds, and antihistamines have only a minimal effect in reducing nasal secretions.[41] Until truly effective and specific treatment becomes available, there will continue to be fads in the use of unproven cold remedies. The ingestion of large doses of vitamin C has been widely used as a preventive or therapeutic measure for colds. In some instances, controlled studies have shown a modest beneficial effect of vitamin C for colds. However, a careful analysis of the studies has indicated that a placebo effect could not be ruled out. Many participants correctly surmised from the taste of the contents of the capsules used whether they were receiving vitamin C or a placebo.[42] In volunteers experimentally infected with rhinovirus, vitamin C in doses of 3 g/day was not effective in preventing infection and illness.[43,44]

PROSPECTS FOR CONTROL

Vaccine development has reached an impasse because of the discovery of the many different cold viruses, particularly the 100 rhinoviruses. Unless ways are found to combine large numbers of viral antigens effectively or to take advantage of minor antigenic cross-relationships that exist, prospects for common cold vaccines are not good. A number of chemical compounds have inhibitory activity against respiratory viruses in tissue culture systems, and attempts are being made to develop antiviral agents for clinical use. The activity of such compounds tends to be relatively group-specific, but some have shown activity against most of the rhinoviruses.

The most promising approach to control of colds has come through the development of interferon. Topically applied intranasal recombinant human interferon-α_2 has a highly effective prophylactic activity against experimental rhinovirus infection.[45–47] When given therapeutically in the same manner, interferon has reduced viral excretion, but its effect on development of illness has been of only minimal to moderate benefit.[48] In addition, topically applied intranasal interferon, when used longer than approximately 1 week, is associated with local side effects in the nose, such as stuffiness, dryness, discomfort, and pinpoint areas of ulceration.[49–51] To avoid these problems associated with the biologic properties of interferon, a strategy has been proposed and tested that employs short-term contact prophylaxis by family members exposed to individuals with colds of recent onset. Using this approach, two field studies have observed an approximately 40 percent reduction of total colds and a virtual elimination of rhinovirus-specific infections in exposed individuals.[52,53] Side effects were avoided by the short duration of application of the interferon. The success of these studies is a cause for optimism, although topical interferon-α_2 apparently failed to prevent colds due to viruses other than those in the rhinovirus group. The failure of a "broad spectrum" antiviral agent, such as interferon, to be effective for all cold viruses emphasizes the reality of the need to develop individual approaches for the different virus groups.

Another approach under investigation is to develop ways to interrupt the transmission of colds. Since spread of some viruses may occur by direct hand contact/self-inoculation, handwashing and avoiding finger-to-nose and finger-to-eye contact should be practiced, particularly with exposure to a cold sufferer. It may be possible to develop virucidal preparations for use on the hands that interrupt transmission of infection.[23] Also, covering coughs and sneezes with disposable nasal tissues is recommended as a means of controlling aerosol transmission.

REFERENCES

1. Rice DP, Feldman JJ, White KL. The current burden of illness in the United States. Occasional Papers of the Institute of Medicine. Washington, DC: National Academy of Sciences; 1976:1.
2. Chanock RM. Association of a new type of cytopathogenic myxovirus with infantile croup. J Exp Med. 1956;104:55.
3. Pelon W, Mogabgab WJ, Phillips IA, et al. A cytopathogenic agent isolated from naval recruits with mild respiratory illness. Proc Soc. Exp Biol Med. 1957;94:262.
4. Price WH. The isolation of a new virus associated with respiratory clinical disease in humans. Proc Natl Acad Sci USA. 1956;43:892.
5. Chanock RM, Roizman B, Myers R. Recovery from infants with respiratory illness of a virus related to Chimpanzee Coryza Agent (CCA). I. Isolation, properties, and characterization. Am J Hyg. 1957;66:281.
6. Lennette EH, Fox VL, Schmidt NJ, et al: The COE virus: an apparently new virus recovered from patients with mild respiratory disease. Am J Hyg. 1958;68:272.
7. Tyrrell DAJ, Bynoe ML. Cultivation of a novel type of common-cold virus in organ cultures. Br Med J. 1965;1:1467.
8. Hamre D, Procknow JJ: A new virus isolated from the human respiratory tract. Proc Soc Exp Biol Med. 1966;121:190.
9. Gwaltney JM Jr. Virology of middle ear. Ann Otol Rhinol Laryngol 1971;80:365.
10. Stuart-Harris CH, Andrewes C, Andrews BE, et al. A collaborative study of the aetiology of acute respiratory infection in Britain 1961–4. A report of the Medical Research Council working party on acute respiratory virus infections. Br Med J. 1965;2:319.
11. Hamre D, Connelly AP Jr, Procknow JJ. Virologic studies of acute respiratory disease in young adults. IV. Virus isolations during four years of surveillance. Am J Epidemiol. 1966;83:238.
12. Monto AS, Ullman BM. Acute respiratory illness in an American community; the Tecumseh study. JAMA. 1974;227:164.
13. Monto AS. Coronaviruses. In Evans AS, ed. Viral Infections of Humans: Epidemiology and Control. New York: Plenum; 1982:151.
14. Dingle JH, Badger GF, Jordan WS Jr. Illness in the Home: Study of 25,000 Illnesses in a Group of Cleveland Families. Cleveland: The Press of Western Reserve University; 1964:1.
15. Gwaltney JM Jr, Hendley JO, Simon G, et al. Rhinovirus infections in an industrial population. I. The occurrence of illness. N Engl J Med. 1966;275:1261.
16. Douglas RG Jr, Lindgren KM, Couch RB. Exposure to cold environment and

rhinovirus common cold: failure to demonstrate effect. N Engl J Med. 1968;279:743.
17. Gwaltney JM Jr. The Jeremiah Metzger Lecture. Climatology and the common cold. Trans Am Clin Climatol Assoc. 1984;96:159.
18. Hendley JO, Gwaltney JM Jr, Jordan WS Jr. Rhinovirus infections in an industrial population. IV. Infections within families of employees during two fall peaks of respiratory illness. Am J Epidemiol. 1969;89:184.
19. Gwaltney JM Jr, Hendley JO, Simon G, et al. Rhinovirus infections in an industrial population. II. Characteristics of illness and antibody response. JAMA. 1967;202:494.
20. Beem MO. Acute respiratory illness in nursery school children: a longitudinal study of the occurrence of illness and respiratory viruses. Am J Epidemiol. 1969;90:30.
21. Gwaltney JM Jr. Epidemiology of the common cold. Ann NY Acad Sci. 1980;353:54.
22. Gwaltney JM Jr, Moskalski PB, Hendley JO. Hand-to-hand transmission of rhinovirus colds. Ann Intern Med. 1978;88:463.
23. Hendley JO, Gwaltney JM Jr. Mechanisms of transmission of rhinovirus infections. Epidemiol Rev. 1988;10:242.
24. Dick EC, Jennings LC, Mink KA, et al. Aerosol transmission of rhinovirus colds. J Infect Dis. 1987;156:442.
25. Cate TR, Couch RB, Johnson KM. Studies with rhinoviruses in volunteers: production of illness, effect of naturally acquired antibody, and demonstration of a protective effect not associated with serum antibody. J Clin Invest. 1964;43:56.
26. Winther B, Gwaltney JM Jr, Mygind N, et al. Sites of rhinovirus recovery after point inoculation of the upper airway. JAMA. 1986;256:1763.
27. Hamre D, Rhinoviruses. In: Melnick JL, ed. Monographs in Virology 1. Basel: Karger;1968:1.
28. Frank AL, Taber LH, Wells CR, et al. Patterns of shedding of myxoviruses in children. J Infect Dis. 1981;144:433.
29. Bryan WTK, Bryan MP, Smith CA. Human ciliated epithelial cells in nasal secretions. Transactions of the 85th Annual Meeting of the American Laryngological Association. 1964:145.
30. Turner RB, Hendley JO, Gwaltney JM Jr. Shedding of infected ciliated epithelial cells in rhinovirus colds. J Infect Dis. 1982;145:849.
31. Douglas RG, Jr, Alford BR, Couch RB. Atraumatic nasal biopsy for studies of respiratory virus infection in volunteers. Antimicrob Agents Chemother. 1968;8:340.
32. Hamory BH, Hendley JO, Gwaltney JM Jr. Rhinovirus growth in nasal polyp organ culture. Proc Soc Exp Biol Med. 1977;155:577.
33. Winther B, Brofeldt S, Christensen B, Mygind N. Light and scanning electron microscopy of nasal biopsies from patients with naturally acquired common colds. Acta Otolarungol. 1984;97:309.
34. Douglas RG Jr, Cate TR, Gerone PJ, et al. Quantitative rhinovirus shedding patterns in volunteers. Am Rev Respir Dis. 1966;94:159.
35. Naclerio RM, Proud D, Lichtenstein LM, et al. Kinins are generated during experimental rhinovirus colds. J Infect Dis. 1988;157:133.
36. Evans FO Jr, Sydnor JB, Moore WEC, et al. Sinusitis of the maxillary antrum. N Engl J Med. 1975;293:735.
37. Doyle WJ, McBride TP, Skoner DP, et al. A double blind placebo-controlled clinical trial of the effect of chlorpheniramine on the response of the nasal airway, middle ear and eustachian tube to provocative rhinovirus challenge. Pediatr Infect Dis J. 1988;7:222.
38. Straker E, Hill AB, Lovell RA. A study of the nasopharyngeal bacterial flora of different groups of persons observed in London and south-east England during the years 1930 to 1937. Reports on Public Health and Medical Subjects, no. 90. London: His Majesty's Stationery Office; 1939:7.
39. Brimblecombe FSW, Cruickshank R, Master P, et al. Family studies of respiratory infections. Br Med J. 1958;1:119.
40. Borum P, Olsen L, Winther B, and Mygind N. Ipratropium nasal spray: a new treatment for rhinorrhea in the common cold. Am Rev Respir Dis. 1981;123:418.
41. Howard JC Jr, Kantner TR, Lilienfield LS, et al. Efféctiveness of antihistamines in the symptomatic management of the common cold. JAMA. 1979;242:2414.
42. Chalmers TC. Effects of ascorbic acid on the common cold. An evaluation of the evidence. Am J Med. 1975;58:532.
43. Walker GH, Bynoe ML, Tyrrell DAJ. Trial of ascorbic acid in prevention of colds. Br Med J. 1967;1:603.
44. Schwartz AR, Togo Y, Hornick RB, et al. Evaluation of the efficacy of ascorbic acid in prophylaxis of induced rhinovirus 44 infection in man. J Infect Dis. 1973;128:500.
45. Scott GM, Phillpotts RJ, Wallace J, et al. Purified interferon as protection against rhinovirus infections. Br Med J. 1982;284:1822.
46. Hayden FG, Gwaltney JM Jr. Intranasal interferon-alpha$_2$ for prevention of rhinovirus infection and illness. J Infect Dis. 1983;148:543.
47. Samo T-C, Greenberg SB, Couch RB Jr, et al. Evaluations of efficacy and tolerance to intranasally applied recombinant leukocyte A interferon in normal volunteers. J Infect Dis. 1983;148:535.
48. Hayden FG, Gwaltney JM Jr. Intranasal interferon-α_2 treatment of experimental rhinoviral colds. J Infect Dis. 1984;150:174.
49. Farr BM, Gwaltney JM Jr, Adams KF, et al. Intranasal interferon-α_2 for prevention of natural rhinovirus colds. Antimicrob Agents Chemother. 1984;26:31.
50. Douglas RM, Albrecht JK, Miles HB, et al. Intranasal interferon-α_2 prophylaxis of natural respiratory virus infection. J Infect Dis. 1985;151:731.
51. Hayden FG, Gwaltney JM Jr, Johns ME. Prophylactic efficacy and tolerance of low-dose intranasal interferon-alpha$_2$ in natural respiratory viral infections. Antiviral Res. 1985;5:11.
52. Hayden FG, Albrecht JK, Kaiser DL, et al. Prevention of natural colds by contact prophylaxis with intranasal alpha$_2$-interferon. New Engl J Med. 1986;314:71.
53. Douglas RM, Moore BW, Miles HB, et al. Prophylactic efficacy of intranasal alpha$_2$-interferon against rhinovirus infections in the family setting. N Engl J Med. 1986;314:65.

43. PHARYNGITIS

JACK M. GWALTNEY, JR.

Acute pharyngitis is an inflammatory syndrome of the pharynx caused by several different groups of microorganisms. Most cases are of viral etiology and occur as part of common ccold and influenzal syndromes. The most important of the bacterial infections is due to the group A β-hemolytic streptoccoccus (*Streptococcus pyogenes*). It is important to differentiate streptococcal from viral pharyngitis because of the response of streptococcal infection to penicillin therapy and the ineffectiveness of antibiotic therapy in the viral infections. Also streptococcal pharyngitis may be complicated by acute rheumatic fever and acute glomerulonephritis. There are other uncommon or rare types of pharyngitis that are of clinical importance, and the list of these conditions continues to grow as new etiologic associations are established.

ETIOLOGY

The known microbial causes of pharyngitis are shown in Table 1. The relative importance of the different agents is not fully defined, and it is still not possible to determine the cause of a sizable proportion of cases. The results of epidemiologic investigations are influenced by the season of the year, the age of the population, the severity of illness, and the diagnostic methods used in the various studies. The importance of the various agents listed in Table 1 are known to cause acute respiratory illness[1–4] and on the results of specific studies of the cause of pharyngitis.[5,6] A large amount of mild pharyngitis is associated with rhinovirus and coronavirus colds. Adenovirus and herpes simplex virus pharyngitis, although less common, are important because of their clinical severity. Others of the known respiratory viruses each account for a small proportion of cases. Primary human immunodeficiency syndrome (HIV) infection has joined the list of viral infections associated with acute pharyngitis.[7]

Approximately 15 percent of all cases of pharyngitis are due to *S. pyogenes*. In children with sore throat, *S. pyogenes* may cause up to half of the cases during some periods. The importance of non-group A β-hemolytic streptococci as a cause of pharyngitis is not entirely clear. While non-group A β-hemolytic streptococci, especially strains in groups C and G, have been associated with food-borne outbreaks of pharyngitis,[8,9] non-group A strains have not been clearly implicated in the nonepidemic setting.[10–12] Mixed anaerobic bacterial infection (Vincent's angina) causes an occasional case of acute pharyngitis as does *Corynebacterium diphtheriae, Corynebacterium hemolyticum, Yersinia entero colitica*, and *Neisseria gonorrhoeae*.

Mycoplasma pneumoniae has been associated with pharyngitis since the late 1950s,[13] but in epidemiologic studies of unselected patients, *M. pneumoniae* has not been an important cause of the disease.[5,6,10,11,14] The role of chlamydial infections in pharyngitis is under continuing investigation. A report of an association with *C. trachomatis*[15] was not confirmed,[11,16,17] but

TABLE 1. Microbial Causes of Acute Pharyngitis

	Syndrome/Disease	*Estimated Importance*[a]
Viral		
Rhinovirus (89 types and 1 subtype)	Common cold	20
Coronavirus (4 or more types)	Common cold	≥5
Adenovirus (types 3, 4, 7, 14, 21)	Pharyngoconjunctival fever, ARD	5
Herpes simplex virus (types 1 and 2)	Gingivitis, stomatitis, pharyngitis	4
Parainfluenza virus (types 1–4)	Common cold, croup	2
Influenza virus (types A and B)	Influenza	2
Coxsackievirus A (types 2, 4–6, 8, 10)	Herpangina	<1
Epstein-Barr virus	Infectious mononucleosis	<1
Cytomegalovirus	Infectious mononucleosis	<1
Human immunodeficiency virus	Primary HIV infection	<1
Bacterial		
Streptococcus pyogenes (group A β-hemolytic streptococcus)	Pharyngitis/tonsillitis, scarlet fever	15–30
Mixed anaerobic infection	Gingivitis, pharyngitis (Vincent's angina)	<1
	Peritonsillitis/peritonsillar abscess (quinsy)	<1
Neisseria gonorrhoeae	Pharyngitis	<1
Corynebacterium diphtheriae	Diphtheria	≥1
Corynebacterium ulcerans	Pharyngitis, diphtheria	<1
Corynebacterium hemolyticum (*Arcanobacterium hemolyticum*)	Pharyngitis, scarlatiniform rash	<1
Yersinia enterocolitica	Pharyngitis, enterocolitis	<1
Treponema pallidum	Secondary syphilis	<1
Chlamydial		
Chlamydia psittaci	ARD, pneumonia	Unknown
Mycoplasmal		
Mycoplasma pneumoniae	Pneumonia/bronchitis/pharyngitis	<1
M. hominis (type 1)	Pharyngitis in volunteers	Unknown
Unknown		40

[a] Estimated percentage of cases of pharyngitis due to indicated organism in civilians of all ages.

the TWAR strain of *C. psittaci* has recently been isolated from patients who have pharyngitis associated with febrile bronchitis and pneumonia.[18]

EPIDEMIOLOGY

Most pharyngitis occurs during the colder months of the year, during the respiratory disease season. Viral agents such as rhinoviruses tend to have annual periods of peak prevalence, which are most important in the fall and spring; coronaviruses have been found most often in the winter. Influenza appears in epidemics, which in the United States usually occur between December and April. In military recruits adenoviruses cause the syndrome acute respiratory disease (ARD) during the colder months. In civilians wintertime ARD occurs as well as epidemics of pharyngoconjunctival fever in the summer. Streptococcal pharyngitis occurs during the respiratory disease season, with peak rates of infection in late winter and early spring. The reservoir for the agents that cause pharyngitis is in humans. For details on the epidemiologic behavior of these organisms, the reader is referred to the chapters dealing with each.

PATHOGENESIS

Symptoms of sore or scratchy throat occur in approximately 50 percent of people with rhinovirus colds[19] and in 20–70 percent of people with respiratory illness due to coronavirus.[20,21] Pharyngeal complaints are present in up to 80 percent of people with parainfluenza virus illness[22] and in approximately 50 percent of people with type A influenza[19] and adenovirus illness.[22] Other viral respiratory illnesses with pharyngitis occur with coxsackievirus A21, echoviruses 6 and 20,[22] herpes simplex virus,[23] Epstein-Barr (EB) virus, and cytomegalovirus infections.

The pathogenic mechanisms are undoubtedly different for the various organisms. Nasal epithelial biopsies obtained from volunteers with experimental rhinovirus infections have shown little or no evidence of viral cytopathic effect.[24,25] However, it has recently been discovered that bradykinin and lysylbradykinin are generated in the nasal passages of persons with experimental rhinovirus colds.[26] These inflammatory mediators are potent stimulators of pain nerve endings. Also, volunteers given experimental intranasal challenge with bradykinin have developed symptoms of sore throat.[27] With other respiratory virus infections, such as adenovirus and coxsackievirus, there is evidence that direct invasion of pharyngeal mucosa occurs.

The events leading to invasive streptococcal infection of the pharynx and tonsil are also not well understood. Pharyngeal carriage of *S. pyogenes* is commonly observed in asymptomatic people. Factors that influence the balance between colonization and invasive infection may include natural and acquired host immunity and interference among the bacteria present in the oropharynx. *Streptococcus pyogenes* elaborates a number of extracellular factors, including erythrogenic toxin, hemolysins, streptokinase, deoxyribonuclease, proteinase, and hyaluronidase, which are of known or possible pathogenic importance.

The usual pathologic changes occurring in viral pharyngitis are edema and hyperemia of the tonsils and the pharyngeal mucous membrane. An inflammatory exudate may be present with adenovirus and EB virus infections; with the latter, nasopharyngeal lymphoid hyperplasia also occurs. Vesiculation and mucosal ulceration may occur with herpes simplex virus and some coxsackievirus A infections. With streptococcal pharyngitis there is an intense, inflammatory response in the pharyngeal membrane, and there may be exudate and hemorrhage of the tonsils and pharyngeal walls. With diphtheria a fibrous pseudomembrane containing necrotic epithelium, leukocytes, and bacterial colonies develops on the epithelial surface.

CLINICAL PRESENTATION

Pharyngitis with the Common Cold

Mild-to-moderate pharyngeal discomfort is frequently present during a cold but is often not the primary complaint. The symptom is characterized as soreness, scratchiness, or irritation. Severe pharyngeal pain and dysphagia are not characteristic of this type of pharyngitis. Nasal symptoms and cough are also usually present. Systemic complaints of feverishness, chilliness, malaise, and myalgia are not prominent, and a temperature elevation is unusual in adults and older children. On examination, the pharynx may appear normal or show a mild amount of edema and erythema. Rhinorrhea and postnasal discharge are usually present, but pharyngeal and tonsillar exudates and painful lymphadenopathy are not seen. Pharyngeal complaints usually subside over 3 or 4 days, and most patients have recovered by the end of a week (see Chapter 42).

Pharyngitis with Influenza

Sore throat is a major complaint in some patients with influenza. It is usually associated with other manifestations of the disease, such as myalgia, headache, and cough.[10,19] Coryzal symptoms and hoarseness may also be present. Temperature elevations are common in both adults and children, reaching levels of 38.3°C or higher. Edema and erythema of the pharyngeal mucosa may be present but are not marked. Pharyngeal exudates and painful cervical adenopathy are not present. Defervescence occurs in 3–4 days on the average, but in some uncomplicated cases fever may last up to a week (see Chapter 142).

Pharyngoconjunctival Fever

The clinical presentation of adenoviral pharyngitis is usually more severe than pharyngitis associated with the common cold. Malaise, myalgia, headache, chills, and dizziness often accompany adenovirus infections. Temperature elevations persist for 5–6 days in studies of recognized cases. Sore throat is often marked. On examination, pharyngeal erythema and exudate may be present, mimicking streptococcal pharyngitis. A distinguishing feature of adenovirus pharyngitis, when present, is conjunctivitis, which occurs in one-third to one-half of cases. The conjunctivitis is of the follicular type and is bilateral in about one-fourth of the cases when it occurs. Cough, hoarseness, and substernal pain occur in ARD in military recruits but are usually not prominent features of pharyngoconjunctival fever (see Chapter 122).

Acute Herpetic Pharyngitis

Primary infection with herpes simplex virus may present as an acute pharyngitis. Mild cases are indistinguishable from those caused by other respiratory viruses. In severe cases of herpetic pharyngitis, the presence of inflammation and exudate may mimic full-blown streptococcal pharyngitis. Vesicles and shallow ulcers of the palate are characteristic of herpetic infection and when present are helpful in the differential diagnosis. Tender cervical adenopathy and fever are seen in some cases. Vesicles or ulcers are present on the labial and buccal mucosa when there is an associated gingivostomatitis. Acute primary herpetic infection should be distinguished from chronic mucocutaneous infection of the oropharynx due to herpes simplex virus. The chronic form of the disease is seen exclusively in patients with impaired immunity and is characterized by large shallow, painful ulcers that slowly progress unless the patient's immune status improves or antiviral therapy is given (see Chapter 118).

Herpangina

This uncommon type of pharyngitis caused by coxsackieviruses is distinguished by the presence of small vesicles (1–2 mm) on the soft palate, uvula, and anterior tonsillar pillars. The lesions rupture to become small white ulcers. Herpangina has been recognized primarily in children, in whom it may manifest as a severe febrile illness with marked sore throat and dysphagia. In some cases anorexia and abdominal pain mimic acute appendicitis (see Chapter 150).

Infectious Mononucleosis

Exudative tonsillitis or pharyngitis occurs in approximately one half the cases of infectious mononucleosis due to the EB virus. Fever and cervical adenopathy are usually present. The pharyngeal complaints of mononucleosis are usually associated with other characteristic features of the disease, such as headache and persistent malaise and fatigue. Generalized adenopathy may be present, and there is enlargement of the spleen in approximately half the cases. The mononucleosis syndrome is also associated with cytomegalovirus infection. Some patients with cytomegalovirus mononucleosis have pharyngeal soreness, but examination of the pharynx is usually unremarkable (see Chapters 120 and 121).

HIV Infection

Febrile pharyngitis is a characteristic feature of primary infection with human immunodeficiency virus (HIV).[12,28] Following an incubation period of 3–5 weeks, patients have developed fever and pharyngitis associated with varying amounts of myalgia, arthralgia, lethargy, and in some cases nonpruritic maculopapular rash. This has been followed in approximately 1 week by the development of lymphadenopathy. Pharyngeal hyperemia, sometimes marked, has been noted as well as mucosal ulcerations, but exudate has not been described (see Chapter 108).

Streptococcal Pharyngitis

The severity of illness associated with *S. pyogenes* infection of the pharynx varies greatly. In a severe case, there is marked pharyngeal pain, dysphagia, and a temperature of 39.4°C or greater. The pharyngeal membrane is a fiery red, and a thick exudate covers the posterior pharynx and tonsillar area. Edema of the uvula is often pronounced. Tender, enlarged cervical nodes and a leukocyte count of over 12,000/mm^3 complete the picture of an acute suppurative bacterial infection. At the other extreme are those streptococcal infections that are so mild as to go unrecognized by the patient or that are indistinguishable from pharyngitis caused by the common respiratory viruses. Infection with strains of *S. pyogenes* that produce erythrogenic toxin results in the characteristic erythematous rash of scarlet fever (see Chapter 176).

The clinical features of pharyngeal infection with strains of groups C and G streptococci are similar to those of *S. pyogenes*, including the occurrence of purulent exudates.[14] Most identified cases occur in the setting of a common source food epidemic; cold hard-boiled eggs are recognized as an important vehicle.

Anaerobic Pharyngitis (Vincent's Angina) / Peritonsillitis/Peritonsillar Abscess (Quinsy)

Pharyngeal and tonsillar infection with a mixture of anaerobic bacteria and spirochetes, while uncommon, still occurs. *Streptococcus pyogenes* and *Staphylococcus aureus* may play a role in some cases. With this infection, a purulent exudate coats the membrane, and there may be a foul odor to the breath. Postanginal septicemia (Lemierre's disease) is a specific form of the condition caused by *Fusobacterium necrophorum*.[29] It is associated with jugular vein septic thrombophlebitis and metastatic infection to the lung and other sites. The disease is most common in adolescents and young adults. Exudative tonsillitis or peritonsillar abscess may be present but in some patients will have subsided by the time the patient is seen. With jugular vein thrombophelebitis, there is pain, swelling, neck stiffness, and dysphagia.

With development of an abscess, pharyngeal pain is usually severe, and dysphagia and low grade fever are common. On examination, there is inflammation and swelling of the peritonsillar area with medial displacement of the tonsil. The infection is usually limited to one side, but when the condition is bilateral, partial obstruction of the pharynx occurs. Rarely, there is extension of the infection along the carotid sheath and into the mediastinum.[30] (see Chapter 49).

Gonorrheal Pharyngitis

The incidence of gonococcal infections of the pharynx has increased in recent years. Most infections are asymptomatic, but gonorrheal infection may be responsible for an occasional case of mild pharyngitis[190] (see Chapter 190).

Diphtheria

Although uncommon today, diphtheria still occurs in unvaccinated populations in the United States. The disease characteristically has a slow onset, and pharyngeal discomfort is usually not marked. Temperature elevation is present but is low grade. The characteristic tonsillar or pharyngeal membrane varies from light to dark gray and is firmly adherent to the tonsil and pharyngeal mucosa. Human infection with *Corynebacterium ulcerans* is a rare cause of human pharyngeal infection. It is associated with the consumption of raw milk and has presented as mild pharyngitis but in one case presented as serious diphtheria[32] (see Chapter 183).

Corynebacterium hemolyticum has been increasingly identified as a cause of exudative pharyngitis.[33–35] Characteristically, the infection has been recognized in adolescents and young adults and is associated with a diffuse, sometimes pruritic, erythematous maculopapular skin rash on the extremities and trunk. Cases of *C. hemolyticum* with membranous pharyngitis that mimics diphtheria[36] and with peritonsillar abscess[37] have also been reported.

Yersinial Pharyngitis

Yersinia enterocolitica causes exudative pharyngitis, which in adults may occur without the typical enterocolitis seen in children. Fever, prominent cervical lymphadenopathy, and abdominal pain with or without diarrhea have been reported.[38] A fulminant course with high mortality has been associated with reported cases of yersinial pharyngitis, making recognition important.

Mycoplasmal Pharyngitis

Epidemiologic studies of pharyngitis have associated some cases with *Mycoplasma pneumoniae* infection. The illnesses observed have been relatively mild and have had no distinguishing clinical features. *Mycoplasma pneumoniae* characteristically causes bronchitis and primary atypical pneumonia (see Chapter 162).

Noninfectious Pharyngitis

Occasional cases presenting as an inflammatory pharyngitis may have noninfectious causes. These include conditions such as bullous pemphigoid, systemic lupus erythematosis, Behçet's disease, and paraquat ingestion. Kawasaki syndrome may present as a febrile sore throat without exudate. It occurs in children and is associated with characteristic findings of the lips, tongue, and skin.

DIAGNOSIS

The primary objectives in the diagnosis of acute pharyngitis are to distinguish cases of common viral etiology from those due to *S. pyogenes* and to detect and identify the occasional case due to an unusual or rare cause. In the majority of cases, an etiologic diagnosis is not possible on clinical grounds alone. The presence of pharyngeal or tonsillar exudates, skin rash, or conjunctivitis aids in the differential diagnosis, but these findings are not present with sufficient frequency to be helpful in most cases.

The list of etiologic agents associated with the presence of pharyngeal exudate include groups A, C, and G streptococci; the anaerobic bacteria; *C. diphtheriae; C. hemolyticum; Y. enterocolitica*; adenovirus; herpes simplex virus; and EB virus. However, pharyngeal exudate is not always present with these infections so that its absence does not exclude them from consideration. On the other hand, exudate is rarely, if ever, seen in the large group of cases of pharyngitis due to the common cold viruses and influenza. The presence of skin rash suggests the possibility of infection with *S. pyogenes, C. hemolyticum,* HIV, and EB virus. Toxic shock syndrome should also be considered. The presence of conjunctivitis suggests adenovirus infection.

The development of rapid antigen detection tests, using a specimen collected by throat swab, has been a significant advance in the diagnosis of streptococcal pharyngitis. Tests employing a latex agglutination system are highly specific (95–99%) and moderately sensitive (70–90%), compared with throat culture.[39–41] Also, newer solid phase enzyme immunoassay tests, which give similar results, are becoming available.[42] The performance characteristics of the antigen detection tests have dictated a strategy in which a positive test establishes the diagnosis of streptococcal pharyngitis, while a negative test should be followed by a standard throat culture on sheep blood agar. Among the advantages of routinely performing an antigen detection test and/or culture in patients with pharyngitis are that the test results may influence the management of family members and other close contacts who subsequently become ill, and a negative test should prompt consideration of the more unusual, and sometimes serious, causes of pharyngeal infection, especially in patients with fever and exudative disease.

The patient's history and a consideration of epidemiologic factors may be helpful in suggesting a specific etiologic diagnosis in cases in which the antigen detection test is negative. Other family members frequently have common colds and influenzal illnesses. The season of the year and the occurrence of known epidemics may provide clues of diagnosis. Rhinovirus infections predominate in the fall and spring and coronavirus infections in the winter. The occurrence of an influenza epidemic in the community is usually known to the physician. Patients with pharyngoconjunctival fever, a summer illness, may give a history of swimming, and they or a family member may have conjunctivitis. The diagnosis of infectious mononucleosis, primary HIV infection, and diphtheria may be suggested by the nonpharyngeal manifestations of these infections.

Examination of the structures of the pharynx should be thorough and should include mirror examination of the nasopharynx and larynx when diphtheria is suspected. In children under the age of 3 years, the presence of an exudate is a less reliable indicator of streptococcal infection than it is in older children and adults. Diphtheria produces a pseudomembrane that may be mistaken for an exudate. The presence of small vesicles or ulcers suggests herpes simplex virus infection or herpangina. The mucosal lesions of herpangina are less numerous and more confined to the area of the palate than those of herpes simplex virus, which may involve the entire oropharynx. Aphthous stomatitis, a benign condition of unknown cause, produces small painful mucosal ulcers that are sometimes confused with those of herpetic infection. Aphthosis tends to be recurrent, in contrast to acute herpetic pharyngitis, and with the usual case of aphthosis there are fewer lesions, which are usually located in the anterior part of the mouth.

Medial displacement of one or both tonsils is seen with peritonsillitis or peritonsillar abscess, and dysphagia may be present. Patients with postanginal septicemia with jugular vein thrombophlebitis will have malaise, fever, and chills, suggestive of serious illness. Also pain, tenderness, and swelling at the angle of the jaw and stiff neck are characteristic, but these findings may be subtle. Patients with infectious mononucleosis usually have generalized adenopathy and may have enlargement of the spleen. Severe sore throat and odynophagia in an adult in the absence of findings in the pharynx should suggest epiglottitis (Chapter 48).

Laboratory tests are available to help in the diagnosis of some of the above-mentioned infections. *Neisseria gonorrhea* may be detected on Thayer-Martin or other suitable media. Vincent's angina is diagnosed by a crystal violet stained smear of the pharyngeal or tonsillar exudate showing the presence of numerous fusobacteria and spirochetes. Blood cultures should be obtained in cases of suspected postanginal septicemia, and radiographic examination of the lungs, bones, and large joint may detect metastatic infection. A throat culture using Loeffler's medium should be obtained on all suspected cases of diphtheria (see Chapter 182). The hemolysis associated with *C. hemolyticum* becomes maximal at 48–72 hours and is more prominent on rabbit and human blood agar than sheep blood agar; thus this organism may be missed on standard throat culture.[34] The diagnosis of infectious mononucleosis can be confirmed by specific serologic tests (see Chapter 121). Serum antigen has been detected in cases of pharyngitis due to primary HIV infection.[28] Also, suspected cases of this infection should be followed for appearance of serum antibody to HIV (see Chapter 108). Cultures and serologic tests for influenza virus, adenovirus, herpes simplex virus, cytomegalovirus, and *M. pneumoniae* are now available in some large laboratories. Acute and convalescent (3-week) serum specimens are necessary for serologic tests for these agents. Laboratory tests for the common cold viruses are not readily available.

Pharyngitis due to noninfectious causes may sometimes present a diagnostic problem. Pemphigus, bullous pemphigoid, and systemic lupus erythematosus are among the diseases that can cause pharyngeal inflammation and discomfort. Also drug reactions are sometimes manifest by pharyngeal soreness, as is agranulocytosis. The presence of other manifestations of these diseases, particularly involvement of the skin, is helpful in leading to the diagnosis.

TREATMENT AND PREVENTION

Antimicrobial Therapy

Streptococcal Pharyngitis. Patients with pharyngitis due to *S. pyogenes* should receive a 10-day course of penicillin or an equivalent antibiotic if the patient is allergic to penicillin. The recommended oral dose of penicillin V in adults is 200,000 or 250,000 units every 6–8 hours and in children 50,000 units/kg/24 hours divided into three or four equal doses. An injection of long-acting benzathine penicillin is an excellent, although painful, form of therapy because it does not require patient compliance. The adult dose of benzathine penicillin is 1.2 million units. In patients who are allergic to penicillin, a 10-day course of erythromycin is recommended. The availability of rapid antigen detection tests for *S. pyogenes* has reduced, but not eliminated, the dilemma of when to begin antimicrobial therapy in the suspected case. In patients with a positive antigen test, treatment should be started immediately, with the goals of providing maximal symptomatic relief for the acute illness, eradicating or suppressing the infection to prevent transmission, and preventing suppurative and nonsuppurative complications.[43–47] In patients with a negative test in which the clinical diagnosis of streptococcal pharyngitis is still entertained, either of two strategies is recommended. One strategy is to await the results of throat culture before starting treatment; the other is to begin therapy when the patient is originally seen and to discontinue treatment if the culture is negative. Both of these approaches have advantages and disadvantages. Withholding treatment until culture results are known limits the immediate therapeutic benefit of antimicrobial therapy but reduces unnecessary drug use. Beginning treatment before the results of culture are known provides maximal therapeutic benefit but exposes many patients to an antimicrobial drug unnecessarily. Initiation of treatment within 1 week of the onset of streptococcal pharyngitis will prevent subsequent acute rheumatic fever,[48] and either of the two approaches will achieve this goal (see Chapter 177).

Reports of therapeutic failure with penicillin therapy as manifested by recurrent symptomatic illness[49,50] do not warrant the abandonment of penicillin as the drug of choice for streptococcal pharyngitis at the present time.[47] It has long been known that a 10-day course of penicillin does not necessarily eradicate carriage of the organism from the pharynx. However, the clinical importance of these bacteriologic failures in asymptomatic persons has not been established. Patients with recurrent clinical illness associated with the documented presence of *S. pyogenes* in the pharynx require antimicrobial therapy. It is unavoidable that some "cases" of streptococcal pharyngitis, initial or recurrent, which are diagnosed by currently available means in reality represent persons with viral pharyngitis who are merely colonized with *S. pyogenes*.

Because the incidence of acute rheumatic fever declined to a low level in the United States, the need for *any* antimicrobial treatment of streptococcal pharyngitis has been questioned. However, the recent resurgence of rheumatic fever in some areas of the United States[51–53] and its continuing prevalence in other areas of the world are sufficient reasons not to abandon the general policy of using antimicrobials in the treatment of streptococcal pharyngitis. Discounting the benefit in rheumatic fever prevention and in reduction of acute morbidity, treatment is still important for prevention of suppurative complications of streptococcal pharyngitis, which include sinusitis, otitis media, mastoiditis, lateral sinus thrombosis, bacteremia, and pneumonia.

Anaerobic Pharyngitis/Peritonsillitis/Peritonsillar Abscess. Oral penicillin in the doses recommended for streptococcal pharyngitis has been successfully used in the treatment of anaerobic pharyngitis and peritonsillitis. The use of early antimicrobial therapy has reduced but not eliminated the cases that require surgical drainage of an abscess. Suspected cases of postanginal septicemia require hospitalization and appropriate diagnostic evaluation.[29] Parenteral treatment with high doses of penicillin or another antimicrobial with activity against *F. necrophorum* should be given for a prolonged course.

Diphtheria. The treatment of diphtheria is described in Chapter 183. *Corynebacterium hemolyticum* pharyngitis has been reported not to respond to a standard 10-day course of penicillin V but did respond to one injection of benzathine penicillin or a course of oral erythromycin.[33,34]

Yersinial Pharyngitis. *Yersinia enterocolitica* is usually susceptible to aminoglycosides, trimethoprim-sulfamethoxazole, and third-generation cephalosporins but resistant to penicillin (see Chapter 207).

Gonorrheal Pharyngitis. The treatment of gonococcal infections is described in Chapter 190.

Mycoplasmal Pharyngitis. The treatment of *M. pneumoniae* is described in Chapter 162.

Viral Pharyngitis. Amantadine, if given early in the course of illness, has a therapeutic effect for type A influenza. It is recommended for cases of presumed influenzal pharyngitis occurring during a known influenza type A epidemic (see Chapter 34). Chronic oropharyngeal herpetic infection in an immunosuppressed patient should be treated with acyclovir. Acyclovir is not recommended for acute herpetic pharyngitis in otherwise healthy people (see Chapter 34).

Symptomatic Therapy

Treatment is directed at relieving pharyngeal discomfort and associated systemic or respiratory symptoms. Warm saline gargles and supportive measures such as rest, aspirin, and liquids are sufficient in most cases of viral pharyngitis. Symptomatic therapy is also helpful in relieving symptoms of streptococcal pharyngitis. Patients with severe streptococcal pharyngitis or peritonsillitis may be in extreme discomfort and require liberal use of analgesics during the early course of illness. Hospitalization is rarely necessary unless supportive care is unavailable or dehydration results from diminished fluid intake.

Prevention

Tonsillectomy has been shown to reduce the incidence of throat infections in children who were severely affected with recurrent pharyngitis.[54] However, it is not recommended as a routine practice.[55] Active immunization is available for types A and B influenza and for diphtheria (see Chapters 142, 296). The prophylactic administration of amantadine is also effective against type A influenza. Liver adenovirus vaccines have been used successfully in military populations but are not available for civilian use (see Chapter 122). There has been work on experimental vaccines for a number of the agents that cause pharyngitis, including *S. pyogenes*, but these vaccines are still in the experimental stage of development.

REFERENCES

1. Stuart-Harris CH, Andrewes C, Andrews BE, et al. A collaborative study of the aetiology of acute respiratory infection in Britain 1961–4. A report of the Medical Research Council working party on acute respiratory virus infections. Br Med J 1965;2:319.
2. Gwaltney JM Jr. Virology of middle ear. Ann Otol Rhinol Laryngol. 1971;80:365.
3. Hamre D, Connelly AP Jr, Procknow JJ. Virologic studies of acute respiratory disease in young adults. IV. Virus isolations during four years of surveillance. Am J Epidemiol. 1966;83:238.
4. Monto AS, Ullman BM: Acute respiratory illness in an American community: The Tecumseh study. JAMA 1974;227:164.
5. Evans AS, Dick EC. Acute pharyngitis and tonsillitis in University of Wisconsin students. JAMA. 1964;190:699.
6. Glezen WP, Clyde WA Jr, Senior RJ, et al. Group A streptococci, mycoplasmas, and viruses associated with acute pharyngitis. JAMA 1967;202:455.
7. Valle, S-L. Febrile pharyngitis as the primary sign of HIV infection in a cluster of cases linked by sexual contact. Scand J Infect Dis. 1987;19:13–17.
8. Stryker WS, Fraser DW, Facklam RR. Foodborne outbreak of group G streptococcal pharyngitis. Am J Epidemiol. 1982;116:533–40.
9. Cohen D, Ferne M, Rouach T, et al. Foodborne outbreak of group G streptococcal sore throat in an Israeli military base. Epidemiol Infect. 1987;99:249–55.
10. McMillan JA, Sandstrom C, Weiner LB, et al. Viral and bacterial organisms associated with acute pharyngitis in a school-aged population. J Pediatr. 1986;109:747–52.
11. Reed BD, Huck W, Lutz LJ, et al. Prevalence of *Chlamydia trachomatis* and *Mycoplasma pneumoniae* in children with and without pharyngitis. J Fam Prac. 1988;26:387–92.
12. Hofkosh D, Wald ER, Chiponis DM. Prevalence of non-group-A β-hemolytic streptococci in childhood pharyngitis. South Med J. 1988;81:329–31.
13. Denny FW. Current problems in managing streptococcal pharyngitis. J Pediat. 1987;111:797–806.
14. Gwaltney JM Jr, Hendley JO, Simon G, et al. Rhinovirus infections in an industrial population. I. The occurrence of illness. N Engl J Med. 1966;275:1261.
15. Komaroff AL, Aronson MD, Pass TM, et al: Serologic evidence of chlamydial and mycoplasmal phyaryngitis in adults. Science. 1983;222:927–9.
16. Gerber MA, Ryan RW, Tilton RC, et al. Role of *Chlamydia trachomatis* in acute pharyngitis in adults. J Clin Microbiol. 1984;20:993–4.
17. Huss H, Jungkind D, Amadio P, et al. Frequency of *Chlamydia trachomatis* as the cause of pharyngitis. J Clin Microbiol. 1985;22:858–60.
18. Grayston JT, Kuo C-C, Wang S.-P, et al. A new *Chlamydia psittaci* strain, TWAR, isolated in acute respiratory tract infections. N Engl J Med. 1986;315:161–8.
19. Gwaltney JM Jr. Rhinoviruses. In: Evans AS, ed. Viral Infections of Humans: Epidemiology and Control. New York: Plenum; 1982:491.
20. Hendley JO, Fishburne HB, Gwaltney JM Jr. Coronavirus infections in working adults. Am Rev Respir Dis. 1972;105:805.
21. Wenzel RP, Hendley JO, Davies JA, et al. Coronavirus infections in military recruits. Three-year study with coronavirus strains OC43 and 229E. Am Rev Respir Dis 1974;109:621.
22. Tyrrell DAJ: Common Colds and Related Diseases. Baltimore: Williams & Wilkins; 1965.
23. Glezen WP, Fernald GW, Lohr JA. Acute respiratory disease of university students with special reference to the etiologic role of herpesvirus hominis. Am J Epidemiol. 1975;101:111.
24. Douglas RG Jr, Alford BR, Couch RB: Atraumatic nasal biopsy studies of respiratory virus infections in volunteers. Antimicrob Agents Chemother. 1968;8:340–2.
25. Winther B, Farr B, Turner RB, et al. Histopathologic examination and enumeration of polymorphonuclear leukocytes in the nasal mucosa during experimental rhinovirus colds. Acta Otolaryngol [Suppl] (Stockh) 1984;413:19–24.
26. Naclerio RM, Proud D, Lichtenstein, et al. Kinins are generated during experimental rhinovirus colds. J Infect Dis. 1988;157:133–142.
27. Proud D, Reynolds CJ, Lacapra S, et al. Nasal provocation with bradykinin induces symptoms of rhinitis and a sore throat. Am Rev Respir Dis. 1988;137:613–16.
28. Kessler HA, Blaauw B, Spear J, et al. Diagnosis of human immunodeficiency virus infection in seronegative homosexuals presenting with an acute viral syndrome. JAMA. 1987;258:1196–9.
29. Seidenfeld SM, Sutker WL, Luby JP. *Fusobacterium necrophorum* septicemia following oropharyngeal infection. JAMA. 1982;248:1348.
30. Scully RE, Galdabini JJ, McNeely BU: Case records of the Massachusetts General Hospital. N Engl J Med. 1978;298:894.
31. Hutt DM, Judson FN. Epidemiology and treatment of oropharyngeal gonorrhea. Ann Intern Med. 1986;104:655.
32. Hart RJC. *Corynebacterium ulcerans* in humans and cattle in North Devon. J Hyg Camb. 1984;92:161–4.
33. Banck G, Nyman M. Tonsillitis and rash associated with *Corynebacterium haemolyticum*. J Infect Dis. 1986;154:1037–40.
34. Miller RA, Brancato F, Holmes KK. *Corynebacterium hemolyticum* as a cause of phyaryngitis and scalatiniform rash in young adults. Ann Intern Med. 1986;105:867–72.
35. Greenman JL. *Corynebacterium hemolyticum* and pharyngitis. Ann Intern Med. 1987;106:633.
36. Green SL, LaPeter KS. Pseudodiphtheritic membranous pharyngitis caused by *Corynebacterium hemolyticum*. JAMA. 1981;245:2330.
37. Kovatch AL, Schuit KE, Michaels RH. *Corynebacterium hemolyticum* peritonsillar abscess mimicking diphtheria. JAMA. 1983;249:1757.
38. Rose FB, Camp CJ, Antes EJ. Family outbreak of fatal *Yersinia enterocolitica* pharyngitis. Am J Med. 1987;82:636–7.
39. Berkowitz CD, Anthony BF, Kaplan EL, et al. Cooperative study of latex agglutination to identify group A streptococcal antigen on throat swabs in patients with acute pharyngitis. J Pediatr. 1985;107:89.
40. Schwartz RH, Hayden GF, McCoy P, et al. Rapid diagnosis of streptococcal pharyngitis in two pediatric offices using a latex agglutination kit. Pediatr Infect Dis. 1985;4:647.
41. Roddy OF, Clegg HW, Clardy LT, et al. Comparison of a latex agglutination kit and four culture methods for identification of group A streptococci in a pediatric office laboratory. J Pediatr. 1986;108:347.
42. Radetsky M, Solomon JA, Todd JK. Identification of streptococcal pharyngitis in the office laboratory: reassessment of new technology. Pediatr Infect Dis J. 1987;6:556.
43. Nelson JD. The effect of penicillin therapy on the symptoms and signs of streptococcal pharyngitis. Pediatr Infect Dis. 1984;3:10.
44. Krober MS, Bass JW, Michels GN. Streptococcal pharyngitis. Placebo-controlled double-blind evaluation of clinical response to penicillin therapy. JAMA. 1985;253:1271.
45. Randolph MF, Gerber MA, DeMeo KK, et al. The effect of antibiotic therapy on the clinical course of streptococcal pharyngitis. J Pediatr. 1985;106:870.
46. Denny FW. Effect of treatment on streptococcal pharyngitis: is the issue really settled? Pediatr Infect Dis. 1985;4:352.
47. McCracken GH Jr. Diagnosis and management of children with streptococcal pharyngitis. Pediatr Infect Dis. 1986;5:754.
48. Caranzaro FJ, Stetson CA, Morris AJ, et al: The role of the streptococcus in the pathogenesis of rheumatic fever. Am J Med. 1954;17:749.
49. Brook I. The role of beta-lactamase-producing bacteria in the persistence of streptococcal tonsillar infection. Rev Infect Dis. 1984;6:601.
50. Gastanaduy AS, Kaplan EL, Hume BB, et al. Failure of penicillin to eradicate Group A streptococci during an outbreak of pharyngitis. Lancet. 1980;2:498.
51. Wald ER, Dashefsky B, Feidt C, et al. Acute rheumatic fever in western Pennsylvania and the tristate area. Pediatrics. 1987;80:371.
52. Congeni B, Rizzo C, Congeni J, et al. Outbreak of acute rheumatic fever in northeast Ohio. J Pediatr. 1987;111:176.
53. Papadimos T, Escamilla J. Acute rheumatic fever at a Navy training center—San Diego, California. Leads from the MMWR. JAMA. 1988;259:1782.
54. Paradise JL, Bluestone CD, Bachman RZ, et al. Efficacy of tonsillectomy for recurrent throat infection in severely affected children. Results of parallel randomized and nonrandomized clinical trials. New Engl J Med. 1984;310:674.
55. Hendley JO. Tonsillectomy: justified but not mandated in special patients. New Engl J Med. 1984;310:717.

44. ACUTE LARYNGITIS

JACK M. GWALTNEY, JR.

Acute laryngitis usually occurs in association with the common cold and influenzal syndromes. Lowering of the normal pitch of the voice, hoarseness, and occasionally aphonia are the characteristic complaints[1,2]; obstruction of the airway is rare in adults. In young children, airway obstruction due to infection of the larynx and tracheobronchial tree is more common, and acute laryngitis must be distinguished from acute bacterial supraglottitis (epiglottitis) (see Chapter 48). Acute supraglottitis has been recognized with increasing frequency in adults, but is still unusual.

Hoarseness is present in 20 percent of cases of common respiratory illness.[3] It occurs most frequently with midwinter illnesses and correlates with the occurrence of cough and, to a lesser extent, sore throat. All the major respiratory viruses have been reported to cause hoarseness (Table 1).[3–6] Influenza virus, rhinovirus, and adenovirus have most often been the cause of laryngitis in reported studies. The role of secondary bacterial invasion in acute laryngitis is not clear; however, *Branhamella catarrhalis* has been recovered from the nasopharynx of 50 to 55 percent of adults with acute laryngitis compared with 6 to 14 percent of controls.[7,8] Hoarseness was also reported by approximately 10 percent of adults with streptococcal pharyngitis.[4] Unusual causes of laryngitis include syphilis, tuberculosis,[9] herpes zoster,[10] histoplasmosis, blastomycosis, and candidiasis. Candidal laryngitis has been recognized chiefly in patients with impaired immunity.[11,12]

Diagnosis of acute laryngitis is usually apparent from the history and clinical characteristics of the illness. Eighty-seven percent of patients with laryngitis reporting to an otolaryngology clinic had preceding upper respiratory tract infection symptoms, and 13 percent reported prior voice abuse.[8] Examination of the larynx reveals hyperemia, edema, or vascular injection of the vocal cords, and there may be superficial mucosal ulcerations. The presence of an exudate or membrane on the pharyngeal or laryngeal mucosa should arouse the suspicion of streptococcal infection, mononucleosis, or diphtheria. In acute epiglottitis, the epiglottis is characteristically intensely red and greatly swollen. Patients with traumatic aphonia usually give a history of excessive use of the voice.

Treatment consists primarily of resting the voice until hoarseness and aphonia have subsided. Inhalation of moistened air on a regular basis may also give relief. A recent double-blind study failed to show a beneficial effect of penicillin V in the treatment of adults with acute laryngitis.[8] Until there is evidence for the value of antimicrobials in the treatment of acute laryngitis, they are not recommended for what is usually a benign self-limited disease. Diphtheritic laryngitis and acute bacterial epiglottitis require specific antimicrobial therapy. Patients with hoarseness persisting longer than 10 days to 2 weeks should have a laryngoscopic examination to exclude tumors and other chronic diseases of the larynx.

TABLE 1. Occurrence of Hoarseness with Acute Respiratory Infections

Infectious Agent	Percentage of Cases
Viruses	
Influenza virus	22–37 (3,4)[a]
Rhinovirus	10–25 (4,5)
Adenovirus	6–25 (5,6)
Parainfluenza virus	2–18 (5)
Respiratory syncytial virus	10 (5)
Coxsackievirus A21	9 (5)
Coronavirus	Not determined[b]
Bacteria	
Streptococcus pyogenes	10 (4)

[a] Reference numbers.
[b] In one small study of hospitalized Marine recruits, hoarseness was present in 7 of 11 patients with coronavirus infection diagnosed by seroconversion to coronavirus OC43.[13]

REFERENCES

1. Proctor DF: The upper airways. II. The larynx and trachea. Am Rev Respir Dis. 1977;115:315.
2. Vaughan CW. Current concepts in otolaryngology. Diagnosis and treatment of organic voice disorders. N Engl J Med. 1982;307:863.
3. Dingle JH, Badger GF, Jordan WS Jr: Illness in the Home. A study of 25,000 Illnesses in a Group of Cleveland Families. Cleveland: The Press of Western Reserve University; 1964:66.
4. Gwaltney JM Jr: Rhinoviruses. In: Evans, AS, Ed. Viral Infections of Humans: Epidemiology and Control. 2nd ed. New York: Plenum; 1982:507.
5. Tyrrell DAJ: *Common Colds and Related Diseases*. Baltimore: Williams & Wilkins; 1965:95.
6. McNamara MJ, Pierce WE, Crawford YE, et al. Patterns of adenovirus infection in the respiratory diseases of naval recruits. A longitudinal study of two companies of naval recruits. Am Rev Respir Dis. 1962;86:485.
7. Schalén L, Christensen P, Kamme C, et al. High isolation rate of *Branhamella catarrhalis* from the nasopharynx in adults with acute laryngitis. Scand J Infect Dis. 1980;12:277.
8. Schalen L, Christensen P, Eliasson I, et al. Inefficacy of penicillin V in acute laryngitis in adults. Evaluation from results of double-blind study. Ann Otol Laryngol. 1985;94:14.
9. Bachman AL, Zizmor J, Noyek AM. Tuberculosis of the larynx. Semin Roentgenol. 1979;14:325.
10. Lederer FJ, Soboroff BJ. Medical problems related to diseases of the larynx. Otolaryngol Clin North Am. 1970;3:599.
11. Lawson R, Bodey G, Luna M. *Candida* infection presenting as laryngitis. Am J Med Sci. 1980;280:173.
12. Dudley JP, Byrne WJ, Kobayashi R, et al. *Candida* laryngitis in chronic mucocutaneous candidiasis. Its association with *Candida* esophagitis. Ann Otol Rhinol Laryngol. 1980;89:574.
13. Wenzel RP, Hendley JO, Davies JA, et al. Coronavirus infections in military recruits. Three-year study with coronavirus strains OC43 and 229E. Am Rev Respir Dis. 1974;109:621.

45. ACUTE LARYNGOTRACHEOBRONCHITIS (CROUP)

CAROLINE BREESE HALL

> . . . the sharp stridulous voice which I can resemble to nothing more nearly than the crowing of a cock . . . is the true diagnostic sign of the disease.—Francis Home, 1765[1]

Croup or acute laryngotracheobronchitis is an age-specific viral infection of the upper and lower respiratory tract that produces inflammation in the subglottic area and results in the striking picture of dyspnea accompanied on inspiration by the characteristic stridulous notes of croup. Croup demonstrates perhaps best the piquant interaction of host and microorganism. Age, sex, an undefined predisposition of the child, and the type of virus all appear to influence the susceptibility and severity of the infection.

Francis Home of Edinburgh first introduced the word *croup* in his famous treatise "An Inquiry into the Nature, Causes and Cure of the Croup" in which he describes 12 patients with croup.[1] Croup was derived from the old Scottish term *roup*, which meant "to cry out in a shrill voice."

Croup at that time and for the next century was the term often applied to a number of disease entities including diphtheria. John Cheyne, however, appeared to describe not only diphtheria, cynanche trachealis, but also croup that appeared most similar to the viral laryngotracheobronchitis of today.[2] Bretonneau in 1859 argued that diphtheria was a separate and specific disease.[3] However, the confusion between "membranous," or "true croup," and "spasmodic," or "false croup," continued. Differentiation awaited Klebs' discovery of *Corynebacterium diphtheriae* in 1883. In 1948 Rabe[4] classified the forms of infectious croup according to etiology—bacterial or nonbacterial—and suggested that the latter, larger group might be viral in origin. In only 15 percent of his 347 patients was he able to identify a pathogen, namely, *C. diphtheriae* or *Haemophilus influenzae* type b.

INCIDENCE

Croup occurs mostly in children between the ages of 3 months and 3 years, with a peak occurrence in the second year of life.[5–8] In a Seattle prepaid group practice the annual incidence of croup per 1000 children under 6 years of age was 7.[5] In the first 6 months of life the rate was 5.2, and in the second 6 months of life, the rate was 11. The peak incidence was 14.9 in the second year of life, and fell to half that rate in the third year of life. In a group practice in North Carolina, the incidence was about three to five times higher, with a peak of 47 per 1000 each year for children in the second year of life.[8] Even in the first 6 months of life the incidence was 24, and after 6 years of age it was 4.6. In series of hospitalized or outpatient cases of croup, boys predominate, although the attack rates of upper respiratory illnesses by these same viral agents show no sex preference.[5,7–11]

ETIOLOGY

Acute laryngotracheobronchitis may be caused by a variety of viral agents and occasionally by *Mycoplasma pneumoniae* (Table 1).[5,6,8–14] Parainfluenza type 1 virus is the most common cause of croup in the United States and Great Britain (Table 1). Parainfluenza type 3 virus is usually the second most frequently associated agent. In infants this virus more commonly tends to cause bronchiolitis and pneumonia. However, the more frequent manifestation in children 2–3 years of age is croup, and in older children it is tracheobronchitis.[9] Influenza A virus is also a major cause of croup, but its annual incidence varies because of its unpredictable nature and fluctuating seasonal occurrence. Although croup caused by influenza A virus may be less frequent than that from the parainfluenza viruses, some studies have reported it to be more severe,[15–17] while others have not.[8] Influenza A virus may produce croup in a broader age range of children and sometimes with a higher frequency of hospitalization. In Washington, D.C., between 1957 and 1976, 14.3 percent of the croup patients had influenza A or B viral infection.[12] Influenza A more commonly caused croup than did influenza B virus, and interestingly, the frequency of croup appeared to be related to the particular strain of influenza. Croup was more frequently observed in H3N2 than in H2N2 epidemics.[17]

Only a small proportion (approximately 5 percent) of respiratory syncytial viral infections result in croup, but anywhere from 1 to 11 percent of the reported croup cases have been associated with this virus (Table 1). Similarly, croup is an unusual manifestation of adenoviral infection, but these viruses may contribute a small proportion of cases. In contrast, croup is the characteristic manifestation of parainfluenza type 2 viral infection. The total proportion of croup cases produced by parainfluenza type 2 virus is, however, less than that associated with its relatives, types 1 and 3. This is because type 2 virus tends to be a less frequent visitor to a community and sizable outbreaks of infection with parainfluenza type 2 virus are unusual in comparison to outbreaks with type 1.[7–9] Rhinoviruses, enteroviruses, and *M. pneumoniae* all contribute a small, but variable proportion of cases. At all ages the parainfluenza viruses are the major agents. Respiratory syncytial virus (RSV), however, rarely causes croup in children older than 5 years, and the influenza viruses and *M. pneumoniae* predominately cause croup in this older age group.[8]

Of all these agents, only parainfluenza type 1 virus, influenza viruses, and sometimes RSV and parainfluenza type 2 virus occur in epidemics and have a great enough predilection for causing croup as to produce an appreciable rise in the occurrence of croup cases when they are prevalent in a community.[5,8,11,17,18] An appreciable proportion of parainfluenza type 3 infections are also manifested as croup, but this virus is usually more sporadic in its appearance.[8] When epidemic, however, parainfluenza type 3 virus may also cause a discernable increase in the number of croup cases observed.[5,8,11]

EPIDEMIOLOGY

The epidemiologic patterns of croup mainly reflect the seasonal personalities of the major agents. Since parainfluenza type 1 virus causes the largest proportion of croup cases, the major peak of cases occurs when this virus is prevalent in the community. In recent years parainfluenza type 1 virus has tended to cause outbreaks of infection every other year in the fall.[7,9,11] Outbreaks of croup that occur in the winter to early spring are most apt to be related to influenza A viral activity and, to a lesser extent, to respiratory syncytial viral activity.[7–9,18] Sporadic cases of croup are commonly associated with parainfluenza type 3 virus. This virus had been isolated throughout much of the year, but more recently has been observed to have swells

TABLE 1. Percentage of Croup Cases Associated with Various Agents

	Reported Series								
Agent	Cramblett 1977[12] (%)	Parrott et al. 1962[13] (%)	Loda et al. 1968[14] (%)	Glezen et al. 1971[9] (%)	Foy et al. 1973[5] (%)		Buchan et al. 1974[11] (%)	Downham et al. 1974[6] (%)	Denny et al. 1983[8] (%)
Parainfluenza virus									
Type 1	8	21	39	21	13[a]	6.4[b]	25	26	18
Type 2	6	8	1.6	4	1.4	7.3	1.7	6	3
Type 3	14	10	1.6	9	3	13	8	10	6.6
Influenza A	6	} 8		2	1	3.7	10	6	1.4
Influenza B				1	1	2			1.2
Respiratory syncytial		8	11.4	6	1	9	1.7	6	3.8
Adenovirus	4	9	3	1	4	4.6	1.7	3	
Rhinovirus				0.6	2		1	6	
Enterovirus	12			1	1		1		
Other viruses							5		2
Mycoplasma pneumoniae			5	1.4	0.5	2		1	1.4
Total percentage of cases with identified agent	50	64	62	47	56		54	64	37.6

[a] Identified by isolation of agent.
[b] Identified by serology.

of activity during the warmer months of late spring and summer.[6,9,11] Sporadic cases of croup may also be caused by any of the less common agents such as the adenoviruses, rhinoviruses, and *M. pneumoniae*, which may be prevalent through many months of the year. Croup from enteroviruses, although uncommon, tends to occur in the summer and early fall. Parainfluenza type 2 virus tends to produce smaller outbreaks of infection at less predictable intervals, commonly in the fall and early winter.[6–8,11]

PATHOPHYSIOLOGY

The viral infection initially affects the upper respiratory tract, usually producing inflammation of the nasal passages and nasopharynx. Subsequently the infection spreads downward to involve essentially all levels of the respiratory tract. The classic signs of croup—the stridor, hoarseness, and cough—arise mostly from the inflammation occurring in the larynx and trachea. However, involvement of the lower respiratory tract is also present in most cases requiring hospitalization.[19] The inflammation and obstruction are greatest at the subglottic level. This is because it is the least distensible part of the airway since it is encircled by the cricoid cartilage with the narrow anterior ring and the larger posterior quadrangular lamina.

Inflammation at the subglottic level results in the characteristic obstruction observed in viral croup. The impeded flow of air through this narrowed area produces the classic high-pitched vibratory sounds, or stridor. This is most apparent on inspiration since the negative pressure tends to narrow the extrathoracic airway further, much as sucking on a partially occluded paper straw causes it to collapse inwardly. This is enhanced in young children since their airway walls are relatively compliant.[20] In 1836 Ley[21] descriptively expressed this as

> The shrill sonorous inspiration so characteristic of this complaint, marks very unequivocally its seat. . . . From some cause there is an unusual approximation of the sides of the glottis . . . the influence being very analogous to that produced by too strong compression of the reed against the mouthpiece of the clarionet by the lips of one who has made no great proficiency in that instrument, when a harsh, squeaking sound is produced abundantly discordant and grating to the ear.

In histologic sections, inflammatory changes may be seen in the epithelium, the mucosa, and the submucosa of the larynx, trachea, and the linings of the bronchi, bronchioles, and even the alveoli.[22] Small areas of atelectasis may also be present.

Why children in the second year of life are particularly prone to develop croup is not entirely clear. However, this may be partly explained by the fact that most of these children are experiencing primary infection with the viral agent, which is more likely to be manifested by spread of the virus to involve the lower respiratory tract and also by the anatomy. The diameters of the larynx and glottis are relatively smaller in the young child, and inflammation of the membranes lining these passages causes a relatively greater degree of obstruction. Airway resistance is highly sensitive to even small changes in the diameter of the airway. In fact, the resistance to airflow is inversely related to the fourth power of the radius of the airway. Furthermore, the mucous membrane is relatively looser and more vascular and the cartilage ring less rigid. Also, nasal obstruction and crying can aggravate the dynamic narrowing of the child's airway.

Immunologic mechanisms may also be involved in the pathogenesis of croup. Urquhart and colleagues[23] have suggested that the pathogenesis of croup may be different in children with abrupt vs. gradual onset. Noting a different serologic response in such children, they hypothesized that croup of sudden onset resulted from a hypersensitivity reaction to parainfluenza type 1 virus in children with previous infection with a closely related paramyxovirus such as parainfluenza type 3. In the children with a more gradual onset of prodromal upper respiratory tract symptoms for more than 1 day, antibody to the parainfluenza viruses in the acute-phase serum was less often present and in lower titers than in the acute sera of patients with a sudden onset of croup.

Greater concentrations of IgE antibody to parainfluenza viral antigen and histamine have been detected in children with parainfluenza viral infections whose illness was manifested as croup, wheezing, or both in comparison to those with only upper respiratory tract illness.[24] Furthermore, the lymphoproliferative responses of peripheral blood lymphocytes from children with parainfluenza viral croup were significantly greater than those from children with upper respiratory tract illness, and their histamine-induced suppression of the lymphoproliferative response was diminished.[25] From these findings, Welliver et al.[24,25] have suggested that a defect in immunoregulation, similar to that found in atopic subjects, contributes to the pathogenesis of croup.

Physiologic Correlations

When the infection produces obstruction at the subglottic level, the child's tidal volume initially declines. This, however, is compensated by an increase in the respiratory rate to maintain adequate alveolar ventilation (Fig. 1). If, however, the degree of obstruction increases, the work of breathing may increase such that the child tires and can no longer maintain the necessary compensatory respiratory effort. The tidal volume may then further decrease, and as the respiratory rate declines, hy-

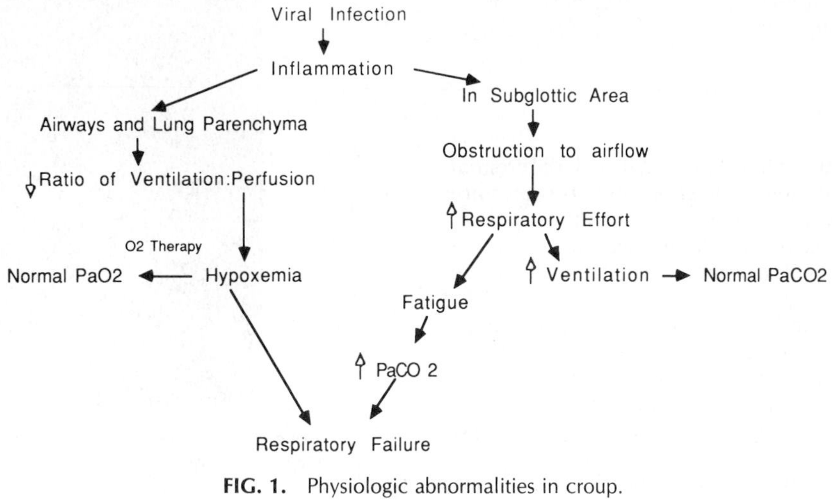

FIG. 1. Physiologic abnormalities in croup.

percarbia and secondary hypoxemia ensue. The subglottic obstruction does not result in hypoxemia until this stage, when respiratory failure occurs.

Hypoxemia, however, occurs in 80 percent of the children hospitalized with croup.[19] The hypoxemia arises from the inflammation in the lung parenchyma, which results in an abnormally low ratio of ventilation to perfusion and an increased alveolar-to-arterial gradient (Fig. 1).

CLINICAL MANIFESTATIONS

> The disease generally comes on in the evening after the little patient has been exposed to the weather during the day and often after a slight catarrh of some days' standing. At first his voice is observed to be hoarse and pulling . . . he awakens with a most unusual cough, rough and stridulous. And now his breathing is laborious, each inspiration being accompanied by a harsh, shrill noise."— John Cheyne, 1814[2]

Most children with croup have a history of an upper respiratory tract infection for 1 to several days previously. Commonly the child has had rhinorrhea, a sore throat, and mild cough. Most children have fever, either initially during the upper respiratory tract infection or at the onset of croup. Children with croup from influenza A and parainfluenza viruses commonly have fevers with temperatures ranging from 38–40°C.[26] Fever with respiratory syncytial viral infection tends not to be as high.

The onset of croup is commonly heralded by hoarseness and a deepening cough. The cough is usually not productive but has the striking brassy tone that has earned it the sobriquet "seal's bark." The child may awaken at night with this distinctive cough, tachypnea, and the characteristic inspiratory stridor. In 1836, Ley[21] described the stridor as "the crowing of a cock, the yelping of a fox, the barking of a dog, the braying of an ass, or a ringing sound, as if the voice came from a brazen tube." The child may sit forward in bed and appear apprehensive. Commonly accompanying the stridor are retractions of the chest wall, usually most marked in the supraclavicular and suprasternal area.

In children who are more severely affected, auscultation of the chest commonly reveals not only the inspiratory stridor but also rales, rhonchi, and/or wheezing. Occasionally, a markedly distressed child will have stridor on expiration as well as inspiration. The respiratory rate is commonly elevated to 35–45/min. However, respiratory rates much above 50/min are uncommon in children with croup, in contrast to the marked tachypnea often evident in bronchiolitis. With progression of the disease, auscultation of the chest may reveal poor exchange of air with diminished breath sounds.

One of the hallmarks of croup is its fluctuating course. A child may clinically appear to worsen or improve within an hour. In milder cases of croup, children commonly improve in the morning, only to worsen again at night. In most children the course of croup is 3–4 days, although the cough may persist for a longer period.

LABORATORY FINDINGS

In most cases of croup the white blood cell and differential counts are not particularly abnormal or helpful. In the more severely stressed child the white blood cell count may be somewhat elevated, and if hypoxemia is present, an increase in the proportion of immature polymorphonuclear cells may be observed.

Hypoxemia (PaO_2 <85 mmHg) occurs in most hospitalized children, and hypercapnea is present in over half.[19] In the study of Newth et al.,[19] most children hospitalized with croup had PaO_2 values between 50 and 80 mmHg, and about half had $PaCO_2$ values in the normal range below 40 mmHg. The rest had $PaCO_2$ levels between 40 and 50 mmHg. Only 1 of the 35 children manifested hypercarbia of greater then 50 mmHg. Few other pulmonary function studies have been obtained in children with croup, but in five out of six children in one study the functional residual capacity was found to be increased.[27]

DIAGNOSIS

The diagnosis of croup is usually based on the characteristic clinical picture. However, differentiation from noninfectious causes of stidor such as foreign body aspiration or an allergic reaction, and from *H. influenzae*-induced epiglottis usually may be made on the basis of both the history and the anterior–posterior and lateral roentgenograms of the neck.[28]

Characteristically the course of epiglottitis is much more rapidly progressive, and the children appear to be in a more toxic state. The history of an upper respiratory tract infection with rhinorrhea and laryngitis is usually not present in epiglottitis. The absence of the distinctive cough or "seal's bark" and the presence of marked dysphagia with drooling are often two of the more helpful differentiating clinical signs. In viral laryngotracheobronchitis the anterior–posterior view of the neck (Fig. 2) shows the characteristic subglottic swelling, sometimes described as the "hourglass" or "steeple" sign. In epiglottitis, the lateral neck view may show the edematous epiglottis without subglottic narrowing (see Chapter 48). The roentgenographic picture may not, however, always be diagnostic for croup or epiglottitis, and controversy exists about their reliability and usefulness in the acute situation.[29–31]

Identification of the specific viral agent may be accomplished by isolation in tissue culture or by one of the newer techniques of rapid viral diagnosis.[32] Serologic diagnosis generally may be made only retrospectively, and for some of the major agents of croup serologic rises are variable and unreliable. With parainfluenza viral infections, heterotypic antibody rises are frequent among the various types of the parainfluenza viruses and the related viruses such as mumps.[13,33] Furthermore, during reinfection no measurable antibody response may occur.[33]

In reported series the cause has been determined in approximately one-third to two-thirds of the cases of croup (Table 1), which is higher than that generally reported for other respiratory tract syndromes. Viral isolation has usually been accomplished from throat, tracheal, and nasal wash specimens.[5,6,8,9,11,14,26] Rapid diagnostic techniques, mostly the enzyme-linked im-

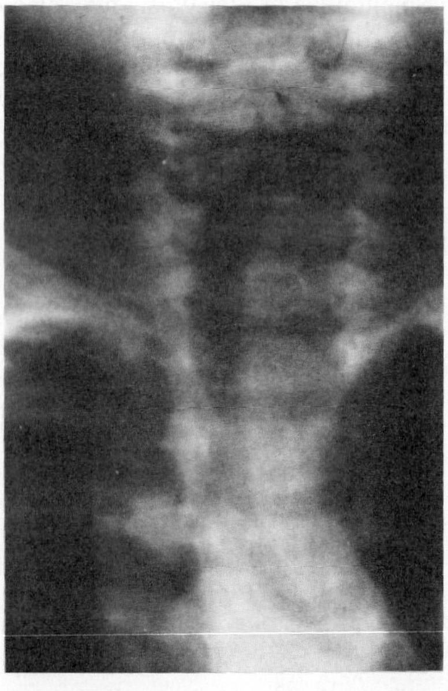

FIG. 2. Roentgenogram of the neck of a child with viral croup that shows the characteristic narrowing of the air shadow of the trachea in the subglottic area.

munosorbent assay (ELISA) and immunofluorescent techniques, have also been successfully used.[6,32,34–38]

COMPLICATIONS

The severity of croup appears to be influenced by both virus and host factors. Some children appear predisposed to croup, with repetitive episodes from a variety of agents. John Cheyne[2] noted ". . . the first attack establishes a predisposition to the disease. I have observed, that after the first attack, a slighter cause will produce Croup a second time than is required originally."

Children with repeated episodes of croup are sometimes diagnosed as having *spasmodic croup*.[39] An allergic diathesis or hyperreactivity of the airway may contribute to the illness in these children since positive intradermal skin tests and family members with allergy have been frequently seen in children with recurrent versus single episodes of croup.[40–42] A tendency toward lower serum IgA levels has also been noted in children with recurrent croup.[43] Nevertheless, a viral infection initiates the croup even in these children, and the disease cannot be distinguished clinically.

Boys are particularly prone to develop croup for reasons that are not entirely clear.[7–9,11,40,44] However, recently Taussig[45] has shown that young girls had significantly larger flow rates than did boys. This suggests that there are differences anatomically or in intrinsic airway resistance that are related to sex, which might in part explain why young boys tend to develop lower respiratory tract disease more frequently or more severely than do young girls.

Severe croup has sometimes been reported as more frequent with influenza A viral infection than with the other viral agents.[15,16] In the study of Howard et al.[15] made during an outbreak of influenza A infection, 10 out of 25 infants hospitalized with croup required tracheotomy. This complication has been estimated to occur in about 5–12 percent of the cases of croup.[44,46,47] In Adair and coworkers'[46] review of reported cases of laryngotracheobronchitis, the percentage requiring tracheotomy varied between 0 and 13 percent. The associated mortality rate in these series ranged from 0 to 2.7 percent. Of the major acute complications, respiratory failure necessitating such airway intervention is the most frequent. Subglottic stenosis after intubation occasionally occurs in children with complicated and prolonged courses.[44,46–49]

Pneumonia cannot truly be considered a complication of croup but should rather be thought of as a part of the disease. Parenchymal involvement, as evidenced by hypoxemia, is present in most hospitalized children, whether it is visible on the chest roentgenogram or not. Less common complications include pneumothorax, pulmonary edema, and aspiration pneumonia. Aspiration of gastric contents is most likely to occur during emergency intubation. Transient pulmonary edema without evidence of cardiac enlargement has been described in children with croup.[49–51] The mechanism leading to this complication is not completely understood, but it may arise from a neurogenic effect on the pulmonary vasculature, as a direct result of alveolar hypoxia, or possibly from an increased alveolar-capillary gradient causing a leakage of intravascular fluids.

Whether long-term complications can follow croup is currently speculative. The disease is self-limited, and recovery appears clinically to be complete. However, several follow-up studies of children with croup early in life have shown an increased frequency of hyperreactivity of the airways and altered pulmonary function that, in some children, may be clinically occult.[27,47,52,53] In one study of 12-year-old children who had a history of hospitalization for croup, elevated residual volumes and significant reductions in forced vital capacity (FVC), forced expiratory volume in 1 second (FEV_1), and maximal expiratory flow between 25 and 75 percent of vital capacity ($FEF_{25-75\%}$) were found.[53] Hyperreactivity of the airways has been observed in each of these follow-up studies of children with croup.[27,47,52,53]

THERAPY

Despite a Pandora's box of home therapies for croup, none has proved to be consistently effective. The natural fluctuations in the course of croup make evaluation of many therapies difficult. Vaporizers and other means of producing steam or mist in the home have long been advised. The beneficial effects of these devices have not actually been proved, and in one small controlled trial humidification provided no benefit.[54] These methods certainly provide humidification of the upper airway, but the droplet size produced is generally too large to reach the lower respiratory tract. The advantages of such home humidification devices must be balanced against the discomfort or fear they may produce in the child. Crying and lack of rest may aggravate the condition.

In hospitalized patients, the essence of successful management is close observation and good supportive care based on a thorough understanding of the physiologic changes associated with croup. Clinical estimation of the severity of croup is difficult. Cyanosis may not be present despite compromising degrees of hypoxemia.[55] Of the clinical signs, an increasing respiratory rate is often the best indication of hypoxemia. The severity of the stridor and retractions reflect more the degree of subglottic obstruction and are not indicative of the arterial oxygen saturation. Hence, in all children ill enough to require hospitalization the objective criteria of determining arterial blood gases should be used initially in the management. Capillary as well as arterial blood gases may be used, but oximetry offers a simple, noninvasive means of following the child's arterial oxygen saturation.[56]

In children with hypoxemia, supplemental oxygen becomes the mainstay of therapy.[48,57,58] Children with PaO_2 values of less than 60 mmHg will benefit from supplemental oxygen. Since the hypoxemia in children without marked hypercarbia results from an abnormal ratio of ventilation to perfusion, the hypoxemia will respond to oxygen therapy, usually at relatively low concentrations (Fig. 1).

Humidification of the airway may be administered by an ultrasonic nebulizer fitted to a mask or an oxygen tent. Although humidification of the lower airway theoretically may be achieved by this means, the value of such therapy has not been proved.

In one of the few animal studies of croup, cold-dry, cold-moist, and dry air were more effective in the dog model in decreasing airway resistance.[59] All of these types of air contain little humidification as compared with warm-moist air, which was least effective.

A variety of pharmacologic agents have been evaluated in the treatment of croup. The only one that currently appears to be of possible benefit is racemic epinephrine. L-Epinephrine has also been suggested as being as efficient since it contains only the active isomer.[60] The reported results with racemic epinephrine, however, have not been consistent.[61–65] Gardner and colleagues in a controlled double-blind study administered nebulized racemic epinephrine by face mask to croup patients and evaluated their response clinically.[62] The racemic epinephrine proved to be no more effective than the saline. In a subsequent double-blind study by Westley and coworkers,[63] racemic epinephrine was delivered by intermittent positive-pressure breathing and resulted in significant clinical improvement. In both of these studies the response was evaluated clinically. Taussig and colleagues,[64] however, evaluated the effect of racemic epinephrine by intermittent positive-pressure breathing clinically and with concurrent determinations of the blood gases. The racemic epinephrine resulted in clinical improvement in terms of stridor and retractions but did not alter the arterial PO_2. It would appear, therefore, that such therapy may have benefit by providing clinical improvement and thus deterring fatigue. Such therapy should, however, be used with the understanding that the amelioration of clinical signs is transient, continued observation is necessary, and despite the clinical appearance, the degree of hypoxemia is unchanged.

Corticosteroid therapy generally has not been shown to be beneficial and remains controversial.[61,66–68] The many studies evaluating steroid use in croup have been recently reviewed, and most all have been noted to have faults in their design or methods.[66] Despite this, some continue to recommend steroids for selected cases of severe croup.[44] Antibiotic therapy in viral croup is not indicated, and secondary bacterial infection is uncommon.

A few children, despite adequate supportive therapy, may fatigue and develop respiratory failure, demonstrated by a climbing $PaCO_2$ level. If a mechanical airway becomes necessary, nasotracheal intubation is the preferred method, provided personnel skilled in this technique are available.[47–49] Complications with nasotracheal intubation are less than with tracheostomies. In Schuller and Birck's[47] 8-year follow-up study of children receiving nasotracheal intubation for croup and epiglottitis, the rate of immediate and reversible complications was 7 percent, and for the delayed, irreversible complications the rate was 1.6 percent. The average period of intubation for the children with croup was 88 hours as compared with 55 hours for those with epiglottitis.

BACTERIAL TRACHEITIS

Recently, an atypical form of croup has been described and designated as *bacterial tracheitis*.[69–72] This uncommon entity tends to affect somewhat older children but may affect any age and produce a dramatic, acute onset marked by high fever, stridor, and dyspnea with copious amounts of purulent sputum. The clinical picture may resemble epiglottitis and progress rapidly, requiring endotracheal intubation or tracheotomy. The area of inflammation and obstruction, however, is subglottic and is covered with a thick exudate. The lateral soft tissue roentgenogram of the neck characteristically reveals a normal epitlottis with subglottic narrowing within which a shaggy membrane may sometimes be visible.

The organisms most commonly recovered from this exudate are *Staphylococcus aureus*, group A β-hemolytic streptococci, and *H. influenzae* type b.[69–72] The pathogenesis of this entity, nevertheless, is not clear. The syndrome appears to develop in children who are predisposed by previous conditions, especially those associated with injury to the trachea. Children who have been recently intubated and sometimes those with a preceding viral infection appear to be at risk. In one reported case *Chlamydia trachomatis* was isolated from the tracheal exudate along with *S. aureus*.[72]

The rapidly progressive course of this disease demands its prompt diagnosis and differentiation from viral croup by its clinical and roentgenographic picture. Direct laryngoscopy can confirm the diagnosis and provide specimens of the localized exudate for culture. Initial antibiotic therapy should be broad enough to cover the associated major pathogens.

REFERENCES

1. Home F. An Inquiry into the Nature, Cause and Cure of Croup. Edinburgh, 1765.
2. Cheyne J. Essays on the Diseases of Children, with Cases and Dissections. Philadelphia 1802–1808. Philadelphia: Anthony Finley Merritt; 1814:20.
3. Semple RH. Memoirs on diphtheria. From the Writings of Bretonneau, Guersant, Trousseau, Bouchut, Empis, Daviot. London: New Sydenham Society Publications; 1859:5.
4. Rabe EF. Infectious croup: I. Etiology. Pediatrics. 1948;2:255–65.
5. Foy HM, Cooney MK, Maletzky AJ, et al. Incidence and etiology of pneumonia, croup and bronchiolitis in pre-school children belonging to a prepaid medical care group over a four year period. Am J Epidemiol. 1973;97:80–92.
6. Downham MAPS, McQuillan J, Gardner PS. Diagnosis and clinical significance of parainfluenza virus infections in children. Arch Dis Child. 1974; 49:8–15.
7. Glezen WP, Denny FW. Epidemiology of acute lower respiratory disease in children. N Engl J Med. 1973;288:498–505.
8. Denny FW, Murphy TF, Clyde WA Jr, et al. Croup: An 11 year study in a pediatric practice. Pediatrics. 1983;71:871–6.
9. Glezen WP, Loda FA, Clyde WA Jr, et al. Epidemiogical patterns of acute lower respiratory disease of children in a pediatric group practice. J Pediatr. 1971;78:397–406.
10. Loda FA, Glezen WP, Clyde WA Jr. Respiratory disease in group day care. Pediatrics. 1972;49:428–37.
11. Buchan KA, Marten KW, Kennedy DH. Aetiology and epidemiology of viral croup in Glasgow, 1966–72. J Hyg (Camb). 1974;73:143–50.
12. Cramblett HG. Croup (epiglottitis, laryngitis, laryngotracheobronchitis). In: Kendig EL Jr, Chernick V, eds. Disorders of the Respiratory Tract in Children. 3rd ed. Philadelphia: WB Saunders; 1977:353.
13. Parrott RH, Vargosko AJ, Kim HW, et al. Acute respiratory diseases of viral etiology. III. Myxoviruses: Parainfluenza. Am J Public Health. 1962;52:907–17.
14. Loda FA, Clyde WA Jr, Glezen WP, et al. Studies of the role of viruses, bacteria, and *M. pneumoniae* as causes of lower respiratory tract infections in children. J Pediatr. 1968;72:161–76.
15. Howard JB, McCracken GH Jr, Luby JP. Influenza A 2 virus as a cause of croup requiring tracheotomy. J Pediatr. 1972;81:1148–50.
16. Eller JJ, Fulginiti VA, Plunket DC, et al. Attack rates for hospitalized croup in children in a military population: Importance of A_2 influenza infection. Pediatr Res. 1972;6:126.
17. Kim HW, Brandt CD, Chanock RM, et al. Influenza A and B virus infection in infants and young children during the years 1957–1976. Am J Epidemiol. 1979;109:464–79.
18. Hall CB, Douglas RG Jr. Respiratory syncytial virus and influenza: Practical community surveillance. Am J Dis Child. 1976;130:615–20.
19. Newth CJ, Levison H, Bryan AC. The respiratory status of children with croup. J Pediatr. 1972;81:1068–73.
20. McBride JT. Stridor in childhood. J Fam Pract. 1984;19:782–90.
21. Ley H. An Essay on the Laryngismus Stridulus or Croup-like Inspiration of Infants. London: Churchill; 1836:6.
22. Szpunar J, Glowacki J, Laskowski A, et al. Fibrinous laryngotracheobronchitis in children. Arch Otolaryngol. 1971;93:173–8.
23. Urquhart GED, Kennedy DH, Ariyawansa JP. Croup associated with parainfluenza type 1 virus: Two subpopulations. Br Med J. 1979;1:1604.
24. Welliver RC, Wong DT, Middleton E Jr, et al. Role of parainfluenza virus-specific IgE in pathogenesis of croup and wheezing subsequent to infection. J Pediatr. 1982;101:889–96.
25. Welliver RC, Sun M, Rinaldo D. Defective regulation of immune responses in croup due to parainfluenza virus. Pediatr Res. 1985;19:716–20.
26. Hall CB, Geiman JM, Breese BB, et al. Parainfluenza viral infections in children: Correlation of shedding with clinical manifestations. J Pediatr. 1977;91:194–8.
27. Loughlin G, Taussig LM. Pulmonary function in children with a history of laryngotracheobronchitis. J Pediatr. 1979;94:365–9.
28. Rapkin RH. The diagnosis of epiglottitis: Simplicity and reliability of radiographs of the neck in the differential diagnosis of the croup syndrome. J Pediatr. 1972;80:96–8.
29. Currarino G, Williams B. Lateral inspiration and expiration radiographs of the neck in children with laryngotracheobronchitis (croup). Radiology. 1982;195:365–6.
30. Jones JL. False positives in lateral neck radiographs used to diagnose epiglottitis (Letter). Ann Emerg Med. 1983;12:797.
31. Stankiewicz JA, Bowes AK. Croup and epiglottitis: A radiologic study. Laryngoscope. 1985;95:1159–60.
32. Richman D, Schmidt N, Plotkin S, et al. Summary of a workshop on new and useful methods in rapid viral diagnosis. J Infect Dis. 1984;150:941–51.
33. Bloom HH, Johnson KM, Jacobsen R, et al. Recovery of parainfluenza viruses from adults with upper respiratory illness. Am J Hyg. 1961;74:50–9.
34. McIntosh K, Wilfert C, Chernesky M, et al. Summary of a workshop on new and useful techniques in rapid viral diagnosis. J Infect Dis. 1980;142:793–802.
35. Grauballe PC, Johnsen NJ, Hornsleth A. Rapid diagnosis by immunofluorescence of viral infections associated with the croup syndrome in children. Acta Pathol Microbiol Scand [B]. 1974;82:41–7.
36. Gardner PS, McQuillin J, McGuckin R, et al. Observations on clinical and immunofluorescent diagnosis of parainfluenza virus infections. Br Med J. 1971;2:7–12.
37. Gardner PS, McGuckin R, McQuillin J. Adenovirus demonstrated by immunofluorescence. Br Med J. 1972;3:175.
38. Marks MI, Nagahama H, Eller JJ. Parainfluenza virus immunofluorescence. In vitro and clinical application of the direct method. Pediatrics. 1971; 48:73–8.
39. McLain LG. Croup syndrome. Am Fam Physician. 1987;36:207–14.
40. Hide DW, Guyer BM. Recurrent croup. Arch Dis Child. 1985;60:585–6.
41. Laufer P. The relationship of respiratory allergies to croup. J Asthma. 1986;23:9–10.
42. Zach M, Erban A, Olinsky A. Croup, recurrent croup, allergy, and airways hyper-reactivity. Arch Dis Child. 1981;56:336–41.
43. Zach M. Serum IgA in recurrent croup. Am J Dis Child. 1983;137:184–5.

44. Postma DS, Jones RD, Pillsbury HC III. Severe hospitalized croup: Treatment trends and prognosis. Laryngoscope. 1984;94:1170–5.
45. Taussig LM. Maximal expiratory flows at functional residual capacity: A test of lung function for young children. Am Rev Respir Dis. 1977;116:1031–8.
46. Adair JC, Ring WH, Jordan WS, et al. Ten year experience with IPPB in the treatment of acute laryngotracheobronchitis. Anesth Analg (Cleve). 1971;50:649–55.
47. Schuller DE, Birck HG. The safety of intubation in croup and epiglottitis: An eight-year follow-up. Laryngoscope. 1975;85:33–46.
48. Hen J Jr. Current management of upper airway obstruction. Pediatr Ann. 1986;15:274–94.
49. Kilham H, Gillies J, Benjamin B. Severe upper airway obstruction. Pediatr Clin North Am. 1987;34:1–14.
50. Broniatowski M. Croup. Ear Nost Throat J. 1985;64:12–21.
51. Travis KW, Todres ID, Shannon DC. Pulmonary edema associated with croup and epiglottitis. Pediatrics. 1977;59:695–8.
52. Zach MS, Schnall RP, Landau LI. Upper and lower airway hyperreactivity in recurrent croup. Am Rev Respir Dis. 1980;121:979–83.
53. Gurwitz D, Corey M, Levison H. Pulmonary function and bronchial reactivity in children after croup. Am Rev Respir Dis. 1980;122:95–9.
54. Bourchier D, Dawson KP, Fergusson DM. Humidification in viral croup: A controlled trial. Aust Paediatr J. 1984;20:289–91.
55. Hall CB, Hall WJ, Speers DM. Clinical and physiological manifestations of bronchiolitis and pneumonia: Outcome of respiratory syncytial virus. Am J Dis Child. 1979;133:798–802.
56. Gussack GS, Tacchi EJ. Pulse oximetry in the management of pediatric airway disorders. South Med J. 1987;80:1381–4.
57. Barker GA. Current management of croup and epiglottitis. Pediatr Clin North Am. 1979;26:565–79.
58. Newth CJL, Levison H. Diagnosing and managing croup and epiglottitis. J Respir Dis. 1981;2:22–41.
59. Wolfsdorf J, Swift DL. An animal model simulating acute infective upper airway obstruction of childhood and its use in the investigation of croup therapy. Pediatr Res. 1978;12:1062–5.
60. Davis HW, Gartner JC, Galvis AG, et al. Acute airway obstruction: Croup and epiglottitis. Pediatr Clin North Am. 1981;28:859–80.
61. Cherry JD. The treatment of croup: Continued controversy due to failure of recognition of historic, ecologic, etiologic, and clinical perspectives. J Pediatr. 1979;94:352.
62. Gardner HG, Powell KR, Roden VJ, et al. The evaluation of racemic epinephrine in the treatment of infectious croup. Pediatrics. 1973;52:52–5.
63. Westley CR, Cotton EK, Brooks JG. Nebulized racemic epinephrine by IPPB for the treatment of croup: A double-blind study. Am J Dis Child. 1978;132:484–87.
64. Taussig LM, Castro O, Beaudry PH, et al. Treatment of laryngotracheobronchitis (croup). Use of intermittent positive-pressure breathing and racemic epinephrine. Am J Dis Child. 1975;129:790–3.
65. Bass JW, Bruhn FW, Merrit WT. Corticosteroids and racemic epinephrine with IPPB in the treatment of croup. J Pediatr. 1980;96:173–4.
66. Tunnessen WW Jr, Feinstein AR. The steroid-croup controversy: An analytic review of methodologic problems. J Pediatr. 1980;96:751–6.
67. Asher MI, Beaudry PH. Croup and corticosteroid therapy. J Pediatr. 1981;97:506–7.
68. Leipzig B, Oski FA, Cummings CW, et al. A prospective randomized study to determine the efficacy of steroids in treatment of croup. J Pediatr. 1979;94:194–6.
69. Jones R, Santos JI, Overall JC. Bacterial tracheitis. JAMA. 1979;242:721–6.
70. Liston SL, Gehrz RC, Jarvis CW. Bacterial tracheitis. Arch Otolaryngol. 1981;107:561–4.
71. Davidson S, Barzilay Z, Yahav J, et al. Bacterial tracheitis: A true entity? J Laryngol Otol. 1982;96:173–5.
72. Miller BP, Arthur JD, Parry WH, et al. Atypical croup and chlamydia trachomatis (Letter). Lancet. 1982;1:1022.

46. OTITIS EXTERNA, OTITIS MEDIA, MASTOIDITIS

JEROME O. KLEIN

OTITIS EXTERNA

Infection of the external auditory canal (otitis externa) is similar to infection of skin and soft tissue elsewhere. Unique problems occur because the canal is narrow and tortuous; fluid and foreign objects enter, are trapped and cause irritation and maceration of the superficial tissues. The pain and itching that results may be severe because of the limited space for expansion of the inflamed tissue. Infections of the external canal may be subdivided into four categories: acute localized otitis externa, acute diffuse otitis externa, chronic otitis externa, and malignant otitis externa. Recent reviews by Senturia et al.[1] and Bergstrom[2] provide more complete information.

Pathogenesis

The external auditory canal is approximately 2.5 cm long from the concha of the auricle to the tympanic membrane. The lateral half of the canal is cartilaginous; the medial half tunnels through the temporal bone. A constriction, the isthmus, present at the juncture of the osseous and cartilaginous portions, limits entry of wax and foreign bodies to the area near the tympanic membrane. The skin of the canal is thicker in the cartilaginous portion and includes a well-developed dermis and subcutaneous layer. The skin lining the osseous portion is thinner and firmly attached to the periosteum and lacks a subcutaneous layer. Hair follicles are numerous in the outer third and sparse in the inner two-thirds of the canal.

The microbial flora of the external canal is similar to the flora of skin elsewhere. There is a predominance of *Staphylococcus epidermidis, S. aureus*, diphtheroids, and to a lesser extent, anaerobic bacteria such as *Propionibacterium acnes*.[3–5] Pathogens responsible for infection of the middle ear, *Streptococcus pneumoniae, Haemophilus influenzae*, or *Branhamella (Moraxella) catarrhalis*, are uncommonly found in cultures of the external auditory canal when the tympanic membrane is intact.

The epithelium absorbs moisture from the environment. Desquamation and denuding of the superficial layers of the epithelium may follow. In this warm, moist environment, the organisms in the canal may flourish and invade the macerated skin. Inflammation and suppuration follow. Invasive organisms include those of the normal skin flora and gram-negative bacilli, particularly *Pseudomonas aeruginosa*. Malignant otitis media is a necrotizing infection frequently associated with *P. aeruginosa*. The organism gains access to the deeper tissues of the ear canal and causes a localized vaculitis, thrombosis, and necrosis of tissues. Diabetic microangiopathy of the skin overlying the temporal bone results in poor local perfusion and a milieu for invasion by *P. aeruginosa*.[6]

Clinical Manifestations and Management

Acute localized otitis externa may occur as a pustule or furuncle associated with hair follicles; it is due to *Staphylococcus aureus*. Erysipelas caused by group A *Streptococcus* may involve the concha and the canal. Pain may be severe. Bluish, red hemorrhagic bullae may be present on the osseous canal walls and also on the tympanic membrane. Adenopathy in the lymphatic drainage areas is often present. Local heat and systemic antibiotics are usually curative. Incision and drainage may be necessary to relieve severe pain.

Acute diffuse otitis externa (swimmer's ear) occurs mainly in hot, humid weather. The ear itches and becomes increasingly painful. The skin of the canal is edematous and red. Gram-negative bacilli, mainly *P. aeruginosa*, may play a significant role. A severe hemorrhagic external otitis due to *P. aeruginosa* was associated with mobile redwood hot tub systems.[7] Gentle cleansing to remove debris including irrigation with hypertonic saline (3%) and cleansing with mixtures of alcohol (70–95%) and acetic acid should be used initially. Hydrophilic solutions such as 50% Burrow solutions may be used for 1–2 days to reduce inflammation. Ear drops of topical antibiotics (including neomycin and polymyxin) combined with a steroid in an acid vehicle serve to diminish local inflammation and infection. Systemic antibiotics may be necessary if there is significant tissue infection.

Chronic otitis externa is due to irritation of drainage from the middle ear in patients with chronic suppurative otitis media. Itching may be severe. Management is directed to treatment of the middle ear disorder. Rare causes of chronic otitis externa include tuberculosis, syphilis, yaws, leprosy, and sarcoidosis.

Malignant otitis externa is a severe, necrotizing infection that spreads to adjacent areas of soft tissue, cartilage, and bone. Severe pain and tenderness of the tissues around the ear and mastoid is accompanied by drainage of pus from the canal. The elderly, diabetic, and debilitated patient is at particular risk. Life-threatening disease may result from spread to the sigmoid sinus, jugular bulb, base of the skull, meninges, and brain. Permanent facial paralysis is frequent. Diagnostic tests for underlying disease should be instituted. The canal should be cleansed, devitalized tissue removed, and ear drops with antipseudomonal antibiotics combined with steroid instilled. Systemic therapy with antimicrobial regimens including coverage for *Pseudomonas* sp. (such as gentamicin and/or ticarcillin or piperacillin) should be used for 4–6 weeks.

Fungal otitis may be part of a general or local fungal infection. *Aspergillus* sp. are responsible for most cases of fungal otitis. *Candida albicans* is a frequent cause of external otitis in children with chronic mucocutaneous candidiasis.

OTITIS MEDIA

Otitis media, or inflammation of the middle ear, is defined by the presence of fluid in the middle ear accompanied by signs or symptoms of illness. A survey of the office practice of physicians who provided medical care to children showed that otitis media was the most frequent diagnosis recorded for illness.[8] The peak incidence occurs in the first 3 years of life. The disease is less common in the school-age child, adolescent, and adult. Nevertheless, infection of the middle ear may be the cause of fever, significant pain, and impaired hearing in these age groups. In addition, adults suffer from the sequelae of otitis media of childhood: hearing loss, cholesteatoma, adhesive otitis media, and chronic perforation of the tympanic membrane. A comprehensive review of otitis media is included in a recent text, *Otitis Media in Infants and Children*.[9]

Epidemiology

By 3 years of age, more than two-thirds of children have had one or more episodes of acute otitis media, and one-third have had three or more episodes.[10] The highest incidence of acute otitis media occurs between 6 and 24 months of age. Subsequently, the incidence declines with age except for a limited reversal of the downward trend between 5 and 6 years of age, the time of school entry. Although considered uncommon in adults, a survey identified almost 4 million visits to physicians by adults each year for middle ear infection.

Some racial groups such as American Indians and Canadian and Alaskan Eskimos have high rates of infection and severe middle ear disease. Poverty with its accompanying factors of crowding, poor sanitation, and inadequate medical facilities is common to these groups. Whether other factors specifically related to race or culture are involved remains unknown. Other epidemiologic factors of importance identified in a recent study of Boston children[10] include the following: age at first episode is an important predictor of recurrent otitis media in that infants who have otitis media during the first year of life are at increased risk of recurrent disease, males have more episodes of acute otitis media and are at increased risk for recurrent disease, breast-feeding is associated with decreased risk for recurrent otitis media during the first year of life, and recurrent otitis media in a sibling is an important risk feature. Children in group and day care are more likely than are children cared for at home to experience recurrent episodes of acute otitis media.[11]

Pathogenesis

The middle ear is part of a continuous system that includes, medially and anteriorly, the nares, nasopharynx, and eustachian tube and, posteriorly, the mastoid air cells. These structures are lined with a respiratory epithelium that contains ciliated cells, mucus-secreting goblet cells, and cells capable of secreting local immunoglobulins.

Anatomic or physiologic dysfunction of the eustachian tube appears to play a critical role in the development of otitis media. The eustachian tube has at least three physiologic functions with respect to the middle ear: protection of the ear from nasopharyngeal secretions, drainage into the nasopharynx of secretions produced within the middle ear, and ventilation of the middle ear to equilibrate air pressure with that in the external ear canal. When one or more of these functions is compromised, the results may be development of fluid and infection in the middle ear. Congestion of the mucosa of the eustachian tube may result in obstruction. Secretions that are constantly formed by the mucosa of the middle ear accumulate behind the obstruction, and if a bacterial pathogen is present, a suppurative otitis media may result.

Microbiology

Bacteria. The microbiology of otitis media has been documented by appropriate cultures of middle ear effusions obtained by needle aspiration. Many studies of the bacteriology of acute otitis media have been performed. The results are remarkably consistent in demonstrating the importance of *S. pneumoniae* and *H. influenzae* in all age groups[9] (Table 1).

Streptococcus pneumoniae is the most important bacterial cause of otitis media. Relatively few types are responsible for most disease. The most common types in order of decreasing frequencies are 19, 23, 6, 14, 3, and 18.[11–13] All are included in the currently available 23-type pneumococcal polysaccharide vaccine.

Otitis media due to *H. influenzae* is associated with nontypable strains in the vast majority of patients. In approximately 10 percent, the otitis is due to type b; some of these patients appear to be in a very toxic state, and about one-quarter have concomitant bacteremia or meningitis.[14] Until recently, *H. influenzae* appeared to be limited in importance to preschool children; however, recent studies indicate that *H. influenzae* is a significant cause of otitis media in older children, adolescents, and adults.

Recent studies indicate an increasing importance of *B. catarrhalis*.[15,16] The organism was isolated from the middle ear fluids of 19 percent of 200 middle ear specimens from 146 Pittsburgh children with acute otitis media.[16] Prior to 1970 almost all strains of *B. catarrhalis* were sensitive to penicillin. Today most strains produce β-lactamase and are resistant to penicillin G, ampicillin, and amoxicillin.

Viruses. Virologic and epidemiologic data suggest that viral infection is frequently associated with acute otitis media.[17–19]

TABLE 1. Bacterial Pathogens Isolated from Middle Ear Fluid in 4675 Children with Acute Otitis Media[a]

Microorganism	*Mean Percentage of Children with Pathogen*
Streptococcus pneumoniae	33
Haemophilus influenzae	21
Streptococcus, group A	8
Staphylococcus aureus	2
Branhamella catarrhalis	3
Gram-negative enteric bacilli	1
Miscellaneous bacteria	1
None or nonpathogens	31

[a] Twelve reports from centers in the United States, Finland, and Sweden, 1952–1981.[9]

In a study of children attending a day care program, isolation of viruses from the upper respiratory tract was correlated with a clinical diagnosis of otitis media. Virus outbreaks coincided with epidemics of otitis media. Recent studies identify respiratory viruses[17] or viral antigens[18] in approximately one-quarter of middle ear fluids of children with acute otitis media. Respiratory syncytial virus, influenza virus, enteroviruses, and rhinoviruses were the most common viruses found in middle ear fluids.

Mycoplasma, Chlamydia, and Unusual Organisms. *Mycoplasma pneumoniae* was responsible for hemorrhagic bullous myringitis in a study of nonimmune volunteers inoculated with the organism.[20] However, the middle ear fluid of a large number of patients (771) has been studied, and *M. pneumoniae* was isolated in only one case.[21,22] Although mycoplasmas do not appear to play a significant role in acute otitis media, some patients with lower respiratory tract disease due to *M. pneumoniae* may have concomitant otitis media.

Chlamydia trachomatis is associated with acute respiratory infections in infants under age 6 months and is a cause of acute infection of the middle ear in this age group. The organism has been isolated from middle ear fluid of infants with acute infection.[23]

Uncommon forms of otitis include diphtheritic otitis, tuberculous otitis, otogenous tetanus, and otitis due to *Ascaris lumbricoides*.

Immunology

The middle ear is the site of a secretory immune system similar to those of other areas of the respiratory tract. Local and systemic immune responses occur in patients with acute or chronic otitis media with effusion. In the middle ear, immunologically active antigen interacts with immunocompetent cells in the lamina propria to produce a local immune response. The middle ear effusion that results from acute or chronic infection contains all the major classes of immunoglobulins, complement, cells, immune complexes of antigen and antibody, and various chemical mediators of inflammation. The role of these substances in the course of otitis media is uncertain. The immune response to various antigens may prevent subsequent infection, assist in clearance of fluid during the acute episode, or contribute to the accumulation and persistence of fluid in the middle ear cavity.

Diagnosis and Clinical Course

Acute otitis media is defined by the presence of fluid in the middle ear along with signs or symptoms of acute illness. Signs and symptoms may be specific, such as ear pain, ear drainage, or hearing loss, or may be nonspecific, such as fever, lethargy, or irritability. Vertigo, nystagmus, and tinnitus may occur. Redness of the tympanic membrane is an early sign of otitis media, but erythema alone is not diagnostic of middle ear infection since it may be caused by inflammation of the mucosa throughout the upper respiratory tract.

The presence of fluid in the middle ear is determined by the use of pneumatic otoscopy, a technique that permits an assessment of the mobility of the tympanic membrane. The motion of the tympanic membrane is proportional to the pressure applied by gently squeezing and then releasing the rubber bulb attached to the head of the otoscope. Normal mobility is apparent when positive pressure is applied and the tympanic membrane moves rapidly inward; with release of the bulb and the resulting negative pressure, the membrane moves outward. Fluid or high negative pressure in the middle ear dampens the mobility of the tympanic membrane. Tympanometry uses an electroacoustic impedance bridge to record compliance of the tympanic membrane and middle ear pressure. This technique presents objective evidence of the status of the middle ear and the presence or absence of fluid.

Fluid persists in the middle ear for prolonged periods after the onset of acute otitis media even though symptoms usually resolve within a few days after initiation of antimicrobial therapy. About 70 percent of children with otitis media have fluid in the middle ear 2 weeks after the onset of disease, 40 percent still have fluid 1 month after onset, and 10 percent still have fluid 3 months after the first signs of middle ear infection.[10]

Patients with middle ear effusion suffer from hearing loss of variable severity. On average, a patient with fluid in the middle ear has a 25 db (pure tone average) loss.[24] Since development is dynamic during infancy when the incidence of acute otitis media is highest, there is concern that any impediment to reception or interpretation of auditory stimuli might have an adverse effect. Recent studies suggest that children with histories of recurrent episodes of acute otitis media score lower in tests of speech, language, and cognitive abilities than do their disease-free peers.[25–26]

The results of microbiologic studies of middle ear effusions in patients with otitis media are so consistent that the choice of antimicrobial agents may be based on knowledge of the bacteriology acquired from the many investigations rather than the results of cultures from other sites such as the throat or nasopharynx (Table 1). If the patient is toxic or has focal infection elsewhere, culture of the blood and culture of the focus are warranted. Needle aspiration of the middle ear effusion (tympanocentesis) to define the microbiology should be considered in selected patients: the patient who is critically ill at the onset, the patient who has not responded to initial antimicrobial therapy in 48–72 hours and is toxic, and the patient with altered host defenses (e.g., immunologic defect, including the newborn infant).

Management

Acute Otitis Media. ANTIMICROBIAL AGENTS. The preferred antimicrobial agent for the patient with otitis media must be active against *S. pneumoniae, H. influenzae*, and in some areas, *B. catarrhalis*. Group A streptococci and *S. aureus* are infrequent causes of acute otitis media and need not be considered in initial therapeutic decisions. Gram-negative enteric bacilli must be considered when otitis media occurs in the newborn infant, in the patient with a depressed immune response, and in the patient with suppurative complications of chronic otitis media. Amoxicillin or ampicillin are the current drugs of choice for initial treatment since they are effective against the two major pathogens and are less expensive than alternative regimens are. The current incidence of ampicillin-resistance *H. influenzae* and *B. catarrhalis* is not high enough to require a change in initial therapy. Other drugs that are satisfactory include amoxicillin-clavulanate, cefuroxime-axetil, trimethoprim-sulfamethoxazole (TMP-SMZ), the fixed combination preparation of erythromycin and sulfisoxazole, cefaclor, and combinations of a sulfonamide and penicillin G (administered by mouth or as a single intramuscular dose of the benzathine salt), penicillin V, or erythromycin. Trimethoprim-sulfamethoxazole, cefaclor, or the combination of erythromycin and a sulfonamide provide antimicrobial coverage for *H. influenzae* and *S. pneumoniae* and are acceptable regimens for the child with an allergy to penicillin. If the child has had a major reaction to a penicillin (an immediate or accelerated reaction with urticaria, bronchospasm, or hypotension), cross-reactivity of penicillins and cephalosporins must be considered possible, and the use of a cephalosporin should be avoided.

Some children with acute otitis media due to a bacterial pathogen improve without the use of antimicrobial agents. Clinical resolution may occur because the contents of the middle ear are discharged through the eustachian tube or after spontaneous perforation of the tympanic membrane. The cases of spontaneous resolution of acute otitis media are important to the investigator who must consider this factor in an analysis of the results of new therapeutic regimens, but they do not weigh against the use of appropriate antimicrobial agents for the treatment of acute otitis media to uniformly resolve the clinical signs and prevent suppurative complications.

With appropriate antimicrobial therapy, most children with acute otitis media are significantly improved within 48–72 hours. If there is no improvement, the patient should be examined. Toxicity with persistent or recurrent fever or otalgia should prompt consideration of tympanocentesis to identify the causative organism; the appropriate antimicrobial agent may then be chosen on the basis of results of Gram staining and culture of the middle ear fluid. If signs persist but the child is not toxic and aspiration is not performed, the initial antimicrobial regimen should be changed to one that is effective for less common organisms, including β-lactamase–producing *H. influenzae* and *B. catarrhalis*. If ampicillin or amoxicillin was given initially, then amoxicillin-clavulanate, TMP-SMZ, erythromycin-sulfisoxazole, or cefaclor should be administered.

DECONGESTANTS AND ANTIHISTAMINES. Nasal and oral decongestants, administered either alone or in combination with an antihistamine, are used extensively for treatment of otitis media with effusion. The use of the drugs is based on the consideration that they reduce congestion of the respiratory mucosa and relieve the obstruction of the eustachian tube that results from inflammation caused by respiratory infection. The results of clinical trials, however, indicate no significant evidence of efficacy of any of these preparations, used alone or in combination, for relief of signs of disease or decrease in time spent with middle ear effusion.[27] A recent symposium reviewed the efficacy and safety of antihistamines in the treatment of upper respiratory tract infections.[28]

Chronic Otitis Media. The term *chronic otitis media* includes recurrent episodes of acute infection and prolonged duration of middle ear effusion usually resulting from a previous episode of acute infection. For the prevention of recurrent episodes of acute otitis media, management includes the consideration of chemoprophylaxis (the use of antimicrobial agents) and immunoprophylaxis (the use of pneumococcal vaccine). For the management of persistent middle ear efflusions, three surgical methods are considered: myringotomy, adenoidectomy, and placement of tympanostomy tubes.

Chemoprophylaxis has been shown to be of value in the prevention of acute illness in children who have suffered from recurrences of middle ear infections.[29–31] Although the results are inadequate to provide conclusive evidence of the efficacy of chemoprophylaxis, they are persuasive in that a reduction of episodes of acute febrile illnesses due to otitis media occurred. On the basis of available information,[31] a protocol has been suggested that uses a once-a-day regimen of amoxicillin or sulfisoxazole during winter and spring, the periods of high incidence of infections of the respiratory tract. Chemoprophylaxis may suppress symptoms of otitis media, but middle ear effusion may persist (though without apparent symptoms). The physician who chooses to use chemoprophylaxis to prevent acute recurrent disease must examine the patient at approximately 1-month intervals for middle ear effusion.

Pneumococcal vaccines have been evaluated for the prevention of recurrences of acute otitis media in children.[32–34] As in previous studies, children less than 2 years of age had unsatisfactory responses to single-dose regimens. The vaccine reduced the number of episodes of acute otitis media due to types of *S. pneumoniae* present in the vaccine, but the reduction was not sufficient to alter the experience of the children with middle ear infections. The basis for failure of the vaccine was due to the poor immunologic response to the polysaccharide antigens in the young infants enrolled in the trials. The data suggested that the vaccine was likely to be more effective in children over the age of 2 years.[34]

Surgical management of the persistent effusion of the middle ear includes the use of myringotomy, adenoidectomy, and the placement of tympanostomy tubes. Myringotomy, or incision of the tympanic membrane, is a method of draining middle ear fluid. Before the introduction of antimicrobial agents, myringotomy was the major method of managing suppurative otitis media. Today, the use of myringotomy is limited to the relief of intractable ear pain, hastening resolution of mastoid infection, and drainage of persistent middle ear effusion that is unresponsive to medical therapy.

Enlarged adenoids may obstruct the orifice of the eustachian tube in the posterior portion of the nasopharynx and interfere with adequate ventilation and drainage of the middle ear. Recent studies of the use of adenoidectomy in children with prolonged effusions in the middle ear identify in selected children a beneficial effect in reducing time spent with effusion.[35,36]

Tympanostomy tubes resemble small collar buttons. They are placed through an incision in the tympanic membrane to provide drainage of fluid and ventilation of the middle ear. The placement of these tubes is now one of the most common surgical procedures in children. The criteria for the placement of tubes include persistent middle ear effusions unresponsive to adequate medical treatment over a period of 3 months and persistent negative pressure. Hearing improves dramatically after placement of the ventilating tubes. The tubes have also been of value in patients who have difficulty maintaining ambient pressure in the middle ear such as would occur due to barotrauma in airline personnel. The liabilities of the placement of tubes include those of anesthesia associated with the procedure, persistent perforation, scarring of the tympanic membrane, development of cholesteatoma, and otitis media caused by swimming with ventilating tubes in place, but these occur infrequently.

MASTOIDITIS

The proximity of the mastoid to the middle ear cleft suggests that most cases of suppurative otitis media are associated with inflammation of the mastoid air cells (Fig. 1). The incidence of clinically significant mastoiditis, however, is low since the introduction of antimicrobial agents. Nevertheless, acute and chronic disease still occurs and may be responsible for significant morbidity and life-threatening disease.

Pathogenesis

At birth, the mastoid consists of a single cell, the antrum, connected to the middle ear by a small channel. Pneumatization of the mastoid bone takes place soon after birth and is extensive by 2 years of age. The clinical importance of the mastoid is related to contiguous structures including the posterior cranial fossa, the middle cranial fossa, the sigmoid and lateral sinuses, the canal of the facial nerve, the semicircular canals, and the petrous tip of the temporal bone. The mastoid air cells are lined with modified respiratory mucosa, and all are connected with the antrum.

Infection in the mastoid follows middle ear infection. Initially, there is hyperemia and edema of the mucosal lining of the air cells. Serous, then purulent exudate collects in the cells. Necrosis of bone due to pressure of the purulent exudate on the thin bony septa follows. Coalescence of pus in contiguous areas results in abscess cavities.

Clinical Manifestations

Acute mastoiditis is usually accompanied by acute infection in the middle ear. During early stages, the signs are those of acute otitis media with hearing loss, otalgia, and fever. Subsequently,

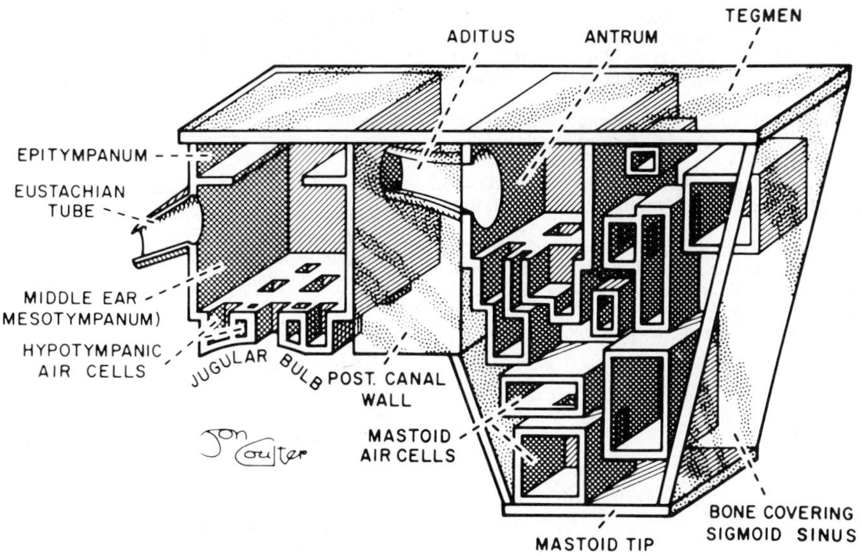

FIG. 1 Diagrammatic representation of the anatomy of the middle and mastoid air cell system showing the narrow connection (aditus and antrum) between the two.

swelling, redness, and tenderness is present over the mastoid bone. The pinna is displaced outward and downward. A purulent discharge may emerge through a perforation in the tympanic membrane.

Diagnosis

Roentgenographs of the mastoid area may show a loss of sharpness of the shadows of cellular walls due to demineralization of bony septa and cloudiness of areas of pneumatization due to inflammatory swelling of the air cells.

Cultures for bacteria from ear drainage fluid must be taken with care to distinguish fresh drainage fluid from material in the external canal. The canal must be cleaned and fresh pus obtained as it exudes from the tympanic membrane. If the tympanic membrane is not perforated, tympanocentesis should be performed to obtain material from the middle ear.

Management

The antimicrobial drugs of choice for acute infection are similar to those for acute otitis media: antibiotics with activity against *S. pneumoniae* and *H. influenzae*. If the disease in the mastoid has had a prolonged course, coverage for *S. aureus* and gram-negative enteric bacilli may be considered for initial therapy until the results of cultures become available.

A mastoidectomy is performed when an abscess has formed in the mastoid bone. The procedure should be performed at a time when sepsis has been controlled by antimicrobial agents.

References

1. Senturia BH, Marcus MD, Lucente FE. Diseases of the External Ear. An OtologicDermatologic Manual. 2nd ed. New York: Grune & Stratton; 1980.
2. Bergstrom L. Diseases of the external ear. In Bluestone CD, Stool SE eds. Pediatric Otolaryngology, Philadelphia, WB Saunders, 1983;347.
3. Riding KH, Bluestone CD, Michaels RH, et al. Microbiology of recurrent and chronic otitis media with effusion. J Pediatr 1978;93:739–43.
4. Pelton SI, Teele DW, Shurin PA, et al. Disparate cultures of middle ear fluids. Am J Dis Child. 134:951–953, 1980;134:951–3.
5. Brook I, Schwartz R. Anaerobic bacteria in acute otitis media. Acta Otolaryngol. 1981;91:111–4.
6. Otitis due to *Pseudomonas aeruginosa* serotype 0:10 associated with mobile redwood hot tub system—North Carolina. MMWR. 1982;31:541–2.
7. Doroghazi RM, Nadol JB, Hyslop NE, et al. Invasive external otitis. Am J Med. 1981;71:603–13.
8. Koch H, Dennison NJ. Office visits to pediatricians. National Ambulatory Medical Care Services, National Center for Health Statistics, 1974.
9. Bluestone CD, Klein JO, eds. Otitis Media in Infants and Children. Philadelphia: WB Saunders; 1987.
10. Wald ER, Dashefsky B, Byers C, et al. Frequency and severity of infections in day care. J Pediatr. 1968;112:540–6.
11. Kamme C, Ageberg M, Lundgren K. Distribution of *Diplococcus pneumoniae* types in acute otitis media in children and influence of the types on the clinical course in penicillin V therapy. Scand J Infect Dis. 1970;2:183–90.
12. Austrian R, Howie VM, Ploussard JH. The bacteriology of pneumococcal otitis media. Johns Hopkins Med J. 1977;141:104–11.
13. Gray BM, Converse GM, Dillion, HC. Serotypes of *Streptococcus pneumoniae* causing disease. J Infect Dis. 1979;140:979–83.
14. Harding AL, Anderson P, Howie VM, et al. *Haemophilus influenzae* isolated from children with otitis media. In: Sell SHW, Karzon DT, eds. *Haemophilus influenzae*. Nashville: Vanderbilt University Press; 1973:21.
15. Van Hare GF, Shurin PA, Marchant CD, et al. Acute otitis media caused by *Branhamella catarrhalis*: Biology and therapy. Rev Infect Dis 1987;9:16–27.
16. Kovatch AL, Wald ER, Michaels RH: β-Lactamase–producing *Branhamella catarrhalis* causing otitis media in children. J Pediatr. 1983;102:261–4.
17. Chonmaitree T, Howie VM, Truant AL. Presence of respiratory viruses in middle ear fluids and nasal wash specimens from children with acute otitis media. Pediatrics. 1986;77:698–702.
18. Klein BS, Dallette ER, Volken RH. The role of respiratory syncytial virus and other viral pathogens in acute otitis media. J Pediatr. 1982;101:16–20.
19. Henderson FW, Collier AM, Sanyal MA, et al. A longitudinal study of respiratory viruses and bacteria in the etiology of acute otitis media with effusion. N Engl J Med. 1982;306:1377.
20. Rifkind DR, Chanock RM, Kravetz H, et al. Ear involvement (myringitis) and primary atypical pneumonia following inoculation of volunteers with Eaton agent. Am Rev Respir Dis. 1962;85:479–89.
21. Klein JO, Teele DW. Isolation of viruses and mycoplasma from middle ear effusions: A review. Ann Otol Rhinol Laryngol. 1976;85:140–44.
22. Sobeslavsky O, Syrucek L, Bruckoya M, et al. The etiological role of *Mycoplasma pneumoniae* in otitis media in children. Pediatrics. 1965;35:652–7.
23. Tipple MA, Beem MO, Saxon EM. Clinical characteristics of the afebrile pneumonia associated with *Chlamydia trachomatis* infection in infants less than 6 months of age. Pediatrcs. 1979;63:192–7.
24. Fria TJ, Cantekin EI, Eichler JA. Hearing acuity of children with effusion. Arch Otolaryngol. 1985;111:10–6.
25. Holm VA, Kunze LH: Effects of chronic otitis media on language and speech development. Pediatrics. 1969;43:833–9.
26. Teele DW, Klein JO, Rosner BA. Otitis media with effusion during the first three years of life and development of speech and language. Pediatrics. 1984;74:282–7.
27. Cantekin EI, Mandel EM, Bluestone CD. Lack of efficacy of a decongestant–antihistamine combination for otitis media with effusion ("secretory" otitis media) in children. N Engl J Med. 1983;308:297–301.
28. Bluestone CD, Connell JT, Doyle WJ, et al. Symposium: Questioning the efficacy and safety of antihistamines in the treatment of upper respiratory infection. Pediatr Infect Dis J. 1988;7:15–42.
29. Perrin JM, Charney E, MacWhinney JB, et al. Sulfisoxazole as chemoprophylaxis for recurrent otitis media: A double-blind crossover study in pediatric practice. N Engl J Med. 1974;291:664–7.
30. Maynard JE, Fleshman JK, Tschopp CF. Otitis media in Alaskan Eskimo children: Prospective evaluation of chemoprophylaxis. JAMA. 1972;219:597–9.

31. Klein JO, Bluestone CD. Acute otitis media: Management of pediatric infectious diseases in office practice. Pediatr Infect Dis. 1982;1:66–73.
32. Teele DW, Klein JO, the Greater Boston Collaborative Study Group Use of pneumococcal vaccine for prevention of recurrent acute otitis media in infants in Boston. Rev Infect Dis. 1981;3 (Suppl):113.
33. Sloyer JL, Ploussard JH, Howie VM. Efficacy of pneumococcal polysaccharide vaccine in preventing acute otitis media in infants in Huntsville, Alabama. Rev Infect Dis. 1981;3(Suppl):119.
34. Makela PH, Leinonen M, Pukander J, et al. A study of the pneumococcal vaccine in prevention of clinically acute attacks of recurrent otitis media. Rev Infect Dis. 1981;3(Suppl):124.
35. Paradise JL, Bluestone CD, Rogers KD, et al. Efficacy of adenoidectomy in recurrent otitis media: Historical overview and preliminary results from a randomized, controlled trial. Ann Otol Rhinol Laryngol. 1980;89:319–21.
36. Gates GA, Avery CA, Prihoda TJ, et al. Effectiveness of adenoidectomy and tympanostomy tubes in the treatment of chronic otitis media with effusion. N Engl J Med. 1987;317:1444–51.

47. SINUSITIS

JACK M. GWALTNEY, JR.

Acute sinusitis is an infection of one or more of the paranasal sinuses that usually complicates a common cold or other viral infection of the upper respiratory tract. A minor proportion of cases are associated with dental infection. Acute sinusitis may also occur in patients with allergic rhinitis or anatomic abnormalities of the nose that interfere with normal mucociliary function in the sinus cavity. Sinusitis in turn may be complicated by serious intracranial infections such as bacterial meningitis, epidural and subdural abscess, and brain abscess.

ETIOLOGY

The infectious agents responsible for most cases of acute maxillary sinusitis are listed in Table 1. The information is from studies in which specimens for culture were obtained by direct sinus puncture and aspiration to avoid contamination by nasopharyngeal flora.[1,2,5–10] *Streptococcus pneumoniae* and unencapsulated strains of *Haemophilus influenzae* accounted for approximately one-half of all cases. Mixtures of anaerobic bacteria were associated with 6 percent of infections in adults. Sinusitis due to anaerobic bacteria was usually found in patients with associated dental disease. *Staphylococcus aureus, Streptococcus pyogenes, Branhamella catarrhalis*, and other gram-negative bacteria were each associated with a proportion of the total cases. α-Hemolytic streptococci have also been recovered in pure culture in high titers from aspirates of acute infected sinuses. In children, anaerobic infections were not seen, presumably due to less frequent dental infections, and *B. catarrhalis* was recovered almost as frequently as *H. influenzae*.[10]

Rhinovirus, influenza virus, and parainfluenza virus were recovered alone or in combination with bacteria in approximately one-fifth of the adult cases. Whether the sequence was for the viral infection to precede the bacterial infection or for a simultaneous invasion by both organisms was not clear.

Nosocomial sinusitis has been most often associated with *Pseudomonas aeruginosa, Klebsiella pneumoniae, Enterobacter* sp. and *Proteus mirabilis* and was often polymicrobic.[3] *Pseudomonas aeruginosa* was also the most frequent isolate in sinus aspirates from patients with cystic fibrosis.[11]

A small proportion of sinus disease results from fungal infections. The list of fungal infections associated with sinus disease continues to grow and includes aspergillosis.[12,13] phaeohyphomycosis,[14,15] mucormycosis, pseudallescharіasis, and many other mycoses.[16–18] Whereas acute fungal sinusitis occurs in patients with serious underlying diseases, most patients with chronic fungal sinusitis are otherwise healthy.

TABLE 1. The Microbial Etiology of Acute Community-Acquired Antral Sinusitis

	Percent of Cases Mean (Range)	
Microbial Agent	*Adults*	*Children*
Bacteria		
S. pneumoniae	31 (20–35)	36
H. influenza (unencapsulated)	21 (6–26)	23
S. pneumoniae and *H. influenzae*	5 (1–9)	—
Anaerobic bacteria (*Bacteroides, Peptostreptococcus, Fusobacterium* sp., and so forth)	6 (0–10)	—
S. aureus	4 (0–8)	—
S. pyogenes	2 (1–3)	2
B. catarrhalis	2	19
Gram-negative bacteria[a]	9 (0–24)	2
Viruses		
Rhinovirus	15	—
Influenza virus	5	—
Parainfluenza virus	3	2
Adenovirus	—	2

[a] One study had a 24 percent isolation of gram-negative bacteria, but in four other studies the recovery rate was not over 5 percent. Gram-negative bacteria recovered included *P. aeruginosa, K. pneumoniae*, and *E. coli*.

EPIDEMIOLOGY

Approximately 0.5 percent of common upper respiratory infections are complicated by acute sinusitis.[19] The incidence of sinusitis parallels the incidence of acute infections of the upper respiratory tract, being most prevalent during the fall, winter, and spring months. Sinus infection in the summer is often associated with swimming. Sinusitis is more common in adults than in children. Full development of the maxillary, frontal, and sphenoidal sinuses is not reached until adolescence. Some physicians have the clinical impression that the incidence of acute sinusitis is increased in cigarette smokers, but studies of this risk factor are not available.

PATHOGENESIS

Most acute sinusitis is thought to be a bacterial complication of viral colds. This idea is supported by studies in which viruses were recovered from sinus aspirates of patients with maxillary sinusitis.[1,2] The exact pathogenic mechanisms involved are unknown. The sinuses are normally sterile as a result of continuous mucociliary cleansing of particulate matter that enters the sinus cavity. However, respiratory viruses are efficient in eluding the protection provided by the mucous blanket of normal respiratory epithelium and in initiating infection. When viral infection occurs in a sinus there is presumed disruption of the normal cleansing mechanism, opening the way for secondary bacterial invasion. From 5 to 10 percent of the cases of acute maxillary sinusitis result from infection originating from a dental source. The floor of the maxillary sinus is close to the roots of the molars and bicuspids, and infection at these sites may spread to the sinus cavity.

During acute sinusitis, the sinus mucosal lining is characteristically inflamed and swollen. Mucosal erosion may occur with some viral infections, such as influenza, but pathologic descriptions of the findings in specific infections are not available. An exudate develops in the sinus cavity containing polymorphonuclear leukocytes that are usually present in concentrations greater than 5000 cells/mm^3.[1] The bacterial titers in exudates from acutely infected sinuses are usually greater than 10^5 cfu/ml and may reach levels of 10^8 cfu/ml.

Noninfectious conditions that predispose to acute sinusitis include anatomic abnormalities such as congenital choanal atresia, septal deviation, foreign bodies, and tumors. Allergic reactions in the nose cause mucosal swelling and polyp formation that also may lead to infection. Recently, attention has been called to nosocomial sinusitis in hospitalized patients, resulting from indwelling nasal tubes of various types, or nasal packing.[3]

Prolonged and repeated episodes of infection in untreated or inadequately treated patients probably lead to irreversible changes in the mucosal lining of the sinus, resulting in chronic sinusitis. The normal ciliated epithelium is replaced by stratified squamous epithelium that may eventually fill the sinus lumen. Sterility is no longer maintained in the sinus cavity. Cultures of surgical specimens obtained aseptically from patients with chronic sinus disease have grown a wide variety of gram-positive and gram-negative bacteria.[4] Anaerobic bacteria, *Staphylococcus aureus*, and *Streptococcus* of the *viridans* group were recovered most often. The ongoing bacterial growth is secondary to the structural damage, which leads to a loss of the sinus membranes' capacity for self-cleansing. Thus, infection is not thought to be the basic problem in chronic sinusitis, although acute infectious exacerbations due to organisms such as *Streptococcus pneumoniae* and *H. influenzae* sometimes occur.

CLINICAL PRESENTATION

Acute sinusitis usually develops during the course of a common cold or influenzal illness. Facial pain and purulent nasal discharge are the most constant features of the disease. Other complaints include headache, nasal obstruction, disorders of smell, and a nasal quality to the voice. A purulent nasal and/or postnasal discharge is usually present; with maxillary sinusitis pus is characteristically observed in the middle meatus on examination of the nose. In a small proportion of cases, erythema and tenderness are present over the involved sinus, but the absence of such external manifestations of inflammation should not exclude the diagnosis of acute sinusitis. Edema of the eyelids and excessive tearing occur with ethmoid sinusitis. Appearance of chemosis, proptosis, or limited extraocular movement should suggest the possibility of orbital extension from the ethmoidal infection. In maxillary sinusitis of dental origin, the findings of caries and signs of associated dental infection may be present. Temperature elevation has been reported in only approximately one-half of adults and children with acute maxillary sinusitis diagnosed by sinus puncture. In children, cough was the most common complaint; also fetid breath was a frequent sign.[10] In both children and adults the clinical features of acute sinusitis are often difficult to distinguish from those of a prolonged cold. In some studies, patients with acute sinusitis have become asymptomatic despite the persistence of pus and active infection in the sinus cavity as determined by sinus puncture.[1]

Maxillary sinusitis frequently occurs alone. Infection of the other sinuses is more often associated with concomitant infection of another sinus. Patients who develop intracranial extension of infection, such as meningitis and brain abscess, usually show the characteristic signs of these infections. It may be difficult to determine when acute frontal sinusitis has progressed to a frontal lobe abscess of the brain. Inflammation and tenderness over the frontal sinus is often lacking with this infection. Patients may become apathetic and have a minimum of complaints because of destruction of the frontal lobe cortex (Fig. 1).

Osteomyelitis of the frontal bone may occur by spread from the frontal or ethmoid sinuses. Pus may collect under the periosteum of the frontal bone causing swelling and edema over the forehead, a condition known as Pott puffy tumor.[20]

Nosocomial sinusitis resulting from indwelling nasal tubes has occurred most often during the second week of hospitalization.[3] Unilateral maxillary sinusitis was most common, followed by bilateral maxillary disease and pansinusitis. Fever and leukocytosis were common. Unexplained fever in patients with indwelling nasal tubes is an indication for evaluation for sinus infection.

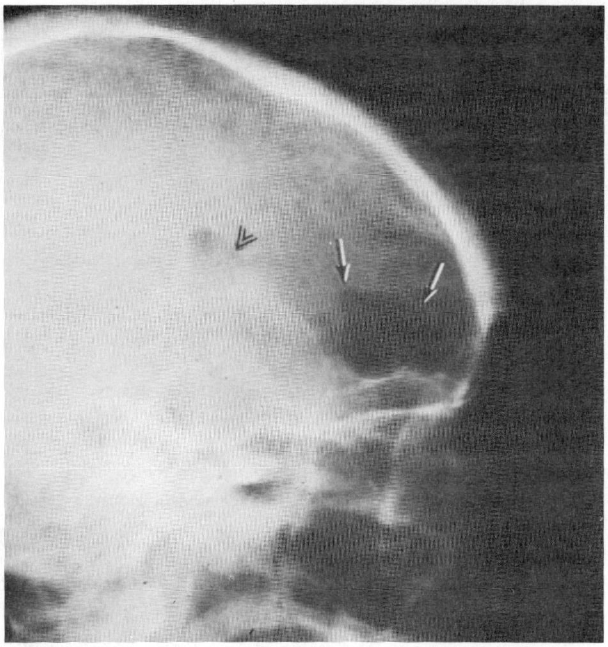

FIGURE 1. Lateral sinus roentgenogram of a patient with acute frontal sinusitis complicated by abscess of the frontal lobe of the brain. Destruction of the posterior wall of the frontal sinus resulted in air in the abscess cavity (→) and in the lateral ventricle (⩔). The infection was caused by *S. aureus*.

DIAGNOSIS

Diagnostic evaluation should include a history and an examination of the pharynx, nose, ears, sinuses, and teeth. Information should be obtained on the occurrence of coryzal and influenzal illness and of respiratory allergies. Because the ''typical'' complaints of acute sinusitis frequently overlap those of a prolonged but uncomplicated common cold, it is not possible to make a diagnosis of sinusitis on history and physical examination alone in many patients.

Valuable information may be obtained from transillumination of the maxillary and frontal sinuses although this method is less used than in the past. Transillumination should be performed in a completely darkened room. In patients with previously normal sinuses, the finding of complete opacity of the sinus on transillumination is strong evidence for the presence of active infection.[1] Conversely, the finding of normal light transmission is equally good evidence that no infection is present. The finding of diminished light tránsmission, ''dullness'' but not complete opacity, is less helpful. Approximately one-quarter of the patients with this finding were found to have active infection as determined by sinus puncture, while the remaining three-quarters were normal. It should be emphasized that sinus transillumination is less helpful in patients with chronic sinusitis in whom absent or reduced light transmission may be a persistent finding.

The most sensitive routine test for the diagnosis of acute sinusitis in adults and children over 1 year of age is radiologic examination of the sinuses. The presence of radiologic opacity, an air–fluid level, or of mucosal thickening is strong evidence for the presence of active infection (Fig. 2)[1,2,21,22] In children under 1 year of age, sinus radiographs appear to be of limited utility.[22] Also, the value of sinus radiology in diagnosing active infection is limited in patients with chronic sinusitis because of persistent radiologic abnormalities in such patients.

While not practical for routine diagnosis of community-acquired sinusitis, (computed tomography (CT)) and magnetic resonance imaging (MRI) provide very sensitive methods for evaluating abnormalities of the paranasal sinuses. These techniques

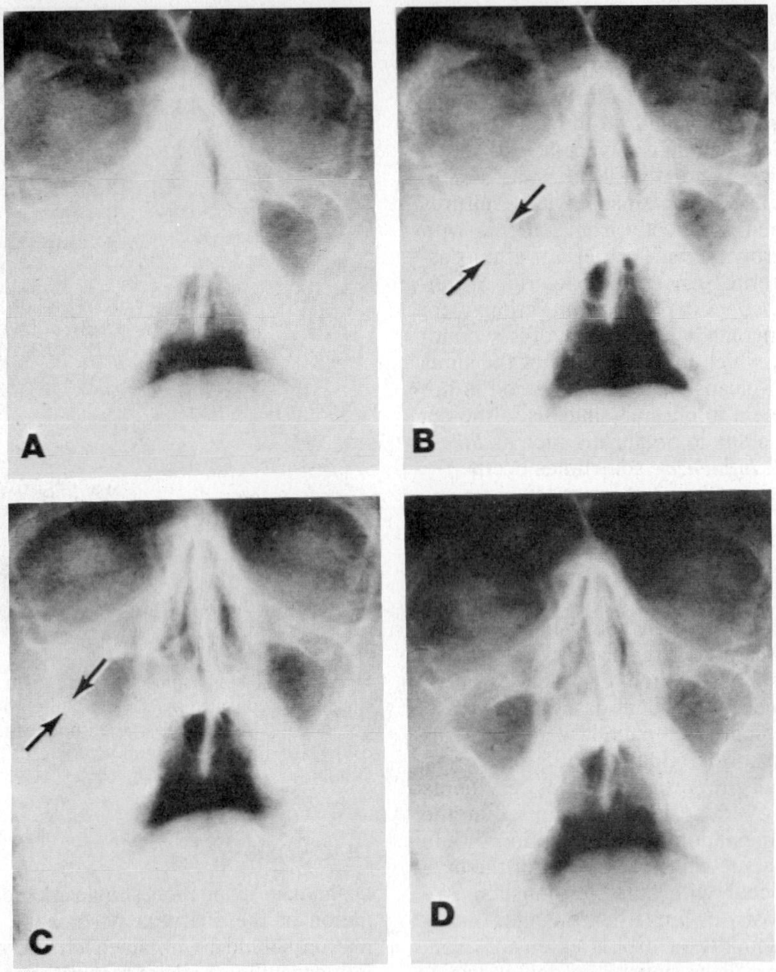

FIGURE 2. Serial roentgenograms of a patient with acute infection of the right maxillary antrum (occipitomental views). **(A)** February 18, complete opacity of the antrum. Culture of sinus aspirate yielded *H. influenzae* in a titer of 10^6 cfu/ml. **(B)** February 25, marked thickening of the mucosal lining. **(C)** March 4, diminished thickening of the mucosal lining. **(D)** March 18, normal. The patient received ampicillin from February 18 to February 26.

are particularly useful for examination of the ethmoid and sphenoid sinuses, since conventional radiography lacks optimal sensitivity here. CT or MRI is also useful whenever orbital extension of ethmoid sinusitis is expected.

The specific microbial etiology of acute sinusitis can be determined only by culture of an exudate or a rinse obtained directly from the sinus by puncture and aspiration. Cultures of nasal pus or of sinus exudates obtained by rinsing through the natural sinus ostium give unreliable information because of contamination with resident bacterial flora in the nose. Since the microbial etiology of acute sinusitis has been well described in studies using direct puncture,[1–3,5–10] there is no indication for using sinus puncture in the management of the average case of acute sinusitis. However, sinus puncture should be performed for bacterial diagnosis in patients with unusually severe sinusitis, particularly if intracranial extension of the infection is suspected. Also, sinus puncture is of value in patients who have not responded to empiric antimicrobial therapy, those with severe immunosuppression, and those with nosocomial sinusitis when it is not possible to predict the identity and antimicrobial sensitivity of the causative agent.

The antral sinus is punctured below the inferior turbinate of the nose and the frontal sinus below the infraorbital rim of the eye. Thorough cleansing of the puncture site with an antiseptic solution such as povidone–iodine is important to prevent contamination of the specimen with surface bacteria. Specimens for culture should be aspirated through the puncture needle or through a plastic catheter and should not be obtained by collecting material that has been rinsed through the natural sinus ostium. When free fluid cannot be obtained from the sinus cavity, 1 ml of antibiotic-free normal saline or Ringer's lactate solution can be instilled and aspirated to provide a specimen. The syringe containing the specimen should be transported to the laboratory for examination by gram stain and aerobic and anaerobic bacterial culture. When available, quantitative culture of the specimen is useful to help to detect bacterial contaminants accidentally introduced into the specimen. Most bacteria causing active sinus infection are present in titers of $\geq 10^5$ cfu/ml, while titers of contaminants in a freshly processed specimen are usually less.

In patients with acute sinusitis in whom intracranial complications, such as bacterial meningitis and brain abscess, are suspected appropriate diagnostic evaluations should be conducted promptly (see Chapters 66 and 70).

Noninfectious causes of persistent sinus disease which enter the differential diagnosis of sinusitis include Wegener's granulomatosis, lethal midline granuloma, and its variant polymorphic reticulosis.

TREATMENT

Antimicrobial Therapy

Although viruses may play a role in the initiation of acute sinusitis, the disease should be treated as a bacterial infection. The

TABLE 2. Antimicrobials Effective in the Therapy of Acute Sinusitis

Antimicrobial Agent	*Recommended Oral Dose in Adults*
Ampicillin	500 mg q6h
Amoxicillin	500 mg q8h
Cyclacillin	500 mg q8h
Bacampicillin	800 mg bid
Trimethoprim-sulfamethoxazole (80 mg/400 mg)	2 tablets bid
Cefaclor	500 mg q6h
Cefuroxime axetil	250 mg q12h

efficacy of antimicrobials for treating acute sinusitis has been established in studies employing pre- and posttreatment sinus aspirations.[23,24] Antimicrobial therapy must be selected on an empiric basis since in the usual case, sinus puncture to determine a specific microbial diagnosis is not indicated. Therapy should ideally cover all the bacteria listed in Table 1, but primarily it should be effective for both *S. pneumoniae* and *H. influenzae*. Antimicrobials shown to be effective in acute sinusitis in studies employing pre- and posttreatment sinus aspirations[24–27] and the doses recommended are listed in Table 2. A 10-day course of therapy is recommended based on findings in the sinus puncture studies. Ampicillin or amoxicillin is recommended for the initial treatment of uncomplicated community-acquired sinusitis. In evaluating the response to these drugs, it should be remembered that they are not effective against β-lactamase-producing bacteria. For the penicillin-allergic patient, trimethoprim-sulfamethoxazole is an alternative that provides adequate coverage against both *S. pneumoniae* and *H. influenzae*. Sinusitis due to penicillin-resistant strains of bacteria requires treatment with a penicillinase-resistant antimicrobial agent. In areas where *Haemophilus* and *Branhamella* isolates are often β-lactamase producers, a third-generation cephalosporin may be an appropriate choice when parenteral therapy is indicated.

Supportive Therapy

Nasal decongestants should be used in the supportive treatment of acute sinusitis. Phenylephrine nose drops, 0.25 or 0.5%, are recommended for use on a regular basis as described in Chapter 42. If pain is severe, codeine may be required. Most patients with acute sinusitis can be successfully treated as outpatients. For patients with severe infection and for those in whom intracranial extension of infection is a consideration, hospitalization is advisable for parenteral antimicrobial therapy, close observation and prompt initiation of diagnostic tests when needed. Antihistamines may thicken purulent sinus fluid and impair drainage. Their use for acute sinusitis is to be discouraged.

Surgical Therapy

Patients with severe sinus infection or those suspected of developing intracranial or orbital complications should be evaluated with computerized tomography for emergency or early surgical drainage. Infection of the orbit frontal[28] and sphenoid[29] sinuses should be recognized as conditions in which surgical intervention may be required.

SUBACUTE AND CHRONIC SINUSITIS

Sinus lavage has been used traditionally for the treatment of patients with acute sinusitis in whom complaints have persisted. A series of irrigations of the affected sinus appears to be beneficial. When lavage is performed via direct sinus puncture, a sample of the sinus contents should be aspirated and cultured quantitatively for bacterial identification and antibiotic sensitivities.

Once sinusitis has reached a chronic state, there is no evidence that it is primarily an infectious problem, although patients with permanent mucosal damage of the sinuses may have acute infectious exacerbations. Infectious exacerbations, which are recognized in patients with chronic sinus disease, should be treated in the same way as described above for the treatment of an acute infection. Surgical procedures, such as creation of an artificial ostium to facilitate sinus drainage and submucous resection, are used in the treatment of patients with chronic sinusitis.

Measures to Prevent Acute or Chronic Sinusitis

There are no proven ways to prevent acute sinusitis. When control of colds and influenzal illness becomes practical, the incidence of sinusitis should decline. For the present, prompt and regular use of vasoconstrictors in nasal drops or sprays for the treatment of colds may help to reduce the incidence of secondary bacterial infection of the sinuses, but this is unproven. Control of nasal allergies and corrective surgery for nasal abnormalities may promote normal sinus drainage and thus lessen the risk of sinus infection. Good dental hygiene and prompt treatment of tooth root infection may help reduce the incidence of acute infection of the maxillary sinus secondary to dental disease.

Effective antimicrobial therapy for patients with acute sinusitis may help to reduce the incidence of chronic sinus disease, although this is not established. The diversity of bacteria responsible for acute sinusitis limits the choice of antimicrobials that have an adequate spectrum of activity, particularly for both *S. pneumoniae* and *H. influenzae*. Penicillin, tetracyclines, and cephalosporins, which have been widely used in the past to treat acute sinusitis, do not provide optimum coverage for both these organisms. Undoubtedly, many patients with acute sinusitis who were given one of these drugs did not receive effective treatment. This may have resulted in the infection causing permanent damage to the sinus and may have been a preventable cause of chronic sinusitis.

REFERENCES

1. Evans FO, Sydnor JB, Moore WEC, et al. Sinusitis of maxillary antrum. N Engl J Med. 1975;293:735.
2. Hamory BH, Sande MA, Sydnor A Jr, et al. Etiology and antimicrobial therapy of acute maxillary sinusitis. J Infect Dis. 1979;139:197.
3. Caplan ES, Hoyt NJ. Nosocomial sinusitis. JAMA. 1982;247:639.
4. Frederick J, Braude AI. Anaerobic infection of the paranasal sinuses. N Engl J Med 1974;290:135.
5. Urdal K, Berdal P. The microbial flora in 81 cases of maxillary sinusitis. Acta Otolaryngol. 1949;37:20.
6. Björkwall T. Bacteriologic examinations in maxillary sinusitis: bacterial flora of the maillary antrum. Acta Otolaryngol. 1950;83(Suppl):33.
7. Lystad A, Berdal P, Lung-Iversen L. The bacterial flora of sinusitis with in vitro study of the bacterial resistance to antibiotics. Acta Otolaryngol. 1964;188(Suppl):390.
8. Rantanen T, Arvilommi H. Double-blind trial of doxycycline in acute maxillary sinusitis; a clinical and bacteriological study. Acta Otolaryngol. 1973; 76:58.
9. Axelsson A, Broson JE. The correlation and maxillary sinus in acute maxillary sinusitis. Laryngoscope. 1973;83:2003.
10. Wald ER, Milmoe GJ, Bowen A'D, et al. Acute maxillary sinusitis in children. N Engl J Med. 1981;304:749.
11. Shapiro ED, Milmoe, Wald ER, et al. Bacteriology of the maxillary sinuses in patients with cystic fibrosis. J Infect Dis. 1982;146:589.
12. McGuirt WF, Harril JA. Paranasal sinus aspergillosis. Laryngoscope. 1979;89:1563.
13. Rinaldi MG. Invasive aspergillosis. Rev Infect Dis. 1983;5:1061.
14. Padhye AA, Ajello L, Wieden MA, et al. Phaeohyphomycosis of the nasal sinuses caused by a new species of *Exserohilum*. J Clin Microbiol. 1986;24:245.
15. MacMillan RH III, Cooper PH, Body BA, et al. Allergic fungal sinusitis due to *Curvularia lunata*. Hum Pathol. 1987;18:960.
16. Parfrey NA. Improved diagnosis and prognosis of mucormycosis. A clinicopathologic study of 33 cases. Medicine 1986;65:113.

17. Kern ME, Uecker FA. Maxillary sinus infection caused by the homobasidiomycetous fungus *Schizophyllum commune*. J Clin Microbiol. 1986;23:1001.
18. Washburn RG, Kennedy AW, Begley MG, et al. Chronic fungal sinusitis in apparently normal hosts. Medicine. 1988;67:231–47.
19. Dingle JH, Badger GF, Jordan WS Jr. Illness in the Home. A Study of 25,000 Illnesses in a Group of Cleveland Families. Cleveland: The Press of Western Reserve University; 1964;292.
20. Wells RG, Sty JR, Landers AD. Radiological evaluation of Pott puffy tumor. JAMA. 1986;255:1331–1333.
21. Lusted LB, Keats TE. Atlas of Roentgenographic Measurement. 4th ed. Chicago: Year Book Medical Publishers; 1978.
22. Kovatch AL, Wald ER, Ledesma-Medina J, et al. Maxillary sinus radiographs in children with non-respiratory complaints. Pediatrics. 1984;73:306.
23. Carenfelt C, Eneroth C-M, Lundberg C, et al. Evaluation of the antibiotic effect of treatment of maxillary sinusitis. Scand J Infect Dis. 1984;73:306.
24. Gwaltney JM Jr, Sydnor A Jr, Sande MA. Etiology and antimicrobial treatment of acute sinusitis. Ann Otol Rhinol Laryngol. 1981;90:68.
25. Farr B, Scheld M, Gwaltney JM Jr, et al: Bacampicillin HCl in the treatment of acute maxillary sinusitis. Bull NY Acad Med. 1983;59:477.
26. Scheld WM, Sydnor A Jr, Farr B, et al. Comparison of cyclacillin and amoxicillin for therapy of acute maxillary sinusitis. Antimicrob Agents Chemother. 1986;30:250.
27. Sydnor A Jr, Gwaltney JM Jr, Scheld WM. Cefuroxime axetil vs. cefaclor therapy of acute maxillary sinusitis. Presented at the 28th Interscience Conference on Antimicrobial Agents and Chemotherapy, Los Angeles, October 24, 1988.
28. Middleton WG, Briant TDR, Fenton RS. Frontal sinusitis—a 10 year experience. J Otolaryngol. 1985;14:197.
29. Lew D, Southwick FS, Montogomery WW, et al. Sphenoid sinusitis. A review of 30 cases. N Engl J Med. 1983;309:1149.

48. EPIGLOTTITIS

JAMES E. BURNS
J. OWEN HENDLEY

Acute epiglottitis (supraglottitis) is a rapidly progressive cellulitis of the epiglottis and adjacent structures that has the potential for causing abrupt, complete airway obstruction.

The typical patient is a 2- to 4-year-old boy having at any time of the year a 6- to 12-hour history of fever and dysphagia. Sore throat is the most prominent symptom in older children and adults. At the time medical attention is sought, varying degrees of respiratory distress may be evident. The patient usually prefers to sit leaning forward while drooling oral secretions. Respirations tend to be tentative and careful without marked tachypnea. Tachycardia is usually commensurate with fever but may be related to hypoxia and be out of proportion to fever.[1] Inspiratory stridor and hoarseness occur frequently, but the barking cough and aphonia that may occur in croup syndrome are rare. The diagnosis is established by finding an edematous "cherry red" epiglottis. The course of acute epiglottitis may be fulminating, as emphasized by the report of a patient who progressed from being completely asymptomatic to having complete airway obstruction in 30 minutes.[2] The course may be more languid in adults, but the disease is potentially no less serious.[3]

Laboratory data include moderate leukocytosis with a "shift to the left," positive cultures of blood and the epiglottis, and evidence of pneumonia on chest x-ray films in up to 25 percent of cases.[4,5] A roentgenogram of the lateral neck may show an enlarged epiglottis, ballooning of the hypopharynx, and normal subglottic structures (Fig. 1).[6] However, the use of x-ray films in the diagnosis of epiglottitis is questionable both because of the delay in securing an airway while the films are being obtained and the poor sensitivity (as low as 31 percent) and specifity (as low as 44 percent) of this procedure.[3,7,8] The epiglottis should be visualized directly, even if the x-ray findings are negative, in those patients in whom there is a strong suspicion of epiglottitis. This examination should be performed only when prepared to immediately secure the airway. In adults, examination of the epiglottis may be safer than in children.[3] *Haemophilus influenzae* type b is isolated from cultures of blood and/or epiglottis in most pediatric and up to 26 percent of adult patients with epiglottitis,[9] an association first demonstrated by Le Mierre and associates in 1936.[10] Other agents occasionally implicated are pneumococci, staphylococci, streptococci, and *H. paraphrophilus*.[2,11,12] The role of viruses in epiglottitis is not established.

H. influenzae bacteremia occurs in up to 100 percent of children with epiglottitis.[1,13] Significantly, this bacteremia has been associated with only a small number of metastatic infections such as meningitis and arthritis.[1,4,14,15]

DIFFERENTIAL DIAGNOSIS

The croup syndrome is the most frequent differential consideration in epiglottitis. Although the barking cough typical of croup is an infrequent feature of epiglottitis, differentiation from croup is sometimes difficult unless the epiglottis is visualized. In contrast to epiglottitis, croup is frequently preceded by an upper respiratory infection, has a more gradual onset, involves somewhat younger children (aged 3 months to 3 years), and may last up to a week. The etiology is usually viral, and the area of obstruction is subglottic while the epiglottis is normal. Children with croup are more likely to prefer to lie supine and do not have the dysphagia and drooling that are characteristic of epiglottitis. In croup, x-ray films of the lateral aspect of the neck are more likely to reveal a normal epiglottis and may show the airway narrowed in the sublottic region (Fig. 1),[6] but they may have up to a 24 percent false-positive rate for readings consistent with epiglottitis.[7]

Diphtheria can be differentiated from epiglottitis by the presence of a pseudomembrane in the respiratory tract and the presence of typical organisms on direct smear and culture of the membrane. Allergic laryngeal edema (angioneurotic edema) and foreign body aspiration lack the toxic manifestations of epiglottitis and often have a history that is helpful in suspecting the correct diagnosis. Retropharyngeal abscess, peritonsillar abscess, and lingual tonsillitis are other rare causes of upper airway obstruction; these can usually be differentiated from epiglottitis on physical examination.

THERAPY

Maintenance of an adequate airway should be the primary concern as soon as the diagnosis of epiglottitis is even suspected in a child or an adult.

There has been discussion over the years about whether all patients with epiglottitis should have an artificial airway (tracheostomy or endotracheal tube) inserted as soon as the diagnosis is made or whether a period of observation before insertion of an airway is justifiable. In recent years there has been agreement among most authors that provision of an airway immediately is the safest course.[2,3,16–20] Observation of a child with epiglottitis for signs of airway obstruction cannot be recommended since the mortality is up to 6–25 percent in those observed and 33–80 percent in those in whom obstruction occurs.[2,21]

The use of an endotracheal tube rather than a tracheostomy for provision of the artificial airway is preferred as therapy for acute epiglottitis by most authors.[5,17–19,22] In spite of theoretic difficulties with insertion of an endotracheal tube through the region of the inflamed epiglottis, this has not proved to be a problem. An advantage to the use of an endotracheal tube is the ease of its removal after the 36–48 hours required for the inflammation and edema to subside after institution of appropriate antimicrobial therapy.

Because of the potential for rapid deterioration to complete respiratory obstruction, patients even suspected of having acute epiglottitis should be handled as a medical emergency. Patients

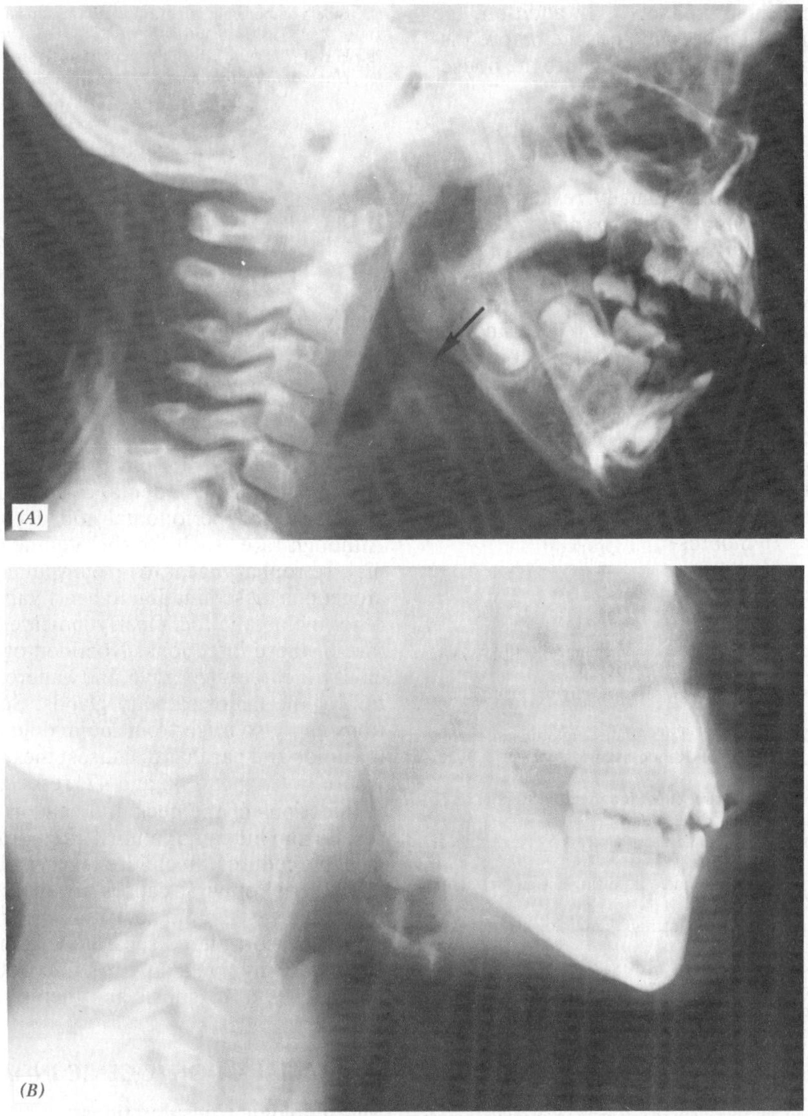

Fig. 1. Lateral neck roentgenograms. **(A)** Enlarged epiglottis—the thumb sign[6]—in a patient with acute epiglottitis. Arrows indicate epiglottitis. **(B)** Normal epiglottis—the little finger sign—in a patient with croup syndrome. (Courtesy of Dr. Caroline B. Hall, University of Rochester School of Medicine, Rochester, NY.)

being transported between medical facilities and within such facilities must be accompanied by personnel capable of securing the airway should obstruction occur.

The epiglottis can be visualized in most patients by depressing the tongue with a depressor placed as far posteriorly as the tonsillar pillars. However, it is unwise to examine the epiglottis of a pediatric patient suspected of having epiglottitis because of the possibility of precipitating complete airway obstruction or vagally mediated cardiopulmonary arrest. It is also unwise to restrain pediatric patients in the supine position because this may also lead to airway obstruction.[20] As a consequence, it is safer to transfer a patient thought to have acute epiglottitis to an operating room and then visualize the epiglottis with a laryngoscope or bronchoscope after all is in readiness for insertion of an artificial airway under controlled conditions. As soon as the diagnosis is made, by visualization of the "cherry red" epiglottis, an uncuffed endotracheal tube should be inserted or a tracheostomy performed. If the epiglottis is normal, the patient may be managed in a manner appropriate for croup or laryngotracheobronchitis. If difficulty is encountered or if obstruction occurs while trying to establish the airway, the possibility of ventilating the apneic patient by bag and mask or mouth-to-mouth ventilation should not be overlooked.[16,17]

After establishment of an airway, samples of blood and the epiglottis should be cultured, and the patient should be administered intravenous antibiotic therapy directed at *H. influenzae*. In view of the risk of infection with ampicillin-resistant *H. influenzae,* ampicillin, 200 mg/kg/day, and chloramphenicol, 75–100 mg/kg/day, both in four divided doses intravenously, have been conventional therapy.[23] At present, intravenous cefuroxime (100–200 mg/kg/day in three divided doses) or a third-generation cephalosporin such as cefotaxime (100–150 mg/kg/day in four doses) may be used for initial therapy.

Patients with acute epiglottitis are usually improved 36–48 hours after initiation of appropriate antibiotic therapy. Depending on the patient's progress, the artificial airway can usually be removed in 48 hours. Before extubation the patient should be afebrile and alert with either a leak around the endotrachael tube or evidence of resolution by direct visualization with a fiber-optic laryngoscope.[19,24] Antibiotics should be continued for 7–10 days. The route by which the antibiotic is administered after extubation should be dictated by the clinical response and status of the patient.

If the patient with epiglottitis has household contacts who are younger than 4 years old, rifampin prophylaxis given once daily for 4 days in a dose of 20 mg/kg/day (maximum of 600 mg/day) is recommended for all household contacts.[25] In addition, the patient should receive rifampin in the same dosage before discharge to prevent reintroduction of the organism into the household (see Chapter 184).

IMMUNITY

An episode of *H. influenzae* epiglottis usually results in high levels of serum antibody to capsular polysaccharide.[26] This response appears to provide immunity since second cases of epiglottitis are extremely rare. The presence of maternally derived serum antibody at birth explains the infrequent occurrence of *H. influenzae* infections in infants. After the disappearance of this maternal antibody there is an inverse relationship between rising levels of naturally acquired antibody and the declining incidence of epiglottitis.[27]

Widespread use of *H. influenzae* type b polysaccharide vaccine should decrease the incidence of epiglottitis.[28] However, since approximately one-third of cases occur in children under 18 months of age, the disease will not disappear with the current conjugated vaccine given at 18 months.[29]

REFERENCES

1. Sendi K, Crysdale WS. Acute epiglottitis: Decade of change—a 10-year experience with 242 children. J Otolaryngol. 1987;16:196–202.
2. Bass JW, Steele RW, Wiebe RA. Acute epiglottitis: A surgical emergency. JAMA. 1974;229:671–5.
3. MayoSmith MF, Hirsch PJ, Wodzinski SF, et al. Acute epiglottitis in adults: An eight-year experience in the state of Rhode Island. N Engl J Med. 1986;314:1133–9.
4. Molteni RA. Epiglottitis: Incidence of extraepiglottic infection: Report of 72 cases and review of the literature. Pediatrics. 1976;58:526–31.
5. Battaglia JD, Lockhart CH. Management of acute epiglottitis by nasotracheal intubation. Am J Dis Child. 1975;129:334–6.
6. Podgore JK, Bass JW. The "thumb sign" and "little finger sign" in acute epiglottitis. J Pediatr. 1976;88:154–5.
7. Stankiewicz JA, Bowes AK. Croup and epiglottitis: A radiologic study. Laryngoscope. 1985;95:1159–60.
8. Jones JL, Holland P. False positives in lateral neck radiographs used to diagnose epiglottitis. Ann Emerg Med. 1983;12:797.
9. Mustoe T, Strome M. Adult epiglottitis. Am J Otolaryngol. 1983;4:393–9.
10. Le Mierre A, Meyer A, Laplane R. Les septicemies a bacille de pfeiffer. Ann Med. 1936;39:97–119.
11. Berenberg W, Kevy S. Acute epiglottitis in childhood. N Engl J Med. 1958;258:870–4.
12. Jones RN, Slepack J, Bigelow J. Ampicillin-resistant *Haemophilus paraphrophilus* laryno-epiglottitis. J Clin Microbiol. 1976;4:405–7.
13. Alexander HE, Ellis C, Leidy G. Treatment of type-specific hemophilus infections in infancy and childhood. J Pediatr. 1942;20:673–98.
14. Dajani AD, Asmar BI, Thirumoorthia MC. Systemic *Haemophilus influenzae* disease: An overview. J Pediatr. 1979;94:355–64.
15. Branfors-Helander P, Jeppsson P-H. Acute epiglottitis: A clinical, bacteriological, and serological study. Scand J Infect Dis. 1975;7:103–11.
16. Adair JC, Ring WH. Management of epiglottitis in children. Anesth Analg. 1975;54:622–5.
17. Blanc VF, Weber ML, Ludec C, et al. Acute epiglottitis in children: Management of 27 consecutive cases with nasotrachael intubation with special emphasis on anaesthetic considerations. Can Anaesth Soc J. 1977;24:1–11.
18. Rapkin RH. Nasotrachael intubation in epiglottitis. Pediatrics. 1975;56:110–2.
19. Baines DB, Wark H, Overton JH. Acute epiglottitis in children. Anaesth Intensive Care. 1984;13:25–8.
20. Bass JW, Fajardo JE, Brien JH, et al. Sudden death due to acute epiglottitis. Pediatr Infect Dis. 1985;4:447–9.
21. Rapkin RH. Tracheostomy in epiglottitis. Pediatrics. 1973;52:426–9.
22. Schuller DE, Brick HG. The safety of intubation in croup and epiglottitis: An eight year follow-up. Laryngoscope. 1975;85:33–46.
23. McCracken GH Jr. Commentary. J Pediatr. 1979;94:987.
24. Gonzalez C, Reilly JS, Kenna MA, et al. Duration of intubation in children with acute epiglottitis. Otolaryngol Head Neck Surg. 1986;95:477–81.
25. Committee on Infectious Diseases, American Academy of Pediatrics. In Peter G, ed. Report of the Committee on Infectious Diseases. Evanston, IL: American Academy of Pediatrics; 1986:169–74.
26. Whisnant JK, Rogentine GN, Gralnick MA, et al. Host factors and antibody response in *Haemophilus influenzae* type b meningitis and epiglottitis. J Infect Dis. 1976;133:448–55.
27. Schneerson R, Rodrigues LP, Parke JC Jr, et al. Immunity to disease caused by *Hemophilus influenzae* type b. J Immunol. 1971;107:1081–9.
28. Petola H, Käyhty H, Virtanen M, et al. Prevention of *Hemophilus influenzae* type b bacteremic infections with the capsular polysaccharide vaccine. N Engl J Med. 1984;310:1561–6.
29. Hay JW, Daum RS. Cost-benefit analysis of two strategies for prevention of *Haemophilus influenzae* type b infections. Pediatrics. 1987;80:319–29.

49. INFECTIONS OF THE ORAL CAVITY, NECK, AND HEAD

ANTHONY W. CHOW

Infections of the oral cavity most commonly are odontogenic in origin and include dental caries, pulpitis, periapical abscess, gingivitis, and periodontal and deep fascial space infections. Although rare, such life-threatening complications as intracranial, retropharyngeal, or pleuropulmonary extension and hematogenous dissemination to heart valves, prosthetic device, and other metastatic foci clearly indicate the potentially serious nature of these infections. Nonodontogenic infections of the oral cavity include ulcerative and gangrenous stomatitis and infection of the major salivary glands. Suppurative orofacial infections can also arise from the middle ear, oronasopharynx, and mastoids and paranasal sinuses; these have been discussed elsewhere in Chapters 46 and 47, respectively.

Infections of the neck and head in the adult most commonly result from human or animal bites, trauma, irradiation, and surgical procedures. In children, cervical adenitis or thyroiditis due to bacterial or viral causes are more common. Rarely do embryologic cysts in the neck region become secondarily infected. These are considered separately from oral infections since they frequently involve a different microflora and require alternative approaches to diagnosis and therapy.

OROFACIAL ODONTOGENIC INFECTIONS

Microbiologic Considerations

The microbiota associated with odontogenic infections is complex and generally reflects the indigenous oral flora. Despite this complexity, recent evidence strongly supports a causative role of specific microorganisms in different forms of odontogenic infections. This emerging concept of specific microbial cause has created considerable dilemma in our traditional approach to the diagnosis and management of such infections. Since the microflora associated with these infections is typically polymicrobial, it does not necessarily follow that each component of this complex flora has equal pathogenic potential or that the numerically predominant cultivable microflora are the most important. Furthermore, it may not be necessary to eradicate the complete microflora for effective therapy. An appreciation of the indigenous oral flora and the host factors that may modify its composition and knowledge of the specific microorganisms implicated in different odontogenic infections should therefore greatly assist in a more rational approach to such infections arising from the oral cavity.

Indigenous Oral Flora. The oral cavity cannot be regarded as a single, uniform environment. Although representative species of microorganisms can be isolated from most areas of the mouth, certain sites such as the tongue, tooth surface, gingival crevice, and saliva tend to favor colonization by specific organisms[1–3] (Table 1). Quantitative studies indicate that obligate anaerobes constitute a large and important part of the

TABLE 1. Predominant Cultivable Bacteria from Various Sites of the Oral Cavity

		Total Viable Count (Mean %)			
Type	*Predominant Genus or Family*	*Gingival Crevice*	*Dental Plaque*	*Tongue*	*Saliva*
Facultative					
Gram-positive cocci	*Streptococcus*	28.8	28.2	44.8	46.2
	S. mutans	(0–30)	(0–50)	(0–1)	(0–1)
	S. sanguis	(10–20)	(40–60)	(10–20)	(10–30)
	S. mitior	(10–30)	(20–40)	(10–30)	(30–50)
	S. salivarius	(0–1)	(0–1)	(40–60)	(40–60)
Gram-positive rods	*Lactobacillus* *Corynebacterium*	15.3	23.8	13.0	11.8
Gram-negative cocci	*Branhamella*	0.4	0.4	3.4	1.2
Gram-negative rods	Enterobacteriaceae	1.2	ND	3.2	2.3
Anaerobic					
Gram-positive cocci	*Peptostreptococcus*	7.4	12.6	4.2	13.0
Gram-positive rods	*Actinomyces* *Eubacterium* *Lactobacillus* *Leptotrichia*	20.2	18.4	8.2	4.8
Gram-negative cocci	*Veillonella*	10.7	6.4	16.0	15.9
Gram-negative rods		16.1	10.4	8.2	4.8
	Fusobacterium	1.9	4.1	0.7	0.3
	Bacteroides, pigmented	4.7	ND	0.2	ND
	Bacteroides, nonpigmented	5.6	4.8	5.1	2.4
	Campylobacter	3.8	1.3	2.2	2.1
Spirochetes	*Treponema*	1.0	ND	ND	ND

Abbreviations: ND: not detected.
(Data from Chow et al.,[1] Hardie,[2] and Hamada et al.[3])

residential oral flora. In the gingival crevice of healthy adults, for example, the total microscopic counts averaged 2.7×10^{11} microorganisms per gram wet weight.[4] The total cultivable anaerobic bacteria averaged 1.8×10^{11} microorganisms per gram, whereas facultative bacteria averaged 2.2×10^{10} microorganisms per gram, an eightfold difference. Overall, *Streptococcus, Peptostreptococcus, Veillonella, Lactobacillus, Corynebacterium*, and *Actinomyces* account for more than 80 percent of the total cultivable oral flora. Facultative gram-negative rods are uncommon in healthy adults but may be more prominent in seriously ill, hospitalized, and elderly patients.[5,6] Unique ecologic niches are observed. For example, *Streptococcus sanguis, S. mutans*, and *S. mitis* as well as *Actinomyces viscosus* preferentially colonize the tooth surface.[7] In contrast, *S. salivarius* and *Veillonella* sp. have a predilection for the tongue and buccal mucosa.[2] *Fusobacterium*, pigmented *Bacteroides*, and anaerobic spirochetes appear concentrated in the gingival crevice.[2] Factors that appear to govern these localization patterns include selective adherence characteristics of certain bacteria for various types of cells, local environmental conditions such as oxygen tension, oxidation–reduction potential (Eh) and pH, interbacterial coaggregation, and microbial inhibition.[2,8,9] Apart from anatomic considerations, numerous factors such as age, diet and nutrition, eruption of deciduous dentition, oral hygiene, smoking habits, the presence of dental caries or periodontal disease, antimicrobial therapy, hospitalization, pregnancy, as well as genetic and racial factors may influence the composition of the oral flora.[2,7–9]

Microbial Specificity in Odontogenic Infections. Although it had been recognized for some time that odontogenic infections are initiated by microorganisms through the establishment of dental plaques, the microbial specificity of these infections was not fully appreciated until recently. This breakthrough was brought about by technological advances in sampling and anaerobic culture of specimens as well as by improved methods for species identification and taxonomy. Important differences in bacterial compositions have been noted for dental caries, gingivitis, and different forms of periodontitis when compared with cultures from healthy tissues.[10–12] An etiologic association of *S. mutans* in dental caries has been firmly established.[13,14] *Streptococcus mutans* is the only organism consistently isolated from all decayed dental fissures and is the only organism consistently found in greater numbers in carious teeth as compared with noncarious teeth. The infectious and transmissable nature of this organism in dental caries has been demonstrated in both experimental animals and longitudinal studies in humans. Similarly, in gingivitis and periodontitis, a unique and specific bacterial composition of the subgingival plaque has been identified. In the healthy periodontium, the microflora is sparse and consists mainly of gram-positive organisms such as *S. sanguis* and *Actinomyces* sp. In the presence of gingivitis, the predominant subgingival flora shifts to a greater proportion of anaerobic gram-negative rods, and *Bacteroides intermedius* is most commonly isolated.[11,12,15] With established periodontitis, the flora further increases in complexity with a preponderance of anaerobic gram-negative and motile organisms. *Bacteroides gingivalis* (formerly *B. asaccharolyticus* and *B. melaninogenicus* ssp. *asaccharolyticus*) is most commonly isolated. In juvenile periodontitis, a clinical variant seen primarily in adolescents, the subgingival plaque mainly consists of saccharolytic organisms, with *Actinobacillus actinomycetemcomitans* and *Capnocytophaga* sp. as the most common identifiable species. *Bacteroides gingivalis* is rarely found in this condition.[12,16] In suppurative odontogenic infections such as periapical abscesses or deep fascial space infections, a polymicrobial flora is usually present, with *Fusobacterium nucleatum*, pigmented *Bacteroides, Peptostreptococcus, Actinomyces*, and *Streptococcus* as the most predominant isolates.[1,17] Except in selected patients with serious underlying illnesses, facultative gram-negative bacilli and *Staphylococcus aureus* are uncommonly isolated.[18,19]

This microbial specificity demonstrated for different odontogenic infections probably reflects the acquisition of a unique microflora during the development of a supragingival dental plaque and its progression to a subgingival dental plaque.[20] Plaques that accumulate above the gingival margin are composed mainly of gram-positive facultative and microaerophilic cocci and rods; plaques that accumulate below the gingival margin are composed mainly of gram-negative anaerobic rods and motile forms including spirochetes (Fig. 1). Microorganisms residing within the supragingival plaque are characterized by their ability to adhere to the tooth surface and by their saccharolytic activity. Microorganisms in the subgingival plaque are frequently asaccharolytic and need not be adherent.

Pathogenetic Mechanisms

Suppurative orofacial infections are usually preceded by dental caries or periodontal disease. The pathogenetic mechanisms of cariogenesis remain poorly defined. The most universally accepted theory is that originated by W. D. Miller in 1882, which proposes that bacterial action on carbohydrates produces acidic substances that cause demineralization and dissolution of the hard tissues of the tooth.[21,22] In order for dental caries to develop three factors need to be present: (*1*) a susceptible tooth surface (host factors), (*2*) acidogenic (acid-producing) and aciduric (able to grow at low pH) bacteria within a dental plaque (microbial factors), and (*3*) carbohydrates and simple sugars (dietary factors). In the healthy host, at least three mechanisms serve to protect the tooth from carious decay: (*1*) the cleaning action of the tongue and buccal membranes which acts to re-

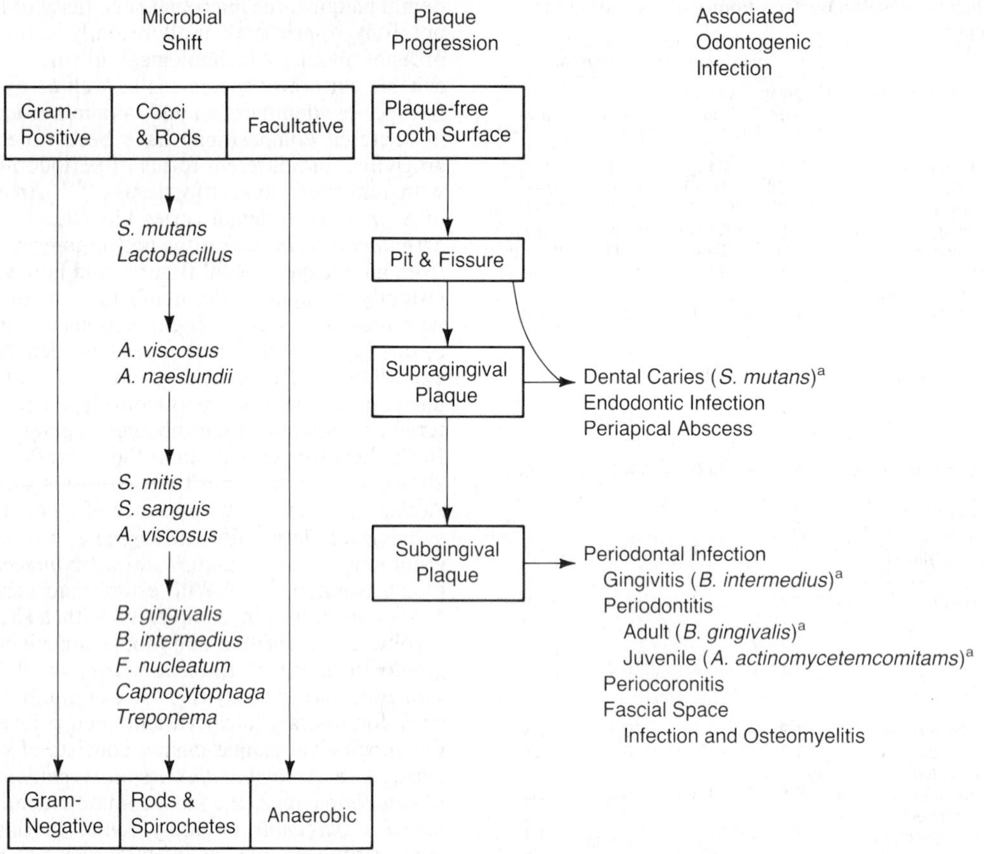

FIG. 1. Microbial specificity in odontogenic infections. A unifying hypothesis demonstrating a microbial shift from a plaque-free tooth surface and progression to supragingival and subgingival plaque organisms. (From Chow,[21] with permission.)

move any food particles from the proximity of the tooth; (*2*) the buffering effect of saliva, which has a neutral pH, washes away bacterial acids, and provides essential substrates for remineralization and repair of damaged tooth surfaces; and (*3*) the protective effect of an acellular bacteria-free coating of salivary origin on the tooth surface, known as the acquired pellicle, which acts as a surface barrier to most dietary and bacterial acids and other proteolytic substances. In the absence of tooth brushing and flossing, the acquired pellicle becomes rapidly colonized and is replaced by the bacterial plaque. It is not surprising, therefore, that carious lesions occur most often in areas inaccessible to the self-cleaning mechanisms of the mouth and on the occlusal surfaces and interproximal sites that are protected from the reaches of the toothbrush.

Unlike dental caries, diet does not appear to have a significant role in the pathogenesis of periodontal disease. The periodontal microflora associated with the subgingival plaque elicits an inflammatory host response that ultimately results in destruction of the periodontium.[11,16,20,22] Two major predisposing factors are poor oral hygiene and increasing age. Other factors include hormonal effects, with exacerbation of disease activity during puberty, menstruation, and pregnancy. Diabetes causes an increased incidence, particularly in juvenile diabetics. Finally, various genetic disorders are associated with an increased incidence of periodontal disease. In particular, those with neutrophil defects (such as Chédiak-Higashi syndrome, agranulocytosis, cyclic neutropenia, and Down syndrome) have a higher incidence of periodontal disease.[22]

It is a tribute to the local defenses in the healthy host that infections within the oral cavity are not more common. Establishment of the normal resident flora appears to be particularly important in providing a strong mucosal defense against colonization and invasion by potential pathogens ("colonization resistance").[23,24] Other nonspecific local defenses include the continuous cell shedding and turnover of the mucosal epithelium and the constant flow of saliva containing lysozyme, lactoferrin, β-lysin, lactoperoxidase, and other antimicrobial systems.[23] Various salivary glycoproteins and histidine-rich polypeptides have been reported to inhibit bacteria and fungi and may prevent infection by the inhibition of microbial attachment to oral epithelium by way of competition for cellular receptor sites or clumping of microorganisms. The epithelial barrier may be affected by radiation therapy, cancer chemotherapy, or trauma. A reduced turnover rate of the epithelial cells will allow retention of adherent organisms. A reduction in saliva volume will also have significant effects on the oral environment and predispose to microbial invasion. In addition to nonspecific host defenses, specific humoral and cellular immune mechanisms are also important. Specific antibodies are present in saliva, with secretory IgA as the predominant immunoglobulin.[25] Salivary antibodies may affect the oral flora by aggregation of organisms and prevention of their attachment to mucosal epithelium. Cell-mediated immunity is important in oral defense against intracellular pathogens including viruses, fungi, and bacteria. In the severely immunocompromised patient, a reactivation of viral infection involving the oral cavity is common, often with potentially life-threatening complications.[26] In addition to humoral and cellular immunity, various phagocytic cells in the oral mucosa also appear important. Phagocytic cells such as lymphocytes, granulocytes, and macrophages are abundant in the lamina propria and presumably contribute to the removal of foreign matter that has breached the epithelial barrier. Unique defects in host defenses have been identified in periodontal infections.[20] For example, impairment of neutrophil chemotaxis has been demonstrated in patients with juvenile periodontitis.[27,28] A number of oral anaerobes and streptococci implicated in periodontitis including *B. gingivalis*, *B. intermedius*, *B. melaninogenicus*, *Capnocytophaga* sp., *S. sanguis*, and *S. mitis* are found to secrete IgA proteases.[29,30] The pathogenic significance of this finding is uncertain at present; it has been suggested that cleavage of IgA by microbial IgA proteases may impair local mucosal immunity of the host. It remains to be seen if similar or other defects of host resistance can be identified in different forms of destructive odontogenic infections.

Anatomic Considerations

Soft tissue infections of odontogenic origin tend to spread along planes of least resistance from the supporting structures of the affected tooth to various potential spaces in the vicinity. Accumulated pus, therefore, must generally perforate bone at the site where it is thinnest and weakest before it extends into the periapical areas or deeper fascial spaces. In the mandible, this is usually in the region of the molar teeth on the lingual aspect and more anterior on the buccal aspect.[31,32] In the maxilla, the bone is weakest on the buccal aspect throughout and relatively thicker on the palatal aspect. If pus perforates through either the maxillary or mandibular buccal plate, it will present intraorally if inside the attachment of the buccinator muscle to the maxilla or mandible and extraorally if outside this muscle attachment (Fig. 2). When a mandibular infection perforates lingually, it presents in the sublingual space if the apices of the involved teeth lie above the attachment of the mylohyoid muscle (e.g., mandibular incisor, canines, premolars, and first molars) and in the submandibular space if below the attachment of this muscle (e.g., second and third molars) (Fig. 2). Thus, these local anatomic barriers of bone, muscle, and fascia predetermine the routes of spread, extent, and clinical manifestations of many orofacial infections of odontogenic origin. The clinically important "fascial spaces" most often involved are illustrated in Figures 3 and 4. These are potential spaces between layers of fascia normally bound together by loose connective tissue. The breakdown of these attachments by a spreading infective process results in a fascial space infection. These spaces intercommunicate with one another to varying degrees, and the potential pathways of extension from one space to another are illustrated in Figure 5. A thorough understanding of the potential *anatomic routes* of infection will not only provide valuable information on the nature and extent of infection but will also suggest the optimum surgical approach for effective drainage.

Clinical Presentations

Odontogenic infections originate in either the dental pulp or the periodontium. The most common site is the dental pulp and results in dentoalveolar infections.

Dentoalveolar Infections. Pulpal infection most frequently results from carious exposure, rarely from physical or chemical injury. The carious process most frequently begins in pits and fissures on the occlusal surfaces of molars and premolars, which encourage food retention. Interproximal sites and the gingival margin are the next most common. Demineralization of the enamel results in discoloration, the first visible evidence of carious involvement. Destruction of the enamel and dentin and invasion of the pulp produce either a localized or generalized pulpitis. If drainage from the pulp is obstructed, a rapid progression with pulpal necrosis and proliferation of endodontic microorganisms leads to invasion of the periapical areas (periapical abscess) and alveolar bone (acute alveolar abscess).

Clinically, the tooth is sensitive to percussion and to both heat and cold during early or reversible pulpitis, although the

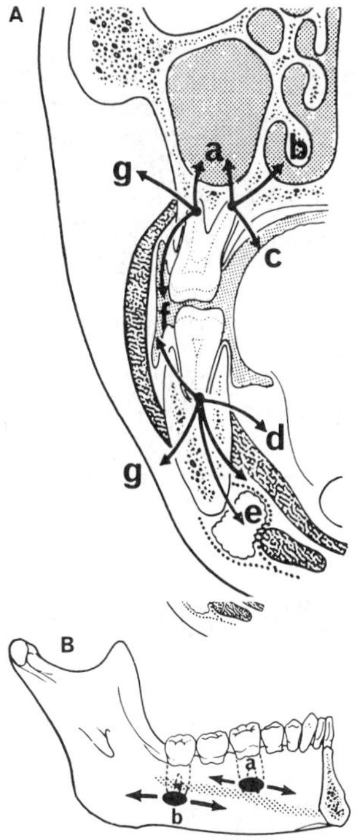

FIG. 2. Routes of spread of odontogenic orofacial infections along planes of least resistance. **(A)** Coronal section in the region of the first molar teeth: a: maxillary antrum; b: nasal cavity; c: palatal plate; d: sublingual space (above the mylohyoid muscle); e: submandibular space (below the mylohyoid muscle); f: intraoral presentation with infection spreading through the buccal plates inside the attachment of the buccinator muscle; g: extraoral presentation to buccal space with infection spreading through the buccal plates outside the attachment of the buccinator muscle. **(B)** Lingual aspect of the mandible: a: apices of the involved tooth above the mylohyoid muscle, with spread of infection to the sublingual space; b: apices of involved tooth below the mylohyoid muscle, with spread of infection into the submandibular space. (From Chow et al.,[1] with permission.)

painful response will stop abruptly when the stimulus is withdrawn. During late or irreversible pulpitis, the tooth is exquisitely painful to a hot stimulus, with prompt relief by the application of cold. If drainage is established through the tooth before extension into the periapical region, chronic irritation from the necrotic pulp may result in periapical granuloma or cyst formation that may be relatively asymptomatic. Dental radiographs are particularly helpful for the detection of silent lesions, particularly those caused by interproximal caries, which are difficult to detect clinically.

The principles of treatment in dentoalveolar infections include prompt elimination of the infected pulp, deep periodontal scaling, or extraction of the affected tooth. Dentoalveolar abscess should be surgically drained at the same time. Other supportive measures include hydration, a soft diet, analgesics, and oral hygiene. Antibiotic therapy is indicated primarily if drainage cannot be adequately established or when infection has perforated the cortex and spread into surrounding soft tissue.

Gingivitis and Periodontal Infections. *Periodontal disease* is a general term that refers to all diseases involving the supporting structures of the teeth (periodontium), which include the gingiva, periodontal ligament, alveolar bone, and cementum. In the early phase of periodontal disease, infection is confined to the gingiva (gingivitis). Later, the underlying supporting tissues are affected (periodontitis), ultimately leading to complete destruction of the periodontium and a permanent loss of teeth. Periodontal infections tend to localize in intraoral soft tissues and seldom spread into deeper structures of the face or neck.

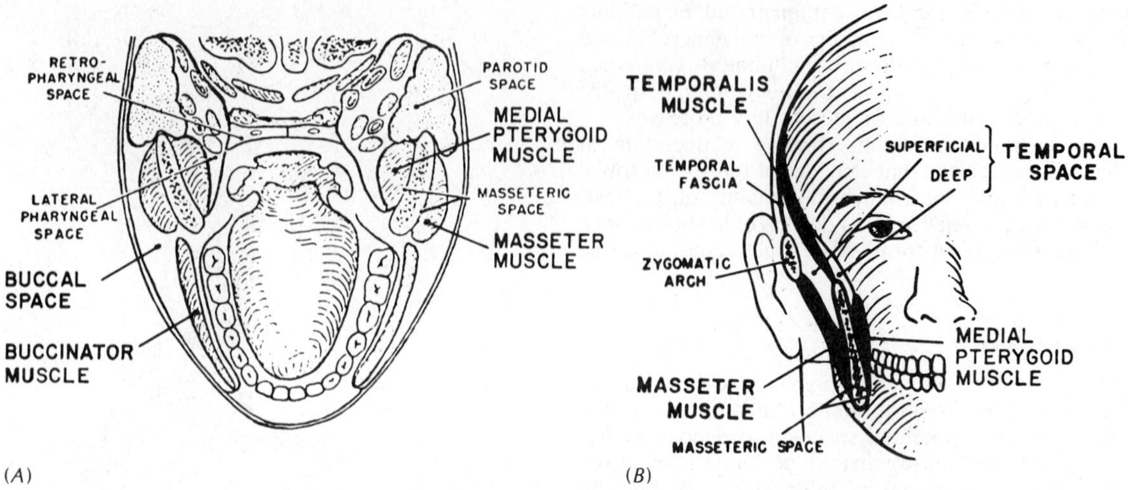

FIG. 3. Fascial spaces around the mouth and face. **(A)** Horizontal section at the level of the occlusal surface of the mandibular teeth. **(B)** Frontal view of the face. (From Chow et al.,[1] with permission.)

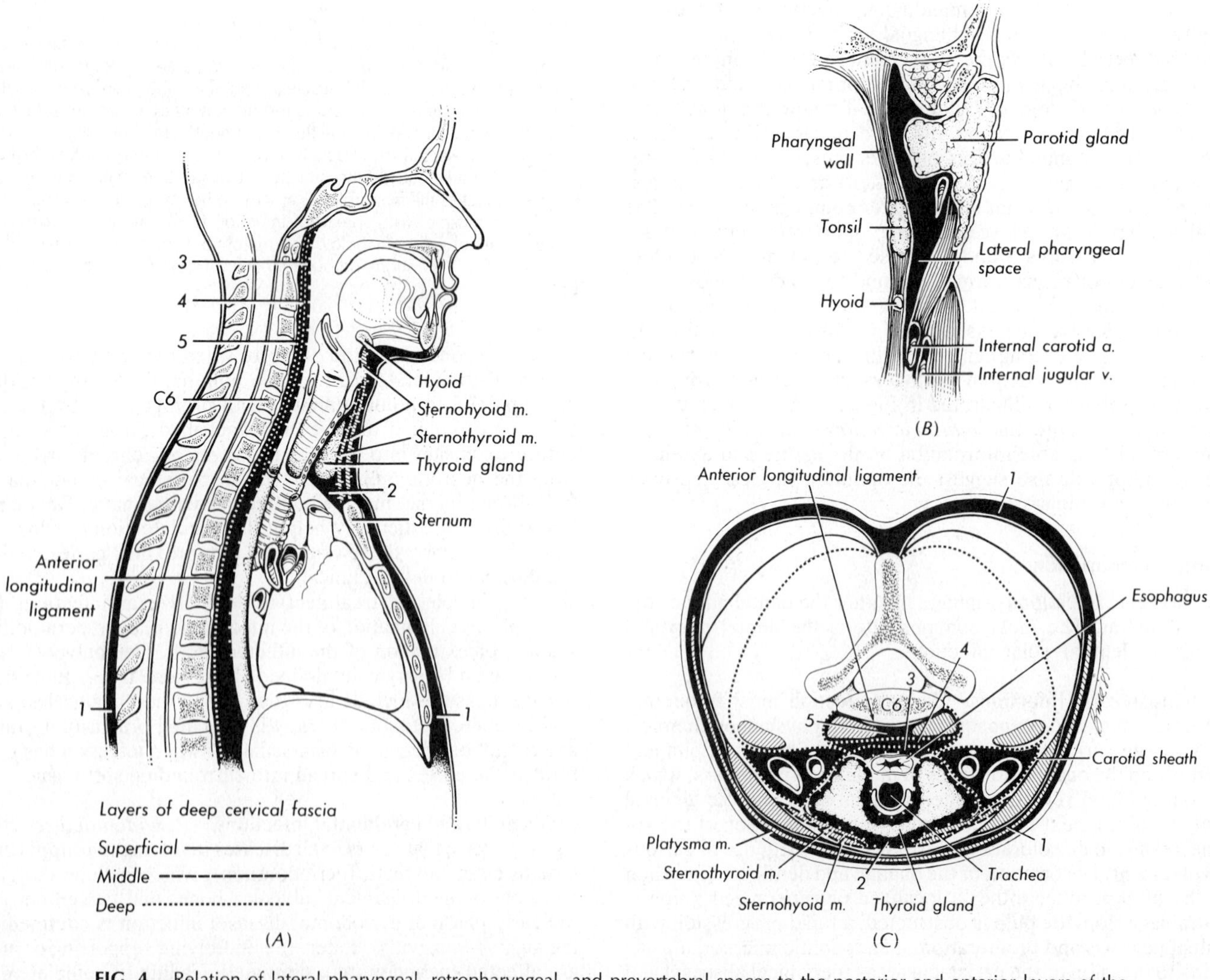

FIG. 4. Relation of lateral pharyngeal, retropharyngeal, and prevertebral spaces to the posterior and anterior layers of the deep cervical fascia (DCF). 1: Superficial space; 2: pretracheal space; 3: retropharyngeal space; 4: "danger" space; 5: prevertebral space. **(A)** Midsagittal section of the head and neck. **(B)** Coronal section in the suprahyoid region of the neck. **(C)** Cross section of the neck at the level of the thyroid isthmus.

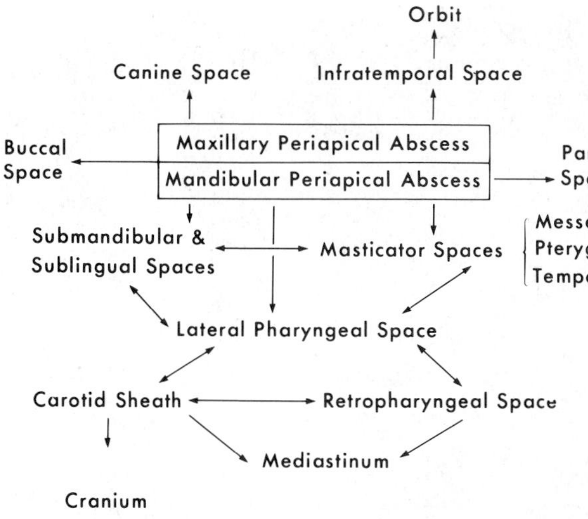

FIG. 5. Potential pathways of extension in deep fascial space infections.

GINGIVITIS. Acute and chronic inflammation of the gingiva is initiated by local irritation and microbial invasion.[11,16,22] Subgingival plaque is always present. In simple gingivitis, there is a bluish red discoloration, with swelling and thickening of the free gingival margin. A tendency for bleeding of the gums after eating or toothbrushing may be one of the earliest findings. There is usually no pain, but a mild fetor oris may be noticed. In acute necrotizing ulcerative gingivitis (Vincent's disease, or trench mouth), the patient typically experiences a sudden onset of pain in the gingiva that interferes with normal mastication. Necrosis of the gingiva occurs mainly in the interdental papilla and results in a marginated, punched-out, and eroded appearance. A superficial grayish pseudomembrane is formed, and a characteristic halitosis with altered taste sensation is present. There is usually associated fever, malaise, and regional lymphadenopathy. Treatment includes local débridement and lavage with oxidizing agents, which usually brings relief from pain within 24 hours. Antibiotic therapy with penicillin or metronidazole is indicated and is highly effective.[33,34]

PERIODONTITIS. Chronic inflammation of the periodontium is the major cause of tooth loss in adults. The destructive process proceeds insidiously, usually beginning in early adulthood. Subgingival plaque is always present, and both supragingival and subgingival calculi are usually abundant. Unlike pulpal infection in which drainage is frequently obstructed, periodontal infections drain freely, and patients experience little or no discomfort. Associated sensations include pressure and an itchy feeling in the gums and between the teeth, a bad taste in the mouth, hot and cold sensitivity, and vague pains in the jaws. The gingiva is inflamed and discolored, bleeds readily, and presents as periodontal pockets around the affected teeth. Frank pus can be readily expressed by digital pressure or may exude freely from the pockets. As periodontitis advances, the supporting tissues are destroyed, ultimately leading to loosening and exfoliation of teeth. Localized juvenile periodontitis is a particularly destructive form of periodontitis seen in adolescents and is characterized by rapid vertical bone loss affecting the first molar and incisor teeth. Plaque is usually minimal, and calculus is absent. A specific defect with impaired neutrophil chemotaxis has been demonstrated in this condition. Recent experience suggests excellent therapeutic results with systemic tetracycline or metronidazole combined with local periodontal treatment involving root débridement and surgical resection of inflamed periodontal tissues.[20,35–37]

PERIODONTAL ABSCESS. Periodontal abscesses may be focal or diffuse and present as red, fluctuant swelling of the gingiva, which is extremely tender to palpation. These abscesses are always in communication with a periodontal pocket from which pus can be readily expressed after probing. Treatment is surgical and aimed at drainage of loculated pus.

PERICORONITIS. Pericoronitis is an acute localized infection associated with gum flaps overlying a partially erupted or impacted wisdom tooth. Food debris and microorganisms become entrapped under the affected gingival tissues. If drainage is interrupted due to sudden swelling or trauma, infection extends along fascial planes of least resistance into adjacent soft tissues. The underlying alveolar bone is usually not involved. Clinically, the pericoronal tissues are erythematous and swollen. Digital pressure will produce a small amount of exudate from under the infected flap. Since the masticator spaces are often involved, marked trismus secondary to irritation of the masseter or medial pterygoid muscle is a prominent presenting feature. Treatment of pericoronitis includes gentle débridement and irrigation under the tissue flap. The use of antibiotics and incision and drainage may be necessary if cellulitis of fascial planes occurs. Excision of the operculum or extraction of the involved tooth may also be considered.

Deep Fascial Space Infections. Infections of either odontogenic or oropharyngeal origin may extend to potential fascial spaces of the lower part of the head and upper portion of the neck. These "space infections" can be conveniently divided into those around the face (masticator, buccal, canine, and parotid spaces), those in the suprahyoid region (submandibular, sublingual, and lateral pharyngeal spaces), and those involving the infrahyoid region or the total neck (retropharyngeal, "danger," and pretracheal spaces).[19,31,32]

MASTICATOR SPACES. Masticator spaces consist of the masseteric, pterygoid, and temporal spaces, all of which are well differentiated but intercommunicate with each other as well as with the buccal, submandibular, and lateral pharyngeal spaces (Fig. 3). Infection of the masticator spaces occurs most frequently from molar teeth, particularly the third molars (wisdom teeth). Clinically, the hallmark of masticator space infection is trismus and pain in the area of the body or ramus of the mandible. Swelling may not be a prominent finding, especially in the masseteric compartment, since infection exists deep in large muscle masses, which obscures or prevents clinically apparent swelling. When present, swelling tends to be brawny and indurated, which suggests the possibility of cervicofacial actinomycosis or mandibular osteomyelitis. If infection extends internally, it can involve an area close to the lateral pharyngeal wall and result in dysphagia. A true lateral pharyngeal space infection, however, is accompanied by displacement of the lateral pharyngeal wall toward the midline, a finding not present in masticator space infections. Infection of the deep temporal space usually originates from involvement of the posterior maxillary molar teeth. Very little external swelling is observed early in the course; if present, it usually affects the preauricular region and an area over the zygomatic arch. As infection progresses, the cheek, eyelids, and whole side of the face may be involved (Fig. 6). Infection may extend directly into the orbit via the inferior orbital fissure and produce proptosis, optic neuritis, and abducens nerve palsy.

BUCCAL, CANINE, AND PAROTID SPACES. As noted previously, infections arising from mandibular or maxillary bicuspid and molar teeth tend to extend in a lateral or buccal direction. The relation of the root apices to the origins of the buccinator muscle determines whether infection will exit intraorally into the buccal vestibule or extraorally into the buccal space (Fig. 2). Infection of the buccal space is readily diagnosed because of marked cheek swelling with minimal trismus and systemic symptoms. There is a great tendency to resolution with antibiotic therapy alone. Drainage, if required, is superficial and should be performed extraorally. Involvement of the maxillary incisors and canines may result in a canine space infection, which presents as dramatic swelling of the upper lip, canine fossa, and frequently the periorbital tissues. Pain is usually moderate, and

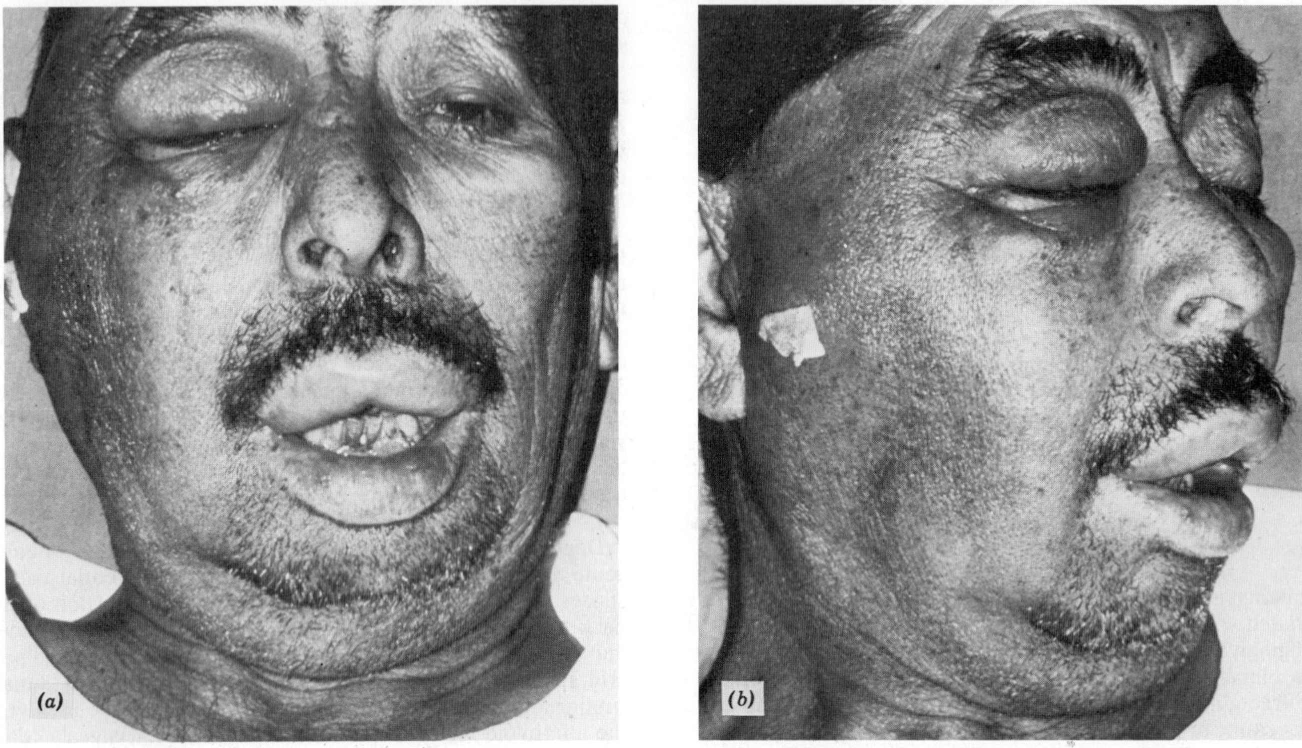

FIG. 6. Deep temporal space infection with spread to the right parotid space and the orbit. This patient developed right optic neuritis with permanent loss of vision in that eye. **(A)** Frontal view. **(B)** Lateral view. (From Chow, et al.,[1] with permission.)

systemic signs are minimal. Occasionally, a purulent maxillary sinusitis may result due to direct extension of infection into the adjoining antrum. Treatment consists of antibiotics and drainage, which can be accomplished intraorally. Parotid space infection from an odontogenic cause generally represents secondary spread from a masseteric space infection in the area of the ramus of the mandible (Fig. 3). There is marked swelling of the angle of the jaw without associated trismus. Pain may be intense and accompanied by high fever and chills. Because of its close relationship with the posterior aspect of the lateral pharyngeal space, a parotid space infection carries the potential risk of direct extension into the "danger" and visceral spaces and hence to the posterior mediastinum (Fig. 4).

SUBMANDIBULAR AND SUBLINGUAL SPACES. These two spaces are separated by the mylohyoid muscle (Fig. 2), and the submandibular space is further divided into the submaxillary and submental spaces. Infection in these spaces usually arises from the second and third mandibular molar teeth since their root apices lie inferior to the mylohyoid muscle. There is typical swelling, although much less trismus in contradistinction to masseteric space infection since the major muscles of mastication are usually not involved. Submandibular odontogenic infection should be distinguished from submandibular sialadenitis and lymphadenitis that are due to other causes. Therapy includes antibiotics, dental extraction, and extraoral surgical drainage. Infection of the sublingual space generally arises from mandibular incisors since their root apices lie above the mylohyoid muscle. Clinically, this space infection presents as a brawny, erythematous, tender swelling of the floor of the mouth that begins close to the mandible and spreads toward the midline or beyond. Some elevation of the tongue may be noted in late states. Surgical drainage of the sublingual space should be performed intraorally by an incision through the mucosa parallel to Wharton's duct. If the submandibular space is also to be drained, both spaces can be reached through a submandibular approach.

The term *Ludwig's angina* has been loosely applied to a heterogenous array of infections involving the sublingual, submaxillary, and submandibular spaces.[38] However, for therapeutic and prognostic purposes, it is desirable to restrict this diagnosis to cases that conform to the following classic description: (*1*) the infection is always bilateral, (*2*) both the submandibular and sublingual spaces are involved, (*3*) the infection is a rapidly spreading indurated cellulitis without abscess formation of lymphatic involvement, and (*4*) the infection begins in the floor of the mouth. A dental source of infection has been found in 50–90 percent of reported cases. The second and third mandibular molars are most commonly involved. Clinically, patients present with a brawny boardlike swelling in the submandibular spaces that does not pit on pressure (Fig. 7). The mouth is usually held open and the floor elevated, which pushes the tongue to the roof of the mouth. Eating and swallowing are difficult, and respiration may be impaired by obstruction from the tongue. A rapid progression of the infection will result in edema of the neck and glottis and may precipitate asphyxiation. Fever and systemic toxicity are usually present and may be severe. Treatment requires high doses of parenteral antibiotics, airway monitoring, early intubation or tracheostomy when required, soft tissue decompression, and surgical drainage.

LATERAL PHARYNGEAL SPACE. The lateral pharyngeal space (also known as the pharyngomaxillary space) in the lateral aspect of the neck is shaped like an inverted cone, with its base at the skull and its apex at the hyoid bone (Fig. 4). Its medial wall is contiguous with the carotid sheath, and it lies deep to the pharyngeal constrictor muscle. Infection of the lateral pharyngeal space may result from pharyngitis, tonsillitis, parotitis, otitis, mastoiditis, as well as odontogenic infection, especially if the masticator spaces are primarily involved. If the anterior compartment is infected, the patient will exhibit fever, chills, marked pain, trismus, swelling below the angle of the mandible, dysphagia, and medial displacement of the lateral pharyngeal wall. Although not prominent, dyspnea can occur. Posterior compartment infection is characterized by septicemia with little pain or trismus. Swelling is usually internal and deep and can often be missed because it is behind the palatopharyngeal arch.

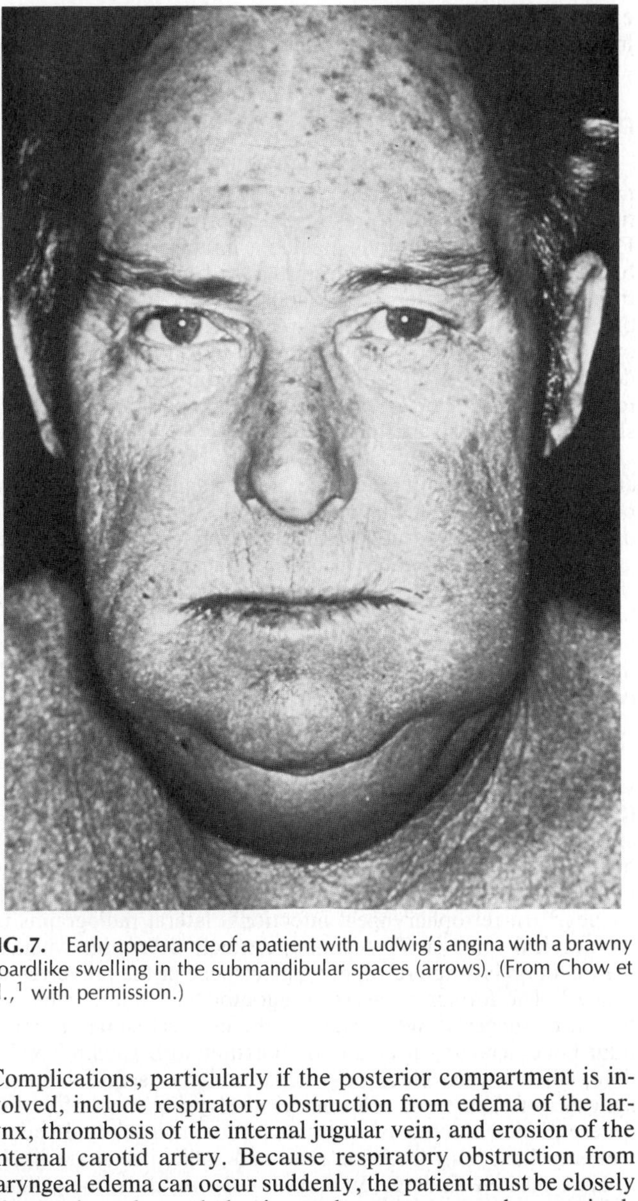

FIG. 7. Early appearance of a patient with Ludwig's angina with a brawny boardlike swelling in the submandibular spaces (arrows). (From Chow et al.,[1] with permission.)

Complications, particularly if the posterior compartment is involved, include respiratory obstruction from edema of the larynx, thrombosis of the internal jugular vein, and erosion of the internal carotid artery. Because respiratory obstruction from laryngeal edema can occur suddenly, the patient must be closely observed, and prophylactic tracheostomy may be required. Treatment includes high levels of antibiotics and surgical drainage. It is usually prudent to wait for the infection to localize before drainage is attempted unless respiratory obstruction or hemorrhage necessitates early surgical intervention.

RETROPHARYNGEAL, DANGER, AND PRETRACHEAL SPACES. The retropharyngeal space comprises the posterior part of the visceral compartment in which the esophagus, trachea, and thyroid glands are enclosed by the middle layer of deep cervical fascia (Fig. 4). It lies behind the hypopharynx and the esophagus and extends inferiorly into the superior mediastinum to about the level from T1 to T2. Posterior to this compartment lies the "danger" space, which descends directly into the posterior mediastinum to the level of the diaphragm. Infection of the retropharyngeal space may result from contiguous infection of the lateral pharyngeal space or from lymphatic spread from more distant sites to involve the retropharyngeal lymph nodes. Dysphagia, dyspnea, nuchal rigidity, esophageal regurgitation, as well as high fever and chills may be present. Bulging of the posterior pharyngeal wall may be observed. Lateral soft tissue radiographs of the neck may reveal marked widening of the retropharyngeal space. Infection of the retropharyngeal space is potentially life-threatening and requires prompt surgical drainage. Complications include hemorrhage and spontaneous rupture into the airway with asphyxiation, laryngeal spasm, bronchial erosion, and thrombosis of the jugular vein. The pretracheal space comprises the anterior portion of the visceral compartment and completely surrounds the trachea. Most commonly, infections reach this space through perforations of the anterior esophageal wall, occasionally through contiguous extension from a retropharyngeal space infection. The clinical presentation is characterized by severe dyspnea, but hoarseness may be the first complaint. Swallowing is difficult, and regurgitation of fluids through the nose may occur. A pretracheal space infection is always serious because of possible extension into the mediastinum, and prompt surgical drainage is critically important.

Complications of Odontogenic Infections

Complications of odontogenic infections can occur either by hematogenous spread or by direct extension. Transient bacteremia is common during or after various dental procedures, especially extraction of infected teeth.[39] The temporal relationship between these procedures and subsequent bacterial endocarditis and cardiovascular prosthetic infections is well documented.[10] Reports of infected total hip replacements after dental procedures add further concern.[22,40] Prophylactic antibiotic treatment during dental procedures, although frequently used, remains a controversial issue, especially in the absence of pre-existing valvular heart disease. Complications of odontogenic infections secondary to direct extension include mediastinal spread,[41] intracranial suppuration (especially cavernous sinus thrombosis),[42] suppurative jugular thrombophlebitis, carotid artery erosion,[43] maxillary sinusitis,[1] and osteomyelitis.[44] Acute mediastinitis and intracranial suppuration secondary to odontogenic infections are relatively uncommon in the postantibiotic era.

Suppurative Jugular Thrombophlebitis and Carotid Artery Erosion. These are uncommon complications of oropharyngeal or odontogenic infections in the postantibiotic era. Extension of infection to the carotid sheath, which encloses both the internal jugular vein and the internal carotid artery, usually arises from the lateral pharyngeal space.[43] Since the carotid sheath space in this area is relatively compact with little areolar connective tissue, there is little tendency of spread up and down this vascular sheath, with the exception of possible retrograde thrombophlebitis and intracranial extension. The major concern is protracted septicemia and erosion of the carotid artery or one of its branches.

The onset of suppurative jugular thrombophlebitis is acute, with shaking chills, spiking fevers, and profound prostration. Localizing signs of pain and swelling at the angle of the jaw, tenderness and induration along the sternocleidomastoid muscle, and swelling of the lateral pharyngeal wall with dysphagia and neck ridigity are usually present. However, these findings may be subtle, and their clinical significance may not be fully recognized until postmortem. Systemic evidence of infection such as septic pulmonary emboli and metastatic abscesses to the brain, lungs, kidneys, and joints is not infrequent. The usual recommended treatment consists of external drainage of the lateral pharyngeal space and ligation of the internal jugular vein. *Fusobacterium necrophorum* has been the organism most frequently isolated from blood cultures,[45,46] and mortality remains high. Important warning signals that may herald major hemorrhage due to erosion of the carotid artery include multiple episodes of minor bleeding from the oral cavity or ear and ecchymosis of oral and cervical tissue. With the onset of major hemorrhage, primary considerations are maintenance and protection of the airway because death may occur more rapidly from asphyxiation than from hemorrhagic shock. Appropriate treatment consists of emergency carotid ligation after the restoration of blood volume and pressure. Hemorrhage is controlled by local compression until ligation can be attempted.

The mortality for emergency ligation ranges from 30 to 50 percent. Cerebrovascular accident is a significant complication in survivors.

Septic Cavernous Sinus Thrombosis. This dreaded complication is fortunately rare in the postantibiotic era. Facial furuncles and purulent paranasal sinusitis were the major predisposing conditions. Infection of the maxillary teeth was the most common dental cause. Eagleton[47] described six criteria for the diagnosis of septic cavernous sinus thrombosis to help distinguish it from other less lethal infections, particularly those of the ethmoid sinus and the orbit: (*1*) a known site of infection; (*2*) evidence of blood stream invasion; (*3*) early signs of venous obstruction in the retina, conjunctiva, and eyelid; (*4*) paresis of the third, fourth, and sixth cranial nerves resulting from inflammatory edema; (*5*) abscess formation in neighboring soft tissue; and (*6*) evidence of meningeal irritation. Before the antibiotic era, septic cavernous sinus thrombosis was virtually always fatal. Mortality since 1970 has been markedly reduced to 15–30 percent.[43,48,49] Treatment requires early recognition, high-dose intravenous antibiotics, and surgical decompression of the underlying predisposing infection. Anticoagulation and steroids are not indicated.

Maxillary Sinusitis. In many people, the roots of the maxillary molars lie proximate to the maxillary antrum. At times, congenital bony defects occur, with the root adjacent to the sinus membrane. In these cases, sinusitis can result from direct extension of an odontogenic infection or from perforation of the sinus floor during extraction of a maxillary tooth.[1] The clinical presentation of secondary sinus involvement is similar to that of primary sinus disease.

Osteomyelitis of the Jaws. The mandible is much more susceptible to osteomyelitis than is the maxilla, mainly because the cortical plates of the latter are thin and its medullary tissues are relatively poor in vascular supply.[44] In view of the large number of odontogenic infections and the intimate relationship of teeth to the medullary cavity, it is surprising that osteomyelitis of the jaws is not more frequent. When osteomyelitis occurs, there is usually a predisposing condition that affects host resistance such as a compound fracture, previous irradiation, osteopetrosis, Paget's disease, diabetes mellitis, or steroid therapy. With initiation of infection, the intramedullary pressure markedly increases, further compromising blood supply and leading to bone necrosis. Pus travels through the haversian and perforating canals, accumulates beneath the periosteum, and elevates it from the cortex. If pus continues to accumulate, the periosteum is eventually penetrated, and mucosal and cutaneous abscesses and fistulas may develop. As the inflammatory process becomes more chronic, granulation tissue is formed. Spicules of necrotic and nonviable bone may become either totally isolated (sequestrum) or encased in a sheath of new bone (involucrum). Severe mandibular pain is a common symptom and may be accompanied by anesthesia or hypoesthesia on the affected side. In protracted cases, mandibular trismus may develop. A clinical variant is chronic sclerosing osteomyelitis associated with a proliferative periostitis. Clinically, it is characterized by a localized, hard, nontender swelling over the mandible. Actinomycosis and radiation necrosis are two common causes of this form of osteomyelitis of the jaws.

Treatment of osteomyelitis of the jaws is complicated by the presence of teeth and persistent exposure to the oral environment. Antibiotic therapy needs to be prolonged, often requiring weeks to months. Adjunctive therapy with hyperbaric oxygen may prove beneficial in hastening the healing process, particularly for the chronic sclerosing variety.[44,50] Surgical management including sequestrectomy, saucerization, decortication, and closed-wound suction irrigation may occasionally be necessary. Rarely, in advanced cases the entire segment of the infected jaw may have to be resected.

Diagnostic Approaches

Specimen Collection and Processing. It is imperative that the normal resident oral flora be excluded during specimen collection in order that culture results be appropriately interpreted. For closed-space infections, needle aspiration of loculated pus by an extraoral approach is desirable, and specimens should be transported immediately to the laboratory under anaerobic conditions. For intraoral lesions, direct microscopic examination of stained smears often provides more useful information than do culture results from surface swabs. Gram and acid-fast stains for bacteria and potassium hydroxide preparations for fungi should be routinely performed. Tissue biopsy specimens examined for typical histopathology and the presence of microbial antigens by immunofluorescence are particularly useful in suspected mycobacterial, fungal, and viral infections. In chronic osteomyelitis, soft tissue swelling and draining fistulas are frequently present. Aspirates from the adjacent soft tissue swellings may be valuable, but cultures from the sinus tracts may be misleading since these sinus tracts are often colonized by organisms that do not reflect what is actually occurring within the infected bone.[51] Bone biopsies for histopathology and culture are often required for a definitive diagnosis.

Imaging Techniques for the Localization of Infection. Ultrasonography, radionuclide scanning, and computed tomography (CT) are particularly useful for the localization of deep fascial space infections of the head and neck.[52,53] A lateral radiograph of the neck may demonstrate compression or deviation of the tracheal air column or the presence of gas within necrotic soft tissues.[54] In retropharyngeal infections, lateral radiographs of the cervical spine or CT scanning can help determine whether the infection is in the retropharyngeal space or the prevertebral space.[55] The former suggests an odontogenic source, whereas the latter suggests involvement of the cervical spine. Technetium bone scanning used in combination with gallium- or indium-labeled white blood cells is particularly useful for the diagnosis of acute or chronic osteomyelitis and for the differentiation of infection or trauma from malignancy. In acute osteomyelitis, both the bone scan and gallium scan are likely to have positive findings. In chronic osteomyelitis, the gallium or indium scans may be negative, but the technetium may be positive. Similarly, both scans may be positive during infection and trauma, while neoplasms in the bone may be associated only with a positive bone scan but negative gallium or indium scan results.

Therapeutic Considerations

Dental Caries and Periodontitis. For both caries prevention and treatment of periodontitis, the clinical goal must continue to be control of the supragingival and subgingival plaques. With the emerging concept of microbial specificity in these infections, the prospect of specific antimicrobial therapy appears increasingly promising.[10,20,37,56] In localized juvenile periodontitis, for example, systemic tetracycline therapy directed against *A. actinomycetemcomitans* and combined with local periodontal treatment has yielded excellent results.[35,36] Unfortunately, the administration of tetracycline to children under 5 years of age can cause staining of the permanent dentition and is not generally recommended. Similarly, in advanced periodontitis, several double-blind studies have indicated that systemic metronidazole plus mechanical débridement of the root surfaces is more effective than placebo treatment plus mechanical débridement.[37] The successful treatment of acute necrotizing ulcerative gingivitis with metronidazole has been well documented, and in fact such treatment by Shinn et al.[33] led to the discovery of metronidazole as a unique anaerobicidal agent.

Several topical agents appear to have cariostatic effects in humans. By far the most effective is fluoride. Fluoride forms a complex with the apatite crystals in dentin by replacing the hydroxyl group, thereby lending strength to the entire structure.[10] Further, fluoride promotes remineralization of the carious lesions and also exerts a bacteriostatic effect. Topical chlorhexidine is another compound with useful anticariogenic properties. It acts as a cationic detergent killing a wide range of bacteria and is retained on the oral surfaces for prolonged periods to prevent plaque advancement.[22] Unfortunately, it has a bitter taste and stains the enamel and tongue. Prolonged application may also promote the emergence of resistant microorganisms. Among the antibiotics, although both penicillin and tetracycline have cariostatic effects in animal models, only topical application of vancomycin has been shown to reduce dental caries with some degree of success in humans.[10] Other important approaches to caries and periodontitis prevention include the adoption of improved oral hygiene through more effective educational programs,[13] a reduction of cariogenic oral flora by diet modification with sucrose substitutes, and active immunization against caries by the use of vaccines prepared from *S. mutans*.[57–59]

Suppurative Odontogenic Infections. The most important therapeutic modality for pyogenic odontogenic infections is surgical drainage and removal of necrotic tissue. Needle aspiration by the extraoral route can be particularly helpful both for microbiologic sampling and for evacuation of pus. The need for definitive restoration or extraction of the infected tooth, the primary source of infection, is readily apparent. Deep periodontal scaling and endodontic treatments with root filling may be required in most instances. Effective surgical management requires a thorough understanding of the most likely anatomic routes of spread. The neighboring potential fascial spaces should be carefully and systematically surveyed. The optimum timing for incision and drainage is equally important. Premature incision into an unlocalized cellulitis in an ill-conceived search for pus can disrupt the normal physiologic barriers and cause further diffusion and extension of infection.

Antibiotic therapy is important in halting the local spread of infection and in preventing hematogenous dissemination. Antimicrobial agents are generally indicated if fever and regional lymphadenitis are present or when infection has perforated the bony cortex and spread into surrounding soft tissue. Severely immunocompromised patients are particularly at risk for unhalted and spreading orofacial infections, and empirical broad-spectrum antimicrobial therapy in these patients is warranted.[60,61] The choice of specific antibiotics for the treatment of odontogenic infections requires not so much the results of bacterial culture and sensitivity as knowledge of the indigenous organisms that colonize the teeth, gums, and mucous membranes. By far most of these organisms, including both anaerobes and aerobes, are sensitive to penicillin.[60–63] Thus, penicillin monotherapy in doses appropriate for the severity of infection remains a good choice. The problem of β-lactamase production and penicillin resistance among *Bacteroides* sp., particularly B. *melaninogenicus*, has been increasingly recognized, and treatment failure with penicillin in odontogenic infections due to such β-lactamase–producing strains has been reported.[64–66] Thus, in patients with life-threatening deep fascial space infections and in patients who have had an unfavorable or delayed response to penicillin, alternative therapy with a broader spectrum against anaerobes as well as facultative gram-negative bacilli may be considered. Penicillin-allergic patients may be treated with either clindamycin or cefoxitin. Ambulatory patients with less serious odontogenic infections may be treated with amoxicillin, ampicillin, or doxycycline. Erythromycin and tetracycline are not preferred in orofacial odontogenic infections because of emergence of resistance among oropharyngeal anaerobes and some strains of streptococci.[60] Metronidazole, although highly active against anaerobic gram-negative bacilli and spirochetes, is only moderately active against anaerobic cocci and is not active against aerobes, including streptococci.[1,61,67] Except in acute necrotizing gingivitis and in advanced periodontitis,[33,34,37] it should not be used as a single agent in odontogenic infections. In the compromised host such as the patient with leukemia and severe neutropenia after chemotherapy, it is prudent to cover for facultative gram-negative bacilli as well, and agents with broad-spectrum activity against both aerobes and anaerobes are desirable (Table 2).

TABLE 2. Empirical Antibiotic Regimens for Odontogenic Soft Tissue Infections

Normal host
Penicillin G, 1–4 million units iv q4–6h
Clindamycin, 600 mg iv q6–8h
Cefoxitin, 1–2 g iv q6h
Compromised host (each of following ± an aminoglycoside)
Piperacillin, 3 g iv q4h
Cefoxitin, 1–2 g iv q6h
Cefotetan, 2 g iv q12h
Imipenem/cilastatin, 500 mg iv q6h
Ticarcillin/clavulanate, 3.0 g/0.1 g iv q4–6h

OROFACIAL NONODONTOGENIC INFECTIONS

Nonodontogenic infections of the oral cavity most frequently occur secondary to chemical, thermal, or traumatic injury. Virtually all infectious microorganisms can present with intraoral manifestations, particularly sexually transmitted agents and childhood viral enanthems. Cancer patients with mucositis from cytotoxic drugs are especially prone to acute and chronic opportunistic infections of the oral cavity, particularly candidiasis, aspergillosis, mucormycosis, herpetic gingivostomatitis, and mixed gram-negative infections.[68,69] In this section, some of the conditions affecting primarily the oral mucosa and salivary glands in which an infectious cause is either proved or suspected will be briefly discussed.

Infections of the Oral Mucosa

Noma, or Gangrenous Stomatitis. Noma, or gangrenous stomatitis, also known as cancrum oris, is an acute, fulminating, and gangrenous infection of the oral and facial tissues. It usually occurs in the presence of severe debilitation and malnutrition, and children are most often affected. The earliest lesion is a small, painful, red spot or vesicle on the attached gingiva in the premolar or molar regions of the mandible. A necrotic ulcer rapidly develops and undermines the deeper tissue. Painful cellulitis of the lips and cheeks is observed as the lesion extends outward in a conelike fashion. Within a short period, sloughing of necrotic soft tissues occurs and exposes underlying bone, teeth, and deeper tissues.

Fusospirochetal organisms such as *Borrelia vincentii* and *Fusobacterium nucleatum* are consistently cultured from noma lesions. *Bacteroides melaninogenicus* may also be present. Biopsy specimens of tissue from the advancing lesion show a mat of predominantly gram-negative threadlike bacteria that cannot be positively identified.[70] Thus, this lesion bears a similarity to acute necrotizing ulcerative gingivitis in several respects but appears to be more focal and destructive, involving deeper tissues beyond the gingiva. Treatment of noma requires high doses of intravenous penicillin. Every effort should be directed to correct the dehydration and underlying malnutrition and debility. Loose teeth and sequestra may be removed, but saucerization should be avoided. Healing is by secondary intention. Serious mutilation and facial deformity may require subsequent cosmetic surgery.

Apthous Stomatitis. Aphthous ulcers are the most common cause of recurrent oral lesions. This entity must be distinguished from oral ulceration due to herpes simplex, coxsackievirus, agranulocytosis, and Behçet's and other diseases. Three major clinical variants are recognized: (*1*) minor aphthous ulcers, (*2*) major aphthous ulcers, and (*3*) herpetiform aphthous ulcers.[71] The true cause of aphthous ulcerations is not known, although a number of infectious agents including viruses have been implicated. The most prevailing hypothesis suggests that the mechanism causing the ulceration is autoimmune in nature. Circulating humoral antibodies and sensitized T lymphocytes active against oral mucosa have been demonstrated in patients with aphthous ulcers.[71] Furthermore, the active T lymphocytes undergo a phase of rapid proliferation just before the onset of ulceration. The origin of the autoantibodies is not clear, and no common antigenic factor between oral epithelium and the indigenous microflora has been demonstrated.

In their most characteristic form, minor aphthous ulcers appear as a number of small ulcers on the buccal and labial mucosa, the floor of the mouth, or the tongue. The palatal soft tissues are rarely involved. Moreover, the ulcers are concentrated in the anterior part of the oral cavity, whereas the pharynx and tonsillar fauces are rarely implicated. A prodromal stage is usually present. The ulcers appear gray-yellow, often with a raised and erythematous margin, and are exquisitely painful. Lymph node enlargement is seen only with secondary bacterial infection. The course of ulceration varies from a few days to a little over 2 weeks and is followed by spontaneous healing. Major aphthous ulcers are more protracted and last up to several months. All areas of the oral cavity including the soft palate and tonsillar areas may be involved. Long periods of remission may be followed by intervals of intense ulcer activity. Herpetiform aphthous ulcers are small and multiple and characteristically affect the lateral margins and tip of the tongue. The ulcers are gray, without a delineating erythematous border, and are extremely painful, which makes eating and speaking difficult. Despite its name, there is little clinical resemblance to an acute herpetic gingivostomatitis. Although intranuclear inclusions have been demonstrated in herpetiform aphthous ulcers, there is no evidence to suggest that these inclusions bear any relationship to presence of viruses.

The treatment of aphthous ulcers is primarily symptomatic. Strict oral hygiene should be maintained, and the use of antiseptic mouthwashes may be helpful in temporarily reducing secondary infection. Local anaesthetic lozenges or gels may be used as a last resort for brief periods of pain relief. Topical or systemic steroids may be beneficial in selected people with extensive disease, but caution must be exercised in their administration.

Mucositis and Stomatitis in the Severely Immunocompromised. Much of what is known about management of oromucosal infections has been studied in cancer patients being treated with radiotherapy, chemotherapy, and bone marrow transplantation.[68,72] Other patient groups that develop oromucosal complications include those undergoing solid organ transplantation, patients with the acquired immunodeficiency syndrome (AIDS),[73] and those with autoimmune diseases associated with xerostomia and systemic immunosuppression. The underlying mechanism appears to be a breakdown of the mucosal epithelium that leads to mucositis, secondary bacterial or fungal infection, or reactivation of latent viral infection. Oral candidiasis, herpes simplex, varicella-zoster, and cytomegalovirus infections are the most common manifestations. Mucositis that complicates radiation or chemotherapy most commonly involves the nonkeratinized oral epithelium, including the buccal and labial mucosa, soft palate, oropharynx, floor of the mouth, and ventral and lateral surfaces of the tongue. Ulceration and pseudomembrane formation are evident usually between 4 and 7 days after the initiation of chemotherapy when the rate of destruction of the basal epithelium exceeds that of proliferation of new cells. The clinical manifestations may be quite variable. The lesions are often protracted in duration and may not be associated with an inflammatory reaction, thereby masking the usual signs and symptoms. Pain or tenderness may be the only abnormal finding. Since the etiologic agents of infection cannot be readily predicted on clinical grounds alone in such patients, specific microbiologic diagnosis by culture, histopathology or antigen detection techniques is critical for appropriate treatment. Topical as well as systemic antimicrobial agents may be indicated along with antiseptic (e.g., chlorhexidine) and anesthetic (e.g., benzydamine, viscous lidocaine, etc.) applications.[74] Frequent saline rinses may reduce mucosal irritation, remove thickened secretions or debris, and increase moisture in the mouth.[68] Coating agents such as milk of magnesia or aluminum hydroxide gel (Amphojel) have been useful for the symptomatic relief of painful oral lesions. Topical or oral cytoprotective agents (e.g., sucralfate) or nonsteroidal anti-inflammatory analgesics (e.g., benzydamine, salicylates, etc.) may provide additional benefit, but further controlled clinical trials are required to assess their appropriate indications and efficacy.[74,75] Meticulous oral and dental hygiene, effective management of xerostomia, selective suppression of oropharyngeal microbial colonization, and early control of reactivation by latent viral infections appear to be the critical steps to prevent and reduce the overall morbidity of oromucosal infections in the severely immunocompromised.[68,76]

Infections of the Salivary Gland

Sialadenitis, or infection of salivary tissue, is a relatively common disease. Sialolithiasis in elderly patients leads to ductal obstruction and secondarily to suppuration of the salivary gland and appears to be a major predisposing condition. In this regard, stones of Wharton's duct are much more common than are those of Stensen's duct, and obstructive sialadenitis is much more frequent with the submandibular than the parotid gland.[77] Other predisposing factors for sialadenitis include dehydration, general debility, sialogogic drugs, and trauma.

Suppurative Parotitis. Acute bacterial parotitis is a specific clinical entity primarily affecting the elderly, malnourished, dehydrated, or postoperative patient. Clinically, there is a sudden onset of firm, erythematous swelling of the pre- and postauricular areas that extends to the angle of the mandible. This is associated with exquisite local pain and tenderness. Systemic findings of high fevers, chills, and marked toxicity are generally present. Progression of the infection may lead to massive swelling of the neck, respiratory obstruction, septicemia, and osteomyelitis of the adjacent facial bones. Staphylococci have been the predominant isolates, and antibiotic therapy should include an antistaphylococcal agent. Early surgical drainage and decompression of the gland are generally required since spontaneous drainage is uncommon.

Chronic Bacterial Parotitis. In this condition, parotitis is recurrent with intermittent acute exacerbations. There is chronic, low-grade, bacterial infection resulting in functional destruction of the salivary gland. Pus, when obtained directly from the gland, usually reveals the growth of staphylococci or mixed oral aerobes and anaerobes. Sialography during remission may reveal a sialectatic pattern of pooling of contrast medium that suggests multiple cystic cavities in place of the normal acinar pattern. Chronic parotitis may be confused with Sjögren syndrome, a noninfectious illness characterized by the triad of xerostomia, keratoconjunctivitis, and systemic autoimmune disease such as rheumatoid arthritis, lupus erythematosus, scleroderma, periarteritis nodosa, and polymyositis. The presence of associated temporomandibular arthritis or arthralgia should strongly suggest Sjögren syndrome rather than chronic bacterial parotitis.

Therapy for chronic parotitis should initially be conservative and consist of systemic antibiotics and ductal saline or antibiotic irrigations. Parotidectomy may eventually be required for people with long-standing infection.

Viral Parotitis. Mumps parotitis is characterized by the rapid, painful swelling of one or both parotid glands within 2–3 weeks after exposure. A prodromal phase of preauricular pain, fever, chills, and headache may be present. Other viral causes of parotitis include influenza and enteroviruses, and specific neutralizing antibody titers may be required for distinguishing these from true mumps. Mumps parotitis usually resolves spontaneously in 5–10 days. Symptomatic relief of pain and fever is necessary, and prevention of dehydration and secondary bacterial infection is essential.

MISCELLANEOUS INFECTIONS OF THE NECK AND HEAD

In the antibiotic era, dental causes have surpassed oropharyngeal and tonsillar sources of deep neck infections.[78] Other miscellaneous infections of the neck and head include suppurative cervical adenitis, infected embryologic cysts of the neck, various infections secondary to human and animal bites, maxillofacial trauma, irradiation, and surgical procedures of the head and neck.

Cervical Adenitis

Cervical adenitis, which presents unilaterally in association with warm, tender, enlarged, and fluctuant lymph nodes, is usually due to pyogenic infections. Its anatomic location in relationship to major cervical landmarks will provide the clinical clues to the primary source of infection.[31,79] Bilateral acute cervical adenitis generally suggests a nonspecific or viral cause, toxoplasmosis, or group A streptotoccal infection. A more chronic or recurrent cervical adenitis should suggest the possibility of typical or atypical mycobacteriosis, human immunodeficiency virus infection, Epstein-Barr virus or cytomegalovirus mononucleosis, cat-scratch fever, actinomycosis, sarcoidosis, as well as lymphoproliferative and neoplastic disorders.

Infected Embryologic Cysts

Three distinct embryologic abnormalities can present with infection in the neck. They are (*1*) cystic hygroma or lymphangioma, (*2*) pharyngeal and bronchial cleft cysts, and (*3*) thyroglossal duct cysts.[78,79] Cystic hygroma is associated with a diffuse tumor mass usually evident within the first 2 years of life. It commonly involves the lower aspect of the neck, but it can appear anywhere in the cervical region. It is probably an abnormal development of lymphatic vessels from the jugular lymphatic sacs. Sudden enlargement by infection or hemorrhage into a lymphangioma may cause obstruction of the upper airways. Pharyngeal cleft cysts can develop from the first, second, or third pharyngeal clefts, although the second is most common. They usually present in childhood as fistulas or masses just posterior to the angle of the mandible along the anterior border of the sternocleidomastoid muscle. The mass can fluctuate in size, and enlargement can be associated with upper respiratory infection. Thyroglossal duct cysts originate from the foramen cecum of the tongue and descend through the body of the hyoid bone into the anterior portion of the neck. Any residual secretory lining may give rise to a thyroglossal duct cyst that is midline in location. It can cause respiratory obstruction or fistula formation if secondarily infected. Treatment of these congenital abnormalities during secondary bacterial infection requires broad-spectrum antibiotics such as a cephalosporin. Definitive surgical excision to prevent recurrence should be performed after complete resolution of the acute process.

Suppurative Thyroiditis

Although infections of the thyroid gland are rare, they are potentially life-threatening. Such infections may arise by a variety of pathways including hematogenous dissemination, direct spread from an adjacent deep fascial space infection, an infected thyroglossal fistula, or anterior perforation of the esophagus. Pre-existing diseases of the thyroid gland such as a goiter or adenoma are frequently present.[80,81] Acute suppurative thyroiditis is characterized by fever, local pain, tenderness, warmth, erythema, and symptoms of dysphagia, dysphonia, hoarseness, or pharyngitis. The infection may involve single or both lobes, and fluctuance may not be apparent until late in the course. Subacute thyroiditis may have similar local findings, but systemic manifestations are not as severe and tend to be more self-limiting. Laboratory investigation of thyroid infections should include ultrasonography, radionuclide scanning, and lateral radiographs or CT scanning of the neck for evidence of peritracheal extension; thyroid function tests; and diagnostic needle aspiration for microbiologic diagnosis. *Staphylococcus aureus, S. pyogenes*, and *S. pneumoniae* are most frequently isolated. Other pathogens include *H. influenzae*, viridans streptococci, *Eikonella corrodens, Bacteroides, Peptostreptococcus*, and *Actinomyces* species. Treatment requires specific antimicrobial agents and appropriate surgical drainage.

Infections from Bites, Maxillofacial Trauma, Irradiation, and Surgical Wounds

Human and Animal Bites. Human and animal bite wounds to the head and neck are relatively common. Although they may look innocuous initially, serious complications can occur. For this reason, empirical antibiotic therapy is recommended when the bite wound involves the face, head, or neck. Recent studies that used adequate anaerobic culture techniques indicate indigenous oral flora rather than the skin flora to be the major source of bite wound infections.[82] Streptococci, *Eikenella corrodens*, and *S. aureus* are the most prevalent facultative organisms, and *Bacteriodes*, and *Peptostreptococcus* are the most common anaerobic isolates. Penicillin-resistant gram-negative rods are infrequent. *Eikenella corrodens* is unique in that it is susceptible to penicillin and ampicillin but resistant to oxacillin, methicillin, nafcillin, and clindamycin.[63] In animal bite wounds, *Pasteurella multocida* has been a common cause of infection.[83] It is susceptible to penicillin. In view of these findings, penicillin remains the antibiotic of choice for initial therapy for both human and animal bite wounds.

Maxillofacial Trauma. Automobile and motorcycle accidents cause the most severe maxillofacial trauma. Particular attention should be paid to fractures that may traverse sinus cavities and teeth-bearing areas of the maxilla or mandible since secondary infection rates at these sites are particularly high. Treatment is aimed not only at correcting the fracture but also at prevention of infection and subsequent osteomyelitis. Early stabilization of the fracture and the jaws is generally required to protect the airway. Tracheostomy with use of inflated, cuffed endotracheal tubes may prevent aspiration of blood and other foreign materials. The occurrence of otorrhea or rhinorrhea with a persistent cerebrospinal fluid leak should be carefully observed.

Irradiation and Postsurgical Wounds. Malignancies of the head and neck are frequently treated with a combination of irradiation, chemotherapeutic agents, and surgical resection. Infectious complications are particularly common after such procedures. Pharyngocutaneous fistulas, osteonecrosis of the mandible, or radionecrosis of the laryngeal cartilage may occur. *Staphylococcus aureus* and *Pseudomonas aeruginosa* are frequent pathogens. Prolonged courses of intravenous antibiotics selected according to culture and sensitivity data as well as frequent wound débridement and cleansing are indicated. Although some controversy still exists, immunocompromised patients undergoing oropharyngeal surgery for cancer should receive perioperative antibiotics since they are at particular high risk for infection.[78,83,84] A broad-spectrum antibiotic such as cefazolin, cefuroxime, or cefoxitin appears appropriate in this setting.[18,84,85]

REFERENCES

1. Chow AW, Roser SM, Brady FA. Orofacial odontogenic infections. Ann Intern Med. 1978;88:392.
2. Hardie J. Microbial flora of the oral cavity. In: Schuster GS, ed. Oral Microbiology and Infectious Disease. Baltimore: Williams & Wilkins; 1983:162.
3. Hamada S, Slade HD. Biology, immunology and cariogenicity of *Streptococcus mutans*. Microbiol Rev. 1980;44:331.
4. Gordon DF, Stutman M, Loesche WJ. Improved isolation of anaerobic bacteria from the gingival crevice area of man. Appl Microbiol. 1971;21:1046.
5. Valenti WM, Trudell RB, Bentley DW. Factors predisposing to oropharyngeal colonization with gram-negative bacilli in the aged. N Engl J Med. 1978; 298:1108.
6. Rosenthal S, Tager IB. Relevance of gram-negative rods in the normal pharyngeal flora. Ann Intern Med. 1975;83:355.
7. Schuster GS, Burnett GW. The microbiology of oral and maxillofacial infections. In: Topazian RG, Goldberg MH, eds. Management of Infections of the Oral and Maxillofacial Regions. Philadelphia: WB Saunders; 1981:39.
8. Hardie JM, Bowden GH. The normal microbial flora of the mouth. In: Skinner FA, Carr JG, eds. The Normal Microbial Flora of the Mouth. London: Academic Press; 1974:47.
9. Geddes DAM, Jenkins GN. Intrinsic and extrinsic factors influencing the flora of the mouth. In: Skinner FA, Carr JG, eds. The Normal Microbial Flora of the Mouth. London: Academic Press; 1974:85.
10. Schachtele CF. Dental caries. In: Schuster GS, ed. Oral Microbiology and Infectious Diseases. Baltimore: Williams & Wilkins; 1983:197.
11. Patters MR. Periodontal disease. In: Schuster GS, ed. Oral Microbiology and Infectious Diseases. Baltimore: Williams & Wilkins; 1983:234.
12. Van Palenstein, Helderman WH. Microbial etiology of periodontal disease. J Clin Periodont. 1981;8:261.
13. Shaw JH. Causes and control of dental caries. N Engl J Med. 1987;317:996.
14. Loesche WJ. Role of *Streptococcus mutans* in human dental decay. Microbiol Rev. 1986;50:353.
15. Moore WEC, Holdeman LV, Smibert RM, et al. Bacteriology of experimental gingivitis in young adult humans. Infect Immun. 1982;38:651.
16. Socransky SS, Tan ACR, Haffajee AD, et al. Present status of studies on the microbial etiology of periodontal disease. In: Genco RJ, Mergenhagen SE, eds. Host–Parasite Interactions in Periodontal Diseases. Washington DC: American Society for Microbiology; 1982:1.
17. Willams BL, McCann GF, Schoenknecht FD. Bacteriology of dental abscesses of endodontic origin. J Clin Microbiol. 1983;18:770.
18. Greenberg RN, James RB, Marier RL, et al. Microbiologic and antibiotic aspects of infections in the oral and maxillofacial region. J Oral Surg. 1979;37:873.
19. Baker AS, Montgomery WW. Oropharyngeal space infections. Curr Clin Top Infect Dis. 1987;8:227.
20. Newman MG. Anaerobic oral and dental infection. Rev Infect Dis. 1984;6:107.
21. Chow AW. Odontogenic infections. In: Schlossberg D, ed. Infections of the Head and Neck. New York: Springer Publishing; 1987:148.
22. Kureishi K, Chow AW. The tender tooth—dentoalveolar, pericoronal, and periodontal infections. Infect Dis Clin North Am. 1988;2:163.
23. Roscoe DL, Chow AW. Normal flora and mucosal immunity of the head and neck. Infect Dis Clin North Am. 1988;2:1.
24. Sutter VL. Anaerobes as normal oral flora. Rev Infect Dis. 1984;6(Suppl):62.
25. McGhee JR, Michalek SM. Immunobiology of dental caries—microbial aspects and local immunity. Annu Rev Microbiol. 1981;35:595.
26. Saral R, Ambinder RF, Burns WH, et al. Acyclovir prophylaxis against recrudescent herpes simplex virus infections in leukemia patients. A randomized double-blind placebo controlled study. Ann Intern Med. 1983;99:773.
27. Van Dyke TE, Horoszewicz HU, Cianciola LJ, et al. Neutrophil chemotaxis dysfunction in human periodontitis. Infect Immun. 1980;27:124.
28. Cianciola LJ, Genco RJ, Patters MR, et al. Defective polymorphonuclear leukocyte function in human periodontal disease. Nature. 1977;265:445.
29. Genco RJ, Plaut AG, Moellering RC Jr. Evaluation of human oral organisms and pathogenic *Streptococcus* for production of IgA protease. J Infect Dis. 1975;131(Suppl):17.
30. Kilian M. Degradation of immunoglobulins A1, A2, and G by suspected principal periodontal pathogens. Infect Immun. 1981;34:757.
31. Goldberg MH, Topazian RG. Odontogenic infections and deep fascial space infections of dental origin. In: Topazian RG, Goldberg MH, eds. Management of Infections of the Oral and Maxillofacial Regions. Philadelphia: WB Saunders; 1981:173.
32. Thadepalli H, Mandal AK. Anatomic basis of head and neck infections. Infect Dis Clin North Am. 1988;2:21.
33. Shinn DLS, Squires S, McFadzean JA. The treatment of Vincent's disease with metronidazole. Dent Pract. 1965;15:275.
34. Stephen KW, McLatchie MF, Mason DK, et al. Treatment of acute ulcerative gingivitis (Vincent's type). Br Dent J. 1966;121:313.
35. Lindhe J. Treatment of localized juvenile periodontitis. In: Genco RJ, Mergenhagen SE, eds. Host–Parasite Interactions in Periodontal Disease. Washington DC: American Society for Microbiology; 1982:382.
36. Slots J, Reynolds HS, Genco RJ. *Actinobacillus actinomycetemcomitans* in human periodontal disease: A cross-sectional microbiological investigation. Infect Immun. 1980;29:1013.
37. Loesche WJ. The therapeutic use of antimicrobial agents in patients with periodontal disease. Scand J Infect Dis Suppl. 1985;46:106.
38. Finch RG, Snider GE, Sprinkle PM. Ludwig's angina. JAMA. 1980;243:1171.
39. Crawford JJ, Sconyers JR, Moriarty JD, et al. Bacteremia after tooth extractions studied with the aid of prereduced anaerobically sterilized culture media. Appl Microbiol. 1974;27:927.
40. Rubin R, Solvate EA, Lewis R. Infected total hip replacement after dental procedures. Oral Surg. 1976;41:18.
41. McCurdy JA, MacInnis EL, Hays LL. Fatal mediastinitis after a dental infection. J Oral Surg. 1977;35:726.
42. Yoshikawa TT, Quinn W. The aching head—intracranial suppuration due to head and neck infections. Infect Dis Clin North Am. 1988;2:265.
43. Blomquist IK, Bayer AS. Life-threatening deep fascial space infections of the head and neck. Infect Dis Clin North Am. 1988;2:237.
44. Topazian RG. Osteomyelitis of the jaws. In: Topazian RG, Goldberg MH, eds. Management of Infections of the Oral and Maxillofacial Regions. Philadelphia: WB Saunders; 1981:232.
45. Chow AW, Guze LB. Bacteroidaceae bacteremia—clinical experience with 112 patients. Medicine (Baltimore). 1974;53:93.
46. Vogel LC, Boyer KM. Metastatic complications of *Fusobacterium necrophorum* sepsis: Two cases of Lemierre's postanginal septicemia. Am J Dis Child. 1980;134:356.
47. Eagleton WP. Cavernous Sinus Thrombophlebitis and Allied Septic and Traumatic Lesions of the Basal Venous Sinuses. A Clinical Study of Blood Stream Infection. New York: Macmillan; 1926.
48. Harbour RC, Trobe JD, Ballinger WE. Septic cavernous sinus thrombosis associated with gingivitis and parapharyngeal abscess. Arch Ophthalmol. 1984;102:94.
49. Yarington CT Jr. Cavernous sinus thrombosis revisited. Proc R Soc Med. 1977;70:456.
50. Sanders B. Current concepts in the management of osteomyelitis of the mandible. J Oral Med. 1978;33:40.
51. Mackowiak PA, Jones SR, Smith JW. Diagnostic value of sinus-tract cultures in chronic osteomyelitis. JAMA. 1978;239:2772.
52. Salit IE. Diagnostic approaches to head and neck infections. Infect Dis Clin North Am. 1988;2:35.
53. Holt GR, McManus K, Newman RK, et al. Computed tomography in the diagnosis of deep-neck infections. Arch Otolaryngol. 1982;108:693.
54. Wholey MH, Bruwer AJ, Baker HL. The lateral roentgenogram of the neck. Radiology. 1958;71:350.
55. Bryan CS, King BG Jr, Bryant RE. Retropharyngeal infection in adults. Arch Intern Med. 1974;134:127.
56. Loe H, Kornman K. Strategies in the use of antibacterial agents in periodontal disease. In: Genco RJ, Mergenhagen SE, eds. Host–Parasite Interactions in Periodontal Disease. Washington DC: American Society for Microbiology; 1982:376.
57. Danish Medical Research Council Consensus Report. Prevention and control of dental caries. Dan Med Bull. 1986;33:199.
58. Gregory RL, Filler SJ. Protective secretory immunoglobulin A antibodies in humans following oral immunization with *Streptococcus mutans*. Infect Immun. 1987;55:2409.
59. Russell RRB, Johnson NW. The prospects of vaccination against dental caries. Br Dent J. 1987;162:29.
60. Heimdahl A, Nord CE. Treatment of orofacial infections of odontogenic origin. Scand J Infect Dis Suppl. 1985;46:101.
61. Hill MK, Sanders CV. Principles of antimicrobial therapy for head and neck infections. Infect Dis Clin North Am. 1988;2:57.
62. Busch DF, Kureshi LA, Sutter VL, et al. Susceptibility of respiratory tract anaerobes to orally administered penicillins and cephalosporins. Antimicrob Agents Chemother. 1976;10:713.
63. Tami TA, Parker GS. *Eikenella corrodens*—an emerging pathogen in head and neck infections. Arch Otolaryngol. 1984;110:752.
64. Edson RS, Rosenblatt JE, Lee DT, et al. Recent experience with antimicrobial susceptibility of anaerobic bacteria—increasing resistance to penicillin. Mayo Clin Proc. 1982;57:737.

65. Heimdahl A, von Konow L, Nord CE. Isolation of β-lactamase producing *Bacteroides* strains associated with clinical failures with penicillin treatment of human orofacial infections. Arch Oral Biol. 1980;25:687.
66. Murray PR, Rosenblatt JE. Penicillin resistance and penicillinase production in clinical isolates of *Bacteroides melaninogenicus*. Antimicrob Agents Chemother. 1977;11:605.
67. Hood FJC. The place of metronidazole in the treatment of acute orofacial infection. Antimicrob Agents Chemother. 1978;15:71.
68. Epstein JB. The painful mouth—mucositis, gingivitis and stomatitis. Infect Dis Clin North Am. 1988;2:183.
69. Barrett AP. A long-term prospective clinical study of oral complications during conventional chemotherapy for acute leukemia. Oral Surg. 1987;63:313.
70. Topazian RG. Uncommon infections of the oral and maxillofacial regions. In: Topazian RG, Goldberg MH, eds. Management of Infections of the Oral and Maxillofacial Regions. Philadelphia: WB Saunders; 1981:293.
71. Tyldesley WR, ed. Recurrent oral ulcerations. In: Oral Medicine. Oxford: Oxford University Press; 1981:49.
72. Epstein JB, Gangbar SJ. Oral mucosal lesions in patients undergoing treatment for leukemia. J Oral Med. 1987;42:132.
73. Lee PL, Kiviat N, Truelove EL, et al. Oral manifestations in patients with AIDS or AIDS-related disorders. J Dent Res. 1987;66:183.
74. Epstein JB, Stevenson-Moore P. Benzydamine hydrochloride in prevention and management of pain in oral mucositis associated with radiation therapy. Oral Surg. 1986;62:145.
75. Adams S, Toth B, Dudley BS. Evaluation of sucralfate as a compounded oral suspension for the treatment of stomatitis. Clin Pharmacol Ther. 1985;2:178.
76. Epstein JB, Schubert MM. Synergistic effects of sialogogues in management of xerostomia following radiation therapy. Oral Surg. 1987;64:179.
77. Goldberg MH. Infections of the salivary glands. In: Topazian RG, Goldberg MH, eds. Management of Infections of the Oral and Maxillary Regions. Philadelphia: WB Saunders; 1981:293.
78. Adams GL. Infections of the head and neck. In: Simmons RL, Hoeard RF, eds. Surgical Infectious Diseases. New York: Appleton-Century-Crofts; 1982:593.
79. Brook I. The swollen neck—cervical lymphadenitis, parotitis, thyroiditis and infected cysts. Infect Dis Clin North Am. 1988;2:221.
80. Berger SA, Zonszein J, Villanema P, et al. Infectious diseases of the thyroid gland. Rev Infect Dis. 1983;5:108.
81. Freidig EE, McClure SP, Wilson WR, et al. Clinical-histologic-microbiologic analysis of 419 lymph node biopsy specimens. Rev Infect Dis. 1986;8:322.
82. Goldstein EJC, Citron DW, Wield B, et al. Bacteriology of human and animal bite wounds. J Clin Microbiol. 1978;8:667.
83. Herzon FS. The prophylactic use of antibiotics in head and neck surgery. Otolaryngol Clin North Am. 1976;9:781.
84. Seagle MB, Duberstein LE, Gross CW, et al. Efficacy of cefazolin as a prophylactic antibiotic in head and neck surgery. Otolaryngology. 1978;86:568.
85. Zide MF, Sanders CV, Marier RL, et al. Cefuroxime therapy for maxillofacial infections. Curr Ther Res. 1986;40:278.

SECTION C. PLEUROPULMONARY AND BRONCHIAL INFECTIONS

50. ACUTE BRONCHITIS

JACK M. GWALTNEY, JR.

Acute bronchitis is an inflammatory condition of the tracheobronchial tree that is usually associated with a generalized respiratory infection. It occurs most commonly during the winter months when acute respiratory tract infections are prevalent. Patients seen in general practices in Great Britian had annual attack rates of acute bronchitis that varied between 40 and 54 percent 100,000.[1] Weekly attack rates peaked (117–171/100,000) in January and February and fell to trough levels (26–42/100,000) in August. The diagnosis was made most often in children under 5 years of age.

The syndrome of acute bronchitis is associated with infection with both common cold viruses, such as rhinovirus and coronavirus, and lower respiratory tract pathogens, such as influenza virus, adenovirus, and *Mycoplasma pneumoniae*. Secondary bacterial invasion may play a role in the etiology of the syndrome, but this is not well established.

ETIOLOGY

Cough occurs in approximately 50 percent of the cases of common respiratory illness in persons of all ages.[2] Cough is the localizing symptom in the respiratory tract that is most frequently associated with fever and is also highly associated with the occurrence of hoarseness. Infection with members of all the major respiratory virus groups causes cough (Table 1).[2–9] Cases of acute bronchitis are particularly common during influenza epidemics. While rhinovirus infections do not produce as severe an involvement of the tracheobronchial tree as influenza, rhinovirus infections, because of their frequency, are an important cause of acute bronchitis. In populations of military recruits, adenovirus infections are a major cause of acute bronchitis. Among the other respiratory viruses that cause acute bronchitis, measles virus has been recognized as causing a particularly severe form of the disease.

A small proportion of cases are of known nonviral etiology. *Mycoplasma pneumoniae* and *Bordetella pertussis* are among the nonviral causes of acute bronchitis. Recently, a new *Chlamydia psittaci* strain, TWAR, has been associated with acute respiratory tract infections that include cases with the clinical features of acute bronchitis.[10,11] The etiologic role of *Streptococcus pneumoniae* and *Haemophilus influenzae* in acute bronchitis is not clear. Since these bacteria are carried in the resident flora of the upper respiratory tract of normal persons, it is difficult to evaluate studies in which expectorated sputum specimens have been cultured. To examine the role of secondary bacterial infection in the pathogenesis of acute bronchitis, it is

TABLE 1. Cough Associated with Acute Viral Infections of the Respiratory Tract

Virus	*Percent of Cases with Cough (References)*
Influenza	75–93 (2, 3)
Adenovirus	45–90 (4, 6)
Rhinovirus	32–60 (3, 5)
Coronavirus	10–50 (7, 8)
Parainfluenza virus	2–45 (5)
Respiratory syncytial virus	61 (9)
Coxsackievirus A21	26 (5)
Miscellaneous (rubeola, rubella, and so forth)	—

necessary to conduct studies in which samples are collected from the tracheobronchial tree without contamination from nasopharyngeal flora.

PATHOGENESIS

The pathogenesis of acute bronchitis has not been investigated for all the causative agents. During acute bronchial infection, the mucous membrane of the tracheobronchial tree is hyperemic and edematous, and there are increased bronchial secretions. Destruction of respiratory epithelium may be extensive in some infections, such as influenza,[12] but appears to be minimal in others, such as rhinovirus colds.[13,14] Bronchial mucociliary function may be diminished in infections in which overt mucosal damage is limited.[15] With *M. pneumoniae* infection, bronchial irritation results from the attachment of the organism to the respiratory mucosa, with eventual sloughing of affected cells.[16]

It is also possible that severity of attacks of acute bronchitis may be increased by exposure to cigarette smoke and air pollutants. These substances, in association with recurrent acute bronchial infection, may result in permanent injury to the bronchial tree. Epidemiologic studies support the idea that acute respiratory infections play a role in the pathogenesis of chronic obstructive lung disease.[17,18] Also, studies of pulmonary function in previously healthy adults with acute infection due to some viruses, such as respiratory syncytial virus, have shown prolonged abnormalities in airway resistance and reactivity.[19]

There has been recent interest in examining the relationship between acute bronchitis and heightened airway reactivity. Mild bronchial asthma was found to be increased in patients with a history of recurrent acute bronchitis over that seen in the general population.[20] Also, in a case control study, patients with acute bronchitis were more likely to have a previous history of asthma and a history, or diagnosis, of atopic disease.[21] These findings have raised the question of the possible role of bronchospasm in some cases of prolonged cough associated with acute respiratory infection.

CLINICAL PPRESENTATION

Cough begins early in the course of many acute respiratory infections and tends to become more prominent as the illness progresses (Fig. 1). In the usual cold and influenzal illness, nasal and pharyngeal complaints subside after 3 or 4 days, while the cough tends to persist and to achieve greater prominence.[3] Persons presenting for medical care who are diagnosed as having acute bronchitis probably represent a subset of all patients with acute respiratory infection. In one prospective study of such patients, 45 percent were still coughing 2 weeks after presentation and 25 percent were still coughing after 3 weeks.[22] With a variety of different respiratory virus infections, sputum production was reported in approximately one-half of the cases in which cough was occurring.[4,5] An initially dry cough may later result in mucoid sputum, which characteristically develops a more purulent character in the later stages of illness. A study of natural rhinovirus infections in young adults has shown that the frequency and duration of cough is prolonged in cigarette smokers.[22]

With pronounced tracheal involvement, there may be burning substernal pain associated with respiration and coughing. Dyspnea and cyanosis are not seen in adults unless the patient has underlying chronic obstructive pulmonary disease or other conditions that impair lung function. Rhonchi and coarse rales may be heard on examination of the chest. Signs of consolidation and alveolar involvement are not present in uncomplicated bronchitis. The frequency with which fever occurs depends on the specific infectious agent involved and the age of the patient. In adults, influenza virus, adenovirus, and *M. pneumoniae* infections are commonly associated with temperature elevations.

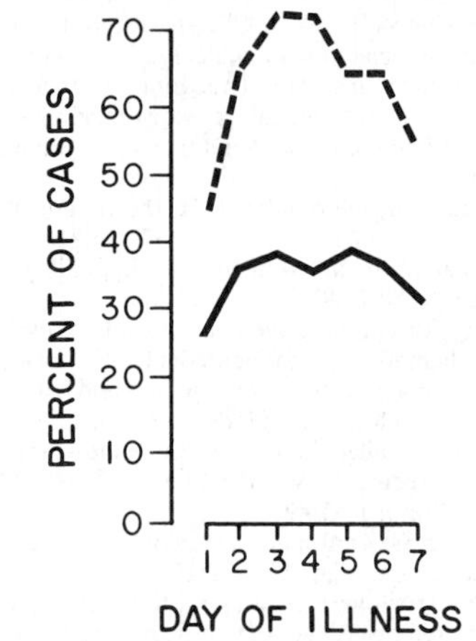

FIG. 1. Occurrence of cough in rhinovirus colds (139 cases) (solid line) and type A_2 influenza (33 cases) (broken line) in young adults. (Modified from Gwaltney,[3] with permission.)

Fever is unusual in adults with bronchitis associated with cold viruses, like rhinovirus and coronavirus.

DIAGNOSIS

Bronchitis may be suspected in the patient with an acute respiratory infection with cough, but because a large number of more serious diseases of the lower respiratory tract cause cough, bronchitis must be considered a diagnosis of exclusion. A complete history should be obtained, including information on exposure to toxic substances and cigarette use. Complaints involving other organ systems should be sought. Epidemiologic considerations and vaccination history may aid in the diagnosis of specific causes of bronchitis, such as influenza, *M. pneumoniae*, and whooping cough.

Included in a complete physical examination should be a careful evaluation of the chest for evidence of pneumonia and signs of cardiovascular and thromboembolic diseases. Radiologic examination of the chest may be required in the occasional patient in whom the question of parenchymal disease of the lung remains after the physical examination. Cultures of respiratory secretions for influenza virus, *M. pneumoniae*, and *B. pertussis* should be obtained when these diseases are suspected. Cultures for the common cold viruses are usually not available. Bacterial cultures of expectorated sputum are not helpful because of the sampling problem of avoiding nasopharyngeal flora and because of the unknown importance of bacterial infection in the etiology of acute bronchitis. Patients in whom cough persists beyond the expected duration of the acute illness should have further diagnostic examinations, including chest x-ray films, sputum cytology, and bronchoscopy to exclude foreign body aspiration, tuberculosis, tumors, and other chronic diseases of the tracheobronchial tree and lungs.

TREATMENT

Treatment of acute bronchitis is symptomatic and is directed primarily at the control of cough. Otherwise, healthy patients do not require hospitalization except in cases of unusual severity. Patients with underlying chronic cardiopulmonary diseases who contract influenzal bronchitis may develop serious ventilatory abnormalities that require hospitalization with ventilatory assistance and oxygen therapy. In the average case, cough suppressants such as dextromethorphan 15 mg po every 6 hours are the main form of treatment required. With severe cough, preparations containing codeine are most useful.[23] The value of expectorants is not well established,[24] and in patients with a good cough reflex, maintaining hydration is probably the most effective way to prevent drying of bronchial secretions. Aspirin and bed rest are beneficial in influenzal syndromes in which malaise and fever are prominent.

The value of antibiotics in the treatment of unselected patients with acute bronchitis is uncertain, and the use of these agents is not recommended as a general practice. Controlled trials[25–29] have given conflicting results, which could result from a number of variables, including type of antibiotic and dosage schedule used, duration of follow-up, season of the year (reflecting prevalence of different pathogens), and adequacy of subject blinding related to drug side effects. *Mycoplasma pneumoniae* infection should be treated with erythromycin or tetracycline (see Chapter 162) and *B. pertussis* infection with erythromycin (see Chapter 208). During epidemics known to be due to influenza A virus, treatment with amantadine (100 mg po bid) is recommended for patients with suspected influenza if the illness is less than 48 hours in duration. Also annual immunization with influenza vaccine or prophylaxis with amantadine is recommended in patients with chronic cardiopulmonary problems (see Chapter 142). Children should receive pertussis vaccine as part of their routine immunizations. It is particularly important to discourage cigarette smoking in patients in whom acute respiratory tract infections are associated with protracted cough and sputum production.

REFERENCES

1. Ayres JG. Seasonal pattern of acute bronchitis in general practice in the United Kingdom 1976–83. Thorax. 1986;41:107–110.
2. Dingle JH, Badger GF, Jordon WS Jr. Illness in the Home: A Study of 25,000 Illnesses in a Group of Cleveland Families. Cleveland: The Press of Western Reserve University; 1964;68.
3. Gwaltney JM Jr. Rhinoviruses. In: Evans AS, ed. Viral Infections of Humans: Epidemiology and Control. 2nd ed. New York: Plenum; 1982:507.
4. Dascomb HE, Hilleman MR. Clinical laboratory studies in patients with respiratory disease caused by adenovirus (RI-APC-ARD agents). Am J Med. 1956;21:161.
5. Tyrrell DAJ. Common Colds and Related Diseases. Baltimore: Williams & Wilkins; 1965.
6. Bloom HH, Forsyth BR, Johnson KM, et al. Patterns of adenovirus infections in Marine Crops personnel. I. A 42-month survey in recruit and nonrecruit populations. Am J Hyg. 1964;80:328.
7. Kaye HS, Marsh HB, Dowdle WR. Seroepidemiologic survey of coronavirus (strain OC43) related infections in a children's population. Am J Epidemiol. 1971;94:43.
8. Hendley JO, Fishburne HB, Gwaltney JM Jr. Coronavirus infections in working adults, Eight-year study with 229E and OC43. Am Rev Respir Dis 1972;105:805.
9. Knight V, Kapikian AZ, Kravetz MH, et al. Ecology of a newly recognized common respiratory agent RS-virus. Ann Intern Med. 1961;55:507.
10. Grayston JT, Kuo C-C, Wang S-P, et al. A new *Chlamydia psittaci* strain, TWAR, isolated in acute respiratory tract infections. N Engl J Med. 1986;315:161–168.
11. Grayston JT, Kuo C-C, Wang S-P, et al. Clinical findings in TWAR respiratory tract infections. In: Oriel JD, Ridgway G, Schacter J, et al. eds. Chlamydial Infections. Cambridge: Cambridge University Press; 1986;337–340.
12. Loosli CG, Stinson SF, Ryan DP, et al. The destruction of type 2 pneumocytes by airborne influenza PR8-A virus: its effect on surfactant and lecithin content of the pneumonic lesions of mice. Chest. 1975;67(Suppl):7S.
13. Douglas RG Jr, Alford BR, Cough RB: Atraumatic nasal biopsy for studies of respiratory virus infection in volunteers. Antimicrob Agents Chemother. 1968;8:340.
14. Winther B, Farr B, Turner RB, et al. Histopathologic examination and enumeration of polymorphonuclear leukocytes in the nasal mucosa during experimental rhinovirus colds. Acta Otoaryngol [Suppl] (Stockh) 1984;413:19–24.
15. Sasaki Y, Togo Y, Wagner NH Jr, et al. Mucociliary function during experimentally induced rhinovirus infection in man. Ann Otol. 1973;82:203.
16. Powell DA, Hu PC, Wilson M, et al. Attachment of *Mycoplasma pneumoniae* to respiratory epithelium. Infect Immun 1976;13:959.
17. Lebowitz MD, Burrows B. The relationship of acute respiratory illness history to the prevalence and incidence of obstructive lung disorders. Am J Epidemiol. 1977;105:544.
18. Monto AS, Ross HW. The Tecumseh study of respiratory illness. X. Relation of acute infections to smoking, lung function and chronic symptoms. Am J Epidemiol. 1978;107:57.
19. Hall WJ, Hall CB, Speers DM. Respiratory syncytial virus infection in adults. Clinical, virologic, and serial pulmonary function studies. Ann Intern Med. 1978;88:203.
20. Hallett JS, Jacobs RL. Recurrent acute bronchitis: the association with undiagnosed bronchial asthma. Ann Allergy. 1985;55:568–570.
21. Williamson HA, Jr, Schultz P. An association between acute bronchitis and asthma. J Fam Prac. 1987;24:35–38.
22. Gwaltney JM Jr, Hendley JO, Simon G, et al. Rhinovirus infections in an industrial population. II. Characteristics of illness and antibody response. JAMA. 1967;202:494.
23. Eddy NB. Codeine and its alternates for pain and cough relief. Ann Intern Med. 1969;71:1209.
24. Kuhn JJ, Hendley JO, Adams KF, Antitussive effect of guaifenesin in young adults with natural colds. Objective and subjective assessment. Chest. 1982;82:713.
25. Stott NC, and West RR. Randomized controlled trial of antibiotics in patients with cough and purulent sputum. Br Med J. 1976;2:556.
26. Franks P, Gleiner JA. The treatment of acute bronchitis with trimethoprim and sulfamethoxazole. J Fam Prac. 1984;19:185–190.
27. Williamson HA Jr. A randomized, controlled trial of doxycycline in the treatment of acute bronchitis. J Fam Pract. 1984;19:481–486.
28. Brickfield FX, Carter WH, Johnson RE. Erythromycin in the treatment of acute bronchitis in a community practice. J Fam Pract. 1986;23:119–122.
29. Dunlay J, Reinhardt R, Roi LD. A placebo-controlled, double-blind trial of erythromycin in adults with acute bronchitis. J Fam Prac 1987;25:137–141.

51. CHRONIC BRONCHITIS AND ACUTE INFECTIOUS EXACERBATIONS

HERBERT Y. REYNOLDS

Chronic bronchitis is a condition in which cough and excessive secretion of mucus are present in the tracheobronchial tree that are not due to other specific diseases such as bronchiectasis, asthma, or tuberculosis. The label "chronic bronchitic" is often loosely applied to patients and is very much a clinical diagnosis. By definition, the diagnosis is given to patients who report to have coughed up sputum on most days during at least 3 consecutive months for more than 2 successive years.[1,2] Some clinical surveys have added to the definition the occurrence of attacks of cough with sputum in the previous 2 years that have prevented the patient from working for a total of at least 3 weeks. If wheezing and bronchospasm occur with the disease, the designation chronic or recurrent asthmatic bronchitis may be used. Emphysema often complicates the clinical presentation. Although the precise diagnosis of emphysema is a morbid and anatomic one, its coexistence is usually inferred. The two diagnoses are usually lumped together and used to identify patients as having "chronic obstructive lung disease with bronchitis and emphysema."

ETIOLOGY AND PATHOLOGY

Although the causes of chronic bronchitis have not been elucidated completely, three factors seem to be of particular importance: cigarette smoking, infection, and inhalation of dust or fumes in the workplace environment. Chronic bronchitis is common and affects about 10–25 percent of the adult population. Bronchitis is more common in men than in women and more common after the age of 40 than before. Smoking, cigarette smoking in particular, is the most important factor associated with the disease. Related diseases that impair mucociliary transport in the lung may be important in susceptible people. The clinician must be alert for the possibility that recurrent respiratory infections and persistent chronic bronchitis might signal that the patient has an immunodeficiency syndrome. This association may become evident in teenagers or young adults and not in young children as generally expected.[3] Investigation for cystic fibrosis, an intrinsic defect in the structure of epithelial cilia, immunoglobulin deficiency involving IgA or selective IgG subclasses,[4,5] and rarely abnormal polymorphonuclear (PMN) granulocyte function should be considered.

Cigarette smoking is a significant airway irritant for most patients. Not all patients with chronic bronchitis, however, have a history of smoking; an average of 6–10 percent of nonsmoking men will have persistent cough and phlegm production. In light-to-moderate smokers (20 or fewer cigarettes per day), the frequency of chronic bronchitis is approximately 25 percent; for heavy smokers (greater than a 40–60 pack-year history) it increases to almost 50 percent. The frequency is less in ex-smokers. Investigators who have performed bronchoalveolar lavage to obtain respiratory cells from human lungs have uniformly found a tremendous increase in the recovery of alveolar macrophages from cigarette smokers as compared with nonsmokers.[6] "Normal" smokers usually yield a small percentage of inflammatory cells (PMN granulocytes) as well. A modest degree of smoking (2–5 pack-years) induces cellular and lavage fluid immunoglobulin changes similar to those found in heavy smokers. Postmortem examination of lungs obtained from young accident victims showed evidence of inflammation involving respiratory bronchioles in smokers but not in nonsmokers. The lesion consisted of clusters of pigmented macrophages in association with edema, fibrosis, and epithelial hyperplasia of the bronchiolar and aveolar walls.[7] Thus, cigarette users, even those who smoke minimally, initiate irritative stimuli that may insidiously culminate years later as chronic bronchitis and possibly other forms of degenerative lung diseases. The realization that cigarette smoke can inactivate the antiprotease function of α_1-antitrypsin in lung secretions further supports this sequence of destructive lung disease.[8,9]

One striking change noted in the lungs of patients with chronic bronchitis is the increase in the number of goblet (mucus-secreting) cells in the surface epithelium of major and smaller bronchi. Whereas goblet cells normally account for one-fourth of the epithelial cells lining the larger bronchi and are virtually absent from the smaller ones, particularly bronchioles,[10] in chronic bronchitis the epithelium may consist almost entirely of such cells. In addition, mucous glands in the walls of the larger bronchi undergo hypertrophy. Normally, the ratio of the mucous glands compared with the bronchial wall (the latter measured from the surface of the epithelium to the inner surface of the cartilaginous plates) is about 0.3, but with enlargement of the mucous glands, as found in chronic bronchitis, the ratio is greater and on the order of 0.6 (Reid index).[11] Besides mucous gland enlargement, chronic bronchitics have irritation of the airway mucosa and more mucus in their peripheral airways. The irritated airways respond by producing extra secretions, exposing sensitive stretch receptors (which aggravates cough), and developing bronchospasm. Inflammation of the mucosa gives rise to swelling and edema, infiltration of PMNs, hyperplasia of goblet cells, and enlargement of bronchial mucus glands as observed in the pathology. However, mechanisms that produce these changes have only been investigated recently.[12]

Explants of human airways (2–10 mm in diameter from the second- to fifth-generation bronchi) can be established and cultured for 2–3 days. Such explants contain normal-appearing mucosal surfaces and goblet cells and intact submucosal glands.[13] In this in vitro system, secretion of mucous glycoproteins can be stimulated with a variety of factors: histamine, slow-reacting substance of anaphylaxis (leukotrienes C, D, and E), IgE antibody, and methacholine. Products of mast cell degranulation and pharmacologic agents can enhance the output of mucous glycoproteins as well as neuropeptides that stimulate cyclic guanosine monophosphate (GMP). Other products of arachidonic acid metabolism can also stimulate these explants to produce mucus.[14] In addition, human blood monocytes and alveolar macrophages produce a mucus secretagogue, after a phagocytic stimulus, that causes the release of mucous glycoprotein from cultured human airways.[15,16]

CLINICAL PRESENTATION

Incessant cough marks most advanced bronchitics. The patient may clear his throat frequently, and during conversation, an outburst of laughter or animated speech can precipitate a loud, raspy, coughing episode. Many patients expectorate sputum throughout the day, but most cough up the largest amount in the morning on arising. Sputum may be tenacious and sticky and vary in appearance from mucoid or whitish to yellowish green and obviously purulent. Many patients have associated nasal problems and often complain of a postnasal drip or sinus congestion. A bad taste in the mouth and halitosis are frequent complaints. Most patients with chronic bronchitis are not incapacitated by their respiratory disorder unless an acute infection or some other illness occurs.

As mentioned, emphysema is often present, and some patients with advanced chronic bronchitis have complications that are determined for the most part by the degree and type of associated emphysema. The use of descriptive terms to separate patients with chronic obstructive lung disease into groups such as "blue bloaters" (or type B) and "pink puffers" (or type A) is often an oversimplification.[17] However, the separation may be useful in understanding the clinical course of the patient with chronic bronchitis and recurrent respiratory infections.

The blue bloater is characterized by severe obstructive lung disease with serious and persistent blood gas abnormalities and an impaired air flow that is worse than predicted from the forced expiratory volume of the first second (FEV_1). Frequent tracheobronchial infections (bacterial and viral) occur and occasionally lead to bronchopneumonia. Dyspnea, although a prominent symptom, is less intense than in the pink puffer. As a consequence of the blood gas derangements, a number of associated features may follow. Somnolence and lethargy can develop. Pulmonary vasospasm induced by the combination of hypoxemia and respiratory acidosis increases pulmonary vascular resistance, which in turn increases the work load of the right ventricle of the heart. Cor pulmonale with peripheral edema and its other attendant consequences may occur. Patients often cough up copious amounts of sputum and do not show radiologic evidence of emphysema. These patients are thought primarily to be severe bronchitics with little evidence of emphysema. In contrast, pink puffers, despite severe airway obstruction, maintain relatively normal blood gases because of high minute ventilation. These patients, frequently underweight and barrel chested, do not appear cyanotic or plethoric and do not develop cor pumonale except terminally. Radiologically emphysema is present. These are considered patients with severe emphysema and little bronchitis. It is now apparent that the clinical distinction between these two syndromes is not clear-cut and that many patients (perhaps the majority) have features of both.

The bronchitic maintains normal body weight and tends to be obese. Normal vesicular breath sounds are diminished, and inspiratory and expiratory rales, rhonchi, and mild wheezing may be heard instead. The chest is noisy rather than quiet, as is observed with emphysema. If pulmonary artery pressure is elevated, cardiac signs may reflect it. With advanced bronchitis and emphysema, the patient may have acrocyanosis, plethoric complexion, and manifestations of overt heart failure. Digital clubbing is not a finding in the uncomplicated bronchitic.

Evidence of an Acute Infectious Exacerbation

Objective signs that bronchitis has worsened in temporal relationship to a documented infection are not always evident. Reliance is placed on the patient's observation that his sputum has changed in color and consistency or has increased in amount. In some patients the development of an increased amount of noneosinophilic purulent sputum is presumptive evidence of infection. However, other patients consistently produce purulent sputum without other evidence of infection. Patients may note increasing cough and dyspnea, but during an acute illness, most will not have symptoms suggesting systemic toxicity such as chills and fever, nor will they develop a blood leukocytosis. Patients often experience chest tightness and increased fatigue. No uniform definition for an acute exacerbation of chronic bronchitis exists.

Sputum Analysis

Cellular analysis[18,19] of a fresh sputum specimen (early morning sample) is necessary in the evaluation of every patient with chronic bronchitis. Continual bronchial irritation is indicated by the presence of many PMN granulocytes, even during quiescent periods of the disease. It is important to determine the number of eosinophils. Ciliated epithelial cells can be recognized, and their number correlates reasonably well with the degree of vigorous coughing that was needed to produce the sputum specimen. A few alveolar macrophages may be identified that in the cigarette smoker characteristically contain yellowish brown cytoplasmic inclusions. Gram stain will often show a mixture of gram-positive and gram-negative bacteria that is consistent with contamination by normal mouth flora or with tracheal colonization by *Haemophilus influenzae* and *Streptococcus pneumoniae*.

The mucus secreted in chronic bronchitis contains various glycoproteins, mucopolysaccharide acids, and albumin. Small amounts of a number of immunoglobulin species are present including secretory IgA, IgG, occasionally IgM and IgE, or proteolytic fragments derived from them. Other proteins present include transferrin, complement components, and enzyme inhibitors such as α_1-antiprotease. With high degrees of bronchial irritation and inflammation, any of the intravascular proteins may be identified in purulent mucus; however, the protein is likely to be fragmented or denatured because of the effect of pH or the action of lysosomal enzymes and other degradative substances in sputum.[20,21] Immunologic analysis of IgA in sputum may help in diagnosing the presence of infection in patients with a flare-up of chronic bronchitis. With active infection, the content of 7S IgA is increased, and free-secretory component is all used; without infection, 11S IgA is increased, and excess secretory component exists.[22]

Radiologic Evidence

Standard chest films contribute little to the definitive diagnosis of chronic bronchitis, but they serve the essential purpose of excluding other diseases that may mimic or contribute to chronic bronchitis. The chest film can appear normal in chronic bronchitis and may not undergo change during infectious exacerbations; therefore, it is not a very sensitive or helpful way of following most patients.

RELATIONSHIP OF INFECTION TO ACUTE EXACERBATIONS

The most enigmatic problem in chronic bronchitis is the role of bacterial infection. Although its exact place is uncertain, bacterial infection does not appear to initiate the disease except possibly in the patient with a history of frequent childhood respiratory infections.[23] However, bacteria are probably significant in perpetuating the disease and may be critical in producing the characteristic exacerbations.

It is generally accepted that the bronchi of nonbronchitics who are free of other lung diseases are almost always sterile, although methods of culture are not perfect and may not exclude oral flora.[24–26] Pathogenic bacteria can be cultured from the bronchi in up to 82 percent of chronic bronchitics. Pathogenic organisms have also been cultured from the airways of nonbronchitics who have carcinoma of the lung or tuberculosis or after radiation to the lung. Thus, various forms of damage to the lung may predispose to bacterial infection. Routine sputum cultures from patients with chronic bronchitis commonly contain nonencapsulated *H. influenzae, S. pneumoniae,* and other oropharyngeal commensal flora. In most clinical series, one or both of these species is recovered from approximately 30–50 percent of the sputum specimens and rightfully can be considered as the baseline microbial flora of many patients with chronic bronchitis. Anaerobic bacteria could be recovered in only 17 percent of transtracheal aspirate specimens.[27] However, sputum carriage of *H. influenzae* and pneumococci does seem to be of particular significance. These bacteria tend to persist in sputum during quiescent intervals, and the frequency of recovery is not greatly increased during acute infectious episodes. The development of purulent sputum is not correlated specifically with the presence of one or the other of these bacteria. However, evidence suggests that purulence is associated with a quantitative increase in the number of pneumococci cultured from sputum.[28] *Mycoplasma pneumoniae* does not seem to be of great importance, for some studies[28,29] attribute only 1–10 percent of acute infections to this organism.

As mentioned, it is often impossible to judge when an acute infection has supervened, microbiologically as well as clinically. This is particularly true of patients who always experience symptoms of cough and produce sputum that is purulent. One study[28] that monitored infectious episodes on the basis of changes in monthly serum antibody titers to a large number of microorganisms indicated that infection could occur frequently without a clinical exacerbation of bronchitis. This was especially true of viral infections. Of those viral infections documented to have occurred by significant changes in serum antibody titers, 40 percent were not associated with a clinical exacerbation.

The following statements summarize the relationship between causative agents[30] and acute flare-ups of infection in chronic bronchitis: (*1*) Chronic colonization of the airways and sputum with unencapsulated strains of *H. influenzae* and with pneumococci occurs in at least one-half of the affected patients. Microbiologically, it is difficult to incriminate one or both these bacteria as the specific cause of an acute infection. However, many physicians usually attribute acute infectious exacerbation to one of these bacteria, and antibiotic selection is often based on this probability. (2) Other bacteria such as hemolytic species of streptococci, *Staphylococcus aureus,* and gram-negative enteric bacilli are infrequent causes of acute infection in chronic bronchitis. Only 5–10 percent of the sputum specimens will contain significant numbers of these other bacteria. Since sputum may be contaminated by oropharyngeal flora, it is uncertain whether these bacteria originate in the lower airways. Other sampling methods such as transtracheal aspiration may be necessary to make this distinction.[27] (*3*) *Mycoplasma pneumoniae* infections can be sporadic and may be responsible for some acute exacerbations. (*4*) Viruses are frequent causes of acute infection. Fully 25–50 percent of acute exacerbations are related to these agents, including influenza, parainfluenza, respiratory syncytial virus, rhinovirus, and coronavirus. Viral infections are seasonal and occur more frequently in winter.

MANAGEMENT

General Considerations

Attempts should be made to have the patient stop smoking or at least reduce the amount of smoking. During the patient's initial evaluation, analysis of the cellular content of a sputum specimen is indicated; if eosinophils are among the inflammatory cells present, an allergic component to the illness should be investigated. Some asthmatics cough instead of wheeze, so it is not infrequent to encounter an asthmatic who has symptoms of chronic cough rather than audible wheezing.[31] Since excessive mucus secretion is common to both asthma and bronchitis, eosinophils in the sputum and in the peripheral blood can be a diagnostic clue. Initial pulmonary function tests to assess expiratory airflow should also include tests performed after the aerosol administration of a bronchodilator, unless a contraindication exists. It is useful to establish whether the patient has a reversible component of bronchospasm to the airway obstruction. Appropriate bronchodilator therapy may improve breathing and may improve exercise tolerance. Patients who develop wheezing during acute infectious exacerbation may profit from a bronchodilator as well. Consultation with an ear, nose, and throat specialist and x-ray films of the sinuses may help to identify a deviated nasal septum, nasal polyps, or chronic sinusitis. A program of weight reduction and a suitable exercise regimen can be considered. Patients should receive a yearly immunization with the current influenza vaccine. Indications for the use of pneumococcal vaccine need individual consideration.

The accumulation and clearance of secretions can be a real problem for some patients, and postural drainage maneuvers are indicated, especially during acute infections. The yield of secretions from postural drainage can sometimes be improved by the addition of two procedures: (*1*) the initial use of an aerosol bronchodilator to achieve maximum dilatation and opening of the airways and then (*2*) humidification or wetting of respiratory secretions. Patients who are plagued with copious secretions and gain benefit from postural drainage ought to receive instruction in the technique from a qualified respiratory therapist. Other therapy aimed at liquifying respiratory secretions or controlling cough are not of particular value. Mucolytic agents designed to loosen and dissolve tenacious secretions are often irritative and actually may serve to increase mucus production. Cough-suppressant drugs are rarely indicated. The effect of sedatives contained in many preparations is generally not desirable, especially for patients with chronic obstructive lung disease. Cough is an efficient way of removing secretions. The use of an intermittent positive-pressure breathing device is rarely justified; if aerosol administration of medications is deemed necessary, a hand-held or motorized nebulizer will provide adequate drug distribution in the airways.

Spirometry and expiratory airflow values may not improve even though the patient has achieved a quiescent and "infection-free" stage. Actually, bronchiolar inflammation and airway resistance may have decreased, but the routine pulmonary tests are generally insensitive to this improvement.

Since most chronic bronchitics continue to be cigarette smokers, they remain in a group that is statistically at increased risk to develop primary lung cancer. Early detection of cancer that is still localized provides the best hope for cure. Therefore, periodic sputum specimens for cytology and chest films are indicated.

Finally, the use of corticosteroid therapy should be mentioned. At some point the bronchitic patient will not rebound from an acute infection despite a vigorous and optimal treatment regimen that includes antibiotics and other ancillary drugs in maximal doses. In such a circumstance, a trial of corticosteroids may be indicated with moderate doses of the drug (20–30 mg/day equivalent of prednisone, for example). Current preference still favors the use of a systemically administered drug instead of a topical aerolized preparation. Because mucus plugging and diffuse areas of obstruction are present in the airways, a systemically absorbed steroid will achieve more even distribution throughout the lung tissue. The steroid effect is often not immediate, so a drug course of 3–6 weeks may be necessary. For many patients with chronic obstructive lung disease, a trial of corticosteroids and inhaled β_2-agonist drugs is worthwhile and may improve dyspnea and the FEV_1 value.[32] Moreover, the use of inhaled atropine can be helpful also, not only for bronchospasm but also to inhibit the formation of mucus and secretions.

Antimicrobial Therapy

Prophylactic treatment with tetracycline decreased the number of exacerbations in patients who had many episodes, but it did nothing for those who ordinarily had few exacerbations. Antibiotic treatment did not alter the rate of decline in pulmonary function.[33] Prophylactic antibiotic therapy may have some usefulness in highly selected patients who experience frequent exacerbations. Either tetracycline (250–500 mg qid po), ampicillin (250–500 mg qid po), amoxicillin (500 mg qid po), or erythromycin (250 mg qid or 500 mg bid po) is an acceptable drug. Trimethoprim-sulfamethoxazole is also effective. Because bacteria such as *Haemophilus influenzae* can inactivate β-lactam antibiotics by secreting β-lactamases, inhibitors such as clavulanate have been combined with amoxicillin. The use of such a combination is appropriate if β-lactamase–producing bacteria are causing infection. Several different strategies appear to be effective. Patients may receive antibiotics daily during the winter months, 4 days/wk during the winter, or a 7-day course at the first sign of a "chest cold."

The effectiveness of the short-term use of antibiotics for acute exacerbations is difficult to assess.[28,29,34,35,36] Infection can cause acute decompensation and is the most common identifiable cause of death in these patients. The usual strategy is to institute a course of antimicrobial therapy for a 7- to 10-day period and hope that the acute flare-up subsides; an objective end point for success is usually lacking. Erythromycin may be prescribed as an alternative on the assumption that it (like tetracycline) is effective for *Mycoplasma* infection. The oral administration of antibiotics is sufficient for most of the acute bacterial flare-ups. Questions exist about the overall benefit of antimicrobial therapy in exacerbations of chronic bronchitis, although they may improve symptoms and reduce disability.

REFERENCES

1. Ciba Guest Symposium. Terminology, definitions and classification of chronic pulmonary emphysema and related conditions. Thorax. 1959;14:286.
2. Medical Research Council. Definition and classification of chronic bronchitis for clinical and epidemiological purposes. A report to the Medical Research Council by their committee on the etiology of chronic bronchitis. Lancet. 1965;1:775.
3. Reynolds HY. Respiratory infections may reflect deficiencies in host defense mechanisms. DM. 1985;31:1–98.
4. Beck GS, Heiner DC. Selective immunoglobulin G4 deficiency and recurrent infections of the respiratory tract. Am Rev Respir Dis. 1981;124:94.
5. Reynolds HY. Immunoglobulin G and its function in the human respiratory tract. Mayo Clin Proc. 1988;63:161–74.
6. Reynolds HY, Merrill WW. Airway changes in young smokers that may antedate chronic obstructive lung disease. Med Clin North Am. 1981;65:667–89.
7. Nieworehner DE, Kleinerman J, Rice DB. Pathologic changes in the peripheral airways of young cigarette smokers. N Engl J Med. 1974;291:755.
8. Gadek JE, Fellis GA, Crystal RG. Cigarette smoking induces functional antiprotease deficiency in the lower respiratory tract of humans. Science. 1979;206:1315.
9. Carp H, Miller F, Hoidal J, et al. Alpha 1-proteinase inhibitor purified from lungs of cigarette smokers contains oxidized methionine and has decreased elastase inhibitory capacity. Proc Natl Acad Sci USA. 1982;779:2041–5.
10. Gail DB, Lenfant CJM. Cells of the lung: Biology and clinical implications. Am Rev Respir Dis. 1983;127:366–87.
11. Reid L. Measurement of the bronchial mucous gland layer: A diagnostic yardstick in chronic bronchitis. Thorax. 1960;15:132.
12. Reynolds HY. Lung Inflammation: Normal host defense or a complication of some diseases? Annu Rev Med. 1987;38:295–323.
13. Shelhamer JH, Marom Z, Kaliner M. Immunologic and neuropharmacologic stimulation of mucous glycoprotein release from human airways in vitro. J Clin Invest. 1980;66:1400–6.
14. Marom Z, Shelhamer JH, Bach NK, et al. Slow-reacting substances (LTC_4 and LTD_4) increase the release of mucus from human airways in vitro. Am Rev Respir Dis. 1982;126:449–51.
15. Marom Z, Shelhamer JH, Kaliner M. Human pulmonary macrophage-derived mucus secretagogue. J Exp Med. 1984;159:844–60.
16. Marom Z, Shelhamer JH, Kaliner M. Human monocyte-derived mucus secretagogue. J Clin Invest. 1985;75:191–98.
17. Burrows B, Niden AH, Fletcher CM, et al. Clinical types of chronic obstructive lung disease in London and Chicago. Am Rev Respir Dis. 1964;90:14.
18. Chodosh S. Examination of sputum cells. N Engl J Med. 1970;282:854.

19. Baigelman W, Chodosh S. Sputum "wet preps": Window on the airways. J Respir Dis 1984;59–70.
20. Wiggins J, Hill SL, Stockley RA. The secretory IgA system of lung secretions in chronic obstructive bronchitis: Comparison of sputum with secretions obtained during fiberoptic bronchoscopy. Thorax. 1984;39:517–23.
21. Niederman MS, Merrill WW, Polomski LM, et al. Influence of sputum IgA and elastase on tracheal cell bacterial adherence. Am Rev Respir Dis. 1986;133:255.
22. Stockley RA, Afford SC, Burnett D. Assessment of 7S and 11S immunoglobulin A in sputum. Am Rev Respir Dis. 1980;122:956.
23. Leeder SR. Role of infection in the cause and course of chronic bronchitis and emphysema. J Infect Dis. 1975;131:731.
24. Laurenzi GG, Potter RT, Kass EH. Bacterial flora of the lower respiratory tract. N Engl J Med. 1961;265:1273.
25. Potter RT, Totman F, Fernandez R, et al. The bacteriology of the lower respiratory tract. Bronchoscopic study of 100 clinical cases. Am Rev Respir Dis. 1968;97:1051.
26. Halperin SA, Suratt PM, Gwaltney JM Jr, et al. Bacterial cultures of the lower respiratory tract in normal volunteers with and without experimental rhinovirus infection using a plugged double catheter system. Am Rev Respir Dis. 1982;125:678.
27. Hass H, Morris JF, Samson S, et al. Bacterial flora of the respiratory tract in chronic bronchitis: Comparison of transtracheal, fiber-bronchoscopic and oropharyngeal sampling methods. Am Rev Respir Dis. 1977;116:41.
28. Gump DW, Phillips CA, Forsyth BR, et al. Role of infection in chronic bronchitis. Am Rev Respir Dis. 1976;113:465.
29. Tager I, Speizer FE. Role of infection in chronic bronchitis. N Engl J Med. 1975;292:583.
30. Reynolds HY. Bacterial adherence to respiratory tract mucosa—a dynamic interaction leading to colonization. Semin Respir Infect. 1987;2:8–19.
31. Corrao WM, Bramen SS, Irwin RS. Chronic cough as the sole presenting manifestation of bronchial asthma. N Engl J Med. 1979;300:633.
32. Mendella LA, Manfreda J, Warren CPW, et al. Steroid response in stable chronic obstructive lung disease. Ann Intern Med. 1982;96:17.
33. Fletcher CM, Oldham PD. Value of chemoprophylaxis and chemotherapy in early chronic bronchitis. A report to the medical research council by their working party on trials of chemotherapy in early chronic bronchitis. Br Med J. 1966;1:1317.
34. Nicotra MB, Rivera M, Awe RJ. Antibiotic therapy of acute exacerbations of chronic bronchitis. Ann Intern Med. 1982;97:18.
35. Bates JH. The role of infection during exacerbations of chronic bronchitis. Ann Intern Med. 1982;97:130.
36. Anthonisen NR, Manfreda J, Warren CPW, et al. Antiobiotic therapy in exacerbations of chronic obstructive pulmonary disease. Ann Intern Med. 1987;106:196.

52. BRONCHIOLITIS

CAROLINE BREESE HALL
WILLIAM J. HALL

In bronchiolitis we must now contend
with both the disease of the "now" and the "then";
For many such infants a mold has been cast,
perhaps by their unborn and unknown past,
which destines that they shall in time wheeze again.
For them this disease
is the distant, boding knell
Of vulnerable lungs
to a microbe's mystic spell.

C.B.H.

Bronchiolitis is an acute viral lower respiratory tract illness occurring within the first 2 years of life. The characteristic clinical findings include an acute onset of wheezing and hyperaeration, most commonly associated with cough, rhinorrhea, tachypnea, and respiratory distress. The entity "bronchiolitis" appears to have been born from a long lineage of confusing sobriquets, including acute catarrhal bronchitis, interstitial bronchopneumonia, spastic bronchopneumonia, capillary or obstructive bronchiolitis, and asthmatic bronchiolitis.[1] Bronchiolitis, however, did not become recognized as a separate entity until the 1940s.[2]

ETIOLOGY

Although bronchiolitis was initially thought to be caused by bacteria, viruses and occasionally *Mycoplasma pneumoniae* are now known to be the instigators of bronchiolitis. Respiratory syncytial virus (RSV) is clearly the major cause, with the parainfluenza viruses being the second most commonly isolated agent (Table 1, Fig. 1).[3–11] A long-term study of respiratory illnesses associated with wheezing in children from a private practice in Chapel Hill, North Carolina, showed that RSV, parainfluenza viruses type 1 and type 3, adenoviruses, rhinoviruses, and *Mycoplasma pneumoniae* make up 87 percent of the isolates obtained from children of all ages.[3] Within the first 2 years of life, RSV accounted for 44 percent of the isolates, with the parainfluenza viruses type 1 and type 3 and adenoviruses each accounting for about 13 percent. Similarly, RSV was in 55 percent of the isolates obtained from children with bronchiolitis from two group practices in Rochester, New York, over a 6-year period.[12] The second most frequently identified agent was parainfluenza type 3, accounting for 11 percent of the cases. The proportion of these agents may change, depending on the population and whether the cases occur as part of an epidemic. In hospitalized cases, the contribution of RSV is even higher, as demonstrated by the Newcastle-upon-Tyne studies in which 74 percent of the infants hospitalized with bronchiolitis had infection with this agent.[10]

EPIDEMIOLOGY

Bronchiolitis shows a definite seasonal pattern in temperate climates, with a yearly upsurge of cases in winter to early spring.[3,7–10,12,13] This pattern mirrors that of its prime agent, RSV. Lesser swells of activity are seen during the fall and spring when the parainfluenza viruses are active.

Bronchiolitis is a common illness during the first year of life, with the peak attack rate occurring between 2 and 10 months of age.[3,5,10,13–16] In the Chapel Hill studies, the incidence of bronchiolitis was about 11 cases per hundred children for both the first and second 6 months of life.[3,13] In the second year of life the incidence fell to approximately one-half. A much higher incidence, however, has been reported[16] in long-term studies of children in a day care center who were examined regularly. Since even the mildest cases were detected, the rate rose to 115 cases per 100 children aged 6 months or less per year. By the second year of life this rate had declined to 32 cases per 100 children per year.

An appreciable proportion of hospital admissions for infants within the first year of life are caused by bronchiolitis, especially that resulting from RSV. In the review by Breese et al.[17] of their group practice, 4 percent of their patients of all ages requiring hospitalization for medical illnesses were bronchiolitis cases. In the Seattle prepaid medical care group, the rate of infants hospitalized with bronchiolitis during the first 6 months of life was 6 per 1000 children per year.[5] Bronchiolitis is more

TABLE 1. Agents Causing Bronchiolitis

Agent	*Cases (%)*	*Epidemiology*
Respiratory syncytial virus	45–75	Yearly epidemics winter to spring
Parainfluenza viruses		
Type 3	8–15	Predominantly spring to fall
Type 1	5–12	Epidemics in the fall every other year
Type 2	1–5	Fall
Rhinoviruses	3–8	Endemic, all seasons
Adenoviruses	3–10	Endemic, all seasons
Influenza viruses	5–8	Epidemic, winter to spring
Mycoplasma pneumoniae	1–7	Endemic, all seasons
Enteroviruses	1–5	Summer to fall

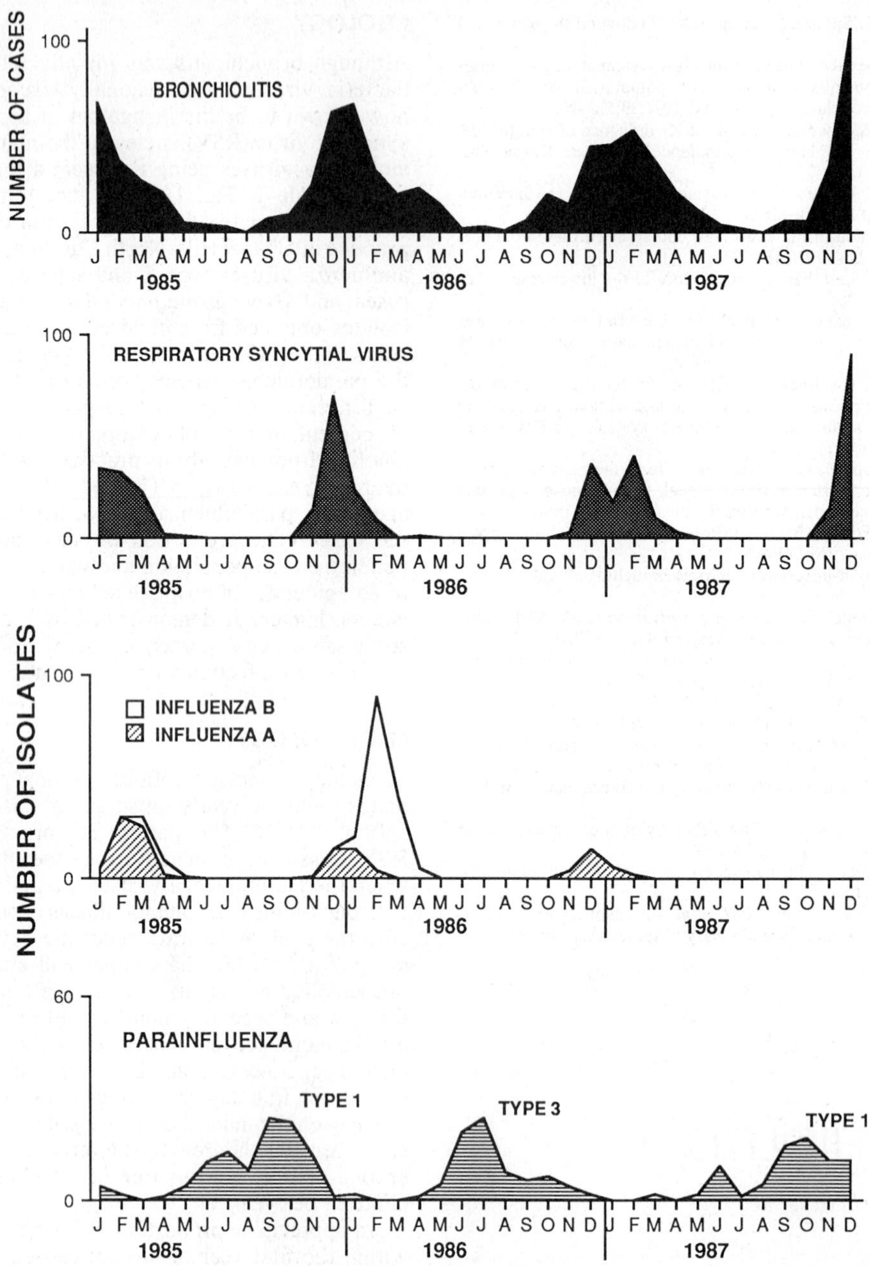

FIG. 1. Patterns of reported cases of bronchiolitis shown in relation to the activity of the major respiratory viruses in Monroe County, New York. Data are obtained from a weekly community surveillance program for infectious diseases.

common in boys, especially in those requiring hospitalization, with a ratio of about 1.5 to 1.[3,15,18]

PATHOPHYSIOLOGY

Engle and Newns[2] in 1940 carefully described the pathologic findings of bronchiolitis, which have subsequently been expanded and further delineated.[1,19–22] The characteristic initial findings are inflammation and necrosis of the respiratory epithelium. Subsequently, the epithelium may proliferate and demonstrate cuboidal cells without cilia. Peribronchiolar infiltration, mostly with mononuclear cells, and edema of the submucosa and adventitia are observed. Necrosis of the bronchiolar epithelium and sloughing subsequently results (Figs. 2 and 3).

Inflammation of the small bronchi and bronchioles is generalized but of varying severity. Since resistance to the flow of air is inversely related to the cube of the radius, this inflammation and edema make the small lumens of an infant particularly vulnerable to obstruction. Plugs of necrotic material and fibrin may completely or partially obstruct the small airways. Smooth muscle constriction does not appear to be important in the obstruction.[22] In areas peripheral to sites of partial obstruction, air becomes trapped by a process similar to a "ball–valve" mechanism. The negative intrapleural pressure during inspiration allows air to flow beyond the point of partial obstruction. However, on expiration, the size of the lumen decreases with the positive pressure, thereby resulting in increased obstruction and hyperinflation. Thus, although airflow is impeded during both inspiration and expiration, the latter is more affected and prolonged. In areas peripheral to complete obstruction, the trapped air eventually becomes absorbed, which results in multiple areas of focal atelectasis. The degree of atelectasis or hy-

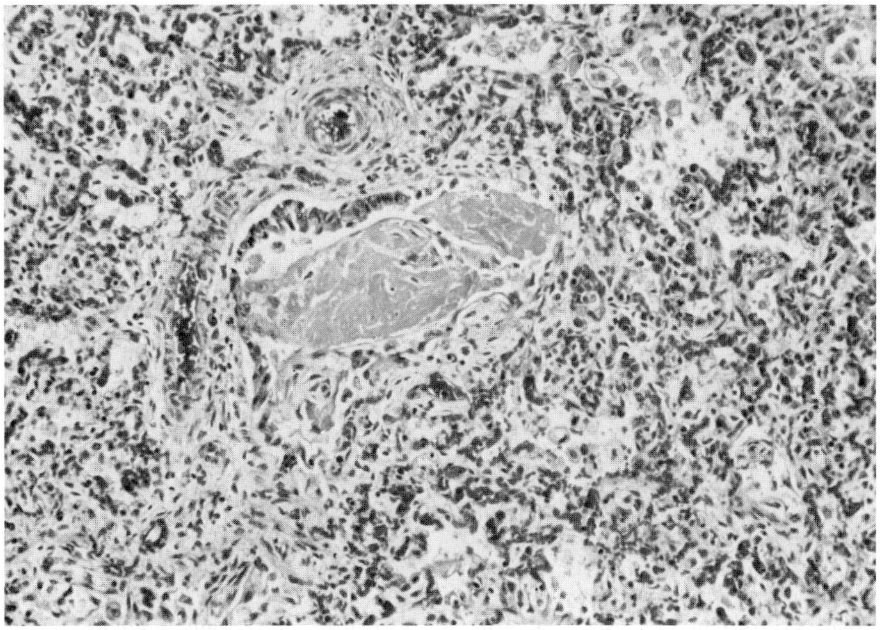

FIG. 2. Inflammation and necrosis in bronchiolitis resulting in obliteration of the bronchiolar lumen.

perinflation that develops is related to the amount of collateral ventilation present.

The physiologic correlates of this resistance to air flow are dyspnea, tachypnea, and a diminished tidal volume. The distribution of ventilation within the infant's lung is also markedly altered. The low ratio of ventilation to perfusion of the lung parenchyma produces arterial hypoxemia. With progression of the disease, hypercarbia ensues. The pathologic process may progress to involve the alveolar walls and spaces and produce an interstitial pneumonitis. Recovery tends to be slow, requiring several weeks.

An abnormal immune response may contribute to the pathogenesis of bronchiolitis and to the subsequent hyperreactivity of the airways that is frequently seen in children who have been hospitalized with bronchiolitis. In infants infected with RSV, specific IgE antibody and histamine have been found to be present in the nasopharyngeal secretions more frequently and in higher titer in those patients whose illness was associated with wheezing.[23,24] Furthermore, the amount of specific IgE antibody and histamine in the secretions correlated with severity of illness as determined by the degree of hypoxia. Infants with RSV-induced wheezing also tended to demonstrate higher degrees of whole blood lymphocyte transformation to RSV.[25] The number of suppressor cells (OKT8 antigen–positive cells) has also been reported to be diminished in convalescing bronchiolitis patients and was associated with higher titers of specific IgE antibody in the secretions.[24] In patients with infection from one of the parainfluenza viruses, similar correlations have been made between illness manifested by wheezing and increased titers of virus-specific IgE antibody in the secretions

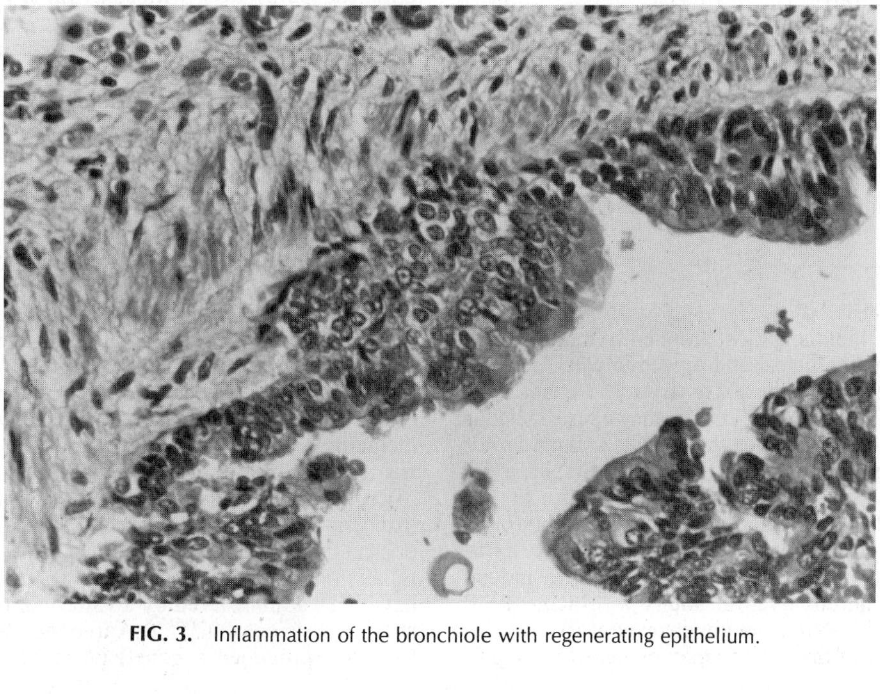

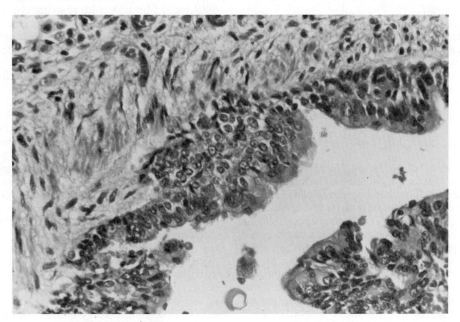

FIG. 3. Inflammation of the bronchiole with regenerating epithelium.

and an increased lymphocyte transformation response to parainfluenza virus.[26]

CLINICAL MANIFESTATIONS

Upper respiratory tract signs, especially coryza and cough, usually herald the onset of bronchiolitis. During a prodromal period of 1–7 days mild fever is common. Lower respiratory tract involvement may appear relatively acute with deepening cough, an increased respiratory rate, and restlessness. With progression, the tachypnea and tachycardia may be marked, although fever may no longer be present. Retractions of the chest wall, flaring of the nasal alae, and grunting are evidence of the increased work of breathing. Cyanosis is rarely evident even though moderate to severe hypoxemia may be present.[22,27] Auscultation, which may vary from hour to hour, reveals wheezing with or without crackles. Increasing dyspnea with decreasing auscultatory findings and movement of air may indicate progressive obstruction and impending respiratory failure.

Dehydration is a common accompaniment of bronchiolitis that results from paroxysms of coughing that may trigger vomiting and from a poor oral intake related to the respiratory distress and lethargy. The tachypnea further increases the fluid requirements. Otitis media, occurring in 10–30 percent of infants, mild conjunctivitis, and occasionally diarrhea may also be present.

For most infants the acute course lasts 3–7 days. Most show improvement within 3–4 days, with a gradual recovery period of 1–2 weeks, but in some it may be prolonged.[27,28]

LABORATORY FINDINGS

The total white blood cell count is usually within the normal range or slightly elevated.[28,29] In hospitalized infants, however, who are more seriously ill and hypoxemic, the white blood cell count may be elevated, and the differential may show a left shift.[27,29] Almost all hospitalized infants with bronchiolitis are hypoxemic, but the degree of hypoxemia is difficult to assess clinically.[27] The degree of wheezing and retractions also cannot be assumed to be indicative of the level of oxygenation. An inverse correlation, however, appears to exist between the respiratory rate and the arterial oxygen saturation.[27,30] Only the most severely ill children develop hypercarbia because most are able to compensate for the increased work of breathing with an elevated respiratory rate.[27,30,31]

The classic findings on chest roentgenogram films are those of hyperinflation, depressed diaphragms, hyperlucency of the parenchyma, and decreased costophrenic angles.[32–35] The bronchovascular markings are usually prominent, with linear densities radiating out from the hila.[36] Multiple areas of atelectasis of varying degrees are also commonly present and difficult to differentiate from the infiltrates of pneumonia. Indeed, both bronchiolitis and pneumonia are frequently present, especially with RSV infection.

DIAGNOSIS

The diagnosis of bronchiolitis is most frequently made on the basis of the characteristic clinical and epidemiologic findings. However, considerable confusion exists over the exact definition of bronchiolitis.[37] A variety of entities may cause a similar picture of dyspnea and wheezing in the infant. Asthma is not easily differentiated, particularly if it is the infant's first episode. Furthermore, the two diseases may be combined. An appreciable proportion of wheezing episodes occurring in a child with an atopic diathesis may arise from viral infections.[38] Respiratory syncytial virus in particular has a propensity to induce wheezing in young children. Even in adults with acute RSV infection clinically manifested as an upper respiratory tract infection, hyperreactivity of the airways may be detected by pulmonary function testing, which lasts for 1 or 2 months.[39] Children who first wheeze during an epidemic of RSV infection may therefore be less likely to have an atopic predisposition than do children who appear to develop bronchiolitis during nonepidemic periods.[40]

Gastric reflux may also produce a picture that is clinically indistinguishable from acute bronchiolitis. Other considerations include obstruction of the airway from a foreign body, vascular rings, retropharyngeal abscess, and even enlarged adenoids. Congestive heart failure may also occasionally cause a similar picture in young infants.

A specific diagnosis of the agent of acute bronchiolitis can be made in an appreciable proportion of infants by viral isolation from respiratory secretions, preferably from a nasal wash.[3,5–10,41] In most cases the viruses associated with bronchiolitis may be identified in tissue culture within 3–7 days. Newer rapid viral diagnostic techniques are available, especially for RSV, that allow identification of the viral antigen in the respiratory secretions within hours to 1 day.[42–44] Serologic determination of the etiologic agent is rarely helpful. Not only does the time required to obtain a convalescent serum preclude its being of help in the clinical management, but also maternally acquired antibody to many of the viral agents of bronchiolitis will be present in these young infants.

THERAPY

Over 2 decades ago Reynolds and Cook[45] noted that "oxygen is vitally important in bronchiolitis, and there is little convincing evidence that any other therapy is consistently or even occasionally useful." Today the mainstay of therapy remains oxygen administration with careful supportive care.[1] Although mist therapy is also commonly employed, its use has not been proved beneficial, and chest physiotherapy has been shown to be of no help.[46]

A variable but sometimes high proportion of infants, especially those with RSV infection, who are admitted to the hospital may require mechanical ventilation,[47,48] which has necessitated high tidal volumes with high peak inspiratory pressures and low respiratory rates to achieve a high minute ventilation.[47] Even though infants with bronchiolitis generally have hyperexpanded lungs, most benefit from positive end-expiratory pressure.

Specific therapy has recently become available for bronchiolitis caused by RSV with ribavirin (1-β-D-ribafuranysol-1,2,4-triazole-3-carboxamide), a synthetic nucleoside.[49] This broad-spectrum antiviral agent has only been approved for infants hospitalized with RSV infections and is administered as a small particle aerosol for 12–18 hours each day, usually for 2–5 days.[50–59] In all of the controlled studies thus far reported, clinical benefit has been demonstrated, with a faster rate of improvement in the severity of illness and the arterial blood gases and with no evidence of toxicity.[49–59] Ribavirin administered via a ventilator, however, requires careful monitoring. The drug can precipitate in the lines of the ventilator, which could cause obstruction of the expiratory valve. The use of one-way valves and filters in the inspiratory and expiratory lines will prevent this potential complication. The aerosolized drug does not appear in these infants to aggravate the wheezing or any airway hyperreactivity as evidenced by the improvement in the arterial blood gases and, second, by serial pulmonary function testing, including carbachol challenge, of RSV-infected volunteers treated with ribavirin or placebo.[60]

Bronchodilator therapy for infants with bronchiolitis is controversial. In most young infants the major cause of the airway obstruction is the inflammation caused by the viral infection rather than smooth muscle contraction.[1,22] Bronchodilators have been administered by a variety of routes and usually have not been successful.[1,61] β-Adrenergic agents in most studies have not produced a beneficial response, as documented by pulmonary function studies,[62–66] and may even produce a detrimental effect.[67]

A few infants, however, may appear to improve with careful bronchodilator therapy.[22,68] A trial of aerosolized or parenteral bronchodilators, therefore, has been recommended by some for those infants who require hospitalization and who may be carefully monitored.[68,69]

Several studies have evaluated the use of steroids in bronchiolitis but have generally not found them to be of benefit.[70–73] The Committee of Drugs of the American Academy of Pediatrics has thus advised against the use of steroids in bronchiolitis. However, a recent study showed a beneficial effect of nebulized beclomethasone dipropionate in infants who, after bronchiolitis, had persistent wheezing.[74] Antibiotics should not be routinely administered to infants with bronchiolitis since bacteria have no role in the etiology. Furthermore, secondary bacterial infection is rarely observed after bronchiolitis.[75]

COMPLICATIONS

With the currently available methods of respiratory support, the mortality from bronchiolitis is very low. The most severe and complicated courses tend to occur in children with underlying conditions such as cardiopulmonary diseases and prematurity.[22,47] Even previously healthy infants, however, tend to have prolonged pulmonary function abnormalities despite clinical improvement.[27,76] Apnea may complicate the course of bronchiolitis, especially in very young infants with RSV infection.[27,77–79]

The long-term effects of bronchiolitis on the immature and developing lung have not been entirely clarified.[22,80] Infants who have been hospitalized with bronchiolitis do, however, appear to be at risk for recurrent wheezing and long-term pulmonary function abnormalities.[81–88] Children who had milder bronchiolitis not requiring hospitalization do not appear to be at the same degree of risk.[81,89] Abnormalities in function of the small airways appear to persist for years but may be clinically silent. The pathogenesis of these long-term effects is not clear. A variety of factors in different studies have been associated with increasing the infant's risk of later pulmonary abnormalities, including passive smoking, lack of breast-feeding, prematurity, crowded homes, and young age at time of the initial respiratory infections.[81,83,84,86–88,90] Controversy exists as to the relative roles of a genetic predisposition toward atopy or hyperreactivity of the lung vs. the direct effect of the virus on the lung during critical stages of development that result in subsequent functional abnormalities.[1,81,90]

BRONCHIOLITIS OBLITERANS

Rarely, a chronic type of bronchiolitis, bronchiolitis obliterans, may develop in infants and young children initially having acute bronchiolitis. This unusual disease appears to develop most commonly after infections with adenovirus, in infants with a certain undefined genetic predisposition, and in bone marrow transplant patients with graft-vs.-host diseases.[22,91–94] The disease has appeared to be particularly prevalent in Indian populations in central Canada and in Polynesians in New Zealand.[91–93] Such infants commonly have bronchopneumonia along with the signs of bronchiolitis that continue for weeks to months with fluctuating severity. Approximately 60 percent of these children develop chronic disease with atelectasis, bronchiectasis, intermittent pneumonia, and hyperinflation. These sequelae are accompanied by severe pathologic abnormalities involving the occlusion and destruction of the bronchi and bronchioles.

REFERENCES

1. Wohl MEB, Chernick V. Bronchiolitis. Am Rev Respir Dis. 1978;118:759–81.
2. Engle S, Newns GH. Proliferative mural bronchiolitis. Arch Dis Child. 1940;15:219–29.
3. Henderson FW, Clyde WA Jr, Collier AM, et al. The etiologic and epidemiologic spectrum of bronchiolitis in pediatric practice. J Pediatr. 1979;95:183–90.
4. Chanock R, Chambon L, Chang W, et al. WHO respiratory disease survey in children. A serologic study. Bull WHO. 1967;37:363–9.
5. Foy HM, Cooney MK, Maletzky AJ, et al. Incidence and etiology of pneumonia, croup and bronchiolitis in preschool children belonging to a prepaid medical care group over a four year period. Am J Epidemiol. 1973;97:80–92.
6. Glezen WP, Loda FA, Clyde WA Jr, et al. Epidemiologic patterns of acute lower respiratory tract disease of children in a pediatric group practice. J Pediatr. 1971;78:397–406.
7. Kim HW, Arrobio JO, Brandt CD, et al. Epidemiology of respiratory syncytial virus infection in Washington, D.C. I. Importance of the virus in different respiratory disease syndromes and temporal distribution of infection. Am J Epidemiol. 1973;98:216–25.
8. Loda FA, Glezen WP, Clyde WA Jr. Respiratory disease in group day care. Pediatrics. 1972;49:428–37.
9. Macasaet FF, Kidd PA, Bolano CR, et al. The etiology of acute respiratory infections. II. The role of viruses and bacteria. J Pediatr. 1968;72:829–39.
10. Gardner PS. How etiologic, pathologic, and clinical diagnosis can be made in a correlated fashion. Pediatr Res. 1977;11:254–61.
11. Chang Tzu-ching, Wang Chih-liang, Han Hsu-lau. Etiologic and clinical investigation of bronchiolitis. Chinese Med J. 1978;4:135–41.
12. Hall CB. Infectious Diseases Newsletter. 1983;31:1 and 1982;29:1.
13. Denny FW, Clyde WA Jr. Acute lower respiratory tract infections in nonhospitalized children. J Pediatr. 1986;108:635–46.
14. Glezen WP. Pathogenesis of bronchiolitis. Epidemiologic considerations. Pediatr Res. 1977;11:239–43.
15. Parrott RH, Kim HW, Arrobio JO, et al. Epidemiology of respiratory syncytial virus infection in Washington, D.C. II. Infection and disease with respect to age, immunologic status, race and sex. Am J Epidemiol. 1973;98:289–300.
16. Denny FW, Collier AM, Henderson FW, et al. The epidemiology of bronchiolitis. Pediatr Res. 1977;11:234–6.
17. Breese BB, Disney FA, Talpey W. The nature of a small pediatric group practice, Part I. Pediatrics. 1966;38:264–77.
18. Kravits H. Sex distribution of hospitalized children with acute respiratory diseases, gastroenteritis and meningitis. Clin Pediatr (Phila). 1965;4:484–91.
19. Aherne W, Bird T, Court SDM, et al. Pathological changes in virus infections of the lower respiratory tract in children. J Clin Pathol. 1970;23:7–18.
20. McLean KH. The pathology of bronchiolitis. A study of its evolution. I. The exudative phase. Aust Ann Med. 1956;5:254.
21. McLean KH. The pathology of bronchiolitis. A study of its evolution. II. The repair phase. Aust Ann Med. 1957;6:29.
22. Wohl MEB. Bronchiolitis. Pediatr Ann. 1986;15:307–13.
23. Welliver RC, Wong DT, Sun M, et al. The development of respiratory syncytial virus specific IgE and the release of histamine in nasopharyngeal secretions after infection. N Engl J Med. 1981;305:841–6.
24. Welliver RC, Kaul TN, Sun M, et al: Defective regulation of immune responses in respiratory syncytial virus infection. J Immunol. 1984;133:1925–30.
25. Welliver RC, Kaul A, Ogra PL. Cell-mediated immune response to respiratory syncytial virus infection: Relationship to the development of reactive airway disease. J Pediatr. 1979;94:370–5.
26. Welliver RC, Wong DT, Sun M, et al. Parainfluenza virus bronchiolitis: Epidemiology and pathogenesis. Am J Dis Child. 1986;14:34–40.
27. Hall CB, Hall WJ, Speers DM. Clinical and physiologic manifestations of bronchiolitis and pneumonia. Am J Dis Child. 1979;133:798–802.
28. Ackerman BD. Acute bronchiolitis: A study of 207 cases. Clin Pediatr (Phila). 1962;1:75–81.
29. Portnoy B, Haynes B, Salvatore MA, et al. The peripheral white blood count in respirovirus infection. J Pediatr. 1966;68:181–8.
30. Reynolds EOR. Arterial blood gas tensions of babies with bronchiolitis. Br Med J. 1963;1:1192–5.
31. Downes JJ, Wood DW, Striker TW, et al. Acute respiratory failure in infants with bronchiolitis. Anesthesiology. 1968;29:426–34.
32. Simpson W, Hacking PM, Court SDM, et al. The radiological findings in respiratory syncytial virus infection in children. Pediatr Radiol. 1974;2:97–100.
33. Simpson W, Hacking PM, Court SDM, et al. The radiological findings in respiratory syncytial virus infection in children. Part II. The correlation of radiological categories with clinical and virological findings. Pediatr Radiol. 1974;2:155–60.
34. Rice RP, Loda F. A roentgenographic analysis of respiratory syncytial virus pneumonia in infants. Radiology. 1966;87:1021–7.
35. Koch DA. Roentgenologic considerations of capillary bronchiolitis. Am J Roentgenol Rad Ther Nucl Med. 1959;82:433–6.
36. Khamapirad T, Glezen WP. Clinical and radiographic assessment of acute lower respiratory tract disease in infants and children. Semin Respir Infect. 1987;2:130–44.
37. McConnochie K. Bronchiolitis: What's in the name? Am J Dis Child. 1983;137:11–3.
38. McIntosh K, Ellis EF, Hoffman LS, et al. The association of viral and bacterial respiratory infections with exacerbations of wheezing in young asthmatic children. J Pediatr. 1973;82:578–90.

39. Hall WJ, Hall CB, Speers DM. Respiratory syncytial virus infections in adults: Clinical, virologic and serial pulmonary function studies. Ann Intern Med. 1978;88:203–5.
40. Polmar SH, Robinson LD Jr, Minnefor AB. Immunoglobulin E in bronchiolitis. Pediatrics. 1972;50:279–84.
41. Hall CB, Douglas RG Jr. Clinically useful method for the isolation of respiratory syncytial virus. J Infect Dis. 1975;131:1–5.
42. Richman D, Schmidt N, Plotkin S, et al: Summary of a workshop on new and useful methods in rapid viral diagnosis. J Infect Dis. 1984;150:941–51.
43. Chonmaitree T, Bessette-Henderson BJ, Hepler RE, et al. Comparison of three rapid diagnostic techniques for detection of respiratory syncytial virus from nasal wash specimens. J Clin Microbiol. 1987;25:746–7.
44. Anestad G, Breivik N, Thoressen T. Rapid diagnosis of RSV and influenza A virus infections by immunofluorescence: Experience with a simplified procedure for the preparation of cell smears from nasopharyngeal secretions. Acta Pathol Microbiol Immunol Scand. 1983;91:267–71.
45. Reynolds EOR, Cook CD. The treatment of bronchiolitis. J Pediatr. 1963;63:1205–7.
46. Webb MSC, Martin GA, Cartlidge PHT, et al. Chest physiotherapy in acute bronchiolitis. Arch Dis Child. 1985;60:1078–9.
47. Frankel LR, Lewiston NJ, Smith DW, et al. Clinical observations on mechanical ventilation for respiratory failure in bronchiolitis. Pediatr Pulmonol. 1986;2:307–11.
48. Outwater KM, Crone RK. Management of respiratory failure in infants with acute viral bronchiolitis. Am J Dis Child. 1984;138:1071–5.
49. Knight V, Gilbert BE. Chemotherapy of respiratory viruses. Adv Intern Med. 1986;31:95–118.
50. Hall CB, McBride JT, Walsh EE, et al. Aerosolized ribavirin treatment of infants with respiratory syncytial virus infection: A randomized double-blind study. N Engl J Med. 1983;308:1443–7.
51. Taber LH, Knight V, Gilbert BE, et al. Ribavirin aerosol treatment of bronchiolitis due to respiratory syncytial virus infection in infants. Pediatrics. 1983;72:613–8.
52. Hall CB, Walsh EE, Hruska JF, et al. Ribavirin aerosol treatment of experimental respiratory syncytial viral infection in young adults: A controlled double-blind study. JAMA. 1983;249:2666–70.
53. Rodriquez WJ, Kim HW, Brandt CD, et al. Aerosolized ribavirin in the treatment of patients with respiratory syncytial virus disease. Pediatr Infect Dis J. 1987;6:159–63.
54. Conrad DA, Christenson JC, Waner JL, et al. Aerosolized ribavirin treatment of respiratory syncytial virus infection in infants hospitalized during an epidemic. Pediatr Infect Dis J. 1987;6:152–8.
55. Caramia G, Palazzini E. Efficacy of ribavirin aerosol treatment for respiratory syncytial virus bronchiolitis in infants. J Int Med Res. 1987;15:227–33.
56. Barry W, Cockburn F, Cornall R, et al. Ribavirin aerosol for acute bronchiolitis. Arch Dis Child. 1986;61:593–4.
57. Frankel LR, Wilson CW, Demers RR, et al. A technique for the administration of ribavirin to mechanically ventilated infants with severe respiratory syncytial virus. Crit Care Med. 1987;15:1051–4.
58. Demers RR, Parker J, Frankel LR, et al. Administration of ribavirin to neonatal and pediatric during mechanical ventilation. Respir Care. 1986;31:1188–96.
59. Outwater KM, Meissner C, Peterson MB. Ribavirin administration to infants receiving mechanical ventilation. Am J Dis Child. 1988;142:512–5.
60. Hall CB, Walsh EE, Hruska JF, et al. Ribavirin treatment of experimental respiratory syncytial virus infection in young adults: A controlled double blind study. JAMA. 1983;249:2666–70.
61. Silverman M. Bronchodilators for wheezy infants? Arch Dis Child. 1984;59:84–7.
62. Phelan PD, Williams HE. Sympathomimetic drugs in acute viral bronchiolitis. Their effect on pulmonary resistance. Pediatrics. 1969;44:493–7.
63. Rutter N, Milner AD, Hiller EJ. Effect of bronchodilators on respiratory resistance in infants and young children with bronchiolitis and wheezy bronchitis. Arch Dis Child. 1975;50:719–22.
64. Henry RL, Milner AD, Stokes GM. Ineffectiveness of ipratropium bromide in acute bronchiolitis. Arch Dis Child. 1983;58:925–6.
65. Lenney W, Milner AD. Alpha and beta adrenergic stimulants in bronchiolitis and wheezy bronchitis in children under 18 months of age. Arch Dis Child. 1978;53:707–9.
66. Radford M. Effect of salbutamol in infants with wheezy bronchitis. Arch Dis Child. 1975;50:535–8.
67. Hughes DM, Lesouef PN, Landau LI. Effect of salbutamol on respiratory mechanics in bronchiolitis. Pediatr Res. 1987;22:83–6.
68. Soto M, Sly PD, Uren E, et al. Bronchodilator response in acute viral bronchiolitis. Pediatr Pulmonol. 1985;2:85–90.
69. Ellis EF. Therapy of acute bronchiolitis. Pediatr Res. 1977;11:263–4.
70. Stecenko MA. Treatment of viral bronchiolitis: Do steroids make sense? Contemp Pediatr 1987;April:121–30.
71. Connolly JH, Field CMB, Glasgow JFT, et al. A double blind trial of prednisolone in epidemic bronchiolitis due to respiratory syncytial virus. Acta Paediatr Scand 1969;58:116.
72. Leer JA, Green JL, Heimlich EM, et al. Corticosteroid treatment in bronchiolitis. A controlled collaborative study in 297 infants and children. Am J Dis Child. 1969;117:495–503.
73. Yaffe SJ, Weiss CF, Cann HM, et al. Should steroids be used in treating bronchiolitis? Pediatrics. 1970;46:640–642.
74. Maayan C, Itzhaki T, Bar-Yishay E, et al. The functional response of infants with persistent wheezing to nebulized beclamethasone dipropionate. Pediatr Pulmonol. 1986;2:9–14.
75. Hall CB, Powell KR, Schnabel KC, et al. The risk of secondary bacterial infection in infants hospitalized with respiratory syncytial viral infection. J Pediatr. 1988;113:266–71.
76. Wohl MEB, Stigol LC, Mead J. Resistance of the total respiratory system in healthy infants and infants with bronchiolitis. Pediatrics. 1969;43:495–509.
77. Bruhn FW, Mokrohisky ST, McIntosh K. Apnea associated with respiratory syncytial virus infection in young infants. J Pediatr. 1977;90:382–6.
78. Anas N, Boettrich C, Hall CB, et al. The association of apnea and respiratory syncytial virus in infants. J Pediatr. 1982;101:65–8.
79. Church NR, Anas NG, Hall CB, et al. Respiratory syncytial virus related apnea in infants: Demographics and outcome. Am J Dis Child. 1984;138:247–50.
80. Workshop on bronchiolitis, sponsored by the National Heart, Blood and Lung Institute Division of Lung Diseases, National Institutes of Health. Pediatr Res. 1977;11:209–70.
81. Twiggs JT, Larson LA, O'Connell EJ, et al. Respiratory syncytial virus infection: Ten-year follow up. Clin Pediatr (Phila). 1981;20:187–90.
82. Kattan M, Keens TG, Lapierre JG, et al. Pulmonary function abnormalities in symptom free children after bronchiolitis. Pediatrics. 1977;59:683–8.
83. Sims DG, Gardner PS, Weightman D, et al. Atopy does not predispose to RSV bronchiolitis or postbronchiolitic wheezing. Br Med J. 1981;282:2086–8.
84. McConnochie KM, Roughman KJ. Bronchiolitis as a possible cause of wheezing in childhood: New evidence. Pediatrics. 1984;74:1–10.
85. Duiverman EJ, Neijens HJ, van Strik R, et al. Lung function and bronchial responsiveness in children who had infantile bronchiolitis. Pediatr Pulmonol. 1987;3:38–44.
86. Hall CB, Hall WJ, Gala CL, et al. A long term prospective study of children following respiratory syncytial virus infection. J Pediatr. 1984;105:358–64.
87. Carlsen KH, Larsen S, Bjerve O, et al. Acute bronchiolitis: Predisposing factors and characterization of infants at risk. Pediatr Pulmonol. 1987;3:153–60.
88. Webb MSC, Henry RL, Milner AD, et al. Continuing respiratory problems three and a half years after acute viral bronchiolitis. Arch Dis Child. 1985;60:1064–7.
89. McConnochie KM, Mark JD, McBride JT, et al. Normal pulmonary function measurements and airway reactivity in childhood after mild bronchiolitis. J Pediatr. 1985;107:54–8.
90. McConnochie KM, Roughman KJ. Breast feeding and maternal smoking as predictors of wheezing in children age 6 to 10 years. Pediatr Pulmonol. 1986;2:260–7.
91. Lang WR, Howden CW, Lars J, et al. Bronchopneumonia with serious sequelae in children with evidence of adenovirus type 21 infections. Br Med J. 1969;1:73–9.
92. Chernick V, Macpherson RI. Respiratory syncytial and adenovirus infections of the lower respiratory tract in infancy. Clin Notes Respir Dis. 1971;10:3.
93. Gold R, Wilt JC, Adhikari PK, et al. Adenoviral pneumonia and its complications in infancy and childhood. J Can Assoc Radiol. 1969;20:218–24.
94. Ralph DD, Springmeyer SC, Sullivan KM, et al: Rapidly progressive airflow obstruction in marrow transplant recipients. Am Rev Respir Dis. 1984;129:641–4.

53. ACUTE PNEUMONIA

GERALD R. DONOWITZ
GERALD L. MANDELL

In 1901, Sir William Osler noted in the fourth edition of his book *The Principles and Practice of Medicine* that "the most widespread and fatal of all acute diseases, pneumonia, is now Captain of the Men of Death."[1] Almost 90 years later, the prominence of pneumonia as a clinical entity remains. It is the sixth most common cause of death in the United States and the most common cause of infection-related mortality.[2] The challenge confronting most clinicians is not in detecting the presence of the disease but rather in identifying its etiology. Since a wide array of microbial agents may cause acute pneumonia (Table 1), and since no single antimicrobial regimen can be expected to cover all the possibilities, specific diagnosis remains a prerequisite for proper therapy. To this end, the pathogenesis of the disease should be understood and information from the his-

TABLE 1. Etiologic Agents of Acute Pneumonia

- Bacterial
  - Common
    - *Streptococcus pneumoniae*
    - *Staphylococcus aureus*
    - *Haemophilus influenzae*
    - Mixed anaerobic bacteria (aspiration)
      - *Bacteroides* spp.
      - *Fusobacterium* spp.
      - *Peptostreptococcus* spp.
      - *Peptococcus* spp.
    - Enterobacteriaceae
      - *Escherichia coli*
      - *Klebsiella pneumoniae*
      - *Enterobacter* spp.
      - *Serratia* spp.
    - *Pseudomonas aeruginosa*
    - *Legionella* spp. (including *L. pneumophila* and *L. micdadei*)
  - Uncommon
    - *Acinetobacter* var. *anitratus*
    - *Actinomyces* and *Arachnia* spp.
    - *Aeromonas hydrophilia*
    - *Bacillus* spp.
    - *Branhamella catarrhalis*
    - *Campylobacter fetus*
    - *Eikenella corrodens*
    - *Francisella tularensis*
    - *Neisseria meningitidis*
    - *Nocardia* spp.
    - *Pasteurella multocida*
    - *Proteus* spp.
    - *Pseudomonas pseudomallei*
    - *Salmonella* spp.
    - *Enterococcus faecalis*
    - *Streptococcus pyogenes*
    - *Yersinia pestis*
- Viral
  - Children
    - Common
      - Respiratory syncytial virus
      - Parainfluenza virus types 1, 2, 3
      - Influenza A virus
    - Uncommon
      - Adenovirus types 1, 2, 3, 5
      - Influenza B virus
      - Rhinovirus
      - Coxsackievirus
      - Echovirus
      - Measles virus
  - Adults
    - Common
      - Influenza A virus
      - Influenza B virus
      - Adenovirus types 4 and 7 (in military recruits)
    - Uncommon
      - Rhinovirus
      - Adenovirus types 1, 2, 3, 5
      - Enteroviruses
        - Echovirus
        - Coxsackievirus
        - Poliovirus
      - Epstein-Barr virus
      - Cytomegalovirus
      - Respiratory syncytial virus
      - Varicella-zoster virus
      - Parainfluenza virus
      - Measles virus
      - Herpes simplex virus
- Fungal
  - *Aspergillus* spp.
  - *Candida* spp.
  - *Coccidioides immitis*
  - *Cryptococcus neoformans*
  - *Histoplasma capsulatum*
  - Agents of mucormycosis
    - *Rhizopus* spp.
    - *Absidia* spp.
    - *Mucor* spp.
- Rickettsial
  - *Coxiella burnetii*
  - *Rickettsia rickettsiae*
- Bacteria-like agents
  - *Mycoplasma pneumoniae*
  - *Chlamydia* spp.
    - *C. psittaci*
    - *C. trachomatis*
    - TWAR
- Mycobacterial
  - *Mycobacterium tuberculosis*
- Parasitic
  - *Ascaris lumbricoides*
  - *Pneumocystis carinii*
  - *Strongyloides stercoralis*
  - *Toxoplasma gondii*
  - *Paragonimus westermani*

tory and physical examination, as well as from the microbiology laboratory, must be used.

PATHOGENESIS

In the absence of disease, normal pulmonary defense mechanisms maintain essentially sterile infralaryngeal airways and parenchyma. The development of acute pulmonary infection indicates either a defect in host defenses, challenge by a particularly virulent microorganism, or an overwhelming inoculum. Infectious agents gain entry to the lower respiratory tract through inhalation of aerosolized material or aspiration of upper airway resident flora. Less frequently, pneumonia results from metastatic seeding of the lungs from the blood stream.

Lung defense mechanisms important in the prevention of infection include (*1*) filtration and humidification of inspired air in the upper airways, (*2*) intact epiglottic and cough reflexes, (*3*) tracheobronchial secretions (the mucous blanket) and mucociliary transport via the ciliated epithelium, (*4*) cell-mediated immunity (alveolar macrophages, T lymphocytes), (*5*) humoral immunity (B lymphocytes, immunoglobulin, complement), and (*6*) polymorphonuclear neutrophils.[3,4]

A number of factors are known to interfere with normal host defenses and to predispose to infection.[3] Alterations in the level of consciousness from any cause (stroke, seizures, drug intoxication, anesthesia, alcohol abuse, and even normal sleep) can compromise epiglottic closure and lead to aspiration of oropharyngeal flora into the lower respiratory tract.[5,6] Cigarette smoke, perhaps the most common agent involved in compromising natural pulmonary defense mechanisms, disrupts both mucociliary function and macrophage activity.[7] Other factors that impair pulmonary clearance of pathogens include hypoxemia,[8] acidosis, alcohol,[9] toxic inhalations,[10,11] pulmonary edema,[12] uremia, malnutrition, corticosteroids,[9] immunosuppressive agents,[13] viral infection,[14] and mechanical obstruction.[4]

Recurrent episodes of bacterial pneumonia suggest the presence of specific predisposing factors,[15,16] which have been categorized by Roth and Gleckman according to the age of the patient.[16] In children and young adults, recurrent pneumonias are associated with congenital defects in host defenses, including leukocyte function[17] and immunoglobulins.[17–20] Congenital defects in cilia activity including the immotile-cilia syndrome,[21] Kartagener syndrome[22] (ciliary dysfunction, situs inversus, sinusitis, bronchiectasis), Young syndrome (azospermia, sinusitis, pneumonia),[23] and cystic fibrosis are other clinical entities associated with recurrent pneumonia in the young. Structural lung abnormalities such as bronchiectasis and pulmonary sequestration[24] are also important predisposing factors for both younger and older patient populations.

In adults, factors predisposing to recurrent pneumonia include acquired defects in host defenses (chronic lymphocytic leukemia, myeloma, hypogammaglobulinemia, the acquired immunodeficiency syndrome [AIDS]), bronchial obstruction due to intrinsic compression (adenomas, carcinomas) or extrinsic compression (lymph node enlargement due to sarcoid or malignancy), and esophageal abnormalities (reflux, stricture).[25] Episodes of altered mental states due to alcohol, trauma, or neurologic disorders are also important factors predisposing to recurrent pneumonia.

CLINICAL EVALUATION

History

The history should attempt to define (*1*) the clinical setting in which the pneumonia is taking place, (*2*) defects in host resistance that could predispose to the development of pneumonia, and (*3*) possible exposure to specific pathogens. Although age and race are usually of little diagnostic value, it should be remembered that mycoplasma pneumonia occurs more often in younger people,[26,27] that gram-negative pneumonia tends to occur in the elderly,[28] and that tuberculosis appears to be more prevalent in nonwhite populations.[29]

Pneumonia has been noted to occur with increased frequency in patients with a variety of underlying disorders such as congestive heart failure, diabetes, alcoholism, and chronic obstructive pulmonary disease.[28,30,31] In one series of 292 patients with pneumonia, only 18 percent were found to have no underlying disease.[28] A history of upper respiratory tract infection has been elicited in 36–50 percent of patients with acute pneumonia, especially in those with pneumococcal disease.[30,32] Recent dental manipulations, sedative overdoses, seizures, alcoholism, or loss of consciousness for any reason should raise the suspicion of anaerobic infection due to aspiration of oral contents.[5]

Specific etiologic agents of pneumonia have been associated with certain underlying diseases. An increased incidence of staphylococcal pneumonia has been noted during epidemics of influenza.[33] Patients with chronic obstructive pulmonary disease are frequently colonized with *Streptococcus pneumoniae* and *Haemophilus influenzae* and are at increased risk for the development of pneumonia caused by these agents.[34] Cystic fibrosis is associated with pseudomonas and staphylococcal pulmonary infection.[35] Pulmonary alveolar proteinosis has been associated with *Nocardia* infection.[36] Patients with AIDS are at high risk for the development of pneumonia caused by *Pneumocystis carinii,* cytomegalovirus, and mycobacteria, as well as more common pulmonary pathogens.[37–39] Pneumonia developing in hospitalized patients often involves enteric gram-negative bacilli, *Pseudomonas aeruginosa,* and *Staphylococcus aureus,* agents that are unusual in nonhospitalized populations.[40] Similarly, pneumonia in the elderly, especially those living in nursing homes or extended care facilities, is more often associated with gram-negative bacilli than is pneumonia in younger populations.[40–42]

Occupational history, history of exposure to animals, travel history, and sexual history are all important in suggesting specific potential infectious agents (Table 2). The presence of noninfectious pulmonary disease such as tumors or pulmonary emboli, which may masquerade as pneumonia, may also be suggested by a careful history.

Physical Examination

Fever is usually present and may be sustained, remittent, or at times hectic. Fever patterns per se, however, are not useful for establishing a specific diagnosis. The temperature should be taken rectally to reduce error due to rapid mouth breathing. Recording of postural changes in blood pressure and pulse rate is useful in assessing hydration and intravascular fluid volume. The pulse usually increases by 10 beats/min for every degree (C) of temperature elevation. A pulse temperature deficit (i.e., a relative bradycardia for the amount of fever) should suggest viral infection, mycoplasmal infection, chlamydial infection, tularemia, or infection with *Legionella* spp. Cyanosis, rapid respiratory rate, the use of accessory muscles of respiration, sternal retraction, and nasal flaring suggest serious respiratory compromise.

Furuncles are rarely secondary to staphylococcal pneumonia acquired by the respiratory route but may signal a source of bacteremia with subsequent hematogenous pneumonia. Herpes labialis is seen in up to 40 percent of the patients with pneumococcal pneumonia.[43] Bullous myringitis is an infrequent although significant finding in mycoplasmal pneumonia.[27] The presence of poor dentition should suggest a mixed infection due to aspiration of anaerobes and aerobes that colonize the oropharynx. While edentulous people may develop anaerobic pneumonia due to aspiration, it is uncommon.[44]

Examination of the thorax may reveal "splinting" or an inspiratory lag on the side of the lesion that is suggestive of bacterial pneumonia. Early in the disease process, definite signs of pulmonary involvement may be lacking or may be manifest only as fine, crackling rales. Chest examination may reveal these early signs of pneumonia even though the chest film is normal. Evidence of consolidation (dullness on percussion, bronchial breath sounds, and E to A changes) is highly suggestive of bacterial infection. Patients with mycoplasmal or viral infection may exhibit few abnormalities on physical examination despite the presence of impressive infiltrates on the chest film.

TABLE 2. Important Environmental Factors in Pneumonia

Pneumonia Associated with	Environmental History
Anthrax	Exposure to cattle, swine, horses, goat hair, wool, hides
Brucellosis	Exposure to cattle, goats, pigs; employment as abattoir worker or veterinarian
Melioidosis	Travel to W. Indies, Australia, Guam, S.E. Asia, South and Central America
Plague	Exposure to ground squirrels, chipmunks, rabbits, prairie dogs, rats
Tularemia	Exposure to tissue or body fluids of infected animals (rabbits, hares, foxes, squirrels) or to bites of an infected arthropod (flies, ticks) Handling or ingesting poorly cooked meat from an infected animal
Psittacosis	Exposure to birds (parrots, budgerigars, cockatoos, pigeons, turkeys)
Leptospirosis	Exposure to wild rodents, dogs, cats, pigs, cattle, horses, or exposure to water contaminated with animal urine
Coccidioidomycosis	Travel to San Joaquin Valley, S. California, S.W. Texas, S. Arizona, New Mexico
Histoplasmosis	Exposure to bat droppings or dust from soil enriched with bird droppings
Q fever	Exposure to infected goats, cattle, sheep and their secretions (milk, amniotic fluid, placenta, feces)
Legionnaires' disease	Exposure to contaminated aerosols (e.g., air coolers, hospital water supply)

SPUTUM EXAMINATION

Microscopic examination and culture of expectorated sputum remain the mainstays of the laboratory evaluation of pneumonia despite ongoing controversy concerning their sensitivity and specificity.[45–48] Procurement of expectorated sputum is a noninvasive technique that can be carried out at no risk to the patient, provides samples of lower respiratory tract secretions for immediate evaluation, and in the majority of cases allows the clinician to make a presumptive diagnosis.

Examination of the sputum should include observation of the color, amount, consistency, and odor of the specimen. Mucopurulent sputum is most commonly found with bacterial pneumonia or bronchitis. Sputum of similar nature has been described in one-third to one-half of patients with mycoplasma[27] or adenovirus infections.[49,50] However, scant or watery sputum is more often noted with these and other atypical pneumonias. "Rusty" sputum suggests alveolar involvement and has been most commonly (although not solely) associated with pneumococcal pneumonia.[51] Dark red, mucoid sputum (currant-jelly sputum) suggests Friedlander's pneumonia caused by encapsulated *Klebsiella pneumoniae*.[52] Foul-smelling sputum is associated with mixed anaerobic infections most commonly seen with aspiration.[44]

Where possible, frankly purulent material should be selected for microscopic examination. In all cases of acute pneumonia, a Gram stain of the sputum should be prepared. In order to maximize the diagnostic yield of the sputum examination, only samples free of oropharyngeal contamination should be reviewed. As a guide, the number of neutrophils and epithelial cells should be quantitated under low power (100×), with further examination reserved for samples containing ≥25 neutrophils and ≤10 epithelial cells. Such samples contain minimal oropharyngeal contamination.[53] Samples with more epithelial cells and fewer neutrophils are nondiagnostic and should be discarded. The morphologic and staining characteristics of any bacteria seen should be recorded and an estimate made of the predominant organisms (Figs. 1–4). Where no bacterial predominance exists, this should be noted as well.

In the appropriate clinical setting, a predominance of gram-positive, lancet-shaped diplococci should suggest pneumococ-

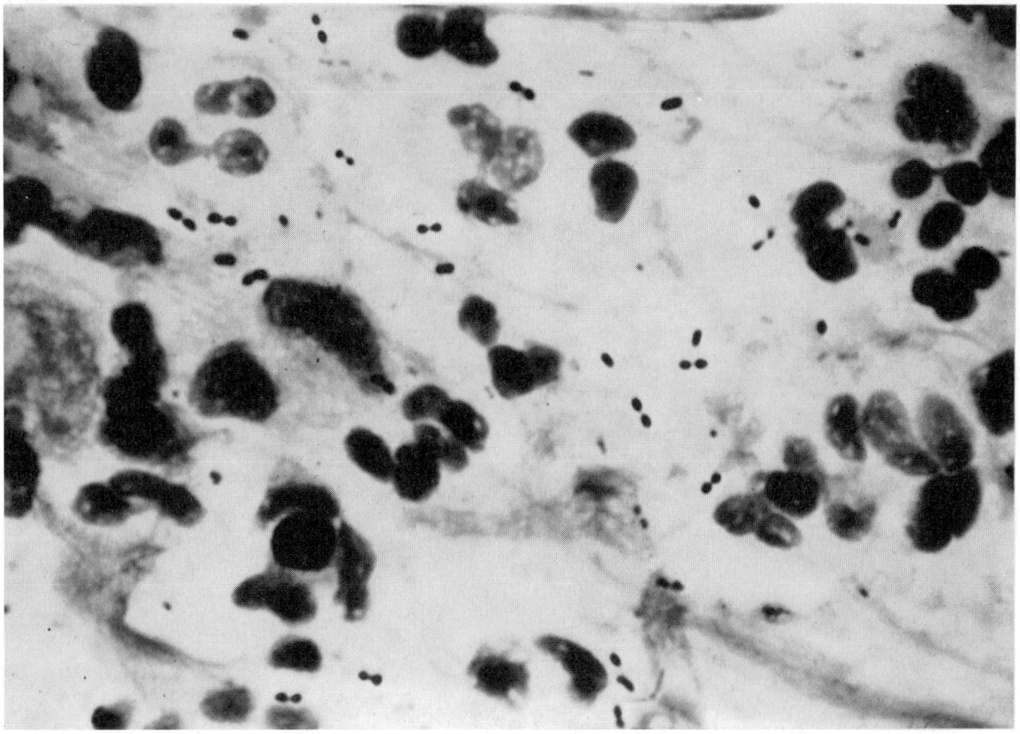

FIG. 1. Expectorated sputum with gram-positive, lancet-shaped diplococci from a patient with pneumococcal pneumonia.

cal infection (Fig. 1). When strict criteria for Gram stain positivity are used (predominant flora and/or more than 10 gram-positive, lancet-shaped diplococci per oil immersion field [100×]), the specificity of the Gram stain for identifying pneumococci has been shown to be 85 percent, with a sensitivity of 62 percent.[54] The diagnostic yield of the sputum examination for pneumococci can be maximized by the use of the quellung reaction. Anticapsular antiserum reacts with capsular polysaccharide, and this may be seen as a distinctly outlined capsule. Rare false-positive results may occur with α-hemolytic streptococci. Occasional false-negative results may occur as well. An 89 percent correlation between pneumococcal isolation by culture and a positive sputum quellung test has been demonstrated.[46]

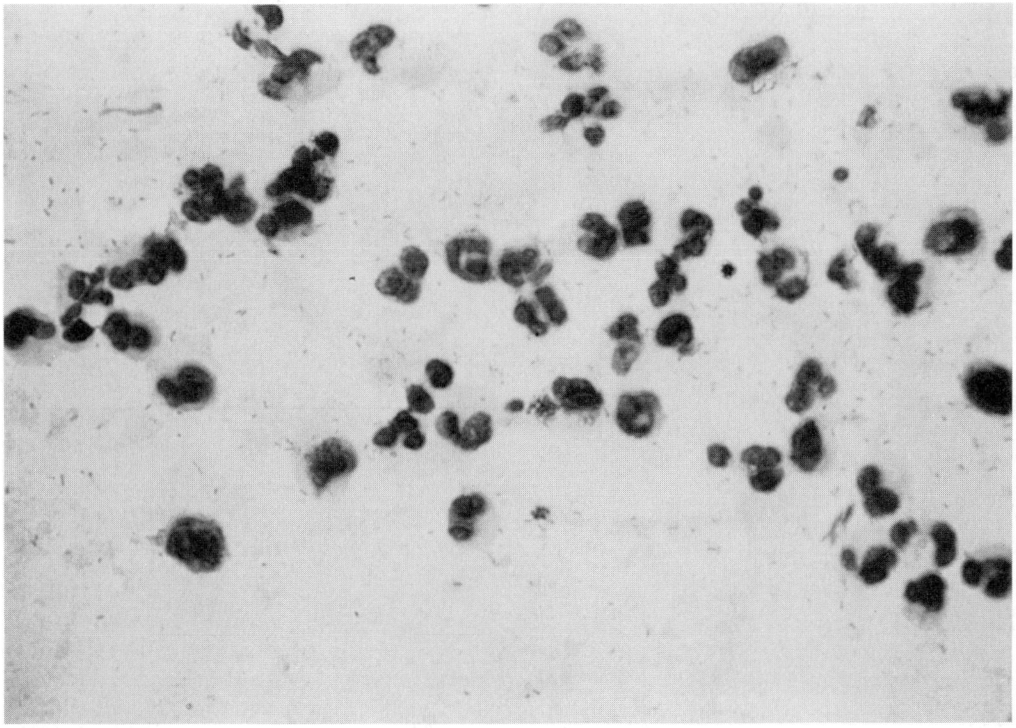

FIG. 2. Expectorated sputum with gram-negative coccobacillary forms from a patient with *Haemophilus influenzae* pneumonia.

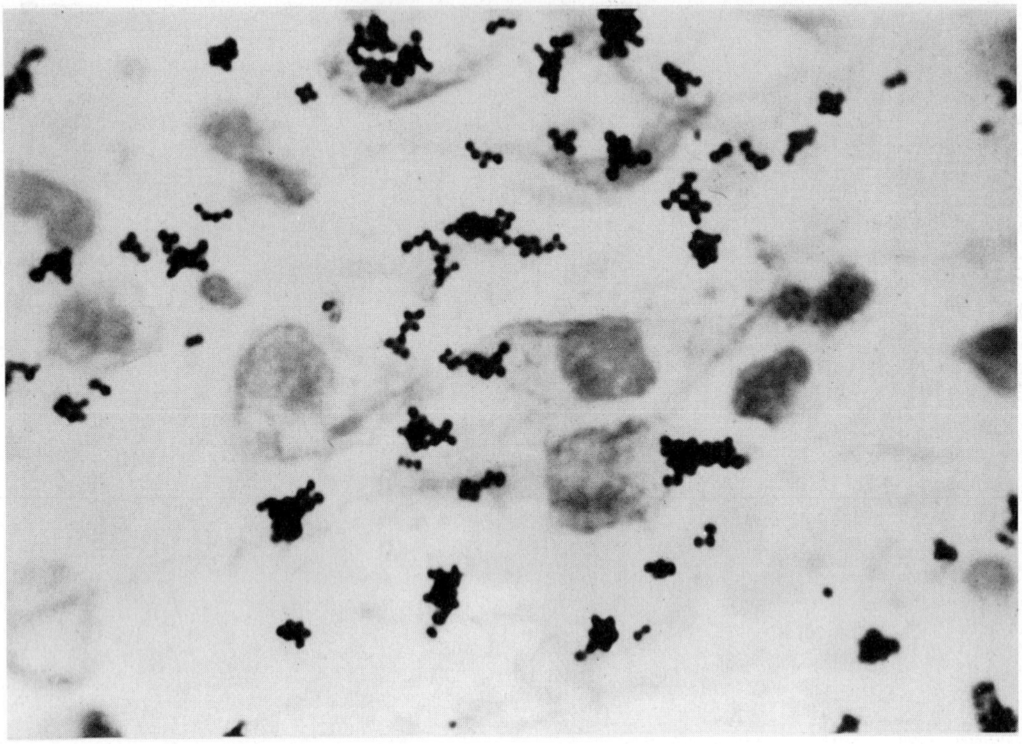

FIG. 3. Expectorated sputum with gram-positive cocci in clumps from a patient with staphylococcal pneumonia.

Since pneumococci may be part of the nasopharyngeal flora in up to 50 percent of healthy adults and may colonize the lower airways in patients with chronic bronchitis, identification of the organism does not always mean that it is the cause of disease.[55–57] However, it is our belief that the large number of pneumococci necessary to produce a positive Gram stain or quellung reaction is unusual in carriers.

The sputum Gram stain is helpful to identify organisms other than the pneumococcus. Small gram-negative coccobacillary organisms are characteristic of *H. influenzae* (Fig. 2). Staphylococci appear as gram-positive cocci in tetrads and grapelike clusters (Fig. 3). Organisms of mixed morphology are characteristic of anaerobic infection. Few bacteria are seen with legionnaires' disease, mycoplasma pneumonia, and viral pneumonia. Sputum examination has been a useful means of diagnosing *P. carinii* pneumonia in patients with AIDS. Use of

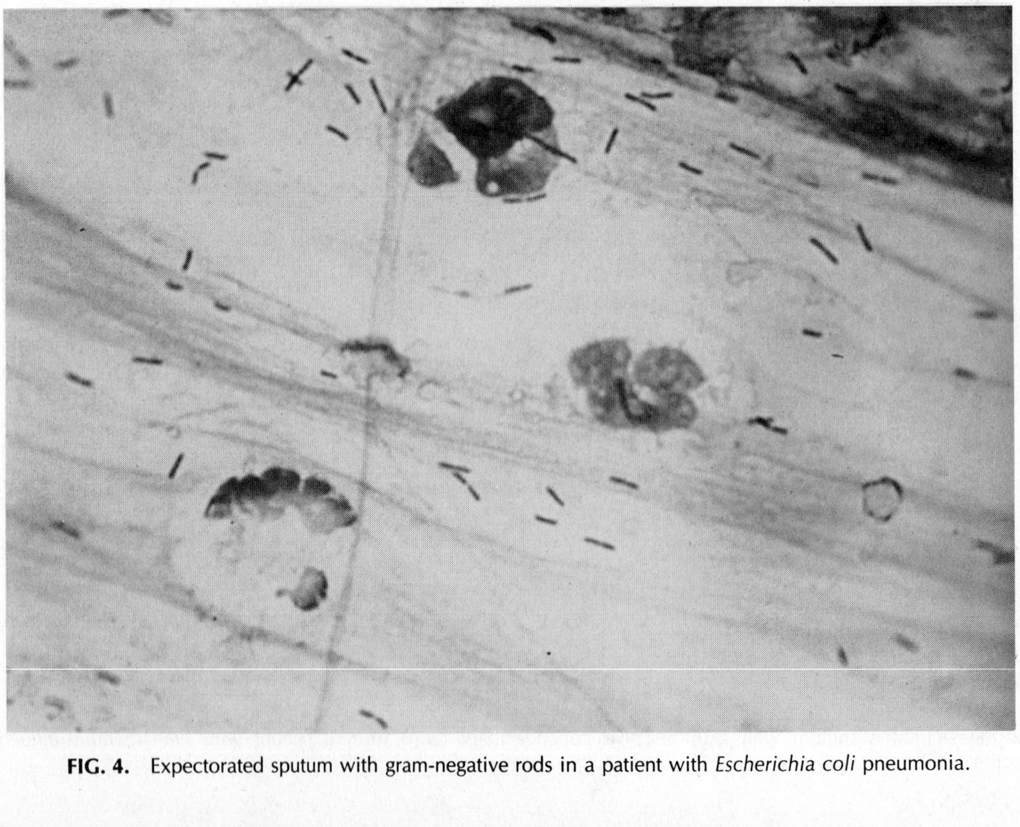

FIG. 4. Expectorated sputum with gram-negative rods in a patient with *Escherichia coli* pneumonia.

the Giemsa or Gomori methanamine silver stain has led to a diagnosis in over 50 percent of cases, making more aggressive diagnostic procedures unnecessary.[58,59]

A variety of diagnostic techniques have been recently introduced that provide the potential for more accurate and rapid identification of the etiologic agents of pneumonia. Nucleic acid hybridization techniques have been used to detect herpes simplex virus, cytomegalovirus, mycoplasma, *Legionella* spp., *Mycobacterium tuberculosis,* and nontuberculosis mycobacterium. Monoclonal antibodies in the immunofluorescence assay and the enzyme-linked immunosorbent assay (ELISA) have been used to rapidly detect a variety of viruses and *Legionella* spp. in respiratory secretions.[60–62] While many of these techniques are of great interest, their general applicability has yet to be determined.

The utility of the sputum culture as a means of diagnosing pneumonia has been questioned. Patients with bacteremic pneumococcal pneumonia have been reported to have negative sputum cultures in 45–50 percent of cases, even when large numbers of organisms have been noted on Gram stain.[63,64] Similarly, 34–47 percent of sputum cultures are negative with proven *H. influenzae* pneumonia.[65,66] Further, sputum cultures have frequently been shown to yield more bacterial species than more invasive methods of obtaining respiratory tract secretions.[67,68] Contamination with gram-negative bacilli from the oropharynx has been noted in 32 percent of sputum cultures.[69]

Several key parameters have been identified in efforts to maximize the diagnostic yield from sputum culture. Procurement of adequate sputum samples is an essential first step. Where fewer than 10 epithelial cells and more than 25 neutrophils per low-power field are noted, oropharyngeal contamination is minimal and sputum samples are comparable to transtracheal aspirates in terms of the number of bacterial species isolated.[53] With increasing numbers of epithelial cells and decreasing numbers of neutrophils, an increased amount of oropharyngeal contamination is present, as indicated by the isolation of more bacterial species.

The presence of alveolar macrophages does not alter the bacteriologic findings when substantial numbers of epithelial cells are present, indicating that otherwise adequate samples of sputum can be contaminated with oropharyngeal contents and thereby rendered nondiagnostic. This type of initial screening has proven helpful in differentiating adequate sputum samples from saliva, thereby increasing the diagnostic yield of sputum culture.

When culture of sputum is delayed, isolation of pneumococci is less likely due to overgrowth of the organism by oropharyngeal flora. Rapid processing of samples is therefore another important factor leading to higher diagnostic yields.

Laboratory techniques for maximizing the useful information from sputum cultures have included quantitative cultures, washing of samples to remove contaminating mouth flora, and the use of mucolytic agents. The varying results noted have not warranted the increased efforts required. Further, washing samples does not guarantee that adequate samples of lower respiratory tract secretions are present.[70] Some reports suggest that with adequate sputum samples and prompt culture of specimens, the diagnostic yield of the sputum culture may approach 100 percent.[45,71,72]

TRANSTRACHEAL ASPIRATION

Although the sputum examination should always be included in the initial evaluation of patients with pneumonia, it may be inadequate for a presumptive diagnosis. In cases in which either (*1*) no sputum is produced, (*2*) no clear predominance of a potential pathogen exists on sputum Gram stain or culture, (*3*) there has been a poor response to antibiotics chosen on the basis of expectorated sputum, (*4*) gram-negative rods or yeast forms are found in the sputum, or (*5*) the possibility of superinfection exists, a more direct method of obtaining lower respiratory tract secretions may be necessary. Transtracheal aspiration should be considered, although this is a potentially dangerous procedure and is now uncommonly performed in patients with acute pneumonia.

Comparative studies have shown that less oropharyngeal contamination occurs in sputum obtained by transtracheal aspiration as compared with expectorated sputum.[67,69,73,74] In patients with chronic obstructive pulmonary disease, fewer yeast forms and fewer species of bacteria (especially anaerobes) were noted in cultures of transtracheal aspirates as compared with cultures of aspirates from fiberoptic bronchoscopy.[75] Furthermore, if anaerobes are to be isolated from the lower respiratory tract, the oropharynx, with its abundant resident flora of anaerobes, must be bypassed.[76] Several authors have reported the clinical usefulness of transtracheal aspiration in defining the etiology of acute bacterial pneumonia.[68,74,77]

False-negative results of cultures of transtracheal aspirate have been reported in 11 percent of samples. Theoretically, false-negative transtracheal aspirates can occur if infection involves the periphery of the lung only or if the involved bronchi are obstructed. In practice, false-negative aspirates seem to be most common in patients treated with antibiotics before the procedure. A false-positive rate of approximately 21 percent has been noted and is thought to be due to oropharyngeal contamination or tracheobronchial colonization, especially in patients with chronic lung disease.[77]

Transtracheal aspiration is carried out by having the patient lie with a pillow under the shoulders so that the neck is hyperextended. The cricothyroid membrane at the base of the thyroid cartilage is located, and the area is prepared and draped (Fig. 5A). After local anesthesia is applied to the skin over the cricothyroid membrane, a large-bore needle containing a 17- or 18-gauge indwelling catheter is inserted through the cricothyroid space in the midline with the needles angled downward toward the coccyx (Fig. 5B). After the trachea has been entered (Fig. 5C), the catheter is advanced several inches and the needle is removed, leaving the catheter in place. With a syringe attached to the catheter, the sputum is aspirated (Fig. 5D). If no material is obtained, 2–3 ml of sterile saline (without antibacterial additives) is injected and aspiration is again attempted. Once the material is obtained, the catheter is removed and firm pressure is applied to the puncture site. Material obtained from transtracheal aspiration should be Gram stained and cultured anaerobically and aerobically.

Transtracheal aspiration is not without risk. Significant hemoptysis,[69,74,78] subcutaneous and mediastinal emphysema,[69,74] aspiration of oral contents,[79] soft tissue infection,[80,81] and pneumothoraces[82] have occurred in association with the procedure. Bradycardia, thought to be due to stimulation of the vagus nerve in the presence of hypoxia and hypercapnia, has been observed and has been associated with cardiorespiratory arrest.[79] Coagulation abnormalities (especially thrombocytopenia) and significant hypoxemia or hypercapnia should be contraindications for the procedure. Patients who are coughing violently are probably at greater risk for mediastinal emphysema. In patients who cannot cooperate, the procedure should be carried out with great care, if at all.

FIBEROPTIC BRONCHOSCOPY

Initial studies concerning the usefulness of fiberoptic bronchoscopy for the diagnosis of bacterial pneumonia demonstrated that the procedure was limited by contamination of specimens by oropharyngeal flora. Cultures obtained via the bronchoscope averaged two to three more bacterial isolates than samples from paired transtracheal aspirates.[75] In patients without lower respiratory tract infections, cultures of aspirates obtained at bronchoscopy produced an average of five different

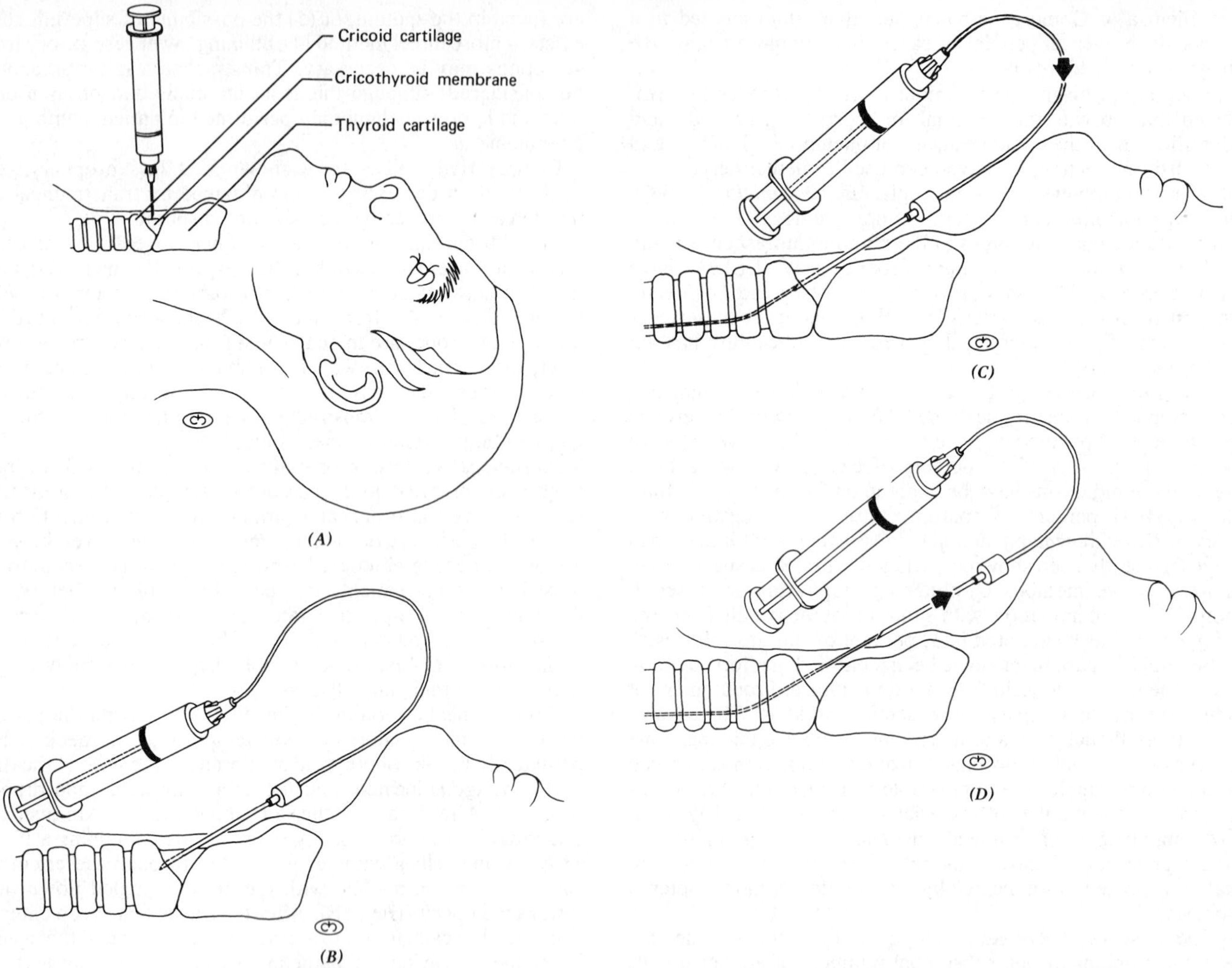

FIG. 5. Transtracheal aspiration. **(A)** The patient's neck is hyperextended, and local anesthesia is applied to the area over the cricothyroid membrane. **(B)** A large-bore needle with an indwelling catheter is inserted through the cricothyroid membrane into the trachea. **(C)** The catheter is advanced several inches into the trachea. **(D)** The needle is carefully withdrawn. Secretions are obtained by aspiration.

bacterial strains.[83] The development of the protected brush catheter (a brush within two catheters sealed at the end with a polyethylene glycol plug) has significantly decreased but not eliminated this problem[84,85] Quantitative culturing has been used to differentiate contaminants from true infecting agents.[84,86,87] Using $\geq 10^3$ colony-forming units per milliliter as a "breakpoint" for determination of the clinical significance of an isolate, studies employing the protected brush catheter have proven experimentally and clinically to be both sensitive (70–97 percent) and specific (95–100 percent) for the diagnosis of bacterial pneumonia.[86–89] However, not all series using this technique have produced impressive results,[90–92] and in some patient groups this technique is not useful. One group consists of patients receiving prior antibiotics, and another includes patients with underlying structural disease, in whom over 50 percent of bronchoscopic specimens yield significant numbers of organisms even in the absence of pneumonia.[86,89] Detection of the antibody coating of organisms found at bronchoscopy has been used in an attempt to differentiate colonization from true infection. Experience has been limited and results have been mixed, with a high false-positive rate noted in patients with chronic bronchitis.[93,94]

Bronchoalveolar lavage, in which a segment of lung is "washed" with sterile fluid, has proved to be an excellent means of diagnosing *P. carinii* and cytomegalovirus pneumonia. In patients with AIDS, the sensitivity of the procedure for detecting these pathogens ranges from 89 to 98 percent.[95,96] By using immunofluorescent monoclonal antibodies to viral antigens or centrifuging lavage material onto tissue culture preparations, the diagnosis of cytomegalovirus pneumonia may be made within hours.[97,98] While bronchoalveolar lavage may detect other pathogens (fungi, mycobacteria) in patients with AIDS, and may be useful in defining the etiology of pneumonia in other immunosuppressed patients, lower sensitivities than those noted above have been observed.[99,100]

By using cytologic screening and microbiologic quantitation of bronchoalveolar lavage fluid, bacterial etiologies of pneumonia have been identified. Criteria of <1 percent squamous epithelial cells and $>10^5$ colony-forming units of a bacterial isolate have been used to diagnose bacterial pneumonias with sensitivities of up to 86 percent and specificities of up to 100 percent.[101,102] Most series have involved patients who were immunocompromised; the applicability of this procedure to general patient populations has not yet been thoroughly evaluated.

LUNG BIOPSY

Direct means of obtaining diagnostic material in patients with pneumonia include percutaneous lung aspiration, transbronchial lung biopsy, thoracoscopy, and open lung biopsy.[103] These procedures are usually reserved for cases of pneumonia in pediatric populations, in which sputum is not routinely available and transtracheal aspiration is dangerous, or in patients who are immunosuppressed, in whom routine diagnostic procedures are often unsuccessful in providing a diagnosis and where unusual pathogens may be present. Biopsy procedures are rarely indicated in the normal person with acute pneumonia. The indications and usefulness of these invasive procedures remain controversial. Lung aspiration has provided a diagnostic yield of 30–82 percent in adults and children, though false-negative rates of up to 18 percent have been reported.[104–107] Bleeding and pneumothorax have been reported as the major complications in 5–39 percent of procedures.[107–109] The use of transbronchial biopsy in the diagnosis of pneumonia has been reviewed recently, revealing similar diagnostic yields though somewhat lower complication rates.[110]

Thoracoscopy, in which the pleura and underlying lung are visualized through a thorascope before biopsy, has been used in several series of children and adults with pneumonia. Despite a diagnostic yield of over 90 percent and low complication rates, there has not been extensive experience with this procedure.[111,112]

Open lung biopsy remains the definitive invasive procedure for making an etiologic diagnosis of pneumonia in immunosuppressed patients.[109,110,113] Review of the recent literature has noted diagnostic yields of 60–100 percent. The incidence of pneumothorax and bleeding is usually less than 10 percent, even in patients who are thrombocytopenic.[110] Some have questioned whether open lung biopsy provides meaningful information that significantly affects patients' clinical outcome.[114,115]

Examination of Pleural Effusions

The characteristics of pleural effusions and their importance in the differential diagnosis of pulmonary disease are discussed in Chapter 54. It should be noted that the incidence of pleural effusions associated with pneumonia varies with the etiologic agent, from approximately 10 percent with pneumococci to 50–70 percent with gram-negative bacilli to up to 95 percent with group A streptococcal disease.[51,116,117] Pleural fluid cultures, when positive, are specific for the etiology of the underlying pneumonia. Furthermore, analysis of pleural fluid may play a major role in differentiating other causes of pulmonary infiltrates that may mimic pneumonia, including tuberculosis, tumors, pulmonary emboli, and collagen vascular diseases. Pleural biopsy specimens from patients with acute bacterial pneumonia are nonspecific and are therefore of little use in the differential diagnosis. Analysis of pleural fluid may be of prognostic significance. A pleural fluid pH of less than 7.0 or a pleural fluid glucose level below 40 mg/100 ml has been associated with the presence of a complicated parapneumonic effusion and the need for a tube thoracostomy.[118]

Blood Culture, Serologic Studies, and Antigen Detection

Approximately 20–30 percent of patients with bacterial pneumonia are bacteremic. Positive blood cultures offer definitive proof of the etiology of an associated pneumonia, and blood should be cultured from all patients suspected of having bacterial pneumonia.

Since the demonstration by Dorff et al. that pneumococcal capsular antigen could be detected by counterimmunoelectrophoresis (CIE),[119] a variety of techniques have been used to identify antigen in urine, serum, and plural fluid. None, including CIE, latex agglutination, and ELISA, have proven to be definitive. Sensitivities vary from 20 to 90 percent, and false-positive rates vary from 8 to 20 percent.[120–123] In a small number of cases, CIE of pleural fluid has been helpful in defining the etiology of empyema in patients with previous antibiotic therapy and negative pleural fluid cultures.[124]

CIE of sputum in patients with bacteremic pneumococcal pneumonia has been positive in 75–100 percent of cases but appears to be less sensitive than either the quellung reaction or culture.[125–127] This test is less helpful in detecting disease caused by pneumococcal types 7 and 14, which contain neutral polysaccharides not easily detected by CIE.[128] Further, although a positive sputum CIE will detect the presence of pneumococcal antigen, it cannot distinguish colonization from true infection.[129,130]

CIE and latex agglutination techniques have been used for the detection of *H. influenzae* and pseudomonas antigens in patients with pneumonia, though clinical experience has been limited and the results disappointing.[131]

Serologic tests have been used to diagnose a variety of other pulmonary pathogens, including *Legionella pneumophila, Legionella micdadei, Mycoplasma pneumoniae, Chlamydia* spp., and *Coxiella burnetii*.[132] The sensitivity and specificity of these assays are variable, and many assays have not been completely standardized. Since many of these tests are not routinely done, their usefulness in making a rapid diagnosis is limited. They are of more help in confirming a clinical diagnosis.

RADIOLOGIC EXAMINATION

The chest film most frequently shows a bronchopneumonia pattern that is not very helpful in making a specific etiologic diagnosis (Fig. 6). However, certain features may be of some diagnostic aid. Lobar consolidation, cavitation, and large pleural effusions support a bacterial etiology (Fig. 7). In cases in which bilateral diffuse involvement is noted, *P. carinii* pneumonia, *Legionella* pneumonia, or a primary viral pneumonia should be suspected. Staphylococcal pneumonia may result from infection metastasizing from a primary focus unrelated to the lung. In these cases, multiple nodular infiltrates throughout the lung may be seen. Staphylococci may cause marked necrosis of lung tissue with ill-defined thin-walled cavities (pneumatoceles), bronchopleural fistulas, and empyema, especially in children[133–135] (Fig. 8). Although pneumatoceles are diagnostically significant findings in staphylococcal pneumonia, they may be seen in pneumonias of other etiologies, including

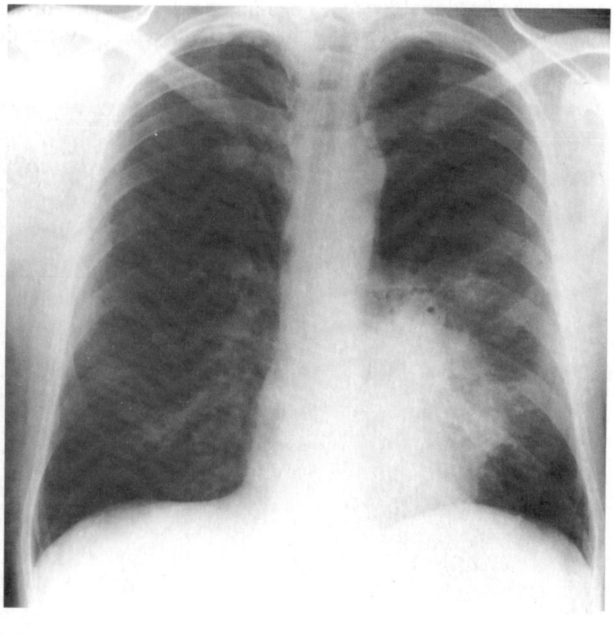

FIG. 6. Patchy infiltrate representing a bronchopneumonia in a patient with *S. pneumoniae* infection.

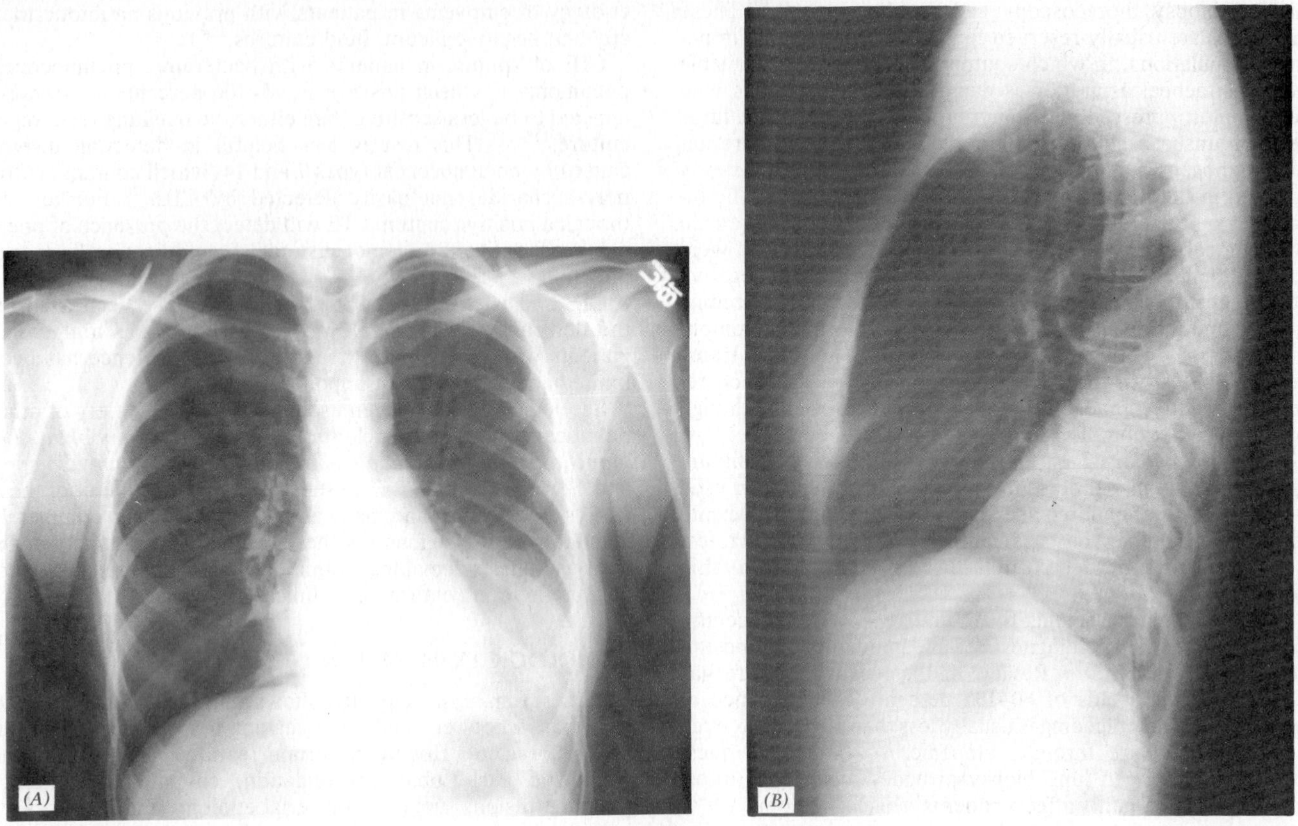

FIG. 7. **(A)** Posteroanterior film showing dense left lower lobe consolidation consistent with a bacterial pneumonia, in this case caused by *S. pneumoniae.* **(B)** Lateral film of patient with left lower lobe pneumococcal pneumonia.

K. pneumoniae, H. influenzae, S. pneumoniae, and, more rarely, *P. carinii.*[136–138] Pulmonary infections due to *Pseudomonas* have a marked tendency toward cavitation. Although its initial manifestation is that of patchy bronchopneumonia, microabscesses form quickly and coalesce to form one or several large abscesses. *Pseudomonas* and other gram-negative bacilli cause lower lobe pneumonia most commonly.[139]

Aspiration pneumonia should be considered along with gram-negative and staphylococcal pneumonias as a source of necrotizing pneumonia, cavitation, and empyema. Aspiration

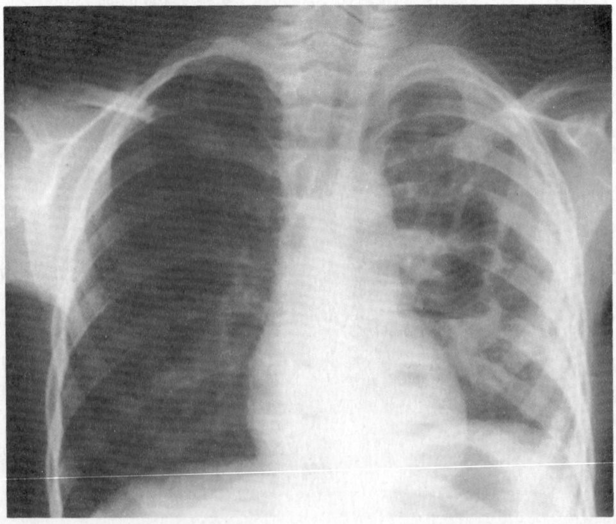

FIG. 8. Pneumatocele formation in the left upper lobe of a patient with staphylococcal pneumonia.

pneumonia commonly involves either the superior segment or the basilar segment of either lower lobe or the posterior segment of the upper lobes, depending on whether aspiration occurred in the dependent or upright position.[140] Chronic aspiration most commonly results in a bilateral lower lobe pneumonia, although it often may appear to involve one side more than the other.[139]

Many viral pneumonias produce generalized destruction of ciliated epithelium with little radiologic distinction between the various viral etiologies. Initially, ciliated epithelial cells, goblet cells, and bronchial mucous gland cells are destroyed. Subsequent involvement may include terminal bronchioles and alveoli. Diffuse hemorrhagic congestion of alveolar septa with red blood cells and inflammatory edema fluid may be seen, especially with primary influenza pneumonia.[141] The x-ray film concomitants of these pathologic findings are varied and may be confusing if a secondary bacterial infection complicates the initial process. Diffuse and localized involvement with both interstitial and alveolar patterns have been noted[142] (Fig. 9). Peribronchial involvement with nodular infiltrates is a pattern often seen with varicella.

Mycoplasmal pneumonia often manifests with an interstitial pattern in a peribronchial distribution. As more edema fluid is elaborated, there may be rapid progression to lobar or sublobar consolidation. Once this consolidation stage is reached, radiologic differentiation between bacterial and myocplasmal pneumonia is difficult. *Mycoplasma* is usually associated with lower lobe disease. Cavitation is rare, although pleural effusion may be seen in 20 percent of the cases.[143]

Legionnaires' disease may initially present with an x-ray picture similar to that of mycoplasmal pneumonia. A patchy interstitial or finely nodular pattern is seen in the lower lobes.[144] However, unlike mycoplasmal pneumonia, pneumonia with more than two-lobe involvement is commonly seen. Rapid progression and pleural effusions are also common.[145] Pneumonia

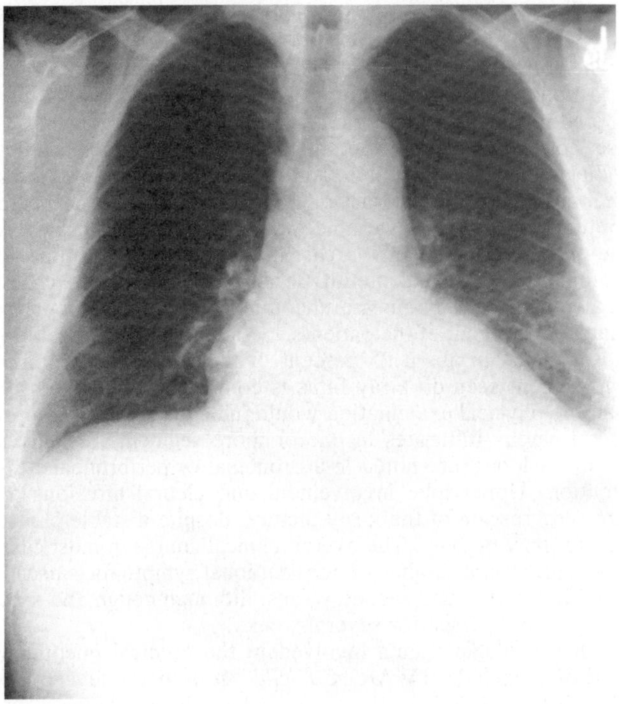

FIG. 9. Bilateral involvement with a mixed interstitial-alveolar pattern in a patient with viral pneumonia.

caused by *L. micdadei* (Pittsburgh pneumonia agent) may present with pulmonary nodules, either single or multiple, as well as with segmental infiltrates. As in pneumonia caused by *L. pneumophila,* rapid radiologic progression of the disease is characteristic.[146]

It must be recognized that x-ray films are most helpful in conjunction with the clinical history and physical examination. This point was clearly shown by Tew et al.,[147] who evaluated readings of x-ray films of patients with pneumonia made without clinical information. Pneumonia was correctly identified as bacterial only 67 percent of the time and as viral only 65 percent of the time. Mycoplasmal pneumonia was incorrectly identified as bacterial 81 percent of the time.

PNEUMONIA SYNDROMES

Acute Community-Acquired Pneumonia

Review of large numbers of patients with community-acquired pneumonia have provided an epidemiologic and clinical profile of this syndrome.[28,30,31,148–150] Typically, patients are in their mid-50s to 60s and usually become ill in midwinter or early spring. Although the onset of pneumonia symptoms is acute and represents a marked change from their usual health, most patients have one or more chronic underlying diseases, including chronic obstructive lung disease, cardiovascular disease, diabetes, or alcoholism.

The onset of disease is usually marked by a sudden chill. Sustained temperature elevations to approximately 40°C, pleuritic chest pain, and cough productive of mucopurulent sputum usually follow.

Physical examination reveals fever, tachypnea, and tachycardia. Localized pulmonary findings with rales are noted early in the disease, and signs of lobar consolidation are noted as the disease progresses. Laboratory evaluation is significant. Most commonly, the white blood cell count is in the range of 15–35,000/mm^3, and the differential cell count reveals an increased number of juvenile forms.[151] Leukopenia may be noted and is a poor prognostic sign.[152] The hematocrit and the red blood cell indices are usually normal. Examination of the sputum reveals thick, purulent material that may be rust colored. The sputum Gram stain reveals numerous neutrophils and bacteria, usually with a single organism predominating. Chest films reveal areas of parenchymal involvement, usually in a bronchopneumonic pattern. Arterial blood gas determinations reveal a moderate degree of hypoxemia due to ventilation perfusion abnormalities.

With the diagnostic tests presently available, a microbiologic diagnosis may be made in 50–70 percent of cases of pneumonia.[150,151] In the past, 50–90 percent of the cases of acute community-acquired pneumonia were caused by *S. pneumoniae*.[30,31,153] More recently, the relative importance of this pneumococcus has decreased. At present, it causes 25–60 percent of the cases of acute community-acquired pneumonia.[149,150,154–156] Advanced age, cigarette smoking, institutionalization, dementia, seizures, and the presence of chronic illnesses such as chronic obstructive pulmonary disease, congestive heart failure, and cerebrovascular disease have been identified as significant risk factors for the development of pneumococcal pneumonia.[157] Severe pneumococcal infections, including pneumonia, have been associated with splenectomy due to trauma or staging for Hodgkin's disease.[158,159]

An estimated 4–15 percent of the cases of acute community-acquired pneumonia are caused by *H. influenzae*.[28,31,150,154–156,160,161] The true incidence of this organism is obscured by the difficulty in isolating it from sputum and identifying it in sputum Gram stain, and by the failure of early studies to differentiate colonization from true infection. *Staphylococcus aureus* accounts for 2–10 percent of acute community-acquired pneumonia,[162] and takes on increased importance as a cause of pneumonia in the elderly and in patients recovering from influenza.[163,164] Patients developing postinfluenza pneumonia are usually younger and have less underlying disease than most other patients with community-acquired pneumonia. Clinical signs and symptoms of influenza are present but appear to resolve over several days. After a variable period of time ranging from 2 to 14 days, symptoms suddenly reappear, with the onset of shaking chills, pleuritic chest pain, and cough productive of purulent sputum. An elevated white blood cell count with a shift to the left, physical signs of pulmonary consolidation and radiographic evidence of focal parenchymal disease appear. The sputum Gram stain is consistent with bacterial pneumonia. Although the pneumococcus still represents the most common etiologic agent, staphylococcal disease occurs with a higher frequency than that noted in non-influenza-related, community-acquired pneumonia.[163,164]

Aerobic gram-negative bacteria, exclusive of *H. influenzae,* and mixed aerobic and anaerobic infections cause most of the remaining cases of acute community-acquired pneumonia. Gram-negative rods may cause 7–18 percent of pneumonia[154–156] and are particularly important pathogens in the elderly. The importance of *Legionella* spp. in causing pneumonia varies greatly in different geographic areas. While incidences as high as 17–22.5 percent have been reported,[153,165] many centers report significantly lower rates[155,156] Recently, *Branhamella catarrhalis* has been identified as a cause of pneumonia.[166–168] The overall incidence of disease due to this bacterium is low, but it is an important pathogen in elderly patients with chronic obstructive pulmonary disease and various forms of immunosuppression. In contrast to disease patterns in adults, viruses are the most important cause of pneumonia in young children. Respiratory syncytial virus and parainfluenza virus type 3 are the major pathogens. Other parainfluenza viruses and low-numbered adenovirus serotypes are also important.

Two clinical entities differ significantly from the above description of community-acquired pneumonia and therefore deserve special mention. Pneumonia in the elderly is a major cause of morbidity and mortality and in some series represents the leading cause of death[169] (see Chapter 295). The clinical presentation may be more subtle than in younger populations, with less frequent complaints of chills and rigor and less fever.[41,170] Bacteremia, metastatic foci of infection, and death are more frequent in older populations.[28,41,152] While the etiologies of pneumonia in the elderly follow the general pattern noted in younger patients, aerobic gram-negative bacilli and *Staph. aureus* play a more important role, especially in patients in nursing homes and extended care facilities.[170–174] Of the gram-negative organisms, *K. pneumoniae* and *H. influenzae,* including nontypable strains, appear especially important. The elderly also appear to be at high risk of infection from organisms such as group B streptococci and *B. catarrhalis*.[42,166–168] Increased oropharyngeal colonization with aerobic gram-negative bacilli has been documented in the elderly, with an increase in colonization paralleling the level of care needed by the patient.[175] Other factors that have been associated with increased colonization include prior use of antibiotics, serious underlying disease, and decreased activity.[171,175]

The etiology of community-acquired pneumonia in patients with AIDS is also different from that noted in other populations. *Pneumocystis carinii* pneumonia occurs in approximately 85 percent of patients at some time during their course.[176,177] In addition to the more common bacterial agents usually associated with community-acquired pneumonia, cytomegalovirus, *Mycobacterium tuberculosis,* and *Cryptococcus neoformans* also play important roles as etiologic agents (see Chapter 108).

Pneumonia in the Setting of Aspiration

The clinical setting in which aspiration occurs involves any disease state in which consciousness is altered and the normal gag and swallowing reflexes are abnormal.

Three major syndromes are recognized as a consequence of aspiration: chemical pneumonitis, bronchial obstruction secondary to aspiration of particulate matter, and bacterial aspiration pneumonia.[178,179] Although chemical pneumonitis and mechanical obstruction usually cause acute symptoms, aspiration pneumonia is more insidious, with symptoms usually occurring gradually several days after the initial episode of aspiration. Pneumonitis, necrotizing pneumonia, abscess, and empyema are common. Symptoms often include fever, weight loss, and productive cough. Putrid sputum is produced in 50 percent of the cases.[44,140] Anemia and an elevated white blood cell count are frequently associated findings. The bacteriologic findings in aspiration pneumonia reflect the flora of the oropharynx, and the importance of periodontal disease in this regard has been noted. Anaerobic bacteria, alone (45–58 percent of the cases) or in combination with aerobes (41–46 percent), are most commonly seen when adequate culture techniques are used.[5,44]

Bacteroides melaninogenicus. *Fusobacterium* spp., and anaerobic gram-positive cocci are the predominant anaerobes isolated. In community-acquired aspiration pneumonia, *Streptococcus* spp. are the most common aerobic isolates.[179,180] In contrast, gram-negative bacilli, and *Staph. aureus* are the most commonly isolated aerobes from nosocomial aspiration pneumonia.[179,180]

Atypical Pneumonia Syndrome

The atypical pneumonia syndrome is a symptom complex representing disease caused most commonly by *Myocplasma pneumoniae*. The older child (>5 years of age), the adolescent, or the young adult is at greatest risk of developing the disease. Increased incidence of disease and true epidemics have been documented in relatively enclosed populations of young adults at military bases, colleges, and boarding schools.[181–183] Mycoplasmal infection occurs throughout the year, although a relative increase in incidence is noted in the late summer and fall. In contrast, adenovirus infection, another cause of atypical pneumonia, most commonly occurs between January and April, outbreaks occurring primarily in military recruit camps.[181,183,184]

The course of the atypical pneumonias is characterized by a 3- to 4-day history of symptoms. Constitutional symptoms seem to predominate over specific respiratory findings. Fever, malaise, coryza, headache, and cough represent the major clinical findings. Pleuritic chest pain, splinting, and respiratory distress are not usually seen. Moist or crepitant rales may be heard. Sputum production is variable, and although it is purulent in one-third to one-half of the cases, Gram stain and culture of sputum usually reveal mouth flora. White blood cell counts greater than 10,000/mm^3 are uncommon, occurring in approximately 20 percent of the patients.[50] An elevated sedimentation rate is noted in about 25 percent of the cases.[185] Pulmonary involvement seen on x-ray films is commonly more extensive than the physical examination would indicate. Unilateral or bilateral patchy infiltrates in one or more segments, usually in the lower lobes, are noted in a bronchial or peribronchial distribution. Upper lobe involvement and pleural effusions are rare. Progression of the x-ray picture, despite a stable clinical picture, may be seen. The overall clinical course in most cases is benign. Disappearance of constitutional symptoms is usually noted in the first and second weeks, although cough and x-ray changes may persist for several weeks.

Other etiologic agents involved in the atypical pneumonia syndrome include TWAR, *Coxiella burnetti* (Q fever), and *Chlamydia psittaci* (psittacosis). Chlamydia trachomatis has been described as a pulmonary pathogen in immunocompromised as well as healthy hosts.[186,187] Productive cough, myalgias, and fever associated with diffuse nonsegmental infiltrates appear most commonly. The agent has also been associated with chronic pneumonia in neonates and infants. Onset occurs at 2–3 weeks of age and is associated with tachypnea, a staccato cough with periods of cyanosis and emesis, lack of fever, and diffuse interstitial and patchy alveolar infiltrates on chest films. Elevated IgG and IgM levels and absolute eosinophilia have also been noted.

The TWAR strain of *Chlamydia* has been identified by culture and serology as the cause of pneumonia presenting both as an atypical pneumonia as well as an acute community-acquired pneumonia.[190,191] Mild to moderate illness with prolonged symptoms and frequent relapses have been characteristic (see Chapter 160).

Of the viral agents associated with atypical pneumonia in adults, influenza A and B and adenovirus types 3, 4, and 7, especially in military recruits, are the most common. Reports of other viral agents causing pneumonia are scant but have included rhinovirus,[192] enterovirus,[193] parainfluenza virus,[194] and respiratory syncytial virus.[195]

Respiratory syncytial virus, the predominant respiratory pathogen in infants and children, is now recognized as an etiology of pneumonia in adults.[195–197] While the number of cases is small, groups at particular risk appear to be the elderly and patients who are immunosuppressed.

Legionnaires' disease may present as either an acute, community-acquired pneumonia or an atypical pneumonia. Although early symptoms of malaise, muscle aches, headache, and nonproductive cough resemble the onset of a "viral syndrome," the rapid progression of pulmonary symptoms is noteworthy. Abdominal pain and gastrointestinal symptoms, especially diarrhea, have been noted. Physical examination reveals only rales; x-ray films show patchy interstitial or nodular infiltrates that may progress rapidly to more widespread consolidation. Approximately 50 percent of cases have bilateral involvement. Transient impairment of renal function, abnormally low serum phosphorus levels, and elevated serum creatinine phosphokinase levels have been described.[144,145,198,199] For the most part, it is not possible to clinically distinguish legionnaires' disease from other bacterial pneumonias.[165]

Pulmonary Infiltrates with Eosinophilia

Pulmonary infiltrates with eosinophilia (PIE) is a syndrome associated with a variety of clinical entities, only some of which are infectious in etiology.[200] Pulmonary eosinophilia with transient, peripheral pulmonary infiltrates and minimal symptoms has been associated with *Ascaris* and *Strongyloides* infections. Prolonged pulmonary eosinophilia associated with weight loss, fever, cough, and dyspnea may be due to tuberculosis, brucellosis, psittacosis, coccidioidomycosis, and parasitic infections including ascariasis, strongyloidiasis, paragonomiasis, echinococcosis, visceral larva migrans, cutaneous larva migrans, *Schistosoma Dirofilaria immitus, Entamoeba histolytica* and infection with *Ancylostoma* spp. Noninfectious etiologies include drug allergy, sarcoidosis, eosinophilic leukemia, and hypersensitivity pneumonitis (i.e., pigeon breeders' disease).[200,201]

It has recently been suggested that chronic eosinophilic pneumonia may represent a unique clinical entity that is a form of collagen-vascular disease or an infection in a hyperimmune patient.[202–204] Interstitial infiltrates, focal interstitial fibrosis, bronchiolitis obliterans, microabscesses, and sarcoid-like granulomas are characteristic pathologic features. A rapid response to steroids has been reported.[204]

Tropical eosinophilia consists of myalgia, fatigue, weight loss, and anorexia associated with cough, frequently with nocturnal exacerbations, dyspnea, and peripheral eosinophilia in patients who have lived in or visited the tropics. X-ray film changes are distinctive and include increased interstitial markings with 2- to 4-mm nodules throughout the lungs with preferential involvement of the bases. Most cases represent microfilarial infection and can be treated with diethylcarbamazine.

Nosocomial Pneumonia and Pneumonia in the Immunosuppressed Host

Nosocomial pneumonia accounts for approximately 10–20 percent of all nosocomial infections and is the leading cause of infection-related mortality in hospitalized patients.[205,206] Important risk factors for the development of disease include advanced age, severity of underlying disease, intubation, use of respiratory equipment, surgery, and previous use of antibiotics.[207–209] Use of antacids and histamine type 2 blockers that raise the gastric pH have been shown to increase stomach colonization with aerobic gram-negative rods and may be another risk factor for the development of pulmonary infection.[210–212]. Approximately 60 percent of cases of nosocomial pneumonia are caused by aerobic gram-negative bacilli, with members of the family Enterobacteriaceae (*K. pneumoniae, E. coli, Serratia marcescens, Enterobacter* spp.) and *Pseudomonas* spp. accounting for the majority of these. *Staphylococcus aureus* causes approximately 13 percent of nosocomial pneumonia, with *S. pneumoniae* causing only 8 percent.[40]

Pneumonia in the immunosuppressed host represents an important subset of nosocomial pneumonia and deserves special emphasis.[213] In patients with nonlymphocytic leukemia, 25 percent of all documented infections are pulmonary.[214] In patients with acute leukemia, 64 percent of fatal bacteremias of known cause originate in the lung, the majority of episodes caused by enteric gram-negative bacilli.[214] Approximately one-fourth of renal transplant recipients,[216,217] as well as one-half of bone marrow transplant patients,[218] will develop pneumonia at some time during their course. Again, the most common bacterial pathogens are gram-negative bacilli. As with other nosocomial pneumonias, pneumonias in the compromised host are most commonly caused by *K. pneumoniae, E. coli,* or *Pseudomonas aeruginosa*. In some series these organisms cause 50 percent of all infections, with mixed gram-negative infections accounting for another 20 percent.[219,220]

In addition to bacterial pathogens, a variety of nonbacterial agents are of etiologic importance. These include fungi (*Aspergillus* spp., agents of mucormycosis, *Candida* spp.), protozoa (*Pneumocystis carinii, Toxoplasma gondii*), parasites (*Strongyloides*), and viruses (herpes zoster virus, cytomegalovirus). Chapter 280 and Part IV, Section B discuss more fully nosocomial pneumonia and infections in the compromised host, respectively.

THERAPY FOR PNEUMONIA

Once the etiologic agent is identified, selection of appropriate therapy is relatively straightforward. (In-depth discussions are provided in the sections dealing with specific antibiotics and etiologic agents.) The choice of antibiotics becomes more difficult when sputum cannot be obtained or when the sputum examination is nondiagnostic. In these cases, empiric therapy should be designed to treat the most likely and/or the most potentially lethal possibilities.

Patients with a mild illness, no history of cigarette abuse, and a nondiagnostic sputum test who present with a sudden onset of fever, a pulmonary infiltrate, and leukocytosis are likely to have pneumococcal pneumonia and may be treated empirically with penicillin. When an atypical pneumonia presentation is noted, empiric use of erythromycin will provide adequate therapy against the pneumococcus as well as against *M. pneumoniae,* the most likely cause of atypical pneumonia. Where *H. influenzae* is suspected, cefuroxime axetil (Ceftin), trimethoprimsulfamethoxazole (Bactrim, Septra) or amoxicillin/clavulanic acid (Augmentin) are appropriate oral regimens.

A seriously ill patient with acute community-acquired pneumonia and a nondiagnostic sputum examination should be treated for the most likely pathogens. Therapy should include coverage for *S. pneumoniae, H. influenzae, Staph. aureus,* and, in some cases, *L. pneumophila*. Selection of antibiotics should take into account the possibility of ampicillin-resistant *H. influenzae* unless it is known that no such resistant organisms have been isolated from the community. While third-generation cephalosporins and broad-spectrum penicillins are not usually needed for therapy of community-acquired pneumonia, they are indicated for therapy of life-threatening disease when gram-negative aerobes are suspected.[221] Erythromycin is the drug of choice for *Legionella* pneumonia and should be added to the above regimens if the diagnosis is suspected.

The therapy for aspiration pneumonia is dependent on whether the episode of aspiration occurs in the community or in the hospital. Penicillin is effective for most cases of community-acquired aspiration pneumonia, since the predominant organisms are usually penicillin sensitive.[222] However, an increased incidence of in vitro penicillin resistance has been observed in several *Bacteroides* spp.[223–226] Clindamycin[227,228] or other agents with potent antianaerobic plus aerobic activity may be used for seriously ill patients and those who do not respond promptly to penicillin. Therapy for nosocomial pneumonia is discussed in Chapter 280.

REFERENCES

1. Osler W. The Principles and Practice of Medicine. 4th ed. New York: D. Appleton; 1901:108.
2. Statistical Abstract of the United States, 104th ed. Washington, DC: US Government Printing Office, 1984.
3. Johanson WG Jr, Gould KG Jr. Lung defense mechanisms. Basics of RD. 1977;6:(2)1–6.
4. Green G. In defense of the lung. Am Rev Respir Dis. 1970;102:691–703.
5. Bartlett J, Gorbach S, Finegold S. The bacteriology of aspiration pneumonia. Am J Med. 1974;56:202–7.
6. Huxley EJ, Viroslav J, Gray WR, et al. Pharyngeal aspiration in normal adults and patients with depressed consciousness. Am J Med. 1978;64: 564–8.
7. Green GM, Carolin D. The depressant effect of cigarette smoke on the in

vitro antibacterial activity of alveolar macrophages. N Engl J Med. 1967; 276:421–7.
8. Green GM, Kass EH. The influence of bacterial species on pulmonary resistance to infection in mice subjected to hypoxia, cold stress and ethanolic intoxication. Br J Exp Pathol. 1965;46:360–6.
9. Green GM, Kass EH. The role of the alveolar macrophage in the clearance of bacteria from the lung. J Exp Med. 1964;119:167–76.
10. Coffin DL, Gardner DE, Holzman RS, et al. Influence of ozone on pulmonary cells. Arch Environ Health. 1968;16:633–6.
11. Ehrlich R, Henry MC. Chronic toxicity of nitrogen dioxide. I. Effect on resistance to bacterial pneumonia. Arch Environ Health. 1968;17:860–5.
12. LaForce FM, Mullane JF, Boehme RF, et al. The effect of pulmonary edema on antibacterial defenses of the lung. J Lab Clin Med. 1973;82:634–48.
13. Huber GL, LaForce FM, Mason RJ, et al. Impairment of pulmonary bacterial defense mechanisms by immunosuppressive agents. Surg Forum. 1970;21:285–6.
14. Warshauer D, Goldstein E, Akers T, et al. Effect of influenza viral infection on the ingestion and killing of bacteria by alveolar macrophages. Am Rev Respir Dis. 1977;115:269–77.
15. Winterbauer RH, Bedon GA, Bal WC Jr. Recurrent pneumonia: Predisposing illness and clinical patterns in 158 patients. Ann Intern Med. 1969;70:689–700.
16. Roth RM, Gleckman RA. Recurrent bacterial pneumonia: A contemporary perspective. South Med J. 1985;78:573–9.
17. Donowitz GR, Mandell GL. Clinical presentation and unusual infections. In: Advances in Host Defense Mechanisms. v. 3. Gallin JI, Fauci AS, eds. New York: Raven Press; 1983;55–75.
18. Donabedian H, Gallin JI. The hyperimmunoglobulin E recurrent infection (Jobs) syndrome. Medicine. 1983;62:195–208.
19. Beck S, Heiner DC. Selective immunoglobulin G_4 deficiency and recurrent infections of the respiratory tract. Am Rev Respir Dis. 1981;124:94–96.
20. Ammann AJ, Hong R. Selective IgA deficiency: Presentation of 30 cases and a review of the literature. Medicine. 1971;50:223–36.
21. Eliasson R, Mossberg B, Camner P, et al. The immotile-cilia syndrome. N Engl J Med. 1977;297:1–6.
22. Kartagener M. Zur Pathologie der Bronchiektasien: Bronkiectasien lei situs inversus. Beitr Klin Tuberk. 1933;83:489–501.
23. Handelsman DJ, Conway AJ, Boylan LM, et al. Young's syndrome: Obstructive azospermia and chronic sinopulmonary infections. N Engl J Med. 1984;310:3–9.
24. Savic B, Birtel FJ, Tholen W, et al. Lung sequestration: Report of seven cases and review of 540 published cases. Thorax. 1979;34:96–101.
25. Iverson LIG, May IA, Samson PC. Pulmonary complications in benign esophageal disease. Am J Surg. 1973;126:223–8.
26. Grayston JT, Alexander ER, Kenny GE, et al. Mycoplasma pneumoniae infections: Clinical and epidemiological studies. JAMA. 1965;191:369–74.
27. Murray HW, Masur H, Senterfit L, et al. The protean manifestations of mycoplasma pneumoniae infection in adults. Am J Med. 1975;58:229–42.
28. Dorff GJ, Rytel MW, Farmer SG, et al. Etiologies and characteristic features of pneumonias in a municipal hospital. Am J Med Sci. 1973;266:349–58.
29. MacGregor RR. A year's experience with tuberculosis in a private urban teaching hospital in the postsanitorium era. Am J Med. 1975;58:221–8.
30. Fekety FR, Caldwell J, Grump D, et al. Bacteria, viruses, and mycoplasmas in acute pneumonia in adults. Am Rev Respir Dis. 1971;104:499–507.
31. Sullivan RJ, Dowdle WR, Marine WM, et al. Adult pneumonia in a general hospital: Etiology and host risk factors. Arch Intern Med. 1972;129:935–42.
32. Lepow ML, Balassanian N, Emmerich J, et al. Interrelationships of viral, mycoplasmal and bacterial agents in uncomplicated pneumonia. Am Rev Respir Dis. 1968;97:533–45.
33. Martin CM, Kunin CM, Gottlieb LS, et al. Asian influenza A in Boston, 1957–1958. II. Severe staphylococcal pneumonia complicating influenza. Arch Intern Med. 1959;103:532–42.
34. Sprunt K. Infection in chronic lung disease. Bull NY Acad Med. 1972;48:698–703.
35. Hoiby N. Epidemiological investigations of the respiratory tract bacteriology in patients with cystic fibrosis. Acta Pathol Microbiol Scand B. 1974;82:541–50.
36. Burbank B, Morrione TG, Cutler SS. Pulmonary alveolar proteinosis and nocardiosis. Am J Med. 1960;28:1002–7.
37. Murray JF, Felton CP, Garay SM, et al. Pulmonary complications of the acquired immunodeficiency syndrome: Report of a National Heart Lung and Blood Institute Workshop. New Engl J Med 1984;310:1682–8.
38. Stover DE, White DA, Romano PA, et al. Spectrum of pulmonary diseases associated with the acquired immunodeficiency syndrome. Am J Med. 1985;78:429–37.
39. Witt DJ, Craven DE, McCabe WR. Bacterial infections in adult patients with the acquired immune deficiency syndrome (AIDS) and AIDS-related complex. Am J Med. 1987;82:900–6.
40. Gross PA. Epidemiology of hospital-acquired pneumonia. Semin in Respir Infect. 1987;2:2–7.
41. Marrie TJ, Haldane EV, Faulkner RS, et al. Community acquired pneumonia requiring hospitalization: Is it different in the elderly? J Am Geriatr Soc. 1985;33:671–80.
42. Verghese A, Berk SL, Boelen LJ, et al. Group B streptococcal pneumonia in the elderly. Arch Intern Med. 1982;142:1642–5.
43. Heffron R. Pneumonia. New York: Commonwealth Fund; 1939:505.
44. Bartlett JG, Finegold SM. Anaerobic infections of the lung and pleural space. Am Rev Respir Dis. 1974;110:56–77.
45. Thorsteinsson SB, Musher DM, Fagan T. The diagnostic value of sputum culture in acute pneumonia. JAMA. 1975;233:894–5.
46. Merrill C, Gwaltney JM, Hendley JO, et al. Rapid identification of pneumococci. N Engl J Med. 1973;288:510–2.
47. Drew WL. Value of sputum culture in diagnosis of pneumococcal pneumonia. J Clin Microbiol. 1977;6:62–5.
48. Bartlett RC, Melnick A. Usefulness of Gram stain and routine and quantitative culture of sputum in patients with and without acute respiratory infection. Conn Med. 1970;34:347–51.
49. Bryant RE, Rhoades ER. Clinical feature of adenoviral pneumonia in Air Force recruits. Am Rev Respir Dis. 1967;96:717–23.
50. George RB, Ziskind MM, Rasch JR, et al. Mycoplasma and adenovirus pneumonias—comparison with other atypical pneumonias in a military population. Ann Intern Med. 1966;65:931–42.
51. Reimann H. The Pneumonias. Philadelphia: WB Saunders; 1938:67.
52. Solomon S. Primary Friedlander pneumonia. JAMA. 1937;108:937–47.
53. Murray PR, Washington JA III. Microscopic and bacteriologic analysis of expectorated sputum. Mayo Clin Proc. 1975;50:339–44.
54. Rein MF, Gwaltney JM, O'Brien WM, et al. Accuracy of the Gram's stain in identifying pneumococci in sputum. JAMA. 1978;239:2671–3.
55. Hendley JO, Sande MA, Stewart PM, et al. Spread of *Streptococcus pneumoniae* in families. I. Carriage rates and distribution of types. J Infect Dis. 1975;132:55–61.
56. Finland M. Recent advances in the epidemiology of pneumococcal infections. Medicine. 1942;21:307–44.
57. Lees AW, McNaught W. Bacteriology of lower-respiratory tract secretions, sputum and upper-respiratory tract secretions in "normals" and "chronic bronchitis." Lancet. 1959;2:1112–5.
58. Bigby TD, Margolskee D, Curtis JL, et al. The usefulness of induced sputum in the diagnosis of *Pneumocystis carinii* pneumonia in patients with the acquired immunodeficiency syndrome. Am Rev Respir Dis. 1986;133:515–8.
59. Pitchenik AE, Ganjei P, Torres A, et al. Sputum examination for the diagnosis of *Pneumocystis carinii* pneumonia in the acquired immunodeficiency syndrome. Am Rev Respir Dis. 1986;133:226–9.
60. Tenover FC. Diagnostic deoxyribonucleic acid probes for infection. Dis Clin Microbiol Rev. 1988;1:82–101.
61. Peterson LR, Shanholtzer CJ. Using the microbiology laboratory in the diagnosis of pneumonia. Semin Respir Infect. 1988;3:106–12.
62. Sullivan CJ, Joran ML. Diagnosis of viral pneumonia. Semin Respir Infect. 1988;3:148–61.
63. Barrett-Connor E. The non-value of sputum culture in the diagnosis of pneumococcal pneumonia. Am Rev Respir Dis. 1971;103:845–8.
64. Rathburn HK, Govani I. Mouse inoculation as means of identifying pneumococci in the sputum. Johns Hopkins Med J. 1967;120:46–8.
65. Wallace RJ, Musher DM, Martin RR. *Hemophilus influenzae* pneumonia in adults. Am J Med. 1978;64:87–93.
66. Levin D, Schwarz M, Matthay R, et al. Bacteremic *Hemophilus influenzae* pneumonia in adults. A report of 24 cases and a review of the literature. Am J Med. 1977;62:219–24.
67. Davidson M, Tempest B, Palmer DL, Bacteriologic diagnosis of acute pneumonia, comparison of sputum, transtracheal aspirates, and lung aspirates. JAMA. 1976;235:158–63.
68. Geckeler RW, Gremillion DH, McAllister CK, et al. Microscopic and bacteriological comparison of paired sputa and transtracheal aspirates. J Clin Microbiol. 1977;6:396–9.
69. Kalinske RW, Parker RH, Brandt D, et al. Diagnostic usefulness and safety of transtracheal aspiration. N Engl J Med. 1967;276:604–8.
70. Hoeprich PD. Etiologic diagnosis of lower respiratory tract infections. Calif Med. 1970;112:1.
71. Tillotson JR, Lerner AM. Pneumonias caused by gram negative bacilli. Medicine. 1966;45:65–76.
72. Saadah HA, Nasr FL, Shagoury ME. Washed sputum gram stain and culture in pneumonia. J Okla State Med Assoc. 1980;73:354–9.
73. Ries K, Levison ME, Kaye D. Transtracheal aspiration in pulmonary infection. Arch Intern Med. 1974;133:453–8.
74. Hahn HH, Beaty HN. Transtracheal aspiration in the evaluation of patients with pneumonia. Ann Intern Med. 1970;72:183–7.
75. Jordan GW, Wong GA, Hoeprich PD. Bacteriology of the lower respiratory tract as determined by fiber-optic bronchoscopy and transtracheal aspiration. J Infect Dis. 1976;134:428–35.
76. Bartlett JG, Rosenblatt JE, Finegold SM. Percutaneous transtracheal aspiration in the diagnosis of anaerobic pulmonary infection. Ann Intern Med. 1973;79:535–40.
77. Bartlett JG. Diagnostic accuracy of transtracheal aspiration bacteriologic studies. Am Rev Respir Dis. 1977;115:777–82.
78. Schillaci RF, Iacovoni VE, Conte RS. Transtracheal aspiration complicated by fatal endotracheal hemorrhage. N Engl J Med. 1976;295:488–90.
79. Spencer CD, Beaty HN. Complications of transtracheal aspiration. N Engl J Med. 1972;286:304–6.
80. Lourie B, McKinnon B, Kibler L. Transtracheal aspiration and anaerobic abscess. Ann Intern Med. 1974;80:417–8.
81. Deresinski SC, Steven DA. Anterior cervical infections: Complications of transtracheal aspirations. Am Rev Respir Dis. 1974;110:354–6.

82. Parsons GH, Price JE, Auston PW. Bilateral pneumothorax complicating transtracheal aspiration. West J Med. 1976;125:73–5.
83. Bartlett JG, Alexander J, Mayhew J, et al. Should fiberoptic bronchoscopy aspirates be cultured? Am Rev Respir Dis. 1976;114:73–8.
84. Wimberly N, Faling LJ, Bartlett JG. A fiberoptic bronchoscopy technique to obtain uncontaminated lower airway secretions for bacterial cultures. Am Rev Respir Dis. 1979;119:337–42.
85. Meden G, Hall GS, Ahmad M. Retrieval of microbiological specimens through the fiberoptic bronchoscope. Cleve Clin Q. 1985;52:495–502.
86. Wimberly NW, Bass JB, Boyd BW, et al. Use of a bronchoscopic protected catheter brush for the diagnosis of pulmonary infections. Chest. 1982; 81:556–82.
87. Hays DA, McCarthy LC, Friedman M. Evaluation of two bronchofiberscopic methods of culturing the lower respiratory tract. Am Rev Respir Dis. 1980;122:319–23.
88. Higuchi JH, Coalson JJ, Johanson, WG. Bacteriologic diagnosis of nosocomial pneumonia in primates. Am Rev Respir Dis. 1982;125:53–7.
89. Pollock HM, Hawkins EL, Bonner JR, et al. Diagnosis of bacterial pulmonary infections with quantitative protected cathether cultures obtained during bronchoscopy. J Clin Microbiol. 1983;17:255–9.
90. Halperin SA, Suratt PM, Gwaltney JM, et al. Bacterial cultures of the lower respiratory tract in normal volunteers with and without experimental rhinovirus infection using a plugged double catheter system. Am Rev Respir Dis. 1982;125:678–80.
91. Bordelon JY Jr, Legrand P, Gewin WL, et al. The telescoping plugged catheter in suspected anaerobic infections: A controlled series. Am Rev Respir Dis. 1983;128:465–8.
92. Wimberly NW, Bass JR Jr, Boyd DW, et al. Bronchial brush specimens from patients with stable chronic bronchitis. Chest. 1986;90:534–6.
93. Winterbauer RH, Hutchinson JF, Reinhardt GN, et al. The use of quantitative culture and antibody coating of bacteria to diagnose bacterial pneumonia by fiberoptic bronchoscopy. Am Rev Respir Dis. 1983;128: 98–103.
94. Vereen L, Smart LM, George RB. Antibody coating and quantitative cultures of bacteria in sputum and bronchial brush specimens from patients with stable chronic bronchitis. Chest. 1986;90:534–6.
95. Broaddus C, Dake MD, Stulburg MS, et al. Bronchoalveolar lavage and transbronchial biopsy for the diagnosis of pulmonary infections in the acquired immunodeficiency syndrome. Ann Intern Med. 1986;102:747–52.
96. Orenstein M, Webber CA, Cash M, et al. Value of bronchoalveolar lavage in the diagnosis of pulmonary infection in acquired immune deficiency syndrome. Thorax. 1986;41:345–9.
97. Crawford SW, Bowden RA, Hackman RC, et al. Rapid detection of cytomegalovirus pulmonary infection by bronchoalveolar lavage and centrifugation culture. Ann Intern Med. 1988;108:180–5.
98. Emmanuel D, Peppard J, Stover D, et al. Rapid diagnosis of cytomegalovirus pneumonia by bronchoalveolar lavage using human and murine monoclonal antibodies. Ann Intern Med. 1986;104:476–81.
99. Stover DE, Zaman MB, Hajdu SI, et al. Bronchoalveolar lavage in the diagnosis of diffuse pulmonary infiltrates in the immunosuppressed host. Ann Intern Med. 1984;101:1–7.
100. Martin WJ, Smith TF, Sanderson DR, et al. Role of bronchoalveolar lavage in the assessment of opportunistic pulmonary infections: Utility and complications. Mayo Clin Proc. 1987;62:549–57.
101. Kahn FW, Jones JM. Diagnosing bacterial respiratory infection by bronchoalveolar lavage. J Infect Dis. 1987;155:862–9.
102. Thorpe JE, Baughman RP, Frame PT, et al. Bronchoalveolar lavage for diagnosing acute bacterial pneumonia. J Infect Dis. 1987;155:855–61.
103. Busk MF, Rosenow EC III, Wilson WR. Invasive procedures in the diagnosis of pneumonia. Semin Respir Infect. 1988;3:113–22.
104. Mimica I, Donoso E, Howard JE, et al. Lung puncture in the etiological diagnosis of pneumonia. Am J Dis Child. 1971;122:278–82.
105. Klein JO. Diagnostic lung puncture in the pneumonias of infants and children. Pediatrics. 1969;44:486–92.
106. Bartlett JG. Invasive diagnostic techniques in respiratory infections. In: Pennington JE, ed. Respiratory Infections: Diagnosis and Management. New York: Raven Press; 1983:55–77.
107. Palmer DL, Davidson M, Lusk R. Needle aspiration of the lung in complex pneumonias. Chest. 1980;78:16–21.
108. Bandt PD, Blank N, Castellino RA. Needle diagnosis of pneumonitis, value in high risk patients. JAMA. 1972;220:1578–80.
109. Greenman RL, Goodall PT, King D. Lung biopsy in immune compromised hosts. Am J Med. 1975;59:488–96.
110. Cockerill FR III, Wilson WR, Carpenter HA, et al. Open lung biopsy in immunocompromised patients. Arch Intern Med. 1985;145:1398–1404.
111. Dijkman JH, van der Meer JWM, Bakker W, et al. Transpleural lung biopsy by the thoracoscopic route in patients with diffuse interstitial pulmonary disease. Chest. 1982;82:76–83.
112. Rodgers BM. Thoracoscopy in children. Poumon-Coeur. 1981;37:301–6.
113. Springmeyer SC, Silvestri RC, Sale GE, et al. The role of transbronchial biopsy for the diagnosis of diffuse pneumonias in immunocompromised marrow transplant recipients. Am Rev Respir Dis. 1982;116:763–5.
114. McCabe RE, Brooks RG, Mark JBD, et al. Open lung biopsy in patients with acute leukemia. Am J Med. 1985;78:609–16.
115. McKenna RJ, Mountain CF, McMurtrey MJ. Open lung biopsy in immunocompromised patients. Chest. 1984;86:671–4.
116. Lowell JR. Pleural Effusions—A Comprehensive Review. Baltimore: University Park Press; 1977:96.
117. Unger JD, Rose HD, Unger GF. Gram-negative pneumonia. Diagn Radiol. 1973;107:283–91.
118. Light RN, Girard WM, Jenkinson SG, et al. Parapneumonic effusions. Am J Med. 1970;69:507–12.
119. Dorff GJ, Coonrod JD, Rytel MW. Detection by immunoelectrophoresis of antigen in sera of patients with pneumococcal bacteremia. Lancet. 1971;1:578–9.
120. Cerosalette KM, Roghmann MC, Bentley DW. Comparison of latex agglutination and counterimmunoelectrophoresis for the detection of pneumococcal antigen in elderly pneumonia patients. J Clin Microbiol. 1985; 22:553–7.
121. Ajello GW, Bolan GA, Hayes PS, et al. Commercial latex agglutination tests for detection of *Haemophilus influenzae* Type B and *Streptococcus pneumoniae* antigen in patients with bacteremic pneumonia. J Clin Microbiol. 1987;25:1388–91.
122. Palmer DL, Jones CC. Diagnosis of pneumococcal pneumonia. Semin Respir Infect. 1988;3:131–9.
123. Perlino CA. Laboratory diagnosis of pneumonia due to *Streptococcus pneumoniae*. J Infect Dis. 1985;150:139–144.
124. Coonrod JD, Wilson HD. Etiologic diagnosis of intrapleural empyema by counterimmunoelectrophoresis. Am Rev Respir Dis. 1976;113:637–41.
125. Krook A, Homberg H. Pneumococcal antigens in sputa: ELISA for the detection of pneumococcal C-polysaccharide in sputa from pneumonia patients. Diagn Microbiol Infect Dis. 1987;7:73–5.
126. Sands RL, Green ID. The diagnosis of pneumococcal chest infection by counter-current immunoelectrophoresis. J Appl Bacteriol. 1980;49:471–8.
127. Tugwell P, Greenwood BM. Pneumococcal antigen in lobar pneumonia. J Clin Pathol. 1975;28:118–23.
128. Congeni BL, Nankervis GA. Diagnosis of pneumonia by counterimmunoelectrophoresis of respiratory secretions. Am J Dis Child. 1978;132:684–7.
129. Downes BA, Ellner PD. Comparison of sputum counterimmunoelectrophoresis and culture in diagnosis of pneumococcal pneumonia. J Clin Microbiol. 1979;10:662–5.
130. Schmid RE, Anhalt JP, Wold AD, et al. II. Sputum counterimmunoelectrophoresis in the diagnosis of pneumococcal pneumonia. Am Rev Respir Dis. 1979;119:345–8.
131. Martin SJ, Hogansan DA, Thomas ET. Detection of *Streptococcus pneumoniae* and *Haemophilus influenzae* Type B antigens in acute nonbacteremic pneumonia. J Clin Microbiol. 1987;25:248–50.
132. Campbell JF, Spika JS. The serodiagnosis of nonpneumococcal bacterial pneumonia. Semin Respir Infect. 1988;3:123–30.
133. Lerner AM, Jankauskas K. The classic bacterial pneumonias. Disease-A-Month. Feb 1975:1–46.
134. Willman VL, Lewis JE, Hanlon CR. Staphylococcal pneumonia—surgical considerations in cases in infants and children. Arch Surg. 1961;83:93–7.
135. Highman JH. Staphylococcal pneumonia and empyema in childhood. Am J Roentgenol. 1969;106:103–8.
136. Dines DE. Diagnostic significance of pneumatocoeles of the lung. JAMA. 1968;204:1169–72.
137. Warner JO, Gordon I. Pneumatocoeles following *Haemophilus influenzae* pneumonia. Clin Radiol. 1981;32:99–105.
138. Luddy RE, Champion LA, Schwartz AD. *Pneumocystis carinii* pneumonia with pneumatocele formation. Am J Dis Child. 1977;131:470.
139. Scanlon GT, Unger JD. The radiology of bacterial and viral pneumonias. Radiol Clin North Am. 1973;11:317–38.
140. Bartlett JG, Finegold SM. Anaerobic pleuropulmonary infections. Medicine. 1972;51:413–50.
141. Lindsay MI, Morrow GW. Primary influenzal pneumonia. Postgrad Med. 1971;49:173–8.
142. Conte P, Heitzman ER, Markarian B. Viral pneumonia. Roentgen pathological correlations. Radiology. 1970;95:267–72.
143. Fine NL, Smith LR, Sheedy PF. Frequency of pleural effusions of mycoplasma and viral pneumonias. N Engl J Med. 1970;283:790–3.
144. Fraser DW, Tsai TR, Orenstein W, et al. Legionnaire's disease. Description of an epidemic of pneumonia. N Engl J Med. 1977;297:1189–97.
145. Kirby BD, Snyder KM, Meyer RD, et al. Legionnaire's disease—A cluster of cases (Abstract). Clin Res. 1978;26:A399.
146. Pope TL, Armstrong P, Thompson R, et al. Pittsburgh pneumonia agent chest film manifestations. AJR. 1982;138:237–41.
147. Tew J, Calenoff L, Berlin BS. Bacterial or nonbacterial pneumonia: Accuracy of radiographic diagnosis. Radiology. 1977;124:607–12.
148. Pennington JE. Community-acquired Pneumonia and Acute Bronchitis in Respiratory Infections: Diagnosis and Management. New York: Raven Press; 1973:125–34.
149. Garibaldi RA. Epidemiology of community acquired respiratory tract infections in adults: Incidence, etiology, and impact. Am J Med. 1985;78(Suppl 6B):32–7.
150. Kerttula Y, Leinonen M, Koskela M, et al. The aetiology of pneumonia. Application of bacterial serology and basic laboratory methods. J Infect. 1987;14:21–30.
151. Chatard JA. The leukocytes in acute lobar pneumonia. Johns Hopkins Hosp Rep. 1910;15:89–98.
152. Austrian R, Gold J. Pneumococcal bacteremia with especial reference to bacteremic pneumococcal pneumonia. Ann Intern Med. 1964;60:759–76.

153. MacFarlane JT, Finch RG, Ward MJ, et al. Hospital study of adult community acquired pneumonia. Lancet. 1982;2:255–8.
154. Klimek JJ, Ajemian E, Fontecchio S, et al. Community acquired bacterial pneumonia requiring admission to hospital. Am J Infect Cont. 1983;11:79–82.
155. Levy M, Dromer F, Brion N, et al. Community-acquired pneumonia: Importance of initial non-invasive bacteriologic and radiographic investigations. Chest. 1988;92:43–8.
156. Stratton CW. Bacterial pneumonia. An overview with emphasis on pathogenesis, diagnosis and treatment. Heart Lung. 1986;15:226–44.
157. Lipsky BA, Boyko EJ, Inui TS, et al. Risk factors for acquiring pneumococcal infections. Arch Intern Med. 1986;146:2179–85.
158. Rosner F, Zarrabi MH. Late infections following splenectomy in Hodgkin's disease. Cancer Invest. 1983;1:57–65.
159. Zarrabi MH, Rosner F. Serious infections in adults following splenectomy for trauma. Arch Intern Med. 1984;144:1421–4.
160. Crofton J. The chemotherapy of bacterial respiratory infections. Am Rev Respir Dis. 1970;101:841–59.
161. Hirschmann JV, Everett ED. *Haemophilus influenzae* infections in adults: Report of nine cases and a review of literature. Medicine. 1979;58:80–94.
162. Hausmann W, Karlish AJ. Staphylococcal pneumonia in adults. Br Med J. 1956;2:845–7.
163. Schwarzmann SW, Adler JL, Sullivan RJ, et al. Bacterial pneumonia during the Hong Kong influenza epidemic of 1968–1969. Experience in a city-county hospital. Arch Intern Med. 1971;127:1037–41.
164. Louria DB, Blumenfeld HL, Ellis JT, et al. Studies on influenza. J Clin Invest. 1959;38:213–65.
165. Yu VL, Kroboth FJ, Shonnard J, et al. Legionnaire's disease: New clinical perspective from a prospective pneumonia study. Am J Med. 1982;73:357–61.
166. Nicotra B, Rivera M, Luman I, et al. *Branhamella catarrhalis* as a lower respiratory tract pathogen in patients with chronic lung disease. Arch Intern Med. 1986;146:890–3.
167. Slevin NJ, Aitken J, Thornleg PE. Clinical and microbiological features of *Branhamella catarrhalis* bronchopulmonary infections. Lancet. 1987;1: 782–3.
168. Wallace RJ Jr, Musher DM. In honor of Dr. Sarah Branham. A star is born: The realization of *Branhamella catarrhalis* as a respiratory pathogen. Chest. 1986;90:447–50.
169. Gross JS, Neufeld RR, Libon LS, et al. Autopsy study of the elderly institutionalized patients: Review of 234 autopsies. Arch Intern Med. 1988;148:173–6.
170. Verghese A, Berk SL. Bacterial pneumonia in the elderly. Medicine. 1983;62:271–85.
171. Garb JL, Brown RB, Garb JR, et al. Differences in etiology of pneumonias in nursing home and community patients. JAMA. 1978;240:2169–72.
172. Ebright JR, Rytel MW. Bacterial pneumonia in the elderly. J Am Geriatr Soc. 1980;28:220–3.
173. Gleckman RA, Esposito AL. Bacterial pneumonia in the elderly: A reappraisal of conventional therapy with a note on cefamandole. J Am Geriatr Soc. 1979;27:345–7.
174. Berk KC, Holtsdan SA, Wiener SL, et al. Nontypeable *Haemophilus influenzae* in the elderly. Arch Intern Med. 1982;142:532–9.
175. Valenti WM, Trudell RG, Bentley DW. Factors predisposing to oropharyngeal colonization with gram-negative bacilli in the aged. N Engl J Med. 1978;298:1108–11.
176. Murray JF, Felton CP, Garay SM, et al. Pulmonary complications of the acquired immunodeficiency syndrome. Report of a National Heart, Lung and Blood Institute Workshop. N Engl J Med. 1984;310:1682–8.
177. Stover DE, White DA, Romano PA, et al. Spectrum of pulmonary diseases associated with the acquired immune deficiency syndrome. Am J Med. 1985;78:429–37.
178. Bartlett JG, Gorbach SL. The triple threat of aspiration pneumonia. Chest. 1979;68:560–6.
179. Wynne JW, Modell JH. Respiratory aspiration of stomach contents. Ann Intern Med. 1977;87:466–74.
180. Lorber B, Swenson RM. Bacteriology of aspiration pneumonia. A prospective study of community and hospital-acquired cases. Ann Intern Med. 1974;81:329–31.
181. Mogabgab WJ. *Mycoplasma pneumoniae* and adenovirus respiratory illness in military and university personnel 1959–1966. Am Rev Respir Dis. 1968;97:345–58.
182. Forsyth BR, Bloom HH, Johnson KM, et al. Etiology of primary atypical pneumonia in a military population. JAMA. 1965;191:364–8.
183. Wenzel RP, McCormick DP, Smith EP, et al. Acute respiratory disease: Clinical and epidemiologic observations of military trainees. Military Med. 1971;136:873–80.
184. Grayston JT, Kenny GE, Foy HM, et al. Epidemiological studies of *Mycoplasma pneumoniae* infections in civilians. Ann NY Acad Sci. 1967;143:436–46.
185. Mufson MA, Manko MA, Kingston JR, et al. Eaton agent pneumonia—clinical features. JAMA. 1961;178:369–74.
186. Tack KJ, Peterson PK, Rasp FL, et al. Isolation of *Chlamydia trachomatis* from the lower respiratory tracts of adults. Lancet. 1980;1:116–20.
187. Komaroff AL, Aronson MD, Schachter J. *Chlamydia trachomatis* infections in adults with community acquired pneumonia. JAMA. 1981;245:1319–22.
188. Beem MO, Saxon EM. Respiratory tract colonization and a distinctive pneumonia syndrome in infants infected with *Chlamydia trachomatis*. N Engl J Med. 1977;296:306–10.
189. Frommell GT, Bruhn FW, Schwartzman JD. Isolation of *Chlamydia trachomatis* from infant lung tissue. N Engl J Med. 1977;296:1150–2.
190. Cranston JT, Juo C, Wang S, et al. A new *Chlamydia psittaci* strain, TWAR, isolated in acute respiratory tract infection. N Engl J Med. 1986;315:161–8.
191. Marrie TJ, Grayston JT, Wang S, et al. Pneumonia associated with the TWAR strain of *Chlamydia*. Ann Intern Med. 1987;106:507–11.
192. George RB, Mogabgab WJ. Atypical pneumonia with rhinovirus infections. Ann Intern Med. 1969;71:1073–8.
193. Jahn CL, Felton OL, Cherry JD. Coxsackie B1 pneumonia in an adult. JAMA. 1964;189:236–7.
194. Wenzel RP, McCormick DP, Beam WE Jr. Parainfluenza pneumonia in adults. JAMA. 1972;221:294–5.
195. Respiratory syncytial virus—Missouri. Morbid Mortal Wkly Rep. 1977; 26:351.
196. Sorvillo FJ, Huie SF, Strassburg MA, et al. An outbreak of respiratory syncytial virus pneumonia in a nursing home for the elderly. J Infect. 1984;9:252–6.
197. Kasupski GJ, Leers WD. Presumed respiratory syncytial virus pneumonia in three immunocompromised adults. Am J Med Sci. 1983;285:28–33.
198. Legionnaire's disease: Diagnosis and management. Ann Intern Med. 1978;88:363–5.
199. Helms CM, Viner JP, Sturm RH. Comparative features of pneumococcal, mycoplasmal, and legionnaire's disease pneumonias. Ann Intern Med. 1979;90:543–7.
200. Ludmerer KM, Kissare JM. Pulmonary infiltrates and eosinophilia in a young man. Am J Med. 1986;81:533–40.
201. Schatz M, Wasserman S, Patterson R. Eosinophils and immunologic lung disease. Med Clin North Am. 1981;65:1055–71.
202. Citro LA, Gordon ME, Miller WT. Eosinophilic lung disease (or how to slice P.I.E.). Am J Roentgenol. 1973;117:787–97.
203. Liebow AA, Carrington CB. The eosinophilic pneumonias. Medicine. 1969;48:251–85.
204. Jederlinic PJ, Sicilian L, Graensler EA. Chronic eosinophilic pneumonia. Medicine. 1988;67:154–62.
205. Haley RW, Culver DH, White JW, et al. The nationwide nosocomial infection rate: A new need for vital statistics. Am J Epidemiol. 1985;121:159–67.
206. Simmons BP, Wong ES. CDC guidelines for the prevention and control of nosocomial infections: Guideline for prevention of nosocomial pneumonia. Am J Infect Control. 1983;11:230–3.
207. Haley RN, Hooton TM, Culver DH, et al. Nosocomial infections in U.S. hospitals 1975–1976. Am J Med. 1981;70:947–59.
208. Toews GB. Nosocomial pneumonia. Clin Chest Med. 1987;8:467–79.
209. Hooten TM, Haley RW, Culver DH, et al. The joint association of multiple role factors with the occurrence of nosocomial infection. Am J Med. 1981;70:960–70.
210. Donowitz LG, Page MC, Mileur BL, et al. Alteration of normal gastric flora in critical care patients receiving antacid and cimetidine therapy. Infect Control. 1986;7:23–6.
211. Snepar R, Poporad GA, Romano JM, et al. Effect of cimetidine and antacid on gastric microbial flora. Infect Immun. 1982;36:518–24.
212. Driks MR, Craven DE, Celli BR, et al. Nosocomial pneumonia in intubated patients given sucralfate as compared with antacids or histamine type-2 blockers. The role of gastric colonization. N Engl J Med. 1987;317:1376–82.
213. Wilson WR, Cockerill FR, Rosenow EC III. Pulmonary disease in the immunocompromised host. Mayo Clin Proc. 1985;60:610–31.
214. Schimpff SC, Young VM, Greene WH, et al. Origin of infection in acute nonlymphocytic leukemia: Significance of hospital acquisition of potential pathogens. Ann Intern Med. 1972;77:707–14.
215. Chang HY, Rodriguez V, Narboni G, et al. Causes of death in adults with acute leukemia. Medicine. 1976;55:259–68.
216. Peterson PK, Ferguson R, Fryd DS, et al. Infectious disease in hospitalized renal transplant recipients: A prospective study of a complex and evolving problem. Medicine. 1982;61:360–72.
217. Ramsey PG, Rubin RH, Tolkoff-Rubin NE, et al. The renal transplant patient with fever and pulmonary infiltrates: Etiology, clinical manifestations and management. Medicine. 1980;59:206–22.
218. Winston DJ, Gale RP, Meyer DV, et al. Infectious complications of human bone marrow transplantation. Medicine. 1979;58:1–31.
219. Valdivieso M, Gil-Extremera G, Zoronoza J, et al. Gram-negative bacillary pneumonia in the compromised host. Medicine. 1977;56:241–4.
220. Sickles EA, Young VM, Greene WH, et al. Pneumonia in acute leukemia. Ann Intern Med. 1973;79:528–34.
221. Donowitz GR, Mandell GR. Beta-lactam antibiotics (parts 1 and 2). N Engl J Med. 1988;318:419–26, 490–500.
222. Finegold SM, Wexler HM. Therapeutic implications of bacteriologic findings in mixed aerobic-anaerobic infections. Antimicrob Agents Chemother. 1988;32:611–16.
223. Murray PR, Rosenblatt JE. Penicillin resistance and penicillinase production in clinical isolates of *Bacteroides melaninogenicus*. Antimicrob Agents Chemother. 1977;11:605–8.
224. Kirby BD, George WL, Sutter VL, et al. Gram-negative anerobic bacilli: Their role in infection and patterns of susceptibility to antimicrobial agents. I. Little known *Bacteroides* species. Rev Infect Dis. 1980;2:914–51.

225. Bawdon RE, Crane LR, Palchaudhuri S. Antibiotic resistance in anaerobic bacteria: Molecular biology and clinical aspects. Rev Infect Dis. 1982; 4:1075–95.
226. Aldridge KE, Sanders CV, Janney A, et al. Comparison of the activities of penicillin G and new beta-lactam antibiotics against clinical isolates of *Bacteroides* species. Antimicrob Agents Chemother. 1984;26:410–3.
227. Levison ME, Mangura CT, Lorber B, et al. Clindamycin compared with penicillin for the treatment of anaerobic lung abscess. Ann Intern Med. 1983;98:466–71.
228. Bartlett JG, Gorbach SL. Penicillin or clindamycin for primary lung abscess. Ann Intern Med. 1983;98:546–8.

54. PLEURAL EFFUSION AND EMPYEMA

RICHARD E. BRYANT

Although the clinical course and need for surgical drainage of pleural empyema were known to Hippocrates, most of the changes in its recognition and treatment are of recent origin.[1,2] Microbial contamination of the pleural space is usually secondary to pneumonia but may arise from extrapulmonic infection and complicate neoplasm, collagen vascular disease, trauma, or medical or surgical procedures involving the pleura.[2] The mode of presentation is modified by the origin of the infection, the infecting microorganisms, and the patient's underlying disease(s).

ETIOLOGY

Medical and societal changes have modified the types of organisms causing empyema.[3–5] In 1935 acute bacterial empyema at the Boston City Hospital was caused by *Streptococcus pneumoniae* (46 percent), hemolytic streptococci (18 percent), *Staphylococcus aureus* (9 percent), gram-negative bacilli (3 percent), mixed aerobes (6 percent), and anaerobes (13 percent).[3] The cause of bacterial empyema from that institution in 1965 was *S. pneumoniae* (12 percent), hemolytic streptococci (5 percent), *Staph. aureus* (15 percent), gram-negative bacilli (25 percent), mixed aerobes (14 percent), and anaerobes (24 percent).[3] A report from Iowa described a 4-fold fall in the frequency of pneumococcal empyema and a 1.5- and 5-fold increase in staphylococcal and gram-negative bacillary empyema, respectively, in a comparable period.[4] These changes in microbial etiology may be explained by the changes in the types of patients developing empyema. In otherwise healthy patients with pneumonia, the most common causes of pleural empyema may still be *Staph. aureus, S. pneumoniae*, and *Streptococcus pyogenes*.[5] Staphylococcal empyema is especially common in children.

The recent increase in recognition of anaerobic empyema is due to improved microbiologic techniques and recognition of anaerobic infection associated with aspiration pneumonia, putrid lung abscess, and pleural infection arising from oropharyngeal or gastrointestinal sites.[6,7] Bartlett and coworkers found that pleural empyema was caused by aerobic bacteria in 24 percent, anaerobic bacteria in 35 percent, and both aerobic and anaerobic bacteria in 41 percent of 83 medical service patients without prior antibiotic therapy or surgical procedures.[6] Empyema secondary to subdiaphragmatic disease is often polymicrobial and anaerobic in origin.[8]

There is a high frequency of *Staph. aureus* and aerobic gram-negative bacillary infection in patients with post-traumatic or nosocomial empyema.[5,9] Empyema complicating hemothorax is often staphylococcal, while that associated with pneumothorax or serous effusion is often caused by gram-negative aerobic bacilli.[9] Immunocompromised patients have a higher frequency of empyema caused by fungi and gram-negative bacilli.[10] Organ transplant recipients and patients with the acquired immunodeficiency syndrome may reactivate pleural foci of mycobacterial or fungal infection but will rarely present with empyema without disseminated disease. Unsuccessful resection of cavitary coccidioidomycosis may be complicated by empyema from that organism. The association of fistulous tracts from the pleura suggests the possibility of actinomycosis, nocardiosis, or tuberculosis. Less common causes of empyema include extension of extrapulmonic infection caused by salmonella, clostridia, or *Entamoeba histolytica*.

PATHOGENESIS

Pleural effusions are caused by altered oncotic or capillary pressure from renal, cardiac, hepatic, or metabolic diseases. Pleural effusions may occur in 40–50 percent of patients with pneumonia.[2] However, only a small percentage (≈5 percent) of parapneumonic effusions become exudates with the associated microbiologic, chemical, and physical features of empyema.[2,11] Microorganisms gain access to the pleura by direct extension from the lung; from blood or lymphatics; by extension from subdiaphragmatic, mediastinal, pericardial, or cervical infection; and by transthoracic entry from trauma, surgery, or manipulative procedures. Patients with trauma to the esophagus, mediastinum, or heart or those who have had surgery in those areas are at increased risk of infection extending to the pleura. Similarly, patients with retropharyngeal or paravertebral suppurative disease may present with pleural empyema. As the efficiency of trauma rescue programs increase, the frequency of empyema associated with chest and head trauma will increase.[9,10]

Empyema fluid is deficient in opsonins and complement needed for optimal phagocytic function and ultimately develops extremes of hypoxia and acidity that further impair local neutrophil activity.[12,13] Endotoxins and other toxic factors elaborated by bacteria suppress the leukocyte host defense function and permit the growth of bacteria to concentrations of 10^8 bacteria per milliliter of empyema fluid.[14]

Inflammatory exudates may become loculated in a relatively small area or may extend to involve virtually the entire hemithorax, leading to ventilatory dysfunction and to the signs and symptoms of overwhelming sepsis and multiple organ failure. The exuberant inflammatory response can on occasion lead to erosion of the chest wall and to spontaneous drainage of the empyema.

Empyema fluid inhibits antimicrobial efficacy by a number of means. Aminoglycoside activity is suppressed by acid pH (minimum inhibitory concentration [MIC] is increased ≥64-fold by a 1-unit drop in pH), hypoxia (membrane transport of aminoglycosides is an oxygen-dependent step), increased concentrations of divalent cations, and binding of aminoglycosides to the DNA present in pleural pus.[14,15] β-Lactamase from microorganisms can degrade β-lactamase-susceptible β-lactam antibiotics, and chloramphenicol may be degraded by microbial enzymes in pus.[14] Moreover, late in the course of the disease, the growth of organisms within empyema fluid is suppressed to the extent that bacteria become refractory to antibiotic therapy.

By convention, the phases of empyema formation are divided into the *exudate phase*, during which leukocytes increase until pus is formed; the *fibropurulent phase*, during which fibrin formation begins to limit expansion of the lung; and the *organizing phase*, during which fibroblast formation and scarring produce a thick, leathery encasement that traps the lung.[16]

Microbe specific factors affect the pathophysiology of pleural space infection. Induction of experimental empyema in guinea pigs requires inoculation of $>10^6$ organisms per milliliter of

Escherichia coli, or *Staph. aureus* plus *Bacteroides fragilis*, in order to infect >50 percent of animals.[17] Use of umbilical tape as a foreign body does not increase lethality, but addition of blood greatly enhances the lethality of challenge with *E. coli* and *B. fragilis* mixtures.[17]

CLINICAL PRESENTATION

The clinical presentation of empyema is largely nonspecific and reflects the findings of the underlying disease. Patients may have chest pain, dyspnea, weight loss, chills, fever, or night sweats.[4] Development or persistence of fever and leukocytosis in a patient at risk of having a pleural empyema is frequently a clue to its presence. Physical examination often reveals signs of an effusion, but may be unchanged except for altered vital signs. A high index of suspicion and recognition of factors that predispose patients to the development of pleural empyema are the keys to its recognition.

Pleural effusion is demonstrated radiologically when at least 300–500 cc of fluid causes blunting of the costophrenic angles[11]

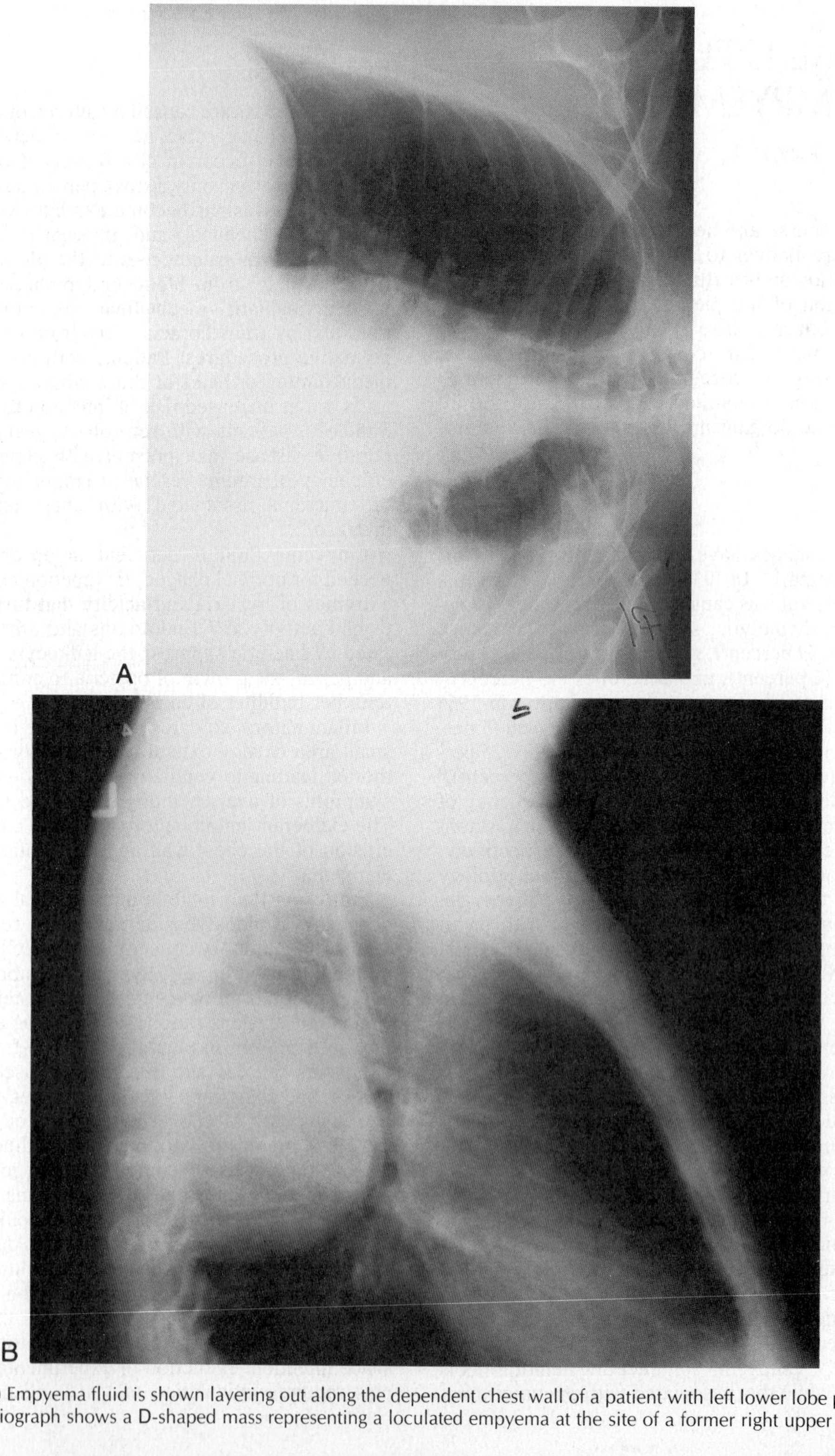

FIG. 1 **(A)** Empyema fluid is shown layering out along the dependent chest wall of a patient with left lower lobe pneumonia. **(B)** The radiograph shows a D-shaped mass representing a loculated empyema at the site of a former right upper lobectomy.

(Fig. 1). Lateral views often show a fluid meniscus and loss of distinct margins of the diaphragm. Lateral decubitus views permit detection of smaller volumes of fluid (100–200 cc) and verify the absence of loculation as fluid ''layers out'' along the dependent chest wall.[11] Conventional x-ray films may not distinguish effusions developing in interlobar or subpulmonic spaces. Similarly, loculated empyema with a bronchopleural fistula may resemble a lung abscess.

Empyema complicating extensive pneumonia may be difficult to recognize when the lung densities and pleural fluid overlap. Similarly, small volumes of pleural fluid may not be apparent on conventional x-ray films. Fortunately, both ultrasound and computer tomography provide more sensitive techniques for pleural fluid detection.[18,19] Pleural fluid aspiration under ultrasound guidance provides an accurate and safe means of obtaining infected pleural fluid and is especially helpful when fluid volumes are small or loculated.[20,21] However, it is not necessary to tap all parapneumonic effusions if the volume of fluid is small (less than 1 cm in depth on lateral decubitus films), the patient is doing well, and the x-ray picture is improving.[11,22,23]

Computed tomography (CT) is especially helpful for demonstrating pleural fluid accumulation due to extension from mediastinal or subdiaphragmatic disease[19,20] (Fig. 2). This technology can also distinguish between loculated pleural effusions

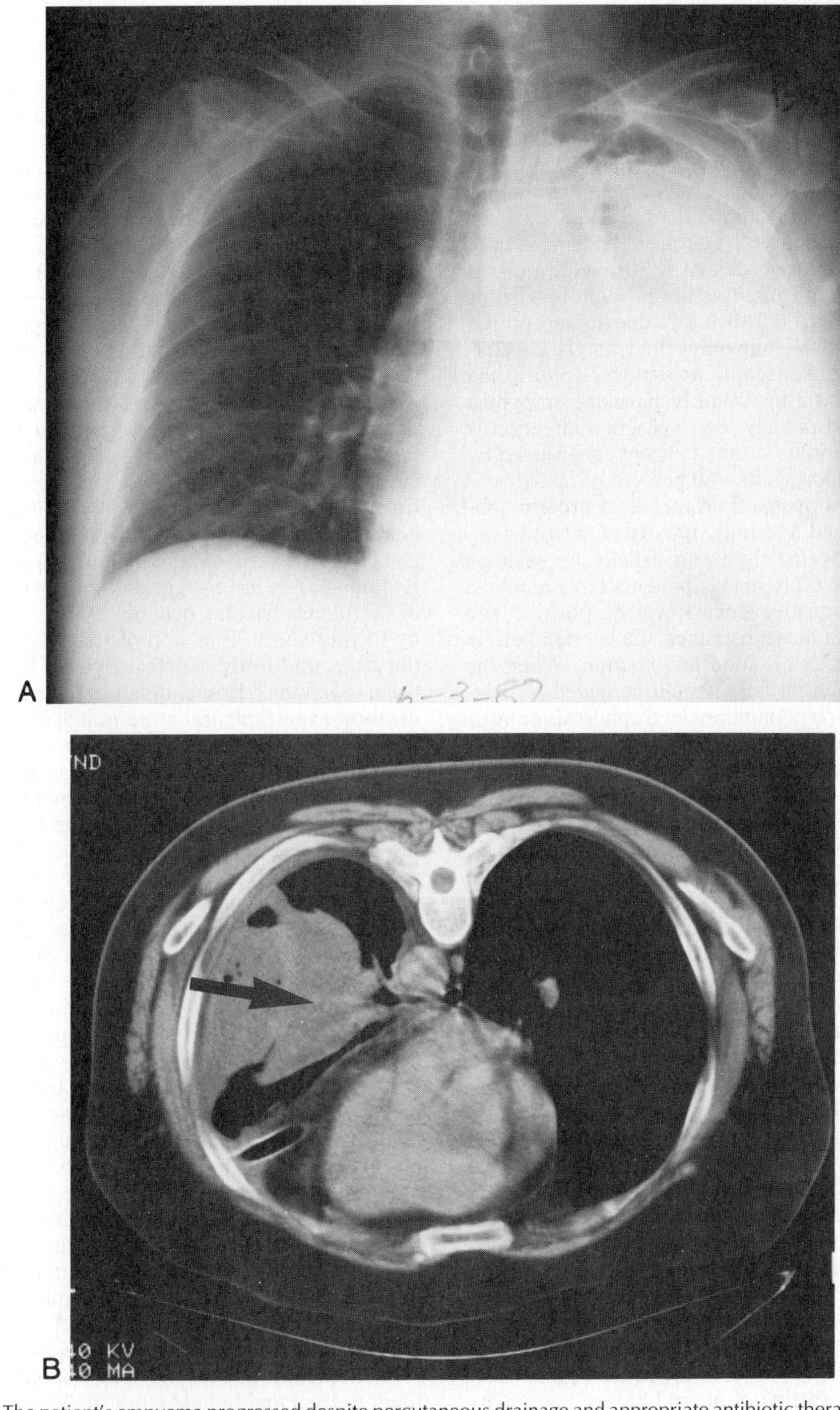

FIG. 2 **(A)** The patient's empyema progressed despite percutaneous drainage and appropriate antibiotic therapy. **(B)** Computed tomography showed malposition of chest tubes, but all attempts at tube drainage failed. The arrow designates the loculated empyema. The patient responded promptly to surgical decortication.

with bronchopleural fistulas and lung abscesses. CT has largely replaced the need for bronchograms to demonstrate bronchopleural fistulas. However, bronchoscopy and bronchography may be needed to define the cause of pleural empyema in patients in whom the etiology of infection is unexplained.[1]

Empyema is documented by finding pus and/or high concentrations of microorganisms in exudative pleural fluid obtained by thoracentesis. The character of the fluid depends on the type and duration of the infection and the associated trauma, surgery, malignancy, or other underlying disease. Initially, the fluid is thin and serous, but it becomes thick and purulent as neutrophil accumulation occurs. The poor correlation between the white blood cell counts in empyema fluid and the clinical features of infection may be due to lysis of neutrophils in pus. However, the status of the infection can be assessed by measuring pleural fluid pH, glucose, and lactic dehydrogenase.[11,22] Empyema fluid characteristically has a pH of less than 7.2, glucose less than 40 mg/dl, and lactic dehydrogenase activity of ≥600–1000 mg/dl.[11,22] Demonstration of these features or the presence of large numbers of bacteria on Gram stain suggests that drainage procedures are necessary. The pH of empyema fluid has the best correlation with the extent of the inflammatory process. Acid pH is primarily metabolic in origin and is caused secondarily by local CO_2 retention.[23] The mean lactic acid concentration of pus from human abscesses is 30 mg/dl, and pH values may be as low as 5.5. Thus, it is not prudent to assume that an empyema fluid pH of 6.0 to 6.5 is due to a ruptured esophagus unless tests like an empyema fluid amylase determination and radiologic or endoscopic procedures confirm the diagnosis. At the other extreme, frankly purulent empyema fluid can have a disproportionately high pH when infection is caused by urea-splitting *Proteus* strains.[24] Empyema caused by anaerobic bacteria is malodorous in ≈60 percent of instances.[6] Less specific findings of empyema fluid include a protein concentration of >3.0 mg/dl and a specific gravity of >1.018.[2]

Microorganisms in empyema fluid can usually be seen on Gram stain and grown in culture unless patients have received antibiotic therapy. Occasionally, smears will be positive and cultures will be negative. In those instances, the bacterial origin should be sought by cultures of blood and sputum. When the diagnosis is in question, pleural fluid should be tested for bacterial antigen by countercurrent immunoelectrophoresis or latex agglutination studies. In addition, fluid should be tested for *Legionella* by direct fluorescent antibody stains and culture because that organism will not be seen on conventional Gram stains. Empyema fluid devoid of microorganisms should also be examined for anaerobes, fungi, mycobacteria, and amoebae. Patients thought to have pleural or pulmonary amebiasis should have serologic tests for *E. histolytica*. Patients at risk of developing nocardiosis should have modified acid-fast stains. Acridine orange may permit visualization of organisms in abscess fluid that is smear negative by Gram stain. It should be noted that chylous pleural effusions may resemble purulent material, but lack white cells or microorganisms and remain opaque after centrifugation.[2]

Potts and coworkers found no bacteria on microscopic examination of 4 of 10 empyema fluids.[23] Two were sterile by culture. Smear-negative sterile empyema fluid has been reported in 6 to 15 percent[4,25] of patients, and culture-negative empyema has been described in up to 37 percent of patients.[25] Although improper culture technique, fastidious microorganisms, and prior antibiotic therapy may account for many cases of sterile empyema. It is likely that certain organisms are killed in pus. However, by the time bacterial empyemas become frankly purulent, they must be drained, whether sterile or not.

Pleural tuberculosis may be diagnosed by pleural fluid cultures or stains in 18 to 23 percent of patients or by cultures, stains, and histologic examination of pleural biopsy specimens in up to 95 percent of patients.[26] Liquid culture media are preferable to solid culture media, and it is rarely necessary to culture more than a single biopsy specimen. Radiometric culture detection methods may increase the speed of diagnosis in patients with pleural tuberculosis. A history of exposure, skin test conversion, or symptoms of weight loss, night sweats, and fever are helpful clues to the diagnosis of tuberculosis. However, patients may be both afebrile and anergic.

The pleural fluid of patients with rheumatoid arthritis, pancreatitis, or malignancy will occasionally have features suggestive of empyema.[2] The rare malignant effusion with a pH of <7.0 is readily diagnosed by cytologic examination and is associated with a worse prognosis than that of alkaline pleural fluid.[22] Exudates of rheumatoid or pancreatic origin only rarely have a pH of <7.2 and can be identified by serologic tests or increased pleural fluid amylase levels, respectively.[2]

TREATMENT

The goals for treatment of pleural empyema are eradication of infection, drainage of pus, and expansion of the lung. The primary treatment of empyema is drainage and will be necessary for patients with pleural fluid containing gross pus, a heavy growth of organisms visible by microscopy, a pH <7.2, glucose <40 mg/dl, and lactic dehydrogenase >1000 mg/dl.[11,22] Those with smear-negative serous pleural fluid with a pH ≥7.2 and intermediate lactic dehydrogenase and glucose levels may be treated with antibiotics and repeat thoracentesis in 12–18 hours to reassess the need for drainage procedures.[11] Those with improving pleural fluid parameters may be followed and reassessed.[11,22]

Repeated thoracentesis is rarely adequate unless the empyema fluid is quite thin and present in small volume. Percutaneous drainage of thin or serous fluid with small-bore catheters early in the course of empyema has been successful. Closed chest tube drainage with an underwater-sealed system is successful in two-thirds of patients, and the system can be placed by the surgeon, the radiologist, or the pulmonologist.[27,28] Recent studies have suggested that thoracoscopy and irrigation of the pleura hastens healing.[29] This needs to be substantiated by further study. Injection of streptokinase into the pleura has not been uniformly satisfactory and has been associated with toxic reactions.[2] Bronchopleural fistula is an absolute contraindication to intrapleural streptokinase.

The need for continued vacuum or water-sealed drainage is assessed by measuring the volume of fluid drained daily and by the size of the residual pleural cavity. Tubes can usually be withdrawn gradually when drainage is less than 50 ml/day and the cavity is less than 50 ml in size.[1,28]

Drainage of thick pleural pus is largely the province of the chest surgeon, who should be involved early in the course of such patients.[28–34] Closed chest tube drainage fails in approximately one-third of patients, who often have more extensive disease or prior chest surgery.[9,10,28] In addition, immunocompromised patients may require more extensive drainage procedures, including early rib resection and open drainage.[10] Management of open drainage tubes with daily irrigation and convalescence for 3–4 months is a tedious and time-consuming but time-honored method. In young adults who are otherwise healthy and are good operative candidates, decortication may be preferable.[27] This procedure provides more rapid recovery and more complete restoration of pulmonary function in adults but may be needed less frequently in children.[1,27] Decortication is traditionally advocated during the second or third week or after the sixth week of the disease in order to minimize the risk of tearing the poorly demarcated pleural peel during the 3–6 weeks of illness. The importance of surgical timing for the decortication procedure has been questioned.[31] Although small bronchopleural fistulas may close spontaneously, many are difficult to treat and require surgical closure. There is considerable variation in the frequency with which surgeons at different centers use rib resection, decortication, or empyectomy to manage empyema.[1,10,32,33] Similarly, several methods are used to treat chronic empyema or empyema that occurs after pneumonectomy. These operative approaches are selected on the basis of expected benefits and risks. Tube drainage has the fewest side effects, is tried first, and is rarely successful in that setting. Alternatives include permanent drainage, obliteration of the empyema space by muscle flaps, sterilization by instillation of antibiotics, and thoracoplasty.[34] The open window thoracostomy procedure devised by Eloesser was adapted to manage postpneumonectomy empyema. It can be used as permanent therapy for patients unable to undergo more extensive surgery.[31,32,34] Patients with bronchopleural fistulas that do not close with tube drainage are often treated successfully with muscle flap transposition by suturing the muscle directly to the bronchus or adjacent to the closed bronchial stump and using the muscle mass to obliterate the empyema cavity.[34] Patients with empyema and residual lung but without bronchopleural fistulas may respond to decortication or, if that fails, to myoplasty. Those without residual lung may respond to placement or irrigation with 0.25% neomycin in the closed chest cavity.[34] However, the risk of noemycin toxicity is substantial and makes this approach less desirable. Thoracoplasty is usually the procedure of last resort.[34]

Tuberculous pleural effusions rarely require more than antibiotic therapy unless a bronchopleural fistula is present. Special care should be taken not to introduce a secondary bacterial infection while performing a diagnostic or therapeutic thoracentesis of a tuberculosis pleural effusion.

The guidelines for optimal antibiotic therapy of bacterial empyema differ little from the recommendations for treatment of suppurative disease at other sites. Antibiotics are selected on the basis of their activity against microorganisms causing or presumed to be causing infection. There is virtually no problem in achieving adequate levels of antibiotics in empyema fluid with parenteral agents.[35] However if the empyema is caused by β-lactamase-producing organisms, β-lactamase-susceptible antibiotics should not be used. β-Lactam antibiotics should be used in high doses for prolonged periods, i.e., usually 2–4 weeks for bacterial infection. Patients with nocardiosis, actinomycosis, tuberculosis, or fungal empyema require even more prolonged therapy. In addition, patients with long-standing bacterial empyema may require prolonged therapy. Aminoglycosides should not be used as single-drug therapy of bacterial empyemas because they are toxic drugs with poor activity in the abscess milieu.[13] However, aminoglycosides may be combined with β-lactam antibiotics to achieve synergistic activity against empyema caused by *Pseudomonas aeruginosa, Enterobacter cloacae, Acinetobacter calcoaceticus*, and *Serratia marcescens*. Ciprofloxacin will probably play a major role in the long-term treatment of gram-negative empyema because it is a potent drug that can be given orally. At present, experience with this agent is too limited to permit it to be recommended as an initial drug of choice for therapy of empyema.

Anaerobic pleural empyema can be treated adequately with clindamycin, β-lactamase-stable β-lactams, or combinations of β-lactam and β-lactamase inhibitors. Although metronidazole is an excellent agent for anaerobic infection, it may be ineffective in anaerobic lung abscesses or partially drained empyemas because the drug is not reduced to its active metabolite in a partially oxygenated environment. Chloramphenicol or tetracycline should not be used to treat empyema caused by anaerobes.

PROGNOSIS

The mortality rate of pleural empyema is affected by the type and severity of infection, the patient's health or associated underlying diseases, and the adequacy of antibiotic therapy and drainage. The complexity of this picture is shown by the fact that the mortality due to empyema at Boston City Hospital rose from 38 percent in 1935 to 49 percent in 1965 despite the availability of antibiotics during the latter year.[3] Although mortality rates of 8 to 15 percent have been reported in otherwise healthy young patients,[27,33] rates of 40 to 70 percent have been reported in the elderly and in groups with severe underlying disease.[10,27] Mortality is increased in patients with nosocomial infection or empyema caused by polymicrobial or resistant gram-negative bacteria.[4] Patients with inadequately drained empyemas often die.[6] There are no criteria validating the superiority of a single technique, but in general, the more fragile or compromised patient may need more rapid achievement of adequate drainage by rib resection, lysis of adhesions, and use of a large-bore drainage tube earlier in the illness because such patients are more vulnerable to the serious sequelae of malnutrition, chronic sepsis, and multiple organ failure associated with delayed drainage of pus.[10] Post-traumatic empyema has a worse prognosis and should be considered for early decortication if (*1*) sepsis is not contained despite adequate antibiotic therapy, (*2*) fluid levels persist, (*3*) ventilatory function is compromised by inadequate lung expansion, or (*4*) pleural drainage is inadequate after 2 weeks of therapy.[9,10] An infected hemothorax rarely responds to tube drainage alone because clots obstruct the tube. Polymicrobial or nosocomial infection carries a worse prognosis because such patients have multiple underlying diseases and poor host defense.[4,5,32] In addition, these patients have an increased frequency of colonization and infection with multiply resistant gram-negative bacilli.[5] Thus, the sickest and most infirm patients often have pus that is hard to drain and organisms that are difficult to treat.

REFERENCES

1. Sherman MM, Subramanian V, Berger RL. Management of thoracic empyema. Am J Surg. 1977;133:474–9.
2. Light RW. Clinical manifestations and useful tests. In: Light RW, ed. Pleural Diseases. Philadelphia: Lea & Febiger; 1983:33–60.
3. Finland M, Barnes MW. Changing ecology of acute bacterial empyema. J Infect Dis. 1978;137:274–91.
4. Weese WC, Shindler ER, Smith IM, et al. Empyema of the thorax then and now. Arch Intern Med. 1973;131:516–20.
5. Vianna NJ. Nontuberculous bacterial empyema in patients with and without underlying disease. JAMA. 1971;215:69–71.
6. Bartlett JG, Finegold SM. Anaerobic infections of the lung and pleural space. Am Rev Resp Dis. 1974;110:56–77.
7. Barlett JG, Thadepalli H, Gorbach SL, et al. Bacteriology of empyema. Lancet. 1974;1:338–40.
8. Ballantyne KC, Sethia B, Reece IJ, et al. Empyema following intra-abdominal sepsis. Br J Surg. 1984;71:723–5.
9. Caplan ES, Hoyt NJ, Rodriguez A, et al. Empyema occurring in the multiply traumatized patient. J Trauma. 1984;24:785–98.
10. Lemmer JH, Botham MJ, Orringer MD. Modern management of adult thoracic empyema. J Thorac Cardiovasc Surg. 1985;90:849–55.
11. Light RW. Parapneumonic effusions and infections of the pleural space. In: Light RW, ed. Pleural Diseases. Philadelphia: Lea & Febiger; 1983:101–18.
12. Lew P, Zubler R, Vaudauz P. Decreased heat-labile opsonic activity and complement levels associated with evidence of C3 breakdown products in infected pleural effusions. J Clin Invest. 1979;63:326–34.
13. Bryant RE. Pus: Friend or foe? In: Root RK, Trunkey D, Sande MD, eds. Contemporary Issues in Infectious Diseases. v. V: New Surgical and Medical Approaches. New York: Churchill Livingstone, 1987;31–48.
14. Bryant RE. Effect of the suppurative environment on antibiotic activity. In: Root RK, Sand MD, eds. Contemporary Issues in Infectious Diseases. v. 1: New Dimensions in Antimicrobial Therapy. New York: Churchill Livingstone, 1984;313–37.
15. Vaudaux P, Waldvogel FA. Gentamicin inactivation in purulent exudates; role of cell lysis. J Infect Dis. 1980;142:586–93.
16. Andrews NC, Parker EF, Shaw RP, et al. Management of nontuberculous empyema. Am Rev Respir Dis. 1963;3:935–6.
17. Mavroudis C, Ganzel BL, Cox SK, et al. Experimental aerobic-anaerobic thoracic empyema in the guinea pig. Ann Thorac Surg. 1987;43:298–302.
18. O'Moore PV, Mueller PR, Simeone JF. Sonographic guidance in diagnostic and therapeutic interventions in the pleural space. AJR. 1987;149:1–5.
19. Mirvis SE, Tobin KD, Kostrubiak I, et al. Thoracic CT in detecting occult disease in critically ill patients. AJR. 1987;148:685–9.
20. Van Sonnenberg E, Nakamoto SK, Mueller PR, et al. CT and ultrasound guided catheter drainage of empyemas after chest-tube failure. Radiology. 1984;151:349–53.
21. Webb WB, La Berge JM. Radiographic recognition of chest tube malposition in the major fissure. Chest. 1984;85:81–3.

22. Good JA, Taryle DA, Maulitz RM, et al. The diagnostic value of pleural fluid pH. Chest. 1980;78:55–9.
23. Potts DE, Levin DC, Sahn SA. Pleural fluid pH in parapneumonic effusions. Chest. 1976;70:328–31.
24. Pine JR, Hollman JL. Elevated pleural fluid pH in *Proteus mirabilis* empyema. Chest. 1983;84:99–111.
25. Yeh TJ, Hall DP, Ellison RG. Empyema thoracis: A review. Am Rev Respir Dis. 1963;88:785–90.
26. Levine H, Metzger W, Lacera D, et al. Diagnosis of tuberculous pleurisy by culture of pleural biopsy specimen. Arch Intern Med. 1970;126:269–71.
27. Mandal AK, Thadepalli H. Treatment of spontaneous bacterial empyema thoracis. J Thorac Cardiovasc Surg. 1987;94:414–8.
28. Miller KS, Sahn SA. Chest tubes. Chest. 1987;91:258–64.
29. Hutter JA, Harari D, Braimbridge MV. The management of empyema thoracis by thoracoscopy and irrigation. Ann Thorac Surg. 1985;39:517–20.
30. Mittapalli MR. Successful treatment of empyema with thoracenteses and intrapleural antibiotics. South Med J. 1980;73:533–4.
31. Hoover EL, Ross MJ, Webb H, et al. Reappraisal of empyema thoracis. Chest. 1986;90:511–5.
32. Grant DR, Finley RJ. Empyema: Analysis of treatment techniques. Can J Surg. 1985;28:449–52.
33. Mayo P. Early thoracotomy and decortication for nontuberculous empyema in adults with and without underlying diseases. Am Surg. 1985;4:230–6.
34. Le Roux BT, Mohlala ML, Odell JA, et al. Suppurative diseases of the lung and pleural space. Part 1: Empyema thoracis and lung abscess. Curr Probl Surg. 1986;23:4–38.
35. Taryle DA, Good JT, Morgan EJ, et al. Antibiotic concentrations in human parapneumonic effusions. Antimicrob Chemother. 1981;7:171–7.

55. LUNG ABSCESS

SYDNEY M. FINEGOLD

Lung abscess is a suppurative pulmonary infection involving the destruction of lung parenchyma to produce one or more large cavities with an air–fluid level. A similar process with multiple small cavitations (less than 2 cm in diameter) has been designated *necrotizing pneumonia* by some clinicians. The distinction is arbitrary since lung abscess and necrotizing pneumonia are different expressions of the same fundamental pathologic process. The earliest manifestation of this type of problem is pneumonia without excavation or abscess formation. In the absence of effective therapy, the disease may progress to lung abscess or to necrotizing pneumonia, with or without pleural empyema. Generally, the specific infecting organisms and the predisposing conditions do not influence the type of clinical disease that results. However, the size of the inoculum of organisms and the defense mechanisms of the host are likely to influence the outcome. Most often lung abscess follows aspiration, and anaerobic bacteria are the major organisms involved.

PREDISPOSING CAUSES

By far the most important background factor for abscess of the lung is aspiration,[1] usually related to altered consciousness. Common causes of altered consciousness in such patients are alcoholism, cerebral vascular accident, general anesthesia, drug overdose or addiction, seizure disorder, diabetic coma, shock, and other serious illness. Other factors in aspiration include dysphagia due to either esophageal disease or neurologic disease, intestinal obstruction, and tonsillectomy or tooth extraction. A study by Huxley et al.[2] using a sensitive radioactive tracer technique determined that 70 percent of patients with depressed consciousness and 45 percent of healthy subjects in deep sleep aspirated. Aspiration occurred more frequently and extensively in patients with depressed consciousness. Impairment of normal clearance mechanisms or the overwhelming of such mechanisms by large volumes of aspirated secretions may result in pulmonary infection. Alcoholics and patients who are acutely or chronically ill (whether or not they are hospitalized or in a nursing home) often demonstrate oropharyngeal colonization with gram-negative bacilli, particularly if they undergo endotracheal intubation and especially if they also receive histamine type 2 blockers or antacids.[3,4]

Next to aspiration, the most important factor predisposing to lung abscess or to necrotizing pneumonia is periodontal disease or gingivitis. Lung abscess is rare in an edentulous person and suggests the possibility of an associated bronchogenic carcinoma.[5] Other underlying processes include bronchiectasis, secondary infection of a bland pulmonary embolus with infarction, septic embolization, bacteremia, inhalation of bacteria-containing aerosols, and intra-abdominal infection. Suppurative inflammation behind an obstruction in a bronchus is another important mechanism. Patients receiving immunosuppressive therapy may develop multiple lung abscesses due to *Nocardia* or other organisms.

PATHOGENESIS AND PATHOLOGIC CHARACTERISTICS

Lung abscess is primarily of endogenous origin. Most of the bacteria involved are elements of the normal flora of the upper respiratory tract. Infections involving *Staphylococcus aureus, Klebsiella,* and other organisms may be of nosocomial origin.

The primary site of lung abscess is the posterior segment of the right upper lobe, with the same segment on the left less commonly affected. Next in frequency of involvement are the apical segments of the lower lobes. These segments are dependent in location when the subject is in a horizontal position, and the distribution relates to the fact that aspiration or inhalation is the primary background factor. Normally, aspirated material is handled effectively by ciliary action, cough, and alveolar macrophages. If the protective mechanisms are not effective, as with ethanol ingestion or viral disease, infection may result. Endotracheal tubes impair coughing, impede pulmonary clearance mechanisms, and allow leakage of oropharyngeal secretions into the tracheobronchial tree. Thick or particulate matter and foreign bodies are not easily removed and thus may lead to bronchial obstruction and atelectasis. With aspiration, gastric acid and enzymes may be the primary offending agents.

Subdiaphragmatic infection may extend to the lung or to the pleural space by way of lymphatics, directly through the diaphragm or defects in it, or by way of the blood stream. Most amebic lung abscesses are located in the right lower lobe adjacent to the diaphragm since they typically arise by direct extension of hepatic abscesses through the diaphragm.

Infection may arise in or behind an obstruction (neoplasm, foreign body, or enlarged mediastinal lymph node). Septic emboli from bacterial endocarditis of the right side of the heart or from pelvic or other deep vein thrombophlebitis may result in a metastatic lung abscess.

Although the virulence of the infecting organism(s) may be a factor determining the nature and extent of the infectious process, this is not usually important in the case of the anaerobes except for *Fusobacterium necrophorum*. However, the number of organisms aspirated may well be an important factor. With certain of the nonanaerobes such as *Klebsiella, Staphylococcus,* and group A *Streptococcus,* virulence may play an important role.

The pathologic characteristic is essentially that of necrosis supervened on inflammation with cavitation and abscess formation. The abscess cavity may become partially lined with regenerated epithelium, and localized bronchiectasis and emphysema may develop. There is usually no significant vascular involvement in lung abscess. However, a septic or bland pulmonary embolus may be the initial event. Once underway, the infection itself may give rise to pulmonary arteritis as in infection caused by *Pseudomonas aeruginosa*.

CLINICAL MANIFESTATIONS

Anaerobic Lung Abscess

In patients with lung abscess admitted to a hospital, symptoms have generally been present for at least 2 weeks. At times the patient will have had several weeks or even months of malaise, low-grade fever, and productive cough before seeking medical attention. Weight loss and anemia are common and confirm that the infection is indolent. Often the patient runs a low-grade fever; that is, a temperature about 101–102°F. Sputum production is usually copious. Foul-smelling sputum or empyema fluid occurs in only about one-half of the patients.[1,5,6]

In patients in whom the course of the infection has been followed radiologically, pneumonia appears first and cavitation subsequently. The earliest time of appearance of a cavity is about 7 days after aspiration; the average is about 12 days. Mediastinal adenopathy occasionally accompanies the parenchymal disease in patients with lung abscess or with other types of anaerobic pulmonary infection.[6] There may be a history of a period of unconsciousness, evidence of alcoholism, diseased gums, absence of the gag reflex, or other indications of the predisposing condition.

The physical findings are those of a pneumonia, with or without pleural effusion, early in the course of the illness. Later there may be amphoric or cavernous breath sounds. Clubbing of the fingers is noted on occasion.

Anaerobic Necrotizing Pneumonia

Usually anaerobic necrotizing pneumonia is confined primarily to one pulmonary segment or lobe. However, it may extend to involve an entire lung or even both lungs (Fig. 1). This type of anaerobic pulmonary infection is the most severe of all. There may be an associated empyema. The disease often spreads rapidly and produces destruction that is characterized by ragged, greenish discoloration of the lung and large putrid sloughs of tissue. This process culminates in "pulmonary gangrene."[5–7]

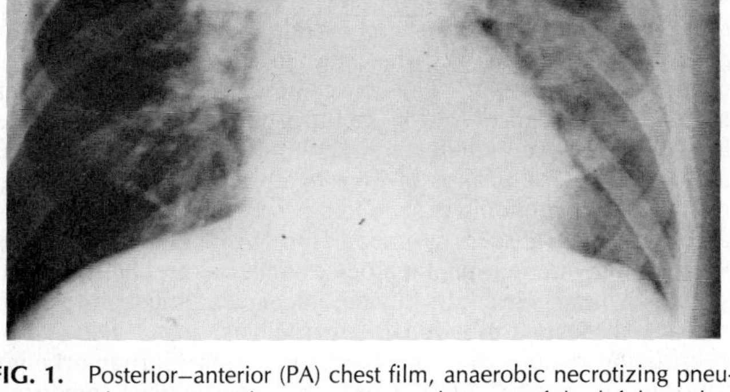

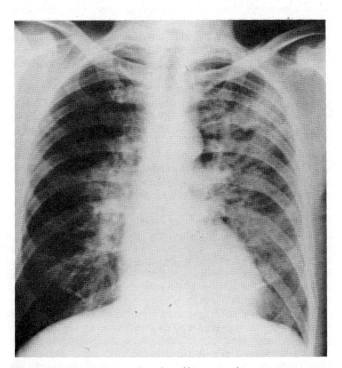

FIG. 1. Posterior–anterior (PA) chest film, anaerobic necrotizing pneumonia, and empyema. There is major involvement of the left lung, less involvement of the right. Note the multiple small excavations and one larger cavity in the left lung and blunting of the left costophrenic angle.

The patients are generally quite ill, with a temperature of 102–103°F. Leukocytosis is usually pronounced; for example, more than 20,000/mm^3. Most of these patients have putrid sputum or empyema fluid when first seen.

Pulmonary actinomycosis may be manifested as a necrotizing pneumonia; a number of cases will be complicated by extension of the process to the pleural space and to the chest wall.

Nonanaerobic Lung Abscess and Necrotizing Pneumonia

In primary infections due to organisms such as *S. aureus, Streptococcus pyogenes, Nocardia,* or *Klebsiella pneumoniae,* the symptoms are those of a severe pneumonia.

Secondary Lung Abscess and Necrotizing Pneumonia

In cases of secondary lung abscess, the basic process (bacteremia, endocarditis, septic thrombophlebitis, subphrenic infection, and so forth) will usually be evident in addition to the pulmonary process. The most characteristic hematogenous lung abscess is seen in staphylococcal bacteremia, especially in children. These abscesses are commonly multiple and peripheral in location. Empyema is frequently seen in this situation (Fig. 2). Repeated septic emboli should be suspected when multiple lesions appear over an extended period.

Less than 5 percent of bland pulmonary infarcts become secondarily infected. Secondary infection of infarcts should be suspected if fever is persistent, if the temperature rises above 103°F for more than 48 hours, or if the white blood cell count rises to more than 20,000 cells/mm^3. Abscess formation may occur within a necrotic pulmonary tumor or behind an obstructing tumor.

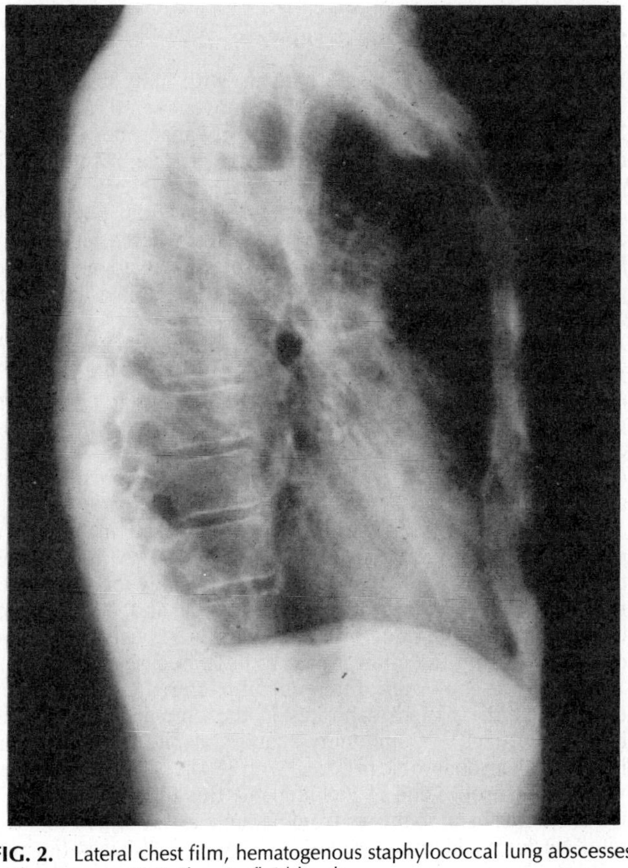

FIG. 2. Lateral chest film, hematogenous staphylococcal lung abscesses and empyema. Note the air–fluid levels.

The syndrome of tonsillitis or pharyngitis (Vincent's angina) with septicemia due to *F. necrophorum,* followed by widespread metastatic disease involving the lungs and other organs, is not commonly seen any longer, probably as a result of early antibiotic therapy for upper respiratory tract infections. However, it is important to be aware of this serious illness that occurs in children and young adults.

Amebic Lung Abscess

In patients with amebic lung abscess, the symptoms of the associated liver abscess will often have been present before the rupture through the diaphragm. After perforation of the liver abscess into the lung, there is a gradually developing cough and expectoration of a peculiar chocolaty or anchovy saucelike sputum. There is no odor to the sputum. The development of a pulmonary amebic abscess varies from a very insidious phenomenon to a dramatic onset with a sudden attack of severe cough productive of a large amount of brownish red sputum.[8] There may be a history of diarrhea, and an appropriate travel history may be elicited.

Complications

Approximately one-third of lung abscesses are complicated by empyema. This may be seen with or without bronchopleural fistulas. Brain abscess (via vertebral veins as a rule) may also be a complication in patients not receiving appropriate therapy early. A brain abscess is typically solitary. There is virtually never dissemination to other organs. Localized bronchiectasis may occur. Amyloidosis is no longer seen.

Complications of amebic abscess[9] include spontaneous perforation creating a cutaneous sinus, hepatobronchial fistula, empyema, secondary bacterial infection, and amebic abscess of the brain.

MICROBIOLOGIC CHARACTERISTICS

In a prospective study of 26 patients with lung abscesses by Bartlett et al.,[1] anaerobic bacteria were recovered in 24 of the 26 transtracheal aspirate specimens. Only anaerobes (including microaerophilic streptococci) were recovered from 16 of the 24 patients, whereas aerobic or facultative bacteria were recovered along with anaerobes in the other 8. Four patients had a single anaerobe recovered in pure culture, whereas 20 patients had multiple isolates, averaging 3.1 bacteria (2.6 anaerobes) per patient. The most commonly encountered anaerobes were gram-negative rods and gram-positive cocci.

Among 28 cases of anaerobic necrotizing pneumonia,[5] 20 yielded only anaerobes. Overall, there was an average of 2.3 anaerobes and 0.4 aerobes per case. *Fusobacterium nucleatum,* pigmented and other *Bacteroides,* and anaerobic and microaerophilic streptococci and cocci predominated among the anaerobes. Another distinctive cause of necrotizing pneumonia is actinomycosis.

The anaerobes most commonly encountered in anaerobic pleuropulmonary infection are listed in Table 1. Although clostridia, including *Clostridium perfringens,* may be recovered from patients with necrotizing pneumonia and empyema or other anaerobic pulmonary infections, there is usually nothing distinctive about the clinical picture in such cases.

There is an important difference in bacterial cause in terms of whether the patient aspirates in the community or in the hospital setting.[6,12] Community-acquired aspiration pneumonia is primarily an anaerobic process, with 35 out of 38 cases studied yielding anaerobes and 25 yielding only this type of organism.[12] On the other hand, cultures from patients aspirating in the hospital setting yielded anaerobes in 26 out of 32 cases (in pure culture in only 7 cases) and, most importantly, as part of the other infecting flora yielded important nosocomial pathogens such as *S. aureus* and various aerobic and facultative gram-negative bacilli such as *Klebsiella, Pseudomonas,* and *Proteus.*

TABLE 1. Anaerobes Most Commonly Encountered in Pleuropulmonary Infection

Gram-negative bacilli
Pigmented *Bacteroides* or *Porphyromonas*
Bacteroides oralis
B. buccae
B. ureolyticus group (especially *B. gracilis*)
B. bivius
B. oralis group
B. fragilis group
Fusobacterium nucleatum
F. necrophorum
F. naviforme
F. gonidiaformans
Gram-positive cocci
Peptostreptococcus (especially *P. anaerobius, P. magnus, P. asaccharolyticus, P. prevotii, P. intermedius*[a], *P. micros*)
Microaerophilic streptococci
Gram-positive spore-forming bacilli
Clostridium perfringens, C. ramosum
Gram-positive non-spore-forming bacilli
Actinomyces sp.
Arachnia sp.
Bifidobacterium dentium (*eriksonii*)

[a] This organism officially belongs in the genus *Streptococcus.*
(Data from Kirby et al.,[10] George et al.,[11] Sutter et al.[20])

Nichols and Smith[13] have shown that patients with bleeding or obstructing duodenal ulcers or with gastric ulcers or malignancy commonly have a much more profuse microflora in the stomach than do people without such pathologic conditions. This flora includes various organisms from the oral flora such as streptococci and anaerobes of various types but also coliform bacilli and, on occasion, *B. fragilis.* Thus, aspiration of gastric contents in people with the aforementioned pathologic conditions would carry with it a greater risk of bacterial infection, and the infecting flora might be different from what would ordinarily be expected. Histamine type 2 blockers or antacids have commonly been used to prevent upper gastrointestinal bleeding due to stress ulcers in critically ill patients. This leads to an elevated gastric pH and gastric and pharyngeal (by the retrograde route) colonization with gram-negative bacilli. This can likely be avoided by the use of sucralfate in lieu of antacids or H2 blockers.[3]

There are also several major aerobic causes of necrotizing pneumonia: *S. aureus, S. pyogenes, K. pneumoniae,* and *P. aeruginosa.* It is said that, on rare occasion, pneumococci (type 3) may cause a lung abscess. Infrequently, other gram-negative bacilli such as *Escherichia coli, Legionella pneumophila,* and perhaps *Proteus* sp. may cause pulmonary necrosis. Uncommon but important causes of cavitating pneumonia are *Nocardia* infection, melioidosis, and glanders. In acute Friedländer's (*Klebsiella*) pneumonia, 25–50 percent of the patients will develop one or more lung abscesses. Lung abscess due to *Pseudomonas cepacia* was reported by Poe et al.[14] The patient was a diabetic and developed the lung abscess after therapy with ultrasonic nebulization. The source of the organism was determined to be the reservoir of the ultrasonic nebulizer. Such nebulizers have been implicated in gram-negative bacillary pneumonia by several groups of investigators. However, although necrotizing pneumonia is seen in a proportion of these groups, a solitary lung abscess is uncommon. In infants with staphylococcal pneumonia, pneumatoceles occur as frequently as abscesses, whereas in adults the radiolucencies almost always represent abscess formation. Tuberculosis may also cause necrotizing pneumonia, and fungal infection (particularly histoplasmosis, coccidioidomycosis, and aspergillosis) sometimes produces this lesion.

Three major groups of bacteria are involved in hematogenous spread to the lungs: gram-positive cocci, notably staphylococci;

gram-negative enteric bacilli; and anaerobic bacteria. Multiple abscesses are likely to be of hematogenous origin, either as a result of bacteremia or of septic embolization. The most characteristic hematogenous lung abscess is seen in staphylococcal bacteremia. Hematogenous pulmonary infection with gram-negative enteric bacilli occurs in association with urinary tract infection or manipulation, after bowel surgery, after septic abortion, or as a nosocomial infection (usually in relation to vascular or urinary tract catheterization). Anaerobic or microaerophilic streptococci and gram-negative anaerobic bacilli may also produce hematogenous necrotizing pulmonary infection secondary to intra-abdominal or pelvic infections. In all of these anaerobic infections, there may be only bacteremia or else a septic thrombophlebitis that results in septic embolization. Uncommon hematogenous necrotizing pulmonary processes are those seen with anthrax, plague, and *Salmonella choleraesuis* infection.

Metastatic lung abscess may occur as a result of septic emboli from bacterial endocarditis of the right side of the heart (*S. aureus* is the major pathogen in this setting) or from pelvic or other deep vein thrombophlebitis. Various anaerobic bacteria and also pyogenic cocci such as *S. aureus* and streptococci not infrequently cause septic thrombophlebitis. As noted earlier, the anaerobes may be involved in this type of process in association with pelvic or intra-abdominal infection or, uncommonly now, with jugular vein thrombophlebitis in association with tonsillopharyngeal infections. Thrombophlebitis of the cavernous sinus most often involves *S. aureus* or streptococci. *Staphylococcus aureus* may also produce septic thrombophlebitis in association with superficial skin or soft tissue infections or in relation to intravenous catheters. The latter setting also may lead to septic thrombophlebitis involving gram-negative bacilli. Various organisms may be involved in secondary infection of bland pulmonary infarcts including staphylococci, streptococci, pneumococci, gram-negative enteric bacilli, and anaerobes of various types. Infection within a necrotic pulmonary tumor or behind an obstructing tumor may lead to abscess formation. Anaerobic bacteria of various types are commonly involved in such infections, but various other infecting organisms including *Mycobacterium tuberculosis* and fungi as well as a variety of bacteria may also be involved.

Unusual organisms may be involved in immunocompromised patients. Thus, there is a report[15] of a lung abscess due to *Rhodococcus* (*Corynebacterium*) *equi* in a renal transplant recipient.

DIAGNOSIS

The typical lung abscess can be suspected on clinical grounds. Most diagnoses are made from the chest roentgenogram, specifically from the presence of a cavity with an air–fluid level or pneumonitis with multiple small excavations located in a dependent segment. Diagnosis of the specific cause as well as differentiation from similar lesions depends on definitive bacteriologic studies. Because of the presence of large numbers of anaerobes as indigenous flora in the mouth and the common presence in hospitalized people of potential pathogens such as *S. aureus* and *K. pneumoniae* as colonizers in the mouth or the upper respiratory tract, it is necessary to obtain a specimen other than expectorated sputum for bacteriologic diagnosis. Empyema fluid, if available, provides an excellent specimen. On occasion, particularly with a mestatic lung abscess, blood cultures may be positive; however, blood cultures may reveal only part of the infecting flora. In the absence of the aforementioned sources of specimens for diagnosis, percutaneous transtracheal aspiration is an easy, safe, and dependable way of establishing the specific cause of the lung abscess or necrotizing pneumonia in patients who are able to cooperate.[16] This procedure should not be used in people with a significant bleeding tendency or in those in whom it is difficult to provide adequate oxygenation. Subcutaneous emphysema is an occasional complication of transtracheal aspiration, usually in patients with a severe cough, and may dissect into the mediastinum. Percutaneous transthoracic aspiration may be useful, particularly in children, but provides a smaller, less satisfactory specimen. Obtaining specimens during fiber-optic bronchoscopy by means of a bronchial brush within a plugged double-lumen catheter has been recommended.[17] It is absolutely essential that the techniques as outlined in detail by Broughton et al.[18] be used exactly as described and that cultures be done quantitatively. Growth at a 10^{-3} dilution is considered significant. The amount of the secretions collected by the brush is 0.001–0.01 ml, so the 10^{-3} dilution represents 10^5–10^6 organisms/ml of lower respiratory tract secretions. The small volume of material obtained and the difficulty one would encounter to arrange for anaerobic transport are a concern; nevertheless, good results appear to have been obtained in a small number of cases of anaerobic pulmonary infection. Recently quantitative culture of fluid obtained by bronchoalveolar lavage (during bronchoscopy) has been stated to provide reliable results in bacterial pneumonia.[19] Studies to date are limited, not fully controlled, and did not include anaerobic cultures but appear promising.

It is essential that material obtained for culture be placed under anaerobic conditions promptly before transport to the laboratory. It is usually desirable to aspirate the material to be cultured into a syringe, to expel all bubbles of air or gas from the syringe and needle, and then to transfer the specimen to a tube that has been gassed out with oxygen-free gas for transport to the laboratory.[20]

Demonstration of the usual underlying liver abscess is basic to the diagnosis of amebic lung abscess, but one may be able to demonstrate *Entamoeba histolytica* in the patient's sputum. Charcot-Leyden crystals in the sputum are suggestive of amebic infection. The usual procedures for the diagnosis of intestinal or hepatic amebiasis should be undertaken. The vast majority of patients with extraintestinal amebiasis will have high titers of hemagglutinating or complement-fixing antibodies.

Differential Diagnosis

Factors that would suggest a cavitating carcinoma rather than lung abscess include the absence of predisposing factors for an aspiration abscess (including an edentulous patient), location of an abscess in a nondependent segment, irregular abscess wall, and failure to respond to antibacterial therapy. Tuberculosis may also simulate a lung abscess or necrotizing pneumonia. Patients with infected lung cysts typically lack the systemic symptoms that may be seen in lung abscess, the cavity wall is thin, and there is no surrounding pneumonitis.

THERAPY AND PROGNOSIS

The primary mode of therapy is the administration of antimicrobial agents. Treatment may need to be continued for 2–4 months to achieve cure without relapse.

The anaerobes involved in lung abscess or in necrotizing pneumonia are increasingly resistant to penicillin G. Reports have appeared of less than optimum response or even frank failure to cure anaerobic lung abscesses or necrotizing pneumonia with penicillin therapy,[21,22] primarily because of β-lactamase producing *Bacteroides*. Metronidazole, or clindamycin, supplemented with penicillin G, represents the treatment of choice for serious anaerobic pulmonary infections. Thus, penicillin G (or penicillin V, ampicillin, or amoxicillin) is no longer used by the author as the sole initial therapy for patients with a suspected or proven anaerobic lung abscess or necrotizing pneumonia who are seriously ill. Penicillin is still favored as the initial therapy for patients who are mildly to moderately ill. Since some of the anaerobic cocci may require 8 units/ml or more of penicillin G for inhibition, one should use large doses of this agent (10–20 million units/day intravenously). After there has been a good clinical response, the regimen can usually be changed to a lower dosage. Patients who are not very ill may be treated satisfactorily with one of the aforementioned oral penicillins. Other penicillins are often considerably less active than is penicillin G. Oral cephalosporins such as cephalexin or cephradine may be used with good effect in patients who are not very ill.

A significant percentage of strains of most anaerobes are resistant to tetracyclines. Accordingly, these compounds should be used only when susceptibility data are available or when the patient's illness is minor so that a therapeutic trial in the patient can be undertaken safely. Clindamycin is active against most anaerobes with the exception of some strains of *Peptostreptococcus, Bacteroides gracilis, Fusobacterium varium,* and some strains of clostridia other than *C. perfringens*; 20 percent of the *B. fragilis* group are resistant in some centers. The addition of penicillin G would increase the spectrum of coverage except for the *B. fragilis* group and *B. gracilis*. Metronidazole is active against all gram-negative anaerobes including the *Bacteroides fragilis* group and other β-lactamase producers. It is also always active against all clostridia. Some anaerobic cocci and most microaerophilic streptococci, *Actinomyces,* and *Arachnia* are resistant. For this reason, metronidazole should ordinarily be used together with penicillin G (or erythromycin) in the treatment of anaerobic pulmonary infections. Certain β-lactam agents are quite active against the *B. fragilis* group and other β-lactamase-producing *Bacteroides* and most other anaerobes, although increasing resistance has been encountered in some centers. Included are cefoxitin, the carboxy penicillins (carbenicillin and ticarcillin), and the piperazine and ureidopenicillins (piperacillin and mezlocillin). Cefoxitin is inactive against one-third of clostridia other than *C. perfringens*. These agents, especially the piperazine and ureidopenicillins and cefoxitin, also have significant activity against various Enterobacteriaceae. Cefoxitin is also active against *S. aureus*, and the penicillins mentioned have activity against *P. aeruginosa*. The third-generation cephalosporins and related new compounds all have less activity against anaerobes, especially the *B. fragilis* group, than do cefoxitin and the broad-spectrum penicillins just discussed. One exception is imipenem, which is active against essentially all anaerobes. Combinations of β-lactam drugs and β-lactamase inhibitors such as ticarcillin plus clavulanic acid and ampicillin plus sulbactam are active against essentially all anaerobes and have good activity vs. *S. aureus* and many gram-negative bacilli. Chloramphenicol is active against essentially all anaerobes of all types and represents another option in a seriously ill patient with necrotizing pneumonia or lung abscess in whom β-lactamase-producing anaerobes may be present.

For staphylococcal infections, a penicillinase-resistant penicillin is preferable, but one of the parenteral cephalosporins or vancomycin may be used in the event of significant allergy. Vancomycin is the drug of choice for methicillin-resistant *S. aureus*. Penicillin G is the drug of choice for group A streptococcal infection. For infections due to *K. pneumoniae* or other facultative or aerobic gram-negative bacilli that may be involved in the type of pulmonary infection under discussion, one of the aminoglycosides would represent a drug of choice, but the extended-spectrum penicillins and combinations of β-lactam drugs and β-lactamase inhibitors have very good activity against some of these organisms. This is also true of imipenem. Gentamicin is ordinarily suitable, but in certain hospitals significant numbers of gram-negative bacilli are resistant to gentamicin; amikacin would then be the drug of choice. In seriously ill patients, particularly those who may be immunosuppressed, the use of appropriate β-lactam agents along with the aminoglycoside is desirable.

Postural drainage is an important aspect of the therapy for a lung abscess. Bronchoscopy may be helpful in effecting drainage and for removal of foreign bodies and biopsy diagnosis of tumors. Surgical resection of lung abscesses is rarely required unless there is a coexisting malignant process. Indeed, surgery is contraindicated because of the hazard of the spread of infection or asphyxiation from spillage of abscess contents. Surgical drainage of a lung abscess through the chest wall is rarely indicated.

Prognosis

The prognosis varies with the type of underlying or predisposing pathologic process, if any, and in the case of acute severe necrotizing pneumonias, the speed with which appropriate therapy is instituted. The mortality in anaerobic lung abscess is 15 percent or less. In anaerobic necrotizing pneumonia it is 25 percent. The mortality may be significantly higher in acute pneumonias caused by *S. aureus, K. pneumoniae,* and other facultative or aerobic gram-negative bacilli. The prognosis in amebic lung abscess is good when the diagnosis and treatment are prompt. Nocardiosis often has a relatively poor prognosis, especially when it complicates a serious underlying disease.

REFERENCES

1. Bartlett JG, Gorbach SL, Tally FP, et al. Bacteriology and treatment of primary lung abscess. Am Rev Respir Dis. 1974;109:510.
2. Huxley EJ, Viroslav J, Gray WR, et al. Pharyngeal aspiration in normal adults and patients with depressed consciousness. Am J Med. 1978;64:564.
3. Driks MR, Craven DE, Celli BR, et al. Nosocomial pneumonia in intubated patients given sucralfate as compared with antacids or histamine type 2 blockers. N Engl J Med. 1987;317:1376–82.
4. Tryba M. Risk of acute stress bleeding and nosocomial pneumonia in ventilated intensive care unit patients: Sucralfate versus antacids. Am J Med. 1987;83(Suppl 3B):117–24.
5. Bartlett JG, Finegold SM. Anaerobic infections of the lung and pleural space. Am Rev Respir Dis. 1974;110:56.
6. Finegold SM. Anaerobic Bacteria in Human Disease. New York: Academic Press; 1977.
7. Bartlett JG, Finegold SM. Anaerobic pleuropulmonary infections. Medicine (Baltimore). 1972;51:413.
8. Craig DF. The Etiology, Diagnosis and Treatment of Amebiasis. Baltimore: Williams & Wilkins; 1944.
9. Ochsner A, DeBakey ME. Pleuropulmonary complications of amebiasis: An analysis of 153 collected and 15 personal cases. J Thorac Surg. 1936;5:225.
10. Kirby BD, George WL, Sutter VL, et al. Gram-negative anaerobic bacilli: Their role in infection and patterns of susceptibility to antimicrobial agents. I. Little-known *Bacteroides* species. Rev Infect Dis. 1980;2:914.
11. George WL, Kirby BD, Sutter VL, et al. Gram-negative anaerobic bacilli: Their role in infection and patterns of susceptibility to antimicrobial agents. II. Little-known *Fusobacterium* species and miscellaneous genera. Rev Infect Dis. 1981;3:599.
12. Bartlett JG, Gorbach SL, Finegold SM. The bacteriology of aspiration pneumonia. Am J Med. 1974;56:202.
13. Nichols RL, Smith JW. Intragastric microbial colonization in common disease states of the stomach and duodenum. Ann Surg. 1975;182:557.
14. Poe RH, Marcus HR, Emerson GL. Lung abscess due to *Pseudomonas cepacia*. Am Rev Respir Dis. 1977;115:861.
15. Savdie E, Pigott P, Jennis F. Lung abscess due to *Corynebacterium equi* in a renal transplant recipient. Med J Aust. 1977;1:817.
16. Bartlett JG, Rosenblatt JE, Finegold SM. Percutaneous transtracheal aspiration in the diagnosis of anaerobic pulmonary infection. Ann Intern Med. 1973;79:535.
17. Wimberly NW, Bass JB Jr, Boyd BW, et al. Use of a bronchoscopic protected catheter brush for the diagnosis of pulmonary infections. Chest. 1982;81:556.
18. Broughton WA, Bass JB, Kirkpatrick MB. The technique of protected brush catheter bronchoscopy. J Crit Ill. 1987;2:63–70.
19. Kahn FW, Jones JM. Diagnosing bacterial respiratory infection by bronchoalveolar lavage. J Infect Dis. 1987;155:862–9.
20. Sutter VL, Citron DM, Edelstein MAC, et al. Wadsworth Anaerobic Bacteriology Manual. 4th ed. Belmont, CA: Star Publishing; 1985.
21. Levison ME, Mangura CT, Lorber B, et al. Clindamycin compared with penicillin for the treatment of anaerobic lung abscess. Ann Intern Med. 1983;98:466.
22. Panwalker AP. Failure of penicillin in anaerobic necrotizing pneumonia. Chest. 1982;82:500.

56. CHRONIC PNEUMONIA

WILLIAM E. DISMUKES

For purposes of this chapter, chronic pneumonia syndrome is defined as a pulmonary parenchymal process that may be caused by either an infectious or a noninfectious agent, has been present for weeks to months rather than for days, and is manifested by abnormal chest x-ray findings and by chronic or progressive pulmonary symptoms. The abnormal chest film, which may reveal any one of several radiologic patterns, is probably the most important criterion. In many patients, the diagnosis of chronic pneumonia may be based more on the pulmonary roentgenographic findings than on the pulmonary symptoms. However, asymptomatic patients who have abnormal chest x-ray findings, for example, a solitary nodule, on routine evaluation should not be considered to have chronic pneumonia.

The major emphasis in this chapter will be on the chronic pneumonias caused by infectious agents; however, it is important to keep in mind that there are noninfectious causes of chronic pneumonia, including collagen-vascular diseases, neoplasia, drugs, radiation, bronchiolitis obliterans organizing pneumonia,[1] and the various types of interstitial fibrosis.

ETIOLOGY

The infectious causes of chronic pneumonia can be divided into two main groups: (*1*) infectious agents that typically cause acute pneumonia and uncommonly cause chronic pneumonia and (*2*) infectious agents that typically cause chronic pneumonia. Among the agents that typically cause acute pneumonia, the anaerobes, *Staphylococcus,* the Enterobacteriaceae, and *Pseudomonas aeruginosa* are the organisms most likely to produce a persistent chronic pneumonia infection. This is usually a necrotizing process that most commonly occurs in patients with underlying disease such as alcoholism, diabetes mellitus, or chronic obstructive lung disease or in hospitalized patients.[2,3] Acute pneumonias caused by *Streptococcus pneumoniae, Mycoplasma pneumoniae, Legionella* sp., *Coxiella burnetii,* or most viruses rarely progress to a chronic pulmonary illness.

Table 1 shows the various causes of chronic pneumonia. In the normal host, tuberculosis,[4] other mycobacterial infections,[5] histoplasmosis,[6] coccidioidomycosis (in the appropriate geographic area),[7] mixed aerobic–anaerobic bacterial infection,[8] actinomycosis,[9] blastomycosis,[10] cryptococcosis,[11] and sporotrichosis[12] are the infections deserving prime consideration. Adiaspiromycosis, caused by *Emmonsia,* is a rare occurrence.[13] In the compromised host, chronic pneumonia should raise the possibility of tuberculosis, nocardiosis, cryptococcosis, and in the appropriate geographic areas, coccidioidomycosis and histoplasmosis.[14,15] In persons with acquired immunodeficiency syndrome (AIDS), a special immunocompromised population, these same infections are frequently seen. In addition, in these individuals, chronic pneumonia may be associated with atypical mycobacteria, *Pneumocystis carinii,* and cytomegalovirus plus noninfectious disorders such as Kaposi sarcoma, lymphoma, and nonspecific interstitial pneumonitis.[16–19] The protozoa and worms listed in Table 1 are uncommon causes of chronic pneumonia disease among people living in the United States, but the diseases caused by these organisms are important considerations in patients who live in or have traveled in areas in which these agents are endemic.

No studies have been done to determine the approximate frequency of the various causes of chronic pneumonia in a large series of patients. This lack of perspective on the incidence of the various etiologies of chronic pneumonia is in contrast to our better overall understanding of the *acute* pneumonia syndrome. In addition, since the introduction of antibiotics in the 1940s, the overall spectrum of pneumonia has changed; new pathogens have emerged, organisms that were previously considered harmless commensals now cause disease, and powerful immunosuppressive therapies render some patients more susceptible to certain microorganisms. Consequently, in considering the differential diagnosis in an individual patient, emphasis on specific entities must, in general, be based less on statistical likelihood and more on a thorough and methodic analysis of all available clinical, epidemiologic, and laboratory data.

TABLE 1. Etiology of Chronic Pneumonia Syndrome

Infectious agents that *typically* cause chronic pneumonia
Bacteria and actinomycetes
Mixed aerobic–anaerobic bacteria
Actinomyces sp.
Arachnia propionica
Nocardia sp.
Pseudomonas pseudomallei
Mycobacteria
M. tuberculosis
M. kansasii
M. avium-intracellulare complex
Fungi
Blastomyces dermatitidis
Coccidioides immitis
Cryptococcus neoformans
Emmonsia
Histoplasma capsulatum
Sporothrix schenckii
Paracoccidioides brasiliensis
Protozoa
Entamoeba histolytica
Worms
Echinococcus granulosus
Schistosomes—*S. hematobium, S. japonicum, S. mansoni*
Paragonimus westermani
Noninfectious causes
Neoplasia
Carcinoma (primary or metastatic)
Lymphoma
Lymphomatoid granulomatosis
Sarcoidosis
Vasculitis
Systemic lupus erythematosus
Polyarteritis nodosa
Allergic angiitis and granulomatosis (Churg-Strauss syndrome)
Progressive systemic sclerosis
Rheumatoid arthritis
Mixed connective tissue syndrome
Wegener's granulomatosis
Chemicals, drugs, or inhalation
Radiation
Recurrent pulmonary infarction
Pulmonary infiltration with eosinophilia (PIE) syndrome
Löffler syndrome—usually transient
Tropical eosinophilia
Pneumonia plus asthma, e.g., allergic bronchopulmonary aspergillosis
Vasculitis
Eosinophilic pneumonia—chronic
Pneumoconiosis
Chronic form of extrinsic allergic alveolitis or hypersensitivity pneumonitis
Other lung disease—unknown cause
Bronchiolitis obliterans organizing pneumonia
Interstitial pneumonia (fibrosing alveolitis, idiopathic pulmonary fibrosis)
Usual interstitial pneumonia (UIP)
Desquamative interstitial pneumonia (DIP)
Lymphoid interstitial pneumonia (LIP)
Giant cell interstitial pneumonia (GIP)
Eosinophilic granuloma
Lymphangioleiomyomatosis
Goodpasture syndrome
Pulmonary alveolar proteinosis (phospholipidosis)
Pulmonary alveolar microlithiasis
Idiopathic pulmonary hemosiderosis

EPIDEMIOLOGY

Age, Sex, Race

Although pulmonary tuberculosis over the past several decades has changed from a disease of the young to a disease of the middle-aged and elderly,[20] the significance of the age and sex of a particular patient usually relates more in an indirect manner to other epidemiologic factors. For example, an elderly patient is at higher risk of having a cerebrovascular accident, which in turn might predispose to an aspiration episode and subsequent pneumonia and abscess. Likewise, older, debilitated patients are at higher risk of developing chronic gram-negative necrotizing pneumonia. In a similar manner, the sex of a given patient is more likely to determine occupation or avocation and, ultimately, the likelihood of exposure to certain infectious agents or other etiologic vehicles. The race of the patient may be a more important factor. For example, pulmonary tuberculosis should be the presumptive diagnosis in a black patient with bilateral upper lobe cavitary disease[21]; coccidioidomycosis is more likely to be severe in dark-skinned persons, including blacks and Filipinos, who have lived or have traveled in the southwestern United States, the endemic area for the disease,[7] and chronic cavitary histoplasmosis is less likely to occur in the black population.[6]

Occupation and Avocation

Certain occupations or hobbies should arouse the suspicion of certain diseases. Despite the presence of *Cryptococcus neoformans* in pigeon droppings, the vast majority of patients with pulmonary cryptococcosis have no unusual exposure to pigeons. Occupational exposure to plant materials predisposes to cutaneous and, according to some authorities, pulmonary sporotrichosis.[22] Examples of occupationally or avocationally related conditions include coccidioidomycosis among rock collectors, archeologists conducting excavations, construction workers, or others exposed to desert dust in the endemic area[23,24]; histoplasmosis among persons who are exposed to starling roosts,[25] who clean out old chicken houses with dirt floors,[26] who cut and clear fallen oak trees,[27] or who explore caves inhabited by bats[28]; echinococcosis in those who tend sheep[29]; the pneumoconioses, for example, silicosis and asbestosis, among sandblasters and shipyard workers[30]; and chronic as well as acute pulmonary disease resulting from repeated occupational exposure to agents of allergic alveolitis or to irritant gases such as phosgene, ammonia, ozone, and nitrogen dioxide.[31]

Travel

Since the initial exposure to the agents of many chronic and indolent infectious diseases may have occurred months or years before disease, it is necessary to inquire whether a patient has lived in or has traveled to another part of the United States or the world at any time. For example, a patient with bilateral upper lobe infiltrates with or without cavitation who has never traveled or lived in Central America, Mexico, South America, or west of the Mississippi River is unlikely to have coccidioidomycosis. The exceptions include the occasional worker handling dusty material from the endemic area such as cotton bales. On the other hand, if the patient has lived in the Central, Southeast or mid-Atlantic area of the United States, chronic pulmonary histoplasmosis should be considered since histoplasmosis is endemic in these locations. Paracoccidioidomycosis is acquired only during residence in Mexico and in South or Central America. In addition to identifying a state or country visited, there may be a need for detailed questioning about rural or urban exposure, type of lodging, source of drinking water, exposure to native foods, and so forth. For example, any person who has lived or traveled extensively in Southeast Asia, particularly in low-lying or rice-growing areas, and who subsequently develops chronic pneumonia with pulmonary roentgenographic abnormalities resembling tuberculosis or the respiratory mycoses should be suspected of having melioidosis.[32] Similarly, a businessperson who makes frequent trips to Japan and the Philippines, who admits to eating raw or partly cooked crayfish, and who has chronic pulmonary symptoms plus dense, nodular lung opacities and ring shadows should be suspected of having pulmonary paragonimiasis.[33]

Contacts, Habits, and Drugs

In patients in whom tuberculosis is suspected, contacts among friends or relatives with tuberculosis should be sought. Inquiry should be made into the patient's smoking and drinking history as well as other personal habits. The likelihood of cancer of the lung in a patient with coal worker's pneumoconiosis is greater in a smoker than in a nonsmoker. Aspiration pneumonia, chronic gram-negative bacillary pneumonia, and tuberculosis are more likely to occur in an alcoholic than in a nondrinker. Intravenous drug users who inject heroin or similar agents are not only at risk of developing infection with human immunodeficiency virus (HIV) and subsequently AIDS but also acute pulmonary edema,[34] septic pulmonary emboli followed by necrotizing pneumonia and single or multiple abscesses, or an interstitial granulomatous reaction with pulmonary hypertension.[35] Similarly, frequent use of free-base cocaine has been reported to cause bronchiolitis obliterans organizing pneumonia.[36]

Certain drugs may cause acute and chronic pulmonary symptoms as well as radiographic abnormalities.[37] Early in the course of drug-induced pulmonary disease, the chest roentgenogram findings may be normal; later, an interstitial, nodular, and/or alveolar pattern may be present. Still later, the chest x-ray film may reveal only a fibrotic pulmonary process. The drugs that are more likely to cause chronic pulmonary disease include cytotoxic agents such as bleomycin, busulfan, chlorambucil, methotrexate, and mitomycin and noncytotoxic agents such as amiodarone, gold salts, nitrofurantoin, and penicillamine. Since drug-induced pulmonary disease may develop after drug therapy has been discontinued, the physician should inquire not only about all drugs the patient is presently taking but also about those taken in the recent past.

Similarly, important questions arise in regard to any previous or current antimicrobial therapy. Did the antimicrobial result in roentgenographic or clinical improvement? If not, was the antimicrobial used in sufficient quantity to cure the suspected process or alter its course? Was the appropriate agent used? What effect does the antimicrobial have on the results of cultures? Is the report of "normal flora" on the sputum culture the result of antimicrobial therapy eliminating a specific pathogen?

Underlying Disease

Pulmonary complications including both acute and chronic or refractory pneumonia are especially common in persons with AIDS (see Chapter 108). Patients with diabetes mellitus or preexisting chronic obstructive pulmonary disease are at high risk for developing chronic or persistent bacterial pneumonia. Similarly, chronic obstructive lung disease commonly precedes fibrocavitary histoplasmosis or *M. intracellulare* infection. Recurrent or persistent pneumonia in the same area of the lung raises the suspicion of a local endobronchial lesion that may not be apparent on routine chest x-ray films. Since aspiration may predispose to chronic pneumonia, inquiry should be made into any history of recent dental problems or manipulation, sinusitis with chronic postnasal drip, disorders of swallowing resulting from neurologic or esophageal disease, seizure disorders, recent anesthesia, quantity and effect of alcohol, or any illness leading to an unconscious state. Finally, is the chronic pneumonia community or hospital acquired?

CLINICAL FEATURES

Symptoms

Since there are multiple causes of chronic pneumonia, no single symptom complex is common to all causes. Often, constitutional symptoms including fever, chills, and malaise are present initially. A history of progressive anorexia and weight loss usually indicates chronic illness. Pulmonary symptoms may be present early but frequently appear later in the course of the illness. Any patient with a prolonged illness and nonspecific constitutional complaints plus pulmonary symptoms including a new or persistent cough, sputum production, hemoptysis, chest pain (especially pleuritic pain), or dyspnea deserves medical evaluation, including a chest x-ray.

Inquiries should be made to determine whether there is involvement of extrapulmonary organs. For example, skin lesions might suggest coccidioidomycosis, cryptococcosis, blastomycosis, nocardiosis, or Kaposi sarcoma, whereas mucous membrane lesions would suggest histoplasmosis, paracoccidioidomycosis, or Kaposi sarcoma. Mono- or polyarticular arthritis, polyarthralgias, or localized bone tenderness or pain might indicate a collagen-vascular disease. A history of persistent headache together with the documentation of an abnormal cerebrospinal fluid should raise the suspicion of tuberculosis, cryptococcosis, or coccidioidomycosis involving both the lungs and central nervous system. The presence of focal neurologic symptoms and signs argues strongly for a space-occupying lesion in the central nervous system; such findings in a patient with a cavitary infiltrate seen on a chest film suggest the possibility of a brain abscess associated with chronic suppurative lung disease or pulmonary nocardiosis.

Signs

Although the findings on physical examination of the chest are usually not helpful in differentiating specific causes of chronic pneumonia, the presence of generalized wheezing or other signs of bronchospasm, in the absence of underlying lung disease, indicates an asthmatic component to the pulmonary illness and raises the possibility of a disorder causing both pneumonia and asthma such as extrinsic allergic alveolitis, allergic bronchopulmonary aspergillosis, or allergic granulomatosis and angiitis (Churg-Strauss syndrome). Similarly, localized wheezes suggest the presence of an endobronchial obstructing lesion. The findings of tachycardia, cardiomegaly, gallop rhythm, and ankle edema provide evidence of cardiac disease and suggest that the pulmonary symptoms and signs are at least in part due to cardiovascular causes. The presence of skin lesions, clubbing, cyanosis, or phlebitis are not specific for any single pulmonary disorder but may help to narrow the differential diagnosis, especially when considered along with other clinical and epidemiologic information. Similarly, the findings of jaundice, adenopathy, hepatomegaly, splenomegaly, or ascites suggest that a systemic disorder involving multiple organs is the cause.

DIAGNOSTIC PROCEDURES

Initial Laboratory Studies

Routine laboratory studies may provide some important clues to diagnosis. Pancytopenia may suggest miliary tuberculosis, disseminated histoplasmosis, or metastatic tumor in the bone marrow. Anemia alone is consistent with too many disorders to suggest a cause. A normal white blood cell count does not exclude infection. In particular, mycotic chronic pneumonia is usually associated with a normal or minimally elevated white blood cell count. Leukopenia and/or lymphopenia should raise the suspicion of infection with HIV. In addition, leukopenia should suggest sarcoidosis, systemic lupus erythematosus, tuberculosis, histoplasmosis, or tumor. A leukemoid reaction may be seen in disseminated mycobacteriosis. Leukocytosis is suggestive of but not specific for a bacterial cause.

Laboratory tests that measure the function of other organs may provide more helpful information. Liver function studies including bilirubin, alkaline phosphatase, and serum aspartate aminotransferase determinations and prothrombin time should be obtained in all patients. Urinalysis, with particular attention to the urinary sediment, plus tests of renal function including measure of the blood urea nitrogen and creatinine should also be done. Abnormalities of either liver function, especially elevated enzyme levels, kidney function, or both, should raise the suspicion of disorders that are not limited to the lung but are known to involve multiple organs including lung, liver, and kidney. Such disorders include disseminated histoplasmosis and disseminated mycobacteriosis as well as the collagen-vascular diseases, sarcoidosis, and certain neoplastic diseases, especially the lymphoproliferative types.

An elevated serum globulin level is usually nonspecific and indicates chronic inflammation, although it may indicate an underlying myeloma or another gammopathy predisposing to chronic or recurrent infection. If myeloma is suspected, immunoelectrophoresis of urine and serum is indicated. Similarly, in a patient with an abnormally low serum globulin level, a quantitative serum immunoglobulin determination should be obtained to evaluate the patient for hypogammaglobulinemia.

Studies to Establish an Etiology

A basic core of studies should usually be performed on all patients with chronic pneumonia, regardless of suspected etiology, but there should be flexibility in choosing additional tests or procedures to confirm a specific diagnosis. The orderly sequence of diagnostic studies that is given below necessarily results in oversimplification and consequently overlooks the unique aspects of a given patient's illness.

Chest X-ray Studies. The chest roentgenogram, including a posteroanterior and a lateral film, is probably the single most important diagnostic study. Because of the singular importance of the chest x-ray, Table 2 is provided to emphasize the major radiologic patterns that may be seen. In Table 2 the disorders have been grouped according to the type of radiologic abnormality that is characteristic of the disease. Because there are some disorders in which there is a spectrum of radiologic manifestations, these disorders appear more than once in the table. In selected patients, a computed tomographic examination of the chest may provide additional useful information, especially about the presence and extent of mediastinal, hilar, and pleural disease. For example, documentation of *anterior* mediastinal involvement argues strongly in favor of neoplasia including lymphoma and metastatic carcinoma as the etiology of chronic pneumonia syndrome and argues against an infectious cause.

Tuberculosis and nontuberculous mycobacterial diseases, histoplasmosis, coccidioidomycosis, sporotrichosis, melioidosis, paragonimiasis, and the pneumoconioses, especially silicosis, characteristically produce fibrocavitary disease—a contracted area of lung with linear fibrosis, nodular or rounded densities, and cavitation. In addition, mycobacterial diseases, histoplasmosis, and silicosis characteristically involve the upper lobes. A thin-walled cavity is suggestive of coccidioidomycosis, sporotrichosis, and paragonimiasis, whereas a thick-walled cavity surrounded by an area of pneumonitis is more typical of tuberculosis, nontuberculous mycobacterial diseases, histoplasmosis, melioidosis, nocardiosis, actinomycosis, and pyogenic lung abscess. Cavitation is less common in blastomycosis and cryptococcosis. Ecchinococcal lung lesions occasionally show a crescent of air between the pericyst and endocyst or a collapsed membrane floating on cyst fluid (water

TABLE 2. Radiologic Patterns of Diseases That Commonly Cause Chronic Pneumonia Syndrome

Disease	*Radiologic Characteristics*
Diseases that cause patchy infiltrates and/or bronchopneumonia or lobar consolidation	
Infectious	
Aspiration pneumonia secondary to mixed aerobic and anaerobic infection	Usually dependent portions: superior or basilar segments of lower lobes or posterior segments of upper lobes Pleural involvement with empyema common
Necrotizing pneumonia secondary to Enterobacteriaceae, *P. aeruginosa*, or *S. aureus*	Any lobe or segment Chronic *Klebsiella* pneumonia commonly involves upper lobes May be multiple sites of pulmonary infection secondary to septic embolization
Actinomycosis	Commonly involves lower lobes Cavitation frequently present Pleural involvement with empyema common
Nocardiosis	No distinctive pattern May involve single or multiple lobes Cavitation may be present Pleural involvement may occur
Tuberulous exudative pneumonia	Not restricted to upper lobes Often bilateral with perihilar distribution
Blastomycosis	Often a dense area of lobar or segmental consoliation Cavitation infrequent
Cryptococcosis	Single or multiple patchy infiltrates; less commonly, lobar consolidation Occasionally, single or diffuse nodular lesions
Paracoccidioidomycosis	Asymptomatic bilateral fluffy infiltrates May be extremely indolent
Noninfectious	
Chronic eosinophilic pneumonia	Rapidly progressive, dense infiltrates Usually peripheral (reverse pattern of pulmonary edema)
Bronchiolitis obliterans organizing pneumonia	Focal, patchy ground glass densities
Diseases that cause pulmonary cavitation	
Infectious	
Pyogenic lung abscess	
Complicating aspiration pneumonia	Usually single cavity Location—same as aspiration pneumonia Air–fluid level common
Complicating necrotizing pneumonia	May involve any lobe Often multiple and bilateral, depending on route of acquisition of pneumonia
Tuberculosis—reactivation or adult type	Usually upper lobes Often bilateral May be multiple Fibrosis and calcification common
Atypical mycobacterial disease	Radiologically indistringuishable from tuberculosis, except that cavitation may be more frequent
Melioidosis	Simulates tuberculosis, but may involve any lobe
Histoplasmosis, chronic cavitary	Mimics tuberculosis Upper lobes frequently involved but can involve any lobe Unilateral or bilateral
Coccidioidomycosis	Usually single thin-walled cavity with minimum involvement of surrounding lung Occasionally thick-walled cavity surrounded by extensive parenchymal disease
Sporotrichosis	May mimic tuberculosis but can involve any lobe Cavitation is frequent; thin-walled cavity more likely than thick-walled cavity
Aspergillosis	Single or multiple areas of pneumonia with or without central cavitation Not to be confused with intracavitary fungus ball
Paragonimiasis	Cystlike lesions as well as cavities, usually associated with linear or patchy infiltrates, fibrosis, and/or calcification
Echinococcosis	Single or multiple discrete, sharply defined round lesions (cysts) with little surrounding inflammatory response Cavitation and/or calcification may occur
Noninfectious	
Wegener's granulomatosis and lymphomatoid granulomatosis	Often multiple nodules with cavitation May be unilateral or bilateral
Silicosis	Associated with conglomerate nodular densities, frequently in upper lobes Usually superimposed on background of diffuse nodulation Rarely, eggshell calcification of hilar nodes
Bronchogenic carcinoma	Eccentric cavitation more common in squamous cell type
Lymphoma, especially Hodgkin's disease	Cavitation typically occurs in peripheral parenchymal nodules
Infectious and noninfectious diseases that cause chronic diffuse pulmonary infiltration and fibrosis	
Alveolar cell carcinoma Intrapulmonary bleeding, e.g., Goodpasture syndrome Pulmonary alveolar proteinosis	Alveolar pattern
Sarcoidosis Early asbestosis or berylliosis Bronchiolitis obliterans organizing pneumonia	Ground-glass interstitial pattern

(*Continued*)

TABLE 2. *(Continued)*

Disease	*Radiologic Characteristics*
Granulomatous infectious diseases, e.g., miliary tuberculosis and disseminated histoplasmosis Sarcoidosis Bronchiolitis obliterans organizing pneumonia Lymphangitic carcinomatosis Wegener's granulomatosis Lymphomatoid granulomatosis Allergic angiitis and granulomatosis Rheumatoid lung disease Pneumoconioses including asbestosis, silicosis, and berylliosis	Nodular interstitial pattern, including miliary spherical nodules
Chronic form of hypersensitivity pneumonitis Idiopathic pulmonary hemosiderosis Radiation injury—chronic Progressive systemic sclerosis Sarcoidosis	Linear interstitial pattern including fine reticular markings and dense fibrosis
Advanced form of fibrosing alveolitis Bronchiectasis Eosinophilic granuloma Sarcoidosis	Honeycombing (coarse reticular pattern with cystic air spaces)

lily sign).[38] Calcification is typical of tuberculosis, histoplasmosis, and coccidioidomycosis but is rare in actinomycosis, nocardiosis, blastomycosis, and cryptococcosis. Abscess of the chest wall or osteomyelitis of a rib adjacent to the pneumonia and/or pleural effusion may be seen in actinomycosis and nocardiosis. Representative x-ray films are shown in Figures 1–15.

Studies in Patients with X-ray Evidence of Localized Infiltrates and/or Cavitation. In all patients with x-ray evidence of localized infiltrates and/or cavitation, examination of the sputum is essential. The specimen of sputum must be a representative sample. If the expectorated sputum is a deep, coughed specimen, of adequate volume, and acceptable after cytologic screening,[39] other procedures to obtain sputum may not be necessary. *Microscopic* examination of sputum should include the following:

1. Gram stains for bacteria and actinomyces
2. Acid-fast or fluorochrome stains for *Mycobacteria* and modified acid-fast stain for *Nocardia*
3. Wet mounts for fungi and eggs of *Paragonimus*
4. Gomori methenamine silver (GMS) stain or periodic acid–Schiff (PAS) stain for fungi.
5. Cytologic preparations for neoplastic cells, eosinophils, fungi

Generous volumes of expectorated sputum (but not 24-hour collections) should also be obtained and sent to the microbiology laboratory for *culture* for bacteria, fungi, and mycobacteria. In addition, it is often diagnostically rewarding if the clinician speaks directly with the personnel in the microbiology laboratory to alert them to specific etiologic considerations. Then the specimens will be inoculated on the most appropriate media, and the microbiologists will be more aware of the suspected pathogens.

In all patients in whom an infectious cause is considered, cultures from sources other than sputum should be obtained. These sources might include the following:

1. Blood
2. Urine
3. Pleural fluid in all patients with pleural effusion. Pleural tissue should also be obtained for culture
4. Cerebrospinal fluid in all patients with central nervous system symptoms or signs
5. Synovial fluid in all patients with joint effusion
6. Skin, mucous membrane, or any tissue obtained at biopsy

To obtain sputum, if adequate sputum cannot be readily produced via spontaneous expectoration by the patient, consider the following:

1. Inducing sputum by the use of hypertonic aerosols or ultrasound, hydration, chest physiotherapy, or postural drainage
2. Bronchoscopy for bronchial washings, transbronchial biopsy, bronchoalveolar lavage, or protected catheter sampling of lower respiratory tract secretions while minimizing upper airway contamination of the sample[40]

Skin tests should be made in all cases in which an infectious cause is considered. The tuberculin skin test is the single most important test. If a patient has never had a tuberculin skin test

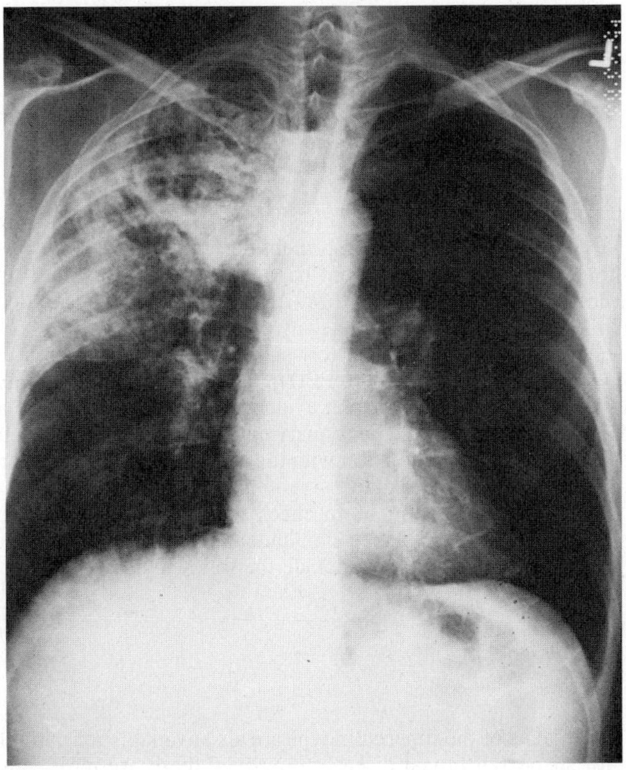

FIG. 1. Mixed aerobic–anaerobic chronic bacterial pneumonia in a 46-year-old alcoholic man with a 3-week history of malaise, nausea, fever, chills, and cough productive of copious amounts of foul-smelling sputum. Note the multiple small cavities throughout the right upper lobe. Long-term penicillin therapy was curative.

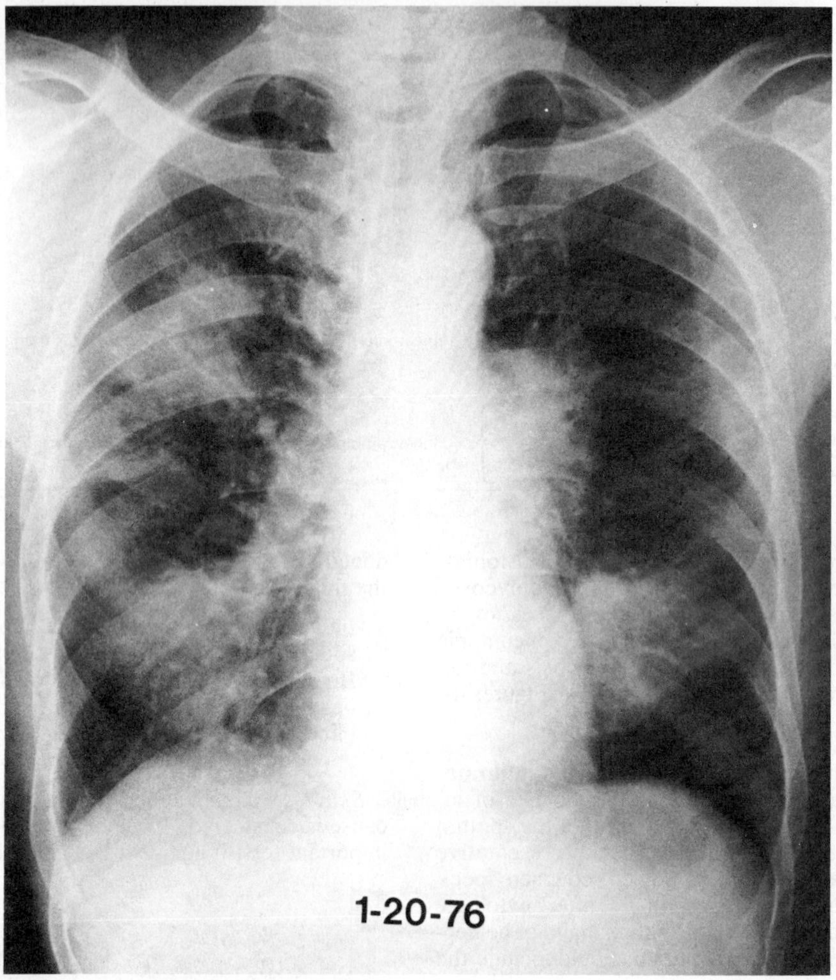

FIG. 2. Pulmonary actinomycosis in a 49-year-old with a 3-month history of chronic productive cough, anorexia, and weight loss. The x-ray film was taken during the initial clinic evaluation. Note the bilateral bronchopneumonia, more marked in the lower lobes. There was no cavitation.

or has had a previously negative response, a 5 tuberculin unit (TU) (intermediate) purified protein derivative (PPD) skin test should be used. If the patient has a history of a positive tuberculin skin response, a TU (first-strength) PPD may be applied. If the intermediate PPD is negative after 48 hours, a 250 TU (second-strength) PPD skin test should then be performed. A nonreactive second-strength PPD in a patient who is shown not to be anergic provides strong evidence against tuberculosis as the cause of the chronic pulmonary disease.[41] Skin test antigens for the detection of infection with the atypical mycobacteria are not commercially available.

Other skin test antigens to check for intact delayed hypersensitivity should be placed simultaneously with a PPD antigen. These "control" antigens include the following:

1. Mumps antigen
2. *Trichophyton* antigen
3. *Candida* antigen

Skin tests of the tuberculin type are also available for patients with suspected fungal disease; however, these are most valuable when used for epidemiologic studies to determine the prevalence of infection in a given population or in a certain geographic area. Like the tuberculin test, fungal skin tests do not distinguish between current and previous infection. Unlike the tuberculin test, a negative result is common with active disease. Hence, fungal skin tests are of little diagnostic value in the individual patient. Of the tests available, the coccidioidin antigen is the best, although a negative response does not exclude coccidioidomycosis. The blastomycin and histoplasmin antigens should not be used for diagnostic purposes in individual patients because of the high incidence of cross-reactions and false-negative results. In addition, histoplasmin may cause a false elevation of serum antibody to the mycelial antigen of *Histoplasma capsulatum*.

Serologic tests for antibodies and antigens are often used when infectious causes, especially fungi, are considered. However, there are problems that include long delays in obtaining results, false-positive results because of cross-reactions to other antigens, and false-negative results. Serologic tests are most helpful in patients when pulmonary mycoses including coccidioidomycosis, cryptococcosis, histoplasmosis, and paracoccidioidomycosis are suspected. Similarly, in patients in whom hypersensitivity pneumonitis is suspected, serum should be examined for precipitating antibodies to various inhalant antigens.

Invasive Procedures. Certain clinical situations dictate that a more aggressive diagnostic approach be used. In patients who are unable to raise sputum spontaneously and in whom attempts to induce sputum production are unsuccessful, invasive procedures may become necessary. Bronchoscopy with a flexible fiber-optic bronchoscope usually is the initial procedure and is diagnostically helpful when accompanied by bronchial washings and transbronchial biopsy with appropriate microbiologic

FIG. 3. X-ray film taken 12 days after that in Figure 2. Note the large loculated pleural effusion on the right.

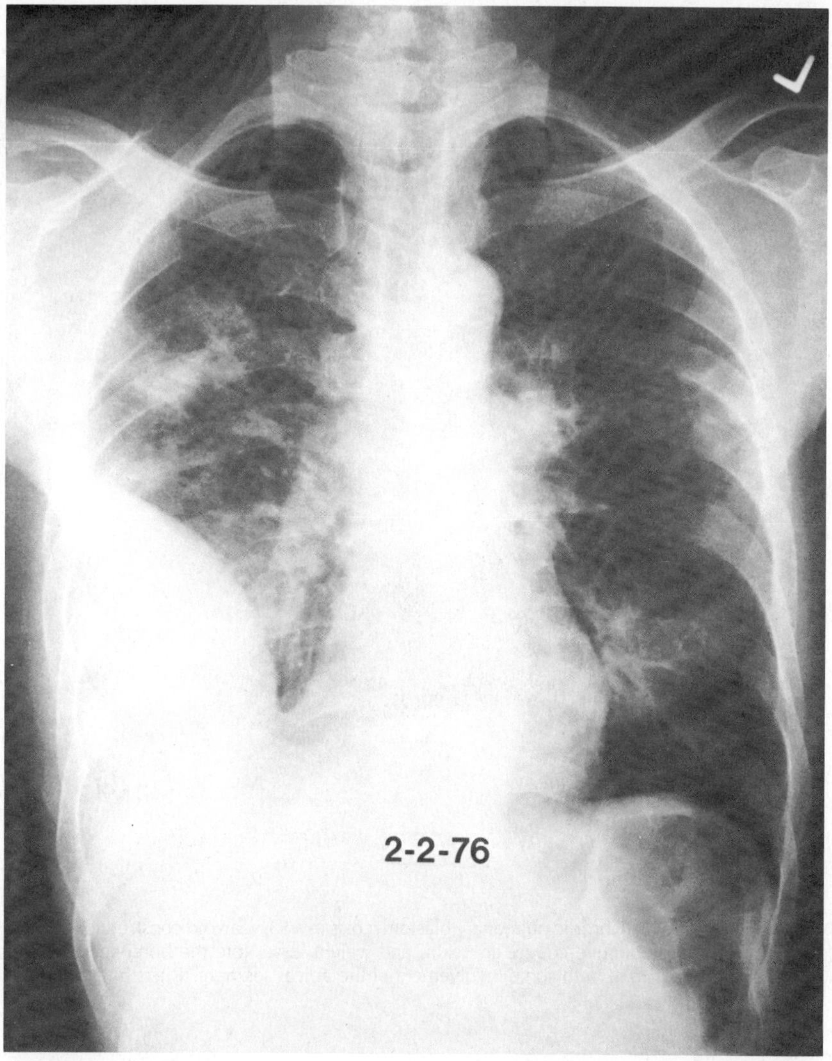

FIG. 4. Pulmonary nocardiosis in a 38-year-old after a renal transplant who was taking corticosteroids and had symptoms of malaise, fever, and a productive cough. Note the extensive consolidation of the right upper lobe with central cavitation.

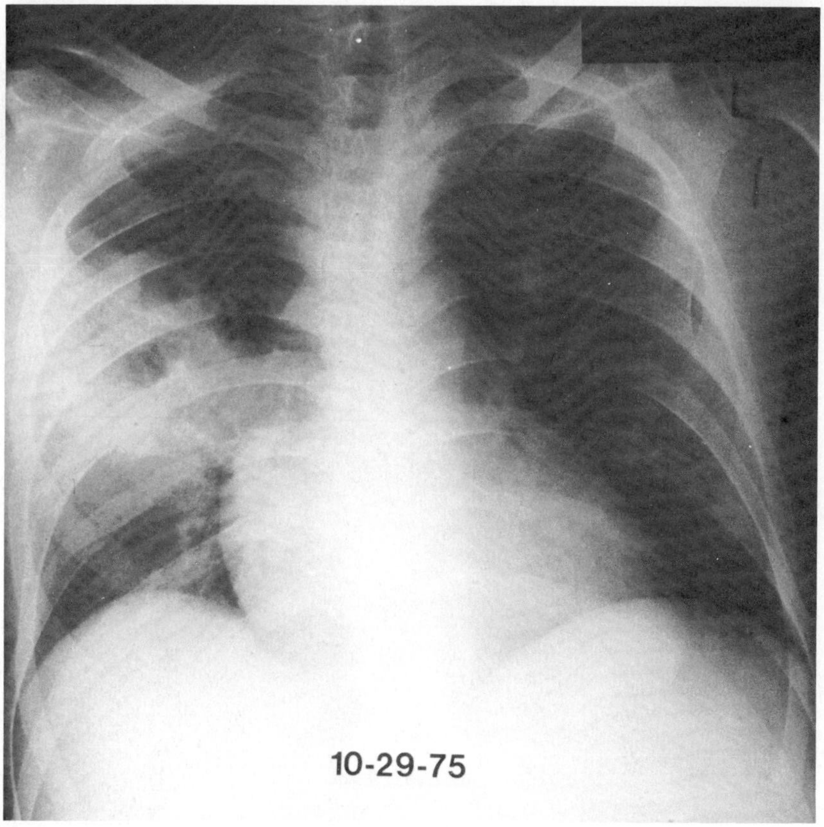

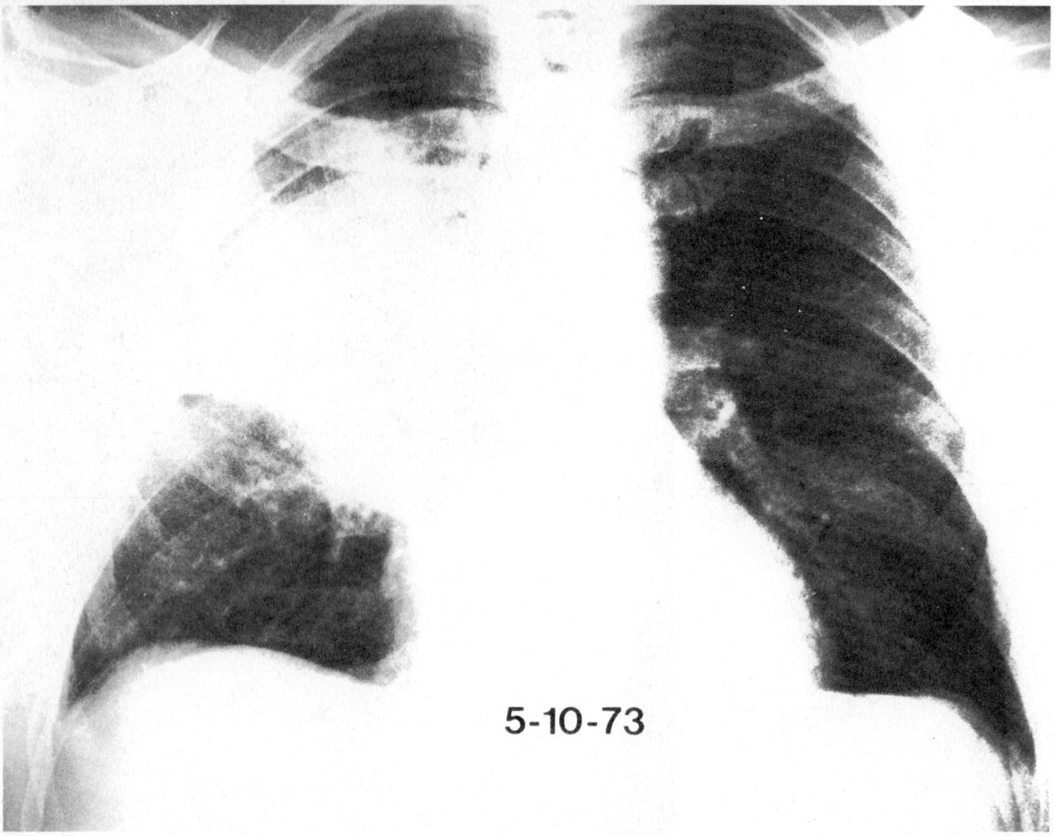

FIG. 5. Chronic pulmonary blastomycosis in a 53-year-old construction worker with a 4-week illness of fever, chills, myalgias, nonproductive cough, anorexia, and weight loss. Note the homogeneous consolidation of the anterior segment of the right upper lobe with some involvement of the apical segment. Right hilar adenopathy is also present.

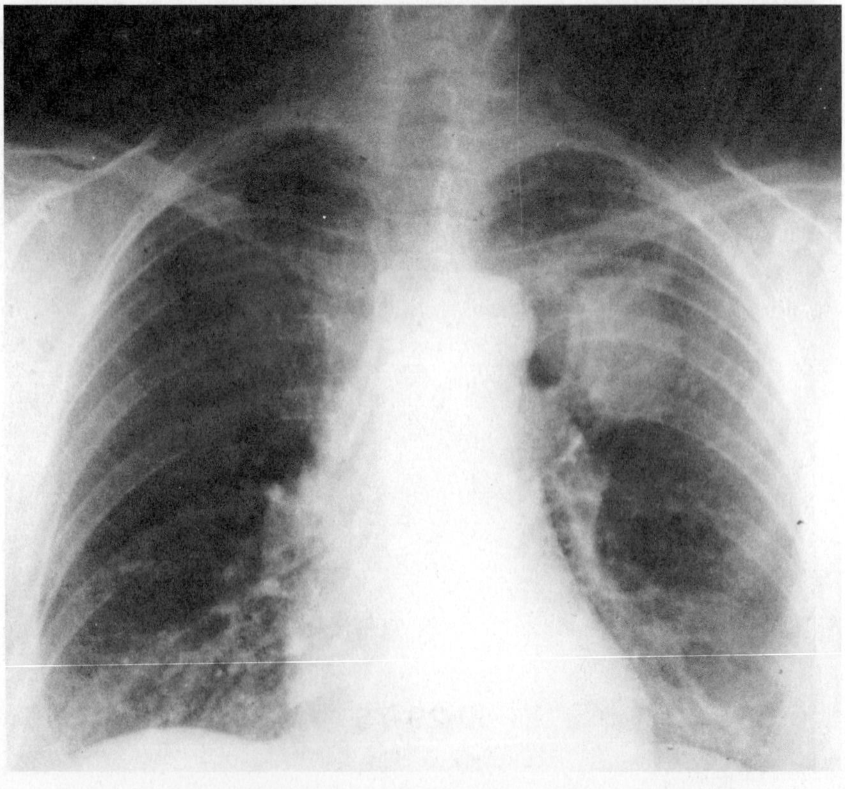

FIG. 6. Pulmonary cryptococcosis in a 54-year-old woman with a 2-month history of headache and chronic cough. Note the large, sharply circumscribed mass in the left upper lobe. She also had culture-proven cryptococcal meningitis.

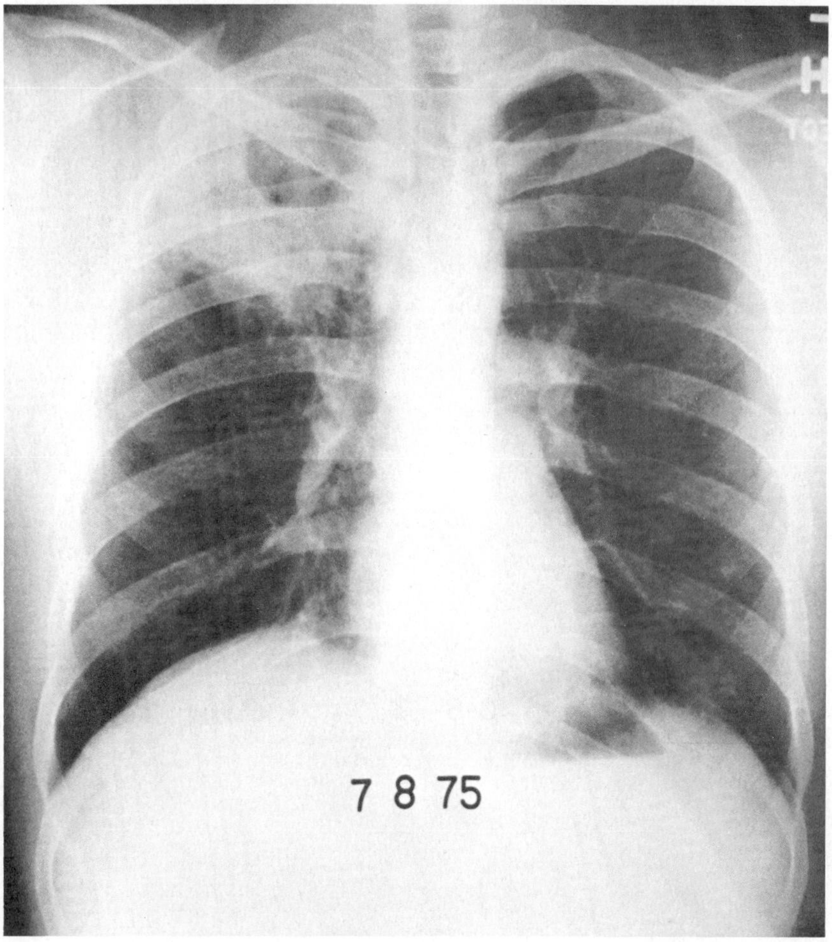

FIG. 7. Cavitary tuberculosis in a 30-year-old man with symptoms of cough, sputum production, and weight loss for 10 months. Note the thick-walled cavity in the right upper lobe with surrounding parenchymal infiltrate. The patient was originally diagnosed as having a nonspecific lung abscess.

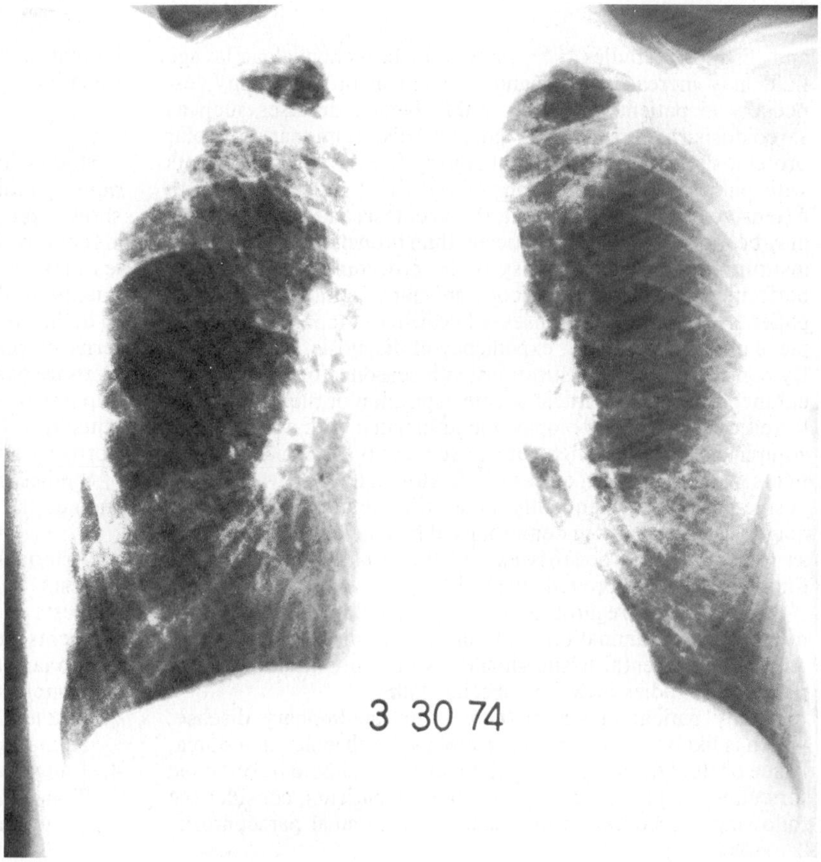

FIG. 8. Atypical tuberculosis caused by *M. avium-intracellulare* in a 68-year-old with chronic obstructive pulmonary disease. At time of this x-ray film, the patient had been symptomatic for 1 year with malaise, anorexia, weight loss, and progressive dyspnea. Note the fibrocavitary appearance of the right upper lung.

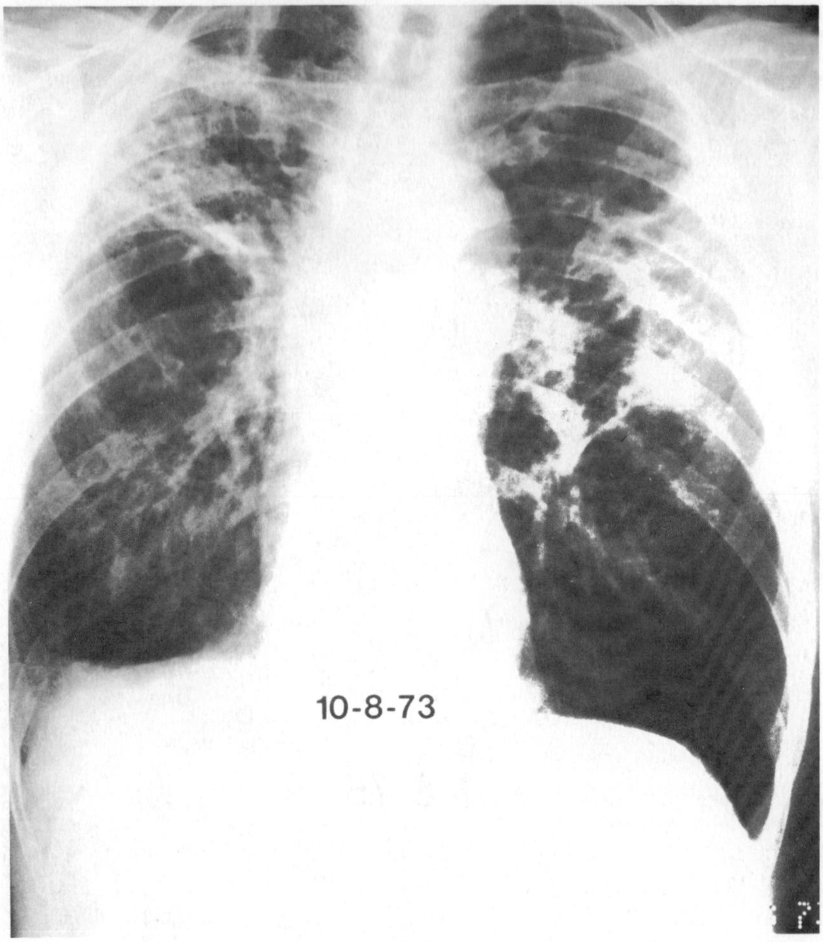

FIG. 9. Chronic cavitary pulmonary histoplasmosis in a 67-year-old with chronic obstructive pulmonary disease and a 4-month history of night sweats, low-grade fever, chronic cough, and weight loss. Note the bilateral fibrocavitary disease primarily involving the upper lobes.

and histologic studies.[42,43] Analysis of bronchoaveloar lavage fluid may increase the diagnostic yield of bronchoscopy, especially in patients with interstitial/alveolar diseases such as sarcoidosis, hypersensitivity pneumonitis, pulmonary alveolar proteinosis, and idiopathic pulmonary fibrosis and in patients with pulmonary complications of AIDS.[44,45] In a patient with extensive pleural involvement, thoracentesis and pleural biopsy may be more helpful diagnostically than bronchoscopy. In some institutions, open lung biopsy is the procedure of choice and performed before bronchoscopy in many immunosuppressed patients with pulmonary disease because of the relatively large piece of tissue obtained, expediency of diagnosis, and safety.[46] By contrast, in other institutions with seasoned operators, percutaneous or transthoracic needle aspiration of the lung is preferred over open lung biopsy and associated with a low risk of complications and a high rate of sensitivity, especially in patients with neoplastic disease.[47,48] Although these various invasive procedures frequently are used to obtain lung tissue for diagnosis, especially in compromised hosts, controversy exists as to whether the benefits exceed the risks and whether the findings lead to improved survival.[49]

All specimens, regardless of source, should be submitted for microscopic examination and culture, as already described. Any lung or pleural tissue should also be submitted for histopathologic studies including special stains.

In any patient in whom there is extrapulmonary disease, which is likely due to the same cause as the chronic pneumonia, tissue or fluid from the extrapulmonary sites should be obtained for culture and histologic studies. In such patients, consider the following procedures: arthrocentesis, abdominal paracentesis, lumbar puncture, bone marrow biopsy, liver biopsy, lymph node biopsy, and skin and muscle biopsy.

Studies in Patients with X-ray Film Evidence of Diffuse Pulmonary Infiltration and Fibrosis. In patients whose x-ray films show a predominately diffuse infiltrative pattern, either of the alveolar or interstitial type (Table 2), pulmonary function studies may be of greater importance. These studies will not only quantitate the degree of pulmonary insufficiency but may help to delineate the disease processes by virtue of the different patterns of pulmonary function impairment. Accordingly, these tests are particularly useful in characterizing those diseases that impair gas transfer and predispose to ventilation—perfusion inequalities, for example, sarcoidosis, interstitial pneumonia, or fibrosing alveolitis.

Studies that may be especially useful in this group of patients include the following:

1. Arterial blood gas studies, including resting and postexercise tests
2. Tests of pulmonary function including spirometric measurements, measurements of lung volume, measurement of pulmonary diffusing capacity and measurement of pulmonary compliance
3. Studies on sputum as previously outlined. Cytologic examination is especially important
4. Lung biopsy to make an accurate morphologic diagnosis. Transbronchial biopsy via the fiberoptic bronchoscope or open lung biopsy are the procedures of choice

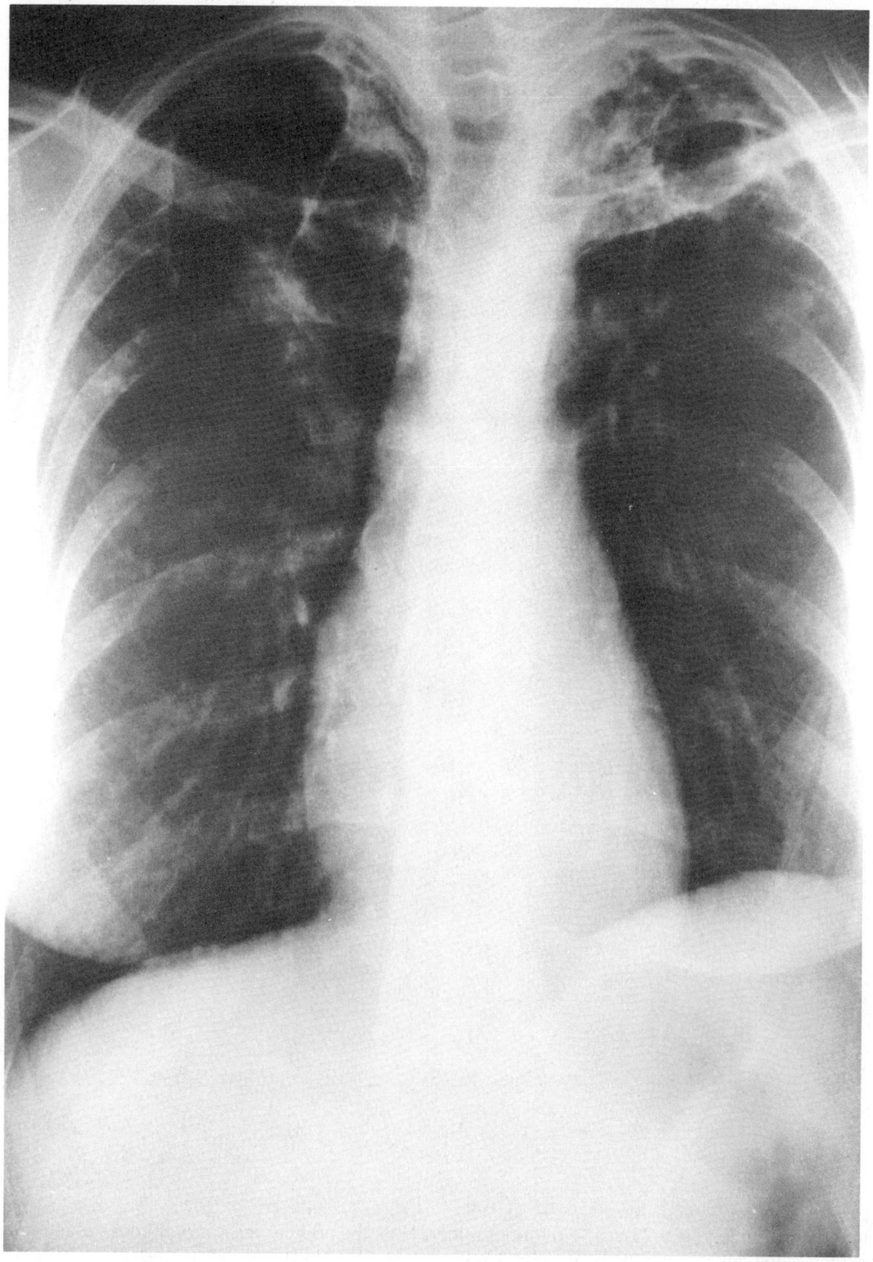

FIG. 10. Cavitary coccidioidomycosis in a 44-year-old woman who had previously lived in El Paso, Texas. She had been previously treated for tuberculosis that was never culture proven. At the time of this x-ray film she complained of hemoptysis. Note the bilateral upper lobe infiltrates with contracted lobes plus large thin-walled cavities as well as smaller thick-walled cavities.

THERAPY

Antimicrobial Agents

If a specific infectious agent is readily identified as the cause of the chronic pneumonia, the appropriate antimicrobial agent(s) should be administered. In many patients, no etiologic agent will be identified on the basis of the initial stains and cultures, and a definitive diagnosis must await the completion of serologic, histologic, and bacteriologic studies as well as other diagnostic tests. In such situations, if immediate empirical therapy is advisable, the choice of antimicrobial agents must be based on the available epidemiologic, clinical, and microbiologic data.

For example, if an otherwise healthy young patient has been ill for a relatively short period (2–3 weeks), the chest x-ray film shows a lobar or patchy pneumonia, especially in the lower lobes, Gram stain of the sputum reveals few-to-moderate polymorphonuclear leukocytes and organisms resembling normal flora, and the patient acquired the infection outside the hospital, the patient may have persistent or chronic pneumonia as a complication of one or more common acute pneumonia syndromes, namely, pneumococcal pneumonia, aspiration pneumonia, *Mycoplasma*-caused pneumonia, or legionnaires' disease. Reasonable empirical therapy in such a patient is erythromycin since this drug, in general, provides effective treatment of these four pneumonias. If, on the other hand, a patient has chronic pneumonia after thoracotomy, initial antimicrobial therapy should provide broad-spectrum coverage against normal mouth flora including anaerobes, *Staphylococcus aureus,* and aerobic gram-negative bacteria. In both of the above cases, once the path-

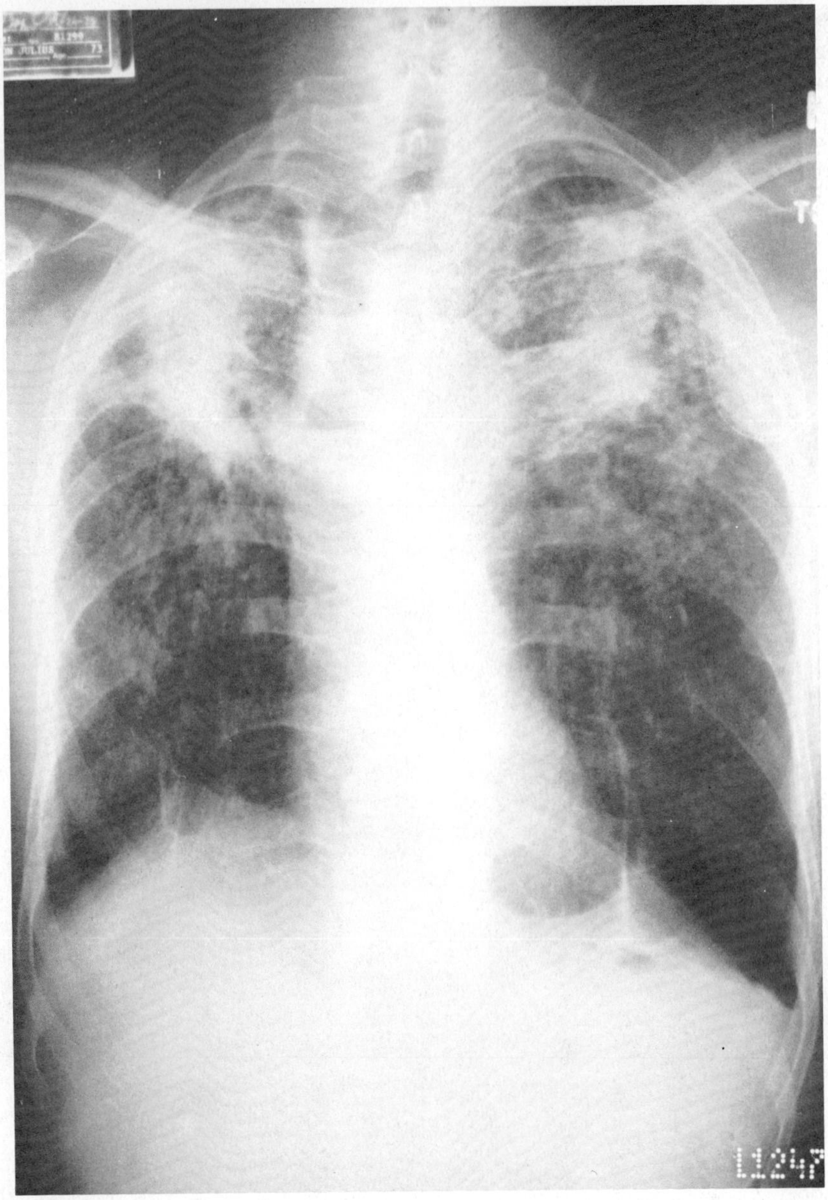

FIG. 11. Conglomerate silicosis in a 73-year-old former miner. Note the nodular masses of fibrous tissue in upper lung fields with upper lobe retraction and cavitation. Tuberculosis was searched for but not found.

ogen(s) has (have) been identified and sensitivity testing completed, appropriate changes in the antibiotic regimen should be made.

If a patient has a more chronic indolent illness, is stable, and does not require immediate empirical therapy, a methodic and thorough diagnostic evaluation is the initial priority. In a patient with bilateral upper lobe cavitary disease in whom the initial microscopic examinations are nonrevealing, the leading considerations include tuberculosis, histoplasmosis, and coccidioidomycosis. In general, in every such patient with a positive tuberculin test response, tuberculosis should be presumed to be the diagnosis until proved otherwise, and antituberculous therapy should be initiated and continued for at least 8 weeks, pending the final results of the mycobacterial cultures. Similarly, disseminated tuberculosis should be strongly suspected in any patient with unexplained fever and a chest film showing a nodular interstitial pattern; prompt institution of antituberculous therapy may be lifesaving in this otherwise fatal condition. In contrast, rarely should antifungal therapy be given empirically to a patient with chronic pneumonia since fungal pulmonary diseases usually progress slowly and the most commonly used agents, amphotericin B and ketoconazole, may be associated with significant toxicity.

Corticosteroids

The question of when to use corticosteroids in the treatment of a patient with chronic pneumonia frequently arises. If the cause of the illness is an infectious agent, particularly a bacterium or a fungus, steroids are usually not indicated. In contrast, corticosteroids may be helpful in chronic pneumonia due to noninfectious causes such as the vasculitidies, sarcoidosis, chronic eosinophilic pneumonia, and many of the fibrotic lung diseases including chronic hypersensitivity pneumonitis (along with avoidance of exposure to the offending antigen).

Supportive Measures

Vigorous measures aimed at good bronchopulmonary hygiene should be instituted. Generous fluid intake and humidified air

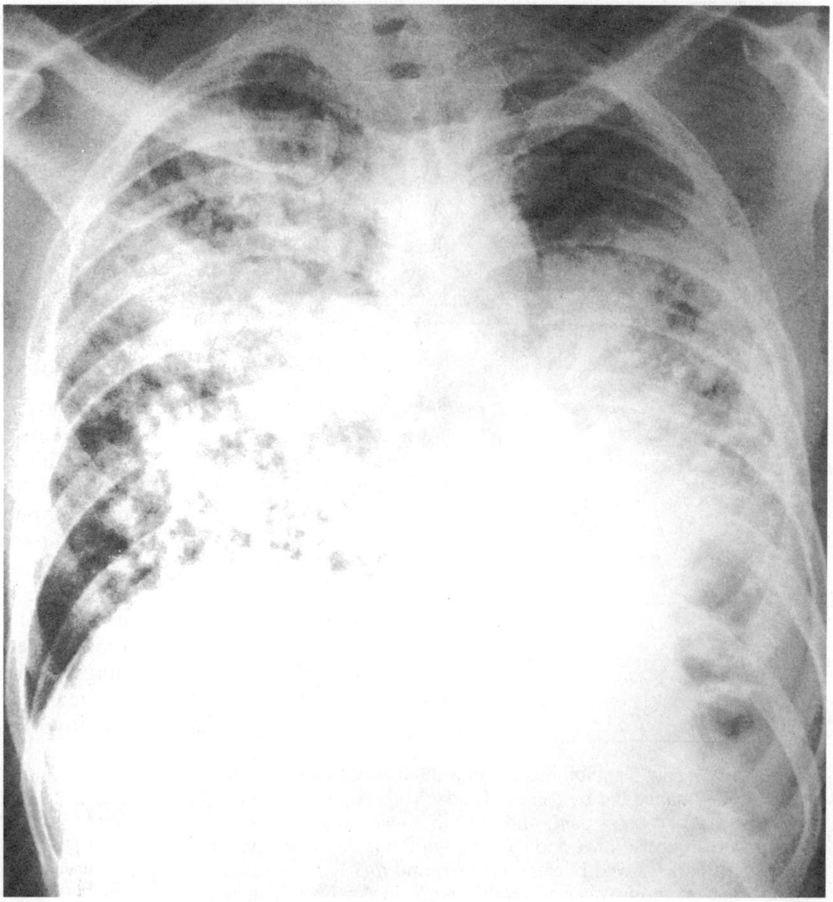

FIG. 12. Alveolar cell carcinoma in a 46-year-old man with a minimal smoking history. His symptoms of 6 months' duration included progressive dyspnea, cough with copious sputum production, and fever. Note the bilateral alveolar filling pattern.

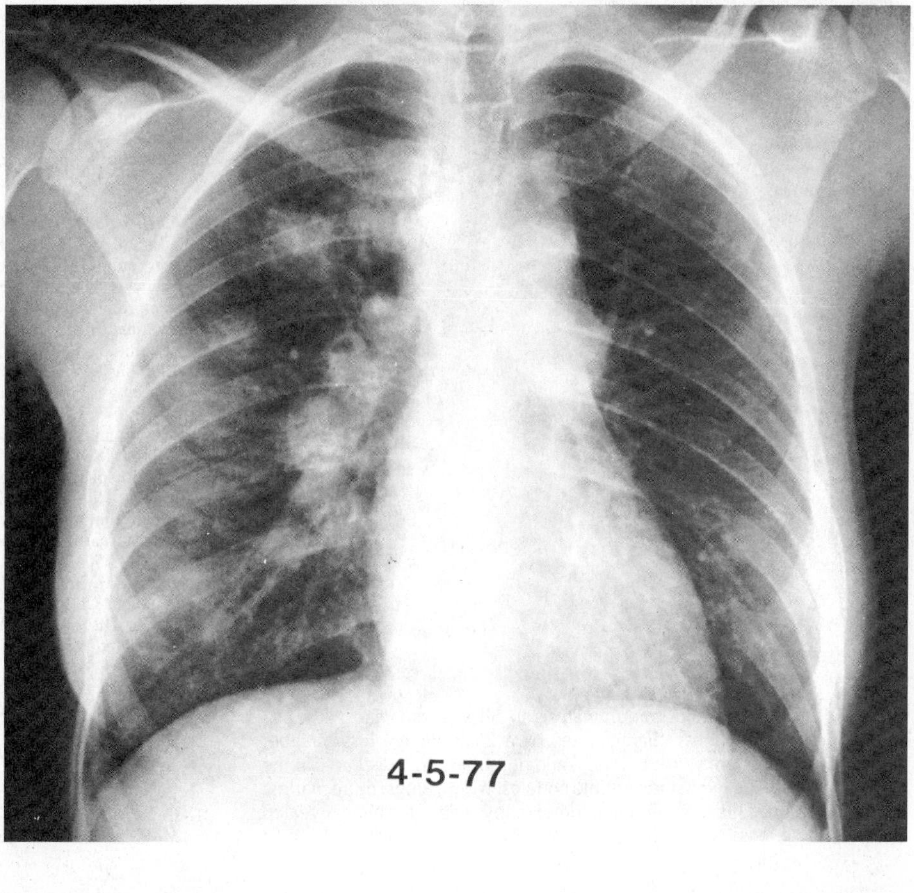

FIG. 13. Pulmonary sarcoidosis in a 22-year-old woman. Note the spherical, nodular opacities in the right lung and prominent right hilar adenopathy.

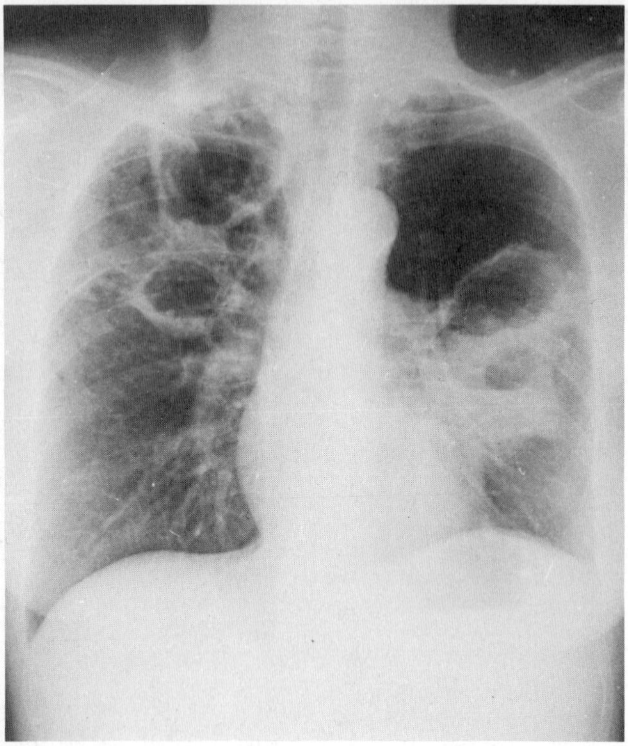

FIG. 14. Wegener's granulomatosis in a 55-year-old woman with a 4-month illness manifested by "sinus" headaches, cough, intermittent hemoptysis, pleuritic chest pain, and a 30 lb weight loss. Note the large cavities in both upper lobes and the subpleural nodule in the right upper lobe. Sinus films showed bilateral ethmoid and maxillary opacification. A pathologic diagnosis was made on tissue obtained at open lung biopsy.

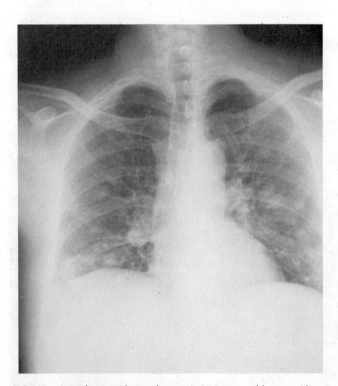

FIG. 15. Lymphomatoid granulomatosis in 54-year-old man with a 2-month progressive illness characterized by a 25 lb weight loss, fatigue, nonproductive cough, slurred speech, and numbness and weakness of the right side of his face. Note the multiple nodules in both lungs, more marked in the lower lung fields. A computed tomography scan of the head revealed an enhancing mass within the pons.

may promote easier expectoration. In patients with chronic cavitary disease or bronchiectasis and in whom there is copious sputum production, postural drainage and chest vibropercussion are important adjuncts. However, these procedures must be carried out with caution in an attempt to prevent infection from spreading to the noninvolved lung. Hypoxia may be a feature of chronic pneumonia; the severity will depend on the cause and the distribution of the pulmonary parenchymal process. Appropriate means of administering oxygen should be used to ensure adequate oxygen supply to the tissues, and alterations in delivery should be made on the basis of sequential arterial blood gas studies.

Bronchoscopy and Surgery

Bronchoscopy may be used as a therapeutic adjunct, especially in patients who have thick tenacious secretions that cannot be raised by noninvasive techniques. In other patients, mucous plugs or foreign bodies may predispose to atelectasis and chronic pneumonia; therapeutic bronchoscopy may be necessary to expand the collapsed lung.

Lobectomy or pneumonectomy should be considered in a patient with chronic destructive pneumonia and multiple macro- or microabscesses involving an entire lobe or lung and a ventilation–perfusion scan indicating nonfunction of the involved lung.[8] Thoracotomy may also be indicated for purposes of decortication of the pleura in patients whose chronic pneumonia has involved the pleura with resulting restrictive lung disease.

REFERENCES

1. Epler GR, Colby TV, McLoud TC, et al. Bronchiolitis obliterans organizing pneumonia. N Engl J Med. 1985;312:152–8.
2. Bartlett JG, Finegold SM. Anaerobic infections of the lung and pleural space. Am Rev Respir Dis. 1974;110:56–77.
3. Lerner AM. The gram-negative bacillary pneumonias. DM. 1980;27:1–56.
4. Khan MA, Kovnat DM, Bachus B, et al. Clinical and roentgenographic spectrum of pulmonary tuberculosis in the adult. Am J Med. 1977;62:31–8.
5. Rosenzweig DU. Pulmonary mycobacterial infections due to *Mycobacterium intracellulare avium* complex—clinical features and course in 100 consecutive cases. Chest. 1979;75:115–9.
6. Goodwin RA, Owens FT, Snell JD, et al. Chronic cavitary histoplasmosis. Medicine (Baltimore). 1976;55:413–52.
7. Bayer AS. Fungal pneumonias; pulmonary coccidioidal syndromes. Part 1 and Part 2. Chest. 1981;79:575–83,686–91.
8. Cameron EWJ, Appelbaum PC, Pudifin D, et al. Characteristics and management of chronic destructive pneumonia. Thorax. 1980;35:340–6.
9. Farrell GE, ed. Actinomycosis of the Thorax. St Louis: Warren H. Green; 1981:1–90.
10. Cush R, Light RW, George RB. Clinical and roentgenographic manifestations of acute and chronic blastomycosis. Chest. 1976;69:345–9.
11. Kerkering TM, Duma RJ, Shadomy S. The evolution of pulmonary cryptococcosis. Clinical implications from a study of 41 patients with and without compromising host factors. Ann Intern Med. 1981;94:611–6.
12. Zvetina JR, Rippon JW, Daum V. Chronic pulmonary sporotrichosis. Mycopathologia. 1978;64:53–7.
13. Emmons CW, Binford CH, Utz JP, et al., eds. Adiaspiromycosis. In: Medical Mycology. Philadelphia: Lea & Febiger; 1977:493–505.
14. Rosenow EC III, Wilson WR, Cockerill FR. Pulmonary disease in the immunocompromised host. Mayo Clin Proc. 1985;60:473–87,610–31.
15. Cairns MR, Durack DT. Fungal pneumonia in the immunocompromised host. Sem Respir Infect 1986;1:166–85.
16. Murray JF, Garay SM, Hopewell PC, et al. Pulmonary complications of the acquired immunodeficiency syndrome: An update. Report of the Second National Heart, Lung and Blood Institute Workshop. Am Rev Respir Dis. 1987;135:504–9.
17. Garay SM, Belenko M, Fazzini E, et al. Pulmonary manifestations of Kaposi's sarcoma. Chest. 1987;91:39–43.
18. Stover DE, White DA, Romano PA, et al. Spectrum of pulmonary diseases associated with the acquired immunodeficiency syndrome. Am J Med. 1985;78:429–37.
19. Suffredini AF, Ognibene FP, Lack EE, et al. Nonspecific interstitial pneumonitis: A common cause of pulmonary disease in the acquired immunodeficiency syndrome. Ann Intern Med. 1987;107:7–13.
20. Stead WW, Lofgren JP, Warren E, et al. Tuberculosis as an endemic and nosocomial infection among the elderly in nursing homes. N Engl J Med. 1985;312:1483–7.
21. Centers for Disease Control. Tuberculosis in minorities—United States. MMWR. 1987;36:77–80.

22. Baum GL, Donnerberg RL, Stewart D, et al. Pulmonary sporotrichosis. N Engl J Med. 1969;280:410–3.
23. Werner SB, Pappagianis D, Heindl I, et al. An epidemic of coccidioidomycosis among archeology students in northern California. N Engl J Med. 1972;286:507–12.
24. Rao S, Biddle M, Balchum OJ, et al. Focal endemic coccidioidomycosis in Los Angeles County. Am Rev Respir Dis. 1972;105:410–6.
25. Latham RH, Kaiser AB, DuPont WD, et al. Chronic pulmonary histoplasmosis following the excavation of a bird roost. Am J Med. 1980;68:504–8.
26. Seward CW. Outbreak of histoplasmosis in Oklahoma. Am Rev Respir Dis. 1970;102:950–8.
27. Ward JI, Weeks M, Allen D, et al. Acute histoplasmosis: Clinical, epidemiologic and serologic findings of an outbreak associated with exposure to a fallen tree. Am J Med. 1979;66:587–95.
28. Hasenclever HF, Shacklette MH, Young RV, et al. The natural occurrence of *H. capsulatum* in a cave. I. Epidemiologic aspects. Am J Epidemiol. 1967;886:238–45.
29. Kahn JB, Spruance C, Harbottle J, et al. Ecchinococcosis in Utah. Am J Trop Med Hyg. 1972;21:185–8.
30. Bristol LJ, Pneumoconioses caused by asbestos and by other siliceous and nonsiliceous dusts. Semin Roentgenol. 1967;2:283–305.
31. Parkes WR, ed. Nonneoplastic disorders due to metallic, chemical and physical agents. In: Occupational Lung Disorders. 2nd ed. London: Butterworths; 1982:454–98.
32. Everett ED, Nelson RA. Pulmonary melioidosis. Am Rev Respir Dis. 1975;112:331–40.
33. Warren KS, Mahmoud AAF. Algorithms in the diagnosis and management of exotic diseases. XXI. Liver, intestinal and lung flukes. J Infect Dis. 1977;135:692–6.
34. Frand UI, Shim CS, Williams MH Jr. Heroin-induced pulmonary edema. Sequential studies of pulmonary function. Ann Intern Med. 1972;77:29–35.
35. Robertson CH, Reynolds RC, Wilson JE. Pulmonary hypertension and foreign body granulomas in intravenous drug abusers. Documentation by cardiac catheterization and lung biopsy. Am J Med. 1976;61:657–64.
36. Patel RC, Dutta D, Schonfeld SA. Free-base cocaine use associated with bronchiolitis obliterans organizing pneumonia. Ann Intern Med. 1987;107:186–7.
37. Cooper JAD, White DA, Matthay RA. Drug-induced pulmonary disease. Part 1: Cytotoxic drugs. Part 2: Noncytotoxic drugs. Am Rev Respir Dis. 1986;133:321–40,488–505.
38. Reeder MM. Radiological Pathological Conference of the Month from Armed Forces Institute of Pathology: Hydatid cyst of the lung. Radiology. 1970;95:429–37.
39. Bartlett JG, Ryan KJ, Smith TF, et al. Cumitech 7A. In: Washington JA II, ed. Laboratory Diagnosis of Lower Respiratory Tract Infections. Washington, DC: American Society for Microbiology; 1987:1–18.
40. Wimberly NW, Bass JB, Boyd BW, et al. Use of bronchoscopic protected catheter brush for the diagnosis of pulmonary infections. Chest. 1982;81:556–62.
41. Stead WW. Second-strength PPD test (Letter). N Engl J Med. 1972;286:844.
42. Fulkerson WJ. Fiberoptic bronchoscopy. N Engl J Med. 1984;311:511–5.
43. Hanson RR, Zavala DC, Rhodes ML, et al. Transbronchial biopsy via flexible fiberoptic bronchoscope: Results in 164 patients. Am Rev Respir Dis. 1976;114:67–72.
44. Crystal RG, Reynolds HY, Kalica AR. Bronchoalveolar lavage: The report of an international conference. Chest. 1986;90:122–31.
45. Stover DE, Zaman MB, Hajdn SI, et al. Bronchoalveolar lavage in the diagnosis of diffuse pulmonary infiltrates in the immunosuppressed host. Ann Intern Med. 1984;101:1–7.
46. Cockerill FR III, Wilson WR, Carpenter HA, et al. Open lung biopsy in immunocompromised patients. Arch Intern Med. 1985;145:1398–1404.
47. Zavala DC, Schoell JE. Ultrathin needle aspiration of the lung in infectious and malignant disease. Am Rev Respir Dis. 1981;123:125–31.
48. Wang KP, Kelly SJ, Britt JE. Percutaneous needle aspiration biopsy of chest lesions: New instrument and new technique. Chest. 1988;93:993–7.
49. Robin ED, Burke CM. Lung biopsy in immunosuppressed patients. Chest. 1986;89:276–8.

57. CYSTIC FIBROSIS

MICHAEL R. KNOWLES
PETER GILLIGAN
RICHARD C. BOUCHER

Because the molecular basis of this genetic disorder is unknown, cystic fibrosis (CF) remains in strict terms a syndrome rather than a disease, and the diagnosis rests on a compatible clinical picture. Diagnostic criteria include chronic obstructive lung disease and/or pancreatic exocrine insufficiency; the presence of characteristic sputum microbiologic flora (i.e., mucoid *Pseudomonas aeruginosa* and *Staphylococcus aureus*); and a family history of CF. The diagnosis is supported by the hallmark laboratory abnormality, an elevated sweat chloride concentration. Although CF is generally regarded as a disease of children, about one-third of currently identified CF patients are adults. It should be noted that the normal range for sweat chloride values in adults is greater than for children. Whereas values must be less than 40 mEq/liter to be clearly normal in children, healthy adults may have values of up to 70 mEq/liter.[1]

CLINICAL MANIFESTATIONS

The clinical manifestations of CF reflect obstruction of organs by viscous secretions and the presence of a chronic bacterial infection in the lung. Although multiple organ systems are involved, chronic airway infection accounts for most disease-related morbidity and mortality. Chronic suppurative airway disease is present in more than 98 percent of adults who have CF, and 95 percent of CF deaths are related to progressive pulmonary insufficiency.[1–3] Most respiratory infections in CF adults are caused by *S. aureus, P. aeruginosa*, and *Haemophilus influenzae*, whereas the incidence of infections with other infectious agents (e.g., *Mycoplasma pneumoniae*, and viruses) is believed to be similar to that of the general population.[4,5]

The clinical picture of CF is dominated by a chronic cough punctuated by episodes of clinical deterioration that are characterized by an increased volume and purulence of sputum, dyspnea, and sometimes anorexia and weight loss. Although adults with CF may exhibit low-grade fever with these exacerbations, high fever is unusual and sepsis or bacteremia is extraordinarily uncommon despite the large number of bacteria in the airways (10^8 organisms per milliliter of sputum). Clinical exacerbations are also associated with modest elevations of white blood cell counts and worsening spirometric values. The chest radiography typically is dominated by cystic bronchiectatic changes and diffuse roentgenographic shadowing that reflects airway wall thickening and retained secretions. Many adult CF patients exhibit an upper lung zone predominance of these roentgenographic abnormalities, which raises the diagnostic possibility of tuberculosis. Hypoxemia and carbon dioxide retention are uncommon in CF adults during acute exacerbations until the forced expired volume in one second (FEV_1) is less than 50 percent of the predicted value. Thus, significant gas exchange abnormalities usually occur only near the terminal stages of the disease and herald a relatively rapid downhill course.

The pulmonary manifestations of CF in adults are frequently complicated by hemoptysis and pneumothorax. Minor hemoptysis occurs in more than 50 percent of CF patients, and massive hemoptysis occurs in 5–10 percent of adult CF patients. Fortunately, medical (nonsurgical) intervention is usually sufficient for the treatment of pulmonary hemorrhage. The presence of CF epithelial defects in the mucosa of the nasal sinuses, and the frequent occurrence of nasal polyps in adults, make symptoms of subacute/chronic sinusitis a major problem in many adult patients. It is important to note that the microbiology of sinusitis is not reflected by the flora identified in expectorated sputum.[6]

Because most CF patients have progressive destruction and loss of pancreatic function, the prevalence of diabetes mellitus in adult CF populations may be as high as 15 percent.[8] The presence of glucose intolerance may add further difficulty to the treatment of pulmonary infection.

PATHOGENESIS

The clinical syndrome of CF reflects an autosomal recessive genetic disorder. Although the CF defect has not been identified in molecular terms, it has been localized to the Cen-q22 region of chromosome 7 with studies using restriction length fragment polymorphisms.[8–10] Linkage analysis allows accurate genetic counseling for the parents of most CF patients.[11]

Two general features characterize the pathogenesis of CF at the cellular level: (*1*) the affected cells in target organs are epithelia; and (*2*) the abnormality in epithelial cells appears to involve regulation of ion transport. The most prevalent defect is abnormal regulation of the activation state of plasma membrane Cl^- channels. Defective Cl^- channel activation has been detected in the epithelia of airways,[12–14] sweat ducts,[15] and the small intestine.[16] In airway epithelia, the Cl^- defect principally reflects abnormalities in cAMP-dependent mechanisms for channel activation.[17,18] A second major defect in ion transport has been detected in CF airway epithelia. The rate of absorption of Na^+ ions from the airway lumen to the interstitium is raised threefold compared to normal.[17] In contrast to the failure of cAMP to activate Cl^- channels in airway epithelia, cAMP further increases the accelerated rate of Na^+ absorption in CF airway epithelia.[17]

Because the ion transport activities of airway epithelia regulate the volume and composition of the liquids (secretions) that line airway surfaces, the ion transport abnormalities that characterize CF affect these liquids. Both accelerated Na^+ absorption and reduced Cl^- channel permeability, by inhibiting Cl^- ion secretion, would be expected to reduce the water content of secretions. The depletion of water, perhaps by changing the viscoelastic properties of secretions and/or the linkage between the mucous component of secretions and cilia, projects reductions in mucociliary and cough clearance. Whether reduced clearance of thickened secretions from the airways is sufficient to lead to persistent staphylococcal and pseudomonal infection is not clear. A role for increased bacterial adherence, perhaps through a change in the $SO_4^{=}$ content of the airway cell surface glycocalyx, has recently been postulated.[19]

The development of persistent bacterial infection generates a complex series of events that lead to airway wall damage and ultimately to destroyed or bronchiectatic airways. Bacterial exoproducts from both *S. aureus* and *P. aeruginosa* have been implicated in airway destruction. In adults, lipopolysaccharides, exotoxin A, and a cell wall-associated rhamnolipid from *P. aeruginosa* have been implicated as important bacterial toxins.[20] The host inflammatory response appears intact in CF, and the vigorous host response may contribute to airway damage. Chemotactic agents, both bacterial and locally derived (e.g., arachidonic acid metabolites from airway epithelia), attract inflammatory cells into the airway lumen. Polymorphonuclear cell-derived enzymes (e.g., elastase) likely damage airway wall structures. In addition, it has been reported that the chronic antigenic stimulus of persistent airway infections generates immunologically mediated airway wall destruction. The best-documented response of this type is antigen–antibody complex-mediated damage.[21] Eventually, the combination of retained secretions and airway damage deranges gas exchange, perturbs cardiac function, and leads to death.

MICROBIOLOGY

Staphylococcus aureus and *P. aeruginosa* are the primary etiologic agents of pulmonary infection in patients with CF.[22] *Staphylococcus aureus* often colonizes the respiratory tract in the first 2 years of life and can be found in up to 50–60 percent of patients with CF in the United States. Before the advent of effective antistaphylococcal therapy, lung infection due to this organism was the leading cause of death. Antistaphylococcal penicillins such as oxacillin and nafcillin control infections with this organism, and resistance to these agents is very unusual. In patients receiving long-term (>3 months) prophylactic trimethoprim/sulfamethoxazole therapy, approximately 50 percent of *S. aureus* isolated is thymidine dependent.[23] Because thymidine-dependent organisms grow poorly on most commonly used isolation media, and because mucoid *P. aeruginosa* may obscure recognition of its growth, mannitol salts agar must be used to ensure reliable recovery of *S. aureus*.

In childhood or early adolescence, patients with CF become chronically infected with *P. aeruginosa*. Up to 70 percent of patients with CF, primarily adolescents and adults, are infected with this organism. The *P. aeruginosa* isolates recovered from these patients appear to evolve from a smooth, serum-resistant, serotypable organism to a rough, serum-sensitive, nonserotypable one.[24] The latter form of *P. aeruginosa* is characterized by its ability to produce large amounts of an extracellular cell-associated mucoid polysaccharide referred to as *alginate*.[25] Mucoid colonies that result from alginate production are predominant in infected CF patients but are rarely seen in other patients with chronic airway disease.[26] This mucoid variant is believed to be responsible for the formation of microcolonies that are believed to be resistant to both mechanical and immunologic clearance from the airways.

When first isolated, *P. aeruginosa* is usually susceptible to all antipseudomonal β-lactams, imipenem, quinolones, and aminoglycosides. With increasing antimicrobial pressure due to repeated antimicrobial treatment of pulmonary exacerbations, resistance to these agents may develop, especially if each one is used alone. In patients repeatedly treated for *P. aeruginosa*, the organism may remain susceptible only to polymixin b and colistin.

A third organism, *Pseudomonas cepacia*, which has been recovered from up to 20 percent of patients at selected CF centers,[27] has recently been recognized as a potentially important agent in the lung disease of adults with CF. This organism has been associated with significantly increased mortality and presents difficult problems for the clinician. First, *P. cepacia* is usually resistant (>90 percent of isolates) to ticarcillin and aminoglycosides on initial isolation and, after therapy with antipseudomonal β-lactams or trimethoprim/sulfamethoxazole, will often become resistant to them as well. Imipenem and the quinolones are only marginally active against this organism. Second, the organism may be difficult to recover from airway secretions unless specific isolation media[28] are used because the organism grows slowly and may be obscured by other airway flora, particularly mucoid *P. aeruginosa*. Finally, unlike *P. aeruginosa*, *P. cepacia* produces few easily identifiable virulence factors,[29] making the mechanism by which it produces lung disease obscure.

Other microbes, such as *Haemophilus influenzae, Branhamella catarrhalis, Xanthamonas maltophilia, Achromobacter xylosoxidans*, and Enterobactericeae, may play a role in the pulmonary disease observed in CF patients. Of these organisms, the recovery of *H. influenzae* is particularly difficult because other organisms, particularly *P. aeruginosa*, may overgrow the isolation medium. This obstacle can be overcome by incubating enrichment medium under anaerobic conditions in order to inhibit the growth of *P. aeruginosa*.[30]

Mycobacteria, including *M. tuberculosis, M. avium-intracellulare*, and Runyon group IV mycobacteria, have infrequently been recovered from patients with CF.[31] One of the difficulties in isolating mycobacteria in this population is that proteases present in CF sputa may liquify the Lowestein-Jensen agar slants.

Aspergillus fumigatus may be cultured from CF patients,[32] and elevated titers of IgG antibody may be found in serum from these patients. Unless the patient has pre-existing asthma, he or she does not fulfill the diagnostic criteria for the clinical syndrome of allergic bronchopulmonary aspergillosis.

The exact role of viral infection in pulmonary deterioration of patients with CF has not been clearly defined. In a prospective study, no virus could be recovered from nasopharyngeal washings of symptomatic patients with CF, although some of these patients had serologic evidence of viral infection.[33]

TREATMENT

The goal of therapy is to retard progressive lung damage by controlling bacterial infection with antibiotics, by removing viscous/purulent airway secretions, and by providing proper nutrition for host defense. Antibiotics have played a key role in improved survival, and indications for antimicrobial therapy continue to evolve.[2–5,34]

Broad-spectrum oral antibiotics (amoxicillin, cephalexin, dicloxacillin, tetracycline, trimethoprim/sulfamethoxazole) can provide successful therapy for acute pulmonary exacerbations despite the presence of *P. aeruginosa* that is resistant to these agents. The clinical benefit may reflect antibiotic activity against pathogens that are difficult to culture in the presence of mucoid *P. aeruginosa* (*S. aureus, H. influenzae*) or against airway infection with high concentrations of bacteria ($>10^5$ organisms/per milliliter) that are not typical pathogens.[2] High doses and prolonged therapy (3–4 weeks) are recommended for treatment of acute illnesses (exacerbations) with oral agents. Oral antibiotics are also of benefit in chronic bacterial sinusitis, which results from pathogens that are frequently sensitive to broad-spectrum antimicrobials.[6] The use of oral antibiotics for prophylactic (maintenance) therapy is controversial but may have a useful role in some patients.

Ciprofloxacin is an oral antipseudomonal drug that is useful for intermittent therapy. The emergence of bacterial resistance during monotherapy with this drug limits its usefulness for chronic treatment,[35–37] and the duration of periodic treatment should be limited to 2–4 weeks.[34]

Aggressive parenteral therapy is indicated for clinical exacerbations that do not respond to oral antimicrobials.[2–4,34] Although sterilization of airway secretions rarely occurs and is not the goal of parenteral therapy, the bacterial burden in conducting airways can be reduced[38] and irreversible lung damage presumably retarded. Whereas parenteral therapy should be guided by sputum bacteriology and drug sensitivity, treatment in adult CF patients usually focuses on *P. aeruginosa*. A combination of antibiotics is indicated because thickened airway secretions present a barrier to drug penetration and because aminoglycoside activity can be reduced by suppurative secretions.[39] A combination of antibiotics also protects against the emergence of resistant strains. Therapy usually includes an aminoglycoside (gentamicin, tobramycin, amikacin), plus another agent effective against *P. aeruginosa,* such as antipseudomonal penicillins, cephalosporins (e.g., ceftazidime[40,41]), or imipenem. If *S. aureus* is clinically suspected or cultured from sputum, addition of a specific antistaphylococcal agent should be considered if the antipseudomonal drug therapy is not adequate for *S. aureus*. Increased plasma clearance of almost all effective antibiotics in CF patients dictates the use of large, frequent doses of antimicrobials.[42] For example, CF adults require 6–15/mg/kg/day of gentamicin to achieve desired peak serum levels of 10 μg/ml in a q8h dosing regimen. Aminoglycoside toxicity is uncommon in CF patients, but trough serum levels should be carefully monitored. Parenteral therapy should be continued for a minimum of 10–14 days or until a full clinical and pulmonary functional response has been achieved. Recent experience suggests that effective parenteral antibiotic therapy can be administered on an outpatient basis.[43]

Aerosolized antibiotics can be used for subacute pulmonary exacerbations and to assist in the maintenance of a stable clinical status in some patients.[44] Effective aerosol delivery techniques are essential if this approach is to be successful.[45,46] Colistin is an attractive agent for inhalation therapy.[47] The development of bacterial resistance during prolonged aerosol therapy with colistin does not reduce the response to parenteral alternatives.

Interestingly, despite intensive antibiotic exposure, symptomatic disease with *Clostridium difficile* is uncommon in CF patients despite the presence of the organism in fecal samples.[48,49] The asymptomatic carriage of *C. difficile* may reflect the absence of the capacity of the CF intestinal epithelium to response to *C. difficile*-derived toxins.[16]

The presence of a large bacterial burden in the bronchiectatic airways of patients dictates that airway clearance techniques be combined with antibacterial therapy to achieve optimal results.[3–5] Chest percussion and postural drainage is the time-honored method, but deep breathing, exercise, and voluntary coughing are also effective. Bronchodilators may assist in clearing retained secretions in some patients, but a paradoxical reduction in airflow in some patients,[50] and potential acceleration of abnormal Na^+ transport,[17] suggest that these agents should be used intermittently and with caution in adult CF patients. Anti-inflammatory agents may occasionally be useful in reducing mucosal edema and assisting in airway clearance, but the indications for these agents are poorly defined.[4] There is little role for the use of inhaled mucolytic agents or bronchial lavage.[3]

Chronic malabsorption, coupled with increased caloric requirements due to chronic infection and increased respiratory activity, can induce malnourishment and impaired host–defense mechanisms in CF patients. High caloric intake with supplemental pancreatic digestive enzymes is therefore essential in the treatment of these patients.[51]

Although *A. fumigatus* is frequently cultured from the sputum of CF adults, treatment with systemic corticosteroids is usually not indicated, unless the syndrome of allergic bronchopulmonary aspergillosis is established. The increasing number of adults in the CF patient population is associated with increasing recovery of nontuberculous mycobacteria from sputum cultures.[22] The clinical and radiographic patterns should be monitored for evidence of pathogenic mycobacterial activity.

Annual influenza vaccinations are recommended, but the pneumococcal vaccine is not routinely indicated because of the relative absence of *S. pneumoniae* as a pathogen.

Finally, heart-lung transplants are a novel therapeutic strategy in patients with CF. Of 6 long-term (23 months) surviving patients, 3 had airway infection, 1 with *H. influenzae*, 1 with *P. aeruginosa*, and 1 with *S. aureus* and *P. aeruginosa*.[52]

REFERENCES

1. Davis PB. Cystic fibrosis in adults. In: Lloyd-Still JD, ed. Textbook of Cystic Fibrosis. V. 9. Littleton, Mass: John Wright-PSG; 1983:351–66.
2. Myers MG, Koontz FP, Weinberger M. Lower respiratory infections in patients with cystic fibrosis. In: Lloyd-Still JD, ed. Textbook of Cystic Fibrosis. V. 90. Littleton, Mass: John Wright-PSG; 1983;91–107.
3. Taussig LM, Landau LI, Marks MI. Respiratory system. In: Taussig LM, ed. Cystic Fibrosis. V. 5. New York: Thieme-Stratton; 1984;115–74.
4. Mischler EH. Treatment of pulmonary disease in cystic fibrosis. Semin Respir Med. 1985;6(4):271–84.
5. Thomassen MJ, Demko CA, Doershuk CF. Cystic fibrosis: A review of pulmonary infections and interventions. Pediatr-Pulmonol. 1987;3(5):334–51.
6. Shapiro ED, Milmoe GJ, Wald ER, et al. Bacteriology of the maxillary sinuses in patients with cystic fibrosis. J Infect Dis. 1982;146(5):589–93.
7. Knowles MR, Fernald GW. Diabetes and cystic fibrosis: New questions emerging from increased longevity. J Pediatr. 1988;101:415–16.
8. Egberg H, Mohr J, Schmiegelow K, et al. Linkage relationships of paraoxonase (PON) with other markers: Indication of PON-cystic fibrosis synteny. Clin Genet. 1985;28:265–71.
9. Tsui L-C, Buchwald M, Barker D, et al. Cystic fibrosis locus defined by a genetically linked polymorphic DNA marker. Science. 1985;230:1054–7.
10. Wainwright BJ, et al. Localization of cystic fibrosis locus to human chromosome 7cen-q22. Nature. 1985;318:384–5.
11. Beaudet A, Spence J, O'Brien W, et al. Experience with new DNA markers for the diagnosis of cystic fibrosis. N Engl J Med. 1988;318:50–1.
12. Knowles MR, Stutts MJ, Spock A, et al. Abnormal ion permeation through cystic fibrosis respiratory epithelium. Science. 1983;221:1067–70.
13. Frizzell RA, Rechkemmer G, Shoemaker RL. Altered regulation of airway epithelial cell chloride channels in cystic fibrosis. Science. 1986;233:558–60.

14. Case M. Cl^- impermeability in cystic fibrosis. Nature. 1986;322:407.
15. Quinton PM. Chloride impermeability in cystic fibrosis. Nature. 1983;301:421–2.
16. Berschneider HM, Knowles MR, Azizkhan RG, et al. Altered intestinal chloride transport in cystic fibrosis. FASEB J. 1988;2(10):2625–9.
17. Boucher RC, Stutts MJ, Knowles MR, et al. Na^+ transport in cystic fibrosis respiratory epithelia: Abnormal basal rate and response to adenylate cyclase activation. J Clin Invest. 1986;78:1245–52.
18. Shoumacher RA, Shoemaker RL, Halm DR, et al. Phosphorylation fails to activate chloride channels from cystic fibrosis airway cells. Nature. 1987;330:752–4.
19. Cheng P-W, Boucher RC, Yankaskas JR, et al. Glycoconjugates secreted by cultured human nasal epithelial cells. In: Mastella G, Quinton PM, eds. Cellular and Molecular Basis of Cystic Fibrosis. San Francisco: San Francisco Press; 1988:233–8.
20. Stutts MJ, Schwab JH, Chen MG, et al. Effects of *Pseudomonas aeruginosa* on bronchial epithelial ion transport. Am Rev Respir Dis. 1986;134:17–24.
21. Lewiston NJ, Moss RB. Circulating immune complexes decrease during corticosteroid therapy in cystic fibrosis. Pediatr Res. 1982;16:354.
22. Friend PA. Pulmonary infection in cystic fibrosis. J Infect. 1986;13:55–72.
23. Gilligan PH, Gage PA, Welch DF, et al. Prevalence of thymidine-dependent *Staphylococcus aureus* in patients with cystic fibrosis. J Clin Microbiol. 1987;25:1258–61.
24. Penketh A, Pitt T, Roberts D, et al. The relationship of phenotype changes in *Pseudomonas aeruginosa* to the clinical conditions of patients with cystic fibrosis. Am Rev Respir Dis. 1983;127:605–8.
25. Pier GB. Pulmonary disease associated with *Pseudomonas aeruginosa* in cystic fibrosis: Current status of the host–bacterium interaction. J Infect Dis. 1985;151:575–80.
26. McCarthy VP, Rosenberg G, Rosenstein BJ, et al. Mucoid *Pseudomonas aeruginosa* from a patient without cystic fibrosis: Implications and review of the literature. Pediatr Infect Dis. 1986;5:256–8.
27. Tablan OC, Chorba TH, Schidlow DV, et al. *Pseudomonas cepacia* colonization in patients with cystic fibrosis: Risk factors and clinical outcome. J Pediatr. 1985;107:382–7.
28. Gilligan RH, Gage PA, Bradshaw LM, et al. Isolation medium for the recovery of *Pseudomonas cepacia* from respiratory secretions of patients with cystic fibrosis. J Clin Microbiol. 1985;139:805–8.
29. McKevitt AI, Woods DE. Characterization of *Pseudomonas cepacia* isolates from patients with cystic fibrosis. J Clin Microbiol. 1984;19:291–3.
30. Roberts DE, Cole P. Use of selective media in bacteriological investigation of patients with chronic respiratory infections. Lancet. 1980;1:796–7.
31. Smith MJ, Efthimou J, Hodson ME, et al. Mycobacterial isolations in young adults with cystic fibrosis. Thorax. 1984;39:369–75.
32. Brueton MJ, Ormerod LP, Shah KJ, et al. Allergic bronchopulmonary aspergillosis complicating cystic fibrosis in childhood. Arch Dis Child. 1980;55:348–53.
33. Wang EEH, Prober GC, Munson B, et al. Association of respiratory viral infections with pulmonary deterioration in patients with cystic fibrosis. N Engl J Med 1984;311:1653–8.
34. Michel BC. Antibacterial therapy in cystic fibrosis: A review of the literature published between 1980 and February 1987. Chest. 1988;94(2S):129S–40S.
35. Scully BE, Nakatomi M, Ores C, et al. Ciprofloxacin therapy in cystic fibrosis. Am J Med. 1987;82(4A):196–201.
36. Goldfarb J, Stern RC, Reed MD, et al. Ciprofloxacin monotherapy for acute pulmonary exacerbations of cystic fibrosis. Am J Med. 1987;82(4A):174–9.
37. Stutman HR. Summary of a workshop on ciprofloxacin use in patients with cystic fibrosis. Pediatr Infect Dis J. 1987;6(10):932–5.
38. Smith AL, Redding G, Doershuk C, et al. Sputum changes associated with therapy for endobronchial exacerbation in cystic fibrosis. J Pediatr. 1988;112:547–54.
39. Mendelman PM, Smith AL, Levy J, et al. Aminoglycoside penetration, inactivation, and efficacy in cystic fibrosis sputum. Am Rev Respir Dis. 1985;132:761–5.
40. Blumer JL, Stern RC, Yamashita TS, et al. Cephalosporin therapeutics in cystic fibrosis. J Pediatr. 1986;108(5 Pt 2):854–60.
41. Reed MD, Stern RC, O'Brien CA, et al. Randomized double-blind evaluation of ceftazidime dose ranging in hospitalized patients with cystic fibrosis. Antimicrob Agents Chemother 1987;31(5)698–702.
42. de Groot R, Smith AL. Antibiotic pharmacokinetics in cystic fibrosis: Differences and clinical significance. Clin Pharmacokinet. 1987;13:228–53.
43. Donati MA, Guenette G, Auerbach H. Prospective controlled study of home and hospital therapy of cystic fibrosis pulmonary disease. J Pediatr. 1987;111:28–33.
44. Stead RJ, Hodson ME, Batten JC. Inhaled ceftazidime compared with gentamycin and carbenicillin in older patients with cystic fibrosis infected with *Pseudomonas aeruginosa*. Br J Dis Chest. 1987;81:272–9.
45. Newman SP, Pavia D. Aerosol deposition in man. In: Moren F, Newhouse MT, eds. Aerosols in Medicine: Principles, Diagnosis and Therapy. V. 7. Amsterdam: Elsevier, 1986:193–218.
46. Newman SP, Woodman G, Clarke SW. Deposition of carbenicillin aerosols in cystic fibrosis: Effects of nebulizer system and breathing pattern. Thorax. 1988;43:318–22.
47. Jensen T, Pedersen SS, Garne S, et al. Colistin inhalation therapy in cystic fibrosis patients with chronic Pseudomonas aeruginosa lung infection. J Antimicrob Chemother. 1987;19:831–8.
48. Welkon CJ, Long SS, Thompson CM, et al. *Clostridium difficile* in patients with cystic fibrosis. Am J Dis Child. 1987;139:805–8.
49. Peach SL, Borriello SP, Gaya H, et al. Asymptomatic carriage of *Clostridium difficile* in patients with cystic fibrosis. J Clin Pathol. 1986;39:1013–8.
50. Shapiro GG, Bamman J, Kanarek P, et al. The paradoxical effect of adrenergic and methylxanthine drugs in cystic fibrosis. Pediatrics. 1976;58(5):740–3.
51. Hubbard VS. Nutritional considerations in cystic fibrosis. Semin Respir. Med. 1985;6(4):308–13.
52. Scott J, Higenbottam T, Hutter J, et al. Heart–lung transplantation for cystic fibrosis. Lancet. 1988;2:192–4.

SECTION D.

58. URINARY TRACT INFECTIONS

JACK D. SOBEL
DONALD KAYE

Bacteriuria is a frequently used term and literally means bacteria in the urine. The probability of the presence of infected urine in the bladder can be ascertained by means of quantitating numbers of bacteria in voided urine and in urine obtained via urethral catheterization. *Significant bacteriuria* is a term that has been used to describe the numbers of bacteria in voided urine that exceed the numbers usually due to contamination from the anterior urethra (i.e., $\geq 10^5$ bacteria/ml). The implication is that in the presence of $\geq 10^5$ bacteria/ml urine, infection must be seriously considered. *Asymptomatic bacteriuria* refers to significant bacteriuria in a patient without symptoms.

Urinary tract infection may only involve the lower urinary tract or may involve both the upper and lower tracts. The term *cystitis* has been used to describe the syndrome involving dysuria, frequency, urgency, and occasionally suprapubic tenderness. However, these symptoms may be related to lower tract inflammation without bacterial infection and can be caused by urethritis (for example, gonorrhea or chlamydial urethritis). Furthermore, the presence of symptoms of lower tract infection without upper tract symptoms by no means excludes upper tract infection, which is also often present.

Acute pyelonephritis describes the clinical syndrome characterized by flank pain and/or tenderness and fever, often associated with dysuria, urgency, and frequency. However, these symptoms can occur in the absence of infection (for example, in renal infarction or renal calculus). A more rigorous definition of acute pyelonephritis is the above syndrome accompanied by significant bacteriuria and acute infection in the kidney.

Urinary tract infection may occur de novo or may be a recurrent infection. Recurrences may be either *relapses* or *reinfections*. Relapse of bacteriuria refers to recurrence of bacteriuria with the same infecting microorganism that was present before therapy was started. This is due to persistence of the organism in the urinary tract. Reinfection is a recurrence of bacteriuria with a microorganism different from the original infecting bacterium. It is a new infection. Occasionally reinfection may occur with the same microorganism, which may have persisted in the vagina or feces. This can be mistaken for a relapse.

The term *chronic urinary tract infection* has little meaning in many patients. True chronic infection should really mean persistence of the same organism for months or years with relapses after treatment. Reinfections do not mean chronicity any more than repeated episodes of pneumonia indicate chronic pneumonia. However, in spite of the questionable application of the term, many authorities have grouped patients with relapsing infections and reinfections together as having "chronic infection."

The term *chronic pyelonephritis* is difficult to define and means different things to different authors. To some, chronic pyelonephritis refers to pathologic changes in the kidney due to infection only. However, identical pathologic alterations are found in several other entities such as chronic urinary tract obstruction, analgesic nephropathy, hypokalemic nephropathy, vascular disease, and uric acid nephropathy. Pathologic descriptions do not (and cannot) differentiate between the changes produced by infection versus those produced by these other entities.

Papillary necrosis from infection is an acute complication of pyelonephritis usually in the presence of diabetes mellitis, urinary tract obstruction, sickle cell disease, or analgesic abuse. Papillary necrosis can occur in the absence of infection in some of these conditions. The necrotic renal papillae may slough and cause unilateral or bilateral ureteral obstruction. *Intrarenal abscess* may result from bacteremia or may be a complication of severe pyelonephritis. *Perinephric abscess* occurs when microorganisms from either the renal parenchyma or blood are deposited in the soft tissues surrounding the kidneys.

PATHOLOGIC CHARACTERISTICS

Acute Pyelonephritis

In severe acute pyelonephritis the kidney is somewhat enlarged, and discrete, yellowish, raised abscesses are apparent on the surface (Fig. 1). The pathognomonic histologic feature is suppurative necrosis or abscess formation within the renal substance.[1]

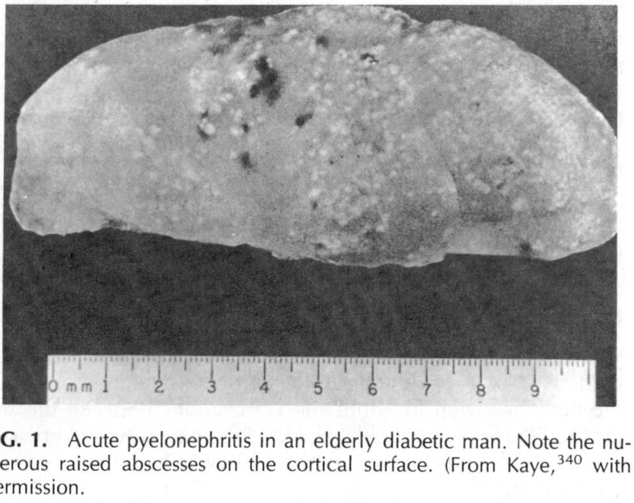

FIG. 1. Acute pyelonephritis in an elderly diabetic man. Note the numerous raised abscesses on the cortical surface. (From Kaye,[340] with permission.

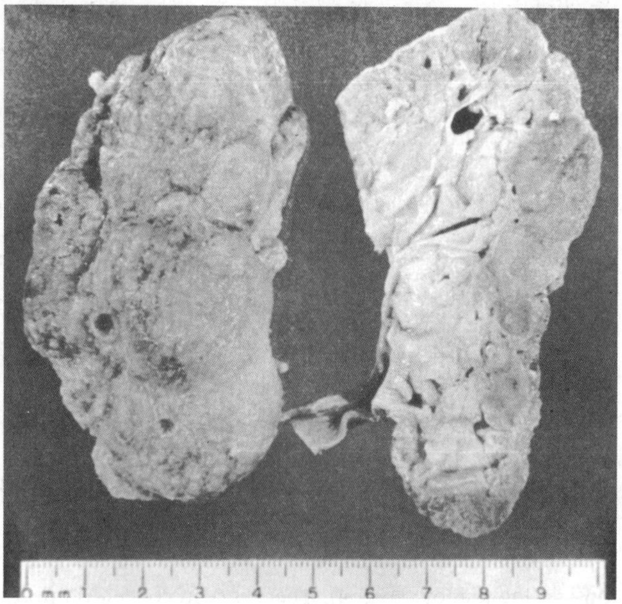

FIG. 2. Chronic pyelonephritis. The kidney is contracted and coarsely scarred, weighing 80 g. Note the thinned cortex and the poorly defined corticomedullary demarcation. (From Kaye,[340] with permission.)

Chronic Pyelonephritis (Chronic Interstitial Nephritis)

The pathologic picture of "chronic pyelonephritis" can be described as follows.[1] One or both kidneys contain gross scars, but even when involvement is bilateral, the kidneys are not equally damaged. This uneven scarring is useful in differentiating chronic pyelonephritis from diseases that cause symmetrical contracted kidneys, for example, chronic glomerulonephritis (Fig. 2). There are inflammatory changes in the pelvic wall with papillary atrophy and blunting. The parenchyma shows interstitial fibrosis with an inflammatory infiltrate of lymphocytes, plasma cells, and occasionally neutrophils (Fig. 3). The tubules are dilated or contracted with atrophy of the lining epithelium. Many of the dilated tubules contain colloid casts, which suggest the appearance of thyroid tissue ("thyroidiza-

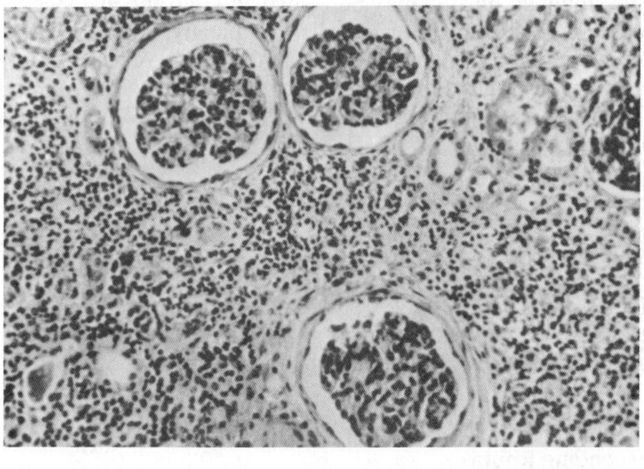

FIG. 3. Chronic pyelonephritis with interstitial and periglomerular fibrosis. Tubules within these scarred areas are atrophic and surrounded by a dense infiltrate of lymphocytes and plasma cells. Glomeruli are well preserved (H&E, ×160). (From Kaye,[340] with permission.)

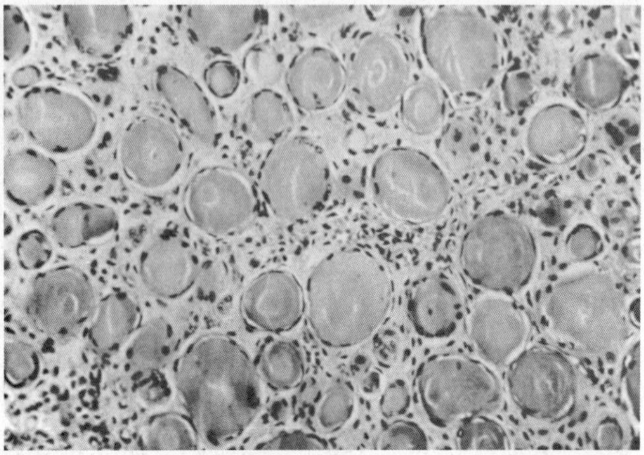

FIG. 4. Chronic pyelonephritis. Tubules are closely packed and filled with eosinophilic casts. Their resemblance to thyroid is striking (H&E, ×160). (From Kaye,[340] with permission.)

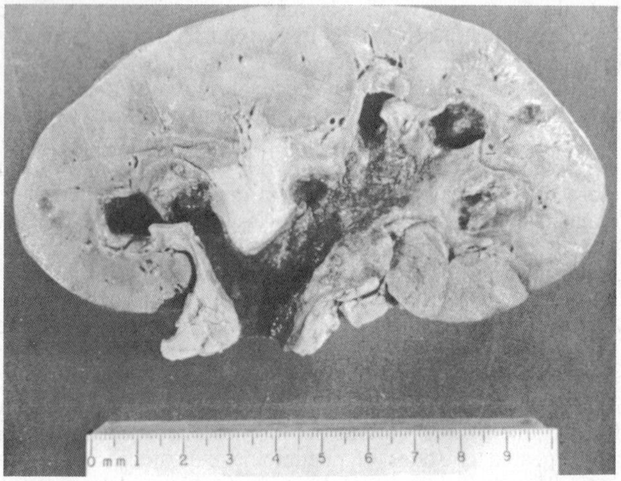

FIG. 5. Papillary necrosis. Necrosis of the renal papillae has resulted in large and irregular defects. The pelvis is hemorrhagic and covered by a granular exudate. (From Kaye,[340] with permission.)

tion'' of the kidney) (Fig. 4). There is also concentric fibrosis about the parietal layer of Bowman capsule (termed *periglomerular fibrosis*) and vascular changes similar to those of benign or malignant arteriolar sclerosis.

Several studies[2–4] have found little correlation between these pathologic findings and evidence for past or present urinary tract infection. Clearly a better term for this pathologic entity would be *chronic interstitial nephritis* to encompass all the clinical states that can cause these changes. To incriminate infection as the sole cause of chronic interstitial nephritis, evidence is required of past or present urinary tract infection and the absence of any other condition that can cause the pathologic picture of chronic interstitial nephritis. These criteria are seldom met, and even if they are, it is frequently impossible to establish whether or not infection is complicating interstitial nephritis of some unrecognized etiology. For example, analgesic nephropathy was not recognized until the 1950s.

Papillary Necrosis Caused by Infection

Frequently both kidneys are affected, and one or more pyramids may be involved[1] (Fig. 5). The pyramids are replaced by wedge-shaped areas of yellow necrotic tissue with the base located at the corticomedullary junction. As the lesion progresses, a portion of the necrotic papilla may break off, producing a calyceal deformity that results in a recognizable radiologic filling defect. The sloughed portion may be voided and in some instances can be recovered from the urine. Microscopically, edema is initially seen of the interstitium. Eventually the lesion resembles an infarct with coagulation necrosis involving the entire pyramid. The collecting tubules are filled with bacteria and polymorphonuclear leukocytes.

PATHOGENESIS OF URINARY TRACT INFECTION

There are three possible routes by which bacteria can invade and spread within the urinary tract. These are the ascending, hematogenous, and lymphatic pathways.

Ascending Route

The urethra is usually colonized with bacteria. Studies[5] using suprapubic puncture techniques have revealed the occasional presence of small numbers of microorganisms in the urine of uninfected persons. Massage of the urethra in women[6] and presumably sexual intercourse[7–11] can force bacteria into the bladder. Furthermore, just one catherization of the bladder will result in urinary tract infection in about 1 percent of ambulatory patients,[12] and infection will develop within 3 or 4 days in essentially all patients with indwelling catheters with open drainage systems.[13] Both the diaphragm in women and condom catheter in men have been shown to predispose to infection.[10,14–18]

The fact that urinary tract infection is much more common in women than men gives support to the importance of the ascending route of infection. The female urethra is short and is in proximity to the warm moist vulvar and perirectal areas, making contamination likely. It has been shown[19] that the organisms that cause urinary tract infection in women colonize the vaginal introitus and periurethral area before urinary infection results. Once within the bladder, bacteria may multiply and then pass up the ureters, especially if vesicoureteral reflux is present, to the renal pelvis and parenchyma. Animal studies[20] have also confirmed the importance of ascending infection. If bladder bacteriuria is established after unilateral ureteral ligation, only the unligated kidney develops pyelonephritis.

Hematogenous Route

Infection of the renal parenchyma by blood-borne organisms clearly occurs in humans. The kidney is frequently the site of abscesses in patients with staphylococcal bacteremia and/or endocarditis.[21] Experimental pyelonephritis can be produced by intravenous injection of several species of bacteria and even *Candida*.[22–26] However, production of experimental pyelonephritis by the intravenous route with gram-negative enteric bacilli, the common pathogens in urinary tract infection, is difficult. Additional manipulations such as creation of ureteral obstruction are often necessary.[24,25,27] It would appear that in humans, infection of the kidney with gram-negative bacilli rarely occurs by the hematogenous route.

Lymphatic Route

Evidence for a significant role for renal lymphatics in the pathogenesis of pyelonephritis is unimpressive and consists of the demonstration of lymphatic connections between the ureters and kidneys in animals, and the fact that increased pressure in the bladder can cause lymphatic flow to be directed toward the kidney.[28,29]

Thus, it would seem at the present level of understanding that the ascending pathway of infection is the most important.

Host Parasite Interaction

The Organism. Although urinary tract infections are caused by many species of microorganisms, most are due to *Escherichia coli*. However, only a few serogroups of *E. coli*—01, 02, 04, 06, 07, 075—cause a high proportion of infections.[30] This has led to the concept of uropathogenic *E. coli*, whereby certain strains of *E. coli* are selected from the fecal flora by the presence of virulence factors that enhance both colonization and invasion of the urinary tract and the capacity to produce disease.[31] Recognized virulence factors include increased adherence to uroepithelial cells,[31] resistance to serum bactericidal activity,[32] higher quantity of K antigen,[30] presence of aerobactin,[33] and hemolysin production.[33] These factors are less frequently observed among serotypes of *E. coli* in the fecal flora that are less likely to produce infection.[31]

In particular, adhesive properties have been suggested to select bacteria capable of reaching and colonizing the normal urinary tract and to influence the level of infection in the urinary tract (i.e., upper versus only lower tract).[31,34] Accordingly, bacteria with enhanced adherence to vaginal and periurethral cells would be selected to colonize the anatomic regions adjacent to the urethral orifice. Human studies and the mouse model of nonobstructive ascending pyelonephritis have confirmed the significance of the adhesive capacity of the urinary pathogen in causing lower and upper tract infection.[35–38] Svanborg-Eden et al. demonstrated that *E. coli* pyelonephritis isolates adhere better than *E. coli* cystitis isolates, and urinary isolates tend to adhere more strongly to uroepithelial cells than random fecal *E. coli* isolates.[38] The major types of surface adhesins on uropathogenic *E. coli* are fimbrial in nature and may be differentiated by the effect of α-methyl-mannoside. The binding of *E. coli* to epithelial cell receptors containing globoseries glycolipid accounts for the attachment of most strains causing kidney infection and is not inhibited by mannose (MR—for mannose-resistant).[39,40] Fimbriae attaching to globoseries receptors are termed *P fimbriae*. The globoseries glycolipid receptors are distributed throughout the urinary tract, particularly in the kidney.[40] Binding of *E. coli* to mannose-containing receptors occurs with most uropathogenic strains. In fact, strains from cystitis patients are more likely to bind than those from pyelonephritis patients.[38] Fimbriae attaching to mannosides are the common type 1 fimbriae (pili), and attachment is inhibited in the presence of mannose (MS—for mannose sensitive). Urinary mucus or slime is rich in mannose residues, and hence *E. coli* possessing MS adhesins adhere avidly to urinary slime.[41] The biologic significance of this phenomenon is unclear. Currently, in addition to type 1 and P fimbriae, a variety of adhesins including S, type 1c and G fimbriae, and M and X adhesins,[42] with differing molecular binding specificities and serologic properties, have been identified on uropathogenic strains of *E. coli* and are expressed in vivo in urine.[42] Adherent bacteria not only persist within the urinary tract but have growth advantages and enhanced toxicity due to restricted diffusion of products secreted by eukaryotic cells.[43]

Currently, a two-phase concept is postulated regarding adherence kinetics in the pathogenesis of urinary tract infection.[34,35] After entry into the lower urinary tract, MS adhesins, present on the majority of Enterobacteriaceae, are thought to be important for colonization of the bladder and lower urinary tract.[44] Mannose-resistant P fimbriae, on the other hand, appear to be critical for the organisms to reach the pelvis and renal parenchyma.[40] There is evidence to suggest that in vivo a urinary pathogen may alter its surface expression or presentation of adhesins so as to ensure survival.[44,45] Type 1 fimbriae increase the susceptibility of *E. coli* to neutrophil phagocytosis.[34] Therefore, not surprisingly, *E. coli* cease to express these fimbriae on reaching the renal parenchyma.[34] This phenomenon is called *phasic variation*. In contrast to type 1 fimbriae, polymorphonuclear leukocytes lack receptors for P fimbriae, and the latter block phagocytosis.[46]

Studies with other species of bacteria have similarly demonstrated the significance of adherence in the pathogenesis of urinary infections. Silverblatt,[45] confirmed the role of fimbriae in *Proteus mirabilis* attachment to the renal pelvic mucosa, and similar observations have been made with *Klebsiella* sp.[47] *Staphylococcus aureus* uncommonly causes cystitis and ascending pyelonephritis; in contrast, *Staphylococcus saprophyticus* is a frequent cause of lower urinary tract infections. *Staphylococcus saprophyticus* adheres significantly better to uroepithelial cells than *S. aureus* or *Staphylococcus epidermidis*.[48] The significance of adherence has been emphasized by inhibition of experimental ascending *E. coli* urinary tract infection by the use of epithelial cell–surface receptor analogues.[49,50] Trimethoprim—sulfamethoxazole, extensively used to prevent urinary infection, at concentrations well below the minimum inhibitory concentration (MIC) reduces synthesis, expression, and adhesive function of type 1 fimbriae.[51]

Evaluation of urinary isolates for virulence characteristics in the presence of underlying structural abnormalities (e.g., severe reflux) frequently fails to demonstrate the typical bacterial virulence factors. Therefore, in complicated urinary tract infections virulence factors are often absent, and a natural selection of uropathogens is not apparent.[34] Similarly, *E. coli* blood isolates obtained from patients with urosepsis following bladder instrumentation lack virulence factors.[52]

The importance of adherence as a virulence factor is not complete without consideration of the role of the host. A difference in receptor density linked to variable susceptibility to infection has been proposed. In women and children with recurrent urinary tract infection, an increased avidity of bacterial attachment has been found to vaginal,[53] periurethral,[54] and uroepithelial[55,56] cells. However, several other authors have failed to corroborate these findings.[57] Thus, the role of receptors as biologic risk factors in uncomplicated urinary tract infections remains unsettled.

Certain other characteristics of bacteria may be important in the production of upper tract infection. Motile bacteria can ascend in the ureter against the flow of urine,[58] and the endotoxins of gram-negative bacilli have been shown to decrease ureteral peristalsis,[59] but contribute to the renal parenchymal inflammatory response by phagocytic cell activation.[60] Production of urease by infecting microorganisms such as *Proteus* species has been related to ability to cause pyelonephritis.[61]

Several experimental studies[23,27] have shown that the greater the number of organisms delivered to the kidneys, the greater the chance of producing infection. The kidney itself is not uniformly susceptible to infection, since very few organisms are needed to infect the medulla, whereas 10,000 times as many are needed to infect the cortex.[22,62] The greater susceptibility of the medulla may be due to the high concentration of ammonia, which may inactivate complement,[63] and to poor chemotaxis of polymorphonuclear leukocytes into an area of high osmolality, low pH, and low blood flow.[64]

The Host. With the exception of urethral mucosa, the normal urinary tract is resistant to colonization by bacteria and for the most part efficiently and rapidly eliminates both pathogenic and nonpathogenic microorganisms that gain access to the bladder. This is achieved by the presence of several lower urinary tract antibacterial defense mechanisms.

Although urine is generally considered to be a good culture medium for most bacteria, it does possess antibacterial activity. Anaerobic bacteria and other fastidious organisms that make up most of the urethral flora generally do not multiply in urine. It has been shown that extremes of osmolality, high urea concentration, and low pH levels are inhibitory for the growth of some of the bacteria that cause urinary tract infection.[65] Furthermore, the pH and osmolality of urine from pregnant women tend to be more suitable for bacterial growth than those of nonpregnant women, which in turn are more suitable for bacterial growth than urine from men.[66] The presence of glucose makes urine a better culture medium, whereas the addition of prostatic fluid to urine inhibits bacterial growth.[66,67] Furthermore, urine has been shown to inhibit the migrating, adhering, aggregating, and killing functions of polymorphonuclear leukocytes.[68]

The flushing mechanism of the bladder apparently exerts a protective effect. When bacteria are introduced into the bladders of humans, there is a tendency for spontaneous clearance.[69] Since "flushing" alone would probably not completely clear the bacteria, there must be additional protective factors. Host factors including bladder catheterization influence susceptibility of uroepithelial cells to attachment by uropathogens, and this in turn increases susceptibility to bacteriuria.[70]

Parsons et al., in a study of bladder defense mechanisms in dogs, demonstrated an active antiadherence mechanism of bladder mucosa.[71] Pretreatment of the bladder with acid was shown to increase bacterial adherence 20- to 50-fold. The increased adherence was independent of the bacterial species employed.[72] Histochemical studies revealed that bacterial adherence was increased by the removal of a surface mucopolysaccharide, glycosaminoglycan, which seems to be responsible for the natural resistance to adherence.[73] Thus, normally small inocula of bacteria are probably unable to adhere, remain suspended in urine, and are removed by voiding. In the presence of a larger bladder inoculum of bacteria, especially with good adhesive qualities, the primary defense of antiadherence may be overcome, colonization can occur, and subsequent bladder infection may result.[74] With the occurence of bladder infection, secondary defense mechanisms such as mobilization of leukocytes, phagocytosis, and bacterial destruction are called on to remove bacteria.[74,75]

Colonization of the vaginal introitus and periurethral region by Enterobacteriaceae is thought by some to be important in the pathogenesis of urinary tract infections in women.[19] Several authors have shown that periurethral colonization with the same organism almost invariably precedes episodes of significant bacteriuria.[19,76,77] Microbiologic studies have demonstrated that the urethra, periurethral region, and vaginal vestibule of women with recurrent urinary tract infections tends to be more commonly colonized with coliform bacteria.[53,54,76] Stamey has postulated that such colonization is often the prelude to new infection[76] and that women with recurrent urinary tract infection have a biologic predisposition to infection. The hypothesis is that these women have defective local perineal and vaginal defense mechanisms that result in increased susceptibility to introital and perineal colonization with urinary pathogens such as coliform bacteria.[76] In a series of studies, the effects of several factors in vaginal secretions on colonization were examined.[53,78–83] It appeared that a low vaginal pH level was the most important factor related to lack of colonization. Furthermore, serogroups of *E. coli* that were more likely to cause urinry tract infection were more resistant to low pH levels than serogroups that did not commonly cause infection. It was also found in these studies that *E. coli* was less susceptible to the inhibitory effects of vaginal fluid than *P. mirabilis* or *Pseudomonas aeruginosa*. Finally, it was noted that *E. coli* adhered more avidly to vaginal epithelial cells of women with recurrent urinary tract infection, and this was attributed to reduced local production of antibodies in vaginal secretions.[53] Kallenius et al. similarly showed that the periurethral cells of young girls prone to recurrent urinary tract infections were more susceptible to bacterial attachment,[54] and other authors found enhanced attachment of *E. coli* to uroepithelial cells of patients with recurrent urinary tract infections.[55,56] Not all authors agree that introital colonization is the most important factor in the pathogenesis of recurrent urinary tract infection.[77,84–87] They point out that introital colonization with Enterobacteriaceae is as common in women not prone to infection. Furthermore, Parsons et al. found no enhanced bacterial adherence to vaginal epithelial cells in women with recurrent urinary tract infection,[57] and Kurdydyk et al. found no difference in IgG and IgA levels in cervicovaginal washings between women prone to infection and those with no past history of urinary tract infection.[88] These studies failed to confirm the hypothesis that women with recurrent bacteriuria possess a local periurethral and vaginal defect in host resistance. Kunin et al.[77] stated the view that all women who do not have a structural or neurologic problem in the voiding mechanism are approximately at the same risk of having a first urinary tract infection. In their view, once established, each infection sets the stage for the next episode, since infection itself may lead to colonization unless periurethral colonization is eradicated by therapy. Antimicrobial therapy per se may alter periurethral flora in favor of colonization with enteric organisms. The longer the interval between infections, the less likelihood there is for recurrences. The antagonists to Stamey's hypothesis have concluded that the decisive factor is not the colonization of the periurethral area per se but rather the ability of these organisms to ascend the urethra including the ability of infecting organisms to adhere to mucosal cells and withstand normal host defense mechanisms.

The role of humoral immunity in the host's defense against infection of the urinary tract, although extensively studied, is poorly understood, as summarized in several reviews.[89–100] During acute pyelonephritis, there is a systemic antibody response. Antibodies against the O antigen and occasionally the K antigen of the infecting strain have been found, and recently antibodies to type 1 and P fimbriae were described.[93,101] IgM antibodies dominate in the response to the first upper tract infection but not to subsequent episodes. Of note is the observation that high levels of IgG antibodies to lipid A correlate with the severity of renal infection and progression of renal parenchyma destruction.[94] An antibody response consisting of IgG and secretory IgA antibodies can be detected in the urine. In contrast to upper tract infection, lower urinary infection is usually associated with a reduced or nondetectable serologic response reflecting the superficial nature of the infection. However, recently Hopkins et al., using a monkey model, reported the production of systemic and urinary IgG and IgA that accompanied experimental cystitis.[102]

In particular, antipili antibodies are absent in the urine in lower tract infection.[99] Systemic serologic response has been used to distinguish between upper and lower urinary tract infection, but is not practical because of too many false-negative and false-positive results. However, local coating of bacteria with antibodies within the kidney (and prostate) has formed the basis of modern localization techniques.

In spite of the impressive systemic and local urinary antibody production that follows acute pyelonephritis, the protective role of these antibodies is unclear. When bacteria persist in the kidney for several months, antigenic drift may occur.[95] Nevertheless, antibodies against several bacterial structures including O and K antigen and more recently fimbrial antigens have been found to protect against hematogenous or ascending pyelonephritis in experimental animals.[92,93,96]

Antibodies may be of value in limiting the damage incurred within the kidney or preventing colonization preceeding recurrence. Svanborg-Eden et al. reported that the urine of patients with pyelonephritis inhibited the adherence of *E. coli* to uroepithelial cells and that this activity was removed by absorption with O antigen.[97] Antibodies have not been shown to protect against bladder infection.[98,99] Cell-mediated immunity has not been shown to play a major role in host defenses against urinary tract infection.[90]

During pyelonephritis, an acute inflammatory exudate consisting predominantly of polymorphonuclear leukocytes is present. Although the inflammatory reaction is directed at limiting bacterial spread and persistence within the kidney, it has been suggested that the infiltrating phagocytic cells may contribute to tissue damage and renal scarring. Using experimental animals, Bille and Glauser were able to reduce parenchymal kidney destruction by inducing neutropenia as well as by interfering with leukocyte migration.[103] The clinical significance of these observations is unclear, since any interference with the normal inflammatory response may possibly contribute to bacteremia.

Several studies[1] have demonstrated persistence of bacterial antigens in kidneys of experimental animals following renal infection. This suggests the possibility of autoimmunity as an explanation for progression of the lesion in "chronic pyelonephritis." An interesting observation is that patients with acute pyelonephritis have increased serum antibody titers against Tamm-Horsfall protein.[104] This protein is formed in the tubular region and is excreted in the urine. It has been speculated that these act as autoantibodies in the renal parenchyma. Cross-reactivity between the Tamm-Horsfall protein and gram-negative bacteria has been reported by Fasth et al., raising the possibility of antibody induced by gram-negative bacilli injuring renal cells containing Tamm-Horsfall protein even after elimination of the bacteria.[100] On the other hand, the highest concentrations of serum IgG and IgA antibodies against Tamm-Horsfall protein were seen in patients with vesicoureteral reflux even in the absence of bacteriuria, suggesting that after tubular–interstitial damage, Tamm-Horsfall antigen could act as an independent antigen unrelated to the presence of bacterial antigens.[100]

Aoki and colleagues,[105] examined kidney tissue from patients with proven pyelonephritis and others with renal scarring suggestive of pyelonephritis who had no history of bacteriuria. Bacterial antigen was found in all patients in the first group and was present in biopsy specimens from most in the second group. They concluded that there might be a group of patients with cryptogenic renal scarring of a pyelonephritic type in whom the pathologic process was related not to the presence of viable bacteria but to an ongoing destructive interaction between bacterial antigen and antibody. Subsequent work[106] has not confirmed the observations of Aoki et al.

There are several abnormalities of the urinary tract that interfere with its natural resistance to infection. Obstruction to urine flow is the most important of these. Extrarenal obstruction can result from congenital anomalies of the ureter or urethra such as valves, stenosis, or bands; calculi; extrinsic ureteral compression from a variety of causes; benign prostatic hypertrophy; and others. Intrarenal obstruction may be produced by entities such as nephrocalcinosis, uric acid nephropathy, analgesic nephropathy, polycystic kidney disease, hypokalemic nephropathy, and the renal lesions of sickle cell trait or disease.[107] Obstruction inhibits the normal flow of urine, and the resulting stasis is probably important in increasing susceptibility to infection.

In animals, obstruction of a ureter markedly increases susceptibility to hematogenous infection.[27] Intrarenal obstruction, experimentally produced by scars in a variety of ways, also increases susceptibility of the kidney to infection. Medullary scars, which produce greater amounts of obstruction than cortical scars, increase the susceptibility of animals to infection more than cortical scars.[108] Furthermore, the intravenous injection of *E. coli* in animals with renal scars from prior staphylococcal pyelonephritis produces pyelonephritis in the regions of intrarenal hydronephrosis caused by the old scars.[109] Men of any age and pregnant women are the most prone to lesions that result in obstruction to the free flow of urine.

Calculi may increase susceptibility to urinary tract infection by producing obstruction. However, not all stones obstruct, and local irritative phenomena may also be important. Furthermore, calculi may develop secondary to infection. It has been observed clinically and experimentally that *Proteus* species and other urea-splitting organisms (e.g., *Klebsiella*) are most likely to produce calculi.[110] Furthermore, bacteria survive deep within the calculi and are extremely difficult to eradicate even by artificial means such as by incubating in solutions containing antibiotics or iodine and alcohol.[111] This may account for the well-known difficulties encountered clinically in trying to cure urinary tract infection in the presence of stones.

Vesicoureteral reflux and urinary tract infection are also intricately related. Reflux due either to a congenital abnormality, bladder overdistension, or unknown etiology, probably contributes to upper tract infection via the ascending route. On the other hand, clinical observations have demonstrated that infection may, in itself, produce reflux especially in children.[112] Reflux tends to perpetuate infection by maintaining a residual pool of infected urine in the bladder after voiding. It is probable that reflux, especially in young children, plays an important role in the production of upper tract infection and subsequent scarring.[113] Patients with incomplete emptying of the bladder for either mechanical reasons (bladder neck obstruction, urethral valves, urethral strictures, prostatic hypertrophy) or neurogenic malfunctions (poliomyelitis, tabes dorsalis, diabetic neuropathy, cord injuries) are prone to frequent urinary tract infections. These patients are subject to bladder overdistension, which may interfere with local defense mechanisms, and, most importantly, frequent instrumentation of the urinary tract.

EPIDEMIOLOGY OF URINARY TRACT INFECTION

Infecting Organisms

There is a great difference between the bacterial flora of the urine in patients with an initial episode of urinary tract infection as compared with the flora from those with frequent recurrences of infection. *Escherichia coli* is by far the most frequent infecting organism in acute infection.[114] In so called "chronic" urinary tract infection, especially in the presence of structural abnormalities of the urinary tract (such as obstructive uropathy, congenital anomalies, neurogenic bladder, and fistulous communication involving the urinary tract), the relative frequency of infection caused by *Proteus, Pseudomonas, Klebsiella Enterobacter* species, and by enterococci and staphylococci increases greatly. In the presence of structural abnormalities, it is also relatively common to isolate multiple organisms from the urine. Since instrumentation and repeated courses of antimicrobial therapy are common in these patients, antibiotic-resistant isolates might be expected.

The hospital environment is an important determinant of the nature of the bacterial flora in urinary tract infection. *Proteus, Klebsiella, Enterobacter, Pseudomonas*, staphylococci, and enterococci are more often isolated from inpatients, as compared with a greater preponderance of *E. coli* in an outpatient population.[115,116] Cross-infections are important in the pathogenesis of hospital-related urinary tract infections, especially with indwelling catheters.[116,117]

Anaerobic organisms are rarely pathogens in the urinary tract.[118] A variety of bacteria may be found in the urine in specific clinical settings. For example, *Salmonella* species are found with *Salmonella* bacteremia.[119] Fungi (particularly *Candida* species) occur in patients with indwelling catheters who are receiving antimicrobial therapy. Coagulase-negative staphylococci are a common cause of urinary tract infection in some reports.[120] *Staphylococcus saprophyticus* tends to cause infection in young, sexually active females.[121,122] Coagulase-positive staphylococci most often invade the kidney from the hematogenous route resulting in intrarenal or perinephric abscesses.[21] Serotyping of *E. coli* has substantially aided in the epidemologic study of urinary tract infection. Using these techniques, it has been demonstrated that only a relatively small number of serologically distinct strains (e.g., 04, 06, 075, and secondarily 01, 02, and 07) are responsible for a major proportion of *E. coli* urinary tract infections.[123,124]

Adenoviruses (particularly type 11) have been strongly implicated as causative agents in hemorrhagic cystitis in pediatric patients, especially boys.[125,126] Cell-wall deficient bacteria have been demonstrated in urine from patients with pyelonephritis, particularly in association with therapy using cell-wall active antibiotics.[127] However, these forms have not been consistently isolated from either urine or renal tissue despite the use of adequate techniques and are probably not of major importance.

Bacteriuria in Children

The problem of urinary tract infection spans all age groups beginning with neonates. The incidence of urinary tract infection in infants up to 6 months is about 2 cases per 1000 live births and is much more common in boys.[128,129] Bacteremia is often present. Autopsy series have also revealed a predominance of infant boys with pyelonephritis.[130]

During the preschool years, urinary tract infection is more common in girls than in boys.[128] When infection occurs in preschool boys it is frequently associated with serious congenital abnormalities. With repeated study over a period of 1 year, the period prevalance of significant bacteriuria in this age group was reported to be 4.5 percent for girls and about 0.5 percent for boys.[131] Infections during this period often are symptomatic, and it is believed that much of the renal damage that occurs from urinary tract infection takes place at this time.[113,132]

Much information on the natural history and epidemiology of urinary tract infection has been gleaned from the studies of Kunin and associates with school children from central Virginia.[133–135] It was found that bacteriuria is common in girls in this population, is often asymptomatic, and frequently recurs. For example, the prevalence of bacteriuria among school girls was about 1.2 percent, and about 5 percent of the girls had significant bacteriuria at some time before leaving high school. About one-third of these patients had some symptom referable to the urinary tract when the bacteriuria was first detected. It was shown that each year about 0.3 to 0.4 percent of the female population (25 percent of those infected) was either cured spontaneously or with antimicrobial agents and was replaced by an equal number who developed bacteriuria. Bacteriuria was rare in school boys (prevalence 0.03 percent).

These studies also provided an opportunity to treat the patients and follow their clinical course. Patients were initially treated for 10 days to 2 weeks. Girls with frequent infections were given longer courses of therapy (1–3 months). Caucasian girls tended to have frequent reinfections, whereas black girls became reinfected less frequently. With each course of therapy, about 20 percent of white girls went into long-term remission. However, when many of these girls were married or became pregnant, bacteriuria recurred at a rate far above that expected for the general population. Over 50 percent developed bacteriuria within 3 months after marriage. Thus, the presence of bacteriuria in childhood defines a population at higher risk for the development of bacteriuria in adulthood.

Bacteriuria in Adults

Once adulthood is reached, the prevalence of bacteriuria increases in the female population. The prevalence of bacteriuria in young nonpregnant women is about 1–3 percent.[136,137] Each year about 25 percent of bacteriuric women clear their bacteriuria and are replaced by an equal number who have become infected (often women who have had urinary infection previously). At least 10–20 percent of the female population experience a symtomatic urinary tract infection at some time during their life.[137,138] Both sexual intercourse and diaphragm use are risk factors for urinary infection in women.[10,14–16,18] The diaphragm can cause urinary obstruction in some women, but its main effect may be a change in vaginal flora.[16]

The prevalence of bacteriuria in adult men is low (0.1 percent or less) until the later years, when it rises. The increase in bacteriuria in older men is probably mainly related to prostatic disease and the resultant instrumentation. Men with bacteriuria frequently have anatomic abnormalities of the urinary tract.

Bacteriuria in the Elderly

At least 10 percent of men and 20 percent of women over 65 have bacteriuria. In contrast to young adults, in whom bacteriuria is 30 times more frequent in women than men, over the age of 65 the ratio alters dramatically, with a progressive decrease in the female–male ratio.[139–141] In both sexes, the prevalance of bateriuria rises substantially. Possible reasons for the high frequency of urinary infection in the elderly include obstructive uropathy from the prostate and loss of bactericidal activity of prostatic secretions in men, poor emptying of the bladder due to prolapse in women, soiling of the perineum from fecal incontinence in demented women, and neuromuscular diseases and increased instrumentation and bladder catheter usage in both sexes.[139,140,142] There is a high rate of spontaneous cure and reinfection in both women and men.[141] The spectrum of microorganisms is unaltered in the elderly.

Bacteriuria in Patients with Other Conditions

Several studies[143,144] have reported a higher prevalence of bacteriuria in hospitalized patients as compared with outpatients. It is stated that the general ill health of hospitalized patients as well as the higher probability of urinary tract instrumentation are the major contributors to these differences.

A single catheterization causes urinary tract infection in only about 1 percent of ambulatory persons.[12] However, after catheterization of hospitalized patients, infection occurs in at least 10 percent.[12] Race apparently does not appreciably affect the prevalence of bacteriuria. However, socioeconomic status is important, with pregnant women from lower socioeconomic groups having a higher prevalence of bacteriuria.[145]

Various underlying diseases have also been associated with an increased frequency of urinary tract infection. While diabetic women have been found to have a higher prevalence of bacteriuria in some studies, others have found no difference in the prevalence between normals and diabetics.[146] The higher prevalence of bacteriuria in diabetics in some series may be attributed, at least in part, to more frequent catheterization.

Black women with sickle cell trait have a higher prevalence of bacteriuria during pregnancy than black women without sickle trait.[147] Other conditions stated to be associated with urinary tract infection (but without documentation) include chronic potassium deficiency, gout, hypertension, and other conditions causing interstitial renal disease.

CLINICAL MANIFESTATIONS

Symptoms

Urinary tract infection in children tends to manifest with different symptoms depending on the age of the child.[128,129,148,149] Symptoms in neonates and children less than 2 years of age are nonspecific.[128,129,148,149] Failure to thrive, vomiting, and fever seem to be the major manifestations. When children over 2 years of age (and more consistently above 5) develop infection, they are more likely to display localizing symptoms such as frequency, dysuria, and abdominal or flank pain.

The manifestations of urinary tract infection in adults are usually easy to recognize. The lower tract symptoms result from bacteria producing irritation of urethral and vesical mucosa causing frequent and painful urination of small amounts of turbid urine. Patients sometimes complain of suprapubic heaviness or pain. Occasionally the urine is grossly bloody or shows a bloody tinge at the end of micturition. Fever tends to be absent in infection limited to the lower tract.

The classic clinical manifestation of upper urinary tract infection includes fever (sometimes with chills), flank pain, and frequently lower tract symptoms (e.g., frequency, urgency, and dysuria). At times the lower tract symptoms antedate the appearance of fever and upper tract symptoms by 1 or 2 days. It should be recognized that the symptoms described, while classic, may vary greatly. In fact, pyelonephritis may show protean clinical manifestations in adults as well as in children. Flank tenderness or discomfort is frequent in upper tract infection in adults and is more intense when there is obstructive disease. Severe pain with radiation into the groin is rare in acute pyelonephritis per se and suggests the presence of a renal calculus. The pain from the kidney is occasionally felt in or near the epigastrium and may radiate to one of the lower quadrants. These manifestations may offer difficulties in differential diagnosis and suggest gallbladder disease or appendicitis.

The vast majority of elderly patients with urinary infection are asymptomatic; in addition, pyuria may be absent.[139,140] Symptoms, when present, are often not diagnostic since noninfected elderly patients often experience frequency, dysuria, hesitancy, and incontinence. Nevertheless, typical symptoms may occur, and less frequently acute pyelonephritis develops, usually necessitating hospitalization. Gleckman et al. found a much higher frequency of bacteremia (61 percent) associated with pyelonephritis in the elderly than is found in the young, and shock commonly supervened.[150] Most of the patients had significant urologic abnormalities. The effect of asymptomatic bacteriuria on the general sense of well-being, appetite, and urinary continence has been studied, and in one investigation no association could be demonstrated.[151]

The clinical manifestations of recurrent or persistent urinary tract infection are more difficult to define. Patients with lower urinary tract involvement tend to have repeated bouts of transient symptomatic or asymptomatic infection. Patients with upper tract infection may have episodes of fever, pain in the renal regions, and dysuria during acute exacerbations or new bouts of infection. However, upper tract infection may result in only lower tract symptoms or no symptoms at all. Patients with urinary tract infection in the presence of an indwelling urinary catheter usually have no lower tract symptoms, but flank pain or fever are common. Urinary tract infection is the most common source of bacteremia produced by gram-negative bacilli. Bacteremia may occur with no urinary symptoms, especially in the presence of an indwelling catheter.

Alterations in Renal Function

In experimentally produced pyelonephritis, the only consistent abnormality of renal function is the inability to concentrate the urine maximally.[152] The mechanism of the concentrating defect is not clear but seems to be related in experimental animals to inflammation and perhaps to increased production of prostaglandins.[153,154] The concentrating defect occurs early in the course of experimental infection and is rapidly reversible with antimicrobial therapy and following the administration of prostaglandin inhibitors.[152,153] The same phenomenon occurs in humans.[155]

Progressive destruction of the kidney (particularly in the presence of obstruction) may occur and give rise to clinical manifestations of renal insufficiency. Bilateral papillary necrosis occasionally can lead to rapidly progressive renal failure.[156]

DIAGNOSIS

Presumptive Diagnosis of Urinary Tract Infection

Microscopic examination of the urine is the first step in laboratory diagnosis of urinary tract infection. A clean-catch midstream urine specimen is centrifuged for 5 minutes at 2000 rpm, and then the sediment is examined under high power. Each leukocyte seen represents about 5–10 cells/mm^3 of urine; 10–50 white cells/mm^3 have been stated to be the upper limit of normal.[157] With this criterion 5–10 leukocytes per high-power field in the sediment from a clean-catch midstream urine specimen is the upper limit of normal, as they represent 50–100 cells/mm^3. Although more elaborate and precise methods for determining the urinary concentration of leukocytes have been evaluated, it is generally not necessary to use these clinically.[157] It should be emphasized that the finding of pyuria is nonspecific, and patients with and without pyuria may or may not have infection.[158] However, the vast majority of patients with symptomatic infection have significant pyuria.[159] Using a stricter definition of pyuria (at least 10 leukocytes per mm^3 of midstream urine by counting chamber), the vast majority of patients with either symptomatic or asymptomatic bacteriuria will have pyuria. However, pyuria without infection remains common.[160]

Microscopic or sometimes gross hematuria is occasionally seen in patients with urinary tract infection (i.e., hemorrhagic cystitis). However, red blood cells may be indicative of other disorders such as calculi, tumor, vasculitis, glomerulonephritis, and renal tuberculosis. White cell casts in the presence of an acute infectious process are strong evidence for pyelonephritis, but the absence of white cell casts does not rule out upper tract infection. White cell casts can also be seen in renal disease in the absence of infection.

Proteinuria is a common although not universal finding in urinary tract infection. Most patients with urinary tract infection excrete less than 2 g of protein in 24 hours; excretion of 3 g or more suggests glomerular disease.

One of the most useful tests for presumptive diagnosis of urinary tract infection is the microscopic examination of a specimen for bacteria. The ability to identify bacteria in the urine depends on whether or not the specimen has been centrifuged and on whether or not it has been stained with Gram or methylene blue stain[161] (Table 1). Smaller numbers of bacteria can be detected microscopically in a stained than in an unstained specimen, and smaller numbers can be detected in a centrifuged than in uncentrifuged urine. Presence of at least one bacterium per oil-immersion field in a midstream, clean-catch, Gram-stained, uncentrifuged urine correlates with $\geq 10^5$ bacteria/ml of urine. As this titer is regarded to represent significant bacteriuria, Gram staining of an uncentrifuged specimen is an easy, rapid, and relatively reliable way to detect significant numbers of organisms. The absence of bacteria in several fields in a stained sedimented specimen indicates the probability of less than 10^4 bacteria/ml.

Several biochemical tests have been devised to detect bacteriuria for presumptive diagnosis. The many variations of the griess test (a diazotization reaction) detect the presence of nitrite in the urine that is formed when bacteria reduce the nitrate that is normally present.[161,162] Bacteria that possess dehydrogenase activity are able to reduce triphenyltetrazolium chloride (TTC), causing a color reaction to occur if these bacteria are present.[161,162] Both tests unfortunately often give false-negative results, but a combination of the two is more accurate. The detection of subnormal urinary glucose in patients with urinary tract infections is another test that has been used with very few false-positive and false-negative results.[163] Because of their general lack of specificity, biochemical tests for bacteriuria should not be routinely used in management of patients with urinary tract infection. Recently, automated rapid screening tests have become available that may be cost-effective for processing large numbers of samples.[164]

TABLE 1. Correlation of Methods of Direct Examination of Urine for Bacteria with Quantitative Cultures

	Unstained	*Stained*
Uncentrifuged	$\geq 10^6$(400×)	$\geq 10^5$(1000×)
Centrifuged	$\geq 10^5$(400×)	$\geq 10^4$(1000×)

Diagnosis of Urinary Tract Infection by Culture

Urine in the bladder is normally sterile. Since the urethra and periurethral areas are very difficult to sterilize, even the most carefully collected specimens (including those obtained by catheterization) are frequently contaminated. By quantitating bacteria in midstream, clean-voided urine, it is possible statistically to separate contamination from urinary tract infection. Patients with infection usually have $\geq 10^5$ bacteria/ml in urine in the bladder, and therefore voided urine usually contains $\geq 10^5$ bacteria/ml.[13] Patients without infection have sterile bladder urine and with proper collection, voided urine usually contains $<10^4$ bacteria/ml. However, it is important to remember that about one-third of young women with symptomatic lower tract infection have $<10^5$ bacteria per ml urine (see below under "Urethral Syndrome"). It is likely that a significant proportion of other patients with both symptomatic and asymptomatic infection have $<10^5$ bacteria per ml urine.

Several methods can be employed to quantitate bacteria present in urine. The serial dilution and pour plate method is the most accurate[165] but is cumbersome and not suitable for routine use in a busy clinical laboratory. Calibrated loops serve as a simple inexpensive way to examine quantitatively the bacteriologic characteristics of urine specimens.[166] Platinum loops that deliver 0.01 ml and 0.001 ml are used to streak urine onto agar plates. After incubating at 37°C for 24 hours the number of colony-forming units are counted, and the total number of organisms originally present in the specimen is estimated by multiplying the colony count by 10^2 or 10^3, respectively. A further refinement of the technique involves the use of differential agars to allow isolation from mixed cultures and more rapid identification.

Other methods of quantitative culture include (*1*) the flood plate method, which is similar to the calibrated loop method but involves pipetting a volume of urine onto a plate[165]; (*2*) the filter paper method[165] in which a given volume of urine is absorbed in a piece of filter paper and then put on a plate; and (*3*) the dip inoculum method[167] in which an agar-coated glass slide is dipped into urine. The dip inoculum method and its variants have excellent correlation with pour plate techniques and are available for office use at inexpensive prices.[149]

Acceptable methods for urine collection include (*1*) midstream clean catch, (*2*) catheterization, and (*3*) suprapubic aspiration. The clean-catch method is preferred for routine collection of urine for culture. It avoids the risk of infection inherent in catheterization. The patient must be instructed in the proper technique of obtaining the urine; this is especially important in women. The woman should wash her hands, straddle the commode (facing the back of the commode), wash the vulva from front to back four times with four different sterile gauze pads soaked in green soap or another appropriate cleansing agent and then rinse with two more sponges soaked in sterile distilled water. She should then spread the labia and void, discarding the first portion of urine and collecting the second. The urine should be processed immediately or, if refrigerated at 4°C, can be cultured within 24 hours. In men the prepuce should be retracted, and thereafter the technique is similar. In infants and small children sterile bags have been used for collection of urine, but contamination is common.[168]

In patients unable to cooperate, such as those with an altered sensorium, or those who are unable to void for neurologic or urologic reasons, catheterization may be necessary. When catheterization is performed, scrupulous aseptic technique should be observed.

The suprapubic aspiration method has been established as a safe technique in premature infants, neonates, children, adults, and even pregnant patients.[5,128,149,169] With this method the bladder must be full. The patient refrains from voiding until the bladder can be percussed above the pubic and suprapubic pressure causes the urge to void. After preparation of the skin, the bladder is then punctured above the symphysis pubis with a 22-gauge needle on a syringe (local anesthesia is not required). Following the procedure self-limited hematuria may be observed. Suprapubic aspiration may be indicated in special clinical situations such as in pediatric practice when urine is difficult to obtain. Another situation is the rare adult in whom infection is suspected, results obtained from more routine procedures have been confusing or equivocal, and diagnosis is critical.

If there are more than 10^5 bacteria/ml in a clean-catch urine specimen from an asymptomatic woman, there is an 80 percent probability that this represents true bacteriuria. If two different specimens demonstrate at least 10^5 of the same bacterium per ml, the probability increases to 95 percent. Thus two clean-catch specimens should be obtained in an asymptomatic woman to confirm the diagnosis. When the number of bacteria per ml is between 10^4 and 10^5 in an asymptomatic woman, a confirmatory second specimen will contain $\geq 10^5$ bacteria/ml in only 5 percent of instances. Thus in asymptomatic women 95 percent of the time 10^4–10^5 bacteria/ml represents contamination, with occasional infection manifested by $<10^5$ bacteria per ml urine. In men, in whom contamination is less likely, 10^4 organisms/ml is more suggestive of infection.[170] False-positive cultures are caused by contamination or incubation of urine before processing. False-negative cultures may be due to use of antimicrobial agents, soap from the preparation falling in the urine, total obstruction below the infection, infection with a fastidious organism, renal tuberculosis, and diuresis.[171]

These criteria apply only to the Enterobacteriaceae. Gram-positive organisms, fungi, and bacteria with fastidious growth requirements may not reach titers of 10^5/ml in patients with infection and may be in the 10^4–10^5/ml range.[165] The organism recovered often helps distinguish contamination from true bacteriuria. Samples with counts of less than 10^4 organisms/ml often contain saprophytic skin organisms such as diphtheroids, *Neisseria*, and staphylococci. Pure growth of Enterobacteriaceae is uncommonly found in low-titer specimens but is present in over 90 percent of the urines containing more than 10^5 bacteria/ml. High colony counts containing more than one species of bacteria from urine of asymptomatic persons often represent contamination but may be more significant in the presence of symptoms. Mixed infection occurs in about 5 percent of the cases.

In patients with symptoms of urinary tract infection, one titer of $\geq 10^5$ bacteria per ml urine carries a 95 percent probability of true bacteriuria. With titers of $<10^5$/ml but in the presence of frequency, urgency, and dysuria, women have a one-third chance of having bacterial infection (see "Urethral Syndrome" below). Presence of low numbers of Enterobacteriaceae (i.e., 10^2–10^5/ml) in such women correlates highly with infection. Presence of $<10^2$/ml Enterobacteriaceae is evidence against urinary tract infection.[172]

Samples obtained by catheterization from noninfected patients are less likely to become contaminated enough to demonstrate 10^5 bacteria/ml. For example, one catheterized specimen in an asymptomatic patient that contains 10^5 or more organisms/ml has a 95 percent chance of indicating infection, and counts between 10^4 and 10^5/ml (which are uncommon) are significant at least 50 percent of the time. The contamination is presumably from the urethra. Bladder urine obtained by suprapubic aspiration is either sterile or contains significant growth even if bacterial numbers are below 10^5 ml. The practice of forcing fluids before the procedure tends to reduce titers.[173] In fact, almost 50 percent of such specimens contain $<10^5$ organisms/ml. However, small numbers of bacteria may be found in aspirated urine from presumably noninfected persons.[5] This suggests that bladder urine may be occasionally contaminated from the urethra.

Urethral Syndrome. Most women with acute onset of frequency, urgency, and/or dysuria have urinary tract infection with $\geq 10^5$ bacteria per ml urine (Fig. 6). However, about 40 percent are found to have $<10^5$ bacteria per ml urine and the term *urethral syndrome* has been used to refer to this entity.[174] Stamm et al.[175] have shown that about one-third of young female patients with the urethral syndrome have bacteria in bladder urine as demonstrated by suprapubic puncture. Thus they have urinary infections that are probably mainly restricted to the lower tract. Furthermore, about a quarter of young women with symptomatic infection localized to the lower urinary tract have $<10^5$/ml bacteria in urine. Pyuria (defined as ≥ 8 leukocytes/mm^3 uncentrifuged urine) is found in these patients with bacteria in the bladder but $<10^5$ ml in voided urine. In a prospective double-blind placebo controlled study such patients were shown to benefit from antimicrobial therapy, confirming the relevance of bacterial pathogens in low titer.[176]

The remaining patients with the urethral syndrome (after excluding those with bacteria in the bladder and those with genital herpes infection or vaginitis) can be divided into two groups: (*1*) those with sterile pyuria from urethritis due to *Chlamydia trachomatis*, less frequently *Neisseria gonorrhoeae* infection, and (*2*) those without pyuria in whom all cultures are negative. The pathogenesis of this symptom complex is unknown, but *Ureaplasma urealyticum* as well as noninfectious factors (traumatic, psychological, allergic, and chemical) have been suggested as causes. Patients with *C. trachomatis* and *N. gonorrhoeae* urethritis respond to antimicrobial therapy. Komaroff et al. reported that vaginitis was a common cause of dysuria, and, accordingly, patients should be questioned regarding vaginal symptoms particularly if the complaint of burning is external, such as pain felt in the inflamed vaginal labia during micturition.[177] Dysuria has also been described in 10 percent of women with initial genital herpes infection.[178]

While symptoms and the clinical setting cannot reliably distinguish between causes of frequency, urgency, and dysruia, they can be suggestive. Bacterial urinary tract infections tend to have a sudden onset of symptoms; suprapubic pain and hematuria may be present. Clinical clues to chlamydial infection include a gradual onset of internal dysuria, a sexually active patient with a recent new sexual partner, and no hematuria.

Strong consideration should be given to performing a pelvic examination in sexually active women with dysuria to evaluate for vaginitis and herpes virus infection. Although the diagnosis of chlamydial infection is best confirmed by culture, chlamydial cultures are expensive and do not give prompt results. Immunofluorescent methods for immediate diagnosis are also expensive. In the absence of a culture or immunofluorescent methods, the findings of pyuria, $<10^5$/ml bacteria in urine, a negative gonococcal culture, and a negative pelvic examination in a sexually active woman with frequency/dysuria should suggest consideration of therapy for *C. trachomatis* urethritis. Tetracycline would also constitute adequate therapy for the other major possibility—urinary tract infection with $<10^5$/ml bacteria in urine.

Localization of Site of Infection

Several methods have been used to determine if infection is restricted to the urinary bladder or if the upper tract is also involved. Needle biopsy specimens of the kidney have been cultured.[179] However, this is an unreliable approach because pyelonephritis is a focal disease and specimens obtained by needle biopsy may miss the area of infection.

The most reliable method of localization of infection involves obtaining urine directly from the ureter for quantitative cultures. In one study[170] using this method 95 women and 26 men with bacteriuria were evaluated. Approximately one-half had infection limited to the bladder. History and physical examination were of little value in predicting the site of infection. Turck et al.[180] using similar techniques demonstrated that in women with recurrent urinary tract infection, relapse was associated with upper tract involvement and reinfection with lower tract infection.

Fairley and colleagues[181] devised a technique for assessing ureteral bacteriuria that involves Foley catheterization only. However, results are equivocal in about 10–20 percent of patients.[138,182] As in the ureteral catheterization studies, about 50 percent of the patients have renal infection regardless of signs or symptoms.[182] Methods are also available for localization of bacteria in the prostate gland[183] and are discussed later.

Several studies[184,185] have reported the association of a defect in renal concentrating ability with upper tract infection. As might be expected, patients with unilateral bacteriuria have an ipsilateral defect in concentrating ability.[185] However, there are too many false-positive and false-negative responses to allow the use of concentrating ability for localization of urinary tract infection.

The immune response has been used as a means of localizing the site of infection. The presence of high titers of serum antibody directed against the infecting organism has been correlated with the presence of upper tract infection in patients undergoing ureteral catheterization.[186] Although there is a good

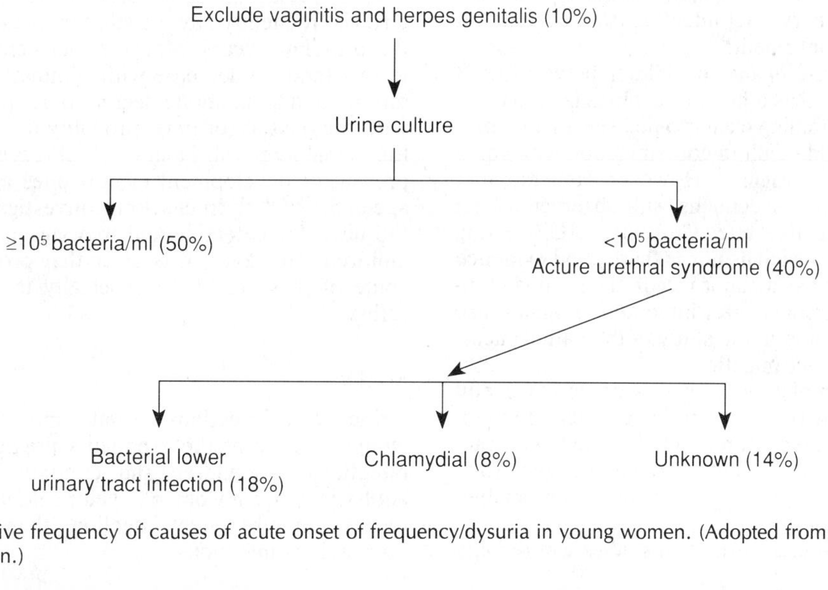

FIG. 6. Relative frequency of causes of acute onset of frequency/dysuria in young women. (Adopted from Stamm et al.,[175] with permission.)

association of high antibody titers and renal infection, there is a high incidence of false-positive and false-negative results (about 20 percent each).

Some investigators have hypothesized that measurement of urinary enzymes may be useful in detection of urinary tract infections and the differentiation of upper versus lower tract involvement. Various enzymes such as lactic dehydrogenase, alkaline phosphatase, β-glucuronidase, catalase, transaminase, leucine amino peptidase, and lysozyme have been evaluated.[187] From these studies, it is apparent that determination of urinary enzyme activity adds little if anything to the diagnostic approach or localization of infection, because a number of inflammatory processes as well as upper or lower tract infection can result in increased enzyme activity.[187,188]

Detection of antibody coating of bacteria (ACB) in urine has been used to localize infection.[189,190] This technique, which uses an immunofluorescent method, appears to be a relatively sensitive, reliable, and noninvasive way of detecting renal bacteriuria. Fluorescein-conjugated anti-human globulin is added to urine containing bacteria, and the bacteria are examined for fluorescence. The sensitivity of the test for ACB has been established collectively by several studies as 88 percent (range 72–100) with a specificity of 76 percent (range 50–100 percent). The predictive value of associating a positive test result for ACB with upper tract infection is 79 percent; the predictive value of associating a negative test result for ACB with bladder bacteriuria is 86 percent.[191] Discrepancies have resulted from lack of standardization of criteria of what constitutes a positive test result. False-negative results occur in 20 percent of patients with early acute pyelonephritis, because it may take several days for adequate antibody titers to develop.[191] An additional cause is the inability of the antibody to combine with certain infecting organisms such as mucoid-coated pseudomonads.[191] False-positive ACB test results occur in approximately 20–30 percent of patients with lower urinary infection. In men, the most important cause of false-positive results is the presence of bacterial prostatitis.[191] In women, false-positive results may be the consequence of contamination of urine samples by small numbers of ACB and yeast from the vaginal vestibule of patients without urinary tract infections. Yeast and pseudomonads may fluoresce even if not coated.[192] Proteinuria, hemorrhagic cystitis—probably because of tissue invasion—bladder tumors, and bladder stones may also be associated with false-positive ACB tests.[191]

Several studies have observed high false-positive and false-negative results in catheterized paraplegics.[191,193] ACB testing has been found to be accurate during pregnancy, and one-half the patients with asymptomatic bacteriuria are ACB-positive.[194,195] Although patients with renal transplants demonstrate an immune response to urinary tract infection, the reliability of ACB testing is as yet unconfirmed.[196]

There has been a major discrepancy in children between ACB localization and direct as well as other indirect localization techniques.[197–199] Difficulty obtaining clean-voided specimens, particularly in small girls, could result in contamination with small numbers of ACB of perineal origin.[197] However, Hellerstein et al.,[198] using catheter-obtained specimens, still observed a high false-positive and false-negative rate. Currently, ACB testing is not widely available to physicians nor is there good evidence to conclude that this assay has a major role in the routine management of patients with urinary tract infections. Its main use is as an epidemiologic tool and in the study of the pathogenesis and treatment of urinary tract infection.

Outcome of therapy can also be used in a crude but useful manner to separate those with upper and lower tract infection. Virtually all patients with infection restricted to the lower tract can be cured with a short course of antimicrobial therapy. However, the relapse rate with upper tract infection is appreciable, even with 7–10 days of therapy.

At present, only ureteral catheterization studies can reliably predict the site of infection in the urinary tract. However, this procedure is not without risk and cannot be justified for routine use. The Fairley bladder washout procedure is also quite reliable but gives equivocal results in about 10–20 percent of the patients. However, it also involves catheterization. The determination of presence of antibody-coated bacteria in the urine is practical and is noninvasive. However, in the clinical management of patients, it is rarely important to localize infection to either the upper tract or the lower tract other than by symptoms.

NATURAL HISTORY OF URINARY TRACT INFECTION

Children

In general, children with urinary tract infections without obstruction or vesicoureteral reflux have a very good prognosis.[113,129,132] In the presence of obstruction (e.g., urethral valves), severe destruction of renal parenchyma can occur.

Reflux is found in 30–50 percent of the children with asymptomatic or symptomatic bacteriuria (Fig. 7).[128,200] Reflux can be caused by obstruction with increased pressure in the bladder, delayed development of the ureterovesical junction, a short intravesical ureter, and/or inflammation of the vesicoureteral junction. Reflux in the presence of infection is associated with the development of scarring detected by intravenous pyelography.[129,132,200] Infants and young children (preschool age group) are at the highest risk for the development of progressive renal scarring.[128,129,132,200–202] These children frequently have severe degrees of reflux with repeated infections, and some develop end-stage renal disease and hypertension. Obstruction (most common in infant boys with congenital anomalies) is likely to be associated with marked reflux.[200–204]

It should be emphasized that the contribution of reflux alone as compared with reflux plus infection in the progression of renal scarring has not been clearly delineated. Reflux alone can apparently lead to renal damage and insufficiency.[188,205,206] Studies in uninfected animals[207] have demonstrated that reflux alone and in particular *intrarenal reflux* can produce "pyelonephritic" scars. It has also been shown that the immature kidneys of infants are more prone to intrarenal reflux.[208] The term *reflux nephropathy*, infected or uninfected, has been suggested to emphasize the primary role of reflux in scarring.[202] However, it is probable that reflux is more likely to lead to severe damage and scarring when infection is also present.[207] It is also clear that infection tends to produce reflux or at least to make it more severe.

After the age of 5, children (predominantly girls) with bacteriuria frequently have renal scars presumably acquired during the preschool years. Many of these children also have reflux. Reflux tends to decrease with elimination of bacteriuria. In addition, mild to moderate degrees of reflux are likely to disappear with the passage of time, probably in relation to maturation of the vesicoureteral junction.[209] Progression of scar already present or development of new ones are uncommon after the age of 5.[135,209–211] In fact, some investigators[212] have questioned the need for detecting and treating bacteriuria in school-aged children. However, it is clear that progression does occur in some of these children, especially in the presence of severe reflux.[209]

Adults

Urinary tract infections are much more common in women than in men. Many of these patients previously had urinary tract infections as children and continue to have infections as adults.[135] Once a woman develops infection, she is more likely to develop subsequent infections than a patient who has had no previous infections.

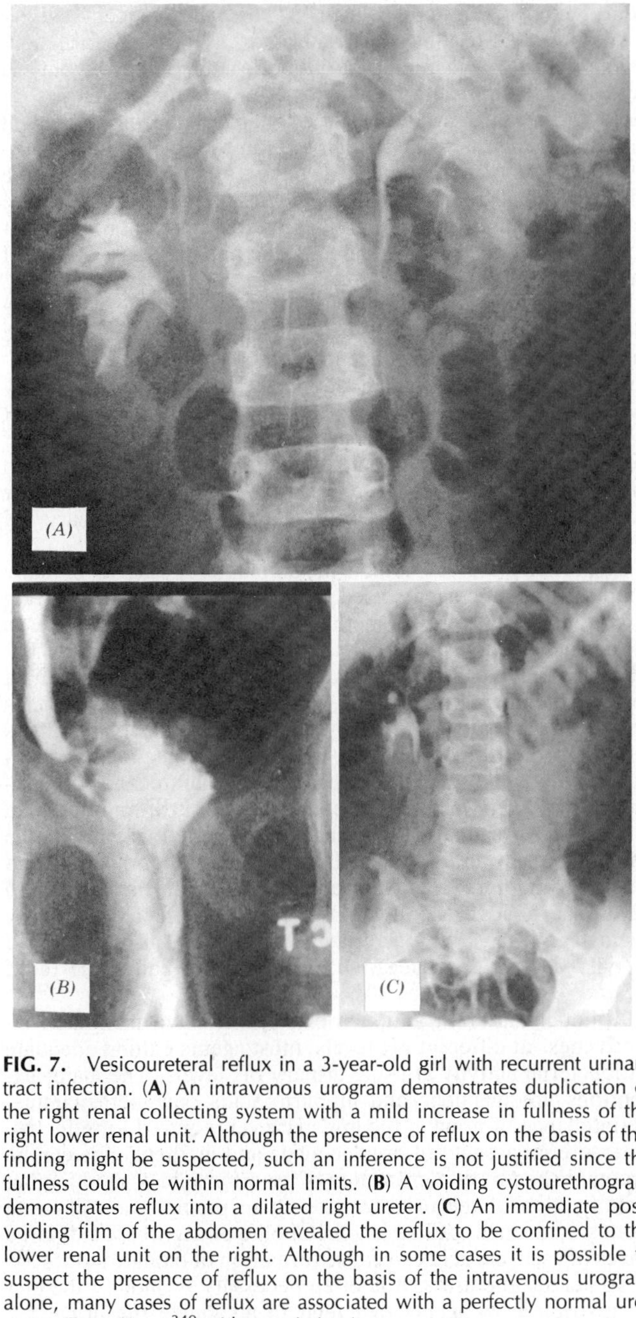

FIG. 7. Vesicoureteral reflux in a 3-year-old girl with recurrent urinary tract infection. (**A**) An intravenous urogram demonstrates duplication of the right renal collecting system with a mild increase in fullness of the right lower renal unit. Although the presence of reflux on the basis of this finding might be suspected, such an inference is not justified since the fullness could be within normal limits. (**B**) A voiding cystourethrogram demonstrates reflux into a dilated right ureter. (**C**) An immediate post-voiding film of the abdomen revealed the reflux to be confined to the lower renal unit on the right. Although in some cases it is possible to suspect the presence of reflux on the basis of the intravenous urogram alone, many cases of reflux are associated with a perfectly normal urogram. (From Kaye,[340] with permission.)

The courses of women with symptomatic recurrent urinary tract infections were described by Kraft and Stamey.[213] However, it was not defined whether these recurrences were reinfections or relapses. Twenty-three patients were followed over a period of 800 months, and each episode of urinary tract infection was treated. The overall attack rate was about 0.2 infections per month. Of interest is that even in these women (i.e., with recurrent urinary tract infections), significant bacteriuria (i.e., $\geq 10^5$ bacteria per ml urine) was present in only 70 percent of symptomatic episodes. Infections tended to occur in clusters with an increased attack rate of 0.5 percent per month. These periods of more frequent infection were followed by a remission or infection-free interval that averaged about 13 months. However, most remissions were followed by further clusters of infection. Thus, in many women it is more correct to use the term *remission* rather than *cure* of urinary tract infection. It may be a simple matter to cure an individual episode, but recurrence is common.

It is clear that urinary tract infection in adults can lead to progressive renal damage in the presence of obstruction.[4] However, recurrent infection in adults in the absence of obstruction rarely, if ever, leads to renal failure.

Autopsy studies[2,214] have shown that it is difficult to implicate infection per se (i.e., in the absence of other renal abnormalities) as an important pathogenetic factor in the production of severe renal disease in adults. One exception might be severe papillary necrosis secondary to infection. In fact, some authors[215] have been unable to find any cases of uncomplicated pyelonephritis that progressed to end-stage renal disease among 173 patients admitted to dialysis programs. In prospective studies,[135,216–221] hundreds of patients have been followed for years with persistent or recurrent infections without documenting progression of renal disease from infection alone.

The role of infection in the progression of clinically or radiographically diagnosed interstitial renal disease has also been examined.[3,222,223] In general, these studies indicate that infection is rarely, if ever, the major factor leading to further renal decompensation. However, infection may occasionally accelerate the progression of the primary underlying disease process.[222] In summary, except for perhaps rare instances there is no evidence to indicate that uncomplicated urinary tract infection alone produces renal failure in adults.[4]

Some studies have demonstrated decreased survival among elderly people with bacteriuria.[224,225] However, other studies have not confirmed this association.[225,226] At present, it is not known if asymptomatic bacteriuria in the elderly has any deleterious effects. Furthermore, there is no evidence to suggest that treatment of asymptomatic bacteriuria in the elderly has any beneficial effects. Therefore, routine treatment of asymptomatic bacteriuria in the elderly is not advocated by most experts.

Hypertension

It is clear that severe renal disease may cause hypertension. The entity of chronic interstitial renal disease (not necessarily related to infection) has also been related to hypertension.[3] It has been suggested that patients with bacteriuria in the absence of other renal disease are more likely to have hypertension, but the data have not shown a clear-cut relationship.[4] No definite cause and effect relationships have been documented.

MANAGEMENT OF URINARY TRACT INFECTION

General Considerations

Ideally antimicrobial agents should only be administered when there is reasonable evidence of infection in the urinary tract. Symptoms are not a reliable indication of infection.[13,175] The diagnosis of infection in the asymptomatic patient should be made on no fewer than two cultures of clean-voided, midstream urine in which the same microorganism is present in significant titers. If the patient is symptomatic, one specimen will suffice, and therapy should be started.

There has been much controversy as to how vigorously chemotherapy should be pursued.[227] A rational approach to the treatment of urinary tract infection depends on an appreciation of the prognosis of the untreated infection and the long-term results to be expected from therapy. The side effects, cost, and inconvenience of different therapeutic regimens must also be considered. As the prognosis of urinary tract infection in nonpregnant adult women seems to be quite good and reinfection is common, therapy probably makes little contribution to the patient's well-being other than eradicating symptoms.

While bacteriuria in the elderly is associated with degenerative and debilitating diseases and in some reports with mortality, there is no convincing evidence for a cause and effect relationship.[225,228] There certainly is no evidence that treatment of the urinary tract infection alters the patient's course. Urinary tract infection serves as a marker for debilitating diseases, which in turn may contribute to mortality. In addition, urinary tract infection is very common in the elderly, and many of these patients become reinfected or relapse after antimicrobial therapy. Furthermore, a higher frequency of side effects from chemotherapy would be expected in an older age group because of pre-existing renal, auditory, and other diseases. Considering the large numbers of patients involved, intensive antimicrobial therapy may lead to an unwarranted financial burden and the danger of drug toxicity and thus may do more harm than good in elderly patients.

In contrast, bacteriuria in preschool children with vesicoureteral reflux (especially if congenital anomalies are present) can result in stunted growth of the kidney, scar formation, and, rarely, renal failure. Bacteriuria in pregnancy may also have serious implications. Treatment of children and pregnant women is most likely to be beneficial. Furthermore, it is feasible to treat all these patients since the prevalence of bacteriuria is relatively low in these groups.

Hospitalized patients with bacteriuria have higher mortality rates than those without bacteriuria.[229,230] This observation may be related to deaths from bacteremia in patients with indwelling urinary catheters.

It is usually necessary to treat all symptomatic patients regardless of age, even when infection is likely to recur. Some patients have such frequent symptomatic episodes (either relapses or reinfections) that they are almost chronically incapacitated. In these patients it may be necessary to give prolonged therapy or prophylaxis to prevent recurrent symptoms.

Nonspecific Therapy

Hydration. Forcing fluids has been advocated in the therapy for urinary tract infection. There is some theoretical support for this modality of treatment. Hydration produces rapid dilution of the bacteria and removal of infected urine by frequent bladder emptying, which in the presence of minimal residual volume may offset the logarithmic growth of gram-negative bacilli. Forcing fluids usually results in a rapid reduction of bacterial counts. Permanent loss of bacteriuria has been reported in a few patients with rapid hydration, but in most patients bacterial counts return to original levels when hydration is stopped (e.g., overnight when urine flow rate and frequency of micturition are reduced).[231]

Medullary hypertonicity tends to inhibit leukocytic migration into the renal medulla, and the high concentration of ammonia tends to inactive complement.[63,64] Abolition of medullary hypertonicity by diuresis would be expected to reverse these effects. In addition, a reduction in bacterial counts in the urine by hydration would enhance the effect of factors otherwise overwhelmed by large numbers of bacteria (e.g., bladder mucosal defenses or the effect of relatively low concentrations of antimicrobial drugs).

Hydration may also have some disadvantages. Increased fluid intake could theoretically result in increased vesicoureteral reflux and possibly cause acute urinary retention in the partially obstructed bladder. The larger urine output results in dilution of antibacterial substances normally present in the urine as well as lower urinary concentrations of antimicrobial agents. Water diuresis also decreases urinary acidification, which enhances the antibacterial activity of urine and certain antimicrobial agents.

As there is no evidence that hydration improves the results of appropriate antimicrobial therapy, and because continuous hydration is inconvenient, we are not in favor of this approach.

Urinary pH. Antibacterial activity of urine results mainly from high urea concentration and osmolality and is pH-dependent, being greater at a lower pH.[65] The pH-dependent activity may be related to a high concentration of various weakly ionizable organic acids, such as hippuric and β-hydroxybutyric acids.[232] The antibacterial activity of these organic acids is related to the concentration of the undissociated molecule that probably penetrates better than the ionized form into the bacterial cell. As these organic acids have a relatively low pKa (the pH at which 50 percent of the molecules are undissociated), the lower the urinary pH, the greater the concentration of undissociated molecules and the greater the antibacterial activity of the organic acid.

Hippuric acid is a common constituent of urine, being the glycine conjugate of dietary benzoic acid, and is bacteriostatic in proportion to the concentration of undissociated molecules.[227] The production of antibacterial activity in urine by ingestion of large volumes of cranberry juice (if the urinary pH level is kept low) results from the appearance in the urine of high concentrations of hippuric acid derived from precursors in the berry. The successful use of mandelic acid, another organic acid, is also dependent on maintenance of a low urinary pH level.

The urinary pH level affects the antibacterial activity of many chemotherapeutic agents used in the treatment of urinary tract infections. The activity of methenamine results from the release of formaldehyde as the urinary pH level is decreased below 5.5. Clinically, methenamine is used in the form of its mandelic acid salt (methenamine mandelate) or its hippuric acid salt (methenamine hippurate). The antibacterial activity of these salts is related to the formation of the unionized organic acid and formaldehyde, which is highly dependent on maintenance of a urinary pH of 5.5 or less. The effectiveness of nitrofurantoin (pKa 7.2) is also greater at low urinary pH level. In contrast, the aminoglycoside antibiotics such as gentamicin, tobramycin, and amikacin are more effective in alkaline urine. Erythromycin and other macrolides, generally considered to be effective primarily against gram-positive bacteria, are known to have increased activity against gram-negative bacilli at an alkaline pH (e.g., 8.5).[233]

Although different antimicrobial agents have maximum effectiveness at different pH levels, most agents exhibit adequate antibacterial activity at usual urinary pH levels. The major exceptions are mandelic and hippuric acids and methenamine. Maintenance of urine at the low pH level required for effective antibacterial activity of organic acids and methenamine can be accomplished by administration of ascorbic acid or methionine. Acidification of the urine can result in precipitation of urate stones, and since oxalate is a metabolite of ascorbic acid, large doses of ascorbic acid can cause formation of oxalate stones.[227]

To acidify the urine, it is often necessary to modify the diet by restriction of agents that tend to alkalinize the urine, for example, milk, fruit juices (except cranberry juice), and sodium bicarbonate. Another major problem with acidification is that patients with renal insufficiency are unable to excrete an acid load and may become systemically acidotic when urinary acidification is attempted. It may be impossible to acidify urine infected with urea-splitting organisms such as *Proteus* species because of production of ammonia from urea. Acidification for long-term antimicrobial therapy should only be used with concomitant use of organic acids or methenamine. Urinary acidification is frequently difficult to achieve[234] and is rarely if ever necessary at present.

Analgesics. Urinary analgesics such as phenazopyridine hydrochloride (Pyridium) have little place in the routine management of symptomatic infections. The dysuria of urinary tract infection usually responds rapidly to antibacterial therapy and requires no local analgesia. If flank pain or dysuria is severe, systemic analgesics can be used. Analgesics such as phenazopyridine hydrochloride may be useful in the management of certain patients with dysuria but without infection.

Principles of Antimicrobial Therapy

Selection of an appropriate antimicrobial agent has become complex because of the increasing number of compounds available, each with its characteristic spectrum and toxic properties. However, in most cases, any of many available agents are perfectly satisfactory. Given two or more drugs with equivalent activity against the infecting microorganism, the agent with the least toxicity should be chosen.

There is no evidence to support any superiority of bactericidal drugs over bacteriostatic agents in urinary tract infection. However, there may be theoretical reasons for using bactericidal drugs in the treatment of relapsing urinary tract infection.

Serum, Tissue, and Urine Concentrations of Antimicrobial Agents. A poor correlation exists between response of bacteriuria and blood levels of antimicrobial agents.[170,235,236] Many oral antimicrobial agents, in the dosages commonly used for urinary tract infection, do not achieve serum levels above the minimal inhibitory concentration for most urinary pathogens.

Disappearance of bacteriuria is closely correlated with the sensitivity of the microorganism to the concentration of the antimicrobial agent achieved in the urine.[170,235,236] Inhibitory urinary concentrations are achieved after oral administration of essentially all commonly used antimicrobial agents. While blood levels do not seem to be important in treatment of urinary tract infection, they may be critical in patients with bacteremia and may be important in the cure of patients with renal parenchymal infection who relapse.

In patients with renal insufficiency, dosage modifications are necessary for agents that are excreted primarily by the kidneys and cannot be cleared by any other mechanism. In renal failure, the kidney may not be able to concentrate an antimicrobial agent in the urine, and difficulty in eradicating bacteriuria may occur. This may be an important factor in failure of therapy for urinary tract infection with aminoglycosides.

In addition, high concentrations of magnesium and calcium as well as a low pH level can raise the minimal inhibitory concentrations of aminoglycosides for gram-negative bacilli to levels above those achievable in the urine of patients with renal failure.[237] In general the penicillins and cephalosporins attain adequate urine concentrations despite severely impaired renal function and are the agents of choice in renal insufficiency.[238]

Response to Therapy. The objective of antimicrobial therapy is to eliminate bacteria from the urinary tract. Symptoms usually abate spontaneously without chemotherapy, even though bacteriuria may persist. Therefore, the results of therapy can only be determined by follow-up urine cultures.

There are four patterns of response of bacteriuria to antimicrobial therapy: cure, persistence, relapse, and reinfection. Quantitative bacterial counts in urine should decrease within 48 hours after initiation of an antimicrobial agent to which the microorganism is sensitive in vitro. If titers do not decrease within this time, the therapy being given will almost invariably be unsuccessful.

Cure is defined as negative urine cultures on chemotherapy and during the follow-up period (usually 1–2 weeks). However, it must be understood that some of these patients will develop reinfection at a later time.

Persistence has been used in two ways to describe response to therapy: (*1*) persistence of significant bacteriuria after 48 hours of treatment and (*2*) persistence of the infecting organism in low numbers in urine after 48 hours. Significant bacteriuria usually persists only if urinary levels of the antimicrobial agent are below the concentration of the drug needed to inhibit the microorganism. This can occur when the infecting strain is resistant to the urinary levels usually attained (i.e., a resistant organism) or because levels are inordinately low (i.e., from not taking the agent, insufficient dosage, poor intestinal absorption, or poor renal excretion as in renal insufficiency). Persistence of the infecting microorganism in low titers in voided urine may mean persistence in the urinary tract or contamination from the urethra or vagina. Bladder puncture cultures would be needed to evaluate the significance of low titers of bacteria obtained on therapy, and we do not routinely recommend this procedure. Also worth noting is the fact that bacteria may persist within the urinary tract during therapy without excretion of organisms in the urine. Sites of persistence within the urinary tract are the renal parenchyma, calculi, and the prostate. The simplest way of determining the significance of persistence of the organism in low titers in the urine is to obtain follow-up urine cultures after therapy has been stopped. Prompt relapse of significant bacteriuria usually follows persistence of the organism in the urinary tract.

Relapse usually occurs within 1–2 weeks after cessation of chemotherapy and is often associated with renal infection, with structural abnormalities of the urinary tract, or with chronic bacterial prostatitis. Relapse indicates that the infecting microorganism has persisted in the urinary tract during therapy. However, an apparent relapse can be related to reinfection (new infection) with the same microorganism. In spite of eradication from the urinary tract, the original infecting organism may still be present in the intestine, vagina, or external urethra and then may cause a new infection. Markedly delayed relapses (more than 1 month after stopping therapy) are much more likely due to this phenomenon or to chronic bacterial prostatitis than to true relapse. Relapses occurring within 1–2 weeks are usually true relapses. One postulated but unsubstantiated mechanism of relapse following treatment with cell-wall active antibiotics (e.g., penicillins and cephalosporins) is persistence of osmotically fragile, cell-wall-deficient forms in the hypertonic renal medulla during therapy, with reversion to normal bacterial forms after therapy is stopped.[127]

After initial sterilization of the urine, *reinfection* may occur during administration of chemotherapy (also called superinfection) or at any time thereafter. Reinfection is easy to identify when there is a change in bacterial species. However, there may be reinfection with a different serotype of the same species (usually *E. coli*) or even the same serotype.

Classification and Antimicrobial Therapy for Different Groups

Symptomatic Urinary Tract Infection. The majority of patients classified as having symptomatic urinary tract infection are women, usually of child-bearing age. The onset of symptoms is frequently related to sexual intercourse. The patient may have upper urinary tract symptoms, lower urinary tract symptoms, or both. As mentioned previously, patients with only lower urinary tract symptoms may also have upper urinary tract infection.

ACUTE PYELONEPHRITIS. Patients who are severely ill with pyelonephritis should be hospitalized. Although mild to moderate illness responds well to orally administered antimicrobial agents, nausea and vomiting may preclude oral treatment, necessitating parenteral therapy. If the patient is reliable, compliant, and tolerates oral therapy, the patient may be treated with a variety of oral antimicrobial agents. At the time of antibiotic selection, a Gram stain of the urine should have indicated the morphology of the infecting organism (e.g., gram-negative bacillus, gram-positive coccus), but the precise identity and antimicrobial susceptibility pattern are usually unknown. Therefore, selection of antimicrobial therapy is usually empiric. When streptococci are seen on Gram stain, ampicillin or amoxicillin is probably the agent of choice. When staphylococci are implicated on Gram stain, cephalosporins (such as cephalexin) are appropriate agents.

Although sulfonamides and ampicillin or amoxicillin have been mainstays of oral therapy for gram-negative bacillus infection for many years, these agents can no longer be recommended as reliable agents, since 25–35 percent of *E. coli* are now resistant.[239] Accordingly, oral antimicrobial agents currently advocated for gram-negative bacillus urinary infection include: trimethoprim, trimethoprim–sulfamethoxazole, cephalexin, amoxicillin–clavulanic acid, and the recently introduced quinolones (norfloxacin and ciprofloxacin). The doses are listed under "Lower Urinary Tract Infection" below. In all patients with symptoms of upper tract infection, therapy should be preceded by culture of a clean-catch midstream urine sample.

In hospitalized patients, particularly those with suspected gram-negative bacillary bacteremia complicating pyelonephritis (high fever, shaking chills, hypotension), parenteral therapy should be used and is directed at the life-threatening bacteremia. In these seriously ill patients the spectrum of antibacterial activity of the initial agents should include all potential pathogens. In seriously ill patients with community-acquired acute pyelonephritis, when the Gram stain reveals gram-negative bacilli, empiric therapy includes a wide selection of antimicrobial agents, e.g., parenteral trimethoprim–sulfamethoxazole, aminoglycosides (e.g., gentamicin 3–5 mg/kg/day), aztreonam 3–6 g/day, ureido-penicillins (mezlocillin, azlocillin, or piperacillin 18 g/day, the ampicillin–sulbactam combination (as 12 g ampicillin/day) or the ticarcillin–clavulanic acid combination (as 18 g ticarcillin/day) and third-generation cephalosporins, e.g., cefotaxime or ceftriaxone, etc. In patients with hospital-acquired gram-negative bacillary infection, particularly when seriously ill, the initial selection of antibiotics should not leave any hiatus in the spectrum of activity and should anticipate the possibility of resistant microorganisms. Under these circumstances ceftazidine (3–6 g/day), ticarcillin–clavulanic acid, aztreonam, or imipenem (2 g/day), often used in combination with aminoglycosides, are recommended. When the susceptibility pattern of the infecting organism is known, therapy can be altered to less expensive single-agent therapy, and oral treatment can be used once response has occurred.

Effective therapy results in a marked decrease in bacterial titers in the urine within 48 hours after onset of treatment. Antimicrobial agents are sometimes effective in vivo even when disk sensitivity tests indicate drug resistance, because most antimicrobials are excreted in the urine in concentrations much higher than tested for by disk sensitivity testing.

If bacteriologic response does not occur by 48 hours, there is no point in continuing the same regimen. Therapy is then changed to an alternate drug on the basis of susceptibility tests (e.g., from the initial isolate). The finding of continuing positive blood cultures or persistent fever and toxicity past the first 3 days suggests the need for investigation to exclude urinary obstruction or intrarenal or perinephric abscess formation. Investigation should include renal ultrasound, computed tomographic scan, and, according to the findings, perhaps an intravenous pyelogram (IVP) examination. The availability of sensitive noninvasive studies has resulted in early diagnosis of intrarenal or perinephric abscess formation that may respond to antibiotic therapy alone. In uncomplicated pyelonephritis after clinical response and defervesence occurs, oral therapy is initiated and should be continued to complete a course of 14 days of antimicrobial therapy.[240] When upper tract infection is complicated by abscesses, more prolonged therapy and perhaps drainage is indicated (see "Perinephric Abscess" and "Intrarenal Abscess" below). All patients with acute pyelonephritis should have at least an ultrasound examination to evaluate for obstruction and/or stones. Follow-up urine cultures are mandatory within 1–2 weeks of completion of therapy in pregnant women, children, and patients with recurrent symptomatic pyelonephritis in whom suppressive maintenance therapy is planned. In the majority of nonpregnant adults who remain asymptomatic, follow-up cultures are optional.

Renal infection is a special problem in adults with hereditary polycystic disease. Although parenchymal infections respond well to appropriate antibiotics, cyst infections frequently fail to improve, and may require lipid-soluble antibiotics, e.g., trimethoprim–sulfamethoxazole[241] or surgical aspiration/drainage. Emphysematous pyelonephritis is most often seen in elderly female diabetics with chronic urinary infections and renal vascular disease. Because of the extraordinary high mortality rate of 70 percent in spite of appropriate antibiotic and supportive therapy, immediate nephrectomy is indicated for this condition[242] (Fig. 8).

LOWER URINARY TRACT INFECTION. *Conventional Therapy*. In the past, 7–10 days of therapy was routinely recommended for patients with lower tract symptoms. However, in recent years it has become apparent that most women with lower tract infection have only a superficial mucosal infection and can be cured with much shorter courses of therapy and in fact with only a single dose of an antimicrobial agent.

Single-Dose Vs. Three-Day Therapy. Single-dose therapy achieves high urinary concentrations that are prolonged for at least 12–24 hours and eliminate infection when confined to the bladder. Cure rates have ranged from 61–100 percent in women with symptoms of lower urinary tract infection.[243–254] In many of these studies methods were used to select patients with infection localized to the lower tract. The regimens used were sulfadoxine 2 g orally, sulfamethoxypyridazine 2 g orally, sulfisoxazole 2 g orally, kanamycin 0.5 g intramuscularly, amoxicillin 3 g orally, trimethoprim–sulfamethoxazole 2 single-strength tablets orally, trimethoprim 400 mg orally, tetracycline 2 g orally, nitrofurantoin 200 mg orally, and cefonicid 1 g intramuscularly. In the studies in which the ACB test was used,

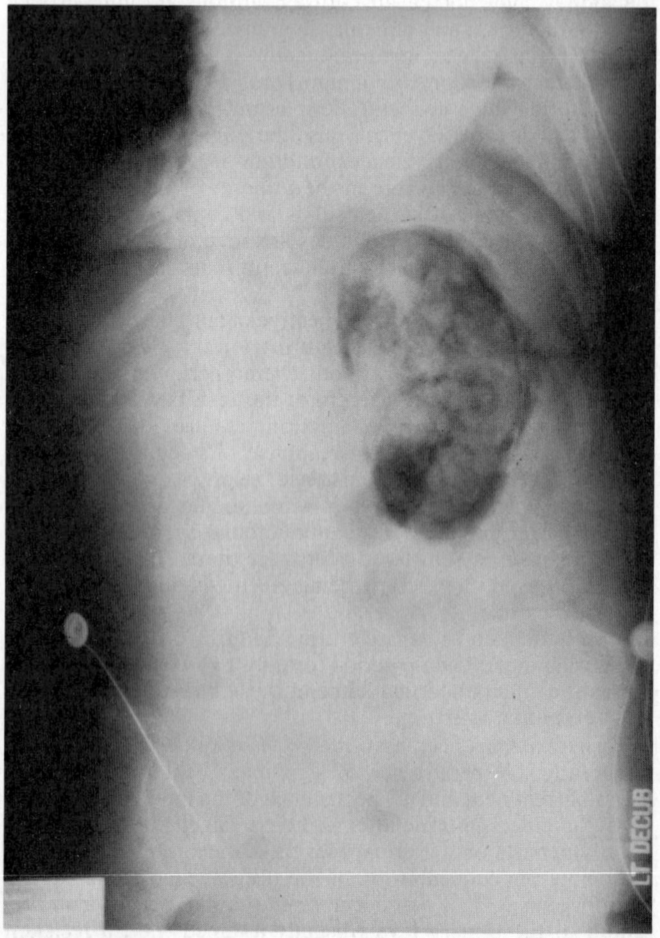

FIG. 8. Flat plate roentgenogram of abdomen showing emphysematous pyelonephritis.

clinical cure was almost always achieved in patients with negative ACB tests.

The advantages of single-dose therapy include lesser expense, assured compliance, fewer side effects, and perhaps less intense selective pressure for emergence of resistant organisms in gut, urinary, or vaginal flora. Possible deleterious effects include a poorer outcome of infections that are actually in the upper tract and are first treated with single-dose therapy, for example, a delay in appropriate therapy may result in more deeply seated infection and impair the response to subsequent more prolonged therapy. Finally, it should not be assumed that every antibiotic administered as a single dose will be effective even with regard to susceptible organisms. Results depend on high sustained urinary concentrations of the antimicrobial agent. For example, a 2 g oral dose of cefaclor resulted in a 57 percent failure rate.[255] Before using single-dose therapy, certain factors should be evaluated, including frequency of attacks, poor response to single-dose therapy in the past, known structural abnormalities, history of childhood infection, symptoms longer than 7 days, pyelonephritis during the past year, diabetes, etc. Any of these factors increases the likelihood of upper tract infection and might mitigate against using single-dose therapy.

A by-product of single-dose therapy is that failure to eradicate a urinary tract infection after a single dose of an agent may indicate in which patient further investigation should be considered. Response to single-dose therapy appears comparable with the ACB test in localizing the site of infection.[256]

Single-dose therapy gives basically 1 day of therapy with regard to antimicrobial activity in the urine. The same results should be achievable with 1 day of standard-dose antimicrobial therapy; however, the data to support this do not exist. Two reviews concluded that 3 days of therapy may be superior to single-dose therapy.[257,258] It is our preference to advocate the concept of short-course therapy, which may constitute single-dose or 3 days of therapy using standard doses. Some of the preferred agents for 3 days of therapy are trimethoprim–sulfamethoxazole (one double-strength tablet twice a day), trimethoprim (100 mg twice a day), cephalexin (250–500 mg four times a day), amoxicillin–clavulanic acid (250–500 mg amoxicillin three times a day), norfloxacin (400 mg twice a day), or ciprofloxacin (500 mg twice a day). With present knowledge, our preference is single-dose trimethoprim–sulfamethoxazole, or trimethoprim alone, or 3 days of these or other agents.

We do not advocate use of sulfonamides, ampicillin, or amoxicillin because of the relatively high frequency of *E. coli* resistant to these agents among community-acquired urinary tract infections.[239]

The approach to management of lower urinary tract infection has evolved to where short-course therapy should become the standard for most female patients with suspected lower tract infection. Preliminary studies in pediatric populations have shown similar good results.[259] Short-course therapy has not been adequately evaluated in men and is not recommended at present. Short-course therapy is not appropriate for women who have a history of previous urinary infection caused by antibiotic-resistant organisms, or more than 7 days of symptoms.[239] In these patients (who have an increased likelihood of upper tract infection) and in males, 7–10 days of therapy are recommended.

If symptoms do not respond or if they recur, a urine culture should be obtained. In pregnant women, children, and patients at high risk for renal damage who remain asymptomatic, follow-up cultures should be obtained 1–2 weeks after discontinuation of therapy to detect relapses.

OFFICE STRATEGY FOR FREQUENCY, URGENCY, AND DYSURIA SYNDROME. When a sexually active woman is first seen with frequency, urgency, and dysuria, urine culture is not mandatory, and the therapeutic decision is based on the clinical presentation and the presence or absence of pyuria. If pyuria (defined as ≥ 10 leukocytes/mm^3) is present, antimicrobial therapy is warranted for urinary tract infection. Short-course therapy is a reasonable first approach in adult females except in settings in which occult pyelonephritis is more likely, as described above. An agent likely to be effective against most pathogens (e.g., trimethoprim, trimethoprim–sulfamethoxazole, amoxicillin–clavulanic acid, norfloxacin, ciprofloxacin) should be used. If clinical response does not occur, a culture should be obtained (for the possibility of a resistant organism), and therapy should be changed and directed at chlamydia, with 500 mg tetracycline four times a day for 7 days.

In the nonsexually active female with symptoms of lower tract infection and pyuria, there is a high probability of urinary tract infection; lack of response to therapy probably indicates a resistant organism and mandates a urine culture.

In the absence of pyuria, symptomatic urinary tract infection is unlikely in any patient. Symptomatic response followed by recurrence after therapy is discontinued indicates the probability of upper tract infection and the need for a culture and at least 2 weeks of therapy. Men and children should have a urine culture, and males should receive 7–10 days of treatment.

Asymptomatic Bacteriuria. Most patients with asymptomatic bacteriuria are women and are in the older age groups. Although cure may result following treatment, relapse and especially reinfection are common. The approach to asymptomatic bacteriuria depends on the age of the patient. In children, therapy should be given as described for symptomatic infection. A trial of single-dose or short-course therapy is reasonable. In contrast, therapy for asymptomatic bacteriuria in the adult is by no means mandatory in the absence of obstruction except during pregnancy. Nonpregnant women can be treated providing that a nontoxic antimicrobial agent is used. If the infecting microorganism is resistant to all but toxic agents, then treatment should not be instituted in the nonobstructed patient.

At present, most physicians believe that asymptomatic bacteriuria in the elderly is a benign disease and need not be treated, especially since with vigorous treatment a great many people will be exposed to drug toxicity.

When dealing with asymptomatic bacteriuria, there is no urgency in treating. Therapy should be delayed until two cultures have been obtained for confirmation of presence of bacteriuria. By that time, the identity and antimicrobial susceptibility pattern of the infecting organism will have been determined.

Relapsing Urinary Tract Infection. If the patient relapses after therapy for symptomatic urinary tract infection or for asymptomatic bacteriuria, the most likely possibilities are that the patient has (*1*) renal involvement, (*2*) a structural abnormality of the urinary tract (for example, calculi), or (*3*) chronic bacterial prostatitis.

Relapses, especially in the absence of structural abnormalities, may be related to renal infection that may require a longer duration of therapy. Patients who relapse after a short course or 7–10 days of therapy should be considered for a 2-week course. Turck and colleagues[180] demonstrated that a 6-week course of therapy resulted in a higher cure rate than a 2-week course in patients who relapsed after 2 weeks of therapy.

Structural abnormalities of the urinary tract predispose to relapse. Urinary tract infection in the presence of obstruction is likely to be associated with renal involvement, a tendency for renal functional impairment, and bacteremia. Obstructive lesions can be corrected surgically and should be sought in the evaluation of patients with relapsing infection. Calculi may be a cause of relapse of urinary tract infection. Ultimate success of chemotherapy is dependent on the removal of stones.

Some patients continue to relapse despite surgical correction of urologic abnormalities. In others, surgical correction may not be indicated or feasible, or no abnormalities may be found. In these patients who relapse after 2 weeks of chemotherapy, a repeat course of 2 weeks should be considered. Following another relapse a 4–6-week course should be considered. In men, chronic bacterial prostatitis should first be ruled out.

If relapse occurs after a 6-week course, therapy lasting 6 months or even longer may be considered. Only carefully selected patients, such as children, adults who have continuous symptoms, or adults who are at high risk of developing progressive renal damage (for example, those with obstruction not amenable to surgery), should be considered for 4-week or longer courses of therapy. Asymptomatic adults without obstruction should not receive these longer courses. Some of the agents that can be used for long-term therapy are amoxicillin (250 mg three times a day), cephalexin, trimethoprim–sulfamethoxazole, trimethoprim, norfloxacin, and ciprofloxacin, in usual doses, nitrofurantoin in full dosage for 1 week and then half the usual dose, and carbenicillin indanyl sodium (2 tablets four times daily in adults).

An antimicrobial agent being used for long-term therapy is continued only as long as significant bacteriuria is absent. If bacteriuria persists or relapses during chemotherapy (indicating that the infecting organism is now resistant to that agent), the agent is altered. The aim is to achieve continuous suppression of bacteriuria for the entire course of therapy. If relapse occurs after discontinuation of the antimicrobial agent, therapy is reinstituted with the same or another drug. If deemed necessary, this agent is administered for an additional 6 to 12 months (if bacteriuria remains suppressed). All patients are followed with urine cultures at least monthly while on therapy.

Long-term therapy or even repeated 2-week courses should be reserved for children, symptomatic patients of any age, and patients at high risk of developing progressive renal damage. A creatinine clearance determination and an intravenous pyelogram initially and yearly (or at least every 2 years) should be obtained on patients receiving long-term therapy to determine glomerular filtration rate and structural changes in the kidneys. Blood counts, urinalyses, and liver chemistries (when indicated) are also obtained periodically as tests for drug toxicity.

Reinfection of the Urinary Tract. Patients with reinfection can generally be divided into two groups: (*1*) those who have relatively infrequent reinfections, perhaps only once every 2 or 3 years to several times a year and (*2*) those who develop frequent reinfections. An extreme example of the latter group is patients who become reinfected during or shortly after each course of antimicrobial therapy. With infrequent reinfections, each episode can be approached with therapy as if it were a new episode of either symptomatic or asymptomatic infection. Single-dose or short-course therapy should be used in women with lower tract symptoms. Women with reinfections associated with lower tract symptoms can be managed with self-administration of short-course therapy with onset of symptoms.[260]

Many patients with frequent reinfections after therapy are middle-aged or elderly women in whom infection is limited to the lower urinary tract. Most asymptomatic reinfections in this group should not be treated, because the frequent use of antimicrobial agents in this group is apt to result in toxic side effects, and because progressive destruction of the kidneys is rare. If, however, the episodes are symptomatic or if the likelihood of renal damage is increased, these patients should be treated.

Occasionally patients of any age develop symptomatic reinfection so frequently that they can be incapacitated. In some women, these symptomatic reinfections are associated with sexual activity. Voiding immediately after intercourse may help prevent reinfection. However, single-dose prophylactic chemotherapy taken after sexual intercourse is a more effective method of decreasing episodes.[261]

In other patients with frequent symptomatic reinfections, no precipitating event is apparent; in these patients, when symptoms are severe, long-term chemoprophylaxis may be instituted. Although these courses seem to decrease the frequency of reinfections and symptoms in most patients, it is impossible to prevent completely reinfection in many patients. When reinfection occurs on therapy, the prophylactic agent must be changed.

Long-term chemoprophylaxis should be considered for asymptomatic patients who reinfect frequently and are at risk of developing renal parenchymal damage with each reinfection (for example, young children with vesicoureteral reflux and children and adults with obstructive uropathy). In these groups, keeping the patient abacteriuric helps to protect the kidneys. Several studies in patients with frequent reinfections indicate that such prolonged chemotherapy reduces the frequency of reinfections.

Long-term prophylactic antimicrobial agents have reduced the frequency of symptomatic infections of the urinary tract in older men, women, and children.[262–268] Before prophylaxis is initiated, the patient should receive a course of therapy with an appropriate antimicrobial agent. Trimethoprim–sulfamethoxazole, nitrofurantoin, or trimethoprim alone are particularly useful for long-term prophylaxis, because these drugs are unlikely to allow the emergence of antimicrobial-resistant bacteria with prolonged use.[264,268–270]

Full antimicrobial dosage is not necessary for successful prophylaxis. One 50-mg tablet of nitrofurantoin or one-half tablet of trimethoprim–sulfamethoxazole (40 mg trimethoprim, 200 mg sulfamethoxazole) nightly will suffice. Sulfisoxazole, nalidixic acid, methenamine mandelate, and other agents have been used with good results.[227]

A single dose of an antimicrobial agent immediately before or after coitus can reduce the incidence of urinary tract infection that is related to sexual activity.[261]

Patients receiving long-term prophylaxis should be followed with urine cultures monthly or more often if interim symptomatic episodes develop. Thereapy is continued with the same agent as long as the patient remains abacteriuric. If bacteriuria persists or recurs during administration of an antimicrobial agent, therapy is altered using response of bacteriuria as a parameter of adequacy of therapy. Long-term prophylaxis can be undertaken only if urine cultures are obtained periodically and therapy altered if bacteriuria recurs.

URINARY TRACT INFECTION IN PREGNANCY

Physiologic Alterations in the Urinary Tract

During pregnancy there is dilatation of the ureters and renal pelves with markedly decreased ureteral peristalsis. These changes begin as early as the seventh week of gestation and progress to term.[271] The bladder also decreases in tone so that late in gestation it can contain twice its normal contents without causing discomfort. These changes vary from patient to patient. They are more marked on the right side and are more likely to occur during the first pregnancy or when pregnancies occur in rapid succession (Fig. 9). The urinary tract tends to revert to normal by the second month following delivery.[271,272]

Changes similar to those of pregnancy have been described in the urinary tracts of women taking oral contraceptives.[273] Because of this observation, it has been suggested that the urinary tract alterations may be at least in part related to "hyperestrogenism."[271] Other possible explanations for the alterations are obstruction of the ureters by the gravid uterus and hypertrophy of muscle bundles at the lower end of the ureter.[271] To investigate the effects of estrogens on these changes, Andriole and Cohn[274] treated nonpregnant female and male rats with estrogens and obtained intravenous pyelograms before and during treatment. Hydroureter and marked increased susceptibility to *E. coli* pyelonephritis are observed in both male and female animals.

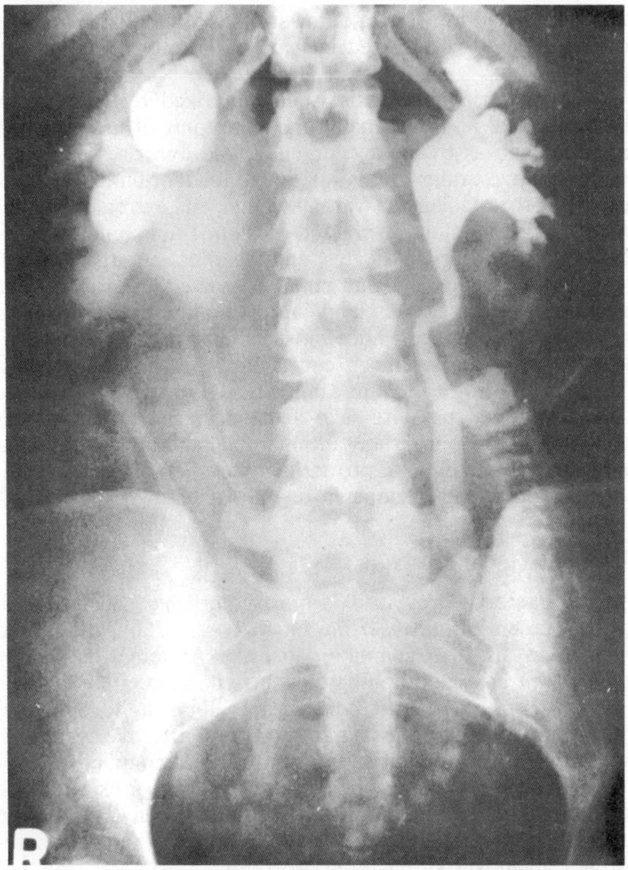

FIG. 9. Urogram in pregnancy. Urography was performed during the seventh month of pregnancy because of severe right-sided pyelonephritis. Although the right hydronephrosis is pronounced, no cause for it other than pregnancy could be found. Following delivery the urogram reverted to normal. Physiologic changes such as these make it difficult to detect superimposed pathologic disorders such as small ureteral calculi when they occur during pregnancy. (From Kaye[340] with permission.)

Epidemiology

The prevalence of asymptomatic bacteriuria in pregnancy ranges from 4 to 7 percent.[275,276] It is unclear if *U. urealyticum* and *Gardnerella vaginalis*, reported by some to be in bladder urine of an additional 10–15 percent of pregnant women, play a significant pathogenic role.[271,277] Pregnant women of higher socioeconomic status have a lower frequency of bacteriuria of pregnancy than women of lower socioeconomic status.[145] The prevalence of bacteriuria also rises with parity and age.[278] For example, in low-income populations, the prevalence of bacteriuria is about 2 percent in primiparas under age 21 as compared with 8–10 percent in grandmultiparas over age 35.[276] Most women who develop bacteriuria during pregnancy have infection at the first prenatal visit. However, 1–1.5 percent of pregnant women or about 25 percent of those with bacteriuria of pregnancy develop infection in the later trimesters.[275,276] The development of symptomatic pyelonephritis late in pregnancy is usually an expression of asymptomatic bacteriuria that was present early in parturition. The marked dilatation of the ureters and pelves during the later stages apparently allows bacteria in the bladder to reach the upper tract and to produce symptomatic pyelonephritis.

About 20–40 percent of the patients with bacteriuria early in gestation develop acute symptomatic pyelonephritis later in pregnancy.[277–280] In contrast, less than 1 percent of patients whose urine is uninfected early in gestation develop acute infection. Therefore, over 75 percent of the cases of acute pyelonephritis can be prevented by eliminating asymptomatic bacteriuria in the early stages of pregnancy.[271,275,276] It has also been noted that those whose bacteriuria fails to respond to treatment are at highest risk of developing symptomatic infection.[281] Lack of cure is probably an indication of upper versus lower tract infection.

An association between acute pyelonephritis of pregnancy and premature delivery was well known in the preantibiotic era.[271] The rate of prematurity can be as high as 20–50 percent. Kass[278] in 1959 reported that there was an association between asymptomatic bacteriuria and prematurity, and that the eradication of bacteriuria significantly reduced the rate of premature delivery. Since then there have been conflicting studies both supporting and denying these observations.[271,276,281] In general, it seems that prematurity is increased in patients with asymptomatic bacteriuria. However, it does not necessarily follow that asymptomatic bacteriuria is a cause of prematurity. It is possible that certain patients are predisposed to both bacteriuria and to deliver premature infants. Some investigators have reported that elimination of bacteriuria decreases the frequency of prematurity.[271,276,281] However, other studies have failed to show a decrease in prematurity or fetal wastage with elimination of asymptomatic bacteriuria.[271,276,281] Neonates of patients refractory to multiple courses of therapy have been reported to have a significantly lower birth weight than infants of those who respond; this phenomenon may be related to the presence of upper tract infection in these patients.[194,281,282] There have been several studies that have attempted to relate asymptomatic bacteriuria to the development of hypertension in pregnancy, but results have been unclear.[276]

Even though the data relating bacteriuria of pregnancy to prematurity are not clear-cut, the relationship of asymptomatic bacteriuria to later development of acute pyelonephritis is indisputable. As acute pyelonephritis has possible serious consequences for both mother and fetus, screening for, and treatment of bacteriuria of pregnancy seems justified. Quantitative urine cultures should be obtained in all pregnant patients at the initial prenatal visit.

Postpartum studies of patients with bacteriuria of pregnancy demonstrate a high frequency of bacteriuria even with treatment during the pregnancy.[283] Postpartum intravenous pyelography of these patients has shown that 10–30 percent have radiologic changes of "chronic pyelonephritis" and other abnormalities.[221,283] These abnormalities are most common in patients in whom renal bacteriuria has been demonstrated or in whom bacteriuria during pregnancy was difficult to eradicate with antimicrobial therapy.[283,284] However, pyelographic abnormalities should not necessarily be attributed to the infection that occurred during the pregnancy. In fact, these abnormalities probably antedate the pregnancy and in most cases are related to childhood infection. Treatment of bacteriuria of pregnancy has little effect on the long-term course of the patient. When patients who had bacteriuria of pregnancy were studied 10–14 years later, there were no differences between those who were treated and those who were not. About 25 percent of the women in each group had bacteriuria at time of follow-up.[221]

Management of Bacteriuria of Pregnancy

Treatment with an appropriate antimicrobial agent is recommended for all pregnant patients found to have significant bacteriuria.[188,271,276,277,280] The goal of therapy is to maintain sterile urine throughout gestation and thereby to avoid the complications associated with urinary tract infection during pregnancy. The administration of a relatively nontoxic drug for 7 days (e.g., a sulfonamide, ampicillin, cephalexin, nitrofurantoin) eradicates bacteriuria in 70–80 percent of patients.[188,271,276] Failure of treatment is most commonly seen in patients with renal infection or radiologic abnormalities of the urinary tract.[188,271,276] Sulfonamides should not be administered in the last few weeks of gestation because of hyperbilirubinemia and kernicterus in the newborn. Tetracyclines should be avoided during pregnancy.

There are relatively few studies evaluating the efficacy of single-dose or 3 days of antimicrobial therapy for asymptomatic bacteriuria during pregnancy. In general, results appear to be inferior to conventional therapy.[271] However, single-dose or 3 days of therapy may be a reasonable first option both in symptomatic and in asymptomatic infection in an attempt to decrease drug administration in pregnancy.

Urine cultures should be obtained 1–2 weeks after discontinuing therapy and at regular intervals (e.g., monthly) for the remainder of gestation. If bacteriuria recurs, therapy should be given for relapse or reinfection, as already discussed. Catheterization should be avoided at the time of delivery. If relapses or multiple reinfections occurred during pregnancy, radiologic evaluation should be considered postpartum.

PROSTATITIS

Bacterial prostatitis can manifest as either an acute or chronic disease. Although the manner by which bacteria reach the prostate is unknown,[285] possibilities include the hematogenous route, ascending infection from the urethra, and lymphatic spread from the rectum. Reflux of infected urine may also play a role in the pathogenesis of bacterial prostatitis.[286] Urethral instrumentation and prostatic surgery are known causes of prostatitis, but many patients have no history of a precipitating event.

Stamey and colleagues[287] have noted that male sex partners of women with vaginal colonization by gram-negative bacilli may develop transient urethral colonization with the same organisms. They postulated that sexual intercourse might play an important role in infection of the prostate.Prostatic fluid normally has substantial antibacterial properties.[67,288] However, the prostatic secretions of some patients with chronic bacterial prostatitis have been shown to lack such activity.[288]

The syndromes of acute and chronic bacterial prostatitis are different and distinct. Acute prostatitis does not usually result in chronic prostatitis, and chronic bacterial prostatitis is not usually antedated by acute prostatitis. Acute prostatitis is an acute infectious disease and is similar to an acute localized infection in any other organ, producing local heat, tenderness, and fever. In contrast, chronic bacterial prostatitis often produces few or no symptoms related to the prostate, which just serves as a nidus of low-grade infection. Some patients with chronic bacterial prostatitis have persistent symptoms such as perineal pressure, low back pain, or difficulty urinating. Symptoms of acute cystitis or pyelonephritis occur when bacteria, which are repeatedly invading the bladder, overcome the defense mechanisms of the bladder.

Bacteria originating in the prostate may be coated with antibody and, therefore, are a cause of a false-positive ACB test.[191,192] Following acute bacterial prostatitis, a serum and local immune response is elicited, with the presence of IgA and IgG bacteria-specific immunoglobulins being detected in prostatic secretions. More prolonged prostatic secretion of IgA is observed in chronic bacterial prostatitis.[289]

Acute Prostatitis

Most cases of acute bacterial prostatitis in the preantibiotic era were caused by *N. gonorrhoeae*. Gram-negative enteric organisms are now the most frequent pathogens.[285] *Neisseria gonorrhoeae* is currently an unusual cause.

Pathologically, acute bacterial prostatitis is characterized by inflammation of part or all of the gland with marked cellular infiltrate (predominantly polymorphonuclear leukocytes), diffuse edema, and hyperemia of the stroma. Microabscesses may occur and may be followed by large, clinically apparent collections of pus.

Acute bacterial prostatitis is characterized by high fever, chills, perineal and back pain, and symptoms of urinary tract infection such as frequency, urgency, and dysuria.[285] The patient may have urinary retention due to bladder outlet obstruction. The prostate gland is warm, swollen, and extremely tender on rectal examination. Expressed prostatic fluid contains many polymorphonuclear leukocytes, and the infecting organism can frequently be seen on Gram stain. However, massage of the acutely infected prostate gland can precipitate bacteremia and should be discouraged. Since most patients also have bacteriuria, the infecting organism can usually be isolated by midstream urine culture. Many antibiotics diffuse well into the acutely inflamed prostate, and acute bacterial prostatitis responds well to appropriate antimicrobial therapy. Complications such as bacteremia, prostatic abscess, epididymitis, seminal vesiculitis, and pyelonephritis may occur.

Chronic Bacterial Prostatitis

Chronic bacterial prostatitis is most commonly caused by *E. coli* (80 percent), but *Klebsiella, Enterobacter, P. mirabilis*, and enterococci are also common causes.[285] Although *S. epidermidis, S. aureus*, and diphtheroids have been frequent isolates in some series,[290] there is considerable doubt as to their real pathogenic role, and most gram-positive bacteria cultured in association with prostatitis represent urethral commensals.[291]

The histologic findings of chronic bacterial prostatitis are focal, nonacute inflammation. similar findings may be noted in patients without evidence of bacterial infection and are therefore not diagnostic of bacterial prostatitis.

Many men with chronic infection of the prostate are totally asymptomatic. However, some have perineal discomfort, low back pain, or dysuria. Symptoms of acute urinary tract infection may appear periodically. In fact, chronic bacterial prostatitis is probably the most common cause of relapsing urinary tract infection in men. Fever, if present, tends to be low grade unless pyelonephritis occurs. The results of rectal examination and intravenous pyelogram are unremarkable unless the patient also has an enlarged prostate gland from benign prostatic hypertrophy or carcinoma.

Because of the focal nature of chronic bacterial prostatitis, needle biopsy of the prostate gland for culture of tissue is unreliable.[292] Demonstration of leukocytes in prostatic fluid is not specific for bacterial prostatitis. Most clinicians agree that >15 leukocytes per high-power field represents an abnormal number of leukocytes in prostatic fluid.[291] Provided that simultaneous urethral and midstream specimens show insignificant pyuria, this finding would indicate prostatic inflammation irrespective of the etiology. Meares and Stamey[183] have described a quantitative localization technique for making the bacteriologic diagnosis. Because bacteria present in the urethra can contaminate prostatic secretions obtained by prostatic massage, accurate diagnosis requires simultaneous quantitative cultures of (*1*) urethral urine (VB_1), (*2*) midstream urine (VB_2), (*3*) prostatic secretions expressed by massage (EPS), and (*4*) the urine voided after massage (VB_3). An ejaculate is probably preferable to the EPS.

The specimens must be cultured immediately after collection, and methods of quantitating small numbers of bacteria must be used. The study should be done at a time the patient does not have significant bacteriuria. If bacteriuria is present, ampicillin, cephalexin, or nitrofurantoin should be given for 2–3 days to sterilize the urine; these agents will not affect bacterial counts in the prostate in chronic bacterial prostatitis. If chronic bacterial prostatitis is present, the number of bacteria in EPS or ejaculate will exceed those in VB_1 or VB_2 urine by at least 10-fold. If no EPS or ejaculate can be obtained, the bacterial counts in the VB_3 specimen should be at least 10-fold higher than the VB_1 or VB_2 samples.

Chronic bacterial prostatitis is very difficult to cure since few antimicrobial agents penetrate well into the noninflamed prostate. Furthermore, the nidus of infection in some patients may be small prostatic calculi or abscesses that presumably are difficult to sterilize. Chronic bacterial prostatitis is therefore likely to persist and cause relapsing urinary tract infection. Unlike classic urinary tract infection, relapses may occur after long periods without bacteriuria (e.g., months). Management may be difficult (see "Therapy," below).

Nonbacterial Prostatitis

This syndrome is the most common type of prostatitis and represents an inflammatory condition of unknown cause.[291] The symptoms are perineal pressure, dysuria, urgency, and/or low back pain, symptoms that can also be caused by chronic bacterial prostatitis. However, bacterial pathogens cannot be demonstrated using sequential quantitative cultures. Urinary tract infection does not occur, although prostatic secretions contain excessive numbers of leukocytes and fat-laden macrophages. The most controversial putative agent of nonbacterial prostatitis is *C. trachomatis*. The problem has been in distinguishing urethral colonization with *Chlamydia* from prostatic infection.[291,293] Similarly, the role of *U. urealyticum* is obscure. The term prostadynia or prostatosis refers to a similar clinical syndrome in the absence of any objective signs of prostatic inflammation. Some feel that the symptoms may be caused by spasm of the pelvic floor musculature.[294] Others feel that there may be a major psychological component. Because the etiology of both entities is unknown, therapy is difficult (see "Therapy," below).

Therapy

A dog model has been used to measure diffusion of antimicrobial agents into the noninflamed prostate.[295] In this system, antimicrobial agents are infused, giving high and constant plasma levels, and prostatic secretions are simultaneously collected. Although the basic macrolides such as erythromycin prenetrated well into prostatic secretions, penicillins, cephalosporins, tetracyclines, nitrofurantoin, and vancomycin did not. The explanation given was that only lipid-soluble and basic compounds are capable of entering the acid milieu of the prostate gland. Trimethroprim has been shown to diffuse into prostatic fluid in high concentrations.[296]

Acute bacterial prostatitis frequently responds dramatically to antibacterial therapy. It is thought that the intense diffuse inflammatory reaction of acute bacterial prostatitis allows the passage of antimicrobial agents from plasma into the prostate.[285] Therefore, in management of acute prostatitis, antimicrobial agents should be given to the patient in doses that achieve therapeutic concentrations in the blood. Measures such as hydration, analgesics, best rest, and stool softeners may be helpful. Urethral instrumentation should be avoided. If acute urinary retention occurs, suprapubic drainage of urine is required through a suprapubic catheter. Prostatic abscess is rarely cured by antimicrobial agents alone and requires surgical drainage. Computed tomography (CT) studies or transrectal ultrasonography are important advances in diagnosis of abscess formation.[297] Drainage can often be achieved by an ultrasound guided needle.

Chronic bacterial prostatitis is very difficult to cure. Partial transurethral prostatectomy is curative only if all the infected tissue is removed; about one-third of the patients are cured by this procedure.[285] However, a higher percentage is cured if a complete transurethral prostatectomy is performed.[291] Complete prostatectomy is contraindicated because of the complications of sexual impotence and incontinence.

The primary approach to chronic bacterial prostatitis is an attempt at cure with antimicrobial therapy. Although occasional cures have been achieved with penicillins, cephalosporins, tetracyclines, or aminoglycosides, the focus of infection in the prostate has usually persisted, resulting in relapse after therapy was discontinued. Better results have been reported in limited trials with trimethoprim–sulfamethoxazole (2 tablets twice a day), oral carbenicillin indanyl sodium, and rifampin in combination with trimethoprim.[298–300] Cure rates have varied from one-third to most of the patients treated with these agents for 1–3 or more months. The sulfonamide component of trimethroprim–sulfamethoxazole probably contributes little, and rifampin may be more suitable than sulfamethoxazole as a partner for trimethroprim. Rifampin has an excellent antibacterial spectrum, but has the unfortunate property of rapid development of resistance. Trimethoprim prevents emergence of resistance to rifampin.[300] Recently preliminary studies with oral quinolones have produced encouraging results.[301] At present, our initial regimen of choice is trimethoprim–sulfamethoxazole, or a quinolone. If therapy fails on these regimens, the patient should be managed either with treatment of acute exacerbations of urinary tract infection or with chronic suppressive therapy using low daily doses (e.g., half-normal doses) of an antimicrobial agent. Nonbacterial prostatitis can be treated empirically with erythromycin or tetracycline relying on clinical response to justify a further trial of therapy. Reassurance is important.

PERINEPHRIC ABSCESS AND INTRARENAL ABSCESS

Perinephric Abscess

Perinephric abscess is an uncommon complication of urinary tract infection.[302] The most common predisposing factors are urinary tract calculi and diabetes mellitus. It usually occurs secondary to obstruction of an infected kidney or calyx or occasionally secondary to bacteremia. It may occur insidiously, and up to one-third of cases may not be diagnosed until autopsy. The infecting bacteria are usually gram-negative enteric bacilli and occasionally gram-positive cocci when the infection is of hematogenous origin.

The patients have a syndrome suggestive of acute pyelonephritis, with fever, abdominal and flank pain (usually unilateral), and often symptoms of lower tract infection. The patient has often been ill for 2 or more weeks. The diagnosis should be strongly considered in any patient with a febrile illness and unilateral flank pain who does not respond to therapy for acute pyelonephritis. A palpable mass may or may not be present. About one-half of the patients have an abnormal plain film of the abdomen (e.g., abdominal mass, a calculus, a poorly defined renal shadow), and 85 percent have abnormal intravenous pyelograms.

Intrarenal Abscess

Intrarenal abscess may occur as a consequence of bacteremia (often caused by coagulase-positive staphylococci). However, these lesions are being recognized with increasing frequency as a complication of classic acute pyelonephritis. The clinical setting is usually that of acute pyelonephritis with high fever, severe flank pain, and tenderness, but with no response or very slow response to appropriate antimicrobial therapy. Most patients with intrarenal abscess respond, although slowly, to antimicrobial therapy, but fever and severe flank pain may persist for days. Occasionally drainage becomes necessary.

Diagnosis and Therapy

The introduction of renal ultrasound and in particular CT scans have added a new dimension of sensitivity and specificity permitting the early diagnosis of intrarenal and perinephric

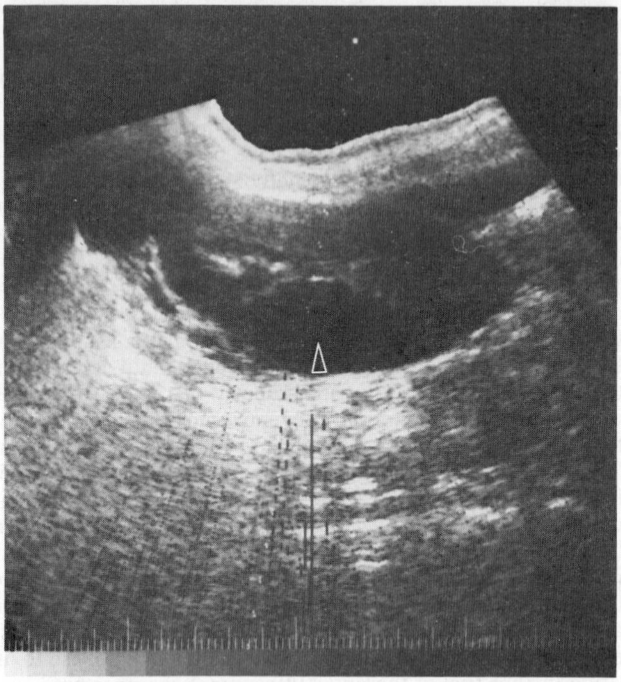

FIG. 10. Ultrasound examination of the kidney showing an intrarenal abscess (arrow). (Courtesy of Dr. George Popky, Philadelphia, PA.)

abscesses[303,304] (Figs. 10 and 11). The most common CT findings include thickening of Gerota's fascia, renal enlargement, focal parenchymal decreased attenuation, and fluid and/or gas in and around the kidney.[305]

In patients with a clinical or radiographic suspicion of perinephric abscess, diagnostic needle aspiration can be safely performed by using ultrasound or CT scan quidance. When an abscess is confirmed, small catheters can be introduced percutaneously via the diagnostic aspiration route to provide immediate decompression as well as continuous and definitive drainage without need for surgery.[303,304] Advantages to guided percutaneous drainage compared with open surgical drainage include earlier diagnosis and treatment, avoidance of general anesthesia and surgery, less expensive therapy, easier nursing

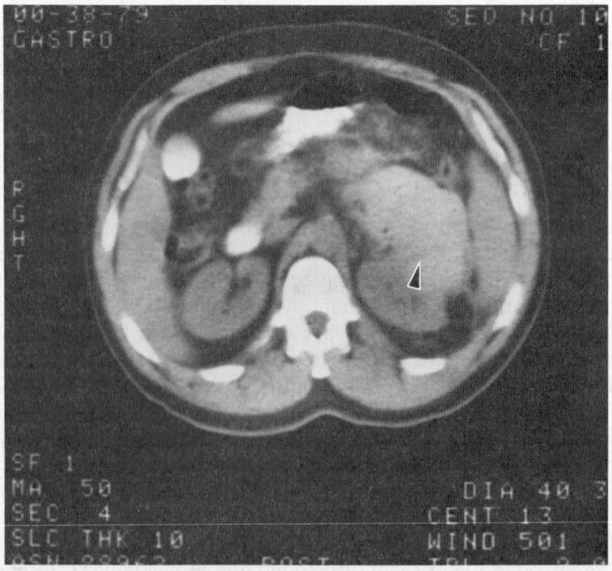

FIG. 11. CT scan showing a perinephric abscess (arrow). (Courtesy of Dr. George Popky, Philadelphia, PA.)

care, and greater patient acceptance of closed drainage. Accordingly, it is now recommended that after starting antimicrobial therapy directed against the most likely pathogens, a trial of percutaneous drainage should be the initial mode of therapy for perinephric abscess. Surgical intervention should be undertaken only when percutaneous drainage fails or is contraindicated. While parenteral antimicrobial therapy directed against the infecting organism isolated from blood or urine should be initiated before drainage, if additional organisms are isolated at the time of surgery, treatment directed against these organisms must be added. Therapy must also be used for the underlying disease (for example, staphylococcal bacteremia or obstructive uropathy).

Percutaneous drainage has been equally effective in drainage of renal abscesses and infected renal cysts, often avoiding the previous approach of open surgical drainage or nephrectomy.[303,306,307]

RADIOLOGIC EVALUATION OF PATIENTS WITH URINARY TRACT INFECTION

Radiologic procedures play an important role in the management of patients with urinary tract infection,[308,309] both in control of complicated episodes of acute pyelonephritis as well as in the investigation of patients of all ages in whom the clinician suspects the presence of underlying structural abnormalities that may be surgically correctable.

Radiologic assessment should commence with a plain film of the abdomen for detection of urinary tract calculi, calcification, soft tissue masses, and abnormal gas collections. In the past, excretory urography in the form of intravenous pyelography was the initial and definitive investigatory study but has been largely replaced by both ultrasonography and CT scans. In general, sonography serves as a rapid, noninvasive, and relatively inexpensive means of evaluating the renal collecting system, parenchyma, and surrounding retroperitoneum.[308] Ultrasound is more sensitive than intravenous pyelography for detecting parenchymal changes associated with renal infection; CT, however, is the most sensitive technique of all. Compared with CT, sonography offers several advantages, including no irradiation, portability, and relative accessibility.[309] Both CT and ultrasound are sensitive in diagnosing intrarenal and perirenal suppuration. Similarly, both these procedures may be used for guidance of percutaneous needle aspiration. Intravenous pyelography remains useful for detecting lesions of the collecting system and ureters. Contrast-enhanced CT provides physiologic information similar to that obtained with IV pyelography, with much better parenchymal delineation but less optimal delineation of the collecting system.[305] All studies requiring parenteral administration of contrast material are associated with some risk of allergy or contrast-induced renal insufficiency. Predisposing factors for renal insufficiency include myeloma, diabetes mellitus, pre-existing renal failure, severe intravascular volume depletion, and recent administration of large doses of iodinated contrast material. Radioisotope studies play only a small role, if any, in the investigation of the urinary tract. Gallium-67 citrate scanning and indium-111-labeled white blood cell studies occasionally prove useful in localizing inflammation or infection to the kidneys in patients with fever of unknown origin and may be of value, after ultrasound or CT scans have identified a solid renal mass, in suggesting the inflammatory nature of the lesion.

Radiologic or ultrasound investigation may be indicated in patients with nonresponsive pyelonephritis (particularly if bacteremic) to identify local complications such as renal and perinephric abscess formation. The most important contribution provided by these modalities is the detection of surgically correctable abnormalities of the urinary tract. Investigation should be considered in patients at greatest risk of having surgically correctable abnormalities. Persons with urinary tract infection included in this high-risk category are all children, men of any age, patients who relapse after therapy, and patients whose infection has been complicated by bacteremia. In the past excretory urography was indicated for all these categories and for adult women only after multiple episodes of urinary tract infection. As mentioned above, given the value of ultrasonography, its availability, and its safety, it is reasonable to study all patients with upper tract infection. Women with bacteriuria of pregnancy in whom eradication of infection is difficult should be evaluated. Whereas ultrasonography can be safely performed during pregnancy, accurate delineation of the urinary tract should be delayed until at least 2 months after delivery, by which time the physiologic alterations of the urinary tract that occur during pregnancy should be reversed.[271,272] Ultrasound examination is also useful in diagnosing lower urinary tract obstruction and detecting residual urine in the bladder. A radionuclide DTPA scan with furosemide to increase urine flow is useful in determining if there is structural as opposed to functional ureteropelvic junction obstruction.

In addition to delineating lesions amenable to surgical correction, urography frequently provides information previously unknown to the patient or physician. For example, unsuspected renal scarring may be seen, suggesting the presence of undiagnosed urinary tract infection in childhood (Fig. 12). Occasionally an unusual or unsuspected type of renal infection such as tuberculosis, papillary necrosis (Figs. 13 and 14), or xanthogranulomatous pyelonephritis may be discovered.[310] The last is a severe and chronic form of kidney inflammation in which areas of renal parenchyma are replaced by an inflammatory granulomatous reaction characterized by lipid-laden macrophages (foam cells).[310] Renal calculi and obstruction are often associated with this lesion.[272] Two major radiologic patterns are seen: that of a localized mass and that of diffuse nodularity. When a mass lesion is present, differentiation from pyogenic abscess, tuberculous abscess, or avascular carcinoma may not be possible.

Excretory urography and voiding cystourethrography are recommended in all boys after the first episode of urinary infection and in preschool girls at least after the second infection.[311] Investigation is indicated since the incidence of vesicoureteral reflux in this population has been reported to be 20–35 percent. Reflux is associated with renal scar formation, and

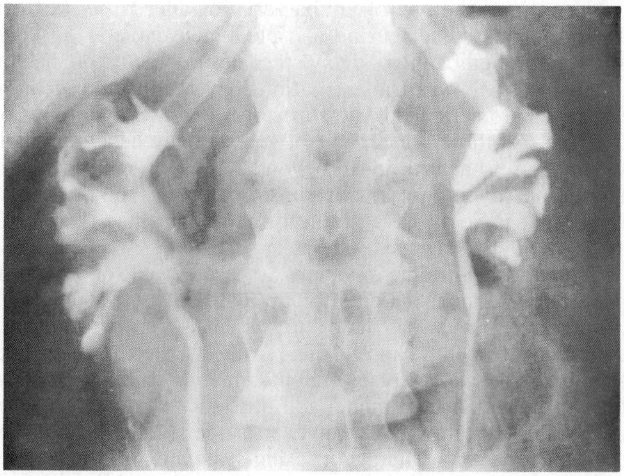

FIG. 12. Bilateral chronic pyelonephritis (retrograde pyelogram). Severe renal insufficiency precluded adequate visualization by excretory urography. Note the severe caliectasis bilaterally with marked left renal atrophy. There is moderate atrophy on the right.

While retrograde pyelography is not infrequently required to demonstrate the collecting system in severely diseased kidneys, it is probably best to avoid the performance of bilateral simultaneous retrograde pyelography in the azotemic patient. (From Kaye,[340] with permission.)

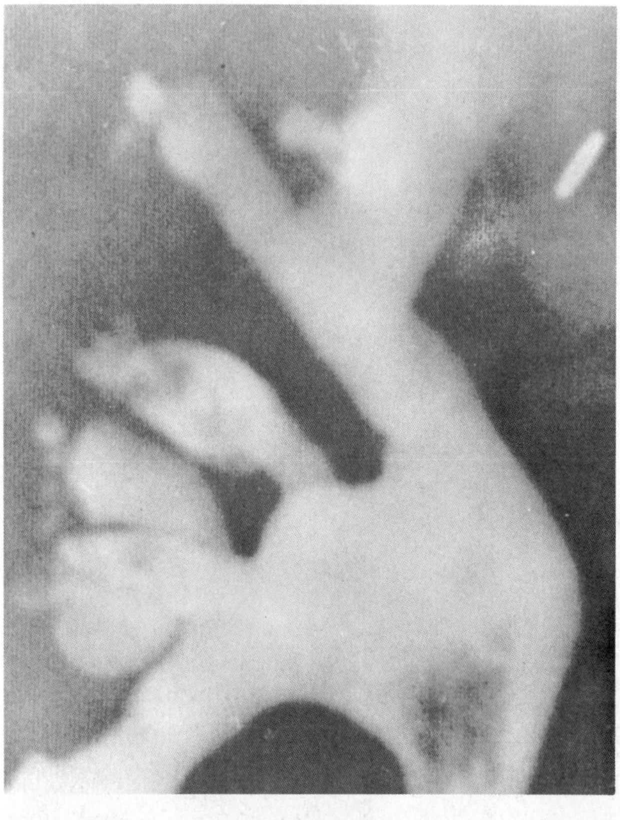

FIG. 13. Renal papillary necrosis (medullary type). Medullary cavities are seen involving almost all the visualized calyces. The cavities tend to be located within the central portion of the medulla rather than at the calyceal fornices. This is the medullary type of papillary necrosis so frequently associated with sickle cell disease, as was the case in this patient. Filling defects within the renal pelvis are attributable to a combination of sloughed papillas, mucus, and pus. (From Kaye,[340] with permission.)

surgery may be indicated in some of these children and infants. There is, however, growing evidence that ultrasonography is as sensitive and may replace intravenous pyelography as the initial study in evaluating children with urinary tract infections[312,313] and detecting children who require corrective surgery.[314,315] In children, intravenous pyelography should be used when other imaging methods show an abnormality and more detailed anatomic visualization of the upper tract is required.[312] As an elective procedure for detection and evaluation of vesicoureteral reflux, conventional cystourethrography or, more commonly, high-resolution radionuclide voiding cystography is still required, especially since reflux with urinary tract dilatation is frequently undetected by ultrasonography and intravenous pyelography. The use of radionuclide cystography involves less irradiation and is better tolerated than conventional contrast material introduced by bladder catheterization.[312] Cystourethrography should be avoided in older children unless intravenous pyelography shows evidence of renal scars. However, even with scars, if serial urographic evaluation demonstrates stability of upper tract lesions, the need for studying the lower tract is questionable. Fairly[316] has suggested that it may be possible to avoid cystourethrography by taking a late roentgenogram (4–6 hours) after intravenous pyelography. By this time the ureters should no longer contain contrast material, but the bladder will be filled. A voiding film taken at this time may then demonstrate presence or absence of reflux. Fairley feels that if no reflux is demonstrated by this method, it is doubtful that cystourethrography will add much in older children and adults. When reflux is found, it should be graded as minimal (grade I) to severe (grade IV), so progression or improvement can be quantitated and decisions on surgery can be made.[200]

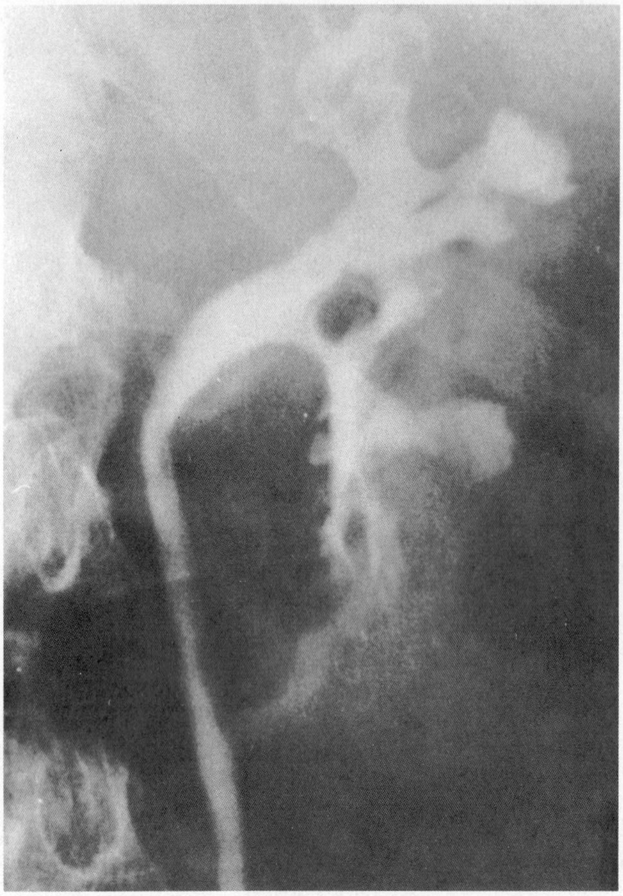

FIG. 14. Renal papillary necrosis (papillary type). The filling defects in the upper calyces represent sloughed papillas that have completely detached from the medulla. This has been referred to as the *ring sign* and indicates the papillary type of renal papillary necrosis. (From Kaye,[340] with permission.)

SURGICAL MANAGEMENT

Surgical therapy in the management of urinary tract infection consists of the elimination of obstructive lesions or calculi and the reimplantation of ureters in the bladder for reflux. An obstruction may be intrinsic (such as renal cysts), or it may be extrinsic anywhere along the urinary conduit from the ureteropelvic junction to the external urethral meatus. Surgical therapy should be directed toward eliminating the obstruction and preserving renal function. After the obstruction is eliminated, the patient should be followed with urine cultures. Urinary tract infection should be treated before surgery to render the urine sterile at the time of surgery; this decreases the possibility of bacteremia occurring in association with the surgery. For management of perinephric or intrarenal abscess see "Perinephric Abscess" and "Intrarenal Abscess," above.

CATHETER-ASSOCIATED URINARY TRACT INFECTION

The urinary tract is one of the most common sites of nosocomial infection, and most of these hospital-acquired infections occur in patients who have undergone urologic manipulation (frequently catheterization).[116] It has been estimated that 10–15 percent of the patients in community hospitals have indwelling urinary catheters. Proper catheter care and management is essential for prevention of infection (see Chapter 281).

Bacteria may enter the bladder at the time of catheterization especially if faulty technique is used. Two pathways have been postulated by which bacteria invade the bladder through indwelling catheters. The most important pathway with open-drainage systems is probably through the catheter lumen via the upward movement of air bubbles, by motility of the bacteria, or by capillary action.[58,317–319] The second route by which bacteria can reach the bladder is through the exudative sheath that surrounds the catheter in the urethra, and this route is probably more important with closed-drainage systems.[320]

The "open system" of indwelling catheters consists of a catheter with two lumens—one for balloon inflation and one for urine that drains into an open receptacle. Fifty percent of the patients with sterile urine before catheterization develop significant bacteriuria within 24 hours with this system; virtually all are infected at 4 days.[13] Furthermore, many of these patients also develop acute pyelonephritis and life-threatening gram-negative bacillary bacteriemia.[321–323]

Bacteria that produce catheter-associated urinary tract infection can be acquired from the patient's fecal flora, or by cross-infection (i.e., transfer of bacteria from patient to patient by hospital personnel).[117]

The incidence of catheter-associated urinary tract infection depends on the method and duration of catheterization. The risk of infection after a single catheterization is about 1 percent,[12] but it is higher in elderly or debilitated patients, in patients with urologic abnormalities, and in pregnant women.[12,324] Patients with indwelling catheters have a much greater risk of infection.

Prevention

Most patients who require indwelling urethral catheters need them for only short periods (less than 1 week).[319] Several systems of bladder drainage have been studied in an attempt to keep bladder urine sterile for this period of time. Administration of systemic antimicrobial agents to patients with open drainage systems does not prevent the development of bacteriuria but does predispose to infection with antibiotic-resistant organisms, such as *Pseudomonas* and *Serratia*.[325] The application of antibiotic ointments to the external urethral meatus, the incorporation of antibiotics into lubricants, and the impregnation of the catheter itself with antibiotics have met with little success in preventing infection with an open drainage system.[317]

In contrast, the use of antibacterial bladder rinses with the open-drainage system using a triple-lumen catheter has been shown to significantly delay the development of bacteriuria.[317,321,322] Several rinse solutions have been used including 0.25 percent acetic acid, nitrofurazone, and neomycin plus polymyxin. All three are capable of substantially delaying the development of bacteriuria (to beyond 10 days in most patients), but the neomycin–polymyxin rinse is probably the most effective. Most patients have sterile urine after catheterization for up to 10 days using this system.[326]

Sterile closed-drainage systems are also capable of preventing bacteriuria in most patients for up to 10 days without the use of antibiotic rinses provided the system is kept closed.[326] Indiscriminant opening and flushing of the sterile closed-catheter system are common causes of contamination and infection. Antibiotic rinses and ointments add little to the protective effect of a closed system.[327–330] However, some studies indicate that there may be an advantage in using systemic antibiotics when the closed system is used for only a few days.[319,327,331]

Closed drainage systems and three-way catheter systems with a neomycin–polymyxin rinse are comparable in preventing infection. However, our preference is for the closed drainage system, because (*1*) it is less expensive; (*2*) it is easier to maintain; and (*3*) if infection occurs, there is a reasonable chance that it will be with an antibiotic-susceptible organism. However, if for some reason frequent irrigation of the catheter is needed, an antibiotic drip is preferable. When catheters are required for many months or permanently, no system prevents infection.

In one study, the outlet tube of the closed urinary drainage set was kept full of 3% hydrogen peroxide at all times, and there was no evidence of bacterial growth in the urine of the collection bag in 92 percent of patients.[332] While this observation is of interest, it does not necessarily mean that there would be a major decrease in infection, as the more important pathway for infection with closed systems is probably via the urethra around the catheter.

Recommendations for urinary catheter care are listed in Table 2.

Treatment

Butler and Kunin,[335] using a closed sterile drainage system, showed that with systemic antimicrobials the initial infecting organism could usually be eradicated even though the catheter remained in place. However, when the catheter remained in place, subsequent reinfection was common, usually with more

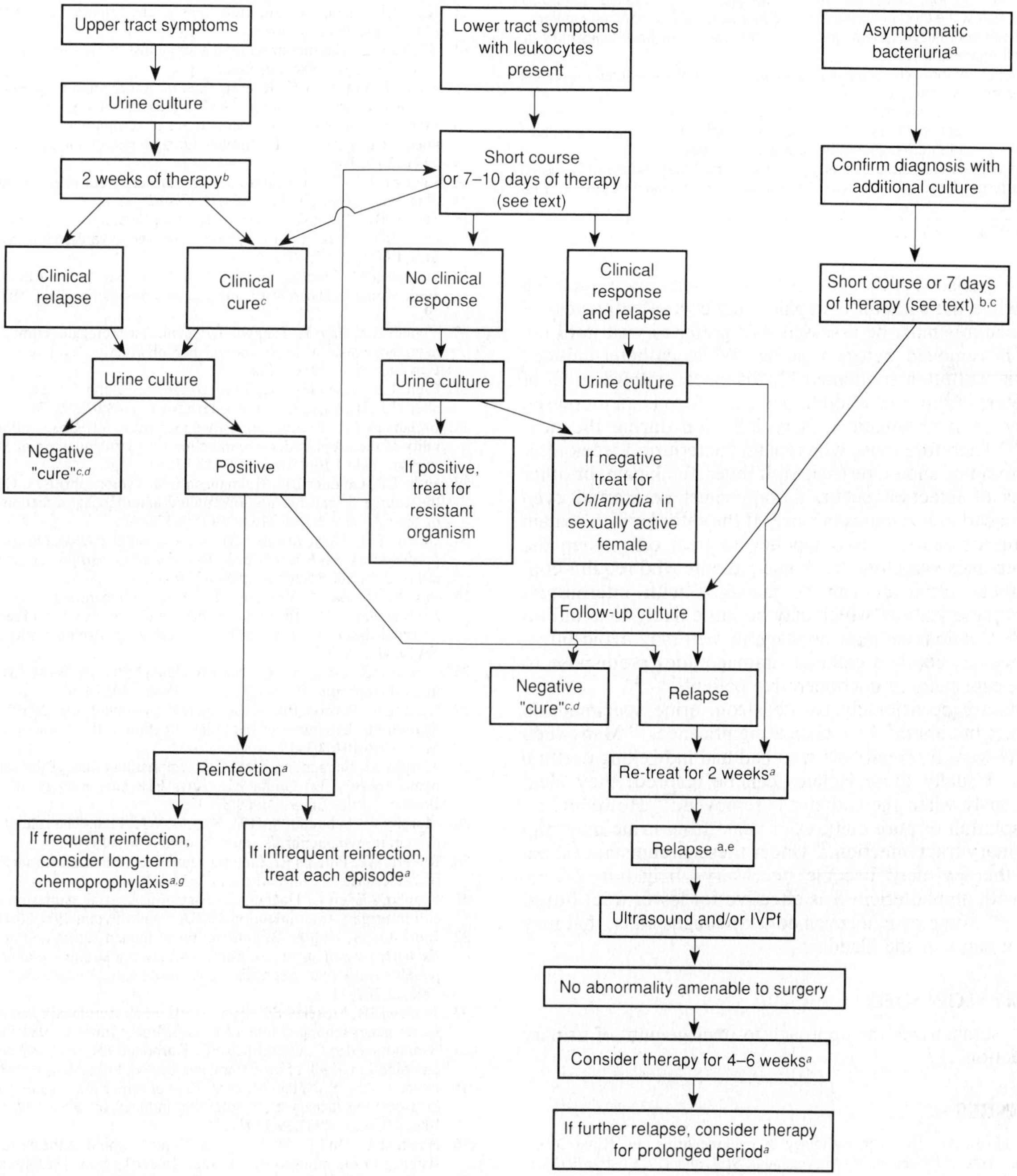

FIG. 15. Management of urinary tract infection.
[a] Consider no therapy in nonpregnant adults without obstructive uropathy or symptoms of urinary tract infection.
[b] Consider ultrasound and/or intravenous pyelogram (IVP) in all children and men with correction of significant lesions.
[c] Follow-up culture required only in pregnancy, in children, and in adults with obstructive uropathy.
[d] Follow-up cultures monthly in pregnant women and at 6 weeks and 6 months in children.
[e] Evaluate men for chronic bacterial prostatitis.
[f] Delay 2 months postpartum in pregnant women.
[g] Consider ultrasound and/or IVP after three to four reinfections in women.

TABLE 2. Guidelines for Indwelling Catheter Care[a]

1. Use only when absolutely necessary—not for convenience. Remove as soon as possible.
2. Catheters should be inserted and maintained by trained personnel only. Catheter teams are preferable.
3. Catheters must be inserted using stringent aseptic technique.
4. Perineal care should be administered twice daily. Antimicrobial ointment can be applied to the meatal-catheter junction.
5. When a sterile closed-drainage system is used, it is mandatory to keep it closed. The catheter and drainage tube must never be disconnected except when irrigation is necessary for obstruction. Sterile technique must be used under these circumstances.
6. Urine for culture should be obtained by aspirating the catheter with a 21-gauge needle after the catheter is prepared with povidone–iodine.
7. "Downhill," nonobstructed flow must be maintained. The catheter should always be below the level of the bladder and the bag should be emptied regularly.
8. Closed sterile drainage systems that have been opened or have leaks must be replaced immediately.
9. Replacement of indwelling catheters is not necessary unless concretions are felt or the system is obstructed.
10. Personnel and patients must be routinely educated on catheter care.
11. Catheterized patients should be separated from each other whenever possible.
12. Postcatheterization urine should be obtained for culture.
13. Patients with cardiac diseases that predispose to bacterial endocarditis should receive prophylactic antibiotics at the time of both catheter insertion and removal.

[a] See Stamm[333] and Fincke et al.[334]

resistant organisms. Although some experts may favor initiating therapy while the catheter is in place, the cost effectiveness of such procedures must be assessed. We prefer to wait until the catheter is removed before treating. While catheter-induced bacteriuria will often spontaneously disappear with removal of the catheter, in those in whom it persists, there is an increased frequency of symptomatic urinary infection during the next year.[319,336] Therefore those who remain bacteriuric 1 week after catheter removal should be treated. If fever, flank pain, or other symptoms of infection occur, therapy must be started even though the catheter remains in place. If the catheter is to remain for months or years, it is our policy to treat only when the patient becomes symptomatic. Some patients who require constant catheter drainage can be managed with intermittent straight catheterization, which may be more likely to avoid infection.[337] Condom catheter drainage in men may avoid infection. However, condom catheter drainage does predispose to infection, especially in uncooperative patients.[17,319]

Candida are occasionally isolated from urine specimens in pure culture but are rarely of clinical significance.[338] Many such specimens were from patients who had had indwelling urethral catheters. Usually these isolates can be ignored; they clear spontaneously when the catheter is removed.[338] However, repeated isolation of pure cultures of yeast from urine may represent urinary tract infection.[26] Under these circumstances, antifungal therapy may become necessary. Irrigation of the bladder with amphotericin B is effective for lower tract fungal infection.[339] Some patients even develop fungus balls, that may obstruct a calyx or the bladder.

SUMMARY FLOW SHEET

Figure 15 summarizes the approach to management of urinary tract infection.

REFERENCES

1. Susin M, Becker EL. The pathology of pyelonephritis. In: Kaye D, ed. Urinary Tract Infection and its Management. St. Louis: CV Mosby; 1972:65–83.
2. Freedman L. Chronic pyelonephritis at autopsy. Ann Intern Med. 1967; 66:697–710.
3. Murray T, Goldberg MD: Etiologies of chronic interstitial nephritis. Ann Intern Med. 1975;82:453–9.
4. Freedman LR. Natural history of urinary tract infection in adults. Kidney Int. 1975;8:S96–S100.
5. Monzon OT, Ory EM, Dobson HL, et al: A comparison of bacterial counts of the urine obtained by needle aspiration of the bladder, catheterization and midstream-voided methods. N Engl J Med. 1958;259:764–7.
6. Bran JL, Levison ME, Kaye D: Entrance of bacteria into the female urinary bladder. N Engl J Med. 1972;286:626–9.
7. Buckley RM, McGuckin M, MacGregor RR. Urine bacterial counts following sexual intercourse. N Engl J Med. 1978;298:321–4.
8. Kelsey MC, Mead MG, Gruneberg RN, et al. Relationship between sexual intercourse and urinary tract infection in women attending a clinic for sexually transmitted diseases. J Med Microbiol. 1979;12:511–2.
9. Nicolle LE, Harding GKM, Preiksaitis J, et al: The association of urinary tract infection with sexual intercourse. J Infect Dis. 1982;146:579–83.
10. Foxman B, Frerichs RR. Epidemiology of urinary tract infection: I. Diaphragm use and sexual intercourse. Am J Public Health. 1985;75:1308–13.
11. Leibovici L, Alpert G, Laor A, et al. Urinary tract infections and sexual activity in young women. Arch Intern Med. 1987;147:345–7.
12. Turck M, Goffe B, Petersdorf RG. The urethral catheter and urinary tract infection. J Urol. 1962;88:834–7.
13. Kass EH. Asymptomatic infections of the urinary tract. Trans Assoc Am Physicians. 1956;69:56–64.
14. Gillespie L. The diaphragm: an accomplice in recurrent urinary tract infections. Urology. 1984;24:25–30.
15. Fihn SD, Latham RH, Roberts P, et al. Association between diaphragm use and urinary tract infection. JAMA. 1985;254:240–5.
16. Fihn SD, Johnson C, Pinkstaff C, et al. Diaphragm use and urinary tract infections: analysis of urodynamic and microbiological factors. J Urol. 1986;136:853–6.
17. Johnson ET. The condom catheter: urinary tract infection and other complications. South Med J. 1983;76:579–82.
18. Strom, BL, Collins, M, West SL, et al. Sexual activity, contraceptive use, and other risk factors for symptomatic and asymptomatic bacteremia. Ann Intern Med. 1987;107:816–23.
19. Stamey TA, Timothy M, Millar M, et al. Recurrent urinary infections in adult women. The role of introital enterobacteria. Calif Med. 1971;115:1–19.
20. Vivaldi E, Cotran R, Zangwill DP, et al. Ascending infection as a mechanism in pathogenesis of experimental non-obstructive pyelonephritis. Proc Soc Exp Biol Med. 1959;102:242–4.
21. Cluff LE, Reynolds RC, Page DL, et al. Staphylococcal bacteremia and altered host resistance. Ann Intern Med. 1968;69:859–73.
22. Freedman LR. Experimental pyelonephritis. VI. Observation on susceptibility of the rabbit kidney to infection by a virulent strain of *Staphylococcus aureus*. Yale J Biol Med. 1960;32:272–9.
23. Guze LB, Goldner BH, Kalmanson GM. Pyelonephritis. I. Observations on the course of chronic non-obstructed enterococcal infection in the kidney of the rat. Yale J Biol Med. 1961;33:372–85.
24. Gorrill RH, DeNavasquez SJ. Experimental pyelonephritis in the mouse produced by *Escherichia coli, Pseudomonas aeruginosa* and *Proteus mirabilis*. J Pathol Bacteriol. 1964;87:79–87.
25. Prat V, Hatala M, Venesova D, et al. Pathogenicity of various strains of *Escherichia coli* for the intact rabbit kidney and the effect of repeated passage on renal tissue. In: Kass EH, ed. Progress in Pyelonephritis. Philadelphia: FA Davis; 1965:135.
26. Louria DB, Finkel G. *Candida* pyelonephritis. In: Kass EH, ed. Progress in Pyelonephritis. Philadelphia: FA Davis; 1965:179.
27. Guze LB, Beeson PB. Experimental pyelonephritis. I. Effect of ureteral ligation on the course of bacterial infection in the kidney of the rat. J Exp Med. 1956;104:803–15.
28. Murphy JJ, Schoenberg HW. The lymphatic system of the urinary tract and pyelonephritis. In: Quinn EL, Kass EH, eds. Biology of Pyelonephritis. Boston: Little, Brown; 1960:89–109.
29. Murphy JJ, Schoenberg HW, Rattner WH, et al. The role of the lymphatic system in pyelonephritis. Surg Forum. 1960;10:880–3.
30. Roberts AP, Phillips R. Bacteria causing symptomatic urinary tract infection or bacteriuria. J Clin Pathol. 1979;32:492–6.
31. Svanborg-Eden C, Hagberg L, Hanson LA, et al. Adhesion of Escherichia coli in urinary tract infection. CIBA Found Symp. 1981;80:161–87.
32. Bjorksten B, Kaijser B. Interaction of human serum and neutrophils with *Escherichia coli* strains: differences between strains isolated from urine of patients with pyelonephritis or asymptomatic bacteriuria. Infect Immun. 1978;22:308–11.
33. Johnson JR, Moseley SL, Roberts PL, et al. Aerobactin and other virulence factor genes among strains of *E. coli*. Infect Immun. 1988;56:405–12.
34. Svanborg-Eden C, Gotschlich EC, Korhonen TK, et al. Aspects of structure and function of pili of uropathogenic *E. coli*. Prog Allergy. 1983;33:189–202.
35. Iwahi T, Abe Y, Nakao M, et al. Role of type 1 fimbriae in the pathogenesis of ascending urinary tract infection induced by *Escherichia coli* in mice. Infect Immun. 1983;39:1307–15.
36. Hagberg L, Hull R, Hull S, et al. Contribution of adhesin to bacterial persistence in the mouse urinary tract. Infect Immun. 1983;40:265–72.
37. Hagberg L, Jodal U, Korhonen TK, et al. Adhesion, haemagglutination and virulence of *Escherichia coli* causing urinary tract infections. Infect Immun. 1981;31:564–70.
38. Svanborg-Eden C, Eriksson B, Hanson LA. Adhesion of *Escherichia coli* to human uroepithelial cells in vitro. Infect Immun. 1977;18:767–74.
39. Kallenius G, Mollby R, Svensson SB, et al. Occurence of P-fimbriated *Escherichia coli* in urinary tract infections. Lancet. 1981;ii:1369–72.
40. Leffler, H, Svanborg-Eden C. Glycolipid receptors for uropathogenic *Escherichia coli* binding to human erythrocytes and uroepithelial cells. Infect Immun. 1981;34:920–9.

41. Orskov I, Ferencz A, Orskov F. Tamm-Horsfall protein or uromucoid is the normal urinary slime that traps type 1 fimbriated *Escherichia coli*. Lancet. 1980;i:887.
42. Pere A, Nawicki B, Saxen H, et al. Expression of P_1 type-1, and type 1c fimbriae of *Escherichia coli* in the urine of patients with acute urinary tract infection. J Infect Dis. 1987;156:567–74.
43. Zafriri D, Gron Y, Eisenstein BI, et al. Growth advantages and enhanced toxicity of *Escherichia coli* adherent to tissue culture cells due to restricted diffusion of products secreted by the cells. J Clin Invest. 1987;79:1210–6.
44. Schaeffer AJ, Schwan WR, Hultgren SJ, et al. Relationship of type 1 pilus expression in *Escherichia coli* to ascending urinary tract infections in mice. Infect Immun. 1987;55:373–80.
45. Silverblatt FS. Host-parasite interaction in the rat renal pelvis: a possible role of pili in the pathogenesis of pyelonephritis. J Exp Med. 1974;140: 1696.
46. Svanborg-Eden C, Bjursten LM, Hull R, et al. Influence of adhesins on the interaction of *Escherichia coli* with human phagocytes. Infect Immun. 1984;44:672–80.
47. Fader RC, Davis CP. Effect of piliation on *Klebsiella pneumoniae* infection in rat bladders. Infect Immun. 1980;30:554–61.
48. Mardh PA, Colleen S, Hovelius B. Attachment of bacteria to exfoliated cells from the urogenital tract. Invest Urol. 1979;16:322–6.
49. Svanborg-Eden C, Freter R, Hagberg L, et al. Inhibition of experimental ascending urinary tract infection by an epithelial cell-surface analogue. Nature. 1982;298:560–2.
50. Aronson M, Medalia O, Schori L, et al. Prevention of colonization of the urinary tract of mice with *Escherichia coli* by blocking of bacterial adherence with methyl-α-D-mannopyranoside. J Infect Dis. 1979;139:329–32.
51. Schifferli DM, Abraham SN, EH Beachey. Influence of trimethoprim and sulfamethoxazole on the synthesis, expression and function of type 1 fimbriae of *Escherichia coli*. J Infect Dis. 1986;154:490–6.
52. Johnson JR, Roberts PL, WE Stamm. P fimbriae and other virulence factors in *Escherichia coli* urosepsis: association with patient's characteristics. J Infect Dis. 1987;156:225–9.
53. Fowler JE, Jr, Stamey TA. Studies of introital colonization in women with recurrent infections. VII. The role of bacterial adherence. J Urol. 1977;117:472–6.
54. Kallenius G, Winberg J. Bacterial adherence to periurethral epithelial cells in girls prone to urinary tract infection. Lancet. 1978;2:540–3.
55. Svanborg-Eden C, Jodal U: Attachment of *Escherichia coli* to urinary sediment epithelial cells from urinary tract infection prone and healthy children. Infect Immun. 1979;26:837–40.
56. Jacobson S, Carstensen A, Kallenius G, et al. Fluorescence-activated cell analysis of P-fimbriae receptor accessibility on uroepithelial cells of patients with renal scarring. Eur J Clin Microbiol. 1986;5:649–54.
57. Parsons CL, Schmidt JD. In vitro bacterial adherence to vaginal cells of normal and cystitis prone women. J Urol. 1980;123:184–7.
58. Weyrauch HM, Bassett JB. Ascending infection in an artificial urinary tract. An experimental study. Stanford Med Bull. 1951;9:25–9.
59. Boyarsky S, Labay P. Ureteral motility. Annu Rev Med. 1969;20:383–94.
60. Svanborg-Eden C, Hagberg L, Hull R, et al. Bacterial virulence versus host resistance in the urinary tracts of mice. Infect Immun. 1987;55:1224–32.
61. Musher DM, Griffith DP, Yawn D, et al. Role of urease in pyelonephritis resulting from urinary tract infection with *Proteus*. J Infect Dis. 1975; 131:177–81.
62. Freedman LR, Beeson PB. Experimental pyelonephritis. IV. Observations on infections resulting from direct inoculation of bacteria in different zones of the kidney. Yale J Biol Med. 1958;30:406–14.
63. Beeson PB, Rowley D. The anticomplimentary effect of kidney tissue. Its association with ammonia production. J Exp Med. 1959;110:685–97.
64. Rocha H, Fekety FR. Acute inflammation in the renal cortex and medulla following thermal injury. J Exp Med. 1964;119:131–8.
65. Kaye D. Antibacterial activity of human urine. J Clin Invest. 1968;47:2374–90.
66. Asscher AW, Sussman M, Weiser R. Bacterial growth in human urine. In: O'Grady F, Brumfitt W, eds. Urinary Tract Infection. London: Oxford University Press; 1968:3–13.
67. Stamey TA, Fair WR, Timothy MM, et al. Antibacterial nature of prostatic fluid. Nature. 1968;218:444–7.
68. Bryant RE, Sutcliffe MC, McGee FA. Human polymorphonuclear leukocyte function in urine. Yale J Biol Med. 1973;46:113–24.
69. Cox CE, Hinman F Jr. Experiments with induced bacteriuria, vesical emptying and bacterial growth on the mechanism of bladder defense to infection. J Urol. 1961;86:739–48.
70. Daifuku R, Stamm WE. Bacterial adherence to bladder uroepithelial cells in catheter associated urinary tract infections. N Engl J Med. 1986;314:1208–13.
71. Parsons CL, Greenspan C, Mulholland SG. The primary antibacterial defense mechanism of the bladder. Invest Urol. 1975;13:72–6.
72. Parsons CL, Schrom SH, Hanno P, et al. Bladder surface mucin: examination of possible mechanism for its antibacterial effect. Invest Urol. 1978;6:196–200.
73. Parsons CL, Mulholland SG, Anwar H. Antibacterial activity of bladder surface mucin duplicated by exogenous glycosaminoglycan (Heparin). Infect Immun. 1979;24:552–7.
74. Mulholland SG. Lower urinry tract antibacterial defense mechanisms. Invest Urol. 1979;17:93–7.
75. Cobbs CG, Kaye D. Antibacterial mechanisms in the urinary bladder. Yale J Biol Med. 1967;40:93–108.
76. Stamey TA. The role of introital enterobacteria in recurrent urinary infections. J Urol. 1973;109:467–72.
77. Kunin CM, Polyak F, Postel E. Periurethral bacterial flora in women. Prolonged intermittent colonization with *Escherichia coli*. JAMA. 1980; 243:134–9.
78. Stamey TA, Timothy MM. Studies of introital colonization in women with recurrent urinary infections. I. The role of vaginal pH. J Urol. 1975;114:261–63.
79. Stamey TA, Kaufman MF. Studies of introital colonization in women with recurrent urinary infections. II. A comparison of growth in normal vaginal fluid of common versus uncommon serogroups of *E. coli*. J Urol. 1975;114:264–7.
80. Stamey TA, Timothy MM. Studies of introital colonization in women with recurrent urinary infections. III. Vaginal glycogen concentrations. J Urol. 1975;114:268–70.
81. Stamey TA, Howell JJ. Studies of introital colonization in women with recurrent urinary infections. IV. The role of local vaginal antibodies. J Urol. 1976;115:413–5.
82. Stamey TA, Mihara G. Studies of introital colonization in women with recurrent urinary infections. V. The inhibitory activity of normal vaginal fluid on *Proteus mirabilis* and *Pseudomonas aeruginosa*. J Urol. 1976;115:416–7.
83. Stamey TA, Mihara G. Studies of introital colonization in women with recurrent urinary infections. VI. Analysis of segmented leukocytes on the vaginal vestibule in relation to enterobacterial colonization. J Urol. 1976;116:72–3.
84. Marsh FP, Murray M, Panchamia P. The relationship between bacterial cultures of the vaginal introitus and urinary infection. Br J Urol. 1972;44:368–75.
85. Elkins IB, Cox CE. Vaginal and urethral bacteriology of young women. I. Incidence of gram negative colonization. J Urol. 1974;111:88–92.
86. Cattell WR, McSherry MA, Northeast A, et al. Periurethral enterobacterial carriage in pathogenesis of recurrent urinary infection. Br Med J. 1974;4:136–9.
87. Brumfitt W, Gargan RA, Hamilton-Miller JMT, Periurethral enterobacterial carriage preceding urinary infection. Lancet. 1987;i:824–6.
88. Kurdydyk LM, Kelly K, Harding GKM, et al. Role of cervicovaginal antibody in the pathogenesis of recurrent urinary tract infection in women. Infect Immun. 1980;29:76–82.
89. Hanson LA. Host parasite relationships in urinary tract infections. J Infect Dis. 1973;127:726–30.
90. Miller TE, North JD. Host response in urinary tract infections. Kidney Internat. 1974;5:179.
91. Hanson LA, Ahlstedt S, Fasth A, et al. Antigens of *Escherichia coli*, human immune response, and the pathogenesis of urinary tract infections. J Infect Dis. 1977;136:S144–9.
92. Kaijser B, Larson P, Olling S, et al. Protection against acute pyelonephritis caused by *Escherichia coli* in rats, using isolated capsular antigen conjugated to bovine serum albumin. Infect Immun. 1983;39:142–6.
93. Hanson LA, Fasth A, Jodal U, et al. Biology and pathology of urinary tract infection. J Clin Pathol. 1981;34:695–700.
94. Mattsby-Baltzer I, Claesson I, Hanson LA, et al. Antibodies to lipid A during urinary tract infection. J Infect Dis. 1981;144:319–28.
95. Mattsby-Baltzer I, Hanson LA, Kaijser B, et al. Experimental *Escherichia coli* ascending pyelonephritis in rats: changes in bacterial properties and the immune response to surface antigens. Infect Immun. 1982;35:639–46.
96. Mattsby-Baltzer I, Hanson LA, Olling S, et al. Experimental *Escherichia coli* ascending infection in rats: active peroral immunization with live *Escherichia coli*. Infect Immun. 1982;35:647–53.
97. Svanborg-Eden C, Svennerholm AM. Secretory immunoglobulin A and G antibodies prevent adhesion of *Escherichia coli* to human urinary tract epithelial cells. Infect Immun. 1978;22:790–7.
98. Rene P, Dinolfo M, Silverblatt FJ. Serum and urogenital antibody response to *Escherichia coli* pili in cystitis. Infect Immun. 1982;38:542–7.
99. Rene P, Silverblatt FJ. Serological response to *Escherichia coli* pili in pyelonephritis. Infect Immun. 1982;37:749–52.
100. Fasth A, Ahlstedt S, Hanson LA, et al. Cross reaction between Tamm-Horsfall glycoprotein and *Escherichia coli*. Int Arch Allergy Appl Immunol. 1980;63:303–11.
101. DeRee JM, Van DenBosch JF. Serological response to the P fimbriae of uropathogenic *Escherichia coli* in pyelonephritis. Infect Immun. 1987; 55:2204–7.
102. Hopkins WJ, Uehling DT, Balish E. Local and systemic antibody responses accompany spontaneous resolution of experimental cystitis in cynomolgus monkeys. Infect Immun. 1987;55:1951–6.
103. Bille J, Glauser MP. Protection against chronic pyelonephritis in rats by suppression of acute suppuration. Effect of colchicine and neutropenia. J Infect Dis. 1982;146:220–6.
104. Hanson LA, Fasth A, Jodal U. Autoantibodies to Tamm-Horsfall protein, a tool for diagnosing the level of urinary-tract infection. Lancet. 1976;1:226–8.
105. Aoki S, Imamura S, Aoki M, et al. Abacterial and bacterial pyelonephritis. Immunofluorescent localization of bacterial antigen. N Engl J Med. 1969; 281:1375–82.
106. Schwartz MM, Cotran RS. Common enterobacterial antigen in human

chronic pyelonephritis and interstitial nephritis. N Engl J Med. 1973; 289:830–5.
107. Rocha H. Pathogenesis and clinical manifestations of urinary tract infection. In: Kaye D, ed. Urinary Tract Infection and Its Management. St. Louis: CV Mosby; 1972:6–27.
108. Rocha H, Guze LB, Freedman LR, et al, Experimental pyelonephritis. III. The influence of localized injury in different parts of the kidney on susceptibility to bacillary infection. Yale J Biol Med. 1958;30:341–54.
109. DeNavasquez SJ. Further studies in experimental pyelonephritis produced by various bacteria, with special reference to renal scarring as a factor in pathogenesis. J Pathol Bacteriol. 1956;71:27–32.
110. Cotran TS, Vivaldi E, Zangwill DP, et al. Retrograde pyelonephritis in rats. Am J Pathol. 1963;43:1–31.
111. Rocha H, Santos LCS. Relapse of urinary infection in the presence of urinary tract calculi: the role of bacteria within the calculi. J Med Microbiol. 1969;2:372–6.
112. Smellie JM, Normand ICS. Experience of followup of children with urinary tract infection. In: O'Grady F, Brumfitt W, eds. Urinary Tract Infection. London: Oxford University Press; 1968:123–38.
113. Smellie JM, Normand ICS. Bacteriuria, reflux, and renal scarring. Arch Dis Child. 1975;50:581–5.
114. Gould JC. The comparative bacteriology of acute and chronic urinary tract infection. In: O'Grady F, Brumfitt W, eds. Urinary Tract Infection. London: Oxford University Press; 1968:43–50.
115. Teles E, Rocha H. Epidemiologia de bacteriuria: prevalencia em pacientes hospitalizados e de ambulatorio. In: Rocha H, ed. Temas de Nefrologia. Salvador: Fundacao Goncalo Moniz, 1967:51.
116. Turck M, Stamm WE. Nosocomial infection of the urinary tract. Am J Med. 1981;70:651–4.
117. Kippax PW. A study of proteus infections in a male urological ward. J Clin Pathol. 1957;10:211–214.
118. Finegold SM, Miller LG, Merrill SL, et al. Significance of anaerobic and capnophilic bacteria isolated from the urinary tract. In: Kass EH, ed. Progress in Pyelonephritis. Philadelphia: FA Davis; 1965:159.
119. Mitchell RG. Urinary tract infections caused by salmonellae. Lancet. 1965;1:1092–3.
120. Paed L, Crump J, Maskell R. Staphylococci as urinary pathogens. J Clin Pathol. 1977;30:427–31.
121. Jordan PA, Iravani A, Richard GA, et al. Urinary tract infection caused by *Staphylococcus saprophyticus*. J Infect Dis. 1980;142:510–5.
122. Hovelius B, Mardh P. *Staphylococcus saprophyticus* as a common cause of urinary tract infections. Rev Infect Dis. 1984;6:328–37.
123. Gruneberg RN, Leigh DA, Brumfitt W. *Escherichia coli* serotypes in urinary tract infection: studies in domicillary, antenatal and hospital practice. In: O'Grady F, Brumfitt W, eds. Urinry Tract Infection. London: Oxford University Press; 1968:68–79.
124. Olling S, Hanson LA, Holmgren J, et al. The bactericidal effect of normal human serum on *E. coli* strains from normals and from patients with urinary tract infections. Infection. 1973;1:24–8.
125. Mufson MA, Zollar IM, Mandad VN, et al. Adenovirus infection in acute hemorrhagic cystitis: a study in 25 children. Am J Dis Child. 1971; 121:281–5.
126. Numazaki YN, Kumasaka T, Yana N, et al. Further study on acute hemorrhagic cystitis due to adenovirus 11. N Engl J Med. 1973;289:344–7.
127. Gutman LT, Turck M, Petersdorf RG, et al. Significance of bacterial variants in urine of patients with chronic bacteriuria. J Clin Invest. 1965;44:1945–2.
128. Boineau, FG, Lewy, JE. Urinary tract infection in children: an overview. Pediatr Ann 1975;4:515–26.
129. McCracken GH. Diagnosis and management of acute urinary tract infections in infants and children. Pediatr Infect Dis. 1987;6:107–12.
130. Neumann CG, Pryles CV. Pyelonephritis in infants and children. Autopsy experience at the Boston City Hospital, 1933–1960. Am J Dis Child. 1962;104:215–29.
131. Randolph MF, Greenfield M. The incidence of asymptomatic bacteriuria and pyuria in infancy. J Pediatr. 1964;65:57–66.
132. Huland H, Busch R. Pyelonephritic scarring in 213 patients with upper and lower urinary tract infections: Long-term followup. J Urol. 1984;132: 936–9.
133. Kunin CM. The natural history of recurrent bacteriuria in school girls. N Engl J Med. 1970;282:1443–8.
134. Kunin CM. Urinary tract infections in children. Hosp Pract. 1976;11:91–8.
135. Gillenwater JY, Harrison RB, Kunin CM. Natural history of bacteriuria in schoolgirls. A long-term case-control study. N Engl J Med. 1979;301: 396–9.
136. Freedman LR, et al. The epidemiology of urinary tract infections in Hiroshima. Yale J Biol Med. 1965;37:262–82.
137. Kass EH, Savage W, Santamarina BAG. The significance of bacteriuria in preventive medicine. In: Kass EH, ed. Progress in Pyelonephritis. Philadelphia: FA Davis; 1965:3.
138. Sanford JP: Urinary tract symptoms and infection. Annu Rev Med. 1975;26:485–98.
139. Kaye D. Urinary tract infection in the elderly. Bull NY Acad Med. 1980;56:209–20.
140. Romano JM, Kaye D. UTI in the elderly: common yet atypical. Geriatrics. 1981;36:113–5.
141. Boscia JA, Kobasa WD, Knight RA, et al. Epidemiology of bacteriuria in an elderly ambulatory population. Am J Med. 1986;80:208–214.
142. Boscia JA, Kaye D. Asymptomatic bacteriuria in the elderly. Infect Dis Clin North Am. Dec, 1987:893–905.
143. Kaitz AL, Williams EJ. Bacteriuria and urinary tract infections in hospitalized patients. N Engl J Med. 1960;262:425.
144. Kass EH. The role of asymptomatic bacteriuria in the pathogenesis of pyelonephritis. In: Quinn EL, Kass EH, eds. Biology of Pyelonephritis. Boston: Little, Brown; 1960:399.
145. Turck M, Goffe B, Petersdorf RG. Bacteriuria of pregnancy. N Engl J Med. 1962;266:857.
146. Forland M, Thomas V, Shelokov A. Urinary tract infections in patients with diabetes mellitus: studies on antibody-coating of bacteria. JAMA. 1977; 238:1924.
147. Whalley PJ, Pritchard JA, Richards JR. Sickle cell trait and pregnancy. JAMA. 1963;186:1132.
148. Govan D. Investigation and management of urinary tract infections in children. Urol Clin North Am. 1974;1:397.
149. Margileth AM, Pedreira FA, Hirschman GH, et al. Urinary tract bacterial infections. Symposium on Pediatric Nephrology. Pediatr Clin North Am. 1976;23:71.
150. Gleckman R, Blagg N, Hibert D, et al. Acute pyelonephritis in the elderly. South Med J. 1982;75:551–4.
151. Boscia JA, Kobasa WB, Abrutyn E, et al. Lack of association between bacteriuria and symptoms in the elderly. Am J Med. 1986;81:979–82.
152. Kaye D, Rocha H. Urinary concentrating ability in early experimental pyelonephritis. J Clin Invest. 1970;49:1427–37.
153. Levison SP, Levison ME. The effect of indomethacin and sodium meclofenamate on the renal concentrating defect in experimental enterococcal pyelonephritis in rats. J Lab Clin Med. 1976;88:958–64.
154. Levison SP, Pitsakis PG, Levison ME. Free water reabsorption during saline diuresis in experimental enterococcal pyelonephritis in rats. J Lab Clin Med. 1982;99:474–80.
155. Norden CW, Tuttle EP. Impairment of urinary concentrating ability in pregnant women with asymptomatic bacteriuria. In: Kass EH, ed. Progress in Pyelonephritis. Philadelphia: FA Davis; 1965:73.
156. Hellebusch AA. Renal papillary necrosis. A urological emergency. JAMA. 1969;210:1098–100.
157. Brumfitt W. Urinary cell counts and their value. J Clin Pathol. 1965;18: 550–5.
158. Thysell H. Evaluation of chemical and microscopical methods for mass detection of bacteriuria. Acta Med Scand. 1969;185:393–400.
159. Brumfitt W, Percival A. Pathogenesis and laboratory diagnosis of non-tuberculous urinary tract infection: a review. J Clin Pathol. 1964;17:482–91.
160. Boscia JA, Levison ME, Abrutyn E, et al. Correlation of pyuria and bacteriuria in elderly ambulatory women. Ann Intern Med. 1989;110:404–5.
161. Cobbs CG. Presumptive tests for urinary tract infections. In: Kaye D, ed. Urinary Tract Infection and Its Management. St. Louis: CV Mosby; 172:43–51.
162. James GP, Paul KL, Fuller JB. Urinary nitrite and urinary tract infection. Am J Clin Pathol. 1978;70:671–8.
163. Fritz H, Kohler L, Schersten B. Assessment of subnormal urinary glucose as an indicator of bacteriuria in population studies. Acta Med Scand. 1969;504(Suppl):256.
164. Pezzlo MT. Automated methods for detection of bacteriuria. Am J Med. 1983;75(1B):71–8.
165. Andriole VT. Diagnosis of urinary tract infection by culture. In: Kaye D, ed. Urinary Tract Infection and Its Management. St. Louis: CV Mosby; 1972:28–42.
166. Hoeprich P. Culture of the urine. J Lab Clin Med. 1960;56:899.
167. Kunin CM. New methods of detecting urinary tract infections. Urol Clin North Am. 1975;2:423–32.
168. Hardy JD, Furnell PM, Brumfitt W. Comparison of sterile bag, clean catch, and suprapubic aspiration in the diagnosis of urinary tract infection in early childhood. Br J Urol. 1976;48:279–83.
169. McFadyen IR, Eykyn SS. Suprapubic aspiration of urine in pregnancy. Lancet. 1968;1:1112–4.
170. Stamey TA, Govan DE, Palmer JM. The localization and treatment of urinary tract infections: the role of bactericidal urine levels as opposed to serum levels. Medicine. 1965;44:1–36.
171. Cattel WR, Sardeson JM, Sutcliffe MB, et al. Kinetics of urinary bacterial response to antibacterial agents. In: O'Grady F, Brumfitt W, eds. Urinary Tract Infection. London: Oxford University Press; 1968:212–26.
172. Stamm WE, Counts GW, Running KR, et al. Diagnosis of coliform infection in acutely dysuric women. N Engl J Med. 1982;307:463–8.
173. Goldberg LM, Vosti KL, Rantz LA. Microflora of the urinary tract examined by voided and aspirated urine culture. In: Kass EH, ed. Progress in Pyelonephritis, Philadelphia: FA Davis; 1965:545.
174. Gallager DJ, Montgomerie JZ, North JD. Acute infections of the urinary tract and the urethral syndrome in general practice. Br Med J. 1965;1:622–6.
175. Stamm WE, Wagner KF, Amsel R, et al. Causes of the acute urethral syndrome in women. N Engl J Med. 1980;303:409–15.
176. Stamm WE, Running K, McKuvitt M, et al. Treatment of the acute urethral syndrome. N Engl J Med. 1981;304:956–8.
177. Komaroff AL, Pass TM, McCue JD, et al. Management strategies for urinary and vaginal infections. Arch Intern Med. 1978;138:1069–73.
178. Stamm WE. Management of the acute urethral syndrome. Drug Ther. 1982;12:155–9, 162–3, 166.

179. Brun C, Raschou F, Eriksen KR. Simultaneous bacteriologic studies or renal biopsies and urine. In: Kass EH, ed. Progress in Pyelonephritis. Philadelphia: FA Davis; 1965:461.
180. Turck M, Ronald AR, Petersdorf RG. Relapse and reinfection in chronic bacteriuria. II. The correlation between site of infection and pattern of recurrence in chronic bacteriuria. N Engl J Med. 1968;278:422–7.
181. Fairley KF, Bond AG, Brown RB, et al. Simple test to determine the site of urinary tract infection. Lancet. 1967;2:427–8.
182. Fairley KF, Carson NE, Gutch RC, et al. Site of infection in acute urinary tract infection in general practice. Lancet. 1971;2:615–8.
183. Meares EM, Stamey TA. Bacteriologic localization patterns in bacterial prostatitis and urethritis. Invest Urol. 1968;5:492–518.
184. Clark H, Ronald AR, Cutler RE, et al. The correlation between site of infection and maximal concentrating ability in bacteriuria. J Infect Dis. 1969;120:47–53.
185. Ronald AR, Cutler RE, Turck M. Effect of bacteriuria on renal concentrating mechanisms. Ann Intern Med. 1969;70:723–30.
186. Reeves DS, Brumfitt W. Localization of urinary tract infection. In: O'Grady F, Brumfitt W, eds. Urinary Tract Infection. London: Oxford University Press; 1968:53–67.
187. Turck M. Localization of the site of recurrent urinary tract infection in women. Urol Clin North Am. 1975;2:433–41.
188. Andriole VT. Advances in the treatment of urinary infections. J Antimicrob Chemother. 1982;(Suppl A):163–72.
189. Thomas V, Shelokov A, Forland M. Antibody-coated bacteria in the urine and the site of urinary tract infection. N Engl J Med. 1974;290:588–90.
190. Jones SR, Smith JW, Sanford JP. Localization of urinary tract infections by detection of antibody-coated bacteria in urine sediment. N Engl J Med. 1974;290:591–3.
191. Thomas VL, Forland M. Antibody coated bacteria in urinary tract infections. Kidney Int. 1982;21:1–7.
192. Jones SR. The current status of urinary tract infection localization by the detection of antibody-coated bacteria in the urinary sediment. In: Gilbert DA, Sanford JP, eds. Infectious Diseases. Current Topics. vol. 1. New York: Grune & Stratton; 1979:97.
193. Merritt JL, Keys TF. Limitations of the antibody-coated bacteria test in patients with neurogenic bladders. JAMA. 1982;247:1723–5.
194. Harris RE, Thomas VL, Shelokov A. Asymptomatic bacteriuria in pregnancy: antibody-coated bacteria, renal function and intrauterine growth retardation. Am J Obstet Gynecol. 1975;126:20–5.
195. Thomas VL, Harris RE, Gilstrap LC III, et al. Antibody-coated bacteria in the urine of obstetrical patients with acute pyelonephritis. J Infect Dis. 1975;131(Suppl):557–61.
196. Riedasch G, Ritz E, Dreikorn K, et al. Antibody-coating of urinary bacteria in transplanted patients. Nephron. 1978;20:267–72.
197. Montplaisir S, Cote P, Martineall B, et al. Localization du site de l'infection urinaire chez l'enfant par la recherche des bacteries recouvretes d'anticorps. Can Med Assoc J. 1976;115:1096–9.
198. Hellerstein S, Kennedy E, Nussbaum L, et al. Localization of the site of urinary tract infections by means of antibody-coated bacteria in the urinary sediment. J Pediatr. 1978;92:188–93.
199. Kwasnik I, Klauber G, Tilton RC. Clinical and laboratory evaluation of the antibody-coated bacteria test in children. J Urol. 1979;121:658–61.
200. Smellie J, Edwards D, Hunter N, et al. Vesico-ureteral reflux and renal scarring. Kidney Int. 1975;8:S65–S72.
201. MacGregor ME, Freeman P. Childhood urinary infection associated with vesicoureteric reflux. Q J Med. 1975;44:481–9.
202. Bailey RR. The relationship of vesico-ureteric reflux to urinary tract infection and chronic pyelonephritis-reflux nephropathy. Clin Nephrol 1973; 1:132–41.
203. Cohen M. The first urinary tract infection in male children. Am J Dis Child. 1976;130:810–3.
204. Siegel SR, Sokoloff B, Siegel B. Asymptomatic and symptomatic urinary tract infection in infancy. Am J Dis Child. 1973;125:45–7.
205. Bakshandeh K, Lynne C, Carrion H. Vesicoureteral reflux and end stage renal disease. J Urol. 1976;557–8.
206. Salfatierra O, Tangaho E. Reflux as a cause of end stage kidney disease. Report of 32 cases. J Urol. 1977;117:441–3.
207. Hodson J, Maling TMJ, McManamon PS, et al. Reflux nephropathy. Kidney Int. 1975;8:S50–8.
208. Rolleston GI, Maling TMJ, Hodson CJ. Intrarenal reflux and the scarred kidney. Arch Dis Child. 1974;49:531–9.
209. Edwards D, Normand ICS, Prescod N, et al. Disappearance of vesicoureteric reflux during long-term prophylaxis of urinary tract infection in children. Br Med J. 1977;2:285–8.
210. Blank E. Caliectasis and renal scars in children. J Urol. 1973;110:225–6.
211. Cardiff-Oxford Bacteriuria Study Group. Sequelae of covert bacteriuria in school-girls. A four year follow-up study. Lancet. 1978;1:889–93.
212. Dodge WF, West EF, Travis LB. Bacteriuria in school children. Am J Dis Child. 1974;127:364–70.
213. Kraft JK, Stamey TA. The natural history of symptomatic recurrent bacteriuria in women. Medicine (Baltimore): 1977;56:55–60.
214. Pawlowski JM, Bloxdorf JW, Kimmelstiel P. Chronic pyelonephritis: a morphologic and bacteriologic study. N Engl J Med. 1963;268:965–9.
215. Schechter H, Leonard CD, Scribner BH. Chronic pyelonephritis as a cause of renal failure in dialysis candidates. JAMA. 1971;216:514–7.
216. Freedman LR, Andriole VA. The long term follow-up of women with urinary tract infections. Proc 5th Int Congr Nephrol (Mexico City) 1974;3:230.
217. Bullen M, Kincaid-Smith P. Asymptomatic pregnancy bacteriuria: a follow-up study 4–7 after years delivery. In: Renal Infection and Renal Scarring. Melbourne: Mercedes Publishing; 1970:33.
218. Gower PE, Haswell B, Sidaway ME, et al. Follow-up of 164 patients with bacteriuria of pregnancy. Lancet. 1968;1:990–4.
219. Asscher AW, Chick S, Radford N, et al. Natural history of asymptomatic bacteriuria in non-pregnant women. In: Brumfitt W, Asscher AW, eds. Urinary Tract Infection. London: University Press; 1973:51.
220. Gaches CGC, Miller KW, Roberts BM, et al. The Bristol pyelonephritis registry: 10 years on. Br J Urol. 1976;47:721–5.
221. Zinner S, Kass EH. Long term (10 to 14 years) follow-up of bacteriuria of pregnancy. N Engl J Med. 1971;285:820–4.
222. Gower PE. A long-term study of renal function in patients with radiological pyelonephritis and other allied radiological lesions. In: Brumfit W, Asscher AW, eds. Urinary Tract Infection. London: Oxford University Press; 1973:74.
223. Johnson CW, Smythe CM. Renal function in patients with chronic bacteriuria. South Med J. 1969;62:81–9.
224. Dontas AS, Kasviki-Charvati P, Panayiotis CL, et al. Bacteriuria and survival in old age. N Engl J Med. 1981;304:939–43.
225. Boscia JA, Abrutyn E, Kaye D. Asymptomatic bacteriuria in elderly persons. Treat or do not treat? Ann Intern Med. 1987;106:764–6.
226. Nordenstam GR, Brandberg CA, Oden AS, et al Bacteriuria and mortality in an elderly population. N Engl J Med. 1986;314:1152–6.
227. Levison ME, Kaye D. Management of urinary tract infection. In: Kaye D, ed. Urinary Tract Infections and Its Management. St Louis: CV Mosby; 1972:188–226.
228. Boscia JA, Kaye D. Asymptomatic bacteriuria in the elderly. Infect Dis Clin North Am. 1987;1893–905.
229. Platt R, Polk BF, Murdock B, et al. Reduction of mortality associated with nosocomial urinary tract infection. Lancet. 1983;i:893–7.
230. Platt R. Adverse consequences of asymptomatic urinary tract infections in adults. Am J Med. 1987;82(Suppl 6B):47–52.
231. O'Grady F, Gauci CL, Watson BW, et al. In vitro models simulating conditions of bacterial growth in the urinary tract. In: O'Grady F, Brumfitt W, eds. Urinary Tract Infection. London: Oxford University Press; 1968:80–92.
232. Kass EH, Zangwill DP. Principles in the long-term management of chronic infection of the urinary tract. In: Quinn EL, Kass EH eds. Biology of Pyelonephritis. Boston: Little, Brown; 1960:663–72.
233. Zinner SH, Sabath LD, Casey JI, et al. Erythromycin plus alkalinization in treatment of urinary infections. Antimicrob Agents Chemother. 1969: 413–6.
234. Vainrub B, Musher DM. Lack of effect of methenamine in suppression of, or prophylaxis against, chronic urinary infection. Antimicrob Agents Chemother. 1977;12:625–9.
235. McCabe WR, Jackson GG. Treatment of pyelonephritis: bacterial drug and host factors in success or failure among 252 patients. N Engl J Med. 1965;272:1037–44.
236. Stamey TA, Fair WR, Timothy MM, et al. Serum versus urinary antimicrobial concentrations in case of urinary tract infections. N Engl J Med. 1974;291:1159–63.
237. Minuth JN, Masher DM, Thorsteinsonn, SB. Inhibition of the antibacterial activity of gentamicin by urine. J Infect Dis. 1976;133:14–21.
238. Kunin CM, Finkelberg Z. Oral cephalexin and ampicillin: antimicrobial activity, recovery in urine, and persistence in blood of uremic patients. Ann Intern Med. 1970;72:349–56.
239. Johnson J, Stamm W, Diagnosis and treatment of acute urinary tract infection. In: Andriole V, ed. Infect Dis Clin North Am. 1987;1:773–91.
240. Stamm WE, McKevitt M, Counts GW. Acute renal infection in women: treatment with trimethoprim-sulfamethoxazole or ampicillin for two or six weeks. A randomized trial. Ann Intern Med. 1987;106:341–5.
241. Schwab SJ, Bander SJ, Klahr S. Renal infection in autosomal dominant polycystic kidney disease. Am J Med. 1987;82:714–8.
242. Michaeli J, Mogle D, Perlberg S, et al. Emphysematous pyelonephritis. J Urol. 1984;131:203–8.
243. Fang LST, Tolokoff-Rubin NE, Rubin RH. Efficacy of single-dose and conventional amoxicillin therapy in urinary-tract infection localized by the antibody-coated bacteria technic. N Engl J Med. 1978;298:413–6.
244. Gruneberg RN, Brumfitt W. Single-dose treatment of acute urinary tract infection. a controlled trial. Br Med J. 1967;3:649–51.
245. Slade N, Crowther ST. Multicenter survey of urinary tract infections in general practice. Br J Urol. 1972;44:105–9.
246. Ronald AR, Boutrous P, Mourtada H. Bacteriuria localization and response to single-dose therapy in women. JAMA. 1976;235:1854–6.
247. Rubin RH, Fang LST, Jones SR, et al. Single-dose amoxicillin therapy for urinary tract infection. JAMA. 1980;244:561–4.
248. Bailey RR, Abbott GD. Treatment of urinary tract infection with a single dose of trimethoprim-sulfamethoxazole. Can Med Assoc J. 1978;118: 551–2.
249. Souney P, Polk BF. Single antimicrobial therapy for urinary tract infections in women. Rev Infect Dis. 1982;4:29–34.
250. Pontzer RE, Krieger RE, Boscia JA, et al. Single-dose cefonicid therapy for urinary tract infections. Antimicrob Agents Chemother. 1983;23:814–6.
251. Rosenstock J, Smith LP, Gurney M, et al. Comparison of single-dose tet-

racycline hydrochloride to conventional therapy of urinary tract infection. Antimicrob Agents Chemother. 1985;27:652–4.
252. Harbord RB, Gruneberg RN. Treatment of urinary tract infection with a single dose of amoxycillin, cotrimoxazole or trimethoprim. Br Med J. 1981;283:1301–2.
253. Grossius G. Single dose nitrofurantoin therapy for urinary tract infections in women. Curr Ther Res 1984;35:925–31.
254. Carlson KJ, Mulley AG. Management of acute dysuria. Ann Intern Med. 1985;102:244–9.
255. Greenberg RN, Sanders CV, Lewis AC. Single-dose therapy for urinary tract infection with cefaclor. Am J Med. 1981;71:841–5.
256. Stamm WE. Single-dose treatment of cystitis. JAMA. 1980;244:591–2.
257. Philbrick JT, Bracikowski JP. Single-dose antibiotic treatment for uncomplicated urinary infections. Less for less? Arch Intern Med. 1985;145: 1672–8.
258. Stamey TA. Recurrent urinary tract infections in female patients: an overview of management and treatment. Rev Infect Dis. 1987;9(Suppl 2):S195–S208.
259. Shapiro ED, Wald ER. Single-dose amoxicillin treatment of urinary tract infection. J Pediatr. 1981;99:989–92.
260. Wong ES, McKevitt M, Running K, et al. Management of recurrent urinary tract infections with patient-administered single-dose therapy. Ann Intern Med 1985;102:302–7.
261. Vosti K. Recurrent urinary tract infection: prevention by prophylactic antibiotics after sexual intercourse. JAMA. 1975;231:934–40.
262. Bailey RR, Roberts AP, Gower PL, et al. Prevention of urinary-tract infection with low-dose nitrofurantoin. Lancet. 1971;2:1112.
263. Freeman RB, Smith WM, Richardson JA, et al. Long-term therapy for chronic bacteriuria in men: U.S. Public Health Service Cooperative Study. Ann Intern Med. 1975;83:133–47.
264. Stamey TA, Condy M, Mihara G. Prophylactic efficacy of nitrofurantoin macrocrystals and trimethoprim-sulfamethoxazole in urinary infection. N Engl J Med. 1977;296:780–3.
265. Smellie JM, Gruneberg RN, Leakey A, et al. Long-term low-dose, co-trimoxazole in prophylaxis of childhood urinary tract infection: Clinical aspects. Br Med J. 1976;2:203–6.
266. Stamm WE, Counts GW, Wagner KF, et al. Antimicrobial prophylaxis of recurrent urinary tract infections. Double-blind placebo control trial. Ann Intern Med. 1980;92:770–5.
267. Harding GKM, Buckwold FJ, Marrie TJ, et al. Prophylaxis of recurrent urinary tract infection in female patients. JAMA. 1979;242:1975–7.
268. Light RB, Ronald AR, Harding GKM, et al. Trimethoprim alone in the treatment and prophylaxis of urinary tract infection. Arch Intern Med. 1981;141:1807–10.
269. Grüneberg RN, Smellie JM, Leaky A, et al. Long-term low-dose, co-trimoxazole in prophylaxis of childhood urinary tract infection: Bacteriologic aspects. Br Med. J. 1976;2:206–8.
270. Brumfitt W, Smith GW, Hamilton-Miller JMT, et al. A clinical comparison between macrodantin and trimethoprim for prophylaxis in women with recurrent urinary infections. J Antimicrob Chemother. 1985;16:111–20.
271. Patterson TF, Andriole VT. Bacteriuria in pregnancy. Infect Dis Clin North Am. 1987;1:807–22.
272. Popky GL, Pollack HW. Radiologic evaluation of patients with urinary tract infection. In: Kaye D, ed. Urinary Tract Infection and Its Management. St. Louis: CV Mosby, 1972:84–123.
273. Guyer PB, Delaney D. Urinary tract dilatation and oral contraceptives. Br Med J. 1970;4:588–90.
274. Andriole VT, Cohen GL. The effect of diethylstilbestrol on the susceptibility of rats to hematogenous pyelonephritis. J Clin Invest 1973;43:1136–45.
275. Norden CW, Kass EH. Bacteriuria of pregnancy: a critical appraisal. Annu Rev Med. 1968;19:431–70.
276. Norden CW. Significance and management of bacteriuria of pregnancy. In: Kaye D, ed. Urinary Tract Infection and Its Management. St. Louis: CV Mosby; 1972:171–87.
277. Pedler SJ, Bint AJ. Management of bacteriuria in pregnancy. Practical Therapeutics. 1987;33:413–21.
278. Kass E. Bacteriuria and pyelonephritis of pregnancy. Trans Assoc Am Physicians. 1959;72:257–64.
279. Kincaid-Smith P, Bullen M. Bacteriuria in pregnancy. Lancet. 1965;1: 395–9.
280. Krieger JN. Complications and treatment of urinary tract infections during pregnancy. Urol Clin North Am. 1986;13:685–93.
281. Condie AP, Williams JD, Reeves DS, et al. Complications of bacteriuria in pregnancy. In: O'Grady F, Brumfitt W, eds. Urinary Tract Infection. London: Oxford University Press; 1968:148–59.
282. Gruneberg R, Leigh D, Brumfitt W. Relation of bacteriuria to acute pyelonephritis, prematurity and fetal mortality. Lancet. 1969;2:1–3.
283. Leigh D, Gruneberg R, Brumfitt W. Long term followup of bacteriuria in pregnancy. Lancet. 1968;1:603–5.
284. Williams JD, Reeves DS, Condie AD, et al. The treatment of bacteriuria in pregnancy. In: O'Grady F, Brumfitt W, eds. Urinary Tract Infection. London: Oxford University Press; 1968:160–9.
285. Meares EM. Prostatitis: a review. Urol Clin North Am. 1975;2:3–27.
286. Kirby RS, Lowe D, Bultitude MI, et al. Intraprostatic urinary reflux: an aetiological factor in abacterial prostatitis. Br J Urol. 1982;54:729–31.
287. Stamey TA. Urinary infections in males. In: Pathogenesis and Treatment of Urinary Tract Infections. Baltimore: Williams & Wilkins; 1980:342–429.
288. Fair WR, Couch J, Wehner N. The purification and assay of the prostatic antibacterial factor (PAF). Biochem Med. 1973;8:329–39.
289. Shortliffe LM, Wehner N. The characterization of bacterial and nonbacterial prostatitis by prostatic immunoglobulins. Medicine. 1986;65:399–414.
290. Drach GW. Prostatitis: man's hidden infection. Urol Clin North Am. 1975;2:499–520.
291. Meares EM Jr. Acute and chronic prostatitis. Infect Dis Clin North Am. 1987;1:855–73.
292. Kohnen PW, Drach GW. Patterns of inflammation in prostatic hyperplasia: a histologic and bacteriologic study. J Urol. 1979;121:755–60.
293. Weidner W, Brunner H, Krause W. Quantitative culture of *Ureaplasma urealyticum* in patients with chronic prostatitis or prostatosis. J Urol. 1980;124:62–7.
294. Segura JW, Opitz J, Green LF. Prostatosis, prostatitis, or pelvic floor tension myalgia? J Urol. 1979;122:168–9.
295. Winningham DF, Nemoy NJ, Stamey TA. Diffusion of antibiotics from plasma into prostatic fluid. Nature 1968;219:139–43.
296. Stamey TA, Bushby SRM, Bragonse J. The concentration of trimethoprim in prostatic fluid: nonionic diffusion or active transport. J Infect Dis. [Suppl] 1973;128:S686–90.
297. Meares EM Jr. Editorial: Prostatic abscess. J Urol. 1986;136:1281–2.
298. Meares EM. Long-term therapy of chronic bacterial prostatitis with trimethoprim-sulfamethoxazole. Can Med Assoc J. 1975:112(spec. no):22–25.
299. Mobley DF. Bacterial prostatitis: treatment with carbenicillin indanyl sodium. Invest Urol. 1981;19:31–3.
300. Giamarellou H, Kosmidis J, Leonidas M, et al. A study of the effectiveness of rifaprim in chronic prostatitis caused mainly by *Staphylococcus aureus*. J Urol. 1982;128:321–4.
301. Weidner W, Schiefer HG, Dalhoff A. Treatment of chronic bacterial prostatitis with ciprofloxacin: results of one year follow-up studies. Am J Med. 1987;82(4):280–3.
302. Thorley JD, Jones SR, Sanford JP. Perinephric abscess. Medicine (Baltimore). 1974;53:441–51.
303. Gerzof SG, Gale ME. Computed tomography and ultrasonography for diagnosis and treatment of renal and retroperitoneal abscesses. Urol Clin North Am. 1982;9:185–93.
304. Rauschkolb EN, Sandler CM, Patel S, et al. Computed tomography of renal inflammatory diseases. J Comp Assist Tomogr. 1982;6:502–6.
305. Bova JG, Potter JL, et al. Renal and perirenal infection. The role of computerized tomography. J Urol. 1985;133:375–8.
306. Costello AJ, Blandy JP, Hately W. Percutaneous aspiration of renal cortical abscess. Urology. 1983;21:201–4.
307. Finn DJ, Palestrant AM, DeWolf WC. Successful percutaneous management of renal abscess. J Urol 1982;127:425–6.
308. Filly R. Ultrasonography. In Friedland GW, Filly R, Goris ML, et al, eds. Uroradiology: An Integrated Approach. New York: Churchill Livingstone; 1983:311.
309. Piccirello M, Rigsby C, Rosenfield AT. Contemporary imaging of renal inflammatory disease. Infect Dis Clin North Am. 1987;1:927–64.
310. Grainger RG, Longstaff AJ. Xanthogranulomatous pyelonephritis: a reappraisal. Lancet. 1982;1:1398–401.
311. Hellerstein S, Wald ER, Winberg J, et al. Consensus: roentgenographic evaluation of children with urinary tract infections. Pediatr Infect Dis. 1984;3:291–3.
312. Honkinen O, Ruuskanen O, Rikalairen H, et al. Ultrasonography as a screening procedure in children with urinary tract infection. Pediatr Infect Dis. 1986;5:633–5.
313. Leonidas JC, McCauley RG, Klauber G, et al. Sonography as substitute for excretory urography in children with urinary tract infection. Am J Roentgenol. 1985;144:815–9.
314. Mason WG Jr. Urinary tract infections in children: renal ultrasound evaluation. Radiology. 1984;153:109–11.
315. Kangarloo H, Gold RH, Fine RN, et al. Urinary tract infection in infants and children evaluated by ultrasound. Radiology. 1985;154:367–73.
316. Fairley KF. The investigation and treatment of urinary tract infection. Med J Aust. 1976;2:305–7.
317. Andriole VT. Care of the indwelling catheter. In: Kaye D, ed. Urinary Tract Infection and Its Management. St. Louis: CV Mosby; 1972:256–66.
318. Gillespie WA, Linton KB, Miller A, et al. The diagnosis, epidemiology and control of urinary infection in urology and gynecology. J Clin Pathol. 1960;13:187–94.
319. Warren JW. Catheter-associated urinary tract infections. Infect Dis Clin North Am. 1987;1:823–54.
320. Garibaldi RA, Burke JP, Britt MR, et al. Meatal colonization and catheter associated bacteriuria. N Engl J Med. 1980;303:316–8.
321. Martin CM, Bookrajian EN. Bacteriuria prevention after indwelling urinary catheterization: a controlled study. Arch Intern Med. 1962;110:703–11.
322. Martin CM, Vaquer F, Meyers MS, et al. Prevention of gram-negative rod bacteremia associated with indwelling urinary tract catheterization. In: Sylvester JC, ed. Antimicrobial Agents and Chemotherapy—1963. Washington, DC: American Society for Microbiology; 1964:617–23.
323. Miller A, Linton KB, Gillespie WA, et al: Catheter drainage and infection in acute retention of urine. Lancet. 1960;1:310–2.

324. Brumfitt W, Davies BL, Rosser E. The urethral catheter as a cause of urinary tract infection in pregnancy and puerperium. Lancet. 1961;2:1059–62.
325. Sanford JP. Hospital-acquired urinary tract infections. Ann Intern Med. 1964;60:903–14.
326. Andriole VT. Hospital acquired urinary tract infections and the indwelling catheter. Urol Clin North Am. 1975;2:451–69.
327. Garibaldi RA, Burke JP, Dickman ML, et al. Factors predisposing to bacteriuria during indwelling urethral catheterization. N Engl J Med. 1974; 291:215–19.
328. Butler HK, Kunin CM. Evaluation of polymyxin catheter lubricant and impregnated catheters. J Urol. 1968;100:560–6.
329. Gladstone JL, Robinson CG. Prevention of bacteriuria resulting from indwelling catheters. J Urol. 1968;99:458–61.
330. Warren JH, Platt R, Thomas RJ, et al. Antibiotic irrigation and catheter-associated urinary tract infection. N Engl J Med. 1978;299:570–73.
331. Platt R, Polk BF, Murdock B, et al. Risk factors for nosocomial urinary tract infection. Am J Epidemiol. 1986;124:977–85.
332. Desautels RE, Chibaro EA, Lang RJ. Maintenance of sterility in urinary drainage bags. SGO. 1982;154:838–40.
333. Stamm WE. Guidelines for prevention of catheter-associated urinary tract infections. Ann Intern Med. 1975;82:386–90.
334. Fincke BG, Friedland G. Prevention and management of infection in the catheterized patient. Urol Clin North Am. 1976;3:313–21.
335. Butler HK, Kunin CM. Evaluation of specific antimicrobial therapy in patients while on closed catheter drainage. J Urol. 1968;100:567–72.
336. Andersen JT, Heisterberg L, Hebjorn S, et al. Suprapubic versus transurethral bladder drainage after colposuspension/vaginal repair. Acta Obstet Gynecol Scand. 1985;64:139–143.
337. Van Den Broek PJ, Dahha TJ, et al. Bladder irrigation with povidone-iodine in prevention of urinary tract infections associated with intermittent urethral catheterization. Lancet. 1985;1:563–5.
338. Thornton GF, Lytton B, Andriole VT. Bacteriuria during indwelling catheter drainage. JAMA. 1966;195:179–183.
339. Dudley MN, Barriere SL. Antimicrobial irrigations in the prevention and treatment of catheter-related urinary tract infections. Am J Hosp Pharm. 1981;38:59–65.
340. Kaye D. Urinary Tract Infection and Its Management. St. Louis: CV Mosby; 1972.

SECTION E

59. GRAM-NEGATIVE SEPSIS

LOWELL S. YOUNG

Bacteremic infections caused by gram-negative bacilli remain one of the major if not the principal infectious disease problem encountered in modern medical centers. These blood stream infections usually represent the most serious extension of a process that initially involves local sites such as the integument, urinary tract, respiratory tract, and mucous membranes of the gastrointestinal tract. While bacteremia can be transient, self-limited, and therefore of little clinical significance (as sometimes occurs spontaneously or with instrumentation of some organs), severe gram-negative rod bacteremia constitutes a medical emergency. It calls for an organized diagnostic approach and aggressive implementation of a therapeutic program directed at terminating blood stream invasion by the infecting microbe and, equally important, correction of the pathophysiologic sequelae to that event.

Gram-negative bacilli are a major component of humans' abundant native microbial flora. Thus it may seem paradoxical that these organisms have assumed such a major role in the modern practice of infectious diseases. There are a number of explanations for this apparent paradox, but one factor seems mainly responsible, namely, microbial opportunism in the face of significant depression of host defenses. This disturbance of the host–parasite relationship assumes many forms, and it would be naive to regard all the major categories of gram-negative bacilli as the cause of only one type of clinical syndrome. Indeed, there are quite clear-cut clinical differences between the fulminating bacteremic infections caused by the plague bacillus or by *Pseudomonas aeruginosa* and the more indolent blood stream infections caused by some *Salmonella* and *Haemophilus* species. The diseases caused by certain important gram-negative organisms are dealt with in individual sections of this book. This chapter will focus on the syndrome of gram-negative rod bacteremia.

HISTORICAL PERSPECTIVE

Diseases such as plague and typhoid fever are caused by well-known organisms, *Yersinia pestis* and *Salmonella typhi*, that are properly classified as gram-negative bacilli. Many of the signs and symptoms of the overwhelming gram-negative rod infections that are seen as nosocomial complications bear similarities to the catastrophic illnesses that have been identified with plague and typhoid that usually affect normal hosts. While the latter are classic examples of gram-negative rod bacteremia, it seems appropriate from an epidemiologic and clinical view to distinguish them from the syndrome of systemic gram-negative bacteremia that appears as a common nosocomial complication of current therapy for medical, surgical, and pediatric disorders.

Clinical descriptions of a "shock" syndrome after infections can be inferred from the work of physicians such as Laennec,[1] but the description of gram-negative rod bacteremia in the form that we appreciate it today is probably most correctly ascribed to work just before the beginning of the present century.[2] In fact, fewer than 100 cases appear to have been reported in the medical literature before 1920.[3] The current upsurge in the problem of gram-negative rod bacteremia is a development that has followed the introduction of antimicrobial agents. Waisbren, in 1951, can be properly credited with the first major report of cases of superinfection caused by gram-negative bacilli after the use of penicillins and tetracyclines to treat gram-positive infection.[4] Since that report many important clinical studies[5–7] have documented the role of gram-negative rods as a cause of bacteremic infection in patients often afflicted with a serious underlying disease. The increase in all types of nosocomial gram-negative bacillary infections that coincides with the introduction of a large number of antibacterial agents need not indicate a causal relationship inasmuch as the availability of new antimicrobial agents can be interpreted as paralleling other advances in medical and surgical practice. Among these developments has been the tendency to use increasingly more immunosuppressive therapy for various disorders and more aggressive surgical intervention. Viewed in this light, gram-negative rod infections can be properly regarded as diseases of medical progress.

INCIDENCE AND EPIDEMIOLOGIC TRENDS

The magnitude of the problem and its economic cost have been difficult to assess. Part of the problem in the United States seems related to the fact that gram-negative rod bacteremia is not an officially reportable disease. The bulk of available data derive from relatively few hospitals that have kept records on infections long enough to discern meaningful trends. The experience of one institution, that of Boston City Hospital, has been unique in that epidemiologic data have been collated by one technique and by one group of observers for a period of almost 40 years, from 1935 to 1972.[8] Bacterimas due to *Escherichia coli* and *Salmonella* species were the only ones that were seen with any frequency before the widespread use of sulfonamides. Between 1957 and 1972 the incidence of *E. coli* bacteremia per 1000 admissions rose fivefold at the Boston City Hospital. Community-acquired cases of *E. coli* bacteremia were usually more common than was hospital-acquired disease, but the case-fatality ratios were higher for the latter group. In 1972 *Klebsiella-Enterobacter* species were the second most common cause of bacteremic gram-negative bacillary infections (after *E. coli*), almost 4 cases/1000 admissions, a higher incidence actually than for *E. coli*. Remarkably, there were no cases of *Klebsiella-Enterobacter* bacteremia (excluding bacteremic Friedländer's pneumonia) identified at this hospital in 1935 and 1941.

Because it is often a complication and the final lethal event in the course of an underlying disease, identification of bacteremia per se may be omitted from an attributable cause of death in a patient with extensive burns or with an advanced hematologic malignancy. Statistical data derived from death certificates probably underestimate the magnitude of the problem, and incidence data from surveys of community or university hospitals, while filling an important gap in present knowledge, have provided little information on the disease-specific incidence of this complication, that is, the frequency in time of gram-negative rod bacteremia associated with underlying disorders such as collagen-vascular disease or lymphoma. It has been shown, for instance, in one cancer treatment center that *P. aeruginosa* represented two-thirds of all gram-negative rod bacteremias and 84 percent of all fatal gram-negative rod bacteremias in patients with acute myelocytic leukemia.[9] *Pseudomonas aeruginosa* has also been shown to be the most lethal bacteremic infection complicating renal, hepatic, cardiac, and bone marrow transplantation.[10–13] There are only limited data, however, on the disease-specific incidence for other gram-negative pathogens.

By extrapolating data obtained at one university hospital, McCabe estimated that as many as 300,000–500,000 cases of systemic gram-negative rod infections had recently occurred each year in the United States and that perhaps one-third to one-half of these cases were fatal.[14] A special task force appointed by the Director of the National Institute of Allergy and Infectious Disease in collaboration with the Centers for Disease Control reviewed much of the reported data on the incidence and mortality from gram-negative rod bacteremia and concluded that the correct figure for incidence in the United States was probably between 100,000 and 300,000 cases per year.[15] Many series have reported that mortality has ranged anywhere from 20 to 50 percent, with a clear-cut increase for those with the most adverse host factors such as neutropenia and immunosuppression (Table 1). However, in recent series this mortality appears to be decreasing.

A major goal of the Centers for Disease Control has been to obtain basic epidemiologic data on the magnitude of this problem and has led to the creation of the National Nosocomial Infections Surveillance.[27,28] The analysis of this information is divided into categories of "primary" and "secondary" bacteremia, the former being those cases in which no source could be identified and the latter being those infections in which the source of infection was secondary to an identifiable source. The 1976 survey[27] indicated that between 49 and 56 percent of all bacteremias were caused by Enterobacteriaceae and *P. aeruginosa*. When fungemias and miscellaneous blood-borne pathogens were deleted from the total, gram-negative rod bacteremia outnumbered all other causes of bacteremic infection. The 1984 survey[28] reflected the overall importance of gram-negative bacilli in nosocomial infections but also underscored the resurgence of gram-positive organisms as causes of bacteremia. Still, the mortality from gram-positive bacteremia has tended to be lower than from gram-negative bacteremia and case fatality ratios for *P. aeruginosa* bacteremia remain high.[29]

RELATIVE FREQUENCY OF GRAM-NEGATIVE BACTERIAL PATHOGENS AND ASSOCIATED MORTALITY

Table 1 summarizes the relative incidence of various aerobic gram-negative pathogens in a number of large series of bacteremic infections that have been reported since 1965.[16–26] This type of information seems valuable only in discerning the broadest trends and associations inasmuch as differences in mortality are likely related to the types of patients cared for at each in-

TABLE 1. Distribution of Gram-Negative Bacteremic Isolates Excluding Polymicrobial Infections

Author	Period of Observation	*E. coli*	*Klebsiella*	*Enterobacter*	*Serratia*	*P. aeruginosa*	*Proteus* Species	Total Episodes/ Mortality
EORTC[16]	1983–1986	63	9			34		129 (12)
Klastersky[17]	1981–1983	38	8			23		83 (17)
Weinstein[18]	1975–1977	76 (35)[a]	25 (48)			22 (72)		123 (39.8)
Spengler[19]	1968–1974	127 (38.6)	233 (31.8)	67 (35.8)	37 (32.4)	74 (68.9)[b]	30 (36.7)	568 (38.9)
Kreger[20]	1965–1974	189 (19.5)	74 (24.3)	47 (17.0)	11 (18.0)	60 (36.6)	49 (16.3)	430 (22.1)
Singer[21]	1972–1973	86 (17.4)	37 (43.2)		4 (0)	30 (60)	14 (35.7)	171 (31.6)
McHenry[22]	1967–1972	68 (26.4)	72 (26.9)	35 (14.3)	8 (25)	29 (48.3)	11 (27.3)	233 (27.3)
Myerowitz[23]	1968–1969	58 (18)	23 (13)	9 (0)	27 (54)	21 (57)[b]	13 (16)	151 (27.8)
Bryant[24]	1965–1968	83 (21)	57 (33)[b]			45 (71)	19 (16)	204 (34.8)
Dupont[25]	1958–1966	190 (42)	138 (55)[b]			67 (67)[b]	63 (33)	458 (50.7)
Altemeier[26]	1955–1967	93 (48)	68 (66)[b]			39 (77)	42 (67)	242 (61.2)
Usual rank order for frequency		1	2	5[c]	4[c]	3	6[c]	
Usual rank order for mortality		4[c]	2	6[c]	5[c]	1	3[c]	

[a] Values are numbers of isolates; mortality is in parentheses.
[b] Species grouped together.
[c] No significant difference in rank order.

stitution and the time each study was carried out. It has usually been observed that *E. coli* is the most common pathogen and that *K. pneumoniae* is the second most frequent. Some centers have not until recently differentiated among *Klebsiella, Enterobacter*, and *Serratia* species. *Pseudomonas* species are usually the third most common and are often grouped together. When speciated, most of these strains are identified as *aeruginosa*. The relative frequency of *Enterobacter, Serratia*, and *Proteus* bacteremias is probably not significantly different. It is noteworthy that *P. aeruginosa* has been consistently associated with the highest mortality of all bacteremic infections. In all likelihood this is a manifestation of the association of *P. aeruginosa* with neutropenia and clinical conditions like leukemia and extensive burns that have the more adverse clinical prognosis. Systemic *K. pneumoniae* infections appear to be associated with the next highest mortality after *P. aeruginosa*. When the outcome of gram-negative bacteremia is assessed in terms of the nature of underlying disease (such as in leukemia and burns), the mortality associated with specific pathogens (*P. aeruginosa, Klebsiella* species, and so on) appears more similar.

EPIDEMIOLOGY AND GRAM-NEGATIVE BACTEREMIC INFECTIONS

The gastrointestinal tract is the obvious reservoir of gram-negative bacilli, although many other sources of infection exist. Quantitative studies of healthy subjects have indicated that the endogenous fecal flora is predominantly anaerobic and that *E. coli* accounts for the largest proportion of aerobic gram-negative bacilli. Not surprisingly, *E. coli* is often the most common aerobic organism isolated from blood cultures. Additionally, *Bacteroides fragilis* is one of the most common anaerobic constituents of the fecal flora and by analogy is also commonly implicated in anaerobic gram-negative rod bacteremia. Most *E. coli* isolated from healthy people tend to be susceptible to most commonly used antimicrobial agents. Numerous studies, however, have indicated that organisms isolated from the fecal flora of hospitalized patients and those previously receiving antimicrobial therapy tend to have a larger proportion of organisms that are resistant to one or more antimicrobial agents.[30]

The finding that *E. coli* is the most frequently encountered organism in gram-negative rod septicemia seems related to its role in intra-abdominal trauma, postabdominal surgical infections, and pyelonephritis. It is widely accepted that initial fecal contamination of the lower urinary tract is the usual primary event in the pathogenesis of acute pyelonephritis. Thus, it would be expected that *E. coli* is the predominant organism in bacteremic genitourinary infections. Interestingly, *Bacteroides* species are rarely implicated in ascending pyelonephritis, and there must be a significant factor between the ability of aerobes and anaerobes to cause bacteremic infection via the urinary tract.

The dynamic interaction between the native, endogenous fecal flora and sources of gram-negative rods acquired from environmental sources have been the subject of several interesting studies. For instance, with *P. aeruginosa* it is now quite clear from selective microbial sampling surveys of many healthy subjects including medical students and nonhospitalized personnel that the prevalence of fecal carriage, defined as any isolation of *P. aeruginosa* from the stool, is less than 10 percent.[31,32] Fecal carriage increased fivefold with increasing debility or treatment of underlying diseases to neutropenia. Additionally, antimicrobial therapy with broad-spectrum agents predisposes to colonization by *P. aeruginosa*.[33] Careful prospective epidemiologic studies indicate that specific serotypes isolated from stool correlate very well with serotypes of *P. aeruginosa* that are subsequently cultured from blood.[34] Although it is usually possible to define the source of a gram-negative bacteremia, a certain number of intensely immunosuppressed patients may develop bacteremia without an obvious source. It has been postulated that the latter situation represents bacteremia originating from small ulcerations of the gastrointestinal tract. This is supported by some autopsy data and the epidemiologic data indicating a correlation between strains isolated from the blood and the organisms colonizing stool.[35]

It seems plausible that the normal host possesses mechanisms for resisting colonization by these potential pathogens or that the normal flora has an inhibiting effect on some potential pathogens (bacterial interference). Both normal and debilitated subjects are continuously exposed to *P. aeruginosa* from many environmental sources including food and water. Given the setting of the altered host, resistance to colonization by an as yet undefined factor (but perhaps relating to bacterial interference) is lost. Bacteremia ensues after the onset of neutropenia, disruption of mechanical barriers to microbial invasion, development of anatomic obstruction, or a combination of these factors. The evidence for a role of the normal flora in resistance to colonization lies in studies where normal volunteers fed large quantities of *P. aeruginosa* could not be colonized except when oral ampicillin was given concomitantly.[33]

Information on the epidemiology of *P. aeruginosa* infections is relatively more available because this organism can be easily differentiated from *E. coli* in environmental or fecal sampling surveys. Assessment of the epidemiology of *E. coli* bacteremia is more difficult because these organisms are components of the normal fecal flora. Some serotypes of *E. coli* seem more commonly involved in upper urinary tract infections which suggests that there may be some virulence factors that affect bacteremic urinary tract infection.[36] On the other hand, *Klebsiella, Serratia*, and *Proteus* are probably not part of the normal fecal flora of humans, and the same factors promoting *P. aeruginosa* colonization of stool may result in gastrointestinal acquisition. In one study there was a strong correlation between the serotype of *K. pneumoniae* isolated from stool and what appeared in a variety of infected sites including the blood stream.[37] For *Proteus* and *Serratia* infections, less information is available. There are data showing that irrespective of medical therapy the oropharynx of patients with serious underlying diseases becomes readily colonized by gram-negative rods; this parallels the deterioration in overall host status.[38] Thus the oropharynx is another site for colonization by gram-negative rods that precedes other organ involvement or systemic infection. It has been observed that organisms colonization the oropharynx correlate with some bacteremic isolates even when stool cultures are negative for the same organism.[39] This has occurred when some chemotherapeutic agents have caused ulceration of the upper gastrointestinal tract. The gastric mechanisms for elimination or reduction of organisms entering the small and large intestines may be a factor limiting colonization of the lower gastrointestinal tract in these patients.

Besides the gastrointestinal route there are clearly other pathways to invasion of the host. One of the most obvious mechanisms involves acquisition via exposure to contaminated inhalation therapy equipment and by gram-negative rods like *S. marcescens* and *P. aeruginosa*. This can lead to bacteremic gram-negative pneumonia, which has a mortality among the highest observed in gram-negative infections. A wide variety of other sources for gram-negative rods' invasion are possible including indwelling vascular catheters, monitoring devices, urinary tract catheters, drainage tubes, percutaneous reservoirs, contaminated intravenous fluids, and so forth. Instruments used for diagnostic procedures may be contaminated and may introduce infection into a relatively sterile area or may disrupt mucosal barriers in an area with its own microbial flora (like the lower gastrointestinal tract). Decubitus ulcers can be readily colonized by gram-negative rods and can be a source of bacteremic infection.

The plethora of gram-negative bacilli and the wide variety of serogrouping or serotyping systems that are available for organisms such as *E. coli* (more than 160 O types), *K. pneumoniae* (over 80 serotypes), and even *S. marcescens* (almost 20 serotypes) reflects the formidable task involved in defining the epidemiology of certain infections. Within the *E. coli* and *K. pneumoniae* strains there may be certain types that predispose to serious systemic infection. Extensive studies of *K. pneumoniae* infections have indicated that a relatively large proportion of infections are caused by a certain limited number of serotypes.[40] This suggests that certain organisms have selective advantages in some epidemiologic settings.

It is also apparent that antimicrobial usage has a very definite relationship to epidemiologic patterns of gram-negative infections. In immunologically impaired subjects, the bacteremias encountered early in the clinical course tend to be due to *Staphylococcus aureus* or *E. coli*, possibly because of the predominance of these organisms in the native flora. Repeated courses of antimicrobial therapy, such as in the patient receiving antineoplastic therapy, tend to select out for systemic infection due to more antibiotic-resistant bacilli such as *P. aeruginosa, Proteus* species, and *Serratia* species. Thus the association of certain organisms with high mortality may reflect the effect of antimicrobial selection rather than intrinsic virulence.

The role of human carriers in the spread of gram-negative rod infections has been described in some situations such as some clusters of *Proteus* infections[41] or *Salmonella* infections. However, the bulk of current information suggests that a carrier situation similar to what has been observed with staphylococci is probably not relevant to the vast majority of gram-negative infections that occur in the hospital setting.

THE CLINICAL SYNDROME: SIGNS AND SYMPTOMS OF GRAM-NEGATIVE ROD BACTEREMIA

There are no specific clinical findings in gram-negative rod bacteremia that distinguish it from systemic infection caused by gram-positive cocci (and for that matter some viral hemorrhagic fevers). Table 2 summarizes some of the clinical findings that suggest the diagnosis and should prompt a careful culture of blood, cultures of likely sources of infection, and possible initiation of therapy. The distinction between primary manifestations and complications is arbitrary; indeed, such complications as hypotension, bleeding, hypoxia, acidosis, and jaundice may be the major clues that first suggest the diagnosis. Although fever and chills are typically encountered, many patients who develop bacteremic infection are debilitated and may not exhibit striking changes in symptomatology early during the course of infection. Paradoxically, hypothermia rather than hyperthermia occasionally can be a manifestation of gram-negative rod infection and is associated with poor prognosis. While neutropenia definitely predisposes to gram-negative bacillary infection, a precipitous decline in the neutrophil count from a normal or an already depressed level is also commonly seen. The clinician should be alert to the possibility that hypotension, a fall in urine output, a decrease in circulating platelet levels, and evidence for bleeding even in the absence of fever and chills could be manifestations of bacteremia.

TABLE 2. Signs and Symptoms Suggesting Gram-Negative Rod Bacteremia

Primary	*Complications*
Fever	Hypotension
Chills	Bleeding
Hyperventilation	Leukopenia
Hypothermia	Thrombocytopenia
Skin lesions	Organ failure
Change in mental status	Lung: cyanosis, acidosis
	Kidney: oliguria, anuria, acidosis
	Liver: jaundice
	Heart: congestive failure

Even before temperature elevation or the onset of chills, bacteremic patients will often begin to hyperventilate. Continuous monitoring of patients in intensive care units has indicated that the earliest clinical finding is apprehension and hyperventilation; thus the earliest metabolic change in septicemia and particularly gram-negative rod infections is a resultant respiratory alkalosis. In the critically ill patient the sudden onset of hyperventilation should lead to drawing blood for culture and to carefully evaluating the patient for the possibility of infection. Change in mental status can be an important clinical clue: while the most common pattern is lethargy or obtundation, an occasional patient may become excited, agitated, or combative or may display bizarre behavior.

Cutaneous manifestations of gram-negative rod bacteremia, usually colorful skin lesions, were described as early as the previous century.[42] Skin lesions have been most commonly associated with *P. aeruginosa* bacteremia. The so-called pathognomonic skin lesion of *P. aeruginosa* bacteremia was described and given the name *ecthyma gangrenosum*.[43] Ecthyma gangrenosum lesions are round or oval, vary from 1 to 5 cm, and have a raised halo or rim of erythema and induration that surround a central are that may begin as vesicle but usually evolves into a necrotic ulcer (Fig. 1). The appearance of these "bull's-eye"–type lesions strongly suggests *P. aeruginosa* infection and has been observed in 5–25 percent of all *Pseudomonas* bacteremias. In the thrombocytopenic patient, the periphery of these lesions may become ecchymotic. Biopsy specimens of the lesions indicate that the underlying process is

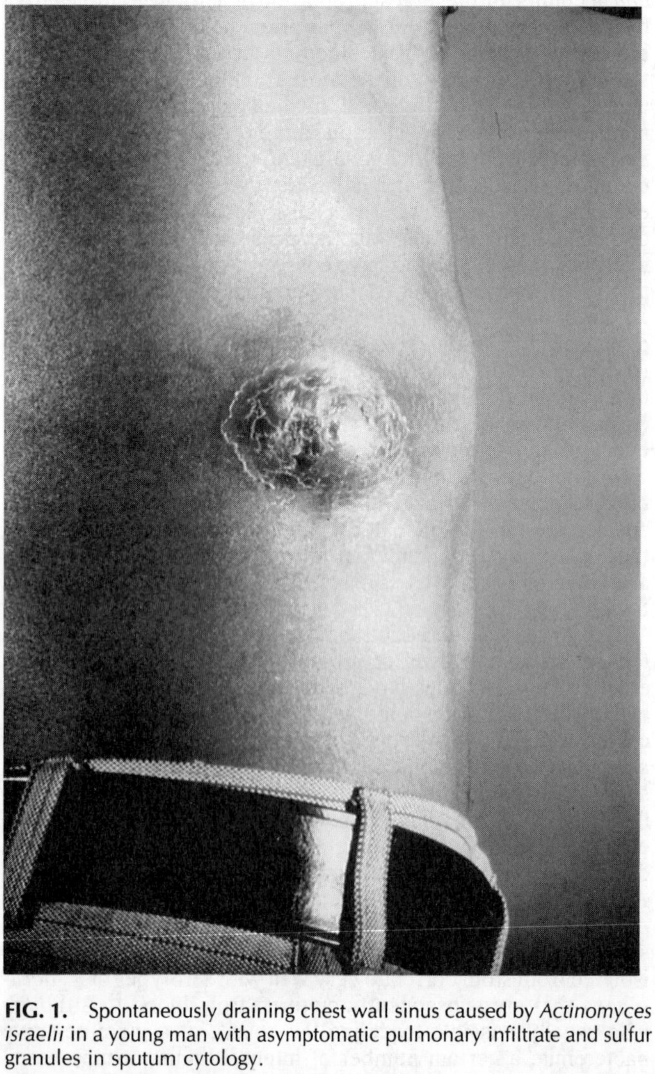

FIG. 1. Spontaneously draining chest wall sinus caused by *Actinomyces israelii* in a young man with asymptomatic pulmonary infiltrate and sulfur granules in sputum cytology.

infectious, with direct vascular invasion by bacilli and thrombosis on the venous side of the capillary bed.[43] It seems likely that extracellular products of bacteria such as proteases (elastases) and/or exotoxins are responsible for tissue damage. Nonetheless, there are some reports attributing this phenomenon to local manifestations of Shwartzman reactions in the skin, that is, a localized area of consumption coagulopathy where venous thrombosis triggered perhaps by endotoxin is the initiator of tissue injury. By and large, however, most of these ecthyma lesions appear to be infectious because organisms can be directly aspirated or cultured from these lesions and histopathologic sections reveal organisms invading blood vessel walls. Since bacteria are involved in a demand vasculitis, the presence of ecthyma lesions can be considered tantamount to bacteremia.

It has become clear that, while ecthyma-type lesions are strongly suggestive of *P. aeruginosa* infection, the latter are not the only organisms that can cause this characteristic lesion. *Aeromonas hydrophila* can produce a clinical picture similar to that of *P. aeruginosa* infection, and a large proportion of bacteremic patients have had ecthymalike skin lesions.[44,45] Additionally, cutaneous lesions have been observed in *E. coli*,[46] *Klebsiella, Enterobacter*, and *Serratia* septicemia. Besides ecthyma lesions, colorful vesicular or bullous lesions, cellulitis, diffuse erythematous reactions (similar to scarlet fever), or showers of petechial lesions (not unlike meningococcemia) can be cutaneous manifestations of gram-negative bacteremia.[47] Thus, cutaneous lesions should not lead the clinician to make a specific etiologic diagnosis (although ecthyma-type lesions in the neutropenic patient are most often due to *P. aeruginosa*) but to alert medical personnel to the possibility of a systemic gram-negative bacillary infection, the need for diagnostic measures, and therapeutic intervention. The availability of a lesion from which a biopsy specimen can be obtained and that is easily aspirated, cultured, and processed with Gram stain may provide the basis for an initial microbiologic diagnosis before the isolation and characterization of organisms from blood cultures.

Some patients may have a fulminating bacteremia manifested by shock or rapidly progressing to the stage of shock in a matter of hours. The latter course may be indistinguishable from meningococcemia and is often due to *P. aeruginosa* or *Aeromonas* infection. More typically, however, the onset of shock is slower and follows a period of several hours of hemodynamic instability. A reasonable working definition of shock is hypotension manifested by systolic blood pressures less than 90 mmHg and diastolic pressure less than 60 mm Hg accompanied by tachycardia, peripheral vasoconstriction, and oliguria or anuria. Oliguria is defined by hourly urine outputs of less than 20 ml. The hallmark of shock is tissue hypoperfusion resulting from a decrease in intravascular fluid volume, diminished vascular resistance, or both. Both vasodilatation and increased vascular permeability of some compartments of the circulation may be an initial manifestation of certain pathophysiologic processes (see the section on pathophysiology), and the net effect is a reduction in circulating blood volume.

Many patients may have transient hypotension or oliguria that is quickly ameliorated by prompt corrective measures such as fluid challenge. Others progress from an initial phase of hypotension, tachycardia, and peripheral vasodilatation ("warm shock") to a moribund phase of deep pallor, intense vasoconstriction, and anuria ("cold shock"). The latter state clearly reflects the inability of compensatory mechanisms to maintain perfusion even to vital organs. The onset of shock is seen in perhaps 20–35 percent of the patients with gram-negative rod bacteremia and increases the mortality to perhaps twice that figure.

While clinical findings are likely to reflect the severity and stage of shock rather than a specific microbial etiology, there exists some evidence for hemodynamic differences between shock complicating gram-positive bacteremia and gram-negative bacillemia. Gunnar and colleagues[48] have conducted prospective hemodynamic studies in patients proven to have shock associated with both gram-positive cocci and gram-negative rods. Patients were hospitalized in the intensive care unit of a large municipal hospital, and most had procedures involving urinary tract instrumentation. As shown in Table 3, a number of variables were monitored including heart rate, cardiac index, left ventricular end-diastolic pressure, systemic vascular resistance, and mean arterial pressure. Of these parameters, the cardiac rate and cardiac index (which parallels the former) were significantly lower in patients developing shock secondary to gram-negative bacillary infection. These findings were felt to be consistent with release of a vasodilator substance early during the course of gram-negative bacteremia, but ultimately vasoconstriction was more common in patients with gram-negative infections. Myocardial function also appeared depressed. While both changes in cardiac rate and index reflect decreased tissue perfusion, it should be noted, nonetheless, that the differences were small, with considerable overlap between the two groups. In the individual patient, a single measurement of either heart rate or cardiac index is likely to be of limited value in distinguishing whether the patient has gram-negative or gram-positive infection. For this reason, it still seems prudent in the critically ill patient with septic shock to initiate empirical antimicrobial therapy aimed at both gram-positive and gram-negative causes until the results of cultures are known.

There has been increasing interest focused on pulmonary complications of gram-negative rod bacteremia.[49,50] Some patients, although probably a minority, have bacteremia originating from the lung. These subjects develop infection secondary to aspiration (bronchial embolism) whereby material from the upper respiratory tract that contains gram-negative rods is aspirated into the lung parenchyma and subsequent pneumonitis and bacteremia develops.[51,52] More commonly, however, diffuse pneumonitis can develop secondary to bacteremia and is often of overwhelming severity. The attention of pulmonary physiologists and clinicians has been focused on this complication, which is often referred to as the adult respiratory distress syndrome (ARDS) or "shock lung." It is likely that ARDS reflects a wide variety of pathophysiologic mechanisms and clearly has no single etiology, but gram-negative rod bacteremia is one of them.[49] The mechanism for the diffuse infiltrates may entail direct involvement of the lung by a bacteremic necrotizing pneumonitis or a combination of pulmonary edema (diffuse alveolar/capillary leak) associated with evidence for macro- and microembolization to the lung (consumption coagulopathy).

TABLE 3. Comparison Between Hemodynamic Values during Septic Shock in 19 Patients with Gram-Positive Organisms and 31 Patients with Gram-Negative Organisms Cultured from Blood

	MAP (mmHg)	*CVP* (mmHg)	*HR* (per min)	*CI* (liter/min/m²)	*SVR* (mmHg/liter/min)	*LVEDP* (mmHg)
Gram-positive	57 ± 2[a]	3.5 ± 0.06	119 ± 4	3.8 ± 0.3	8.5 ± 1.1	6.7 ± 1.3
Gram-negative	57 ± 3	5.1 ± 0.7	100 ± 4	2.9 ± 0.2	11.5 ± 0.9	9.8 ± 1.6
p (unpaired)	NS	NS	<.01	<.05	NS	NS

Abbreviations: MAP: mean arterial pressure; CVP: central venous pressure; HR: heat rate; CI: cardiac index; SVR: systemic vascular resistance; LVEDP: left ventricular end-diastolic pressure; NS: not significant.
[a] Mean ± SE.
(From Gunnar et al.,[48] with permission.)

TABLE 4. Factors Affecting the Outcome of Gram-Negative Bacteremia

Underlying disease
Neutropenia
Hypogammaglobulinemia
Diabetes
Alcoholism ± cirrhosis
Renal failure
Respiratory failure
Complications of the bacteremic event at the onset of treatment (e.g., shock, anuria)
Antimicrobial chemotherapy
Grade of severity of bacteremia (polymicrobial bacteremia)
Source of infection
Interval to initiation of treatment
Age

That bacterial products can trigger intrinsic clotting and (pari passu) that the body has mechanisms for resorption of thrombi (activation of the fibrinolytic system) is well known. The complexity of the clinical situation probably relates to the multiple events that are triggered by bacterial invasion of the blood stream and ensuing host responses. Included in this concept is a role for endotoxin-triggered mediators such as tumor necrosis factor (TNF) in the pathophysiologic changes leading to ARDS. The characteristic clinical findings include hypoxia, evidence for a right-to-left shunt, and diffuse pulmonary infiltrates. The most important finding is the relatively normal pulmonary wedge pressure (left ventricular end-diastolic pressure) in the face of a high pulmonary arterial pressure and marked hypoxia (PaO_2 <60 mmHg). This indicates that the diffuse pulmonary capillary leak syndrome and mechanical alterations in lung function are not secondary to left-sided cardiac failure, that is, represent "noncardiogenic" pulmonary edema.

Clearly, it is not the bacteremic event per se but the status of host defense mechanisms and the ability to maintain function of vital organs that are the factors deciding the outcome of any blood stream infection. Table 4 summarizes, in order of estimated importance, some of the factors commonly accepted as affecting prognosis. In addition to underlying disease and complications, other factors can have a significant effect. Although quantitative blood cultures are now less frequently performed, several studies indicate that mortality is greater with high-grade bacteremia and with polymicrobial bacteremia.[28,53] The source of infection may be important because people with leukemia often (with an overall poorer prognosis) have no discernible focus of a primary infection. Age is linked in a biphasic manner to outcome, with poorer survival in the very young and older age groups. The selection of antimicrobial therapy and the urgency with which it is implemented has a definite effect on outcome and will be dealt with later in this chapter.

MICROBIAL PROPERTIES THAT UNDERLIE VIRULENCE AND INVASIVENESS

Despite the extraordinary numbers of organisms with which humans have intimate contact, relatively few types cause significance disease. An important and recurring question is "What are those properties possessed by certain microorganisms that are responsible for their ability to cause disease and that differentiate them from mere saprophytes?" Much of the work in microbial pathogenesis has focused on two areas: first, the characterization of cell wall structures, several of which appear antigenic, that are associated with properties of invasiveness and give the organism some advantage in the face of host defense mechanisms; second, a variety of products that are either released or are closely associated with the microorganism that causes tissue damage such as enzymes, toxins, and metabolic by-products. Some of these microbial properties were recognized in the previous century, but there has been an upsurge of new information on the specific antigenic components of the bacterial cell wall and in the case of certain species, such as species of *Aeromonas* and *Pseudomonas*, new work on the characterization of microbial exotoxins.

Table 5 summarizes some of the implicated mechanisms underlying the ability of certain gram-negative bacilli to cause human disease. Since infection must start at some local site, the property of adherence to a mucosal surface may be important in the initiation of infection such as in the urinary or gastrointestinal tract. Most invasive gram-negative bacilli are serum resistant, that is, not lysed by complement-mediated reactions. Further, some are heavily encapsulated or have surfaces that enable them to resist phagocytosis. Some bacterial cell walls have an antigenic composition similar to host tissue such as blood group substances or sialic acid. As will be discussed, some cell wall constituents are clearly "toxic" and elicit a variety of inflammatory and pyrogenic reactions; there may be differences in the ability of these cell wall constituents to trigger pathophysiologic events. It has been demonstrated that some gram-negative organisms like *Brucella* and the typhoid bacillus survive intracellular and thus can evade host defense mechanisms. Finally, the aforementioned enzymes and toxins can clearly have a deleterious effect on host tissue and an effect on the initiation and propagation of infection as well as "lethal" sequelae.

Figure 2 is a schema of the cell wall antigens of gram-negative bacilli. There are three layers to this cell wall. The so-called outer membrane contains protein, lipid, and carbohydrate, with substantial amounts of the latter arranged in polymeric units or polysaccharides. The heat-stable serologic specificity of gram-negative bacilli, which is the basis for the "O," or somatic, antigen typing scheme, is principally related to the polysaccharide component of the other membrane.[67] The original serologic typing schemata for enteric bacilli proposed by Kauffman[68] and Edwards and Ewing[69] used tube or slide agglutination techniques on antisera produced against boiled organisms. Thus, major antigenic differences were determined by producing antisera (usually in rabbits) against boiled whole cell cultures and the similarities or differences between strains deduced by the pattern of agglutination with test organisms that were similarly boiled. The O antisera produced in this manner react with polysaccharide antigens that are constituents of the outer membrane. In the past, the O antigens of gram-negative organisms have been referred to as synonymous with lipopolysaccharide (LPS) or endotoxin, but as will be discussed subsequently, endotoxic activity appears to be lipid and not polysaccharide associated. The intermediate or murein layer of the gram-negative bacterial cell wall is rigid material composed predominantly of peptidoglycan or mucopeptide. The peptidoglycans of gram-negative bacteria are chemically and antigenically similar if not identical: they are composed of alternating *N*-acetyl glucosamine and *N*-acetyl neuraminic acid residues linked to a tetrapeptide.[70] It is primarily at this site that agents that inhibit cell wall synthesis, such as the penicillins and cephalosporins, have effect and result in osmotically unstable microbial forms, the so-called spheroplasts or L-forms. In that circumstance the structure responsible for retention of the integrity of the microbe is the inner or cytoplasmic membrane. In addition to these basic structures a wide variety of organisms such as *P. aeruginosa* and *E. coli* appear to have one or more flagellar structures that confer properties of motility. Not all

TABLE 5. Probable Mechanisms for "Virulence" of Disease-Causing Gram-Negative Organisms

Mechanisms	*References*
Adherence	54, 55
Serum resistance	56–58
"Antiphagocytic" surfaces	58–60
Have capsular or surface antigens similar to host tissue	61
Capsular or endotoxin type has special trophism	62
Survive intracellularly or are killed slowly	63
Elaborate extracellular factors, e.g., enzymes and toxins	64, 65

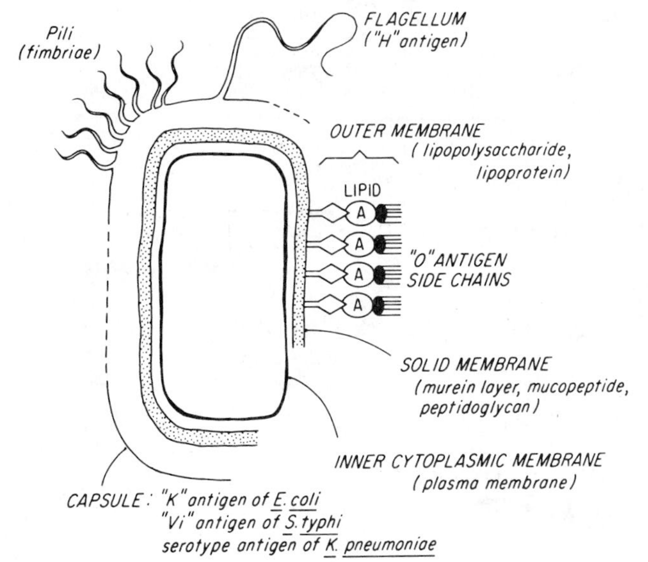

FIG. 2. Major cell wall antigens of gram-negative bacilli. See Figure 3 for details of the outer membrane. (From Young et al.,[66] with permission.)

gram-negative rods are motile or flagellated; *K. pneumoniae* is a notable exception. Additionally, many of these organisms contain structures that lie exterior to the outer membrane. These structures include pili or fimbriae, which are protein in nature and seem important for the attachment or adherence of microbes to mucosal surfaces. Other protein surface structures include porins, literally porelike structures that regulate the entry of nutrients, macromolecules, and antimicrobial agents into the bacterial cell.[71] Finally, a number of organisms, particularly *E. coli* or *Klebsiella* species, have a capsular or envelope antigen, the so-called K antigen, that lies exterior to the O antigen. These antigens are normally highly negatively charged polysaccharides, although a few are protein in nature. Also, *Salmonella typhi* has polysaccharide K-type capsular antigen that has been designated as the so-called Vi antigen.

One of the more confusing aspects of bacterial cell wall composition is the structural interrelationship of previously described components, the assessment of their pathogenic role, and the interaction of these factors with host defense mechanisms. Physicochemical methods for the isolation of cell wall components require large masses of cultured bacteria and result in products that are difficult to purify to homogeneity. Three-dimensional structural analysis of cell wall fractions reveals that there is no clear-cut demarcation between one structure and another, that is, a separation between somatic (O) antigen and capsular (K) antigen. In a broad sense, the schematic representation of Figure 3 can be misleading because it supports the concept of the bacterial cell wall as a multilamellar structure rather than a mosaic of interdigitating antigens that may or may not be exposed on the surface.

One of the greatest areas of confusion is the relationship between the O and K antigens. Originally, K, or capsular, antigens were discovered when it was found that some strains of *E. coli* could not be serotyped by O antiserum unless they were first boiled for approximately an hour.[68] This led to the suggestion that there was a structure exterior to the O antigen that inhibited agglutination; it was inferred that boiling removed or changed the surface characteristics in such a way as to permit reaction with O antiserum. A large series of K antigens of *E. coli* were described in the early work of Kauffman and his coworkers,[68] but more recently, Orskov et al. and have reassessed the concept of the K antigen.[74] These antigens appear to be highly negatively charged acidic polysaccharides whose effect is, indeed, to block agglutination by O antiserum. However, K antigens are not actually destroyed by heating, and the agglutinability that is observed after heating is probably due to rearrangement or alteration of microbial surface structures. Some of the K antigens that were described by Kauffman and his associates do not appear to be acidic polysaccharides but were probably O antigens. Further, the functional definition of the K antigen has now been extended to include some protein structures like the K-88 and K-99 types.[74] The latter protein K antigens have been associated with diarrheal syndromes in animals and appear to facilitate the attachment of these microbes to mucosal surfaces. For the great majority of strains of enteric bacilli, a functional definition of the K antigen encompasses the original concept that K antigen inhibits agglutination by O antiserum. In addition to this, a specific K antigen must be identified as a highly negatively charged surface polysaccharide by biochemical and immunoelectrophoretic techniques.[74] A K antigen may also be a factor promoting adherence to host cells and thus may be responsible for giving an infecting microbe some advantage in the initial contact with the host. Both O (somatic) and K antigens have been associated with the microbial properties of resistance to phagocytosis,[67,75] in effect permitting the microbe to evade engulfment unless specific antibodies are present.

There are several other antigenic structures that have been identified in the gram-negative cell wall. One is an antigen common to Enterobacteriaceae that was originally described by Kunin et al. and Makela and Mayer[76,77] and often referred to as the "common antigen." This appears to be polysaccharide in nature[78] and antigenic. Another antigenic material is lipoprotein in composition and is both covalently linked to the lipid portion of the outer membrane and covalently bound to the murein layer.[79] A large proportion of humans infected by enteric bacilli form antibodies against the "common antigen"[80] and lipoprotein,[81] but it has not been determined whether these antigens are true virulence factors and whether or not the antibody response confers protection against reinfection or death.

From the viewpoint of the pathophysiology of gram-negative rod septicemia, much interest has focused on the "core" region of the outer membrane. As illustrated in Figure 3A, the sequence of constituents from the exterior to the interior of the outer membrane is O antigen, outer "core," and inner "core."[72,73,82] The core region is an acidic hetero-oligosaccharide that in turn is linked to a lipoidal acylated glucosamine disaccharide termed *lipid A*. The innermost constituent of the core region, lipid A, has been chemically characterized[72,73] and exhibits all the hemodynamic, pyrogenic, and inflammatory properties associated with "endotoxicity." The inner "core" linked to lipid A has also been termed *core glycolipid*. Major clues to unraveling of the structure of the outer membrane and its core region and the evidence that lipid A is, indeed, the "toxic" moiety of the gram-negative cell wall have resulted from exhaustive investigative work on both naturally occurring and induced mutants of certain gram-negative bacilli.[67,72,82] Colonies of organisms that have O polysaccharide or somatic antigens tend to be smooth and glistening in their appearance on agar and are often referred to as "smooth." These organisms are often resistant to the killing of complement-mediated bacteriolysis in fresh human serum. Some organisms, however, appear to have a "rough" or coarse irregular appearance in colonial growth, do not grow homogeneously in broth culture media, and tend to autoaggulutinate. These so-called rough organisms are hydrophobic because of their lipid content, and immunochemical analysis has revealed that the roughness is associated with a lack of O-specific polysaccharide. A series of mutants have been studied that lack one or more of the sugar moieties normally present in the core region (Fig. 3A). There is progressing roughness associated with cell wall structures that successively lack certain sugar moieties. Because most Enterobacteriaceae have similar inner core regions, a chemotype designation has evolved for identifying the rough mutants that

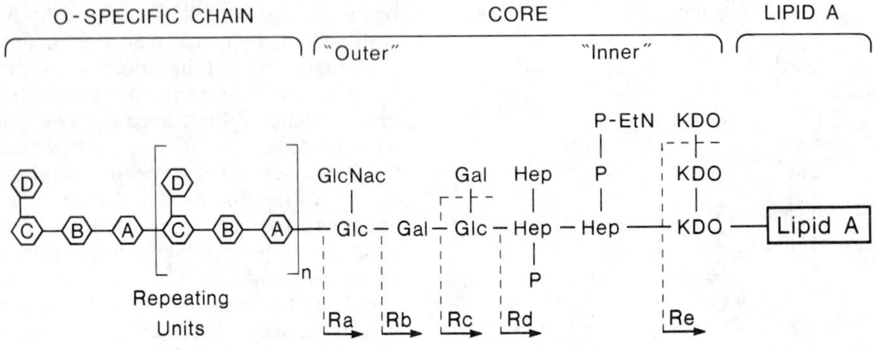

A

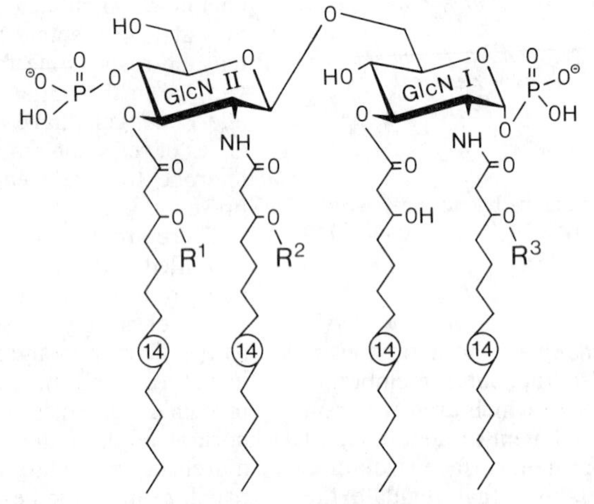

Source of Lipid A	Chemical Nature of:		
	R^1	R^2	R^3
E. coli	14:0	12:0	H
S. minnesota	14:0	12:0	H, 16:0
P. mirabilis	14:0	14:0	H, 16:0

B

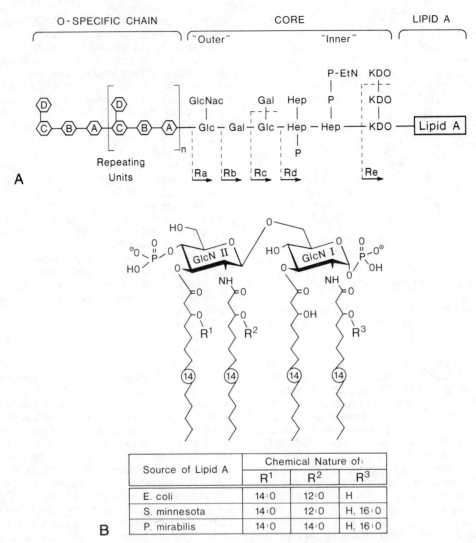

FIG. 3. (A) Biochemical structure of the outer membranes (lipopolysaccharides) of enteric bacteria, based primarily on work involving "rough" mutants of *Salmonella* species.[72,73] The "O" antigen side chains of repeating monosaccharide units are linked to lipid A through a "core" structure consisting of *N*-acetylglucosamine (GLcNaC), glucose, (Glu), galactose (gal), heptose (hep), phosphate (P), ethanolamine (ETN), and 2-keto, 3-deoxyoctonate (KDO, also known as manno-octulosonic acid). Chemotype mutants of increasing "roughness" such as "Ra", . . . "Rc" result from the progressive deletion of sugars from the outer to the inner core. The *E. coli* core region contains two KDOs. (Modified from Young et al.,[66] Rietschel et al.,[72] and Brade et al.[73]) **(B)** The chemical structure of the lipid A component of *E. coli, S. minnesota,* and *P. mirabilis* contains two *N*-acetyl glucosamine residues. (Modified from Rietschel et al.[72] and Brade et al.[73]). The numbers in circles indicate the number of carbon atoms in the acyl chains. The distribution of normal fatty acids (with chain lengths of 12 to 16 carbon atoms) at hydroxyl groups (R1, R2, R3) is highly specific and characteristic for the bacterial genus. (Modified from Brade et al.,[73] with permission.)

lack specific, sequential inner core constituents. The "Ra" rough chemotype designates mutants that merely lack attachment to an O-specific antigen, while the designations "Rb, Rc, Rd, and Re" represent mutants containing cell walls with the progressive deletion of individual sugars as one progresses to the inner core. The so-called Re mutants contain only 2-keto, 3-deoxyoctonate (KDO or manno-octulosonic acid) linked to lipid A.

The *E. coli* core region contains two KDOs, while the *Salmonella* core possesses three of these moieties. Lipid A is the most highly conserved component of the aerobic gram-negative LPS structure and appears to be absent in *B. fragilis*.[83] Figure 3B shows the variation in fatty acid composition for lipid A derived from *E. coli, S. minnesota*, and *P. mirabilis*[73]; *Pseudomonas* lipid A also shows differences.[84]

The precise chemical structure of lipid A several biologically active variants and the preparation of a totally synthetic lipid A have been reported in detail.[72,73] Full endotoxicity is expressed by a molecule containing two β-(1-6)D-glucosamine residues, two phosphoryl groups, and five or six fatty acids. Slight modifications in lipid A architecture result in significant changes in biologic activity, thus suggesting that endotoxicity is not dependent on a single lipid A constituent but by several factors including three-dimensional conformation. This knowledge may be of critical importance in devising means for competing with lipid A (lipid A is a nontoxic analogue) as a therapeutic or prophylactic approach[85] or as an antimicrobial in blocking lipid A synthesis.

Recent modifications overall, however, in the limulus gelation reaction that are based on spectrophotometric measurements of the process have improved its sensitivity and reliability.[86] This test, however, should not be used as a substitute for blood cultures. Endotoxin or perhaps more appropriately the lipid A of gram-negative bacilli plays a critical role in the pathophysiology of gram-negative rod infections and is an important cause of the clinical manifestations of disease. Some of the evidence supporting this association is summarized in Table 6. It should be recognized, however, that the toxicity attributed to LPS is not unique to gram-negative organisms since certain cell wall antigens of gram-positive bacteria such as hemolytic group A streptococci have an M protein that has similar "toxic" effects.[98] Nonetheless, in primates there do not appear to be significant differences between the cardiovascular and metabolic effects of viable gram-negative bacilli and those of bacterial endotoxin.

With such circumstantial evidence it has been commonly assumed that endotoxin may be circulating in the blood of humans or animals with bacteremic infections caused by gram-negative bacilli. Certain large-molecular-weight polysaccharide antigens of organisms such as *K. pneumoniae* or *S. typhi* have been found circulating in the blood of humans in the acute stages of bacteremia,[99,100] but it has not been possible to demonstrate consistently circulating endotoxin in bacteremic subjects. A number of endotoxin assay systems have been reported, virtually all using some biologic end point such as the epinephrine skin test in rabbits[101] or the limulus gelation reaction.[86,102] The latter is perhaps the most sensitive assay for endotoxin-like activity in vitro and is based on the observation that endotoxin or LPS causes gelation of fluid extracts from the amebocyte of the horseshoe crab *Limulus polyphemus*. The amebocyte has a plateletlike function; hence, what is observed in a positive reaction is coagulation triggered by quantities as small as a nanogram or picogram of endotoxin. Unfortunately, both false-positive and false-negative limulus gelation test results have been well documented in gram-negative bacteremia, and fungal and gram-positive functions have been associated with positive responses.[103,104] There are several explanations for this including (*1*) inherent problems in the biologic variability of reagent materials and maintaining test materials free of contamination by endotoxin, (*2*) demonstration that fresh human serum contains factors that detoxify or inactivate endotoxin,[105,106] and (*3*) the observation that circulating antibodies may bind or complex with endotoxins and thus give a negative test result.[107,108]

Conflicting reports on the feasibility of detecting endotoxin by the limulus gelation or other tests probably do not rule out a role in human bacteremic infections.[109] The presence of exposed antigen on the bacterial cell wall with or without bacteremia might be sufficient to trigger pathophysiologic sequelae that are observed in certain human disease states (see below). Further, experimental animal studies show that the clearance of infused bacteria by reticuloendothelial cells and circulating phagocytes leads to a rapid reduction in the number of microorganisms within minutes. Some 10^6 organisms/ml/min must be infused at a constant rate to yield a sustained bacteremia of 100–1000 circulating organisms per milliliter.[110] By inference, many more organisms may have actually been introduced into the blood stream than are revealed by quantitative blood cultures of venous blood. The significance of this observation is that endotoxemia may be transient, organisms may be rapidly cleared, after which adverse effects on the host are observed, and the sequelae of certain gram-negative infections may be triggered by far greater numbers of bacteria than are present when an attempt is made to actually document bacteremia or endotoxemia. Conversely, it is conceivable that absorption of bacterial toxins (both endotoxins and exotoxins) may occur from local sites of infection in the absence of bacteremia.[109]

TABLE 6. Evidence Implicating a Role for Bacterial Endotoxins in the Pathophysiology of Gram-Negative Septicemia

Evidence	*References*
1. Similarity in clinical manifestations between infection and administration of LPS to humans or animals	87, 88
2. Common pattern of hematologic changes after LPS administration and infection	89, 90
3. Generation of kinins and activation of Hageman factor in clinical infection and after LPS administration to animals	91, 92
4. Consumption of complement (C3 and alternative-pathway factors) in human infection complicated by shock and in animals given LPS	93, 94
5. Antibody against the "core" glycolipid antigens of LPS protects humans and experimental animals against sequelae of shock and death	95, 96
6. Administration of LPS to human volunteers results in the liberation of TNF; TNF mimics all of the pathophysiologic changes seen in gram-negative sepsis and can be detected in body fluids of septic patients	94, 97

Besides endotoxin, attention has been focused on other bacterial products that might be important in pathogenesis. The proteolytic enzymes might be such factors as are suggested by work with the elastases of *P. aeruginosa*. These elastases are dermonecrotic, cornea damaging, and possibly responsible for some of the changes seen in vasculitic lesions.[65] A correlation with proteolytic activity and virulence for mice has been reported for *P. aeruginosa*.[111]

Some of the other extracellular virulence factors that have been studied include the extracellular toxins of *Aeromonas* species[112] and *P. aeruginosa*.[64] The latter species produces a variety of exotoxins, perhaps the best characterized of which is exotoxin A. This toxin is produced by most clinical isolates of *P. aeruginosa*,[113] is lethal for mammalian cells,[114] and being analogous to diphtheria toxin is a potent inhibitor of protein synthesis.[115] In murine test systems toxin-producing strains are considerably more virulent than are nontoxigenic organisms.[116] In humans, high levels of antibodies directed against exotoxin A correlate with recovery from bacteremic *P. aeruginosa* infection.[117]

The tendency of investigators to usually focus on one microbial disease-producing mechanism has probably led to too narrow a view of the pathogenesis of gram-negative bacillary infection. The factors listed in Table 5 are certainly not mutually exclusive. It seems likely that organisms that are adherent, serum resistant, heavily encapsulated, and producers of extracellular proteolytic enzymes are likely to be more virulent than are those that are rough, serum sensitive, poorly adherent, and nonproteolytic. Not to be underestimated is the capacity of the microbe to survive in the environment of the hospital where seriously ill patients are managed. *Serratia marcescens* and *P. aeruginosa* have few nutritional requirements and can persist in a host of environmental reservoirs. Thus, a "unifying view" of the pathogenesis of gram-negative rod infections culminating in bacteremia takes into account a wide variety of epidemiologic, host, and microbial factors. Epidemiologic factors (types of exposure, antimicrobial usage) involve disruption of what might be termed *colonization immunity*. Microbial factors such as adherence and production of enzymes like proteases help to establish infection in local sites. Bacteremia is abetted by microbial properties of serum resistance and resistance to phagocytosis, but host factors such as numbers and function of phagocytic cells and humoral opsonins are likely to be deficient. Persistence of infection may be due to sequestration of infection in sites relatively protected from host defense mechanisms (deep abscesses, renal medulla, bone), and some phagocytic cells may actually become "sanctuaries" for microbes that survive intracellularly. The adverse sequelae of bacteremia—hypotension, shock, and death—may result from endotoxin, exotoxins, or other microbial products that are either directly lethal or can "trigger" pathophysiologic processes through various mediators or enzymatic reactions. The latter will be reviewed in the ensuing section.

PATHOPHYSIOLOGY OF GRAM-NEGATIVE ROD BACTEREMIA

The pathophysiologic events in gram-negative rod bacteremia are complex, and there are major reasons for our current problems in understanding what actually occurs in humans. First, there is the problem in human studies of trying to relate cause and effect, particularly with regard to the complications of gram-negative bacteremia such as septic shock. For instance, the role of complement activation and consumption of certain components is well documented in septic shock,[93,118] but in all likelihood the depression of levels of certain complement components is a result of bacteremia and the activation of the complement system. Whether or not complement activation can be regarded as a cause of septic shock remains speculative, although a large body of experimental evidence suggests that by-products of complement activation such as anaphylatoxins enhance vascular permeability and thus may affect both the hemodynamic status of the patient[119] and the functional capability of critical organs like the lung.[120]

Shock associated with gram-negative sepsis represents the extreme aspect of the spectrum of disease manifestations that result from a relative excess of systemically absorbed endotoxin. The complex pattern of pathophysiologic events now appears to be the result of activation or release of various mediators rather than direct endotoxin toxicity.

A second major problem in understanding the pathophysiology of gram-negative bacteremia is the fact that many of the changes that are observed either clinically or histopathologically may not be the manifestations of the infection itself but of a primary disease that is complicated by an infection. In the advanced stages of neoplasia or collagen-vascular disease it may be difficult to distinguish between primary or secondary changes. For instance, bleeding is a major potential complication of leukemias and lymphomas, but demonstration of a hemorrhagic diathesis or histologic evidence of bleeding (or clotting) may be difficult to attribute to the underlying disease, to the treatment of that underlying disease, or to a supervening infection. Finally, there is a major problem in translating the results of animal studies to the human clinical setting because of major species differences in the susceptibility of laboratory animals to gram-negative bacillary infections and the marked discrepancy between what has been observed in such common laboratory animals as dogs and rabbits to what has been seen both clinically and histologically in humans.[121]

Based on the administration of small, fairly nonlethal doses of bacterial endotoxin to humans, it appears that humans are one of the most susceptible species to the pyrogenic effects of bacterial endotoxin.[122] The administration of endotoxins to dogs produces some changes that have been uncommonly observed in human disease such as a diarrheal phase and an acute hypotensive phase that can be blocked by antihistamines.[42] Similarly, there has been a tendency to ascribe the changes of repeated endotoxin administration in rabbits to the reaction originally described by Sanarelli and subsequently elaborated on by Shwartzman and Gerber.[123,124] In the "local" Shwartzman reaction, an initial preparatory dose of endotoxin is injected intracutaneously, and hemorrhagic necrosis is produced by a second intravenous dose. The intravenous doses of endotoxin at 24-hour intervals results in bilateral renal cortical necrosis in rabbits. Hemorrhagic necrosis of the skin has been observed as a manifestation of gram-negative rod bacteremia in humans, although organisms have been recovered from such lesions and might reflect the concurrent bacteremia in contrast to circulating endotoxemia. Clinical and histopathologic findings consistent with a generalized Shwartzman reaction in humans has been reported in women with *E. coli* pyelonephritis, but findings of bilateral renal cortical necrosis in human material that is analogous to that observed in rabbits with the generalized Shwartzman reaction have been relatively rare.[125]

Current evidence favors the concept that the damage exerted by endotoxins is the direct result of the release of various mediators (which, although toxic, can by themselves have a role in host defense) and the triggering of humoral enzymatic mechanisms involving the complement, intrinsic clotting, fibrinolytic, and kinin pathways (Fig. 4). The most important set of developments in our understanding the pathophysiology of gram-negative sepsis is the identification of various mediators or cytokines[126] that are synthesized and released by macrophages and other mononuclear cells after exposure to endotoxin.[127] These cytokines include interleukin-1 (IL-1) (endogenous pyrogen), γ-interferon, a variety of colony-stimulating factors, and TNF (also known as cachectin). Of these biochemically defined substances. TNF appears to be an important if not the most

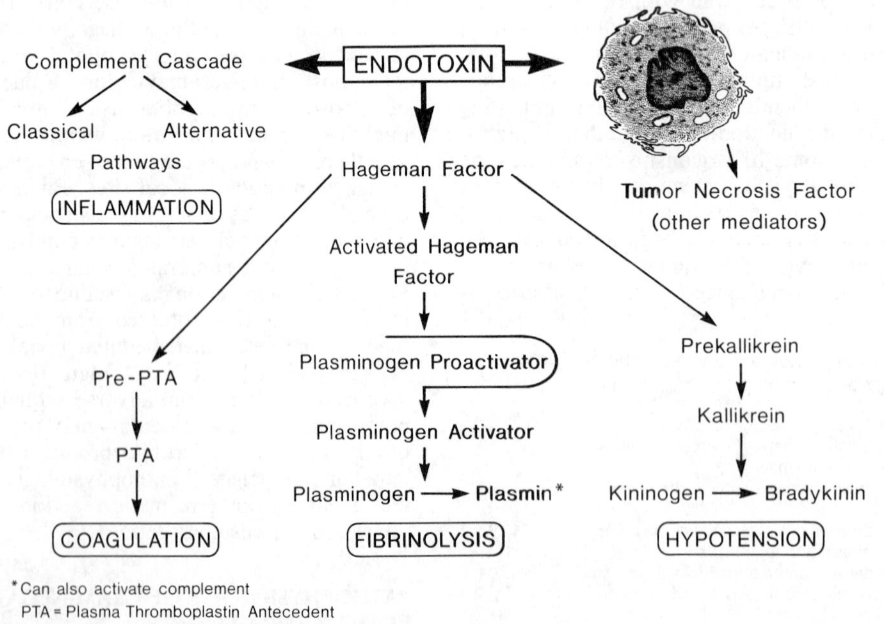

FIG. 4. The biologic effect of gram-negative bacillary endotoxins (lipopolysaccharides) are complex and interrelated. The intravenous administration of tumor necrosis factor (TNF, also known as cachectin) reproduces most of the pathophysiologic events observed in gram-negative sepsis, including the most extreme state, shock. Other mediators (cytokines) and pharmacologically active substances (e.g., prostaglandins) can act in concert with TNF. Lipopolysaccharides have other, diverse biologic effects: they can activate the complement, coagulation, and fibronolytic systems and can trigger a series of enzymatic reactions leading to the release of bradykinins and possibly other vasoactive peptides that cause hypotension.

potent mediator of the pathophysiology of gram-negative sepsis.[128–130] Evidence for this view is derived from studies showing that (*1*) mice that are genetically unresponsive to endotoxin lack the capacity to produce murine TNF from their macrophages[131]; (*2*) the administration of endotoxin to human volunteers results in the liberation of free TNF in plasma accompanied by many symptoms typical of gram-negative infection.[88] Interleukin-1 and γ-interferon were not detected at challenge doses of 4 ng/kg. (*3*) High levels of free TNF in plasma have been associated with morbidity and increased mortality in human meningococcemia[132]; (*4*) the administration of purified recombinant TNF to humans[88,130,133] and animals[134–137] mimics most of the clinical, laboratory, and histopathologic findings seen in gram-negative sepsis and septic shock; and (*5*) antibodies directed against TNF, particularly when given before endotoxin challenge, significantly increased the survival of experimental animals.[128] Protection studies have now employed monoclonal antibodies specific for TNF epitopes.[138] Infusion of anti-TNF murine monoclonal antibodies into primates who were bacteremic abrogated the development of signs of endotoxicity. TNF can also act directly on cellular components of blood and vascular epithelium,[135,139] and it has pyrogenic properties per se.[140] TNF appears to trigger the release of prostaglandins that can act as "second messengers" of systemic toxicity.[141] TNF appears to act synergistically with IL-1[142] or γ-interferon[143] to trigger inflammation and reactions such as the Shwartzman reaction, which have been associated with endotoxemia.[144] An overall conceptual picture would involve an inflammatory cascade of reactions, with TNF as the principal mediatory working synergistically with other biologically active products released by host cells. Clearly, other infectious processes such as parasitic infection can lead to TNF release,[145] so its detection is not specific for gram-negative infection. Furthermore, in some experimental models TNF alone has limited toxicity, but the full range of toxicity seen in clinical infection results from the combined use of TNF and bacterial products[141] (see Table 6). Thus, the identification of TNF as an important mediator of septic shock suggests that the sepsis syndrome is an example of immune system "overresponsiveness" to invading pathogens[137,146] or large doses of provocative antigens (e.g., LPS) in a manner analogous to anaphylaxis.

As shown in Figure 4, gram-negative bacilli and cocci that possess bacterial endotoxins have been shown to activate Hageman factor (factor XII), which in turn directly leads to the activation of the complement, coagulation, fibrinolytic, and bradykinin systems. Not shown in this diagram is the presence, at major stages in these reactions, of inhibitory or regulatory factors such as the inhibitor of the first component of complement, α_2-macroglobulin, and α_1-antitrypsin that can have an important modulating effect on these reactions. What happens in vivo is the result, perhaps quantitatively related, between the stimulus (such as endotoxin or other bacterial factors) and countervening or modulating influences.

Endotoxin can activate the complement system[93,118,147] and it is now appreciated that complement activation may take place through two different mechanisms, the classic and alternative pathways, that appear to have different antibody requirements. To produce thrombocytopenia, experimental studies suggested that activation through the classic pathway is obligatory.[147] There may be both complement-dependent and complement-independent mechanisms that are activated during the course of gram-negative bacteremia.[148] Complement activation results in the release of factors that attract the migration of phagocytic cells into tissue, that is, leukotaxis. Phagocytosis is abetted by activation of C3b and the release of chemotactic factors (C5a); this also leads to the release of anaphylatoxins that increase vascular permeability and enhance or potentiate the inflammatory reaction. It seems important to place this series of events into its proper perspective: complement appears vital for enhancing phagocytosis and lysis of serum-sensitive organisms, thus promoting blood stream clearance of microorganisms. The inflammatory reactions seem beneficial to the host, but excessive complement activation, possibly related to a large bacterial challenge, may well have a deleterious effect.

Activated Hageman factor can initiate the intrinsic clotting cascade through the conversion of plasma thromboplastin antecedent (pre-PTA) to PTA. Eventually, fibrinogen (factor I) is converted to fibrin, and clotting ensues. Uncontrolled activation of coagulation, usually accompanied by shock, will result in thrombosis and consumption of platelets and clotting factors II, V, and VIII. The term *acute disseminated intravascular coagulation* (DIC) has been used synonymously with consumption coagulopathy, defibrination syndrome, and coagulation-fibrinolytic syndrome. In this syndrome the use of coagulation factors II, V, and VIII as well as platelets significantly exceeds production rates and results in levels less than those required for hemostasis. The activation of clotting through an endotoxin-triggered mechanism thus may paradoxically result in clinical bleeding due to the consumption of clotting factors. The end results of disseminated coagulation depend on the target organ. Severe clinical bleeding, thrombosis, tissue ischemia and necrosis, hemolysis, and organ failure (lung, kidney, liver) are common complications.

At the same time as clotting appears to be initiated, countervening mechanisms also appear to be activated by clotting, namely, activation of the fibrinolytic system.[119] Activated Hageman factor appears to effect the conversion of plasminogen proactivator to plasminogen activator. An α_2-macroglobulin influenced by the latter subsequently affects the conversion of plasminogen to plasmin, a potent fibrinolytic substance that mediates clot lysis. The activation of plasmin fibrinolytic systems may thus also contribute to bleeding tendencies. Fibrinolytic mechanisms act to lyse fibrin into soluble peptides called fibrin split products or degradation products, which provide substantial diagnostic evidence for the presence of DIC. Additionally, evidence for a prolonged prothrombin time (PT) and partial thromboplastin time (PTT) is usually present because fibrin split products have anticoagulant activity. It is also of interest that plasmin, the end product of the fibrinolytic system, also has the capacity to initiate the complement cascade, again indicating the interrelationship of the inflammatory reactions that appear to be triggered by a bacterial gram-negative product.

The complication of DIC is not unique to gram-negative infections and has been observed in gram-positive, fungal, and viral infections as well. Furthermore, the pattern of abnormalities in laboratory findings should be assessed rather than relying on one or two laboratory values. Although factor II (prothrombin) is consumed during coagulation, it is a vitamin K dependent factor and can be affected by vitamin K deficiency such as in liver disease. Depression of vitamin K dependent factors with resultant prolongation in PT and PTT have been observed in 25 percent of normotensive septicemic patients without other evidence of DIC.[149] Additionally, patients may develop evidence of thrombocytopenia without DIC. In hypotensive patients, however, prolonged PT and PTT seem to be related to consumption coagulopathy irrespective of the levels of vitamin K dependent factors.[149]

It has been proposed that, in subjects without liver disease, the minimum criteria for the diagnosis of DIC includes thrombocytopnia, detection of fibrin split products, and a reduction in one or more of the coagulation factors II, V, or VII. If hepatic disease is present at the time of infection, reduced factor VIII levels are necessary to confirm the diagnosis of DIC.[149] Table 7 summarizes the general clotting parameters observed in normotensive or hypotensive patients. The levels of factors II, V, and VI may in fact be elevated in patients without hemodynamic alterations. The timing of clotting studies also seems important since levels of some factors and platelets may be initially depressed and then show a "rebound" response.

Demonstration of coagulation defects in conditions such as

TABLE 7. Effect of Bacteremic Infections on Levels of Platelets and Clotting Factors

Condition	*Platelets*	*Factor II*	*Factor V*	*Factor VIII*	*Fibrinogen*	*Fibrin Split Products*
Normotensive	—, ↓	—, ↓	↑	↑	↑	±
Hypotensive	↓	↓	↓	↓	↓	+

Key: —: normal; ↑: elevated; ↓: reduced; +: present.

typhoid fever has not correlated with clinical bleeding; thus, mere detection of laboratory abnormalities is not synonymous with alterations of clinical significance.[150] Further, the pathway via activated Hageman factor is not the only means by which endotoxin or bacterial products may initiate the clotting or bleeding. There are three other mechanisms that have been reported: (*1*) complexes of bacterial antigen with antibody can interact with human leukocytes and result in the release of a procoagulant that can trigger clotting.[151] (*2*) Circulating granulocyte proteases have been detected in gram-negative rod bacteremia, and these substances are capable of digesting clotting proteins in a manner distinct from DIC.[152] (*3*) Endotoxin can cause intimal vascular injury, thereby triggering or aggravating both clotting and bleeding, and this effect is probably mediated by TNF.[135,139]

Renal glomerular microclots as observed in rabbits after injections of endotoxin (generalized Shwartzman-type reaction) appear to be related to endotoxin-activated DIC.[153] Further, this experimental model of DIC suggests a role for both neutrophils and platelets in the initiation or augmentation of the reaction.[144] A reduction in numbers of circulating granulocytes through the use of cytotoxic agents may actually abort the generalized Shwartzman reaction.

The injection of small quantities of bacterial endotoxins into human volunteers indicates that the inflammatory and pyrogenic effects are manifested at low doses such as 5 ng.[87,88,122] The sequence of events appears similar to what has been observed in the monkey with the onset of hypotensive changes within an hour or 2.[154] Similar changes have also been observed after the intravenous injection of bacilli in dogs, although the hypotensive changes observed in the latter animal appear to be biphasic, with the initial phase aborted by the use of antihistamines.[96]

The effect of endotoxin on the kinin system is a direct result of the action of Hageman factor on the conversion of prekallikrein to kallikrein. Kallikrein in turn catalyzes the conversion of kininogen to bradykinin. Bradykinin is a vasoactive peptide whose primary effect is vasodilatation and increased vascular permeability. Tissue damage results from the margination of leukocytes, smooth muscle relaxation, leakage of fluid into the interstitial space, and an "effective" intravascular hypovolemia. Because bradykinin causes decreased peripheral vascular resistance secondary to vasodilatation, hypotension and septic shock ensue, with the result being hypoperfusion of critical organs.

In hypotensive patients with gram-negative bacteremia, Mason and coworkers demonstrated decreased prekallikrein and kallikrein inhibitor levels in blood.[155] Similar studies were also reported by Robinson and associates.[156] These findings were interpreted as indirect evidence for kinin release during severe episodes of infection, presumably by conversion of kininogen to kinins by plasma kallikrein. Infusion of synthetic bradykinin into animals results in hypotension followed by an elevation of cardiac output in response to reduced peripheral vascular resistance.[154] This sequence of events, including an increase in pulmonary vascular resistance, is similar to the circulatory and respiratory responses of humans to sepsis.

In human volunteer studies direct evidence that endotoxin triggers the release of bradykinin was obtained by Kimball and coworkers, who reported elevations of bradykinin levels to as high as 6 ng/ml as measured by radioimmunoassay in subjects given 3 or 5 ng/kg of endotoxin.[91] At these doses, bradykinin reached its maximum level at 1 hour without producing hypotension. These experiments were complicated by the relationship between the formation of angiotensin II and the inactivation of bradykinin since the hypotensive effects of bradykinin may be counteracted by the action of angiotensin II. O'Donnell and colleagues measured the blood prekallikrein levels in human infections and assessed the results with respect to hepatic synthesis since bradykinin is rapidly destroyed by plasma kininases and 90 percent of kinin is removed by single passage through the lung.[157] The highest mortality was observed in groups of patients who were hypotensive and had liver dysfunction. Blood prekallikrein levels were below normal in all groups studied, were significantly less in patients with liver dysfunction, and were reduced proportionally in hypotensive patients to less than 30 percent of the values noted in normotensive groups. These findings suggest that prekallikrein consumption in the hypotensive groups is the result of the process of activating kallikrein and the conversion of kininogen to bradykinin. Circulating kinin levels were elevated in hypotensive patients with or without liver disease.

A further extension of these studies of the kinin-generating system has included human volunteers serially followed after ingestion of 10^5 *Salmonella typhi*.[158] Although none of the clinical illnesses were severe and neither endotoxemia nor hypotension could be documented, the onset of positive blood cultures and fever was accompanied by a fall in platelet count, a reduction in prekallikrein esterase activity, a drop in levels of kallikrein inhibitor, and a rise in high-molecular-weight kininogen clotting activity. These findings plus electrophoretic evidence for the formation of a complex between kallikrein and a C1 esterase inhibitor provide further evidence for activation of the kinin system in gram-negative bacillary infections such as typhoid.

A variety of vasoactive substances including serotonin, endogenous catecholamines, adrenal corticosteroids, lysosomal enzymes, platelet-activating factor (PAF), and endorphins have been found circulating in the blood of animals after endotoxin administration.[121,159,160] In humans with gram-negative bacteremia, alterations in serum lipid profiles[161] and elevations in plasma thromboxane and prostaglandin levels have been observed.[162] These changes may be a result of TNF or a response secondary to bradykinin generation.

If bacteremia is transient, the result may only be a mild fever with little if any hemodynamic changes. The short-lived bacteremia that has been observed after instrumentation of the urinary or gastrointestinal tract indicates that bacteremia can occur without severe sequelae. On the other hand, activation of these inflammatory processes by a substantial inoculum of organisms in the debilitated patient may produce the clinical manifestations observed in severe gram-negative infections, particularly septic shock. Septic shock arises when cardiac output is unable to compensate for a falling blood pressure secondary to vasodilatation, an increased volume of the intravascular bed, and peripheral pooling of blood. The net result of inadequate tissue perfusion is cellular hypoxia and a shift of cellular metabolism from aerobic to anaerobic glycolysis followed by lactic acidosis, lysosomal injury, failure of essential cellular metabolism, and cell death.

The histopathologic changes in gram-negative septicemia include microthromboses of blood vessels on the venous side of the circulation, tissue necrosis, and hemorrhages. With gram-negative infections there appears to be a higher incidence of pulmonary hemorrhages than in other forms of shock,[163] and it is felt that these hemorrhages can aggravate fatal respiratory insufficiency (ARDS). Signs of metastatic pneumonia are found in patients with bacteremia arising from an extrapulmonary source. With a long period of ventilatory support for prolonged hypoxia, evidence of a superimposed aspiration-type pneumonia and hyaline membranes are often observed, but the latter are possibly related to pulmonary oxygen toxicity. Fibrin thrombi in small pulmonary vessels are almost invariably found if the patient dies in shock within 24 hours.[163] Microthrombi are difficult to identify after 48 hours, possibly because of the activation of fibrinolytic systems. After the lungs, the intestine has been most frequently affected, with lesions corresponding to acute ischemic enterocolitis. The liver at necropsy has occasionally shown zonal necrosis, which is not unique to gram-negative infection. Somewhat comparable to the findings in the lung, patients dying early in septic gram-negative shock (within 24 hours) may have fibrin thrombi in the hepatic vasculature. However, extensive necrosis and thrombi are not frequently observed in patients who succumb at longer intervals after the onset of infection.

Much work has been carried out to characterize the renal changes in gram-negative septicemic patients. Evidence for Shwartzman-type reactions has been presented by McKay and associates.[125] Classic lesions of the Shwartzman reaction with cortical necrosis are found infrequently, but other changes have been described that include scattered necrosis, hemorrhage, and tubular necrosis as well.[163]

Adrenal complications of gram-negative septicemia have long been the subject of interest among clinicians and pathologists. Bilateral adrenal cortical hemorrhages are an essential component of the Waterhouse-Friedricksen syndrome associated with meningococcemia, but these changes have been also found in a variety of shock states. They are commonly associated with fibrin thrombi that extend from the cortical sinusoids in the central vein of the adrenals and result in necrosis. Functionally, adrenal cortical necrosis has resulted in increased levels of circulating corticosteroid hormones, and there is little to support the belief that severe meningococcemia or gram-negative rod bacteremia complicated by shock is a functionally hypoadrenal state.

HOST DEFENSES AGAINST GRAM-NEGATIVE BACTERIA

Mechanical barriers are one of the most important factors limiting the systemic invasion of the host by gram-negative bacilli. Because the alimentary canal is clearly the largest reservoir of gram-negative rods in the body, the gastrointestinal mucosa has an important function in restricting entry of these organisms into the blood stream. Bacteremia may result from trauma, penetrating wounds, small surface ulcerations, mechanical obstruction such as caused by tumors, and ischemic necrosis of the bowel. Immunosuppressed people may have multiple small ulcerations of the gastrointestinal mucosa as the apparent source of entry of microorganisms; such ulcerations may be the effect of antineoplastic agents.

Irrespective of whether the organisms are aerobic or anaerobic, the complement-mediated serum bacteriolytic system is an important factor limiting invasion of the host by the great majority of gram-negative organisms that colonize the gastrointestinal tract. Most studies show these colonizing or saprophytic organisms to be serum sensitive, that is, they are killed or lysed by fresh human serum containing functional active components of the classic or alternative complement pathway.[56–58] Nonetheless, it appears that organisms causing bacteremic disease in humans and higher mammals are usually serum resistant or fairly resistant to the native serum bacteriolytic activity. There have been some reports of depressed serum bactericidal activity associated with bacteremic human infection.[164] It is possible that serum-sensitive organisms tend to cause a self-limited bacteremia, and this may well account for the finding that patients who have intermittent portal bacteremia (such as those with ulcerative colitis) or hepatic cirrhosis (where there may be impaired clearance of bacteria) have a wide variety of antibodies against enteric bacteria.[165] The susceptibility of strains to complement-mediated lysis appears to be related to structural defects in the trilamellar cell wall of the organisms rather than to variations in the bacteriolytic power of human serum.[59] Serum resistance seems related to the structural integrity of the LPS and probably quantity of polysaccharide. The amount and structure of capsular (K) antigens may also account for serum resistance.[166] Thus, serum sensitivity is related to microbial structure rather than to a variation in levels of specific antibodies or complement in human serum. While most serum-resistant organisms are "smooth" and most "rough" organisms are serum sensitive, it has been observed that some smooth strains can be used by fresh serum.[167] For some time it has been debated whether or not complement alone can kill serum-sensitive gram-negative bacilli or whether serum bacteriocidal activity has an obligatory requirement for antibodies of the IgG and IgM classes. Since the alternative complement pathway now appears to be activated in the absence of specific antibody, lysis without antibody is possible.[168] However, the presence of antibodies can enhance alternative-pathway activation through the so-called amplification loop.

Complement deficiency states are associated with increased susceptibility to infection, and this has been best documented with genetic deficiencies in certain complement components.[169] Early in life such as in the neonatal period, the alternative pathway is functionally deficient, and this may explain some of the increased susceptibility of newborn infants to gram-negative bacteremia.[170] It has also been reported that functional deficiencies of the alternative pathway are present in such diseases as sickle cell anemia and systemic lupus erythematosus, and this could be a predisposing factor to gram-negative bacillary systemic infections in these conditions.[171,172]

The basis for the presence of "natural" antibodies in normal serum, that is, detection of circulating antibodies against a number of bacteria that have not caused clinical disease, has been the matter of some speculation.[173] Such antibodies could result from low-grade or inapparent infection and would thus be engendered by specific antigenic exposure. Another mechanism by which humans could acquire natural antibodies against specific O or K antigens would be by exposure to organisms that bear similar or identical antigenic determinants but are relatively avirulent.[174] For instance, immunochemical studies now indicate identity between polyribose phosphate, the capsular polysaccharide of *Haemophilus influenzae* type B, and the capsular polysaccharide of *E. coli* K-100.[175] The group-specific B and C polysaccharides of *Neisseria meningitis* are similarly identical to the K-1 and K-92 *E. coli* polysaccharides, respectively.[176,177] *Bacillus pumilis* is an organism with exceedingly low pathogenicity that has cell wall material identical to the group A meningococcal polysaccharide.[178] Only a few scattered cases of group A meningococcal disease have occurred in the United States in the last few decades, yet the majority of the adult population has bactericidal antibody against group A meningococci.[179] Exposure to *B. pumilis* or similar organisms may account for the prevalence of these antibodies in the absence of epidemic meningococcal disease. By analogy, cross-protective immunity against a variety of other bacterial pathogens may derive from antecedent exposure to antigens borne by microorganisms in the human environment with considerbly less pathogenic potential.

Since the great majority of organisms that cause bacteremic disease in humans are resistant to the bactericidal activity of fresh human serum, the burden for clearing organisms from the blood stream must fall to phagocytic cells, whether they are the fixed phagocytes of the reticuloendothelial system or the circulating phagocytes such as the neutrophil or monocyte.[58] There is good correlation between susceptibility to bacterial and in particular gram-negative infections and depressed levels of circulating neutrophils. Since it is commonly observed that bacteremia follows neutropenia,[180] the neutropenic patient might still develop systemic infection in spite of the presence of high levels of antibodies against cell wall antigens. In actual clinical or experimental circumstances antibody levels seem to fall in parallel with levels of circulating phagocytes,[180,181] thus suggesting binding or consumption of antibody before or near the onset of bacteremia.

The humoral opsonic system of humans is complex. Antibodies of both IgG and IgM classes can serve as opsonins, and they are primarily directed against O or K polysaccharide antigens. There is evidence to suggest that K antibodies can be more protective than O antibodies are. Since K antigens lie more exteriorly on the bacterial cell surface than do somatic (O) antigens, K antibodies on a molar basis may be more effective as opsonins than O antibodies are.[182]

Complement activation may play an important role in deciding the pathways to C3b, the critical opsonic protein of the circulating humoral system. Opsonization via the classic complement pathway appears to have an obligatory requirement for specific antibody of either the IgG or IgM type.[183] IgM, in turn, has an obligatory requirement for complement, but IgG may opsonize gram-negative organisms in the absence of complement, although at a slower rate than in the presence of a normally functioning complement system.[184] It has been well demonstrated that phagocytes bind and engulf antibody-coated particles 100 times more efficiently when these particles are also coated with activated complement components.[185] Confirmation of the existence of the properdin or alternative complement pathway has given rise to considerable speculation about the phylogenetic and evolutionary role of this series of enzymatic reactions. Quite logically, the alternative pathway may have preceded the classic pathway since the former seems a more premordial, "nonspecific" mechanism for the recognition of microbial pathogens in the absence of specific antibody.[186] The alternative pathway appears to have an important function in providing nonspecific opsonic support before the availability of the specific antibody.[171] While specific antibody provides the most rapid and efficient opsonization,[187] the myriad numbers of different microbial antigens make it quite unlikely that normal subjects will have natural antibodies to every potential pathogen. Activation of components of the alternative pathway seems to serve an antibody-like function leading toward the activation of C3b. In the initial encounter between host and microbe, the opsonization via the alternative pathway may be important for serum-resistant organisms in the absence of specific antibody. Not all organisms activate the alternative pathway efficiently[75,188,189] and thus require type-specific antibody for efficient opsonization. The absence of type-specific antibody could give rise to relative or absolute deficiencies in the opsonic activity of serum. The finding that some organisms such as *E. coli* or *K. pneumoniae* are not readily phagocytosed in the presence of even normal serum[189] and the further documentation that these strains do not efficiently activate the alternative complement pathway[72] give rise to speculation that the more virulent strains causing human gram-negative rod bacteremia may be restricted in their complement-activating properties.

After gram-negative bacillary infections or immunization with cell wall antigens, specific antibodies of the IgM and IgG classes appear in the circulation; additionally, IgG may be locally secreted. IgM is primarily intravascular, whereas IgG is widely distributed throughout the intra- and extravascular spaces. The relative protective roles of these antibodies have also differed depending on the assay system.[190,191] In in vitro studies using antibodies against *P. aeruginosa* and in opsonophagocytic and bactericidal assays, IgM antibodies were found to be more protective than IgG antibodies.[192] The opposite conclusion was derived from mouse passive protection experiments, that is, IgG antibodies were more protective. This led to the hypothesis that while IgM is more protective in the presence of complement the wider distribution of IgG is the basis for its superior protective activity because such antibodies are present not only in the intravascular space but extravascularly as well. In addition to the aspect of superior tissue distribution, such results may reflect the fact that murine hosts have immature complement systems and actually negligible serum complement activity as compared with nonhuman primates or humans.[193] Such an assay system would tend to overemphasize the activity of IgG antibodies relative to IgM.

Besides passive protection assays, many other techniques have been used to measure antibodies against gram-negative bacillary antigens.[182,190–192] If passive hemagglutination with human or ovine erythrocytes is used, primarily IgM activity is measured. When indirect fluorescent antibody measurements are used, both IgG and IgM antibodies have been associated with protection against shock and death in human infections.[191] It is clear that both IgM and IgG have opsonic and bactericidal activities, particularly in the presence of complement. Fresh serum from healthy patients is efficient in promoting uptake of *P. aeruginosa* by neutrophils. In normal fresh serum, 2-mercaptoethanol reduction, which destroys IgM activity, effectively abolishes the opsonic activity against most bacteremic strains of *P. aeruginosa*.[58]

Whatever the activities of IgM or IgG antibodies as measured by indirect techniques (e.g., hemagglutination, immunofluorescence), functional assays such as opsonophagocytic tests also implicate depressed levels of heat-stable opsonins (humoral factors such as IgG and IgM[55,180] near the onset of bacteremia. Further, there has been some correlation between low levels of these opsonins, the presence of circulating endotoxin-like activity, and poor clinical prognosis.[108]

Antibodies may also play a role on toxin neutralization. Whereas antibodies against O-specific polysaccharide and K antigens appear to have opsonic activity, those directed against the inner "core" regions of the gram-negative cell wall appear to have endotoxin-neutralizing or "antitoxic" capabilities.[94,95] The evidence for this stems from experiments in which the hemodynamic and pathophysiologic effects of injected bacterial endotoxins or live bacilli have been neutralized by antibodies directed against a core glycolipid antigen.[95] Confirmatory studies include the ability of such anti-core antibodies to prevent generalized and local Shwartzman reactions as well as the ability to abort the complications of DIC.[194–196] The protection has been demonstrated both actively and passively. Antibodies against whole bacterial cells (outer cell wall membrane) have the capability of promoting phagocytosis as well as aborting the pathophysiologic sequelae of gram-negative bacteremia.[95] Antibodies against the core regions (Rc, Re structure, lipid A) appear to function mainly by aborting endotoxic activity.

After gram-negative bacillary infection, the bulk of antibody response is directed to somatic (O) antigens, with smaller amounts of antibody directed against core glycolipid antigens.[14] There are many reports that anti-core antibodies appear to protect humans and animals against the sequelae of gram-negative bacteremia and appear to have a broad cross-protective activity.[14,94,95,197–201] In contrast, some investigators have not been able to discern a cross-protective effect for anti-core glycolipid antibodies,[202,203] and even those who find anti-Re antibodies to be protective find little protection with lipid A antibodies.[204] There is evidence from immunization studies in humans that the protective antibody against endotoxin core is IgM rather than IgG.[205] In addition, the failure to observe any cross-protective activity may be related to the nature of the challenge, that is, more heavily encapsulated organisms may not have rough antigenic determinants exposed for neutralization. The failure to find protection with lipid A antisera, even though lipid A appears to be the "toxic" moiety of LPS, suggests that KDO is the immunodominant component of the Re antigen and protective antibodies are best engendered when both KDO and lipid A are linked (as they occur naturally).

How core antibody may exert its cross-protective effect is suggested schematically in Figure 5. Antibody directed against the toxic or core portion of the LPS (e.g., Rc or Re antigen) molecule acts to neutralize a moiety common to most enteric bacilli in a manner analogous to a master key capable of fitting many locks. This protection seems less than type-specific (O antibody) protection and may be considerably less against the more encapsulated bacilli whose core regions are relatively less exposed.

Little information is available on the protective activity of antibodies directed against extracellular toxins such as the exotoxin A of *P. aeruginosa*. It seems clear that antibodies are synthesized in response to infection,[117,206] and in experimental settings such antibodies are protective.[116] Further, the simultaneous presence of antibodies against both exotoxins and somatic antigens may provide enhanced protective activity.[207]

In addition to specific and cross-reactive antibodies, there appear to be a variety of other humoral substances that have endotoxin binding properties, and they may be significant in host defense.[105] These include high-density lipoproteins,[208] serum inactivators of LPS,[106] serum esterases, α-globulins, and transferrin.[209] A specific endotoxin binding protein has been described[210] that has been purified and is protective in animal models. The availability of large quantitites of these materials produced by recombinant techniques may permit an assessment of their relative protective role.

Many patients with serious gram-negative infections, including bacteremia, are neutropenic, and it seems obvious that phagocytic and intraleukocytic microbicidal function is necessary to clear serum-resistant organisms from the blood stream and body fluids.

Except for a few relatively unusual genetic disorders of leukocyte microbicidal activity, impaired killing by phagocytic

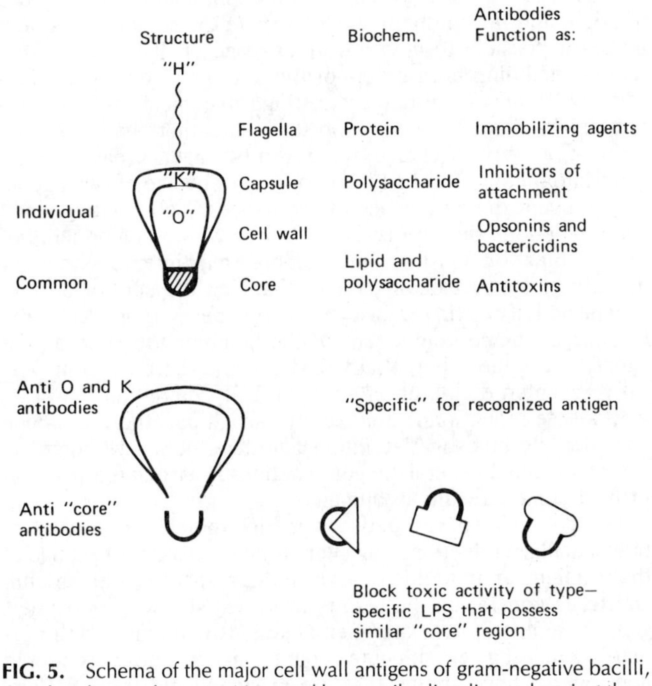

FIG. 5. Schema of the major cell wall antigens of gram-negative bacilli, their biochemical composition, and how antibodies directed against three antigens may function. Multiple functions are possible, that is, opsonin and antitoxin. O and K antibodies have limited specificities, while antibodies directed against the toxic "core" region cross react with most enteric bacilli.

cells is rare. This does not exclude defects in leukocyte motility (either congenital or drug induced) that predispose to infection, and this has certainly been suggested by several reports.[211,212]

DIAGNOSIS AND ANTIMICROBIAL THERAPY FOR GRAM-NEGATIVE ROD BACTEREMIA

Early clinical suspicion, rigorous diagnostic measures, aggressive initiation of appropriate antimicrobial therapy, comprehensive supportive care, and measures aimed at reversing predisposing causes are the cornerstones of successful management. While diagnostic microbiologic techniques are covered elsewhere in more detail, it is obvious that the clinical suspicion of bacteremia should be promptly confirmed by rapid identification and antimicrobial susceptibility testing of disease-causing organisms. Without confirmation of infection, the clinician will face the dilemma of whether or not to continue therapy with potentially toxic or sensitizing antimicrobial agents. Good liaison between the practicing clinician and the microbiology laboratory may be helpful in selecting methods for the rapid identification of causative organisms and for adjustment of antimicrobial therapy according to some initial biochemical reaction patterns even before the results of in vitro susceptibility tests are available.

In most hospitals it has become a common practice to use commercially available culture systems that aerobic and anaerobic bacterial growth. In untreated patients who are eventually shown to be bacteremic, the very first blood culture set that is taken will be positive more than 75 percent of the time, and the cumulative rate of positivity by the third blood culture set approaches 98 percent.[213] Further, recent analysis of the time interval to positivity of positive blood cultures indicates that for most gram-negative bacilli growth of microorganisms in blood culture bottles or on subcultures is revealed usually by 72 hours of incubation. The use of radiometric or lysis centrifugation techniques may result in even faster results. Thus, three sets of blood cultures and 3 days of careful observation have been sufficient to document of gram-negative bacteremia in more than 90 percent of previously untreated patients who are eventually shown to have blood stream infections.[79] Observation for signs of growth in blood culture bottles for periods of up to 10 days is still recommended for the detection of fastidious organisms or if the patient is receiving antimicrobials when the culture material was obtained.

The rapid isolation of some organisms poses special problems. *Pseudomonas aeruginosa* is an obligate aerobe and may not be rapidly detected just by the conventional technique of examining blood culture bottles for turbidity. One procedure that has been developed to enhance the detection of both aerobic and anaerobic sepsis is that of "blind" subculturing of apparently clear broth culture bottles. After incubation for 24 and 72 hours, blood culture bottles that are not turbid are nonetheless subcultured to aerobic and anaerobic media. The rationale for this approach is that as many as 10^5 organisms can be present and yet a broth suspension may appear to be clear. Particularly for *P. aeruginosa*, the subculture technique is advantageous because the aerobic environment that the subcultured plates are incubated in supports more rapid, uninhibited growth.

Because of the occurrence of polymicrobial bacteremia in a significant number of cases, the blind subculture technique also permits the identification of variants of bacterial types (two types of the same species such as *E. coli*) as well as mixed cultures before there is overgrowth by one predominant component. In intra-abdominal sepsis, blind subcultures of both aerobic and anaerobic bottles may enhance the yield of multiple pathogens that are likely to be present.

Antimicrobial therapy remains the mainstay of treatment of gram-negative rod bacteremia, but approaches aimed at correcting the predisposition to this complication have a critical bearing on the outcome of the infection. Amelioration of an underlying disease such as achievement of remission in leukemia is usually the major factor determining recovery irrespective of the choice of antimicrobial agents. The removal of foreign bodies that predispose to or potentiate infection, such as intravascular or urinary catheters, may by themselves cause resolution of symptoms and lead to a cure. Transient gram-negative rod bacteremia is a well-documented event, particularly with urinary tract manipulation, and the latter accounts for a number of instances where bacteremic patients have been cured either with inappropriate antibiotics or with no antimicrobial therapy at all.[20,214] A major corollary of the latter observation is that attempts to drain abscesses or to remove obvious sources of infection such as obstructed abdominal viscera are of paramount importance in determining recovery. Antimicrobial sterilization of large abscesses seems futile, although it is possible that small foci of infection could be sterilized by aggressive antimicrobial therapy.

The focus of much of the clinical work in the area of gram-negative sepsis over the last decades has been placed on the evaluation of new antimicrobial agents. There have been relatively few well-controlled, comparative human clinical trials of the efficacy of new antimicrobial regimens as well as definitive studies of the adjunctive measures that have been advocated to support patients during complications of sepsis. Clearly, it is not possible to conduct clinical trials of antibacterial therapy vs. no therapy, but what is lacking are comparisons of the efficacy and toxicity of some of the popular therapeutic regimens.

An analysis of the status of host factors, the severity of underlying disease, and the outcome of gram-negative rod bacteremia has consistently demonstrated increasing mortality in patients with "nonfatal," "ultimately fatal," and "rapidly fatal" diseases.[7,24,66] The classification of underlying disease as proposed by McCabe and Jackson[7] and as modified by others[25] assumes critical importance in attempting to compare treatment results due to the heterogeneity of predisposing or underlying conditions. It is clearly unfair and unscientific to compare therapeutic results in patients with transient bacteremia secondary to a kidney stone (usually these are patients with nonfatal underlying disease) with results in patients developing bacteremia during chemotherapy for acute unremitting leukemia (the usual example of a rapidly fatal disease). Classifying patients with postsurgical or post-traumatic conditions is more difficult, but for the most part intra-abdominal infections complicating surgical procedures or traumatic injury occur in nonimmunosuppressed patients without obvious derangement in host defense mechanisms.

During the 1960s, several major published reports indicated that appropriate antimicrobial therapy (as defined by antimicrobials that inhibited the infecting strain) significantly reduced mortality in patients with nonfatal or ultimately fatal disease.[7,24] It was not possible, however, to show that appropriate antimicrobial therapy significantly improved the chances of recovery in patients with the most adverse host factors, namely, those with rapidly fatal diseases such as acute leukemia in relapse.[24,66] For instance, mortality in three combined series[7,24,215] for patients with rapidly fatal disease who were treated appropriately (the antimicrobial inhibited their infecting strain) was 84 percent vs. 85 percent for patients treated "inappropriately." In contrast, the results of studies carried out since 1968 in patients with cancer and neutropenia have shown a general overall improvement in clinical response rates.[66,216,217] Most of the studies of patients with neutropenia reported since 1968 show survival rates ranging from 40 to 85 percent, especially with some of the most potent modern treatment regimens.[16,17,217,218] There also appears to be some decrease in overall mortality if the series of gram-negative rod bacteremias summarized in Table 1 are viewed chronologically from the oldest to the more recent. Few of these studies, however, assessed the adequacy of therapy by determining whether adequate blood levels of antimicrobial agents were actually achieved in vivo. It should be further recalled that there have been no comparative studies of the relative clinical efficacy of antimicrobial agents available since 1968 and now widely used vs. agents that were commonly used to treat gram-negative infections before that date. The reason for selecting this temporal dividing point is that 1968–1969 marks the beginning (in the United States at least) of the availability of two groups of compounds with activities different from those previously available: both aminoglycosides and β-lactam compounds (broad-spectrum penicillins and cephalosporins) that are active against *P. aeruginosa, Enterobacter* species, indole-positive *Proteus* species, and *Serratia*.

Many factors besides the introduction of new antimicrobial agents could account for the improved therapeutic results observed in certain classes of patients or within the experience of a single institution. These factors would include more aggressive approaches to diagnosis and the initiation of treatment, overall improvements in supportive care, and many of the adjunctive measures detailed in subsequent sections of this chapter. Because of institutional and demographic differences, it seems most fair to assess trends within the experience of a single institution or single observers, and these in selected instances have shown a reduction in mortality.[19,20]

One attitude that has become widely prevalent in the therapeutic approaches to gram-negative rod infection, particularly in the critically ill, has been the willingness to begin empirical broad-spectrum therapy before the results of cultures are obtained.[219] This approach has inherent dangers such as the selection for antimicrobial resistance as well as the risk of drug toxicity. There are some patients with apparently intact host defenses in whom empirical therapy may not be indicated because there is adequate time to obtain material for culture and sensitivity testing. Nonetheless, one definite change in attitude in the last two decades in the approach to the critically ill patient with presumed infection has been to initiate empirical therapy with the intention of making subsequent therapeutic adjustments.

It is only logical that clinicians have used combinations of antimicrobial agents for serious gram-negative rod infections, particularly for those patients with the most adverse prognostic factors. The supporting arguments for combination therapy are multiple and not mutually exclusive: (*1*) Combination therapy makes it possible to cover a broad range of diagnostic possibilities including both gram-positive and gram-negative infection, which may be difficult to distinguish clinically. (*2*) Polymicrobial bacteremia may be present, so rather than being an "either/or" type of choice, the use of two agents may give appropriate therapy for dual infections. (*3*) The use of two agents may prevent the emergence of resistance by eliminating small subpopulations that are resistant to one of the components of the combination. (*4*) Two antimicrobials may interact either additively or synergistically, thus enhancing the sum of antimicrobial activity or (in the case of synergy) permitting a reduction in dosage of one component of the combination such as the agent that is more potentially toxic. While there is no universally accepted definition of antimicrobial synergy and in practice dosage reduction is not usually carried out, there has been considerable investigative interest in determining whether the use of so-called synergistic combinations is associated with improved clinical results in humans.

The role of synergy between antimicrobial agents used to treat bacillary infections has been difficult to assess because of the problems in initiating randomized, prospective human clinical trials comparing the results of synergistic with nonsynergistic combinations. Experimental studies in animals with normal circulating granulocyte counts or in those rendered neutropenic have shown that use of synergistic combinations leads to a more favorable outcome in *P. aeruginosa* infections.[220–222] Several human studies have shown an association between the use of combinations that interact synergistically against infecting strains and improved clinical results.[214,223] In one study, an association was noted between the use of synergistic combinations and improved clinical results in the face of adverse clinical factors such as neutropenia, rapidly fatal underlying disease, and shock.[214] Because multiple agents are usually given on different dosage schedules, it has been difficult to ensure that the drug concentrations that are achieved in vivo reflect test concentrations used in in vitro studies. The finding of serum inhibitory titers by one group equal to or exceeding 1:8 has been associated with favorable clinical outcome.[224] Still, it is possible that good clinical results obtained when using combinations of antimicrobial agents may not be related to synergistic interactions. For instance, with such commonly used agents as aminoglycosides and penicillins, which often interact synergistically in vitro, "peak" blood levels that are used to gauge in vitro susceptibility are actually maintained for rather short periods of time followed by periods of rapid "decay." The use of a broad-spectrum penicillin with an aminoglycoside may merely ensure a more sustained interval of serum inhibitory or bactericidal activity or may avoid too low "trough" levels of such activity. Some investigators believe the latter is a cause of treatment failure and have given continuous infusions of antibiotics to maintain a "constant" blood level.[225] However, it is still unclear whether continuous vs. intermittent administration of antimicrobial agents is superior for a variety of infectious conditions. Factors such as tissue penetration, protein binding, rapidity of killing, and postantibiotic effects are likely to influence the outcome as well as the timing and duration of drug infusion. For critically ill patients with septicemia it is implicit that the administration of all pharmacologic agents should be via the intravenous route.

In selecting antimicrobial therapy, the severity of the underlying disease and the possibility of synergistic interactions are still important considerations. Table 8 summarizes recommendations for initial empirical therapy for presumed gram-negative rod bacteremia. First- and second-generation cephalosporins alone may be justified for community-acquired bacteremia secondary to urinary tract infection in the non-neutropenic host where *E. coli* and *Klebsiella* are the main concerns. For the patient with nosocomial infection, initial therapy should consist of an aminoglycoside initially paired with a β-lactam agent. Preference is expressed for a cephalosporin as the β-lactam agent in the non-neutropenic patient because of the greater likelihood of *Klebsiella* vs. *P. aeruginosa*. The regimen of an aminoglycoside paired with a penicillin or cephalosporin having antipseudomonal activity is preferred for the neutropenic patient, the patient receiving assisted ventilation, or the patient with an extensive burn injury.

Amikacin and netilmicin are semisynthetic aminoglycosides that are less susceptible to attack by bacterial exoenzymes known to inactivate gentamicin and tobramycin.[226] Consideration of these as primary therapy in presumed gram-negative rod bacteremia should be based on the prevalence of resistance to gentamicin or to tobramycin in the institution or on the likelihood of resistance in high-risk patients such as those with neutropenia or thermal injury. If organisms are equally susceptible to all aminoglycosides and adequate therapeutic levels are achieved, the clinical results are likely to be similar. Recommended doses of gentamicin, tobramycin, or netilmicin are 1.7 mg/kg q8h and for amikacin either 5 mg/kg q8h or 7.5 mg/kg q12h. The carbenicillin dose should probably be on the order of 70 mg/kg intravenously q4h with a total dose limited to 36 g/day. More potent semisynthetic penicillins like ticarcillin, mezlocillin, azlocillin, and piperacillin may be given in doses varying from 40 mg/kg q4h to 60 mg/kg q6h.

The third-generation cephalosporins, related β-lactam agents like moxalactam, carbapenems like imipenem, and monobactam agents like aztreonam have markedly augmented activity against enteric bacteria but variable bactericidal effect against *P. aeruginosa*. The potency of cefotaxime, ceftizoxime, and moxalactam against *E coli* and *Klebsiella* (minimum inhibitory concentrations [MICs], often 0.5 μg/ml or less with achievable blood levels 100-fold or more higher) suggests that single-agent therapy directed against those bacteria may be quite successful even in severely compromised hosts. In contrast, resistance among *Pseudomonas, Serratia*, and *Enterobacter* species may emerge rapidly on monotherapy. Ceftazidime and cefsulodin appear most active against *P. aeruginosa*, but the latter is only active against *Pseudomonas*. Clinical trials in which third-generation cephalosporins are combined with an aminoglycoside show results similar to penicillin/aminoglycoside combinations.[227] Monotherapeutic regimens (e.g., ceftazidime, imipenem, or intravenous quinolones) may be effective for fevers of undetermined origin in neutropenic patients and for documented infections due to highly susceptible gram-negative bacteria.[218] However, successful treatment for bacteremic patients with profound persistent neutropenia (e.g., neutrophil counts less than 100/μl) still appears to be linked to the use of two agents that inhibit the infecting strain (irrespective of synergistic interactions.[16,228] In view of excellent responses associated with the initial use of combination therapy it still seems prudent to begin treatment of the critically ill patient with two agents that are likely to be active[216,217] and to modify treatment on the basis of antibiotic susceptibility test results and changes in the status of the host.

There is no evidence that a three-drug regimen, for example, aminoglycoside/penicillin/cephalosporin, is superior to an aminoglycoside/β-lactam combination.[229] Combining bactericidal with bacteristatic agents is generally avoided because some clinical evidence argues against their combined use.

Clinicians should not assume that the administration of apparently adequate doses of antimicrobial agents consistently ensures therapeutic levels. Aminoglycosides have a marrow therapeutic ratio, and there is marked individual variability in the individual peak blood levels of gentamicin.[230] Studies of patients with recurrent or breakthrough bacteremia have indicated an association with subinhibitory blood levels of agents such as gentamicin.[231] In view of the variations in blood pharmacokinetics of aminoglycosides, it would seem prudent in the critically ill patients to monitor blood levels frequently. There is some evidence that such monitoring may also avert potentially toxic complications.[232] The measurement of aminoglycoside blood levels is usually not indicated in patients with bacteremia from the genitourinary tract inasmuch as the levels of many agents excreted in the urine are high. The average duration of treatment in normal hosts experiencing gram-negative sepsis is 10–14 days, but this may be longer if the patient has persistent infection at the source of bacteremia. Treatment of the neutropenic or immunocompromised patient may require an even longer duration. Patients in the latter group should be afebrile for a minimum of 4–7 days and have evidence of resolving infection at the source of bacteremia, and the neutrophil count should be rising and in excess of 500/μl before drug ther-

TABLE 8. Recommended Antimicrobial Regimens for Empirical (Presumptive) Therapy for Gram-Negative Rod Bacteremia

1. Community-acquired infection in the non-neutropenic subject (neutrophil count ≥1000/mm³)
   a. Suspected urinary tract source: ampicillin plus an aminoglycoside
   b. Nonurinary tract source: a third-generation cephalosporin plus/minus an aminoglycoside
2. Hospital-acquired infection, non-neutropenic subject: a third-generation cephalosporin plus an aminoglycoside
3. Neutropenic patient with hospital-acquired infection: antipseudomonal penicillin plus an aminoglycoside or a third-generation cephalosporin plus an aminoglycoside
4. Thermal injury to at least 20 percent of the body surface area: same as 3
5. Pulmonary source associated with inhalation therapy equipment: same as 3
6. Established or suspected gentamicin resistance: use amikacin as the aminoglycoside
7. Nosocomial infection in the setting of resistance to penicillins and cephalosporins: imipenem plus/minus an aminoglycoside

apy is stopped. The exception to this guideline would be patients with marrow failure syndromes who are unlikely to generate white counts as high as 500/μl; in these subjects clinical defervescence alone should suffice.

Oral therapy is ill advised for the bacteremic patient with fever, hemodynamic instability, and factors that might limit absorption of antimicrobial agents from the gut. On the other hand, a change to an effective oral agent (as determined by in vitro testing) is often justified after defervescence if the patient's overall condition is improving. Potentially useful agents include the quinolones, oral cephalosporins or penicillins, and trimethoprim-sulfamethoxazole.

ADJUNCTIVE MEASURES IN THERAPY FOR GRAM-NEGATIVE ROD BACTEREMIA

Maintenance of Adequate Tissue Perfusion with Volume Replacement

Management of fluid and electrolyte balance is a crucial aspect of the care of the patient with gram-negative bacteremia, particularly the person whose course is complicated by shock. Perfusion of vital organs such as the brain and kidney must be maintained. It is clear that the body has an order of priorities that result in distribution of blood preferentially to vital organs; this causes splanchnic vasoconstriction as well as a marked reduction of circulation to the skin. When these compensatory changes are inadequate to maintain adequate perfusion, central arterial pressures will fall. The first goal of management of the patient with bacteremia, particularly in the incipient stages of shock, is adequate monitoring of vital signs so that any hemodynamic changes can be readily counteracted. Insertion of a central venous pressure monitoring device, an arterial catheter, and Swan-Ganz catheters to determine the left atrial end-diastolic pressure are useful measures in the critically ill patient, although it is clear that they present certain infection hazards per se. These monitoring devices are not used to determine optimal therapy but rather the limits of therapy. In other words, normal or low central venous pressure and left atrial end-diastolic pressures (pulmonary wedge pressures) in the presence of a declining systemic arterial blood pressure are an indication for further volume replacement. On the other hand, it is clear that these parameters may rise to dangerously elevated levels without being able to restore adequate arterial perfusion. In the presence of cardiac failure, cautious digitalization with a rapidly acting intravenous digitalis preparation is indicated. Digitalis toxicity may be manifested at relatively lower doses of digitalis in septic shock, and this risk is further enhanced by the administrator of sympathomimetic amines.

There are a number of solutions that can be used to expand intravascular fluid volume and colloid oncotic pressure, including fresh frozen plasma, albumin of the regular type or salt depleted, and various dextran preparations. If the patient is anemic, thrombocytopenic, as well as hypotensive, the transfusion of whole blood in the face of a low central venous pressure is justified. If there is no need for erythrocytes, one of the plasma fractions will suffice. With evidence for bleeding and consumption coagulopathy, the use of fresh frozen plasma may be indicated. There has been a tendency to avoid dextran preparations because of an association with hemorrhagic tendencies. Other authorities have preferred to use crystalloid solutions in preference to colloid.[233]

Use of Sympathomimetic Amines

Sympathomimetic amines have been widely used to treat the hemodynamic complications of shock, but there have been no controlled or comparative studies of the efficacy of different compounds. For many years norepinephrine and epinephrine were the principal agents available. Norepinephrine has intense peripheral vasoconstricting activity, and extravasation around iv infusion sites has led to ischemic necrosis of tissues. There is justifiable concern that its use compromises the perfusion of vital organs. Both norepinephrine and epinephrine increase myocardial irritability. Alternative agents like isoproterenol, dopamine, and dobutamine have largely supplanted norepinephrine. They have an inotropic effect on myocardial function but because of β-adrenergic activity are capable of enhancing peripheral tissue perfusion. Isoproterenol increases the cardiac index but has little effect on mean arterial pressure.[234] Dopamine causes vasodilatation of renal, coronary, and cerebral blood flow while causing an increase in systolic blood pressure and heart rate and an effective reduction in the blood supplied to skeletal muscle. Dobutamine has little chronotropic activity and is otherwise quite similar to dopamine. Presently norepinephrine should be reserved only for those patients in whom it is not possible to support systemic blood pressure and vascular perfusion with dopamine or isoproterenol. Table 9 is a summary of recommended doses and techniques for administering sympathomimetic amines.

Sympathomimetic agents have a wide range of effects, particularly on pulmonary airway passages, regulation of blood sugar, and so forth. None of these considerations is as important as perfusion of vital organs during septic shock. Perhaps the critical factor that is often neglected in the management of patients with sympathomimetic amines is the relationship between fluid therapy and the use of these agents. It is inappropriate to use dopamine and isoproterenol before aggressive volume replacement. If they are used in the presence of a reduced intravascular fluid volume, the vasodilatation secondary to β-adrenergic stimulation can cause a paradoxical decline in blood pressure and decreased tissue perfusion because of the sudden drop in effective intravascular volume. Because of this danger, constant monitoring of central venous pressure and pulmonary wedge pressure is indicated; some authors advocate fluid replacement to the point that either or both of the latter begin to rise to the upper limits of normal. At that juncture it would be appropriate to use an agent such as dopamine, dobutamine, or isoproterenol if the patient remains hypotensive.

In spite of volume replacement, digitalization, and sympathomimetic amine administration, significant metabolic acidosis may ensue. While primary efforts should still be aimed at enhancing tissue perfusion, temporary correction of acidosis may be achieved with infusions of sodium bicarbonate.

Role of Corticosteroids in the Treatment of Gram-Negative Rod Septicemia and Its Complications

Since the clinical availability of corticosteroids, there has been controversy over their effectiveness as adjunctive therapy in the management of infection. Corticosteroids have a variety of metabolic, anti-inflammatory, and immunosuppressive effects, and it is commonly observed that the short-term administration often results in defervescence, thus leading to a clinical impression of improvement. Weitzman and Berger emphasized the

TABLE 9. Sympathomimetic Amines for Support of the Circulation in Septic Shock

Listed in order of preference, to be used after volume replacement and with careful ECG, CVP, and BP monitoring:

1. Dopamine, 2–25 μg/kg/min: increase the rate of infusion (D_5W or saline) q15–20 min until systolic blood pressure exceeds 90 mmHg and the urine output exceeds 30 ml/hr
2. Dobutamine, 2–25 μg/kg/min: titrate as with dopamine
3. Isoproterenol, 5 μg/ml/min: observe the effect within 15–25 min and double the rate of infusion if necessary
4. Norepinephrine: give a test dose of 0.1–0.2 μg/kg and observe the response (usually in minutes). The normal maintenance dose is 0.05 μg/kg/min delivered via a plastic catheter into a large peripheral or central vein

Abbreviations: ECG: electrocardiographic; CVP: central venous pressure; BP: blood pressure; D_5W: 5% dextrose in water.

lack of convincing evidence from controlled studies that corticosteroids accelerate the rate of recovery or lower mortality from sepsis.[235] Nonetheless, there has been widespread belief that corticosteroids are beneficial as adjunctive therapy in gram-negative infections, particularly those complicated by shock. Much of the belief is derived from animal studies wherein healthy experimental subjects of varying susceptibility to the effects of bacterial endotoxin were given large doses of these substances to induce shock. Such doses are questionably associated with the pathogenesis of the complications of shock in humans. Furthermore, the animals used in such studies have almost always been immunologically intact or physiologically normal before the induction of shock.

One of the major issues relating to the efficacy of corticosteroids in human sepsis complicated by shock has been that of dosage. Since relatively low doses (up to 1 mg/kg betamethasone or roughly 25–30 mg/kg equivalent of hydrocortisone) were used in one well-controlled, prospective study[236] and showed no beneficial effect, advocates of corticosteroid therapy have escalated their recommendations so that one study reported a beneficial effect of corticosteroids in doses of 30 mg/kg of methylprednisolone or 2 mg/kg of dexamethasone.[237] Doses in this range were found to improve survival in one controlled clinical trial in patients with typhoid fever.[238] Another comparative study found that large doses of corticosteroids (2 g methylprednisolone for the 70 kg patient) actually reversed septic shock in a significant number of patients. While a transient, "early" effect in increased survival was noted, mortality at the conclusion of the study was similar in both groups, and steroid recipients had a higher incidence of superinfection.[239] Despite these aforementioned studies, however, the largest and most comprehensive, controlled clinical trials in the United States have failed to confirm the beneficial effect of corticosteroids in septic shock. This conclusion was reached in the final report of a multicenter collaborative trial involving the Veterans Administration Hospitals[240] and a multihospital collaborative group[241] involving some of the same investigators who earlier had noted a beneficial effect.[239] Additionally, two other controlled human trials employed similar doses of corticosteroids for ARDS patients and obtained negative results.[242,243] In view of these findings, large doses of prednisone/prednisolone/dexamethasone cannot be recommended as adjunctive therapy for sepsis or shock. Replacement doses of corticosteroids are clearly justified in suspected adrenal insufficiency.

Anticoagulation

The use of anticoagulation, particularly heparinization, to treat septicemic states associated with DIC is logical because there is strong experimental and human clinical evidence that coagulopathy can be terminated by heparinization. At present, however, it is unclear whether anticoagulation has any effect in prolonging survival, however desirable it may be to abolish the sequence of events leading to clotting, consumption of clotting factors, and the onset or aggravation of bleeding. In both human and experimental studies the use of agents such as heparin has failed to significantly decrease the mortality from bacteremic gram-negative infections.[244,245] In human infection the failure to show a difference may be related to the overall poor prognosis of the underlying disease that is complicated by bacteremia. Until it can be shown that a reduction in mortality is consistent, the use of routine anticoagulation in the management of patients with DIC should be avoided. This is particularly true for normotensive people. If bleeding in such patients is associated with depressed levels of platelets or a specific factor, replacement therapy may be required to control the hemorrhage.

For hypotensive septicemic patients, measures aimed at controlling the infection and correcting hemodynamic alterations (volume replacement and sympathomimetic amines) are of primary importance. If the blood pressure responds to such measures (an effect is usually observed within 4 hours), consumption coagulopathy will usually cease. If the patient has bleeding because of the coagulopathy and not from another cause such as an associated gastrointestinal ulcer, replacement therapy is indicated. This should consist of platelet transfusions for thrombocytopenia, cryoprecipitate preparations for hypofibrinogenemia, and fresh frozen plasma for depleted coagulation factors. While this approach theoretically could aggravate coagulopathy by providing additional substrate for clotting, this complication is not commonly observed when replacement therapy is used in conjunction with measures aimed at controlling shock and infection.[149]

For patients with refractory shock and coagulopathy in spite of the preceding measures, heparin therapy may be beneficial in terminating DIC (without evidence that this prolongs life). Other patients who should be considered for anticoagulation are those who appear to have pulmonary embolic phenomena. This includes patients with pelvic thrombophlebitis. Heparin may be given by either intermittent or continuous infusion. The dose for intermittent infusion is 50–100 units/kg of aqueous heparin given by bolus infusion every 4 hours. For continuous infusion the recommended dose of heparin in adult therapy is 10,000 units made up in 500 ml of 5% dextrose in water (D_5W) delivered over a period of approximately 4–6 hours. Since reversal of coagulation tendencies has an immediate effect, it would appear judicious to terminate therapy as soon as possible after the subsidence of fever. Other anticoagulants such as coumadin-type drugs have been shown in experimental model systems to obviate some of the manifestations of endotoxemia such as generalized Shwartzman reaction. On the other hand, there appears to be little indication for coumadin in gram-negative sepsis in view of the slow onset of the defect. Heparin is preferable, and prolonged anticoagulation should be avoided.

Therapeutic Role of Granulocyte Transfusion

Transfusion of granulocytes is a logical strategy to counteract the functional or absolute neutropenia present in many patients who develop gram-negative rod bacteremia. The rationale and techniques for granulocyte transfusion therapy are discussed elsewhere (Chapter 7).

At least four controlled studies have suggested that there may be a benefit for transfused subjects evaluated with regard to short-term survival and resolution of fever.[246–249] Unfortunately, these studies were small, and the nature of both the underlying infection and type of antimicrobial therapy was often unclear. Subsequently, a much larger study randomizing patients with documented gram-negative bacteremia to receive or not to receive neutrophil transfusions showed no difference in recovery rates or survival, even in the subset of patients without evidence of bone marrow recovery.[250] Survival was quite good in the control group as compared with previous studies, and this may have been due to better antimicrobial therapy. The complications of white cell transfusion, particularly viral infections and pulmonary complications, plus the outcome of this more recent study should discourage routine granulocyte transfusions in septicemic, neutropenic patients if appropriate antimicrobial therapy is given. Recent granulocyte transfusion studies have delivered small numbers of neutrophils relative to the normal daily production and the anticipated granulocyte "requirement" in the face of infection.[251] Thus it is conceivable that improvements in techniques for procuring granulocytes so that much larger numbers of cells may be given safely could improve the efficacy of the approach. Presently, it appears that patients who are most likely to benefit from white cell transfusions are those with the potentially reversible defect in granulocyte production such as transient bone marrow aplasia or a neoplastic disorder where there is evidence for an early remission. If appropriate antimicrobial therapy fails in this setting, then granulocyte transfusions might be considered. Candidates least likely to benefit from transfusions are patients who have had multiple courses of unsuccessful therapy for refractory underlying disease such as marrow aplasia or acute leukemia.

Diuretics

Diuretics are commonly used in the management of the early oliguric or anuric phases of bacteremic shock. The use of agents such as furosemide or ethacrynic acid is controversial, however, since there is no controlled study demonstrating that acute renal failure may be avoided by the aggressive use of such agents. The action of potent loop diuretics such as furosemide or ethacrynic acid usually results in a significant increase in the output of dilute urine, but it is unclear whether the aggressive use of diuretics in the early oliguric phases of shock makes the ensuing renal failure less severe. What has been observed is that some of these agents, including both ethacrynic acid and furosemide, may cause deafness and there may be enhanced toxicity when these agents are simultaneously used with agents that can damage eighth nerve or renal function such as aminoglycoside antibiotics. In view of these effects it seems prudent to monitor the patient's vital signs and central venous or left atrial pressure and to use diuretics only when volume expansion is not adequate to maintain urine output.

Other Pharmacologic Agents Used to Treat Patients in Septic Shock

Naloxone, an antagonist of opiates and β-endorphins, has been shown to reverse the course of endotoxic and hypovolemic shock in experimental animals.[252–253] In a small study of humans with prolonged hypotension, an intravenous dose of 0.4–1.2 mg of naloxone resulted in a 45 percent increase in systolic blood pressure that lasted at least 45 minutes.[254] Before naloxone infusion, patients had been treated with fluids, dopamine, and appropriate antibiotics. Nonresponders were subjects who had previously been treated with corticosteroids or phenothiazines. Thus, it appears that naloxone has a transient pressor effect in human shock with the added appeal of no immunosuppressive complications (unlike corticosteroids). However, a small controlled study of naloxone therapy in gram-negative infections complicated by shock failed to demonstrate any benefit.[255]

A wide variety of pharmacologic agents including phenothiazines, antihistamines, anti-inflammatory agents such as indomethacin and phenylbultazone, glucagon, α-adrenergic blocking agents, and vasodilators have been used experimentally as adjunctive therapy for septic shock complicating gram-negative infections. Among the more interesting recent observations is the finding that cyclooxygenase inhibitors can inhibit the effects of TNF.[141,143] Other pharmacologic agents such as pentoxyphylline can inhibit the effect of TNF on neutrophils.[256] However, no controlled studies support the clinical use of any of these pharmacologic agents in humans.

THERAPEUTIC ANTISERUM IN GRAM-NEGATIVE SEPSIS

The use of antiserum to treat bacterial infections antedates the antimicrobial era, but was all but abandoned more than four decades ago. Resurgent interest in the therapeutic applications of antibody stems for the persistently high mortality associated with sepsis often complicated by shock in spite of the use of appropriate antimicrobials. There have been anecdotal reports of the successful use of convalescent serum for *P. aeruginosa* bacteremia[257] or *Pseudomonas* immune globulin in surgical patients,[258] but the latter study was uncontrolled. More recently, Ziegler and associates reported the results of a large multicenter, double-blind trial of therapeutic antiserum prepared by immunizing donors with the "J5" mutant of *E. coli* 0111 (a "rough mutant" with an endotoxin core analogous to an Rc mutant). Mortality was 22 percent in 103 bacteremic recipients of antiserum as opposed to 39 percent in 109 subjects randomized to control serum therapy.[201] An even more significant difference was noted in the ability of antiserum to reverse profound shock. Therapeutic antiserum did not, however, significantly affect survival in patients with cancer and/or neutropenia, and no protective antibody titer or level could be inferred. The encouraging results of Ziegler's group have spurred efforts to prepare human antiserum by active immunization with other core endotoxin antigens,[257] harvest IgG antibodies from high-titer human serum lots and modify them for intravenous use,[260] and produce monoclonal antibodies of murine[199,261] or human origin.[200] A clinical trial of intravenous IgG was unsuccessful, possibly because of low titer or because IgG antibodies are not protective.[205] Murine monoclonals of IgM isotype have been produced that can abrogate the effect of endotoxins and can increase survival above that obtained with antimicrobial therapy.[199,261] Human clinical trials with these antibodies indicate that they are generally well tolerated.[262] It is possible that their benefit may derive from their action on endotoxins liberated during the course of antimicrobial therapy, as has been documented by some investigators.[263] Greater species compatibility and fewer hypersensitivity reactions may be anticipated with the use of human monoclonal antibodies than have been described to date.[200,264] Clinical trials to critically assess these concepts are now underway.

PROPHYLAXIS OF GRAM-NEGATIVE ROD BACTEREMIA

Measures to prevent gram-negative rod bacteremia have ranged from meticulous efforts aimed at limiting the spread of infection within the hospital, the use of prophylactic antimicrobial agents of a topical or systemic form, management of high-risk patients in so-called protective environments, active or passive immunoprophylaxis with type-specific or cross-reactive antibodies, and augmentation of the host granulocyte pool with prophylactic granulocyte transfusions. These measures have been applied to patients with different underlying diseases of varying degrees of severity. The validity of many of these approaches has not been rigorously tested in controlled studies in humans.

It seems reasonable that the simplest and most cost-effective measures for the prophylaxis of gram-negative bacillary infections would involve minimizing the infection hazard associated with such procedures as Foley catheterizations and prolonged intravascular catheterization. The value of antimicrobial prophylaxis of either a topical or systemic nature is highly controversial, but there is emerging evidence that it may be beneficial in certain well-defined circumstances.

Logical applications of antimicrobial prophylaxis include topical application to the skin, the use of an oropharyngeal spray, and orally ingested nonabsorbable antibiotics to suppress the fecal flora. The application of topical agents like silver nitrate, silver sulfadiazine, or sulfamylon to burned skin appears to have significantly reduced the incidence of burn wound sepsis caused by organisms like *P. aeruginosa*[265] The application of a polymyxin spray to the posterior portion of the pharynx appears to have limited gram-negative bacillary colonization of the oropharynx and prevented some cases of nosocomial gram-negative pneumonia.[266] However, such efforts offer the potential hazard of selecting for the emergence of organisms resistant to the prophylactic agent, as has been amply documented with the use of polymyxin sprays.[267]

Since the gastrointestinal tract is a vast reservoir of gram-negative bacilli, an essentially topical approach to prophylaxis is the use of oral nonabsorbable antimicrobial agents. Sterilization of bowel contents is unrealistic, but suppression of the aerobic fecal flora has been achieved to varying degrees with regimens that use polymyxin[268] or gentamicin[269] normally with vancomycin and nystatin. Randomized studies have shown a significant reduction in bacterial sepsis in neutropenic subjects given a polymyxin-containing regimen as compared with placebo.[268] The efficacy of gentamicin-vancomycin-nystatin has been assessed in a three-arm study with management of neutropenic patients in "protected environments" with laminar airflow and under regular ward care.[269] The reduction in infection was similar for both groups receiving oral antimicrobials and was not significantly greater for those additionally managed in laminar airflow rooms.

Regimens containing oral nonabsorbable agents are unpalatable, and patient compliance has been variable. Better-tolerated alternatives include trimethoprim-sulfamethoxazole[270,271] and the newer quinolones. Trimethoprim-sulfamethoxazole has been used to prevent both *Pneumocystis carinii* pneumonia and bacterial infection. Unfortunately, it has no effect against *P. aeruginosa* and may predispose to superinfection with fungi and resistant bacilli. Recent studies suggest a significant reduction in gram-negative infections occurring in neutropenic patients given prophylactic norfloxacin[272] or ciprofloxacin.[273]

AUGMENTATION OF HOST DEFENSES: PROPHYLACTIC GRANULOCYTE TRANSFUSIONS AND IMMUNOPROPHYLAXIS

Patients about to receive intense cytotoxic therapy for leukemia or marrow transplants have been considered candidates for prophylactic white cell transfusions. Although one report was favorable to this approach,[274] a large multicentered study clearly pointed out the dangers associated with prophylactic transfusion.[275] Some studies have shown a reduction in the incidence of gram-negative infections,[274,275] but this was offset by a high incidence of pulmonary complications in the transfused recipients.[275,276] Many of the lung infiltrates were probably due to cytomegalovirus infections. Perhaps most important, there has been no evidence of increased survival in any group receiving daily prophylactic transfusions and having a high incidence of sensitization. In the absence of better methods for reducing complications such as sensitization[277] and transfusion-associated viral infections, there are no indications of prophylactic transfusions outside of an investigative setting.

Augmentation of levels of circulating granulocytes will correct only one component of altered host defenses in the immunosuppressed person. Deficiencies in the levels of circulating immunoglogulins or opsonins might be anticipated in such a person.[55,180] A study of the efficacy of transfused granulocytes demonstrated that therapeutic failures were associated with deficiencies in humoral opsonins.[278] These findings suggest a need to supplement both phagocytes and opsonic factors (including antibody) in the prophylaxis of serious infections in the immunosuppressed host.

With respect to the feasibility of immunoprophylaxis in the prevention of gram-negative bacteremia, the impetus for this approach is the convincing evidence that some bacterial infections can be prevented by active or passive immunization with either cell wall components of certain bacteria or toxoid preparations of extracellular toxins. Particularly with toxoid immunization, as in the case of tetanus, immunity appears to be lifelong. With some of the polysaccharide bacterial vaccines there is evidence that active immunization prevents disease in immunodeficient patients.[279]

Evidence that initial titers of circulating antibodies against either type-specific, cross-reacting, or exotoxin antigens of gram-negative bacilli provide some protection against shock and death in bacteremic human infections raises the possibility that even in states of altered immunity it may be possible to enhance host resistance against certain gram-negative infections.[14,191,207] One of the major obstacles to the development of immunizing preparations has been the multiplicity of somatic antigens of gram-negative organisms. The fact that more than 160 serotypes of *E. coli* and 80 serotypes of *K. pneumoniae* have been identified makes a somatic antigen preparation based on those known antigenic types somewhat akin to trying to develop the vaccine for the common cold. On the other hand, it is true that perhaps 10 serotypes of *E. coli* account for 60 percent of bacteremic coliform infections.[280] It has been demonstrated that with *P. aeruginosa*, one of the most common pathogens in the neutropenic host, approximately seven somatic antigens account for 90 percent of the bacteremic infections.[281] Immunization of experimental animals or healthy people with a *Pseudomonas* LPS vaccine has led to some augmentation of circulating antibody levels against these seven LPS antigens.[180] Some evidence exists, from the study of patients with burn injuries, that this vaccine is protective, but definitive double-blind controlled studies are lacking.[282] Other *Pseudomonas* LPS antigens have been used in controlled studies in burn patients and the results have been significantly in favor of immunization.[283] A randomized, prospective study of *Pseudomonas* immunization in cancer patients showed some overall reduction in *Pseudomonas* infections as well as *Pseudomonas*-associated mortality but no significant reduction in bacteremic *P. aeruginosa* infections.[180] An analysis of the results of that study indicated that many immunosuppressed cancer patients failed to show a significant antibody response to vaccine antigens and that in those who did manifest a significant humoral antibody response elevated antibody titers were short-lived. Most of the *P. aeruginosa* infections that were subsequently documented in the vaccinated or control group were associated not only with neutropenia but also with low levels of circulating opsonizing antibodies against the patient's infecting strains. Thus, it appears that immunization alone is not likely to be successful in the prevention of gram-negative bacteremia in markedly immunosuppressed patients, particularly those who are neutropenic. On the other hand, immunization may provide opsonic support for the function of phagocytic cells, and measures other than active immunization, that is, passive immunization, would be more promising, particularly in those neutropenic subjects who receive granulocyte transfusions. Combined immunization and granulocyte transfusion therapy has been shown to be beneficial in animal model systems.[284] Since infused granulocytes are short-lived and most passive immunization is with IgG preparations (Cohn's fraction II) the administration of passive antibody will require new developments such as stable, nonaggregated immunoglobulins that can be given intravenously.

Interest in the so-called core or cross-reactive antigens of the outer cell wall membrane of enteric bacteria stems from the fact that most Enterobacteriaceae share a common core region that this common core region contains an antigen, lipid A, that is responsible for the properties of "endotoxicity." Evidence from human serologic studies and from experimentally produced infections suggests that antibodies directed against core antigens are protective and that such an immunogen would be more versatile than type-specific antigens.[13,96,191,259]

Antibodies directed against the Re and Rc antigenic determinants would appear to have antitoxin activity (endotoxin neutralizing) and possibly activity as opsonins. From the animal studies, however, one would not anticipate a degree of protection as complete as that observed with O antigen immunization. Baumgartner and colleagues have presented evidence from a controlled clinical trial that J5 antiserum produced in human volunteers (similar to the material studied by Ziegler et al.[201]) prevented gram-negative shock and death.[285] In contrast, the use of a single dose of similar product was ineffective in preventing bacteremic gram-negative infections in patients with prolonged neutropenia.[286] Other prophylactic studies now underway have used pooled immune IgG that has been modified for intravenous use.

The possibility that exposure to "avirulent" organisms that share antigens with disease-causing bacteria might be a feasible technique for engendering active immunity has been assessed experimentally and in healthy people. Human volunteers fed live *E. coli* possessing the K-100 capsular antigen develop circulatory antibodies to the apparently identical *H. influenzae* type B antigen.[287] From the viewpoint of active immunization in the altered host such an approach may face the risk of causing active disease secondary to a live immunogen. It has been shown that there are a number of cross-reactions between antigens contained in the licensed (in the United States) pneumococcal polysaccharide vaccines and the capsular or cell wall antigens of *E. coli* and *Klebsiella*. Antecedent polysaccharide administration has been shown to protect against death from experimental *E. coli* and *Klebsiella* infections, and the administration of the purified antigens could have an effect on the incidence of some gram-negative bacillary infections.[288]

REFERENCES

1. Kwaan HM, Weil MH. Differences in the mechanism of shock caused by bacterial infections. Surg Gynecol Obstet. 1969;128:37.
2. Brill NE, Libman E. Pyocaneus bacillaemia. Am J Med Sci. 1899;118:153.
3. Felty AR, Keefer CS. *Bacillus coli* sepsis. Clinical study of 28 cases of bloodstream invasion by colon bacillus. JAMA. 1924;82:1430.
4. Waisbren BA. Bacteremia due to gram-negative bacilli other than the *Salmonella*. A clinical and therapeutic study. Arch Intern Med. 1951;88:467.
5. Rogers DE. The changing pattern of life-threatening microbial disease. N Engl J Med. 1959;261:677
6. Finland M, Jones WF Jr, Barnes MW. Occurrence of serious bacterial infections since introduction of antibacterial agents. JAMA. 1959;170:2188.
7. McCabe WR, Jackson GG. Gram-negative bacteremia. II. Clinical, laboratory and therapeutic observations. Arch Intern Med. 1962;110:856.
8. McGowan JE, Barnes MW, Finland MW. Bacteremia at Boston City Hospital. Occurrence and mortality during 12 selected years (1935–1972) with special reference to hospital-acquired cases. J Infect Dis. 1975;132:316.
9. Armstrong D, Young LS, Meyer RD, et al. Infectious complications of neoplastic disease. Med Clin North Am. 1971;55:729.
10. Leigh DA. Bacteraemia in patients receiving human cadeveric renal transplants. J Clin Pathol. 1971;24:295.
11. Hill RB, Dahrling BE II, Starzl TE, et al. Death after transplantation: An analysis of sixty cases. Am J Med. 1967;42:327.
12. Montgomery JR, Barrett FF, Williams TW Jr. Infectious complications in cardiac transplant patients. Transplant Proc. 1973;5:1239.
13. Winston DJ, Gale RP, Meyer DV, et al. Infectious complications of human bone marrow transplantation. Medicine Baltimore. 1979;58:1.
14. McCabe WR, Kreger BE, Johns M. Type-specific and cross reactive antibodies in gram-negative bacteremia. N Engl J Med. 1972;287:262.
15. Wolff SM, Bennett JV. Gram-negative rod bacteremia, (Editorial). N Engl J Med. 1974;291:733.
16. EORTC Antimicrobial Therapy Project Group. Ceftazidime combined with a short or long course of amikacin for empirical therapy of gram-negative bacteremia in cancer patients with granulocytopenia. N Engl J Med. 1987;317:1692–98.
17. Klastersky J, Glauser MP, Schimpff SC, et al. Prospective randomized comparison of three antibiotic regimens for empirical therapy of suspected bacteremia infection in febrila granulocytopenic patients. Antimicrobial Agents Chemother. 1986;29:263–70.
18. Weinstein MP, Murphy JR, Reller LB, et al. The clinical significance of positive blood culture: Comprehensive analysis of 500 episodes of bacteremia and fungemia in adults. II. Clinical observations, with special reference to factors influencing prognosis. Rev Infect Dis. 1983;6:54.
19. Spengler RF, Geenough WB III, Stolley PD. A descriptive study of nosocomial bacteremias at The Johns Hopkins Hospital, 1968–1974. Johns Hopkins Med J. 1978;142:77.
20. Kreger BE, Craven DE, Carling P, et al. Gram-negative bacteremia. III. Reassessment of etiology, epidemiology, and ecology in 612 patients. Am J Med. 1980;68:332.
21. Singer C, Kaplan M, Armstrong D. Bacteremia and fungemia complicating neoplastic disease. A study of 364 cases. Am J Med. 1977;62:731.
22. McHenry MC, Gavan TL, Hawk WA, et al. Gram-negative bacteremia: variable clinical course and useful prognostic factors. Cleve Clin Q. 1975;42:15.
23. Myerowitz RL, Medeiros AA, O'Brien TF. Recent experience with bacillemia due to gram-negative organisms. J Infect Dis. 1971;124:239.
24. Bryant RE, Hood AF, Hood CE, et al. Factors affecting mortality of gram-negative rod bacteremia. Arch Intern Med. 1971;127:120.
25. DuPont HL, Spink WW. Infections due to gram-negative organisms: An analysis of 860 patients with bacteremia at the University of Minnesota Medical Center, 1958–1966. Medicine Baltimore. 1969;48:307.
26. Altemeier WA, Todd JC, Inge WW. Gram-negative septicemia: A growing threat. Ann Surg. 1967;166:530.
27. Centers for Disease Control. National nosocomial infectious study report, annual summary 1976. February, 1978;1.
28. Centers for Disease Control. Nosocomial infection surveillance, 1984. CDC Surveillance Summary. MMWR. 1986;35:19–29.
29. Young LS. Treatment of infections due to gram-negative bacilli: A perspective of past, present and future. Rev Infect Dis. 1985;7(Suppl 4):572–8.
30. Pollack M, Charache P, Nieman RE, et al. Colonization and antibiotic resistance patterns of gram-negative bacteria in hospitalized patients. Lancet. 1972;2:668
31. Shooter RA, Walter KA, Williams VR, et al. Faecal carriage of *Pseudomonas aeruginosa* in hospital patients. Possible spread from patient to patient. Lancet. 1966;2:1331.
32. Shooter RA, Cooke EM, Gaya H, et al. Food and medicaments as possible sources of hospital strains of *Pseudomonas aeruginosa*. Lancet. 1969;1:1227
33. Buck AC, Cooke EM. The fate of ingested *Pseudomonas aeruginosa* in normal persons. J Med Microbiol. 1969;2:521.
34. Schimpff SC, Young VM, Greene WH, et al. Origin of infection in acute nonlymphocytic leukemia: Significance of hospital acquisition of potential pathogens. Ann Intern Med. 1972;77:707.
35. Young LS. Nosocomial infections in the immunocompromised adult. Am J Med. 1981;70:398–402.
36. Kaijser B. Immunology of *Escherichia coli:* K antigen and its relation to urinary tract infection. J Infect Dis. 1973;127:670.
37. Selden R, Lee S, Wang WL, et al. Nosocomial *Klebsiella* infections. Intestinal colonization as a reservoir. Ann Intern Med. 1971;74:657.
38. Johanson WG, Pierce AK, Sanford JP. Changing pharyngeal bacterial flora of hospitalized patients. Emergency of gram-negative bacilli. N Engl J Med. 1969;281:1137.
39. Schimpff SC, Greene WH, Young VM, et al. *Pseudomonas* septicemia: Incidence, epidemiology, prevention, and therapy in patients with advanced cancer. Eur J Cancer. 1973;9:449.
40. Steinhauer BW, Eickhoff TC, Kislak JW, et al. The *Klebsiella-Enterobacter-Serratia* division: Clinical and epidemiologic characteristics. Ann Intern Med. 1966;65:1180.
41. Burke JP, Ingall D, Klein JO, et al. *Proteus mirabilis* infections in a hospital nursery traced to a human carrier. N Engl J Med. 1971;284:115.
42. Waisbren BA. Gram-negative shock and endotoxin shock. Am J Med. 1964;36:819.
43. Dorff GJ, Geimer NF, Rosenthal DR, et al. *Pseudomonas* speticemia. Arch Intern Med. 1971;128:591.
44. Ketover BP, Young LS, Armstrong D. Septicemia due to *Aeromonas hydrophilia:* Clinical and immunologic aspects. J Infect Dis. 1973;127:284.
45. Davis II WA, Kane JG, Garagusi VF. Human *Aeromonas* infections: A review of the literature and a case report of endocarditis. Medicine (Baltimore). 1978;57:267.
46. Fisher KW, Berger B, Keusch GT. Subepidermal bullae due to *E. coli*. Arch Dermatol. 1974;110:105.
47. Forkner CE, Frei III E, Edgcomb JH, et al. *Pseudomonas* septicemia. Observations on twenty-three cases. Am J Med. 1958;25:877.
48. Gunnar RM, Loeb HS, Winslow EJ, et al. Hemodynamic measurements in bacteremic and septic shock in man. J Infect Dis. 1973;128:287.
49. Hopewell PC, Murray JS. The adult respiratory distress syndrome. Annu Rev Med. 1976;181:343.
50. Rothstein JL, Schreiber H. Synergy between tumor necrosis factor and bacterial products causes hemorrhagic necrosis and lethal shock in normal mice. Proc Natl Acad Sci USA. 1988:85:607–11.
51. Tillotson JR, Lerner AM. Characteristics of nonbacteremic *Pseudomonas* pneumonia. Ann Intern Med. 1968;68:308.
52. Tillotson JR, Lerner AM. Characteristics of pneumonias caused by *Bacillus proteus*. Ann Intern Med. 1968;68:287.
53. Dietzman DE, Fischer GW, Schoenknecht FD. Neonatal *E. coli* septicemia: Bacterial counts in blood. J Pediatr. 1974;85:128.
54. Silverblatt FJ. Host parasite interactions in the rat renal pelvis. A possible role for pili in the pathogenesis of pyelonephritis. J Exp Med. 1974;140: 1696.
55. Svanborg-Eden C, Hausson S, Jodal U, et al. Host–parasite interaction in urinary tract. J Infect Dis. 1988;157:421–6.
56. Roantree RJ, Rantz LA. A study of the relationship of the normal bactericidal activity of human serum to bacterial infection. J Clin Invest. 1960;39:72.
57. Fierer J, Finley J, Braude E. A plaque assay on agar for detection of gram-negative bacilli sensitive to complement. J Immunol. 1972;109:1156.
58. Young LS, Armstrong D. Human immunity to *Pseudomonas aeruginosa*. I. In vitro interaction of bacteria, polymorphonuclear leukocytes, and serum factors. J Infect Dis. 1972;126:257.
59. Rowley O: Endotoxins and bacterial virulence. J Infect Dis. 1971;123:317.
60. Sjostedt S. Pathogenicity of certain serological types of *B. coli*. Their mouse toxicity, hemolytic power, capacity for skin necrosis and resistance to phagocytosis and bactericidal faculties of human serum. Acta Pathol Microbiol Scand. 1946;63(Suppl):148.
61. Drach GH, Reed WP, Williams RC Jr. Antigens common to human and bacterial cells. II. *E. coli* 014. The common Enterobacteriacae antigen, blood groups A and B and *E. coli* 086. J Lab Clin Med. 1972;79:38.
62. Davis CE, Arnold K. Role of meningococcal endotoxin in meningococcal purpura. J Exp Med. 1974;140:159.
63. Miller RM, Garbus J, Hornick RB. Lack of enhanced oxygen consumption by polymorphonuclear leukocytes on phagotycosis of virulent *Salmonella typhi*. Science. 1972;175:1010.
64. Liu PV. Extracellular toxins of *Pseudomonas aeruginosa*. J Infect Dis. 1974;130(Suppl):94.
65. Wretlind B, Wadstrom T. Purification and properties of a protease with

elastase activity from *Pseudomonas aeruginosa*. J Gen Microbiol. 1977;103:319.
66. Young LS, Martin WJ, Meyer RD, et al. Gram-negative rod bacteremia: Microbiologic immunologic, and therapeutic considerations. Ann Intern Med. 1977;86:456.
67. Stevens P, Huang S, Welch WD, et al. Restricted complement activity by *Escherichia coli* with the K 1 capsular serotype. J Immunol. 1978;121:2174.
68. Young LS. Role of antibody in infections due to *Pseudomonas aeruginosa*. J Infect Dis. 1974;130(Suppl):111.
69. Zinner SH, McCabe WR. The effects of IgM and IgG antibody in patients with bacteremia due to gram-negative bacilli. J Infect Dis. 1976;133:37.
70. Bjornson AB, Michael JG. Biological activities of rabbit immunoglobulin M and immunoglobulin G antibodies to *Pseudomonas aeruginosa*. Infect Immun.
71. Hancock REW. Role of porins in outer membrane permeability. J Bacteriol. 1987;169:929–33.
72. Rietschel ETH, Wollenweber HW, Russa R, et al. Concepts of the chemical structure of lipid A. Rev Infect Dis. 1986;6:432–8.
73. Brade H, Brade L, Schade U, et al. Structure, endotoxicity, immunogenicity and antigenicity of bacterial lipopolysaccharides (endotoxins, O-antigens). In: Levin J, Buller HR, tenCate JW, et al., eds. Bacterial Endotoxins: Pathophysiological Effects, Clinical Significance, and Pharmacological Control. New York: Alan R Liss; 1988.
74. Orskov I, Orskov F, Jann E, et al. Serology, chemistry and genetics of O and K antigens of *Escherichia coli*. Bacteriol Rev. 1977;41:667
75. Stevens P, Huang S, Welch W, et al. Restricted complement activation by *E. coli* with the K-1 capsular serotype: A possible role in pathogenicity. *J Immunol*. 1978;121:2714.
76. Kunin CM, Beard MV, Halmagyi NE. Evidence for a common hapten associated with endotoxin fractions of *E. coli* and other Enterobacteriaceae. Proc Soc Exp Biol Med. 1962;111:160.
77. Makela PH, Mayer H. Enterobacterial common antigen. Bacteriol Rev. 1976;40:591.
78. Mannel D, Mayer H. Isolation and chemical characterization of the enterobacterial common antigen. Eur J Biochem. 1978;86:361.
79. Braun V, Bosch V, Klumpp ER, et al. Antigenic determinants of murein lipoprotein and its exposure at the surface of Enterobacteriaceae. Eur J Biochem. 1976;62:555.
80. McCabe WR, Johns M, Genio TD. Common enterobacterial antigen. III. Initial titers and antibody response in bacteremia caused by gram-negative bacilli. Infect Immun. 1973;7:393.
81. Griffiths EK, Yoonessi, Neter E. Antibody response to enterobacterial lipoprotein of patients with varied infections due to Enterobacteriacaea. Proc Soc Exp Biol Med. 1977;154:246.
82. Nikaido A, Nikaido K, Subbaiah TV, et al. Rough mutants of *Salmonella typhimurium*. Nature. 1964;201:1298.
83. Kasper DL, Seiler MW. Immunochemical characterization of the outer membrane complex of *Bacteroides fragilis* subspecies *fragilis*. J Infect Dis. 1975;132:440.
84. Meadow P. Wall and membrane structures in the genus *Pseudomonas*. In: Clarke PH, Richmond MH, eds. Genetics and biochemistry of Pseudomonas. London: John Wiley; 1975:6.
85. Golenbock DT, Will JA, Ratez CRH, et al. Lipid X ameliorates pulmonary hypertension and protects sheep from death due to endotoxin. Infect Immun. 1987;55:2471–6.
86. van der Meer JWM, Barza M, Wolff SM, et al. A low dose of recombinant interleukin 1 protects granulocytopenic mice from lethal gram-negative infection. Proc Natl Acad Sci USA. 1988;85:1620–3.
87. Wolff S. Biological effects of bacterial endotoxins in man. J Infect Dis. 1973;128(Suppl):259.
88. Michie HR, Manogue KR, Spriggs DR, et al. Detection of circulating tumor necrosis factor after endotoxin administration. N Engl J Med. 1988;318:1481–6.
89. Corrigan JJ, Walker LR, May N. Changes in the blood coagulation system associated with septicemia. N Engl J Med. 1968;279–851.
90. McKay DG, Shapiro SS. Alterations in the blood coagulation system induced by bacterial endotoxin. I. In vivo (generalized Shwartzman reaction). J Exp Med. 1958;107:353.
91. Kimball HR, Melmon KL, Wolff SM. Endotoxin-induced kinin production in man. Proc Soc Exp Biol Med. 1972;139:1078.
92. Nies AS, Forsyth RP, Williams HE, et al. Contribution of kinins to endotoxin shock in unanesthetized rhesus monkeys. Circ Res. 1968;22:155.
93. Fearon DT, Ruddy S, Schur PH, et al. Activation of the properdin pathway of complement in patients with gram-negative bacteremia. N Engl J Med. 1975;292:937.
94. Ulevitch RJ, Cochran CG, Henson PM, et al. Mediation systems in bacterial lipopolysaccharide-induced hypotension and disseminated intravascular coagulation. I. The role of complement. J Exp Med. 1975;142:1570.
95. Ziegler EJ, Douglas H, Sherman JE, et al. Treatment of *E. coli* and *Klebsiella* bacteremia in agranulocytic animals with antiserum to a UDP-GAL epimerase-deficient mutant. J Immunol. 1973;111:433.
96. Young LS, Ingram J, Stevens P. Functional role of antibody against core glycolipid of Enterobacteriaceae. J Clin Invest. 1975;56:850.
97. Tracey KJ, Wei H, Manogue KR, et al. Cachectin/tumor necrosis factor induces cachexia, anemia, and inflammation. J Exp Med. 1988;167:1211–27.
98. Ginsberg I. Mechanisms of cell and tissue injury induced by group A streptococci: Relation to poststreptococcal sequelae. J Infect Dis. 1972;126:294.
99. Pollack M. Significance of circulating capsular antigen in *Klebsiella* infections. Infect Immun. 1976;13:1543.
100. Dennis EW, Saigh AS. Precipitable typhoid somatic antigen in the serum of typhoid fever patients. Science. 1945;102:208
101. Kass E, Porter P, McGill M, et al. Clinical and experimental observations on the significance of endotoxemia. J Infect Dis. 1973;128(Suppl):299.
102. Levin J, Poore TE, Zauber NP, et al. Detection of endotoxin in the blood of patients with sepsis due to gram-negative bacteria. N Engl J Med. 1970;283:1313.
103. Stumacher RJ, Kovnat MJ, McCabe WR. Limitations of the usefulness of the limulus assay for endotoxin. N Engl J Med. 1973;288:1261.
104. Elin RJ, Hosseini J. Clinical utility of the limulus amebocyte updated test. In: Watson SW, Levin J, Novitsky TJ, eds. Detection of Bacterial Endotoxins with Limulus Amebocyte Lysate Test. New York: Alan R Liss; 1985:307–24.
105. Tesh VL, Vukajlovich SW, Morrison DC. Endotoxin interactions with serum proteins—relationship to biological activity. In: Levin J, Buller HR, tenCate JW, et al., eds. Bacterial Endotoxins: Pathophysiological Effects, Clinical Significance, and Pharmacological Control. New York: Alan R Liss, 1988.
106. Johnson KJ, Ward PA, Goralnick S, et al. Isolation from human serum of an inactivator of bacterial lipopolysaccharide. Am J Pathol. 1977;88:559.
107. Koster F, Levin J, Walter L, et al. Hemolytic uremic syndrome after shigellosis: Relation to endotoxemia and circulating immune complexes. N Engl J Med. 1978;298:927.
108. Young LS. Opsonizing antibodies, host factors, and the limulus assay for endotoxin. Infect Immun. 1975;12:88.
109. Young LS. The complex challenge of bacteremia and endotoxemia. In: Levin J, Buller HR, tenCate JW, et al., eds. Bacterial Endotoxins: Pathophysiological Effects, Clinical Significance, and Pharmacological Control. New York: Alan R Liss; 1988:209–12.
110. Postel J, Schloerb PR, Furtado D. Pathophysiologic alterations during bacterial infusions for the study of bacteremic shock. Surg Gynecol Obstet. 1975;141:683.
111. Muszynski Z. Enzymatic and toxinogenic activity of culture filtrates of high and low virulent strains of *Pseudomonas aeruginosa* on mice. Pathol Microbiol. 1973;39:135.
112. Wretlind B, Mollby R, Wadstrom T. Separation of two hemolysins from *Aeromonas hydrophila* by isoelectric focusing. Infect Immun. 1971;4:503.
113. Pollack M, Taylor NS, Callahan LT III. Exotoxin production by clinical isolates of *Pseudomonas aeruginosa*. Infect Immun. 1977;15:776.
114. Middlebrook JL, Dorland RB. Response of cultured mammalian cells to exotoxins of *Pseudomonas aeruginosa* and *Corynebacterium diphtheriae:* Differential cytotoxicity. Can J Microbiol. 1977;23:183.
115. Iglewski BH, Kabat D. NAD-dependent inhibition of protein synthesis by *Pseudomonas aeruginosa* toxin. Proc Natl Acad Sci USA. 1975;72:2284
116. Pavlovskis OR, Pollack M, Callahan LT III, et al. Passive protection by antitoxin in experimental *Pseudomonas aeruginosa* burn infections. Infect Immun. 1977;18:596.
117. Young LS. Role of exotoxins in the pathogenesis of *Pseudomonas aeruginosa* infections. J Infect Dis. 1980;142:626.
118. McCabe WR. Serum complement levels in bacteremia due to gram-negative organisms. N Engl J Med. 1973;288:21.
119. Schreiber AD, Austen KF. Interrelationships of the fibrinolytic, coagulation, kinin generating, and complement systems. Semin Hematol. 1973;6:4.
120. Jacob HS. Granulocyte-complement interaction. A beneficial antimicrobial mechanism that can cause disease. Arch Intern Med. 1978;138:461.
121. McCabe WR. Gram-negative bacteremia. Adv Intern Med. 1974;19:135.
122. Greisman SE, Hornick RB. Comparative pyrogenic reactivity of rabbit and man to bacterial endotoxin. Proc Soc Exp Biol Med. 1969;131:1154.
123. Sanarelli G: De la pathogenié du choléra (Neuvième mémoirè) Le choléra expérimental. Ann Inst Pasteur Lille. 1924;38:11.
124. Shwartzman G, Gerber LE. Hemorrhagic manifestations of bacterial and virus infections: Experimental studies and pathological interpretations. Ann NY Acad Sci. 1948;49:627.
125. McKay DG, Jewett JF, Reid DE. Endotoxin shock and the general Shwartzman reaction in pregnancy. Am J Obstet Gynecol. 1959;78:546.
126. Dinarello CA, Mier JW. Current Concept: Lymphokines. N Engl J Med. 1987;317:940–5.
127. Morrison DC, Ryan JL. Endotoxins and disease mechanisms. Annu Rev Med. 1987;38:417–32.
128. Beutler B, Milsark IW, Cerami A. Passive immunization with cachectin/tumor necrosis factor (TNF) protects mice from the lethal effects of endotoxin. Nature. 1985;229:869–71.
129. Tracey KJ, Lowry SF, Cerami A. Cachectin: A hormone that triggers acute shock and chronic cachexia. J Infect Dis. 1988;157:413–20.
130. Tracey KJ, Lowry SF, Cerami A. Cachectin/TNF mediates the pathophysiological effects of bacterial endotoxin/lipopolysaccharide (LPS). In: Levin J, Buller HR, tenCate JW, et al., eds. Bacterial Endotoxins: Pathophysiological Effects, Clinical Significance, and Pharmacological Control. New York: Alan R Liss; 1988.
131. Beutler B, Krochin N, Milsark IW, et al. Control of cachectin (tumor necrosis factor) synthesis: Mechanisms of endotoxin resistance. Science. 1986;232:977–80.
132. Waage A, Halstensen A, Espevik T. Association between tumor necrosis factor in serum and fatal outcome in patients with meningococcal disease. Lancet. 1987;1:355–7.

133. Blick M, Sherwin SA, Rosenblum M, et al. Phase I study of recombinant tumor necrosis factor in cancer patients. Cancer Res. 1987;47:2986–9.
134. Mathison JC, Wolfson E, Ulevitch RJ. Participation of tumor necrosis factor in the mediation of gram-negative bacterial lipopolysaccharide-induced injury in rabbits. J Clin Invest. 1988;81:1925–37.
135. Remick DG, Kunkel RG, Larrick JW, et al. Acute in vivo effects of human recombinant tumor necrosis factor. Lab Invest. 1987;56:583–90.
136. Stephens KE, Ishizaka A, Larrick JW, et al. Tumor necrosis factor causes increased pulmonary permeability and edema. Am Rev Respir Dis. 1988;137:1364–70.
137. Tracey KJ, Beutler B, Lowry SF, et al. Shock and tissue injury induced by recombinant human cachectin. Science. 1986;234:470–4.
138. Tracey KJ, Fong Y, Hesse DG, et al. Anti-cachectin/TNF monoclonal antibodies prevent septic shock during lethal bacteremia. Nature. 1987;330:662–4.
139. Nawroth PP, Bank I, Handley D, et al. Tumor necrosis factor/cachectin interacts with endothelial cell receptors to induce release of interleukin-1. J Exp Med. 1986;163:1363–75.
140. Dinarello CA, Cannon JG, Solff SM, et al. Tumor necrosis factor (cachectin) is an endogenous pyrogen and induces production on interleukin 1. J Exp Med. 1986;163:1433–50.
141. Kettelhut IC, Fiers W, Goldberg AL. The toxic effects of tumor necrosis factor in vivo and their preventive by cyclooxygenase inhibitors. Proc Natl Acad Sci USA. 1987;84:4273–7.
142. Okusawa S, Gelfand JA, Ikejima T, et al. Interleukin 1 induces shock-like state in rabbits: Synergism with tumor necrosis factor and the effect of cyclooxygenase inhibition. J Clin Invest. 1988;81:1162–72.
143. Talmadge JE, Bowersox O, Tribble H, et al. Toxicity of tumor necrosis factor is synergistic with gamma-interferon and can be reduced with cyclooxygenase inhibitors. Am J Pathol. 1987;128:410–25.
144. Billiau A. Gamma-interferon: The match that lights the fire? Immunol Today. 1988;9:37–40.
145. Scuderi P, Sterling KE, Lam KS, et al. Raised serum levels of tumor necrosis factor in parasitic infections. Lancet. 1986;2:1364–5.
146. Ulich TR, Kaizhi G, del Castillo J. Rapid communication. Endotoxin-induced cytokine gene expression *in vivo*. I. Expression of tumor necrosis factor mRNA in visceral organs under physiologic conditions and during endotoxemia. Am J Pathol. 1989;134:11–14.
147. Frank MM, May JE, Kane MA. Contributions of the classical alternative complement pathways to the biological effects of endotoxin. J Infect Dis. 1973;128(Suppl):176.
148. Ulevitch RJ, Cochrane CG. Role of complement in lethal bacterial lipopolysaccharide-induced hypotensive and coagulative changes. Infect Immun. 1978;20:204.
149. Corrigan JJ. Heparin therapy in bacterial septicemia. J Pediatr. 1977;91:695.
150. Butler T, Bell WR, Levin J, et al. Studies of blood coagulation, bacteremia, endotoxemia. Arch Intern Med. 1978;138:407.
151. Rothberger H, Zimmerman TS, Spiegelberg HL, et al. Leukocyte procoagulant activity: Enhancement of production in vitro by IgG and antigen–antibody complexes. J Clin Invest. 1977;59:549.
152. Egbring R, Schmidt W, Fuchs G, et al. Demonstration of granulocytic proteases in plasma of patients with acute leukemia and septicemia with coagulation defects. Blood. 1977;49:219.
153. Brown DL, Lachmann PJ. The behaviour of complement and platelets in lethal endotoxin shock in rabbits. Int Arch Allergy. 1973;45:193.
154. Miller RL, Reichgott MJ, Melmon KL. Biochemical mechanisms of generation of bradykinin by endotoxin. J Infect Dis. 1973;128(Suppl):144.
155. Mason JW, Kleeberg U, Dolan P, et al. Plasma kallikrein and Hageman factor in gram-negative bacteremia. Ann Intern Med. 1970;73–545.
156. Robinson JA, Klodnycky ML, Loeb HS, et al. Endotoxin, prekallikrein, complement and systemic vascular resistance: Sequential measurement in man. Am J Med. 1975;59:61.
157. O'Donnell TF, Clowes GHA, Talamo RC, et al. Kinin activation in the blood of patients with sepsis. Surg Gynecol Obstet. 1976;143:539.
158. Colman RW, Edelman R, Scott CF, et al. Plasma kallikrein activation and inhibition during typhoid fever. J Clin Invest. 1978;61:287.
159. Jacobs ER, Bone RC, Wilson JB, et al. Naloxone blockage of endorphins in canine endotoxin shock. Microcirculation. 1982;2:19.
160. Doebber TW, Wu MS, Robbins JC, et al. Platelet activating factor (PAF) involvement in endotoxin-induced hypotension in rats. Biochem Biophys Res Commun. 1985;127:799–808.
161. Gallin JI, Kaye D, O'Leary WM. Serum lipids in infection. N Engl J Med. 1969;281:1081.
162. Reines HD, Halushka PV, Cook JA. Plasma thromboxane concentrations are raised in patients dying with septic. Lancet. 1982;2:174.
163. McGovern VJ. The pathology of shock. In: Sommers S, ed. Pathology Annual. New York: Appleton-Century-Crofts; 1971:279.
164. Waisbren BA, Brown I. A factor in the serum of patients with persisting infection that inhibits the bactericidal activity of normal serum against the organism that is causing the infection. J Immunol. 1966;97:431.
165. Bjornboe M, Prytz H, Orskov F. Antibodies to intestinal microbes in serum of patients with cirrhosis of the liver. Lancet. 1972;1:58.
166. Howard CJ, Glynn AA. The virulence for mice of strains of *Escherichia coli* related to the effects of K antigens on their resistance to phagocytosis and killing by complement. Immunology. 1971;20:767.
167. Vosti KL, Randall E. Sensitivity of serologically classified strains of *Escherichia coli* of human origin to the serum bactericidal system. Am J Med Sci. 1970;259:114.
168. Kierszenbau F, Weinman D. Antibody-independent activation of the alternative complement pathway in human serum by parasitic cells. Immunology. 1977;32:245.
169. Agnello V. Complement deficiency states. Medicine (Baltimore). 1978;57:1.
170. Feinstein PA, Kaplan SR. The alternative pathway of complement activation in the neonate. Pediatr Res. 1975;9:803.
171. Johnston RB, Newman MS, Struth AG. An abnormality of the alternate pathway of complement activation in sickle-cell disease. N Engl J Med. 1973;288:803.
172. Jasin HE, Orozco JH, Ziff M. Serum heat-labile opsonins in systemic lupus erythematosus. J Clin Invest. 1974;53:343.
173. Michael JG, Rosen FS. Association of natural antibodies to gram-negative bacteremia with the gamma macroglobulins. J Exp Med. 1963;118:619.
174. Robbins JB, Myerowitz RL, Whisnant JK, et al. Enteric bacteria cross-reactive with *Neisseria meningitidis* groups A and C and *Diplococcus pneumoniae* types I and III. Infect Immun. 1972;6:651.
175. Schneerson R, Bradshaw M, Whisnant JK, et al. An *Escherichia coli* antigen cross reactive with the capsular polysaccharide of *Hemophilus influenzae* type b. J Immunol. 1972;108:1551.
176. Kasper DL, Winkelhake JL, Zollinger WD, et al. Immunochemical similarity between polysaccharide antigens of *Escherichia coli* 07:K1:NM and group B. *Neisseria meningitidis*. J Immunol. 1973;110:262.
177. Glode MP, Robbins JB, Liu TY, et al. Cross antigenicity and immunogeneicity between capsular polysaccharides of Group C *Neisseria* meningitidis and *Escherichia coli* K 92. J Infect Dis. 1977;135:94.
178. Robbins JB, Gotschlich EC, Liu TY, et al. Bacterial antigens cross-reactive with the capsular polysaccharides of *Hemophilus influenzae* type b, *Neisseria meningitidis* groups A and C, *Diplococcus pneumoniae* types I and III. In: Robbins JB, Horton RE, Krause RM, eds. Proceedings of the Symposium on New Approaches for Inducing Natural Immunity to Pyogenic Organisms. Washington, DC: Department of Health, Education and Welfare; Publication No (NIH) 74–553, 1973:45.
179. Goldschneider I, Gotschlich EC, Artenstein MS. Human immunity to the meningococcus. I. The role of humoral antibodies. J Exp Med. 1969;129:1307.
180. Young LS, Meyer RD, Armstrong D. *Pseudomonas aeruginosa* vaccine in cancer patients. Ann Intern Med. 1973;79:518.
181. Harvath L, Andersen BR. Evaluation of type-specific and nontype-specific pseudomonas vaccine for treatment of pseudomonas sepsis during granulocytopenia. Infect Immun. 1976;13:1139.
182. Kaijser B, Ahlstedt S. Protective capacity of antibodies against *Escherichia coli* O and K antigens. Infect Immun. 1977;17:286.
183. Ruddy S, Gigli I, Austen KF. The complement system of man. N Engl J Med. 1972;287:489.
184. Dossett JH, Williams RC, Quie PG. Studies on interaction of bacteria, serum factors, and polymorphonuclear leukocytes in mothers and newborns. Pediatrics. 1969;44:49.
185. Ehlenberger AG, Nussenzweig V. The role of membrane reception for C_3B and C_3D in phagocytosis. J Exp Med. 1977;145:357.
186. Gotze O, Muller-Eberhard JH. The alternative pathway of complement activation. In: Kunkeland HJ, Dixon FJ, eds. Advances in Immunology. v. 24. New York: Academic Press; 1976:1.
187. Jasin HE. Human heat labile opsonins: Evidence for their mediation via the alternate pathway of complement activation. J Immunol. 1972;109:26.
188. Guckian JC, Christensen WP, Fine DP. Evidence for quantitative variability of bacterial opsonic requirements. Infect Immun. 1978;19:882.
189. Weinstein RJ, Young LS. Neutrophil function in gram-negative rod bacteremia: The interaction between phagocytic cells, infecting organisms, and humoral factors. J Clin Invest. 1976;58:190.
190. Young LS. Role of antibody in infections due to *Pseudomonas aeruginosa*. J Infect Dis. 1974;130(Suppl):111.
191. Zinner SH, McCabe WR. The effects of IgM and IgG antibody in patients with bacteremia due to gram-negative bacilli. J Infect Dis. 1976;133:37.
192. Bjornson AB, Michael JG. Biological activities of rabbit immunoglobulin M and immunoglobulin G antibodies to *Pseudomonas aeruginosa*. Infect Immun. 1970;2:453.
193. Inoue K. Immune bacteriolytic and bactericidal reactions. In: Kwapinski JBG, ed. Research in Immunochemistry and Immunobiology. Baltimore: University Park Press; 1972:177.
194. Young LS. Gram-negative septicemia: Antibody deficiency and specific protection. In: Bayer-Symposium VIII. The Pathogenesis of Bacterial Infections. Berlin: Springer-Verlag; 1985:138–45.
195. Braude A, Douglas H, Davis C. Treatment and prevention of intravascular coagulation with antiserum to endotoxin. J Infect Dis. 1973;128(Suppl):157.
196. Ziegler EJ, Douglas H, Braude A. Human antiserum for prevention of the local Shwartzman reaction and death from bacterial lipopolysaccharides. J Clin Invest. 1973;52:3236.
197. McCabe WR. Immunization with R mutants of *S. minnesota*. I. Protection against challenge with heterologous gram-negative bacilli. J Immunol. 1972;108:601.
198. McCabe WR. Immunoprophylaxis of gram-negative bacillary infections. Annu Rev Med. 1976;27:335.
199. Young LS. Immunoprophylaxis and serotherapy of bacterial infections. Am J Med. 1984;76:664–71.

200. Teng NH, Kaplan HS, Hebert JM, et al. Protection against gram-negative bacteremia and endotoxemia with human monoclonal IgM antibodies. Proc Natl Acad Sci USA. 1985;82:1790–4.
201. Ziegler EJ, McCutchan JA, Fierer J, et al. Treatment of gram-negative bacteremia and shock with human antiserum to a mutant *Escherichia coli*. N Engl J Med. 1982;307:1225.
202. Ng AK, Chen CL, Chang CM, et al. Relationship of structure to function in bacterial endotoxins: Serologically cross-reactive components and their effect on protection of mice against some gram-negative infections. J Gen Microbiol. 1976;94:107.
203. Ziegler EJ. Protective antibody to endotoxin core: The emperor's new clothes? J Infect Dis. 1988;158:286–90.
204. Bruins SC, Stumacher R, Johns MA, et al. Immunization with R mutants of *Salmonella minnesota*. III. Comparison of the protective effect of immunization with lipid A and the Re mutant. Infect Immun. 1977;17:16.
205. McCabe WR, DeMaria A Jr, Berberich H, et al. Immunization with rough mutants of *Salmonella minnesota:* Protective activity of IgM and IgG antibody to the R595 (Re chemotype) mutant. J Infect Dis. 1988;158:291–300.
206. Pollack M, Taylor NS. Serum antibody to *Pseudomonas aeruginosa* exotoxin measured by a passive hemagglutination assay. J Clin Microbiol. 1977;6:58
207. Pollack M, Young LS. Protective activity of antibodies to exotoxin A and lipopolysaccharide at onset of *Pseudomonas aeruginosa* septicemia in man. J Clin Invest. 1979;63:276.
208. Freudenberg MA, Bog-Hansen TC, Back U. Interaction of lipopolysaccharides with plasma high density lipoprotein. Infect Immun. 1980;28:373–80.
209. Berger D, Beger HG. Quantification of the endotoxin-binding capacity of human transferrin. In: Levin J, Buller HR, tenCate JW, et al., eds. Bacterial Endotoxins: Pathophysiological Effects, Clinical Significance, and Pharmacological Control. New York: Alan R Liss; 1988.
210. Ulevitch RJ, Tobias PS. Interactions of bacterial lipopolysaccharides with serum proteins. In: Levin J, Buller HR, tenCate JW, et al., eds. Bacterial Endotoxins: Pathophysiological Effects, Clinical Significance, and Pharmacological Control. New York: Alan R Liss; 1988:309–18.
211. Quie PG, Cates KL. Clinical conditions associated with defective polymorphonuclear leukocyte chemotaxis. Am J Pathol. 1977;88:711.
212. Warden GD, Mason AD, Pruitt BA. Evaluation of leukocyte chemotaxis in vitro in thermally injured patients. J Clin Invest. 1974;54:1001.
213. Washington II JA. Blood cultures: Principles and techniques. Mayo Clin Proc. 1975;50:91.
214. Anderson ET, Young LS, Hewitt WL. Antimicrobial synergism in the therapy of gram-negative bacteremia. Chemotherapy. 1978;24:45.
215. Freid MA, Vosti KL. Importance of underlying disease in patients with gram-negative bacteremia. Arch Intern Med. 1968;121:418.
216. Young LS. Combination or single drug therapy for gram-negative sepsis. In: Remington JS, Swartz MN, eds. Curr Clin Topics Infect Dis. 1982;3:177.
217. Young LS. Empirical antimicrobial therapy in the neutropenic host. N Engl J Med. 1986;315:580.
218. Pizzo PA, Hawthorn JW, Hiemenz J, et al. A randomized trial comparing ceftazidime alone with combination antibiotic therapy in cancer patients with fever and neutropenia. N Engl J Med. 1986;315:552–8.
219. Schimpff S, Satterlee W, Young VM, et al. Therapy with carbenicillin and gentamicin in febrile cancer patients. N Engl J Med. 1971;284:1061.
220. Lumish RM, Norden CW. Therapy of neutropenic rats infected with *Pseudomonas aeruginosa*. J Infect Dis. 1976;133:538.
221. Andriole VT. Synergy of carbenicillin and gentamicin in experimental infection with pseudomonas. J Infect Dis. 1971;124(Suppl):460.
222. Robson HG. Synergistic activity of carbenicillin and gentamicin in experimental pseudomonas bacteremia in neutropenic rats. Antimicrob Agents chemother. 1976;10:646.
223. Klastersky J, Meunier-Carpentier F, Prevost JM. Significance of antimicrobial synergism for the outcome of gram-negative sepsis. Am J Med Sci. 1977;273:157.
224. Sculier JP, Klastersky J. Significance of serum bactericidal activity in gram-negative bacillary bacteremia in patients with and without granulocytopenia. Am J Med. 1984;76:429–35.
225. Feld R, Valdivieso M, Bodey GP, et al. A comparative trial of sisomicin therapy by intermittent versus continuous infusion. Am J Med Sci. 1977;274:179.
226. Price KE, DeFuria MD, Pursiano TA. Amikacin, an aminoglycoside with marked activity against antibiotic-resistant clinical isolates. J Infect Dis. 1976;134(Suppl):249.
227. DeJongh CA, Wade JC, Schimpff SC, et al. Empiric antibiotic therapy for suspected infection in granulocytopenic cancer patients. Am J Med. 1982;73:89.
228. DeJongh CA, Joshi JH, Newman KA, et al. Antibiotic synergism and response in gram-negative bacteremia in granulocytopenic cancer patients. Am J Med. 1986;80:96–100.
229. International Antimicrobial Therapy Project Group of the European Organization for Research and Treatment of Cancer. Combination of amikacin and carbenicillin with or without cefazolin as empirical treatment of febrile neutropenic patients. J Clin Oncol. 1983;1:597–603.
230. Kaye D, Levison ME, Labovitz ED. The unpredictability of serum concentrations of gentamicin. Pharmacolinetics of gentamicin in patients with normal and abnormal renal function. J Infect Dis. 1974;130:150.
231. Anderson ET, Young LS, Hewitt WL. Simultaneous antibiotic levels in "breakthrough" gram-negative rod bacteremia. Am J Med. 1976;61:493.
232. Smith CR, Maxwell RR, Edwards CQ, et al. Nephrotoxicity induced by gentamincin and amikacin. Johns Hopkins Med. J. 1978;142:85.
233. Shine K, Silver M, Young LS, et al. Aspects of the management of shock. Ann Intern Med. 1980;93:723–34.
234. Winslow EJ, Loeb HS, Pahimtoola SH, et al. Hemodynamic studies and results of therapy in 50 patients with bacteremic shock. Am J Med. 1973;54:421.
235. Weitzman S, Berger S. Clinical trial design in studies of corticosteroids for bacterial infections. Ann Intern Med. 1974;81:36.
236. Klastersky J, Cappel R, Debusscher L. Effectiveness of betamethasone in management of severe infections. N Engl J Med. 1971;284:1248.
237. Schumer W. Steroids in the treatment of clinical septic shock. Ann Surg. 1976;184:333.
238. Hotfman SL, Punjabi NH, Kumala S, et al. Reduction of mortality in chloramphenicol-treated severe typhoid fever by high-dose dexamethasone. N Engl J Med. 1981;310:456–7.
239. Sprung CL, Caralis PV, Marcial EH, et al. The effects of high-dose corticosteroids in patients with septic shock: A prospective controlled study. N Engl J Med. 1984;311:1137–43.
240. Veterans Administration Systemic Sepsis Cooperative Study Group. Effect of high dose glucocorticoid therapy on mortality in patients with clinical signs of systemic sepsis. N Engl J Med. 1987;317:659–65.
241. Bone RC, Fisher CJ, Clemmer TP, et al. A controlled clinical trial of high-dose methylprednisolone in the treatment of severe sepsis and septic shock. N Engl J Med. 1987;317:653–8.
242. Bernard GR, Luce JM, Sprungs CL, et al. High-dose corticosteroids in patients with the adult respiratory distress syndrome. N Engl J Med. 1987;317:1565–70.
243. Luce JM, Montgomery AB, Marks JD, et al. Ineffectiveness of high-dose methylprednisolone in preventing parenchymal lung injury and improving mortality in patients with septic shock. Am Rev Respir Dis. 1988;138:62–8.
244. Corrigan JJ Jr, Ray WL, May N. Change in blood coagulation system associated with septicemia. N Engl J Med. 1968;279:851.
245. Corrigan JC, Kiernat JF. Effect of heparin in experimental gram-negative septicemia. J Infect Dis. 1975;131:138.
246. Higby DJ, Yates JW, Henderson ES. Filtration leukopheresis for granulocyte transfusion therapy. N Engl J Med. 1975;292:761.
247. Herzig RH, Herzig GP, Graw RG Jr, et al. Successful granulocyte transfusion therapy for gram-negative septicemia. N Engl J Med. 1977;296:701.
248. Alavi JB, Root RK, Djerassi I, et al. A randomized clinical trial of granulocyte transfusions for infection in acute leukemia. N Engl J Med. 1977;296:706.
249. Vogler WR, Winston EF. A controlled study of the efficacy of granulocyte transfusions in patients with neutropenia. Am J Med. 1977;63:548.
250. Winston DJ, Ho WG, Gale RP. Therapeutic granulocyte transfusions for documented infections. Ann Intern Med. 1982;97:509.
251. Young LS. The role of granulocytes transfusions in treating and preventing infection. Cancer Treat Rep. 1983;67:109.
252. Faden AI, Holaday JW. Experimental endotoxin shock. The pathophysiologic function of endorphins and treatment with opiate antagonists. J Infect Dis. 1980;142:229.
253. Faden AI, Holaday JW. Opiate antagonists: A role in the treatment of hypovolemic shock. Science. 1979;205:317.
254. Peters WP, Johnson MW, Friedman PA, et al. Pressor effect of naloxone in septic shock. Lancet. 1981;1:529.
255. DeMaria A, Craven DE, Heffernan JJ, et al. Naloxone versus placebo in treatment of septic shock. Lancet. 1985;1:1363–5.
256. Sullivan GW, Carper HT, Novick WJ, et al. Inhibition of the inflammatory action of interleukin-1 and tumor necrosis factor (alpha) on neutrophil function by pentoxifylline. Infect Immun. 1988;56:1722–9.
257. Feingold DS, Oski F. *Pseudomonas* infection. Treatment with immune human plasma. Arch Intern Med. 1965;116:326.
258. Jones CE, Alexander JW, Fisher MW. Clinical evaluation of *Pseudomonas* hyperimmune globulin. J Surg Res. 1973;14:87.
259. DeMaria A Jr, Johns MA, Berberich H, et al. Immunization with rough mutants of *Salmonella minnesota:* Initial studies in human subjects. J Infect Dis. 1988;158:301–11.
260. Calandra T, Glauser MP, Schellekens J, et al. Treatment of gram-negative septic shock with human IgG antibody to *Escherichia coli* J5: A prospective, double-blind, randomized trial. J Infect Dis. 1988;158:312–9.
261. Young LS, Gascon R, Alam Soosan, et al. Monoclonal antibodies for treatment of gram-negative infections. Rev Inf Dis. In press.
262. Harkonen S, Scannon P, Mischak RP, et al. Phase I study of a murine monoclonal anti-lipid A antibody in bacteremic and nonbacteremic patients. Antimicrob Agents Chemother. 1988;32:710–6.
263. Shenep JL, Flynn PM, Barrett FF, et al. Serial quantitation of endotoxemia and bacteremia during therapy for gram-negative bacterial sepsis. J Infect Dis. 1988;157:565–8.
264. Pollack M, Ranbitschek, Larrick J. Human monoclonal antibodies that recognize conserved epitopes in the core-lipid A region of lipopolysaccharides. J Clin Invest. 1987;79:1421–30.
265. Lindberg RB, Moncrief JA, Mason AD Jr. Control of experimental and clinical burn wound sepsis by topical application of sulfamylon compounds. Ann NY Acad Sci. 1968;50:950.

266. Greenfield S, Teres D, Bushnell LS, et al. Prevention of gram-negative bacillary pneumonia using aerosol polymixin as prophylaxis. J Clin Invest. 1973;52:2935.
267. Feeley TW, du Moulin GC, Hedley-Whyte J, et al. Aerosol polymixin and pneumonia. N Engl J Med. 1975;293:471.
268. Storring RA, McElwain TJ, Jameson B, et al. Oral non-absorbed antibiotics prevent infection in acute non-lymphoblastic leukaemia. Lancet. 1977;2:837.
269. Schimpff SC, Greene WH, Young VM, et al. Infection prevention in acute nonlymphocytic leukemia. Laminar air flow room reverse isolation with oral, nonabsorbable antibiotics prophylaxis. Ann Intern Med. 1975;82:351.
270. Young LS. Trimethorprim-sulfamethoxazole and bacterial infections during leukemic therapy. Ann Intern Med 1981;95:508.
271. Young LS. Antimicrobial prophylaxis against infection in neutropenic patients. J Infect Dis. 1983;147:611.
272. Karp JE, Merz WG, Hendricksen C, et al. Oral norfloxacin for prevention of gram-negative bacterial infections in patients with acute leukemia and granulocytopenia: A randomized, double-blind, placebo-controlled trial. Ann Intern Med. 1987;106:1–7.
273. Dekker AW, Rozenberg-Arska M, Verhoef J. Infection prophylaxis in acute leukemia: A comparison of ciprofloxacin with trimethoprim-sulfamethoxazole and colistin. Ann Intern Med. 1987;106:7–12.
274. Clift RA, Sanders JE, Thomas ED, et al. Granulocyte transfusions for the prevention of infection in patients receiving bone marrow transplants. N Engl J Med. 1978;298:1052.
275. Strauss RG, Connett JE, Gale RP, et al. A controlled trial of prophylactic granulocyte transfusions during initial induction of chemotherapy for acute myelogenous leukemia. N Engl J Med. 1981;305:597.
276. Winston DJ, Ho WG, Young LS, et al. Prophylactic granulocyte transfusions during human bone marrow transplantation. Am J Med. 1980;68:893.
277. Schiffer CA, Aisner J, Daly A, et al. Alloimmunization following prophylactic granulocyte transfusion. Blood. 1979;54:766.
278. Keusch GT, Ambinder EP, Kovacs I, et al. Role of opsonins in clinical response to granulocyte transfusion in granulocytopenic patients. Am J Med. 1982;73:552.
179. Ammann AJ, Addiego J, Wara D, et al. Polyvalent pneumococcal polysaccharide immunization of patients with sickle cell anemia and patient with splenectomy. N Engl J Med. 1977;297:897.
280. Orskov F, Orskov I. *Escherichia coli* O:H serotypes isolated from human blood. Acta Pathol Microbiol Scand LB 1975;83:595.
281. Moody MR, Young VM, Kenton DM, et al. *Pseudomonas aeruginosa* in a center for cancer research. I. Distribution of intraspecies types from human and environmental sources. J Infect Dis. 1972;125:95.
282. Alexander JW, Fisher MW, MacMillan BG. Immunological control of *Pseudomonas* infection in burn patients. A clinical evaluation. Arch Surg. 1971;102:31.
283. Jones RJ, Roe EA, Gupta JL. Low mortality in burned patients in a *Pseudomonas* vaccine trial. Lancet. 1978;2:401.
284. Harvath L, Andersen B, Zander AR, et al. Combined preimmunization and granulocyte transfusion therapy for treatment of *Pseudomonas* septicemia in neutropenic dogs. J Lab Clin Med. 1976;87:840.
285. Baumgartner JD, Glauser MP, McCutchan JA, et al. Prevention of gram-negative shock and death in surgical patients by antibody to endotoxin core glycolipid. Lancet. 1985;1:59–63.
286. McCutchan JA, Wolf JL, Ziegler EF, et al. Ineffectiveness of single-dose human antiserum to core glycolipid (*E. coli* J5) for prophylaxis of bacteremic, gram-negative infections in patients with prolonged neutropenia. Schweiz Med Wochenschr [Suppl] 1983;14:40–5.
287. Schneerson R, Robbins JB. Induction of serum *Haemophilus influenzae* type B capsular antibodies in adult volunteers fed cross-reacting *Escherichia coli* 075:K100:H5. N Engl J Med. 1975;292:1093.
288. Young LS, Stevens P. Cross-protective immunity against gram-negative bacilli: Studies with "core" glycolipid and pneumococcal antigens. J Infect Dis. 1977;136(Suppl):174.

SECTION F

60. PERITONITIS AND OTHER INTRA-ABDOMINAL INFECTIONS

MATTHEW E. LEVISON
LARRY M. BUSH

Intra-abdominal infection may take several forms.[1] Infection may be in the retroperitoneal space or within the peritoneal cavity. Intraperitoneal infection may be diffuse or localized into one or more abscesses. Intraperitoneal abscesses may form in dependent recesses such as the pelvic space or Morison's pouch, in the various perihepatic spaces, within the lesser sac, and along the major routes of communication between intraperitoneal recesses, such as the right paracolic gutter. In addition, infection may be contained within the intra-abdominal viscera, such as hepatic, pancreatic, splenic, tuboovarian, or renal abscesses. Abscesses also frequently form about diseased viscera—pericholecystic, periappendiceal, pericolic, and tuboovarian—and between adjacent loops of bowel, i.e., interloop abscesses.

ANATOMY

The anatomic relationships within the abdomen are important in determining possible sources as well as routes of spread of infection. The peritoneal cavity extends from the undersurface of the diaphragm to the floor of the pelvis. In men the peritoneal cavity is a closed space. In women it is perforated by the free ends of the fallopian tubes. The stomach, jejunum, ileum, cecum, appendix, transverse and sigmoid colons, liver, gallbladder, and spleen lie within the peritoneal cavity, some being suspended by a mesentery.

The peritoneal reflections and mesenteric attachments compartmentalize the intraperitoneal space and route spreading exudate to sites that are often distant from their source (Fig. 1). The transverse mesocolon (14, in Fig. 1) divides the peritoneal cavity horizontally into an upper and a lower space. The greater omentum, extending from the transverse mesocolon and lower border of the stomach, covers the lower peritoneal cavity and further separates the upper from the lower peritoneal cavity (Fig. 2). The small bowel mesentery divides the lower peritoneal space.

The peritoneal cavity has several recesses into which exudate may become loculated. The most dependent recess of the peritoneal cavity in the supine position is in the pelvis. Between the rectum and bladder in men is a pouch of peritoneal cavity that extends slightly below the level of the seminal vesicles. In women, the uterus and fallopian tubes project into the pelvic recess. Between the rectum and body of the uterus is the pouch of Douglas, which lies above the posterior fornix of the vagina. On either side of the rectum and bladder are the pararectal and paravesical fossae. The pelvic recess is continuous with both the right and left paracolic gutters.

The phrenicocolic ligament, which fixes the splenic flexure of the colon to the diaphragm, partially bridges the junction between the left paracolic gutter and the left perihepatic space. In contrast, the right paracolic gutter is continuous with the right subhepatic space and the right subphrenic space. A posterior superior extension of the right subhepatic space, Mori-

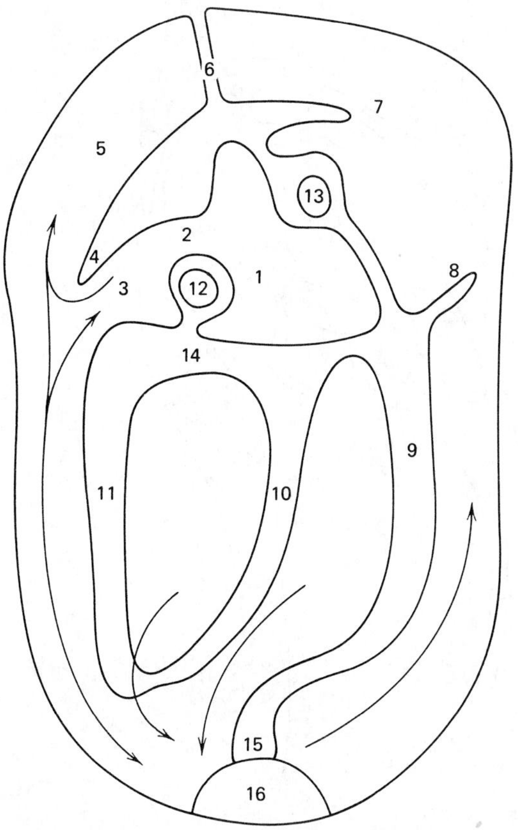

FIG. 1. Schema of the posterior peritoneal reflections and recesses of the peritoneal cavity. 1: Lesser sac; 2: foramen of Winslow; 3: Morison's pouch; 4: right triangular ligament; 5: right subphrenic space; 6: falciform ligament; 7: left subphrenic space; 8: phrenico-colic ligament; 9: bare area of the descending colon; 10: root of the small bowel mesentery; 11: bare area of ascending colon; 12: duodenum; 13: esophagus; 14: root of the transverse mesocolon; 15: bare area of rectum; 16: bladder.

son's pouch, is the most dependent portion in the supine position of the right paravertebral groove and lies just above the beginning of the transverse mesocolon. The horizontal posterior reflection of the serosal surface of the liver onto the diaphragm (the right triangular and coronary ligaments) and vertical reflection (the falciform ligament) divide the right perihepatic space into a right subphrenic and right subhepatic spaces[2] (Figs. 1 and 2A). The left subphrenic and subhepatic spaces communicate freely around the smaller left lobe of the liver and its more superiorly placed left triangular ligament[3,4] (Figs. 1 and 2B). The right and left subphrenic spaces are separated by the falciform ligament, which probably prevents the spread of pus to the opposite side and explains why only about 5–15 percent of subphrenic abscesses are bilateral.[4] The left subhepatic space is divided by the gastrohepatic omentum into an anterior space and the lesser sac (Fig. 2B). Abscesses within the perihepatic spaces become localized by pyogenic membranes. In the right subphrenic space they lie anteriorly or posteriorly and in the subhepatic space superiorly or inferiorly.[3,4] Abscesses of the left perihepatic space are either in the single left subphrenic space or in the lesser sac.[3,4]

The lesser sac, the largest recess of the peritoneal cavity, is connected to the main peritoneal space by the foramen of Winslow, an opening situated between the free border of the gastrohepatic omentum and the posterior parietal peritoneum. The lesser sac is surrounded posteriorly by the pancreas and kidneys, anteriorly by the stomach, and laterally by the liver and spleen. It may also extend to a variable extent between the folds of the greater omentum. Because of the limited communication from the lesser sac to the major cavity via the foramen of Winslow, suppuration in the lesser sac may exist with little or no involvement of the major cavity. Abscesses in the lesser sac lie between the stomach and pancreas but may spread to the right and lie anterior to the right kidney and inferior to the liver.

After intraperitoneal injection of water-soluble contrast material selectively into various intraperitoneal spaces, Meyers has demonstrated that the right paracolic gutter is the main communication between the upper and lower peritoneal cavities.[5] Fluid introduced into the right upper peritoneal space gravitates toward Morison's pouch and then into the right subphrenic space and along the right paracolic gutter into the pelvic recess (Fig. 3). Flow of fluid in the left upper peritoneal space is mainly into the left subphrenic space. The phrenicocolic ligament limits flow inferiorly into the left paracolic gutter. Fluid introduced into the lower peritoneal cavity first gravitates to the pelvic recess and then ascends, whether in the supine or erect position, along the right paracolic gutter into the right subhepatic space, especially into Morison's pouch, and into the right subphrenic space. Ascension of fluid from the pelvic space along the left paracolic gutter is minimal and limited by the phrenicocolic ligament. Although gravity would account for the pooling of fluid in the dependent peritoneal recesses, such as the pelvic recess and Morison's pouch, ascension of fluid from the pelvis to the subphrenic space is probably due to hydrostatic pressure differences between the upper and lower peritoneal cavities created by diaphragmatic motion. Normal intestinal and abdominal wall motion would also account for some spread of intraperitoneal fluid.

The retroperitoneal space lies between the posterior peritoneal membrane and the transversalis fascia, extending from the diaphragm to the pelvic brim. In the anterior retroperitoneal space between the peritoneum and anterior renal fascia lie the ascending and descending colons, duodenum, and pancreas. The kidneys and ureters lie within the posterior retroperitoneal (perinephric) space, between the anterior and posterior renal fasciae. The renal fascia encloses the kidneys and adrenals superiorly and laterally, but not inferiorly, favoring spread of infection in this space inferiorly.[6]

The parietal peritoneum, mainly the anterior portion, is well supplied by somatic afferent nerves and is sensitive to all forms of stimuli. The ability of the anterior parietal peritoneum to sense sharp, well-localized pain in response to local inflammation is of primary importance in diagnosing abdominal infection and may be associated with involuntary abdominal muscle contraction, tenderness, and rebound tenderness. Irritation of the peripheral diaphragmatic peritoneum is felt as pain near the adjacent body wall, and irritation of the central portion is felt as pain referred to the shoulder. Stimulation of the visceral peritoneum, usually due to distension of an organ, causes poorly localized, somewhat dull, pain.

The peritoneal cavity is lined by a serous membrane. The surface area of this membrane approximates that of the skin. The membrane consists of a monolayer of flat polygonal cells beneath which are lymphatics, blood vessels, and nerve endings. Normally, the peritoneal space contains only sufficient fluid to maintain moistness of the surface, facilitating movements of the viscera. Noninflamed serous fluid is clear yellow with a low specific gravity (<1.016) and low protein content (usually <3 g/dl). The protein is predominantly albumin. Fibrinogen is not present and serous fluid will not clot. Solute concentrations are nearly identical to those in plasma. A few leukocytes ($<300/mm^3$), mostly mononuclear cells, and desquamated serosal cells may be found.

The peritoneal membrane is highly permeable. Bidirectional transfer of substances across this membrane is rapid and, because of the large surface area involved, is potentially great in quantity. In fact, the peritoneal surface has been used extensively as a dialyzing membrane for the treatment of uremia and has also been used for the administration of fluid, electrolytes,

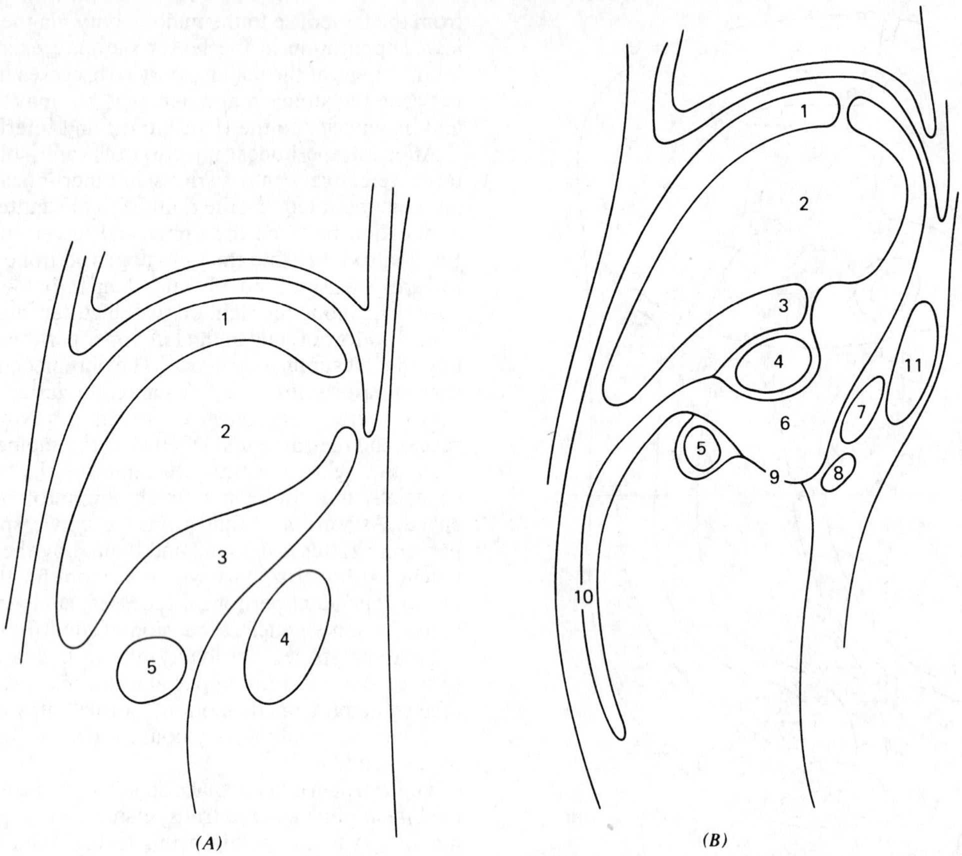

FIG. 2. Schema of a sagittal section of the peritoneal cavity. (**A**) Right upper quadrant. 1: Subphrenic space; 2: liver; 3: subhepatic space; 4: right kidney; 5: transverse colon. (**B**) Left upper quadrant. 1: Subphrenic space; 2: liver—left lobe; 3: subhepatic space; 4: stomach; 5: transverse colon; 6: lesser sac; 7: pancreas; 8: duodenum; 9: transverse mesocolon; 10: omentum; 11: left kidney.

antibiotics, and even blood.[7] The effective serum oncotic pressure and the hydrostatic pressure in the portal veins and lymphatics are major determinants of the rate and direction of fluid movement. The rate of movement of water and solutes between blood and peritoneal fluid is also dependent on concentration gradients between these compartments and has been studied in detail.[8,9] Water and solutes diffuse via blood capillaries and to a lesser extent by lymphatics. Lymphatics are primarily involved in removal of nonirritating colloids and particles into the blood stream. Absorption into lymphatics of particulate matter is thought to take place mostly from the diaphragmatic surface and is aided by the pumping action of diaphragmatic motion.[10] Following infusion of ^{51}Cr-labeled red blood cells into the peritoneal cavity of dogs, Rochlin et al.[11] reported absorption of about 70 percent of the labeled red blood cells by 48–96 hours. This absorption occurred mostly via the lymphatics. In humans, two-thirds of intraperitoneally injected red blood cells in anticoagulated blood have been found in the circulation 8–12 days after infusion.[12] The quantity of resorbed cells was less when no anticoagulant was used with the transfused cells, presumably due to trapping of red blood cells in intraperitoneal clots.[12] Transport of other particulate matter, such as intraperitoneal bacteria, may be similarly impeded because of trapping in fibrinous intraperitoneal exudate.[13]

In addition, there are communications between the peritoneal and pleural cavities that are independent of the blood stream. In patients with Meigs syndrome, for example, radioactive colloidal gold instilled into the peritoneal cavity appears in the pleural space probably as a result of transdiaphragmatic lymphatic transport.[14]

PERITONITIS

Inflammation of the peritoneum may be the result of contamination of the peritoneal cavity with microorganisms, irritating chemicals, or both. There are two major types of infective peritonitis: (*1*) the primary (so-called spontaneous or idiopathic) variety, in which no primary focus of infection is evident, and (*2*) the secondary variety, in which a primary intra-abdominal process such as ruptured appendix or perforated peptic ulcer is evident.

Primary Peritonitis

Etiology. Primary peritonitis is probably not a specific entity with a common cause but represents a group of diseases with different causes having in common only infection of the peritoneal cavity without an evident source. Primary peritonitis occurs at all ages. The prevalence of primary peritonitis in children apparently has been decreasing.[15] In the preantibiotic era, primary peritonitis occurred in about 10 percent of all pediatric abdominal emergencies; it now accounts for less than 1–2 percent.[16,17] The decline has been attributed to widespread use of antibiotics for minor upper respiratory tract illness. Although primary peritonitis may occur in children without predisposing disease,[15] it is known to occur particularly in children with postnecrotic cirrhosis[16,18] and in 2 percent of children with the nephrotic syndrome.[15,19] In one study, it was also frequently associated with urinary tract infections.[16] In some nephrotic children, repeated episodes of peritonitis occur and peritonitis may precede other manifestations of nephrosis.[15]

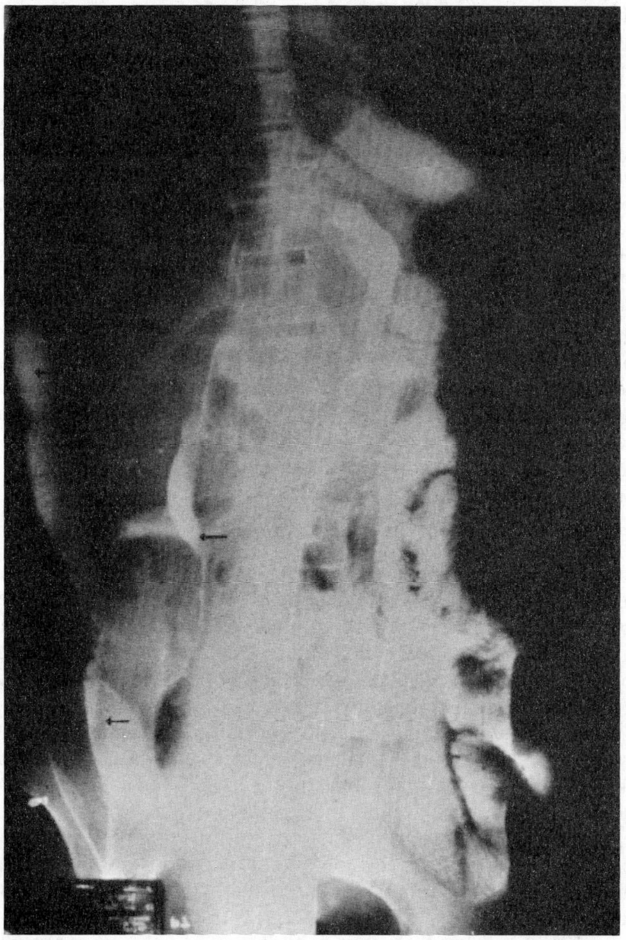

FIG. 3. Abdominal x-ray film (right decubitis) after oral administration of gastrografin to a patient with dehiscence of an esophageal-gastric anastomosis. Radiopaque gastrografin (arrows) can be seen in the subhepatic space, right paracolic gutter, and right subphrenic space, as well as within the lumen of the intestinal tract.

In adults, primary peritonitis usually has been reported in patients with alcoholic cirrhosis and ascites. In 1971 Conn and Fessel summarized their experience with 32 episodes in 28 patients and, in addition, reviewed 46 episodes in 42 patients reported in the literature.[20] Subsequent reports have confirmed and extended their initial findings.[21–28] Primary peritonitis was found to occur in about 10 percent of the patients with alcoholic cirrhosis collected retrospectively.[20,21] Among 63 consecutive patients with cirrhosis and ascites studied prospectively, using optimal aerobic and anaerobic bacteriologic techniques, primary peritonitis was found in 5.[25] Primary peritonitis has also been reported in adults with postnecrotic cirrhosis,[18] chronic active hepatitis,[29] acute viral hepatitis,[30] congestive heart failure,[31] metastatic malignant disease,[32] systemic lupus erythematosus,[33] lymphedema,[34] and, rarely, with no underlying disease.[35] The presence of ascites appears to be the common link among these various conditions.

Bacteriologic Characteristics. Several decades ago, the organisms reported to cause primary peritonitis in children were *Streptococcus pneumoniae* and group A streptococci.[15–17] More recently, the number of nephrotic children with streptococcal peritonitis has declined, and the relative frequency of peritonitis due to gram-negative enteric bacilli[16,17,19] and staphylococci[15,17] apparently has increased.

In cirrhotic patients, microorganisms presumably of enteric origin account for up to 69 percent of the pathogens.[36] *Escherichia coli* is the most frequently recovered pathogen, followed by *Klebsiella pneumoniae, S. pneumoniae*, and other streptococcal species, including enterococci.[20,24,36–38] *Staphylococcus aureus* is an unusual isolate in primary peritonitis, accounting for 2–4 percent of the cases in most series, and has been noted to occur in patients with an erosion of an umbilical hernia.[37] Anaerobes and microaerophilic organisms are infrequently reported.[24,28] Possible explanations include the intrinsic bacteristatic activity of ascites against *Bacteroides* species,[39] the relatively high PO_2 of ascitic fluid,[40] and the lack of optimal anaerobic bacteriologic techniques used to study patients with primary peritonitis in the past. In a review of 126 cases of primary peritonitis in cirrhotic patients recorded in the literature, only 6 percent (eight patients) were due to anaerobic or microaerophilic bacteria, including *Bacteroides* spp., *Bacteroides fragilis, Clostridium perfringens, Peptostreptococcus* spp., *Peptococcus* spp., and *Campylobacter fetus*.[24] Polymicrobial infection was present in four of these eight cirrhotic patients with peritonitis due to anaerobes, in contrast to the relatively low frequency of polymicrobial infection (only 10 of 118 cases of peritonitis) when aerobes alone were involved.

Ascitic fluid with positive cultures but few leukocytes in patients without clinical findings of peritonitis has been noted and called *bacterascites*.[38] This may represent early colonization before a host response.[28] However, patients with a low leukocyte response have the same mortality as those with a greater response.[27] Conversely, several series have identified cases of primary peritonitis with negative ascitic fluid cultures.[20,28] A recent series reported negative cultures in 35 percent of patients with clinical findings consistent with primary peritonitis, ascitic fluid leukocyte counts of $>500/mm^3$, and no evident source of intra-abdominal infection.[41] Blood cultures were positive in one-third of these patients. This variant of primary peritonitis has been termed *culture-negative neutrocytic ascites*.[41] The frequency of culture-negative ascitic fluid may be decreased by inoculating blood culture bottles with ascitic fluid at the bedside.[42]

Bacteremia is present in up to 75 percent of patients with primary peritonitis due to aerobic bacteria,[36] but is rarely found in those with peritonitis due to anaerobes.[24] Usually the same organisms isolated from the peritoneal fluid are recovered from the blood.[20,24]

Occasionally, primary peritonitis may be caused by *Mycobacterium tuberculosis, Neisseria gonorrhoeae*, or *Chlamydia trachomatis*.

Pathogenesis. The route of infection in primary peritonitis is usually not apparent and often it is presumed to be either hematogenous, lymphogenous, transmural migration through an intact gut wall from the intestinal lumen, or, in women, from the vagina via the fallopian tubes. Conn and Fessel[20] have postulated that the hematogenous route is most likely in cirrhotic patients: either (*1*) organisms removed from circulation by the liver may contaminate hepatic lymph and pass through the permeable lymphatic walls into the ascitic fluid or (*2*) portosystemic shunting greatly diminishes hepatic clearance of bacteremia in the portal circulation, which would tend to perpetuate bacteremia and increase the opportunity to cause metastic infection at susceptible sites such as the ascitic collection. The infrequency of primary peritonitis in all forms of ascites except that secondary to liver disease emphasizes the importance of intrahepatic shunting in the pathogenesis of this disease. The hepatic reticuloendothelial system is known to be a major site for removal of bacteria from blood,[43] and animal studies have suggested that destruction of blood-borne bacteria by the reticuloendothelial system is impaired in experimental cirrhosis[44] and in alcoholic liver disease.[45] The decrease in phagocytic activity seen in alcoholic cirrhosis is proportional to the severity of the liver disease.[46] Additionally, alcohol abuse and cirrhosis have been reported to be associated with impaired intracellular killing by monocytes and neutrophils,[47] as well as impaired opsonization[48] and low levels of serum complement.[49] The characteristics of ascitic fluid in nephrosis and cirrhosis predispose to infection. Opsonic activity, as reflected by low levels of complement and immunoglobulins, is reduced in the ascitic fluid of patients with the nephrotic syndrome and cirrhosis.[50,51] Primary bacteremia, usually due to coliforms, is a common complication in cirrhosis,[52] and metastatic infection in the pleural space has also been reported in cirrhotic patients.[53] An increased frequency of gram-negative endocarditis has also been noted in cirrhotics.[54]

Enteric bacteria may also gain access to the peritoneal cavity by directly traversing the intact intestinal wall. This has been demonstrated in animals[55]: Schweinburg et al. demonstrated that in dogs ^{14}C-labeled *E. coli* passed from the bowel into the peritoneal cavity after the introduction of hypertonic solutions into the peritoneum. A similar mechanism may explain the enteric bacterial peritonitis that frequently complicates peritoneal dialysis.[56] The infrequent occurrence of bacteremia and the multiplicity of species in peritoneal fluid when anaerobic bacteria are involved suggest that transmural migration of bacteria is the probable route of infection of ascitic fluid in the majority of these patients.[24] In addition, the occurrence of polymicrobial anaerobic peritonitis in two patients after infusion of vasopressin into the superior mesenteric or gastroduodenal arteries suggests that arterial vasoconstriction decreased the intestinal mucosal barrier and permitted transmural migration of enteric organisms.[22] Colonic microorganisms have been reported to colonize the upper small bowel in cirrhotic patients.[57]

The simultaneous presence of pneumococci in vaginal secretions and peritoneal fluid in girls[58] makes an ascending infection of genital origin likely in these patients. The alkaline vaginal secretions of prepubertal girls may be less inhibitory to bacterial growth than the acidic secretions of postpubertal females. Transfallopian spread is also suggested by the development of primary peritonitis in women with intrauterine devices (IUDs).[59,60] The route of spread in women with gonococcal or chlamydial perihepatitis (Fitz-Hugh-Curtis syndrome) is presumably from the fallopian tubes and paracolic gutters to the subphrenic space, but may also be hematogenous. In the one man with this syndrome, *Neisseria gonorrhoeae* was recovered from a liver biopsy specimen, and the route of spread was presumably via bacteremia.[61]

Although tuberculous peritonitis may result from direct entry into the peritoneal cavity of tubercle bacilli (from the lymph nodes, intestine, or genital tract in patients with active disease of these organs), it is more likely to be disseminated hematogenously from remote foci of tuberculosis, most commonly in the lung. Tuberculous peritonitis may become clinically evident after the initial focus has completely healed.

Clinical Manifestations. Primary peritonitis is an acute febrile illness often confused with acute appendicitis in children. Fever, abdominal pain, nausea, vomiting, and diarrhea are usually present with diffuse abdominal tenderness, rebound tenderness, and hypoactive or absent bowel sounds. In cirrhotic patients with primary peritonitis, preexisting ascites is present. In some patients, the clinical manifestations may be atypical. The onset, for example, may be insidious, and findings of peritoneal irritation may be absent in an abdomen distended with ascites. Fever (>100°F) is the most common presenting sign, occurs in 50–80 percent of cases,[20,27] and may be present without abdominal signs or symptoms or the process may be completely silent. Primary peritonitis in cirrhotic patients is generally associated with other features of end-stage liver disease (hepatorenal syndrome, progressive encephalopathy, and variceal bleeding).

The ascitic fluid protein concentration may be low[20] in abdominal inflammation for the following reasons: (*1*) hypoalbuminemia[62] and (*2*) dilution of ascitic fluid with transudate from the portal system when there is cirrhosis or the portal vein is obstructed.[63] The leukocyte count in peritoneal fluid usually is greater than 300/mm^3 (in 85 percent of cases, >1000/mm^3), with granulocytes predominating in >80 percent of cases.[26] However, the total leukocyte count of some patients with ascites uncomplicated by infection may be similarly elevated.[25] Indeed, an increase in ascites leukocyte counts has been noted during diuresis in patients with chronic liver disease.[64] Recent studies of other parameters of ascitic fluid that may help in diagnosing primary bacterial peritonitis have found the lactate concentration and pH to be useful.[65–67] Ascitic fluid pH <7.35 and lactate >25 mg/dl were more specific but less sensitive than a leukocyte count of >500/mm^3, and using all three parameters together increased the diagnostic accuracy.[66,67] Gram stain of the sediment when positive is diagnostic, but it may be negative in about 60–80 percent of cases with cirrhosis and ascites.[20,26]

Gonococcal perihepatitis (Fitz-Hugh-Curtis syndrome) most often occurs in women. It manifests with sudden onset of pain in the right upper quandrant of the abdomen, at times referred to the right shoulder. There may be low-grade fever, right upper quadrant tenderness, guarding, and a friction rub over the liver.[68] Gonococcal cervicitis and/or salpingitis may or may not be clinically evident. Chlamydial and gonococcal perihepatitis are clinically indistinguishable.

Primary tuberculous peritonitis usually is gradual in onset, with fever, weight loss, malaise, night sweats, and abdominal distension. The abdomen may not be rigid and is often characterized as being "doughy" on palpation. The findings at operation or laparoscopy consist of multiple nodules scattered over the peritoneal surface and omentum. Adhesions and a variable amount of peritoneal fluid are usually present. Ascitic fluid may have an elevated protein concentration (>3 g/dl) and a lymphocytic pleocytosis, but neither may be present, especially in cirrhotic patients.[69] Similarly, *Coccidioides immitis* can cause a granulomatous peritonitis with a variable clinical manifestation.[70]

Diagnosis. The diagnosis of primary peritonitis is one of exclusion of a primary intra-abdominal source of infection and can be made with certainty only after a thorough laparotomy. However, under certain circumstances, laparotomy may be avoided on the basis of findings in peritoneal fluid obtained by paracentesis. For example, if gram-positive organisms are obtained after paracentesis, a diagnosis of primary peritonitis can usually be made and exploratory laparotomy deferred. In children, if gram-negative organisms, a mixed flora, or no organisms are obtained, full exploratory laparotomy is indicated to rule out possible intra-abdominal sources of continuing peritoneal contamination. However, in end-stage cirrhotic patients, exploratory laparotomy may be life-threatening, and the likelihood of finding a primary intra-abdominal focus may be small. Laparotomy performed on cirrhotic patients with sepsis in an attempt to find the source of infection has been reported to have a mortality rate of 80 percent.[71] Surgery in these patients can be deferred while awaiting the response to antimicrobial therapy. Patients with primary peritonitis usually respond within 48 hours to appropriate antimicrobial therapy. The observation of an exponential rate of decline in the number of ascitic fluid leukocytes after the initiation of antimicrobial therapy for primary peritonitis has also been found to help differentiate primary from secondary bacterial peritonitis.[72]

Recovery of pneumococci from peritoneal fluid may not indicate primary peritonitis, as illustrated by a case report of appendicitis and secondary peritonitis due to pneumococci.[73] For this reason, some surgeons have considered the differential diagnosis in children between appendicitis and primary peritonitis too difficult to make without operative examination, even when gram-positive bacteria are identified in peritoneal fluid.[17] Paracentesis for smear and culture is indicated in all cirrhotic patients with ascites and in children with gross proteinuria and abdominal pain, whether or not the diagnosis of nephrotic syndrome was previously established. However, paracentesis is not without hazard, especially in patients with hemorrhagic tendencies or bowel distension. In a retrospective analysis of 242 consecutive diagnostic abdominal paracenteses in patients with liver disease and ascites, major complications were reported in 7, including perforation of the bowel with generalized peritonitis or abdominal wall abscess and serious hemorrhage.[74]

The diagnosis of tuberculous peritonitis can usually be made at operation or laparoscopy and confirmed by the histologic characteristics of the peritoneal biopsy specimen[75] and by bacteriologic examination of the peritoneal biopsy specimen and fluid.[76] The diagnosis of *C. immitis* peritonitis can be made on a wet mount of ascitic fluid, by finding *C. immitis* by culture and by histologic examination.[70]

Prognosis. The treatment of primary peritonitis has been reported to be successful in more than one-half of the cirrhotic patients, but because of the frequency of accompanying end-state cirrhosis, the overall mortality in cirrhotic adults has been as high as 95 percent.[20,23] However, more recent studies have reported lower mortality rates of 70 and 57 percent, with 28 and 40 percent dying from the primary peritonitis, respectively.[26,27] Those patients with the poorest prognosis were found to have renal insufficiency, hypothermia, hyperbilirubinemia, and hypoalbuminemia. The lower mortality rates in these series can perhaps be explained by the less frequent occurrence of hepatic encephalopathy in these later series. Treatment of peritonitis caused by gram-positive organisms, as well as early infections, has been more frequently successful than treatment of gram-negative or late infections. In nephrotic patients with gram-positive infections or in patients who do not have a preterminal underlying illness, the survival rate is over 90 percent.[15]

Treatment. Because the Gram stain is frequently negative in primary bacterial peritonitis, the initial choice of antimicrobial drug is often empiric, based on the most likely pathogens. The antimicrobial regimen can be modified once the results of the culture and susceptibility tests are available.

Some of the third-generation cephalosporin antibiotics have been demonstrated to be as efficacious as the combination of ampicillin plus an aminoglycoside in primary bacterial peritonitis.[77] They also avoid the risk of nephrotoxicity, which is sufficiently frequent in this group of patients to warrant the avoidance of aminoglycosides if an equally effective alternative antimicrobial regimen can be used.[27,78] Other antimicrobial agents such as the broad-spectrum penicillins (e.g., mezlocillin, ticarcillin, piperacillin), carbapenems (e.g., inipenem), and β-lactam antibiotic/β-lactamase inhibitor combinations (e.g., ticarcillin-clavulanate, ampicillin-sulbactam) are potential alternatives.

Primary bacterial peritonitis due either to *S. pneumoniae* or group A streptococci is best treated with penicillin G. Peritonitis suspected of being due to *Staph. aureus* should be treated with a penicillinase-resistant penicillin (e.g., nafcillin) or with a first-generation cephalosporin (e.g., cefazolin). If *Pseudomonas aeruginosa* is isolated, an aminoglycoside antibiotic plus an antipseudomonal penicillin or cephalosporin should be used together. For those situations in which the Gram stain is suggestive of *Bacteroides* or polymicrobial peritonitis is evident, antimicrobials with activity against *B. fragilis* and other anaerobic organisms should be added (e.g., metronidazole, clindamycin).

In those cases where there is a strong clinical suspicion of primary bacterial peritonitis but all cultures are sterile, antimicrobial therapy should be continued. Clinical improvement together with a significant decline in the ascitic fluid leukocyte count should occur after 24 to 48 hours of antimicrobial therapy if the diagnosis is correct.[72,79] The lack of the expected clinical response or the persistence of an elevated ascitic fluid leukocyte count should make other diagnoses a consideration. Antimicrobial therapy should be continued for 10 to 14 days if improvement is noted. The administration of intraperitoneal antimicrobials is not necessary.

Secondary Peritonitis

Etiology. The primary intra-abdominal processes that may give rise to peritonitis are numerous. These include diseases or injuries of the gastrointestinal tract such as perforation of a peptic ulcer; traumatic perforation of the uterus, urinary bladder, stomach, or small or large bowel; spontaneous perforation associated with typhoid, tuberculous,[80] amebic, *Strongyloides*, and cytomegalovirus ulcers; appendicitis, diverticulitis, or intestinal neoplasms; gangrene of the bowel either from strangulation, bowel obstruction, or mesenteric vascular obstruction; suppurative cholecystitis; bile peritonitis; pancreatitis; operative contamination of the peritoneum or disruption of a surgical anastomosis site; lesions of the female genital tract such as septic abortion, puerperal sepsis, postoperative uterine infection, endometritis complicating an IUD,[81] and gonococcal salpingitis or gonococcal vulvovaginitis in children; lesions of the male genital tract such as suppurative prostatitis; and rupture of an intraperitoneal or visceral abscess (e.g., renal or perinephric, tuboovarian, liver, splenic, or pancreatic abscess). Peritonitis is a major hazard of peritoneal dialysis used in the management of renal failure, fluid and electrolytic imbalance, and certain intoxications.[56] Not uncommonly, bacterial peritonitis can occur secondary to the use of peritoneovenous and ventriculoperitoneal shunts.[82,83]

Microbiologic Characteristics. Infrequently, secondary peritonitis is caused by exogenous microorganisms, for example, *Staph. aureus, N. gonorrhoeae*, or *M. tuberculosis*, which have caused infection in intra-abdominal or adjacent viscera and have spread to involve the peritoneum. Most cases of secondary peritonitis, however, are endogenous in origin due to the large number and variety of microorganisms that normally colonize mucous membranes lining certain viscera within the abdominal cavity. Although forming a continuous surface, the mucous membranes of the stomach, upper small bowel, lower small bowel, and large bowel each has a characteristic microflora. The vagina also has a distinct microflora. Normally, invasive activities of indigenous bacteria are controlled by the intact mucosa of the gastrointestinal tract and vagina. Disturbances in this mucosal barrier may occur as a result of spontaneous disease, trauma, or surgical operations that permit escape of indigenous bacteria and may result in infection of the peritoneum, the abdominal viscera, or the retroperitoneal space. The frequency with which various indigenous organisms are recovered from intra-abdominal infection varies according to the site of the primary process and whether the primary process is associated with an alteration of the indigenous microflora.[84]

The stomach normally contains $\leq 10^3$ cfu of microorganisms/ml in the fasting state. If bacteria are present, they are mostly facultative, gram-positive, salivary microorganisms, such as lactobacilli and streptococci. The numbers of these organisms in stomach contents transiently increase after a meal.[85] Gastric flora is more numerous and may be composed of different organisms when there is achlorhydria (e.g., from cimetidine) or blood in the stomach.[85,86] The flora of the upper small intestine is normally sparse and consists of salivary microorganisms.[87] But in the presence of achlorhydria,[85] intestinal obstruction, or other processes affecting motility or absorption, the flora of the small intestine is more profuse and varied. Conditions that favor small bowel stasis include scleroderma, regional enteritis, small bowel strictures, nontropical sprue, tropical sprue, duodenal and jejunal diverticula, presence of an afferent loop of the Billroth II gastrojejunostomy, and intestinal pseudo-obstruction.[88] Large bowel flora has been found in the proximal small bowel of cirrhotic patients.[57] The ileum normally contains *E. coli*, enterococci, and an equal number of microorganisms that are obligately anaerobic, such as *B. fragilis*.[87] It is the colon, however, in which a profuse microflora exists in concentrations of about 10^{11} bacteria/ml of feces, a wet sludge of practically pure bacteria.[89] The colonic flora is predominantly composed of the obligate anaerobes, *B. fragilis*, and *Bifidobacterium* spp., which outnumber facultative microorganisms, primarily *E. coli*, by 10^3–10^4 to 1. Other colonic bacteria are viridans streptococci, enterococci, *Eubacterium* spp., *Klebsiella* spp., *Proteus* spp., *Enterobacter* spp., and *C. perfringens*. The large bowel flora is relatively stable[89] but may be significantly altered by antibiotic therapy.[90]

As would be anticipated from the nature of the gastrointestinal flora, Altemeier[91] reported anaerobes in 96 percent of 100 cases of peritonitis secondary to acute appendicitis with perforation. *Bacteroides melaninogenicus* and anaerobic gram-positive cocci were the most frequent isolates. Recent studies of the bacteriologic characteristics of intra-abdominal infections,[92–94] using modern bacteriologic techniques that provide an anaerobic environment during collection, transport, and incubation, have confirmed the findings of Altemeier that anaerobes play a major role. Finegold reported that in a series of 73 intra-abdominal infections including 16 cases of peritonitis, there were an average of 4.5 isolates per case (range, 1–12 organisms), with 2.5 anaerobes and 2 aerobes or facultatives.[92] The most frequent isolate was *E. coli*, followed by *B. fragilis* (the most common anaerobic isolate), enterococci, other *Bacteroides* spp., *Fusobacterium, C. perfringens*, other clostridia, *Peptococcus, Peptostreptococcus*, and *Eubacterium*. Similar findings have been reported by Gorbach et al. in a series of 43 patients, which included 10 cases of peritonitis, in 93 percent of whom anaerobes or a mixture of anaerobes and facultatives were recovered,[93] and by Swenson et al. in a series of 64 patients, which included 26 cases of peritonitis, in 81 percent of whom anaerobes were recovered.[95]

In these series, bacteremia was reported in about 20–30 percent of patients. Organisms recovered from blood frequently included *B. fragilis* or *E. coli*. In series of patients with *Bacteroides* bacteremia, 14–62 percent had a gastrointestinal source.[101–104]

Together with highly antibiotic-resistant strains of *Serratia* and *Acinetobacter, P. aeruginosa* is more frequently isolated from patients who develop their intra-abdominal infection while in the hospital, after having received broad-spectrum parenteral antimicrobials.[96] However, two recent studies have noted that *P. aeruginosa* comprises a more significant portion of the aerobic isolates in community-acquired intra-abdominal infection[97,98] than had been noted in previous series.[99]

Penetrating injuries to the liver and spleen are rarely followed by infection due to the usual sterility of these organs.[100]

Recent quantitative studies[105–107] in sexually active women during the childbearing period have revealed that the predominant vaginal microflora is composed of five to seven different microorganisms, and that anaerobes are approximately 10 times more numerous than facultative organisms. There are about 10^8–10^9 cfu of anaerobes and about 10^7–10^8 cfu of facultatives per milliliter of vaginal secretions. The most frequent isolates in titers of $\geq 10^5$/ml are obligate or facultative anaerobic lactobacilli, nonenterococcal streptococci, anaerobic gram-positive cocci, Bacteroidaceae other than *B. fragilis* (e.g., *B. melaninogenicus, B. bivius, B. ruminicola*), and a group of unidentified catalase-negative facultative bacilli. Diphtheroids and *S. epidermidis* have also been reported to be frequent vaginal isolates.[107] When specifically looked for, *Gardnerella vaginalis* in high counts has also been found to be only slightly less frequent than lactobacilli in the vaginal secretions of normal women.[105,106] Colonic organisms, such as *B. fragilis*, Enterobacteriaceae, and enterococci are rarely found as predominant components of the normal vaginal flora and probably proliferate at this site only under exceptional circumstances. For example, these organisms have been reported to appear in vaginal secretions in the immediate postoperative periods after vaginal operations,[108] and *C. perfringens* has been reported more frequently in vaginal secretions after difficult labor or abortions.[109] Hite et al.[110] noted the relative infrequency of *Bacteroides* and anaerobic gram-positive cocci in the vagina of normal prenatal women, whereas during the puerperium in both women with postpartum endometritis and noninfected women, these organisms were found to be more prevalent.[110,111] Factors favoring colonization by these anaerobes after surgery and in the puerperium are unknown but are possibly related to blood or necrotic tissue that provides the reduced, enriched environment required by these anaerobes.

Sequential sampling of vaginal secretions during the menstrual cycle has been reported to show constant levels of anaerobes, although recovery of specific organisms varies from specimen to specimen in each woman.[107] By contrast, levels of facultatives decrease 100-fold in the premenstrual week.[107] This variation in microflora may reflect cyclic fluctuation in the vaginal environment due to changes in hormonal activity during the menstrual cycle. Because the vaginal flora varies under certain conditions and members of this flora have differing pathogenicity, the frequency of endogenous intra-abdominal infections of gynecologic origin, as well as the types of pathogens involved, vary accordingly. For example, the frequency of vaginal colonization with group B streptococci increases during pregnancy, and infections due to these organisms are relatively common in the postpartum period.[112] In addition, in women with trichomoniasis, *Bacteroides* species more frequently may be found in vaginal secretions.[106,110] Postpartum infection, presumably due to anaerobes, has been reported to be more frequent in women who have trichomoniasis during pregnancy.[113]

The bacteriologic characteristics of intra-abdominal infection that complicates female genital tract infections is quite similar to secondary peritonitis due to a gastrointestinal source, except for the occurrence of *N. gonorrhoeae* in cul-de-sac aspirates.[114] Data compiled by Swenson et al.,[115] Thadepalli et al.,[116] and Chow et al.[117] indicate that anaerobes were found in 72 percent of 200 gynecologic infections. Anaerobes were especially frequent (92 percent) in closed-space infections such as tuboovarian and pelvic abscesses. *Bacteroides*, in particular *B. fragilis* and *B. melaninogenicus*, and anaerobic gram-positive cocci were the most frequently isolated anaerobes. *Escherichia coli* and streptococci were the most prevalent facultatives. Apparently, even in acute salpingitis, recent bacteriologic studies have demonstrated in the majority of patients the presence of anaerobes, usually gram-positive cocci in cul-de-sac aspirates, despite the recovery of gonococci from the endocervix.[118–120] The data are interpreted as supporting the concept of superinfection with anaerobes after initial infection with *N. gonorrhoeae* late in the course of this disease.[121] In children, gonococcal peritonitis has been rarely reported with gonococcal vulvovaginitis.[122,123]

Intraperitoneal rupture has been reported in 10 percent of the cases of amebic liver abscess and may cause acute generalized peritonitis or a less commonly localized intraperitoneal abscess with a mortality of about 18 percent.[124] Perforation of the colon with bacterial peritonitis due to fulminant amebic colitis is also unusual but often fatal.[125] Similarly, *Strongyloides stercoralis* infestation of the small bowel may rarely cause fatal peritonitis, with or without concurrent bacterial contamination.[126] *Candida* has been isolated from the abdominal fluid in patients undergoing peritoneal dialysis, as has *Staph. aureus*, Enterobacteriaceae, and *P. aeruginosa*.[127] *Candida* peritonitis has also been observed as a complication of gastrointestinal surgery or in perforation of a viscus,[128,129] and its occurrence is related to numerous factors that increase the rate of *Candida* colonization in the gastrointestinal tract. These include immunosuppression, prolonged hospitalization, and antimicrobial and/or antacid therapy. *Candida* is most commonly isolated from the peritoneum after perforation of a gastric or duodenal peptic ulcer, or after spillage of colonic contents into the peritoneum due to trauma, mesenteric artery occlusion, or dehiscence of a surgical anastomosis.

Pathogenesis. The virulence of the bacteria that cause peritonitis is enhanced when certain microorganisms either are combined intraperitoneally with substances such as mucus, enzymes, or hemoglobin or are combined with certain other microorganisms.

Chemical peritonitis can be produced by escape of bile or of gastric or pancreatic secretions into the peritoneal cavity. When gastric acid escapes into the peritoneal cavity, there is an outpouring of serum protein and electrolytes from the blood into the peritoneal cavity. The acidity is quickly neutralized by these buffers and by diffusion of hydrogen ions into the body fluids.[130,131] Widespread necrosis may result from enzymatic digestion after intraperitoneal spillage of potent pancreatic enzymes. Escape of bile into the peritoneal cavity is generally considered to be a very grave, often fatal situation.[132,133] The severity of peritonitis after escape of these intestinal secretions is due in part to subsequent bacterial peritonitis. Indeed, in the dog with experimentally produced partial biliary diversion into the peritoneal cavity, fatal effects were reduced by oral nonabsorbable or parenteral antibiotics.[134] Bacteria may enter the peritoneal cavity with contaminated intestinal secretions through perforations in the gastrointestinal wall, as well as by migration through the wall of the intact gastrointestinal tract, in response to the irritation of bile and possibly other intestinal tract secretions on the serosal surface.[55]

Nemir et al. demonstrated that after experimental strangulation obstruction of a loop of bowel in the dog, the animal usually died within 36 hours, and the peritoneal fluid at first was light pink and eventually became black. When this black fluid was removed and injected into the peritoneal cavity of a normal animal, the recipient also developed a similar fatal peritonitis, but the early peritoneal fluid was nontoxic.[135–137] The toxicity could be largely counteracted by instilling antibiotics into the obstructed loop of intestine or by giving antibiotics simultaneously when the fluid was injected into normal animals.[138,139] Many workers in the past have shown that intraperitoneal injection of large numbers of organisms in pure culture is incapable of producing peritonitis unless some additional factor is present, such as gum tragacanth, talc, mucin, turpentine, or other irritants. It seemed unlikely, therefore, that the toxicity of strangulation obstruction fluid was due to its bacterial content alone. Evidence has been reported that viable bacteria in addition to the presence of free hemoglobin in the peritoneal fluid are necessary to account for the lethality both of bowel strangulation and of the fluid that collects in the peritoneal cavity after bowel strangulation.[140–142] The mechanism by which free hemoglobin enhances peritoneal infection is unknown but perhaps is related to free iron. Iron is required for bacterial metabolism and, in amounts that leave an excess of free iron after having saturated transferrin, may greately enhance infections due to certain microorganisms, such as Enterobacteriaceae and *C. perfringens*.[143] Hau et al. demonstrated that intraperitoneal hemoglobin depresses the influx of granulocytes into the peritoneal cavity in response to intraperitoneal bacteria, and hemoglobin depresses in vitro the chemotactic response of granulocytes and monocytes.[144]

Intraperitoneal fluid and fibrin that enter the peritoneal cavity as a result of the increased vascular permeability due to local trauma or bacterial infection are important components of the inflammatory response and play adjuvant roles. It has been shown that low numbers of *E. coli* in small volumes of saline infused intraperitoneally are innocuous, but these numbers of *E. coli* can become lethal in direct proportion to the increase in the volume of saline infused. This is thought to be related to the resultant dilution of opsonic proteins.[145] Trapping of bacteria beneath layers of fibrin may limit their spread but may also lead to abscess formation and isolation of bacteria from host defense mechanisms.[146]

A number of other substances such as hog gastric mucin, bile salts,[147] and barium sulfate[148,149] have been used as adjuvants in producing lethal intraperitoneal infections. The mechanisms of their respective effects have been the subject of numerous studies. It has been postulated that hog gastric mucin coats bacteria, thus protecting them from intraperitoneal phagocytosis.[150]

Cuevas and Fine[151] have attributed the lethality of bowel strangulation and infectious or chemical irritation of the serosal surface of the bowel to endotoxemia. Endotoxin was thought to escape from the gut lumen, to cross the intact bowel wall into the peritoneal cavity, and then to be absorbed into the systemic circulation. Within minutes after experimental superior mesenteric artery occlusion, endotoxin has been detected in the systemic circulation, before its appearance in the portal vein.[151]

Secondary peritonitis is usually a mixed infection involving predominantly obligate and facultative anaerobes. Obligate anaerobes are sensitive to oxygen in the molecular form and also to bound oxygen, as in organic peroxides. Survival and growth of anaerobes are also dependent on the oxidation-reduction potential, that is, the oxidizing capacity of their environment. Most pathogenic anaerobes require a negative potential of at least -150 mV. Low oxidation-reduction potentials are thought to occur in many abscesses,[152] and oxidation-reduction potentials ≤ -150 mV are measured in abscesses from which anaerobes are recovered.[153] Some anerobic organisms have additional requirements, such as vitamin K, arginine, serum, blood pigments, or bile, before growth is obtained. Thus, establishment of an anaerobic infection requires an environment in which the oxygen tension is very low, the oxidation-reduction potential is low, and abundant nutrients are available to support anaerobic fermentative metabolism. These requirements are usually met by devitalized tissue as a consequence of ischemia, trauma, or neoplastic growth. Once proper conditions are obtained, anaerobic organisms can achieve doubling rates equivalent to those seen with aerobic enteric bacilli. In vivo, the rapidly expanding bacterial and inflammatory cell mass, frequently accompanied by gas production, can interrupt the blood supply to the immediately surrounding tissue and cause further tissue necrosis.

Gram-negative anaerobic cocci and bacilli (including *B. fragilis* and *B. melaninogenicus*) possess endotoxins with much weaker biologic activity in comparison to those extracted from their aerobic counterparts and have low or absent 2-keto-3-deoxyoctanoate content.[153a] In addition, certain anaerobes elaborate collagenase,[155] other proteolytic enzymes, and deoxyribonuclease.[154] Certain Bacteroidaceae are capable of degrading heparin,[156] which may be responsible for the suppurative thrombophlebitis frequently seen in infections due to these microorganisms.[157] These factors tend to provide more areas well adapted to the growth requirements of the anaerobe, with the result that the infection progresses.

In addition, anaerobes may be resistant to host defenses. For example, although leukocytes have been shown to have bactericidal activity under both aerobic and anaerobic conditions against several anaerobic species, including *B. fragilis*, presumably by mechanisms other than those dependent on the superoxide anion O_2^- or H_2O_2,[158] Keusch and Douglas[159] found that granulocytic killing of *C. perfringens* was impaired under anaerobic conditions. Also, a capsule has been demonstrated on *B. fragilis*[160] and *B. asaccharolyticus* (formerly *B. melaninogenicus ss. asaccharolyticus*),[161] which might protect the organisms from phagocytosis and favor abscess formation.[162–164] Some anaerobes, especially *B. fragilis*, may be resistant to the normal bactericidal activity of serum.[158]

Many anaerobic infections appear to be synergistic. Although it is probable that the majority of bacteria isolated in mixed infections are nonpathogenic by themselves, their presence may nevertheless be essential for the pathogenicity of the bacterial mixture. Such examples of bacterial synergism in infection have been demonstrated in periodontal infection by Socransky and Gibbons[165] and in peritonitis by Altemeier.[166]

Facultative organisms in mixed infections may be essential by providing a sufficiently reduced environment for the growth of obligate anaerobic organisms. Another mechanism of bacterial synergy is the generation of a substance by one organism, which is essential for the growth of another, for example, the production of vitamin K (a required growth factor for *B. melaninogenicus*) by diphtheroids. Anaerobes such as *Bacteroides* spp. have also demonstrated the ability to protect aerobic bacteria from phagocytic killing[167,168] and from otherwise effective antibiotic therapy (e.g., via β-lactamase production).[169]

In addition, each component of the pathogenic mixture may contribute in different ways to the clinical picture. After implantation of fecal contents intraperitoneally into rats. Onderdonk et al. observed that *E. coli* initially predominated in the peritoneal exudate.[170] Bacteremia, due to *E. coli* during this phase, was uniformly present and frequently fatal. In rats that survived, indolent intra-abdominal abscesses developed in which *B. fragilis* predominated. Elimination of *E. coli* by early administration of gentamicin reduced early mortality but did not prevent late intra-abdominal abscess due to obligate anaerobes, whereas elimination of obligate anaerobes with clindamycin did not prevent early mortality due to *E. coli* bacteremia but reduced late abscess formation in survivors. These findings indicate that although *E. coli* is responsible for early mortality, anaerobes are responsible for late abscess formation in this model.[171,172]

Pathophysiologic Responses. Whatever the initiating cause of peritonitis, a similar series of reactions takes place, both locally and systemically.

LOCAL RESPONSE. The local inflammatory response of the peritoneum is similar to that in other tissues, but the peritoneal lining presents a large exudative and absorptive surface. At sites of irritation, there is an outpouring of fluid into the peritoneal cavity that, in contrast to normal serous fluid, has a high protein content (>3 g/dl) and many cells, primarily granulocytes, that phagocytize and kill organisms. The exudate contains fibrinogen that polymerizes, and plaques of fibrinous exudate form on the inflamed peritoneal surfaces. This exudate glues adjacent bowel, mesentery, and particularly omentum to each other. Localization is further aided by inhibition of motility in involved intestinal loops. Experimentally, radiopaque medium injected intraperitoneally at one locus can be demonstrated to have spread over much of the greater peritoneal sac within a short time. The extent and rate of intraperitoneal spread of contamination are undoubtedly dependent on the volume and nature of the exudate[13] and on the effectiveness of the localizing processes.

If peritoneal defenses aided by appropriate supportive measures control the inflammatory process, the disease may resolve spontaneously. A second possible outcome is a confined abscess. A third course results when the peritoneal and systemic defense mechanisms are unable to localized the inflammation, which then progresses to spreading diffuse peritonitis. Some of the factors favoring spread of the inflammatory process are (*1*) greater virulence of bacteria, (*2*) greater extent and duration of contamination, or (*3*) impaired host defenses.

SYSTEMIC RESPONSE. Peritonitis leads to changes not only locally in the peritoneal cavity but throughout the body.

Gastrointestinal Tract. Initially in peritonitis there is hypermotility, followed by paralysis of the bowel. Accumulation of fluid and electrolytes in the lumen of the adynamic bowel continues until distension is sufficient to inhibit capillary inflow and secretion ceases.

Cardiovascular. Because of the large surface area of the peritoneum, shifts of fluid into the peritoneal cavity, combined with fluid shifts into the bowel lumen, can produce a profound fall in circulating blood volume and elevation of the hematocrit.[173,174] Fluid and electrolyte loss is further exaggerated by coexistent fever, vomiting, diarrhea, and loss of aspirated gastrointestinal fluid. As the process continues, the decreased venous return to the right side of the heart results in a drop in cardiac output, with resulting hypotension.[174] In addition, the patient may be exposed to the circulatory effects of endotoxin, namely, progressive pooling of blood within tissue capillary beds, producing a further decrease in venous return. Usually, there is evidence of increased adrenergic activity—sweating, tachycardia, and cutaneous vasoconstriction (i.e., cold moist skin, mottled and cyanotic extremities).

With adequate replacement of blood volume, cardiac output may be maintained above normal.[174] Cardiac output of two or even three times normal may be required to satisfy the increased metabolic needs of the body in the presence of infection. Failure to sustain increased cardiac output results in progressive lactic acidosis, oliguria, hypotension, and ultimately death if the infection cannot be controlled.

Respiratory. The intraperitoneal inflammation results in relatively high and fixed diaphragms and considerable pain on respiration. This results in basilar atelectasis with intrapulmonary shunting of blood. Satisfactory compensation is possible only if the increase in energy demands does not exceed the respiratory reserve. Heavy cigarette smoking, chronic bronchitis, emphysema, and obesity compound the problem. With decompensation in respiratory function, hypoxemia is accompanied first by hypocapnia (respiratory alkalosis) and later by hypercapnia (respiratory acidosis). In some patients, pulmonary edema develops, due not to left ventricular failure but perhaps to increased pulmonary capillary leakage as a consequence of hypoalbuminemia or direct effects of bacterial toxins (adult respiratory distress syndrome). In these patients, progressive hypoxemia develops with decreasing pulmonary compliance. This requires volume-cycled ventilatory assistance with increasingly higher concentrations of inspired oxygen and positive end-expiratory pressure.

Renal. Low renal perfusion may be followed by acute tubular necrosis and progressive azotemia.

Metabolic. During the first few days, the excretion of cortisol is increased and subsequently returns to normal.[175] The increased energy demands of infection rapidly deplete body stores of glycogen, followed by catabolism of protein (muscle) and fat, thus accounting for the rapid weight loss of severely infected patients. Prolonged intra-abdominal infection is associated with extreme wasting. Heat production may eventually fail, and body temperature then falls. Exhaustion and death may ensue.

Clinical Manifestations. SYMPTOMS. The early manifestations of peritonitis secondary to disease of abdominal viscera are frequently those of the primary disease process. Moderately severe abdominal pain is almost always the predominant symptom. The pain is aggravated by any motion, even respiration. The progression of abdominal pain is a function of the rate of dissemination of the material producing the pain stimulus. Rupture of a peptic ulcer with massive spillage of gastric contents produces severe epigastric pain that, within minutes, may spread to involve the entire abdomen. In contrast, the spread of pain from a lesion such as a ruptured appendix is much more gradual. Decreased intensity and extent of pain with time usually suggest localization of the inflammatory process.

Anorexia, nausea, and vomiting commonly accompany abdominal pain. Patients may also complain of feverishness, sometimes with chill, thirst, scanty urination, inability to pass feces or flatus, and abdominal distension.

The formation and progression of an intraperitoneal abscess is often gradual: The patient who seemed to be recoving from peritonitis or an abdominal operation stops improving; fever returns, and localizing symptoms may develop.

PHYSICAL FINDINGS. Patients with fully developed peritonitis have a characteristic appearance, the *Hippocratic* facies, including "a sharp nose, hollow eyes, collapsed temples; the ears cold, contracted and their lobes turned out; the skin about the forehead being rough, distended and parched; the color of the whole face being brown, black, livid, lead-colored." Patients with peritonitis characteristically lie quietly in bed, supine, with the knees flexed and with frequent limited intercostal respirations, since any motion intensifies the abdominal pain. Early in the course the patient is alert, restless, and irritable, but later may become apathetic or delerious.

Body temperatures may reach 42°C. Subnormal temperatures in the range of 35°C often seen in the early stages of chemical peritonitis and late in the course of patients with continuing intra-abdominal sepsis or septic shock and are a grave sign.

Increasing tachycardia with weak, thready peripheral pulses reflects decreased effective blood volume. The blood pressure is maintained within normal limits early in the disease process. As peritonitis progresses, the blood pressure lowers to shock levels. Respiration is increasingly rapid and shallow.

Marked abdominal tenderness to palpation is present, usually maximally over the organ in which the process originated. Rebound tenderness, both direct and referred, signifies parietal peritoneal irritation. This finding is sometimes more accurate than direct palpation in locating the point of maximal tenderness as well as in delineating the extent of peritoneal irritation.

Muscular rigidity of the abdominal wall is produced both by voluntary guarding and by reflex muscular spasm. Hyperresonance due to gaseous intestinal distension can usually be demonstrated by percussion. Pneumoperitoneum from a ruptured hollow viscus may produce decreased liver dullness to percussion. Bowel sounds, initially hypoactive, later disappear. Rectal and vaginal examination may reveal tenderness and the presence of a pelvic abscess and may indicate a primary focus in the female pelvic organs.

Abdominal pain and muscle spasm may be deceptively absent in some patients. Those with lax abdominal musculature (e.g., patients in the postpartum period, patients with ascites due to cirrhosis, patients with marked cachexia) may not have abdominal rigidity. Similarly, patients in shock, on glucocorticosteroid therapy, or in whom loculated intra-abdominal abscesses are not in contact with the anterior abdominal wall (e.g., subphrenic, lesser sac, pelvic) may not exhibit marked abdominal pain and spasm. Absent bowel sounds may be the only manifestation of peritonitis in such patients, and a high index of suspicion is necessary.

Diagnostic Studies. The differential diagnosis in patients with symptoms and signs of peritonitis includes pneumonia, sickle cell anemia, herpes zoster, diabetic ketoacidosis, tabes dorsalis, porphyria, familial Mediterranean fever, plumbism, lupus erythematosus, and uremia.

A peripheral blood leukocyte count of 17,000–25,000 white blood cells/mm^3 is usual in acute peritonitis, the differential count showing polymorphonuclear predominance and a moderate to marked shift to the left. However, reliance on the significance of the total white blood cell count may be misleading. Massive peritoneal inflammation may mobilize leukocytes into the diseased area, so there may be, for example, fewer than 5000 white blood cells/mm^3 in the circulating blood, but the differential smear in this situation may show an extreme shift to immature polymorphonuclear forms.

Hemoconcentration and dehydration are reflected by elevated hematocrit and blood urea nitrogen values. Hyperglycemia and glycosuria usually are not present in peritonitis but may be seen in diabetic acidosis and acute pancreatitis, which may manifest with signs suggesting peritonitis. Hematuria and pyuria without bacteriuria may reflect intra-abdominal inflammatory disease such as appendicitis adjacent to the urinary tract. Elevated serum amylase levels may be seen in peritonitis due to almost any cause, but very high levels are only seen in acute pancreatitis. Hyponatremia may be seen in patients given water to replace isotonic fluid losses but is also characteristic of porphyria. Acidosis, both metabolic and respiratory, is present in severe and late peritonitis. Supine, upright, and lateral decubitis x-ray films of the abdomen may reveal distension of both the small intestine and the colon with adynamic loops of bowel or features of mechanical intestinal obstruction, volulus, intussusception, or vascular occlusion. Inflammatory exudate and edema of the intestinal wall produces a widening of the space between adjacent loops. Peritoneal fat lines and psoas shadows may be obliterated. Free air may be visible if there is a ruptured viscus. Chest x-ray films should always be taken to rule out a pulmonary or thoracic problem as the cause of the abdominal distress. The presence of air beneath the diaphragm may be best defined in these pictures. Trapped gas with a fluid level or mottling due to gas may also be visible in intraperitoneal or visceral abscesses. Calcification in the gallbladder or other organs may also be noted on x-ray films.

Needle aspiration of the peritoneal cavity is often helpful. If no fluid can be aspirated, peritoneal lavage with Ringer's lactate solution should be done to obtain fluid for examination. In performing a tap, the region of abdominal scars where bowel may be adherent to the underside of the scar should be avoided. The aspirate is examined grossly for content of blood, pus, bile, or digested fat; chemically, for amylase content; and microscopically, with Gram stain, for bacteria. A positive tap is meaningful; a dry or negative tap is of little significance. Guidance for the tap may be obtained by ultrasound or CT scan.

Prognosis. Survival of a patient with secondary peritonitis depends on many factors, including the age of the patient, the duration of peritoneal contamination, the presence of foreign material (bile or pancreatic secretions, barium), the primary intra-abdominal process, and the microorganisms involved.[176] Altemeier[91] has shown that the more organisms present in peritoneal exudate, the worse the prognosis, although there was no correlation between severity of infection and any particular organism. Mortality increases with more distal gastrointestinal sources of contamination.[177] The age of the patient also influences the mortality from peritonitis. In the very young patient, because of the relatively small omentum, the walling-off process is less effective, so diffuse peritonitis occurs more frequently than in the adult. In the elderly, preexisting conditions such as emphysema, diabetes, or cardiovascular disease reduce the capacity of the patient to meet the demands on the cardiovascular, respiratory, and renal systems during this period of intense metabolic activity.[176] Mortality rates range from 3.5 percent in those with early infection following penetrating abdominal trauma to more than 60 percent in patients with established intra-abdominal infection and secondary organ failure.[178] Persistent peritoneal contamination, leakage of pancreatic enzymes, septicemia, fluid and electrolyte abnormalities, and cardiovascular, renal, and respiratory failure are the principal causes of death.

Treatment. ANTIMICROBIAL THERAPY. Secondary peritonitis is typically polymicrobial, and the pathogens in the majority of patients with secondary peritonitis are derived from the gastrointestinal tract even in patients with a primary gynecologic process. Typically, the facultative microorganisms are *E. coli, Klebsiella/Enterobacter* spp., *Proteus* spp., and enterococci, and the obligate anaerobes are *B. fragilis, B. melaninogenicus,*

Peptococcus, Peptostreptococcus, Fusobacterium, Eubacterium lentum, and *Clostridium*. Other less commonly isolated pathogens include *Staph. aureus, P. aeruginosa,* and *Candida*.

The role of antimicrobial therapy in the outcome of infection due to anaerobes or due to a mixture of anaerobes and facultative microorganisms is extremely difficult to assess. This is primarily because of the often dramatic response to surgical drainage and débridement alone when there is localized infection. Nevertheless, appropriate antimicrobial therapy has been shown to reduce significantly mortality among patients with bacteremic infections due to Bacteroidaceae or Enterobacteriaceae.[104,179,180] Antimicrobial drugs are expected to control bacteremia and early metastatic foci of infection, to reduce suppurative complications if given early, and to prevent local spread of existing infection. Once suppuration has occurred, it may be difficult to cure the infection if antimicrobial drugs are used without drainage; also, antimicrobial drugs used alone may mask some of the clinical manifestations of abscess formation. Evidence is accumulating, however, that some intra-abdominal abscesses can be treated successfully with antibiotics alone.[181,182]

Antimicrobial therapy should be started immediately after appropriate specimens (e.g., blood and peritoneal fluid) are obtained for culture. This means that antimicrobial therapy is often started before the completion of in vitro antimicrobial sensitivity testing of the specific facultative pathogens. In addition, rapid isolation, identification, and in vitro sensitivity testing of anaerobes, in contrast to testing of facultatives, are often not possible in many community hospitals. Several factors account for the delay in obtaining anaerobic bacteriologic results. For example, infections due to anaerobes are frequently caused by mixtures of five or more microorganisms, and cultures require long periods for growth and isolation. In addition, in vitro sensitivity testing by the conventional disk diffusion technique has not been standardized for anaerobes.[153] Such tests are influenced to a large extent by the growth rate of the bacteria, inoculum size, pH and type of medium, duration of incubation, and CO_2 concentration in the atmosphere.[183,184] In vitro studies of the stability of the β-lactam antibiotics when exposed to reducing agents such as mercaptoamines (cysteine), which are frequently incorporated in media used for the growth of anaerobes, have shown that these compounds are able to open the β-lactam ring and to inactivate penicillins.[185] However, susceptibility of anaerobic organisms can be reliably determined by the broth or agar dilution techniques with appropriate media.[186] Because these tests are generally performed by research laboratories, knowledge of the antimicrobial susceptibility of anaerobes is gained from periodically published reports on anaerobic isolates by centers that specialize in performing these tests. Therefore, initial chemotherapy is usually empiric, based on the use of the most reliable and least toxic antimicrobial agents for the most probable anaerobic and facultative pathogens. In vitro sensitivity reports (usually reliable only for the facultative or aerobic organisms) allows subsequent adjustment of the initial regimen to more specific therapy.

Because these infections are commonly polymicrobial, a broad spectrum of antimicrobial activity is required. Drugs active against anaerobic bacteria may be quite inactive against the accompanying aerobic or facultative pathogens in the mixed infections, and vice versa. For this reason, combinations of usually two or three drugs are used. These combinations of antimicrobial agents are selected for their activity against most of the more virulent pathogens in the infective mixture (e.g., the Enterobacteriaceae and *B. fragilis*). The Enterobacteriaceae in the mixture are significant and frequently cause bacteremia in these patients, as in the rat model of intra-abdominal infection of Onderdonk et al.[170] However, antibiotics need not be active against every pathogen isolated. It is apparent that if only some of the organisms can be eliminated, the synergistic effect may be removed, and the patient's defenses may be able to eradicate the remaining organisms. For example, clindamycin alone (which has no activity against Enterobacteriaceae and enterococci) has been reported to be sufficient treatment for some patients with infections resulting from a mixture of Enterobacteriaceae, enterococci, and anaerobes.[187] Experimental evidence in the rat model of intraperitoneal infection suggests that the enterococcus is not a primary pathogen, although in the presence of anaerobes it may aid in abscess formation.[188] In several clinical studies of anaerobic infections, patients were treated successfully with both gentamicin and clindamycin despite absence of activity of this therapeutic regimen against enterococci.[189,190] However, more recent reviews emphasize the role of the enterococcus in intra-abdominal infections.[191] In some reports, this organism has been noted to emerge as the sole intra-abdominal pathogen, at times associated with enterococcal bacteremia,[192,193] especially if patients with polymicrobial intra-abdominal infection were treated with an antimicrobial agent that lacked activity against the enterococcus.[194,195]

When combinations of antibiotics are used, synergism or antagonism may occur. Chloramphenicol has been shown to impair early bactericidal activity of gentamicin in vitro, and antagonism was demonstrated in mice with experimental *Proteus mirabilis* infection when phagocytic function was impaired (i.e., in neutropenic mice).[196] Two recent studies suggest that clindamycin inhibits early in vitro killing of *E. coli* and *K. pneumoniae* by gentamicin.[197] However, in an in vivo study of aminoglycoside therapy of *E. coli* peritonitis and bacteremia in normal and neutropenic mice, prior or simultaneous administration of clindamycin with the aminoglycoside did not inhibit the therapeutic effect of the aminoglycoside.[198] Clindamycin combined in vitro with gentamicin has been reported to have indifferent or synergistic activity against Enterobacteriaceae after 18 hours of incubation.[199] The activities of various antimicrobial agents against the usual peritoneal pathogens and the results of various clinical trials are discussed in the sections that follow.

Chloramphenicol. At a concentration of 16 μg/ml, chloramphenicol has activity against over 99 percent of the anaerobic pathogens involved in intra-abdominal infection, especially *B. fragilis*.[200] However, resistant strains may inactivate chloramphenicol, so no chloramphenicol is present in abscesses containing these organisms.[201] Up to 15 percent of the strains of *Bacteroides* may require 16 μg/ml for inhibition, a concentration close to the maximum attainable therapeutic serum levels without encountering the dose-related bone marrow suppressive effect.[200] For this reason, chloramphenicol may be difficult to use because of its toxicity for the hematopoietic tissues, especially with the doses and duration of therapy required for severe anaerobic bacterial infection. In addition, patients treated with chloramphenicol have been reported to have persistent bacteremia due to chloramphenicol-sensitive organisms.[202] Chloramphenicol is active against facultative microorganisms involved in polymicrobial anaerobic infections, such as most *E. coli*, other Enterobacteriaceae, and enterococci, but lacks activity against *P. aeruginosa*. The availability of equally effective and potentially less toxic antimicrobial agents to treat anaerobic infections (e.g., clindamycin, metronidazole, imipenem) has all but eliminated the need for chloramphenicol.[203]

Clindamycin. Clindamycin has been reported to inhibit over 95 percent of the anaerobes, including *B. fragilis*, at a concentration of 8 μg/ml.[200] About 15 percent of the strains of *Clostridium* spp. other than *C. perfringens, Peptococci* spp., and rare strains of *Fusobacterium* spp., have been reported to be resistant to clindamycin. Most strains of *B. fragilis* have remained highly susceptible to clindamycin during the past decade.[204,205] Recently, plasmid-mediated, transferable clindamycin resistance in *B. fragilis* has been demonstrated,[204] and clindamycin resistance among *B. fragilis* may have become a problem at certain medical centers. Clindamycin is active against only certain facultative gram-positive cocci, such as

Staph. aureus and *S. pyogenes*, but not *S. faecalis*, and has virtually no activity against Enterobacteriaceae.

Diarrhea is reported to be the most frequent side effect of clindamycin therapy and occurs at an incidence of 2 to 20 percent.[206] The severity of the diarrhea varies but may be associated with pseudomembranous colitis in up to one-half of the patients with diarrhea, as reported in one study.[207] Toxic megacolon, colonic perforation, and death on rare occasions have been reported. The cause has been attributable to an exotoxin produced by clindamycin-resistant strains of *Clostridium difficile*.[206]

Metronidazole. Metronidazole is active against strict anaerobes, inhibits most *B. fragilis*. *Fusobacterium* spp., and *Clostridium* spp., and has unique bactericidal action against *B. fragilis* and *C. perfringens*.[208] Its in vitro activity, however, is poor against aerobes, microaerophiles, and anaerobes that may become somewhat aerotolerant on subculture (i.e., certain anaerobic gram-positive cocci and sporeless gram-positive rods).[200,209] Despite the poor in vitro activity demonstrated against aerobic and microaerophilic organisms, there is now some in vivo evidence in animal models and humans that metronidazole has activity against *E. coli* and other aerobes in mixed aerobic-anaerobic infections.[210,211] The mechanism for this is poorly understood but may be related to the conversion by *B. fragilis* of metronidazole into active metabolites with activity against *E. coli* and other aerobes.[210] Nonetheless, metronidazole should be used clinically in combination with other antimicrobial agents in the treatment of mixed infections.

Tetracyclines. Sutter et al.[212] noted that while 14 of 15 strains of *B. fragilis* isolated before 1960 were sensitive to tetracycline, only 24 of 63 strains isolated after 1970 were susceptible. Tetracycline similarly has poor activity against many other anaerobes.

Doxycycline and minocycline[213] have been reported to be more active than tetracycline against anaerobic bacteria. However, their activity is relatively poor against *B. fragilis, Clostridum* spp., and anaerobic gram-positive cocci.[213] The large number of resistant anaerobes, especially *B. fragilis*, precludes the use of these drugs as initial therapy.

Cephalosporin. *Bacteroides fragilis* and other *Bacteroides* species are usually resistant to the so-called first-generation cephalosporins (e.g., cefazolin) and to some second-generation cephalosporins (e.g., cefamandole, cefuroxime). However, cefoxitin is distinctly more active than any of the other second-generation cephalosporins against *Bacteroides* species.[200,214,215] Cefotetan has activity similar to that of cefoxitin, except that it is less active against the *B. fragilis* group (not including *B. fragilis*).[214,215] These first- and second-generation cephalosporins are also active against the majority of the strains of *E. coli*, *P. mirabilis*, and *K. pneumoniae*. The third-generation cephalosporins (e.g., cefotaxime, ceftizoxime, cefoperazone, ceftriaxone, and ceftazidime) have demonstrated significantly better activity against the Enterobacteriaceae, including *Enterobacter* and *Serratia* species. Only ceftazidime, and less so cefoperazone, have activity against *P. aeruginosa*. With a few exceptions, the third-generation cephalosporins have relatively poor activity against *B. fragilis* and other *Bacteroides* species.[216] Moxalactam, an oxacephem with good activity against *B. fragilis*, has been found to be an effective single agent in the treatment of intra-abdominal infections.[217,218] The potential for bleeding secondary to the use of moxalactam has greatly limited its utility.[219] Ceftizoxime is reported to have good in vitro activity against *B. fragilis* and other *Bacteroides* species in some studies,[215,220] but has been found to be inadequate against *Bacteroides* species, including *B. fragilis*, in other in vitro studies.[214,221] Because the activity of ceftizoxime is greatly affected by the inoculum of *Bacteroides* in in vitro studies,[200] this antibiotic would most likely be inadequate in treating severe intra-abdominal infections where the inoculum of organisms is great.

Penicillins. Penicillin G and ampicillin have excellent activity against all anaerobes, with the exception of *Bacteroides* spp. (especially *B. fragilis*) and *Fusobacterium* spp. other than *F. nucleatum*. Ampicillin also is active against 70–80 percent of the strains of *E. coli* and almost all *P. mirabilis*. Although *B. fragilis* has been considered to be resistant to penicillins, in vitro sensitivity testing reveals that over 90 percent of *B. fragilis* isolates may be sensitive to carbenicillin, ticarcillin, mezlocillin, and piperacillin in concentrations of ≤125 μg/ml. In fact, these antibiotics have been reported to be rapidly bactericidal against *B. fragilis*.[222,223] The clinical experience with these broad-spectrum penicillins in the treatment of anaerobic bacterial infection has been reported to be favorable.[224,225] A prospective controlled study has shown that the therapeutic response to ticarcillin was similar to that of clindamycin or chloramphenicol, each in combination with an aminoglycoside in the therapy of intra-abdominal infection.[226]

Because sensitive strains of *B. fragilis* may require up to 125 μg of the broad-spectrum penicillins per milliliter for inhibition, these antibiotics should be used in high dosages (300–500 mg/kg/day) to treat these infections. However, because up to 20 percent of the strains of *B. fragilis* are resistant to concentrations of the broad-spectrum penicillins[227] that can be achieved in serum, use of the broad-spectrum penicillins as the initial therapy for suspected *B. fragilis* infection should be undertaken with caution. In addition, there is some evidence to suggest that penicillin G may fail to achieve concentrations at the site of *B. fragilis* infection, because of both a reduction in penetration of penicillin into infected sites and inactivation of the drug by *B. fragilis*.[228] It is unknown if this is also true for broad-spectrum penicillins. Therapeutic failures despite high doses of penicillin for *B. fragilis* bacteremia have been well documented.[101] Resistance of *B. fragilis* to penicillins is frequently due to production of β-lactamase.[229]

The spectrum of antibacterial activity of the older broad-spectrum penicillins (e.g., carbenicillin, ticarcillin) includes the majority of aerobic gram-negative bacilli (including *P. aeruginosa*) commonly isolated from patients with intra-abdominal infections with the exception of most *Klebsiella* and many *Serratia* spp. However, these penicillins are considerably less active than ampicillin and penicillin G against enterococci. The newer broad-spectrum penicillins (e.g., mezlocillin, azlocillin, piperacillin) are more active than carbenicillin and ticarcillin against the Enterobacteriaceae group, including many strains of *Klebsiella*, and against *P. aeruginosa* and enterococci.[230]

The combination of a β-lactamase inhibitor, such as clavulanic acid or sulbactam, with a penicillin increases the activity of the penicillin against certain β-lactamase producers.[231,232] Ticarcillin-clavulanic acid inhibits 60–80 percent of ticarcillin-resistant strains of Enterobacteriaceae, including most *E. coli* and *Klebsiella* spp., as well as all β-lactamase-producing *Bacteroides* species.[233] However, the combination will not inhibit the inducible β-lactamase produced by *P. aeruginosa, Serratia* spp., *Citrobacter freundii* or *Enterobacter cloacae*.[234] Ampicillin-sulbactam is active against many bacteria resistant to ampicillin, including *E. coli, Klebsiella*, and *Bacteroides* spp.[235,236]

Other β-Lactams. Imipenem, a carbapenem antibiotic, has the broadest antimicrobial spectrum of any current antibiotic,[237] with activity against almost all aerobic and anaerobic bacteria. It is resistant to most β-lactamases except those produced by rare strains of *B. fragilis*.[238] Aztreonam, a monobactam antibiotic, has a spectrum of activity limited to aerobic gram-negative bacilli.[239] It would be necessary to use an antibiotic with anaerobic activity (e.g., clindamycin, metronidazole) along with aztreonam in the treatment of secondary intra-abdominal infections.

Aminoglycosides. Aminoglycosides, except for their excellent spectrum of activity against Enterobacteriaceae and *P. aeruginosa*, do not have much advantage over penicillins or cephalosporins against sensitive strains of these organisms for many reasons. For example, the serum concentrations of gentamicin are unpredictable after a dose based on the body weight, so peak and trough serum levels must be confirmed by any of various assay methods available.[240] In addition, the therapeutic range of peak serum concentrations of 4–8 μg/ml is narrow: levels below 4 μg/ml may likely be below the inhibiting concentration for the pathogen, and levels greater than 10–12 μg/ml may be toxic. Thus, the peak serum levels are either equal to or only slightly greater than the minimum inhibitory concentration (MIC) for the aminoglycoside in vitro.

Aminoglycosides are inactive against obligate anaerobes, and their activity against sensitive pathogens is antagonized by an anaerobic environment.[241] and by reducing substances such as sulfhydryl compounds. Aminoglycosides are also not active in acidic conditions. Both anaerobic and acidic conditions are frequently present in intra-abdominal abscesses. The penicillins and cephalosporins, by contrast, are relatively nontoxic, can be used in concentrations that are many times the MIC for the pathogen, and are active under anaerobic or acidic conditions. For these reasons, the penicillins and cephalosporins are probably more reliable antibiotics than the aminoglycosides against sensitive pathogens. Therefore, if indicated on the basis of in vitro sensitivity testing, penicillins or cephalosporins should be used in preference to aminoglycosides.

Quinolones. The fluoroquinolones (e.g., norfloxacin, ciprofloxacin, enoxacin, ofloxacin) are a new class of antimicrobial agents related to nalidixic acid.[242] They are active against almost all aerobic gram-negative bacilli and most gram-positive cocci, including some enterococci.[243] Their ability to kill bacteria in the stationary phase of growth, along with the lack of development of plasmid-mediated resistance, make the fluoroquinolones potentially valuable antimicrobial agents for the treatment of intra-abdominal infections including abscesses. Current limitations of these agents include the need to administer them orally (though parenteral forms will be available in the future) and the relatively low serum drug concentrations in relation to the potency of some of these agents (e.g., norfloxacin). The addition of an antimicrobial agent active against anaerobic bacteria would be required if the use of a quinolone was considered for secondary intra-abdominal infection.

Controlled Clinical Trials. There is no one antimicrobial regimen applicable to every clinical situation. However, it is clear that for an antimicrobial regimen to be efficacious in the treatment of secondary peritonitis and other intra-abdominal infections, the agents chosen must have significant antibacterial activity against *B. fragilis* and enteric gram-negative bacilli.[244–246] Therapy with an agent with activity against *P. aeruginosa* would be desired if the infectious process developed while in the hospital or after a course of broad-spectrum antibiotics. The need to add specific agents active against the enterococcus remains controversial.[191] Although the results of many antimicrobial trials for treatment of intra-abdominal infections have been published, caution must be exercised when interpreting these studies because of the possibility of inadequate study design and analysis of data.[247] Some of the variables that must be considered are (*1*) differences in patient populations, (*2*) types and severity of underlying illnesses, (*3*) community- vs. hospital-acquired infection, and (*4*) the pathogens isolated.

The standard antimicrobial regimen against which most new regimens are compared is an aminoglycoside in combination with clindamycin.[248–250] The risk of renal toxicity and ototoxicity, along with the need to monitor serum aminoglycoside levels, may limit the use of aminoglycosides as newer agents prove to be useful alternatives.[251] Table 1 lists many of the antimicrobials regimens that have been found to be efficacious for the treatment of intra-abdominal infections in clinical trials. The majority of second- or third-generation cephalosporins have limited activity against the *B. fragilis* group, and their use as single antimicrobial agents for the treatment of intra-abdominal infections has had variable results.[97,262–265] However, combining one of these cephalosporins with clindamycin or metronidazole would likely be an adequate antimicrobial regimen in this setting.[266]

TABLE 1. Comparative Antimicrobial Trials for Treatment of Intra-Abdominal Infections

Regimen	*Reference*
Cefoxitin ± aminoglycoside vs. clindamycin + aminoglycoside	252–254
Moxalactam vs. clindamycin + aminoglycoside	218
Moxalactam vs. cefoxitin + aminoglycoside	255
Ticarcillin + aminoglycoside vs. clindamycin + aminoglycoside	217
Piperacillin vs. cefoxitin	256
Ampicillin-sulbactam vs. clindamycin + aminoglycoside	257
Imipenem vs. clindamycin + aminoglycoside	258–260
Aztreonam + clindamycin vs. clindamycin + aminoglycoside	261

Although the need for treatment is controversial,[267,268] clearly *Candida* species, either as part of a polymicrobial peritoneal infection or as a single isolate, have the potential to cause peritonitis, intraperitoneal abscesses, and subsequent candidemia.[128,269] The dominant clinical view today favors aggressive early therapy of all intra-abdominal isolates of *Candida* species in symptomatic patients with peritonitis, usually with the parenteral administration of at least 375–500 mg amphotericin B over 10–14 days.[270]

The duration of therapy is usually prolonged to prevent relapse because host defenses cannot be relied on to eradicate completely the pathogens from sequestered areas of extensive tissue necrosis and abscess formation. Not all these areas are accessible to adequate surgical drainage. Antibiotic therapy should be given before, during, and after surgery to ensure tissue and blood drug levels that can combat local and metastatic spread of the infection. The dose, the frequency, and usually the route of administration of the antimicrobial agents are maintained to achieve adequate blood and tissue drug concentrations during the entire treatment period and are not necessarily changed as the patient improves.

The intravenous route of antibiotic administration is preferred, especially in shock, when poor perfusion of the gut and muscle preclude use of the oral or intramuscular routes. Blood levels may be less satisfactory after intramuscular administration of certain antibiotics, for example, chloramphenicol. Although some surgeons use antibiotics intraperitoneally at the time of operation in irrigating fluid,[271] others do not.[272] Decreases in the rate of wound infection but not in the rate of intraperitoneal sepsis have been shown with the use of intraperitoneal irrigation.[273] Respiratory arrest may occur after peritoneal absorption of aminoglycosides, and lavage of the peritoneal cavity at the time of surgery with large amounts of saline alone may be sufficient.[274] Also, intravenous or intramuscular antibiotics in adequate doses reach the peritoneum without additional intraperitoneal administration.

The effect of irrigation of the peritoneal cavity with agents such as povidone-iodine has also been studied. In one study, there was a decreased frequency of intra-abdominal abscess formation in the povidone-iodine group compared to that of the saline group.[275] However, povidone-iodine has been shown to be a potent inactivator of such neutrophil functions as chemotaxis and phagocytosis, and thus may have a detrimental effect.[276]

Another technique is to place a plastic catheter through the abdominal wall at the time of the operation so that antibiotics can be injected directly postoperatively into the peritoneal cavity. The method is said to be beneficial clinically,[277] but its superiority over intravenous antibiotics alone has not been proven in clinical peritonitis. Recent comparative studies showed no significant difference in clinical outcome between patients who had irrigation of the peritoneal cavity and those who did not.[278,279] However, when peritoneal dialysis is being done in the presence of peritonitis, antibiotics in therapeutic doses should be included in the dialysis fluid to maintain antibiotic levels in the rapidly exchanged peritoneal fluid.[280] If intraperitoneal antibiotics are used, systemic antibiotics may be necessary as well to maintain adequate blood levels.

HYPERBARIC OXYGEN. Increased oxygen tension attainable with hyperbaric oxygen therapy inhibits and kills *C. perfringens*[281] and reduces the production of *C. perfringens* α-toxin. Hyperbaric oxygenation has been used clinically and experimentally for clostridial myonecrosis, with some reported success.[282] Because *C. perfringens* is a relatively oxygen-tolerant anaerobe in comparison to other obligate anaerobic pathogens, it would be reasonable to assume that hyperbaric oxygen therapy would be at least equally efficacious with anaerobic infections due to these more oxygen-sensitive anaerobes. Except for a few reports[283] almost no clinical or experimental data, however, are available. Hill[284] reported suppression of experimental liver abscesses due to anaerobes in mice treated with hyperbaric oxygen therapy alone. In a more recent study, it appeared that the use of hyperbaric oxygen therapy favorably affected the outcome of experimental sepsis in a rat model, perhaps by enhancing host defense mechanisms.[285] Consideration should also be given to the hazards of hyperbaric oxygen therapy.

GASTROINTESTINAL DRAINAGE. In the presence of peritonitis, the patient should receive nothing by mouth. If no distension is present when treatment is instituted, continuous gastric suction is usually sufficient. For those patients who are distended when treatment is started and for those who become distended in spite of gastric drainage, small intestinal intubation should be instituted.

WATER AND ELECTROLYTE ADMINISTRATION. The type of fluid replacement is determined in large part by the chemical abnormalities found. In general, hypovolemia, dehydration, and metabolic acidosis predominate, so plasma or albumin, Ringer's lactate solution, and 5% dextrose in water usually suffice. The amount to be given in the 2- to 4-hour period before anticipated surgery is determined by watching vital signs, hematocrit values, hourly urinary output, and central venous pressure.

BLOOD AND PLASMA TRANSFUSION. Although many patients recover from an illness satisfactorily with a hemoglobin of 8 or 10 g/dl, some surgeons recommend that the patient be transfused to maintain levels as high as 12–13 g/dl in order to provide a margin of safety should some complication such as septic shock or upper gastrointestinal hemorrhage supervene.

RESPIRATORY SUPPORT. Fluid sequestered in the abdomen and loops of bowel distended by gas may elevate the diaphragm. Inflammation of the parietal peritoneum, including the diaphragmatic surface, leads to guarding and splinting of the muscular wall, which interferes with deep breathing or coughing. A subphrenic abscess may be responsible for splinting of the diaphragm. Retained bronchial secretions may lead to atelectasis and subsequent pneumonitis. These factors that impair the ability to augment respiratory exchange in the face of the increased expenditure of energy required by the inflammatory process produce hypoxemia and respiratory alkalosis. When the patient tires, the combination of metabolic and respiratory acidosis may develop and prove fatal.

Arterial blood gas studies are necessary to detect and quantitate respiratory decompensation. Measures aimed primarily at gastrointestinal decompression, elevation of the head of the bed, and control of the inflammation may sufficiently improve respiration. Administration of oxygen may improve arterial oxygen saturation. If these measures are inadequate, endotracheal intubation or tracheostomy should be done without delay. A volume-cycled respirator should be used and adjusted to give a P_{O_2} of 80–100 mmHg and a normal pH. If the P_{CO_2} is not then normal, metabolic acidosis or alkalosis may need to be treated. As the intra-abdominal process subsides, the patient may be able to breathe spontaneously again and may be weaned from the ventilator. In certain severe cases, positive end-expiratory pressure may also be necessary.

OPERATIVE APPROACH. The aims of an operation for spreading peritonitis are to stop continuing contamination, to remove foreign material from the peritoneal cavity, and to provide drainage of purulent collections. Operation is generally not indicated (*1*) in primary peritonitis, (*2*) in moribund patients who continue to deteriorate despite vigorous supportive therapy, (*3*) in patients in whom the disease process subsides and localizes while they are being prepared for surgery, (*4*) in patients with peritonitis secondary to hemorrhagic pancreatitis, and (*5*) in patients with peritonitis secondary to pelvic inflammatory disease, since this usually responds to nonsurgical therapy.

There is general agreement as to the necessity of (*1*) removing all material, such as necrotic tissue, feces, and blood, from the operative field, since the virulence of peritoneal infections is enhanced by the presence of these substances, (*2*) eliminating any possible anaerobic conditions, and (*3*) reducing the bacterial count to a minimum. Also, in acute diffuse peritonitis, recent studies have clearly shown that copious peritoneal irrigation with isotonic saline or Ringer's lactate solution significantly reduces mortality and morbidity.[274] In localized infection, local drainage alone is adequate because the risk of disseminating infection outweighs any possible benefit of removing foreign material that may have escaped mechanical removal.

Use of multiple drains for drainage of the general peritoneal cavity is physically impossible since exudate and adhesions rapidly isolate and occlude the drains and may increase secondary infections.[286] However, drains are often placed in a dependent point to which fluid can be expected to gravitate or in an area of devitalized tissue that cannot be removed.

Prevention. Prevention of postoperative peritonitis requires avoiding contamination of the peritoneum with gastrointestinal or vaginal secretions. In addition to using good surgical technique, this can be accomplished by early treatment of a primary intra-abdominal infection. For example, Leigh et al. noted that the rate of wound infection in patients with perforated appendix was over 50 percent if no antimicrobial therapy was used and 15 percent in the group given appropriate therapy.[287] Similarly, two studies demonstrate the efficacy of early use of antibiotics in penetrating wounds of the abdomen, especially involving the colon.[288,289] Surgeons have also used various means to reduce the complex gastrointestinal or vaginal flora before clean, contaminated surgery. Mechanical cleansing of the bowel with a low-residue diet and then a liquid diet, cathartics, and enemas can reduce the total fecal mass and coliform count in the colon, although not necessarily the predominant anaerobic flora.[290] The use of oral antibiotics preoperatively to reduce bowel flora is well accepted. *Escherichia coli* in the colonic flora is sensitive to either oral neomycin or kanamycin, whereas *B. fragilis* frequently is sensitive to erythromycin or metronidazole. Thus, combinations such as neomycin-erythromycin base have been shown to be effective in reducing total bowel flora preoperatively and decreasing the incidence of postoperative infection.[291]

Parenteral antibiotics have also been used in gastrointestinal and vaginal surgery prophylactically when there is a chance of contamination with normal microflora at the operative site (clean, contaminated surgery). Up to 30 percent of these types of operations may be complicated by infections. These involve cutting through the large bowel without significant spillage; compromising the blood supply of the large bowel; cutting through stomach or small bowel when there is anticipated intraluminal bacterial overgrowth; appendectomy for appendicitis without rupture; penetrating wounds of the abdomen; gallbladder surgery in the elderly; cesarian section after rupture of the membranes and labor; vaginal hysterectomy in the premenopausal woman; and radical pelvic surgery for gynecologic malignancy.[292] Several studies have shown significant reduction in the frequency of postoperative infection from about 20–30 percent to about 4–8 percent after prophylactic antibiotic use in clean, contaminated surgery.[293,294] The basic principle of antibiotic prophylaxis is to provide adequate tissue levels at the site of contamination and blood levels during the procedure and for possibly up to 24 hours after the procedure.

Peritonitis During Peritoneal Dialysis

Chronic Peritoneal Dialysis. Peritoneal dialysis has been used successfully to treat uremia in patients with end-stage renal disease since the mid-1940s. Peritonitis was a frequently associated side effect that hindered the acceptance of chronic peritoneal dialysis until an improved access catheter was developed by Tenckhoff in 1968. This catheter significantly decreased the incidence of peritonitis, but initial reports of patients undergoing chronic ambulatory peritoneal dialysis (CAPD) with this catheter had peritonitis rates of more than six episodes per patient-year.[295,296] This rate has appeared to decline with the introduction of collapsible plastic bags, improved adapters, and better techniques. However, peritonitis remains the major complication of CAPD today.[297] It occurs at a rate of about one episode per patient a year, with a range from three or more episodes a year to less than one every 2 years. Forty-five percent of CAPD patients develop peritonitis at least once during their initial 6 months on CAPD. This increases to 60–70 percent during the first year.[298–300] Recurrent peritonitis occurs in 20–30 percent of patients and is one of the most common reasons for discontinuation of CAPD.[301] A small proportion of patients seem to have an unusually high frequency of peritonitis.[302] This disparity in the frequency of infection has been attributed, at least in part, to faulty sterile technique on the part of the patient when self-administering CAPD.

The origin of infection in most cases appears to be contamination of the catheter by common skin organisms.[296] Alterations of skin flora in CAPD patients[303] may lead to peritoneal contamination with enteric pathogens. A higher incidence of peritonitis has been reported in dialysis patients who are nasal carriers of *Staph. aureus*.[304] Pathogens may also contaminate the peritoneum from exit-site and subcutaneous-tunnel infections, transient bacteremia, and contamination of the dialysate delivery system during bag exchanges. As mentioned previously, it has been demonstrated that enteric bacteria may also gain access to the peritoneal cavity by transmural migration through an intact intestinal wall after the introduction of hypertonic solutions into the peritoneum.[55] This mechanism may account for enteric bacterial peritonitis in dialysis patients.[56] Polymicrobial infection with fecal organisms suggests perforation of the bowel as a complication of catheter placement.

Alterations in peritoneal defenses may increase the risk of peritonitis in CAPD patients. The antimicrobial function of peritoneal macrophages and polymorphonoclear cells generally requires the presence of opsonins. A reduction in the levels of IgG and C3 has been noted in peritoneal dialysis effluents when compared with serum, and the levels of these crucial opsonizing agents are inversely related to the frequency of peritonitis.[305] The addition of IgG to peritoneal dialysis fluid has been found to have a prophylactic effect.[306] Other important factors that impair host defense mechanisms are the low pH and high osmolality of peritoneal dialysis fluid, both of which can impair polymorphonuclear function and antibiotic efficacy.[307]

Gram-positive organisms compose 60–80 percent of isolates, most commonly *Staph. epidermidis* followed by *Staph. aureus, Streptococcus* spp., and diphtheroids. Staphylococcal isolates have been noted to grow on polymer surfaces and frequently produce an extracellular slime substance or biofilm that may protect these bacteria from host defenses.[308] Gram-negative organisms are obtained from 15–30 percent of isolates. *Escherichia coli* is the most common, followed by *Klebsiella/Enterobacter, Proteus*, and *Pseudomonas* spp. Less common pathogens include *Acinetobacter* spp., *C. albicans*, and anaerobic bacteria. Rare isolates include *Mycobacterium tuberculosis, Candida parapsilosis, Aspergillus fumigatus, Nocardia asteroides*, and *Fusarium* spp.[302,309–311]

Diagnosis of peritonitis is made when microorganisms and an increased number of leukocytes are present in the dialysate combined with a constellation of clinical findings that include abdominal pain and tenderness (found in 60–80 percent of patients), nausea and vomiting (in 30 percent), fever (in 10–20 percent), and diarrhea (in 10 percent).[296,302,310,311] However, not all these criteria need to be met to fulfill the diagnosis.

The dialysate is almost always cloudy, and microscopic examination reveals a leukocyte count greater than $100/mm^3$, approximately 85 percent being more than $500/mm^3$, with neutrophils predominating.[302] Gram stain of the fluid reveals organisms in 9–50 percent of cases.[296,302] Peripheral leukocytosis has been reported to be a poor indicator for peritonitis in this group of patients.[310] Blood cultures are rarely positive, in contrast to the 30–50 percent positive rate in other types of intra-abdominal infection.

Peritonitis with negative cultures occurs in 5–10 percent of cases. Constant flow of dialysis fluid into and out of the peritoneal cavity dilutes the microbial density and may falsely lower the rate of positive dialysate culture results. Negative cultures may also be due to infection with fastidious organisms, previous antimicrobial treatment, or inadequate culture technique. One method that has been used to improve the yield of dialysate cultures is the filtration method. A 100 ml aliquot of peritoneal fluid is filtered through a 0.45 μm filter. The filter is then washed with sterile saline and incubated in thioglycolate broth.[310] Rubin et al. compared the filtration method with direct inoculation of blood culture bottles and found no significant difference in positive culture rates.[296] Still others found the inoculation of 2–3 ml of dialysate into thioglycolate broth to be the most sensitive culture technique.[310] A recent study comparing direct inoculation of dialysate into a biphasic blood culture system, direct inoculation of dialysate into routine blood culture bottles, and centrifugation of 50 ml of dialysate and culture of the sediment failed to demonstrate a significant difference among these methods in the recovery of a pathogen.[312] All cultures should be performed aerobically. Fungal, mycobacterial, and anaerobic cultures should be performed if clinically indicated (e.g., negative aerobic cultures).

The prognosis of peritonitis in dialysis patients is generally favorable. A recent large series reported less than 1 percent mortality attributed directly to infection.[302] The duration of illness and positive peritoneal fluid cultures after institution of antimicrobial therapy is usually 1–4 days. However, some infections, especially those due to *Staph. aureus, Pseudomonas*, or fungus, resolve more slowly and may cause relapse more frequently.[310]

Adequate levels of antimicrobial agents necessary to treat peritonitis successfully can be obtained in the peritoneal fluid by both systemic and intraperitoneal routes.[302,309,310,313] However, because CAPD peritonitis is a localized infection, the intraperitoneal route is preferred, as no therapeutic advantage of intravenously administered antibiotic has been demonstrated.[314] Although a variety of doses can be found in the literature, the initial doses recommended in Table 2 for intraperitoneal administration result in effective peritoneal fluid drug concentrations. Subsequent dosing is used to maintain these levels. The aim of the dosing regimen is to maintain a concentration of the drug in the peritoneal cavity fluid above the MIC of the offending pathogen for most if not all of the dosing interval. Caution must be exercised when reviewing the MIC and minimum bactericidal concentration (MBC) data, since these concentrations have been demonstrated to be markedly increased when peritoneal dialysis effluent is used as the in vitro growth medium.[315]

Because of the lack of comparative, prospective clinical trials, no one antimicrobial regimen can be called superior to

TABLE 2. Antibiotic Dosage for Peritonitis during Peritoneal Dialysis

Drug	Intraperitoneal Dosage (mg/liter dialysate)	Intraperitoneal Maintenance Dosage (mg/liter dialysate)
Amphotericin B[a]	0.007 mg/kg[b]	0.07 mg/kg
Ampicillin	7 mg/kg	0.7 mg/kg
Cefazolin	5 mg/kg	1.3 mg/kg
Ceftazidime	7 mg/kg	3.5 mg/kg
Clindamycin	4.3 mg/kg	0.7 mg/kg
Gentamicin	0.9 mg/kg	0.5 mg/kg q24h
Piperacillin	14 mg/kg	1.5 mg/kg
Trimethoprim-sulfamethoxazole	80 mg/400 mg/kg	16 mg/80 mg/kg
Vancomycin	9 mg/kg	0.2 mg/kg

[a] A low dose is used initially with progression to a maintenance dose, guided by tolerance to abdominal pain.
[b] Body weight.
(Adapted from Petersen et al.,[311] with permission.)

another. After cultures are obtained, initial antimicrobial therapy should be based on the Gram stain results or the most likely pathogens if the Gram stain is not helpful. A reasonable initial empiric regimen would be vancomycin in combination with an aminoglycoside. Vancomycin is preferable to a cephalosporin because of the frequency of β-lactam resistance (i.e., methicillin resistance) in staphylococci, which predicts resistance to cephalosporins as well. Initial antibiotic choices should be modified, if necessary, after culture results are obtained. The minimum length of therapy needed for dialysis-related peritonitis has not been determined, but the usual duration ranges from 10 days to 3 weeks. Most patients with CAPD peritonitis show clinical improvement within 48–96 hours of the initiation of antimicrobial therapy. If the signs and symptoms of peritonitis persist after 96 hours of therapy, reevaluation is warranted, with consideration given to the possibilities of resistant pathogens, unusual organisms (e.g., mycobacterial, fungal), and other intra-abdominal processes, as recommended by Keane et al.[314]

Fungal peritonitis, usually caused by *C. albicans*, should be treated with amphotericin B.[316–319] If CAPD is continued, amphotericin B should be given intraperitoneally, but it can cause appreciable abdominal pain when given by this route. However, most patients with fungal CAPD infection will fail to respond unless the catheter is removed. Once the catheter is removed, amphotericin B should be given intravenously (30 mg/day). Flucytosine has also been recommended. However, this drug may be difficult to use in end-stage renal disease because of dose-dependent bone marrow toxicity. If this drug is used, serum levels should be monitored closely to prevent the development of toxic levels (>100 μg/ml). There is limited experience with the use of miconazole and ketoconazole in treating fungal peritonitis.[319–322]

Removal of the catheter may be necessary in 10–20 percent of patients. The indications for removal of the catheter include persistent skin exit site or tunnel infection; fungal, fecal, and mycobacterial peritonitis; *P. aeruginosa* peritonitis; persistent peritonitis; recurrent peritonitis with the same organism; and catheter malfunction (e.g., poor flow). The catheter should also be removed in patients with intraperitoneal abscess. Use of oral or intraperitoneal antibiotics has not been shown to be effective in preventing peritonitis during peritoneal dialysis.[56,323]

Acute Peritoneal Dialysis. The incidence of peritonitis during acute peritoneal dialysis has remained stable during the past 20 years. Innovations in technique, which began during the 1960s, reduced the rate of peritonitis from as high as 50 percent to acceptably low levels. These innovations included closed-drainage systems, small-bore catheters, limitation of dialysis to no longer than 48–72 hours, the incorporation of a millipore filter into the tubing, and the development of closed automatic systems. Also, the use of dry-heat incubators to warm the dialysate decreases the risk of contamination that may occur when water baths are used for this purpose.[324]

Some authorities have recommended that cultures of dialysate be obtained every 8–24 hours during acute peritoneal dialysis and at its termination. Culture of dialysate from the last exchange is more useful than culture of the catheter tip at the end of dialysis because of the frequent contamination of the catheter tip at the time of its removal. However, results of such routine cultures, in the absence of symptoms or cloudy fluid, provide a guide of doubtful value for initiation of therapy. More importantly, dialysate samples should be cultured and examined microscopically (cell count, Gram stain) if the dialysate becomes cloudy or the patient develops signs or symptoms of peritonitis (e.g., fever, abdominal pain). Cultures are best obtained by syringe from the port closest to the catheter.

Peritonitis during acute peritoneal dialysis is frequently caused by antibiotic-resistant, hospital-acquired, gram-negative bacilli. Therefore, it is recommended that therapy be initiated with intraperitoneal vancomycin and gentamicin (or tobramycin), with or without concurrent or subsequent addition of the same antibiotics parenterally, depending on the severity of the illness and the response to initial therapy (see Table 2 for dosages). Modification of the antibiotic regimen should be made when the culture results become available.

The clinical manifestations, prognosis, and response to therapy are similar to those described above for peritonitis associated with chronic peritoneal dialysis.

INTRAPERITONEAL ABSCESSES

Etiology

Intraperitoneal abscess may complicate either primary or secondary peritonitis.[325,326] Diseases causing secondary intraperitoneal abscesses include appendicitis, diverticulitis, biliary tract lesions, pancreatitis, perforated peptic ulcers, inflammatory bowel disease, trauma, and abdominal surgery. The relative frequency of abscess formation associated with appendicitis may be declining, and that of trauma and diverticulitis may be increasing.[326,327] The location of an abscess is generally related to the site of primary disease and the direction of dependent peritoneal drainage. For example, appendicitis has been reported to be most commonly associated with right lower quadrant and pelvic abscesses; colonic diverticulitis with left lower quadrant and pelvic abscesses; and pancreatitis with lesser sac abscesses.[325] In one large series[325] of 194 intraperitoneal abscesses, about 44 percent were in the right lower quadrant, 14 percent in the left lower quadrant, and 14 percent in the pelvis, whereas 20 percent were perihepatic. In a more recent series reported by Saini et al.[326] the frequency of various abscess locations had changed somewhat, perhaps reflecting the change in the relative frequency of the various etiologic diseases.

Of the various perihepatic (right subphrenic, right subhepatic, left perihepatic, and lesser sac) abscesses, the most common continues to be in the right subphrenic space, but the difference in numbers between the right and left sides has been falling. In fact, in one large series of 267 cases of intra-abdominal abscesses, about one-half were in the subphrenic space, 60 percent of which were noted in the left perihepatic space.[328] This increased frequency of left perihepatic space abscess has also been noted by Ozeran,[329] Sherman et al.,[330] and Sanders.[331] This is in contrast to the series of Ochsner-DeBakey in 1938[332] when right subphrenic abscesses were the most frequent, due to the numerous ruptured appendices.

In children, appendicitis is still responsible for more than 50 percent of the cases of subphrenic abscesses.[333] In contrast, in adults, perihepatic abscesses currently are seen mainly as postoperative complications[329–331,334] rather than in neglected primary intra-abdominal infections, such as appendicitis or perforated peptic ulcer. This may explain the increasing frequency of subphrenic abscesses, especially on the left, in comparison to other intraperitoneal sites.[328] Usually, the surgery has been in the gastroduodenal and biliary tracts. One group of investigators[335] has noted that abscesses that followed gastric operations were left subphrenic if incidental splenectomy had been performed but right subhepatic if splenectomy had not been done. The subhepatic space is less frequently involved than the subphrenic spaces. Lesser sac abscesses generally follow pancreatitis or perforation of the stomach or duodenum. Multiple perihepatic space abscesses have been reported in 5–26 percent of the patients.[329–331,334,335]

Bacteriologic Findings

These infections are typically polymicrobial. In studies in which bacteriologic techniques permitted isolation of anaerobes, anaerobes were found in 60–70 percent of cases.[325,326,334,336] In one study,[334] anaerobes were recovered in 20 of 24 subphrenic abscesses, and *B. fragilis* was the most common pathogen, with anaerobic cocci and clostridia in 50 percent of the patients. Other bacteria frequently recovered are *E. coli, Klebsiella/Enterobacter* group, *Proteus* spp., *P. aeruginosa, Staph. aureus*, and enterococci.[325,329,330,334]

Pathogenesis

Intraperitoneal abscesses develop as a result of localization of diffuse peritonitis usually in the pelvis, perihepatic spaces, and paracolic gutters. In addition, abscess may develop about diseased organs such as periappendiceal or pericholecystic abscesses, through a penetrating wound (from a stab, gunshot, auto accident, or other trauma), or after a surgical procedure. These abscesses are termed *secondary* and account for the majority of these cases. In contrast, the pathogenesis of primary abscesses is unknown and is presumably similar to that of primary peritonitis.

Clinical Manifestations

An acute course, with a high intermittent fever, shaking chills, abdominal pain, and tenderness over the involved area, is characteristic. The clinical pattern may be that of an acute secondary illness occurring after surgery for primary abdominal disease or a prolonged recuperative course in a patient who has been receiving antibiotics after abdominal surgery. Various authors[330–335] have emphasized the occasional chronicity of subphrenic abscesses and have speculated that the course is often modified by antibiotics. Subphrenic abscesses have been described with 6 months or more of an indolent illness.[337]

Local symptoms and signs vary widely with the location and source of the abscess. Subphrenic abscesses are usually accompanied by chest findings with costal tenderness and pleural or pulmonary involvement, whereas subhepatic abscesses have more dominant signs of upper abdominal or subcostal involvement and fewer pulmonary changes.

Diagnosis

New noninvasive diagnostic procedures including ultrasonography and computed tomography have provided greater sensitivity and specificity than the more traditional methods of radiography and radionuclide scanning.[338,339] However, these older techniques remain useful, and often a combination of diagnostic tests is the optimal approach to confirm the diagnosis of intra-abdominal abscess.[340]

Plain radiographs of the abdomen can suggest the location of abscesses in as many as 50 percent of patients.[341] Radiologic findings associated with a subphrenic abscess may include pleural effusion, elevation of the hemidiaphragm, and/or loss of diaphragmatic movement on fluoroscopy. Routine radiography may also reveal displacement of viscera by an abscess. These findings can be enhanced by contrast radiology. The stomach, for example, may be outlined with barium or air to indicate displacement due to a left perihepatic or lesser sac abscess. The presence of gas, either as a single air-fluid level or mottling within the abscess, may aid localization on routine abdominal radiography.

Combined radionuclide scanning of the lungs and liver with ^{99m}Tc may be especially useful to evaluate the right subphrenic space.[342,343] Normally, the image of the lung and liver blend uniformly in all views. With subphrenic collections, there is a clear separation of the liver from the right lung base. The liver is displaced medially and/or inferiorly, and its superior margins may be locally flattened or indented.[4] Separation of the lung and liver image may also occur in patients with a right pleural effusion or pulmonary perfusion defect or in patients with ascites. These later lesions, however, should not cause defects in the contour of the liver. Subcapsular hematomas and certain hepatic tumors, though, may distort the liver contour and separate the lung from the liver image.

^{67}Ga and ^{111}In-tagged leukocytes are two other radionuclide scans that at times are helpful in detecting intra-abdominal abscesses. Unlike the ^{99m}Tc sulfur colloid liver-spleen scan, which visualizes the entire organ and delineates abnormal areas as "cold" spots due to decreased uptake of the isotope, ^{67}Ga and ^{111}In actually accumulate in areas of inflammation, such as abscesses, and appear as areas of increased radioactivity or "hot" spots[344–347] (Fig. 4). Gallium is excreted into the intestinal tract and can accumulate in any inflammatory process, as well as in certain neoplasms. For these reasons, false-positive scan readings may occur when radioactivity within the lumen of the bowel, within the wall of an inflamed bowel, or within a non-

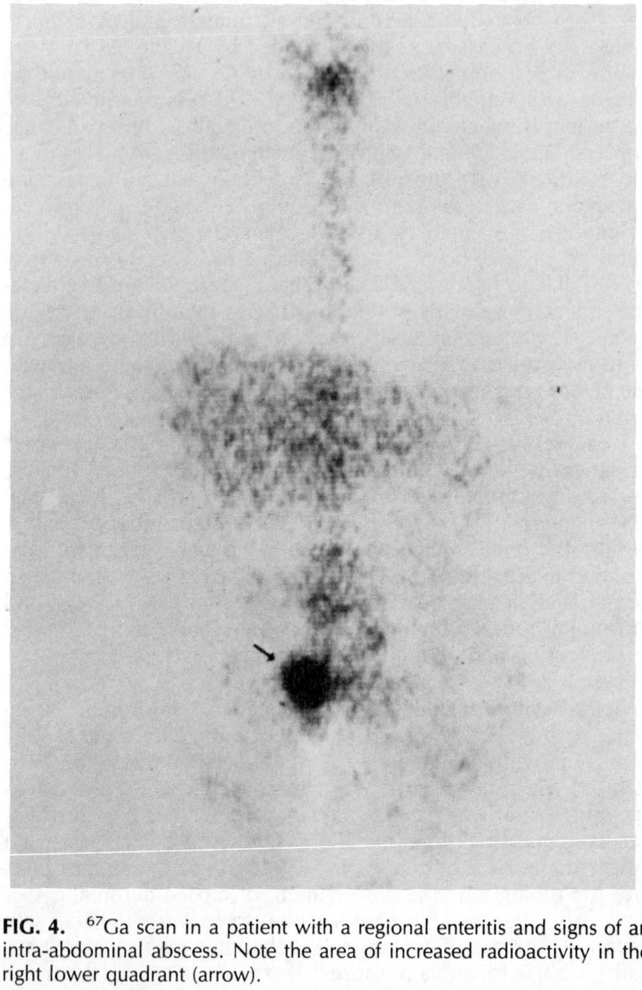

FIG. 4. ^{67}Ga scan in a patient with a regional enteritis and signs of an intra-abdominal abscess. Note the area of increased radioactivity in the right lower quadrant (arrow).

infected operative site in the process of healing is misinterpreted as an intra-abdominal abscess.

^{111}In scans are as sensitive as but more specific than ^{67}Ga scans because the labeled leukocytes tend to concentrate only in areas of inflammation, since, unlike ^{67}Ga, ^{111}In is not secreted into the bowel.[348,349] Approximately one-third of the ^{111}In-labeled leukocytes normally localized in the spleen. For this reason, ^{67}Ga is the preferred agent for detecting left-sided subphrenic abscesses because its less intense splenic uptake allows more accurate discrimination between normal splenic activity and that due to an abscess.

The diagnostic use of ultrasound is a noninvasive technique that is helpful in the determination of the size, shape, consistency, and anatomic relationships of an intra-abdominal mass.[349,351] A pulsed, focused, beam of high-frequency sound is directed into the suspect area of the patient's body by means of a transducer. Echoes are received by the same transducer from skin and tissue planes. The echo pattern is displayed on an oscilloscope as the transducer is moved along the surface of the body. The appearance of abscesses may vary widely from echo-free lesions to highly echo-genic masses, but typically appear as a fluid collection with an irregular wall and the presence of a few internal echoes. Ultrasound images may be obscured by overlying gas-filled viscera and by postoperative wounds and drains.

Computed tomography has proven especially well suited for the diagnosis of intra-abdominal abscess. Definition is unimpeded by intraluminal gas and postoperative changes, except in the presence of surgical metallic clips or residual barium that may disrupt the image. Observed findings consistent with abscess include a low-density tissue mass and a definable capsule. Computed tomography can detect extraluminal gas, a finding highly suggestive of abscess.[339] Contrast material is commonly administered orally, rectally, and intravenously when attempting to diagnose intra-abdominal abscess. The intraluminal contrast material helps to distinguish loops of bowel from abscess cavities, and the parenteral contrast material may enhance a surrounding capsule thus allowing for easier identification.

Magnetic resonance imaging (MRI) has the potential to display normal anatomy and to show abnormal conditions in many of the body's organ systems and anatomic regions.[352,353] However, only a few trials have compared MRI to older radiologic procedures. In one study, MRI demonstrated a clearer delineation of the extent of inflammatory changes than did computed tomography and better distinguished the abscess from the surrounding structures.[354] In addition, the use of MRI does not require the administration of contrast medium and eliminates exposure to radiation, but it may be more costly than other radiologic techniques.

Arteriographic localization has also been helpful.[355] However, overreliance on any one of these techniques is dangerous and should be confirmed by other methods and the clinical findings (Fig. 5).

Prognosis

The period of morbidity is unusually prolonged in patients with intraperitoneal abscesses. Altemeier et al. reported average hospital stays of 21–47 days.[325] The presence of residual or recurrent infection due to inadequate surgical drainage, more common in patients with multiple or bilateral abscesses, is associated with significantly greater mortality.[356]

Treatment

Although conflicts exist in the literature regarding the proper form of drainage of subphrenic abscesses, all agree that the main

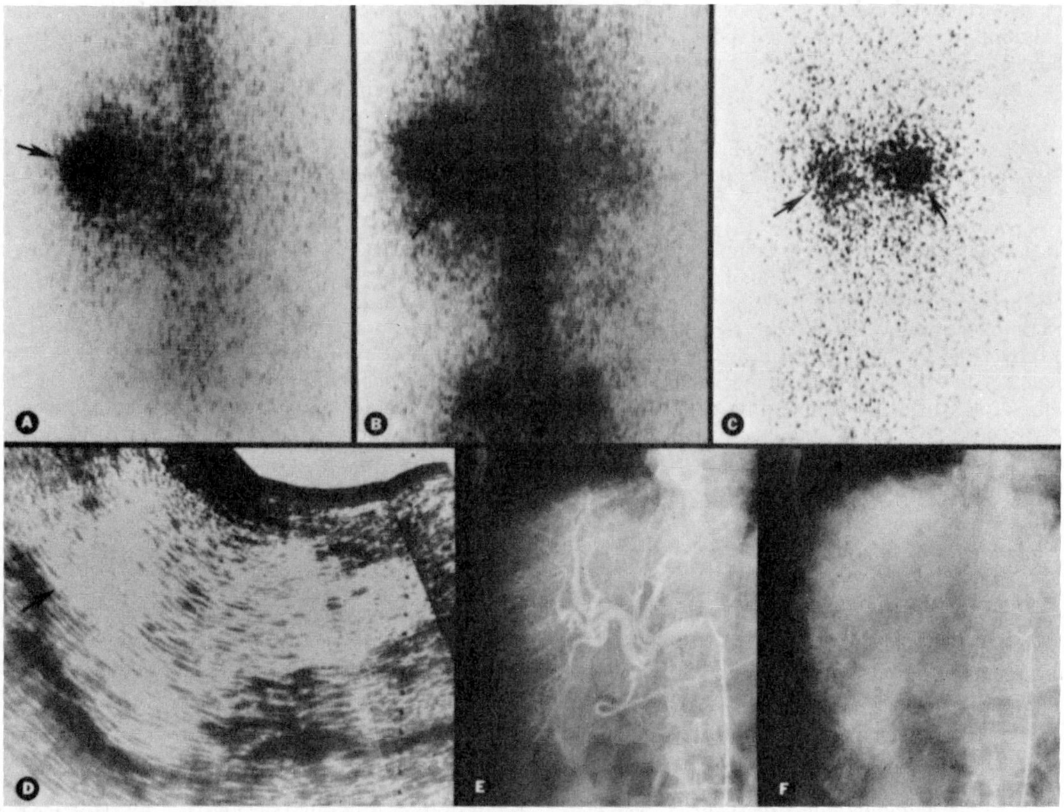

FIG. 5. ^{67}Ga scan in anterior view (**A**), posterior view (**B**), and right lateral view (**C**), shows increased radioactivity in a dumbell-shaped abscess (arrows) in the right lobe of the liver. Ultrasound examination in this patient (**D**) reveals an echo-free area in the right lobe of the liver (arrow), but both the arterial phase (**E**) and hepatogram (**F**) after selective celic axis arteriography were normal. At laparotomy a large abscess in the right lobe of the liver was drained.

therapy for any intraperitoneal abscess is drainage. Effective management is dependent on accurate localization of the abscess, discrimination between single and multiple abscesses, and early and adequate drainage. Conventional therapy for intraperitoneal abscesses has usually included surgical drainage. However, in recent years, successful therapy has been accomplished using percutaneous catheter drainage as an alternative to surgery.[357–359] This method has become possible with the use of refined imaging techniques, especially ultrasonography and computed tomography. The general requirements for percutaneous catheter drainage include (*1*) an abscess that can be adequately approached via a safe percutaneous route; (*2*) an abscess that is unilocular; (*3*) an abscess that is not vascular and the patient has no coagulopathy; (*4*) joint radiologic and surgical evaluation, with surgical backup for any complication or failure; and (*5*) the possibility of dependent drainage via the percutaneously placed catheter. Of the patients who fit these criteria, percutaneous drainage has been successful in 80–90 percent.[359,360] In most series, the frequency of complications ranges from 5 to 15 percent[357,361] and include septicemia, hemorrhage, peritoneal spillage, and fistula formation. In addition, failure may occur due to undrained abscesses or pus too viscid to drain via the catheter. Recent reports indicate that the morbidity and mortality associated with percutaneous drainage may be less than with surgical treatment.[358,362]

Antimicrobial therapy should be started immediately after appropriate specimens (e.g., blood) are obtained for culture, usually this occurs before drainage. Because the pathogens usually are similar to those involved in secondary peritonitis, initial antibiotic therapy is similarly directed at the anaerobes (especially *B. fragilis* and the Enterobacteriaceae. The antimicrobial regimens discussed above in the section on treatment of secondary peritonitis would be appropriate initial therapy. This antibiotic regimen should be adjusted to conform to results of in vitro testing of the infecting organisms isolated from blood or from purulent material obtained at surgery. During the course of a prolonged illness, repeated cultures of blood and purulent collections, when clinically indicated, should provide a basis for change in antimicrobial therapy.

VISCERAL ABSCESS: PANCREATIC ABSCESS

Etiology

Most pancreatic abscesses develop as a complication of pancreatitis, which may be either biliary, alcoholic, postsurgical, or post-traumatic in origin. More recently, pancreatitis has been found to be a complication of endoscopic retrograde cholangiopancreatography (ERCP).[363] Pancreatic abscess occurs in about 1–9 percent of the patients after acute pancreatitis.[364–368] The preceding attack of acute pancreatitis has been noted to be frequently severe.[369,370] Occasionally, penetration of a peptic ulcer or secondary infection of a pancreatic pseudocyst may be the cause of a pancreatic abscess.

Bacteriologic Findings

About one-third to one-half of pancreatic abscesses have been reported to be polymicrobial with mainly enteric facultative microorganisms, such as *E. coli* and other Enterobacteriaceae, enterococci, and viridans streptococci, and occasionally *Staph. aureus*.[366–369] However, since most studies have not used modern anaerobic bacteriologic techniques, it is unknown how frequently anaerobes are involved. More recent series have documented the presence of anaerobic bacteria in pancreatic abscesses.[365,366,371,372] *Mycobacterium tuberculosis* has also been cultured from pancreatic abscesses[373] and more recently in a patient with acquired immunodeficiency syndrome. (Joseph F. John, Jr., M.D., Medical University of South Carolina, 1988: personal communication).

Pathogenesis

The release of enzymes from an acutely damaged pancreas results in pancreatic necrosis. Infection of pancreatic necrosis is most likely a secondary event.[374,375] The mixed enteric bacterial etiology of many pancreatic abscesses suggests that bacteria may reach the pancreas by reflux of contaminated bile. The frequency of bactobilia increases with biliary obstruction and with the patient's age, occurring in approximately 50 percent of those over 70 years of age.[376] The hematogenous route may account for some of the monomicrobial infections, especially those due to *Staph. aureus*.

Clinical Manifestations

The clinical manifestations are varied. The patient may fail to respond to therapy for pancreatitis, or 1–3 weeks after the onset of pancreatitis the patient may suddenly deteriorate after an initial response.[366–369] Abdominal pain that frequently radiates to the back, nausea, and vomiting are present in more than 80–90 percent of patients. Temperature of more than 101°F and abdominal tenderness are usually present, although fever may be absent. Less frequently, jaundice, abdominal distension, or an abdominal mass may be present, or the patient may have generalized peritonitis. The serum amylase level is elevated in 21–66 percent of cases and may remain elevated.

Diagnosis

Radiologic, ultrasonic, radionuclide, and computed tomography studies reveal the lesion in 80–90 percent of the cases. Plain films may show diaphragmatic elevation, pleural effusion, presence of a retrogastric mass, forward displacement of the gastric air shadow on cross-table lateral views of the abdomen, widening of the gastrocolic omentum as seen by an increase in the distance between the gastric and colon gas, or mottling and the presence of gas bubbles in the gastrocolic or retrogastric region. Barium studies may show the visceral displacement (e.g., pressure effects in the posterior gastric wall or displacement and enlargement of the duodenal sweep). Ultrasonography and computed tomography are also useful in the diagnosis of pancreatic abscess.[377,378] Computed tomography appears to be superior to ultrasonography because the images are unaffected by overlying bowel gas and can better demonstrate pancreatic gas collections. It is, however, difficult to discern infected from noninfected pseudocysts by both methods, and diagnostic needle aspiration under ultrasound or CT guidance is often helpful.[377] ^{67}Ga and ^{111}In radionuclide scans have not been found to be very helpful in differentiating pancreatitis or a pseudocyst from an abscess.[379,380] To date, neither has MRI been a very helpful modality in imaging pancreatic abscesses.[381] Spleen scans, angiography, and retrograde duodenoscopic pancreatography may also be useful.[382]

Prognosis

The presence of proteolytic enzymes within the abscess may cause erosion of major blood vessels with intra-abdominal hemorrhage.[368,369] Spread of infection may occur in the retroperitoneum, along the roots of the transverse mesocolon and small bowel mesentery, and may involve suppuration in the lesser sac with extension into the perihepatic spaces. Fistulas may form between the abscess cavity and the stomach, duodenum, or transverse colon. Patients with undrained abscesses seen in surgical practice have a 100 percent mortality.[367] About 53–86 percent of those operated on survive. Survival has been dependent on early surgical drainage.[366,369,371] Higher mortality has occurred in those with biliary tract disease or in those who developed pancreatic abscess postoperatively. These were usually older patients who had ultimately fatal underlying disease.

Death may result from septicemia, peritonitis, pleuropulmonary complications, or hepatic or renal failure.

Treatment

Early surgical drainage is most important. Percutaneous drainage alone appears to be inadequate for the majority of pancreatic abscesses. However, it may do until the patient can be stabilized for surgical drainage.[383,384] Optimal treatment appears to require effective surgical débridement and drainage.[385,386] Also, prompt reoperation is often necessary for persistent infection. The prophylactic use of antibiotics early in the course of pancreatitis has been shown to be ineffective in preventing the subsequent development of pancreatic abscess.[387] Initial antibiotic therapy should have adequate activity against *E. coli*, other Enterobacteriaceae, and anaerobic gram-negative bacilli. The regimens discussed in the section on the treatment of secondary peritonitis would be appropriate choices. Antibiotic therapy should be adjusted according to the results of in vitro sensitivity testing. Routine therapy for pancreatitis should also be used.

VISCERAL ABSCESS: HEPATIC ABSCESS

Etiology

Bacterial abscesses of the liver are relatively uncommon lesions, despite the frequency of cholecystitis, appendicitis, diverticulitis, and peritonitis, which frequently are the source for bacterial infections of the liver. More recently, pyogenic liver abscess has been noted to be one of the infectious complications following liver transplantation,[388] and there is a high frequency of liver abscesses in patients with chronic granulamatous disease.[388] Bacterial abscesses have been reported to be more frequent than amebic liver abscess, especially in the northern United States.[389–392]

Liver abscesses due to *E. histolytica* complicate about 3–9 percent of the cases of amebic colitis.[389] Although there is no sex predominance in bacterial liver abscesses, over 90 percent of amebic liver abscesses occur in men, and patients with amebic liver abscesses are generally younger than those with bacterial abscesses.[389,392] Pyogenic abscesses have been reported in patients with sickle cell anemia.[393] Liver abscesses occur at all ages but are especially rare in children, when they have been noted to follow umbilical vein catheterization in neonates.[394]

Bacteriologic Findings

Pyogenic hepatic abscess is frequently polymicrobial.[392,395–397] Enteric gram-negative bacilli, usually *E. coli*, have been cultured from the majority of pyogenic hepatic abscesses.[392,397,398] The high frequency of "sterile" abscesses, reported in some series to be about 50 percent, is probably due to inadequate anaerobic cultivation.[397,399,400] Recently, as a result of modern anaerobic bacteriologic techniques, anaerobic bacteria have become recognized as a major cause of hepatic abscesses. In reports in which modern anaerobic techniques were used, about 50 percent of all pyogenic liver abscesses were caused by anaerobes, and blood cultures were positive for anaerobes in up to 54 percent of these cases.[399,401] These anaerobes included anaerobic gram-positive cocci, *Bacteroides* spp., *Fusobacterium* spp., and *Actinomyces* spp. Although the frequency of recovery of *Staph. aureus* or group A streptococci from liver abscesses varies among reports, these organisms occur in 20 percent or less of the cases.[389,397,400] *Staph. aureus* is noted to be more frequently isolated in children, primarily in those under 5 years of age[397,402] and is presumably of hematogenous origin.

Staphylococcus aureus microabscesses in the liver may be associated with microabscesses in other organs as part of generalized hematogenous dissemination in children with impaired host defenses (e.g., in acute leukemia).[403]

On rare occasion, *Yersinia enterocolitica* has been isolated from liver abscesses.[404] It most commonly produces an acute gastroenteritis, especially in children, and a right iliac fossa syndrome due to inflammation of the terminal ileum, mesenteric lymphadenitis, or both.

Candida may also invade the liver as part of a systemic infection. However, recently, a marked increase in cases has been observed in which the infection is confined to the liver and/or the spleen.[405,406] Most of these patients have acute leukemia, usually granulocytic, and the microabscesses in the liver are probably secondary to intestinal candida colonization and portal fungemia.[270] The diagnosis is most often delayed because of a nonspecific clinical presentation while the patient is neutropenic. Fever occurs with right upper quadrant abdominal pain and abdominal distension. During this phase of the illness, ultrasound and computed tomography are not helpful, and blood and liver biopsy cultures are usually negative. The diagnosis can be made by histopathologic findings in the liver biopsy. Even when the patient's neutropenia resolves, fever and abdominal pain persist. At this point, ultrasonography or computed tomography may reveal characteristic "bull's-eye" lesions.[406] The response to amphotericin therapy has been noted to be poor, sometimes requiring 2 or 3 months for defervescence.

The specific types of microorganisms that cause hepatic abscess probably vary with the underlying disease. For example, anaerobic abscesses are more frequently cryptogenic or portal in origin, whereas gallbladder disease has been noted in one series in only 2 of 25 patients with anaerobic liver abscesses.[399] Group A streptococcal and *Staph. aureus* abscesses probably result from bacteremia due to these organisms. In the past, it was believed that about 10–20 percent of amebic liver abscesses were secondarily infected with bacteria, usually of enteric origin.[391] However, in more recent series, superinfection was found to have occurred in 0–4 percent of cases.[392] Echinococcal hepatic cysts may also become secondarily infected.

Pathogenesis

The source of infection in the liver may be (*1*) biliary, in which disease of the extrahepatic biliary tract is due to a calculus, stricture, or malignancy and results in ascending cholangitis; (*2*) portal, in which a pathologic process such as appendicitis, diverticulitis,[407] or inflammatory bowel disease[408] is in the bed of the portal venous circulation and may be associated with pylephlebitis (acute suppurative thrombophlebitis in the portal venous system; (*3*) infection in a contiguous structure, such as the gallbladder, which spreads directly to the liver; (*4*) infected foci anywhere in the body via the hepatic artery; (*5*) infection secondary to penetrating wounds and even nonpenetrating trauma to the liver; or (*6*) cryptogenic, in which no source is evident. About one-fourth of the liver abscesses are cryptogenic and are thought to be caused by infection of infarcted portions of the liver.[409] Although a portal venous source, mainly appendicitis, was a common cause of liver diseases in the past, biliary disease in recent series is now the most common source.[397,410]

Pyogenic abscesses may be single or multiple. Multiple abscesses are more apt to be due to biliary tract disease,[400] whereas abscesses arising via the portal vein are usually solitary[400]; the right lobe is more commonly involved than the left. Amebic abscesses are predominantly solitary in the right lobe.

Clinical Manifestations

The predominant symptoms of pyogenic hepatic abscess include fever and chills of several days' to weeks' duration. Characteristically, multiple abscesses associated with ascending cholangitis give rise to spiking temperatures. Right upper quadrant pain may be dull, and abscesses high in the right lobe may cause respiratory symptoms such as cough and pleuritic pain with radiation to the right shoulder and an associated pleural rub. Tender hepatomegaly is present in 50–70 percent of the patients. Jaundice is not often present unless ascending cholangitis is a cause of the abscesses or there is extensive hepatic involvement usually associated with multiple abscesses.[389,397,399] Either the indolence of the illness in some patients or the minimal physical findings (no hepatomegaly or abdominal tenderness) may account for these patients having a "fever of unknown origin."[397]

Clinical differentiation of an amebic from a pyogenic abscess is difficult; a history of diarrhea, the presence of chest findings, or the lack of spiking temperatures has been reported in some series to be more common in patients with amebic abscesses, but these characteristics have not been especially frequent in other series of patients with amebic abscesses. Pain in the left upper quadrant of the abdomen in patients with amebic abscess is infrequent but may indicate a left lobe abscess that can extend into the pericardium.[124] Swelling may occur over the right chest wall or there may be point tenderness that localizes abscesses due to ameba.[124]

The serum alkaline phosphatase is the most frequently elevated serum liver enzyme test. Blood cultures have been reported in recent studies to be positive in about one-half of the patients with pyogenic abscesses.[399,400] The presence of viridans streptococcus in several blood cultures in patients with an indolent clinical course and elevated hepatic enzymes without evidence of endocarditis may be an important clue to the diagnosis of liver abscess[411] (Fig. 6). Persistent recovery of viridans streptococci from liver also has been reported in the absence of bacteremia in a patient with an indolent clinical course and persistent serum alkaline phosphatase elevation.[412]

Diagnosis

Elevation and limitation of motion of the right diaphragm, basilar atelectasis, right pleural effusion, or gas within the abscess cavity may be noted on plain films of the abdomen or chest.[413] Scintigraphy with either ^{99m}Tc or ^{67}Ga, ultrasonography, computed tomography and MRI are highly sensitive techniques for the detection of liver abscesses.[414] ^{99m}Tc sulfur colloid liver scan is capable of detecting about 85 percent of lesions greater than 2 cm in diameter.[414] Anteroposterior and lateral views should reveal decreased isotope concentration in both pygenic and amebic abscesses (Fig. 6). ^{67}Ga or ^{111}In scans should reveal areas of increased isotope concentration of pyogenic abscesses (Fig. 5). Because the amebic abscess is not really a purulent lesion, it may show decreased central gallium concentration and may be surrounded by a zone of increased activity in the hypervascular abscess rim.[414]

The hepatic angiographic findings in liver abscess are the mass effect with stretching or displacement of blood vessels and an avascular area surrounded by a blush of contrast seen during the capillary-venous phase of the angiogram.[415]

The effectiveness of ultrasonography for the detection of liver abscess is now well documented.[398,410,416] It has proven especially useful for the evaluation of right upper quadrant structures, primarily because of the absence of air-filled viscera that often impede visualization in other areas of the abdomen. As mentioned previously, the appearance of abscesses may vary from echo-free lesions to highly echogenic masses within the liver. Sonography, as opposed to ^{99m}Tc scintigraphy, can often distinguish abscess from tumor and other solid focal lesions. Computed tomography is also a highly sensitive technique for the diagnosis of liver abscess.[398,417,418] Abscesses produce areas of decreased attenuation on computed tomography (Fig. 7). Both ultrasound and CT may be used to guide needle aspiration for diagnostic and therapeutic purposes.[358,418,419] The aspirated material should be cultured aerobically and anaerobically.

Ultrasound- or CT-guided percutaneous aspiration in patients suspected of having amebic abscess has been recommended to rapidly rule out a pyogenic etiology. Aspiration of sterile fluid that is brownish and without a foul odor is characteristic of an amebic abscess. However, fluid in amebic abscesses may frequently be yellow or green, and possibly is secondarily infected with enteric bacteria. Diagnosis is confirmed by finding *E. histolytica* on direct microscopy or culture of the aspirate or wall of the abscess. In endemic areas, aspiration is usually not performed if amebic abscess is suspected clinically because of the favorable response to drug therapy. Serologic tests indicative of past or present amebiasis are positive in over 90 percent of amebic liver abscesses but may be misleading in endemic areas.[392]

Prognosis

The prognosis of pyogenic liver abscesses depends on the rapidity with which the diagnosis is made and treatment is started. High mortality is also associated with advanced age and serious underlying disease. In the past, the mortality from pyogenic abscesses ranged from about 24 to 79 percent,[397,399,400] and un-

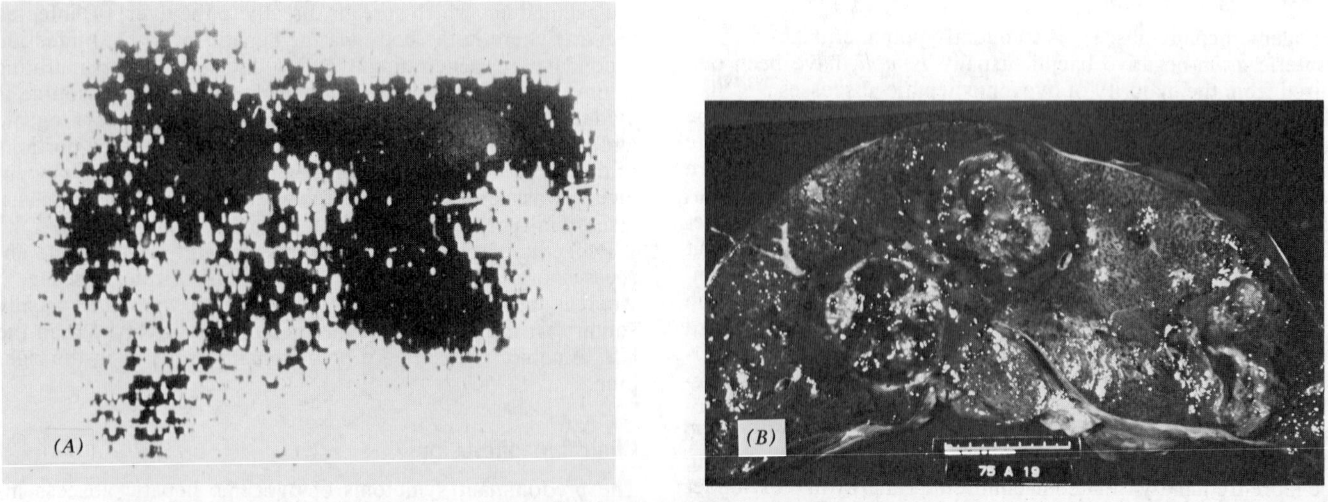

FIG. 6. **(A)** ^{99m}Tc scan of the liver in a patient who had an α-hemolytic streptococcal bacteremia. **(B)** At autopsy, cut section of the liver revealed several large abscesses that corresponded to areas of decreased radionuclide uptake in Figure 6A. At laparotomy, needle aspiration failed to yield pus, perhaps because of its viscosity, as evidenced at necropsy.

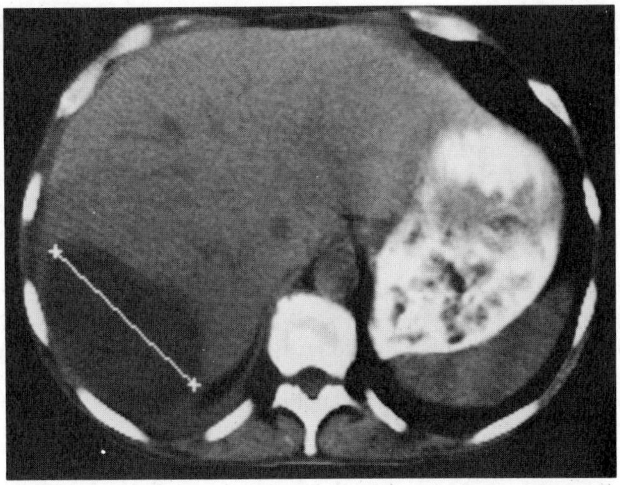

FIG. 7. Abdominal CT scan reveals a liver abscess (arrow) due to a mixture of anaerobic and aerobic pathogens. The abscess developed following drainage of an appendiceal abscess.

drained abscesses had a reported mortality of up to 100 percent.[420,421] Recent series, however, have shown an improvement in prognosis, with cure rates of 88–100 percent.[181,182,419] Traditional therapy for pyogenic liver abscesses has been surgical drainage and antibiotics; however, the recently reported high success rates have occurred in patients treated with either antibiotics plus percutaneous drainage or antibiotics alone. The older series reporting high mortality for undrained abscesses may have included patients who were not candidates for surgical drainage because of poor clinical condition or extensive infection (i.e., multiple small abscesses). The apparent improvement in prognosis during recent years may be related to earlier diagnosis afforded by the use of ultrasonography and computed tomography. Mortality of uncomplicated amebic abscesses is reported to be less than 1 percent in recent series.[124,392] However, amebic abscesses that rupture into the peritoneal or pericardial cavity carry an 18 or 30 percent mortality, respectively, and amebic abscesses that rupture into the bronchi or pleura carry a 6 percent mortality.[124]

Treatment

The treatment of pyogenic liver abscesses has changed during recent years as the use of ultrasonography and computed tomography has become common for diagnosis and therapy. These imaging procedures offer the ability to follow closely the resolution of the abscess during therapy and allow precise placement of percutaneous catheters for single or continuous drainage. Some series have reported high cure rates after antibiotic treatment without concomitant percutaneous drainage.[181,182] However, most other reports have emphasized the necessity of some drainage procedure to ensure a good outcome.[419,420,422,423] Most patients will defervesce within 2 weeks of the start of medical therapy and drainage.[392] However, some patients who are cured by medical and drainage therapy may still take up to 4 weeks to defervescence.[392] It has been recommended that surgery be considered for patients whose fever persists for more than 2 weeks despite percutaneous catheter drainage and appropriate antimicrobial therapy.[392]

The abscess should decrease in size following percutaneous catheter drainage. Should the patient's condition not improve and fever not resolve within 48 hours after catheter drainage, repeat ultrasound or CT scan should be performed to assess for undrained loculations of pus. Surgery is required for hepatic abscesses secondary to biliary obstruction. Loculated or highly viscous abscesses also usually require surgical incision and drainage.

Antibiotic therapy should be started as soon as the diagnosis is suspected and should be directed at the expected pathogens. Because the pathogens usually are similar to those involved in secondary peritonitis, initial antibiotic therapy is similarly directed at the anaerobes (especially *B. fragilis*) and the Enterobacteriaceae. The antimicrobial regimens outlined earlier in the section on treatment of secondary peritonitis would be appropriate initial therapy. At the time of drainage, cultures are taken of the abscess for aerobic and anaerobic incubation, and specific antibiotic therapy is instituted on the basis of the culture results. Therapy should be prolonged, usually for more than 1 month. Up to 4 months of antibiotic therapy for multiple pyogenic abscesses has been recommended to prevent relapses.[399]

Amebic abscess is usually treated with a tissue amebicide, such as metronidazole or parenteral dehydroemetine.[424] Metronidazole has cure rates similar to those of dehydroemetine and has the advantage of being active for both the hepatic and intestinal phase of the disease and of being less toxic. Aspiration of the cavity has been recommended not only for diagnosis but also for therapeutic drainage by some authors.[124] However, others have found aspiration to be unnecessary, except in the occasional patient who responds poorly to medical therapy or in patients with large left lobe abscesses that may rupture into the pericardium and cause death.[392] Aspiration may also be indicated to evacuate an expanding abscess in an attempt to prevent imminent rupture. Repeated aspiration has been recommended if more than 250 ml is obtained initially.[124] If a solitary right lobe abscess occurs in a male, despite the finding of bacteria in the aspirate, additional antiamebic therapy has been recommended initially because of the likelihood of a secondarily infected amebic abscess.

VISCERAL ABSCESS: SPLENIC ABSCESS

Etiology

Splenic abscesses are uncommon lesions and may occur in patients with sickle hemoglobinopathies, trauma, or bacteremia, or in intravenous drug abusers.[425] Usually multiple small abscesses develop as a complication of hematogenous dissemination. One-quarter of these abscesses have been reported to be solitary.[426]

Bacteriologic Characteristics

Splenic abscesses that develop during the course of bacterial endocarditis are usually due to *Staph. aureus* or streptococcus. Enterobacteriaceae (e.g., *Salmonella*) and anaerobic microorganisms have also been recovered.[425–427] In one series, the bacteriology of the abscess was polymicrobial in 25 percent and included anaerobes.[425] The proportion of splenic abscesses reported to have sterile cultures has declined as anaerobic culture techniques have improved. Fungi (mostly *Candida* species) have been isolated from splenic abscesses with greater frequency during the past decade as the population with conditions predisposing to infections with *Candida* has increased (e.g., patients on high-dose corticosteroids or cancer chemotherapy). Fungal splenic abscesses are often part of the syndrome of heptosplenic candidiasis.[405,407] Blood cultures have been reported to be positive in 70 percent of patients with multiple splenic abscesses but in only 14 percent with solitary abscesses.[425]

Pathogenesis

Splenic abscesses most likely develop as a metastatic process. Some are related to infection in contiguous organs and others from infected traumatic hematomas or infarcts, for example, in patients with sickle hemoglobinopathies.

Manifestations

Left upper quadrant abdominal pain is usual. Irritation of the adjacent diaphragm may result in pain referred to the left shoulder. Splenic enlargement and tenderness are often present, with high, spiking temperatures and perhaps a splenic rub. No clinical findings to suggest splenic involvement may occur in some patients with multiple small splenic abscesses.[425,426]

Diagnosis

Radiographic examination may reveal an elevated left hemidiaphragm, basilar pulmonary infiltrates, atelectasis, or a left pleural effusion. Shift of the colon and stomach down and to the right, and extraintestinal gas, either diffusely mottled or producing an air-fluid level in the left upper quadrant, may also be seen.[425,426] Radionuclide imaging with ^{99m}Tc sulfur colloid may also be helpful. However, ^{67}Ga may have relatively low sensitivity, in part due to the inherent normal splenic uptake of this isotope.[427,428] Ultrasonography, computed tomography, and MRI are the preferred diagnostic techniques for the evaluation of suspected splenic abscess[429,430] (Fig. 8). Computed tomography appears to be somewhat superior to ultrasound for visualization of splenic structure because of adjacent gas-filled viscera and inconstant position in the left upper quadrant.[428]

Treatment

In untreated cases, the mortality rate with splenic abscess is 100 percent.[428] Initial antibiotic therapy should have a broad spectrum of activity. A combination of antibiotics that has activity against streptococci and both aerobic and anaerobic gram-negative bacilli would be appropriate initial antimicrobial ther-

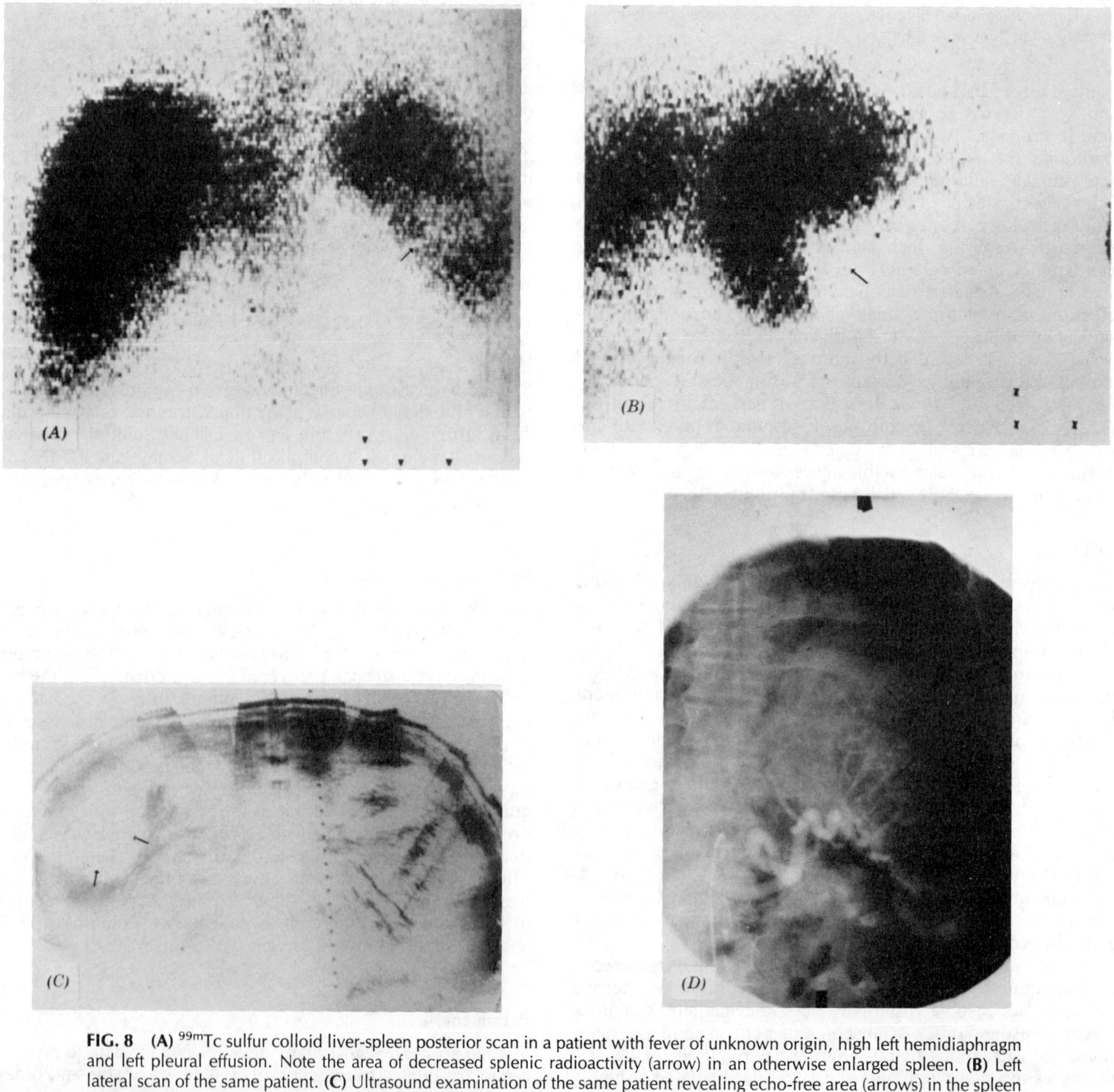

FIG. 8 **(A)** ^{99m}Tc sulfur colloid liver-spleen posterior scan in a patient with fever of unknown origin, high left hemidiaphragm and left pleural effusion. Note the area of decreased splenic radioactivity (arrow) in an otherwise enlarged spleen. **(B)** Left lateral scan of the same patient. **(C)** Ultrasound examination of the same patient revealing echo-free area (arrows) in the spleen surrounded by an echo-dense border due to increased transmission of the sound. **(D)** Splenic arteriography in the same patient. Note the avascular area (arrows) and surrounding area of increased vascularity.

apy. Subsequent modifications of antibiotic therapy may be based on results of blood cultures or cultures of material obtained at the time of surgery. With multiple, small abscesses, and with some large solitary abscesses when feasible, splenectomy is the treatment of choice; otherwise when the spleen is surrounded by extensive adhesions, incision and drainage may be preferred.[425–427,431] Percutaneous drainage was successful in 15 of 22 patients in one series,[425] but its indications, efficacy, and safety remain to be determined.[432]

SPECIFIC SOURCES OF INTRA-ABDOMINAL INFECTION

Acute Appendicitis

Appendicitis manifests as right lower quadrant abdominal pain accompanied by anorexia, nausea, and vomiting. When the inflamed appendix lies in the anterior position, tenderness is often maximal at or near McBurney's point with low-grade fever, rebound tenderness, voluntary guarding at first, and then abdominal rigidity. Variations in the anatomic location of the appendix may result in variations in the location of the pain and physical findings. For example, a retrocecal appendix may cause principally flank or back pain and tenderness; a pelvic appendix may cause suprapubic pain; and on rectal examination pain may be felt locally and suprapubically.

Persistent obstruction of the appendiceal lumen, usually due to a fecalith, leads to gangrene and rupture of the pus-filled organ. During the several hours between onset of acute appendicitis and rupture, adjacent viscera and omentum may wall off and confine the subsequent spill to the periappendiceal area, with development of an inflammatory mass felt in the right lower quadrant. If the walling-off process is incomplete, spreading diffuse peritonitis occurs. The two sites for loculation of intraperitoneal spread are the pelvic recess and the right subhepatic space. Pylephlebitis and liver abscess may complicate the picture. Colonic microflora, namely a mixture of *B. fragilis*, *B. melaninogenicus*, anaerobic gram-positive cocci, and Enterobacteriaceae, are the primary pathogens in appendicitis and its complications.

The therapy for appendicitis without rupture and for ruptured appendicitis with local or diffuse peritonitis is surgery. If perforation is suspected to have occurred, antibiotic therapy is initiated while the patient is being prepared for surgery. For recommendation of specific antimicrobial agents, see the section on therapy for secondary peritonitis. The severity of appendicitis is related to the development of the rupture of the appendix, which is more common in children and the elderly. Meckel's diverticulitis may manifest in a manner identical to that of acute appendicitis, and the therapeutic approach is similar.

Although not a source of intra-abdominal infection, nonspecific mesenteric lymphadenitis is often confused with appendicitis in children and may account for the symptoms suggestive of appendicitis in up to 20 percent of these patients. It is a self-limited, sometimes recurrent illness in childhood of unknown etiology that primarily involves mesenteric nodes in the right iliac fossa. The nodes are enlarged and discrete. The adjacent bowel and peritoneum are at most mildly inflamed, and a small amount of clear serous peritoneal fluid is frequently present. The patient has fever, poorly localized right lower quadrant tenderness, rebound tenderness, and voluntary guarding, but rarely abdominal rigidity. On occasion, leukocytosis is present.

Since the clinical manifestation of nonspecific mesenteric lymphadenitis is so similar to that of acute appendicitis, the therapeutic approach is surgical to rule out appendicitis. Even though the appendix may appear normal, an appendectomy should be done, since a recurrent episode of mesenteric adenitis may again lead to misinterpretation. An identical clinical picture can be caused by rubeola, infectious mononucleosis, and *Yersinia* spp.

Diverticulitis

Diverticula of the colon are herniations of the mucosa and submucosa through the circular muscular layer. Diverticula are usually located in the sigmoid and descending colons, and usually occur after 35 years of age. Inflammation is the most frequent complication of diverticulosis. The pathogenesis is similar to that of appendicitis. Diverticulitis is more frequent in patients with widespread diverticulosis, and the frequency of the complication increases with age. The inflammation may remain localized to the bowel wall as a simple diverticulitis. Complications such as confined perforation with pericolic abscess to which adjacent viscera and omentum are adherent,[433] fistula formation, or, less commonly, free perforation with spreading peritonitis may occur.[434] The clinical picture of uncomplicated sigmoid diverticulitis resembles that of appendicitis, but with findings on the left side of the abdomen. Urinary symptoms are sometimes present as a result of inflammation close to the bladder or ureter and may be followed by fistulization. Pneumaturia and fecaluria often accompanied by chills and fever indicate fistulization between the colon and urinary tract. Passage of flatus and feces through the vagina indicates fistulas into the uterus or vagina. With uncomplicated diverticulitis, low-grade fever and mild leukocytosis are usually found with tenderness, some rigidity in the left lower quadrant and/or suprapubic area, and normal bowel sounds. Perforation produces clinical findings of an intraperitoneal abscess or of diffuse peritonitis.

It is advisable to defer the barium enema until the process has abated with conservative therapy. Nonoperative therapy should be tried for the first few attacks of acute uncomplicated diverticulitis or for well-localized pericolic abscesses. For confined perforation, conservative treatment may resolve an inflammatory mass sufficiently to permit a one-stage resection of the diseased portion of the colon.[435] Operative therapy for recurrent acute diverticulitis is indicated if the patient does not respond promptly within about 48 hours, if there is free perforation with diffuse peritonitis, and if carcinoma cannot be ruled out. Initial nonoperative treatment consists of parenteral fluids, broad-spectrum antibiotics, and nasogastric suction. Antibiotic recommendations are similar to those discussed in the section on therapy for secondary peritonitis.

Regional Enteritis

The onset of regional enteritis may be acute, especially in the young, and may mimic acute appendicitis. The correct diagnosis of early regional enteritis may be made only at operation, which reveals a thickened bowel wall and mesenteric lymph node involvement. Usually, however, the diagnosis is established by contrast radiography.

Perforation as the result of an ulcer burrowing through the entire thickness of the bowel wall may occur.[436] Usually the perforation is confined and may result in abscesses or internal fistulas. Rarely does the ulcer perforate freely into the peritoneal cavity. Perianal or perirectal abscesses and fistulas are also common manifestations of regional enteritis.

Systemic antibiotics are often of value in the management of suppurative complications (see the section on antimicrobial therapy for secondary peritonitis). Surgery is indicated to drain abdominal abscesses, to correct fistulas, and for free perforation. The principal complications of surgery are enterocutaneous fistula, intraperitoneal or wound sepsis, and prolonged postoperative ileus.

Necrotizing Enterocolitis in Neutropenic Patients (Typhlitis)

Necrotizing enterocolitis occurs in patients who are severely granulocytopenic from any cause, including acute leukemia, aplastic anemia, cyclic neutropenia, Felty's syndrome, and chemotherapy for various neoplasms.[437–439]

Pathologically, the bowel is edematous, with marked thickening of the wall. The luminal surface has discrete areas of punctate ulceration, which at times may coalesce. There is also transmural inflammation with hemorrhagic necrosis and degeneration of the muscularis mucosae. The inflammatory cells found in histologic specimens are almost always mononuclear. It is thought that bacteria found in the normal gut flora opportunistically invade the ulcerations in the bowel during periods of profound neutropenia. Due to the lack of granulocytes, these organisms proliferate and cause local destruction by elaboration of exotoxins.[437]

Initially, the signs and symptoms are similar to those of acute appendicitis. These patients present with a new fever, abdominal pain, rebound tenderness in the right lower quadrant (because of the predominance of cecal involvement), and diarrhea. Rapid progression to the development of an acute abdomen is not uncommon.

Plain radiographs of the abdomen may demonstrate a boggy, thickened cecum and possibly the presence of gas within the wall of the colon.[440]

The mortality rate with neutropenic enterocolitis is greater than 50 percent.[441] Although the management of this disease is somewhat controversial,[442,443] antimicrobial therapy with activity against the aerobic and anaerobic gut bacteria, together with surgical resection of the necrotic bowel, is generally recommended.

Actinomycosis

Actinomycosis is an uncommon suppurative infection produced by the anaerobe *Actinomyces israelii* or one of several closely related species. The cecal area is most frequently the site of abdominal actinomycosis. Typically, the history begins with an attack of acute appendicitis or with recurrent bouts of right lower quadrant pain and fever, which prompts surgery for a presumptive diagnosis of appendicitis. At surgery an indurated pericecal mass is found with sinus tracts. After appendectomy, persistent draining sinuses form. The diagnosis of actinomycosis is made by demonstration of "sulfur granules" in the purulent sinus discharge and by histologic examination of the tissues. Treatment is discussed in Chapter 233.

ACUTE CHOLECYSTITIS

Pathogenesis

In over 90 percent of patients with acute cholecystitis, gallstones are impacted in the cystic duct.[444] Thus, it is generally assumed that a sudden change in the degree of obstruction leads to a sudden increase in intraductal pressures, which produces distension of the gallbladder, compromising the blood supply and lymphatic drainage. This is followed by tissue necrosis and proliferation of bacteria present in calculous gallbladders. Although infection may not be a primary cause of acute cholecystitis, it develops in over half of the cases. Infective complications include empyema or gangrene of the gallbladder, emphysematous cholecystitis, pericholecystic abscess, intraperitoneal abscess, peritonitis, cholangitis, liver abscess, and bacteremia. A detailed schema for the proposed pathogenesis of acute cholecystitis is shown in Figure 9.

Pathologic Findings

Acute cholecystitis is usually superimposed on a histologic picture of chronic cholecystitis. Ninety-five percent of the gallbladders removed for acute cholecystitis exhibit fibrosis, flattening of the mucosa, and clusters of chronic inflammatory cells as sequelae of previous disease. Rokitansky-Aschoff sinuses are present in 56 percent of the cases. These sinuses represent mucosal herniations presumably related to increased hydrostatic pressure during previous episodes of cystic duct obstruction. The early acute changes may be only edema and venous congestion. This is followed by focal necrosis and an influx of neutrophils as secondary bacterial proliferation occurs. This may then be followed by actual gangrene or perforation (Table 3).

Symptoms and Signs

Initial obstruction of the cystic duct may be accompanied by only mild epigastric pain followed by reflex nausea and vomiting. If the obstruction is transient, these symptoms subside within 1–2 hours. With persistent obstruction the findings of acute cholecystitis evolve. Pain shifts to the right upper quad-

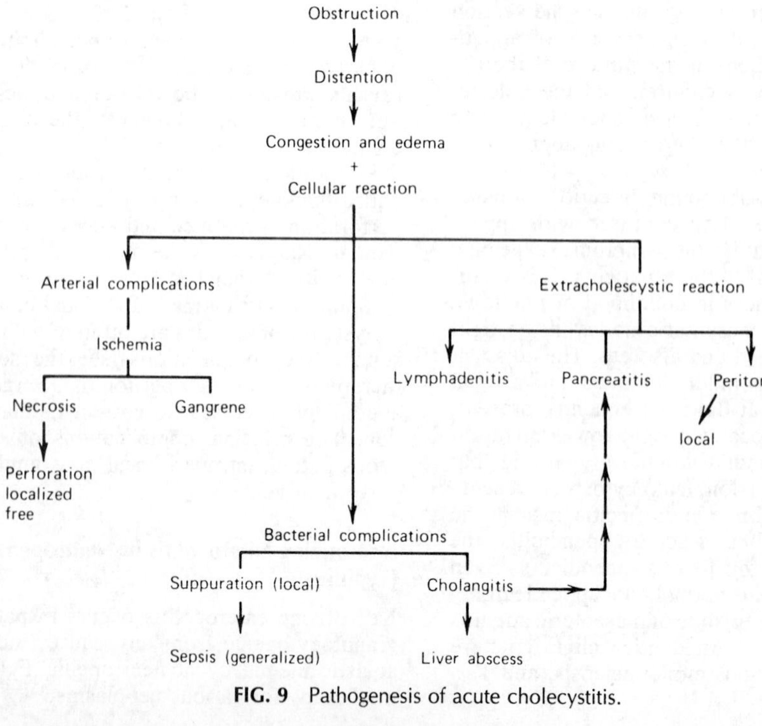

FIG. 9 Pathogenesis of acute cholecystitis.

TABLE 3. Pathologic Classification of Acute Cholecystitis

Edema	
Edema and congestion	
Focal necrosis	
Suppuration	Intramural Intraluminal Pericholecystic
Gangrene	
Perforation	Localized Free

rant and becomes increasingly severe. Signs of peritoneal irritation may be present, and in a small number of patients the pain may radiate to the right shoulder or scapula. The gallbladder is palpable in 30–40 percent of the cases.[445] Moderate temperature elevations and minimal icterus occur in two-thirds of patients. However, repeated chills and fever, jaundice, or hypotension would suggest suppurative cholangitis as a consequence of common duct obstruction (see below under "Bacteriologic Findings"). Most patients with acute cholecystitis have a complete remission within 1–4 days. However, approximately 25–30 percent of patients require surgery or develop some complication.

Laboratory Findings

The laboratory data obtained rarely are required to make the diagnosis of acute obstructive cholecystitis, but they may be indicative of further complications (see the next section). The leukocyte count is usually moderately elevated, with a slight increase in early segmented forms. Fifty percent of the patients have mild hyperbilirubinemia; forty percent have a mild elevation of serum aspartate aminotransferase (AST) levels; twenty-five percent have elevated alkaline phosphatase levels; and only ten percent have mild elevations of serum amylase levels.[446]

Bacteriologic Findings

In the presence of cholecystitis and cholelithiasis, appreciable numbers of various bacteria may be found in the bile and walls of the gallbladder, even in the absence of symptoms. The frequency of bactobilia is higher (*1*) the longer the duration and severity of symptoms, (*2*) in the elderly (>60–70 years of age), (*3*) in the jaundiced patient, (*4*) in acute cholecystitis (up to 94 percent of patients) in comparison to chronic cholecystitis, and (*5*) especially when the common duct is obstructed.[376,447]

The organisms found in the biliary tract are commonly the same as the normal intestinal flora, namely, the enteric gram-negative bacilli, including *E. coli, Klebsiella/Enterobacter*, and *Proteus* spp., as well as the enterococci.[376,448] In addition, recent studies have demonstrated the frequent recovery of anaerobic organisms including *Bacteroides, Clostridia*, and *Fusobacterium* spp.[448] When present, these anaerobes are frequently involved in polymicrobic infections, mixed with other anaerobes and aerobic gram-negative bacilli.[449]

Patients from whom anaerobes have been recovered were reported more likely to have had prior multiple, complex, biliary tract surgical procedures, especially biliary-intestinal anastomoses and common duct manipulations. These patients often have severe symptoms and a high incidence of postoperative infectious complications, especially wound infections.[450]

The source of bactobilia is unknown, but has been assumed to be the duodenum, and spread is assumed to occur via an ascending route.[449] Although the duodenum normally has a sparse flora in the fasting state, higher counts occur transiently after meals and in conditions that allow bacterial overgrowth in the stomach (achlorhydria or gastric obstruction) or in the small bowel (obstruction, diverticula, or blind loops).

Roentgenographic and Related Studies

An upright chest film is of limited value. In two-thirds of the cases the right hemidiaphragm is elevated. Since subdiaphragmatic free air cannot originate in the biliary tract, if present, it indicates another disease process. In only about 10–15 percent of cases are calcified gallstones seen on plain films of the abdomen, but this finding in any case indicates only cholelithiasis. Occasionally, a diffusely calcified gallbladder ("porcelainized gallbladder") may be seen. Since this rarely, if ever, develops into acute cholecystitis, its presence should strongly suggest another diagnosis. The demonstration of gas limited to the gallbladder wall or lumen is diagnostic of emphysematous cholecystitis.

Oral cholecystography is of little value in diagnosing acute cholecystitis because it requires too long a preparation time and is not applicable in jaundiced or vomiting patients. Intravenous cholangiography has been replaced by more sensitive and specific techniques. Recent advances in ultrasonography and nuclear medicine have made these modalities the diagnostic studies of choice for acute cholecystitis. Both imaging modalities are noninvasive, with little reported morbidity, and have been reported to have sensitivity and specificity values of greater than 90 percent. Sonographic findings consistent with acute cholecystitis include the presence of stones, thickened gallbladder wall, dilated lumen of the gallbladder, or a pericholecystic collection.[451,452] Hepatobiliary scanning with one of the ^{99m}Tc-labeled acetanilide iminodiacetic acid derivatives (IDA) is also a sensitive and rapid study for the diagnosis of acute cholecystitis.[451–453] Even in the presence of moderately severe liver dysfunction,[453] the IDA nuclide is concentrated in the liver and excreted into the bile, resulting in visualization of the functioning hepatobiliary system, including the gallbladder and duodenum, within the first hour. In acute cholecystitis, however, since the cystic duct is occluded by a stone or mucosal inflammation, the gallbladder is not visualized, despite common duct and small bowel visualization. During the first hour, nonvisualization of the gallbladder also occurs in more than 50 percent of patients with chronic cholecystitis, but usually the gallbladder is visualized in delayed images obtained up to 4 hours after IDA administration. In chronic cholecystitis and cholelithiasis, a normal cholescintigram may also occur if the cystic duct is patent.

Findings consistent with acute cholecystitis may also be demonstrated with computed tomography, but this technique should not be used for initial screening.[454]

Recently, MRI was found to provide both functional and anatomic information, and was sensitive in detecting gallbladder disease in patients with suspected cholecystitis.[455]

Complications

Perforation occurs in 10–15 percent of the cases. A small percentage of these are acute free perforations into the peritoneal cavity. These cases are readily recognizable, since they have the catastrophic symptoms and signs of diffuse peritonitis. More frequently, the omentum and serosa of contiguous viscera localize the perforation early. In such cases, there is persistent fever, often a palpable mass that may be in a somewhat atypical location, and occasionally a friction rub. Acute emphysematous cholecystitis is seen most commonly in elderly diabetic men. Systemic symptoms are more severe, and the classic x-ray picture of the abdomen reveals gas within the gallbladder lumen, frequently with a gas-fluid level, and gas in a ring along the contours of the gallbladder wall.[456] Cholangitis is described in detail below. Pancreatitis may also complicate cholecystitis.

Here the pain is more midline and may radiate to the back. Urine and serum amylase are often elevated.

Differential Diagnosis

In addition to the complications noted above, the differential diagnosis should include myocardial infarction, perforating ulcer, right lower lobe pneumonia, intestinal obstruction, hepatitis, perihepatitis, and acute disease involving the right kidney. Radiographs of the chest and abdomen, electrocardiograms, and urinalysis can exclude these in the majority of cases.

Antimicrobial Therapy in Acute Obstructive Cholecystitis

Certainly in severely ill or elderly patients or in patients with infectious complications such as emphysematous cholecystitis, perforation with peritonitis or a pericholecystic collection and cholangitis should be treated early for infection possibly due to enteric gram-negative bacilli and anaerobic bacteria, including *B. fragilis*.[367,447,448] An appropriate initial antibiotic regimen includes an aminoglycoside (gentamicin or tobramycin) or a cephalosporin in addition to an agent such as clindamycin or metronidazole, to treat for *B. fragilis*. The antimicrobial regimens discussed in the section on treatment of secondary peritonitis would be appropriate alternatives. A more specific antibiotic regimen should be substituted when results of antimicrobial sensitivity testing of the isolated pathogens become available.

The role of antibiotics for the treatment of uncomplicated acute cholecystitis remains unclear. A large retrospective study has demonstrated that routine antibiotic therapy for acute cholecystitis did not appear to affect the outcome of the attack or to decrease the incidence of local infectious complications such as empyema or pericholecystic abscess formation.[457] These results could be due to the fact that although high concentrations of antibiotics may be present in blood, tissues, and common duct bile, these levels do not appear in the gallbladder bile, blocked by the almost universal presence of cystic duct obstruction in acute cholecystitis, and thus are unable to eradicate bactobilia.

Available evidence suggests that perioperative antibiotics are a helpful adjunct to surgery to prevent postoperative infectious complications.[458] Because wound infection is thought to be due to contamination of the incision with infected bile at the time of operation, prophylactic antibiotics should be given in a manner that will achieve high blood and tissue concentrations at the time of surgery.

Perioperative antibiotics have been recommended in situations in which the frequency of bactobilia is high (such as in the elderly and in those with either a history of jaundice or jaundice at operation, common duct obstruction from stones, chills and fever, or previous biliary tract surgery). Also, it has been recommended that administration of prophylactic antibiotics be dependent on the results of an intraoperative Gram stain of bile.[376] Although ineffective against enterococci and some anaerobes, a cephem antibiotic appears to be a reasonable choice.[458]

Surgery

Immediate surgery is indicated for gangrenous (emphysematous) cholecystitis, perforation with peritonitis, and suspected pericholecystic abscess. In these patients, cholecystectomy with intraoperative cholangiography is the procedure of choice. However, in patients with severe clinical deterioration, a cholecystostomy and removal of cystic duct stones may prove to be a temporizing life-saving measure until a second definitive procedure can be performed,[459,460] provided there is no evidence of suppurative cholangitis (i.e., repeated chills, fever, jaundice, and hypotension), which would require immediate decompression of the common bile duct. Cholecystostomy is not an adequate operation for acute suppurative cholangitis unless the common duct is clearly decompressed through a large patent cystic duct.

The timing of surgery in patients with uncomplicated acute cholecystitis has been controversial. Supporters of delayed surgery after the acute attack has subsided following conservative management feel that morbidity is decreased and that the delay may lower the frequency of unnecessary surgery when the diagnosis is unclear.[461] However, many recent series have supported early surgery reporting that a deceptively benign presentation, especially in the elderly, may actually mask the presence of complications and prompt an inappropriate delay in surgery. Also, no difference in morbidity has been reported between early and delayed surgery, and recent advances in diagnostic studies have markedly decreased the incidence of misdiagnosis.[462,463] The disadvantages of delayed surgery include prolonged hospitalization and a significant incidence of recurrent symptoms that may precipitate urgent surgery under less favorable conditions.

CHOLANGITIS

Cholangitis may be defined as varying degrees of inflammation and/or infection involving hepatic and common bile ducts. Since the mucosa of the gallbladder is continuous with that of the common bile duct via the cystic duct, it is not surprising that varying degrees of choledochitis occur as a limited cholangitis with cholecystitis. In fact, specimens of the common duct taken at the time of cholecystectomy for acute cholecystitis usually show localized edema and inflammation. However, this disease is indistinguishable from uncomplicated acute cholecystitis. In this section, we focus on the more severe entities of ascending cholangitis and acute obstructive suppurative cholangitis.

Pathogenesis

In a manner similar to that described for cholecystitis, obstruction of the common duct results in increased pressure, edema, congestion, and necrosis of the walls of the biliary tree followed by rapid proliferation of bacteria within the biliary tree. In most instances, obstruction is due to gallstones.[464] However, obstruction may be due to prior biliary tract surgery, tumor, chronic calcific pancreatitis, and parasitic infections. Fulminant cholangitis has also been reported as a complication of ERCP.[465]

Pathogenic Findings

Microscopic examination of the common duct reveals marked fibrous thickening and focal areas of chronic inflammation. Superimposed on this is necrosis of the mucosa and dense infiltration of acute inflammatory cells. In the liver, portal inflammation is uniformly seen. Usually, this is a dense neutrophilic infiltrate. In 40 percent of the cases, numerous microabscesses are present. Bile duct dilatation and cholestasis are also present.

Symptoms and Signs

Patients usually have an antecedent history compatible with gallbladder disease. The onset is usually acute, with high fever, chills, and diffuse pain and tenderness over the liver. Jaundice is usually prominent. In some cases, shock and other findings of gram-negative bacteremia may be present; altogether 85 percent of the patients fulfill Charcot's triad of fever, chills, and jaundice.[466]

Laboratory Findings

There is usually marked leukocytosis with an increase in immature forms. The serum bilirubin level is often higher than 4 mg/dl and the serum alkaline phosphatase level is significantly higher than that encountered in acute cholecystitis. Serum AST level is modestly elevated. Biochemical and even clinical evidence of disseminated intravascular coagulation may be present.

Bacteriologic Findings

Little adequate data are available on the bacteriologic findings in cholangitis. Recent studies using detailed aerobic and anaerobic culture techniques suggest that the bacteriologic findings in cholangitis are similar to those in acute obstructive cholecystitis. Gram-negative enteric bacilli and anaerobic bacteria are the most common isolates. Those patients with a stent in their bile duct may harbor resistant flora such as *P. aeruginosa*. Unlike uncomplicated cholecystitis, bacteremia occurs in approximately 50 percent of the cases. *Escherichia coli* (52 percent of the isolates), *B. fragilis* (22 percent), and *C. perfringens* (16 percent) are the most frequent isolates from blood cultures.

Roentgenographic and Related Studies

An upright chest film is of limited value. The right hemidiaphragm is frequently elevated. Other findings are similar to those described above for acute cholecystitis and are nonspecific. Oral cholecystography is of no value. Intravenous cholangiography is usually not helpful since the serum bilirubin level is frequently higher than 4.0 mg/dl and has been replaced by less morbid and more sensitive techniques. Ultrasonography can easily be used to evaluate gallbladder size, the presence of stones, and the degree of bile duct dilatation. Marked bile duct dilatation in a patient with the clinical picture described above corroborates this diagnosis. It is important to note that not all patients with obstructive cholangitis have a grossly dilated biliary tree, and ultrasonography is unlikely to be helpful in these cases. Obstruction of the common bile duct can be diagnosed by hepatobiliary scanning with one of the ^{99m}Tc-labeled derivatives of IDA. In this case, no component of the biliary system or small bowel is visualized, despite adequate hepatic uptake. In obstructive cholangitis, however, ultrasonography is the preferred study due to its ability to visualize dilated ducts and the decreased dependability of IDA scintigraphy in the presence of severe jaundice.[467] Percutaneous transhepatic cholangiography and endoscopic retrograde cholangiography are extremely valuable in evaluating bile duct obstruction. However, it is seldom feasible to use these techniques in the acutely ill patient with cholangitis.

Complications

Bacteremia and shock occur commonly and perhaps are best included as part of the clinical picture of obstructive cholangitis. Perforation of the gallbladder may occur and is described under complications of acute cholecystitis. In some less acute cases, macroscopic hepatic abscesses may develop. This clinical picture may be similar to cholangitis alone. However, ultrasonography, computed tomography, or technetium or gallium scans may visualize multiple defects in the hepatic parenchyma. Finally, pancreatitis may occur as a complication.

Differential Diagnosis

Acute cholecystitis and its complications, hepatic abscess, perforating ulcer, pancreatitis, intestinal obstruction, right lower lobe pneumonia, acute disease involving the right kidney, and bacteremic shock related to another focus of infection should all be considered in the differential diagnosis. In acute cholecystitis the patient is usually less ill; in addition, the serum bilirubin level is usually less than 4.0 mg/dl, the serum alkaline phosphatase level is not markedly elevated, and ultrasonography of cholescintigraphy usually demonstrate a patent, nondilated hepatic and common duct. Patients with hepatic abscesses not due to obstructive cholangitis are usually not as acutely ill; hepatic tenderness, when present, is also not as severe, and liver function tests may be only minimally abnormal. Diagnostic studies usually detect a macroscopic parenchymal defect. In pancreatitis, the pain and tenderness are more midline and may radiate to the back. Serum and urine amylase levels are significantly elevated, but liver function tests are not markedly abnormal. Finally, radiographs of the chest and abdomen and urinalysis exclude the majority of other possibilities.

Antimicrobial Therapy in Cholangitis

Prompt institution of appropriate antibiotic therapy is mandatory, since these severe infections are frequently complicated by bacteremia and shock. Based on the bacteriologic findings described above and on the known in vitro susceptibilities of these organisms, an appropriate regimen would be clindamycin or metronidazole plus an aminoglycoside or cephalosporin antibiotic. The antimicrobial regimens discussed in the section on treatment of secondary peritonitis would be alternative choices. This antibiotic regimen is directed primarily at the complicating bacteremia, since antibiotics alone will not sterilize the biliary tract in the face of obstruction.[448]

Surgery

Prompt operative intervention with decompression of the common duct is mandatory in all but those few patients who respond promptly to antibiotics.[468] In all patients who undergo surgery, regardless of the procedure, operative cholangiography should be performed. The simplest but least satisfactory procedure is simple cholecystostomy if patency of the cystic duct is assured. However, if at all possible, a cholecystectomy should be performed, followed by common duct exploration and T-tube drainage. In more complicated cases, choledochoduodenostomy or cholecystoduodenostomy may have to be performed.

REFERENCES

1. Altemeier WA, Culbertson WR, Fullen WD. Intra-abdominal sepsis. In: Welch CE, Hardy JD, eds. Advances in Surgery. Chicago: Year Book Medical Publishers; 1971:281–333.
2. Boyd DP. The subphrenic spaces and the emperor's new robes. N Engl J Med. 1966;275:911–7.
3. Whalen JP, Bierny JP. Classification of perihepatic abscesses. Radiology. 1969;92:1427–37.
4. Sanders RC, James AE Jr, Fischer K. Correlation of liver scans and images with abdominal radiographs in perihepatic sepsis. Am J Surg. 1972;124:346–52.
5. Myers MA. The spread and localization of acute intraperitoneal effusions. Radiology. 1970;95:547–54.
6. Altemeier WA, Culbertson WR, Fullen WD, et al. Intra-abdominal abscesses. Am J Surg. 1973;125:70–9.
7. Henderson LW, Nolph KD. Altered permeability of the peritoneal membrane using hypertonic peritoneal dialysis fluid. J Clin Invest. 1969;48:992–1001.
8. Shear L, Swartz C, Shinaberger JA, et al. Kinetics of peritoneal fluid absorption in adult men. N Engl J Med. 1965;272:123–7.
9. Boen ST. Kinetics of peritoneal dialysis: A comparison with artificial kidney. Medicine. 1961;40:243–87.
10. Tsilibury EC, Wissig SL. Absorption from the peritoneal cavity: SEM study of the mesothelium covering the peritoneal surface of the muscular portion of the diaphragm. Am J Anat. 1977;149:127–33.
11. Rochlin DB, Zill H, Blakemore WS. Studies of the resorption of chromium-51 tagged erythrocytes from the peritoneal cavity; the absorption of fluids and particulate matter from the peritoneal cavity. Int Abstr Surg. 1958;107:1–14.
12. Pritchard JA, Adams RH. The fate of blood in the peritoneal cavity. Surg Gynecol Obstet. 1957;105:621–9.

13. Zinsser HH, Pryde AW. Experimental study of physical factors, including fibrin formation, influencing the spread of fluids and small particles within and from the peritoneal cavity of the dog. Ann Surg. 1952;136:818–27.
14. Macbeth RA, Mackenzie WC. The abdominal wall, umbilicus, peritoneum, mesenteries, and retroperitoneum. In: Sabiston DC Jr, ed. Davis-Christopher Textbook of Surgery. 10th ed. Philadelphia: WB Saunders; 1972:773–95.
15. Nohr CW, Marshall DG. Primary peritonitis in children. Can J Surg. 1984;27(2):179–81.
16. McDougal WS, Izant RJ, Zollinger RM Jr. Primary peritonitis in infancy and childhood. Ann Surg. 1975;181:310–3.
17. Golden GT, Shaw A. Primary peritonitis. Surg Gynecol Obstet. 1972;135:513–6.
18. Epstein M, Calia FM, Gabuzda GJ. Pneumococcal peritonitis in patients with postnecrotic cirrhosis. N Engl J Med. 1968;278:69–71.
19. Speck WT, Dresdale SS, McMillan RW. Primary peritonitis and the nephrotic syndrome. Am J Surg. 1974;127:267–9.
20. Conn HO, Fessel JM. Spontaneous bacterial peritonitis in cirrhosis: Variations on a theme. Medicine. 1971;50:161–97.
21. Conn HO. Spontaneous bacterial peritonitis, multiple revisitations. Gastroenterology. 1976;70:455–7.
22. Bar-Meir S, Conn HO. Spontaneous bacterial peritonitis inducecd by intra-arterial vasopressin therapy. Gastroenterology. 1976;70:418–21.
23. Curry N, McCallum RW, Guth PH. Spontaneous peritonitis in cirrhotic ascites: A decade of experience. Am J Dig Dis. 1974;19:685–92.
24. Targan SR, Chow AW, Guze LB. Role of anaerobic bacteria in spontaneous peritonitis of cirrhosis: Report of two cases and review of the literature. Am J Med. 1977;62:397–403.
25. Kline MM, McCallum RW, Guth PH. The clinical value of ascitic fluid culture and leukocyte count studies in alcoholic cirrhosis. Gastroenterology. 1976;70:408–12.
26. Weinstein MP, Iannini PB, Stratton CW, et al. Spontaneous bacterial peritonitis: A review of 28 cases with emphasis on improved survival and factors influencing prognosis. Am J Med. 1978;64:592–8.
27. Hoefs JC, Canawati HN, Sapico FL, et al. Spontaneous bacterial peritonitis. Hepatology. 1982;2:399–407.
28. Pinzello G, Simonetti R, Craxi A, et al. Spontaneous bacterial peritonitis: A prospective investigation in predominantly nonalcoholic cirrhotic patients. Hepatology. 1983;3:545–9.
29. Conn HO. Cirrhosis. In: Schiff L, Schiff ER, eds. Diseases of the Liver. 5th ed. Philadelphia: JB Lippincott; 1982:847–977.
30. Thomas FB, Fromkes JJ. Spontaneous bacterial peritonitis associated with acute viral hepatitis. J Clin Gastroenterol. 1982;4:259–62.
31. Runyon BA. Spontaneous bacterial peritonitis with cardiac ascites. Am J Gastroenterol. 1984;79:796.
32. Isner J, MacDonald JS, Schein PS. Spontaneous *Streptococcus pneumoniae* peritonitis in a patient with metastatic gastric cancer. Cancer. 1979;39:2306–9.
33. Shesol BF, Rosato EF, Rosato FE. Concomitant acute lupus erythematosus and primary pneumococcal peritonitis. Am J Gastroenterol. 1975;63:324–6.
34. Friedland JA, Harris MN. Primary pneumococcal peritonitis in a young adult. Am J Surg. 1970;119:737–9.
35. Golden GT, Stevenson TR, Ritchie WP Jr. Primary peritonitis in adults. South Med J. 1975;68:413–4.
36. Wilcox CM, Dismukes WE. Spontaneous bacterial peritonitis: A review of pathogenesis, diagnosis and treatment. Medicine. 1987;66:447–56.
37. Correia JP, Conn HO. Spontaneous bacterial peritonitis in cirrhosis: Endemic or epidemic? Med Clin North Am. 1975;59:963–81.
38. Hoefs JC, Runyon BA. Spontaneous bacterial peritonitis. Dis Mon. 1985;31(9):1–48.
39. Fromkes JJ, Thomas FB, Mekhjian HS, et al. Antimicrobial activity of human ascitic fluid. Gastroenterology. 1977;73:668–72.
40. Scheckman P, Onderdonk AB, Bartlett JG. Anaerobes in spontaneous peritonitis. Lancet. 1977;2:1223.
41. Runyon BA, Hoefs JC. Culture-negative neutrocytic ascites: A variant of spontaneous peritonitis. Hepatology. 1984;4:1209–11.
42. Runyon BA, Umland ET, Merlin T. Inoculation of blood culture bottles with ascitic fluid: Improved detection of spontaneous bacterial peritonitis. Arch Intern Med. 1987;147:73–75.
43. Beeson PB, Brannon ES, Warren JU. Observations on the sites of removal of bacteria from the blood in patients with bacterial endocarditis. J Exp Med. 1945;81:9–23.
44. Rutenburg AM, Sonnenblick F, Koven I, et al. Comparative response of normal and cirrhotic rats to intravenously injected bacteria. Proc Soc Exp Biol Med. 1959;101:279–81.
45. Lahnborg G, Friman L, Berghem L. Reticuloendothelial function in patients with alcoholic liver disease. Scand J Gastroenterol. 1981;16:481–9.
46. Rimola A, Soto R, Bory F, et al. Reticuloendothelial system phagocytic activity in cirrhosis and its relation to bacterial infections and prognosis. Hepatology. 1984;4:53–8.
47. Rajkovic IA, Williams R. Abnormalities of neutrophilic phagocytosis, intracellular killing and metabolic activity in alcoholic cirrhosis and hepatitis. Hepatology. 1986;6:252–62.
48. Wyke RJ, Rajkovic IA, Eddleston WF, et al. Defective serum opsonization in patients with chronic liver disease (Abstract). Gut. 1979;20:A931.
49. Yousif-Kadura AGM, Rajkovic IA, Wyke RJ, et al. Defects in serum attractant activity in different types of chronic liver disease. Gut. 1984;25:79–84.
50. Simberkoff MS, Moldover NH, Weiss G. Bactericidal and opsonic activity of cirrhotic ascites and nonascitic peritoneal fluid. J Lab Clin Med. 1978;91:831–9.
51. Runyon BA, Hoefs JC. Ascitic fluid analysis in the differentiation of spontaneous bacterial peritonitis from gastrointestinal performation into ascitic fluid. Hepatology. 1984;4:447–50.
52. Whipple RL Jr, Harris JF. *E. coli* septicemia in Laennec's cirrhosis of the liver. Ann Intern Med. 1950;33:462–9.
53. Murray HW, Marks SJ. Spontaneous bacterial empyema, pericarditis and peritonitis in cirrhosis. Gastroenterology. 1977;72:772–3.
54. Snyder N, Atterbury CE, Correia JP, et al. Increased concurrence of cirrhosis and bacterial endocarditis. Gastroenterology. 1977;73:1107–13.
55. Schweinburg FB, Seligman AM, Fine J. Transmural migration of intestinal bacteria: A study based on the use of radioactive *Escherichia coli.* N Engl J Med. 1950;242:747–51.
56. Schwartz FD, Kallmeyer J, Durea G, et al. Prevention of infection during peritoneal dialysis. JAMA. 1967;199:79–81.
57. Gorbach SL, Lai D, Levitan R. Intestinal microflora in Laennec's cirrhosis. J Clin Invest. 1970;49:36a.
58. McCartney JE, Fraser J. Pneumococcal peritonitis. Br J Surg. 1922;9:479–89.
59. Herbert TJ, Mortimer PP. Recurrent pneumococcal peritonitis associated with an intrauterine contraceptive device. Br J Surg. 1974;61:901–2.
60. Brinson RR, Kolts BE, Monif GRG. Spontaneous bacterial peritonitis associated with an intrauterine device. J Clin Gastroenterol. 1986;8:82–4.
61. Kimball MW, Knee S. Gonococcal perihepatitis in a male. The Fitz-Hugh-Curtis syndrome. N Engl J Med. 1970;282:1082–4.
62. Luetscher JA Jr. Electrophoretic analysis of the proteins of plasma and serous effusions. J Clin Invest. 1941;20:99–106.
63. Witte MH, Witte CL, Davis WM, et al. Peritoneal transudate: A diagnostic clue to portal system obstruction in patients with intra-abdominal neoplasms or peritonitis. JAMA. 1972;221:1380–3.
64. Hoefs JC. Increase in ascites white blood cell and protein concentrations during diuresis in patients with chronic liver disease. Hepatology. 1981;1:249–54.
65. Stassen WN, McCullough AJ, Bacon BR, et al. Immediate diagnostic criteria for bacterial infection of ascitic fluid: Evaluation of ascitic fluid polymorphonuclear leukocyte count, pH, and lactate concentration, alone and in combination. Gastroenterology. 1986;90:1247–54.
66. Garcia-Tsao G, Conn HO, Lerner E. The diagnosis of bacterial peritonitis: Comparison of pH, lactate concentration and leukocyte count. Hepatology. 1985;5:91–6.
67. Yang C-Y, Liaw F, Chu E-M, et al. White count, pH and lactate in ascites in the diagnosis of spontaneous bacterial peritonitis. Hepatology. 1985;5:85–90.
68. Vickers FN, Maloney PJ. Gonococcal perihepatitis: Reports of three cases with comments on diagnosis and treatment. Arch Intern Med. 1964;114:120–3.
69. Burack WR, Hollister RM. Tuberculous peritonitis: A study of forty-seven proved cases encountered by a general medical unit in twenty-five years. Am J Med. 1960;28:510–23.
70. Saw EC, Shields SJ, Comer TP, et al. Granulomatous peritonitis due to *Coccidioides immitis*. Arch Surg. 1974;108:369–71.
71. Harrison RN, Cryer HM, Howard DA, et al. Clarification of risk factors for abdominal operations in patients with hepatic cirrhosis. Ann Surg. 1984;199:648–65.
72. Runyon BA, Hoefs JC. Spontaneous vs. secondary bacterial peritonitis: Differentiation by response of ascitic fluid neutrophil count to antimicrobial therapy. Arch Intern Med. 1986;146:1563–5.
73. Dimond M, Proctor HJ. Concomitant pneumococcal appendicitis, peritonitis and meningitis. Arch Surg. 1976;111:888–9.
74. Mallory A, Schaefer JW. Complications of diagnostic paracentesis in patients with liver disease. JAMA. 1978;239:628–30.
75. Levine H. Needle biopsy of peritoneum in exudative ascites. Arch Intern Med. 1967;120:542–5.
76. Dineen P, Homan WP, Grafe WR. Tuberculous peritonitis: 43 years experience in diagnosis and treatment. Ann Surg. 1976;184(6):717–22.
77. Felisart J, Rimona A, Arroyo V, et al. Cefotaxime is more effective than is ampicillin-tobramycin in cirrhotics with severe infections. Hepatology. 1985;5:457–62.
78. Cabrera J, Arroyo V, Ballesta AM, et al. Aminoglycoside nephrotoxicity in cirrhosis: Value of urinary β_2-microglobulin to discriminate functional renal failure from acute tubular damage. Gastroenterology. 1982;82:97–105.
79. Runyon BA, Hoefs JC. Ascitic fluid chemical analysis before, during and after spontaneous bacterial peritonitis. Hepatology. 1985;5:257–9.
80. Porter JM, Snowe RJ, Silver D. Tuberculous enteritis with perforation and abscess formation in childhood. Surgery. 1972;71:254–7.
81. Rowland TC Jr. Severe peritonitis complicating an intrauterine contraceptive device. Am J Obstet Gynecol. 1971;110:786–7.
82. Prokesch RC, Rimland D. Infectious complications of the peritoneovenous shunt. Am J Gastroenterol. 1983;78:235–40.
83. Reynold M, Sherman JO, Mclone DG. Ventriculoperitoneal shunt infections masquerading as an acute abdomen. J Pediatr Surg. 1983;18:951–4.

84. Nichols RL. Intra-abdominal infections: An overview. Rev Infect Dis. 1985;7(Suppl 4):S709–15.
85. Drasar BS, Shiner M, McLeod GM. Studies on the intestinal flora. I. The bacterial flora of the gastrointestinal tract in healthy and achlorhydric persons. Gastroenterology. 1969;56:71–9.
86. Nichols RL, Smith JW. Intragastric microbial colonization in common disease states of the stomach and duodenum. Ann Surg. 1975;182:557–61.
87. Gorbach SL, Plaut AG, Nahas L, et al. Studies of intestinal microflora. II. Microorganisms of the small intestine and their relations to oral and fecal flora. Gastroenterology. 1967;53:856–67.
88. Drasar BS, Shiner M. Studies on the intestinal flora. Part II. Bacterial flora of the small intestine in patients with gastrointestinal disorders. Gut. 1969;10:812–9.
89. Gorbach SL, Nahas L, Lerner PI, et al. Studies of intestinal microflora. I. Effects of diet, age, and periodic sampling of numbers of fecal microorganisms in man. Gastroenterology. 1967;53:845–55.
90. Finegold SM. Interaction of antimicrobial therapy and intestinal flora. Am J Clin Nutr. 1970;23:1466–71.
91. Altemeier WA. The bacterial flora of acute perforated appendicitis with peritonitis. Ann Surg. 1938;107:517–28.
92. Finegold SM. Abdominal and perineal infections. In: Finegold SM, ed. Anaerobic Bacteria in Human Disease. New York. Academic Press; 1977;257–313.
93. Gorbach SL, Thadepalli H, Norsen J. Anaerobic microorganisms in intraabdominal infections. In: Balows A, de Haan RM, Dowell VR Jr, et al, eds. Anaerobic Bacteria: Role in Disease. Springfield, Ill: Charles C. Thomas; 1974:399–407.
94. Lorber B, Swenson RM. The bacteriology of intra-abdominal infections. Surg Clin North Am. 1975;55:1349–54.
95. Swenson RM, Lorber B, Michaelson TC, et al. The bacteriology of intraabdominal infections. Arch Surg. 1974;109:398–9.
96. Tally FP, McGowan K, Kellum JM, et al. A randomized comparison of cefoxitin with or without amikacin and clindamycin plus amikacin in surgical sepsis. Ann Surg. 1981;193:318–23.
97. Aronoff SC, Olson MM, Gaudierer MWL, et al. *Pseudomonas aeruginosa* as a primary pathogen in children with bacterial peritonitis. J Pediatr Surg. 1987;22:861–4.
98. Heseltine PNR, Yellin AE, Applebaum MD, et al. Perforated and gangrenous appendicitis: An analysis of antibiotic failures. J Infect Dis. 1983;148:322–9.
99. Dunn DL, Simmons RL. The role of anaerobic bacteria in intra-abdominal infections. Rev Infect Dis. 1984;6(Suppl 1):S139–46.
100. Nichols RL, Smith JW, Klein DB, et al. Risk of infection after penetrating abdominal trauma. N Engl J Med. 1984;311:1065–70.
101. Bodner SJ, Koenig MG, Goodman JS. Bacteremic *Bacteroides* infections. Ann Intern Med. 1970;73:537–44.
102. Gelb EF, Seligman SJ. Bacteroidaceae bacteremia. Effect of age and focus of infection upon clinical course. JAMA. 1970;212:1038–41.
103. Fry DE, Garrison RN, Polk HC Jr. Clinical implications in *Bacteroides* bacteremia. Surg Gynecol Obstet. 1979;149:189–92.
104. Chow AW, Guze LB. Bacteroidaceae bacteremia: Clinical experience with 112 patients. Medicine. 1974;53:93–126.
105. Levison ME, Korman LC, Carrington ER, et al. Quantitative microflora of the vagina. Am J Obstet Gynecol. 1977;127:80–5.
106. Levison ME, Trestman I, Quach R, et al. Quantitative bacteriology of the vaginal flora in vaginitis. Am J Obstet Gynecol. 1979;133:139–44.
107. Bartlett JG, Onderdonk AB, Drude E, et al. Quantitative bacteriology of the vaginal flora. J Infect Dis. 1977;136:271–7.
108. Ohm M, Galask RP. The effect of antibiotic prophylaxis on patients undergoing vaginal operations: II. Alteration of microbial flora. Am J Obstet Gynecol. 1975;123:597–604.
109. Ramsay AM. The significance of *C. welchii* in the cervical swab and blood serum in postpartum and postabortum sepsis. J Obstet Gynecol. 1949;56:247–58.
110. Hite KE, Hesseltine HC, Goldstein L. A study of the bacterial flora of the normal and pathologic vagina and uterus. Am J Obstet Gynecol. 1947;53:233–40.
111. Gibbs RS, O'Dell TN, MacGregor RR, et al. Puerperal endometritis: A prospective microbiologic study. Am J Obstet Gynecol. 1975;121:919–25.
112. Baker CJ, Barrett FF, Yow MD. The influence of advancing gestation on group B streptococcal colonization in pregnant women. Am J Obstet Gynecol. 1975;122:820–3.
113. Penza JF. Moniliasis and trichomoniasis. In: Charles D, Finland M, eds. Obstetric and Perinatal Infections. Philadelphia: Lee & Febiger; 1973:209.
114. Finegold SM. Female genital tract infections. In: Finegold SM, ed. Anaerobic Bacteria in Human Disease. New York: Academic Press; 1977: 350–85.
115. Swenson RM, Michaelson TC, Daly MJ, et al. Anaerobic bacterial infections of the female genital tract. Obstet Gynecol. 1973;42:538–41.
116. Thadepalli H, Gorbach SL, Keith L. Anaerobic infections of the female genital tract: Bacteriologic and therapeutic aspects. Am J Obstet Gynecol. 1973;117:1034–40.
117. Chow AW, Marshall JR, Guze LB. Anaerobic infections of the female genital tract: Prospects and perspectives. Obstet Gynecol Surg. 1975;30:477–94.
118. Chow AW, Malkasian KI, Marshall JR, et al. The bacteriology of acute pelvic inflammatory disease. Value of cul-de-sac cultures and relative importance of gonococcal and other aerobic or anaerobic bacteria. Am J Obstet Gynecol. 1975;122:876–9.
119. Eschenbach DA, Buchanon TM, Pollock HM, et al. Polymicrobial etiology of acute pelvic inflammatory disease. N Engl J Med. 1975;293:166–71.
120. Wasserheit JN, Bell TA, Kiviat NB, et al. Microbial causes of proven pelvic inflammatory disease and efficacy of clindamycin and tobramycin. Ann Intern Med. 1986;104:187–93.
121. Monif GRG, Welkos SI, Baer H, et al. Cul-de-sac isolates from patients with endometritis-salpingitis-peritonitis and gonococcal endocervicitis. Am J Obstet Gynecol. 1976;126:158–61.
122. Burry VF. Gonococcal vulvovaginitis and possible peritonitis in prepubertal girls. Am J Dis Child. 1971;121:536–7.
123. Fuld GL. Gonococcal peritonitis in a prepubertal child. Am J Dis Child. 1968;115:621–2.
124. Adams EB, MacLeod IN. Invasive amebiasis. II. Amebic liver abscess and its complications. Medicine. 1977;56:325–34.
125. Turner GR, Millikan M, Carter R, et al. Surgical significance of fulminating amebic colitis. Report of perforation of the colon with peritonitis. Am Surg. 1965;31:759–63.
126. Lintermans JP. Fatal peritonitis, an unusual complication of *Strongyloides stercoralis* infestation. Clin Pediatr. 1975;14:974–5.
127. Eisenberg ES, Leviton I, Soeiro R. Fungal peritonitis in patients receiving peritoneal dialysis: Experience with 11 patients and review of the literature. Rev Infect Dis. 1986;3:309–21.
128. Bayer AS, Blumenkrantz MJ, Montgomerie JZ, et al. Candida peritonitis: Report of 22 cases and review of the English literature. Am J Med. 1976;61:832–40.
129. Solomkin JS, Flohr AB, Quie PG, et al. The role of candida in intraperitoneal infections. Surgery. 1980;88:524–30.
130. Howard JM, Singh LM. Peritoneal fluid pH after perforation of peptic ulcers. Arch Surg. 1963;87:483–4.
131. Mortez WH, Erickson WG. Neutralization of hydrochloric acid in the peritoneal cavity. Arch Surg. 1957;75:834–7.
132. Santschi DR, Huizenga KA, Scudamore HH, et al. Bile ascites. Arch Surg. 1963;87:851–6.
133. Diamonon JS, Barnes JP. Choleperitoneum. Am Surg. 1964;30:331–4.
134. Cohn I, Cotlar AM, Atik M, et al. Bile peritonitis. Ann Surg. 1960;152:827–35.
135. Nemir P Jr, Hawthorne HR, Cohn I, et al. I. The cause of death in strangulation obstruction. An experimental study. Ann Surg. 1949;130:857–73.
136. Nemir P Jr, Hawthorne HR, Cohn I, et al. II. The lethal action of the peritoneal fluid. Ann Surg. 1949;130:874–80.
137. Barnett WO, Hardy JD. Observations concerning the peritoneal fluid in experimental strangulated intestinal obstruction: The effects of removal from the peritoneal cavity. Surgery. 1958;43:440–4.
138. Barnett WO, Doyle RS. The effects of neomycin upon the toxicity of peritoneal fluid resulting from strangulation obstruction. Surgery. 1958;44:442–6.
139. Barnett WO, Messina AJ. The influence of massive antibiotics in experimental strangulation obstruction. Gastroenterology. 1959;36:534–6.
140. Davis JH, Yull AB. A possible toxic factor in abdominal surgery. J Trauma. 1962;2:291–300.
141. Filler RM, Sleeman HK, Hendry WS, et al. Lethal factors in experimental peritonitis. Surgery. 1966;60:671–8.
142. Lee JT Jr, Ahrenholz DN, Nelson RD, et al. Mechanisms of the adjuvant effect of hemoglobin in experimental peritonitis. V. The significance of the coordinated iron component. Surgery. 1979;86:41–8.
143. Weingerg ED. Roles of iron in host–parasite interactions. J Infect Dis. 1971;124:401–10.
144. Hau T, Nelson RD, Fiegel VD, et al. Mechanisms of the adjuvant action of hemoglobin in experimental peritonitis—2. Influence of hemoglobin on human leukocyte chemotaxis in vitro. J Surg Res. 1977;22:174–80.
145. Dunn DL, Barke RA, Ahrenholz DH, et al. The adjuvant effect of peritoneal fluid in experimental peritonitis. Ann Surg. 1984;199:37–43.
146. Rotstein OD, Pruett TL, Simmons RD. Fibrin in peritonitis. V. Fibrin inhibits phagocytic killing of *Escherichia coli* by human polymorphonuclear leukocytes. Ann Surg. 1986;203:413–9.
147. Schneierson SS, Amsterdam D, Perlman E. Enhancement of intraperitoneal staphylococcal virulence for mice with different bile salts. Nature. 1961;190:829–30.
148. Sisel RJ, Donovan AJ, Yellin AE. Experimental fecal peritonitis. Influence of barium sulfate or water-soluble radiographic contrast material on survival. Arch Surg. 1972;104:765–8.
149. Westfall RH, Nelson RH, Musselman MM. Barium peritonitis. Am J Surg. 1966;112:760–3.
150. Olitzki L. Mucin as a resistance-lowering substance. Bacteriol Rev. 1948;12:149–72.
151. Cuevas P, Fine J. Role of intraintestinal endotoxin in death from peritonitis. Surg Gynecol Obstet. 1972;134:953–7.
152. Bieluch VM, Tally FP. Pathophysiology of abscess formation. Clin Obstet Gynecol. 1983;10:93–103.
153. Gorbach SL, Bartlett JG. Anaerobic infections (third of three parts). N Engl J Med. 1974;290:1289–94.
153a. Hofstad T. Endotoxins of anaerobic gram-negative microorganisms. In: Balows A, de Haan RM, Dowell VR Jr., et al., eds. Anaerobic Bacteria: Role in Disease. Springfield, IL: Charles C. Thomas; 1974:295.

154. Bjornson HS. Enzymes associated with the survival and virulence of gram-negative anaerobes. Rev Infect Dis. 1984;6(Suppl 1):S21–4.
155. Gibbons RJ, MacDonald JB. Degradation of collagenous substrates by *Bacteroides melaninogenicus*. J Bacteriol. 1961;81:614–21.
156. Gesner BM, Jenkin CR. Production of heparinase by bacteroides. J Bacteriol. 1961;81:595–604.
157. Bjornson H, Hill EO. Bacteroidaceae in thromboembolic disease. Effects of cell wall components on blood coagulation in vivo and in vitro. Infect Immun. 1974;9:337–41.
158. Casciato DA, Rosenblatt JE, Goldberg LS, et al. In vitro interaction of *Bacteroides fragilis* with polymorphonuclear leukocytes and serum factors. Infect Immun. 1975;11:337–42.
159. Keusch GT, Douglas SD. Intraleukocytic survival of anaerobic bacteria. Clin Res. 1974;22:445A.
160. Kasper DL. The polysaccharide capsule of *Bacteroides fragilis* subspecies fragilis: Immunochemical and morphologic definition. J Infect Dis. 1976;133:79–87.
161. Mansheim BJ, Orderdonk AB, Kasper DL. Immunochemical characterization of surface antigens of *Bacteroides melaninogenicus*. Rev Infect Dis. 1979;1:263–77.
162. Onderdonk AB, Kasper DL, Cisneros RL, et al. The capsular polysaccharide of *Bacteroides fragilis* as a virulence factor: Comparison of the pathogenic potential of encapsulated and unencapsulated strains. J Infect Dis. 1977;136:82–9.
163. Ingham HR, Tharagonnet D, Sisson PR, et al. Inhibition of phagocytosis in vitro by obligate anaerobes. Lanct. 1977;2:1252–4.
164. Simon GL, Klempner MS, Kasper DL, et al. Alterations in opsonophagocytic killing by neutrophils of *Bacteroides fragilis* associated with animal and laboratory passage: Effect of capsular polysaccharide. J Infect Dis. 1982;145:72–7.
165. Socransky SS, Gibbons RJ. Required role of *Bacteroides melaninogenicus* in mixed anaerobic infections. J Infect Dis. 1965;115:247–53.
166. Altemeier WA. The pathogenicity of the bacteria of appendicitis peritonitis. Surgery. 1942;11:374–84.
167. Namavar FA, Verweij MJ, Bal M, et al. Effects of anaerobic bacteria on killing of *Proteus mirabilis* by human polymorphonuclear leukocytes. Infect Immun. 1983;40:930–5.
168. Rotstein OD, Nasmith PE, Grinstein S. The bacteroides by-product succinic acid inhibits neutrophil respiratory burst by reducing intracellular pH. Infect Immun. 1987;55:864–70.
169. Brook I. Anaerobic infections in childhood. Rev Infect Dis. 1984;6(Suppl 1):S187–92.
170. Onderdonk AB, Weinstein WN, Sullivan NM, et al. Experimental intra-abdominal abscess in rats: Quantitative bacteriology of infected animals. Infect Immun. 1974;10:1256–9.
171. Weinstein WM, Onderdonk AB, Bartlett JG, et al. Antimicrobial therapy of experimental intraabdominal sepsis. J Infect Dis. 1975;132:282–6.
172. Onderdonk AB, Bartlett JG, Louie T, et al. Microbial synergy in experimental intra-abdominal abscess. Infect Immun. 1976;13:22–6.
173. Rosoff L. Weil M, Bradely EC, et al. Hemodynamic and metabolic changes associated with bacterial peritonitis. Am J Surg. 1967;114:180–9.
174. MacLean LD, Mulugan WG, McLean APH, et al. Patterns of septic shock in man: A detailed study of 56 patients. Ann Surg. 1967;166:543–62.
175. Davis JH. Current concepts of peritonitis. Am Surg. 1967;33:673–81.
176. Pine RW, Wertz MJ, Lennard ES, et al. Determinants of organ malfunction or death in patients with intra-abdominal sepsis. Arch Surg. 1983;118:242–9.
177. Dellinger EP, Wertz MJ, Meakins JL, et al. Surgical infection stratification system for intra-abdominal infection. Arch Surg. 1985;120:21–9.
178. Meakins JL, Solomkin JS, Allo MD, et al. A proposed classification of intra-abdominal infections. Stratification of etiology and risk for future therapeutic trials. Arch Surg. 1984;119:1372–8.
179. Nobles ER Jr. Bacteroides infections. Ann Surg. 1973;177:601–6.
180. Young LS, Martin WJ, Meyer RD, et al. Gram-negative rod bacteremia. Microbiologic, immunologic and therapeutic considerations. Ann Intern Med. 1977;86:456–71.
181. Maler JA Jr, Reynolds TB, Yellin AE. Successful medical treatment of pyogenic liver abscess. Gastroenterology. 1979;77:618–22.
182. Herbert DA, Fogel DA, Rothman J, et al. Pyogenic liver abscesses: Successful nonsurgical therapy. Lancet. 1982;1:134–36.
183. Stalons DR, Thonsberry C, Dawell VR. Effect of culture medium and carbon dioxide concentration on growth of anaerobic bacteria commonly encountered in clinical specimens. Appl Microbiol. 1974;27:1098–1104.
184. Rosenblatt JE, Schoenknecht F. Effect of several components of anaerobic incubation on antibiotic susceptibility test results. Antimicrob Agents Chemother. 1972;1:433–40.
185. Wagoner ES, Gorman M. The reaction of cysteine and related compounds with penicillins and cephalosporins. J Antibiot. 1971;24:647–58.
186. Wilkins TD, Chalgren S. Medium for use in antibiotic susceptibility testing of anaerobic bacteria. Antimicrob Agents Chemother. 1976;10:926–8.
187. Gorbach SL, Thadepalli H. Clindamycin in pure and mixed anaerobic infections. Arch Intern Med. 1974;134:87–92.
188. Bartlett JG, Louie TJ, Onderdonk AB, et al. Whither the enterococcus? 15th ICACC. Abstract No. 297. Washington, DC; September 24–26, 1975.
189. Fass RJ, Scholand JF, Hodges GR, et al. Clindamycin in the treatment of serious anaerobic infections. Ann Intern Med. 1973;78:853–9.
190. Levison ME, Santoro J, Bran JL, et al. In vitro activity and clinical efficacy of clindamycin in the treatment of infections due to anaerobic bacteria. J Infect Dis. 1977;135:S49–53.
191. Dougherty SH. Role of enterococcus in intra-abdominal sepsis. Am J Surg. 1984;148:303–12.
192. Weinstein MP, Reller LB, Murphy J, et al. The clinical significance of positive blood cultures: A comprehensive analysis of 500 episodes of bacteremia and fungemia in adults. I. Laboratory and epidemiologic observations. Rev Infect Dis. 1983;5:35–53.
193. Shales DM, Levy J, Wolinsky E. Enterococcal bacteremia without endocarditis. Arch Intern Med. 1981;141:578–81.
194. Dougherty SH, Flohr AB, Simmons RL. Breakthrough enterococcal septicemia in surgical patients. Arch Surg. 1983;118:232–7.
195. Salzer W, Pegram PS, McCan CE. Clinical evaluation of moxalactam: Evidence of decreased efficacy in gram-positive aerobic infection. Antimicrob Agents Chemother. 1983;23:565–70.
196. Sande MA, Overton JW. In vivo antagonism between gentamicin and chloramphenicol in neutropenic mice. J Infect Dis. 1973;128:247–50.
197. Zinner SH, Provonchee RB, Elias KS. Effect of clindamycin on the in vitro activity of amikacin and gentamicin against gram negative bacilli. Antimicrob Agents Chemother. 1976;9:661–4.
198. Ekwo E, Peter G. Effect of clindamycin on aminoglycoside activity in murine model of *Escherichia coli* infection. Antimicrob Agents Chemother. 1976;10:893–8.
199. Fass RJ, Rotilie CA, Prior RB. Interaction of clindamycin and gentamicin in vitro. Antimicrob Agents Chemother. 1974;6:582–7.
200. Cuchural GJ Jr, Tally FB, Jacobus NV, et al. Susceptibility of the *Bacteroides fragilis* group in the United States: Analysis by site of isolation. Antimicrob Agents Chemother. 1988;32:717–22.
201. Louis TJ, Bartlett JG, Onderdonk AB, et al. Failure of chloramphenicol therapy of experimental intra-abdominal sepsis. 17th ICAAC. Abstract No. 25. New York; October 12–14, 1977.
202. Thadepalli H, Gorbach SL, Bartlett JG. Apparent failure of chloramphenicol in anaerobic infections. 13th ICAAC. Abstract No. 117. Washington DC; September 19–21, 1973.
203. Van Scoy RE, Wilkowske CJ, O'Fallon WM, et al. Clindamycin versus chloramphenicol in treatment of anaerobic infections: A prospective, randomized double-blind study. Mayo Clin Proc. 1984;59:842–6.
204. Tally FB, Sosa A, Jacobus NV, et al. Clindamycin resistance in *Bacteroides fragilis*. J Antimicrob Chemother. 1981;8(Suppl):43–8.
205. Tally FP, Cuchural GH Jr, Jacobus NV, et al. Nationwide study of the susceptibility of the *Bacteroides fragilis* group in the United States. Antimicrob Agents Chemother. 1985;28:675–7.
206. Wilson WR, Cockerhill FR III. Tetracyclines, chloramphenicol, erythromycin and clindamycin. Mayo Clin Proc. 1987;62:906–15.
207. Tedesco FJ, Barton RW, Alpers DH. Clindamycin associated colitis: A prospective study. Ann Intern Med. 1974;81:429–33.
208. Ralph ED, Kirby WMM. Unique bactericidal action against *Bacteroides fragilis* and *Clostridium perfringens*. Antimicrob Agents Chemother. 1975;8:409–14.
209. Chow AW, Patten V, Guze LB. Susceptibility of anaerobic bacteria to metronidazole: Relative resistance of non-spore-forming gram-positive bacilli. J Infect Dis. 1975;131:182–5.
210. Onderdonk AB, Louie TJ, Tally FP, et al. Activity of metronidazole against *Escherichia coli* in experimental intra-abdominal sepsis. J Antimicrob Chemother. 1979;5:201–10.
211. Bartlett JG, Louie TJ, Gorbach SL, et al. Therapeutic efficacy of 29 antimicrobial regimens in experimental intra-abdominal sepsis. Rev Infect Dis. 1981;3:535–42.
212. Sutter VL, Kwoh Y-Y, Finegold SM. Standardized antimicrobial disc susceptibility testing of anaerobic bacteria. I. Susceptibility of *Bacteroides fragilis* to tetracyclines. Appl Microbiol. 1972;23:268–75.
213. Sutter VL, Finegold SM. Susceptibility of anaerobic bacteria to 23 antimicrobial agents. Antimicrob Agents Chemother. 1976;10:736–52.
214. Wexler HM, Finegold SM. In vitro activity of cefotetan compared with that of other antimicrobial agents against anaerobic bacteria. Antimicrob Agents Chemother. 1988;32:601–4.
215. O'Keefe JP, Vlenezio FR, Divincenzo CA, et al. Activity of newer beta-lactam agents against clinical isolates of *Bacteroides fragilis* and other *Bacteroides* species. Antimicrob Agents Chemother. 1987;31:2002–4.
216. Rolfe RD, Finegold SM. Comparative in vitro activity of new beta-lactam antibiotics against anaerobic bacteria. Antimicrob Agents Chemother. 1981;200:600–9.
217. Tally FP, Kellum JM, Ho TF, et al. Randomized prospective study comparing moxalactam and cefoxitin with or without tobramycin for treatment of serious surgical infections. Antimicrob Agents Chemother. 1986;29:244–9.
218. Schentag JJ, Wells PB, Reitberg DP, et al. A randomized clinical trial of moxalactam alone versus tobramycin plus clindamycin in abdominal sepsis. Ann Surg. 1983;198:35–41.
219. Andrassy K, Bechtold H, Ritz F. Hypoprothrombinemia caused by cephalosporins. J Antimicrob Chemother. 1985;15:133–6.
220. Aldridge KE. Comparison of the activities of penicillin G and new beta-lactam antibiotics against clinical isolates of *Bacteroides* species. Antimicrob Agents Chemother. 1984;26:410–3.
221. Chow AW, Finegold SM. In vitro activity of ceftizoxime against anaerobic bacteria and comparison with other cephalosporins. J Antimicrob Chemother. 1982;10(Suppl c):45–50.

222. Schoutens E, Yourassowsky E. Speed of bactericidal action of penicillin G, ampicillin and carbenicillin on *Bacteroides fragilis*. Antimicrob Agents Chemother. 1974;6:227–31.
223. Trestman I, Kaye D, Levison ME. Activity of semisynthetic penicillins and synergism with mecillinam against *Bacteroides* species. Antimicrob Agents Chemother. 1979;16:283–6.
224. Swenson RM, Lorber B. Clindamycin and carbenicillin in treatment of patients with intra-abdominal and female genital tract infections. J Infect Dis. 1977;135:S40–5.
225. Winston DJ, Murphy W, Young LS, et al. Piperacillin therapy for serious bacterial infections. Am J Med. 1980;69:255–61.
226. Harding GKM, Buckwalk FJ, Ronald AR, et al. Prospective, randomized comparative study of clindamycin, chloramphenicol, and ticarcillin, each in combination with gentamicin, for therapy of intra-abdominal and female genital tract sepsis. J Infect Dis. 1980;142:384–93.
227. Levison ME, Trestman I, Egert J, et al. Evaluation of ticarcillin in anaerobic infections. 17th ICAAC. Abstract No. 176. New York; October 12–14, 1977.
228. O'Keefe JP, Tally FP, Barza M, et al. Inactivation of penicillin G during experimental infection with *Bacteroides fragilis*. J Infect Dis. 1978;137:437–42.
229. Sykes RB, Squibb Institute for Medical Research. The classification and terminology of enzymes that hydrolyze beta-lactam antibiotics. J Infect Dis. 1982;145:762–5.
230. Eliopoulos GM, Moellering RC Jr. Azlocillin, mezlocillin and piperacillin: New broad-spectrum penicillins. Ann Intern Med. 1982;97:755–60.
231. Gould IM, Wise R. Beta-lactamase inhibitors. In: Peterson PK, Verhoef J, Amsterdam BV, eds. The Antimicrobial Agents Annual. 2nd ed. New York: Elsevier; 1987:58–69.
232. Wise R, Andrews JM, Bedford KA. Clavulanic acid and CP-45, 899: A comparison of their in vitro activity in combination with penicillins. J Antimicrob Chemother. 1980;6:197–206.
233. Donowitz GR, Mandell GL. Beta-lactam antibiotics (first of two parts). N Engl J Med. 1988;313:419–26.
234. Bansal MB, Chuah SK, Thadepalli H. In vitro activity and in vivo evaluation of ticarcillin plus clavulanic acid against aerobic and anaerobic bacteria. Am J Med. 1985;79(Suppl 5B):33–8.
235. Retsema JA, English AR, Girard A, et al. Sulbactam/ampicillin: In vitro spectrum, potency and activity in models of acute infection. Rev Infect Dis. 1986;8(Suppl 5):S528–42.
236. Reinhardt JF, Johnston L, Ruane P, et al. A randomized double blind comparison of sulbactam/ampicillin and clindamycin for the treatment of aerobic and aerobic-anaerobic infections. Rev Infect Dis. 1986;8(Suppl 5): S569–75.
237. Jones RN. Review of the in vitro spectrum of activity of imipenem. Am J Med. 1985;78(Suppl 6A):22–32.
238. Yotsuji A, Minami S, Inoue M, et al. Properties of a novel beta-lactamase produced by *Bacteroides fragilis*. Antimicrob Agents Chemother. 1983;24:925–9.
239. Jacobus NV, Ferreira MC, Barza M. In vitro activity of aztreonam, a monobactam antibiotic. Antimicrob Agents Chemother. 1982;22:832–8.
240. Kaye D, Levison ME, Labovitz ED. The unpredictability of serum concentrations of gentamicin: Pharmacokinetics of gentamicin in patients with normal and abnormal renal function. J Infect Dis. 1974;130:150–4.
241. Verklin RM Jr, Mandell GL. Alteration of effectiveness of antibiotics by anaerobiosis. J Lab Clin Med. 1977;89:65–71.
242. Wolfson JS, Hooper DC. The fluoroquinolones: Structures, mechanisms of action and resistance, and spectra of activity in vitro. Antimicrob Agents Chemother. 1985;28:581–86.
243. Neu HE. New antibiotics: Areas of appropriate use. J Infect Dis. 1987;155:403–17.
244. Finegold SM, Wexler HM. Therapeutic implications of bacteriologic findings in mixed aerobic-anaerobic infections. Antimicrob Agents Chemother. 1988;32:611–6.
245. David IB, Buck JR, Filler RM. Rational use of antibiotics for perforated appendicitis in childhood. J Pediatr Surg. 1982;17:494–500.
246. Norwegian Study Group for Colorectal Surgery. Should antimicrobial prophylaxis in colorectal surgery include agents effective against both anaerobic and aerobic microorganisms? A double blind multicenter study. Surgery. 1984;97:402–7.
247. Solomkin JS, Meakins JC, Allo MD, et al. Antibiotic trials in intra-abdominal infections. A critical evaluation of study design and outcome reporting. Ann Surg. 1984;200:29–39.
248. Stone HH. Metronidazole in the treatment of surgical infections. Surgery. 1983;93(2):230–4.
249. Aoki FY, Biron S, Doris PJ, et al. Prospective, randomized comparison of metronidazole and clindamycin, each with gentamicin, for the treatment of serious intra-abdominal infection. Surgery. 1983;93(2):217–20.
250. Canadian Metronidazole-Clindamycin Study Group: Prospective, randomized comparison of metronidazole and clindamycin, each with gentamicin, for the treatment of serious intra-abdominal infections. Surgery. 1983;93:221–9.
251. Ho JL, Barza M. Role of aminoglycoside antibiotics in the treatment of intra-abdominal infection. Antimicrob Agents Chemother. 1987;31:485–91.
252. Drusano GL, Warren WJ, Saah AJ, et al. A prospective randomized controlled trial of cefoxitin versus clindamycin-aminoglycoside in mixed aerobic-anaerobic infections. Surg Gynecol Obstet. 1982;154:715–20.
253. Tally FP, McGowan K, Kellum JM, et al. A randomized comparison of cefoxitin with or without amikacin and clindamycin plus amikacin in surgical sepsis. Ann Surg. 1981;193:318–23.
254. Nichols RL, Smith JW, Klein DB, et al. Risk of infection after penetrating abdominal trauma. N Engl J Med. 1984;311:1065–70.
255. Harding GKM, Buckwold FJ, Ronald AR, et al. Prospective, randomized, comparative study of clindamycin, chloramphenicol, and ticarcillin, each in combination with gentamicin, in therapy for intra-abdominal and female genital tract sepsis. J Infect Dis. 1980;142:384–93.
256. Najem AZ, Kaminski CR, Spiller CR, et al. Comparative study of parenteral piperacillin and cefoxitin in the treatment of surgical infections of the abdomen. Surgery. 1983;157:423–5.
257. Study Group of Intra-Abdominal Infections: A randomized controlled trial of ampicillin plus sulbactam vs gentamicin plus clindamycin in the treatment of intra-abdominal infections. Rev Infect Dis. 1986;8(Suppl 5):S533–88.
258. Scandinavian Study Group. Imipenem-cilastatin versus gentamicin-clindamycin for treatment of serious bacterial infections. Lancet. 1983;1:868–71.
259. Solomkin JS, Fant WK, Rivera JO, et al. Randomized trial of imipenem-cilastatin versus gentamicin and clindamycin in mixed flora infections. Am J Med. 1985;78(Suppl 6A):85–91.
260. Guerra JG, Casaline GE, Plomina JC, et al. Imipenem-cilastatin versus gentamicin-clindamycin for treatment of moderate to severe infections in hospitalized patients. Rev Infect Dis. 1985;7(Suppl 3):463–70.
261. Birolini D, Moraes MF, Soare de Souza O. Aztreonam plus clindamycin vs tobramycin plus clindamycin for the treatment of intra-abdominal infections. Rev Infect Dis. 1985;7(Suppl 4):S724–8.
262. Harding GJ, Vincelette A, Rachlis I, et al. A preliminary report on the use of ceftizoxime vs clindamycin/tobramycin for the therapy of intra-abdominal and pelvic infections. J Antimicrob Chemother. 1982;10(Suppl C):191–2.
263. Lou MA, Chen DF, Bansal M, et al. Evaluation of ceftizoxime in acute peritonitis. J Antimicrob Chemother. 1982;(Suppl C):183–9.
264. Berne TV, Yellin AW, Applebaum MC, et al. Antibiotic management of surgically treated or perforated appendicitis: Comparison of gentamicin and clindamycin versus cefamandole versus cefoperazone. Am J Surg. 1982;144:8–12.
265. Lau WY, Fan ST, Chu KW, et al. Randomized, prospective and double-blind trial of new beta-lactams in the treatment of appendicitis. Antimicrob Agents Chemother. 1985;28:639–42.
266. Saurio IH, Aruilommi C, Silvola H. Comparison of cefuroxime and gentamicin in combination with metronidazole in the treatment of peritonitis due to perforation of the appendix. Acta Chir Scand. 1983;149:423–6.
267. Peoples JB. *Candida* and perforated peptic ulcers. Surgery. 1986;100:758–64.
268. Rutledge R, Mandel SR, Wilde RE. *Candida* species. Insignificant contaminant or pathogenic species? Am Surg. 1986;52:299–302.
269. Marsh PK, Tally FP, Kellum J, et al. *Candida* infections in surgical patients. Ann Surg. 1983;198:42–7.
270. Sobel JD. *Candida* infections in the intensive care unit. Crit Care Clin North Am. 1988;4:325–44.
271. Hau T, Nishilawa R, Phuangsab A. Irrigation of the peritoneal cavity and antibiotics in the treatment of peritonitis. Surg Gynecol Obstet. 1983;156:25–30.
272. Rambo WM. Irrigation of the peritoneal cavity with cephalothin. Am J Surg. 1972;123:192–5.
273. Nichols RL. Management of intra-abdominal sepsis. Am J Med. 1985;80(Suppl 6B):204–9.
274. Hudspeth AS. Radical surgical debridement in the treatment of advanced generalized bacterial peritonitis. Arch Surg. 1975;110:1233–6.
275. Sindelar WF, Mason GR. Intraperitoneal irrigation with povidone-iodine solution for the prevention of intra-abdominal abscess in the bacterially contaminated abdomen. Surg Gynecol Obstet. 1979;148:409–11.
276. Ahrenholz DH, Simmons RL. Povidone-iodine in peritonitis. I. Adverse effects of local instillation in experimental *E. coli* peritonitis. J Surg Res. 1979;26:458–63.
277. Bhushan C, Mital VK, Elhence IP. Continuous postoperative peritoneal lavage in diffuse peritonitis using balanced saline antibiotic solution. Int Surg. 1975;60:526–8.
278. Hallerback B, Anderson C, Englund N, et al. A prospective randomized study of continuous peritoneal lavage postoperatively in the treatment of purulent peritonitis. Surg Gynecol Obstet. 1986;163:433–6.
279. Leiboff AR, Soroff HS. The treatment of generalized peritonitis by closed postoperative peritoneal lavage: A critical review of the literature. Arch Surg. 1987;122:1005–10.
280. Smithivas T, Hyams PJ, Matalon R, et al. The use of gentamicin in peritoneal dialysis. I. Pharmacologic results. J Infect Dis. 1971;124:S77–83.
281. Hill GB, Osterhout S. Experimental effects of hyperbaric oxygen on selected clostridial species. In vitro studies. J Infect Dis. 1972;125:17–25.
282. Holland JA, Hill GB, Wolfe WG, et al. Experimental and clinical experience with hyperbaric oxygen in the treatment of clostridial myonecrosis. Surgery. 1975;77:75–85.
283. Schreiner A, Tonjum S, Digranes A. Hyperbaric oxygen therapy in bacteroides infections. Acta Chir Scand. 1974;140:73–6.
284. Hill GB. Hyperbaric oxygen exposures for intrahepatic abscesses produced in mice by nonsporeforming anaerobic bacteria. Antimicrob Agents Chemother. 1976;9:312–7.
285. Thom SR, Lavermann MW, Hart GB. Intermittent hyperbaric oxygen therapy for reduction of mortality in experimental polymicrobial sepsis. J Infect Dis. 1986;154:504–10.

286. Haller JA Jr, Shaker IJ, Donahoo JS, et al. Peritoneal drainage versus non-drainage for generalized peritonitis from ruptured appendicitis in children: A prospective study. Ann Surg. 1973;177:595–600.
287. Leigh DA, Simmons K, Norman E. Bacterial flora of the appendix fossa in appendicitis and postoperative wound infection. J Clin Pathol. 1974;27:997–1000.
288. Follen WD, Hunt J, Altemeier WA. Prophylactic antibiotics in penetrating wounds of the abdomen. J Trauma. 1972;12:282–8.
289. Fabian TC, Boldreghini SJ. Antibiotics in penetrating abdominal trauma. Comparison of ticarcillin plus clavulanic acid with gentamicin plus clindamycin. Am J Med. 1985;79(Suppl 5B):157–60.
290. Nichols RL, Gorbach SL, Condon RE. Alteration of intestinal microflora following preoperative mechanical preparation of the colon. Dis Colon Rectum. 1971;14:123–7.
291. Condon RE, Bartlett JG, Greenlee H, et al. Efficacy of oral and systemic antibiotic prophylaxis in colorectal operations. Arch Surg. 1983;118:496–502.
292. Kaiser AB. Antibiotic prophylaxis in surgery. N Engl J Med. 1986;315:1129–38.
293. Baum ML, Anish Ds, Chalmers TC, et al. A survey of clinical trials of antibiotic prophylaxis in colon surgery: Evidence against further use of non-treatment controls. N Engl J Med. 1981;305:795–9.
294. Guglielmo BJ, Hohn DC, Koo PJ, et al. Antibiotic prophylaxis in surgical procedures: A critical analysis of the literature. Arch Surg. 1983;118:943–55.
295. Holph KD, Sorkin M, Rubin J, et al. Continuous ambulatory peritoneal dialysis: Three-year experience at one center. Ann Intern Med. 1980;92:609–13.
296. Rubin J, Rogers WA, Taylor HM, et al. Peritonitis during continuous ambulatory peritoneal dialysis. Ann Intern Med. 1980;92:7–13.
297. Fenton SSA, Pei Y, Delmore T, et al. The CAPD peritonitis rate is not improving with time. Trans Am Soc Artif Intern Organs. 1986;32:546–9.
298. Vas SL. 2. Peritonitis of peritoneal dialysis patients: Pathogenesis and treatment. Med Microbiol. 1986;5:21–63.
299. Peterson PK, Matzke GR, Keane WF. Current concepts in the management of peritonitis in continuous ambulatory peritoneal dialysis patients. Rev Infect Dis. 1987;9(3):604–12.
300. Everett ED. Diagnosis, prevention and treatment of peritonitis. Perit Dialy Bull. 1984;4(Suppl):139–42.
301. Steinberg SM, Cutler SJ, Novak JK, et al. Report of the national CAPD registry of the National Institutes of Health: Characteristics of participants and selected outcome measures for the period January 1, 1981 through August 31, 1984. In: National CAPD Registry of the National Institute of Arthritis, Diabetes, and Digestive and Kidney Diseases. Washington, DC: US Public Health Services; 1985.
302. Kraus ES, Spector DA. Characteristics and sequelae of peritonitis in diabetics and non-diabetics receiving chronic intermittent peritoneal dialysis. Medicine. 1983;62:52–7.
303. Fenton S, Wu G, Cattran D, et al. Clinical aspects of peritonitis in patients on CAPD. Perit Dialy Bull. 1981;1(Suppl):4–8.
304. Sewell CM, Clarridge J, Lacke C, et al. Staphylococcal nasal carriage and subsequent infection in peritoneal dialysis patients. JAMA. 1982;248:1493–5.
305. Keane WJ, Comty CM, Verbrugh HA, et al. Opsonic deficiency of peritoneal dialysis effluent in CAPD. Kidney Int. 1984;25:539–43.
306. Lamperi S, Carozzi S, Nasini MG. Intraperitoneal immunoglobulin treatment in prophylaxis of bacterial peritonitis in CAPD. In: Khanna R, Nolph KD, Provant B, et al, eds. Advances in CAPD. Toronto: University of Toronto Press; 1986:110.
307. Duwe AK, Vas SI, Weatherhead IW. Effects of composition of peritoneal dialysis fluid on chemiluminescence, phagocytosis and bacterial activity in vitro. Infect Immun. 1981;33:130–5.
308. Marrie TJ, Noble MA, Costerton JW. Examination of the morphology of bacteria adhering to peritoneal dialysis catheters by scanning and transmission electron microscopy. J Clin Microbiol. 1983;18:1388–98.
309. Arfania D, Everett ED, Nolph KD, et al. Uncommon causes of peritonitis in patients undergoing peritoneal dialysis. Arch Intern Med. 1981;141:61–4.
310. Vas SI. Microbiologic aspects of chronic ambulatory dialysis. Kidney Int. 1983;23:83–92.
311. Peterson PK, Keane WF. Infections in chronic peritoneal dialysis patients. In: Remington JS, Swartz MN, eds. Current Clinical Topics in Infectious Diseases. New York: McGraw-Hill; 1985:239–60.
312. Woods GL, Washington JA II. Comparison of methods for processing dialysate in suspected continuous ambulatory peritoneal dialysis-associated peritonitis. Diagn Microbiol Infect Dis. 1987;7:155–7.
313. Gokal R, Ramos JM, Francis DM, et al. Peritonitis in continuous ambulatory peritoneal dialysis: Laboratory and clinical studies. Lancet. 1982;2:1388–91.
314. Keane WF, Everett ED, Fine RN, et al. CAPD related peritonitis management and antibiotic therapy recommendations: Travenol Peritonitis Management Advisory Committee. Perit Dialy Bull. 1987;7:55–68.
315. Verbrogh HA, Keane WF, Conroy WE, et al. Bacterial growth and killing in chronic ambulatory peritoneal dialysis fluids. J Clin Microbiol. 1984;20:199–203.
316. Eisenberg ES, Leviton I, Soeiro R. Fungal peritonitis in patients receiving peritoneal dialysis: Experience with 11 patients and review of the literature. Rev Infect Dis. 1986;8:309–21.
317. Rubin J, Kirchner K, Walsh D, et al. Fungal peritonitis during continuous ambulatory peritoneal dialysis: A report of 12 cases. Am J Kidney Dis. 1987;10:361–8.
318. Kerr CM, Perfect JR, Craven PC, et al. Fungal peritonitis in patients on continuous ambulatory peritoneal dialysis. Ann Intern Med. 1983;99:334–7.
319. Vargemezis V, Papadopoulov ZL, Llamos H, et al. Management of fungal peritonitis during continuous ambulatory peritoneal dialysis (CAPD). Perit Dialy Bull. 1986;6:17–20.
320. McNeely DJ, Vas SI, Dambros N, et al. *Fusarium* peritonitis: An uncommon complication of continuous ambulatory peritoneal dialysis. Perit Dialy Bull. 1981;1:94–6.
321. Chapman JR, Warnock DW. Ketoconazole and fungal CAPD peritonitis. Lancet. 1983;2:510–1.
322. McGuire NM, Port FK, Kauffman CA. Ketoconazole pharmacokinetics in continuous peritoneal dialysis. Perit Dialy Bull. 1984:4:199–201.
323. Axelrod J, Meyers BR, Hirschman SZ, et al. Prophylaxis with cephalothin in peritoneal dialysis. Arch Intern Med. 1973;132:368–71.
324. Abrutyn E, Goodhart GL, Roos K, et al. *Acinetobacter calcoaceticus* outbreak associated with peritoneal dialysis. Am J Epidemiol. 1978;107:328–35.
325. Altemeir WA, Culbertson WR, Fullen WD, et al. Intra-abdominal abscesses. Am J Surg. 1973;125:70–9.
326. Saini S, Kellum JM, O'Leary MP, et al. Improved localization and survival in patients with intra-abdominal abscesses. Am J Surg. 1983;145:136–42.
327. Gibson DM, Feliciano DV, Mattox KL, et al. Intra-abdominal abscess after penetrating abdominal trauma. Am J Surg. 1981;142:699–703.
328. Patterson HC. Left subphrenic abscesses. Am Surg. 1977;43:430–3.
329. Ozeran RS. Subdiaphragmatic abscess: Diagnosis and treatment. Am Surg. 1967;33:64–7.
330. Sherman NJ, Davis JR, Jesseph JE. Subphrenic abscess: A continuing hazard. Am J Surg. 1969;117:117–23.
331. Sanders RC. The changing epidemiology of subphrenic abscess and its clinical and radiological consequences. Br J Surg. 1970;57:449–55.
332. Ochsner A, DeBakey M. Subphrenic abscess. Collective review of 3608 collected and personal cases. Surg Gynecol Obstet. 1939;66:426.
333. Mackenzie M, Fordyle J, Young DG. Subphrenic abscess in children. Br J Surg. 1975;62:305–8.
334. Wang SMS, Wilson SE. Subphrenic abscess. The new epidemiology. Arch Surg. 1977;112:934–6.
335. DeCosse JJ, Poulin TL, Fox PS, et al. Subphrenic abscess. Surg Gynecol Obstet. 1974;138:841–6.
336. Gorbach SL. Treatment of intra-abdominal infection. Am J Med. 1984;76(Suppl 5A):107–10.
337. Milne GAC, Geere IIW. Chronic subphrenic abscess: The missed diagnosis. Can J Surg. 1977;20:162–5.
338. Mueller PR, Simeone JF. Intra-abdominal abscesses: Diagnosis by sonography and computed tomography. Radiol Clin North Am. 1983;21:425–43.
339. Ferrucci JT Jr, Van Sonnenberg E. Role of ultrasound and computed tomography in the diagnosis and treatment of intraabdominal abscess. In: Remington JS, Swartz MN, eds. Current Clinical Topics in Infectious Diseases. New York: McGraw-Hill; 1982:136–59.
340. Kerlan RK Jr, Pogany AC, Jeffrey RB, et al. Radiologic management of abdominal abscesses. AJR. 1985;144:145–9.
341. Connell TR, Stephens DH, Carlson HC, et al. Upper abdominal abscess: A continuing and deadly problem. AJR. 1980;134:759–65.
342. Middleton HM, Patton DD, Hoyumpa AM, et al. Liver-lung scan in the diagnosis of right subphrenic abscess. Dig Dis Sci. 1976;21:215–22.
343. Gold RP, Johnson PM. Efficacy of combined liver-lung scintillation imaging. Radiology. 1975;117:105–11.
344. Caffee HH, Watts G, Mena I. Gallium 67 citrate scanning in the diagnosis of intra-abdominal abscess. Am J Surg. 1977;133:665–9.
345. Tsan M. Mechanism of gallium 67 accumulation in inflammatory lesions. J Nucl Med. 1985;26:88–92.
346. Disbro M, Datz F, Cook P, et al. Indium-111 labeled leukocytes: Clinical utility and accuracy. Clin Nucl Med. 1982;7:44–6.
347. Froelich JW, Krasicky GA. Radionuclide imaging of abdominal infections. Curr Concepts Diag Nucl Med. 1985;2:12–6.
348. Coleman RE, Brack RE, Welch DM, et al. Indium-111 labeled leukocytes in the evaluation of suspected abdominal abscess. Am J Surg. 1980;139:99–104.
349. Sfakianakis GN, A-Sheitch W, Heal A, et al. Comparisons of scintigraphy with In-111 leukocytes and Ga^{67} in the diagnosis of occult sepsis. J Nucl Med. 1982;23:618–26.
350. Hill BA, Yamaguchi K, Flynn JJ, et al. Diagnostic sonography in general surgery. Arch Surg. 1975;110:1089–94.
351. Goudie E, Andrew WK. The role of diagnostic ultrasound in the assessment of masses in the left upper quadrant of the abdomen. S Afr Med J. 1976;50:1391–4.
352. Baker HL Jr, Berquist TN, Kispert DB, et al. Magnetic resonance imaging in a routine clinical setting. Mayo Clin Proc. 1985;60:75–90.
353. Cammoun D, Hendee WR, Davis KA. Clinical applications of magnetic resonance imaging—current status. West J Med. 1985;143:793–803.
354. Wall SD, Fisher MR, Amparo EG, et al. Magnetic resonance imaging in the evaluation of abscesses. AJR. 1985;144:1217–21.
355. Jacobs JB, Hammond WG, Poppman JL. Arteriographic localization of suprahepatic abscesses. Radiology. 1969;93:1299–300.
356. Halasz NA. Subphrenic abscess: Myths and facts. JAMA. 1970;214:724–6.

357. Gerzof SG, Robbins AH, Johnson WC. Percutaneous catheter drainage of abdominal abscesses. N Engl J Med. 1981;305:653–7.
358. Mandel SR, Boyd D, Jaques PF, et al. Drainage of hepatic, intra-abdominal and mediastinal abscesses guided by computerized axial tomography: Successful alternative to open drainage. Am J Surg. 1983;145:120–5.
359. Pruett TL, Simmons RL. Status of percutaneous catheter drainage of abscesses. Surg Clin North Am. 1988;68:89–105.
360. Brolin RE, Nosher JL, Leiman S, et al. Percutaneous catheter versus open surgical drainage in the treatment of abdominal abscesses. Am Surg. 1984;50:102–8.
361. Van Sonnenberg E, Ferruci JT Jr, Mueller PR, et al. Percutaneous drainage citrate in acute pancreatitis. Appl Radiol. 1978;1:163–5.
diology. 1982;142:1–10.
362. Olak J, Christov NV, Stein LA, et al. Operative vs percutaneous drainage of intra-abdominal abscesses. Arch Surg. 1986;121:141–6.
363. Hurley JE, Vargish T. Early diagnosis and outcome of pancreatic abscesses in pancreatitis. Am Surg. 1987;53:29–33.
364. Kodesch R, DuPont HL. Infectious complications of acute pancreatitis. Surg Gynecol Obstet. 1973;136:763–8.
365. Becker JM, Pemberton JH, Diamgno EP, et al. Prognostic factors in pancreatic abscess. Surgery. 1984;96:455–60.
366. Shi ECP, Yeo BW, Ham JM. Pancreatic abscesses. Br J Surg. 1984;71:689–91.
367. Altemeier WA, Alexander JW. Pancreatic abscess. A study of 32 cases. Arch Surg. 1963;87:80–9.
368. Holden JL, Berne TV, Rosoff LSR. Pancreatic abscess following acute pancreatitis. Arch Surg. 1976;111:858–61.
369. Miller TA, Lindenauer SM, Frey CF, et al. Pancreatic abscess. Arch Surg. 1974;108:545–51.
370. Ransom JHC, Balthazar E, Caccavale R, et al. Computed tomography and the prediction of pancreatic abscess in acute pancreatitis. Ann Surg. 1985;201:656–63.
371. Aranha GU, Prinz RA, Greenlee HB. Pancreatic abscess: An unresolved surgical problem. Am J Surg. 1982;144:534–8.
372. Bradley EL, Fulenwider JT. Open treatment of pancreatic abscess. Surg Gynecol Obstet. 1984;159:509–13.
373. Stambler JB, Klibaner MI. Tuberculous abscess of the pancreas. Gastroenterology. 1982;83:922–5.
374. Sostre CF, Flournoy JG, Bova P, et al. Pancreatic phegmon: Clinical features and course. Dig Dis Sci. 1985;30:918–27.
375. Berger HG, Krautzberger W, Bittner R, et al. Results of surgical treatment of necrotizing pancreatitis. World J Surg. 1985;9:972–9.
376. Keighley MRB, Drysdale RB, Quoraiski AH, et al. Antibiotic treatment of biliary sepsis. Surg Clin North Am. 1975;55:1379–90.
377. Crass RA, Meyer AA, Jeffrey RB, et al. Pancreatic abscess: Impact of computerized tomography on early diagnosis and surgery. Am J Surg. 1985;150:127–31.
378. Williford ME, Foster WL Jr, Halversen RA, et al. Pancreatic pseudocyst: Comparative evaluation of sonography and computed tomography. Am J Roentgenol. 1983;140:53–7.
379. Bicknell TA, Kohatsu S, Goodwin DA. Use of indium-111 labeled autologus leukocytes in differentiating pancreatic abscess from pseudocyst. Am J Surg. 1981;142:312–6.
380. Tanaka T, Miskin FS, Buozas DJ, et al. Pancreatic uptake of gallium-67 citrate in acute pancreatitis. Appl Radiol. 1978;1:163–5.
381. Paushter DM, Modic MT, Borkowski GP, et al. magnetic resonance: Principles and applications. Med Clin North Am. 1984;68:1393–1421.
382. Weiss HD, Anacker H, Kramann B, et al. The diagnosis of necrotizing pancreatic lesions by means of duodenoscopic pancreatography. Its value for the surgical procedure. Am J Gastroenterol. 1975;64:26–33.
383. Karlson KB, Martia EC, Fankochen EL, et al. Percutaneous drainage of pancreatic pseudocysts and abscesses. Radiology. 1982;142:619–24.
384. Pruett TC, Rotstein OD, Crass J, et al. Percutaneous aspiration and drainage for selected abdominal infections. Surgery. 1984;96:731–7.
385. Ranson JH, Spencer FC. Prevention, diagnosis and treatment of pancreatic abscess. Surgery. 1977;82:99–106.
386. Warshaw AL, Jin G. Improved survival in 45 patients with pancreatic abscess. Ann Surg. 1985;202:408–15.
387. Finch WT, Sawyers JL, Schenker S. A prospective study to determine the efficacy of antibiotics in acute pancreatitis. Ann Surg. 1976;183:667–71.
388. Kusne S, Dummer JS, Singh N, et al. Infections after liver transplantation. An analysis of 101 consecutive cases. Medicine. 1988;67:132–43.
389. Barbour GL, Juniper K Jr. A clinical comparison of amebic and pyogenic abscesses of the liver in sixty-six patients. Am J Med. 1972;53:323–34.
390. Dietrich RB. Experience with liver abscess. Am J Surg. 1984;147:288–91.
391. Ribaudo JM, Ochsner A. Intrahepatic abscesses: Amebic and pyogenic. Am J Surg. 1973;125:570–4.
392. Barnes PF, DeLock KM, Reynolds TN, et al. A comparison of amebic and pyogenic abscess of the liver. Medicine. 1987;66:472–83.
393. Shulman ST, Beem MO. A unique presentation of sickle cell disease. Pyogenic hepatic abscess. Pediatrics. 1971;47:1019–22.
394. Williams JW, Rittenberry A, Dillard R, et al. Liver abscess in newborn: Complications of umbilical vein catheterization. Am J Dis Child. 1973;125:111–3.
395. Gyorffy EJ, Frey CF, Silva J Jr, et al. Pyogenic liver abscess. Diagnostic and therapeutic strategies. Ann Surg. 1987;206:699–705.
396. Sabbaj J, Anaerobes in liver abscess. Rev Infect Dis. 1984;6(Suppl 1):152–5.
397. Rubin RH, Swartz MN, Malt R. Hepatic abscess: Changes in clinical, bacteriologic and therapeutic aspects. Am J Med. 1974;57:601–10.
398. McDonald MI, Corey GR, Gallis HA, et al. Single and multiple pyogenic liver abscesses. Medicine. 1984;63:291–302.
399. Sabbaj J, Sutter VL, Finegold SM. Anaerobic pyogenic liver abscess. Ann Intern Med. 1972;77:629–38.
400. Lazarchick J, de Souza E, Silva NA, et al. Pyogenic liver abscess. Mayo Clin Proc. 1973;48:349–55.
401. Perera MR, Kirk A, Noone P. Presentation, diagnosis and management of liver abscess. Lancet. 1980;2:629–32.
402. Loh R, Wallace G, Thong Y. Successful non-surgical management of pyogenic liver abscess. Scand J Infect Dis. 1987;19:137–40.
403. Kaplan SL. Pyogenic liver abscess. In: Feigin RD, Cherry JD, eds. Textbook of Pediatric Infectious Disease. Philadelphia: Saunders; 1981:537–40.
404. Rabson AR, Koornhof HJ, Notman J, et al. Hepatosplenic abscesses due to *Yersinia enterocolitica*. Br Med J. 1972;4:341.
405. Haron E, Feld R, Tuffnell P, et al. Hepatitic candidiasis: An increasing problem in immunocompromised patients. Am J Med. 1987;83:17–26.
406. Thaler M, Pastakia B, Shawker T, et al. Hepatic candidiasis in cancer patients: The evolving picture of the syndrome. Ann Intern Med. 1988;108:88–100.
407. Wallack MK, Brown AS, Austrian R, et al. Pyogenic liver abscess secondary to asymptomatic sigmoid diverticulitis. Ann Surg. 1976;184:241–3.
408. Sparberg M, Gottschalk A, Kirsner JB. Liver abscess complicating regional enteritis: Report of two cases. Gastroenterology. 1965;49:548–51.
409. Lee JF, Block GE. The changing clinical pattern of hepatic abscesses. Arch Surg. 1972;104:465–70.
410. Miedema BW, Dineen P. The diagnosis and treatment of pyogenic liver abscesses. Ann Surg. 1984;200:328–35.
411. Williams RA, Finegold SM. Pyogenic and amebic liver abscess and splenic abscess. In: Wilson SE, Finegold SM, Williams RA, eds. Intra-Abdominal Infection. New York: McGraw-Hill; 1982:139–56.
412. Weinstein L. Bacterial hepatitis: A case report on an unrecognized cause of fever of unknown origin. N Engl J Med. 1978;299:1052–4.
413. Foster SC, Schneider B, Seaman WB. Gas-containing pyogenic intra-hepatic abscesses. Radiology. 1970;94:613–8.
414. Stenson WF, Eckert T. Pyogenic liver abscess. Arch Intern Med. 1983;143:126–8.
415. Madayag MA, LeFleur RS, Braunstein P, et al. Radiology of hepatic abscesses. NY State J Med. 1975;75:1417–23.
416. Reynolds TB. Medical treatment of pyogenic liver abscesses. Ann Intern Med. 1982;96:373–4.
417. Callen PW. Computed tomographic evaluation of abdominal and pelvic abscesses. Radiology. 1979;131:171–5.
418. Koehler PR, Moss AA, Diagnosis of intraabdominal and pelvic abscesses by computerized tomography. JAMA. 1980;244:49–52.
419. Gerzof SG, Johnson WC, Robbins AH, et al. Intrahepatic pyogenic abscesses: Treatment by percutaneous drainage. Am J Surg. 1985;149:487–94.
420. Altemeier WA, Schowenserdt CG, Whiteby DH. Abscesses of the liver: Surgical consideration. Arch Surg. 1970;101:258–66.
421. DeBakey ME, Jordan GL Jr. Hepatic abscesses, both intra- and extra-hepatic. Surg Clin North Am. 1977;57:325–37.
422. Attar B, Levendoglu H, Cuasay N. CT-guided percutaneous aspiration and catheter drainage of pyogenic liver abscesses. Am J Gastroenterol. 1986;81:550–5.
423. McCorkell SJ, Niles NC. Pyogenic liver abscess: Another look at medical management. Lancet. 1985;1:803–6.
424. Drugs for parasitic infections. Med Let. 1988;30:15–24.
425. Nelken N, Isnatius J, Skinner M, et al. Changing clinical spectrum of splenic abscess. A multicenter study and review of the literature. Am J Surg. 1987;154:27–34.
426. Gadacz T, Way LW, Dunphy JE. Changing clinical spectrum of splenic abscess. Am J Surg. 1974;128:182–7.
427. Chun CH, Raff MJ, Contreras L, et al. Splenic abscess. Medicine. 1980;59:50–63.
428. Linos DA, Nagorney DM, McIlrath DC. Splenic abscess: The importance of early diagnosis. Mayo Clin Proc. 1983;58:261–4.
429. Grant E, Mertens MA, Mascatello VJ. Splenic abscess: Comparison of four imaging methods. AJR. 1979;132:465–6.
430. Pawar S, Kay CJ, Gonzalez R, et al. Sonography of splenic abscess. AJR. 1982;138:259–62.
431. Sarr MG, Zuidema GD. Splenic abscess: Presentation, diagnosis and treatment. Surgery. 1982;92:480–5.
432. Quinn SF, von Sonnenberg E, Casola G, et al. Interventional radiology in the spleen. Radiology. 1986;161:289–91.
433. Byrne RV. Localized perforated diverticulitis. Arch Surg. 1964;88:552–5.
434. Lozon AA, Duff JH. Acute perforation of the colon. Can J Surg. 1976;19:48–51.
435. Rodkey GV, Welch CE. Colonic diverticular disease with surgical treatment. A study of 338 cases. Surg Clin North Am. 1974;54:655–74.
436. Tugwell P, Southcott D, Walmesley P. Free perforation of the colon in Crohn's disease. Br J Clin Pract. 1972;26:44–5.
437. Prolla JC, Kirsner JB. The gastrointestinal lesions and complications of the leukemias. Ann Intern Med. 1964;61:1084–1103.

438. Pokorney BH, Jones JM, Skaikh BS, et al. Typhlitis: A treatable cause of recurrent septicemia. JAMA. 1980;243:682–3.
439. Mulholland MW, Delaney JP. Neutropenic colitis and aplastic anemia: A new association. Ann Surg. 1983;197:84–90.
440. Archibald RG. Nelson JA. Necrotizing enterocolitis in acute leukemia: Radiographic findings. Gastrointest Radiol. 1987;3:63–5.
441. Alt B, Glass NR, Sallinger H. Neutropenic enterocolitis in adults: Review of the literature and assessment of surgical intervention. Am J Surg. 1985;149:405–8.
442. Shaked A, Shinar E, Freund H. Neutropenic typhlitis: A plea for conservatism. Dis Colon Rectum. 1983;26:351–2.
443. Varki AP, Armitage JO, Feagler JR. Typhlitis in acute leukemias: Successful treatment by early surgical intervention. Cancer. 1979;43:695–7.
444. Berk JE, Zinbers SS. Acute Cholecystitis: Medical Aspects. In: Berk JE, Haubrich WS, Kalser MH, et al, eds. 4th ed. Gastroenterology. Philadelphia: WB Saunders; 1985;6:3597–3616.
445. Bailey HA, Thrush LB. Consideration of acute cholecystitis: An analysis of seventy-six cases. Am J Surg. 1951;82:328–33.
446. Schein CJ. Acute Cholecystitis. New York: Harper & Row; 1972:63–5.
447. Truedson H, Elmros T, Holm S. The incidence of bacteria in gallbladder bile at acute and elective cholecystectomy. Acta Chir Scand. 1983;149:307–13.
448. Pitt HA, Postier RG, Cameron JC. Biliary bacteria: Significance and alteration after antibiotic therapy. Arch Surg. 1982;117:445–9.
449. Finegold S. Anaerobes in biliary tract infection. Arch Intern Med. 1979;139:1338–9.
450. Bourgalt AM, England DM, Rosenblatt JE, et al. Clinical characteristics of anaerobic bactibilia. Arch Intern Med. 1979;139:1346–9.
451. Samuels BI, Freitas JE, Bree RL, et al. A comparison of radionuclide hepatobiliary imaging and real-time ultrasound for the detection of acute cholecystitis. Radiology. 1983;147:207–10.
452. Gill PT, Dillon E, Leahy AL, et al. Ultrasonography, HIDA scintigraphy or both in the diagnosis of acute cholecystitis? Br J Surg. 1985;72:267–8.
453. Johnson DG, Coleman RE. New techniques in radionuclide imaging of the alimentary system. Radiol Clin North Am. 1982;20:635–51.
454. Kane RA, Costello P, Duszlak E. Computed tomography in acute cholecystitis: New observations. AJR. 1983;141:697–701.
455. McCarthy S, Hricak H, Cohen M, et al. Cholecystitis: Detection with MR imaging. Radiology. 1986;158:333–6.
456. Mentzer RM, Golden CT, Chandler JG, et al. A comparative appraisal of emphysematous cholecystitis. Am J Surg. 1975;125:10–5.
457. Kune GA, Burdon JGW. Are antibiotics necessary in acute cholecystitis? Med J Aust. 1975;2:627–30.
458. Hirschmann JV, Inui TS. Antimicrobial prophylaxis: A critique of recent trials. Rev Infect Dis. 1980;2:1–23.
459. Bulow S, Dronberg O, Lung-Kristenson K. Reappraisal of surgery for suppurative cholecystitis. Arch Surg. 1977;112:282–4.
460. Moore EE, Kelly GL, Driver T, et al. Reassessment of simple cholecystostomy. Arch Surg. 1979;114:515–8.
461. Naitove A. When cholecystectomy? Hosp Pract. 1978;13:121–8.
462. Jarvinen HJ, Hastbacka J. Early cholecystectomy for acute cholecystitis: A prospective randomized study. Ann Surg. 1980;191:501–5.
463. Morrow DJ, Thompson J, Wilson SE. Acute cholecystitis in the elderly: A surgical emergency. Arch Surg. 1979;113:1149–52.
464. Thompson JE Jr, Tompkins RK, Longmire WP Jr. Factors in the management of acute cholangitis. Ann Surg. 1982;117:437–44.
465. Bilboa MK, Dotter CT, Lee TG, et al. Complications of endoscopic retrograde cholangiopancreatography. A study of 10,000 cases. Gastroenterology. 1976;70:314–20.
466. Hinshaw DB. Acute obstructive cholangitis. Surg Clin North Am. 1973;53:1089–94.
467. Ralls PW, Colletti PM, Halls JM, et al. Prospective evaluation of ^{99m}TC-IDA cholescintigraphy and gray-scale ultrasound in the diagnosis of acute cholecystitis. Radiology. 1982;144:369–71.
468. Welch JP, Donaldson G. The urgency of diagnosis and surgical treatment of suppurative cholangitis. Am J Surg. 1976;131:527–32.

SECTION G. CARDIOVASCULAR INFECTIONS

61. ENDOCARDITIS AND INTRAVASCULAR INFECTIONS

W. MICHAEL SCHELD
MERLE A. SANDE

INFECTIVE ENDOCARDITIS

The term *infective endocarditis* (IE) denotes infection of the endocardial surface of the heart and implies the physical presence of microorganisms in the lesion. Although the heart valves are most commonly affected, the disease may also occur on septal defects or on the mural endocardium. Infection of arteriovenous shunts, arterioarterial shunts (patent ductus arteriosus), and coarctation of the aorta are also included under this heading since the clinical manifestations are similar. The term *infective endocarditis,* first used by Thayer in the Gibson lectures of 1930 and later popularized by Lerner and Weinstein,[1,2] is preferable to the old term *bacterial endocarditis* since chlamydiae, rickettsiae, fungi, and perhaps even viruses may be responsible for the syndrome.

In the past, the disease has been classified as "acute" or "subacute." This was based on the usual progression of the untreated disease and is mainly of historic interest. The acute form follows a fulminant course, usually with high fever, systemic toxicity, and leukocytosis, with death occurring in several days to less than 6 weeks. It is classically associated with infection caused by *Staphylococcus aureus, Streptococcus pyogenes, Streptococcus pneumoniae,* and *Neisseria gonorhoeae.* The subacute (death in 6 weeks to 3 months) and "chronic" (death in greater than 3 months) forms are usually considered together. They commonly occur in the setting of prior valvular disease and are characterized by a slow, indolent course with a low-grade fever, night sweats, weight loss, and vague systemic complaints. This form of the disease is classically caused by the viridans streptococci. Although useful conceptually, this classification ignores the nonbacterial forms of IE and the frequent overlap in manifestations by individual organisms such as the enterococci. A classification based on the etiologic agent responsible is preferable since it has implications for the course usually followed, the likelihood of pre-existing heart disease, and the appropriate antimicrobial agent(s) to employ.

Although relatively uncommon, IE has received considerable attention by both clinicians and scientists for the past century. The clinical manifestations of the disease are so varied that they may be encountered in any of the medical subspecialities. Successful management is dependent on the close cooperation of medical and surgical disciplines. This collaboration has markedly improved the outlook of a disease that was universally fatal 45 years ago. The disease has attracted considerable investigative interest. Although the factors that influence its development are now more clearly identified, many questions remain about the unique aspects of this infection. For example, (*1*) why do organisms lodge specifically on the cardiac valves rather than elsewhere in the vascular tree; (*2*) what enables the microorganisms to survive on the valve surface after colonization; (*3*) why do only a relatively small number of strains of bacteria produce the vast majority of cases of endocarditis, while many others produce only bacteremia; (*4*) what factors are responsible for the marked variations in the manifestation of the disease; and (*5*) why is the infection so difficult to eradicate with antibiotics even though the infecting organisms are often exquisitely sensitive to the drugs in vitro? These questions will be discussed in detail in the following sections.

Epidemiology

The incidence of IE is difficult to determine since the criteria for diagnosis and the methods of reporting vary with different series.[3] An analysis based on strict case definitions often reveals that only a small proportion ($\approx$20 percent) of clinically diagnosed cases are categorized as definite. Nevertheless, IE accounted for approximately 1 case/1000 hospital admissions with a range of 0.16–5.4 cases/1000 admissions in a review of 10 large surveys.[3,4] This incidence has not changed in the past 30 years.[5] The mean annual incidence was 3.8/100,000 person-years in Olmstead County, Minnesota, from 1950 to 1981 with no significant change during this interval.[6] A similar figure of 1.7/100,000 person-years was reported from a prospective survey in Louisiana[7] and is analogous to results from the United Kingdom.[8] In an autopsy study[9] there was no change in the yearly number of cases of IE in the United Kingdom from 1939 to 1967. The proportion of acute cases has increased from approximately 20 percent in the pre-antibiotic era to 33 percent.[4,5] Despite these changes in the disease spectrum, IE remains a prevalent disease with a significant mortality in the antibiotic era.[10]

The mean age of patients with IE has gradually increased in the antibiotic era. In 1926, the median age was less than 30 years;[11] this had increased to 39 years by 1943, and currently over 50 percent of the patients are older than 50 years.[5,12,13] At the present time, 54 percent (range, 41–69 percent) of the cases occur in patients aged 31–60, 26 percent (range, 12–40 percent) in patients less than 30 years of age, and 21 percent (range, 8–38 percent) in people older than 60 years.[2] The mean age of patients with IE caused by group D streptococci is even higher: 61–67 years.[14] The disease remains uncommon in children. The mean age for men is 6–7 years older than that for women, and men are more commonly affected (54–69 percent of the cases, the mean male:female ratio is 1.7:1 with a range of 1.2–3.0:1 in 17 large series). In patients under the age of 35, more cases occur in women. A number of factors may relate to this shift in age distribution. First, there has been a change in the substrate of the underlying heart disease due to a decline in the incidence of acute rheumatic fever and rheumatic heart disease countered by the increasing importance of degenerative heart disease in elderly patients. Second, the age of the population has been steadily increasing, and people with rheumatic or congenital heart disease are surviving longer. A new form of the disease (nosocomial endocarditis) secondary to new therapeutic modalities (intravenous catheters, hyperalimentation lines, pacemakers, dialysis shunts, and so forth) has emerged.[3] Of 125 cases of endocarditis recently reviewed in Seattle, 35 were nosocomial in origin (28 percent).[15] Although nosocomial endocarditis accounted for only 14.3 percent of cases in another recent study, 64 percent of patients were over 60 years of age, and mortality was high.[16] It is interesting, however, that the age-adjusted incidence for the most common organisms (viridans streptococci) has not appreciably changed.[17]

The heart valve involved by the infection varies considerably with the proportion of acute cases reported in each series. The distribution ranges from 28 to 45 percent for the mitral valve alone, 5 to 36 percent for the aortic valve alone, and 0 to 35 percent for the aortic and mitral valves combined. The tricuspid valve is rarely involved (0–6 percent), and the pulmonary valve even less (<1 percent).[12,14,15,18] Both right- and left-sided disease is present in 0–4 percent.[2] Involvement of the aortic valve alone is increasing in frequency and correlates with the increase in acute cases; the incidence was 5 percent in 1938 and rose to 39 percent by 1978.[12] The aortic valve is involved in 61 percent of the male cases but in only 31 percent of the female cases.[15]

Almost any type of structural heart disease may predispose to IE, especially when the defect results in turbulence of blood flow. Rheumatic heart disease has been the underlying lesion in 37–76 percent of the infections in the past, and the mitral valve is involved in more than 85 percent of these cases.[4] If the mitral valve is solely involved, women outnumber men by 2:1. The aortic valve is affected in approximately 50 percent of these cases, and if involved alone, men outnumber women by 4:1. Right-sided endocarditis is a rare and accounts for fewer than 10 percent of all cases occurring in patients with rheumatic heart disease. The proportion of cases related to rheumatic heart disease has continued to decline to $\leq$25 percent in the past two decades.[19]

Congenital heart disease (especially patent ductus arteriosus, ventricular septal defect, coarctation of the aorta, bicuspid aortic valve, tetralogy of Fallot, and pulmonic stenosis) is responsible in 6–24 percent of the cases.[4] Endocarditis is uncommon in the secundum atrial septal defects, probably because this lesion results in a low-pressure shunt with little turbulence. The congenitally bicuspid aortic valve, erroneously attributed to rheumatic carditis in the past,[20] is now recognized as an important condition in elderly patients (especially men), is the underlying lesion in over 20 percent of the cases occurring over the age of 60, and is associated with a poor prognosis despite rapid valve replacement.[21] Marfan's syndrome, when associated with aortic insufficiency, has also been associated with IE.

The "degenerative" cardiac lesions (calcified mitral annulus, calcific nodular lesions secondary to arteriosclerotic cardiovascular disease, post-myocardial infarction thrombus, and so forth) assume the greatest importance in the 30–40 percent of the patients without any demonstrable underlying valvular disease. The actual contribution made by these lesions is unknown, but they occur with an increased incidence in the elderly. In one series, degenerative lesions were present in 50 percent of patients over 60 years old with native valve endocarditis.[22] The contribution of these degenerative cardiac lesions to the development of IE is apparent in an analysis of 148 patients treated in London since 1970.[23,24] The underlying structural cardiac defects were as follows: rheumatic heart disease, 39; congenital defects, 13; and normal or degenerate valves, 65. Similarly, only 31 percent of patients with IE in a recent series[25] had known cardiac disease. Although a calcified mitral annulus is fairly frequent in elderly women, this lesion is rarely complicated by IE (only 3 of 80 in one report).[26] When acute cases of IE are considered separately, over 50 percent have no recognized underlying cardiac disease.

Many other conditions such as luetic heart disease, arterioarterial fistulas, hemodialysis shunts or fistulas, intracardiac pacemaker wires, and intracardiac prostheses may predispose to endocarditis. Prosthetic valve endocarditis is rising in incidence in proportion to other forms of endocarditis and is discussed in Chapter 62. Infective endocarditis also occurs more frequently in seriously ill hospitalized patients who are compromised hosts and who are subjected to invasive intravascular access procedures (intravenous catheters including central venous pressure monitoring lines, hyperalimentation lines, intracardiac pacemaker wires, and so on).[12] Another group with an increased risk of IE are intravenous ("mainlining") drug abusers. (This group will be considered in detail in a later section.)

Although idiopathic hypertrophic subaortic stenosis (IHSS) or asymetric hypertrophy of the interventricular septum has not classically been recognized as a condition leading to bacterial endocarditis, by 1982, 32 such cases had been reported in the literature.[27–29] In seven cases examined histologically the infection was found on the aortic valve in three cases, mitral valve in two, both valves in one, and the subaortic endocardium in one. This distribution is likely related to the associated mitral regurgitation due to the displacement of the anterior leaflet by the abnormal ventricular architecture and by the turbulence of the jet stream affecting the aortic valve distal to the intraventricular obstruction. The age of patients developing endocarditis ranged from 20 to 66 years, and in most cases (70 percent) the disease was produced by viridans streptococci. Approximately 5 percent of patients with IHSS develop IE.[29] Infective endocarditis is more common in the subset of patients with IHSS who have hemodynamically severe forms of the disease manifested by a higher peak systolic pressure gradient and a high prevalence of symptoms. New murmurs develop in 36 percent of patients with IHSS complicated by IE, and this new physical finding correlates with a higher mortality rate.[29]

The association of the mitral prolapse syndrome and endocarditis has also been only recently recognized. Of 87 consecutive cases of IE reported from Stanford University, 10 (11 percent) occurred in patients with well-documented mitral valve prolapse.[30] These 10 cases represented over one-third of the 28 cases in which isolated mitral regurgitation was the predisposing condition. Four additional cases occurred in patients who were not studied by echocardiography or angiography but who had clinical evidence of the mitral prolapse syndrome. Thus, 40–50 percent of the cases of IE associated with isolated insufficient mitral valves probably occurred in patients with the mitral prolapse syndrome. In a recent series[22] of 63 cases of native valve endocarditis diagnosed in Memphis from 1980 to 1984, mitral valve prolapse was the most common underlying lesion (29 percent). In another study,[31] 5 of 58 patients with mitral valve prolapse followed prospectively for 9–22 years developed endocarditis. This syndrome should be suspected in patients with midsystolic clicks with or without a late systolic murmur. The condition is common and has been recognized in 0.5–20 percent of otherwise healthy people, especially young women. It has become apparent that mitral valve prolapse is only one component of a developmental syndrome. This lesion is often associated with a distinct habitus in women,[32] von Willebrand's disease, or ophthalmoplegia. Some of these characteristics may be useful in identifying patients at high risk for IE. It is important to emphasize that all 25 patients who developed IE on a prolapsing mitral valve had a holosystolic murmur, and none had the isolated click without a murmur.[30] The risk of IE appears to be increased in the subset of patients with mitral valve prolapse who exhibit valvular redundancy.[22] Nevertheless, the risk of IE is clearly higher in patients with mitral valve prolapse. In a careful retrospective epidemiologic matched case control analysis, the odds ratio (8.2; 95 percent confidence interval, 2.4–28.4) indicates a substantially higher risk for the development of IE in these patients when compared with controls.[33] It appears that once IE develops in people with mitral valve prolapse, the symptoms and signs are more subtle and the mortality rate less when compared with left-sided IE of other types.[34]

Pathogenesis

In vitro observations and studies in experimental animals have demonstrated that the development of IE most likely requires the simultaneous occurrence of several independent events, each of which may be influenced by a host of separate factors. The valve surface must first be altered to produce a suitable site for bacterial attachment and colonization. Surface changes may be produced by various local and systemic stresses, including blood turbulence. These alterations result in the deposition of platelets and fibrin and in the formation of so-called nonbacterial thrombotic endocarditis (NBTE). Bacteria must then reach this site and adhere to the NBTE to produce colonization. Certain strains appear to have a selective advantage in adhering to platelets and/or fibrin and thus produce the disease with a lower inoculum. After colonization, the surface is rapidly covered with a protective sheath of fibrin and platelets to produce an environment conducive to further bacterial multiplication and vegetation growth. The interaction of these events is depicted in Figure 1. In the following sections, these factors will be considered independently (see Scheld[35] and Freedman[36] for in-depth discussions).

Nonbacterial Thrombotic Endocarditis. Luschka, in 1852, first suggested that endocarditis resulted when septic coronary emboli lodged in the vessels of the cardiac valve.[37] This hypothesis was discarded since cardiac valves are poorly vascularized and only in the proximal portion, which does not coincide with the area of infection.[38–40] It is now clear that the initial colonization occurs on the endothelial surface of the valve. In experimental animals it is nearly impossible to produce IE with intravenous injections of bacteria unless the valvular surface is first damaged or otherwise altered. When a polyethylene catheter is passed across the aortic valve of a rabbit, endocarditis is readily produced with intravenously injected bacteria or fungi.[41,42] Microscopic examination of this early lesion demonstrates the organisms intimately adherent to fibrin–platelet deposits overlying interstitial edema and mild cellular distortion that have formed in areas of valvular trauma.[43] Scanning electron micrographs of the damaged valvular surface confirm the adhesion of microorganisms to these areas of fibrin–platelet deposition early in the disease course.[44] The organisms are rapidly covered by fibrin.[45] Opossums and pigs are the only animals known to develop endocarditis readily without experimentally induced valvular alteration.[46] The stress of captivity is apparently sufficient in these animals to produce subtle valvular changes that lead to both spontaneous endocarditis and a markedly increased susceptibility to the disease after the intravenous injection of bacteria. In other animals and probably in humans, alteration of the valve surface is a prerequisite for bacterial colonization. Angrist first recognized the importance of these deposits as the critical factor in allowing bacterial colonization of

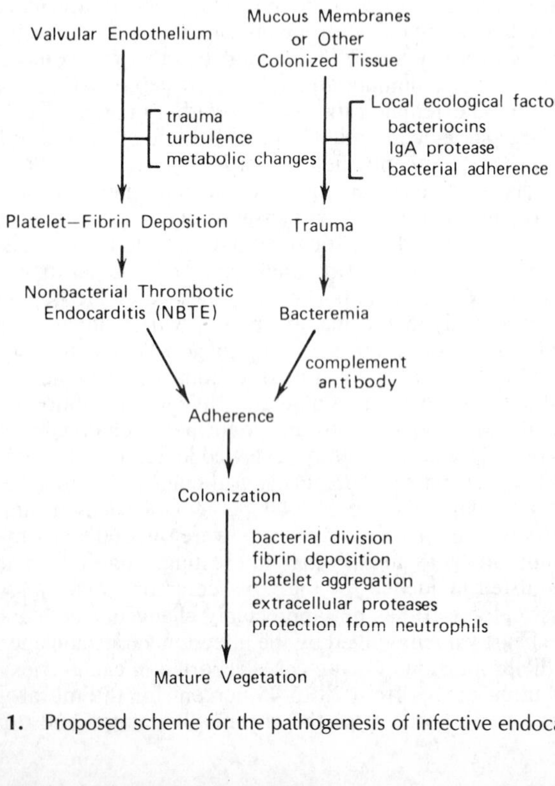

FIG. 1. Proposed scheme for the pathogenesis of infective endocarditis.

valve surfaces and suggested the term *nonbacterial thrombotic endocarditis*. Many forms of exogenous stress produce these lesions experimentally including infection, hypersensitivity states, cold exposure, simulated high altitude, high cardiac output states, cardiac lymphatic obstruction, and hormonal manipulations.[47] These procedures all increase the susceptibility of the animals to IE.

Nonbacterial thrombotic endocarditis has been found in patients with malignancy (particularly pancreatic, gastric, or lung carcinoma) or other chronic wasting diseases, rheumatic or congenital heart disease,[39] uremia, connective tissue diseases such as systemic lupus erythematosus, after the placement of intracardiac catheters (e.g., Swan-Ganz), and even after a self-limited acute illness. In a careful analysis performed in Japan, NBTE was found in 2.4 percent of 3404 autopsies, especially in elderly people with chronic wasting disease.[48] Importantly, NBTE was most frequent on the low-pressure side of the cardiac valves along the line of closure, precisely the site most often involved in IE. Whether this lesion is always essential for the development of endocarditis in humans is unknown.

Hemodynamic Factors. Infective endocarditis characteristically occurs on the atrial surface of the mitral valve and the ventricular surface of the aortic valve when associated with valvular insufficiency. Rodbard[49] showed that this localization is related to a decrease in lateral pressure (presumably with decreased perfusion of the intima) immediately "downstream" from the regurgitant flow. Lesions with high degrees of turbulence (small ventricular septal defect with a jet lesion, valvular stenosis < insufficient valves) readily create conditions that lead to bacterial colonization, whereas defects with a large surface area (large ventricular septal defect), low flow (ostium secundum atrial septal defect), or attenuation of turbulence (chronic congestive heart failure with atrial fibrillation) are rarely implicated in IE. Cures of IE achieved with ligation alone of an arteriovenous fistula or patent ductus arteriosus also stress the importance of hemodynamic factors. A hyperdynamic circulation itself, such as that created after experimentally induced arteriovenous fistulas in dogs or fistulas and shunts in hemodialysis patients, indirectly may lead to IE by producing NBTE.[38]

The degree of mechanical stress exerted on the valve also affects the location of the endocarditis.[50] In 1024 autopsy cases of IE reviewed through 1952, the incidence of valvular lesions was as follows: mitral, 86 percent; aortic, 55 percent; tricuspid, 19.6 percent; and pulmonic, 1.1 percent. This correlates with the pressure resting on the closed valve: 116, 72, 24, and 5 mmHg, respectively.

Transient Bacteremia. In the setting of pre-existent NBTE, transient bacteremia may result in the colonization of these lesions and to the development of IE.[51] Transient bacteremia occurs whenever a mucosal surface heavily colonized with bacteria is traumatized, such as with dental extractions and other dental procedures and gastrointestinal, urologic, and gynecologic procedures[51,52] (Table 1). The degree of bacteremia is proportional to the trauma produced by the procedure and to the number of organisms inhabiting the surface, and the organisms isolated reflect the resident microbial flora. The bacteremia is usually low grade (≤10 colony-forming units [cfu]/ml) and transient; the blood stream is usually sterile in less than 15–30 minutes. It is noteworthy that in two studies where blood cultures were drawn from patients with severe gingival disease before the dental procedure, spontaneous bacteremia was identified in 9–11 percent. Other studies have demonstrated an even higher frequency of spontaneous bacteremia. Of the blood cultured from healthy people, 60–80 percent were positive when filters and anaerobic techniques were used.[53] The degree of bacteremia, however, was low, with only 2–10 cfu/5 ml of blood isolated. "Nonpathogenic" organisms such as *Propionibacterium acnes, Actinomyces viscosus, Staphylococcus epidermidis,* and other *Actinomyces* or streptococcal species were responsible. Frequent episodes of silent bacteremia are also suggested by the identification of circulating humoral antibodies to the resident oral flora and by the noted increase in sensitized peripheral T cells to the flora of dental plaque.

TABLE 1. Incidence of Bacteremia after Various Procedures

Procedure/Manipulation	*Percentage of Positive Blood Cultures*
Dental	
Dental extraction	18–85
Periodontal surgery	32–88
Chewing candy or paraffin	17–51
Tooth brushing	0–26
Oral irrigation device	27–50
Upper airway	
Bronchoscopy (rigid scope)	15
Tonsillectomy	28–38
Nasotracheal suctioning/intubation	16
Gastrointestinal	
Upper GI endoscopy	8–12
Sigmoidoscopy/colonoscopy	0–9.5
Barium enema	11
Percutaneous needle biopsy of liver	3–13
Urologic	
Urethral dilatation	18–33
Urethral catheterization	8
Cystoscopy	0–17
Transurethral prostatic resection	12–46
Obstetric/Gynecologic	
Normal vaginal delivery	0–11
Punch biopsy of the cervix	0
Removal/insertion of an IUD	0

(From Everett et al.,[52] with permission.)

Another factor of critical importance during the transient bacteremia stage is susceptibility of the potential pathogen to complement-mediated bactericidal activity. Only "serum-resistant" gram-negative aerobic bacilli (e.g., *Escherichia coli, Pseudomonas aeruginosa, Serratia marcescens*) reliably produce experimental IE in rabbits,[54,55] and this property is found in all isolates from human cases of IE. Although experimental IE can be induced in rats with "serum-sensitive" *E. coli,* the organisms are eliminated rapidly upon catheter removal.[55]

Microorganism–Nonbacterial Thrombotic Endocarditis Interaction. The ability of certain organisms to adhere to NBTE is a critical early step in the development of endocarditis. Gould et al[56] showed that organisms frequently associated with IE (enterococci, viridans streptococci, *Staphylococcus aureus, S. epidermidis, P. aeruginosa*) adhered more avidly to normal canine aortic leaflets in vitro than did organisms uncommon in IE (*Klebsiella pneumoniae, E. coli*). In addition, *S. aureus* and the viridans streptococci produce IE more readily than does *E. coli* in the rabbit model of IE.[57] This observation correlates with the relative frequency with which these organisms produce the disease in humans. The rarity of IE due to gram-negative aerobic bacilli may also be related to their "serum sensitivity," as above.

Recent studies with an elegant experimental model of IE after dental extraction in rats with periodontitis, which closely resembles the presumed pathogenetic sequence in humans, also suggest an important role for bacterial adhesion to NBTE in the early events. Although viridans streptococci were much more commonly isolated than were group G streptococci in blood cultures obtained 1 minute postextraction, the latter strains caused 83 percent of the IE episodes in this rat model.[58,59] This propensity to cause IE was associated with an increased adhesion of group G streptococci to fibrin–platelet matrices in vitro.[59]

The adherence of oral streptococci to NBTE may depend on

the production of a complex extracellular polysaccharide, dextran. This polymer plays an essential role in the pathogenesis of dental caries by *Streptococcus mutans*.[60] It allows the organism to adhere tightly to the surface of dental enamel. The enhanced ability to adhere to inert surfaces may also be important in IE. In an analysis of 719 cases of streptococcal infections in the United Kingdom, 317 cases of IE were found.[61] The most common etiologic agents were *S. sanguis* (16.4 percent of the cases), previously called "streptococcus SBE," and *S. mutans* (14.2 percent). When a ratio denoting endocarditis to nonendocarditis bacteremia was derived (Table 2), the relative propensity for a particular organism to cause endocarditis could be predicted. The ratios range from 14.2:1 for *S. mutans* to a reversed ratio of 1:32 for *S. pyogenes*. Only the first four organisms listed in Table 2 (all with ratios greater than 3:1) produce extracellular dextran. This suggests that dextran production may also be a virulence factor in the pathogenesis of IE.

The role of dextran in the adherence of oral streptococci to NBTE has also been studied in vitro by using artificial fibrin–platelet matrices (simulating NBTE). The amount of dextran produced by the organism in broth correlated with adherence and was increased by incubating the organism in sucrose (which stimulates dextran production) and was decreased by the addition of dextranase (which removes the dextran from the cell surface). The addition of exogenous dextran to *S. sanguis* grown in sucrose-free media increased adherence. Dextran production also correlated directly with the ability of these organisms to produce endocarditis in vivo in the rabbit model.[62] The strain of *S. sanguis* produced endocarditis less readily when incubated in dextranase than did control strains, and a strain that produced large quantities of dextran produced endocarditis more easily than did a strain that produced relatively small quantities of dextran. Dextran production also increases the adherence of *S. mutans* to traumatized canine aortic valves in vitro,[63] an effect dependent on polymers of higher molecular weight.[64] Thus, dextran formation by oral streptococci may be a virulence factor for the production of IE by these organisms.[65] It is clear, however, that non-dextran-producing streptococci may produce endocarditis in humans and adhere to artificial fibrin–platelet surfaces in vitro,[66] which suggests that other microbial surface characteristics are instrumental for this early event. Whatever the role of the extracellular glycocalyx in microbial adhesion, its presence may retard antimicrobial therapy for streptococcal endocarditis[67] (see below).

A similar important role of adhesion to NBTE in the pathogenesis of IE has also been shown for yeasts. *Candida albicans* adheres readily to NBTE in vitro and produces IE in rabbits more readily than does *C. krusei*, a nonadherent yeast rarely implicated in IE in humans.[68] Although microbial adhesion is a crucial early event in the pathogenesis of IE, the precise intracardiac loci are unknown and may differ among organisms.

TABLE 2. Ratio of Infective Endocarditis Cases to Nonendocarditis Bacteremia for Various Streptococci

Bacteria	Endocarditis: Nonendocarditis
S. mutans	14.2:1
S. bovis I	5.9:1
DX + *S. mitior*[a]	3.3:1
S. sanguis	3.0:1
S. mitior	1.8:1
Unclassified "viridans"	1.4:1
Enterococcus faecalis	1:1.2
Miscellaneous streptococci	1:1.3
S. bovis II	1:1.7
S. anginosus	1:2.6
Group G streptococci	1:2.9
Group B streptococci	1:7.4
Group A streptococci	1:32.0

[a] DS +: dextran-positive.
(Modified from Parker et al.,[61] with permission.)

Most organisms probably adhere initially to a constituent of NBTE; some evidence implicates fibronectin as the host receptor within NBTE.[69] Other normal constituents of damaged endothelium or NBTE (e.g., fibrinogen, laminin, type 4 collagen, etc.[70]) may also serve to bind circulating bacteria. Other organisms may bind directly to, or become ingested by endothelial cells as the initial event[71–73]; this sequence appears important in the initiation of IE by *S. aureus* on "normal" cardiac valves. Although the specific microbial surface–host receptor ligand relationship remain obscure, this is an active area of investigation because inhibition of these events may provide novel prophylactic strategies.

The importance of adherence characteristics in the development of endocarditis has also been examined by using preincubation of organisms with antibiotics. Many classes of drugs, after incubation even at subinhibitory concentrations, decrease the adhesion of streptococcal species to fibrin–platelet matrices and damaged canine valves in vitro.[74] Several elegant studies in animal models have verified the significance of this in vitro observation since preincubation of the organism in subinhibitory antibiotic concentrations prevents the development of endocarditis in vivo.[75,76] This has direct relevance to the chemoprophylactic prevention of IE (see Chapter 63). In one study, subinhibitory concentrations of penicillin were found to result in a loss of streptococcal lipoteichoic acid with reduced adhesion to NBTE and an impaired ability to produce IE in vivo.[77] Thus, antibiotics may prevent IE by at least two mechanisms: (*1*) bacterial killing and (*2*) inhibition of adhesion to NBTE.[78]

Since platelets are (with fibrin) the major constituents of NBTE, the role of the platelet in the pathogenesis of endocarditis has also been studied. Some strains of bacteria have been found to be potent stimulators of platelet aggregation and the release reaction.[79] Endocarditis-producing strains of staphylococci and streptococci more actively aggregate platelets than do other bacteria that less frequently produce IE. Platelet–bacterial aggregates have been found in the peripheral blood in patients with bacteremia. The importance of these bacterial–platelet aggregates in the formation of the vegetation or, conversely, in the effect of the aggregation on the rate of removal of organisms from the circulation is unknown. Even small numbers of platelets greatly increased the adherence of oral streptococci to fibrin in vitro.[62] Recent studies[80] have shown that *S. sanguis*, an important cause of IE, aggregates platelets and adheres to these blood components by protease-sensitive components, not dextrans. A platelet receptor for ligands on certain strains of *S. sanguis* was suggested. This platelet aggregation by viridans streptococci, however, requires both direct platelet binding and plasma components.[81] Recent experiments implicate IgG in this specific streptococcal–platelet interaction and suggest that platelet activation is mediated through the platelet surface, 40,000 molecular weight Fc receptor.[82]

Once the colonization of the valve occurs and a critical mass of adherent bacteria develops, the vegetation enlarges by further platelet–fibrin deposition and continued bacterial proliferation. The bacterial colonies are found beneath the surface of the vegetation (variable, depending on the intracardiac location[83]), and infiltration by phagocyte cells is minimal; hence the vegetation creates an environment of impaired host resistance. These conditions allow for unimpaired bacterial growth resulting in extremely high colony counts of 10^9–10^{10} bacteria/g of tissue. Bacteria deep within the fibrin matrix have been shown by autoradiography to reach a state of reduced metabolic activity.[84] Recent studies by Freedman and others suggest that impairment of host defenses (e.g., neutropenia, corticosteroids) potentiates progression of the disease when the tricuspid but not the aortic valve is involved[85,86] but is largely dependent on the intracardiac location of the vegetation.[87] The role of granulocytes within the vegetation is unsettled. When vegetation formation is retarded with anticoagulants in experimental animals with IE, the organisms appear to divide on the surface, total bacterial titers are lower, and the clinical disease is more explosive.[68,69] In addition, it has been suggested that phagocytosis of microorganisms by monocytes on or within the vegetation generates tissue thromboplastin formation that then acts as a stimulant to fibrin deposition and growth of the vegetation.[90] The best evidence, however, suggests that coagulation activation initiated by tissue factor,[91] with subsequent local thrombus formation, is responsible for the initiation of vegetation growth and persistence on the cardiac valve. It appears that some organisms (i.e., *S. aureus*) induce tissue factor production by endothelium without the necessity for host cytokines.[92]

Immunopathologic Factors. Infective endocarditis causes the stimulation of both humoral and cellular immunity as manifested by hypergammaglobulinemia, splenomegaly, and the presence of macrophages in the peripheral blood. The possibility that preformed antibody increased the likelihood of the development of IE was suggested by the spontaneous occurrence of IE in animals receiving repeated immunizations with live pneumococci.[93] It was suggested that these antibodies produced bacterial agglutination in vivo that increased the chances of valvular colonization. Recent studies in animals have suggested a protective role for circulating antibody. Rabbits preimmunized with heat-killed streptococci plus Freund's adjuvant had a significantly higher median infective dose (ID_{50}) than did nonimmunized controls after aortic valve trauma.[94] Others have found similar results with *S. sanguis, S. mutans,* and *S. pneumoniae*.[95] In other experiments, we demonstrated that antibody directed against cell surface components (including mannan) reduced the adhesion of *Candida albicans* to fibrin and platelets in vitro and endocarditis production in vivo.[96] This effect may be dependent on the infecting organism, however, since antibody to *Staphylococcus epidermidis* and *Staphylococcus aureus* does not prevent the development of endocarditis in immunized animals or result in reduced bacterial concentrations in infected vegetations or kidneys,[97] perhaps due to the inability of immune sera to enhance opsonophagocytosis of staphylococci. Therefore, the role of preformed antibody in the pathogenesis of IE remains unclear. Intravascular agglutination of bacteria may, in fact, decrease the frequency of endocarditis by reducing the actual number of circulating organisms.

Rheumatoid factor (anti-IgG IgM antibody) develops in about 50 percent of patients with IE of greater than 6 weeks' duration.[98] Rheumatoid factors have been found at the time of admission in 24 percent of the patients with acute staphylococcal endocarditis (less than 6 weeks' duration), and the frequency increased to 40 percent if fever persisted for 2 weeks after the initiation of antibiotic therapy.[99] Over two-thirds of the patients became seronegative after 6 weeks of therapy, and two patients with a second episode of acute IE promptly redeveloped positive rheumatoid factors. The titers correlate with the level of hypergammaglobulinemia and decrease with therapy. Rheumatoid factor may play a role in the disease process by blocking IgG opsonic activity (by reacting with the Fc fragment), stimulating phagocytosis, and/or accelerating microvascular damage. Rheumatoid factor (IgM) has not been eluted from the immune complex glomerulonephritis associated with IE.[100] Antinuclear antibodies also occur in IE and may contribute to the musculoskeletal manifestations, low-grade fever, or pleuritic pain.[101]

Infective endocarditis, like malaria, schistosomiasis, syphilis, kala-azar, and leprosy, is associated with a constant intravascular antigenic challenge; therefore, the development of several classes of circulating antibody is not unexpected. Opsonic (IgG), agglutinating (IgG, IgM), and complement-fixing (IgG, IgM) antibodies, cryoglobulins (IgG, IgM, IgA, C3, fibrinogen), and macroglobulins have all been described in IE.[102,103] By using the sensitive Raji cell or Clq deviation techniques, circulating immune complexes have been found in high titer in virtually all patients with IE.[104] Circulating immune complexes are found with increased frequency in connection with a long duration of illness, extravalvular manifestations, hypocomplementemia, and right-sided IE. Levels fall and become undetectable with successful therapy. Patients with IE and circulating immune complexes may develop a diffuse glomerulonephritis that is analogous to the nephritis seen with infected ventriculoatrial shunts.[105] Immune complexes plus complement are deposited subepithelially along the glomerular basement membrane to form a "lumpy-bumpy" pattern. Immunoglobulin eluted from these lesions has been shown to cross react with bacterial antigens.[106] In addition, bacterial antigens have actually been demonstrated within circulating immune complexes.[107] Some of the peripheral manifestations of IE, such as Osler nodes, may also result from a deposition of circulating immune complexes. Pathologically these lesions resemble an acute Arthus reaction. However, the finding of positive culture aspirates in Osler nodes[108] suggests that they may in fact be due to septic emboli rather than immune complex deposition. In some diffuse purpuric lesions in IE, immune complex deposits (IgG, IgM, and complement) have been demonstrated in the dermal blood vessels by immunofluorescence.[109] Quantitative determinations of serum immune complex concentrations are useful in gauging the response to therapy. Effective treatment leads to a prompt decrease, with eventual disappearance of circulating immune complexes.[110] Conversely, therapeutic failures or relapses are characterized by rising titers or a reappearance of circulating immune complexes.[111]

Pathologic Changes

Heart. The classic vegetation of IE is usually located along the line of closure of a valve leaflet on the atrial surface for atrioventricular valves or the ventricular surface for semilunar valves. Vegetations may be single or multiple, are a few millimeters to several centimeters in size, and vary in color, consistency, and gross appearance. Microscopically, the lesion consists primarily of fibrin, platelet aggregates, and bacterial masses; neutrophils and red blood cells are rare. Destruction of the underlying valve may coexist. With treatment, healing occurs by fibrosis and occasionally calcification. The vegetation in acute cases is larger, softer, and more friable and may be associated with suppuration, more necrosis, and less healing than in subacute cases.[37,112] This infection may lead to perforation of the valve leaflet, rupture of the chordae tendinae, interventricular septum, or papillary muscle. Staphylococcal endocarditis frequently results in valve ring abscesses[113] with fistula formation into areas of the myocardium or pericardial sac. Aneurysms of the valve leaflet or sinus of Valsalva are also common. Valvular stenosis may result from large vegetations. Myocarditis, myocardial infarction, and pericarditis[112,113] are frequently found at autopsy. Myocardial abscesses are found in 20 percent of the autopsy cases and are associated primarily with acute staphylococcal endocarditis with hectic fever, a rapid onset of congestive heart failure, and conduction disturbances. Myocardial infarcts are found in as many as 40–60 percent of the autopsied cases, often without diagnostic changes in the electrocardiogram. Pericarditis is much more common in acute IE.

Embolic phenomena are common in IE. In the pre-antibiotic era, 70–95 percent of the patients had clinically demonstrable embolic events, but this has decreased to 15–35 percent today. Pathologic evidence of embolization is still detected in 45–65 percent of autopsies, most frequently involving the renal, splenic, coronary, or cerebral circulation. Emboli and immune complex deposition contribute to the extracardiac manifestations of IE and may involve virtually any organ system. When large emboli occlude major vessels, fungal endocarditis, marantic endocarditis, or an intracardiac myxoma should be suspected.

Kidney. Three pathologic processes may be found in the kidney in IE: abscess, infarction, or glomerulonephritis. Abscesses are infrequent, but infarctions have been seen in 56 percent of the autopsy cases.[1] The kidney is usually normal in size but may be slightly swollen, and petechiae may be found in the capsule. When renal biopsies are done during active IE, the renal architecture is abnormal in *all* cases,[114] even in the absence of clinical or biochemical evidence of renal disease. "Focal" glomerulonephritis is found in 48–88 percent of the cases but is rare in acute IE. It is a focal, local, and segmental process characterized by endothelial and mesangial proliferation, hemorrhage, neutrophilic infiltration, fibrinoid necrosis, crescent formation, and healing by fibrosis. Diffuse glomerulonephritis is found in 17–80 percent of the cases and consists of generalized cellular hyperplasia in all glomerular tufts. A less common condition called membranoproliferative glomerulonephritis is associated with endocarditis due to *S. epidermidis* and characterized by marked mesangial proliferation and by splitting of the glomerular basement membrane. Renal interstitial cellular infiltration is common.[114]

Of the patients with IE, 10–15 percent will exhibit an immune complex glomerulonephritis similar to that seen in lupus erythematosus.[105,106,110,111] The evidence for immune complex deposition rather than recurrent embolic phenomenon as the primary pathogenic mechanism includes the following:

1. Bacteria are rarely if ever seen in the lesions.
2. Glomerulonephritis occurs with right-sided IE.
3. Glomerulonephritis is rare in acute IE even though large, friable vegetations result in widespread metastatic abscess formation.
4. Immunofluorescent staining with anti-immunoglobulin antibody reveals the typical lumpy-bumpy distribution seen in other forms of immune complex nephritis.
5. In diffuse glomerulonephritis, subepithelial electron-dense deposits are seen by electron microscopy, with IgG, IgM, IgA, and/or complement demonstrated in these deposits by immunofluorescence.
6. Specific antibacterial antibody can be eluted from the lesions.[106]
7. Anti-glomerular basement membrane antibody has been found in a single case of IE with nephritis.
8. The glomerulonephritis is often accompanied by hypocomplementemia and a positive rheumatoid factor in serum.
9. All these abnormalities usually resolve with successful antimicrobial therapy as the concentration of circulating immune complexes declines.

Mycotic Aneurysms. Mycotic aneurysms usually develop during active IE but are occasionally detected months or years after successful treatment. They are more common with viridans streptococcal infections and are found in 10–15 percent of the autopsied cases. They may arise by any of the following mechanisms: (*1*) direct bacterial invasion of the arterial wall with subsequent abscess formation and/or rupture, (*2*) septic or bland embolic occlusion of the vasa vasorum, or (*3*) immune complex deposition with resultant injury to the arterial wall. The aneurysms tend to occur at bifurcation points. They are found in the cerebral vessels (primarily the peripheral branches of the middle cerebral artery), but they also occur in the abdominal aorta, sinus of Valsalva, a ligated patent ductus arteriosus, and the splenic, coronary, pulmonary, and superior mesenteric arteries. Myoctic aneurysms are usually clinically silent until rupture occurs; consequently, their true incidence in active IE is unknown.[115]

Central Nervous System. Cerebral emboli occur in at least one-third of all cases[37] and most commonly affect the middle cerebral artery and its branches. Three percent of the cerebral emboli from all causes are secondary to IE. Cerebral infarction, arteritis, abscesses, mycotic aneurysms, intracerebral or subarachnoid hemorrhage, encephalomalacia, cerebritis, and meningitis have all been reported.[116] True acute purulent meningitis is rare except in pneumococcal endocarditis, but multiple microabscesses (cerebritis) are relatively common in acute staphylococcal endocarditis.

Spleen. Spenic infarctions have been reported in 44 percent of the autopsy cases but are rarely detected clinically.[37] Abscess formation and rupture have been described but are uncommon. Splenic enlargement is common, and virtually all cases are associated with hyperplasia of the lymphoid follicles, an increase in secondary follicles, proliferation of reticuloendothelial cells, and scattered focal necrosis.[112]

Lung. When right-sided IE is present, pulmonary emboli with or without infarction, acute pneumonia, pleural effusion, or empyema are common and are due to septic or bland emboli.

Skin. Petechiae are found in 20–40 percent of the cases (Fig. 2) (see below). Osler nodes microscopically consist of arteriolar intimal proliferation with extension to venules and capillaries and may be accompanied by thrombosis and necrosis. A diffuse perivascular infiltrate consisting of neutrophils and monocytes surrounds the dermal vessels. Immune complexes have been demonstrated in the dermal vessels. Janeway lesions consist of bacteria, neutrophilic infiltration, necrosis, and subcutaneous hemorrhage (Fig. 3). Janeway lesions are due to septic emboli and reveal subcutaneous abscesses on histologic examination.[117]

Eye. "Roth spots" consist microscopically of lymphocytes surrounded by edema and hemorrhage in the nerve fiber layer of the retina (Fig. 4).[118]

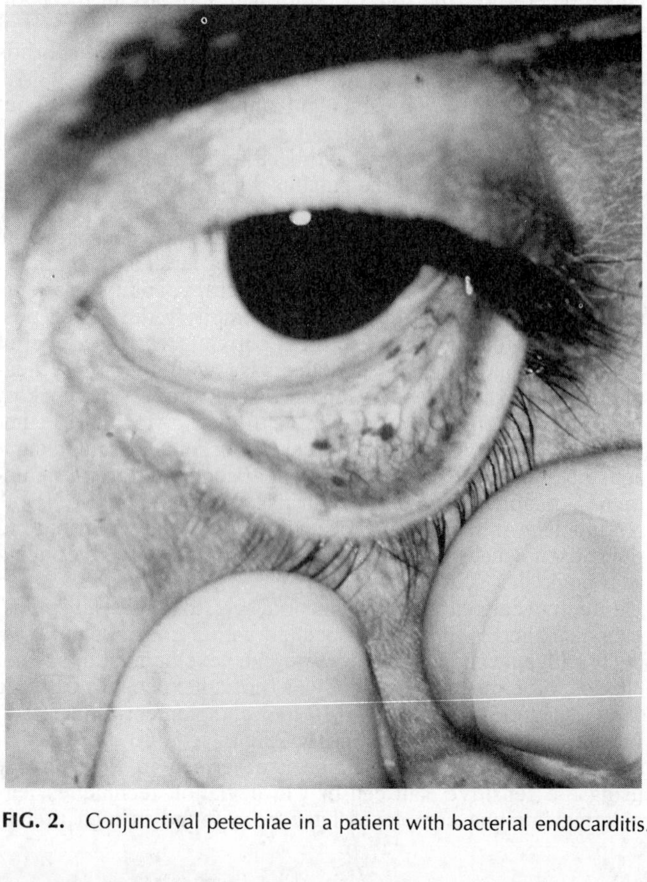

FIG. 2. Conjunctival petechiae in a patient with bacterial endocarditis.

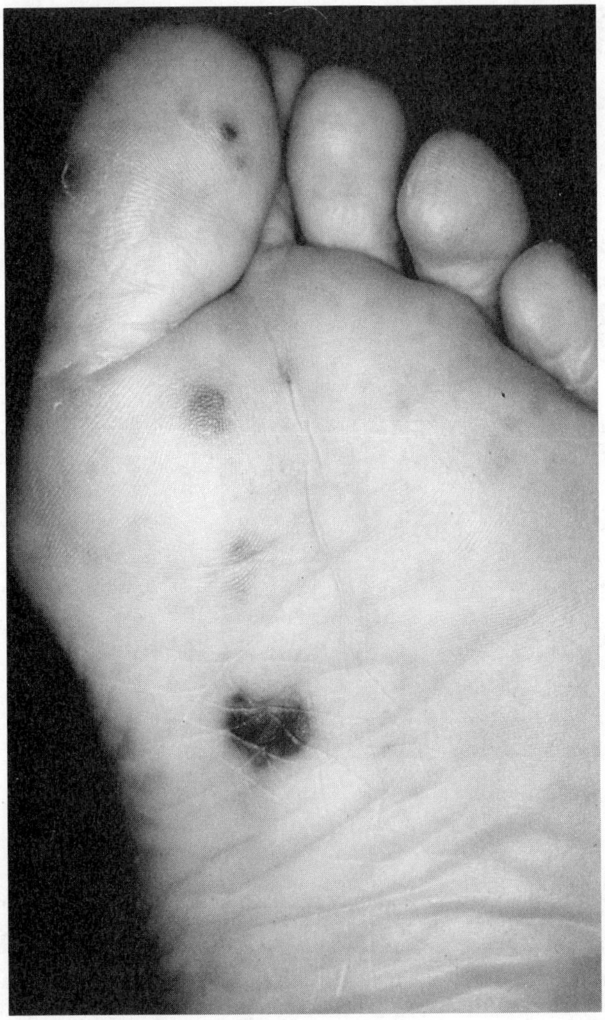

FIG. 3. Janeway lesions in a patient with Staphylococcus aureus endocarditis. (From Hook et al.,[483] with permission.)

Clinical Manifestations

The interval between an event likely to produce bacteremia (e.g., dental extraction) and the onset of symptoms of IE, contrary to older estimates, is actually quite short. The so-called "incubation period" in 84 percent of 76 cases of streptococcal endocarditis was less than 2 weeks.[119] However, the time from the onset of symptoms to diagnosis in the subacute form of IE is quite long, with a median interval of approximately 5 weeks.

The symptoms and signs (Table 3) are protean, and essentially any organ system may be involved. Four processes contribute to the clinical picture[37]: (*1*) the infectious process on the valve including the local intracardiac complications; (*2*) bland or septic embolization to virtually any organ; (*3*) constant bacteremia, often with metastatic foci of infection; and (*4*) circulating immune complexes and other immunopathologic factors.[36,121] As a result, the clinical presentation of patients with IE is highly variable and the differential diagnosis often broad.[122]

Fever is common but may be absent (5 percent of the cases), especially in the setting of congestive heart failure (CHF), renal failure, a terminal disease, old age,[123] or previous antibiotic therapy. The fever pattern is usually remittent, and the patient's temperature rarely exceeds 103°F except in acute IE.[120] Nonspecific symptoms such as anorexia, weight loss, malaise, fatigue, chills, weakness, nausea, vomiting, and night sweats are common, especially in subacute cases.[15] These nonspecific symptoms often result in an incorrect diagnosis of malignancy,

TABLE 3. Clinical Manifestations of Infective Endocarditis

Symptoms	*Percentage*	*Physical Findings*	*Percentage*
Fever	80	Fever	90
Chills	40	Heart murmur	85
Weakness	40	Changing murmur	5–10
Dyspnea	40	New murmur	3–5
Sweats	25	Embolic phenomenon	>50
Anorexia	25	Skin manifestations	18–50
Weight loss	25	Osler nodes	10–23
Malaise	25	Splinter hemorrhages	15
Cough	25	Petechiae	20–40
Skin lesions	20	Janeway lesion	<10
Stroke	20	Splenomegaly	20–57
Nausea/vomiting	20	Septic complications	20
Headache	15	(pneumonia,	
Myalgia/arthralgia	15	meningitis, etc.)	
Edema	15	Mycotic aneurysms	20
Chest pain	15	Clubbing	12–52
Abdominal pain	10–15	Retinal lesion	2–10
Delirium/coma	10	Signs of renal failure	10–15
Hemoptysis	10		
Back pain	10		

(Data from Lerner et al.,[1] Pelletier et al.,[15] Venezio et al.,[25] and Weinstein et al.[120])

collagen vascular disease, tuberculosis, or other chronic diseases.

Heart murmurs occur in over 85 percent of the cases but may be absent with right-sided or mural infection. The classic "changing murmur" and the development of a new murmur (usually aortic insufficiency) are uncommon and occur in 5–10 percent and in 3–5 percent of the cases, respectively. When present, these are diagnostically useful signs and usually complicate acute staphylococcal disease. New or changing murmurs are less common in the elderly and often lead to diagnostic confusion.[123,124] Over 90 percent of patients who demonstrate a new regurgitant murmur will develop CHF. The incidence of CHF appears to be increasing (approximately 25 percent in 1966 and 67 percent in 1972)[15] and is now the leading cause of death in IE. Pericarditis is rare but, when present, is usually accompanied by myocardial abscess formation as a complication of staphylococcal infection.

The classic peripheral manifestations are found in up to one-half of the cases but the prevalence has decreased in recent years. Clubbing is present in 10–20 percent, especially if the disease is of long duration, and may recede with therapy. The complete syndrome of hypertrophic osteoarthropathy is rare. Splinter hemorrhages are linear red to brown streaks in the fingernails or toenails and are commonly found in IE. They are a nonspecific finding and are often seen in the elderly or in people experiencing occupation-related trauma. These lesions are most suggestive of IE when located proximally in the nail bed. Petechiae are found in 20–40 percent of the cases, particularly after a prolonged course, and usually appear in crops on the conjunctivae (Fig. 2), buccal mucosa, palate, and extremities. These lesions are initially red and nonblanching but become brown and barely visible in 2–3 days. Petechiae may result from either local vasculitis or emboli. Osler nodes are small, painful, nodular lesions usually found in the pads of fingers or toes and occasionally in the thenar eminence. They are 2–15 mm in size and are frequently multiple and evanescent, disappearing in hours to days. Osler nodes are rare in acute cases of IE but occur in 10–25 percent of all the cases. They are not specific for IE since they may be seen in systemic lupus erythematosus, marantic endocarditis, hemolytic anemia, and gonococcal infections and in extremities with cannulated radial arteries. Janeway lesions (Fig. 3) are hemorrhagic, macular, painless plaques with a predilection for the palms or soles. They persist for several days and are thought to be embolic in origin and occur with greater frequency in staphylococcal endocarditis. Roth spots (Fig. 4) are oval, pale, retinal lesions surrounded by hemorrhage and are usually located near the optic disk. They occur in less than 5 percent of the cases of IE and may also be found in

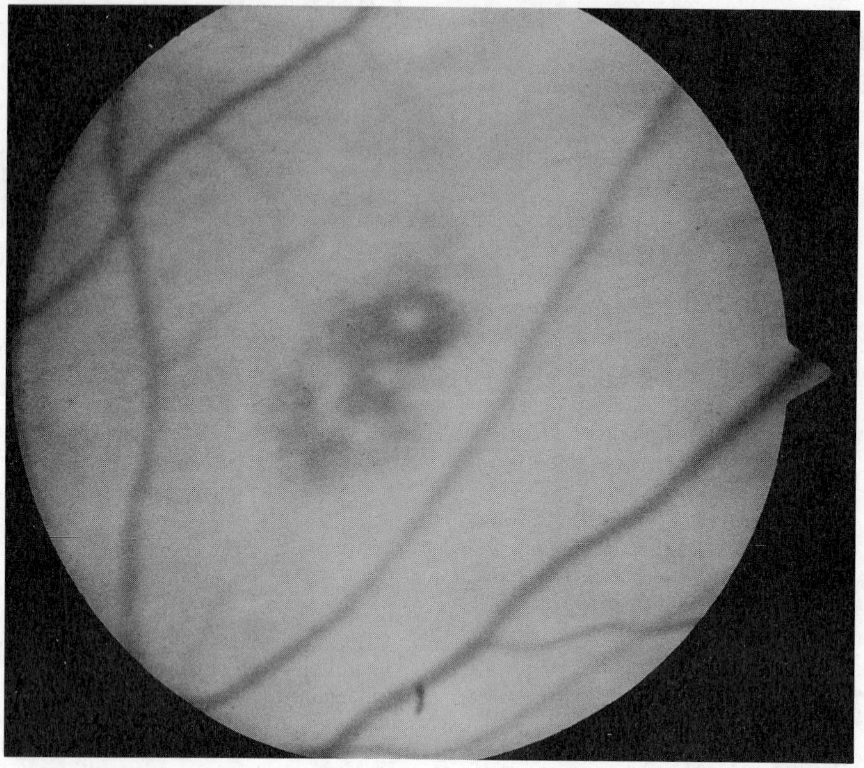

FIG. 4. Retina from a patient with viridans streptococcal endocarditis showing Roth spots. (From Hook et al.,[483] with permission.)

anemia, leukemia, and connective tissue disorders such as systemic lupus erythematosus.

Splenomegaly has been reported in 25–60 percent of all the cases and is more common in patients with endocarditis of prolonged duration. The incidence of splenomegaly appears to be progressively decreasing since the advent of antibiotics.

Musculoskeletal manifestations are common in IE. In a review of 192 cases,[125] 44 percent of the patients had musculoskeletal symptoms. These symptoms usually occur early in the disease and were the only initial complaint in 15 percent of the cases. They included proximal oligo- or monoarticular arthralgias (38 percent), lower extremity mono- or oligoarticular arthritis (31 percent), low back pain (23 percent), and diffuse myalgias (19 percent). These findings may mimic rheumatic disease and result in a diagnostic delay.

Major embolic episodes, as a group, are second only to congestive heart failure as a complication of IE and occur in at least one-third of cases. Splenic artery emboli with infarction may result in left upper quadrant abdominal pain with radiation to the left shoulder, a splenic or pleural rub, or a left pleural effusion. Renal infarctions may be associated with microscopic or gross hematura, but renal failure, hypertension, and edema are uncommon. Retinal artery emboli are rare (fewer than 2 percent of the cases) and may be manifested by a sudden complete loss of vision. A panophthalmitis has been reported with pneumococcal endocarditis. Pulmonary emboli arising from right-sided endocarditis is a common feature in narcotic addicts (see below). Coronary artery emboli usually arise from the aortic valve and may cause myocarditis with arrythmias or myocardial infarction. Major vessel emboli (femoral, brachial, popliteal, or radial arteries) are more frequent in fungal endocarditis.

Neurologic manifestations occur in 20–40 percent of the cases and may dominate the clinical picture, especially in staphylococcal endocarditis. A sudden neurologic event in a young person should suggest IE. Major cerebral emboli afflict 10–30 percent of the patients and may result in hemiplegia, sensory loss, ataxia, aphasia, or an alteration in mental status.[116,126] Mycotic aneurysms of the cerebral circulation occur in 2–10 percent of the cases. They are usually single, small, and peripheral and may lead to devastating subarachnoid hemorrhage. Other features include seizures, severe headache, visual changes, choreoathetoid movements, mononeuropathy, and cranial nerve palsies. A toxic encephalopathy with symptoms ranging from a mild change in personality to frank psychosis may occur, especially in elderly patients.

Patients with IE may have symptoms of uremia. In the preantibiotic era, renal failure developed in 25–35 percent of the cases, but presently fewer than 10 percent are affected. When uremia does develop, diffuse glomerulonephritis with hypocomplementia is usually found, but focal glomerulonephritis has also been implicated. Renal failure is more common with longstanding disease but usually subsides with appropriate antimicrobial treatment alone. IE may be confused with thrombotic thrombocytopenic purpura when neurologic signs, fever, renal failure, anemia, and thrombocytopenia are present.[127]

Infective Endocarditis in Drug Addicts. Acute infection accounts for ≈60 percent of hospital admissions among intravenous drug abusers; IE is implicated in 5–8 percent of these episodes.[128] It has proved difficult to accurately predict the presence of IE in the febrile drug addict,[129] although cocaine use by the intravenous drug user should heighten the suspicion of IE.[130] Cocaine use was strongly associated with the presence of IE in 102 intravenous drug users in San Francisco when analyzed by logistic regression analysis in comparison with febrile addicts from other causes. Although may of the aforementioned clinical manifestations are seen in addicts with endocarditis, several distinctions are worthy of emphasis. In this group of patients, two-thirds have no clinical evidence of underlying heart disease, and there is a predilection for the infection to affect the tricuspid valve. Only 35 percent of addicts ultimately proven to have IE demonstrate heart murmurs on admission.[128] The frequency of valvular involvement is as follows: tricuspid alone or in combination with others, 52.2 percent; aortic alone, 18.5 percent; mitral alone, 10.8 percent; and aortic plus mitral, 12.5 percent.[2] Of these patients with tricuspid valve infection, 30 percent have pleuritic chest pain, pulmonary findings may dominate the clinical picture, and the chest roentgenogram will document abnormalities (infiltrates, effusion, etc.) in 75–85 percent of patients.[131] Roentgenographic evidence of septic pulmonary emboli is eventually present in 87 percent of cases.[132] Signs of tricuspid insufficiency (gallop rhythm, systolic regurgitant murmur louder with inspiration, large V waves, or a pulsatile liver) are present in only one-third of the cases. Most of these patients are 20–40 years old (80 percent), and men predominate 4–6:1. The course of acute staphylococcal endocarditis in the addict tends to be less severe than in nonaddicts.[131] Almost two-thirds of these patients have extravalvular sites of infection that are helpful in the diagnosis.[131–133]

Laboratory Findings

Hematologic parameters are often abnormal in IE, but none are diagnostic. Anemia is nearly always present (70–90 percent of the cases) and has the characteristics of the anemia of chronic disease with normochromic, normocytic indices, a low serum iron concentration, and a low iron-binding capacity. The anemia tends to worsen with the duration of the illness. Thrombocytopenia occurs in 5–15 percent of the cases but is common in neonatal IE. Leukocytosis is present in 20–30 percent of cases but is rare in the subacute variety, whereas counts of 15,000–25,000/mm^3 are not uncommon in acute IE. The differential count is usually normal, but there may be a slight shift to the left. Leukopenia is uncommon (5–15 percent) and, when present, is usually associated with splenomegaly. Large mononuclear cells can be detected in the peripheral blood in approximately 25 percent of the patients, but the yield is higher in blood taken from an earlobe puncture. This finding is nonspecific since similar cells have been found in malaria, typhus, typhoid fever, and tuberculosis.

The erythrocyte sedimentation rate (ESR) is nearly always (90–100 percent) elevated, with a mean value of 57 mm/hr found in one large series.[15] In the absence of renal failure, congestive heart failure, or disseminated intravascular coagulation, a normal ESR is evidence against a diagnosis of IE. Hypergammaglobulinemia is detected in 20–30 percent of the cases and may be accompanied by a plasmacytosis in the bone marrow aspirate. A positive rheumatoid factor is found in 40–50 percent of the cases, especially when the duration of the illness is greater than 6 weeks.[98] Hypocomplementemia (5–15 percent) parallels the incidence of abnormal renal function test results (elevated creatinine level in 5–15 percent). A false-positive Venereal Disease Research Laboratory (VDRL) test is uncommon (0.2 percent).

The urinalysis is frequently abnormal; proteinuria occurs in 50–65 percent of the cases and microscopic hematuria in 30–50 percent. Red cell casts may be seen in as many as 12 percent of the cases[15]; gross hematura, pyuria, white cell casts, and bacteriuria may also be found.

Circulating immune complexes can be detected in most cases of IE but are also found in 32 percent of the patients with septicemia but without endocarditis, in 10 percent of the healthy controls, and in 40 percent of noninfected narcotic addicts.[98] However, levels greater than 100 μg of aggregated human γ-globulin equivalent per milliliter were found only in IE (35 percent of the cases). Detection of high levels of immune complexes may be useful in the diagnosis of right-sided IE in narcotic addicts or in culture-negative cases. In addition, since the levels fall with appropriate treatment, serial measurement of immune complexes may assist in management of the disease.[110,111] Mixed-type cryoglobulins are detectable in 84–95 percent of the patients with IE but are also a nonspecific finding. Although nonspecific and virtually always elevated in IE, serial determination of the serum C-reactive protein concentration may be useful to monitor therapy and detect intercurrent complications or infections.[134]

The detection of vegetations by ^{67}Ga myocardial imaging initially appeared to be a useful diagnostic tool. Of 11 patients in one study,[135] 7 had infected vegetations localized by scans including one culture-negative case that was confirmed at autopsy. Further studies are needed to determine the potential value of noninvasive imaging of cardiac vegetations by using a radiolabeled compound, for example, ^{99m}Tc-labeled antibacterial antibody[136] or ^{111}In-labeled platelets[137] because both have shown promise in experimental endocarditis. At present, these techniques must be considered investigational. Radiographic techniques are occasionally useful in the diagnosis or decisions regarding surgical intervention. For example, computed tomography (CT) of the abdomen detected splenic infarcts in 6 of 25 (24 percent) consecutive patients with IE in one series[138]: 2 of 6 were asymptomatic.

The blood culture is the single most important laboratory test performed in a diagnostic work-up of IE. The bacteremia is usually continuous and low grade (80 percent of the cases have less than 100 cfu/ml of blood).[139] In approximately two-thirds of the cases, all the blood cultures drawn will be positive.[15] When bacteremia is present, the first two blood cultures will yield the etiologic agent more than 90 percent of the time. In a review of 206 cases of IE seen over a 15-year period at The New York Hospital,[140] 95 percent of the blood cultures were positive. In streptococcal endocarditis, the first blood culture was positive in 96 percent of cases, and one of the first two cultures was positive in 98 percent. When antibiotics had been administered in the previous 2 weeks, the rate of positive cultures declined from 97 to 91 percent ($p < .02$). The influence of outpatient antibiotic administration on blood culture positivity was more significant in another retrospective analysis;[141] 64 percent of 88 cultures were positive in 17 patients receiving antibiotics before hospitalization vs. 100 percent in 15 patients without antibiotic exposure. In nonstreptococcal endocarditis, the first blood culture was positive in 86 percent of the cases and when two cultures were taken, in 100 percent. Most blood cultures contained only a few organisms; over 50 percent of the cultures contained 1–30 bacteria/ml. Only 17 percent of the cultures yielded more than 100 bacteria/ml. The bacteremia was also constant with little variation in quantitative culture determinations in any individual patient. The sensitivity of blood cultures for the detection of streptococci is particularly susceptible to prior antibiotic therapy and/or the media employed.[142]

On the basis of these studies, the following procedures for culturing blood are recommended. At least three blood culture sets (no more than two bottles per venipuncture) should be obtained in the first 24 hours. More cultures may be necessary if the patient has received antibiotics in the preceding 2 weeks. At least 10 ml of blood (where feasible) should be injected into both trypticase soy (or brain–heart infusion) and thioglycollate broth.[143,144] Trypticase soy bottles should be transiently "vented." Pour plates may be made at the bedside for an estimate of the degree of bacteremia. Supplementation with 15% sucrose (in an attempt to isolate cell wall-deficient forms) or the use of prereduced anaerobic media is unrewarding.[145] The newer commercial media are also effective, but comparative data are few. In general, culture of arterial blood offers no advantage over venous blood. Inspection for macroscopic growth should be performed daily and routine subcultures done on days 1 and 3. The cultures should be held for at least 3 weeks. When gram-positive cocci grow on the initial isolation but fail to grow on subculture, nutritionally variant (thiol-dependent) streptococci should be suspected.[146] In this event, subculture should be onto media supplemented with either 0.05–0.1% L-cysteine or 0.001% pyridoxal phosphate.

Intraleukocytic bacteria have been visualized in peripheral blood in approximately 50 percent of the cases[147] by a simple "monolayer" technique. This may be helpful in culture-negative cases or when patients have been receiving antibiotics.[148]

Ribitol teichoic acids are major constituents of the cell wall of staphylococci. Gel diffusion and counterimmunoelectrophoresis techniques have been used to detect teichoic acid antibodies in the serum of patients suspected of having *Staphylococcus aureus* endocarditis. Teichoic acid antibodies can be detected by counterimmunoelectrophoresis in over 95 percent of the patients,[149] but the rate of false-positive tests may exceed 10 percent. Serial titrations of serum by using the double-agar diffusion technique can be used to detect the low titers found in some healthy people. Antibody titers ≥1:4 are indicative of disseminated staphylococcal disease (endocarditis, multiple metastatic abscesses, or hematogenous osteomyelitis). Since these conditions all require prolonged antimicrobial therapy, this test may be of practical value if the results are positive. The value of a negative result is controversial; some authorities suggest that a short course of antimicrobial therapy is justified in this instance,[150] while others find a negative test response helpful only if all clinical signs are indicative of "benign" (i.e., superficial) staphylococcal bacteremia.[151] This issue is unresolved; we view this test as confirmatory of clinical suspicions only. The detection of other circulating staphylococcal antigens (e.g., capsular polysaccharide by enzyme-linked immunosorbent assay [ELISA]) has been documented in experimental animal models of IE,[152] but experience in humans in scant.

Special Diagnostic Tests. These tests are not routinely used (with the exception of echocardiography) in all cases of IE but may be useful in two situations: (*1*) in the diagnostic approach to culture-negative IE and (*2*) in decisions about surgical intervention during active infection.

The incidence of so-called blood culture-negative endocarditis has varied from 2.5 to 31 percent in published series.[153] If the patients have not received previous antibiotic therapy and the blood cultures are obtained as outlined, these cases should represent fewer than 5 percent of the total. Some of the aforementioned tests (rheumatoid factor, teichoic acid antibodies, earlobe histiocytes, monolayer technique for intraleukocytic bacteria) may be helpful in identifying such cases, but other procedures are often necessary. If the patient has received antibiotics, blood cultures in hypertonic media may allow detection of cell wall-defective organisms. Supplementation of media with vitamin B_6 or with cysteine may assist the recovery of nutritionally variant streptococci. The lysis–centrifugation blood culture technique assists in the detection of staphylococci and fungi, but nutritionally variant streptococci do not survive this procedure, and yields of pneumococci and anaerobes are decreased.[155] Routine use of this technique is not indicated, but it may be helpful in suspected culture-negative cases of IE. Since some anaerobes, *Brucella* sp., and members of the HACEK group (see below) are slow-growing organisms, holding cultures for 4 weeks may increase the recovery rate. Cultures of bone marrow or urine may rarely be positive when blood cultures are negative. Serologic studies are necessary for the diagnosis of Q fever, murine typhus,[156] or psittacosis endocarditis. Special culture techniques (e.g., for *Legionella* sp.[157]) are indicated in patients with suspected prosthetic valve endocarditis when initial cultures are "negative" (Chapter 62). Other tests to exclude collagen vascular diseases are usually necessary in patients undergoing evaluation for culture-negative, native-valve IE.[158]

Blood cultures are negative in over 50 percent of the cases of fungal endocarditis.[159] The lysis–centrifugation method of blood culture is also useful in detecting fungi. This disease is increasing in frequency and usually affects narcotic addicts, patients with prosthetic valves, or hospitalized patients receiving antibiotics and/or hyperalimentation. Use of the Castaneda principle (a culture of blood in a bottle containing both agar and liquid broth) has been shown to increase the yield of fungal cultures.[145] Blastospores and pseudohyphae have been found in Wright-stained peripheral blood in at least one case of *Candida*-induced endocarditis.[160] Various serologic procedures have been used in an attempt to substantiate a diagnosis of fungal endocarditis. Tests for the determination of antifungal antibody are poorly standardized, variably sensitive, often nonspecific, and difficult to interpret.[161] In a rabbit moddel of *Candida*-induced endocarditis, both precipitating and agglutinating antibodies were detected after 12 days of active infection, and titers rose progressively until death of the animals.[162] In contrast, animals without endocarditis developed only a transient rise in antibody titers after a single intravenous injection of viable *Candida albicans*. Newer tests for detecting fungal antigen in serum are more promising as indicators of invasive fungal disease. Tests for mannan antigenemia (a constituent of the cell wall of *Candida*) by hemagglutination inhibition, by gas–liquid chromatography, or by the ELISA method[163,164] have been reported as helpful in the diagnosis of disseminated candidiasis. In addition, a reliable radioimmunoassay for the detection of *Aspergillus* antigenemia is currently under investigation. When embolism to major vessels occurs, an embolectomy should be performed, and the material should be examined by both special fungal stains and culture. Identification of the fungus by either technique is diagnostic of fungal endocarditis even when blood cultures are sterile.

The use of echocardiography in the diagnosis of IE was first reported in 1973.[165] To date, echocardiograms have correctly identified vegetations on all valves. Most reports have focused on left-sided disease. The sensitivity and specificity of this technique is uncertain; however, two studies correctly identified 33 of 52 vegetations documented surgically or at autopsy.[166,167] The characteristic finding is a shaggy dense band of irregular echoes in a nonuniform distribution on one or more leaflets with full unrestricted motion of the valve. The smallest vegetation detected was approximately 2 mm, but the acoustic impedance of the mass relative to the surrounding structures is a more important factor than size is in identifying the vegetation. The use of two-dimensional cross-sectional real-time techniques improves the diagnostic accuracy over M-mode methods.[168] If the vegetation is calcified (which may occur early and independent of the healing process), the sensitivity of echocardiography may be increased. Echocardiography has correctly localized vegetations in culture-negative cases. Echocardiography may be of special value in the detection of the large friable vegetations characteristic of fungal endocarditis. However, its use with prosthetic heart valves has been disappointing because of the difficulty in resolution around the prosthetic device. Many reports have appeared[169] that have evaluated the role of echocardiography in the diagnosis and management of suspected IE and were summarized in a cogent analysis.[170] These studies suggest the following: (*1*) variable sensitivity for the detection of vegetations (<50 to >90 percent positive), and therefore a negative study does not exclude IE; (*2*) the echocardiogram is useless in excluding IE; (*3*) false-positive results are extremely rare; (*4*) only technically adequate studies are really valuable, a characteristic heavily dependent on the experience of the person performing the examination; (*5*) echocardiography is extremely valuable in assessing local complications of IE, especially surrounding the aortic valve; (*6*) patients with a "vegetation" identified by echocardiography are at an increased risk for subsequent systemic emboli, congestive heart failure, the need for emergency surgery, and death, especially with aortic valve involvement. This influence on prognosis has hastened earlier surgery in some cases,[171] but this point remains controversial.[172] A positive echocardiogram in a patient with IE should serve as an adjunctive piece of evidence, together with clinical parameters, in indicating surgical intervention. Visualization of vegetations by echocardiography is not sufficient alone to prompt early surgery.[173] Serial echocardiograms often reveal the persistence of vegetations after successful therapy, but sequential studies may be useful in the timing of surgical intervention. Esophageal lead echocardiograms have been especially useful in detecting vegetations. Short-term changes in vegetation size during therapy do not correlate well with clinical outcome.[174] However, a new technique, digital image processing of two-dimensional echocardiograms, may differentiate active from healed lesions.[175] If substantiated, this method may be useful in "culture-negative" cases (particularly with suspected recurrent IE) or when the response to therapy is suboptimal or inconclusive.

In conjunction with the physical examination, phonocardiography, and electrocardiography, the echocardiogram may play an important role in assessing the severity of acute aortic insufficiency in cases of active IE.[176] In this setting, classic physical findings such as a wide pulse pressure and bounding pulses are often absent; however, there is usually a reduction in intensity of the first heart sound and Austin Flint murmurs may be audible. The chest roentgenogram and electrocardiogram may be normal. The degree of mitral valve preclosure (as determined by echocardiography) correlates with the elevation of the left ventricular end-diastolic pressure. If this event occurs before the Q wave on the electrocardiogram, rapid surgical intervention is recommended.

Cardiac catheterization with quantitative blood cultures proximal and distal to suspected sites of infection has been useful in the localization of vegetations in both right-sided and left-sided IE.[177] Multiple specimens from identical sites are necessary since minor fluctuations in bacteremia do occur. However, this technique is potentially dangerous and has been associated with rapid clinical deterioration when used in the setting of acute aortic insufficiency complicated by progressive congestive heart failure.[177] Cardiac catheterization does provide valuable hemodynamic and anatomic information in patients with IE when considering surgical intervention.[133] Properly performed, the procedure is safe as demonstrated by the lack of postcatheterization emboli or hemodynamic deterioration in 35 consecutive patients in one series.[178]

Cineangiography is the definitive procedure in determining the anatomic alterations resulting from the infection. If is of value in determining the degree of aortic regurgitation, in assessing the contribution of left ventricular dysfunction in congestive heart failure, in visualizing ventricular and aortic aneurysms, and in gauging the patency of the coronary arteries. This information may be critically important in determining a surgical approach, especially if multivalvular involvement is documented. The additional information gained from obtaining right- and left-heart pressures with complete cardiac catheterization are not useful in decisions on therapy in acute IE.[177]

Etiologic Agents

Streptococci. A plethora of microorganisms have been implicated in IE, but streptococci and staphylococci account for 80–90 percent of the cases in which identification is made. The most common etiologic agents are outlined in Table 4. The streptococci still cause most of the cases of IE,[25] especially in the community hospital setting. The disease usually runs a classic subacute course with multiple nonspecific symptoms as outlined in Table 3. Over 80 percent of these patients have underlying heart disease. Infective endocarditis in a young woman with isolated mitral valve involvement is almost universally caused by streptococci. Approximately 20 percent of the cases are seen because of embolic phenomena. With modern medical and surgical management, the cure rate should exceed 90 percent in cases of nonenterococcal streptococcal endocarditis, although complications may ensue in more than 30 percent of cases.[179]

TABLE 4. Etiologic Agents in Infective Endocarditis

Agent	*Percentage of Cases*
Streptococci	60–80
Viridans streptococci	30–40
Enterococci	5–18
Other streptococci	15–25
Staphylococci	20–35
Coagulase-positive	10–27
Coagulase-negative	1–3
Gram-negative aerobic bacilli	1.5–13
Fungi	2–4
Miscellaneous bacteria	<5
Mixed infections	1–2
"Culture negative"	<5–24

The nomenclature of the streptococci is confusing, and various authors differ in terminology used. Streptococci of the viridans group (not a true species) are α-hemolytic and usually nontypeable by the Lancefield system. The most common streptococci isolated from cases of endocarditis are *S. sanguis, S. bovis, S. mutans,* and *S. mitior.*[61] In a series of 317 cases of streptococcal endocarditis, the breakdown was as follows: α-hemolytic, 45 percent; nonhemolytic, nongroup D, 21 percent; group D, 25 percent; pyogenic (groups A, B, C, G), 5 percent; miscellaneous, 3 percent; and aerococci, 1.3 percent. The α-hemolytic strains included *S. sanguis* (16.4 percent of all cases of IE), non-dextran-producing *S. mitior* (13.2 percent), dextran-positive *S. mitior* (7.3 percent), and an unclassified group (7.9 percent). Some isolates of *S. sanguis,* formerly called "streptococcus SBE," are in Lancefield group H, however, most are nontypeable. *Streptococcus mutans* (14.2 percent), *S. anginosus* (5.4 percent), and *S. salivarius* (1.3 percent) comprised the nonhemolytic, non-group D strains. Group D organisms included the enterococci (8 percent) and *S. bovis* (17 percent). In another analysis,[180] viridans streptococci caused 58 percent of cases of IE at the New York Hospital from 1970 to 1978. The various responsible species were as follows: *S. mitior,* 31 percent; *S. bovis,* 27 percent; *S. sanguis,* 24 percent; *S. mutans,* 7 percent; vitamin B_6 dependent *S. mitior,* 5 percent; *S. anginosus,* 4 percent; and others, 2 percent—all of which are slightly different from the experience in the United Kingdom. A similar species distribution was observed in 48 patients (with 51 episodes of IE) reported from Washington, D.C.[181] There appears to be no correlation, however, between the clinical outcome and the species involved[179,181] with the exception of nutritionally deficient strains (see below). Viridans streptococci remain the most commonly isolated pathogens in IE cases associated with mitral valve prolapse.[182] The relative role of each species overall is problematic, however, since species designations of identical strains among laboratories are often disparate.[179]

Streptococcus mutans, the etiologic agent in 14.2 percent of the cases in the review of Parker and Ball,[61] is microaerophilic, pleomorphic, and fastidious. Two-thirds of strains will hydrolyze bile-esculin,[183] a test used to identify group D organisms, and thus may be confused with enterococci. Other characteristics of *S. mutans* include the absence of group D antigen (some strains are positive for group E), production of acid from mannitol, a failure to hydrolyze hippurate, and the formation of gelatinous deposits (dextran) in media containing 5% sucrose. This organism may be difficult to isolate and to identify. It often requires over 3 days for primary isolation, grows best on horse blood agar in 5–10% CO_2 on subculture, and is very pleomorphic, resulting in confusion with diphtheroids. *Streptococcus mutans* was first isolated in 1924 by Clark from dental caries lesions of humans and was first reported in 1928 to cause IE.

The central importance of this organism in dental caries has been amply documented.

Streptococcus bovis is a normal inhabitant of the gastrointestinal tract of humans and many animal species. It is important to separate this organism from the other members of group D (the enterococci) because their respective therapeutic approaches are different (see below). Group D organisms are presumptively identified by bile-esculin hydrolysis.[184,185] However, only the enterococci (*E. faecalis* and its varieties *zymogenes* and *liquifaciens, E. faecium, E. durans*) grow in 6.5% NaCl whereas *S. bovis* and *S. equinus* (a very rare cause of IE) are salt sensitive. Seventy-five percent of strains of *S. bovis* are heat tolerant, and they may also grow and produce acid in "*E. faecalis* broth"; therefore, these methods are unreliable for separation.[186] Arginine hydrolysis by enterococci and starch hydrolysis by *S. bovis* are other means for reliable separation. The association of bacteremia due to *S. bovis* with carcinoma of the colon and other lesions of the gastrointestinal tract suggests that colonoscopy and/or a barium enema be performed when this organism is isolated from blood cultures.[187,188]

Enterococci are normal inhabitants of the gastrointestinal tract and occasionally the anterior urethra or mouth. All enterococci are in Lancefield's group D; are catalase-negative and nonmotile; and may exhibit α-, β-, or γ-hemolysis on blood agar. They grow well in sodium azide ("SF broth"), 40% bile, 6.5% NaCl, and 0.1% methylene blue and can survive at 56°C for 30 minutes or at a pH of 9.6.[189] They should be separated from *S. bovis*. The enterococcus group is responsible for 5–18 percent of the cases of IE, and the incidence appears to be increasing,[190] especially in intravenous drug addicts. The disease usually runs a subacute course and affects older (mean age, 59) men after genitourinary manipulation or younger (mean age, 37) women after obstetric procedures. The mean duration of nonspecific symptoms such as malaise, fatigue, anorexia, and weight loss was 140 days in one review. Over 40 percent of the patients have no underlying heart disease although >95 percent develop a heart murmur during the course of the illness. Classic peripheral manifestations are uncommon (fewer than 25 percent of the cases). Bacteriuria with enterococci is a helpful diagnostic clue and was found in 4 of 15 patients[189] in one study. Cure is difficult because of resistance to antibiotics, and a high mortality persists in this disease. With the increasing usage of third-generation cephalosporins and other factors, recent reports[191–193] emphasize an alarming increase in enterococcal bacteremias during the past two decades. Most enterococcal bacteremias are nosocomial in origin, often polymicrobial (42 percent in one large series[193]) and are associated with serious underlying disorders. Factors that suggest IE in patients with enterococcal bacteremia include (*1*) community acquisition, (*2*) pre-existent valvular heart disease, (*3*) a cryptogenic source, and (*4*) the absence of polymicrobial bacteremia.[193] Antibiotic usage patterns, the aging of the population, and more invasive procedures in hospitalized adults all portend a continued increase in serious enterococcal infections, including IE, in the future.

Before 1945, *S. pneumoniae* was responsible for approximately 10 percent of cases of IE, but this has decreased to approximately 1–3 percent currently.[120] The course is usually fulminant and is often (in approximately one-third of cases) associated with perivalvular abscess formation and/or pericarditis. Left-sided involvement is the rule, and there is a predilection for the aortic valve (≈70 percent). Many patients with pneumococcal endocarditis are alcoholics (≈40 percent), and concurrent meningitis is present in ≈70 percent of cases.[194,195] The overall mortality remains at approximately 50 percent, usually due to rapid valvular destruction and hemodynamic compromise.

Nutritionally variant streptococci (usually *S. mitior*) may cause difficulties in isolation and were implicated in 5.4 percent of the cases of streptococcal endocarditis at The New York Hospital.[196] The organisms do not grow on subculture unless L-cysteine or pyridoxal (vitamin B_6) is supplemented. Infective endocarditis due to nutritionally deficient streptococci is virtually always indolent in onset and associated with prior heart disease.[197] Therapy remains difficult because systemic embolization, relapse, and death are not infrequent (17–27 percent of cases). A closely related species, *S. mitis,* although not nutritionally deficient, also causes serious infections, including IE, in adults[198] and has emerged as an important causative agent of IE among drug addicts in some areas (i.e., New York City[199]). Group B streptococci (*S. agalactiae*) are normal inhabitants of the mouth, vagina, and anterior urethra in 5–12 percent of the general population. In 149 patients with group B streptococcal infections, the serotypes isolated were Ia in 46 percent, II in 22 percent, and III in 11 percent.[200] Although long recognized as a cause of bacteremia and meningitis in neonates, serious *S. agalactiae* infections in adults have been emphasized recently.[201] Risk factors for group B streptococcal sepsis and IE in adults include diabetes mellitus, carcinoma, alcoholism, hepatic failure, and intravenous drug use.[201–203] Like *S. bovis,* occasional cases occur in association with villous adenomas of the colon.[204] Over 70 cases of group B streptococcal IE have been reported.[202,203] Underlying heart disease is common, the male-to-female ratio is 1.4:1, the mean age is approximately 54 years, and left-sided involvement predominates. The overall mortality is nearly 50 percent. The organism does not produce fibrinolysin, which may be responsible for the large crumbling vegetations and frequent major systemic emboli. A similar clinical picture with a destructive process, left-sided predominance, frequent complications, and high mortality (≈40 percent) has been observed in the 47 cases of group G streptococcal endocarditis reported in the literature.[205,206]

Streptococcus anginosus is a rare cause of IE (≈6–7 percent of cases) but is unusual among these streptococci in that it has a predilection for suppurative complications including brain, liver, perinephric and other abscesses, cholangitis, peritonitis, and empyema,[207] although evidence for pathogenicity in these infections is circumstantial. Some of these complications occur during IE with this organism and may require surgical attention. Approximately 50 percent of *S. anginosus* strains carry the group F antigen,[208] but most strains are nongroupable, and the nomenclature is confusing,[209] with substantial differences between American and British classification schemes. Although some strains display α- or β-hemolysis, most isolates (≈60 percent) are nonhemolytic. Many previously reported cases of *S. intermedius* or *S. milleri* infections are now considered in the *S. anginosus* group.[209] Infective endocarditis caused by *S. anginosus* may result in "virulent" intracardiac complications (e.g., myocardial abscess, purulent pericarditis) more typical of *S. aureus* infections.[210]

Infective endocarditis due to *Gemella haemolysans* was recognized recently.[211] This organism is now placed in genus V of the family Streptococcaceae. *Gemella* should be suspected if blood cultures reveal a variable morphology (resembling diphtheroids) and an indeterminate Gram stain. The antimicrobial susceptibility of *Gemella* sp. is similar to that of the viridans streptococci.

Staphylococci. Staphylococci cause 20–30 percent of the cases of IE, and 80–90 percent of these are due to coagulase-positive *S. aureus*. *Staphylococcus aureus* is the causative agent in most cases of acute IE, but only a minority of patients with *S. aureus* bacteremia seen currently have IE.[212,213] The organism attacks normal (no clinically detectable cardiac disease) heart valves in approximately one-third of the patients. The course is frequently fulminant with widespread metastatic infection and results in death in approximately 40 percent of the cases.[214–217]

Myocardial abscesses (with conduction disturbances), purulent pericarditis, and valve ring abscesses are more common in staphylococcal endocarditis than in other forms. Peripheral foci of suppuration (lung, brain, spleen, kidney, and so forth) are common and afflict over 40 percent of these patients.[214,217] These extravascular sites of involvement may offer clues for an early diagnosis, especially in addicts.[131,132] This disease is often unsuspected and therefore not clinically recognized in elderly patients, and mortality rates often exceed 50 percent in patients over 50 years of age, especially when nosocomially acquired.[124,218] The rare entity of neonatal endocarditis is also often caused by *S. aureus*[219]; survival is unusual.

Infective endocarditis in narcotic addicts is often due to *S. aureus,* but the disease tends to be less severe, with mortality rates of 2–6 percent.[131,132] The recent emergence of methicillin-resistant strains (MRSA) in addicts with staphylococcal IE in the Detroit area is disturbing.[128,220] Among 180 bactermic addicts admitted to the Detroit Medical Center in 1 year, 24 percent grew MRSA, and 41 percent of the patients overall had IE. Previous hospitalizations, long-term addiction (particularly in males), and nonprescribed antibiotic use were predictive of MRSA acquisition (odds ratio, 8.6:1[220]).

Staphylococcus epidermidis is an important agent in prosthetic valve endocarditis (see Chapter 62) and in infants with umbilical venous catheters in neonatal intensive care units.[221] Although still rare, recent reports[222–224] have emphasized the importance of coagulase-negative staphylococci in native-valve IE, particularly in patients with mitral valve prolapse.[222] Approximately two-thirds of patients have pre-existent valvular disease. Although indolent in onset, complications of IE were frequent; despite this, medical and/or surgical therapy was usually successful. Separation of IE from uncomplicated bacteremias due to *S. epidermidis* (implicated in ≈50 percent of native-valve coagulase-negative staphylococcal endocarditis) may be difficult, but a solid-phase radioimmunoassay for the detection of IgG antibodies is promising.[225] Extensive laboratory evaluation[226] reveals that most *S. epidermidis* endocarditis isolates are distinct and do not represent common-source outbreaks despite the frequent shift to a small-colony variant by many strains in vivo.[227]

Gram-Negative Bacilli. Gram-negative aerobic bacilli have been reported to cause 1.3–4.8 percent of the cases of IE, but in two reports,[228,229] they accounted for over 10 percent of the cases. In the latter reports, approximately two-thirds of the cases coexisted with or followed serious gram-positive infections. In spite of an increasing incidence of gram-negative bacillary septicemia, IE due to these organisms remains uncommon, but the incidence is increasing. Only 1.7 percent of 452 valvular infections reported in the 1960s were caused by gram-negative organisms vs. 7 percent in more recent series.[230] A total of 56 cases of IE due to gram-negative bacteria were seen at the Mayo Clinic from 1958 to 1975, 35 in the last decade alone.[231] Most cases were due to "fastidious" nonenteric organisms (see below); this group caused 10 percent of the IE cases seen at this institution. Narcotic addicts, prosthetic valve recipients, and patients with cirrhosis[232] appear to be at an increased risk for the development of gram-negative bacillary endocarditis. The duration of illness is usually less than 6 weeks, most patients are aged 40–50 years, and the sex distribution is equal.[233] In gram-negative septicemia, the blood stream is usually cleared readily with appropriate antimicrobial agents. In contrast, in gram-negative bacillary endocarditis persistent bacteremia is common even with high levels of antimicrobial activity. Congestive heart failure is common, and the prognosis is poor. Most series report a mortality approaching 75–83 percent,[15,233] but recent experience indicates a better prognosis[231] with a cure rate of 62 percent in 21 patients infected with aerobic enteric bacilli. A heart murmur noted during an episode of gram-negative sepsis with unexplained anemia or the persistence of positive blood cultures despite adequate antibiotics may indicate endocarditis. In the early postoperative period after prosthetic valve replacement, sustained gram-negative bacillary bacteremia does not necessarily imply IE,[234] and other foci of infection (sternal wound, pneumonia, urinary tract, iv catheters, and so forth) should be carefully sought (see Chapter 62).

Among the Enterobacteriaceae, *Salmonella* sp. were most common in early reports. These organisms have an affinity for abnormal cardiac valves, usually on the left side of the heart.[233,235] Although many serotypes have been implicated, most cases are due to *S. chloraesuis, S. typhimurium,* and *S. enteritidis.* Valvular perforation and/or destruction, atrial thrombi, myocarditis, and pericarditis are common, and the outlook is grave. Salmonellae may also produce endarteritis in aneurysms of major vessels (see below).

In a review of 44 cases of Enterobacteriaceae endocarditis due to species other than *Salmonella,*[233] the following organisms were identified: *E. coli,* 17; *Citrobacter* sp., 1; *Klebsiella-Enterobacter* sp., 9; *Serratia marcescens,* 13; *Proteus* sp., 2; and *Providencia* sp., 2. There were 19 additional cases of endocarditis due to *Serratia marcescens* reported from San Francisco[236]; 17 occurred in narcotic addicts. Two-thirds of these patients had previously normal heart valves, and most of the infections occurred on the aortic and mitral valves. The cases are characterized by large vegetations with near-total occlusion of the valve orifice in the absence of significant underlying valvular destruction. The overall mortality ranges from 68 to 73 percent since a cure of left-sided IE due to the Enterobacteriaceae is uncommon with medical therapy alone. Since 1974, 17 more cases of IE due to *S. marcescens* have been observed in the San Francisco area; 15 occurred in intravenous drug abusers. As above, only 3 of 10 patients with left-sided involvement survived despite antimicrobial combination therapy and high serum bactericidal activity. Valve replacement after ≈7–10 days of antibiotics was recommended for these difficult infections.[237] Approximately a dozen cases of IE due to *Campylobacter fetus* have been reported since the first case in 1955.[238]

The first case of *Pseudomonas*-induced endocarditis was recognized in 1899; over 110 cases have subsequently been reported.[128,220,230,239–241] Most (95 percent) of the patients have abused intravenous drugs.[128,239–241] Males predominate by a ratio of 2.5:1, and the mean age is 30 years. The organism affects normal valves in most cases. Major embolic phenomena and rapidly progressive congestive heart failure are common. Ecthyma gangrenosum, the necrotizing cutaneous lesion characteristic of *Pseudomonas* bacteremia, has occasionally been noted, especially in cases of IE due to *Pseudomonas cepacia.*[242] The disease carries the highest mortality in patients over 30 years of age (73 percent mortality vs. 33 percent in younger patients), when the duration of illness is less than 5 days (raises the mortality from 41 percent to 76 percent), and when there is left-sided cardiac involvement.[240,243] Due to the gloomy outlook and frequent complications,[128] early surgery is recommended by many authorities for *Pseudomonas* endocarditis.[241] Nearly all addicts with *P. aeruginosa* endocarditis in recent reports[128,220,241] have abused pentazocine and tripelennamine ("T's and blues").

Unusual Gram-Negative Bacteria. Endocarditis produced by several other gram-negative species has received recent attention. *Neisseria gonorrhoeae* was responsible for 5–10 percent of the cases of IE before the introduction of penicillin but is now rarely implicated. In the older series, one-half of the patients with gonococcal endocarditis had involvement of the right side of the heart and exhibited the characteristic double quotidian fever pattern. Of the 34 cases of gonococcal endocarditis reported since 1949,[244] 23 occurred in men. Skin manifestations consistent with the gonococcal arthritis–dermatitis syndrome or endocarditis are documented in only 20 percent of cases. Most of the cases of gonococcal endocarditis now follow an indolent course, in contrast to the often fulminant progression in the pre-antibiotic era. Nonpathogenic *Neisseria* sp. (*N. perflava, N. flava, N. pharyngis, N. mucosa, N. sicca, N. flavesceus* and especially *Branhamella* [*Neisseria*] *catarrhalis*) are now isolated more frequently in IE than are gonococci, but they usually produce infection on abnormal or prosthetic heart valves.[245,246] *Haemophilus* sp., predominantly *H. paraphrophilus, H. parainfluenzae,* and *H. aphrophilus,* account for 0.8–1.3 percent of all cases of IE.[247–250] This disease usually runs a subacute course and occurs in the setting of pre-existing valvular disease. Emboli to major peripheral arteries were recently found in six of seven cases of *H. parainfluenzae* endocarditis,[247] and major central nervous system complications are relatively frequent.[250] *Haemophilus aphrophilus* produced a similar clinical pattern and has been transmitted from dogs to humans. Single cases of IE due to *H. segnis* and *H. aegyptius* have been reported from Denmark and Israel, respectively.[251,252] A closely related organism, *Actinobaccillus actinomycetemcomitans,* is a rare cause of subacute endocarditis (35 cases reported) with a mortality of 34 percent.[253,254] Infective endocarditis due to *Cardiobacterium hominis*[255] resembles the disease caused by Haemophilus sp.; 26 cases of IE due to this organism were reported by 1983. Only one extravascular infection due to *C. hominis* has been documented (meningitis during IE). At least 28 cases of *Kingella* endocarditis (*K. kingae,* 25; *K. denitrificans,* 2; *K. indologenes,* 1) have been reported.[256] Approximately 50 percent develop complications, including acute stroke in ≈25 percent of cases. A dozen cases of IE due to *Eikenella corrodens* have been reported; intravenous drug use (especially amphetamines) was implicated in five patients.[257] All these organisms (the HACEK group) are fastidious and may require 2–3 weeks for primary isolation. Routine subculturing onto supplemented chocolate agar or incubation in atmospheres of 5–10% CO_2 is necessary for the isolation of these organisms and should be performed in all culture-negative cases of IE. Granular growth in broth is characteristic and should suggest their presence. In addition, the clinical syndrome produced by this group is virtually identical with a subacute course of IE: large friable vegetations, frequent emboli, and the development of congestive heart failure and often eventual valve replacement.[258]

Gram-Positive Bacilli. Infective endocarditis due to various species of corynebacteria (diptheroids) is uncommon and usually occurs on damaged or prosthetic valves,[259] although native-valve infections (e.g., *C. haemolyticum* in an addict) are rarely reported. *Listeria monocytogenes* has been isolated from 44 cases of IE.[260,261] Most cases of IE due to *Listeria* have occurred in patients without any underlying defect in host defenses, although pre-existent heart disease is present in ≈50 percent. The mean age was 51 years and the overall mortality 48 percent.[261] Lactobacilli have also been reported to cause a subacute form of IE and are rare, with only 24 cases reported.[262] Despite an initial response to therapy, relapse of this infection is not unusual (≈40 percent of cases). These organisms also may take several weeks for isolation on blood culture. Over 90 percent of 49 serious infections caused by *Erysipelothrix rhusiopathiae* were characterized as endocarditis.[263] Occupational or vocational animal or fish exposure is a major risk factor, and approximately one-third of patients are alcoholics. Most patients are male, a characteristic erysipeloid skin lesion is present in ≈40 percent of cases, and the organism exhibits significant aortic valve tropsim (involved in 70 percent of patients).[263] The overall mortality was 38 percent. Nearly all cases of *Bacillus* endocarditis involve the tricuspid valve in addicts. *Rothia dentocariosa* is a rare cause of IE (five reported cases) but has led to significant central nervous system complications.[264]

Anaerobic Bacteria. Nonstreptococcal anaerobic bacteria were responsible for 1.3 percent of all the cases of IE in 1970.[265] *Bacteroides fragilis* was the predominant pathogen in a review of 67 cases from the literature.[266] The following organisms were isolated: *B. fragilis,* 35.8 percent; *B. oralis,* 3.0 percent; *B. melaninogenicus,* 3.0 percent; *Fusobacterium necrophorum,* 13.4 percent; *Fusobacterium nucleatum,* 9.0 percent; *Clostridium* sp., 13.4 percent; *Propionibacterium acnes,* 7.5 percent; *Dialister granuliformans,* 1.5 percent; and unidentified, 16.4 percent. Over one-third of the unidentified cases were also thought by the authors to represent *B. fragilis*. Approximately 25 percent of these cases were polymicrobial, usually mixed with anaerobic or microaerophilic streptococci. The portal of entry for *B. fragilis* was most likely the gastrointestinal tract, while *B. oralis, B. melaninogenicus,* or fusobacteria originated from the mouth or upper resiratory tract. Two-thirds of the patients were over 40 years of age and had pre-existing heart disease. The course is usually subacute except for *F. necrophorum,* which characteristically produces a more fulminant disease. These organisms usually cause extensive valve destruction, congestive heart failure, and major systemic emboli (in 60–70 percent of the cases). Thromboembolic episodes are especially common in cases caused by *B. fragilis,* a phenomena that may be related to the heparinase produced by this organism. The mortality in cases of anaerobic endocarditis has ranged from 21 to 46 percent,[266] but one series from California noted no deaths in seven patients with anaerobic or microaerophilic endocarditis,[267] which constituted 10.6 percent of the IE cases seen. This is similar to a 7.7 percent incidence reported by others[3] and suggests that anaerobic endocarditis may be more prevalent now than it was in 1970.[268] Isolation of these organisms may be improved by the newer culture techniques currently in use.

Other Bacteria. Many other genera of bacteria have been described in cases of IE; however, consideration of these organisms separately is beyond the scope of this review. These include *Acinetobacter, Alcaligenes, Bordetella, Flavobacterium, Micrococcus, Moraxella, Paracolon, Streptobacillus, Vibrio,* and *Yersinia*. *Brucella* sp. continue as important etiologic agents in Spain and in Saudi Arabia where these organisms are responsible for ≈10 percent of IE cases.[269] Aggressive medical therapy with valve replacement is usually necessary for a cure of *Brucella* endocarditis.

Etiology of Infective Endocarditis in Addicts. The organisms responsible for IE in narcotic addicts require separate consideration since the distribution differs from other patients with IE. The frequency of the etiologic agents isolated before 1977 in seven major series were as follows[2]: *S. aureus,* 38 percent; *Pseudomonas aeruginosa,* 14.2 percent; *Candida* sp., 13.8 percent; enterococci, 8.2 percent; viridans streptococci, 6.0 percent; *S. epidermidis,* 1.7 percent; gram-negative aerobic bacilli, 1.7–15 percent; other bacteria, 2.2 percent; mixed infections, 1.3 percent; and culture-negative, 12.9 percent. In addition, there appears to be an unexplained geographic variation in the causal agents of narcotic-associated IE. *Staphylococcus aureus* predominated in New York City, Washington, D.C., Chicago, and Cincinnati; *Pseudomonas aeruginosa* was commonly isolated in Detroit, but methicillin-resistant *S. aureus* now predominates.[128,220] The most recent compilation from Detroit[128] indicates the distribution of causative agents in addicts with IE (n = 74) as follows: *S. aureus,* 60.8 percent; streptococci, 16.2 percent; *P. aeruginosa,* 13.5 percent; polymicrobial, 8.1 percent; and *Corynebacterium* JK, 1.4 percent. Although *S. aureus* IE in this population was usually tricuspid, streptococci infected left-sided valves significantly more often than the other pathogens. Biventricular and multiple-valve infections occurred most commonly in *Pseudomonas* endocarditis; all of these addicts abused "T's and blues." There is an increased incidence of enterococcal endocarditis in Cleveland. *Serratia marcescens* was once an important pathogen in San Francisco,[237] but currently *S. aureus* is the most common (≈85 percent) etiologic agent (M. Sande, personal communication). These differences do not correlate with contamination of "street" heroin.[270] The high incidence of staphylococcal endocarditis may be partially explained by an increase in nasal and/or oral carriage of this organism.[271] Heroin usage in the previous week was associated with an *S. aureus* isolation rate of 35 percent from skin, nose, or throat cultures; this declined to 11 percent (not significantly different from controls) if heroin had not been injected in the preceding 2 weeks. This suggests an endogenous source for the infecting organism since *S. aureus* is infrequently (<5 percent) isolated from street heroin or injection paraphernalia. The exact incidence of IE in narcotic addicts is unknown. A conservative estimate is 1.5–2 cases of IE per 1000 addicts at risk per year.[128,272] Moreover, intravenous drug use is the most common risk factor for the development of recurrent native-valve IE; 43 percent of 281 patients surveyed from 1975 to 1986 with this syndrome were addicts.[273]

Fungi. Most of the cases of fungal endocarditis can be grouped into three categories: (*1*) narcotic addicts, (*2*) patients after reconstructive cardiovascular surgery, and (*3*) patients after prolonged intravenous and/or antibiotic therapy. In a review of 24 patients with fungal endocarditis seen at the New York University Medical Center from 1968 to 1973,[159] 11 were heroin addicts, 9 had undergone cardiac surgery, and 5 had other serious illnesses requiring antibiotics or hyperalimentation. Underlying heart disease and a tendency for major systemic embolization were noted in two-thirds of these patients. *Candida parapsilosis* and *C. tropicalis* predominated in the addicts, whereas *C. albicans* and *Aspergillus* sp. caused most cases in nonaddicts. In 23 addicts reviewed, *C. parapsilosis* was responsible in 12 patients (52 percent), and other *Candida* sp. (*C. guillermondii, C. stellatoidea, C. krusei, C. tropicalis*) caused most of the remaining cases. *Candida albicans* was isolated in only 1 of the 23 addicts. In contrast, in 82 patients who developed fungal endocarditis after cardiac surgery, the reported distribution of causative organisms was different. *Candida albicans* and *Aspergillus* sp. each accounted for approximately one-third of the isolates. *Candida parapsilosis* was found in fewer than 10 percent. Fungal endocarditis was documented in 29 patients after prolonged intravenous therapy, and in 17 it developed during the treatment of bacterial endocarditis. One-half of this group of patients was infected with *C. albicans*. The overall cure rate in cases of fungal endocarditis is poor (14.5 percent in cases treated since 1968). The poor prognosis may be due to (*1*) the large bulky vegetations, (*2*) the tendency for fungal invasion of the myocardium, (*3*) widespread systemic septic emboli, (*4*) the poor penetration of antifungal agents into the vegetation,[274] (*5*) the low toxic/therapeutic ratio of the available antifungal agents, and (*6*) the usual lack of fungicidal activity with these compounds. A cure is virtually impossible without surgical intervention (see below). Fatal endocarditis due to *Candida* sp. has also followed Swan-Ganz catheterization.

In a review of 25 cases of *Aspergillus*-induced endocarditis in which cultures were made,[275] the organisms isolated were as follows: *A. fumigatus*, 14; *A. flavus*, 4; *A. niger*, 3; and *A. ustus, A. sydowi, A. terreus*, and *A. glaucus*, 1 each. Only 5 of 34 patients in this series had positive blood cultures, and only 1 patient survived. A few cases, usually fatal, of *Aspergillus* endocarditis after coronary artery bypass surgery have been described. *Aspergillus clavatus* was isolated in one case. Other fungi that have caused IE include *Histoplasma, Blastomyces, Coccidioides, Cryptococcus, Hansenula, Hormodendrum, Mucor, Paecilomyces, Phialophora*, and *Oerskovia*. Fungal endocarditis was unknown before 1945, and the incidence is increasing; currently 1.2–2.6 percent of all cases of IE are due to fungi. Endocarditis has also been caused by higher bacteria such as *Actinomyces, Arachnida, Nocardia*, and *Mycobacterium* species.

Other Microorganisms. Five cases of IE due to *Spirillum minor*, a spirochete, have been reported.[276] This organism is widely distributed in nature, especially in fresh or salt water with organic debris. *Spirillum minor* is the etiologic agent of "rat-bite fever" (sodoku), but rodent transmission was not documented in the cases of endocarditis. Pre-existent heart disease or severe underlying disease (e.g., aplastic anemia) is usually present, although one case occurred in an otherwise healthy person.

Infective endocarditis due to *Coxiella burnetii* (the cause of Q fever) is well documented in the United Kingdom and Australia with over 200 recognized cases and was recently reported in the United States.[277] Ten cases of Q fever endocarditis were recognized in four Dublin teaching hospitals in only 3 years.[278] Q fever is usually a self-limited respiratory illness due to the inhalation of infected aerosols, especially from animal products. The first endocarditis cases were reported in 1959. Males outnumber females by a ratio of 6:1, and 90 percent have preexisting heart disease. Most cases of IE are chronic with a history of an influenza-like illness occurring 6–12 months previously. Risk factors may include exposure to parturient cats or rabbits. The aortic valve is involved in over 80 percent of the cases. Hematuria is uncommon even though it is frequently observed in acute Q fever. Hepatosplenomegaly and hepatitis, common features in other types of Q fever, are usual in IE caused by this organism. Other important clues are thrombocytopenia (90 percent) and hypergammaglobulinemia. Immune complex-mediated glomerulonephritis develops in ≈25 percent of cases.[278] The rickettsiae were demonstrated histologically in the valve tissue in 62 percent of the cases, and the organism was isolated in 83 percent. The diagnosis is best made serologically; a positive antibody titer by complement fixation to the phase I antigen is indicative of chronic infection, whereas a fourfold rise in titer to the phase II antigen is associated with active current infection. A phase I antibody titer greater than 1:200 is considered virtually diagnostic of Q fever endocarditis. Isolation of *Coxiella burnetii* by inoculation of valve suspensions into a human fetal diploid fibroblast cell line appears to be a promising technique.[279] The prognosis with medical therapy alone is poor, and valve replacement is often necessary for a cure (see below). This agent may also cause endarteritis. A single case of IE due to the causative agent of murine typhus has been reported.[156]

Chlamydia psittaci, the agent of psittacosis, has been implicated in at least 10 well-documented cases of IE.[280] This organism may also cause myocarditis or pericarditis. Most of the cases have been associated with psittacine bird exposure; in one case, chlamydiae were found in the liver of the suspected budgerigar. However, transmission from pet cats has also been proposed. The course is subacute, and the diagnosis is often made retrospectively. Most patients had pre-existing heart disease. A diagnosis can be established with the demonstration of complement-fixing antibodies. Cure usually requires valve replacement and prolonged antibiotic therapy. The mortality in this small group was 40 percent. Two well-documented cases of IE due to *C. trachomatis* have been reported.[281] Microimmunofluorescence tests are necessary for a diagnosis. A single case of IE due to *Mycoplasma pneumoniae* was proposed in a case report, but cultural confirmation was lacking.[282]

The role of viruses in IE is unknown. Experimentally, Coxsackie B virus has been shown to produce valvular and mural endocarditis in mice and cynomologus monkeys.[283] In these studies the viral antigen was demonstrated in the valvular tissue by immunofluorescent techniques. Although the enteroviruses are commonly implicated in cases of myocarditis or pericarditis in humans, there is no proof that viral infections produce IE in the human. Adenoviruses are also capable of producing IE in mice.[284] Persand has described a case of "cytomegalovirus endocarditis," but bacteria were also cultured from a mural lesion.

"Culture-Negative" Endocarditis. As discussed earlier, sterile blood cultures have been noted in 2.5–31 percent of the cases of IE.[153,158,285,286] This may be due to several factors: (*1*) subacute right-sided endocarditis; (*2*) cultures taken toward the end of a chronic course (longer than 3 months); (*3*) if uremia supervenes in a chronic course, a higher percentage of cases may be culture-negative; (*4*) mural endocarditis as in ventricular septal defects, post-myocardial infarction thrombi, or pacemaker wires; (*5*) slow growth of fastidious organisms such as anaerobes, *Haemophilus* sp., *Actinobacillus* sp., *Cardiobacterium* sp., nutritionally variant streptococci, or *Brucella* sp; (*6*) the prior administration of antibiotics[285,286]; (*7*) fungal endocarditis; (*8*) endocarditis caused by obligate intracellular parasites such as rickettsiae, chlamydiae, and perhaps viruses; or (*9*) noninfective endocarditis or an incorrect diagnosis. Attention to the proper collection of blood cultures, serologic tests, and newer diagnostic techniques may reduce the proportion of "culture-negative" cases.

THERAPY FOR INFECTIVE ENDOCARDITIS

The response to antimicrobial therapy for IE is unique among bacterial infections. Although the organisms may be exquisitely sensitive to the antibiotics used, complete eradication takes weeks to achieve, and relapse of disease is not unusual. There are a few possible explanations for these phenomena: (*1*) the infection exists in an area of impaired host resistance and is tightly encased in a fibrin meshwork where the bacterial colonies are free to divide without interference from phagocytic cells, and (*2*) the number of bacteria in these vegetations reaches tremendous population densities (10^9–10^{10} cfu/g). At these high populations, the organisms may exist in a state of reduced metabolic activity and cell division as was suggested by Durack and Beeson in studies of L-alanine incorporation into bacterial cell walls.[84] A similar finding is observed in broth in vitro after 18 hours of incubation. In both situations the bacteria are less susceptible to the bactericidal action of penicillin or other drugs that require cell wall synthesis and division for maximum activity. The relative importance of antimicrobial penetration into vegetations and the response to therapy is unresolved. Although multiple studies have examined antibiotic concentrations in human cardiac valve tissue obtained during surgery,[287] usually in close agreement with concurrent serum concentrations, the relevance of these data to therapy for IE is unknown and has not altered current recommendations. Information on antimicrobial concentration in vegetations, either in experimental models or in humans with IE, is sparse. Agents that are selectively localized in vegetations (vs. normal endocardium), such as porphyrins,[288] may be useful in the diagnosis and/or drug delivery to the site of infection as carriers for other compounds. Studies in animals have confirmed that when vegetation formation is inhibited with anticoagulants the organisms are eradicated more rapidly with penicillin treatment than in control animals with larger vegetations.[88] Furthermore, enzymatic modification of the glycocalyx in the vegetations of experimental streptococcal endocarditis by in vivo dextranase administration facilitates the bactericidal activity of penicillin by more rapid sterilization of the lesion.[289] In contrast, tissue-type plasminogen activator produced a concentration-dependent lysis of fibrin clots or vegetations infected with *S. epidermidis* or *S. sanguis* but did not enhance antimicrobial activity in in vitro models.[290,291]

Certain general principles have been accepted that provide the framework for the current recommendations for treatment of endocarditis. Parenteral antibiotics are recommended over oral drugs because of the importance of sustained antibacterial activity. Erratic absorption makes oral drugs less desirable. Short-term therapy has been associated with relapse of disease, and all current recommendations emphasize extended drug administration. Early studies by the British Medical Research Council[292] first emphasized the necessity for prolonged treatment. Bacteriostatic antibiotics are generally ineffective in the treatment of bacterial endocarditis. Their use has been associated with frequent relapses and/or a failure to control the infection. A symptomatic response to such agents as tetracycline, erythromycin, or in some cases, clindamycin should not be accepted as indicative of successful treatment since once treatment with these agents is discontinued relapse is common. Likewise, antibiotic combinations should produce a rapid bactericidal effect. This is seen with synergistic combinations such as penicillin plus an aminoglycoside against most viridans streptococci or enterococci. In experimental animals it has been shown that the rate of bactericidal action expressed by a drug or combination of drugs in broth is predictive of the relative rate that the organisms will be eradicated from the cardiac vegetations in vivo. Antagonistic combinations such as penicillin plus chloramphenicol, which are less rapidly bactericidal, are less effective in experimental endocarditis than is the single bactericidal drug (penicillin) alone.[293]

Patients with IE may have an associated myocarditis complicated by cardiac arrhythmias and congestive heart failure and require close observation in an intensive care environment with electrocardiographic monitoring. As discussed below, the selection of antibiotics should be based on antimicrobial susceptibility tests and the treatment monitored with periodic determinations of serum bactericidal activity and/or antimicrobial blood levels when indicated. Blood cultures should be obtained during the early phase of therapy to ensure eradication of the bacteremia. The use of anticoagulants during therapy for endocarditis has been associated with fatal subarachnoid hemorrhage and other bleeding complications. Most authorities agree that anticoagulant administration is this setting is contraindicated, but this area remains controversial.

All patients with IE should be managed in facilities with rapid access to cardiothoracic surgery. Although persistent or recurrent fever despite appropriate antimicrobial therapy may be due to pulmonary or systemic emboli or drug hypersensitivity, the most common cause is extensive valve ring or adjacent structure infection.[294] These patients and many others with IE require surgery, often emergently. Close monitoring and early surgical consultation is therefore essential.

Tests Useful for Antimicrobial Treatment Monitoring

Management of IE demands careful considerations of the choice, dose, and duration of antimicrobial therapy. The following laboratory tests can help the physician to monitor treatment and can aid in rational therapeutic decisions. In every case of bacterial endocarditis, the etiologic agent must be isolated in pure culture, and the minimum inhibitory concentration (MIC) and the minimum bactericidal concentration (MBC) must be determined for the usual antibiotics used (see below). Standard disk sensitivity testing is unreliable, and results may be misleading without the quantitative information provided by determining the MICs and MBCs. During therapy the serum can be monitored for bactericidal activity against the offending organism as originally described by Schlicter and Macllean.[295] The performance of this test varies greatly, and consequently there are disagreements in interpretation. The inoculum size, composition of the broth, timing of samples ("peak" vs. "trough"), methods of dilution and subculture, and criteria for determination of the bactericidal end point are among the important variables. Perhaps because of these problems and the frequent adverse events unrelated to bactericidal effects, the serum bactericidal titer (SBT) often correlates poorly with the clinical outcome in patients with IE. There is still intense disagreement regarding the value of this test in monitoring therapy for IE. A retrospective review[296] of 17 reports published between 1948 and 1980 failed to confirm any correlation between and SBT $\geq$1:8 and therapeutic success.[297] Controversy regarding the usefulness of "peak" vs. "trough" SBTs abounds.[298] When all of these variables are standardized,[299,300] the SBT test may be useful in selected patients with IE. A recent prospective multicenter study[301] evaluated a standardized SBT method in 129 patients with bacterial endocarditis. Peak and trough SBT ratios of ≥1:64 and 1:32 predicted bacteriologic cure in all patients, but specific levels could *not* be used to accurately predict bacteriologic failure or clinical outcome. Although there are problems with this study,[297] recent data[302] support a role for the SBT when standarized and performed in the presence of 50% human serum: all patients with peak SBTs ≥1:32 were cured, whereas 7 of 21 (33 percent) with SBTs ≤1:16 failed treatment.[302] Unless precluded by drug toxicity, it seems reasonable to attempt to achieve this level (1:8–1:16) of activity in patients, although this goal may be unattainable in some forms (e.g., gram-negative bacillary, enterococcal) of IE. Performance of the SBT test is usually unnecessary in patients with viridans streptococcal endocarditis but may be useful when (*1*) the organism is inherently resistant or tolerant to one of the drugs administered or (*2*) the response to therapy is suboptimal.

In some forms of IE, combinations of antibiotics are used routinely.[303] These regimens are based on synergy studies performed in vitro and results obtained in experimental animal models of IE. In difficult cases with a slow therapeutic response or in those due to unusual organisms, a determination of synergistic combinations of antibiotics may be helpful. In these cases, tests for bactericidal synergism may be undertaken by standard techniques such as broth dilution, microtiter "checkerboards," or "time–kill" curves in broth. Proper attention to standardized techniques, especially inoculum size, are critically important for a meaningful interpretation of the results.

When aminoglycosides are used in therapy, the concentration of antibiotic in the serum should be periodically determined. These agents have a low toxic–therapeutic ratio, especially in elderly patients or in those with renal disease. Peak and trough concentrations should be measured, and the dose should be altered accordingly. This method is superior to reliance solely on nomograms for dosage changes. When synergy with another agent is demonstrable, serum concentrations of the aminoglycosides lower than those generally considered "therapeutic" may be adequate, thus lessening the potential for toxicity. Levels can be determined by microbiologic assays using agar well diffusion (±15 percent accuracy), radioimmunoassay, or enzyme assay with equally satisfactory results.

Antimicrobial Therapy

"Penicillin-Sensitive" Streptococcal Endocarditis. Most strains of viridans streptococci, "other" streptococci (including *S. pyogenes*), and nonenterococcal group D streptococci (primarily *S. bovis*) are exquisitely sensitive to penicillins with an MIC of <0.2 μg/ml. However, 15–20 percent of viridans streptococci are "resistant" to this arbitrary concentration of penicillin.[180,196] In addition,[183] approximately 15 percent of the strains of *S. mutans* demonstrate a low MIC to penicillin (<0.1 μg/ml), but the MBC is considerably higher (1.25–50 μg/ml). These organisms should probably be considered "penicillin-tolerant" and should be treated accordingly. Although dependent on the in vitro methodology employed, recent studies suggest that tolerance to penicillin among viridans streptococci is more prevalent than previous reports suggested.[304] For example, 19 percent of viridans streptococci cultured from gingiva and blood after dental procedures were tolerant,[305] especially among *S. mutans* (27 percent) and *S. mitior* (20 percent) isolates. Almost identical figures were reported among blood culture isolates of viridans streptococci,[306] with tolerance defined as a penicillin MBC-to-MIC ratio exceeding 10:1. Nearly all strains of nutrionally dependent streptococci are tolerant to penicillin.[307,308] The influence of the tolerance phenomenon on the response to penicillin therapy in experimental endocarditis is not known; two recent studies yielded conflicting results.[309,310] Data on human infections with tolerant strains and the therapeutic results are unavailable. Except for nutritionally variant streptococci, we do not believe that the demonstration of tolerance by an isolate of viridans streptococci influences therapeutic decisions.

By broth dilution susceptibility tests, the usual MBC for these so-called penicillin-sensitive streptococci is as follows: penicillin, 0.1–1.0 μg/ml; cephalothin, 0.15–1.25 μg/ml; vancomycin, 0.15–0.4 μg/ml; streptomycin, 6.25–50 μg/ml; and gentamicin, 1.56–3.12 μg/ml.[311,312] *Streptococcus bovis* is 10–5000 times more susceptible to penicillin than are the other group D species (enterococci). They are also relatively susceptible to oxacillin, methicillin, and lincomycin, while the enterococci are resistant.[185] Virtually all streptococci in this group demonstrate synergism in vitro between penicillin or vancomycin and streptomycin, gentamicin, or kanamycin[313,314] (see below). The first strains of viridans streptococci with high-level streptomycin resistance (MIC ≥1000 μg/ml) were reported in 1982 from Paris. Although these strains are rare (2–8 percent of isolates in some locales[315]) the documentation of aminoglycoside-modifying enzymes and the lack of penicillin–streptomycin synergy in vitro and in experimental animal models[315,316] is alarming. These penicillin-susceptible strains are killed synergistically by penicillin–gentamicin combinations. Significant antibiotic antagonism has been shown with the combination of clindamycin and gentamicin for *S. mutans*. The in vitro synergism between penicillin and aminoglycosides has been found to correlate with a more rapid rate of eradication of bacteria from cardiac vegetations in vivo in the rabbit endocarditis model[315,317,318] for the common viridans streptococci. All of these studies have been summarized in recent reviews.[179,198,319–321]

The combination of penicillin and streptomycin has been used in over 200 cases at the New York Hospital–Cornell Medical Center since 1959 without a documented relapse.[313] This clinical experience has been confirmed elsewhere,[2] but the overall reported relapse rate is 1.4 percent.[320] This regimen is as follows: aqueous penicillin G, 10–20 million units iv qd, or procaine penicillin G, 1.2 million units im q6h for 4 weeks, combined with streptomycin, 0.5 g im q12h for the first 2 weeks. Studies by Wilson and colleagues at the Mayo Clinic[322,323] demonstrated that a 2-week course of intramuscular procaine penicillin (1.2 million units q6h) and streptomycin (0.5 g q12h) cured ≥99 percent of patients with penicillin-sensitive streptococcal endocarditis. These results are similar to those obtained with therapy consisting of β-lactams alone for a total of 4 weeks[324,325] but significantly better than penicillin alone for 2 weeks; the latter regimen was associated with a 50 percent relapse rate when low doses of penicillin were used and improved to 17 percent with higher penicillin dosages. The 2-week penicillin–streptomycin regimen is the most cost-effective and is the preferred therapy in uncomplicated penicillin-sensitive (MIC ≤0.1 μg/ml) streptococcal endocarditis in young patients. Four weeks of penicillin alone is recommended in patients with impaired renal function or those particularly susceptible to the low risk of streptomycin-induced ototoxicity (the elderly). The "Cornell regimen" of 4 weeks of penicillin plus an initial 2 weeks of streptomycin is recommended in patients with a complicated course, a history of disease exceeding 3 months' duration, or prosthetic valve endocarditis due to these sensitive strains or when susceptibility testing reveals the rare penicillin-resistant streptococci.[326] The preferred regimen for IE due to penicillin-"tolerant" streptococci is unsettled. These concepts have been recently summarized[320,321] and serve as a basis for the recommendations of the American Heart Association on therapy for penicillin-sensitive streptococcal endocarditis.[327] We believe that gentamicin, at a dosage of 1.0 mg/kg (not to exceed 80 mg) im or iv q8h, can be substituted for streptomycin in the aforementioned regimens when combination therapy is deemed advisable. A penicillin–gentamicin regimen is indicated for viridans streptococcal endocarditis if high-level streptomycin resistance is present[315,316] or for strains with a penicillin MIC ≥0.2 and <0.5 μg/ml.[327] Strains with a penicillin MIC >0.5 μg/ml should be treated as for enterococcal endocarditis (see below). Due to the enhanced rate of bacterial killing in animal models[328,329] and the high relapse rates of ≈17 percent,[330] we also believe the "Cornell regimen" should be employed for all patients with IE due to nutritionally variant streptococci. Other regimens for the treatment of this disease (e.g., vancomycin plus rifampin) deserve further study.[330] In the penicillin-allergic patient when a cephalosporin is deemed safe, several regimens are acceptable: cephalothin, 2 g iv q4h, or cefazolin, 1–2 g im or iv q8h for 4 weeks, combined with streptomycin, 0.5 g im q12h, or gentamicin, 1 mg/kg (≤80 mg) im or iv q8h for the initial 2 weeks. Although ceftriazone at a dosage of 2 g daily for 4 weeks has been successfully employed in 49 cases of streptococcal endocarditis (M.P. Glauser, personal communication) and the prolonged half-life of this agent may facilitate outpatient therapy, the first-generation agents are preferred pending further data. When treatment with β-lactams are contraindicated, the regimen of choice is vancomycin, 1 g iv q12h (or 500 mg iv q6h) for 4 weeks; experience with teicoplanin or daptomycin is too preliminary.

"Penicillin-Resistant" Streptococcal Endocarditis (e.g., MIC for penicillin ≥0.5 μg/ml).[327] Infective endocarditis due to the enterococcus is the third most common form of the disease and is the most resistant to therapy. The mortality still approximates 20 percent,[189] and relapses are not uncommon. By broth dilution susceptibility tests, the MIC determinations for most enterococci are as follows: penicillin, 0.4–12.5 μg/ml; ampicillin, <0.4–3.1 μg/ml; cephalothin, 12.5–25 μg/ml; vanomycin, 0.78–3.1 μg/ml; streptomycin, 3.1–>50 μg/ml; and gentamicin, 6.25–25 μg/ml. Ampicillin is approximately twice as active as penicillin by weight. In contrast, the usual MBCs are as follows: penicillin, >6.25 μg/ml (80 percent are >100 μg/ml); cephalothin, >100 μg/ml; streptomycin, >25 μg/ml; vancomycin, >100 μg/ml; and gentamicin, ≤25 μg/ml.[331] *Enteroccus faecium* strains are more resistant to β-lactams than *E. faecalis* strains.[332] Thus, in general these agents are bacteriostatic against the enterococci and should not be administered alone in this disease. This bacteriostatic action of agents known to inhibit cell wall synthesis is due to a defective bacterial autolytic enzyme system.[333,334] As stated before, all β-lactams, including imipenem, are bacteriostatic against enterococci in vitro. However, a new mechanism of penicillin-resistance among *E. faecalis* was described in 1983: plasmid-mediated β-lactamase production. At least two strains have been isolated,[335] both demonstrating, in addition, high-level resistance to all aminoglycosides (see below). β-Lactamase production by *E. faecium* has not been demonstrated to date. Patients with IE due to these strains should receive vancomycin plus an aminoglycoside, although animal experiments with penicillin–β-lactamase inhibitor combinations appear promising.[336]

Cell wall–active antibiotics plus an aminoglycoside are synergistic and produce a bactericidal effect in vitro against most enterococcal strains. Successful treatment of enterococcal endocarditis requires such combinations. Studies in experimental models[337] suggest that "low-dose" streptomycin (peak serum concentrations of 9.1 μg/ml) in combination with penicillin is sufficient to treat streptomycin-susceptible enterococcal endocarditis. "High-level" streptomycin resistance (MIC >2000 μg/ml) is demonstrable in 40 percent of the enterococcal strains. This resistance correlates with an inability to demonstrate in vitro synergism between penicillin and streptomycin.[190,338] These highly resistant strains demonstrate synergism between a penicillin and gentamicin in vitro[339,340] at clinically achievable serum concentrations. Enhanced activity with the penicillin and gentamicin combination was seen in vivo for both streptomycin-resistant and streptomycin-sensitive enterococci in the rabbit model of IE.[341] No differences in results were seen when penicillin was combined with low- vs. high-dose gentamicin (peak serum levels of 3.06 and 8.05 μg/ml, respectively) in the treatment of experimental streptomycin-resistant enterococcal endocarditis.[342] Early reports[343,344] revealed high-level gentamicin resistance among enterococci in up to 14 percent of isolates. This phenomenon has become prevalent in some areas[345,346] among *E. faecalis* strains. Although the strains infrequently cause IE, resistance to multiple aminoglycosides is common. High-level gentamicin (and other aminoglycoside) resistance has been recently documented for clinical isolates of *E. faecium* as well.[347] This resistance mechanism is plasmid mediated through the production of aminoglycoside-modifying enzymes and can be transferred among strains. In addition, penicillin– or vancomycin–aminoglycoside synergy is not apparent against these organisms in vitro. The optimal therapy for IE due to these highly resistant strains has not been established. None of the currently recommended regimens in current use is bactericidal against these isolates, and valve replacement[348] may be necessary for a cure. When these isolates are encountered, all available aminoglycosides must be tested separately because the organism may be susceptible to one while resistent to others. Some isolates are sensitive to quinolones or daptomycin, but these agents have received scant attention in human infections. At this time, we favor long-term therapy (8–12 weeks) with high dosages of penicillin (20–40 million units iv daily in divided doses) or ampicillin (2–3 g iv q4h) for IE due to these multiply aminoglycoside-resistant enterococci, pending further data.

Vancomycin is also bacteriostatic against enterococci and exhibits synergy with the aminoglycosides in vitro. The vancomycin–streptomycin combination synergistically kills 40–80 percent of enterococcal strains, whereas the vancomycin–gentamicin combination demonstrates synergy against 93–98 percent.[349] Vancomycin therapy alone was ineffective in eradicating enterococci from cardiac vegetations in the rabbit model of endocarditis, but the combination of vancomycin plus gentamicin rapidly achieved a bactericidal effect.[341] Vancomycin combined with rifampin has an indifferent effect against enterococci (43/48 strains) in vitro; antagonism is observed rarely.[350] Of some concern, outbreaks of infection due to vancomycin-resistant enterococci have been described recently.[351] The resistance is plasmid mediated (at least for two well-studied strains of *E. faecium*[352]) for glycopeptide antibiotics (e.g., vancomycin and teicoplanin but not LY146032), but the biochemical mechanism is unknown. Enterococci are no longer uniformly susceptible to glycopeptide antibiotics, but the impact of this development on therapy for IE is unclear presently. The cephalosporins are relatively inactive against enterococci, even in combination with an aminoglycoside, and should not be used in this disease. The quinolones (i.e., ciprofloxacin) and daptomycin (LY146032) do not appear promising for the treatment of enterococcal endocarditis.[353,354]

Although controlled trials are lacking, clinical experience would dictate that enterococcal endocarditis be treated with combination antimicrobial therapy for at least 4–6 weeks.[320,321,327] The recommended regimen is as follows: aqueous penicillin G, 20 million units iv qd combined with streptomycin, 0.5 g im q12h, or gentamicin, 1 mg/kg im or iv q8h, for 4–6 weeks. If toxicity (vestibular, aural, or renal) occurs, the streptomycin dose is divided into a q6h regimen. If the streptomycin MIC determined for the infecting strain is ≥2000 μg/ml, gentamicin should be substituted for streptomycin, although relapses or therapeutic failures are unusual with penicillin plus streptomycin. Some authorities recommend penicillin plus gentamicin as the initial therapy. If the peak serum bactericidal level is <1:8, the penicillin dose may be increased, or the aminoglycoside drug may be changed in accordance with in vitro tests. Wilson et al. have recently analyzed the experience at the Mayo Clinic of 56 patients treated for 4 weeks with aqueous penicillin G (20 million units iv qd) combined with either streptomycin, 0.5 g im q12h, for enterococcal IE due to streptomycin-sensitive strains or with gentamicin (1 mg/kg im q8h) for IE due to streptomycin-resistant strains.[355] Relaps rates were high (12.5 percent) for both regimens; however, all patients who relapsed had had symptoms suggestive of IE for longer than 3 months. Relapses also only occurred in patients with mitral valve involvement. All patients who received over 3 mg/kg qd of gentamicin developed reversible nephrotoxicity (defined as a twofold increase in serum creatinine concentration) and 19 percent of patients receiving streptomycin for 4 weeks developed irreversible vestibular toxicity. Although this was not a prospective randomized trial, we believe that selected patients with enterococcal endocarditis may be treated with 4 weeks of combination therapy. The exceptions include mitral valve involvement, symptomatic illness exceeding 3 months, enterococcal prosthetic valve endocarditis (PVE), and patients with a relapse(s) of enterococcal endocarditis.

The penicillin-allergic patient presents the clinician with a difficult therapeutic dilemma. Vancomycin as a single drug at 1 g iv q12h has been used in the treatment of enterococcal endocarditis. However, experience is limited, and because of its lack of bactericidal activity in vitro and poor performance in experimental endocarditis, vancomycin should be combined with streptomycin or gentamicin. Unfortunately, this combination is potentially more nephrotoxic, and clinical proof of the superiority of this regimen over vancomycin alone is not available. The other therapeutic option in the allergic patient is "penicillin desensitization" followed by the administration of penicillin and an aminoglycoside.

Staphylococcal Endocarditis. The mortality in acute staphylococcal endocarditis still approximates 40 percent, and the preferred antibiotic regimen is controversial. Mortality is highest for men, patients over 50 years of age, and patients with left-sided involvement and/or central nervous system manifestations. In addition, narcotic addicts appear to have a lower mortality than do nonaddicts. Most *S. aureus* isolates, whether community or hospital acquired, are now resistant to penicillin G (MIC >0.2 μg/ml). The current recommended regimen includes a penicillinase-resistant penicillin (nafcillin or oxacillin, 1.5–2 g iv q4h) or a cephalosporin (cephalothin, 2 g iv q4h, or cefazolin, 2 g im q8h) given for 4–6 weeks.[214,215,356] The addition of gentamicin produces a synergistic effect against *S. aureus* in vitro and in experimental staphylococcal endocarditis in rabbits.[357] However, the combination did not improve the survival rate (60 percent) over that observed with a penicillin derivative alone in a small group of patients.[217] Combination therapy did not improve the results of therapy for staphylococcal IE in addicts,[358] but the mortality rate is low in this subgroup of patients (≃2–8 percent) with this disease. Combination therapy may permit a shorter duration of therapy in addicts with *S. aureus* endocarditis. Two weeks of nafcillin plus tobramycin (1 mg/kg iv q8h) cured 47 of 50 (94 percent) intravenous drug abusers with right-sided endocarditis[359] without evidence of renal failure, extrapulmonary metastatic infectious complications, aortic or mitral involvement, meningitis, or infection by MRSA. In addition, anecdotal case reports in nonaddicts with staphylococcal endocarditis suggest a beneficial response by the addition of gentamicin in patients failing to respond to nafcillin therapy.[360] This issue was addressed in a multicenter prospective trial comparing nafcillin alone with nafcillin plus gentamicin (for the initial 2 weeks) in the treatment of endocarditis due to *S. aureus*.[361] Although the combination resulted in a more rapid rate of eradication of the bacteremia, the incidence of nephrotoxicity was increased, and no improvement in mortality was achieved. Despite these results, many authorities still use combination therapy for short periods (e.g., 3–5 days), especially in fulminant cases. If the organism is susceptible to penicillin (MIC, <0.1 μg/ml), then this agent in a dose of 20 million units iv qd should be used. The response to treatment may be slow, often with fever and positive blood cultures lasting up to 1 week.[214] In penicillin-allergic patients or if the staphylococcus is "methicillin-resistant," vancomycin, 1 g iv q12h for 6 weeks, is recommended.[327,356,362] Clindamycin has been used to treat over 60 cases of staphylococcal endocarditis but is associated with an unacceptable relapse rate, and its use is not recommended.[363] The optimal therapy for IE due to "tolerant" strains of *S. aureus* is controversial.[364,365] One retrospective study[366] suggested that patients with IE due to these tolerant strains had a more complicated course; however, combination therapy did not appear to be of benefit. Another controversial area is the adjunctive role of rifampin, the most active antibiotic currently available against *S. aureus* in vitro, in therapy for IE. Due to the emergence of resistant strains, this drug is ineffective alone. Unfortunately, in vitro studies on rifampin combinations with either β-lactam agents or vancomycin are frequently contradictory, and the results in experimental IE induced by *S. aureus* are dependent on which drug in the combination exerts the greatest bactericidal activity in vivo.[367] At present, rifampin should be reserved for patients demonstrating poor serum bactericidal activity during therapy with a β-lactam or vancomycin, or in those with suppurative complications (e.g., valve-ring abscesses). Several new agents including teicoplanin, fosfomycin, and quinolones (e.g., ciprofloxacin, enoxacin, difloxacin, etc.) are active against MRSA in vitro and are as rapidly bactericidal as vancomycin in experimental animal models of IE due to MRSA,[368] although resistance to the quinolones has emerged during therapy. Experience with these drugs in humans with *S. aureus* endocarditis is scant.

Some authors[369] have felt that when *S. aureus* bacteremia occurs in a patient with a removable focus of infection the risk of concurrent endocarditis is low, and treatment schedules may be shortened to 2–3 weeks, thus avoiding the high costs, risks of suprainfection, and/or antibiotic reactions associated with prolonged therapy. In another study, 8 of 21 patients with an infected intravenous catheter as the suspected source of *S. aureus* bacteremia developed endocarditis.[370] We concur with the findings of Bayer et al.[371] who identified four parameters predictive of the presence of IE in 72 patients with *S. aureus* bacteremia in a prospective study: (*1*) the absence of a primary site of infection; (*2*) community acquisition of infection; (*3*) metastatic sequelae; and (*4*) valvular vegetations detected by echocardiography. Therefore, short-term therapy should be used only if endocarditis can be reasonably excluded by methods previously discussed.

Staphylococcus epidermidis is the most common etiologic agent in cases of prosthetic valve endocarditis. Most of these strains (87 percent) are methicillin resistant when isolated within 1 year of valve implantation. Recent studies[372] suggest that the optimal antimicrobial therapy of these infections is vancomycin plus rifampin, perhaps with the addition of an aminoglycoside as well. The recent emergence of vancomycin resistance among coagulase-negative staphylococci[373] is cause for concern. These concepts are discussed further in Chapter 62.

Endocarditis Due to Enterobacteriaceae or Pseudomonas Species. Of 125 cases of IE reported from Seattle, 4.8 percent were due to gram-negative aerobic bacilli.[15] These patients had a mortality of 83 percent, and none treated without surgery survived. The prognosis is especially poor with left-sided cardiac involvement. Determination of tube dilution MBCs are necessary to guide therapy. Certain combinations of penicillins or cephalosporins and aminoglycosides have been shown to be synergistic against many of these strains and are usually recommended. For IE due to most strains of *E. coli* or *Proteus mirabilis* a combination of a penicillin, either ampicillin (2 g iv q4h) or penicillin (20 million units iv qd) with an aminoglycoside, usually gentamicin (1.7 mg/kg q8h), is suggested. Third-generation cephalosporins are extremely active against *E. coli* in vitro, and some (e.g., ceftriaxone) have proved effective in experimental animal models of *E. coli* endocarditis,[374] even when long dosing intervals were used. This group of agents deserves further evaluation in humans for IE due to susceptible gram-negative bacilli. A combination of a third generation cephalosporin and an aminoglycoside (either gentamicin or amikacin) is recommended for *Klebsiella* endocarditis. Left-sided IE due to *S. marcescens* is refractory to medical therapy alone; valve replacement is invariably required to effect a cure.[237]

Pseudomonas aeruginosa remains an important pathogen in addicts with IE. Medical therapy may be successful in *P. aeruginosa* endocarditis involving the right side of the heart. If the disease is refractory to antibiotics, tricuspid valvulectomy or "vegetectomy"[375] without valve replacement is indicated.[240,376] Although valve replacement is often necessary for a cure of left-sided IE due to *P. aeruginosa*,[240,377] recent experience[128] with 10 patients (7 with left-sided involvement alone or in combination with tricuspid disease) suggests that medical therapy alone is occasionally curative. Studies in animals with experimental *Pseudomonas* endocarditis[378] offer an explanation for these disparate results: the penetration into vegetations and the time antibiotic concentrations exceeded the MBC were both significantly greater in tricuspid than in aortic vegetations for both ceftazidime and tobramycin.

The optimal antimicrobial regimen for *P. aeruginosa* endocarditis is evolving; the most extensive experience has been at the Detroit Medical Center. Problems have emerged with all potential regimens in animal models of this disease, as extensively studied by Bayer, Levison, and colleagues: (*1*) therapy with β-lactams (e.g., ceftazidime) has failed due to the constitutive hyperproduction of type Id β-lactamase[379]; (*2*) aminoglycoside-resistant isolates due to permeability defects emerge during therapy[380] and (*3*) no postantibiotic effect of β-lactams against *P. aeruginosa* is evident in vivo,[381] thus necessitating frequent (or continuous) drug administration. Treatment failures of *Pseudomonas* endocarditis in humans have been due to the selection of isolates with an enhanced production of type Id β-lactamase.[382] Based on clinical experience,[128,220,239,240] however, the preferred regimen for IE due to *P. aeruginosa* is high-dose tobramycin (8 mg/kg/day iv or im in divided doses q8h) with maintenance of peak and trough concentrations of 15–20 and ≤2 μg/ml, respectively, in combination with an extended-spectrum penicillin (e.g., ticarcillin, piperacillin, azlocillin) or ceftazidime in full doses. The toxicity associated with this regimen is surprisingly low; treatment should be combined for a minimum of 6 weeks. The quinolones are promising for the treatment of *Pseudomonas* endocarditis on the basis of favorable results in animal models[379] and in humans,[383] but the development of stepwise resistance during therapy may limit the efficacy of this class of drugs in the future.

Infective endocarditis due to *Haemophilus* sp. is usually responsive to ampicillin alone[231] administered for 3 weeks. However, therapy for IE due to these (and other) fastidious gram-negative organisms must be individualized on the basis of in vitro susceptibility data; in practice, β-lactam–aminoglycoside combinations are usually employed for approximately 1 month. The role of the newer third-generation cephalosporins in the treatment of IE due to gram-negative bacilli is unknown despite excellent in vitro activity and the potential for the avoidance of aminoglycoside-induced toxicity. It is important to emphasize that the above recommendations offer a rough guide for initial treatment. However, it is imperative that each isolate be subjected to sensitivity testing in vitro to ensure the optimal selection of antibiotics.

Endocarditis Due to Anaerobic Bacilli. Although IE caused by anaerobic bacilli is uncommon, the mortality is high. *Bacteroides fragilis* is isolated in many of these cases and is responsible for most fatalities. Most strains of anaerobic bacilli, with the exception of *B. fragilis,* are sensitive to penicillin in vitro, and this agent, in a dose of 20 million units iv qd, is the recommended therapy.[266,267] In addition, 33 percent of the strains of *B. fragilis* demonstrate an MIC of penicillin that is less than 25 μg/ml, and increasing resistance to penicillin among multiple anaerobic genera is evident. However, penicillin is only bacteriostatic against these strains (MBC invariably greater than 100 μg/ml), and relapse of the disease is common. Although clindamycin, carbenicillin, and chloramphenicol readily inhibit most strains of *B. fragilis,* they lack bactericidal activity, and they are poor therapeutic choices even though several patients have been cured with either high-dose penicillin, chloramphenicol (1 g iv q6h), clindamycin (600 mg iv q6h), or carbenicillin (5 g iv q3h). Due to excellent bactericidal activity in vitro and the serum concentrations attained, metronidazole, ticarcillin plus clavulanic acid, or imipenem are reasonable choices for therapy for anaerobic endocarditis.[268]

Pneumococcal, Gonococcal, and Meningococcal Endocarditis. Infective endocarditis caused by these organisms is now very rare. Pneumococcal endocarditis must be considered in any patient with pneumococcal bacteremia, especially if meningitis is present. Most common in alcoholics, the organism generally attacks the aortic valve and results in valvular insufficiency, often with perivalvular abscess formation and/or pericarditis. Type 12 pneumococci cause over 20 percent of the cases of pneumococcal endocarditis but are a rare (5 percent of the cases) cause of pneumococcal pneumonia. Penicillin, 20 million units iv qd for 4 weeks, is recommended for the treatment of pneumococcal endocarditis.

The gonococci that cause systemic infection are usually susceptible to penicillin.[384] These organisms as well as the meningococci can be effectively treated with the same penicillin regimen recommended for pneumococcal endocarditis. Although endocarditis due to penicillin-resistant gonococci (PPNG or chromosomally mediated) has not been reported, ceftriaxone has been used successfully to treat gonococcal endocarditis.[385]

Fungal Endocarditis. The incidence of IE caused by fungi has undergone a striking increase in the past decade. Fungal endocarditis occurs principally in a setting of narcotic addiction, after cardiac surgery, after the prolonged intravenous administration of drugs (especially "broad-spectrum" antibiotics), and in the compromised host. The overall survival rate in patients treated since 1968 is only 14.5 percent.[159] The preferred mode of therapy is unknown. The use of antifungal agents alone has been almost universally unsuccessful in achieving a cure of this disease. The addition of surgical measures to antifungal therapy may result in an improvement in prognosis, but to date there is insufficient clinical experience. When fungal endocarditis is diagnosed, a combined medical/surgical approach should be undertaken.

The mainstay of antifungal drug therapy is amphotericin B. This agent is toxic and produces multiple side effects including fever, chills, phlebitis, headache, anorexia, anemia, hypokalemia, renal tubular acidosis, nephrotoxicity, nausea, and vomiting. Drug toxicity is frequent and commonly necessitates alterations in the regimen. Dosages and the technique of administration are given in Chapter 33.

After 1–2 weeks of amphotericin B therapy at "full" dosages, surgery should probably be performed. If isolated tricuspid endocarditis is present, as in a narcotic addict, total tricuspid valvulectomy can usually be performed. Rarely, removal of the vegetation alone is curative. Most of these patients tolerate the valvulectomy without the development of significant right-sided heart failure. Valve replacement is necessary for left-sided fungal endocarditis. The duration of antifungal therapy after surgery is empirical, but 6–8 weeks is usually recommended.

It is possible that combination antifungal therapy may improve the poor survival from fungal endocarditis. Some strains of *Candida* sp. and *Cryptococcus neoformans* are inhibited in vitro by concentrations of 5-fluorocytosine achieved with the oral administration of 150 mg/kg/day in six divided doses. Synergism between 5-fluorocytosine and amphotericin B has been documented for these yeasts in vitro and in the treatment of cryptococcal meningitis. This combination was fungicidal and perhaps instrumental in the cure of one case of *Aspergillus* endocarditis. However, in the rabbit model of endocarditis due to *Candida albicans,*[162] the addition of 5-fluorocytosine did not improve the rate of eradication of fungal organisms from the vegetation when compared with amphotericin B alone. Potentiation of amphotericin B activity by rifampin has been noted for virtually all strains tested of *Candida* sp. and for a few isolates of *Histoplasma capsulatum*. The therapeutic advantage of the addition of 5-fluorocytosine or rifampin to amphotericin for fungal endocarditis requires further investigation, but initial results in animal models of disseminated candidiasis are not encouraging.[386] The role of triazoles and imidazoles in the treatment of fungal endocarditis has received scant attention. On the basis of animal model data,[387] high-dose intraconazole may be of value in the treatment of *Aspergillus* endocarditis, but valve replacement will likely remain imperative for a cure.

Q Fever Endocarditis. More than 200 well-documented cases of this form of IE have been reported, and the mortality exceeds 65 percent.[277–279] The only antibiotics effective in acute Q fever, chloramphenicol and the tetracyclines, are rickettsiostatic. In addition, chloramphenicol cannot be administered for the prolonged periods of time necessary in this disease. The mortality with tetracycline therapy alone is at least 70 percent, and the recovery of *Coxiella burnetii* from valve tissue after 4 years of tetracycline therapy[277] both argue against medical therapy alone. Thus, most authorities agree that valve replacement is probably required for cure. Based on in vitro data and anecdotal experience,[279,388,389] the following approach is suggested: doxycycline (100 mg po q12h) or tetracycline (500 mg po q6h) plus trimethoprim-sulfamethoxazole (approximately 480 mg trimethoprim plus 2400 mg sulfisoxazole daily in four divided doses) in combination with valve replacement. The duration of therapy is empirical but should usually exceed 1 year; treatment can be stopped when there is no clinical evidence of infection and phase I antibody titers are <1:128 by complement fixation.[279] Rifampin plus cotrimoxazole is not recommended for Q fever endocarditis. A careful follow-up for recrudescence of infection is essential.

Infective Endocarditis Due to Chlamydiae. Albeit based on limited experience, a combination of valve replacement and prolonged (greater than 3 months) tetracycline therapy seems justified in these cases. Rifampin has cured at least one case of chlamydial IE after therapy with tetracyclines had failed, but exposure to this agent rapidly induces the emergence of rifampin resistance of *C. trachomatis* in tissue culture.[390] The role of combination regimens (e.g., rifampin plus erythromycin or tetracycline) deserves further study.

Culture-Negative Endocarditis. The therapy for this entity is controversial, but the regimen usually used will "cover" the enterococcus and fastidious gram-negative bacilli and consists of a combination of penicillin, 20 million units iv qd in divided doses, or ampicillin, 2 g iv q4h, plus streptomycin, 0.5 g im q12h, or gentamicin, 1.7 mg/kg im or iv q8h. When staphylococcal endocarditis is a strong consideration (narcotic addicts or after cardiac surgery), a penicillinase-resistant penicillin or a cephalosporin in full dosage should be added to this regimen. If clinical improvement occurs, some authorities recommend discontinuation of treatment with the aminoglycoside after 2 weeks. The other agent(s) should be continued for a full 6 weeks of treatment. Continued surveillance for an etiologic agent and careful follow-up are mandatory. An analysis of any correlation between the response to empirical antimicrobial therapy and survival was performed in 52 patients with culture-negative endocarditis[286]: 92 percent of the patients who became afebrile within the first week of therapy survived vs. only 50 percent if fever persisted longer than 7 days. Most deaths were caused by major systemic emboli or uncontrollable congestive heart failure due to valvular insufficiency.

Surgical Therapy

In recent years, valve replacement has become an important adjunct to medical therapy in the management of IE and is now used in ≥25 percent of the cases. The generally accepted indications for surgical intervention during active IE are as follows: (*1*) refractory congestive heart failure; (*2*) more than one serious systemic embolic episode; (*3*) uncontrolled infection; (*4*) valve dysfunction as demonstrated by fluoroscopy; (*5*) ineffective antimicrobial therapy (e.g., fungal endocarditis); (*6*) resection of mycotic aneurysms; (*7*) most cases of prosthetic valve endocarditis; and (*8*) local suppurative complications including perivalvular or myocardial abscesses with conduction system abnormalities, heart block, etc. The major indications in the past have been persistent infection and congestive heart failure.[391–393] For example, congestive heart failure during active IE was the indication for surgery in 86 percent of 108 patients undergoing valve replacement at Stanford from 1963 to 1984.[393]

The most frequent causes of death in IE, in approximate order, are congestive heart failure, embolic phenomena, rupture of a mycotic aneurysm, complications of cardiac surgery, lack of response to antimicrobial therapy, and prosthetic valve endocarditis.[2–15] Failure to make a diagnosis or renal failure are rare causes of death. In a recent review from Seattle,[15] congestive heart failure was present in 91 percent of the patients who died. Overall, two-thirds of the patients in this series of 125 cases developed congestive heart failure, and this complication appears to be increasing in frequency. The overall mortality in this group of patients was 37 percent.

When acute aortic regurgitation complicated by congestive heart failure supervenes in IE, the mortality still exceeds 50 percent. The classic physical findings of chronic aortic regurgitation are often absent in these patients.[176] The current trend is to advise early surgery in this group of patients since nothing is gained by delay. In a series of 28 patients from Birmingham, Alabama, with acute aortic regurgitation, 4 had no congestive heart failure and were treated medically, and all survived. In contrast, 7 of 11 patients with mild congestive heart failure and 7 of 8 with moderate to severe congestive heart failure died during medical therapy, often suddenly and with pathologic evidence of coronary emboli and myocardial infarction. Four of five patients with moderately severe congestive heart failure who underwent surgery survived. This suggests that early surgical intervention may improve the survival statistics in this setting. Similar results were obtained at the Mayo Clinic (3/11 deaths). The hemodynamic status of the patient, not the activity of the infection, is the critical determining factor in the timing of cardiac valve replacement.[394] The hemodynamic severity of the acute aortic regurgitation may be assessed by determining the degree of mitral valve preclosure by echocardiography. If premature closure of the mitral valve occurs before the Q wave of the electrocardiogram, then the left ventricular end-diastolic pressure is very high, and surgical intervention is urgently required. Nothing is gained by temporizing, even if only a few hours of antibiotics can be administered. When congestive heart failure persists despite digoxin, diuretics, and other therapeutic modalities, surgery is also indicated. In 80 patients subjected to aortic valve replacement for IE, the surgical cure rate was 72 percent. There were no instances of subsequent infection of the prosthesis, but 16 percent developed paravalvular regurgitation. This latter complication was usually easily controlled medically. Organisms visible on Gram stain, positive cultures or annular abscesses at the time of surgery are associated with late complications.[393] When left-sided IE is present and the clinical assessment implicates more than one valve or extravalvular extension of the disease, then cardiac angiography is useful in delineating the proper surgical approach (see above).

In contrast to left-sided IE where congestive heart failure is the usual indication for surgical intervention, in right-sided IE persistent infection is the indication for surgery in over 70 percent of the patients. Most of the patients are narcotic addicts, with IE caused by organisms that are difficult to eradicate with antimicrobial therapy alone (e.g., fungi, gram-negative aerobic bacilli). Tricuspid valvulectomy is now the procedure of choice for refractory right-sided IE.[395] Subsequent valve replacement, at a second operation, is advised only when medical management fails to control the hemodynamic manifestations and the patient has ceased using illicit drugs. Combination antimicrobial therapy with optimal serum bactericidal activity should be continued for 4–6 weeks postoperatively. These patients may develop mild to moderate right-sided heart failure, but this is easily tolerated, and the success rate of this approach is over 70 percent. Persistent fever, recurrent pulmonary emboli, or vegetations demonstrable by echocardiography usually do not require tricuspid valvulectomy in this setting.[396] In addition, many surgeons contend that a return to the use of illicit drugs and reinfection of the valve after initial cure is a contraindication to reoperation.[397]

Outstanding reviews on the indications for surgery during therapy for IE are available.[392,398] The rationale for surgical intervention, including major and minor criteria for valve replacement, are discussed in detail. A point system weighting multiple factors has been devised by Alsip and colleagues to assist in decision making concerning surgery in patients with active IE.[398] The value of this system remains to be defined. It has become apparent that virtually all patients with prosthetic valve endocarditis (except those with late disease caused by penicillin-sensitive viridans streptococci) require valve replacement for consistent cures (see Chapter 62).

SUPPURATIVE THROMBOPHLEBITIS

Suppurative thrombophlebitis is an inflammation of the vein wall due to the presence of microorganisms and is frequently associated with thrombosis and bacteremia. Suppuration of the vein wall is usually absent in intravenous catheter-related sepsis and bacteremia secondary to contaminated intravenous fluid and will not be discussed here. Suppurative thrombophlebitis may be classified into four forms: superficial, central (including pelvic), cavernous sinus, and infection of the portal vein (pylephlebitis). The last two conditions have become rare since the introduction of antibiotics. In contrast, superficial suppurative thrombophlebitis has been steadily increasing in incidence since the introduction of the plastic intravenous cannula. Superficial suppurative thrombophlebitis secondary to intravenous fluid therapy was first described in 1947[399] when 93 cases were reported, 43 of which were amenable to surgical therapy.

Epidemiology

In 1973, approximately one of every four hospitalized patients received intravenous therapy for a total of over 10 million patients annually in the United States.[400] Suppurative thrombophlebitis accounts for up to 10 percent of all nosocomial infections and is a particular problem in burned patients where it represents a common cause of death due to infection. In several large series of burned patients,[401–404] suppurative thrombophlebitis developed in 4–8 percent and increased in frequency if cutdowns were performed. Suppurative thrombophlebitis is also found in other hospitalized patients (especially those with cancer and/or those receiving steroid therapy).[405,406] Seven such cases were recognized in a recent 18-month period in Charleston, South Carolina,[407] and 35 cases were identified in 7 years in Louisville, Kentucky. Suppurative thrombophlebitis may also be increasing in frequency. Eight cases were encountered during an 8-month period in Johannesburg; suppurative thrombophlebitis was estimated to represent a minimum incidence of 0.12 percent of all admissions.[408] When using strict criteria, 29 episodes of suppurative thrombophlebitis in 27 patients were identified in a large Air Force hospital within 4 years.[409] Based on data from the National Nosocomial Infection Study, Rhame and associates estimate the overall incidence of suppurative thrombophlebitis as 88 per 100,000 discharges, but this disease is underreported.[410] Suppurative thrombophlebitis is also common in abusers of intravenous drugs.[411] This condition is unusual during childhood[412] but may occur as a complication related to intravenous therapy. Catheter-related sepsis without suppurative thrombophlebitis is more common and affects at least 25,000 patients per year in the United States.[413] The risk of this complication is approximately 40 times higher with plastic cannulas (8 percent) than with steel or "scalp vein" cannulas (0.2 percent). Irritation to the vein wall and the subsequent development of suppurative thrombophlebitis is greater with polyethylene catheters when compared with those constructed of Teflon or Silastic materials. Central venous catheterization has been employed for over 30 years for hemodynamic monitoring, total parenteral nutrition (TPN), and infusion of drugs. The exact incidence of suppurative thrombophlebitis of the central veins commonly cannulated (i.e., jugulars, subclavian, venae cavae) is unknown. Catheter-induced thrombosis is relatively common. Autopsy series have revealed central venous thrombosis in 37 percent of catheterized subjects, but this diagnosis is rarely recognized because most patients are asymptomatic. When examined by phlebography at the time of catheter withdrawal, 42 percent of catheters have sleeve thrombi, and another 8 percent revealed veno-occlusive thrombi.[414] In addition, sepsis has been reported in ≈7 percent of patients receiving TPN and other medications by the central route. When thrombosis and bacterial or fungal contamination/sepsis coexist, suppurative thrombophlebitis may intervene. At least 50 cases of suppurative thrombophlebitis of the great thoracic veins have been reported in the literature,[415–417] but this is almost certainly a gross underestimate of the problem. Eight cases in 8 years due to *Candida* sp. alone were observed at the University of Wisconsin.[418] Septic atrial thrombosis, occasionally with a coexistent Budd-Chiari syndrome, has complicated Broviac catheter insertion in infants.[419]

Superficial suppurative thrombophlebitis is a complication of either a dermal infection and/or an indwelling intravenous catheter. Pelvic suppurative thrombophlebitis is associated with parturition, abortion, gynecologic surgery, or a pelvic abscess. Therefore, this is a disease of women of the childbearing age, with most cases occurring between the ages of 15 and 40 years (mean, 20 years). In 123 cases in two reports,[420,421] the predisposing conditions were as follows: vaginal delivery, 39 cases; cesarean section, 19 cases; abortion, 33 cases; and major gynecologic surgery, 32 cases. During a 9-year period in Atlanta, 27 cases of postpartum septic pelvic thrombophlebitis were identified in over 54,000 deliveries.[421] The relative risk for this condition was as follows: parturition, 1/2000 (highest in the inner-city population); septic abortion, 1/200; and major gynecologic surgery, 1/800. The incidence of suppurative thrombophlebitis rises proportionally with the degree of trauma to the pelvic tissues.

Pathogenesis

The pathogenesis of suppurative thrombophlebitis is poorly understood. A thrombus may act as a nidus for local entrapment and colonization of bacteria that gain access to the site from another focus. This is analogous to the proposed role of nonbacterial thrombotic endocarditis in the pathogenesis of IE.

When superficial suppurative thrombophlebitis is associated with intravascular cannulae, the route of infection may be (*1*) migration from the skin between the catheter wall and perivascular tissue, (*2*) from contaminated IV fluid, and (*3*) hematogenous dissemination from an infected focus elsewhere. The relative contribution(s) of these three routes is unknown. The observation that the predominant organism in burn wounds, *Pseudomonas aeruginosa,* is a rare cause of suppurative thrombophlebitis and that suppurative thrombophlebitis usually develops days to weeks after the cutdown incision is healed[402,404] argues against a local cutaneous source in burn patients.

The venous system draining the pelvis includes the intervertebral venous plexus, the lumbar venous plexus, the superficial and deep veins of the abdominal wall, and the hemorrhoidal plexus. Any component of this system may be affected in pelvic suppurative thrombophlebitis, but the veins draining the uterus, including the ovarian veins and the inferior vena cava, are most often involved.[422] Thrombus formation may result from stasis of blood flow due to the gravid uterus and by the hypercoagulable state of parturition. Normal residents of the vaginal or perineal bacterial flora gain access to the thrombus via the blood stream and/or regional lymphatics. There is often an associated endometritis or parametritis. Septic pulmonary emboli and metastatic abscess formation are common.

Pathologic Changes

Regardless of the vein involved, the pathologic changes are similar. The vein is enlarged, tortuous, and thickened. There may be associated perivascular suppuration and/or hemorrhage, and the vein lumen usually contains both pus and thrombus. Microscopically, endothelial damage, fibrinoid necrosis, and thickening of the vein wall are evident. Microabscesses may be present in the vein wall or in the surrounding tissue.[407,423] Gross periphlebitic abscesses are not unusual and may be evident on physical examination. Thrombi frequently extend beyond the area of suppuration. In an autopsy series of peripheral suppurative thrombophlebitis in burned patients, extension of the clot into the great central veins was found in 18 percent of the cases.[402,404] Metastatic abscess formation and septic pulmonary emboli with infarction are found in over 50 percent of the fatal cases. This may result from bacterial liquefaction and fragmentation of affected thrombi within the vein since clot liquefaction is noted commonly in autopsy series.

Clinical Manifestations

Superficial suppurative thrombophlebitis is often difficult to identify since local findings of inflammation may be absent. The disease occurs more frequently when plastic catheters are inserted in the lower extremities, a common practice in burn patients. In 132 cases reported from the burn center at Fort Sam Houston, Texas, the distribution of superficial suppurative thrombophlebitis was as follows: lower extremity (predominantly saphenous system), 100; upper extremity (predominantly antecubital fossa), 32; jugular, 7; and iliac, 4. The mean duration of preceding venous cannulation was 4.81 days, and the latent interval from removal of the catheter to the development of symptoms ranged from 2 to 10 days.[401,403] Fever was present in over 70 percent of the cases, but rigors were rare. Local findings such as warmth, erythema, tenderness, swelling, or lymphangitis were present in only 32 percent of these patients; however, bacteremia with signs of systemic sepsis were found in 84 percent. Septic pulmonary emboli with secondary pneumonia occurred in 44 percent and were often the first diagnostic clue. Thus, pneumonia, sepsis, or metastatic abscess formation was the only manifestation of this disease in two-thirds of the cases. These authors emphasize that the late onset of pneumonia or sepsis in a burned patient demands the careful inspection of all previously cannulated veins since untreated suppurative thrombophlebitis is associated with a high mortality. In these series, fewer than 50 percent of the cases were diagnosed antemortem.[402]

In contrast to the experience with suppurative thrombophlebitis in burn patients, most medical and postoperative patients develop superficial suppurative thrombophlebitis in the upper extremities, and signs of local inflammation are more commonly present (94 percent in one series).[411] Many of these patients are elderly (20/35 over 50 years old) with debilitating diseases and are often receiving antibiotics when superficial suppurative thrombophlebitis intervenes. As above, the duration of intravenous catheterization is an important risk factor; 68 percent of implicated cannulae had been left in place for ≥5 days in patients reported recently.[405,411]

Subperiosteal abscesses of adjacent long bones may complicate superficial suppurative thrombophlebitis in children.[424] The local findings of this condition, including bone tenderness, erythema, warmth, and limitation of motion with occasional extension into the joint space, may overshadow the suppurative thrombophlebitis iself. Septic deep vein thrombosis of the femoral vessels with swollen, tender, and inflamed inguinal areas has been described in intravenous users of heroin and cocaine. Contiguous pelvic bone osteomyelitis is unusual.

Suppurative thrombophlebitis of the thoracic central veins occurs in critically ill patients with central catheters in place, in those receiving TPN, or in patients after long-term cannulation with Broviac, Hickman, and other devices. The systemic findings of sepsis overshadow any local findings of venous occlusion (e.g., superior vena cava syndrome), which are rare in this setting. This syndrome should be suspected in any septic patient when bacteremia and/or fungemia fail to resolve upon removal of the central catheter and institution of appropriate antimicrobial therapy.

Pelvic suppurative thrombophlebitis usually develops 1–2 weeks postpartum or postoperatively and is associated with high fever, chills, anorexia, nausea, vomiting, abdominal pain, and a protracted course.[421] Flank pain may result from ureteral obstruction by enlarged veins. Abdominal tenderness, usually in the right lower quadrant, may be mild to severe. Approximately 80 percent of cases are unilateral on the right side, 14 percent are bilateral, and only 6 percent are unilateral and left sided. This distribution is thought to result from compression of the right ovarian vein at the pelvic brim by the enlarged uterus with retrograde flow on the left and protection from ascending infection. However, the physical examination may be normal. A tender vein can be palpated in 30 percent of the cases on pelvic or abdominal examination.[407] The uterus is usually freely movable. Spread of the process to the femoral vein with edema and tenderness of the lower extremity is unusual. Many of these patients are extremely ill with an acute or chronic course characterized by little or no response to antibiotics and the development of multiple, small, septic pulmonary emboli. Since many of the manifestations are nonspecific, the differential diagnosis is broad and includes acute appendicitis, ureteral obstruction, torsion of an ovarian cyst, pyelonephritis, broad ligament hematoma, parametritis, endometritis, perinephric abscess, pelvic abscess, small bowel volvulus, pelvic inflammatory disease, sickle cell crisis, and ectopic pregnancy.

Laboratory Findings

Bacteremia occurs in 80–90 percent of the cases of superficial suppurative thrombophlebitis. Gross pus within the vein lumen is found in about one-half of the cases, and this finding establishes a diagnosis of suppurative phlebitis. When infection of a venous catheter is suspected, it should be removed and cultured. The results, however, may be misleading since even though bacteria will be isolated in up to 60 percent of the cases a positive culture does not correlate with inflammation.[425] The following semiquantitative culture technique has recently been developed in an attempt to differentiate catheter-related sepsis from suppurative thrombophlebitis. After preparing the skin with alcohol, the catheter is removed with sterile forceps (avoiding skin contact) and is placed in a sterile tube for transport. The catheter is then aseptically cut into 5.7 cm pieces, and each section is rolled across the surface of a 5% sheep blood agar plate. The growth of more than 15 colonies on the plate correlates well[425] with the presence of venous infection. In the few cases of suppurative thrombophlebitis studied by this technique, all catheters have yielded confluent growth. Since the standard 5.7 cm catheter retains approximately 0.7–1.5 mg of moisture on its surface and the plate growth has exceeded 1000 colonies in every case of suppurative thrombophlebitis, bacterial counts must exceed 10^6 organisms/g in the catheter wound. These titers are similar to those found in other types of infected wounds. This technique is simple, rapid, and inexpensive and may prove useful in establishing the need for exploratory venotomy. Simple needle aspiration of the suspected vein may also be diagnostic. ^{111}In-labeled leukocyte imaging studies have detected superficial suppurative thrombophlebitis, but experience is limited.

Other laboratory findings in patients with superficial suppurative thrombophlebitis, for example, leukocytosis, are nonspecific. The chest x-ray film may reveal multiple peripheral densities or a pleural effusion consistent with pulmonary emboli, infarction, abscess, or empyema. The diagnosis of an associated subperiosteal abscess is difficult: bone and gallium scans usually reveal hyperperfusion without definite osteomyelitis, routine x-ray films are virtually always negative, and CT often demonstrates only soft tissue swelling with obliteration of tissue planes. High-resolution CT scans may improve these results.[424] The diagnosis of deep central vein suppurative thrombophlebitis in the thorax is established by venography with the demonstration of thrombi in a patient with positive blood cultures, but CT with contrast enhancement is probably as sensitive and is noninvasive. Experience with magnetic resonance imaging and ^{111}In-labeled leukocytes is meager.

In most cases of pelvic suppurative thrombophlebitis there is a peripheral blood leukocytosis, and the urinalysis is usually normal. The chest x-ray film may reveal multiple septic pulmonary emboli, and abdominal x-ray films may show a pelvic mass. Intravenous pyelography can be useful in disclosing ureteral obstruction. Real-time ultrasonography is very helpful in delineating the location and extent of the thrombus, but the ileus that is often associated with this infection may render interpretation difficult. Computed tomography reveals low attenuation with contrast enhancement in suppurative venous thrombosis and is very sensitive in the diagnosis of pelvic suppurative thrombophlebitis.[426,427] Magnetic resonance imaging may be even more sensitive and can differentiate fresh (≤1 week old) from organizing or subacute thrombosis, but experience is limited.[428] These sensitive and noninvasive techniques may lead to an increased recognition of pelvic suppurative thrombophlebitis, earlier diagnosis, and improved outcome. The role of newer diagnostic techniques such as pelvic venography, transuterine phebography, ^{111}In-labeled leukocyte scanning, and laparoscopy is still undefined. Since bacteremia is demonstrated in only 20–30 percent[420,421,429] of cases of pelvic suppurative thrombophlebitis, negative blood cultures do not exclude the diagnosis.

Etiologic Agents

Staphylococcus aureus was the causative agent of 65–78 percent of the cases of superficial suppurative thrombophlebitis reported before 1968. In recent years, most have been due to the Enterobacteriaceae, especially *Klebsiella-Enterobacter* sp.[405,411] These agents are acquired nosocomially and are often resistant to multiple antibiotics. Nearly all patients with superficial suppurative thrombophlebitis due to gram-negative aerobic bacilli or fungi are receiving broad-spectrum antibiotics at the time the disease becomes manifested. In a review of 86 cases compiled from the literature reported since 1970, the organisms isolated were as follows: *Klebsiella-Enterobacter* sp., 34; *Providencia* sp., 5; *Proteus* sp., 5; *Serratia* sp., 3; *E. coli,* 6; *P. aeruginosa,* 3; *S. aureus,* 15; *C. albicans,* 9; *S. epidermidis,* 4; and enterococci, 2.[405,411] Suppurative thrombophlebitis due to gram-negative pathogens and *E. faecalis* is more common (than *S. aureus*) in patients with significant intra-abdominal pathology.[409] *Staphylococcus aureus,* other gram-positive cocci, and *Candida* sp. were more frequent when this risk factor was absent. Multiple organisms are isolated in up to 14 percent of cases. Anaerobic isolates are extremely rare. An increase in incidence of superficial suppurative thrombophlebitis due to *Candida* sp. was reported recently[430,431]; all patients were receiving antibiotics without hyperalimentation. None were neutropenic or receiving corticosteroids. In one series of seven patients observed in a 15-month interval,[431] all had concomitant or preceding bacterial infections and had received a median of five antibiotics for at least 2 weeks. Preceding candidal colonization at other sites (e.g., sputum, urine) was often present. Although not documented by culture, histopathologic evidence suggests that cytomegalovirus may cause suppurative thrombophlebitis in patients with the acquired immunodeficiency syndrome (AIDS) despite therapy with ganciclovir.[432]

The responsible agents in pelvic suppurative thrombophlebitis are poorly defined since blood cultures are often negative and most investigators did not use adequate anaerobic techniques. The organisms isolated in approximate order of frequency are *Bacteroides* sp., microaerophilic or anaerobic streptococci, *E. coli* and other coliforms, and β-hemolytic streptococci. The predominance of *Bacteroides* sp. may be related to the heparinase produced by this organism. A prolonged latent period (up to 3 weeks) may occur before blood cultures become positive. The more extensive use of anaerobic isolation techniques and the routine culturing of surgical specimens may serve to clarify the role of anaerobic bacteria in this entity.

Presumptive Therapy

Superficial suppurative thrombophlebitis is a lethal iatrogenic disease, and surgery is usually necessary for cure. The first reported successful cure of suppurative thrombophlebitis followed surgical ligation of the vein by John Hunter in 1784.[433] All investigators strongly endorse surgical excision as an integral part of the management. In a review of 24 patients,[402] 14 were treated medically alone, and all died either directly from suppurative thrombophlebitis with persistent bacteremia or secondary to metastatic complications. However, of 10 patients who underwent surgical exploration, 7 survived, and only 1 of the 3 deaths was attributable to suppurative thrombophlebitis. Antibiotics should also be used in the treatment of this disease; initial treatment with a semisynthetic penicillin (e.g., nafcillin, 2 g iv q4–6h) plus an aminoglycoside (e.g., gentamicin, 1.0–1.7 mg/kg iv or im q8h) is recommended since the Enterobacteriaceae and/or staphylococci are the usual etiologic agents. The duration of therapy is unknown and largely empirical. The role of antifungal therapy for superficial suppurative thrombophlebitis due to *Candida albicans* is controversial.[430,431] Although most of these infections can be cured by vein excision, a short course of amphotericin B (approximately 200 mg) is advised postoperatively, pending further data. Antifungal therapy is mandatory in the immunosuppressed patient or if signs of metastatic complications (e.g., endophthalmitis) develop.

When superficial suppurative thrombophlebitis is considered, an exploratory venotomy is necessary. This procedure should be performed proximal to the suspected site; the vein should be ligated and then "milked" in an attempt to express purulent material for inspection by Gram stain and culture. If no pus is apparent, an exploratory venotomy is necessary to establish the diagnosis. Simple ligation was thought to be sufficient 30 years ago, but the rate of relapse with ongoing sepsis was high. Therefore, the segment of vein and all its involved tributaries should be totally excised. Radical surgery from the ankle to the groin may be required in some burn patients. Nevertheless, local or regional anesthesia alone is often sufficient (approximately 90 percent of cases) for vein excision. Backbleeding, indicative of a patent lumen, should be evident at the point of vein transection. Vein excision is usually followed by prompt (≤24 hours) defervescence. If systemic symptoms, bacteremia, and/or marked local findings persist after vein excision, reexploration is necessary with careful attention to total removal of all involved veins and drainage of contiguous (e.g., periphlebitic, subperiosteal) abscesses. It should be stressed, however, that the role of less radical surgery in therapy for superficial suppurative thrombophlebitis has not been addressed adequately. Although the literature supports vein excision, this experience stems largely from burn centers. Despite infection with gram-negative bacilli or *Candia* sp., six of eight children with superficial suppurative thrombophlebitis were cured by local incision and drainage of the involved site plus parenteral antimicrobials.[408] Radical surgery with extensive excision can perhaps be reserved for patients failing these measures. Delayed closure is preferred over primary wound closure. If osteomyelitis is documented in the adjacent long bones, antimicrobial therapy should be continued for a least 6 weeks. Resection of the involved vasculature in most patients with suppurative thrombophlebitis of the great central veins is technically impossible. Fortunately, medical therapy is usually sufficient.[415–418,434] The recommmended approach is catheter removal, full-dose anticoagulation with heparin,[418,434] and parenteral antibiotics. The duration of therapy is unsettled; 2–3 weeks after catheter removal is suggested. The antibiotics employed are the same as for superficial suppurative thrombophlebitis. Experience with more potent agents (e.g., third-generation cephalosporins) for suppurative thrombophlebitis due to gram-negative bacilli is scant, but trials are indicated. Because heparin may precipitate vancomycin with a partial loss of antibacterial activity at concentrations present in intravenous lines,[435] these drugs should not be administered simultaneously by the same intravenous access when MRSA, *S. epidermidis, E. faecalis,* etc., are suspected or grown. Unlike *Candida* IE, suppurative thrombophlebitis of the great central veins due to *Candida* sp. is curable medically, but antifungal regimens must be continued longer than those usually adequate for superficial suppurative thrombophlebitis. Based on limited data,[418] amphotericin B at a daily dose of 0.7 mg/kg to a total dosage ≥22 mg/kg plus 5-fluorocytosine (100–150 mg/kg/day in four divided doses, if tolerable) is recommended after catheter removal. Surgery may, however, be essential in patients with suppurative thrombophlebitis of the thoracic or neck veins when perivascular collections are present.[418]

The optimal therapy for pelvic suppurative thrombophlebitis is still controversial. Because anaerobic streptococci and *Bacteroides* sp. predominante, the initial antibiotics of choice are aqueous penicillin G, 20 million units iv qd, plus either clindamycin, 450–600 mg iv q6h, metronidazole, 500–750 mg iv q8h, or chloramphenicol, 1 g iv q6h. The use of heparin is debated. The addition of heparin after several days of unsuccessful treatment with antibiotics may itself produce an antipyretic effect.[429] In one series of 46 patients with pelvic suppurative thrombophlebitis[421] including 7 with massive ovarian vein involvement and 15 with septic pulmonary emboli, 42 patients become afebrile within 7 days (mean, 2.5 days) while receiving penicillin, chloramphenicol, and heparin. Four patients required exploratory laparotomy, and pelvic abscesses were found in three. These results argue strongly that medical therapy alone is often effective, but no controlled studies on the use of heparin have been done. When medical therapy is unsatisfactory, surgery with drainage of abscesses and usually ligation of the implicated venous system must be performed. Some authorities[422] feel that inferior vena cava and/or ovarian vein ligation should be performed in all these cases, but the evidence for this approach is inconclusive.

Prevention

The incidence of superficial suppurative thrombophlebitis can be reduced by the same preventive procedures that are used for intravenous cannulae in general. These include the use of "scalp vein" cannulae whenever possible, the avoidance of lower extremity cannulations, insertion under aseptic conditions, secure anchoring of the cannula, and frequent replacement (at least every 48–72 hours) of intravenous fluid bottles, cannulae, and connecting tubing. Although neomycin-polymixin B-bacitracin ointment is effective in reducing the incidence of cutdown infections,[436] this modality has not demonstrated consistent benefit with intravenous cannulae.[437] When clinical signs of bacteremia occur in a patient receiving intravenous fluids, the following steps should be taken: (*1*) blood cultures should be obtained, (*2*) intravenous administration should be discontinued and all cannulae removed, (*3*) the intravenous fluid itself should be cultured, (*4*) the cannula should be cultured semiquantitatively on blood agar as described by Maki et al.,[425] and (*5*) appropriate antibiotic therapy should be initiated. If clinical signs of sepsis and bactermia persist despite appropriate antibiotic therapy, then an intravascular focus (including suppurative thrombophlebitis at a previously cannulated vein) should be sought as discussed above.

INFECTIVE ENDARTERITIS AND "MYCOTIC ANEURYSMS"

The term "mycotic aneurysm" was coined by Osler in the Gulstonian lectures of 1885, to describe a mushroom-shaped aneurysm that developed in a patient with subacute bacterial endocarditis. At that time mycotic was used to refer to all microorganisms. Presently, the use of myocotic has been restricted specifically to fungal infections, but the term mycotic aneurysm is still used for all extra- (or intra-) cardiac aneurysms of infectious etiology except for syphilitic aortitis. Unfortunately, this term has also been used to describe pre-existing aneurysms secondarily infected from contiguous or distant foci or pseudoaneurysms arising from trauma or iatrogenic causes. "Endarteritis" refers to inflammation of the arterial wall, which may occur with or without coexistent aneurysmal dilatation. Unless an aneurysm or coarctation of the aorta is present, infective endarteritis is usually a postmortem diagnosis. Since infected aneurysms differ in their pathogenesis, the various classifications, given in Table 5, will be examined separately.[438] Infections of arterial prosthetic devices are dealt with in detail in Chapter 62 and are not considered here.

Epidemiology

Although incidence figures are unavailable, a localized suppurative process of the arterial wall is rare. Estimates derived

TABLE 5. Classification of "Mycotic Aneurysms"

Pre-existent Arterial Status	*Source of Infection*
Normal	Intravascular
Atherosclerotic	Embolism
Aneurysm	Bacteremia with "seeding"
Arterial prosthesis	Extension from adjacent endocardial focus or erosion
	Extravascular
	Contiguous site of infection
	Iatrogenic

from autopsy series of aortic aneurysms are available but ignore infections at other locations in the arterial tree. In a review of over 22,000 autopsies performed at the Boston City Hospital from 1902 to 1951,[439] aortic aneurysms were found in 1.5 percent. However, mycotic aneurysms constituted only 2.6 percent of these lesions. In another review of 178 aneurysms found among more than 20,000 autopsies at the Mayo Clinic from 1925 to 1954,[440] only 6 were felt to be of infectious origin. In the preantibiotic era, infected aneurysms were predominantly confined to patients with IE; in a series of 217 cases reported in 1923,[441] 86 percent were associated with IE. With the advent of antibiotics, mycotic aneurysms in IE have become less prevalent, and hematogenous seeding of a previously damaged arteriosclerotic vessel constitutes the most common mechanism. There is also evidence to suggest that this entity is increasing in frequency. In reviewing four large series,[115,442–444] 78 lesions of this type were discovered from 1946 to 1975. Only eight of these were reported before 1957. Because most of these lesions arise in areas of severe atherosclerosis, males predominate by a ratio of 3:1, and the average age has been 65 years. The mean age for mycotic aneurysms that occur with IE is younger (approximately 40 years), and the sex distribution is nearly equal. Estimates of the incidence of mycotic aneurysms in patients with IE range up to 15 percent.[115,445] Approximately 3–4 percent of IE patients develop intracranial mycotic aneurysms.[446] These lesions remain a significant cause of morbidity and mortality due to intracerebral and subarachnoid hemorrhage, especially in young people in developing countries where acute rheumatic fever, rheumatic heart disease, and resultant IE are still prevalent.[447] Nine intracranial mycotic aneurysms associated with IE were treated in one neurosurgical unit in South Africa in a recent 18-month period, with five deaths.[447]

Pathogenesis

Four different mechanisms have been postulated to produce infection of the arterial wall: (*1*) embolomycotic aneurysms secondary to septic microemboli to the vasa vasorum, (*2*) extension from a contiguous infected focus, (*3*) hematogenous seeding of the intima during bacteremia originating from a distant infection, and (*4*) trauma to the arterial wall with direct contamination.[448] Embolomycotic aneurysms usually occur in patients with active IE, and the incidence of this type has declined in the antibiotic era. The source of infection is the cardiac vegetation with production of arterial emboli that lodge in the vasa vasorum, often at points of bifurcation of the affected artery. Contiguous foci of infection such as a caseous tuberculous lymph node or pyogenic vertebral osteomyelitis may extend directly to major vessels with subsequent aneurysm formation. The normal arterial intima is very resistant to infection. However, when this lining is altered by congenital malformations (e.g., coarctation of the aorta) or acquired disease (especially atherosclerotic plagues and/or ulcers), resistance to infection is lowered, and the surface may become colonized by blood-borne organisms. This hypothesis is analogous to the central role of nonbacterial thrombotic endocarditis in the pathogenesis of IE. An intraluminal thrombus associated with an atherosclerotic vessel may also serve as a nidus for colonization. Atherosclerosis accounts for over 74 percent of secondarily infected aneurysms. Luetic arteritis and cystic medical necrosis have also been associated with secondary infection.[442] Trauma to the arterial wall with subsequent infection has been associated with narcotic addicts due to needle trauma[449] as well as with gunshot wounds, vascular surgery, cardiac catheterization, and even puncture of a femoral artery for analysis of arterial blood gases.[438] These events, if associated with contamination, usually lead to pseudoaneurysm formation in a peripheral artery and a contiguous abscess in extravasated blood.

Pathologic Changes

Infection of the arterial tree has been recognized by pathologists for more than a century. Virchow first demonstrated local dilatation of the arterial wall at the site of a septic embolus in 1847. Infection superimposed on an atherosclerotic aorta was first reported by Koch in 1851. Stengel and Wolfroth[441] collected 217 cases of mycotic aneurysms in 1923. Since these lesions are probably underreported, pathologic material has been scant in recent years.

Most mycotic aneurysms that develop during the course of IE are situated in the sinus of Valsalva or in the supravalvular proximal thoracic aorta (>70 percent develop proximal to the aortic arch). Aneurysms are more frequent in the right and/or posterior sinus and may be complicated by acquired shunts (rupture into the right ventricle is most common site), tamponade, coronary artery occlusion, or an atrioventricular conduction block.[450] Less commonly major visceral, intracranial, and peripheral arteries are involved. Fewer than 10 percent are found in the upper extremities, but these arteries are usually not examined adequately by pathologic or radiologic techniques. Multiple lesions are identified in many IE patients with mycotic aneurysms.[451] Saccular forms appear to be more common than fusiform ones are.[440] The aneurysms vary in size from 1 mm to more than 10 cm. As mentioned before, many of these aneurysms arise from emboli to the vasa vasorum, and occasionally the embolus can be demonstrated grossly and microscopically. Acute and chronic inflammation is found diffusely through the arterial wall; necrosis, hemorrhage, abscess formation, and bacterial colonies may all be present in the sections. The elastica and muscularis layers are usually obliterated, but the intima is often intact. Rupture with surrounding hemorrhage and infection may be present.

Secondary infection of a pre-existing aneurysm is most commonly found in the abdominal aorta (70 percent of the cases) since this is the area most frequently and severely damaged by atherosclerosis. Ascending and descending aortic aneurysms each account for about 15 percent of the cases. The primary bacteremia most commonly originates from distal infections in soft tissue, lung, bone, or joint. The arterial infection usually begins in the distal abdominal aorta or iliac arteries as a focus of inflammation on an ulcerated atheromatous plaque. The wall of the aneurysm is thinned, and there is focal acute and chronic inflammation that may lead to arterial rupture. Even "bland" aortic aneurysms commonly have some mild inflammation (predominantly lymphocytes and mononuclear cells) in the wall; however, infected atherosclerotic aneurysms are characterized by acute polymorphonuclear inflammation, necrosis, abscess formation, hemorrhage, and visible bacterial colonies. This lesion is probably underreported since the focal suppuration may be limited in extent and overlooked unless routine culture and histologic sections are examined on every aortic aneurysm specimen. Erosion and rupture may be present without aneurysmal dilatation. Lumbar or thoracic osteomyelitis is present in up to one-third of the cases[442] and may either precede the aneurysm or develop secondary to contiguous spread from the vascular infection.

When contamination accompanies arterial injury, an infected pseudoaneurysm may result. These lesions are located in the extremities in over 80 percent of the cases and are characterized by more extensive local tissue inflammation than are the two types mentioned previously. Infection as a cause of pseudoaneurysm formation is increasing; 17 of 57 (30 percent) such lesions seen in the past decade[452] were infected.

Of special interest are mycotic aneurysms in renal transplant patients. In 640 renal transplants performed at the University of Minnesota over a period of 8 years, perinephric infections developed in 28 patients, and 8 of these developed mycotic aneurysms.[453] These lesions were evident clinically 1½–4 months post-transplant. Six were located in the external iliac artery, with one each in the internal iliac artery and aorta. All these lesions were secondary to contiguous foci of infection in the deep tissues of the transplant wound.[453,454]

Clinical Manifestations

When mycotic aneurysms occur during the course of IE, manifestations of the underlying disease may be evident. Peripheral middle cerebral artery aneurysms constitute 2.5–6.2 percent of all intracranial aneurysms[445–447,455] and are usually secondary to infection. Intracranial mycotic aneurysms are usually clinically silent. When hemorrhage occurs, a sudden onset of severe headache with rapid deterioration in the level of consciousness is noted. The time interval from the diagnosis of IE to the onset of hemorrhage is variable (0–35 days) with a mean of 18 days.[446] Some of these lesions produce premonitory or "herald" neurologic findings including focal deficits and seizures. Unfortunately, these symptoms are relatively common in patients with IE without intracranial aneurysms, and the differential diagnosis as well as decisions regarding arteriography are difficult.[456] A sudden focal deficit consistent with embolism is seen in ≈23 percent of patients and should prompt arteriography.[456] Mycotic aneurysms tend to occur more commonly in females of a younger age than does IE in general. They must be differentiated from aneurysms secondary to tumor emboli (especially choriocarcinoma or atrial myxoma), trauma, arteritis, or moyamoya disease and from congenital aneurysms. Visceral artery aneurysms are uncommon but, when present, are almost uniformly due to infection[448] or polyarteritis nodosa. The most common location is in the superior mesenteric artery. Although superior mesenteric artery aneurysms account for only 8 percent of visceral artery aneurysms overall, most are of infectious etiology.[457] Symptoms include an acute onset of colicky abdominal pain, but the presentation is variable. Hepatic artery aneurysms may produce colicky right upper quadrant pain, fever, jaundice, and gastrointestinal hemorrhage.[458] There are over 190 cases of this entity reported in the literature; 75 percent were extrahepatic and 25 percent intrahepatic. When the external iliac artery is involved, a triad of clinical signs may be present: pain in the lower extremity (especially the anterior aspect of the thigh) with quadriceps muscle wasting and a depressed knee jerk, arterial insufficiency of the extremity with coolness, pallor, and depressed pulses, and bacteremia.[459] Distal aneurysms (e.g., femoral) occasionally present with unusual manifestations including arthritis and purpura in the affected limb.

When more peripheral arteries are involved (usually with a pseudoaneurysm), a tender diffusely indurated mass is present in 92 percent of cases. The mass is pulsatile with an associated bruit in 50–60 percent of patients, and approximately 20–30 percent are associated with decreased peripheral pulses, skin changes, or even frank gangrene.[454] Local suppuration, petechiae, and purpura are often present, and the lesion may be confused with localized cellulitis or an abscess without consideration of vascular involvement. In abusers of illicit drugs, 80 percent of mycotic aneurysms occur in the lower extremity, with the remainder in the radial, brachial, or occasionally carotid arteries. Only 50 percent of these patients are febrile on admission. A superimposed septic arthritis may also be present.[460]

Although most infected aortic atherosclerotic aneurysms occur in elderly men, there are no pathognomonic findings to separate these patients from those with bland uninfected aneurysms. Fever is a helpful differentiating sign (present in over 70 percent of the patients) since it is uncommon in patients with bland aneurysms. Back pain or abdominal pain each occur in about one-third of the cases. A draining cutaneous sinus may be present. Separation of an infected aneurysm from the entity of inflammatory abdominal aortic aneurysms may be difficult. Inflammatory abdominal aortic aneurysms were first described in 1935 and account for 5–10 percent of abdominal aortic aneurysms; the lesions are usually infrarenal and often lead to ureteral obstruction due to the densely adherent fibrotic mass surrounding the vessel.[461] In a large series of 2816 patients undergoing repair of abdominal aortic aneurysms, 127 (4.5 percent) had inflammatory abdominal aortic aneurysms.[462] Most patients (123/127) were men and heavy smokers. Inflammatory abdominal aortic aneurysms are associated with an elevated erythrocyte sedimentation rate (73 percent), weight loss, symptoms (back and/or abdominal pain in 30–50 percent), and a higher operative mortality. Continuing bacteremia despite "appropriate" antimicrobial therapy in an elderly (especially diabetic) patient with no signs of IE is suggestive of an infected intravascular site. The aneurysm is palpable in 50–60 percent of the cases.[444,448] In most cases, the onset is insidious, and a low-grade fever may be present for several months before diagnosis. The nonspecificity of the clinical manifestations is reflected by the 75 percent preoperative rupture rate for this entity. Rupture may occur into the retroperitoneal space or peritoneal cavity (56 percent), pleural cavity (9 percent), duodenum (12 percent), esophagus (6 percent), mediastinum (3 percent), or the pericardium (3 percent). The most common site of aortoenteric fistulas is between the aorta and the third portion of the duodenum. Short periods of "herald" bleeding are common warning signs before exsanguinating hemorrhage occurs.[463] Severe pain and the rapid onset of shock usually accompany rupture of the aneurysm.

Laboratory Findings

There are no characteristic laboratory abnormalities in this group of diseases. When mycotic aneurysms occur with IE, alterations suggesting the underlying disease may be present. Patients with infected aortic aneurysms usually demonstrate a leukocytosis (65–83 percent), but this is nonspecific and may be present when the aneurysm is bland. Bacteremia is found in 53 to >90 percent of the cases, is continuous, and usually does not clear with antibiotic therapy alone. Evidence for a primary source of bacteremia (e.g., pneumonia, osteomyelitis) may be evident but is absent in up to 46 percent of the cases.[442] The abdominal aorta is noted to be calcified on abdominal x-ray films in 47 percent,[444] and anterior vertebral body erosion has been demonstrated in 18 percent. A lack of calcification is suggestive of infection since 70–80 percent of bland aneurysms demonstrate this finding on abdominal x-ray films. Certain procedures (e.g., intravenous pyelography, sonography, computed tomography) may reveal the presence of an aneurysm but are often not satisfactory for preoperative detail. The absence of intimal calcification, an associated perianeurysmal fluid collection or osteomyelitis, or the sudden appearance of an aneurysm in a septic patient are all suggestive features of an infected abdominal aortic aneurysm by computed tomography.[464] Gas in the aortic wall is diagnostic, but rare. Although the sensitivity is unknown, ^{67}Ga and ^{111}In leukocyte imaging have been used to localize intra-arterial infections.[465] Nevertheless, preoperative angiography is often preferred to precisely delineate the extent of aneurysmal involvement.[466] This information may alter the operative approach and may minimize the complications. Two-dimensional or M-mode echocardiography is a very useful noninvasive technique for documenting mycotic aneurysms in the vicinity of the aortic valve, (e.g., sinus of Valsalva, supravalvular, subvalvular), and this technique is adjunctive to aortic root angiography preoperatively.[467] Intraoperative epicardial echocardiography has also been used to facilitate the surgical approach. When a hepatic aneurysm is suspected, liver scans and ultrasonography may be helpful before angiography.[458]

Etiologic Agents

Before the antibiotic era, mycotic aneurysms associated with IE were usually due to the more "virulent" organisms such as the β-hemolytic group A streptococci, pneumococci, or *H. influenzae*. With the decline of these organisms as causal agents in IE, most of these lesions are now due to streptococci or staphylococci and follow the incidence patterns outlined in Table 4 for the underlying disease.

When bacteria "seed" a pre-existing atherosclerotic vessel, the etiologic agents are markedly different from those found in mycotic aneurysms associated with IE. Gram-positive organisms cause approximately 60 percent of these lesions, but gram-negative (chiefly *Salmonella*) bacilli are isolated in 35 percent. Staphylococci are implicated in 40 percent of the cases overall,[444] and over two-thirds of these are *S. aureus*. Salmonellae cause 20 percent of the cases and involve, in order of frequency, the aorta and femoral and iliac arteries. Only 1 of 24 cases reported before 1974 was above the renal arteries.[468] Lumbar osteomyelitis due to *Salmonella* was present in one-third of cases. The presumed portal of entry is the gastrointestinal tract. *Salmonella enteritidis* strains are isolated in 40 percent of cases, which is proportional to their overall rate of isolation in the United States. *Salmonella chloreaesuis,* an uncommon clinical isolate, appears to be particularly pathogenic for this condition since this species was isolated in 32 percent of the cases.[469] *Salmonella typhi* is very rarely implicated in this disorder (one case report). *Salmonella* infections of aortic aneurysms were first reported in 1948. The predilection for involvement by this organism is not understood, but *Salmonella* organisms tend to "seed" abnormal tissues during bacteremia, e.g., hematomas, malignant tumors, cysts, gallstones, bone infarcts, and altered endothelium (aortic aneurysms). It has been estimated that 25 percent of patients over 50 years of age with *Salmonella* bacteremia have an intravascular focus of infection.[470] *Arizona* species (especially *A. hinshawii*) are closely related to *Salmonella* sp., cause similar clinical syndromes, and also infect aortic aneurysms in elderly diabetic males.[471] The following organisms also produce infection in atherosclerotic aneurysms: *E. coli, P. aeruginosa, Proteus* sp., *Citrobacter freundii, Klebsiella-Enterobacter* sp., *S. marcescens, Campylobacter fetus,*[472] *Listeria monocytogenes, Bacteroides fragilis,* gonococci, group A or C streptococci, diphtheroids, enterococci, and pneumococci. Fungal mycotic aneurysms are rare in the intracranial compartment, with only 13 definite cases reported by 1981.[473] The most common etiologic agents are *Aspergillus* sp., agents of mucormycoses, and *Candida* sp. The first two agents may involve intracranial arteries by direct extension from foci of sinusitis. One case of multiple intracranial aneurysms due to *Coccidioides immitis* that occurred during therapy for basilar meningitis has been described. Fungal mycotic aneurysms tend to involve larger, more proximal vessels at the base of the brain (11/18 [61 percent] carotid or basilar) than do bacterial causes with IE.[474] Tuberculous aneurysms are now uncommon and when present are due to contiguous foci of infection.

Pseudoaneurysms resulting from intra-arterial or perivascular injection of illicit street drugs, often in addicts with sclerosed veins due to repeated intravenous inoculation, are associated with contiguous abscesses. The causative agents are *S. aureus* (76 percent), *P. aeruginosa* (18 percent), and many others.[449]

Therapy

No uniformly acceptable approach has been devised for the treatment of mycotic aneurysms in IE. The treatment of intracranial mycotic aneurysms is particularly controversial. Some of these lesions appear to resolve with antimicrobial therapy alone. In a review of 56 aneurysms occurring in 45 patients,[475] 3 of 20 patients died when treated with antibiotics alone. Mild to moderate neurologic deficits were observed in 8 of the 17 survivors. Likewise, 6 of 25 patients treated with both antibiotics and surgery died, and 9 of 19 survivors were left with mild to moderate neurologic deficits. Others report a different experience with a higher mortality in the nonsurgical group,[446] but patients were selected only after subarachnoid hemorrhage had occurred. For example, in a review of 13 intracranial mycotic aneurysms,[446] 6/8 patients treated with antibiotics alone died, and no deaths were observed in the surgically treated group. In a review of 85 cases treated between 1954 and 1978, 20 of 38 patients treated solely with antibiotics died vs. 8 of 30 operated upon.[445] The distal location of most intracranial mycotic aneurysms associated with IE may permit ligation and excision with fewer complications when compared with surgery for berry aneurysms in the circle of Willis. Interestingly, the mortality rate was low in patients with multiple aneurysms (4/15) treated with antibiotics alone. In one series, the mortality was 29 percent after rupture of an intracranial mycotic aneurysm. The use of serial angiography may be useful in following these patients since the aneurysm(s) may change in size or new lesions may develop. In 21 patients subjected to serial angiography, the mycotic aneurysm increased in size in 5, did not change in 1, became smaller in 6, and completely resolved in 11, and new aneurysms developed in 2. Therefore, over 50 percent of these peripheral intracranial aneurysms resolved with antibiotic therapy alone during the treatment of IE.[475] Surgery is indicated for aneurysms increasing in size on repeat angiography[476,477] but may be deferred for 4–6 weeks for those remaining the same size (if the patient is an acceptable medical risk). The definitive treatment for aneurysms decreasing in size on repeat serial angiography every 2 weeks is unclear. Computed tomograpy is not helpful in localizing the aneurysm but provides important information if hematomas, infarcts, or abscesses develop. The antibiotics used are governed by the etiologic agent of the IE (see above).

Peripheral vessels are usually involved when arterial trauma (narcotic addict, gunshot wound, iatrogenic) results in pseudoaneurysm formation with infection. Therapy with antibiotics, proximal ligation of the vessel, resection of the pseudoaneurysm, and appropriate drainage result in cures in 75 percent of the cases. Vascular reconstruction through uninfected tissue planes with autogenous grafts is necessary when limb viability is dependent on the affected vessel. This is encountered more frequently in the lower extremity. For example, severe ischemia developed in 9 of 28 patients after excision of mycotic aneurysms of the common femoral artery[449] in one series of 52 cases. Amputation was required in only 11 percent of a large series of 54 aneurysms among drug addicts recently seen at the Henry Ford Hospital; there were no deaths.[478]

The mortality for patients with infected atherosclerotic aneurysms still exceeds 90 percent; approximately 40-long-term survivors have been reported since 1962.[469,479,482] A high index of suspicion is necessary to intervene surgically before rupture occurs since this complication is uniformly fatal and occurs in about 80 percent of the cases. When gram-negative bacilli are the cause of the infection, "early" (e.g., within 2 weeks after the first positive blood culture) rupture occurs much more frequently (84 percent) than if gram-positive bacteria are isolated (10 percent). Survival after surgery is also more common (75 percent) for patients with aneurysms infected with gram-positive cocci than for those with gram-negative bacilli (25 percent). Antibiotics should be used in this disease; but even if the lesion is sterilized (only one reported case), the aneurysm may still continue to enlarge and rupture, so therefore surgery is required. At surgery, the aneurysm and any intraluminal thrombus must be sectioned, Gram stained, and cultured. If infection is present, all aneurysmal tissue and surrounding inflammation must be resected before grafting. Basic principles of grafting in this situation include the use of autogenous rather than synthetic grafts and insertion only in clean noninfected tissue planes. If the graft is placed in the infected area, then continued infection, leakage, thrombus formation, abscess formation, and rupture usually result. Although some authorities have achieved a successful result by restoration of vascular continuity in situ after radical débridement,[479,481] this approach is not recommended in most cases. In a review of 24 patients with abdominal aortic aneurysms infected with *Salmonella* sp., 10 died after rupture without surgery, and another 7 patients survived grafting only to succumb to continued leakage from the anastomosis (only 5 were long-term survivors). If a graft is inserted in situ and persistent fever and bacteremia or emboli to the lower extremities ensue, reoperation with extra-anatomic grafting is mandatory. Since the resected area is contaminated, special bypass techniques (especially thoracoiliac, transpublic, or axillofemoral) are usually required. When an axillofemoral approach is used, a single graft should be inserted for both lower extremities since long-term patency is prolonged under these circumstances.[480,482] Bactericidal antibiotics should be continued for 6–8 weeks postoperatively, and peak serum bactericidal levels of at least 1:8 should be achieved. The actual agents used are dependent on the isolated organism (or the morphologic characteristics of the organisms in the surgical specimen) and on the results of in vitro susceptibility testing.

REFERENCES

1. Lerner PI, Weinstein L. Infective endocarditis in the antibiotic era. N Engl J Med. 1966;274:199.
2. Watanakunakorn C. Changing epidemiology and newer aspects of infective endocarditis. Adv Intern Med. 1977;22:21.
3. Von Reym CF, Levy BS, Arbeit RD, et al. Infective endocarditis: An analysis based on strict case definitions. Ann Intern Med. 1982;94:505.
4. Kaye D. Definitions and demographic characteristics. In: Kaye D, ed. Infective Endocarditis. Baltimore: University Park Press; 1976:1.
5. Durack DT, Petersdorf RG. Changes in the epidemiology of endocarditis. In: Kaplan EL, Taranta AV, eds. Infective Endocarditis. An American Heart Association Symposium. Dallas: American Heart Association; 1977:3.
6. Griffin MR, Wilson WR, Edwards WD, et al. Infective endocarditis. Olmsted County, Minnesota, 1950 through 1981. JAMA. 1985;254:1199–202.
7. King JW, Nguyen VQ, Conrad SA. Results of a prospective statewide reporting system for infective endocarditis. Am J Med Sci. 1988;295:517–27.
8. Shulman ST. Infective endocarditis: 1986. Pediatr Infect Dis. 1986;5:691–4.
9. Hayward GW. Infective endocarditis: A changing disease. Br Med J. 1973;2:706.
10. Anonymous (Editorial). Infective endocarditis. Br Med J. 1981;1:677.
11. Thayer WS. Studies on bacterial (infective) endocarditis. Johns Hopkins Hosp Rep. 1926;22:1.
12. Garvey GJ, Neu HC. Infective endocarditis: An evolving disease. Medicine (Baltimore). 1978;57:105.
13. Lien EA, Solberg CO, Kalager T. Infective endocarditis 1973–1984 at the Bergen University Hospital: Clinical feature, treatment and prognosis. Scand J Infect Dis. 1988;20:239–46.
14. Come PC. Infective endocarditis: Current perspectives. Compr Ther. 1982;8:57.
15. Pelletier LL, Petersdorf RG. Infective endocarditis: A review of 125 cases from the University of Washington Hospitals, 1963–72. Medicine (Baltimore). 1977;56:287.
16. Terpenning MS, Buggy BP, Kaufmann CA. Hospital-acquired infective endocarditis. Arch Intern Med. 1988;148:1601–3.
17. Cherubin CE, Neu HC. Infective endocarditis at the Presbyterian Hospital in New York City from 1938–1967. Am J Med. 1971;51:83.
18. Roberts WC, Buchbinder NA. Right-sided valvular infective endocarditis. A clinicopathologic study of 12 necropsy patients. Am J Med. 1972;53:7.
19. Kaye D. Changing pattern of infective endocarditis. Am J Med. 1985;78(Suppl 6B):157–62.
20. Roberts WC, Perloff JK, Constantin T. Severe valvular aortic stenosis in patients over 65 years of age. Am J Cardiol. 1971;27:497.
21. Delahaye JP, Loire R, Milon H, et al. Infective endocarditis on stenotic aortic valves. Eur Heart J. 1988;9(Suppl E):43–9.
22. McKinsey DS, Ratts TE, Bisno AL. Underlying cardiac lesions in adults with infective endocarditis. The changing spectrum. Am J Med. 1987;82:681–8.
23. Lowes JA, Hamer J, Williams G, et al. Ten years of infective endocarditis at St. Bartholomew's hospital: Analysis of clinical features and treatment in relation to prognosis and mortality. Lancet. 1980;1:133.
24. Moulsdale MT, Eykyn SJ, Phillips I. Infective endocarditis, 1970–1979. A study of culture-positive cases in St. Thomas' Hospital. Q J Med. 1980;49:315.
25. Venezio FR, Westenfelder GO, Cook FV, et al. Infective endocarditis in a community hospital. Arch Intern Med. 1982;142:789.
26. Fulkerson PK, Beaver BM, Avseon JC, et al. Calcification of the mitral annulus: Etiology, clinical associations, complications and therapy. Am J Med. 1979;66:967.
27. Cardelia JV, Befeler B, Hildner FJ, et al. Hypertrophic subaortic stenosis complicated by aortic insufficiency and subacute bacterial endocarditis. Am Heart J. 1971;81:543.
28. Wang K, Gobel FL, Gleason DF. Bacterial endocarditis in idiopathic hypertrophic subaortic stenosis, Am Heart J. 1975;89:359.
29. Chagnac A, Rudniki C, Loebel H, et al. Infectious endocarditis in idiopathic hypertrophic subaortic stenosis. Report of three cases and review of the literature. Chest. 1982;81:346.
30. Corrigan D, Bolen J, Hancock EW, et al. Mitral valve prolapse and infective endocarditis. Am J Med. 1977;63:215.
31. Jeresaty RM. Mitral valve prolapse—click syndrome. Prog Cardiovasc Dis. 1973;15:623.
32. Schutte JE, Gaffney FA, Blend L, et al. Distinctive anthropometric characteristics of women with mitral valve prolapse. Am J Med. 1981;71:533.
33. Clemens JD, Horwitz RI, Jaffe CC, et al. A controlled evaluation of the risk of bacterial endocarditis in persons with mitral-valve prolapse. N Engl J Med. 1982;307:776.
34. Nolan CM, Kane JJ, Grunow WA. Infective endocarditis and mitral prolapse. A comparison with other types of endocarditis. Arch Intern Med. 1981;141:447.
35. Scheld WM. Pathogenesis and pathophysiology of infective endocarditis. In: Sande MA, Kaye D, Root RK, eds. Endocarditis. v. 1. Contemporary Issues in Infectious Diseases. London: Churchill Livingston; 1984:1–32.
36. Freedman LR. The pathogenesis of infective endocarditis. J Antimicrob Chemother. 1987;20(Suppl A):1–6.
37. Weinstein L, Schlesinger JJ. Pathoanatomic, pathophysiologic, and clinical correlations in endocarditis (first of two parts). N Engl J Med. 1974;291:832.
38. Levison ME. Pathogenesis of infective endocarditis. In: Kaye D, ed. Infective Endocarditis. Baltimore: University Park Press; 1976:29.
39. Angrist AA, Oka M. Pathogenesis of bacterial endocarditis. JAMA. 1963;183:249.
40. Durack DT, Beeson PB. Pathogenesis of infective endocarditis. In: Rahimtoola SH, ed. Infective Endocarditis. New York: Grune & Stratton, 1978:1.
41. Durack DT, Beeson PB. Experimental bacterial endocarditis. I. Colonization of a sterile vegetation. Br J Exp Pathol. 1972;53:44.
42. Durack DT, Beeson PB, Petersdorf RG. Experimental endocarditis. III. Production and progress of the disease in rabbits. Br J Exp Pathol. 1973;54:142.
43. Durack DT. Experimental bacterial endocarditis. IV. Structure and function of very early lesions. J Pathol. 1975;115:81.
44. McGowan DA, Gillett R. Scanning electron microscopic observations of the surface of the initial lesion in experimental streptococcal endocarditis in the rabbit. Br J Exp Pathol. 1980;61:164.
45. Ferguson DJP, McColm AA, Ryan DM, et al. Experimental staphylococcal endocarditis and aortitis. Morphology of the initial colonization. Virchows Arch [A] 1986;410:43–8.
46. Sherwood BF, Rowlands DT, Vakilzadeh J, et al. Experimental bacterial endocarditis in the opossum (*Didelphis virginiana*). Am J Pathol. 1971;64:513.
47. Sande MA: Experimental endocarditis. In: Kaye D, ed. Infective Endocarditis. Baltimore: University Park Press; 1976:11.
48. Chino F, Kodama A, Otake M, et al: Nonbacterial thrombotic endocarditis in a Japanese autopsy sample. A review of 80 cases. Am Heart J. 1975;90:190.
49. Rodbard S. Blood velocity and endocarditis. Circulation. 1963;27:18.
50. Lepeschkin E. On the relation between the site of valvular involvement in endocarditis and the blood pressure resting on the valve. Am J Med Sci. 1952;224:318.
51. Okell CC, Elliott SD. Bacteraemia and oral sepsis. With special reference to the aetiology of subacute endocarditis. Lancet. 1935;2:869.
52. Everett ED, Hirschmann JV. Transient bacteremia and endocarditis prophylaxis: A review. Medicine (Baltimore). 1977;56:61.
53. Loesche WJ. Indigenous human flora and bacteremia. In: Kaplan EL, Taranta AV, eds. Infective Endocarditis. An American Heart Association Symposium. Dallas: American Heart Association; 1977:40.
54. Durack DT, Beeson PB. Protective role of complement in experimental *Escherichia coli* endocarditis. Infect Immun. 1977;16:213.
55. Yersin B, Glauser M-P, Guze L, et al. Experimental *Escherichia coli* endocarditis in rats: Roles of serum bactericidal activity and duration of catheter placement. Infect Immun. 1988;56:1273–80.
56. Gould K, Ramirez-Ronda CH, Holmes RK, et al. Adherence of bacteria to heart valves in vitro. J Clin Invest. 1975;56:1364.
57. Freedman LR, Valone J Jr. Experimental infective endocarditis. Prog Cardiovasc Dis. 1979;22:169.
58. Overholser CD, Moreillon P, Glauser MP. Experimental bacterial endocarditis after dental extractions in rats with periodontitis. J Infect Dis. 1987;155:107–12.
59. Moreillon P, Overholser CD, Malinverni R, et al. Predictors of endocarditis in isolates from cultures of blood following dentral extractions in rats with periodontal disease. J Infect Dis. 1988;157:990–5.
60. Gibbons RJ, Nygaard M. Synthesis of insoluble dextran and its significance in the formation of gelatinous deposits by plaque-forming streptococci. Arch Oral Biol. 1968;13:1249.
61. Parker MT, Ball LC. Streptococci and aerococci associated with systemic infection in man. J Med Microbiol. 1976;9:275.
62. Scheld WM, Valone JA, Sande MA. Bacterial adherence in the pathogenesis

of endocarditis. Interaction of bacterial dextran, platelets, and fibrin. J Clin Invest. 1978;61:1394.
63. Ramirez-Ronda CH. Adherence of glucan-positive and glucan-negative streptococcal strains to normal and damaged heart valves. J Clin Invest. 1978;62:805.
64. Ramirez-Ronda CH. Effects of molecular weight of dextran on the adherence of *Streptococcus sanguis* to damaged heart valves. Infect Immun. 1980;29:1.
65. Pelletier LL Jr, Coyle M, Petersdorf R. Dextran production as a possible virulence factor in streptococcal endocarditis. Proc Soc Exp Biol Med. 1978;158:415.
66. Crawford I, Russell C. Comparative adhesion of seven species of streptococci isolated from the blood of patients with subacute bacterial endocarditis to fibrin-platelet clots in vitro. J Appl Bacteriol. 1986;60:127–33.
67. Dall L, Barnes WG, Lane JW, et al. Enzymatic modification of glycocalyx in the treatment of experimental endocarditis due to viridans streptococci. J Infect Dis. 1987;156:736–40.
68. Scheld WM, Calderone RA, Alliegro GM, et al. Yeast adherence in the pathogenesis of *Candida* endocarditis. Proc Soc Exp Biol Med. 1981;168:208.
69. Scheld WM, Strunk RW, Balian G, et al. Microbial adhesion to fibronectin in vitro correlates with production of endocarditis in rabbits. Proc Soc Exp Biol Med. 1985;180:474–82.
70. Becker RC, DiBello PM, Lucas FV. Bacterial tissue tropism: An in vitro model for infective endocarditis. Cardiovasc Res. 1987;21:813–20.
71. Vercellotti G, Lussenhop D, Peterson PK, et al. Bacterial adherence to fibronectin and endothelial cells: A possible mechanism for bacterial tissue tropism. J Lab Clin Med. 1984;103:34–43.
72. Ogawa SK, Yurberg ER, Hatcher VB, et al. Bacterial adherence to human endothelial cells in vitro. Infect Immun. 1985;50:218–24.
73. Hamill RJ, Vann JM, Proctor RA. Phagocytosis of *Staphylococcus aureus* by cultured bovine aortic-endothelial cells: Model for post adherence events in endovascular infections. Infect Immun. 1986;54:833–6.
74. Scheld WM, Zak O, Vosbeck K, et al. Bacterial adhesion in the pathogenesis of endocarditis. Effect of subinhibitory antibiotic concentrations on streptococcal adhesion in vitro and the development of endocarditis in rabbits. J Clin Invest. 1981;68:1381.
75. Bernard J-P, Francioli P, Glauser MP, et al. Vancomycin prophylaxis of experimental *Streptococcus sanguis* endocarditis: Inhibition of bacterial adherence rather than bacterial killing. J Clin Invest. 1981;68:1113.
76. Glauser MP, Francioli P. Successful prophylaxis against experimental streptococcal endocarditis with bacteriostatic antibiotics. J Infect Dis. 1982;146:806.
77. Lowry FD, Chang DS, Neuhaus EG, et al. Effect of penicillin on the adherence of *Streptococcus sanguis* in vitro and in the rabbit model of endocarditis. J Clin Invest. 1983;71:668.
78. Glauser MP, Bernard JP, Moreillon P, et al. Successful single-dose amoxicillin prophylaxis against experimental streptococcal endocarditis. Evidence for two mechanisms of protection. J Infect Dis. 1983;147:568.
79. Clawson CC, Rao Gunda HR, White JG. Platelet interaction with bacteria. IV. Stimulation of the release reaction. Am J Pathol. 1975;81:411.
80. Herzberg MC, Brintzenhofe KL, Clawson CC. Aggregation of human platelets and adhesion of *Streptococcus sanguis*. Infect Immun. 1983;39:1457.
81. Sullam PM, Valone FH, Mills J. Mechanisms of platelet aggregation by viridans group streptococci. Infect Immun. 1987;55:1743–50.
82. Sullam PM, Jarvis GA, Valone FH. Role of immunoglobulin G in platelet aggregation by viridans group streptococci. Infect Immun. 1988;56:2907–11.
83. Ferguson DJP, McColm AA, Ryan DM, et al. A morphological study of experimental staphylococcal endocarditis and aortitis II. Inter-relationship of bacteria, vegetation and cardiovasculature in established infections. Br J Exp Pathol. 1986;67:679–86.
84. Durack DT, Beeson PB. Experimental bacterial endocarditis. II. Survival of bacteria in endocardial vegetations. Br J Exp Pathol. 1972;53:50.
85. Yersin BR, Glauser MP, Freedman LR. Effect of nitrogen mustard on natural history of right-sided streptococcal endocarditis: Role of cellular host defenses. Infect Immun. 1982;35:320.
86. Meddens MJM, Thompson J, Eulderink F, et al. Role of granulocytes in experimental *Streptococcus sanguis* endocarditis. Infect Immun. 1982;36:325.
87. Meddens MJM, Thompson J, Mattie H, et al. Role of granulocytes in the prevention and therapy of experimental *Streptococcus sanguis* endocarditis in rabbits. Antimicrob Agents Chemother. 1984;25:263–7.
88. Hook EW III, Sande MA. Role of the vegetation in experimental *Streptococcus viridans* endocarditis. Infect Immun. 1974;10:1433.
89. Thorig L, Thompson J, Eulderink F, et al. Effects of monocytopenia and anticoagulation in experimental *Streptococcus sanguis* endocarditis. Br J Exp Pathol. 1980;61:108.
90. van Ginkel CJW, Thorig L, Thompson J, et al. Enhancement of generation of monocyte tissue thromboplastin by bacterial phagocytosis: Possible pathway for fibrin formation on infected vegetations in bacterial endocarditis. Infect Immun. 1979;25:388.
91. Drake TA, Rodgers GM, Sande MA. Tissue factor is a major stimulus for vegetation formation in enterococcal endocarditis in rabbits. J Clin Invest. 1984;73:1750–3.
92. Drake TA, Pang M. *Staphylococcus aureus* induces tissue factor expression in cultured human cardiac valve endothelium. J Infect Dis. 1988;157:749–56.
93. Mair W. Pneumococcal endocarditis in rabbits. J Pathol Bacteriol. 1923;26:426.
94. Scheld WM, Thomas JH, Sande MA. Influence of preformed antibody on experimental *Streptococcus sanguis* endocarditis. Infect Immun. 1979; 25:781.
95. Durack DT, Gilliland BC, Petersdorf RG. Effect of immunization on susceptibility to experimental *Streptococcus mutans* and *Streptococcus sanguis* endocarditis. Infect Immun. 1978;22:52.
96. Scheld WM, Calderone RA, Brodeur JP, et al. Influence of preformed antibody on the pathogenesis of experimental *Candida albicans* endocarditis. Infect Immun. 1983;40:950.
97. Greenberg DP, Ward JI, Bayer AS. Influence of *Staphylococcus aureus* antibody on experimental endocarditis in rabbits. Infect Immun. 1987; 55:3030–4.
98. Williams RC, Kunkel HG. Rheumatoid factors and their disappearance following therapy in patients with SBE. Arthritis Rheum. 1962;5:126.
99. Sheagren JN, Tuazon CV, Griffin C, et al. Rheumatoid factor in acute bacterial endocarditis. Arthritis Rheum. 1976;19:887.
100. Phair JP, Clarke J. Immunology of infective endocarditis. Prog Cardiovasc Dis. 1979;22:137.
101. Bacon PA, Davidson C, Smith B. Antibodies to *Candida* and autoantibodies in subacute bacterial endocarditis. Q J Med. 1974;43:537.
102. Laxdal T, Messner RP, Williams RC. Opsonic, agglutinating, and complement-fixing antibodies in patients with subacute bacterial endocarditis. J Lab Clin Med. 1968;71:638.
103. Horwitz D, Quismorio FP, Friou GJ. Cryoglobulinemia in patients with infectious endocarditis. Clin Exp Immunol. 1975;19:131.
104. Bayer AS, Theofilopoulos AN, Eisenberg R, et al. Circulating immune complexes in infective endocarditis. N Engl J Med. 1976;295:1500.
105. Gutman RA, Striker GE, Gilliland BC, et al. The immune complex glomerulonephritis of bacterial endocarditis. Medicine (Baltimore). 1972;51:1.
106. Levy RL, Hong R. The immune nature of subacute bacterial endocarditis (SBE) nephritis. Am J Med. 1973;54:645.
107. Inman RD, Redecha PB, Knechtle SJ, et al. Identification of bacterial antigens in circulating immune complexes of infective endocarditis. J Clin Invest. 1982;70:271.
108. Alpert JS, Krous HF, Dalen JE, et al. Pathogenesis of Osler's nodes. Ann Intern Med. 1976;85:471.
109. Lowenstein MB, Urman JD, Abeles M, et al. Skin immunofluorescence in infective endocarditis. JAMA. 1977;238:1163.
110. Cabane J, Godeau P, Herreman G, et al. Fate of circulating immune complexes in infective endocarditis. Am J Med. 1979;66:277.
111. Kauffman RH, Thompson J, Valentijn RM, et al. The clinical implications and the pathogenetic significance of circulating immune complexes in infective endocarditis. Am J Med. 1981;71:17.
112. Krause JR, Levison SP. Pathology of infective endocarditis. In: Kaye D, ed. Infective Endocarditis. Baltimore: University Park Press; 1976:55.
113. Roberts WC. Characteristics and consequences of infective endocarditis (active or healed or both) learned from morphologic studies. In: Rahimtoola SH, ed. Infective Endocarditis. New York: Grune & Stratton: 1978;55.
114. Morel-Maroger L, Sraer JD, Herreman G, et al. Kidney in subacute endocarditis. Pathological and immunofluorescence findings. Arch Pathol. 1913;94:205.
115. Anderson CB, Butcher HR, Ballinger WF. Mycotic aneurysms. Arch Surg. 1974;109:712.
116. Greenlee JE, Mandell GL. Neurological manifestations of infective endocarditis: A review. Stroke. 1973;4:958.
117. Kerr A Jr, Tan JS. Biopsies of the Janeway lesion of infective endocarditis. J Cutan pathol. 1979;6:124.
118. Silverberg HH. Roth spots. Mt Sinai J Med. 1970;37:77.
119. Starkebaum M, Durack D, Beeson P. The "incubation period" of subacute bacterial endocarditis. Yale J Biol Med. 1977;50:49.
120. Weinstein L, Rubin RH. infective endocarditis—1973. Progr Cardiovasc Dis. 1973;16:239.
121. Freedman LR. Infective endocarditis and other intravascular infections. In: Braude AI, David CE, Fierer J, eds. Medical Microbiology and Infectious Diseases. Philadelphia: WB Saunders; 1981:1511.
122. Hermans PE. The clinical manifestations of infective endocarditis. Mayo Clin Proc. 1982;57:15.
123. Terpenning MS, Buggy BP, Kauffman CA. Infective endocarditis: Clinical features in young and elderly patients. Am J Med. 1987;83:626–34.
124. Espersen F, Frimodt-Moller N. *Staphylococcus aureus* endocarditis. A review of 119 cases. Arch Intern Med. 1986;146:1118–21.
125. Churchill MA, Geraci JE, Hunder GG. Musculoskeletal manifestations of bacterial endocarditis. Ann Intern Med. 1977;87:754.
126. Lerner PI. Neurologic complications of infective endocarditis. Med Clin North Am. 1985;69:385–98.
127. Bayer AS, Theofilopaulos AN, Eisenberg R, et al. Thrombotic thrombocytopenic purpura-like syndrome associated with infective endocarditis. A possible immune complex disorder. JAMA. 1977;238:408.
128. Levine DP, Crane LR, Zervos MJ. Bacteremia in narcotic addicts at the Detroit Medical Center II. Infectious endocarditis: A prospective comparative study. Rev Infect Dis. 1986;8:374–96.
129. Marantz PR, Linzer M, Feiner CJ, et al. Inability to predict diagnosis in febrile intravenous drug abusers. Ann Intern Med. 1987;106:823–8.

130. Chambers HF, Morris DL, Tauber MG, et al. Cocaine use and the risk for endocarditis in intravenous drug users. Ann Intern Med. 1987;106:833–6.
131. Chambers HF, Korzeniowski OM, Sande MA, et al. *Staphylococcus aureus* endocarditis: Clinical manifestations in addicts and nonaddicts. Medicine (Baltimore). 1983;62:170.
132. Sklaver AR, Hoffman TA, Greenman RL. Staphylococcal endocarditis in addicts. South Med J. 1978;71:638.
133. Thadepalli H, Francis CK. Diagnostic clues in metastatic lesions of endocarditis in addicts. West J Med. 1978;128:1.
134. McCartney AC, Orange GV, Pringle SD, et al. Serum C reactive protein in infective endocarditis. J Clin Pathol. 1988;41:44–8.
135. Wiseman J, Rouleau J, Rigo P, et al. Gallium-67 myocardial imaging for the detection of bacterial endocarditis. Radiology. 1976;120:135.
136. Wong DW, Dhawan VK, Tanaka T, et al. Imaging endocarditis with technitium 99m-labeled antibody—an experimental study: Concise communication. J Nucl Med. 1982;23:229.
137. Riba AL, Thakur ML, Gottschalk A, et al. Imaging experimental infective endocarditis with indium-111-labeled blood cellular components. Circulation. 1979;59:336.
138. Haft JI, Altieri J, Smight LG, et al. Computed tomography of the abdomen in the diagnosis of splenic emboli. Arch Intern Med. 1988;148:193–7.
139. Beeson PB, Brannon ES, Warren JV. Observations on the sites of removal of bacteria from the blood of patients with bacterial endocarditis. J Exp Med. 1945;81:9–23.
140. Werner AS, Cobbs CG, Kaye D, et al. Studies on the bacteremia of bacterial endocarditis. JAMA. 1967;202:199.
141. Pazin GJ, Saul S, Thompson ME. Blood culture positivity. Suppression by outpatient antibiotic therapy in patients with bacterial endocarditis. Arch Intern Med. 1982;142:263.
142. McKenzie R, Reimer LG. Effect of antimicrobials on blood cultures in endocarditis. Diagn Microbiol Infect Dis. 1987;8:165–72.
143. Aronson MD, Bos DH. Blood cultures. Ann Intern Med. 1987;106:246–53.
144. Washington JA II, Ilstrup DM. Blood cultures: Issues and controversies. Rev Infect Dis. 1986;8:792–802.
145. Washington JA II. The role of the microbiology laboratory in the diagnosis and antimicrobial treatment of infective endocarditis. Mayo Clin Proc. 1982;57:22.
146. Carey RB, Gross KC, Roberts RB. Vitamin-B_6-dependent *Streptococcus mitior (mitis)* isolated from patients with systemic infections. J Infect Dis. 1975;131:722.
147. Powers DL, Mandell GL. Intraleucocytic bacteria in endocarditis patients. JAMA. 1974;227:313.
148. Whitcomb DC. Bugs in the blood: Acute staphylococcal septicemia and endocarditis diagnosed by staining the buffy coat. NC Med J. 1986;47:293–5.
149. Tuazon CU, Sheagren JW. Teichoic acid antibodies in the diagnosis of serious infections with *Staphylococcus aureus*. Ann Intern Med. 1976;84:543.
150. Bayer AS, Tillman DB, Concepcion M, et al. Clinical value of teichoic acid antibody titers in the diagnosis and management of staphylococcemias. West J Med. 1980;132:294.
151. Kaplan JE, Palmer DL, Tung KSK. Teichoic acid antibody and circulating immune complexes in the management of *Staphylococcus aureus* bacteremia. Am J Med. 1981;70:769.
152. Arbeit RD, Nelles MJ. Capsular polysaccharide antigenemia in rats with experimental endocarditis due to *Staphylococcus aureus*. J Infect Dis. 1987;155:242–6.
153. Cannady PB, Sanford JP. Negative blood cultures in infective endocarditis. A review. South Med J. 1976;69:1420.
154. Walker RC, Henry NK, Washington JA II, et al. Lysis-centrifugation blood culture technique. Clinical impact in *Staphylococcus aureus* bacteremia. Arch Intern Med. 1986;146:2341–3.
155. Washington JA II. The microbiological diagnosis of infective endocarditis. J Antimicrob Chemother. 1987;20(Suppl A):29–36.
156. Austin SM, Smith SM, Co B, et al. Case report: Serologic evidence of acute murine typhus infection in a patient with culture-negative endocarditis. Am J Med Sci. 1987;293:320–3.
157. Tompkins LS, Roessler BJ, Redd SC, et al. *Legionella* prosthetic-valve endocarditis. N Engl J Med. 1988;318:530–5.
158. Walterspiel JN, Kaplan SL. Incidence and clinical characteristics of "culture-negative" infective endocarditis in a pediatric population. Pediatr Infect Dis. 1986;5:328–32.
159. Rubenstein E, Noreiga ER, Simberkoff MS, et al. Fungal endocarditis: Analysis of 24 cases and review of the literature. Medicine (Baltimore). 1975;54:331.
160. Kobza K, Steenblock U. Demonstration of candida in blood smears. Br Med J. 1977;1:1640.
161. Merz WG, Evans GL, Shadomy S, et al. Laboratory evaluation of serological tests for systemic candidiasis: A cooperative study. J Clin Microbiol. 1977;5:596.
162. Sande MA, Bowman CR, Calderone RA. Experimental *Candida albicans* endocarditis: Characterization of the disease and response to therapy. Infect Immun. 1977;17:140.
163. Warren RC, Bartlett A, Bidwell DE, et al. Diagnosis of invasive candidosis by enzyme immunoassay of serum antigen. Br Med J. 1977;1:1183.
164. Scheld WM, Brown RS Jr, Harding SA, et al. Detection of circulating antigen in experimental *Candida albicans* endocarditis by an enzyme-linked immunosorbent assay. J Clin Microbiol. 1980;12:679.
165. Dillan JC, Feigenbaum H, Konecke LL, et al. Echocardiographic manifestations of valvular vegetations. Am Heart J. 1973;86:698.
166. Boucher CA, Fallion JT, Myers GS, et al. The value and limitations of echocardiography in recording mitral valve vegetations. Am Heart J. 1977;94:37.
167. Thomson KR, Nanda NC, Gramiak R. The reliability of echocardiography in the diagnosis of infective endocarditis. Radiology. 1977;125:473.
168. Melvin ET, Berger M, Lutzker LG, et al. Noninvasive methods for detection of valve vegetations in infective endocarditis. Am J Cardiol. 1981; 47:271.
169. Mintz GS, Kotler MN. Clinical value and limitations of echocardiography. Its use in the study of patients with infectious endocarditis. Arch Intern Med. 1980;140:1022.
170. Popp RL. Echocardiography and infectious endocarditis. In: Remington JS, Swartz MN, eds. Current Clinical Topics in Infectious Diseases. v. 4. New York: McGraw-Hill; 1983:98.
171. Davis RS, Strom JA, Frishman W, et al. The demonstration of vegetations by echocardiography in bacterial endocarditis. An indication for early surgical intervention. Am J Med. 1980;57:69.
172. Martin RP, Mettzer RS, Chia EL, et al. Clinical utility of two-dimensional echocardiography in infective endocarditis. Am J Cardiol. 1980;46:379.
173. Bayer AS, Blomquist IK, Bello E, et al. Tricuspid valve endocarditis due to *Staphylococcus aureus*. Correlation of two-dimensional echocardiography with clinical outcome. Chest. 1988;93:247–53.
174. Manolis AS, Melita H. Echocardiographic and clinical correlates in drug addicts with infective endocarditis. Implications of vegetation size. Arch Intern Med. 1988;148:2461–5.
175. Tak T, Rahimtoola SH, Kumar A, et al. Value of digital image processing of two-dimensional echocardiograms in differentiating active from chronic vegetations of infective endocarditis. Circulation. 1988;78:116–23.
176. Mann T, McLaurin L, Grossman W, et al. Assessing the hemodynamic severity of acute aortic regurgitation due to infective endocarditis. N Engl J Med. 1975;293:108.
177. Mills J, Abbott J, Utley JR, et al. Role of cardiac catheterization in infective endocarditis. Chest. 1977;72:576.
178. Welton DE, Young JB, Raizner AE, et al. Value and safety of cardiac catheterization during active infective endocarditis. Am J Cardiol. 1979;44:1306.
179. Sussman JI, Baron EJ, Tenenbaum MJ, et al. Viridans streptococcal endocarditis: Clinical, microbiological, and echocardiographic correlations. J Infect Dis. 1986;154:597–603.
180. Roberts RB, Krieger AG, Schiller NL, et al. Viridans streptococcal endocarditis: The role of various species, including pyridoxal-dependent streptococci. Rev Infect Dis. 1979;1:955.
181. Tuazon CV, Gill V, Gill F. Streptococcal endocarditis: Single vs. combination antibiotic therapy and the role of various species. Rev Infect Dis. 1986;8:54–60.
182. Baddour LM, Bisno AL. Infective endocarditis complicating mitral valve prolapse: Epidemiologic, clinical, and microbiologic aspects. Rev Infect Dis. 1986;8:117–37.
183. Harder EJ, Wilkowske CJ, Washington JA, et al. *Streptococcus mutans* endocarditis. Ann Intern Med. 1974;80:364.
184. Watanakunakorn C. *Streptococcus bovis* endocarditis. Am J Med. 1974;56:256.
185. Moellering RC, Watson BK, Kunz LJ. Endocarditis due to group D streptococci. Comparison of disease caused by *Streptococcus bovis* with that produced by the enterococci. Am J Med. 1974;57:239.
186. Hoppes WL, Lerner PI. Nonenterococcal group D streptococcal endocarditis caused by *Streptococcus bovis*. Ann Intern Med. 1974;81:588.
187. Klein RS, Reuco RA, Catalano MT, et al. Association of *Streptococcus bovis* with carcinoma of the colon. N Engl J Med. 1977;297:800.
188. Steinberg D, Naggar CZ. *Streptococcus bovis* endocarditis with carcinoma of the colon. N Engl J Med. 1977;297:1354.
189. Mandell GL, Kaye D, Levison ME, et al. Enterococcal endocarditis: An analysis of 38 patients observed at the New York Hospital–Cornell Medical Center. Arch Intern Med. 1970;125:258.
190. Serra P, Brandimarte C, Martino P, et al. Synergistic treatment of enterococcal endocarditis. Arch Intern Med. 1977;137:1562.
191. Malone DA, Wagner RA, Myers JP, et al. Enterococcal bacteremia in two large community teaching hospitals. Am J Med. 1986;81:601–6.
192. Hoffmann SA, Moellering RC Jr. The enterococcus: "Putting the bug in our ears." Ann Intern Med. 1987;106:757–61.
193. Maki DG, Agger WA. Enterococcal bacteremia: Clinical features, the risk of endocarditis, and management. Medicine (Baltimore).1988;67:248–69.
194. Ugolini V, Pacifico A, Smitherman TC, et al. Pneumococcal endocarditis update: Analysis of 10 cases diagnosed between 1974 and 1984. Am Heart J. 1986;112:813–19.
195. Powderly WG, Stanley SL Jr, Medoff G. Pneumococcal endocarditis: Report of a series and review of the literature. Rev Infect Dis. 1986;8:786–91.
196. Carey RB, Brause BD, Roberts RB: Antimicrobial therapy of vitamin B_6-dependent streptococcal endocarditis. Ann Intern Med. 1977;87:150.
197. Stein DS, Nelson KE. Endocarditis due to nutritionally deficient streptococci: Therapeutic dilemna. Rev Infect Dis. 1987;9:908–16.
198. Catto BA, Jacobs MR, Shlaes DM. *Streptococcus mitis*. A cause of serious infection in adults. Arch Intern Med. 1987;147:885–8.
199. Rapeport KB, Giron JA, Rosner F. *Streptococcus mitis* endocarditis. Report of 17 cases. Arch Intern Med. 1986;146:2361–3.
200. Hager WD, Speck EL, Mathew PK, et al. Endocarditis with myocardial

abscesses and pericarditis in an adult. Group B streptococcus as a cause. Arch Intern Med. 1977;137:1725.
201. Opal SM, Cross A, Palmer M, et al. Group B streptococcal sepsis in adults and infants. Contrasts and comparisons. Arch Intern Med. 1988;148:641–5.
202. Gallagher PG, Watanakunakorn C. Group B streptococcal endocarditis: Report of seven cases and review of the literature, 1962–1985. Rev Infect Dis. 1986;8:175–88.
203. Scully BE, Spriggs D, Neu HC. *Streptococcus agalactiae* (Group B) endocarditis—a description of twelve cases and review of the literature. Infection. 1987;15:169–76.
204. Wiseman A, Rene P, Crelinsten GL. *Streptococcus agalactiae* endocarditis: An association with villous adenonas of the large intestine. Ann Intern Med. 1985;103:893–4.
205. Venezio FR, Gullberg RM, Westenfelder GO, et al. Group G streptococcal endocarditis and bacteremia. Am J Med. 1986;81:29–34.
206. Smyth EG, Pallett AP, Davidson RN. Group G streptococcal endocarditis: Two case reports, a review of the literature and recommendations for treatment. J Infect. 1988;16:169–76.
207. Murray HW, Gross KC, Masur H, et al. Serious infections caused by *Streptococcus milleri*. Am J Med. 1978;64:759.
208. Shlaes DM, Lerner PI, Wolinsky E, et al. Infections due to Lancefield group F and related streptococci (*S. milleri, S. anginosus*). Medicine (Baltimore). 1981;60:197.
209. Gossling J. Occurence and pathogenicity of the *Streptococcus milleri* group. Rev Infect Dis. 1988;10:257–85.
210. Hosea SW: Virulent *Streptococcus viridans* bacterial endocarditis. Am Heart J. 1981;101:174.
211. Buu-Joi A, Sapoetra A, Branger C, et al. Antimicrobial susceptibility of *Gemella haemolysans* isolated from patients with subacute endocarditis. Eur J Clin Microbiol. 1982;1:102.
212. Mylotte JM, McDermott C, Spooner JA. Prospective study of 114 consecutive episodes of *Staphylococcus aureus* bacteremia. Rev Infect Dis. 1987;9:891–908.
213. Eykyn SJ. Staphylococcal sepsis. The changing pattern of disease and therapy. Lancet. 1988;1:100–4.
214. Watanakunakorn C, Tan JS, Phair JP. Some salient features of *Staphylococcus aureus* endocarditis. Am J Med. 1973;54:473.
215. Musher DM, McKenzie SO. infection due to *Staphylococcus aureus*. Medicine (Baltimore). 1977;56:383.
216. Bayer AS. Staphylococcal bacteremia and endocarditis. State of the art. Arch Intern Med. 1982;142:1169.
217. Thompson RL. Staphylococcal infective endocarditis. Mayo Clin Proc. 1982;57:106.
218. Julander I. Unfavourable prognostic factors in *Staphylococcus aureus* septicemia and endocarditis. Scand J Infect Dis. 1985;17:179–87.
219. O'Callaghan C, McDougall P. Infective endocarditis in neonates. Arch Dis Child. 1988;63:53–7.
220. Crane LR, Levine DP, Zervos MJ, et al. Bacteremia in narcotic addicts at the Detroit Medical Center. I. Microbiology, epidemiology, risk factors, and empiric therapy. Rev Infect Dis. 1986;8:364–73.
221. Noel GJ, O'Loughlin JE, Edelson PJ. Neonatal *Staphylococcus epidermidis* right-sided endocarditis: Description of five catheterized infants. Pediatrics. 1988;82:234–9.
222. Baddour LM, Phillips TN, Bisno AL. Coagulase-negative staphylococcal endocarditis. Occurrence in patients with mitral valve prolapse. Arch Intern Med. 1986;146:119–21.
223. Harris LF, O'Shields H. Coagulase-negative staphylococcal endocarditis: A view from the community hospital. South Med J. 1986;79:1379–86.
224. Caputo GM, Archer GL, Calderwood SB, et al. Native valve endocarditis due to coagulase-negative staphylococci. Clinical and microbiologic features. Am J Med. 1987;83:619–25.
225. Espersen F, Wheat LJ, Bemis AT, et al. Solid-phase radio-immunoassay for IgG antibodies to *Staphylococcus epidermidis:* Use in serious coagulase-negative staphylococcal infections. Arch Intern Med. 1987;147:689–93.
226. Etienne J, Brun Y, El Solh N, et al. Characterization of clinically significant isolates of *Staphylococcus epidermidis* from patients with endocarditis. J Clin Microbiol. 1988;26:613–7.
227. Baddour LM, Simpson WA, Weems JJ Jr, et al. Phenotypic selection of small-colony variant forms of *Staphylococcus epidermidis* in a rat model of endocarditis. J Infect Dis. 1988;157:757–63.
228. Finland M, Barnes MW. Changing etiology of bacterial endocarditis in the antibacterial era. Experiences at Boston City Hospital 1933–1965. Ann Intern Med. 1970;72:341.
229. Pedersen FK, Petersen EA. Bacterial endocarditis of Blegdamshospitalet in Copenhagen 1944–1973. Scand J Infect Dis. 1976;8:99.
230. Cohen PS, Maquire JH, Weinstein L. Infective endocarditis caused by gram-negative bacteria: A review of the literature, 1945–1977. Prog Cardiovasc Dis. 1980;22:205.
231. Geraci JE, Wilson WR. Endocarditis due to gram-negative bacteria. Report of 56 cases. Mayo Clin Proc. 1982;57:145.
232. Snyder N, Atterbury CE, Correia JP, et al. Increased occurrence of cirrhosis and bacterial endocarditis. Gastroenterology. 1977;73:1107.
233. Carruthers M. Endocarditis due to enteric bacilli other than salmonellae: Case reports and literature review. Am J Med Sci. 1977;273:203.
234. Sande MA, Johnson WD, Hook EW, et al. Sustained bacteremia in patients with prosthetic cardiac valves. N Engl J Med. 1972;286:1067.
235. Schneider PJ, Nernoff J, Gold JA. Acute salmonella endocarditis. Report of a case and review. Arch Intern Med. 1967;120:478.
236. Mills J, Drew D. *Serratia marcescens* endocarditis. Ann Intern Med. 1976;85:397.
237. Cooper R, Mills J. *Serratia* endocarditis. A follow-up report. Arch Intern Med. 1980;140:199.
238. Caramelli B, Mansur AJ, Grinberg M, et al. *Campylobacter fetus* endocarditis on a prosthetic heart valve. South Med J. 1988;81:802–3.
239. Reyes MP, Brown WJ, Lerner AM. Treatment of patients with *Pseudomonas* endocarditis with high dose aminoglycoside and carbenicillin therapy. Medicine (Baltimore). 1978;57:57.
240. Reyes MP, Lerner AM. Current problems in the treatment of infective endocarditis due to *Pseudomonas aeruginosa*. Rev Infect Dis. 1983;5:314.
241. Wieland M, Lederman MM, Kline-King C, et al. Left-sided endocarditis due to *Pseudomonas aeruginosa*. A report of 10 cases and review of the literature. Medicine (Baltimore). 1986;65:180–9.
242. Noriega ER, Rubinstein E, Simberkoff M, et al. Subacute and acute endocarditis due to *Pseudomonas cepacia* in heroin addicts. Am J Med. 1975;59:29.
243. Reyes MP, Palutke WA, Wylin RF, et al. *Pseudomonas* endocarditis in the Detroit Medical Center 1969–1972. Medicine (Baltimore). 1973;52:173.
244. Jurica JV, Bomzer CA, England AC III. Gonococcal endocarditis: A case report and review of the literature. Sex Trans Dis. 1987;14:231–3.
245. Dover D, Danzinger Y, Pinkhaus J. *Neisseria catarrhalis* endocarditis. Ann Intern Med. 1977;86:116.
246. Davis CL, Towns M, Henrich WL, et al. *Neisseria mucosus* endocarditis following durg abuse. Case report and review of the literature. Arch Intern Med. 1983;143:583.
247. Chunn CJ, Jones SR, McCutchan JA, et al. *Haemophilus parainfluenzae* infective endocarditis. Medicine (Baltimore). 1977;56:99.
248. Lynn DJ, Kane JG, Parker RH. *Haemophilus parainfluenzae* and influenzae endocarditis: A review of forty cases. Medicine (Baltimore). 1977;56:115.
249. Geraci JE, Wilkowske CJ, Wilson WR, et al. *Haemophilus* endocarditis. Report of 14 cases. Mayo Clin Proc. 1977;52:209.
250. Parker SW, Apicella MA, Fuller CM. *Hemophilus* endocarditis. Two patients with complications. Arch Intern Med. 1983;143:48.
251. Bangsborg JM, Tuede M, Skinhoj P. *Haemophilus seguis* endocarditis. J Infect. 1988;16:81–5.
252. Porath A, Wanderman K, Simu A, et al. Case report: Endocarditis caused by *Haemophilus aegyptius*. Am J Med Sci. 1986;292:110–11.
253. Vandepitte J, DeGeest H, Jousten P. Subacute bacterial endocarditis due to *Actinobacillus actinomycetemcomitans*. Report of a case with a review of the literature. J Clin Pathol. 1977;30:842.
254. AhFat LNC, Patel BR, Pickens S. *Actinobacillus actinomycetemcomitans* endocarditis in hypertrophic obstructive cardiomyopathy. J Infect Dis. 1983;6:81.
255. Lane T, MacGregor RR, Wright D, et al. *Cardiobacterium hominis:* An elusive cause of endocarditis. J Infect. 1983;6:75.
256. Jenny DB, Letendre PW, Iverson G. Endocarditis due to *Kingella* species. Rev Infect Dis. 1988;10:1065–6.
257. Decker MD, Graham BS, Hunter EB, et al. Endocarditis and infections of intravascular devices due to *Eikinella corrodens*. Am J Med Sci. 1986;292:209–12.
258. Ellner JJ, Rosenthal MS, Lerner PI, et al. Infective endocarditis caused by slow-growing, fastidious, gram-negative bacteria. Medicine (Baltimore). 1979;58:145.
259. Gerry JL, Greenough WB. Diptheroid endocarditis: Report of nine cases and review of the literature. Johns Hopkins Med J. 1976;139:61.
260. Bayer AS, Chow AW, Guze LB. *Listeria monocytogenes* endocarditis: Report of a case and review of the literature. Am J Med Sci. 1977; 273:319.
261. Carvajal A, Frederiksen W. Fatal endocarditis due to *Listeria monocytogenes*. Rev Infect Dis. 1988;10:616–23.
262. Sussman JI, Baron EJ, Goldberg SM, et al. Clinical manifestations and therapy of *Lactobacillus* endocarditis: Report of a case and review of the literature. Rev Infect Dis. 1986;8:771–6.
263. Gorby GL, Peacock JE Jr. *Erysipelothrix rhusiopathiae* endocarditis: Microbiologic, epidemiologic, and clinical features of an occupational disease. Rev Infect Dis. 1988;10:317–25.
264. Shands JW Jr. *Rothia dentocariosa* endocarditis. Am J Med. 1988;85:280–1.
265. Felner JM, Dowell UR. Anaerobic bacterial endocarditis. N Engl J Med. 1970;283:1188.
266. Nastro LJ, Finegold SM. Endocarditis due to anaerobic gram-negative bacilli. Am J Med. 1973;54:482.
267. Nastro FL, Sarma RJ. Infective endocarditis due to anaerobic and microaerophilic bacteria. West J Med. 1982;137:18.
268. Jackson RT, Dopp AC. *Bacteroides fragilis* endocarditis. South Med J. 1988;81:781–2.
269. Al-Kasab S, Fagih MR, Al-Yousef S, et al. *Brucella* infective endocarditis. Successful combined medical and surgical therapy. J Thorac Cardiovasc Surg. 1988;95:862–7.
270. Tuazon CW, Hill R, Sheagren JW. Microbiologic study of street heroin and injection paraphenalia. J Infect Dis. 1974;129:327.
271. Tuazon CW, Sheagren JW. Increased rate of carriage of *Staphylococcus aureus* among narcotic addicts. J Infect Dis. 1974;129:725.

272. Reisberg BE. Infective endocarditis in the narcotic addict. Prog Cardiovasc Dis. 1979;22:193.
273. Baddour LM. Twelve-year review of recurrent native-valve infective endocarditis: A disease of the modern antibiotic era. Rev Infect Dis. 1988;10:1163–70.
274. Rubenstein E, Noreiga ER, Simberkoff MS, et al. Tissue penetration of amphotericin B in *Candida* endocarditis. Chest. 1974;66:376.
275. Carrizosa J, Levison ME, Lawrence T, et al. Cure of *Aspergillus ustus* endocarditis of prosthetic valve. Arch Intern Med. 1974;133:486.
276. McIntosh CS, Nickers PJ, Isaqacs AJ. *Spirillum* endocarditis. Postgrad Med J. 1975;51:645.
277. Applefield MM, Billingsley LJ, Tucker HJ, et al. Q fever endocarditis—a case occurring in the United States. Am Heart J. 1977;93:669.
278. Tobin MJ, Cahill N, Gearty G, et al. Q fever endocarditis. Am J Med. 1982;72:396.
279. Fernandez-Guerrero ML, Muelas JM, Aquado JM. Q fever endocarditis on porcine bioprosthetic valves. Ann Intern Med. 1988;108:209–13.
280. Jones RB, Priest JB, Kuo C-C. Subacute chlamydial endocarditis. JAMA. 1982;247:655.
281. Brearley BF, Hutchinson DN. Endocarditis associated with *Chlamydia trachomatis* infection. Br Heart J. 1981;46:220.
282. Popat K, Barnardo D, Webb-Peploe M. *Mycoplasma pneumoniae* endocarditis. Br Heart J. 1980;44:111.
283. Burch GE, Tsui CY. Evolution of coxsackie viral valvular and mural endocarditis in mice. Br J Exp Pathol. 1971;52:360.
284. Persand V. Two unusual cases of mural endocarditis with a review of the literature. Am J Clin Pathol. 1970;53:832.
285. Van Scoy RE. Culture-negative endocarditis. Mayo Clin Proc. 1982;57:149.
286. Pesanti EL, Smith IM. Infective endocarditis with negative blood cultures. An analysis of 52 cases. Am J Med. 1979;66:43.
287. Daschner FD, Frank V. Antimicrobial drugs in human cardiac valves and endocarditis lesions. J Antimicrob Chemother. 1988;12:776–82.
288. Spokojny AM, Sinclair IN, Schnitt S, et al. Uptake of hematoporphyrin derivative by valvular vegetations in experimental infective endocarditis. Circulation 1985;72:1087–91.
289. Dall L, Barnes WG, Lane JW, et al. Enzymatic modification of glycocalyx in the treatment of experimental endocarditis due to viridans streptococci. J Infect Dis. 1987;156:736–40.
290. Buiting AGM, Thompson J, Emeis JJ, et al. Effects of tissue-type plasminogen activator on *Staphylococcus epidermidis*–infected plasma clots as a model of infected endocardial vegetations. J Antimicrob Chemother. 1987;19:771–80.
291. Buiting AG, Thompson J, Emeis JJ, et al. Effects of tissue-type plasminogen activator (t-PA) on *Streptococcus sanguis*–infected endocardial vegetations in vitro. J Antimicrob Chemother. 1988;21:609–20.
292. Cates JE, Christie RV. Subacute bacterial endocarditis. Q J Med. 1951;20:93.
293. Carrizosa J, Kobasa WD, Kaye D. Antagonism between chloramphenicol and penicillin in streptococcal endocarditis in rabbits. J Lab Clin Med. 1975;85:307.
294. Douglas A, Moore-Gillon J, Eykyn S. Fever during treatment of infective endocarditis. Lancet. 1986;1:1341–3.
295. Schlicter JG, MacIlean H. A method of determining the effective therapeutic level in the treatment of subacute bacterial endocarditis with penicillin. Am Heart J. 1947;34:209.
296. Coleman DL, Horwitz RI, Andriole VT. Association between serum inhibitory and bactericidal concentrations and therapeutic outcome in bacterial endocarditis. Am J Med. 1982;73:260.
297. Mellors JW, Coleman DL, Andriole VT. Value of serum bactericidal test in management of patients with bacterial endocarditis. Eur J Clin Microbiol. 1986;5:67–70.
298. Rahal JJ, Chan Y-K, Johnson G. Relationship of staphylococcal tolerance, teichoic acid antibody, and serum bactericidal activity to therapeutic outcome in *Staphylococcus aureus* bacteremia. Am J Med. 1986; 81:43–52.
299. Wolfson JS, Swartz MN. Serum bactericidal activity as a monitor of antibiotic therapy. N Engl J Med. 1985;312:968–75.
300. Reller LB. The serum bactericidal test. Rev Infect Dis. 1986;8:803–8.
301. Weinstein MP, Stratton CW, Ackley A, et al. Multicenter collaborative evaluation of a standardized serum bactericidal test as a prognostic indicator in infective endocarditis. Am J Med. 1985;78:262–9.
302. Stratton CW. The role of the microbiology laboratory in the treatment of infective endocarditis. J Antimicrob Chemother. 1987;20(Suppl A):41–9.
303. Sande MA, Scheld WM. Combination antibiotic therapy of bacterial endocarditis. Ann Intern Med. 1980;92:390.
304. Meylan PR, Francioloi P, Glauser MP. Discrepancies between MBC and actual killing by viridans group streptococci by cell-wall-active antibiotics. Antimicrob Agents Chemother. 1986;29:418–23.
305. Holloway Y, Pankert J, Hess J. Penicillin tolerance and bacterial endocarditis. Lancet. 1980;1:589.
306. Pulliam L, Inokuchi S, Hadley WK, et al. Penicillin tolerance in experimental streptococcal endocarditis. Lancet. 1979;2:957.
307. Gephart JF, Washington JA II. Antimicrobial susceptibilities of nutritionally variant streptococci. J Infect Dis. 1982;146:536.
308. Holloway Y, Dankert J. Penicillin tolerance in nutritionally variant streptococci. Antimicrob Agents Chemother. 1982;22:1073.
309. Lowry FD, Neuhas EG, Chang DS, et al. Penicillin therapy of experimental endocarditis caused by tolerant *Streptococcus sanguis* and nontolerant *Streptococcus mitis*. Antimicrob Agents Chemother. 1983;23:67.
310. Brennan RO, Durack DT. Therapeutic significance of penicillin tolerance in experimental streptococcal endocarditis. Antimicrob Agents Chemother. 1983;23:273.
311. Baker CW, Thornsberry C. Antimicrobial susceptibility of *Streptococcus mutans* isolated from patients with endocarditis. Antimicrob Agents Chemother. 1974;5:268.
312. Thornsberry C, Baker CN, Facklam RR. Antibiotic susceptibility of *Streptococcus bovis* and other group D streptococci causing endocarditis. Antimicrob Agents Chemother. 1974;5:228.
313. Wolfe JC, Johnson WD. Penicillin-sensitive streptococcal endocarditis. In vitro and clinical observations on penicillin-streptomycin therapy. Ann Intern Med. 1974;81:178.
314. Watanakunakorn C, Glotzbecker C. Synergism with aminoglycosides of penicillin, ampicillin, and vancomycin against nonenterococcal group D streptococci and viridans streptococci. J Med Microbiol. 1977;10:133.
315. Enzler MJ, Rouse MS, Henry NK, et al. In vitro and in vivo studies of streptomycin-resistant, penicillin-susceptible streptococci from patients with infective endocarditis. J Infect Dis. 1987;155:954–8.
316. Farber BF, Yee Y. High-level aminoglycoside resistance mediated by aminoglycoside-modifying enzymes among viridans streptococci: Implications for the therapy of endocarditis. J Infect Dis. 1987;155:948–53.
317. Sande MA, Irvin RG. Penicillin-aminoglycoside synergy in experimental *Streptococcus viridans* endocarditis. J Infect Dis. 1974;129:572.
318. Durack DT, Pelletier LL, Petersdorf RG. Chemotherapy of experimental streptococcal endocarditis. II. Synergism between penicillin and streptomycin against penicillin-sensitive streptococci. J Clin Invest. 1974; 53:929.
319. Drake TA, Sande MA. Studies of the chemotherapy of endocarditis: Correlation of in vitro, animal model, and clinical studies. Rev Infect Dis. 1983;5(Suppl):345.
320. Wilson WR, Geraci JE. Treatment of streptococcal infective endocarditis. Am J Med. 1985;78(Suppl 6B):128–137.
321. Scheld WM. Therapy of streptococcal endocarditis: Correlation of animal model and clinical studies. J Antimicrob Chemother. 1987;20(Suppl A):71–85.
322. Wilson WR, Geraci JE, Wilkowske CJ, et al. Short-term intramuscular therapy with procaine penicillin plus streptomycin for infective endocarditis due to viridans streptococci. Circulation. 1978;57:1158.
323. Wilson WR, Thompson RL, Wilkowske CJ, et al. Short-term therapy for streptococcal infective endocarditis. Combined intramuscular administration of penicillin and streptomycin. JAMA. 1981;245:360.
324. Karchmer AW, Mollering RC Jr, Maki DG, et al. Single antibiotic therapy for streptococcal endocarditis. JAMA. 1979;241:1801.
325. Malacoff RF, Frank E, Andriole VT. Streptococcal endocarditis (nonenterococcal, non-group A). Single vs. combination therapy. JAMA. 1979; 241:1807.
326. Parillo JE, Borst GC, Mazur MH, et al. Endocarditis due to resistant viridans streptococci during oral penicillin chemoprophylaxis. N Engl J Med. 1979;300:296.
327. Bisno AL, Dismukes WE, Durack DT, et al. Antimicrobial treatment of infective endocarditis due to viridans streptococci, enterococci, and staphylococci. JAMA. 1989;261:1471–7.
328. Bouvet A, Cremieux AC, Contrepois A, et al. Comparison of penicillin and vancomycin, individually and in combination with gentamicin and amikacin, in the treatment of experimental endocarditis induced by nutritionally variant steptococci. Antimicrob Agents Chemother. 1985;28:607–11.
329. Henry NK, Wilson WR, Roberts RB, et al. Antimicrobial therapy of experimental endocarditis caused by nutritionally variant viridans group streptococci. Antimicrob Agents Chemother. 1986;30:465–7.
330. Stein DS, Nelson KE. Endocarditis due to nutritionally deficient streptococci: Therapeutic dilemma. Rev Infect Dis. 1987;9:908–16.
331. Watanakunakorn C. Penicillin combined with gentamicin or streptomycin: Synergism against enterococci. J Infect Dis. 1971;124:581.
332. Moellering RC Jr, Korzeniowski OM, Sande MA, et al. Species-specific resistance to antimicrobial synergism in *Streptococcus faecium* and *Streptococcus faecalis*. J Infect Dis. 1979;140:203.
333. Krogstad DJ, Parquette AR. Defective killing of enterococci: A common property of antimicrobial agents acting on the cell wall. Antimicrob Agents Chemother. 1980;17:965.
334. Storch GA, Krogstad DA, Parquette AR. Antibiotic-induced lysis of enterococci. J Clin Invest. 1981;68:639.
335. Murray BE, Church DA, Wanger A, et al. Comparison of two β-lactamase–producing strains of *Streptococcus faecalis*. Antimicrob Agents Chemother. 1986;30:861–4.
336. Ingerman M, Pitsakis PG, Rosenberg A, et al. β-Lactamase production in experimental endocarditis due to aminoglycoside-resistant *Streptococcus faecalis*. J Infect Dis. 1987;155:1226–32.
337. Henry NK, Wilson WR, Geraci JE. Treatment of streptomycin-susceptible enterococcal experimental endocarditis with combinations of penicillin and low- or high-dose streptomycin. Antimicrob Agents Chemother. 1986;30:725–8.
338. Harwick HJ, Kalmanson GM, Guze LB. In vitro activity of ampicillin or vancomycin combined with gentamicin or streptomycin against enterococci. Antimicrob Agents Chemother. 1973;4:383.

339. Weinstein AJ, Moellering RC. Penicillin and gentamicin therapy for enterococcal infections. JAMA. 1973;223:1030.
340. Moellering RC, Wennersten C, Weinberg AW. Synergy of penicillin and gentamicin against enterococci. J Infect Dis. 1971;124(Suppl):207.
391. Hook EW III, Roberts RB, Sande MA. Antimicrobial therapy of experimental enterococcal endocarditis. Antimicrob Agents Chemother. 1975;8:564.
392. Wright AJ, Wilson WR, Matsumoto JY, et al. Influence of gentamicin dose size on the efficacies of combinations of gentamicin and penicillin in experimental streptomycin-resistant enterococcal endocarditis. Antimicrob Agents Chemother. 1982;22:972.
343. Murray BE, Tsao J, Panida J. Enterococci from Bangkok, Thailand, with high-level resistance to currently available aminoglycosides. Antimicrob Agents Chemother. 1983;23:799.
344. Mederski-Samoraj BD, Murray BE. High-level resistance to gentamicin in clinical isolates of enterococci. J Infect Dis. 1983;147:751.
345. Zervos MJ, Dembinski S, Mikesell T, et al. High-level resistance to gentamicin in *Streptococcus faecalis:* Risk factors and evidence for exogenous acquisition of infection. J Infect Dis. 1986;153:1075–83.
346. Zervos MJ, Terpenning MS, Schaberg DR, et al. High-level aminoglycoside-resistant enterococci. Arch Intern Med. 1987;147:1591–4.
347. Eliopoulos GM, Wennersten C, Zighelboim-Daum S, et al. High-level resistance to gentamicin in clinical isolates of *Streptococcus* (*Enterococcus*) *faecium*. Antimicrob Agents Chemother. 1988;32:1528–32.
348. Fernandez-Guerrero ML, Barros C, Rodriquez Tudela JL, et al. Aortic endocarditis caused by genamicin-resistant *Enterococcus faecalis*. Eur J Clin Microbiol. 1988;7:525–7.
349. Watanakunakorn C, Bakie C. Synergism of vancomycin-gentamicin and vancomycin-streptomycin against enterococci. Antimicrob Agents Chemother. 1973;4:120.
350. Watanakunakorn C, Tisone JC. Effects of a vancomycin-rifampin combination on enterococci. Antimicrob Agents Chemother. 1982;22:915.
351. Uttley AH, Collins CH, Naidoo J, et al. Vancomycin-resistant enterococci. Lancet. 1988;1:57–8.
352. Leclercq R, Derlot E, Dural J, et al. Plasmid-mediated resistance to vancomycin and teichoplanin in *Enterococcus faecium.* N Engl J Med. 1988;319:157–61.
353. Fernandez-Guerrero M, Rouse MS, Henry NK, et al. In vitro and in vivo activity of ciprofloxacin against enterococci isolated from patients with infective endocarditis. Antimicrob Agents Chemother. 1987;31:430–3.
354. Bush LM, Boscia JA, Kaye D. Daptomycin (LY146032) treatment of experimental enterococcal endocarditis. Antimicrob Agents Chemother. 1988;32:877–81.
355. Wilson WR, Wilkowski CJ, Wright AJ, et al. Treatment of streptomycin-susceptible and streptomycin-resistant enterococcal endocarditis. Ann Intern Med. 1984;100:816–23.
356. Karchmer AW. Staphylococcal endocarditis. Laboratory and clinical basis for antibiotic therapy. Am J Med. 1985;78(Suppl B):116–27.
357. Sande MA, Courtney KB. Nafcillin-gentamicin synergism in experimental staphylococcal endocarditis. J Lab Clin Med. 1976;88:118.
358. Abrams B, Sklaver A, Hoffman T, et al. Single or combination therapy of staphylococcal endocarditis in intravenous drug abusers. Ann Intern Med. 1979;90:789.
359. Chambers HF, Miller RT, Newman MD. Right-sided *Staphylococcus aureus* endocarditis in intravenous drug abusers: Two week combination therapy. Ann Intern Med. 1988;109:619–24.
360. Murray HW, Wigley FM, Mann JJ, et al. Combination antibiotic therapy in staphylococcal endocarditis: The use of methicillin sodium–gentamicin sulfate therapy. Arch Intern Med. 1976;136:480.
361. Korzeniowski OM, Sande MA, The National Collaborative Endocarditis Study Group. Combination antimicrobial therapy for *Staphylococcus aureus* endocarditis in patients addicted to parenteral drugs and in nonaddicts. A prospective study. Ann Intern Med. 1982;97:496.
362. Craven DE, Kollisch MR, Hsieh CR, et al. Vancomycin treatment of bacteremia caused by oxacillin-resistant *Staphylococcus aureus:* Comparison with β-lactam antibiotic treatment of bacteremia caused by oxacillin-sensitive *Staphylococcus aureus*. J Infect Dis. 1983;147:137.
363. Watanakunakorn C. Clindamycin therapy of *Staphylococcus aureus* endocarditis. Clinical relapse and development of resistance to clindamycin, lincomycin, and erythromycin. Am J Med. 1976;60:419.
364. Kaye D. The clinical significance of tolerance of *Staphylococcus aureus*. Ann Intern Med. 1980;93:924.
365. Jackson MA, Hicks RA. Vancomycin failure in staphylococcal endocarditis. Pediatr Infect Dis J. 1987;6:750–2.
366. Rajashekaraiah KR, Rice T, Rao VS, et al. Clinical significance of tolerant strains of *Staphylococcus aureus* in patients with endocarditis. Ann Intern Med. 1980;93:796.
367. Zak O, Scheld WM, Sande MA. Rifampin in experimental endocarditis due to *Staphylococcus aureus* in rabbits. Rev Infect Dis. 1983;5(Suppl):481.
368. Fernandez-Guerrero M, Rouse M, Henry N, et al. Ciprofloxacin therapy of experimental endocarditis caused by methicillin-susceptible or methicillin-resistant *Staphylococcus aureus*. Antimicrob Agents Chemother. 1988;32:747–51.
369. Iannini PB, Crossley K. Therapy of *Staphylococcus aureus* bacteremia associated with a removable focus of infection. Ann Intern Med. 1976;84:558.
370. Watanakunakorn C, Baird IM. *Staphylococcus aureus* bacteremia and endocarditis associated with a removable infected intravenous device. Am J Med. 1977;63:253.
371. Bayer AS, Lam K, Ginzton L, *Staphylococcus aureus* bacteremia. Clinical, serologic, and echocardiographic findings in patients with and without endocarditis. Arch Intern Med. 1987;147:757–62.
372. Karchmer AW, Archer GL, Dismukes WE. *Staphylococcus epidermidis* causing prosthetic valve endocarditis: Microbiologic and clinical observations as guides to therapy. Ann Intern Med. 1983;98:447.
373. Schwalbe RS, Stapleton JT, Gilligan PH. Emergence of vancomycin resistance in coagulase-negative staphylococci. N Engl J Med. 1987;316:927–31.
374. Joly V, Parigon B, Vallois J-M, et al. Value of antibiotic levels in serum and cardiac vegetations for predicting antibacterial effect of ceftriaxone in experimental *Escherichia coli* endocarditis. Antimicrob Agents Chemother. 1987;31:1632–9.
375. Hughes CF, Noble N. Vegetectomy: An alternative surgical treatment for infective endocarditis of the atrioventricular valves in drug addicts. J Thorac Cardiovasc Surg. 1988;95:857–61.
376. Arbulu A, Thomas NW, Chiscano A, et al. Total tricuspid valvulectomy without replacement in the treatment of *Pseudomonas* endocarditis. Surg Forum. 1971;22:162.
377. Mammana RB, Levitsky S, Sernaque D, et al. Valve replacement for left-sided endocarditis in drug addicts. Ann Thorac Surg. 1983;35:436.
378. Bayer AS, Crowell DJ, Yih J, et al. Comparative pharmacokinetics and pharmacodynamics of amikacin and ceftazidine in tricuspid and aortic vegetations in experimental *Pseudomonas* endocarditis. J Infect Dis. 1988;158:355–9.
379. Bayer AS, Hirano L, Yih J. Development of β-lactam resistance and increased quinolone MIC's during therapy of experimental *Pseudomonas aeruginosa* endocarditis. Antimicrob Agents Chemother. 1988;32:231–5.
380. Parr TR Jr, Bayer AS. Mechanisms of aminoglycoside resistance in variants of *Pseudomonas aeruginosa* isolated during treatment of experimental endocarditis in rabbits. J Infect Dis. 1988;158:1003–10.
381. Hessen MT, Pitsakis PG, Levison ME. Absence of a post-antibiotic effect in experimental *Pseudomonas* endocarditis treated with imipenem, with or without gentamicin. J Infect Dis. 1988;158:542–8.
382. Jimenez-Lucho VE, Saravolatz LD, Medeiros AA, et al. Failure of therapy in *Pseudomonas* endocarditis: Selection of resistant mutants. J Infect Dis. 1986;154:64–8.
383. Daikos GL, Kathopalia SB, Lolans VT, et al. Long-term oral ciprofloxacin: Experience in the treatment of incurable infective endocarditis. Am J Med. 1988;84:786–90.
384. Weisner PJ, Handsfield HH, Holmes KK. Low antibiotic resistance of gonococci causing disseminated infection. N Engl J Med. 1973;288:1221.
385. Black JR, Brint JM, Reichart CA. Successful treatment of gonococcal endocarditis with ceftriaxone. J Infect Dis. 1988;157:1281–2.
386. Ernst JD, Rusmak M, Sande MA. Combination antifungal chemotherapy for experimental disseminated candidiasis: Lack of correlation between in vitro and in vivo observations with amphotericin B and rifampin. Rev Infect Dis. 1983;5(Suppl):626.
387. Longman LP, Martin MV. A comparison of the efficacy of intraconazole, amphotericin B and 5-fluorocytosine in the treatment of *Aspergillus fumigatus* endocarditis in the rabbit. J Antimicrob Chemother. 1987;20:719–24.
388. Haldane EV, Marrie TJ, Faulkner RS, et al. Endocarditis due to Q fever in Nova Scotia: Experience with five patients in 1981–1982. J Infect Dis. 1983;148:978–85.
389. Street AC, Durack DT. Experience with trimethoprim-sulfamethoxazole in treatment of infective endocarditis. Rev Infect Dis. 1988;10:915–22.
390. Jones JB, Ridgeway GL, Boulding S, et al. In vitro activity of rifamycins alone and in combination with other antibiotics against *Chlamydia trachomatis*. Rev Infect Dis. 1983;5(Suppl):556.
391. McAnulty JH, Rahimtoola SH. Surgery for infective endocarditis. JAMA. 1979;242:77.
392. Dinubile MJ. Surgery in active endocarditis. Ann Intern Med. 1980;96:650.
393. D'Agostino RS, Miller DC, Stinson EB, et al. Valve replacement in patients with native valve endocarditis: What really determines operative outcome? Ann Thorac Surg. 1985;40:429–38.
394. Wilson WR, Danielson GK, Giuliani ER, et al. Valve replacement in patients with active infective endocarditis. Circulation. 1978;58:585.
395. Arbulu A, Asfaw I. Tricuspid valvulectomy without prosthetic replacement. Ten years of clinical experience. J Thorac Cardiovasc Surg. 1981;82:684.
396. DiNubile M. Surgery for addiction-related tricuspid valve endocarditis: Caveat emptor. Am J Med. 1987;82:811–3.
397. Arbulu A, Asfaw I. Management of infective endocarditis: Seventeen years' experience. Ann Thorac Surg. 1987;43:144–9.
398. Alsip SG, Blackstone EH, Kirklin JW, et al. Indications for cardiac surgery in patients with active infective endocarditis. Am J Med. 1985;78(Suppl 6B):138–48.
399. Neuhof H, Seley GP. Acute suppurative phlebitis complicated by septicemia. Surgery. 1947;21:831.
400. Goldman DA, Maki DG, Rhame FS, et al. Guidelines for infection control in intravenous therapy. Ann Intern Med. 1973;79:848.
401. O'Neill JA, Pruitt BA, Foley FD, et al. Suppurative thrombophlebitis—a lethal complication of intravenous therapy. J Trauma. 1968;8:256.
402. Stein JM, Pruitt BA. Suppurative thrombophlebitis: A lethal iatrogenic disease. N Engl J Med. 1970;282:1452.
403. Pruitt BA, Stein JM, Foley FD, et al. Intravenous therapy in burn patients.

Suppurative thrombophlebitis and other life-threatening complications. Arch Surg. 1970;100:399.
404. Pruitt BA, McManus WF, Kim SH, et al. Diagnosis and treatment of cannularelated intravenous sepsis in burn patients. Ann Surg. 1980;191:546.
405. Garrison RN, Richardson JD, Fry DE. Catheter-associated septic thrombophlebitis. South Med J. 1982;75:917.
406. Sacks-Berg A, Strampfer MJ, Cunha BA. Suppurative thrombophlebitis caused by intravenous line sepsis. Heart Lung. 1987;16:318–20.
407. Munster AM. Septic thrombophlebitis. A surgical disorder. JAMA. 1974;230:1010.
408. Berkowitz FE, Argent AC, Baise T. Suppurative thrombophlebitis: A serious nosocomial infection. Pediatr Infect Dis J. 1987;6:64–7.
409. Johnson RA, Zajac RA, Evans ME. Suppurative thrombophlebitis: Correlation between pathogen and underlying disease. Infect Control. 1986;7:582–5.
410. Rhame FS, Maki DG, Bennett JV. Intravenous cannula-associated infections. In: Bennett JV, Brachman PS, eds. Hospital Infections. Boston: Little, Brown; 1979:433–42.
411. Baker CC, Peterson SR, Sheldon GF. Septic phlebitis: A neglected disease. Am J Surg. 1979;138:97.
412. Sears N, Grosfeld JL, Weber TR, et al. Suppurative thrombophlebitis in childhood. Pediatrics. 1981;68:630.
413. Zinner MJ, Zuidema GD, Lowery BD. Septic nonsuppurative thrombophlebitis. Arch Surg. 1976;111:122.
414. Brismar B, Hardstedt C, Jacobson S. Diagnosis of thrombosis by catheter phlebography after prolonged central venous catheterization. Ann Surg. 1981;194:779–83.
415. Slagle DC, Gates RH Jr. Unusual case of central vein thrombosis and sepsis. Am J Med. 1986;81:351–4.
416. Kaufman J, Demas C, Stark K, et al. Catheter-related septic central venous thrombosis—current therapeutic options. West J Med. 1986;145:200–3.
417. Veghese A, Widrich WC, Arbeit RD. Central venous septic thrombophlebitis—the role of medical therapy. Medicine (Baltimore). 1985;64:394–400.
418. Strinden WD, Helgerson RB, Maki DG. *Candida* septic thrombosis of the great central veins associated with central catheters. Clinical features and management. Ann Surg. 1985;202:653–8.
419. Haddad W, Idowu J, Georgeson K, et al. Septic atrial thrombosis: A potentially lethal complication of Broviac catheters in infants. Am J Dis Child. 1986;140:778–80.
420. Collins CG, MacCallum EA, Nelson EW, et al. Suppurative pelvic thrombophlebitis. I. Incidence, pathology, and etiology. Surgery. 1951;30:298.
421. Josey WE, Staggers SR. Heparin therapy in septic pelvic thrombophlebitis: A study of 46 cases. Am J Obstet Gynecol. 1974;120:228.
422. Collins CG. Suppurative pelvic thrombophlebitis. A study of 202 cases in which the disease was treated by ligation of the vena cava and ovarian vein. Am J Obstet Gynecol. 1970;108:681.
423. Barenholtz L, Kaminsky NI, Palmer DL. Venous intramural microabscesses: A cause of protracted sepsis with intravenous cannulas. Am J Med Sci. 1973;265:335.
424. Jupiter JB, Ehrlich MG, Novelline RA, et al. The association of septic thrombophlebitis with subperiosteal abscesses in children. J Pediatr. 1982;101:690.
425. Maki DG, Weise CE, Sarafin HW. A semiquantitative culture method for identifying intravenous-catheter-related infection. N Engl J Med. 1977;296:1305.
426. Angel JL, Knuppel RA. Computed tomography in diagnosis of puerperal ovarian vein thrombosis. Obstet Gynecol. 1984;63:61–4.
427. Isada NB, Landy HJ, Larson JW Jr. Postabortal septic pelvic thrombophlebitis diagnosed with computed tomography. J Reprod Med. 1987;32:866–8.
428. Martin B, Molopulos GP, Bryan PJ. MRI of puerperal ovarian vein thrombosis. AJR. 1986;147:291–2.
429. Josey WE, Cook CC. Septic pelvic thrombophlebitis. Report of 17 patients treated with heparin. Obstet Gynecol. 1970;35:891.
430. Torres-Rojas JR, Stratton CW, Sanders CV, et al. Candidal suppurative peripheral thrombophlebitis. Ann Intern Med. 1982;96:431.
431. Walsh TJ, Bustamente CI, Vlahov D, et al. Candidal suppurative peripheral thrombophlebitis: Recognition, prevention, and management. Infect Control. 1986;7:16–22.
432. Peterson P, Stahl-Bayliss CM. Cytomegalovirus thrombophlebitis after successful DHPG therapy. Ann Intern Med. 1987;106:632–3.
433. Miller CJ. Ligation and excision of pelvic veins in treatment of puerperal pyaemia. Surg Gynecol Obstet. 1917;25:431.
434. Topiel MS, Bryan RT, Kessler CM, et al. Treatment of Silastic catheter-induced central vein septic thrombophlebitis. Am J Med Sci. 1986;291:425–8.
435. Barg NL, Supena RB, Fekety R. Persistent staphylococcal bacteremia in an intravenous drug abuser. Antimicrob Agents Chemother. 1986;29:209–11.
436. Moran JM, Atwood RP, Rowe MI. A clinical and bacteriologic study of infections associated with venous cutdowns. N Engl J Med. 1965;272:554.
437. Norden CW. Application of antibiotic ointment to the site of venous catheterization—a controlled trial. J Infect Dis. 1969;120:611.
438. Patel S, Johnston KW. Classification and management of mycotic aneurysms. Surg Gynecol Obstet. 1977;144:691.
439. Parkhurst GF, Decker JP. Bacterial aortitis and mycotic aneurysms of the aorta. A report of 12 cases. Am J Pathol. 1955;31:821.
440. Sommerville RL, Allen EV, Edwards JE. Bland and infected arteriosclerotic abdominal aortic aneurysms: A clinicopathologic study. Medicine (Baltimore). 1959;38:207.
441. Stengel A, Wolfroth CC. Mycotic (bacterial) aneurysms of intravascular origin. Arch Intern Med. 1923;31:527.
442. Bennett DE, Cherry JK. Bacterial infection of aortic aneurysms. A clinicopathologic study. Am J Surg. 1967;113:321.
443. Cliff MM, Soulen RL, Firestone AJ. Mycotic aneurysms: A challenge and a clue. Arch Intern Med. 1970;126:977.
444. Jarrett F, Darling C, Mundth ED, et al. Experience with infected aneurysms of the abdominal aorta. Arch Surg. 1975;110:1281.
445. Bohmfalk GL, Story JL, Wissenger JP, et al. Bacterial intracranial aneurysm. J Neurosurg. 1978;48:369.
446. Frazee JG, Cahan LD, Winter J. Bacterial intracranial aneurysms. J Neurosurg. 1980;53:633.
447. Bullock R, Van Dellen JR, Van den Heever CM. Intracranial mycotic aneurysms. A review of 9 cases. S Afr Med J. 1981;60:970.
448. Jarrett F, Darling RC, Mundth ED, et al. The management of infected arterial aneurysms. J Cardiovasc Surg. 1977;18:361.
449. Johnson JR, Ledgerwood AM, Lucas CE. Mycotic aneurysm. New concepts in therapy. Arch Surg. 1983;118:577.
450. Feigl D, Feigl A, Edwards JE. Mycotic aneurysms of the aortic root. A pathologic study of 20 cases. Chest. 1986;90:553–7.
451. Dean RH, Mecham PW, Weaver FA, et al. Mycotic embolism and embolomycotic aneurysms. Neglected lessons of the past. Ann Surg. 1986;204:300–7.
452. Sedwitz MM, Hye RJ, Stabile BE. The changing epidemiology of pseudoaneurysm. Therapeutic implications. Arch Surg. 1988;123:473–6.
453. Kyriakides GK, Simmons RL, Najarian JS. Mycotic aneurysms in transplant patients. Arch Surg. 1976;111:472.
454. Smith EJ, Milligan SL, Filo RS. *Salmonella* mycotic aneurysms after renal transplantation. South Med J. 1981;74:1399.
455. Olmsted WW, McGee TP. The pathogenesis of peripheral aneurysms of the central nervous system: A subject review from the AFIP. Radiology. 1977;123:661.
456. Salgado AV, Furlan AJ, Keys TF. Mycotic aneurysm, Subarachnoid hemorrhage, and indications for cerebral angiography in infective endocarditis. Stroke. 1987;18:1057–60.
457. Friedman SG, Pogo GJ, Moccio CG. Mycotic aneurysm of the superior mesenteric artery. J Vasc Surg. 1987;6:87–90.
458. Sukerkar AN, Dulay CC, Anandappa E, et al. Mycotic aneurysm of the hepatic artery. Radiology. 1977;124:444.
459. Feinsod FM, Norfleet RG, Hoehn JL. Mycotic aneurysm of the external iliac artery. A triad of clinical signs facilitating early diagnosis. JAMA. 1977;238:245.
460. Merry M, Dunn J, Weissmann R, et al. Popliteal mycotic aneurysm presenting as septic arthritis and purpura. JAMA. 1972;221:58.
461. Plate G, Forsley N, Stigsson L, et al. Management of inflammatory abdominal aortic aneurysm. Acta Chir Scand. 1988;154:19–24.
462. Pennell RC, Hollier LH, Lie JT, et al. Inflammatory abdominal aortic aneurysms: A thirty year review. J Vasc Surg. 1985;2:859–69.
463. Morrow C, Safi H, Beall AC Jr. Primary aortoduodenal fistula caused by *Salmonella* aortitis. J Vasc Surg. 1987;6:415–8.
464. Vogelzang RL, Sohaey R. Infected aortic aneurysms: CT appearance. J Comput Assist Tomogr. 1988;12:109–12.
465. Rivera JV, Blanco G, Perez M, et al. Gallium-67 localization in a mycotic aneurysm of the thoracic aorta. Clin Nucl Med. 1985;10:814–6.
466. Brewster DC, Retana A, Waltman AC, et al. Angiography in the management of aneurysms of the abdominal aorta. N Engl J Med. 1972;292:822.
467. Griffiths BE, Petch MC, English TAH. Echocardiographic detection of subvalvular aortic root aneurysm extending to mitral valve annulus as complication of aortic valve endocarditis. Br Heart J. 1982;47:392.
468. Kanwar YS, Malhotra U, Anderson BR, et al. Salmonellosis associated with abdominal aortic aneurysm. Arch Intern Med. 1974;134:1095.
469. Cohen JI, Bartlett JA, Corey GR. Extra-intestinal manifestations of *Salmonella* infections. Medicine (Baltimore). 1987;66:349–88.
470. Cohen OS, O'Brien TF, Schoenbaum SC, et al. The risk of endothelial infection in adults with *Salmonella* bacteremia. Ann Intern Med. 1978;89:931.
471. McIntyre KE Jr, Malone JM, Richards E. Mycotic aortic pseudoaneurysm with aortoenteric fistula caused by *Arizona hinshawii*. Surgery. 1982;91:173.
472. Anolik JR, Mildvan D, Winter JW, et al. Mycotic aortic aneurysm. A complication of *Campylobacter fetus* septicemia. Arch Intern Med. 1983;143:609.
473. Mielke B, Weir B, Oldring D, et al. Fungal aneurysm: Case report and review of the literature. Neurosurgery. 1981;9:578.
474. Hadley MN, Martin NA, Spetzler RF, et al. Multiple intracranial aneurysms due to *Coccidioides immitis* infection. J Neurosurg. 1987;66:453–6.
475. Bingham WF: Treatment of mycotic intracranial aneurysms. J Neurosurg. 1977;46:428.
476. Leipzig MJ, Brown FD. Treatment of mycotic aneurysms. Surg Neurol. 1985;23:403–7.
477. Rodesch G, Noterman J, Thys JP, et al. Treatment of intracranial mycotic aneurysm: Surgery or not. Acta Neurochir. 1987;85:63–8.
478. Reddy DJ, Smith RF, Elliott JP Jr, et al. Infected femoral artery false aneurysms in drug addicts: Evolution of selective vascular reconstruction. J Vasc Surg. 1986;3:718–24.
479. Johansen K, Devin J. Mycotic aortic aneurysms. A reappraisal. Arch Surg. 1983;118:583.

480. Parsons R, Gregory J, Palmer DL. *Salmonella* infections of the abdominal aorta. Rev Infect Dis. 1983;5:227.
481. Bitseff EJ, Edwards WH, Mulherin JL Jr, et al. Infected abdominal aortic aneurysms. South Med J. 1987;80:309–12.
482. Taylor LM Jr, Deitz DM, McConnell DB, et al. Treatment of infected abdominal aneurysms by extra anatomic bypass, aneurysm excision, and drainage. Am J Surg. 1988;155:655–8.
483. Sande MA, Strausbaugh LJ. Infective endocarditis. In: Hook EW, Mandell GL, Gwaltney JM Jr, Sande MA, eds. Current Concepts of Infectious Diseases. New York: John Wiley & Sons; 1977;55–68.

62. INFECTIOUS DISORDERS OF PROSTHETIC VALVES AND INTRAVASCULAR DEVICES

MICHAEL G. THRELKELD
C. GLENN COBBS

PROSTHETIC VALVE ENDOCARDITIS

Infection of the intracardiac prosthesis is a serious complication of valve replacement surgery. The intravascular foreign body is inherently more susceptible to bacterial colonization than is native valve tissue, and established infection on a prosthetic device is often difficult to eradicate. Although clinical outcome has improved during the past decade, prosthetic valve endocarditis (PVE) remains a significant cause of morbidity and mortality.

Epidemiology

Early and Late Prosthetic Valve Endocarditis. By convention, PVE occurring within 60 days of valve insertion has been termed "early PVE" and endocarditis occurring more than 60 days after valve replacement, "late PVE." However, illness characteristic of early disease may not always become apparent until 6 months or more after the operation. Some investigators have therefore recommended that the time limit for early disease be extended to 6 months or even 1 year.[1,2]

Incidence. A number of authors have described their experiences with PVE during the past two decades.[1–22] Among 25,923 patients undergoing valve replacement, 740 episodes of PVE were observed (an incidence of 2.9 percent). If one uses the traditional 60-day time limit, approximately 37 percent of reported episodes represented "early PVE," while 63 percent were "late PVE." Of the 459 patients identified by sex, 64 percent were male.

Valves in the aortic position were once believed to be more susceptible to infection than are valves in the mitral position. However, more recent studies have failed to confirm this finding.[21] Of 603 reported cases of PVE, 55 percent involved an aortic prosthesis; 32 percent, a mitral prosthesis; and 12 percent, other valves or combinations of valves.[3,4,6–14,18,19,21,22] These differences presumably reflect the frequency of surgery at the different sites.

Types of Prostheses Involved. There are currently more than two dozen varieties of artificial valves in use.[23] They can be classified as mechanical valves (including ball valves, disk valves, hinged leaflet valves, and tilting disk valves) and bioprosthetic tissue valves (including homografts and porcine heterografts). Based on data from several recent series, the incidence of PVE in patients receiving porcine heterografts is 3.1 percent, and the incidence for mechanical valve recipients is 3.8 percent.[2,19,20]

Microorganisms Responsible. Table 1 lists the microbial etiology of PVE in 272 patients with early infection and 429 patients with late.[4–7,13,19,21,22,24] The most common etiologic microorganism was *Staphylococcus epidermidis,* which accounted for 29 percent of episodes. Viridans streptococci accounted for 17 percent and *Staphylococcus aureus* for 14 percent. These frequencies vary substantially from those seen in native valve endocarditis (NVE), in which the viridans streptococci and *S. aureus* account for approximately 50 and 20 percent of episodes, respectively. Aerobic gram-negative bacilli and fungi (especially *Candida* sp. and *Aspergillus* sp.), uncommon in NVE, are important causes of early PVE.

Diphtheroids, a term used to describe corynebacteria other than *Corynebacterium diphtheriae,* are important causes of early PVE.[25] Recognition of their role in PVE has served to emphasize the pathologic potential of these usually avirulent bacteria. Group JK corynebacteria, in particular, are important pathogens of prosthetic devices. A wide variety of other bacterial and fungal species has been reported in individual patients with PVE.

Pathogenesis of Early Prosthetic Valve Endocarditis

Staphylococcus epidermidis is the most common cause of early PVE. Of 16 patients with *S. epidermidis* PVE seen at one center, 11 became ill within 6 months of surgery, with a median time of onset of 2 months.[2] These data suggest that *S. epidermidis* PVE may result from valve contamination occurring in the perioperative period. Several studies have emphasized the potential role of intraoperative contamination in the pathogenesis of early PVE. Kluge et al.[26] during an investigation of microbial contamination occurring during open heart surgery found tissue surfaces and the valvular prostheses to be the most common sites from which microorganisms could be recovered. An important observation was the frequent recovery of *S. epidermidis* and diphtheroids, presumably shed from the skin of the patient or operating room personnel. Another possible mode of contamination was suggested by Blakemore et al.,[27] who found bacteria contaminating blood in the bypass pump. Identical microorganisms were isolated from the air in the operating room, which suggests that suctioning devices used in the operative field inoculated microorganisms into the blood.

TABLE 1. Microorganisms Responsible for Prosthetic Valve Endocarditis

Organism	*Early PVE*[a] *(%)*	*Late PVE (%)*	*Overall (%)*
Staphylococci			
S. epidermidis	35	26	29
S. aureus	17	12	14
Streptococci			
Group D streptococci (including enterococci)	3	9	7
S. pneumoniae	1	<1	1
Other (including viridans streptococci)	4	25	17
Gram-negative bacilli	16	12	13
Diphtheroids	10	4	7
Other bacteria	1	2	2
Candida	8	4	5
Aspergillus	2	1	1
Other fungi	1	<1	1
Culture-negative	1	4	3
Total number			
Microorganisms	292	445	737
Patients	272	429	701

[a] Occurring less than 2 months after surgery.
(Data from Refs. 4–7, 13, 19, 21, 22, and 24.)

In the immediate postoperative period, the prosthetic valve and sewing ring are not yet endothelialized and are apparently quite susceptible to microbial colonization. Bacteria or fungi originating from infected intravascular catheters, cardiac pacemakers, or pressure monitoring devices may seed the prosthesis. One study of patients undergoing open heart surgery demonstrated that 29 percent of intravenous catheters were contaminated.[28] This rate was reduced to 12 percent when catheters were removed sooner. Another study suggested that *S. epidermidis* is readily introduced into the blood stream during thermodilution cardiac output determinations unless careful aseptic technique is practiced.[29] Bacteremia may also result from postoperative infections at extracardiac sites. Dismukes et al.[3] noted pneumonia, wound infection, or contaminated intravascular catheters in 12 patients who subsequently developed early PVE. Another potential (but uncommon) source of infection is contamination of the prosthesis before implantation such as the contamination of glutaraldehyde-fixed porcine prosthetic valves by *Mycobacterium chelonae*.[30,31]

Pathogenesis of Late Prosthetic Valve Endocarditis

The pathogenesis of late PVE appears similar to that of NVE, with microorganisms from a source of transient bacteremia localizing on a prosthesis or area of damaged endocardium. This is reflected in the much higher incidence of infection due to viridans streptococci in late disease. Late PVE caused by *S. epidermidis* or other organisms that typically cause early PVE may result from a delayed onset of the infection acquired in the perioperative period.

Pathology of Prosthetic Valve Endocarditis

Valve ring abscess is a serious complication of PVE in both mechanical and bioprosthetic valves.[3,6,12,32,33] Valve ring abscesses occur when infection involves the sutures used to secure the sewing ring to the periannular tissue; this may result in dehiscence of the valve (Fig. 1). The clinical finding of a paravalvular leak in a patient with PVE is presumptive evidence of a valve ring abscess. Arnett and Roberts described the precise pathologic findings in 22 patients with valve ring abscess. The infectious process involved the entire valve circumference in 14 patients; there was partial involvement in the other 8.[33] Extension of the abscess beyond the valve ring may result in myocardial abscess formation, septal perforation, or purulent pericarditis. In addition to sewing ring abscesses, PVE of bioprostheses may cause leaflet destruction with resulting valvular incompetence.[14,34] Large vegetations occasionally obstruct blood flow and lead to functional valvular stenosis or a combination of stenosis and insufficiency. This complication appears to be more common in mitral PVE than in aortic disease.[14,33,35]

Extracardiac pathologic features classically associated with NVE may also be seen in PVE. Embolic events are common in patients with PVE. Septic emboli to the carotid circulation may lead to a brain infarct, brain abscess, mycotic aneurysm, or hemorrhagic infarct (especially in patients who are excessively anticoagulated). LePort et al. noted that 7 of 17 deaths from their series of patient with late PVE were due to neurologic complications.[36] Peripheral emboli may lead to deep tissue abscesses and mycotic aneurysms.

Immune complex–mediated glomerulonephritis manifested by abnormal urinalysis with or without elevations of serum creatinine levels has been described in patients with PVE.[37–39] Renal pathologic findings are variable but often mimic the diffuse proliferative changes found in poststreptococcal glomerulonephritis. Immunoglobulin and complement deposits can frequently be demonstrated along the glomerular basement membrane (by immunofluorescent staining).

Diagnosis of Prosthetic Valve Endocarditis

Clinical Manifestations. The symptoms and signs of PVE are protean.[6,11,40–42] As shown in Table 2, fever is the most common

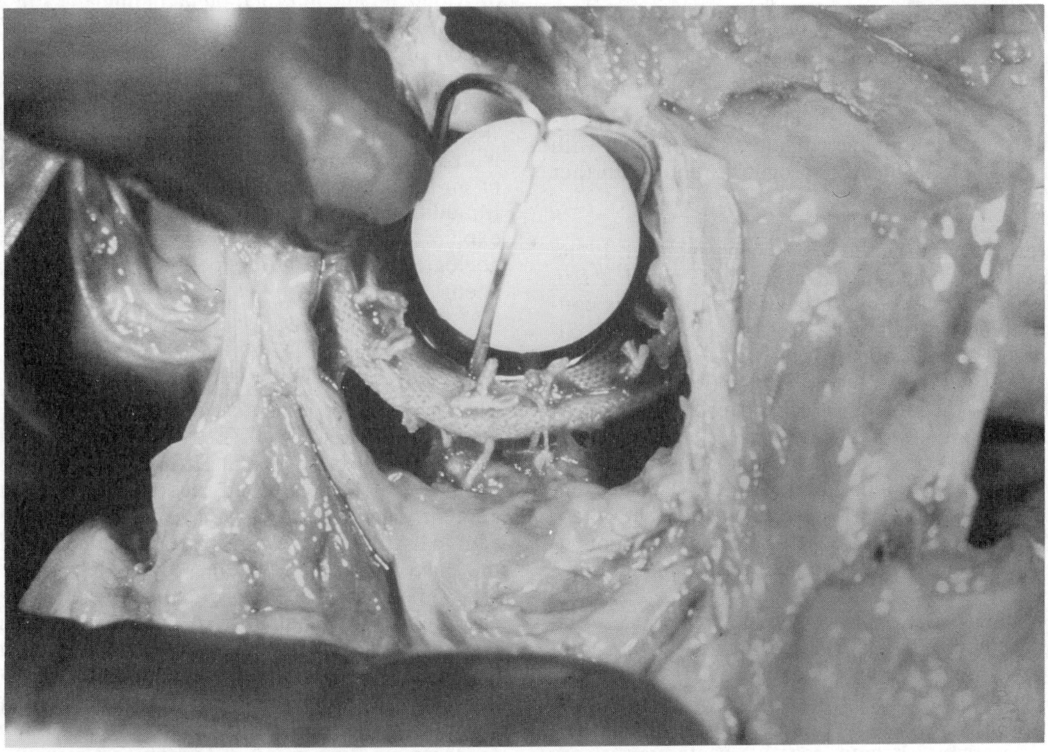

FIG. 1. Autopsy specimen demonstrates valve dehiscence complicating prosthetic valve endocarditis.

TABLE 2. Clinical Findings in Prosthetic Valve Endocarditis (228 Patients)

Finding	%
Fever	97
New or changing murmur	56
Systemic embolus	40
Petechiae	39
Splenomegaly	32
Peripheral signs (Osler nodes, Janeway lesions, Roth spots)	15
Anemia (Hct <35)	74
Hematuria	57
Leukocytosis (WBC >12,000)	54

(Data from Refs. 6, 11, 40, and 42.)

sign and occurs in almost all patients. Clinical evidence of systemic embolization has been reported in 40 percent of patients. The frequency of various organ system involvement by emboli is similar to NVE. Embolization to the central nervous system (CNS) commonly presents as an acute focal neurologic deficit. Splenomegaly is reported in one-third of patients and may be more common in late PVE, presumably reflecting more prolonged antigenemia. Petechiae have been noted in 39 percent, but other peripheral signs due to small emboli or small vessel vasculitis (Osler nodes, Janeway lesions, Roth spots) are less frequently encountered.

New or changing cardiac murmurs have been reported in 56 percent of patients with PVE. Regurgitant murmurs reflect the hemodynamic consequences of valvular insufficiency due to a paravalvular leak, while muffling of heart sounds or stenosis murmurs result from occlusion or malfunction of the prosthetic valve. Although cardiac murmurs may frequently suggest the diagnosis of PVE, in general it is difficult to accurately predict the extent of valvular pathology by auscultation alone.

Laboratory Findings. Anemia is present in many patients with PVE. In late PVE, the degree of anemia is probably a function of the duration of infection. The packed cell volume is a less useful finding in the diagnosis of early PVE. Leukocytosis occurs in only 50 percent of the patients; it may be more frequently seen in those with early PVE. Hematuria (secondary to glomerulonephritis) can be a helpful diagnostic sign in the patient with suspected late PVE but is difficult to interpret in a postoperative patient who may have recently required urethral catheterization. A number of investigators have reported elevated levels of circulating immune complexes in patients with PVE, but their utility for diagnosis or prognosis requires further evaluation.[37,38]

Blood Cultures. The cornerstone of diagnosing PVE is the isolation of an etiologic microorganism from the blood. As in the case of NVE, the bacteremia associated with PVE is continuous. Ninety percent of blood cultures obtained in such patients should reveal the infecting pathogen.[43] Negative blood cultures in a patient who has not received antibiotics is quite unusual in PVE unless the infection is caused by organisms such as *Legionella, Mycobacterium, Rickettsia, Histoplasma capsulatum,* or *Aspergillus* species, which do not grow readily in routine blood cultures. Fastidious microorganisms such as *Haemophilis* species may require prolonged incubation before appearing in blood cultures; therefore, all blood cultures from patients with suspected PVE should be held for a minimum of 3 weeks.

On the other hand, not all instances of bacteremia occurring after valve replacement indicate PVE.[44] Infected wounds and contaminated intravascular catheters may lead to transient bacteremia. Prosthetic valves seem relatively resistant to colonization by gram-negative bacilli, and PVE is rare after transient gram-negative bacteremia. If gram-negative bacteremia clears after the extracardiac source is removed, patients who have no other manifestations of PVE can usually be treated with 2 weeks of intravenous antibiotics.[45] If bacteremia fails to clear or the source of infection is not apparent, the patient should be assumed to have PVE and be treated accordingly. Because gram-positive bacteria are more adherent, their presence in blood cultures usually reflects colonization of the prosthetic device. However, if there is doubt about the significance of a positive blood culture (e.g., a single blood culture growing *S. epidermidis* in the absence of clinical manifestations), antimicrobial therapy may reasonably be withheld while additional cultures are obtained.

Special Studies. Myocardial damage from ischemia, an abscess, or pericarditis may cause a variety of arrhythmias or conduction defects in patients with PVE. In one series, atrioventricular conduction defects occurred in 44 percent of patients with prosthetic aortic valve infection due to extension of the abscess into the conduction system.[41] Serial electrocardiograms or continuous cardiac monitoring may be important for some patients.

Standard echocardiography, which is useful in the management of patients with NVE, has been less helpful in patients with PVE. Echoes generated by the prosthesis are intense, and subtle abnormalities such as small vegetations may be obscured. Bioprosthetic valves are more easily assessed by two-dimensional echocardiography than are mechanical valves.[46] In contrast, Doppler echocardiography does appear to be a valuable technique for the assessment of valvular dysfunction of mechanical as well as bioprosthetic valves. In one series, Doppler echocardiography correctly identified significant regurgitation or obstruction in 15 of 17 patients with malfunctioning prosthetic valves.[47]

Cardiac cinefluoroscopy is a useful procedure for detecting prosthetic valve instability due to loosening of the sewing ring.[6,48] A thrombus or vegetation on the prosthesis may also be suggested by impaired motion of a radiopaque poppet. Cardiac catheterization is often unnecessary in the evaluation of patients with PVE, even when surgical intervention is anticipated. In some circumstances, however, catheterization can provide valuable information including an estimation of the degree of valvular dysfunction, the location of the fistula, an evaluation of left ventricular function, delineation of coronary artery anatomy, or an assessment of possible multiple valve involvement.[49]

Computed tomography of the head is indicated in all patients with PVE and neurologic symptoms. Infarction, hemorrhage, or an abscess can usually be differentiated by this technique. In addition, all patients with neurologic symptoms not readily explained by computed tomography should undergo cerebral angiography to exclude the possibility of an intracranial mycotic aneurysm.[50]

Mortality of Prosthetic Valve Endocarditis

The mortality of patients with PVE remains high. Dismukes analyzed 105 cases of PVE treated between 1976 and 1979 at the Massachusetts General Hospital and the University of Alabama Medical Center and reported an overall mortality of 29 percent. The mortality was 41 percent in early PVE and 21 percent in late disease.[51] More recently, Calderwood et al. reported the outcomes of 116 patients with PVE; in-hospital mortality was 23 percent. The authors applied logistic regression analysis and found that "complicated" infection (defined as persistent fever while receiving antibiotics, changing murmurs heard on physical examination, worsening heart failure, or new conduction abnormalities) was the best predictor of death.[1]

The mortality of PVE varies somewhat with the etiologic microorganism. In a group of 184 patients reviewed by Wilson et al.[52] significantly higher mortality was seen in PVE caused by fungi, gram-negative bacilli, or staphylococci.

Management of Prosthetic Valve Endocarditis

General Principles. Successful management of patients with PVE depends on the same principles used in treating patients with NVE. All patients should be hospitalized, confined to bed during the acute phase of the illness, and monitored carefully for hemodynamic deterioration and arrhythmias. Patients should undergo careful daily physical examination to detect heart failure, changes in murmurs, or evidence of embolization or a mycotic aneurysm.

Antibiotic Therapy. Antimicrobial therapy is based on laboratory identification of the etiologic microorganism and in vitro susceptibility testing; bactericidal antibiotics are necessary. In an effort to enhance in vivo activity, combinations of antibiotics that demonstrate synergistic killing of the pathogen in vitro are often used. Whenever possible, intravenous medications should be administered via scalp vein needles rather than indwelling intravenous catheters to reduce the risk of bacteremia from a contaminated intravascular device. Recommended antibiotic regimens are shown in Table 3.

The combination of aqueous penicillin G plus gentamicin[53,54] is recommended to treat patients with PVE caused by penicillin-susceptible streptococci (minimum inhibitory concentration [MIC] ≤0.1 μg/ml). Streptomycin may be used in place of gentamicin if the MIC for streptomycin is less than 1000 μg/ml. The combination of penicillin G (or ampicillin) and gentamicin is the preferred regimen for PVE due to enterococci[54,55] or other resistant streptococci. The aminoglycoside susceptibility of enterococci should be routinely determined since some strains are highly resistant to all aminoglycosides (MIC, ≥2000 μg/ml).[54,56] There is currently no proven satisfactory treatment regimen for endocarditis caused by aminoglycoside-resistant enterococci (see Chapter 179).

For PVE caused by *S. aureus*, penicillin G is the treatment of choice if the isolate is penicillinase-negative and the MIC for penicillin G is 0.1 μg/ml or less. If penicillinase is produced, a semisynthetic antistaphylococcal penicillin (e.g., nafcillin) should be used instead. Because in vitro studies have demonstrated enhanced killing of *S. aureus* by certain antibiotic combinations, many authorities advocate the addition of gentamicin for the first 2 weeks of therapy. Prosthetic valve endocarditis caused by methicillin-resistant isolates of *S. aureus* must be treated with vancomycin plus gentamicin.

In one study, approximately 80 percent of *S. epidermidis* isolates from patients with PVE were resistant to methicillin.[57] Resistance is not due to β-lactamase production but to alterations in penicillin-binding proteins. Resistance of *S. epidermidis* to methicillin or cephalosporins may not always be apparent by routine in vitro susceptibility testing. Consequently, the use of β-lactam antibiotics alone to treat *S. epidermidis* PVE has resulted in high failure rates.[58] On the basis of currently available data, the combination of vancomycin and rifampin with gentamicin added for the first 2 weeks of therapy appears to be the most effective regimen for *S. epidermidis* PVE.[54,59]

Selection of an antimicrobial regimen for the treatment of diphtheroid PVE is somewhat controversial. If the diphtheroid strain is susceptible to penicillin and gentamicin, therapy with this combination is recommended. The clinical efficacy of penicillin plus gentamicin has also been demonstrated even when the diphtheroid isolate is penicillin resistant,[25] although some would recommend vancomycin in this circumstance. Vancomycin is the therapy of choice for PVE caused by diphtheroid strains (such as group JK corynebacteria) which are resistant to both penicillin and gentamicin.

The design of an antibiotic regimen for PVE caused by aerobic gram-negative bacilli must be based on identification of the organism and careful in vitro susceptibility and synergy studies. Therapy will usually include a β-lactam antibiotic (penicillin, cephalosporin, carbapenem, or monobactam) plus an amino-

TABLE 3. Antimicrobial Therapy for Patients with Bacterial Infections of Prosthetic Valves

Organism	*Regimen*	*Duration of Therapy (wk)*	*Regimen in Penicillin-Allergic Patients[a,b]*
Susceptible streptococci (MIC <0.1 μg/ml Pen G)	Aqueous Pen G[c] plus gentamicin[d,e]	4–6 2	Vancomycin[f] plus gentamicin[d,e] or Cephalothin[g] plus gentamicin[d,e]
Resistant streptococci (MIC >0.1 μg/ml Pen G), enterococci	Aqueous Pen G[c] or ampicillin[h] plus gentamicin[d]	6–8 6–8	Vancomycin[f] plus gentamicin[d]
Staphylococcus aureus			
Methcillin susceptible	Nafcillin[i] plus gentamicin[d]	6–8 2	Cephalothin[g] plus gentamicin[d]
Methcillin resistant	Vancomycin[f] plus gentamicin[d]	6–8 2	Not applicable
Staphylococcus epidermidis	Vancomycin[f] plus rifampin[j] and gentamicin[d]	6–8 6–8 2	Not applicable
Diphtheroids	Aqueous Pen G[c] plus gentamicin[d] or Vancomycin[f,k]	6 6	Vancomycin[f,k] Not applicable
Aerobic gram-negative bacilli	β-Lactam[l] plus aminoglycoside—based on in vitro data	6–8 6–8	Consider aztreonam[l] plus aminoglycoside
Empirical regimen, bacteria not identified	Vancomycin[f] plus gentamicin[d]		Not applicable

[a] The duration of therapy is similar to that recommended for non-penicillin-allergic patients.
[b] Cephalosporins are contraindicated when there is history of penicillin anaphylaxis.
[c] Aqueous penicillin G, 24 million units daily in divided doses q4h.
[d] Gentamicin, 1 mg/kg iv q8h.
[e] Streptomycin may be used for sensitive organisms (MIC <1000 μg/ml).
[f] Vancomycin, 0.5 g iv q6h.
[g] Cephalothin, 2 g iv q4h (or equivalent cephalosporin).
[h] Ampicillin, 2 g iv q4h.
[i] Nafcillin, 2 g iv q4h.
[j] Rifampin, 300 mg po q8h.
[k] Preferred agent for gentamicin-resistant strains.
[l] For strains resistant to all β-lactams, consider ciprofloxacin as a single agent.

glycoside. Newer quinolones may be useful in therapy for resistant organisms, but their efficacy in endocarditis has not yet been established in large-scale clinical trials.[60,61]

Fungal PVE is a very serious disorder that requires combined medical and surgical therapy. For *Candida* endocarditis, high doses of intravenous amphotericin B (up to 1 mg/kg/day) is given in combination with oral flucytosine (dose adjusted for renal function). A preoperative induction course of amphotericin B does not seem to improve outcome; prompt valve replacement is mandatory.[62]

When PVE seems clinically apparent but blood cultures are not yet positive, therapy with vancomycin plus gentamicin should be initiated. For patients in whom infection has been demonstrated at an extracardiac site (e.g., wound infection, pneumonia, urinary tract infection), initial antimicrobial therapy should include drugs active against the microorganism present at that site as well. When PVE is considered but the level of clinical suspicion is low, three or four blood cultures should be obtained by separate venipunctures and the patient observed. If valve replacement is imminent, it is reasonable to initiate empirical antimicrobial therapy with vancomycin and gentamicin. The diagnosis of PVE can usually be confirmed or excluded at the time of surgery.

Serum bactericidal activity should be measured during the first few days of therapy to demonstrate the in vivo activity of the antimicrobial regimen being used. Controversy exists regarding the usefulness of the test, the best method of testing, the optimal antimicrobial activity desired, and the timing of testing (peak vs. trough). In general, a serum bactericidal titer of greater than 1:32 against the infecting bacteria (measured at the time of peak antibiotic concentration) appears to correlate with a more favorable clinical response.[63,64] If a titer of at least 1:8 is not achieved, an increase in dosage or change in antibiotics should be considered, particularly if the patient is not responding clinically.

After the initiation of antimicrobial therapy, blood cultures should be obtained daily for the first 3–4 days and weekly thereafter until the completion of therapy. Usually blood cultures will be sterile within 3–5 days of initiating appropriate antimicrobial therapy. After the completion of therapy, blood cultures should be obtained weekly for 1 month. A relapse necessitates reinstitution of antimicrobial therapy, retesting of the microorganism for antimicrobial susceptibility, and strong consideration of valve replacement. Occasionally, a relapse may be due to persistent infection at an extracardiac site; careful consideration should be given to the possibility of an occult abscess or mycotic aneurysm.

Surgical Therapy. Several general observations can be made regarding the increasingly important role of surgery in the management of PVE. First, the mortality of patients with PVE who undergo valve replacement during active infection is no greater (and may be less) than is the mortality of patients who receive medical therapy alone. Mortality statistics may underestimate the value of surgical intervention in the management of PVE since many of the patients in the medical–surgical treatment group were critically ill and underwent surgery only after failing medical therapy. Second, the risk of recurrent PVE after the surgical removal of an infected prosthesis is real but usually acceptable. The incidence in published series has ranged from 0 to 15 percent, and the microorganisms causing PVE after valve replacement for NVE are usually different from those infecting the native valve.[2,12,65] This perhaps reflects the more complex techniques necessary for repair in these patients. Third, when valve replacement is clinically indicated, there is little to be gained by delaying surgery despite an incomplete course of antibiotic therapy. A delay only increases the chances for serious complications such as refractory heart failure, renal failure, or emboli.[2,12,66]

The objectives of cardiac surgery in PVE are to remove infected tissues and materials and to restore hemodynamic integrity.[67] Other goals include the repair of acquired defects (such as abscesses) and elimination of sources of emboli.[63,68] The decision to proceed with cardiac surgery in the seriously ill patient with PVE is seldom an easy one. To provide some guidelines for physicians and surgeons caring for these patients, we have used a point system to assess the need for valve replacement. If assessment of a patient results in the accumulation of five or more points by the system described in Table 4, we would recommend surgery—emergent surgery in the case of severe heart failure and urgent surgery in the case of other complications.

TABLE 4. Indications for Valve Replacement during Active Prosthetic Valve Endocarditis

Disorder	*Point Rating*[a]
Heart failure due to valve dysfunction	
Severe	5
Moderate	5
Mild	2
Acute valve obstruction	5
Fungal etiology	5
Persistent bacteremia	5
Organism other than penicillin-susceptible *Streptoccus*	2
Relapse after appropriate therapy	3
One major embolus	2
Two or more emboli	4
Vegetations by echocardiogram	1
Heart block	3
Ruptured ventricular septal defect or sinus of Valsalva	4
Early PVE (<60 days)	2
Unstable prosthesis by fluoroscopy	5
Paravalvular leak	2
Prior prosthetic valve replacement	−2

[a] The accumulation of 5 or more points suggests the need for valve replacement.
(From Alsip et al.,[69] with permission.)

The severity of heart failure is a leading prognostic factor in patients with PVE. In patients with moderate to severe heart failure secondary to valvular dysfunction, emergency valve replacement may be lifesaving. Two large series reported by Richardson et al.[12] and Karchmer et al.[13] contain a total of 52 PVE patients with moderate to severe heart failure. The mortality in the medical therapy group was 100 percent, while the combined medical–surgical therapy group had a 49 percent mortality. Valve replacement is therefore recommended in all PVE patients with moderate to severe heart failure. Emergency valve replacement is also required in patients who develop acute prosthetic obstruction due to large vegetations. Hemodynamically stable patients who may later require valve replacement for mild heart failure or a paravalvular leak should receive a full course of antimicrobial therapy before elective surgery.

Valve replacement within 48–72 hours is recommended in cases of fungal PVE because of the poor response to medical therapy and high frequency of major emboli.[62] In patients with bacterial PVE, valve replacement should be considered whenever bacteremia persists for more than a few days after the initiation of the best antimicrobial therapy.

Anticoagulation. Most patients with mechanical heart valves require long-term anticoagulation to prevent thromboembolic complications. However, the theoretic risks of bleeding at the site of a mycotic aneurysm or embolic infarction raises important questions about the use of anticoagulants in patients with active PVE. Carpenter et al. described 14 patients who received anticoagulants during therapy for PVE. Thirty-six percent had symptomatic episodes of CNS hemorrhage.[70] In contrast, Wilson et al. noted a higher frequency of neurologic complications in PVE patients who did not receive adequate anticoagulation.[71] Although the proper use of anticoagulants remains controversial, most authorities do continue anticoagulation in patients with PVE. However, it may be prudent to monitor patients closely and maintain clotting parameters at the lower end of the therapeutic range.

Prophylaxis

Although there have been no adequate placebo-controlled trials to assess the value of prophylactic antibiotics in valve replacement surgery, they are routinely employed. Prophylaxis, usually with a first-generation cephalosporin, is directed at the prevention of wound infection and PVE due to staphylococci and streptococci; the duration of administration should not exceed 2 days. Vancomycin is an appropriate alternative drug. After discharge from the hospital, the patient should be aware of the importance of prophylactic antimicrobial agents before any procedure likely to cause transient bacteremia (see Chapter 63).

INDWELLING RIGHT ATRIAL CATHETERS

Broviac and Hickman catheters are silicone elastomer intravenous devices designed to permit long-term vascular access for hyperalimentation, drug or blood product administration, and blood sampling[72,73] (see Chapters 61 and 279). The catheters are similar in design, but the Hickman device has a larger diameter, which facilitates aspiration of blood samples. The distal, intravascular portion of the catheter is inserted into the superior vena cava or right atrium via the external jugular or cephalic vein. The extravascular portion, with a Dacron felt cuff in place, is drawn through a subcutaneous chest wall tunnel that exits between the nipple and sternum. The Dacron cuff is designed to permit fibroblast ingrowth to anchor the catheter and prevent microorganisms from tracking along the outside.

Four varieties of infectious complication of Broviac or Hickman catheters include (*1*) exit site infections, (*2*) tunnel infectoins, (*3*) septic thrombophlebitis, and (*4*) isolated bacteremia or fungemia. Press et al. reviewed the courses of 992 oncology patients with a total of 1088 Hickman catheter placements. One hundred forty-three catheter infections were documented (incidence, 0.14 infections/100 catheter days). Exit site infections, isolated bacteremia, tunnel infections, and septic thrombophlebitis accounted for 46, 31, 20, and 4 percent of all infections, respectively.[74]

Microbiology

Presently, gram-positive cocci are responsible for most silicone elastomer catheter infections in the United States.[74–79] *Staphylococcus epidermidis* accounted for 54.1 percent and *Staphylococcus aureus* for 20 percent of the clinical isolates in the review of 143 catheter infections by Press et al. Gram-negative bacilli, gram-positive bacilli, and fungi such as *Candida albicans* respectively accounted for 9, 5, and 7 percent of all clinical isolates.[74]

Pathogenesis

The precise pathogenesis of catheter-related infections is unclear. However, the frequency with which *S. epidermidis* is isolated suggests that microorganisms may track along the catheter from the skin or perhaps are introduced at the time of catheter placement. The risk of hematogenous seeding of the catheter during bacteremia from a distant focus appears to be low.[74]

Clinical Manifestations

The clinical manifestations of catheter infections vary with the sites of involvement. (*1*) Exit site infections are characterized by local warmth, erythema, and tenderness at the site where the catheter exits from the skin. Purulent drainage around the catheter may or may not be evident. (*2*) Tunnel infections may resemble exit site infections, but tenderness and erythema extend up the chest along the subcutaneous tract of the proximal portion of the catheter. Both exit site and tunnel infections may be complicated by the presence of concomitant bacteremia (three of four and three of eight patients, respectively, in one series.[74] (*3*) The manifestations of septic thrombophlebitis reflect bacterial invasion and subsequent thrombosis of the vein that the catheter enters. Patients are almost always bacteremic, and there are local signs of venous insufficiency such as edema of the upper extremity. (*4*) Finally, patients may be bacteremic in the absence of localizing signs or symptoms. This type of infection may be particularly important in neutropenic individuals who are unable to mount a local inflammatory response to infection.

Diagnosis

The early diagnosis of catheter-related infections requires regular examination of the catheter exit site and the skin overlying the tunnel for signs of tenderness and erythema. If infection is suspected, Gram stain and culture should be performed on any purulent material expressed from around the catheter. In addition, blood cultures should be routinely obtained. Cultures drawn through the catheter will occasionally be positive even though peripheral blood cultures are negative.

Therapy

Therapy for indwelling right atrial catheter infections has changed significantly in the 1980s. Previously, clinicians believed that all infected catheters required removal, especially if bacteremia was documented. Many catheters can now be salvaged. Exit site infections with or without associated bacteremia are the type most responsive to antibiotic therapy, with cure rates as high as 85 percent in one series.[74] Bacteremia without evidence of localized catheter infection may also be successfully managed with parenteral antibiotics (see Chapter 61 and 280). Tunnel infections and septic thrombophlebitis are more difficult to eradicate and usually require catheter removal. Similarly, catheters infected with resistant organisms such as gram-negative bacilli or fungi are difficult to salvage. In any case, catheter removal should be considered whenever patients fail to respond to antibiotics as indicated by persistent fever or continued positive blood cultures while receiving therapy. The empirical treatment of catheter-related infections should generally include vancomycin and gentamicin to treat *S. epidermidis*. The therapeutic regimen can be altered on the basis of the antimicrobial susceptibility patterns of organisms isolated. All cases other than mild exit site infections should be treated with approximately 14 days of parenteral antibiotics. Some investigators have advocated the instillation of fibrinolytic agents (streptokinase or urokinase) into the catheter if there is evidence of partial occlusion by a clot. Shuman et al. reported a 90 percent catheter salvage rate when using local fibrinolytic therapy and systemic antimicrobial agents in 28 episodes of bacteremia occuring in 24 patients with indwelling right atrial catheters.[80]

INFECTION OF VASCULAR GRAFTS

Incidence

The reported incidence of vascular prosthesis infection ranges from less than 1 percent to more than 5 percent and varies with the site of graft placement.[81–83] Grafts implanted in the inguinal area (e.g., aortofemoral or femoropopliteal grafts) have a higher rate of infection than do grafts that lie entirely within the abdomen. In one series of 3652 patients receiving primarily aortic, aortoiliac, or aortofemoral grafts, a groin incision was associated with a threefold increase in the incidence of graft infection (1.34 vs. 0.43 percent).[84] Infection rates for grafts in the upper extremities and other sites are less well documented.

Pathogenesis

The mechanisms by which microorganisms colonize vascular grafts include (*1*) contamination at the time of surgery, (*2*) direct extension from an adjacent tissue site, and (*3*) hematogenous seeding during an episode of bacteremia.

Lower extremity grafts are at greatest risk for infection, which may reflect higher rates of perioperative contamination with microorganisms from the skin at the relatively superficial lower extremity graft site. Preoperative extremity infections, postoperative wound infections, and underlying disorders, such as diabetes mellitus may also contribute to the high incidence of infections in femoral and popliteal grafts.

Abdominal aortic grafts have a relatively high incidence of infection with gram-negative enteric bacilli, probably reflecting contamination of the graft by bowel microorganisms. Several investigators have suggested that unsuspected infections in aortic aneurysms may be responsible for some cases of postrepair graft infections. In two recent reports, cultures were obtained from 266 clinically uninfected aneurysmectomy specimens. Bacteria were isolated in 33 instances, with *S. epidermidis* the most common organism.[85,86] However, the incidence of subsequent infections in these individuals was quite low, and the significance of these data remains unclear.

Graft infections may result from bacteremia, but the risk of infection diminishes as the graft becomes incorporated in the host tissue.[87] After an initial inflammatory reaction, fibrous tissue accumulates on the outer surface of the graft, and a pseudointima composed of connective tissue and fibrin begins to form on the inner surface of the graft.[88] A true endothelial lining extends from the native artery but rarely grows more than 10 mm beyond the anastomosis.[89] In animal models, resistance of an implanted graft to blood-borne infection correlates with the degree of pseudointima formation.[90,91]

Microbiology

Table 5 lists by site the etiologic mocroorganisms recovered from 85 patients with graft infections.[82,92,93] *Staphylococcus aureus* and *S. epidermidis* are the most commonly reported causes of graft infections, particularly sites involving the lower extremity.[81,94] Intra-abdominal graft infections are most commonly caused by *E. coli* or other gram-negative enteric bacilli. Data from several large series show that two or more microorganisms were isolated from 37 percent of graft infections; multiple isolates were found in 60 percent of abdominal graft infections and 23 percent of groin infections.[82,92,93,95] Polymicrobial infections most often included a staphylococcus and a gram-negative bacillus or combinations of gram-negative bacilli.

TABLE 5. Microbial Etiology of Vascular Graft Infections

	Anatomic Location of Infection			
Organism	*Abdominal* (%)	*Groin* (%)	*Popliteal* (%)	*Overall* (%)
S. aureus	14	40	33	33
S. epidermidis	7	13	17	12
Streptococci	14	8	25	11
E. coli	42	9	0	16
Proteus sp.	3	11	0	8
Other aerobic gram-negative bacilli	0	8	17	7
Other bacteria	10	5	0	6
Candida sp.	3	1	0	1
Unknown	7	5	8	6
Total number				
Microorganisms	29	85	12	126
Patients	17	60	8	85

(Data from Szilagyi et al.,[82] Becker et al.,[92] and Hoffert et al.[93])

Clinical Features

The local and systemic manifestations of graft infections vary with the location of the prosthesis. Over 70 percent of infections involving groin and popliteal vascular prostheses develop within 2 months of surgery, whereas 70 percent of intra-abdominal graft infections do not become clinically apparent until more than 1 year after surgery.[92,96] The most common presentations of graft infection in the groin or leg are the formation of a localized abscess or draining sinus, the formation of a false aneurysm (which may be associated with pain and a new bruit), thrombosis of the graft, or septic emboli to the distal extremity.[96] Erythema, warmth, or tenderness at a graft site is highly suggestive of infection. Rapid swelling over an area of vascular repair of a hemorrhage from a graft site suggests disruption of the suture line with bleeding or false aneurysm formation. Ischemic changes and a loss of pulses in the distal part of the extremity indicate thrombosis of the arterial implant. Exteriorization of the graft due to a breakdown of overlying tissues is pathognomonic of infection.

The presentation of intra-abdominal graft infections may be subtle. Fever is usually present but may be low grade. Specific findings in aortic graft infections can include abdominal tenderness, retroperitoneal hemorrhage, an abdominal mass due to a false aneurysm, graft thrombosis, ureteral obstruction with hydronephrosis, and septic emboli.[97] Petechiae and spinter hemorrhages similar to those in endocarditis may also occur. Aortoenteric fistula formation due to erosion of the graft into the bowel occurred in 0.36 percent of patients in one series.[84] In 80 percent of cases of aortoenteric fistula, the proximal anastomosis erodes into the third portion of the duodenum[98] A breakdown of the suture line results in upper or lower gastrointestinal bleeding that may be massive. Melena or hematemesis in a patient with an aortic graft should immediately arouse suspicion of a developing aortoenteric fistula.[92,99]

Diagnosis

A variety of diagnostic techniques are useful in evaluating patients with suspected vascular graft infection. If a draining sinus is present, a careful sinogram may reveal the extent of an underlying infectious process. Abscesses and aneurysms may also be demonstrated by noninvasive techniques such as sonography and computerized tomography. Magnetic resonance imaging may prove to be a sensitive technique for diagnosing graft infections. In one report of three patients, magnetic resonance imaging clearly delineated the extent of perigraft infection. Abscesses have a high signal intensity that contrasts strongly with the signal of flowing blood.[100] Gallium scanning has not generally been found to be useful; indium-labeled leukocyte scanning may be a sensitive diagnostic technique, but its specificity appears to be low, at least in the perioperative period.[101] Arteriography is the most precise method for documenting false aneurysm formation, suture line leakage, or graft thrombosis.

Cultures and Gram stains should be obtained on all draining wounds, although cultures obtained at the time of surgical inspection provide more reliable microbiologic data. Routine venous blood cultures should also be obtained. No good estimation of the frequency of positive blood cultures is available, but negative blood cultures do occur in an appreciable number of cases when infection has not yet extended to the graft lumen. Material removed at embolectomy, however, should always be cultured.

Morbidity and Mortality

Morbidity and mortality vary with the position of the graft. In a review of 84 patients with vascular graft infection, O'Hara et al. found an overall 30-day mortality rate of 28 percent. The same authors reported a 1-year mortality rate among the 43 patients who received grafts since 1980 of 46 percent.[84] In another series of infected aortobifemoral prostheses, mortality was 23 percent.[102] Mortality rates are lower for distal graft infections (14 percent[96] in one series of femoropopliteal grafts), largely due to the ease of earlier diagnosis and the decreased severity of bleeding relative to proximal grafts.

The major morbidity associated with graft infection is loss of the extremity supplied by the prosthesis. In one recent review, the amputation rate among 13 patients with aortofemoral infections was 38 percent.[102]

Management

Successful treatment usually requires a combination of systemic antibiotic administration and surgery. Removal of the entire graft and débridement of infected tissue is almost always necessary for cure. Most attempts to treat graft infection with antibiotics and local wound care alone are unsuccessful. Infections occurring at midpoints of long grafts (e.g., axillofemoral) may be temporarily managed by drainage and antibiotics, but graft removal will ultimately be required for a successful outcome. The viability of distal structures depends upon the adequacy of collateral vessels and the feasibility of additional bypass procedures. If the extremity or organ is totally dependent upon flow through the graft, some form of revascularization that bypasses the site of infection should be attempted. For example, axillofemoral grafts may be used to bypass an infected aortic bifurcation graft. If a new graft must be placed in the infected field, some authors have recommended use of autogenous artery or vein grafts, which may be less suceptible to infection than are grafts made of synthetic materials. The only common situation in which removal of a portion of the graft is acceptable occurs when infection involves the distal anastamosis of one branch of an aortofemoral graft; the infected limb may sometimes be removed and the opposite limb preserved. Identification of the infecting microorganism and in vitro susceptibility testing are also essential for successful therapy. Some graft infections may be temporarily managed by drainage and antibiotics, but graft removal will ultimately be required for a successful outcome. Recommended initial antimicrobial regimens for graft infections are generally the same as those recommended for PVE (Table 3). Antibiotics should be administered parenterally for 4 weeks after the prosthetic device is removed.

Prevention

Strict adherence to principles of asepsis, vigorous preoperative skin decontamination, and meticulous surgical technique are the most important factors in preventing wound and graft infections. Simultaneous procedures that could result in bacteremia or wound contamination should be avoided.

Prophylactic antibiotics are routinely employed in vascular operations. A double-blind study of cefazolin vs. placebo demonstrated a significantly lower rate of postoperative wound and graft infections in patients who receive cefazolin.[103] Some surgeons routinely instill antibiotic solutions into the wound before closure, but the value of this practice is unproved.[104] Grafts containing antibiotics incorporated into the material have been developed but remain investigational.[105]

Little information is available to assess the value of prophylactic antibiotics in patients with vascular grafts who undergo manipulations likely to result in bacteremia. Graft infection resulting from such bacteremia appears to be rare, but some authors have recommended that prophylactic antibiotics be given before dental, genitourinary, or other procedures.[106,107] This may have the greatest value in the first few months after graft placement.[108]

INFECTIONS OF DIALYSIS-ACCESS ARTERIOVENOUS FISTULAS

Because of lower rates of infection and thrombosis, surgically created subcutaneous arteriovenous fistulas (AVFs) have generally replaced external arteriovenous cannulas for vascular access in chronic dialysis patients.[109,110] An AVF may be created by direct artery-to-vein anastomosis (native AVF) or by implantation of a prosthetic conduit. Expanded polytetrafluoroethylene is the most commonly used material.

Infectious complications of native vessel AVFs appear to be uncommon. The incidence of infection has averaged less than 2 percent in several recent studies with follow-ups as long as 5 years.[111,112] Infection occurs more frequently in prosthetic AVFs. In three recent studies, infections developed in 11, 23, and 25 percent of patients receiving expanded polytetrafluoroethylene grafts.[111–113]

Microbiology

Staphylococcus aureus is the most common etiologic microorganism and accounts for 60–90 percent of access site infections.[109,110,114–116] Gram-negative bacilli, especially *Pseudomonas aeruginosa* are also commonly encountered.[110,114,116] A prosthetic AVF may become infected through a variety of mechanisms. Contamination may occur at the time of implantation, or a relatively superficial wound infection may extend to involve the graft. In addition, access sites are subjected to multiple needle punctures during dialysis, which may result in direct inoculation of the prosthesis. Hematomas or false aneurysms occurring at puncture sites may also become infected. Bacteremia is a possible but apparently uncommon source of AVF infection.

Clinical Manifestations

Arteriovenous fistula infections may present with local pain, tenderness, erythema, abscess formation, or bacteremia. However, as many as a third of AVF infections have no clinically apparent local findings.[114,117] As with other types of vascular graft infections, involvement of the suture line may result in disruption of the anastomosis and subsequent hemorrhage. Approximately 30 percent of AVF infections are associated with bacteremia. Metastatic infections such as endocarditis or septic pulmonary thromboembolism may occur, especially with staphylococcal AVF infections.[109,117]

Therapy

Management of infected AVFs almost always necessitates the combination of antibiotic administration and surgery. However, there are reports of graft salvage when antimicrobial therapy and surgical débridement are combined. This may be more effective when the infectious process involves only a localized site distant from suture lines.[118] Infection involving native vessel AVFs may respond to antimicrobial therapy alone.[94,114]

Initial empirical antimicrobial therapy for an infected AVF should include agents active against staphylococci and aerobic gram-negative bacilli (e.g., vancomycin, an antipseudomonal β-lactam, and an aminoglycoside). Subsequent therapy must be based upon the susceptibility pattern(s) of the isolated pathogen(s). The doses of all agents must be carefully adjusted for the patient's renal function.

PERMANENT PACEMAKER INFECTIONS

Infection is second only to problems with pacing or sensing as a complication of permanent pacemaker insertion. In one series of 457 patients, the reported incidence of pacemaker infections was 3.6 and 2 percent for epicardial and transvenous devices, respectively.[119] Pacemaker infections may involve any portion of the implanted hardware from the generator box to the pacing electrode. Concomitant bacteremia or endocarditis may also be present.

The most common location for pacemaker infections is the subcutaneous pocket containing the generator box. Most such infections present soon after surgery but may not become evident for 2 years or more. Staphylococci are the most common causes of generator box infections. In one large review, *S. epidermidis* was responsible for 44 percent of pacemaker infections while *S. aureus* was isolated from 29 percent.[120] The most likely pathogenesis of generator box infections is contamination of the device by skin flora at the time of implantation. Wound infection or erosion of the box through the overlying skin may also lead to microbial contamination.

The other major category of pacemaker infection is involvement of the epicardial or transvenous electrodes. This usually results from the direct spread of microorganism along the wires from an infected generator box, but hematogenous seeding occasionally occurs.[121]

The clinical manifestations of pacemaker infection depends upon the site of involvement. Generator box infections typically present with fever and local warmth, erythema, and tenderness over the generator pocket. Isolated lead infections are less common but may present similarly to bacterial endocarditis with fever and positive blood cultures. A definite diagnosis of pacemaker infection depends upon the isolation of an etiologic microorganism from the pacemaker pocket or the blood stream.

Treatment of pacemaker infections remains controversial. All hardware should be removed in both generator box and electrode infections, particularly when these disorders are accompanied by bacteremia. Occasional cures have been reported in generator box infections with parenteral antibiotics and local irrigation alone. Parenteral antimicrobial agents must be chosen carefully on the basis of the identification and susceptibility of the isolated pathogen. The proper duration of therapy is not well established. If any foreign material is left in place, antibiotic administration should be continued for at least 6 weeks, perhaps followed by long-term suppressive therapy. Antimicrobial therapy should continue for approximately 4 weeks after the hardware is removed if bacteremia is documented. Two weeks of antimicrobial therapy may be adequate for nonbacteremic infection if the device is removed.

REFERENCES

1. Calderwood SB, Swinski LA, Karchmer AW, et al. Prosthetic valve endocarditis: Analysis of factors affecting outcome of therapy. J Thorac Cardiovasc Surg. 1986;92:776–83.
2. Ivert TSA, Dismukes WE, Cobbs CG, et al. Prosthetic valve endocarditis. Circulation. 1984;69:223.
3. Dismukes WE, Karchmer AW, Buckley MJ, et al. Prosthetic valve endocarditis: Analysis of 38 cases. Circulation. 1973;48:365.
4. Rossiter SJ, Stinson EB, Oyer PE, et al. Prosthetic valve endocarditis: Comparison of heterograft tissue valves and mechanical valves. J Thorac Cardiovasc Surg. 1978;76:795.
5. Grignon A, Spencer H, Robson HG, et al. Prosthetic valve infections. Can J Surg. 1981;24:615.
6. Masur H, Johnson WD Jr. Prosthetic valve endocarditis. J Thorac Cardiovasc Surg. 1980;80:31.
7. Auger P, Marquis G, Dyrda I, et al. Infective endocarditis update: Experience from a heart hospital. Acta Cardiol. 1981;36:105.
8. Aintablian A, Hilsenrath J, Hamby RJ, et al. Endocarditis in prosthetic valves. NY State J Med. 1976;76:673.
9. Wilson WR, Jaumin PM, Danielson GK, et al. Prosthetic valve endocarditis. Ann Intern Med. 1975;82:751.
10. Slaughter L, Morris JE, Starr A. Prosthetic valvular endocarditis: A 12-year review. Circulation. 1973;47:1319.
11. Petheram IS, Boyce JMH. Prosthetic valve endocarditis: A reiew of 24 cases. Thorax. 1977;32:478.
12. Richardson JV, Karp RB, Kirklin JW, et al. Treatment of infective endocarditis: A 10 year comparative analysis. Circulation. 1978;58:589.
13. Karchmer AW, Dismukes WE, Buckley MJ, et al. Late prosthetic valve endocarditis: Clinical features influencing therapy. Am J Med. 1978;64:199.
14. Bortotti U, Thiene G, Milano A, et al. Pathological study of infective endocarditis on Hancock porcine bioprostheses. J Thorac Cardiovasc Surg. 1981;81:934.
15. Magilligan DJ, Quinn EL, Davila JC. Bacteremia, endocarditis, and the Hancock valve. Ann Thorac Surg. 1977;24:508.
16. Isom OW, Spencer FC, Glassman E, et al. Long-term results in 1375 patients undergoing valve replacement with the Starr-Edwards cloth-covered steel ball prosthesis. Ann Surg. 1977;186:310.
17. Downham WH, Rhoades ER. Endocarditis associated with porcine valve xenografts. Arch Intern Med. 1979;139:1350.
18. Gallo JI, Ruiz B, Carrion MF, et al. Heart valve replacement with the Hancock bioprosthesis: A 6-year review. Ann Thorac Surg. 1981;31:444.
19. Rutledge R, Kim BJ, Applebaum RE. Actuarial analysis of the risk of prosthetic valve endocarditis in 1,598 patients with mechanical and bioprosthetic valves. Arch Surg. 1985;120:469.
20. Hammond GL, Geha AS, Kopf GS, et al. Biological versus mechanical valves: Analysis of 1,116 valves inserted in 1,012 adult patients with a 4,818 patient-year and a 5,327 valve-year follow-up. J Thorac Cardiovasc Surg. 1987;93:182.
21. Calderwood SB, Swinski LA, Waternaux CM, et al. Risk factors for the development of prosthetic valve endocarditis. Circulation. 1985;72:31.
22. Horstkotte D, Korfer R, Loogen F, et al. Prosthetic valve endocarditis: Clinical findings and management. Eur Heart J. 1984;5:17.
23. Chun PKC, Nelson WP. Common cardiac prosthetic valves: Radiologic identification and associated complications. JAMA. 1977;238:401.
24. Delgado DG, Cobbs CG. Infections of prosthetic valves and intravascular devices. In: Mandell GL, Douglas RG Jr, Bennett JE, eds. Principles and Practice of Infectious Diseases. New York: Churchill Livingstone; 1979;690.
25. Murray BE, Karchmer AW, Moellering RC Jr. Diphtheroid prosthetic valve endocarditis: A study of clinical features and infecting organisms. Am J Med. 1980;69:838.
26. Kluge RM, Calia FM, McLaughlin JS, et al. Sources of contamination in open heart surgery. JAMA. 1974;230:1415.
27. Blakemore WS, McGarrity GJ, Thurer RJ, et al. Infection by airborne bacteria with cardiopulmonary bypass. Surgery. 1971;70:830.
28. Freeman R, King B. Analysis of results of catheter tip cultures in open-heart surgery patients. Thorax. 1975;30:26.
29. Stiles GM, Singh L, Imazaki G, et al. Thermodilution cardiac output studies as a cause of prosthetic valve bacterial endocarditis. J Cardiovasc Surg. 1984;88:1035.
30. Centers for Disease Conttrol. Follow-up on mycobacterial contamination of porcine heart valve prostheses—United States. MMWR. 1978;27:92.
31. Rumisek JD, Albus RA, Clarke JS. Late *Mycobacterium chelonei* bioprosthetic valve endocarditis: Activation of implanted contaminant? Ann Thorac Surg. 1985;39:277.
32. Anderson DJ, Bulkley BH, Hutchins GM. A clinicopathologic study of prosthetic valve endocarditis in 22 patients: Morphologic basis for diagnosis and therapy. Am Heart J. 1977;94:325.
33. Arnett EN, Roberts WC. Prosthetic valve endocarditis: Clinicopathologic analysis of 22 necropsy patients with comparison of observations in 74 necropsy patients with active infective endocarditis involving natural left-sided cardiac valves. Am J Cardiol. 1976;38:281.
34. Ferrans VJ, Boyce SW, Billingham ME, et al. Infection of glutaraldehyde-preserved porcine valve heterografts. Am J Cardiol. 1979;43:1123.
35. Karchmer AW, Stinson EB. The role of surgery in infective endocarditis. In Swartz M, Remington J, eds. Current Clinical Topics in Infectious Diseases. McGraw-Hill, New York: 1980:124.
36. Leport C, Vilde JL, Bricaire F, et al. Fifty cases of late prosthetic valve endocarditis: Improvement in prognosis over a 15 year period. Br Heart J. 1987;58:66.
37. Hooper DC, Bayer AS, Karchmer AW, et al. Circulating immune complexes in prosthetic valve endocarditis. Arch Intern Med. 1983;143:2081.
38. Kauffmann RH, Thompson J, Valentijn RM, et al. The clinical implications and the pathogenetic significance of circulating immune complexes in infective endocarditis. Am J Med. 1981;71:17.
39. Neugarten J, Baldwin DS. Glomerulonephritis in bacterial endocarditis. Am J Med. 1984;77:297.
40. Watanakunakorn C. Prosthetic valve infective endocarditis: A review. Prog Cardiovasc Dis. 1979;22:181.
41. Madison J, Wang K, Gobel FI, et al. Prosthetic aortic valvular endocarditis. Circulation. 1975;51:940.
42. Quenzer RW, Edwards LD, Levin S. A comprehensive study of 48 host valve and 24 prosthetic valve endocarditis cases. Am Heart J. 1976;92:15.
43. Washington JA II. The role of the microbiology laboratory in the diagnosis and antimicrobial treatment of infective endocarditis. Mayo Clin Proc. 1982;57:22.
44. Sande MA, Johnson WD Jr, Hook EW, et al. Sustained bacteremia in patients with prosthetic cardiac valves. N Engl J Med. 1972;286:1067.
45. Dismukes WE, Karchmer AW. The diagnosis of infected prosthetic heart valves: Bacteremia versus endocarditis. In Duma RJ, ed. Infections of Prosthetic Heart Valves and Vascular Grafts. Baltimore, University Park Press; 1977:61.
46. Martin RP, French JW, Popp RL. Clinical utility of two-dimensional echocardiography in patients with bioprosthetic valves. Adv Cardiol. 1980;27:294.
47. Panidis IP, Ross J, Mintz GS. Normal and abnormal prosthetic valve func-

tion as assessed by Doppler echocardiography. J Am Coll Cardiol. 1986;8:317.
48. Ellis K, Jaffe C, Malm JR, et al. Infective endocarditis: Roentgenographic considerations. Radiol Clin North Am. 1973;11:415.
49. Welton DE, Young JB, Raizner AE, et al. Value and safety of cardiac catheterization during active infective endocarditis. Am J Cardiol. 1979;44:1306.
50. Dean RH, Waterhouse G, Meacham PW, et al. Mycotic embolism and embolomycotic aneurysms: Neglected lessons of the past. Ann Surg. 1986;204:300.
51. Dismukes WE. Prosthetic valve endocarditis: Factors influencing outcome and recommendations for therapy. In Bisno AL, ed. Treatment of Infective Endocarditis. New York: Grune & Stratton; 1981:67.
52. Wilson WR, Danielson GK, Giuliani ER, et al. Prosthetic valve endocarditis. Mayo Clin Proc. 1982;57:155.
53. Bisno AL, Dismukes WE, Durack DT, et al. Treatment of infective endocarditis due to viridans streptococci. JAMA. 1989;261:1471.
54. Bisno AL, Dismukes WE, Durack DT, et al. Antimicrobial treatment of infectious endocarditis due to viridans streptococci, enterococci, and staphylococci. Submitted for publication.
55. Carrizosa J, Kaye D. Antibiotic synergism in enterococcal endocarditis. J Lab Clin Med. 1976;88:132.
56. Mederski-Samoraj BD, Murray BE. High-level resistance to gentamicin in clinical isolates of enterococci. J Infect Dis. 1983;147:751.
57. Archer GL. Antimicrobial susceptibility and selection of resistance among *Staphylococcus epidermidis* isolates recovered from patients with infections of indwelling foreign devices. Antimicrob Agents Chemother. 1978;14:353.
58. Karchmer AW, Archer GL, Dismukes WE. *Staphylococcus epidermidis* causing prosthetic valve endocarditis: Microbiologic and clinical observations as guides to therapy. Ann Intern Med. 1983;98:447.
59. Karchmer AW, Archer GL, Dismukes WE. *Staphylococcus epidermidis* causing prosthetic valve endocarditis: Microbiologic and clinical observations as guides to therapy. Ann Intern Med. 1983;98:447.
60. Sande MA, Brooks-Fournier RA, Gerberding JL. Efficacy of ciprofloxacin in animal models of infection: Endocarditis, meningitis, and pneumonia. Am J Med. 1987;82:63.
61. Fernandez-Guerrero M, Rouse M, Henry N, et al. Ciprofloxacin therapy of experimental endocarditis caused by methicillin-susceptible or methicillin-resistant *Staphylococcus aureus*. Antimicrob Agents Chemother. 1988;32:747.
62. McLeod R, Remington JS. Fungal endocarditis. In: Rahimtoola SH, ed. Infective Endocarditis. New York: Grune & Stratton; 1978:211.
63. Reller LB. The serum bactericidal test. Rev Infect Dis. 1986;8:803.
64. Weinstein MP. Am J Med. 1985;78:262.
65. Baumgartner WA, Miller DC, Reitz BA, et al. Surgical treatment of prosthetic valve endocarditis. Ann Thorac Surg. 1983;35:87.
66. Mayer KH, Schoenbaum SC. Evaluation and management of prosthetic valve endocarditis. Prog Cardiovasc Dis. 1982;25:48.
67. Dinubile MJ. Surgery in active endocarditis. Ann Intern Med. 1982;96:650.
68. Karp RB. Role of surgery in infective endocarditis. Cardiovasc Clin. 1981;12:157.
69. Alsip SG, Blackstone EH, Kirklin JW, et al. Indications for cardiac surgery in patients with infective endocarditis. Am J Med. 1985;78:138.
70. Carpenter JL, McAllister CK, US Army Collaborative Group. Anticoagulation in prosthetic valve endocarditis. South Med J. 1983;76:1372.
71. Wilson WR, Geraci JE, Danielson GK, et al. Anticoagulant therapy and central nervous system complications in patients with prosthetic valve endocarditis. Circulation. 1978;57:1004.
72. Broviac JW, Cole JJ, Scribner BH. A silicone rubber atrial catheter for prolonged parenteral alimentation. Surg Gynecol Obstet. 1973;136:602.
73. Hickman RO, Buckner CD, Cliff RA, et al. A modified right atrial catheter for access to the venous system in marrow transplant recipients. Surg Gynecol Obstet. 1979;148:871.
74. Press OW, Ramsey PG, Larson EB, et al. Hickman catheter infections in patients with malignancies. Medicine (Baltimore). 1984;63:189.
75. Begala JE, Maher K, Cherry JD. Risk of infection associated with the use of Broviac and Hickman catheters. Am J Infect Control. 1982;10:17.
76. Wade JC, Newman KA, Schimpff SC, et al. Two methods for improved venous access in acute leukemia patients. JAMA. 1981;246:140.
77. Abrahm JL. A prospective study of prolonged central venous access in leukemia. JAMA. 1982;248:2868.
78. Thomas JH, MacArthur RI, Pierce GE, et al. Hickman-Broviac catheters: Indications and results. Am J Surg. 1980;140:791.
79. Lowder JN, Lazarus HM, Herzig RH. Bacteremias and fungemias in oncologic patients with central venous catheters. Arch Intern Med. 1982;142:1456.
80. Schuman ES, Winters V, Gross GF, et al. Management of Hickman catheter sepsis. Am J Surg. 1985;149:627.
81. Liekweg WG, Greenfield LJ. Vascular prosthetic infections: Collected experience and results of treatment. Surgery. 1977;81:335.
82. Szilagyi DE, Smith RF, Elliott JP, et al. Infection in arterial reconstruction with synthetic grafts. Ann Surg. 1972;176:321.
83. Goldstone J, Moore WS. Infection in vascular prostheses: Clinical manifestations and surgical management. Am J Surg. 1974;128:225.
84. O'Hara PJ, Hertzer NR, Beven EG, et al. Surgical management of infected abdominal aortic grafts: Review of a 25-year experience. J Vasc Surg. 1986;3:725.
85. Ilsenfritz FM, Jordan FT. Microbiological monitoring of aortic aneurysm wall and contents during aneurysmectomy. Arch Surg. 1988;123:506.
86. Schwartz JA, Powell TW, Burnham SJ, et al. Culture of abdominal aortic aneurysm contents. An additional series. Arch Surg. 1987;122:777.
87. Moore WS, Malone JM, Keown K. Prosthetic arterial graft material: Influence on neointimal healing and bacteremic infectibility. Arch Surg. 1980;115:1379.
88. DeBakey ME, Jordan GL Jr, Abbott JP, et al. The fate of Dacron vascular grafts. Arch Surg. 1964;89:757.
89. Berger K, Sauvage LR, Rao AM, et al. Healing of arterial prostheses in man: Its incompleteness. Ann Surg. 1972;175:118.
90. Malone JM, Moore WS, Campagna G, et al. Bacteremic infectibility of vascular grafts: The influence of pseudointimal integrity and duration of graft function. Surgery. 1975;78:211.
91. Roon AJ, Malone JM, Moore WS, et al. Bacteremic infectibility: A function of vascular graft material and design. J Surg Res. 1977;22:489.
92. Becker RM, Blundell PE. Infected aortic bifurcation grafts: Experience with 14 patients. Surgery. 1976;80:544.
93. Hoffert PW, Gensler S, Haimovici H. Infection complicating arterial grafts: Personal experience with 12 cases and review of the literature. Arch Surg. 1965;90:427.
94. Wilson SE, Van Wagenen P, Passaro E Jr. Arterial infection. Curr Probl Surg. 1978;15:1.
95. Casali RE, Tucker WE, Thompson BW, et al. Infected prosthetic grafts. Arch Surg. 1980;115:577.
96. Liekweg WG Jr, Levinson SA, Greenfield LJ. Infections of vascular grafts: Incidence, anatomic location, etiologic agents, morbidity, and mortality. In: Duma RJ, ed. Infections of Prosthetic Heart Valves and Vascular Grafts. Baltimore: University Park Press; 1977:239.
97. Rich NM, Collins GJ Jr, Andersen CA. Infected grafts: Clinical presentation and diagnosis. In Duma RJ, ed. Infections of Prosthetic Heart Valves and Vascular Grafts. Baltimore: University Park Press; 1977:253.
98. Elliott JP Jr, Smith RF, Szilagyi DE. Aortoenteric and paraprostheticenteric fistulas. Arch Surg. 1974;108:479.
99. Willwerth BM, Waldhausen JA. Infection of arterial prostheses. Surg Gynecol Obstet. 1974;139:446.
100. Justich E, Amparo EG, Hricak H, et al. Infected aortoiliofemoral grafts: Magnetic resonance imaging. Radiology. 1985;154:133.
101. Sedwitz MM, Davies RJ, Pretorius HT, et al. Indium 111-labeled white blood cell scans after vascular prosthetic reconstruction. J Vasc Surg. 1987;6:476.
102. Schellack J, Stewart MT, Smith RB III, et al. Infected aortobifemoral prosthesis—a dreaded complication. Am Surg. 1988;54:137.
103. Kaiser AB, Clayson KR, Mulherin JL, et al. Antibiotic prophylaxis in vascular surgery. Ann Surg. 1978;188:283.
104. Pitt HA, Postier RG, MacGowan WA, et al. Prophylactic antibiotics in vascular surgery: Topical, systemic, or both? Ann Surg. 1980;192:356.
105. Moore WS, Chvapil M, Seiffert G, et al. Development of an infection-resistant vascular prosthesis. Arch Surg. 1981;116:1403.
106. Moore WS, Malone JM. Vascular infection. In: Simmons RL, Howard RJ, eds. Surgical Infectious Diseases. New York: Appleton-Century-Crofts; 1982:777.
107. Sweeney TF, Kerstein MD. Management of peripheral vascular infections. In: Kerstein MD, ed. Management of Surgical Infections. New York: Futura; 1980:117.
108. Threlkeld MG, Cobbs CG: Questions and Answers: Arterial graft infections—Is antibiotic prophylaxis necessary? JAMA. 1988;259:2608.
109. Ralston AJ, Harlow GR, Jones DM, et al. Infections of Scribner and Brescia arteriovenous shunts. Br Med J. 1971;3:408.
110. Kuruvila KC, Beven EG. Arteriovenous shunts and fistulas for hemodialysis. Surg Clin North Am. 1971;51:1219.
111. Winsett OE, Wolma FJ. Complications of vascular access for hemodialysis. South Med J. 1985;78:513.
112. Kheriakian GM, Roedersheimer LR, Arbaugh JJ. Comparison of autogenous fistula versus expanded polytetrafluoroethylene graft fistula for angioaccess in hemodialysis. Am J Surg. 1986;152:238.
113. Munda R, First MR, Alexander JW, et al. Polytetrafluoroethylene graft survival in hemodialysis. JAMA. 1983;249:219.
114. Dobkin JF, Miller MH, Steigbigel NH. Septicemia in patients on chronic hemodialysis. Ann Intern Med. 1978;88:28.
115. Nsouli KA, Lazarus M, Schoenbaum SC, et al. Bacteremic infection in hemodialysis. Arch Intern Med. 1979;139:1255.
116. Kaslow RA, Zellner SR. Infection in patients on maintenance hemodialysis. Lancet. 1972;2:117.
117. Cross AS, Steigbigel RT. Infective endocarditis and access site infections in patients with hemodialysis. Medicine (Baltimore). 1978;55:453.
118. Bhat DJ, Tellis VA, Kohlberg WI, et al. Management of sepsis involving expanded polytetrafluoroethylene grafts for hemodialysis access. Surgery. 1980;87:445.
119. Oldershaw PJ, Sutton MG, Ward D, et al. Ten-year experience of 359 epicardial pacemaker systems: complications and results. Clin Cardiol. 5:515, 1982.
120. Bluhm G. Pacemaker infections: A clinical study with special reference to prophylactic use of some isoxazolyl penicillins. Acta Med Scand Suppl. 1985;699:1.
121. Wade JS, Cobbs CG. Infections in cardiac pacemakers. In: Remington JS, Swartz MN, eds. Current Clinical Topics in Infectious Diseases. v. 9. New York: McGraw-Hill; 1988:44.

63. PROPHYLAXIS OF INFECTIVE ENDOCARDITIS

DAVID T. DURACK

Infective endocarditis is a serious disease. Even though the etiologic organisms usually can be eradicated by antibiotic treatment, they often leave an unwelcome legacy of permanent valvular damage. Only a minority of patients die during the active phase of infection, but many more suffer further complications and have a shortened life span after being "cured." Therefore, prevention of infective endocarditis has universally been accepted as a worthwhile goal.

It is important to appreciate at the outset that only a small proportion (perhaps 15 percent) of all cases of infective endocarditis can be attributed to bacteremias caused by previous medical, surgical, or dental procedures.[1–6] It follows that the proportion of potentially preventable cases is also small.

Attempted prevention of bacterial infections with antibiotics is most likely to succeed when a single antimicrobial drug is directed against a single pathogen and when the disease occurs with fairly high frequency in the absence of prophylaxis.[5,6] Prevention of endocarditis does not meet these ideals because a variety of antibiotics are used against a variety of organisms and because the disease occurs rarely even if prophylactic antibiotics are not given.

Developments in this field have been hampered by a serious lack of information on which to base recommendations. For example, reliable data are not available to answer even these basic questions: what is the risk of developing infective endocarditis after procedures that cause bacteremia? What procedures and operations should be covered by antibiotics? Is antibiotic prophylaxis effective? If so, which prophylactic antibiotic regimens give the best results? Thus, this area is characterized by uncertainties and controversy.

It is doubtful that sufficient epidemiologic data will ever be accumulated to answer these questions definitively. Random bacteremias occur commonly, probably daily[7,8]; thus patients with underlying heart disease are continually at some risk of developing endocarditis, and it is not possible to determine with certainty which one of many bacteremias, including those caused by health care practitioners, is responsible for an episode of endocarditis.

Clinical investigations of the prophylactic efficacy of antibiotics are also unlikely to provide the answers because an excessively large number of patients would be required to reach a significant conclusion, as the following example illustrates. Let us make the following assumptions: that the risk of acquiring bacterial endocarditis after dental extraction is approximately 1 in 500,[9] that approval for a randomized trial of antibiotic vs. placebo could be obtained from an ethics review committee, and that an antibiotic regimen 100 percent effective in preventing endocarditis is available. An imaginary clinical trial under these admittedly arbitrary conditions might yield the following figures:

Treatment Group		*Number of Patients*	*Cases of Endocarditis*
Placebo		3000	6
Antibiotic		3000	0
	Total	6000	$\chi^2 = 4.2$ $p < .05$

At least 6000 patients with pre-existing valvular heart disease would have to be studied during dental procedures for the results to reach statistical significance. Although these figures are only approximations, it is obvious that it would be difficult or impossible to carry out such a large study. However, it may be possible to demonstrate the efficacy of prophylaxis by selecting subgroups of patients at highest risk for endocarditis. Among patients with prosthetic heart valves undergoing various surgical procedures, it was recently reported that no cases of endocarditis followed 287 procedures for which antibiotic prophylaxis was given, while 6 occurred after 390 procedures for which it was omitted.[10] This interesting result, which needs to be confirmed, just reaches statistical significance.

We must conclude that attempted prevention of infective endocarditis at present remains an empirical practice. Nevertheless, most authorities agree that prophylaxis should be offered to susceptible patients during certain procedures known to be associated with bacteremia.[1,3–6,11–15]

ESTIMATES OF RISK FOR INFECTIVE ENDOCARDITIS

To determine when antibiotic prophylaxis for infective endocarditis should be given, it is necessary to estimate the relative risk of developing endocarditis after certain procedures. Many investigators have reported on the incidence of transient bacteremia after various manipulations.[3–5,7,8,16–25] It should be noted that incidence of bacteremia varies quite widely between studies and that the frequency with which certain species (especially streptococci) enter the blood may correlate better than the overall incidence of bacteremia with risk of endocarditis. Some representative figures from selected studies are presented in Table 1.

Several hundred cases of endocarditis that were attributed to prior dental procedures have been recorded in the literature. In many of these, the first symptoms of endocarditis appeared within less than 2 weeks.[2] Although the incubation period of endocarditis is not known precisely, the onset of symptoms soon after dental operations in these cases makes a causal relationship seem likely. These case reports provide the basis for the belief that dental procedures often cause endocarditis—a belief that is widely but not universally accepted. The risk of developing infective endocarditis due to a dental extraction certainly must be low because bacteremia is common after this operation and endocarditis is relatively rare. It has been variously estimated that the risk is as high as 1 in 533,[9] as low as 1 in 115,500,[26] or even zero.[27] Most authorities would agree that dental operations do indeed pose a significant risk to susceptible patients, but it appears that the risk of acquiring infective endocarditis is probably *less than 1 percent* for each procedure, even if antibiotic prophylaxis is not given.

Similarly, more than 100 case reports provide reasonably good evidence that bacteremias originating from the genitourinary tract may cause endocarditis, especially when urologic or gynecologic operations are carried out in the presence of urinary or pelvic infections.[28] Evidence that other medical and surgical procedures cause infective endocarditis is rather sketchy. For example, only a handful of cases after miscellaneous operations such as drainage of soft tissue infections, abdominal surgery,

TABLE 1. Incidence of Transient Bacteremia after Various Procedures

Extraction of 1 or more teeth	82%
Periodontal surgery	88%
Brushing teeth	40%
Tonsillectomy	38%
Catheter removal after urologic surgery	50%
Prostatectomy (sterile urine)	11%
Prostatectomy (infected urine)	57%
Normal delivery	4–11%
Diagnostic procedures	
Bronchoscopy	0–15%
Barium enema	10%
Liver biopsy	10%
Upper GI endoscopy	4%
Sigmoidoscopy	0–5%
Colonoscopy	5%

(Data from Refs. 7, 16–18, 22–24.)

TABLE 2. Estimate of Risk of Developing Infective Endocarditis after Various Procedures That May Cause Bacteremias

Significant Risk	*Very Low or Negligible Risk*[a]
Dental procedures likely to cause bleeding (e.g., detailed examinations, scaling, extractions)	Minor dental procedures not causing bleeding (e.g., superficial examinations, simple fillings above the gum line, adjustment of orthodontic appliances)
Oral surgery involving teeth and gums	Spontaneous loss of deciduous teeth
Delivery, abortion, insertion or removal of IUD, dilatation and curettage (*in the presence of pelvic infection*)	Normal delivery, therapeutic abortion, insertion or removal of IUD, dilatation and curettage (*in absence of pelvic infection*)
Tonsillectomy, adenoidectomy	Cardiac catheterization
Urinary catheterization, passage of urethral dilators, cystoscopy, prostatectomy (especially with infected urine or bacterial prostatitis)	Insertion of cardiac pacemaker
Drainage of abscesses, operations involving infected soft tissue	Endotracheal intubation
	Diagnostic procedures Endoscopy of upper and lower GI tract Barium meal, barium enema Liver biopsy Bronchoscopy (with flexible bronchoscope)

[a] The risk for some of these procedures may be significant in patients with prosthetic valves.

diagnostic cardiac catheterization, and the use of oral irrigation devices have been recorded.[29,30] The frequency of bacteremia during normal delivery is very low,[31] and very few cases of endocarditis have been recorded in the setting.[32] Although bacteremias may occur during the performance of common diagnostic procedures such as endoscopies, barium enemas, and liver biopsies, very few cases of endocarditis attributable to these common procedures have been reported.[23,24] Some estimates of the risk related to procedures that may cause bacteremia are offered in Table 2.

Underlying Cardiac Conditions

An assessment of risk in relation to the patient's underlying cardiac condition must also be made (Table 3). These estimates are based on the frequency with which various pre-existing cardiac defects are found in patients with infective endocarditis. Certain conditions strongly predispose to endocardial infection; thus a patient with uncorrected patent ductus arteriosus runs approximately a 30 percent risk of developing the disease during his lifetime.[33] Similarly, congenital or acquired aortic valve disease, interventricular septal defects, mitral stenosis or incompetence, and especially prosthetic valves are known to present a relatively high risk of infection.[29,34,35] At the other end of the spectrum, uncomplicated secundum-type atrial septal defects carry such a low risk for infective endocarditis[29] that prophylaxis is probably not indicated for these patients.[13] Mitral valve prolapse presents a special problem. This condition increases a person's risk for endocarditis by five- to eightfold,[36] and it underlies a significant proportion of cases of subacute bacterial endocarditis.[37–39] The risk appears to be greater for those with a precordial systolic murmur.[38] Nevertheless, because mitral valve prolapse is so common in the general population while endocarditis is relatively uncommon, a prolapse cannot be regarded as a high-risk lesion,[36] even when a murmur is present. Most authorities currently recommend prophylaxis for patients with prolapse, especially those with mitral regurgitation. On the other hand, a study of benefits vs. costs by decision analysis indicates that prophylaxis for prolapse would not be cost-effective.[40] This study also indicated that, because the incidence of endocarditis when a patient with prolapse undergoes a dental procedure without prophylaxis is very low, the years of life lost from anaphylaxis due to parenteral penicillin could exceed the years of life saved by prevention of endocarditis.

What are the implications of the above for prophylaxis? In the author's opinion, patients with prolapse should receive prophylaxis because (for the individual) the costs and risks of taking two oral doses of amoxicillin are very low, and a serious disease may occasionally be prevented. However, the use of antibiotics could be considered optional rather than mandatory in this setting, and parenteral prophylaxis should be avoided.

TABLE 3. Estimate of Risk of Developing Infective Endocarditis as Related to Underlying Conditions

Relatively High Risk	*Intermediate Risk*	*Very Low or Negligible Risk*
Prosthetic valves	Mitral valve prolapse	Arteriosclerotic plaques
Previous infective endocarditis	Tricuspid valve disease	Coronary artery disease
Patent ductus arteriosus	Pulmonary valve disease	Atrial septal defects
Fallot's tetralogy	Asymmetric septal hypertrophy	Cardiac pacemakers
Ventricular septal defect		Surgically corrected lesions (without prosthetic implants)
Coarctation of the aorta		
Aortic valve disease		
Mitral stenosis and/or insufficiency		
Marfan syndrome		
Intra-atrial alimentation catheters		
Arteriovenous fistulas		

INDIRECT EVIDENCE OF EFFICACY OF PROPHYLAXIS

In the absence of definitive data, recommendations for the prophylaxis of infective endocarditis must be based on secondary sources of information. These include anecdotal experience with patients, in vitro study of the organisms that cause bacteremia and endocarditis, and evaluation of the prevention of infective endocarditis in experimental animals.

Uncontrolled Clinical Observations

Case reports describing patients who developed endocarditis after a procedure known to cause bacteremia despite the administration of antibiotics provide anecdotal evidence that attempts to prevent endocarditis are not uniformly successful.[4,41] From 1979 to 1982 an American Heart Association committee collected and recorded examples of apparent prevention failures.[39] Among 52 such cases, mitral valve prolapse was the single most common underlying cardiac lesion (33 percent), followed by various congenital abnormalities (29 percent) and rheumatic heart disease (21 percent). Nineteen percent had prosthetic valve endocarditis. Forty-eight cases (92 percent) followed a dental procedure, and 75 percent of cases were caused by viridans streptococci. Symptoms began fairly soon after the procedure suspected to have caused endocarditis: within 2 weeks in 50 percent and within 5 weeks in 79 percent. Most patients received oral penicillin as prophylaxis. Sixty percent of organisms for which antimicrobial susceptibility was known were sensitive to the antibiotic(s) used for prophylaxis. This experience, although anecdotal, indicates that endocarditis prophylaxis failures are not rare and that failures may occur even when the infecting organism is susceptible to the antibiotics used. It confirms that mitral valve prolapse is a common underlying lesion in patients with streptococcal endocarditis.

In Vitro Studies

A variety of organisms may be found in the blood stream after dental, surgical, and diagnostic procedures, including many strains of anaerobes.[8,17] However, only gram-positive cocci such as viridans streptococci, enterococci, and staphylococci commonly cause infective endocarditis in this setting. It is therefore appropriate to focus on the antibiotic susceptibilities of these organisms in attempting to formulate rational prophylactic programs. Most of the bacteria in the oral flora that are likely to cause endocarditis are sensitive to penicillin G.[1,4,42] In fact, it is widely believed that all strains of viridans streptococci are exquisitely sensitive to penicillin. This is not entirely correct; in some series up to one-third of the strains are partially resistant, with minimal bactericidal concentrations (MBC) for penicillin G of 0.1–1.0 μg/ml or more.[43,44] Ampicillin and amoxicillin both possess good in vitro activity against most streptococci associated with endocarditis[42] and provide high serum concentrations.[11] Almost all strains of viridans streptococci, irrespective of their MBCs, are killed more rapidly and completely by a combination of a penicillin and an aminoglycoside than by a penicillin alone.[45] Similarly enterococci, although more likely to be resistant to both penicillins and aminoglycosides, are usually killed synergistically by these drugs in combination, in vitro and in vivo.[46,47]

Experimental Infective Endocarditis

Study of the prevention of experimental infective endocarditis in animal models has provided another secondary source of information. In 1970 Garrison and Freedman[48] reported that placement of a polyethylene catheter in the rabbit heart led to the development of small sterile vegetations at points of contact between the catheter and endocardium. If staphylococci were placed in the lumen of the catheter, staphylococcal endocarditis resulted. Modification of this model by injecting organisms intravenously[49] provided a suitable in vivo system for examining the efficacy of various antibiotic regimens for the prophylaxis of endocarditis.[47,50–53] A similar model in rats has also been used to investigate antibiotic prophylaxis.[56–60] Under experimental conditions, the time of onset of infective endocarditis is known exactly. Another important advantage is that the incidence of infection in untreated animals can be adjusted easily by altering the inoculum size; thus the problem of very low infection rates in patients can be overcome in animals by choosing an inoculum large enough to infect most of the subjects for the organism under investigation. Significant differences among antibiotic regimens can then be demonstrated with manageable numbers of animals in each group.[47,50–60]

Early experiments comparing the success of various antibiotic regimens against viridans streptococci in this model system showed that bacteriostatic antibiotics were usually ineffective, that penicillin in low doses or in high doses of brief duration was often ineffective, that high penicillin concentrations in serum for 12 hours or more were desirable for effective prophylaxis, that the combination of a penicillin plus an aminoglycoside was synergistic against viridans streptococci as well as enterococci, and that vancomycin provided an excellent alternative to regimens using penicillins.[47,50–52,54] Other antibiotics that proved effective under controlled experimental conditions were ampicillin, amoxicillin,[53,59,60] erythromycin,[60] and rifampin.[58]

Further experiments have modified the view that bactericidal antibiotic activity is essential for prophylaxis. Streptomycin proved surprisingly effective in the prevention of experimental infection by some strains of enterococci, even though the serum concentrations of streptomycin were far too low to kill them.[47] Subinhibitory concentrations of certain antibiotics, especially vancomycin, can inhibit the adherence of streptococci to fibrin surfaces in vitro.[61] More recent experiments have demonstrated successful prophylaxis for various streptococci with sublethal doses of vancomycin, clindamycin, erythromycin, and even a tetracycline.[54,55,60] Penicillin was much less effective in the prevention of experimental streptococcal endocarditis if the strain was tolerant to penicillin.[62] However, penicillin exhibited some prophylactic activity even if the strain was so tolerant that bactericidal concentrations of penicillin could not be achieved in serum.[62] All these findings suggest that prevention can sometimes be achieved by antibiotic effects that fall short of total bacterial killing, perhaps by an alteration of surface structures that mediate adherence to fibrin or by other unknown mechanisms. In other words, bactericidal action may be sufficient but not always necessary for prevention. The implications of these findings for humans are uncertain. At present, it still seems prudent to choose bactericidal drugs for the prophylaxis of infective endocarditis whenever possible.

To place these experimental findings in perspective, it is important to emphasize that direct extrapolations to humans should not be made from the extensive experimental data. If the results are applied too literally, stringent prophylactic regimens that are impractical for general use may be recommended. Although in vivo models provide a closer simulation of human endocarditis than any in vitro system could, there are two important differences. First, a foreign body was present throughout many of these experiments because the intracardiac catheter often was left in place. The presence of a foreign body in tissue lowers the inoculum required to initiate infection and then makes infection harder to eradicate. Therefore, the animal models probably simulate patients with prosthetic valves more closely than they do patients with congenital or rheumatic valvular disease. Second, in many of the experiments a high inoculum was chosen deliberately to make statistical comparisons possible with a relatively small number of animals. Both the presence of a foreign body and the use of a high inoculum would tend to make prevention harder to achieve, so any regimen that proved effective under these rigorous experimental conditions should provide a margin of safety in clinical use.

With these reservations in mind, what has been the real contribution of experimental studies of prevention? Animal models provide a convenient in vivo method for *ranking* prophylactic antibiotic regimens in order of efficacy, but they cannot be used to determine whether any particular antibiotic regimen will or will not prevent endocarditis in patients. For example, experimental findings do not exclude the possibility that tetracycline may prevent endocarditis in some patients. They do support the conclusion that one of the optimal regimens such as vancomycin, or penicillin plus streptomycin, should provide a much wider margin of safety than does a lower-ranking regimen such as tetracycline.[52]

CARDIAC SURGERY

Most cardiovascular surgeons believe that the use of prophylactic antibiotics has reduced the incidence of postcardiotomy endocarditis.[35,63] While this is may be true, it should be noted that numerous technical improvements, introduced during the period when the incidence of postoperative endocarditis was falling, also may have contributed significantly. In fact, the efficacy of antibiotics for the prevention of postcardiotomy endocarditis has not yet been subjected to an adequate, critically controlled trial.[63] The clinical impression that antibiotic prophylaxis during cardiac surgery is effective is now so widely accepted that ethical consent to perform a placebo-controlled trial probably could no longer be obtained.[63]

Early-onset postcardiotomy endocarditis may be caused by a wide variety of organisms including staphylococci, gram-negative bacteria, and fungi. No single antibiotic regimen is effective against all these, and the use of broad-spectrum antibiotics may itself predispose to superinfection with resistant organisms. Therefore, attempts to prevent endocarditis with antibiotics during open heart surgery should probably be limited to a short course of an antistaphylococcal agent such as a cephalosporin or vancomycin.[5,13] Many practitioners add an aminoglycoside in the hope of taking advantage of possible synergism.

Diagnostic cardiac catheterizations (including Swan-Ganz catheters), insertion of pacemakers, coronary artery surgery, pericardial surgery, and the use of the aortic balloon pump all appear to present little risk, and the administration of antibiotics specifically for the prevention of infective endocarditis is not usually recommended during these operations. However, it should be noted that in patients with severe burns (who often develop bacteremias) pulmonary artery catheters have been reported to predispose to both nonbacterial and bacterial endocarditis.[64]

Prosthetic Heart Valves

Extensive clinical experience has established that patients with prosthetic heart valves are at a relatively high risk for infective endocarditis.[10,34,35,65] The high mortality and morbidity associated with prosthetic valve endocarditis and the frequent necessity for repeated valve replacement in later years make its prevention of primary importance. Although the incidence of endocarditis after cardiac surgery has fallen steadily since these operations became commonplace, the risk of endocarditis in the first year remains in the region of 1 percent and thereafter approximates 1 percent per year.[34,35,65] For comparison, the incidence of endocarditis is approximately 0.4 percent per year in patients with rheumatic heart disease.[66] It is important to recognize this risk and to take all possible steps to minimize it. Before cardiac surgery, the dental health of every patient should be evaluated. Any necessary dental work should be completed under close observation and with appropriate antibiotic coverage before valve replacement. Healthy teeth should not be extracted, but if advanced dental or periodontal disease is present, extraction of all teeth should be considered. Thereafter, the patient should maintain good oral hygiene. Consultation between the patient's dentist and physician is important to ensure optimal antibiotic coverage during routine dental procedures. Practitioners may choose to administer prophylaxis to cover certain procedures (such as colonoscopy) that present very little risk in patients without prosthetic valves (see Tables 1 and 2).

Late-onset prosthetic valve endocarditis (later than 60 days after the operation) is more likely to be caused by organisms originating in the oral cavity, just as for native valve endocarditis. Attempted prophylaxis for endocarditis in this setting should be directed against streptococci, not staphylococci and gram-negative bacilli.

Many cardiac patients receive anticoagulant therapy, which may alter the choice of prophylactic antibiotics. Intramuscular injections are contraindicated in patients receiving heparin and should be avoided if possible in patients being administered coumadin. For some patients an oral regimen may suffice, but for patients with prosthetic valves, an intravenous regimen should be chosen.

COMMON ERRORS IN ATTEMPTED PREVENTION OF ENDOCARDITIS

Starting Antibiotic Treatment Too Early

Antibiotics should be administered so as to provide the highest serum levels at the time the procedure causing the bacteremia is performed. There is no rationale to support the common practice of beginning antibiotic therapy earlier than is necessary to meet this criterion. Indeed, if antibiotics are given more than a few hours before the procedure, penicillin-sensitive oral flora may be replaced by penicillin-resistant organisms, and endocarditis, should it occur, may be caused by resistant organisms.[41] For most regimens, the administration of antibiotics 30–60 minutes before the procedure is suitable. If the operation is delayed unexpectedly, doses may have to be repeated.

Continuing Antibiotic Therapy Too Long

As with most other forms of antibiotic prophylaxis, a short course is indicated. Experimental studies provide some evidence that even a single dose may be adequate, providing an optimal antibiotic regimen is chosen.[49,50–52,59] However, many practitioners continue prophylaxis for days.[39,67,68] This wastes antibiotic, may lead to the emergence of resistant organisms, and places the patient at an additional risk of adverse reactions. In any case, a patient who is feeling perfectly well is unlikely to adhere to an unnecessarily prolonged regimen.

Use of Low-Dose Antibiotics

Low-dose prophylactic regimens are often used for the prevention of endocarditis, even though both theoretic considerations and experimental studies indicate that a fairly high serum level of antibiotic is advisable.[39,50,52] Oral therapy is not ideal for this purpose since variability of intestinal absorption may result in relatively low and unreliable serum levels. For this reason I prefer to use parenteral prophylaxis when circumstances allow, for example, when the patient is in the hospital. However, it must be accepted that oral regimens will continue to be used in a great majority of cases because they are more convenient for both patient and practitioner. The full dose should always be given.

Prophylaxis for Tooth Extraction but Not for Lesser Dental Procedures

Much of the literature on infective endocarditis after dental procedures has emphasized tooth *extraction*. However, bacteremias may occur after almost any form of dental manipulation.[1,3,7] One reasonable criterion is to use antibiotic prophylaxis for all procedures likely to cause gingival bleeding.[13] This will exclude many routine check-ups, simple fillings above the gum line, and adjustment of orthodontic appliances but will usually include detailed examination, scaling and cleaning of the teeth by a dentist or hygienist, and more extensive dental operations.

Confusion between Prevention of Rheumatic Fever and Prevention of Infective Endocarditis

One frequently hears that antibiotics were not given to a patient with rheumatic heart disease before dental extractions "because he was already receiving penicillin prophylaxis." Whereas the administration of continuous, low-dose penicillin effectively prevents rheumatic fever, it is *inadequate* to prevent infective endocarditis. The incidence of infective endocarditis in children receiving penicillin for the prevention of rheumatic fever is no less than in those with rheumatic heart disease who are not receiving prophylaxis.[66] Because patients taking low-dose oral penicillin for the prevention of rheumatic fever often carry moderately penicillin-resistant streptococci in the mouth, attempted prevention of infective endocarditis with an oral penicillin regimen in these patients is not advisable. They should receive one of the parenteral regimens or an alternative regimen that does not include penicillin (Table 4).

Failure to Use Prophylaxis for Children

Because bacteremia during dental procedures appears to be somewhat less common in children than in adults, it has been suggested that antibiotic prophylaxis for infective endocarditis is unnecessary in children.[69] However, careful studies indicate that bacteremia does indeed occur in a significant proportion of children after dental procedures,[40] and cases of endocarditis following soon after dental extraction have been reported.[71] The present consensus, therefore, is that children should receive antibiotic prophylaxis for infective endocarditis, with appropriate adjustment of dosages.

TABLE 4. Author's Current Recommendations for Prophylaxis of Endocarditis[a]

Standard regimen	For dental procedures; oral or upper respiratory tract surgery; minor GI or GU tract procedures	Amoxicillin, 3.0 g orally 1 hr before, then 1.5 g 6 hr later[b]
Special regimens	Oral regimen for penicillin-allergic patients (oral and respiratory tract only)	Erythromycin, 1.0 g orally 1–2 hr before, then 0.5 g 6 hr later[b]
	Parenteral regimen for high-risk patients; also for GI or GU tract procedures	Ampicillin 2.0 g im or iv, *plus* gentamicin 1.5 mg/kg im or iv, 0.5 hr before[b]
	Parenteral regimen for penicillin-allergic patients	Vancomycin, 1.0 g iv slowly over 1 hr, starting 1 hr before; *add* gentamicin, 1.5 mg/kg im or iv, if GI or GU tract involved[b]
	Cardiac surgery including implantation of prosthetic valves	Cefazolin, 2.0 g iv, at induction of anesthesia, repeated 8 and 16 hr later[b,c]
		or vancomycin, 1.0 g iv slowly over 1 hr starting at induction, then 0.5 g iv 8 and 16 hr later[b,c,d]

[a] These regimens are empirical suggestions; no regimen has been *proved* effective for the prevention of endocarditis, and prevention failures may occur with any regimen. These regimens are not intended to cover all clinical situations; the practitioner should use his own judgment on safety and cost–benefit issues in each individual case. One or two additional doses may be given if the period of risk for bacteremia is prolonged.

[b] Pediatric dosages: ampicillin, 50 mg/kg; cefazolin, 30 mg/kg; erythromycin, 20 mg/kg for first dose, then 10 mg/kg; gentamicin, 2.0 mg/kg; amoxicillin, for children who weigh more than 60 lb, use the same as for adults; for children less than 60 lb, use half the adult dose; vancomycin, 20 mg/kg.

[c] Gentamicin, 1.5 mg/kg iv, may be given with each dose if postoperative gram-negative infections have occurred with significant frequency at that hospital.

[d] This regimen is recommended for units where *Staphylococcus epidermidis* prosthetic valve infection is a problem.

THE MALPRACTICE DILEMMA

The question of professional liability in the prophylaxis of endocarditis has led to allegations of negligence and malpractice suits. In today's litigious social climate, such claims have become increasingly common. It should be obvious that the lack of basic information referred to earlier makes evaluation of such cases exceedingly difficult. For example, it is hard to establish that any single procedure known to cause bacteremia was the "proximate cause" in a case of endocarditis. It is even harder to prove that the failure of a physician or dentist to administer antibiotics was the direct cause of a patient acquiring endocarditis. If a strict demonstration of proximate cause were always required, it is doubtful that any claim based on the failure to administer prophylaxis could succeed, but juries are sometimes capricious in deciding liability in malpractice cases. Another common problem for the defense in claims based on a failure to administer prophylaxis is our ignorance of the precise duration of the incubation period of infective endocarditis. Damages have been claimed when the first symptoms of endocarditis did not appear for 3 months or more after tooth extractions without antibiotic cover. The likelihood of proximate cause here is remote, because review of case reports indicates that the incubation period is 2 weeks or less in most cases.[2]

In the light of present knowledge, the health care professional can reasonably be expected to appreciate the risk that infective endocarditis may occur under certain circumstances. He should question the patient about underlying conditions that may predispose to endocarditis and should inform susceptible patients of the small risk that they may develop the disease. An antibiotic regimen should be administered to these patients before selected dental, surgical, and genitourinary tract manipulations that might cause bacteremia. Indications for prophylaxis outside these areas are less firmly established at present. A failure to use any recognized antibiotic regimen in preference to another should not be construed as negligence because many different regimens have been published over the past 25 years. Although some authorities recognize evidence that certain antibiotic regimens probably provide a wider margin of efficacy than do others,[11–13,44–60] this evidence is not yet firm enough to make the choice of any particular regimen mandatory.

The risks of toxicity from any prophylactic regimen must be considered carefully. Allergic reactions may occur even after low doses of penicillin; this risk is common to all regimens using penicillins as drugs of choice. However, the risk of anaphylaxis to penicillin is higher for parenteral than for oral administration. Other side effects such as ototoxicity and nephrotoxicity from aminoglycosides or vancomycin are extremely unlikely to occur after the very short courses (1 day or less) now used for the prophylaxis of infective endocarditis.

CURRENT RECOMMENDATIONS

The *Medical Letter*[12] and an American Heart Association Committee[13] have published recommendations for the prophylaxis of infective endocarditis. Such recommendations for prophylaxis[12,13,77] are rather lengthy and complex; while widely known, they are not well understood, and they are often ignored in practice.[39,68,73,74] Therefore, an American Heart Association committee and other advisory bodies are presently developing recommendations for simplified regimens in an attempt to improve compliance. My current suggestions are listed in Table 4.

REFERENCES

1. Hood EW, Kaye D. Prophylaxis of bacterial endocarditis. J Chronic Dis. 1963;15:635.
2. Starkebaum M, Durack D, Beeson P. The "incubation period" of subacute bacterial endocarditis. Yale J Biol Med. 1977;50:49.
3. Everett ED, Hirschmann JV. Transient bacteremia and endocarditis prophylaxis. A review. Medicine (Baltimore). 1977;56:61.
4. Bisno AL. Antimicrobial prophylaxis of endocarditis. In: Bisno AL, ed. Treatment of Infective Endocarditis. New York: Grune & Stratton; 1981:281.
5. Sanford JP. Prophylactic use of antibiotics: Basic considerations. South Med J. 70(Suppl) No. 1, p 2, 1977.
6. Freedman LR. Prophylaxis of intravascular infection. In: Infective Endocarditis and Other Intravascular Infections. New York: Plenum; 1982:63.
7. Cobe HM. Transient bacteremias. Oral Surg. 1954;7:609.
8. Loesche WJ. Indigenous human flora and bacteremia in infective endocarditis. Am Heart Assoc Monogr. 1977;52:40.
9. Kelson SR, White PD. Notes on 250 cases of subacute bacterial (streptococcal) endocarditis studied and treated between 1927 and 1939. Ann Intern Med. 1945;22:40.
10. Horstkotte D, Friedrichs W, Pippert H, et al. Benefit of prophylaxis for infectious endocarditis (IE) in patients with prosthetic heart valves. Z Kardiol. 1986;75:8.
11. Shanson DC. The prophylaxis of infective endocarditis. J Antimicrob Chemother. 1978;4:2.
12. Prevention of bacterial endocarditis. Med Let. 1986;28:22.
13. American Heart Association Committee on Rheumatic Fever and Infective Endocarditis. Prevention of bacterial endocarditis (Abstract). Circulation. 1984;70:1123.
14. Kaye D. Prophylaxis for infective endocarditis: An update. Ann Intern Med. 1986;104:419.
15. McGowan DA. A dental view of controversies in the prophylaxis of infective endocarditis. J Antimicrob Chemother. 1987;20(Suppl A):105.
16. Elliott SD. Bacteriaemia and oral sepsis. Proc R Soc Med. 1939;32:747.
17. Rogosa M, Hampp EG, Nevin TA, et al. Blood sampling and cultural studies in the detection of postoperative bacteremias. J Am Dent Assoc. 1960;60:171.
18. Slade N. Bacteriaemia and septicaemia after urologic operations. Proc R Soc Med. 1958;51:331.
19. LeFrock JL, Ellis CA, Turchik JB, et al. Transient bacteremia associated with sigmoidoscopy. N Engl J Med. 1973;289:467.
20. LeFrock JL, Ellis CA, Klainer AS, et al. Transient bacteremia associated with barium enema. Arch Intern Med. 1975;135:835.
21. Hoffman BI, Kobasa W, Kaye D. Bacteremia after rectal examination. Ann Intern Med. 1978;88:658.
22. Creevy CD, Feeney MJ. Routine use of antibiotics in transurethral prostatic resection. A clinical investigation. J Urol. 1954;71:615.
23. Sande MA. Prophylactic antibiotics during diagnostic procedures of the gastrointestinal tract. Am Heart Assoc Monogr. 1977;52:73.
24. Shorvon PJ, Eykyn SJ, Cotton PB. Gastrointestinal instrumentation, bacteraemia, and endocarditis. Gut. 1983;24:1078.
25. Baltch AL, Pressman HL, Schaffer C, et al. Bacteremia in patients undergoing oral procedures. Study following parenteral antimicrobial prophylaxis as rec-

ommended by the American Heart Association, 1977. Arch Intern Med. 1988;148:1084.
26. Pogrel MA, Welsby PD. The dentist and prevention of infective endocarditis. Br Dent J. 1975;139:12.
27. Schwartz SP, Salman I. The effect of oral surgery on the course of patients with diseases of the heart. Am J Orthodont. 1942;28:331.
28. Vosti KL. Special problems in prophylaxis of endocarditis following genitourinary tract and obstetrical and gynecological procedures. Am Heart Assoc Monogr. 1977;52:75.
29. Kerr AJ Jr. Subacute Bacterial Endocarditis. Springfield, Il: Charles C Thomas; 1955.
30. Drapkin MS. Endocarditis after the use of an oral irrigation device. Ann Intern Med. 1977;87:455.
31. Sugrue D, Blake S, Troy P, et al. Antibiotic prophylaxis against infective endocarditis after normal delivery—is it necessary? Br Heart J. 1980;44:499.
32. Seaworth BJ, Durack DT. Infective endocarditis in obstetric and gynecologic practice. Am J Obstet Gynecol. 1986;154:180.
33. Wood P. Diseases of the Heart and Circulation. 3rd ed. London: Eyre & Spottiswoode; 1968:465.
34. Rossiter SJ, Stinson EB, Oyer PE, et al. Prosthetic valve endocarditis. J Thorac Cardiovasc Surg. 1978;76:795.
35. Braimbridge MV, Eykyn SJ. Prosthetic valve endocarditis. J Antimicrob Chemother. 1987;20(Suppl A):173.
36. Clemens JD, Horwitz RI, Jaffee CC, et al. A controlled evaluation of the risk of bacterial endocarditis in persons with mitral valve prolapse. N Engl J Med. 1982;307:776.
37. Nolan CM, Kane JJ, Grunow WA. Infective endocarditis and mitral prolapse. A comparison with other types of endocarditis. Arch Intern Med. 1981;131:477.
38. MacMahon SW, Hickey AJ, Wilcken DEL, et al. Risk of infective endocarditis in mitral valve prolapse with and without precordial systolic murmurs. Am J Cardiol. 1986;58:105.
39. Durack DT, Disno AL, Kaplan EL. Apparent failures of endocarditis prophylaxis: Analysis of 52 cases submitted to a national registry. JAMA. 1983;250:2318.
40. Clemens JD, Ransohoff DF. A quantitative assessment of pre-dental antibiotic prophylaxis for patients with mitral-valve prolapse. J Chronic Dis. 1984;37:531.
41. Garrod LP, Waterworth PM. The risks of dental extraction during penicillin treatment. Br Heart J. 1962;24:39.
42. Basker MJ, Sutherland R. Activity of amoxycillin, alone, and in combination with aminoglycoside antibiotics against streptococci associated with bacterial endocarditis. J Antimicrob Chemother. 1977;3:273.
43. Blount JG. Bacterial endocarditis. Am J Med. 1965;38:909.
44. Wilson WR, Garaci JE, Wilkowske CJ, et al. Short-term intramuscular therapy with procaine penicillin plus streptomycin for infective endocarditis due to viridans streptococci. Circulation. 1978;57:1158.
45. Wolfe JC, Johnson WD. Penicillin-sensitive streptococcal endocarditis. In vitro and clinical observations on penicillin-streptomycin therapy. Ann Int Med. 1974;81:178.
46. Russell EJ, Sutherland R. Activity of amoxicillin against enterococci and synergism with aminoglycoside antibiotics. J Med Microbiol. 1975;8:1.
47. Durack DT, Starkebaum MK, Petersdorf RG. Chemotherapy of experimental streptococcal endocarditis. VI. Prevention of enterococcal endocarditis. J Lab Clin Med. 1977;90:171.
48. Garrison PK, Freedman LR. Experimental endocarditis. 1. Staphylococcal endocarditis in rabbits resulting from placement of a polyethylene catheter in the right side of the heart. Yale J Biol Med. 1970;42:394.
49. Durack DT, Beeson PB, Petersdorf RG. Experimental bacterial endocarditis. III. Production and progress of the disease in rabbits. Br J Exp Pathol. 1973;54:142.
50. Durack DT, Petersdorf RG. Chemotherapy of experimental streptococcal endocarditis. I. Comparison of commonly recommended prophylactic regimens. J Clin Invest. 1973;52:592.
51. Pelletier LL, Durack DT, Petersdorf RG. Chemotherapy of experimental streptococcal endocarditis. IV. Further observations on prophylaxis. J Clin Invest. 1975;56:319.
52. Durack DT. Experience with prevention of experimental endocarditis. Am Heart Assoc Monogr. 1977;52:28.
53. McGowan DA, Nair S, MacFarlane TW, et al. Prophylaxis of experimental endocarditis in rabbits using one or two doses of amoxycillin. Br Dent J. 1983;155:88.
54. Bernard JP, Francioli P, Glauser MP. Vancomycin prophylaxis of experimental *Streptococcus sanguis*; inhibition of bacterial adherence rather than bacterial killing. J Clin Invest. 1981;68:1113.
55. Glauser MP, Francioli P. Successful prophylaxis against experimental streptococcal endocarditis with bacteriostatic antibiotics. J Infect Dis. 1982;146:806.
56. Moreillon P, Francioli P, Overholser D, et al. Mechanisms of successful amoxicillin prophylaxis of experimental endocarditis due to *Streptococcus intermedius*. J Infect Dis. 1986;154:801.
57. Overholser CD, Moreillon P, Glauser MP. Experimental bacterial endocarditis after dental extractions in rats with periodontitis. J Infect Dis. 1987;155:107.
58. Malinverni R, Bille J, Glauser MP. Single-dose rifampin prophylaxis for experimental endocarditis induced by high bacterial inocula of viridans streptococci. J Infect Dis. 1987;156:151.
59. Malinverni R, Francioli PB, Glauser MP. Comparison of single and multiple doses of prophylactic antibiotics in experimental streptococcal endocarditis. Circulation. 1987;76:376.
60. Malinverni R, Overholser CD, Bille J, et al. Antibiotic prophylaxis of experimental endocarditis after dental extractions. Circulation. 1988;77:182.
61. Scheld WM, Zak O, Vosbeck K, et al. Bacterial adhesion in the pathogenesis of infective endocarditis. Effect of subinhibitory antibiotic concentrations on streptococcal adhesion in vitro and the development of endocarditis in rabbits. J Clin Invest. 1981;68:1381.
62. Hess J, Dankert J, Durack DT. Significance of penicillin tolerance in vivo of experimental *Streptococcus sanguis* endocarditis. J Antimicrob Chemother. 1983;11:555.
63. Schaffner W. Antibiotic prophylaxis in valvular replacement surgery. In: Duma RJ, ed. Infections of Prosthetic Heart Valves and Vascular Grafts. Baltimore: University Park Press; 1977:313.
64. Ehrie M, Alfred PM, Moore FD, et al. Endocarditis with the indwelling balloon-tipped pulmonary artery catheter in burn patients. J Trauma. 1978;18:664.
65. Wilson WR. Prosthetic valve endocarditis: Incidence, anatomic location, cause, morbidity and mortality. In: Duma RJ, ed. Infections of Prosthetic Heart Valves and Vascular Grafts. Baltimore: University Park Press; 1977:3.
66. Doyle EF, Spagnuolo M, Taranta A, et al. The risk of bacterial endocarditis during antirheumatic prophylaxis. JAMA. 1967;201:129.
67. Durack DT. Current practice in prevention of bacterial endocarditis. Br Heart J. 1975;37:478.
68. Brooks SL. Survey of compliance with American Heart Association guidelines for prevention of bacterial endocarditis. J Am Dent Assoc. 1980;101:41.
69. Hurwitz GA, Speck WT, Keller GD. Absence of bacteremia in children after prophylaxis. Oral Surg. 1971;32:891.
70. Peterson LJ, Peacock R. The incidence of bacteremia in pediatric patients following tooth extraction. Circulation. 1976;53:676.
71. Johnson DH, Rosenthal A, Nadas AS. A forty-year review of bacterial endocarditis in infancy and childhood. Circulation. 1975;51:581.
72. Working Party of the British Society for Antimicrobial Chemotherapy. The antibiotic prophylaxis of infective endocarditis. Lancet. 1982;2:1323.
73. Murrah VA, Merry JW, Little JW, et al. Compliance with guidelines for management of dental school patients susceptible to infective endocarditis. J Dent Educ. 1987;51:229.
74. Sadowsky D, Kunzel C. Recommendations for prevention of bacterial endocarditis: Compliance by dental general practitioners. Circulation. 1988;77:1316.

64. MYOCARDITIS, PERICARDITIS AND MEDIASTINITIS

MARIA C. SAVOIA
MICHAEL N. OXMAN

Inflammatory processes affecting the heart frequently involve both the myocardium (myocarditis) and the pericardium (pericarditis). However, involvement of one or the other usually predominates, and the syndromes of myocarditis and pericarditis are sufficiently distinct in clinical presentation, etiology, and pathophysiology to warrant separate consideration.

MYOCARDITIS

Myocarditis, literally inflammation of the myocardium, is a protean disease with a wide variety of infectious and noninfectious etiologies. Postmortem examinations reveal evidence of previously unsuspected myocarditis in 2–10 percent of unselected cases,[1,2] with a higher incidence in young persons who have died suddenly.[3,4] The diagnosis of infectious myocarditis is generally considered when unexplained heart failure or arrhythmias occur in the setting of a systemic febrile illness or after symptoms of an upper respiratory tract infection. The inflammatory process may affect myocytes, vascular elements, the conducting system, autonomic nerves, and/or the interstitium. One or more of at least four mechanisms appear to be involved: (*1*) direct damage to cells by an infectious agent; (*2*) cytotoxicity caused by a circulating toxin; (*3*) cytotoxicity caused by infection-induced immune reactions; and (*4*) nonspecific damage to myocytes as a result of the inflammatory process.

Etiologic Agents

Viruses are the most important infectious cause of myocarditis in the United States and Western Europe. Long before the era of modern virology, pericardial and myocardial involvement was recognized during outbreaks of mumps,[5] influenza,[6] measles,[7,8] poliomyelitis,[9] and enterovirus-associated pleurodynia.[10] In modern times, enteroviruses[11,12] and especially group B coxsackieviruses[13,14] have been the major agents implicated. These small, nonenveloped, single-stranded RNA viruses belonging to the picornavirus family attach to specific receptors on myocardial cells.[11] Though uncommon, symptomatic myocarditis or myopericarditis is also observed in persons infected with many other viruses, particularly arboviruses and arenaviruses (Table 1).

Myocardial involvement is the most common cause of death in diphtheria[45]; the toxin produced by *Corynebacterium diphtheriae* severely damages the myocardium and conduction system. The cardiac damage seen in patients with *Clostridium perfringens* may be the result of toxin, metastatic abscess formation, or both.[46,47] The immunologically mediated carditis associated with acute rheumatic fever[48] is discussed in Chapter 177.

Invasion of the blood stream by any bacterial pathogen may result in metastatic foci in the myocardium, and myocarditis has been recognized in the course of meningococcemia,[49] salmonellosis,[50] brucellosis,[51] and streptococcal and staphylococcal bacteremia.[52] More commonly, bacteria invade the myocardium as a complication of endocarditis by contiguous spread from valvular tissue or via septic embolization of the coronary arteries.[72]

Myocarditis has been observed in the course of *Mycoplasma pneumoniae*[53,54] and *Chlamydia psittaci*[55] infections and is commonly seen in rickettsial infections,[56] especially scrub typhus.[44,57,58] Approximately 10 percent of patients with Lyme disease develop cardiac abnormalities, most commonly conduction system disturbances.[59,60] In South America, the principal agent responsible for myocarditis is *Trypanosoma cruzi*, the protozoan that causes Chagas disease. The initial infection is often asymptomatic but it sometimes results in an acute illness complicated by myocarditis.[65] Myocarditis is the principal manifestation of chronic Chagas disease, which occurs in approximately 30% of infected individuals. These patients typically have cardiomegaly, congestive heart failure (often predominantly right-sided), and conduction disturbances.[66,67] *Trypanosoma gambiense* and *rhodesiense*, the agents of African trypanosomiasis, may also affect the heart with similar results, but central nervous system findings usually predominate.[68] Myocarditis is also observed in trichinosis[69,70] and is responsible for the occasional deaths that occur in severe infections.

In immunocompromised patients, myocarditis occurs as a consequence of a number of disseminated infections. Overt myocarditis is common in disseminated toxoplasmosis,[71] and systemic aspergillosis and candidiasis may also involve the heart.[61,62] Cryptococcal myocarditis has been reported in patients with the acquired immunodeficiency syndrome (AIDS).[63,64] Cardiac abnormalities in AIDS are common but are usually clinically silent.[73–76] In a retrospective review, mild focal myocarditis was found at necropsy in 37 of 71 AIDS cases examined.[77] A potential pathogen was identified in only seven. Heart failure with biventricular dilatation was the most common clinical correlate, occurring in 6 percent of patients. Human immune deficiency virus (HIV) has been cultured from endomyocardial biopsies,[78,79] but the effect of the virus on myocytes is not known. Patients with AIDS may also be infected with known cardiotropic viruses.[79] The full spectrum of diseases associated with HIV infection remains to be elucidated.

TABLE 1. Infectious Causes of Myocarditis

Viruses	
Coxsackie A[11–13]	Yellow fever[28]
Coxsackie B[11–14]	Argentina hemorrhagic fever[29]
Echoviruses[15,16]	Bolivian hemorrhagic fever[29]
Polio[9,17,18]	Lymphocytic choriomeningitis[30]
Mumps[5,19,20]	Adenovirus[31,32]
Rubeola[7,8]	Varicella-zoster[33–35]
Influenza A and B[6,21,22]	Cytomegalovirus[36]
Rabies[23]	Epstein-Barr[37,38]
Rubella[24,25]	Vaccinia[39]
Dengue[26,27]	Variola[40]
Chikungunya[27]	Hepatitis B[41–43]
Bacteria and Rickettsia	
Corynebacterium diphtheriae[44,45]	*Staphylococcus aureus*[52]
Clostridium perfringens[46,47]	*Mycoplasma pneumoniae*[53,54]
Streptococcus pyogenes[44,48]	*Chlamydia psittaci*[55]
Neisseria meningitidis[49]	*Rickettsia rickettsii*[56]
Salmonella[50]	*Rickettsia tsutsugamushi*[44,57,58]
Brucella[51]	*Borrelia burgdorferi*[59,60]
Fungi	
Aspergillus[61,62]	*Cryptococcus*[62–64]
Candida[62]	
Parasites	
Trypanosoma cruzi[65–67]	*Trichinella spiralis*[69,70]
Trypanosoma gambiense[68]	*Toxoplasma gondii*[71]
Trypanosoma rhodesiense[68]	

Pathology and Pathogenesis

Myocardial pathology depends upon the infecting agent, the mechanism of pathogenesis, and the duration of the process. The hallmarks of myocarditis are an inflammatory infiltrate and injury to adjacent myocardial cells. Pathologic changes may be acute or chronic and vary markedly in severity, depending upon the nature of the disease and the point in its course at which tissue is obtained. Some agents, like the coxsackie B viruses, infect the myocytes themselves, while agents like varicella-zoster virus and hepatitis B virus appear to injure vascular endothelial cells. Although routine histology may help in the differential diagnosis, it rarely provides definitive information regarding the etiologic agent. Early in many viral infections, scattered hypereosinophilic myofibers, widespread edema, and only a few inflammatory cells may be present. Later, there is loss of striation, nuclear degeneration, and fragmentation of myofibers. The degenerating or partially necrotic myofibers are usually surrounded by lymphocytes, plasma cells, and macrophages.[13] Polymorphonuclear cells are occasionally seen[3] (Fig. 1). The acute process may resolve completely; healing and chronicity are reflected by the development of interstitial fibrosis and loss of myofibers.[80]

Mouse models of myocarditis induced by infection with either coxsackievirus B3 or encephalomyocarditis virus have revealed several possible pathogenetic mechanisms. Susceptibility to coxsackievirus B-induced myocarditis is age-dependent and genetically determined.[81] Mechanisms of injury vary in different mouse strains.[82–85] In susceptible animals acute myocarditis results from direct infection and cytolysis of myocytes.[3] In surviving animals, neutralizing antibody, perhaps in conjunction with macrophages[86,87] and natural killer (NK) cells,[88] appears to terminate virus replication by 7–9 days after infection.[11,89,90] Exercise[3,11] and corticosteroids[91] markedly enhance mortality during the early stages of infection. Nonsteroidal anti-inflammatory agents may also have deleterious effects.[92] Mice surviving the acute replicative phase of the virus infection may go on to develop severe myocarditis in the absence of recoverable virus. This second phase of virus-induced myocardial destruction is dependent upon the presence of cytolytic T cells,[13] which appear as virus replication ceases. Some of these cytolytic T cells recognize and lyse both infected and uninfected myocytes,[93] and their presence correlates with myocardial damage.[94,95] The severity of myocardial damage caused by this im-

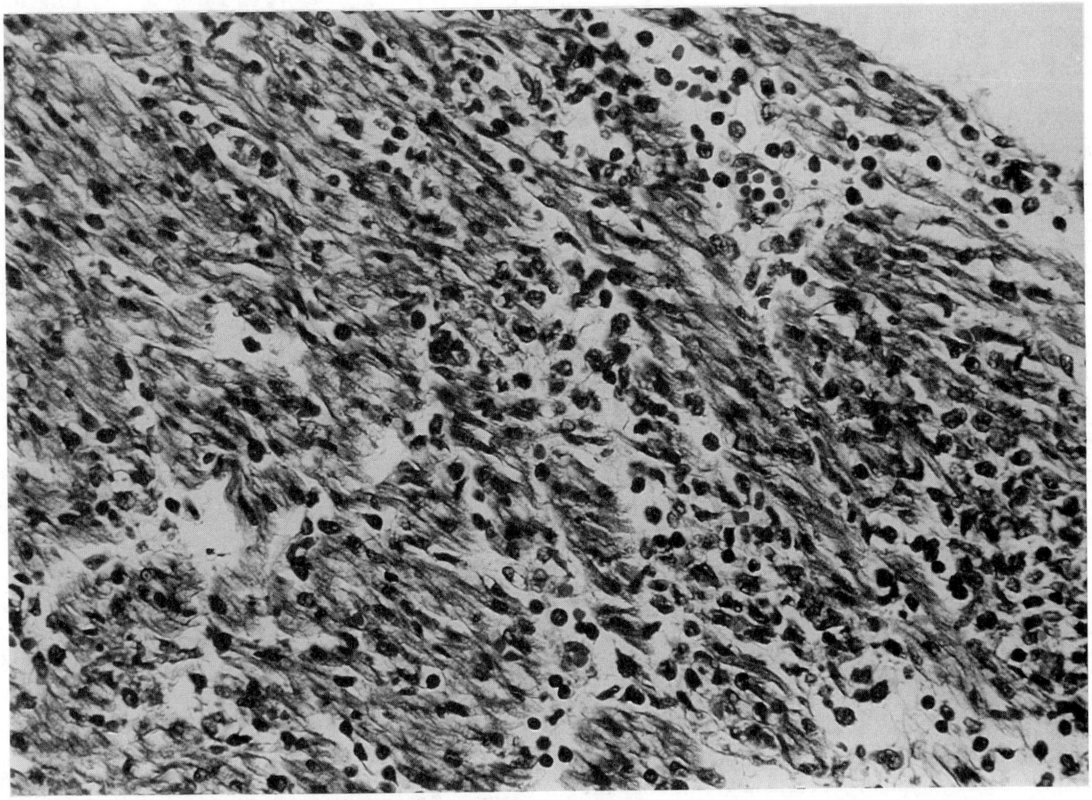

FIG. 1. Coxsackievirus myocarditis with extensive infiltration of mononuclear cells, plasma cells, lymphocytes, and some eosinophils in the interstitial tissue. (×250) (From Bloor,[3] with permission.)

mune mechanism is greatest in male and in pregnant female mice.[96] In some strains of mice less prone to myocarditis, the cytolytic T-cell response appears to be inhibited by suppressor cells.[97] Variants of coxsackievirus B3 that do not evoke cytolytic T cells directed against both infected and uninfected myocytes fail to cause myocarditis even though they are indistinguishable from myocarditic strains in their ability to replicate and stimulate neutralizing antibodies.[98] Mice infected with coxsackievirus B3 also develop heart reactive antibodies,[99,100] which do not cross react with the virus,[101] and these may contribute to myocyte destruction in some strains.[83,102] Certain strains of mice infected with coxsackievirus B3 may go on to develop a picture resembling chronic dilated cardiomyopathy[11,103]—primarily as a result of ongoing immunopathology in the absence of detectable virus. Enterovirus-associated myocarditis in humans appears to present a comparable spectrum of pathogenetic mechanisms and outcomes.

In acute Chagas disease, pathologic examination often reveals parasites within cardiac myocytes. When rupture of the cysts occurs, there is a marked inflammatory infiltrate consisting of lymphocytes, plasma cells, macrophages, and some eosinophils.[65,104] In chronic Chagas disease, the heart is often enlarged and flabby. Aneurysm formation may be present at the apex. The conduction system is often also involved, and this is reflected by a high frequency of rhythm disturbances. Microscopic examination reveals focal mononuclear cell infiltrates and fibrosis.[66,104] In this stage, parasites can only be identified in 25% of patients.[66] The heart, as well as the central nervous system, is often prominently involved in disseminated toxoplasmosis. *Toxoplasma* pseudocysts containing numerous organisms may be readily identified in cardiac tissue, and there is a striking absence of cellular response around them (Fig. 2). Rupture of parasitized fibers is followed by infiltration of neutrophils and eosinophils.[104]

Myocardial microabscesses, affecting both myocytes and the conducting system, may occur in the course of systemic bacterial infections with organisms such as *Staphylococcus aureus*, but heart failure is rarely a direct consequence of such lesions.[72]

Rickettsia and most fungi produce vasculitic lesions with surrounding inflammation. Damage to myocytes may be caused by the adjacent inflammatory process or may reflect anoxia due to occlusion of small blood vessels.

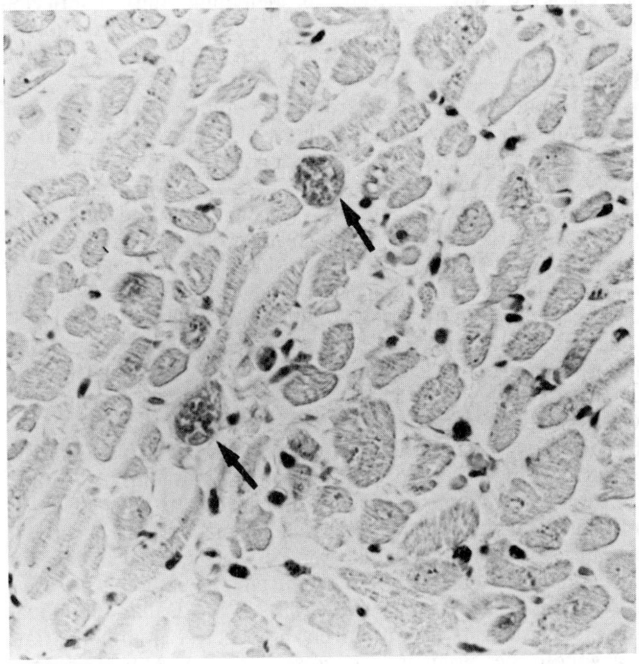

FIG. 2. Cysts of *Toxoplasma gondii* (arrows) are easily visible in the heart of this immunosuppressed patient who died with disseminated toxoplasmosis.

Diphtheria toxin inhibits cellular protein synthesis. This results in hyaline degeneration and necrosis of myocardial fibers, with a secondary inflammatory response.[3,45]

Clinical Manifestations

Patients with myocarditis may be asymptomatic or may have a rapidly progressive fatal disease. The diagnosis of infectious myocarditis is generally considered when a young person develops unexplained heart failure or arrhythmias, or when cardiac abnormalities occur in the course of a recognized systemic infection. Fever, malaise, arthralgias, upper respiratory tract symptoms, and chest pain may precede or accompany coxsackievirus myocarditis,[103,105] but these symptoms are not specific. Supraventricular tachycardia and ventricular extrasystoles are common.[106] Arrhythmias provide early evidence of involvement of the conduction system and are responsible for the occurrence of sudden death in patients with myocarditis. Myocarditis may mimic acute myocardial infarction,[107–110] but care should be taken not to mistake myocardial infarction occurring in a patient with infection for myocarditis.[111] In acute myocarditis, cardiac enzymes may be elevated and remain so for several days.[112] Symptomatic pericarditis may or may not be present.

Diagnosis

In fulminant myocarditis caused by any agent, the diagnosis is usually obvious; signs and symptoms of cardiac dysfunction are plentiful. When findings are more subtle, establishing a firm diagnosis may be difficult. Nonspecific ST- and T-wave abnormalities on the electrocardiogram are frequently cited as presumptive evidence of myocardial involvement, but they may also be seen with fever, hypoxia, electrolyte disturbances, and tachycardia. Failure to reverse T-wave abnormalities with beta blockade has been cited by some as indicative of myocarditis,[112] but physicians should approach the diagnosis of myocarditis based only on the presence of nonspecific ST- and T-wave abnormalities with skepticism,[113] especially in the absence of cardiomegaly on chest radiograph or signs of cardiac failure. Echocardiography may be useful in detecting and quantifying impairment in systolic function.[114,115] Gallium scans may be positive in myocarditis,[116–119] but this technique may lack sensitivity.

At present, the gold standard for the premortem diagnosis of myocarditis is endomyocardial biopsy.[120] Biopsy confirmation of the clinical diagnosis of myocarditis, however, has been highly variable, ranging from 17 to 100 percent in different reports.[120–123] Conversely, in some series, patients undergoing endomyocardial biopsy for the evaluation of congestive cardiomyopathy have shown a surprisingly high incidence of myocarditis,[124–126] while in other series this has not been the case.[127,128] Several factors undoubtedly contribute to this variability and make interpretation of the literature difficult. Most important, perhaps, is the lack of uniform clinical or histologic criteria for the diagnosis of myocarditis.[80] A recent study in which slides from biopsies of 16 patients with dilated cardiomyopathy were submitted to seven experienced pathologists revealed a high degree of interobserver variability.[129] Some question whether sparse focal inflammatory infiltrates have any prognostic significance.[130] Others cite sampling error as an explanation for the poor correlation between clinical and histologic findings.[131] Recent agreement among pathologists on a classification scheme for myocarditis (''the Dallas classification'')[130,132] and its use in current prospective treatment trials is a hopeful development. At present, endomyocardial biopsy may be useful in diagnosis, but practitioners should be aware of its limitations. Gallium 57[119] and indium 111-labeled antimyosin antibody scanning[133] may be useful noninvasive tests to screen patients in whom myocarditis is suspected, but experience with these modalities is limited.

Except in neonates, viruses have rarely been isolated from the hearts of patients who have died with myocarditis or from myocardial biopsies.[134] Diagnosis of viral myocarditis is often based on serologic criteria (fourfold or greater rise in antibody titer from acute to convalescent sera) or isolation of the putative agent from other body sites (e.g., stool). At best, such data provide circumstantial evidence for causation of myocardial disease and must be interpreted cautiously, since in a prospective study 26 percent of patients without myocarditis demonstrated serologic evidence of infection with agents known to cause myocarditis.[106] The application of in situ hybridization techniques, which detect virus-specific nucleic acid within cells,[135] and methods that detect or amplify viral nucleic acids[136,137] in biopsy and necropsy specimens may prove useful in the future.

As suggested by data in the mouse model, idiopathic dilated cardiomyopathy may represent the end stage of viral myocarditis.[13,126,138] Serial biopsies have demonstrated progression of fibrosis and scarring in humans,[123,139,140] but the role that viruses play in idiopathic congestive cardiomyopathy remains to be elucidated.[80,141,142]

A wide variety of noninfectious diseases and agents may mimic infectious myocarditis and produce identical clinical syndromes (see Table 2).

Treatment

Treatment of myocarditis should be directed at the specific etiologic agent involved whenever possible. Based on inferences from the murine model of coxsackievirus B3 myocarditis, bed rest remains an important part of therapy. Ensuring adequate oxygenation, avoiding and treating fluid overload if it develops, and monitoring for the development of ventricular arrhythmias constitute usual adjunctive care. In severe cases, cardiac assist devices may be lifesaving.

Most patients with viral myocarditis recover completely[151]; the factors that predispose certain patients to a poor outcome are not clear. Glucocorticoids administered during the acute phase of viral myocarditis have been associated with rapid clinical deterioration, and their deleterious effects have been clearly demonstrated in the acute phase of coxsackievirus infection in mice.[91,152] In some uncontrolled trials, patients with myocarditis on endomyocardial biopsy[119,153] or with positive gallium scans[118] who have been given immunosuppressive agents have shown improvement, but others have not.[127,154] In animal models, early therapy with cyclosporine[155] or anti-inflammatory

TABLE 2. Noninfectious Causes of Myocarditis

Collagen vascular disease[143,144]
Systemic lupus erythematosis
Rheumatoid arthritis
Still's disease
Thyrotoxicosis[143]
Pheochromocytoma[145]
Radiation-induced[146]
Drug-induced (direct toxic)[145]
Cocaine
Alcohol
Emetine
Catecholamines
Arsenic
Cyclophosphamide
Daunorubicin
Adriamycin
Drug-induced (hypersensitivity)[147]
Methyldopa
Sulfonamides
Tetracycline
Scorpion, wasp, and spider stings[145,148]
Agent(s) not yet identified
Kawasaki disease[149]
Giant cell myocarditis[150]

agents[92] increases myocardial damage. Because of the potentially deleterious effects of immunosuppressive therapy, treatment with these agents should await the results of controlled clinical trials now in progress.

PERICARDITIS

Pericarditis may result from either infectious or noninfectious processes. It may be clinically silent or may result in severe hemodynamic compromise and death. In 1892, Sir William Osler called attention to the frequency with which pericarditis was overlooked by the practitioner.[156] In this century the spectrum of organisms causing pericardial inflammation has changed somewhat, and methods of diagnosis have improved. Viral pericarditis appears to predominate and is usually a benign, self-limited disease. Bacterial and tuberculous pericarditis, while now infrequent, still cause significant morbidity and mortality and remain diagnostic challenges.

Etiologic Agents

Because of the difficulties encountered in establishing a specific etiologic diagnosis, most cases of acute self-limited pericarditis are classified as *idiopathic*. Many of these are likely to be caused by viruses.

Most viruses infecting the heart affect both the myocardium and the pericardium (see above). Of the many viruses associated with heart disease, the enteroviruses, especially the coxsackieviruses, are most frequently implicated in pericarditis.[14,157,158] The association of myopericarditis with coxsackieviruses was first recognized in neonates with overwhelming fatal systemic infections.[159] Pericarditis has also been recognized in the setting of epidemic coxsackievirus infection.[160] Coxsackieviruses have been isolated from pericardial fluid[161] infrequently; as with myocarditis, most diagnoses have been based upon the isolation of virus from other body sites (e.g., stool) and/or the demonstration of at least a fourfold rise in antibody titer after the acute illness. Viruses known to cause pericarditis are listed in Table 3.

A wide variety of bacteria can cause pericarditis. In the preantibiotic era, purulent pericarditis occurred primarily as a complication of pneumonia in previously healthy individuals.[172,173,175] Of the 425 cases of purulent pericarditis reported in 1961 by Boyle,[172] 43 percent were associated with pleuropulmonary infections. *Streptococcus pneumoniae* and *Staph. aureus* accounted for more than half of the cases. With the advent of antibiotics, the incidence of purulent pericarditis has decreased markedly. Although staphylococci and streptococci are still etiologic in a substantial number of cases, the incidence of pneumococcal pericarditis has declined substantially, and gram-negative bacilli have assumed a much more important role.[173,175] Patients with purulent pericarditis are now often older and have an underlying predisposing condition. Purulent pericarditis may occur as a complication of meningococcal meningitis or fulminant meningococcemia, but *Neisseria meningitidis*, especially serogroup C, also causes primary pericarditis.[176] *Mycoplasma pneumoniae* can cause pericarditis, and, although uncommon, this manifestation has been observed in nearly 1 percent of patients hospitalized with this infection.[181–183] *Legionella pneumophila* has been isolated from the pericardial fluid,[184,185] and pericarditis has occurred in association with pneumonia[184–186] and endocarditis.[187] Bacterial infections account for proportionately more pericarditis in children, and after *S. aureus, Haemophilus influenzae* is the second most common etiologic agent.[177]

Acute or chronic pericarditis is reported to occur in approximately 1 percent of patients with pulmonary tuberculosis.[188] Because of the declining incidence of primary tuberculosis and the use of effective chemotherapy, *Mycobacterium tuberculosis* now accounts for fewer than 5 percent of cases of acute pericarditis.[189,211] Nevertheless, diagnosis is difficult, and mortality remains high.[190] *Mycobacterium tuberculosis* remains an important treatable cause of chronic pericardial effusion and constrictive pericarditis.[191,212]

Fungi are infrequently recognized as a cause of pericarditis. However, in large recent outbreaks, pericarditis occurred in 6 percent of patients with acute symptomatic histoplasmosis.[194] In the majority, it appeared to represent a sterile inflammatory response to infection in adjacent mediastinal lymph nodes, and it resolved spontaneously without specific therapy. In disseminated histoplasmosis the pericardium itself may be infected with *Histoplasma capsulatum*.[195] Pericarditis is rarely recognized in acute coccidioidomycosis. Spontaneously resolving cases resembling those seen in acute histoplasmosis have been described,[196] but most reported cases have occurred in the setting of disseminated coccidioidomycosis and represent *Coccidioides immitis* infection of the heart.[197] Fungal pericarditis, (resulting from direct inoculation or extension of mediastinal infection), is seen with increasing frequency as a complication of cardiothoracic surgery.[175] Pericarditis caused by *Candida* sp., *Aspergillus* sp., *Cryptococcus neoformans*, and other fungi occurs as a consequence of disseminated infection in severely debilitated and immunocompromised patients, especially those with prolonged neutropenia receiving multiple courses of antibiotics.[198–202] The rare parasitic causes of pericarditis are referenced in Table 3.

TABLE 3. Infectious Causes of Pericarditis

Viruses	
Coxsackie A[162]	Epstein-Barr[166,167]
Coxsackie B[14,157,158,161]	Varicella-zoster[168]
Echovirus[163]	Cytomegalovirus[169]
Mumps[164]	Herpes simplex[170]
Influenza[165]	Hepatitis B[171]
Bacteria	
Streptococcus pneumoniae[172–174]	*Actinomyces*[180]
Staphylococcus aureus[172,173,175]	*Mycoplasma pneumoniae*[181–183]
Neisseria meningitidis[176]	*Legionella pneumophila*[184–187]
Haemophilus influenzae[172,177,178]	*Mycobacterium tuberculosis*[188–193]
Enteric gram-negative rods[173,179]	*Borrelia burgdorferi*[59,60]
Salmonella[172]	
Fungi	
Histoplasma capsulatum[194,195]	*Cryptococcus neoformans*[198]
Coccidioides immitis[196,197]	*Candida* species[199–201]
Blastomyces dermatitidis[172]	*Aspergillus* species[175,202,203]
Parasites	
Toxoplasma gondii[204,205,211]	Schistosomes[210]
Entamoeba histolytica[206–209]	

Pathology, Pathogenesis, and Pathophysiology

The pericardium has two opposing mesothelial surfaces. The parietal pericardium forms a flask-shaped sac that encloses the heart and the origins of the great vessels. It consists of a 1 mm thick layer of dense collagen lined by a single layer of mesothelial cells. The mesothelial cell layer is reflected onto the epicardial surface of the heart to form the visceral pericardium. The parietal pericardium has firm attachments to the sternum, the diaphragm, and the adventitia of the great vessels. The function of the normal pericardium has been a matter of considerable investigation and speculation.[213] It normally contains 15–50 ml of clear fluid, which may act as a lubricant. The pericardium reacts to acute injury by exuding fluid, fibrin, and cells in various combinations.[212] Acute pericarditis may resolve completely or progress to fibrous thickening, with or without constriction.

Cardiotropic viruses generally spread to the myocardium and pericardium hematogenously. Inflammation occurs in both visceral and parietal portions; effusion may develop and be serous, serofibrinous, or serosanguinous. Concomitant myocarditis may or may not be evident. Although most patients with viral pericarditis recover completely, occasional patients have repeated disabling recurrences.[214] The pathophysiology of these recurrences has not been established, but it probably involves immunologic mechanisms and not recurrent or persistent virus replication. Rarely, viral pericarditis leads to constriction as a late complication.[215]

Bacterial pericarditis generally results from (*1*) spread from a contiguous focus of infection within the chest, either de novo or after surgery or trauma; (*2*) spread from a focus of infection within the heart, most commonly from endocarditis; or (*3*) hematogenous infection. The incidence of purulent pericarditis arising from a contiguous pneumonia has steadily decreased and now generally occurs only when there has been significant delay in antibiotic therapy.[173,174] Pericarditis after cardiothoracic or esophageal surgery often occurs in patients with sternal wound infections and/or mediastinitis[175] and may be overlooked. Mortality is high. Pericarditis not infrequently accompanies fatal endocarditis,[72] especially that caused by *S. aureus*.[52] It often results from extension of a perivalvular abcess into the pericardium.[72] However, pericardial effusions in endocarditis may also be hemorrhagic[216] or sympathetic and sterile.[217] The presence of pre-existing nonbacterial pericardial effusion may predispose to the development of purulent pericarditis in bacteremic patients. Although the pericardial fluid may initially be clear,[172,175] it is usually grossly purulent and may be loculated by the time the disease is clinically apparent. Subsequent organization with adhesions, obliteration of the pericardial space, and calcification may occur and result in constrictive pericarditis.

Tuberculous pericarditis may develop from a hematogenous focus present from the time of primary infection, as a result of lymphatic spread from peritracheal, peribronchial, or mediastinal lymph nodes, or by contiguous spread from a focus of infection in lung or pleura. Four pathologic stages in tuberculous pericarditis have been described.[212,218] In the first stage, there is diffuse fibrin deposition, and granulomas with viable mycobacteria are present (Fig. 3). A serous or serosanguinous pericardial effusion then develops, usually quite slowly and often without symptoms. Lymphocytes, monocytes, and plasma cells replace the polymorphonuclear cells present early in infection. In the third stage, the effusion is absorbed, the pericardium thickens, granulomas proliferate, and a thick coat of fibrin is deposited on the parietal pericardium. Acid-fast bacilli become difficult to find as dense fibrous tissue and collagen are deposited. In stage four, which is associated with constriction, the pericardial space is obliterated by dense adhesions, the parietal pericardium is markedly thickened, and many granulomas are replaced by fibrous tissue. This is often followed by the accumulation of cholesterol crystals and calcification. Constrictive pericarditis appears to develop in half of patients with tuberculous pericarditis despite the use of antituberculous chemotherapy.[193,219] Although the incidence of tuberculosis has declined, it remains an important cause of constrictive pericarditis, especially in underdeveloped countries.[212]

Irrespective of etiology, if fluid accumulates rapidly in the pericardium and intrapericardial pressure rises, cardiac tamponade may result. Tamponade implies a progressive limitation of ventricular diastolic filling, with resultant reduction in stroke volume and cardiac output. In a recent series of medical patients with early cardiac tamponade, the etiology was infectious in 12.5 percent, noninfectious in 74 percent, and undetermined in the remainder.[220]

Clinical Manifestations

The presentation of acute pericarditis varies depending on the etiology. In viral or idiopathic pericarditis, chest pain is an important feature. This pain is often retrosternal, radiating to the shoulder and neck, and typically is aggravated by breathing, swallowing, and lying supine. In Smith's review of coxsackievirus B heart disease in adults,[158] 67 percent of patients had chest pain. Fever was present in 59 percent. A concurrent or prodromal flulike illness with malaise, arthralgias, myalgias,

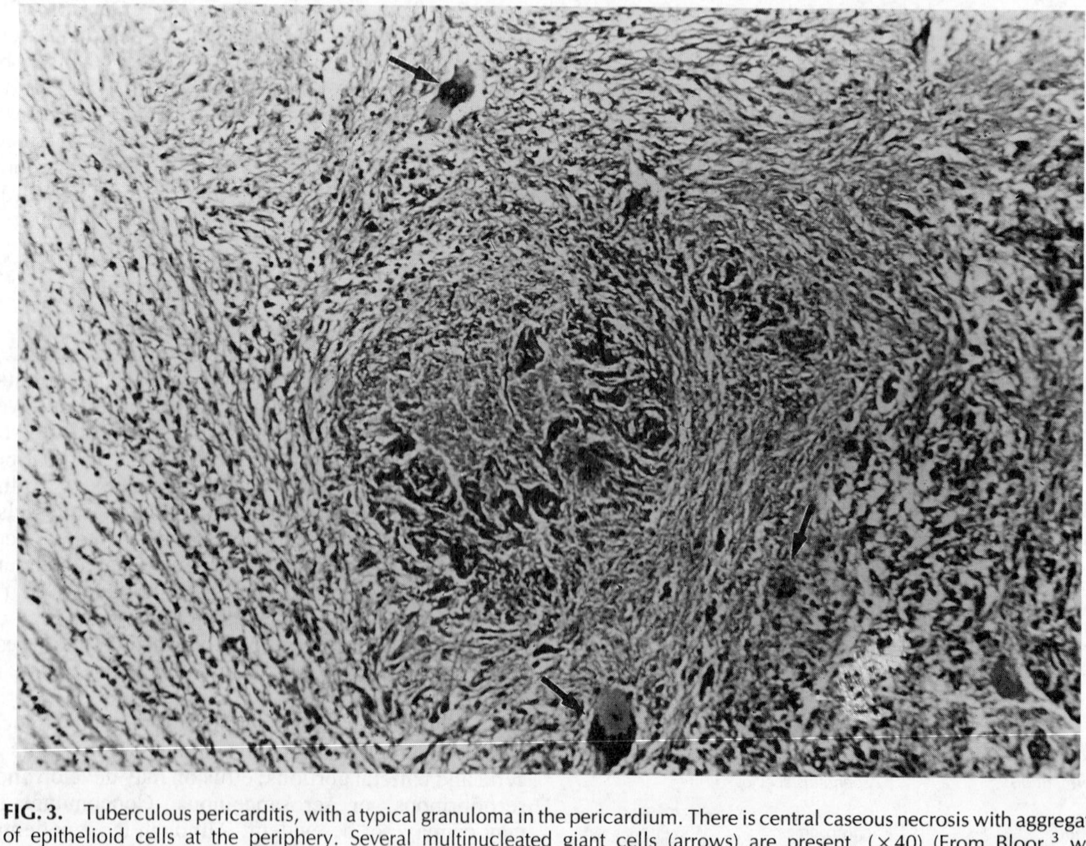

FIG. 3. Tuberculous pericarditis, with a typical granuloma in the pericardium. There is central caseous necrosis with aggregates of epithelioid cells at the periphery. Several multinucleated giant cells (arrows) are present. (×40) (From Bloor,[3] with permission.)

and occasionally cough with sputum was present in 36 percent. Patients with bacterial pericarditis are often acutely ill but frequently do not complain of chest pain.[175] Fever is almost invariably present and dyspnea is common. Bacterial pericarditis is rarely an isolated disease, and the symptoms and signs of the accompanying systemic or local infection may take clinical precedence. Tuberculous pericarditis most often has an insidious onset. Chest pain is present in 39–76 percent[193] but may be vague in nature. Weight loss, night sweats, cough, and dyspnea are common.

The classic physical finding in acute pericarditis is the three-component pericardial friction rub, which reflects cardiac motion during atrial systole, ventricular systole, and rapid ventricular filling in early diastole. This three-component rub was present in 50 percent of patients with acute pericarditis reported by Spodick.[221] The ventricular systolic component is often the loudest and most frequently appreciated. Rubs are often evanescent and may vary in quality; they are characteristically high-pitched, scratching, or grating. In the presence of significant pericardial effusion, there may be jugular venous distension, the most common physical finding in acute cardiac tamponade. Enlargement of the cardiac silhouette usually does not occur until at least 250 ml of fluid have accumulated in the pericardial space[222]; if fluid accumulates rapidly, tamponade may occur without detectable cardiomegaly. A pulsus paradoxus of more than 10 mmHg and a prominent x descent with loss of the y descent in the jugular venous pressure may be present. Dyspnea is common, but signs of left heart failure are usually absent in cardiac tamponade, and clear lung fields may help to differentiate tamponade from cardiogenic shock.

Although the pericardium produces no electrical activity, the electrocardiogram (ECG) is abnormal in 90 percent of patients with acute pericarditis,[222] reflecting diffuse subepicardial inflammation. Characteristic ECG changes are seen in approximately 50 percent of patients.[223] Early in pericarditis, ST segment elevation without change in QRS morphology typically occurs in multiple leads. Several days later, the ST segment returns to baseline, and there is T-wave flattening. During these early stages, there may also be depression of the PR segment. In contrast to myocardial infarction, the T-wave inversions in pericarditis do not generally occur until after the ST segment has returned to baseline. These T-wave inversions may last for weeks or months. Large pericardial effusions may be associated with reduced QRS voltage and electrical alternans. Sinus tachycardia is common, but the presence of other arrhythmias suggests pre-existing underlying heart disease or significant myocardial involvement.[224]

Echocardiography has been proved to be an extremely useful tool for diagnosis of pericardial effusion and should be performed if the situation is not immediately life-threatening. The size of the effusion can be roughly quantitated, and early hemodynamic compromise can often be detected.[222] Computerized tomography has been useful in demonstrating pericardial thickening and, in some cases, in differentiating an uncomplicated transudate from a high-density exudate.[236,237] Magnetic resonance imaging techniques also can easily detect pericardial fluid and thickening[238] but at present have no particular advantage over more conventional methods.

Diagnosis

A wide variety of agents and diseases may cause pericarditis and pericardial effusion (see Tables 3 and 4). Low-grade fever is common to many. A careful history, knowledge of the clinical setting in which the pericarditis occurs, and a search for clues outside the cardiovascular system are helpful in establishing a diagnosis. In a young person without underlying illness who presents with acute pericardial pain, the most likely diagnosis is viral or idiopathic pericarditis. However, establishing a specific viral diagnosis is difficult, costly, and often possible only in retrospect. Virus isolation can be attempted from throat and stool, and acute and convalescent sera can be tested for antibodies to potential pathogens (e.g., the coxsackie B viruses and any other enteroviruses prevalent locally at the time), but these approaches frequently fail to yield a specific diagnosis. Viruses are rarely isolated from pericardial fluid, even in patients in whom the diagnosis of viral myocarditis is highly probable. However, new techniques that permit the detection and identification of minute quantities of viral nucleic acid in the absence of infectious virus may revolutionize the diagnosis of viral and idiopathic pericarditis.

TABLE 4. Major Noninfectious Causes of Acute Pericarditis

Acute myocardial infarction[225]
Uremia[226]
Neoplasia[222]
Primary
Metastatic
Postirradiation[227]
Postcardiac injury
Trauma (penetrating or blunt)[222]
Postmyocardial infarction (Dresslers)[228]
Postpericardiotomy[229]
Dissecting aortic aneurysm[222]
Sarcoidosis[230]
Collagen vascular diseases
Systemic lupus erythematosis[231]
Rheumatoid arthritis[232]
Scleroderma[233]
Rheumatic fever[222]
Drug-induced[222]
Procainamide
Hydralazine
Other
Myxedema[234]

If the clinical suspicion of viral or idiopathic pericarditis is strong in an otherwise healthy patient with uncomplicated pericarditis, pericardiocentesis or other invasive procedures add little diagnostically[211] and carry a small but definite risk.[235] After excluding patients with postpericardiotomy syndrome, myocardial infarction, renal failure, known neoplastic disease, trauma, and irradiation, Permanyer-Miralde et al.[211] prospectively evaluated 231 patients with primary acute pericardial disease. After thorough diagnostic evaluation, 199 were felt to have acute idiopathic pericarditis. Unsuspected neoplastic pericarditis was found in 13, tuberculosis in 9, and collagen vascular disease in 4. Purulent pericarditis, viral pericarditis, and *Toxoplasma gondii* infection were each found in two patients. The diagnostic yield was substantial when pericardiocentesis or pericardiectomy with biopsy were done to relieve cardiac tamponade (39 percent and 54 percent, respectively), but it was only 5 percent when these procedures were done solely for the purpose of diagnosis. The authors concluded that the presence of a pericardial effusion per se is not an indication for an invasive procedure; in patients with pericardial effusion that has persisted for more than 3 weeks, an invasive procedure may be indicated.

Untreated purulent pericarditis is usually rapidly fatal.[175] In acutely ill patients in whom purulent pericarditis is suspected, the diagnosis should be pursued quickly and aggressively. When possible, pericardiotomy with biopsy and drainage is preferable to pericardiocentesis because of greater diagnostic yield and fewer complications.[222] Noninfectious diseases predominate as causes of significant pericardial effusion and cardiac tamponade,[220] but bacterial and tuberculous effusions are more likely to have serious hemodynamic consequences.[235]

Treatment

Bed rest, symptomatic therapy for pain, and careful monitoring for the developmentof hemodynamic compromise are the mainstays of treatment for presumed viral or idiopathic pericarditis. Nonsteroidal anti-inflammatory agents are often successful in relieving symptoms. Because myocarditis often accompanies viral pericarditis and steroids enhance myocardial injury during active virus replication, we believe that steroids should be avoided during the acute illness. Viral or idiopathic pericarditis is generally benign and self-limited, but recurrences[214] and late constriction[215] do occur.

Surgical drainage of the pericardium, in addition to appropriate antibiotic therapy, is essential in almost all patients with purulent pericarditis.[172,175,177] Initial pericardiocentesis may be lifesaving, but fluid often reaccumulates, and constriction can develop rapidly.[175,177] There is little rationale for irrigating the pericardium with antibiotics, because penetration from serum is excellent.[239] With early diagnosis and aggressive therapy, *H. influenzae* pericarditis in young patients has a good prognosis.[177] However, overall mortality in bacterial pericarditis remains high, especially when it develops after surgery or occurs in the course of endocarditis.[175]

The treatment of tuberculous pericarditis remains controversial. Antituberculous therapy has reduced mortality substantially.[240] The addition of steroids to reduce inflammation and avoid late constriction is favored by many, including the authors, but it remains unproved.[190,240,241] Early surgical intervention is advocated in patients with hemodynamic compromise from recurrent effusion or progressive pericardial thickening.[219,240]

MEDIASTINITIS

Infections in the mediastinum may be divided into two categories, acute and chronic, which differ markedly in their microbiology, pathogenesis, presentation, and treatment. Acute mediastinitis is a rare but dreaded disease that complicates oropharyngeal infection,[242,243] perforation of the esophagus,[244] cardiac surgery,[245,246] or infection of contiguous structures. In the preantibiotic era, acute mediastinitis often resulted from infection of the pharynx or the second or third mandibular molars, with dissection downward along anatomic planes. Currently, only a small proportion of cases result from retropharyngeal or odontogenic infections. Rupture of the esophagus is also uncommon; it may occur spontaneously, from erosion with tumor, after sclerotherapy for varicies or esophageal dilatation, or as a postoperative complication. Most cases of acute mediastinitis now occur as a complication of cardiac surgery. The reported incidence of mediastinitis after surgery ranges from 0.4 to 5 percent,[245] with mortality rates from 8.6 to 77 percent.[246] Factors that have been associated with higher rates of infection include serious underlying noncardiovascular diseases, increased complexity of surgery, sternal dehiscence, and emergency reoperation.[246,247]

Patients with acute mediastinitis are often severely ill with fever and tachycardia, and the infection may progress rapidly. There may be crepitus, brawny edema of the neck or chest wall, purulent pleural and/or pericardial effusions, pneumonitis, and mediastinal widening visible on chest radiograph. Postoperative mediastinitis generally occurs within 2 weeks following sternotomy. Patients often first develop fever and bacteremia followed by an abnormal-appearing wound. However, mediastinal widening and sternal instability are infrequent.[246]

The origin of the infection is predictive of its bacteriology. Mouth organisms, especially anaerobes, play an important role in mediastinitis following esophageal perforation and oropharyngeal infection.[248] *Staphylococcus aureus* and gram-negative bacilli, including *Pseudomonas aeruginosa*, are found after surgical procedures. *Staphylococcus epidermidis*, although usually not a pathogen, cannot be ignored in the postsurgical setting if signs of infection are present.[249] Not unexpectedly, pathogens encountered are frequently resistant to the antibiotic used in perioperative prophylaxis.[246]

Computed tomography has proved a very useful aid in the diagnosis of acute mediastinitis and its management.[250,251] Aggressive débridement and drainage in conjunction with appropriate antibiotic therapy are essential, but mortality remains high (24–40 percent).[242,243,246,248]

A more indolent form of mediastinitis, termed fibrosing mediastinitis, may occur as a complication of granulomatous infections such as histoplasmosis or tuberculosis. Fibrosing mediastinitis has been postulated to result from rupture of mediastinal lymph nodes with release of caseous material, which provokes an intense inflammatory reaction. Patients may present with symptoms of occlusion of major mediastinal structures (e.g., superior vena cava syndrome) or with an asymptomatic mass detected on routine chest radiograph. Granulomatous and fibrous mediastinitis may account for up to 10 percent of all primary mediastinal masses and 20 percent of cases of superior vena cava syndrome.[252,253] *Histoplasma capsulatum* is the etiologic agent most commonly implicated.[253] The organism is visible with appropriate staining techniques in from 35 to 73 percent of cases.[254,255] The process is often located near the bifurcation of the trachea or the hilum of the lung. The pathology is variable but generally consists of caseous necrosis with granuloma formation surrounded by dense fibrosis. Organisms are generally not abundant and attempts to grow the organism are usually not successful.[254,256] As the lesions age, the fibrous capsule extends and may invade surrounding tissues, but why this occurs in the individuals so afflicted is a matter of conjecture. Early in disease, surgical resection may be attempted, but during the latter stages, surgery is technically difficult and at best palliative.[253–255]

REFERENCES

1. Saphir O. Myocarditis: a general review with an analysis of two hundred and forty cases. Arch Pathol. 1941;32:1000–51 and 1942;33:88–137.
2. Stevens PJ, Underwood Ground KE. Occurrence and significance of myocarditis in trauma. Aerospace Med. 1970;41:776–80.
3. Bloor CM. Pericarditis and myocarditis. In: Cardiac Pathology. Philadelphia: JB Lippincott; 1978:265–95.
4. Bandt CM, Staley NA, Noren GR. Acute viral myocarditis: clinical and histological changes. Minn Med. 1979;62:234–7.
5. Bengtsson E, Orndahl G. Complications of mumps with special reference to the incidence of myocarditis. Acta Med Scand. 1954;149:381–8.
6. Lucke B, Wight T, Kime E. Pathologic anatomy and bacteriology of influenza: epidemic of autumn 1918. Arch Intern Med. 1919;24:154–237.
7. Degen JA Jr. Visceral pathology in measles; clinicopathologic study of 100 fatal cases. Am J Med Sci. 1937;194:104–11.
8. Lucke B. Postmortem findings in measles bronchopneumonia and other acute infections. JAMA. 1918;70:2006–11.
9. Saphir O, Wile SA. Myocarditis in poliomyelitis. Am J Med Sci. 1942;203:781–8.
10. Sylvest E. Epidemic Myalgia: Bornholm Disease. London: Oxford University Press; 1934.
11. Reyes MP, Lerner AM. Coxsackievirus myocarditis—with special reference to acute and chronic effects. Prog Cardiovasc Dis. 1985;27:373–94.
12. Hirschman SZ, Hammer GS. Coxsackie virus myopericarditis. A microbiological and clinical review. Am J Cardiol. 1974;34:224–32.
13. Woodruff JF. Viral myocarditis. Am J Pathol. 1980;101:427–78.
14. Grist NR, Bell EJ. A six-year study of coxsackievirus B infections in heart disease. J Hyg Camb. 1974;73:165–72.
15. Russell SJM, Bell EJ. Echoviruses and carditis. Lancet. 1970;1:784–5.
16. Bell EJ, Grist NR. ECHO viruses, carditis and acute pleurodynia. Am Heart J. 1971;82:133–8.
17. Jungeblut CW, Edwards JE. Isolation of poliomyelitis virus from the heart in fatal cases. Am J Clin Pathol. 1951;21:601–23.
18. Weinstein L, Shelokov A. Cardiovascular manifestations in acute poliomyelitis. N Engl J Med. 1951;244:281–5.
19. Roberts WC, Fox III SM. Mumps of the heart: clinical and pathological features. Circulation. 1965;32:342–5.
20. Baandrup U, Mortensen SA. Fatal mumps myocarditis. Acta Med Scand. 1984;216:331–3.
21. Hamburger WW. The heart in influenza. Med Clin North Am. 1938;22:111–21.
22. Verel D, Warrack AJN, Potter CW, et al. Observations on the A2 England influenza epidemic. A clinicopathological study. Am Heart J. 1976;92:290–6.
23. Ross E, Armentrout SA. Myocarditis associated with rabies. Report of a case. N Engl J Med. 1962;266:1087–9.
24. Ainger LE, Lawyer NG, Fitch CW. Neonatal rubella myocarditis. Br Heart J. 1966;28:691–7.

25. Kriseman T. Rubella myocarditis in a 9 year old patient. Clin Pediatr. 1984;23:240–1.
26. Chuah SK. Transient ventricular arrhythmia as a cardiac manifestation in dengue haemorrhagic fever—a case report. Singapore Med J. 1987;28:569–72.
27. Obeyesekere I, Hermon Y. Myocarditis and cardiomyopathy after arbovirus infections (dengue and chikingunya fever). Br Heart J. 1972;34:821–7.
28. Cannell DE. Myocardial degenerations in yellow fever. Am J Pathol. 1928;4:431–43.
29. Milei J, Bolomo NJ. Myocardial damage in viral hemorrhagic fevers. Am Heart J. 1982;104:1385–91.
30. Thiede WH. Cardiac involvement in lymphocytic choriomeningitis. Arch Intern Med. 1962;109:50–4.
31. Henson D, Mufson MA. Myocarditis and pneumonitis with type 21 adenovirus infection: association with fatal myocarditis and pneumonitis. Am J Dis Child. 1971;121:334–6.
32. Karjalainen J, Heikkila J, Nieminen MS, et al. Etiology of mild acute infectious myocarditis. Relation to clinical features. Acta Med Scand. 1983;213:65–73.
33. Hackel DB. Myocarditis in association with varicella. Am J Pathol. 1953;29:369–79.
34. Woolf PK, Chung T-S, Stewart J, et al. Life-threatening dysrhythmias in varicella myocarditis. Clin Pediatr. 1987;26:480–2.
35. Coppack SW, Doshi R, Ghose AR. Fatal varicella in a healthy young adult. Postgrad Med J. 1985;61:529–31.
36. Tiula E, Leinikki P. Fatal cytomegalovirus infection in a previously healthy boy with myocarditis and consumption coagulopathy as presenting signs. Scand J Infect Dis. 1972;4:57–60.
37. Webster BH. Cardiac complications of infectious mononucleosis: a review of the literature and report of five cases. Am J Med Sci. 1957;234:62–70.
38. Hudgins JM. Infectious mononucleosis complicated by myocarditis and pericarditis. JAMA. 1976;235:2626–7.
39. Matthews AW, Griffiths ID. Post vaccinal pericarditis and myocarditis. Br Heart J. 1974;36:1043–5.
40. Anderson T, Foulis MA, Grist NR, et al. Clinical and laboratory observations in a smallpox outbreak. Lancet. 1951;1:1248–52.
41. Mahapatra RK, Ellis GH. Myocarditis and hepatitis B virus. Angiology. 1985;36:116–9.
42. Bell H. Cardiac manifestations of viral hepatitis. JAMA. 1971;218:387–91.
43. Ursell PC, Habib A, Sharma P, et al. Hepatitis B virus and myocarditis. Hum Pathol. 1984;15:481–4.
44. Gore I, Saphir O. Myocarditis. A classification of 1402 cases. Am Heart J. 1947;34:827–30.
45. Gore I. Myocardial changes in fatal diphtheria; summary of observations in 221 cases. Am J Med Sci. 1948;215:257–66.
46. Roberts WC, Berard CW. Gas gangrene of the heart in clostridial septicemia. Am Heart J. 1967;74:482–8.
47. Guneratne F. Gas gangrene (abscess) of heart. NY State J Med. 1975;75:1766.
48. Joshi MK, Kandoth PW, Barve RJ, et al. Rheumatic fever: clinical profile of 339 cases with long term follow up. Indian Pediatr. 1983;20:849–53.
49. Brasier AR, Macklis JD, Vaughan D, et al. Myopericarditis as an initial presentation of meningococcemia. Unusual manifestation of infection with serotype W135. Am J Med. 1987;82:641–4.
50. Cohen JI, Bartlett JA, Corey GR. Extra-intestinal manifestations of *Salmonella* infections. Medicine. 1987;66:349–88.
51. Lubani M, Sharda D, Helin I. Cardiac manifestations in brucellosis. Arch Dis Child. 1986;61:569–72.
52. Watanakunakorn C, Tan JS, Phair JP. Some salient features of *Staphylococcus aureus* endocarditis. Am J Med. 1973;54:473–81.
53. Chen S-C, Tsai CC, Nouri S. Carditis associated with *Mycoplasma pneumoniae* infection. AJDC. 1986;140:471–2.
54. Lind K. Manifestation and complications of *Mycoplasme pneumoniae* disease: a review. Yale J Biol Med. 1983;56:461–8.
55. Dymock IW, Lawson JM, MacLennan WJ, et al. Myocarditis associated with psittacosis. Br J Clin Pract. 1971;25:240–2.
56. Marin-Garcia J, Mirvis DM. Myocardial disease in Rocky Mountain spotted fever: clinical, functional, and pathologic findings. Pediatr Cardiol. 1984;5:149–54.
57. Brown GW, Shirai A, Jegathesan M, et al. Febrile illness in Malaysia—an analysis of 1629 hospitalized patients. Am J Trop Med Hyg. 1984;33:311–5.
58. Ognibene AJ, O'Leary DS, Czarnecki SW, et al. Myocarditis and disseminated intravascular coagulation in scrub typhus. Am J Med Sci. 1971;262:233–9.
59. Steere AC, Batsford WP, Weinberg M, et al. Lyme carditis: cardiac abnormalities of Lyme disease. Ann Intern Med. 1980;93:8–16.
60. McAlister HF, Klementowicz PT, Andrews C, et al. Lyme carditis: an important cause of reversible heart block. Ann Intern Med. 1989;110:339–45.
61. Williams AH. *Aspergillus* myocarditis. Am J Clin Pathol. 1974;61:247–56.
62. Atkinson JB, Connor DH, Robinowitz M, et al. Cardiac fungal infections: review of autopsy findings in 60 patients. Hum Pathol. 1984;15:935–42.
63. Lewis W, Lipsick J, Cammarosano C. Cryptococcal myocarditis in acquired immune deficiency syndrome. Am J Cardiol. 1985;9:1240.
64. Lafont A, Wolff M, Marche C, et al. Overwhelming myocarditis due to *Cryptococcus neoformans* in an AIDS patient. Lancet. 1987;2:1145–6.
65. Rosenbaum MB. Chagasic myocardiopathy. Prog Cardiovasc Dis. 1964;7:199–255.
66. Mott KE, Hagstrom JWC. The pathologic lesions of the cardiac autonomic nervous system in chronic Chagas' myocarditis. Circulation. 1965;31:273–86.
67. Mendoza I, Camardo J, Moleiro F, et al. Sustained ventricular tachycardia in chronic Chagasic myocarditis. Am J Cardiol. 1986;57:423–7.
68. Poltera AA, Owor R, Cox JN. Pathological aspects of human African trypanosomiasis in Uganda. Virchows Arch [A] 1977;373:249–65.
69. Barr R. Human trichinosis: report of 4 cases with emphasis on central nervous system involvement and a survey of 500 consecutive autopsies at the Ottawa Civic Hospital. Can Med Assoc J. 1966;95:912–7.
70. Grey DF, Morse BS, Phillips WF. Trichinosis with neurologic and cardiac involvement. Review of the literature and report of three cases. Ann Intern Med. 1962;57:230–44.
71. Yermakov V, Rashid RK, Vuletin JC, et al. Disseminated toxoplasmosis. Case report and review of the literature. Arch Pathol Lab Med. 1982;106:524–8.
72. Buchbinder NA, Roberts WC. Left-sided valvular active infective endocarditis. A study of 45 necropsy patients. Am J Med. 1972;53:20–35.
73. Welch K, Finkbeiner W, Alpers CE, et al. Autopsy findings in the acquired immune deficiency syndrome. JAMA. 1984;252:1152–9.
74. Baroldi G, Carallo S, Moroni M, et al. Focal lymphocytic myocarditis in acquired immunodeficiency syndrome (AIDS): a correlative morphologic and clinical study in 26 consecutive fatal cases. J Am Coll Cardiol. 1988;12:463–9.
75. Cammarosano C, Lewis W. Cardiac lesions in acquired immune deficiency syndrome (AIDS). J Am Coll Cardiol. 1985;5:703–6.
76. Fink L, Reichek N, St. John Sutton MG. Cardiac abnormalities in acquired immune deficiency syndrome. Am J Cardiol. 1984;54:1161–3.
77. Anderson DW, Virmani R, Reilly JM, et al. Prevalent myocarditis at necropsy in the acquired immunodeficiency syndrome. J Am Coll Cardiol. 1988;11:792–9.
78. Calabrese LH, Proffitt MR, Yen-Lieberman B, et al. Congestive cardiomyopathy and illness related to the acquired immunodeficiency syndrome (AIDS) associated with isolation of retrovirus from myocardium. Ann Intern Med. 1987;107:691–2.
79. Dittrich H, Chow L, Denaro F, et al. Human immunodeficiency virus, coxsackievirus, and cardiomyopathy. (Letter) Ann Intern Med. 1988;108:308–9.
80. Edwards WD. Myocarditis and endomyocardial biopsy. Cardiol Clin. 1984;2:647–56.
81. Lyden D, Olszewski J, Huber S. Variation in susceptibility of BALB/c mice to coxsackievirus group B type 3-induced myocarditis with age. Cell Immunol. 1987;105:332–9.
82. Herskowitz A, Wolfgram LJ, Rose NR, et al. Coxsackievirus B_3 murine myocarditis: a pathologic spectrum of myocarditis in genetically defined inbred strains. J Am Coll Cardiol. 1987;9:1311–9.
83. Huber SA, Lodge PA. Coxsackievirus B-3 myocarditis. Identification of different pathogenic mechanisms in DBA/2 and BALB/c mice. Am J Pathol. 1986;122:284–91.
84. Wolfgram LJ, Beisel KW, Herskowitz A, et al. Variations in the susceptibility to Coxsackievirus B_3-induced myocarditis among different strains of mice. J Immunol. 1986;136:1846–52.
85. Khatib R, Probert A, Reyes MP, et al. Mouse strain-related variation as a factor in the pathogenesis of coxsackievirus B3 murine myocarditis. J Gen Virol. 1987;68:2981–8.
86. Rager-Zisman B, Allison AC. The role of antibody and host cells in the resistance of mice against infection by coxsackie B-3 virus. J Gen Virol. 1973;19:329–38.
87. Woodruff JF. Lack of correlation between neutralizing antibody production and suppression of coxsackievirus B-3 replication in target organs: evidence for involvement of mononuclear inflammatory cells in host defense. J Immunol. 1979;123:31–6.
88. Godeny EK, Gauntt CJ. *In situ* immune autoradiographic identification of cells in heart tissue of mice with coxsackievirus B3-induced myocarditis. Am J Pathol. 1987;129:267–76.
89. Godeny EK, Gauntt CJ. Murine natural killer cells limit coxsackievirus B3 replication. J Immunol. 1987;139:913–8.
90. Godeny EK, Gauntt CJ. Involvement of natural killer cells in coxsackievirus B3-induced murine myocarditis. J Immunol. 1986;137:1695–702.
91. Kilbourne ED, Wilson CB, Perrier D. The induction of gross myocardial lesions by a coxsackie (pleurodynia) virus and cortisone. J Clin Invest. 1956;35:362–70.
92. Rezkalla S, Khatib G, Khatib R. Coxsackievirus B3 murine myocarditis: deleterious effects of nonsteroidal anti-inflammatory agents. J Lab Clin Med. 1986;107:393–5.
93. Huber SA, Lodge PA. Coxsackievirus B-3 myocarditis in BALB/c mice. Evidence for autoimmunity to myocyte antigens. Am J Pathol. 1984;116:21–9.
94. Guthrie M, Lodge PA, Huber SA. Cardiac injury in myocarditis induced by coxsackievirus group B, type 3 in BALB/c mice is mediated by Lyt 2^+ cytolytic lymphocytes. Cell Immunol. 1984;88:558–67.
95. Kishimoto C, Kuribayashi K, Masuda T, et al. Immunologic behavior of lymphocytes in experimental viral myocarditis: significance of T lymphocytes in the severity of myocarditis and silent myocarditis in BALB/c-nu/nu mice. Circulation. 1985;71:1247–54.
96. Lyden DC, Huber SA. Aggravation of coxsackievirus, group B, type 3-induced myocarditis and increase in cellular immunity to myocyte antigens

in pregnant BALB/c mice and animals treated with progesterone. Cell Immunol. 1984;87:462–72.
97. Job LP, Lyden DC, Huber SA. Demonstration of suppressor cells in coxsackievirus group B, type 3 infected female BALB/c mice which prevent myocarditis. Cell Immunol. 1986;98:104–13.
98. Huber SA, Job LP. Differences in cytolytic T cell response of BALB/c mice infected with myocarditic and non-myocarditic strains of coxsackievirus group B, type 3. Infect Immun. 1983;39:1419–27.
99. Wolfgram LJ, Beisel KW, Rose NR. Heart-specific autoantibodies following murine coxsackievirus B_3 myocarditis. J Exp Med. 1985;161:1112–21.
100. Neu N, Beisel KW, Traystman MD, et al. Autoantibodies specific for the cardiac myosin isoform are found in mice susceptible to coxsackievirus B_3-induced myocarditis. J Immunol. 1987;138:2488–92.
101. Neu N, Craig SW, Rose NR, et al. Coxsackievirus induced myocarditis in mice: cardiac myosin autoantibodies do not cross-react with the virus. Clin Exp Immunol. 1987;69:566–74.
102. Neu N, Rose NR, Beisel KW, et al. Cardiac myosin induces myocarditis in genetically predisposed mice. J Immunol. 1987;139:3630–6.
103. Kishimoto C, Tomioka N, Kawai C. Clinical findings in acute viral myocarditis. With special attention to experimental and immunological evidence. Herz. 1985;10:15–20.
104. Bloor CM. Protozoal, helminthic and fungal heart disease. In: Cardiac Pathology. Philadelphia: JB Lippincott; 1978:335–366.
105. Abelmann WH. Virus and the heart. Circulation. 1971;44:950–6.
106. Vikerfors T, Stjerna A, Olcen P, et al. Acute myocarditis. Serologic diagnosis, clinical findings and follow-up. Acta Med Scand. 1988;223:45–52.
107. Stratmann HG. Acute myocarditis versus myocardial infarction: evaluation and management of the young patient with prolonged chest pain-case reports. Angiology. 1988;39:253–8.
108. Miklozek CL, Crumpacker CS, Royal HD, et al. Myocarditis presenting as acute myocardial infarction. Am Heart J. 1988;115:768–76.
109. Spodick DH. Infection and infarction. Acute viral (and other) infection in the onset, pathogenesis, and mimicry of acute myocardial infarction. Am J Med. 1986;81:661–8.
110. Beaufils P, Slama R. Myocarditis confirmed by biopsy presenting as acute myocardial infarction. Br Heart J. 1986;4:420.
111. Griffiths PD, Hannington G, Booth JC. Coxsackie B virus infections and myocardial infarction. Results from a prospective, epidemiologically controlled study. Lancet. 1980;1:1387–9.
112. Heikkila J, Karjalainen J. Evaluation of mild acute infectious myocarditis. Br Heart J. 1982;47:381–91.
113. Scott LP III, Gutelius MF, Parrott RH. Children with acute respiratory tract infections. An electrocardiographic survey. Am J Dis Child. 1970;119:111–3.
114. Weinhouse E, Wanderman KL, Sofer S, et al. Viral myocarditis simulating dilated cardiomyopathy in early childhood: evaluation by serial echocardiography. Br Heart J. 1986;56:94–7.
115. Nieminen MS, Heikkila J, Karjalainen J. Echocardiography in acute infectious myocarditis: relation to clinical and electrocardiographic findings. Am J Cardiol. 1984;53:1331–7.
116. Alpert LI, Welch P, Fisher N. Gallium-positive Lyme disease myocarditis. Clin Nucl Med. 1985;9:617.
117. Shulkin BL, Wahl RL. SPECT imaging of myocarditis. Clin Nucl Med. 1987;12:841–2.
118. Robinson JA, O'Connell J, Henkin RE, et al. Gallium-67 imaging in cardiomyopathy. Ann Intern Med. 1979;90:198–9.
119. O'Connell JB, Robinson JA, Henkin RE, et al. Immunosuppressive therapy in patients with congestive cardiomyopathy and myocardial uptake of gallium-67. Circulation. 1981;64:780–6.
120. Fowles RE, Mason JW. Endomyocardial biopsy. Ann Intern Med. 1982;97:885–94.
121. Nippoldt TB, Edwards WD, Holms DR, et al. Right ventricular endomyocardial biopsy. Clinicopathologic correlates in 100 consecutive patients. Mayo Clin Proc. 1982;57:407–18.
122. Parrillo JE, Aretz HT, Palacios I, et al. The results of transvenous endomyocardial biopsy can frequently be used to diagnose myocardial diseases in patients with idiopathic heart failure. Endomyocardial biopsies in 100 consecutive patients revealed a substantial incidence of myocarditis. Circulation. 1984;69:93–101.
123. Takahashi O, Kamiya T, Echigo S, et al. Myocarditis in children—clinical findings and myocardial biopsy findings. Jpn Circ J. 1983;47:1298–303.
124. Dec GW, Palacios IF, Fallon JT, et al. Active myocarditis in the spectrum of acute dilated cardiomyopathies. Clinical features, histologic correlates, and clinical outcome. N Engl J Med. 1985;312:885–90.
125. Zee-Cheng C-S, Tsai CC, Palmer DC, et al. High incidence of myocarditis by endomyocardial biopsy in patients with idiopathic congestive cardiomyopathy. J Am Coll Cardiol. 1984;3:63–70.
126. Fenoglio JJ, Ursell PC, Kellogg CF, et al. Diagnosis and classification of myocarditis by endomyocardial biopsy. N Engl J Med. 1983;308:12–8.
127. Mason JW, Billingham ME, Ricci DR. Treatment of acute inflammatory myocarditis assisted by endomyocardial biopsy. Am J Cardiol. 1980;45:1037–44.
128. Chow LC, Dittrich HC, Shabetai R. Endomyocardial biopsy in patients with unexplained congestive heart failure. Ann Intern Med. 1988;109:535.
129. Shanes JG, Ghali J, Billingham ME, et al. Interobserver variability in the pathologic interpretation of endomyocardial biopsy results. Circulation. 1987;75:401–5.
130. Billingham M. Acute myocarditis: a diagnostic dilemma. Br Heart J. 1987;58:6–8.
131. Kereiakes DJ, Parmley WW. Myocarditis and cardiomyopathy. Am Heart J. 1984;108:1318–26.
132. Aretz HT, Billingham ME, Edwards WD, et al. Myocarditis, a histopathologic definition and classification. Am J Cardiovasc Pathol. 1987;1:3–14.
133. Yasuda T, Palacios IF, Dec GW, et al. Indium 111-monoclonal antimyosin antibody imaging in the diagnosis of acute myocarditis. Circulation. 1987;76:306–11.
134. Weinstein C, Fenoglio JJ. Myocarditis. Hum Pathol. 1987;18:613–8.
135. Easton AJ, Eglin RP. The detection of coxsackievirus RNA in cardiac tissue by *in situ* hybridization. J Gen Virol. 1988;69:285–91.
136. Rotbart HA, Eastman PS, Ruth JL, et al. Nonisotopic oligomeric probes for the human enteroviruses. J Clin Microbiol. 1988;26:2669–71.
137. Erlich HA, Gelfand DH, Saiki RK. Specific DNA amplification. Nature. 1988;331:461–2.
138. Kawai C, Matsumori A, Fujiwara H. Myocarditis and dilated cardiomyopathy. Annu Rev Med. 1987;38:221–39.
139. Lowry PJ, Edwards CW, Nagle RE. Herpes-like virus particles in myocardium of patient progressing to congestive cardiomyopathy. Br Heart J. 1982;48:501–3.
140. Daly K, Richardson PJ, Olsen EGJ, et al. Acute myocarditis. Role of histological and virological examination in the diagnosis and assessment of immunosuppressive treatment. Br Heart J. 1984;51:30–5.
141. Kopecky SL, Gersh BJ. Dilated cardiomyopathy and myocarditis: natural history, etiology, clinical manifestations, and management. In: O'Rourke RA, Crawford MH, eds. Current Problems in Cardiology. Chicago: Year Book Medical Publishers, Inc.; 1987:569–647.
142. Lowry BS. Viruses and heart disease: a problem in pathogenesis. Ann Clin Lab Sci. 1986;16:358–64.
143. Fowler NO. The secondary cardiomyopathies. In: Fowler NO. Myocardial Disease. New York: Grune & Stratton; 1973:337–59.
144. Bank I, Marboe CC, Redberg RF, et al. Myocarditis in adult Still's disease. Arthritis Rheum. 1985;28:452–4.
145. Myocarditis. In: Braunwald E, ed. Heart Disease, a Textbook of Cardiovascular Medicine. 3rd ed. Philadelphia: WB Saunders; 1988:1440–69.
146. Ikaheimo MJ, Niemela KO, Linnaluoto MM, et al. Early cardiac changes related to radiation therapy. Am J Cardiol. 1988;56:943–6.
147. Taliercio CP, Olney BA, Lie JT. Myocarditis related to drug hypersensitivity. Mayo Clin Proc. 1985;60:463–8.
148. Brand A, Keren A, Kerem E, et al. Myocardial damage after a scorpion sting: long-term echocardiographic follow-up. Pediatr Cardiol. 1988;9:59–61.
149. Matsuura H, Ishikita T, Yamamoto S, et al. Gallium-67 myocardial imaging for the detection of myocarditis in the acute phase of Kawasaki disease (mucocutaneous lymph node syndrome): the usefulness of single photon emission computed tomography. Br Heart J. 1987;58:385–92.
150. Humbert P, Faivre R, Fellman D, et al. Giant cell myocarditis: an autoimmune disease? Am Heart J. 1988;115:485–7.
151. Hayakawa M, Inoh T, Yokota Y, et al. A long-term follow-up study of acute viral and idiopathic myocarditis. Jpn Circ J. 1983;47:1304–9.
152. Tomioka N, Kishimoto C, Matsumori A, et al. Effects of prednisolone on acute viral myocarditis in mice. J Am Coll Cardiol. 1986;7:868–72.
153. Ettinger J, Feucht H, Gartner R, et al. Cyclosporine A (CyA) for successful treatment of myocarditis (Letter). Eur Heart J. 1986;7:452.
154. Hosenpud JD, McAnulty JH, Niles NR. Lack of objective improvement in ventricular systolic function in patients with myocarditis treated with azathioprine and prednisone. J Am Coll Cardiol. 1985;6:797–801.
155. Monrad ES, Matsumori A, Murphy JC, et al. Therapy with cyclosporine in experimental murine myocarditis with encephalomyocarditis virus. Circulation. 1986;73:1058–64.
156. Osler, W. The Principles and Practice of Medicine. New York: D Appleton; 1892.
157. Koontz CH, Ray CG. The role of coxsackie group B virus infections in sporadic myoparicarditis. Am Heart J. 1971;82:750–8.
158. Smith WG. Coxsackie B myopericarditis in adults. Am Heart J. 1970;80:34–46.
159. Montgomery J, Gear JHS, Prinslou FR, et al. Myocarditis of the newborn. An outbreak in a maternity home in Southern Rhodesia associated with coxsackie group-B virus infection. S Afr Med J. 1955;29:608–12.
160. Helin M, Savola J, Lapinleimu K. Cardiac manifestations during a coxsackie B5 epidemic. Br Med J. 1968;2:97–9.
161. Brodie HR, Marchessault V. Acute benign pericarditis caused by coxsackie virus group B. N Engl J Med. 1960;262:1278–80.
162. Grist NR, Bell EJ. Coxsackie viruses and the heart. Am Heart J. 1969;77:295–300.
163. Russell SJM, Bell EJ. Echoviruses and carditis. Lancet. 1970;1:784–5.
164. Kleinfeld M, Milles S, Lidsky M. Mumps pericarditis: review of the literature and report of a case. Am Heart J. 1958;55:153–6.
165. Proby Cm, Hacket D, Gupta S, et al. Acute myopericarditis in influenza A infection. Q J Med. 1986;60:887–92.
166. Cheng TC. Severe chest pain due to infectious mononucleosis. Postgrad Med. 1983;73:149–52.
167. Shugoll GI. Pericarditis associated with infectious mononucleosis. Arch Intern Med. 1957;100:630–4.
168. Williams AJ, Freemont AJ, Barnett DB. Pericarditis and arthritis complicating chickenpox. Br J Clin Pract. 1983;37:226–7.

169. Kassab A, Demoulin JC, Vanlancker MA, et al. Cytomegalovirus hemopericarditis. Report of 1 case with histologic confirmation. Acta Cardiol. 1987;42:69–72.
170. Freedberg RS, Gindea AJ, Dieterich DT, et al. Herpes simplex pericarditis in AIDS. NY State J Med. 1987;87:304–6.
171. Adler R, Takahashi M, Wright, Jr. HT. Acute pericarditis associated with hepatitis B infection. Pediatrics. 1978;61:716–9.
172. Boyle JD, Pearce ML, Guze LB. Purulent pericarditis: review of literature and report of eleven cases. Medicine. 1961;40:119–44.
173. Klacsmann PG, Bulkley BH, Hutchins GM. The changed spectrum of purulent pericarditis. An 86 year autopsy experience in 200 patients. Am J Med. 1977;63:666–73.
174. Kauffman CA, Watanakunakorn C, Phair JP. Purulent pneumococcal pericarditis. A continuing problem in the antibiotic era. Am J Med. 1973;54:743–50.
175. Rubin RH, Moellering RC. Clinical, microbiologic and therapeutic aspects of purulent pericarditis. Am J Med. 1975;59:68–78.
176. Blaser MJ, Reingold AL, Alsever RN, et al. Primary meningococcal pericarditis: a disease of adults associated with serogroup C *Neisseria meningitidis*. Rev Infect Dis. 1984;6:625–32.
177. Fyfe DA, Hagler DJ, Puga FJ, et al. Clinical and therapeutic aspects of *Haemophilus influenzae* pericarditis in pediatric patients. Mayo Clin Proc. 1984;59:415–22.
178. Schwartz KV, Guercio CA, Katz A. *Haemophilus influenza* pericarditis. Conn Med. 1987;51:423–4.
179. Corachan M, Poore P, Hadley GP, et al. Purulent pericarditis in Papua New Guinea: report of 12 cases and review of the literature in a tropical environment. Trans R Soc Trop Med Hyg. 1983;77:341–3.
180. Ramsdale DR, Gautam PC, Perera B, et al. Cardiac tamponade due to actinomycosis. Thorax. 1984;39:473–4.
181. Linz DH, Tolle SW, Elliot DL. *Mycoplasma pneumoniae* pneumonia. Experience at a referral center. West J Med. 1984;140:895–900.
182. Ponka A. The occurrence and clinical picture of serologically verified *Mycoplasma pneumoniae* infections with emphases on central nervous system, cardiac and joint manifestations. Ann Clin Res. 1979;24:1–60.
183. Sands MJ, Satz JE, Turner WE Jr, et al. Pericarditis and perimyocarditis associated with active *Mycoplasma pneumoniae* infection. Ann Intern Med. 1977;86:544–8.
184. Maycock R, Skale B, Kohler RB. *Legionella pneumophila* pericarditis proved by culture of pericardial fluid. Am J Med. 1983;75:534–6.
185. Reyes RR, Noble RC. Legionnaires' pericarditis. J Ky Med Assoc. 1983;81:757–8.
186. Svendsen JH, Jonsson V, Niebuhr U. Combined pericarditis and pneumonia caused by *Legionella* infection. Br Heart J 1987;58:663–4.
187. Friedland L, Snydman DR, Weingarden AS, et al. Ocular and pericardial involvement in Legionnaires' disease. Am J Med 1984;77:1105–7.
188. Larrieu AJ, Tyers GFO, Williams EH, et al. Recent experience with tuberculous pericarditis. Ann Thorac Surg. 1980;29:464–468.
189. Sagrista-Sauleda J, Permanyer-Miralda G, Soler-Soler J. Tuberculous pericarditis: ten year experience with a prospective protocol for diagnosis and treatment. J Am Coll Cardiol. 1988;11:724–8.
190. Rooney JJ, Crocco JA, Lyons HA. Tuberculous pericarditis. Ann Intern Med. 1970;72:73–8.
191. Desai HN. Tuberculous pericarditis. A review of 100 cases. S Afr Med J. 1979;55:877–80.
192. Dalli E, Quesada A, Juan G, et al. Tuberculous pericarditis as the first manifestation of acquired immunodeficiency syndrome. Am Heart J. 1987;114:905–6.
193. Ortbals DW, Avioli LV. Tuberculous pericarditis. Arch Intern Med. 1979;139:231–4.
194. Wheat LJ, Stein L, Corya BC, et al. Pericarditis as a manifestation of histoplasmosis during two large urban outbreaks. Medicine. 1983;62:110–9.
195. Young EJ, Vainrub B, Musher DM. Pericarditis due to histoplasmosis. JAMA. 1978;240:1750.
196. Larson R, Scherb RI. Coccidioidal pericarditis. Circulation. 1953;7:211–7.
197. Chapman MG, Kaplan L. Cardiac involvement in coccidioidomycosis. Am J Med. 1957;23:87–98.
198. Duvall CP, Carbone PP. *Cryptococcus neoformans* pericarditis associated with Hodgkin's diseases. Ann Intern Med. 1966;64:850–6.
199. Kraus WE, Valenstein PN, Corey GR. Purulent pericarditis caused by *Candida:* report of three cases and identification of high-risk populations as an aid to early diagnosis. Rev Infect Dis. 1988;10:34–41.
200. Eng RHK, Sen P, Browne K, et al. Candida pericarditis. Am J Med. 1981;70:867–9.
201. Kaufman LD, Seifert FC, Eilbott DJ, et al. *Candida* pericarditis and tamponade in a patient with systemic lupus erythematosus. Arch Intern Med. 1988;148:715–7.
202. Walsh TJ, Bulkley BH. *Aspergillus* pericarditis: clinical and pathologic features in the immunocompromised patient. Cancer. 1982;49:48–54.
203. Cooper JAD, Weinbaum DL, Aldrich TK, et al. Invasive aspergillosis of the lung and pericardium in a nonimmunocompromised 33 year old man. Am J Med. 1981;71:903–7.
204. Theologides A, Kennedy BJ. Editorial: Toxoplasmic myocarditis and pericarditis. Am J Med. 1969;47:169–74.
205. Sagrista-Sauleda J, Permanyer-Miralda G, Juste-Sanchez C, et al. Huge chronic pericardial effusion caused by *Toxoplasma gondii*. Circulation. 1982;66:895–7.
206. Ibarra-Perez C, Green LS, Calvello-Juarez M, et al. Diagnosis and treatment of rupture of amebic abscess of the liver into the pericardium. J Thorac Cardiovasc Surg. 1972;64:11–7.
207. Rab SW, Alam N, Hoda AN, et al. Amoebic liver abscess. Some unique presentations. Am J Med. 1967;43:811–6.
208. Baid CS, Varma AR, Lakhotia M. A case of subacute effusive constrictive pericarditis with a probable amoebic aetiology. Br Heart J. 1987;58:296–8.
209. Strang JIG. Two-dimensional echocardiography in the diagnosis of amoebic pericarditis. A case report. S Afr Med J. 1987;71:328–9.
210. Van der Horst R. Schistosomiasis of the pericardium. J R Soc Trop Med Hygiene. 1979;73:243–4.
211. Permanyer-Miralda G, Sagrista-Sauleda J, Soler-Soler J. Primary acute pericardial disease: a prospective series of 231 consecutive patients. Am J Cardiol 1985;56:623–30.
212. Roberts WC, Spray TL. Clinical and morphologic spectrum of pericardial heart disease. Curr Probl Cardiol. 1977;2:1–71.
213. Shabetai R. Function of the pericardium. In: Fowler NO, ed. The Pericardium in Health and Disease. Mount Kisco, NY: Futura; 1985:19–50.
214. Fowler NO, Harbin AD. Recurrent acute pericarditis: follow-up study of 31 patients. J Am Coll Cardiol. 1986;7:300–5.
215. Matthews JD, Cameron SJ, George M. Constrictive pericarditis following coxsackie virus infection. Thorax. 1970;25:624–6.
216. Utley JR, Mills J. Annular erosion and pericarditis. Complications of endocarditis of the aortic root. J Thorac Cardiovasc Surg. 1972;64:76–81.
217. Ribeiro P, Shapiro L, Nihoyannopoulos P, et al. Pericarditis in infective endocarditis. Eur Heart J. 1985;6:975–8.
218. Peel AAF. Tuberculous pericarditis. Br Heart J. 1948;10:195–207.
219. Carson TJ, Murray GF, Wilcox BR, et al. The role of surgery in tuberculous pericarditis. Ann Thorac Surg. 1974;17:163–7.
220. Guberman BA, Fowler NO, Engel PJ, et al. Cardiac tamponade in medical patients. Circulation. 1981;64:633–40.
221. Spodick DH. Pericardial rub: prospective multiple observer investigation of pericardial friction rub in 100 patients. Am J Cardiol. 1975;35:357–62.
222. Lorell BH, Braunwald E. Pericardial disease. In: Braunwald E, ed: A Textbook of Cardiovascular Medicine. 3rd ed. Philadelphia: WB Saunders; 1988:1484–534.
223. Spodick DH. Electrocardiogram in acute pericarditis. Distributions of morphologic and axial changes by stages. Am J Cardiol. 1974;33:470–4.
224. Spodick DH. Frequency of arrhythmias in acute pericarditis determined by holter monitoring. Am J Cardiol. 1984;53:842–5.
225. Krainin FM, Flessas AP, Spodick DH. Infarction associated pericarditis. Rarity of diagnostic electrocardiogram. N Engl J Med. 1984;311:1211–4.
226. Renfrew R, Buselmeier TJ, Kjeilstrand CM. Pericarditis and renal failure. Annu Rev Med. 1980;31:345–60.
227. Brosius FC, Waller BF, Roberts WC. Radiation heart disease. Am J Med. 1981;70:519–30.
228. Dressler W. Post-myocardial infarction syndrome. JAMA. 1956;160:1379–83.
229. Engle MA, Gay WA Jr, Zabriskie JB, et al. The post pericardiotomy syndrome: 25 years experience. J Carijovasc Med. 1984;4:321–32.
230. Silverman KJ, Hutchins GM, Bulkley BH. Cardiac sarcoid: a clinicopathologic study of 84 unselected cases with systemic sarcoidosis. Circulation. 1978;58:1204–11.
231. Ansari A, Larson PH, Bates HD. Cardiovascular manifestations of systemic lupus erythematosis: current perspective. Prog Cardiovasc Dis. 1985;27:421–34.
232. Lebowitz WB. The heart in rheumatoid arthritis (rheumatoid disease). A clinical and pathological study of sixty-two cases. Ann Intern Med. 1963;58:102–23.
233. McWhorter JE, LeRoy RC. Pericardial disease in scleroderma (systemic sclerosis). Am J Med. 1974;57:566–75.
234. Zimmerman J, Yahalom J, Bar-On H. Clinical spectrum of pericardial effusion as the presenting feature of hypothyroidism. Am Heart J. 1983;106:770–1.
235. Krikorian JG, Hancock EW. Pericardiocentesis. Am J Med. 1978;65:808–14.
236. Isner JM, Carter BL, Bankoff MS, et al. Computed tomography in the diagnosis of pericardial heart disease. Ann Intern Med. 1982;97:473–9.
237. Tomoda H, Hoshiai M, Furuya H, et al. Evaluation of pericardial effusion with computed tomography. Am Heart J. 1980;99:701–6.
238. Sechtem U, Tscholakoff D, Higgins CB. MRI of the abnormal pericardium. AJR. 1986;147:245–52.
239. Tan JS, Holmes JC, Fowler NO, et al. Antibiotic levels in pericardial fluid. J Clin Invest. 1974;53:7–12.
240. Quale JM, Lipschik GY, Heurich AE. Management of tuberculous pericarditis. Ann Thorac Surg. 1987;43:653–5.
241. Strang JIG, Kakaza HHS, Gibson DG, et al. Controlled trial of prednisolone as adjuvant in treatment of tuberculous constrictive pericarditis in Transkei. Lancet. 1987;11:1418–22.
242. Levine TM, Wurster CF, Krespi YP. Mediastinitis occurring as a complication of odontogenic infections. Laryngoscope. 1986;96:747–50.
243. Estrera AS, Landay MJ, Grisham JM, et al: Descending necrotizing mediastinitis. Surg Gynecol Obstet. 1983;157:545–52.
244. Bennett DJ, Deveridge RJ, Wright JS. Spontaneous rupture of the esophagus: a review with reports of six cases. Surgery 1970;68:766–70.
245. Sarr MG, Gott VL, Townsend TR. Mediastinal infection after cardiac surgery. Ann Thorac Surg. 1984;38:415–23.

246. Bor DH, Rose RM, Modlin JF, et al. Mediastinitis after cardiovascular surgery. Rev Infect Dis. 1983;5:885–97.
247. Ottino G, De Paulis R, Pansini S, et al. Major sternal wound infection after open-heart surgery: a multivariate analysis of risk factors in 2,579 consecutive operative procedures. Ann Thorac Surg. 1987;44:173–9.
248. Murray PM, Finegold SM. Anaerobic mediastinitis. Rev Infect Dis. 1984;6:S123–7.
249. Kauffman CA, Sheagren JN, Quie PG. *Staphylococcus epidermis* mediastinitis and disseminated intravascular coagulation. Ann Intern Med. 1984;100:60–1.
250. Breatnach E, Nath PH, Delany DJ. The role of computed tomography in acute and subacute mediastinitis. Clin Radiol. 1986;37:139–45.
251. Kay HR, Goodman LR, Teplick SK, et al. Use of computed tomography to assess mediastinal complications after median sternotomy. Ann Thorac Surg. 1983;36:706–14.
252. Schowengerdt CG, Suyemoto R, Beachley Main F. Granulomatous and fibrous mediastinitis. A review and analysis of 180 cases. J Thorac Cardiovasc Surg. 1969;57:365–79.
253. Wieder S, Rabinowitz JG. Fibrous mediastinitis: a late manifestation of mediastinal histoplasmosis. Radiology. 1977;125:305–12.
254. Hewlett TH, Steer A, Thomas DE. Progressive fibrosing mediastinitis. Ann Thorac Surg. 1966;2:345–57.
255. Gryboski WA, Crutcher RR, Holloway JB, et al. Surgical aspects of histoplasmosis. Arch Surg. 1963;87:590–9.
256. Scully RE, Galdabini JJ, McNeely BU. Case records of the Massachusetts General Hospital. Weekly clinicopathological exercises. N Engl J Med. 1976;295:381–8.

SECTION H. CENTRAL NERVOUS SYSTEM INFECTIONS

65. ANATOMIC CONSIDERATIONS IN CENTRAL NERVOUS SYSTEM INFECTIONS

JOHN E. GREENLEE

The pathogenesis and course of central nervous system infections are greatly influenced by the anatomy of the brain and spinal cord and by the relationships of brain and cord to vessels, cranial nerves, spinal nerve roots, meninges, and overlying skeletal structure.

ANATOMIC RELATIONSHIPS OF THE BRAIN AND SPINAL CORD

Relationships of Brain, Meninges, and Skull

The brain is suspended in cerebrospinal fluid (CSF) and is surrounded by three layers of meninges: the pia mater and arachnoid, which constitute the leptomeninges, and the dura mater or pachymeninges (Fig. 1).[1] The pia mater is continuous with the external surface of the brain and cord, forming a cuff of meningeal tissue around penetrating vessels and merging with the ependymal lining of the fourth ventricle at the foramina of Luschka and Magendie. The arachnoid encloses the brain more loosely, and between the pia and arachnoid, completely surrounding the brain and cord and communicating with the fourth ventricle, is the CSF-filled subarachnoid space. The outward pressure of brain and CSF holds the arachnoid in contact with the most superficial layer of meninges, the dura mater. The dura mater is adherent to the periosteum and skull except where it invaginates into the cranial cavity to form four rigid septa: the falx cerebri, falx cerebelli, tentorium cerebelli, and diaphragma selli.

Under normal conditions, the only meningeal compartment within the skull is the subarachnoid space. Infection within this space may involve the entire surface of the leptomeninges around the brain and cord and may also cross the foramina of Luschka and Magendie to produce ventriculitis.[2] During leptomeningitis, intracranial pressure may rise markedly, but this increase in pressure, even if severe, tends to be transmitted to the entire subarachnoid space around the brain and cord (Fig. 1). Unless concomitant abscess or empyema is present, or unless severe edema has developed, there is little displacement of cerebral structures and little risk of brain herniation after lumbar puncture.[2] Infection may also develop between the arachnoid and dura or between the dura and skull by dissecting along tissue planes. Because the arachnoid and dura are attached at only a few points, subdural infection will spread rapidly over the surface of one hemisphere to produce a subdural empyema. Infection outside the dura, on the other hand, will be contained by the attachment of dura to periosteum and bone to form a more localized epidural abscess. Both subdural empyema and epidural abscess behave as mass lesions, and lumbar puncture may precipitate brain herniation.[3]

Relationship of Brain and Meninges to Cranial Structures

The undersurface of the brain rests within the anterior, middle, and posterior cranial fossae. Each fossa abuts on structures from which infection may spread (Fig. 2). The anterior fossa forms the roof of the frontal and ethmoidal sinuses. Infection within either sinus may produce a frontal epidural abscess, subdural empyema over the frontal lobes or falx, or a frontal lobe brain abscess.[3–5] The sella turcica, located between the left and right middle fossae, forms the roof of the sphenoid sinuses. Infection within these sinuses can spread centrally to cause not only epidural abscess and subdural empyema but also palsies of extraocular muscles, optic neuritis, and cavernous sinus thrombophlebitis.[6]

Infections of the middle ear or mastoid within the petrous bone may extend into the middle fossa to involve the temporal lobe or may extend into the posterior fossa to involve the cerebellum or brain stem.[4,5] Rarely, infection within the maxillary sinus may cause temporal lobe abscess.

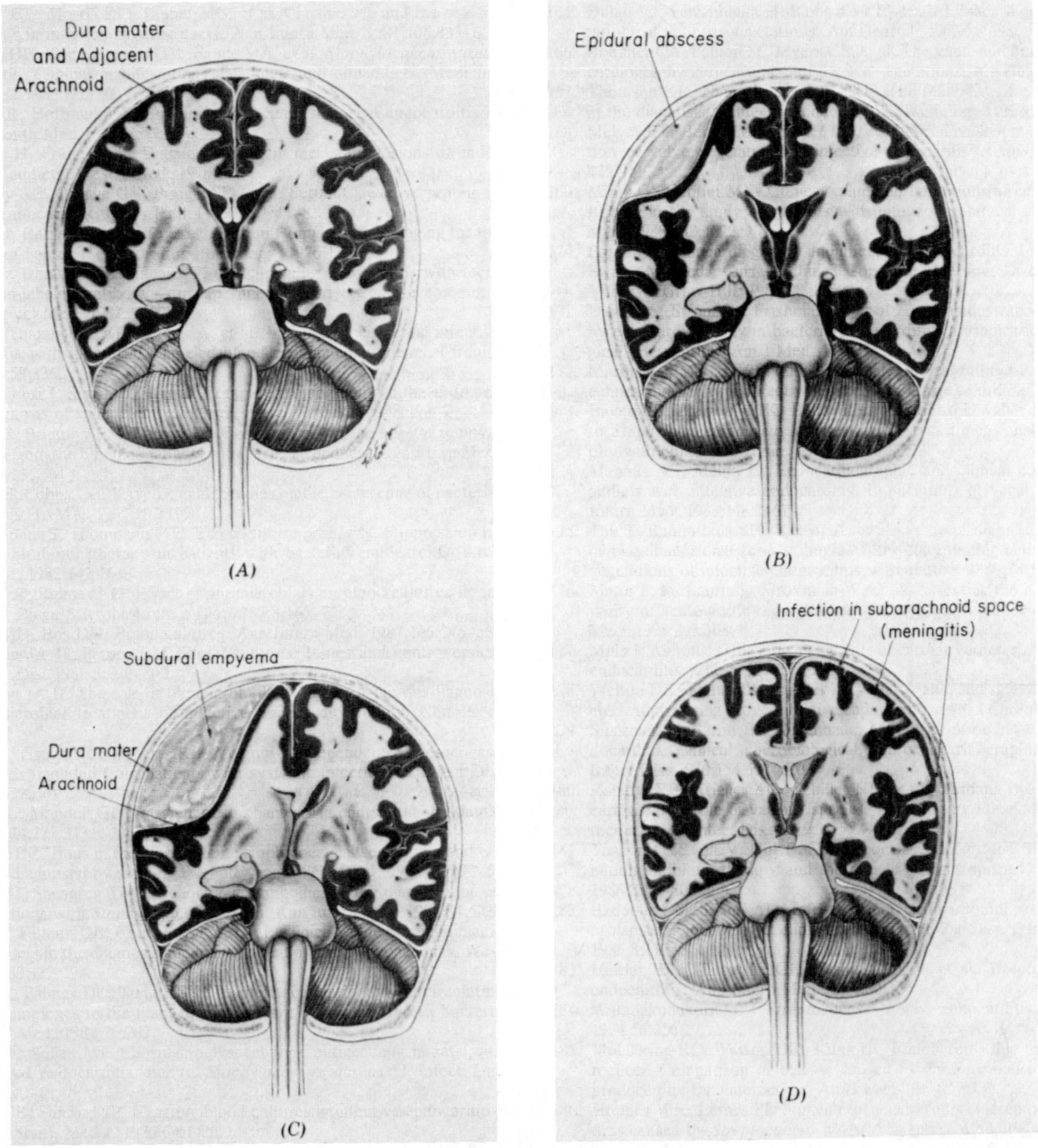

FIG. 1. The cranial meninges: normal anatomic relationships **(A)** and alterations in epidural abscess **(B)**, subdural empyema **(C)**, and meningitis **(D)**.

Injury to Cranial Nerves During Infections

All 12 cranial nerves exit through the meninges at the base of the brain and may be injured during meningitis. Cranial nerve deficits are particularly common in chronic infections of the basilar meninges such as those caused by *Mycobacterium tuberculosis, Cryptococcus neoformans*, or sarcoidosis.[7–9] Cranial nerves VII and VIII are most often affected, followed by cranial nerves III, IV, VI, IX, and X. Cranial nerve II may also be involved. If meningeal infection is protracted, multiple cranial nerve deficits may develop and may fluctuate during the course of the illness.[10]

Several of the cranial nerves have anatomic characteristics that predispose them to damage during infections or during states of increased intracranial pressure (see Table 1). Of particular importance is the close relationship of cranial nerve III to the tentorium: compression of the third nerve by the uncus of the temporal lobe is often the initial indication of transtentorial herniation. Cranial nerve VI has the longest intracranial course of any cranial nerve. An isolated paresis of the sixth

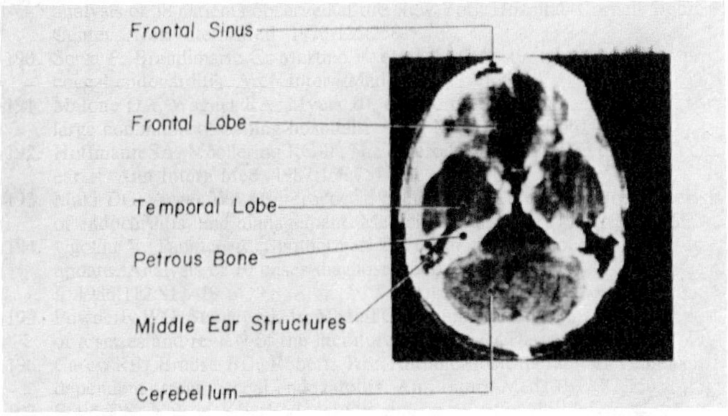

FIG. 2. Anatomic relationships of anterior, middle, and posterior tossa structures as seen on computed tomography. The frontal sinuses lie at the anterior pole of the cerebrum. The petrous bone, containing middle ear structures, lies between temporal lobe and cerebellum. An abscess, arising from the left frontal sinus, is faintly seen within the frontal lobe. (Courtesy of Dr. Frederick Vines, Jacksonville, FL.)

TABLE 1. Cranial Nerve Involvement in CNS Infections

Cranial Nerve or Nerves	*Anatomic Features*	*Significance*	*Consequence*
I	Traverses dura mater and ethmoid bone, surrounded by a cuff of arachnoid; terminates in free nerve endings within the nasal mucosa and nasopharynx.	Is the only cranial nerve in direct contact with the external environment.	May provide a route of direct CNS inoculation for neurotropic viruses.
II	1. Develops as a part of the brain and is contained within the subarachnoid space up to its point of entry into the eye.	1. Increased intracranial pressure causes papilledema. Chronic increased pressure results in optic atrophy.	1. Early signs are retinal vascular engorgement, followed by blurring of the optic disk, with hemorrhages appearing later. Initial visual change is enlargement of the physiologic blind spot. If intracranial hypertension persists, transient visual blurring and concentric constriction of visual fields occur. Chronic papilledema progresses to optic atrophy and blindness. Central scotomas may occur but are rare.
	2. Myelin sheath is composed of central myelin.	2. May be the target of immune response against central myelin in postinfectious encephalitis or encephalomyelitis.	2. Visual field deficit (usually central or centrocecal scotoma).
III	Passes directly beneath the edge of the tentorium cerebelli below the uncus of the temporal lobe.	Is almost always the first structure compressed by the uncus during transtentorial herniation.	Paresis of CN III parasympathetic fibers causes pupillary dilatation. Interruption of nerve supply to all extraocular muscles except lateral rectus and superior oblique causes lateral deviation of the eye and ptosis.
III, IV, V, VI	Travel together in the wall of the cavernous sinus.	All may be affected by cavernous sinus thrombosis.	Total ophthalmoplegia, mid-position fixed pupil, loss of corneal reflex and ipsilateral facial sensation.
V, VI	Travel in close proximity to the tip of the petrous bone.	May be injured in the course of chronic otitis media, especially where osteomyelitis of the petrous tip has developed.	Abducens palsy (lateral rectus weakness) and ipsilateral facial pain or sensory loss (Gradenigo's syndrome).
IX–XI	Exit from skull through jugular foramen.	May be injured by thrombosis of the internal jugular vein at the jugular foramen.	Ipsilateral palatal weakness and diminished gag reflex; weakness of trapezius and sternomastoid muscles on the involved side (jugular foramen syndrome).
III–XII	Myelin sheaths composed of peripheral myelin.	May be involved with peripheral nerves and spinal nerve roots in postinfectious polyneuritis (Landry-Guillain-Barré syndrome).	Deficits of any cranial nerve except I or II may occur. Cranial nerve VII is most often involved.

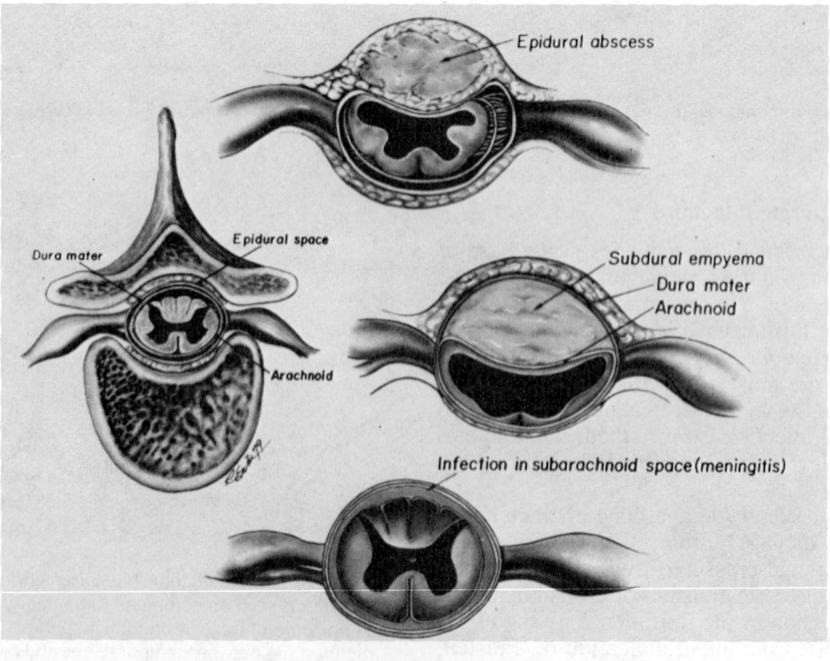

FIG. 3. The spinal meninges and epidural space: normal anatomic relationships and alterations in epidural abscess, subdural empyema, and meningitis.

nerve may indicate either direct involvement of the nerve anywhere along its length or compression due to elevated intracranial pressure.

Anatomic Relationships of the Spinal Cord

The spinal cord extends from the foramen magnum to the level of the L1-L2 intervertebral disk.[11] Below L2 the spinal canal contains the nerve roots, which form the cauda equina. Unlike the cerebral hemispheres, where gray matter is most external, the spinal cord has a central core of gray matter and an external layer of white matter containing ascending and descending nerve tracts. Lesions developing within the cord (intramedullary lesions) often produce neuronal injury at one or more spinal cord segments early in their course and only later expand laterally to involve motor and sensory nerve tracts. Lesions external to the cord, on the other hand, (extramedullary lesions) produce symptoms of nerve root irritation early in their course, followed by long tract signs; injury to central gray matter occurs only later.

The relationships of pia mater, arachnoid, and dura are essentially the same for the spinal cord as for the brain (Fig. 3), and the interface between spinal arachnoid and dura, like its intracranial counterpart, provides a plane along which infection can easily dissect. In contrast to the close adherence of the dura mater to the cranial periosteum and skull, however, the spinal dura and periosteum diverge at the foramen magnum, and by the level of the seventh cervical vertebra are separated by a fat-filled epidural space that offers little resistance to the longitudinal spread of infection. Both spinal subdural empyema and spinal epidural abscess may thus extend over many vertebral segments. Both are usually posterior to the cord and may be inadvertently entered during lumbar puncture (see Fig. 3).

ROLE OF THE INTRACRANIAL CIRCULATION IN CENTRAL NERVOUS SYSTEM INFECTIONS

Vascular Anatomy

Arteries. The brain is supplied by two internal carotid arteries and two vertebral arteries that join to form the basilar artery (Fig. 4).[12–14] Each internal carotid supplies the retina via the ophthalmic artery and bifurcates into an anterior cerebral artery that supplies the medial surface of the cerebrum and a middle cerebral artery that supplies the frontal, parietal, and temporal lobes over the cerebral convexity. The vertebrobasilar system supplies the rostral spinal cord, the brain stem, and the cerebellum before terminating in two posterior cerebral arteries. These angle sharply backward over the tentorium cerebelli to supply the occipital lobes, the posterior parietal lobes, and the posterior and mesial portions of temporal lobes. Because the ophthalmic artery is a branch of the internal carotid, emboli within the anterior circulation may produce monocular visual loss or retinal lesions visible by ophthalmoscopy and may give indirect evidence of an embolic source of central nervous system infection.

The major intracranial arteries differ in both caliber and volume of flow. The middle cerebral arteries receive the greatest volume of blood, followed by the anterior cerebrals and vertebrobasilar system. The likelihood of septic embolization, with resultant brain abscess or mycotic aneurysm, is thus greatest in the branches of the middle cerebral and least in the smaller branches of the posterior circulation.[15] The choroid plexuses also receive a large volume of blood.[16]

The major arteries of the brain are connected at the circle of Willis by anterior and posterior communicating branches and are also connected by smaller anastomotic vessels at the meningeal surface. The intracranial circulation communicates with the external carotid system through anastomoses between the

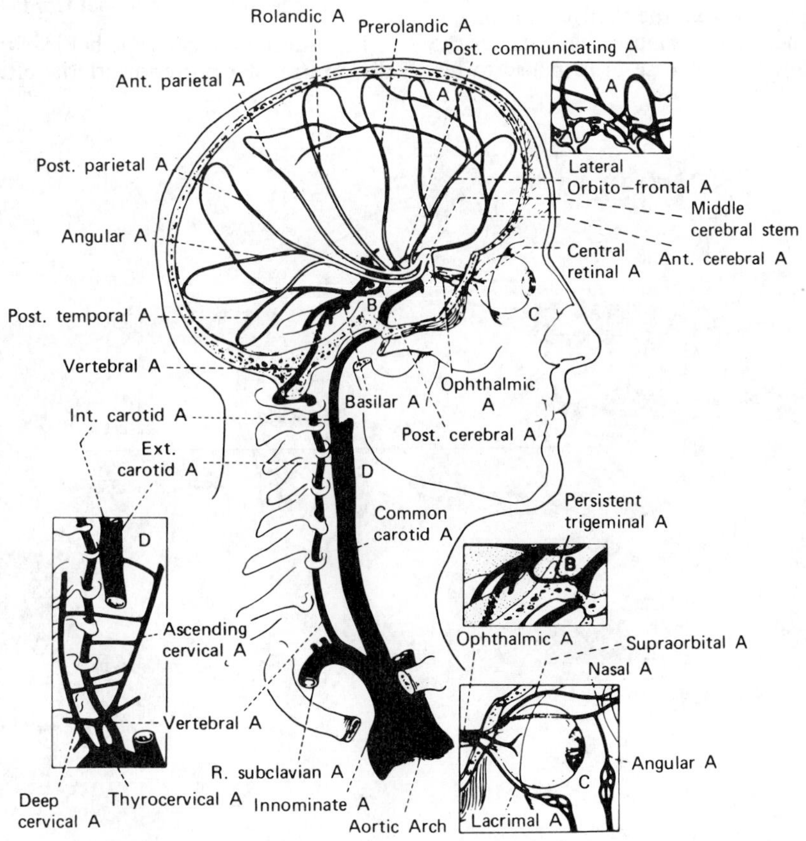

FIG. 4. Arterial supply of central nervous system. (From Adams and Victor,[62] with permission.)

ophthalmic and maxillary arteries and between branches of the vertebrals and the occipital arteries. There is also extensive communication with the meningeal branches of the external carotid via the rete mirabile, a network of small vessels that cross the meninges and anastomose with arteries on the surface of the brain.[12–14] Despite this collateral circulation, however, certain parts of the brain are arterial border zones or "watershed areas," receiving their arterial supply from terminal branches of two or more vessels. The most important of these watershed areas lies between middle and posterior cerebral arteries at the junction of parietal, occipital, and temporal lobes. Similar watershed areas exist on the medial surface of the hemispheres, within the internal capsule, and over the cerebellum. These areas, particularly in the elderly patient with extensive vascular disease, are particularly vulnerable to ischemic injury if any of their supplying vessels becomes compromised. The signs and symptoms produced by watershed infarcts often extend beyond the usual distribution of the vessel involved. Cerebral white matter also forms a watershed area, receiving terminal arterial flow from both penetrating cortical and ventricular vessels. For this reason, white matter is more easily rendered ischemic than is gray matter, and abscesses arising within devitalized brain are most common in white matter or at the gray-white junction.[17]

Veins. The intracranial venous system is composed of three groups of vessels: superficial veins that drain the external portions of cerebrum and brain stem; deep veins that drain central white matter, basal ganglia, and thalamus; and venous sinuses within the dura mater (Fig. 5).[14] The superficial veins of the cerebrum are divided about a watershed area above the Sylvian fissure into veins that empty upward into the superior sagittal sinus and veins emptying downward into the basilar venous sinuses.[18] The superficial and deep cerebral veins are extensively interconnected, and anastomoses exist as well among the venous sinuses. There is also communication of superficial veins and venous sinuses with the extracranial venous system via numerous emissary veins that cross the skull and meninges. Neither intracranial veins nor venous sinuses have valves, so the direction of venous flow may reverse in response to hemodynamic changes. Because of these extensive anastomoses, cortical vein thrombosis or even occlusion of a venous sinus may at times be silent or may produce only transient neurologic abnormalities. If infarction results, clinical findings often evolve slowly and in fluctuating fashion as the thrombotic process involves increasing numbers of venous collaterals. Venous infarcts are frequently hemorrhagic, with irregular borders that are determined by remaining collateral venous drainage.[19] Thrombosis of the posterior portion of the superior sagittal sinus may produce cortical venous thrombosis of both hemispheres, causing bilateral lower extremity weakness. Cortical blindness may be present if both occipital lobes are involved. Because the hand area on the cerebral convexity has two routes of venous drainage, neurologic deficits referable to this area in venous thrombosis frequently resolve.

The cerebral venous sinuses not only drain venous blood but also reabsorb CSF through arachnoid villi, most of which are located along the anterior third of the superior sagittal sinus. Thrombosis of the superior sagittal sinus may block CSF reabsorption and produce communicating hydrocephalus, at times without other symptoms. Impairment of CSF reabsorption may also occur if venous outflow from the superior sagittal sinus is blocked by occlusion of both lateral sinuses or of one lateral sinus where the other is hypoplastic.[14,19]

Capillaries. The capillaries of the brain and cord, except for those of the pituitary, the choroid plexuses, and several circumventricular structures within the brain stem, differ from capillaries elsewhere in the body in that they do not have fenestrations or intercellular clefts.[20] Molecules thus cross cerebral capillaries less by diffusion than on the basis of lipid solubility or by active transport. This relative impermeability of brain capillaries is the basis of the barrier systems that sequester brain and CSF from the extracranial environment and is a major factor in the selection of antibiotics for intracranial infections (see below).

Vascular Supply of the Spinal Cord

The posterior columns and horns of the spinal cord are supplied by an irregular posterior arterial plexus that is virtually never

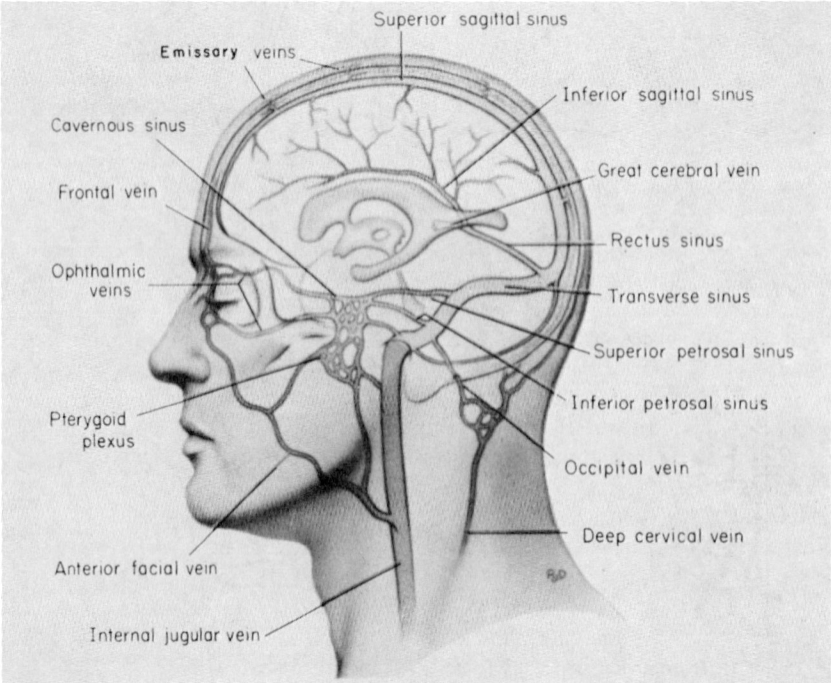

FIG. 5. Venous supply of the central nervous system. (From Truax and Carpenter,[59] with permission.)

involved in infections. The remainder of the cord is supplied by the anterior spinal artery system, which arises from the vertebrals and receives contributory branches from cervical and intercostal arteries and from the descending aorta.[21] In many but not all patients there is a predominant tributary vessel from the aorta, the artery of Adamkiewicz, which joins the anterior spinal artery between cord segments T8 and L4. The thoracic cord above the artery of Adamkiewicz, particularly in the region around T4, may act as a watershed area much like those within the brain and may suffer ischemic injury during systemic hypotension or if vessels above or below it are occluded. The veins of the spinal cord are roughly similar in distribution to the spinal arteries.

Role of Central Nervous System Vessels in Infections

The vessels of the central nervous system provide the most frequent route by which infection reaches the meninges, brain, or cord (see below). In addition, involvement of the vessels themselves may produce ischemic or hemorrhagic injury to the brain or cord, with or without accompanying suppuration. Arteries may be occluded by septic emboli. If the embolus breaks up before irreversible ischemia has occurred, it may produce symptoms of a transient ischemic attack; more protracted ischemia results in infarction. Arterial thrombosis may occur if the vessel wall becomes involved by meningeal inflammation, as in tuberculous meningitis.[7] Multiplication of organisms within vascular endothelial cells, as in Rocky Mountain spotted fever, may cause thrombosis of small vessels.[22] Vasculitis and thrombosis of vessels may also occur as a complication of hepatitis B antigenemia[23,24] and is responsible for the syndrome of ipsilateral cerebral infarction occasionally seen during ophthalmic herpes zoster infections.[25] Similar but more chronic virus-induced vasculitis may be the major pathogenetic mechanism in progressive rubella encephalitis.[26] Occasionally, in bacterial endocarditis or other states of prolonged bacteremia, hyperplasia of vascular endothelial cells or obliterative endarteritis may occur and may occlude the vessel lumen.[27–29] In addition to causing vascular occlusion, arteritis may produce necrosis of the vessel wall and/or formation of a mycotic aneurysm. Rupture of the affected vessel with intracranial hemorrhage may occur during or even after successful therapy for the infection.[15] Spontaneous resolution of mycotic aneurysms may occur,[30] but the likelihood of rupture or spontaneous resolution cannot be predicted in a given case.

The veins of the central nervous system may also thrombose in response to internal or extramural inflammation and may provide a source of sterile or septic emboli to other parts of the nervous system or to the lungs. The infarcted tissue produced by either arterial or venous occlusion may become the site of single or multiple abscesses.

Injury to central nervous capillaries may allow escape of organisms into ischemic brain and may produce transudation of fluid from the vascular compartment and cerebral edema (see below). Loss of integrity of the blood-brain barrier also permits radioisotopes or radiological contrast media to leak into involved brain, allowing localization of lesions by radionuclide, computed tomography (CT), or magnetic resonance (MR) scans (Figs. 2 and 6). Antibiotics normally unable to cross cerebral or meningeal capillaries penetrate the brain or CSF across such injured vessels. As inflammation subsides, capillary integrity is restored, edema resolves, and CSF antibiotic concentrations fall, even if no alteration is made in antibiotic dose or route of administration.

Spinal vessels are rarely involved by infection. Spinal artery occlusion may occur during bacterial endocarditis, Rocky Mountain spotted fever, or tertiary syphilis. Spinal veins may be involved by epidural abscess or subdural empyema and may produce cord injury more extensive than would be expected on the basis of compression alone.

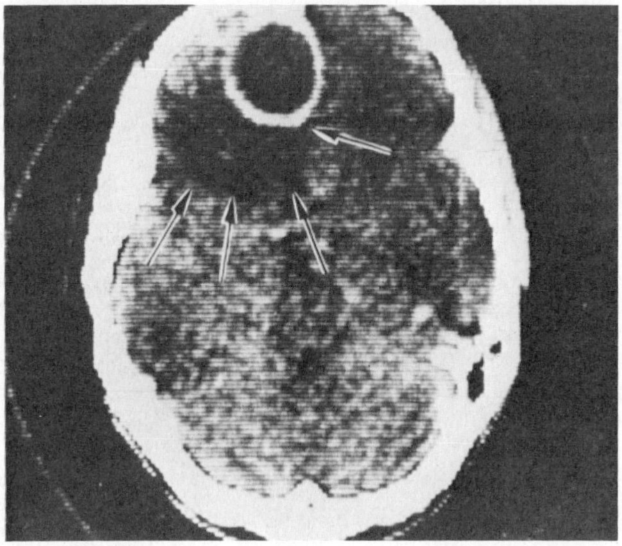

FIG. 6. Brain abscess as seen on computed tomography. The arrows outline an area of cerebral edema equal in size to the abscess itself. This is a more rostral view of the abscess faintly seen in Figure 2. (Courtesy of Dr. Frederick Vines, Jacksonville, FL.)

CEREBROSPINAL FLUID CIRCULATION IN NERVOUS SYSTEM INFECTIONS

Eighty-five percent of the CSF is produced within the lateral, third, and fourth ventricles by the choroid plexuses (see Fig. 7), the remainder forming by diffusion across the meninges.[31] The choroid plexuses resemble renal tubules histologically and produce CSF by secretion rather than passive diffusion. Like renal tubules, the choroid plexuses also contain probenecid-sensitive and other transport mechanisms and are capable of removing weak organic acids including penicillin and gentamicin from the CSF against a concentration gradient.[31] The direction of the CSF circulation is outward through the foramina of Luschka and Magendie into the subarachnoid space, where it circulates around the brain and cord by bulk flow. Reabsorption of CSF occurs by vesicular transport through cells of the arachnoid villi along the superior sagittal sinus. A small amount of CSF may be absorbed directly across the meninges. Complete exchange of CSF occurs every 3 to 4 hours.

The CSF circulation is important in the diagnosis, treatment, and complications of central nervous system infections. Chemical and cellular changes in CSF may provide accurate information about infections within the subarachnoid space and, in extensive leptomeningeal infections, may contain the infectious agent in large numbers.[32] However, lumbar CSF may not always give precise information in chronic basilar or other localized meningeal infections and, unless very large volumes of lumbar CSF are studied,[33,34] may not allow recovery of the infectious agent or contain diagnostic antigens at a time when the causative agent may be isolated by high cervical or cisternal puncture.[34,35] In subdural or epidural infection or in brain abscess, where infection occurs outside the subarachnoid space, the CSF may be normal or may reveal only a mild, nonspecific lymphocytosis, with a slight elevation of the protein concentration and a normal sugar level; organisms are only rarely present.[4,36]

The physiology of the CSF circulation is important in the treatment of ventriculitis with aminoglycosides or other antibiotics that penetrate into CSF poorly. Although it is possible, under experimental conditions, to produce high ventricular levels of agents by the instillation of large volumes,[37] intrathecal administration of antibiotics in conventional volumes produces

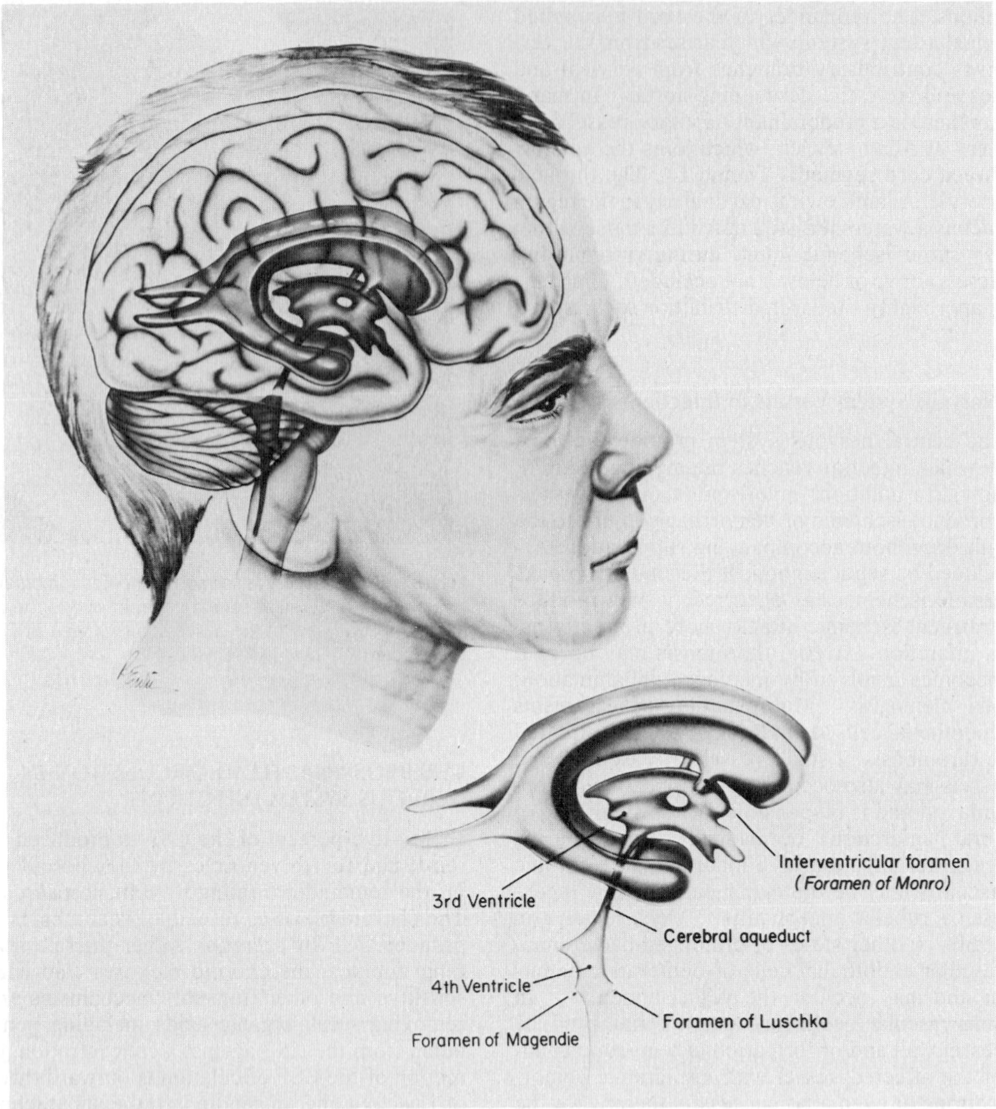

FIG. 7. The cerebral ventricles. The ventricular system is narrowest and hence most easily obstructed at the foramen of Monro, the cerebral aqueduct (aqueduct of Sylvius), and the foramina of Luschka and Magendie.

unreliable ventricular concentrations, and lumbar administration does not allow measurement of the ventricular concentrations achieved.[38] Because of these factors, therapy for ventriculitis with agents that must be instilled directly into the CSF requires direct administration into the ventricles through a subcutaneous reservoir.[38–40]

Infections involving the nervous system may produce communicating or obstructive hydrocephalus. Communicating hydrocephalus follows impairment of CSF reabsorption across the arachnoid villi and may be due to blood within the subarachnoid space, chronic meningitis, or occlusion of the superior sagittal or lateral sinuses. In communicating hydrocephalus, although ventricular dilatation occurs, the increase in pressure is distributed equally throughout the subarachnoid space and ventricular system. Obstructive hydrocephalus develops when there is compromise of CSF circulation within the ventricles and most often represents occlusion of the ventricular system at its narrowest points: the foramina of Luschka and Magendie, the aqueduct of Sylvius, or, rarely, the foramina of Monro. Occlusion may be due to inflammation within the ventricular system or subarachnoid space or to external compression by abscess, mass, or hemorrhage. In obstructive hydrocephalus, ventricular dilatation occurs rostral to the point of obstruction, and the trapped CSF behaves as a mass lesion. Brain herniation may occur and may be precipitated by lumbar puncture. Although lumbar puncture may theoretically be safely used to lower intracranial pressure in communicating hydrocephalus, both communicating and obstructive components are frequently present in central nervous system infections. For this reason, lumbar puncture in the face of papilledema, suspected space-occupying lesion, or increase in ventricular size must be approached with great caution.[41]

ROUTES OF CENTRAL NERVOUS SYSTEM INVOLVEMENT BY INFECTIOUS AGENTS

Most infectious agents reach the central nervous system by hematogenous spread from extracranial foci or by retrograde propagation of infected thrombi within emissary veins. Possible sites for invasion of the CNS by blood-borne bacteria or viruses include vessels within the choroid plexuses, meninges, and brain parenchyma.[26,42,43] Tuberculous meningitis develops by seeding of the cerebrospinal fluid space from subependymal or submeningeal granulomas.[44] Intracranial epidural or subdural infection is usually of venous origin but may occasionally follow spread of organisms through bone. Spinal subdural and epidural infections more often follow bacteremia with or without accompanying osteomyelitis. Brain abscess may be of arterial or venous origin.

The central nervous system itself has no lymphatic system, but lymphatics are present within the spinal epidural space and form a route by which infections of the retropharyngeal, posterior mediastinal, or retroperitoneal spaces may produce spinal epidural abscess. Under experimental conditions, organisms can be shown to enter the subarachnoid space from lymphatics within peripheral nerves, but the spread of infection by this route has never been documented clinically.[26]

Because viruses have been shown experimentally to replicate in Schwann cells surrounding nerves or to ascend within nerves at a rate equal to reverse axoplasmic flow, infection of the nervous system by neurotropic spread of viruses has received a great deal of attention. In clinical situations, however, neurotropism has been shown to be important only for herpes simplex and zoster, which produce latent infection of sensory ganglia, and rabies, which may bind to or near acetylcholine receptors at the neuromuscular junction[45] and reaches the central nervous system by spread within axons. Rare cases of rabies have been reported after exposure to infected aerosols.[26,46] In these instances, the virus is believed to have penetrated free olfactory nerve endings within the nasal cavity, with rapid entry into the central nervous system[26] (see Table 1). Infection of the nervous system via cranial nerve I has also been postulated in herpes simplex encephalitis, because of the frequent involvement of olfactory brain, but has never been proven.

RESPONSE OF THE CENTRAL NERVOUS SYSTEM TO INFECTION

The central nervous system is unlike other organs in its unique cellular composition, its sequestration from the rest of the body by physiologic barriers, and its close confinement within rigid skeletal structures. These properties greatly influence the course of infection.[17] Widespread infection of the brain, involving all tissue elements, is characteristic of many viral encephalitides and of the diffuse cortical inflammation that accompanies bacterial meningitis. The functional specialization of different cell populations and of specific neuroanatomic regions, however, enables infections that involve specific cell types or anatomic areas to produce characteristic neurologic syndromes. Cellular specificity is seen in poliomyelitis, in which infection of motor neurons within spinal cord and medulla produces flaccid paralysis; in rabies, which is almost exclusively an infection of neurons; and in progressive multifocal leukoencephalopathy, in which destruction of oligodendrocytes results in multifocal, scattered areas of demyelination. Predilection for particular anatomic areas is seen in herpes simplex encephalitis, in which involvement of the temporal lobes may produce psychosis, impairment of recent memory, and uncinate seizures. Focal infection may also be seen in the localized encephalitis that precedes brain abscess, in brain abscess itself, or in granulomatous infections of tuberculous, fungal, or other origins. Certain viral agents, such as rabies virus, produce severe neurologic dysfunction in the absence of extensive necrosis or other pathologic changes. The ability of rabies virus to bind to the acetylcholine receptor has been discussed above. Work by Tsiang has shown that acetylcholine binding in brain is progressively impaired during experimental rabies.[47] These observations suggest that rabies virus may produce its clinical effects by interfering with neurotransmitter function. Central nervous system infection by human immune deficiency virus (HIV) in human acquired immunodeficiency syndrome (AIDS) has been associated with a progressive encephalopathy (AIDS-related dementia), a vacuolar myelopathy, and a subacute meningitis. HIV genomic material within brains has been identified predominantly in macrophages. It is not yet known whether neurologic injury by HIV is the result of viral replication per se or is due to virus-induced perturbations of neuronal metabolic activities or neurotransmitter function.[48,49]

Organisms producing acute infection, such as most bacteria, elicit a polymorphonuclear inflammatory response. Subacute or chronic infections such as those caused by *M. tuberculosis*, fungi, or viruses result in a predominantly lymphocytic infiltrate, although large numbers of polymorphonuclear cells may be present if tissue destruction is extensive. Subacute and chronic inflammatory infiltrates often contain plasma cells, and antibody production may occur at the site of infection. The inflammatory response within the brain or spinal cord differs from that in other organs in that it may be less intense and includes infiltration by microglial cells and proliferation of astrocytes. Although abscesses within the brain develop in much the same way that they do in other organs, encapsulation of brain abscesses occurs for the most part not by fibrosis but by the slower, less complete process of gliosis. When the brain has suffered previous ischemic injury, the inflammatory response may be minimal, and reactive gliosis may fail to occur.

Recovery from central nervous system infection involves antibody, cell-mediated immunity, and complement. Antibody is normally excluded from the central nervous system. The presence of antibody in brain or spinal fluid thus indicates diffusion of immunoglobulin molecules across an injured blood-brain barrier or local synthesis of antibody by immunocompetent cells that have gained entry into brain parenchyma.[50] Antibody produced within the central nervous system is oligoclonal, suggesting that the plasma cells responsible for local antibody synthesis are derived from a limited number of B cells.[26] Systemic humoral immunity plays a major protective role against bacterial infections of the central nervous system and may play a role in determining survival in bacterial meningitis.[51] Demonstration of a rise in antibody titers between acute and convalescent sera is an important retrospective means of identifying infections caused by viruses or other agents that are poorly recovered by culture techniques. Determination of CSF antibody titers to specific agents is of more limited value. Because the blood-CSF barrier is poorly permeable to immunoglobulins, the serum:CSF antibody ratio is normally above 200.[52] Injury to the blood-brain barrier can lower this ratio nonspecifically, and intrathecal synthesis of antibody directed against a particular infectious agent may selectively alter the ratio for that agent. Detection of CSF antibody or proof of intrathecal antibody synthesis has proved useful in the diagnosis of chronic or slow infections such as Lyme disease, subacute sclerosing panencephalitis, or progressive rubella encephalitis.[26,53] Investigation of CSF antibody titers has also been employed in epidemiologic studies of central nervous system involvement by HIV.[54] Penetration of antibody across the blood-brain barrier and intrathecal antibody synthesis develop over time, however, and are not reliable initial diagnostic tests in acute infections such as herpes simplex virus encephalitis.[55,56] Cell-mediated immunity comprises the major defense of the central nervous system against infections due to fungi or to intracellular parasites such as viruses, *M. tuberculosis*, *Listeria monocytogenes*, and *Toxoplasma gondii*. Where cell-mediated immunity is impaired, these organisms are particularly likely to involve the central nervous system and may cause fatal disease despite extremely high titers of specific antibody. Humoral and cell-mediated immune responses are closely related, and severe compromise of T-cell-mediated immune response, as in AIDS, may be accompanied by blunting of humoral immune response.[57] Complement has a number of functions, including the ability to lyse infectious agents or cells expressing viral or other foreign antigens on their surfaces. Complement may thus serve as an important mechanism of host defense against infection, but, in experimental circumstances at least, the action of complement on infected cells may be a major cause of neurologic injury.[58]

In certain infections due to virus or *Mycoplasma* or after immunization, the host may develop an immune response not only against the causative agent but also against the basic protein of peripheral or central myelin. Reaction against peripheral myelin produces segmental demyelination and at times axonal loss within nerve roots and peripheral nerves, causing an ascending motor paralysis (Landry-Guillain-Barre syndrome). Reaction to central myelin results in a monophasic illness characterized by perivascular inflammation and multifocal demyelination of brain, spinal cord, and optic nerve.[26] In severe cases, necrosis and/or hemorrhage of white matter may occur.

The Role of Edema and Brain Herniation in Central Nervous System Infections

Infection and inflammation produce not only local injury to nervous system parenchyma but also loss of capillary integrity with transudation of intravascular fluid into brain or cord.[60] The resultant edema is an almost invariable part of infection of the central nervous system, occurring not only around brain abscess (Fig. 6) but also in viral encephalitis, as a part of the diffuse cortical encephalitis that accompanies bacterial meningitis and as a complication of both infarction and hemorrhage. In meningitis, encephalitis, or ischemia, additional brain swelling may result from entry of extracellular water into injured cells. Interstitial edema of periventricular structures may develop in hydrocephalus. Although a small amount of edema may be asymptomatic, larger amounts frequently act as a space-occupying lesion.

Inflammation, hemorrhage, hydrocephalus, and edema may all produce displacement of brain or cord. In infections of the nervous system any or all of these conditions may be present simultaneously. Although the nervous system is able to deform greatly beneath gradual compression, both brain and spinal cord are poorly compliant beneath rapidly expanding lesions and, within the rigid confines of the skull or spinal column, have little room in which to be displaced before significant compression occurs. Displacement of one cerebral hemisphere will force brain tissue beneath the falx cerebri and over the tentorium cerebelli (Fig. 8).[61] Herniation beneath the falx is usually asymptomatic. Herniation of the temporal lobe over the tentorium, however, initially produces paresis of cranial nerve III and may cause corticospinal tract signs ipsilateral to the lesion as the contralateral cerebral peduncle is compressed against the tentorium (Fig. 8). Coma follows, and there is progressive loss of brain stem reflexes culminating in respiratory arrest as the medullary respiratory centers are affected. The characteristic neurologic syndromes that result at successively lower levels of brain stem function are described in detail in the monograph by Plum and Posner[61] and an understanding of these syndromes is crucial to the management of the patient with central nervous system infection. It should be kept in mind, however, that posterior fossa mass lesions such as a cerebellar abscess or hemorrhage may produce rapid compression of the medulla and

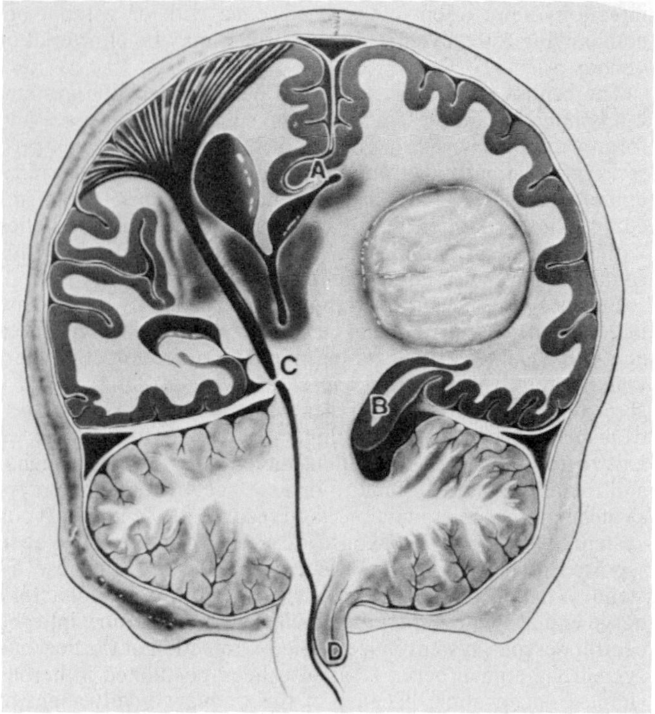

FIG. 8. Consequences of brain displacement by a mass lesion: herniation of cingulate gyrus beneath the falx cerebri (*A*); herniation of the uncus of the temporal lobe over the tentorium cerebelli (*B*), with compression of the contralateral corticospinal tract against the tentorium (*C*) and development of false localizing signs; herniation of the cerebellar tonsils through the foramen magnum (*D*).

pons without antecedent midbrain signs. Compressive lesions may also occur within the spinal column. Because of the narrow diameter of the spinal canal, even a small intrinsic or extrinsic lesion may rapidly progress to cord necrosis and effective cord transection.

The treatment of mass lesions within the skull or spinal canal requires prompt therapy in addition to antibiotics and is of particular urgency in patients with lesions of the posterior fossa or spinal canal because of the rapidity with which brain stem or cord compression may develop. Treatment of cerebral edema should be begun as soon as suspected (see Table 2).[60] Osmotic agents are effective in all types of edema but are most useful acutely since their continued administration may cause a rebound in intracranial pressure. Dexamethasone is effective in brain abscess[60] but is of less certain value in meningitis, encephalitis, or ischemia. The benefits of corticosteroids in edema due to infection must always be weighed against their possible

TABLE 2. Short-Term Therapy for Cerebral Edema[a]

Therapy	*Mechanism of Action*	*Dosage or Therapeutic End-Point*	*Remarks*
Hyperventilation	Decreases intracranial vascular volume	PCO_2 should be lowered to 25–30 torr	Produces almost immediate fall in intracranial pressure (ICP) but requires intubation and mechanical ventilation unless the patient is spontaneously hyperventilating.
Mannitol	Hyperosmolar effect	Give as a 20% solution IV 1–1.5 g/kg over 10 min and a total of 2.5–3 g/kg over 1–1.5 hours	Produces rapid fall in ICP. Rebound of ICP may occur due to diffusion of mannitol into brain tissue but may be minimized by fluid restriction or diuretic therapy with furosemide or ethacrynic acid. Patient should undergo urinary catheterization at initiation of therapy. Mannitol produces transient intravascular hypervolemia and may precipitate congestive heart failure. Protracted use of mannitol necessitates measurement of intake and output, serum electrolytes, and serum osmolality.
Corticosteroids	Mechanism uncertain	Dexamethasone, 10 mg IV followed by 4 mg IV at 6-hour intervals	Produces fall in intracranial pressure over several hours, without rebound. Most effective in edema associated with brain abscess. Efficacy in meningitis or ischemic infarction is less well established.

[a] Medical therapy of increased intracranial pressure is never a substitute for evacuation of loculated infection or relief of hydrocephalus. Intracranial pressure monitoring may be essential in assessing efficacy of treatment. Other less proven measures have been employed when the therapeutic measures listed above have been unsuccessful.[60]

deleterious effects on host immune response. At no time is medical treatment of cerebral edema a substitute for evacuation of a surgically approachable abscess, empyema, or hemorrhage, nor does it obviate the need for shunting in the presence of hydrocephalus. Appropriate neuroradiologic studies should be begun as soon as a mass lesion is suspected, and plans should be made for immediate surgery if indicated.

ACKNOWLEDGMENTS

Work on this chapter was supported in part by the Veterans Administration.

REFERENCES

1. Bargmann W, Oksche A, Fix JD, et al. Meninges, choroid plexuses, ependyma, and their reactions. In: Haymaker W, Adams RD, eds. Histology and Histopathology of the Nervous System. Springfield, IL: Charles C Thomas; 1982:560–714.
2. Schwartz MN, Dodge PR. Bacterial meningitis—a review of selected aspects. N Engl J Med. 1965;272:725.
3. Kaufman DM, Litman N, Miller MH. Sinusitis: induced empyema. Neurology. 1983;33:123.
4. Kaplan RJ. Neurological complications of infections of the head and neck. Otol Clin N Am. 1976;9:729.
5. Beckhuis GJ, Taylor M. Ear and sinus aspects of intracranial suppurative disease. In: Gurdjian ES, ed. Cranial and Intracranial Suppuration. Springfield, IL: Charles C Thomas; 1969:42–58.
6. Dale BAB, Mackenzie J. The complications of sphenoid sinusitis. J Laryngol Otol. 1983;97:661–70.
7. Tandon PN. Tuberculous meningitis. In: Vinken PJ, Bruyn GW, Klawans HL, eds. Handbook of Clinical Neurology. Part 1. Amsterdam: North Holland; 1978:195–262.
8. Lewis JL, Rabinovich S. The wide spectrum of cryptococcal infections. Am J Med. 1972;53:315.
9. Delaney P. Neurologic manifestations in sarcoidosis. Review of the literature with a report of 23 cases. Ann Intern Med. 1977;87:336.
10. Symonds C. Recurrent multiple cranial nerve palsies. J Neurol Neurosurg Psychiatr. 1959;21:95.
11. DeMyer W. Anatomy and clinical neurology of the spinal cord. In: Baker AB, Joynt RJ, eds. Clinical Neurology. v. 3. Philadelphia: Harper & Row; 1987:1–24.
12. Toole JF. Applied anatomy of the brain arteries. In: Toole JF, ed. Cerebrovascular Disorders. 3rd ed. New York: McGraw-Hill; 1984:1–18.
13. Dudley AW. Cerebrospinal blood vessels normal and diseases. In: Haymaker W, Adams RD, eds. Histology and Histopathology of the Nervous System. Springfield, IL: Charles C Thomas; 1982:714–97.
14. Stehbens WE. Pathology of the cerebral blood vessels. In: Anatomy of the Blood Vessels of the Brain and Spinal Cord. St Louis: CV Mosby; 1972:1–59.
15. Roach MR, Drake CG. Ruptured cerebral aneurysms caused by microorganisms. N Engl J Med. 1956;273:240.
16. Csaky TZ. Choroid plexus. In Lajtha A, ed. Handbook of Neurochemistry. v. 2. London: Plenum; 1969:49–69.
17. Slager UT. Infections and parainfectious inflammations. In: Basic Neuropathology. Baltimore: Williams & Wilkins; 1970:89–135.
18. Merwarth HR. The syndrome of the rolandic vein. Am J Surg. 1942;56:526.
19. Toole JF. Anatomy and diseases of the venous system. In: Cerebrovascular Disorders. 3rd ed. New York: McGraw-Hill; 1984:391–404.
20. Oldendorf WH. Permeability of the blood-brain barrier. In: Tower DB, ed. The Nervous System. v. 1. New York: Raven Press; 1975:279–89.
21. Moossy J. Vascular diseases of the spinal cord. In: Baker AB, Joynt RJ, eds. Clinical Neurology. v. 3. Philadelphia: Harper & Row; 1987:1–19.
22. Miller JQ, Price TR. The nervous system in Rocky Mountain spotted fever. Neurology. 1972;22:561.
23. Duffy J, Lidsky M, Sharp JT, et al. Polyarthritis, polyarteritis, and hepatitis B. Medicine. 1976;55:19.
24. Sergent JS, Lockshin MD, Christian CL, et al. Vasculitis with hepatitis B antigenemia. Medicine. 1976;55:1.
25. Reshef E, Greenberg SB, Jankovic J. Herpes zoster ophthalmicus followed by contralateral hemiparesis: report of two cases and review of the literature. J Neurol Neurosurg Psychiatr. 1985;48:122–7.
26. Johnson RT. Viral Infections of the Nervous System. New York: Raven Press; 1982.
27. Winkelman NW, Eckel JL. Productive endarteritis of the small cortical vessels in severe toxemias. Brain. 1927;50:608.
28. Winkelman NW, Eckle JL. The brain in bacterial endocarditis. Arch Neurol Psychiatr. 1930;23:1161.
29. Woollam DHM, Miller JW. Vascular tissues in the central nervous system. In: Minckler J, ed. Pathology of the Nervous System. v. 1. New York: McGraw-Hill; 1968:486–98.
30. Moskowit MA, Rosenbaum AE, Tyler HR. Angiographically monitored resolution of cerebral mycotic aneurysms. Neurology. 1974;24:1103.
31. Fishman RA. Cerebrospinal Fluid in Diseases of the Nervous System. Philadelphia: WB Saunders; 1980.
32. DeJong RN. Spinal puncture and the examination of the cerebrospinal fluid. In: The Neurological Examination. 4th ed. Hagerstown: Harper & Row; 1976:741.
33. Ellner JJ, Bennett JE. Chronic meningitis. Medicine. 1976;55:341.
34. Gonyea EF. Cisternal puncture and cryptococcal meningitis. Arch Neurol. 1973;28:200.
35. Berger MP, Paz. Diagnosis of cryptococcal meningitis. JAMA. 1976;236:2517.
36. Samson DS, Clark K. A current review of brain abscess. Am J Med. 1973;54:201.
37. Rieselback RE, DiChiro G, Freireich EJ, et al. Subarachnoid distribution of drugs after lumbar injection. N Engl J Med. 1962;267:1273.
38. Kaiser AB, McGee ZA. Aminoglycoside therapy of gram-negative bacillary meningitis. N Engl J Med. 1975;293:1215.
39. McCracken GH, Mize SG. A controlled study of intrathecal antibiotic therapy in gram-negative enteric meningitis of infancy. J Pediatr. 1976;89:66.
40. Salmon JH. Ventriculitis complicating meningitis. Am J Dis Child. 1972;124:35.
41. Duffy GP. Lumbar puncture in the presence of raised intracranial pressure. Br Med J. 1969;1:407.
42. Netsky MG, Shuangshoti S. The choroid plexus in health and disease. In: Inflammatory Disorders of the Chroid Plexus and Ependyma. Charlottesville: University of Virginia Press; 1975:249–64.
43. Moxon ER, Smith AL, Averill DR, et al. *Haemophilus influenzae* meningitis in infant rats after intranasal inoculation. J Infect Dis. 1974;129:154.
44. Rich AR, McCordock HA. The pathogenesis of tuberculous meningitis. Bull Johns Hopkins Hosp. 1933;52:5.
45. Rupprecht CE, Dietzschold B. Perspectives on rabies virus pathogenesis. Lab Invest. 1987;57:603.
46. Winkler WG, Fashinell TR, Leffingwell L, et al. Airborne rabies transmission in a laboratory worker. JAMA. 1973;266:1219.
47. Tsiang H. Neuronal function impairment in rabies-infected rat brain. J Gen Virol. 1982;61:277.
48. McArthur JC. Neurologic manifestations of AIDS. Medicine. 1987;66:407.
49. Pert CB, Smith CC, Ruff MR, et al. AIDS and its dementia as a neuropeptide disorder: role of VIP receptor blockade by human immunodeficiency virus envelope. Ann Neurol. 1987;32(Suppl):S71.
50. Greenlee JE, Johnson RT. Virology and neurological disease. In: Swash M, Kennard C, eds. The Scientific Basis of Clinical Neurology. London: Churchill Livingstone; 1985:619.
51. Oppenheimer SI, O'Toole RD, Petersdorf RG. Bacterial meningitis. In: Goldensohn ES, Appel SH, eds. Scientific Approaches to Clinical Neurology. v. 1. Philadelphia: Lea & Febiger; 1977:434–51.
52. Tourtellotte W. On cerebrospinal fluid immunoglobulin-G (IgG) quotients in multiple sclerosis and other diseases. J Neurol Sci. 1970;10:279.
53. Finkel MF. Lyme disease and its neurological complications. Arch Neurol. 1988;45:99–104.
54. McArthur JC, Cohen BA, Farzedegan, et al. Cerebrospinal fluid abnormalities in homosexual men with and without neuropsychiatric findings. Ann Neurol. 1988;32(Suppl):S34.
55. Nahmias AJ, Whitley RJ, Visintine AN, et al. Herpes simplex encephalitis: laboratory evaluations and their diagnostic significance. J Infect Dis. 1982;145:829.
56. Koskiniemi M, Vaheri A, Taskinen E. Cerebrospinal fluid alterations in herpes simplex virus encephalitis. Rev Infect Dis. 1984;6:608.
57. Bowen DL, Lane HC, Fauci AS. Immunopathogenesis of the acquired immunodeficiency syndrome. Ann Intern Med. 1985;103:704.
58. Hirsch RL, Griffin DE, Winkelstein JA. The effect of complement depletion on the course of Sindbis virus infection in mice. J Immunol. 1978;121:1276.
59. Truax RC, Carpenter MB. Human Neuroanatomy. 6th ed. Baltimore: Williams & Wilkins; 1969.
60. Ropper AH, Kennedy SK, Zervas NT. Neurological and Neurosurgical Intensive Care. Baltimore: University Park Press; 1982.
61. Plum F, Posner JB. The Diagnosis of Stupor and Coma. 3rd ed. Philadelphia: FA Davis; 1980.
62. Adams RD, Victor M. Principles of Neurology. 2nd ed. New York: McGraw-Hill; 1981:532.

66. ACUTE MENINGITIS

ZELL A. McGEE
J. RICHARD BARINGER

Acute meningitis is a medical emergency that requires the utmost in diagnostic and therapeutic skills. The death rate, about 30 percent, has changed little in the last 25 years. To lower the death rate further will require: (*1*) earlier recognition of meningitis, (*2*) more rapid determination of the most likely etiologic agent, (*3*) more rapid initiation of appropriate antimicrobial therapy (within 30 minutes in acutely ill patients), (*4*) earlier recognition of those conditions in which cerebrospinal fluid (CSF) bacterial cultures are negative (aseptic meningitis syndrome) but in which antimicrobial therapy is required, and (*5*) earlier recognition and treatment of the consequences (e.g., acidosis, disseminated intravascular coagulation) of the septicemia that frequently accompanies bacterial meningitis. This chapter, in addition to providing information about specific types of meningitis, focuses on how the physician can most easily recognize meningitis and can best approach the patient with known or suspected meningitis to minimize the risk of neurologic damage or death.

EPIDEMIOLOGY

In bacterial meningitis caused by *Streptococcus pneumoniae, Neisseria meningitidis*, and *Haemophilus influenzae*, the immediate source of the invading pathogen is usually the bacterial flora that colonizes the nasopharynx. Although there is great variability in the duration of colonization before invasion, the greatest risk of meningitis seems to be in patients who have recently been colonized. Approximately 25 percent of healthy people acquire new strains of pneumococci each year[1] and 6 percent acquire new strains of meningococci.[2] *Haemophilus influenzae* colonization, which occurs in less than 3 percent of normal infants and seldom in adults,[3] occurs much more frequently in case contacts (in about 50 percent of children <5 years old and in about 20 percent of adults and children 5 years or older.[4] Pneumococci and meningococci usually require several weeks to spread among a family unit following the initial nasopharyngeal acquisition by one family member.[1,2] Colonization and secondary cases of meningococcal meningitis and *H. influenzae* meningitis usually follow close contact (sleeping together, eating together, kissing, and so on).[5] However, acquisition of one of these meningeal pathogens usually results in the asymptomatic carrier state. Although asymptomatic carriers can spread meningeal pathogens, the likelihood of spread of a particular pathogen may vary with the presence or absence of disease, the type of disease, and probably other factors. For instance, colonization rates of *H. influenzae* in children younger than 5 years old are 20 percent if the index case has epiglottitis versus 55 percent if the index case has meningitis.[4] The epidemiology of other types of bacterial meningitis as well as viral, fungal, and amebic meningitis are discussed below in sections dealing with these specific agents.

PATHOPHYSIOLOGY

The pathogenesis of most cases of meningitis almost certainly involves at least six steps. These steps include (*1*) attachment to epithelial cells of nasopharyngeal and oropharyngeal mucosa, (*2*) transgression of the mucosal barrier, (*3*) survival in the bloodstream (avoiding phagocytic cells and bacteriolytic activity), (*4*) entry into the CSF, (*5*) survival in the CSF, and (*6*) production of disease in the meninges and brain.

It seems likely that in meningitis at least some of the damage to the meninges and brain is effected by various cytokines, which are biologic mediators that can cause severe tissue damage and death.[6] Although Waage et al.[7] did not show that cytokines per se produce brain damage in meningitis, they did demonstrate in patients with meningococcal meningitis, septicemia, or both that the serum concentration of tumor necrosis factor, a potent cytokine elicited by lipopolysaccharide (endotoxin)[6] correlates directly with the likelihood of death.[7]

The bacteria that most frequently cause meningitis are capable of doing so because they have a variety of virulence mechanisms, each one of which may play a unique role in one or more of the successive steps of the pathogenic process. Our knowledge of these mechanisms is incomplete but is best worked out for *N. meningitidis*.

The bacteria that cause meningitis usually attach to and colonize host mucosal surfaces in the nasopharynx. Both *H. influenzae* and *N. meningitidis* have pili that appear to mediate attachment.[8,9] Host cell-surface receptors for meningococcal pili appear to be concentrated on certain cells in the oro- and nasopharynx.[9–11] The distribution of these receptors appears to determine the sites of meningococcal colonization.

Meningococci are ingested by certain epithelial cells of the nasopharyngeal mucosa.[10] Whether meningococci and other meningeal pathogens are passed through such cells to the subepithelial tissues where they have access to the bloodstream is not yet known. However, such a mechanism results in transgression of mucosal barriers by other human pathogens.[11]

Once in the bloodstream, the most frequently successful meningeal pathogens appear to avoid phagocytosis by polymorphonuclear leukocytes and cells of the reticuloendothelial system by virtue of having antiphagocytic capsules.[12,13] The available pneumococcal and meningococcal vaccines probably intervene in this pathogenesis by eliciting antibodies that neutralize the antiphagocytic capsules and enhance phagocytosis. Gram-negative meningeal pathogens may avoid being killed by antibody and complement by having special lipopolysaccharides on their surfaces or by having outer membrane proteins that deter bacteriolysis or combine with blocking IgA antibodies.[14,15]

How bacteria cross from the bloodstream into the CSF is not known. Many bacteria, encapsulated and unencapsulated, from the oropharynx and other sites cause bacteremia but not meningitis.[16] The possible role of polysaccharides is suggested by the observation that only certain capsular types of pneumococci, meningococci, *H. influenzae*, *Escherichia coli*, and group B streptococci have a particular predilection for causing meningitis.[12,13]

Bacteria probably enter the CSF space from the blood via the choroid plexuses of the lateral ventricles and then spread to the extracerebral CSF space along normal paths of CSF flow.[17–20] They also may enter the CSF space directly through defects of congenital or traumatic origin or from parameningeal suppurative foci. The CSF is generally devoid of sufficient humoral factors or phagocytic cells to repel successfully the initial invasion of pathogens.[20,21] The ingress of antibody, complement, and phagocytic cells that occurs during the course of meningitis may ablate infections with some bacterial strains but may be ineffective in halting the lethal progression of infection with other strains.

Meningeal pathogens are generally limited to the subarachnoid space.[22,23] Thus, the disordered function of the nervous system in meningitis is likely to result from occlusion of blood vessels traversing the subarachnoid space and from the intense inflammatory process with attendant necrosis of nerve roots, cerebral edema, cerebral ischemia and possible hydrocephalus.

If there are defects in host defenses, bacteria that do not ordinarily have the virulence factors necessary to complete all steps of the pathogenic process may do so and cause meningitis, or bacteria that can complete all steps may do so more easily and more often. Lack of humoral immunity, the presence of complement defects, loss of integrity of the CSF space, and other, less well-defined factors, such as the stress of boot camp and viral infections, all predispose to meningitis.[24–26]

In viral meningitis and meningoencephalitis, the etiologic agents reach the nervous system by one or more of three major routes: neural pathways, the olfactory tract, and the blood stream. Most viruses causing meningitis use the hematogenous route after undergoing multiplication of the site of entry or in regional lymph nodes draining the entry site. The precise mechanisms by which most viruses enter the CSF and produce neurologic damage are still under investigation.[27]

The mechanisms of pathogenicity in fungal infections are less well studied but seem to be similar to those in bacterial meningitis.

SPECIFIC CAUSES OF MENINGITIS AND THEIR TREATMENT

The specific causes of meningitis (Table 1) can be divided into two major diagnostic groups, bacterial meningitis and the aseptic meningitis syndrome. Bacterial meningitis, which may have an acute presentation (symptoms of less than 24 hours' duration) or a subacute presentation (symptoms of 1–7 days' duration), can generally be diagnosed quickly by examining a Gram stain of the sediment of the CSF. Those patients with negative Gram stains and negative bacterial cultures may be considered to have the aseptic meningitis syndrome. However, the absence of bacteria on Gram strain and negative bacterial cultures do not exclude an etiologic role for bacteria or other treatable agents.

Bacterial Meningitis

Pneumococcal Meningitis. In adults *Streptococcus pneumoniae* is the most frequent bacterial species causing meningitis. Pneumococcal meningitis occurs in the very young, the old, and those of any age with a predisposing factor. Pneumonia, sinusitis, endocarditis, old or recent head trauma, CSF leak, splenectomy, sickle hemoglobinopathy, bone marrow transplantation, and alcoholism predispose to or accompany meningitis caused by pneumococci more often than meningitis caused by meningococci or *H. influenzae*.[26,28–30] Also, patients with pneumococcal meningitis are somewhat more likely to have alterations of consciousness or focal neurologic defects than are patients with meningococcal or *H. influenzae* meningitis. The most critical element in therapy appears to be early administration of adequate amounts of the optimal antimicrobial (i.e., crystalline penicillin G, 70,000 units/kg iv q8h for neonates and 50,000 units/kg iv q4th in adults). In penicillin-allergic patients, chloramphenicol (25 mg/kg iv q6h in adults) is the best alternative to penicillin. The mortality is 30–60 percent. Some patients die despite apparently optimal antimicrobial therapy with sterilization of the CSF and other body fluids. In those who survive, residual defects of hearing, convulsions, hemiparesis, or other more selective nerve deficits may persist. Although penicillin is the drug of choice, it may not provide adequate therapy for meningitis caused by the approximately 2 percent of pneumococcal strains that are relatively resistant to penicillin (MIC $\geq$ 0.1 μg/ml). Therefore the Centers for Disease Control now recommend that all clinically significant pneumococcal isolates be screened for penicillin susceptibility with oxacillin disks.[31]

TABLE 1. Conditions Presenting as Acute Meningitis

Infectious diseases
Bacteria and spirochetes
Streptococcus pneumoniae
Neisseria meningitidis
Haemophilus influenzae
Streptococcus (particularly group B)
Listeria monocytogenes
Treponema pallidum
Leptospires
Staphylococcus aureus
Pseudomonas aeruginosa
Enteric gram-negative bacilli
Staphylococcus epidermidis
Propionibacterium acnes
Viruses
Echovirus
Coxsackievirus types A and B
Enterovirus
Mumps virus
Herpes simplex virus types 1 and 2
Epstein-Barr virus
Human Immunodeficiency virus
Herpes zoster virus
Cytomegalovirus
California encephalitis virus
St. Louis encephalitis virus
Colorado tick fever virus
Lymphocytic choriomeningitis virus
Poliovirus
Parasites
Naegleria
Angiostrongylus
Strongyloides stercoralis (hyperinfection syndrome)
Infections resembling acute meningitis
Rickettsiosis and ehrlichiosis
Brain abscess (see Chapter 70)
Epidural or subdural abscess (see Chapter 71 and 72)
Tuberculosis, cryptococcosis, and other forms of chronic meningitis (see Chapter 67)
Viral and other causes of encephalitis (see Chapter 68)
Noninfectious causes of acute meningitis syndrome
Mollaret's meningitis
Drug induced
Epidermoid cyst of the meninges

Meningococcal Meningitis. In contrast to pneumococcal meningitis, meningococcal meningitis is primarily a disease of children and young adults; less than 10 percent of the cases occur in patients over age 45.[32] A majority of cases occur in the winter or spring, a time when viral meningitis is relatively infrequent. Four meningococcal serogroups are responsible for a majority of the disease: serogroups A and C are most often associated with epidemics of meningococcal meningitis; serogroup B is the primary cause of sporadic cases; and serogroup Y causes sporadic cases of pneumonia, sometimes associated with meningitis.[33] Meningococcal meningitis may be rapidly progressive. Approximately 50 percent of those hospitalized within the first 24 hours of their illness subsequently die, some within a few hours of the onset of symptoms.[30,34] Thus, early suspicion, performance of a lumbar tap, and prompt therapy are critical. The presence of petechiae in a patient with meningitis most likely indicates the presence of meningococcemia, although petechiae are sometimes seen in meningitis due to echovirus type 9, in pneumococcal meningitis in asplenic patients, or with concomitant endocarditis caused by pneumococci or staphylococci.[32,35] About half the patients with meningococcal meningitis have petechiae, purpuric lesions, or both.[30,34] Subclinical or clinical disseminated intravascular coagulation, which frequently accompanies meningococcemia, may progress to hemorrhagic infarction of the adrenal glands, renal cortical necrosis, widespread pulmonary microvascular thrombosis, shock, and death. Therefore early antimicrobial therapy (crystalline penicillin G, 50,000 units/kg iv q4h) must be accompanied by efforts to control acidosis, tissue hypoxia, shock, adrenal insufficiency, and disseminated intravascular coagulation if these complications occur (Ch. 189). An approach to prevention of meningococcal meningitis in contacts of cases is discussed in the last section of this chapter.

Haemophilus Influenzae Meningitis. *Haemophilus influenzae* type b is the most common bacterial cause of meningitis between the neonatal period and age 6 years.[34] The occurrence of *H. influenzae* meningitis in older patients should prompt efforts to exclude the presence of otitis media, other parameningeal foci of infection, CSF leak, or an immunodeficiency disease, since these often accompany *H. influenzae* meningitis in older patients. Pharyngitis and otitis media are associated with *H. influenzae* meningitis in one-half and two-thirds of the cases, respectively.[30] In contrast to meningococcal meningitis, petechiae rarely occur in *H. influenzae* meningitis. A substantial proportion of *H. influenzae* isolates are resistant to ampicillin. Most of these strains are infected with a plasmid (Ch. 201) that mediates production of β-lactamase, an enzyme that destroys penicillins and some cephalosporins. Because approximately 20 percent of the cases of *H. influenzae* meningitis are caused by these ampicillin-resistant strains, ampicillin plus chloramphenicol is currently recommended by some authorities as therapy for meningitis known or likely to be caused by *H. influenzae*.

The chloramphenicol is stopped if the organism is ampicillin susceptible. The third-generation cephalosporins are very active against β-lactamase producing and nonproducing strains and are considered by many to be the drugs of choice for serious ampicillin-resistant *H. influenzae* infections (see Chapter 201).[36,37] The continuation or recurrence of decreased mentation or fever after antimicrobial therapy may indicate the presence of subdural effusions, a relatively frequent complication in *H. influenzae* meningitis. The death rate is approximately 3–8 percent.[34] Intelligence testing has revealed mental deficits in 30–50 percent of the children who have had *H. influenzae* meningitis, and this infection is thought to be the leading cause of acquired mental retardation in the United States.[3] The evidence that *H. influenzae* meningitis occurs in clusters and that chemoprophylaxis may stop contact spread is reviewed in the section on prevention of meningitis.

Gram-Negative Bacillary Meningitis. Whereas pneumococci, meningococci, and *H. influenzae* combined have continued to cause approximately 40 percent of the cases of bacterial meningitis in adults over the last 20 years, the proportion of cases of meningitis caused by gram-negative bacilli (exluding neonatal meningitis and that caused by *H. influenzae*) has increased significantly, and the proportion caused by staphylococci and streptococci has decreased.[38,39] This trend is not surprising since gram-negative bacillary meningitis is usually hospital acquired, and the proportion of hospital-acquired infections caused by gram-negative bacilli remains substantial.

Approximately 30 percent of the cases of gram-negative bacillary meningitis occur in conjunction with head trauma (especially in association with CSF rhinorrhea), about 50 percent of cases occur after neurosurgical procedures, and 20 percent are "medical" (e.g., in patients with accompanying gram-negative sepsis, ruptured brain abscess, impaired host defenses, or strongyloidiasis).[39,40] The most likely gram-negative bacilli causing meningitis at any time after the neonatal period are *Klebsiella* (approximately 40 percent of the cases), *E. coli* (15–30 percent), and *Pseudomonas* (10–20 percent).[39,41] However, the flora causing this type of meningitis may vary somewhat from hospital to hospital.

The presence of meningitis is less likely to be suspected in patients with gram-negative bacillary meningitis because most of them have had head trauma or a neurosurgical procedure and already have altered consciousness, signs of meningeal irritation, and an elevated CSF protein or WBC count. Thus, the presence of fever, the readiness of the physician to do a spinal tap, and a low CSF glucose concentration may be the most useful keys to the diagnosis. Although it is important to start therapy early, initial Gram stains may be negative in up to 50 percent of the patients.[41] In these patients the CSF lactic acid determination and the limulus lysate assay[42,43] may be useful.

The third-generation cephalosporins have provided a significant advance in the therapy of gram-negative bacillary meningitis. Although older cephalosporins were usually not effective in treating bacterial meningitis of any etiology owing to inadequate CSF concentrations, intravenous therapy with the third-generation cephalosporins usually results in CSF concentrations many times the MBC for the most frequently infecting bacteria. For example, CSF concentrations of cefotaxime (at 12 g/day iv) for therapy of *E. coli* meningitis usually exceeds the MBC for the infecting organism by 50- to 60-fold.[37,44] This high ratio of CSF drug concentration to the MBC is similar to that seen during high-dose penicillin therapy of pneumococcal meningitis. Use of third-generation cephalosporins is discussed further in a separate section below.

The optimal antimicrobial, route of administration, and duration of therapy of gram-negative bacillary meningitis have never been defined in a systematic trial. If the patient is not severely ill, therapy for meningitis can be begun with a third-generation cephalosporin in high doses (e.g., cefotaxime, 50 mg/kg iv q6h or ceftazidime 2 g q8h) plus a systemic aminoglycoside (e.g., amikacin 5 mg/kg iv q8h). With *Pseudomonas aeruginosa* meningitis, ceftazidime plus an aminoglycoside might be selected (see below). Use of an aminoglycoside is largely to aid in treatment of extracerebral manifestations. If the organism is initially resistant or becomes resistant to the third-generation cephalosporin during therapy, the physician should consider intraventricular administration of an aminoglycoside given with systemic aminoglycoside plus systemic ticarcillin or piperacillin (75 mg/kg iv q6h).[45–49] If there is reason to belive that the infection may be limited to the extracerebral CSF space (e.g., meningitis associated with spinal surgery), a trial of intralumbar aminoglycoside—0.03 mg of tobramycin or gentamicin per ml of estimated CSF volume or 0.1 mg of amikacin per ml of estimated CSF volume every 24 hours—may be warranted. The total CSF volume in individuals without hydrocephalus has been estimated to be 40–60 mol in infants and 60–100 ml in young children; for older children and adults of average build, estimate 1 ml of CSF per pound body weight.[20,49] If there is no reason to suspect that the infection is limited to the extracerebral CSF space, most data suggest that intraventricular aminoglycoside offers a better chance of cure than lumbar intrathecal drug.

Intravenous trimethoprim-sulfamethoxazole has been used occasionally in gram-negative bacillary meningitis.[50] Its use in *Listeria* meningitis will be discussed later.

If the patient is critically ill—has an altered sensorium or is in a coma—and there is no reason to suspect that the gram-negative bacilli present are unlikely to respond to third-generation cephalosporins, these are the drugs of choice. If, however, epidemiologic, cultural, or susceptibility data suggest that the organism is unlikely to respond to third-generation cephalosporins an Ommaya or Rickham reservoir should be put in place immediately, and intraventricular and systemic therapy should be begun in the operating room with gentamicin, tobramycin, or amikacin along with systemic ticarcillin or piperacillin in the doses suggested above. As soon after emplacement of the reservoir as possible, computed axial tomography or simple injection of a bolus of air through the catheter with subsequent skull x-ray films should be performed to ensure that the catheter is actually in the cerebral ventricles. The reservoir and catheter can be used immediately after their emplacement. After the first dose of aminoglycoside into the ventricle, the concentration should be monitored in the lumbar CSF to ensure adequate distribution of the drug throughout the CSF space. In addition, ventricular levels of aminoglycoside should be measured just before the next intraventricular dose every 2 or 3 days, and the dose altered to maintain this "trough" level in an approximate range of 2–10 μg/ml.

Regardless of the drug chosen for treatment of the meningitis per se, the patient should also be treated intravenously with antimicrobials appropriate for gram-negative bacteremia that is present in 70 percent or more of the patients with gram-negative meningitis.[51] Therapy for the meningitis should be maintained for 10 days after cultures of the CSF become sterile. Spinal fluid cultures may be positive for 10 days or more on a regimen that will eventually result in a cure. During this time colony counts of organisms in the CSF, which are performed every 2 to 3 days, should show a progressive decrease in the number of organisms if therapy is effective.

Meningeal irritation with radiculitis occasionally occurs with intralumbar and intraventricular administration of aminoglycosides, but ototoxicity has not been a problem. In seven patients observed by one of the authors, serial audiograms have been normal despite CSF concentrations of aminoglycosides as high as 200 μg/ml.

Third-Generation Cephalosporins. Some of the third-generation cephalosporins, particularly cefotaxime and ceftazidime, have become the drugs of choice for meningitis caused by most aerobic gram-negative bacilli. Response rates of 80–90 percent have been reported for meningitis caused by *E. coli*, *Klebsiella pneumoniae*, and *Serratia* sp.[52,53] Somewhat lower responses have been reported for *Enterobacter* and *Salmonella*. In every case, the patient's isolate must be tested for susceptibility to the third-generation caphalosporin to be used. Drug resistance arising during therapy has also been encountered.[54] With *P. aeruginosa*, activity of third-generation cephalosporins is quite variable. Cefotaxime, ceftizoxime, moxalactam, and ceftriaxone are not indicated in meningitis caused by *Ps. aeruginosa*. Some of the cephalosporins that have antipseudomonal activity in vitro, such as cefoperazone, are not sufficiently active to be used in meningitis. With ceftazidime, the rate of response has been reported to be as high as 80 percent in *Ps. aeruginosa* meningitis.[55] However, drug resistance arising during therapy is a problem of sufficient magnitude that we believe that the preferred therapy is intraventricular and systemic aminoglycoside in conjunction with systemic ticarcillin or piperacillin.[45–49] Also notable is that a substantial portion of patients with gram-negative bacillary meningitis have recently had neurosurgical procedures. The bleeding tendency induced by moxalactam, cefoperaxone, and other cephalosporins with a methyltetrazolethiol group raises concern about the use of these drugs in such patients. Activity of third-generation cephalosporins against gram-positive cocci is variable. Moxalactam has too little activity against gram-positive cocci and should not be used for meningitis caused by gram-positive cocci, including pneumococcus or streptococcus. With *S. aureus*, none of the third-generation cephalosporins would be the drug of choice for meningitis. Patients with staphylococcal meningitis who are allergic to penicillin and therefore cannot be given nafcillin, oxacillin, or methicillin can be treated with vancomycin.

Against the usual pathogens of acute bacterial meningitis of childhood, *H. influenzae*, *N. meningitidis* and *S. pneumoniae*, cefotaxime and ceftazidime have given rates of cure that are comparable but not superior to those of other regimens.[56,57] However, experience is still small compared with that with older agents, and the ability to prevent the long-term sequelae such as deafness or mental retardation will take time to assess. Penicillin G remains the drug of choice for meningitis caused by *N. meningitidis* and susceptible strains of *S. pneumoniae*. Activity of the third-generation cephalosporins against *Enterococcus* and *Listeria* is poor. None of these drugs should be used as sole agents in initial therapy of meningitis when one of these pathogens is suspect, such as in neonatal meningitis.

Use of Corticosteroids in Acute Bacterial Meningitis. A recent placebo-controlled study of 200 infants and older children with bacterial meningitis evaluated the efficacy of dexamethasone, 0.15 mg/kg every 6 hours for the first 4 days of therapy.[58] The antibacterial antibiotic was changed from cefuroxime to ceftriaxone during the study. Aside from the expected effects on fever and spinal fluid analysis (protein, glucose, and lactate), the only statistically significant benefit of dexamethasone was on deafness. Of the children not receiving dexamethasone, 15.5 percent lost auditory acuity, while only 3.3 percent of dexamethasone recipients experienced hearing loss. Follow-up of these children for assessment of long-term neurologic sequelae is needed to see whether other differences may appear. Additionally, too few patients with meningitis caused by organisms other than *H. influenzae* were included to determine how these results apply more generally to bacterial meningitis of childhood. At present, no firm recommendation for dexamethasone can be made for children with meningitis due to organisms other than *H. influenzae* or for adults.

Group B Streptococcal Meningitis. Group B streptococci seldom cause meningitis in adults except in conjunction with endocarditis. The features of neonatal meningitis caused by group B streptococci are discussed later in this chapter.

Listeria Meningitis. *Listeria monocytogenes* can cause meningitis in normal adults[59] but most often causes meningitis in neonates, in the aged, or in immunosuppressed patients.[59,60] In some centers *Listeria* is the primary cause of meningitis in renal transplant patients.[60] In neonates the source of *Listeria* is the genital tract or subclinical infection of the mother, which is transferred to the baby during birth; the source in adults is probably other adults, food,[61] or the patient's own flora. Gram stains of the CSF are often negative, but the cultures are positive. The organisms, which are gram-positive rods, may be mistaken for diphtheroids and considered skin contaminants unless the physician is alert to this possibility and asks the laboratory to make a special effort to test for *Listeria*. β-hemolysis (clear) on blood agar and motility of such organisms strongly suggests *Listeria*. The therapy of choice is ampicillin (100 mg/kg iv q8h in neonates, 200 mg/kg per day divided into doses every 4 hours for adults). An aminoglycoside is usually added. However, a number of therapeutic successes with trimethoprim-sulfamethoxazole[62] suggest that this drug combination may be as effective or more effective than ampicillin plus an aminoglycoside. Therapy should be continued for 3 weeks or longer as indicated clinically.

Other Causes of Bacterial Meningitis. *Staphylococcus aureus* may cause meningitis, especially in conjunction with brain abscesses, paranasal sinusitis, endocarditis, or severe staphylococcal septicemia. The drug of choice is nafcillin or oxacillin, 2 g iv q4h. Infection with *S. aureus* or *S. epidermidis* in conjunction with CSF shunts presents special problems dealt with in a subsequent section of this chapter. A wide variety of other bacteria occasionally cause meningitis.[30,34]

Partially Treated Bacterial Meningitis. At the time the diagnosis of bacterial meningitis is considered and a lumbar puncture is obtained, 25–50 percent of the patients already will have received antimicrobial therapy.[63,64] The Gram stains and cultures of CSF from such patients are more often negative than those of untreated patients,[65] so an erroneous diagnosis of viral meningitis may be made. However, the CSF white cell and differential counts and the protein and glucose levels are generally not significantly altered by prior therapy; several days are required to decrease the number of polymorphonuclear leukocytes and to reverse the high-protein and low-glucose levels of bacterial meningitis. Counterimmunoelectrophoresis (CIE) and latex agglutination tests are routinely used in many hospitals and may detect antigens of pneumococci, meningococci, *H. influenzae* and group B streptococci in spinal fluid when Gram stain and culture have been rendered negative by prior therapy.[43,66] These tests are not sensitive enough to exclude a bacterial etiology when a negative result is obtained. Other tests such as the limulus lysate assay or lactic acid concentration may also point to a bacterial etiology in this situation.[42,43] If a search for a bacterial etiology is negative, the physician should not necessarily conclude that the meningitis is "partially treated" and initiate antibacterial therapy. Work-up of other causes of the aseptic meningitis syndrome, such as brain abscess, tuberculous meningitis, and cryptococcal meningitis (Table 1), should be initiated even if a decision to begin antibacterial therapy is made. When no treatment is given, a repeat lumbar puncture in 8–12 hours may be useful.

Other Causes of the Syndrome

Parameningeal Suppurative Foci. Suppurative foci adjacent to the meninges may cause signs of meningeal irritation and CSF abnormalities indistinguishable from those observed in the aseptic meningitis syndrome when it is caused by viruses. If not misinterpreted, the finding of the aseptic meningitis syndrome can be a valuable clue to the presence of a focus of life-threatening infection that may require antimicrobials, surgery, or both. All patients with meningitis should have sinus and mastoid x-ray studies; this is of particular importance if there is a history of sinusitis, mastoiditis, of middle ear infection. The finding of abnormalities on these x-ray studies, the finding of alterations of mentation, focal nerve deficits (excluding ophthalmoplegias), or the presence of diseases that predispose to brain abscess such as endocarditis or lung abscess should prompt the performance of a computed axial tomography (CAT) scan or magnetic resonance imaging to detect a brain abscess (see Chapter 70). Especially in the setting of a recent superficial staphylococcal infection, the finding of localized back pain and peripheral nerve abnormalities should suggest spinal epidural abscess and prompt consideration of a spinal CAT scan or magnetic resonance imaging.[67,68] Foci of dermal sinus infection (Fig. 1), cranial osteomyelitis, mastoiditis, and middle ear or paranasal sinus infection may also be detectable by a thorough physical examination. Other suppurative foci, such as subdural empyema or suppurative intracranial phlebitis, require special diagnostic procedures (see Chapters 71, 72).

Tuberculous Meningitis. Although tuberculous meningitis is more often subacute or chronic (see Chapter 229), it may have a rapid onset and progression, especially in immunosuppressed hosts. It usually occurs in the course of miliary tuberculosis or with rupture of a subependymal tubercle. Thus, x-ray and other signs of tuberculosis may or may not be present. In this acute form, the WBCs in the CSF may be primarily polymorphonuclear leukocytes. Other features of the laboratory diagnosis are discussed later in the chapter.

Amebic Meningitis. Free-living amebas of the genus *Naegleria*, which are widely distributed in water, soil, air, and decomposing organic matter, occasionally cause acute, purulent meningoencephalitis in humans. Most patients give a history of swimming in a warm, freshwater lake or indoor swimming pool and of severe, persistent frontal headache.[69,70] The diagnosis can be made by observing motility of the amebas (often mistaken for macrophages) on wet mount or hanging drop suspensions of CSF. Since centrifugation or refrigeration destroys the amebas, the tests should be performed on fresh, uncentrifuged CSF. The organisms can be cultured on a lawn of *E. coli* on agar or observed histologically in cytologic studies of CSF.[69] Although progression to death is the rule, high doses of amphotericin B administered systemically and intraventricularly[71] have been associated with recovery.[72]

Syphilitic Meningitis. Acute meningitis is an infrequent manifestation of syphilis (Chapter 213). It can mimic completely other causes of the aseptic meningitis syndrome; but papilledema may occur in conjunction with hydrocephalus. Cranial or

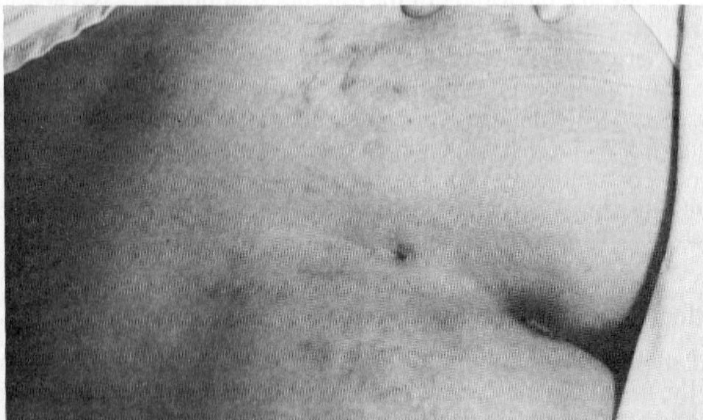

FIG. 1. Midline dermal sinus in the coccygeal area of a patient with recurrent gram-negative bacillary meningitis.

peripheral nerve signs, mental deterioration, and convulsions occur more frequently in syphilitic than in viral meningitis.[73,74] Meningitis may occur months to years after primary infection, but a majority of cases occur within the first year, probably in conjunction with the dissemination of spirochetes that occurs in the secondary stage of syphilis. Central nervous system invasion is now known to be more common than appreciated previously. In one study, 30 percent of 40 patients with untreated primary or secondary syphilis had *Treponema pallidum* isolated from their CSF.[75] In 25 percent of the patients with acute syphilitic meningitis, the meningitis is the first manifestation of infection with *T. pallidum*.[73] Thus, serum and CSF serologic testing are most important in evaluating the possibility of syphilis in a patient with the aseptic meningitis syndrome. Intramuscular penicillin regimens for neurosyphilis and syphilitic meningitis may be inadequate; optimal therapy is aqueous penicillin G, 3.5 million units iv q4h for 2 weeks.

Viral Meningitis. Patients with viral meningitis have rapid onset of headache, low-grade fever, stiff neck, and photophobia. Despite their obvious discomfort, they are usually alert and oriented. Most are children or young adults. Patients with encephalitis have early onset of lethargy, obtundation, confusion, seizures, and focal neurologic signs.

Distinction between viral and bacterial meningitis is best made by lumbar puncture. In viral meningitis, the CSF usually contains 50 to 500 leukocytes/mm^3, predominantly lymphocytes. Early in the course of the disease, the CSF may have a predominance of neutrophils, but rarely exceeding 90 percent, as is seen in bacterial meningitis. Repeat lumbar puncture in 12 to 24 hours can be helpful in borderline cases by showing a shift to lymphocyte predominance in viral meningitis. CSF glucose is above 40 mg/dl in viral meningitis, with the exception of some patients with mumps, herpes simplex, or lymphocytic choriomeningitis virus. Protein is elevated but rarely beyond 200 mg/dl. Cultures of CSF and blood for bacteria should be obtained in every case. Early in the course of enteroviral meningitis, the virus may be recovered from the CSF, but yields are low. If a viral diagnosis is to be pursued, throat washings and stool should be tested as well as CSF. Both acute and convalescent serum should be obtained for serology. These studies may be useful in outbreaks but not facilitate the management of individual cases.

The etiology of viral meningitis varies with the season of the year, the age of the patient, and the geographic location. In the United States, about 70 percent of cases are due to enteroviruses, especially echovirus types 4, 6, 9, 11, 16, and 30 and coxsackievirus types A7, A9, and B2-5. Most of these cases occur in children in the late summer and early fall, but a few cases may continue to occur well into the winter months. Arbovirus meningitis also occurs in the summer months, contributing to the frequency of viral meningitis during the months of July, August, and September.

Mumps virus, in contrast, tends to be more frequent in the late winter and early spring. The herpesvirus and human immunodeficiency virus infections[76] occur sporadically year round. Poliovirus and lymphocytic choriomeningitis virus cause remarkably few cases of viral meningitis in the United States but remain important causes worldwide. Viral meningitis caused by adenovirus and cytomegalovirus may be seen in immunocompromised patients.

Meningitis of subacute or chronic onset may be considered acute if the early symptoms are not elicited or understood by the clinician. In this way, tuberculous, cryptococcal, and carcinomatous meningitis appear in the differential diagnosis of acute meningitis. Acid-fast smear of centrifuged CSF should be done when tuberculosis is a possibility, in addition to culturing several milliliters of CSF for mycobacteria. Rapid diagnosis of cryptococcal meningitis can be afforded by testing CSF and serum for cryptococcal antigen and by India ink smear of centrifuged CSF sediment. Confirmation of the diagnosis requires recovery of *Cryptococcus neoformans* from CSF. The best test for carcinomatous meningitis is CSF cytology.

Imaging by CAT or magnetic resonace imaging (MRI) can be helpful in detecting parameningeal infection, brain abscess, intracerebral neoplasm, epidural or subdural abscess, and herpes simplex virus encephalitis. Patients who are severely ill with fever, peripheral leukocytosis, polymorphonuclear predominance in the CSF, altered consciousness, papilledema, or focal neurologic signs deserve aggressive investigation and use of these imaging techniques. Antibacterial antibiotic therapy may be required in such patients, even in the absence of a firm diagnosis. However, many patients with the typical features of viral meningitis are not very ill and can be observed in the hospital. Improvement often begins in 24 to 72 hours.

Leptospiral Meningitis. Leptospires have been implicated in about 5 percent of cases of the aseptic meningitis syndrome.[77] About half the patients with leptospirosis have meningeal signs, and over 80 percent have abnormal CSF findings.[78] In leptospirosis an acute septicemic phase, characterized by the rapid onset of fever, chills, nausea and vomiting, myalgia, conjunctival suffusion, headache, and meningismus, either blends with or is followed in a few days by a phase in which rash, renal and hepatic damage, and meningitis may dominate the clinical picture.[78,79] In many cases the disease is mild, and the patient has a vague history of flulike prodromal illness followed by the septic meningitis syndome. The meningitis is occasionally accompanied by varying degrees of encephalitis or spinal involvement.[78] Thus, the illness may be indistinguishable from viral meningitis, including the early predominance of polymorphonuclear leukocytes in the CSF and CSF glucose concentrations seldom less than 40 mg/100 ml. There are two major clues to the specific etiology: (*1*) the history of contact with water frequented by domestic animals or rodents and (*2*) the occurrence of meningitis in conjunction with the clinical illness like that described for leptospirosis. The diagnosis is confirmed by documenting a fourfold or greater rise in agglutination titers. Although the disease is usually self-limited and does not require therapy, some authors suggest using 10 million units of penicillin per day in especially severe cases.

Neoplastic Meningitis. The presence in the CSF of tumor cells from a variety of neoplasms can produce the aseptic meningitis syndrome. Among patients with the syndrome, the usually modest elevation of cells and protein, at times in association with marked hypoglycorrhachia, should suggest the diagnosis, which can be confirmed by cytologic examination of the CSF.[34]

Cyst-Related Meningitis. Cells and other debris released from dermoid or epidermoid cysts into the subarachnoid space can cause meningitis, which tends to be recurrent.[34,80]

Chemical Meningitis. The onset of the aseptic meningitis syndrome in temporal proximity to spinal anesthesia or to diagnostic radiologic studies that involve the subarachnoid space (e.g., myelograms or pneumoencephalograms) should suggest not only bacterial meningitis but also chemical meningitis. The chemicals implicated include procaine and various soaps or disinfections in which syrings or needles are treated. Chemical meningitis may produce marked hypoglycorrhachia—glucose level less than 1 mg/dl.[81]

Drug-Induced Meningitis. A variety of pharmaceutical products that are administered orally or intravenously are capable of causing meningitis. To compound the problem, the settings in which the offending products are given are frequently ones in which the host is immunocompromised so that a microbial etiology of the meningitis is likely to be suspected and antibiotic or antiviral therapy given unnecessarily.

Drug-induced meningitis has clinical and laboratory features that suggest an acute aspetic meningitis syndrome, in that no bacteria or fungi are detected by culture, by microscopic examination of the centrifuged CSF sediment, or by antigen detection tests. Nevertheless, the patients often appear acutely ill, with a stiff neck, temperature over 103°F (39.4°C), and CSF findings that suggest a bacterial etiology because the CSF leukocyte counts frequently exceed 1000/mm^3, of which over 80 percent are polymorphonuclear neutrophils. The protein concentration in the CSF is usually over 150 mg/dl, but the glucose concentration is usually within the normal range.

Co-trimoxazole (trimethoprim-sulfamethoxazole [TMP-SMX]) can cause aseptic meningitis.[82,83] It is not clear which of the two components is the major offender; the syndrome has been reproduced by readministration of the drugs, but only in combination.[82,83] Drug-induced meningitis can occur during TMP-SMX treatment of *Pneumocystis carinii* pneumonia in AIDS patients and simulate either AIDS meningitis or an opportunistic infection of the central nervous system. Such an event might necessitate switching the therapy of the pneumocystis infection from TMP-SMX to pentamidine.

A recently marketed murine monoclonal antibody preparation, Orthoclone OKT3, which is often given for acute kidney allograft rejection, has also been associated with an aseptic meningitis syndrome that usually comes on within 72 hours of administration and resolves with cessation of administration of the product.[84]

Another drug that immunocompromises a host, azathioprine, can also cause acute aseptic meningitis. In one of the reported cases the patient had papilledema in addition to headache, meningismus, and CSF pleocytosis.[85] Because papilledema rarely occurs in acute meningitis, the findings in this patient might have suggested chronic meningitis or a space-occupying lesion (e.g., a tumor or brain abscess). Whereas in a patient with papilledema the need to exclude space occupying lesions is not obviated by getting a history of their taking azathioprine, the possibility that azathioprine is causing the meningitis must be considered and administration of the drug discontinued if no alternative cause of the papilledema and meningitis is found.

The nonsteroidal anti-inflammatory agents ibuprofen,[86,87] tolmetin,[88] naproxen,[89] and sulindac have also been reported to cause an aseptic meningitis syndrome; ibuprofen-associated meningitis has occurred primarily in patients with systemic lupus erythematosus or mixed connective tissue disease. Although a number of the patients have developed meningitis on first exposure to the drugs, the circumstances of the reported cases favor a hypersensitivity etiology of the meningitis.

A careful drug history and chart review in a patient with the aseptic meningitis syndrome may identify recent exposure to one of the drugs discussed above and, in conjunction with laboratory tests which fail to indicate the presence of a microbial agent in the CSF, may help avoid unnecessary antibiotic or antiviral therapy.

Other Nonantimicrobial-Requiring Causes of Meningitis. Mollaret's meningitis is characterized by recurrent febrile episodes in which signs and symptoms of meningitis begin abruptly, reach maximal intensity within 12 hours, and diminish over 1–4 days without therapy. The CSF usually shows a polymorphonuclear pleocytosis; mononuclear cells and large ''epithelial cells'' may also be seen. The patients are free of symptoms between episodies.[90] A variety of other conditions that may produce apparently noninfectious, often recurrent meningitis include Behçet syndrome, Vogt-Koyanagi-Harada syndrome, sarcoidosis, and systemic lupus erythematosus.[34]

STRATEGY FOR DIAGNOSIS AND THERAPY

Recognition of Meningitis

Some patients seek medical attention early in the course of their infection and have only subtle signs of meningitis; these are the patients who have the best chance of recovery if the diagnosis is made promptly and therapy is instituted early. Carpenter and Petersdorf[30] comment on the recognition of meningitis as follows:

> Meningeal infection should be considered in every patient with a history of infection of the upper respiratory tract interrupted by one of the "meningeal" symptoms—vomiting, headache, lethargy, confusion or stiff neck. When first seen, some of the patients present a rather unimpressive picture with no more than low-grade fever, mild headache or occasional vomiting. Nevertheless, the possibility of meningeal infection must be carefully considered.

In neonates, infants, and the aged, the signs and symptoms of meningitis may be especially subtle. There may be no more to suggest meningitis than the presence of fever plus irritability, lassitude, confusion, poor feeding, unstable or low temperature, or the occurrence of seizures. Stiff neck or full fontanelles may be relatively late signs of meningitis in infants. Whereas clinical judgment is certainly called for, the adage "If you think of doing a spinal tap, do one" still holds. The diagnostic value of a lumbar puncture far outweights the small risk of harm.[91]

Acute Versus Subacute Presentation of Meningitis

Most patients with meningitis have some clear-cut signs and symptoms of meningitis when they are first seen by a physician. There is often fever, heahache, vomiting, photophobia, and mental dysfunction ranging from lethargy to coma. Seizures and cranial nerve deficits are not uncommon, but papilledema oc-

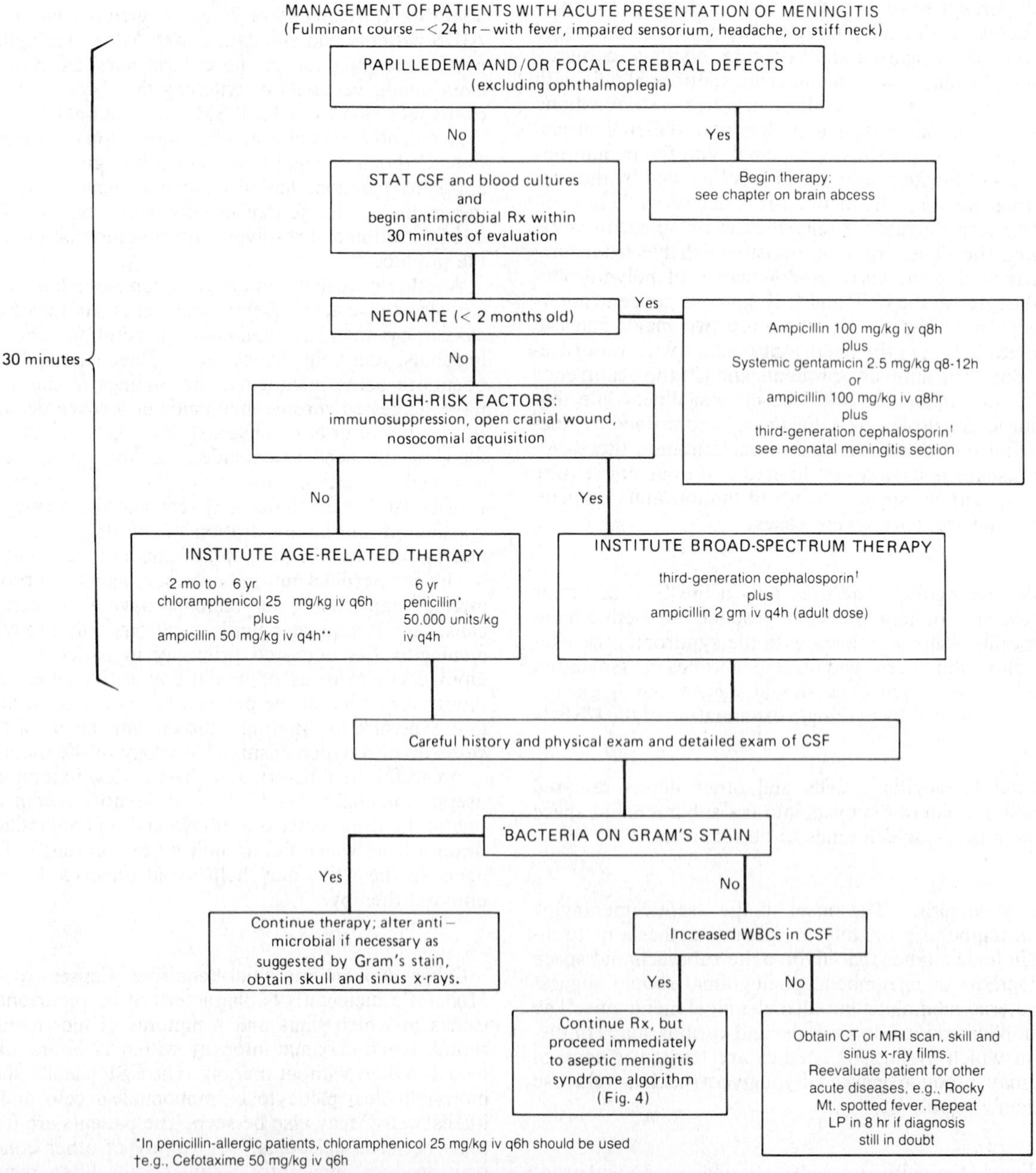

*In penicillin-allergic patients, chloramphenicol 25 mg/kg iv q6h should be used
†e.g., Cefotaxime 50 mg/kg iv q6h
**Third generation cephalosporin is an alternative to chloramphenicol-ampicillin.

FIG. 2. Algorithm for management of patients with acute presentation of meningitis.

curs so infrequently that its presence should prompt a search for a mass lesion such as a brain abscess.[34,91] In patients with such clear-cut signs of meningitis, the examining physician should immediately make the determination of whether the patient has an *acute* or a *subacute* presentation of meningitis. The signs and symptoms may be similar in the two groups. However, in the *acute presentation* (Fig. 2), signs and symptoms have been present less than 24 hours and are rapidly progressive; the most likely etiology is pyogenic bacteria (Table 1); and the death rate is approximately 50 percent. An acute presentation of meningitis will be seen in approximately 10 percent of the patients with infectious meningitis. In the *subacute presentation* (Fig. 3), signs and symptoms have usually been present for 1–7 days before evaluation; there are a number of possible etiologic agents or conditions (e.g., viruses, pyogenic bacteria, leptospires, tubercle bacilli, fungi, parameningeal foci); and the death rate, even in the presence of pyogenic bacterial meningitis, is less than half that of the acute presentation. Almost all patients with viral meningitis and 75 percent of the patients with bacterial meningitis exhibit a subacute presentation of meningitis.[30,34,92]

The first consideration in a patient with the acute presentation of meningitis is therapy, not specific diagnosis, as outlined in Figure 2. The brief physical examination before lumbar puncture should include a check for papilledema or focal neurologic defects (excluding ophthalmoplegia); these findings are a contraindication to a lumbar puncture until a CAT or MRI scan has excluded a mass lesion because of the increased risk of uncal herniation. In this situation, cultures of blood and other appropriate sites should be obtained and therapy initiated immediately thereafter, before getting the CAT scan. If papilledema is not present, blood cultures and CSF are obtained and intravenous antimicrobial therapy is begun with 30 minutes of encountering the patient. Examination of a Gram stain of the CSF before giving therapy would be a waste of potentially valuable therapeutic time. Only the most elementary data are necessary to make an adequate choice of an antimicrobial regimen. (Fig. 21). The need for prompt antimicrobial therapy is emphasized by the occurrence of death within hours of the onset of symptoms in some patients. Especially in acutely ill patients, the goal of therapy is to treat before the pathologic processes of the meningitis are irrevocably committed to lethal progression.

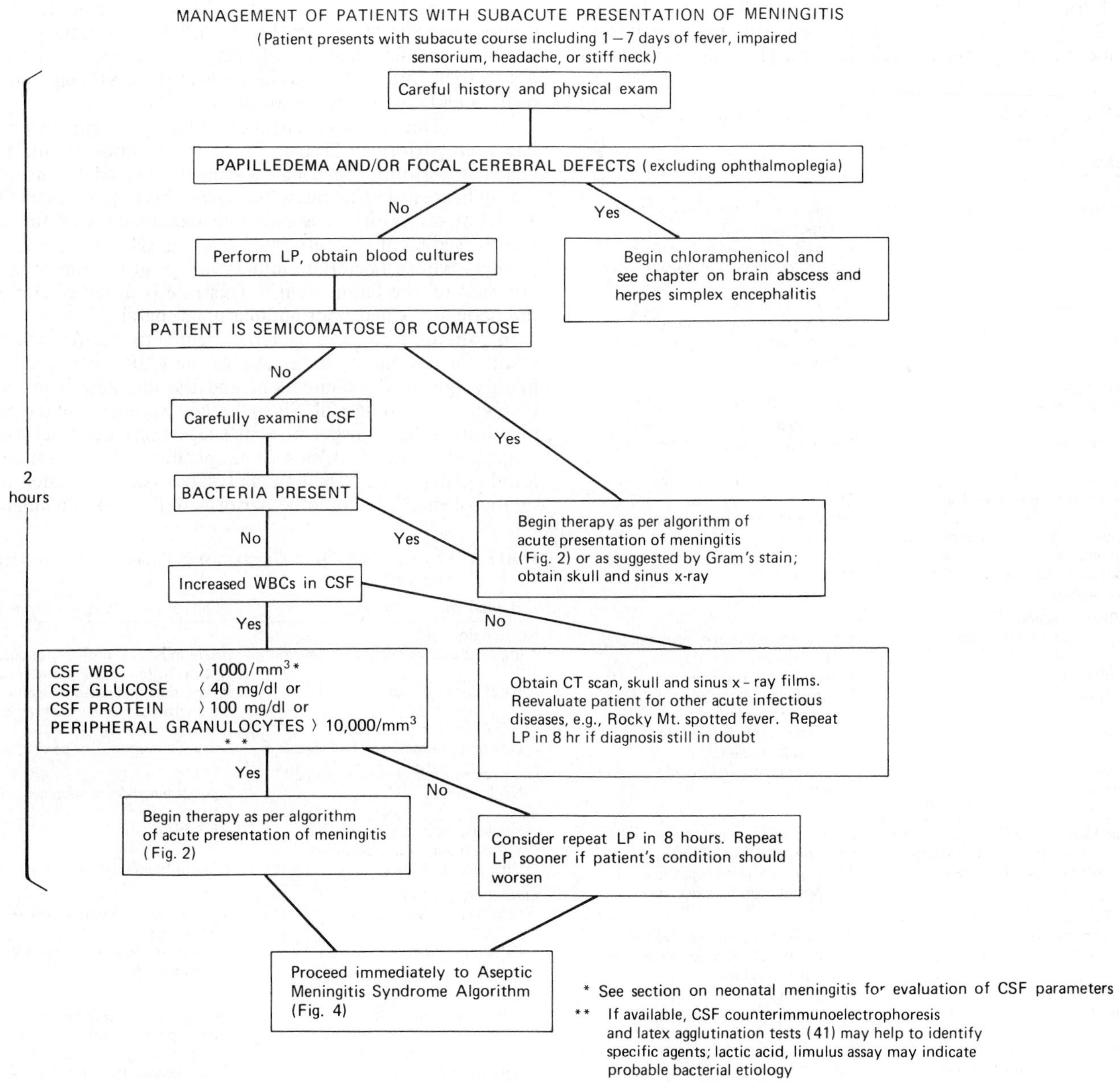

FIG. 3. Algorithm for management of patients with subacute presentation of meningitis.

In a patient with the subacute presentation of meningitis early emphasis is on diagnosis (Fig. 3).

Diagnosis. Once therapy has been initiated in patients with an acute presentation of meningitis (Fig. 2), or once it has been determined that a patient has a subacute presentation of meningitis (Fig. 3), attention should be focused on determining the most likely organism. A decision on the need for a change of therapy in the former group or on the design of optimal therapy in the latter group should be made within 2 hours of first seeing the patient. This generally provides ample time for performing history and physical examinations, for obtaining cultures of blood and CSF, for a complete examination of the CSF (cell count, differential count, protein and glucose level determinations, and special stains), and, if necessary, for tests to detect antigens of specific meningeal pathogens.[43]

As noted in Table 1, the etiologic agent may be bacterial, viral, fungal, protozoan, parasitic, neoplastic, or chemical. Despite this variety of potential causes, the physician who uses an organized approach to the problem can rapidly and correctly predict the etiology agent in a majority of patients. Thus, there are elements of the history (e.g., the season of the year, previous skull fracture) and the physical examination (e.g., a search for midline dermal sinuses [Fig. 1]) that should be systematically considered because they may point to or away from specific microorganisms (Table 2). The physical examination may not only provide clues to the etiology but also may indicate the need for surgery to provide adequate primary therapy or to prevent relapse (Table 3). In addition, the physical examination provides important baseline data to serve as a reference for any changes in the patient's condition. *There is no substitute for the same physician performing a complete initial neurologic examination and carefully reexamining the patient periodically for changes in the neurologic status.*

To decide the most likely etiologic agent, the CSF cell count, differential count, and protein and glucose level determinations may be of limited value. If the cell count is over 1000/mm^3, the protein concentration is over 150 mg/dl, and the glucose concentration less than 30 mg/dl, a bacterial etiology is likely and tuberculous or viral meningitis is quite unlikely (an exception is mumps or lymphocytic choriomengitis).[92] However, for each of these parameters there are 30–40 percent of the cases of bacterial meningitis that overlap the range of values for tuberculous, fungal, and viral meningitis. Although the differential count is more likely to show a predominance of polymorphonuclear leukocytes (PMNs) in bacterial meningitis and a predominance of lymphocytes in nonbacterial meningitis, there is overlap of these groups (e.g., one-third of the cases of tuberculous and viral meningitis have a predominance of PMNs, and about 10 percent of the cases of bacterial meningitis have greater than 80 percent lymphocytes).[92] Therefore the physician is seldom justified in excluding bacterial meningitis and deciding not to treat for it solely on the basis of the CSF cell count and protein and glucose concentrations.

After the history has been taken and the physical examination has been performed (Tables 2 and 3), attention should be focused on performing in a logical sequence those laboratory tests that indicate a specific microbial agent or group of agents (Table 4). Of first priority is a thorough examination of the Gram stained sediment of centrifuged CSF. In 80–90 percent of the patients whose bacterial cultures are positive, the organisms are seen on the Gram stain.[92] This rate is about 60 percent if the patient has had prior antimicrobial therapy.[34,65]

In patients who have bacterial meningitis but for whom the results of the initial Gram stain of the CSF are negative, the history, physical examination, and the characteristics of the CSF can be most helpful. Since therapy cannot await the results of culture, other nonspecific tests suggesting a bacterial etiology (e.g., CSF lactic acid), as well as specific tests for certain bacterial agents (e.g., CIE, limulus lysate assay, and latex agglutination tests,[43,66] should be performed if they are available.

TABLE 2. Historical and Other Data Suggesting Specific Etiologic Agents

Historical Data	*Microorganisms*
Age	
Neonates	*E. coli*, group B streptococci, *Listeria*, herpes simplex 2
Infants <2 months	Group B streptococci, *Listeria, E. coli*
Children <10 years	Viruses, *H. influenzae*, pneumococci, meningococci
Young adults	Viruses, meningococci
Adults	Pneumococci, meningococci
Elderly	Pneumococci, gram-negative bacilli, *Listeria*
Epidemiology	
Summer and fall	Coxsackievirus or echovirus, leptospires
Hospital acquired	Gram-negative bacilli, staphylococci, *Candida*
Sibling with meningitis	Meningococci, *H. influenzae*
Swimming in freshwater lake	Amebas
Handling hamsters or mice	Lymphocytic choriomeningitis
Contact with water frequented by rodents or domestic animals	Leptospires
Exposure to tuberculosis	*M. tuberculosis*
Prior meningitis	Pneumococci
Associated infection	
Upper respiratory infection	Viruses, *H. influenzae*, pneumococci, meningococci
Pneumonia	Pneumococci, meningococci
Sinusitis	Pneumococci, *H. influenzae*, anaerobic bacteria
Otitis	Pneumococci, *H. influenzae*, anaerobic bacteria
Cellulitis	Streptococci, staphylococci
Brain abscess	Anaerobes
Trauma	
Close skull fracture	Pneumococci, gram-negative bacilli
Open skull fracture or craniotomy	Gram-negative bacilli, staphylococci
CSF otorrhea and rhinorrhea	Pneumococci, gram-negative bacilli, staphylococci, *H. influenzae*
Underlying Condition	
Diabetes mellitus	Pneumococci, gram-negative bacilli, staphylococci, *Cryptococcus*, agents of mucormycosis
Alcoholism	Pneumococci
Leukemia, lymphoma	Pneumococci, gram-negative bacilli, *Cryptococcus, M. tuberculosis*
Steroid therapy	*Cryptococcus, M. tuberculosis*
Acquired immunodeficiency syndrome	HIV, *Cryptococcus*

TABLE 3. Physical Findings of Importance in Patients With Suspected Meningitis

Abnormal Physical Findings	*Clinical and Etiologic Interpretation*
Neurologic	
Impaired higher integrative function	Severe infection, probably pyogenic bacteria; rule out viral encephalitis
Focal cerebral signs	Severe, uncomplicated pyogenic meningitis; rule out brain abscess, herpes encephalitis
Late onset of focal cerebral signs	Delayed thrombosis of cortical veins
Head, eyes, ears, neck, and throat	
Neck stiffness	Suggests infection of subarachnoid space
Sinusitis, otitis, CSF otorrhea or rhinorrhea, skull fracture	See Table 2
Early papilledema	Rule out brain abscess
Cardiac–respiratory	
Pulmonary rales	Pneumococci, meningococci, *H. influenzae*
Pathologic heart murmur	Bacterial endocarditis—pneumococci, *S. aureus*
Skin	
Petechiae and/or rashes	Meningococci, echovrius type 9, leptospires, *S. aureus, Haemophilus aegyptius*
Midline dermal sinuses	Gram-negative bacilli, staphylococci
Herpes progenitalis or labialis	Herpes simplex 2

The designation "aseptic meningitis syndrome" is helpful because it circumscribes a number of specific causes of meningitis that should be pursued by the examining physician. It is critical to note that even if the routine bacterial cultures are, or are likely to be, negative, *many of the causes of the aseptic meningitis syndrome require antimicrobial therapy, surgical intervention, or both.* Although the initiation of specific therapy in such patients may be delayed for a few hours pending appropriate diagnostic procedures, complete failure to administer such therapy may result in death or severe morbidity. Thus, the "aseptic meningitis syndrome" cannot be equated solely with aseptic meningitis of viral origin. It is useful to direct the work-up of the aseptic meningitis syndrome to two groups of diagnostic possibilities: (*1*) antimicrobial-requiring causes and (*2*) nonantimicrobial-requiring causes, in that order of priority. A systematic examination of these possible causes of meningitis should aid the physician in reaching an optimal therapeutic decision as rapidly as possible (Fig. 4).

The physician may decide to administer antimicrobial therapy for partially treated meningitis, but this decision should be ac-

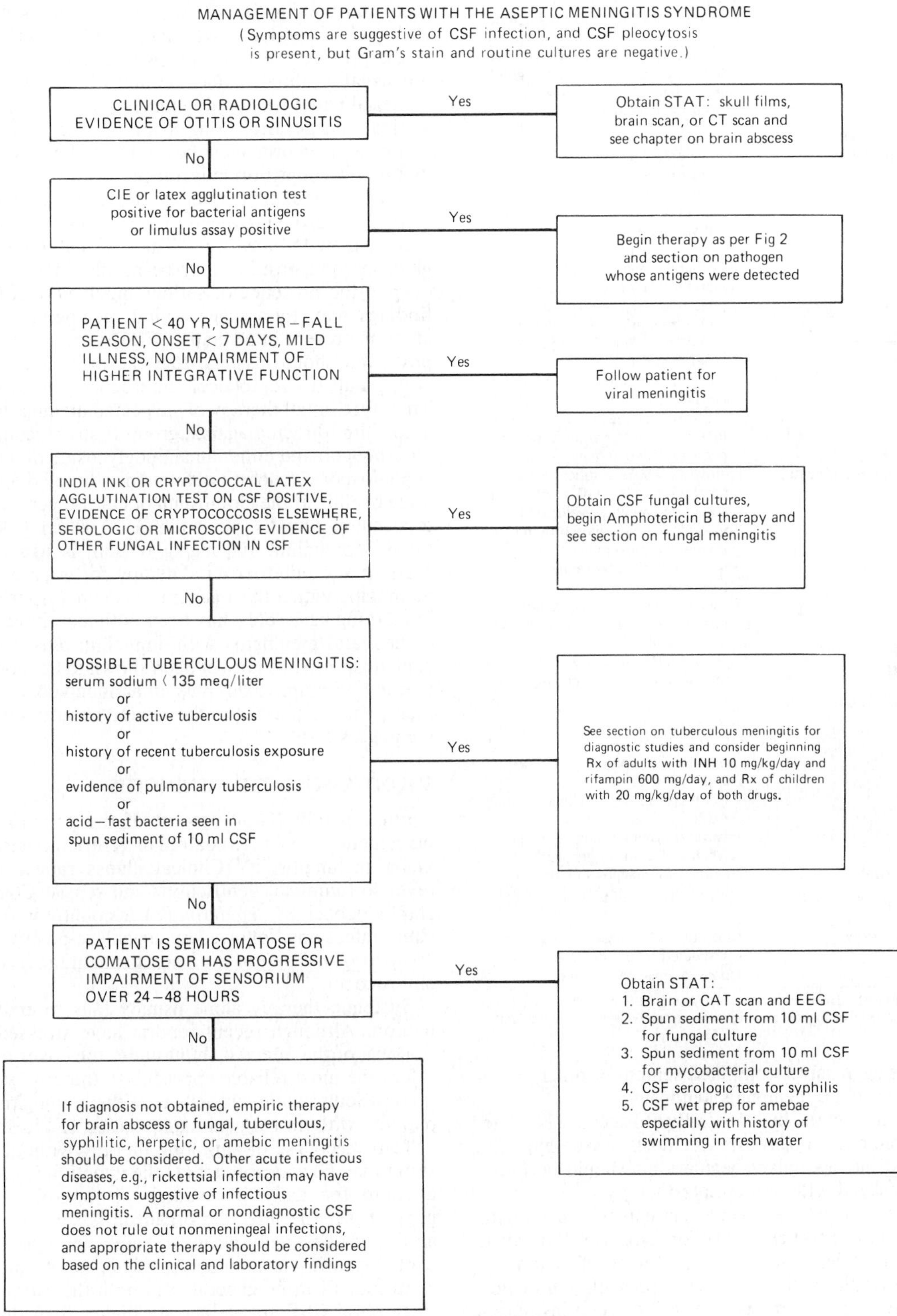

FIG. 4. Algorithm for management of patients with the aseptic meningitis syndrome.

TABLE 4. Laboratory Features in Patients with Suspected Infectious Meningitis

Laboratory Tests	Interpretation
Routine CSF evaluation	
Gram stain of centrifuged sediment	Usually positive in bacterial meningitis; more often negative in partially treated bacterial meningitis; always negative in nonbacterial meningitis; should be performed even with no increase in CSF white cells
Culture (include chocolate agar plates)	As above
White blood cell count	Greater than 1200[a] WBC/mm^3 suggests bacterial meningitis
Percent neutrophils	Less than 50%[a] suggests nonbacterial meningitis—but significant overlap
Glucose	Less than 30 mg/dl suggests bacterial, fungal, or tuberculous meningitis[a]
Protein	Greater than 150[a] mg/dl suggests bacterial meningitis
Special CSF evaluations (indicated when Gram stain is negative)	
Observations of supernatant	Orange color suggests subarachnoid hemorrhage
Counterimmunoelectrophoresis (CIE)	Specific for antigens of pneumococci, meningococci, or *H. influenzae*; test not very sensitive, false-negative results frequent
Lactic acid	>35 mg/dl suggests bacterial infection
Latex agglutination	Generally specific for antigens of pneumococci, meningococci, *H. influenzae*, group B streptococci and cryptococci; more sensitive and rapid than CIE
Limulus lysate assay	Positive indicates infection with gram-negative bacteria
Chloride	<110 mEq/liter suggests tuberculous infection if bacterial infection has been excluded
Acid-fast examination of sediment	Positive in >80% of tuberculous meningitis when >10 ml of CSF is spun and carefully evaluated
India ink	Cryptococci are diagnosed by this test; if ameboid movement is seen, *Naegleria* infection should be suspected
Tumor cytology	Tumor cells indicate CNS tumor—does not exclude infectious cause for meningitis
Wet mount	Ameboid movement of what look like monocytes may be amebas
Evaluation of peripheral blood	
Granulocyte count	>10,000 granulocytes/mm^3 suggest bacterial infection
Glucose	A baseline is helpful for comparison with CSF glucose
Serum sodium	<135 mEq/liter suggests inappropriate ADH
Culture	May yield agent causing meningitis when CSF cultures are sterile
Acute and convalescent sera	Important for diagnosis of viral and leptospiral meningitis
Other	
Sputum and bone marrow	Tuberculosis or fungal etiology often suspected by positive sputum or bone marrow examination

[a] Do not assume the converse of CSF parameters (For example, a WBC of <1200 does not imply viral infection since bacterial meningitis is also frequently associated with <1200 WBCs).

companied by an aggressive, continued search for other potential causes of the aseptic meningitis syndrome.

In any case of meningitis, but especially those caused by bacteria, the systemic effects of sepsis—acidosis, tissue hypoxia, and disseminated intravascular coagulation—should be monitored for and managed with appropriate therapy.

For those physicians who encounter patients with meningitis but who refer them to another facility (or for those who advise such physicians by telephone), the best course of action, regardless of whether the patient has acute presentation or not, is to follow those steps outline in Figure 2 through institution of empirical therapy. After intravenous therapy has been begun, the patient, accompanied by the physician's notes (history, physical findings, precise therapy), blood culture bottles, and at least one tube of CSF, should be sent by ambulance to the facility where definitive care can be given. Ideally CSF bacterial cultures, Gram stain, cell count, and protein and glucose level determinations should be performed at the referring facility after the patient has left, and the results of the tests phoned ahead. If this is not possible, the blood culture bottles and all tubes of CSF can be sent with the patient.

NEONATAL MENINGITIS

Neonatal meningitis differs from meningitis in older children and adults in at least two fundamental ways: (*1*) as described in the previous section, the signs and symptoms of meningitis are usually muted or lacking and (*2*) a different spectrum of bacterial pathogens predominates, the origin of these being the vaginal and perineal flora of the mother. The CSF laboratory values in newborns must be interpreted with caution. The CSF white cell count normally ranges from 0 to 30 with polymorphonuclear leukocytes accounting for over 50 percent of the cells. CSF protein concentration normally may be elevated to greater than 150 mg/dl.[13,20] The CSF cell count and protein or glucose concentration may be normal or only slightly altered despite the presence of serious meningitis. Although the CSF findings may thus suggest viral meningitis, when meningitis alone is present in neonates, viruses are seldom the cause; the physician should assume that the most likely pathogen is *E. coli*, group B streptococci, enterococci, or *L. monocytogenes*. Therefore initial therapy of suspected meningitis should include ampicillin (directed against group B streptococci, *Listeria*, and enterococci) and either an aminoglycoside or a third-generation cephalosporin (such as cefotaxime, directed against gram-negative bacilli). If the Gram stain or culture verifies group B streptococcal meningitis, penicillin G, 70,000 units/kg iv q8h, is optimal. Ampicillin, 100 mg/kg iv q8h, is usually adequate for *Listeria* and enterococci. Therapy for gram-negative bacillary meningitis with a third-generation cephalosporin (e.g., cefotaxime 50 mg/kg iv q6h) has been outlined above. Initial therapy of neonatal meningitis with ampicillin plus a third-generation caphalosporin has not yet been shown to be more effective than therapy with ampicillin plus an aminoglycoside. Details of this therapy are discussed in the section on gram-negative bacillary meningitis.

SHUNT-ASSOCIATED MENINGITIS

Approximately 10–30 percent of the patients who have emplacement of a ventriculoatrial or ventriculoperitoneal shunt develop meningitis.[93,94] Clinical illness ranges from low-grade fever to fulminant ventriculitis and sepsis. Coagulase-negative staphylococci (*S. epidermidis*) account for over half of the shunt infections, followed by coagulase-positive staphylococci, *Propionibacterium acnes*, gram-negative bacilli, and enterococci.[93,95]

Systemic therapy alone usually fails to eradicate shunt infection. Although recent reports have stressed that complete removal of the infected shunt under the cover of antimicrobials offers the most reliable approach to therapy, systemic plus intraventricular antimicrobials cure the meningitis in some of the patients without surgical manipulation of the shunt.[96]

Thus, a course of antibiotic therapy without removal of the shunt may be warranted if (*1*) the infection is not fulminant, (*2*) a route for daily intraventricular antimicrobial therapy is present, (*3*) the infecting organism is sensitive to bactericidal antibiotics that may be given safely into the ventricles (e.g., cephalosporins or aminoglycosides), or (*4*) antimicrobial concentrations can be generated in both the intracerebral and extracerebral CSF space that are higher than the mimimal bactericidal concentration for the infecting organisms during most of the interval between doses.

RECURRENT MENINGITIS

Recurrent bacterial meningitis most often signals the presence of a communication of the subarachnoid space with the paranasal sinuses, nasopharynx, middle ear, or skin. Communications with the skin are usually associated with congenital defects of the skull or dura such as cranial or lumbosacral midline dermal sinuses (Fig. 1), dermoid cysts, or myelomeningoceles. The meningitis that results from such lesions if often caused by gram-negative bacilli.[34] Communications with the paranasal sinuses, nasopharynx, and middle ear usually result from fractures of the paranasal sinuses, cribriform plate, or petrous bone, respectively. Some patients have experienced over 10 episodes of meningitis in association with such lesions.[29,34] The causative agent in over 80 percent of such instances is *S. pneumoniae*.[29] If the patient has received antimicrobial prophylaxis, especially with ampicillin, gram-negative bacilli are the more likely causative organisms. The value of such antimicrobial prophylaxis in skull fractures associated with CSF leak is not clear. The occurrence of meningitis in any patient with a history of head trauma—even years previously—should prompt a search for CSF rhinorrhea or otorrhea. This can be done by injecting metrizamide or radioactive tracer into the lumbar CSF and monitoring its appearance in the nose or ear. Testing for rhinorrhea can be done by measuring with glucose oxidase tape the glucose content of nasal secretions, which should be low relative to CSF. Note that this test may falsely indicate that rhinorrhea is only nasal secretions if the patient has a CSF leak with meningitis and hypoglycorrhachia. Any communications that are discovered should be repaired surgically after meningitis has resolved.

In patients with recurrent meningitis, a search should also be made for a parameningeal focus of infection such as those discussed in a previous section. In many cases surgical drainage or removal of such foci is a critical adjunct to antimicrobial therapy.

In diseases such as brucellosis, cryptococcosis, and leptospirosis there may be CNS manifestations; the fluctuation in intensity of clinical manifestations that characterize these diseases can be mistaken for recurrent meningitis.[79,90]

The defects of the immune system most frequently associated with recurrent meningitis include splenectomy, hypogammaglobulinemia, leukemia and lymphoma, sickle and other hemoglobinopathies, and selected defects of the complement system.[25,26,28,34] In some patients with recurrent meningitis no anatomic or functional defects can be found.[97]

A variety of other conditions, such as Mollaret's meningitis, that can cause recurrent meningitis are reviewed in an earlier section.

PREVENTION OF MENINGITIS

The two primary means of preventing meningitis are with antimicrobial prophylaxis (chemoprophylaxis) and with vaccination. They are applied in selected patients who are at increased risk of acquiring meningitis.

Chemoprophylaxis

In meningitis caused by meningococci, the risk to case contacts and the efficacy of chemoprophylaxis has been proved. The avoidance of panic in all the people casually exposed to a case of meningococcal meningitis requires a well-planned strategy on the part of the physician. As soon as the diagnosis is firm and therapy is under way, the physician should notify appropriate public health authorities about the case and work out a program for announcing promptly and aggressively *who should* and *who should not* receive antimicrobial prophylaxis. Prophylaxis should be administered only to intimate contacts of the patient (e.g., family, girlfriends or other intimates, and roommates). Unless there has been intimate contact, it generally is not necessary to provide prophylaxis for classmates, fellow office workers, or members of the bridge club. However, a recent report indicates that school-aged children may be at risk of secondary infection particularly when classrooms are crowded (average midchair distance ≤30 inches), when contact during lunch and recess is frequent, or both.[98] In the absence of prolonged intimate contact, such as might occur during mouth-to-mouth resuscitation, prophylaxis is not necessary for medical personnel caring for a case.[99]

The risk of *H. influenzae* spreading among case contacts in households and day care centers and resulting in serious secondary disease including meningitis approximates similar risks with meningococcal infection.[4,98,100] Rifampin should be given to adults and children in households and day care centers containing children 4 years old or younger, other than the index case, providing that exposure to *H. influenzae* type b was within the week before prophylaxis. The index case may still be a carrier despite successful therapy and should receive rifampin prophylaxis.

The drug of choice for chemoprophylaxis of contacts of patients with meningococcal or *H. influenzae* meningitis is rifampin; for *H. influenzae* prophylaxis of children and adults, one dose of 20 mg/kg (not to exceed 600 mg per dose) a day for each of 4 successive days is most effective.[4] For meningococcal case contacts, one dose of 10 mg/kg (not to exceed 600 mg per dose) twice a day for 2 days appears adequate.

Vaccination

Vaccines are available for protection against selected strains of three of the bacteria that most frequently cause meningitis—*S. pneumoniae* (pneumococcus), *N. meningitidis* (meningococcus), and *H. influenzae* (see Chapter 296).

The meningococcal polysaccharide vaccines licensed are monovalent serogroup A, monovalent serogroup C, bivalent A-C, and quadrivalent A/C/Y/W-135. Monovalent A or C vaccines are recommended for use in epidemics of serogroup A or C meningococcal disease. With the use of serogroup C vaccine in army recruits, the incidence of meningococcal meningitis decreased approximately 90 percent in immunized men as compared with those who received control injections.[101,102] Quadrivalent vaccine is recommended for military personnel and for persons traveling to countries where meningococcal disease is epidemic (e.g., Nigeria). Although there is no effective capsular vaccine for serogroup B, which causes a majority of serious meningococcal disease in the United States, a vaccine composed of type 2 outer membrane protein I, a porin protein, appears promising.[103] Note that meningococcal vaccine should not be used in place of chemoprophylaxis in persons exposed to a case; the protection from immunization is too group specific and too slowly generated in this situation. There is no firm evidence that vaccination is a useful adjunct to chemoprophylaxis. For help in determining whether an epidemic of meningococcal meningitis exists or in obtaining and planning administration of the vaccine, call the Centers for Disease Control ([404]639-3687).

Pneumococcal vaccine, originally released in 1978 composed of 14 capsular serotypes, has been reformulated to include 23 serotypes.[104] Although the spectrum of immunity elicited is broader, the new vaccine is still not expected to prevent all pneumococcal infections.[105] Pneumococcal vaccine is recommended for persons over 2 years of age who are at special risk because of (*1*) functional asplenia (e.g., sickle cell disease) or traumatic asplenia, (*2*) diabetes, and (*3*) cardiorespiratory, hepatic, or renal disease.[106] The vaccine is also recommended for persons over age 50—especially when entering chronic care institutions where pneumococcal infections are endemic or epidemic. For adults, polyvalent pneumococcal vaccine is given in a dose of 0.5 ml intramuscularly. No serious complications have been observed. The optimal interval for a booster is unknown, but booster injections should not be given at less than 3-year intervals.

Although children less than 1 year of age are at particular risk from meningitis caused by pneumococci, meningococci, *H. influenzae*, or *E. coli*, vaccines that protect against these microorganisms currently are not available or are ineffective in this age group. Two different vaccines are available for *H. influenzae* type b, both licensed for use in children 18 months of age or older.[107] One (HbPV) contains the polysaccharide polyribosephosphate (PRP) alone. In the other (HbCV), the PRP is conjugated to diphtheria toxoid. HbCV is currently the preferred vaccine because it elicits higher antibody titers than HbPV.

REFERENCES

1. Suhs RH, Feldman HA. Pneumococcal types detected in throat cultures from a population of "normal" families. Am J Med Sci. 1965;250:424.
2. Greenfield S, Sheehe PR, Feldman HA. Meningococcal carriage in a population of "normal" families. J Infect Dis. 1971;123:67.
3. Robbins JB, Schneerson R, Argaman M, et al. *Haemophilus influenzae* type b: Disease and immunity in humans. Ann Intern Med. 1973;78:259.
4. Glode MP, Daum RS, Halsey NA, et al. Rifampin alone and in combination with trimethoprim in chemoprophylaxis for infections due to *Haemophilus influenzae* type b. Rev Infect Dis. 1983;5:549S.
5. Kaiser AB, Hennekens CH, Saslaw MS, et al. Seroepidemiology and chemoprophylaxis of disease due to sulfonamide-resistant *Neisseria meningitidis* in a civilian population. J Infect Dis. 1974;130:217.
6. Beutler B, Cerami A. Cachectin: More than a tumor necrosis factor. N Engl J Med. 1987;316:379–85.
7. Waage A, Halstensen A, Espevik T. Association between tumour necrosis factor in serum and fatal outcome in patients with meningococcal disease. Lancet. 1987;1:355–7.
8. Guerina NG, Langermann S, Clegg HW, et al. Adherence of piliated *Haemophilus influenzae* type b to human oropharyngeal cells. J Infect Dis. 1982;146:564.
9. Stevens DS, McGee ZA. Attachment of *Neisseria meningitidis* to human mucosal surfaces: Influence of pili and type of receptor cell. J Infect Dis. 1981;143:525.
10. Stephens DS, Hoffman LH, McGee ZA. Interaction of *Neisseria meningitidis* with human nasopharyngeal mucosa: Attachment and entry into columnar epithelial cells. J Infect Dis. 1983;148:369.
11. McGee ZA, Stephens DS, Hoffman LH, et al. Mechanisms of mucosal invasion by pathogenic Neisseria. Rev Infect Dis. 1983;5:708S.
12. Robbins JB, McCracken GH Jr, Gotschlich EC, et al. *Escherichia coli* K1 capsular polysaccharide associated with neonatal meningitis. N Engl J Med. 1974;290:1216.
13. McCracken GH Jr. Neonatal septicemia and meningitis. Hosp Pract. 1976;2:89.
14. Stephens DS, McGee ZA. Association of virulence of *Neisseria meningitidis* with transparent colony type and low-molecular-weight outer membrane proteins. J Infect Dis. 1983;147:282.
15. Griffiss JM, Bertram MA. Immunoepidemiology of meningeal disease in military recuits. II. Blocking of serum bactericidal activity by circulating IgA in the course of invasive disease. J Infect Dis. 1977;136:733.
16. Hook EW, Kaye D. Prophylaxis of bacteria endocarditis. J Chronic Dis. 1962;15:635.
17. Feldman WE. Relation of concentrations of bacteria and bacterial antigen in cerebrospinal fluid to prognosis in patients with bacterial meningitis. N Engl J Med. 1977;296:433.
18. Moxon ER, Smith AL, Averill DR, et al. *Haemophilus influenzae* meningitis in infant rats after intranasal inoculation. J Infect Dis. 1974;129:154.
19. Gregorius FK, Johnson BL Jr, Stern WE, et al. Pathogenesis of hematogenous bacterial meningitis in rabbits. J Neurosurg. 1976;45:561.
20. Conly JM, Ronald AR: Cerebrospinal fluid as a diagnostic body fluid. Am J Med. 1983;75(1B):102.
21. Rahal JJ, Simberkoff MS. Host defense and antimicrobial therapy in adult gram-negative bacillary meningitis. Ann Intern Med. 1982;96:468.
22. Berman PH, Banker BQ: Neonatal meningitis: A clinical and pathological study of 29 cases. Pediatrics. 1966;38:6.
23. Rorke LB, Pitts FW: Purulent meningitis: The pathological basis of clinical manifestations. Clin Pediatr. 1963;2:64.
24. Young LS, LaForce FM, Head JJ, et al. A simultaneous outbreak of meningococcal and influenza infections. N Engl J Med. 1972;287:5.
25. Petersen BH, Lee TJ, Snyderman R, et al. *Neisseria meningitidis* and *Neisseria gonorrhoeae* bacteremia associated with C6, C7 or C8 deficiency. Ann Intern Med. 1979;90:917.
26. Griessmer DA, Winkelstein JA, Luddy R. Pneumococcal meningitis in patients with a major sickle hemoglobinopathy. J Pediatr. 1978;92:82.
27. Johnson RT, Mims CA. Pathogenesis of viral infections of the nervous system. N Engl J Med. 1968;278:23, 84.
28. Winston DJ, Schiffman G, Wang DC, et al. Pneumococcal infections after human bone-marrow transplantation. Ann Intern Med. 1979;91:835.
29. Hand WL, Sanford JP. Posttraumatic bacterial meningitis. Ann Intern Med. 1970;72:869.
30. Carpenter RR, Petersdorf RG: The clinical spectrum of bacterial meningitis. Am J Med. 1962;33:262.
31. Centers for Disease Control. Multiply resistant pneumococcus—Colorado. MMWR. 1981;30:197.
32. Bell WE, Silber DL. Meningococcal meningitis: Past and present concepts. Milit Med. 1971;136:601.
33. Koppes GM, Ellenbogen C, Gebhart RJ. Group Y meningococcal disease in United States Air Force recruits. Am J Med. 1977;62:661.
34. Swartz MN, Dodge PR. Bacterial meningitis: A review of selected aspects. N Engl J Med. 1965;272:725.
35. Gopal V, Bisno AL. Fulminant pneumococcal infections in "normal" asplenic hosts. Arch Intern Med. 1977;137:1526.
36. Dabernat HJ, Delmas C. Comparative activity of cefotaxime and selected β-lactam antibiotics against *Haemophilus influenzae* and aerobic gram-negative bacilli. Rev Infect Dis. 1983;4:401S.
37. Cherubin CE, Corrado ML, Nair SR, et al. Treatment of gram-negative bacillary meningitis: Role of the new cephalosporin antibiotics. Rev Infect Dis. 1983;4:453S.
38. Eigler JOC, Wellman WE, Rooke ED, et al. Bacterial meningitis. I. General review. Proc Mayo Clin. 1961;36:357.
39. Kaiser AB, McGee ZA. Unpublished results.
40. Bradley SL, Dines DE, Brewer NS. Disseminated *Strongyloides stercoralis* in an immunosuppressed host. Mayo Clin Proc. 1978;53:332.
41. Mangi RJ, Quintiliani R, Andriole VT: Gram-negative meningitis. Am J Med. 1975;59:829.
42. Ross S, Rodriguez W, Controni G, et al. Limulus lysate test for gram-negative bacterial meningitis: Bedside application. JAMA. 1975;233:1366.
43. Martin WJ. Rapid and reliable techniques for the laboratory detection of bacterial meningitis. Am J Med. 1983;75(1B):119.
44. Landesman SH, Shah PM, Armengaud M, et al. Past and current roles for cephalosporin antibiotics in treatment of meningitis. Am J Med. 1981;71:693.
45. Kaiser AB, McGee ZA: Aminoglycoside therapy of gram-negative bacillary meningitis. N Engl J Med. 1975;293:1215.
46. Wright PF, Kaiser AB, Bowman CM, et al. The pharmacokinetics and efficacy of an aminoglycoside administered into the cerebral ventricles in neonates: Implications for further evaluation of this route of therapy in meningitis. J Infect Dis. 1981;143:141.
47. Mangi RJ, Holstein LL, Andriole VT. Treatment of gram-negative bacillary meningitis with intrathecal gentamicin. Yale J Biol Med. 1977;50:31.
48. Lee EL, Robinson MJ, Thong ML, et al. Intraventricular chemotherapy in neonatal meningitis. J Pediatr. 1977;91:991.
49. Wirt TC, McGee ZA, Oldfield EH, et al. Intraventricular administration of amikacin for complicated gram-negative meningitis and ventriculitis. J Neurosurg. 1979;50:95.
50. Velvis H, Carrasco N, Hetherington S. Trimethoprim-sulfamethoxazole therapy of neonatal *Proteus mirabilis* meningitis unresponsive to cefotaxime. Pediatr Infect Dis. 1986;5:591–3.
51. McCracken GH Jr, Mize SG. A controlled study of intrathecal antibiotic therapy in gram-negative enteric meningitis of infancy. J Pediatr. 1976;89:66.
52. Lecour H, Sears A, Miranda AM, et al. Treatment of 160 cases of acute bacterial meningitis with cefotaxime. J Antimicrob Chemother. 1984;14(Suppl B):195–202.
53. Norrby SR. Role of cephalosporins in the treatment of bacterial meningitis in adults: Overview with special emphasis on ceftazidime. Am J Med. 1985;79(Suppl 2A):56–61.
54. Ralph ED, Behma RJ. Enterobacter meningitis—treatment complicated by emergence of mutants resistant to cefotaxime. Scand J Infect Dis. 1987;19:577–9.
55. Fong IW, Tompkins KB. Review of *Pseudomonas aeruginosa* meningitis with special emphasis on treatment with ceftazidime. Rev Infect Dis. 1985;7:604–12.
56. Barson WJ, Miller MA, Brady MT, et al. Prospective comparative trial of ceftriaxone vs conventional therapy for treatment of bacterial meningitis in children. Pediatr Infect Dis. 1986;4:362–8.
57. Jacobs RJ, Wells TG, Steele RM, et al. A prospective randomized comparison of cefotaxime vs ampicillin and chloramphenicol for bacterial meningitis in children. J Pediatr. 1985;107:1290–133.
58. Lebel MH, Freij BJ, Syrogiannopoulos GA, et al. Dexamethasone therapy for bacterial meningitis. Results of two double-blind, placebo-controlled trials. N Engl J Med. 1988;319:964–71.
59. Iwarson S, Lidin-Janson G, Svensson R. Listeric meningitis in the noncompromised host. Infection. 1977;5:204.
60. Schröter GPJ, Weil R III. *Listeria monocytogenes* infection after renal transplantation. Arch Intern Med. 1977;137:1395.
61. Schlech WF III. Listeriosis: New pieces to an old puzzle. Arch Intern Med. 1986;146:459–60.

62. Scheer MS, Hirschman SZ. Oral and ambulatory therapy of *Listeria* bacteremia and meningitis with trimethoprim-sulfamethoxazole. Mt Sinai J Med. 1982;49:411.
63. Converse GM, Gwaltney JM Jr, Strassburg DA, et al. Alteration of cerebrospinal fluid findings by partial treatment of bacterial meningitis. Pediatrics. 1973;83:220.
64. Dalton HP, Allison MJ. Modification of laboratory results by partial treatment of bacterial meningitis. Am J Clin Pathol. 1968;49:410.
65. Jarvis CW, Saxena KM. Does prior antibiotic treatment hamper the diagnosis of acute bacterial meningitis? Clin Pediatr. 1972;11:201.
66. Rytel MW: Counterimmunoelectrophoresis in diagnosis of infectious disease. Hosp Pract. 1975;10:75.
67. Baker AS, Ojemann RG, Swartz MN, et al. Spinal epidural abscess. N Engl J Med. 1975;293:463.
68. Schlossberg D, Shulman JA. Spinal epidural abscess. South Med J. 1977;70:669.
69. Nicoll AM. Fatal primary amoebic meningoencephalitis. NZ Med J. 1973;78:108.
70. Cerva L, Novak K. Amoebic meningoencephalitis: Sixteen fatalities. Science. 1968;160:92.
71. Goodman JS, Koenig MG. Amphotericin B: Specifics of administration. Mod Treat. 1970;7:581.
72. Anderson K, Jamieson A. Primary amoebic meningoencephalitis. Lancet. 1972:1:902.
73. Merritt HH, Moore M. Acute syphilitic meningitis. Medicine. 1935;14:119.
74. Tramont EC. Persistence of *Treponema pallidum* following penicillin G therapy. JAMA. 1976;236:2206.
75. Lukehart SA, Hook EW, Baker-Zander SA, et al. Invasion of the central nervous system by *Treponema pallidum*: Implications for diagnosis and treatment. Ann Intern Med. 1988;109:855–62.
76. Cooper DA, Gold J, Maclean P, et al. Acute AIDS retrovirus infection: Definition of a clinical illness associated with seroconversion. Lancet. 1985;1:537–40.
77. Meyer HM Jr, Johnson RT, Crawford IP, et al. Central nervous system syndromes of "viral" etiology: A study of 713 cases. Am J Med. 1960;29:334.
78. Pierce JF, Jabbari B, Shraberg D. Leptospirosis: A neglected cause of nonbacterial meningoencephalitis. South Med J. 1977;70:150.
79. Edwards GA, Domm BM. Human leptospirosis. Medicine. 1960;39:117.
80. Schwartz JF, Balentine JD. Recurrent meningitis due to an intracranial epidermoid. Neurology. 1978;28:124.
81. Gibbons RB. Chemical meningitis following spinal anesthesia. JAMA. 1969;210:900.
82. Kremer I, Ritz R. Aseptic meningitis as an adverse effect of co-trimoxazole. N Engl J Med. 1983;308:1481.
83. Derbes SJ. Trimethoprim-induced aseptic meningitis. JAMA. 1984; 252:2865–6.
84. Centers for Disease Control. Aseptic meningitis among kidney transplant recipients receiving a newly marketed murine monoclonal antibody preparation. MMWR. 1986;35:551–2.
85. Lockshin MD, Kagen LJ. Meningitic reactions after azathioprine. N Engl J Med. 1972;286:1321–2.
86. Jensen S, Torben KG, Bacher T, et al. Ibuprofen-induced meningitis in a male with systemic lupus erythematosus. Acta Med Scand. 1987;221:509–11.
87. Giansiracusa DF, Blumberg S, Kantrowitz FG. Aseptic meningitis associated with ibuprofen. Arch Intern Med. 1980;140:1553.
88. Ruppert GB, Barth WF. Tolmetin-induced aseptic meningitis. JAMA. 1981;245:67–8.
89. Sylvia LM, Forlenza SW, Brocavich JM. Aseptic meningitis associated with naproxen. Drug Intell Clin Pharm. 1988;22:399.
90. Hermans PE, Goldstein NP, Wellman WE. Mollaret's meningitis and differential diagnosis of recurrent meningitis. Am J Med. 1972;52:128.
91. Dillon HC, Gray BM. Bacterial meningitis in children. Guidelines Antibiot Ther. 1977;2:3.
92. Karandanis D, Shulman JA. Recent survey of infectious meningitis in adults: Review of laboratory findings in bacterial, tuberculous, and aseptic meningitis. South Med J. 1976;69:449.
93. Schoenbaum SC, Gardner P, Shillito J. Infections of cerebrospinal fluid shunts: Epidemiology, clinical manifestations and therapy. J Infect Dis. 1975;131:543.
94. Shurtleff DB, Christie D, Foltz EL. Ventriculoauriculostomy-associated infection: A 12-year study. J Neurosurg. 1971;35:686.
95. Simpson PB Jr, Warren GC, Smith RR. Intraventricular cephalothin in childhood ventriculitis. Surg Neurol. 1975;4:279.
96. McLaurin RL. Infected cerebrospinal fluid shunts. Surg Neurol. 1973;1:191.
97. Whitecar JP Jr, Reddin JL, Spink WW. Recurrent pneumococcal meningitis: A review of the literature and studies on a patient who recovered from eleven attacks caused by five serotypes of *Diplococcus pneumoniae*. N Engl J Med. 1966;274:1285.
98. Feigin RD, Baker CJ, Herwaldt LA, et al. Epidemic meningococcal disease in an elementary-school class room. N Engl J Med. 1982;307:1255.
99. Artenstein MS, Ellis RE. The risk of exposure to a patient with meningococcal meningitis. Milit Med. 1968;133:474.
100. Ward JI, Fraser DW, Baraff LJ, et al. *Hemophilus influenzae* meningitis: A national study of secondary spread in household contacts. N Engl J Med. 1979;301:122.
101. Gotschlich EC, Goldschneider I, Artenstein MS. Human immunity to the meningococcus. V. The effect of immunization with meningococcal group C polysaccharide on the carrier status. J Exp Med. 1969;129:1385.
102. Artenstein MS, Gold R, Zimmerly JG, et al. Prevention of meningococcal disease by group C polysaccharide vaccine. N Engl J Med. 1970;282:417.
103. Craven DE, Frasch CE. Protection against group B meningococcal disease: Evaluation of serotype II protein vaccines in a mouse bacteremia model. Infect Immun. 1979;26:110.
104. An expanded pneumococcal vaccine. Med Lett. 1983;25:91.
105. Kaiser AB, Schaffner W. Prospectus: The prevention of bacteremic pneumococcal pneumonia. JAMA. 1974;230:404.
106. Advisory Committee on Immunization Practices: Pneumococcal polysaccharide vaccine. MMWR. 1978;27:25.
107. Gilsdorf JR. *Haemophilus influenzae* type b vaccine efficacy in the United States. Pediatr Infect Dis. 1988;7:147–8.

67. CHRONIC MENINGITIS

MICHAEL KATZMAN
JERROLD J. ELLNER

A large number of infectious and noninfectious diseases can cause the clinical syndrome of chronic meningitis. The onset of symptoms in such cases typically is subacute to chronic with signs of meningoencephalitis such as fever, headache, lethargy, confusion, nausea, vomiting, and stiff neck. Cerebrospinal fluid (CSF) is abnormal with elevated protein concentrations, a pleocytosis that usually is predominantly lymphocytic, and sometimes a low glucose level. The major difficulty during initial evaluation is in distinguishing the rare patient with chronic meningitis from individuals with the more common syndromes of acute meningitis and encephalitis. If the neurologic symptoms and signs either persist or progress clinically and the CSF remains abnormal for a period of at least 4 weeks, the diagnosis of chronic meningitis is appropriate.[1–3] This duration of symptoms was derived empirically to optimize the distinction between patients with chronic progressive disease and those with self-limited processes. In practice, patients frequently are seen by a physician within 1–4 weeks of the onset of symptoms. Prompt diagnosis and institution of appropriate treatment, therefore, may abort the neurologic process before the criteria for chronic meningitis are fulfilled. The diagnosis of chronic meningitis has a number of implications; particularly important are those relating to etiology, management, and prognosis.

Central nervous system (CNS) involvement by most diseases causing chronic meningitis has a high morbidity and mortality. Successful intervention requires the early administration of specific, often potentially toxic forms of therapy. Furthermore, drugs appropriate for treating one cause of chronic meningitis may be contraindicated in others. Therefore, a precise etiologic diagnosis is critical in modifying the course of this syndrome, and broad empirical therapeutic regimens are a poor and sometimes hazardous substitute. While exact diagnosis may prove difficult, certain aspects of the presentation can be helpful in determining causality or at least in limiting the differential diagnosis.

HISTORY

The exposure history may be important in suggesting certain infectious diseases such as tuberculosis, coccidioidomycosis, histoplasmosis, brucellosis, cysticercosis, syphilis, Lyme disease, or the acquired immunodeficiency syndrome (AIDS) with its distinctive spectrum of pathogens. The exposure history should direct the evaluation to include specific serologic studies and other diagnostic tests.

The history also is of importance in distinguishing chronic meningitis from two superficially similar syndromes, acute men-

TABLE 1. Differential Diagnosis of Recurrent Meningitis

Parameningeal focus
Infection
Epidermoid cyst, craniopharyngioma
Post-traumatic (bacterial meningitis)
Aseptic meningitis
Mollaret's meningitis[5]
Systemic lupus erythematosus
Migrainous syndrome with pleocytosis[6]

ingitis or encephalitis with a protracted recovery and recurrent meningitis. In chronic meningitis, onset is insidious and symptoms chronic, although they may wax and wane. Episodes of acute neurologic deterioration sometimes punctuate the clinical course and may be caused by cerebral edema, hydrocephalus, cerebrovascular occlusions, and seizures. Even when symptoms temporarily regress, CSF abnormalities persist and reflect continued disease activity. One confusing syndrome that must be distinguished from chronic meningitis is that of a protracted recovery period that sometimes follows pyogenic or aseptic meningitis and viral encephalitis. In these patients, actual progression of disease is confined to the acute stages of the illness; clearing of the signs, symptoms, and CSF abnormalities, although gradual, may occur during observation. The second syndrome that must be differentiated from chronic meningitis is recurrent meningitis.[4] Patients with recurrent meningitis usually have repeated episodes of acute disease followed by symptom free periods during which signs and symptoms are absent and the CSF is normal (Table 1).

The history also is important in defining the cause of meningitis in those instances in which CNS extension typically occurs as a late manifestation of a previously diagnosed systemic disease. These conditions include acute leukemia, lymphoma, blastomycosis, and Behçet's disease. The history sometimes reveals an underlying disease associated with disordered cellular immunity. In such cases, the differential diagnosis shifts as considered below.

PHYSICAL EXAMINATION

Diagnostic physical findings are rare. However, physical examination may delineate signs of an associated systemic disease that provide a potential source of rapid diagnosis. Skin lesions, although infrequent, are particularly important for their diagnostic value. Even benign-appearing superficial lesions, subcutaneous nodules and abscesses, or draining sinuses should be cultured and biopsy specimens obtained. India ink preparations also should be prepared from expressed material. The eye examination may be helpful if such lesions as choroidal tubercles, sarcoid granulomas, or uveitis are demonstrable. The finding of papilledema also is of significance since it alters the course of the neurologic work-up and contraindicates lumbar puncture. Hepatomegaly may reflect systemic disease involving the liver and increases the potential diagnostic yield of a liver biopsy.

Neurologic examination is of obvious importance in delineating the extent of CNS involvement. However, it is of limited use in differentiating among specific etiologies since mental status changes, meningismus, oculomotor palsies, and less frequently, focal findings, evidence of increased intracranial pressure, and spinal cord signs may be caused by most processes associated with chronic meningitis. Focal signs, however, often reflect a parenchymal mass such as an abscess or granuloma that would dictate specific diagnostic and therapeutic maneuvers. Hydrocephalus may complicate chronic meningitis, and appropriate neuroradiographic evaluation should be initiated when the constellation of headache, nausea, vomiting, mental changes, ataxia, incontinence, and papilledema is present. The finding of hydrocephalus, particularly with associated cranial neuropathies, is suggestive of an infectious etiology with basilar leptomeningitis, although hydrocephalus also may complicate sarcoidosis and CNS tumor. Peripheral neuropathy is noted uncommonly in chronic meningitis and is suggestive of sarcoidosis or Lyme disease.

LABORATORY EVALUATION

The etiology of chronic meningitis ultimately must be established in the laboratory. Abnormalities on chest x-ray films may reflect systemic involvement by the underlying infectious process, carcinoma, or sarcoidosis. These findings should be pursued in an attempt to define the etiology of the meningitis. In more enigmatic cases, thoracotomy may be indicated and is associated with less morbidity and greater yield than a brain biopsy is.

The CSF formula is never itself diagnostic.[7] However, certain abnormalities and patterns are more characteristic of a restricted group of causes of chronic meningitis. A pleocytosis of fewer than 50 cells may occur in most diseases associated with chronic meningitis but is typical of sarcoidosis, carcinoma, and "chronic benign lymphocytic meningitis." Persistence of a neutrophilic pleocytosis suggests infection with *Nocardia, Actinomyces, Brucella*, or several fungi, especially *Candida, Aspergillus*, and the Zygomycetes,[8] although these agents all may present with a lymphocytic pattern. Hypoglycorrhachia limits the differential diagnosis of chronic meningitis somewhat to certain infectious diseases (tuberculosis, fungal infection, syphilis, toxoplasmosis, cysticercosis), sarcoidosis, and carcinoma. However, decreased CSF glucose levels may be found in lymphocytic choriomeningitis virus infection, in mumps meningoencephalitis, after subarachnoid bleeds, occasionally in "chronic benign lymphocytic meningitis," and in diseases associated with recurrent meningitis. Hypoglycorrhachia also may develop during the course of herpes simplex encephalitis, although it is uncommon (5 percent) during the first 3–5 days of hospitalization. Therefore, the finding of depressed CSF glucose early in the course of a patient with presumed herpes simplex virus encephalitis increases the likelihood of an alternative treatable infectious disease such as cryptococcosis or tuberculosis.[9]

Lumbar puncture needs to be repeated periodically both for culture and to follow the course of meningeal inflammation. India ink preparations should be prepared from the sediment of 3–5 ml of CSF. The entire slide must be examined since cryptococci may be present in small numbers. As opposed to artifacts that are seen commonly, encapsulated yeast has a regular, round, distinct capsule and a refractile central structure; budding yeast forms also may be found. The India ink preparation is more likely to be positive in patients with relatively acute presentations and/or immunosuppressed patients with lymphoma or AIDS. In the latter setting, yeast organisms often far outnumber leukocytes in the CSF. Cerebrospinal fluid cytologic studies are indicated in all patients with chronic meningitis. Multiple specimens may be necessary for the diagnosis of CNS involvement by tumor, and negative cytologic studies do not preclude this possibility. The demonstration of a clonal origin of CSF lymphocytes also is useful in the diagnosis of lymphomatous meningitis.[10]

Serologic studies of serum and CSF are extremely important in evaluating the patient for coccidioidomycosis, cryptococcosis, and syphilis and should be performed routinely. In the case of cryptococcal meningitis, relevant testing is for cryptococcal polysaccharide antigen. Serum antibodies to *Brucella* and *Toxoplasma* also may suggest these infections when they are present in high or increasing titers. Serum antibodies to *Histoplasma* are found in fewer than one-half of patients with *Histoplasma* meningitis. Complement-fixing antibodies to *Histoplasma* are found in most patients with CNS histoplasmosis, but there is an unacceptably high (25–50 percent) rate of false-positive test results in other fungal meningitides.[11,12] More promising is the detection of *H. capsulatum* antigen in serum, urine, or CSF by radioimmunoassay.[13] Recent studies indicate selective compartmentalization of lymphocytes and antibody-producing cells in the CNS. Cerebrospinal fluid lymphocytes may be more reactive to specific antigens than blood lymphocytes.[14] A relative or absolute increase in antibody levels in the CSF as compared with serum, indicative of local production rather than passive diffusion, may prove important in the diagnosis of tuberculosis[15] and other chronic infections as it has in herpes simplex encephalitis. Ultimately, the demonstration of constituents of the causative organism in CSF, so useful in the diagnosis of cryptococcal disease, may be extended to other infections; for example, tuberculostearic acid in CSF might be indicative of tuberculous meningitis.[16]

Skin testing should be limited to tuberculin purified protein derivative (PPD) and antigens to test for anergy. Repeated skin testing may be helpful when tuberculosis is a possibility. Fungal skin test antigens are of no use diagnostically and may cause confusion by altering the fungal serologies, particularly in the case of histoplasmosis.

Cultures are mandatory even when a specific diagnosis is suggested by serologies or other studies. Cerebrospinal fluid should be cultured at least three times for bacteria, acid-fast bacilli, and fungi and more numerous samples obtained and cultured in their entirety when the cause of the meningitis remains uncertain after the initial diagnostic evaluation is complete. The low density of fungi in the CSF and difficulty in culturing certain organisms may delay the diagnosis of some mycotic infections. In such cases, the yield can be improved by inoculating Sabouraud agar layered on the bottom of Erlenmeyer flasks with large volumes of CSF. The finding of even a single colony of an organism capable of causing chronic meningitis such as *Sporothrix schenckii* should never be disregarded as a contaminant.[17] In fact, it may be useful to continue to examine fungal cultures for at least 4–6 weeks because the growth of such organisms can be exceedingly slow. Ventricular CSF may have a higher cultural yield than lumbar CSF in certain infections.[18] Urine, sputum, gastric washings, stool, and blood cultures should be obtained and processed routinely and for mycobacteria and fungi even in the absence of clinical evidence of extraneural infection. These ancillary cultures frequently are positive in cases of cryptococcosis, tuberculosis, histoplasmosis, and blastomycosis. Special culture techniques such as anaerobiosis or increased carbon dioxide tension also are appropriate in the search for certain pathogens such as *Actinomyces* species and *Brucella abortus*, respectively.

Biopsy of specific tissues should be directed by abnormal findings on physical examination. Skin, lymph node, and liver biopsy specimens may demonstrate granulomas, sometimes with caseation and occasionally with an organism demonstrable on special staining. Caseation is suggestive of tuberculosis, histoplasmosis, and coccidioidomycosis. Focal necrosis may be found in brucellosis. All biopsy specimens should be cultured for bacteria, fungi, and mycobacteria. Bone marrow biopsy and culture are particularly useful in tuberculosis and histoplasmosis. Liver biopsy is indicated when miliary tuberculosis is suspected, even in the absence of hepatomegaly or abnormal liver function. Meningeal and brain biopsies should be performed and ventricular fluid sampled at the time of craniotomy for exploration of a mass or other focal lesion or indicated ventricular shunting procedures. In addition, despite the relatively low yield of nondirected meningeal and brain biopsies, these are indicated in patients with undiagnosed clinically progressive meningitis or in individuals with marked functional limitation.

Additional Radiographic Techniques

Computed axial tomography (CT) should be performed on all patients with chronic meningitis and allows a demonstration of inflammation at the base of the brain. The basal cisterns may be obscured, at least partly, by inflammatory tissue with attenuation similar to brain.[19] Areas of granulomatous inflammation show contrast enhancement. Similar findings occur with leptomeningeal infiltration by tumor. CT scanning also is useful to search for focal parenchymal lesions and hydrocephalus. The demonstration of hydrocephalus is not itself a sufficient indication for ventricular shunting since neurosurgical procedures have a high morbidity and failure rate in chronic meningitis. Furthermore, hydrocephalus may clear spontaneously with treatment of the underlying condition. Nonetheless, if clinical deterioration attributable to hydrocephalus occurs, a surgical approach must be considered. In enigmatic cases, magnetic resonance imaging has the potential to add further information, although the abnormalities often are not specific or diagnostic.

Ancillary procedures such as mammography and gastrointestinal radiographic series may be appropriate in the search for a primary carcinoma when meningeal carcinomatosis is suspected.

THERAPEUTIC TRIALS

Therapeutic trials are indicated when the specific etiology remains uncertain despite comprehensive evaluation. However, further attempts at establishing a diagnosis should be continued actively during such trials. The interpretation of the response to empirically administered drugs may be quite difficult since clinical improvement is often slow, even when the agent selected is appropriate. When the patient is stable, sequential trials are indicated, reserving amphotericin B for last and avoiding corticosteroids, which may have a disastrous effect on undiagnosed fungal infection.

An empirical trial of antituberculous drugs clearly is appropriate when the presentation and CSF formula are consistent with tuberculosis and there is evidence of active or prior tuberculous infection. Recent studies suggest that initial tuberculin skin test results are negative in up to 35 percent of patients with tuberculous meningitis.[20] Therefore, empirical antituberculous therapy in fact is indicated in most cases of undiagnosed chronic meningitis. Adequate cultures of CSF, urine, sputum, or gastric aspirates must be obtained before starting therapy and should include biopsy specimens of liver and bone marrow if miliary disease is suspected. Repeat intermediate-strength PPD skin testing after 2–4 weeks also may be of value if the initial studies are negative. The second-strength tuberculin skin test is less frequently negative than intermediate tests are and may be helpful. Positive cultures or a clinical response to antituberculous treatment despite negative cultures would be an indication to complete a full course of therapy.

An empirical trial of penicillin, 20 million units/day, or tetracycline, 2 g/day for 1 month, should be effective for meningitis due to actinomycosis and Lyme disease or brucellosis, respectively. Such treatment is indicated in the presence of a parameningeal focus suggesting actinomycosis when chronic meningitis occurs in late summer or early fall, particularly with confirmatory *Brucella* serologies and exposure history or in an area endemic for Lyme disease.

Empirical use of amphotericin B should be withheld as long as possible in view of its toxicity and the difficulty in determining the duration of administration even when the causative fungus is known. However, when chronic meningitis is caused by certain fungi (*Histoplasma, Blastomyces, Sporothrix*), cultures of lumbar CSF typically are negative. Generally empirical treatment with amphotericin B should be reserved for patients with progressive chronic meningitis who remain undiagnosed despite meningeal biopsy. Once initiated empirically, amphotericin B should be administered for 10–12 weeks intravenously. The development of nephrotoxicity should indicate a reduction in daily dose rather than discontinuation of the trial. Shorter-term trials of this drug are of little value. If patients respond to amphotericin B but relapse, a pattern suggestive of coccidioidal or cryptococcal meningitis, intrathecal therapy must be considered.

Empirical trials of corticosteroids are contraindicated because of potential catastrophic adverse effects on unrecognized fungal meningitis. In addition, the efficacy of this form of therapy has not been established in those forms of chronic meningitis generally considered to be corticosteroid responsive such as sarcoidosis.

DIFFERENTIAL DIAGNOSIS

A number of conditions may cause syndromes resembling chronic meningitis superficially but are usually distinguishable from it on clinical grounds at presentation or during evaluation and observation of the patient (Table 2). In addition, a careful history is important to differentiate between recurrent and chronic meningitis since the former syndrome connotes a different spectrum of diseases (Table 1).

Those infections causing the syndrome of chronic meningitis (Table 3) are discussed in detail in other chapters. Features that are important in establishing the cause of the chronic meningitis are reviewed here.

Tuberculous Meningitis

Tuberculous meningitis[20–29] results from rupture of a superficial infective focus into the subarachnoid space. In younger patients, this event typically is associated with active, progressive systemic disease. Stigmata of miliary tuberculosis may be present on physical examination and on chest x-ray films. Tuberculin skin test results frequently are negative initially, but "conversion" is noted on repeated skin testing. The diagnosis of tuberculosis usually is confirmed by smear, biopsy, and cultures obtained from extraneural specimens as well as CSF culture. In contrast, tuberculous meningitis in the adult more frequently results from the discharge of an old tuberculous focus into the subarachnoid space. As a result, physical examination, chest x-ray films, and extraneural cultures often are not helpful; despite presumably long-standing tuberculous infection, recent series indicate that the initial tuberculin skin test result is negative in up to 35 percent of patients. The diagnosis rests on the outcome of CSF cultures. As a result of the frequent early use of antituberculous therapy empirically, more cases now are "unproved" culturally, but the diagnosis of tuberculosis is suggested by an apparent response to treatment.[25] Overall there is nothing about the clinical syndrome of tuberculous meningitis that distinguishes it from other etiologies of chronic meningitis. About one-half of the patients have had symptoms for over 2 weeks. Ocular palsies, particularly due to involvement of nerve VI, are found in 30–70 percent of the cases. The typical CSF findings consist of a lymphocytic pleocytosis, usually of 100–500 cells, increased protein concentration and depressed glucose levels in two-thirds of the patients on the initial lumbar puncture. This formula also is not specific for tuberculous meningitis. However, in unclear cases, progressive decrease in CSF glucose in the absence of specific treatment may be useful in distinguishing tuberculosis from aseptic meningitis and viral encephalitis. Cytologic examination of CSF often shows activated monocytoid cells and rarely Langhans cells.[27] It should be noted that neutrophils may predominate, particularly during the first 10 days of symptoms. Cerebrospinal fluid smears contain acid-fast bacilli in 10–22 percent of the cases; a smear of the pellicle formed on standing may increase the diagnostic yield. Cerebrospinal fluid cultures are positive in 38–88 percent of the cases and sputum and gastric washings each in about 50 percent. Cerebrospinal fluid tests under evaluation for the presumptive diagnosis of tuberculous meningitis include adenosine deaminase levels (elevated due to release by T lymphocytes), bromide partitioning (abnormal due to alterations in the blood-brain barrier), and various antibody and antigen detection assays.[28] Conversion of the tuberculin skin test result from negative to positive is a supportive finding. In view of the 4- to 6-week delay often inherent in interpreting cultural results, empirical antituberculous therapy is appropriate in the patient with unexplained chronic meningitis. The duration of therapy needs to be individualized, with attention to the clinical course and results of repeat tuberculin skin testing if all cultures are negative after 6 weeks.

TABLE 2. Diseases That Sometimes Resemble Chronic Meningitis

Infectious etiologies
Aseptic meningitis
Viral and nonviral encephalitis
Partially treated bacterial meningitis
Parameningeal infections
Infective endocarditis
Noninfectious diseases
Metabolic and other encephalopathies
Brain tumor
Subarachnoid hemorrhage
Subdural hematoma
Multiple sclerosis
Systemic lupus erythematosus
Postinfectious encephalitis
Giant cell arteritis
Thrombotic thrombocytopenic purpura

TABLE 3. Infectious Diseases That May Be Manifest as Chronic Meningitis

Tuberculosis	Actinomycosis[a]
Cryptococcosis	Phaeohyphomycosis (chromomycosis)[a]
Coccidioidomycosis	Toxoplasmosis[a]
Histoplasmosis	Cysticercosis[a]
Candidiasis	Rarer infectious etiologies
Blastomycosis[a]	*Pseudallescheria boydii*
Syphilis	*Sporothrix schenckii*
Brucellosis	Agents of mucormycosis
Toxoplasmosis[a]	*Coenurus cerebralis*
Nocardiosis[a]	*Leptospira icterohaemorrhagiae*
Lyme disease	*Angiostrongylus cantonensis*

[a] More commonly occur as brain abscesses or focal lesions.

Cryptococcal Meningitis

Cryptococcal meningitis[20,29–34] presents in several different fashions, but the most characteristic, that of a subacute to chronic meningoencephalitis, is not at all distinctive among the etiologies of chronic meningitis. Exposure history is of little value clinically since this yeastlike fungus is a widespread saprophyte. Although one-half of patients in the pre-AIDS era lacked gross immunologic deficits, an underlying cellular immune dysfunction was known to predispose to this infection. The development of chronic meningitis in patients with Hodgkin's disease or lymphosarcoma, in persons receiving high-dose daily corticosteroid therapy, or in individuals at risk for AIDS, suggests this diagnosis. In the previously healthy person, cryptococcal meningitis may cause an extremely indolent illness with gradual progression of dementia. The India ink preparation frequently is negative in such cases. More commonly, the onset of disease is subacute, at times mimicking a brain tumor, particularly when signs of increased intracranial pressure are present. In patients with hematologic malignancies or AIDS, the initial manifestations of cryptococcosis may be unexplained fever. However, CNS involvement often evolves rapidly. Cerebrospinal fluid abnormalities include a lymphocytic pleocytosis, generally with 40–400 cells, and a depressed glucose level in 55 percent of the cases. In patients with AIDS, the CSF often shows little evidence of an inflammatory response.[33,34] Overall, the India ink preparation suggests the diagnosis of cryptococcal meningitis in over one-half of cases. The yield is highest in patients with an acute syndrome. More than 85 percent of patients have cryptococcal polysaccharide antigen in the CSF. However, serum also should be processed for this antigen; the overlap between significant antigen titers in the serum and CSF allows a presumptive diagnosis of cryptococcosis in 94 percent of the cases. Negative serologies do not exclude a diagnosis of cryptococcal meningitis. Cultural confirmation of the diagnosis is mandatory. The initial CSF culture is positive in three-quarters of patients; additional CSF cultures increase this yield and are indicated. Cultures of urine, sputum, stool, and blood also should be obtained. They have both diagnostic and prognostic value and frequently are positive in the absence of overt signs of extraneural infection. CSF cultures and serologies also are indicated in all patients with extraneural cryptococcal infection since they may have subclinical CNS disease.

Coccidioidal Meningitis

Exposure history is important in the diagnosis of coccidioidal meningitis since this infection is endemic in certain arid and semiarid areas of the Western Hemisphere.[35–40] Central nervous system infection may be a part of generalized coccidioidomycosis or may represent the sole extrapulmonary site of active clinical disease. Headache is the most prominent finding in patients with coccidioidal meningitis; the clinical syndrome is, however, in no way distinctive from the other causes of chronic meningitis. Skin tests with coccidioidin usually are negative in patients with meningitis. However, complement-fixing antibody to the causative organism is found in the CSF of 75–95 percent of such patients. A presumptive diagnosis is possible when chronic meningitis occurs in the presence of demonstrated systemic coccidioidomycosis or a serum complement fixation titer to *Coccidioides immitis* of at least 1:16. Cerebrospinal fluid findings resemble those of cryptococcal meningitis; CSF cultures are positive in one-third to one-half of the cases, and rarely, spherules of *C. immitis* may be present on a smear.

Histoplasma Meningitis

Although demonstrable spread to the CNS occurs in about one-quarter of the autopsied cases of disseminated histoplasmosis, neurologic symptoms usually are not prominent. *Histoplasma* meningitis[41–44] has been reported rarely and usually occurs without overt signs of extraneural infection. The clinical syndrome of *Histoplasma* meningitis is not differentiable from the other causes of chronic meningitis. A diagnosis of this entity may be extremely difficult in view of the absence of reliable serologic and skin tests and the paucity of viable fungi in the CSF. Nonetheless, serologies for antibody and *Histoplasma* antigen as discussed above and the repeated culture of large volumes of CSF sometimes have allowed a diagnosis to be made when initial cultures were negative.

Other Infectious Etiologies

Involvement of the CNS is common in disseminated candidiasis, but the clinical syndrome of chronic meningitis is less frequent. Most patients developing *Candida* meningitis[45,46] have significant underlying disease, although hematologic malignancy has not been prominent. Rather, *Candida* meningitis occurs in some of the other settings associated with disseminated candidiasis, i.e., prior antibiotic and corticosteroid therapy, indwelling bladder or venous catheters, and recent abdominal surgery. One-third of the patients are under 2 years of age. The expression of the meningitis is variable, but the average delay between the onset of symptoms and diagnosis has been 17 weeks. The mean CSF pleocytosis in one series was 600 cells; about one-half of the patients had lymphocytes predominating. Hypoglycorrhachia is present in 60 percent of the cases. Yeast cells have been noted on CSF smears in 43 percent of the cases, and results of CSF cultures usually are diagnostic. Overall, 71 percent of the patients with meningitis have active extraneural *Candida* infection, and an additional 14 percent have had antecedent invasive CNS procedures such as ventricular shunting or lumbar puncture, which are presumably responsible for introduction of the yeast into the subarachnoid space. Although spontaneous recovery has been recorded, antifungal therapy clearly seems indicated.

Syphilitic meningitis[47,48] is a rare but easily diagnosed and treated form of secondary syphilis. The disease is usually subacute, with the symptoms persisting for over 1 month in about one-quarter of the cases. Meningitis is the first overt sign of syphilis in 25 percent of meningitic patients. When extraneural manifestations have occurred, they generally preceded CNS involvement by less than 2 years. The clinical presentation and CSF abnormalities resemble those of the other causes of chronic meningitis. Hypoglycorrhachia is present in 55 percent of the cases. The diagnosis of syphilitic meningitis is suggested by positive CSF and serum serologies for syphilis. Transient dramatic deterioration of patients with meningitis after the initiation of penicillin therapy should suggest a Jarisch-Herxheimer reaction and the possibility of syphilis.

Borrelia burgdorferi, the cause of Lyme disease, is another spirochete associated with chronic meningitis. After the bite of an infected tick, the characteristic skin lesion of erythema chronicum migrans may or may not occur and is followed by neurologic symptoms in approximately one-third of cases. Cranial or peripheral neuropathies may be prominent.[49] The diagnosis is made by appropriate serologies in serum and CSF,[50] especially in the setting of tick exposure in an endemic area in late summer or early fall.

A meningoencephalomyelitis may follow the initial manifestations of brucellosis by 2 months to 2 years in fewer than 5 percent of cases.[51–55] Exposure to unpasteurized milk products or contact with cows, goats, sheep, swine, or their carcasses suggests the diagnosis. The patient also may have or have had symptoms and signs of systemic brucellosis such as night sweats, unexplained fever, orchitis, and hepatosplenomegaly. The clinical presentation of the meningitis and CSF abnormalities usually are nonspecific. However, transient episodes of hemianesthesia or paresthesia can be prominent in neurobrucellosis. Serologic studies often suggest the diagnosis of brucellosis. In chronic cases, calcified foci may be noted in the liver and spleen on abdominal x-ray films. Cultures should be maintained in an increased carbon dioxide atmosphere for 3 weeks. Cerebrospinal fluid cultures are positive for *Brucella* in fewer than one-half of the cases. Blood cultures are occasionally positive. *Sporothrix schenckii* has been described as a cause of chronic meningitis, and the CSF may demonstrate *Sporothrix* antibody before the fungus is recovered by culture.[56]

Central nervous system involvement by a large number of infections commonly is expressed as brain abscesses or other focal lesions occurring by hematogenous seeding or direct extension from clinically apparent extraneural sites. Rarely, the syndrome of chronic meningitis may be caused by these agents, sometimes without other stigmata of the infection. Infectious diseases belonging in this category include North American blastomycosis,[18,57,58] paracoccidioidomycosis,[59] cerebral dematiomycosis,[60] actinomycosis,[61–64] nocardiosis,[65,66] and toxoplasmosis.[67–69] One-half of patients with cerebral cysticercosis have the clinical syndrome of chronic meningitis; the frequent finding of hypoglycorrhachia is a somewhat confusing feature.[70–72]

Several infectious agents have been documented to cause chronic meningitis in unique epidemiologic circumstances (*Angiostrongylus cantonensis, Coenurus cerebralis*)[1] or in isolated case reports (*Leptospira icterohaemorrhagiae*, mucormycosis)[1,73] and will not be discussed. Other infections in which CNS involvement is a late manifestation with few related symptoms or leptomeningitis is noted pathologically but not clinically, also will not be reviewed.

Neoplastic Meningitis

The noninfectious diseases causing chronic meningitis may be difficult to diagnose and distinguish from occult infections (Table 4). Primary and metastatic, hematologic, and solid tumors all may involve the meninges diffusely to cause a similar clinical syndrome. In the case of acute leukemia and lymphoma,[74–76] CNS involvement usually occurs in the setting of known underlying malignancy. The major diagnostic problem involves distinguishing CNS involvement by the tumor from superimposed CNS infection and the uncommon paraneoplastic syndromes. Primary brain tumors including gliomas, pinealomas, ependymomas, and choroid plexus tumors may involve the meninges diffusely,[77] sometimes without gross parenchymal involvement. A diagnosis can be difficult in such cases. In metastatic "meningeal carcinomatosis,"[78–82] the nature of the meningeal process also may be difficult to ascertain. In one large series, the primary tumor had not been diagnosed at the onset of neurologic symptoms in 75 percent of the patients,[80] although the figure was 8 percent in patients selected by admission to an oncology center.[81] Typically, the onset of symptoms is subacute, with an intractable headache a prominent complaint along with mental changes. Cranial neuropathy occurs in 50 percent of the cases, and meningismus in about 20 percent. Fever usually is absent or when it occurs is associated with an intercurrent infection. Characteristically, neurologic signs far exceed symptoms and indicate widespread neurologic dysfunction; cerebral, cranial nerve, and spinal involvement are noted in one-half of the patients on initial physical examination. Cerebrospinal fluid is abnormal; 72 percent of the patients have a pleocytosis, often minimal, although occasional patients have a marked cellular response. The glucose content is depressed in 38 percent of the patients initially and in 72 percent during serial examinations. The finding of marked hypoglycorrhachia in the presence of minimal pleocytosis should suggest this diagnosis. In one series, CSF cytologies were diagnostic in 42 percent of patients on the first study and in 74 percent when multiple specimens were processed.[81] Of the ancillary neurodiagnostic tests, the myelogram was particularly helpful diagnostically and revealed multiple nodular deposits on nerve roots in 39 percent of the cases. The finding of markedly elevated CSF levels of β-glucuronidase is suggestive of meningeal carcinomatosis.[83] The most frequent primary sites of malignancy causing this syndrome are the breast, lung, stomach, pancreas, and skin (melanoma). Although neurologic signs may fluctuate and even partly regress, the course of meningeal carcinomatosis usually is rapidly progressive with involvement of all parts of the neuraxis. Since the primary tumor may be occult and extraneural metastatic sites lacking, cytologic examination of multiple CSF specimens is appropriate in all patients with undiagnosed chronic meningitis.

Sarcoid Meningitis

The neurologic manifestations of sarcoidosis are protean.[84–89] Chronic basilar granulomatous meningitis frequently occurs in the setting of characteristic systemic sarcoidosis. However, CNS involvement may be the presenting feature or the sole clinical manifestation of the disease. The clinical syndrome of sarcoid meningitis often includes cranial nerve palsies, long-tract and cerebellar abnormalities, and changes in mentation. The predilection for the basilar meninges with extension to the hypothalamus results in diabetes insipidus in 14–30 percent of the cases; this is of diagnostic significance because it rarely occurs in other forms of chronic meningitis. In addition, peripheral neuropathies accompany CNS sarcoidosis in 14 percent of patients but generally are unusual in chronic meningitis except for Lyme disease. Characteristic CSF abnormalities consist of a minimal lymphocytic pleocytosis in 60 percent of the patients and hypoglycorrhachia in 18 percent. The diagnosis of CNS sarcoidosis in patients with classic systemic manifestations of the disease is complicated by the necessity of excluding superimposed tuberculosis or cryptococcosis that occur with increased frequenty in sarcoidosis and in patients receiving corticosteroid therapy. The diagnosis is more difficult when disease is limited to the CNS. Even the demonstration of granulomas in meningeal biopsy specimens is not specific. Although corticosteroids are recommended for the treatment of CNS sarcoidosis, their efficacy has not been established rigorously. Low-dose irradiation of the CNS has been used with apparent advantage in one patient.[89]

TABLE 4. Noninfectious Causes of Chronic Meningitis

Neoplasm
Sarcoidosis
Granulomatous angiitis
Uveomeningoencephalitis
Behçet's disease
Chronic benign lymphocytic meningitis[a]
Chronic meningitis of unknown etiology[a]

[a] Some cases may be due to infecious agents.

Other Noninfectious Etiologies

Granulomatous angiitis is a necrotizing vasculitis of small leptomeningeal and perforating arteries and veins.[90–94] The process is usually manifested as a subacute meningoencephalitis in patients over 45 years of age. Cerebrospinal fluid findings include minimal lymphocytic pleocytosis and elevated protein levels. The major involvement by this syndrome has been limited to the CNS, although one patient developed a generalized granulomatous angiitis. The diagnosis can only be made from brain biopsy specimens or at autopsy. Corticosteroids may have had a saluatory effect in some cases, but the disease has been invariably fatal. On clinical and pathologic grounds, this syndrome is distinct from sarcoidosis, giant cell arteritis, and Wegener's granulomatosis. Central nervous system vasculitis also may accompany or follow ophthalmic zoster; in some instances, varicella-zoster virus has been cultured from involved cerebral blood vessels.

A subacute meningoencephalitis usually occurs early in the course of the Vogt-Koyanagi-Harada syndrome.[95–97] The diagnosis is established by the development of severe, protracted, granulomatous uveitis and depigmentary skin changes such as poliosis (whitening of the eyebrows and eyelashes) and vitiligo. The CNS disease gradually resolves spontaneously.

Of the patients with Behçet's disease (recurrent oral and genital ulcerations and iridocyclitis) 10–25 percent develop CNS involvement.[98] The neurologic manifestations are variable, severe, and progressive in most cases. Occasionally, they precede other features of the syndrome. All parts of the neuraxis may be involved. Cerebrospinal fluid abnormalities include a slight elevation of protein levels and minimal pleocytosis.

The syndrome of "chronic benign lymphocytic meningitis"[99] defines a small group of patients with unexplained headache and lymphocytic pleocytosis but no focal signs. In one series, clinical remission occurred in all patients within 7–25 weeks. The relationship of this syndrome to aseptic meningitis and benign intracranial hypertension is not clear. However, it seems likely that a small group of patients with unexplained chronic meningitis—chosen to exclude those with focal signs, progressive neurologic involvement, and marked CSF abnormalities—have a self-limited illness.

In contrast to the patients with unexplained minimal, self-limited disease, an additional group of patients have an enigmatic chronic meningitis with significant neurologic involvement, a high CSF protein concentration, and sometimes a depressed glucose level.[1] The prognosis in this group is poor. Therapeutic trials may alter the course of the disease, the cultures, and the pathologic findings. A specific diagnosis may be apparent at autopsy, but this is not always the case. A temporal response to antifungal therapy in some cases has implicated an infectious etiology, and mycotic meningitis too often is associated with negative CSF cultures (as discussed above) and only diagnosed postmortem. Therefore a thorough diagnostic evaluation followed ultimately by meningeal and brain biopsy and, if appropriate, an empirical trial of emphotericin B therapy is indicated in this type of patient.

THE IMMUNOCOMPROMISED PATIENT

Chronic meningitis in the immunosuppressed patient with impaired cellular immunity requires special consideration because of the distinctive differential diagnosis. Among renal transplant recipients and patients with lymphoma and leukemia, *Cryptococcus neoformans* is the most common etiology of chronic meningitis.[100] *Listeria monocytogenes, M. tuberculosis, Toxoplasma gondii, Nocardia, Histoplasma*, and *Coccidioides* also cause chronic meningitis more often in such patients.

In the severely immunocompromised patient, progressive multifocal leukoencephalopathy (caused by papovaviruses) may produce profound focal neurologic deficits with minimal or no abnormalities in the CSF. Computed tomographic scans in such cases demonstrate low-density, nonenhancing, progressive lesions in the white matter without mass effect. The list of opportunistic pathogens associated with chronic meningitis in patients with AIDS is long and continues to increase.[101,102] *Cryptococcus neoformans, Toxoplasma gondii, Mycobacterium avium-intracellulare*, and cytomegalovirus were noted early during the AIDS epidemic; they were followed later by papovavirus, *Mycobacterium tuberculosis, Treponema pallidum, Candida* sp., and others including the human immunodeficiency virus (HIV) itself. Aseptic meningitis may be associated with the initial seroconversion to HIV or may occur later in the course of HIV infection; occasionally it may be chronic or recurrent and involve cranial nerves V–VIII and XII.[103] The CSF usually shows a mononuclear pleocytosis, normal glucose, and mildly elevated protein levels. It is possible that infection of the meninges is a usual concomitant of HIV infection, even when asymptomatic.[104] Of greater concern is the AIDS dementia complex, a progressive decline in mentation and motor function that ultimately occurs in up to two-thirds of AIDS patients. Pathologic studies have demonstrated HIV in the brain, in particular in macrophages, microglia, and multinucleated cells derived from these, thus implicating the blood monocyte as a vehicle for entry of HIV into the CNS.

Patients with AIDS are also at risk for primary CNS lymphoma as well as metastatic neoplasms.[101,102] Recognition that a patient is at increased risk of AIDS, therefore, becomes crucial in considering the differential diagnosis of chronic meningitis.

REFERENCES

1. Ellner JJ, Bennett JE. Chronic meningitis. Medicine (Baltimore). 1976;55:341.
2. Wilhelm C, Ellner JJ. Chronic meningitis. Neurol Clin. 1986;4:115.
3. Salaki JS, Louria DB, Chmel H. Fungal and yeast infections of the central nervous system: A clinical review. Medicine (Baltimore). 1984;63:108.
4. Hermans PE, Goldstein NP, Wellman WE. Mollaret's meningitis and differential diagnosis of recurrent meningitis. Am J Med. 1972;52:128.
5. Haynes BF, Wright R, McCracken JP. Mollaret's meningitis: A report of three cases. JAMA. 1976;236:1967.
6. Bartleson JD, Swanson JW, Whisnant JP. A migrainous syndrome with cerebrospinal fluid pleocytosis. Neurology (NY). 1981;31:1257.
7. Swartz M. Chronic meningitis—many causes to consider. N Engl J Med. 1987;317:957.
8. Peacock JE Jr, McGinnis MR, Cohen MS. Persistent neutrophilic meningitis: Report of four cases and review of the literature. Medicine (Baltimore). 1984;63:379.
9. Sawyer J, Ellner J, Ransohoff DF. To biopsy or not to biopsy in suspected herpes simplex encephalitis: A quantitative analysis. Med Decis Making. 1988;8:95.
10. Goodson JD, Strauss GM. Diagnosis of lymphomatous leptomeningitis by cerebrospinal fluid lymphocyte cell surface markers. Am J Med. 1979;66:1057.
11. Plouffe JF, Fass RJ. *Histoplasma* meningitis. Diagnostic value of cerebrospinal fluid serology. Ann Intern Med. 1980;92:189.
12. Wheat J, French M, Batteiger B, et al. Cerebrospinal fluid *Histoplasma* antibodies in central nervous system histoplasmosis. Arch Intern Med. 1985;145:1237.
13. Wheat LJ, Kohler RB, Tewari RP. Diagnosis of disseminated histoplasmosis by detection of *Histoplasma capsulatum* antigen in serum and urine specimens. N Engl J Med. 1986;314:83.
14. Plouffe JF, Silva J, Fekety R, Baird I. Cerebrospinal fluid lymphocyte transformations in meningitis. Arch Intern Med. 1979;139:191.
15. Radin SB, Phair JP, Shaughnessy M, et al. Production of specific IgG antibody to purified protein derivative in the central nervous system in a patient with tuberculous meningitis (Abstract). Clin Res. 1982;30:738.
16. Mardh P-A, Larsson L. Hoiby N, et al. Tuberculostearic acid as a diagnostic marker in tuberculous meningitis. Lancet. 1983;1:367.
17. Ewing GE, Bose GJ, Petersen PK. *Sporothrix schenckii* meningitis in a farmer with Hodgkin's disease. Am J Med. 1980;68:455.
18. Kravitz GR, Davies SF, Eckman MR, et al. Chronic blastomycotic meningitis. Am J Med. 1981;71:501.
19. New FJ, Davis KR. The role of CT scanning in diagnosis of infections of the central nervous system. In: Remington JS, Swartz MN, eds. Current Clinical Topics in Infectious Diseases. v. 1. New York: McGraw-Hill; 1980:1.
20. Stocksill MT, Kauffman CA. Comparison of cryptococcal and tuberculous meningitis. Arch Neurol. 1983;40:81.
21. Rich AR, McCordock HA. The pathogenesis of tuberculous meningitis. Bull Johns Hopkins Hosp. 1933;52:5.
22. Merritt HH, Fremont-Smith F. Cerebrospinal fluid in tuberculous meningitis. Arch Neurol Psychol. 1935;33:516.
23. Lepper MH, Spies HW. The present status of the treatment of tuberculosis of the central nervous system. Ann NY Acad Sci. 1963;106:106.
24. Weiss W, Flippin HF. The changing incidence and prognosis of tuberculous meningitis. Am J Med Sci. 1965;50:46.
25. Barrett-Connor EB. Tuberculous meningitis in adults. South Med J. 1967;60:1061.
26. Kennedy DH, Fallon FJ. Tuberculous meningitis. JAMA. 1979;241:264.
27. Jeren T, Beus I. Characteristics of cerebrospinal fluid in tuberculous meningitis. Acta Cytol (Baltimore). 1982;26:678.
28. Daniel TM. New approaches to the rapid diagnosis of tuberculous meningitis. J Infect Dis. 1987;155:599.
29. Spickard A, Butler WT, Andriole V, et al. The improved prognosis of cryptococcal meningitis with amphotericin B therapy. Ann Intern Med. 1963;58:66.
30. Butler WT, Alling DW, Spickard A, et al. Diagnostic and prognostic value of clinical and laboratory findings in cryptococcal meningitis. A follow-up study of forty patients. N Engl J Med. 1964;270:59.
31. Littman ML, Walter JE. Cryptococcosis: Current status. Am J Med. 1968;45:922.
32. Diamond RD, Bennett JE. Prognostic factors in cryptococcal meningitis. A study of 111 cases. Ann Intern Med. 1974;80:176.
33. Kovacs JA, Kovacs AA, Polis M, et al. Cryptococcosis in the acquired immunodeficiency syndrome. Ann Intern Med. 1985;103:533.
34. Zuger A, Louie E, Holzman RS, et al. Cryptococcal disease in patients with the acquired immunodeficiency syndrome: Diagnostic features and outcome of treatment. Ann Intern Med. 1986;104:234.
35. Smith CE, Saito MT, Simons SA. Pattern of 39,500 serologic tests in coccidioidomycosis. JAMA. 1956;160:546.
36. Winn WA. The treatment of coccidioidal meningitis. The use of amphotericin B in a group of 25 patients. Calif Med. 1964;101:75.
37. Winn WA. Coccidioidal meningitis: A follow-up report. In: Ajello L, ed. Coccidioimycosis. Tucson: University of Arizona Press; 1967:55.
38. Candill RG, Smith CE, Reinarz JA. Coccidioidal meningitis. A diagnostic challenge. Am J Med. 1970;49:360.
39. Deresinski SC, Stevens DA. Coccidioidomycosis in compromised hosts. Medicine (Baltimore). 1974;54:377.
40. Bouza E, Dreyer JS, Hewitt WL, et al. Coccidioidal meningitis. An analysis of 31 cases and review of the literature. Medicine (Baltimore). 1981:60:139.
41. Tynes BS, Crutcher JC, Utz JP. Histoplasma meningitis. Ann Intern Med. 1963;59:615.
42. Smith JW, Utz JP. Progressive disseminated histoplasmosis. Ann Intern Med. 1972;76:557.
43. Gilden DH, Miller EM, Johnson WG. Central nervous system histoplasmosis after rhinoplasty. Neurology (Minn). 1974;24:874.
44. Gelfand JA, Bennett JE. Active *Histoplasma* meningitis of 22 years duration. JAMA. 1975;233:1294.
45. DeVita VT, Utz JP, Williams T, et al. *Candida* meningitis. Arch Intern Med. 1966;117:527.
46. Bayer AS, Edwards JE Jr, Seidel JS, et al. *Candida* meningitis. Medicine (Baltimore). 1976;55:477.
47. Merritt HH, Adams RD, Solomon HC. Neurosyphilis. New York: Oxford University Press; 1946:24.

48. Hooshmand H, Escobar MR, Kopf SW. Neurosyphilis, a study of 241 patients. JAMA. 1972;219:726.
49. Pachner AR, Steere AC. The triad of neurologic manifestations of Lyme disease: Meningitis, cranial neuritis, and radiculoneuritis. Neurology (NY). 1985;35:47.
50. Wilske B, Schierz G, Preac-Mursic V, et al. Intrathecal production of specific antibodies against *Borrelia burgdorferi* in patients with lymphocytic meningoradiculitis (Bannworth's syndrome). J Infect Dis. 1986;153:304.
51. Nelson-Jones A. Neurologic complications of undulant fever. Lancet. 1951;1:495.
52. Nichols E. Meningoencephalitis due to brucellosis. Ann Intern Med. 1951;35:673.
53. Fincham RW, Sahs AL, Joynt RJ. Protean manifestations of nervous system brucellosis. JAMA. 1963;184:97.
54. Reddin JL, Anderson RK, Jenness R, et al. Significance of 7S and macroglobulin brucella agglutinins in human brucellosis. N Engl J Med. 1965;272:1263.
55. Bouza E, Garcia de la Torre M, Parras F, et al. Brucellar meningitis. Rev Infect Dis. 1987;9:810.
56. Scott EN, Kauman L, Brown AC, et al. Serologic studies in the diagnosis and management of meningitis due to *Sporothrix schenckii*. N Engl J Med. 1987;317:935.
57. Wilhelmj CM. The primary meningeal form of systemic blastomycosis. Am J Med Sci. 1925;169:172.
58. Buechner HA, Clawson CM. Blastomycosis of the central nervous system. II. A report of nine cases from the Veterans Administration Cooperative Study. Am Rev Respir Dis. 1967;95:820.
59. Pereira WC, Raphael A, Tehuto RA, et al. Localizacao encefalica da blastomicose sul-Americana: Consideracoes a proposito de 9 casos. Arq Neuropsiquiat. 1965;23:113.
60. Bennett JE, Bonner H, Jennings AE, et al. Chronic meningitis caused by *Cladosporium trichoides*. Am J Clin Pathol. 1973;59:398.
61. Bolton CF, Ashenhurst EM. Actinomycosis of the brain. Case report and review of the literature. Can Med Assoc J. 1964;90:922.
62. Brown JR: Human actinomycosis. Hum Pathol. 1973;4:319.
63. Albright L, Toczek S, Brenner VJ, et al. Osteomyelitis and epidural abscess caused by *Arachnia proprionica*. J Neurosurg. 1974;40:115.
64. Smego RA Jr. Actinomycosis of the central nervous system. Rev Infect Dis. 1987;9:855.
65. King RB, Stoops WL, Fitzgibbons J, et al. *Nocardia asteroides* meningitis. A case successfully treated with large doses of sulfadiazine and urea. J Neurosurg. 1966;24:749.
66. Richter RW, Silva M, Neu HC, et al. The neurological aspects of *Nocardia asteroides* infection. Infect Nervous System. 1968;44:424.
67. Kramer W. Frontiers of neurological diagnosis in acquired toxoplasmosis. Psychiatr Neurol Neurochirg. 1966;69:43.
68. Townsend JJ, Wolinsky JS, Baringer JR, et al. Acquired toxoplasmosis. A neglected cause of treatable nervous system disease. Arch Neurol. 1975;32:335.
69. Grines C, Plouffe JF, Baird IM, et al. *Toxoplasma* meningoencephalitis with hypoglycorrhachia. Arch Intern Med. 1981;141:935.
70. Denti JH. Cysticercosis cerebri-cestode infestation of the human brain. JAMA. 1957;164:401.
71. Lombardo LL, Mateos JH. Cerebral cysticercosis in Mexico. Neurology (Minn). 1961;11:824.
72. Loo L, Braude A. Cerebral cysticercosis in San Diego. A report of 23 cases and a review of the literature. Medicine (Baltimore). 1982;61:341.
73. Jones PG, Gilman RM, Medeiros AA, et al. Focal intracranial mucormycosis presenting as chronic meningitis. JAMA. 1981;24:2063.
74. Moore EW, Thomas LB, Shaw RK, et al. The central nervous system in acute leukemia. Arch Intern Med. 1960;105:451.
75. Hyman CB, Boyle JM, Brubaker CA, et al. Central nervous system involvement by leukemia in children. Blood. 1965;25:1.
76. Griffin JW, Thompson RW, Mitchinson MJ, et al. Lymphomatous leptomeningitis. Am J Med. 1971;51:200.
77. Berg L. Hypoglycorrhachia of noninfectious origin: Diffuse meningeal neoplasia. Neurology (Minn). 1953;3:811.
78. Fischer-Williams M, Bosanquet FD, Daniel P. Carcinomatosis of the meninges. Brain. 1955;78:42.
79. Dinsdale HB, Taghavy A. Carcinomatosis of the meninges. Can Med Assoc J. 1964;90:505.
80. Vital C, Bruno-Martin F, Henry P, et al. La carcinomatose méningée. Bordeaux Med. 1970;12:2927.
81. Olson ME, Cherniak NL, Posner JB. Infiltration of the meninges by systemic cancer: A clinical and pathologic study. Arch Neurol. 1974;30:122.
82. Gonzalez-Vitale JC, Garcia-Bunvel R. Meningeal carcinomatosis. Cancer. 1976;37:2906.
83. Shuttleworth E, Allen N. CSF β-glucuronidase assay in the diagnosis of neoplastic meningitis. Arch Neurol. 1980;37:684.
84. Wiederholt WC, Siekert RB. Neurological manifestations of sarcoidosis. Neurology (Minn). 1965;15:1147.
85. Mathews WB. Sarcoidosis of the nervous system. J Neurol Neurosurg Psychiatry. 1965;28:23.
86. Gaines JD, Eckman PB, Remington JS. Low CSF glucose level in sarcoidosis involving the central nervous system. Arch Intern Med. 1970;125:333.
87. Douglas AC, Maloney AFJ. Sarcoidosis of the central nervous system. J Neurol Neurosurg Psychiatry. 1973;36:1024.
88. Delaney P. Neurological manifestations in sarcoidosis. Ann Intern Med. 1977;87:336.
89. Grizzanti JN, Knapp AB, Schecter AJ, et al. Treatment of sarcoid meningitis with radiotherapy. Am J Med. 1982;73:605.
90. Kolodny EM, Rebeiz JJ, Caviness VS, et al. Granulomatous angiitis of the central nervous system. Arch Neurol. 1968;19:510.
91. Nurick S, Blackwood W, Mair WGP. Giant cell granulomatous angiitis of the central nervous system. Brain. 1972;95:133.
92. Mohr JP, Powell HC. Clinicopathologic conference. Headache and progressive mental deterioration in a 45-year-old man. N Engl J Med. 1976;295:944.
93. Cupps TR, Moore PM, Fauci AS. Isolated angiitis of the central nervous system. Prospective diagnostic and therapeutic experience. Am J Med. 1983;74:97.
94. Reik L, Grunnet ML, Spencer RP, et al. Granulomatous angiitis presenting as chronic meningitis and ventriculitis. Neurology (NY). 1983;33:1609.
95. Cowper AR. Harada's disease and Vogt-Koyanagi syndrome. AMA Arch Ophthal. 1951;45:367.
96. Pattison EM. Uveomeningoencephalitis syndrome. Arch Neurol (Chicago). 1965;12:197.
97. Riehl J-L, Andrews JM. The uveomeningoencephalitis syndrome. Neurology (Minn). 1966;16:603.
98. Schotland DL, Wolf SM, White HH, et al. Neurologic aspects of Behçets disease. Am J Med. 1963;34:544.
99. Hopkins AP, Harvey PKP. Chronic benign lymphocytic meningitis. J Neurol Sci. 1973;18:443.
100. Hooper DC, Pruitt AA, Rubin RH. Central nervous system infection in the chronically immunosuppressed. Medicine (Baltimore). 1982;61:166.
101. Gopinathan G, Laubenstein LJ, Mondale B, et al. Central nervous system manifestations of the acquired immunodeficiency syndrome. (Abstract). Neurology (NY). 1983;33(Suppl):105.
102. Snider WD, Simpson DM, Nielsen S, et al. Neurological complications of the acquired immunodeficiency syndrome. Ann Neurol. 1983;14:403.
103. Bredesen DE, Lipkin WI, Messing R. Prolonged recurrent aseptic meningitis with prominent cranial nerve abnormalities: A new epidemic in gay men (Abstract). Neurology (NY). 33(Suppl):85.

68. ENCEPHALITIS, MYELITIS, AND NEURITIS

DIANE E. GRIFFIN
RICHARD T. JOHNSON

Encephalitis, myelitis, and *neuritis* mean inflammations of brain, spinal cord, and peripheral nerves, respectively. If sensory or motor spinal roots are specifically involved, the term *radiculitis* may be used. Since meningeal inflammation often accompanies these inflammatory processes, compounded terms such as *meningoencephalitis* and *meningoencephalomyelitis* are sometimes used. None of these terms, however, differentiates between the inflammatory diseases caused by direct invasion of agents and the post- or parainfectious demyelinating processes that may involve the brain, spinal cord, or peripheral nerve. Because of the diversity of clinical symptoms and signs that can occur with these inflammatory diseases, infectious or parainfectious causes must be entertained in the differential diagnosis of a great variety of neurologic diseases. As in the diagnosis of all neurologic disease, the differential diagnosis will be determined by the temporal evolution of signs and symptoms and by the localization of the disease process to one or more anatomic sites by physical findings. Systemic involvement of skin, lung, salivary glands, gastrointestinal tract, and so forth, or fever may suggest an infectious cause, but these may also be absent.

ENCEPHALITIS AND MYELITIS

This section will deal with infectious and postinfectious encephalitis and myelitis together since they are often considered in the same differential diagnosis and have considerable overlap in manifestation and causation. Peripheral neuropathies due to infectious agents are rare and will be considered, along with tetanus, in a separate section.

Pathogenesis and Pathologic Characteristics

Infectious agents can produce clinical symptoms and signs within the central nervous system (CNS) by either direct or indirect involvement of neural tissue. Infectious agents can invade the CNS by several pathways. The most common is via the blood. This is best documented for viral infections but probably is also important in rickettsial, bacterial, and fungal infections.[1–3] The initial site of entry of a pathogen and the primary site of replication may be the respiratory tract (measles, mumps, influenza, varicella-zoster, *Mycobacterium tuberculosis, Cryptococcus neoformans*), gastrointestinal tract (poliovirus, coxsackievirus, echovirus) or subcutaneous tissue (togaviruses, *Rickettsia rickettsia, R. typhi*, trypanosomes). Involvement of the CNS is, for the most part, an infrequent consequence of common infections.[1]

In certain viral infections, entry into the CNS occurs by way of the peripheral nerves. Transport systems within motor and sensory axons carry substances from the cell body to the periphery (anterograde transport) and from the periphery to the cell body (retrograde transport). The neural route of entry is important in viral infections such as rabies[4] and occasionally poliomyelitis.[5] Retrograde transport from the skin or mucous membranes moves herpes simplex and varicella-zoster viruses into sensory ganglia at the time of primary infection, and anterograde transport carries reactivated virus from the ganglia to the periphery during exacerbations.[6] On occasion reactivated virus may also be carried retrograde to the CNS. Retrograde transport of herpes simplex virus by nerves innervating the dura from the trigeminal ganglion may contribute to the unique temporal lobe localization of herpes simplex virus encephalitis.[7]

Entry of infectious agents into the CNS by way of the exposed olfactory nerves in the nasal mucosa has been demonstrated in experimental animals[8] but is of proven clinical importance only in the entry of free-living amebas into the olfactory and frontal lobes through the nasal mucosa and across the cribiform plate.[9]

Once within the CNS, only selected cells may be infected, giving rise to variations in clinical manifestations. Neuronal infection may cause seizure activity, which, depending on the areas involved, may be focal or generalized. Infection of oligodendroglia may cause demyelination alone. Cortical infection or reactive parenchymal swelling may give rise to changes in the state of consciousness,[10] and infection of specific brain stem neurons can cause coma or respiratory failure.[11]

In fatal viral encephalitis an inflammatory reaction is usually prominent in the meninges and in a perivascular distribution within the brain. Although the perivascular inflammatory reaction is composed predominantly of mononuclear cells, polymorphonuclear cells may be evident. Neural cells may show degenerative changes, and apparent phagocytosis of neurons by macrophages or microglial cells (neuronophagia) is often found. Myelin pallor, glial nodules, and giant cells containing viral antigen are found in the brain of patients with acquired immunodeficiency syndrome (AIDS)-related dementia.[12,13] Spinal cord lesions in human immunodeficiency virus infections may include vacuolar myelopathy[14] and gracile tract degeneration.[15] Whether these pathologic changes are direct or indirect consequences of virus infection is not yet clear. Intranuclear inclusion bodies are seen in herpesvirus,[6] adenovirus,[16] and subacute and chronic forms of measles virus infections.[17] Cytomegalovirus infections produce characteristic pathologic changes with the induction of cytomegalic cells containing inclusion bodies.[18] Negri bodies are found in rabies virus encephalitis.[19]

Rickettsiae tend to invade and to multiply in vascular endothelial cells, resulting in widespread vasculitis of capillaries, arterioles, and small arteries,[20] including the retina.

Infectious agents can give rise to signs or symptoms suggesting encephalitis or myelitis without actually invading CNS parenchyma. One mechanism is by the development of adhesive meningitis and vasculitis during the course of subacute or chronic leptomeningeal infections. In chronic tuberculosis, fungal or syphilitic meningitis, or in untreated or partially treated bacterial meningitis, the chronic meningeal reaction may cause obstruction of cerebrospinal fluid (CSF) flow, causing hydrocephalus, cranial nerve palsies, or gliosis in the underlying cerebral cortex. In addition, the vasculitis involving large vessels may lead to infarctions of brain and focal neurologic deficits. This sequence of events is frequently observed in tuberculosis,[21] aspergillosis,[22] and meningovascular neurosyphilis.[23] Syphilis of the meningovascular type appears relatively early in the course of this disease, and, in contrast to the parenchymatous manifestations (tabes dorsalis and paresis) that appear later, is inflammatory and often reversible. *Cryptococcus*, produces a chronic meningitis with little inflammatory reaction.[24] In chronic bacterial or fungal meningitis, organization of a subarachnoid exudate at the base of the brain may lead to communicating hydrocephalus and cranial nerve palsies.[25]

In the acute demyelinating diseases complicating viral exanthems or respiratory infections, it is not known whether invasion into the CNS is a prerequisite to disease. These diseases involve either central myelin (postinfectious myelitis or encephalomyelitis) or peripheral myelin (Guillain-Barré syndrome), and the pathogenesis of these syndromes is thought to be related to a sensitization of the infected person to central or peripheral myelin.[26] This mechanism is analogous to neurologic complications of neural tissue-derived rabies vaccines.[27,28]

The pathologic changes of postinfectious and postvaccinal encephalomyelitis are characterized by perivascular infiltration of mononuclear inflammatory cells and perivenous demyelination.[29,30] Acute hemorrhagic leukoencephalitis, characterized by fibrinoid necrosis of arterioles and hemorrhage as well as the perivenular demyelination, is thought to represent a more severe form of postinfectious encephalomyelitis.[30]

On the other hand, Reye syndrome is a distinct acute encephalopathy of unknown cause that usually follows a viral infection. This syndrome affects children and is characterized by acute fatty liver and a noninflammatory cerebral edema. Reye syndrome has been most commonly associated with influenza A and B virus infections, although cases have been reported after varicella and many other viral infections.[31] The pathogenesis of this disease and its relationship to the prior infection and/or medications taken during the prior illness are not completely understood.[32] Likewise, the role of the organism in the encephalopathy associated with cat-scratch disease is unknown.[33].

Clinical Findings

Infections limited to the leptomeninges manifest with signs and symptoms of meningeal irritation: headache, stiff neck, and pleocytosis. If the meningeal process is chronic, as in tuberculosis, manifesting symptoms and signs may be of a communicating hydrocephalus (headache, nausea and vomiting, mental deterioration, or spastic paraparesis) and/or of localized infarction secondary to vasculitis.[34] The chronic form of cryptococcal meningitis may manifest as progressive mental deterioration and headache, rather than with fever and meningismus, as seen in the more acute form.[25,35]

Patients with viral encephalitis usually have signs and symptoms of meningeal inflammation, but in addition to headache, fever, and nuchal rigidity, encephalitis is characterized by alterations of consciousness: Mild lethargy may progress to confusion, stupor, and coma. Focal neurologic signs usually develop, and seizures are common. Motor weakness, accentuated deep tendon reflexes, and extensor plantar responses may be observed. Abnormal movements are seen in some cases of encephalitis, and, rarely, a tremor characteristic of Parkinson's disease may develop. The hypothalamic pituitary area may be involved, causing severe hyperthermia or poikilothermia, diabetes insipidus, and inappropriate antidiuretic hormone secretion. Involvement of the spinal cord can lead to flaccid paralysis, depression of tendon reflexes, and paralysis of bowel and bladder. Increased intracranial pressure can cause papilledema and third and sixth cranial nerve palsies.

In herpes simplex encephalitis signs often include bizarre behavior, hallucinations, and aphasia, suggesting the temporal lobe localization typical of that infection.[36] Rabies may begin with local paresthesia at the site of the bite.[37] A parkinsonian syndrome is common in Japanese encephalitis.[38] Acute contralateral hemiparesis may occur after herpes zoster ophthalmicus related to a localized cerebral angiitis, causing frontal lobe infarction.[39] With Lyme disease, both peripheral and CNS complications occur, ranging from severe meningoencephalitis to isolated cranial nerve palsies.[40,41]

Myelitis can occur, with or without encephalitis. Transverse myelitis simulates acute transection of the cord with rostral limb weakness, sensory level, and the loss of control of bowel and bladder. Ascending myelitis leads to an ascending flaccid paralysis and rising sensory deficit and is characterized by early bowel and bladder involvement. Poliomyelitis, where anterior horn cells are involved primarily, typically causes flaccid paralysis and muscular pain without sensory loss or bladder dysfunction.

In postinfectious encephalomyelitis the time lapse between the primary viral infection, rash in measles, varicella, rubella, or parotid swelling in mumps, and the onset of symptoms referable to the nervous system ranges between 2 and 12 days. The onset is often abrupt, with depression of consciousness or seizure.[26,30,31]

Systemic findings of particular importance are the rashes of Lyme disease, Rocky Mountain spotted fever (palms and soles), typhus, varicella, and herpes zoster. An exanthem is also occasionally seen with *Mycoplasma*, coxsackievirus, and echovirus infections. A history of tick bite is usually obtained in Rocky Mountain spotted fever, Lyme disease, ehrlichiosis, and Colorado tick fever. A history of animal or bat bite may be obtained in rabies, although most patients in the United States never give such a history.[42]

Mycobacterial and fungal infections often present as chronic and, on occasion, fluctuating disease, but in certain cases (mucormycosis) they may progress very rapidly.

Bacterial infections usually manifest with an acute onset, but certain infections such as neurosyphilis, Lyme disease, relapsing fever, brain abscess, and Whipple's disease may have an insidious onset and an indolent, chronic, or even fluctuating course. The neurologic features of Whipple's disease may include dementia, supranuclear ophthalmoplegia, myoclonus, spastic paresis, ataxis, and papilledema. The patient may have neurologic signs and symptoms without significant manifestations of malabsorption.[43] The rickettsial diseases are usually acute in onset with fever, headache, and myalgias. Rocky Mountain spotted fever is associated with a rash before or after neurologic disease,[44] while there is no rash in ehrlichiosis.[45]

Viral infections also may be acute, subacute, or chronic. Encephalitis due to adenovirus and enteroviruses has occurred both as acute disease in immunologically healthy individuals[1,46] and as subacute disease in immunologically compromised individuals.[16,47] Certain of the "slow virus infections" such as Creutzfeldt-Jakob disease, subacute sclerosing panencephalitis, rubella panencephalitis, AIDS encephalopathy, tropical spastic paraparesis, and progressive multifocal leukoencephalopathy are slowly progressive disease with an insidious onset and absence of fever.[1,48–50]

Laboratory Findings

Peripheral blood counts are rarely helpful in this group of diseases since they may be normal or show a moderate leukocytosis or leukopenia. Peripheral blood smears may show atypical lymphocytes in Epstein-Barr virus infections, the diagnostic gametocytes of *Plasmodium falciparum* malaria, the morulae of *Ehrlichia*, the borreliae in relapsing fever, or the trypanosomes in trypanosomiasis. The serum amylase level may be elevated in mumps virus infection. Pulmonary infiltrates may accompany lymphocytic choriomeningitis virus, typhus, and *Mycoplasma* infections.

CSF examination is essential. The pleocytosis of viral encephalomyelitis is variable (10–2000 cells/mm^3), and mononuclear cells usually predominate, although early in any of these diseases, there may be no cells or polymorphonuclear cells may be present in considerable numbers. Repeat examination of the CSF in 24 hours is often useful.[51] Significant numbers of red blood cells may be found in herpesvirus,[52] acute necrotizing hemorrhagic leukoencephalitis,[53] and *Naegleria* encephalitis.[54] In the chronic fungal and bacterial meningitides a moderate mononuclear pleocytosis is usually found. Meningoencephalitis due to the free-living amebas, *Nocardia, Actinomyces, Candida,* and *Aspergillus* elicit a polymorphonuclear response.[54,55]

The CSF protein level is usually elevated, and in chronic infections an increased proportion of this protein is IgG (normal is $<$12 percent).[56] Under normal conditions CSF IgG is derived primarily from the serum, but antibodies are present at about $\frac{1}{200}$ the concentration.[57] During acute inflammatory reactions a transudate of protein occurs, including serum immunoglobulins. During convalescence plasma cells may produce a specific IgG within the CNS, as seen after mumps meningitis,[58] herpes simplex,[52] and zoster[59] encephalitis. In chronic infection examination of the CSF for specific antibody can be diagnostic in syphilis[60] Lyme disease,[61] tropical spastic paraparesis,[43] subacute sclerosing,[62] and rubella panencephalitis[63] and may be useful, when compared with serum levels, in the viral, rickettsial, and bacterial encephalitides for which antibody tests are available. If antibody to a particular pathogen is present at a comparable or higher amount in CSF compared with serum and the CSF protein is only moderately elevated, it is indicative of CNS infection with the agent.

For diagnosis by serum antibodies, it is important to obtain serum early in the course (acute phase) for comparison with serum taken after 1–3 weeks of illness to demonstrate a significant antibody increase.[64] This diagnosis is often of more than academic interest since presumptive therapy begun early may then be discontinued if a diagnosis is established. Tests for cold agglutinins and heterophile antibody may be suggestive but may yield false negatives in the diagnosis of *Mycoplasma* and Epstein-Barr virus infections, respectively; therefore, organism-specific antibody tests need to be done. Myelin basic protein may be present in diseases associated with central demyelination.[65]

The CSF glucose level is usually within the normal range during viral or rickettsial infections of CNS, although a mild depression may be seen. The glucose level is usually low in tuberculous,[66] fungal,[25] bacterial, or amoebic infections.[54]

Direct examination of the CSF by Gram stain for bacteria, by acid-fast stain for mycobacteria, and by India ink for *Cryptococcus* should be performed and may be diagnostic. Wet preparation of CSF may reveal *Naegleria*, and Giemsa stain will identify trypanosomes. Bacteria, mycobacteria, fungi, and viruses may also be recovered from the CSF by appropriate culture techniques, Microbial antigen detection methods are sometimes more sensitive than cultures and have proved particularly useful in cryptococcal meningitis.[35] Brain biopsy is necessary to diagnose herpes simplex virus encephalitis definitively.[36]

Etiology of Encephalomyelitis

Table 1 lists the viruses known to cause acute encephalitis or myelitis in the United States, as well as the viruses associated with postinfectious encephalomyelitis. Many of these infections have distinct seasonal variations that are helpful in narrowing the differential diagnosis (Fig. 1). The togavirus, flavivirus, and bunyavirus encephalitides (except rubella) are arthropod borne and therefore occur when their insect vectors are biting, generally in spring and summer. The mosquito-borne California and western equine encephalitides peak in August, and St. Louis encephalitis peaks somewhat later.[67,68] The tick-borne diseases occur most often in spring and early summer.[69–71] Enterovirus infections, and therefore their complications, are more common in late summer and fall, and mumps is most common in the winter and spring. In contrast, the herpesvirus encephalitides occur throughout the year. Lymphocytic choriomeningitis virus is most frequent in the winter when rodents come indoors, and leptospirosis is more common in the warm months when rodents and people are in contact with ponds and streams.[64]

In addition to the season, geographic occurrence and travel histories may be helpful in the diagnosis of vector-borne encephalitides. For instance, eastern equine encephalitis is confined to the Atlantic and Gulf Coast states, and California and St. Louis encephalitides are found primarily in the Midwestern United States. Colorado tick fever and western equine encephalitis are most common in the Western states.[1] Lyme disease is endemic in the Northeast and the upper Midwestern United States, Northern California, and Europe.[72] Japanese encephalitis is found in most of Asia,[73] and tick-borne encephalitis occurs over a wide area of Europe and the Soviet Union.[74]

Infections with eastern equine encephalitis virus produce clinically evident encephalitis with high frequency in all age groups,[75] in contrast to the other alphaviruses, in which the majority of the infections are subclinical. Clinical disease with St. Louis encephalitis virus occurs in about 1 percent of infections, and infants and adults over age 50 are most likely to develop encephalitis.[76] California and western equine encephalitis viruses infect persons of all ages but produce encephalitis predominantly in children.[77,78] Venezuelan equine encephalitis virus primarily causes a flulike illness in humans but can produce encephalitis in any age group.[79]

Nonviral causes of encephalomyelitis are listed in Table 2. Some of these diseases are of known and others of unknown

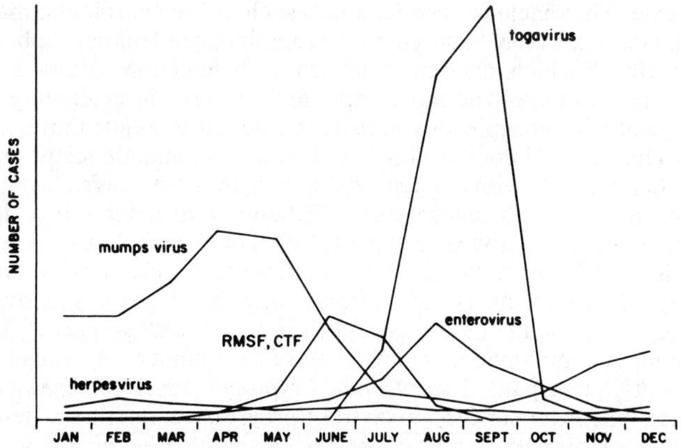

FIG. 1. Seasonal variation in the encephalitides caused by togaviruses, enteroviruses, mumps virus, herpesvirus, Rocky Mountain spotted fever (RMSF), and Colorado tick fever (CTF).

TABLE 1. Viral Causes of Acute Encephalomyelitis

Direct Infection	*Postinfection*
TOGAVIRIDAE	TOGAVIRIDAE
Alphaviruses	Rubivirus
Eastern equine	Rubella
Western equine	MYXOVIRIDAE
Venezuelan equine	Influenzavirus
FLAVIVIRIDAE	Influenza A and B
St. Louis	PARAMYXOVIRIDAE
Murray Valley	Paramyxovirus
West Nile	Mumps
Japanese	Morbillivirus
Dengue	Measles
Tick-borne complex	POXVIRIDAE
BUNYAVIRIDAE	Orthopoxvirus
Bunyavirus	Vaccinia
California	HERPETOVIRIDAE
Rift Valley	Herpesvirus
PARAMYXOVIRIDAE	Varicella-zoster
Paramyxovirus	Epstein-Barr
Mumps	
Morbillivirus	
Measles	
ARENAVIRIDAE	
Arenavirus	
Lymphocytic choriomeningitis	
Machupo	
Lassa	
Junin	
PICORNAVIRIDAE	
Enterovirus	
Poliovirus	
Coxsackievirus	
Echovirus	
REOVIRIDAE	
Colorado tick fever	
RHABDOVIRIDAE	
Lyssavirus	
Rabies	
FILOVIRIDAE	
Ebola	
Marburg	
RETROVIRIDAE	
Lentivirus	
Human immunodeficiency	
HERPETOVIRIDAE	
Herpesvirus	
Herpes simplex types 1 and 2	
Varicella-zoster	
Epstein-Barr	
Cytomegalovirus	
ADENOVIRIDAE	
Adenovirus	

TABLE 2. Nonviral Causes of Encephalomyelitis

Rocky Mountain spotted fever
Typhus
Ehrlichia canis
Mycoplasma
Brucellosis
Subacute bacterial endocarditis
Listeria
Syphilis (meningovascular)
Relapsing fever
Lyme disease
Leptospirosis
Nocardia
Actinomycosis
Tuberculosis
Cryptococcus
Histoplasma
Naegleria
Acanthamoeba
Toxoplasma
Plasmodium falciparum
Trypanosomiasis
Whipple's disease
Behçet's disease
Cat-scratch disease
Vasculitis
Drug reactions

cause. They include drug reactions such as the neuroleptic malignant syndrome[80] and chemotherapy-induced leukoencephalopathy,[81] which may be confused with infection. Many are treatable. One of the most important concerns in evaluating a patient with encephalomyelitis is to rule out treatable entities.

The cause of encephalitis is different in immunodeficient patients. Patients with hypogammaglobulinemia may have chronic encephalitis with enterovirus.[47] Patients with defects in cell-mediated immunity have unusual forms of encephalitis or myelitis with herpesviruses,[18,82–84] a subacute inclusion body encephalitis with measles,[17] chronic encephalitis with adenovirus,[16] and granulomatous encephalitis with *Acanthamoeba*.[85] In acquired immunodeficiency disease a number of unusual agents, principally *Toxoplasma, Cryptococcus*, cytomegalovirus, *Nocardia*, and papovavirus (progressive multifocal leukoencephalopathy), may cause CNS disease, either singly or in combination.[42,86]

Transverse myelitis caused by a vasculitis of the anterior spinal artery has been seen in tuberculosis, syphilis, and schistosomiasis.[87] Postinfectious transverse myelitis has been associated with measles, rubella, mumps, and upper respiratory diseases, as well as with immunizations.[88,89] Direct involvement with varicella-zoster virus may also produce a transverse myelitis or an ascending necrotizing myelitis.[90] Infection with human T-lymphotropic virus type I causes disease primarily in the thoracic cord, leading to progressive spastic paraparesis.[49,50] Infection with human immunodeficiency virus causes myelopathy manifest by spastic paraparesis and sensory ataxia.[48] Dumb rabies after lower extremity bites by rabid vampire bats has also been described as producing an ascending myelitis.[91] The lower motor neuron variety of myelitis may be produced by poliovirus, coxsackievirus, or echovirus.

Presumptive Treatment

Specific therapy is available for most of the diseases listed in Table 2 and should be instituted as soon as possible if a presumptive diagnosis can be made. Tuberculous meningitis is, unfortunately, often a diagnosis of exclusion, and if the clinical picture is compatible and other diagnoses have been excluded, antituberculous therapy should be instituted.

For viral diseases vidarabine and acyclovir are of proven efficacy in herpes simplex virus encephalitis. They are equally efficacious in neonatal infection,[92] but acyclovir is superior in older individuals.[93] In immunocompromised patients acyclovir prevents visceral dissemination of varicella-zoster virus, including encephalitis.[94]

Patients in coma caused by encephalitis or postinfectious encephalomyelitis may make remarkable recoveries even after prolonged periods of unconsciousness. For this reason vigorous supportive treatment is indicated, and the complications of ventilator therapy, catheters, intravenous lines, and so forth, should be avoided if possible and should be treated vigorously if present. Blood glucose levels and electrolytes should be monitored closely, since the hypothalamic area may be involved in the encephalitic process. Seizures should be controlled, if they occur, with diphenylhydantoin. Some fever may be beneficial, but extreme hyperthermia, as well as hypoxia, may aggravate seizures. Cerebral edema can be damaging in itself and should be controlled with glycerol or mannitol, if possible, but steroids should be used if necessary for this purpose.

NEURITIS

Neuritis is an inflammatory disease involving the peripheral nerves. Only leprosy and trypanosomes are known to cause a direct infection leading to clinical signs of peripheral neuropathy, although human immunodeficiency virus and cytomegalovirus may cause disease directly as well.[95] Lyme disease is frequently associated with radiculoneuritis and cranial neuritis.[96] Herpes simplex virus and varicella-zoster virus infect sensory ganglia. Reactivation of herpes simplex virus type 2 has been associated with radiating radicular pain, which may mimic lumbar disk disease.[97] Radicular pain and segmental motor paralysis may accompany herpes zoster, and this may be followed by a postherpetic pain syndrome along the distribution of nerves supplied by the affected ganglia. Three bacterial toxins affect peripheral nerves either directly (diphtheria) or indirectly (tetanus, botulism), each causing distinct syndromes. The Guillain-Barré syndrome may represent a postinfectious inflammatory demyelinating process of peripheral nerves predominantly involving anterior roots.

Pathologic Characteristics and Pathogenesis

In lepromatous leprosy there is little if any immunologic response to the infection. There is a widespread distribution of *Mycobacterium leprae*. Nerves in the skin may exhibit only minor changes, but larger peripheral nerves contain many leprosy bacilli demonstrable in Schwann cells on acid-fast stains. These nerves show little inflammation. The organisms grow best in the cooler parts of the body, and nerves close to skin surface and distal nerves are affected preferentially. In late stages of the disease extensive axonal degeneration may occur.[98]

Tuberculoid leprosy is characterized by a marked granulomatous reaction to the infection and few demonstrable bacilli. Cutaneous nerves beneath the depigmented skin macules are destroyed, producing anesthesia. The peripheral nerves are nodular and thickened, with destruction of the normal architecture. Segmental demyelination and axonal degeneration result in nerve destruction and severe fibrosis.[98] *Trypanosoma cruzi, T. gambiense*, and *T. rhodesiense* all can invade and replicate in tissue of the peripheral as well as the central nervous system. *Trypanosoma cruzi* preferentially damages cells of the autonomic nervous system by replication in the supporting Schwann cells, satellite cells, and capsular fibroblasts rather than in the neurons. In African trypanosomiasis patients dying with encephalomyelitis often have evidence of neuritis.[99]

Tetanus toxin, produced by *Clostridium tetani* under anaerobic conditions, is transported up the axon and binds to the presynaptic endings on motor neurons in the anterior horns of the spinal cord blocking inhibitory input.[100,101] This results in uncontrolled motor input to skeletal muscle and the spasms typical of this disease. Because of this transport mechanism for entry into the CNS, patients may have only localized disease in the area of the *Clostridium*-containing wound.

Botulinum toxin is produced during anaerobic metabolism of *Clostridium botulinum* and may either be ingested as performed toxin or produced by organisms in the intestine (infant botulism) or introduced into a wound (wound botulism). Botulinum toxin binds to the presynaptic axon terminal of the neuromuscular junction, preventing release of acetylcholine and thus producing a flaccid paralysis.[101,102] Little, if any, histologic abnormality is seen in either tetanus or botulism.

Diphtheria toxin is produced by *Corynebacterium diphtheriae* lysogenized by a phage coding for this toxin. The toxin is a protein with two subunits; one (A) inhibits protein synthesis by blocking the adenosine diphosphate (ADP) ribosylation of elongation factor 2, whereas the second (B) binds to cell membranes and therefore enables the active subunit A to enter the cell.[103] The effect of this toxin on peripheral nerves is to cause a noninflammatory demyelination. Both cranial and peripheral nerves may be demyelinated, although cranial nerves are more frequently affected.

The Guillain-Barré syndrome often follows within 4 weeks of a respiratory or gastrointestinal infection, immunization, trauma, or metabolic insult. Infections with a wide spectrum of viruses as well as *Mycoplasma pneumoniae* have been associated with this syndrome. There is an increased incidence in individuals infected with human immunodeficiency virus.[95,104] A history of a nonspecific upper respiratory illness is, however, most common.[105] Nerves show segmental inflammation and demyelination. The inflammatory lesions are composed of mononuclear cells that are perivascular and focal. If nerve destruction has occurred, Wallerian degeneration may be present. Low-grade perivascular inflammation may persist for months to years after the episode.[106] Clinically and pathologically, the Guillain-Barré syndrome closely resembles experimental allergic neuritis, a disease induced in animals by immunization with peripheral nerve myelin.[107] The mechanism of the induction of this sensitization and whether the actual effector mechanism is humoral or cellular are unknown.

Clinical Findings

Leprosy has two distinctive manifestations, depending on whether the disease is of the tuberculoid or the lepromatous type. Tuberculoid leprosy produces a mononeuropathy beneath the sharply demarcated, hypopigmented skin patches. Peripheral nerves may be palpably and visibly enlarged, and the neurologic involvement is a prominent part of the disease. In lepromatous leprosy a distal hypesthesia with a selective loss of pain and temperature is most common, although a mononeuropathy may be present. Cooler areas of the body are more strikingly affected, and the loss of pain sensation results in mutilation and eventual loss of digits.[98]

Tetanus usually manifests with rigidity of muscles, which may be painful. The initial manifestation may be of ''local tetanus'' in which the rigidity affects only one limb or area of the body in which the *Clostridium*-containing wound is located. Stiffness of the jaw muscles causes trismus, and stiffness of the facial muscles may cause a change of expression. This mild picture may progress to generalized rigidity with reflex spasms and dysphagia. The history of a soil-contaminated puncture wound should be sought. The wound may have seemed insignificant at the time of the injury and may appear well healed at the time of the neurologic disease.[108]

Botulism characteristically manifests 12–36 hours after the ingestion of the toxin with weakness, dizziness, and dryness of the mouth. Neurologic symptoms follow within 12–72 hours with blurred vision, diplopia, dysphonia, dysphagia, and muscle weakness. On examination sensation is preserved, the tendon reflexes are depressed or absent, and the paralysis flaccid.[109] The same picture can develop more gradually in a patient with wound botulism. The original wound is usually of a rather severe traumatic nature and may appear to be healing well at the time of neurologic disease.[110]

The earliest sign of pharyngeal diphtheria (5–12 days) is paralysis of the palate, which produces a nasal quality of the voice and an increasing tendency to regurgitate fluids through the nose. Other cranial nerves (particularly the third, sixth, seventh, ninth and tenth) may become involved, with blurring of vision and inability to accommodate as early symptoms. Later in the course of the disease, when previous symptoms may have subsided (4–8 weeks), a predominantly motor polyneuropathy involving initial symmetrical weakness of distal extremities may appear similar to Guillain-Barré syndrome. There is a flaccid paralysis with loss of deep tendon reflexes that may be accompanied by the signs and symptoms of a diphtheritic myocarditis.[111]

Neuropathies associated with human immunodeficiency virus infection include acute and chronic inflammatory demyelinating polyneuropathies, sensory ganglioneuritis and polyradiculopathy early in infection, and a distal symmetrical polyneuropathy later when AIDS has developed.[95]

In approximately 60 percent of the cases, Guillain-Barré syndrome follows an infection or immunization. Clinically it manifests with subjective paresthesias and/or weakness, which may continue to progress for up to 4 weeks.[112] Examination typically reveals a flaccid paralysis with loss of deep tendon reflexes. Involvement of the autonomic nervous system resulting in lability of blood pressure, inappropriate antidiuretic hormone (ADH) secretion, and inability to compensate for volume changes occurs in approximately 20 percent of the cases.[113] These problems frequently necessitate the management of patients in an intensive care unit even though they may not require ventilatory assistance. The condition of an individual patient may change rapidly either during progression or during recovery. Improvement is often slow, however, and may continue for up to 12 months.[112]

Laboratory Findings

Routine blood chemistries are not helpful in this group of diseases. If botulinism is suspected serum for mouse inoculation should be procured. Cerebrospinal fluid should also be obtained. In Guillain-Barré syndrome or diphtheritic polyneuritis an increased protein level with few cells (albuminocytologic dissociation) in the CSF is the characteristic finding; some patients, however may have a normal protein level particularly early in the disease and others, particularly those with human immunodeficiency virus infection, will have a moderate pleocytosis.[104,114] The CSF findings are normal in tetanus, botulism, and leprosy. Neurometric tests that aid in localization of the pathologic changes and thus the diagnosis are (*1*) the measurement of nerve conduction times to look for the slowed conduction found in the peripheral nerve lesions of Guillain-Barré syndrome and diphtheria (F wave measurements may allow the identification of abnormalities if lesions are very proximal) and (*2*) the recording from muscle during repetitive nerve stimulation to look for the incremental response characteristic of botulism[109] and not found in Guillain-Barré syndrome. Nerve biopsies may be useful in identifying the granulomas and/or acid-fast bacilli of leprosy and the inflammatory demyelination of Guillain-Barré syndrome.[115]

Presumptive Treatment

In this group of clinically distinctive diseases it is important to recognize the disease and to treat it appropriately. Most patients with Guillain Barré syndrome benefit from plasmapheresis, especially when performed early in the disease.[104,116] Patients must be closely monitored for vital capacity, electrolytes, blood pressure, temperature, and heart rate and those with respiratory failure should be ventilated mechanically. Patients with autonomic nervous system dysfunction should be treated with short-acting drugs, since autonomic function in these patients may be very labile. A patient who is hypertensive in the morning may be distressingly hypotensive in the evening and vice versa. Patients may not adjust to abrupt changes in intravascular volume, so intravenous fluids should be carefully controlled.

REFERENCES

1. Johnson RT. Viral Infections of the Nervous System. New York: Raven Press; 1982.
2. Mims CA. The Pathogenesis of Infectious Diseases. 2d ed. London: Academic Pres; 1982.
3. Moxon ER, Murphy PA. *Hemophilus influenzae* bacteremia and meningitis resulting from survival of a single organism. Proc Natl Acad Sci USA. 1978;75:1534–6.
4. Murphy FA. Rabies pathogenesis: A brief review. Arch Virol. 1977;54:279.
5. Bodian D, Howe HA, Experimental studies on intraneural spread of poliomyelitis virus. Bull Johns Hopkins Hosp. 1941;68:248–67.

6. Baringer JR. Herpes simplex virus infection of nervous tissue in animals and man. Prog Med Virol. 1975;20:1–26.
7. Davis LE, Johnson RT. A possible explanation for the localization of herpes simplex encephalitis. Ann Neurol. 1979;5:2–5.
8. Monath TP, Cropp CP, Harrison AK. Mode of entry of a neurotropic arbovirus into the central nervous system. Reinvestigation of an old controversy. Lab Invest. 1983;48:399–410.
9. Martinez AJ, Duma RJ, Nelson EC, et al. Experimental *Naegleria* meningoencephalitis in mice. Penetration of the olfactory mucosal epithelium by *Naegleria* and pathologic changes produced: A light and electron microscopic study. Lab Invest. 1973;29:121.
10. Johnson RT. Selective vulnerability of neural cells to viral infection. Brain. 1980;103:447.
11. Johnson RT, Burke DS, Elwell M, et al. Japanese encephalitis: Immunocytochemical studies of viral antigen and inflammatory cells in fatal cases. Ann Neurol. 1985;18:567–73.
12. Navia BA, Cho ES, Petito CK, et al. The AIDS dementia complex II. Neuropathology. Ann Neurol. 1986;19:525–35.
13. Koenig S, Gendelman HE, Orenstein JM, et al. Detection of AIDS virus in macrophages in brain tissue from AIDS patients with encephalopathy. Science. 1986;233:1089–93.
14. Petito CK, Navia BA, Cho ES, et al. Vacuolar myelopathy pathologically resembling subacute combined degeneration in patients with the acquired immunodeficiency syndrome. N Engl J Med. 1985;312:874–9.
15. Rance NE, McArthur JC, Cornblath DR, et al. Gracile tract degeneration in patients with sensory neuropathy and AIDS. Neurology. 1988;38:265–71.
16. Chou SM, Roos R, Burrell R, et al. Subacute focal adenovirus encephalitis. J Neuropathol Exp Neurol. 1973;32:34.
17. Roos RP, Graves MC, Wollmann RL, et al. Immunologic and virologic studies of measles inclusion body encephalitis in an immunosuppressed host: The relationship to subacute sclerosing panencephalitis. Neurology. 1981;31:1263–70.
18. Dorfman LJ, Cytomegalovirus encephalitis in adults. Neurology. 1973;23:136.
19. Dupont JR, Earle KM. Human rabies encephalitis: A study of forty-nine fatal cases with a review of the literature. Neurology. 1965;15:1023.
20. Miller JQ, Price TR. The nervous system in Rocky Mountain spotted fever. Neurology. 1972;22:561.
21. Dastur DK, Lalitha VS, Udani PM, et al. The brain and meninges in tuberculous meningitis: Gross pathology in 100 cases and pathogenesis. Neurol India. 1970;18:86.
22. Young RC, Bennett JE, Vogel CL, et al. Aspergillosis: The spectrum of disease in 98 patients. Medicine. 1970;49:147–73.
23. Greenfield JG. Infectious diseases of the central nervous system: Neurosyphilis. In: Blackwood W, McMenemey WH, Meyer A, et al, eds. Greenfield's Neuropathology. Baltimore: Williams and Wilkins; 1963:164.
24. Baker RD, Haugen RK. Tissue changes and tissue diagnosis in cryptococcosis: A study of 26 cases. J Clin Pathol. 1955;25:14.
25. Ellner JJ, Bennett JE. Chronic meningitis. Medicine. 1976;55:341.
26. Johnson RT, Griffin DE, Hirsch RL, et al. Measles encephalomyelitis—Clinical and immunologic studies. N Engl J Med. 1984;310:137–41.
27. Hemachudha T, Griffin DE, Giffels JJ, et al. Myelin basic protein as an encephalitogen in encephalomyelitis and polyneuritis following rabies vaccination. N Engl J Med. 1987;316:369–74.
28. Hemachudha T, Phanuphak, Johnson RT, et al. Neurological complications of Semple type rabies vaccine: Clinical and immunologic studies. Neurology. 1987;37:550–6.
29. Miller HG, Stanton JB, Gibbons JL. Para-infectious encephalomyelitis and related syndromes: A critical review of the neurological complications of certain specific fevers. Q J Med. 1956;25:427–505.
30. Hart MN, Earle KM. Haemorrhagic and perivenous encephalitis: A clinical pathologic review of 38 cases. J Neurol Neurosurg Psychiatry. 1975;38:585–91.
31. Morens DM, Sullivan-Bolyai JZ, Slater JE, et al. Surveillance of Reye syndrome in the United States, 1977. Am J Epidemiol. 1981;114:406.
32. Hurwitz ES, Barrett MJ, Bregman D, et al. Public health service study on Reye's syndrome and medications: Report of the pilot phase. N Engl J Med. 1985;313:849–57.
33. Lewis DW, Tucker SH. Central nervous system involvement in cat scratch disease. Pediatrics. 1986;77:714–21.
34. Osuntokun BO, Adeuja AOG, Familusi JB. Tuberculous meningitis in Nigerians: A study of 194 patients. Trop Geogr Med. 1971;23:225.
35. Kovacs JA, Kovacs AA, Polis M, et al. Cryptococcosis in the acquired immunodeficiency syndrome. Ann Intern Med. 1985;103:533–8.
36. Whitley RJ, Soong S-J, Linneman C, et al. Herpes simplex encephalitis: Clinical assessment. JAMA. 1982;247:317.
37. Hattwick MAW. Human rabies. Public Health Rep. 1981;96:580–4.
38. Dickerson RB, Newton JR, Hansen JE. Diagnosis and immediate prognosis of Japanese B encephalitis. Am J Med. 1952;12:277–88.
39. Hilt DC, Buchholz D, Krumholz A, et al. Herpes zoster ophthalmicus and delayed contralateral hemiparesis due to cerebral angiitis: Diagnosis and management approaches. Ann Neurol. 1983;14:543.
40. Reik L, Steere AC, Bartenhagen NH, et al. Neurologic abnormalities of Lyme disease. Medicine. 1979;58:281.
41. Reik L, Burgdorfer W, Donaldson JO. Neurologic abnormalities in Lyme disease without erythema chronicum migrans. Am J Med. 1986;81:73–8.
42. Centers for Disease Control. Human rabies—California, 1987. MMWR. 1988;37:305–8.
43. Knox DL, Bayless TM, Pittman FE. Neurologic disease in patients with treated Whipple's disease. Medicine. 1976;55:467–76.
44. Helmick CG, Bernard KW, D'Angelo LJ. Rocky Mountain spotted fever: Clinical, laboratory, and epidemiological features of 262 cases. J Infect Dis. 1984;150:480–8.
45. Fishbein DB, Sawyer LA, Holland CJ, et al. Unexplained febrile illnesses after exposure to ticks. Infection with an *Ehrlichia*? JAMA. 1987;257:3100–4.
46. Kelsey DS. Adenovirus meningoencephalitis. Pediatrics. 1978;61:291.
47. McKinney RE Jr, Katz SL, Wilfert CM. Chronic enteroviral meningoencephalitis in agammaglobulinemic patients. Rev Infect Dis. 1987;9:334–56.
48. McArthur JC. Neurologic manifestations of human immunodeficiency virus infection. Medicine. 1987;66:407–37.
49. Osame M, Matsumoto M, Usuku K, et al. Chronic progressive myelopathy associated with elevated antibodies to human T-lymphotropic virus type 1 and adult T-cell leukemia-like cells. Ann Neurol. 1987;21:117–22.
50. Vernant JC, Maurs L, Gessain A, et al. Endemic tropical spastic paraparesis associated with human T-lymphotropic virus type I: A clinical and seroepidemiological study of 25 cases. Ann Neurol. 1987;21:123–30.
51. Feigin RD, Shackelford PG. Value of repeat lumbar puncture in the differential diagnosis of meningitis. N Engl J Med. 1973;289:571.
52. Koskiniemi M, Vaheri A, Taskinen E. Cerebrospinal fluid alterations in herpes simplex virus encephalitis. Rev Infect Dis. 1984;6:608–18.
53. Adams RD, Victor M. Multiple sclerosis and demyelinating disease: Acute hemorrhagic encephalomyelitis. In: Principles of Neurology. New York: McGraw-Hill; 1977:690.
54. Carter RF. Primary amoebic meningoencephalitis: An appraisal of present knowledge. Trans R Soc Trop Med Hyg. 1972;66:193–208.
55. Peacock JE Jr, McGinnis MR, Cohen MS. Persistent neutrophilic meningitis: Report of four cases and review of the literature. Medicine. 1984;63:379–95.
56. Link H, Muller R. Immunoglobulins in multiple sclerosis and infections of the nervous system. Arch Neurol. 1971;25:326–44.
57. Tourtellotte W. On cerebrospinal fluid immunoglobulin-G (IgG) quotients in multiple sclerosis and other diseases. J Neurol Sci. 1970;10:279.
58. Vandvik B, Nilsen RE, Vartdal F, et al. Mumps meningitis: Specific and nonspecific antibody responses in the central nervous system. Acta Neurol Scand. 1982;65:468–87.
59. Vartdal F, Vandvik B, Norrby E. Intrathecal synthesis of virus-specific oligoclonal IgG, IgA, and IgM antibodies in a case of varicella-zoster meningoencephalitis. J Neurol Sci. 1982;57:121–32.
60. Vartdal F, Vandvik B, Michaelson TE, et al. Neurosyphilis: Intrathecal synthesis of oligoclonal antibodies to *Treponema pallidum*. Ann Neurol. 1982;11:35.
61. Ackermann R, Rehese-Kupper B, Gollmer E, et al. Chronic neurologic manifestations of erythema migrans borreliosis. Ann NY Acad Sci. 1989;539:16–23.
62. Salmi AA, Norrby E, Panelius M. Identification of different measles virus-specific antibodies in the serum and cerebrospinal fluid from patients with subacute sclerosing panencephalitis and multiple sclerosis. Infect Immun. 1972;6:248.
63. Townsend JJ, Baringer JR, Wolinsky JS, et al. Progressive rubella panencephalitis: Late onset after congenital rubella. N Engl J Med. 1975;292:99.
64. Meyer HM, Johnson RT, Crawford IP, et al. Central nervous system syndromes of "viral" etiology: A study of 713 cases. Am J Med. 960;29:334–47.
65. Cohen SR, Herndon RM, McKhann GM. Radioimmunoassay of myelin basic protein in spinal fluid: An index of active demyelination. N Engl J Med. 1976;295:1455.
66. Ogawa SK, Smith MA, Brennessel DJ, et al. Tuberculous meningitis in an urban medical center. Medicine. 1987;66:317–26.
67. Lennette EH, Longshore WA. Western equine and St. Louis encephalitis in man. California 1945–1950. Calif Med. 1951;75:189.
68. Calisher CH, Thompson WE, eds. California Serogroup Viruses. New York: Alan R. Liss; 1983.
69. Spruance SL, Bailey A. Colorado tick fever: A review of 115 laboratory confirmed cases. Arch Intern Med. 1973;131:288.
70. Wilfert CM, MacCormack JN, Kleeman K, et al. Epidemiology of Rocky Mountain spotted fever as determined by active surveillance. J Infect Dis. 1984;150:469–79.
71. Ciesielski CA, Hightower AW, Horsley R, et al. The geographic distribution of Lyme disease in the United States. Ann NY Acad Sci. 1989;539:283–8.
72. Schmid GP. The global distribution of Lyme disease. Rev Infect Dis. 1985;7:41–50.
73. Rosen L. The natural history of Japanese encephalitis virus. Ann Rev Microbiol. 1986;40:395–414.
74. Monath TP. Flaviviruses. In: Fields BN, ed. Virology. New York: Raven Press; 1985:955–1004.
75. Goldfield M, Sussman O. The 1959 outbreak of Eastern encephalitis in New Jersey. I. Introduction and description of outbreak. Am J Epidemiol. 1968;87:1.
76. Southern PM, Smith JW, Luby JP, et al. Clinical and laboratory features of epidemic St. Louis encephalitis. Ann Intern Med. 1969;71:681.
77. Hilty HD, Haynes RE, Azimi PH, et al. California encephalitis in children. Am J Dis Child. 1972;124:530.

78. Earnest MP, Goolishian HA, Calverley JR, et al. Neurologic, intellectual and psychologic sequelae following western encephalitis. Neurology. 1971;21:969–74.
79. Ventura AK, Buff EE, Ehrenkranz NJ. Human Venezuelan equine encephalitis virus infection in Florida. Am J Trop Med Hyg. 1974;23:507.
80. Guze BH, Baxter LR Jr. Neuroleptic malignant syndrome. N Engl J Med. 1985;313:163–6.
81. Glass JP, Lee YY, Bruner J, et al. Treatment-related leukoencephalopathy: A study of three cases and literature review. Medicine. 1986;65:154–62.
82. Jemsek J, Greenberg SB, Taber L, et al. Herpes zoster-associated encephalitis: Clinicopathologic report of 12 cases and review of the literature. Medicine. 1983;62:81–96.
83. Linnemann CC, First MR, Alvira MM, et al. Herpes virus hominis type 2 meningoencephalitis following renal transplantation. Am J Med. 1976;61:703.
84. Morgello S, Cho ES, Nielson S, et al. Cytomegalovirus encephalitis in patients with acquired immunodeficiency syndrome: An autopsy study of 30 cases and a review of the literature. Human Pathol. 1987;18:289–97.
85. Martinez AJ. Is *Acanthamoeba* encephalitis an opportunistic infection? Neurology. 1980;30:567–74.
86. Elder GA, Sever JL. Neurologic disorders associated with AIDS retroviral infection. Rev Infect Dis. 1988;10:286–302.
87. Cohen J, Capildeo R, Rose FC, et al. Schistosomal myelopathy. Br Med J. 1977;1:1258.
88. Altrocchi PH. Acute transverse myelopathy. Arch Neurol. 1963;9:111.
89. Lipton HL, Teasdall RD. Acute transverse myelopathy in adults. Arch Neurol. 1973;28:252.
90. Hogan EL, Krigman MR. Herpes zoster myelitis: Evidence for viral invasion of spinal cord. Arch Neurol. 1973;29:309.
91. Hurst EW, Pawan JL. A further account of the Trinidad outbreak of acute rabic myelitis: Histology of the experimental disease. J Pathol Bacteriol. 1932;35:301.
92. Whitley R, Arvin A, Corey L, et al. Clinical factors which influence morbidity and mortality of herpes simplex virus. Pediatr Res. 1988;23:386A.
93. Whitley RJ, Alford CA, Hirsch MS, et al. Viradabine versus acyclovir therapy in herpes simplex encephalitis. N Engl J Med. 1986;314:144–9.
94. Balfour HH, Bean B, Laskin O, et al. Acyclovir halts progression of herpes zoster in immunocompromised patients. N Engl J Med. 1983;308:1448.
95. Parry GJ. Peripheral neuropathies associated with human immunodeficiency virus infection. Ann Neurol. 1988;23(Suppl):S49–S53.
96. Pachner AR, Steere AC. The triad of neurologic manifestations of Lyme disease: Meningitis, cranial neuritis, and radiculoneuritis. Neurology. 1985;35:47–53.
97. Hinthorn DR, Baker LH, Romig DA, et al. Recurrent conjugal neuralgia caused by herpes virus hominis type 2. JAMA. 1976;236:587.
98. Sabin TD, Swift TR. Leprosy. In: Dyck PJ, Thomas PK, Lambert EH, et al, eds. Peripheral Neuropathy. 1984;1955–87.
99. Palmieri JR, LaChance MA, Connon DH. Parasitic infection of the peripheral nervous system. In: Peripheral Neuropathy. Dyck PJ, Thomas PK, Lambert EH, et al, eds. 1984:1988–2009.
100. Prince DL, Griffin J, Young A, et al. Tetanus toxin: Direct evidence for retrograde intraaxonal transport. Science. 1975;188:945.
101. Simpson LL. Molecular pharmacology of botulinum toxin and tetanus toxin. Ann Rev Pharmacol Toxicol. 1986;26:427–53.
102. Black JD, Dolly JO. Interaction of ^{125}I-labelled botulinum neurotoxins with nerve terminals. II. Autoradiographic evidence for uptake into motor nerves by acceptor-mediated endocytosis. J Cell Biol. 1986;103:535–44.
103. Pappenheimer AM. Diphtheria toxin. Ann Rev Biochem. 1977;46:69–94.
104. Cornblath DR, McArthur JC, Kennedy PGE, et al. Inflammatory demyelinating peripheral neuropathies associated with human T-cell lymphotropic virus type III infection. Ann Neurol. 1987;21:32–40.
105. Server AC, Johnson RT. Guillain-Barré syndrome. In: Remington JS, Schwartz MN, eds. Current Clinical Topics in Infectious Diseases. vol. 3. New York: McGraw-Hill; 1982:74–96.
106. Asbury AK, Arnason BG, Adams RD. The inflammatory lesion in idiopathic polyneuritis: Its role in pathogenesis. Medicine. 1969;48:173–215.
107. Waksman BH, Adams RD. Allergic neuritis: An experimental disease of rabbits induced by the injection of peripheral nervous tissue and adjuvants. J Exp Med. 1955;102:213.
108. Weinstein L. Tetanus. N Engl J Med. 1973;289:1293.
109. Cherington M. Botulism: Ten-year experience. Arch Neurol. 1974;30:432.
110. Merson MH, Dowell VR Jr. Epidemiologic, clinical and laboratory aspects of wound botulism. N Engl J Med. 1973;289:1005.
111. McDonald WI, Kocen PS. Diphtheritic neuropathy. In: Dyck PJ, Thomas PK, Lambert EH, et al, eds. Peripheral Neuropathy. 1984:2010–7.
112. Masucci EF, Kurtzke JF. Diagnostic criteria for the Guillain-Barré syndrome: An analysis of 50 cases. J Neurol Sci. 1971;13:483.
113. Lichtenfeld P. Autoimmune dysfunction in the Guillain-Barré syndrome. Am J Med. 1971;50:772–80.
114. Wiederholt WC, Mulder DW, Lambert EH. The Landry-Guillain-Barré-Strohl syndrome or polyradiculoneuropathy: Historical review, report on 97 patients, and present concepts. Mayo Clin Proc. 1964;39:427.
115. McLeod JG, Walsh JC, Prineas JW, et al. Acute idiopathic polyneuritis: A clinical and electrophysiological follow-up study. J Neurol Sci. 1976;27:145–62.
116. The Guillain-Barré Syndrome Study Group: Plasmapheresis and acute Guillain-Barré syndrome. Neurology. 1985;35:1096–1104.

69. SLOW INFECTIONS OF THE CENTRAL NERVOUS SYSTEM

JAMES R. LEHRICH
KENNETH L. TYLER

The concept of "atypically slow infections" was introduced in 1954 by Sigurdsson,[1] an Icelandic pathologist who was particularly interested in visna, maedi, and scrapie, three diseases of sheep. By adapting his criteria, a slow infection may be defined as a progressive pathologic process caused by a transmissible agent that remains clinically silent during a prolonged incubation period of months to years, after which progressive clinical disease appears, usually ending months later in profound disability or death.[2]

Interest in slow infections of the human central nervous system (CNS) has been particularly keen since the experimental transmission of kuru from humans to chimpanzees. Several CNS diseases of humans can be classified as slow infections (Table 1), and there are diseases of other organ systems (e.g., infectious hepatitis) that might be considered slow infections as well. Two CNS diseases of known viral etiology (subacute sclerosing panencephalitis and progressive multifocal leukoencephalopathy) are described in Chapters 124 and 138. The transmissible spongiform encephalopathies (kuru and Creutzfeldt-Jakob disease), diseases caused by unnamed agents that may be viruses, and a common CNS disease for which a viral causation has been proposed (multiple sclerosis) are discussed in this chapter. The subject of prions, a putative agent of the transmissible spongiform encephalopathies, is discussed in Chapter 156.

The term *slow infection* is used rather than *slow virus* for two reasons: (*1*) for some of these diseases, the transmissible spongiform encephalopathies, the causative agent does not fit the conventional definition of virus, and (*2*) even in those slow infections that are caused by conventional viruses, it is the disease process and not the virus that is slow.

UNNAMED AGENTS OF CREUTZFELDT-JAKOB DISEASE AND KURU

Kuru, a neurologic disease found only among the primitive Fore tribes of the New Guinea highlands, was the first chronic, "degenerative" CNS disease of humans shown to be a transmissible slow infection. When intensive study began in 1956,[8] kuru was thought to be of genetic origin. In 1959, Hadlow[9] pointed out clinical and histopathologic similarities between kuru and scrapie, a disease of sheep that had been shown to be transmissible as long ago as 1936.[10] In both diseases, the CNS shows spongiform degeneration of gray matter, with severe loss of neurons, vacuolization of neuronal cytoplasm, marked proliferation of astrocytes, and little inflammation. Hadlow's suggestion led to intensified efforts to transmit kuru to experimental animals, and in 1965 Gajdusek and his colleagues reported that a kurulike disease developed in chimpanzees 20 months after intracerebral inoculation with suspensions of brain tissue from kuru patients.[11]

Creutzfeldt-Jakob disease (CJD),[12] a relatively uncommon dementing illness of humans that is found throughout the world, has spongiform neuropathologic changes that are similar to those seen in kuru. The successful transmission of kuru prompted similar attempts to transmit CJD to chimpanzees, and this was accomplished in 1968.[13] The most recent addition to the list of transmissible spongiform encephalopathies in humans is the Gerstmann-Straussler syndrome, an adult-onset chronic cerebellar ataxia in which dementia is a late feature.[14]

TABLE 1. Slow Infections of the Central Nervous System

Disease	Virus	Nucleic Acid
Subacute sclerosing panencephalitis (SSPE) (Chapter 138)	Measles	RNA
Progressive congenital rubella encephalomyelittis[3]	Rubella	RNA
Chronic progressive rubella panencephalitis[4,5]	Rubella	RNA
Rabies (Chapter 140)	Rabies	RNA
Acquired immune deficiency syndrome (AIDS) encephalopathy and vacuolar myelopathy (Chapter 108)[6,7]	HIV (HTLV-III)	RNA
Progressive multifocal leukoencephalopathy (PML) (Chapter 124)	JC and SV40-PML	DNA
Congenital cytomegalic inclusion disease (Chapter 120)	Cytomegalovirus	DNA
Transmissible spongiform encephalopathies Kuru (humans) Creutzfeldt-jakob disease (humans) Scrapie (sheep) Transmissible mink encephalopathy (mink) Chronic wasting disease (mule, elk, deer)	Unnamed	?
Multiple sclerosis (possibly a slow infection)	?	?

The transmissible spongiform encephalopathies—kuru, Creutzfeldt-Jakob disease, scrapie, transmissible mink encephalopathy, and chronic wasting disease of mule, elk, and deer (Table 1)—are caused by transmissible agents that share the unusual properties of extremely small size, great resistance to chemical and physical agents, failure to induce either an inflammatory or an immune response, and a lack of demonstrable nucleic acid or non-host protein. Gajdusek[15] has called this group of unnamed agents "unconventional viruses," but it is still uncertain whether they are best considered viruses or some new group of microorganisms.

DESCRIPTION OF THE PATHOGEN

Much of the information about this group of agents comes from research on the more readily studied scrapie agent, which has been adapted to mice[16] and hamsters.[17] The agents of kuru and CJD had been transmissible only to primates until adaptation of the CJD agent to cats, mice, and guinea pigs and adaptation of the kuru agent to mink during the 1970s.

The infectivity of the agents of scrapie and transmissible mink encephalopathy are filterable to a 25 nm average pore diameter. The kuru and CJD agents are filterable to an average pore diameter of 100 nm. γ-Radiation inactivation studies of the scrapie agent indicate an equivalent target molecular mass of 150,000 daltons or less.[18] All replicate to 50 percent lethal dose (LD_{50}) titers of 10^5–10^{11}/g in infected brain tissue and can be assayed in either end point titration or incubation time interval bioassays. Infectivity is closely associated with cell membrane elements,[19] and complete destruction of the membrane is required to destroy infectivity. Thus, the agents are unusually resistant to inactivation by physical and chemical means, including formaldehyde, β-propiolactone, ethylenediamine tetraacetic acid (EDTA), proteases, nucleases, heat to 80°C, ultraviolet radiation (>20,000 J/m^2 at 254 nm), γ-radiation, and ultrasonic energy. They remain stable for many years at −70°C or after lyophilization. The agents can, however, be inactivated by autoclaving (121°C, 15 lb/in^2, 4.5 hours), or by three treatments with 1 N sodium hydroxide for 30 minutes at room temperature.[20]

The unusual properties of these agents, particularly their small size and resistance to inactivation, have raised questions as to whether they should be considered viruses. There are no detectable humoral or cellular immune responses to the agents,[21] and the scrapie agent does not influence interferon induction in mice.[22] No virions have been recognized in infected cells in tissue culture.[15] However, transmission experiments have shown that the agents of scrapie, kuru, and CJD persist in vitro in tissue culture explants from infected brain and that the scrapie agent replicates in cell culture.[23,24] Hunter[25] has postulated that the scrapie agent is an integral part of the cell membrane, possibly a replicable glycoprotein. Diener has suggested that these agents may be similar to viroids,[26] very small, naked, single-stranded RNA viruses of plants that are also extremely resistant to inactivation by ionizing and ultraviolet irradiation. Prusiner has introduced the term *prion* to denote small, proteinaceous infectious particles that resist inactivation by most procedures that modify nucleic acids.[27,28] (The subject is discussed in detail in Chapter 156).

It was not until recently that reliable and confirmed reports have appeared of characteristic fibrillar or rod-shaped particles specifically found in material prepared from the brains of humans infected with CJD or animals infected with scrapie. Previous reports[29–31] of virus-like or spiroplasma-like organisms have not been confirmed. In 1981, Merz and her colleagues described abnormal fibrils seen by electron microscopy in lysosomal fractions prepared from scrapie-infected brains.[32] They subsequently found similar fibrils in preparations of brain material from patients with CJD[33] and felt that these fibrils represented "infection specific particles" from the unconventional slow virus diseases.[34] Morphologically, the scrapie-associated fibrils (SAFs) resemble both the paired helical filaments of neurofibrillary tangles and the fibrils of amyloid. Rod-shaped particles can also be seen in purified preparations of prions made from the brains of scrapie-infected animals. These rods are typically 10–20 nm in diameter and 100–200 nm in length and appear to be composed almost exclusively of the prion protein PrP 27-30.[35,36] Extensive controversy continues about the relationship between SAFs and prion rods and whether or not they are in fact identical or closely related structures.[28,37]

EPIDEMIOLOGY

Kuru has been confined to a few primitive tribes in the mountainous highlands of eastern New Guinea. More than 80 percent of the cases have occurred among tribes of the Fore linguistic group. During the 1950s[8] there were more than 200 kuru deaths per year in that population, a prevalence rate that approached 1 percent per year. The disease affected all ages beyond infants, with an equal sex ratio among preadolescents but a striking excess in female adults. The number of deaths per year resulting from kuru has been declining gradually but steadily since 1957–8 when accurate statistics first became available. Since 1985 there have been fewer than 15 kuru-related deaths per year. This decline has been attributed to the cessation of ritual cannibalism, the consumption of dead kinsmen that had been practiced as a rite of mourning. No one born since cannibalism ceased in a given village has died of kuru. Gajdusek[38] has suggested that kuru was transmitted by autoinoculation of infected tissue through skin cuts, nasal mucosae, or ocular conjunctivae, thus infecting women and small children, the main participants in these ceremonies. The kuru agent has been shown to be transmissible to experimental animals orally as well as by peripheral routes of inoculation (see the section on "Pathogenesis"). The incubation period of kuru in humans can be more than 30 years.[39,40] The disease appears not to be contagious; there have been no secondary cases among contacts of kuru emigrants and no cases in immigrants to the endemic area.[41]

Creutzfeldt-Jakob disease has been found throughout the world, with a prevalence, annual incidence, and yearly mortality rate of about one per million reported from large population centers where the disease is more readily diagnosed.[15] A 30-fold higher incidence has been noted in Libyan Jews who had migrated to Israel, as compared with the incidence in Jews of European origin.[42] Other small geographic and temporal clusters of cases have been reported,[43,44] and there are two reports of a husband and wife dying of CJD within a few years of each other.[44,45] About 15 percent of the cases have been familial, and a pattern of occurrence that suggests autosomal dominant transmission has been described.[43,46] Most cases occur during the fifth to seventh decades of life, and men and women are affected equally. A study of cases in the United States[47] found no apparent relationship to occupation or exposure to other patients or animals. A possible association with the eating of animal brains or sheep eyeballs has been suggested but not confirmed to date.[47–49]

PATHOGENESIS

There is clear evidence that both kuru and CJD are caused by transmissible agents. In 1965, kuru was transmitted to chimpanzees, and they developed an ataxic illness quite similar to the human disease 18–30 months after the intracerebral inoculation of brain suspensions from kuru patients.[11] Subsequent studies have shown that kuru can be transmitted by peripheral or intracerebral inoculation to several species of new-world and old-world monkeys and to the mink and ferret; incubation periods vary from 8 months in the smaller animals to more than 8 years in the monkeys. CJD has been transmitted to new-world and old-world monkeys, goats, cats, guinea pigs, mice, and hamsters. Both agents can be passaged serially in experimental animals inoculated with infected tissues. Scrapie, kuru, and CJD have recently been orally transmitted by feeding infected tissues to squirrel monkeys.[50] Spongiform encephalopathy has been induced in monkeys inoculated with brain tissue suspensions from two patients with familial Alzheimer's disease, although subsequent attempts to confirm this result have not been successful.[51]

The agents are found in brain in 50 percent infective dose (ID_{50}) titers of over 10^8/g[15] and also in lower titers in the liver, lymph nodes, and spleen; in addition, the CJD agent has been found in the lung, kidney, cornea, and cerebrospinal fluid (CSF) and also in leukocytes of infected guinea pigs.[52]

Creutzfeldt-Jakob disease has been transmitted from human to human through corneal transplants,[53] contaminated stereotactic brain electrodes,[57] dura mater grafts,[55,56] and the administration of human growth hormone derived from pools of pituitary glands obtained at autopsy and contaminated by tissue from patients who had CJD.[57–59] Thus CJD is transmissible from human to human, but probably only via direct inoculation. Of possible relevance are the increased incidence of recent brain or eye surgery that has been noted in CJD patients[44] and the experimental spongiform encephalopathy that has been produced in primates inoculated with brain tissue from a neurosurgeon who died after an atypical encephalopathy accompanied by vasculitis in skin and peripheral nerves and whose brain also showed pathologic changes of CJD.[62] No cases of CJD have been observed among virologists working with the disease or in pathologists, and there does not appear to be an excess of cases among medical personnel.[43] However, the unusual resistance of the agent to inactivation necessitates special precautions in dealing with patients and tissues, although special isolation procedures do not appear to be necessary.[63] Kuru is thought to be transmitted by autoinoculation during ritual cannibalism, as discussed previously.

The actual mechanisms by which the agents cause neurologic disease are unknown. There is no evidence of an inflammatory response in kuru- and CJD-infected brains and no significant humoral or cell-mediated immune response to any known infectious agent.[21] Autoantibodies that react with neurofilaments and with the paired helical filaments found in neurofibrillary tangles have been found not only in the sera of patients and animals afflicted with kuru, CJD, and scrapie[64,65] but also in some patients with other neurologic diseases and in some normal subjects. Reactivity is directed primarily against the 150 and 200 kD proteins of the neurofilament triplet and against the 62 kD neurofilament-associated protein.[66] Studies of the pathogenesis of mouse scrapie suggest that after inoculation at peripheral sites the scrapie agent replicates in spleen and lymphoid tissue before spreading via nerves to reach the CNS.[67] Neural spread may be mediated by slow axonal transport.[37] Neural spread of the scrapie agent within the CNS and from the CNS to the peripheral nervous system has also been reported.[68,69] Whether these pathways of spread also occur in human spongiform encephalopathies remains to be established.

PATHOLOGIC FINDINGS

Both kuru and CJD are spongiform encephalopathies; pathologic findings are limited to the CNS. Brains show diffuse losses of neurons, intense astrocytic proliferation with fibrous gliosis, and swelling and intracytoplasmic vacuolation of neuronal and astroglial processes that correspond to the spongy state.[70] The severity and distribution of the vacuolation has been variable in cases of kuru; in CJD it is most prominent in the early stage of the disease.[71] There are no inflammatory phenomena and no demyelination, although rare cases may show large areas of diffuse degeneration of white matter.[72] In 70 percent of kuru and 10 percent of CJD cases, argyrophilic, periodic acid–Schiff (PAS)-positive amyloid-like plaques are found, especially in the cerebellum. In kuru, the most severe changes are in the cerebellum and the areas to which it has afferent and efferent connections. In CJD, the frontal cortex is usually most severely affected, although there are some cases in which the occipitoparietal regions of the cerebral cortex are involved almost exclusively (Heidenhain type) and others in which there is severe granule cell atrophy of the cerebellum. The electron microscope has demonstrated the vacuoles within neurons and cytoplasmic processes of astrocytes as well as rupture of plasma membranes with accumulation of curled membrane fragments.[70,73] Golgi impregnations have shown a loss of dendritic spines of pyramidal neurons and unusual focal spherical distensions of dendritic and axonal processes.[73]

CLINICAL MANIFESTATIONS

Kuru

Almost all cases of this increasingly rare disease have occurred in individuals between the ages of 5 and 60 years.[8,20,38,40,51,74] The core syndrome is one of a rapidly progressive cerebellar degeneration to which features of cortical and brain stem dysfunction are conjoined. The disease is characterized by an insidious onset (without fever or evidence of systemic illness), cerebellar ataxia of gait and limbs, and a shivering tremor that involves the head, trunk, and legs more than the arms. Some patients experience a prodrome of headache or limb or joint pain that may last several months. *Kuru* is the Fore term for shivering. Dysarthria, signs of pyramidal and extrapyramidal involvement, strabismus, and mood changes are also found. These worsen progressively until the patient is unable to walk and cannot move without the ataxic tremors. During this stage, involuntary movements resembling chorea or athetosis and an exaggerated response to being startled ("startle myoclonus") may be found. A dementia may supervene and can be associated with frontal release signs. Dysphagia develops, and patients usually die of inanition, pneumonia, or respiratory failure 3–12 months after onset.

The diagnosis is usually made based on the occurrence of the appropriate clinical findings in the correct epidemiologic setting. Laboratory tests have not been useful as aids to diagnosis. The electroencephalogram (EEG), electromyogram (EMG), CSF examination, blood count, and serum chemistries and electrolytes are typically normal. There are no reports to date of the use of computed tomography (CT) or magnetic resonance imaging (MRI).

Creutzfeldt-Jakob Disease

CJD is a relatively uncommon, rapidly evolving cerebral disease of late middle age, in which profound dementia is combined with ataxia and diffuse myoclonic jerking; rare cases in teenagers and octogenarians have been reported.[12,41,51,60,61,75–77] A presenile dementia with myoclonus is almost invariably CJD. The distribution is worldwide and the occurrence sporadic. In the early stages, there are changes in behavior, emotional responses, memory, and reasoning together with visual distortions or impaired visual acuity; patients often are delerious. Progression is rapid, and obvious deterioration can be detected from week to week. Most patients are profoundly demented within 6 months. Myoclonic contractions of various muscle groups appear eventually and can be triggered by sudden stimuli (noise, bright lights) or can occur spontaneously. Ataxia, dysarthria, and delerium progress to eventual stupor and coma. Death usually occurs in less than a year, often as a result of intercurrent infection. About 5–10 percent of patients have a clinical course of 2 years or more.

Certain laboratory tests may aid in the diagnosis. More than 50 percent of patients will have characteristic EEG findings at some point during their illness.[78] The most characteristic pattern is one of periodic-appearing (1 Hz), biphasic or triphasic, high-amplitude sharp waves, which may appear time locked to myoclonic jerks. This EEG appearance is quite different from what is seen in subacute sclerosing panencephalitis (SSPE) (see Chapter 138). A number of patients will never develop classic periodic sharp waves but instead show diffuse, polymorphic, high-amplitude, irregular slow (delta) waves. It is often helpful to obtain repeat EEGs at regular intervals because the characteristic periodic changes may become apparent only as the disease progresses. Even in patients without these changes, the EEG will often show progressive disorganization and deterioration with each successive recording.

The CSF is almost always normal. A mild elevation in protein levels is occasionally encountered. Significant pleocytosis, hypoglycorrachia, or an elevation in protein levels should prompt a search for other disorders or concomitant processes. A recent two-dimensional gel analysis report of the detection of abnormal proteins in the CSF of patients with CJD awaits confirmation.[79]

It has recently been reported that a 27 kD protein can be identified on Western blots of preparations of infected brain tissue from patients with CJD and kuru by using an antibody directed against a purified fraction of scrapie-infected hamster brain.[80] Whether this procedure will turn out to be sensitive and specific enough to aid in the diagnosis of CJD remains to be established.

Cerebral and cerebellar atrophy, sometimes rapidly progressive, may be shown by CT and MRI, although CT scans show normal anatomy in most cases.[81] The diagnosis may be confirmed by finding the characteristic neuropathologic features in a brain biopsy specimen or at autopsy. Cases with typical neuropathologic features ("spongiform encephalopathy") should be distinguished from similar cases that have been successfully transmitted to animals ("transmissible spongiform encephalopathy") and from cases of dementing diseases that lack the typical pathology but are transmissible to animals (which can be grouped under the more general label of "transmissible dementia").

PREVENTION AND TREATMENT

Kuru has been disappearing since the practice of cannibalism was eliminated among the Fore people between 1957 and 1962; cases are no longer seen among children or adolescents.[14] Our knowledge of the epidemiology of CJD is still incomplete, and little can be said about prevention of the disease as it occurs in nature. However, the evidence that CJD can be transmitted from person to person by corneal transplantation and accidental inoculation (see the section on pathogenesis) indicates that precautions are necessary in caring for patients and handling infected materials.[48,68] Certainly, demented patients should not be used as donors for tissue transplantation or blood or as sources of tissue for the preparation of biologic products to be used in humans (e.g., corneal transplants, dura mater, pituitary hormone, interferon). Needles, needle electrodes, scalpels, ophthalmic tonometers, autopsy instruments, and all other potentially contaminated materials should be sterilized, preferably by autoclaving at 121°C at 15 lb/in^2 for 4–5 hours or by three successive 30-minute immersions in 1 N sodium hydroxide at 25°C. Shorter treatment periods, lower dilutions of sodium hydroxide, or even the use of undiluted bleach are not consistently effective. Special isolation of CJD patients does not appear necessary, but clinical and pathologic laboratory specimens must be clearly marked, disposable gloves should be worn, and any skin contact with potentially infectious materials (especially blood, urine, or CSF), should be followed by washing with 1 N sodium hydroxide for several minutes.[20,63]

There is no treatment known to be effective for kuru or CJD, although there are unconfirmed reports of improvement in humans or experimental animals treated with amantidine, vidaribine, amphotericin B, high-molecular-weight dextran sulfate, and other agents.

AGENTS OF MULTIPLE SCLEROSIS

Multiple sclerosis (MS) is the most common and best known demyelinating disease of the human CNS. Demyelinating diseases are characterized by foci of destruction of the myelin sheaths of nerve fibers, with relative sparing of axons, nerve cell bodies, and the other elements of nervous tissue. It is important to use the term *demyelination* in this restricted sense since myelin is damaged in any disease in which there is necrosis or degeneration of white matter. Thus, progressive multifocal leukoencephalopathy (PML) (Chapter 124) is a demyelinating disease caused by papovavirus infection of oligodendrocytes. Subacute sclerosing panencephalitis (SSPE) (Chapter 138) and the acquired immunodeficiency syndrome (AIDS)-dementia complex (Chapter 108) are not considered demyelinating diseases, although there may be considerable damage to CNS myelin. A classification of the demyelinating diseases is given in Table 2.

The myelin sheath is formed from the cytoplasmic membrane of oligodendrocytes (central nervous system) or Schwann cells (peripheral nervous system) wrapped around the axon to form concentric layers of lipid and protein. Thus, demyelination could result from attacks on the oligodendrocyte or Schwann cell, attacks on the myelin itself, or disordered metabolism of myelin lipid or protein.

The pathogenesis of MS remains unknown, but a viral causation has often been proposed. The evidence in favor of the viral hypothesis remains indirect and incomplete but includes epidemiologic data, the inflammatory pathologic changes of MS, the oligoclonal immunoglobulins found in the CSF and synthesized within the neuraxis in MS, and the humoral and cell-mediated immunity to certain viral agents that have been detected in MS patients. The current evidence for and against a viral etiology of MS is summarized in this chapter. Several reviews of the subject are also available.[82–85]

TABLE 2. Central Nervous System Demyelinating Diseases of Humans

Multiple sclerosis
Acute disseminated encephalomyelitis (after viral infections or vaccination)
Acute necrotizing hemorrhage leukoencephalopathy
Schilder's disease (diffuse cerebral sclerosis)
Progressive multifocal leukoencephalopathy

EPIDEMIOLOGY

A relationship between the occurrence of MS and geographic latitude has been well established.[86] Rates of death, incidence, and prevalence increase with increasing latitudes, proceeding north or south from the equator, with especially high rates found above latitude 35 degrees in the northern hemisphere. For example, the prevalence in Rochester, Minnesota (latitude 45 degrees) is 60–70/100,000, while in New Orleans, Louisiana (latitude 30 degrees), it is 6/100,000. Similar gradients have been found in northern Europe and in the southern hemisphere, but there is a low prevalence of MS in Japan, latitudes at which North American and European cities have high prevalence.

It has also been shown that a person who migrates from a high-risk to a low-risk zone after early adolescence carries with him a high risk of developing MS, although the disease may not become apparent until 20 years after migration. Studies of immigrants from northern Europe to South Africa or Israel have indicated that there is a critical age of migration of 15 years.[86] If migration from the high-risk to the low-risk country takes place before the age of 15, the risk of MS equals that in the low-risk country; a person who migrates after the age of 15 carries with him the high risk of the native country. Patients with MS tend to have had measles and rubella later than the usual age.[87,88] A point-source epidemic of 24 cases of MS occurring between 1943 and 1960 in natives of the Faroe Islands and temporally related to the occupation of the Islands by British troops between 1940 and 1945 has also been described.[89] These data suggest that environmental factors, possibly related to an infectious agent, are significant in the genesis of MS. Studies of families have also been interpreted as consistent with exposure to an environmental factor before puberty.[86] MS is 15–20 times more common in first-degree relatives of MS patients than in unrelated persons, but there is increased prevalence in spouses of MS patients.

Clusters of extremely high prevalence have also been found. In the Shetland and Orkney islands off the north coast of Scotland (latitude 59 degrees) there are 128 cases of MS per 100,000 population.

Certain histocompatibility antigens are overrepresented in patients with MS as compared with controls.[90] These antigens are believed to provide markers for immune response genes and may affect susceptibility to an infectious agent or to an autoallergic mechanism in the causation of MS.

Reports of a possible association of MS with cats, dogs, and canine distemper have not been confirmed.[83,91–93]

These epidemiologic data do not establish which factors in the environment are significant in MS. Those lines of evidence that implicate viral infection are being considered here, but it should be recognized that the viral hypothesis may prove incorrect in the long run.

Humoral Antibodies to Viruses

In 1962, Adams and Imagawa[94] reported higher levels of serum antibodies to measles virus in patients with MS than in control subjects and the presence of measles antibodies in CSF from patients with MS but not controls. Since that time, there have been numerous investigations of measles antibodies in MS utilizing a variety of techniques. Although not all results have reached a level of statistical significance, most of these studies have shown elevations of mean antibody titer when larger numbers of MS and control sera were compared.[83] There has been particular interest in measles virus because a measleslike virus is the causative agent of subacute sclerosing panencephalitis (SSPE) (see Chapter 138). In MS, as in SSPE, the most impressive data have emerged from determinations of antibodies against the ribonucleoprotein components of measles virus, which are found elevated more consistently and to higher titers than are antibodies to the viral envelope.

The presence and probable local synthesis of measles antibodies in CSF in MS strongly imply a connection between the virus and the CNS disease. When antibody levels in CSF are compared with those in serum, there is a significantly lower serum:CSF ratio for measles antibodies than for several other viral antibodies tested.[95,96] This suggests the synthesis of measles antibodies within the CNS-CSF compartment; however, low serum:CSF ratios for other antibodies (for example, rubella, mumps, herpes simplex type 1, and vaccinia) have been reported in some patients with MS,[95,96] so the specificity of these findings is unclear.

Another observation consistent with local CNS production of viral antibodies is the presence in 35–100 percent of patients with MS (depending on the laboratory) of oligoclonal immunoglobulin G (IgG) appearing as multiple discrete γ-bands on agar gel electrophoresis of MS CSF.[97] These oligoclonal immunoglobulins suggest that a process of hyperimmunization goes on in MS. Their presence has been correlated with CSF lymphocytosis, CSF measles antibody titers, and reduced serum:CSF measles antibody ratios, and some investigators have been able to elute measles antibodies from the oligoclonal CSF IgG bands.[98,99] However, most of the immunoglobulins found in MS CSF have not been shown to be directed against specific viral antigens.[99] These observations should be compared with similar data from studies of SSPE (see Chapter 138), a disease in which levels of serum and CSF measles antibodies are much higher than in MS and in which dense oligoclonal IgG bands in serum, CSF, and brain tissue have been shown to contain antibodies to measles ribonucleoprotein antigens.[100]

Although most antibody studies of MS patients have concentrated on the measles virus, there have been data implicating herpes simplex type-2, varicella-zoster, vaccinia, rubella, and some other viruses.[82–84,99] By using highly sensitive radioimmunoassays, antibodies to more than one virus can be detected in the CSF in 67 percent of MS patients and 26 percent of controls.[101] It has been suggested that the antibodies to multiple viruses found in MS CSF are produced by preprogrammed B lymphocytes that enter the CNS and are then activated nonspecifically or released from normal immune regulation.[102]

The retrovirus human T-lymphotropic virus I (HTLV-I) has been implicated in patients with MS who were reported to have antiviral antibodies in serum and CSF; in four patients there were rare cells in the CSF that reacted with HTLV-I antigen by in situ hybridization under conditions of low stringency.[103] Using the polymerase chain reaction (PCR) technique, a recent study has identified DNA sequences related to HTLV-I in the peripheral blood mononuclear cells of 6 MS patients and in 1 of 20 healthy controls.[103a] Other neurologic syndromes have been associated with retroviruses: HTLV-I with tropical spastic paraparesis, HTLV-I–associated myelopathy in Japan,[104] the chronic leukoencephalitidies in sheep and goats caused by the visna and caprine arthritis-encephalitis viruses, as well as the encephalopathy (AIDS-dementia complex), myelopathy, and peripheral neuropathies that are common in patients infected with HIV (see Chapter 108). Several subsequent serologic and in situ hybridization studies have failed to confirm an association of retrovirus infection and MS, however,[104,105] and further studies in other laboratories are needed.[105a]

Some of the conflicting results reported in studies of humoral antibodies in MS may be accounted for by differences in control groups and in the viral antigens and antibody assay techniques used. Moreover, there is an increased prevalence in the MS population of the histocompatibility antigens HLA-A3, HLA-B7, HLA-BW18, and possibly others and of the mixed lymphocyte culture determinant HLA-Dw2 (present in up to 60 percent of MS patients in some studies); there is also evidence that persons carrying HLA-A3, HLA-B7, or HLA-BW18 have higher levels of serum antibodies to measles virus and to herpes simplex virus types 1 and 2, but not to parainfluenza virus type

1, than do persons lacking these HLA antigens, whether they suffer from MS or not.[82,90] It may be that the elevated levels of antibodies to measles and other viruses that are sometimes found in patients with MS reflect the overrepresentation in this disease of certain immune response (Ir) genes for which histocompatibility antigens and the HLA-Dw2 determinant provide a marker. Thus, persons carrying these antigens and an Ir gene linked to them may react to viral or to CNS antigens in a manner different from members of a control population. We do not know whether this difference is relevant to susceptibility to demyelinating disease.

Cell-Mediated Hypersensitivity to Viruses

Several studies of cell-mediated immunity to measles and other viruses in MS have been reported, but the results have been conflicting.[82–84,96] Some investigators have found impaired reactivity of lymphocytes to measles and other viral antigens, while others have found normal responses. Some of the apparent conflicts in these observations are, again, probably methodologic. Definite conclusions about cell-mediated hypersensitivity to viruses in MS have to await additional information.

Multiple sclerosis patients differ from controls in the distribution of T and B lymphocytes and their subpopulations. Suppressor T-cell activity as identified by suppression of lymphocyte mitogen responsiveness and numbers of suppressor-cytotoxic T cells labeled by monoclonal antibodies to phenotypic cell markers are in the low normal range in patients with stable disease. During acute attacks, suppressor activity and suppressor T-cell numbers are subnormal, rising to high normal levels as remission commences.[106,107] A relationship between suppressor activity and interferon production has also been described,[108] and decreased production of interferon by peripheral blood leukocytes in response to viruses and other interferon inducers have been found in some MS patients.[109]

Viral Isolation

Direct evidence of a viral causation of MS would require consistent and reproducible isolation of a viral agent from MS CNS tissue or body fluids and induction of demyelinating disease in experimental animals infected with that virus.

Early and unconfirmed reports[82] have included those of a rabies virus isolated in the Soviet Union and herpes simplex type 2 isolated in Iceland. Since then, there have been reports of isolation of virus or identification of virus antigen in brain and other tissues for a variety of agents, including parainfluenza type 1, measles, herpes simplex type 1, coronavirus and HTLV-I (see above). All these studies await confirmation.

There have also been many unsuccessful attempts to transmit disease to experimental animals by means of inoculation of affected CNS tissue. Reports of induction of a scrapielike disease in sheep and mice[110] and an MS-associated agent that caused a polymorphonuclear leukopenia in mice have not been reproducible.[111]

Electron Microscopic Studies

There have been numerous reports of "paramyxovirus-like" intranuclear and cytoplasmic filamentous rodlike profiles seen under the electron microscope within inflammatory cells near lesions in MS brains. Further study has led to general agreement that the profiles have the electron density of nuclear chromatin, are of homogeneous density, lack an inside tubular structure, and have an irregular diameter. This is in contrast to measles virus nucleocapsids (as observed in SSPE tissue, for example) and parainfluenza virus nucleocapsids, which are clearly tubular with a helical configuration, have a constant diameter (16 and 18 nm, respectively), and show clear-cut periodic striations. It is probable that the fuzzy rods seen in MS tissue are dispersed nuclear chromatin in damaged nuclei, similar to profiles seen in a wide variety of unrelated diseases and even in normal tissue.[112] A report of coronavirus-like particles seen within the cisterns of the rough endoplasmic reticulum of one patient has not been confirmed.[113]

PATHOGENESIS

The pathogenesis of MS is unknown. As noted earlier, demyelination could result from attacks on the oligodendrocyte, attacks on the myelin itself, or disordered metabolism of myelin lipid or protein. The ways in which viral infection or autoallergy may relate to MS remain to be elucidated. There is considerable indirect evidence indicating an autoallergic mechanism of cell-mediated destruction of myelin sheaths in MS. Multiple sclerosis has many histopathologic similarities to postinfectious or postvaccinal acute disseminated encephalomyelitis of humans and to experimental autoallergic encephalomyelitis (EAE), a disease induced in experimental animals by immunization with CNS myelin encephalitogenic basic protein in adjuvant. There have also been many studies of cell-mediated immunity to myelin encephalitogenic protein, cerebrosides, and oligodendrocytes in MS patients, but the results have been as confusing and conflicting as have the studies of delayed hypersensitivity to viral antigens. It is possible that an initial or persistent viral infection incites the disease and that the destruction of myelin is mediated by sensitized lymphocytes. Variations in the distribution of T and B lymphocytes, particularly suppressor-cytotoxic T cells, have been described (see above) and may be involved in the pathogenesis of the disease.

Several hypotheses concerning an infectious or immunologic pathogenesis of MS have been suggested: (*1*) suppressor cells may be damaged by viral infection or by some antigen or toxin released from CNS tissue during attacks; (*2*) a loss of suppressor cell function may permit autoallergic damage to tissue by effector lymphocytes or by antibodies; (*3*) the decreased numbers of suppressor-cytotoxic cells in peripheral blood during acute attacks may result from migration of cytotoxic effector lymphocytes into the CNS where they may damage myelin or oligodendrocytes directly; (*4*) suppressor cells may share an antigen, possibly viral-induced, with myelin or oligodendrocytes, and suppressor cells may thus be attacked as part of the disease; and (*5*) the inability of some MS patients to produce interferon in response to viral antigens may increase their susceptibility to persistent viral infection. It remains to be determined whether suppressor cell function or viral infection play any role in the pathogenesis of MS, however.

The reader should recall that, in contrast to MS, the viral etiology of progressive multifocal leukoencephalopathy (PML), another demyelinating disease, has been well substantiated (see Chapter 124). In PML, the mechanism of myelin destruction appears to be via direct infection and destruction of oligodendrocytes by a polyomavirus. That pathogenesis is unlikely in MS.

PATHOLOGIC FINDINGS

The characteristic lesion is the MS plaque, a zone of destruction of myelin that can be seen with the naked eye in the white matter of sectioned brain and spinal cord.[114] Plaques are especially common in the spinal cord, optic nerves, and paraventricular areas of the cerebrum, especially in proximity to veins. Under the microscope, recent lesions show a considerable degree of inflammation with perivenous infiltrates of mononuclear cells and lymphocytes. Later lesions contain microglial phagocytes and reactive astrocytes. Older "sclerotic" plaques contain relatively acellular fibroglial tissue (gliosis); at this stage, axis cylinders may no longer remain intact. As has been mentioned earlier, this sequence of pathologic changes has been interpreted as reflecting lymphocyte-mediated destruction of myelin, with late glial "scarring" in inactive lesions.

CLINICAL MANIFESTATION

The reader is referred to textbooks of neurology[86,115] for a detailed discussion of the clinical presentation of MS. The disease is characterized by episodes of focal disorder of the spinal cord, brain, and optic nerves that remit and recur, usually over a period of 20–30 years. Lesions are distributed in the CNS, although certain regions are affected preferentially. In the typical case, attacks and lesions are disseminated in time and space within the CNS. The more common sites of disease are the following:

1. *Optic nerve:* Optic neuritis is the initial episode in about 40 percent of patients with MS; probably about 40–60 percent of patients with acute optic neuritis eventually develop MS.
2. *Spinal cord:* Spinal cord lesions result in sensory symptoms and deficits (especially of posterior column function) and in pyramidal tract and bladder and bowel dysfunction.
3. *Brain stem and cerebellar connections:* Lesions may cause diplopia, nystagmus, internuclear ophthalmoplegia, gaze palsy, dysarthria, vertigo, facial anesthesia, facial weakness, trigeminal neuralgia, and cerebellar ataxia.
4. *Cerebrum:* Depression, euphoria, and dementia may appear as MS lesions accumulate.

Although the usual case is one of exacerbations and remissions, with gradually accumulating neurologic deficit and disability, MS may also be chronic and progressive, without remissions. Multiple sclerosis may also occur as an acute, fulminating disease, especially in childhood, as transverse myelitis or as neuromyelitis optica (myelitis plus optic neuritis), or it may be found incidentally at autopsy or by MRI, without a history of neurologic disease during life.

The CSF may contain increased numbers of mononuclear cells, especially in cases of acute onset or in exacerbation.[116] There are usually fewer than 10 cells/mm^3, rarely as many as 50/mm^3. The number of cells may correlate with the activity of the disease. Cerebrospinal fluid total protein levels are usually normal or slightly elevated; more than 100 mg/100 ml is highly unusual. Cerebrospinal fluid IgG levels are elevated (above 10–12 percent) in about 70 percent of the cases but do not correlate with the activity or severity of the disease; once elevated, the IgG level usually remains elevated. The CSF IgG/albumin ratio, the IgG/albumin index (derived from the CSF/serum ratio for both Ig and albumin), and the level of free κ-chains[117] are also abnormal in most patients with MS. In many patients (35–100 percent, depending on the laboratory), oligoclonal IgG bands can be demonstrated by agarose electrophoresis of CSF.[98] The IgG is probably synthesized within the CNS-CSF compartment. (The subject of CSF immunoglobulins in MS is reviewed by Desmond et al.[3] and Johnson and Nelson.[116]) Myelin basic protein components are often present in MS CSF, especially after acute exacerbations,[118,119] but also in other diseases in which there is active destruction of myelin. CSF glucose levels and pressure are normal.

Magnetic resonance imaging is quite sensitive in detecting the presence of plaques in the brain and less so in the spinal cord; the findings are not specific for MS, however.[120] Computed cranial tomography (CT scanning), especially delayed, contrast-enhanced scans, may reveal large MS plaques, although the test findings are normal in most cases.[121] Recordings of visual-, auditory-, and somatosensory-evoked responses have proved quite useful in documenting the presence of multiple CNS lesions that may be undetected by the neurologic examination.[122]

PREVENTION AND TREATMENT

Unfortunately, nothing is known about prevention. Moving from a higher latitude to a more tropical climate would have a theoretically protective effect, but only if the move were made in childhood (see the section on epidemiology).

Because of the usually unpredictable, exacerbating-remitting course of MS, the results of any therapeutic regimen are difficult to evaluate. Treatment with adrenocorticotrophic hormone (ACTH) or corticosteroids is used commonly, especially for acute exacerbations of the disease, and there are data indicating some benefit.[123,124] It has been presumed that these drugs act by suppressing lymphocyte-mediated myelin destruction in MS, although this is difficult to prove. Azathioprine, cyclophosphamide, cyclosporine A, anti-lymphocyte globulin, plasmapheresis, total lymphoid irradiation, and other immunosuppressive therapies have also been used in MS, but most studies have been uncontrolled or unconfirmed or are still in progress. Intensive immunosuppression with intravenous cyclophosphamide and ACTH has been reported in controlled studies to bring about 1 or 2 years of stabilization or improvement in most patients with severe, progressive MS.[125,126] Additional controlled studies are required for confirmation and extension of these findings.[127] Intrathecal interferon-β (IFN-β)[128] and subcutaneous IFN-α[129] have been reported to reduce exacerbation rates in relapsing-remitting MS. Interferon-γ administered intravenously has increased exacerbation rates, possibly as a result of its ability to augment the immune response.[130] The role of IFN in MS treatment remains unclear and subject to confirmation by further studies.[131]

At the present time, symptomatic and supportive measures such as drugs to treat spasticity, bladder dysfunction, and neuralgia continue to play a major role in the management of multiple sclerosis.

REFERENCES

1. Sigurdsson B. Observation on three slow infections of sheep. Br Vet J. 1954;110:255,307,341.
2. Johnson RT. Viral Infections of the Nervous System. New York: Raven Press; 1982.
3. Desmond MM, Wilson GS, Melnick JL, et al. Congenital rubella encephalitis: Course and early sequelae. J Pediatr. 1967;71:311.
4. Townsend JJ, Baringer JR, Wolinsky JS, et al. Progressive rubella panencephalitis: Late onset after congenital rubella. N Engl J Med. 1975;292:990.
5. Weil ML, Itabashi HH, Cremer NE, et al. Chronic progressive panencephalitis due to rubella virus simulating SSPE. N Engl J Med. 1975;292:994.
6. Price RW, Sidtis J, Rosenblum M. The AIDS dementia complex: Some current questions. Ann Neurol. 1988;23(Suppl):27–33.
7. Petito CK, Navia BA, Cho E-S, et al. Vacuolar myelopathy pathologically resembling subacute combined degeneration in patients with acquired immunodeficiency syndrome (AIDS). N Engl J Med. 1985;312:874–9.
8. Gajdusek DC, Zigas V. Degenerative disease of the central nervous system in New Guinea. The endemic occurrence of "kuru" in the native population. N Engl J Med 1957;257:974.
9. Hadlow WJ. Scrapie and kuru. Lancet 1959;2:289.
10. Cuille J, Chelle PL. La maladie dite tremblante du mouton est-elle inoculable? CR Acad Sci (Paris) 1936;203:1552.
11. Gajdusek DC, Gibbs CJ, Alpers M. Experimental transmission of a kuru-like syndrome to chimpanzees. Nature. 1966;209:794.
12. Kirschbaum WR. Jakob-Creutzfeldt Disease, New York: Elsevier Science Publishing; 1968.
13. Gibbs CJ, Gajdusek DC, Asher DM, et al. Creutzfeldt-Jakob disease (subacute spongiform encephalopathy): Transmission to the chimpanzee. Science. 1968;161:388.
14. Masters CL, Gajdusek DC, Gibbs DC Jr. Creutzfeldt-Jakob disease virus isolations from the Gerstmann-Straussler syndrome, with an analysis of the various forms of plaque deposition in the virus-induced spongiform encephalopathies. Brain. 1981;104:559–88.
15. Gajdusek DC. Unconventional viruses and the origin and disappearance of kuru. Science. 1977;197:943.
16. Chandler RL. Encephalopathy in mice produced with scrapie material. Lancet. 1961;2:1378.
17. Zlotnik I, Rennie JC. Experimental transmission of mouse passaged scrapie to goats, sheep, rats and hamsters. J Comp Pathol. 1965;75:147.
18. Gibbs CJ Jr, Gajdusek DC, Latarjet R. Unusual resistance to ionizing ra-

diation of the viruses of kuru, Creutzfeldt-Jakob disease and scrapie. Proc Natl Acad Sci USA. 1978;75:6268.
19. Millson GC, Hunter GD, Kimberlin RH. An experimental examination of the scrapie agent in cell membrane mixtures. II. The association of scrapie activity with membrane fractions. J Comp Pathol. 1971;81:255.
20. Prusiner SB. The biology of prion transmission and replication. In: Prusiner SB, McKinley M, eds. Prions. San Diego: Academic Press, 1987:83–112.
21. Brown P, Hooks J, Roos R, et al. Attempt to identify the agent of Creutzfeldt-Jakob disease by antibody relationship to known viruses. Nature. 1972;235:149.
22. Katz M, Koprowski H. Failure to demonstrate a relationship between scrapie and production of interferon in mice. Nature. 1968;219:639.
23. Gajdusek DC, Gibbs CJ, Rogers NG, et al. Persistence of viruses of kuru and Creutzfeldt-Jakob disease in tissue cultures of brain cells. Nature. 1972;235:104.
24. Clarke MC, Haig DA. Evidence for the multiplication of scrapie agent in cell culture. Nature. 1970;225:100.
25. Hunter GD. Scrapie. Prog Med Virol. 1974;18:289.
26. Diener TO. Viroids: The smallest known agents of infectious disease. Annu Rev Microbiol. 1974;28:23.
27. Prusiner SB. Prions and neurodegenerative diseases. N Engl J Med. 1987;317:1571–81.
28. Fields BN. Powerful prions? (Editorial). N Engl J Med. 1987;317:1597–8.
29. Baringer JR, Prusiner SB. Experimental scrapie in mice: Ultrastructural observations. Ann Neurol. 1970;4:205.
30. Cho HJ. Is the scrapie agent a virus? Nature. 1976;262:411.
31. Siakotos AN, Raveed D, Longa G. The discovery of a particle unique to brain and spleen subcellular fractions from scrapie-infected mice. J Gen Virol. 1979;43:417.
32. Merz PA, Somerville RA, Wisniewski HM, et al. Abnormal fibrils from scrapie infected brain. Acta Neuropathol (Berl). 1981;54:63–74.
33. Merz PA, Somerville RA, Wisniewski HM, et al. Scrapie associated fibrils in Creutzfeldt-Jakob disease. Nature. 1983;306:474–6.
34. Merz PA, Rohwer RG, Kascak R, et al. An infection specific particle from the unconventional slow virus diseases. Science. 1984;225:437–40.
35. Prusiner SB, Bolton DC, Groth DF, et al. Further purification and characterization of scrapie prions. Biochemistry. 1982;21:6942–50.
36. Prusiner SB, McKinley MP, Bowman KA, et al. Scrapie pions aggregate to form amyloid-like birefringent rods. Cell. 1983;35:349–58.
37. Gajdusek DC. Hypothesis: Interference with axonal transport of neurofilament as a common pathogenetic mechanism in certain disease of the central nervous system. N Engl J Med. 1985;312:714–9.
38. Gajdusek DC. Kuru in the New Guinea highlands. In: Spillane JD, ed. Tropical Neurology. V. 29. London: Oxford University Press; 1973:376.
39. Klitzman RL. Alpers MP, Gajdusek DC. The natural incubation period of kuru and the episodes of transmission in three clusters of patients. Neuroepidemiology. 1984;3:3–20.
40. Alpers M. Epidemiology and clinical aspects of Kuru. In: Prusiner SB, McKinley MP, eds. Prions. San Diego: Academic Press; 1987:451–65.
41. Brody JA, Gibbs CJ. Chronic neurological diseases: Subacute sclerosing panencephalitis, progressive multifocal leukoencephalopathy, kuru, Creutzfeldt-Jakob disease. In: Evans AS, ed. Viral Infections of Humans. New York: Plenum; 1976:519.
42. Kahana E, Alter M, Braham J, et al. Creutzfeldt-Jakob disease: A focus among Libyan Jews in Israel. Science. 1974;183:90.
43. Masters CL, Harris JO, Gajdusek DC, et al. Creutzfeldt-Jakob disease: Patterns of worldwide occurrence and the significance of familial and sporadic clustering. Ann Neurol. 1979;5:177.
44. Matthews WB. Epidemiology of Creutzfeldt-Jakob disease in England and Wales. J Neurol Neurosurg Psychiatry. 1975;38:210.
45. Jellinger VK, Seitelberger F, Heiss WD, et al. Konjugale Form der subakuten spongiosen Enzephalopathie (Jakob-Creutzfeldt-Erkrankung). Wein Klin Wochenschr. 1972;84:245.
46. Masters CL, Gajdusek DC, Gibbs CR Jr, et al. Familial Creutzfeldt-Jakob disease and other familial dementias: An inquiry into possible modes of transmission of virus-induced familial diseases. In: Prusiner SB, Hadlow WJ, eds. Slow Transmissible Diseases of the Nervous System. New York: Academic Press; 1979:143.
47. Bobowick AR, Brody JA, Matthews MR, et al. Creutzfeldt-Jakob disease: A case control study. Am J Epidemiol. 1971;98:381.
48. Herzberg L, Herzberg BW, Gibbs CJ, et al. Creutzfeldt-Jakob disease: Hypothesis for high incidence in Libyan Jews in Israel. Science. 1974;186:848.
49. Cavanipour Z, Alter M, Sobel E, et al. A case control study of Creutzfeldt-Jakob disease. Dietary risk factors. Am J Epidemiol. 1985;122:443–51.
50. Gibbs CJ Jr, Amyx HL, Bacote A, et al. Oral transmission of kuru. Creutzfeldt-Jakob disease and scrapie to nonhuman primates. J Infect Dis. 1980;142:205.
51. Brown P, Salazar AM, Gibbs CJ Jr, et al. Alzheimer disease and transmissible virus dementia (CJD). Ann NY Acad Sci. 1982;396:131–43.
52. Gajdusek DC, Gibbs CJ, Asher DM, et al. Precautions in medical care of, and in handling materials from, patients with transmissible virus dementia (Creutzfeldt-Jakob disease). N Engl J Med. 1977;297:1253.
53. Duffy P, Wolf J, Collins G, et al. Person-to-person transmission of Creutzfeldt-Jakob disease. N Engl J Med. 1974;299:692.
54. Bernoulli C, Siegfried J, Baumgartner G, et al. Danger of accidental person-to-person transmission of Creutzfeldt-Jakob disease by surgery. Lancet. 1977;1:478.
55. Rapidly progressive dementia in a patient who received a cadaveric dura mater graft. MMWR. 1987;36:49–55.
56. Update: Creutzfeldt-Jakob disease in a patient receiving a cadaveric dura mater graft. MMWR. 1987;36:324–5.
57. Brown P, Gajdusek DC, Gibbs CJ Jr, et al. Potential epidemic of Creutzfeldt-Jakob disease from human growth hormone therapy. N Engl J Med. 1985;313:728–31.
58. Bannister BA, McCormick A. Creutzfeldt-Jakob disease with reference to the safety of pituitary growth hormone. J Infect Dis. 1987;14:7–12.
59. Brown R. Human growth hormone therapy and Creutzfeldt-Jakob disease: A drama in three acts. Pediatrics. 1988;81:85–92.
60. Traub RD, Gajdusek DC, Gibbs CJ. Transmissible virus dementia: The relation of transmissible spongiform encephalopathy to Creutzfeldt-Jakob disease. In: Kinsbourne M, Smith L, eds. Aging, Dementia and Cerebral Function. New York: Spectrum Publications; 1977:91.
61. Nevin S, McMenemy WH, Behrman D, et al. Subacute spongiform encephalopathy: A subacute form of encephalopathy attributable to vascular dysfunction (spongiform cerebral atrophy). Brain. 1960;83:519.
62. Schoene WC, Masters CL, Gibbs CJ Jr, et al. Transmissible spongiform encephalopathy (Creutzfeldt-Jakob disease): Atypical clinical and pathological findings. Arch Neurol. 1981;38:473.
63. Committee on Health Care Issues, American Neurological Association. Precautions in handling tissues, fluids, and other contaminated materials from patients with documented or suspected Creutzfeldt-Jakob disease. Ann Neurol. 1986;19:75–7.
64. Sotelo J, Gibbs CJ Jr, Gajdusek DC. Autoantibodies against axonal neurofilaments in patients with kuru and Creutzfeldt-Jakob disease. Science. 1981;210:190.
65. Aoki T, Gibbs CJ Jr, Sotelo J, et al. Heterogeneic autoantibody against neurofilament protein in the sera of animals with experimental kuru and Creutzfeldt-Jakob disease and natural scrapie infection. Infect Immun. 1982;38:316.
66. Toh BH, Gibbs CJ Jr, Gajdusek DC, et al. The 200- and 150-kDa neurofilament proteins react with IgG autoantibodies from chimpanzees with kuru or Creutzfeldt-Jakob disease; a 62-kDa neurofilament-associated protein reacts with sera from sheep with natural scrapie. Proc Natl Acad Sci USA. 1985;82:3894–6.
67. Kimberlin RH, Walker CA. Pathogenesis of mouse scrapie: Evidence for neural spread of infection to the CNS. J Gen Virol. 1980;51:183–87.
68. Kimberlin RH, Field HJ, Walker CA. Pathogenesis of mouse scrapie: Evidence for spread of infection from central to peripheral nervous system. J Gen Virol. 1983;64:713–6.
69. Fraser H. Neuronal spread of scrapie agent and targeting of lesions within the retino-tectal pathway. Nature. 1982;295:149–50.
70. Lampert PW, Gajdusek DC, Gibbs CJ. Subacute spongiform virus encephalopathies. Scrapie, kuru and Creutzfeldt-Jakob disease. Am J Pathol. 1972;68:626.
71. Masters CL, Richardson EP Jr. Subacute spongiform encephalopathy (Creutzfeldt-Jakob disease): The nature and progression of spongiform change. Brain. 1978;101:333.
72. Park TS, Kleinman GM, Richardson EP Jr. Creutzfeldt-Jakob disease with extensive degeneration of white matter. Acta Neuropathol (Berl). 1980;52:239–42.
73. Landis DMD, Williams RS, Masters CL. Golgi and electron-microscopic studies of spongiform encephalopathy. Neurology (NY). 1981;31:538.
74. Hornabrook RW. Slow virus infections of the central nervous system. In: Vinken PJ, Bruyn GW, Klawans HL, eds. Infections of the Nervous System. part II. Handbook of Clinical Neurology. V. 34. Amsterdam: Elsevier North Holland; 1978:275–90.
75. May WW. Creutzfeldt-Jakob disease. I. Survey of the literature and clinical diagnosis. Acta Neurol Scand. 1968;44:1.
76. Roos R, Gajdusek DC, Gibbs Jr. The clinical characteristics of transmissible Creutzfeldt-Jakob disease. Brain. 1973;96:1–20.
77. Brown P, Cathala F, Castaigne P, et al. Creutzfeldt-Jakob disease: Clinical analysis of a consecutive series of 230 neuropathologically verified cases. Ann Neurol. 1986;20:597–602.
78. Chiappa KH, Burke CJ, Young RR. Early evolution and incidence of electroencephalographic abnormalities in Creutzfeldt-Jakob disease. J Clin Neurophysiol. 1986;3:1–21.
79. Harrington MG, Merrill CR, Asher DM, et al. Abnormal proteins in the cerebrospinal fluid of patients with Creutzfeldt-Jakob disease. N Engl J Med. 1986;315:279–83.
80. Brown P, Coter-Vann M, Pomeroy K, et al. Diagnosis of Creutzfeldt-Jakob disease by Western blot identification of marker protein in human brain tissue. N Engl J Med. 1986;314:547–51.
81. Kovanen J, Erkinjuntti T, Iivanainen M, et al. Cerebral MRI and CT imaging in Creutzfeldt-Jakob disease. J Comput Assist Tomogr. 1985;9:125–128.
82. Lehrich JR, Arnason BGW. Virology of multiple sclerosis. In: Vinken PJ, Bruyn GW, eds. Handbook of Clinical Neurology. V. 34. New York: Elsevier Science Publishing; 1978:435.
83. Cook SD, Dowling PC. Multiple sclerosis and viruses: An overview. Neurology (NY). 1980;30:80.
84. McFarlin DE, McFarland HF. Multiple sclerosis. N Engl J Med. 1982;307:1183,1246.
85. Johnson RT. Viral Infections of the Nervous System. New York: Raven Press; 1982:263.

86. Matthews WB, Acheson ED, Batchelor JR, et al. McAlpine's Multiple Sclerosis. Edinburgh: Churchill Livingstone; 1985.
87. Sullivan CB, Visscher BR, Detels R. Multiple sclerosis and age at exposure to childhood diseases and animals: Cases and their friends. Neurology (NY). 1984;34:1144–8.
88. Compston DA, Vakarelis BN, Paul E, et al. Viral infection in patients with multiple sclerosis and HLA-DR matched controls. Brain. 1986;109:325–44.
89. Kurtzke JF, Hyllested K. Multiple sclerosis in the Faroe Islands: I. Clinical and epidemiological features. Ann Neurol. 1979;5:6.
90. Fog T. International symposium on the histocompatibility system in multiple sclerosis. Acta Neurol Scand. 1977;55(suppl 63):6.
91. Cook SD, Dowling PC. A possible association between house pets and multiple sclerosis. Lancet. 1977;1:980.
92. Alter M, Berman M, Kahana E. The year of the dog. Neurology (NY). 1979;29:1023.
93. Anderson LJ, Kibler RF, Kaslow RA, et al. Multiple sclerosis unrelated to dog exposure. Neurology (NY). 1984;34:1149–54.
94. Adams JM, Imagawa DT. Measles antibodies in multiple sclerosis. Proc Soc Exp Biol Med. 1962;111:562.
95. Salmi AA. Virus antibodies in patients with multiple sclerosis. Ann Clin Res. 1973;5:319.
96. Norrby E, Link H, Olsson JE, et al. Comparison of antibodies against different viruses in cerebrospinal fluid and serum samples from patients with multiple sclerosis. Infect Immun. 1974;10:688.
97. Link H, Müller R. Immunoglobulins in multiple sclerosis and infections of the nervous system. Arch Neurol. 1971;25:326.
98. Panelius M, Salmi A. Association of measles antibody activity with electrophoretic fractions of CSF in a patient with multiple sclerosis. Acta Neurol Scand. 1973;49:266.
99. Norrby E. Viral antibodies in multiple sclerosis. Prog Med Virol. 1978;24:1.
100. Salmi AA, Norrby E, Panelius M. Identification of different measles virus-specific antibodies in the serum and cerebrospinal fluid from patients with subacute sclerosing panencephalitis and multiple sclerosis. Infect Immun. 1972;6:248.
101. Forghani B, Cremer NE, Johnson KP, et al. Viral antibodies in cerebrospinal fluid of multiple sclerosis and control patients: Comparison between radioimmunoassay conventional standards. J Clin Microbiol. 1978;7:63.
102. Cremer NE, Johnson KP, Fein G, et al. Comprehensive viral immunology of multiple sclerosis. II. Analysis of serum and CSF antibodies by standard serologic methods. Arch Neurol. 1980;37:610.
103. Koprowski H, DeFreitas E, Harper M, et al. Multiple sclerosis and human T cell lymphotropic retroviruses. Nature. 1985;318:154–60.
103a. Reddy EP, Sandberg-Wollheim M, Mettus RV, et al. Amplification and molecular cloning of HTLV-I sequences from DNA of multiple sclerosis patients. Science. 1989;243:529–533
104. Johnson RT. Myelopathies and retroviral infections. Ann Neurol. 1987;21:113–6.
105. Madden DL, Mundon FK, Tzan NR, et al. Antibody to human and simian retrovirus, HTLV-I, HTLV-II, HIV, STLV-III, and SRV-I not increased in patients with multiple sclerosis. Ann Neurol. 1988;23(Suppl):171–3.
105a. Waksman BH. Multiple sclerosis: Relationship to a retrovirus? Nature. 1989;337:599
106. Antel JP, Arnason BGW, Medof ME. Suppressor cell function in multiple sclerosis: Correlation with clinical disease activity. Ann Neurol. 1978;5:338.
107. Reinherz EL, Weiner HL, Hauser SL, et al. Loss of suppressor T cells in active multiple sclerosis. N Engl J Med. 1980;303:125.
108. Kadish AS, Tansey FA, Yu GSM, et al. Interferon as a mediator of human lymphocyte suppression. J Exp Med. 1980;151:637.
109. Neighbor PA, Miller AE, Bloom BR. Interferon responses of leukocytes in multiple sclerosis. Neurology (NY). 1981;31:561.
110. Palsson PA, Pattison IH, Field EJ. Transmission experiments with multiple sclerosis. In: Gajdusek DC, Gibbs CJ, Alpers M, eds. Slow, Latent and Temperate Virus Infections. NINDB Monograph No. 2. Washington, DC: US GPO; 1965:19.
111. Carp RI, Licursi PC, Merz PA, et al. Decreased percentage of polymorphonuclear neutrophils in mouse peripheral blood after inoculation with material from multiple sclerosis patients. J Exp Med. 1972;136:618.
112. Lampert F, Lampert P. Multiple sclerosis. Morphologic evidence of intranuclear paramyxovirus or altered chromatin fibers? Arch Neurol. 1975;32:425.
113. Tanaka R, Iwasaki Y, Koprowski H. Intracisternal virus-like particles in brain of a multiple sclerosis patient. J Neurol Sci. 1976;28:121.
114. Adams RD, Kubik CS. The morbid anatomy of the demyelinative diseases. Am J Med. 1977;12:510.
115. Adams RD, Victor M. Principles of Neurology. 3rd ed. New York: McGraw-Hill; 1985:699–717.
116. Johnson KP, Nelson BJ. Multiple sclerosis: Diagnostic usefulness of cerebrospinal fluid. Ann Neurol. 1977;2:425.
117. DeCarli C, Menegus MA, Rudick RA. Free light chains in multiple sclerosis and infections of the CNS. Neurology (NY). 1987;37:1334–8.
118. Cohen SR, Herndon RM, McKhann GM. Radioimmunoassay of myelin basic protein in spinal fluid: An index of active demyelination. N Engl J Med. 1976;295:1455.
119. Whitaker JN. Myelin encephalitogenic protein fragments in cerebrospinal fluid of persons with multiple sclerosis. Neurology (NY). 1977;27:911.
120. Uhlenbrock D, Seidel D, Gehlen W, et al. MR imaging in multiple sclerosis: Comparison with clinical, CSF, and visual evoked potential findings. AJNR. 1988;9:56–67.
121. Vinuela FV, Fox AJ, Debrun GM, et al. New perspectives in computed tomography of multiple sclerosis. AJNR. 1982;3:277.
122. Chiappa KH. Pattern shift visual, brainstem auditory, and short-latency somatosensory evoked potentials in multiple sclerosis. Neurology (NY). 1980;30:110.
123. Miller HG, Newell DJ, Ridley A. Multiple sclerosis. Treatment of acute exacerbations with corticotrophin (ACTH). Lancet 1961;2:1120.
124. Rose AA, Kuzma JW, Kurtzke JF, et al. Cooperative study in the evaluation of therapy in multiple sclerosis: ACTH vs. placebo: Final report. Neurology (NY). 1970;20:1.
125. Hauser SL, Dawson DM, Lehrich JR, et al. Intensive immunosuppression in progressive multiple sclerosis: A randomized, three-arm study of high-dose intravenous cyclophosphamide, plasma exchange, and ACTH. N Engl J Med. 1983;308:173.
126. Goodkin DE, Plencner S, Palmer-Saxerud J, et al. Cyclophosphamide in chronic progressive multiple sclerosis. Maintenance vs nonmaintenance therapy. Arch Neurol. 1987;44:823–7.
127. McFarlin DE. Treatment of multiple sclerosis (Editorial). N Engl J Med. 1983;308:215.
128. Jacobs L, Salazar AM, Herndon R, et al. Multicenter double-blind study of effect of intrathecally administered natural human fibroblast interferon on exacerbations of multiple sclerosis. Lancet. 1986;2:1411–3.
129. Knobler RL, Panitch HS, Braheny SL, et al. Systemic alpha interferon therapy of multiple sclerosis. Neurology (NY). 1984;34:1273–9.
130. Panitch HS, Hirsch RL, Schindler J, et al. Treatment of multiple sclerosis with gamma interferon. Exacerbations associated with activation of the immune system. Neurology (NY). 1987;37:1097–102.
131. McFarlin DE. Use of interferon in multiple sclerosis (Editorial). Ann Neurol. 1985;18:432–3.

70. BRAIN ABSCESS

BRIAN WISPELWEY
W. MICHAEL SCHELD

Brain abscess is a focal suppurative process within the brain parenchyma that continues to challenge the diagnostic acumen and therapeutic skill of the clinician. Despite the presence of potent and specific antimicrobial agents and improved neurosurgical technique, the mortality and morbidity from brain abscesses remained as high as in the preantibiotic era until relatively recently. A description of the disease together with a therapeutic proposal was found in an article dating back to the sixteenth century[1]; however, it was not until the late nineteenth century that the first encouraging results of surgical intervention were reported. MacEwen[2] reported the remarkable figure of a 80 percent (8 of 10) survival rate after neurosurgical drainage of temporal lobe abscesses.

Since that time, surgical techniques have continued to improve, and antibiotics have been introduced, but diagnostic delay has continued to be the major obstacle in the success of therapeutic intervention. Significant improvement in the mortality and moribidity of brain abscess has only occurred within the last 10–15 years. These improvements reflect advances in noninvasive diagnostic techniques allowing earlier diagnosis and more precise localization before mass effect leads to intracranial shifts, which result in irreversible brain damage or death. A combined medical–surgical approach is advisable; optimal management of a brain abscess requires cooperation between the medical physician and neurosurgeon.

EPIDEMIOLOGY

The incidence of brain abscess has remained relatively stable in the antibiotic era.[3–5] Although some series report a mild increase,[6] this may represent a bias of more sensitive diagnostic techniques.[7] It is estimated that brain abscess accounts for approximately 1 in 10,000 general hospital admissions and that 4–

10 cases are seen yearly on active neurosurgical services in hospitals of developed countries.[8,9] The etiology and incidence of brain abscesses varies among different geographic areas. In China, 65 percent of brain abscesses are thought to be secondary to otitis media but only 0.5 percent secondary to paranasal sinusitis.[10] This is contrasted to a 20–40 percent incidence secondary to otitis media and a 15–25 percent incidence secondary to paranasal sinusitis reported in series from Northern European countries.[11,12] Several authors[5,6,13] reported a male predominance (3:1) among patients with brain abscesses; more recently a series of 45 patients diagnosed between 1970 and 1983 revealed a male-to-female ratio of 2.7:1.[7] In another series of 257 patients (1973–1977), the ratio was only 1.2:1.[14,15] The median age of patients is 30–40 years[10,16,17]; however, the predominant age may vary somewhat by etiology. In some series, brain abscess due to otitis media displays a bimodal age distribution, with peaks in the pediatric age group and after 40 years of age,[18] whereas abscesses secondary to paranasal sinusitis more commonly occur between 10 and 30 years of age.[18,19] Approximately 25 percent of all brain abscesses occur in children less than 15 years of age,[6] with a peak incidence between ages 4 and 7.[20] A brain abscess before the age of 2 years is extremely rare.[21]

PATHOGENESIS

Brain abscesses develop in four clinical settings: (*1*) in association with a contiguous suppurative focus, (*2*) after hematogenous spread from a distant focus, (*3*) after trauma (e.g., open cranial fracture with a dural breach, postneurosurgery, pencil-tip injuries to the eye in children,[22] and more recently after lawn dart injuries to the head,[23] and (*4*) cryptogenic (no focus is recognized in approximately 20 percent of cases).[3,5,6,13,17] In approximate decreasing order of frequency a solitary abscess may involve various regions: frontal ≈ temporal > frontoparietal > parietal > cerebellar > occipital.[6] This distribution reflects the associated, often contiguous, focus of infection. Understanding the predisposing condition(s) in a given brain abscess case has important implications for its therapy (Table 1). Intrasellar, brain stem, basal ganglia, and thalamic abscesses are rare. Intrasellar abscesses are most common in the setting of pre-existing pituitary adenomas; however, cases have occurred in their absence.[25] Sinusitis, particularly sphenoid sinusitis, is a most important predisposing condition, with one series revealing pituitary abscesses in 16 of 126 patients with sphenoid sinusitis.[26] Brain stem abscesses arise most often from hematogenous spread from a distant focus; rare cases occur in association with a contiguous infection. In one-third of the 48 reported cases, no source was defined. These abscesses are often fusiform and extend over several levels of the brain stem; therefore, the clinical findings can be confusing. Before 1974, brain stem abscesses were uniformly fatal, but recent improvements in diagnosis and aggressive neurosurgical drainage have led to occasional survival.[27]

Most patients with brain abscesses demonstrate a contiguous focus of infection, usually sinusitis or otitis. Approximately 40 percent of brain abscesses were associated with otitis media and/or mastoiditis in earlier series; this is decreasing in most parts of the world. However, in areas where otitis media continues to be neglected or therapy is delayed, intracranial complications still present a serious threat.[28] As stated, a bimodal age distribution of brain abscess as a complication of otitis media is often seen, with cases in the youngest age groups often secondary to acute otitis media as opposed to the overwhelming preponderance of associated chronic otitis media in the older age group.[18] Overall, chronic otitis media and/or mastoiditis leads to intracranial extension four to eight times more frequently than does acute disease. Before the availability of antibiotic therapy it was estimated that about 3–6 percent of patients with otogenic suppuration developed an intracranial complication, with approximately 15 percent of those presenting as brain abscesses.[21,29] Current risk estimates are more difficult to assess; however, epidemiologic data from Scotland suggest that only 1 in 3500 cases of otitis media are complicated by intracranial spread.[30] Most otogenic brain abscesses are located in the temporal lobe, next is the cerebellum, but cases of frontal lobe and rare brain stem localizations have been reported. Most otogenic brain abscesses are solitary lesions.[3–6,9,13,17]

Brain abscess secondary to paranasal sinusitis also appears to be decreasing in incidence; however, sinusitis continues to be the major predisposing condition leading to subdural empyema. In a recent British review, sinusitis accounted for 15 percent of brain abscesses over a 30-year period.[19] The frontal lobe is almost exclusively involved as a complication of sinusitis; however, particularly with sphenoid sinusitis, the temporal lobe or sella turcica have been affected. Sphenoid sinusitis, despite its relative rarity when compared with frontoethmoidal or maxillary disease, has seemingly more frequent and severe complications. This stems from the difficulty in making this diagnosis and/or the lack of appropriately aggressive therapy for this condition.[31] Dental infection is a less frequent site of infection that can be complicated by brain abscess. Brain abscess appears more likely after infection of the molar teeth. A large majority of intracranial infections in this setting follow a recent tooth extraction. The site of the abscess is most com-

TABLE 1. Brain Abscess: Predisposing Condition, Site of Abscess, and Microbiology

Predisposing Conditions[a]	*Site of Abscess*	*Usual Isolate(s) from Abscess*
Contiguous site or primary infection		
Otitis media and mastoiditis	Temporal lobe or cerebellar hemisphere	Streptococci (anaerobic or aerobic), *Bacteroides fragilis*, Enterobacteriaceae
Frontoethmoidal sinusitis	Frontal lobe	Predominantly streptococci; *Bacteroides*, Enterobacteriaceae, *S. aureus*, and *Haemophilus* species
Sphenoidal sinusitis	Frontal or temporal lobe	Same as in frontoethmoidal sinusitis
Dental sepsis	Frontal lobe	Mixed *Fusobacterium*, *Bacteroides*, and *Streptococcus* species
Penetrating cranial trauma or postsurgical infection	Related to wound	*S. aureus*; streptococci, Enterobacteriaceae, *Clostridium*
Distant site of primary infection		
Congenital heart disease	Multiple abscess cavities; middle cerebral artery distribution common but may occur at any site	Viridans, anaerobic, and microaerophilic streptococci; *Haemophilus* species
Lung abscess, empyema, bronchiectasis	Same as in congenital heart disease	*Fusobacterium*, *Actinomyces*, *Bacteroides*, streptococci, *Nocardia asteroides*
Bacterial endocarditis	Same as in congenital heart disease	*S. aureus*, streptococci
Compromised host (immunosuppressive therapy or malignancy)	Same as in congenital heart disease	*Toxoplasma*, fungi, Enterobacteriaceae, *Nocardia*

[a] Predisposing conditions are identified in approximately 80 percent of cases.
(Data from Dacey et al.[24])

monly frontal, but temporal lobe localization can also occur by direct extension.[32] Many cases of cryptogenic brain abscess may be secondary to dental foci of infection. Facial or scalp infections are also important since they may lead to cavernous sinus thrombosis and attendant intracranial complications. Brain abscess rarely complicates meningitis; however, it should be strongly considered as an associated possibility in the neonate with meningitis, particularly meningitis due to gram-negative organisms. Abscess formation has been associated with >70 percent of cases of *Citrobacter diversus* meningitis in the infant.[33]

Brain abscesses from contiguous infection may occur by two major mechanisms: (*1*) direct extension through areas of associated osteitis or osteomyelitis and (*2*) retrograde thrombophlebitic spread via diploic or emissary veins into the intracranial compartment. Additional possibilities in the case of otogenic infection include spread through pre-existing channels (such as the internal auditory canal, cochlear and vestibular aqueducts, or between temporal suture lines). Hematogenous dissemination is occasionally implicated, particularly in cases of sinus or odontogenic origin.[8,9,32,34,35] None of these hypotheses explain the relative rarity of intracranial infection with sinusitis or otitis, how bacteria traverse an intact dura, the striking age and sex predominance of subdural empyema, or what determines the form of intracranial complication that eventually evolves (e.g., epidural abscess vs. brain abscess vs. subdural empyema) in the individual case with the same predisposing condition.

Hematogenous brain abscesses often share the following characteristics: (*1*) distant foci of infection, most often within the chest; (*2*) location in the distribution of the middle cerebral artery; (*3*) initial location at the gray-white matter junction where brain capillary flow is slowest; (*4*) poor encapsulation; and (*5*) high mortality. These abscesses are more commonly multiple and multiloculated as compared with those that have an origin in foci of contiguous infection.[3–6,8,9,13,17,35,36] Chronic pyogenic lung diseases (especially lung abscess, bronchiectasis, empyema, and cystic fibrosis) remain important diagnostic considerations.[6,8,9,37] Other distant foci of infection may be associated with brain abscesses and include wound and skin infections, osteomyelitis, pelvic infection, cholecystitis, and other forms of intra-abdominal sepsis. More recently, brain abscess has been described as a complication of esophageal dilation of caustic strictures and endoscopic sclerosis of varices, both of which can produce bacteremia.[38,39] Brain abscess rarely develops after bacteremia in the presence of a normal blood-brain barrier. Thus, brain abscess is rare in bacterial endocarditis, despite the presence of persistent bacteremia. In a series of 218 patients with infective endocarditis, only 9 cases of brain abscess were noted. In 8 of these cases, the brain abscesses were less than 1 cm^3, and in all cases multiple lesions were found.[40] In addition, only 4 of 148 brain abscesses in two large series were due to endocarditis.[5,17] Hereditary hemorrhagic telangiectasia is complicated by brain abscess with striking regularity, almost always presenting in those patients with pulmonary arteriovenous malformations. These abnormalities presumably allow septic microemboli to pass through the pulmonary circulation and avoid the normal pulmonary capillary filter, thereby affording direct access to the cerebral circulation. Cyanosis, clubbing, polycythemia, and hypoxemia were also found in those patients most likely to develop a brain abscess[41] and may be a necessary substrate. Cyanotic congenital heart disease (CCHD) is found in 5–10 percent of brain abscess cases, with some pediatric series revealing that it is the most common underlying condition in children. As many as 25 percent of all brain abscesses are attributable to this condition in this age group. Between 2 and 6 percent of children with CCHD develop a brain abscess, with tetralogy of Fallot and transposition of the great vessels being the most commonly cited.[1,6,21,42,43] The polycythemia associated with CCHD increases the viscosity, thus reducing brain capillary flow and perhaps leading to microinfarction and reduced tissue oxygenation. This may be the final common pathway of brain abscess from many etiologies. These insults can be caused by polycythemic thrombosis and hypoxia (as described), septic emboli, or a suppurative vasculitis from a contiguous infection. Experimental data suggest that infection is extremely difficult to establish in normal brain tissue.[44]

PATHOLOGY

Established infection recruits inflammatory cells and alters local vascular permeability. The evolution of an abscess includes four somewhat arbitrary histopathologic stages.[45] This staging process, described in animal models of brain abscess, correlates well with human brain abscess evolution.[46] An important feature of this description is its correlation with computed tomographic (CT) findings, which has direct implications for subsequent therapy. The four stages include early cerebritis (days 1–3), late cerebritis (days 4–9), early capsule formation (days 10–13), and late capsule formation (day 14 on). This sequence of events may be altered in the immunosuppressed host. Dogs immunosuppressed by azathioprine and prednisone therapy showed a decreased early inflammatory response and edema formation followed by a delayed increase in abscess size as compared with healthy controls.[47] Two repeated observations regarding encapsulation deserve special attention. First, capsule formation is frequently more complete on the cortical than on the ventricular side of the abscess.[35,45] Second, encapsulation is less extensive in abscesses from hematogenous spread as compared with those arising from a contiguous focus of infection.[48] These observations may be related to the requirement of oxygen for pro-α chains of collagen to form triple-helix strands.[49] Normal cortical gray matter is more vascular than is adjacent white matter, perhaps allowing greater fibroblast proliferation and collagen helix formation. This discrepancy probably explains the propensity for abscesses to rupture medially into the ventricles rather than into the subarachnoid space. Similarly, the infarct resulting from a septic embolus might impede optimal collagen formation by fibroblasts.[45] Two experimental models using organisms other than α-hemolytic streptococci, however, indicate that this view of abscess evolution may be overly stereotyped. In a model of *Bacteroides fragilis* brain abscess,[50] the same stages of evolution were observed, but the early and late capsule stages could not be differentiated due to a delay in encapsulation. *Staphylococcus aureus* inoculation in the same experimental model[51] resulted in larger lesions, earlier ependymitis, and delayed progress toward healing. Again, separation of the previously described stages was not as distinct. Additionally, the abscess reached maximum size in the late cerebritis stage, which suggests that the host was able to contain the infection before capsule formation and thereby contradicts the assumption that the capsule serves to contain infection.

Therefore, brain abscess formation is a continuum from cerebritis to a collagen-encapsulated necrotic focus; however, its maturity of development is dependent on many factors including local oxygen concentration, the offending organism, and the host immune response.

ETIOLOGIC AGENTS

In the preantibiotic era, analysis of intracranial pus revealed *Staphylococcus aureus* in 25–30 percent of cases, streptococci in 30 percent, coliforms in 12 percent, and no growth in about 50 percent.[14,15] With proper attention to techniques, the role of anaerobic agents in brain abscesses has become apparent. In one earlier study,[52] 14 of 18 abscesses grew anaerobes on culture, predominately streptococci in 66 percent with *Bacteroides* sp. in 60 percent. Recent series from the United Kingdom have stressed the role of anaerobic bacteria in brain abscesses, especially of otic origin.[14,15,53] In addition, some reports suggest that the proportion of abscesses due to staphylococci are decreasing in frequency, whereas those due to Enterobacteriaceae are now more prevalent.[3,6]

The current pattern of microbial isolates from brain abscesses is shown in Table 2.[14,15,53–57] *Staphylococcus aureus* causes 10–15 percent of brain abscesses, usually in pure culture, and is the most common pathogen in abscesses after trauma. The Enterobacteriaceae are found, usually in mixed culture, in 23–33 percent of cases.[14,15,60] *Proteus* sp., *Escherichia coli,* and *Pseudomonas* sp. appear in approximate order of decreasing frequency. Bacteria associated with pyogenic meningitis (*S. pneumoniae, H. influenzae*) cause fewer than 1 percent of brain abscesses. Various streptococci are implicated in 60–70 percent of cases. These streptococci are often microaerophilic but yield aerobic patterns by gas liquid chromotographic analysis.[14,15] The *S. milleri* group (*S. anginosus* and *S. intermedius*) has a predilection for causing focal suppurative disease, including brain abscesses.[61,62] These organisms were found in 13 of 16 (approximately 80 percent) cases in one recent analysis.[63] Most of the *S. milleri* group are placed within Lancefield group F and possess the group O III antigen,[14,15,62] a potential virulence factor for the suppuration characteristic of these organisms. *Bacteroides* sp., including *B. fragilis,* are isolated in 20–40 percent of cases of brain abscess, often in mixed culture.[14,15,53,57] Many other bacteria are occasionally found in brain abscess pus,[15,58] including *Clostridium* sp. (often trauma related), *Haemophilus* sp., *Fusobacterium* sp., other anaerobes,[9,14,15,59,64] *Actinomyces* sp., *Listeria monocytogenes,*[65,66] *Nocardia asteroides,*[67] and others. When *Citrobacter* sp.[68] and *Eikenella corrodens*[36] invade the central nervous system (CNS), abscess formation is very commonly present. *Citrobacter diversus* is the most common pathogen isolated from cerebral abscesses of neonates.[69] *Salmonella* brain abscess is rare, with the most common serotypes being typhi, typhimurium, and enteritidis.[70] It occurs more commonly in adults, with precipitating factors being meningitis, trauma, and intracranial hematoma. *Streptobacillus moniliformis,* the cause of the streptobacillary form of rat-bite fever, has also been reported as a rare cause of brain abscess.[71]

Yeasts and dimorphic fungi have assumed an increasing role, causing 9–17 percent of cases in a recent series from San Francisco.[72] Most cases occur in immunocompromised patients, and mortality remains extremely high.[73] A partial list of fungi causing intracerebral mass lesions includes *Aspergillus* sp.,[74] agents of mucormycosis, *Candida* sp.,[75] *Cryptococcus neoformans, Coccidioides immitis, Cladosporium trichoides, C. bantianum,*[76] *Pseudallescheria* (*Petriellidium*) *boydii, Bipolaris* sp., *Curvularia* sp., agents of chromoblastomycosis, *Blastomyces dermatitidis,* and rarely *Histoplasma capsulatum*. In addition to the rhinocerebral form found in diabetes with ketoacidosis or leukopenic hosts, cerebral mucormycosis with brain abscess formation also occurs in parenteral drug abusers.

Various protozoa and helminths may cause brain abscesses. In a well-documented case of multiple abscesses caused by *Strongyloides stercoralis,*[77] bacteria carried within the gut of the nematode were implicated in the abscesses found in the distribution of the middle cerebral artery. Brain abscesses caused by *Entamoeba histolytica, Schistosoma japonicum,* and *Paragonimus* species remain uncommon in the United States but are seen in other countries.[78,79] Cysticercosis is a major cause of brain lesions in the developing world. For example, cysticercosis accounted for 85 percent of all brain infections in Mexico City; tuberculomas were responsible in 11 percent, and only 3 percent were pyogenic abscesses.[9]

The patient's immune status is an important determinant of the microbiology of a brain abscess. The infecting organism can be predicted with some degree of certainty, or the differential diagnosis can be narrowed significantly by knowing which arm of the immune system is more severely altered.[80] Patient's with T-lymphocyte or mononuclear phagocytic defects are commonly encountered in most hospital settings. Common causes of brain abscess in this patient group are *Toxoplasma gondii* and *Nocardia asteroides*. Less common but still possible etiologies are *Cryptococcus neoformans, Mycobacterium* spp., and *Listeria monocytogenes*. *Nocardia asteroides* infection almost always has a pulmonary portal of entry, so patients with nocardial brain abscesses usually have a concomitant pulmonary lesion.[80,81] Central nervous system involvement with this organism has been reported in 18–44 percent of patients with nocardial infection elsewhere in the body. Nocardial abscesses are most often single, but multiple abscesses have been reported. *Toxoplasma gondii* is the most common cause of brain abscess in patients with the acquired immunodeficiency syndrome (AIDS)[81] (see below). *Cryptococcus neoformans* more commonly causes meningitis in the compromised host, but mass lesions have been described. *Listeria monocytogenes* is also more commonly associated with meningitis or meningoencephalitis, but single large abscesses as well as disseminated small abscesses with this organism have also been reported.[66,83] Neutrophil defects are most often due to chemotherapy-induced neutropenia. An increased incidence of brain abscess secondary to Enterobacteriaceae and *Pseudomonas aeruginosa* is seen to parallel their increased presence as a cause of meningitis in this group of patients.[80] Neutrophil abnormalities also lead to an increased occurrence of CNS fungal disease. Multiple agents have been described, as seen above, and prominent among these are infections with *Aspergillus* spp., Mucoraceae, or *Candida* spp. A fungal etiology of a brain abscess should be suspected in a patient with a protracted hospital course who has been neutropenic for more than 1 week and has been treated with broad-spectrum antibiotics.[81]

Focal CNS lesions of several etiologies can occur in patients with AIDS (Table 3), and multiple pathologic processes commonly coexist.[84] In one series, CNS toxoplasmosis occurred in 103 of 366 (28 percent) AIDS patients with CNS complications.[85] Single or multiple abscesses are characteristic and are difficult to distinguish from pyogenic lesions by CT. Unlike the situation in non-AIDS patients, serologic studies are rarely helpful; cases of CNS toxoplasmosis have been documented even in serology-negative patients.[84] In the same series, primary CNS lymphoma was the next most prevalent complication and occurred in 11 percent. Progressive multifocal leukoencephalopathy occurs in a significant minority, and abnormal focal CT findings are observed; however, the lack of mass effect, surrounding edema, or contrast enhancement and the confinement of the lesions to white matter helps differentiate this process

TABLE 2. Microbiologic Etiology of Brain Abscess

Organism	Isolation Frequency (%)
S. aureus	10–15
Enterobacteriaceae	23–33
S. pneumoniae	<1
H. influenzae	<1
Streptococci (*S. milleri* group, including *S. intermedius* and *S. anginosus*)	60–70
Bacteroides sp.	20–40
Fungi	10–15
Protozoa, helminths[a]	<1

[a] Heavily dependent on geographic locale (see the text).
(Data from Nielsen et al.,[6] Carey,[9] de Louvois et al.,[14,15,57,58] Ingham et al.,[53] and Brook.[59])

TABLE 3. Differential Diagnosis of Focal CNS Lesions in Patients with AIDS

Toxoplasmosis	*Candida* spp.
Primary CNS lymphoma	*Listeria monocytogenes*
Mycobacterium tuberculosis	*Nocardia asteroides*
Mycobacterium avium-intracellulare	*Salmonella* group B
Progressive multifocal leukoencephalopathy	*Aspergillus* spp.
Cryptococcus neoformans	

from toxoplasmosis or lymphoma. Additional less common infectious etiologies of mass lesions in this patient population include *Mycobacterium tuberculosis,*[86] *Mycobacterium avium-intracellulare, C. neoformans, Candida* spp., *Aspergillus* spp., *N. asteroides, L. monocytogenes,* and *Salmonella* group B.[84,87]

Location within the brain can predict the etiologic agent(s) (Table 1). For example, a frontal lobe abscess in association with sinusitis often yields one of the *S. milleri* group in pure culture.[14,15,57] Post-traumatic abscesses are usually caused by staphylococci, and abscesses from otitis media are virtually always polymicrobial in origin, with streptococci, *Bacteroides* sp., and gram-negative aerobic bacilli (particularly *Proteus* sp.) most often isolated in combination.[14,15,53,57] Thus, the location of the abscess may have important implications for antimicrobial therapy.

CLINICAL MANIFESTATIONS AND DIFFERENTIAL DIAGNOSIS

The course for a brain abscess patient may range from indolent to fulminant; in approximately 75 percent of patients, the duration of symptoms is 2 weeks or less.[13] Only a minority (≤50 percent) of patients display the classic triad of fever, headache, and focal neurologic deficit. The prominent clinical manifestations of brain abscesses are due to the space-occupying mass rather than to infection. A moderate to severe headache, often hemicranial but also generalized, is the most common symptom (approximately 70 percent of cases).[5,6,13,53] Fever occurs in only 45–50 percent of patients.[4,6,13] A change in mental status ranging from lethargy to frank coma occurs in most patients.[5,7,13] Focal neurologic findings are present in approximately 50 percent of cases and are dependent on the location and size of the lesion and concurrent surrounding edema; hemiparesis is the most common manifestation.[3–6,8,9,13] Nausea and vomiting afflict one-half of patients, presumably due to raised intracranial pressure. Seizures occur in 25–35 percent of patients; they most often appear generalized and are common with frontal lobe lesions.[6,8,9,13] Nuchal rigidity and papilledema each are present in about 25 percent of cases.[6,8,9,13,17] The clinical manifestations of a brain abscess, on rare occasions, may closely mimic pyogenic meningitis with a rapidly fulminant course. Other symptoms and signs are dependent on the intracranial location. Abscesses of the cerebellar hemispheres (10–18 percent of intracranial abscesses) often produce nystagmus, ataxia, vomiting, and dysmetria.[54,60] The clinical presentation of frontal lobe abscesses is often dominated by headache, drowsiness, inattention, and a generalized deterioration in mental function. Hemiparesis with unilateral motor signs and a motor speech disorder are the most common focal neurologic signs. A temporal lobe abscess may present with an early ipsilateral headache. If the abscess is in the dominant hemisphere, aphasia may be present. An upper homonymous quadrantanopia may also be demonstrated and may be the only sign of a right temporal lobe abscess.[88] Intrasellar abscesses often simulate a pituitary tumor and present with headache, visual field defects, and various endocrine disturbances.[25,89] Brain stem abscesses most frequently present with facial weakness, fever, headache, hemiparesis, dysphagia, and vomiting.[27] The symptoms and signs of the extracerebral focus of infection may be present and dominate the clinical picture. Neurologic findings, however subtle, in a patient with a predisposing condition outlined in Table 1, mandate investigation of the CNS to exclude a brain abscess and other intracranial complications of these disorders.[6,8,11,13]

The differential diagnosis of brain abscesses is broad and includes subdural empyema, epidural abscess, pyogenic meningitis, primary or metastatic cerebral neoplasms, viral (especially herpes simplex) encephalitis, hemorrhagic leukoencephalitis, echinococcosis, cysticercosis, cryptococcosis, cerebral infarction, CNS vasculitis, mycotic aneurysms, and chronic subdural hematoma. Computed tomography is often necessary but frequently not sufficient to accomplish this differentiation.

LABORATORY FINDINGS AND DIAGNOSIS

A moderate peripheral blood leukocytosis may be present in patients with abscesses but exceeds 20,000/mm^3 in only 10 percent of patients, while 40 percent display a completely normal leukocyte concentration.[5,6,64] The erythrocyte sedimentation rate is usually elevated with a mean of 45–50 mm/hr. Hyponatremia may be seen as a reflection of the syndrome of inappropriate antidiuretic hormone secretion.

Lumbar puncture is contraindicated in patients with a suspected or proven cerebral abscess since the diagnostic yield is poor and the procedure is dangerous. The cerebrospinal fluid (CSF) profile is nonspecific in patients with brain abscesses: hypoglycorrhachia in 25 percent; elevated protein in 67–81 percent; and a pleocytosis, usually <500/mm^3 and predominantly mononuclear, in 60–70 percent of cases.[5,6,9,13] Fewer than 10 percent of CSF cultures are positive, only increasing to 20 percent after ventricular rupture.[7] In addition, the removal of CSF may result in herniation. In one series,[3] 41 of 140 patients subjected to lumbar puncture deteriorated clinically in less than 48 hours; 25 of these 41 patients died (11 of these were fully alert or only mildly drowsy at the time of the procedure). Similarly, 7 of 44 patients deteriorated in less than 24 hours after lumbar puncture and 6 died.[65] In the analysis of Samson and Clark,[13] 22 of 44 patients with brain abscesses underwent lumbar puncture; 5 of the 22 developed signs of midbrain compression within 2 hours of the procedure. These sobering figures have been recently confirmed in a series of patients observed from 1970 to 1983. Sixty percent (27/45) of these patients were subjected to a lumbar puncture, and 4 of these 27 patients died within 24 hours of the procedure.[7] For these reasons, a lumbar puncture should be delayed in patients with a febrile CNS disorder with focal neurologic signs.[24,90] However, if pyogenic meningitis is also a strong consideration, blood cultures should be obtained and appropriate antibiotics started parenterally before obtaining the CT scan. In this case, if the CT scan findings are negative, a lumbar puncture is then performed.

The skull roentgenogram is usually normal in patients with brain abscesses but may show a pineal shift, signs of raised intracranial pressure, an effaced dorsum sellae (with intrasellar abscess), or pathognomonic collections of air within a cavity.[3–6,8,9,13,17] The electroencephalogram (EEG) is usually abnormal in patients with brain abscess and lateralizes to the side of the lesion.[5,6,13,17,64] In developing countries, the EEG is a useful (and often the only) screening procedure for the detection of brain abscesses.[9]

Arteriography and ventriculography are rarely necessary in the evaluation of patients with suspected brain abscesses since the advent of CT. Arteriograms are abnormal in about 80 percent of brain abscess patients and may show a "ring shadow" in 20–40 percent; the usual pattern is an avascular mass with surrounding hyperemia.[3–6,8,9,13,91] The absence of neovascularity may be helpful in excluding a necrotic tumor. Arteriography is essential if mycotic aneurysms due to endocarditis are suspected.

A technetium 99 brain scan is a very sensitive test for the detection of brain abscess and remains the procedure of choice in areas where CT scanning is unavailable. The results are abnormal in >95 percent of patients, and a "doughnut" lesion is detected in 25–35 percent.[92] Unfortunately, this radiographic appearance is also compatible with a necrotic tumor or infarction. The results of some series suggest that the brain scan is more sensitive than CT is in the early cerebritis stage of a brain abscess, but more information is necessary.[93] Compared with CT, localization is not as accurate; posterior fossa lesions are more difficult to visualize, and postoperative uptake can obscure the recognition of persistent or recurrent abscesses.[94] A

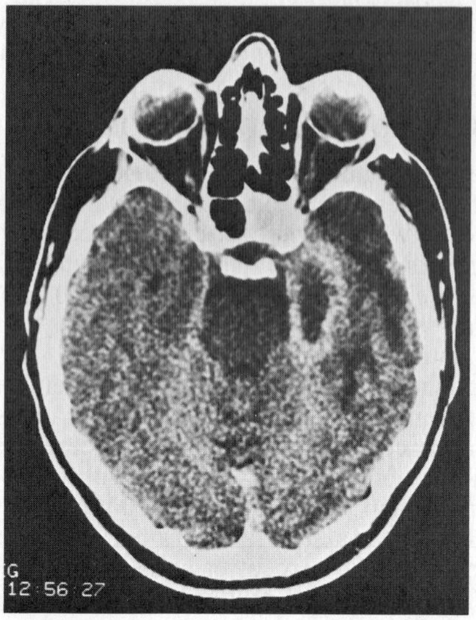

FIG. 1. CT scan after contrast administration in the axial projection of a 44-year-old woman with a history of chronic otitis media and documented sphenoid sinusitis. Note the ring enhancement around a hypodense lesion in the left medial temporal lobe with hypodense edema in the white matter. Aspiration revealed *S. anginosus* in pure culture.

brain scan or magnetic resonance imaging (MRI) (see below) should be performed when a brain abscess is suspected and CT findings are negative to exclude early cerebritis and alterations in the blood-brain barrier.

The introduction of CT revolutionized the diagnostic (and perhaps therapeutic) approach to brain abscess. CT has been shown to be superior to standard radiologic procedures for the evaluation of the paranasal sinuses, mastoids, and the middle ear; scans of these areas should be obtained, along with chest x-ray films, in all patients with suspected brain abscesses.[95] This technique is more sensitive (95–99 percent) than are traditional brain scans beyond the cerebritis stage and yields more information—the extent of surrounding edema, the presence of a midline shift, hydrocephalus, or imminent ventricular rupture.[96,97] The characteristic appearance (Figs. 1 and 2) is a hypodense center (leukocytes and necrotic debris) with an outlying uniform ring enhancement surrounded by a variable hypodense region of brain edema. Contrast enhancement is essential. The impressive sensitivity of CT is not paralleled by an equivalent specificity; a similar appearance is seen with neoplasms, granulomas, cerebral infarction, or resolving hematoma.[98,99] In addition, this characteristic appearance may be lost after ventricular rupture (Fig. 3). Features thought to discriminate abscesses from malignant tumors (thinner, more regular contrast-enhancing rim, and homogeneous enhancement of the capsule after infusion of contrast medium) do not always permit a precise diagnosis. Ependymal enhancement, when present, is indicative of ventriculitis and favors a diagnosis of brain abscess.[7] Holtas et al.[100] reported a series of 26 patients with brain abscesses wherein the CT and clinical findings in 8 were interpreted as representing a malignant tumor instead of abscess. In an effort to improve the diagnostic accuracy of CT, Coulam and associates[101] selected six parameters that could be used to differentiate between abscess and tumor, including patient age, ring thickness variability, outside ring diameter, lesion-to-ring ratio, maximum ring thickness, and CT mean value in the ring center. The overall classification accuracy in his study was still only 86 percent (84 percent for abscesses, 96 percent for tumors).

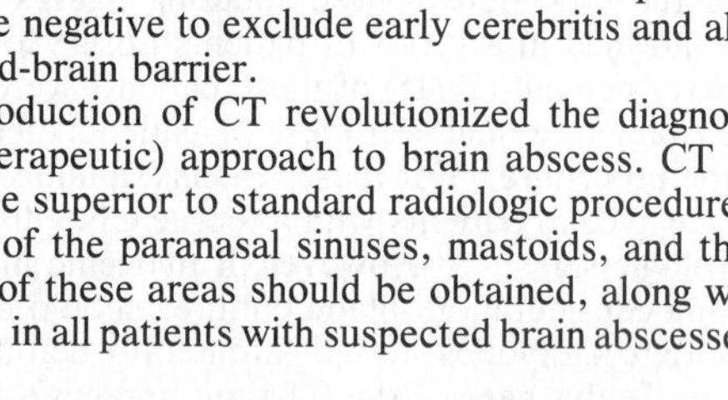

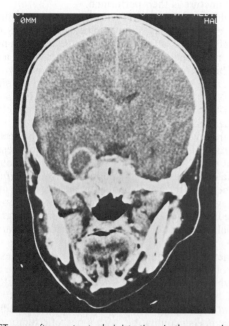

FIG. 2. CT scan after contrast administration, in the coronal projection, of the same patient shown in Fig. 1. Note the ring enhancement of the inferomedial left temporal lobe abscess, edema in the temporal lobe white matter, and effacement of the left lateral ventricle. Also note the proximity of the abscess to the petrous ridge and cavernous sinus. After abscess aspiration, drainage of sphenoid sinusitis, and 4 weeks of parenteral penicillin, the patient made a complete recovery without sequelae.

A diagnostic modality that may prove to be complimentary to CT is indium 111 labeled leukocyte scintigraphy, which has been useful in the diagnosis of occult abscesses elsewhere in the body and has been recently evaluated in the diagnosis of brain abscess. Radiolabeled leukocytes migrate to and accumulate in a focus of active inflammation, thus differentiating a brain abscess from other causes of mass lesions in the brain. In a study of 16 patients where CT was felt to be inconclusive in making a differentiation between tumor or abscess, leukocyte scintigraphy correctly predicted tumor in 10 of 11 patients and abscess in 4 of 5 patients for an overall diagnostic accuracy of 88 percent.[102] A second study of 20 patients yielded a sensitivity of 100 percent, specificity of 94 percent, and overall accuracy of 96 percent in making this differentiation.[103] Potential problems illustrated in these studies are that necrotic tumors can occasionally yield a false-positive result and that the concomitant use of steroids may be responsible for a false-negative scan finding.

Data regarding the utility of MRI (Fig. 4) in the diagnosis of a brain abscess is preliminary but encouraging. MRI appears to be more sensitive than CT is in the early detection of cerebritis as well as in detecting cerebral edema in healthy brain tissue adjacent to a cerebritic focus.[104–106] This increased sensitivity may be of limited clinical usefulness since there is already an obvious CT lesion when most brain abscess patients seek help. However, MRI may detect satellite lesions earlier. Contrast-enhanced MRI scans using the paramagnetic agent gadolinium diethylenetriamine penta-acetic acid (Gd-DTPA) increase the information obtained by MRI. This agent crosses a damaged blood-brain barrier and enhances proton relaxation, which in turn increases T1 signal intensity at the site of its accumulation. Gd-DTPA yields consistently increased enhancement of lesions relative to that seen with enhanced CT scans. Additionally, it differentiates three regions with greater accuracy: (*1*) the central abscess, (*2*) the surrounding enhancing rim, and (*3*) cerebral edema around the abscess.[105–107] Preliminary reports indicate that MRI may be superior to CT for the detection and characterization of a cerebral abscess, particularly in early stages of evolution. Its lack of ionizing radiation, greater tissue characterization, lack of bone artifact (which improves its sensitivity in posterior fossa lesions), and the decreased toxicity of Gd-

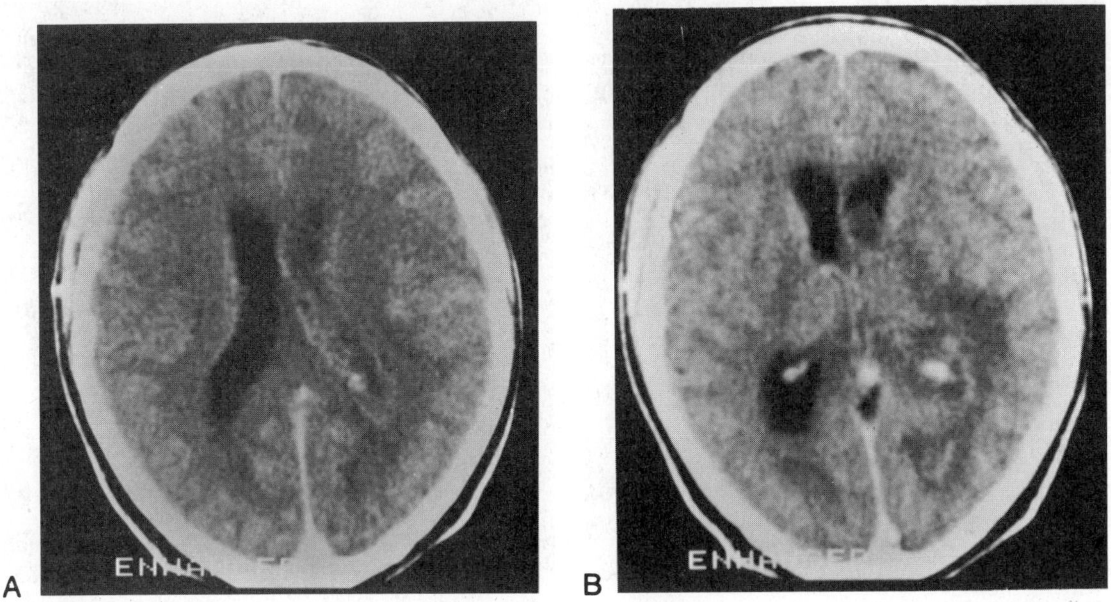

FIG. 3. CT scan after contrast administration in the axial projection. Note the loss of contrast enhancement in the original right hemispheric abscess after rupture into the right lateral ventricle. (A) Abscess enhancement is replaced by ependymal enhancement. (B) Abscess fluid/CSF interface in the right lateral ventricle.

DTPA as compared with CT contrast agents may make MRI the procedure of choice in the evaluation of brain abscesses.

ANTIBIOTIC THERAPY

Antibiotic Entry into Brain Abscess Pus

The various factors that determine the presentation of an antibiotic into the CSF[108] may not predict entry into brain tissue or abscess pus. The blood-brain barrier is altered in proximity to areas of cerebritis or an encapsulated abscess[109] and permits increased permeation of normally excluded antibiotics such as penicillin into the brain parenchyma. Few studies have addressed this issue in the treatment of brain abscesses.

An early study[110] examined brain tissue, CSF, and serum antibiotic concentrations in 27 patients subjected to a prefrontal lobotomy, presumably with an intact blood-brain barrier. After collection at various intervals after dosing, tetracycline entered both the CSF and the brain, streptomycin and erythromycin were found in the CSF but not in the brain, and penicillin was not present at either site, perhaps reflecting the low dose (600,000 units) and serum concentrations attained (0.06–2.0 μg/ml) 4 hours later when brain samples were analyzed. In patients undergoing excision of an intracranial neoplasm, a parenteral bolus of 2 g led to the following calculated brain-blood ratios: chloramphenicol, 9:1; cephalothin, 1:10; penicillin G, 1:23; and ampicillin, 1:56.[111] On the basis of this evidence and activity against anaerobic bacteria, chloramphenicol has often been included in recommended regimens for the treatment of brain abscesses.

Black et al.[112] analyzed antibiotic concentrations in brain abscess pus from 6 patients. Chloramphenicol, methicillin, and penicillin were detectable in the pus after standard dosages, whereas nafcillin was not. All six patients deteriorated clinically during medical treatment, and all cultures were still positive at surgery, thus indicating the need for surgical intervention. In the best analysis to date, de Louvois et al.[113] examined antibiotic concentrations in brain abscess pus obtained from 32 patients. Penicillin G was detectable consistently if the dose exceeded 24 million units daily (adults); however, the drug was ≥90 percent inactivated after incubation in pus for 1 hour in vitro[114] in 4 of 22 specimens. Fusidic acid entered the brain abscess pus readily, but concentrations of various cephalosporins and cloxacillin were low.[113] CSF and brain concentrations of clindamycin are low after conventional dosages[114]; however, potentially therapeutic concentrations in abscess fluid may be attainable.[115] Metronidazole attains high concentrations (approximately 35–45 μg/g) in brain abscess pus,[53] often exceeding serum concentrations after a dose of 400–600 mg every 8 hours. Due to these results and the bactericidal activity of metronidazole against strict anaerobes, this agent is often a component of antimicrobial regimens for brain abscesses.[116]

Trimethoprim-sulfamethoxazole, effective in cerebral nocardiosis[117,118] and gram-negative meningitis,[119] may have a role where susceptible organisms are present. In two studies, this drug combination was found to attain adequate brain abscess pus concentrations for the organisms being treated (*Proteus mirabilis* and *Nocardia asteroides*) and yielded successful results when combined with surgery.[118,120] In a recent report[121] vancomycin also attained acceptable concentrations in a single brain abscess.

Little information is currently available on the penetration of newer antimicrobial agents into brain abscesses or their clinical efficacy in this infection. Cefotaxime, ceftizoxime, ceftriaxone, ceftazidine and moxalactam have been shown to penetrate the CSF in therapeutic concentrations, but this does not necessarily predict activity in a brain abscess. A recent report demonstrated good penetration of moxalactam into brain abscess fluid,[122] and this agent has been used successfully in the treatment of neonatal brain abscess.[123] Aztreonam, a new monobactam derivative, has recently been shown to be effective in the treatment of experimental cerebritis,[124] but its penetration into brain tissue has not been evaluated, and it has not yet been evaluated in human brain abscesses.

Any study evaluating antibiotic penetration into the CNS must be interpreted cautiously. Considerable variation in tissue concentrations among different patients is often present as well as conflicting results between studies. A single tissue concentration may not represent the dynamics of antibiotic movement into the brain in the presence of inflammation.[125,126] The relevance of brain and abscess pus antibiotic concentrations or the necessity of bactericidal activity at the site of infection remains unknown.

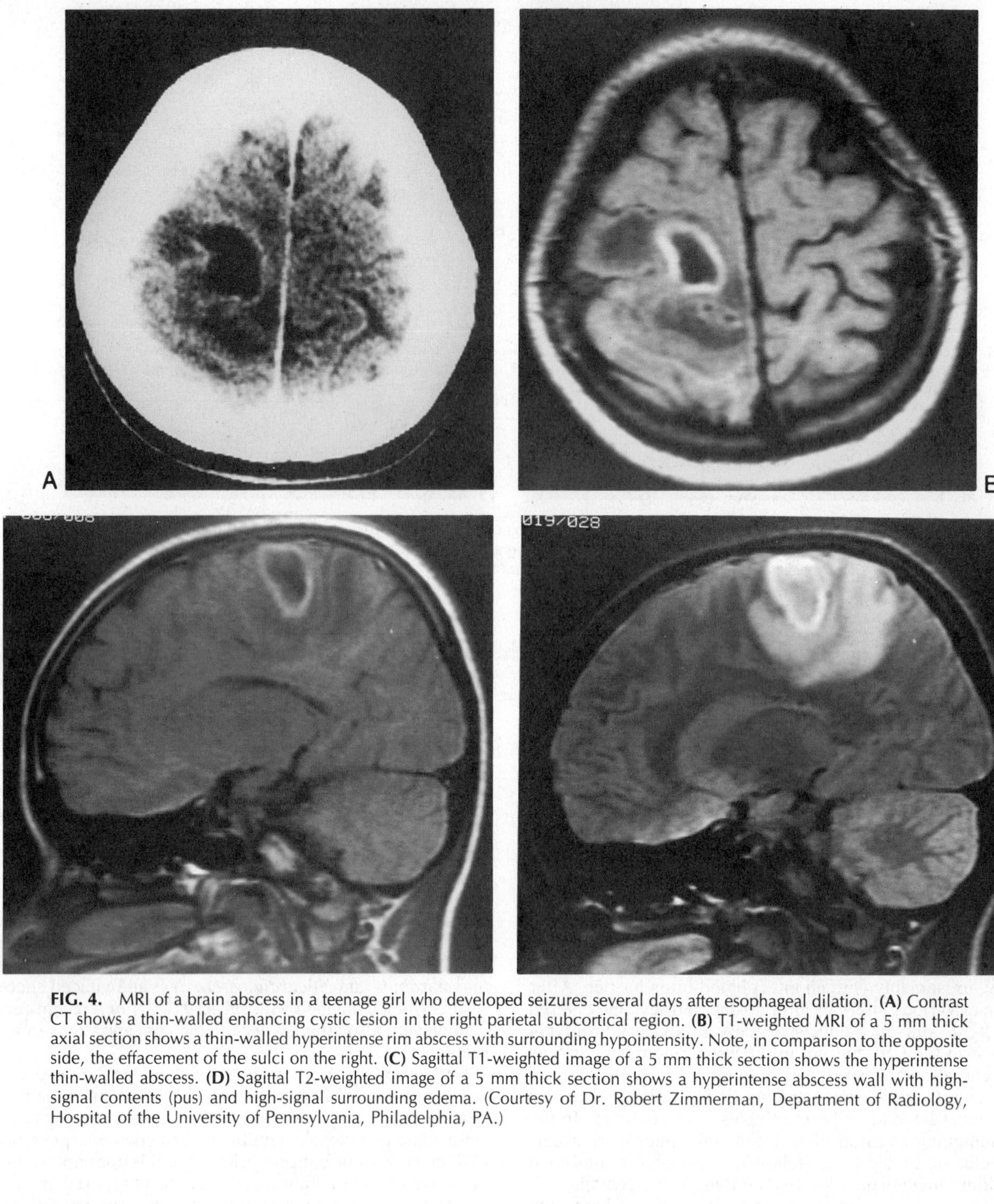

FIG. 4. MRI of a brain abscess in a teenage girl who developed seizures several days after esophageal dilation. **(A)** Contrast CT shows a thin-walled enhancing cystic lesion in the right parietal subcortical region. **(B)** T1-weighted MRI of a 5 mm thick axial section shows a thin-walled hyperintense rim abscess with surrounding hypointensity. Note, in comparison to the opposite side, the effacement of the sulci on the right. **(C)** Sagittal T1-weighted image of a 5 mm thick section shows the hyperintense thin-walled abscess. **(D)** Sagittal T2-weighted image of a 5 mm thick section shows a hyperintense abscess wall with high-signal contents (pus) and high-signal surrounding edema. (Courtesy of Dr. Robert Zimmerman, Department of Radiology, Hospital of the University of Pennsylvania, Philadelphia, PA.)

Choice of Antibiotic

The antimicrobial regimens commonly recommended for therapy for brain abscesses are empirical and reflect the considerations already noted as well as their in vitro activity against the usual pathogens. No controlled trials on the relative efficacy of various regimens have been performed. Since the early 1960s, a combination of penicillin G (20–24 million units/day) plus chloramphenicol (1.0–1.5 g intravenously q6h) has been advocated. Penicillin remains a mainstay of therapy[14,15,57] due to its excellent activity against streptococci in vitro and the favorable results obtained in experimental models of brain abscess.[127] The introduction of penicillin in the 1940s may have been instrumental in reducing brain abscess mortality from 50–80 percent to 20–30 percent by 1950.[128–131] Due to the important role of streptococci (especially the *S. milleri* group) in brain abscesses complicating contiguous foci of infection and pyogenic lung disease, penicillin should be employed in all such cases. Most anaerobes are also susceptible to penicillin with the notable exception of *Bacteroides fragilis*. Chloramphenicol is often administered concurrently with penicillin because its high lipid solubility results in concentrations in brain tissue often exceeding those in serum and its activity against anaerobic bacteria is significant. The use of metronidazole in brain abscesses has increased greatly in recent years because (*1*) metronidazole is bactericidal against *B. fragilis*, where chloramphenicol is frequently bacteriostatic; (*2*) metronidazole attains reproducibly excellent concentrations in brain abscess pus[53]; (*3*) metronidazole's entry into brain abscess pus is not affected by concomitant steroid treatment, unlike several other antibiotics[131];

(*4*) chloramphenicol may be degraded by deacetylation in pus (shown in experimental intra-abdominal abscesses); and (*5*) metronidazole may have a salutary effect on mortality as suggested by retrospective experience.[109] Metronidazole, when substituted for chloramphenicol, may lead to more rapid healing and lower mortality[40,116,132]; however, these two agents have never been compared in a prospective, randomized trial. Additionally, metronidazole may cause CNS side effects that are difficult to differentiate from clinical deterioration in brain abscess patients. An antianaerobic agent (e.g., chloramphenicol or metronidazole) is indicated in brain abscesses complicating otitis media, mastoiditis, or pyogenic lung disease since anaerobes (particularly *B. fragilis*) are often present. These agents may not be required in abscesses secondary to frontoethmoidal sinusitis because *B. fragilis* is an uncommon isolate.

When staphylococci are suspected (see Table 1) or grown, nafcillin (1.5 g q4h) is indicated.[133] Vancomycin should be substituted if the patient is either allergic to penicillin or a methicillin-resistant strain is isolated. European investigators favor fusidic acid for this indication,[14,15] but experience with this agent by physicians in the United States is limited.

The frequent isolation of Enterobacteriaceae in brain abscesses of otitic origin prompts many authorities to add a third-generation cephalosporin or trimethoprim-sulfamethoxazole to the regimen pending culture results. This approach appears to be reasonable, but the pathogenetic role of these organisms remains unsettled. Finally, the duration of therapy with any of the regimens as outlined remains unknown.

SURGICAL THERAPY

Although some patients with brain abscess respond to prolonged medical therapy alone, most require surgery for optimal management. The timing and type of surgical procedure remains controversial. Aspiration of the abscess after burr hole placement and complete excision after craniotomy have both been advocated, but no prospective randomized trial has ever been performed. By retrospective analysis, the two procedures appear to be equivalent as judged by outcome.[3–5,15] However, patients considered for excision are more often in a satisfactory neurologic condition, whereas aspiration is more often performed in the deteriorating neurologically compromised patient or for the drainage of inaccessible lesions (brain stem, thalamus, basal ganglia, etc.) where mortality is significant.[9] The procedure employed must be individualized in each patient and is dependent on the clinical course, size and location of the abscess, CT scan appearance, and other factors. Emergent surgery is mandatory when there is a progression of neurologic signs. Young and Frazee[134] advocate that abscesses exhibiting gas by CT or plain film should be considered for complete excision. In a review of five such patients, three of whom had unsuccessful aspiration procedures, a total excision was required, and a persistent extracranial communication was discovered. A brain abscess in a comatose patient carries a grave prognosis regardless of the form of treatment,[6,135] and surgery is indicated before this stage. Incomplete drainage of a multiloculated abscess is a major disadvantage of aspiration and is an important reason why reoperation is required more frequently after this procedure.[9] Excision is preferred for posterior fossa lesions and in fungal brain abscesses where antifungal therapy is limited. The incidence of postoperative seizures or other deficits is not clearly different after excision as compared with aspiration[9,136]; however, since the advent of CT, the data appear to favor more conservative surgical procedures, i.e., aspiration.[137] Instillation of antibiotics into the abscess cavity during aspiration (often bacitracin or penicillin) is frequently employed, although its efficacy has never been clearly established. Antibiotics given in this manner may potentially diffuse into surrounding brain tissue in high concentrations and cause seizures.[15,112,129,138] In cases where *Pseudomonas* spp. are complicated, direct instillation of specific antibiotics is probably warranted because adequate local antibiotic concentrations for this organism after systemic administration are difficult to obtain.[7]

Aspiration may be accomplished by stereotaxic CT guidance,[139] an extremely promising technique. This procedure affords the surgeon rapid, accurate (within 1 mm), and safe access to virtually any intracranial point. In a recent review of its use in 80 patients, recovery of tissue specific to establish a histologic diagnosis or the etiologic factors related to each disease process was realized in 94 percent of cases. There was no associated mortality and only 4 percent transient morbidity. The diagnosis of 20 cases of infection was made, 6 of which were pyogenic brain abscess, and in most instances the choice of antimicrobial therapy was significantly affected. In addition, this procedure allowed for successful drainage, even in two cases of multicompartment abscesses.[140] A second series of 102 patients[141] showed a diagnostic yield of 96 percent by this technique. There was no mortality and a 5.9 percent transient morbidity. The five abscesses that were encountered were definitively drained. Several recent evaluations confirm the efficacy and low morbidity of this procedure.[142–144] The risk of stereotaxic aspiration may be less than the risk of incorrect diagnosis and suboptimal choice of antibiotics, which makes it, in many cases, more difficult to support empirical therapy. Serial CT is useful in individual cases and may permit improved decisions regarding the need, timing, and type of surgery.

GENERAL MANAGEMENT

The CT scan, as noted earlier, has dramatically altered the diagnosis and treatment of brain abscesses. The results in animal models and humans suggest that focal bacterial infections of the brain parenchyma may be "staged" by sequential CT scans.[45,145] Cerebritis is characterized by an area of low density surrounded by ring enhancement (often thick and diffuse) that does not decay on delayed contrast scans obtained 60 minutes later (Table 4). In contrast, encapsulation is characterized by a faint ring on the unenhanced scan and ring enhancement that decays in the delayed CT scan. These parameters may prove useful in planning the combined medical–surgical approach.

Since 1971 it has been recognized that early antibiotic therapy alone could cure cerebritis without the later development of an encapsulated abscess.[146] Between 1975 and 1985, 67 cases of presumably established brain abscesses were reported to be cured by medical therapy alone.[147] These studies share the following features: (*1*) the initial diagnosis and resolution of brain abscess(s) were documented by sequential CT scans, (*2*) prolonged courses of high-dose antibiotic therapy (8 weeks or longer parenterally) were administered, and (*3*) there was a lack of surgical or histopathologic evidence of encapsulation.[9,137,148–153] Careful studies in animal models of brain abscess[45,154] and clinical observations[46,99,145,155] have clearly shown, however, that ring enhancement on the CT scan may be observed during the cerebritis stage. Thus, it is possible that these results with antimicrobial therapy represent successful resolution of bacterial cerebritis rather than a well-encapsulated abscess in some cases. This problem requires further study.

No general management guidelines can be formulated to en-

TABLE 4. "Staging" of Brain Abscesses with Computed Tomography

Stage[a]	Precontrast	Contrast Enhancement at 10 min	Contrast Enhancement at 60 min
Cerebritis	Low density	Ring enhancement	No decay
Abscess	Capsule-faint ring around low density	Ring enhancement	Decay in contrast enhancement

[a] Both lesions may be surrounded by low-density areas of edema.
(Data from Britt et al.[46])

sure optimal results in the individual patient with a brain abscess. If the scanning suggests cerebritis and the patient is neurologically stable, antibiotic therapy (usually penicillin plus chloramphenicol or metronidazole) can be started and the patient observed. Criteria for nonoperative management also generally include (*1*) medical conditions that greatly increase the risk of surgery; (*2*) the presence of multiple abscesses, especially remotely distant from one another; (*3*) abscesses in a deep or dominant location; (*4*) concomitant meningitis or ependymitis; (*5*) early abscess reduction and clinical improvement attributable to antibiotic therapy; and (*6*) abscess size under 3 cm.[20,98,150,151] As noted, these criteria may be altered by the availability of stereotaxic CT guided aspiration. Neurologic deterioration mandates surgery, usually aspiration.[9] If the patient remains stable and the abscess is accessible, aspiration (CT guided, if possible) is desirable to make a specific bacteriologic diagnosis and narrow the antimicrobial regimen. Although this delay may render cultures negative, aspiration during the cerebritis stage may be dangerous with resultant hemorrhage.[155] Certain poor prognostic parameters, clinical or radiographic, may necessitate earlier aspiration.[135] If the lesion appears encapsulated by CT scan criteria, antibiotic treatment can be started and aspiration (for diagnosis and drainage) performed without delay.[46,145] Subsequent management is dependent on clinical and radiographic (CT) parameters. Later neurologic deterioration or failure of the abscess to decrease in size as detected by CT scan are indications for further surgery, often excision, if feasible. The duration of antimicrobial therapy remains unsettled. Many authorities treat parenterally for 4–6 weeks, often followed by prolonged oral therapy if a suitable agent is available against the isolated pathogens, for 2–6 months. It must be stressed that such regimens are empirical and may not be necessary; a cured brain abscess may continue to appear as nodular contrast enhancement on CT scans for 4–10 weeks to up to 6 months[46,98,99] after completion of successful therapy.

Steroids are often employed as adjunctives in the management of brain abscess, but their role remains controversial. These agents may be deleterious by reducing antibiotic entry into the CNS,[156,157] decreasing collagen formation and glial response,[158] or altering the CT scan appearance of ring enhancement as inflammation subsides,[159,160] which may obscure information from sequential studies or an assessment of cure. However, steroids may prove lifesaving in the patient with rapid neurologic deterioration and raised intracranial pressure. In this circumstance, intracranial pressure monitoring is advisable, and elevations in pressure should be controlled with steroids, forced hyperventilation, and mannitol if necessary. Anticonvulsants are appropriate in the patient having seizures.

PROGNOSIS

The mortality of brain abscesses was 40–60 percent in the preantibiotic era; some series report a decline after the introduction of penicillin.[3-6,8,9,13,17,64] An adverse prognosis is associated with (*1*) delayed or missed diagnosis; (*2*) poor localization, especially in the posterior fossa before the availability of CT scans; (*3*) multiple, deep, or multiloculated lesions; (*4*) ventricular rupture (80–100 percent mortality); (*5*) coma (Table 5) (80–100 percent mortality); (*6*) fungal etiology; and (*7*) inappropriate antibiotics.[6,9,135] Additional negative factors often cited include extremes of age, large abscesses, and metastatic abscesses.[7] More recently, a decreased mortality ranging between 0 and 24 percent has been reported in numerous series and is attributed to the introduction of CT scanning.[18,94,116,161] The incidence of neurologic sequelae ranges between 30 and 55 percent.[7] Most sequelae are mild, but up to 17 percent of patients may be incapacitated, with the severity of sequelae more often correlating with the patient's neurologic condition on admission than the form of treatment employed.[7,13,43,94] The likelihood of seizures is variable and ranges from 35 to >90 percent; these differences may relate to the length of follow-up. Anticonvulsant therapy appears to reduce this complication.[162] There is some recent suggestion that lesions treated conservatively (i.e., with antibiotics and/or aspiration vs. complete excision) have a lower incidence of post-treatment sequelae, correlating with less visible abnormalities on follow-up CT scans.[137] Earlier diagnosis, refinements in technology, and an aggressive medical–surgical approach may lead to a more consistent reduction in the morbidity and mortality of this still serious disease.

TABLE 5. Brain Abscess: Influence of Preoperative Mental Status on Mortality

Mental Status	*Patients (No.)*	*Mortality (%)*
Grade I (fully alert)	33	0
Grade II (drowsy)	55	4
Grade III (response to pain only)	61	59
Grade IV (coma, no pain response)	51	82

(Data from Nielsen et al.[6])

REFERENCES

1. Theophilo F, Markakis E, Theophilo L, et al. Brain abscess in childhood. Child Nerv Syst. 1985;1:324.
2. MacEwen W. Pyogenic Infective Diseases of the Brain and Spinal Cord. Glasgow: James MacLehose & Sons; 1893.
3. Garfield J. Management of supratentorial intracranial abscess: A review of 200 cases. Br Med J. 1969;2:7.
4. Beller AJ, Sahar A, Praiss I. Brain abscess. Review of 89 cases over 30 years. J Neurol Neurosurg Psychiatry. 1973;36:757.
5. Morgan H, Wood M, Murphy F. Experience with 88 consecutive cases of brain abscess. J Neurosurg. 1973;38:698.
6. Nielsen H, Glydensted C, Harmsen A. Cerebral abscess. Aetiology and pathogenesis, symptoms, diagnosis and treatment. Acta Neurol Scand. 1982;65:609.
7. Chun CH, Johnson JD, Hofstetter M, et al. Brain abscess. A study of 45 consecutive cases. Medicine (Baltimore). 1986;65:415.
8. Garvey G. Current concepts of bacterial infections of the central nervous system. Bacterial meningitis and bacterial brain abscess. J Neurosurg. 1983;59:735.
9. Carey ME. Brain abscesses. Contemp Neurosurg. 1982;3:1.
10. Yang SH. Brain abscess: A review of 400 cases. J Neurosurg. 1981;55:794.
11. Bradley PJ, Shaw MDM. Three decades of brain abscess in Merseyside. J R Coll Surg Edinb. 1983;28:223.
12. Van Alphen HAM, Driessen JJR. Brain abscess and subdural empyema. J Neurol Neurosurg Psychiatry. 1976;39:481.
13. Samson DS, Clark K. A current review of brain abscess. Am J Med. 1973;54:201.
14. de Louvois J, Gortvai P, Hurley R. Bacteriology of abscesses of the central nervous system. A multicentre prospective study. Br Med J. 1977;2:981.
15. de Louvois J. The bacteriology and chemotherapy of brain abscess. J Antimicrob Chemother. 1978;4:395.
16. Harrison MJG. The clinical presentation of intracranial abscesses. Q J Med. 1982;51:461.
17. Brewer NS, MacCarty CS, Wellman WE. Brain abscess: A review of recent experience. Ann Intern Med. 1975;82:571.
18. Small M, Dale BAB. Intracranial suppuration 1968–1982—a 15 year review. Clin Otolaryngol. 1984;9:315.
19. Bradley PJ, Manning KP, Shaw MDM. Brain abscess secondary to paranasal sinusitis. J Laryngol Otol. 1984;98:719.
20. Kaplan K: Brain abscess. Med Clin North Am. 1985;69:345.
21. Spires JR, Smith RJH, Catlin FI. Brain abscesses in the young. Otolaryngol Head Neck Surg. 1985;93:468.
22. Foy P, Skarr M. Cerebral abscesses in children after pencil-tip injuries. Lancet. 1980;2:662.
23. Tay JS, Garland JS. Serious head injuries from lawn darts. Pediatrics. 1987;79:261.
24. Dacey RG Jr, Winn HR. Brain abscess and perimeningeal infections. In: Stein JH, Cline MJ, Daly WJ, eds. Internal Medicine. Boston: Little, Brown; 1983:1213.
25. Berger SA, Edberg SC, David G. Infectious disease of the sella turcica. Rev Infect Dis. 1986;8:747.
26. Teed RW. Meningitis from the sphenoid sinus. Arch Otolaryngol. 1938;28:589.
27. Dake MD, McMurdo SK, Rosenblum ML, et al. Pyogenic abscess of the medulla oblongata. Neurosurgery. 1986;18:370.
28. Samuel J, Fernandes CMC, Steinberg JL. Intracranial otogenic complications: A persisting problem. Laryngoscope. 1986;96:272.

29. Gower D, McGuirt WF. Intracranial complications of acute and chronic infectious ear disease: A problem still with us. Laryngoscope. 1983;93:1028.
30. Browning GG. The unsafeness of safe ears. J Laryngol Otol. 1984;98:23.
31. Lew D, Southwick FS, Montgomery WW, et al. Sphenoid sinusitis. A review of 30 cases. N Engl J Med. 1983;309:1149.
32. Hollin SA, Hayashi H, Gross SW. Intracranial abscesses of odontogenic origin. Oral Surg. 1967;23:277.
33. Foreman SD, Smith EE, Ryan NJ, et al. Neonatal *Citrobacter* meningitis: Pathogenesis of cerebral abscess formation. Ann Neurol. 1984;16:655.
34. Brand B, Caparosa RJ, Lubic LG. Otorhinological brain abscess therapy—past and present. Laryngoscope. 1984;94:483.
35. Waggener JD. The pathophysiology of bacterial meningitis and cerebral abscesses: An anatomical interpretation. Adv Neurol. 1974;6:1.
36. Bronitsky R, Heim CR, McGee ZA. Multifocal brain abscesses: Combined medical and neurosurgical therapy. South Med J. 1982;75:1261.
37. Kline MW. Brain abscess in a patient with cystic fibrosis. Pediatr Infect Dis. 1985;4:72.
38. Schlitt M, Mitchem L, Zorn G, et al. Brain abscess after esophageal dilation for caustic stricture: Report of three cases. Neurosurgery. 1985;17:947.
39. Cohen FL, Koerner RS, Taub SJ. Solitary brain abscess following endoscopic injection sclerosis of esophageal varices. Gastrointest Endosc. 1985;31:331.
40. Pruit AA, Rubin RHJ, Karchmer AW, et al. Neurologic complications of bacterial endocarditis. Medicine (Baltimore). 1978;57:329.
41. Press OW, Ramsey PG. Central nervous system infections associated with hereditary hemorrhagic telangiectasia. Am J Med. 1984;77:86.
42. Fischbein CA, Rosenthal A, Fischer EG, et al. Risk factors for brain abscess in patients with congenital heart disease. Am J Cardiol. 1974;34:97.
43. Fischer EG, McLennan JE, Suzuki Y. Cerebral abscess in children. Am J Dis Child. 1981;135:746.
44. Molinari GF, Smith L, Goldstein MN, et al. Brain abscess from septic cerebral embolism: An experimental model. Neurology (NY). 1973;23:1205.
45. Britt RH, Enzmann DR, Yeager AS. Neuropathological and computerized tomographic findings in experimental brain abscess. J Neurosurg. 1981;55:590.
46. Britt RH, Enzmann DR. Clinical stages of human brain abscesses on serial CT scans after contrast infusion. Computerized tomographic, neuropathological, and clinical correlations. J Neurosurg. 1983;59:972.
47. Obana WG, Britt RH, Placone RC, et al. Experimental brain abscess development in the chronically immunosuppressed host. Computerized tomographic and neuropathological correlations. J Neurosurg. 1986;65:382.
48. Wood JH, Doppman JL, Lightfoote WE. Role of vascular proliferation on angiographic appearance and encapsulation of experimental traumatic and metastatic brain abscesses. J Neurosurg. 1978;48:264.
49. Prockop DJ, Kivirikko KI, Tuderman L, et al. The biosynthesis of collagen and its disorders. Part I. N Engl J Med. 1979;301:13.
50. Britt RH, Enzmann DH, Placone RC, et al. Experimental anaerobic brain abscess. J Neurosurg. 1984;60:1148.
51. Enzmann DR, Britt RH, Obana WG, et al. Experimental *Staphylococcus aureus* brain abscess. AJNR. 1986;7:395.
52. Heinnemann HS, Braude AI. Anaerobic infection of the brain. Observations on eighteen consecutive cases of brain abscess. Am J Med. 1963;35:682.
53. Ingham HR, Selkon JB, Roxby CM. Bacteriological study of otogenic cerebral abscesses: Chemotherapeutic role of metronidazole. Br Med J. 1977;2:991.
54. Arseni C, Ciurea AV. Cerebellar abscesses. A report on 119 cases. Zentralbl Neurochir. 1982;43:359.
55. Arseni C, Ciurea AV. Etiological data on cerebral abscesses. Zentralbl Neurochir. 1982;43:1.
56. Arseni C, Ciurea AV. Rhinogenic cerebral abscesses. Zentralbl Neurochir. 1982;43:12.
57. de Louvois J. Antimicrobial chemotherapy in the treatment of brain abscess. J Antimicrob Chemother. 1983;11:205.
58. de Louvois J. Bacteriological examinations of pus from abscesses of the central nervous system. J Clin Pathol. 1980;33:66.
59. Brook I. Bacteriology of intracranial abscess in children. J Neurosurg. 1981;54:484.
60. Shaw MDM, Russell JA. Cerebellar abscess—a review of 47 cases. J Neurol Neurosurg Psychiatry. 1975;38:429.
61. Murray HW, Gross KC, Masur H, et al. Serious infections caused by *Streptococcus milleri*. Am J Med. 1978;64:759.
62. Shlaes DM, Lerner PM, Wolinsky E, et al. Infections due to Lancefield group F and related streptococci (*S. milleri, S. anginosus*). Medicine (Baltimore). 1981;60:197.
63. Parker MT, Ball LC. Streptococci and aerococci associated with systemic infection in man. J Med Microbiol. 1976;9:275.
64. Carey ME, Chou SN, French LA. Experience with brain abscesses. J Neurosurg. 1972;36:1.
65. Lechtenberg R, Sierra MF, Pringle GF, et al. *Listeria monocytogenes:* Brain abscess or meningoencephalitis: Neurology (NY). 1979;29:86.
66. Nieman RE, Lorber B. Listeriosis in adults: A changing pattern. Report of eight cases and review of the literature. Rev Infect Dis. 1980;2:207.
67. Norden CW, Ruben FL, Selker R. Nonsurgical treatment of cerebral nocardiosis. Arch Neurol. 1983;40:594.
68. Levy RL, Saunders RL. *Citrobacter* meningitis and cerebral abscess in early infancy: Cure by moxalactam. Neurology (NY). 1981;31:1575.
69. Curless RG: Neonatal intracranial abscess: Two cases caused by *Citrobacter* and a literature review. Ann Neurol. 1980;8:269.
70. Rodriquez RE, Valero V, Watanakunakorn C. *Salmonella* focal intracranial infections: Review of the world literature (1884–1984) and report of an unusual case. Rev Infect Dis. 1986;8:31–41.
71. Dijkmans BAC, Thomeer RTWM, Vielvoye GJ, et al. Brain abscess due to *Streptobacillus moniliformis* and *Actinobacterium meyerii*. Infection. 1984;12:262.
72. Bell WE. Treatment of fungal infections of the central nervous system. Ann Neurol. 1981;9:417.
73. Chernik NL, Armstrong D, Posner JB. Central nervous system infections in patients with cancer. Medicine (Baltimore). 1973;52:563.
74. Beal MF, O'Carroll CP, Kleinman GM, et al. Aspergillosis of the nervous system. Neurology (NY). 1982;32:473.
75. Parker JC Jr, McCloskey JJ, Lee RS. The emergence of candidosis. The dominant postmortem cerebral mycosis. Am J Clin Pathol. 1978;70:31.
76. Sandhyamani S, Bhalia R, Mohapatra LN, et al. Cerebral cladosporiosis. Surg. Neurol. 1981;15:431.
77. Masdeu JC, Tantulavanich S, Gorelick PP, et al. Brain abscess caused by *Strongyloides stercoralis*. Arch Neurol. 1982;39:62.
78. Becker GL Jr, Knep S, Lance KP, et al. Amebic abscess of the brain. Neurosurgery. 1980;6:192.
79. Schmutzhard E, Mayr U, Rumpl E, et al. Secondary cerebral amebiasis due to infection with *Entamoeba histolytica*. Eur Neurol. 1986;25:161.
80. Armstrong D. Central nervous system infections in the immunocompromised host. Infection. 1984;12(Suppl 1):58.
81. Hooper DC, Pruitt AA, Rubin RH. Central nervous system infection in the chronically immunosuppressed. Medicine (Baltimore). 1982;61:166.
82. Horowitz SL, Bentson JR, Benson F, et al. CNS toxoplasmosis in acquired immunodeficiency syndrome. Arch Neurol. 1983;40:649–52.
83. Stamm SM, Dismukes WE, Simmons BP, et al. Listeriosis in renal transplant recipients: Report of an outbreak and review of 102 cases. Rev Infect Dis. 1982;4:589.
84. McArthur JC. Neurologic manifestations of AIDS. Medicine (Baltimore). 1987;66:407.
85. Levy RM, Bredesen DE, Rosenblum ML. Neurological manifestations of the acquired immunodeficiency syndrome (AIDS): Experience at UCSF and review of the literature. J Neurosurg. 1985;62:475.
86. Bishburg E, Sunderan EG, Reichman LB, et al. Central nervous system tuberculosis with the acquired immunodeficiency syndrome and its related complex. Ann Intern Med. 1986;105:210.
87. Helweg-Larsen S, Jakobsen J, Boesen F, et al. Neurological complications and concomitants of AIDS. Acta Neurol Scand. 1986;74:467.
88. Adams RD, Victor M. Nonviral infections of the nervous system. In: Adams RD, Victor M, eds. Principles of Neurology. New York: McGraw-Hill, 1985:552.
89. Domingue JN, Wilson CB: Pituitary abscesses. Report of seven cases and review of the literature. J Neurosurg. 1977;46:601.
90. Yoshikawa TT, Goodman SJ. Brain abscess. West J Med. 1974;121:207.
91. Nielsen H, Halaburt H. Cerebral abscess with special reference to the angiographic changes. Neuroradiology. 1976;12:73.
92. Crocker EF, McLaughlin AF, Morris JG, et al. Technetium brain scanning in the diagnosis and management of cerebral abscess. Am J Med. 1974;56:192.
93. Mascucci EF, Sauerbrunn BJL. The evolution of a brain abscess. The complementary roles of radionuclide and computed tomography scans. Clin Nucl Med. 1982;7:166.
94. Rosenblum ML, Hoff JT, Norman D, et al. Decreased mortality from brain abscesses since advent of computerized tomography. J Neurosurg. 1978;49:658.
95. Potter GD, ed. CT of the ear, nose and throat. Radiol Clin North Am. 1984;22:1.
96. New PFJ, Davis KR, Ballantine HT Jr. Computed tomography in cerebral abscess. Radiology. 1976;121:641.
97. Whelan MA, Hilal SK. Computed tomography as a guide in the diagnosis and follow-up of brain abscesses. Radiology. 1980;135:663.
98. Weisberg L. Clinical-CT correlations in intracranial suppurative (bacterial) disease. Neurology (NY). 1984;34:509.
99. Dobkin JF, Healton EB, Dickinson T, et al. Nonspecificity of ring enhancement in medically cured brain abscess. Neurology (NY). 1984;34:139.
100. Holtas S, Tornquist C, Cronqvist S. Diagnostic difficulties in computed tomography of brain abscesses. J Comput Assist Tomogr. 1982;6:683.
101. Coulam CM, Seshul M, Donaldson J. Intracranial ring lesions: Can we differentiate by computed tomography? Invest Radiol. 1980;15:103.
102. Rehncrona S, Brismar J, Holtas S. Diagnosis of brain abscesses with indium-111 labeled leukocytes. Neurosurgery. 1985;16:23.
103. Bellotti C, Aragno MG, Medina M, et al. Differential diagnosis of CT-hypodense cranial lesions with indium-111-oxine–labeled leukocytes. J Neurosurg. 1986;64:750.
104. Brant-Zawadzki M, Enzmann DR, Placone RC, et al. NMR imaging of experimental brain abscess: Comparison with CT. AJNR. 1983;4:250.
105. Runge VM, Clanton JA, Price AC, et al. Evaluation of contrast-enhanced MR imaging in a brain-abscess model. AJNR. 1985;6:139.
106. Grossman RI, Joseph PM, Wolf G, et al. Experimental intracranial septic infarction: Magnetic resonance enhancement. Radiology. 1985;155:649.

107. Davidson MD, Steiner RE. Magnetic resonance imaging in infections of the central nervous system. AJNR. 1985;6:499.
108. Scheld WM. Experimental animal models of bacterial meningitis. In: Zak O, Sande MA, eds. Experimental Models in Antimicrobial Chemotherapy. v. 1. Orlando, FL: Academic Press; 1986:139.
109. Oftedahl PR, Winn G, Rodeheaver G, et al. Changes in regional cerebral blood flow and blood brain barrier permeability in experimental brain abscess. J Cereb Blood Flow Metab. 1981;1(Suppl):38.
110. Wellman WE, Dodge HW, Heilmann FR, et al. Concentration of antibiotics in the brain. J Lab Clin Med. 1954;43:275.
111. Kramer PW, Griffith RS, Campbell RL. Antibiotic penetration of the brain. A comparative study. J Neurosurg. 1969;31:295.
112. Black P, Graybill JR, Charache P. Penetration of brain abscess by systemically administered antibiotics. J Neurosurg. 1973;38:705.
113. de Louvois J, Gortvai P, Hurley R. Antibiotic treatment of abscesses of the central nervous system. Br Med J. 1977;2:985.
114. Picardi JL, Lewis HP, Tan JS, et al. Clindamycin concentrations in the central nervous system of primates before and after head trauma. J Neurosurg. 1975;43:717.
115. de Louvois J, Hurley R. Inactivation of penicillin by purulent exudates. Br Med J. 1977;1:998.
116. Alderson D, Strong AJ, Ingham HR, et al. Fifteen year review of the mortality of brain abscess. Neurosurgery. 1981;8:1.
117. Smego R, Moeller MS, Gallis HA. Trimethoprim-sulfamethoxazole therapy for *Nocardia* infections. Arch Intern Med. 1983;143:711.
118. Maderazo EG, Quintiliani R. Treatment of nocardial infection with trimethoprim and sulfamethoxazole. Am J Med. 1974;57:671.
119. Levitz R, Quintiliani R. Trimethoprim-sulfamethoxazole for bacterial meningitis. Ann Intern Med. 1984;100:881.
120. Greene BM, Thomas FE Jr, Alford RH. Trimethoprim-sulfamethoxazole and brain abscess. Ann Intern Med. 1975;82:812.
121. Levy RM, Gutin PH, Baskin DS, et al. Vancomycin penetration of a brain abscess: Case report and review of the literature. Neurosurgery. 1986;18:633.
122. Preheim LC, McCracken GH, Jubeliver DP. Moxalactam penetration into brain abscess (abstract 738). In: Proceedings of the 21st Interscience Conference on Antimicrobial Agents and Chemotherapy. Chicago: American Society for Microbiology (ASM);1981.
123. Marcus MG, Atluru VL, Epstein N, et al. Conservative management of *Citrobacter diversus* meningitis with brain abscess. NY State J Med. 1984;84:252.
124. Scheld WM, Brodeur JP, Foresman PA, et al. Comparative evaluation of aztreonam in therapy for experimental bacterial meningitis and cerebritis. Rev Infect Dis. 1985;7(Suppl 4):635.
125. Neu HC. Uses of antimicrobial agents in brain abscesses. In: Nelson JD, Grassi C, eds. Current Chemotherapy and Infectious Disease. v. 1. Washington DC: American Society for Microbiology; 1980:41.
126. Norrby R. A review of the penetration of antibiotics into CSF and its clinical significance. Scand J Infect Dis. 1978;14(Suppl):296.
127. Haley EC Jr, Costello GT, Rodeheaver GT, et al. Treatment of experimental brain abscess with penicillin and chloramphenicol. J Infect Dis. 1983;148:737.
128. Ballantine HJ, White JC. Brain abscess. Influence of the antibiotic on therapy and morbidity. N Engl J Med. 1953;248:14.
129. Jooma OV, Pennybacker JB, Tutton GT. Brain abscess: Aspiration, drainage or excision? J Neurol Neurosurg Psychiatry. 1951;14:308.
130. Tutton GK: Cerebral abscess. The present position. Ann R Coll Surg Engl. 1953;13:281.
131. Holm S, Kourtopoulos H. Penetration of antibiotics into brain tissue and brain abscesses. An experimental study in steroid treated rats. Scand J Infect Dis. 1985;44(Suppl):68.
132. Warner J, Perkins RL, Cordero L. Metronidazole therapy of anaerobic bacteremia, meningitis, and brain abscess. Arch Intern Med. 1979;139:167.
133. Frame PT, Watanakunakorn C, McLaurin RL, et al. Penetration of nafcillin, methicillin, and cefazolin into human brain tissue. Neurosurgery. 1983;12:14.
134. Young RF, Frazee J. Gas within intracranial abscess cavities: An indication for surgical excision. Ann Neurol. 1984;16:35.
135. Karandanis D, Shulman JA. Factors associated with mortality in brain abscess. Arch Intern Med. 1975;135:1145.
136. Ohaegbulam SC, Saddeqi NU. Experience with brain abscesses treated by simple aspiration. Surg Neurol. 1980;13:289.
137. Rousseaux M, Lesoin F, Destee A, et al. Long term sequelae of hemispheric abscesses as a function of the treatment. Acta Neurochir. 1985;74:61.
138. LeBeau J, Creissard P, Harispe L, et al. Surgical treatment of brain abscess and subdural empyema. J Neurosurg. 1973;38:198.
139. Lunsford LD, Nelson PB. Stereotactic aspiration of a brain abscess using the therapeutic CT scanner. Acta Neurochir. 1982;62:25.
140. Apuzzo MLJ, Sabshin JK. Computed tomographic guidance stereotaxis in the management of intracranial mass lesions. Neurosurgery. 1983;12:277.
141. Lunsford D, Martinez AJ. Stereotactic exploration of the brain in the era of computed tomography. Surg Neurol. 1984;22:222.
142. Nauta HJW, Conteras FL, Weiner RL, et al. Brain stem abscess managed with computed tomography–guided stereotactic aspiration. Neurosurgery. 1987;20:476.
143. Itakura T, Yokote H, Ozaki F, et al. Stereotactic operation for brain abscess. Surg Neurology (NY). 1987;28:196.
144. Hall WA, Martinez AJ, Dummer JS, et al. Nocardial brain abscess; diagnostic and therapeutic use of stereotactic aspiration. Surg Neurol. 1987;28:114.
145. Enzmann DR, Britt RH, Placone R. Staging of human brain abscess by computed tomography. Radiology. 1983;146:703.
146. Heinnemann HS, Braude AI, Osterholm JL. Intracranial suppurative disease. Early presumptive diagnosis and successful treatment without surgery. JAMA. 1971;218:1542.
147. Rosenblum ML, Mampalam TJ, Pons VG. Controversies in the management of brain abscesses. Clin Neurosurg. 1986;33:603.
148. Berg B, Franklin G, Cuneo R, et al. Nonsurgical cure of brain abscess: Early diagnosis and follow-up with computerized tomography. Ann Neurol. 1978;3:474.
149. Rotheram EB Jr, Kessler LA. Use of computerized tomography in nonsurgical management of brain abscess. Arch Neurol. 1979;36:25.
150. Rosenblum ML, Hoff JT, Norman D, et al. Nonoperative treatment of brain abscesses in selected high-risk patients. J Neurosurg. 1980;52:217.
151. Boom WH, Tuazon CU. Successful treatment of multiple brain abscesses with antibiotics alone. Rev Infect Dis. 1985;7:189.
152. Daniels SR, Price JK, Towbin RB, et al. Nonsurgical cure of brain abscess in a neonate. Child Nerv Syst. 1985;1:346.
153. Keren G, Tyrrell DLJ. Nonsurgical treatment of brain abscesses: Report of two cases. Pediatr Infect Dis. 1984;3:331.
154. Enzmann DR, Britt RH, Yeager AS. Experimental brain abscess evolution: Computed tomographic and neuropathologic correlation. Radiology. 1979;133:113.
155. Epstein F, Whelan M. Cerebritis masquerading as brain abscess: Case report. Neurosurgery. 1982;10:757.
156. Scheld WM, Brodeur JP. Effect of methylprednisolone on entry of ampicillin and gentamicin into the cerebrospinal fluid in experimental pneumococcal and *E. coli* meningitis. Antimicrob Agents Chemother. 1983;23:108.
157. Kourtopoulos H, Holm SE, Norrby SR. The influence of steroids on the penetration of antibiotics into brain tissue and brain abscesses. An experimental study in rats. J Antimicrob Chemother. 1983;11:245.
158. Neuwelt EA, Lawrence MS, Blank NK. Effect of gentamicin and dexamethasone on the natural history of the rat *Escherichia coli* brain abscess model with histopathologic correlation. Neurosurgery. 1984;15:475.
159. Enzmann DR, Britt RH, Placone RC Jr, et al. The effect of short-term corticosteroid treatment on the CT appearance of experimental brain abscesses. Radiology. 1982;145:79.
160. Black KL, Farhat SM. Cerebral abscess: Loss of computed tomographic enhancement with steroids. Neurosurgery. 1984;14:215.
161. Gruszkiewicz J, Doron Y, Peyser E, et al. Brain abscess and its surgical management. Surg Neurol. 1982;18:7.
162. Calliauw WL, dePraetere P, Verbeke L. Postoperative epilepsy in subdural suppurations. Acta Neurochir. 1984;71:217.

71. SUBDURAL EMPYEMA

JOHN E. GREENLEE

The outer two layers of meninges, the dura and arachnoid, enclose a potential subdural space crossed by numerous small veins. Anatomic barriers to extension of infection within this space exist only at the falx cerebri, the tentorium cerebelli, the base of the brain, the foramen magnum, and the anterior spinal canal where arachnoid and dura are joined by penetrating nerves and vessels.[1] These structures divide the subdural space into several large compartments, within each of which subdural infection can spread but in which the infection will be confined to behave as a rapidly expanding mass lesion. Infection of the spinal subdural space is rare, but subdural empyema constitutes 13–23 percent of localized intracranial bacterial infections.[2,3] LeBeau has described subdural empyema as "the most imperative of all neurosurgical emergencies."[4]

ETIOLOGY AND PATHOGENESIS

In most cases, infection reaches the subdural space through emissary veins or by extension of an osteomyelitis of the skull, with accompanying epidural abscess.[5–9] In over half the cases, the source of infection is the paranasal sinuses, with the frontal and ethmoidal sinuses involved in 50–80 percent of the cases.[3,5–11] The middle ear and mastoid are the source in 10–

20 percent. In 5 percent of the cases, the infection is metastatic, principally from the lung.[2,8] Subdural empyema may also follow skull trauma, surgical procedures, or infection of a pre-existing subdural hematoma.[10–13]

BACTERIOLOGIC CHARACTERISTICS

Aerobic streptococci have been isolated in 35 percent of reported cases and staphylococci in 17 percent. A variety of other organisms including *Streptococcus pneumoniae, Haemophilus influenzae*, and gram-negative organisms have been recovered in 14 percent of cases.[2,7] Anaerobic organisms, particularly anaerobic and microaerophilic streptococci (including *Streptococcus anginosus*) and *Bacteroides fragilis*, have been reported in 12 percent of cases.[14] When careful anaerobic culturing is performed, however, these organisms are isolated in 33–100 percent of cases.[15] Polymicrobial infections are common.

PATHOLOGIC CHARACTERISTICS

The infection may involve one or both hemispheres and may occur at the base of the brain, over the convexity, or along the falx cerebri.[1,5–9] The posterior fossa is rarely involved. The subdural space contains an inflammatory exudate that is largest over the frontal lobes if the empyema follows sinusitis or over the temporal and occipital lobes if it follows otitis.[3] The empyema may be multiloculated and may be contralateral to the associated sinusitis. A focal, inflammatory reaction is frequently present within the subarachnoid space, but purulent meningitis occurs in only 14 percent of the cases. Focal osteomyelitis and/or epidural abscess is present in as many as 50 percent of the cases.[5–9] Septic thrombosis of veins within the empyema may extend into venous sinuses or cortical veins, causing hemorrhagic infarction and superficial abscess formation. Cerebral edema rapidly develops and may contribute greatly to mass effect early in the course of infection. Transtentorial herniation occurs unless there is prompt surgical intervention and may be precipitated by lumbar puncture.[2,5]

CLINICAL FEATURES

Subdural empyema may develop at any age but is most common in the second and third decades. Males are affected four times more frequently than are females.[2,3,5] In 60–90 percent of the cases there is an accompanying, frequently asymptomatic sinusitis or otitis. Extension of infection into the subdural space produces fever, focal headaches that later become generalized, vomiting, and signs of meningeal irritation.[2,6,9] Alteration in mental status may be insidious in onset and is present in 50 percent of the patients early in the infection.[3] Within 24–48 hours focal neurologic signs appear and progress rapidly to those of dysfunction of an entire cerebral hemisphere,[2] with hemiparesis, hemisensory deficit, and hemianopsia. Seizures, usually focal,[2] occur in 50 percent of the cases, and aphasia is common when the dominant hemisphere is involved.[3] Unless treatment is instituted, neurologic signs worsen, and signs of increased intracranial pressure appear, with transtentorial and tonsillar herniation. The course of the illness is sufficiently rapid that papilledema develops in less than 50 percent of the patients.[2,3]

Several exceptions exist to this clinical picture. Symptoms may be fulminant in onset or may develop over a period of several weeks. Development of symptoms in cases arising after craniotomy may be extremely insidious.[16] Prior antibiotic therapy may minimize systemic symptoms and may mask sinusitis or otitis, to make the clinical presentation that of brain abscess.[11] Infections metastatic to the subdural space or to a pre-existing subdural hematoma may fail to produce sinus tenderness or systemic symptoms. In such cases, particularly in the alcoholic with an infected subdural hematoma, the patient often is seen late in the illness, and mortality is higher.

DIAGNOSIS

Subdural empyema should be suspected in any patient with meningeal signs and a focal neurologic deficit, particularly where the deficit indicates extensive dysfunction of one cerebral hemisphere. Sinusitis followed by meningeal signs should also suggest the diagnosis, for bacterial meningitis per se is rarely due to sinusitis.[17]

Sinusitis or otitis is present on skull x-rays or computed tomography (CT) in over two-thirds of patients.[18–20] Spinal fluid changes are nonspecific, and the danger of transtentorial herniation represents an absolute contraindication to lumbar puncture.[2,3] Magnetic resonance imaging (MRI) and CT with contrast enhancement are the diagnostic procedures of choice.[18–20] Both procedures are useful not only for identifying the empyema but also for detecting cerebral edema and concomitant brain abscess. MRI provides greater clarity of morphologic detail and may detect empyemas not clearly seen by CT scan.[20] The ability of MRI to view the brain in coronal and sagittal sections make it of particular value in identifying empyemas located at the base of the brain, along the falx cerebri, or in the posterior fossa. CT may show a poorly circumscribed extra-axial region of diminished density, often with a thin rim of contrast enhancement (Fig. 1; see also Chapter 72, Fig. 1).[18–20] CT, unlike currently available MRI, can be used to image bone and should be employed to supplement MRI when there are questions of penetrating injury or osteomyelitis. It must be kept in mind that CT early in the course of infection or with older equipment may show only loss of normal cortical markings or unilateral hemispheric swelling.[18–20] For this reason, failure of CT to demonstrate an empyema does not exclude the diagnosis. Angiography should be considered on an emergency basis when MRI is not available and subdural empyema is suspected despite a normal CT scan.[20] Because artifacts produced by patient movement may obscure positive findings on both MRI and CT, sedation should be used if required to achieve an optimal study. Occasionally, a subdural empyema may be diagnosed only by burr holes or craniotomy.

THERAPY

Aerobic and anerobic cultures of blood and other material should be obtained and antibiotics should be begun as described

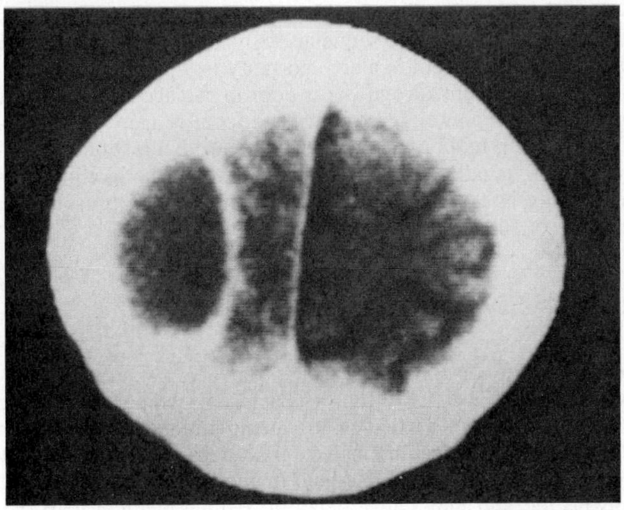

FIG. 1. Computed tomogram of subdural empyema overlying the left cerebral hemisphere. (Courtesy of Dr. Leon Morris, Charlottesville, VA.)

TABLE 1. Bacterial Etiology and Initial Antibiotic Therapy of Subdural Empyema, Epidural Abscess, and Septic Intracranial Thrombophlebitis

			Initial Therapy for Adults With Normal Renal Function	
Condition	*Site of Primary Infection*	*Probable Organisms*	*Suggested Initial Therapy (Intravenous)*	*Suggested Initial Therapy if Penicillin Allergy Present*
Subdural empyema, epidural abscess, or septic intracranial thrombophlebitis in adults[a]	Paranasal sinuses	Aerobic and anaerobic streptococci Other anaerobes *Staphylococcus aureus* (rarely facultative gram-negative bacilli)	Nafcillin 1.5 g q4h with either metronidazole or chloramphenicol[b]	Vancomycin 500 mg. IV q6h with either metronidazole or chloramphenicol[b]
	Otitis media or mastoiditis	*Staphylococcus aureus* Aerobic and anaerobic streptococci Other anaerobes Facultative gram-negative bacilli		
	Following cranial surgery	*Staphylococcus aureus* Facultative gram-negative bacilli	For suspected gram-negative bacilli infections see therapy for gram-negative meningitis (Chapter 66)	
	Hematogenous from distant and/or unknown site	Above organisms or organisms isolated from primary site		
Spinal or epidural abscess or subdural empyema	Extension of osteomyelitis or paravertebral infection Hematogenous spread	*Staphylococcus aureus* Aerobic and anaerobic streptococci Organisms isolated from distant source of sepsis	Nafcillin (1.5 g iv q4h) or antibiotic determined by organism isolated previously	Vancomycin (500 mg IV q6h)

[a] Subdural empyema in young children is almost always a complication of meningitis. See Chapter 66 for appropriate therapy.
[b] Metronidazole therapy is initiated with a loading dose of 1 g. The drug must be diluted and neutralized before intravenous use and is administered by slow intravenous infusion as 500 mg q6h. Chloramphenicol succinate is given intravenously as 1 g q6h.

in Table 1. Increased intracranial pressure may necessitate the preoperative use of mannitol, 1–1.5 g/kg infused over 10–15 minutes; hyperventilation to a P_{CO_2} of 30 torr; or dexamethasone, 10 mg iv, to be followed postoperatively by 4 mg every 6 hours (see Chapter 65). In rare cases, resolution of subdural empyemas has been reported with antibiotic therapy alone.[21] In most instances, however, the rapidly progressive nature of the infection and the fact that neuroradiologic studies may understate the actual size of the empyema necessitate emergency surgical as well as medical intervention. Craniotomy is believed by many workers to have a lower rate of complications than use of burr holes and may be essential in posterior fossa subdural empyema.[7,22–25] Use of burr holes and irrigation of the subdural space may be possible in early cases.[26] Empyema fluid should be submitted for culture, including culture for anaerobes. Otitis or sinusitis may require simultaneous surgery. The possibility of multiloculated or parafalcine infection must be kept in mind. Postoperative recurrence of the empyema may necessitate further surgery. Antibiotic therapy should be continued for at least 3 weeks.

PROGNOSIS

When treatment is prompt, there is good likelihood of neurologic recovery, but delay in therapy greatly increases the risk of permanent neurologic sequelae.[22] Overall mortality is 14–18 percent. If the patient is alert, mortality is 9 percent but if comatose, 75 percent. Prognosis is poor in the aged or when the infection is precipitous in onset. Late focal or generalized seizures develop in 42 percent of patients surviving subdural empyema and usually appear within 16 months. The likelihood of developing late seizures is not influenced by the presence or absence of seizures during the acute illness.[24]

SUBDURAL EMPYEMA IN INFANTS AND YOUNG CHILDREN

In children under 5 years of age,[27,28] intracranial subdural empyema almost invariably follows bacterial meningitis, and the causative organism is that of the meningitis itself, most often *H. influenzae*, or, in neonates, gram-negative bacilli. Early signs of irritability, poor feeding, or increase in head size are nonspecific and may cause delay in seeking medical help. By the time the child is seen by a physician, hemiparesis, convulsions, stupor, and coma are common, but fever may be absent. Examination may reveal increased head size and bulging fontanelle. Papilledema is unusual. The empyema fluid is often too turbid to allow transillumination. In infants, the diagnosis may be made by subdural taps, although this procedure will not detect a parafalcine empyema. Radiographic diagnosis and surgical therapy are as described for adults. Initial antibiotic therapy is that of the meningitis itself: a third-generation cephalosporin such as cefotaxime or alternatively ampicillin and gentamicin in neonates or ampicillin plus chloramphenicol in older infants and small children when *H. influenzae* is suspected (see Chapter 61).

SPINAL SUBDURAL EMPYEMA

Spinal subdural empyema is rare and virtually always metastatic.[29–32] Etiologic organisms are *Staphylococcus aureus* and less often, the streptococci. The empyema is usually posterior to the cord and involves the thoracic and lumbar cord more often than the cervical. Radicular pain and symptoms of cord compression may occur at multiple levels. Spinous process tenderness is often absent and vertebral osteomyelitis rare. High-resolution computed tomography may detect the lesion at one level but cannot, with equipment presently available, give accurate information as to the extent of the empyema. MRI is the diagnostic procedure of choice. Myelography should be employed when MRI is not available. Both MRI and myelography will reveal cord compression, block, or multiple extra-axial defects. Myelography, however, may not delineate the entire length of the empyema if complete obstruction of the subarachnoid space is present at multiple levels. If lower thoracic or lumbar empyema is suspected, myelography should be performed using a lateral cervical or cisternal route to avoid producing infection of the subarachnoid space. Therapy involves surgical drainage and antibiotics against penicillinase-producing staphylococci and streptococci (see Table 1). Unless therapy is begun early, cord necrosis is likely, and prognosis for recovery is poor.

REFERENCES

1. Courville CB. Subdural empyema secondary to purulent frontal sinusitis. Arch Otolaryngol. 1944;39:211–30.
2. Kaufman DM, Miller MH, Steigbigel NH. Subdural empyema: analysis of 17 recent cases and review of the literature. Medicine. 1975;54:485–98.
3. Hitchcock E, Andreadis A. Subdural empyema: a review of 29 cases. J Neurol Neurosurg Psychiatr. 1964;27:422–34.
4. LeBeau J, Creissard P, Harispe L, et al. Surgical treatment of brain abscess and subdural empyema. J Neurosurg. 1973;38:198–203.
5. Kaufman DM, Litman N, Miller MH. Sinusitis: induced empyema. Neurology. 1983;33:123–32.

6. Stephanov S, Joubert MJ, Welchman JM. Combined convexity and parafalx subdural empyema. Surg Neurol. 1979;11:147–51.
7. Mauser HW, Van Houwelingen HC, Tuleken CAF. Factors affecting the outcome in subdural empyema. J Neurol Neurosurg Psychiatr. 1987;50:1136–41.
8. Kubik CS, Adams RD. Subdural empyema. Brain. 1943;66:18–42.
9. Schiller F, Cairns H, Russell DS. The treatment of purulent pachymeningitis and subdural empyema with special reference to penicillin. J Neurol Neurosurg Psychiatr. 1948;11:143–82.
10. McLaurin RL. Subdural infection. In: Gurdjian ES, ed. Cranial and Intracranial Suppuration. Springfield, IL: Charles C Thomas; 1969:73–88.
11. Coonrod JD, Dans PE. Subdural empyema. Am J Med. 1972;53:85–91.
12. Balch RE. Wound infections complicating neurosurgical procedures. J Neurosurg. 1967;26:26:41–7.
13. Casson IR, Petel P, Blair D, et al. Subdural empyema caused by infection of a preexisting subdural hematoma. NY State Med J. 1981;81:389–91.
14. Blayney AW, Frootko NJ, Mitchell RG. Complications of sinusitis caused by *Streptococcus milleri*. J Laryngol Otol. 1984;98:895–9.
15. Yoshikawa TT, Chow AW, Guze LB. Role of anaerobic bacteria in subdural empyema. Am J Med. 1975;58:99–104.
16. Post EM, Modesti LM. "Subacute" postoperative subdural empyema. J Neurosurg. 1981;55:761–5.
17. Biehl JP. Subdural empyema secondary to acute frontal sinusitis: a neglected but curable emergency complication. JAMA. 1955;721–4.
18. Hodges J, Anslow P, Gillett G. Subdural empyema—continuing diagnostic problems in the CT scan era. Q J Med. 1986;228:387–93.
19. Weisberg L. Subdural empyema: clinical and computed tomographic correlations. Arch Neurol. 1986;43:497–500.
20. Moseley IF, Kendall BE. Radiology of intracranial empyemas, with special reference to computed tomography. Neuroradiology. 1984;333–45.
21. Mauser HW, Ravjist RAP, Elderson A, et al. Nonsurgical treatment of subdural empyema. J Neurosurg. 1985;63:128–30.
22. Bannister G, Williams B, Smith S. Treatment of subdural empyema. J Neurosurg. 1981;55:82–8.
23. Borzone M, Capuzzo T, Rivano C, et al. Subdural empyema: fourteen cases surgically treated. Surg Neurol. 1980;13:449–52.
42. Cowie R, Williams B. Late seizures and morbidity after subdural empyema. J Neurosurg. 1983;58:569–73.
25. Morgan DW, Williams B. Posterior fossa subdural empyema. Brain. 1985;108:983–92.
26. Miller ES, Dias PS, Uttley D. Management of subdural empyema: a series of 24 cases. J Neurol Neurosurg Psychiatr. 1987;50:1415–8.
27. Jacobsen PL, Farmer TW. Subdural empyema complicating meningitis in infants: improved prognosis. Neurology. 1981;31:190–6.
28. Farmer TW, Wise GR. Subdural empyema in infants, children and adults. Neurology. 1973;23:254–62.
29. Fraser RAR, Ratzan K, Wolpert SM, et al. Spinal subdural empyema. Arch Neurol. 1973;28:235–8.
30. Abbott KH. Acute pyogenic spinal epidural abscess. Bull Los Angeles Neurol Soc. 1952;17–18:91–103.
31. Dacey RG, Winn HR, Jane JA, et al. Spinal subdural empyema: report of two cases. Neurosurgery. 1978;3:400–3.
32. Heindel CC, Ferguson JP, Kumarasamy T. Spinal subdural empyema complicating pregnancy. J Neurosurg. 1974;40:654–6.

72. EPIDURAL ABSCESS

JOHN E. GREENLEE

An epidural abscess represents localized infection between the outermost layer of the meninges, the dura mater, and the overlying skull or vertebral column. Within the skull, the dura forms the inner layer of the cranial periosteum, and an intracranial epidural abscess must form by stripping periosteum from bone: such an abscess is almost always sharply confined and accompanied by focal osteomyelitis. Because of the ease with which infection can cross the cranial dura along emissary veins, subdural empyema is often present. Within the spinal canal, however, the dura mater is separated from the vertebrae by an epidural space filled with fat and vascular areolar tissue. Although the spinal dura itself is only rarely breached by bacteria, the spinal epidural space offers little resistance to the longitudinal spread of infection. For this reason, a spinal epidural abscess often occupies several vertebral segments and, within the narrow confines of the vertebral canal, may cause extensive cord compression and necrosis.

INTRACRANIAL EPIDURAL ABSCESS

The etiology, pathogenesis, and bacteriology of intracranial epidural abscess are identical to those described for intracranial subdural empyema (see Chapter 71).[1–4] Virtually all cases follow frontal sinusitis, craniotomy, or mastoiditis.[1,4] Epidural abscess may also develop during rhinocerebral mucormycosis.[5]

Pathologic Characteristics

Epidural abscess most often arises adjacent to the frontal sinuses. In almost all cases, osteomyelitis is present within overlying bones, and there is septic thrombosis of veins bridging skull and meninges. Subdural empyema is present in 81 percent of autopsied cases, with 38 percent of the cases also having meningitis and 17 percent brain abscess.[6] Rarely, infection of the bridging veins may produce venous necrosis and epidural hemorrhage rather than abscess.[7]

Clinical Features

The onset of symptoms may be insidious[4] and at first may be overshadowed by sinusitis or otitis. The abscess produces local pain followed by generalized headache, at times with alteration of mental state.[1,2,4] Focal neurologic signs and focal or generalized seizures then appear. An epidural abscess near the petrous bone may involve cranial nerves V and VI, with unilateral facial pain and lateral rectus weakness (Gradenigo syndrome).[8] As the abscess enlarges, papilledema and other signs of intracranial hypertension develop. Extension of the infection into the subdural space is accompanied by rapid neurologic deterioration.

Diagnosis

Persistent fever, leukocytosis, and focal or generalized neurologic signs in the setting of sinusitis or otitis suggest intracranial infection. Edema or cellulitis of face or scalp may be

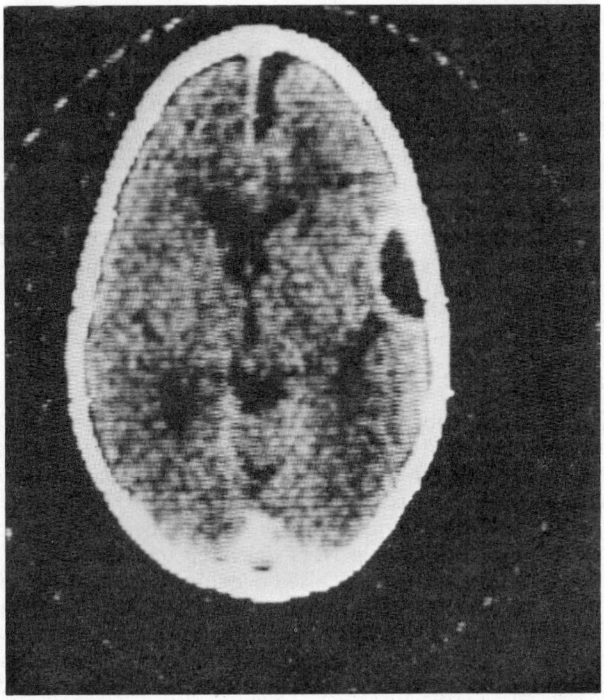

FIG. 1. Computed tomography of right-sided epidural abscess. A subdural empyema is also present between the falx cerebri and the medial aspect of the right frontal lobe. (Courtesy of Drs. D. M. Kaufman, N. E. Leeds and I. Kricheff; from Kaufman and Leeds,[9] with permission.)

present.[4] Skull x-ray films may demonstrate the sinusitis or otitis. Osteomyelitis may not be radiologically discernible if the infection is of recent onset. Magnetic resonance imaging (MRI) or computed tomography (CT)[8,9] (Fig. 1) will show a superficial, circumscribed area of diminished density; arteriography will outline an avascular mass, with inward displacement of cortical vessels and venous sinuses. Spinal fluid is usually sterile and CSF changes are nonspecific; the danger of tonsillar herniation contraindicates lumbar puncture. Successful medical therapy of intracranial epidural abscess without surgical intervention may be possible in lesions detected early in their course and followed closely by CT or MRI scans throughout treatment.[10] In general, however, intracranial epidural abscess should be drained as a neurosurgical emergency to avoid development of subdural empyema. Antibiotic therapy should be directed against aerobic and anaerobic streptococci and against *Staphylococcus aureus*, as outlined in Table 1 in Chapter 71. Concomitant surgery of infected sinuses or bone may be necessary.

SPINAL EPIDURAL ABSCESS

Etiology and Pathogenesis

Both acute and chronic spinal epidural abscess follow infection elsewhere in the body.[11–23] In most cases, infection reaches the epidural space by hematogenous spread, either by direct metastasis or by production of a vertebral osteomyelitis with extension into the spinal epidural space. Infection of the epidural space may also be caused by penetrating injuries or by extension of decubitus ulcers or paraspinal abscesses.[13] Epidural abscess has been reported following back surgery, lumbar puncture, and epidural anesthesia.[12,13,15] Rarely, infection may spread along a persistent dermal sinus. In 10–30 percent of the cases there is a history of back trauma and, less often, a history of diabetes mellitus, intravenous drug abuse, or pregnancy.[12,13,19,23]

Bacteriology

Staphylococcus aureus is the agent in 60–90 percent of both the acute and chronic cases and in some series is the only organism recovered.[11–14,16,17,19,23] Aerobic and anaerobic streptococci cause approximately 18 percent of the cases and gram-negative organisms, especially *Escherichia coli* and *Pseudomonas aeruginosa*, 13 percent.[13] Isolation of *Staphylococcus epidermidis*, pneumococcus, *Actinomyces israelii*, and gram-negative anaerobes has been reported.[13,18] Chronic epidural infection may occur during tuberculosis, frequently without other detectable evidence of infection, and may occasionally develop as a complication of echinococcosis.[19] In 10 percent of the cases, multiple organisms are present.[17]

Pathology

The abscess involves thoracic spine in 50–80 percent of the cases, lumbar in 17–38 percent, and cervical in 10–25 percent.[11–18] In children, cervical and lumbar spine are more often involved.[20] The abscess is posterior to the cord in 80–90 percent of the cases[13,21]; anterior abscesses usually occur at cervical levels, except in tuberculosis, in which the anterior thoracic or lumbar epidural spaces may also be involved. Vertebral osteomyelitis is present in 15 percent of acute and in over 50 percent of chronic epidural abscesses.[12,13,18] Acute abscesses consist of granulation tissue containing loculated pus; in chronic abscesses there may be a prominent fibroblastic component. The abscess usually occupies four or five vertebral segments but may extend the length of the cord. Enlargement of the abscess produces myelomalacia or cord necrosis both by compression and by invasion of the spinal venous plexus.[13,18] Extension of the infection into the subdural or subarachnoid spaces is unusual, except in anterior abscesses where meningitis may develop.[12,21]

Clinical Features

Epidural abscess is more common in males and may occur at any age. The abscess may develop acutely within hours to days or may pursue a chronic course over months. Most abscesses, however, pass through four clinical stages, differing only in time course: focal vertebral pain, root pain, deficits of motor, sensory, or sphincter function, and paralysis.[11] Acute metastatic infection of the epidural space produces rapid progression with prominent systemic symptoms and severe, focal pain. Patients usually seek medical help within the first few days of illness when radicular signs are already present. When epidural abscess arises following vertebral osteomyelitis, vertebral pain may develop over 2–3 weeks, but progression is rapid once radicular symptoms appear. Chronic epidural abscess may manifest with a course indistinguishable from that of an extrinsic neoplasm and without systemic signs. Where cervical cord is involved, respiratory function may be impaired.[22]

Diagnosis

Epidural abscess is a diagnostic consideration in any patient with localized back pain and radicular symptoms, especially when a source of infection is evident. Headache is a common additional complaint.[23] Nuchal rigidity and focal tenderness to percussion are almost universal.[11–13] In acute cases the white blood cell count and the erythrocyte sedimentation rate are elevated. X-ray films of the spine may show osteomyelitis but may also be normal. Magnetic resonance imaging is the diagnostic procedure of choice (Fig. 2), since it can visualize the cord and epidural space in both sagittal and transverse sections and can identify not only epidural abscess but also osteomyelitis, intra-

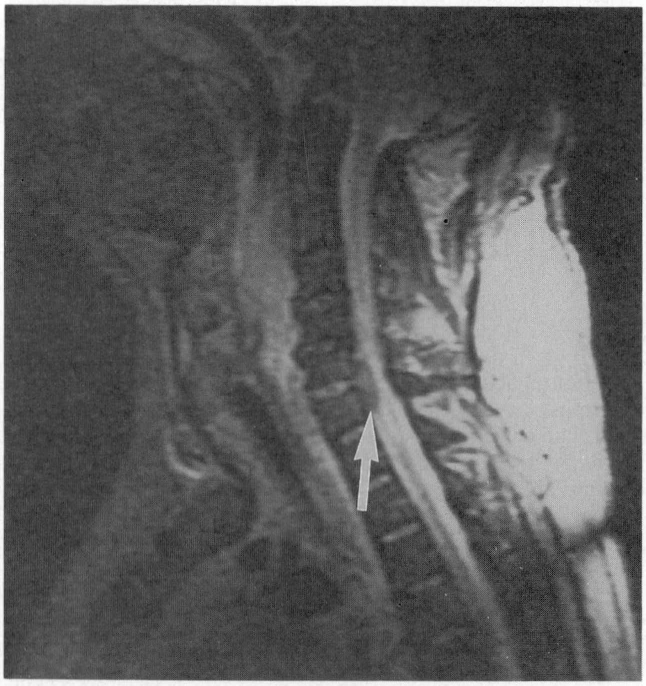

FIG. 2. Magnetic resonance scan of patient with anterior cervical epidural abscess. The abscess is seen as an area of diminished attenuation bulging into the spinal canal and compressing the spinal cord (arrow). The infection also involves the adjacent disc space. (Courtesy of Dr. J. Richard Baringer, Salt Lake City, UT.)

medullary spinal cord lesions, and joint space infection.[23,24] Myelography should be employed if MRI is not available or cannot be performed. Computed tomography with contrast enhancement may be helpful in differentiating subdural from epidural infections or in identifying osteomyelitis. CT is less sensitive than MRI, however, and may fail to define the longitudinal extent of the abscess. MRI should precede lumbar puncture when epidural abscess is suspected. In the absence of MRI, lumbar puncture should never be attempted without provision to introduce dye and carry out myelography before the needle is withdrawn. Spinal puncture, if indicated, should be performed well above or below the suspected area of involvement, and the needle should be advanced slowly with frequent aspiration to avoid contaminating the subdural or subarachnoid space. Artifacts produced by patient movement may obscure positive findings on MRI, CT, or myelography, and adequate sedation should be employed if required to achieve an optimal study. Spinal fluid is usually sterile, with nonspecific changes in cells, protein, and glucose. Blood and abscess material should be submitted for aerobic and anaerobic culture.

Therapy

The danger of spinal cord necrosis requires laminectomy and drainage as soon as the diagnosis is made. Antibiotic therapy should begin before surgery and, in the absence of a known causative organism, should be directed against penicillin-resistant *S. aureus*, with modification of antibiotic therapy based on Gram stain and culture. In certain carefully selected cases, the availability of highly sensitive, noninvasive methods of imaging the spine and epidural space has made it possible to treat spinal epidural abscess with antibiotics alone.[25,26] Such cases have included those who represent unacceptable surgical risks and also occasional patients without neurologic deficit in whom it is decided to defer surgery while monitoring the patient's neurologic status closely and following abscess size with serial MRI or CT scans. In such patients, surgery should be carried out immediately if neurologic findings appear despite antibiotic therapy. Antibiotic therapy should be continued for 3–4 weeks in spinal epidural abscess per se or for 8 weeks when there is an accompanying osteomyelitis. Prognosis for neurologic recovery is excellent if therapy is begun before or during the stage of radicular symptoms but worsens rapidly as evidence of cord injury appears. Mortality is 10–20 percent[13] but is higher, as is the likelihood of permanent neurologic deficit, if cervical cord is involved.[22,23]

HYPERTROPHIC SPINAL PACHYMENINGITIS

Rarely, chronic inflammation or infection within the spinal canal involves the dura mater alone, to produce a diffuse, fibrosing pachymeningitis. Cases have been attributed to syphilis and also to tuberculosis, but in many cases no etiologic organism can be identified.[27–29] The fibrosis compresses nerve roots and if extensive may injure the spinal cord. Early symptoms are pain, muscle weakness, and muscle atrophy occurring in a radicular pattern. Spinal fluid contains elevated protein but no cells. Electromyography may localize the process to nerve roots. In most cases, diagnosis has been made by myelography with lateral views. Newer techniques, however, such as myelography followed by CT or, in particular MRI with and without contrast enhancement with gadolinium may give much more precise information.[27,29] Treatment consists of surgical removal of the hypertrophied dura and antibiotic therapy of any diagnosed causative infection.

ACKNOWLEDGMENTS

Work on this chapter was supported in part by the Veterans Administration.

REFERENCES

1. Handel SF, Klein WC, Kim YW. Intracranial epidural abscess. Radiology. 1974;11:117–20.
2. Koenig RP, Craigmile TK. Epidural intracranial abscess. USAF Med J. 1957;8:120–4.
3. Norrell HA, Wilson CB. Primary intracranial extradural abscess diagnosed by carotid angiography. J Kentucky Med Assoc. 1967;65:1186–7.
4. French LA, Chou SN. Osteomyelitis of the skull and epidural abscess. In: Gurdjian ES, ed. Cranial and Intracranial Suppuration. Springfield, IL: Charles C Thomas; 1969:59–72.
5. Muresan A. A case of cerebral mucormycosis diagnosed in life, with eventual recovery. J Clin Pathol. 1960;13:34–6.
6. Slager UT. Infection and parainfectious inflammations. In: Basic Neuropathology. Baltimore: Williams & Wilkins; 1970:89–135.
7. Rajput AJ, Rozdilsky B. Extradural hematoma following frontal sinusitis. Arch Otolaryngol. 1971;94:83–5.
8. Lott T, El Gammal T, Dasilva R, et al. Evaluation of brain and epidural abscesses by computed tomography. Radiology. 1977;122:371–6.
9. Kaufman DMA, Leeds NE. Computed tomography (CT) in the diagnosis of intracranial abscesses. Neurology. 1977;27:1069–73.
10. Leys D, Destee A, Warot P. Empyeme extra-dural en fosse posterieure: traitement medical exclusif. Presse Med. 1983;12:1549.
11. Heusner AP. Nontuberculous spinal epidural infections. N Engl J Med. 1948;239:845–54.
12. Hulme A, Dott NM. Spinal epidural abscess. Br Med J. 1954;1:64–5.
13. Baker AS, Ojemann RG, Swartz MN, et al. Spinal epidural abscess. N Engl J Med. 1975;293:463–8.
14. Dandy WE. Abscesses and inflammatory tumors in the spinal epidural space (so-called pachymeningitis externa). Arch Surg. 1926;13:477–94.
15. Ferguson JF, Kirsch WM. Epidural empyema following thoracic extradural block. J Neurosurg. 1974;41:762–4.
16. Russell NA, Vaughan R, Morley TP. Spinal epidural infection. Can J Neurol Sci. 1979;6:325–8.
17. Dus V. Spinal peripachymeningitis (epidural abscess). J Neurosurg. 1960;17:972–83.
18. Browder J, Meyers R. Pyogenic infections of the spinal epidural space. Surgery. 1941;10:296–308.
19. Kaufman DM, Kaplan JG, Litman N. Infectious agents in spinal epidural abscess. Neurology. 1980;30:844–50.
20. Baker CJ. Primary spinal epidural abscess. Am J Dis Child. 1971;121:337–9.
21. Mixter WJ, Smithwick RH. Acute intraspinal epidural abscess. N Engl J Med. 1932;207:126–36.
22. Durity F, Thompson GB. Localized cervical extradural abscess. J Neurosurg. 1968;28:387–90.
23. Lasker BR, Harter DH. Cervical epidural abscess. Neurology. 1987;37:1747–53.
24. Modic MT, Feiglin DH, Piranio DW. Vertebral osteomyelitis: assessment using MRI. Radiology. 1985;157:157–66.
25. Leys D, Lesoin F, Viaud C, et al. Decreased morbidity from acute bacterial spinal epidural abscesses using computed tomography and nonsurgical treatment in selected patients. Ann Neurol. 1985;17:350–5.
26. Messer HD, Lenchner GS, Brust JCM, et al. Lumbar spinal abscess managed conservatively. J Neurosurg. 1977;46:825–9.
27. Bucy PC, Freeman W. Hypertrophic spinal pachymeningitis. J Neurosurg. 1952;9:564–78.
28. Guidetti B, LaTorre E. Hypertrophic spinal pachymeningitis. J Neurosurg. 1967;26:496–503.
29. Oonishi T, Ishiko T, Arai M, et al. Pachymeningitis cervicalis hypertrophica. Acta Pathol Jpn. 1982;32:163–71.

73. SUPPURATIVE INTRACRANIAL PHLEBITIS

JOHN E. GREENLEE

Septic intracranial thrombophlebitis most frequently follows infection of paranasal sinuses, middle ear, mastoid, face, or oropharynx. The infection spreads centrally along emissary veins.[1–5] Septic thrombophlebitis may also occur in association with epidural abscess, subdural empyema, or meningitis. Occasionally, the infection is metastatic from lungs or other distant sites.[3] The likelihood of thrombosis is increased by states altering blood viscosity or coagulability, including dehydration, polycythemia, pregnancy, oral contraceptive use, sickle cell disease, malignancy, or trauma.[4,6,7] *Staphylococcus aureus* is the most frequent isolate.[1] A minority of cases are due to *Staphylococcus epidermidis*, streptococci including *S. pneumoniae*, gram-negative bacilli,[1,2] and anaerobic organisms. Multiple infecting organisms may be present.[8]

PATHOLOGIC CHANGES

Septic intracranial thrombophlebitis may begin within veins or venous sinuses and may involve additional vessels by propagation or discontinuous spread.[1,9] The pathologic changes are those of both venous thrombosis and suppuration. Venous occlusion may produce no local injury, but if collateral veins are compromised, edema and hemorrhagic infarction result. The most common sites of infarction are the area of venous watershed immediately above the Sylvian fissue (see Chapter 65)[3] and the medial surfaces of the cerebral hemispheres.[3,4] Thrombosis of the anterior portion of the superior sagittal sinus or of the lateral sinuses may block reabsorption of cerebrospinal fluid with resultant communicating hydrocephalus. Local suppuration may produce venous necrosis and hemorrhage or may cause epidural abscess, subdural empyema, meningitis, or brain abscess.[1–4] Septic embolization may produce pulmonary infarction, abscesses in lungs or other organs, or mycotic aneurysm.[2–4,9]

CLINICAL FEATURES

Cortical Vein Thrombosis

If collateral venous drainage is adequate, septic venous thrombosis may produce only transient neurologic findings or may be silent except for its metastatic consequences. If the thrombus outstrips collateral flow, however, a progressive neurologic deficit will result and may mimic brain abscess, with impairment of consciousness, focal or generalized seizures, and increased intracranial pressure.[2,3] Focal neurologic findings include hemiparesis, which involves the face and hand if veins over the cerebral convexity are involved.[3] Thrombosis of veins along the falx cerebri may produce unilateral leg weakness, which becomes bilateral if propagation of the thrombus involves the veins of the contralateral hemisphere.[2,3] Aphasia is common when the dominant hemisphere is involved. Transient hemodynamic variation in venous collateral flow may cause considerable fluctation in neurologic signs.

Venous Sinus Thrombosis

The clinical findings vary with the sinus involved and are summarized in Table 1 (see Chapter 65, Fig. 5). Cavernous sinus, lateral sinus, and superior sagittal sinus are most often involved. Cavernous sinus thrombosis most commonly follows infections of the face or of the sphenoid and ethmoid sinuses.[1,9] Onset is abrupt, with diplopia, photophobia, orbital edema, and progressive exophthalmos.[9,10] Involvement of cranial nerves III, IV, V, and VI produces ophthalmoplegia, a midposition fixed pupil, loss of corneal reflex, and diminished sensation over the upper face. Obstruction of venous return from the retina results in papilledema, retinal hemorrhages, and visual loss. Similar findings appear in the opposite eye as the infection spreads to the contralateral cavernous sinus. Engorgement or thrombosis of facial veins may occur.

Thrombosis of the superior sagittal sinus produces bilateral leg weakness and may cause communicating hydrocephalus.[2,3,5] Occlusion of the lateral sinus produces pain over the ear and mastoid and may cause edema over the mastoid (Griesinger's sign).[4,11,12] Impairment of veins supplying cranial nerves V and VI produces ipsilateral facial pain and lateral rectus weakness (Gradenigo syndrome). Septic cortical vein or venous sinus occlusion may produce subdural empyema, meningitis, or brain abscess. The danger of septic pulmonary embolization is always present.

DIAGNOSIS

Septic intracranial thrombophlebitis may manifest as sepsis without neurologic signs or with stupor and focal neurologic signs in the presence of cranial infection. In the latter instance, septic thrombophlebitis may be indistinguishable from brain abscess or subdural empyema. Fever, leukocytosis, and elevated erythrocyte sedimentation rate are usually present. Skull x-rays should be evaluated for the presence of sinusitis or mastoiditis, with particular attention to frontal, ethmoidal, and sphenoidal sinuses. Lumbar puncture may reveal increased pressure, slight

TABLE 1. Symptoms of Intracranial Venous Sinus Occlusion

Venous Sinus Involved	*Associated Infection*	*Anatomic Structures Affected*	*Clinical Findings*
Cavernous sinus	Paranasal sinusitis, especially of frontal, ethmoidal or sphenoidal sinuses, infection of face or mouth	Venous drainage from orbit and eye. Cranial nerves III, IV, V, and VI within the cavernous sinus [venous supply of frontal lobe and pituitary]	Unilateral periorbital edema, exophthalmos, and chemosis; examination shows papilledema, ocular palsies, diminished pupillary reactivity, frequently diminished corneal reflex, and impaired sensation in the first and second divisions of V; extension to the contralateral sinus may duplicate these findings in the opposite eye [seizures, frontal lobe, deficits, hypopituitarism]
Lateral sinus	Otitis media or mastoiditis; rarely pharyngitis	Cranial nerves V and VI Venous route of CSF reabsorption [venous supply of temporal lobe, jugular bulb, cranial nerves IX, X, XI at jugular foramen]	Lateral rectus weakness; facial pain and altered facial sensation; increased intracranial pressure with papilledema if the other lateral sinus is also compromised [temporal lobe seizures; jugular foramen syndrome with ipsilateral palatal weakness, diminished gag reflex, and weakness of trapezius and sternomastoid]
Superior sagittal sinus	Infections of face, scalp, subdural or epidural spaces; meningitis	Venous drainage from medial portion of cerebral hemispheres; CSF reabsorption	Bilateral leg weakness; intracranial hypertension
Superior petrosal sinus	Otitis media or mastoiditis	Trigeminal ganglion [venous drainage from temporal lobe]	Ipsilateral pain or sensory deficit [temporal lobe seizures]
Inferior petrosal sinus	Otitis media or mastoiditis	Cranial nerves V and VI at tip of petrous bone	"Gradenigo syndrome"; ipsilateral facial pain and sensory deficit; ipsilateral lateral rectus palsy

Note: Brackets indicate structures affected or symptoms produced by extension of the sinus thrombus into cortical veins.

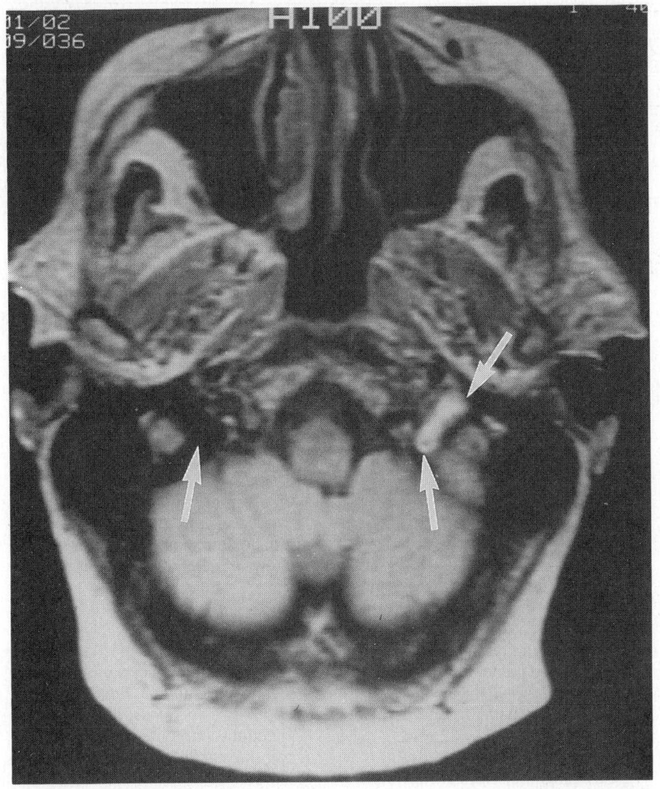

FIG. 1. Magnetic resonance scan in patient with left internal jugular vein thrombosis. There is bright signal, consistent with vessel occlusion, arising from the left internal jugular vein (double arrows). In contrast, the right internal jugular vein exhibits diminished signal (flow void) consistent with normal blood flow (single arrow). (Courtesy of Dr. Anne Osborn, Salt Lake City, UT.)

lymphocytic pleocytosis, and mild elevation of protein. Evidence of subarachnoid blood detectable by lumbar puncture is present in less than 15 percent of cases,[1,2] and cerebrospinal fluid is usually sterile. Magnetic resonance imaging (MRI), because of its ability to visualize vessels and to differentiate between normally flowing blood and thrombus, is the diagnostic procedure of choice (Fig. 1).[13–16] Computed tomography (CT) scanning, although considerably less sensitive and reliable than MRI, permits diagnosis of venous sinus thrombosis in many cases and should be employed as the initial diagnostic test when MRI is not available.[17–19] Magnetic resonance imaging and CT also provide information about concomitant subdural or epidural infections and allow visualization of brain infarction, hemorrhage, and edema. Angiography with close attention to the venous phase should be employed when venous sinus thrombosis is suspected despite negative MRI or CT.[20] Retrograde venography or digital subtraction angiography may prove useful in selected cases. Blood, spinal fluid, and all infected material should be cultured for both aerobic and anaerobic organisms.

TREATMENT

Appropriate antibiotic therapy, reversal of elevated intracranial pressure, and control of seizures are the goals of therapy. Initial antibiotics should be directed against *Staphylococcus aureus*, aerobic streptococci, and anaerobes (see Chapter 71, Table 1). Control of infection may require urgent surgery of infected cranial structures or drainage of intra- or extracranial abscess. Intracranial hypertension may require glucocorticoids, osmotic diuretics, or hyperventilation; an intracranial pressure monitor may be essential in assessing efficacy of therapy. Communicating hydrocephalus may require serial lumbar punctures or ventricular drainage. The use of anticoagulants is controversial[2,7,14] but may be necessary when there is progressive thrombosis or overt embolization in the face of antibiotic therapy. If anticoagulation is used, the danger of intracranial hemorrhage should always be kept in mind. Internal jugular vein ligation has been used with lateral sinus thrombosis,[11,12] and in a few instances thrombectomy has been successful.[21]

PROGNOSIS

Even when an apparently fixed neurologic deficit is present, intracranial venous infarction carries a better likelihood of functional recovery than does arterial infarction, but permanent deficits may occur. Overall mortality in suppurative intracranial thrombophlebitis is 34 percent. Mortality in complete occlusion of the superior sinus, however, is 78 percent.[1,22] Ominous prognostic signs are coma, progression of focal seizures to generalized ones, generalized seizures as an initial symptom, and bilateral signs, particularly bilateral flaccid hemiplegia.[1,2,21,23]

ACKNOWLEDGMENTS

Work on this chapter was supported in part by the Veterans Administration.

REFERENCES

1. Southwick FS, Richardson EP, Swartz MN. Septic thrombosis of the dural venous sinuses. Medicine. 1986;65:82–106.
2. Krayenbuhl HA. Cerebral venous and sinus thrombosis. Clin Neurosurg. 1967;14:1–24.
3. Stuart EA, O'Brien FH, McNally WJ. Cerebral venous thrombosis. Ann Otolaryngol. 1951;406–38.
4. Courville CB, Nielsen JM. Fatal complications of otitis media. Arch Otolaryngol. 1934;19:451–9.
5. Strauss SI, Stern NS, Mendelow H, et al. Septic superior sagittal sinus thrombosis after oral surgery. J Oral Surg. 1973;31:560–5.
6. Stehbens WE, ed. Pathology of the Cerebral Blood Vessels. St. Louis: CV Mosby; 1972:188–92.
7. Parsons M. Intracranial venous thrombosis. Postgrad Med J. 1967;43:409–14.
8. Pallares R, Santamaria J, Ariza X, et al. Polymicrobial anaerobic septicemia due to lateral sinus thrombophlebitis. J Laryngol Otolaryngol. 1984;98:895–9.
9. Shaw RE. Cavernous sinus thrombophlebitis: a review. Br J Surg. 1952;40:40–8.
10. Pascarelli E, Lemlich A. Diplopia and photophobia as premonitory symptoms in cavernous sinus thrombosis. Ann Rhinol Laryngol. 1964;73:210–7.
11. Jahrsdoerfer RA, Fitz-Hugh GS. Lateral sinus thrombosis. South Med J. 1968;61:1271–5.
12. Teichgraeber JF, Per-Lee JH, Turner JS. Lateral sinus thrombosis: a modern perspective. Laryngoscope. 1982;92:744–51.
13. Marchi PJ, Grossman RI, Gomori JM, et al. High field MR imaging of cerebral venous thrombosis. J Comput Assist Tomogr. 1986;10:10–5.
14. McArdle CB, Mirfakhraee M, Amparo EG, et al. MR imaging of transverse/sigmoid dural sinus and jugular vein thrombosis. J Comput Assist Tomogr. 1987;11:831–8.
15. Sze G, Simmons B, Krol G, et al. Dural sinus thrombosis: verification with spin-echo techniques. AJNR. 1988;9:679–86.
16. Snyder TC, Sachdev HS. MR imaging of dural sinus thrombosis. J Comput Assist Tomogr. 1986;10:889–92.
17. Goldberg AL, Rosenbaum AE, Wang H, et al. Computed tomography of dural sinus thrombosis. J Comput Assist Tomogr. 1986;10:16–20.
18. Virapongse C, Cazenave C, Quisling R, et al. The empty delta sign: frequency and significance in 76 cases of dural sinus thrombosis. Radiology. 1987;162:779–85.
19. Shinohara Y, Yoshitoshi M, Yoshii F. Appearance and disappearance of the empty delta sign in superior sagittal sinus thrombosis. Stroke. 1986;17:1282–4.
20. Askenasy HM, Kosary IZ, Braham J. Thrombosis of the longitudinal sinus. Neurology. 1962;12:288–92.
21. Kinal Me, Jaeger RM. Thrombophlebitis of dural sinuses following otitis media. J Neurosurg. 1960;17:81–9.
22. Kalbag RM, Woolf AL. Cerebral Venous Thrombosis. London: Oxford University Press; 1967:242–3.
23. Weber G. Treatment of cerebral venous and sinus thrombosis. Thromb Diath Haemorrh. 1966;21(Suppl):435–55.

SECTION I. SKIN AND SOFT TISSUE INFECTIONS

74. CELLULITIS AND SUPERFICIAL INFECTIONS

MORTON N. SWARTZ

Major attention should be directed to determination of the specific microbial cause of any infection involving the skin. In this chapter, bacterial and mycotic (exclusive of those due to the common dermatophytes) infections are considered. Classification of cutaneous infections on morphologic and clinical grounds can be most helpful in providing initial clues as to the most likely responsible infectious agents (Table 1).

PRIMARY PYODERMAS

Impetigo

Imeptigo is an initially vesicular, later crusted, superficial infection of the skin, usually due to group A streptococci. The majority of cases occur in children. *Staphylococcus aureus* is the etiologic agent in less than 10 percent of the cases, although it has been suggested recently that this figure may be increasing[1]; frequently, mixtures of streptococci and *S. aureus* are isolated from lesions, but in this situation the staphylococci are usually secondary invaders.

Pathologic Characteristics and Pathogenesis. Histopathologically, impetigo consists of a superficial, intraepidermal, unilocular vesicopustule. In epidemiologic studies, group A streptococcal acquisition on normal skin antedates the appearance of impetigo by about 10 days.[2] During that time, minor trauma (insect bites, abrasions) predisposes to the development of infected lesions. Impetigo is most common during hot, humid summer weather. Two to three weeks after skin acquisition of streptococci, pharyngeal colonization by the same organism occurs in about 30 percent of the children with skin lesions. (The sporadic cases of facial impetigo occurring in cooler climates probably result from contiguous spread from an initial nasopharyngeal infection, and the serotypes involved are those commonly causing pharyngeal disease.) In contrast, in the less common cases of staphylococcal impetigo (where *S. aureus* is the only pathogen), nasal colonization precedes that of the normal skin; skin lesions then follow such colonization.[3,4]

Impetigo is a highly communicable infection; spread in families (particularly among preschool children) is facilitated by crowding and poor hygiene.

Clinical Findings. Streptococcal impetigo begins as small vesicles, sometimes with narrow inflammatory halos, that rapidly pustulate and readily rupture. The purulent discharge dries, forming the characteristic thick, golden-yellow "stuck-on" crusts. Exposed areas are the most common sites of lesions. Pruritus is common, and scratching of lesions can spread infection. Occasionally, large crusts are produced by coalescence of smaller pustules. The lesions remain superficial and do not ulcerate or infiltrate the dermis. Mild regional lymphadenopathy is common. Healing occurs without scarring. The lesions are painless, and constitutional manifestations are minimal.

TABLE 1. Classification of Bacterial and Mycotic Infections of the Skin

Type of Lesion	*Etiologic Agents*
Primary pyodermas	
Impetigo	Group A streptococcus; *S. aureus*
Folliculitis	*S. aureus; Candida ; P. aeruginosa; Pityrosporum ovale*
Furuncles and carbuncles	*S. aureus*
Paronychia	*S. aureus*; Group A streptococcus; *Candida; P. aeruginosa*
Ecthyma	Group A streptococcus
Erysipelas	Group A streptococcus
Chancriform lesions	*T. pallidum; H. ducreyi; Sporothrix; B. anthracis; F. tularensis; M. ulcerans; M. marinum*
Membranous ulcers	*Corynebacterium diphtheriae*
Cellulitis	Group A streptococcus; *S. aureus*; rarely, various other organisms
Infectious gangrene and gangrenous cellulitis	
Streptococcal gangrene and necrotizing fasciitis	Group A streptococcus
Progressive bacterial synergistic gangrene	Anaerobic streptococci plus a second organism (*S. aureus, Proteus*)
Gangrenous balanitis and perineal phlegmon	Group A streptococcus; mixed infections with enteric bacteria (*E. coli, Klebsiella*, etc.) and anaerobes
Gas gangrene; crepitant cellulitis	*Clostridium perfringens* and other clostridial species; *Bacteroides*, peptostreptococci, *Klebsiella, E. coli*
Gangrenous cellulitis in immunosuppressed patients	*Pseudomonas, Aspergillus*, agents of mucormycosis
Erythrasma	*Corynebacterium minutissimum*
Nodular lesions	*Candida; Sporothrix; S. aureus* (botryomycosis); *M. marinum*
Hyperplastic (pseudoepitheliomatous) and proliferative lesions (mycetomas, etc.)	*Nocardia; Pseudoallescheria boydii, Blastomyces dermatitidis; Paracoccidioides brasiliensis; Phialophora; Cladosporium*
Annular erythema (erythema chronicum migrans)	*B. burgdorferi*
Secondary bacterial infections complicating pre-existing skin lesions such as the following:	
Burns	*P. aeruginosa; Enterobacter*; various other gram-negative bacilli; various streptococci; *S. aureus; Candida; Aspergillus*
Eczematous dermatitis and exfoliative erythrodermas	*S. aureus*; group A streptococcus
Chronic ulcers (varicose, decubitus)	Coliform bacteria; *P. aeruginosa*; peptostreptococci; enterococci, *Bacteroides, C. perfringens*
Dermatophytosis	*S. aureus*; group A streptococcus
Traumatic lesions (abrasions, animal bites, insect bites, etc.)	*P. multocida; C. diphtheriae; S. aureus*; group A streptococcus
Vesicular or bullous eruptions (varicella, pemphigus)	*S. aureus*; group A streptococcus
Acne conglabata	*Propionibacterium acnes*
Hidradenitis suppurativa	*S. aureus, Proteus* and other coliforms, streptococci, peptostreptococci, *Bacteroides*
Intertrigo	*S. aureus*, coliforms, *Candida*
Pilonidal and sebaceous cysts	Peptostreptococci; *Bacteroides*; coliforms
Pyoderma gangrenosa	*S. aureus*; peptostreptococci; *Proteus* and other coliforms; *P. aeruginosa*
Cutaneous involvement in systemic bacterial and mycotic infections	
Bacteremias	*S. aureus*; group A streptococcus (also other groups such as D); *N. meningitidis; N. gonorrhoeae; P. aeruginosa; S. typhi; H. influenzae*
Endocarditis	Viridans streptococci; *S. aureus*; group D streptococci, etc.
Fungemias	*Candida; Cryptococcus; B. dermatitidis*

(Continued)

TABLE 1. *(Continued)*

Type of Lesion	*Etiologic Agents*
Listeriosis	*Listeria monocytogenes*
Leptospirosis (Weil's disease and pretibial fever)	*L. interrogans* serotypes
Rat-bite fever	*Streptobacillus moniliformis; Spirillum minor*
Melioidosis	*P. pseudomallei*
Glanders	*P. mallei*
Carrion's disease (verruga peruana)	*Bartonella bacilliformis*
Scarlet fever syndromes	
Scarlet fever	Group A streptococcus; rarely *S. aureus*
Scalded skin syndrome	*S. aureus* (phage group II)
Toxic shock syndrome	*S. aureus* (pyrogenic toxin-producing strains)
Para- and postinfectious nonsuppurative complications	
Purpura fulminans	Group A streptococcus; *S. aureus*; pneumococcus
Erythema nodosum	Group A streptococcus; *M. tuberculosis; M. leprae; C. immitis; L. autumnalis; Y. Enterocolitica; L. pneumophila*
Erythema multiforme-like lesions (rarely)	Group A streptococcus

Laboratory Findings. Gram-stained smear of vesicles shows gram-positive cocci, usually streptococci. Culture of exudate beneath an unroofed crust reveals group A streptococci or a mixture of streptococci and *S. aureus*. The antistreptolysin O (ASLO) titer after streptococcal impetigo is scant, probably related to the inhibition of streptolysin O by skin lipids at the infection site. In contrast, the anti-DNase B response readily occurs (elevated titers in 90 percent of patients with nephritis complicating streptococcal skin infections).[5]

Etiologic Agents. Group A streptococci responsible for impetigo usually belong to different M serotypes (e.g., 2, 49, 52, 55, 57, 59–61) than the strains producing pharyngitis (e.g., 1, 2, 4, 6, 25). Group C and G streptococci rarely may cause impetigo; group B streptococci have been associated with impetigo in the newborn.

Differential Diagnosis. Although the initial vesicular lesions may resemble early varicella, the crusts of the latter are darker brown and harder. The central clearing of a confluent cluster of lesions of impetigo may suggest tinea circinata but can be distinguished by the thick crusts that are not formed in the fungus infection. When the vesicles of herpes simplex become turbid, they may look like impetigo.

Presumptive Therapy. Penicillin is the drug of choice in the treatment of ordinary impetigo because of the role of group A streptococci in the majority of cases and the possible occurrence of acute glomerulonephritis as a sequela. Whether penicillin therapy is effective (because of the delay in seeking medical attention for such a mild infection) in reducing the incidence of pyoderma-associated nephritis remains unclear. Penicillin is administered either as a single intramuscular injection of benzathine penicillin (300,000–600,000 units for children; 1,200,000 units for adults) or as oral penicillin (25,000–90,000 units/kg/day in divided doses every 6 hours for 10 days). Erythromycin (30–50 mg/kg/day in divided doses every 6 hours for 10 days for children; 250–500 mg orally every 6 hours for adults) is an alternative for the penicillin-allergic patient. Local care (removal of crusts by soaking with soap and water) is helpful.

Mixed streptococcal-staphylococcal impetigo has the same crusted lesions and clinical course as streptococcal impetigo and responds well to treatment with penicillin G.[6]

Topical antibiotic-containing (bacitracin-neomycin-polymyxin) ointments are inferior to systemic antibiotics in the treatment of impetigo, since they sterilize the lesions less rapidly and prevent transmission less promptly. However, among young children in close contact (e.g., in a day care center) during the peak impetigo season, application of such a topical antibiotic ointment several times daily to insect bites and minor abrasions can be effective in preventing the subsequent development of streptococcal pyoderma.[7]

A newer topical antibiotic, mupirocin, appears to be as effective in the topical treatment of impetigo as other more established topical agents. It has also been used topically to eradicate methicillin-resistent *S. aureus* from secondarily infected skin lesions and from colonized patients. However, since resistance in *S. aureus* strains has emerged sooner than anticipated after its introduction, particularly where long-term therapy has been employed, prolonged use should probably be avoided.

Bullous Impetigo

Clinical Findings. This form of impetigo is due to *S. aureus* of phage group II (usually type 71), occurs principally in the newborn and younger children, and comprises about 10 percent of all cases of impetigo. The lesions begin as vesicles that turn into flaccid bullae, initially containing clear yellow fluid. There is no erythematous areola, and the Nikolsky sign is absent. The bullae quickly rupture, leaving a moist red surface, and then form thin, "varnish-like" light brown crusts. Bullous impetigo, like the "staphylococcal scalded skin syndrome" (SSSS) and the staphylococcal scarlatiniform syndrome, represents a form of cutaneous response to the extracellular exfoliative toxins (ET) produced by *S. aureus* of phage group II. Staphylococci are regularly isolated from the skin lesions of bullous impetigo. Streptococcal superinfection rarely complicates bullous impetigo, probably because type 71 strains of *S. aureus* produce a bacteriocin that inhibits streptococci. Fever and constitutional symptoms are uncommon. Healing occurs without scarring.

Presumptive Therapy. Extensive bullous impetigo responds to treatment with a penicillinase-resistant penicillin (e.g., in the child, oxacillin, 50 mg/kg/day in divided doses orally every 6 hours) or erythromycin in the penicillin-allergic patient.

Staphylococcal Scalded Skin Syndrome

This is the most severe manifestation of infection with *S. aureus* strains producing an exfoliative exotoxin and is characterized by widespread bullae and exfoliation.[8–11] Pemphigus neonatorum (Ritter's disease) is the SSSS in the newborn. The more general term *toxic epidermal necrolysis* (*TEN*) is often used to encompass both SSSS and a morphologically identical syndrome due to various etiologies (drug reactions, viral illnesses). (See Chapter 173.)

Clinical Findings. SSSS usually occurs in younger children, but rarely it can develop in adults. Epidemics have occurred in neonatal nurseries.[12] It begins abruptly (sometimes a few days after a recognized staphylococcal infection) with fever, skin tenderness, and a scarlatiniform rash. The Nikolsky sign can be demonstrated. Large, flaccid, clear bullae form and promptly rupture, resulting in the separation of sheets of skin. New bullae appear over 2–3 days. Exfoliation exposes large areas of bright red skin surface (Fig. 1). With appropriate fluid replacement and antimicrobial therapy, the skin lesions heal within 2 weeks, in contrast to drug-induced TEN, where recovery is more prolonged, since the entire epidermis must be replaced, and where scarring is more frequent.

Presumptive Therapy. Intravenous use of a penicillinase-resistant penicillin (e.g., nafcillin, 50–100 mg/kg/day in the newborn, 100–200 mg/kg/day for older children) is indicated in the initial treatment of SSSS because of the presence of active staphylococcal infection and the rapid progression of the skin lesions. Topical treatment consists of cool saline compresses.

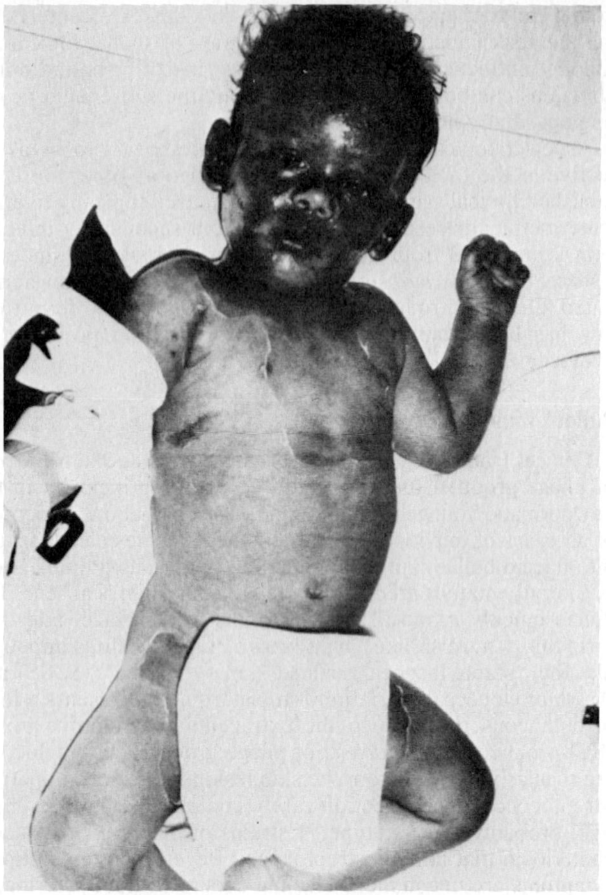

FIG. 1. Staphylococcal scalded skin syndrome in a young infant. Exfoliation has occurred on the face, chest, and groin, exposing areas of bright red skin surface.

Systemic corticosteroids alone should not be used in the treatment of SSSS, although they may be indicated in the therapy of drug-induced TEN.

Staphylococcal Scarlet Fever

This is fundamentally a forme fruste of SSSS (due to ET) that does not progress beyond the initial stage of a generalized erythematous eruption. At that stage the rash is indistinguishable from that of scarlet fever, and Pastia's lines can develop. However, pharyngitis is usually not present, and an enanthem does not develop. Desquamation, beginning on the face and involving most of the body, occurs 2–5 days after the onset of the scarlatiniform rash. Antibiotic treatment with penicillinase-resistant penicillins is indicated.

Toxic Shock Syndrome

The toxic shock syndrome (TSS) is another acute febrile illness with a generalized scarlatiniform eruption associated with *S. aureus* infection. Other elements of the syndrome include (*a*) hypotension (or shock), (*2*) functional abnormalities of three or more organ systems, and (*3*) desquamation in the evolution of the skin lesions[13–15] (see Chapter 173).

Folliculitis

Folliculitis is a pyoderma located within hair follicles and the apocrine regions. The lesions consist of small (2–5 mm) erythematous, sometimes pruritic, papules often topped by a central pustule. Sycosis barbae is a distinctive form of deep folliculitis, often chronic, occurring on the bearded areas. *Staphylococcus aureus* is the usual etiology of folliculitis. *Pseudomonas aeruginosa* (most often serotype 0–11) has been responsible for folliculitis acquired from swimming pools and whirlpools contaminated with large numbers of these organisms.[16] This type of skin infection produces pruritic papulourticarial lesions (appearing within 48 hours of exposure) that go on to pustule formation. Lesions in different stages of development are present simultaneously. Sites of predilection include the buttocks, hips, and axillae; the palms and soles are spared. Otitis externa is also a common manifestation. Healing occurs spontaneously, either by drainage or regression, within 5 days. Scarring develops rarely when an occasional pustule has progressed to furuncle formation. When acquired in a whirlpool, the lesions are sharply limited to the trunk below the upper chest or neck. Inadequate chlorine levels in whirlpools, hot tubs, and swimming pools have been responsible for many of the reported outbreaks. *Pseudomonas aeruginosa* can also cause superinfection in acne. In granulocytopenic or immunosuppressed hospitalized patients, *P. aeruginosa* 0–11 from tap water used for washing has been implicated in folliculitis that has rapidly progressed to ecthyma gangrenosum.[17]

Folliculitis due to Enterobacteriaceae can occur as a complication in patients with acne, usually during prolonged courses of oral antibiotic therapy.[18]

Candida is sometimes the etiology of folliculitis, producing pruritic satellite lesions surrounding areas of intertriginous candidiasis, particularly in patients on prolonged antibiotic or corticosteroid therapy. *Malassezia furfur*, common skin saprophytes, may also produce a folliculitis with pruritic erythematous papules and papulopustules on the trunk, upper extremities, and face, particularly in the setting of diabetes mellitus, corticosteroid administration, or granulocytopenia.[19,20] These lesions, particularly the early papular nodular ones, may suggest those of systemic candidiasis, a diagnosis that may seem to be supported by the presence of budding yeasts on Gram-stained material from unroofed lesions. Unlike *Candida, Malassezia furfur* requires lipid-supplemented media for primary isolation.

A rare pruritic dermatosis, eosinophilic pustular folliculitis, characterized by recurrent crops of follicular papules and pustules with eosinophilic infiltration of perifollicular dermis, resembles bacterial or mycotic folliculitis but is a sterile process.[21]

Local measures (saline compresses and topical antibacterials or antifungals such as clotrimazole) are usually sufficient to control the infection.

Furuncles and Carbuncles

Definition and Pathologic Characteristics. A furuncle is a deep inflammatory nodule, usually developing from a preceding folliculitis. A carbuncle is a more extensive process extending into the subcutaneous fat in areas covered by thick, inelastic skin. In the latter, multiple abscesses develop, separated by connective tissue septae, and drain to the surface along hair follicles. *Staphylococcus aureus* is almost invariably the etiologic agent (see also Chapter 173).

Clinical Findings. Furuncles occur in skin areas subject to friction and perspiration and containing hair follicles (neck, face, axillae, buttocks). Predisposing factors include obesity, blood dyscrasias, treatment with corticosteroids, defects in neutrophil function, and probably diabetes mellitus. A furuncle begins as a firm, tender, red nodule that soon becomes painful and fluctuant. Spontaneous drainage of pus commonly occurs and the lesion subsides. A carbuncle is a larger, deeper, indurated, more serious lesion, usually located at the nape of the neck, on the back, or on the thighs. Fever and malaise are frequent, and some patients are acutely ill. As the lesion progresses, drainage occurs externally along the course of multiple hair follicles. A leukocytosis occurs, particularly when the lesion contains a large amount of undrained pus or when there is a complicating cellulitis or bacteremia.

Blood stream invasion may occur unpredictably (but is sometimes precipitated by manipulation of the lesions), resulting in osteomyelitis, endocarditis, or other metastatic foci. Lesions about the upper lip and nose present the special problem of spread of infection via the facial and angular emissary veins to the cavernous sinus.

Presumptive Therapy. Most furuncles are satisfactorily treated by the application of moist heat, which promotes localization and drainage of the process. A carbuncle or a furuncle with surrounding cellulitis and/or fever, or if located about the midface, should be treated with an antistaphylococcal antibiotic (e.g., oxacillin, 0.5–0.75 g orally every 4–6 hours for an adult). In the penicillin-allergic adult, clindamycin (150–300 mg orally every 6 hours) or erythromycin (0.25–0.5 g orally every 6 hours) are alternatives. If the lesions are large and fluctuant, surgical drainage is indicated. Antibiotic treatment should be continued until evidences of acute inflammation have subsided.

Management of patients with recurrent furunculosis presents a troublesome problem. This disease does not appear to be due to specific staphylococcal strains with special biologic properties, and most patients do not have definable underlying defects in host defenses. Prophylaxis of recurrent episodes involves several measures:

1. *Antibiotic treatment*. Systemic antibiotic treatment, as described above, should be administered for the most recent episode. Prolonged treatment (2 months) is no more effective than a 10- to 14-day course in preventing recurrences.[22]
2. *General skin care*. Soap and water should be used to reduce the number of *S. aureus* organisms on the body surface, and careful handwashing should be performed after contact with lesions. A separate towel and washcloth (carefully washed in hot water before reuse) should be reserved for the patient. Some physicians prefer hexachlorophene or chlorhexidine to soap.
3. *Care of clothing*. Sheets and underclothing should be laundered at high temperatures and should be changed daily in problem patients.
4. *Care of dressings*. Draining lesions should be covered at all times with sterile dressings to prevent autoinoculation, and the dressings should be wrapped and promptly disposed of after removal.

Local (nasal) application of antibiotic ointments (bacitracin or neomycin) is sometimes used in refractory cases with the aim of reducing nasal carriage and subsequent shedding of *S. aureus* onto the skin. Occasionally, recurrent furunculosis occurs in a family, or sometimes other members of the family carry the same strain of *S. aureus* in their nares. Prophylaxis with antibiotic ointment in the nares twice daily for every fourth week for the patient and family members who are nasal carriers of the infecting strain has been employed.[22] Rifampin (600 mg orally daily for 10 days) is effective in eradicating coagulase-positive staphylococci from the majority of nasal carriers for periods of up to 12 weeks.[23] The use of rifampin for such a short period to eliminate nasal carriage of *S. aureus* and interrupt a continuing cycle of recurrent furunculosis might be considered in the patient in whom other measures have failed. However, selection of rifampin-resistant *S. aureus* strains can occur with such therapy. Thus we suggest cloxacillin, 500 mg po qid, along with the rifampin to reduce the emergence of rifampin-resistant organisms. Various staphylococcal vaccines have not proven effective in preventing recurrent furunculosis.

Ecthyma

Clinical Findings. The lesions of ecthyma begin in a fashion similar to those of impetigo but penetrate through the epidermis. Group A streptococci either produce the lesions de novo or secondarily infect pre-existing superficial lesions (insect bites, excoriations), resulting in the same clinical picture.[24] It is important to note that lesions with the same ultimate appearance can be produced in the course of *Pseudomonas* bacteremia (see below). The lesions most frequently occur on the lower extremities, particularly of children and the elderly. They consist of "punched-out" ulcers, covered by greenish yellow crusts, extending deeply into the dermis and surrounded by raised violaceous margins. Treatment is the same as for impetigo. Very extensive involvement with complicating bacteremia has occurred in a patient with the acquired immunodeficiency syndrome (AIDS).[25]

Chancriform Lesions

A variety of infections, often with systemic consequences, are characterized by an initial chancriform lesion (Table 1). Of the nonvenereal infections, anthrax has one of the most prominent chancriform lesions.

Anthrax. See Chapter 186 for a detailed discussion.

PATHOGENESIS. Anthrax is a very rare disease in the United States. Infections are limited to persons working with raw imported wool and other animal products contaminated with highly resistant spores of *Bacillus anthracis*. Routine safety measures for employees in wool plants and so forth virtually have eliminated anthrax from this group; sporadic cases still occur in transient workers in factories (e.g., ventilation repairmen) and in persons directly importing wool for their own weaving. Most infections occur on the face, neck, or arms in an area of a minor abrasion. Rarely, pulmonary infection follows inhalation of *B. anthracis*, or intestinal anthrax results from ingestion of the organism.

CLINICAL FINDINGS. After an incubation period of 1–3 days, a painless papule develops on an exposed area. The lesion enlarges, vesiculates ("malignant pustule"), and is surrounded by a wide zone of brawny, erythematous, gelatinous, nonpitting edema.[26] Malaise and low-grade fever are present. As the lesion evolves, the vesicle becomes hemorrhagic, necrotic, and covered by an eschar of variable dimensions (Fig. 2). At all stages the lesion remains painless. Bacteremic dissemination of infection from a skin site may occur, accompanied by high fever and

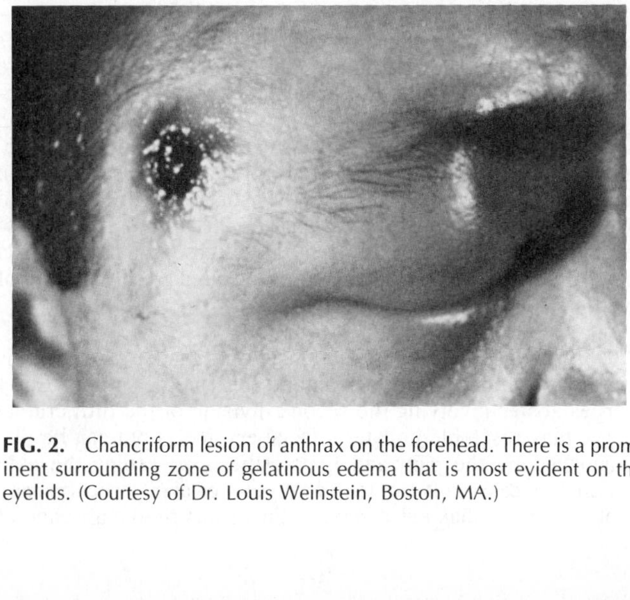

FIG. 2. Chancriform lesion of anthrax on the forehead. There is a prominent surrounding zone of gelatinous edema that is most evident on the eyelids. (Courtesy of Dr. Louis Weinstein, Boston, MA.)

hypotension. Meningitis may complicate either such a bacteremic infection or primary pulmonary anthrax.

The epidemiologic background and the striking appearance of extensive gelatinous edema serve to distinguish anthrax from other types of chancriform lesion. A staphylococcal pustule or carbuncle with a necrotic eschar may be mistaken for early anthrax. However, the former is very painful and tender, and the etiologic agent can usually be demonstrated on a Gram-stained smear of material from the lesion.

PRESUMPTIVE TREATMENT. Incision and débridement should be avoided, since they increase the likelihood of bacteremia. Parenteral penicillin G (1 million units every 4–6 hours) is used. In the penicillin-allergic patient, tetracycline (1.0–2.0 g/day intravenously in the adult) is an alternative.

Erysipelas

Erysipelas is a distinctive type of superficial cellulitis of the skin with prominent lymphatic involvement. It is almost always due to group A streptococci (uncommonly, group C or G). Group B streptococci have produced erysipelas in the newborn. Very rarely, a similar skin lesion is caused by *S. aureus*.

Clinical Findings. Erysipelas is more common in infants, young children, and older adults. Formerly, the face was most commonly involved, and an antecedent streptococcal respiratory tract infection preceded cutaneous involvement in about one-third of patients even though streptococci might not be found on culture at the time the skin lesion became evident. Now the localization of erysipelas has changed: 70–80 percent of the lesions are on the lower extremities and 5–20 percent are on the face.[27] Portals of entry are commonly skin ulcers, local trauma or abrasions, psoriatic or eczematous lesions, or fungal infections; in the neonate, erysipelas may develop from an infection of the umbilical stump. Predisposing factors include venous stasis, paraparesis, diabetes mellitus, and alcohol abuse. Patients with the nephrotic syndrome are particularly susceptible. Erysipelas tends to occur in areas of pre-existing lymphatic obstruction or edema (e.g., after a radical mastectomy). Also, because erysipelas itself produces lymphatic obstruction, it tends to recur in an area of earlier infection. Over a 3-year period, the recurrence rate is about 30 percent,[27] predominantly in individuals with venous insufficiency or lymphedema.

Streptococcal bacteremia occurs in about 5 percent of patients with erysipelas; group A, C, or G streptococci can be isolated on throat culture from about 20 percent of cases.[27]

Erysipelas is a painful lesion with a bright red, edematous, indurated ("peau d' orange") appearance and an advancing, raised border that is sharply demarcated from the adjacent normal skin (Fig. 3). Fever is a feature. A common form of erysipelas involves the bridge of the nose and the cheeks. Uncomplicated erysipelas remains confined primarily to the lymphatics and the dermis. Occasionally, the infection extends more deeply, producing cellulitis, subcutaneous abscess, and necrotizing fasciitis.

A leukocytosis is common with erysipelas. Group A streptococci usually cannot be cultured from the surface of the skin lesion, and only rarely can they be isolated from tissue fluid aspirated from the advancing edge of the lesion. In cases of erysipelas complicating infected ulcers, group A streptococci have been isolated from the ulcerated area in 30 percent of patients.[27]

Differential Diagnosis. The diagnosis is made on the basis of the appearance of the lesion and the clinical setting. Early herpes zoster involving the second division of the fifth cranial nerve may resemble unilateral facial erysipelas but can be distinguished by the pain and hyperesthesia preceding the skin lesions. Occasionally contact dermatitis or giant urticaria may look like erysipelas but can be distinguished by the absence of fever and the presence of pruritus. Lesions closely resembling erysipelas, but apparently not due to streptococcal infection, may occur recurrently in patients with familial Mediterranean fever. Diffuse inflammatory carcinoma of the breast may mimic a low-grade erysipelas. Erythema chronicum migrans, the cutaneous lesion of Lyme disease, resembles erysipelas but is not painful and progresses much more slowly, and the associated fever is less marked.

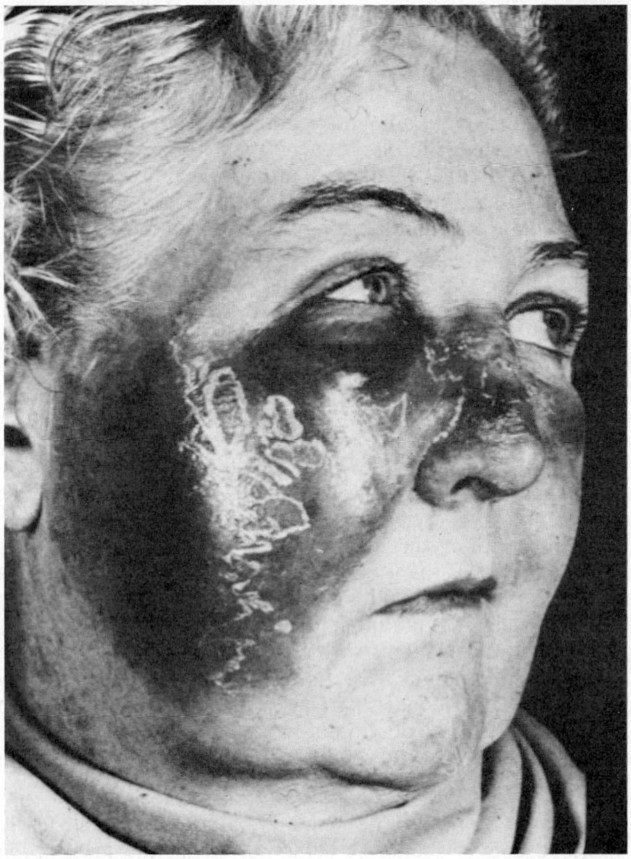

FIG. 3. Facial erysipelas involving both cheeks and the bridge of the nose. The sharp demarcation between the bright red area of erythema and the normal surrounding skin is evident. (From Fitzpatrick et al.,[28] with permission.)

Presumptive Therapy. Mild early cases of erysipelas in the adult may be treated with intramuscular procaine penicillin (600,000 units once or twice daily) or with oral penicillin V (250–500 mg every 6 hours). Erythromycin (250–500 mg orally every 6 hours) is a suitable alternative. For more extensive erysipelas, patients should be hospitalized and receive parenteral aqueous penicillin G (600,000–2,000,000 units every 6 hours).

Cellulitis

Cellulitis is an acute spreading infection of the skin extending deeper than erysipelas to involve the subcutaneous tissues. Group A streptococcus or *S. aureus* is most frequently the etiologic agent.

Clinical Findings. Previous trauma (laceration, puncture wound) or an underlying skin lesion (furuncle, ulcer) predisposes to the development of cellulitis; rarely, the latter may result from blood-borne spread of infection to the skin and subcutaneous tissues. Within several days of the inciting trauma, local tenderness, pain, and erythema develop and rapidly intensify. Malaise, fever, and chills develop. The involved area is often extensive and the lesion is very red, hot, and swollen. In contrast to erysipelas, the borders of an area of cellulitis are not elevated and sharply demarcated. Regional lymphadenopathy is common, and bacteremia can occur. Local abscesses may develop; small patches of overlying skin may subsequently undergo necrosis. Superinfection with gram-negative bacilli may supervene.

Cellulitis due to group A streptococci may occur as a postoperative wound infection. Although uncommon today, it is particularly noteworthy because of the rapidity with which it can spread and invade the blood stream. Such infection may manifest itself within 6–48 hours of surgery (comparable to the short incubation period of postoperative clostridial myonecrosis), earlier than the usual postoperative staphylococcal infection, which is not evident for at least several days after operation. Hypotension, often due to bacteremia, may be the initial sign of infection before significant erythema is evident about the incision. A thin serous discharge may be expressed on compression of the wound margins, and streptococci can be identified on a Gram-stained smear.

Cellulitis is a serious disease because of the propensity of infection to spread via the lymphatics and blood stream. Cellulitis of the lower extremities in older patients may be complicated by thrombophlebitis. In patients with chronic dependent edema, cellulitis may spread extremely rapidly.

A distinctive (by virtue of the clinical setting) form of cellulitis occurs in the lower extremities of patients whose saphenous veins have been removed for coronary artery bypass surgery.[29] Occasionally, an associated lymphangitis is present. In some patients, episodes of cellulitis are recurrent. Systemic manifestations such as chills, high fever, and toxicity are prominent. The area of cellulitis extends along the course of the saphenous venectomy. Edema, erythema, and tenderness are marked. Occasionally, the involved areas are somewhat similar to those of erysipelas (''pseudoerysipelas''). Although the bacterial etiology has not been defined in most cases, the available isolates from involved skin or blood implicate non-group A β-hemolytic streptococci (groups C, G, B) as major etiologies.[30] The portal of entry of the infection is often an associated area of tinea pedis. The combination of compromised lymphatic drainage and minor venous insufficiency secondary to saphenous venectomy may result in lower leg edema, a favorable setting for cellulitis. The inflammation from an initial episode of cellulitis, erysipelas, or lymphangitis obstructs lymphatic drainage, thus enhancing the predisposition to further episodes of infections.

Similar recurrent episodes of cellulitis or pseudoerysipelas due to group B and G streptococci have occurred in patients with lower extremity lymphedema secondary to radical pelvic surgery, radiation therapy, or neoplastic involvement of pelvic lymph nodes.[31] Typically, the cellulitis involves the vulva, inguinal areas, and both lower extremities. In this setting, recurrent episodes have occurred in association with recent coitus.[32]

An uncommon but distinctive form of cellulitis, perianal streptococcal (group A) cellulitis, occurs principally in children.[33] The clinical features consist of intense perianal erythema, pain on defecation, blood-streaked stools from anal fissures, and chronicity (months) if not treated with penicillin.

A rare but particularly troublesome, chronic, and progressive form of cellulitis, known as *dissecting cellulitis of the scalp* or *perifolliculitis capitis*, is probably similar to hydradenitis suppurativa and acne conglobata in pathogenesis. The clinical features consist of recurrent painful, fluctuant dermal and subcutaneous nodules, purulent drainage from burrowing interconnecting abscesses, scarring, and alopecia. The pathogenesis, as in hydradenitis suppurativa, is probably related to follicular plugging, secondary infection, and deep dissecting inflammation. *Staphylococcus aureus* is most commonly isolated. Effective treatment has involved wide excision and skin grafting.[34]

Lymphatic cutaneous metastases from neoplasms, particularly adenocarcinoma, may produce a localized, edematous, erythematous lesion resembling cellulitis. Inflammatory carcinoma of the breast, carcinoma erysipeloides, involves the skin overlying the site of the primary tumor.

A polymorphonuclear leukocytosis is usually present, regardless of the bacterial etiology.

Etiologic Agents. Group A streptococci and *S. aureus* are responsible for the overwhelming majority of cases of cellulitis, but other organisms may be involved occasionally. Streptococci belonging to other groups (group C, group G, and in neonates particularly, group B) are sometimes the etiologic agents.

Erysipelothrix rhusiopathiae is the etiologic agent of erysipeloid, a cellulitis occurring principally in persons handling saltwater fish, shellfish, poultry, meat, and hides (see Chapter 188). The infection, usually occurring in the summer, is introduced through an abrasion on the hands. A painful violaceous area appears within a week of the injury. As the process spreads peripherally with distinct raised borders, the central portion of the lesion clears. Ulceration is not a feature. Occasionally an adjacent joint is involved, and rarely, bacteremia and endocarditis may follow. The causative organism is generally not observed on Gram-stained drainage from the lesion but may be isolated on culture of a biopsy specimen taken from the advancing margin of the lesion. The development of a typical lesion in a person handling fish or meat products suggests the diagnosis. Other forms of bacterial cellulitis or erysipelas may resemble erysipeloid, particularly when the lesion is on the hand. A somewhat similar lesion of unknown etiology, ''seal finger,'' occurs in aquarium workers and veterinarians secondary to seal bites or trauma sustained in caring for these animals. While penicillin is the antibiotic of choice in the treatment of erysipeloid, it appears that seal finger responds to tetracycline.[35]

Rare cases of pneumococcal cellulitis acquired through the bacteremic route have been reported.[36] Soft tissue infections due to the pneumococcus can bear a striking resemblance to streptococcal erysipelas. A variety of bacteria (*Serratia, Proteus*, and other Enterobacteriaceae) and fungi (*Cryptococcus neoformans*) that are not the cause of cellulitis in normal individuals may produce cellulitis in the immunocompromised or granulocytopenic patient. Spontaneous *Escherichia coli* cellulitis occurs in children with the nephrotic syndrome in relapse.[37]

An environmental gram-negative bacillus, *Aeromonas hydrophila*, found particularly in lakes, rivers, and soil, may produce an acute cellulitis after introduction of the organism through a laceration acquired during swimming in fresh water.[38]

Cellulitis, bullous lesions, or necrotic ulcers may complicate infection of a traumatic wound sustained in salt water (or brackish inland waters) or exposed to drippings from raw seafood. Such infections, due to *Vibrio* spp. (e.g., *V. vulnificus, V. alginolyticus, V. parahaemolyticus*) can result in bacteremia and progress to necrosis, requiring extensive surgical débridement.[39] These vibrios are generally susceptible to chloramphenicol and tetracycline in vitro; most isolates are also susceptible to the aminoglycoside antibiotics.

Although needle aspiration of the lesion of erysipelas is commonly unsuccessful in providing a bacteriologic diagnosis (by Gram stain or culture), it is sometimes very helpful in defining the pathogen in cases of cellulitis. Using aspirates from the advancing edge of cellulitis, skin biopsy, and blood cultures, potential pathogens are isolated in only about 25 percent of patients.[40] When a site of origin (abrasion, ulcer) for the infection is present, isolates of potential pathogens (*S. aureus*, group A streptococci) can be obtained in about one-third of cases. The yield of potential pathogens may be higher if aspirates are obtained from the point of maximum inflammation (commonly the center) of areas of cellulitis rather than from the leading edge.[41]

The appearance and clinical features of a noninfectious process, eosinophilic cellulitis, may suggest the appearance of bacterial cellulitis on the extremities or trunk.[42] The involved area is moderately erythematous and edematous. The lesion develops rapidly, is often accompanied by fever, and enlarges over several days. It can be distinguished from the usual bacterial cellulitis by its minimal tenderness, lack of local heat, and its failure to respond to antibiotics. Biopsy of the early lesion shows marked infiltration of the dermis with eosinophils. The lesions resolve in several weeks but frequently recur.

Presumptive Therapy. If a mild early cellulitis is suspected to be of streptococcal etiology, it may be treated with an initial injection of aqueous penicillin G (600,000 units) followed by intramuscular procaine penicillin (600,000 units every 8–12 hours). When staphylococcal infection is suspected, or when there are no initial clues to the etiology, a penicillinase-resistant penicillin (e.g., oxacillin, 0.5–1.0 g orally every 6 hours) should be used. In adults allergic to penicillin, erythromycin (0.5 g orally every 6 hours) is an alternative. For more severe infections where both streptococcal and staphylococcal etiologies are considered, parenteral administration of a penicillinase-resistant penicillin (e.g., nafcillin, 1.0–1.5 g intravenously every 4 hours) should be used. Vancomycin (1.0–1.5 g/day intravenously) is an alternative for the highly penicillin-allergic patient. If the clinical setting suggests a gram-negative bacillus as a possible etiology of a serious cellulitis, an aminoglycoside such as gentamicin may be added to the semisynthetic penicillin initially while awaiting definitive bacteriologic results. Gentamicin, along with a penicillinase-resistant penicillin, is probably indicated in the initial treatment of a rapidly progressive cellulitis developing after a freshwater injury. *Aeromonas hydrophila* is usually susceptible to gentamicin and chloramphenicol (and to tetracycline to a slightly lesser degree).

Initial local care of cellulitis includes immobilization and elevation of the involved limb to reduce swelling and cool sterile saline dressing to decrease local pain. Subsequently, application of moist heat may aid in localization of the infection.

Patients with cellulitis at the saphenous site after coronary bypass surgery who have fungal infection in the intergidital spaces should be treated topically for the latter with miconazole or clotrimazole. The initial antibiotic (penicillin or nafcillin) should be given in high dosage by the intravenous route for 6–7 days to ensure prompt resolution before switching to other routes of therapy. Attention to the problem of tinea pedis before bypass surgery can prevent this form of cellulitis. Similar prompt attention to pedal epidermophytosis in patients who have had one such episode of cellulitis can obviate subsequent episodes.

Recurrent episodes of cellulitis usually occur in patients with peripheral edema. The use of support stockings and good skin hygiene can reduce its frequency or eliminate recurrences. In the occasional patient who continues to have frequent episodes of cellulitis or erysipelas despite such measures, prophylactic penicillin G (250–500 mg orally twice daily) may be indicated.

Membranous Ulcers

Infected ulcers of varied or mixed bacterial etiology may be covered at their base by a layer of necrotic debris resembling a membrane. The latter usually is not strongly adherent and can be removed without much difficulty. In addition, such a lesion has abundant purulent drainage attributable to infection with pyogenic bacteria. Membrane-covered lesions (both superficial and deep ulcers) also are produced by cutaneous infection with *Corynebacterium diphtheriae*.

Cutaneous Diphtheria. Cutaneous diphtheria (see Chapter 165) is uncommon in developed countries; most cases occur in unimmunized persons in overcrowded, underdeveloped parts of the world, particularly in tropical areas, and are associated with skin trauma and poor hygiene. Recent increases in cutaneous diphtheria have been noted in the Pacific Northwest and the South.

CLINICAL FINDINGS. Three types of cutaneous lesions have been described in cutaneous diphtheria: (*a*) *Wound diphtheria*—secondary infection with *C. diphtheriae* of a pre-existing wound, which becomes partially covered by a membrane and encircled by a zone of erythema; (*2*) *primary cutaneous diphtheria*—a disease of the tropics, which begins as a single or several pustules, usually on a lower extremity, and progresses to form a punched-out ulcer covered by a gray-brown membrane; and (*3*) *superinfection of eczematized skin lesions*—a superficial membranous infection; *C. diphtheriae* also have been isolated from lesions resembling impetigo, ecthyma, and infected insect bites, where they may represent true infections or merely a cutaneous carrier state.[43] Cutaneous diphtheria may be as contagious as the respiratory form of the disease among school children.

Occasionally, membranous pharyngitis may accompany cutaneous diphtheria. However, 20–40 percent of the patients with cutaneous diphtheria carry *C. diphtheriae* in their upper respiratory tract.[43,44] Myocarditis is extremely rare as a complication of cutaneous diphtheria, but cranial nerve palsies and Guillain-Barré syndrome occur in 3–5 percent of the patients with membranous diphtheritic skin ulcers.

LABORATORY FINDINGS. Characteristic beaded, metachromatically staining bacilli can be found in methylene blue-stained smears of the edge of the membrane. However, the diagnosis can be established only by isolation of *C. diphtheriae* from a suggestive skin lesion. Selective media (Loeffler's or tellurite agar) are necessary for isolation in order to inhibit other bacteria in skin ulcers. In addition to isolation of the organism, toxigenicity should be demonstrated by an Elek plate (agar diffusion precipitin reaction) or by guinea pig inoculation (dermonecrosis).

DIFFERENTIAL DIAGNOSIS. Pyogenic infection of ulcerated traumatic lesions is usually purulent, and the lesions are not covered by a membrane. Cutaneous fungal infections have more proliferative and irregular margins. The early stages of primary cutaneous diphtheria and of secondary infection of insect bites and abrasions with *C. diphtheriae* may closely resemble impetigo.

PRESUMPTIVE THERAPY. If a presumptive diagnosis of ulcerative cutaneous diphtheria is made on clinical grounds and on the basis of preliminary bacteriologic findings, antitoxin is administered (20,000–40,000 units intramuscularly or intravenously) after testing for sensitivity to horse serum. Antibiotic administration (erythromycin, 2.0 g/day orally, or procaine penicillin, 1.2–2.4 million units/day intramuscularly in the adult for 7–10 days) also assists elimination of the convalescent carrier state. Removal of necrotic debris aids in healing of the lesions.

Infectious Gangrene (Gangrenous Cellulitis)

Infectious gangrene is a cellulitis that has rapidly progressed, with extensive necrosis of subcutaneous tissues and overlying skin. Several different clinically distinguishable pictures may be produced, depending to varying extents on the specific causative organism, the anatomic location of the infection, and the predisposing conditions. Such clinical entities include (*1*) necrotizing fasciitis (streptococcal gangrene), (*2*) gas gangrene (clostridial myonecrosis and anaerobic cellulitis), (*3*) progressive bacterial synergistic gangrene, (*4*) synergistic necrotizing cellulitis (perineal phlegmon) and gangrenous balanitis, (*5*) gangrenous cellulitis in the immunosuppressed patient, and (*6*) very localized areas of skin necrosis complicating conventional cellulitis.

Pathologic Characteristics and Pathogenesis. The pathologic changes of gangrenous cellulitis are those of necrosis and some hemorrhage in skin and subcutaneous tissues. In most types of gangrenous cellulitis an abundant polymorphonuclear leukocytic exudate is present, but in clostridial gas gangrene the exudate is thin, consisting of fluid, fibrin, and gas, but with few leukocytes. In most types of gangrenous cellulitis (particularly streptococcal gangrene), fibrin thrombi are present in small arteries and veins of the dermis and subcutaneous fat.[45] In most instances, gangrenous cellulitis has developed secondary to introduction of the infecting organism at the infected site. It also may result from extension of infection from a deeper site to involve the subcutaneous tissues and skin (as in clostridial myonecrosis after intestinal surgery or in perineal phlegmon after dissection of infection from a perirectal abscess). Occasionally, gangrenous cellulitis may begin at a site of metastatic infection in the course of a bacteremia (gas gangrene due to *Clostridium septicum* at a peripheral site secondary to spread from an associated colonic neoplasm; *Pseudomonas* gangrenous cellulitis).

Clinical Findings. STREPTOCOCCAL GANGRENE. This is a rare form of gangrene, due to group A (or C or G) streptococci, which usually develops at a site of trauma on an extremity but may occur in the absence of an obvious portal of entry. The lesion begins as a local painful area of erythema and edema. Over the next 1–3 days the skin becomes dusky. Bullae containing yellowish to red-black fluid develop and rupture.[46] The lesion evolves into a sharply demarcated area covered by a necrotic eschar and surrounded by a border of erythema. The process at this point resembles a third-degree burn, for which it could be mistaken if a history were not available. Lymphangitis is rarely evident. Extensive necrotic sloughs can result because of deep penetration of the infection along fascial planes. Bacteremia, metastatic abscesses, and death may result from this life-threatening illness if appropriate antibiotic therapy is not initiated promptly. Secondary thrombophlebitis may be a complication when the lower extremities are involved. Streptococci can usually be cultured from the early bullous lesions and frequently from the blood.

PROGRESSIVE BACTERIAL SYNERGISTIC GANGRENE. This distinctive lesion usually follows infection at an abdominal operative wound site (frequently when wire sutures have been used), about an ileostomy or colostomy, at the exit of a fistulous tract, or in proximity to a chronic ulceration on an extremity.[47,48] It beings as a local tender area of swelling and erythema that subsequently ulcerates. The painful, shaggy ulcer gradually enlarges and is characteristically encircled by a margin of gangrenous skin (Fig. 4). Surrounding the latter is a violaceous zone that fades into an outer pink edematous border area. If untreated, the process extends slowly but relentlessly, ultimately producing an enormous ulceration. A related lesion, Meleney's ulcer, is essentially bacterial synergistic gangrene with the additional feature of burrowing necrotic tracts through tissue planes emerging at distant skin sites.

Microaerophilic or anaerobic streptococci can be recovered from aspirates of the advancing margin of the lesion, and *S. aureus* (or occasionally *Proteus* or other gram-negative bacilli) are present in the ulcerated area. Meleney has reproduced the same type of lesions by injecting both microaerophilic streptococci and *S. aureus* (but not either alone) into the skin of experimental animals.

GAS GANGRENE, ANAEROBIC CELLULITIS, AND OTHER FORMS OF CREPITANT CELLULITIS. See Chapters 75 and 76.

GANGRENOUS CELLULITIS IN THE PREDISPOSED HOST. The etiologic considerations in cellulitis occurring in the compromised host include agents that produce such infections in healthy persons, as well as a variety of other organisms not ordinarily regarded as causes of cellulitis, Mucormycotic gangrenous cellulitis may be engrafted on an extensive burn wound, or it may develop rarely in patients with diabetes mellitus or in those who are receiving immunosuppressive therapy. Local factors (open fracture sites, ileostomy stomas, fistulous tracts) also play a predisposing role in this type of infection. Spores of *Rhizopus* spp. (member of the Mucoraceae) contaminating Elastoplast tape used for occlusive dressings have resulted in progressive local and disseminated infection in immunosuppressed patients.[50] The infection may exhibit an indolent course with minimal fever and a slowly enlarging black ulcer, or it may follow a rapidly progressive febrile course. The characteristic lesion consists of a central anesthetic black necrotic area with a surrounding raised zone of violaceous cellulitis and edema.[51] Superficial vesicles may occur in the gangrenous area. Hematogenous dissemination is not ordinarily demonstrable, and the skin infection usually does not result from an initial pulmonary or rhinocerebral focus. Cultures of the necrotic skin or aspirates from the advancing margin usually do not reveal the fungus. Definition of the etiology is best obtained on biopsy specimens: fungal wet mount on a crushed tissue preparation, tissue sections stained with hematoxylin and eosin (showing tissue and vascular invasion by characteristic broad hyphae), and culture.

Pseudomonas bacteremia may also produce a gangrenous cellulitis (see the section on "Cutaneous Involvement in Systemic Bacterial and Mycotic Infections" later in this chapter) in immunocompromised hosts, patients with thermal burns, and so forth. In similar settings, gangrenous skin lesions may occur with disseminated aspergillosis.

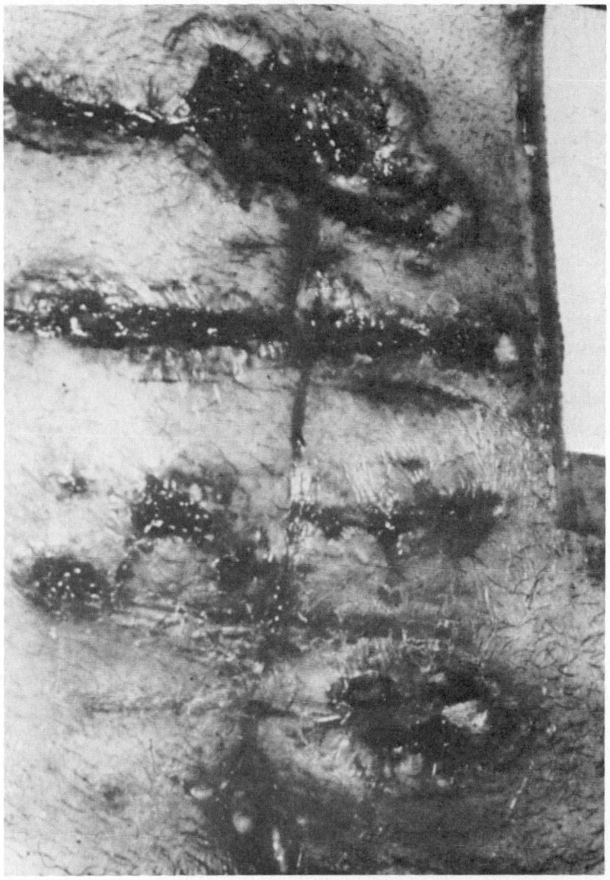

FIG. 4. Progressive bacterial synergistic gangrene of the abdominal wall. Ulcerated areas had developed about wire stay sutures that have since been removed. (From Bornstein et al.,[49] with permission.)

Differential Diagnosis. See Table 2. The bite of the brown recluse house spider can produce a necrotizing skin lesion that resembles infectious gangrenous cellulitis. The occurrence of fever and chills 24–48 hours after the bite enhances the mimicry.

TABLE 2. Differential Diagnosis of Infectious Gangrene and Gangrenous Cellulitis

	Progressive Bacterial Synergistic Gangrene	*Synergistic Necrotizing Cellulitis*	*Streptococcal Gangrene*	*Gas Gangrene*	*Necrotizing Cutaneous Mucormycosis*	*Bacteremic Pseudomonas Gangrenous Cellulitis*	*Pyoderma Gangrenosum*
Predisposing conditions	Surgery; draining sinus	Diabetes common	Occasionally diabetes or myxedema; after abdominal surgery	Local trauma	Diabetes; corticosteroid therapy	Burns, immunosuppression	Ulcerative colitis; rheumatoid arthritis
Pain	Prominent	Prominent	Prominent	Prominent	Minimal	Mild	Moderate
Systemic toxicity	Minimal	Marked	Marked	Very marked	Variable	Marked	Minimal
Course	Slow	Rapid	Very rapid	Extremely rapid	Rapid	Rapid	Slow
Fever	Minimal or absent	Moderate	High	Moderate or high	Low grade	High	Low grade
Anesthesia of lesion	–	–	±	–	+	±	–
Crepitus	–	Often present	–	+	–	–	–
Appearance of the involved area	Central shaggy, necrotic ulcer surrounded by dusky margin and erythematous periphery	Crepitant cellulitis; thick, copious, foul-smelling "dishwater" drainage from scattered areas of skin necrosis	Necrosis of subcutaneous tissue and fascia; black necrotic "burned" appearance of overlying skin	Marked swelling; yellow-bronzed discoloration of skin; brown bullae; green-black patches of necrosis; serosanguinous discharge	Usually a central black necrotic area with purple raised margin; also may present as just a black ulcer	A sharply demarcated necrotic area with black eschar and surrounding erythema, resembling a decubitus ulcer; may evolve from initial hemorrhagic bulla	Begin as bullae, pustules, or erythematous nodules that ulcerate deeply; often multiple, large and coalesce; usually on lower extremities or abdomen
Etiology	Microaerophilic streptococcus plus *S. aureus* (or *Proteus* sometimes)	Usually a mixture of organisms (e.g., *Bacteroides*, peptostreptococci, *E. coli*, etc.)	Primarily group A streptococci; when develops secondary to abdominal surgery, enteric bacteria also involved	*C. perfringens* (occasionally other clostridia)	*Rhizopus, Mucor, Absidia*	*P. aeruginosa*	Not an infection primarily; may be confused with such due to secondary colonization by Enterobacteriaceae, microaerophilic streptococci, *P. aeruginosa, S. aureus*

(Modified from Wilson et al.[51] with permission.)

Presumptive Therapy. Treatment of streptococcal gangrene consists of immediate surgical drainage with longitudinal incisions extending through the deep fascia and beyond the involved gangrenous and undermined areas.[46] Areas of cutaneous necrosis are excised. Antibiotic therapy consists of parenteral aqueous penicillin G (600,000–2,000,000 units every 4–6 hours). If there is any question as to the etiologic agent (e.g., possibly *S. aureus* rather than group A streptococcus), then nafcillin (1.5–2.0 g intravenously every 4–6 hours) should be used. The etiology of necrotizing fasciitis due to mixed anaerobes and facultative organisms (synergistic necrotizing cellulitis) can usually be suspected at the outset from the foul odor and the appearance of the exudate on a Gram-stained smear. After surgery the wound is treated with elevation and moist dressings. Skin grafting is usually required later.

Progressive bacterial synergistic gangrene is very difficult to treat. Local irrigations with bacitracin and systemic therapy with parenteral penicillin (4–6 million units/day intravenously) and a second drug (based on antibiotic susceptibility testing of bacteria other than microaerophilic streptococci isolated from the lesion) is sometimes helpful. However, wide excision of all necrotic tissue (extending well into normal tissue) combined with antibiotic treatment usually is required.

Erythrasma

Clinical Findings. Erythrasma is a common superficial bacterial infection of the skin characterized by slowly spreading, pruritic, reddish-brown macular patches, usually located in the genitocrural area.[52] The lesions are finely scaled and finely wrinkled, and they are more common in men and in obese individuals with diabetes mellitus. The disease may be asymptomatic or may undergo periodic exacerbations. The etiology appears to be bacterial: *Corynebacterium minutissimum*, a species that can be grown aerobically. Gram-stained imprints of the skin surface show large numbers of small gram-positive bacilli. Examination of the lesions under a Wood's lamp reveals a distinctive coral red fluorescence.

The principal superficial skin infections to be considered in the differential diagnosis are tinea versicolor lesions on the trunk and tinea cruris (a deeper, more inflammatory, and more rapidly progressive process).

Treatment with oral erythromycin (1.0 g/day orally for 5–7 days) is usually efficacious, clearing the lesions within several weeks. Topical treatment with an aqueous solution of 2% clindamycin hydrochloride can also be effective.[53]

SECONDARY BACTERIAL INFECTIONS COMPLICATING PRE-EXISTING SKIN LESIONS

A variety of skin lesions (burns, eczematous dermatitides, traumatic lesions, and so on) may become secondarily infected (Table 1). Such infected lesions usually do not exhibit distinctive morphologic characteristics based on the infecting organism; rather, the appearance of the lesions is determined to a large measure by the nature of the pre-existing injury or dermatosis. Several of these processes are considered in detail elsewhere (Chapters 75–77). Others are cared for primarily by dermatologists (dermatophytosis, acne conglabata). Several of the other secondarily infected dermatoses have some distinctive clinical and bacteriologic features and merit brief consideration here.

Chronic Superficial Skin Ulcers

A variety of aerobic and facultative organisms (*Pseudomonas, Proteus*, enterococci, and so on) colonize and secondarily infect decubitus ulcers. Only in recent years has the prominent role of anaerobic bacteria in such infections been recognized.[54] The character of the ulcers (extensive undermining and necrosis of tissue) and their location, frequently in proximity to the anus, provide the opportunity for invasion by anaerobes. *Bacteroides fragilis* and other Bacteroidaceae and *Clostridium perfringens* have commonly been isolated from infected decubitus ulcers. Such lesions have been the sources of symptomatic bacteremias.

Chronic foot infections in patients with diabetes mellitus are common and difficult problems. They usually begin after minor trauma in patients with peripheral neuropathy and arterial vascular insufficiency, and take the form of cellulitis, soft tissue necrosis, or osteomyelitis with a draining sinus. They are usually polymicrobial in etiology.[55,56] Deep tissue cultures provide the most reliable bacteriologic information. When these are not available, cultures and Gram-stained smears of material obtained from curettage of the base of the ulcer or from a purulent exudate may provide the needed information to guide antimicrobial therapy. Among the facultative bacteria involved in these infections, those most commonly isolated are *S. aureus*, enterococci, group B streptococci, and members of the Enterobacteriaceae (most commonly *Proteus* spp.).[56] Peptostreptococci, *B. fragilis*, and other *Bacteroides* spp. are the most frequently isolated anaerobes. When gas is present in surrounding tissues on radiologic examination, it may represent air introduced through the ulcer or gas generated in the soft tissues by the infecting anaerobic or coliform organisms.

Antibiotic treatment of infected diabetic foot ulcers is based on bacteriologic data. Initial treatment in a previously untreated patient with a mild infection might use a broad-spectrum cephalosporin such as cefoxitin. In patients with more severe infections, broader coverage with clindamycin and an aminoglycoside might be indicated, provided that renal function is not impaired. The oral route and broad spectrum of activity of the newer quinolones such as ciprofloxacin against the facultative bacteria involved in this process suggest that they will have an important role in the treatment of such chronic infections, either alone or in combination with another drug with activity against anaerobes.

Occupationally related contaminated traumatic wounds often involve loss of skin and subcutaneous tissues, with ensuing cellulitis and deeper infections. Comparison of the bacteriology of initial wounds sustained in factories with those on farms (associated with corn-harvesting machinery) indicates that gram-negative bacilli (particularly *Enterobacter* spp. and *Pseudomonas maltophilia*) are 10 times commoner in the latter.[57]

Post-Traumatic Opportunistic Skin Infections in Immunocompromised Patients

A variety of unusual pathogens may invade the skin of immunocompromised patients after some local, often minor laceration or abrasion. Such pathogens include fungi (*Paecilomyces, Penicillium, Trichosporon, Fusarium, Alternaria*), mycobacteria (*M. marinum*), and even algae (*Prototheca wickerhamii*).[50] The lesions are usually ulcerative but, in the case of *M. marinum*, may take the form of a nodular lymphangitis extending from the original focus. A typical dermatophyte, *Trichophyton rubrum*, which ordinarily produces only superficial skin infections, may invade the deeper subcutaneous tissues of immunosuppressed hosts and produce multiple nodular or fluctuant masses.[58]

Hydradenitis Suppurativa

This is an extremely troublesome, chronic, suppurative, cicatricial disease of apocrine glands in the axillary, genital, and perianal areas. The primary lesion appears to be an unexplained keratinous plugging of the ducts of the apocrine glands resulting in dilation and eventual rupture of the gland and surrounding tissue inflammation. The initial lesions are reddish-purple nodules that slowly become fluctuant and drain. Irregular sinus tracts are formed with repeated crops of lesions; reparative processes are only partially successful. Ultimately the involved areas show a mixture of burrowing, draining tracts, and cicatricial scarring. In some patients, hydradenitis suppurativa is associated with acne conglobata or dissecting cellulitis of the scalp. In such patients, a distinctive spondyloarthropathy may occur.[59]

Although not initially infected, the lesions frequently become so secondarily. Staphylococci, nonhemolytic streptococci, *E. coli, Proteus*, and *Pseudomonas* are often isolated from draining lesions. Anaerobic organisms (*Bacteroides*, anaerobic gram-positive cocci) also have been reported from such lesions.[54] The foul odor of the discharge from such lesions would suggest the presence of anaerobes.

Treatment of hidradenitis suppurativa is difficult, particularly when the process is chronic and extensive, because of the multiple deep-seated sites of secondary infection that are inaccessible to antibiotics. Antimicrobial therapy (based on Gram-stained smears and culture results) and local moist heat to establish drainage are helpful in the treatment of the initial phases of infection. Surgical drainage is required in the management of large abscesses. In very severe, resistant cases exhibiting chronicity and scarring, radical excision of most of the involved area followed by skin grafting may become necessary.

Self-Induced Skin Infections

Rarely, persisting unexplained skin ulcers are self-induced. Their colonization with a variety of gram-negative and gram-positive bacteria is inevitable. However, the continuing ulceration is the result of repeated, self-induced trauma rather than of bacterial infection per se. Very rarely, unexplained continuing or recurrent polymicrobial (oral or intestinal flora) cellulitis or a subcutaneous abscess is the result of injection of foreign material containing saliva or contaminated fluids into subcutaneous tissue. Examination of biopsy specimens from the involved area by polarizing microscopy may reveal the presence of birefringent foreign bodies, suggesting the true diagnosis.

CUTANEOUS INVOLVEMENT IN SYSTEMIC BACTERIAL AND MYCOTIC INFECTIONS

Cutaneous manifestations may be a feature of a variety of bacteremias, fungemias, and systemic bacterial infections[60] (Table 1). In leptospirosis, rat-bite fever, and listeriosis cutaneous manifestations are a small part of the total clinical picture and are considered elsewhere in chapters dealing with the responsible organisms. In some systemic infections cutaneous manifestations are noninfectious complications of the illness (erythema nodosum, purpura fulminans).

Bacteremias

Staphylococcus aureus. The occurrence of skin lesions (pustules, subcutaneous abscesses, purulent purpura) in the course of bacteremia or endocarditis due to *S. aureus* can provide a clue to the nature of the infecting organism. The most distinctive of these lesions is that of purulent purpura. This is a small area of purpura with a white, purulent center. Aspiration of the contents of the central portion reveals staphylococci and polymorphonuclear leukocytes. Rarely, scattered tender subcutaneous nodules may develop during *S. aureus* bacteremia.

Pseudomonas aeruginosa. Four types of skin lesion have been described in the course of *Pseudomonas* septicemia:

1. *Vesicles and bullae*. These occur as isolated bullae, or occasionally in small clusters, anywhere on the skin surface.

They rapidly become hemorrhagic and have a narrow encircling zone of dusky erythema. Occasionally, in infants, the lesions are surrounded by large, erythematous halos resembling insect bites or erythema multiforme.
2. *Ecthyma gangrenosum*. This is a round, indurated, ulcerated, painless area with a central gray-black eschar and a surrounding narrow zone of erythema. The lesions may develop de novo or may evolve from an initial bullous lesion.
3. *Gangrenous cellulitis*. This is either a superficial, sharply demarcated necrotic area that may resemble a decubitus ulcer or an area of cellulitis with edema and some necrosis of the overlying skin.
4. *Macular or maculopapular lesions*. These are small, oval, erythematous macules, located predominantly over the trunk, resembling the "rose spots" of typhoid fever. Such lesions have been reported, particularly in the tropics, in association with fever and diarrhea, the syndrome described as *Shanghai fever*.

The foregoing types of metastatic lesion contain numerous gram-negative bacilli but relatively few polymorphonuclear leukocytes. The development of such lesions in a febrile patient with leukemia undergoing induction chemotherapy or on uninvolved skin areas of a patient with extensive thermal burns should strongly suggest the presence of *Pseudomonas* bacteremia. Presumptive antibiotic management should be aimed at *P. aeruginosa* and includes a combination of ticarcillin with tobramycin or a similar aminoglycoside. Rarely, ecthyma gangrenosum occurs in the course of bacteremia due to other gram-negative bacilli or in disseminated candidiasis; or it may occur in the absence of bacteremia as progression of *Pseudomonas* folliculitis in an immunocompromised patient.[61]

Neisseria meningitidis. The skin lesions of acute meningococcemia consist of erythematous macules (initially), petechiae, purpura, and ecchymoses located on the extremities and trunk. Extensive gun-metal gray, hemorrhagic, necrotic patches can develop by confluence of petechial and purpuric lesions in fulminant meningococcemia. Symmetric peripheral gangrene and purpura fulminans occur with prominent disseminated intravascular coagulation. Occasionally, gram-negative diplococci can be observed on smears of serum obtained from the skin lesions of acute meningococcemia.

Skin lesions are an important feature of the unusual syndrome of chronic meningococcemia, characterized by recurrent cycles of fever, arthralgias, and rash over a period of 2–3 months.[62] The rash appears in crops, each consisting of a small number of individual lesions during febrile episodes. The lesions are generally located on the extremities, particularly about joints. They may consist of erythematous maculopapules, petechiae, petechiae with vesiculopustular centers, petechiae with small areolas of pale erythema, suggilations or tender erythema nodosum-like nodules. Biopsy specimens of the lesions reveal the histologic picture of leukocytoclastic angiitis, a finding that may erroneously direct attention toward a diagnosis of a small vessel hypersensitivity vasculitis and away from that of vasculitis secondary to systemic infection.

Neisseria gonorrhoeae. The skin lesions of gonococcemia consist of pustules surrounded by a thin zone of purpura, macules, papules, purpuric vesicles and bullae, and/or purpuric infarcts. The lesions are few, scattered over the distal extremities particularly, and frequently painful. They are part of the gonococcemic dermatitis-arthritis syndrome. In addition to arthralgias and frank arthritis, tenosynovitis may be a conspicuous feature.

Salmonella typhi. "Rose spots" frequently appear 7–10 days into the febrile course of untreated typhoid fever. The lesions are slightly raised, small (1–3 mm), pink papules that tend to occur in crops of 10–20 lesions. They are found most commonly on the upper abdomen, lower chest, and back. Rose spots are less frequently found in enteric fevers due to *Salmonella* spp. other than *S. typhi*. Early treatment with ampicillin or chloramphenicol will prevent the appearance of these skin lesions. *Salmonella typhi* can sometimes be found on Gram-stained preparations from the papules and isolated on culture.

Haemophilus influenzae. Cellulitis involving the face, neck, or upper extremities occasionally occurs with bacteremic *Haemophilus influenzae* type b infections in children, particularly under the age of 3 years. Although commonly described as having a peculiar purple-red or blue-red hue, the lesion most often is erythematous, indurated, and indistinguishable from cellulitis due to streptococci or staphylococci. The site of primary infection is in the pharynx, the middle ear, or elsewhere in the upper respiratory tract. Direct invasion across traumatized buccal mucous membranes by *H. influenzae* type b colonizing the respiratory tract has been suggested as the pathogenesis of most cases of buccal cellulitis in children.[63] Until very recently, this uncommon lesion had been described only in pediatric practice, but now cases have been reported in adults with epiglottitis and other forms of upper respiratory disease due to *H. influenzae*.[64] In view of the increasing incidence of ampicillin resistance in clinical strains of *H. influenzae* type b, provisional antibiotic therapy should use a third-generation cephalosporin (chloramphenicol, either alone or in combination with ampicillin), until the isolate can be tested for β-lactamase activity.

Infective Endocarditis

The cutaneous lesions of subacute bacterial endocarditis consist of petechiae, subungual "splinter" hemorrhages, Osler's nodes, and Janeway's lesions. Petechiae tend to occur in small crops, particularly in the conjunctivae, on the palate, and on the upper chest and extremities. These are the most common skin lesions of endocarditis. Rarely, petechiae are extremely numerous, particularly on the lower extremities, and suggest a primary vasculitis. Osler's nodes are split-pea sized, erythematous, tender nodules located principally on the pads of the fingers and toes. They are few at any given time and occur in about 15 percent of the patients with subacute bacterial endocarditis. The lesions are usually transient, clearing in 1–2 days. Similar lesions may also occur in acute endocarditis (e.g., due to *S. aureus*). Histologic examination of such lesions in several cases of acute endocarditis has suggested septic embolization in their pathogenesis.[65] The genesis of Osler's nodes in subacute bacterial endocarditis may have a different basis, perhaps an allergic vasculitis. Janeway's lesions are painless, small, erythematous macules or minimally nodular hemorrhages in the palms or soles occuring in either acute or subacute endocarditis (more commonly in the former, particularly when *S. aureus* is the etiology).

Fungemias

Candida albicans. Systemic candidiasis developing in the setting of leukemia, immunosuppression, extensive antibiotic therapy, hyperalimentation, heroin addiction, cardiac surgery, and so on may be difficult to diagnose clinically until the organism is isolated from routine blood cultures—often not until 5–7 days of incubation (more rapidly with lysis-centrifugation culture methods). The portal for disseminated candidiasis (or aspergillosis) may be an area of skin injured in the course of intravenous therapy (or trauma induced by adhesive tape or extravasation of intravenous fluid).[50] Examination of the optic fundi (for evidence of candidal ophthalmitis) and the search for *Candida* pseudohyphae and yeast forms on a smear of buffy coat of venous blood are sometimes helpful in making an early diagnosis of candidal fungemia while awaiting isolation of the organism from blood cultures. In occasional patients, the appearance of multiple discrete (2–5 mm) pink maculopapules (sometimes with pale centers) on the trunk or extremities can suggest the diagnosis.[66] In some of these patients severe diffuse muscle tenderness has been present, and muscle biopsy specimens have shown necrosis with yeast and pseudohyphal forms.[67] Occasionally, subcutaneous abscesses due to *Candida* may develop in the course of fungemia. Aspiration of such abscesses reveals the etiology on stained smear. Punch biopsy specimens of the maculopapular lesions provide a more accurate diagnosis than simple culture, since histologic sections can reveal *Candida* emboli in blood vessels and pseudohyphae in adjacent soft tissues. The isolation of *Candida* from an unroofed lesion may only represent surface colonization or may be consistent with *Candida* folliculitis rather than disseminated candidiasis.

REFERENCES

1. Schachner L, Taplin D, Scott GB, et al. A therapeutic update of superficial skin infections. Pediatr Clin North Am. 1983;30:397.
2. Ferrieri P, Dajani AS, Wannamaker LW, et al. Natural history of impetigo. I. Site sequence of acquisition and familial patterns of spread of cutaneous streptococci. J Clin Invest. 1972;51:2851.
3. Dajani AS, Ferrieri P, Wannamaker LW. Natural history of impetigo. II. Etiologic agents and bacterial interactions. J Clin Invest. 1972;51:2863.
4. Dillon HC. Impetigo contagiosa: Suppurative and non-suppurative complications. I. Clinical bacteriologic, and epidemiologic characteristics of impetigo. Am J Dis Child. 1968;115:530.
5. Dillon HC. Post-streptococcal glomerulonephritis following pyoderma. Rev Infect Dis. 1979;1:935.
6. Baltimore RS. Treatment of impetigo: A review. Pediatr Infect Dis. 1985;4:597.
7. Maddox JS, Ware JC, Dillon HC Jr. The natural history of streptococcal skin infection: Prevention with topical antibiotics. J Am Acad Dermatol. 1985;13:207.
8. Dajani AS. The scalded-skin syndrome: Relation to phage group II staphylococci. J Infect Dis. 1972;125:548.
9. Melish ME, Glascow LA, Turner MD, et al. The staphylococcal epidermolytic toxin: Its isolation, characterization, and site of action. Ann NY Acad Sci. 1974;236:317.
10. Elias PM, Fritsch P, Epstein EH Jr. Staphylococcal scalded skin syndrome: Clinical features, pathogenesis, and recent microbiological and biochemical developments. Arch Dermatol. 1977;113:207.
11. O'Reilly M, Dougan G, Foster TJ, et al. Plasmids in epidermolytic strains of *Staphylococcus aureus*. J Gen Microbiol. 1981;124:99.
12. Curran JP, Al-Salihi FL. Neonatal staphylococcal scalded skin syndrome: Massive outbreak due to an unusual phage type. Pediatrics. 1980;66:285.
13. Shands KN, Schmid GP, Dan BB, et al. Toxic-shock syndrome in menstruating women: Its association with tampon use and *Staphylococcus aureus* and the clinical features in 52 cases. N Engl J Med. 1980;303:1436.
14. Institute of Medicine, National Academy of Science: Conference on the Toxic Shock Syndrome. Ann Intern Med. 1978;96:835.
15. Todd JT, Fishaut M, Kapral F, et al. Toxic shock syndrome associated with phage-group-I staphylococci. Lancet. 1978;2:1116.
16. Gustafson LT, Band JD, Hutcheson RH, et al. *Pseudomonas* folliculitis: An outbreak and review. Rev Infect Dis. 1983;5:1.
17. El Baze P, Thyss A, Caldini C, et al. *Pseudomonas aeruginosa* 0-11 folliculitis: Development into ecthyma gangrenosum in immunosuppressed patients. Arch Dermatol. 1985;121:873.
18. Blankenship MI. Gram negative folliculitis. Arch Dermatol. 1984;120:1301.
19. Klotz SA, Drutz DJ, Huppert M, et al. *Pityrosporum* folliculitis. Its potential for confusion with skin lesions of systemic candidiasis. Arch Intern Med. 1982;142:2126.
20. Bufill JA, Lum LG, Caya JG, et al. Pityrosporum folliculitis after bone marrow transplantation. Ann Intern Med. 1988;108:560.
21. Buchness MR, Lim HW, Hatcher VA, et al. Eosinophilic pustular folliculitis in the acquired immunodeficiency syndrome. N Engl J Med. 1988;318:1183.
22. Hedstrom SA. Treatment and prevention of recurrent staphylococcal furunculosis: Clinical and bacteriologic follow-up. Scand J Infect Dis. 1985;17:55.
23. Wheat LJ, Kohler RB, Luft FC, et al. Long-term studies of the effect of rifampin on nasal carriage of coagulase-positive staphylococci. Rev Infect Dis. 1983;5:459S.
24. Allen AM, Taplin D, Twigg L. Cutaneous streptococcal infections in Vietnam. Arch Dermatol. 1971;104:271.
25. Hewitt WD, Farrar WE. Case report: Bacteremia and ecthyma caused by *Streptococcus pyogenes* in a patient with acquired immunodeficiency syndrome. Am J Med Sci. 1988;295:52.
26. Gold H. Anthrax: A report of 117 cases. Arch Intern Med. 1955;96:387.
27. Jorup-Ronstrom C. Epidemiological, bacteriological and complicating features of erysipelas. Scand J Infect Dis. 1986;18:519.
28. Fitzpatrick TB, Eisen AZ, Wolff K, et al, eds. Dermatology in General Medicine. New York: McGraw-Hill; 1971: PlateXXXVII.
29. Baddour LM, Bisno AL. Recurrent cellulitis after saphenous venectomy for coronary bypass surgery. Ann Intern Med. 1982;97:493.
30. Baddour LM, Bisno AL. Non-group A beta-hemolytic streptococcal cellulitis. Association with venous and lymphatic compromise. Am J Med. 1985;79:155.
31. Chmel H, Hamdy M. Recurrent streptococcal cellulitis complicating radical hysterectomy and radiation therapy. Obstet Gynecol. 1984;63:862.
32. Ellison RT III, McGregor JA. Recurrent postcoital lower extremity streptococcal erythroderma in women. Streptococcal-sex syndrome. JAMA. 1987;257:3260.
33. Spear RM, Rothbaum RJ, Keating JP, et al. Perianal streptococcal cellulitis. J Pediatr. 1985;107:557.
34. Williams CN, Cohen M, Ronan SG, et al. Dissecting cellulitis of the scalp. Plastic Reconstruct Surg. 1986;77:378.
35. Markham RB, Polk BF. Seal Finger. Rev Infect Dis. 1979;1:567.
36. Miyais S, Uwaydah M. Pneumococcal cellulitis. Infection. 1983;11:173.
37. Asmar BI, Bashour BN, Fleischmann LE. *Escherichia coli* cellulitis in children with idiopathic nephrotic syndrome. Clin Pediatr. 1987;26:592.
38. Hanson PG, Standridge J, Jarrett F, et al. Freshwater wound infection due to *Aeromonas hydrophila*. JAMA. 1977;238:1053.
39. Bonner JR, Coker AS, Berryman CR, et al. Spectrum of *Vibrio* infections in a gulf coast community. Ann Intern Med. 1983;99:464.
40. Hook EW III, Hooton TM, Horton CA, et al. Microbiologic evaluation of cutaneous cellulitis in adults. Arch Intern Med. 1986;146:295.
41. Howe PM, Fajardo JE, Orcutt MA. Etiologic diagnosis of cellulitis: Comparison of aspirates obtained from the leading edge and the point of maximal inflammation. Pediatr Infect Dis. 1987;6:685.
42. Saulsbury FT, Cooper PH, Bracikowski A, et al. Eosinophilic cellulitis in a child. J Pediatr. 1983;102:266.
43. Belsey MA, Sinclair M, Roder MR, et al. *Corynebacterium diphtheriae* skin infections in Alabama and Louisiana. A factor in the epidemiology of diphtheria. N Engl J Med. 1969;280:135.
44. Koopman JS, Campbell J. The role of cutaneous diphtheria infections in a diphtheria epidemic. J Infect Dis. 1975;131:239.
45. Barker FG, Leppard BJ, Seal DV. Streptococcal necrotizing fasciitis: Comparison between histological and clinical features. J Clin Pathol. 1987;40:335.
46. Strasberg SM, Silver MS. Hemolytic streptococcus gangrene. An uncommon but frequently fatal infection in the antibiotic era. Am J Surg. 1968;115:763.
47. Meleney FL. Bacterial synergism in disease processes with a confirmation of the synergistic bacterial etiology of a certain type of progressive gangrene of the abdominal wall. Ann Surg. 1931;94:961.
48. Husseinzadeh N, Nahas WA, Manders EK, et al. Spontaneous occurrence of synergistic bacterial gangrene following external pelvic irradiation. Obstet Gynecol. 1984;63:859.
49. Bornstein DL, Weinberg AN, Swartz MN, et al. Anaerobic infections. Review of current experience. Medicine. 1964;43:207.
50. Wolfson JS, Sober AJ, Rubin RH. Dermatologic manifestations in the compromised host. Ann Rev Med. 1983;14:205.
51. Wilson CB, Siber GR, O'Brien TF, et al. Phycomycotic gangrenous cellulitis. Arch Surg. 1976;111:532.
52. Sarkany I, Taplin D, Blank H. The etiology and treatment of erythrasma. J Invest Derm. 1961;37:283.
53. Sindhuphak W, MacDonald E, Smith EB. Erythrasma: Overlooked or misdiagnosed. Int J Dermatol. 1985;24:95.
54. Finegold SM. Infections of skin, soft tissue and muscle. In: Anaerobic Bacteria in Human Diseases. New York: Academic Press; 1977:386.
55. Sapico FL, Witte JL, Canawati HN, et al. The infected foot of the diabetic patient: Quantitative microbiology and analysis of clinical features. Rev Infect Dis. 1984;6(Suppl 1):S171.
56. Wheat LJ, Allen SD, Henry M, et al. Diabetic foot infections: Bacteriologic analysis. Arch Intern Med. 1986;146:1935.
57. Agger WA, Cogbill TH, Busch H Jr, et al. wounds caused by corn-harvesting machines: An unusual source of infection due to gram-negative bacilli. Rev Infect Dis. 1986;8:927.
58. Novick NL, Tapia L, Bottone EJ. Invasive *Trichophyton rubrum* infection in an immunocompromised host. Am J Med. 1987;82:321.
59. Rosner IA, Richter DE, Huettner TL, et al. Spondyloarthropathy associated with hydradenitis suppurativa and acne conglobata. Ann Intern Med. 1982;97:520.
60. Kingston ME, Mackey D. Skin clues in the diagnosis of life-threatening infections. Rev Infect Dis. 1986;8:1.
61. Huminer D, Siegman-Igra Y, Morduchowicz G, et al. Ecthyma gangrenosum without bacteremia: Report of six cases and review of the literature. Arch Intern Med. 1987;147:299.
62. Benoit FL. Chronic meningococcemia. Am J Med. 1963;35:103.
63. Chartrand SA, Harrison CJ. Buccal cellulitis reevaluated. Am J Dis Child. 1986;140:891.
64. Drapkin MS, Wilson ME, Shrager SM, et al. Bacteremic *Hemophilus influenzae* type B cellulitis in the adult. Am J Med. 1977;63:449.
65. Alpert JS, Krous HF, Dalen JE. Pathogenesis of Osler's nodes. Ann Intern Med. 1976;85:471.
66. Balandral L, Rothschild H, Pugh N, et al. A cutaneous manifestation of systemic candidiasis. Ann Intern Med. 1973;78:400.
67. Jarowski CI, Fialk MA, Murray HW, et al. Fever, rash, and muscle tenderness. A distinctive clinical presentation of disseminated candidiasis. Arch Intern Med. 1978;138:544.

75. SUBCUTANEOUS TISSUE INFECTIONS AND ABSCESSES

MORTON N. SWARTZ

Exact categorization of some bacterial infections of the soft tissues (skin, subcutaneous tissues, fascia, and skeletal muscle) may be difficult. While the differences between a superficial pyoderma and a necrotizing myositis like gas gangrene are readily apparent, distinctions between many other types of soft tissue infection are sometimes blurred. Classification is usually based on features such as the anatomic structure involved, the infecting organism(s), and the clinical picture. Unfortunately for convenience in categorization, some infections may involve several components of the soft tissues, and multiple bacterial species may produce infections with the same clinical appearance.

To compound the problem of classification further, a variety of designations have been given to closely related or virtually identical processes. For example, *streptococcal gangrene* has also been referred to as *necrotizing fasciitis*. Subsequent to the initial descriptions of this condition, it became apparent that it was sometimes caused by other bacteria than group A streptococci.[1] Thus, streptococcal gangrene can be considered the major subset of necrotizing fasciitis. For convenience, because a major feature of its manifestation is cutaneous gangrene, streptococcal gangrene has been considered in the preceding chapter with cellulitis and infectious cutaneous gangrene. Necrotizing fasciitis is reconsidered in this chapter on subcutaneous tissue infections, particularly in relation to its nonstreptococcal etiologies. Another example of the problems in nomenclature is that presented by infections that involve multiple soft tissue strata and that can be caused by a variety of bacterial species. Thus, the condition known as *synergistic necrotizing cellulitis* has also been described as *gram-negative anaerobic cutaneous gangrene* and *synergistic nonclostridial anaerobic myonecrosis*.[2,3] Because of the prominence of subcutaneous tissue involvement in this condition, it is considered primarily in this chapter, although it could be considered almost as readily in chapters on cellulitis or myositis.

CLOSTRIDIAL ANAEROBIC CELLULITIS

This is a necrotizing clostridial infection of devitalized subcutaneous tissues. Deep fascia is not appreciably involved, and ordinarily there is no associated myositis. Gas formation is common and often extensive. Anaerobic cellulitis is several times more common than gas gangrene in war wounds.

Pathogenesis and Pathologic Characteristics

Clostridial species, usually *Clostridium perfringens*, are introduced into subcutaneous tissues either through a dirty or inadequately debrided traumatic wound, through contamination at operation, or from a pre-existing localized infection. The last is frequently located in the perineum, abdominal wall, buttocks, and lower extremities, areas that are readily contaminated with fecal flora. The presence of foreign debris and necrotic tissue in the depths of a wound provides a suitable anaerobic milieu for clostridial proliferation.

Clinical Findings

The incubation period is several days, longer than the 1–2 days for clostridial myonecrosis. The onset is gradual but the process subsequently may spread rapidly.[4] Local pain, tissue swelling, and systemic toxicity are not prominent features, and the relative mildness of the process helps to distinguish it from true gas gangrene. The dark blebs and bronzing of the skin seen in gas gangrene are not usually features of clostridial cellulitis. A thin, dark, sometimes foul-smelling drainage (often containing fat globules) from the wound is characteristic, as is extensive tissue gas formation, more prominent than that observed in clostridial myonecrosis. Frank crepitus is present in the involved area and may extend very widely, even beyond the limits of the active infection.

Gram-stained smears of the drainage shows numerous blunt-ended, thick, gram-positive bacilli and variable numbers of polymorphonuclear leukocytes. Soft tissue x-ray films show abundant gas, but usually not in the feathery linear pattern in muscles observed in gas gangrene.

Etiologic Agents

Clostridium perfringens is the most common clostridial species responsible for this infection, but *C. septicum* and other species have been isolated. Sometimes, the clostridia are present in mixed culture with facultative organisms.

Differential Diagnosis

When crepitus is observed in a wound, a variety of possibilities must be considered in the differential diagnosis (Table 1). The first is gas gangrene because of the fulminant nature of the infection and the requirement for emergency surgery. At the same time, distinguishing between clostridial gas gangrene and anaerobic cellulitis is essential to avoid performing unnecessarily extensive surgery. Ultimately, the two processes are differentiated in the operating room when the wound is laid open and the viability and appearance of the muscle are observed. The muscle is normal (pink) in clostridial cellulitis but distinctly abnormal (discolored, fails to contract on stimulation, does not bleed from cut surface) in clostridial myonecrosis (see Chapter 76).

Presumptive Therapy

Surgical exploration is essential to determine the presence of any muscle involvement. If no myonecrosis is found, treatment should be limited to débridement of necrotic tissue and drainage of pus after the wound is opened widely. Penicillin in high dosage intravenously is indicated in management. Based on Gram-stained smears of exudate and tissue, an additional drug may be indicated for initial treatment of a potentially mixed infection.

NONCLOSTRIDIAL ANAEROBIC CELLULITIS

A clinical picture very similar to that of clostridial anaerobic cellulitis can be produced by infection with a variety of non-spore-forming anaerobic bacteria (various *Bacteroides* spp., peptostreptococci, peptococci—either alone or as mixed infections).[3] The anaerobic bacteria may be present along with facultative species (coliform bacilli, various streptococci, staphylococci) in a mixed infection. Gas-forming soft tissue infections have been produced by *Escherichia coli, Klebsiella, Aeromonas*, and perhaps other facultative bacteria.[5,6]

The surgical approach used is the same as in the treatment of clostridial anaerobic cellulitis. Antimicrobial therapy is initially based on the findings on Gram-stained smears of wound exudate. In view of the frequently mixed nature of the infections (and the spectrum of organisms involved), several antimicrobials (e.g., penicillin or ampicillin plus chloramphenicol) are probably indicated while awaiting the results of cultures.

TABLE 1. Differential Diagnosis of Crepitant Soft Tissue Wounds[a]

	Clostridial Cellulitis	*Nonclostridial Anaerobic Cellulitis*	*Gas Gangrene*	*Streptococcal Myositis*	*Necrotizing Fascitis*[b]	*Infected Vascular Gangrene*	*Synergistic Necrotizing Cellulitis*[c]	*Noninfectious Causes of Gas in Tissues*
Predisposing conditions	Local trauma or surgery	Diabetes mellitus; preexisting localized infection	Local trauma or surgery	Local trauma	Diabetes mellitus; abdominal surgery; perineal infection	Peripheral arterial insufficiency	Diabetes mellitus; cardiorenal disease; obesity; perirectal infection	Mechanical effects of penetrating trauma; injuries involving use of compressed air; entrapment of air under loosely sutured wounds or under ulcers; irrigation of wounds with hydrogen peroxide; intravenous catheter placement
Incubation period	Usually over 3 days	Several days	1–2 days	3–4 days	1–4 days	>5 days	3–14 days	Less than an hour
Onset	Gradual	Gradual or rapid	Acute	Not as rapid as gas gangrene	Acute	Gradual	Acute	Usually present immediately after trauma or manipulation; may not be recognized until examined several hours later
Pain	Mild	Mild	Marked	Occurs late; marked	Moderate or severe	Variable	Severe	Mild
Swelling	Moderate	Moderate	Marked	Moderate	Marked	Moderate or marked	Moderate or marked	Slight or absent
Skin appearance	Minimal discoloration	Minimal discoloration	Yellow-bronze; dark bullae; green-black patches of necrosis	Erythema	Erythematous cellulitis; areas of skin necrosis	Discolored or black	Scattered areas of skin necrosis	Only those due to initiating trauma
Exudate	Thin, dark	Dark pus	Serosanguinous	Abundant seropurulent	Seropurulent	0	"Dishwater" pus	0
Gas	+ + + +	+ + + +	+ +	±	+ +	+ + +	+ +	Variable but present; does not extend
Odor	Sometimes foul	Foul	Variable; slightly foul or peculiar sweet	Slight; "sour"	Foul	Foul	Foul	0
Systemic toxicity	Minimal	Moderate	Marked	Only late in course	Moderate or marked	Minimal	Marked	0
Muscle involvement	0	0	+ + + +	+ + +	0	Dead	+ +	0

Key: ±: rarely present; + +: present to mild extent; + + +: present to moderate extent; + + + +: extensive.
[a] In addition to the causes of crepitant infections listed in this table, *Aeromonas hydrophila* myositis may be associated with gas in soft tissues.
[b] The term *necrotizing fascitis* is employed here to designate forms of this syndrome of streptococcal gangrene.
[c] Synergistic necrotizing cellulitis is essentially the same process as Type I necrotizing fasciitis. Since the former occasionally extends to involve muscle it is given a separate designation here; however, the two processes are clinically indistinguishable in most instances.
(Modified from Finegold,[3] with permission.)

NECROTIZING FASCIITIS

The term *necrotizing fasciitis* encompasses two bacteriologic entities[7,8]: *Type I* is the first entity, in which at least one anaerobic sp. (most commonly *Bacteroides* and *Peptostreptococcus* spp.) is isolated in combination with one or more facultative anaerobic sp. such as streptococci (other than group A) and members of the Enterobacteriaceae (e.g., *E. coli, Enterobacter, Klebsiella, Proteus*). An obligate aerobe such as *Pseudomonas aeruginosa* is only rarely a component of such a mixed infection. Cases in which only anaerobes are present appear to be rare.[8] *Type II* is the second entity (corresponding to the entity known also as *hemolytic streptococcal gangrene*) in which group A streptococci, either alone or in combination with other species, *Staphylococcus aureus* most commonly, are isolated. Streptococcal gangrene has been considered in Chapter 74 as a form of gangrenous cellulitis; the more general feature of necrotizing fasciitis will be considered here.

Clinical Findings

Necrotizing fasciitis is an uncommon severe infection involving the subcutaneous soft tissues, particularly the superficial (and often the deep) fascia. It usually is an acute process but rarely may follow a subacute progressive course. It can affect any part of the body but is most common on the extremities, particularly the legs. Other sites of predilection are the abdominal wall, perianal and groin areas, and postoperative wounds.[9] The portal of entry is usually a site of trauma (laceration, abrasion, burn, insect bite), a laparotomy performed in the presence of peritoneal soiling (penetrating abdominal trauma or perforated viscus) or other surgical procedure (e.g., hemorrhoidectomy or vasectomy), perirectal abscess, decubitus ulcer, or an intestinal perforation. The last may be secondary to occult diverticulitis,[10,11] rectosigmoid neoplasm, or a foreign body such as chicken bone or toothpick. Necrotizing fasciitis from such intestinal sources may occur in the lower extremity (extension along the psoas muscle), as well as in the groin or abdominal wall (via a colocutaneous fistula). Particular clinical settings in which necrotizing fasciitis may develop include diabetes mellitus, alcoholism, and parenteral drug abuse.[12]

In the newborn necrotizing fasciitis can be a serious complication of omphalitis. Initial swelling and erythema about the umbilicus can progress over several hours to several days, resulting in purplish discoloration and periumbilical necrosis.[13] Involvement of the anterior abdominal wall frequently extends to the flanks and even onto the chest wall.

The affected area initially is erythematous, swollen, without sharp margins, hot, shiny, exquisitely tender, and painful.[14] Lymphangitis and lymphadenitis are infrequent. The process progresses rapidly over several days, with sequential skin color changes from red-purple to patches of blue-gray. Within 3–5 days of onset, skin breakdown with bullae (containing thick pink or purple fluid) and frank cutaneous gangrene (resembling a thermal burn) occurs. By this time, the involved area is no longer tender but has become anesthetic secondary to thrombosis of small blood vessels and destruction of superficial nerves located in the necrotic undermined subcutaneous tissues. The development of anesthesia may antedate the appearance of skin necrosis, and this may provide a clue that the process is necrotizing fasciitis and not a simple cellulitis. Subcutaneous gas is often present in the polymicrobial form of necrotizing fasciitis, particularly in patients with diabetes mellitus. Systemic toxicity is prominent, and the temperature is elevated in the 102–105°F range. On probing of the lesion with a hemostat through a limited incision, easy passage of the instrument along a plane just superficial to the deep fascia occurs. This would not occur with ordinary cellulitis.

A leukocytosis is commonly present. Gram-stained smears of the exudate usually reveal a mixture of organisms or, in the case of streptococcal gangrene, chains of gram-positive cocci. In one instance, we observed numerous long gram-positive bacilli with subterminal spores (along with gram-negative bacilli) in the foul-smelling, purulent exudate of a patient with crepitant necrotizing fasciitis after a lower leg amputation for peripheral vascular disease. The presence of numerous spores in the wound exudate indicated that the gram-positive bacilli were unlikely to be *C. perfringens*. Before surgery the patient had had *Clostridium difficile* enterocolitis, and *C. difficile* was isolated, along with several members of the Enterobacteriaceae, from the wound drainage.

Blood cultures are frequently positive. Hypocalcemia (without tetany) may occur when necrosis of subcutaneous fat is extensive.

Fournier's Gangrene. A form of necrotizing fasciitis occurring about the male genitals is known as *Fournier's gangrene*[3] (*idiopathic gangrene of the scrotum, streptococcal scrotal gangrene, perineal phlegmon*). It may be confined to the scrotum or may extend to involve the perineum, penis, and abdominal wall. Predisposing factors include diabetes mellitus, local trauma, paraphimosis, periurethral extravasation of urine, perirectal or perianal infections, and surgery in the area (circumcision, herniorrhaphy). In cases originating in the genitalia, the infecting bacteria probably pass through Buck's fascia of the penis and spread along the dartos fascia of the scrotum and penis, Colles' fascia of the perineum, and Scarpa's fascia of the anterior abdominal wall. In view of the typical foul odor associated with this form of necrotizing fasciitis, a major role for anaerobic bacteria is likely. Mixed cultures containing facultative organisms (*E. coli, Klebsiella*, enterococci), along with anaerobes (*Bacteroides, Fusobacterium, Clostridium*, anaerobic or microaerophilic streptococci), have been obtained from the lesions in the limited number of cases studied. Group A streptococcal gangrene can, on rare occasions, also involve the male genital area.

The infection commonly starts as cellulitis adjacent to the portal of entry. Early on, the involved area is swollen, erythematous, and tender as the infection begins to involve the deep fascia. Pain is prominent; fever and systemic toxicity are marked.[15] The swelling and crepitus of the scrotum quickly increase, and dark purple areas develop and progress to extensive scrotal gangrene. If the abdominal wall becomes involved in an obese patient with diabetes, the process can spread like wildfire.

Differential Diagnosis

See Table 1.

Presumptive Therapy

Prompt diagnosis is of paramount importance because of the rapidity with which the process can progress. The mortality rate of necrotizing fasciitis ranges from 20 to 47 percent overall (13 and 22 percent for Fournier's gangrene).[14,15] Among patients (including those with either type I or type II necrotizing fasciitis) in whom the diagnosis is made within 4 days of appearance of the initial symptoms, the mortality rate is reduced to 12 percent.[16] Early clinical differentiation of necrotizing fasciitis from cellulitis may be difficult, since the initial signs, including pain, edema, and erythema, are not distinctive. However, the presence of marked systemic toxicity out of proportion to the local findings should alert the physician. Frozen section examination of biopsy specimens (including dermis, infected subcutaneous tissue, fascia, and underlying muscle) has been found to be helpful for early diagnosis.[16] Once the diagnosis is made, immediate surgical débridement is essential. In the patient in whom the diagnosis is clearly suspected on clinical grounds—deep pain with patchy areas of surface hypesthesia, or crepitation, or bullae and skin necrosis—direct operative intervention is indicated. Extensive incisions should be made through the skin and subcutaneous tissues, going beyond the area of involvement until normal fascia is found. Necrotic fat and fascia should be excised, and the wound should be left open. A second-look procedure may be necessary 24–48 hours later if there is any question as to the adequacy of the initial débridement. In the case of Fournier's gangrene, orchiectomy is almost never required, since the testes have their own blood supply independent of the compromised fascial and cutaneous circulation of the scrotum. Initial antimicrobial therapy is based on the evidence for prominent roles for anaerobic bacteria, Enterobacteriaceae, and various streptococci in this process and on the specific findings on Gram-stained smears. Antibiotics employed before obtaining bacteriologic data include combinations of ampicillin, gentamicin, and clindamycin; or ampicillin, gentamicin, and metronidazole.

SYNERGISTIC NECROTIZING CELLULITIS

Clinical Findings

Synergistic necrotizing cellulitis (gram-negative anaerobic cutaneous gangrene, necrotizing cutaneous myositis, synergistic nonclostridial anaerobic myonecrosis) is a variant of necrotizing fasciitis, one in which there is prominent involvement of skin and muscle as well as of subcutaneous tissue and fascia. Some cases of Fournier's gangrene extending onto the abdominal wall represent this condition. Predisposing factors include diabetes mellitus, obesity, advanced age, and cardiorenal disease. Most infections are located on the lower extremities or near the perineum (e.g., originating in a perirectal abscess).[2]

The lesion may first manifest with small skin ulcers draining foul-smelling reddish-brown ("dishwater") pus. Circumscribed areas of blue-gray gangrene surround these draining sites, but the intervening skin appears normal despite necrosis of underlying subcutaneous tissues, fascia, and muscle. Local pain and tenderness are marked. Tissue gas is noted in about a quarter of the patients. Systemic toxicity is a feature; about half the patients have bacteremia.

Etiologic Agents

Cultures consistently show mixtures of anaerobic (anaerobic streptococci and/or *Bacteroides*) and facultative bacteria (*Klebsiella-Enterobacter, E. coli, Proteus*).[2] *Bacteroides* has been reported as the major pathogen on occasion.[17]

Presumptive Therapy

Initial surgery involves incision and drainage, but radical débridement is often necessary because of extensive involvement of deep fascia and muscle.[2,17] Amputation may be required. Antibiotic management initially is based on the results of Gram-stained smears of wound exudates, but it should include an antimicrobial effective against *Bacteroides* (see "Presumptive Therapy" above for type I necrotizing fasciitis).

MISCELLANEOUS INFECTIONS SECONDARY TO TRAUMA

Bite Infections

See Chapter 80.

Burn Infections

See Chapter 79.

Injection Site Abscesses

Subcutaneous and intramuscular abscesses infrequently occur after therapeutic injections. *Staphylococcus aureus*, facultative gram-negative bacilli, and anaerobic bacteria are usually implicated. Hematomas may be the site of delayed infections. Gas gangrene has followed various injections, particularly epinephrine in oil.[5] Subcutaneous and intramuscular abscesses due to a variety of oral anaerobes and streptococci have occurred after "skin popping" or attempted intravenous injections by narcotic addicts.[3] In the case of subcutaneous abscesses secondary to intravenous drug abuse, appropriate débridement and drainage should include excision of involved veins, which often contain pus or an infected thrombus.[18]

Factitial Disease (Self-Induced Abscesses)

Occasionally, subcutaneous abscesses and cellulitis are produced when a patient deliberately injects or inserts into the skin contaminated substances.[19,20] Such abscesses often are recurrent and may be of mono- or polymicrobial etiology (often consisting of oral or fecal flora). Sterile abscesses may be induced by introduction of foreign material without bacterial contamination. Such foreign material may be identified by examination of biopsy specimens with polarizing microscopy.

SUBCUTANEOUS INFECTIONS ORIGINATING IN CONTIGUOUS FOCI

Osteomyelitis

In an occasional patient, most commonly a child, acute hematogenous osteomyelitis may manifest as a subcutaneous abscess. Under these circumstances, a subperiosteal abscess has ruptured through intervening tissues into the subcutaneous tissues. *Staphylococcus aureus* is the most common etiologic agent in such infections. It is important to recognize the nature of the process because of the different therapeutic programs required for osteomyelitis in contrast to a subcutaneous abscess of cutaneous origin. Involvement of subcutaneous tissues as a consequence of osteomyelitis may also occur in the form of a draining sinus associated with chronic osteomyelitis and sequestrum formation. Multiple draining sinuses may occur as a result of multiple foci of osteomyelitis in disseminated blastomycosis.

Actinomycosis

Subcutaneous abscesses frequently develop in the course of cervical, thoracic, or sometimes abdominal actinomycosis. Draining sinuses ultimately result (see Chapter 233).

Primary Pyodermas

On occasion, more superficial skin infections, beginning as folliculitis, furunculosis, or cellulitis, may progress into the deeper subcutaneous tissues and form a subcutaneous (sometimes "cold") abscess. *Staphylococcus aureus* is commonly the etiology. Such progression repeatedly might suggest certain underlying phagocytic cell defects such as chronic granulomatous disease of childhood or hyperimmunoglobulin E syndrome (Job syndrome).[21,22]

SUBCUTANEOUS ABSCESSES IN THE COURSE OF BACTEREMIC INFECTIONS

Metastatic pyogenic infections can occur during the course of bacteremias or endocarditis due to invasive organisms (e.g., *S. aureus*) in subcutaneous tissues as well as a variety of other organs and tissues. These abscesses are tender and fluctuant.

Rarely, multiple, firm, nodular subcutaneous lesions, clinically resembling those of Weber-Christian disease, occur in the course of a staphylococcal bacteremia. If promptly identified and treated, the process may be aborted before frank abscess formation occurs.

MYCETOMA

See Chapter 240.

REFERENCES

1. Wilson HD, Haltalin KC. Acute necrotizing fasciitis in childhood. Am J Dis Child. 1973;125:591.
2. Stone HH, Martin JJ Jr. Synergistic necrotizing cellulitis. Ann Surg. 1972;175:702.
3. Finegold SM. Anaerobic Bacteria in Human Disease. New York: Academic Press; 1977:Chap. 13.
4. MacLennan JD. The histotoxic clostridial infections of man. Bact Rev. 1962;26:177.
5. Bornstein DL, Weinberg AN, Swartz MN, et al. Anaerobic infections: A review of current experience. Medicine. 1964;43:207.
6. Bessman AN, Wagner W. Nonclostridial gas gangrene. JAMA. 1975;233:958.
7. Rea WJ, Wyrick WJ Jr. Necrotizing fasciitis. Ann Surg. 1970;172:957.
8. Giuliano A, Lewis F Jr, Hadley K, et al. Bacteriology of necrotizing fasciitis. Am J Surg. 1977;134:52.
9. Casali RE, Tucker WE, Petrino RA, et al. Postoperative necrotizing fasciitis of the abdominal wall. Am J Surg. 1980;140:787.
10. Galbut DL, Gerber DL, Belgraier AH. Spontaneous necrotizing fasciitis. Occurrence secondary to occult diverticulitis. JAMA. 1977;238:2302.
11. Barza MJ, Proppe KH. Case records of the Massachusetts General Hospital. N Engl J Med. 1979;301:370.
12. Schecter W, Meyer A, Schecter G, et al. Necrotizing fasciitis of the upper extremity. J Hand Surg. 1982;7:15.
13. Lally KP, Atkinson JB, Woolley MM, et al. Necrotizing fasciitis: A serious sequela of omphalitis in the newborn. Ann Surg. 1984;199:101.
14. Sudarsky LA, Laschinger JC, Coppa GF, et al. Improved results from a standardized approach in treating patients with necrotizing fasciitis. Ann Surg. 1987;206:661.
15. Nickel JC, Morales A. Necrotizing fasciitis of the male genitalia (Fournier's gangrene). Can Med Assoc J. 1983;129:445.
16. Stamenkovic I, Lew PD. Early recognition of potentially fatal necrotizing fasciitis: Use of frozen-section biopsy. N Engl J Med. 1984;310:1689.
17. Baxter CR. Surgical management of soft tissue infections. Surg Clin North Am. 1972;52:1483.
18. Biderman P, Hiatt JR. Management of soft-tissue infections of the upper extremity in parenteral drug abusers. Am J Surg. 1987;154:526.
19. Aduan RP, Fauci AS, Dale DC, et al. Factitious fever and self-induced infection: A report of 32 cases and review of the literature. Ann Intern Med. 1979;90:230.
20. Reich P, Gottfried LA. Factitious disorders in a teaching hospital. Ann Intern Med. 1983;99:240.
21. Dreskin SC, Gallin JI. Evolution of the hyperimmunoglobulin E and recurrent infection (HIE, JOB'S) syndrome in a young girl. J Allergy Clin Immunol. 1987;80:746.
22. Curnutte JT, Boxer LA. Clinically significant phagocytic cell defects. In: Remington JS, Swartz MN, eds. Current Clinical Topics in Infectious Diseases. v. 6. New York: McGraw-Hill; 1985:103–156.

76. MYOSITIS

MORTON N. SWARTZ

Infection of skeletal muscle (infectious myositis) is uncommon. When it occurs, a wide range of organisms may be responsible: bacteria, mycobacteria, fungi, viruses, and parasitic agents. Bacteria invade muscle either from contiguous sites of infection (skin and subcutaneous abscesses, penetrating wounds, decubitus ulcers, osteomyelitis) or by hematogenous spread from a distant focus. It is helpful to categorize infectious myositis on the basis of clinical manifestations. These may be very distinctive, as in clostridial gas gangrene, and suggest the specific etiologic agent; or they may be very nonspecific, as in the myalgias of viral infections and infective endocarditis (Table 1). In certain instances (e.g., psoas abscess), it is the anatomic location rather than the morphologic characteristics of the lesion or the nature of the infecting agent that distinguishes the particular type of muscle infection.

PYOMYOSITIS

Pyomyositis is an acute bacterial infection of skeletal muscle usually due to *Staphylococcus aureus*. The accumulation of pus is always intramuscular initially. Clinically, it is characterized by localized muscle pain, swelling, and tenderness.

Pathogenesis and Pathologic Characteristics

Bacterial infections of muscle usually occur after a penetrating wound, prolonged vascular insufficiency in an extremity, or a contiguous infection. Bacteremic spread of infection to skeletal muscle is extremely uncommon. Of fatal cases of staphylococcal septicemia, abscesses in skeletal muscle are found in less than 1 percent.[1] Pyomyositis (primary muscle abscess) is a bacterial infection of muscle occurring in the absence of a predisposing site of infection. *Staphylococcus aureus* is the most common etiology.[2] Blood cultures are positive in less than 5 percent of the cases at the time of clinical manifestation; metastatic infections in tissue other than muscle are rare.

Most cases of pyomyositis occur in the tropics, hence the term *tropical pyomyositis*. It accounts for 1–4 percent of hospital admissions in some tropical areas.[2,3] In the United States pyomyositis is very rare (only 31 cases reported up to 1984), occurring both in persons who have recently immigrated from the tropics and in those who have always resided in a temperate climate.[4–6] As yet, no convincing evidence to relate pyomyositis causally to predisposing circumstances peculiar to the tropics (malaria, filariasis, arbovirus infection) has been developed. Migration of the guinea worm, *Dracunculus medinensis*, in the deep connective tissues of the lower extremities may be complicated by staphylococcal abscesses. However, these are located between muscle groups and are not the intramuscular abscesses typical of pyomsitis. Staphylococcal myositis has been reported in immunosuppressed hosts in the temperate zone.[7,8]

Clinical Findings

Pyomyositis occurs at all ages. In 20–50 percent of cases, there has been recent trauma to the involved area. The onset is most often subacute, with localized muscle pain, then swelling, with induration and tenderness, developing over several days. Fever generally follows the onset of localizing symptoms by a few days. In an occasional patient the onset is acute, with malaise, chills, and high fever. In a rare patient, the clinical picture is combined with that of toxic shock syndrome.[9] The most frequent sites of involvement are the lower limb and trunk muscles.

Since the muscle abscesses are contained by the overlying fascia, local erythema and heat may be minimal until the process extends through to the subcutaneous tissues some days or weeks later. The initial local swelling is "woody" on palpation and pain may not be striking, directing attention away from an infectious etiology. Regional lymphadenitis is not prominent. Only a single muscle group is usually involved, but multiple muscle abscesses occur in up to 40 percent of the patients.

In addition to producing an occasional case of typical pyomyositis with abscess formation, on rare occasions group A streptococci cause a fulminant form of pyomyositis (peracute streptococcal pyomyositis, streptococcal necrotizing myositis, spontaneous streptococcal gangrenous myositis).[10,11] The entire clinical course may be telescoped to 2–3 days. Bacteremia and toxemia are prominent features and contribute to the very high mortality. Intramuscular pressure may lead to muscle necrosis,

TABLE 1. Classification of Infectious Myositis

Type of Process	*Clinical Pattern*	*Principal Specific Etiologies*
Pyogenic and predominantly localized (spreading by contiguity)	Pyomyositis	*S. aureus*; group A streptococcus (rarely)
	Gas gangrene	*C. perfringens;* occasionally other histotoxic clostridial species
	Nonclostridial (crepitant) myositis	
	Anaerobic streptococcal gangrene	*Peptostreptococcus* (plus group A streptococci or *S. aureus*)
	Synergistic nonclostridial anaerobic myonecrosis	Mixed infections: *Bacteroides* and other anaerobic non-spore-forming gram-negative bacilli; *Peptostreptococcus* and various streptococci; *E. coli*; *Klebsiella*; *Enterobacter*
	Infected vascular gangrene	Same as for synergistic nonclostridial anaerobic myonecrosis
	Aeromonas hydrophila myonecrosis	*Aeromonas hydrophila*
	Psoas abscess	Gram-negative bacilli; *S. aureus*; mixed infections; *M. tuberculosis*
Nonpyogenic and predominantly generalized	Myalgias	Viral infections (e.g., influenza, dengue); infective endocarditis; bacteremias (e.g., meningococcemia); rickettsioses (e.g., Rocky Mountain spotted fever); toxoplasmosis
	Pleurodynia	Coxsackievirus B
	Myalgias with eosinophilia	
	Trichinosis	*Trichinella spiralis*
	Cysticercosis (also subcutaneous nodules)	*Taenia solium*
	Muscle degeneration and destruction associated with infections elsewhere	
	Acute rhabdomyolysis	Viral influenza, echovirus, coxsackie and Epstein-Barr viruses, *Legionella*

much as in a compartment syndrome. This process differs from necrotizing fasciitis in that the skin and fascia are minimally if at all involved.[12,13]

A leukocytosis occurs. Eosinophilia is common in patients (even in the presence of a prominent leukocytosis) with tropical pyomyositis and appears to reflect the prevalence of parasitic infestation. Serum muscle enzyme levels may be elevated but frequently are normal despite gross muscle destruction. However, marked rhabdomyolysis with myoglobinuria and acute renal failure has developed in a patient with pyomyositis.[14]

Etiologic Agents

Staphylococcus aureus is responsible for 95 percent of the cases. Group A streptococci account for 1–5 percent of the cases. Other rare bacterial causes include *Streptococcus pneumoniae, Haemophilus influenzae, Escherichia coli, Klebsiella* spp., *Yersinia enterocolitica*, and other *Pseudomonas* spp. *Pseudomonas mallei* and *Pseudomonas pseudomallei* occasionally cause abscesses in muscle in the septicemic or chronic suppurative forms of the diseases they produce, glanders and meliodosis, respectively. *Aspergillus fumigatus* has caused localized myositis in a patient with myelodysplasia. Other causes of fungal myositis include disseminated cryptococcal and candidal infections.

Differential Diagnosis

Early in the course of pyomyositis, other diagnoses may be suspected, particularly in nontropical areas: osteomyelitis, septic arthritis, muscle hematoma, muscle rupture, and thrombophlebitis. Streptococcal necrotizing fasciitis, like gangrenous streptococal myositis, produces localized swelling, tenderness, and erythema, but it is less common and produces necrosis of fascia and skin. In the patient with multiple sites of muscle involvement and eosinophilia (from incidental parasitic infestation), the picture may suggest trichinosis. This resemblance ends when localized swellings become prominent and markedly tender. Rupture of the muscle abscess through the fascia into subcutaneous tissues may suggest the diagnosis of cellulitis. Radionuclide (^{67}Ga) scanning shows diffuse uptake in the involved area but does not distinguish an intramuscular abscess from necrotizing myositis or necrotizing fasciitis. Computed tomography can reveal low-density areas with loss of muscle planes characteristic of pyomyositis.

Presumptive Therapy

Surgical (open or ultrasound-guided percutaneous) drainage of all abscesses is essential. Initial antibiotic therapy should consist of intravenous administration of a β-lactamase-resistant penicillin because of the preponderance of penicillin-resistant *S. aureus* isolates from such abscesses. If a group A streptococcus is isolated, treatment should be changed to penicillin G. Continued fever after surgical drainage of a muscle abscess while the patient is receiving appropriate antimicrobial therapy should suggest the presence of other undrained suppurative foci. Streptococcal necrotizing myositis requires prompt radical débridement of all necrotic muscles.

GAS GANGRENE (CLOSTRIDIAL MYONECROSIS)

Gas gangrene is a rapidly progressive, life-threatening, toxemic infection of skeletal muscle due to clostridia (principally *Clostridium perfringens*). It usually follows muscle injury and contamination, as in a dirty traumatic wound, or sometimes surgery.

Pathogenesis and Pathologic Characteristics

Gas gangrene occurs in settings having in common muscle injury and contamination with soil or other foreign material containing spores of *C. perfringens* or other histotoxic clostridial species: (*1*) accidental traumatic civilian injuries such as compound fractures,[15] (*2*) penetrating war wounds,[16] (*3*) surgical wounds, particularly after bowel or biliary tract surgery,[17] and (*4*) arterial insufficiency in an extremity.[17] Rare cases of gas gangrene have occurred after parenteral injection of medication, particularly epinephrine in oil. A fulminant case has been described beginning at the site of a simple venipuncture in a granulocytopenic patient.[17] *Clostridium perfringens* are usually present in large numbers as normal flora in human feces and thus can endogenously contaminate skin surfaces. Despite a high frequency (up to 88 percent) of clostridial contamination of major traumatic, open wounds, the incidence of gas gangrene in this setting is only 1–2 percent,[18] emphasizing the importance of devitalized tissue and the presence of foreign bodies in the pathogenesis of gas gangrene. The minimal dose of *C. perfringens* needed to produce fatal gas gangrene in the experimental animal is reduced by a factor of 10^6 when injected into devitalized muscle contaminated with sterile dirt rather than into normal muscle. The policy of prompt, thorough débridement and of leaving wounds open has decreased the incidence of gas gangrene in wartime injuries; only 22 cases among 139,000 combat casualties in Vietnam have been reported.[19]

Gas gangrene may occasionally develop in the absence of an obvious external wound. It may manifest in the buttocks or flanks as the consequence of an intra-abdominal catastrophe, with extension of infection along the iliopsoas or other deep muscle groups. Such "idiopathic" gas gangrene may occur at a greater distance from the original intra-abdominal focus, spreading by the bacteremic route. *Clostridium septicum* has been involved, often with documented bacteremia, in clostridial infections occurring in the setting of neoplastic disease (particularly leukemia and carcinoma of the colon).[20,21] The primary source of the organism is probably mucosal ulceration or perforation of the intestinal tract.

The involved muscle undergoes rapid disintegration. Initially, it may exhibit only pallor, edema, and loss of elasticity. When examined in the operating room, it fails to contract on stimulation and does not bleed from a cut surface. Later it becomes discolored (reddish purple, then greenish purple and gangrenous) and friable. Histologically, the muscle fibers show coagulation necrosis, and the supporting connective tissue is destroyed; numerous gram-positive bacilli are present.

Clinical Findings

The usual incubation period between injury and the development of clostridial myonecrosis is 2–3 days, but it may be as short as 6 hours. The onset is acute. Pain is the earliest and most important symptom. It rapidly increases in intensity and is more severe than the pain that is generally associated with the preceding injury or surgical procedure. The patient soon appears severely ill, pale, and sweaty. The pulse is rapid, the blood pressure falls, and shock and renal failure follow. The patient may be apathetic or may be apprehensive and restless but mentally clear. Delirium, stupor, and unconsciousness may supervene. Fever is frequently present, but often with temperature elevations of less than 38.3°C (101°F). Hypothermia is a poor prognostic sign and is usually associated with shock. Jaundice may become evident. The process may rapidly progress over a period of hours, with a fatal outcome if not properly treated.

Appearance of the Local Lesion. Very early, tense edema and local tenderness may be the only findings. If an open wound is present, swollen muscle may herniate through. A serosanguineous, dirty-appearing discharge, containing numerous organisms but few leukocytes, escapes from the wound. The wound has a peculiar foul odor. Gas bubbles may be visible in the discharge. Crepitus is usually present but not prominent; sometimes it is completely obscured by very marked edema. The skin adjacent to the wound is initially swollen and white, but rapidly takes on a yellowish or bronze discoloration (Fig. 1). Tense blebs containing thin serosanguineous or dark fluid develop in the overlying skin, and areas of green-black cutaneous necrosis appear. In fulminant cases, progression of the

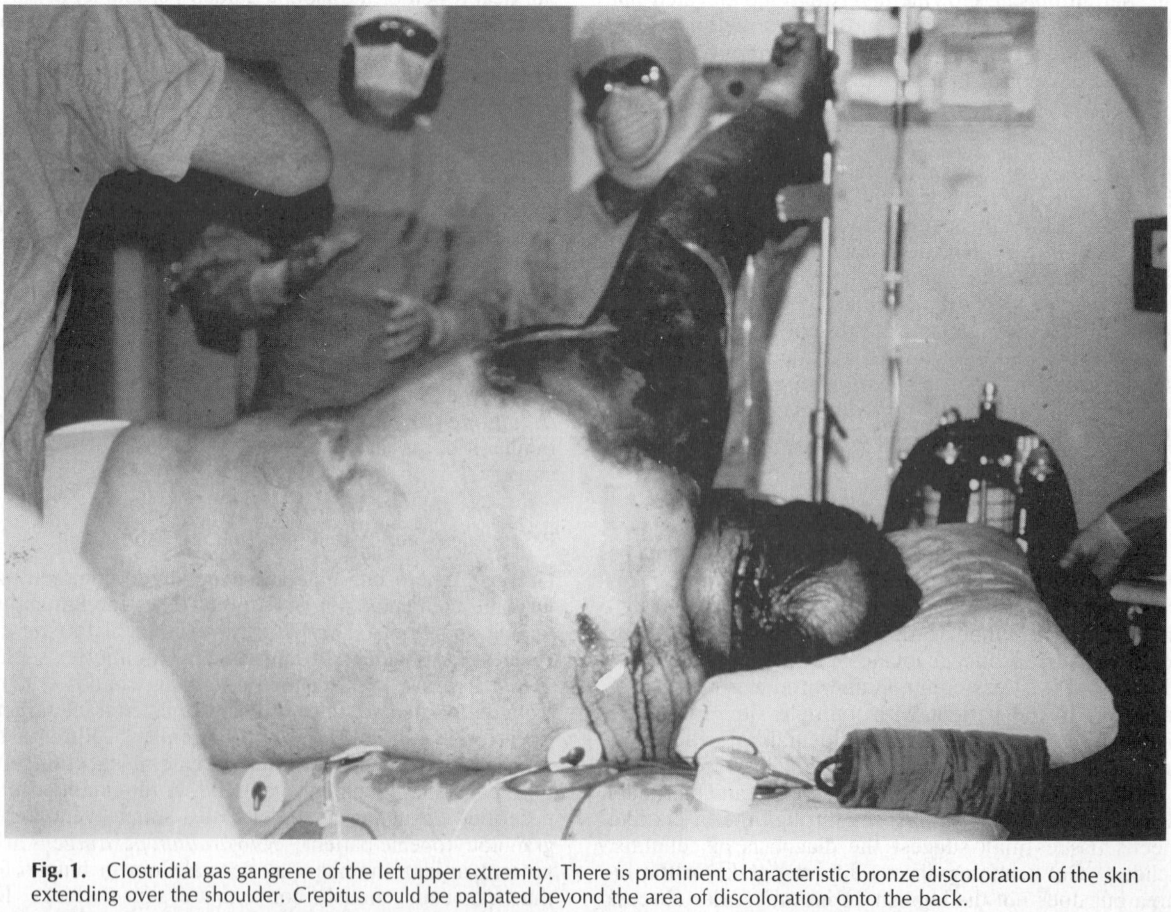

Fig. 1. Clostridial gas gangrene of the left upper extremity. There is prominent characteristic bronze discoloration of the skin extending over the shoulder. Crepitus could be palpated beyond the area of discoloration onto the back.

changes occurs over 2–4 hours, as indicated by the advance of the area of edema and crepitation.

Laboratory Findings

The hematocrit level is usually reduced. *Clostridium perfringens* bacteremia occurs in about 15 percent of the patients with gas gangrene.[22] Intense bacteremia (with associated intravascular hemolysis) is more likely to occur as a complication of uterine infection. A leukocytosis is common.

Gram-stained smear of the wound exudate or of an aspirate from one of the blebs reveals many large, gram-positive bacilli with blunt ends but few polymorphonuclear leukocytes (see Chapter 222, Fig. 1). In almost all cases, spores are not evident. Not infrequently, scattered gram-negative bacilli are also present, particularly in grossly contaminated wounds.

X-ray films of the involved areas show extensive and progressive gaseous dissection of muscle and fascial planes.

Etiologic Agents

Clostridium perfringens is most commonly isolated from the lesions of gas gangrene (80–95 percent of the cases).[15,19] *Clostridium novyi* is involved in 10–40 percent of the cases and *C. septicum* in 5–20 percent. Other clostridial species (*C. bifermentans, C. histolyticum, C. fallax*) have been implicated on rare occasions. In addition to clostridia, other organisms (*E. coli, Enterobacter*, enterococci, and so forth) are sometimes isolated from the lesions of gas gangrene, reflecting the contaminated character of the initiating trauma or lesion.[22]

Differential Diagnosis

The major considerations in differential diagnosis ae gas-forming infections of the soft tissues (clostridial anaerobic cellulitis, nonclostridial crepitant myositis, nonclostridial crepitant cellulitis). Clostridial anaerobic cellulitis (Chapter 74) is more gradual in onset and progression, and the systemic manifestations of illness are much milder than in gas gangrene. Local pain is relatively mild, and the skin lesions of gas gangrene (bronzing, dark blebs) do not develop. Gas formation is often much more extensive in clostridial cellulitis than in gas gangrene. Clinically, it is often difficult to distinguish between early clostridial cellulitis and myonecrosis. Definitive evaluation requires examination in the operating room for the characteristic changes of myonecrosis described earlier. The clinical picture of nonclostridial crepitant cellulitis is very similar to that of clostridial cellulitis. Although contamination of an operative or traumatic wound may be the source of infection in both types of cellulitis, nonclostridial crepitant cellulitis frequently develops in the setting of vascular insufficiency or perirectal infection. Bacteria isolated from nonclostridial crepitant cellulitis include facultative species (*E. coli, Klebsiella*, various streptococci) and anaerobic bacteria (*Bacteroides, Peptostreptococcus*, and so forth). Commonly, these are present in mixed culture and can be seen on Gram-stained smear of a wound aspirate.

Presumptive Therapy

Treatment includes emergency surgical exploration both to define the nature of the process (gas gangrene vs. crepitant cellulitis) by direct examination of muscles at the site of infection and to carry out appropriate débridement. Prompt and extensive surgery is the principle element in the treatment of gas gangrene. This includes excision of involved muscles (or amputation when necessary) and fasciotomies to decompress and to drain the swollen fascial compartments. Antibiotic therapy is an important adjunct to surgical management. Penicillin G is the antibiotic of choice and is administered intravenously in a dosage for the adult of 1–2 million units every 2–3 hours. A second antibiotic, such as chloramphenicol, is sometimes added initially when Gram-stained smears of the wound exudate show gram-negative bacilli as well as the predominant gram-positive bacilli. Chloramphenicol is also a good alernative drug in the highly penicillin-allergic patient; it is preferable to tetracycline or clindamycin in view of the resistance of some clostridia to these agents. Although the majority of *C. perfringens* isolates ae susceptible in vitro to first-, second-, and third-generation cephalosporins, the minimum inhibitory concentrations for at least 10 percent of isolates are above levels readily achievable in vivo.[23] The demonstration of plasmids mediating transferable drug resistance (tetracycline and chloramphenicol; perhaps erythromycin and clindamycin) in *C. perfringens*[24] suggests the need for periodic monitoring of antibiotic susceptibilities of clinical isolates. Recent evidence suggests that some strains of this organism may be showing somewhat less susceptibility in vitro to penicillin than was formerly the case.[23] *Clostridium perfringens* are susceptible in vitro to metronidazole, but experience with the use of this drug in clostridial myonecrosis is lacking.

The role of hyperbaric oxygen therapy is still under debate. Its most appropriate role at present would appear to be in the management of patients with extensive involvement of the trunk in whom surgical excision would be mutilating.[25] Initial hyperbaric oxygen therapy may reduce the extent of débridement necessary under these circumstances. The efficacy of intravenously administered polyvalent gas gangrene antitoxin has never been established clinically. It is no longer available. Ancillary therapy is essential in the management of gas gangrene. This includes attention to fluid and electrolyte replacement and maintenance of adequate hematocrit levels by transfusions.

NONCLOSTRIDIAL (CREPITANT) MYOSITIS

Nonclostridial (crepitant) myositis includes four relatively distinct entities, differing from gas gangrene in their clinical picture and bacteriologic characteristics: (*1*) anaerobic streptococcal myonecrosis, (*2*) synergistic nonclostridial anaerobic myonecrosis, (*3*) infected vascular gangrene and (*4*) *Aeromonas hydrophila* myonecrosis.

Anaerobic Streptococcal Myonecrosis

This is an acute interstitial myositis that clinically resembles subacute clostridial gas gangrene. The initial manifestations are swelling and a copious seropurulent exudate occurring 3–4 days after injury. Pain develops subsequently, unlike the early occurrence of pain in gas gangrene. Tissue gas is present in muscle and fascial planes but is not extensive. The wound has an unpleasant sour odor. The involved muscles are discolored but do react to stimulation. In contrast to gas gangrene, early cutaneous erythema is prominent. If not adequately treated, the infection progresses, with the development of toxemia, frank gangrene, and shock.

Numerous streptococci and polymorphonuclear leukocytes are present in the exudate. The infection is usually mixed (anaerobic streptococci with group A streptococci or *S. aureus*). A mixed infection of muscle with both peptostreptococci and *Bacillus subtilis* has been observed on several occasions in the setting of vascular injury. The clinical picture, along with the appearance of the Gram-stained smear, initially might suggest the diagnosis of clostridial myonecrosis.[26] Treatment involves the use of large doses of penicillin and surgical debridement.

Synergistic Nonclostridial Anaerobic Myonecrosis. This severe infection, also known as *synergistic necrotizing cellulitis* (Chapter 75), involves skin, subcutaneous tissue, fascia, and muscle. The most extensive involvement is in the subcutaneous tissues and fascia; changes in the overlying skin and underlying muscle are usually secondary.

Infected Vascular Gangrene[27]

This is a mixed infection developing in a group of muscles or in a limb devitalized as a result of arterial insufficiency, particularly in patients with diabetes mellitus. *Proteus, Bacteroides*, and anaerobic streptococci are among the bacteria found in such lesions. Gas formation and foul-smelling pus are prominent. The infection does not extend beyond the area of vascular gangrene to involve healthy muscle. *Bacillus cereus* infection has been associated with myonecrosis with slight crepitance after thrombosis of arterial grafts.[28]

Aeromonas Hydrophila Myonecrosis

Rapidly progressivve myonecosis due to *Aeromonas hydrophila*, a facultative, anaerobic, gram-negative bacillus, may follow penetrating trauma either in a freshwater environment or associated with fish or other aquatic animals.[29,30] In a few instances, myonecrosis has been accompanied by gas spreading extensively in soft tissue planes. The rapid onset (24–48 hours) and rapid progression after trauma resemble those of clostridial gas gangrene. The prominence of pain, marked edema, serosanguineous bullae, and toxicity, as well as the presence of gas in fascial planes, adds to the similarity of these conditions. Baceremia is frequently present. Treatment consists of extensive surgical débridement and prompt initiation of antimicrobial therapy. Most isolates of *Aeromonas* are susceptible in vitro to chloramphenicol, tetracyclines, gentamicin, tobramycin, and trimethoprim-sulfamethoxazole. Cefotaxime and moxalactam also appear to be active.[31]

PSOAS ABSCESS

Infection of the psoas muscle takes the form of either an abscess or a phlegmon. It is usually the consequence of spread of infection from an adjacent structure. Rarely, it develops by the hematogenous route; in children particularly, there may be no prior inciting event such as trauma or preceding infection, and *S. aureus* is the most common etiology in this setting. Psoas abscess usually is confined within the psoas fascia, but occasionally, due to anatomic relations, infection extends to the buttock, hip, or upper thigh. Psoas abscess may complicate pyogenic or tuberculous vertebral osteomyelitis. The latter was formerly the principle cause of a psoas abscess; now psoas abscesses most commonly result from direct extension of intraabdominal infections (diverticulitis, appendicitis, Crohn's disease, and so on).[32] Occasionally, a psoas abscess results from extension of a perinephric abscess or from secondary infection of a retroperitoneal hematoma. The organisms involved in spread of infection from an intestinal site are usually members of the aerobic and anaerobic bowel flora. *Staphylococcus aureus* is the most common cause of psoas abscess secondary to vertebral osteomyelitis.

The iliacus muscle, applied to the ilium in the iliac fossa, forms a conjoined tendon with the lower portion of the psoas muscle. Osteomyelitis of the ilium or septic arthritis of the sacroiliac joint can penetrate the sheathes of either or both muscles in this location, producing an iliacus or psoas abscess.[33]

Clinical manifestations of a psoas abscess include fever, lower abdominal or back pain, or pain referred to the hip or knee. A limp may be evident and flexion deformity of the hip may develop from reflex spasm, suggesting septic arthritis of the hip. The psoas sign is evident. Often a tender mass can be palpated in the groin.

Roentgenograms may show a bulge produced by a psoas muscle abscess or the presence of gas within the psoas sheath. Calcification in a psoas abscess strongly suggests a tuberculous etiology.

Of the four noninvasive techniques currently available for visualization of the psoas (and iliacus) muscles, computed tomography (CT) scanning is the most rapid and sensitive. Ultrasound is less reliable for detecting small lesions or a phlegmon. Gallium scanning does not provide as sharp a localization and takes up to 72 hours; indium-labeled white blood cell scanning may be preferable to the latter. CT scanning may show diffuse enlargement of the psoas (phlegmon) or sharply circumscribed, low-density fluid collections (abscess) within the muscle, or may demonstrate the presence of gas within the muscle (indicative of abscess).[34]

Pyogenic psoas abscesses are treated by surgical drainage and provisional initial antibiotic therapy based on knowledge of the origin of the infection. CT scanning maybe of considerable value for guidance of direct needle aspiration of an abscess for culture or for drainage when the direct surgical approach is not preferable or warranted. When the process appears to be a phlegmon, repeated CT scanning during the course of antibiotic therapy can confirm resolution of the anatomic changes.

MYALGIAS

Myalgias are prominent features of a variety of infections such as dengue, influenza, and Rocky Mountain spotted fever. Little information is available on the presence of specific histologic findings indicative of myositis.

Influenza

Muscle aches are common early in the course of influenza. Occasionally, severe bilateral muscle pains in the lower limbs may develop in the recovery phase, particularly in young children.[35,36] Muscle tenderness, principally in the gastrocnemius and soleus muscles, is demonstrable and calf swelling may be present. Deep tendon reflexes and muscle strength are normal, but there is considerable difficulty in walking. The leg pains and muscle tenderness subside in less than a week. Mild elevations of serum levels of aldolase and creatine phosphokinase occur. The few biopsies performed have shown either nonspecific degenerative changes or muscle necrosis with polymorphonuclear leukocytic infiltration. Whether this "myositis" is due to direct viral invasion or to some immunologic or other response is unknown. However, influenza A virus has been isolated from the muscle biopsy specimen of an adult with generalized muscle weakness occurring during an influenza A outbreak.[37]

Infective Endocarditis

Prominent myalgias occur in about 15 percent of patients with infective endocarditis.[38] They may be either diffuse or localized. The pathogenesis is not known, but in one instance muscle biopsy specimens showed a small focus of muscle fiber destruction and leukocytic infiltration consistent with embolization to a small artery.[38]

Toxoplasmosis

The major features of acute acquired disseminated toxoplasmosis are those of meningoencephalitis, myocarditis, pneumonitis, skin rash, and occasionally hepatitis (Chapter 252). In rare instances, polymyositis may be a prominent clinical manifestation. Marked myalgias, muscle weakness and swelling, and fasciculations occur in such patients. Muscle biopsy specimens show interstitial myositis with destruction of muscle fibers, and pseudocysts of *Toxoplasma gondii* can be found in areas of muscle free of inflammatory reaction. In several cases *Toxoplasma* have been isolated by animal inoculation.[39,40]

Other Etiologies

Occasionally, the only clinical manifestations of initial infection with human immunodeficiency virus (HIV) retrovirus are those of polymyositis (myalgias, muscle weakness, and increased serum levels of muscle enzymes). HIV viral antigens can be found in OKT4 cells in areas of muscle fiber inflammation and necrosis.[41] Inflammatory myositis with a lymphoplasmacytic cellular response was the major feature in a case of Lyme disease.[42] Spirochetes morphologically similar to *Borrelia burgdorferi* were present on Dieterle silver stain of biopsied muscle. Rarely, *Sarcocystis* (an intracellular sporozoan parasite) infection has been observed in histologic sections of muscle of individuals, mainly from abroad, with muscle pain or weakness.[43] Microsporidia myositis has occurred in a patient with acquired immunodeficiency syndrome (AIDS).[44]

PLEURODYNIA SYNDROMES

Epidemic pleuodynia is an acute, febrile disease due to group B coxsackieviruses and is characterized by the sudden onset of sharp chest pain over the lower ribs or sternum (Chapter 150). Paroxysms of knife-like pain are precipitated by voluntary or respiratory movments. Muscle tenderness may be present. Abdominal pain may also be present in some patients; in others abdominal pain may be the sole manifestation, simulating intraperitoneal processes.

Group B coxsackieviruses produce visceral lesions and also some focal myositis in experimental animals. Myositis has not been demonstrated as a feature pathologically either in the fatal cases of severe neonatal coxsackievirus B infection or in the few biopsy specimens obtained from affected muscles of patients with epidemic pleurodynia.[45,46]

MYALGIAS WITH EOSINOPHILIA (PARASITIC MYOSITIS)

Trichinosis

The prominent clinical manifestations of trichinosis include fever, myositis, periorbital edema, and eosinophilia. An initial intestinal phase during the first week after infection is followed during the second week by larval invasion of skeletal muscle (Chapter 264). Serious complications in the form of myocarditis, meningoencephalitis, and pneumonitis can occur.[47] Myalgias, frequently accompanied by muscle swelling and weakness and occasionally associated with fasciculations, are present in most patients with the disease. Muscles commonly involved include the extraocular muscles, flexor muscles of the extremities, back muscles, and the muscles used in chewing and swallowing. Periorbital edema, chemosis, and conjunctival hemorrhages are related to larval invasion of extraocular muscles. The inflammatory response in muscle produces an elevation of serum levels of muscle enzymes.

Muscle biopsy specimens reveal encysted larval trichinae in necrotic muscle fibers surrounded by inflammatory cells (predominantly eosinophils and neutrophils, but also lymphocytes). Severe skeletal muscle involvement has been reported in a case of trichinosis in an immunosuppressed patient.[48] Although granulomatous reactions have been observed in the heart and lungs of fatal cases, larval encystment does not take place in organs other than skeletal muscle.

Cysticerosis (Cysticerus Cellulosal Myositis)

Human cysticerosis is rare in the United States but is common in Latin America and Asia. It results from the ingestion and subsequent hatching of viable eggs of *Taenia solium* into the larval form of the parasite *Cysticercus cellulosae* (Chapter 266). Eggs reach the upper intestinal tract from food contaminated by feces from a person parasitized by the adult worm. Autoinfection can occur through the fecal-oral route and possibly when reverse peristalsis introduces egg-laden proglottids back into the duodenum or stomach where they hatch. From there they are distributed widely (skeletal muscle, subcutaneous tissues, heart, eye).

Symptomatic involvement of muscle is uncommon. Occasionally, the stage of invasion is characterized by fever, muscle tenderness, and eosinophilia. More characteristically, asymptomatic calcified cysts ("puffed rice" appearance) are detected in muscles on soft tissue x-ray films of patients with neurologic manifestations.

MUSCLE DEGENERATION ASSOCIATED WITH INFECTIONS AT OTHER SITES

Acute Rhabdomyolysis

Myoglobinuria occasionally follows an acute illness with symptoms suggesting an upper respiratory tract infection. Scattered cases in recent years have been shown to follow documented influenza A virus infections in children and adults,[49] legionnaires' disease, echovirus infections,[50] and infections due to coxsackie, Epstein-Barr, and adenovirus.[51] Diffuse muscle pains (especially in the extremities), weakness, swelling, and tenderness are prominent features, along with myoglobinuria. Rhabdomyolysis has occurred in patients who have had no previous episodes and no family history of this condition. Like the myositis after influenza occurring in children, it develops when respiratory symptoms are resolving.

Muscle Proteolysis and Mediators of Fever in Patients with Sepsis

Muscle involvement, in the form of myalgias and weakness, is common in the course of systemic infections. Accelerated catabolism of skeletal muscle contributes to the marked weakness and muscle wasting that can be observed in systemic infections. This appears to be part of a protective "acute-phase" host response to sepsis and trauma. The central role is played by interleukin-1 (IL-1), a polypeptide that appears identical to endogenous leukocytic pyrogen (EP). A polypeptide (possibly a breakdown product of IL-1) that produces a rapid increase in protein degradation in rat or human muscle preparations[52] has been observed in the plasma of patients with sepsis. Similar changes are produced by EP (IL-1) itself.[53] This accelerated proteolysis is effected through increased synthesis in muscle of prostaglandin E_2, which in turn activates proteases in muscle-cell lysosomes. This catabolic activity is accompanied by IL-1-stimulated hepatic protein synthesis (using the newly generated source of amino acids) and other elements of the acute-phase response, such as fever (also generated by IL-1 and mediated by prostaglandin E_2). The important role of prostaglandin E_2 in the generation of the muscle aches and fever of infection is consistent with the amelioration of these symptoms produced by prostaglandin synthesis inhibitors such as aspirin.

REFERENCES

1. Smith IM, Vickers AB. Natural history of 338 treated and untreated patients with staphylococcal septicaemia. Lancet. 1960;1:1318.
2. Levin MJ, Gardner P, Waldvogel FA. "Tropical" pyomyositis. An unusual infection due to *Staphylococcus aureus*. N Engl J Med. 1971;284:196.
3. Horn CV, Master S. Pyomyositis tropicans in Uganda. E Afr Med J. 1968;45:463.
4. Altrocchi PH. Spontaneous bacterial myositis. JAMA. 1971;217:819.
5. Echeverria P, Vaughn MC. "Tropical pyomyositis." A diagnostic problem in temperate climates. Am J Dis Child. 1975;129:856.
6. Gibson RK, Rosenthal SJ, Lukert BP. Pyomyositis: Increasing recognition in temporate climates. Am J Med. 1984;77:768.
7. Jordan GW, Bauer R, Wong GA, et al. Staphylococcal myositis in a compromised host. West J Med. 1976;124:140.
8. Lachiewicz PF, Hadler NM. Spontaneous pyomyositis in a patient with Felty's syndrome: Diagnosis using computerized tomography. South Med J. 1986;79:1047.
9. Immerman RP, Greenman RL. Toxic shock syndrome associated with pyomyositis caused by a strain of *Staphylococcus aureus* that does not produce toxic-shock-syndrome toxin—1. J Infect Dis. 1987;156:505.

10. Svane S. Peracute spontaneous streptococcal myositis. Acta Chir Scand. 1971;137:155.
11. Moore DL, Delage G, Labelle H, et al. Peracute streptococcal pyomyositis: Report of two cases and review of the literature. J Pediatr Orthop. 1986;6:232.
12. Nather A, Wong FYH, Balasubramaniam P, et al: Streptococcal necrotizing myositis: A rare entity. Clin Orthop. 1987;215:206.
13. Yoder EL, Mendez J, Khatib R. Spontaneous gangrenous myositis induced by *Streptococcus pyogenes*: Case report and review of the literature. Rev Infect Dis. 1987;9:382.
14. Armstrong JH. Tropical pyomyositis and myoglobinuria. Arch Intern Med. 1978;138:1145.
15. Altemeier WA, Fullen WD. Prevention and treatment of gas gangrene. JAMA. 1971;217:806.
16. MacLennan JD. The histotoxic clostridial infections of man. Bact Rev. 1962;26:177.
17. Bornstein DL, Weinberg AN, Swartz MN, et al. Anaerobic infections: Review of current experience. Medicine. 1964;43:207.
18. Altemeier WA, Furste WL. Gas gangrene. Surg Gynecol Obstet. 1947;84:507.
19. Finegold SM. Anaerobic Bacteria in Human Disease. New York: Academic Press; 1977:424.
20. Alpern RJ, Dowell VR Jr. *Clostridium septicum* infections and malignancy. JAMA. 1969;209:385.
21. Jendrzejewski JW, Jones SR, Newcombe RL, et al. Nontraumatic clostridial myonecrosis. Am J Med. 1978;65:542.
22. Caplan ES, Kluge RM. Gas gangrene: Review of 34 cases. Arch Intern Med. 1976;136:788.
23. Marrie TJ, Haldane EV, Swantee CA, et al. Susceptibility of anaerobic bacteria to nine antimicrobial agents an demonstration of decreased susceptibility of *Clostridium perfringens* to penicillin. Antimicrob Agents Chemother. 1981;19:51.
24. Brefort G, Magot M, Ionesco H, et al. Characterization and transferability of *Clostridium perfringens* plasmids. Plasmid. 1977;1:52.
25. Shupak A, Halpern P, Ziser A, et al. Hyperbaric oxygen therapy for gas gangrene casualties in the Lebanon War, 1982. Isr J Med Sci. 1984;20:323.
26. Chambers CH, Bond GF, Morris JH. Synergistic necrotizing myositis complicating vascular injury. J Trauma. 1974;14:980.
27. Finegold SM. Anaerobic Bacteria in Human Disease. New York: Academic Press; 1977:425.
28. Johnson DA, Aulicino PL, Newby JG. *Bacillus cereus*-induced myonecrosis. J Trauma. 1984;24:267.
29. Davis WA, Kane JG, Garagusi VF. Human *Aeromonas* infections: A review of the literature and case report of endocarditis. Medicine. 1978;57:267.
30. Heckerling PS, Stine TM, Pottage JC, et al. *Aeromonas hydrophila* myonecrosis and gas gangrene in a nonimmunocompromised host. Arch Intern Med. 1983;143:2005.
31. Fass RJ, Barnishan J. In vitro susceptibilities of *Aeromonas hydrophila* to 32 antimicrobial agents. Antimicrob Agents Chemother. 1981;19:357.
32. Kyle J. Psoas abscess in Crohn's disease. Gastroenterology. 1971;61:149.
33. Simons GW, Sty JR, Starshak RJ, et al. Retroperitoneal and retrofascial abscesses. J Bone Joint Surg. 1983;65-A:1041.
34. Gordin F, Stamler C, Mills J. Pyogenic psoas abscesses: Noninvasive diagnostic techniques and review of the literature. Rev Infect Dis. 1983;5:1003.
35. Middleton PJ, Alexander RM, Szymanski MT. Severe myositis during recovery from influenza. Lancet. 1970;2:533.
36. Mejlszenkier JD, Safran AP, Healy JJ, et al. The myositis of influenza. Arch Neurol. 1973;29:441.
37. Kessler HA, Trenholme GM, Harris AA, et al. Acute myopathy associated with influenza A/Texas/1/77 infection. JAMA. 1980;243:461.
38. Churchill MA, Geraci JE, Hunder GG. Musculoskeletal manifestations of bacterial endocarditis. Ann Intern Med. 1977;87:754.
39. Greenlee JE, Johnson WD, Campa JF, et al. Adult toxoplasmosis presenting as polymyositis and cerebral ataxia. Ann Intern Med. 1975;82:367.
40. Kass EH, Andrus SB, Adams RD, et al. Toxoplasmosis in the human adult. Arch Intern Med. 1952;89:759.
41. Dalakas MC, Pezeshkpour GH, Gravell M, et al. Polymyositis associated with AIDS retrovirus. JAMA. 1986;256:2381.
42. Atlas E, Novak SN, Duray P, et al. Lyme myositis: Muscle invasion by *Borrelia burgdorferi*. Ann Intern Med. 1988;109:245.
43. Beaver PC, Gadgil RK, Morera P. Sarcocystis: A review and report of five cases. Am J Trop Med Hyg. 1979;28:819.
44. Ledford DK, Overman MD, Gonzalvo A, et al. Microsporidiosis myositis in a patient with the acquired immunodeficiency syndrome. Ann Intern Med. 1985;102:628.
45. Adams RD. Diseases of Muscle. A Study in Pathology, Hagerstown, Md.: Harper and Row; 1975:318.
46. Cherry JD. Enteroviruses. In: Remington JS, Klein JO, eds. Infectious Diseases of the Fetus and Newborn Infant. Philadelphia: WB Saunders; 1976:397.
47. Most H. Trichinosis: Preventable but still with us. N Engl J Med. 1978;298:1178.
48. Jacobson ES, Jacobson HG. Trichinosis in an immunosuppressed human host. Am J Clin Pathol. 1977;68:791.
49. Minow RA, Gorbach S, Johnson BL, et al. Myoglobinuria associated with influenza A infection. Ann Intern Med. 1974;80:359.
50. Josselson J, Pula T, Sadler JH. Acute rhabdomyolysis associated with an echovirus 9 infection. Arch Intern Med. 1980;140:1671.
51. Meshkinpour H, Vaziri ND. Acute rhabdomyolysis associated with adenovirus infection. J Infect Dis. 1981;143:133.
52. Clowes GHA Jr, George BC, Villee CA Jr, et al. Muscle proteolysis induced by a circulating peptide in patients with sepsis or trauma. N Engl J Med. 1983;308:545.
53. Baracos V, Rodemann HP, Dinarello CA, et al. Stimulation of muscle protein degradation and prostaglandin E_2 release by leukocytic pyrogen (Interleukin-1). A mechanism for the increased degradation of muscle proteins during fever. N Engl J Med. 1983;308:553.

77. LYMPHADENITIS AND LYMPHANGITIS

MORTON N. SWARTZ

LYMPHADENITIS

Lymphadenitis is an acute or chronic inflammation of lymph nodes. It may be restricted to a solitary node or to a localized group of nodes draining an anatomic area (regional lymphadenitis), or the involvement can be generalized during a systemic infection. The gross features may be those of nonsuppurative, suppurative, or caseous inflammation, depending on the nature of the infecting microorganism.

Pathogenesis and Pathologic Changes

Acute Lymphadenitis. Lymph nodes serve as filters, removing infectious agents from lymphatics draining areas of acute inflammation. The initial histologic response consists of swelling and hyperplasia of sinusoidal lining cells and the infiltration of leukocytes. Depending on the nature of the infecting organism, host defenses, and antimicrobial therapy, the process may or may not progress to abscess formation. With some microorganisms, more distinctive pathologic pictures may be seen—caseation necrosis with infections due to *Mycobacterium tuberculosis, Histoplasma capsulatum, Coccidioides immitis*, and various atypical mycobacteria; stellate abscesses surrounded by palisading epithelioid cells ("granulomatous abscess") with lymphogranuloma venereum and cat-scratch disease; reactive follicular hyperplasia with scattered clusters of epithelioid histiocytes, located in cortical and paracortical zones and characteristically blurring the margins of germinal centers, along with focal distension of subcapsular and trabecular sinuses by monocytoid cells (monocytoid B cells) in toxoplasmosis. The necrotizing granulomatous lymphadenitis that occurs in tularemia can resemble that occurring in cat-scratch disease but often exhibits more granulomatous inflammation. Yersinia (*Y. pseudotuberculosis* or *Y. enterocolitica*) infection in mesenteric lymph nodes can also cause a necrotizing lymphadenitis. Necrotizing nongranulomatous lymphadenitis may be a feature of processes to which an infectious etiology has not yet been ascribed: Kikuchi's necrotizing lymphadenitis, Kawasaki syndrome, and systemic lupus erythematosus.[2]

Chronic Lymphadenitis. Histologically, the response is proliferative with hyperplasia of reticuloendothelial cells, prominent germinal centers, and dilated lymph sinuses filled with mononuclear cells. This picture is nonspecific, can be seen with a variety of infections, and may be observed initially on biopsy in a patient subsequently proven to have a lymphoproliferative disorder.

Dermatopathic lymphadenitis is a distinctive form of chronic lymphadenitis involving lymph nodes draining sites of chronic pruritic dermatitides. Histologically, the enlarged nodes show hyperplasia of reticulum cells in the germinal follicles and of sinusoidal lining cells, as well as the accumulation of lipid and melanin in macrophages (released from the inflammatory process in the skin). The latter feature is the basis for the pathologic designation *lipomelanotic reticuloendotheliosis*. The hyperplastic appearance of such nodes may be so prominent as to suggest erroneously the diagnosis of a lymphoproliferative disorder.

Clinical Findings

Acute Regional Lymphadenitis Due to Pyogenic Bacteria. Palpable lymph nodes do not always indicate serious or ongoing disease. Some degree of inguinal lymphadenopathy is relatively common, reflecting prior episodes of infection on the lower extremities (e.g., interdigital web infections secondary to epidermophytosis); similarly, minor enlargement of cervical nodes may be the residual from previous pharyngeal or dental infections. Lymphadenopathy in certain anatomic areas (preauricular, posterior auricular, supraclavicular, deltoidopectoral, and pectoral) should be viewed with greater suspicion because they are not frequently enlarged as a result of local subclinical infections or minor trauma. Enlargement of superficial lymph nodes along the external jugular vein, as well as of nodes that drain the earlobe and the floor of the external acoustic meatus, is very infrequent but may be associated with superficial infection accompanying recent initial earring insertion. Rarely, a firm mass in the tail or lateral aspect of the breast, suggestive of carcinoma, proves to be an enlarged lymph node in an unusual location due to toxoplasmosis.[1]

Acute suppurative lymphadenitis is more common in children than in adults. In the past three decades, *Staphylococcus aureus* has superseded group A streptococci as the most frequent etiology. The most common sites of involvement are, in order, submandibular (submaxillary), anterior and posterior cervical, inguinal, and axillary lymph nodes. The portal of entry for infection is frequently difficult to determine in children when cervical lymph nodes are involved.

On examination the involved area is swollen and the node(s) is usually at least 3 cm in diameter and tender. Fever is commonly present. The node(s) may be very firm or frankly fluctuant. The overlying skin is warm and often erythematous and edematous.

Syndromes Due to Suppurative Lymphadenitis at Specific Anatomic Sites. CERVICAL LYMPHADENITIS. Acute unilateral adenitis of pyogenic origin occurs most often in pre-school-aged children. The temperature is usually elevated (100–101°F), and local swelling may have been present for some days before the patient is seen by a physician. In only a minority of the cases is there a history of sore throat. However, in the past, group A streptococci have been implicated in about 75 percent of the cases of untreated suppurative cervical lymphadenitis in children.[3,4] *Staphylococcus aureus*, or a combination of *S. aureus* and group A streptococci, is often the etiology of suppurative cervical lymphadenitis associated with pyodermas of the face and scalp.

On examination, there is prominent swelling of the neck or face due to the enlargement usually of a single node, which is often walnut sized. The node is exquisitely tender and firm but may be fluctuant. The swelling may be sufficiently marked to interfere with opening of the mouth. A leukocytosis of 12,000–25,000 white blood cells per cubic millimeter is commonly present.

Acute bilateral cervical adenitis usually involves multiple nodes that are enlarged and somewhat tender in association with viral pharyngitis, infectious mononucleosis, streptococcal pharyngitis, or periodontal infections. Such lymphadenopathy does not ordinarily go on to suppuration unless the symptomatic streptococcal pharyngitis or periodontal infections are ignored.

SUBPECTORAL LYMPHADENITIS. An unusual course may be taken occasionally by infection (usually streptococcal but sometimes staphylococcal) of the thumb or of the interdigital web between the thumb and index finger. Lymphatics from this area do not pass through the epitrochlear nodes but drain directly into the axillary nodes, which in turn communicate with the subpectoral nodes. If infection is not contained in the axillary nodes, subpectoral lymphadenitis develops.[5] Suppuration of these subpectoral nodes can follow. Infection in this area may dissect downward and manifest as cellulitis over the lower chest and upper abdomen or suggest an intra-abdominal infection. The suppurating nodes may drain onto the chest wall.

ACUTE SUPPURATIVE EPITROCHLEAR LYMPHADENITIS. The epitrochlear nodes receive lymphatic drainage from the middle, ring, and little fingers and from the medial portion of the hand and the ulnar aspect of the forearm. Acute suppurative epitrochlear lymphadenitis is uncommon. The predisposing infection in the majority of patients is a primary pyoderma or secondarily infected skin lesions. Unilateral tender swelling, erythema, and induration of the epitrochlear area develop and may subsequently spread along the medial aspect of the arm and forearm. Pain on movement of the elbow is evident. There is often a moderate fever and leukocytosis. The diagnosis is apparent when a discrete, tender nodular swelling can be palpated; but when the area is diffusely swollen and movement at the elbow is limited, the picture may suggest septic arthritis or osteomyelitis.[6] Group A streptococci and *S. aureus* are implicated most commonly.

SUPPURATIVE ILIAC LYMPHADENITIS. The iliac lymph nodes are located along the external and common iliac arteries in the anterior retroperitoneal space. They receive deep lymphatic drainage from the lower abdominal wall and afferents from the superficial and deep inguinal nodes. Iliac lymphadenitis may develop secondary to infection of the lower extremities, lower abdominal wall, perineum, and so forth, or rarely it may result from hematogenous infection. After infection develops, it appears to break through fascial compartments in the iliac fossa and abscess formation ensues. Formerly, most cases occurred in children and young adults, but more recently there appears to be no age predilection. The suppurative lymphadenitis progresses to abscess formation in the space between the posterior peritoneum and the psoas and iliacus fascia.[7] An unexplained limp may be the initial symptom; the acute onset with fever may not occur for some days or weeks. Back and hip pain becomes prominent; extension of the thigh is very painful, but abduction and adduction of the hip evoke minimal discomfort. The symptomatology and clinical findings direct attention to the diagnoses of septic arthritis and osteomyelitis. Only after some days or weeks does lower abdominal pain develop, and the patient becomes acutely ill with high fever and marked leukocytosis. Examination at this point reveals a tightly flexed hip, rectus muscle spasm on the affected side, possibly a tender posterolateral pelvic mass, or a tender inguinal mass suggesting an incarcerated inguinal hernia. By this stage, the abscess may be sizable and may produce elevation and medial displacement of the sigmoid colon and medial displacement of the lower one third of the ureter. When the symptoms are on the right side, the diagnosis of *retrocecal* appendicitis with abscess may be suggested, but the antecedent limp is an important clinical clue. Other diagnoses that may be suggested by the clinical manifestations include tuberculosis of the spine with psoas abscess formation, pelvic inflammatory disease, and tumor of the thigh.[8] Body computed tomography (CT) scanning can be very helpful in defining an inflammatory collection abutting the psoas and iliacus muscles. *Staphylococcus aureus* is the microorganism most commonly implicated, followed in frequency by streptococci.

Acute Regional Lymphadenitis Due to Infecting Agents Other Than Pyogenic Bacteria. A variety of organisms other than the common pyogens may produce localized lymphadenitis (in some cases, going on to abscess and sinus tract formation). These infections resemble pyogenic lymphadenitis but are distinguishable by a prolonged and indolent course, the atypical anatomic areas involved, the lack of prior pyogenic infection, and clues in the history (scratch by a cat, previous tuberculosis, recent sexual exposure, and so forth). Occasionally, the nature of the clinical setting broadens the spectrum of microorganisms to be considered in causing firm or fluctuant lymphadenitis. Mycotic (*Candida albicans, Aspergillus* spp.) cervical lymphadenitis has occurred after oral mucositis in neutropenic children with leukemia.[9] In patients with suppurative lymphadenitis complicating chronic granulomatous disease, the microbial etiology is usually a catalase-positive pathogen. In addition to the commonly involved *S. aureus*, these include Enterobacteriaceae (*Klebsiella, Serratia, Salmonella*), *Pseudomonas* (often *cepacia*), *Aspergillus, Nocardia*, Calmette-Guérin bacillus (BCG), and *Chromobacterium violaceum*.[10–12]

SPECIFIC TYPES OF NONPYOGENIC REGIONAL LYMPHADENITIS. *Scrofula* (Tuberculous Cervical Lymphadenitis). Tuberculous cervical adenitis, formerly a common disease in children and young adults, has become infrequent. It is still occasionally seen in older adults who many years earlier had immigrated to this country from endemic areas (British Isles, Europe, and the Far East) or who lived in rural areas in this country. In this setting it represents breakdown of prior cervical node tuberculosis, acquired either by ingestion of infected milk (bovine tuberculosis) or by lymphohematogenous spread of infection from an initial pulmonary focus to this group of lymph nodes. In this country mycobacterial cervical lymphadenitis (scrofula) is four to five times more frequently due to atypical mycobacteria, commonly *Mycobacterium scrofulaceum*,[13] than to *M. tuberculosis*. In certain areas of the United States, *M. avium-intracellulare* complex is the principal etiology.[14] In parts of the world where BCG vaccination of infants is commonly practiced, subcutaneous abscesses and regional lymphadenitis are not uncommon complications, occurring 2–8 weeks after vaccination, but usually heal spontaneously. Occasionally, the regional (axillary, supraclavicular, or cervical) lymphadenitis progressively enlarges and goes on to caseating suppuration.[15]

The onset of scrofula is insidious, and fever and other systemic manifestations are absent. Several nodes are enlarged and matted together; the mass so formed may develop a swollen fluctuant area, and this brings the patient to medical attention. The process is usually painless. In the majority of cases, clinical evidence of tuberculosis elsewhere is absent. Spontaneous drainage of caseous material onto the skin surface (scrofuloderma) may eventually occur.

Definition of the mycobacterial species involved is important. The atypical mycobacteria causing cervical lymphadenitis are frequently resistant to the usual antituberculous chemotherapy, and surgical excision of the involved fluctuant node(s) is indicated. Antituberculous therapy is usually not needed for BCG nonsuppurative lymphadenitis, but if suppurative lymphadenitis develops, complete excision and antituberculous chemotherapy are indicated.

Granulomatous Lymphadenitis Caused by Nondiphtheria Corynebacteria. Subacute or chronic relapsing lymphadenitis has been reported occasionally to be due to *Corynebacterium pseudotuberculosis* (*C. ovis*).[16] The majority of patients have had extensive contact with animals, particularly sheep. The histologic picture is that of a suppurative or necrotizing granulomatous process. Treatment consists of prolonged antibiotic (erythromycin or penicillin) therapy combined with surgical drainage or excision of the involved nodes.

Oculoglandular (Parinaud) Syndrome. Preauricular lymphadenopathy can occur secondary to granulomatous nodular conjunctival infection caused by the introduction of certain pathogens onto the external eye. Oculoglandular syndromes occur occasionally in tularemia, cat-scratch disease,[17] listeriosis, sporotrichosis, and lymphogranuloma venereum. Epidemic keratoconjunctivitis due to adenoviruses is often associated with an enlarged preauricular lymph node.

Cat-Scratch Disease.[17] This slowly progressive and sometimes chronic form of regional lymphadenitis is presumed to be infectious. Small, pleomorphic, gram-negative bacilli have been identified within the walls of capillaries, in macrophages lining sinuses near germinal centers, and in macrophages in necrotic areas of involved lymph nodes of patients with cat-scratch disease. The organisms have only rarely been noted within neutrophils or free in areas of necrosis. The organisms are most readily demonstrated with the Warthin-Starry silver impregnation stain.[18,19] Convalescent serum from a patient with clinical cat-scratch disease reacted (immunoperoxidase stain) with the bacilli in the lymph nodes of three patients with the same disease, suggesting both a similarity (or identity) of the organisms in these cases and the occurrence of an immune response in these patients. In a recent study, a pleomorphic, as yet unspeciated, gram-negative bacillus has been reported to have been isolated on culture, in biphasic brain-heart infusion medium, of material from lymph nodes of 10 of 19 patients with the clinical diagnosis of cat-scratch disease.[20] Three of seven patients with recent cat-scratch disease had fourfold or greater rises in indirect fluorescent antibody titer against the cultured bacilli. Although the process progresses to suppuration in 10–50 percent of cases, the course is slower than that of suppurative lymphadenitis due to pyogenic bacteria, and most patients are only mildly ill. The nodes are tender, acutely so when there is frank suppuration. Fever is present in only about one-third of patients and is low grade. Almost any peripheral lymph nodes may be involved, but the axillary nodes are most commonly affected. About 90 percent of patients give a history of contact with cats (most often kittens), and most have been scratched. A primary lesion (small papule or vesicle resembling an insect bite) develops at the site of a scratch 7–14 days after contact with the cat. The primary lesion lasts for 1–4 weeks and may be helpful in diagnosis. Lymphadenopathy develops within a week or two of the appearance of the skin papule.[21] There is no lymphangitis.

The diagnosis is made on the basis of a history of appropriate exposure, the clinical picture, the failure to isolate a known etiologic agent from aspirated pus, a bimorphic histologic picture (stellate abscesses with necrotic centers surrounded by epithelioid cells), and a positive intradermal skin test to a known preparation of cat-scratch skin test antigen. The latter (derived from pus from a suppurative node of cat-scratch disease) is not available commercially and must be prepared carefully to ensure complete inactivation of any hepatitis virus. In view of the recent acquired immunodeficiency syndrome (AIDS) epidemic, the use of this type of skin test reagent of human origin must be seriously questioned, particularly if the antigen has been prepared in the past 6 years. We have seen a male homosexual patient with typical cat-scratch disease who some months later developed the characteristic manifestations of AIDS. The preparation and use of cat-scratch skin antigen from such a source might serve as a vehicle for spread of human immunodeficiency virus (HIV) infection.

Inguinal Buboes of Venereal Origin. Inguinal lymphadenopathy due to pyogenic infections or cat-scratch disease is usually unilateral. Prominent bilateral (or unilateral) adenopathy, particularly in the adult man, is suggestive of several venereal diseases (see Chapter 93). The genital chancre of primary syphilis is usually accompanied by one or several discrete, firm, nonsuppurative, painless, enlarged nodes in one or both inguinal areas. Constitutional signs are lacking. The overlying skin is uninflamed. In secondary syphilis the lymphadenopathy is generalized.

In lymphogranuloma venereum (LGV), the primary genital lesion is usually transient and asymptomatic. The initial manifestation of the disease is usually the characteristic inguinal bubo, occurring 10–30 days after sexual exposure. The adenopathy is more commonly unilateral. Initially the node is tender, discrete, and movable, but subsequently the inflammatory process involves multiple nodes in the area. Chills, fever, and constitutional symptoms are common at this stage. As a result of periadenitis, the nodes become fixed and matted into an oval or lobulated mass. The latter is adherent to the overlying skin that is purplish in color. Foci of suppuration develop with multiple fistulous tracts. A central lengthwise linear depression (so-called groove sign of LGV) is produced by involvement of nodes above and below the inguinal ligament. Although characteristic of LGV, the groove sign may rarely be produced by suppurative bacterial lymphadenitis or by lymphomatous involvement of inguinal nodes.

Chancroid is usually accompanied by painful, tender inguinal adenopathy. The primary lesion is a papule or pustule that progresses to form an extremely painful and tender but nonindurated ulceration, quite in contrast to a syphilitic chancre. The adenopathy of chancroid develops about 1 week after the primary lesion appears and, unlike LGV, is present while the ulcer is still active. The chancroidal bubo is typically unilateral, made up of fused inguinal nodes, and is more painful than that of LGV. Unilocular suppuration may develop. However, in the majority of patients, the lymphadenitis subsides without suppuration.

Primary genital herpetic infection in men and women is often associated with tender inguinal adenopathy. Histologically, the nodes show paracortical hyperplasia (with a prominent admixture of immunoblasts, plasma cells, and macrophages), along with sinus histiocytosis, discrete foci of necrosis, and intranuclear inclusions within scattered mononuclear and giant cells. Similar, histologically proven, recurrent, localized herpetic lymphadenitis can occur in immunocompromised patients in the absence of overt mucocutaneous lesions.[22] The "pseudobuboes" of granuloma inguinale are produced by subcutaneous granulomatous infection rather than by suppurative lymphadenitis.

Suppurative inguinal lymphadenitis due to group A streptococci has been superimposed on chronic lymphadenopathy in homosexual males.[23]

Inguinal Buboes of Nonvenereal Origin. Inguinal or femoral buboes occur in bubonic plague, since the flea bite initiating the infection is commonly on a lower extremity.[24] However, involvement of most other peripheral nodes can occur. The disease begins with fever, malaise, headache, and tender regional adenopathy after an incubation period of 2–6 days. Only rarely is a lesion (papule, pustule) at the site of the insect bite evident at the onset of clinical illness. A large, matted collection of lymph nodes with surrounding edema quickly develops and may go on to suppuration and spontaneous drainage. If not treated promptly, the infection rapidly progresses to a septicemic phase. The diagnosis should be suspected in a febrile, acutely ill patient with a large cluster of extremely tender lymph nodes and a history of exposure to fleas, rodents, or rabbits in the western United States. (Tularemia may mimic the epidemiologic and clinical features of bubonic plague but is more likely to produce an *ulceroglandular syndrome* [Table 1], with a primary lesion at the site of inoculation.[25]) Diagnostic procedures include blood cultures (uniformly positive in the septicemic phase of plague), as well as cultures and stained smears (see Chapter 207) of carefully obtained bubo aspirates. Appropriate treatment (see below) should be instituted immediately while awaiting results of cultures if bubonic plague is suspected.

GENERALIZED LYMPHADENITIS ASSOCIATED WITH SYSTEMIC INFECTIONS. Widespread lymphadenitis is a feature of a variety of infections disseminated by the blood stream. In most instances, suppuration of the involved nodes does not occur. Generalized lymphadenopathy is a feature, for example, of secondary syphilis, infectious mononucleosis, leptospirosis, and miliary tuberculosis. Generalized lymphadenopathy associated with infections is commonly due to the presence of the invading microorganism in the nodes. Generalized lymph node enlargement is a feature of a variety of infectious diseases due to bacterial, rickettsial, chlamydial, spirochetal, viral, protozoal, and helminthic agents (Table 1).

Etiologic Agents and Differential Diagnosis

It is helpful for purposes of the differential diagnosis to consider infective lymphadenitis in several categories (Table 1): (*1*) regional lymphadenopathy, (*2*) regional lymphadenopathy with breakdown of nodes, (*3*) inguinal bubo formation, (*4*) ulceroglandular syndrome, (*5*) oculoglandular syndrome, and (*6*) generalized lymphadenopathy.

In distinguishing among the causes of fluctuant cervical lymphadenitis, the history may suggest a streptococcal (preceding tonsillitis), staphylococcal (recent facial or neck infection), tuberculous (prior exposure to tuberculosis), or cat-scratch disease (exposure to cat) etiology. In a study of suppurative cervical adenitis *S. aureus* was the etiology more frequently than group A streptococci (36 percent vs. 26 percent), and in another one-quarter of the cases a bacteriologic diagnosis could not be made.[26] A subacute clinical course with little fever and a normal leukocyte count would be more consistent with cat-scratch disease or tuberculous involvement. Sinus tract formation suggests infection due to *M. tuberculosis* or an atypical mycobacterium. Gram-stained and Ziehl-Neelsen smears and culture (including cultures for mycobacteria) of material aspirated or drained from suppurating nodes provides a diagnosis in about two-thirds of such cases of cervical lymphadenitis. Further information may be provided by skin tests (purified protein derivative; cat-scratch antigen [see earlier comment on the current risk in using this reagent]), serologic tests (antistreptolysin O antibody titer), and histologic examination (caseation necrosis suggesting mycobacterial infection; bimorphic appearance suggesting cat-scratch disease) of an excised node when culture of aspirated material is unrevealing. A variety of noninfectious processes may resemble unilateral cervical lymphadenitis. Lymphoma may be suggested by the indolent course of cat-scratch disease. Acute febrile mucocutaneous lymph node syndrome (Kawasaki syndrome), a disease of infants and young children of unknown etiology, is characterized by nonsuppurative cervical lymphadenopathy.[27] The age of the patient, febrile course, conjunctival injection, erythematous rash, and subsequent desquamation suggest the diagnosis. A recently described benign disorder of lymph nodes, histiocytic necrotizing lymphadenitis or Kikuchi's disease, was first recognized in Japan and now has been observed in the United States.[28] Clinically, its features consist of localized, sometimes tender, cervical lymphadenopathy, often with an upper respiratory prodrome and associated in some patients with fever. Most cases occur in women, commonly under 30 years of age. Mild leukopenia and lymphocytosis may suggest infectious mononucleosis. The illness does not respond to antibiotics, but it usually resolves spontaneously within 1 or 2 months. Histologically, biopsy specimens may be erroneously interpreted as lymphoma, but the principal findings are those of focal reticulum cell hyperplasia combined with patchy areas of necrosis. Although a viral etiology is suspected on the basis of the clinical features, serologic and ultrastructural studies have failed to identify a specific agent.

Bronchial cleft cysts and cystic hygromas may be mistaken for cervical lymphadenitis, particularly if infected; thyroglossal duct cysts may suggest infected submental nodes. Submaxillary sialadenitis or salivary gland tumors may mimic submandibular lymphadenitis. Bimanual (intraoral and submandibular) palpation can be helpful in distinguishing between these processes.

TABLE 1. Clinical Patterns and Microbial Etiologies of Infectious Lymphadenitis

		Form of Lymphadenitis					
Disease	*Infecting Organism*	*Regional*	*Regional with Suppuration (or Caseation)*	*Inguinal Bubo Formation*	*Ulceroglandular*	*Oculoglandular*	*Generalized*
Bacterial							
Pyogenic	Group A strep; S. aureus	+	+				
Scarlet fever	Group A strep.	+	+				+
Diphtheria	*C. diphtheriae*	+					
Fusospirochetal angina	*B. melaninogenicus;* peptostreptococci, etc.	+					
Scrofula	*M. tuberculosis*	+	+				
	M. scrofulaceum; M. avium-intracellulare	+	+				
Miliary tuberculosis	*M. tuberculosis*						+
Brucellosis	*Brucella*						+
Leptospirosis	*Leptospira*						+
Syphilis	*T. pallidum*	+					+
Chancroid	*H. ducreyi*			+			
Plague	*Y. pestis*	+	+	+			
Tularemia	*F. tularensis*		+		+	+	
Rat-bite fever	*Streptobacillus moniliformis;*	+					
	Spirillum minus	+			+		
Anthrax	*B. anthracis*	+			+		
Listeriosis	*L. monocytogenes*					+	
Melioidosis	*P. pseudomallei*	+	+				+
Glanders	*P. mallei*	+	+				+
Cat-scratch	? Unknown gram-negative bacillus	+	+		±	+	
Mycotic							
Histoplasmosis	*H. capsulatum*						+
	H. capsulatum var. duboisii	+					
Coccidioidomycosis	*Coccidioides immitis*	+					
Paracoccidioidomycosis	*P. brasiliensis*	+					
Rickettsial							
Boutonneuse fever, etc.	*R. conori*				+		
Scrub typhus	*R. tsutsugamushi*	+					+
Rickettsialpox	*R. akari*	+					
Chlamydial							
Lymphogranuloma venereum	*C. trachomatis*			+		+	+
Viral							
Measles	Measles virus						+
Rubella	Rubella virus						+
Infectious mononucleosis	EB virus						+
CMV mononucleosis	CMV virus						+
Dengue fever	Dengue virus						+
West Nile fever	West Nile virus						+
Epidemic (Far Eastern) hemorrhagic fevers	?						+
Lassa fever	Lassa virus						+
Genital herpes infection	HSV-type 2	+					
Pharyngoconjunctival fever	Adenovirus (types 3 and 7)	+				+	
Epidemic keratoconjunctivitis	Adenovirus (types 8 and 19)					+	
Cat-scratch	?	+	+		+	+	
Postvaccinial lymphadenitis	Vaccinia virus	+					
AIDS; AIDS-related complex	HIV						+
Protozoan							
Kala azar	*Leishmania donovani*						+
African trypanosomiasis	*Trypanosoma brucei*	+					+
Chagas disease	*T. cruzi*					+	+
Toxoplasmosis	*Toxoplasma gondii*						+
Helminthic							
Filariasis	*Wucheria bancrofti*						+
	Brugia malayi						+
Loiasis	*Loa loa*			+			
Oncocerciasis	*Oncocerca volvulus*			+			

Isolated inguinal lymphadenitis or bubo formation in the adult suggests venereal diseases (syphilis, LGV, chancroid). Distinctive associated primary lesions are usually features of syphilis and chancroid but not of LGV. The inguinal adenopathy of primary syphilis consists of painless, firm, discrete, movable nodes without erythema of the overlying skin. The nodes do not suppurate, whereas spontaneous rupture of the buboes of LGV and chancroid may occur. The groove sign is suggestive of LGV. The buboes of chancroid are characteristically painful. Axillary, cervical, and inguinal buboes may occur with plague and tularemia. In plague an inguinal location is common. The geographic locale and a history of animal exposure are important clues to the diagnosis. Inguinal and femoral nodes can be involved in cat-scratch disease, although much less frequently than axillary or cervical nodes.

Prominent painful lymphadenitis involving cervical, axillary, and particularly supraclavicular nodes (on the left side) occasionally follows smallpox immunization. This may become evident weeks after immunization, and thus this relevant event may be overlooked. The process is self-limited. However, if a node is biopsied because of a suspicion of lymphoma or tuberculosis, the histologic picture may superficially simulate that of a malignant lymphoma. The lymphadenopathy appears to represent a heightened immunoblastic response to the immunizing agent, similar to the changes observed in infectious mononucleosis.[29,30]

Generalized lymphadenopathy is frequently a manifestation of disseminated infection (Table 1). Clues may be provided by the age of the patient and the presence of a characteristic rash (childhood exanthems, secondary syphilis), geographic factors (dengue, filariasis, histoplasmosis), occupational and/or dietary history (brucellosis, toxoplasmosis), exposure to animals (leptospirosis), and the presence of atypical lymphocytes (infectious mononucleosis, cytomegalovirus infection). Diagnosis of toxoplasmic lymphadenitis in the immunocompetent patient is based primarily on serologic testing, although sometimes node biopsy is performed because of initial concern for lymphoma. A negative result in the Sabin-Feldman dye test or in a comparable test for toxoplasma IgG antibody (indirect fluorescent antibody [IFA] or agglutination test) practically excludes the diagnosis. Acute infection is likely if a high IgM antibody titer is present with a high IgG antibody titer (dye test or IFA test titers of >1:1000) in a single serum specimen.[1] Laboratory diagnosis of acute toxoplasmic lymphadenitis can also be made by seroconversion from a negative to a positive IgG antibody test or by demonstration of a fourfold titer rise over 3 weeks.

Widespread suppurative infections of lymph nodes occur as a result of the microbicidal defect characteristic of neutrophils and monocytes of patients with chronic granulomatous disease. Recurrent infections (skin, bones, lungs, and liver, as well as lymph nodes) beginning in childhood and due to *S. aureus* and certain gram-negative bacilli (*Escherichia coli*, salmonella, *Serratia marcescens*) suggest the diagnosis.

Widespread lymphadenopathy may be a feature of many non-infectious diseases, particularly infiltrative processes such as lymphoma and reticuloendothelioses. Prominent peripheral lymphadenopathy may be a feature of rheumatoid arthritis. Lymphadenopathy may occur as an adverse effect of prolonged use of phenytoin. Widespread lymphadenopathy is a feature of the syndrome of immunoblastic lymphadenopathy.

Generalized Lymphadenopathy with AIDS or with the AIDS-Related Complex. Patients with AIDS may have generalized lymphadenopathy in which involvement with opportunistic infection or neoplastic disease (particularly Kaposi sarcoma) is evident on histologic examination. The infections have included those due to cytomegalovirus and *M. avium-intracellulare*.[31] The latter usually show a few poorly formed or no granulomas and a prominent histiocytic reaction. Large clusters ("globi") of acid-fast bacilli are present within the cytoplasm of histiocytes. Kaposi sarcoma in patients with AIDS often follows the pattern of generalized lymph node involvement and a fulminant course with mucosal and visceral lesions.[32] In AIDS other neoplasms, primarily of the B-cell type (B-cell immunoblastic sarcoma; small noncleaved, Burkitt-like lymphoma; plasmacytoid lymphocytic lymphoma) have occurred in lymph nodes and extranodal sites.[33]

Lymphadenopathy occurs in almost 50 percent of patients at risk for AIDS who develop an acute illness after initial exposure to HIV.[34] It often is one feature of a mononucleosis-like syndrome consisting of fever, malaise, myalgias, headaches, sore throat, diarrhea, and a maculopapular rash. After the acute clinical illness subsides, lymphadenopathy may remain as persistant generalized lymphadenopathy (PGL), involving at least several extrainguinal sites, of at least 3 months' duration.[35] PGL may also occur in male homosexuals, intravenous drug abusers, and other individuals in high-risk groups without any history of prior clinically apparent initial HIV infection. The nodes are discrete and nontender; suppuration does not occur. HIV replication takes place in such lymph nodes,[36] which histologically show follicular hyperplasia or mixed follicular and interfollicular hyperplasia. With progression to AIDS, lymphocyte depletion supervenes. PGL is frequently one of the manifestations of what is termed the *AIDS-related complex*, a group of clinical manifestations (including fever, weight loss, diarrhea, fatigue, and night sweats) occurring in individuals at risk for developing AIDS but not as yet having any definable underlying infectious or neoplastic cause for the symptoms. Laboratory findings in this clinical syndrome include two or more of the following: (*1*) lymphopenia, (*2*) decreased numbers of helper T cells, (*3*) depressed helper/suppressor cell ratio, (*4*) increased levels of serum globulins, (*5*) decreased blastogenesis in response to mitogens, and (*6*) anergy to skin test antigens. A sizable number of patients with such chronic generalized lymphadenopathy go on eventually to develop AIDS, with its complicating opportunistic infections and Kaposi sarcoma.[31] Regression of the lymphadenopathy may occur after 8–19 months in some patients. However, opportunistic infections can develop in some patients following such regression.[37]

An abnormal distribution of T-helper and T-suppressor lymphocytes occurs in hyperplastic lymph nodes of homosexual men with lymhadenopathy[38]—a reduced helper/suppressor ratio and an increased number of suppressor cells in the germinal centers and mantle zones (locations in which ordinarily B cells and helper-inducer cells are found). In about 20 percent of cases of PGL in intravenous drug abusers, multinucleate giant cells of the Warthin-Finkeldey type ("mulberry cells") are found in the interfollicular areas.

Presumptive Treatment

Initial treatment of infective lymphadenitis requires some narrowing of the diagnostic possibilities (Table 1). Localized pyogenic lymphadenitis responds well to early antibiotic treatment. When cervical lymphadenitis has developed from a pharyngeal or peridontal portal, initial treatment with penicillin is appropriate (procaine penicillin G, 300,000–600,000 units intramuscularly every 12–24 hours initially to ensure receipt of therapy when the patient may be nauseated; subsequently 250–500 mg of penicillin V may be administered orally every 6 hours for at least 10 days for older children and adults). In patients who are more acutely ill, larger doses of aqueous penicillin G parenterally are indicated. Erythromycin (20–40 mg/kg/day orally in divided doses every 6 hours) is an alternative for patients allergic to penicillin.

Pyogenic lymphadenitis complicating skin infections may be staphylococcal or streptococcal in etiology, and a penicillinase-resistant penicillin is the drug of choice (e.g., oxacillin 0.5 g orally every 4–6 hours for the older child or an adult). In the more acutely ill patient, intravenous administration of the semisynthetic penicillin or a first generation cephalosporin should be employed. Failure to show improvement, or progression to suppuration, is an indication for percutaneous needle aspiration (for bacteriologic diagnosis and treatment) or surgical drainage.

If cat-scratch disease is suspected, the treatment is principally symptomatic; antibiotics are not effective. If the nodes become fluctuant, aspiration is the treatment of choice.

If the diagnosis of bubonic plague is suspected, antibiotic treatment should be instituted promptly. Streptomycin (1.0 g intramuscularly every 12 hours in adults) or tetracycline (0.5 g orally every 6 hours in adults) are the preferred drugs, and treatment is continued for 10 days.

LYMPHANGITIS

Lymphangitis is an inflammation of lymphatic channels, usually in the subcutaneous tissues. It occurs either as an acute process of bacterial origin or as a chronic process of mycotic, mycobacterial, or filarial etiology.

Pathologic Changes and Pathogenesis

The visible red streaking in acute lymphangitis stems from the inflammatory process in the walls (and surrounding tissue spaces) of dilated lymphatic channels. Lymphatic obstruction often occurs on healing, resulting sometimes in persistent lymphedema. Cutaneous lymphatic sporotrichosis, a form of chronic lymphangitis, produces a combined suppurative and granulomatous response.

Clinical Findings

Acute Lymphangitis. Acute lymphangitis develops when an infection, commonly on an extremity, is not contained locally but spreads along lymphatic channels. Such infections are most often due to group A streptococci. Systemic manifestations may develop rapidly before evidence of infection becomes apparent at the site of inoculation of organisms, and they may be more prominent than might be anticipated on the basis of local pain and erythema. Red linear streaks, a few millimeters to several centimeters in width, extend from the initial site of infection toward the regional lymph nodes, which are enlarged and tender. Peripheral edema of the involved extremity often occurs. The time course of this type of infection can be accelerated from initial lesion to lymphangitis to complicating bacteremia in 24–48 hours.

The peripheral white blood cell count is commonly elevated. The etiologic agent often can be identified on Gram-stained smears and cultures obtained from the initial lesion. Blood cultures also may reveal the causative organism.

Acute lymphangitis and/or lymphadenitis, usually involving the lower extremities, is a feature of filariasis due to *Wuchereria bancrofti* (and sometimes to *Brugia malayi*).[39] These mosquito-borne diseases are endemic to Africa, Southeast Asia and the Pacific, and tropical South America. The acute form of disease is characterized by recurrent episodes of headache, backache, lymphangitis, lymphadenitis, epididymitis, and orchitis. Fever is uncommon. The adult filariae reside in lymphatics and lymph nodes and discharge microfilariae into the blood stream. With prolonged exposure in an endemic area, chronic lymphatic obstruction can develop with elephantiasis of the skin and scrotum. In this setting, recurrent episodes of lymphangitis may be the result of both the parasitic infestation and superimposed streptococcal infections (to which the chronic lymphedema predisposes). Serologic tests for filariasis may be helpful in diagnosis if microfilariae are not found, but they are positive in many other filarial infections. Lymph node or lymphatic vessel biopsy may be necessary for diagnosis.

Chronic Granulomatous Lymphangitis. Unlike acute lymphangitis, this is an indolent process with little pain or systemic evidences of infection. Sporotrichosis is most commonly the underlying disease.[40] This infection frequently is introduced by minor trauma (e.g., from a thorn of a barberry or rose bush) into the skin of a gardener. An erythematous subcutaneous nodule (often becoming fluctuant) or a chancriform ulcer subsequently develops at the site of inoculation of *Sporothrix schenckii* (present on some plants and in sphagnum moss used in gardening) on the hand or finger.[41] The lesion does not respond to local treatment or to administration of the common antibacterial agents. Slowly, mutiple subcutaneous nodules appear and extend proximally along the course of regional lymphatics, which become thickened.

Cutaneous infection ("swimming pool granuloma") with *Mycobacterium marinum*, an atypical mycobacterium that grows optimally at 25–32°C and is found in swimming pools and fish tanks, produces a chronic nodular, verrucous or ulcerative lesion at the site of an abrasion, usually about the knees or elbows. The lesion is usually solitary, but in an occasional patient new lesions develop proximally, as in sporotrichosis. Multiple sporotrichoid lesions have occurred in occasional infections due to *Nocardia brasiliensis*[42] and in rare infections due to *Mycobacterium kansasii* and *N. asteroides*.

Etiologic Agents

In the United States acute lymphangitis is most commonly due to group A streptococci, and chronic lymphangitis is usually caused by Sp. *schenckii*. Other infectious agents occasionally produce lymphangitis (Table 2).

Differential Diagnosis

The combination of a peripheral infection or traumatic lesion and the acute onset of fever with proximal red linear streaks directed toward regional lymph nodes is diagnostic of acute lymphangitis. In the legs, thrombophlebitis may produce linear areas of tender erythema, but the absence of an initiating lesion and of tender regional adenopathy is helpful in distinguishing it from lymphangitis. A history of rat bite and the subsequent development of lymphangitis suggest *Spirillum minus* infection. Filariasis is a consideration when an appropriate geographic history is obtained. Sporotrichosis is considered when chronic ulcerative lymphangitis develops in someone working with plants, soil, or timbers. *Mycobacterium marinum* is suggested as the etiology when sporotrichoid lesions develop in a person who has been around swimming pools and fish tanks.

Presumptive Therapy

Penicillin is the initial treatment of acute lymphangitis. In a mildly ill adult, 600,000 units of procaine penicillin G once or twice daily is administered initially, with supplementary oral penicillin V. More acutely ill patients in whom bacteremia may have developed should be hospitalized and treated with parenteral aqueous penicillin G (600,000–2,000,000 units every 4–6 hours). If a staphylococcal etiology is suspected, a penicillinase-resistant penicillin is used.

The initial treatment of presumptive lymphocutaneous sporotrichosis is potassium iodide. If sporotrichoid *M. marinum* infection is suspected, the diagnosis should be confirmed by demonstration of acid-fast bacilli and by isolation of the organism at 30°C on appropriate media. Localized swimming pool granulomas are often treated by surgical excision. Chemotherapy is reserved for more extensive and sporotrichoid forms of infection. On the basis of limited data, the combination of choice would appear to be rifampin and ethambutal.[43] Prolonged tetracycline or minocycline therapy has also been reported as successful in a small number of cases,[44] but in vitro resistance to and treatment failure with doxycycline have been reported.[45] Trimethoprim-sulfamethoxazole has been reported as effective in several studies. However, in vitro activity re-

TABLE 2. Causes of Lymphangitis

Clinical Form	*Etiologic Agent*	*Relative Frequency as Etiology of Lymphangitis*
Acute	Group A streptococcus	Common
	S. aureus	Occasional
	Pasteurella multocida	Occasional
	Spirillium minus (rat-bite fever)	Rare
	W. bancrofti; B. malayi (filariasis)	Rare (only in immigrants from endemic areas)
Chronic	*Sporothrix schenckii* (sporotrichosis)	Occasional
	M. marinum (swimming pool granuloma)	Occasional
	M. kansasii	Rare
	Nocardia brasiliensis	Rare
	W. bancrifti; B. malayi	Rare (only in immigrants from endemic areas)

quires drug concentrations greater than those usually achieved in serum and tissues.[46]

REFERENCES

1. McCabe RE, Brooks RG, Dorfman RF, et al. Clinical spectrum in 107 cases of toxoplasmic lymphadenopathy. Rev Infect Dis. 1987;9:754.
2. Strickler JG, Warnke RA, Weiss LM. Necrosis in lymph nodes. Pathol Annu. 1987;2:253.
3. Scobie WG. Acute suppurative adenitis in children. Scot Med J. 1969;14:352.
4. Dajani AS, Garcia RE, Wolinski E. Etiology of cervical lymphadenitis in children. N Engl J Med. 1963;268:1329.
5. Amren DP. Unusual forms of streptococcal disease. In: Wannamaker LW, Matsen JM, eds. Streptococci and Streptococcal Disease. New York: Academic Press; 1972:545.
6. Currarino G. Acute epitrochlear lymphadenitis. Pediatr Radiol. 1977;6:160.
7. Maull KI, Sachatello CII. Retroperitoneal iliac fossa abscess. A complication of suppurative iliac lymphadenitis. Am J Surg. 1974;127:270.
8. Oliff M, Chuang VP. Retroperitoneal iliac fossa pyogenic abscess. Radiology. 1978;126:647.
9. Shenep JL, Kalwinsky DK, Feldman S, et al. Mycotic cervical lymphadenitis following oral mucositis in children with leukemia. J Pediatr. 1985;106:243.
10. Curnutte JT, Boxer LA. Clinically significant phagocytic cell defects. In: Remington JS, Swartz MN, eds. Current Clinical Topics in Infectious Diseases. v. 4. New York: McGraw-Hill; 1985:103–55.
11. Sorensen RU, Jacobs MR, Shurin SB. *Chromobacterium violaceum* adenitis acquired in the northern United States as a complication of chronic granulomatous disease. Pediatr Infect Dis. 1985;4:701.
12. Kobayashi Y, Komazawa Y, Kobayashi M, et al. Presumed BCG infection in a boy with chronic granulomatous disease. A report of a case and review of the literature. Clin Pediatr. 1984;23:586.
13. Lincoln EM, Gilbert LA. Disease in children due to mycobacteria other than *Mycobacterium tuberculosis*. Am Rev Respir Dis. 1972;105:683.
14. Spark RP, Fried ML, Bean CK, et al. Nontuberculous mycobacterial adenitis of childhood. The ten-year experience at a community hospital. Am J Dis Child. 1988;142:106.
15. Victoria MS, Shah BR. Bacillus Calmette-Guérin lymphadenitis: A case report and review of the literature. Pediatr Infect Dis. 1985;4:295.
16. Lipsky BA, Goldberger AC, Tompkins LS, et al. Infections caused by nondiphtheria corynebacteria. Rev Infect Dis. 1982;4:1220.
17. Carithers HA, Carithers CM, Edwards RO Jr. Cat-scratch disease. Its natural history. JAMA. 1969;207:312.
18. Wear DJ, Margileth AM, Hadfield TL, et al. Cat-scratch disease: A bacterial infection. Science. 1983;221:1403.
19. Hadfield TL, Malaty RH, Van Dellen A, et al. Electron microscopy of the bacillus causing cat-scratch disease. J Infect Dis. 1985;152:643.
20. English CK, Wear DJ, Margileth AM, et al. Cat-scratch disease. Isolation and culture of the bacterial agent. JAMA. 1988;259:1347.
21. Carithers HA. Cat-scratch disease. An overview based on a study of 1,200 patients. Am J Dis Child. 1985;139:1124.
22. Epstein JI, Ambinder RF, Kuhajda, et al. Localized herpes simplex lymphadenitis. Am J Clin Pathol. 1986;86:444.
23. Ho DD, Murata GH. Streptococcal lymphadenitis in homosexual men with chronic lymphadenopathy. Am J Med. 1984;77:151.
24. Reed WB, Palmer DL, Williams RC, et al. Bubonic plague in southwestern United States. Medicine. 1970;49:465.
25. Young LS, Bicknell DS, Archer BG, et al. Tularemia epidemic: Vermont 1968. Forty-seven cases linked to contact with muskrats. N Engl J Med. 1969;280:1253.
26. Barton LL, Feigin RD. Childhood cervical lymphadenitis: A reappraisal. J Pediatr. 1974;84:846.
27. Feigin RD, Schleien CI. Kawasaki's disease. In: Remington J, Swartz MN, eds. Current Clinical Topics in Infectious Disease, v. 4. New York: McGraw-Hill; 1983:30.
28. Unger PD, Rappaport KM, Strauchen JA. Necrotizing lymphadenitis (Kikuchi's disease). Arch Pathol Lab Med. 1987;111:1031.
29. Hartsock RJ. Postvaccinial lymphadenitis. Hyperplasia of lymphoid tissue that simulates malignant lymphomas. Cancer 1968;21:632.
30. Childs CC, Parham DM, Berard CW. Infectious mononucleosis: The spectrum of morphologic changes simulating lymphoma in lymph nodes and tonsils. Am J Surg Pathol. 1987;11:122.
31. Fauci AS, Macher AM, Longo DL, et al. Acquired immunodeficiency syndrome: Epidemiologic, clinical, immunologic, and therapeutic considerations. Ann Intern Med. 1984;100:92.
32. Gottlieb MS, Groopman JE, Weinstein WM, et al. The acquired immunodeficiency syndrome. Ann Intern Med. 1983;99:208.
33. Levine AM, Meyer PR, Begandy MK, et al. Development of B-cell lymphoma in homosexual men: Clinical and immunological findings. Ann Intern Med. 1984;100:7.
34. Tindall B, Barker S, Donovan B, et al. Characterization of the acute clinical illness associated with human immunodeficiency virus infection. Arch Intern Med. 1988;148:945.
35. Biberfeld P, Porwit-Ksiazek A, Böttiger B, et al. Immunohistopathology of lymph nodes in HTLV-III infected homosexuals with persistent adenopathy or AIDS. Cancer Res. 1985;45(Suppl):4665S.
36. Biberfeld P, Chayt KJ, Marselle LM, et al. HTLV-III expression in infected lymph nodes and relevance to pathogenesis of lymphadenopathy. Am J Pathol. 1986;125:436.
37. Metroka CE, Cunningham-Rundles S, Pollack MS, et al. Generalized lymphadenopathy in homosexual men. Ann Intern Med. 1983;99:585.
38. Modlin RL, Meyer PR, Hofman FM, et al. T-lymphocyte subsets in lymph nodes from homosexual men. JAMA. 1983;250:1302.
39. Grove DI, Warren KS, Mahmoud AAF. Algorithms in the diagnosis and management of exotic diseases. VI. The filariases. J Infect Dis. 1975;132:340.
40. Orr ER, Riley HD Jr. Sporotrichosis in childhood: Report of ten cases. J Pediatr. 1971;78:951.
41. Duran RJ, Coventry MB, Weed LA, et al. Sporotrichosis: A report of twenty-three cases in the upper extremity. J Bone Joint Surg. 1957:39(A):1330.
42. Smego RA Jr, Gallis HA. The clinical spectrum of *Nocardia brasiliensis* infection in the United States. Rev Infect Dis. 1984;6:164.
43. Van Dyke JJ, Lake KB. Chemotherapy for aquarium granuloma. JAMA. 1975;233:1380.
44. Izumi AK, Hanke W, Higaki M. *Mycobacterium marinum* infections treated with tetracycline. Arch Dermatol. 1977;113:1067.
45. Ljungberg B, Christensson B, Grubb R. Failure of doxycycline treatment in aquarium-associated *Mycobacterium marinum* infections. Scand J Infect Dis. 1987;19:539.
46. Sanders WJ, Wolinsky E. In vitro susceptibility of *Mycobacterium marinum* to eight antimicrobial agents. Antimicrob Agents Chemother. 1980;18:529.

SECTION J. INFECTIONS RELATED TO TRAUMA

78. PROPHYLAXIS AND TREATMENT OF INFECTION IN TRAUMA

ROGER W. YURT
G. TOM SHIRES

Trauma is the leading cause of death in the first three decades of life in the United States and the fourth leading cause overall. Of the 50 million injuries that occur each year, 10 million of them are disabling.[1] The population at risk for infection associated with trauma is not only quantitatively large but is impressive from the standpoint of a large number of hospitalized patients who are prone to the development of nosocomial infections. The only real prophylaxis of infection in trauma is directed toward nosocomial infection. Initial regimens oriented toward the wound or injured tissue are in fact therapeutic since exogenous and endogenous contamination has already occurred. The magnitude of the infection problem after trauma is most dramatic in patients with severe burns in whom 50 percent of the mortality is related to infection.[2] The hypermetabolic state, depressed immune function, devitalized tissue, specific organ injury, foreign bodies, endogenous and exogenous contamination, and shock, individually or in combination, predispose the injured patient to and may potentiate infection.

THE INJURED PATIENT

The initial approach to the patient with major traumatic injury, that is, to maintain or achieve cardiovascular stability, is not only a lifesaving maneuver but is an attempt to reverse a loss of function on the cellular level. Although cellular dysfunction associated with trauma is reversible,[3] prolonged deficits in tissue perfusion can lead to organ dysfunction. Progressive devitalization of tissue enlarges the niche for infection. In additino, it is anticipated but not shown that the cellular components of the immune system are subject to the same dysfunction that has been documented in tissue and red blood cells.[4] The administration of a balanced salt solution and replacement of lost blood in the hypovolemic injured patient should be considered an integral part of the prophylaxis for infection.

Factors Associated with Infection

Several factors related to the type of injury are associated with the development of infection in the traumatized patient (Table 1). An appreciation for the contribution of devitalized tissue, visceral injury, and extent of contamination guides the therapeutic approach. Injury secondary to a high-velocity missile is anticipated to devitalize tissue, even in the absence of external signs, since cavitation within the wound may destroy large quantities of tissue. In addition, the kinetic energy of a projectile may be transmitted to viscera without obvious violation of body cavities, thereby leading to unsuspected injury. Significant infections related to retained single foreign bodies are rare but do occur. Contamination and infection in such cases are probably more related to the organs the missile passes through than to exogenous sources.[5] On the other hand, injuries caused by multiple fragments are often contaminated by exogenous sources since the wounds may contain pieces of clothing, wadding, and powder in addition to the multiple foreign bodies.

Stab wounds are rarely associated with large amounts of devitalized tissue but are of concern because of the potential for visceral injury and possible contamination with endogenous organisms. Likewise, blunt trauma causes organ injury, and with the rupture of a hollow viscus, endogenous contamination occurs. A high risk of infection is associated with multiple-organ injury and other major injuries, in particular, with an injury to viscera that contain bacteria (Table 2). That this is true is supported by reports that patients sustaining isolated colon injuries have a 12–71 percent chance of infection and a mortality rate of 3–15 percent.[6–9] In 43–100 percent of cases late mortality is due to infectious complications.[10,11] The National Research Council's classification[12] of operative and traumatic wounds, which emphasizes the extent of injury and contamination, includes the criteria outlined here.

TABLE 2. Organ-Specific Factors Associated with a High Risk of Infection

High-Risk Injury	*High Risk on Basis of Contamination*
Multiple organ	Perforated viscus
Pancreatic	Colon/rectum
Liver	Vagina
Esophageal	Biliary tract
	Urinary tract
	Small bowel
	Stomach
	Respiratory tract
	Other
	Mouth
	Anus

Effects of Trauma on Host Defense. In addition to the specific aspects of injury outlined, the trauma patient is at risk for infection due to suppression of the immune response at several levels. Balch studied patients after severe battle trauma and found a decreased ability of neutrophils to phagocytose bacteria in vitro for the first 24 hours after injury.[13] Several studies have shown impaired chemotactic activity, decreased neutrophil lysozomal enzymes, and lower serum immunoglobulin levels subsequent to thermal injury.[14–19] Davis et al.[20] have shown that chemotactic activity and random migration of neutrophils were depressed significantly during days 5–15 after injury. This study confirmed the inverse relationship between neutrophil chemotactic responsiveness and the extent of thermal injury, as well as a correlation between the severity of the neutrophil defect and the decrease in neutrophil lysozyme content. Such findings are consistent with neutrophil degranulation and subsequent depressed neutrophil responsiveness.

Studies from other laboratories[21,22] have demonstrated a cell-directed inhibitor of chemotaxis by serum from burn patients. All of these studies indicate that the burn patient develops a leukocyte chemotactic defect that is thought to predispose to infection. The difficulty in quantitating the extent of injury in other types of trauma contributes to the fact that few data are available in these patients with regard to neutrophil function after injury.

Current studies suggest that defects in human macrophages or function of the reticuloendothelial system (RES) may play a role in postinjury susceptibility to infection. Donovan[23] studied the clearance of iodine 125 microaggregated albumin immediately after surgery. He found a decreased clearance rate in eight out of nine patients, which correlated with the duration of the procedure and with decreased blood pressure. Scovill et al.[24] studied the effect of surgical trauma on the RES of animals. They observed a depressed RES function after surgery and decreased hepatic localization and increased pulmonary localization of labeled test particulate matter. Fibronectin, an α_2-opsonic glycoprotein, has been found to have depressed levels

TABLE 1. Factors Associated with Infection after Traumatic Injury

	Factors Associated with the Development of Infection				
			Contamination		
Type of Trauma	*Devitalized Tissue*	*Foreign Body*	*Exogenous*	*Endogenous*[a]	*Risk of Infection*
Penetrating					
Stab wound	±	–	±	+	+
Projectile					
Low velocity	+ +	+		+ + + +	+ + +
High velocity	+ + + +	+		+ + + +	+ + + +
Multiple fragments (shotgun, shrapnel)	+ + +	+ + +	+ + + +		+ +
Nonpenetrating					
Burn	+ + + +	–	–	–	+ + + +
Blunt	+ +	–	+	+ + +	+ +

[a] Location dependent.

24 hours after major operative procedures in patients who sustain severe trauma. This decrease in opsonic activity was transient and persisted over a 48- to 72-hour period postinjury. The trauma patient who ultimately died had lower levels of this circulating opsonic activity. Preliminary studies suggest that infusion of purified fibronectin may be of some benefit in patients who have depressed RES activity after major injury.

Depressed cellular immune function after major injury has been documented by reports of impaired delayed hypersensitivity reactions,[25,26] a prolongation of allograft and xenograft rejection times,[27–29] and altered mitogen and mixed lymphocyte responses.[30–32] Although these changes are incompletely characterized, there have been reports that T-cell function and numbers are affected such that increased suppressor activity[33] and decreased helper activity[34] may occur. Furthermore, immunologic suppression and fatal outcome have been associated with abnormal monocyte function.[35,36]

The only specific organ injury that has been associated with depressed host resistance is that of a loss of splenic tissue. In 1967, Eraklis and associates[37] reported that 5.4 percent of 467 patients died of postsplenectomy sepsis. Most of these deaths occurred within 4 years of splenectomy, and children seemed to have the greatest risk. Further reports of multicenter studies by Singer[38] suggested that the overall mortality due to sepsis in 2795 patients who underwent splenectomies was 2.52 percent. However, patients who underwent splenectomies for traumatic injury of the spleen had the lowest rate of septic mortality, which was nevertheless almost 60 times higher than that in the healthy population. Additional studies of adult populations suggest that the incidence of sepsis is increased in patients with (4.3 percent) and without (2.2 percent) chronic disease after splenectomy.[39] A more recent retrospective study[40] suggests that trauma patients have a higher rate of sepsis, both early and late after splenectomy, than do injured patients who have not undergone splenectomy. The primary cause of decreased host resistance to encapsulated bacteria after splenic loss is not fully delineated; however, the serum of these patients contains decreased amounts of opsonizing activity for pneumococci[41] and lower levels of IgM,[42] and tuftsin levels have been reported to be decreased.[43] The growing concern for the preservation of splenic tissue will be addressed under prophylaxis.

ACUTE PROPHYLAXIS AND TREATMENT

Coincident with the initiation of fluid resuscitation, systemic antibiotics are administered according to the extent, location, and type of injury. Data to support the use of preoperative antibiotics in the injured patient are based on the use of antibiotics before elective operative procedures (iatrogenic trauma). A recent review of 42 prospective studies of the use of antibiotics in the perioperative period in colon and rectal surgery reaffirms the value of short-term antibiotic administration.[44] These data confirm the necessity of achieving adequate tissue levels of antibiotics at the time of clean–contaminated operative procedures. Since traumatic injuries must be anticipated to equal or exceed this extent of contamination,[45] the standard approach has been to use perioperative antibiotics. However, in most cases contamination has occurred before medical care, and therefore, in a strict sense antibiotic administration must be viewed as therapy rather than as prophylaxis. The importance of the timing of antibiotic therapy is documented by animal studies in which antibiotics given 12 hours before were effective but those given 12 hours after infection were not.[46] Additional studies by Miles et al. and by Burke have indicated that antibiotics administered 4 hours after experimental infection were ineffective.[47,48] The value of preoperative administration of antibiotics after trauma has been shown by Fullen et al.[49] Stone et al.[50] have confirmed these clinical studies. When the interval from injury to the initiation of antibiotics was an average of 64 minutes, the wound infection rate from penetrating colon injuries was 11 percent, and no mortality was reported.[51]

Antibiotics, administered early after injury, are selected on the basis of the organisms that are anticipated to be present. Intra-abdominal contamination–infection is treated with antimicrobials active against aerobic and facultative organisms as well as anaerobes. The typical choice is combination antibiotic therapy; however, some have suggested that cefoxitin may be of equal value if administered soon after injury.[52] Penetrating injuries involving soft tissues are treated with agents that are penicillinase resistant and effective against gram-positive organisms. Injuries likely to be prone to clostridial infection are treated with penicillin. The treatment of soft tissue infections is specifically outlined in Chapters 74 and 75.

Any wound, including burn wounds, has the potential for harboring *Clostridium tetani*; therefore, patients who sustain penetrating injuries need adequate prophylaxis for tetanus. The following outline is a modification from the American College of Surgeons Committee on Trauma as presented by Sandusky[53]:

Immunization completed previously; last booster within 1 year: No additional toxoid required.

Immunization completed within the previous 10 years; no subsequent booster: Give 0.5 ml of Td.*

Immunization completed more than 10 years previously; last booster within the previous 10 years: Give 0.5 ml of Td* if wound is particularly tetanus prone. No booster necessary for minor wounds.

Immunization completed more than 10 years previously; no booster within the previous 10 years; wound minor and relatively clean, treated promptly and adequately: Give 0.5 ml of Td.*

Immunization completed more than 10 years previously; no booster within the previous 5 years; wound other than minor and relatively clean and/or not treated promptly: Give 0.5 ml of Td* and 250 units of TIG(H).† (If wound is considered prone to clostridial infection, give 500 units.)

No history or record of immunization; wound minor and very clean; wound surgery prompt and adequate: Begin immunization using 0.5 ml of Td*; give patient a written record of immunization, and schedule appointments for completion of immunization.

No history or record of immunization; wound other than minor and very clean, or not treated promptly or adequately: Give 250 units of TIG(H).† (If wound is considered prone to clostridial infection, give 500 units.) Begin immunization.

The Surgical Approach

A rapid and complete clinical and laboratory evaluation is essential to detect and anticipate injuries. Undiagnosed and therefore untreated injuries can lead to life-threatening infectious complications in the traumatized patient. For this reason x-ray films are taken to estimate the path of foreign bodies. Blunt trauma to the torso is evaluated clinically, but in the unresponsive patient or in those who are unable to be adequately examined, peritoneal lavage is used to detect intra-abdominal injury.[54] Hematuria demands a full work-up of the genitourinary tract,[55] and elevated serum amylase levels lead to a strong suspection of pancreatic, duodenal, and small bowel injury.[56] The value of computed tomography (CT) scanning in evaluating trauma to the head is well documented, and recent experience suggests that this is a valuable tool in detecting intra-abdominal injury. A comprehensive and quick preoperative evaluation minimizes the chance of infectious complications of missed injuries.

As with all surgical procedures, the goal is to minimize ad-

* Td: tetanus and diphtheria toxoid, adult type.

† TIG(H): tetanus immune globulin (human). When TD and TIG(H) are given concurrently, a separate syringe and needle and separate sites should be used.

ditional tissue injury. Necrotic and contaminated tissues are débrided, and dead space is minimized. Perforation of the gastrointestinal tract requires prompt identification and repair. Even if the secretions released into the abdominal cavity are not contaminated (i.e., bile), chemical peritonitis develops, which leads to ileus, edema of the bowel wall, and ultimately to a leakage of bacteria into the peritoneal cavity. On the other hand, gross contamination of the peritoneal cavity mitigates against primary repair of the violated gastrointestinal tract, particularly in relation to colon injury. The conservative approach in such injuries is to divert the colonic stream or to exteriorize all colonic injuries. Advocates of primary repair without colostomy have sited a significant complication rate related to the colostomy and its closure[57]; this has not been confirmed by additional studies.[58] Attempts to show that primary closure is acceptable in colon injury in highly selected patients have been difficult to interpret due to high baseline infection rates (57 percent wound and 29 percent abdominal) with the conservative approach[59] or the small number of patients studied.[60] The meticulous selection of patients with isolated right colon injuries suggests that primary closure of such injuries is safe without diversion. The study reported by Arango et al.[8] indicated that the mortality is only 3.2 percent and the morbidity 22 percent in 307 right colon cases treated in this manner.

The rationale behind external drainage of injured tissue stems from the high incidence of infection associated with dead space fluid collections, which are isolated from normal defense mechanisms. In addition, if leakage of corrosive material (e.g., pancreatic secretions) or bacteria-laden material is anticipated, drainage is carried out. Furthermore, drainage lessens the chance of the collection of blood from raw surfaces. Concern for draining such collections stems from the long-held belief that blood products potentiate infection in tissues. Current data implicate hemoglobin as a potentiating factor in experimental peritoneal infection and suggest that red blood cell stroma inhibits neutrophil function.[61] Residual blood and bacteria are diluted by irrigation of the peritoneal cavity, but localized contamination may be spread by such procedures, and hypothermia can ensue through the use of large volumes of room temperature fluids.

PROPHYLAXIS AND TREATMENT OF NOSOCOMIAL INFECTION

As already indicated, the early approach to infection in the trauma patient is therapeutic rather than prophylactic. Therefore, prophylaxis in the strict sense is only applicable to the development of hospital-acquired infection in these patients. That nosocomial infection is a substantial problem in severely traumatized patients cared for in critical care units is confirmed by the report of 639 such infections in 381 patients studied over a 2-year period.[62] Bacteremia without an apparent source occurred in 21 percent of these patients. The ability to ascertain whether infection is directly related to trauma or is a secondary occurrence is jaded by the fact that the patient with major injury is predisposed to infection. Cultures obtained initially from the wound or injured viscera assist in defining whether subsequent infection is primarily due to the injury.

If treatment of the injury and associated infection has been appropriate from a surgical standpoint, that is, necrotic tissue débrided, injured viscera repaired, and so on, then the primary concerns in preventing additional infection relate to appropriate antibiotic usage and the environment. The administration of antibiotics for presumed infection initially is limited to a short duration (three doses) unless overwhelming contamination, established infection in the tissue, or surgical débridement has been limited due to concern for removal of vital organs. Concern for the development of infection from resistant organisms selected by prophylactic antibiotics even in cases of major tissue injury such as burns has led to several studies that reveal that the use of such antibiotics in inpatients with major injury is of no benefit.[63] The judicious use of antibiotics for as short a term as possible is advocated to minimize nosocomial infections. Although multiple variables such as severity of the illness and frequency of the use of intravascular catheters contribute to the development of nosocomial infection, it appears that superinfection and especially fungal infection can be attributed to the prolonged use of antibiotics.[64]

There are now sufficient data to support the clinical observation that prolonged immobilization of patients leads to increased rates of infection. In a classic article[65] Seibel et al. have shown that early fixation of long-bone fractures and early mobilization can dramatically decrease the post-trauma complication rate. Not only is the infection rate decreased, but the development of adult respiratory distress syndrome (ARDS) is diminished. Such findings are also supported by studies of early mobilization of patients with disrupted pelvic rings.[66] A less clearly defined factor in these patients was the contribution of enteral feedings. Data are now accumulating to suggest that a decrease in gastrointestinal integrity may contribute to increased infection rates after injury. Enteral nutrition appears to maintain gastrointestinal integrity to a greater degree than does parenteral feeding.[67] Translocation of bacteria across the gastrointestinal barrier after injury has been shown,[68] but whether translocation of bacteria correlates with infection and sepsis is not yet known.

Indwelling Catheters

Infection at the site of intravenous catheters is more often the cause of sepsis than are contaminated intravenous solutions,[69] but contaminated infusion sets due to breaks in aseptic technique may also substantially contribute to sepsis in these immunodepressed patients.[70] The fibrin sheath that forms on the indwelling catheter may be infected from bacteria traveling along the catheter[71] or by hematogenous spread in the patient with prolonged venous cannulation. Most septic phlebitis has been attributed to peripheral intravenous cannulae in surgical patients,[72] especially from those placed in the emergency room.

Additional intravascular devices, including catheters connected to transducers used to measure intra-arterial and intravenous pressures, are sources for septicemia in these patients. Nosocomial outbreaks of bacteremia, candidemia, and hepatitis B have been associated with these devices.[73] Bacterial contamination has been associated with the use of stopcocks[74] and heparin-lock needles left in place for 4 days or longer.[75] Furthermore, ice baths used to cool arterial blood gas and cardiac output syringes have been implicated in outbreaks of infection.[76] Although purulent thrombophlebetis is overall an uncommon occurrence,[72] it carries a high mortality rate in traumatized patients even if appropriately treated.[77] In order to avoid these complications, all catheters are removed after 3 days.[78] A semiquantitative catheter culture technique has been reported that may assist in detecting these infections.[79]

Since the most common site for infection in patients in surgical intensive care units is the urinary tract, attempts should be made to minimize the duration of indwelling urinary catheters.

The Environment

The patient who sustains major trauma and requires intensive care in specialized units has a 50 percent risk of colonization by exogenous bacteria and a 23 percent chance of unit-acquired infection after only 3 days in the unit. This risk increases with time in the unit such that by 10 days colonization occurs in 90 percent of patients and the infection risk is 75 percent.[80] The primary vectors of these infections are personnel in the unit. Additional sources include respiratory equipment, endotracheal tubes, and the catheters listed above. Strict discipline with regard to handwashing, dress policy, cleaning policy, and aseptic technique is essential to minimize the development of nosocomial infection in these patients.[81]

Specific Organ Injury

With the accumulation of data indicating an increased susceptibility to infection in the postsplenectomy patient, emphasis has been placed on the preservation of splenic tissue. Although the risk of postsplenectomy sepsis has been reported to be less after splenectomy for trauma[38] than after splenectomy for other indications, there nevertheless is an increased risk of sepsis in patients after trauma-related splenectomy.[40] Recent studies have supported repair of the injured spleen as an alternative to splenectomy.[82,83] Such an approach is indicated when hemostasis can be obtained and when the abdominal cavity is not contaminated from additional injuries. A more radical approach, applied in children, has been that of nonoperative therapy for splenic injury.[84] This approach has yet to gain general acceptance due to the risks associated with missed additional intra-abdominal injury and the difficulty in applying this approach to the patient with multiple injuries. In general, consideration should be given to long-term prophylactic penicillin administration in patients who have undergone splenectomies as well as to immunization with pneumococcal and perhaps meningococcal vaccines.[85]

REFERENCES

1. Shires GT. Principles of Trauma Care. 3rd ed. New York: McGraw-Hill; 1985:xi.
2. Alexander JW, MacMillian BG. Hospital infections in burns. In: Bennett JV, Brachman P, eds. Nosocomial Infections. Boston: Little, Brown; 1979:335.
3. Shires GT, Cunningham JN, Baker CRF, et al. Alterations in cellular membrane function during hemorrhagic shock in primates. Ann Surg. 1972;176:288–95.
4. Yurt RW. Immunologic and molecular changes associated with trauma. New Dev Med. 1987;2:77–84.
5. Tzeng S, Swan KG, Rush BF. Bullets. A source of infection? Am Surg. 1982;48:239–40.
6. Haygood FD, Polk HC Jr. Gunshot wounds of the colon: A review of 100 consecutive patients with emphasis on complications and their causes. Am J Surg. 1976;131:213–8.
7. Kirkpatrick JR, Rajpal SG. The injured colon: Therapeutic considerations. Am J Surg. 1975;129:187–91.
8. Arango A, Baxter CR, Shires GT. Surgical management of traumatic injuries of the right colon: Twenty years of civilian experience. Arch Surg. 1979;114:703–6.
9. Chilimindris C, Boyd DR, Carlson LE, et al. A critical review of management of right colon injuries. J Trauma. 1971;11:651–60.
10. Mulherin JL, Sawyers JL. Evaluation of three methods for managing penetrating colon injures. J Trauma. 1975;15:580–7.
11. Schrock TR, Christensen W. Management of perforating injuries of the colon. Surg Gynecol Obstet. 1972;135:65–8.
12. Dudrick SJ, Baue AE, Eiseman B, et al. Manual of Preoperative and Postoperative Care: American College of Surgeons. Philadelphia: WB Saunders; 1983:110.
13. Balch HH. The effect of severe battle injury and of post-traumatic renal failure on resistance to infection. Ann Surg. 1955;142:145–63.
14. Warden JD, Mason AD Jr, Pruitt BA Jr. Evaluation of leukocyte chemotaxis in vitro in thermally injured patients. J Clin Invest. 1974;54:1001–4.
15. Grogan JB. Suppressed in vitro chemotaxis of burn neutrophils. J Trauma. 1976;16:985–8.
16. Fikrig SM, Karl SC, Suntharalingam L. Neutrophil chemotaxis in patients with burns. Ann Surg. 1977;136:746–8.
17. Alexander JW. Serum and leukocyte lysosomal enzymes. Arch Surg. 1967;95:482–91.
18. Munster AM, Hoagland HC, Pruitt BA Jr. The effect of thermal injury on serum immunoglobulins. Ann Surg. 1970;172:965–9.
19. Daniels JC, Larson DL, Abston S, et al. Serum protein profiles in thermal burns: I. Serum electrophoretic patterns, immunoglobulins and transport protein. J Trauma. 1974;14:137–52.
20. Davis JM, Dineen P, Gallin JI. Neutrophil degranulation and abnormal chemotaxis after thermal injury. J Immunol. 1980;127:1467–71.
21. Altman LC, Furukawa CT, Klebanoff SJ. Depressed mononuclear chemotaxis in thermally injured patients. J Immunol. 1977;119:199–205.
22. Warden GC, Mason AD, Pruitt BA Jr. Suppression of leukocyte chemotaxis in vitro by chemotherapeutic agents used in the management of thermal injuries. Ann Surg. 1975;181:363–9.
23. Donovan AJ. The effect of surgery on the reticuloendothelial cell function. Arch Surg. 1967;94:247–50.
24. Scovill WA, Saba TM, Blumenstock FA, et al. Opsonic alpha-2 surface binding glycoprotein therapy during sepsis. Ann Surg. 1979;188::521–9.
25. Rapaport FT, Milgrom F, Gesner B, et al. Immunologic sequelae of thermal injury. Ann NY Acad Sci. 1968;150:1004–8.
26. Munster AM, Eurenius K, Katz RM, et al. Cell mediated immunity after thermal injury. Ann Surg. 1973;177:139–43.
27. Polk HC. Prolongation of xenograft survival in patients with pseudomonas sepsis. Surg Forum. 1968;19:514–7.
28. Kay GD. Prolonged survival of a skin homograft in patients with extreme burns. Ann NY Acad Sci. 1957;64:767–74.
29. Ninneman JL, Fisher JC. Prolonged human allograft rejection to the spontaneous immunosuppression following thermal injury. Transplantation. 1978;25:69–72.
30. Miller CL, Baker CC. Changes in lymphocyte activity after thermal injury. J Clin Invest. 1979;63:202–10.
31. Mahler D, Batchelor JR. PHA transformation of lymphocytes in burned patients. Transplantation. 1971;12:409–11.
32. Daniels JC, Sakai H, Cobb ER. Evaluation of lymphocyte reactivity studies in patients with thermal burns. J Trauma. 1971;11:595–601.
33. Munster AM. Post-traumatic immunosuppression is due to activation of suppressor T-cells. Lancet. 1977;1:1319–21.
34. Antonacci AC, Good RA, Gupta S. T-cell subpopulations following thermal injury. Surg Gynecol Obstet. 1982;155:1–8.
35. Miller CL. Effect of surgery on quantity of lymphocyte subpopulations. J Surg Res. 1976;21:155–8.
36. Miller CL, Misholl RT. Differential regulatory effects of accessory cells on CMI. J Immunol. 1975;114:692–5.
37. Eraklis AJ, Kevy SJ, Diamond LK, et al. Hazard of overwhelming infection after splenectomy in childhood. N Engl J Med. 1967;276:1225–9.
38. Singer DB. Postsplenectomy sepsis. Perspect Pediatr Pathol. 1973;1:285–311.
39. O'Neal BJ, McDonald JC. The risk of sepsis in the asplenic adult. Ann Surg. 1981;194:775–8.
40. Sekikawa T, Shatney CH. Septic sequelae after splenectomy for trauma in adults. Am J Surg. 1983;145:667–73.
41. Winkelstein JA, Lambert GH, Swift A. Pneumococcal serum 81: Opsonizing activity in splenectomized children. J Pediatr. 1975;87:430–3.
42. Shumacher MJ. Serum immunoglobulin and transferrin levels after childhood splenectomy. Arch Dis Child. 1970;45:114–7.
43. Constantopoulos A, Najjar VA, Wish JB, et al. Defective phagocytosis due to tuftsin deficiency in splenectomized rats. Am Dis Child. 1973;124:663–5.
44. Bartlett SP, Burton RC. Effects of prophylactic antibiotics on wound infection after elective colon and rectal surgery: 1960 to 1980. Am J Surg. 1983;145:300–9.
45. Shires GT, Dineen P. Sepsis following burns, trauma, and intra-abdominal infections. Arch Intern Med. 1982;142:2012–22.
46. Alexander JW, McGloin JJ, Altemeier WA. Penicillin prophylaxis in experimental wound infections. Surg Forum. 1960;11:299–300.
47. Miles AA, Miles EM, Burke J. The value and duration of defense reactions of the skin to the primary lodgement of bacteria. Br J Exp Pathol. 1957;38:79–96.
48. Burke JF. The effective period of preventive antibiotic action in experimental incisions and dermal lesions. Surgery. 1961;50:161–8.
49. Fullen WD, Hunt J, Altemeier WA. Prophylactic antibiotics in penetrating wounds of the abdomen. J Trauma. 1972;12:282–9.
50. Stone HH, Haney BB, Kolb LD, et al. Prophylactic and preventive antibiotic therapy: Timing, duration and economics. Ann Surg. 1979;189:691–9.
51. Oreskovich MR, Dellinger EP, Lennard ES, et al. Duration of preventive antibiotic administration for penetrating abdominal trauma. Arch Surg. 1982;117:200–5.
52. Nichols RL, Smith JW, Trunkey DD, et al. Clindamycin-gentamicin versus cefoxitin for traumatic fecal soilage of the peritoneum (Abstract). In: Proceedings of the 21st Interscience Conference on Antimicrobial Agents and Chemotherapy. Chicago: 1981.
53. Sandusky WR. Prophylaxis of infection in trauma. In: Mandell GL, Douglas RG, Bennett JE, eds. Principles and Practice of Infectious Diseases. 2nd ed. New York: Churchill Livingstone; 1979:835.
54. Thal ER, Shires GT. Peritoneal lavage in blunt abdominal trauma. Am J Surg. 1973;125:64–71.
55. Shires GT. Trauma. In: Schwartz SI, Shires GT, Spenser FC, et al., eds. Principles of Surgery. New York: McGraw Hill; 1984:202.
56. Olsen WR. The serum amylase in blunt abdominal trauma. J Trauma. 1973;13:200–4.
57. Machiedo GW, Casey KF, Blackwood JM. Colostomy closure following trauma. Surg Gynecol Obstet. 1980;151:58–60.
58. Thal ER, Yeary EL. Morbidity of colostomy closure following colon trauma. J Trauma. 1980;20:287–91.
59. Stone HH, Fabian TL. Management of perforating colon trauma: Randomization between primary closure and exteriorization. Ann Surg. 1979;190:430–6.
60. Flint LM, Vitale GC, Richardson JD, et al. The injured colon: Relationship of management to complications. Ann Surg. 1981;193:619–23.
61. Dunn DL, Nelson RD, Condie RM, et al. Mechanisms of the adjuvant effect of hemoglobin in experimental peritonitis. VI. Effects of stroma-free hemoglobin and red blood cell stroma on mortality and neutrophil function. Surgery. 1983;93:653–9.

62. Caplan ES, Hoyt N. Infection surveillance and control in the severely traumatized patient. Am J Med. 1981;70:638–40.
63. Durtschi MB, Orgain C, Counts GW, et al. A prospective sutdy of prophylactic penicillin in acutely burned hospitalized patients. J Trauma. 1982;22:11–4.
64. Feingold DS. Hospital-acquired infections. N Engl J Med. 1970;283:1384–91.
65. Seibel R, LaDuca J, Hassett JM, et al. Blunt multiple trauma (ISS 36), femur traction, and the pulmonary failure-septic state. Ann Surg. 1985;202:283–93.
66. Goldstein A, Phillips T, Sclafani SJA, et al. Early open reduction and internal fixation of the disrupted pelvic ring. J Trauma. 1986;26:325–33.
67. Alexander JW. Nutrition and infection: New perspectives for an old problem. Arch Surg. 1986;121:966.
68. Deitch EA, Berg RD. Endotoxin but not malnutrition promotes bacterial translocation of the gut flora in burned mice. J Trauma. 1987;27:161–6.
69. Band JD, Maki DG. Safety of changing intravenous delivery systems at longer than 24 hours intervals. Ann Intern Med. 1979;91:173–8.
70. Duma RJ, Warner JF, Dalton HP. Septicemia from intravenous infusions. N Engl J Med. 1971;284:257–61.
71. Maki DG. The prevention and management of device-related infection in infusion therapy. J Med. 1980;11:239–53.
72. Baker CC, Petersen SR, Sheldon GF. Septic phelbitis: A neglected disease. Am J Surg. 1979;138:97–103.
73. Weinstein RA, Stamm WE, Kramer L, et al. Pressure monitoring devices overlooked source of nosocomial infection. JAMA. 1976;236:936–8.
74. Walrath JM, Abbott NK, Caplan E, et al. Stopcock bacterial contamination in invasive monitoring systems. Heart Lung. 1979;8:100–4.
75. Ferguson RL, Rosett W, Hodges GR, et al. Complications with heparin-lock needles. Ann Intern Med. 1976;85:583–6.
76. Stamm WE, Colella JJ, Anderson RL, et al. Indwelling arterial catheters as a source of nosocomial bacteremia: An outbreak caused by *Flavobacterium* species. N Engl J Med. 1975;292:1099–102.
77. Stein JM, Pruitt BA Jr. Suppurative thrombophlebitis: A lethal disease. N Engl J Med. 1976;282:1452–5.
78. Pruitt BA Jr, McManus WR, Kim SH, et al. Diagnosis and treatment of cannula-related intravenous sepsis in burn patients. Ann Surg. 1980;191:546–54.
79. Maki DG, Weise CE, Sarafin HW. A semiquantitative culture method for identifying intravenous catheter-related infections. N Engl J Med. 1977;296:1305–9.
80. Northey D, Adess ML, Hartsuck JM, et al. Microbial surveillance in a surgical intensive care unit. Surg Gynecol Obstet. 1974;139:321–5.
81. Centers for Disease Control. Isolation Techniques for Use in Hospitals. 2nd ed. Washington DC: Government Printing Office; DHEW Publication No. 76-8314. 1976.
82. Ratner M. Surgical repair of the injured spleen. J Pediatr Surg. 1977;12:1019–25.
83. Pachter HL, Hofstetter JR, Spencer FC. Evolving concepts in splenic surgery. Ann Surg. 1981;194:262–9.
84. Wesson DE, Filler RM, Ein SH, et al. Ruptured spleen: When to operate? J Pediatr Surg. 1981;16:324–6.
85. Dickerman JD. Traumatic asplenia in adults. A defined hazard? Arch Surg. 1981;116:361–3.

79. BURNS

ROGER W. YURT
G. TOM SHIRES

The disruption of homeostasis associated with severe burn injury exceeds that of any other injury or disease. With the advent of aggressive early resuscitation measures, mortality in the acute phase after injury is rare.[1] However, the mortality after burns of greater than 40 percent of the body surface area (BSA), which is primarily attributed to infection, continues to be high. Since the risk of developing infection relates directly to the extent of injury, the initial therapeutic approach is oriented toward limiting the progression of the injury by stabilization of the patient and maintenance of blood flow to the wound. The development and progression of the burn wound is well characterized as a dynamic process in which there are irreversible changes in the zone of coagulative necrosis and potentially reversible changes for as long as 3 days in the zones of stasis and hyperemia.[2,3] Since methods of manipulating the inflammatory response that may mediate the progression of the injury are not yet available, the primary goal of early burn therapy is to ensure adequate delivery of oxygen, nutrients, and circulating cells to the wound. Therefore, immediate burn care focuses on prevention of progression of injury and maintenance of a viable interface at which both specific and nonspecific defenses against infection can be mounted.

WOUND AND INFLAMMATORY PATHOPHYSIOLOGY

The evolution of the burn wound is dramatically seen in conversion of partial to full thickness wounds during difficult resuscitations, particularly in patients at the extremes of age in which cardiac output cannot meet the circulatory demand of large surface area injury. In such patients with progressive necrosis and limited defense at the viable tissue interface, early microbial invasion of wounds is to be anticipated. Similarly, decreases in body temperature due to heat loss to the environment or secondary to application of cool solutions or ice to the wound may lead to progressive deterioration of the wounds. Although circulating factors that depress myocardial function after burn injury have been postulated to exist,[4] the primary problem in maintenance of cardiovascular stability is ongoing intravascular volume depletion. Efforts are therefore directed at volume repletion, and α-adrenergic agents in particular are avoided in view of the deleterious result of further diminution of wound blood flow. Likewise, meticulous evaluation of blood flow in extremities with circumferential full thickness injury is necessary to avoid additional compromise of wound and muscular blood flow. When signs of compromised blood flow first appear, escharotomy is performed to diminish the developing pressure in the extremity.

In addition to the culture media provided by the necrotic tissue, the patient with large burns is predisposed to infection due to depression of nonspecific, humoral, and cellular immune function. Circulating levels of immunoglobulins are inversely proportional to the extent of injury,[5] and persistently decreased levels of IgG have been related to mortality.[6] Increased suppressor T-cell activity has been reported,[7,8] the number and function of helper T cells is decreased,[9] and monocyte defects have been reported,[10] leading to the hypothesis that depressed immune response in these patients is due to an imbalance in the cellular immune system. Based on prospective study of patients with large burns, however, it has been suggested that disorders of neutrophil function appear to be the major predisposing factors to the development of sepsis.[11]

That the response of the neutrophil to a site of injury and antigen challenge was depressed in patients with 40 percent or greater total body surface area burn was shown by McCabe et al.[12] using the skin window technique. Such findings of depressed neutrophil response in vivo have been confirmed by quantitating the response to heat-killed *Staphylococcus* in burn-injured patients.[13] The study of the mechanism of decreased neutrophil response to microbial invasion and injury has centered around in vitro study of neutrophil function. The chemotactic response of peripheral blood neutrophils after thermal injury is depressed early after injury in proportion to the extent of tissue damage[14] and correlates with mortality, presumably due to sepsis.[14,15] Although Grogan[15] did not find a factor in burn serum that depressed chemotaxis, others have suggested that such a factor exists and may be related to topical chemotherapy.[16] It has been postulated that consumption of complement components might account for depressed neutrophil response after burn injury[17]; however, even low levels of complement were sufficient to opsonize the invading bacteria.[18] More recent data from an animal model suggests that neutrophils do not respond to the burn wound as well after large burns. However, in vivo evaluation of neutrophil activity indicated that the cells were more responsive than after lesser injury.[19] These findings suggest that "indiscriminant" margination may be occurring after injury. Such a response would lead to depressed appropriate wound response and potentially cause distant tissue damage. Others have described similar events in infected patients and have correlated release of leukocyte enzymes with levels of chemotactic factors produced by complement activation.[20]

PREVENTION OF INFECTION

Although it is common practice to give prophylactic systemic antibiotics (penicillin) to outpatients with burns, current data do not support their general usage in the inpatient population.[21,22] Frequent evaluation of the wound and surrounding tissue allows early and appropriate therapy of cellulitis while sparing a majority of patients exposure to unnecessary antibiotics. However, it is well documented[23] that manipulation of the burn wound leads to bacteremia, and therefore antibiotics are administered immediately before and during burn wound excision. The choice of antibiotics is dictated by knowledge of the current flora in the burn center or more specifically by the burn wound flora of the individual patient. The cyclic nature of particular microorganisms causing burn wound invasion in this center is documented by the results of wound biopsies between January and June of 1982 (Table 1). *Enterobacter cloacae* was frequently isolated but was most prominent in March, April, and June. *Staphylococcus aureus*, which was methicillin-resistant, was most prominent in May, but no isolates were found in April. Based on such data, the current regimen for wound manipulation prophylaxis consists of intravenous vancomycin and amikacin.

The advent of effective topical antimicrobial therapy has decreased the incidence of conversion of partial thickness to full thickness wound by local infection. In addition, these agents may prolong the sterility of the full thickness burn wound; however, they have not eliminated the need for aggressive removal of the necrotic tissue and closure of the wound with autograft. Silver nitrate in a 0.5% solution is an effective topical agent when used before wound colonization. However, since this agent does not penetrate eschar, its broad spectrum gram-negative effectiveness is diminished once bacterial proliferation has occurred in the eschar. Additional disadvantages of this agent include the need for continuous occlusive dressings, which limit evaluation of wounds and range of motion. The black discoloration of the wound, as well as the environment, contributes to a decrease in use of silver nitrate.

The topical burn wound creams allow for open wound therapy and, except in an outpatient setting, are most commonly used without dressings. Mafenide acetate (Sulfamylon) cream has a broad spectrum of activity against gram-negative organisms but little activity against staphylococci. A significant advantage of this agent is that it penetrates the burn eschar and therefore is effective in the colonized wound. The disadvantages of Sulfamylon are transient burning sensation, an accentuation of postinjury hyperventilation, and inhibition of carbonic anhydrase activity. Silver sulfadiazine, on the other hand, is a soothing cream with good activity against gram-negative organisms. Since it does not penetrate the wound, it is best used as a prophylactic antimicrobial. Bacterial resistance to silver sulfadiazine has been reported.[24] Some centers have adopted an approach of alternating agents to take advantage of the attributes of both, such as at Brooke Army Medical Center, where silver sulfadiazine is applied at night and Sulfamylon during the day.[24] The current approach in our center is to initiate topical prophylaxis with silver sulfadiazine and to switch to Sulfamylon if wounds appear to deteriorate based on clinical and laboratory criteria.

TABLE 1. Distribution of Organisms in Burn Wound Biopsies

	Jan	Feb	Mar	Apr	May	June
Number of biopsies	189	141	244	201	162	69
Number of positive biopsies	84[a]	39	85	84	70	41
Enterobacter cloacae	29.8[b]	18.0	37.7	82.1	25.7	39.0
Staphylococcus aureus	27.4	28.2	22.4	0	42.9	17.1
Staphylococcus epidermidis	14.3	5.1	0	3.6	0	0
Enterococcus faecalis	10.7	12.8	4.7	2.4	11.4	17.1
Escherichia coli	7.1	7.6	11.8	6.0	4.3	12.2
Pseudomonas aeruginosa	2.4	5.1	20.0	6.0	8.6	12.2

[a] $\geq 10^5$ organisms/gram tissue.
[b] % of total positive biopsies.

The goal of burn therapy is to prevent burn wound infection by permanent closure of the wound as rapidly as possible. The recognition of the advantages of early removal of necrotic tissue and wound closure has led to an aggressive surgical approach in selected patients.[1] In such cases, full thickness wounds are excised as soon after injury as cardiovascular stability has been achieved. The advantages of this approach include removal of eschar before colonization, which typically is appreciated at 5–7 days after injury, and reduction of the overall extent of injury. The extent of excision of burn wound is usually limited to 20% of the body surface area at any one time, and blood loss is limited to one blood volume. Such an approach is most easily achieved by excision of full thickness injury to the level of the fascia, since blood loss is minimized under these conditions. The open wound is covered with autograft as donor sites are available or with allograft. This is repeated until the entire wound is closed. This aggressive surgical approach is modified by the age of the patient (ideal 15–35 years of age) and factors such as significant pre-existing disease and inhalation injury, which require a more conservative approach to the burn wound.

An additional difficulty with early excisional therapy is that one risks the possibility of excision of burned tissue that may heal if left alone over a 2–3-week period. If such a question arises, initial tangential excision of the eschar or biopsy may assist in evaluating the depth and the possibility of healing of the burn wound. Recent data suggests that a more conservative approach in which operative time is limited to 2 hours and blood loss to four units may contribute to improved survival from extensive burn injury.[25] In an effort to achieve burn wound closure more rapidly, Burke et al.[26] have advocated the use of immunosuppressive therapy to enhance allograft acceptance in children with extensive burns. These patients were kept in bacteria-controlled nursing units to minimize the possibility of infection during immunosuppresion. Attempts to follow a similar protocol in adults have been discouraging.[24]

Throughout the course of hospitalization, efforts are directed toward minimizing contamination of the patient's wounds. Cross-contamination is avoided by use of gowns, gloves, and masks by nursing, medical staff, and visitors. The patient is not touched except with a gloved hand, and each patient is restricted to his or her own monitoring and diagnostic equipment. Concern over the potential for cross-contamination in large burn centers has led to the diminished use of traditional Hubbard tanking of patients. A satisfactory alternative is showering and débridement on a covered or readily disinfected plinth. If adequate nursing care can be provided, it is preferable to isolate patients who have large open wounds in individual rooms. Burke's bacteria-controlled nursing unit[27] has been advocated as a means of protecting the patient and the environment. Such elaborate systems are not generally available.

DIAGNOSIS AND TREATMENT OF INFECTION

Wound Infection

Although surface cultures of burn wounds are helpful from the standpoint of evaluating the potential pathogens that exist on the patient and on a burn ward, they give no indication of the actual status of the wound itself. Biopsy of the wound, however, has been shown to give an accurate indication of the status of the wound.[28] Pruitt and Foley reported that quantitative cultures of 10^5 or more bacteria per gram of tissue or histologic evidence of bacterial invasion of viable tissue correlated with a high (75 percent) mortality rate.[28] In addition, serial biopsies that indicated advancing wound infection were associated with mortality rates of 85 percent, whereas stable or improving wounds were associated with an overall mortality rate of 55 percent. Direct correlation between biopsy and autopsy diagnosis was found in 26 of 32 patients. These data and that of others[29] support systematic evaluation of burn wounds with biopsy of all areas of wound change. Routine biopsy of full thickness burn wound on an every-other-day schedule has allowed detection of progressive wound infections.[30] The rapid fixation technique allows histologic diagnosis of invasive infection within 3 hours, whereas quantitative counts and identification of the organism is available within 24 hours. The combined use of histologic and culture techniques provides early diagnosis as well as identity and sensitivity of the organism to antimicrobials.

A change in wound appearance or character provokes the clinician to modify therapy and stimulates an aggressive diagnostic approach. Hemorrhage, rapid eschar separation, or greenish discoloration of eschar or subeschar fat suggest bacterial colonization or invasion of the wound. If clinical or biopsy data support a diagnosis of colonization, then a change in topical therapy and plans for excision would be entertained (Table 2). However, when the findings are consistent with invasive infection, then more aggressive therapy is instituted. In addition, if bacteremia is documented and other sources are eliminated, urgent surgical intervention is necessary. In the absence of documented bacteremia, signs of sepsis such as hypo- or hyperthermia, hypotension, decreased urinary output, hyperglycemia, thrombocytopenia, or neutropenia or neutrophilia support early intervention. When the wound is invaded with gram-negative organisms, surgical excision to the level of the fascia is the procedure of choice. In preparation for surgery or in those patients who require stabilization before general anesthesia is given, a penetrating topical agent is used (Sulfamylon), and subeschar clysis is initiated using an appropriate antibiotic. The choice of antibiotic is based on previous biopsy sensitivity data or data accumulated on sensitivities of the current flora in the patient population. Such a preoperative approach is based on recent data that indicated that Sulfamylon pulse therapy is effective in decreasing wound colony counts[31] and the previous data of Baxter et al.[30] supporting the efficacy of subeschar clysis. In general, systemic antimicrobials are not necessary, since the full daily dose of antibiotic administered by clysis is absorbed into the circulation. The direct administration of antibiotic into the viable—nonviable tissue interface is supported by concern that systemically administered antibiotics may not reach sufficient levels in the tissues with poor or absent vascularity. There are some data, however, that suggest that antibiotics administered at a distant site are effective[31] and that systemically administered antibiotics reach these tissues. Whether activity of the antimicrobial is maintained in these foci is not known.

In distinction to gram-negative invasion, gram-positive infection often presents as suppurative foci in the tissue or is associated with rapid eschar separation. In such cases, simple débridement with unroofing of involved areas, under the umbrella of appropriate systemic antibiotics, is sufficient acute therapy. Since surgical debridement should arrest this process, topical agents are of lesser importance; however, the wound should not be allowed to dessicate. Silver sulfadiazine, Dakin's solution, and triple antibiotic solutions have been used for this purpose.

Although gram-positive burn wound infection is anticipated to be primarily a suppurative type of infection, there appears to be a growing number of patients who present with primary nonsuppurative gram-positive infections. These infections are caused by methicillin-resistant *Staphylococcus aureus* (personal observation), and whether diminished neutrophil response or a change in the nature or virulence of such organisms[32] may explain this phenomenon is unknown. Burn wound invasion of this type seems to be best treated as are gram-negative invasive infections (Table 2).

Blackened discoloration of the burn wound should arouse suspicion of fungal infection. Such changes are more typical of the phycomycetes.[24] Confirmation of such organisms are best made on histologic sections of wound biopsies, where, in addition, a determination of invasion of viable tissue can be made. Reliance on culture data will prolong the time to diagnosis. Although silver sulfadiazine is active against *Candida* sp., a mixture of this agent or Sulfamylon with Mycostatin may be more effective in the topical therapy of superficial fungal infections. Since fungal infection is often preceded by bacterial infection and multiple antibiotic therapy, the use of Sulfamylon in such a mixture is preferred.[24] The treatment of fungal invasion is surgical excision to the level of noninvaded viable tissue. When invasion extends to the level of the investing fascia, the excision is carried deep to this level to viable muscle.[33] The cytotoxicity of currently available antifungal agents mitigates against their use for preoperative clysis. Recovery of the fungus from the blood mandates systemic therapy, which is often used even without positive blood cultures if invasion is documented and clinical signs are present.

Pulmonary Infection

With the advent of effective topical therapy for the burn wound, pulmonary complications have become a prominent problem in the burned patient.[34] In addition, the ability to salvage an increasing number of patients from the shock phase immediately after injury has led to a greater number of patients surviving to the time (2–3 days postinjury) when the effects of inhalation injury become clinically prominent.[35] In patients without inhalation injury but with large burns, postinjury hyperventilation

TABLE 2. Prophylaxis and Treatment of Burn Wound Infection

Diagnosis	*Topical*	*Clysis*	*Systemic Therapy*	*Surgical*
"Clean" burn	Silver sulfadiazine/ silver nitrate	No	No	Excision/debridement
Superficial/colonization	Silver sulfadiazine/ Sulfamylon	No	No	Excision/debridement
$Gram^-$ invasion	Sulfamylon	Yes	No	Excision to fascia
$Gram^+$ invasion				
Suppurative	Silver sulfadiazine	No	Yes	Unroof
Nonsuppurative		Yes	No	Excision to fascia
Fungus				
Superficial	Sulfamylon/Mycostatin	No	No	Excision
Invasive	Sulfamylon/Mycostatin	No	Yes	Exision to or deep to fascia

and subsequent decreases in tidal volume may lead to atelectasis and subsequent pneumonia. Furthermore, a recognized complication of circumferential full thickness chest burns is a decrease in compliance of the chest wall. Aggressive pulmonary toilet and escharotomy, respectively, are necessary to maintain pulmonary function. Since these patients frequently require large-volume feedings via nasogastric or nasojejunal tubes, aspiration must be guarded against. Diminished mucociliary functions and destruction of airways by inhalation of products of combustion lead to airway obstruction and infection.[36] Frequent diagnostic and therapeutic bronchoscopy are necessary in this group of patients.

Attempts at specific prophylaxis of the sequellae of inhalation injury, such as nebulization of antibiotics[37] and treatment with steroids,[38] have failed to show any benefit. Although hematogenous pneumonia is less frequent than in the past,[34] It remains a significant problem in the patient with burns. When it occurs, the source (most commonly wound or suppurative vein) must be defined and eradicated. Prophylactic antibiotics are not used for either bronchopneumonia or hematogenous pneumonia; specific therapy is based on knowledge of previous endobronchial culture, and sensitivity is substantial by repeat cultures at the time of diagnosis.

Miscellaneous Infections

Several additional types of infection are a significant problem in burned patients and should be mentioned here because of their frequency and peculiarities of clinical presentation. The diagnosis of suppurative thrombophlebitis in the presence of normal tissue (see Ch. 61) is often difficult to make. In the burned patient, the addition of injured and necrotic tissue compounds this difficulty. Less than 35 percent of suppurative veins in burned patients present with local findings.[39] The incidence of this disease in burned patients is at least as high as 5 percent, and the mortality, even in treated suppurative thrombophlebitis, reaches 60 percent.[39] In the absence of a septic venous source, persistent positive blood cultures in the burned patient should be attributed to endocarditis until proven otherwise.

In addition to superficial tissue damaged by direct heat, deeper tissue can be injured and present as a focus of infection. The vascular compromise associated with circumferential full thickness injury if not decompressed early leads to muscle necrosis and subsequent pyomyositis (see Ch. 76). A high index of suspicion is necessary to detect these changes in an already edematous extremity. Direct electrical contact can lead to deep muscular necrosis with delayed infection. Furthermore, significant visceral damage may occur after electrical injury, with subsequent abscess formation.[40]

CONCLUSIONS

The combination of injury-associated immunosuppression and the large area of nonviable tissue in the patient with greater than 30 percent surface area burns inevitably leads to infection. Success in treatment of these patients rests more with removal of necrotic tissue and achieving wound closure than through the use of antimicrobials. Current data support the judicious use of systemic antibiotics for therapy of documented infection and for prophylaxis during burn wound manipulation. The cyclic nature of the rise and fall of various bacteria and the rapid emergence of resistance to antibiotics in the burned patient population supplies ample evidence that there is always a niche that will be filled. Although contamination of the wound must be minimized and surveillance adequate to detect organisms before they invade the wound, closure of the wound is the primary prophylactic and therapeutic maneuver in the care of the burned patient.

REFERENCES

1. Curreri WP, Luterman A, Braun DW, et al. Burn injury analysis of survival and hospitalization time for 937 patients. Ann Surg. 1980;192:472–8.
2. Jackson DM. The diagnosis of the depth of burning. Br J Surg. 1953;40:588–96.
3. Noble HGS, Robson MC, Krizek TJ. Dermal ischemia in the burn wound. J Surg Res. 1977;23:117–25.
4. Baxter CR, Cook WA, Shires GT. Serum myocardial depressant factor of burn shock. Surg Forum. 1966;17:1–2.
5. Arturson G, Hogman CF, Johansson SGO, et al. Changes in immunoglobulin levels in severely burned patients. Lancet. 1969;1:546–8.
6. Munster AM, Hoagland HC, Pruitt BA Jr. The effect of thermal injury on serum immunoglobulins. Ann Surg. 1970;172:965–9.
7. Munster AM. Post-traumatic immunosuppression is due to activation of suppressor T-cells. Lancet. 1977;1:1319–21.
8. Ninnemann JL, Fisher JC. Prolonged human allograft rejection due to the spontaneous immunosuppression following thermal injury. Transplantation. 1978;25:69–72.
9. Antonacci AC, Good RA, Gupta S. T-cell subpopulation following thermal injury. Surg Gyn Obstet. 1982;155:1–8.
10. Shelby J, Merrell SW. In vivo monitoring of postburn immune response. J Trauma. 1987;27:213–6.
11. Alexander JW, Ogle CK, Stinnett JD, et al. A sequential prospective analysis of immunologic abnormalities and infection following severe thermal injury. Ann Surg. 1978;188:809–16.
12. McCabe WP, Rebuck JW, Kelly AP Jr, et al. Leukocyte response as a monitor of immunodepression in burn patients. Arch Surg. 1973;106:155–9.
13. Balch HH, Watters BS, Kelly D. Resistance to infection in burned patients. Ann Surg. 1963;157:1–19.
14. Warden GD, Mason AD Jr, Pruitt BA Jr. Evaluation of leukocyte chemotaxis *in vitro* in thermally injured patients. J Clin Invest. 1974;54:1001–14.
15. Grogan JB. Suppressed *in vitro* chemotaxis of burn neutrophils. J Trauma. 1976;16:985–8.
16. Warden GD, Mason AD Jr, Pruitt BA Jr. Suppression of leukocyte chemotaxis *in vitro* by chemotherapeutic agents used in the management of thermal injuries. Ann Surg. 1975;181:363–9.
17. Bjornson AB, Altemeier WA, Bjornson HS, et al. Host defense against opportunist microorganisms following trauma. I. Studies to determine the association between changes in humoral components of host defense and septicemia in burned patients. Ann Surg. 1978;188:93–101.
18. Bjornson AB, Altemeier WA, Bjornson HS. Complement, opsonins, and the immune response to bacterial infection in burned patients. Ann Surg. 1980;191:323–9.
19. Yurt RW, Pruitt BA. Decreased wound neutrophils and indiscriminate margination in the pathogenesis of wound infection. Surgery. 1985;95:191–8.
20. Solomkin JS, Jenkins MK, Nelson RD, et al. Neutrophil dysfunction in sepsis. II. Evidence for the role of complement activation products in cellular deactivation. Surgery. 1981;90:319–27.
21. Alexander JW: Prophylactic antibiotics in trauma. Am Surg. 1982;48:45–8.
22. Durtschi MB, Orgain C, Counts GW, et al. A prospective study of prophylactic penicillin in acutely burned hospitalized patients. J Trauma. 1982;22:11–4.
23. Sasaki TM, Welch GW, Herndon DN, et al. Burn wound manipulation-induced bacteremia. J Trauma. 1979;19:46–8.
24. Pruitt BA Jr. The burn patient: II. Later care and complications of thermal injury. Curr Probl Surg. 1979;XVI:1–95.
25. Demling RH. Improved survival after massive burns. J Trauma. 1983;23:179–84.
26. Burke JF, Quinby WC, Bondoc CC, et al. Immunosuppression and temporary skin transplantation in the treatment of massive third degree burns. Ann Surg. 1975;182:183–97.
27. Burke JF, Quinby WC, Bondoc CC, et al. The contribution of a bacterially isolated environment to the prevention of infection in seriously burned patients. Ann Surg. 1977;186:377–87.
28. McManus AT, Kim SH, Mason AD, et al. A comparison of quantitative microbiology and histopathology in divided burn wound biopsies. Arch Surg. 1987;122:74–6.
29. Loebl EC, Marvin JA, Heck EL, et al. The method of quantitative burn wound biopsy cultures and its routine use in the care of the burned patient. Am J Clin Pathol. 1974;61:20–4.
30. Baxter CR, Curreri PW, Marvin JA. The control of burn wound sepsis by the use of quantitative bacterial studies and subeschar clysis with antibiotics. Surg Clin North Am. 1973;53:1509–18.
31. McManus WF, Mason AD Jr, Pruitt BA Jr. Subeschar antibiotic infusion in the treatment of burn wound infection. J Trauma. 1980;20:1021–3.
32. Lacey RW, Chopra I. Effect of plasmid carriage on the virulence of *Staphylococcus aureus*. J Med Microbiol. 1975;8:137–47.
33. Levine BA, Sirinek KR, Pruitt BA Jr. Wound excision to fascia in burned patients. Arch Surg. 1978;113:403–7.

34. Pruitt BA Jr, Flemma RJ, DiVincenti FC, et al. Pulmonary complications in burn patients: a comparative study of 697 patients. J Thorac Cardiovasc Surg. 1970;59:7–20.
35. Bingham HG, Gallagher TJ, Powell MD. Early bronchoscopy as a predictor of ventilatory support for burned patients. J Trauma. 1987;27:1286–8.
36. Hunt JL, Agee RN, Pruitt BA Jr. Fiberoptic bronchoscopy in acute inhalation injury. J Trauma. 1975;15:641–9.
37. Levine BA, Petroff PA, Slade CL, et al. Prospective trials of dexamethasone and aerosolized gentamicin in the treatment of inhalation injury in the burned patient. J Trauma. 1978;18:188–93.
38. Welch GW, Lull RJ, Petroff PA, et al. The use of steroids in inhalation injury. Surg Gyn Obstet. 1977;145:539–44.
39. Pruitt BA Jr, McManus WF, Kim SH, et al. Diagnosis and treatment of cannula-related intravenous sepsis in burn patients. Ann Surg. 1980;191:546–54.
40. Newsome TW, Curreri PW, Eurenius K. Visceral injuries: an unusual complication of an electrical burn. Arch Surg 1972;105:494–7.

80. BITES

ELLIE J. C. GOLDSTEIN

Bite wounds are often mistakenly considered innocuous by both patients and physicians. Most data on the incidence of infection, the bacteriology, and the value of various medical and surgical methods of the treatment of bite wounds come from anecdotal case reports and noncomparable and retrospective studies that are further biased by the types of patients who elect to seek medical attention. Consequently, there are diverse approaches to the therapy for these common injuries. Bite wounds consist of lacerations, evulsions, punctures, and scratches. Although many patients never seek or need medical attention, there is a growing awareness of the magnitude of the infectious complications from bites. The bacteria associated with bite infections may come from the environment, from the victim's skin flora, or most frequently, from the "normal" oral flora of the biter.

ANIMAL BITES

It is estimated that 1–2 million people in the United States are bitten by dogs yearly.[1] Although the incidence of bites due to other animals remains undetermined, bite patients account for almost 1 percent of emergency room visits,[2] which results in over $30 million direct medical care costs.[3] Most dog bites are provoked attacks and involve the victim's own pet or a known animal.[4,5] Only 10 percent of attacks are caused by stray animals. Most injuries are caused by large dogs (more than 50 lb)[5] capable of jaw pressures of 200–450 lb/sq in. and result in extensive crush injury.[6] Most victims are men or boys under 20 years old; most incidents occur in the warm-weather months. Over 70 percent of bites are to the extremities, with the right upper extremity the most frequent site. Facial bites are more frequent in children under 10 years old and lead to 5–10 deaths per year, often due to exsanguination.[7]

There appear to be two distinct groups of patients who present for medical care[4]: those who present within 8 to 12 hours after injury and those who present more than 12 hours after injury. The patients in the first group are usually concerned with repair of disfiguring wounds or the need for rabies or tetanus therapy. Most of these patients will have attempted prior therapy, including washing their wounds with soap and water or hydrogen peroxide or applying topical salves. The effect of this first aid on the bacteriology of these wounds or their infection rate, is unknown. These early presenting wounds are almost always contaminated with multiple strains of aerobic and anaerobic bacteria similar to the spectrum found in documented bite infections. Patients who present after 12 hours of injury (often 24–48 hours) usually have established infection.[8–12] It was noted that the risk of infection was increased when the patient was over 50 years old, delayed seeking therapy, or had a puncture wound or a wound to the upper extremity.[8] It was also noted that 16 percent of wounds, including 4 percent of facial wounds, 12 percent of scalp wounds, and 28 percent of hand or arm wounds, later became infected despite various forms of therapy. Other studies note that between 1.6 and 29 percent of "treated" wounds will become infected.[3,4,6,8–14]

Infection is usually manifested by a localized cellulitis, pain at the site of injury, and a purulent discharge, often gray and malodorous. Temperature over 37.2°C, regional adenopathy, and lymphangitis occur in less than 20 percent of patients. Wounds close to bones or joints may penetrate these structures and cause septic arthritis, osteomyelitis, tenosynovitis, or local abscesses in any potential anatomic spaces. Puncture wounds more frequently result in abscess formation. Some patients may develop sepsis, endocarditis, meningitis, or brain abscess secondary to bites.

Several unusual clinical presentations of dog bite infection are recognized. Fiala et al.[15] reported a case of fatal sepsis associated with coagulopathy and renal thrombotic microangiopathy in a compromised host due to *Bacteroides* sp. Several reports have noted fatal infection due to the Centers for Disease Control (CDC)-designated bacteria DF-2 in association with splenectomy or severe hepatic disease.[16–19] This organism may be difficult to isolate and identify and may require up to 14 days of incubation to grow on blood culture. Brucellosis and blastomycosis have also been transmitted by dog bites.[20,21] Women who have undergone modified radical mastectomy may develop lymphangitis and sepsis. Lupus patients and those taking steroids may also have a greater tendency to develop sepsis after bite wounds.

Dog bite wound infections are considered to be predominantly related to the dog's oral flora.[22–25] Studies on the normal canine oral flora note the frequent isolation of *Pasteurella multocida* (12–60 percent), *Staphylococcus aureus* (18–42 percent), coagulase-negative staphylococci (32–40 percent), *Weeksiella zoohelcum* (38–90 percent), EF-4 (up to 74 percent), M5 (10–12 percent), and DF-2 (up to 8 percent). Other species isolated with varying frequency including *Streptococcus, Staphylococcus intermedius, Corynebacterium, Neisseria, Moraxella, Bacillus*, and various gram-negative rods.[26–28, 28a]

In England, Lee and Buhr[11] isolated *P. multocida* in 50 percent of infected dog bites. Other studies note much lower rates of isolation, usually about 20 percent.[4,8,24] Douglas[2] noted *S. aureus, Staphylococcus epidermidis*, and α-hemolytic streptococci to be the most frequently isolated pathogens.

When aerobic and anaerobic cultures are obtained, aerobic (including facultative) and anaerobic bacteria may be isolated from 74 and 41 percent of wounds, respectively.[4] Anaerobic bacteria, when present, were always isolated in mixed culture. Gram stains of the wounds were a specific but nonsensitive predictor of bacterial growth. Sixty-eight percent of noninfected early presenting wounds grew potential pathogens, and 88 percent of infected wounds grew bacterial pathogens. Streptococci were the most frequently isolated bacteria. Other bacteria frequently isolated included *P. multocida* (30 percent), *S. aureus* (30 percent), *Bacteroides* sp. (19 percent), and *Fusobacterium* sp. (19 percent). There was little difference in the types of bacteria isolated from noninfected early-presenting wounds and infected later-presenting wounds. All moderate to severe dog bite wounds, especially to the hands, except those that are not clinically infected and are more than 1 day old should be considered contaminated with potential pathogens.

Wounds inflicted by cats are frequently scratches or tiny punctures located on the lower extremities and are likely to become infected.[29,30] *Pasteurella multocida* has been isolated from the oropharynx of 50–70 percent of healthy cats and is a frequent pathogen in cat-associated wounds.[24,29–31] Tularemia has also been transmitted by cat bites.[32] People are also bitten by a wide variety of other animals, including unusual domestic pets, farm animals, wild animals, and laboratory animals.[2,10,33,34] Monkey bites cause more swelling and infection than do many other animal bites and may transmit B virus (herpesvirus simiae).

Management of Animal Bites

Tear wounds should be copiously irrigated. Puncture wounds may be irrigated by using a 20 ml syringe with a 19 gauge needle attached. Debris should be removed, and skin tags and devitalized tissue should be cautiously, surgically débrided.[35] Whether bite wounds that are clinically uninfected and are seen within 12 hours of injury should be surgically closed remains controversial.[3,4,8,11,35] Hand wounds may present a special situation due to their increased propensity to become infected and the disasterous consequences when infection does occur.

In conflict with most other studies,[4,13,35] one recent prospective study[3] noted the lack of value of early antimicrobial therapy. We feel that since these wounds are usually contaminated with potential pathogens it is advisable to treat hand bites and all bite wounds not trivial in nature with antibiotics. Penicillin (or ampicillin) is the most active agent against *P. multocida* and the other oral aerobic and anaerobic bacteria of dog oral flora. Some feel that amoxicillin/clavulanic acid should be used for empirical therapy since it covers *S. aureus, P. Multocida*, and the anaerobic bacteria likely to be found in bites. Tetracycline is a good alternative for penicillin-allergic patients but should not be used in pregnant women and young children. Erythromycin will be active against only 50 percent of *P multocida* isolates, and anaerobes may be or develop resistance.[36] Clindamycin and the penicillinase-resistant penicillins should be avoided because of their poorer activity against *P. multocida*.[37] Oral first-generation cephalosporins are not as active as penicillin against *P. multocida* and some anaerobes. Cefuroxime axetil, a second-generation oral cephalosporin, and the fluoroquinolones show good activity against *P. multocida* and many other bite isolates.[38] Patients who present early with uninfected wounds should receive antimicrobial therapy for 5 days. Despite the use of the above measures, between 8 and 16 percent of these wounds will become infected.

Patients who present with established infection should be managed similarly. They may need more extensive drainage and surgical débridement. Immobilization and elevation of the injured area is important and even required to achieve optimal healing. Infected wounds should not be closed primarily. Empirical antibiotic therapy should be changed according to specific cultural data and continued for 7–14 days depending on the severity of the infection and patient response.

Tetanus toxoid should be administered to patients requiring a booster. Rabies, cat scratch disease, tularemia, brucellosis, and other animal-associated diseases are discussed in the appropriate chapters.

VENOMOUS SNAKE BITES

Venomous snakes, usually vipers (rattlesnakes, copperheads, cottonmouths, or water moccasins), bite approximately 8000 people in the United States yearly.[39,40] Envenomization can cause extensive tissue destruction and devitalization that predisposes to infection from the snake's "normal" oral flora. Sparse data exist on the incidence and bacteriology of snake bite infections. In rattlesnakes, the oral flora appears to be fecal in nature since their live prey usually defecate in the snake's mouth coincident with ingestion. Common oral isolates include *Pseudomonas aeruginosa, Proteus* sp., coagulase-negative staphylococci, and *Clostridium* sp.[41,42] Other potential pathogens isolated from rattlesnakes mouths include *Bacteroides fragilis* and *Arizona hinshawii*. The role of empirical antimicrobial therapy for noninfected wounds is not well defined. Specific therapy based on cultural data of infected wounds should be instituted.

HUMAN BITES

Human bites have a higher complication and infection rate than do animal bites. Wounds of the lip and paronychia and infections of the structure surrounding the nail account for the majority of self-inflicted bite wounds that come to medical attention. Paronychia are more frequent in children who suck their fingers and result from the direct inoculation of the oral flora into the fingers. Brook[43] took cultures from 33 children with paronychia. Aerobes and anaerobes were each found in pure culture in 27 percent of the cases, whereas mixed infection were found in 46 percent of the cases. The most frequent aerobic organisms isolated were viridans streptococci, group A β-hemolytic streptococci, γ-hemolytic streptococci, *S. aureus, Haemophilus parainfluenzae, Klebsiella pneumoniae,* and *Eikenella corrodens*. The most frequently isolated anaerobic bacteria were *Bacteroides* sp., *Fusobacterium* sp., and anaerobic gram-positive cocci. Therapy should include drainage, appropriate antibiotics, and avoidance of further bacterial contamination.

Occlusional human bites may be to any part of the body but most often involve the distal phalynx of the long and/or index fingers of the dominant hand. Bites to the hand are more serious and more frequently become infected than do bites to other areas.[44–46]

Important prognostic factors for the development of infection include the extent of tissue damage, the depth of the wound and which compartments are entered, and the pathogenicity of the inoculated oral bactera.[45–52] Viridans streptococci were the most common wound isolates. *Staphylococcus aureus* occurred in 40 percent of wounds and was usually present in patients who had attempted self-débridement and presented 3–4 days postinjury. Although *Haemophilus influenzae* was occasionally isolated, no other penicillin-resistant gram-negative rods were isolated. *Bacteroides* sp., excluding *B. fragilis, Peptococcus* sp., *Peptostreptococcus* sp., and *Fusobacterium nucleatum* were also frequent isolates.[48] Up to 45 percent of the *Bacteroides* species isolated from human bite wounds may be penicillin resistant and β-lactamase–positive.[38,53]

Management of Human Bites

A Gram stain and aerobic and anaerobic cultures should be obtained on all infected wounds before any therapy. Wounds should be copiously irrigated, surgically débrided, and diagrammed and/or photographed. Immobilization of the affected area, including splinting if necessary, and elevation should be considered. Empirical antimicrobial therapy should be based on the Gram stain (specific but not sensitive) and/or knowledge of the susceptibility of the oral flora. Patients who present early with uninfected wounds should also be given antimicrobial therapy of shorter duration and may be considered for outpatient management. Penicillin is the drug of choice in bite patients unless *S. aureus* is suspected. In that case amoxicillin/clavulanic acid or penicillin plus a penicillinase-resistant penicillin should be used. First-generation cephalosporins are not as effective as the combination suggested due to resistance of some anaerobic bacteria and *E. corrodens*. Many patients will require hospitalization. Wounds in proximity to the bone should have baseline X-ray films taken to watch for osteomyelitis. Most physicians advise against primary closure even of uninfected human bite wounds, especially those of the hands. Facial wounds may present a special situation due to the possibility of scarring and disfigurement, and many authors recommend primary closure. Approximation of the wound margins or delayed primary closure (3–5 days) is often possible even in infected cases.

CLENCHED-FIST INJURIES

Clenched-fist injuries (CFIs) are traumatic lacerations that occur when one person strikes another in the mouth with a clenched fist. These are most common over the third and fourth metacarpophalangeal joints of the dominant hand, but they may also occur over the proximal interphalangeal joints. These lacerations are often only $\frac{1}{4}$–$\frac{1}{2}$ cm long but, despite their innocuous appearance, frequently lead to serious complications due to the proximity of the skin over the knuckles to the joint capsule and the potential spread of infection into subcutaneous, subfascial, subtendnous, subaponeurotic, and web spaces.

Typically, patients sustain a CFI and attempt to cleanse it or, more usually, ignore it until 3–24 hours postinjury when they awaken with a painful, throbbing, and swollen hand. The swelling usually spreads proximally but not distally and results in a decreased range of motion. A purulent discharge is often present. Lymphangitis, adenopathy, fever, or other signs of systemic infection are infrequent.

The bacteriology of CFIs is similar to that of human bites and usually consists of the normal oral flora. Viridans streptococci are the most frequent isolates, but *S. aureus* may be present in 20–40 percent of cases. Anaerobic bacteria can be recovered in over 55 percent of CFIs including *Bacteroides* sp., *Fusobacterium* sp. and peptostreptococci. *Eikenella corrodens* is an often overlooked but especially important pathogen in CFI infections.[54–59] It has a prevalence rate of 59 percent in human gingival plaque[60] and may be isolated in 25 percent of CFIs.[54] It can act synergistically with viridans streptococci and is a common cause of osteomyelitis. Although *E. corrodens* is susceptible to penicillin, it is resistant to penicillinase-resistant penicillins, clindamycin, and metronidazole and is variably resistant to cephalosporins.[61,62]

Management should include examination by an experienced hand surgeon to evaluate the nerve and muscular function and the extent of injury to tendons, bones, and joints. Débridement and copious irrigation is often required. Elevation and immobilization with a plaster splint from the fingers to the elbow are essential and should be continued until there is marked improvement. Aerobic and anaerobic cultures and x-ray films (to check for fracture and osteomyelitis) should be obtained. Many authors suggest the use of tetanus toxoid or both toxoid and antitoxin when indicated. Secondary débridement to remove necrotic bone and/or tissue or to drain abscesses may be advisable.

Antibimicrobial therapy is often intravenous and should include either cefoxitin or penicillin (or ampicillin) plus a penicillinase-resistant penicillin until cultures return. Failure of first-generation cephalosporins and penicillinase-resistant penicillins, when used alone, have been reported and are often due to *E. corrodens*.[54,55] If *S. aureus* is not present, treatment with the penicillinase-resistant penicillin may be discontinued. If resistant gram-negative rods are isolated, therapy should be altered according to cultural data. What role β-lactamase-positive *Bacteroides* species will have in the selection of antimicrobial therapy remains to be determined.

REFERENCES

1. Klien D. Friendly dog syndrome. NY State J Med. 1966;66:2306.
2. Douglas LG. Bite wounds. Am Fam Physician. 1975;11:93.
3. Elenbaas RM, McNabney WK, Robinson WA. Prophylactic oxacillin in dog bite wounds. Ann Emerg Med. 1982;11:248.
4. Goldstein EJC, Citron DM, Finegold SM. Dog bite wounds and infection: A prospective clinical study. Ann Emerg Med. 1980;9:508.
5. Harris D, Imperato PJ, Oken B. Dog bites—an unrecognized epidemic. Bull NY Acad Med. 1974;50:981.
6. Chambers GH, Payne JF. Treatment of dog-bite wounds. Minn Med. 1969;52:427.
7. Winkle WG. Human deaths induced by dog bites, United States, 1974–1975. Public Health Rep. 1977;92:425.
8. Callaham ML: Treatment of common dog bites: Infection risk factors. J Am Coll Emerg Med 1978;7:83.
9. Graham WP III, Calabretta AM, Miller SH. Dog bites. Am Fam Physician. 1977;15:132.
10. Hubbert WT, Rosen MN. *Pasteurella multocida* infection due to animal bites. Am J Public Health. 1970;60:1103.
11. Lee MLH, Buhr AJ. Dog-bites and local infection with *Pasteurella septica*. Br Med J. 1960;1:169.
12. Schultz RC, McMaster WC. The treatment of dog bite injuries, especially those of the face. *Plast Reconstr Surg*. 1972;49:494.
13. Callaham M. Prophylactic antibiotics in common dog bite wounds: A controlled study. Ann Emerg Med 1980;9:410.
14. Zook EG, Miller M, Van Beek AL, et al. Successful treatment protocol of canine fang injuries. J Trauma. 1980;20:243.
15. Fiala M, Bauer H., Khaleeli M, et al. Dog bite, *Bacteroides* infection, coagulopathy, renal microangiopathy. Ann Intern Med. 1977;87:248.
16. Butler T, Weaver RE, Ramani TKV, et al. Unidentified gram-negative rod infection: A new disease of man. Ann Intern Med. 1977;87:248.
17. Finding JW, Pohlmann GP, Rose H. Fulminant gram-negative bacillemia (DF-2) following dog bite in an asplenic woman. Am J Med. 1980;68:154.
18. Martone WJ, Zuehl RW, Minson GE, et al. Postsplenectomy sepsis with DF-2: Report of a case with isolation of the organism from the patient's dog. Ann Intern Med. 1980;93:457
19. Shankar PS, Scott JH, Anderson CL. Atypical endocarditis due to gram-negative bacillus transmitted by dog bite. South Med J. 1980;73:1640.
20. Swenson RM, Carmichael LE, Cundy KR. Human infection with *Brucella canis*. Ann Intern Med. 1972;76:435.
21. Gann JW Jr, Bressler GS, Bodet CA III, et al. Human blastomycosis after a dog bite. Ann Intern Med. 1983;98:48.
22. Goldstein EJC, Citron DM, Finegold SM. Role of anaerobic bacteria in bite wound infections. Rev Infect Dis. 1984;6(Suppl 1):5177.
23. Branson D, Bunkfeldt F Jr. *Pasteurella multocida* in animal bites of humans. Am J Clin Pathol. 1967;48:552.
24. Francis DP, Holmes MA, Brandon G. *Pasteurella multocida* infections after domestic animal bites and scratches. JAMA. 1975;233:42.
25. Hawkins LG. Local *Pasteurella multocida* infections. J Bone Joint Surg [Am] 1969;55A:363.
26. Baile WE, Stowe EC, Schmitt AM. Aerobic bacterial flora of oral and nasal fluids of canines with reference to bacteria associated with bites. J Clin Microbial. 1978;7:233.
27. Saphir DA, Carter GR. Gingival flora of the dog with special reference to bacteria associated with bites. J Clin Microbiol. 1976;3:344.
28. Nyby MD, Gregory DA, Kuhn DA, et al. Incidence of *Simonsiella* in the oral cavity of dogs. J Clin Microbiol. 1977;6:87.
28a. Talan DA, Goldstein EJC, Staatz D, et al. *Staphylococcus intermedius*: Clinical presentation of a new human dog bite pathogen. Annals Emerg Med. In press (1989).
29. Tindall JP, Harrison CM: *Pasteurella multocida* infections following animal injuries, especially cat bites. Arch Dermatol. 1972;105:412.
30. Lucas GL, Bartlett DH. *Pasteurella multocida* infection in the hand. Plast Reconstr Surg. 1981;67:49.
31. Torpy DE: *Pasteurella multocida* in dog and cat bite infections. Pediatrics. 1969;43:295.
32. Quenzer RW, Mostow SR, Emerson JK. Cat bite tularemia. JAMA. 1977;238:1845.
33. Dawson J, Cockel R. *Actinobacillus lingieresii* infection after a horse bite. Br Med J. 1981;283:583.
34. Marrie TJ, Bent JM, West AB, et al. Extensive gas in tissues of the forearm after horsebite. South Med J. 1979;72:1473.
35. Callaham M: Dog bite wounds. JAMA. 1980;244:2327.
36. Goldstein EJC, Citron DM, Richwald GA. Lack of in vitro efficacy of oral forms of certain cephalosporins, erythromycin and oxacillin against *Pasteurella multocida*. Antimicrob Agent Chemother. 1988;32:213.
37. Stevens DL, Higbee JW, Oberhofer TR, et al. Antibiotic susceptibility of human isolates of *Pasteurella multocida*. Antimicrob Agents Chemother. 1979;16:322.
38. Goldstein EJC, Citron DM. Comparative activity of cefuroxime, amoxicillin/clavulanic acid, ciprofloxacin, enoxacin and ofloxacin against aerobic and anaerobic bite wound bacteria. Antimicrob Agent Chemother. 1988;32:1143.
39. Parish HM. Incidence of treated snake bites in the United States. Public Health Rep. 1966;81:269.
40. Russell FE. Clinical aspects of snake venom poisoning in North America. Toxicon. 1969;7:33.
41. Goldstein EJC, Citron DM, Gonzalez H, et al. Bacteriology of rattlesnake venom and implications for therapy. J Infect Dis. 1979;140:818.
42. Williams FE, Freeman M, Kennedy E. The bacterial flora of the mouths of Australian venomous snakes in captivity. Med J Aust. 1934;2:190.
43. Brook I. Bacteriology study of paronychia in children. Am J Surg. 1981;141:703.
44. Mann RJ, Hoffeld TA, Farmer CB. Human bites of the hand: Twenty years of experience. J Hand Surg. 1977;2:97.
45. Welch CE: Human bite infections of the hand. New Engl J Med. 1936;215:901.
46. Boland FK: Morsus humanis. JAMA. 1941;116:127.
47. Barnes MN, Bibby BG. A summary of reports and a bacteriologic study of infections caused by human tooth wounds. J Am Dent Assoc. 1939;26:1163.
48. Goldstein EJC, Citron DM, Wield B, et al. Bacteriology of human and animal bite wounds. J Clin Microbiol. 1978;8:667.
49. Chuinard RG, D'Ambrosia RD. Human bite infections of the hand. J Bone Joint Surg [Am]. 1977;59:416.

50. Guba AM, Mulliken JB, Hoopes JE. The selection of antibiotics of human bites of the hand. Plast Reconstr Surg. 1975;56:538.
51. Peeples E, Boswick JA Jr, Scott FA. Wounds of the hand contaminated by human and animal saliva. J Trauma. 1980;20:383.
52. Shields C, Patzakis MJ, Meyers MJ, et al. Hand infections secondary to human bites. J Trauma. 1975;15:235.
53. Brook I. Microbiology of human and animal bite wounds in children. Pediatr Infect Dis. 1987;6:29.
54. Goldstein EJC, Miller TA, Citron DM, et al. Infections following clenched-fist injury: A new perspective. J Hand Surg. 1978;3:455.
55. Goldstein EJC, Barone M, Miller TA. *Eikenella corrodens* in hand infections. J Hand Surg. 1983;8:563.
56. Bilos ZJ, Kaucharchuk A, Metzger W. *Eikenella corrodens* in human bites. Clin Orthop. 1978;134:320.
57. Carruthers MM, Sommers HM. *Eikenella corrodens* osteomyelitis. Ann Intern Med. 1973;79:900.
58. Johnson SM, Pankey GA. *Eikenella corrodens* osteomyelitis, arthritis and cellulitis of the hand. South Med J. 1976;69:535.
59. McDonald I: *Eikenella corrodens* infections of the hand. Hand. 1979;11:224.
60. Goldstein EJC, Tarenzi LA, Agyare EO, et al. Prevalence of *Eikenella corrodens* in dental plaque. J Clin Microbiol. 1983;17:636.
61. Goldstein EJC, Sutter VL, Finegold SM. Susceptibility of *Eikenella corrodens* to ten cephalosporins. Antimicrob Agents Chemother. 1978;14:639.
62. Goldstein EJC, Gombert ME, Agyare EO: Susceptibility of *Eikenella ccrrodens* to newer beta-lactam antibiotics. Antimicrob Agents Chemother. 1980;18:832.

SECTION K. GASTROINTESTINAL INFECTIONS AND FOOD POISONING

81. PRINCIPLES AND SYNDROMES OF ENTERIC INFECTION

RICHARD L. GUERRANT

Gastrointestinal infections encompass a wide variety of symptom complexes and recognized infectious agents. With the exception of recently recognized *Campylobacter pylori* gastritis, the term *gastroenteritis* is applied to syndromes of diarrhea or vomiting that tend to involve noninflammatory infection in the upper small bowel or inflammatory infection in the colon. Other enteric infections and infestations cause predominantly systemic symptoms. Infections of the gastrointestinal tract, especially infectious diarrhea, are among the most common debilitating infectious diseases, afflicting people of all ages around the world. In many heavily populated areas, deaths from diarrheal illnesses exceed those from any other single cause.

In the absence of demonstrable causal forces, many descriptive terms have arisen through the years. Names such as "Montezuma's revenge," "Delhi belly," "Aden gut," "gyppi tummy," "Aztec two-step," "Greek gallop," "Rome runs," "Hong Kong dog," "Turkey trots," "La turista," "Basra belly," and "back door sprint" illustrate its widespread occurrence. Although an etiologic agent is not found in many cases, the infectious nature of most acute diarrheal diseases is suggested by their epidemiologic behavior showing case clustering, spread in families and other groups, and occurrence among travelers. In the last two decades, much has been learned about bacterial and viral agents capable of causing acute gastrointestinal illnesses. These include *Escherichia coli* that produce enterotoxins, which cause fluid secretion, other *E. coli* capable of causing tissue destruction and inflammation, newly appreciated and increasingly recognized pathogens such as *Yersinia*, *Campylobacter*, *Clostridium*, *Cryptosporidium*, rotaviruses, and Norwalk-like viruses. With the development of new tools for diagnosis, important information has been gained in our understanding of the etiologies, pathogenesis, epidemiology and control of acute gastrointestinal infections.

OCCURRENCE AND SCOPE OF GASTROINTESTINAL INFECTIONS

On a global scale, diarrheal diseases constitute the greatest single cause of morbidity and mortality,[1] far exceeding that from heart disease, cancer, or strokes in many populous areas.[2] The greatest mortality from diarrheal diseases and enteric infections occurs in infants and small children. Over 13 percent of the children born in certain parts of Latin America die before their fifth birthday. In more than half, diarrhea is the major or associated cause of death.[3] Although the global mortality is decreasing (especially with oral rehydration therapy),[4] some transitional areas have a worsening diarrhea mortality,[5] and prolonged diarrhea is emerging as the major cause of death.[6] In areas such as Bangladesh, Guatemala, and Brazil, the attack rates often exceed seven cases per person per year among children under 2 years of age.[7–10] The attack rate is highest at the time of weaning.[8–11] Studies from rural India reveal an annual death rate of 5.36 percent for children in their second 6 months of life.[11] Enteric infections doubtless account for a much larger submerged iceberg of morbidity, especially in association with malabsorption and malnutrition in the tropical developing world. Over 60 percent of the children dying with diarrhea in Latin America also had nutritional deficiencies as associated causes of death, suggesting that diarrhea may precipitate malnutrition.[3] Acute infectious diarrhea exacerbates nutritional deficiencies in several ways. As with any acute infection, caloric demands are increased and often catabolic steroids, glucagon, and adrenergic amines cause increased breakdown of structural proteins.[11] Through vicious cycles of transient malabsorption and anorexia, repeated bouts of acute diarrhea are major contributors to malnutrition.[12–16] The converse is also true; undernutrition appears to reduce resistance to acute infectious diarrhea. Increased attack rates and increased mortality from acute infectious diarrheal illnesses occur with progressive severity of malnutrition.[16–18] As a specific example, shigellae are shed longer and there is an increased relapse rate in children if they are malnourished.[17] In addition, malnutrition appears to predispose to more prolonged diarrheal illnesses.[19]

Military history indicates that acute diarrheal illnesses have played decisive roles in numerous campaigns. Diarrheal diseases and enteric infections comprised the major nontraumatic cause of hospitalization among U.S. troops in Vietnam and approached the number of hospitalizations resulting from injuries due to hostile action.[20] Although the mortality in the United States from diarrheal disease has been dramatically reduced with economic development and improved sanitation facilities in the last 50 years, diarrhea remains the third most frequent syndrome seen in general practice.[21] In studies of community illness among urban and suburban families in Cleveland, Dingle et al. identified "infectious gastroenteritis" as the second most common class of illnesses after common respiratory diseases.[22] In this community 1.5 bouts of gastroenteritis occurred per person each year and accounted for 16 percent of all illnesses. Although causative agents were not identified, the infectious nature of these diarrheal and febrile vomiting illnesses were confirmed by their passage to volunteers via stool filtrates. Data relevant to the epidemiology of diarrheal illnesses (even when the cause is unknown) can be applied to the prevention and control of the varied syndromes of gastrointestinal infections.[23]

EPIDEMIOLOGIC AND ENVIRONMENTAL FACTORS

The frequency, type, and severity of enteric infections are determined by *who* you are, *where* you are, and *when* you are there.

Who is at risk of acquiring a gastrointestinal infection varies greatly with age, living conditions, personal and cultural habits, and group exposures. Although the infant who is being breast-fed is relatively protected from contaminated food and water and probably to some degree by maternal colostral antibodies and lactoferrin, at weaning there is a great increase in the risk of diarrheal illness. Adults, particularly if living for many years in the same environment, may become asymptomatic reservoirs of microorganisms that cause diarrhea in the immunologically untutored child or visitor. Living conditions often reflect socioeconomic conditions; type of housing, crowding, sanitation facilities, and water sources are major determinants of environmental exposure to enteric pathogens. The quantity of water available for hygienic and sanitation purposes is often as important as the quality of the water supply.[24] Personal hygienic habits determine how many organisms are ingested. Although the infectious dose varies with the organisms, relatively small inocula of certain organisms may result in disease. Shigellae are acquired with an unusually low infectious dose and are often spread by direct contact among children in day care centers. The majority of nonspecific diarrheal illnesses acquired in communities occur in family clusters, often with small children having the first illness. Of great importance whenever a patient has an enteric illness is a careful history of other illnesses in the family or community. Multiple illnesses and common exposure may be clues to a food-borne outbreak or to the causative agent.

The second epidemiologic determinant of risk for enteric infection is *where* one is. The pattern of illnesses and the etiologic agents vary greatly with climate. For example, *E. coli* that produce heat-labile or heat-stable (LT or ST) enterotoxins cause disease primarily in the tropics, where the heaviest burden of parasites also occurs. Viral causes of common enteric illlnesses have recently been found among young children in temperate and tropical climates. Despite their clustering, however, many community cases of diarrhea remain unexplained.

Finally, the third determinant of risk is *when* you are there. The majority of enteric illnesses in temperate climates occur during winter months. The opposite is true in tropical countries, where distinct summer peaks of illnesses are usual. The role of rainfall is uncertain, as some adjacent areas with similar monsoon climates have opposite seasons of major diarrheal illnesses, as illustrated by the peak seasons for cholera in different parts of Bengal. In Dhaka, endemic cholera consistently occurs during the winter dry months, whereas less than 200 miles away, the peak cholera season in Calcutta occurs during the summer monsoon.

HOST FACTORS

Considering the ubiquity of potential enteric pathogens, it is surprising that enteric infections are not even more common. After exposure to infectious agents, several host factors determine who becomes ill. Several enteric host defenses provide substantial protection against many intestinal pathogens (Table 1).

Host Species, Genotype and Age

Host species, genotype, and age are complex but major determinants of susceptibility to colonization and disease with enteric pathogens. While a broad spectrum of animal hosts are infected with pathogens such as *Salmonella enteritidis* and *Campylobacter jejuni*, only primates or humans are characteristically infected with *Salmonella typhi* or *Shigella* spp. In addition, the intestinal cell receptors for the K88, K99, and colonization factor (CF) attachment traits of enterotoxigenic *E. coli* are largely species specific.[25,26] Interspecies variation and host genotype are also important. Certain ABO blood groups in humans are associated with *Vibrio cholerae* infections.[27,28] Furthermore, Rutter et al. have bred a strain of piglets that do not have the single-locus dominant allele for the intestinal receptor for *E. coli* K88 adherence antigen and are consequently resistant to diarrhea caused by these organisms.[29] Such species or even genotype specificities play tremendously important roles in determining the host susceptibility as well as the epidemiology of these infections.

The role of age in determining host susceptibility is complex. In animals a narrow "age window" of susceptibility to specific enteric infections is well recognized. In humans, the tendency of rotaviral and enteropathogenic *E. coli* (EPEC) infections to affect young children is impressive. The explanations likely reside in age-related changes in gut mucus, cell surface factors, microbial flora, environmental exposure, and specific immune factors. In addition, specific receptors for microbial adhesins or toxins may be developmentally regulated, such as that recently described for *Shigella* toxin in rabbits.[30]

Specific receptor components or antagonists such as monosaccharides like *N*-acetyineuraminic acid (NANA) can be added exogenously and compete with intestinal binding sites for *E. coli*.[26,31] Conversely, lectin-like substances that bind to the intestinal cell receptors may compete with the bacterial attachment factors. Positive chemotaxis of *V. cholerae, E. coli* and *S. typhimurium* has been shown toward rabbit ileal mucosa and a role of negative chemotactic factors have been postulated as new types of host defense.[32]

Personal Hygiene

Whether or not we acquire an enteric infection depends first on the number of pathogens ingested. Nearly all agents of concern are acquired by the oral route. The majority of identified enteric pathogens have come from other mammalian intestinal tracts; often a human fecal–oral route can be traced. A plentiful, conveniently located supply of uncontaminated water, in conjunction with improved sanitary facilities, is critically important

TABLE 1. Enteric Host Defenses

Host species, genotype, and age
Personal hygiene
Gastric acidity and other physical barriers
Intestinal motility
Enteric microflora
Specific immunity
Phagocytic
Humoral
Cell mediated
Nonspecific protective factors and human milk
Intestinal receptors

in reducing this mode of spread.[24,33] Studies of presumptive viral agents that have not yet been defined (the "Marcy" and "Family Study" agents) strongly implicate the human fecal–oral route of infection.[34,35] In the cases of bacterial infections, a large number (100,000–100,000,000) of organisms must usually be ingested to overcome host defenses and to cause disease[36] (Table 2). Such numbers may require growth in food that is allowed to stand unrefrigerated for several hours after the initial contaminating inoculum. Exceptions to the large number of organisms usually required for an infecting dose are *Shigella* and cysts of certain parasites, which can be reproducibly transmitted with only 10–100 organisms. This small inoculum can be readily transmitted directly by person-to-person contact (as in day care centers). This is an unusual route of spread for other bacterial enteric pathogens in all but hosts with impaired defenses or newborn infants.

Gastric Acidity and Other Physical Barriers

The majority of bacterial pathogens ingested never reach the intestines because of the normal gastric acid barrier. When this barrier is neutralized with antacids, both the susceptibility and severity of several enteric bacterial and parasitic infections is increased. At the normal gastric pH (<4), over 99.9 percent of the ingested coliform bacteria are killed within 30 minutes. There is no reduction of an experimental bacterial inoculum in achlorhydric stomachs for 1 hour. Not surprisingly then, the gastric coliform flora in fasting subjects (normally fewer than 10/ml) exceed 10,000/ml in the majority of achlorhydric patients.[37] Excessive numbers of normal bacterial flora in the upper small bowel may contribute to malabsorption and diarrheal syndromes.[38,39]

The inoculum of *V. cholerae* required to cause disease can be reduced 10,000-fold (from 10^8 to 10^4 organisms) by neutralizing gastric acid with 2 g of sodium bicarbonate.[40] In an outbreak of cholera in Israel, 25 percent of the patients had had previous gastric resection, whereas none of a comparable control group had had gastric surgery.[41] The similar association of previous gastric surgery or achlorhydria with increased frequency and severity of *Salmonella* infections has also been noted in several studies.[42] Likewise, the frequency of enteric multiplication of a vaccine strain of *Shigella flexneri* increases threefold with sodium bicarbonate neutralization of gastric acid. With *Campylobacter jejuni*, a substantial range in infectious doses has been documented with different strains.[43] Although gastric acidity may enhance the process of excystation and infection by some parasites after ingestion of the ova, it may provide protection against other parasites. The fragile trophozoite of *Giardia lamblia* (requiring a pH of 6.4–7.1) causes more severe symptoms in association with hypochlorhydria or achlorhydria, perhaps by increased survival of trophozoites refluxed to the stomach and proximal duodenum. The association of achlorhydria and hypochlorhydria with symptomatic strongyloidiasis and other helminthic of the gastric mucosa has also been noted. Some have suggested that vitamin B_{12} deficiency occurs more often in association with fish tapeworm (*Diphyllobothrium latum*) in patients who are achlorhydric and who have high jeujunal infestations. Finally, certain parasitic, viral, or bacterial processes such as *Campylobacter pylori* infections may in themselves alter gastric acidity and thus increase host susceptibility to other enteric pathogens. The further importance of gastric acidity in preventing gastric, pharyngeal, and tracheal colonization by gram-negative bacilli and even nosocomial pneumonia has been shown by the increased risk of patients taking antacids or H2 blockers compared to sucralfate, which preserves gastric acidity.[44]

Other physical barriers such as mucus and mucosal tissue integrity are important resistance factors in healthy hosts and work in concert with gastric acidity and intestinal motility to clear many bacteria from the upper small bowel.[45] Continuous removal and renewal of gastrointestinal mucus may bind organisms and toxins and further aid in protecting the intact mucosa from enzymatic and microbial attack.[46]

TABLE 2. Infectious Doses of Enteric Pathogens

Shigella	10^{1-2}
Campylobacter jejuni	10^{2-6}
Salmonella	10^5
Escherichia coli	10^8
Vibrio cholerae	10^8
Giardia lamblia	10^{1-2} cysts
Entamoeba histolytica	10^{1-2} cysts

Intestinal Motility

Intestinal motility plays the following important roles in normal intestinal physiology: (*1*) in the fluid absorptive process, (*2*) in maintaining the appropriate distribution of indigenous enteric microflora, and (*3*) in ridding the host of pathogenic microorganisms. The role of motility in aiding fluid absorption has been demonstrated in a study done on human volunteers by Higgins et al.[47] Using methantheline bromide (Banthine), they showed that inhibition of normal intestinal motility resulted in impaired absorption of radiolabeled water and sodium. Whereas over 90 percent of a labeled saline bolus was normally absorbed in less than 10 minutes, less than 70 percent was absorbed over a half hour after methantheline bromide administration. Intraluminal distribution of a barium bolus in small bowel before and after methantheline bromide suggested that a reasonable explanation for this impaired absorption was a reduction in the absorptive surface area exposed to the intralumenal fluid. In contrast to the distribution within 2–3 minutes of the bolus of barium throughout the small bowel of healthy persons, methantheline bromide caused a puddling of barium near the injection site in the upper small bowel, which often persisted for over 60 minutes.

Motility also helps to maintain normal distribution and flow of microflora. The risk of bowel stasis is evident in the bacterial overgrowth syndromes in the small bowel and in the added risk of "toxic megacolon" in inflammatory bowel disease after antimotility drugs are administered.

In addition, intestinal motility appears to play a role in providing protection from enteric pathogens. Experimental animals are much more easily infected with enteric pathogens after the inhibition of gut motility with opiates.[48] *Salmonella* bacteremia may develop in patients after opiates are taken for relatively mild gastroenteritis.[49] A controlled study of adults with shigellosis treated with diphenoxylate hydrochloride with atropine (Lomotil) revealed that the antimotility drug abolished antibiotic effectiveness in reducing diarrhea and positive cultures and was associated with prolonged fever and shedding of the *Shigella* organisms.[50] Gut motility and diarrhea that help rid the host of offending pathogens may therefore be analogous to the cough in pulmonary infections as a mechanism to expel pathogens.

Normal Enteric Microflora

In recent years, there have been several developments in our understanding of the composition of intestinal microflora. With improved culture techniques[51] we now recognize that 99.9 percent of the normal enteric bacterial flora are anerobes (approximately 10^{11} organisms/g of normal feces). These organisms (*Bacteroides*, clostridia, peptostreptococci, peptococci, and others) far exceed the number of aerobes. The gram-negative aerobic coliform rods follow—*E. coli*: 10^8/g; *Klebsiella*, *Proteus*, enterococci, and other species: approximately 10^{5-7}/g. We are only beginning to appreciate the role of normal flora as an extremely important and often overlooked host defense. In several situations normal bacterial flora can be shown to be highly effective in resisting colonization by potentially pathogenic invaders. The loss of normal flora or a shift in their balance by antibiotics is often attended with their replacement by organisms such as *Pseudomonas*, *Klebsiella*, *Clostridium*, and *Candida*. When these organisms take up residence, there is a risk of their causing serious systemic infections, especially in a nosocomial setting. There are numerous examples of the increased susceptibility to infection of patients with reduced bacterial flora.[52,53] Several enteric infections, such as infant botulism, nosocomial salmonellosis, and enteropathogenic *E. coli*, occur with increased frequency in newborn infants who have not acquired a normal enteric flora. Diarrhea associated with the use of antibiotics is common and, in many cases, is likely related to an alteration in the balance of normal enteric microflora.

The basis for the resistance provided by normal bacterial flora in the intestinal tract has been elucidated in an elegant series of studies by Bohnhoff et al.[54] In experimental mice, the protective effect of normal flora is eradicated by a single injection of streptomycin. They showed that an infecting dose of *Salmonella typhimurium* was reduced over 100,000-fold by the administration of a single dose of streptomycin. This reduced resistance correlated with the reduction in the normal colonic flora and their toxic acidic products. Resistance was restored with the return of enteric flora (especially *Bacteroides*), either by inoculation or naturally. The importance of a reduced pH and volatile fatty acids from the anaerobic flora in colonization resistance has been further shown by Van der Waaj et al.[55] and by Que et al.[56] It has been shown that indigenous microbes such as *Lactobacillus*, *Bacteroides*, and *Clostridium* spp. attach to the intestinal epithelial surface and act synergistically with host immunity to interfere with experimental *S. typhimurium* challenge.[57] Enteric bacteria including *Proteus*, *Enterobacter*, and *E. coli* also act synergistically in mice with vibriocidal immunity from vaccination to antagonize *V. cholerae*.[58] The protective role of normal enteric bacterial flora in humans has been documented by the increased frequency of *Salmonella* infections among Swedish tourists who took a prophylactic antibiotic compared with those who took no antimicrobial agent.[53] In a huge outbreak of antimicrobial-resistant *S. typhimurium* enteritis involving nearly 200,000 people in Illinois in the spring of 1985, there was a significant association of illness with having taken antimicrobials the month before the illness. There was a fivefold increase (from 6 percent of well controls to 30 percent) of persons having taken antibiotics to which the outbreak strain was resistant.[59]

Intestinal Immunity

Enteric immunity is composed of phagocytic, humoral, and cell-mediated elements. Each component has specific contributions to host resistance to enteric infections. The normal intestinal mucosa demonstrates a state of "physiologic inflammation" in the lamina propria with numerous neutrophils, macrophages, plasma cells, and lymphocytes that suggest a constant battle of the host with luminal challenges to maintain the integrity of the mucosa. The importance of intact phagocytic immunity becomes evident when neutrophils are absent in hosts, who then become particularly susceptible to gram-negative rod infections that often originate in the gastrointestinal tract.[60] The importance of immunity is also demonstrated by the potentially severe adenoviral, rotaviral, coxsackieviral, and *Clostridium difficile* infections in bone marrow transplant patients.[61]

Diarrhea in patients with the acquired immunodeficiency syndrome (AIDS) is becoming increasingly common and raises a special set of diagnostic and therapeutic questions. The growing range of severe, recurring enteric infections in immunocompromised patients,[62] especially those with AIDS, demonstrates the critical role of immunity in resisting a broad range of viral, bacterial, parasitic, and fungal enteric infections. The majority of AIDS patients with diarrhea have a documentable infectious etiology such as cytomegalovirus, *Entamoeba histolytica*, *Cryptosporidium*, *Salmonella*, *Giardia*, *C. jejuni*, *Shigella*, *Mycobacterium* or Herpes simplex virus.[63,64] In Haiti and Africa, up to 95 percent of AIDS patients initially present with diarrhea; up to 50 percent may have *Crytosporidium* infections, followed by 15 percent with *Isospora belli*.[65–67] Still other patients may have the human immunodeficiency virus, which infects the bowel epithelium.[68]

Specific active humoral intestinal immunity (so-called coproantibody) arises either from a leakage of serum immunoglobulin (predominantly IgG or IgM) or from the formation of IgA by plasma cells located predominantly in the lamina propria. Secretory IgA (an 11S dimer [MW 390,000] with a secretory piece [MW 60,000] from the mucosal epithelial cells) is found in the lumen.[69] Both serum and secretory antibody responses have been demonstrated in response to parenteral and intraluminal challenge with cholera toxoid.[70] Secretory IgA is resistant to intraluminal degradation by enzymatic proteolysis and sulfhydryl reduction. The dynamics of local intestinal immunity have been elucidated in several experimental models. The most efficient method of eliciting a local antibody response is with a parenteral priming challenge followed by an intestinal booster antigen challenge. Studies of cholera toxoid immunity in rats suggest that the parenteral priming toxoid prepares a widespread distribution of precursor lymphocytes in areas like the Peyer's patches.[71] These cells are then capable of responding to a booster challenge to produce many large IgA-bearing lymphocytes that appear in the thoracic duct before "homing" back to the lamina propria as specific IgA-secreting plasma cells at or distal to this site of booster toxoid. Passively acquired IgA probably accounts for part of the protection against enteric infections in infants who are breast-fed. Colostral antibody against rotaviruses and the enterotoxins of *V. cholerae* and *E. coli* have been demonstrated in breast milk.[72,73]

Intestinal antibodies may be directed at any of a number of different bacterial antigens such as endotoxin, capsular material, or exotoxins and may have bactericidal, opsonic, or neutralizing effects. Although IgA can have hemagglutinating, precipitating, or virus-neutralizing properties, it does not appear capable of fixing complement in order to have the direct bactericidal effect that IgG and IgM may have. Selective IgA deficiency is often associated with a compensatory increase in IgM levels. Hereditary telangiectasia with IgA deficiency is associated with recurrent rhinopulmonary infection but is rarely associated with intestinal infection or dysfunction.[69] Although debated by others,[74] Zinneman and Kaplan[75] and Ament et al.[76] have suggested that patients with giardiasis have lower IgA levels and that hypogammaglobulinemic patients have more malabsorption and diarrhea with giardiasis. Patients with type 2 combined IgA and IgM deficiency and small intestinal lymphoid hyperplasia with a sparsity of plasma cells may have diarrhea, malabsorption, and giardiasis.[77] Crabbe and Heremans have described three patients with another type of selective IgA deficiency with spruelike intestinal symptoms and histopathologic changes.[78] The role of cell-mediated immune processes in the intestine is suggested by adjuvant enhancement of vaccine efficacy against intracellular infections such as *S. typhi*.[79]

Other Protective Factors in Human Milk and Serum

The protection afforded by breast-feeding likely relates to several passively transmitted factors, as well as to reduced exposure to a contaminated environment.[8–13,80,81] In addition to antibody, these include lactoferrin, lysozyme, phagocytes, high lactose, low protein, low phosphate, and low pH (in part from bifidobacteria).[80–85] The role of lactoferrin in human milk is suggested by the abolition of milk's bacteriostatic properties against *V. cholerae* and enteropathogenic *E. coli* by saturation with iron.[85] In addition, patients with chronic iron excess from hemolytic processes such as malaria, sickle cell anemia, and Oroya fever are at increased risk of infection with organisms such as *Salmonella*. Some of the bacteriostatic properties of normal serum were abolished when iron-binding proteins were saturated with iron.[85]

MICROBIAL FACTORS

A number of bacterial virulence traits determine the pathogenic mechanisms responsible for diarrhea. This entire range of traits is demonstrated by the various types of *E. coli*, as summarized in Table 3. This versatile species may represent the predominant normal colonic flora or may be a urinary or enteric pathogen. Depending largely on the transmissible virulence traits encoded on plasmids or phage, *E. coli* may produce one of three families of enterotoxins (LT, STa, or STb), may be invasive (EIEC), may cause hemorrhagic colitis (EHEC), or may exhibit three or four distinct types of adherence (class I and II EPC, with or without the plasmid-encoded focal HEp-2 cell enteroadherence factor, EAF; autoagglutinating enteroadherent *E. coli*, EAEC; and *E. coli* with one of the recognized or new colonization traits, CFAI, CFAII, E8775, 260-1, and 0159:H4). Study of *E. coli* with these varied pathogenic traits have greatly helped to unravel the way that enteric pathogens alter normal intestinal absorptive function to cause diarrheal diseases.[86–88]

Toxins

Toxic microbial components or products are implicated in the disease-producing capacity of several enteric pathogens. Culture filtrates of toxigenic microorganisms are capable of altering gastrointestinal structure or function in the absence of the organisms themselves. Toxins produced by enteric pathogens can be classified as *neurotoxins*, *enterotoxins*, or *cytotoxins* (Table 4). Neurotoxins are usually ingested as preformed toxins that often cause enteric symptoms. These include staphylococcal, *Bacillus cereus*, and botulinal toxins. Although staphylococcal food poisoning is an abrupt upper gastrointestinal syndrome attributed to staphylococcal enterotoxin, the effect appears to be due to the action of this toxin on the central autonomic nervous system rather than to destruction or fluid secretion in the intestine per se.[89] An exotoxin related to entertoxin A may cause fluid accumulation in rabbit ileal loops directly.[90,91] A different staphylococcal α-toxin elicits hyperperistalsis. Certain strains of *B. cereus* isolated from patients with acute food poisoning also produce a highly heat-stable emetic toxin (especially when cultured with rice) that is a small (Mr <5000), nonantigenic polypeptide capable of causing vomiting in monkeys, much like staphylococcal enterotoxin.[92,93] Botulinal toxin has a primary effect on the neuromuscular junction to prevent the release of acetylcholine from the presynaptic vesicle.[89]

True *enterotoxins* are defined as having a direct effect on the intestinal mucosa to elicit net fluid secretion. The classic enterotoxin, choleratoxin, has been extensively studied and causes fluid secretion through the activation of tissue adenylate cyclase to increase intestinal cyclic AMP (cAMP) concentrations.[94,95] Similar toxins both antigenically and mechanistically have been described for other closely related vibrios[96,97] and

TABLE 3. Different Pathogenic Mechanisms of *Escherichia coli* Diarrhea[a]

	Mechanism	*Model*	*Gene Code*	*Predominant Serogroups*
Enterotoxigenic E. coli (*ETEC*)				
LT *E. coli* (LTEC)	Adenylate cyclase-like choleratoxin	Rabbit loops (18h) CHO, Y1 cell immunoassay	Plasmid	LT: 06:K15, 08:K40 LT + St: 011:H27, 015, 020:K79, 025:K7, 027, 063, 080, 085, 0139
STa *E. coli* (STaEC)	Guanylate cyclase	Suckling mice	Plasmid	ST:O groups 12, 78, 115, 148, 149, 153, 159, 166, 167
STb *E. coli* (STbEC)	Noncyclic nucleotide-dependent bicarbonate secretion	Piglet loops	Plasmid	
Enterohemorrhagic E. coli (*EHEC*)				
	Shiga-like (Vero) toxin 1 or 2 inhibits protein synthesis	HeLa cell cytotoxicity	Phage	0157:H7, 026:H11/H^-, 0128, 0139, 0111:K58:H8/H^-, 0113:K75:H7/H21, 0121:H^-, 0145:H^-, rough
Enteroinvasive E. coli (*EIEC*)				
	Local mucosal invasion	Sereny test	Plasmid	O groups 11, 28ac, 29, 115, 124, 136, 144, 147, 152, 164
Enteropathogenic E. coli (*EPEC*)				
Attaching and effacing *E. coli* (AEEC or class I EPEC; EAF-positive EPEC)	Attach to and efface brush border epithelium	Focal HEp-2 cell adherence (EAF)	Plasmid (60 M DA, pMAR2)	055:K59(B5):H^-/H6/H, 0111ab:K58(B4)H^-/H5 H12, 0119:K69(B14), 0125ac:K70(B15)H21, 0126:K71, (B16)H^-/H2, 0127a:K63(B8):H6,[b] 0128ab:K67(B12)H12, 0142, 0158
Class II EPEC (EAF-negative EPEC)	? Close enteroadherence (like class I EPEC)	Diffuse or no HEp-2 cell adherence	? Plasmid	044:K74, 086a:K61(B7), 0114:H2
Autoagglutinating enteroadherent *E. coli* (EAEC)	? Cytotoxic	Aggregative pattern of HEp-2 cell adherence	Plasmid	
Normal enteric flora	? Adherence traits	—	—	O groups 1, 2, 4, 6, 7, 25, 45, 75, 81
Genitourinary, blood stream or meningeal pathogens	? Capsular polysaccharide ± adherence pili	Several animals (mice, rabbits)	—	O groups 1, 2, 4, 6, 7, 11, 18, 22, 25, 62, 75 (K antigens 1, 2, 3, 5, 13)

[a] In addition, nontoxigenic *E. coli* with recognized or new colonization factor fimbriae can cause diarrhea, as documented in experimental animals and in human volunteers.
[b] 0127:H6 is the focally HEp-2 cell adherent strain (E2348) from which the plasmid pMAR-2 was isolated.
(Modified from Guerrant,[87] with permission.)

TABLE 4. Enteric Bacterial Toxins

Neurotoxin group	
	Clostridium botulinum
	Staphylococcus aureus (enterotoxin B)
	Bacillus cereus (emetic toxin)
True enterotoxin group	
	Vibrio cholerae (cAMP)
	Noncholera vibrios
	Escherichia coli—LT (cAMP)
	E. coli—STa (cGMP)
	E. coli—STb
	Salmonella
	Klebsiella
	Clostridium perfringens (A)
	Shigella dysenteriae
	B. cereus
Cytotoxin group	
	Shigella
	C. perfringens (A)
	Vibrio parahemolyticus
	S. aureus
	Clostridium difficile
	E. coli (certain O groups: 26, 39, 128, 157)

E. coli.[98,99] Because there are no reliable markers such as serotype or biotype for enterotoxigenicity, demonstration of the toxin itself is necessary to identify which *E. coli* are enterotoxigenic. The genetic codes for enterotoxigenicity reside on transmissible plasmids that can be lost or transferred to other *E. coli* by conjugation[100,101] or by phage transduction.[102] To recognize which *E. coli* are enterotoxigenic, we must identify enterotoxin activity in culture filtrates of the organisms in question. This has traditionally required inoculation into a ligated rabbit ileal segment[103] or into rabbit skin to test for toxin associated "permeability factor."[104] The ability of the heat-labile enterotoxin of *E. coli* to activate adenylate cyclase has been used in the development of tissue culture bioassays.[105,106] Its similar antigenicity to cholera toxin has provided immunoassay techniques as well.[107–109] Oligonucleotide gene probes for LT and STa are now available with nonradio-active enzyme markers and provide a simple, sensitive, and highly specific detection method for these enterotoxins.[110] The LT-producing *E. coli* are associated with watery diarrhea among adults in Asia,[111,112] travelers to Central America,[113–115] and children in a number of areas.[116–118]

Another plasmid-mediated but smaller, less antigenic, heat-stable toxin may be produced by *E. coli*. The ST-producing *E. coli*, first described as a cause of diarrhea in piglets and calves,[25,119] are capable of causing diarrhea in human volunteers as well.[120] It appears to be significantly associated with diarrhea among tourists to Central America,[121] occasional newborn nursery outbreaks in this country,[122] and among adults with noninflammatory diarrhea on a Navajo reservation[123] or in Brazil.[9,124] The mechanism of action of ST involves the specific activation of intestinal guanylate cyclase.[125–127] Like cyclic AMP, cyclic GMP analogues (such as 8 Br-cyclic GMP) can mimic the secretory effect of the enterotoxin.[125]

Other organisms capable of producing enterotoxic effects by causing fluid secretion in ligated small bowel segments of animal models such as rabbit ileum include *Clostridium perfringens* type A, *Shigella dysenteriae*, and *B. cereus*. A protein neuroenterotoxin isolated from *S. dysenteriae* I (that may be responsible for the headache, meningismus, and seizures) also causes fluid secretion in rabbit ileal loops.[128] Although experimental findings have been contradictory, the activation of adenylate cyclase by this *Shigella* enterotoxin has been demonstrated in rabbit ileal loops.[129] Noninflammatory secretion also occurs in the small bowel of experimental monkeys infected with *S. flexneri* 2A,[130] and 80 percent of the patients infected with *S. flexneri* or *Shigella sonnei* develop neutralizing antibodies to the toxin.[131] However, the toxin alone does not appear to be sufficient to cause *Shigella* diarrhea, because toxigenic, noninvasive opaque colonial mutants of virulent *Shigella* are totally avirulent.[132,133] Certain strains of *B. cereus* have also been reported to produce a heat-labile, adenylate-cyclase-activating rabbit ileal loop-positive, dermonecrotic, and intestinonecrotic enterotoxin.[92,93,134,135]

Certain strains of *S. typhimurium* may cause severe watery cholera-like diarrhea[136,137] that can be prevented in experimental models by indomethacin. As noted in Chapter 83, the products of an inflammatory response could act to cause mucosal secretion.[138] Sandefur and Peterson have described a heat-labile enterotoxinlike effect in rabbit skin and Chinese hamster ovary cell models after separation from an inhibitor.[139] Others have described a heat-stable enterotoxin from *Salmonella*.[140] Other enteric organisms with which enterotoxin-like activity has been reported include *Klebsiella*, *Citrobacter*, *Aeromonas*, and *Enterobacter* spp.[141–145] Both heat-labile and heat-stable toxins have been reported. Although these enterotoxigenic organisms appear to be infrequent at the present time, much needs to be learned about the occurrence and the mechanism of action of enterotoxins from these organisms other than *E. coli*.

Cytotoxic products of several enteric pathogens are responsible for the mucosal destruction that often results in inflammatory colitis. Bacillary dysentery is a colonic mucosal destructive process in which a cytotoxin isolated from *S. dysenteriae* type 1 may play a role.[146,147] Whether this cytotoxin is a component or a digestive product of the larger neuroenterotoxin mentioned above is unknown. *Clostridium perfringens* enterotoxin also produces cytotoxicity similar to that of *S. dysenteriae* toxin in HeLa cell and in animal models.[148] More recent studies have used Vero cells to detect cytotoxicity in fecal filtrates that is neutralized by specific antiserum or toxin fragments.[149–151] These methods have enabled studies to be done that implicate enterocytotoxigenic *C. perfringens* in geriatric institutions and with antibiotic-associated diarrhea.[152–154] Another enteric pathogen for which a cytotoxin has been described is *Vibrio parahemolyticus*. Although some have reported the presence of a true enterotoxin with this organism,[155] others have described a cytotoxin[156]; still others note the tendency of *V. parahemolyticus* to penetrate and cause bacteremia in animal models[157] or an invasive colitis in patients.[158] *Vibrio parahemolyticus* typically causes explosive watery diarrhea in food-borne outbreaks in coastal areas of the United States.[159] *Staphylococcus aureus* produce a nonantigenic Δ-toxin that impairs water absorption and causes cytotoxic disruption of intestinal mucosa or cells in tissue culture.[160] The clindamycin-resistant *C. difficile* isolated from patients with antibiotic-associated pseudomembranous enterocolitis produces a potent cytotoxin capable of causing cytotoxicity in tissue culture and lethality in a hamster model,[161–163] as well as an enterotoxic product that causes hemorrhagic fluid secretion in rabbit ileal loops.[163,164] Data have emerged that associate the capacity to produce one or two *Shiga*-like Vero cell cytotoxins with certain serotypes of *E. coli* that cause hemorrhagic colitis or the hemolytic uremic syndrome (0 groups 26, 39, 111, 113, 121, 128, and 157).[165–169] Two groups have reported the transfer of Vero toxin production to recipient *E. coli* or its association with a large plasmid,[167,169] whereas others have associated the production of Shiga-like toxins I and II with bacteriophages in *E. coli* 0157:H7.[170] The heat-labile Vero cytotoxin, initially found in *E. coli* 026:H11, 0128, and 039, has a slight secretory effect in 18-hour ligated rabbit ileal loops.[166] The multistate outbreak of hemorrhagic colitis with *E. coli* 0157:H7 in 1982[168] was followed by studies showing the near identity (one amino acid difference) of verocytotoxin to Shiga toxin (hence the term *Shiga-like toxin, SLT*) and the association of these enterohemorrhagic *E. coli* (EHEC) with numerous outbreaks and sporadic cases of hemorrhagic colitis or childhood hemolytic uremic syndrome in schools, day care centers, nursing homes, and communities.[168,171–173] Like Shiga toxin, *E. coli* SLT has binding and active subunits, is neutralized by anti-Shiga toxin antibody, and inhibits protein synthesis by cleaving an *N*-glycoside bond at nucleotide position 4324 in the target cell 60S ribosomal RNA, much like the plant lectin ricin. SLT-II acts similarly to SLT but is not neutralized by anti-SLT-I and is about 60 percent homologous by deduced amino acid sequence. The receptor for SLT-I and -II appears to be a globotriosyl ceramide.[174]

Attachment

The ability of many enteric pathogens to cause disease depends not only on the organisms's ability to penetrate the mucosa or to produce enterotoxin or cytotoxin but also on their ability to adhere to and colonize the mucosa. This adherence capacity has been well described with enterotoxigenic *E. coli*, which, in order to cause disease, must not only produce an enterotoxin but also must first adhere to and colonize in the upper small bowel of humans or animals. This adherence capacity for *E. coli* is variously called *K88*, *K99*, or *colonization factor antigen* (*CFA*) for piglet, calf, and human strains, respectively. As with enterotoxigenicity, the production of these adherence antigens also appears to be genetically encoded by transmissible plasmids. These fimbriate bacterial surface adhesins are distinct from type 1 pili and from recognized urinary tract adhesins[175–177] and usually cause hemagglutination that is mannose resistant.[178,179] Although these adhesins hold great promise for immunization against colonization, there are now at least five different types of CFAs among human enterotoxigenic *E. coli* CFAI, CFAII, E8775, 260-1, and O159:H4.[178–183]

In addition, attachment of EPEC to intestinal mucosa appears to be important, and attachment by certain strains has been associated with transferrable plasmids as well.[184–189] Adherence to HEp-2 cells in tissue culture has been helpful as a model of different types of adherence among EPEC strains.[190–196] Focal HEp-2 cell adherence (EAF) is associated with pathogenicity and an approximately 60 MDa plasmid among many EPEC serotypes now being referred to as *class I EPEC*[86,191,192] (see Table 3). These *E. coli* attach and efface the brush border epithelium of human and piglet enterocytes[186,189,197,198] in a manner similar to that seen with HEp-2 cells in culture.[199] Other EPEC serotypes may also attach closely to brush border epithelium but do not exhibit focal HEp-2 adherence ("EAF-negative EPEC"). These *E. coli* exhibit diffuse or no HEp-2 cell adherence and have been called *class II EPEC*.[86,192] Still other *E. coli* (usually not of classically recognized EPEC serotypes) exhibit autoagglutination and a distinct aggregative pattern of adherence to HEp-2 cells that some have referred to as *enteroadherent E. coli* (*EAEC*) and that may be independently associated with diarrhea[86,192,193] (see Table 3). Finally, *E. coli* with the colonization traits mentioned above, but without enterotoxin production, are capable of causing diarrhea in animals[25,200] and in human volunteers fed *E. coli* with the colonization trait as a potential vaccine.[201] Whether such colonizing *E. coli* are responsible, alone or in part, for naturally occurring acute or prolong diarrhea remains to be determined.

The enterohemorrhagic, Shiga toxin-producing *E. coli* (EHEC) 026 has been shown to adhere to the mucosa of human fetal small intestinal tissue in vitro in a mannose-resistant fashion, a trait that is transmissible by a colicinogenic conjugative plasmid.[183] In addition, EHEC strain 0157:H7 has been shown to have a 60 MDa plasmid that encodes a new type of fimbriea that appear to mediate attachment to Henle 407 cells in tissue culture.[195]

Invasiveness

The capacity of organisms such as *Shigella* and certain invasive strains of *E. coli* to invade and destroy epithelial cells is responsible for the inflammatory or dysenteric diarrhea they cause. This capacity is demonstrated in the laboratory by the guinea pig conjunctivitis (Sereny) test.[202] There is cell destruction and superficial inflammatory invasion of the cornea similar to that noted in colonic mucosa. Modifications in the specific components of the O side chain of the cell wall lipopolysaccharide alter this invasive property in *Shigella*.[203,204] There is also evidence that the invasiveness of certain *E. coli* may be reflected in their O antigens or serotype.[205,206] Recent evidence has associated invasiveness with large 120–140-Mdal plasmids in *S. sonnei*,[129] *S. flexneri*,[207] and invasive *E. coli*.[208] HeLa cell, rabbit loop, and Sereny test invasiveness can be genetically constructed by the sequential transfer of defined chromosomal and plasmid genes for *Shigella flexneri* to *E. coli* K12.[209] As discussed above, cytotoxic exotoxins may well play roles in the invasive and destructive properties of certain shigellae, *V. parahemolyticus*, staphylococci, and clostridia.

Other Virulence Factors

In addition to enterotoxin production and adherence, an orchestrated set of additional virulence traits appear to be critical to the ability of pathogen such as *V. cholerae* to succeed in colonizing the intestinal mucosa. These include motility,[210,211] chemotaxis,[32,211] and mucinase production,[212,213] any one of which can be missing and lead to reduced virulence. The virulence of certain enteric pathogens such as *S. typhi* appears to be related to the Vi antigen[214] and to the polysaccharide composition of the O side chain of its lipopolysaccharide cell wall content,[215,216] both of which have been used in vaccine production.[201,217,218] The virulence factors that enable enteric pathogens such as *Yersinia enterocolitica* to cause an enteric fever-like illness or mesenteric adenitis are less clear.

Another potential enteric pathogen that is increasingly recognized with improved culture techniques is *Campylobacter*. *Campylobacter jejuni* tends to cause more diarrhea than *C. fetus*; some *C. jejuni* have been reported to produce an LT-like enterotoxin,[219] or a cytotoxin,[220] and *C. fetus* causes more febrile systemic illness with bacteremia. The mechanisms by which *Campylobacter* cause disease still remain unclear.[221]

Still another way that organisms may cause diarrhea involves the selective destruction of absorptive cells (villus tip cells) in the mucosa, leaving secretory cells (crypt cells) intact.[2,222] Thus it is not surprising that both the rotaviruses and the Norwalk-like viruses, which selectively infect and disrupt the villus tip cells, alter the normal absorptive fluid balance as well as reduce the brush border digestive enzymes present during active infection.[2,223–225] Such an imbalanced disruption of the specialized absorptive surface may also be involved in other small bowel infections that are often associated with villus tip flatening or microvillus destruction, including bacterial overgrowth syndromes, EPEC infections, giardiasis, strongyloidiasis, and cryptosporidiosis.

MAJOR SYNDROMES OF DERANGED GASTROINTESTINAL PHYSIOLOGY

The elements of net fluid balance in the healthy adult intestinal tract are shown diagrammatically in Figure 1. With a daily oral intake of 1.5 liters, salivary, gastric, biliary, and pancreatic secretions contribute a total of approximately 8.5 liters of fluid that enters the upper gastrointestinal tract each day. However, daily fecal fluid excretion is normally less than 150 ml, indicating a net absorption in excess of 8 liters each day by the intestinal tract. Over 90 percent of this net absorption occurs in the small bowel, where there is a massive bidirectional flux that probably exceeds 50 liters a day. We can readily see how a relatively slight shift in the bidirectional flux can result in substantial overload of the colonic absorptive capacity that rarely exceeds 2–3 liters a day. As in the kidney, there are analogous hormonal, physical, and osmotic factors active in the intestinal tract. Aldosterone, for example, enhances intestinal sodium absorption at the expense of potassium.[226,227] Excessive

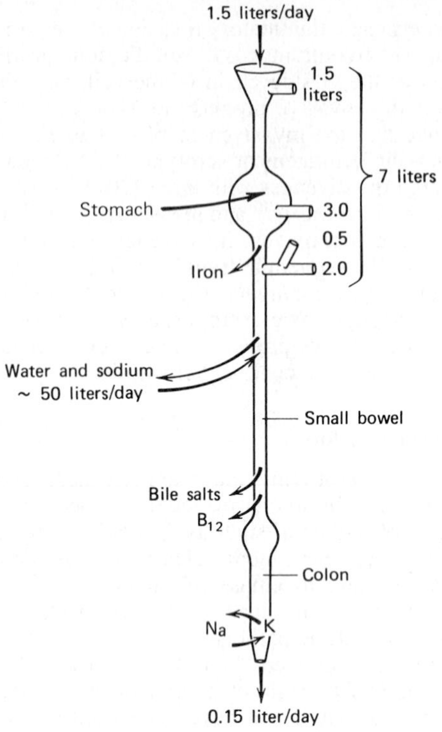

FIG. 1. Diagram of fluid balance in the healthy adult gastrointestinal tract.

fluid volume results in a "third factor" effect that may elicit or prolong diarrhea,[228] and osmotic laxatives are as familiar as osmotic diuretics.

Enteric disease can be produced by the microbe–host interaction that alters normal gastrointestinal physiology in one or more of these three ways: (*1*) a shift in the delicate balance of bidirectional water and electrolyte fluxes in the upper small bowel by intraluminal processes such as enterotoxin action, (*2*) inflammatory destruction of the ileal or colonic mucosa, or (*3*) penetration through an intact mucosa to the reticuloendothelial system. These three types of enteric infections are outlined in Table 5.

They can often be distinguished by a quick, simple examination. Mucus from a fresh stool specimen is mixed with a drop of methylene blue on a slide and examined for the presence of fecal leukocytes.[229,230] In the majority of cases, no leukocytes will be noted. This suggests a noninflammatory process in which diarrhea usually arises from the upper small bowel by the action of a true enterotoxin or by agents such as *Giardia* or viruses. The secretory effects of certain enterotoxins share similar mechanisms with noninfectious endocrine causes of diarrhea such as non-β-cell islet tumors, medullary carcinoma of the thyroid, carcinoid tumors, and other benign or malignant neoplasms that are associated with increased serum prostaglandins, vasoactive intestinal polypeptide, or changes in cyclic nucleotide concentrations.[231] Impaired small bowel absorption is important in tropical sprue, enzyme deficiencies, and solute loads. Enhanced colonic secretion without an inflammatory response characteristic of microbial or ulcerative colitis may result from excessive bile salts or fatty acids or from malignancies such as villous adenomas.

The presence of numerous polymorphonuclear leukocytes documents an inflammatory or invasive process that usually arises from the colon or distal small bowel. Amebic colitis can often be distinguished from bacterial dysenteries by microscopic fecal examination. In addition to the amebic trophozoites or cysts, fecal neutrophils are usually pyknotic or absent with amebiasis, probably because of the cytopathic effect of virulent amebae on mammalian cells, including neutrophils.[232,233] Impaired colonic absorption may contribute to the diarrhea in inflammatory colitis due to shigellosis, pseudomembranous enterocolitis, amebic colitis, or idiopathic ulcerative colitis. In addition, recent evidence suggests that the products of the lipoxygenase pathways in neutrophils may also contribute to a secretory process.[138] Agents that cause an inflammatory colitis may require specific antimicrobial intervention, as well as supportive fluid therapy.[230]

The third type of enteric infection is caused by organisms that penetrate the intact intestinal mucosa, often in the distal small bowel, to multiply in the lymphatic or reticuloendothelial cells. This usually results in a febrile systemic illness with or without diarrhea. If diarrhea is present, mononuclear leukocytes may be found in the stools of these patients.[229] Cultural documentation of the pathogen is important, since a bacteremia that necessitates specific antimicrobial therapy may result in this setting.

DIAGNOSTIC APPROACH TO ENTERIC INFECTIONS

The appropriate diagnostic approach to diarrheal illness is determined by the patient's age, severity of illness, duration of illness, type of illness, and the available facilities. Of greatest importance in patients with diarrhea are a careful history, physical examination, and examination of a fresh stool specimen for fecal leukocytes. A *history* of recent antibiotic use, weight loss, underlying diseases, other illnesses in the family or in other contacts, or of travel outside the United States, to the seacoast, or to rural mountainous areas should elicit a more careful investigation of specific etiologic agents. A prompt evaluation of

TABLE 5. Three Types oe Enteric Infection

	I	*II*	*III*
Mechanism:	Noninflammatory (enterrotoxin)	Inflammatory (invasion ?cytotoxin)	Penetrating
Location	Proximal small bowel	Colon	Distal small bowel
Illness:	Watery diarrhea	Dysentery	Enteric fever
Stool exam:	No fecal leukocytes	Fecal polymorphonuclear leukocytes	Fecal mononuclear leukocytes
Examples	*Vibrio cholerae* *Escherichia coli* (LT) *E. coli* (ST) *Clostridium perfringens* *Bacillus cereus* *Staphylococcus aureus* ?*Salmonella* ?*Vibrio parahemolyticus* *Giardia lamblia* Rotavirus Norwalk-like viruses *Cryptosporidium*	*Shigella* Invasive *E. coli* *Salmonella enteritidis* *V. parahemolyticus* ?*Clostridium difficile* ?*Campylobacter jejuni* *Entamoeba histolytica*[a]	*Salmonella typhi* *Yersinia enterocolitica* ?*Campylobacter fetus*

[a] Although amebic dysentery involves tissue inflammation, the leukocytes are characteristically pyknotic or absent, having been destroyed by the virulent amebae.[232]

physical signs of fever, toxicity, or severe dehydration may result in lifesaving supportive fluid therapy. Particularly worrisome signs of severe dehydration, especially in children, include lethargy, postural hypotension and tachycardia, sunken fontanelles, and dry skin (with decreased turgor), dry eyes, or dry mucous membranes. As noted in Figure 2, if the history of physical findings indicate anything more than a mild, isolated, afebrile illness, examination of a fresh *stool* specimen, preferably collected in a cup, is particularly valuable. First, it provides the physician with an objective determination of the patient's subjective complaints. Second, a gross description of the stool as either watery, mucoid, or bloody will provide important clues about its cause and appropriate management. Third, a microscopic examination for fecal leukocytes, as described above, may reveal heavy parasitic intestinal infestations or maldigested fat or meat fibers, suggesting pancreatic insufficiency, or lipid droplets suggesting malabsorption with steatorrhea. If fever or fecal neutrophils are present, the physician should selectively take a culture for the most commonly recognized invasive pathogens—*C. jejuni*, *Salmonella*, and *Shigella*.[230] Cup specimens, when promptly examined for leukocytes, provide a highly sensitive screen for invasive processes such as shigellosis or *C. jejuni* enteritis.[234,235] Swab or diaper specimens appear to be less sensitive.[235] The history of recent antibiotic use, weight loss, and chronic diarrhea (>10 days), seacoast or other exposures, or immunocompromised states should prompt the physician to consider other agents as noted.

Other diagnostic studies that can be made on fecal specimens include special stains for fat or muscle and determinations of pH and reducing substances. A Sudan stain may reveal many large (10–75 μm) orange-stained globules of fat suggesting malabsorption or smaller (1–4 μm) globules or needle-like crystals

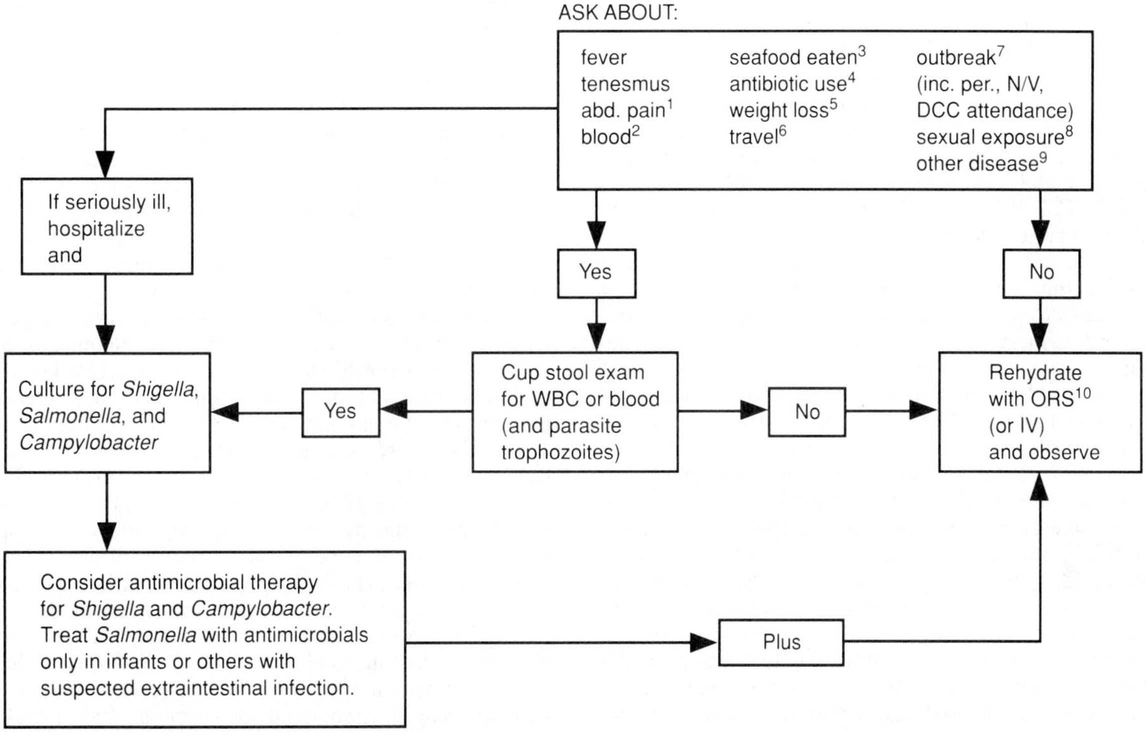

FIG. 2. Initial evaluation and management of diarrhea. Special considerations include the following:

1. If unexpained abdominal pain and fever persist or suggest and appendicitis-like syndrome, culture for *Y. enterocolitica* with cold enrichment.
2. Bloody diarrhea, especially if without fecal leukocytes, suggests enterohemorrhagic (Shiga toxin-producing) *E. coli* 0157 or amebiasis (in which leukocytes are destroyed by the parasite).
3. Ingestion of inadequately cooked seafood should prompt consideration of *Vibrio* infections or Norwalk-like viruses.
4. Associated antibiotics should be stopped if possible and cytotoxigenic *C. difficile* considered.
5. Persistence (>10 days) with weight loss should prompt consideration of giardiasis or cryptosporidiosis.
6. Travel to tropical areas increases the chance of developing enterotoxigenic *E. coli* as well as viral (Norwalk-like or rotaviral), parasite (*Giardia, Entamoeba, Strongyloides, Crytosporidium*), and, if fecal leukocytes are present, invasive bacterial pathogens, as noted in the algorithm.
7. Outbreaks should prompt consideration of *S. aureus, B. cereus,* anisakiasis (incubation period <6 hours), *C. perfringens,* ETEC, *Vibrio, Salmonella, Campylobacter, Shigella,* or EIEC infection. Consider saving *E. coli* for LT, ST, invasiveness, adherence testing, serotyping, and stool for rotavirus, and stool plus paired sera for Norwalk-like virus testing.
8. Sigmoidoscopy in symptomatic homosexual men should distinguish proctitis in the distal 15 cm only (caused by herpesvirus, gonococcal,chlamydial, or syphilitic infection) from colitis (*Campylobacter, Shigella, C. difficile,* or chlamydial [LGV serotypes] infections) or noninflammatory diarrhea (due to giardiasis).
9. In immunocompromised hosts, a wide range of viral (cylomegalovirus, herpes simplex virus, coxsackievirus, rotavirus), bacterial (*Salmonella, M. avium-intracellulare*), and parasitic (*Cryptosporidium, Isospora, Strongyloides, Entamoeba,* and *Giardia*) agents should be considered.
10. ORS can be prepared by adding 3.5 g NaCl (or $\frac{3}{4}$ teaspoon table salt), 2.5 g $NaHCO_3$ (or 2.9 g Na citrate or 1 teaspoon baking soda), 1.5 g KCl (or one cup orange juice or two bananas) and 20 g glucose (or 40 g sucrose or 4 tablespoons sugar) per liter (1.05 qt) of clean water. This makes approximately Na 90, K 20, HCO_3 30, glucose 110 mM/liter.

(Data from Guerrant et al.[230,234])

of fatty acid that may be normal. Numerous undigested muscle fibers may be seen with an aqueous 2% eosin stain that suggest pancreatic insufficiency and maldigestion.

An acidic stool pH may be helpful in the identification of lactose intolerance, especially in children with diarrhea. Although breast-fed infants have a fecal pH ranging from 4.7 to 5.1, stool pH usually exceeds 7.0 if the infant is on a regular milk-containing diet. On a regular diet, a fecal pH less than 5.0 suggests the presence of lactic acid from the action of colonic bacterial flora on unabsorbed lactose. Stool-reducing substances may also be helpful in the detection of carbohydrate malabsorption. A simple test uses copper sulfate (Clinitest) tablets. Mix 1 ml stool with 2 ml water, add 15 drops of this mixture to a test tube, and then add one copper sulfate tablet. A reduction positive for "sugar" indicates reducing substances. Positive tests for blood may suggest an invasive process such as amebiasis or shigellosis. Although this is usually evident from a gross examination of the stool, tests for occult blood are much more sensitive but less specific. Tests for hemoglobin peroxidase use orthotolidine, benzidine, or guaiac reagents in descending order of sensitivity. Some are so sensitive that they may be positive with ingested meat myoglobin. Twenty-four-hour determinations for fecal fat (normal <7.2 g/day fecal fat or <150–200 g/day total stool weight) may also be of value.

For culture of enteric pathogens, the specimen should be inoculated onto culture plates as promptly as possible.[236] The media used are selective and often contain indicator substances that aid in initial identification. Routine techniques must now include selective culture for *C. jejuni*, one of the most common causes of inflammatory diarrhea throughout the world.[237] For optimal results, this requires a highly selective atmosphere of reduced oxygen (4–6 percent) and increased carbon dioxide (6–10 percent) and an increased incubator temperature (42°C). Selective media and means to obtain the proper atmosphere are now available.[237–240] When culturing stool from homosexual men with diarrhea, it should be kept in mind that *Campylobacter cinaedi* and *C. ferinelliae* will not grow at 42°C. Routine stool culture also includes a medium, such as MacConkey's or eosin methylene blue (EMB) agar, that inhibits gram-positive organisms and selects predominantly for aerobic gram-negative rods. In addition more selective media (such as xylose-lysine-deoxycholate [XLD] or *Salmonella–Shigella* [SS] agar) and enrichment broth (such as gram-negative GN, selenite, or tetrathionate) that inhibit most organisms except *Salmonella* and *Shigella* should be used. However, since highly selective media are also more inhibitory, we should also examine the less selective MacConkey's and EMB agar for non-lactose-fermenting (colorless) colonies that may be salmonellae or shigellae. Even the best techniques with fresh specimens may miss fragile organisms such as shigella.[236,239] Fecal cultures failed to yield shigellae in 40 percent of volunteers with inflammatory diarrhea from experimental *Shigella* infection.[229] When immediate culture of specimen is impossible, specimens may be transported to a laboratory in a non-nutrient-holding medium, such as Cary-Blair soft agar, which prevents drying and overgrowth of normal flora.

Culture of vibrios (*V. cholerae*, *V. parahemolyticus*, and others), which should be suspected after any exposure to coastal areas or seafood, requires the highly selective thiosulfate citrate bile salt sucrose (TCBS) agar.[240] Selective culture for *C. difficile* and examination for fecal cytotoxin[158,159,241] may be indicated in patients with refractory antibiotic-associated diarrhea or colitis. Culture of *Y. enterocolitica* may require the selective process of "cold enrichment" on sheep blood agar or phosphate buffered saline for 2–3 weeks.[242]

Escherichia coli that grow readily as dry lactose-fermenting (purple) colonies on EMB or MacConkey's agar are major aerobic constituents of normal fecal flora but should also be considered as potential pathogens. Certain serotypes have been associated with inflammatory diarrhea,[203] recently with bloody diarrhea,[165–170] with outbreaks of diarrhea in newborn nurseries, and even with some enterotoxigenic *E. coli*.[243] However, detection of enterotoxigenicity depends not on serotypes but on detection of the toxin itself. Therefore, routine serotyping of *E. coli* in sporadic cases is of limited value at present and should be considered a special tool for investigating epidemic diarrhea in settings such as nurseries for newborns or unexplained dysentery. Special tests for the cholera-like, heat-labile, adenylate-cyclase-activating enterotoxin may use rabbit ileal loop,[103] rabbit skin permeability,[104] Chinese hamster ovary cell,[105] Y-1 adrenal cell,[106] immunoassay,[107–109] or direct assay for the enterotoxin genome.[110,244] The heat-stable enterotoxin acts through a different mechanism and currently requires the suckling mouse assay for its detection.[245,246] Invasive *E. coli* may be identified by inoculation into the conjunctival sac of guinea pigs (Sereny test).[202]

When diarrhea persists unexplained, especially with blood or weight loss, examinations for *Entamoeba*, *Giardia*, or *Strongyloides* parasites are indicated, using concentration or special staining techniques.[247,248] In immunosuppressed patients with persisting unexplained diarrhea, sugar flotation or modified Kinyoun's acid-fast stains should be done for cryptosporidiosis.[249]

Proctoscopic examination may be very helpful in the differential diagnosis, especially when inflammatory colitis is present. Although necrotic ulcers may be seen in acute shigellosis, discrete ulcers are more suggestive of amebiasis or Crohn's disease. Mucosal friability is more suggestive of inflammatory bowel disease such as ulcerative colitis. The appearance of raised, plaque-like pseudomembranes is diagnostic of pseudomembranous colitis that may be associated with staphylococci or antibiotics such as clindamycin. Large amounts of mucus may be present in "mucous colitis" or with a villous adenoma; melanosis coli may suggest laxative abuse.

Rectal mucosal biopsy specimens, especially when ulcers are present, may be of great help in the identification of the parasite *Entameba histolytica*, granulomata, amyloidosis (with Congo red stain), or Whipple's disease (with periodic acid-Schiff [PAS] stain). Small bowel biopsy specimens may also be diagnostic in Whipple's disease, giardiasis, amyloidosis, a β-lipoproteinemia, lymphoma, coccidiosis, or mast cell disease. Characteristic but not necessarily diagnostic histopathologic changes may be seen in celiac disease, tropical sprue, eosinophilic gastroenteritis, dermatitis herpetiformis, and dysgammaglobulinemia. However, several conditions, including Crohn's disease, bacterial overgrowth syndrome, and pancreatic or bile salt insufficiency, may be associated with normal small bowel histologic findings or with nonspecific changes.

Radiologic studies of the intestinal tract may reveal toxic megacolon, pancreatic calcifications, or nodular adrenal calcifications suggestive of tuberculosis or histoplasmosis. Colonic mucosal edema with a "thumbprint" appearance has been reported on barium enema studies of patients with bloody diarrhea and *E. coli* 0157 infection.[168] Although barium studies may reveal nonspecific changes in the small bowel (giardiasis) or colon (inflammatory colitis), they are less useful in diagnosing microbial diarrheas. Indeed, the barium contrast material renders a microscopic examination of stool virtually useless.

Bacterial overgrowth syndrome may result in deconjugation of bile salts that can be tested with a ^{14}C-glycocholic acid breath test. Carbon-14 labeled carbon dioxide in the breath represents the degradation product of bacterial deconjugation of bile salts.

APPROACH TO PREVENTION, CONTROL, AND THERAPY

The public health measures of improved water supply and sanitation facilities are most important for the control of the majority of enteric infections. Another important area for intervention in the spread of enteric infection lies in the quality control of commercial products such as bottled water and beverages. These may be responsible for outbreaks of significant enteric infections such as those of cholera in Portugal[250] or typhoid fever in Mexico.[251]

Nonspecific host factors should be appreciated to minimize their violation. Examples include careful personal hygiene and limited judicious use of antacids, antimotility drugs, or antimicrobial agents.

Vaccines may be used to boost specific immune processes that may be directed against bacteria themselves, adherence appendages, cytotoxins, or enterotoxins (Chapter 75). Perhaps the most promising are the newly developed live gal-epimerase mutant typhoid vaccine,[214] and the new Vi polysaccaride capsule vaccine against typhoid fever.[217,218] Several additional live and killed bacterial vaccines are currently under study,[201] and new rotavirus vaccines are being studied.[224] To date, there are no effective vaccines against a parasitic enteric infection, and much new work is required to improve the understanding of host defenses against enteric parasitic processes.

New possibilities for pharmacologic antagonists to microbial adherence or to toxin action are now on the horizon. New types of "antibiotics" may work by blocking the formation of bacterial adherence factors, binding bacterial adherence appendages, or lectin-like competitors for the host cell receptors that enable microorganisms to colonize the gastrointestinal tract.[252] Finally, specific competitors for either the binding or the action of enterotoxins hold promise. For example, monosialoganglioside (G_{m1}) successfully binds cholera toxin or the heat-labile enterotoxin of *E. coli* in vitro and in animal experiments. Pharmacologic reversal of the cyclic nucleotide-associated secretory process may also be possible. Such a mechanism has been suggested for bismuth subsalicylate (Pepto-Bismol).[253]

Specific antimicrobial chemotherapy may be indicated, especially in inflammatory processes such as shigellosis or in parasitic diseases such as giardiasis or amebiasis.

Of greatest importance in the treatment of microbial diarrhea, regardless of the cause or category, is fluid replacement. The degree of volume depletion must be first assessed by examining the turgor of the skin and mucous membranes, by noting the amount of lacrimation, and by obtaining a history of urinary output. Postural light-headedness with changes in pulse and blood pressure are helpful objective parameters in volume depletion. Recent observations have documented that, despite the severest form of secretory derangement in cholera, glucose absorption and its coupled sodium and water absorption remain intact in the upper small bowel. Thus, many patients can be completely rehydrated and maintained by a simple oral-glucose-containing electrolyte solution. A controlled study of patients with cholera and other noninflammatory watery diarrhea in Dacca, Bangladesh, documents the efficacy of sucrose (table sugar) as well as glucose in the oral therapy solution.[254] Electrolyte losses in severe watery diarrhea are similar to the electrolyte composition of serum, and fluid replacement should contain approximately these concentrations of electrolytes. A standard oral fluid regimen contains 3.5 g NaCl, 2.5 g $NaHCO_3$, 1.5 g KCl, and 20 g glucose per liter of boiled water. This corresponds to sodium 90, potassium 20, bicarbonate 30, chloride 80, and glucose 110 mM/liter.[255] A similar solution may be prepared with 4 level tablespoons of sugar, $\frac{3}{4}$ teaspoon salt, 1 teaspoon sodium bicarbonate in 1 cup of orange juice to make up 1 liter (1.05 qt) in water. If there is concern about hypertonicity, particularly in children, the salt can be reduced in cases of milder diarrhea or the solution can be given with ad lib water. The electrolyte contents of commonly available soft drinks are quite variable, although solutions of similar electrolyte composition to the ideal as described above can be made in dilute solutions of bouillon or gelatin water. New developments in oral rehydration therapy under study include the use of rice powder or other glucose polymers and the use of amino acids such as glycine, alanine, and glutamine, which enhance sodium absorption independently of glucose.

REFERENCES

1. Walsh JA, Warren KW. Selective primary health care: An interim strategy for disease control in developing countries. N Engl J Med. 1979;301:967.
2. Guerrant RL. Pathophysiology of the enterotoxic and viral diarrheas. In: Chen LC, Scrimshaw NS, eds. Diarrhea and Malnutrition. New York: Plenum Press; 1983:chap 2.
3. Puffer RR, Serrano CV. Patterns of Mortality in Childhood. Washington, DC: Pan American Sanitary Bureau, Regional Office, World Health Organization; 1975.
4. Impact of oral rehydration therapy on hospital admission and case-fatality rates for diarrhoeal disease: Results from 11 countries. WHO Wkly Epidemiol Rec No. 8. 1988;49–52.
5. Yunes J. Evaluation of infant mortality and proportional infant mortality in Brazil. World Health Stats Q. 1981;34:200–19.
6. McAuliffe JF, Shields DS, de Souza MA, et al. Prolonged and recurring diarrhea in the northeast of Brazil: Examination of cases from a community-based study. J Pediatr Gastroenterol Nutr. 1986;5:902–6.
7. Black RE, Brown KH, Becker S, et al. Longitudinal studies of infectious diseases and physical growth of children in rural Bangladesh. Am J Epidemiol. 1982;115:315–24.
8. Mata LJ. The Children of Santa Maria Cauque: A Prospective Field Study of Health and Growth. Cambridge, Mass.: MIT Press; 1978.
9. Guerrant RL, Kirchhoff LV, Shields DS, et al. Prospective study of diarrheal illness in northeastern Brazil: Patterns of disease, nutritional impact, etiologies and risk factors. J Infect Dis. 1983;148:986.
10. Guerrant RL, Hughes JM, Lima NL, et al. Microbiology of diarrhea in developed and developing countries. Rev Infect Dis. In press.
11. Gordon JE, Chitkara ID, Wyon JB. Weanling diarrhea. Am J Med Sci. 1963;245:345.
12. Gordon JE, Scrimshaw NS. Infectious disease in the malnourished. Med Clin North Am. 1970;54:1495.
13. Lindenbaum J. Malabsorption during and after recovery from acute intestinal infection. Br Med J. 1965;2:326.
14. Hirschhorn N, Molla A. Reversible jejunal disaccharidase deficiency in cholera and other acute diarrheal diseases. J Hopkins Med J. 1969;125:291.
15. Lindenbaum J, Kent TH, Sprinz H. Malabsorption and jejunitis in American Peace Corps volunteers in Pakistan. Ann Intern Med. 1966;65:1201.
16. Chen LC, Scrimshaw NS, eds. Diarrhea and Malnutrition: Interactions, Mechanisms and Interventions. New York: Plenum Press; 1983.
17. Gordon JE, Guzman MA, Ascoli W, et al. Acute diarrhoeal disease in less developed countries. 2. Patterns of epidemiological behaviour in rural Guatemalan villages. Bull WHO. 1964;31:9.
18. Bowie MD. Malnutrition and diarrhea. S Afr Med J. 1960;34:344.
19. Black RE, Brown RH, Becker S. Malnutrition is determining factor in diarrheal duration, but not incidence, among young children in a longitudinal study in rural Bangladesh. Am J Clin Nutr. 1984;37:87–94.
20. Sheehy TW. Digestive diseases as a national problem. VI. Enteric disease among United States troops in Vietnam. Gastroenterology. 1968;55:105.
21. Hodgkin K. Towards Earlier Diagnosis. A Family Doctor's Approach. Baltimore: Williams & Wilkins; 1963.
22. Dingle JH, Badger GF, Jordan WS Jr. Illnesses in the Home, A Study of 25,000 Illnesses in a Group of Cleveland Families. Cleveland: The press of Western Reserve University; 1964.
23. Gordon JE, Behar M, Scrimshaw NS. Acute diarrhoeal disease in less developed countries. 1. An epidemiological basis for control. Bull WHO. 1964;31:1.
24. Hollister AC, Beck MD, Gittelsohn AM, et al. Influence of water availability on shigella prevalence in children of farm labor families. Am J Public Health. 1955;45:354.
25. Smith HW, Linggood MA. Observations of the pathogenic properties of the K88, Hly and Ent plasmids of *Escherichia coli* with particular reference to porcine diarrhea. J Med Microbiol. 1971;4:467.
26. Evans DG, Silver RP, Evans DJ, et al. Plasmid-controlled colonization factor associated with virulence in *Escherichia coli* enterotoxigenic for humans. Infect Immun. 1975;12:656.
27. Levine MM, Nalin DR, Rennels MB, et al. Genetic susceptibility to cholera. Ann Hum Biol. 1979;6:369–374.
28. Zisman M. Blood group A and giardiasis. Lancet. 1977;2:1285.
29. Rutter JM, Burrows MR, Sellwood R, et al. A genetic basis for resistance to enteric disease caused by *E. coli*. Nature. 1975;257:135.
30. Mobaselleh M, Donohue-Rolfe A, Jacewicz M, et al. Pathogenesis of *Shigella* diarrhea: Evidence for a developmentally regulated glycolipid receptor for Shiga toxin involved in the fluid secretory response of rabbit small intestine. J Infect Dis. 1988;157:1023–31.
31. Bergman MJ, Evans DG, Sullivan JA, et al. Attachment of *E. coli* to human intestinal epithelial cells: A functional in vitro test for intestinal colonization factor. Trans Assoc Am Physicians. 1978;91:80.
32. Allweiss B, Dostal J, Carey KE, et al. The role of chemotaxis in the ecology of bacterial pathogens of mucosal surfaces. Nature. 1977;266:448.
33. Briscoe J. A role for water supply and sanitation in the child survival revolution. PAHO Bull. 1987;21(2):93–105.

34. Gordon I, Ingraham HS, Korns RF. Transmission of epidemic gastroenteritis to human volunteers by oral administration of fecal filtrate. J Exp Med. 1947;86:409.
35. Jordan WS, Gordon I, Dorrance WR. A Study of Illness in a group of Cleveland families. VII. Transmission of acute nonbacterial gastroenteritis to volunteers: Evidence for two different etiologic agents. J Exp Med. 1953;98:461.
36. Blacklow NR, Dolin R, Fedson DS, et al. Acute infectious nonbacterial gastroenteritis: Etiology and pathogenesis. Ann Intern Med. 1972;76:993.
37. Giannella RA, Broitman SA, Zamcheck N. Gastric acid barrier to ingested microorganisms in man: Studies in vivo and in vitro. Gut. 1972;13:251.
38. Gorbach SL. Progress in gastroenterology: Intestinal microflora. Gastroenterology. 1971;60:1110.
39. Roberts SH, James O, Jarvis EH. Bacterial overgrowth syndrome without "blind loop": A cause for malnutrition in the elderly. Lancet. 1977;2:1193.
40. Hornick RB, Musik SI, Wenzel R, et al. The Broad Street pump revisited: Response to volunteers to ingested cholera vibrios. Bull NY Acad Med. 1971;47:1181.
41. Gitelson S. Gastrectomy, achlorhydria and cholera. Isr J Med Sci. 1971;7:663.
42. Giannella RA, Broitman SA, Zamcheck N. Influence of gastric acidity on bacterial and parasitic enteric infections: A perspective. Ann Intern Med. 1973;78:271.
43. Black RE, Levine MM, Clements ML, et al. Experimental *Campylobacter jejuni* infection in humans. J Infect Dis. 1988;157:472–9.
44. Driks MR, Craven DE, Celli BR, et al. Nosocomial pneumonia in intubated patients given sucralfate as compared with antacids or histamine type 2 blockers. The role of gastric colonization. N Engl J Med. 1987;317:1376.
45. Dixon JMS. The fate of bacteria in the small intestine. J Pathol Bacteriol. 1960;79:131.
46. Schrager J. The chemical composition and function of gastrointestinal mucus. Gut. 1970;11:450.
47. Higgens JA, Code CF, Orvis AL. The influence of motility on the rate of absorption of sodium and water from the small intestine of healthy persons. Gastroenterology. 1956;31:708.
48. Formal SB, Abrams GD, Schneider H, et al. Experimental *Shigella* infections. VI. Role of the small intestine in an experimental infection in guinea pigs. J Bacteriol. 1963;85:119.
49. Sprinz H. Pathogenesis of intestinal infections. Arch Pathol. 1969;87:556.
50. DuPont HL, Hornick RB. Adverse effect of Lomotil therapy in shigellosis. JAMA. 1973;226:1525.
51. Holdeman LV, Cato EP, Moore WEC, eds. Anaerobe Laboratory Manual. Blacksburg, Va.: Virginia Polytechnic and State University Anaerobe Laboratory; 1977.
52. Price DJE, Sleigh JD. Control of infection due to *Klebsiella* aerogenes in a neurosurgical unit by withdrawal of all antibiotics. Lancet. 1970;2:1213.
53. Mentzing LO, Ringertz O. *Salmonella* infection in tourists. 2. Prophylaxis against salmonellosis. Acta Pathol Microbiol Scand. 1968;74:405.
54. Bohnhoff M, Miller CP, Martin WR. Resistance of the mouse's intestinal track to experimental *Salmonella* infections. J Exp Med. 1964;120:805.
55. Van der Waaj D, Berguis JM, Lekkerkerk JEC. Colonization resistance of the digestive tract of mice during systemic antibiotic treatment. J Hyg. 1972;70:605–10.
56. Que JU, Casey SW, Hentges DJ. Factors responsible for increased susceptibility of mice to intestinal colonization after treatment with streptomycin. Infect Immun. 1986;53:116–23.
57. Tannock GW, Savage DC. Indigenous microorganisms prevent reduction in fecal size induced by *Salmonella typhimurium* in vaccinated gnotobiotic mice. Infect Immun. 1976;13:172.
58. Schrank GD, Verwey WF. Distribution of cholera organisms in experimental *Vibrio cholerae* infections: Proposed mechanisms of pathogenesis and antibacterial immunity. Infect Immun. 1976;13:195.
59. Ryan CA, Nickels MK, Hargrett-Bean NT, et al. Massive outbreak of antimicrobial-resistant salmonellosis traced to pasteurized milk. JAMA. 1987;258:3269–74.
60. Bodey GP, Buckley M, Sathe YS, et al. Quantitative relationships between circulating leukocytes and infection in patients with acute leukemia. Ann Intern Med. 1966;64:328.
61. Yolken RH, Bishop CA, Townsend TR, et al. Infectious gastroenteritis in bone-marrow-transplant recipients. N Engl J Med. 1982;306:1009.
62. Bodey GD, Fainstein V, Guerrant RL. Infections of the gastrointestinal tract in the immunocompromised patient. Ann Rev Med. 1986;37:271–81.
63. Smith PD, Lane C, Gill VJ, et al. Intestinal infections in patients with the acquired immunodeficiency syndrome (AIDS). Ann Intern Med. 1988;108:328–33.
64. Sperber SJ, Schlenpner CJ. Salmonellosis during infection with human immunodeficiency virus. Rev Infect Dis. 1987;9:925–34.
65. Soave R, Johnson WD. *Cryptosporidium* and *Isospora belli* infections. J Infect Dis. 1988;157:225–9.
66. Colebunders R, Franastt, Mann J, et al. Persistent diarrhea, strongly associated with HIV infection in Kinshasa, Zaire. Am J Gastroenterol. 1987;82:859–64.
67. Sewankambo N, Mugerwa RD, Goodgame R, et al. Enteropathic AIDS in Uganda. An endoscopic, histological and microbiological study. AIDS. 1987;1:9–13.
68. Nelson JA, Reynolds-Kohler C, Margaretten W, et al. Human immunodeficiency virus detected in bowel epithelium from patients with gastrointestinal symptoms. Lancet. 1988;1:259–62.
69. Bull DM, Tomasi TB: Deficiency of immunoglobulin A in intestinal disease. Gastroenterology. 1968;54:313.
70. Pierce NF, Reynolds HY: Immunity to experimental cholera. II. Secretory and humoral antitoxin response to local and systemic toxoid administration. J Infect Dis. 1975;131:383.
71. Pierce NF, Gowans JL. Cellular kinetics of the intestinal immune responses to cholera toxoid in rats. J Exp Med. 1975;142:1550.
72. Stoliar OA, Pelley RP, Kaniecki-Green E, et al. Secretory IgA against enterotoxins in breast-milk. Lancet. 1976;1:1258.
73. Brown SE III, Sauer KT, Nations-Shields M, et al. Comparison of paired whole milk and dried filter paper samples for antienterotoxin and anti-rotavirus activities. J Clin Microbiol. 1982;16:103.
74. Jones EG, Brown WR. Serum and intestinal fluid immunoglobulins in patients with giardiasis. Am J Dig Dis. 1974;19:791.
75. Zinneman HH, Kaplan AP. The associate of giardiasis with reduced intestinal secretory immunoglobulin A. Am J Dig Dis. 1972;17:793.
76. Ament ME, Ochs HD, Davis SD. Structure and function of the gastrointestinal tract in primary immunodeficiency syndromes: A study of 39 patients. Medicine. 1973;52:227.
77. Hermans PE, Huizenga KA, Hoffman HN, et al. Dysgammaglobulinemia associated with nodular lymphoid hyperplasia of the small intestine. Am J Med. 1966;40:78.
78. Crabbe PA, Heremans JF. Lack of gamma A-immunoglobulin in serum of patients with steatorrhea. Gut. 1966;7:119.
79. Collins FM, Carter PB. Cellular immunity in enteric disease. Am J Clin Nutr. 1974;27:1424.
80. Welsh JK, May JT. Anti-infective properties of breast milk. J Pediatr. 1979;94:1.
81. McClelland DBL, McGrath J, Samson RR. Antimicrobial factors in human milk: Studies of concentration and transfer to the infant during the early stages of lactation. Acta Paediatr Scand. 1978;271(Suppl):1.
82. Arnold RR, Cole MF, McGhee JR. A bactericidal effect for human lactoferrin. Science. 1977;197:263.
83. Griffiths E, Humphreys J. Bacteriostatic effect of human milk and bovine colostrum on *Escherichia coli*: Importance of bicarbonate. Infect Immun. 1977;15:396.
84. Bullen JJ, Rogers HJ, Leight L. Iron-binding proteins in milk and resistance to *Escherichia coli* infection in infants. Br Med J. 1975;1:69.
85. Hanson LA, Winberg J. Breast milk and defence against infection in the newborn. Arch Dis Child. 1972;47:845.
86. Levine MM. *Escherichia coli* that cause diarrhea: Enterotoxigenic enteropathogenic, enteroinvasive, enterohemorrhagic, and enteroadherent. J Infect Dis. 1987;155:377–88.
87. Guerrant RL. *Escherichia coli* and related enteric pathogens. In: Warren KS, Malmoud AAF, eds. *Tropical and Geographical Medicine*. New York: McGraw-Hill; 1989: in press.
88. Schlager TA, Guerrant RL. Seven possible pathogenic mechanisms for *Escherichia coli* diarrhea. Infect Dis Clin North Am. 1988;2:1–18.
89. Lamanna C, Carr CJ. The botulinal, tetanal, and enterostaphylococcal toxins: A review. Clin Pharmacol Ther. 1967;8:286.
90. Koupal A, Deibel RH. Rabbit intestinal fluid accumulation by an enterotoxigenic factor of *Staphylococcus aureus*. Infect Immun. 1977;18:298–303.
91. Freer JH, Arbuthnott JP. Toxins of *Staphylococcus aureus*. In: Dorner F, Drews J, eds. Pharmacology of Bacterial Toxins. Oxford: Pergamon Press; 1986;581–633.
92. Terranova W, Blake PA. *Bacillus cereus* food poisoning. N Engl J Med. 1978;298:143.
93. Turnbull PCB. *Bacillus cereus* toxins. In: Dorner F, Drews J, eds. Pharmacology of Bacterial Toxins. Oxford: Pergamon Press; 1986;397–448.
94. Chen LC, Rohde JE, Sharp GWG. Intestinal adenyl-cyclase activity in human cholera. Lancet. 1971;1:939.
95. Guerrant RL, Chen LC, Sharp GWG. Intestinal adenyl-cyclase activity in canine cholera: Correlation with fluid accumulation. J Infect Dis. 1972;125:377.
96. Honda T, Shimizu M, Takeda Y, et al. Isolation of a factor causing morphological changes of Chinese hamster ovary cells from the culture filtrates of *Vibrio parahemolyticus*. Infect Immun. 1976;14:1028.
97. Blake PA, Weaver RE, Hollis DG. Diseases of humans (other than cholera) caused by vibrios. Ann Rev Microbiol. 1980;34:341.
98. Evans DJ Jr., Chen LC, Curlin GT. Stimulation of adenyl cyclase by *Escherichia coli* enterotoxin. Nature (New Biol). 1972;236:137.
99. Guerrant RL, Ganguly U, Casper AGT, et al. Effect of *Escherichia coli* on fluid transport across canine small bowel: Mechanism and time-course with enterotoxin and whole bacterial cell. J Clin Invest. 1973;52:1707.
100. Skerman FJ, Formal SB, Falkow S. Plasmid-associated enterotoxin production in a strain of *Escherichia coli* isolated from humans. Infect Immun. 1972;5:622.
101. Lathe R, Hirth P. Cell-free synthesis of enterotoxin of *E. coli* from a cloned gene. Nature. 1980;284:473.
102. Takeda Y, Murphy J. Bacteriophage conversion of heat-labile enterotoxin in *Escherichia coli*. J Bacteriol. 1978;133:172.
103. Evans DG, Evans DJ Jr, Pierce NF. Differences in the response of rabbit small intestine to heat-labile and heat-stable enterotoxins of *Escherichia coli*. Infect Immun. 1973;7:873.
104. Craig JP. A permeability factor (toxin) found in cholera stools and culture filtrates and its neutralization by convalescent cholera sera. Nature. 1965;207:614.

105. Guerrant RL, Brunton LL, Schnaitman TC, et al. Cyclic adenosine monophosphate and alteration of Chinese hamster ovary cell morphology: A rapid, sensitive in vitro assay for the enterotoxins of *Vibrio cholerae* and *Escherichia coli*. Infect Immun. 1974;10:320.
106. Donta ST, Moon HW, Whipp SC. Detection of heat-labile *Escherichia coli* enterotoxin with the use of adrenal cells in tissue culture. Science. 1974;183:334.
107. Greenberg HB, Sack DA, Rodriguez W, et al. A microtiter solid-phase radioimmunoassay for detection of *Escherichia coli* heat-labile enterotoxin. Infect Immun. 1977;17:541.
108. Yolken RH, Greenberg HB, Merson MH, et al. Enzyme-linked immunosorbent assay for detection of *Escherichia coli* heat-labile enterotoxin. J Clin Microbiol. 1977;6:439.
109. Honda T, Tage S, Takeda Y, et al. Modified Elek test for detection of heat-labile enterotoxin of enterotoxigenic *E. coli*. J Clin Microbiol. 1981;13:1.
110. Sommerfelt H, Svennerholm AM, Kalland KH, et al. Comparative study of colony hybridizations with synthetic oligonucleotide probes and enzyme-linked immunosorbent assay for identification of *Escherichia coli*. J Clin Microbial. 1988;26:530–4.
111. Gorbach SL, Banwell JG, Chatterjee BD, et al. Acute undifferentiated human diarrhea in the tropics. I. Alterations in intestinal microflora. J Clin Invest. 1971;50:881.
112. Ryder RW, Sack DA, Kapikian AZ, et al. Enterotoxigenic *Escherichia coli* and reovirus-like agent in rural Bangladesh. Lancet. 1976;1:659.
113. Gorbach SL, Kean BH, Evans DG: Traveler's diarrhea and toxigenic *Escherichia coli*. N Engl J Med. 1975;292:933.
114. Merson MH, Morris GK, Sack DA, et al. Travelers' diarrhea in Mexico: A prospective study. Abstract 149 presented at the 15th Interscience Conference on Antimicrobial Agents and Chemotherapy: September 1975.
115. Guerrant RL, Rouse JD, Hughes JM. Turista among members of the Yale Glee Club in Latin America. Am J Trop Med Hyg. 1980;29:895.
116. Gorbach SL, Khurana CM. Toxigenic *Escherichia coli*: A cause of infantile diarrhea in Chicago. N Engl J Med. 1972;287:791.
117. Sack RB, Hirschhorn N, Brownlee I, et al. Enterotoxigenic *Escherichia coli*-associated diarrheal disease in Apache children. N Engl J Med. 1975;292:1041.
118. Guerrant RL, Moore RA, Kirschenfeld PM, et al. Role of toxigenic and invasive bacteria in acute diarrhea of childhood. N Engl J Med. 1975;293:567.
119. Gyles CL. Heat-labile and heat-stable forms of the enterotoxin from *E. coli* strains enteropathogenic for pigs. Ann NY Acad Sci. 1971;176:315.
120. Levine MM, Caplan ES, Waterman D, et al. Diarrhea caused by *Escherichia coli* that produce only heat-stable enterotoxins. Infect Immun. 1977;17:78.
121. Sack DA, Wells JG, Merson MH. Diarrhoea associated with heat-stable enterotoxin-producing strains of *Escherichia coli*. Lancet. 1975;2:239.
122. Ryder RW, Wachsmuth IK, Buxton AE, et al. Infantile diarrhea produced by heat-stable enterotoxin *Escherichia coli*. N Engl J Med. 1976;295:849.
123. Hughes JM, Rouse JD, Barada FA, et al. Etiology of summer diarrhea among the Navajo. Am J Trop Med Hyg. 1980;29:613.
124. Korzeniowski OM, Dantas W, Trabulsi LR, et al. A controlled study of endemic sporadic diarrhoea among adult residents of southern Brazil. Trans R Soc Trop Med Hyg. 1984;78:363–9.
125. Hughes JM, Murad F, Chang B, et al. Role of cyclic GMP in the action of heat-stable enterotoxin of *Escherichia coli*. Nature. 1978;271:755.
126. Field M, Graf LH, Jr, Laird WJ, et al. Heat stable enterotoxin of *E. coli*. In vitro effects on guanylate cyclase activity, cyclic GMP concentration, and ion transportin small small intestine. Proc Natl Acad Sci USA. 1978;75:2800.
127. Guerrant RL, Hughes JM, Chang B, et al. Activation of intestinal guanylate cyclase by heat-stable enterotoxin of *E. coli*: Studies of tissue specificity, potential receptors and intermediates. J Infect Dis. 1980;142:220.
128. Keusch GT, Grady GF, Mata LJ, et al. The pathogenesis of *Shigella* diarrhea. I. Enterotoxin production by *Shigella dysenteriae* 1. J Clin Invest. 1972;51:1212.
129. Charney AN, Gots RE, Formal SB, et al. Activation of intestinal mucosal adenylate cyclase by *Shigella dysenteriae* I enterotoxin. Gastroenterology. 1976;70:1085.
130. Rout WR, Formal SB, Giannella RA, et al. Pathophysiology of *Shigella* diarrhea in the rhesus monkey: Intestinal transport, morphological and bacteriological studies. Gastroenterology. 1975;68:270.
131. Keusch FT, Jacewicz M. Serum enterotoxin neutralizing antibody in human shigellosis. Nature (New Biol). 1973;241:31.
132. Kopecko DJ, Washington O, Formal SB. Genetic and physical evidence for plasmid control of *Shigella sonnei* form I cell surface antigen. Infect Immun. 1980;29:207.
133. Keusch GT. Invasive bacterial diarrhea. In: LC Chen, NS Scrimshaw, eds. Diarrhea and Malnutrition. New York: Plenum Press; 1983: Chap 3, p 45.
134. Turnbull PCB: Studies on the production of enterotoxins by *Bacillus cereus*. J Clin Pathol. 1976;29:941–949.
135. Gilbert RJ, Kramer JM. *Bacillus ceseus* enterotoxins: Present status. Biochem Soc Trans. 1984;12:198–200.
136. Giannella RA, Formal SB, Dammin GJ, et al. Pathogenesis of salmonellosis. Studies of fluid secretion, mucosal invasion, and morphologic reaction in the rabbit ileum. J Clin Invest. 1973;52:441.
137. Giannella RA, Gots RE, Charney AN, et al. Pathogenesis of *Salmonella*-mediated intestinal fluid secretion: Activation of adenylate cyclase and inhibition by indomethacin. Gastroenterology. 1975;69:1238.
138. Musch MW, Miller RJ, Field M, et al. Stimulation of colonic secretion by lipoxygenase metabolites of arachidonic acid. Science. 1982;217:1255.
139. Sandefur PD, Peterson JW. Neutralization of *Salmonella* toxininduced elongation of Chinese hamster ovary cells by cholera antitoxin. Infect Immun. 1977;15:988.
140. Koupal LR, Deibel RH. Assay, characterization and localization of an enterotoxin produced by *Salmonella*. Infect Immun. 1975;11:14.
141. Klipstein FA, Holdeman LV, Corcino JJ. Enterotoxigenic intestinal bacteria in tropical sprue. Ann Intern Med. 1973;79:632.
142. Guerrant RL, Dickens MD, Wenzel RP, et al. Toxigenic bacterial diarrhea: Nursery outbreak involving multiple bacterial strains. J Pediatr. 1976;89:885.
143. Wasdtrom T, Aust-Kettis A, Habte D, et al. Enterotoxin-producing bacteria and parasites in stools of Ethiopian children with diarrhoeal disease. Arch Dis Child. 1976;51:865.
144. Wachsmuth K, Wells J, Shipley P, et al. Heat-labile enterotoxin production in isolates from a shipboard outbreak of human diarrheal illness. Infect Immun. 1979;24:793–7.
145. Ljungh A, Popoff M, Wadstrom T. *Aeromonas hydrophila* in acute diarrhea disease: Detection of enterotoxin and biotyping of strains. J Clin Microbiol. 1977;6:96.
146. Keusch GT, Jacewicz M. The pathogenesis of *Shigella* diarrhea. V. Relationship of Shiga enterotoxin, neurotoxin and cytotoxin. J Infect Dis. 1975:131S:S33.
147. Keusch GT. Invasive bacterial diarrheas. In: Chen LC, Scrimshaw NS, eds. Diarrhea and Malnutrition. New York: Plenum Press; 1983:45–72.
148. McDonel JL, Duncan CL. Histopathological effect of *Clostridium perfringens* enterotoxin in the rabbit ileum. Infect Immun. 1975;12:1214.
149. Bartholomew BA, Stringer MF. Observations on the purification of *Clostridium perfringens* type A enterotoxin and the production of a specific antiserum. Fems Microbiol Lett. 1983;18:43–8.
150. Bartholomew BA, Stringer MF. *Clostridium perfringens* enterotoxin: A brief review. Biochem Soc Trans. 1984;12:195–7.
151. Horiguchi Y, Akai T, Sakaguchi G. Isolation and function of a *Clostridium perfringens* enterotoxin fragment. Infect Immun. 1987;55:2912–5.
152. Borriello SP, Barclay F, Welch AR, et al. Epidemiology of diarrhea caused by enterotoxigenic *Clostridium perfringens*. J Med Microbiol. 1985;20:363–72.
153. Borriello SP, Welch AR, Larson HE, et al. Enterotoxigenic *Clostridium perfringens*: A possible cause of antibiotic associated diarrhea. Lancet. 1984;1:305–7.
154. Larson HE, Borriello SP. Infectious diarrhea due to *Clostridium perfringens*. J Infect Dis. 1988;157:390–2.
155. Bhattacharya S, Bose AK, Ghosh AK: Permeability and enterotoxic factors of nonagglutinable vibrios *V. alcaligenes* and *V. parahaemolyticus*. Appl Microbiol. 1971;22:1159.
156. Carruthers MM. Cytotoxicity of *Vibrio parahemolyticus* in HeLa cell culture. J Infect Dis. 1975;132:555.
157. Calia FM, Johnson DE. Bacteremia in suckling rabbits after oral challenge with *Vibrio parahemolyticus*. Infect Immun. 1975;11:1222.
158. Bolen JL, Zamiska SA, Grennough WB III. Clinical features in enteritis due to *Vibrio parahemolyticus*. Am J Med. 1974;57:638.
159. Barker WH, MacKowiak PA, Fishbein M, et al. *Vibrio parahaemolyticus* gastroenteritis outbreak in Covington, Louisiana in August 1972. Am J Epidemiol. 1974;100:316.
160. Kapral FA, O'Brien AD, Ruff PD, et al. Inhibition of water absorption in the intestine by *Staphylococcal aureus* delta toxin. Infect Immun. 1976;13:140.
161. Bartlett JG, Chang TW, Gurwith M, et al. Antibiotic-associated pseudomembranous colitis due to toxin-producing clostridia. N Engl J Med. 1978;298:531.
162. Rifkin GD, Fekety FR, Silva J Jr, et al. Antibiotic-induced colitis: Implication of a toxin neutralized by *Clostridium sordelli* antitoxin. Lancet. 1977;2:1103.
163. Taylor NS, Thorne GM, Bartlett JG. Comparison of two toxins produced by *Clostridium difficile*. Infect Immun. 1981;34:1036.
164. Lima AAM, Lyerly DM, Wilkins TD, et al. Effects of *Clostridium difficile* toxins A and B in rabbit small and large intestine in vivo and on culltured cells in vitro. Infect Immun. 1988;56:582–8.
165. Konowalchuk J, Speirs JI, Stavric S. Vero response to a cytotoxin of *Escherichia coli*. Infect Immun. 1977;18:775.
166. Konowalchuk J, Dickie N, Stavric S, et al. Properties of an *Escherichia coli* cytotoxin. Infect Immun. 1978;10:575.
167. Scotland SM, Day NP, Willshaw GA, et al. Cytotoxic enteropathogenic *Escherichia coli*. Lancet. 1980;1:90.
168. Riley LW, Remia RS, Helgerson SD, et al. Outbreaks of hemorrhagic colitis associated with a rare *Escherichia coli* serotype. N Engl J Med. 1983;308:681.
169. Johnson WM, Lior H, Bezanson GS. Cytotoxic *Escherichia coli* 0157:H7 associated with hemorrhagic colitis in Canada. Lancet. 1983;1:76.
170. Strockbine NA, Marques LRM, Newland JW, et al. Two toxin-converting phages from *E. coli* 0157:H7 strains 933 encode antigenically distinct toxins with similar biologic activities. Infect Immun. 1986;53:135–40.
171. Karmali MA, Petric M, Lim C, et al. The association between idiopathic hemolytic uremic syndrome and infection by verotoxin producing *E. coli*. J Infect Dis. 1985;151:775–82.
172. Pai CH, Gordon R, Sims HU, et al. Sporadic cases of hemorrhagic colitis associated with *E. coli* 0157:H7. Ann Intern Med. 1984;101:738–42.
173. Carter AO, Borczyk AA, Carlson AK, et al. A severe outbreak of *E. coli* 0157:H7 associated hemorrhagic colitis in a nursing home. N Engl J Med. 1987;317:1496–1500.

174. Edelman R, Karmali, MA, et al. Summary of the International Symposium and Workshop on Infections due to Verocytotoxin (Shiga-like Toxin)-Producing *E. coli*. J Infect Dis. 1988;157:1102–4.
175. Salit IE, Gostchlich EC. Type I *Escherichia coli* pili: Characterization of binding to monkey kidney cells. J Exp Med. 1977;146:1182.
176. Silverblatt FJ. Host parasitic in the rat renal pelvis: A possible role for pili in the pathogenesis of pyelonephritis. J Exp Med. 1974;140:1696.
177. Eden CS, Hausson S, Jodal U, et al. Host–parasite interaction in the urinary tract. J Infect Dis. 1988;157:421–6.
178. Evans DG, Satterwhite TK, Evans DJ Jr, et al. Differences in serological responses and excretion patterns of volunteers challenged with enterotoxigenic *Escherichia coli* with and without the colonization factor antigen. Infect Immun. 1978;19:883.
179. Bergman MJ, Updike WS, Wood SJ, et al. Attachment factors among enterotoxigenic *Escherichia coli* from patients with acute diarrhea from diverse geographic areas. Infect Immun. 1981;32:881.
180. Thomas LV, Cravioto A, Scotland SM, et al. New fimbrial antigenic type E8775 that may represent a colonization factor in enterotoxigenic *E. coli* in humans. Infect Immun. 1982;35:1119–24.
181. Honda T, Arita M, Miwatani T: Characterization of new hydrophobic pili of human enterotoxigenic *Escherichia coli*: A possible new colonization. Infect Immun. 1984;43:959–65.
182. Tacket CO, Maneval DR, Levine MM. Purification, morphology, and genetics of a new fimbrial putative colonization factor of enterotoxigenic *Escherichia coli* 0159:H4. Infect Immun. 1987;55:1063–9.
183. Williams PH, Sedgwick MI, Evans N, et al. Adherence of an enteropathogenic strain of *Escherichia coli* is mediated by a colicinogenic conjugative plasmid. Infect Immun. 1978;22:393.
184. Edelman R, Levine MM. Summary of NIAID workshop on enteropathogenic *E. coli* (EPEC). J Infect Dis. 1983;147:1108.
185. Levine MM, Nalin DR, Hornick RB, et al. *Escherichia coli* strains that cause diarrhea but do not produce heat-labile or heat-stable enterotoxins and are noninvasive. Lancet. 1978;1:1119.
186. Ulshen MH, Rollo JL. Pathogenesis of *Escherichia coli* gastroenteritis in man: Another mechanism. N Engl J Med. 1980;302:99.
187. Polotsky YE, Dragunskaya EM, Seliverstova VG, et al. Pathogenic effect of enterotoxigenic *Escherichia coli* and *Escherichia coli* causing infantile diarrhoea. Acta Microbiol Acad Sci Hung. 1977;24:221.
188. Guerrant RL. Yet another pathogenic mechanism for *Escherichia coli* diarrhea? N Engl J Med. 1980;302:113.
189. Rothbaum R, McAdams AJ, Giannella R, et al. A clinicopathologic study of enterocyte-adherent *Escherichia coli*: A cause of protracted diarrhea in infants. Gastroenterology. 1982;83:441.
190. Cravioto A, Gross RJ, Scotland S, et al. An adhesive factor found in strains of *Escherichia coli* belonging to the traditional infantile enteropathogenic serotypes. Curr Microbiol. 1979;3:95–9.
191. Baldini MM, Kaper JB, Levine MM, et al. Plasmid mediated adhesion of enteropathogenetic *Escherichia coli*. J Pediatr Gastroenterol Nutr. 1983;2:534–8.
192. Nataro JP, Kaper JB, Robins-Browne R, et al. Patterns of adherence of diarrheagenic *Escherichia coli* to HEp-2 cells. Pediatr Infect Dis J. 1987;6:829–31.
193. Mathewson JJ, Johnson PC, Dupont HL, et al. Pathogenicity of enteroadherent *Escherichia coli* in adult volunteers. J Infect Dis. 1986;154:524–7.
194. Bray J, Beavan TED. Slide agglutination of *Bacterium coli* var. *neapolitanum* in summer diarrhoea. J Pathol. 1948;60:395–401.
195. Karch H, Heesemann J, Laufs R, et al. A plasmid of enterohemorrhagic *Escherichia coli* 0157:H7 is required for expression of a new fimbrial antigen and for adhesion to epithelial cells. Infect Immun. 1987;55:455–61.
196. Scaletsky ICA, Silva MLM, Toledo MRF, et al. Correlation between adherence to HeLa cells and serogroups, serotypes, and bioserotypes of *Escherichia coli*. Infect Immun. 1985;49:528–32.
197. Moon HW, Whipp SC, Argenzio RA, et al. Attaching and effacing activities of rabbit and human enteropathogenic *Escherichia coli* in pig and rabbit intestines. Infect Immun. 1983;41:1340–51.
198. Tzipori S, Robins-Browne RM, Gonis G, et al. Enteropathogenic *Escherichia coli* enteritis: Evaluation of the gnotobiotic piglet as a model of human infection. Gut. 1985;26:570–8.
199. Knutton S, Lloyd D, McNeish A. Adhesion of enteropathogenic *Escherichia coli* to human intestinal enterocytes and cultured human intestinal mucosa. Infect Immun. 1987;55:69–77.
200. Wanke C, Guerrant RL. Small-bowel colonization alone is a cause of diarrhea. Infect Immun. 1987;55:1924–6.
201. Levine MM, Kaper JB, Black RE, et al. New knowledge on pathogenesis of bacterial enteric infections as applied to vaccine development. Microbiol Rev. 1983;47:510–50.
202. Sereny B. Experimental *Shigella* keratoconjunctivitis: A preliminary report. Acta Microbiol Acad Sci Hung. 1955;2:293.
203. Gemski P Jr, Sheahan DG, Washington O, et al. Virulence of *Shigella flexneri* hybrids expressing *Escherichia coli* somatic antigens. Infect Immun. 1972;6:104.
204. Keusch GT. *Shigella* infections. Clin Gastroenterol. 1979;8:645.
205. Trabulsi LR, Fernandes MFR. *Escherichia coli* serogroup 0115 isolated from patients with enteritis: Biochemical characteristics and experimental pathogenicity. Rev Inst Med Trop Sao Paulo. 1969;11:358.
206. DuPont HL, Formal SB, Hornick RB, et al. Pathogenesis of *Escherichia coli* diarrhea. N Engl J Med. 1971;285:1.
207. Sansonetti PJ, Kopecko DJ, Formal SB. Involvement of an plasmid in the invasive ability of *Shigella flexneri*. Infect Immun. 1982;35:852.
208. Harris JR, Wachsmuth IK, Davis BR, et al. High-molecular-weight plasmid correlates with *Escherichia coli* invasiveness. Infect Immun. 1982;37:1295.
209. Sansonetti PJ, Hale TL, Oaks EV. Genetics of virulence in enteroinvasive *Escherichia coli*. Microbiology. 1985;74–7.
210. Guentzel MN, Berry LJ. Mortality as a virulence factor for *Vibrio cholerae*. Infect Immun. 1975;2:890–7.
211. Freter R, Allweiss B, O'Brien PCM, et al. Role of chemotaxis in the association of motile bacteria with intestinal mucosa: In vitro studies. Infect Immun. 1981;34:241–9.
212. Schneider DR, Parker CD. Isolation and characterization of protease-deficient mutants of *Vibrio cholerae*. J Infect Dis. 1978;138:143–51.
213. Schneider DR, Parker CD. Purification and characterization of the mucinase of *Vibrio cholerae*. J Infect Dis. 1982;145:474–82.
214. Hornick RB, Greisman SE, Woodward TE, et al. Typhoid fever: Pathogenesis and immunologic control. N Engl J Med. 1970;283:686.
215. Robbins PW, Uchida T. Determinants of specificity in *Salmonella*: Changes in antigenic structure mediated by bacteriophage. Immunochemistry. 1962;21:702.
216. Germanier R, Furer E. Isolation and characterization of Gal E Mutant Ty 21a of *Salmonella typhi*: A candidate strain for a live, oral typhoid vaccine. J Infect Dis. 1975;131:553.
217. Acharva IL, Lowe CU, Thapa R, et al. Prevention of typhoid fever in nepal with the Vi capsular polysaccharide of *Salmonella typhi*. N Engl J Med. 1987;317(18);1102–4.
218. Klugman KP, Koornhof H, Schneerson R, et al. Protective activity of Vi capsular polysaccharide vaccine against typhoid fever. Lancet. 1987;2:1165–7.
219. Ruiz-Palacios GM, Torres J, Torres NI, et al. Cholera-like enterotoxin produced by *Campylobacter jejuni*. Characterization and clinical significance. Lancet. 1983;2:250.
220. Guerrant RL, Wanke CA, Pennie RA, et al. Production of a unique cytotoxin by *Campylobacter jejuni*. Infect Immun. 1987;55:2526–30.
221. Guerrant RL, Lahita RG, Winn WC, Jr, et al. Campylobacteriosis in man: Pathogenic mechanisms and review of 91 bloodstream infections. Am J Med. 1878;65:584.
222. Field M. Cholera toxin, adenylate cyclase, and the process of active secretion in the small intestine. The pathogenesis of diarrhea in cholera. In: Andreoli TE, Hoffman JF, Fauestil DD, eds. Physiology of Membrane Disorder. New York: Plenum Press; 1978.
223. Davidson GP, Barnes GL. Structural and functional abnormalities of the small intestine in infants and young children with rotavirus enteritis. Acta Paediatr Scand. 1979;68:181.
224. Hamilton JR. Viral enteritis. Pediatr Clin North Am. 1988;35:89–102.
225. Agus SG, Dolin R, Wyatt RG, et al. Acute infectious nonbacterial gastroenteritis: Intestinal histopathology, histologic and enzymatic alterations during illness produced by Norwalk agent in man. Ann Intern Med. 1973;79:18.
226. Levitan R, Ingelfinger FJ. Effect of *d*-aldosterone on salt and water absorption from the intact human colon. J Clin Invest. 1965;44:801.
227. Guerrant RL, Chen LC, Rohde JE. Effect of spironolactone on stool electrolyte losses during human cholera. Gut. 1972;13:197.
228. Guerrant RL, Carpenter CCJ. Diarrheagenic effect of volume expansion: Intestinal fluid secretion without mucosal adenyl cyclase stimulation. Johns Hopkins Med J. 1975;136:209.
229. Harris JC, DuPont HL, Hornick RB. Fecal leukocytes in diarrheal illness. Ann Intern Med. 1972;76:697.
230. Guerrant RL, Shields DS, Thorson SM, et al. Evaluation and diagnosis of acute infectious diarrhea. Am J Med. 1985;78:91–8.
231. Said SI, Faloona GR. Elevated plasma and tissue levels of vasoactive intestinal polypeptide in the watery-diarrhea syndrome due to pancreatic, bronchogenic and other tumors. N Engl J Med. 1975;293:155.
232. Guerrant RL, Brush JE, Ravdin JI, et al. The interaction between *Entamoeba histolytica* and human polymorphonuclear leukocytes. J Infect Dis. 1981;143:83.
233. Ravdin JI, Guerrant RL. A review of the parasite cellular mechanisms involved in the pathogenesis of amebiasis. Rev Infect Dis. 1982;4:1185.
234. Guerrant RL. *Campylobacter* enteritis. In: Wyngaarden JB, Smith LH Jr, eds. Cecil Textbook of Medicine. Philadelphia: Saunders; 1988:1648–51.
235. Korzeniowski OM, Basada FA, Rouse JD, et al. Value of examination for fecal leukocytes in the early diagnosis of shigellosis. Am J Trop Med Hyg. 1979;28:1031–5.
236. Rahaman MM, Huq I, Dey CR: Superiority of MacConkey's agar over *Salmonella-Shigella* agar for isolation of *Shigella dysenteria* type 1. J Infect Dis. 1975;131:700.
237. Blaser MJ, Reller LB. Campylobacter enteritis. N Engl J Med. 1981;305:1444.
238. Kaplan RL, Barrett JE: Monograph: Campylobacter. Marion Scientific, Kansas City, Mo.; 1981.
239. Rahaman MM, Khan MM, Azi KMS, et al. An outbreak of dysentery caused by Shigella dysenteriae type I on a coral island in the Bay of Bengal. J Infect Dis. 1975;132:15.
240. Feeley JC, Balows A. Vibrio. In Lennette EH, Spaulding EH, Truant JP eds. Manual of Clinical Microbiology. Washington, DC, American Society for Microbiology; 1974:238.
241. Ryan RW, Kwasnik I, Tilton RC. Rapid detection of *Clostridium difficile* in human feces. J Clin Microbiol. 1980;12:776.

242. Morris GK, Feeley JC, Martin WT, et al. Isolation and identification of *Yersinia enterocolitica*. Public Health Lab. 1977;35:217.
243. Merson MH, Black RE, Gross RJ, et al. Use of antisera for identification of enterotoxigenic *E. coli*. Lancet. 1980;2:222.
244. Moseley SL, Escheverria P, Seriwatana J, et al. Identification of enterotoxigenic *E. coli* by colony hybridization using three enterotoxin fene probes. J Infect Dis. 1982;145:863.
245. Dean AG, Ching Y-C, Williams RG, et al. Test for *Escherichia coli* using infant mice: Application in a study of diarrhea in children in Honolulu. J Infect Dis. 1972;125:407.
246. Giannella RA. Suckling mouse model for detection of heat-stable *Escherichia coli* enterotoxin: Characteristic of the model. Infect Immun. 1976;14:95.
247. Brown HW, Neva FA. Basic Clinical Parasitology. Norwalk, Conn, Appleton-Century-Crofts, 1983.
248. Lima JP, Delgado PG. Diagnosis of stronygloidiasis: Importance of Baermann's method. Am J Dig Dis. 1961;6:899.
249. Current WL, Reese NC, Ernst JV, et al. Human cryptosporidiosis in immunocompetent and immunodeficient persons: Studies of an outbreak and experimental transmission. N Engl J Med. 1983;21:1252.
250. Blake PA, Rosenberg ML, Florencia J, et al. Cholera in Portugal, 1974. Am J Epidemiol. 1977;105:344.
251. Lee JA, Kean BH. International Conference on the Diarrhea of Travelers. New Directions in Research: A summary. J Infect Dis. 1978;137:360.
252. Costerton JW, Geesey GG, Cheng K-J. How bacteria stick. Sci Am. 1977;1:86.
253. Ericsson CD, Evans DG, DuPont HL, et al. Bismuth subsalicylate inhibits activity of crude toxins of *Escherichia coli* and *Vibrio cholerae*. J Infect Dis. 1977;136:693.
254. Palmer DL, Koster FT, Islam AFRM, et al. A comparison of sucrose and glucose in oral electrolyte treatment of cholera and other severe diarrheas. N Engl J Med. 1977;297:1107.
255. Oral glucose/electrolyte therapy for acute diarrhea, editorial. Lancet. 1975;1:79.

82. NAUSEA, VOMITING, AND NONINFLAMMATORY DIARRHEA

RICHARD L. GUERRANT

The vast majority of acute gastrointestinal illnesses do not involve a recognizable inflammatory process.[1–3] Although there is considerable inflammatory enteritis during summer months in warm areas with poor sanitation, most cases of diarrhea in these areas are noninflammatory, which suggests an enterotoxic bacterial, viral, or noninvasive parasitic process.[4–9]

EPIDEMIC DIARRHEA IN NEWBORN NURSERIES

Epidemic infantile diarrhea has long been recognized as a potentially serious problem that occurs in newborn nurseries. Its mortality has been as high as 24–50 percent.[10,11] Epidemic diarrhea among hospitalized newborns has been associated with certain "enteropathogenic" serotypes of *Escherichia coli* (EPEC). Enteropathogenic *E. coli* serotypes have been associated with diarrhea in hospitalized infants under 4 months of age.

The unusual susceptibility of newborns may be explained by their unique host status; they have not yet acquired a normal intestinal flora or specific immunity. Infants in special care nurseries have this situation compounded by severe underlying diseases such as prematurity or congenital cardiac or pulmonary disease. The consequences of diarrhea in the newborn are unusually severe because of poorly developed homeostatic mechanisms and limited water and electrolyte reserves. Nosocomial transmission may occur since the newborn nurseries may be crowded with susceptible infants.[12] A nursery outbreak can go unrecognized since infants may develop diarrhea after being discharged.

The onset is insidious, with the development of listlessness, irritability, and poor feeding over a period of 3–6 days.[11,13,14] Vomiting and fever are infrequent, and the stools tend to be watery, yellow-green, and usually without mucus, pus, or blood. Early signs such as failure to gain weight or a slight weight loss and abdominal distension may be subtle. The disease may progress to more severe signs of dehydration and shock with depressed sensorium, drowsiness, coma, sunken eyes, circumoral cyanosis, and grayish discoloration of the skin. Shock without hyperpnea often occurs in this setting despite the development of severe acidosis. Poorly nourished infants with decreased protein and potassium reserves may have severe hypokalemia, hyponatremic dehydration, and paradoxical edema. The illness usually lasts 5–15 days but may persist or relapse over the course of several weeks. Complications may include intercurrent otitis media, pneumonia, bacteremia, peritonitis, and renal vein or cerebral sinus thrombosis. Dissemination of EPEC to the lungs has been demonstrated by immunofluorescent staining of tissue at autopsy.[15] While the mortality may be quite high as noted above, South and Kaslow et al. have reported a milder illness with lower morbidity and mortality in recent years.[16,17] However, in many areas such as South Africa and southern Brazil, EPEC remain among the most common causes of diarrhea in infants and young children, especially during the summer months.[18–20] Endemic childhood diarrheal illness in areas like England and Canada also remain associated with EPEC in 6–18 percent of cases.[18,19]

Several potentially life-threatening processes may mimic this infantile diarrhea syndrome. So-called parenteral diarrhea is the well-recognized, but poorly understood tendency for systemic or localized infections elsewhere (such as otitis or meningitis) to be manifested clinically with diarrhea. Likewise, a strangulated hernia, intussusception, or torsion of an ovary or testis may be manifested by abdominal pain or diarrhea.

Appropriate antibiotic therapy must be tailored to the specific sensitivity pattern of the organism isolated. While neomycin or colistin have been used successfully, EPEC may develop resistance to these agents as well as to chloramphenicol and gentamicin.[16] Because the illness is often mild, oral nonabsorbable antibiotics such as neomycin or gentamicin are usually adequate. However, if systemic infection is suspected, parenteral therapy should be started and should be tailored to the antibiotic sensitivity pattern of the organism isolated. Appropriate preventive measures include cohorting of nursery admissions, avoidance of overcrowding in nurseries, utilization of individual units and equipment, careful formula preparation, isolation of infants with diarrhea, and careful hand washing by hospital personnel.

The association of a certain strain of *E. coli* with infantile diarrhea was first demonstrated by slide agglutination by Bray and Beavan in 1945 and reported in further detail in 1948.[21] They identified serologically homogeneous *E. coli* in most infants with summer diarrhea (87.5 percent vs. 4 percent of the controls), half of which was hospital acquired. Varela et al.[22] and Olarte and Varela[23] subsequently found this strain (called *E. coli*-"gomez" by Varela) in cases of infantile diarrhea in Mexico. A second serotype, initially designated as "beta" to distinguish it from the earlier serotype called "alpha," was described by Giles and Sangster as the cause of an outbreak of infantile gastroenteritis in Aberdeen.[24]

Escherichia coli strains are classified into a large number of serotypes on the basis of three major types of antigens: the "O" or heat-stable somatic antigen (lipopolysaccharide endotoxin), which forms the basis for 169 serogroups; an outer, heat-labile "capsular" antigen called "K" that may inhibit O agglutination; and for motile organisms, the "H" or flagellar antigen, which is also heat labile. Three different kinds of "K" antigen have been identified; L, A, and B, the latter being of importance in the identification of EPEC serotypes. The original alpha- and beta-serotypes of *E. coli* were subsequently associated with several outbreaks of infantile epidemic gastroenteritis and were classified as serotypes of O111:B4 and O55:B5, respectively, by Kaufmann and Dupont.[25] As shown in Table 1, exclusive of certain invasive serotypes (see Table 2 in Chapter 84), there are some 14 classically recognized EPEC *E. coli* serotypes, beginning with O111:K58 (alpha), O55:K59 (beta), O127:K63, O128:K67, O26:B6, O86:K61, O119:K69, O125:K70, O126:K71, O20:B7, and O44:K74. Additional serotypes recently recognized as causes of epidemic infantile diarrhea include O114,[10,29,30] O142,[12,27] and O158.[28] With the recent association of *E. coli* O157:H7 with hemorrhagic diarrhea in several outbreaks as well as sporadic cases, yet another EPEC serotype (if not another mechanism of pathogenesis) has been introduced.[31–33]

The evidence that EPEC serotypes are responsible for infantile diarrhea has been outlined.[11,18] There is a strong association for these organisms with cases of epidemic infantile diarrhea, and these organisms are infrequently encountered in healthy infants, children, or adults not exposed to cases of diarrhea. However, the mechanism by which most EPEC organisms cause disease is poorly understood. Although most are not invasive and do not produce conventionally recognized heat-labile or heat-stable enterotoxins, these organisms are capable of causing diarrheal disease in human volunteers, from whom the organism can be reisolated and in whom an antibody response can be documented.[13,34] As noted in Table 3 in Chapter 75, these EPEC serotypes differ from those *E. coli* isolated from patients with nonenteric infections.[35]

Epidemic infantile diarrhea may also be caused by enterotoxigenic organisms that are not limited to certain serotypes of *E. coli*. An outbreak has been described in which multiple serotypes of different organisms (*E. coli, Klebsiella*, and *Citrobacter*) that were demonstrated to be transiently enterotoxigenic were isolated,[36] which suggests the transmission of enterotoxigenicity among etiologic strains by plasmids[37] or by bacteriophages.[38] A subsequent outbreak of diarrhea on a cruise ship also documented the association of enterotoxigenic *Klebsiella* and *Citrobacter* as well as *E. coli* with watery diarrhea.[39] Another report of sporadic diarrhea among infants and children in Africa has shown that enteric organisms other than *E. coli* may produce an enterotoxin.[6] Enterotoxigenicity is by no means limited to specific serotypes, and most EPEC serotypes do not produce recognizable enterotoxins.[5–7,40] There do, however, tend to be a number of serotypes of *E. coli* that are more often enterotoxigenic, as shown in Table 2.[26,41] Whether these organisms are better recipients for enterotoxin plasmids or whether they are simply better adapated to maintaining these plasmids is not known.

TABLE 1. Enteropathogenic *E. coli* Serotypes Classically Recognized in Infantile Diarrhea Outbreaks[a]

Serotype	*Difco Serogroup and References*
Class I (EAF-positive) EPEC	
O55:K59(B5):H$^-$/6/7	A (24–26)
O111ab:K58(B4):H$^-$/5/12	A (21–23,25,26)
O127a:K63(B8):H6	A (26)
O119:K69(B14)	B (26)
O125ac:K70(B15):H21	B (26)
O126:K71(B10):H$^-$/H2	B (26)
O128ab:K67(B12)	B (26)
O142	(12,26,27)
O158	(26,28)
Class II (EAF-negative) EPEC	
O44:K74	C (26)
O114	(10,26,29,30)
O86a:K61(B7)	B (26)
Enterohemorrhagic *E. coli* (EHEC)	
O157:H7	(31–33)
O26:B6	A (26)

Abbreviation: EAF: enteroadherence factor probe for focal HEp-2 cell adherence plasmid pMAR2.[a]
[a] See also Table 3, Chapter 81.

TABLE 2. Serotypes of *E. coli* That Appear with Increased Frequency among Enterotoxigenic Isolates

LT *E. coli*	
	O6:K15:H16
	O8:K40:H9, 08:K25:H9
LT + ST *E. coli*	
	O11:H27
	O15:H22
	O20:H—, 020:H11
	O25:K7:H42, 025:K98:H—
	O27:H7
	O63:H12
	O80, 085, 0139
ST *E. coli*	
	O78:H11, 078:H12
	O115:H40
	O128:H7
	O148:H28
	O149:H10
	O153
	O159:H20
	O166, 0167

A 9-month-long outbreak of diarrhea in the special care nurseries of a pediatric hospital has been reported in association with a multiple drug-resistant *E. coli* O78 that produced only the heat-stable type of enterotoxin.[42] Another outbreak of diarrhea lasting 3 months in a newborn nursery in Scotland was related to ST-producing *E. coli* O159.[43]

Shigellosis[44] and epidemic salmonellosis[45,46] may readily spread in the newborn nursery setting. Echoviruses,[47] coxsackieviruses,[48] adenoviruses,[49] and rotaviruses[50–52] are potential viral causes of epidemic infantile diarrhea. Echovirus 18 was isolated from 10 of 12 infants who had watery noninflammatory diarrhea in a 21-patient premature nursery. The virus was also isolated from two nurses, one of whom was implicated in the spread of the agent to five other babies in another ward.[47] While there are conflicting interpretations of the significance of isolation of enteroviruses and adenoviruses among controls as well as patients, some have suspected that they may cause summer or winter gastroenteritis, respectively. Hospital acquisition of rotaviruses may be common among newborns; some suggest that mild diarrhea develops relatively infrequently.[53] However, rotaviruses have been clearly implicated in epidemic neonatal diarrhea[50–52] as well as in sporadic infantile diarrhea after the neonatal period.

WEANLING DIARRHEA

Weanling diarrhea usually occurs in the second year of life in areas where sanitation is poor. In contrast to cases of diarrhea where EPEC are still found in many areas,[18–21] EPEC were not found in the relatively infrequent cases of diarrhea among breast-fed neonates studied in rural Guatemala.[54] The greatest attack rate of diarrhea in the community occurs at the time of weaning, usually between 6 and 24 months of age.[9,11,12,55] As noted in the previous chapter, weanling diarrhea is a major cause of mortality around the world. The increased susceptibility of a recently weaned infant relates to several factors.[56] In areas with poor sanitation the infant ingests large numbers of many new organisms at the time of weaning. A second contributing factor is the deteriorating nutritional status that may occur with weaning in many parts of the world.[57,58] Finally there are cellular and humoral factors passively transferred in human breast milk that convey resistance to agents that commonly cause diarrhea in this age group.[59–63] Weanling diarrhea is manifested clinically as an acute, sporadic, watery diarrheal illness that occurs with increased frequency, especially in the summer months, in areas with poor sanitation. In the well-nourished infant, the disease is usually short-lived and resolves within 2–3 days with adequate hydration. A low-grade fever may be present, and vomiting is common.[5,55] Diarrhea in the malnourished child tends to persist or to recur and is often much more severe.

Weanling diarrhea is usually an acute, noninflammatory process. Acute diarrhea in children 6–24 months of age has been commonly associated with rotaviruses[2–4] and with enterotoxigenic *E. coli*.[5–7] Shigellosis may also occur in this setting. From 16 to 83 percent of acute diarrheal illnesses among infants and young children have been associated with enterotoxigenic *E. coli*.[5–7,64] Most of these reports involve studies of the summer peak of diarrhea in areas with poor sanitation. The presence of antibody to the heat-labile enterotoxin (LT) of *E. coli* in colostrum[59,60] may provide some protection against LT-producing *E. coli* diarrhea among breast-fed infants exposed to unsanitary conditions. The recent demonstration of passive protection against experimental enterotoxigenic *E. coli* infections in human volunteers with immune bovine colostrum further documents the potential protective role of passive antibody in colostrum or milk.[65] The role of enterotoxigenic *E. coli* in causing infantile diarrhea in temperate climates is less clear. Enterotoxigenic *E. coli* serotypes are uncommon among children with diarrhea in Massachusetts and Virginia.[66–68]

The ability of enteric organisms other than *E. coli* to produce enterotoxins has been suggested, but these organisms appear to be considerably less common than enterotoxigenic *E. coli*. Studies from Ethiopia suggested that young children with sporadic diarrhea may have *Klebsiella, Citrobacter, Aeromonas,* or *E. coli* that produce an LT-like toxin.[6] However, in Brazil enterotoxigenic *Klebsiella* organisms were found in only 2 of 40 patients, both of whom also had enterotoxigenic *E. coli*.[5] Diarrhea produced by the heat-labile enterotoxin shares the adenylate cyclase–activating mechanism with cholera toxin,[69–73] while the heat-stable toxin (STa) activates intestinal guanylate cyclase.[74–76]

The major nonbacterial causes of weanling diarrhea are rotaviruses. While most adults have demonstrable antibody to rotaviruses that may protect against symptomatic disease, children less than 2 years of age throughout temperate and tropical climates appear to be highly susceptible to rotavirus diarrhea, which occurs most frequently in the winter or cooler, dry months[2,4,66,77–84] and occasionally in the summer months.[85] Rotavirus diarrhea appears to be associated with low humidity and possibly indoor crowding to a greater extent than with temperature or inadequate sanitation.[86–88] The illness tends to have a more insidious onset and to last slightly longer than bacterial diarrheas do, is slightly more common in males than in females, is usually mild and without fever, and is often associated with vomiting.[2,4,89] Rotaviruses probably account for most cases of "pseudocholera infantum" or hakuri ("white stool diarrhea") in Japan.[80] They have been associated with initial bouts of weanling diarrhea in Aboriginal communities,[90] and anti-rotavirus antibody has been demonstrated in human colostrum among patients in Costa Rica and Brazil.[60,63] There is a high frequency of rotavirus shedding or seroconversion among parents and other household contacts of cases of rotavirus-associated diarrhea.[2,91,92] Up to 40 percent of these infected adult contacts may develop mild abdominal cramps or diarrhea.[93]

The human rotaviruses demonstrate antigenic cross reaction with several animal strains including the Nebraska calf diarrhea virus (NCDV), the agent of epizootic diarrhea of infant mice (EDIM), simian rotavirus (SA-11), and the "O" agent of monkeys.[2,94] However, there are three to five different antigenic types of rotaviruses,[95–98] so multiple attacks may occur.[99]

The laboratory diagnosis of rotavirus diarrhea may be made by examining the stool directly for viruses or the rotaviral RNA genome or by testing for an antibody titer increase in serum. Rotaviruses can be detected in fecal material by direct electron microscopy or by using immunologic techniques such as the enzyme-linked immunosorbent assay (ELISA),[100] radioimmunoassay,[101] counterimmunoelectrophoresis,[102] or fluorescent antibody staining of stool or biopsy specimens.[103,104] Immunoassays for rotaviral antigen are available, with ELISA being the most sensitive. Simple rapid latex agglutination assays with 86 percent sensitivity and 95 percent specificity have been developed.[105] Detection of rotaviral genomic RNA in stools by using "dot" hybridation with labeled RNA probes appears to be sensitive, specific, and convenient.[106] Methods for detecting serum antibody titers to rotaviruses use their cross-reactivity with NCDV, SA-11, or O agents of animals that can be cultivated in bovine embryonic kidney or in African green monkey kidney cells in tissue culture. Serum antibody has been measured by using immune electron microscopy,[79,107] complement fixation,[2,79] and immunofluorescence[66] with one of the substitute antigens.

In vitro studies were initially difficult because rotaviruses do not grow in most widely used tissue culture systems. Human rotaviruses incorporate into human embryonic gut monolayers,[108] guinea pig intestinal monolayers,[109] and human embryonic kidney cells in tissue culture.[110] Gnotobiotic piglets[111] and colostrum-deprived newborn rhesus monkeys[112] also acquire diarrhea after experimental infection with human rotaviruses. After the initial adaptation of human rotavirus type 2 in African green monkey kidney cell cultures after 11 passages through gnotobiotic newborn piglets,[113] several reports demonstrate the primary isolation of two human rotaviral types in MA104 cells in tissue culture with demonstrable cytopathic effects and without requiring animal passage.[114–116]

Much has been learned about the pathogenesis and the pathologic characteristics of intestinal rotavirus infections. Biopsy specimens from confirmed cases have shown transient, patchy, irregular inflammatory responses in the lamina propria and immature, cuboidal epithelium with 70–90 nm rotavirus particles in the distended cisternae of the endoplasmic reticulum.[77] Normal columnar epithelium at the villus tips was replaced by irregular cuboidal cryptlike cells. As would be expected from the destruction of villous tip epithelial cells, a transient brush border disaccharidase deficiency in the duodenal and upper jejunal mucosa and, despite the efficacy of oral therapy with glucose–electrolyte solutions, increased fecal reducing substances have been noted in children with rotavirus diarrhea.[117–120] The degree of microvillus damage parallels the severity of diarrhea and dehydration.[121] As with transmissible gastroenteritis in piglets, experimental rotaviral infections in animals confirm the shortened villi, reduced sucrase activity, increased thymidine kinase activity, no change in cyclic AMP concentrations, and blunted glucose-induced sodium absorption.[122,123] As noted in Chapter 81, this loss of absorptive villus tip cells may be responsible for the fluid imbalance and nutritional impact of rotaviral infections.

The availability, convenience, and cost-effectiveness of enzyme immunoassays or latex agglutination tests for rotavirus infections may enable improved diagnosis and epidemiologic control.[105] Therapy should be directed first at the immediate restoration of fluid balance by intravenous or oral glucose–electrolyte therapy and then at restoring the nutritional state to normal. Although several candidate live oral rotavirus vaccines (including bovine, rhesus monkey, and reassortant rotaviruses) show promise, questions remain about their efficacy in infants (<1 year old), especially in developing countries, and about the optimal means of delivery, age, and serotype to provide protection with minimal side effects.[124,125] Reasonable preventive measures include the provision of improved sanitation facilities and safe water supplies as well as efforts to develop protective antibacterial, antitoxic, or antiviral immunity.

ACUTE NAUSEA AND VOMITING (WINTER VOMITING DISEASE)

The syndrome of acute nausea and vomiting, "intestinal flu," or "viral gastroenteritis" commonly occurs in winter months in temperate climates. While there is some overlap of this syndrome with rotavirus-associated infantile gastroenteritis, rotaviruses appear to be relatively uncommon causes of winter vomiting disease in older children and adults. The Cleveland family studies of Dingle et al.[1] showed that enteritis was second only to upper respiratory infection as a cause of illness in homes. Gastrointestinal illnesses were most common between the ages of 1 and 10 years, when approximately two illnesses occurred per person per year. The peak season of these gastrointestinal illnesses was November through February, with June being the lowest point of the year over this continuous study period. Most illnesses were of less than 1–3 days' duration; 20 percent occurred with respiratory symptoms, and 20 percent involved only diarrhea.

Illnesses tended to occur in one of two patterns: (*1*) mild afebrile illness with watery diarrhea or (*2*) a more severe febrile illness with vomiting, headache, and constitutional symptoms. Although etiologic agents were rarely identified, these two patterns of illness subsequently developed among volunteers who ingested filtrates prepared from the feces of ill patients.[126–128] Studies done in 1975–1977 in Charlottesville, Virginia, confirmed this pattern of winter illnesses with clustering in families, highest attack rates in children, and the absence of identifiable etiologic agents in most cases despite the application of techniques for virologic and enterotoxin studies.[67,68]

Although there has been little consistent documentation of enteroviruses in association with febrile winter vomiting disease, echovirus type 11 has been demonstrated in association with a small laboratory outbreak of febrile vomiting disease.[129] Abdominal pain and vomiting have been described with influenza B infections in children between the ages of 4 and 10 years.[130]

Careful evaluation of specimens from an outbreak of winter vomiting disease in an elementary school revealed a 27 nm parvovirus-like agent.[131–133] Typical winter vomiting disease, first described in 1929 by Zahorsky,[134] occurred over a 2-day period in late October 1968 in Norwalk, Ohio. Fifty percent of 232 students and teachers in an elementary school developed a mild illness characterized by nausea, vomiting, and abdominal cramps that usually lasted only 12–24 hours. Diarrhea occurred in fewer than half, and a low-grade fever occurred in approximately one-third. A remarkable 32 percent secondary attack rate in family contacts occurred approximately 48 hours later. A bacteria-free fecal suspension from a secondary case from the Norwalk outbreak caused an illness with low-grade fever and diarrhea in two of three volunteers. A second passage in volunteers produced either a febrile vomiting disease or an afebrile diarrheal disease, and illness was also produced in one of four volunteers who ingested an inoculum after three passages in human fetal intestinal organ culture.[132] From the stool of a second human passage in these volunteers, Kapikian and his colleagues used convalescent serum to identify a 27 nm agent by immune electron microscopy.[133] Antibody in the convalescent serum of other volunteers and three of five patients with naturally acquired illness was shown to coat and to aggregate these particles. Biopsy specimens revealed an intact small intestinal mucosa but blunted villi, shortened microvilli, and dilatation of the endoplasmic reticulum with intracellular multivesiculate bodies. Dilated mitochondria and intercellular spaces were also observed.[135] There was also a transient decrease in the activities of the brush border enzymes, alkaline phosphatase, sucrase, and trehalase. All changes had returned to normal by 2 weeks after the illness. The colon is relatively spared, and fecal leukocytes are absent in this noninflammatory type of diarrhea.

The pathophysiologic features of winter vomiting disease caused by Norwalk-like agents may be parallel in some respects to that mentioned in the previous section for rotaviruses. Both cause mucosal villus destruction and transient brush border enzyme deficiencies in the upper portion of the small bowel without any alteration in adenylate cyclase activity.[97,136,137] The roles of transient enzyme deficiency, malabsorption of xylose and lactose, and the slight increase in the number of bacteria present during the Norwalk illness remain unclear.[136,138]

Similar outbreaks of vomiting disease have occurred elsewhere with either documented or suspected Norwalk-like agents. In March 1971, all four members of a household in Honolulu, Hawaii, developed a vomiting illness over a 4-day period with an apparent 44- to 48-hour incubation period, and in June 1971, another family of four in Montgomery County, Maryland, developed illnesses at 24- to 48-hour intervals that were characterized by vomiting, diarrhea, and occasional myalgias.[139] Fecal specimens from these patients revealed 27 nm Norwalk-like particles, and subsequent cross-challenge volunteer studies suggested that the Norwalk and Montgomery County agents were antigenically similar and conferred cross-immunity while the Hawaii agent appeared to be antigenically different and failed to confer cross-immunity to the other agents.[139] Other Norwalk-like agents include the Snow Mountain and Taunton agents.[140] Clarke and associates reported an outbreak from a boys' boarding school in Britain. The illness was transmitted to volunteers with filtered extracts of feces from one ill boy (W agent).[141] Another outbreak in a primary school in Ditchling, England, in October 1975 revealed 26 nm particles that aggregated in convalescent serum and appeared to be antigenically similar to the W agent but different from the Hawaii and Norwalk agents.[142] Another 27 nm Norwalk-like agent was associated with an outbreak of gastroenteritis in a winter resort camp in Colorado.[143] From a convalescent hospital in Marin County, California, and a social gathering nearby, outbreaks of acute gastroenteritis have been associated with yet another viral agent capable of causing gastroenteritis, the Marin County agent.[144]

Several small (ranging from 20 to 35 nm in diameter), round (variably structured) viral agents of gastroenteritis have been grouped into four categories.[140,145] The first three categories have a better-defined surface morphology: (*1*) Norwalk-like viruses (including Norwalk or Montgomery County agent, Hawaii, Snow Mountain and Taunton agents); (*2*) caliciviruses, with characteristic "chalicelike" surface hollows (including agents described in the United Kingdom, UK1-4, and Japan); (*3*) astroviruses, with five- or six-pointed starlike surface structure (including Marin County, UK1-5, and Japan agents; and (*4*) Other less well defined, small round viruses (including Wollan, Wor Ditchling agent, Cockle, Paramatta, and other agents). Except for certain astrovirus and calicivirus strains, these have not yet been cultivated in vitro, and the lack of a convenient animal model has restricted their study. The roles of other viral agents, including enteroviruses (especially echovirus types 11, 14, and 18), enteric adenoviruses (said to cause up to 9 percent of pediatric inpatient diarrhea[146]), human coronaviruses (reported from infants with gastroenteritis[147,148], and the recently reported pestiviruses[149] are beyond the scope of this chapter. Over one-third of outbreaks of nonbacterial gastroenteritis in the United States have been associated with the Norwalk virus.[150,151]

Identification of Norwalk-like agents capable of causing winter vomiting disease requires immune electron microscopy[133] or radioimmunoassay for demonstration of a serologic response.[152] It is clear that there are multiple antigenic types of these agents that are capable of causing similar disease and that resistance may relate to individual (genetic) differences rather than to lasting protective immunity after symptomatic infection.[140,153] The detection of other viral causes of gastroenteritis includes monoclonal antibody-based enzyme immunoassay,[149,154] tissue culture,[155] or gene probes.[156]

ACUTE NONINFLAMMATORY DIARRHEA IN ADULTS

In temperate climates, acute noninflammatory diarrhea in adults may be caused by rotaviruses[157,158] or by Norwalk-like viruses.[93,97,132,157] The association of rotaviruses as well as adenoviruses, coxsackieviruses and toxigenic *Clostridium difficile* with diarrhea, abdominal cramps, and a higher mortality among adult bone marrow transplant recipients has also been noted.[159] Additionally, several agents of food poisoning such as *Clostridium perfringens, Bacillus cereus,* or *Staphylococcus aureus* commonly cause noninflammatory diarrheal syndromes in adults (see Chapter 86).

In adults living in areas with poor sanitation, several other agents commonly cause sporadic noninflammatory diarrhea. In certain areas in South Asia, cholera is an endemic cause of severe watery diarrhea. With the increased infection-to-case ratio of El Tor cholera, the seventh pandemic has swept most of the continents of the Eastern Hemisphere including Asia, Africa, and the Mediterranean portions of Europe.[160] Isolated cases have also occurred in the United States.[161,162] Outbreaks have been related to contaminated mineral water[163] or to undercooked shellfish.[164,165] One should suspect cholera in any patient who has severe dehydration and watery diarrhea, especially if the patient has a history of recent travel to a cholera-endemic area. The disease can be so fulminant as to cause hypovolemic shock and death from the outpouring of fluid into the upper portion of the small bowel before the first diarrheal stool occurs.[166] As discussed in detail in Chapter 192, the entire dehydrating syndrome of cholera appears to be related to the activation of intestinal adenylate cyclase by the potent cholera enterotoxin.[69,70] To make the diagnosis of cholera bacteriologically, one should culture stool specimens onto thiosulfate citrate bile salts sucrose agar. Of prime importance in therapy is fluid replacement either intravenously with isotonic fluids or orally with glucose electrolyte solutions.

Patients from whom *Vibrio cholerae* cannot be isolated may also have a cholera-like syndrome. In 1956, De et al. demonstrated that *E. coli* isolated from adults and children with this syndrome caused fluid accumulation similar to that seen with *V. cholerae* in ligated rabbit ileal loops.[167] In the early 1960s Trabulsi, working in São Paulo, reported a similar finding with "toxigenic" *E. coli.*[168] Subsequent studies by Taylor et al.[169,170] demonstrated that enterotoxigenicity correlated poorly with classic serotypes and that viable organisms were not required. Smith and Halls identified several enterotoxigenic strains in association with animal diarrhea.[171] Other workers showed that several adult cases of "acute undifferentiated diarrhea" in tropical Bengal were due to enterotoxigenic *E. coli* strains that were usually not of the classically recognized pathogenic serotypes.[172–175] These strains were transiently present during acute illness and elicited a net jejunal fluid secretion. The toxic material present in the culture filtrate of these *E. coli* strains was demonstrated to be heat labile and nondialyzable and was precipitated in 40% ammonium sulfate. Subsequent studies have demonstrated that two types of enterotoxin are produced by *E. coli,* a heat-labile enterotoxin (LT) and a heat-stable enterotoxin (ST).[176] Like cholera toxin, the *E. coli* heat-labile enterotoxin activates mucosal adenylate cyclase.[58–60] Heat-labile enterotoxin is larger, inactivated by heating at 60°C for 30 minutes, and antigenically and mechanistically similar to cholera toxin with a lag period before the activation of adenylate cyclase. Heat-labile enterotoxin is detected by several bioassay systems that use the adenylate cyclase activating property of this toxin[177–179] or by immunoassay methods.[180] In contrast, ST activates guanylate cyclase,[74–76] has an earlier onset of action,[176] has greater tissue specificity,[76] and has a much lower molecular weight than LT does.[181] It is assayed in suckling mice.[182] The role of yet a different type of enterotoxin, STb, that causes secretion in piglets without altering intestinal cyclic AMP or cyclic GMP remains unclear in humans at present.[183–185]

Methods for demonstrating enterotoxigenic *E. coli* are limited by the lack of a selective culture process (as routinely used, for example, to identify salmonellae or shigellae) and the necessity to pick a few random colonies of *E. coli* for enterotoxin testing. Data from a common-source outbreak of enterotoxigenic *E. coli* diarrhea in Crater Lake National Park in Oregon demonstrate the insensitivity of nonselective culture methods.[186] Fourteen patients in this outbreak had enterotoxigenic *E. coli* diarrhea by epidemiologic and clinical criteria, and each had multiple, random *E. coli* stool isolates tested for enterotoxin as well as paired sera examined for antitoxic immunity. Only 43 percent had enterotoxigenic *E. coli* identified, 36 percent had significant serum antitoxic antibody titer increases, and only 64 percent had either one or the other. Thirty-six percent of the cases could not be confirmed by current, nonselective methods. The lack of a serum antibody response in many patients with this intralumenal toxinosis is not surprising.

Other studies have shown that, in addition to the association with diarrhea in children, LT-only, ST-only, and LT-plus-ST–producing strains are associated with adult diarrhea.[3] Adults living in areas of poor sanitation may often carry LT-producing *E. coli* asymptomatically.[187,188] In contrast, ST-producing *E. coli* strains are significantly associated with diarrheal disease and are less frequently present in asymptomatic control patients living in areas with poor sanitation. However, studies suggest that enterotoxigenic *E. coli* serotypes are uncommonly associated with diarrhea in the United States.[66,67]

A newly recognized cause of acute, noninflammatory, self-limited diarrhea among those exposed to infected animals and patients is cryptosporidiosis.[189–191] This tiny coccidian protozoan parasite causes more severe, watery, prolonged diarrhea in immunocompromised hosts.

Treatment of diarrhea in adults consists primarily of rehydration. If glucose or sucrose accompany the isotonic fluid taken orally, the coupled absorption of sodium and water are often sufficient to replace fluid loss.[192] Pepto-Bismol may reduce enterotoxin action,[193] and if there is no significant febrile or inflammatory process, low doses of antimotility agents may offer some relief with minimum risk if cramping is severe.

DIARRHEA IN AIDS PATIENTS

Patients with the acquired immunodeficiency syndrome (AIDS) often develop or present with diarrhea. Among AIDS patients in the United States, 50–60 percent present with diarrhea,[194,195] a number that reaches 95 percent in tropical developing areas such as Africa or Haiti.[195] In many of these patients, diarrhea becomes prolonged and life-threatening and may present major difficulties in management. Although some have reported an enteropathy without identifiable pathogens[196,197] or with primary human immunodeficiency virus (HIV) infection of enterochromaffin cells in the bowel mucosal crypts and lamina propria,[198] others report one or more enteric pathogens in 55–85 percent of patients with AIDS and diarrhea.[199,200] Sexually promiscuous homosexual males often become infected with *Giardia lamblia, Entamoeba histolytica, Campylobacter jejuni, Shigella, Chlamydia trachomatis, C. difficile,* or (with proctitis) *N. gonorrheae,* herpes simplex virus, or *Treponema pallidum.*[201] As shown in Table 3, the leading agents found in AIDS patients with diarrhea are cytomegalovirus, *Cryptosporidium, E. histolytica, G. lamblia, Salmonella, Campylobacter, Shigella, C. difficile, Vibrio parahaemolyticus, Mycobacterium,* sp.,[199,200] and microsporidia. Even *Pneumocystis carinii* can occasionally involve the intestinal tract in this setting.[202] Although eradicative treatment may be difficult, most of these patients respond to specific antimicrobial or antiparasitic therapy, thus

TABLE 3. Possible Enteric Pathogens in AIDS Patients

Pathogen	*Diarrhea (%)* (n = 69)	*No Diarrhea (%)* (n = 48)
Cytomegalovirus	27–45	0–15
Cryptosporidium	15–16	0
Entamoeba histolytica	0–25	0
Giardia lamblia	4–15	0–5
Salmonella sp.	0–15	0
Campylobacter sp.	10–11	5–8
Shigella sp.	5–10	0
Clostridium difficile toxin	7	0
Vibrio parahaemolyticus	4	0
Mycobacterium sp.	2–5	0
Isospora belli	2	0
Blastocystis hominis	15	0–16
Candida albicans	53	0–24
Herpes simplex	5–18	0–40
Chlamydia trachomatis	11	0–13
Intestinal spirochetes	11	0–11
One or more pathogens	55–85	5–39

(Data from Smith et al.[199] and Laughon et al.[200])

emphasizing the need to specifically diagnose the etiologies of these infections whenever possible. The antiviral agent ganciclovir (DHPG) can transiently reverse intestinal cytomegalovirus infection,[203] and most bacterial and parasitic agents can be treated with some improvement. *Cryptosporidium,* which infects 3–21 percent of AIDS patients in the United States, can be found in as many as 50 percent of patients in Africa and Haiti with AIDS and diarrhea.[195] *Cryptosporidium* may also extend into the biliary tract as well in this setting. The same acid-fast stain that detects *Cryptosporidium* or *Mycobacterium* in fecal specimens may also reveal *Isosora belli* in 2–15 percent of AIDS patients with diarrhea in the United States and Africa, respectively.[195] Nontyphoidal *Salmonella* infections occur with an estimated 20-fold increase in frequency as well as increased severity in AIDS patients.[204–207] Nevertheless, these infections, as those with *Campylobacter jejuni* and other species, are treatable. Other common enteric infections include esophagitis or stomatitis with *Candida* or herpes simplex virus.

DIARRHEA IN INSTITUTIONS

Institutions provide special host and environmental settings for the acquisition of certain enteric pathogens. As with diarrhea in AIDS patients and travelers' diarrhea, most cases are still noninflammatory; however, an increased frequency of certain causes of inflammatory diarrhea should prompt a careful search for fecal leukocytes in sporadic or clustered cases in hospitals, chronic care facilities, or day care centers.[208]

Hospitals

Nosocomial diarrhea is among the most common of reported nosocomial outbreaks to the Centers for Disease Control and accounts for 21 percent of all 223 nosocomial outbreaks reported from 1956 to 1979.[209] However, its frequency is often overlooked, and it has been suggested to be the most common nosocomial infection in some areas.[210] Furthermore, nosocomial diarrhea appears to be a significant predisposing factor to other nosocomial infections such as urinary tract infections.[211] Overall rates range from 2.3 to 4.1 illnesses per 100 admissions on pediatric wards[210,212] and from 7.7 per 100 admissions to 41 percent of adults hospitalized in intensive care units.[210,213] From limited available data, *C. difficile* appears to be associated with most cases with a recognized etiology (45 percent), followed by *Salmonella* (12 percent).[214] *Salmonella* is the commonest cause among reported outbreaks of nosocomial gastroenteritis.[209] In young children and in immunocompromised hosts, viral agents (rotaviruses, adenoviruses, coxsackieviruses, and others) are often found as well.[212,215]

Chronic Care Facilities

Diarrheal illnesses are also significant problems in extended care facilities for the elderly. Conservative estimates based on passively reported illness rates are that one-third of patients in chronic care facilities experience diarrhea each year.[216,217] About one-quarter of these patients have *C. difficile* cytotoxin, one-third of whom are symptomatic with diarrhea.[218] Over 20 percent have fecal cytotoxin on admission, and a comparable number acquire cytotoxigenic *C. difficile* in the institution.[218] When those with diarrhea are studied, 18–53 percent have cytotoxin or *C. difficile,* respectively.[219] The frequency of potentially transmissible enteric pathogens emphasizes the importance of careful hand washing in situations where hygiene is often difficult. Similar problems have been long recognized in mental institutions where hepatitis, *Strongyloides,* and amebiasis are readily acquired.

Day Care Centers

Another special institutional setting where hygiene is difficult and enteric infections are increasingly appreciated is in day care centers. Numerous outbreaks have been reported in association with viruses, bacteria, or parastites. Most common in infants and children <2 years old are rotaviruses, while older toddlers are more likely to acquire *Giardia lamblia.*[220] An identical clinical syndrome of prolonged noninflammatory diarrhea may be seen with *Cryptosporidium* in day care centers.[221–223] Outbreaks of inflammatory diarrhea in the day care center setting include those due to *Shigella, Campylobacter jejuni,* and *Clostridium difficile.*[224,225]

THE DIARRHEA OF TRAVELERS (TURISTA)

Whether it "arouses one from bed with a start at 4 A.M. for a record-breaking race to the bathroom to begin a stacatto ballet"[226] or it produces the poetry of the Psalmist, "I am poured out like water . . . my heart like wax is melted in the midst of my bowels,"[227] travelers' diarrhea has a major impact each year on the 300 million international travelers and probably on the distribution of $100 billion in international tourism receipts.[228] Sixteen million people (8 million from the United States) travel from industrialized to developing countries. It is by far the most common and among the most feared illnesses that threaten the traveler. Many studies have focused on North Americans and northern Europeans who appear to be the groups at greatest risk when they travel to Latin America, Southern Europe, Africa, or Asia.[229–232] Travelers' diarrhea, which may be severe and incapacitating (albeit rarely if ever fatal), is by far the most common health problem encountered with travel to developing countries.[233] The global nature of the problem and some suggested causal forces are illustrated by its more euphemistic names: "Delhi belly," "Gyppi tummy," "GIs," "Rome runs," "Greek gallop," "Turkey trots," "Montezuma's revenge," "Aztec two-step," "Aden gut," "San Franciscitis," "Basra belly," "La turista," "backdoor sprint," "summer complaint," "coeliac flux," "Canary disease," "passion," "Hong Kong dog," "Poona poohs," "Casablanca crud," "tourist trots," "Malta dog," and many more.

The onset of the vast majority of travelers' diarrhea is usually between 5 and 15 days after arrival, with a range from 3 to 31 days in several reported series.[226,234–240] The illness is typically manifested by malaise, anorexia, and abdominal cramps, followed by the sudden onset of watery diarrhea. Nausea and vomiting may accompany 10–25 percent of the illnesses. The diarrhea is usually noninflammatory, without blood or pus. A low-grade fever may be present in approximately one-third of the cases. The duration is usually 1–5 days, but a significant number of people (19–50 percent) have an illness that continues beyond 5–10 days.

TABLE 4. Etiologies of Travelers' Diarrhea

Characteristics	Latin America (15 Studies)	Africa (3 Studies)	Asia (8 Studies)
Duration of stay (days)	21 (2–42)[a]	28 (28–35)	(28–42)
Attack rate (%)	52 (21–100)	54 (36–62)	(39–57)
Percentage with			
Enterotoxigenic *E. coli*	46 (28–72)	36 (31–75)	(20–34)
Shigella	0 (0–30)	0 (0–15)	(4–7)
Salmonella	0 (0–16)	0 (0–0)	(11–15)
C. jejuni	—	—	(2–15)
V. parahaemolyticus	—	—	(1–13)
Rotavirus	23 (0–36)	0 (0–0)	—

[a] Median (range) from 26 studies.[241,242]

The attack rate ranges from 7 percent after 2 weeks in Aden[235] to 54 percent after 8 days in Mexico,[229] and was 4–51 percent over a 14-day period among 17,280 Swiss tourists, depending on where they went.[232] One report of British tourists notes an attack rate ranging from 26 percent in Africa to 7.7 percent in North America. In descending order of risk after Africa in this study were the Middle East, Southern Europe, Central Europe, Asia (including India and Pakistan), South America, Australia, and North America.[240] In general, it appears that one approaches a 50 percent risk of acquiring turista during travel to a tropical country from a temperate climate for 2 weeks or more. The attack rate also appears to decrease with age after 25 years, an observation that may reflect different habits and exposure rather than inherent susceptibility.[226,232]

For many years, the etiology of turista was an enigma; only infrequently have parasites or bacteria such as amebas, *Giardia, Salmonella,* or *Shigella* been identified. Likewise viral studies have failed to elucidate significant viral etiologies of travelers' diarrhea. The first suggestion that an infectious bacterial process was likely came from the effective reduction in the attack rate by the use of prophylactic antimicrobial agents.[185,191,234,240] Studies by Kean suggested that *E. coli* of certain enteropathogenic serotypes might be involved in up to one-third of the cases.[226] The involvement of *E. coli* was further confirmed in an outbreak of travelers' diarrhea among the British troops in Aden, where *E. coli* 0148 was identified among 54 percent of British troops with diarrhea.[235]

Subsequent studies have demonstrated enterotoxigenic *E. coli* (ETEC) in approximately 50 percent (range, 20–75 percent) of cases of travelers' diarrhea in Latin America, Africa, and Asia (Table 4).[241,242] The attack rate ranged from 20 to 100 percent (median, 52–54 percent) in 26 studies reviewed (Table 4).[241,242] Enterotoxigenic *E. coli* organisms were almost never present before the travel; they were acquired by only 14 of 111 (12.6 percent) fellow travelers who did not become ill.[237–239] The type of enterotoxin produced by *E. coli* associated with travelers' diarrhea may be the heat-labile type (LT), the heat-stable type (ST), or both LT and ST (Table 5). In contrast to adults who live in tropical areas and may often carry enterotoxigenic *E. coli* asymptomatically, the traveler appears to be susceptible to illness caused by enterotoxin-producing *E. coli.* Salmonellae, shigellae, or vibrios are present in only 1–16 percent of the patients with travelers' diarrhea. Rotavirus infections have been described in 0–36 percent of cases of travelers' diarrhea, often in association with bacterial or parasitic pathogens.[243] In a study of Panamanian tourists to Mexico, rotavirus or Norwalk viruses were found in 41 percent, *Campylobacter* in 11 percent, and ETEC in only one case of diarrhea.[244] Cholera is rarely a problem for U.S. travelers.[232,245]

In contrast to the frequent identification of potential etiologic agents among travelers to tropical areas who develop diarrhea, careful studies of a group of marines who developed diarrhea upon arrival in temperate South Korea (21 percent in 3 weeks) failed to reveal any evidence of bacterial, parasitic, or rotaviral pathogens.[246] Travelers to certain areas such as Russia and national parks in the United States may be especially prone to the more insidious watery diarrhea seen with giardiasis or cryptosporidiosis.[247–250] Strongyloidiasis may also be acquired in tropical areas and may cause noninflammatory diarrhea, abdominal pain, and eosinophilia.[251]

Several other potentially serious infections may be acquired by travelers whose major complaint is diarrhea or abdominal pain. Malaria may be manifested initially as "gastroenteritis" with nausea, vomiting, diarrhea, or abdominal pain in 30–50 percent of the cases.[252] The physician caring for world travelers should also remember to consider typhoid fever and other infections that may be manifested with a "typhoidal pattern" including plague, meloidosis, typhus, and arboviral hemorrhagic fevers.[252,253]

The desire to control the bothersome problem of diarrhea in travelers has led to extreme and sometimes irrational attempts at its control.[226] Some travelers persist in using iodochlorhydroxquin (Entero-Vioform, clioquinol), which has been shown not only to be ineffective for travelers' diarrhea[229,254] but also to carry a risk of severe subacute myelo-optic atrophy.[255] Other commonly used remedies such as diphenoxylate-atropine (Lomotil) and kaolin-pectin suspension were of no value in treating children with acute diarrhea in Guatemala.[256] The former and other antimotility agents may actually worsen the illness with inflammatory processes such as shigellosis.[257] Bismuth subsalicylate (Pepto-Bismol) has been shown to inhibit enterotoxin activity in experimental animal models[193] and has been recommended for symptomic therapy and, in doses as low as 1.05 g/day (2 tablets bid), for prophylaxis.[258,259]

The mainstay of therapy, as with any diarrheal illness, is adequate hydration with an oral glucose– or sucrose–electrolyte solution.

Prevention of travelers' diarrhea should be directed toward reducing the consumption of infectious agents in food and water. Salads, raw vegetables, and untreated water (or ice) are high-risk foods.[260] Bottled, noncarbonated water cannot be considered safe since outbreaks of cholera[163] and typhoid fever[261,262] have been traced to bottled water and beverages, respectively. It has been suggested that even brief, 10-minute heating to 50–55°C (the temperature of some hot tap water, "too hot for the hand to tolerate") may kill many enteric bacterial

TABLE 5. Frequency of Enterotoxigenic *E. coli* in Association with Travelers' Diarrhea in Latin America, Africa, and Asia

Feature	Study: Gastroenterologists in Mexico[146]	Peace Corps Volunteers in Kenya[147]	Yale Glee Club in Latin America[148]	Japanese Travelers Returning to Tokyo from India, Southeast Asia, Orient[242]	Total
Illness attack rate (%)	49% in 16 days	69% in 5 wk	74% in 1 mon	—	
Type of enterotoxin					
LT only	16%	33%	25%	4.8%	21%
LT and ST	16%	15%	12.5%	11.8%	38%
ST only	9.8%	2%	19%	13.6%	41%
Total	21/51 cases	14/27 cases	9/16 cases	226/749 cases	270/843 cases
(Percentage of illness with ETEC)	(41%)	(52%)	(56%)	(30.2%)	(32%)

Abbreviations: LT: heat-labile; ST: heat-stable.

and parasitic pathogens.[263] Care in eating and drinking may reduce one's risk even in highly endemic areas to <15 percent.[260,264]

The efficacy of prophylactic antimicrobial agents has been documented in several studies.[234,240,265] However, multiple drug-resistant enterotoxigenic *E. coli* occur and have demonstrated cotransfer of enterotoxigenicity and drug resistance.[266,267] The increased risk of acquiring a more severe infection such as salmonellosis,[268] the risk of drug side effects (such as photosensitivity in the tropics), and the emergence of drug-resistant organisms should preclude the widespread use of antibiotic prophylaxis at this time. Until more widespread resistance develops,[269,270] treatment of travelers' diarrhea with trimethoprim, sulfamethoxazole-trimethoprim, bicozamycin, or ciprofloxacin may reduce a 3- to 4- day illness to 1–1½ days.[271–273]

DIFFERENTIAL DIAGNOSIS OF ACUTE NONINFLAMMATORY DIARRHEA

Acute noninflammatory diarrhea may also be the consequence of several noninfectious processes. As with agents that effect an osmotic diuresis, nonabsorbable agents such as sorbitol may cause diarrhea if consumed in excess. Ipecac fluid extract used by mistake instead of ipecac syrup may cause watery diarrhea instead of vomiting. Heavy metal poisoning (As, Sn, Fe, Cd, Hg, Pb) is often associated with diarrhea, probably as a result of toxic effects on the rapidly growing mucosal epithelium. Endocrine causes of diarrhea that may share the adenylate cyclase–activating mechanism with enterotoxins include non-β islet cell tumors, medullary carcinoma of the thyroid, carcinoid tumors, and others that are associated with increased serum prostaglandins or vasoactive intestinal polypeptide (VIP).[274] Patients with thyrotoxicosis and adrenal or parathyroid insufficiency may also have diarrhea. Congenital and acquired enzyme deficiencies include lactase deficiency and pancreatic or biliary insufficiency in which inadequately degraded or absorbed nutrients may promote an osmotic diarrhea. A child with diarrhea as well as with edema, hypertension, or petechiae should be suspected of having hemolytic-uremic syndrome with or without enterohemorrhagic *E. coli* O157:H7. Patients with dermatitis herpetiformis may also have diarrhea that may respond to sulfone or sulfapyridine therapy or to a gluten-free diet.

CHRONIC NONINFLAMMATORY DIARRHEA

Syndromes of chronic noninflammatory diarrhea of infectious etiology include giardiasis, tropical spruelike syndromes, syndromes of bacterial "overgrowth," and *Cryptosporidium* or *Isospora belli* infection (especially in immunocompromised hosts).[189,190,195,249,275]

The patient with weight loss, malaise, and watery or fatty stools should be suspected of having giardiasis or some other cause of a malabsorption syndrome. This syndrome may also be associated with hypocalcemia, with iron or folate deficiency anemia, or with vitamin D, vitamin K, or protein deficiency.

Giardiasis may go undiagnosed for weeks. While it is endemic throughout most of the United States and much of the world, giardiasis received attention when acquired in Rocky Mountain ski resorts and in Leningrad.[247,248] Effective management requires a high index of suspicion followed by a careful search by a competent experienced person for the trophozoite or cyst of *G. lamblia* in multiple stool specimens or in a small bowel aspirate or "string" (Enterotest; Hedeco, Palo Alto, CA) sample. Recommended therapy is quinacrine (Atabrine), 100 mg tid for 5–7 days, with a reported 95 percent cure rate, or metronidazole (Flagyl), 250 mg tid for 7–10 days, with a reported 70 percent cure rate.[275] Higher doses of metronidazole may be more effective. Furazolidone, which is available in liquid form for pediatric use, divided into three daily doses with meals (total, 8 mg/kg/day) for 10 days is often used in children.[276]

The diagnosis of *Cryptosporidium* or *Isospora belli* infection is best made by phase microscopic or modified Kinyoun acid-fast stain examination of fecal specimens with or without sugar floatation.[189,195,277]

BACTERIAL OVERGROWTH SYNDROMES

Many syndromes have been described in which impaired absorption was attributed to abnormal bacterial colonization in the upper segment of the small bowel.[278] Whether these organisms are virulent pathogens or simply normal colonic flora abnormally distributed is currently unclear.

Normally, the upper portion of the small bowel is relatively sparsely populated with fewer than 10^5 organisms/ml that are predominantly facultative gram-positive organisms (diptheroids, streptococci, and lactobacilli).[279] The organisms most often incriminated in bacterial overgrowth syndromes in the small bowel are aerobic enteric coliforms (Enterobacteriaceae) and anerobic gram-negative fecal flora (*Bacteroides* and other genera). Other organisms such as *Plesiomonas shigelloides* may occasionally be responsible.[280] Bacterial colonization in the upper part of the small bowel may be associated with malabsorption or chronic diarrhea in the absence of significant histopathologic changes. Small bowel overgrowth is usually associated with a predisposing bowel abnormality such as achlorhydria, (from gastritis, pernicious anemia, or gastric surgery), blind-loop syndromes, cholangitis, impaired motility (scleroderma, diabetic neuropathy, vagotomy), surgery, strictures, diverticula, or radiation damage.[281,282] Malnutrition, especially with protein, folate, or B_{12} deficiency, may also render the bowel more susceptible to microbial colonization and injury.[279,283] An episode of acute infectious diarrhea may also provide the initiating event in the establishment of small bowel colonization and chronic diarrhea.[279,284,285] Lindenbaum et al. described spruelike morphologic changes in the upper portion of the small bowel in association with increased numbers of bacteria and malabsorption among Peace Corps volunteers living in Pakistan.[286]

The mechanism by which fecal flora in the small bowel cause malabsorption may involve bacterial binding or utilization of nutrients (such as vitamin B_{12} or carbohydrates, respectively), deconjugation of bile salts by bacteria such as enterococci and anerobes,[287] or the toxic effects of bacterial products such as fatty acids or amines.[279] Indeed, colonizing *E. coli* without other recognized virulence traits have been shown to cause prolonged diarrhea in a rabbit model,[288] with an associated impairment in water and electrolyte absorption as well as disaccharidase activity.[289]

The approach to the patient suspected of having bacterial "overgrowth" as a cause of malabsorption or chronic diarrhea should include quantitative aerobic and anerobic cultures of the upper small bowel contents obtained by intubation or "string" passage. Since the critical number of organisms appears to be approximately 10^5 organisms/ml, semiquantitative estimates from a Gram stain analogous to the urine Gram stain may also prove to be of value. Roberts et al. have suggested that unexplained malnutrition in the elderly may be due to clinically inapparent bacterial overgrowth that can be detected by the ^{14}C-glycocholic acid breath test for bacterial deconjugation of bile salts.[284] Tests for urinary indican (from bacterial conversion of tryptophan) have proved to be insensitive and nonspecific for bacterial overgrowth syndromes.[290]

Patients with diarrhea or malabsorption and bacterial overgrowth should be considered for antibiotic therapy, especially if predisposing conditions like achlorhydria, scleroderma, or diabetes are present. Depending on results of quantitative cultures of upper small bowel aspirates, therapy may need to be directed against anerobes as well as aerobic coliform organisms.[279,284] While small amounts of antibiotics have been used to improve the nutritional status of animals and poultry and even of malnourished children,[291] the potential risks of widespread antibiotic use[292] must be weighed against potential benefits.

Noninfectious causes of chronic noninflammatory diarrhea should also be considered in the differential diagnosis. These include congenital deficiency syndromes and food allergies, certain neoplastic and endocrine processes, and less well understood functional disorders. In the first categories one may consider milk allergies, disaccharidase deficiencies, gluten enteropathy, acrodermatitis enteropathica, β-lipoprotein deficiency, familial hyperchloremic alkalosis (congenital "chloridorrhea") Leiner's disease, and Wiskott-Aldrich syndrome. Neoplastic and endocrine causes of diarrhea include carcinoid, Werner syndrome (multiple endocrine adenomatosis), Zollinger-Ellison syndrome (gastrinoma), "pancreatic cholera" syndromes, medullary carcinoma of the thyroid, and thyrotoxicosis. Patients with partial mechanical bowel obstruction or pellagra may also have chronic diarrhea. Finally, frequent small stools may suggest an irritable bowel syndrome of presumed functional etiology. However, a search for treatable infectious agents reviewed in this chapter should always precede this latter diagnosis.

REFERENCES

1. Dingle JH, Badger GF, Jordan WS Jr. Illnesses in the Home: A Study of 25,000 Illnesses in a Group of Cleveland Families. Cleveland: Press of Western Reserve University; 1964.
2. Kapikian AZ, Kim H-W, Wyatt RG, et al. Human reovirus-like agent as the major pathogen associated with "winter" gastroenteritis in hospitalized infants and young children. N Engl J Med. 1976;294:965.
3. Black RE, Merson MH, Huq I, et al. Incidence and severity of rotavirus and *E. coli* diarrhea in rural Bangladesh. Lancet. 1981;1:141.
4. Ryder TW, Sack DA, Kapikian AZ, et al. Enterotoxigenic *Escherichia coli* and reovirus-like agent in rural Bangladesh. Lancet. 1976;1:659.
5. Guerrant RL, Moore RA, Kirschenfeld PM, et al. Role of toxigenic and invasive bacteria in acute diarrhea of childhood. N Engl J Med. 1975;293:567.
6. Wadstrom T, Aust-Kettis A, Habte D, et al. Enterotoxin-producing bacteria and parasites in stools of Ethiopian children with diarrhoeal disease. Arch Dis Child. 1976;51:865.
7. Sack RB, Hirschhorn N, Brownlee I, et al. Enterotoxigenic *Escherichia coli*-associated diarrheal disease in Apache children. N Engl J Med. 1975;292:1041.
8. Black RE, Brown KH, Becker S, et al. Longitudinal studies of infectious diseases and physical growth of children in rural Bangladesh. I. Patterns of morbidity. Am J Epidemiol. 1982;115:305.
9. Guerrant RL, Kirchoff LV, Shields DS, et al. Prospective study of diarrheal illnesses in Northeastern Brazil: Patterns of disease, nutritional impact and risk factors. J Infect Dis. 1983;148:986.
10. Jacobs SI, Holzel A, Wolman B, et al. Outbreak of infantile gastroenteritis caused by *Escherichia coli* 0114. Arch Dis Child. 1970;45:656.
11. Neter E. Enteritis due to enteropathogenic *Escherichia coli:* Present-day status and unsolved problems. J Pediatr. 1959;55:223.
12. Hone R, Fitzpatrick S, Keane C, et al. Infantile enteritis in Dublin caused by *Escherichia coli* 0142. Med Microbiol. 1973;6:505.
13. Levine MM, Nalin DR, Hornick RB, et al. *Escherichia coli* strains that cause diarrhea but do not produce heat-labile or heat-stable enterotoxins and are noninvasive. Lancet. 1978;1:1119.
14. Nelson JD, Haltalin KC. Accuracy of diagnosis of bacterial diarrheal disease by clinical features. J Pediatr. 1971;78:519.
15. Drucker MM, Polliack A, Yeivin R, et al. Immunofluorescent demonstration of enteropathogenic *Escherichia coli* in tissues of infants dying with enteritis. Pediatrics. 1970;46:855.
16. South MA: Enteropathogenic *Escherichia coli* disease: New developments and perspectives. J Pediatr. 1971;79:1.
17. Kaslow RA, Taylor A, Dweck HS, et al. Enteropathogenic *Escherichia coli* infection in a newborn nursery. Am J Dis Child. 1974;128:797.
18. Levine MM, Edelman R. Enteropathogenic *Escherichia coli* of classic serotypes associated with infant diarrhea: Epidemiology and pathogenesis. Epidemiol Rev. 1984;6:31–51.
19. Gurwith M, Hinde D, Gross R, et al. A prospective study of enteropathogenic *E. coli* in endemic diarrheal disease. J Infect Dis. 1978;137:292.
20. Toledo MRF, Alvariza MCB, Murahovschi J, et al. Enteropathogenic *Escherichia coli* serotypes and endemic diarrhea in infants. Infect Immun. 1983;39:586–589.
21. Bray J, Beavan TED. Slide agglutination of *Bacterium coli* var. *Neapolitanum* in summer diarrhea. J Pathol Bacteriol. 1948;60:395.
22. Varela G, Aguirre A, Grillo J. *Escherichia coli*-gomez, nueva especie aislada de un caso mortal de diarrea. Bol Medico del Hospital Infantil Mexico. 1946;3:3.
23. Olarte J, Varela G. A complete somatic antigen common to *Salmonella adelaide, Escherichia coli-gomez* and *Escherichia coli* 0111:B4. J Lab Clin Med. 1952;40:252.
24. Giles C, Sangster G. An outbreak of infantile gastro-enteritis in Aberdeen. J Hyg (Camb) 1948;46:1.
25. Kaufmann F, Dupont A. *Escherichia* strains from infantile epidemic gastroenteritis. Acta Pathol Microbiol Scand. 1950;27:552.
26. Ørskov I, Ørskov F, Jann B, et al. Serology, chemistry and genetics of O and K antigens of *Escherichia coli.* Bacteriol Rev. 1977;41:667.
27. Rowe B, Gion RJ. *Escherichia coli* 0142 and infantile enteritis in Scotland. Lancet. 1971;1:649.
28. Rowe B, Gross J, Lindop R, et al. A new *E. coli* O group 0158 associated with an outbreak of infantile enteritis. J Clin Pathol. 1974;27:832.
29. Rogers KB, Cracknell VM. Epidemic infantile gastro-enteritis due to *Escherichia coli* type 0114. J Pathol Bacteriol. 1956;72:27.
30. Charter RE. *Escherichia coli* type 0114 isolated from infantile diarrhea and calf scours. J Pathol Bacteriol. 1956;72:33.
31. Riley LW, Remis RS, Helgerson SD, et al. Outbreaks of hemorrhagic colitis associated with a rare *Escherichia coli* serotype. N Engl J Med. 1983;308:681.
32. Johnson WM, Lior H, Bezanson GS. Cytotoxic *Escherichia coli* 0157:H7 associated with hemorrhagic colitis in Canada. Lancet. 1983;1:76.
33. Outbreak of hemorrhagic colitis—Ottawa, Canada. MMWR. 1983;32:133.
34. Neter E, Shumway CN: *E coli* serotype D433: Occurrence in intestinal and respiratory tracts, cultural characteristics, pathogenicity, sensitivity to antibiotics. Proc Soc Exp Biol Med. 1950;74:504.
35. Ørskov F. Virulence factors of the bacterial cell surface. J Infect Dis. 1978;137:630.
36. Guerrant RL, Dickens MD, Wenzel RP, et al. Toxigenic bacterial diarrhea: Nursery outbreak involving multiple bacterial strains. J Pediatr. 1976;89:885.
37. Skerman FJ, Formal SB, Falkow S. Plasmid-associated enterotoxin production in a strain of *Escherichia coli* isolated from humans. Infect Immun. 1972;5:622.
38. Takeda Y, Murphy J. Bacteriophage conversion of heat labile enterotoxin in *Escherichia coli.* J Bacteriol. 1978;133:172.
39. Wachsmith K, Wells J, Shipley P, et al. Heat-labile enterotoxin production in isolates from a shipboard outbreak of human diarrheal illness. Infect Immun. 1979;24:793–7.
40. Sack RB. Human diarrheal disease caused by enterotoxigenic *Escherichia coli.* Annu Rev Microbiol. 1975;29:333.
41. Merson MH, Black RE, Gross RJ, et al. Use of antisera for identification of enterotoxigenic *E. coli.* Lancet.. 1980;2:222.
42. Ryder RW, Wachsmuth IK, Buxton AE, et al. Infantile diarrhea produced by heat-stable enterotoxigenic *Escherichia coli.* N Engl J Med. 1976;295:849.
43. Gross RJ, Rowe B, Henderson A, et al. A new *Escherichia coli* O-group, 0159, associated with outbreaks of enteritis in infants. Scand J Infect Dis. 1976;8:195.
44. Haltalin KC. Neonatal shigellosis. Am J Dis Child. 1967;114:603.
45. Schroeder SA, Aserkoff B, Brachman PS. Epidemic salmonellosis in hospitals and institutions. N Engl J Med. 1968;279:674.
46. Rice PA, Craven PC, Wells JG: *Salmonella heidelberg* enteritis and bacteremia. An epidemic on two pediatric wards. Am J Med. 1976;60:509.
47. Eichenwald HF, Ababio A, Arky AM, et al. Epidemic diarrhea in premature and older infants caused by echo virus type 18. JAMA. 1958;166:1563.
48. Yow MD, Melnick JL, Blattner RJ, et al. The association of viruses and bacteria with infantile diarrhea. Am J Epidemiol. 1970;92:33.
49. Moffet HL, Shulenberger HK, Burkholder ER. Epidemiology and etiology of severe infantile diarrhea. J Pediatr. 1968;72:1.
50. Murphy AM, Albrey MB, Crew EB. Rotavirus infections of neonates. Lancet. 1977;2:1149.
51. Cameron DJS, Bishop RF, Davidson GP, et al. New virus associated with diarrhea in neonates. Med J Aust. 1976;1:85.
52. Bishop RF, Hewstone AS, Davidson GP, et al. An epidemic of diarrhea in human neonates involving a reoviruslike agent and "enteropathogenic" serotypes of *Escherichia coli.* J Clin Pathol. 1976;29:46.
53. Chrystie IL, Totterdell BM, Banatvala JE. Asymptomatic endemic rotavirus infections in the newborn. Lancet. 1978;1:1176.
54. Mata LJ, Urrutia JJ. Intestinal colonization of breast-fed children in a rural area of low socioeconomic level. Ann NY Acad Sci. 1971;176:93.
55. Gordon JE, Chitkara ID, Wyon JB. Weanling diarrhea. Am J Med Sci. 1963;245:345.
56. Welsh JK, May JT. Anti-infective properties of breast-milk. J Pediatr. 1979;94:1.
57. Gordon JE, Guzman MA, Ascoli W, et al. Acute diarrhoeal disease in less developed countries. Bull WHO. 1964;31:9.
58. Reddy V, Rashuramulu N, Bhaskaram C. Secretory IgA in protein-calorie malnutrition. Arch Dis Child. 1976;51:871.
59. Stoliar OA, Kaniecki-Green E, Pelley RP, et al. Secretory IgA against enterotoxins in breast milk. Lancet. 1976;1:1258.
60. Brown SE III, Sauer KT, Nations MK, et al. Comparison of paired whole milk and dried filter paper samples for anti-enterotoxin and antirotavirus activities. J Clin Microbiol. 1982;16:103.
61. Bullen CL, Willis AT. Resistance of the breast-fed infant to gastroenteritis. Br Med J. 1971;3:338.
62. Bullen JJ, Rogers HJ, Leigh L. Iron-binding proteins in milk and resistance of *Escherichia coli* infection in infants. Br Med J. 1972;1:69.
63. Simhon A, Mata L. Anti-rotavirus antibody in human colostrum. Lancet. 1978;1:39.

64. Gorbach SL, Khurana CM. Toxigenic *Escherichia coli:* A cause of infantile diarrhea in Chicago. N Engl J Med. 1972;287:791.
65. Tacket CO, Losonsky G, Link H, et al. Protection by milk immunoglobulin concentrate against oral challenge with enterotoxigenic *Escherichia coli.* N Engl J Med. 1988;318:1240–3.
66. Echeverria P, Blacklow NR, Smith DH. Role of heat-labile toxigenic *Escherichia coli* and reovirus-like agent in diarrhea in Boston children. Lancet. 1975;2:1113.
67. Hughes JM, Gwaltney JM, Hughes DH, et al. Acute gastrointestinal illness in Charlottesville: A prospective family study (Abstract). Clin Res. 1978;26:24.
68. Guerrant RL, Hughes JM, Lima NL, et al. Microbiology of diarrhea in developed and developing countries. Rev Inf Dis. 1989. In press.
69. Chen LC, Rohde JE, Sharp GWG. Intestinal adenyl-cyclase activity in human cholera. Lancet. 1971;1:939.
70. Guerrant RL, Chen LC, Sharp GWG. Intestinal adenyl-cyclase activity in canine cholera: Correlation with fluid accumulation. J Infect Dis. 1972;125:377.
71. Evans DJ Jr, Chen LC, Curlin GT, et al. Stimulation of adenyl cyclase by *Escherichia coli* enterotoxin. Nature. 1972;236:137.
72. Guerrant RL, Ganguly U, Casper AGT, et al. Effect of *Escherichia coli* on fluid transport across canine small bowel: Mechanism and time course—with enterotoxin and whole bacterial cells. J Clin Invest. 1973;52:1707.
73. Kantor HS, Tao P, Gorbach SL. Stimulation of intestinal adenyl cyclase by *Escherichia coli* enterotoxin: Comparison of strains from an infant and an adult with diarrhea. J Infect Dis. 1974;129:1.
74. Hughes JM, Murad F, Chang B, et al. Role of cyclic GMP in the action of heat stable enterotoxin of *Escherichia coli.* Nature. 1978;271:755.
75. Field M, Graf LH Jr, Laird WJ, et al. Heat-stable enterotoxin of *Escherichia coli:* In vitro effects on guanylate cyclase activity, cyclic GMP concentration, and ion transport in small intestine. Proc Natl Acad Sci USA. 1978;75:2800.
76. Guerrant RL, Hughes JM, Chang B, et al. Activation of intestinal guanylate cyclase by heat stable enterotoxin of *E. coli:* Studies of tissue specificity, potential receptors, and intermediates. J Infect Dis. 1980;142:220.
77. Bishop RF, Davidson GP, Holmes IH, et al. Virus particles in epithelial cells of duodenal mucosa from children with acute non-bacterial gastroenteritis. Lancet. 1973;2:1281.
78. Flewett TH, Bryden AS, Davies H. Virus particles in gastroenteritis. Lancet. 1973;2:1497.
79. Kapikian AZ, Kim HW, Wyatt RG, et al. Reoviruslike agent in stools: Association with infantile diarrhea and development of serologic tests. Science. 1974;185:1049.
80. Kanno T, Suzuki H, Ishida N. Reovirus-like agent in Japanese infants with gastroenteritis. Lancet. 1975;1:918.
81. Virus of infantile gastroenteritis, editorial. Br Med J. 1975;3:555.
82. Rotaviruses of man and animals, (editorial). Lancet. 1975;1:257.
83. Mata L, Simhon A, Padilla R, et al. Diarrhea associated with rotaviruses, enterotoxigenic *E. coli, Campylobacter,* and other agents in Costa Rican children, 1976–1981. Am J Trop Med Hyg. 1983;32:146.
84. Black RE, Merson MH, Rahman ASMM, et al. A two-year study of bacterial, viral, and parasitic agents associated with diarrhea in rural Bangladesh. J Infect Dis. 1980;142:660.
85. Echeverria P, Ho MT, Blacklow NR, et al. Relative importance of viruses and bacteria in the etiology of pediatric diarrhea in Taiwan. J Infect Dis. 1977;136:383.
86. Paul MO, Erinle EA. Influence of humidity on rotavirus prevalence among Nigerian infants and young children with gastroenteritis. J Clin Microbiol. 1982;15:212.
87. Brandt CD, Kim HW, Rodriguez WJ. Rotavirus gastroenteritis and weather. J Clin Microbiol. 1982;16:478.
88. Gurwith M, Wenman W, Gurwith D, et al. Diarrhea among infants and young children in Canada: A longitudinal study in three Northern communities. J Infect Dis. 1983;147:685.
89. Shepherd RW, Truslow S, Walker-Smith JA. Infantile gastroenteritis: A clinical study of reovirus-like agent infection. Lancet. 1975;2:1082.
90. Sexton M, Davidson GP, Bishop RF, et al. Viruses in gastroenteritis. Lancet. 1974;2:355.
91. Tallett S, MacKenzie C, Middleton P, et al. Clinical, laboratory, and epidemiologic features of a viral gastroenteritis in infants and children. Pediatrics. 1977;60:217.
92. Kim HW, Brandt CD, Kapikian AZ, et al. Human reoviruslike agent infection. Occurrence in adult contacts of pediatric patients with gastroenteritis. JAMA. 1977;238:404.
93. Wenman WM, Hinde D, Feltham S, et al. Rotavirus infection in adults: Results of a prospective family study. N Engl J Med. 1979;301:303.
94. Kapikian AZ, Dienstag JL, Purcell RH. Immune electron microscopy as a method for the detection, identification, and characterization of agents not cultivable in an in vitro system. In: Rose NR, Friedman H, eds.: Manual of Clinical Immunology. Washington, DC: American Society for Microbiology; 1976.
95. Zissis G, Lambert JP. Different serotypes of human rotaviruses. Lancet. 1978;1:38.
96. Beards GM, Pilford JN, Thouless ME, et al. Rotavirus serotypes by serum neutralization. J Med Virol. 1980;5:231.
97. Blacklow NR, Cukor G. Viral gastroenteritis. N Engl J Med. 1981;304:397.
98. Urasawa S, Urasawa T, Taniguchi K. Three human rotavirus serotypes demonstrated by plaque neutralization of isolated strains. Infect Immun. 1982;38:781.
99. Fonteyne J, Zissis G, Lambert JP. Recurrent rotavirus gastroenteritis. Lancet. 1978;1:983.
100. Yolken R, Kim HW, Clem T, et al. Enzyme immunoassay (ELISA) for the detection of human reovirus-like agent in human stools. Lancet. 1977;2:263.
101. Kalica AR, Purcell RH, Sereno NM, et al. Microtiter solid phase radioimmunoassay for detection of the human reovirus-like agent in stools. J Immunol. 1977;118:1275.
102. Middleton PJ, Petrie M, Hewitt CM, et al. Counter-immunoelectroosmophoresis for the detection of infantile gastroenteritis virus (orbi group) antigen and antibody. J Clin Pathol. 1976;29:191.
103. Middleton PJ, Szymanski MT, Abbott GD, et al. Orbivirus acute gastroenteritis of infancy. Lancet. 1974;1:1241.
104. Davidson GP, Goller I, Bishop RF, et al. Immunofluorescence in duodenal mucosa of children with acute enteritis due to a new virus. J Clin Pathol. 1975;28:263.
105. Thomas EE, Puterman ML, Kawano E, et al. Evaluation of seven immunoassays for detection of rotavirus in pediatric stool samples. J Clin Microbiol. 1988;26:1189–93.
106. Flores J, Purcell RH, Perez I, et al. A dot hybridization assay for detection of rotavirus. Lancet. 1983;1:555.
107. Flewett TH, Bryden AS, Davies H, et al. Relation between viruses from acute gastroenteritis of children and newborn calves. Lancet. 1974;2:61.
108. Purdham DR, Purdham PA, Evans N, et al. Isolation of human rotavirus using human embryonic gut monolayers. Lancet. 1975;2:977.
109. Banatvala JE, Totterdell B, Chrystie IL, et al. In vitro detection of human rotaviruses. Lancet. 1975;2:821.
110. Wyatt RG, Gill VW, Sereno MM, et al. Probable in vitro cultivation of human reovirus-like agent of infantile diarrhea. Lancet. 1976;1:98.
111. Middleton PJ, Petric M, Szymanski MT. Propagation of infantile gastroenteritis virus (orbi-group) in conventional and germfree piglets. Infect Immun. 1975;12:1276.
112. Wyatt RG, Sly DL, London WT, et al. Induction of diarrhea in colostrum deprived newborn rhesus monkeys with human reovirus-like agent of infantile gastroenteritis. Arch Virol. 1976;50:17.
113. Wyatt RG, James SD, Bohl EH, et al. Human rotavirus type 2: Cultivation in vitro. Science. 1980;207:189.
114. Sato K, Inaba Y, Shinozuka T, et al. Isolation of human rotavirus in cell cultures. Arch Virol. 1981;69:155.
115. Urasawa T, Urasawa S, Taniguchi K. Sequential passages of human rotavirus in MA-104 cells. Microbiol Immunol. 1981;25:1025.
116. Kutsuzawa T, Konno T, Suzuki H, et al. Isolation of human rotavirus subgroups 1 and 2 in cell culture. J Clin Microbiol. 1982;16:727.
117. Guerrant RL. Pathophysiology of the enterotoxic and viral diarrheas. In Chen LC, Scrimshaw NS, eds. Diarrhea and Malnutrition: Interactions, Mechanisms and Interventions. New York: Plenum; 1983.
118. Middleton PJ, Szymanski MT, Abbott GD, et al. Orbivirus acute gastroenteritis of infancy. Lancet. 1974;1:1241.
119. Davidson GP, Goller I, Bishop RF, et al. Immunofluorescence in duodenal mucosa of children with acute enteritis due to a new virus. J Clin Pathol. 1975;28:263.
120. Sack DA, Chowdhury AMAK, Eusof A, et al. Oral hydration in rotavirus diarrhea: A double blind comparison of sucrose with glucose electrolyte solution. Lancet. 1978;2:280.
121. Davidson GP, Barnes GL. Structural and functional abnormalities of the small intestine in infants and young children with rotavirus enteritis. Acta Paediatr Scand. 1979;68:181.
122. Shepherd RW, Butler DG, Cutz E, et al. The mucosal lesion in viral enteritis: Extent and dynamics of the epithelial response to virus invasion in transmissible gastroenteritis of piglets. Gastroenterology. 1979;76:770.
123. Davidson GP, Gall DG, Petric M, et al. Human rotavirus enteritis induced in conventional piglets: Intestinal structure and transport. J Clin Invest. 1977;60:1402.
124. Vesikari T, Isolauri E, D'Hondt E, et al. Protection of infants against rotavirus diarrhea: RIT 4237 attenuated bovine rotavirus vaccine. Lancet. 1984;1:977–980.
125. Edelman R. Perspective on the development and deployment of rotavirus vaccines. Pediatr Infect Dis. 1987;6:704.
126. Gordon I, Ingraham HS, Korns RF. Transmission of epidemic gastroenteritis to human volunteers by oral administration of fecal filtrates. J Exp Med. 1947;86:409.
127. Jordan WS, Gordon I, Dorrance WR. A study of illness in a group of Cleveland families. VII. Transmission of acute nonbacterial gastroenteritis to volunteers: Evidence for two different etiologic agents. J Exp Med. 1953;98:461.
128. Kojima S, Fukumi H, Kusama H, et al. Studies on the causative agent of the infectious diarrhea; records of the experiments on human volunteers. Jpn Med J. 1948;1:467.
129. Klein JO, Lerner AM, Finland M. Acute gastroenteritis associated with echo virus, type II. Am J Med Sci. 1960;240:749.
130. Kerr AA, McQuillin J, Downham MAPS, et al. Gastric "flu" influenza B causing abdominal symptoms in children. Lancet. 1975;1:291.
131. Adler JL, Zickl R. Winter vomiting disease. J Infect Dis. 1969;119:668.
132. Dolin R, Blacklow NR, DuPont H, et al. Transmission of acute infectious nonbacterial gastroenteritis to volunteers by oral administration of stool filtrates. J Infect Dis. 1971;123:307.

133. Kapikian AZ, Wyatt RG, Dolin R, et al. Visualization by immune electron microscopy of a 27-nm particle associated with acute infectious nonbacterial gastroenteritis. J Virol. 1972;10:1075.
134. Zahorsky J. Hyperemesis hiemis or the winter vomiting disease. Arch Pediatr. 1929;46:391.
135. Agus SG, Dolin R, Wyatt RG, et al. Acute infectious nonbacterial gastroenteritis. Intestinal histopathology. Ann Intern Med. 1973;79:18.
136. Schreiber DS, Trier JS, Blacklow NR. Recent advances in viral gastroenteritis. Gastroenterology. 1977;73:174.
137. Levy AG, Widerlite L, Schwartz CJ, et al. Jejunal adenylate cyclase activity in human subjects during viral gastroenteritis. Gastroenterology. 1976;70:321.
138. Blacklow NR, Dolin R, Fedson DS, et al. Acute infectious nonbacterial gastroenteritis: Etiology and pathogenesis. Ann Intern Med. 1972;76:993.
139. Wyatt RG, Dolin R, Blacklow NR, et al. Comparison of three agents of acute infectious nonbacterial gastroenteritis by cross-challenge in volunteers. J Infect Dis. 1974;129:709.
140. Dolin R, Treanor JJ, Madore HP. Novel agents of viral enteritis in humans. J Infect Dis. 1987;155:365–76.
141. Clarke SKR, Cook GT, Egglestone SI, et al. A virus from epidemic vomiting disease. Br Med J. 1972;3:86.
142. Appleton H, Buckley M, Thom BT, et al. Virus-like particles in winter vomiting disease. Lancet. 1977;1:409.
143. Morens DM, Zweighaft RM, Vernon TM. A waterborne outbreak of gastroenteritis with secondary person-to-person spread. Lancet. 1979;1:964.
144. Oshiro LS, Haley CE, Roberto RR, et al. A 27-nm virus isolated during an outbreak of acute infectious nonbacterial gastroenteritis in a convalescent hospital: A possible new serotype. J Infect Dis. 1981;143:791.
145. Caul EO, Appleton H. The electron microscopical and physical characteristics of small round human fecal viruses: An interim scheme for classification. J Med Virol. 1982;9:257–65.
146. Brandt CD, Kim HW, Rodriguez WJ, et al. Adenoviruses and pediatric gastroenteritis. J Infect Dis. 1985;151:437–43.
147. Gerna G, Passarani N, Battaglia M, et al. Human enteric coronaviruses: Antigenic relatedness to human coronavirus OC43 and possible etiologic role in viral gastroenteritis. J Infect Dis. 1985;151:796–802.
148. Battaglia M, Passarani N, DiMatteo A, et al. Human enteric coronaviruses: Further characterization and immunoblotting of viral proteins. J Infect Dis. 1987;155:140–3.
149. Yolken R, Santosham M, Reid R, et al. Pestiviruses: Major etiological agents of gastroenteritis in human infants and children (Abstract) Clin Res. 1988;36:780.
150. Greenberg HB, Valdesuso J, Yolken RH, et al. Role of Norwalk virus in outbreaks of nonbacterial gastroenteritis. J Infect Dis. 1979;139:564.
151. Kaplan JE, Gary GW Jr, Baron RC, et al. Epidemiology of Norwalk gastroenteritis and the role of the Norwalk virus in outbreaks of nonbacterial gastroenteritis. Ann Intern Med. 1982;96:756.
152. Greenberg HB, Wyatt RG, Valdesuso J, et al. Solid-phase microtiter radioimmunoassay for detection of the Norwalk strain of acute nonbacterial, epidemic gastroenteritis virus and its antibodies. J Med Virol. 1978;2:97.
153. Parrino TA, Schreiber DS, Trier JS, et al. Clinical immunity in acute gastroenteritis caused by Norwalk agent. N Engl J Med. 297:86–89, 1977;297:86–9.
154. Herrmann JE, Perron-Henry DM, Blacklow NR. Antigen detection with monoclonal antibodies for the diagnosis of adenovirus gastroenteritis. J Infect Dis. 1987;155:1167–71.
155. Shinozaki T, Araki K, Ushijima H, et al. Use of Graham 293 cells in suspension for isolating enteric adenoviruses from the stools of patients with acute gastroenteritis. J Infect Dis. 1987;156:246.
156. Neil C, Gomes SA, Leite JPG, et al. Direct detection and differentiation of fastidious and nonfastidious adenoviruses in stools by using a specific nonradioactive probe. J Clin Microbiol. 1986;24:785–9.
157. von Bonsdorff CH, Hovi T, Makela P, et al. Rotavirus associated with acute gastroenteritis in adults. Lancet. 1976;2:423.
158. Wenman WM, Hinde D, Feltham S, et al. Rotavirus infection in adults. Results of a prospective study. N Engl J Med. 1979;301:306.
159. Yolken RH, Bishop CA, Townsend TR, et al. Infectious gastroenteritis in bone-marrow transplant recipients. N Engl J Med. 1982;306:1099.
160. Goodgame RW, Greenough WBIII. Cholera in Africa: A message for the west. Ann Intern Med. 1975;82:101.
161. Weissman JB, DeWitt WE, Thompson J, et al. A case of cholera in Texas, 1973. Am J Epidemiol. 1975;100:487.
162. Blake PA, Allegra DT, Snyder JD, et al. Cholera: A possible endemic focus in the United States. N Engl J Med. 1980;302:305.
163. Blake PA, Rosenberg ML, Florencia J, et al. Cholera in Portugal, 1974. II. Transmission by bottled mineral water. Am J Epidemiol. 1977;105:344.
164. Baine WB, Mazzotti M, Greco D, et al. Epidemiology of cholera in Italy in 1973. Lancet. 1974;2:1370.
165. Gitelson S. Gastrectomy, achlorhydria and cholera. Isr J Med Sci. 1971;7:663.
166. Snow J. On the Mode of Communication of Cholera. 2nd ed. London: Churchill; 1855.
167. De SN, Bhattacharya K, Sarkar JK. A study of the pathogenicity of strains of *Bacterium coli* from acute and chronic enteritis. J Pathol Bacteriol. 1956;71:201.
168. Trabulsi LR. Revelação de colibacilos associados as diarreias infantis pelo metodo da infeccão experimental da alca ligade do intestino do coelho. Rev Inst Med Trop Sao Paulo. 1964;6:197.
169. Taylor J, Wilkins MP, Payne JM. Relation of rabbit gut reaction to enteropathogenic *Escherichia coli*. Br J Exp Pathol. 1961;42:43.
170. Taylor J, Bettlelheim KA. The action of chloroform-killed suspensions of enteropathegenic *Escherichia coli* on ligated rabbit-gut segments. J Gen Microbiol. 1966;42:309.
171. Smith HW, Halls S. Studies on *Escherichia coli* enterotoxin. J Pathol Bacteriol. 1967;93:531.
172. Gorbach SL, Banwell JG, Chatterjee BD, et al. Acute undifferentiated human diarrhea in the tropics. I. Alterations in intestinal microflora. J Clin Invest. 1971;50:881.
173. Banwell JG, Gorbach SL, Pierce NF, et al. Acute undifferentiated human diarrhea in the tropics. II. Alterations in intestinal fluid and electrolyte movements. J Clin Invest. 1971;50:890.
174. Sack RB, Gorbach SL, Banwell JG, et al. Enterotoxigenic *Escherichia coli* isolated from patients with severe cholera-like disease. J Infect Dis. 1971;123:378.
175. DuPont HL, Formal SB, Hornick RB, et al. Pathogenesis of *Escherichia coli* diarrhea. N Engl J Med. 1971;285:1.
176. Evans DG, Evans DJ Jr, Pierce NF. Differences in the response of rabbit small intestine to heat-labile and heat-stable enterotoxins of *Escherichia coli*. Infect Immun. 1973;7:873.
177. Guerrant RL, Brunton LL, Schnaitman TC, et al. Cyclic adenosine monophosphate and alteration of Chinese hamster ovary cell morphology: A rapid, sensitive in vitro assay for the enterotoxins of *Vibrio cholerae* and *Escherichia coli*. Infect Immun. 1974;10:320.
178. Donta ST, Moon HW, Whipp SC. Detection of heat-labile *Escherichia coli* enterotoxin with the use of adrenal cells in tissue culture. Science. 1974;183:334.
179. Guerrant RL, Brunton LL. Characterization of the Chinese hamster ovary cell assay for the enterotoxins of *Vibrio cholerae* and *Escherichia coli* and for antitoxin: Differential inhibition by gangliosides, specific antisera, and toxoid. J Infect Dis. 1977;135:720.
180. Honda T, Arita M, Takeda Y, et al. Further evaluation of the Biken test (modified Elek test) for detection of enterotoxigenic *E. coli* producing heat-labile enterotoxin and application of the test to sampling of heat-stable enterotoxin. J Clin Microbiol. 1982;16:60.
181. Alderete JF, Robertson DC. Purification and chemical characterization of the heat-stable enterotoxin produced by porcine strains of enterotoxigenic *Escherichia coli*. Infect Immun. 1978;19:1021.
182. Dean AG, Ching YC, Williams RG, et al. Test for *Escherichia coli* enterotoxin using infant mice: Application in a study of diarrhea in children in Honolulu. J Infect Dis. 1972;125:407.
183. Gyles CL. Limitations of the infant mouse test for *E. coli* heat-stable enterotoxin. Can J Comp Med. 1979;43:371–9.
184. Kennedy, DJ, Greenberg RN, Dunn JA, et al. Effects of *Escherichia coli* heat stable enterotoxin STb on intestines of mice, rats, rabbits and piglets. Infect Immun 1984;46:639–43.
185. Weikel CS, Mellans HN, Guerrant RL. In vivo and in vitro effects of a novel enterotoxin, STb, produced by *Escherichia coli*. J Infect Dis. 1986;153:893–901.
186. Rosenberg ML, Koplan JP, Wachsmuth IK, et al. Epidemic diarrhea at Crater Lake from enterotoxigenic *Escherchia coli*. A large, waterborne outbreak. Ann Intern Med. 1977;86:714.
187. Korzeniowski OM, Dantas W, Trabulsi LR, et al. A controlled study of endemic sporadic diarrhea among adult residents of southern Brazil. Trans R Soc Trop Med Hyg. 1984;78:363–9.
188. Hughes JM, Rouse JD, Barada FA, et al. Etiology of summer diarrhea among the Navajo. Am J Trop Med Hyg. 1980;29:613.
189. Current WL, Reese NC, Ernst JV, et al. Human cryptosporidiosis in immunocompetent and immunodeficient persons. N Engl J Med. 1983;308:1252.
190. Tzipori S. Cryptosporidiosis in animals and humans. Microbiol Rev. 1983;47:84.
191. Wolfson JS, Richter JM, Waldron MA, et al. Cryptosporidiosis in immunocompetent patients. N Engl J Med. 1985;312:1278–82.
192. Palmer DL, Koster FT, Islam AFMR, et al. A comparison of sucrose and glucose in oral electrolyte therapy of cholera and other severe diarrheas. N Engl J Med. 1977;297:1107.
193. Ericsson CD, Evans DG, DuPont HL, et al. Bismuth subsalicylate inhibits activity of crude toxins of *Escherichia coli* and *Vibrio cholerae*. J Infect Dis. 1977;136:693.
194. Gelb A, Miller S. AIDS and gastroenterology. Am J Gastroenterol. 1986;81:619–22.
195. Soave R, Johnson WD. *Cryptosporidium* and *Isospora belli* infections. J Infect Dis. 1988;157:225–29.
196. Kotler DP, Goetz HP, Lange M, et al. Enteropathy associated with the acquired immunodeficiency syndrome. Ann Intern Med. 1984;101:421–28.
197. Gillin JS, Shike M, Alcock N, et al. Malabsorption and mucosal abnormalities of the small intestine in the acquired immunodeficiency syndrome. Ann Intern Med. 1985;102:619–22.
198. Nelson JA, Reynolds-Kohler G, Margaretten W, et al. Human immunodeficiency virus detected in bowel epithelium from patients with gastro-intestinal symptoms. Lancet 1988;1:259–62.
199. Smith PD, Lance C, Gill VJ, et al. Intestinal infections in patients with the

acquired immunodeficiency syndrome (AIDS). Ann Intern Med. 1988;108:328–33.
200. Laughon BE, Druckman DA, Vernon A, et al. Prevalence of enteric pathogens in homosexual men with and without Acquired Immunodeficiency Syndrome. Gastroenterology. 1988;94:984.
201. Quinn TC, Stamm WE, Goodell SE, et al. The polymicrobial origin of intestinal infections in homosexual men. N Engl J Med. 1983;309:576–82.
202. Carter TR, Cooper PH, Petri WA Jr, et al. *Pneumocystis carinii* infection of the small intestine in a patient with aquired immune deficiency syndrome. Am J Clin Pathol. 1988;89:679–83.
203. Chachoua A, Dieterich D, Krasinski K, et al. 9-(1,3-dihydroxy-2-propoxymethyl) guanine (ganciclovir) in the treatment of cytomegalovirus gastrointestinal disease with the acquired immunodeficiency syndrome. Ann Intern Med. 1987;107:133–7.
204. Celum CL, Chaisson RE, Rutherford GW, et al. Incidence of salmonellosis in patients with AIDS. J Infect Dis. 1987;156:998–1002.
205. Jacobs JL, Gold JWM, Murray HW, et al. *Salmonella* infections in patients with the acquired immunodeficiency syndrome. Ann Intern Med. 1985;102:186–88.
206. Glaser JB, Morton-Kute L, Berger SR, et al. Recurrent *Salmonella typhimurium* bacteremia associated with the acquired immunodeficiency syndrome. Ann Intern Med. 1985;102:189–93.
207. Sperber SJ, Schleupner CJ: Salmonellosis during infection with human immunodeficiency virus. Rev Infect Dis. 1987;9:925–34.
208. Guerrant RL, Hughes JM, Lima NL, et al. Microbiology of diarrhea in developed and developing countries. Rev Infect Dis. 1989. In press.
209. Stamm WE, Weinstein RA, Dixon RE. Comparison of endemic and epidemic nosocomial infections. Am J Med. 1981;70:393–97.
210. Lima N, Searcy M, Guerrant R. Nosocomial diarrhea rates exceed those of other nosocomial infections on ICU and pediatric wards (Abstract 1050). In: Proceedings of the 26th Interscience Conference on Antimicrobial Agents and Chemotherapy, New Orleans, 1986.
211. Lima NL, Guerrant RL, Kaiser DL, et al. Nosocomial diarrhea: A possible risk factor for nosocomial infections (Abstract). Clin Res. 1988;36:580.
212. Welliver RC, McLaughlin S. Unique epidemiology of nosocomial infection in a children's hospital. Am J Dis Child. 1984;138:131–35.
213. Kelly WJ, Patrick MR, Hillman KM. Study of diarrhea in critically ill patients. Crit Care Med. 1983;1:7–9.
214. Hughes JM, Jarvis WR. Nosocomial gastrointestinal infections. In: Wenzel RP, ed. Prevention and Control of Nosocomial Infections. Philadelphia: Williams & Wilkins; 1987.
215. Yolken RH, Bishop CA, Townsend R, et al. Infectious gastroenteritis in bone marrow transplant recipients. N Engl J Med. 1982;306:1009–12.
216. Farber BF, Brennen JC, Puntereri AJ, et al. A prospective study of nosocomial infections in a chronic care facility. J Am Geriatr Soc. 1984;32:499.
217. Nicolle LE, McIntyre M, Zacharias H, et al. Twelve-month surveillance of infections in institutionalized elderly men. J Am Geriatr Soc. 1984;32:513.
218. Bender BS, Laughon BE, Gaydos C, et al. Is *Clostridium difficile* endemic in chronic-care facilities? Lancet. 1986;2:1279.
219. Treolar AJ, Kalra L. Mortality and *Clostridium difficile* diarrhoea in the elderly. Lancet. 1987;2:1279.
220. Pickering LK, Evans DG, Dupont HL, et al. Diarrhea caused by *Shigella*, rotavirus and *Giardia* in day care centers: Prospective study. J Pediatr. 1981;99:51–56.
221. Centers for Disease Control. Cryptosporidiosis among children attending day-care centers: Georgia, Pennsylvania, Michigan, California, New Mexico. MMWR. 1984;33:599.
222. Alpert G, Bell LM, Kirkpatrick CE, et al. Cryptosporidiosis in a day-care center. N Engl J Med. 1984;311:860–1.
223. Taylor JP, Perdue JN, Dingley D, et al. Cryptosporidiosis outbreak in a day-care center. Am J Dis Child. 1985;139:1023–5.
224. Bartlett AV, Moore M, Gary GW, et al. Diarrheal illness among infants and toddlers in daycare centers. I Epidemiology and pathogens. J Pediatr. 1985;107:495–502.
225. Guerrant RL, Lohr JA, Williams EK. Acute infectious diarrhea. I. Epidemiology, etiology, and pathogenesis. Pediatr Infect Dis. 1986;5:353–59.
226. Kean BH. The diarrhea of travelers to Mexico. Summary of five-year study. Ann Intern Med. 1963;59:605.
227. Psalms 22:14.
228. Consensus development conference statement on travelers' diarrhea. Rev Inf Dis. 1986;8(Suppl):227–33.
229. Lowenstein MS, Balows A, Gangarosa EJ. Turista at an international congress in Mexico. Lancet. 1973;1:529.
230. Editorial. The diarrhea of travelers: Turista. JAMA. 1962;180:402.
231. Higgens AR. Observations on the health of United States personnel living in Cairo, Egypt. Am J Trop Med Hyg. 1955;4:970.
232. Steffen R. Epidemiologic studies of travelers' diarrhea, severe gastrointestinal infections, and cholera. Rev Infect Dis. 1986;8(Suppl 2):122–30.
233. Steffen R, Rickernbach M, Wilhelm U, et al. Health problems after travel to developing countries. J Infect Dis. 1987;156:84–91.
234. Kean BH, Schaffner W, Brennan RW. The diarrhea of travelers. V. Prophylaxis with phthalysulfathiazole and neomycin sulphate. JAMA. 1962;180:367–71.
235. Rowe B, Taylor J, Bettelheim KA. An investigation of travelers' diarrhea. Lancet. 1970;1:1.
236. Gorbach SL, Kean BH, Evans DG, et al. Travelers' diarrhea and toxigenic *Escherichia coli*. N Engl J Med. 1975;292:933.
237. Merson MH, Morris GK, Sack DA, et al. Travelers' diarrhea in Mexico, a prospective study of physicians and family members attending a congress. N Engl J Med. 1976;294:1299.
238. Sack DA, Kaminsky DC, Sack RB, et al. Enterotoxigenic *Escherichia coli* diarrhea of travelers: A prospective study of American Peace Corps volunteers. Johns Hopkins Med J. 1977;141:63.
239. Guerrant RL, Rouse JD, Hughes JM. Turista among members of the Yale Glee Club in Latin America. Am J Trop Med Hyg. 1980;29:895.
240. Turner AC. Travelers' diarrhoea: A survey of symptoms, occurrence, and possible prophylaxis. Br Med J. 1967;4:453–4.
241. Black RE. Pathogens that cause travelers' diarrhea in Latin America and Africa. Rev Infect Dis. 1986;8(Suppl 2):131–5.
242. Taylor DN, Echeverria P. Etiology and epidemiology of travelers' diarrhea in Asia. Rev Infect Dis. 1986;8(Suppl 2):136–41.
243. Bolivar R, Conklin RH, Vollet JJ, et al. Rotavirus in travelers' diarrhea: Study of an adult student population in Mexico. J Infect Dis. 1978;137:324.
244. Ryder RW, Oquist CA, Greenberg H, et al. Travelers' diarrhea in Panamanian tourists in Mexico. J Infect Dis. 1981;144:442.
245. Snyder JD, Blake PA. Is cholera a problem for US travelers? JAMA. 1982;247:2268.
246. Echeverria P, Hodge FA, Blacklow NR, et al. Travelers' diarrhea among United States marines in South Korea. Am J Epidemiol. 1978;108:68.
247. Wolfe MS. Current concepts in parasitology. Giardiasis. N Engl J Med. 1978;298:319.
248. Brodsky RE, Spencer HC Jr, Schultz MG. Giardiasis in American travelers to the Soviet Union. J Infect Dis. 1974;130:319.
249. Soave R, Armstrong D. *Cryptosporidium* and cryptosporidiosis. Rev Infect Dis. 1986;8:1012–23.
250. Jokipii L, Pohjola S, Jokipii AMM. *Cryptosporidium:* A frequent finding in patients with gastrointestinal symptoms. Lancet. 1983;2:358–360.
251. Kean BH, Reilly PC. Malaria–the mime. Recent lessons from a group of civilian travelers. Am J Med. 1976;61:159.
252. Pearson RD, Hewlett EL, Guerrant RL. Tropical diseases in North America. DM. 1984;30:1–68.
253. Hill DR, Pearson RD. Health advice for international travel. Ann Intern Med. 1988;108:839–52.
254. Kean BH, Waters SR. Diarrhea of travelers. III. Drug prophylaxis in Mexico. N Engl J Med. 1959;261:71.
255. Oakley GP. The neurotoxicity of the halogenated hydroxyguinolines. JAMA. 1973;225:395.
256. Portnoy BL, DuPont HL, Pruitt D, et al. Antidiarrheal agents in the treatment of acute diarrhea in children. JAMA. 1976;236:844.
257. DuPont HL, Hornick RB. Adverse effect of Lomotil therapy in shigellosis. JAMA. 1973;226:1525.
258. DuPont HL, Sullivan P, Pickering LK, et al. Symptomatic treatment of diarrhea with bismuth subsalicylate among students attending a Mexican university. Gastroenterology. 1977;73:715.
259. Steffen R, Heusser R, DuPont HL. Prevention of travelers' diarrhea by nonantibiotic drugs. Rev Infect Dis. 1986;8(Suppl 2):151–9.
260. Blaser MJ. Environmental interventions for the prevention of travelers' diarrhea. Rev Inf Dis. 1986;8(Suppl 2):142–50.
261. Gonzales-Cortez A, Gangarosa EJ, Parrilla C, et al. Bottled beverages and typhoid fever: The Mexican epidemic of 1972–3. Am J Public Health. 1982;72:844.
262. Harris JR. Are bottled beverages safe for travelers? Am J Public Health. 1982;72:787.
263. Neumann HH. Travellers' diarrhea. Lancet. 1970;1:420.
264. Tjoa W, DuPont HL, Sullivan P, et al. Location of food consumption and travelers' diarrhea. Am J Epidemiol. 1977;106:61.
265. Sack DA, Kaminsky DC, Sack RB, et al. Prophylactic doxycycline for travelers' diarrhea, results of a prospective double-blind study of Peace Corps volunteers in Kenya. N Engl J Med. 1978;298:758.
266. Echeverria P, Verhaert L, Ulyangco CV, et al. Antimicrobial resistance and enterotoxin production among isolates of *Escherichia coli* in the Far East. Lancet. 1978;2:589.
267. Murray BE. Resistance of *Shigella Salmonella* and other selected enteric pathogens. Rev Infect Dis. 1986;8(Suppl 2):172–81.
268. Mentzing LO, Ringertz O. *Salmonella* infection in tourists. 2. Prophylaxis against salmonellosis. Acta Pathol Microbiol Scand. 1968;74:405.
269. Murray BE, Rensimer ER, DuPont HL. Emergence of high level trimethoprim resistance in fecal *E. coli* during oral administration of trimethoprim or trimethoprim/sulfamethoxazole. N Engl J Med. 1982;306:130.
270. Tiemens KM, Shipley PL, Correia RA, et al. Sulfamethoxazole-trimethoprim resistant *Shigella flexneri* in northeastern Brazil. Antimic Ag Chemother. 1984;25:653–54.
271. DuPont HL, Reves RR, Galindo E, et al. Treatment of travelers' diarrhea with trimethoprim/sulfamethoxazole and with trimethoprim alone. N Engl J Med. 1982;307:841–4.
272. Ericsson CD, DuPont HL, Sullivan P, et al. Bicozamycin, a poorly absorbable antibiotic, effectively treats travelers' diarrhea. Ann Intern Med. 1983;98:20.
273. Ericsson CD, Johnson PC, DuPont HL, et al. Ciprofloxacin or trimethoprim-sulfamethoxazole as initial therapy for travelers' diarrhea. Ann Intern Med. 1987;106:216–20.
274. Said SI, Faloona GR. Elevated plasma and tissue levels of vasoactive intestinal polypeptide in the watery diarrhea syndrome due to pancreatic, bronchogenic, and other tumors. N Engl J Med. 1975;293:155.

275. Wolff MS. Giardiasis. JAMA. 1975;233:1362.
276. Murphy TV, Nelson JD. Five vs ten days' therapy with furazolidone for giardiasis. Am J Dis Child. 1983;137:267.
277. Ma P, Soave R. Three-step stool examination for cryptosporidiosis in 10 homosexual men with protracted watery diarrhea. J Infect Dis. 1983;147:824.
278. Donaldson RM Jr. Small bowel bacterial overgrowth. Adv Intern Med. 1970;16:191.
279. Gorbach SL. Intestinal microflora. Gastroenterology. 1971;60:1110.
280. Penn RG, Giger DK, Knoop FC, et al. *Plesiomonas shigelloides* overgrowth in the small intestine. J Clin Microbiol. 1982;15:869.
281. Scott AJ, Khan GA. Partial biliary obstruction with cholangitis producing a blind loop syndrome. Gut. 1968;9:187.
282. Vantrappen G, Janssens J, Hellemans J, et al. Interdigestive motor complex of normal subjects and patients with bacterial overgrowth of the small intestine. J Clin Invest. 1977;59:1158.
283. Heyworth B, Brown J. Jejunal microflora in malnourished Gambian children. Arch Dis Child. 1975;50:27.
284. Roberts SH, James O, Jarvis EH. Bacterial overgrowth syndrome without "blind loop": A cause for malnutrition in the elderly. Lancet. 1977;2:1193.
285. Ruiz-Palacios GM, DuPont HL. Bacterial overgrowth syndrome after acute nonspecific diarrhoea. Lancet. 1978;1:337.
286. Lindenbaum J, Kent TH, Sprinz H. Malabsorption and jejunitis in American Peace Corps Volunteers in Pakistan. Ann Intern Med. 1966;65:1201.
287. Shimada K, Brickenll KS, Finegold SM. Deconjugation of bile acids by intestinal bacteria: Review of literature and additional studies. J Infect Dis. 1969;119:273.
288. Wanke CA, Guerrant RL. Small bowel colonization alone is a cause of diarrhea. Infect Immun. 1987;55:1924–6.
289. Schlager TA, Guerrant RL. Net fluid secretion and impaired villous function induced by small intestinal colonization by non-toxigenic, colonizing *E. coli*. Abst. No. 1133, 28th Intersc Conf Antimic Ag Chemother. 1988;310.
290. Hamilton JD, Dyer NH, Dawson AM, et al. Assessment and significance of bacterial overgrowth in the small bowel. Q J Med. 1970;39:265.
291. MacDougall LG. The effect of aureomycin on undernourished African children. J Trop Pediatr. 1957;3:74.
292. Levy SB, FitzGerald GB, Macone AB. Changes in intestinal flora of farm personnel after introduction of a tetracycline-supplemented feed on a farm. N Engl J Med. 1976;295:583.

83. ANTIBIOTIC-ASSOCIATED COLITIS

ROBERT FEKETY

HISTORICAL PERSPECTIVE

Although antibiotics are the most important precipitating cause of pseudomembranous colitis (PMC), it is noteworthy that this disease was recognized in the preantibiotic era[1]; thus, other factors are important in pathogenesis. Many cases diagnosed soon after antibiotics were introduced were attributed to *Staphylococcus aureus*, but in retrospect many investigators believe that this association may have been coincidental. PMC was rarely recognized from 1960 to 1970, but it was often diagnosed thereafter in patients treated with lincomycin, clindamycin, or broad-spectrum β-lactam antibiotics. In these patients, staphylococci could not be implicated, and many patients died because no effective therapy was known. Furthermore, we now realize that a type of diarrhea unassociated with PMC is common in patients treated with antibiotics. At the University of Michigan Hospitals in 1976, 19 (8 percent) of 242 patients receiving ampicillin or clindamycin developed diarrhea.[2] Only 3 of these 19 patients had PMC, while the rest had a benign diarrhea of unknown cause that was believed to be related to change in the bowel flora.

In order to better understand PMC, investigators administered antibiotics to various species of animals in the hope of producing a model of the human disease. They found that golden Syrian hamsters were highly susceptible to diarrhea and fatal enterocolitis after being given any of many antibiotics either orally or parenterally.[3] After a cytotoxin neutralizable by *Clostridium sordellii* antitoxin was detected in the feces of these hamsters,[4] cultural studies revealed large numbers of *Clostridium difficile* in their feces and showed that this organism produced a cytotoxin neutralizable by *C. sordellii* antitoxin.[1] Hamsters inoculated with cell-free filtrates of broth cultures of *C. difficile* developed enterocolitis,[1] and hamsters passively immunized with *C. sordellii* antitoxin did not develop colitis after being given antibiotics.[5] After *C. difficile* was shown to be susceptible to vancomycin, antibiotic-treated hamsters were given vancomycin prophylactically, and it was found that they did not develop colitis.[6]

When humans with PMC were studied, it was found that *C. difficile* and/or its cytotoxin were almost always present in their stools.[7,8] It was also learned that many patients with antibiotic-associated colitis (AAC) did not have pseudomembranes and that both PMC and AAC could be treated successfully by the oral administration of vancomycin. However, most patients with antibiotic-associated diarrhea had neither colitis nor *C. difficile* or its toxin in their stools. This more common and benign type of diarrhea was found to be treatable by discontinuing antibiotic therapy and replacing fluid and electrolyte losses.

As a result of these studies, *C. difficile* has become recognized as the most frequent cause of AAC. Recently, a comprehensive review and a state-of-the-art book on *C. difficile* and its role in intestinal disease have been published.[9,10]

PATHOLOGY

The important characteristic of the disease is acute colitis. Pseudomembranes may be absent or extensive or consist of small and discrete yellow-white plaques or nodules that are easily dislodged (Fig. 1). The pseudomembrane consists of fibrin, mucus, necrotic epithelial cells, and leukocytes adherent to the underlying inflamed tissues. Colitis usually affects only the epithelium and superficial lamina propria, but in severe cases deeper tissues are involved. In many cases, pseudomembranes are not visible to the naked eye but are detectable microscopically if a biopsy specimen is obtained. These patients are usually categorized as having nonspecific colitis until *C. difficile* and its toxins are detected in their stools. Pseudomembranes occur throughout the colon but are usually most prominent in the rectosigmoid area; the ileum is rarely involved. AAC is uncommon in infants, but cases have been recognized.[12] Some

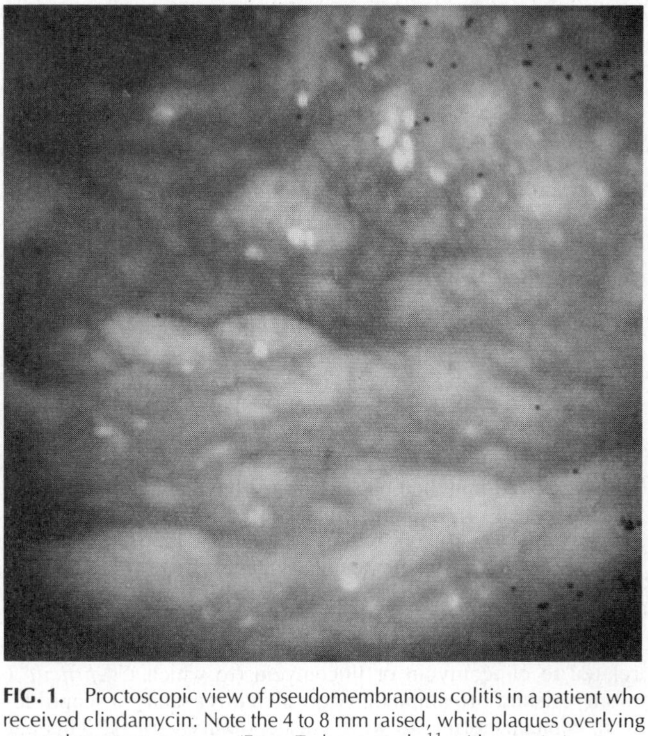

FIG. 1. Proctoscopic view of pseudomembranous colitis in a patient who received clindamycin. Note the 4 to 8 mm raised, white plaques overlying an erythematous mucosa. (From Tedesco et al.,[11] with permission.)

infants with chronic diarrhea and positive stools for *C. difficile* and its toxin have undergone rectal biopsies that revealed cryptitis, and some of them became well after treatment with oral vancomycin.[13]

MICROBIOLOGY, EPIDEMIOLOGY, AND PATHOGENESIS

Clostridium difficile is a spore-forming, gram-positive, obligate anaerobic bacillus. It is part of the normal intestinal flora of about 3 percent of healthy adults. Colonization rates may be much higher in hospitalized persons. We found small numbers of *C. difficile* in the stools of 15 percent of medical patients without diarrhea in our hospital, and 71 percent of asymptomatic infants were positive on a pediatric ward where there was a case of AAC.[14] The organism has been isolated from healthy dogs and cats, waterfowl, horses, camels, donkeys, seals, hamsters, and guinea pigs,[15] but animals are not considered important in transmission to humans. Because the organism was not easily distinguished from *Clostridium sporogenes* and other organisms commonly found in stools, it was difficult to detect with ordinary cultural techniques and was overlooked as a cause of colitis until 1977.[1] In 1979, George and his associates reported that a selective medium that contained cycloserine, cefoxitin, and fructose in agar (CCFA) was helpful in isolating *C. difficile* from stools.[16] The addition of 0.2% highly purified sodium taurocholate to CCFA increased its ability to detect small numbers of spores in stools or on surfaces.[17] *Clostridium difficle* can also be detected on agar because of its production of *p*-cresol from *p*-hydroxyphenylacetic acid.[18] Alcohol shock also facilitates isolation of the organism from stools.[19]

Staphylococcus aureus is now a very rare cause of AAC, and many doubt that it can cause the disease, although our experiences indicate that it can.[20] As observed in earlier times, staphylococcal enterocolitis involved the ileum and cecum more often than it did the colon and rectum, and it usually followed the use of tetracyclines or chloramphenicol, antibiotics that are now rarely associated with colitis. *Clostridium perfringens* type C and salmonellae have been implicated in solitary cases of PMC.[21,22]

Clostridium difficile colitis occurs at all ages but is most frequent in elderly and debilitated patients. Other groups at high risk include women, patients with cancer or burns, and patients undergoing surgery (especially abdominal surgery) or who are in intensive care units.[14] Even short courses of antibiotics given for prophylaxis or treatment of minor infections may permit the organism to overgrow, produce toxin, and cause colitis. AAC may follow oral, intramuscular, intravenous, or topical administration of antibiotics. The list of inciting agents includes penicillin G, ampicillin, amoxicillin, carbenicillin, ticarcillin, cephalothin, cefazolin, cephalexin, cefamandole, cefoxitin, cefotaxime, moxalactam, cefoperazone, ceftizoxime, ceftazidime, ceftriaxone, imipenem-cilastatin, ciprofloxacin, clindamycin, lincomycin, metronidazole, vancomycin, tetracycline, erythromycin, trimethoprim-sulfamethoxazole, chloramphenicol, and rifampin. A few cases have been related to the oral administration of aminoglycosides.[1,14] The relative risk of various antimicrobials in inducing AAC is not known with precision because antibiotic-specific attack rates in well-controlled studies of well-matched patient groups have not been reported. The incidence of AAC in adults treated with clindamycin has ranged from 1 in 10,000 to 1 in 10 in various reports.[2] The high rates reported from some hospitals suggest that the disease can be transmitted nosocomially, either via the hands of personnel or by direct contact with patients or infected surfaces or objects.[14] Most cases reported within the past decade have been related to clindamycin or lincomycin (to which *C. difficile* is often resistant), to ampicillin (to which it is usually susceptible), or to cephalosporins (to which susceptibility varies).[6] This paradox is not completely understood, but β-lactamase production by intestinal bacteria seems important in the pathogenesis of cases associated with ampicillin or cephalosporins.

Since alteration of the intestinal flora is so important in the pathogenesis of AAC, it is not surprising that almost every antibiotic used in treating humans has been implicated at least once. The components of the normal intestinal flora that suppress colonization, overgrowth, or toxin production by *C. difficile* are not known, but the suspects include *Escherichia coli,* enterococci, lactobacilli, *Bacteroides,* and *Clostridium.* Factors predisposing to colitis presumably inhibit or eliminate these competing organisms, but antibiotics may also operate by stimulating toxin production by *C. difficile.* Normal hamsters inoculated orally with large numbers of *C. difficile* remained well, while antibiotic-treated hamseters given only 2 colony-forming units (cfu) of *C. difficile* developed lethal enterocolitis.[8] The effects of antibiotics on stool flora may persist for long periods, and acquisition and overgrowth of *C. difficile* with production of colitis may occur up to 6 weeks after discontinuation of treatment with an antibiotic. Many reported patients with pseudomembranous colitis had received no antibiotics; these cases suggest that dietary changes, anesthesia, uremia, and various nonantibiotic medications (such as methotrexate or gold salts) may precipitate the disease.[23]

Clostridium difficile has been isolated from the hands of hospital personnel caring for colonized patients. The spores of *C. difficile* persist on fomites and surfaces for long periods. They have been found in abundance in the environment of patients with AAC.[14] Instruments inserted into the gastrointestinal tract should be cleaned and disinfected after use on patients with AAC. While vegetative forms of the organism are oxygen-sensitive and easily killed, spores are very resistant to adverse conditions, including most of the disinfectants used in hospitals. Alkaline glutaraldehyde, sodium hypochlorite, and chlorine dioxide are most effective against spores. Enteric isolation precautions and careful handwashing after contact with patients with AAC are recommended.

Colitis results from toxin production by the organism within the intestinal lumen. *Clostridium difficile* is rarely invasive. Isolates from patients with colitis usually produce at least two and possibly more toxins.[24,25] Some isolates are nontoxigenic, but these are never associated with colitis. The two best-characterized toxins are toxins A and B. Because it is difficult to purify these toxins, their characteristics and mechanisms of action are not completely understood. The toxins may attack the membranes or microfilaments of cells and produce contraction, hemorrhage, necrosis, inflammation, and loss of protein into the lumen.[26,27] They also increase intestinal myoelectric responses and peristalsis.[28] They may induce secretion of fluid and electrolytes by purely biochemical mechanisms. The reported molecular weights of toxins A and B have ranged widely (50,000–600,000). Toxin A is lethal for certain rodents and causes intestinal hemorrhage and fluid secretion. Toxin B is detectable by its cytotoxic or actinomorphic effects on cell culture monolayers. Diarrhea associated with *C. difficile* toxins in well-studied humans has almost always been associated with inflammatory mucosal lesions.[1,29]

Newborn infants may be colonized with toxigenic *C. difficile* organisms and yet remain well despite the presence of large amounts of toxins in their stools. Colonization rates as high as 50–60 percent have been reported in newborns.[13,30] In one study, the environment appeared to be the main source of the organism[31]; in another, hand transmissions by nursery personnel from infant to infant seemed responsible (Bacon A, Fekety R: unpublished observations). A glycoprotein found in milk (fetulin) or a subunit of it may interfere with the action of these toxins on the cecum.[32] In addition, the toxins may not bind to the intestinal mucosa.[33] As newborn infants acquire their normal intestinal flora, the rate of isolation of *C. difficile* and its toxins from their stools declines toward the rates in adults.

Hamsters immunized with toxoids prepared from both toxin

A and B (but not those immunized with either one alone) were protected against AAC.[34] Toxin B is a poor immunogen. Neutralizing or other serum antibodies to toxins of *C. difficile* have been detected in adults,[35–37] but their function is unknown. In one report, antibodies against *C. difficile* antigens were found much less often in sera from elderly than young adults[34]; this is of interest because AAC is more common in elderly patients.

CLINICAL MANIFESTATIONS

The range of severity of the symptoms associated with *C. difficile* colitis is wide.[1,29,38–40] Early reports consisted mostly of severe cases documented at the time of surgery or autopsy. Now that there is a high index of suspicion of AAC and noninvasive tests are available to aid in diagnosis, mild cases not only have been documented but also have been shown to be commonplace.

In the typical patient, profuse watery or mucoid green, foul-smelling diarrhea begins along with cramping abdominal pain 4–9 days after starting antibiotics. In some patients, diarrhea does not begin until after antibiotic treatment has been discontinued. Sometimes the diarrhea is guaiac-positive or bloody. *Clostridium difficile* is not reliably identifiable on Gram-stained smears of stools, but leukocytes are found in smears from about 50 percent of patients. High fever (temperatures of 103–105°F), marked abdominal tenderness, a leukocyte count as high as 35,000/mm^3, and hypoalbuminemia are common and point to the diagnosis of colitis rather than benign diarrhea. Sometimes patients with AAC have little or no diarrhea but have an acute abdominal syndrome with toxic megacolon, colonic perforation, or peritonitis. Acute arthritis resembling Reiter syndrome may complicate the illness.[41]

The pseudomembranous nodules or plaques of *C. difficile* colitis are usually most numerous in the distal colon, sigmoid, and rectum and are easily detected by sigmoidoscopy (Fig. 1). In about 10 percent of cases, lesions are present only in the cecum or transverse colon; this form of the illness is difficult to detect without performing colonoscopy but should be suspected when patients with diarrhea and toxin-positive stools have no visible lesions during proctosigmoidoscopy. Diarrhea caused by *C. difficile* without colitis has been postulated but has not been proved to be caused by *C. difficile*.[42] This putative mechanism includes a purely secretory diarrhea or a diarrhea caused by a motility-altering factor.[27,43] Some patients with leukemia or granulocytopenia or who are receiving antineoplastic chemotherapy have ileocecitis (typhlitis) similar to the disease seen in hamsters.[44,45] If *C. difficile* colitis goes unrecognized and untreated, the outcome may be fatal. Death rates of 10–20 percent were reported in untreated elderly or chronically debilitated patients. Hypovolemic shock, cecal perforation, secondary sepsis, and hemorrhage are the most serious complications that can result in death.

Clostridium difficile colitis can cause symptoms that may be eroneously interpreted as an exacerbation of an underlying chronic inflammatory bowel disease. This presentation usually occurs during or within a month of treatment with antibiotics.[46] Some of the diarrhea attributed to the effects of cancer chemotherapeutic agents on the intestinal mucosa may actually be due to *C. difficile* colitis.[47,48]

LABORATORY DIAGNOSIS

The laboratory tests most useful in confirmation of the diagnosis of AAC include CCFA stool cultures for *C. difficile* and tests for the presence of *C. difficile* toxins in stools.

Clostridium difficile has a characteristic chartreuse fluorescence and gross appearance on CCFA. CCFA can detect as few as 100 cfu of *C. difficile* per gram of stool.[16] Patients with AAC usually have many more organisms than that (10^4–10^5/g), but asymptomatic carriers may have only a few organisms per gram. Almost all patients with AAC are culture-positive if the stool is processed properly. Vegetative forms are easily killed by exposure to air or other adverse conditions; spores are hardy but less numerous and harder to detect. Anaerobe jars incubated at 35–37°C provide adequate cultural conditions. When using CCFA, it is possible to isolate *C. difficile* (presumptively) in just a few days. Confirmation is not difficult when using either biochemical reactions, gas–liquid chromatography to detect the production of fatty acids, or tests of toxin production.[49,50] Few fecal organisms that resemble *C. difficile* can grow on CCFA. *Clostridium sporogenes* is similar but does not produce a cytotoxin.[49] While not all isolates of *C. difficile* are toxigenic, those that are not have not caused colitis or diarrhea.[51]

The isolation of *C. difficile* from stools does not in itself prove that the patient has colitis. As mentioned previously, 60–70 percent of healthy newborns can carry it in their stools for a few weeks, and 3 percent or more of healthy adults may be asymptomatic carriers. In some hospitals where AAC is frequent, 20–30 percent of asymptomatic patients carry the organism.[14] Nevertheless, a positive culture may be useful in making therapeutic decisions. In our hospital, about 85 percent of adults with antibiotic-associated diarrhea and positive stool cultures have had colitis. Since the cytotoxin is heat and acid labile, stools from patients with AAC may be toxin-negative but culture-positive. Cultures also are useful in detecting post-treatment carriers who appear to be at an increased risk of relapse, but there is no effective treatment for eradication of the carrier state.

Tests to detect *C. difficile* toxin B usually employ monolayer cultures of fibroblasts or other cell lines.[4,49,50] These are difficult to maintain and are not available in many hospitals. However, demonstration of cytotoxin in stools is very helpful to the clinician. In our hospital, 95 percent of adults with antibiotic-associated diarrhea and *C. difficile* cytotoxin-positive stools have had documentable colitis. When proctosigmoidoscopy performed on patients with toxin titers greater than 1:10 shows normal mucosa, it is likely that they have colitis at a more proximal site. Isolated cecitis (typhlitis) is more common in patients treated with ampicillin or penicillin G or who have leukemia or granulocytopenia.[45] Colonoscopy or radionuclide scans using gallium or indium may be helpful in detecting and localizing colitis in these patients.

With tests for cytotoxin, a cytopathic effects may be seen within 4–6 hours but usually is not definite until 18–24 hours. Nonspecific (false-positive) toxicity can occur with concentrated specimens but is not neutralizable by antitoxin. Thus, it is necessary to confirm all positive results by demonstrating neutralization of cytotoxicity by incubation with *C. difficile* or *C. sordellii* antitoxin (these reagents are equivalent). Patients with AAC usually have large amounts of toxin in their stool filtrates and have positive titers at dilutions of 10^{-3}–10^{-5} or more. However, the value of the toxin B titer in individual patients does not correlate well with the severity of the illness[39,52]; the discrepancy may be either artifactual or indicative of the greater importance of toxin A in determining disease severity.

More than one toxin (or more than one aggregate of toxin subunits) produced by *C. difficile* can be found in stools of patients with AAC.[24,25,53] Enzyme-linked immunosorbent assays (ELISA) for toxin A have been developed and used for research purposes but are not yet available for routine clinical use. Usually both toxins A and B are present when either one is present in stools of patients with colitis.

Clostridium difficile produces other antigenic substances in addition to toxins A and B. One of these is immunologically similar to proteins produced by other microbial species. Counterimmunoelectrophoresis (CIE) has been used as a rapid method for detecting toxin B in fecal extracts. Since this test uses nonspecific antisera, it may detect these other antigens and is therefore subject to frequent false-positive results. False-negative results also occur.[54–56] A rapid and inexpensive latex agglutination test to aid in the diagnosis of diarrhea caused by *C. difficile* has become available recently.[57] The test was originally thought to detect toxin A; it is now known that it actually detects a nontoxic protein that is distinct from toxin A and of unknown function.[58] Nontoxigenic isolates of *C. difficile* produce the antigen, as do several other species of organisms that are found in the intestinal tract.[58] Both false-negative and false-positive latex results occur; the latter are more common. The clinical significance of a positive latex test result is roughly equivalent to that of a positive culture for *C. difficile*.

Staphylococcal toxins can produce cytopathic effects in Walker rat carcinoma cells (as do *C. difficile* toxins) but not in the fibroblast monolayers used to detect *C. difficile* toxins.[20] This difference may be useful in the diagnosis of staphylococcal enterocolitis.

CLINICAL DIAGNOSIS

When patients with antibiotic-associated diarrhea have high fevers, severe abdominal pain and tenderness, bloody stools, or large numbers of leukocytes in their stools, benign diarrhea is ruled out, and colitis is probably present. The diagnosis of AAC is most rapidly and certainly established by endoscopy, which detects evidence of inflammation (colitis) or pseudomembranous lesions. Colonoscopy may be required to detect isolated proximal colonic lesions. Colonic biopsy is not needed when typical gross findings are seen but may aid in the diagnosis of clostridial colitis when so-called nonspecific colitis is visualized because it may reveal pseudomembranes too small to be seen grossly.

Air-contrast barium enema studies may show signs of PMC, but these signs are not specific and are often absent early in the illness. In severe colitis, barium studies may precipitate toxic megacolon, perforation, or other complications, and they are not recommended.

In patients with nonspecific colitis associated with antibiotic usage, it is important also to consider Crohn's disease, idiopathic ulcerative colitis, and ischemic colitis. Infection with other intestinal pathogens such as *Salmonella, Edwardsiella, Shigella,* invasive *E. coli* (especially the 0157:H7 serotype if the colitis is hemorrhagic), *Entamoeba histolytica, Campylobacter, Yersinia,* and *Strongyloides* should be considered. Enterotoxin-producing organisms that can cause diarrhea without colitis include *E. coli, Bacillus cereus, Aeromonas, Vibrio,* and possibly other Enterobacteriaceae and pseudomonads.

TREATMENT

Antibiotics

Clostridium difficile is very susceptible to vancomycin, metronidazole and rifampin, and most isolates are susceptible to bacitracin. The minimal inhibitory concentrations for these are about 1μg/ml or less. Since resistance to rifampin can develop rapidly, this drug is not used alone in the treatment of AAC. Isolates resistant to metronidazole have been reported. Vancomycin-resistant isolates have never been detected. *Clostridium difficile* is often susceptible to tetracycline, erythromycin, ampicillin, cefamandole, cefazolin, and other antibiotics[6,52]; however, all of these except bacitracin have induced AAC and have not been very useful for treating the disease.

Not all patients with AAC need to be treated with antimicrobials. When patients have mild or moderate symptoms, it is sufficient to discontinue treatment with the precipitating antibiotic and give supportive therapy with fluids and electrolytes. If the patient improves within 48 hours, supportive therapy can be continued, and diarrhea usually subsides within 7–10 days. If treatment with the inducing antibiotic must be continued, specific antimicrobial treatment should be started promptly, even if symptoms are mild. Patients with high fever, leukocytosis, marked abdominal pain, and signs of peritoneal inflammation should be treated promptly with specific antibiotics, as should patients who are elderly, toxic, debilitated, or unresponsive to supportive therapy or cholestyramine.

Discontinuation of treatment with the inducing antibiotic, although desirable, is probably not essential if specific therapy for AAC is given. For example, the antibacterial effects of vancomycin on *C. difficile* in vitro are not antagonized by clindamycin, and the continuation of clindamycin therapy in patients treated with oral vancomycin has not been harmful. Furthermore, many of the antibiotics chosen as alternative therapy are capable of inducing AAC.

Vancomycin. Vancomycin given orally is expensive therapy but still the treatment of choice for severe AAC.[38,52,55] Metronidazole[56] and bacitracin[59] are less expensive alternatives for treating mild or moderately severely ill patients or when vancomycin is unavailable. The efficacy of vancomycin has been so well documented in different parts of the world that it must be considered the most reliable treatment. *Clostridium difficile* is usually susceptible to vancomycin at concentrations of less than 5 μg/ml, and no isolate has been identified that required more than 16 μg/ml. Since vancomycin is poorly absorbed from the gastrointestinal tract, it is nontoxic, and concentrations far exceeding 16 μg/ml are easily achieved in stools. When 500 mg is given orally four times daily, stool concentrations average 2000 μg/ml or more. When 125 mg is given four times daily, concentrations reach 300–1000 μg/ml. Even patients with profuse diarrhea achieve adequate concentrations with these regimens. Vancomycin has been detected in the urine of patients treated orally, but only in low concentrations after oral administration. Vancomycin is usually undetectable in serum, but concentrations were 5–30 μg/ml when it was detectable. Systemic toxic reactions have been very rare with oral vancomycin, even in patients with an inflamed colonic mucosa.[38,52,55]

Oral vancomycin was evaluated in a controlled study and was found to be significantly better than placebo in the treatment of *C. difficile* toxin-positive postoperative diarrheal syndromes.[55] The dose was 125 mg every 6 hours for 5 days. Vancomycin-treated patients who had *C. difficile*-negative antibiotic-associated diarrhea fared no better than did placebo-treated patients. Many patients with *C. difficile* colitis have been treated with oral vancomycin in uncontrolled studies. The clinical response almost invariably has been excellent unless the disease was far advanced when treatment was begun or oral therapy was not possible. Antibacterial activity within colonic tissues does not appear necessary; cessation of toxin production within the lumen or at the mucosal surface seems sufficient and indeed essential.

Patients treated with oral vancomycin usually show improvement in fever, diarrhea, abdominal cramps, and malaise within 48 hours. Toxin titers in stools decline shortly after treatment is begun. Treatment should continue until stools no longer contain toxin. Diarrhea and fever may require a week or more to resolve. Treatment should continue for at least 5–7 days but is rarely needed for more than 10 days. Some investigators believe that therapy should not be discontinued until toxin is no longer detected in stools.

The major disadvantages to the use of vancomycin are its expense ($16–$25 or more per day), its short supply in some parts of the world, and its bitter taste. A less expensive tablet form of vancomycin for oral use has recently been made available in the United States.

In about 50 patients entered into a randomized study, there were no significant differences in the overall clinical or bacteriologic responses of those treated with oral vancomycin every 6 hours in dosages of either 500 or 2000 mg/day.[59b] Although diarrhea in very ill patients ceased slightly sooner with the higher dose. The 500 mg/day regimen is less expensive and is therefore preferable except for extremely ill patients. For the treatment of infants and children with AAC, a dose of 500 mg/ 1.73 m^2 every 6 hours orally has been recommended.[12]

Vancomycin is also the drug of choice for the treatment of staphylococcal PMC, which may be suspected when Gram-stained smears of stools show very little except gram-positive cocci.

Patients who are unable to take vancomycin orally should be given it via a nasogastric tube, but patients with adynamic ileus may still not achieve adequate concentrations within the colonic lumen where it is needed to stop toxic production. These patients pose a formidable therapeutic problem since there is no parenteral regimen that is of proven benefit. When healthy adults were given intravenous vancomycin, their stool concentrations ranged from 0 to 100 μg/ml.[60] Thus, some patients with colitis treated intravenously might not achieve adequate concentrations within the bowel lumen. A few patients with colitis appear to have responded to intravenous vancomycin,[61] but other seriously ill patients have failed to respond. Recent evidence suggests that metronidazole given intravenously may also reach therapeutic concentrations in the colonic lumen in some patients. Reliance upon either intravenous metronidazole or vancomycin for the treatment of AAC, to the exclusion of oral therapy, is *not* recommended.

When parenteral therapy is essential (as in patients with paralytic ileus), we recommend treatment with both intravenous vancomycin and metronidazole (see below) supplemented by vancomycin given via nasogastric tube (500 mg four times per day for adults), into ileostomies and colostomies, or by enema. Oral metronidazole plays no role in this setting since, if small amounts of the drug pass down the gastrointestinal tract, they will be absorbed in the small intestine and none will reach the colon.

Metronidazole. Metronidazole is very active against *C. difficile* and has been effective in the treatment of patients with AAC.[56,62,63] It is inactive against staphylococci and has no value in treatment of staphylococcal enterocolitis. In a randomized comparative study, oral metronidazole was associated with a cure rate within 7 days of 92 percent; the rate was 100 percent with vancomycin, but the difference was not statistically significant.[64] Metronidazole was well tolerated, significantly less expensive than vancomycin, and associated with about the same rate of post-treatment carriage and relapse as was vancomycin. The usual oral dose is 500–750 mg three times daily or 250 mg four times daily. The drug is so well absorbed from the small intestine that concerns have been raised about whether the concentrations achieved within the colonic lumen are adequate in all patients, especially seriously ill patients. Some seriously ill patients have failed to respond to metronidazole.[45] We reserve metronidazole for mildly or moderately ill patients with AAC. Metronidazole has a number of side effects, some serious, and is not recommended for use in pregnant women or children. Furthermore, one case of colitis with a metronidazole-resistant organism has been reported.[65] Recent reports have encouraged the use of intravenous metronidazole to treat patients with AAC who are too sick to be treated via the oral route.[66,67] The usual intravenous dose was 500 mg every 6–8 hours. Metronidazole was detected in stools of patients and in rat intestinal tissues when using a chemical assay.[68] However, adequate bioactivity within the colonic lumen of patients has not been documented. Further, it is possible the biliary excretion of metronidazole was responsible for the clinical improvement noted in these patients, most of whom apparently did not have decreased intestinal motility. Since no form of parenteral therapy has been proved to be reliably effective in AAC, it should be used only when oral therapy is not possible. In such patients, both metronidazole and vancomycin should probably be given intravenously. Vancomycin (500 mg four times per day for adults) should also be given via nasogastric tube with intermittent clamping, and the administration of vancomycin by enema or by direct instillation through an ileostomy or colostomy should be considered. A high proportion of these patients ultimately require an emergent colectomy as a lifesaving measure.

Bacitracin. Chang et al. and Tedesco and associates[59,62] reported several patients whose PMC improved with treatment with oral bacitracin. The dosage was 25,000 units (about 500 mg) four times per day for 7–19 days. One patient relapsed after this therapy and then was treated successfully with vancomycin. Bacitracin has a bitter taste and is very nauseating if not given in capsule form (which requires special preparation). Although bacitracin is a useful alternative to vancomycin and metronidazole, the response to bacitracin is slower and less certain than with vancomycin; furthermore, carrier rates and stool toxin titers decline less rapidly, and it is not as reliable.[69,70] More experience with it is needed. Most isolates of *C. difficile* are susceptible to bacitracin, but some require more than 20 units/ml (about 1000 μg/ml) for inhibition, which may indicate resistance since these concentrations may not be achieved in the stools of some patients with diarrhea. Some absorption of the drug occurs when it is given orally. The systemic absorption and safety of bacitracin in patients with an inflamed intestinal mucosa as well as the frequency of relapse after treatment with this drug need better documentation. Bacitracin is often unavailable and is slightly less expensive than vancomycin is. It is also active against staphylococci. It may become available soon in a more palatable oral preparation.

Other Antibiotics. Fusidic acid is highly active against *C. difficile* and has been used successfully for the oral treatment of 15 patients with AAC.[71] It is also active against staphylococci. Tetracycline and erythromycin have been used occasionally in treatment of AAC of unknown cause, but many isolates of *C. difficile* are resistant to these antibiotics, and their use is not recommended.

Cholestyramine

This anion-exchange resin (as well as others) was used in treatment of PMC before the cause of the disease was known and was based on speculation that secretory bile acids might be responsible for antibiotic-associated diarrhea or colitis.[72] Studies in hamsters suggested that secretory bile acids were unlikely to cause antibiotic-associated diarrhea.[73] Cholestyramine binds *C. difficile* toxin B (and probably also toxin A), which is its presumed mechanism of action in this condition. It may also bind vancomycin, so their simultaneous use should be avoided.[74] Since many patients with AAC respond slowly or not at all to cholestyramine and require a change to treatment with antibiotics, it is usually reserved for mild illness. The usual oral dose of cholestyramine for adults is 4 g three or four times per day. Obstipation is the most serious side effect.

Antidiarrheal Agents

Opiates and other antiperistaltic agents should be avoided in patients with AAC. They are especially dangerous in infants. While they often provide symptomatic relief, they may promote more severe damage to the colon because of toxin retention; some patients have become worse when given these drugs.[75]

Adrenal Steroids

These are not of proven value in this disease. Reported mortality is higher in patients who received steroids, but such patients have tended to be sicker on the average before treatment.

Relapse or Recurrence of Colitis

More than one episode of colitis has been observed in 10–20 percent or more of patients treated with vancomycin, metronidazole, or bacitracin.[38,76–79] Recurrences respond to retreatment with vancomycin or, if the organism is susceptible, to metronidazole or bacitracin. Recurrences may be caused by germination of persistent spores or by reinfection from environmental or human contacts; persistence appears more common on the basis of typing studies. Treatment of carriers with oral vancomycin until discharge or transfer in a hospital unit where there is a high rate of the disease may have been useful in terminating outbreaks. The use of sodium hypochlorite diluted 1:500 to disinfect contaminated surfaces has also been recommended for control of nosocomial outbreaks. Careful hand washing by staff after contact with cases or carriers is urged. Not all patients who remain fecal carriers of the organism after treatment relapse. Unfortunately, the carrier state cannot be reliably eradicated with antimicrobials or any other regimen. Most relapses are spontaneous and occur within a few weeks of the first episode. Little is known about local, humoral, or cellular immunity to either the toxins, the organism, or the disease. Serum antibodies to the toxins have been detected in most healthy adults and in a minority of patients who recovered from the disease.[35,37,80] One patient developed neutralizing antibodies to toxin B in serum after eight episodes of colitis. He suffered no further recurrences despite the presence of large amounts of toxin in his stools (Buggy B, Fekety R: Unpublished observations).

Patients who relapse may be treated with oral vancomycin, metronidazole, or bacitracin for 7–10 days or until their diarrhea ceases. Longer courses do not appear more efficacious in preventing recurrences. Indeed, short courses may permit more rapid restoration of the normal fecal flora, which seems inhibitory for *C. difficile*.

Although most patients have only one relapse, some unfortunate persons relapse repeatedly. No reliable way to manage them is known, but anecdotal experiences suggest they may respond to long courses (4–6 weeks) of oral vancomycin or metronidazole, followed by a gradual tapering of the dose[81]; to intermittent short periods (5–7 days) of treatment alternating with periods of nontreatment; to postantibiotic therapy with cholestyramine to suppress symptoms by binding toxin while a normal flora is being reestablished; to recolonization by supplementation of antibiotics with oral lactobacillus preparations; or even to enemas with feces from healthy persons.[82,83] Oral vancomycin plus rifampin has been useful in a few cases[84] in an uncontrolled study. Since recent evidence suggests lactobacilli, enterococci, *Saccharomyces,* and nontoxigenic *C. difficile* isolates are important inhibitors of *C. difficile* within the gut, interest in their use for treatment of patients who relapse is growing.[85–89] A nontoxigenic strain of *C. difficile* has been useful in two patients with relapsing disease in an uncontrolled study.[88]

Surgical Measures

Before specific antibiotic therapy was available for AAC, diversion of the fecal stream or resection of the diseased bowel was often necessary. These drastic measures are now rarely performed except in life-threatening situations such as with toxic megacolon or cecal perforation. Sometimes a colostomy or ileostomy is needed to facilitate instillation of vancomycin or metronidazole into the colonic lumen of patients with ileus.[78]

Prevention

Eventually it may be possible to immunize patients against the toxins or other virulence factors of *C. difficile*, but this is not yet possible. Passive immunization of hamsters with *C. sordellii* antitoxin, which cross reacts with toxin B of *C. difficile*, protected them against clindamycin-induced colitis.[5] However, it has been difficult to purify the toxins and to prepare potent toxoids from them. Ordinary immune serum globulin does not appear useful. Prophylaxis with antibiotics such as vancomycin or metronidazole in patients at high risk of AAC is not of proven value; it is expensive and theoretically undesirable and should not be given.[4] Bacteriophage and bacteriocin typing systems as well as immunologic and antibiogram systems for typing *C. difficile* have recently become available, and their use in epidemiologic studies may lead to new or better preventive measures.[90–94]

REFERENCES

1. Bartlett JG. Antibiotic-associated pseudomembranous colitis. Rev Infect Dis. 1979;1:530.
2. Lusk RH, Fekety FR, Silva J, et al. Gastrointestinal side effects of clindamycin and ampicillin therapy. J Infect Dis. 1977;135(Suppl):111.
3. Lusk RH, Fekety FR, Silva J, et al. Clindamycin-induced enterocolitis in hamsters. J Infect Dis. 1978;137:464.
4. Rifkin GD, Fekety FR, Silva J, et al. Antibiotic-induced colitis: Implication of a toxin neutralized by *Clostridium sordellii* antitoxin. Lancet. 1977;2:1103.
5. Allo M, Silva J, Fekety FR, et al. Prevention of clindamycin-induced colitis in hamsters by *Clostridium sordellii* antitoxin. Gastroenterology. 1979;76:351.
6. Fekety R, Silva J, Toshniwal R, et al. Antibiotic-associated colitis: Effects of antibiotics upon *Clostridium defficile* and the disease in hamsters. Rev Infect Dis. 1979;1:386.
7. Borriello SP, Barclay FE. An in vitro model of colonization resistance to *Clostridium difficile* infection. Med Microbiol. 1986;21:299–309.
8. Larson HE, Price AB, Honour P, et al. *Clostridium difficile* and the aetiology of pseudomembranous colitis. Lancet. 1978;1:1063.
9. Lyerly DM, Krwan HC, Wilkins TD. *Clostridium difficile*: Its disease and toxins. Clin Microbiol Rev. 1988;1:1–18.
10. Rolfe RD, Finegold SM, eds. *Clostridium difficile*: Its role in intestinal disease. San Diego: Academic Press; 1988:408.
11. Tedesco FJ et al. Clindamycin-associated colitis: A prospective study. Ann Intern Med. 1974;81:432.
12. Scapa E. Pseudomembranous colitis in a 5 week old infant. Br Med J. 1982;284:824.
13. Batts DH, Martin D, Holmes R, et al. Treatment of antibiotic-associated *Clostridium difficile* diarrhea with oral vancomycin. J Pediatr. 1980;97:151.
14. Fekety R, Kim K-H, Brown D, et al. Epidemiology of antibiotic-associated colitis. Isolation of *Clostridium difficile* from the hospital environment. Am J Med. 1981;70:906.
15. Borriello SP, Honour P, Turner T, et al. Household pets as a potential reservoir for *Clostridium difficile* infection. J Clin Pathol. 1983;36:84.
16. George WL, Sutter VL, Citron D, et al. Selective and differential medium for isolation of *Clostridium difficile*. J Clin Microbiol. 1979;9:214.
17. Wilson KH, Kennedy MJ, Fekety FR. Use of sodium taurocholate to enhance spore recovery on a medium selective for *Clostridium difficile*. J Clin Microbiol. 1982;15:443.
18. Phillips KD, Rogers PA. Rapid detection and presumptive identification of *Clostridium difficile* by *p*-cresol production on a selective medium. J Clin Pathol. 1981;36:642.
19. Borriello SP, Honour P. Simplified procedure for the routine isolation of *Clostridium difficile* from faeces. J Clin Pathol. 1981;34:1124.
20. Batts DH, Silva J, Fekety R. Staphylococcal enterocolitis, in Nelson JD, Grassi C, eds. Current Chemotherapy and Infectious Disease. v. 2. Washington, DC: American Society for Microbiology; 1980:944.
21. Schwartz JN, Hamilton JP, Fekety R, et al. Ampicillin-induced enterocolitis: Implication of toxigenic *Clostridium perfringens* type C. J Pediatr. 1980;97:661.
22. Hovius SER, Rietra PJ. *Salmonella* colitis clinically presenting as a pseudomembranous colitis. Neth J Surg. 1982;34:81.
23. Peikin SR, Galdibini J, Bartlett JG. Role of *Clostridium difficile* in a case of nonantibiotic-associated pseudomembranous colitis. Gastroenterology. 1980;79:948.
24. Banno Y, Kobayashi T, Watanabe K, et al. Two toxins (D-1 and D-2) of *Clostridium difficile* causing antibiotic-associated colitis: Purification and some characterization. Biochem Int. 1981;2:629.
25. Taylor NS, Thorne GM, Bartlett JG. Comparison of two toxins produced by *Clostridium difficile* Infect Immun. 1981;34:1036.
26. Thelestam M, Bronnegard M. Interaction of cytopathogenic toxin from *Clostridium difficile* with cells in tissue culture. Scand J Infect Dis. 1980;22(Suppl):16.
27. Lima AA, Lyerly DM, Wilkins TD, et al. Effects of *Clostridium difficile* toxins A and B in rabbit small and large intestines in vivo and on cultured cells in vitro. Infect Immun. 1988;56:582–8.

28. Justus TG, Martin JL, Goldberg DA, et al. Myoelectric effects of *Clostridium difficile*: Motility-altering factors distinct from its cytotoxin and enterotoxin in rabbits. Gastroenterology. 1982;83:836.
29. Fekety R, Silva J, Armstrong J, et al. Treatment of antibiotic-associated enterocolitis with vancomycin. Rev Infect Dis. 1981;3(Suppl):273.
30. Welch DF, Marks MI. Is *Clostridium difficile* pathogenic in infants? J Pediatr. 1982;100:393.
31. Delmee M, Verellen G, Avesani V, et al. *Clostridium difficile* in neonates: Serogrouping and epidemiology. Eur J Pediatr. 1988;147:36–40.
32. Griffin GE, Heath J, Knox P. The action of *Clostridium difficile* cytotoxin is inhibited by specific glycoproteins (Abstract 596). Proceedings of the 22nd Interscience Conference on Antimicrobial Agents and Chemotherapy. Washington, DC: American Society for Microbiology; 1982.
33. Chang TW, Sullivan NM, Wilkins TD. Insusceptibility of fetal intestinal mucosa and fetal cells to *Clostridium difficile* toxins. Acta Pharmacol Sin. 1986;7:448–53.
34. Libby JM, Wilkins TD. Production of antitoxins to two toxins of *Clostridium difficile* and immunological comparison of the toxins by cross-neutralization studies. Infect Immun. 1982;35:374.
35. Nakamura S, Mikawa M, Nakashio S, et al. Identification of *Clostridium difficile* from the feces and the antibody in sera of young and elderly adults. Microbiol Immunol. 1981;25:345.
36. Viscidi R, Yolken R, Laughon B, et al. Serum antibody response to toxins A and B of *Clostridium difficile* (Abstract 595). Proceedings of the 22nd Interscience Conference on Antimicrobial Agents and Chemotherapy. Washington, DC: American Society for Microbiology; 1982.
37. Lishman AH, Al-Jumaili IJ, Record CO: Antitoxin production in antibiotic-associated colitis? J Clin Pathol. 1981;34:414.
38. Silva J, Batts DH, Fekety R. Treatment of *Clostridium difficile* colitis and diarrhea with vancomycin. Am J Med. 1981;71:815.
39. Burdon DW, George RH, Mogg G, et al. Faecal toxin and severity of antibiotic-associated pseudomembranous colitis. J Clin Pathol. 1981;34:548.
40. Thompson Jr CM, Gilligan PH, Fisher MC, et al. *Clostridium difficile* cytotoxin in a pediatric population. Am J Dis Child. 1983;137:271.
41. Puddey IB. Reiter's syndrome following antibiotic-associated colitis. Aust NZ J Med. 1982;12:292.
42. Gerding DN, Olson MM, Peterson LR et al. *Clostridium difficile*-associated diarrhea and colitis in adults. A prospective case-controlled epidemiologic study. Arch Intern Med. 1986;146:95–100.
43. Lashner BA, Todorczvk J, Sahm DF, et al. *Clostridium difficile* culture-positive toxin-negative diarrhea. Am J Gastroenterol. 1986;81:940–3.
44. Ikard RW: Neutropenic typhlitis in adults. Arch Surg. 1981;116:943.
45. Rampling A, Warren RE, Berry PJ, et al. Atypical *Clostridium difficile* colitis in neutropenic patients. Lancet. 1982;2:162.
46. Trnka YM, LaMont JT. Associations of *Clostridium difficile* toxin with symptomatic relapse of chronic inflammatory bowel disease. Gastroenterology. 1981;80:693.
47. Cudmore MA, Silva J, Fekety R, et al. *Clostridium difficile* colitis associated with cancer chemotherapy. Arch Intern Med. 1982;142:333.
48. Fainstein V, Bodey GP, Fekety R. *Clostridium difficile* colonization in cancer patients admitted to laminar air-flow units (Abstract). Clin Res. 1982;30:365.
49. Larson L, Holst E, Gemmell CG, et al. Characterization of *Clostridium difficile* and its differentiation from *Clostridium sporogenes* by automatic headspace gas chromatography. Scand J Infect Dis. 1980;22(Suppl):37.
50. Chang TW, Lauermann M, Bartlett JG. Cytotoxicity assay in antibiotic-associated colitis. J Infect Dis. 1979;140:765.
51. Chang TW. *Clostridium difficile* toxin and antimicrobial agent-induced diarrhea. J Infect Dis. 1978;137:854.
52. Tedesco F, Markham R, Gurwith M, et al. Oral vancomycin for antibiotic-associated pseudomembranous colitis. Lancet. 1978;2:226.
53. Aronsson B, Granstrom M, Molby R, et al. Toxin A (enterotoxin) from *Clostridium difficile* in antibiotic-associated colitis. Lancet. 1982;2:1279.
54. Levine HG, Kennedy M, LaMont JT. Counterimmunoelectrophoresis vs. cytotoxicity assay for the detection of *Clostridium difficile* toxin. J Infect Dis. 1982;145:398.
55. Keighley MRB, Burdon DW, Arabi Y, et al. Randomized controlled trial of vancomycin for pseudomembranous colitis and postoperative diarrhea. Br Med J. 1978;2:1667.
56. Pashby NL, Bolton RP, Sherriff RJ. Oral metronidazole in *Clostridium difficile* colitis. Br Med J. 1979;1:1605.
57. Sherman ME, Degirolami PC, Thorne G, et al. Evaluation of a latex agglutination test for diagnosis of *Clostridium difficile* associated colitis. Am J Clin Pathol. 1988;89:228–33.
58. Lyerly DA, Ball DW, Toth J, et al. Characterization of cross-reactive proteins detected by culturette brand rapid latex test for *Clostridium difficile*. J Clin Microbiol. 1988;26:397–400.
59a. Chang T-W, Gorbach SL, Bartlett JG, et al. Bacitracin treatment of antibiotic-associated colitis and diarrhea caused by *Clostridium difficile* toxin. Gastroenterology. 1980;78:1584.
59b. Fekety R, Silva J, Kauffman C, et al. Treatment of *Clostridium difficile* antibiotic-associated colitis with oral vancomycin: Comparison of two dosage regimens. Am J Med. 1989;86:15.
60. Geraci JE, Heilman FR, Nichols DR, et al. Some laboratory and clinical experiences with a new antibiotic, vancomycin. Proc Staff Meet Mayo Clin. 1956;31:564.
61. Donta ST, Lamps GM, Summers KW, et al. Cephalosporin-associated colitis and *Clostridium difficile* Arch Intern Med. 1980;140:574–7.
62. Tedesco FJ. Bacitracin therapy in antibiotic-associated pseudomembranous colitis. Dig Dis Sci. 1980;25:783.
63. Cherry RD, Portnoy D, Jabbari M, et al. Metronidazole: An alternate therapy for antibiotic-associated colitis. Gastroenterology. 1982;82:849.
64. Teasley DG, Gerding DN, Olson MN, et al. Prospective randomized trial of Metronidazole versus vancomycin for the treatment of *Clostridium difficile* asociated diarrhea and colitis. Lancet. 1983;2:1043–6.
65. Saginur R, Hawley CR, Bartlett JG. Colitis associated with metronidazole therapy. J Infect Dis. 1980;141:772.
66. Bolton RF, Culshaw MA. Faecal metronidazole concentrations during oral and intravenous therapy for antibiotic-associated colitis due to *Clostridium difficile* Gut. 1986;27:1169–72.
67. Kleinfeld DI, Sharpe RJ, Donta ST. Parenteral therapy for antibiotic-associated pseudomembranous colitis. J Infect Dis. 1988;157:389.
68. Bergan T, Solhaug JH, Soreide O, et al. Comparative pharmacokinetics of metronidazole and tinidazole and their tissue penetration. Scand J Gastroenterol. 1985;20:945–50.
69. Young GP, Ward PB, Bayley N, et al. Antibiotic-associated colitis due to *Clostridium difficile*: Double-blind comparison of vancomycin with bacitracin. Gastroenterology. 1985;89:1038–45.
70. Dudley MN, McLauglin JC, Carrington G, et al. Oral bacitracin vs vancomycin therapy for *Clostridium difficile*-induced diarrhea. A randomized double-blind trial. Arch Intern Med. 1986;146:1101–4.
71. Cronberg S, Castor B, Thoren A. Fusidic acid for the treatment of antibiotic-associated colitis induced by *Clostridium difficile*. Infection. 1984;12:276–79.
72. Kreutzer EW, Milligan FD. Treatment of antibiotic-associated pseudomembranous colitis with cholestyramine resin. Johns Hopkins Med J. 1978;143:67.
73. Fekety R, Browne RA, Silva J, et al. Fecal bile acids and cholestyramine in hamsters with clindamycin-associated colitis (Abstract 129). Proceedings of the 18th Interscience Conference on Antimicrobial Agents and Chemotherapy. Atlanta: American Society for Microbiology; 1978.
74. King CY, Barriere SL. Analysis of the in vitro interaction between vancomycin and cholestyramine. Antimicrob Agents Chemother. 1981;19:326.
75. Novak E, Lee JG, Seckman E, et al. Unfavorable effect of atropine-diphenoxylate (Lomotil) therapy in lincomycin-caused diarrhea. JAMA. 1976;235:1451–4.
76. George WL, Volpicelli NA, Stiner DB, et al. Relapse of pseudomembranous colitis after vancomycin therapy. N Engl J Med. 1979;301:414.
77. Bartlett JG, Tedesdo FJ, Shull S, et al. Symptomatic relapse after oral vancomycin therapy of antibiotic-associated pseudomembranous colitis. Gastroenterology. 1980;78:431.
78. George WL, Rolfe RD, Finegold SM. Treatment and prevention of antimicrobial agent-induced colitis and diarrhea. Gastroenterology. 1980;79:366.
79. Walters BAJ, Roberts R, Stafford R, et al. Relapse of antibiotic-associated colitis: Endogenous persistence of *Clostridium difficile* during vancomycin therapy. Gut. 1983;24:206.
80. Silva J, Lusk R, Kekety R, et al. Immune responses of hamsters and humans with antibiotic associated colitis. In: Lambe DW Jr, Genco RJ, Mayberry-Carson KJ, eds. Anaerobic Bacteria: Selected Topics. New York: Plenum; 1980:295.
81. Tedesco FJ. Treatment of recurrent antibiotic-associated pseudomembranous colitis. Am J Gastroenterol. 1982;77:220.
82. Schwan A, Sjolin S, Trottestan U. Relapsing *Clostridium difficile* enterocolitis cured by rectal infusion of homologous faeces. Lancet. 1983;2:845.
83. Schwan A, Sjolin S, Trottesam U, et al. Relapsing *Clostridium difficile* enterocolitis cured by rectal infusion of normal faeces. Scand J Infect Dis 1984;16:211–5.
84. Buggy BP, Fekety R, Silva J. Therapy of relapsing *Clostridium difficile*-associated diarrhea and colitis with the combination of vancomycin and rifampin. J Clin Gastroenterol. 1987;9:155–9.
85. Wilson KH, Sheagren JH, Freter R, et al. Gnotobiotic models for study of the microbial ecology of *Clostridium difficile* and *Eschericia coli*. J Infect Dis. 1986;153:547–51.
86. Borriello SP, Barclay FP. An in vitro model of colonisation resistance to *Clostridium difficile* infection. J Med Microbiol. 1986;21:299–309.
87. Elmer G, McFarland LV. Suppression by *Saccharomyces boulardii* of toxigenic *Clostridium difficile* overgrowth after vancomycin treatment of hamsters. Antimicrob Agents Chemother. 1987;31:129–31.
88. Seal D, Borriello SP, Barclay FE, et al. Treatment of relapsing *Clostridium difficile* diarrhoeae by administration of a non-toxigenic strain. Eur J Clin Microbiol. 1987;6:51–3.
89. Wilson KH, Silva J, Fekety FR. Suppression of *Clostridium difficile* by normal hamster cecal flora and prevention of antibiotic-associated cecitis. Infect Immun. 1981;34:626.
90. Wilson KH, Sheagren JN. Antagonism of toxigenic *Clostridium difficile* by non-toxigenic *C. difficile*. J Infect Dis. 1983;147:733.
91. Rolfe RD, Helebian S, Finegold SM. Bacterial interference between *Clostridium difficile* and normal fecal flora. J Infect Dis. 1981;143:470.
92. Malamoa-Lodas H, Tabaqchali S. Inhibition of *Clostridium difficile* by fecal streptococci. J Med Microbiol. 1982;15:569.
93. Wust J, Sullivan NM, Hardegger U, et al. Investigation of an outbreak of antibiotic-associated colitis by various typing methods. J Clin Microbiol. 1982;16:1096.
94. Sell TL, Schaberg DR, Fekety FR. Bacteriophage and bacteriocin typing scheme for *Clostridium difficile*. J Clin Microbiol. 17:1148,1983.

84. INFLAMMATORY ENTERITIDES

RICHARD L. GUERRANT

The acute inflammatory enteritides include several specific distal small bowel and colonic infections such as campylobacteriosis salmonellosis, shigellosis, and amebiasis as well as the syndromes of necrotizing enteritis and antibiotic-associated pseudomembranous enterocolitis. Several other infectious agents cause chronic enteric inflammatory processes that may result in syndromes of abdominal pain, weight loss, diarrhea, or malabsorption. These include such processes as gastrointestinal mycoses, mycobacterioses, bacterial infections, and certain parasitic infections such as coccidiosis.

ACUTE DYSENTERY

Syndromes of acute dysentery with fecal blood and pus have been well recognized since the days of Hippocrates. Dysentery implies frequent, small bowel movements accompanied by blood and mucus with tenesmus or pain on defecation. This syndrome implies an inflammatory invasion of the colonic mucosa resulting from bacterial, cytotoxic, or parasitic destruction.

The pathologic changes of inflammatory colitis range from a superficial intense exudative inflammatory process involving the colonic mucosa by shigellae or invasive *Escherichia coli* to deeper, penetrating, "flask-shaped" ulcers with undermined edges as seen in amebic dysentery. The pathogenesis of the inflammatory colitides may involve cytotoxic products of shigellae,[1] certain *E. coli*,[2] clostridia, or other organisms.

The epidemiologic patterns of acute dysenteric syndromes are influenced by the unusually low inoculum required by organisms such as shigellae or amebae for infection. As few as 10^2 shigellae or as few as 10 cysts of enteric parasites such as *Entamoeba coli* or *Giardia lamblia* may cause infection in adult volunteers.[3,4] Consequently, there is a substantial risk of person-to-person spread in day care centers,[5] institutions, or other areas where nonhygienic conditions may allow direct fecal–oral spread. The cysts of parasites such as *Entamoeba histolytica* or *Balantidium coli* often resist chlorination and therefore may cause water-borne outbreaks of dysenteric illnesses. Saltwater or seafood exposure should lead one to consider *Vibrio parahaemolyticus* as a cause of inflammatory colitis, and farm or domestic animal exposure might lead one to consider nontyphoid *Salmonella* sp., *Campylobacter jejuni*, or *Yersinia enterocolitica*. In addition, when typhoid fever is present with diarrhea in an endemic area, the diarrhea is often inflammatory with many fecal polymorphonuclear leukocytes seen on microscopic examination.[6] Travel to areas of poor sanitation might implicate any of the aforementioned pathogens. Finally, venereal exposure, particularly among male homosexuals, might implicate the gonococcus, herpes simplex virus, *Chlamydia trachomatis*, or *Treponema pallidum* as causes of proctitis or *Campylobacter, Shigella, Chlamydia trachomatis* (lymphogranuloma venereum serotypes), *E. histolytica*, or *Clostridium difficile* as causes of colitis.[7]

Examination for fecal leukocytes often reveals sheets of polymorphonuclear leukocytes in clumps of mucus even in the absence of gross blood in the stool specimen[8,9] (Fig. 1). Fewer, pyknotic leukocytes are reported in amebic dysentery[10–12]; this may be attributable to the deeper, undermining ulcers characteristic of intestinal amebiasis or to a toxic effect of the ameba on leukocytes. A prompt culture of fresh specimens onto appropriate enteric culture media is very important in the isolation of shigellae.[13] Specialized techniques are required to isolate *Vibrio* (thiosulfate citrate bile salt agar),[14] *Yersinia* (cold enrichment),[15] or *Campylobacter jejuni*.[16] Leukocytosis or even a leukemoid reaction has been described. Sigmoidoscopic examination may be useful in the diagnosis of a pseudomembranous enterocolitis or in the identification of parasites such as *E. histolytica* or *B. coli*. Amebic colitis is associated with discrete small ulcerations with undermined edges amid relatively normal mucosa. Acute shigellosis causes more widespread, shallow, 3 to 7 mm ulcers with a more intense inflammatory exudate. Barium studies are unnecessary and are relatively contradicted in toxic patients with acute colitis. Therapy consists of careful supportive fluid management with specific antimicrobial therapy directed at a specific pathogen if suspected by the epidemiologic setting or culture results.

The potential etiologies of acute dysentery are listed in Table 1.

Bacillary Dysentery (Shigellosis and Enteroinvasive E. coli)

Shigella sp. (types A–D: *dysenteriae*, *flexneri*, *sonnei*, and *boydii*) may cause acute bloody dysentery with high fever and systemic manifestations of malaise, headache, and abdominal pain. The incubation period ranges from 6 hours to 9 days but is usually <72 hours. This syndrome may be particularly severe in poorly nourished children. As noted previously, this organism may be spread with relatively small inocula by direct contact as well as in food or water.

Despite the intense superficial destructive process in the colonic epithelium that typifies acute shigellosis, bacteremia and disseminated infection are relatively rare. A complication of severe shigellosis in childhood is a hemolytic-uremic syndrome that may be associated with a leukemoid reaction, pseudomembranous colitis, circulating immune complexes, and circulating endotoxin, usually in the absence of demonstrable bacteremia.[17] Other more common extraintestinal manifestations of shigellosis include headache, meningismus, and even seizures, especially in children.[18] These findings may be attributable to a neurotoxin that has been demonstrated with *Shigella dysenteriae* type I.[1,19] A serous arthritis similar to that seen in Reiter syndrome has been described in up to 10 percent of the patients 2–5 weeks after the dysenteric illness that characteristically occurs in patients with histocompatibility antigen HLA-B27.[20,21] Culture-positive conjunctivitis during acute shigellosis has also been described and may represent autoinoculation of the conjunctiva analogous to that induced in the guinea pigs in the Sereny test.[22] Arthritis syndromes have also been described after inflammatory colitis with *Yersinia enterocolitica* or *Salmonella enteritidis*, again in association with HLA-B27.

Certain *E. coli* strains may produce an identical syndrome to that seen with acute shigellosis. The incubation period is usually 2–3 days after ingestion. Although invasive *E. coli* organisms appear to be limited to certain serotypes[22,23] (Table 2), to identify invasive *E. coli* one should demonstrate that their invasive potential in the guinea pig conjunctivitis (Sereny) test,[26] in Hela cells,[27] or identify the 120–140 megadalton plasmid that is associated with invasiveness in *Shigella* and invasive *E. coli*.[28–30] Invasive *E. coli* organisms were responsible for a single widespread outbreak of dysentery associated with imported French Camembert cheese.[25,31] While they have been identified as occasional causes of diarrhea in Brazil,[22] invasive *E. coli* do not appear to be frequent causes of sporadic diarrhea in the United States. Because they are often slow to ferment lactose in the laboratory, invasive *E. coli* may be initially mistaken for shigellae,[22,25,32] to which it is closely related. Invasive *E. coli* are also usually lysine-negative and often nonmotile.[33] There is also antigenic relatedness among invasive *E. coli* and *Shigella*.[34]

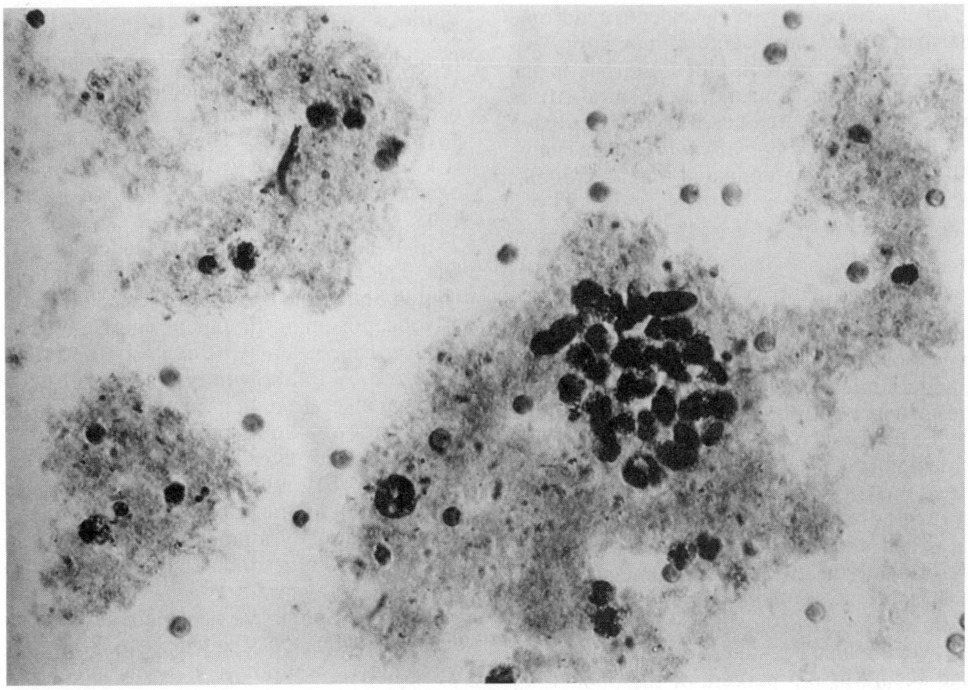

FIG. 1. Methylene blue stain of fecal leukocytes found in colitis. This exudative response may be seen in shigellosis, salmonellosis, *Campylobacter* infection, and colitis due to invasive *E. coli*.

Enterohemorrhagic E. coli Diarrhea

Although the frequency with which it causes inflammatory diarrhea is not clear, a significant cause of bloody diarrhea is now recognized to be enterhemorrhagic *E. coli* (EHEC) that produce relatively large amounts of Shiga-like (Vero) cytotoxin.[2,35] While they account for only 0.8–3.0 percent of all diarrhea in the United States and Canada, EHEC (of serotype 0157) are estimated to account for 15–36 percent of cases of bloody diarrhea.[2,36] The majority of recognized EHEC are of serotype O157; others include O26:K60:H11; O103:H2; O91:H2; O145:H−; O111:K58:H−; O38:H21; O6:H−; O5:H− O128; O139; O113:K75; and O121.[2,24,36] EHEC were the most commonly recognized cause of diarrhea (3 percent) among 5415 patients studied in Calgary in Canada where they showed a summer seasonal peak.[36] In addition to causing 15–36 percent of all cases of bloody diarrhea, including outbreaks of hemorrhagic colitis, EHEC are associated with 75–90 percent of cases of hemolytic-uremic syndrome in North America, a complication that develops in 8 percent of EHEC infections.[2] After binding to a globotriosylceramide receptor, the Shiga-like toxin cleaves adenosine from an *N*-glycoside bond at nucleotide residue 4324 on the 60 S ribosomal RNA to block protein synthesis by inhibiting EF1-dependent aminoacyl t-RNA binding.[2,37,38] The diagnosis is suspected on clinical grounds and confirmed by serotyping sorbitol-negative *E. coli* insolates or by using tissue culture or gene probes to detect the cytotoxin.

TABLE 1. Differential Diagnoses of Acute Dysentery and Inflammatory Enterocolitis

Specific infectious processes
Bacillary dysentery (*Shigella dysenteriae, flexneri, sonnei, boydii;* invasive *E. coli*)
Campylobacteriosis (*Campylobacter jejuni*)
Amebic dysentery (*Entamoeba histolytica*)
Ciliar dysentery (*Balantidium coli*)
Bilharzial dysentery (*Schistosma japonicum, mansoni*)
Other parasites (*Trichinella spiralis*)
Vibriosis (*Vibrio parahaemolyticus*)
Salmonellosis (*Salmonella typhimurium*)
Typhoid fever (*Salmonella typhi*)
Enteric fever (*Salmonella choleraesuis, paratyphi*)
Yersiniosis (*Yersinia enterocolitica*)
Spirillar dysentery (*Spirillum* sp.)
Proctitis
Gonococcal (*Neisseria gonorrhoeae*)
Herpetic (herpes simplex virus)
Chlamydial (*Chlamydia trachomatis*)
Syphilitic (*Treponema pallidum*)
Other syndromes
Necrotizing enterocolitis of the newborn
Enteritis necroticans
Pseudomembraneous enterocolitis (*Chlamydia difficile*)
Syndromes without known infectious etiology
Idiopathic ulcerative colitis
Crohn's disease

Campylobacter Enteritis

Campylobacter jejuni (formerly *C. fetus* or "*Vibrio fetus*") systemic infections have been recognized for many years. While the majority of *Campylobacter* blood stream infections in humans are with *C. fetus* (old subspecies, *intestinalis*),[39] *Campylobacter jejuni* commonly causes an enteric infection in all ages. This organism was recognized many years ago as a cause of swine dysentery.[40] Commercially available techniques of fecal culture have enabled the culture of *C. jejuni* on highly selective media at 42°C from fecal specimens of patients

TABLE 2. Enteroinvasive *E. coli* Serotypes

Serotype	*Difco Serogroup*	*References*
O28 ac	C	22, 23
O29		24
O112 a, c	C	23
O124	B	22, 23, 25
O136	C (Trabulsi's 193-T-64)	23, 25
O143		23
O144		23, 25
O152	(Trabulsi's 185-T-64)	23, 25
O164		23
O167		24

with diarrhea.[16,41] These techniques have revealed a syndrome of severe abdominal pain, fever, and acute inflammatory enteritis that may result in dysentery with blood and pus in the stools.[41–43] Reports from Belgium, England, and central Africa reveal that 5–14 percent of unselected cases of diarrhea have *C. jejuni*,[42–44] and outbreaks of *Campylobacter* enteritis have been associated with ingestion of contaminated water, raw milk, or uncooked meat or poultry.

Amebic Dysentery

Entamoeba histolytica cysts are ingested, pass through the gastric acidity, and have the capsule digested in the small bowel. Trophozoites then invade the colonic mucosa and produce shallow, flasklike undermining ulcers. The capacity of this parasite to invade tissue may be attributed to histolytic enzymes or products that may be delivered on contact of the ameba with cells[45–48] and may depend on associated viable bacteria.[49,50] Amebae may then seed the liver via the portal vein, from which extension may occur to the skin, diaphragm, lung, or pericardium. While extraintestinal amebiasis occurs with less than one-tenth the frequency of symptomatic intestinal amebic dysentery, dissemination is reportedly more common in states of undernutrition, cytotoxic or steroid medication, late pregnancy, carcinoma, or other overwhelming systemic diseases. Asymptomatic cyst carriage occurs in 1–5 percent of the population in the southern United States. The frequency of amebiasis is greater in rural and lower socioeconomic groups and in institutions where fecal–oral spread of this human parasite may occur.[51] The role of amebic infections that are highly prevalent among promiscuous male homosexuals in producing symptoms or invasive disease remain unclear.[52,53]

Ciliar Dysentery

Balantidium coli is the only ciliate parasite that is pathogenic for humans. The most common reservoir is swine. Like *E. histolytica*, this parasite excysts in the small bowel, invades the terminal ileum and colon, and may cause appendicitis or a dysenteric syndrome with rectosigmoid ulceration (with heaped-up 1.5 to 3 cm ulcers) and secondary bacteremia. However, there is no extraintestinal extension of *B. coli* as one may see with amebiasis. The diagnosis is made by scraping the margin of the ulcer and examining microscopically for the ciliate trophozoite. Mucosal invasion is usually limited to the rectal vault. Symptoms may last for 1–4 weeks and may recur several times a year if the diagnosis is not suspected. Treatment is usually successful with tetracycline.

Bilharzial Dysentery

Schistosomiasis may cause acute bloody diarrhea, abdominal pain, and weight loss when the adult schistosomes (usually *S. japonicum* or *S. mansoni*) migrate to the intestinal tract where they begin egg deposition. This occurs 3–8 weeks after initial skin exposure to the cercariae and may last for several weeks. Fecal examination reveals blood, pus, and numerous ova. Fever, leukocytosis, and increasing eosinophilia may be associated with this illness, and hepatosplenic disease may follow. *S. mansoni* may also cause chronic blood or protein loss via inflammatory "polyps."

Other Parasites

Another potential parasitic cause of inflammatory enteritis is acute trichinosis. Approximately 24 hours after the ingestion of infested pork, the larvae excyst and invade the intestinal mucosa, often resulting in nausea, vomiting, diarrhea, and abdominal pain. This precedes the systemic manifestations of periorbital edema, fever, myositis, and eosinophilia by 1–2 weeks.

Vibriosis

In addition to classic and El Tor *Vibrio cholerae* O1, non-O1 *V. cholerae* and several halophilic *Vibrio* species are now recognized to cause diarrhea and occasional wound or blood stream infections.[54,55] The most common and best characterized is *V. parahaemolyticus*. *Vibrio parahaemolyticus* has been recognized since 1950 in Japan and was identified as a *Vibrio* in 1963. *V. parahaemolyticus* is a cause of seafood poisoning 9–25 hours after the ingestion of inadequately cooked fish or shellfish. This has been reported throughout the coastal areas of the United States and on cruise ships and is the most common cause of food poisoning in Japan where raw seafood is commonly eaten.[56] Diarrhea may be explosive and watery or may be characterized by full-blown dysentery with blood and pus and superficial ulceration on proctoscopic examination.[57,58] The latter syndrome may be associated with cramps, nausea, vomiting, headache, and fever. The illness usually is self-limited within 3–4 days. The pathogenic Kanagawa-positive strains from patients produce β-hemolysis on special (Wagatsuma) medium—in contrast to environmental isolates—and are best isolated as blue-green colonies (alkaline) on thiosulfate citrate bile salt sucrose (TCBS) agar.[14]

Other halophilic vibrios include *V. alginolyticus, fluvialis, hollisase, damsella*, and *vulnificus*, which have been associated with enteric, wound, or systemic infections in humans.[54,55] *V. vulnificus* has been associated with life-threatening septicemia within 24 hours of ingesting raw oysters.[55,59]

Salmonellosis

Salmonella enterocolitis is characterized by fever, cramping, abdominal pain, and diarrhea that begins 8–48 hours after ingestion of an infectious dose, usually with food, and usually lasts 3–5 days. The diarrheal stools of patients with salmonellosis often contain a moderate number of polymorphonuclear leukocytes, usually fewer than is typical of shigellosis.

While salmonella enteritis predominantly involves the lamina propria in the small bowel, several reports have noted colitis due to *S. typhimurium*, with crypt abscesses and erosion and ulcerations of the colonic mucosa that resulting in blood and pus in the stool.[60–64] Certain other strains of salmonella (*S. choleraesuis* and *S. paratyphi*), like *S. typhi*, tend to elicit a mononuclear response and cause a bacteremia characteristic of enteric fever.

Typhoid Fever

Typhoid fever may lead to an erosion of the blood vessels in Peyer's patches that, if untreated, may result in gross blood in the feces in 10–20 percent of the patients. Severe intestinal hemorrhage may compliate approximately 2 percent of the cases late in the course of untreated typhoid fever. Such intestinal bleeding may precede perforation, another complication of typhoid fever.[65]

Yersiniosis

Yersinia enterocolitica is another increasingly recognized enteric pathogen that may be responsible for an enteric feverlike illness, mesenteric adenitis, or an inflammatory ileitis or ulcerative colitis syndrome with fecal neutrophils and mononuclear cells.[66–68] *Yersinia* may also be associated with migratory polyarthritis, Reiter syndrome, or erythema nodosum. A syndrome with acute diarrhea and vomiting is especially common in young children.[69] The organism may cause disseminated abscesses in the liver and spleen[70] or an inflammatory colitis.[71] The causative agent, a gram-negative member of the family Enterobacteriaceae, is in the same genus as the plague bacillus *Y.*

pestis and is sometimes mistaken for *Proteus* on initial culture plates. Cultivation may require "cold enrichment."[15]

Gonococcal Proctitis

Neisseria gonorrhoeae may be the cause of ulcerative proctitis, particularly in male homosexuals who may have acquired this infection by venereal exposure.[7] The resultant purulent proctitis appears with an erythematous friable mucous membrane in the rectal vault and occasional abscess or fistula formation. While copious purulent discharge, tenesmus, and burning rectal pain may be noted, two-thirds of the culture-positive patients with anorectal gonococcal infection are asymptomatic.[72,73]

Spirillar Dysentery

"Spirillar" or "spirochetal" dysentery has been reported to occur in southern France and has been attributed to *Spirillum* species.[74] While severe mucoid diarrhea or dysentery has been associated with intestinal spirochetes, their frequency and role in causing enteric disease is unclear.[75]

Approach to Diagnosis and Treatment of Acute Dysentery

Any of the aforementioned microorganisms may cause an acute dysentery syndrome with blood and pus in the stool; examination for leukocytes may suggest one of the above etiologies even if blood is not present in the stool on gross examination. Other diagnoses to be considered in the differential diagnosis of inflammatory colitis are pseudomembranous enterocolitis, which may be associated with antibiotic use, and the potentially rapidly progressive necrotizing enterocolitis syndromes, which are discussed in the subsequent sections. These diagnoses are suspected by clinical course, history, and radiologic and proctoscopic examination. Noninfectious syndromes that may be manifested with acute inflammatory enterocolitis include idiopathic ulcerative colitis and Crohn's disease.

Presumptive therapy for the inflammatory colitides varies greatly with the suspected etiology (see "Algorithm" in Chapter 81). For example, an acute febrile dysenteric illness in a young child with day care exposure or in an area where shigellosis is common should be treated with an appropriate absorbable antimicrobial agent such as ampicillin or sulfamethoxazole-trimethoprim. If the *Shigella* organism is sensitive, prompt therapy can successfully reduce the diarrhea, systemic symptoms, and shedding of the organisms in the feces.[76–78] Nonabsorbable antibiotics such as colistin or aminoglycosides are ineffective, possibly because they do not prevent the spread of shigellae to adjacent epithelial cells.[79] Because shigellae are increasingly antibiotic resistant,[80,81] one must be familiar with the local resistance pattern of shigellae to appropriately treat acute shigellosis early when it is first suspected. The quinolone antibiotics may offer a considerable advance in treating inflammatory diarrhea. Not only are they effective in treating otherwise resistant shigellosis, but they appear to reduce fecal shedding and the duration of illness with *Campylobacter jejuni* and, in preliminary studies, even *Salmonella* infections.[82,83]

Amebic dysentery is usually diagnosed by direct examination of wet mounts of fresh fecal or proctoscopic specimens, which reveal *E. histolytica* trophozoites or cysts in 60–80 percent of the cases. The cysts and trophozoites are characterized by four or fewer delicate nuclei with central karyosomes. Additional patients may be diagnosed by biopsy, where trophozoites or cysts may be found in the undermining ulcer in the lamina propria, or by a serum indirect hemagglutinating antibody (IHA) test, which is positive in approximately 90 percent of the patients with intestinal amebiasis.[84] While the systemic amebacide metronidazole is effective in eradicating hepatic amebiasis and may eradicate intestinal disease, some would use the lumenocide diiodohydroxyquin to eradicate intestinal infection. The therapy for balantidiasis is tetracycline or diiodohydroxyquin. Praziquantel is used for significant schistosomal infections. The optimal therapies for *V. parahaemolyticus, Y. enterocolitica,* and *C. jejuni* infections are not well established and should be tailored to the specific sensitivity pattern of the organism isolated. Gonococcal proctitis may be difficult to eradicate but should first be treated with penicillin or, in areas with significant penicillin resistance (>3 percent), ceftriaxone (250 mg im).

As with all diarrheas, the therapy for *Salmonella* gastroenteritis is supportive fluid management. With the exception of the preliminary experience with ciprofloxacin,[82] oral antibiotics are of no benefit and may actually prolong shedding of the organism and even be associated with increased risk of relapse in children.[85,86]

NECROTIZING ENTEROCOLITIS IN THE NEWBORN

The syndrome of diffuse fulminating necrotizing colitis has been increasingly recognized among infants since reports by Waldhausen et al. in 1963[87] and Mizrahi and colleagues in 1965.[88] This syndrome probably represents the same entity described as "spontaneous" intestinal perforation and peritonitis as early as 1838.[89–91] While milder forms of the syndrome doubtless exist, the syndrome of necrotizing enterocolitis (NEC) is defined by air in the wall of the intestine, portal venous system, or peritoneal cavity or by necrosis of the bowel wall with mucosal sloughing. This fulminant syndrome often leads to intestinal perforation, peritonitis, and bacteremia. It is a major cause of mortality in low-birth-weight infants (<1500 g) after the first week of life.[92] The diffuse necrotic changes that characterize this syndrome most often occur in the terminal ileum but may be seen in the colon or in the proximal portion of the gastrointestinal tract.

The pathogenesis of NEC appears to involve mucosal injury that is most often ischemic from hypoxemic or hypotensive episodes that may occur in premature infants or infants with complicating features such as an umbilical vein exchange transfusion. Ischemia may also result from the effects of endotoxemia followed by the effects of epinephrine, to which the vessels supplying the terminal ileum may be especially sensitive. Other predisposing factors to mucosal ischemia include asphyxia in association with hyaline membrane disease in premature infants or cyanotic heart disease. Increased intraluminal pressures may contribute to ischemia and pneumatosis, a process that may also play a role in previously normal infants who develop necrotizing colitis after protracted periods of diarrhea.[93] Others have suggested a localized Schwarzman reaction to endotoxemia or gram-negative bacteria.[94] The absence of lysozyme (normally present in human breast milk) may allow overgrowth of gram-negative bacilli. McKay and Wahle have reported the association of "enteropathogenic" *E. coli* serotype 0111:B4 with necrotizing enterocolitis.[95] Because of the association with umbilical vein polyvinylchloride catheters and feeding tubes, the toxic effect of plasticizers leached from the polyvinylchloride materials has been suggested.[96] Reports of outbreaks of necrotizing enterocolitis in newborn intensive care units[97–100] have led to a careful search for infectious agents including viral, fungal, or bacterial pathogens.[101–103] Among bacteria, *Pseudomonas*,[88] *Klebsiella*,[101,102] certain *E. coli*,[95,104,105] *Salmonella*,[106] and most recently, *Clostridium butyricum*[99] have been implicated in NEC. The roles of both ischemia and bacteria have been suggested by Barlow et al. with work in an experimental rat model of NEC in which breast milk was also shown to be protective.[107]

Clinical features of this serious condition in newborn infants include apneic spells, vomiting, abdominal distension, and occasionally bloody diarrhea. Most infants are less than 1 week of age, and there is an association with prematurity, maternal infections during delivery (such as anmionitis with prolonged ruptured membranes), and exchange transfusion via the umbilical vein. There is no sexual or seasonal predilection. The disease often progresses rapidly to intestinal perforation, shock, septicemia, and pneumatosis intestinalis. Air may also be evident in the portal venous system or biliary tract on plain roentgenograms. This syndrome is associated with mortality rate that is often in excess of 70 percent.

The diagnosis of NEC should be considered in any premature infant with altered gastrointestinal function, abdominal distension, or apneic spells. It may be further suspected by examination of the stool for occult blood and for the presence of reducing substances.[108] Plain abdominal roentgenograms may reveal air in the bowel wall, peritoneal cavity, or portal venous system, and there may be bloody diarrhea late in the course of the disease. Management must be initiated early and aggressively for any infant suspected of having NEC. Umbilical catheters should be removed, oral feeding should be stopped, and nasogastric aspiration should be initiated. Intravenous fluid therapy is of paramount importance. Laparotomy and excision of the necrotic bowel is often necessary and should be done aggressively if there is any evidence of peritonitis or obstruction.[109]

Prevention of NEC includes avoidance of risk factors and careful infection control measures in newborn intensive care units. Hypertonic elemental formulas have been implicated and should be avoided in high-risk patients.[110] Necrotizing enterocolitis rarely occurs in breast-fed infants. Explanations of the advantage of human breast milk include the presence of lsyozyme, antibodies, and cellular elements that may play a protective role against potential infectious agents. While oral prophylactic nonabsorbable antibiotics have been suggested,[111] serious questions remain about the use of prophylactic antibiotics, even in high-risk newborn infants weighing less than 1500 g.[112]

DARMBRAND, PIG-BEL, NECROTIZING ENTERITIS IN ADULTS (ENTERITIS NECROTICANS)

First described as "Darmbrand" (meaning "fire bowels") in epidemics of enteritis necroticans in northern Germany in the immediate postwar period in the mid-1940s,[113] a severe necrotizing jejunitis has also been recognized in both epidemic and sporadic forms after pork feasting in the highlands of New Guinea.[114] "Pig-bel" was the name given to the syndrome of abdominal discomfort that followed a large pork meal, commonly eaten after a large "pig kill," which takes place every 3–10 years among the highland Melanesians of New Guinea. Sporadic cases have been reported from other parts of the world including the United States.[115,116]

The pathologic findings involved are acute patchy, necrotizing disease of the small bowel in previously healthy people that may proceed rapidly to segmental gangrene with small amounts of gas in the mucosa, mesentery, or nodes.

Several theories of pathogenesis have been suggested, most of which involve the toxic products of *C. perfringens* type C, including α- and β-toxins. Sporadic cases of necrotizing enterocolitis have been noted in association with nutritional disorders, alcoholism, and malabsorption and after pancreatic or gastric resection.[117,118] After gastric surgery, increased numbers of *C. perfringens* and α-toxin have been noted in the upper small bowel and stomach.[119] Whether α- or β-toxins are capable of causing the necrotizing enteritis alone or whether they initiate the invasion of the mucosa by other organisms such as gram-negative rods is currently unclear. An attractive hypothesis has been suggested by Lawrence and Walker that could explain the association of necrotizing enteritis with poor nutrition and episodic dietetic overindulgence.[118] The low-protein diet of New Guinea highlanders is associated with low levels of digestive proteases in the intestinal lumen that can be shown to inactivate the β-toxin. The proteases can be further blocked by the oral intake of trypsin inhibitors, which are found in such dietary staples as sweet potatoes. Proteases return with improved diet,[120] as occurred in postwar Germany. This hypothesis has been confirmed in an animal model that required protease inhibitors for symptomatic infection.[121]

The clinical syndromes of necrotizing enteritis range from anorexia, vomiting, severe abdominal pain, and bloody diarrhea to fulminant toxemia and shock. Acute complications that require emergency surgery include paralytic ileus, strangulation, and bowel perforation with peritonitis. These complications are common in the first 2 weeks of illness. Later complications that may also require surgery include scarring that may lead to stenosis, obstruction, malabsorption, or fistulas. Necrotizing enteritis occurs with greater frequency and greater severity in children under 10 years of age. In contrast to European controls, 70 percent of the healthy adults in New Guinea have demonstrable antibody to clostridial β-toxin.[114,118]

The syndrome is defined pathologically but must be suspected in patients who develop severe abdominal pain, bloody diarrhea, ileus, and toxemia. The course is often too fulminant for detection of air in the bowel wall radiologically to be of any diagnostic value.

Etiologic agents held responsible for necrotizing enteritis include *C. perfringens* type C, once designated as type F in the older classification of *Clostridium welchii*. The majority of surgically resected bowel samples with necrotizing enteritis contain *C. perfringens*, over half of which are type C. Furthermore, 12 of 21 cases described had a significant change in serum β-antitoxin titer after illness with "pig-bel" in New Guinea.[114] While polyvalent gas gangrene antiserum was ineffective, administration of type C antiserum resulted in a 30 percent decrease in the need for surgery and a reduced mortality from 43 to 19 percent.[114] Furthermore, active immuization against the β-toxin has also proved effective in preventing "pig-bel."[122]

Others have suggested that type A *C. perfringens*, staphylococci, or even hepatitis virus may be responsible for necrotizing enteritis.[123] The syndrome of "enteritis gravis" has been described in association with infectious hepatitis, although no viral etiology has been documented.

The differential diagnosis of necrotizing enteritis include acute shigellosis, acute food poisoning syndromes, antibiotic-associated pseudomembranous colitis, and acute ulcerative colitis. The absence of colonic involvement, the epidemiologic setting, especially in poorly nourished patients, and the rapid progression to toxemia and shock are strongly suggestive of necrotizing enteritis.

Therapy for necrotizing enteritis includes careful supportive care and bowel decompression. Fluid requirements may be substantially greater than what is indicated by fecal output. Resection of the involved bowel must be considered if there is a persistence of paralytic ileus, a rapid increase in signs of toxemia, localized or diffuse signs of peritonitis, persistent pain, or a palpable mass lesion. If subacute obstruction or malabsorption is suspected on the basis of weight loss, elective surgery may be required up to 6 months after the acute illness. Raw peanut or soybean diets should be avoided since they contain trypsin inhibitors. *C. perfringens* type C antiserum containing β-antitoxin or the active β-toxin vaccine should be available and should be used in areas where necrotizing enteritis may be expected to occur.

PSEUDOMEMBRANOUS ENTEROCOLITIS (C. DIFFICILE COLITIS)

First reported by Coats in 1883[124] and described by Finney as postoperative diphtheritic enteritis in 1893,[125] the syndrome of pseudomembranous enterocolitis has received increasing attention in recent years as different host and etiologic factors have been unraveled. Pettit and colleagues characterized pseudomembranous entercolitis as occurring typically 4–5 days after abdominal surgery, often for colonic obstruction due to a carcinoma.[126] The association of pseudomembranous enterocolitis with antibiotics was first noted by Reiner et al. in 1952.[127] While this disease occurred in the pre-antibiotic era in association with intestinal obstruction, surgery, uremia, pneumonia, myocardial infarction, and sepsis,[128,129] most reports in the last decade have identified an association with the administration of antimicrobial agents, especially those with a broad antianaerobic spectrum. Diarrhea constitutes a major side effect of many antibiotics. From 4 to 50 percent of the patients taking tetracycline, chloramphenicol, penicillin, ampicillin, lincomycin, and clindamycin will develop diarrhea. Furthermore, each of these antibiotics has also been associated with the potentially life-threatening pseudomembranous enterocolitis.

Pseudomembranous enterocolitis is defined by the protoscopic appearance of small 1 to 5 mm raised whitish yellow plaques of "pseudomembrane" that may become confluent and overlie an erythmatous, minimally friable, colonic mucosa (Fig. 2).[130] It is often necessary to remove a thick layer of mucus to identify the characteristic "pseudomembrane." Ulcers and erosions as seen in amebic, bacillary, or ulcerative colitis are usually absent in pseudomembranous enterocolitis. The "pseudomembrane" is composed microscopically of epithelial debris, fibrin, and polymorphonuclear leukocytes and may be found on biopsy if the whole plaque is obtained (Fig. 2).[131] The appearance of filling defects or "thumb printing" on plain and barium roentgenograms is inconstant and not reliable for diagnosis.

The pathogenesis of pseudomembranous enterocolitis associated with surgery, intestinal obstruction, debilitating diseases, or antibiotics undoubtedly involves multiple factors. Theories have ranged from circulatory failure with intravascular coagulation[132] and localized Schwartzman reaction or lumenal obstruction to toxic substances that are ingested or produced in the intestinal tract by microorganisms locally on the bowel mucosa. However, the pathologic changes are quite distinct from the hemorrhagic lesions of ischemic colitis or vasculitic processes. Some antibiotics such as neomycin have direct effects on binding bowel salts that may result in diarrhea.[133] Other antibiotics that inhibit protein synthesis may have direct effects

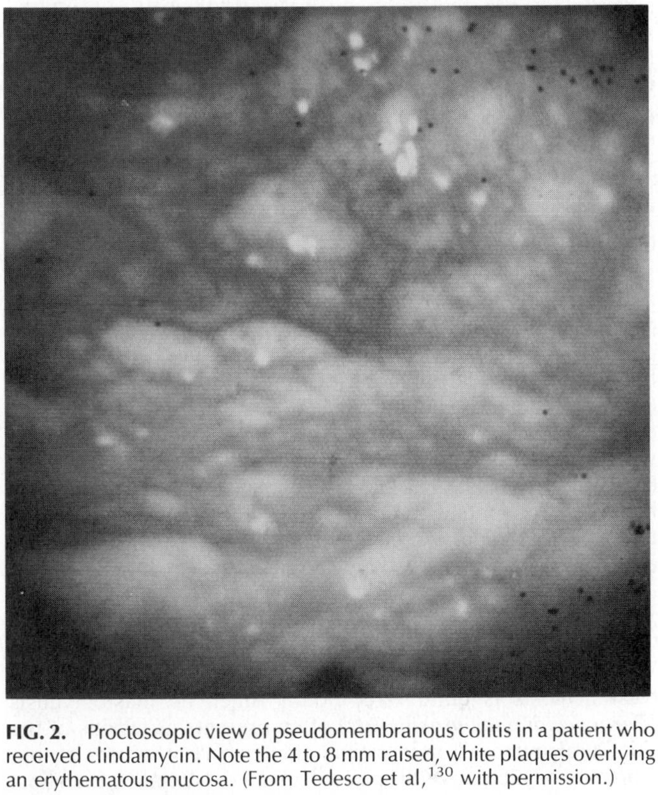

FIG. 2. Proctoscopic view of pseudomembranous colitis in a patient who received clindamycin. Note the 4 to 8 mm raised, white plaques overlying an erythematous mucosa. (From Tedesco et al,[130] with permission.)

on mammalian cells as well. Antibiotics may also induce toxin production by bacteria. Lincomycin enhances enterotoxin productin by *V. cholerae* and enterotoxigenic *E. coli.*[134] Still others have described the appearance of viral particles in the intestinal mucosa of patients with antibiotic-associated colitis.[135] However, the majority of cases involve the alteration of normal bowel flora, especially of anaerobes, which allows the emergence of resistant organisms such as *Clostridium difficile* that are capable of producing cytotoxic substances that alter mucosal function and integrity. While *Candida* often appears in the stools of patients taking broad-spectrum antibiotics and may be associated with diarrhea,[136] a double-blind, controlled trial of antifungal therapy failed to reduce the high frequency of gastrointestinal symptoms with oral tetracycline.[137] Pseudomembranous colitis in humans and animals has been associated with overgrowth of staphylococci in the stool.[138,139] While there is debate about their role in causing colitis,[140] staphylococci are capable of producing a cytotoxic Δ-toxin that causes tissue destruction and cell damage and elicits a net secretory response in animal models.[141]

Most cases of antibiotic-associated pseudomembranous colitis are now associated with cytotoxigenic *C. difficile*[142] (see Chapter 83). Larson et al. reported a nondialyzable heat-labile cytotoxin in the stools of five of six patients with antibiotic-associated pseudomembranous colitis that produced a cytopathic effect.[143] Using a hamster model described by Small in 1968,[144] investigators obtained a heat-labile cytotoxic material from patients with clindamycin-associated pseudomembranous colitis that caused cecal damage and death in hamsters similar to that resulting from administering clindamycin to the animals.[140,141] This effect is neutralized by pentavalent clostridial antiserum, by human immune serum globulin, and by *Clostridium difficile* or *C. sordellii* antiserum but not by specific antisera against *Clostridium perfringens* (*welchii*), *septicum*, *novyi*, or *histolyticum*. Bartlett and colleagues[145] and George et al.[146] have further demonstrated such cytotoxic activity in the broth culture filtrates of strains of *Clostridium difficile* isolated from patients with antibiotic-associated colitis.[147] This organism was described and noted to be pathogenic for guinea pigs and rabbits by Hall and O'Toole in 1935,[148] who found the organism in 4 of 10 newborn infants. Snyder had noted in 1937 that certain strains of this organism produced a thermolabile toxin that was lethal for guinea pigs and that the guinea pigs could be protected with specific antiserum.[149]

The association of pseudomembranous enterocolitis with several antibiotics is well documented.[150,151] Pseudomembranous colitis is said to occur in 0.1–10 percent of the patients given clindamycin irrespective of dose.[152,153] While it occurs more frequently with oral than with parenteral antibiotic, there are several cases in which it has followed intravenous or intramuscular drug administration. There is a slight predominance of females over males and of adults over children in most series. However, children have been reported with the syndrome as well.[154] In one series, clindamycin-associated diarrhea was reported to occur in 46 percent of the patients 60 years old or older.[155] The discrepant incidence figures for pseudomembranous colitis with clindamycin may have their explanation in the apparent clustering of cases in several reports.[156,157] Case clusters suggest that the agent responsible for pseudomembranous colitis may be transmitted in the nosocomial setting.

The onset of clinical illness is usually abrupt, often with fever and abdominal pain. While most patients develop symptoms after receiving antibiotics for 4–9 days, several cases have been reported to begin 2–4 weeks after the discontinuation of clindamycin therapy. Early diagnosis and discontinuation of treatment usually result in resolution of symptoms within 1 week. However, the continuation of the drug or the occurrence of colitis after a full course of antibiotic may lead to diarrhea of 6–10 weeks' duration that may cause severe electrolyte abnormalities and protein loss with significant mortality.

The etiologies of antibiotic-associated diarrhea and of the syndrome pseudomembranous colitis may involve direct effects of antimicrobial agents on gastrointestinal function, effects of antimicrobial agents on microorganisms, or indirect effects of surgery, debilitating disease, or antimicrobial agents on intestinal flora that allow an overgrowth of abnormal, sometimes cytotoxigenic organisms such as staphylococci or clostridia. *Clostridium difficile* colitis is increasingly recognized in immunocompromized patients (those receiving chemotherapy, after marrow transplants, or with human immunodeficiency virus [HIV] infection) and in day care centers or institutions for the elderly.[158]

Any patient who develops diarrhea while taking antibiotics should stop taking the antibiotic immediately if at all possible. If symptoms are severe or persistent or if an inflammatory process is noted by fecal leukocyte examination, one should perform a proctoscopic examination to make the diagnosis of pseudomembranous colitis.

Therapy, after discontinuing treatment with the antibiotic, is mainly supportive. Most patients will improve within a week. The potential risk of *increased* diarrheal symptoms when antimotility drugs are used has been documented with lincomycin-associated colitis.[159] Oral vancomycin or the less expensive metronidazole are used for treating pseudomembranous enterocolitis.[146,160,161] Although vancomycin protects Syrian hamsters against lethal clindamycin-associated enterocolitis,[162] symptoms may recur after vancomycin therapy, and vancomycin itself can cause colitis in experimental animals[163] and should be used only when symptoms persist or worsen. (See Chapter 83 for a complete discussion of diagnosis and therapy.)

CHRONIC INFLAMMATORY PROCESSES

Chronic inflammatory enteritides are often indolent, slowly progressive infections. Often there is a history of weeks or months of fever, abdominal pain, weight loss, or other systemic manifestations. Recurring or relapsing symptoms may be seen with *Campylobacter jejuni* or *Salmonella* gastroenteritis. In addition, 16 percent of cases of shigellosis may become prolonged for 3 weeks or longer.[164] Any diarrheal illness that extends beyond 2 weeks identifies a high-risk child for severe diarrhea and nutritional morbidity in tropical, developing areas.[165]

Chronic E. coli Diarrhea

"Enteropathogenic" *E. coli* organisms that cause acute diarrhea in infants by largely unknown mechanisms may rarely be associated with an insidious persistent or relapsing diarrheal illness.[166] *E. coli* in O groups 1, 2, 4, 7, and 75 that produce hemolysin and necrotoxin have been isolated from patients with ulcerative colitis. These toxic organisms were not present in healthy people or in patients with acute diarrheal syndromes.[167]

Gastrointestinal Tuberculosis

Intestinal tuberculosis, once considered common, has become a relatively rare disease. Intestinal involvement with tuberculosis may be either *primary*, from ingestion of the organism or from spread of miliary tuberculosis, or *secondary*, usually from a pulmonary source.

Primary intestinal tuberculosis without pulmonary disease often results in hypertrophic mucosal changes. Sixty-four percent of the cases of acute miliary tuberculosis may also have gastrointestinal involvement.[168] Primary intestinal tuberculosis may present with abdominal pain, fever, and a tender, fixed palpable mass in the ileocecal area.[169] Primary hypertrophic intestinal tuberculosis continues to occur in the Near East[170] and in India[171] where infection is most often due to the human strain *M tuberculosis*.[172]

Intestinal involvement secondary to pulmonary tuberculosis may result from swallowing infected sputum or from biliary excretion of the organism from an infected liver. The frequency of secondary intestinal tuberculosis increases to 25–80 percent with far-advanced pulmonary disease.[173] Hippocrates stated: "diarrhea attacking a person with phthisis is a mortal symptom."[174]

Tuberculosis may involve any part of the gastrointestinal tract, but most ulcerative and hypertrophic types occur in the ileocecal region where there is a predominance of submucosal lymphatic tissue.[175] The most common features are fever and abdominal pain that is often relieved by defecation or vomiting. Weight loss is more common in secondary intestinal tuberculosis. Only one-third of the patients with gastrointestinal tuberculosis have diarrhea. Diarrhea may be related to exacerbations of abdominal pain and occasionally occurs with extensive involvement of the small intestine that may cause steatorrhea and a malabsorption syndrome. While ulceration and mucous diarrhea are relatively common with secondary intestinal tuberculosis, hemorrhage and the presence of gross blood in the stool are distinctly uncommon, perhaps because of the obliterative endarteritis.

The diagnosis of gastrointestinal tuberculosis may be very difficult radiologically and even histologically. It must be distinguished from regional enteritis, sarcoidosis, actinomycosis, ameboma, carcinoma, and periappendiceal abscess. In contrast to Crohn's disease, gastrointestinal tuberculosis rarely causes anal lesions, fistulas, or perforation; is often associated with miliary nodules on the serosa, rarely causes strictures longer than 3 cm, and may cause circumferential transverse ulcers. Tuberculosis may also cause fibrosis of the muscularis mucosa, pyloric metaplasia, and epithelial regeneration.[176] There may be minimal or no radiologic changes in the bowel mucosa. Small mucosal ulcerations may result in tiny calcified nodules in the mucosa in association with calcified mesenteric lymph nodes analogous to the pulmonary Ghon complex. The ileocecal region often reveals radiologic evidence of irritability and hypermotility, with hypersegmentation of the mucosal folds or poor filling of the ileocecal region detected by barium enema. Occasionally, frank ulcerations can be noted on contrast studies, and late in the course there is scarring. The diagnosis requires a careful examination of involved tissue for acid-fast bacilli by special stain and culture. Caseous necrosis is more frequently found in the mesenteric nodes than in intestinal tissue itself. Complications of intestinal tuberculosis include perforation, peritonitis, and obstruction from either hypertrophy, scarring, or tuberculoma.

Candidiasis

Chronic inflammatory enteritis may be caused by local or disseminated systemic fungal infections, often in association with antibiotic alteration of normal flora or with other host impairment. Candidal involvement of the gastrointestinal tract includes gastric bezoarlike masses after partial gastrectomy.[177] Secondary candidal infection of tumors or ulcerative disease (peptic, amebic, or idiopathic) in the stomach or colon may also occur,[178,179] and *C. albicans* can be seen in over half of patients with diarrhea and the acquired immunodeficiency syndrome (AIDS).[180] Retrosternal pain, dysphagia, or gastrointestinal bleeding in patients with predisposing illnesses should alert one to suspect candidal esophagitis and to proceed with a barium esophagogram and endoscopy for diagnosis.[173]

South American Blastomycosis

While gastrointestinal involvement with the North American blastomycosis is quite rare, South American blastomycosis (*Paracoccidioides brasiliensis*) often presents as lesions of the skin, oral mucosa, or intestinal tract where it causes granulomatous or ulcerative disease.[181] The most common intestinal sites of involvement are the appendix, cecum, and anorectal areas. There is often abscess formation and lymphatic spread to regional nodes and to the spleen, liver, or even the lungs. The major symptoms are abdominal pain and ulcerative, granulomatous lesions, especially in the oropharynx. Palpable, tender abdominal masses in the ileocecal region may be noted on physical examination. Peritoneal signs are often absent. Diagnosis is made by biopsy, stain, and culture of the ulcerative lesion.

Phycomycosis

Other fungi usually involve the intestinal tract only as one feature of disseminated granulomatous disease, some of which may be acquired through a gastrointestinal portal of entry. Phycomycosis (*Absidia, Rhizopus*, and *Mucor* spp.) may invade the predisposed host via the gastrointestinal tract[182] or may involve the gastrointestinal tract by hematogenous spread and cause abdominal pain, diarrhea, gastrointestinal bleeding, and peritonitis.[183]

Histoplasmosis

Histoplasmosis may also involve the intestinal tract as a part of disseminated infection. In the gastrointestinal tract, histoplasmosis presents as ulceration, bleeding, obstruction, or rarely, protein-losing enteropathy.[184–186] Lesions tend to be single and may be considered initially to be neoplastic.

Syphilis

Syphilis can also involve the gastrointestinal tract, usually in the upper part of the small bowel or stomach. An acute erosive and infiltrative gastritis with motile spirochetes and positive specific treponemal immunofluorescence test response has been reported in late secondary syphilis.[187] The initial complaints are upper abdominal pain, vomiting, and weight loss. More classic are the late gastrointestinal manifestations of lues with pyloric obstruction, "hourglass" constriction, or linitis plastica of the stomach. Less commonly, gumma may be seen in the small bowel or colon.

Parasites

Parasitic enteritides that should be considered among causes of chronic inflammatory bowel processes include coccidiosis, chronic or recurrent amebiasis, and the rare invasive, inflammatory form of giardiasis.

Human coccidiosis is an upper small bowel inflammatory process caused by *Isospora belli* that should be considered in patients with obscure chronic diarrhea and eosinophilia,[188,189] especially in AIDS patients.[180,190] Weight loss, fever, headache, and colicky abdominal pain may also be present with steatorrhea and malabsorption. This infection is common in Chile and has occurred in nontraveling United States residents. It is likely that it often is unrecognized. This unicellular sporozoan parasite undergoes asexual schizogony in the intestinal epithelial cells from which merozoites are released. Like malarial plasmodia, the merozoite may then invade other cells and repeat the asexual schizogony cycle or may mature into sexual gametocytes and form a zygote and then a sporulated oocyst that ruptures to yield sporozoites that restart the enterocyte cycle. Sporulated oocysts are the infective form and have caused laboratory-acquired infections. The diagnosis is made by careful examination of multiple serial sections of intestinal biopsy specimens for any stage of the parasite or by examining small bowel contents for oocysts. Stool oocysts may be seen with a modified acid-fast stain as for *Cryptosporidium*[190] or may rarely be demonstrated with some difficulty by incubating a specimen at room temperature for 1–2 days to permit their maturation before examining using a concentration technique such as zinc sulfate flotation. While many therapeutic agents have been used unsuccessfully (including quinacrine, nitrofurantoin, tetracycline, metronadizole), pyramethamine and sulfadiazine in combination have been effective.[189,190]

The related protozoan parasite, *Cryptosporidium*, is a cause of severe chronic diarrhea in immunosuppressed hosts.[190–192] It may also cause diarrhea that is self-limited in normal hosts.[192] Unlike *Isospora*, cryptosporidia usually infect only the surface of the mucosal epithelium, and the process is usually noninflammatory. The organism may be identified by sugar floatation or modified acid-fast stains of fecal specimens.[190,193]

Invasive syndromes may occur over a long period of time or in a recurring pattern with intestinal amebiasis. This syndrome may even extend into an entity called "ulcerative postdysenteric colitis" that may no longer respond to antiamebic therapy.[194]

Inflammatory small bowel disease may occur with unusually severe *Giardia lamblia* infection. This may result in severe villus atrophy, with dense plasma cell infiltration and acute inflammation in the lamina propria.[195]

The differential diagnosis of chronic inflammatory diarrhea includes several syndromes of noninfectious or unknown etiology. Idiopathic inflammatory bowel disease including regional enteritis, granulomatous colitis, and ulcerative colitis may be difficult to distinguish from infectious enteritides. Other processes that often require biopsy and culture to exclude infectious processes are intestinal involvement with sarcoidosis, lymphoma, or carcinoma. Radiation enterocolitis, ischemic colitis, and diverticulitis may also be manifested with chronic inflammatory diarrhea.

Few generalizations can be made about the management of infectious chronic inflammatory enteritides. The causes are so varied that the diagnosis often requires a careful search outside the gastrointestinal tract or surgical biopsy of the involved bowel. Only after the diagnosis is made can specific, effective therapy be instituted.

REFERENCES

1. Keusch GT, Jacewicz M. The pathogenesis of *Shigella* diarrhea. V. Relationship of Shiga enterotoxin, neurotoxin and cytotoxin. J Infect Dis. 1975;131(Suppl):33.
2. Edelman R, Karmali MA, Fleming PA. Summary of the International Symposium and Workshop on Infections due to Verocytotoxin (Shiga-like toxin)-Producing *Escherichia coli*. J Infect Dis. 1988;157:1102–4.
3. Blacklow NR, Dolin R, Fedson DS, et al. Acute infectious nonbacterial gastroenteritis: Etiology and pathogenesis. Ann Intern Med 1972;76:993.
4. Rendtorff RC. The experimental transmission of human intestinal protozoan parasites. Am J Hyg 1954;59:196.
5. Weissman JB, Schmerler A, Gangarosa EJ, et al. Shigellosis in day-care centres. Lancet. 1975;1:88.
6. Roy SK, Speelman P, Butler T, et al. Diarrhea associated with typhoid fever. J Infect Dis. 1985;151:1138–43.
7. Quinn TC, Stamm WE, Goodell SE, et al. The polymicrobial origin of intestinal infections in homosexual men. N Engl J Med. 1983;309:576.
8. Korzeniowski OM, Barada FA, Rouse JD, et al. Value of examination for fecal leukocytes in the early diagnosis of shigellosis. Am J Trop Med Hyg. 1979;28:1031.
9. Pickering LK, DuPont HL, Olarte J, et al. Fecal leukocytes in enteric infections. Am J Clin Pathol. 1977;68:562–5.
10. Haugwout FG. The microscopic diagnosis of the dysenteries at their onset. JAMA. 1924;83:1156.
11. Guerrrant RL, Brush JE, Ravdin JI, et al. Interaction between *Entamoeba histolytica* and human polymorphonuclear neutrophils. J Infect Dis. 1981;143:83–93.
12. Speelman P, McGlaughlin R, Kabir I, et al. Differential clinical features and stool findings in shigellosis and amebic dysentery. Trans R Soc Trop Med Hyg. 1987;81:549–51.
13. Rahaman MM, Khan MM, Azi KMS, et al. An outbreak fo dysentery caused by *Shigella dysenteriae* type I on a coral island in the Bay of Bengal. J Infect Dis. 1975;132:15.
14. Feeley JC, Balows A. *Vibrio*. In: Lennette EH, Spaulding EH, Truant JP, eds. Manual of Clinical Microbiology. Washington, DC: American Society for Microbiology; 1974:238–45.
15. Morris GK, Feeley JC, Martin WT, et al. Isolation and identification of *Yersinia enterocolitica*. Public Health Lab. 1977;35:217.

16. Skirrow MB. *Campylobacter enteritis*: A "new" disease. Br Med J 1977;2:9.
17. Koster F, Levin J, Walker L, et al. Hemolytic uremic syndrome after shigellosis. Relation to endotoxemia and circulating immune complexes. N Engl J Med. 1978;298:927.
18. Barrett-Connor E, Connor JD. Extraintestinal manifestations of shigellosis. Am J Gastroenterol. 1970;53:234.
19. Keusch GT, Grady GF, Mata LJ, et al. The pathogenesis of *Shigella* diarrhea. I. Enterotoxin production by *Shigella dysenteriae* 1. J Clin Invest. 1972;51:1212.
20. Calin A, Fries JF. An "experimental" epidemic of Reiter's syndrome revisted. Follow-up evidence on genetic and environmental factors. Ann Intern Med. 1976;84:564.
21. Aho K, Ahvonen P, Alkio P, et al. HLA-27 in reactive arthritis following infection. Ann Rheum Dis. 1975;34(Suppl):29.
22. Trabulsi LR, Fernandes MFR, Zuliani ME. Noval bacterias pathogenicas para o intestino do homen. Rev Inst Med Trop Sao Paulo. 1967;9:31.
23. Ørskov F. Virulence factors of the bacterial cell surface. J Infect Dis. 1978;137:630.
24. Levine MM. *Escherichia coli* that cause diarrhea: Enterotoxigenic, enteropathogenic, enteroinvasive, enterohemorrhagic, and enteroadherent. J Infect Dis. 1987;155:377–89.
25. Tulloch EF Jr, Ryan KJ, Formal SB, et al. Invasive enteropathic *Escherichia coli* dysentery. An outbreak in 28 adults. Ann Intern Med. 1973;79:13.
26. Sereny B. Experimental shigella keratoconjunctivitis: A preliminary report. Acta Microbiol Acad Sci Hung. 1955;2:293.
27. DuPont HL, Formal SB, Hornick R. Pathogenesis of *E. coli* diarrhea. N Engl J Med. 1971;285:1–9.
28. Harris JR, Wachsmuth IK, Davis BF, et al. High molecular weight plasmid correlates with *E. coli* enteroinvasiveness. Infect Immun. 1982;37:1295–8.
29. Sansonetti PS, d'Hauteville H, Ecobiochon C. Moleculare comparison of virulence in *Shigella* and enteroinvasive *E. coli* (Abstract). Ann Microbiol (Paris). 1983;134:295–318.
30. Silva RM, Toledo MRF, Trabulsi LR. Correlation of invasiveness with plasmids in enteroinvasive strains of *E. coli*. J Infect Dis. 1982;146:706.
31. Marier R, Wells JG, Swanson RC, et al. An outbreak of enteropathogenic *Escherichia coli* foodborne disease traced to imported French cheese. Lancet. 1973;2:1376.
32. DuPont HL, Formal SB, Hornick RB, et al. Pathogenesis of Escherichia coli diarrhea. N Engl J Med 1971;285:1.
33. Silva RM, Toledo MRF, Trabulsi LF. Biochemical and cultural characteristics of invasive Escherichia coli. J Clin Microbiol 1980;11:441.
34. Pal T, Pasca S, Emody L, et al. Antigenic relationship among virulent enteroinvasive E. coli, Shigella flexneri and Shigella sonnei detected by ELISA. Lancet. 1983;2:102.
35. O'Brien AD, Newland JW, Miller SF, et al. Shiga-like toxin-converting phages from *Escherichia coli* strains that cause hemorrhagic colitis or infantile diarrhea. Science. 1984;226:694–6.
36. Pai CH, Ahmed N, Lior H, Johnson WM, Sims HV, Woods DE. Epidemiology of sporadic diarrhea due to Verocytotoxin-producing *Escherichia coli*: A two-year prospective study. J Infect Dis. 1988;157:1054–7.
37. Obrig TG, Moran TP, Brown JE. The mode of action of shigatoxin on peptide elongation of eukaryotic protein synthesis. Biochem J. 1987;244:287–94.
38. Takeda Y, Yutsudo T, Igarashi K, Endo Y. Mode of action of Vero toxins (VT1 and VT2) from *Escherichia coli* and of Shiga toxin. p104. Twenty-third US-Japan Joint Conference on Cholera. Williamsberg, Va., 1987.
39. Guerrant RL, Lahita RG, Winn WC, et al. Campylobacteriosis in man: Pathogenic mechanisms and review of 91 bloodstream infections. Am J Med 1978;65:584.
40. Doyle LP. A vibrio associated with swine dysentery. Am J Vet Res. 1944;5:3.
41. Dekeyser P, Gossuin-Detrain M, Butzler JP, et al. Acute enteritis due to related Vibrio: First positive stool cultures. J Infect Dis 1972;125:390.
42. Butzler JP, Dekeyser P, Detrain M, et al. Related vibrio in stools. J Pediatr. 1973;82:493.
43. Blaser MJ, Reller LB. Campylobacter enteritis. N Engl J Med. 1981;305:1444.
44. DeMol P, Bosmans E. Campylobacter enteritis in Central Africa. Lancet. 1978;1:604.
45. Ravdin JI, Croft BY, Guerrant RL. Cytopathogenic mechanisms of Entamoeba histolytica. J Exp Med. 1980;152:377.
46. Lynch EC, Rosenberg IM, Gitler C. An ion-channel forming protein produced by Entamoeba histolytica. EMBO. 1982;1:801.
47. Young JDE, Young TM, Lu LP, et al. Characterization of a membrane pore-forming protein from Entamoeba histolytica. J Exp Med. 1982;156:1677.
48. Ravdin JI, Guerrant RL. A review of the parasite cellular mechanisms involved in the pathogenesis of amebiasis. Rev Infect Dis. 1982;4:1185–207.
49. Wittner M, Rosenbaum RM. Role of bacteria in modifying virulence of Entamoeba histolytica: Studies of amebae from axenic cultures. Am J Trop Med Hyg. 1970;19:755.
50. Bracha R, Mirelman D. Virulence of *Entamoeba histolytica* trophozoites. Effects of bacteria, microaerobic conditions and metronidazole. J Exp Med. 1984;160:353.
51. Krogstad DJ, Spencer HC Jr, Healy GR, et al. Amebiasis: Epidemiologic studies in the United States, 1971–1974. Ann Intern Med. 1978;88:89.
52. Kean BH. Venereal amoebiasis. NY State J Med. 1967;76:930.
53. Keystone JS, Keystone DL, Proctor LM. Intestinal parasitic infections in homosexual men: Prevalence, symptoms, and factors in transmission. Can Med Assoc J. 1980;123:512.
54. Blake PA. Disease of humans (other than cholera) caused by vibrios. Annu Rev Microbiol. 1980;34:341.
55. Morris JG, Black RE. Colera and other vibrioses in the United States. N Engl J Med. 1985;312:343.
56. Hughes JM, Boyce JM, Aleen ARMA, et al. *Vibrio parahemoliticus* enterocolitis in Bangladesh: Report of an outbreak. Am J Trop Med Hyg. 1978;27:106.
57. Bolen JL, Zamiska SA, Greenough WB III. Clinical features in enteritis due to *Vibrio parahemolyticus*. Am J Med. 1974;57:638.
58. Barker WH. *Vibrio parahemolyticus* outbreaks in the United States. Lancet. 1974;1:551.
59. Blake PA, Merson MH, Weaver RE, et al. Disease caused by a marine vibrio: Clinical characteristics and epidemiology. N Engl J Med. 1979;300:1.
60. Mandal BK, Mani V. Colonic involvement in salmonellosis. Lancet. 1976;1:887.
61. Thomas M, Tillett H. Colonic involvement in salmonellosis. Lancet. 1976;1:1129.
62. Boyd JF. Colonic involvement in salmonellosis. Lancet. 1976;1:1415.
63. Appelbaum PC, Scragg J, Schonland MM. Colonic involvement in salmonellois. Lancet. 1976;2:102.
64. Radsel-Medvescek A, Zargi R, Acko M, et al. Colonic involvement in salmonellosis. Lancet. 1977;1:601.
65. Rowland HAK. The complications of typhoid fever. J Trop Med Hyg. 1961;64:143.
66. Sonnenwirth AC, Weaver RE. *Yersinia enterocolitica*. N Engl J Med. 1970;283:1468.
67. Black RE, Jackson RJ, Tsai T, et al. Epidemic *Yersinia enterocolitica* infection due to contaminated chocolate milk. N Engl J Med. 1978;298:76.
68. Leino R, Kalliomaki JL. Yersiniosis as an internal disease. Ann Intern Med. 1974;81:458.
69. Ahvonen P. Human yersiniosis in Finland. II. Clinical features. Ann Clin Res. 1972;4:39.
70. Rabson AR, Hallett AF, Koornhof HJ. Generalized *Yersinia enterocolitica* infection. J Infect Dis. 1975;131:447.
71. Bradford WD, Noce PS, Gutman LT. Pathologic features of enteric infection with *Yersinia enterocolitica*. Arch Pathol. 1974;98:7.
72. Kilpatrick AM. Medical intelligence—current concepts: Gonorrheal proctitis. N Engl J Med. 1972;287:967.
73. Klein EJ, Fisher LS, Chow AW. Anorectal gonococcal infection. Ann Intern Med. 1977;86:340.
74. Dantec LE. Dysenterie spirillaire. CR Soc Biol. 1903;55:617.
75. Lee FD, Kraszewski A, Gordon J, et al. Intestinal spirochaetosis. Gut. 1971;12:126.
76. Haltalin KC, Nelson JD, Ring R III, et al. Double-blind treatment study of shigellosis comparing ampicillin, sulfadiazine, and placebo. J Pediatr. 1967;70:970.
77. Tong MJ, Martin DG, Cunningham JJ, et al. Clinical and bacteriological elevation of antibiotic treatment in shigellosis. JAMA. 1970;214:1841.
78. Barada FA, Guerrant RL. Sulfamethoxazole-trimethoprim versus ampicillin in treatment of acute invasive diarrhea in adults. Antimicrob Agents Chemother. 1980;17:961.
79. Osada Y, Une T, Ogawa H. Inhibition of cell to cell transfer of *Shigella* by treatment with some antibiotics. Jpn Microbiol. 1973;17:233.
80. Farrar WE Jr, Eidson M: Antibiotic resistance to *Shigella* mediated by R factors. J Infect Dis. 1971;123:477.
81. Ross S, Controni G, Khan W. Resistance of shigellae to ampicillin and other antibiotics. Its clinical and epidemiological implications. JAMA. 1972;221:45.
82. Pichler HET, Diridl G, Sticklerk, et al. Clinical efficacy of ciprofloxacin compared with placebo in bacterial diarrhea. Am J Med. 1987;82(Suppl 4A):329–32.
83. DuPont HL, Ericsson CD, Robinson A, et al. Current problems in antimicrobial therapy for bacterial enteric infection. Am J Med. 1987;82(Suppl 4A):324–8.
84. Healy GR. Laboratory diagnosis of amebiasis. Bull NY Acad Med. 1971;47:478.
85. Aserkoff B, Bennett JV. Effect of antibiotic therapy in acute salmonellosis on the fecal excretion of salmonellae. N Engl J Med. 1969;281:636.
86. Nelson JD, Jusmiesz H, Jackson LH, et al. Treatment of *Salmonella* gastroenteritis with ampicillin, amoxicillin or placebo. Pediatrics. 1980;65:1125.
87. Waldhausen JA, Herendeen T, King H. Necrotizing colitis of the newborn: Common cause of perforation of the colon. Surgery. 1963;54:365.
88. Mizrahi A, Barlow O, Berdon W, et al. Necrotizing enterocolitis in premature infants. J Pediatr. 1965;66:697.
89. Simpson JY. Peritonitis in the fetus in uterus. Edinburgh Med Surg J. 1838;15:390.
90. Genersich A. Bauchfellentzondung beim Neugeboreneh in Folg von Perforation des Ileums. Arch Pathol Anat. 1891;126:485.
91. Thelander HE. Perforation of the gastrointestinal tract of the newborn infant. Am Dis J Child. 1939;58:371.
92. Wilson R, Kanto WP, McCarthy BJ, et al. Epidemiologic characteristics of necrotizing enterocolitis: A population-based study. Am J Epidemiol. 1981;114:880.
93. Fairborn RA. Etiology of necrotising enterocolitis. Lancet. 1977;1:956.
94. Hermann RE. Perforation of the colon from necrotizing colitis in the newborn: Report of a survival and new etiologic concept. Surgery. 1965;58: 436.

95. McKay DG, Wahle GH. Epidemic gastroenteritis due to *Escherichia coli* 0111B4. Arch Pathol. 1955;60:679.
96. Rogers AF, Dunn PM. Intestinal perforation, exchange transfusion and P.V.C. Lancet. 1969;2:1246.
97. Virnig NL, Reynolds JW. Epidemiological aspects of neonatal necrotizing enterocolitis. Am J Dis Child. 1974;128:186.
98. Book LS, Overall JC, Herbst JJ, et al. Clustering of necrotizing enterocolitis. Interruption by infection-control measures. N Engl J Med. 1977;297:984.
99. Howard FM, Flynn DM, Bradley JM, et al. Outbreak of necrotising enterocolitis caused by *Clostridium butyricum*. Lancet. 1977;2:1099.
100. Ryder RW, Buxton AE, Wachsmuth IK. Heat-stable enterotoxigenic *Escherichia coli* and necrotizing enterocolitis: Lack of an association. J Pediatr. 1977;91:302.
101. Olarte J, Ferguson WW, Henderson NI, et al. *Klebsiella* strains isolated from diarrheal infants. Am J Dis Child. 1961;101:763.
102. Frantz ID, L'Heureux P, Engel RR, et al. Necrotizing enterocolitis. J Pediatr. 1975;86:259.
103. Levin SE, Isaacson C. Spontaneous perforation of the colon in the newborn infant. Arch Dis Child. 1960;35:378.
104. Speer ME, Taber LH, Yow MD, et al. Fulminant neonatal sepsis and necrotizing enterocolitis associated with a "nonenteropathogenic" strain of *Escherichia coli*. J Pediatr. 1976;89:91.
105. Drucker MM, Polliack A, Yeivin R, et al. Immunofluorescent demonstration of enteropathogenic *Escherichia coli* in tissue of infants dying with enteritis. Pediatrics. 1970;46:855.
106. Stein H, Beck J, Solomon A, et al. Gastroenteritis with necrotizing enterocolitis in premature babies. Br Med J. 1972;2:616.
107. Barlow B, Santulli TV, Heird WC, et al. An experimental study of acute neonatal enterocolitis—the importance of breast milk. J Pediatr Surg. 1974;9:587.
108. Book LS, Herbst JJ, Jung AL. Carbohydrate malabsorption in necrotizing enterocolitis. Pediatrics. 1975;57:201.
109. Stevenson JK, Oliver TK, Graham CB, et al. Aggressive treatment of neonatal necrotizing enterocolitis: Thirty-eight patients with 25 survivors. J Pediatr Surg. 1971;6:28.
110. Book LS, Herbst JJ, Atherton SO, et al. Necrotizing enterocolitis in low-birth-weight infants fed on elemental formula. J Pediatr. 1975;87:602.
111. Egan EA, Mantilla G, Nelson RM, et al. A prospective controlled trial of oral kanamycin in the prevention of neonatal necrotizing enterocolitis. J Pediatr. 1976;89:467.
112. Nelson JD. Commentary. J Pediatr. 1976;89:471.
113. Hansen K, Jeckeln E, Jochims J, et al. Darmbrand-Enteritis Necroticanss. Stuttgart: Georg Thiem Verlag, 1949.
114. Murrell TGC, Roth L, Egerton J, et al. Pig-bel: Enteritis necroticans. Lancet. 1966;1:217.
115. Patterson M, Rosenbaum HD. Enteritis necroticans. Gastroenterology. 1952;21:110.
116. Fick KA, Wolken AP. Necrotic jejunitis. Lancet. 1949;1:519.
117. Williams MR, Pullan JM. Necrotising enteritis following gastric surgery. Lancet. 1953;2:1013.
118. Lawrence G, Walker PD. Pathogenesis of enteritis necroticans in Papua, New Guinea. Lancet. 1976;1:125.
119. Howie JW, Duncan IBR, Mackie LM. Growth of *Clostridium welchii* in the stomach after partial gastrectomy. Lancet. 1953;2:1018.
120. Kumar R, Banks PA, George PK, et al. Early recovery of exocrine pancreatic function in adult protein-calorie malnutrition. Gastroenterology. 1975;68:1593.
121. Lawrence G, Coake R. Experimental pigbel: The production and pathology of necrotizing enteritis due to *Clostridium welchii* type C in the guinea pig. Br J Exp Pathol. 1980;61:261–71.
122. Lawrence G, Shann F, Frestone DS, et al. Prevention of necrotising enteritis in Papua New Guinea by active immunization. Lancet. 1979;1:227–30.
123. Kravetz RE, Brazenas NV. Viral hepatitis associated with enteritis gravis. Arch Intern Med. 1963;112:179.
124. Coats J. A Manual of Pathology. Philadelphia: Henry C Lea's Sons; 1883:567.
125. Finney JMT. Gastroenterostomy for cicatrizing ulcer of the pylorus. Bull John Hopkins Hosp. 1893;4:53.
126. Pettet JD, Baggenstoss AH, Dearing WH, et al. Postoperative pseudomembranous enterocolitis. Surg Gynecol Obstet. 1954;98:546.
127. Reiner L, Schlesinger MJ, Miller GM. Pseudomembranous colitis following aureomycin and chloramphenicol. Arch Pathol. 1952;54:39.
128. Hardaway RM, McKay DG. Pseudomembranous enterocolitis. Are antibiotics wholly responsible? Arch Surg. 1959;78:446.
129. Goulston SJM, McGovern VJ. Pseudo-membranous colitis. Gut. 1965;6:207.
130. Tedesco FJ, Barton RW, Alpers DH. Clindamycin-associated colitis. Ann Intern Med. 1974;81:429.
131. Sumner HW, Tedesco FJ. Rectal biopsy in clindamycin-associated colitis. Arch Pathol. 1975;99:237.
132. McKay DG, Hardaway RM, Whale GH, et al. Experimental pseudomembranous enterocolitis. Arch Intern Med. 1955;95:779.
133. Antibiotic diarrhea (Editorial). Br Med J. 1975;4:243.
134. Levner M, Wiener FP, Rubin BA. Introduction of *Escherichia coli* and *Vibrio cholerae* enterotoxins by an inhibition of protein synthesis. Infect Immun. 1977;15:132.
135. Steer HW. The pseudomembranous colitis associated with clindamycin therapy—a viral colitis. Gut. 1975;16:695.
136. Kane JG, Chretien JH, Garagusi VF. Diarrhoea caused by *Candida*. Lancet. 1976;1:335.
137. Comparison of side-effects of tetracycline and tetracycline plus nystatin. Report to the Research Committee of the British Tuberculosis Association by the Clinical Trials Subcommittee. Br Med J. 1968;4:411.
138. Dearing WH, Baggenstoss AH, Weed LA. Studies on the relationship of *Staphylococcus aureus* to pseudomembranous enteritis and to postantibiotic enteritis. Gastroenterology. 1960;38:441.
139. Bennett IL, Wood JS Jr, Yardley JH. Staphylococcal pseudomembraneous enterocolitis in chinchillas: A clinico-pathologic study. Trans Assoc Am Physicians. 1956;69:116.
140. Bartlett JG, Gorbach SL. Pseudomembranous enterocolitis (antibiotic-related colitis). Adv Intern Med. 1977;22:455.
141. Kapral FA, O'Brien AD, Ruff PD, et al. Inhibition of water absorption in the intestine by *Staphylococcus aureus* delta toxin. Infect Immun. 1976;13:140.
142. Bartlett JG, Chang TW, Taylor NS, et al. Colitis induced by *Clostridium difficile*. Rev Infect Dis. 1979;1:370.
143. Larson HE, Parry JV, Price AB, et al. Undescribed toxin in pseudomembranous colitis. Br Med J. 1977;1:1246.
144. Small JD. Fatal enterocolitis in hamsters given lincomycin hydrochloride. Lab Anim Care. 1968;18:411.
145. Bartlett JG, Chang TW, Gurwith M, et al. Antibiotic-associated pseudomembranous colitis due to toxin-producing clostridia. N Engl J Med. 1978;298:531.
146. George RH, Symonds JM, Dimock F, et al. Identification of *Clostridium difficile* as a cause of pseusomembranous colitis. Br Med J. 1978;1:695.
147. Rifkin GD, Fekety FR, Silva J, et al. Antibiotic-induced colitis: Implications of a toxin neutralized by *Clostridium sordellii* antitoxin. Lancet. 1977;2:1103.
148. Hall IC, O'Toole E. Intestinal flora in new-born infants with a description of a new pathogenic anaerobe, *Bacillus difficilis*. Am J Dis Child. 1935;49:390.
149. Snyder ML: Further studies on *Bacillus difficilis*. J Infect Dis. 1937;60:223.
150. Silva J, Fekety R, Werk C, et al. Inciting and etiologic agents of colitis. Rev Infect Dis. 1984;6(Suppl):214–21.
151. Aronsson B, Mollby R, Nord CE. Antimicrobial agents and *Clostridium difficile* in acute enteric disease: Epidemiological data from Sweden, 1980–1982. J Infect Dis. 1985;151:476–81.
152. Colitis associated with clindamycin. Med Lett. 1974;16:73.
153. Tedesco FJ, Stanley RJ, Alpers DH. Diagnostic features of clindamycin-associated pseudomembranous colitis. N Engl J Med. 1974;290:841.
154. Buts J-P, Weber AM, Roy CC, et al. Pseudomembranous enterocolitis in childhood. Gastroenterology. 1977;73:823.
155. Tedesco FJ. Clindamycin-associated colitis—review of the clinical spectrum of 47 cases. Am J Digest Dis. 1976;21:26.
156. Kabins SA. Outbreak of clindamycin-associated colitis. Ann Intern Med. 1975;83:830.
157. Keefe EB, Katon RM, Chan TT, et al. Pseudomembranous enterocolitis. Resurgence related to newer antibiotic therapy. West J Med. 1974;121:462.
158. Guerrant RL, Hughes JM, Lima NL, et al. Microbiology of diarrhea in developed and developing countries. Rev Infect Dis. 1989, in press.
159. Novak E, Lee JG, Seckman CE, et al. Unfavorable effect of atropine-diphenoxylate (Lomotil) therapy in lincomycin caused diarrhea. JAMA. 1976;235:1451.
160. Khan MY, Hall WH. Staphylococcal enterocolitis—treatment with oral vancomycin. Ann Intern Med. 1966;65:1.
161. Keighley MRB, Burdon DW, Arabi Y, et al. Randomised controlled trial of vancomycin for pseudomembranous colitis and postoperative diarrhoea. Br Med J. 1978;2:1667.
162. Bartlett JG, Onderdonk AB, Cisneros RL. Clindamycin-associated colitis in hamsters: Protection with vancomycin. Gastroenterology. 1977;73:772.
163. Browne RA, Fekety Jr, Silva J Jr, et al. The protective effect of vancomycin on clindamycin-induced colitis in hamsters. John Hopkins Med J. 1977;141:183.
164. Black RE, Merson MH, Rahaman SMM, et al. Prospective study of bacterial, viral, and parasitic agents associated with diarrhea in rural Bangladesh. J Infect Dis. 1980;142:660.
165. McAuliffe JF, Shields DS, de Souza MA, et al. Prolonged and recurring diarrhea in the northeast of Brazil: Examination of cases from a community-based study. J Pediatr Gastroenterol Nutr. 1986;5:902–6.
166. Nelson JD, Haltalin KC. Accuracy of diagnosis of bacterial diarrheal disease by clinical features. J Pediatr. 1971;78:519.
167. Cooke EM. Properties of strains of *Escherichia coli* isolated from the feces of patients with ulcerative colitis, patients with acute diarrhea and normal persons. J Pathol Bacteriol. 1968;95:101.
168. Cullen JH. Intestinal tuberculosis—a clinic pathologic study. Q Bull Sea View Hosp. 1940;5:143.
169. Davis AA. Hypertrophic intestinal tuberculosis. Surg Gynecol Obstet. 1933;56:907.
170. Hamandi WJ, Thamer MA. Tuberculosis of the bowel in Iraq: A study of 86 cases. Dis Colon Rectum. 1965;8:158.
171. Anand SS. Hypertrophic ileo-cecal tuberculosis in India with a record of fifty hemicolectomies. Ann R Coll Surg Engl. 1956;19:205.
172. Blacklock JWS. Tuberculous diseases in children. Medical Research Council, Spec Rep Ser 1972. London: His Majesty's Stationery Office; 1932.
173. Blumberg A. Pathology of intestinal tuberculosis. J Lab Clin Med. 1928;13:405.

174. Walsh J. Diagnosis of intestinal tuberculosis. Trans Natl Assoc Prev Tuberc London. 1909;5:217.
175. Paustian FF, Monto GL. Tuberculosis of the intestines. In: Bockus HL, ed. Gastroenterology. v. 2. Philadelphia: WB Saunders; 1976:750–77.
176. Tandon HD, Prakach A. Pathology of intestinal tuberculosis and its distinction from Crohn's disease. Gut. 1972;13:260.
177. Borg I, Hejjkenskjold F, Nilehn B, et al. Massive growth of yeasts in resected stomach. Gut. 1966;1:244.
178. Eras P, Goldstein MJ, Sherlock P. *Candida* infection of the gastrointestinal tract. Medicine (*Baltimore*). 1972;51:367.
179. Bensaude A, Breging E. Examen anorecto-sigmoidien au cours des colopathies a *Candida albicans*. Ann Gastroent Hepat. 1972;8:199.
180. Smith PD, Lane C, Gill VJ, et al. Intestinal infections in patients with the acquired immunodeficiency syndrome (AIDS): Etiology and response to therapy. Ann Intern Med. 1988;108:328–33.
181. Restrepo A, Robledo M, Gutierrey F, et al. Paracoccidioidomycosis (South American blastomycosis). Am J Trop Med Hyg. 1970;19:68.
182. Satir AA, Alla MD, Mahgoub S, et al. Systemic phycomycosis. Br Med J. 1971;1:440.
183. Smith JMB. Mycoses of the alimentary tract. Gut. 1969;10:1035.
184. Bank S, Trey C, Gans I, et al. Histoplasmosis of the small bowel with "giant" intestinal villi and secondary protein-losing enteropathy. Am J Med. 1965;39:492.
185. Shull HJ. Human histoplasmosis. Disease with protean manifestations, often with digestive system involvement. Gastroenterology. 1953;25:582.
186. Kirk ME, Lough J, Warner HA. Histoplasma colitis: An electron microscopic study. Gastroenterology. 1971;61:46.
187. Sachar DB, Klein RS, Swerdlow F. Erosive syphilitic gastritis: Dark-field and immunofluorescent diagnosis from biopsy specimen. Ann Intern Med. 1974;80:512.
188. Brandborg LL, Goldberg SB, Breidenbach WC. Human coccidiosis—a possible cause of malabsorption. The life cycle in small-bowel mucosal biopsies as a diagnostic feature. N Engl J Med. 1970;24:1306.
189. Trier JS, Moxey PC, Schimmel EM, et al. Chronic intestinal coccidiosis in man: Intestinal morphology and response to treatment. Gastroenterology. 1974;66:923.
190. Soave R, Johnson WD Jr. *Cryptosporidium* and *Isospora belli* infections. J Infect Dis. 1988;157:225.
191. Tzipori S. Cryptosporidiosis in animals and humans. Microbiol Rev. 1983;47:84.
192. Current WL, Reese NC, Ernst JV, et al. Human cryptosporidiosis in immunocompetent and immunodeficient persons. N Engl J Med. 1983;308:1252.
193. Ma P, Soave R. Three-step stool examination for cryptosporidiosis in homosexual men with protracted watery diarrhea. J Infect Dis. 1983;147:824.
194. Powell SJ, Wilmot AJ. Ulcerative post-dysenteric colitis. Gut. 1966;7:438.
195. Blenkinsopp WK, Gibson JA, Haffenden GP. Giardiasis and severe jejunal abnormality. Lancet. 1978;1:994.

85. ENTERIC FEVER AND OTHER CAUSES OF ABDOMINAL SYMPTOMS WITH FEVER

RICHARD D. PEARSON
RICHARD L. GUERRANT

Several enteric infections are characterized by clinical syndromes of abdominal pain and fever distinct from acute gastroenteritis. The portal of entry of the responsible infectious agents is usually the gastrointestinal tract, but several other infections and some noninfectious conditons may mimic enteric fever. After a systemic phase, these infections may subsequently involve intestinal tissue and are then manifest as one of three clinical syndromes: (*1*) Enteric fever, characterized by sustained fever, headache, abdominal pain, bacteremia, and often skin rash and splenomegaly, is the most serious of these syndromes and may result from infection by several bacteria. A range of systemic bacterial, rickettsial, viral, fungal, and parasitic infections may mimic enteric fever, and these are discussed later in the chapter. (*2*) Mesenteric adenitis, a syndrome that may mimic acute appendicitis, may be caused by several bacteria. (*3*) Eosinophilia, associated with abdominal cramps or diarrhea often accompanied by fever, may be caused by a number of parasites, usually helminths, and several diseases of unknown cause.

This chapter will focus on the differential diagnosis of these syndromes. Important clinical and epidemiologic features, appropriate diagnostic approaches, and antimicrobial therapeutic considerations will be discussed.

ENTERIC FEVER

The classic syndrome of enteric fever is an acute illness, the first typical manifestations of which are fever, headache, abdominal pain, relative bradycardia, splenomegaly, and leukopenia.[1] The prototype of the syndrome is typhoid fever caused by *Salmonella typhi* (see chapter 86), in which fever is present in 75–100 percent of cases[2,3] and is often initially of the remittent type, rising in a stepwise fashion during the first week of illness, after which it becomes sustained.[4,5] Annually, 300–500 cases of typhoid fever are reported in the United States, over half of which are imported, often from Mexico or India.[6,7]

Pathogenesis

Organisms that cause the enteric fever syndrome must be ingested and must survive exposure to gastric acid before gaining access to the small bowel, where they penetrate the intestinal epithelium possibly via microfold (M) cells over Peyer's patches and then multiply in intestinal lymphoid tissue before systemic dissemination via the lymphatic or hematogenous route. Organisms causing enteric fever grow intracellularly, primarily in reticuloendothelial cells in lymph nodes, liver, and spleen. An animal model for this syndrome in which mice are infected orally with *Salmonella enteritidis* has been developed.[8] After multiplication in ileal and distal mesenteric lymphoid tissue, organisms disseminate with the production of microabscesses in the liver and spleen.

Clinical Features

The organisms classically responsible for the enteric fever syndrome is *S. typhi*. Other salmonellae (especially *Salmonella paratyphi* A and B, *S. choleraesuis,* and other salmonella serotypes) may cause a similar clinical illness (Table 1). Other diseases that may mimic enteric fever early in their course and that must be included in the differential diagnosis of enteric fever are also summarized in Table 1; important clinical and epidemiologic clues to these specific diagnoses are indicated.

Symptoms. Classic "typhoidal" fever begins with a remittent fever pattern that becomes sustained over the first few days of illness. The frequencies of reported symptoms from several series of patients infected by *S. typhi* and *S. paratyphi* A and B are summarized in Table 2. Most patients report fever and headache. Although reports from the preantibiotic era suggest that constipation occurs more frequently than diarrhea (79 vs. 43 percent),[5] more recent reports suggest that these symptoms occur with approximately equal frequency[2,9] or that diarrhea may be more common.[10–13] Extraintestinal symptoms reported by patients include cough and conjunctivitis. Although enteric fever caused by salmonellae other than *S. typhi* is usually less severe and of shorter duration than typhoid fever,[14] the syndromes are not sufficiently different to permit clinical separation of the individual case.[9–13]

Physical Findings. In evaluating patients with possible enteric fever syndrome, physical examination should focus on characteristics of the fever curve and accompanying pulse, skin, eyes, oral cavity and oropharynx, chest, abdomen, and lymph

TABLE 1. Clinical, Epidemiologic, and Laboratory Clues to the Causes of Enteric Fever and Conditions That May Mimic Enteric Fever

Etiologic Agent or Disease	*Clinical Clues*	*Epidemiologic Clues*	*Laboratory Clues*
Causes of Enteric Fever			
Salmonella typhi, *Salmonella paratyphi A, B*, *Salmonella choleraesuis*	Relative bradycardia, splenomegaly, rose spots, conjunctivitis	Young adults, travel,[a] exposure to known carrier	Cultures (B, BM, U, F), leukopenia
Yersinia enterocolitica, *Yersinia pseudotuberculosis*	Stigmata of chronic liver disease, arthritis, erythema nodosum	Older adults ± pet exposure	Cultures (B, F. J), serology
Campylobacter fetus	Stigmata or chronic liver disease	Older adults, ± farm or small animal contact	Cultures (B, F), serology
Acute brucellosis	Paucity of physical findings	Occupation (abattoir employee, butcher), animal contact (goats, sheep, cattle), diet (unpasteurized cheese)	Cultures (B, BM), serology, leukopenia
Typhoidal tularemia	Severe prostration, splenomegaly	Animal contact (especially rabbits), vector exposure (ticks)	Serology
Conditions that mimic enteric fever			
Bacterial Infections			
Septicemic plague	Severe prostration	Rodent contact, vector exposure (fleas), travel	Cultures (B), serology
Intestinal anthrax	Severe prostration	Travel,[a] diet (undercooked meat)	Cultures (B, F)
Septicemia melioidosis	Severe prostration, pustular skin lesions	Travel[a]	Cultures (B), serology, chest x-ray
Acute bartonellosis	Severe prostration, renal failure	Travel,[a] vector exposure (sandfly)	Cultures (B), blood smear, acute hemolysis
Leptospirosis	Relative bradycardia, conjunctival suffusion	Occupation (farmers, abattoir and sewer workers, veterinarians), animal contact (especially cattle, dogs) swimming[b]	Cultures (B, CSF, U), serology, hepatorenal dysfunction
Relapsing fever	Fever pattern, conjunctival suffusion, splenomegaly, skin rash	Travel,[a] vector exposure (louse, tick)	Blood smear
Legionellosis	Pneumonia, CNS symptoms	Normal or compromised host	Chest radiogram, purulent sputum, DFA of sputum
Intestinal tuberculosis	Stigmata of tuberculosis	Exposure to known case, ± travel[a] ± diet (unpasteurized milk and milk products), malnourished children	Cultures (S, G, BM, L), x-ray (UGI, SBFT)
Abdominal actinomycosis	Abdominal mass, fistula	Adult males	Culture (FD, A), radiograph (UGI, SBFT)
Intra-abdominal abscess	Spiking daily fever, reduced diaphragmatic excursion, intraabdominal or diaphragmatic pain	Previous surgery, bowel or biliary tract disease	Leukocytosis, computed tomography, gallium scan, sonography, fluoroscopy
Viral Infections			
Hepatitis	Jaundice, arthritis (with hepatitis B)	Exposure to known case, drug abuse, travel[a]	Liver dysfunction, antigen detection
Dengue	Relative bradycardia, conjunctival suffusion, rash, lymphadenopathy	Travel,[a] vector exposure (mosquito)	Culture (B), serology, leukopenia
Infectious mononucleosis	Pharyngitis, lymphadenopathy, splenomegaly, rash	Young adults	Serology, lymphocyte morphology
Rickettsial Infection			
Epidemic typhus	Conjunctival suffusion, rash, severe prostration	Travel,[a] vector exposure (louse)	Serology
Brill-Zinsser disease	Rash	Older adults, remote travel[a] history	Serology
Endemic typhus	Conjunctival suffusion, rash, splenomegaly	Rat contact, vector exposure (flea)	Serology
Scrub typhus	Conjuntival suffusion, rash, lymphadenopathy	Travel,[a] vector exposure (mites)	Serology
Q fever	Pneumonia, hepatitis	Animal contact (especially livestock), ± travel, ± diet (especially unpasteurized milk)	Serology, chest radiograph, liver dysfunction
Mycotic Infections			
Disseminated histoplasmosis	Mucocutaneous lesions, adrenal insufficiency	Travel,[a] animal contact (chicken, birds, bats), hobby (cave exploration)	Culture (B, BM, L, MM), biopsy (BM, L, MM), chest radiograph
Parasitic Infections			
Malaria	Fever pattern, splenomegaly	Travel,[a] vector exposure (mosquito)	Blood smear
Amebiasis	Colitis, liver abscess	Travel[a]	Stool examination, serology, liver scan, sonography, computed tomography, colon biopsy
Babesiosis	Paucity of physical findings	Travel,[a] vector exposure (tick)	Blood smear, serology
Toxoplasmosis	Lymphadenopathy	Animal contact (cat); diet (undercooked pork)	Serology, biopsy (lymph node), lymphocyte morphology
Trichinosis	Periorbital edema, muscle tenderness	Diet (undercooked pork or bear meat)	Serology, eosinophilia, biopsy (muscle)

(*Continued*)

TABLE 1. *(Continued)*

Etiologic Agent or Disease	*Clinical Clues*	*Epidemiologic Clues*	*Laboratory Clues*
Katayama fever (Acute schistosomiasis)	Urticaria, lymphadenopathy	Travel,[a] swimming	Eosinophilia
Visceral larva migrans	Hepatosplenomegaly, rash, bronchospasm, ocular lesions	Young children with history of pica, animal contact (dog, cat)	Serology, biopsy (L), eosinophilia
Noninfectious causes			
Malignancy Hematologic, Intra-abdominal	Adenopathy, anergy, weight loss	Family history or prior malignancy	Sonography, computed tomography, gallium scan, lymphangiography
Vasculitic or granulomatous disease (e.g., sarcoidosis, granulomatous hepatitis, Crohn's disease, Still's disease)	Skin lesions, arthritis, serositis	Family history	Biopsy of involved tissue, serology (ANA, C′), exclusion of other causes

Abbreviations for cultures: B: blood; BM: bone marrow; U: urine; F: feces; J: joint fluid; S: sputum; CSF: cerebrospinal fluid; G: gastric aspirate; L: liver; FD: fistula drainage; A: abscess; T: throat; N: nasal; MM: mucous membrane.
Abbreviations for x-rays: UGI, SBFT: upper gastrointestinal tract with small bowel follow-through.
Abbreviations for serology: ANA: antinuclear antibody; C′: complement; DFA: direct fluorescent antibody test.
[a] Travel to endemic areas, either domestic or foreign.
[b] Swimming in contaminated surface water.

nodes. The frequencies of commonly reported physical findings are summarized in Table 2. Fever is present in most series in over 90 percent of the cases. However, bacteriologic confirmation of typhoid fever has been obtained in patients who were afebrile when the culture was obtained.[10,11] Classically, the fever is remittent during the first week, rising in a stepwise fashion in both naturally acquired infection[5] and volunteer studies[4,15]; after the first week, the fever is usually sustained. Deviations from this classic pattern frequently occur, however, particularly in endemic areas. In two studies from India, fever was remittent in 30 and 60 percent of the case, sustained in 22–25 percent, and intermittent in 15–46 percent.[3,12] Relative bradycardia suggests the diagnosis of enteric fever. The presence of rose spots, although not pathognomonic, is extremely helpful in confirming the impression of enteric fever[16]; however, they are observed in less than half of the patients and are even less frequently in dark-skinned people.[5] Rose spots may be observed more frequently in infection caused by *S. typhi* than in other forms of enteric fever.[9,13,17] Conjunctivitis is reported in up to 44 percent of the patients with enteric fever[9] but is usually less common.[5] Pharyngitis is infrequent and is usually not a prominent feature of the illness. Rales or other auscultatory abnormalities in the chest may be present. Abdominal tenderness may be diffuse or localized, most often in the right lower quadrant. Splenomegaly is noted more frequently than heptomegaly. Two physical findings that may be useful in suggesting alternative diagnoses because they are rarely reported in patients with enteric fever are lymphadenopathy and herpes simplex labialis.

TABLE 2. Frequency of Symptoms and Physical Findings in Patients with Enteric Fever

	Typhoid Fever[a] (%)	*Paratyphoid A and B[b] (%)*
Symptoms		
Fever	39–100	92–100
Headache	43–90	60–100
Nausea	23–36	33–58
Vomiting	24–35	22–45
Abdominal cramps	8–52	29–92
Diarrhea	30–57	17–68
Constipation	10–79	2–29
Cough	11–86	10–68
Physical findings		
Fever	98–100	100
Abdominal tenderness	33–84	6–29
Splenomegaly	23–65	0–74
Hepatomegaly	15–52	16–32
Relative bradycardia	17–50	11–100
Rose spots	2–46	0–3
Rales or rhonchi	4–84	2–87
Epistaxis	1–21	2–13
Meningismus	1–12	0–3

[a] Data from Refs. 2, 3, 5, 9–12.
[b] Data from Refs. 9, 13, 17.

Laboratory Findings. The definitive diagnosis of enteric fever is made by isolating *S. typhi* or another *Salmonella* from blood, bone marrow, stool, or urine. Several cultures of blood, stool, and urine should be obtained from every patient with a syndrome compatible with enteric fever before the initiation of antimicrobial therapy. If multiple blood cultures are obtained, 73–97 percent[5,9] of the cases can be confirmed. Culture of the blood clot after the serum is removed may yield more positive results.[2,9,18] Bone marrow cultures may be positive when blood cultures are negative.[13,19,20] Stool cultures are positive in less than half the patients,[5,19] and urine cultures are even less frequently positive.[5,19] Detection of *S. typhi* antigens in urine by slide coagglutination is a promising rapid diagnostic technique,[21] although lack of specificity may be a problem.[22] When patients have already received antimicrobial therapy, blood cultures may be positive in only 40 percent of the cases. In these cases, cultures of biopsy specimens of rose spots may be useful; these cultures may be positive in nearly two-thirds of the patients, including some who have received previous antimicrobial therapy.[19] Counterimmunoelectrophoresis of serum may reveal circulating *S. typhi* antigen in patients who have received prior antimicrobial therapy.[23,24]

The role of serologic testing (Widal's reaction) in the diagnosis of typhoid fever is controversial. The minimum positive titer must be determined in individual geographic areas and is higher in endemic regions.[10] Cross-reactions occur with both non-*S. typhi* group D salmonellae[25] and salmonellae from other groups .[26] Antibody titers to the O antigen, especially if paired sera demonstrate a fourfold or greater increase, are generally more useful than antibodies to the H antigen that are often elevated after vaccination.[25,27] However, on at least one occasion, antibody titers to the H antigen have been more helpful.[28] Widal's reactions have been reported positive in 46–94 percent of the case of typhoid fever.[3,27,29] The test is most reliable in areas in which data on Widal's titer results in control groups of patients without enteric fever are available; the sensitivity of the test can be improved when diseases such as rheumatoid arthritis associated with false-positive reactions are identified.[27] Although single elevated titers ($O \geq 1{:}40$ and $H \geq 1{:}80$) may suggest the diagnosis of typhoid fever in unvaccinated people in nonendemic areas or in children under 10 years of age in endemic areas,[30] the consensus is that the diagnostic role of Widal's rection is limited.[31] Widal's reaction is not helpful in the diagnosis of enteric fever caused by organisms other than *S. typhi*. The roles of the enzyme-linked immunoabsorbent assay (ELISA) using a cell envelope antigen or lipopolysaccharide (LPS) of *S. typhi*[31–33] or a purified Vi antigen[34,35] and radial counterimmunoelectrophoresis[36] in the serodiagnosis of acute typhoid fever need to be defined.

Additional laboratory tests that may be of value include the white blood cell count and differential, liver function tests, urinalysis, and chest radiograph. Leukopenia is reported in 16–46 percent of the cases.[10,11] In two series, two-thirds of patients had no eosinophils on peripheral smear,[3,9] a finding that may be especially helpful in areas in which parasitic diseases are prevalent and eosinophilia is common. Liver function tests may reveal a mildly elevated bilirubin[9] and a slight to threefold elevation in alkaline phosphatase and transaminase levels in from one-third to two-thirds of the patients[9,11]; on occasion, hepatic manifestations may be prominent.[37] Urinalysis frequently reveals proteinura, pyuria, and casts[5,9]; immune complex glomerulonephritis with red blood cell casts occasionally occurs.[38] Coagulation abnormalities compatible with mild disseminated intravascular coagulation are common, but the syndrome is rarely clinically apparent.[39] Chest radiographic films may reveal pneumonia in 2–11 percent of the cases.[2,5] In patients with diarrhea, a methylene blue stain of a fresh stool specimen for fecal leukocytes may reveal mononuclear cells.[40]

Epidemiology

Certain epidemiologic data may be of value in the diagnosis of enteric fever. Typhoid fever is most common in children and young adults both in the United States[6] and abroad.[9,10] In the United States, cases occur throughout the year. Since humans are the only reservoir for *S. typhi,* history of contact with a known typhoid case or carrier may be extremely useful but is obtained in the minority of cases.[6,7] Over the past 10 years, the proportion of the cases in the United States that were acquired abroad has increased dramatically; during 1977–1979, 62 percent of the cases were acquired abroad, most frequently in Mexico and India.[7] The attack rate was highest for travelers to Pakistan and India.[7] Patients who acquired infection abroad were older than those who acquired disease in the United States.[6] The importance of the microbiology laboratory as a source of domestic *S. typhi* infection has also been recognized.[41,42] In most cases, *S. typhi* had been used for proficiency testing or research.[41] Most patients with enteric fever caused by *S. paratyphi* A or B acquire their infection abroad; *S. paratyphi* B is only occasionally and *S. paratyphi* A is rarely isolated in the United States.

Differential Diagnosis

Enteric Fever-like Syndromes. *Yersinia enterocolitica, Yersinia pseudotuberculosis,* and *Campylobacter fetus* may each produce an enteric fever-like illness characterized by fever, headache, and abdominal pain, which may be clinically indistinguishable from enteric fever caused by *S. typhi* or other salmonellae (see Table 1). However, certain features of these infections may serve to differentiate them from true enteric fever. Acute diarrhea is often a prominent feature of enteric fever-like illnesses caused by *Y. enterocolitica*[43,44] and occasionally *Y. pseudotuberculosis*.[45] Diarrhea is less frequent in enteric fever-like illness caused by *C. fetus*; the acute gastrointestinal symptoms of nausea, vomiting, abdominal cramps, and diarrhea were present in only 27 percent of bacteremic illnesses caused by *C. fetus*.[46] A clue to the diagnosis of *Campylobacter* infection is associated phlebitis.[46,47,48]

The enteric fever-like syndromes caused by *Y. enterocolitica, Y. pseudotuberculosis,* and *C. fetus* more frequently occur in patients with significant underlying disease. Of 31 patients with *Y. enterocolitica* bacteremia for whom information was available 12 had cirrhosis of the liver; 4 others had thalassemia and 1 had kwashiorkor.[44] Only 5 were known to be free of underlying disease. In another series, 5 out of 7 patients with the acute septicemic or typhoidal form of *Y. enterocolitica* infection had evidence of liver disease; in addition all 6 patients with the subacute, localized form of the disease characterized by hepatic and splenic abscesses had cirrhosis of the liver.[43] Of 20 patients with the enteric fever-like syndrome caused by *Y. psuedotuberculosis* 11 had evidence of significant underlying disease; the liver was involved in 10 of these patients.[45] This syndrome has also been reported in a patient with amyloidosis and *Y. pseudotuberculosis* bacteremia.[49] In a series of patients with bacteremic *C. fetus* illness, 73 percent had a significant underlying disease, frequently involving the liver.[46]

Epidemiologic clues in differentiating true enteric fever from these enteric fever-like syndromes include the patient's age, residence, and recent travel history. Patients with *Salmonella*-induced enteric fever are most often less than 30 years of age,[6] whereas the vast majority of patients with non-*Salmonella* enteric fever-like syndromes are over 40.[43–46,50] As in typhoid fever, men are more frequently affected than women. Patients with *Salmonella*-induced enteric fever frequently have a history of recent foreign travel, most often to developing countries. Disease caused by *Y. enterocolitica* and *Y. pseudotuberculosis* appears to be common in Europe, particularly in Scandinavia,[51,52] and in South Africa[41] and is not frequently reported from developing countries. Infections due to both *Y. enterocolitica* and *Y. pseudotuberculosis* may be acquired in the United States as well.[45,53–55] Although bacteremic *C. fetus* infection is relatively rarely documented, the majority of cases have been reported from the United States, and foreign travel has not appeared to be a significant predisposing factor.[46,50]

A pulse–temperature deficit similar to that observed in typhoid fever has been reported in enteric fever-like illness caused by *Y. enterocolitica*[44,55–57] and *Y. pseudotuberculosis*[45,51] but not with *C. fetus*.[46] An additional clue may be provided by the fever pattern. In contrast to *Salmonella*-induced enteric fevers in which sustained fever is common, intermittent fever throughout the illness caused by *Y. enterocolitica* has been reported.[58] Because of the increased frequency of chronic liver disease in patients with these enteric fever-like syndromes, physical examination is more likely to reveal stigmata of chronic liver disease such as spider angiomata, gynecomastia, ascites, and testicular atrophy. In addition, hepatomegaly is frequent and may be more pronounced than in patients with typhoid fever.[44] Both erythema nodosum and polyarthritis occur in patients with illness caused by *Y. enterocolitica* and *Y. pseudotuberculosis*; in one series 55 percent of the patients with yersiniosis had arthritis, and 88 percent of these had multiple joint involvement.[51] Nonsuppurative arthritis is more common in infections caused by *Y. enterocolitica* (43 percent) than in those caused by *Y. pseudotuberculosis* (10 percent).[59] Patients with bacteremic infection caused by *Y. enterocolitica* and *C. fetus* may also have acute septic arthritis,[44,50,55,57] a condition that is infrequently found in patients with classic enteric fever. Erythema nodosum has been reported in 15–24 percent of patients with *Yersinia* and may be slightly more common with *Y. pseudotuberculosis* infection than with *Y. enterocolitica* infection.[51,59] Thrombophlebitis has been reported in patients with *C. fetus* bacteremia and may be an additional diagnostic clue.[60]

As in the *Salmonella* induced enteric fevers, blood cultures are the key to the diagnosis. Each of the three organisms is more frequently isolated from blood than from other specimens.[43–46,50]; the isolation rate from stool cultures may be improved if cold-enrichment techniques are used for *Yersinia*[61] and if special selective media are used for *Campylobacter*.[62,63] However, because of its sensitivity to cephalosporins, *C. fetus* cannot be cultured on commonly used *C. jejuni* selective agars if they contain cephalosporins. In addition, serologic tests are available for documenting infection with *Y. enterocolitica* and *Y. pseudotuberculosis* and appear to be more sensitive and more specific than those for *Salmonella* infection.[52,64] Leukopenia is infrequent in patients with enteric fever-like syndromes; its presence may suggest that *Salmonella* are responsible. Findings on liver, abdominal CT scan, or ultrasound suggestive of hepatic or splenic abscesses may favor the diagnosis of yersioniosis.[43,65] Glomerulitis complicating both typhoid fever and *Y. enterocolitica* has been reported; therefore, the presence of protein, red blood cells, and red blood cell casts in the urine is compatible with either of these syndromes.[38,66]

Patients with typhoidal tularemia may be clinically indistinguishable from those with enteric fever. The epidemiologic history may be of value; a history of rabbit or tick exposure within 7 days before the onset of illness supports the diagnosis of tularemia.[67] Although potentially dangerous, *Francisella tularensis* may be isolated from blood if the appropriate medium is used; serologic tests may confirm the diagnosis of tularemia.

Acute brucellosis may manifest with fever, myalgias, and splenomegaly.[68] As in typhoid fever, white blood cell counts are frequently normal or low. Skin lesions are uncommon in brucellosis. Blood and bone marrow cultures and serologic testing should permit separation of these entities.

Systemic Infections That May Mimic Enteric Fever. A number of other potentially fatal infections such as malaria in travelers or plague in endemic areas such as the southwestern United States may present with fever and abdominal pain or diarrhea and may be initially confused with enteric fever. Similarly, other common extraintestinal infections such as otitis or pneumococcal pneumonia may present with enteric symptoms. These infections are treatable and must be properly considered and diagnosed.

Septicemic plague may mimic enteric fever. The diagnosis of plague may be suggested by the sudden onset and rapid progression of the illness. Epidemiologic history may again provide a clue to the differentiation of these entities; plague is endemic in wild rodents in the southwestern United States, and a history of travel to this area with rodent exposure during the previous 2 weeks would support the diagnosis of plague.[69] In addition, a history of recent foreign travel to countries in which plague is endemic may suggest the diagnosis. Blood cultures, methylene blue stains of peripheral blood,[70] and serologic testing may aid in the separation of these entities.

Intestinal anthrax may be characterized by fever and severe abdominal pain. However, intestinal anthrax is acute in onset and rapid in progression, and patients usually die during the first few days of their illness. A history of ingestion of raw or undercooked meat in an area in which anthrax is endemic should suggest the diagnosis.[71]

Acute septicemic melioidosis may be confused clinically with enteric fever; this disease is endemic in Southeast Asia. Physical findings that may support the diagnosis of septicemic melioidosis are pustular skin lesions.[72] In melioidosis, the chest radiographic film may reveal nodular pulmonary densities. Blood cultures and serologic studies may again permit differentiation of these syndromes.

Acute bartonellosis (Oroya fever) may manifest with fever, headache, and abdominal pain. Since this disease occurs only in certain valleys in the Andes in Peru, Ecuador, and Columbia, a travel history for the preceding month may be helpful in excluding this possibility.[73] Evidence of acute hemolysis may suggest the diagnosis. Since the causative organisms are frequently seen on the stained peripheral blood smear, this procedure may be helpful in ruling out this diagnosis. Since Oroya fever predisposes to *Salmonella* induced bacteremia, both infections may be encountered simultaneously.[74]

Rat-bite fever caused by *Streptobacillus moniliformis* may mimic enteric fever when the rat puncture site is not clinically evident or when the infection is food borne.[75] This illness may also mimic enteric fever-like syndromes since polyarthritis is frequent. History of a recent rat bite may suggest the diagnosis.[75] Cultures of blood and joint fluid may confirm this diagnosis; serologic tests may also be helpful. The other cause of rat-bite fever, *Spirillum minor,* causes subacute fever, headache, nausea, and vomiting, often with an urticarial rash (soduku) 1–4 weeks after an initial rat bite injury that heals with residual regional adenopathy.[76,77] Spirillary fever causes a false-positive serologic test for syphilis in the majority of cases; *Spirillum minor* requires mouse inoculation for its isolation or demonstration of the 2- to 5-μm twisted gram-negative rod in tissue or blood for diagnosis. Like relapsing fever, spirillary fever is often associated with a Herxheimer's reaction when treatment is started with penicillin G.

Leptospirosis frequently manifests with fever and headache and is most frequent in young adults; abdominal pain occurs in approximately 30 percent of cases.[78] Diarrhea and constipation are less frequent. Muscle pain and tenderness occur in nearly 70 percent of the cases, more frequently than in enteric fever. Additional differentiating features are the fever curve and clinical course; leptospirosis is characteristically a biphasic illness.[79] Evidence of liver dysfunction is present in approximately 50 percent of the patients with leptospirosis.[78] Although conjunctival suffusion is characteristic of leptospirosis and is reported in one-third of patients, conjunctivitis occurs in enteric fever as well. Two findings that would favor the diagnosis of leptospirosis are azotemia (26 percent of cases) and cerebrospinal fluid pleocytosis (47 percent of cases).[78] Serologic tests are of value in confirming the diagnosis of leptospirosis.

Relapsing fever due to *Borrelia recurrentis* may simulate enteric fever. The lack of a history of travel during the previous 3 weeks to an area where louse-borne relapsing fever is endemic (Ethiopia, South America, Far East) permits exclusion of this diagnosis. However, tick-borne relapsing fever may be acquired in the western United States.[80] Conjunctivitis, rash, and hepatosplenomegaly are common. However, in contrast to patients with enteric fever, those with tick-borne relapsing fever resolve their fever in a crisis during the first week of their illness.[81] Giemsa or Wright stain of the spirochetes in peripheral blood during a febrile episode may confirm the diagnosis of relapsing fever.

Patients with intestinal tuberculosis may present with fever and findings referable to the gastrointestinal tract. In addition radiologic studies of the terminal ileum may show evidence of a terminal ileitis that can be confused with the terminal ileitis sometimes associated with typhoid fever or *Y. enterocolitica* infection.[82] This disease is currently extremely rare in the United States in the absence of active pulmonary tuberculosis. Abdominal tuberculosis remains an important, treatable disease in developing areas, especially in malnourished children.[83] Evidence of clinical tuberculosis elsewhere or of delayed hypersensitivity to tuberculin would support the diagnosis.

Abdominal actinomycosis may also mimic enteric fever. Physical examination may reveal an abdominal mass; the presence of a draining sinus tract strongly favors this diagnosis.[84]

Intra-abdominal pyogenic abscesses pose difficult diagnostic challenges and remain high on the list of fatal undiagnosed causes of fever of unknown origin.[85] They should be suspected when fever persists or recurs and may be detected by sonography, fluoroscopy of the diaphragms, computed tomography, or gallium scans.

Patients with *Mycoplasma pneumoniae* infection may rarely be confused clinically with those with enteric fever. Fever and headache may be prominent in infection caused by this organism. The presence of pneumonia determined by physical examination or on the chest radiographic film may suggest this diagnosis, although pneumonia may also occur in patients with enteric fever. The presence of bullous myringitis also suggests *M. pneumoniae* infection but is uncommon in naturally acquired infection.[86] The appearance of upper or lower respiratory illness in other members of the patient's family also favors this diagnosis. Serologic studies may be helpful in confirmation of *M. pneumoniae* infection.

Patients with psittacosis frequently have an illness characterized by fever, headache, myalgia, abdominal pain, vomiting, and diarrhea. On physical examination a faint macular rash may be noted; splenomegaly occurs in some patients.[87] A history of exposure to birds may suggest the diagnosis, and serologic testing is helpful in confirmation.

Several rickettsial infections, especially epidemic typhus, Brill-Zinsser disease, endemic typhus, Rocky Mountain spotted fever, scrub typhus, and Q fever are characterized by fever, headache, myalgia, and, except in Q fever, skin rash. Of these, Rocky Mountain spotted fever and endemic typhus are most likely to be encountered in the United States.[88,89] The gastrointestinal manifestations of Rocky Mountain spotted fever include abdominal pain, diarrhea, vomiting and upper gastrointestinal tract bleeding, and an initial diagnosis of appendicitis, cholecystitis, or gastroenteritis is often considered.[90–92] History of recent tick or louse exposure may suggest the diagnosis. Although failure of the characteristic rash to develop may lead to fatal delay in diagnosis and treatment,[93] once the characteristic rashes associated with these illnesses appear, the diagnostic confusion is lessened. Serologic testing may provide documentation of rickettsial infection. In addition, fluorescent antibody techniques may be used to demonstrate the etiologic agent of Rocky Mountain spotted fever in biopsy specimens of involved skin.[94] Q fever may be associated with cat or wild rabbit exposure.[95] Sporadic cases of epidemic typhus associated with flying squirrels have been reported in the United States since 1976.[96,97] The majority of cases have occurred in the southeastern states during the winter months.

Legionella infections in normal or compromised hosts often present with gastrointestinal symptoms of abdominal pain, nausea, vomiting, or diarrhea (usually watery, noninflammatory) in up to 47 percent of patients.[98–100] Patients with disseminated histoplasmosis may have fever, abdominal pain, nausea, vomiting, and diarrhea.[101] The diagnosis may be suggested by the presence of mucous membrane lesions or adrenal insufficiency. Biopsy specimens and cultures of liver, blood, urine, and bone marrow may be useful in confirming the diagnosis.

Several acute viral infections have gastrointestinal manifestations. Abdominal pain, nausea, and vomiting are frequent symptoms in patients with hepatitis. However, the severity of jaundice and extent of transaminase increases are much greater than those observed in enteric fever. Influenza (particularly type B) may manifest with fever, headache, and abdominal pain. Throat cultures and serologic studies may distinguish these illnesses. In dengue, headache, severe myalgias, and leukopenia are common. The maculopapular skin rash that characteristically appears on the trunk on the third to fifth day of illness and subsequently spreads peripherally, the biphasic clinical course, and a history of recent travel to areas in which dengue is endemic may suggest the diagnosis. Infectious mononucleosis may mimic enteric fever, particularly when acute pharyngitis is not a prominent part of the syndrome. Examination of a peripheral blood smear and a heterophil antibody determination are helpful in differentiating this illness from enteric fever.

A number of protozoan and helmintic infections may mimic the enteric fever syndrome. Malaria is endemic in many areas of the world in which enteric fever also occurs. Both may present with fever, headache, abdominal pain, and other gastrointestinal symptoms. Two-thirds of 25 cases of malaria recently reviewed presented with prominent gastrointestinal symptoms (nausea, vomiting, abdominal pain, or diarrhea) that may initially mislead one away from an early diagnosis of malaria.[102] The intermittent fever in malaria is a useful diagnostic clue but may not always be present. Peripheral blood smear may confirm the diagnosis of malaria. Fever chills and hemolytic anemia in an area with the soft tick (nymphal stage of *Ixodes dammini,* the same vector as for Lyme disease) and white-foot mice (*Peromyscus*) or white-tailed deer (*Odocoileus virginianus*) may represent infection with the malaria-like sporozoan *Babesia microti,* especially in an asplenic patient.[103,104] Either intestinal or hepatic amebiasis may mimic acute enteric fever. In patients with hepatic abscesses, documentation of a single abscess cavity somewhat favors the diagnosis of amebiasis.[105] The diagnosis may be confirmed either by demonstration of *Entamoeba histolytica* in stool or colonic mucosal biopsy or by means of the indirect hemagglutination serologic test.

Patients with trichinosis may have fever, headache, myalgias, abdominal pain, and diarrhea; however, the presence of eosinophilia rather than the eosinopenia frequently noted in enteric fever should suggest the diagnosis, which can be confirmed serologically or by muscle biopsy. The history of recent ingestion of raw or undercooked pork may suggest the diagnosis. Patients with acute schistosomiasis (Katayama fever) may be thought to have an enteric fever syndrome. Eosinophilia may again be useful in separating these possibilities; the history of swimming in fresh water during the previous month in areas in which schistosomiasis is endemic also favors this diagnosis. Patients with visceral larva migrans may be confused with those with enteric fever. Patients with visceral larva migrans frequently have fever and hepatomegaly; in more severe infections, splenomegaly, rashes, and pneumonitis may also occur. In contrast to enteric fever, visceral larva migrans is most common in children less than 5 years of age; the diagnosis may be suggested by a history of pica. Serologic tests may confirm the diagnosis of visceral larva migrans.

Noninfectious causes of fever and abdominal pain, such as eosinophilic gastroenteritis, hematologic and other malignancies involving abdominal lymph nodes or organs, and vasculitic and granulomatous diseases, must also be considered. Diagnosis often requires biopsy of involved tissues, scans, serologic tests, or exclusion of other processes.[85] See Chapter 36 for a discussion of the differential diagnosis of fever of unknown origin.

Therapy for Enteric Fever

In some patients with the enteric fever syndrome, antimicrobial therapy may have to be initiated before the diagnosis is documented. Chloramphenicol has been the drug of choice for the treatment of *Salmonella* induced enteric fevers.[106] Alternative drugs are amoxicillin, ampicillin, trimethoprim–sulfamethoxazole, third-generation cephalosporins, and the quinolones.[107–109] Chloramphenicol resistance among *S. typhi* has been reported from Mexico[110] and Southeast Asia[111,112] as well as from the United States, India, and Taiwan. Ampicillin resistance has also been reported, most often from Mexico.[7,113] A patient's recent travel history should be considered before initial empiric antimicrobial therapy is selected. For chloramphenicol-sensitive strains of *S. typhi,* chloramphenicol remains the drug of choice for patients who are seriously ill.[114,115] Strains may occasionally acquire resistance during therapy.[116]

MESENTERIC ADENITIS

Patients with mesenteric adenitis typically have a history of fever and abdominal pain, frequently with localization in the right lower quadrant. The illness closely mimics acute appendicitis. Few data on the incidence of this syndrome are available. In the preantibiotic era, mesenteric adenitis was present in 43 of 2140 patients (2 percent) undergoing appendectomy.[117] In a report from the antibiotic era, 20 of 93 (22 percent) of patients undergoing appendectomy for suspected appendicitis had mesenteric adenitis.[118]

Etiologic Agents and Pathogenesis

In the preantibiotic era, hemolytic streptococci were frequently reported as etiologic agents in this syndrome; in one study, 19 of 36 patients (53 percent) with mesenteric adenitis in whom cultures were obtained grew hemolytic streptococci; 4 (11 percent) grew *Escherichia coli*. Of interest is the fact that 37 of 39 patients (97 percent) had throat cultures positive for hemolytic streptococci, and 35 of these had a history of a recent sore throat.[117] In another report from the preantibiotic era, of 2 patients with mesenteric abscess secondary to suppurative mesenteric adenitis, 1 had enterococci and an unidentified hemolytic bacillus isolated from the abscess, whereas the other had both *Bacteroides* and *Clostridium* species isolated; in both cases the appendix was normal.[119] Hemolytic streptococci appear to be responsible for a few cases of mesenteric adenitis in the antibiotic era as well. Asch et al. reported on one patient from whom β-hemolytic streptococci were isolated from an inflamed mesenteric node and in whom subsequent studies revealed an elevated ASO titer.[120] In another case, both a β-hemolytic streptococcus and a coagulase-positive staphylococcus were isolated from an inflamed mesenteric node in an infant.[120] Of two 9-year-old children, β-hemolytic streptococci were isolated from one and *Staphylococcus aureus* from the other.[121] *Giardia lamblia* has also been reported as a cause of mesenteric adenitis in an adult in Spain.[122] A viral cause has also been suspected for this syndrome; however, 17 well-studied patients in one series had no evidence of viral infection.[118]

At present, the most frequently reported etiologic agents in the syndrome of mesenteric adenitis are *Y. enterocolitica* and *Y. pseudotuberculosis*. Again, few valid data on incidence are available. Of the 20 patients with mesenteric adenitis reported by Mair et al., 17 were adequately studied; 3 (18 percent) had evidence of infection with *Y. pseudotuberculosis*.[118] In another report, 5 of 8 patients (63 percent) who had mesenteric adenitis confirmed at surgery also had serologic evidence of recent *Y. enterocolitica* infection.[123]

In a mouse model after intragastric administration of *Y. enterocolitica*, polymorphonuclear leukocytes appear in Peyer's patches within 24 hours. The infection then spreads to the mesenteric lymph nodes, where abscesses develop.[124] The invasive potential of pathogenic strains of *Y. enterocolitica* has also been demonstrated in HeLa cells in tissue culture[125,126] and in the guinea pig conjunctival (Sereny) test.[126,127] Invasiveness is plasmid-mediated,[128,129] but the correlation of this and other plasmid-mediated traits with the production of human disease is unclear at present.

Clinical Features

Symptoms. *Yersinia enterocolitica* produces a spectrum of disease including acute enterocolitis, terminal ileitis, and mesenteric adenitis. *Yersinia pseudotuberculosis,* which commonly infects animals, is a less frequent cause of human disease. When it infects humans, it usually produces mesenteric adenitis, especially in older children and adults. Patients with mesenteric adenitis have an illness clinically indistinguishable from acute appendicitis.[130] Symptoms reported by ill people in four common-source outbreaks are summarized in Table 3.[131–133] Fever, abdominal pain, vomiting, and diarrhea are frequent. In a series of 37 sporadic cases of *Yersinia*-induced enteritis reported from Belgium, 84 percent of the patients had abdominal pain, 78 percent had diarrhea, 43 percent had fever, and 22 percent reported anorexia; only 13 percent had nausea and 8 percent vomited.[134] Patients with sporadic cases of mesenteric adenitis caused by *Yersinia* may have a history of biphasic illness[135] or experience of similar illnesses in the remote past.[118] Consumption of raw pork in the two weeks before illness has been strikingly associated with *Y. enterocolitica* infection in the most highly endemic country, Belgium.[136]

Physical Examination. Regardless of cause, the clinical syndrome of mesenteric adenitis typically includes fever, right-lower-quadrant tenderness, and rebound tenderness.[59,133] In the setting of a common-source outbreak, rectal tenderness was present in nearly one-third of people examined.[133] In contrast to the enteric fever syndromes, a pulse–temperature deficit is not reported.

Laboratory Findings. Leukocytosis is usually present in patients with mesenteric adenitis[135–140]; white blood cell counts typically are between 10,000 and 15,000/mm^3. A methylene blue examination of fresh feces may reveal polymorphonuclear leukocytes.[141] Blood cultures are rarely positive in this syndrome; however, both *Y. enterocolitica* and *Y. pseudotuberculosis* have been isolated from stool cultures. Frequency of isolation is improved by use of cold enrichment techniques.[61,142] Stool cultures were positive in 56 percent of the hospitalized patients with the syndrome in a recent common-source outbreak[133]; isolation of *Y. pseudotuberculosis* from feces may be less frequent but has been reported.[143] Serologic testing may help in the diagnosis, although agglutinins are rarely present during the first week of illness,[52,134] and cross-reactions can occur with *Brucella* species, *Vibrio* species, and some Enterobacteriaceae. Serologic confirmation was made in 84 percent of the hospitalized patients in one outbreak.[133] The isolation of *Y. enterocolitica* from a stool culture should be considered significant; the organism was isolated from only 1 out of 974 controls in one study and from none of 545 controls in another.[144,145]

Sonographic or radiologic contrast studies of the small bowel may provide a clue to the diagnosis, particularly if ileitis is associated with the mesenteric adenitis. Sonography, using graded compression, may help distinguish appendicitis from mesenteric adenitis. Of 170 patients presenting with a clinical syndrome suggesting acute appendicitis 14 had only enlarged mesenteric nodes with mural thickening of the terminal ileum (without visualization of the appendix); none of the 14 had appendicitis; and 8 (of 9 cultured) had *Y. enterocolitica* in the stool.[146] In a series of 37 adult patients with documented *Y. enterocolitica* infection, 40 percent of whom had symptoms compatible with appendicitis, 21 of the 24 patients studied had a radiologic abnormality of the terminal ileum consisting of coarse mucosal folds in 67 percent, nodularity in 45 percent, and ulceration in 45 percent.[134] Although radiologic studies of the colon were normal in these patients, sigmoidoscopic or colonoscopic examination in 13 revealed evidence of colitis in 6 and aphthoid ulceration in 2, indicating that colonic involvement may occur.[134] In another series of 25 patients with *Yersinia* infection with the clinical diagnosis of acute appendicitis who underwent appendectomy, acute terminal ileitis was confirmed

TABLE 3. Symptoms in Four Outbreaks of Mesenteric Adenitis Caused by *Y. enterocolitica*

Location	Japan (114)	Japan (115)	Japan (115)	United States (116)
Serotype	03	03	03	08
Number ill	198	188	544	38
Percentage with				
Abdominal pain	76	86	64	97
Fever	61	76	50	100
Diarrhea	36	60	32	47
Vomiting	12	4	11	
Percentage undergoing appendectomy	2			42

at surgery. When these patients were examined within 1 week of surgery by a barium contrast study of the small bowel, abnormalities were confined to the distal 20 cm of the ileum. The lesions evolved from an initial nodular pattern to an edematous pattern before resolution within 10 weeks in all cases.[147]

At surgery, patients with mesenteric adenitis may also have evidence of acute appendicitis, but the organ is rarely severely inflamed or ruptured. Patients may also have evidence of acute terminal ileitis.[123,130,137,138,140,147] Culture of the terminal ileum at surgery may yield the organism.[139]

Histopathologic examination of resected mesenteric lymph nodes in cases of *Y. enterocolitica* infection frequently reveals histiocytic infiltration and presence of large pyroninophilic cells; abscesses are typically absent.[148,149] In contrast, although reticulum cell hyperplasia is frequently seen in nodes infected with *Y. pseudotuberculosis*,[118,138,139,150] granulomas, polymorphonuclear leukocyte infiltration, and abscess formation are more frequent.[118,139,148,150] In both infections, tissue Gram's stain may reveal the responsible organisms. Two fatal cases occurred in a *Y. enterocolitica* outbreak among four families in North Carolina.[151] Postmortem examination revealed extensive ulceration and necrosis extending from the stomach or small bowel to the colon. Mesenteric lymph nodes were necrotic in one case, and the sinusoids were filled with leukocytes and mononuclear cells. In the second case, the lymph nodes were large, firm, and edematous. There was reticuloendothelial hyperplasia with abundant histiocytes and plasma cells within the sinusoids.[141]

Epidemiology

Mesenteric adenitis caused by *Y. enterocolitica* or *Y. pseudotuberculosis* is a syndrome of children and young adults,[118] is most frequent in people between 5 and 14 years of age,[59] is more common in boys.[118,144] and is most often encountered during the winter and spring. This seasonal pattern is reported from both the preantibiotic[117] and antibiotic eras.[137,152]

The mode of transmission of *Y. enterocolitica* and *Y. pseudotuberculosis* has not been well defined; outbreaks involving several members of several families[151] have been reported. In these and other episodes of *Yersinia* infection, simultaneous documentation of infection in family pets has been obtained[153]; whether these animals were the source of the human infection or merely acquired the infection simultaneously is unknown. Person-to-person spread to family members does occur.[145] Large common-source outbreaks of mesenteric adenitis have also been reported[131–133,154–155]; in one of these, chocolate milk was the vehicle of transmission.[133] *Yersinia enterocolitica* has been isolated from drinking water,[156,157] but water-borne transmission of these organisms has not been well documented. Results of one study in Wisconsin suggested that *Y. enterocolitica* infection was more common in rural areas.[158]

Differential Diagnosis

The major consideration in the differential diagnosis of mesenteric adenitis is acute appendicitis. Other inflammatory diseases characteristically involving the terminal ileum, such as tuberculosis and actinomycosis, should also be considered. *Angiostrongylus costaricensis* can also produce an appendicitis-like syndrome, but usually is associated with eosinophilia as described below.[159]

Therapy

Mesenteric adenitis is a self-limited illness in the vast majority of cases. Specific antimicrobial therapy is often not required. In patients with the syndrome who are severely ill, the selection of an antimicrobial agent should be based, if possible, on the results of antimicrobial sensitivity tests. When these data are not available, therapeutic agents to be considered include tetracycline, chloramphenicol, trimethoprim–sulfamethoxazole, and third-generation cephalosporins, to which *Y. enterocolitica* is sensitive in vitro.[160,161] The trimethoprim–sulfamethoxazole combination has been shown to be synergistic against 100 percent of 23 human *Y. enterocolitica* isolates.[160] Although *Y. enterocolitica* isolates may also be sensitive in vitro to aminoglycosides[162] these drugs should probably not be the initial choice for treatment of this syndrome because of their toxicity and their reported failure to eradicate effectively systemic infection caused by these organisms.[43] *Y. pseudotuberculosis* is usually sensitive to ampicillin, tetracycline, chloramphenicol, cephalosporins, and aminoglycosides. Persons with septicemic disease should receive antibiotic therapy because of the high mortality.

THE SYNDROME OF ABDOMINAL PAIN AND/OR DIARRHEA WITH EOSINOPHILIA

The differential diagnosis and etiologic considerations for the syndrome of abdominal pain, diarrhea, and eosinophilia as well as useful diagnostic tests are summarized in Table 4. Most cases are caused by helminths. Additional diagnostic considerations include five diseases of unknown cause: eosinophilic gastroenteritis, dermatitis herpetiformis, periarteritis nodosa, regional enteritis, and ulcerative colitis. In addition, lymphomas and some solid tumors may manifest with abdominal pain and eosinophilia. Epidemiologic data, particularly dietary and travel histories, may provide important clues to the diagnosis in patients with this syndrome. Valuable laboratory tests in these patients include examination of stool and small bowel contents for ova and parasites, specific serologic tests, and, in some cases, tissue biopsy and radiologic studies.

Differential Diagnosis

Strongyloides stercoralis is unique among intestinal nematodes in its ability to persist for many years through autoinfection and to produce life-threatening hyperinfection in immunocompromised hosts.[163] It infects people in areas where sanitation is poor. Patients with strongyloidiasis frequently have abdominal pain, diarrhea, or bloating with eosinophilia. In a study of 100 hospitalized adult men, abdominal pain was reported by 79 percent and diarrhea by 36 percent.[164] Pain was most often epigastric, although some patients reported pain in the right-upper and right-lower quadrants and in the periumbilical region. Ninety percent of these patients had eosinophilia. More than 30 cases of severe strongyloidiasis hyperinfection after renal transplantation or in association with Hodgkin's disease or cimetidine use have been reported.[165–167] Hyperinfection is often associated with secondary bacteremia, meningitis, urinary tract infection, or pneumonia due to enteric bacteria.

In the United States, strongyloidiasis is most often found in residents of the southeast, immigrants, or veterans who served in endemic areas. Prolonged infections have been demonstrated in troops and former prisoners of World War II who served in Southeast Asia.[168–171] A prospective study in rural Tennessee documented *S. stercoralis* in 6.1 percent of patients at a Veterans Administration hospital and 2.6 percent of their household contacts.[172] Diagnosis is made by demonstration of larvae in fresh concentrated stool specimens or in duodenal contents obtained either by intestinal intubation or by use of the Enterotest capsule.[173] Serologic tests currently play no role. Eosinophilia is often not present in immunocompromised patients, particularly those taking corticosteroids.[165,166]

Most patients infected with *Ascaris lumbricoides* are asymptomatic. Although ascariasis is not usually associated with diarrhea, severe abdominal pain may occur when patients with heavy worm burdens develop intestinal obstruction, or adult worms occlude the biliary or pancreatic ducts. These compli-

TABLE 4. Etiologic Agents and Useful Laboratory Studies in the Differential Diagnosis of Infectious Causes of the Syndrome of Abdominal Pain and/or Diarrhea with Eosinophilia

Etiologic Agents or Disease	*Stool Examination*	*Small Bowel Fluid Examination or Biopsy*	*Tissue Biopsy*	*Serology*	*Radiologic and Other Studies*
Nematodes					
Strongyloides stercoralis	+	+	−	−	−
Trichinella spiralis	−	−	+ (Muscle)	+	−
Ascaris lumbricoides	+	+	−	−	± (Small bowel)
Visceral larva migrans	−	−	+ (Liver)	+	−
Anisakiasis	−	+	−	−	+ (endoscopy)
Capillaria philippinensis	+	+	−	−	−
Angiostrongylus costaricensis	−	−	+ (Ileum, colon)	−	+ (UGI series; small bowel)
Trematodes					
Schistosomiasis	+	−	+ (Rectum)	+	−
Fasciola hepatica	+	−	−	−	−
Fasciolopsis buski	+	−	−	−	−
Clonorchis sinensis	+	−	−	−	± (Biliary tract abnormalities)
Opisthorchis species	+	−	−	−	± (Biliary tract abnormalities)
Cestodes					
Echinococcosis	−	−	−	±	+ (Chest radiograph, abdominal ultrasound or CT scan)
Protozoa					
Isospora belli	+	+	−	−	−
Dientamoeba fragilis	+	−	−	−	−
Diseases of unknown etiology					
Eosinophilic gastroenteritis	−	+	−	−	+ (UGI series; small bowel)
Periarteritis nodosa	−	−	+ (Skin, muscle, kidney)	−	+ (Angiography)
Inflammatory bowel disease	−	−	+ (Colon)	−	+ (Small bowel, colonoscopy)
Malignancies	−	±	+ (Lymph nodes, liver, bone marrow)	−	+ (UGI Series, barium enema, CT scan)

Key: + : feature present; − : feature absent.

cations are most frequent in young children.[174–175] Ascariasis is most common in areas in which sanitation is poor; the eggs may be ingested in contaminated food or water or, by children, in dirt. In the United States, this infection is most common in the southeastern states,[174] but symptomatic infections are rare. The diagnosis is made by demonstration of the typical eggs in stool specimens. Eosinophilia may or may not be present. Since a single worm produces large numbers of eggs, concentration of feces is not necessary. In patients with intestinal or biliary tract obstruction, radiologic studies and liver or pancreatic enzyme elevations may provide a clue to the diagnosis.

Patients with toxocariasis (visceral larva migrans) caused by animal nematodes such as *Toxocara canis* or *Toxocara cati* may have abdominal pain and eosinophilia. In temperate climates, *T. canis* is the more important etiologic agent.[176] The abdominal pain may be associated with the presence of tender hepatomegaly. Clinical clues to the diagnosis include the simultaneous occurrence of splenomegaly or pneumonitis with bronchospasm.[177–179] Patients may have pruritic rashes on the trunk or lower extremities. The presence of a granuloma in the ocular fundus or other evidence of ocular inflammation, high titers of isoagglutinins, and hypergammaglobulinemia provide additional diagnostic clues. The total white count is often elevated, and eosinophils may exceed 50 percent. Patients are usually young children; additional epidemiologic clues are a history of pica or close contact with dogs or cats. Between 10 and 30 percent of the soil samples in public playgrounds and parks in the United States have been found to be contaminated with *Toxocara* eggs.[176] Serologic tests are available; an ELISA seems to be the most sensitive and specific.[177–179] On occasion, larvae are identified in biopsies of hepatic granulomas.

Infection with *Trichinella spiralis* may be characterized initially by diarrhea, which occurs in approximately 40 percent of the cases; abdominal pain, which occurs in approximately 20 percent; or even by constipation.[180,181] The intestinal symptoms are attributed to the presence of adult worms or invading larvae in the intestinal tract, occur during the first week of illness, and may precede the appearance of eosinophilia. Approximately 100 cases are reported annually in the United States.[182] Infection occurs by the ingestion of raw or undercooked pork or pork products such as sausage, bear meat, and horse meat, and occasionally by other vehicles such as ground beef contaminated during processing with pork.[181–185] Prolonged diarrhea has been the dominant symptom among Inuit inhabitants of northern Canada who acquired *Trichinella nativa* from contaminated, uncooked walrus meat. Myalgia and muscle weakness were less prominent complaints.[186] The presence of myalgias, periorbital edema, muscle tenderness, splinter hemorrhages, and evidence of myocarditis or central nervous system involvement may suggest the diagnosis. The diagnosis may be confirmed serologically with either the bentonite flocculation or immunofluorescence test, which typically do not become positive until several weeks into infection.[187] Definitive diagnosis may be made by demonstration of larvae in specimens from a muscle biopsy, but biopsy is seldom necessary.

Patients with anisakiasis caused by nematodes of the family Anisakidae, ascarid parasites of marine animals, may have an acute illness characterized by epigastric pain, nausea, and vomiting or more commonly a chronic illness characterized by abdominal pain and fever. The disease is caused by larvae that penetrate the gastrointestinal tract. The stomach, small bowel, and colon may be involved. Necrotizing eosinophilic granulomatous inflammation with peripheral eosinophilia may occur.[188] The pathologic and radiologic manifestations may resemble regional enteritis[189]; mass lesions resembling malignancies may also occur.[190] The disease is rarely reported in the United States and is most common in the Netherlands and Japan. The infection is acquired by the ingestion of raw or undercooked marine fish such as cod, salmon, and herring. In Japan, raw or pickled marine fish are common vehicles; in the Netherlands, raw or slightly salted herring is the most common source of infection.[188] Therefore, a travel or a dietary history may suggest the diagnosis. Confirmation is obtained by identification of the larvae by endoscopy or in tissue specimens.

Patients with capillariasis typically give a history of several weeks of vague abdominal pain followed by voluminous watery diarrhea. The illness is characterized by a protein-losing enteropathy and malabsorption. Electrolyte abnormalities and hypoproteinemia are common. Weight loss, muscle wasting, weakness, hyporeflexia, and edema occur.[191,192] The worms are found in the small bowel, especially in the jejunum, and the adults are partially embedded in the mucosa.[193] The intestinal villi are flattened in focal areas.[193] The disease is most common in the Philippines; a few cases have also been reported from Thailand. Although the epidemiology of the disease has not been completely characterized, freshwater fish eaten raw or poorly cooked appear to be the vehicle of transmission.[194] The diagnosis is made by demonstration of the typical eggs of *Capillaria philippinensis* in fecal specimens. The finding of eggs, adult worms, and larvae in the small bowel contents suggest that autoinfection may occur.[193,194] Travel and dietary histories may provide a clue to the diagnosis.

Angiostrongylus costaricensis lives in the lumen of mesenteric arteries of the ileocecal region of rodents and occasionally involves the same site in humans. Eggs form emboli to terminal branches of the mesenteric arteries, where they hatch and invade the intestinal wall. Disease, usually encountered in children, may present as an acute abdominal infection with fever, nausea, vomiting, pain, and sometimes a right lower quadrant mass. Leukocytosis and eosinophilia (11–82 percent) are usually present. It may be impossible to distinguish infection with *A. costaricensis* from acute appendicitis.[159] Other patients experience a visceral larva migrans-like syndrome.[195] Humans are thought to become infected by ingesting material contaminated by infected slugs or snails, which are intermediate hosts. *Angiostrongylus costaricensis* is found in areas of Central and South America.

Patients with trematode infection may occasionally have a syndrome characterized by abdominal pain and/or diarrhea and eosinophilia. Katayama fever, a clinical syndrome characterized by fever, headache, diarrhea, hepatosplenomegaly, generalized lymphadenopathy, urticaria, and eosinophilia, may occur within 4–8 weeks after primary exposure to schistosomes. This syndrome is most common in the presence of heavy infections and occurs most frequently with *Schistosoma japonicum* infection, less frequently with *Schistosoma mansoni* infection, and very rarely with *Schistosoma haematobium* infection.[196] This acute manifestation of schistosomiasis is usually self-limited, although deaths may occur. The diagnosis may be suspected in patients with a serum sickness-like illness accompanied by eosinophilia who have had exposure during the previous 4–8 weeks, through swimming or bathing, to fresh water in an area in which schistosomiasis is endemic.[197,198] As *S. japonicum* is found mainly in China, Japan, and Southeast Asia,[197] a history of recent travel to these areas would suggest the diagnosis. Diagnosis is made by demonstration of the characteristic eggs in either a Kato thick smear of feces[196] or a rectal biopsy specimen. Serologic tests provide suggestive evidence of infection.

Acute infection with the liver fluke *Fasciola hepatica*, which is found in many sheep raising areas of the world, is often characterized by fever and pain in the right upper quadrant, hepatomegaly, and often marked eosinophilia.[199–201] Human infections are acquired by ingestion of encysted metacercariae on aquatic plants such as wild watercress. Infections have been reported from South America, Africa, Europe, China, and Australia. The laboratory diagnosis is based on identification of characteristic ova in the feces or bile. Concentration techniques increase the likelihood of finding eggs.

Another trematode that may be associated with abdominal pain or diarrhea and eosinophilia is the intestinal fluke *Fasciolopsis buski*. Although infection with *F. buski* is usually asymptomatic, patients with heavy infections may have both abdominal pain and diarrhea.[202,203] The diagnosis may be suggested by a history of travel to the Far East and Southeast Asia, where the disease is endemic.[203] Infection is acquired through the ingestion of water chestnuts or the peeling of other freshwater plants with the teeth before ingestion. Diagnosis is made by demonstration of *F. buski* eggs in feces and usually requires a concentration technique.[203]

Acute infections with the liver flukes, *Clonorchis sinensis* and *Opisthorchis* species, may be associated with fever, abdominal pain, diarrhea, hepatomegaly, and eosinophilia. Although at increased risk of ascending cholangitis and cholangiocarcinoma, persons with established infection are usually free of specific symptoms and eosinophilia.[204,205]

Abdominal pain and/or diarrhea and eosinophilia are very uncommon in cestode (tapeworm) infections.[206] Eosinophilia may occur in conjunction with abdominal pain in a few patients with echinococcosis when cysts rupture. Laboratory studies may reveal a cystic lesion(s), in the liver, or other organs. The diagnosis should be suspected in patients who have lived in or traveled to areas in which the disease is endemic. In the United States, endemic areas include California, Utah, and Alaska. Other endemic areas include sheep and cattle raising areas of Australia, South America, South Africa, the Soviet Union, and Mediterranean countries.[207] The diagnosis is usually made on the basis of radiologic or ultrasound findings and serologic tests.[208]

Patients with protozoal infections (e.g., *Entamoeba histolytica*) typically do not have eosinophilia. *Isospora belli* is an important exception.[209,210] It can cause abdominal pain, watery diarrhea, and malabsorption in association with eosinophilia. The disease occurs throughout the world, but it is most prevalent in the tropics where sanitation is poor. In healthy adults, *Isospora belli* produces a self-limited disease. The diagnosis may be suggested by an appropriate history of travel. *Isospora belli* is an important cause of severe, chronic diarrhea and weight loss in Haitians with acquired immunodeficiency syndrome (AIDS).[211] Infection has been documented in a few patients with AIDS in the United States.

The diagnosis of *Isospora belli* is established by the demonstration of oocysts in feces[211]; concentration techniques may be necessary. Examination of duodenal contents or small bowel biopsy specimens are more sensitive diagnostic techniques. Mucosal abnormalities are frequently seen on small bowel biopsy specimens and include blunted villus tips, shortened villi, hypertrophied crypts, and eosinophilic infiltration of the lamina propria.[209] *Dientamoeba fragilis* is another protozoan that can cause diarrhea and abdominal discomfort and has been associated with eosinophilia.[212,213]

Eosinophilic gastroenteritis is a disease of adults with protean clinical manifestations that may include abdominal pain, diarrhea, gastrointestinal bleeding, protein-losing enteropathy, a malabsorption syndrome, and gastric outlet obstruction.[214] Manifestations depend both on the part of bowel involved (stomach, duodenum, jejunum, or ileum) and on the layer of bowel involved (mucosa, muscular layer, or submucosa). The stomach and small intestine are the most common sites of involvement, but eosinophilic ileocolitis has also been reported.[215] Patients frequently have a history compatible with an allergic diathesis.[216] The sedimentation rate is usually normal or mildly elevated. Additional clues to the diagnosis include peripheral blood eosinophilia and presence of Charcot-Leyden crystals in stools.[216–217] Radiologic studies may reveal polypoid gastric or duodenal mucosal folds and rigid dilated loops of jejunum with a sawtooth mucosal pattern.[218] Diagnosis may be made by peroral or endoscopic biopsy. Histologic examination of involved tissue reveals eosinophilia in the absence of both granulomas and vasculitis.[216] Since the involvement may be patchy, multiple biopsies are usually required. All biopsies may be negative if the disease involves only the muscular or subserosal layers. In the latter case, the presence of eosinophils in ascitic fluid may suggest the diagnosis.[216] The disease is chronic and occasionally fatal,[219] but most patients respond to corticosteroid therapy.[214,216]

Gastrointestinal involvement with eosinophilia may occur as manifestations of vasculitis.[220–224] Gastrointestinal involvement appears in up to 25 percent of the patients with periarteritis nodosa and may be the initial manifestation of the disease in 15 percent of the patients.[215,221,222] Abdominal pain is a prominent symptom, and eosinophilia is frequent. The clue to the diagnosis, which may be confirmed by biopsy or angiography, is provided by the systemic nature of the disease with frequent involvement of the kidneys, heart, musculoskeletal, and nervous systems. In allergic angiitis and granulomatosis of the Churg-Strauss syndrome type, lung involvement is pronounced, patients manifest prominent eosinophilia, and there is a strong allergic diathesis, often with asthma.[220] Some of the patients with this syndrome also have abdominal involvement and have been classified as having a polyangiitis overlap syndrome.[223,224]

Abdominal pain and diarrhea accompanied by eosinophilia may occur in patients with regional enteritis, Whipple's disease, and ulcerative colitis.[225] In one series, 32 percent of the patients with radiologically or surgically proven regional enteritis had eosinophilia on more than one occasion.[226] The average elevated eosinophil count was 6.2 percent; the range was from 4 to 22 percent.[226] The characteristic extraintestinal manifestations in patients with these inflammatory bowel diseases may provide clues to their diagnosis.[227]

Patients with solid tumors and lymphomas may also have abdominal pain and eosinopilia.[225] Eosinophilia is most commonly associated with solid tumors after metastasis has occurred.[228,229] Among these solid tumors, frequently implicated malignancies are gastric, colonic, lung, pancreatic, and uterine carcinomas.[228,230] A history of weight loss and the presence of melena or guaiac positive stools and anemia may suggest the diagnosis, which may be confirmed by appropriate radiographic, endoscopic, or cytologic studies. Both Hodgkin's disease and non-Hodgkin's lymphomas may also be associated with eosinophilia and abdominal pain when abdominal or retroperitoneal nodes are involved.

REFERENCES

1. Christie AB. Typhoid and paratyphoid fevers. In: Infectious Diseases: Epidemiology and Clinical Practice, 2nd ed. Churchill Livingstone; New York: 1974:55–130.
2. Walker W, ed. The Aberdeen typhoid outbreak of 1964. Scott Med J 1965;10:466–79.
3. Gulati PD, Saxena SN, Gupta PS, et al. Changing pattern of typhoid fever. Am J Med. 1968;45:544–8.
4. Hornick RB, Greisman SE, Woodward TE, et al. Typhoid fever: Pathogenesis and immunologic control. N Engl J Med. 1970;283:686–91.
5. Stuart BM, Pullen RL: Typhoid, Clinical analysis of three hundred and sixty cases. Arch Intern Med. 1946;78:629–61.
6. Rice PA, Baine WB, Gangarosa EJ. *Salmonella typhi* infections in the United States, 1967–1972: Increasing importance of international travelers. Am J Epidemiol. 1977;106:160–6.
7. Taylor DN, Pollard RA, Blake PA. Typhoid fever in the United States and the risk to international travelers. J Infect Dis. 1983;148:599–602.
8. Carter PB, Collins FM. The route of enteric infection in normal mice. J Exp Med. 1974;139:1189–1203.
9. Kamat SA, Herzog C. Typhoid: Clinical picture and response to chloramphenicol: Prospective study in Bombay (1972). Infection. 1977;5:85–91.
10. Wicks ACB, Holmes GS, Davidson L. Endemic typhoid fever: A diagnostic pitfall. Q J Med. 1971;40:341–54.
11. Hoffman TA, Ruiz CJ, Counts GW, et al. Waterborne typhoid fever in Dade County, Florida: Clinical and therapeutic evaluation of 105 bacteremic patients. Am J Med. 1975;59:481–7.
12. Samantray SK, Johnson SC, Chakrabarti AK. Enteric fever: An analysis of 500 cases. Practitioner. 1977;218:400–8.
13. Wahab MFA, Robertson RP, Raasch FO. Paratyphoid A fever, Cairo, Egypt. Ann Intern Med. 1969;70:913–7.
14. Black PH, Kunz LJ, Swartz MN. Salmonellosis: A review of some unusual aspects. N Engl J Med. 1960;262:811–7.
15. Sprinz H, Gangarosa EJ, Williams M, et al. Histopathology of the upper small intestines in typhoid fever: Biopsy study of experimental disease in man. Am J Dig Dis. 1966;11:615–24.
16. Litwack, KD, Hoke AW, Borchardt KA. Rose spots in typhoid fever. Arch Dermatol. 1972;105:252–5.
17. Meals RA. Paratyphoid fever: A report of 62 cases with several unusual findings and a review of the literature. Arch Intern Med. 1976;136:1422–8.
18. Watson KC. Laboratory and clinical investigation of recovery of *Salmonella typhi* from blood. J Clin Microbiol. 1978;7:122–6.
19. Gilman RH, Terminel M, Levine MM, et al. Relative efficacy of blood, urine, rectal swab, bone-marrow, and rose-spot cultures for recovery of *Salmonella typhi* in typhoid fever. Lancet. 1975;1:1211–3.
20. Guerra-Caceres JG, Gotuzzo-Herencia E, Crosby-Dagnino E, et al. Diagnostic value of bone marrow culture in typhoid fever. Trans R Soc Trop Med Hyg. 1979;73:680–3.
21. Rockhill RC, Rumans LW, Lesmana M, et al. Detection of *Salmonella typhi* D, Vi, and d antigens, by slide coagglutination, in urine from patients with typhoid fever. J Clin Microbiol. 1980;11:213–6.
22. Taylor DN, Harris JR, Barrett TJ, et al. Detection of urinary Vi antigen as a diagnostic test for typhoid fever. J Clin Microbiol. 1983;18:872–6.
23. Tsang RSW, Chau PY. Serological diagnosis of typhoid fever by counter-immunoelectrophoresis. Br Med J. 1981;282:1505–7.
24. Sundararaj T, Ilango B, Subramanian S. A study on the usefulness of counter immuno-electrophoresis for the detection of *Salmonella typhi* antigen in the sera of suspected cases of enteric fever. Trans R Soc Trop Med Hyg. 1983;77:194–7.
25. Schroeder SA. Interpretation of serologic tests for typhoid fever. JAMA. 1968;206:839–40.
26. Reynolds DW, Carpenter RL, Simon WH. Diagnostic specificity of Widal's reaction for typhoid fever. JAMA. 1970;214:2192–3.
27. Senewiratne B, Chir B, Senewiratne K. Reassessment of the Widal test in the diagnosis of typhoid. Gastroenterology. 1977;73:233–6.
28. Brodie J: Antibodies and the Aberdeen typhoid outbreak of 1964:I. The Widal reaction. J Hyg. 1977;79:161–80.
29. Buck RL, Escamilla J, Sangalang RP, et al. Diagnostic value of a single, pre-treatment Widal test in suspected enteric fever cases in the Philippines. Trans R Soc Trop Med Hyg. 1987;81:871–3.
30. Levine MM, Grados O, Gilman RH, et al. Diagnostic value of the Widal test in areas endemic for typhoid fever. Am J Trop Med Hyg. 1978;27:795–800.
31. Editorial: Typhoid and its serology. Br Med J. 1978;1:389.
32. Beasley WJ, Joseph SW, Weiss E: Improved serodiagnosis of *Salmonella* enteric fevers by an enzyme-linked immunosorbent assay. J Clin Microbiol 1981;13:106–114.
33. Petchclai B, Ausavarungnirun R, Manatsathit S. Passive hemagglutination test for enteric fever. J Clin Microbiol. 1987;25:138–41.
34. Nolan CM, Feeley JC, White PC Jr, et al. Evaluation of a new assay for Vi antibody in chronic carriers of *Salmonella typhi*. J Clin Microbiol. 1980;12:22–6.
35. Barrett TJ, Blake PA, Brown SL, et al. Enzyme-linked immunosorbent assay for detection of human antibodies to *Salmonella typhi* Vi antigen. J Clin Microbiol. 1983;17:625–7.
36. Gupta AK, Rao KM. Radial counter-immunoelectrophoresis for rapid serodiagnosis of typhoid fever. J Immunol Methods. 1981;40:373–6.
37. Ramachandran S, Godfrey JJ, Perera MVF. Typhoid hepatitis. JAMA. 1974;230:236–242.
38. Sitprija V, Pipatanagul V, Boonpucknavig V, et al. Glomerulitis in typhoid fever. Ann Intern Med. 1974;81:210–3.
39. Butler W, Bell WR, Levin J, et al. Typhoid fever: Studies of blood coagulation, bacteremia, and endotoxemia. Arch Intern Med. 1978;138:407–10.
40. Harris JC, DuPont HL, Hornick RB. Fecal leukocytes in diarrheal illness. Ann Intern Med. 1972;76:697–703.
41. Blaser MJ, Hickman FW, Farmer JJ III, et al. *Salmonella typhi:* The laboratory as a reservoir of infection. J Infect Dis. 1980;142:934–8.
42. Blaser MJ, Lofgren JP. Fatal salmonellosis originating in a clinical microbiology laboratory. J Clin Microbiol. 1981;13:855–8.
43. Rabson AR, Hallett AF, Koornhof HJ, Generalized *Yersinia enterocolitica* infection. J Infect Dis. 1975;131:447–51.
44. Spira TJ, Kabins SA. *Yersinia enterocolitica* septicemia with septic arthritis. Arch Intern Med. 1976;136:1305–8.
45. Marlon A, Gentry L, Merigan TC. Septicemia with *Pasteurella pseudotuberculosis* and liver disease. Arch Intern Med. 1971;127:947–9.
46. Guerrant RL, Lahita RG, Winn WC Jr, et al. Campylobacteriosis in man: Pathogenic mechanisms and review of 91 bloodstream infections. Am J Med. 1978;65:584–92.
47. Schmidt U, Chmel H, Kaminski Z, et al. The clinical spectrum of *Campylobacter fetus* infection: Report of 5 cases and review of the literature. Q J Med. 1980;49:431–42.
48. Carbone KM, Heinrich MC, Quinn TC. Thrombophlelitis and cellulitis due to *Campylobacter fetus ssp fetus*. Medicine. 1984;64:244–50.
49. Bevanger L. *Yersinia pseudotuberculosis* as the cause of septicemia in a patient with amyloidosis. Acta Pathol Microbiol Scand [B]. 1976;84:461–2.
50. Bokkenheuser, V. *Vibrio fetus* infection in man: I. Ten new cases and some epidemiologic observations. Am J Epidemiol. 1970;91:400–9.
51. Leino R, Kalliomäki JL. Yersiniosis as an internal disease. Ann Intern Med. 1974;81:458–61.
52. Ahvonen P. Human yersiniosis in Finland: I. Bacteriology and serology. Ann Clin Res. 1972;4:30–8.
53. Hubbert WT, Petenyi CW, Glasgow LA, et al. *Yersinia pseudotuberculosis* infection in the United States: Septicemia, appendicitis, and mesenteric lymphadenitis. Am J Trop Med Hyg. 1971;20:679–84.
54. Yamashiro KM, Goldman RH, Harris D, et al. *Pasteurella pseudotuberculosis:* Acute sepsis with survival. Arch Intern Med. 1971;128:605–8.
55. Keet EE. *Yersinia enterocolitica* septicemia: Source of infection and incu-

bation period identified. NY State J Med. 1974;74:2226–30.
56. Sonnenwirth AC. Bacteremia with and without meningitis due to *Yersinia enterocolitica, Edwardsiella tarda, Comamonas terrigena,* and *Pseudomonas maltophilia*. Ann NY Acad Sci. 1970;174:488–502.
57. Taylor BG, Zafarzai MZ, Humphreys DW, et al. Nodular pulmonary infiltrates and septic arthritis associated with *Yersinia enterocolitica* bacteremia. Am Rev Respir Dis. 1977;116:525–9.
58. Bliddal J, Kaliszan S. Prolonged monosymptomatic fever due to *Yersinia enterocolitica*. Acta Med Scand. 1977;201:387–9.
59. Ahvonen P. Human yersiniosis in Finland: II. Clinical features. Ann Clin Res. 1972;4:39–48.
60. Franklin B, Ulmer DD. Human infection with *Vibrio fetus*. West J Med. 1974;120:200–4.
61. Greenwood JR, Flanigan SW, Pickett MJ, et al. Clinical isolation of *Yersinia enterocolitica:* Cold temperature enrichment. J Clin Microbiol. 1975;2:559–60.
62. Skirrow MB. Campylobacter enteritis: A "new" disease. Br Med J. 1977;2:9–11.
63. Lauwers S, DeBoeck M, Butzler JP. Campylobacter enteritis in Brussels. Lancet. 1978;1:604–5.
64. Bokkenheuser V. *Vibrio fetus* infection in man: A serological test. Infect Immun. 1972;5:222–226.
65. Reinicke V, Korner B. Case report: Fulminant septicemia caused by *Yersinia enterocolitica* Scand J Infect Dis. 1977;9:249–51.
66. Forrström J, Viander M, Lehtonen A, et al. Case report: *Yersinia enterocolitica* infection complicated by glomerulonephritis. Scand J Infect Dis. 1977;9:253–6.
67. Guerrant RL, Humphries MK Jr, Butler JE, et al. Tickborne oculoglandular tularemia. Arch Intern Med. 1976;136:811–3.
68. Buchanan TM, Faber LC, Feldman RA. Brucellosis in the United States, 1960–1972: An abattoir-associated disease: I. Clinical features and therapy. Medicine. 1974;53:403–13.
69. Reed WP, Palmer DL, Williams RC Jr, et al. Bubonic plague in the southwestern United States: A review of recent experience. Medicine. 1970;49:465–86.
70. Cantey JR. Plague in Vietnam: Clinical observations and treatment with kanamycin. Arch Intern Med. 1974;133:280–3.
71. Nalin DR, Sultana B, Sahunja R, et al. Survival of a patient with intestinal anthrax. Am J Med. 1977;62:130–2.
72. Brundage WG, Thuss CJ Jr, Walden DG. Four fatal cases of melioidosis in U.S. soldiers in Vietnam: Bacteriologic and pathologic characteristics. Am J Trop Med Hyg. 1968;17:183–91.
73. Schultz MG. A history of bartonellosis (Carrión's disease). Am J Trop Med Hyg. 1968;17:503–15.
74. Cuadra M. Salmonellosis complication in human bartonellosis. Tex Rep Biol Med. 1956;14:97–113.
75. Cole JS, Stoll RW, Bulger RJ. Rat-bite fever: Report of three cases. Ann Intern Med. 1969;71:979–81.
76. Kowal J. Spirillum fever: Report of a case and review of the literature. N Engl J Med. 1961;264:123–8.
77. Anderson LC, Leary SL, Manning PJ. Rat bite fever in animal research laboratory personnel. Lab Anim Sci. 1983;33:292–4.
78. Heath CW Jr, Alexander AD, Galton MM. Leptospirosis in the United States: Analysis of 483 cases in man, 1949–1961. N Engl J Med. 1965;273:857–64.
79. Edwards GA, Domm BM. Human leptospirosis. Medicine. 1960;39:117–56.
80. Boyer KM, Munford RS, Maupin GO, et al. Tick-borne relapsing fever: An interstate outbreak originating at Grand Canyon National Park. Am J Epidemiol. 1977;105:469–79.
81. Southern PM Jr, Sanford JP. Relapsing fever: A clinical and microbiological review. Medicine. 1969;48:129–49.
82. Lewis EA, Kolawole RM. Tuberculous ileo-colitis in Ibadan: A clinico-radiological review. Gut. 1972;13:646–53.
83. Johnson CAC, Hill ID, Bowie MD. Abdominal tuberculosis in children: A survey of cases at the Red Cross War Memorial Children's Hospital. 1976–1985. S Afr Med J. 1987;72:20–2.
84. Weese WC, Smith IM. A study of 57 cases of actinomycosis over a 36-year period: A diagnositc "failure" with good prognosis after treatment. Arch Intern Med. 1975;135:1562–8.
85. Larson EB, Featherstone HJ, Petersdorf RG. Fever of undetermined origin: Diagnosis and follow-up of 105 cases, 1970–1980. Medicine. 1982;61:269–92.
86. Murray HW, Masur H, Senterfit LB, et al. The protean manifestations of *Mycoplasma pneumoniae* infection in adults. Am J Med. 1975;58:229–42.
87. Schaffner W, Drutz DJ, Duncan GW, et al. The clinical spectrum of endemic psittacosis. Arch Intern Med. 1967;119:433–43.
88. Hattwick MAW, O'Brien RJ, Hanson BF. Rocky Mountain spotted fever: Epidemiology of an increasing problem. Ann Intern Med. 1976;84:732–9.
89. Woodward TE. A historical account of the rickettsial diseases with a discussion of unsolved problems. J Infect Dis. 1973;127:583–94.
90. Walker DH. Gastroenterology of Rocky Mountain spotted fever. Practical Gastroenterol. 1986;10:25–39.
91. Jiminez J, Byrne WJ, Seibert JJ, et al. Gastrointestinal symptoms in Rocky Mountain spotted fever: Histopathologic finding of ulcerative enteritis with vasculitis. Clin Pediatr. 1982;21:581–4.
92. Middleton DB. Rocky Mountain spotted fever: Gastrointestinal and laboratory manifestations. South Med J. 1978;71:629–32.
93. Westerman EL. Rocky Mountain spotless fever: A dilemma for the clinician. Arch Intern Med. 1982;142:1106–7.
94. Woodward TE, Pedersen CE Jr, Oster CN, et al. Prompt confirmation of Rocky Mountain spotted fever: Identification of rickettsiae in skin tissues. J Infect Dis. 1976;134:297–301.
95. Marrie TJ, Schlech WF III, Williams JC, et al. Q fever pneumonia associated with exposure to wild rabbits. Lancet 1986;1:427–9.
96. Duma RJ, Sonenshine DE, Bozeman FM, et al. Epidemic typhus in the United States associated with flying squirrels. JAMA. 1981;245:2318–23.
97. Centers for Disease Control. Epidemic typhus associated with flying squirrels: United States. MMWR. 1982;31:555–61.
98. Yu VL, Kroboth FJ, Shonnard J, et al. Legionnaires' disease: New clinical perspective from a prospective pneumonia study. Am J Med. 1982;73:357–61.
99. Kirby BD, Snyder KM, Meyer RD, et al. Legionnaires' disease: Report of 65 nosocomially acquired cases and a review of the literature. Medicine. 1980;59:188–205.
100. Chow JW, Lu VL. New perspectives on *Legionella* pneumonia: Diagnosis, management and prevention. J Crit Illness. 1988;3:17–27.
101. Sturim HS, Kouchonkos NT, Ahlvin RC. Gastrointestinal manifestations of disseminated histoplasmosis. Am J Surg. 1965;110:435–40.
102. Gordon S, Brennessel DJ, Goldstein JA, et al. Malaria: A city hospital experience. Arch Intern Med. 1988;148:1569–71.
103. Steketee RW, Eckman MR, Burgess EC, et al. Babesiosis in Wisconsin: A new focus of disease transmission. JAMA. 1985;253:2675–8.
104. Ruebush TK II, Cassaday PB, Marsh HJ, et al. Human babesiosis on Nantucket Island: Clinical features. Ann Intern Med. 1977;86:6–9.
105. May RP, Lehmann JD, Sanford JP. Difficulties in differentiating amebic from pyogenic liver abscess. Arch Intern Med. 1967;119:69–74.
106. Robertson RP, Wahab MFA, Raasch FO. Evaluation of chloramphenicol and ampicillin in salmonella enteric fever. N Engl J Med. 1968;278:171–6.
107. Butler T, Rumans L, Arnold K. Response of typhoid fever caused by chloramphenicol-susceptible and chloramphenicol-resistant strains of *Salmonella typhi* to treatment with trimethoprim–sulfamethoxazole. Rev Infect Dis. 1982;4:551–61.
108. Bryan JP, Rocha H, Scheld WM. Problems in salmonellosis: Rationale for clinical trials with newer Beta-lactam agents and quinolones. Rev Infect Dis. 1986;8:189–207.
109. Soe GB, Overturf GD. Treatment of typhoid fever and other systemic salmonellosis with cefotaxime, ceftriaxone, cefoperazone and other newer cephalosporins. Rev Infect Dis. 1987;9:719–36.
110. Baine WB, Farmer JJ III, Gangarosa EJ. Typhoid fever in the United States associated with the 1972–1973 epidemic in Mexico. J Infect Dis. 1977;135:649–53.
111. Butler T, Arnold K, Linh NN, et al. Chloramphenicol-resistant typhoid fever in Vietnam associated with R factor. Lancet. 1973;2:983–91.
112. Brown JD, Mo DH, Rhoades ER. Chloramphenicol-resistant *Salmonella typhi* in Saigon. JAMA. 1975;231:162–6.
113. Olarte J, Galindo E. *Salmonella typhi* resistant to chloramphenicol, ampicillin and other antimicrobial agents: Strains isolated during an extensive typhoid fever epidemic in Mexico. Antimicrob Agents Chemother. 1973;4:597–603.
114. Snyder MJ, Gonzalez O, Palomino C, et al. Comparative efficacy of chloramphenicol, ampicillin, and co-trimoaxazole in the treatment of typhoid fever. Lancet. 1976;2:1155–7.
115. Butler T, Linh NN, Arnold K, et al. Therapy of antimicrobial-resistant typhoid fever. Antimicrob Agents Chemother. 1977;11:645–50.
116. Datta N, Richards H, Datta C. *Salmonella typhi* in vivo acquires resistance to both chloramphenicol and co-trimoxazole. Lancet. 1981;1:1181–3.
117. Collins DC. Mesenteric lymphadenitis in adolescents simulating appendicitis. Can Med Assoc J. 1936;34:402–5.
118. Mair NS, Mair HJ, Stirk EM, et al. Three cases of acute mesenteric lymphadenitis due to *Pasteurella pseudotuberculosis*. J Clin Pathol. 1960;13:432–9.
119. Dudley HAF, MacLaren IF. Primary mesenteric abscess. Lancet. 1956;2:1182–4.
120. Asch MJ, Amoury RA, Touloukian RJ, et al. Suppurative mesenteric lymphadenitis: A report of two cases and review of the literature. Am J Surg. 1968;115:570–3.
121. Constantinides CG, Davies MRQ, Cywes S. Suppurative mesenteric lymphadenitis in children: Case reports. S Afr Med J. 1981;60:629–31.
122. Rey C, Escribano JC, Foz M, et al. Mesenteric adenitis secondary to *Giardia lamblia*. Dig Dis Sci. 1980;25:968–71.
123. Winblad S, Nilehn B, Sternby NJ. *Yersinia enterocolitica* (Pasteurella X) in human enteric infections. Br Med J. 1966;2:1363–6.
124. Carter PB. Pathogenicity of *Yersinia enterocolitica* for mice. Infect Immun. 1975;11:164–70.
125. Une T. Studies on the pathogenicity of *Yersinia enterocolitica:* II. Interaction with cultured cells in vitro. Microbiol Immunol. 1977;21:365–77.
126. Kay BA, Wachsmuth K, Gemski P, et al. Virulence and phenotypic characterization of *Yersinia enterocolitica* isolated from humans in the United States. J Clin Microbiol. 1983;17:128–38.
127. Feeley JC, Wells JG, Tsai TF, et al. Detection of enterotoxigenic and invasive strains of *Yersinia enterocolitica*. Contrib Microbiol Immunol. 1979;5:329–34.
128. Zink DL, Feeley JC, Wells JG, et al. Plasmid-mediated tissue invasiveness in *Yersinia enterocolitica*. Nature. 1980;283:224–6.

129. Kay BA, Wachsmuth K, Gemski P. New virulence-associated plasmid in *Yersinia enterocolitica*. J Clin Microbiol. 1982;15:1161–3.
130. Jepsen OB, Korner B, Lauritsen KB, et al. *Yersinia enterocolitica* infection in patients with acute surgical abdominal disease: A prospective study. Scand J Infect Dis. 1976;8:189–94.
131. Zen-Yoji H, Maruyama T, Sakai S, et al. An outbreak of enteritis due to *Yersinia enterocolitica* occurring at a junior high school. Jpn J Microbiol. 1973;17:220.
132. Asakawa Y, Akahane S, Kagata N, et al. Two community outbreaks of human infection with *Yersinia enterocolitica*. J Hyg (Camb). 1973;71:715–23.
133. Black RE, Jackson RJ, Tsai T, et al. Epidemic *Yersinia enterocolitica* infection due to contaminated chocolate milk. N Engl J Med. 1978;298:76–9.
134. Vantrappen G, Agg HO, Ponette E, et al. *Yersinia* enteritis and enterocolitis: Gastroenterological aspects. Gastroenterology. 1977;72:220–7.
135. Jansson E, Wallgren GR, Ahvonen P. *Yersinia enterocolitica* as a cause of acute mesenteric lymphadenitis. Acta Paediatr Scand. 1968;57:448–50.
136. Tauxe RV, Vandepitte J, Wauters G, et al. *Yersinia enterocolitica* infections and pork: The missing link. Lancet. 1987;1:1129–32.
137. Knapp W. Mesenteric adenitis due to *Pasteurella pseudotuberculosis* in young people. N Engl J Med. 1958;259:776–8.
138. Randall KJ, Mair NS. Family outbreak of *Pasteurella pseudotuberculosis* infection. Lancet. 162;1:1042–3.
139. Weber J, Finlayson NB, Mark JBD. Mesenteric lymphadenitis and terminal ileitis due to *Yersinia pseudotuberculosis*. N Engl J Med. 1970;283:172–4.
140. Saari TN, Triplett DA. *Yersinia pseudotuberculosis* mesenteric adenitis. J Pediatr. 1974;85:656–9.
141. Bradford WD, Noce PS, Gutman LT. Pathologic features of enteric infection with *Yersinia enterocolitica*. Arch Pathol. 1974;98:17–22.
142. Weissfeld AS, Sonnenwirth AC. *Yersinia enterocolitica* in adults with gastrointestinal disturbances: Need for cold enrichment. J Clin Microbiol. 1980;11:196–7.
143. Daniëls JJHM. Enteral infection with *Pasteurella pseudotuberculosis:* Isolation of the organism from human feces. Br Med J. 1961;2:997.
144. Niléhn B, Sjöström B. Studies on *Yersinia enterocolitica*. Acta Pathol Microbiol Scand. 1967;71:612–28.
145. Marks MI, Pai CH, Lafleur L, et al. *Yersinia enterocolitica* gastroenteritis: A prospective study of clinical, bacteriologic, and epidemiologic features. J Pediatr. 1980;96:26–31.
146. Puylaert JB. Mesenteric adenitis and acute terminal ileitis: Ultrasound evaluation using graded compression. Radiol. 1986;161:691–5.
147. Ekberg O, Sjöström B, Brahme F. Radiological findings in *Yersinia* ileitis. Radiology. 1977;123:15–9.
148. Ahlqvist J, Ahvonen P, Räsänen JA, et al. Enteric infection with *Yersinia enterocolitica:* Large pyroninophilic cell reproduction in mesenteric lymph nodes associated with early production of specific antibodies. Acta Pathol Microbiol Scand [A]. 1971;79:109–22.
149. Braunstein H, Tucker EB, Gibson BC. Mesenteric lymphadenitis due to *Yersinia enterocolitica:* Report of a case. Am J Clin Pathol. 1971;55:506–10.
150. El-Maraghi NRH, Mair NS. The histopathology of enteric infection with *Yersinia pseudotuberculosis*. Am J Clin Pathol. 1979;71:631–9.
151. Gutman LT, Ottesen EA, Quan TJ, et al. An inter-familial outbreak of *Yersinia enterocolitica* enteritis. N Engl J Med. 1973;288:1372–7.
152. Arvastson B, Damgaard K, Winblad S. Clinical symptoms of infection with *Yersinia enterocolitica*. Scand J Infect Dis. 1971;3:37–40.
153. Wilson HD, McCormick JB, Feeley JC. *Yersinia enterocolitica* infection in a 4-month-old infant associated with infection in household dogs. J Pediatr. 1976;89:767–8.
154. Tacket CO, Narain JP, Sattin R, et al. A multistate outbreak of infections caused by *Yersinia enterocolitica* transmitted by pasteurized milk. JAMA. 1984;251:483–6.
155. Nolan C, Harris N, Ballard J, et al. Outbreak of *Yersinia enterocolitica:* Washington State. MMWR. 1982;31:562.
156. Laasen J. *Yersinia enterocolitica* in drinking-water. Scand J Infect Dis. 1972;4:125–7.
157. Highsmith AK, Feeley JC, Skaliy P, et al. Isolation of *Yersinia enterocolitica* from well water and growth in distilled water. Appl Environ Microbiol. 1977;34:745–50.
158. Snyder JD, Christenson E, Feldman RA. Human *Yersinia enterocolitica* infections in Wisconsin. Am J Med. 1982;72:768–74.
159. Loría-Cortés R, Lobo-Sanahuja JF. Clinical abdominal angiostrongylosis: A study of 116 children with intestinal eosinophilic granuloma caused by *Angiostrongylus costaricensis*. Am J Trop Med Hyg. 1980;29:538–44.
160. Gutman LT, Wilfert CM, Quan T. Susceptibility of *Yersinia enterocolitica* to trimethoprim–sulfamethoxazole. J Infect Dis. 1973;128(Suppl):S538.
161. Hornstein MJ, Jupeau AM, Scavizzi MR, et al. *In vitro* susceptibilities of 126 clinical isolates of *Yersinia enterocolitica* to 21 β-lactam antibiotics. Antimicrob Agents Chemother. 1985;27:806–11.
162. Hammerberg S, Sorger S, Marks MI. Antimicrobial susceptibilities of *Yersinia enterocolitica* biotype 4, serotype 0:3. Antimicrob Agents Chemother. 1977;11:566–8.
163. Grove DI, Warren KS, Mahmoud AAF. Algorithms in the diagnosis and management of exotic diseases: III. Strongyloidiasis. J Infect Dis. 1975;131:755–8.
164. Jones CA. Clinical studies in human strongyloidiasis: I. Semeiology. Gastroenterology. 1950;16:743–56.
165. Purtilo DT, Meyers WM, Connor DH. Fatal strongyloidiasis in immunosuppressed patients. Am J Med. 1974;56:488–93.
166. Morgan JS, Schaffner W, Stone WJ. Opportunistic strongyloidiasis in renal transplant recipients. Transplantation. 1986;42:518–24.
167. Cadranel JF, Eugene C. Another example of *Strongyloides stercoralis* infection associated with cimetidine in an immunosuppressed patient. Gut. 1986;27:1229.
168. Pelletier LL Jr, Baker CB, Gam AA, et al. Diagnosis and evaluation of treatment of chronic strongyloidiasis in ex-prisoners of war. J Infect Dis. 1988;157:573–6.
169. Gill GV, Bell DR. *Strongyloides stercoralis* infection in former Far East prisoners of war. Br Med J [Clin Res]. 1979;2:572–4.
170. Grove DI. Strongyloidiasis in Allied ex-prisoners of war in south-east Asia. Br Med J [Clin Res]. 1980;280:598–601.
171. Pelletier LL Jr. Chronic strongyloidiasis in World War II Far East ex-prisoners of war. Am J Trop Med Hyg. 1984;33:55–61.
172. Berk SL, Verghese A, Alvarez S, et al. Clinical and epidemiologic features of strongyloidiasis: A prospective study in rural Tennessee. Arch Intern Med. 1987;147:1257–61.
173. Beal CB, Viens P, Grant RGL, et al. A new technique for sampling duodenal contents: Demonstration of upper small bowel pathogens. Am J Trop Med Hyg. 1970;19:399–52.
174. Blumenthal DS, Schultz MG. Incidence of intestinal obstruction in children infected with *Ascaris lumbricoides*. Am J Trop Med Hyg. 1975;24:801–5.
175. Krige JEJ, Lewis G, Bornman PC. Recurrent pancreatitis caused by a calcified ascaris in the duct of Wirsung. Am J Gastroenterol. 1987;82:256–7.
176. Schantz PM, Glickman LT. Toxocaral visceral larva migrans. N Engl J Med. 1978;298:436–9.
177. Taylor MRH, Keane CT, O'Connor P, et al. The expanded spectrum of toxocaral disease. Lancet. 1988;1:692–5.
178. Thompson DE, Bundy DAP, Cooper ES, et al. Epidemiological characteristics of *Toxocara canis* zoonotic infection of children in a Caribbean community. *Bull WHO*. 1986;64:283–90.
179. Glickman LT, Magnaval J-F, Domanski LM, et al. Visceral larva migrans in French adults: A new disease syndrome. Am J Epidemiol. 1987;125:1019–34.
180. Grove DI, Warren KS, Mahmoud AAF. Algorithms in the diagnosis and management of exotic diseases: VII. Trichinosis. J Infect Dis. 1975;132:485–8.
181. Campbell WC. Trichinella and Trichinosis. New York: Plenum Press; 1983.
182. Stehr-Green JK, Schantz PM, Chisolm EM. Trichinosis surveillance, 1984. MMWR. 1985;35:11–15SS.
183. Singal M, Schantz PM, Werner SB. Trichinosis acquired at sea: Report of an outbreak. Am J Trop Med Hyg. 1976;25:675–81.
184. Petri WA Jr, Holsinger JR, Pearson RD. Common-source outbreak of trichinosis associated with eating raw home-butchered pork. South Med J. 1988;81:1056–8.
185. Trichinosis outbreaks associated with horsemeat. Parasitol Today. 1986;2:295.
186. Viallet J, MacLean JD, Goresky CA, et al. Arctic trichinosis presenting as prolonged diarrhea. Gastroenterology. 1986;91:938–46.
187. Kagan IG. Serodiagnosis of trichinosis. In: Cohen S, Sadun EH, eds. Immunology of Parasitic Infections. Oxford: Blackwell Scientific; 1976:143–51.
188. Pinkus GS, Coolidge C. Intestinal anisakiasis: First case report from North America. Am J Med. 1975;59:114–20.
189. Richman RH, Lewicki AM. Right ileocolitis secondary to anisakiasis. Am J Roentgen Rad Ther Nucl Med. 1973;119:329–31.
190. Yokogawa M, Yoshimura H. Clinicopathologic studies on larval anisakiasis in Japan. Am J Trop Med Hyg. 1967;16:723–34.
191. Whalen GE, Strickland GT, Cross JH, et al. Intestinal capillariasis: A new disease in man. Lancet. 1969;1:13–6.
192. Watten RH, Beckner WM, Cross JH, et al. Clinical studies of capillariasis philippinensis. Trans R Soc Trop Med Hyg. 1972;66:828–34.
193. Fresh JW, Cross JH, Reyes V, et al. Necropsy findings in intestinal capillariasis. Am J Trop Med Hyg. 1972;21:169–73.
194. Cross JH, Banzon T, Clarke MD, et al. Studies on the experimental transmission of *Capillaria philippinensis* in monkeys. Trans R Soc Trop Med Hyg. 1972;66:819–27.
195. Morera P, Perez F, Mora F, et al. Visceral larva migrans-like syndrome caused by *Angiostrongylus costaricensis*. Am J Trop Med Hyg. 1982;31:67–70.
196. Mahmoud AA. Schistosomiasis. N Engl J Med. 1977;297:1329–31.
197. Warren KS. Schistosomiasis japonicum. In Marsden PD, ed. Clinics in Gastroenterology. v. 17. no. 1: Intestinal Parasites. London: WB Saunders; 1978:77–85.
198. Farid Z, Trabolsi B, Hafez A. Acute schistosomiasis mansoni (Katayama syndrome). Ann Trop Med Parasitol. 1986;80:563–4.
199. Hardman EW, Jones RLH, Davies AH. Fascioliasis—a large outbreak. Br Med J. 1970;3:502–5.
200. Stork MG, Venables GS, Jennings SMF, et al. An investigation of endemic fascioliasis in Peruvian village children. J Trop Med Hyg. 1973;76:231–5.
201. Jones EA, Kay JM, Milligan HP, et al. Massive infection with *Fasciola hepatica* in man. Am J Med. 1977;63:836–42.
202. Plaut AG, Kampanart-Sanyakorn C, Manning GS. A clinical study of *Fasciolopsis buski* infection in Thailand. Trans R Soc Trop Med Hyg. 1969;63:470–8.

203. Warren KS, Mahmoud AAF. Algorithms in the diagnosis and management of exotic diseases. XXI. Liver, intestinal and lung flukes. J Infect Dis. 1977;135:692–6.
204. Lin AC, Chapman SW, Turner HR, et al. Clonorchiasis: An update. South Med J. 1987;80:919–22.
205. Brockelman WY, Upatham ES, Viyanant V, et al. Measurement of incidence of the human liver fluke, *Opisthorchis viverrini*, in northeast Thailand. Trans R Soc Trop Med Hyg. 1987;81:327–35.
206. Warren KS, Mahmoud AAF. Algorithms in the diagnosis and management of exotic diseases: XIV. Tapeworms. J Infect Dis. 1976;134:108–12.
207. Grove DI, Warren KS, Mahmoud AAF. Algorithms in the diagnosis and management of exotic diseases. X. Echinococcosis. J Infect Dis. 1976;133:354–8.
208. Kagan IG. Current status of serologic testing for parasitic diseases. Hosp Pract. 1974;9:157–63.
209. Trier JS, Moxey PC, Schimmel EM, et al. Chronic intestinal coccidiosis in man: Intestinal morphology and response to treatment. Gastroenterology. 1974;66:923–35.
210. Liebman WM, Thaler MM, DeLorimier A, et al. Intractable diarrhea of infancy due to intestinal coccidiosis. Gastroenterology. 1980;78:579–84.
211. DeHovitz JA, Pape JW, Boncy M, et al. Clinical manifestations and therapy of *Isospora belli* infection in patients with the acquired immunodeficiency syndrome. N Engl J Med. 1986;315:87–90.
212. Spencer MJ, Garcia LS, Chapin MR. *Dientamoeba fragilis:* An intestinal pathogen in children? Am J Dis Child. 1979;133:390–3.
213. Yang J, Scholten TH. *Dientamoeba fragilis:* A review with notes on its epidemiology, pathogenicity, mode of transmission, and diagnosis. Am J Trop Med Hyg. 1977;26:16–22.
214. Blackshaw AJ, Levison DA. Eosinophilic infiltrates of the gastrointestinal tract. J Clin Pathol. 1986;39:1–7.
215. Tedesco FJ, Huckaby CB, Hamby-Allen M, et al. Eosinophilic ileocolitis: Expanding spectrum of eosinophilic gastroenteritis. Dig Dis Sci. 1981;26:943–8.
216. Klein NC, Hargrove L, Sleisenger MH, et al. Eosinophilic gastroenteritis. Medicine. 1970;49:299–319.
217. Leinbach GE, Rubin CE. Eosinophilic gastroenteritis: A simple reaction to food allergens? Gastroenterology. 1970;59:874–89.
218. Goldberg HI, O'Kieffe D, Jenis EH, et al. Diffuse eosinophilic gastroenteritis. Am J Roentgen Rad Therapy Nucl Med. 1973;119:342–51.
219. Tytgat GN, Grijm, R, Dekker W, et al. Fatal eosinophilic enteritis. Gastroenterology. 1976;71:479–83.
220. Cupps TR, Fauci AS. The Vasculitides. Philadelphia: WB Saunders; 1981.
221. Mowrey FH, Lundberg EA. The clinical manifestations of essential polyangiitis (periarteritis nodosa), with emphasis on the hepatic manifestations. Ann Intern Med. 1954;40:1145–64.
222. Nightingale EJ. The gastroenterological aspects of periarteritis nodosa. Am J Gastroenterol. 1959;31:152–65.
223. Leavitt RY, Fauci AS. Polyangiitis overlap syndrome. Am J Med. 1986;81:79–85.
224. Churg J, Strauss L. Allergic granulomatosis, allergic angiitis and periarteritis nodosa. Am J Pathol. 1951;27:277–301.
225. Finch SC. Granulocytosis. In: Williams WJ, Beutler E, Erslev AJ, et al. eds. Hematology. New York: McGraw-Hill; 1977:746–755.
226. Haeberle MG, Griffen WO Jr. Eosinophilia and regional enteritis: A possible diagnostic aid. Am J Dig Dis. 1972;17:200–4.
227. Glotzer DJ, Gardner RC, Goldman H, et al. Comparative features and course of ulcerative and granulomatous colitis. N Engl J Med. 1970;282:582–7.
228. Isaacson NJ, Rapoport P. Eosinophilia in malignant tumors: Its significance. Ann Intern Med. 1946;25:893–902.
229. Banerjee RN, Narang RM. Haematological changes in malignancy. Br J Haematol. 1967;13:829–43.
230. Beeson P. Cancer and eosinophilia. N Engl J Med. 1983;309:792–3.

86. FOOD-BORNE DISEASE

JAMES M. HUGHES
ROBERT V. TAUXE

Food-borne disease syndromes result from ingestion of a wide variety of foods contaminated with pathogenic microorganisms, microbial toxins, or chemicals. From 1972 to 1982, between 300 and 600 outbreaks of food-borne disease affecting 10,000–18,000 people in the United States were reported annually to the Centers for Disease Control (CDC).[1–5] These figures certainly underestimate the magnitude of the problem. The actual incidence of food-borne disease is unknown but has been estimated to be 9,000,000 illnesses annually.[6]

Although a wide variety of microorganisms and toxins can cause food-borne disease, this discussion will focus on food-borne disease syndromes that are acute (onset of symptoms usually within 72 hours of ingestion) and whose clinical features include gastrointestinal manifestations. The diseases to be discussed and the frequency with which outbreaks were reported to the CDC from 1972 to 1986 are indicated in Table 1.

TABLE 1. Etiology of Food-borne Disease Outbreaks of Known Etiology Reported to the CDC, 1972–1986

Etiology	*Number of Outbreaks*	*Percentage of Total*
Bacterial		
Salmonella	753	27.4
S. aureus	395	14.4
C. botulinum	220[a]	8.0
C. perfringens	187	6.8
Shigella	99	3.6
B. cereus	52	1.9
C. jejuni	49	1.8
V. parahaemolyticus	25	0.9
Y. enterocolitica	5	0.2
V. cholerae 01	5[b]	0.2
Verotoxigenic *E. coli*	4	0.1
L. monocytogenes	3	0.1
Other	30	1.1
Chemical		
Ciguatera	206	7.5
Histamine fish poisoning (scombroid)	182	6.6
Mushrooms	64	2.3
Heavy metals	53	1.9
Paralytic shellfish poisoning (PSP)	20	0.7
Chinese restaurant syndrome	19	0.7
Neurotoxic shellfish poisoning (NSP)	2	0.1
Other	111	4.0
Parasitic[c]	147	5.4
Viral	114	4.1
	Total 2745	99.8

[a] Excludes cases of infant botulism.
[b] Includes outbreaks on Guam[7] and in Louisiana.[8]
[c] Includes first two reported food-borne outbreaks caused by *Giardia lamblia*.[9,10]

PATHOGENESIS AND CLINICAL FEATURES

The diagnosis of food-borne disease should be considered when an acute illness with gastrointestinal or neurologic manifestations affects two or more persons who have shared a meal during the previous 72 hours. Important clues to the etiologic agent are provided by both the symptoms and incubation period.

Food-borne Disease Due to Microbial Agents or Their Toxins (Table 2)

Nausea and Vomiting within 1–6 Hours. The major etiologic considerations are *Staphylococcus aureus* and *Bacillus cereus*. The relatively short incubation period reflects the fact that these diseases are caused by a preformed enterotoxin. Staphylococcal food poisoning is characterized by vomiting (76 percent of the cases) and diarrhea (77 percent); fever is relatively uncommon (23 percent).[11] Staphylococci responsible for episodes of food poisoning produce one or more enterotoxins; five immunologically distinct heat-stable proteins (A, B, C, D, E) with molecular weights ranging from 28,000 to 35,000 daltons have been identified.[12] Another staphylococcal protein, enterotoxin F, is produced by the majority of *S. aureus* strains causing toxic shock syndrome[13] but has not been reported to cause food-borne disease. Although the mechanism of action of these enterotoxins in humans has not been clarified, studies in monkeys and cats suggest that the enterotoxin produces its emetic action after interaction with abdominal viscera.[14,15] The sensory stimulus is carried to the vomiting center in the brain by the vagus and sympathetic nerves.[14] Other studies suggest that diarrhea may result from inhibition of water and sodium absorption in the small intestine by enterotoxin.[16]

TABLE 2. Pathogenic Mechanisms in Bacterial Food-borne Disease

Preformed Toxin	*Toxin Production in Vivo*	*Tissue Invasion*	*Toxin Production and/or Tissue Invasion*
S. aureus	*C. perfringens*	*C. jejuni*	*V. parahaemolyticus*
B. cereus (short incubation)	*B. cereus* (long incubation)	*Salmonella*	*Y. enterocolitica*
C. botulinum	*C. botulinum* (infant botulism)	*Shigella*	
	Enterotoxigenic *E. coli*	Invasive *E. coli*	
	V. cholerae 01		
	V. cholerae non-01		
	Verotoxigenic *E. coli*		

Enterotoxigenic staphylococci isolated from implicated foods in outbreaks are most often lysed by group III phages; less commonly, they are lysed by both group I and group III phages or by group I phages alone.[17] Over 99 percent of enterotoxigenic staphylococci associated with food poisoning are coagulase positive; occasionally, an outbreak caused by enterotoxigenic *Staphylococcus epidermidis* is reported.[18] In the past, strains producing type A enterotoxin alone accounted for 44–69 percent of the reported outbreaks of staphylococcal food poisoning in the United States and England.[19,20] Strains producing type D enterotoxin, either alone or in combination with type A, were the next most frequently implicated. Strains producing enterotoxins B, C, or E alone accounted for fewer than 10 percent of the outbreaks. During 1979–1981, all reported staphylococcal food-borne outbreaks in the United States of known toxin type were caused by strains producing type A enterotoxin alone.[21]

Bacillus cereus strains can cause two types of food poisoning syndromes: one characterized primarily by nausea and vomiting with an incubation period of 1–6 hours (short-incubation "emetic" syndrome) and a second manifested primarily by abdominal cramps and diarrhea with an incubation period of 8–16 hours (long-incubation "diarrhea" syndrome).[22,23] Recent evidence suggests that the short-incubation syndrome, which is characterized by vomiting (100 percent of the cases), abdominal cramps (100 percent), and, less frequently, diarrhea (33 percent)[24] may be caused by a heat-stable toxin produced by some *B. cereus* strains and capable of causing vomiting when fed to monkeys.[25] The mechanism and site of action of this toxin, which has a molecular weight of less than 5000, are unknown.[26]

Another clue to the cause of both staphylococcal and short-incubation *B. cereus* outbreaks is provided by the fact that the illnesses are of short duration, usually lasting less than 12 hours.[11,24]

Abdominal Cramps and Diarrhea within 8–16 Hours. The major etiologic considerations for this syndrome, which is also enterotoxin mediated, are *Clostridium perfringens* and *B. cereus*. In contrast to staphylococcal food poisoning and the short-incubation *B. cereus* disease, which are caused by ingestion of preformed enterotoxins in food, *C. perfringens* and long-incubation *B. cereus* food poisoning are caused by toxins produced in vivo, accounting for the longer incubation period. In *C. perfringens* food poisoning, the most common symptoms are diarrhea and abdominal cramps. Although nausea may occur, vomiting and fever are uncommon, occurring in less than 10 percent of the patients.[27,28] Only *C. perfringens* type A strains have been associated with this food poisoning syndrome.[28,29] *Clostridium perfringens* enterotoxin is a heat-labile protein with a molecular weight of approximately 35,000 daltons[30] synthesized during sporulation of the vegetative cells of *C. perfringens* in the gastrointestinal tract; the enterotoxin is released during lysis of the sporangium.[31] Studies in rabbits and rats indicate that the enterotoxin is active throughout the small intestine, with greatest activity in the ileum, in which net secretion of sodium and fluid and inhibition of chloride and glucose absorption occur.[32,33] The enterotoxin damages brush borders of epithelial cells at villus tips.[33]

Bacillus cereus strains, which cause a similar syndrome characterized by diarrhea (96 percent) and abdominal cramps (75 percent), sometimes vomiting (33 percent), and rarely fever,[24] elaborate a heat-labile enterotoxin with a molecular weight of approximately 50,000[26] that activates intestinal adenylate cyclase and results in intestinal fluid secretion.[34] This enterotoxin appears to also have cytotoxic properties in rabbit small intestine and guinea pig skin.[26,34]

Although nausea occurs in many patients with *C. perfringens* and long-incubation *B. cereus* food poisoning, vomiting occurs infrequently. In fact, occurrence of vomiting in greater than one-third of affected people suggests that these organisms are not involved. Although these illnesses last longer than staphylococcal and short-incubation *B. cereus* food poisoning, symptoms usually resolve within 24 hours.[24,35] However, in one large long-incubation *B. cereus* outbreak involving elderly patients in a chronic disease hospital, the mean duration of illness was 2.3 days, and one patient was ill for 10 days.[36]

Fever, Abdominal Cramps, and Diarrhea within 16–48 Hours. The major etiologic considerations for this syndrome are salmonellae, shigellae, *Campylobacter jejuni, Vibrio parahaemolyticus*, and invasive *Escherichia coli*. These organisms cause this syndrome after tissue invasion.[37–42] Vomiting occurs in 35–80 percent of the patients.[43–46] These illnesses usually resolve within 2–7 days.

Campylobacter jejuni is the most common food-borne bacterial pathogen.[47,48] The frequency of fecal blood and polymorphonuclear leukocytes[49] and colitis[50] suggests that this organism also causes this syndrome after tissue invasion. In contrast to the illnesses caused by other organisms in this group, *C. jejuni* food poisoning is characterized by vomiting in only 15–25 percent of cases[49,51,52] and a longer incubation period of 1–7 days.[47] The duration of illness is usually less than 1 week, but relapses may occur in untreated patients.[53]

The diarrhea experienced by patients with *Vibrio cholerae* non-01 infection is sometimes bloody, and fever may be present.[54–56]

Abdominal Cramps and Watery Diarrhea within 16–72 Hours. The major etiologic considerations in this syndrome are enterotoxigenic strains of *E. coli, V. parahaemolyticus, V. cholerae* non-01, and in endemic areas, *V. cholerae* 01; *C. jejuni*, salmonellae, and shigellae may also cause this syndrome. Enterotoxins synthesized in vivo are responsible for the syndrome caused by *V. cholerae* 01.[57] *Vibrio cholerae* non-01,[58,59] and enterotoxigenic strains of *E. coli*[60]; enterotoxigenic and/or cytotoxic substances may also play a role in the pathogenesis of this syndrome when caused by salmonellae,[61,62] shigellae,[63–65] and *V. parahaemolyticus*.[66,67]

Fever and vomiting occur in a minority of cases.[68–71] With the exception of cholera, which may last for 5 days, and disease due to *V. cholerae* non-01, which may last for 2–12 days, these illnesses usually resolve within 72–96 hours. However, in one documented enterotoxigenic *E. coli* outbreak, the median duration of illness was 7 days.[72]

Food-borne transmission of the Norwalk agent, a 27-nm virus, may be common.[73–76] In contrast to the illness produced by bacterial agents causing this syndrome, vomiting is a prominent feature of Norwalk agent gastroenteritis and occurs in the majority of cases.[73] The duration of illness is usually 24–48 hours. The occurrence of secondary cases in close contacts not exposed to the suspected food is an important clue to the possibility of a Norwalk agent etiology. A Norwalk-like virus (Snow Mountain agent) has recently been reported to be transmitted by food.[77] The importance of food in transmission of other similar viral agents (e.g., Hawaii, Ditchling, Colorado, and Marin County agents) remains to be determined.[78]

Fever and Abdominal Cramps within 16–48 Hours. *Yersinia enterocolitica* has been incriminated as a cause of food-borne outbreaks in the United States and is a more common cause of food-borne disease in Northern Europe and Canada.[79–82] Although some strains of this organism have been reported to produce a heat-stable enterotoxin,[83,84] the frequent occurrence of fever and mesenteric adenitis suggests that this organism causes disease as a result of tissue invasion. In older children and adults, the clinical illness may closely resemble acute appendicitis; nausea and vomiting are relatively uncommon, occurring in less than 25–40 percent of the cases.[81,85] Diarrhea is the most common symptom in infants.[86] Duration of the illness may range from 24 hours to 4 weeks.[81,85]

Bloody Diarrhea without Fever within 72–120 Hours. The distinctive syndrome of hemorrhagic colitis has been linked to verotoxigenic strains of *E. coli*, most often serotype 0157:H7.[87–89] These strains, which cause diarrhea in infant rabbits,[87,90] produce a cytotoxin for Vero cells, which has been neutralized by antiserum to shiga toxin.[91,92] The illness is characterized by abdominal cramps and diarrhea, which is initially watery but subsequently grossly bloody. Patients with uncomplicated infection usually remain afebrile. The mean incubation period in two outbreaks was 4 days. The duration of uncomplicated illness ranges from 1 to 12 days. The development of fever and leukocytosis may herald complications, which include hemolytic-uremic syndrome, thrombotic thrombocytopenic purpura, and death.[88,93–95] Case fatality rates in two nursing home outbreaks were 16 and 35 percent.[88,93]

Nausea, Vomiting, Diarrhea, and Paralysis within 18–36 Hours. The occurrence of acute gastrointestinal symptoms simultaneously with or just before the onset of descending weakness or paralysis strongly suggests the diagnosis of food-borne botulism. Constipation is common once the neurologic syndrome is well established, but nausea and vomiting occur at onset in 50 percent of the patients, and diarrhea occurs in approximately 20–25 percent.[96–98] The pathogenesis of the acute gastrointestinal symptoms is not understood; the botulinal toxins, which inhibit acetylcholine release from nerve endings,[99,100] do not appear to be responsible. The disease in humans is usually caused by one of three immunologically distinct heat-labile protein neurotoxins designated A, B, and E,[101] which are produced after germination of *Clostridium botulinum* spores in inadequately processed foods. The disease in older children and adults results from ingestion of preformed toxin. The syndrome of infant botulism appears to result from ingestion of spores with subsequent toxin production in vivo.[102–104] Both illnesses last from several weeks to several months. Clinical suspicion is critical if the disease is to be correctly diagnosed.[105]

Food-borne Disease due to Chemicals of Nonmicrobial Origin

Nausea, Vomiting, and Abdominal Cramps within 1 Hour. The major etiologic considerations for this syndrome are heavy metals; copper, zinc, tin, and cadmium have caused food-borne outbreaks.[106–110] Incubation periods most often range from 5 to 15 minutes. Nausea, vomiting, and abdominal cramps result from irritation of the gastric mucosa and usually resolve within 2–3 hours after removal of the offending agent during emesis.

Paresthesias within 1 Hour. When patients have this symptom, fish poisoning, shellfish poisoning (Table 3), and the "Chinese restaurant syndrome," and niacin poisoning are the major possibilities.

Histamine fish poisoning (scombroid) is characterized by symptoms resembling those of a histamine reaction. Burning of the mouth and throat, flushing, headache, and dizziness are common; abdominal cramps, nausea, vomiting, and diarrhea also occur in a majority of the cases.[111] In severe cases, urticaria and bronchospasm may also occur. Symptoms are thought to result from histamine and inhibitors of histamine degradation produced in fish flesh by the enzymatic decarboxylation of histidine by certain marine bacteria.[112–115] In an outbreak traced to tuna sashimi,[116] a strain of *Klebsiella pneumoniae* capable of producing large quantities of histamine was implicated.[117] Symptoms usually resolve in a few hours.

Two types of shellfish poisoning should be considered: paralytic (PSP) and neurotoxic (NSP).[118] PSP is characterized by paresthesias of the mouth, lips, face, and extremities.[119–123] In severe cases, dyspnea, dysphagia, muscle weakness or frank paralysis, ataxia, and respiratory insufficiency may occur.[119,122] Respiratory failure may occur during the first 12 hours of the illness.[122] Some patients also have nausea, vomiting, and diarrhea.[118] The disease is caused by neurotoxic substances in dinoflagellates, one of which is known as *saxitoxin*. Bivalve mollusks feed on these dinoflagellates; the toxins are concentrated in their flesh but do not affect the mollusks.[119] Saxitoxin appears to be the only neurotoxin produced by *Gonyaulax catenella*, whereas *Gonyaulax tamarensis* produces saxitoxin and several additional neurotoxic substances.[124–126] The structure of saxitoxin has been determined[127]; it is heat stable and blocks the propagation of nerve and muscle action potentials by interfering with the increase in sodium permeability by acting at a metal cation binding site in the sodium channels of nerve membranes.[128–130] The mechanism of action of the other neurotoxins is unknown. Duration of the illness ranges from a few hours to a few days.[118]

Although many patients with PSP experience the onset of symptoms within 1 hour of ingestion, the incubation period is often inversely related to the amount of toxin ingested. A European outbreak involved 120 cases after the ingestion of contaminated mussels; the median incubation period in this outbreak was 3.5 hours, with a range of 1–10 hours.[121]

The clinical features of NSP are similar to those of PSP, but

TABLE 3. Fish and Shellfish Poisoning Syndromes

Syndrome	*Incubation Period*	*Duration*	*Geographic Location*[a]	*Season*
Histamine fish poisoning (scombroid)	5 min–1 hr	Few hours	Primarily coastal areas (Hawaii, California)	Year round
Ciguatera	1–6 hr	Few days–few months	35°–35°S latitude (Hawaii, Florida)	Feb.–Sept.
Paralytic shellfish poisoning	5 min–4 hr	Few hours–few days	Above 30°N and below 30°S latitude (New England, West Coast)	May–Nov.
Neurotoxic shellfish poisoning	5 min–4 hr	Few hours–few days	Gulf and Atlantic coasts of Florida (Florida)	Spring, fall

[a] Location of U.S. outbreaks in parentheses.

paralysis does not occur.[118,119] Several poorly characterized neurotoxins responsible for this illness are found in *Gymnodinium breve*, the responsible dinoflagellate.[131–133] One of these neurotoxins stimulates postganglionic cholinergic nerve fibers.[134] Duration of the illness ranges from a few hours to a few days.[118]

The Chinese restaurant syndrome is characterized by a burning sensation in the neck, chest, abdomen, or arms and by a sensation of tightness over the face and chest.[135] Headache, flushing, diaphoresis, lacrimation, weakness, nausea, abdominal cramps, and thirst frequently occur.[135,136] Symptoms appear to be caused by excessive amounts of monosodium L-glutamate in foods, although other undefined substances may also play a role.[135,136] The illness usually resolves within several hours.

Niacin poisoning produces a burning facial erythema within 20 minutes of ingestion, which rapidly resolves.[137]

Paresthesias within 1–6 Hours. The major diagnostic considerations for this syndrome are PSP and ciguatera fish poisoning (Table 3), which is often characterized by the onset of abdominal cramps, nausea, vomiting, and diarrhea preceded or followed by numbness and paresthesias of the lips, tongue, and throat.[138–140] Malaise, headache, pruritus, dry mouth, metallic taste, myalgias, arthralgias, blurred vision, photophobia, and transient blindness have also been reported.[141–143] Sharp shooting pains in the legs and a sensation of looseness and pain in the teeth are characteristic.[139] In severe cases, reversal of hot and cold temperature sensations, sinus bradycardia, hypotension, cranial nerve palsies, and respiratory paralysis may occur.[140,141,144]

The illness is caused by ciguatoxin, a poorly characterized lipid-soluble, relatively heat-stable compound,[145] which is acquired by fish through the food chain.[146] The dinoflagellate, *Gambierdiscus toxicus*, has been identified as the source of the toxin in the food chain.[147] Ciguatoxin inhibits red blood cell cholinesterase activity,[148] increases membrane sodium permeability,[149] and changes the electrical potential of cells through its action on sodium channels.[150,151] Duration of the acute illness ranges from a few days to a few months; pain in the extremities has been reported to occur intermittently for years after an episode of ciguatera.

Miscellaneous Mushroom Poisoning Syndromes within 2 Hours. At least five clinical syndromes may occur within 2 hours of ingestion of toxic mushrooms[152–155] (Table 4). Species containing ibotenic acid and muscimol cause an illness mimicking acute alcoholic intoxication characterized by confusion, restlessness, and visual disturbances followed by lethargy; symptoms resolve within 24 hours. Species containing muscarine cause an illness characterized by evidence of parasympathetic hyperactivity, for example, salivation, lacrimation, diaphoresis, blurred vision, abdominal cramps, and diarrhea. Some patients experience miosis, bradycardia, and bronchospasm. Symptoms usually resolve within 24 hours. Species containing the toxic substances psilocybin and psilocin cause an acute psychotic reaction manifested by hallucinations and inappropriate behavior, which usually resolves within 12 hours. The mushroom *Coprinus atramentarius* contains a disulfiram-like substance that can result in headache, flushing, paresthesias, nausea, vomiting, and tachycardia if alcohol is consumed during the 48-hour period after ingestion. The fifth clinical syndrome is characterized by nausea, vomiting, abdominal cramps, and diarrhea after the ingestion of mushrooms containing gastrointestinal irritants that are not well characterized.

Abdominal Cramps and Diarrhea within 6–24 Hours Followed by Hepatorenal Failure. Species of poisonous mushrooms containing amatoxins and phallotoxins are responsible for this syndrome[152,153,155] (Table 4). The most common implicated species are *Amanita phalloides, A. virosa*, and *A. verna*.[156,157] The illness is typically biphasic; the abdominal cramps and diarrhea, which may be quite severe, usually resolve within 24 hours. The patient then remains well for 1–2 days before evidence of hepatic and renal failure supervenes. A mortality of 30–50 percent has been reported.[158,159]

A similar clinical syndrome follows the ingestion of mushrooms of the *Gyromitra* genus, which contain the toxic substance gyromitrin. However, this toxin does not cause acute renal failure.[160]

Chronic Diarrhea within 1–3 Weeks. A new food-borne disease, chronic watery diarrhea, has recently been described among persons drinking raw milk.[161] After a mean incubation period of 15 days, affected persons developed acute watery diarrhea with marked urgency and abdominal cramps. Diarrhea persisted for a mean period of 2 years. No etiologic agent was identified. A second restaurant-associated outbreak of a similar illness suggests that vehicles other than raw milk may also be involved.[162]

Water-borne Disease. The evaluation of a suspected food-borne outbreak may reveal that water was the vehicle. Pathogens incriminated in water-borne outbreaks are different from those most often responsible for food-borne disease; the responsible etiologic agents for water-borne outbreaks reported to the CDC from 1972 through 1985 are shown in Table 5.[163–176] *Giardia lamblia* is the single most frequently recognized pathogen in the United States and has been responsible for several large outbreaks traced to a municipal water supply.[177–179] This illness is characterized by abdominal pain, bloating, flatulence, and occasionally malabsorption. The incubation period is typi-

TABLE 4. Mushroom Poisoning Syndromes

Syndrome	*Mushroom Species*	*Toxins*
Short incubation		
Delirium	*Amanita muscaria* *A. pantherina*	Ibotenic acid, muscimol
Parasympathetic hyperactivity	*Inocybe* spp. *Clitocybe* spp.	Muscarine
Hallucinations	*Psilocybe* spp. *Panaeolus* spp.	Psilocybin, psilocin
Disulfiram reaction	*Coprinus atramentarius*	Disulfiram-like substance
Gastroenteritis	Many	?
Long incubation		
Gastroenteritis, hepatorenal failure	*Amanita phalloides* *A. virosa* *A. verna* *Galerina autumnalis* *G. marginata* *G. venenata*	Amatoxins, phallotoxins
Gastroenteritis, hepatic failure	*Gyromitra* spp.	Gyromitrin

TABLE 5. Etiology of Water-borne Disease Outbreaks of Known Etiology Reported to the CDC, 1972–1985

Etiology	*Number of Outbreaks*	*Percentage of Total*
G. lamblia	85	38.6
Shigella	26	11.8
Hepatitis A	17	7.7
Norwalk-like agents	15	6.8
C. jejuni	10	4.5
Nontyphoid salmonella	10	4.5
S. typhi	5	2.3
Enterotoxigenic *E. coli*	1	0.5
V. cholerae 01	1	0.5
Y. enterocolitica	1	0.5
Rotavirus	1	0.5
Cryptosporidium	1	0.5
E. histolytica	1	0.5
Miscellaneous chemicals	46	20.9
	Total 220	100.1

TABLE 6. Etiology of Food-borne Disease Outbreaks by Food, Season, and Geographic Predilection

Etiology	*Foods*	*Season*	*Geographic Predilection*
Bacterial			
Salmonella	Beef, poultry, eggs, dairy products	Summer	None
S. aureus	Ham, poultry, egg salads, pastries	Summer	None
C. jejuni	Poultry, raw milk	Spring, summer	None
C. botulinum	Vegetables, fruits, fish, honey (infants)	Summer, fall	West, Northeast
C. perfringens	Beef, poultry, gravy, Mexican food	Fall, winter, spring	None
Shigella	Egg salads, lettuce	Summer	None
V. parahaemolyticus	Crabs	Spring, summer, fall	Coastal states
B. cereus	Fried rice, meats, vegetables	Year round	None
Y. enterocolitica	Milk, tofu, pork	Winter	Unknown
V. cholerae 01	Shellfish	Variable	Tropical, Gulf Coast
V. cholerae non-01	Shellfish	Unknown	Tropical, Gulf Coast
Verotoxigenic *E. coli*	Beef, raw milk	Summer, fall	Unknown
Viral			
Norwalk agent	Shellfish, salads	Year round	Northeast
Chemical			
Ciguatera	Barracuda, snapper, amberjack, grouper	Spring, summer (in Florida)	Tropical
Histamine fish poisoning (scombroid)	Tuna, mackerel, bonito, skipjack, mahi-mahi	Year round	Coastal
Mushroom poisoning	Mushrooms	Spring, fall	Temperate
Heavy metals	Acidic beverages	Year round	None
Monosodium-L-glutamate	Chinese food	Year round	None
Paralytic shellfish poisoning	Shellfish	Summer, fall	Temperate
Neurotoxic shellfish poisoning	Shellfish	Spring, fall	Subtropical

cally 1–4 weeks, and duration of the illness may be several weeks. Large water-borne outbreaks caused by shigellae,[180] hepatitis A,[181] *Salmonella typhi*,[182] nontyphoid salmonellae,[183] enterotoxigenic *E. coli*[184] *C. jejuni*,[185–187] the Norwalk agent,[188,189] and a Norwalk-like virus, the Colorado agent,[190] have been reported. The majority of water-borne outbreaks are of unknown etiology.

Miscellaneous Food-borne Diseases. This discussion has focused on diseases often transmitted by foods and manifested primarily by gastrointestinal or neurologic symptoms and signs. Other infectious diseases with primary symptoms outside the gastrointestinal and neurologic systems, which are occasionally or usually transmitted by foods and their most common vehicles of transmission, include group A β-hemolytic streptococci (potato and egg salds), brucellosis (goat's milk cheese), anthrax (meat), tularemia (water), listeriosis (cole slaw, milk, cheese), *Vibrio vulnificus* (raw oysters), tuberculosis (milk), Q fever (milk), hepatitis A (shellfish, salads), trichinoisis (pork), toxoplasmosis (beef), anisakiasis (fish), and tapeworms (beef, pork, fish).

EPIDEMIOLOGY

In addition to the clinical syndrome and incubation period, additional clues to the cause of an outbreak of food-borne disease may be provided by the type of food responsible and the setting in which it is eaten[191] (Table 6).

Foods

Outbreaks of staphylococcal food poisoning are associated with foods of high protein content, such as ham, poultry, potato and egg salads, and cream-filled pastries, that are thought to be contaminated during preparation by a food handler. The nasal carrier rate for *S. aureus* has been reported to range from 30 to 50 percent, whereas 14–40 percent of healthy people harbor staphylococci on their hands or wrists.[192] Other studies suggest that as many as 38 percent of *S. aureus* isolates from humans are capable of producing an enterotoxin.[193] Although in the classic staphylococcal food-borne outbreak a food handler has a purulent skin lesion on his or her hand, in actuality this is true in only a minority of outbreaks. In contrast, outbreaks of *B. cereus* food poisoning of the short-incubation type are most often associated with fried rice that has been cooked and held warm for extended periods. The growth of *B. cereus* under similar experimental conditions in rice has been well documented.[194] The vehicle in a recently reported outbreak was macaroni and cheese that was mishandled after preparation; investigation revealed that powdered milk was the source of the organism.[195] The short-incubation syndrome is most often caused by serotype 1 strains,[196] possibly because these strains are more heat resistant than strains of other serotypes.[197]

Clostridium perfringens outbreaks usually follow the ingestion of meat (especially beef and poultry) and gravies; organisms have been isolated from 16–85 percent of raw meat, poultry, and fish specimens.[198–200] Outbreaks are more likely to occur when these items are prepared in large quantities for banquets or in institutional settings when food is prepared well in advance without adequate final reheating.[201] Long-incubation *B. cereus* food poisoning is also frequently associated with meat or vegetable dishes. In addition to the frequent contamination of raw meats, vegetables, and milk products with *B. cereus*, the organism has been isolated from 25 percent of dried foods such as seasoning mixes, spices, and dried potatoes[202] and from over 50 percent of dried beans and cereals.[203] A long-incubation *B. cereus* outbreak has also been traced to a "meals-on-wheels" operation in which food was held at and above room temperature for an extended period.[204]

Salmonella food-borne outbreaks most frequently follow the ingestion of poultry, beef, egg, or dairy products. The role of raw milk in the transmission of *Salmonella* infections has recently been re-emphasized.[205–207] Two large international outbreaks have been caused by contaminated chocolate candy.[208,209] A recently recognized contamination of shell eggs is associated with a large number of outbreaks due to *Salmonella enteriditis*.[210] *Shigella* outbreaks are most often associated with cool, moist foods such as potato and egg salads. In a recent outbreak caused by *Shigella dysenteriae* type 2, the vehicle was raw vegetables served at a salad bar.[211] *Campylobacter jejuni* outbreaks most often follow the ingestion of raw milk and poultry.[48,212] *Vibrio parahaemolyticus* outbreaks in the United States are associated with the ingestion of bivalve mollusks and crustaceans[213,214]; in Japan, these outbreaks are more often associated with the ingestion of a variety of saltwater fish.[215] *Vibrio cholerae* 01 and non-01 outbreaks have been traced to contaminated shellfish eaten raw or inadequately cooked.[56,216,217] Crabs, shrimp, and raw oysters have been implicated as the vehicles of transmission of a unique epidemic strain of *V. cholerae* in Louisiana.[8,218–221] Sporadic cases of diarrhea associated with *V. cholerae* non-01 strains in the United States have also been linked to shellfish ingestion.[54,55] Food-borne outbreaks in the United States due to *Y. enterocolitica* were caused by contaminated milk[79,80] and tofu.[81] In Europe, this illness is associated with eating raw pork.[82] The single food-borne outbreak caused by invasive *E. coli* followed the ingestion of cheese.[46] Travelers' diarrhea caused by enterotoxigenic *E. coli* has been associated with consumption of salads in Mexico,[222] a recent food-borne outbreak of enterotoxigenic *E. coli* followed the ingestion of imported cheese,[223]and enterotoxigenic isolates have been obtained from a variety of foods including hamburger, sausage, seafood, and cheese in the United States.[224] Botulism outbreaks are most often associated with the ingestion of low-acid (pH ≥ 4.4) home-canned vegetables, fruits, and fish. Recent outbreaks of botulism followed ingestion of unusual vehicles including baked potatoes, sauteed onions, and chopped garlic.[105,225] Honey may have been the source of *C. botulinum* in some cases of infant botulism.[226] In Norwalk agent outbreaks, oysters[74,227,228] and salads[229] have been implicated. In a recent large outbreak, cake and frosting were implicated.[230] Contamination of food by an ill food handler has been documented.[231] Food-borne transmission of the Snow Mountain agent has been associated with clams.[77]

Outbreaks of heavy metal poisoning are most often associated with acidic beverages such as lemonade, fruit punch, and carbonated drinks that have been stored in corroded metallic containers such as punch bowls[108] or that have been in contact with metallic tubing (e.g., in vending machines)[232] for periods of time sufficient to leach the metallic ions from the container. Histamine fish poisoning outbreaks are associated with scombroid fish, the most common of which are tuna, mackerel, bonito, and skipjack. In addition, the nonscombroid fish mahi-mahi has caused outbreaks of scombroid-like fish poisoning. Ciguatera fish poisoning has been associated with over 400 species of fish. Barracuda, red snapper, amberjack, and grouper are most commonly implicated. The disease is more often associated with large fish; in one study, 69 percent of red snapper weighing 2.8 kg or more was toxic, compared to only 18 percent of smaller fish.[233] PSP and NSP follow the ingestion of bivalve mollusks, most often oysters, clams, and mussels. The most common Chinese food item associated with the Chinese restaurant syndrome is soup, which is frequently the first item ingested at a meal; the absorption of monosodium L-glutamate is most rapid when the stomach is empty.[135]

Seasonality

The time of year may also provide a clue to the cause of a food-borne outbreak. Outbreaks caused by the bacterial pathogens *S. aureus*, *Salmonella*, and *Shigella*, are most common during the summer months. *C. jejuni* outbreaks are more common during the spring and fall, *C. perfringens* outbreaks occur throughout the year but least often during the summer months, and botulism outbreaks are more common during the summer and fall.

In general, chemical food poisoning occurs throughout the year. Exceptions are PSP, which often occurs in association with a red tide[234] and is most common in the summer and fall; ciguatera, which is most common in the spring and summer in Florida;[235] and mushroom poisoning, which is most common in the spring, late summer, and fall.

Geographic Location

The geographic setting may provide a clue to the cause of food-borne disease. *Vibrio parahaemolyticus* outbreaks are most frequently reported from coastal states. The initial 13 outbreaks reported in the United States all occurred in coastal states.[213] An outbreak of cholera and sporadic cases of *V. cholerae* 01 and non-01 infection have been reported from the Gulf Coast of the United States.[8] Type A botulism outbreaks are most common west of the Mississippi River, whereas type B outbreaks are most common in the East, and type E outbreaks are most common in the Great Lakes Region.[101]

Ciguatera outbreaks occur in tropical and subtropical regions between 35°N and 35°S latitudes. Over 90 percent of outbreaks in the United States have been reported from Florida and Hawaii.[118] Ciguatera is common in the West Indies,[237] and travelers who return with the characteristic syndrome should be questioned regarding fish consumption. PSP and NSP outbreaks occur in coastal areas. *Gonyaulax tamarensis* is the dinoflagellate responsible for shellfish contamination along the New England Coast, whereas *G. catenella* is the responsible organism along the Pacific Coast. *Gymnodinium breve* is the dinoflagellate responsible for outbreaks of neurotoxic shellfish poisoning on the Gulf Coast of Florida.

Epidemiologic Assessment

For a food to provide a clue to the cause of a food-borne outbreak, it must be identified. Once a common meal is identified through interviews with ill people, food-specific attack rates should be determined for all foods and beverages served at the meal (see example in Table 7). People who ate the same meal but did not become ill must also be interviewed to serve as controls. Food-specific attack rates may identify the responsible vehicle of transmission. To be adequately incriminated, a food must have a significantly higher attack rate for those who ate it than for those who did not, and most of those who became ill must have eaten the food. On occasion, more than one food

TABLE 7. Example of Use of Food-Specific Attack Rates and Cross-Table Analysis to Identify Food Vehicle in a Food-borne Outbreak

	Food-Specific Attack Rates					
	No. of People Eating Food			*No. of People Not Eating Food*		
Food	*Total*	*Ill*	*Percent Ill*	*Total*	*Ill*	*Percent Ill*
Meat loaf	100	88	88[a]	10	2	20[a]
Gravy	80	80	100[b]	30	10	33[b]
Potatoes	95	78	82	15	12	80
Salad	90	74	82	20	16	80
Water	70	58	82	40	32	80
	Cross-Table Analysis					
	No. of People Eating Meat Loaf			*No. of People Not Eating Meat Loaf*		
	Total	*Ill*	*Percent Ill*	*Total*	*Ill*	*Percent Ill*
No. eating gravy	75	67	89[c]	5	1	20[d]
No. not eating gravy	25	21	84[c]	5	1	20[d]

[a] $p < .05$ (Fisher's exact test).
[b] $p < .05$ (Chi-square analysis).
[c] $p > .05$ (Chi-square analysis).
[d] $p > .05$ (Fisher's exact test).

item may be incriminated. On these occasions, simple cross-table analysis may indicate whether both items were contaminated by the etiologic agent or whether both were eaten by most people at the meal (e.g., meat and gravy) (Table 7). For example, if meat loaf and gravy were both incriminated, subsequent analysis may indicate that attack rates were equally high for those who ate meat loaf, regardless of whether or not they ate gravy, and were similarly low for those who did not eat meat loaf, regardless of whether or not they ate gravy, indicating that the meat loaf alone was responsible for the outbreak.

LABORATORY DIAGNOSIS

Appropriate specimens for laboratory confirmation vary with the etiologic agents but include feces, vomitus, serum, and blood (Table 8). In addition, cultures of the food preparation environment and food handlers may be indicated. The laboratory should be alerted to suspected causes so that special techniques can be used for isolation of *C. perfringens*, vibrios, *C. jejuni, E. coli* 0157:H7 and *Y. enterocolitica* and so that organisms considered part of the normal flora (other *E. coli, B. cereus*) are not overlooked.

Outbreaks of staphylococcal food poisoning may be confirmed by the isolation of *S. aureus* of the same phage type from vomitus or feces of ill people and from the incriminated food or skin lesion or hand of a food handler, by the isolation of more than 10^5 *S. aureus* organisms per gram of incriminated food, or by the demonstration of staphylococcal enterotoxin in the food by gel diffusion, radioimmunoassay (RIA), or the enzyme-linked immunosorbent assay (ELISA), which have sensitivities of 0.1–3 ng/g of food.[238–242] *Bacillus cereus* outbreaks may be documented by the isolation of organisms from the feces of ill people who shared the same meal or by the isolation of 10^5 or more *B. cereus* per gram of incriminated food. Serotyping, if available, may be of value in confirming that isolates were derived from a common source, since 14 percent of healthy adults have been reported to have transient gastrointestinal colonization with *B. cereus*.[243] Plasmid analysis may also be useful.[244]

The laboratory confirmation of *C. perfringens* outbreaks is more difficult. Since both heat-sensitive and heat-resistant strains of *C. perfringens* type A have been implicated as causes of food poisoning, selective isolation procedures involving heat treatment of food and fecal specimens should not be used. Because *C. perfringens* organisms are variably reported as normal flora in 42–100 percent of healthy people,[245,246] organisms of the same serotype[247–249] or bacteriocin type[250] should be demonstrated in stools of ill people and the incriminated food or in stools of ill people and not in those of people who ate the same meal but did not become ill, or median counts of 10^6 or more *C. perfringens* spores per gram of feces obtained within 48 hours after onset of illness should be demonstrated.[247,251] Alternatively, counts of 10^5 or more organisms per gram of food provide etiologic confirmation. For serotyping, approximately 90 *C. perfringens* antisera, including the original 13 Hobbs serotypes, are available, but many isolates cannot be typed. In the United Kingdom, serotyping implicates a specific serotype in nearly two-thirds of outbreaks,[248] whereas in the United States serotyping is helpful in only approximately 20 percent of outbreaks.[252] Alternative confirmatory tests, which remain experimental, are the demonstration of enterotoxin in the stools of ill people and not in control subjects or a fourfold rise in antitoxin titers in serum by counterimmunoelectrophoresis or reverse passive hemagglutination techniques.[253–255] Because 65–100 percent of healthy people have antibody to *C. perfringens* enterotoxin,[253,256] a single elevated titer is inadequate confirmation. Reverse passive hemagglutination (sensitivity 1 ng/ml) is the most sensitive method of enterotoxin detection.[257]

Salmonella, Shigella, C. jejuni, V. cholerae 01 and non-01, *V. parahaemolyticus*, and *Y. enterocolitica* outbreaks may be confirmed by the isolation and serotyping of the organisms from the feces of ill people. In *Salmonella* outbreaks in which it is uncertain whether a common vehicle is responsible, plasmid profiling may be necessary.[258,259] Strains of *V. parahaemolyticus* isolated from patients are hemolytic on special blood agar medium (Kanagawa-positive strains). Isolation and serotyping of salmonellae, shigellae, *C. jejuni*, vibrios, and *Y. enterocolitica* from the incriminated food may also be confirmatory. Because *V. parahaemolyticus* in low numbers are a frequent contaminant of shellfish, counts of 10^5 or more organisms per gram are required for confirmation; food isolates are usually Kanagawa negative. Serologic testing of acute and convalescent sera may be helpful in confirming the diagnosis in patients in *Y. enterocolitica*, cholera, and typhoid fever outbreaks but currently plays no important role in the investigation of nontyphoid *Salmonella, Shigella, C. jejuni*, and *V. parahaemolyticus* outbreaks.

Verotoxigenic *E. coli* may be implicated by isolating sorbitol-negative *E. coli* from stools of ill persons and confirming them

TABLE 8. Appropriate Laboratory Specimens for Documentation of Etiology of a Food-borne Outbreak

	Patient			Food Handler				
	Stools	Vomitus	Blood	Stools	Nose	Hands	Food	Food-Preparation Environment
Bacterial								
Salmonella	C		C	C			C	C
S. aureus	C	C			C	C	C, T	
C. jejuni	C			C			C	C
C. botulinum	C, T	C, T	T				C, T	
C. perfringens	C, T						C	
Shigella	C			C			C	
V. parahaemolyticus	C						C	C
B. cereus	C	C					C	
Y. enterocolitica	C		S	C			C	C
V. cholerae 01 and non-01	C		S	C			C	C
Verotoxigenic *E. coli*	C, T						C, T	
Viral								
Norwalk agent	I		S					
Chemical								
Ciguatera							T	
Histamine fish poisoning (scombroid)							T	
Mushroom	T	T	T				T	
Heavy metals							T	
Monosodium-L-glutamate							T	
Paralytic shellfish poisoning							T	
Neurotoxic shellfish poisoning							T	

Abbreviations: C: culture; T: toxin testing; S: serology; I: immune electron microscopy.

as serotype 0157:H7,[260] by demonstrating free verotoxin in stools, or by isolating other verotoxigenic strains from stools from ill individuals.[95] Enterotoxigenic *E. coli* may be implicated by demonstrating the presence of isolates producing the heat-labile enterotoxin (LT) in tissue culture assays,[261,262] ELISA,[263] or the Biken test[264] or isolates producing the heat-stable enterotoxin (ST) in the suckling mouse assay[265] in ill people and not in control subjects. Invasive strains may be identified using the Sereny test.[266] Since *E. coli* serotypes have been shown to cause diarrhea in volunteers in the absence of detectable enterotoxin production or invasiveness,[267] serotyping of *E. coli* isolates from both patients and controls may also be useful in outbreak settings if cases are found to have a serotype absent from controls.

Botulism outbreaks may be confirmed by the demonstration of botulinal toxin in the serum or stool of ill people or in incriminated food by the mouse neutralization test or by the isolation of *C. botulinum* from the feces of ill people or from the incriminated food.[268,269] Laboratory confirmation by testing of clinical specimens can be obtained in approximately 70–75 percent of the cases of botulism.[268,269] Norwalk agent outbreaks may be confirmed by the demonstration of viral particles in stools of ill people by immune electron microscopy[270] or of a serologic response by a biotin-avidin immunoassay procedure.[271]

Outbreaks caused by heavy metals may be documented by the demonstration of the metallic ion in the incriminated food. Histamine fish poisoning may be confirmed by the demonstration of histamine in the fish; concentrations of 100 mg in 100 g of fish flesh correlate with toxicity. The diagnosis of ciguatera is based on the clinical picture.[272] However, ciguatera outbreaks may be documented by the demonstration of ciguatoxin in the incriminated fish using a bioassay in the mongoose, rat, or cat; RIA and ELISA techniques have been developed but are not generally available.[273,274] Shellfish poisoning may be confirmed either by demonstrating the toxin in mollusks by the mouse bioassay technique or by finding elevated numbers of the responsible dinoflagellate in the water from which the mollusks were obtained. Outbreaks of Chinese restaurant syndrome may be confirmed by the demonstration of elevated monosodium L-glutamate levels in the food. Mushroom poisoning may be confirmed either by the identification of the responsible toxin in gastric contents, blood, urine, or fecal specimens by thin-layer chromatography or RIA or by the identification of the mushroom by a mycologist.

An additional diagnostic tool that may be of value in food-borne disease outbreaks characterized by diarrhea is the fecal leukocyte examination.[275] The presence of leukocytes implies that the responsible organism has invaded the intestinal tract, suggesting that salmonellae, shigellae, *C. jejuni*, invasive *E. coli*, *V. parahaemolyticus*, or *Y. enterocolitica* are responsible for the illness.

Over 50 percent of the reported food-borne disease outbreaks in the United States are of unknown cause. In some cases, appropriate diagnostic procedures are not conducted. In others, no agent is identified, raising the possibility that other etiologic agents are responsible. Possibilities include *Aeromonas hydrophila, Plesiomonas shigelloides*, rotaviruses, and Norwalk-like agents. In several outbreaks in England traced to cockles, 25–26 nm viral particles similar to Norwalk-like agents have been seen in stool specimens.[276] Although enterococci and gram-negative rods (*Klebsiella, Enterobacter, Proteus, Citrobacter*, and *Pseudomonas* spp.) have been reported as causes of food-borne outbreaks on rare occasions, their role in the cause of food-borne outbreaks has not been well documented. Because these latter organisms may be part of the normal fecal flora, documentation of their presence in ill people and their absence from well people will be required to confirm their role in food-borne outbreaks. That the gram-negative organisms might be responsible for some outbreaks is suggested by reports of the production of LT[277,278] and ST enterotoxins[279,280] by some of these organisms.

THERAPY

Supportive measures are the mainstay of therapy in most cases of food poisoning. The majority of these illnesses are self-limited; exceptions are botulism, long-incubation mushroom poisoning, and PSP, which may be fatal in previously healthy people, and listeriosis, which is often fatal in neonates and immunocompromised persons. In addition, fatalities occasionally occur due to staphylococcal and *C. perfringens* food poisoning, salmonellosis, verotoxigenic *E. coli* infections, and shigellosis in infants, the elderly, and debilitated people (Table 9).

Gastrointestinal fluid losses should be replaced either orally or parenterally. Antimicrobial agents may be used in the therapy for shigellosis, cholera, and typhoid fever but should be avoided in uncomplicated gastrointestinal infection caused by nontyphoid salmonellae. Tetracycline shortens both the duration of clinical cholera and the excretion of *V. cholerae* 01. Erythromycin eradicates carriage of *C. jejuni* and can shorten the duration of illness if given early in the disease.[281] The role of antimicrobial agents in the management of food poisoning due to *V. parahaemolyticus*, enterotoxigenic, verotoxigenic, and invasive *E. coli*, and *Y. enterocolitica* is unsettled but probably minimal. Antimicrobial agents are of no value in the management of staphylococcal, *C. perfringens*, or *B. cereus* food poisoning. Antiperistaltic agents appear to be of little if any benefit in controlling diarrhea and are contraindicated in patients with fever or fecal leukocytes, which suggest a syndrome associated with an invasive pathogen. Patients with botulism present several additional therapeutic problems, which are discussed in Chapter 221.

Patients with PSP and occasional patients with ciguatera may require ventilatory support; in these illnesses, this support is usually required for only a few days. A recent report suggests that intravenous mannitol may ameliorate the acute symptoms of ciguatera rapidly.[282] Therapy is otherwise supportive; no antitoxins are available. If not contraindicated by the presence of ileus, enemas or cathartics may be administered to these patients in an effort to remove unabsorbed toxin from the intestinal tract. Because of the severe dysesthesias associated with ciguatera, analgesics may also be required. Symptoms of histamine fish poisoning may be relieved by antihistamines. In severe cases with bronchospasm, epinephrine or aminophylline may be required.

Therapy for short-incubation-period types of mushroom poisoning is primarily supportive.[283] Patients who have ingested species containing pharmacologically active amounts of muscarine and who manifest evidence of parasympathetic hyperactivity may be treated with atropine. Patients who are severely ill after ingestion of species containing ibotenic acid and mus-

TABLE 9. Etiology of Food-borne Disease Deaths Reported to the CDC, 1972–1986

Etiology	Number of Deaths	Percentage of Total
Salmonella	88	28.9
L. monocytogenes	56	18.4
C. botulinum	49	16.1
Unknown	36	11.8
Miscellaneous	18	5.9
C. perfringens	13	4.3
V. cholerae 01	12	3.9
Mushrooms	11	3.6
Trichinella	6	2.0
Verotoxigenic *E. coli*	4	1.3
Shigella	4	1.3
Ciguatera	3	1.0
S. aureus	2	0.7
C. jejuni	2	0.7
Paralytic shellfish poisoning	1	0.3
	Total 305	100.2

cimol may be treated with physostigmine. Therapy for the long-incubation illness includes cathartics and enemas in an effort to remove unabsorbed toxin, as well as a number of specific and supportive measures.[283] Since hypoglycemia often occurs, intravenous glucose may be required. Thioctic acid is an experimental drug that appears to be an effective antidote in these patients[153]; the drug may be obtained from Burton M. Berkson, M.D., Ph.D., in Las Cruces, New Mexico (505-523-3284 or 523-3276). Pyridoxine is indicated in the management of patients poisoned with *Gyromitra* species.

Therapy for acute heavy metal poisoning is supportive. Emesis should be induced if it does not occur spontaneously. Antiemetics are contraindicated, since retention of the toxic ions in the gut with subsequent systemic absorption may result. In severe cases with systemic manifestations of heavy metal toxicity, use of specific antidotes may be considered but is rarely necessary in these outbreaks.

PREVENTION

Food-borne disease can be prevented if food is selected, prepared, and stored properly. In outbreaks reported to the CDC, the most common error is storage of food at inappropriate temperatures; this error is most often identified in staphylococcal, short- and long-incubation *B. cereus, C. perfringens*, and *Salmonella* outbreaks. Bacterial pathogens grow in food at temperatures ranging from 40 to 140°F; growth may be prevented if cold food is adequately refrigerated and if hot food is held at temperatures above 140°F before serving.

Another food-handling deficiency that frequently contributes to staphylococcal, *Shigella*, and typhoid fever outbreaks and appears to be important in some Norwalk agent outbreaks is poor personal hygiene by food handlers. Although thorough cooking of food just before consumption will eliminate the risk of many illnesses, protection against staphylococcal food poisoning is not provided, since the staphylococcal enterotoxins are heat stable. Inadequate heat processing may lead to botulism, and the use of contaminated equipment such as knives and meat slicers may result in nontyphoid salmonellosis.[284] Particular care in handling and cooking raw poultry, raw beef, raw pork, raw shellfish, and raw eggs is important in preventing many food-borne diseases. Avoiding consumption of raw milk is important in preventing *Salmonella* and *C. jejuni* outbreaks.[285]

Food-handling errors resulting in chemical intoxication are different from those leading to bacterial outbreaks. Heavy metal poisoning occurs when acidic beverages are stored in defective metallic containers or when valves in vending machines malfunction. Ciguatera and shellfish poisoning occur when fish or shellfish are obtained from unsafe sources. Items contaminated with these toxins appear and taste normal; in addition, cooking of these items does not provide protection, since the toxins are heat stable.

Food-borne disease outbreaks should be reported to public health authorities. Reporting is essential if investigations are to be conducted to identify the food-handling error so that these deficiencies can be corrected. Prompt reporting may also lead to the prevention of additional cases; there are well-documented episodes of botulism[105,286] and salmonellosis[287] in which recognition and reporting of the initial illness could have prevented subsequent cases. Reporting may lead to recognition of illnesses with the potential for intrafamilial spread (e.g., shigellosis), so secondary transmission can be prevented. Finally, reporting is vital if the 1–2 percent of all reported outbreaks that are caused by commercially distributed foods are to be identified before large numbers of people become ill.

REFERENCES

1. Sours HE, Smith DG. Outbreaks of foodborne disease in the United States, 1972–1978. J Infect Dis. 1980;142:122.
2. Centers for Disease Control. Foodborne Disease Surveillance Annual Summary 1979. April 1981.
3. Centers for Disease Control. Foodborne Disease Surveillance Annual Summary 1980. February 1983.
4. Centers for Disease Control. Foodborne Disease Surveillance Annual Summary 1981. June 1983.
5. MacDonald KL, Griffin PM. Foodborne disease outbreaks, annual summary, 1982. CDC surveillance summaries. Morb Mort Weekly Rep. 1986;35(No 1SS):7–16SS.
6. Bennett JV, Holmberg SD, Rogers MF, et al. Infectious and parasitic diseases. In: Amler RW, Dull HB, eds. Closing the Gap: The Burden of Unnecessary Illness. New York: Oxford University Press; 1987;102–14.
7. Merson MH, Martin WT, Craig JP, et al. Cholera on Guam, 1974: Epidemiologic findings and isolation of non-toxinogenic strains. Am J Epidemiol. 1977;105:349.
8. Blake PA, Allegra DT, Snyder JD, et al. Cholera: A possible endemic focus in the United States. N Engl J Med. 1980;302:305.
9. Osterholm MT, Forfang JC, Ristinen TL, et al. An outbreak of foodborne giardiasis. N Engl J Med. 1981;304:24.
10. Petersen LR, Cartter ML, Hadler JL. A food-borne outbreak of *Giardia lamblia*. J Infect Dis. 1988;157:846–8.
11. Feig M. Staphylococcal food poisoning. A report of two related outbreaks, and a discussion of the data presented. Am J Public Health. 1950;40:279.
12. Bergdoll MS. The enterotoxins. In: Cohen JO, ed. The Staphylococci. New York: Wiley; 1972:301.
13. Bergdoll MS, Crass BA, Reiser RF, et al. A new staphylococcal enterotoxin, enterotoxin F, associated with toxic-shock-syndrome *Staphylococcus aureus* isolates. Lancet. 1981;1:1017.
14. Sugiyama H, Hayama T. Abdominal viscera as site of emetic action for staphylococcal enterotoxin in the monkey. J Infect Dis. 1965;115:330.
15. Clark WG, Vanderhooft GF, Borison HL. Emetic effect of purified staphylococcal enterotoxin in cats. Proc Soc Exp Biol Med. 1962;111:205.
16. Elias J, Shields R. Influence of staphylococcal enterotoxin on water and electrolyte transport in the small intestine. Gut. 1976;17:527.
17. Gilbert RJ. Staphylococcal food poisoning and botulism. Postgrad Med J. 1974;50:603.
18. Breckinridge JC, Bergdoll MS. Outbreak of foodborne gastroenteritis due to a coagulase-negative enterotoxin-producing staphylococcus. N Engl J Med. 1971;284:541.
19. Merson MH. The epidemiology of staphylococcal foodborne disease. Proc Staph in Foods Conf. University Park, PA: Pennsylvania State University; 1973:20.
20. Šimkovičova M, Gilbert RJ. Serological detection of enterotoxin from food-poisoning strains of *Staphylococcus aureus*. J Med Microbiol. 1971;4:19.
21. Holmberg SD, Blake PA. Staphylococcal food poisoning in the United States: New facts and old misconceptions. JAMA. 1984;251:487.
22. Mortimer PR, McCann G. Food-poisoning episodes associated with *Bacillus cereus* in fried rice. Lancet. 1974;1:1043.
23. Midura T, Gerber M, Wood R, et al. Outbreak of food poisoning caused by *Bacillus cereus*. Public Health Rep. 1970;85:45.
24. Terranova W, Blake PA. *Bacillus cereus* food poisoning. N Engl J Med. 1978;298:143.
25. Melling J, Capel BJ, Turnbull PCB, et al. Identification of a novel enterotoxigenic activity associated with *Bacillus cereus*. J Clin Pathol. 1976;29:938.
26. Turnbull PCB, Kramer JM, Jorgensen K. Properties and production characteristics of vomiting, diarrheal, and necrotizing toxins of *Bacillus cereus*. Am J Clin Nutr. 1979;32:219.
27. Hobbs BC, Smith ME, Oakley CL, et al. *Clostridium welchii* food poisoning. J Hyg. 1953;51:75.
28. Shandera WX, Tacket CO, Blake PA. Food poisoning due to *Clostridium perfringens* in the United States. J Infect Dis. 1983;147:167.
29. Smith LDS. *Clostridium perfringens*. The Pathogenic Anaerobic Bacteria. Springfield, Ill: Charles C Thomas; 1975:115.
30. Stark RL, Duncan CL. Purification and biochemical properties of *Clostridium perfringens* type A enterotoxin. Infect Immun. 1972;6:662.
31. Duncan CL. Time of enterotoxin formation and release during sporulation of *Clostridium perfringens* type A. J Bacteriol. 1973;113:932.
32. McDonel JL, Duncan CL. Regional localization of activity of *Clostridium perfringens* type A enterotoxin in the rabbit ileum, jejunum, and duodenum. J Infect Dis. 1977;136:661.
33. McDonel JL. The molecular mode of action of *Clostridium perfringens* enterotoxin. Am J Clin Nutr. 1979;32:210.
34. Turnbull PCB. Studies on the production of enterotoxins by *Bacillus cereus*. J Clin Pathol. 1976;29:941.
35. Loewenstein MS.Epidemiology of *Clostridium perfringens* food poisoning. N Engl J Med. 1972;286:1026.
36. Giannella RA, Brasile L: A hospital food-borne outbreak of diarrhea caused by *Bacillus cereus*. Clinical, epidemiologic, and microbiologic studies. J Infect Dis. 1979;139:366.
37. Giannella RA, Formal SB, Dammin GJ, et al. Pathogenesis of salmonellosis: Studies of fluid secretion, mucosal invasion, and morphologic reaction in the rabbit ileum. J Clin Invest. 1973;52:441.
38. Rout WR, Formal SB, Giannella RA, et al. Pathophysiology of shigella diarrhea in the rhesus monkey: Intestinal transport, morphological, and bacteriological studies. Gastroenterology. 1975;68:270.
39. Bolen JL, Zamiska SA, Greenough WB III. Clinical features in enteritis due to *Vibrio parahaemolyticus*. Am J Med. 1974;57:638.

40. Hughes JM, Boyce JM, Aloem ARMA, et al. *Vibrio parahaemolyticus* enterocolitis in Bangladesh: Report of an outbreak. Am J Trop Med Hyg. 1978;27:106.
41. Boutin BK, Townsend SF, Scarpino PV, et al: Demonstration of invasiveness of *Vibrio parahaemolyticus* in adult rabbits by immunofluorescence. Appl Environ Microbiol. 1979;37:647.
42. Tulloch EF, Ryan KJ, Formal SB, et al. Invasive enteropathic *Escherichia coli* dysentery: An outbreak in 28 adults. Ann Intern Med. 1973;79:13.
43. Horwitz MA, Pollard RA, Merson MH, et al. A large outbreak of foodborne salmonellosis on the Navaho Nation Indian Reservation: Epidemiology and secondary transmission. Am J Public Health. 1977;67:1071.
44. Weissman JB, Williams SV, Hinman AR, et al. Foodborne shigellosis at a country fair. Am J Epidemiol. 1974;100:178.
45. Chatterjee BD, Neogy KN, Gorbach SL. Studies of *Vibrio parahaemolyticus* from cases of diarrhea in Calcutta. Indian J Med Res. 1970;58:234.
46. Marier R, Wells JG, Swanson RC, et al. An outbreak of enteropathogenic *Escherichia coli* foodborne disease traced to imported French cheese. Lancet. 1973;2:1376.
47. Blaser MJ, Reller LB. *Campylobacter* enteritis. N Engl J Med. 1981; 305:1444.
48. Tauxe RV, Bean NH, Patton CH. *Campylobacter* isolates in the United States, 1982–1986. CDC surveillance summaries. MMWR. 1988;37(No SS-2):1–13.
49. Blaser MJ, Wells JG, Feldman RA. *Campylobacter* enteritis in the United States: A multicenter study. Ann Intern Med. 1983;98:360.
50. Lambert ME, Schofield PF, Ironside AG, et al. *Campylobacter* colitis. Br Med J. 1979;1:857.
51. Taylor DN, Porter BW, Williams CA, et al. *Campylobacter* enteritis: A large outbreak traced to commercial raw milk. West J Med. 1982;137:365.
52. Blaser MJ, Checko P, Bopp C, et al. *Campylobacter* enteritis associated with foodborne transmission. Am J Epidemiol. 1982;116:886.
53. Blaser MJ, Berkowitz ID, LaForce FM, et al. *Campylobacter* enteritis: Clinical and epidemiologic features. Ann Intern Med. 1979;91:179.
54. Hughes JM, Hollis DG, Gangarosa FJ, et al. Non-*cholera vibrio* infections in the United States: Clinical, epidemiologic, and laboratory features. Ann Intern Med. 1978;88:602–6.
55. Morris JG Jr, Wilson R, Davis BR, et al. Non-0 group 1 *Vibrio cholerae* gastroenteritis in the United States: Clinical, epidemiologic, and laboratory characteristics of sporadic cases. Ann Intern Med. 1981;94:656.
56. Wilson R, Lieb S, Roberts A, et al. Non-0 group 1 *Vibrio cholerae* gastroenteritis associated with eating raw oysters. Am J Epidemiol. 1981;114:293.
57. Carpenter CCJ Jr. Cholera enterotoxin: Recent investigations yield insights into transport processes. Am J Med. 1971;50:1.
58. Zinnaka Y, Carpenter CCJ Jr. An enterotoxin produced by noncholera vibrios. Johns Hopkins Med J. 1972;131:403.
59. Craig JP, Yamamoto K, Takeda Y, et al. Production of cholera-like enterotoxin by a *Vibrio cholerae* non-01 strain isolated from the environment. Infect Immun. 1981;34:90.
60. Sack RB. Human diarrheal disease caused by enterotoxigenic *Escherichia coli*. Ann Rev Microbiol. 1975;29:333.
61. Sandefur PD, Peterson JW. Neutralization of *Salmonella* toxin-induced elongation of Chinese hamster ovary cells by cholera antitoxin. Infect Immun. 1977;15:988.
62. Sedlock DM, Deibel RH. Detection of *Salmonella* enterotoxin using rabbit ileal loops. Can J Microbiol. 1978;24:268.
63. Keusch GT, Donta ST. Classification of enterotoxins on the basis of activity in cell culture. J Infect Dis. 1975;131:58.
64. Keusch GT, Jacewicz M. The pathogenesis of *Shigella* diarrhea. IV. Toxin and antitoxin in *Shigella flexneri* and *Shigella sonnei* infections in humans. J Infect Dis. 1977;135:552.
65. O'Brien AD, Gentry MK, Thompson MR, et al. Shigellosis and *Escherichia coli* diarrhea: Relative importance of invasive and toxigenic mechanisms. Am J Clin Nutr. 1979;32:229.
66. Honda T, Shimizu M, Takeda Y, et al. Isolation of a factor causing morphological changes of Chinese hamster ovary cells from the culture filtrate of *Vibrio parahaemolyticus*. Infect Immun. 1976;14:1028.
67. Carruthers MM. Cytotoxicity of *Vibrio parahaemolyticus* in HeLa cell culture. J Infect Dis. 1975;132:555.
68. Banwell JG, Gorbach SL, Pierce NF, et al. Acute undifferentiated human diarrhea in the tropics. II. Alterations in intestinal fluid and electrolyte movements. J Clin Invest. 1971;50:890.
69. Barker WH Jr, Mackowiak PA, Fishbein M, et al. *Vibrio parahaemolyticus* gastroenteritis outbreak in Covington, Louisiana, in August 1972. Am J Epidemiol. 1974;100:316.
70. Aldova E, Lázničková K, Stěpánková E, et al. Isolation of nonagglutinable vibrios from an enteritis outbreak in Czechoslovakia. J Infect Dis. 1968;118:25.
71. Carpenter CCJ Jr, Mitra PP, Sack RB. Clinical studies in Asiatic cholera. I. Preliminary observations, November, 1962–March, 1963. Bull Johns Hopkins Hosp. 1966;118:165.
72. Taylor WR, Schell WL, Wells JG, et al. A foodborne outbreak of enterotoxigenic *Escherichia coli* diarrhea. N Engl J Med. 1982;306:1093.
73. Kaplan JE, Gary GW, Baron RC, et al. Epidemiology of Norwalk gastroenteritis and the role of Norwalk virus in outbreaks of acute nonbacterial gastroenteritis. Ann Intern Med. 1982;96:756.
74. Murphy AM, Grohmann GS, Christopher PJ, et al. An Australia-wide outbreak of gastroenteritis from oysters caused by Norwalk virus. Med J Aust. 1979;2:329.
75. Morse DL, Guzewich JJ, Hanrahan JP, et al. Widespread outbreaks of clam- and oyster-associated gastroenteritis: Role of Norwalk virus. N Engl J Med. 1986;314:678–81.
76. Kaplan JE, Feldman R, Campbell DS, et al. The frequency of a Norwalk-like pattern of illness in outbreaks of acute gastroenteritis. Am J Public Health. 1982;72:1329–32.
77. Truman BI, Madore HP, Menegus MA, et al. Snow Mountain Agent gastroenteritis from clams. Am J Epidemiol. 1987;126:516–25.
78. Dolin R, Treanor JJ, Madore HP. Novel agents of viral enteritis in humans. J Infect Dis. 1987;155:365–76.
79. Black RE, Jackson RJ, Tsai T, et al. Epidemic *Yersinia enterocolitica* infection due to contaminated chocolate milk. N Engl J Med. 1978;298:76.
80. Tacket CO, Narain JP, Sattin R, et al. A multistate outbreak of infections caused by *Yersinia enterocolitica* transmitted by pasteurized milk. JAMA. 1984;251:483.
81. Centers for Disease Control. Outbreak of *Yersinia enterocolitica*: Washington State. Morb Mort Wkly Rep. 1982;31:652.
82. Tauxe RV, Vandepitte J, Wauters G, et al. *Yersinia enterocolitica* infections and pork: The missing link. Lancet. 1987;1:1129–32.
83. Pai CH, Mors V. Production of enterotoxin by *Yersinia enterocolitica*. Infect Immun. 1978;19:908.
84. Boyce JM, Doyle DJ Jr, Evans DG, et al. Production off heat-stable, methanol-soluble enterotoxin by *Yersinia enterocolitica*. Infect Immun. 1979;25:532.
85. Asakawa Y, Akahane S, Kagata N, et al. Two community outbreaks of human infection with *Yersinia enterocolitica*. J Hyg (Camb). 1973;71:715.
86. Arvastson B, Damgaard K, Winblad S. Clinical symptoms of infection witih *Yersinia enterocolitica*. Scand J Infect Dis. 1971;3:37.
87. Riley LW, Remis RS, Helgerson SD, et al. Hemorrhagic colitis associated with a rare *Escherichia coli* serotype. N Engl J Med. 1983;308:681.
88. Ryan CA, Tauxe RV, Hosek GW, et al. *Escherichia coli* 0157:H7 diarrhea in a nursing home: Clinical, epidemiological, and pathological findings. J Infect Dis. 1986;154:631–8.
89. Riley L. The epidemiological, clinical, and microbiologic features of hemorrhagic colitis. Ann Rev Microbiol. 1987;41:383–407.
90. Farmer JJ III, Potter ME, Riley LW, et al. Animal models to study *Escherichia coli* 0157:H7 isolated from patients with haemorrhagic colitis. Lancet. 1983;1:702.
91. Johnson WM, Lior H, Bezanson GS. Cytotoxic *Escherichia coli* 0157:H7 associated with haemorrhagic colitis in Canada. Lancet. 1983;1:76.
92. O'Brien AD, Lively TA, Chen ME, et al. *Escherichia coli* 0157:H7 strains associated with haemorrhagic colitis in the United States produce a *Shigella dysenteriae* 1 (shiga) like cytotoxin. Lancet. 1983;1:702.
93. Carter AO, Borczyk AA, Carlson JAK, et al. A severe outbreak of *Escherichia coli* 0157:H7-associated hemorrhagic colitis in a nursing home. N Engl J Med. 1987;317:1496–1500.
94. Centers for Disease Control. Thrombotic thrombocytopenic purpura associated with *Escherichia coli* 0157:H7-Washington. Morb Mort Weekly Rep. 1986;35:549–51.
95. Karmali MA, Petric M, Lim C, et al. The association between idiopathic hemolytic uremic syndrome and infection by verotoxin-producing *Escherichia coli*. J Infect Dis. 1985;151:775–82.
96. Koenig MG, Spickard A, Cardella MA, et al. Clinical and laboratory observations of type E botulism in man. Medicine. 1964;43:517.
97. Barker WH Jr, Weissman JB, Dowell VR Jr, et al. Type B botulism outbreak caused by a commercial food product. JAMA. 1977;237:456.
98. Hughes JM, Blumenthal JR, Merson MH, et al. Clinical features of types A and B food-borne botulism. Ann Intern Med. 1981;95:442.
99. Kao I, Drachman DB, Price DL. Botulinum toxin: Mechanism of presynaptic blockade. Science. 1976;193:1256.
100. Simpson LL. The origin, structure, and pharmacological activity of botulinum toxin. Pharmacol Rev. 1981;33:155.
101. Horwitz MA, Hughes JM, Merson MH, et al. Food-borne botulism in the United States, 1970–1975. J Infect Dis. 1977;136:153.
102. Midura TF, Arnon SS. Infant botulism: Identification of *Clostridium botulinum* and its toxins in feces. Lancet. 1976;2:934.
103. Arnon SS, Midura TF, Clay SA, et al. Infant botulism: Epidemiological, clinical, and laboratory aspects. JAMA. 1977;237:1946.
104. Sugiyama H, Mills DC. Intraintestinal toxin in infant mice challenged intragastrically with *Clostridium botulinum* spores. Infect Immun. 1978;21:59.
105. St Louis ME, Shaun HS, Peck MB, et al. Botulism from chopped garlic: Delayed recognition of a major outbreak. Ann Intern Med. 1988;108:363–8.
106. Semple AB, Parry WH, Phillips DE. Acute copper poisoning: An outbreak traced to contaminated water from a corroded geyser. Lancet 1960;2:700.
107. Brown MA, Thom JV, Orth GL, et al. Food poisoning involving zinc contamination. Arch Environ Health. 1964;8:657.
108. Centers for Disease Control. Illness associated with elevated levels of zinc in fruit punch: New Mexico. Morb Mort Weekly Rep. 1983;32:257.
109. Barker WH Jr, Runte V. Tomato juice-associated gastroenteritis, Washington and Oregon, 1969. Am J Epidemiol. 1972;96:219.
110. Baker TD, Hafner WG. Cadmium poisoning from a refrigerator shelf used as an improvised barbecue grill. Public Health Rep. 1961;76:543.
111. Merson MH, Baine WB, Gangarosa EJ, et al. Scombroid fish poisoning: Outbreak traced to commercially canned tuna fish. JAMA. 1974;228:1268.
112. Kawabata T, Ishizaka K, Miura T. Studies on the allergy-like food poisoning

associated with putrefaction of marine products. III. Physiological and pharmacological action of "saurine," a vagusstimulant of unknown structure recently isolated by the authors, and its characteristics in developing allergy-like symptoms. Jpn J Med Sci Biol. 1955;8:521.
113. Foo, LY. Scombroid poisoning: Recapitulation on the role of histamine. NZ Med J. 1977;85:425.
114. Geiger E, Courtney G, Schnakenberg G. The content and formation of histamine in fish muscle. Arch Biochem. 1944;3:311.
115. Taylor SL. Histamine food poisoning: Toxicology and clinical aspects. CRC Crit Rev Toxicol. 1986;17:91–128.
116. Lerke PA, Werner SB, Taylor SL, et al. Scombroid poisoning: Report of an outbreak. West J Med. 1978;129:381.
117. Taylor SL, Guthertz LS, Leatherwood M, et al. Histamine production by *Klebsiella pneumoniae* and an incident of scombroid fish poisoning. Appl Environ Microbiol. 1979;37:274.
118. Hughes JM, Merson MH. Fish and shellfish poisoning. N Engl J Med. 1976;295:1117.
119. Halstead BW, Courville DA. Poisonous and Venomous Marine Animals of the World. v. 1. Invertebrates. Washington, Government Printing Office; 1965:157.
120. McCollum JPK, Pearson RCM, Ingham HR, et al. An epidemic of mussel poisoning in North-East England. Lancet 1968;2:767.
121. Zwahlen A, Blanc MH, Robert M. Epidémie d'intoxication par les moules ("Paralytic Shellfish Poisoning"). Schweiz Med Wochenschr. 1977;107:226.
122. Acres J, Gray J. Paralytic shellfish poisoning. Can Med Assoc J. 1978; 119:1195.
123. Porkiss MEE, Horstman DA, Harpur D. Paralytic shellfish poisoning: A report of 17 cases in Cape Town. S Afr Med J. 1979;55:1017.
124. Proctor NH, Chan SL, Trevor AJ: Production of saxitoxin by cultures of *Gonyaulax catenella*. Toxicon 1975;13:1.
125. Ghazarossian VE, Schantz EJ, Schnoes HK, et al. Identification of a poison in toxic scallops from a *Gonyaulax tamarensis* red tide. Biochem Biophys Res Comm. 1974;59:1219.
126. Shimizu Y, Buckley LJ, Alam M, et al. Structures of gonyautoxin II and III from the East Coast toxic dinoflagellate *Gonyaulax tamarensis*. J Am Chem Soc. 1976;98:5414.
127. Schantz EJ, Ghazarossian VE, Schnoes HK, et al. The structure of saxitoxin. J Am Chem Soc. 1975;97:1238.
128. Henderson R, Ritchie JM, Strichartz GR. The binding of labelled saxitoxin to the sodium channels in nerve membranes. J Physiol. 1973;235:783.
129. Henderson R, Ritchie JM, Strichartz GR. Evidence that tetrodotoxin and saxitoxin act at a metal cation binding site in the sodium channels of nerve membrane. Proc Natl Acad Sci USA. 1974;71:3936.
130. Catterall WA. Neurotoxins that act on voltage-sensitive sodium channels in excitable membranes. Ann Rev Pharmacol Toxicol. 1980;20:15.
131. McFarren EF, Tanabe H, Silva FJ, et al. The occurrence of a ciguatera-like poison in oysters, clams, and *Gymnodinium breve* cultures. Toxicon. 1965;3:111.
132. Spiegelstein MY, Paster Z, Abbott BC. Purification and biological activity of *Gymnodinium breve* toxins. Toxicon. 1973;11:85.
133. Kim YS, Padilla GM. Purification of the ichthyotoxic component of *Gymnodinium breve* (red tide dinoflagellate) toxin by high pressure liquid chromatography. Toxicon. 1976;14:379.
134. Grunfeld Y, Spiegelstein MY. Effects of *Gymnodinium breve* toxin on the smooth muscle preparation of guinea-pig ileum. Br J Pharmacol. 1974;51:67.
135. Schaumburg HH, Byck R, Gerstl R, et al. Monosodium L-glutamate: Its pharmacology and role in the Chinese restaurant syndrome. Science. 1969;163:826.
136. Reif-Lehrer L. A questionnaire study of the prevalence of Chinese restaurant syndrome. Fed Proc. 1977;36:1617.
137. Hudson PJ, Vogt RL. A foodborne outbreak traced to niacin overenrichment. J Food Protection. 1985;48:249–51.
138. Barkin RM. Ciguatera poisoning: A common source outbreak. South Med J. 1974;67:13.
139. Halstead BW. Fish poisoning: The diagnosis, pharmacology and treatment. Clin Pharmacol Ther. 1964;5:615.
140. Russell FE. Ciguatera poisoning: A report of 35 cases. Toxicon. 1975;13:383.
141. Halstead BW, Courville DA. Poisonous and Venomous Marine Animals of the World, V. 2. Vertebrates. Washington, DC: Government Printing Office; 1967:63.
142. Engleberg NC, Morris JG Jr, Lewis J, et al. Ciguatera fish poisoning: A major common-source outbreak in the U.S. Virgin Islands. Ann Intern Med. 1983;98:336.
143. Bagnis R, Kuberski T, Laugier S. Clinical observations on 3,009 cases of ciguatera (fish poisoning) in the South Pacific. Am J Trop Med Hyg. 1979;28:1067.
144. Morris JG Jr, Lewin P. Hargrett NT, et al. Clinical features of ciguatera fish poisoning: A study of the disease in the U.S. Virgin Islands. Arch Intern Med. 1982;142:1090.
145. Scheuer PJ, Takahashi W, Tsutsumi J, et al. Ciguatoxin: Isolation and chemical nature. Science. 1967;155:1267.
146. Helfrich P, Banner AH. Experimental induction of ciguatera: Toxicity in fish through diet. Nature. 1963;197:1025.
147. Bagnis R, Chanteau S, Chungue E, et al. Origins of ciguatera fish poisoning: A new dinoflagellate, *Gambierdiscus toxicus* Adachi and Fukuyo, definitively involved as a causal agent. Toxicon. 1980;18:199.
148. Li K-M. Ciguatera fish poison: A cholinesterase inhibitor. Science. 1965;147:1580.
149. Halstead BW. Current status of marine biotoxicology: An overview. Clin Toxicol. 1981;18:1.
150. Le Grand AM, Galonnier M, Bagnis R. Studies on the mode of action of ciguateric toxins. Toxicon. 1982;20:311–5.
151. Bidard JN, Vijverberg HPM, Frelin C, et al. Ciguatoxin is a novel type of Na^+ channel toxin. J Biol Chem. 1984;259:8353–7.
152. Lampe KF. Current concepts of therapy in mushroom intoxication. Clin Toxicol. 1974;7:115.
153. Becker CE, Tong TG, Boerner U, et al. Diagnosis and treatment of *Amanita phalloides*-type mushroom poisoning: Use of thioctic acid. West J Med. 1976;125:100.
154. McCormick DJ, Avbel AJ, Gibbons RB. Nonlethal mushroom poisoning. Ann Intern Med. 1979;90:332.
155. Lampe KF. Toxic fungi. Ann Rev Pharmacol Toxicol. 1979;19:85.
156. Paaso B, Harrison DC. A new look at an old problem: Mushroom poisoning. Am J Med. 1975;58:505.
157. Hughes JM, Horwitz MA, Merson MH, et al. Foodborne disease outbreaks of chemical etiology in the United States, 1970–1974. Am J Epidemiol. 1977;105:233.
158. Editorial: Death-cap poisoning. Lancet. 1972;1:1320.
159. Centers for Disease Control: Mushroom poisoning among Laotian refugees: 1981. Morb Mort Weekly Rep. 1982;31:287.
160. Wieland T, Wieland O. The toxic peptides of *Amanita* species. In: Kadis S, Ciegler A, Aji SJ, eds. Microbiol Toxins. v. 8. Fungal Toxins. New York: Academic Press; 1972:249.
161. Osterholm MT, Macdonald KL, White KE, et al. An outbreak of a newly recognized chronic diarrhea syndrome associated with raw milk consumption. JAMA. 1986;256:484–90.
162. Martin DL, Hoberman LJ. A point source outbreak of chronic diarrhea in Texas: No known exposure to raw milk. JAMA. 1986;256:469.
163. Merson MH, Barker WH Jr, Craun GF, et al. Outbreaks of waterborne disease in the United States, 1971–1972. J Infect Dis. 1974;129:614.
164. Hughes JM, Merson MH, Craun GF, et al. Outbreaks of waterborne disease in the United States, 1973. J Infect Dis. 1975;132:336.
165. Horwitz MA, Hughes JM, Craun GF. Outbreaks of waterborne disease in the United States, 1974. J Infect Dis. 1976;133:588.
166. Black RE, Horwitz MA, Craun GF. Outbreaks of waterborne disease in the United States, 1975. J Infect Dis. 1978;137:370.
167. Centers for Disease Control: Foodborne and Waterborne Disease Outbreaks Annual Summary 19876. October 1977.
168. Centers for Disease Control: Foodborne and Waterborne Disease Surveillance Annual Summary 1977. August 1979.
169. Centers for Disease Control: Water-Related Disease Outbreaks Surveillance Annual Summary 1978. May 1980.
170. Centers for Disease Control: Water-Related Disease Outbreaks Surveillance Annual Summary 1979. September 1981.
171. Centers for Disease Control: Water-Related Disease Outbreaks Surveillance Annual Summary 1980. February 1982.
172. Centers for Disease Control: Water-Related Disease Outbreaks Surveillance Annual Summary 1981. September 1982.
173. Centers for Disease Control. Water-Related Disease Outbreaks Surveillance Annual Summary 1982. Centers for Disease Control. 1983;1–15.
174. Centers for Disease Control. Water-Related Disease Outbreaks Surveillance Annual Summary 1983. Centers for Disease Control. 1984;1–15.
175. Centers for Disease Control. Water-Related Disease Outbreaks Surveillance Annual Summary 1984. Centers for Disease Control. 1985;1–15.
176. St Louis ME. Centers for Disease Control. Water-Related Disease Outbreaks, 1985. CDC surveillance summaries. Morb Mort Weekly Rep. 1986;37(No SS-2):15–24.
177. Shaw PK, Brodsky RE, Lyman DO, et al. A community wide outbreak of giardiasis with evidence of transmission by a municipal water supply. Ann Intern Med. 1977;87:426.
178. Lopez CE, Dykes AC, Juranek DD, et al. Waterborne giardiasis: A community-wide outbreak of disease and a high rate of asymptomatic infection. Am J Epidemiol. 1980;112:495.
179. Dykes AC, Juranek DD, Lorenz RA, et al. Municipal waterborne giardiasis: An epidemiologic investigation. Ann Intern Med. 1980;92:165.
180. Weissman JB, Craun GF, Lawrence DN, et al. An epidemic of gastroenteritis traced to a contaminated public water supply. Am J Epidemiol. 1976;103:391.
181. Mosley JW. Water-borne infectious hepatitis. N Engl J Med. 1959;261:703.
182. Feldman RE, Baine WB, Nitzkin JL, et al. Epidemiology of *Salmonella typhi* infection in a migrant labor camp in Dade County, Florida. J Infect Dis. 1974;130:334.
183. A collaborative report. A waterborne epidemic of salmonellosis in Riverside, California, 1965: Epidemiologic aspects. Am J Epidemiol. 1971;93:33.
184. Rosenberg ML, Koplan JP, Wachsmuth IK, et al. Epidemic diarrhea at Crater Lake from enterotoxigenic *Escherichia coli*. A large waterborne outbreak. Ann Intern Med. 1977;86:714.
185. Mentzing LO. Waterborne outbreaks of *Campylobacter* enteritis in central Sweden. Lancet. 1981;2:352.
186. Vogt RL, Sours HE, Barrett T, et al. *Campylobacter* enteritis associated with contaminated water. Ann Intern Med. 1982;96:292.
187. Palmer SR, Gully PR, White JM, et al. Water-borne outbreak of *Campylobacter* gastroenteritis. Lancet. 1983;1:287.
188. Wilson R, Anderson LJ, Holman RC, et al. Waterborne gastroenteritis due to the Norwalk agent: Clinical and epidemiologic investigation. Am J Public Health. 1982;72:72.

189. Kaplan JE, Goodman RA, Schonberger LB, et al. Gastroenteritis due to Norwalk virus: An outbreak associated with a municipal water system. J Infect Dis. 1982;146:190.
190. Morens DM, Zweighaft RM, Vernon TM, et al. A waterborne outbreak of gastroenteritis with secondary person-to-person spread. Lancet. 1979;1:964.
191. Horwitz MA. Specific diagnosis of foodborne disease. Gastroenterology. 1977;73:375.
192. Williams REO. Healthy carriage of *Staphylococcus aureus*: Its prevalence and importance. Bacteriol Rev. 1963;27:56.
193. Wieneke AA. Enterotoxin production by strains of *Staphylococcus aureus* isolated from foods and human beings. J Hyg (Camb). 1974;73:255.
194. Gilbert RJ, Stringer MF, Peace TC. The survival and growth of *Bacillus cereus* in boiled and fried rice in relation to outbreaks of food poisoning. J Hyg (Camb). 1974;73:433.
195. Holmes JR, Plunkett T, Pate P, et al. Emetic food poisoning caused by *Bacillus cereus*. Arch Intern Med. 1981;141:766.
196. Gilbert RJ, Parry JM. Serotypes of *Bacillus cereus* from outbreaks of food poisoning and from routine foods. J Hyg (Lond). 1977;78:69.
197. Parry JM, Gilbert RJ. Studies on the heat resistance of *Bacillus cereus* spores and growth of the organisms in boiled rice. J Hyg (Lond). 1980;84:77.
198. Strong DH, Canada JC, Griffiths BB. Incidence of *Clostridium perfringens* in American foods. Appl Microbiol. 1963;11:42.
199. Hall HE, Angelotti R. *Clostridium perfringens* in meat and meat products. Appl Microbiol. 1965;13:352.
200. Smart JL, Roberts TA, Stringer MF, et al. The incidence and serotypes of *Clostridium perfringens* on beef, pork and lamb carcasses. J Appl Bacteriol. 1979;46:377.
201. Petersen LR, Mshar R, Cooper GH Jr, et al. A large *Clostridium perfringens* foodborne outbreak with an unusual attack rate pattern. Am J Epidemiol. 1988;127:605–11.
202. Kim HU, Goepfert JM. Enumeration and identification of *Bacillus cereus* in foods. I. 24-hour presumptive test medium. Appl Microbiol. 1971;22:581.
203. Blakey LJ, Priest FG. The occurrence of *Bacillus cereus* in some dried foods including pulses and cereals. J Appl Bacteriol. 1980;48:297.
204. Jephcott AE, Barton BW, Gilbert RJ, et al. An unusual outbreak of food-poisoning associated with meals-on-wheels. Lancet. 1977;2:129.
205. Werner SB, Humphrey GL, Kamei I. Association between raw milk and human *Salmonella dublin* infection. Br Med J. 1979;2:238.
206. Small RG, Sharp JCM. A milk-borne outbreak due to *Salmonella dublin*. J Hyg (Lond). 1979;82:95.
207. Galbraith NS, Forbes P, Clifford C. Communicable disease associated with milk and dairy products in England and Wales 1951–80. Br Med J. 1982;284:1761.
208. Gill ON, Bartlett CLR, Sockett PN, et al. Outbreak of *Salmonella napoli* infection caused by contaminated chocolate bars. Lancet. 1983;1:574.
209. Craven PC, Baine WB, Mackel DC, et al. International outbreak of *Salmonella eastbourne* infection traced to contaminated chocolate. Lancet. 1975;1:788.
210. St Louis ME, Morse DL, Potter ME, et al. The emergence of grade A eggs as a major source of *Salmonella enteritidis* infections. JAMA. 1988; 259:2103–7.
211. Centers for Disease Control. Hospital-associated outbreak of *Shigella dysenteriae* type 2: Maryland. Morb Mort Weekly Rep. 1983;32:250.
212. Robinson DA, Jones DM. Milk-borne *Campylobacter* infection. Br Med J. 1981;282:1374.
213. Barker WH Jr. *Vibrio parahaemolyticus* outbreaks in the United States. Lancet. 1974;1:551.
214. Lawrence DN, Blake PA, Yashuk JC, et al. *Vibrio parahaemolyticus* gastroenteritis outbreaks aboard two cruise ships. Am J Epidemiol. 1979;109:71.
215. Kudoh Y, Sakai S, Zen-Yoji H, et al. Epidemiology of food poisoning due to *Vibrio parahaemolyticus* occurring in Tokyo during the last decade. In: Fujino T, Sakaguchi G, Sakazaki R, et al, eds. International Symposium on Vibrio parahaemolyticus. Tokyo: Saikon; 1974:9.
216. Baine WB, Zampieri A, Mazzotti M, et al. Epidemiology of cholera in Italy in 1973. Lancet. 1974;2:1370.
217. Dutt AK, Alwi S, Velauthan T. A shellfish-borne cholera outbreak in Malaysia. Trans R Soc Trop Med Hyg. 1971;65:815.
218. Barrett TJ, Blake PA. Epidemiological usefulness of changes in hemolytic activity of *Vibrio cholerae* biotype El Tor during the seventh pandemic. J Clin Microbiol. 1981;13:126.
219. Kaper JB, Bradford HB, Roberts NC, et al. Molecular epidemiology of *Vibrio cholerae* in the U.S. Gulf Coast. J Clin Microbiol. 1982;16:129.
220. Pavia AT, Campbell JF, Blake PA, et al. Cholera from raw oysters shipped interstate. JAMA. 1987;258:2374.
221. Klontz KC, Tauxe RV, Cook WL, et al. Cholera after the consumption of raw oysters: A case report. Ann Intern Med. 1987;107:846–8.
222. Merson MH, Morris GH, Sack DA, et al. Travelers' diarrhea in Mexico. N Engl J Med. 1976;294:1299.
223. MacDonald KL, Eidson M, Strohmeyer C, et al. A multistate outbreak of gastrointestinal illness caused by enterotoxigenic *Escherichia coli* in imported semisoft cheese. J Infect Dis. 1985;151:716–20.
224. Sack RB, Sack DA, Mehlman IF, et al. Enterotoxigenic *Escherichia coli* isolated from food. J Infect Dis. 1977;135:313.
225. MacDonald KL, Cohen ML, Blake PA. The changing epidemiology of adult botulism in the United States. Am J Epidemiol. 1986;124:794–9.
226. Arnon SS. Infant botulism. Ann Rev Med. 1980;31:541.
227. Linco SJ, Grohmann GS. The Darwin outbreak of oyster-associated viral gastroenteritis. Med J Aust. 1980;1:211.
228. Gunn RA, Janowski HT, Lieb S, et al. Norwalk virus gastroenteritis following raw oyster consumption. Am J Epidemiol. 1982;115:348.
229. Griffin MR, Surowiec JJ, McCloskey DI, et al. Foodborne Norwalk virus. Am J Epidemiol. 1982;115:178.
230. Kuritsky JN, Osterholm MT, Greenberg HB, et al. Norwalk gastroenteritis: A community outbreak associated with bakery product consumption. Ann Intern Med. 1984;100:519.
231. Reid JA, Caul EO, White OG, et al. Role of infected food handler in hotel outbreak of Norwalk-like viral gastroenteritis: Implications for control. Lancet. 1988;2:321–3.
232. Hopper SH, Adams HS. Copper poisoning from vending machines. Public Health Rep. 1958;73:910.
233. Hesse IDW, Halstead BW, Peckham NH. Marine biotoxins. I. Ciguatera poison: Some biological and chemical aspects. Ann NY Acad Sci. 1960;90:788–97.
234. Collins JC, Bicknell WJ. The red tide: A public-health emergency. N Engl J Med. 1974;288:1126.
235. Lawrence DN, Enriquez MB, Lumish RM, et al. Ciguatera fish poisoning in Miami. JAMA. 1980;244:254.
236. Kelly MT, Peterson JW, Sarles HE Jr, et al. Cholera on the Texas Gulf Coast. JAMA. 1982;247:1598.
237. Morris JG Jr, Lewin P, Smith CW, et al. Ciguatera fish poisoning: Epidemiology of the disease on St. Thomas, U.S. Virgin Islands. Am J Trop Med Hyg. 1982;31:574.
238. Casman EP, Bennett RW. Detection of staphylococcal enterotoxin in food. Appl Microbiol. 1965;13:181.
239. Pober Z, Silverman GJ. Modified radioimmunoassay determination for staphylococcal enterotoxin B in foods. Appl Environ Microbiol. 1977;33:620.
240. Saunders GC, Bartlett ML. Double-antibody solid-phase enzyme immunoassay for the detection of staphylococcal enterotoxin. A. Appl Environ Microbiol. 1977;34:518.
241. Stiffler-Rosenberg G, Fey H. Simple assay for staphylococcal enterotoxins A, B, and C: Modification of enzyme-linked immunosorbent assay. J Clin Microbiol. 1978;8:473.
242. Freed RC, Evenson ML, Reiser RF, et al. Enzyme-linked immunosorbent assay for detection of staphylococcal enterotoxins in foods. Appl Environ Microbiol. 1982;44:1349.
243. Ghosh AC. Prevalence of *Bacillus cereus* in the faeces of healthy adults. J Hyg (Lond). 1978;80:233.
244. De Buono BA, Brondum J, Kramer JM, et al. Plasmid, serotypic, and enterotoxin analysis of *Bacillus cereus* in an outbreak setting. J Clin Microbiol. 1988;26:1571–4.
245. Mansson I, Colldahl H. The intestinal flora in patients with bronchial asthma and rheumatoid arthritis: With special reference to *Clostridium perfringens*. Acta Allergy. 1965;20:94.
246. Akama K, Otani S. *Clostridium perfringens* as the flora in the intestine of healthy persons. Jpn J Med Sci Biol. 1970;23:161.
247. Hauschild AHW. Criteria and procedures for implicating *Clostridium perfringens* in food-borne outbreaks. Can J Public Health. 1975;66:388.
248. Stringer MF, Turnbull PCB, Gilbert RJ. Application of serological typing to the investigation of outbreaks of *Clostridium perfringens* food poisoning, 1970–1978. J Hyg (Lond). 1980;84:443.
249. Harmon SM, Kautter DA, Hatheway CL. Enumeration and characterization of *Clostridium perfringens* spores in the feces of food poisoning patients and normal controls. J Food Protection. 1986;49:23–8.
250. Watson GN, Stringer MF, Gilbert RJ, et al. The potential of bacteriocin typing in the study of *Clostridium perfringens* food poisoning. J Clin Pathol. 1982;35:1361.
251. Schiemann DA. Laboratory confirmation of an outbreak of *Clostridium perfringens* food poisoning. Health Lab Sci. 1977;14:35–8.
252. Hatheway CL, Whaley DN, Dowell VR Jr. Epidemiological aspects of *Clostridium perfringens* foodborne illness. Food Technol. 1980;34:77.
253. Naik HS, Duncan CL. Detection of *Clostridium perfringens* enterotoxin in human fecal samples and anti-enterotoxin in sera. J Clin Microbiol. 1978;7:337.
254. Skjelkvåle R, Uemura T. Detection of enterotoxin in faeces and anti-enterotoxin in serum after *Clostridium perfringens* food poisoning. J Appl Bacteriol. 1977;42:355.
255. Birkhead G, Vogt RL, Heun EM, et al. Characterization of an outbreak of *Clostridium perfringens* food poisoning by quantitative fecal culture and fecal enterotoxin measurement. J Clin Microbiol. 1988;26:471–4.
256. Niilo L, Bainborough AR. A survey of *Clostridium perfringens* enterotoxin antibody in human and animal sera in western Canada. Can J Microbiol. 1980;26:1162.
257. Genigeorgis C, Sakaguchi G, Riemann H. Assay methods for *Clostridium perfringens* type A enterotoxin. Appl. Microbiol. 1973;26:111.
258. Taylor DN, Wachsmuth IK, Shangkuan YH. Salmonellosis associated with marijuana: A multistate outbreak traced by plasmid fingerprinting. N Engl J Med. 1982;306:1249.
259. Riley LW, Cohen ML. Plasmid profiles and *Salmonella* epidemiology. Lancet. 1982;1:573.
260. Farmer JJ III, Davis BR. H7 antiserum-sorbitol fermentation medium: A single tube screening medium for detecting *Escherichia coli* 0157:H7 associated with hemorrhagic colitis. J Clin Microbiol. 1985;22:620–5.

261. Guerrant RL, Brunton LL, Schnaitman TC, et al. Cyclic adenosine monophosphate and alteration of Chinese hamster ovary cell morphology: A rapid, sensitive in vitro assay for the enterotoxins of *Vibrio cholerae* and *Escherichia coli*. Infect Immun. 1974;10:320.
262. Donta ST, Moon HW, Whipp SC. Detection of heat-labue *Escherichia coli* enterotoxin with the use of adrenal cells in tissue culture. Science. 1974;183:334.
263. Svennerholm AM, Wiklund G. Rapid GMl-enzyme-linked immunosorbent assay with visual reading for identification of *Escherichia coli* heat-labile enterotoxin. J Clin Microbiol. 1983;17:596.
264. Honda T, Arita M, Takeda Y, et al. Further evaluation of the Biken test (modified Elek test) for detection of enterotoxigenic *Escherichia coli* producing heat-labile entertoxin and application of the test to sampling of heat-stable enterotoxin., J Clin Microbiol. 1982;16:60.
265. Giannella RA. Suckling mouse model for detection of heat-stable *Escherichia coli* enterotoxin: Characteristics of the model. Infect Immun. 1976;14:95.
266. Sereny B. Experimental *Shigella* keratoconjunctivitis: A preliminary report. Acta Microbiol Acad Sci Hung. 1955;2:293.
267. Levine MM, Berquist EJ, Nalin DR, et al. *Escherichia coli* strains that cause diarrhoea but do not produce heat-labile or heat-stable enterotoxins and are non-invasive. Lancet. 1978;1:1119.
268. Dowell VR Jr, McCroskey LM, Hatheway CL, et al. Coproexamination for botulinal toxin and *Clostridium botulinum*. JAMA. 1977;238:1829.
269. Mann JM, Hatheway CL, Gardiner TM. Laboratory diagnosis in a large outbreak of type A botulism. Am J Epidemiol. 1982;115:598.
270. Kapikian AZ, Wyatt RG, Dolin R et al. Visualization by immune electron microscopy of a 27-nm particle associated with acute infectious nonbacterial gastroenteritis. J Virol. 1972;10:1075.
271. Gary GW Jr, Kaplan JE, Stine SE, et al. Detection of Norwalk virus antibodies and antigen with a biotin-avidin immunoassay. J Clin Microbiol. 1985;22:274–8.
272. Morris JG Jr. Ciguatera fish poisoning. JAMA. 1980;244:273.
273. Withers NW. Ciguatera fish poisoning. Annu Rev Med. 1982;33:97.
274. Hokama Y, Abad MA, Kimura LH. A rapid enzyme-immunoassay for the detection of ciguatoxin in contaminated fish tissues. Toxicon. 1983;21:817–24.
275. Harris JC, DuPont HL. Hornick RB. Fecal leukocytes in diarrheal illness. Ann Intern Med. 1972;76:697.
276. Appleton H, Pereira MS. A possible virus etiology in outbreaks of food-poisoning from cockles. Lancet. 1977;1:780.
277. Guerrant RL, Dickens MD, Wenzel RP, et al. Toxigenic bacterial diarrhea: Nursery outbreak involving multiple bacterial strains. J Pediatr. 1976;89:885.
278. Wadström T, Aust-Kettis A, Habte D, et al. Enterotoxin-producing bacteria and parasites in stools of Ethiopian children with diarrhoeal disease. Arch Dis Child. 1976;51:865.
279. Klipstein FA, Engert RF. Purification and properties of *Klebsiella pneumoniae* heat-stable enterotoxin. Infect Immun. 1976;13:373.
280. Klipstein FA, Engert RF. Partial purification and properties of *Enterobacter cloacae* heat-stable enterotoxin. Infect Immun. 1976;13:1307.
281. Salazar-Lindo E, Sack RB, Chea-Woo E, et al. Early treatment with erythromycin of *Campylobacter jejuni*-associated dysentery in children. J Pediatr. 1986;109:355–60.
282. Palafox NA, Jain LG, Pinano AZ, et al. Successful treatment of ciguatera fish poisoning with intravenous mannitol. JAMA. 1988;259:2740–2.
283. Mitchel DH. *Amanita* mushroom poisoning. Annu Rev Med. 1980;31:51.
284. Jordan MC, Powell KE, Corothers TE, et al. Salmonellosis among restaurant patrons: The incisive role of a meat slicer. Am J Public Health. 1973;63:982.
285. Chin J. Raw milk: A continuing vehicle for the transmission of infectious disease agents in the United States. J Infect Dis. 1982;146:440.
286. Horwitz MA, Marr JS, Merson MH, et al. A continuing common-source outbreak of botulism in a family. Lancet. 1975;2:861.
287. Payne DJH, Scudamore JM. Outbreaks of salmonella food poisoning over a period of eight years from a common source. Lancet. 1977;1:1249.

87. TROPICAL SPRUE

FREDERICK A. KLIPSTEIN

Although apparently familiar to medical practitioners in India for centuries, it was not until the colonization of Asia by the European maritime powers early in the eighteenth century that Western physicians first became aware of tropical sprue. The disease was recognized among the British in India, the French in Indochina, the Dutch in Java, and somewhat later, the Americans in the Philippines and West Indies.

EPIDEMIOLOGY

Sprue can afflict visitors to the tropics within weeks, months, or years after arrival, the most common time interval being between 1 and 2 years.[1] It can occur as an isolated case or in epidemic proportions, as happened among British and Indian troops serving in the India–Burma theater of operations during the Second World War.[2] The disorder occurs among both sexes and all age groups, although it is less common in children than in adults. Symptoms of tropical sprue may persist after a return to a temperate climate and, in some instances, first become manifested there.[3]

The geographic regions in which sprue occurs are known (Fig. 1), but the exact prevalence of the disorder among people in these areas is uncertain, due largely to the relatively complex diagnostic procedures required to make the diagnosis. A disorder thought to be sprue was recognized in the southern part of the United States early in this century,[3] and more recently, "temperate sprue" has been described among some people who acquired transient intestinal malabsorption syndrome in temperate climates.[4] Long considered incorrectly to occur principally or even exclusively among European expatriates in the tropics, it is now recognized that sprue occurs more often among native populations of endemic areas. Although the disorder can occur among affluent, well-nourished people, its prevalence among indigenous populations appears to be more common among those living in substandard economic and sanitary conditions.

Abnormalities of small bowel structure and function develop in sprue as sequelae to an episode of acute enteritis; these abnormalities become progressively more severe, cause persistent gastrointestinal symptoms, and eventually result in nutritional deficiencies. In addition to overt sprue, many asymptomatic native residents of the tropics as well as expatriates who have lived in the tropics for more than 6 months are found to have mild-to-moderate small bowel abnormalities that are qualitatively indistinguishable from those present in sprue.[5,6] This condition is referred to as tropical enteropathy; it differs from sprue in a number of aspects: (*1*) the intestinal abnormalities in sprue relentlessly become more severe, whereas those in tropical enteropathy vary over time, either improving or worsening spontaneously. Further, unlike in sprue, the intestinal abnormalities in tropical enteropathy disappear within about a year after either active residents or expatriates move to a temperate climate.[7] (*2*) The intestinal abnormalities in sprue consistently result in nutritional deficiencies, but those in tropical enteropathy contribute to the development of nutritional deficiencies only in people subsiding on marginal or suboptimal diets. (*3*) Treatment with folic acid[8,9] and/or antimicrobials[10,11] either improves or completely heals the intestinal lesion in sprue, but the effect of this form of therapy is variable and usually limited in tropical enteropathy.[12]

ETIOLOGY

The clinical and epidemiologic aspects of sprue strongly suggest that it has an infectious cause: (*1*) It is acquired only by visitors to or residents of endemic areas; (*2*) it can occur in epidemic form among both visitors to and native residents of endemic areas; (*3*) both the epidemics among visitors to India and the occurrence of the disease among the indigenous population of Puerto Rico have a peak seasonal incidence[13]; (*4*) "spruce houses"—dwellings in which there is a high prevalence of the disease among the occupants—have long been recognized in India and Ceylon[14]; and (*5*) treatment with broad-spectrum antibiotics or sulfa preparations is curative.[10,11] Other observations indicate that sprue often occurs as a sequela to epidemics of acute enteritis. During an annual seasonal epidemic of enteritis of unknown cause among Americans in the Philippines,

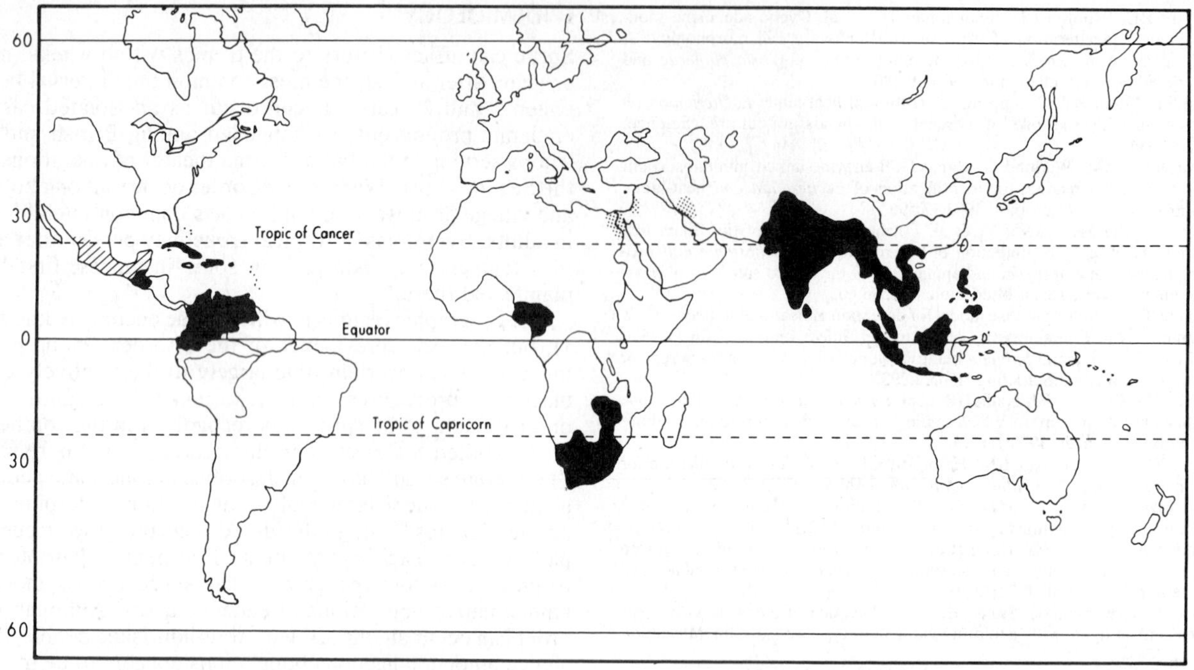

FIG. 1. Geographic distribution of tropical malabsorption. Black indicates those areas where overt tropical sprue occurs; cross-hatching, areas where a disorder resembling sprue occurs; and stippling, areas where only subclinical abnormalities of small intestinal structure or function have been observed.

one-fifth of affected people subsequently developed chronic symptoms and abnormalities of intestinal structure and function characteristic of sprue that were cured by treatment with folic acid or tetracycline.[15] Similar observations have been made after epidemics of acute enteritis that occurred in South Indian villages.[16]

Despite this circumstantial evidence, no single specific infectious agent has been isolated by culture techniques or visualized within the intestinal mucosa by light or electron microscopy. Examinations for fungus or algae with known pathogenic properties have been negative[17,18]; enterovirus- and parovirus-like agents such as the Norwalk and Hawaii agents have not been found, but no studies have been reported in which rotaviruses were searched for; strict anaerobic cultures of jejunal aspirates have not grown any obligate anaerobes,[19] and cultures of *Mycoplasma* have been negative. On the other hand, most patients with sprue who were studied in Calcutta,[20] Puerto Rico,[19] and Haiti[21] as well as expatriates who acquired sprue in Asia[22] have been found to have small intestinal contamination by coliform bacteria, most commonly with *Klebsiella pneumoniae* and less often with *Escherichia coli* and *Enterobacter cloacae*. The evidence suggests that patients with sprue have chronic contamination by a specific coliform strain and that this is not a transient colonization due to constant exposure from an unsanitary environment: (*1*) sprue patients are usually contaminated by a single biotype (as determined by API profile) of a single species; (*2*) the coliforms persist within the small intestine for months in those expatriates who return to a temperate climate,[22] and (*3*) coliforms are rarely isolated from the jejunum of healthy residents of the tropics.[19–21]

The coliform bacteria that are isolated do not have invasive properties; they yield a negative Sereny test response and are not found by immunofluorescent techniques to penetrate the mucosa after instillation with rabbit ileal ligated loops. They do produce two metabolic products that are potentially injurious to the mucosa. The first, ethanol, which is one of the principal fermentation products of coliforms, is found in the jejunal aspirate of most patients with sprue who have coliform overgrowth.[19] The second, enterotoxins, are produced by all three coliform species; these toxins are not produced by similar species of coliform bacteria isolated from the jejunum of people with the blind loop syndrome.[23] These toxins have been identified by the ability of cell-free filtrates to cause fluid secretion in rabbit ligated ileal loops[19] and the ability of semipurified ultrafiltration fractions to cause water secretion when perfused in vivo through the rat jejunum.[23,24] The toxins also impair the absorption of solutes such as xylose and are capable of producing abnormalities of intestinal structure in various experimental animal models.[24] Two toxin forms have been identified: a large-molecular-weight heat-labile form and a low-molecular-weight heat-stable form. Their precise nature remains to be determined; in most cases, they are negative in standard assays for the classic *E. coli* heat-labile (LT) and heat-stable (ST) toxins such as the Y1 adrenal cell tissue culture assay for LT and the suckling mouse assay for ST.[25]

Transient contamination of the small intestine by toxigenic forms of coliform bacteria is a common cause of acute diarrheal episodes among persons in the tropics (see Chapter 81). The finding that toxigenic strains of the same species also chronically colonize the small intestine in tropical sprue has led to the suggestion that sprue is a sequela to acute diarrhea in which failure to eliminate the toxigenic coliform bacteria results in chronic colonization by these organisms during which persistent exposure of the intestinal mucosa to the bacterial toxins results in the development of abnormalities of intestinal structure and function.[26] The milder abnormalities present in those with tropical enteropathy are viewed as sequelae of repeated episodes of transient bowel contamination. In accordance with this concept are the observations that (*1*) intestinal structure is usually normal and transport abnormalities limited to those of water and xylose during the initial phase of sprue,[27] (*2*) postinfective malabsorption is well documented in some cases,[4] and (*3*) eradication of the coliform bacteria by antibiotic treatment in sprue results in cure.[20,22]

The factors responsible for persistent contamination of the small intestine by coliform bacteria are unknown. There is suggestive evidence that the coliforms may be unusually adherent to the intestinal mucosa,[28] but no information is available concerning whether this is due to the presence of plasmid-induced specific fimbrial antigens, as is the case with strains of classic enterotoxigenic *E. coli*. Intestinal motility can be delayed in sprue, and this may contribute to persistent colonization.[29] Immunoglobulins, including mucosal IgA, are normal in people with sprue.[30] Several lines of evidence have suggested that dietary lipids may be of relevance[13]: (*1*) Sprue is endemic in areas in which and among people whose dietary lipid consists principally of long-chain unsaturated fatty acids, but it does not occur in those areas (such as Jamaica) or among those groups (such as Ghurkas) whose dietary lipid is mainly short-chain, saturated fatty acids; (*2*) epidemiologic studies have pointed toward a correlation between the occurrence of outbreaks of sprue and periods of high intake of a diet rich in linoleic acid among the population of Puerto Rico. These observations have led to the suggestion that dietary linoleic acid creates an intestinal milieu favorable for colonization by coliforms by means of its well-recognized capacity to inhibit the growth of the normally resident gram-positive organisms.[13] This sequence of events has been shown to occur in a continuous culture chemostat system,[31] but its relevance to humans remains to be established.

The failure to culture coliform bacteria from the small intestine of some persons with sprue, particularly those in South India[32] and South Africa,[33] raises the possibility that other, unrecognized enteric pathogens such as a virus may be the pathogenic factor in these cases.

The improvement in intestinal structure, particularly of crypt cell morphology, and transport that attends treatment with folic acid indicates that the eventual development of folate deficiency of the intestinal mucosa plays a perpetuating role once the intestinal abnormalities are established in sprue.

CLINICAL MANIFESTATIONS

Diarrhea is usually the first manifestation of tropical sprue and is present in 90 percent of patients; it is usually accompanied by borborygmi, abdominal distension, and cramps. Visitors to the tropics can often date exactly the onset of the disease; in these people, this usually consists of an explosive episode of diarrhea, sometimes accompanied by a flulike illness with malaise, fever, weakness, and nausea, that within a week resolves into chronic gastrointestinal symptoms. Native residents of the tropics who are accustomed to intermittent bouts of gastrointestinal upsets often find it difficult to precisely date the onset of symptoms. Many patients develop milk intolerance due to lactase deficiency, and some develop alcohol intolerance. Within 1–3 months, folate stores become depleted, and this leads to the development of anorexia, decreased dietary intake, and progressive weight loss. After 4–6 months, most develop glossitis and, eventually, symptoms of anemia. Tetany or neurologic manifestations of vitamin B_{12} deficiency are rare.

In those who were well nourished before the onset of the disease, abnormal findings on physical examination are usually confined to pallor, glossitis, increased bowel sounds, evidence of recent weight loss, and in some elderly people with severe anemia, evidence of cardiac decompensation. Among persons who were marginally or poorly nourished before the onset of sprue, signs and symptoms related to the development of nutritional deficiencies develop more rapidly and are often more prominent. These individuals can develop night blindness, stomatitis, hyperpigmentation or a pellagralike rash, koilonychia, edema, and severe emaciation.

INTESTINAL ABNORMALITIES

Function

The function of the stomach and both segments of the small intestine can be impaired in people with chronic sprue. Gastric secretion of both intrinsic factor and hydrochloric acid may be reduced. In the jejunum, there is a net secretion of water and electrolytes; glucose-facilitated water transport remains intact, however, and the administration of glucose reverses water transport to absorption. The absorption of xylose, glucose, minerals such as calcium and magnesium, and both folic acid and its dietary form polyglutamate folate are impaired. Fat absorption is reduced, due in part to a reduced bile salt pool and in part to impaired reesterification within the enterocyte; the absorption of the fat-soluble vitamins A, D, E, and K is commonly reduced. Amino acid absorption is impaired, and there may be an excess loss of albumin into the intestinal lumen. Disaccharidase concentrations of the brush border are reduced with resultant impaired hydrolysis and malabsorption of disaccharides such as lactose. There is malabsorption of vitamin B_{12} and bile salts from the ileum. Vitamin B_{12} absorption returns to normal in most patients only after antibiotic therapy has been given for several months, thus indicating that the basic defect was malabsorption due to ileal disease. In a few, it returns to normal within 1–2 weeks after the institution of antibiotic treatment, which suggests that uptake of this vitamin by the coliform bacteria was the basic abnormality. In vitro studies have shown that the coliform bacteria isolated from sprue patients incorporate vitamin B_{12} but synthesize folate.

Morphology

When observed under the dissecting microscope, the villi are usually thickened and coalesced to form leaves that, in many cases, fuse together to give the more abnormal appearance of ridges and convolutions; the flat pavementlike appearance that is characteristic of biopsy specimens from patients with gluten enteropathy is unusual. Histologic sections of the jejunum (Fig. 2) show changes of variable severity consisting of lengthening of the crypt area, broadening and shortening of the villi, and infiltration by chronic inflammatory cells; fewer than 10 percent have a flat appearance. Abnormalities of the surface epithelial cells and enzymatic activity within these cells, as detected by histochemical stains, are usually directly related to the severity of villus structural abnormality. Crypt cell nuclei often show megalocytic changes. The basement membrane beneath the surface epithelium appears to be thickened on light microscopy; electron microscopy has shown that the basal lamella itself is normal but that directly subjacent to it is a dense collagenous material. The precise identity of this material is unknown, but it has been suggested that it represents an antigen–antibody complex.

DIAGNOSIS

The diagnosis of sprue is based to a degree on the exclusion of other pathologic entities. To be considered are all of those conditions present in a temperate climate that are associated with gastrointestinal symptoms, malabsorption, and the development of nutritional deficiencies. In addition to the usual tests of intestinal function, radiologic examination of the small intestine is helpful in excluding disorders such as blind loops, strictures, and regional enteritis. A jejunal biopsy must be performed to exclude the diagnosis of gluten enteropathy, which is associated with complete villus atrophy (a rare finding in sprue), or infiltrative disease of the submucosa such as lymphoma or Whipple's disease. Conditions that are particularly common in the tropics must also be considered. These include intestinal infestation by parasites including *Giardia lamblia, Strongyloides stercoralis, Capillaria philippensis*, and *Coccidia*. These conditions can be excluded by examination of the stool.

The differential diagnosis among expatriates returning from the tropics who have chronic diarrhea, weight loss, and malabsorption usually rests between sprue and giardiasis.[1] The

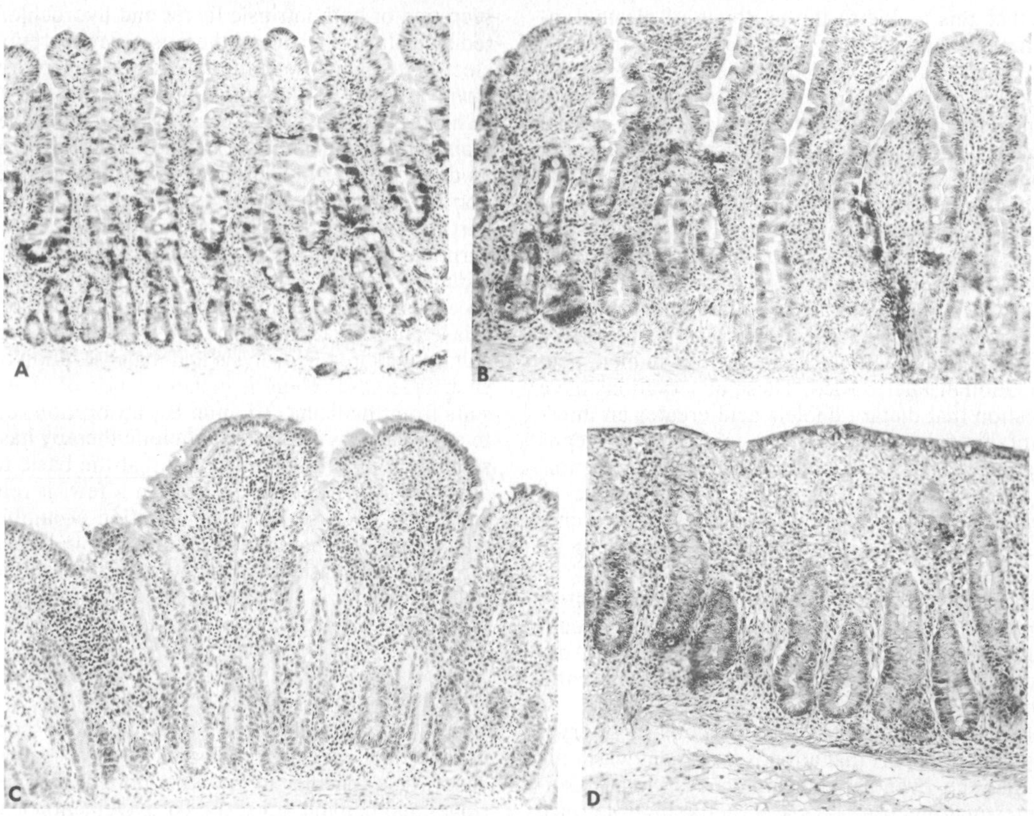

FIG. 2. Jejunal structure in tropical sprue: microscopic changes. (H&E, ×100). (**A**) Mild (1+) abnormality; (**B**) moderate (2+) abnormality; (**C**) severe (3+) abnormality; (**D**) very severe (4+) abnormality, a flat mucosa. (From Gerson,[7] with permission.)

presence of *Giardia* can be confirmed by microscopic examination of stool specimens or jejunal aspirates and biopsy specimens. Some expatriates infected with giardiasis also have small bowel contamination with coliform bacteria.[34]

In our experience with 60 consecutively studied Puerto Ricans with sprue, all had malabsorption of a 25 g oral dose of xylose, 96 percent had reduced absorption of vitamin B_{12} as tested by the Schilling test, and 69 percent had steatorrhea as assessed by fecal fat determination on a 72-hour collection; all had abnormalities of varying degrees of severity of the jejunal mucosa. Patients examined early in the course of the disorder will have none or few nutritional deficiencies. Most of those with chronic sprue have a megaloblastic anemia due to a combined deficiency of folate and vitamin B_{12}; about one-half have reduced serum albumin and cholesterol levels, and one-third mild hypocalcemia. The final confirmatory evidence to the diagnosis of sprue is improvement with the appropriate therapy.

TREATMENT

Supportive measures such as fluid or blood replacement are occasionally required in severely ill patients, but in most cases the institution of specific therapy is all that is required. Before the introduction of liver extract in 1931 and folic acid in 1946, no such therapy was available, and the therapeutic programs used then, such as dietary manipulations, often met with a variable and sometimes fatal result. Treatment with either folic acid or vitamin B_{12} is associated with prompt clinical improvement including a hematologic remission, the disappearance of glossitis, the return of appetite and weight gain, and in some, a progressive decrease in gastrointestinal symptoms. Earlier workers felt that folic acid cures sprue; however, when techniques to examine intestinal function and morphology in detail became available in the early 1960s, it became apparent that such is rarely the case in patients with chronic sprue, most of whom continue to have chronic intestinal abnormalities.[9] An exception to this is that treatment with folic acid alone can be curative in some visitors to the tropics who have been symptomatic for relatively short periods of time.[8,27]

During the Second World War, sulfaguanidine was found to alleviate or halt intestinal symptoms in British military personnel with sprue in India and Burma.[2] Subsequently, workers in England and Puerto Rico showed that combined therapy with a sulfa preparation and tetracycline for 2–3 weeks improved the intestinal abnormalities in most cases. Prolonged antibiotic therapy for 6 months was then shown to result in a complete cure in nearly all Puerto Ricans with sprue.[10] Tetracycline or poorly absorbed sulfonamides are equally effective,[11] erythromycin is said to be ineffective, and the effect of other antimicrobials has not been tested. Since most patients have only been evaluated after 6 months of treatment, it remains uncertain as to whether a shorter course of therapy might be equally effective. Recent studies in Puerto Rico have shown that there is a high rate of recurrence of intestinal abnormalities within several years after the cessation of antibiotic therapy among persons living in the tropics[35]; experience among similarly treated people living in New York City[3] suggests that such is not the case in a temperate zone.

Optimum therapy for chronic sprue consists of folic acid, 5 mg/day by mouth for 6 months, plus tetracycline, 250 mg qid for 1 month followed by the same dose bid for 5 months, and 1000 μg of vitamin B_{12} given intramuscularly several times initially and then at monthly intervals during this period. This therapeutic regimen results in prompt clinical improvement and in eventual healing of the mucosal lesion in nearly all cases.

REFERENCES

1. Klipstein FA. Tropical sprue in travelers and expatriates living abroad. Gastroenterology. 1981;80:590.
2. Keele KD, Bound JP. Sprue in India: Clinical survey of 600 cases. Br Med J. 1946;1:77.
3. Klipstein FA, Falaiye JM. Tropical sprue in expatriates from the tropics living in the continental United States. Medicine (Baltimore). 1969;48:475.
4. Montgomery RD, Beale DJ, Sammons HG, et al. Postinfective malabsorption: A sprue syndrome. Br Med J. 1973;2:265.
5. Lindenbaum J, Kent TH, Sprinz H. Malabsorption and jejunitis in American Peace Corps volunteers in Pakistan. Ann Intern Med. 1966;65:1201.
6. Thomas G, Clain DJ, Wicks ACB. Tropical enteropathy in Rhodesia. Gut. 1976;17:888.
7. Gerson CD, Kent TH, Saha JR, et al. Recovery of small-intestinal structure and function after residence in the tropics. II. Studies in Indians and Pakistanis living in New York City. Ann Intern Med. 1971;75:41.
8. Sheehy TW, Cohen WC, Wallace DK, et al. Tropical sprue in North Americans. JAMA. 1965;194:1069.
9. Sheehy TW, Baggs B, Perez-Santiago E, et al. Prognosis of tropical sprue. A study of the effect of folic acid on the intestinal aspects of acute and chronic sprue. Ann Intern Med. 1962;57:892.
10. Guerra R, Wheby MS, Bayless TM. Long-term antibiotic therapy in tropical sprue. Ann Intern Med. 1965;63:619.
11. Maldonado N, Horta E, Guerra R, et al. Poorly absorbed sulfonamides in the treatment of tropical sprue. Gastroenterology. 1969;57:559.
12. Klipstein FA, Samloff IM, Smarth G, et al. Treatment of overt and subclinical malabsorption in Haiti. Gut. 1969;10:315.
13. Klipstein FA, Corcino JJ. Seasonal occurrence of overt and subclinical tropical malabsorption in Puerto Rico. Am J Trop Med Hyg. 1974;23:1189.
14. Mathan VI, Ignatius M, Baker SJ. A household epidemic of tropical sprue. Gut. 1966;7:490.
15. Jones TC, Dean AG, Parker GW. Seasonal gastroenteritis and malabsorption at an American military base in the Philippines. II. Malabsorption following the acute illness. Am J Epidemiol. 1972;95:128.
16. Mathan VI, Baker SJ. Epidemic tropical sprue and other epidemics of diarrhea in South Indian villages. A comparative study. Am J Clin Nutr. 1968;21:1077.
17. Swanson VL, Haley LD, Wheby MS. Mycological study of jejunal biopsy specimens from patients with tropical sprue. Am J Trop Med Hyg. 1965; 14:1066.
18. Klipstein FA, Schenk EA. Prototheca and sprue. Gastroenterology. 1975;69:1372.
19. Klipstein FA, Holdeman LV, Corcino JJ, et al. Enterotoxigenic intestinal bacteria in tropical sprue. Ann Intern Med. 1973;79:632.
20. Gorbach SL, Banwell JG, Jacobs B, et al. Tropical sprue and malnutrition in West Bengal. I. Intestinal microflora and absorption. Am J Clin Nutr. 1970;23:1545.
21. Klipstein FA, Short HB, Engert RF, et al. Contamination of the small intestine by enterotoxigenic coliform bacteria among the rural population of Haiti. Gastroenterology. 1976;70:1035.
22. Tomkins AM, Drasar BS, James WPT. Bacterial colonisation of jejunal mucosa in acute tropical sprue. Lancet. 1975;1:59.
23. Klipstein FA, Engert RF, Short HB. Enterotoxigenicity of colonising coliform bacteria in tropical sprue and blind-loop syndrome. *Lancet*. 1978;2:342.
24. Klipstein FA, Horowitz IR, Engert RF, et al. Effect of *Klebsiella pneumoniae* enterotoxin on intestinal transport in the rat. J Clin Invest. 1975;56:799.
25. Klipstein FA, Guerrant RL, Wells JG, et al. Comparison of assay of coliform enterotoxins by conventional techniques versus in vivo intestinal perfusion. Infect Immun. 1979;25:146.
26. Klipstein FA. Sprue and subclinical malabsorption in the tropics. Lancet. 1979;1:277.
27. O'Brien W, England NWJ. Tropical sprue amongst British servicemen and their families in South-East Asia. In: Tropical Sprue and Megaloblastic Anaemia. London: Churchill Livingstone; 1971:25.
28. Drasar, BS, Agostini C, Clarke D, et al. Adhesion of enteropathogenic bacteria to cells in tissue culture. Dev Biol Stand. 1980;46:83.
29. Cook GC. Delayed small-intestinal transit in tropical malabsorption. Lancet. 1978;2:238.
30. Ross IN, Mathan VI. Immunological changes in tropical sprue. Q J Med. 1981;50:435.
31. Mickelson MJ, Klipstein FA. Enterotoxigenic intestinal bacteria in tropical sprue. IV. Effect of linoleic acid on growth interrelationships of *Lactobacillus acidophilus* and *Klebsiella pneumoniae*. Infect Immun. 1975;12:1121.
32. Bhat P, Shantakumari S, Rajan D, et al. Bacterial flora of the gastrointestinal tract in southern Indian control subjects and patients with tropical sprue. Gastroenterology. 1972;62:11.
33. Appelbaum PC, Moshal MG, Hift W, et al. Intestinal bacteria in patients with tropical sprue. S Afr Med J. 1980;57:1081.
34. Tomkins AM, Wright SG, Drasar BS, et al. Bacterial colonization of jejunal mucosa in giardiasis. Trans R Soc Trop Med Hyg. 1978;72:33.
35. Rickles FR, Klipstein FA, Tomasini J, et al. Long-term follow-up of antibiotic-treated tropical sprue. Ann Intern Med. 1972;76:203.

88. WHIPPLE'S DISEASE

WILLIAM O. DOBBINS III

Whipple's disease, first described in 1907,[1] is a systemic bacterial illness affecting primarily middle-aged, white men. It is characterized morphologically by the presence of macrophages in virtually all organ systems, and these macrophages are intensely stained by the periodic acid–Schiff (PAS) stain. There may be a subtle cell-mediated immune deficit that predisposes to the infection. Whipple organisms have all the structural characteristics of bacteria.[2–4] Their uniform light and electron microscopic appearance and the antigenic structure of the bacilli as determined by immunofluorescence staining[5,6] strongly suggest that a single microorganism is etiologic. However, this putative microorganism has not been cultured in vitro, and the disease has not been reproduced in animals. Most patients respond to treatment with antibiotics.

PATHOGENESIS AND PATHOLOGIC CHARACTERISTICS

Sieracki and Fine first emphasized the presence of systemic involvement when they found characteristic PAS-positive macrophages in body tissues.[7] The PAS-positive material usually occurred in the form of discrete sickle-shaped masses scattered throughout the cytoplasm of macrophages, described by Sieracki as "characteristic cells containing sickle-form particles" (SPC cells). The PAS reaction has a strong affinity for glycoproteins, and electron microscopic studies have shown that the rod-shaped masses found within macrophages are actually masses of intact and degenerating bacteria, the walls of which are apparently in part composed of glycoproteins.[3,4] Greatest involvement occurs in the lamina propria of the small intestine and its lymphatic drainage, in the heart (with valvular lesions being particularly prominent), and in the central nervous system (CNS).

Electron microscopic studies from many laboratories have documented the presence of bacilli in involved tissues,[3] both intracellularly and extracellularly. The bacilli are usually reported to be gram-positive, but sometimes they have been found to be gram-negative. These bacilli have been remarkably uniform in appearance and are approximately 0.2 μm wide by 1.5–2.5 μm long (Fig. 1). The organism possesses a trilaminar plasma membrane that is surrounded by a homogeneous cell wall approximately 20 nm thick. The cell wall itself is enclosed within an outer trilaminar "membrane."[3] This latter feature is more characteristic of gram-negative bacilli. Tubules and vesicles are located centrally within the bacilli and resemble the mesosomes that are characteristic of gram-positive bacteria. Nucleoids can often be identified within the core of the bacilli. Binary fission is often present. The Whipple bacillus is present within a variety of cells, including macrophages, intestinal epithelial cells, lymphatic and capillary endothelial cells, smooth muscle cells, polymorphonuclear leukocytes, plasma cells, mast cells, and even intraepithelial lymphocytes.[8] The intracellular bacilli are often intact in structure, which suggests that these organisms may be intracellular pathogens.[4] Immunofluorescence studies have shown that the material found within macrophages has a strong antigenic similarity to material found within streptococci groups B and G.[5,6]

Because the disease has not been reproduced in laboratory animals and because the organism has not been convincingly cultured in vitro, the only sure assay for Whipple's disease is the structural characteristic of the organism as seen by electron microscopy and possibly its antigenic structure as defined by immunofluorescence staining. Thus, the remarkable similarity

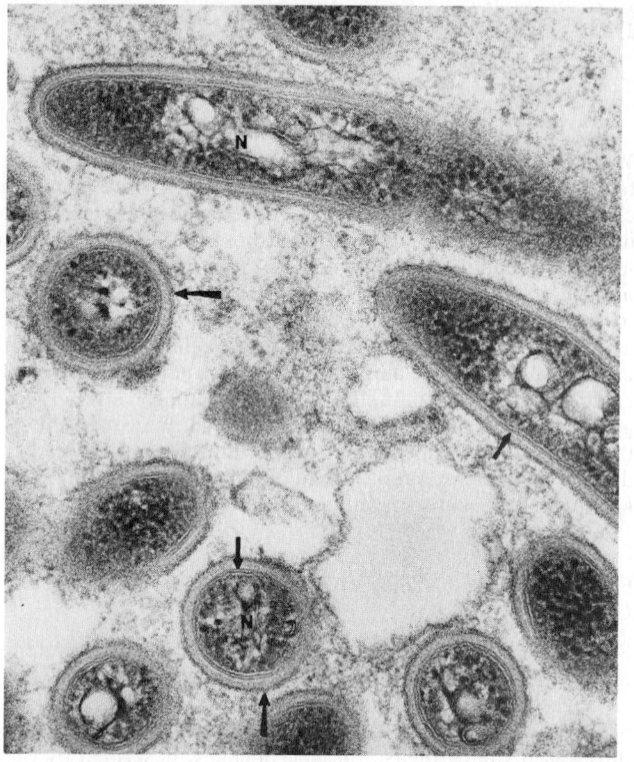

FIG. 1. Electron micrograph showing the characteristic appearance of the Whipple bacilli, many of which have been cut obliquely. These bacilli are up to 0.25 μm wide and, when sectioned lengthwise, up to 2.5 μm long. The nucleoid (N) is enclosed within a typical trilaminar plasma membrane (small arrows). A homogeneous cell wall about 20 nm thick surrounds the plasma membrane, and the cell wall itself is surrounded by a less well characterized "membrane," which has a trilaminar appearance (large arrows). The bacilli have electron microscopic characteristics, therefore, of both gram-positive and of gram-negative bacilli. (× 100,000)

of the Whipple bacillus to the "unidentified erythrocyte-associated bacterium" described by Archer et al. as a cause of human infection suggests that the latter disease may be an unusual presentation of Whipple's disease.[9]

Microscopic pathology in the proximal small intestine shows the presence of typical club-shaped villi containing PAS-positive macrophages. The macrophages are found chiefly in the gastrointestinal tract, the mesenteric and retroperitoneal nodes, the heart, and the CNS. Occasional involvement has been found in the lungs, spleen, pancreas, and peripheral lymph nodes. Minimal changes have been noted in the genitourinary tract, adrenals, joints, skin, bone marrow, and skeletal muscle.

There is evidence supporting the presence of cell-mediated immune deficiency. Even after successful treatment, the cutaneous response to antigens and the responsiveness of lymphocytes to nonspecific mitogens, although improved, are subnormal. There may be an increased association with HLA-B27 (28 percent of Whipple's patients and 10 percent of healthy people).[10]

CLINICAL AND LABORATORY FINDINGS

The patient is usually a middle-aged white man with a history of intermittent arthralgia involving multiple joints over a period of years.[11] The actual illness develops gradually, with diarrhea followed by the development of steatorrhea, weight loss, and finally a progressive downhill course. Rarely, there is no diarrhea, and the illness is characterized by nondescript abdominal pain and low-grade fever. The arthralgias may appear 10–30 years before the development of gastrointestinal symptoms and are usually migratory. Usually the large joints are most prominently involved.

Evidence of weight loss is usual. The abdomen is often distended and tender to palpation, and abdominal nodes may be palpable. Hypotension is often present, and hyperpigmentation of the skin is found in 50 percent of patients. Fever is usually low grade, but on occasion spiking temperatures to 103°F are present. Peripheral lymphadenopathy is often present. Cardiac murmurs (often with marantic endocarditis) have been noted in 25 percent of patients. Ascites is uncommon, and splenomegaly and hepatomegaly occur in less than 5 percent of patients. All of the manifestations of advanced malabsorption may be present in those patients diagnosed late in their clinical course. Neurologic abnormalities are often present and include ophthalmoplegia, dementia, ataxia, myoclonus, hyperreflexia, paresis, and sensory changes such as hearing loss and visual disturbances. The patient may present with neurologic and personality changes as the initial manifestation in the absence of significant gastrointestinal signs or symptoms.[12–14] Exceedingly rarely, Whipple's disease of the CNS has been reported in the absence of involvement of the gastrointestinal tract.

Laboratory findings include a normocytic, normochromic anemia in 90 percent of the patients. Occasional patients have iron deficiency. Megaloblastic anemia is rare. The white blood cell count is usually not elevated, and the differential count is usually normal. Hypoalbuminenia, hypocholesterolemia, hypokalemia, and prolonged prothrombin times are usually present. Steatorrhea is present in 93 percent and decreased D-xylose absorption in 78 percent of patients, whereas decreased vitamin B_{12} absorption is found in only 15 percent of patients.[11]

DIAGNOSIS

Whipple's disease should be suspected in people with the four most prominent symptoms—weight loss, diarrhea, arthralgia, and abdominal pain.[11] If the arthralgias precede the other symptoms, the diagnosis deserves very serious consideration. Histologically, the most severe and consistent changes are seen in the proximal small intestine. Thus, small bowel biopsy is the diagnostic procedure of choice. Rarely, the intestinal mucosa will contain numerous macrophages in patients with diffuse histoplasmosis and in patients with acquired immune deficiency syndrome (AIDS). Macrophages found in these diseases are not intensely PAS-positive and can be easily distinguished from those found in Whipple's disease by using special stains (for *Histoplasma capsulatum* in histoplasmosis and for intracellular *Mycobacterium avium* in AIDS).

PAS-positive macrophages can also be found in most tissues from healthy subjects. This is particularly true in the rectal and colonic mucosa. PAS-positive macrophages in the small intestinal mucosa but not in other tissues are unique and may be considered diagnostic. It is helpful to have electron microscopic confirmation of the presence of the characteristic Whipple bacilli, although these bacilli can be seen by light microscopy in properly prepared specimens.[15]

Occasionally, biopsy specimens of a lymph node or other tissue may permit the diagnosis, but they require electron microscopic confirmation.[16] Even brain biopsy specimens have been used to establish the diagnosis in the rare person with CNS Whipple's disease in the absence of intestinal involvement.[13]

Antibiotics are the treatment of choice, and good responses have been reported to a variety of antibiotics.[17–19] The appropriate duration of the therapy is unclear, but because occasional patients have had a relapse after several weeks to a few months of treatment, antibiotics should be given for 1 year.[11,17–19]

Initial treatment should consist of parenteral penicillin G (1.2 million units) plus streptomycin (1.0 g) daily for 10–14 days followed by one double-strength tablet of trimethoprim–sulfamethoxazole (TMP/SMX) given twice daily for 1 year. TMP/SMX penetrates the blood-brain barrier well. Indeed, two patients who presented with CNS Whipple's disease have responded to treatment with TMP/SMX.[17,18] If the patient is severely ill, the double-strength tablet may be given three times per day for 2 weeks and then given twice daily for 1 year. Folic acid deficiency is a potential complication of such therapy, especially in a malnourished individual. Folinic acid in a dose of 3 mg twice weekly should prevent this complication and should be administered routinely during the 2-week period that patients are given three double-strength tablets on a daily basis.

CNS relapses have not developed in patients treated with the earlier recommended regimen of parenteral penicillin and streptomycin, with or without subsequent administration of oral tetracycline.[17] Thus one could argue that treatment with parenteral penicillin and streptomycin for 10 to 14 days followed by oral tetracycline is appropriate. However, patients so treated do not receive antibiotics that cross the blood-brain barrier. In the patient allergic to or unable to tolerate sulfonamides, treatment with parenteral penicillin and streptomycin for 10–14 days followed by oral penicillin (penicillin V, 250 mg four times per day) for 1 year is recommended. Reed et al.[19] elected to treat their patient with high doses (20 million units per 24 hours) of penicillin initially for 30 days because of the *suspicion* of subclinical cerebral involvement. Because patients with Whipple's disease may be severely malnourished, folate, vitamin B_{12}, vitamin K, iron, and other dietary supplements may be beneficial.

The duration of therapy should not be determined by the presence or absence of PAS-positive macrophages within the intestinal lamina propria. The macrophages may persist within the lamina propria for many years after successful treatment, whereas free bacilli clear very rapidly and have never been reported to last longer than 9 weeks after the initiation of treatment. Routine follow-up intestinal biopsies are thus not necessary. However, it is becoming apparent that many successfully treated patients will develop a clinical relapse years after treatment, with or without intestinal symptoms. Thus, all treated patients should be followed up by careful clinical evaluation on a yearly basis. If a relapse is suspected, then intestinal biopsy specimens should be obtained and the presence or absence of free bacilli determined. An empirical trial of antibiotics may still be appropriate.

Treatment of relapse is the same as that outlined for initial therapy. If a patient with CNS relapse fails to respond to parenteral penicillin and streptomycin followed by oral TMP/SMX, treatment with oral chloramphenicol, 1 g/day (250 mg qid) for 6 to 12 months is indicated. Chloramphenicol, like TMP/SMX, results in a relatively high CNS concentration of the drug. Failure of the patient with non-CNS relapse to respond to TMP/SMX may require trials of oral penicillin (penicillin V, 250 mg four times per day) or oral tetracycline (250 mg four times per day).

REFERENCES

1 Whipple GH. A hitherto undescribed disease characterized anatomically by deposits of fat and fatty acids in the intestinal and mesenteric lymphatic tissues. Johns Hopkins Hosp Bull. 1907;18:382.
2. Dobbins WO III. Whipple's Disease. Springfield, IL: Charles C Thomas; 1987:242.
3. Silva MT, Macedo PM, Moura Nunes JF. Ultrastructure of bacilli and the bacillary origin of the macrophage inclusions in Whipple's disease. J Gen Microbiol. 1985;131:1001.
4. Dobbins WO III, Kawanishi H. Bacillary characteristics in Whipple's disease: An electron microscopic study. Gastroenterology. 1981;80:1468.
5. Keren DF, Weisburger WR, Yardley J, et al. Whipple's disease: Demonstration by immunofluorescence of similar bacterial antigens in macrophages from three cases. Johns Hopkins Med J. 1976;139:51.
6. Kent SP, Kirkpatrick PM. Whipple's disease: Immunological and histochemical studies of eight cases. Arch Pathol Lab Med. 1980;104:544.
7. Sieracki JC, Fine G. Whipple's disease: Observation on systemic involvement. I. Gross and histologic observation. *Arch Pathol.* 1959;67:81.
8. Austin LL, Dobbins WO III. Intraepithelial leucocytes of the intestinal mucosa in normal man and in Whipple's disease: A light and electron microscopic study. Dig Dis Sci. 1982;27:311.
9. Archer GL, Coleman PH, Cole RM, et al. Human infection from an unidentified erythrocyte-associated bacterium. N Engl J Med. 1979;301:897.
10. Dobbins WO III. HLA antigens in Whipple's disease. Arthritis Rheum. 1987;30:102–5.
11. Maizel H, Ruffin JM, Dobbins WO III. Whipple's disease. A review of 19 patients from one hospital and a review of the literature since 1950. Medicine (Baltimore) 1970;49:175.
12. Finelli PF, McEntee WJ, Lessel S, et al. Whipple's disease with predominantly neuroophthalmic manifestations. Ann Neurol. 1977;1:247.
13. Johnson L, Diamond I. Cerebral Whipple's disease: Diagnosis by brain biopsy. Am J Clin Pathol. 1979;74:486.
14. Schmitt BP, Richardson H, Smith E, et al. Encephalopathy complicating Whipple's disease. Ann Intern Med. 1981;94:51.
15. Trier JS, Phelps PC, Eidelman S, et al. Whipple's disease: Light and electron microscope correlation of jejunal mucosal histology with antibiotic treatment and clinical status. Gastroenterology. 1965;48:684.
16. Mansbach CM II, Shelburne FA, Stevens RD, et al. Lymph node bacilliform bodies resembling those of Whipple's disease in a patient without intestinal involvement. Ann Intern Med. 1978;89:64.
17. Keinath RD, Merrell DE, Vlietstra R, et al. Antibiotic treatment and relapse in Whipple's disease: Long-term followup of 88 patients. Gastroenterology. 1985;88:1867–73.
18. Ryser RJ, Locksley RM, Eng SC, et al. Reversal of dementia associated with Whipple's disease by trimethoprim-sulfamethoxazole, drugs that cross the blood-brain barrier. Gastroenterology. 1984;86:745.
19. Reed JI, Sipe JD, Wohlgethan JR, et al. Response of the acute phase reactants to antibiotic treatment of Whipple's disease. Arthritis Rheum. 1985;28:352–5.

SECTION L. BONE AND JOINT INFECTIONS

89. INFECTIOUS ARTHRITIS

JAMES W. SMITH

An inflammatory reaction in the joint space (arthritis) follows infection with many different microorganisms. Bacterial invasion of the joint generally leads to a suppurative arthritis, principally of one joint (monarticular). Certain bacteria, however, may produce symptoms in multiple joints, particularly during the bacteremic stage of their infection, as well as induce inflammation in the neighboring tendon sheaths, for example, *Neisseria gonorrhoeae*. Infections of the joint due to viruses frequently involve multiple joints and demonstrate inflammation without suppuration. A chronic granulomatous monarticular arthritis may be seen with mycobacteria or fungi that must be differentiated from other causes of chronic monarticular arthritis. In addition, a sterile arthritis may be associated with an infection either preceding the typical clinical syndrome, as with hepatitis B, or following the infection as postinfectious arthritis with *Shigella* or *Salmonella*. Infectious arthritis is associated with a low case fatality rate and few residual symptoms if recognized and treated properly. Since a number of other clinical entities may be confused with infectious arthritis, the approach to any person with an inflamed joint must include infection among the differential possibilities.

PATHOGENESIS AND PREDISPOSING FACTORS

Infectious arthritis follows hematogenous inoculation of the pathogenic organism in a great majority of instances since only a few have a history of recent intra-articular injection before infection.[1,2] The infection may develop as a direct infection of the synovial space or may represent extension from infected bone. Infectious arthritis in infants below the age of 1 year may occur secondary to extension from a primary osteomyelitis focus since capillaries still perforate the epiphyseal growth plate.[3] However, children over the age of 1 are more likely to develop infection of the joint alone since the growth plate contains the infection. Many patients with bacterial arthritis give a history of trauma (Table 1) that may enable bacteria, mycobacteria, or fungi to penetrate the synovial space more easily. Extra-articular infections are found in approximately one-quarter of both adults and children with bacterial arthritis (Table 1). In contrast to children, adults frequently have one or more significant systemic conditions predisposing to bacterial arthritis.[1,4] These factors vary from the administration of corticosteroids, either orally or after intra-articular injection, to the presence of a systemic disease as diabetes mellitus or hematologic malignancies. Patients with rheumatoid arthritis and osteoarthritis appear to be predisposed to infectious arthritis more than would be expected by chance alone.[5] Joint infections in rheumatoid patients tend to occur in older people with debilitating arthritis of longer than 10 years' duration.[6]

Endocrine factors appear to be important in the genesis of the disseminated gonococcal syndrome since this syndrome tends to occur in women during a particularly susceptible period in pregnancy (the second or third trimester) and during menstruation.[7,8] Not only is endocervical shedding of the *N. gonorrhoeae* maximal during menstruation, but also access to the blood stream would be greatest at this time. In contrast, infection is rarely seen in the third week of the menstrual cycle when the shedding of *N. gonorrhoeae* is minimal and the pH is not optimal for growth of the bacteria.[8] Arthritis due to particular viral infections also relates to certain endocrine factors since rubella arthritis principally occurs in postpubertal women whereas mumps arthritis is seen exclusively in postpubertal men.[9]

Arthritis that occurs in the convalescent period of infection has been postulated in a number of instances to relate to the immune response to the microorganism. Arthritis has been noted late in the course of infections with meningococci and lymphocytic choriomeningitis virus.[10,11] However, it cannot be clearly established whether these infections represent active infection or are more likely postinfectious arthritis due to the immune response of the organism. Arthritis in patients with hepatitis B infection has been shown to relate to antigen–antibody complexes.[12] Circulating complexes in patients with arthritis have high quantities of IgG, IgM, and IgA, especially IgG1 and IgG3, the complement-fixing globulins. In addition, C3, C4, and C5 have been demonstrated in the immune complexes. As the arthritis disappears with the onset of jaundice, the complement components can no longer be demonstrated in the immune complexes.

The postinfectious arthritis that develops in persons after *Shigella, Salmonella, Campylobacter,* and *Yersinia* infections of the gastrointestinal tract frequently have the specific histocompatibility antigen HLA-B27 (Table 2).[13–16] Persons with arthritis after one outbreak of shigellosis had Reiter syndrome with active disease for up to 10 years.[13] It has been calculated that the likelihood of a B27-positive patient developing Reiter syndrome varies from 16 to 37 percent and that a B27-positive patient has a 50 times greater risk of developing arthritis after *Yersinia* infection than a person who is not B27-positive.[13,14]

TABLE 1. Predisposing Factors in Bacterial Arthritis

Factor	In Adults[a] %	In Children %
Corticosteroid administration	33	
Pre-existing arthritis	24	
Intra-articular injection	23	
Other infection	22	26
Diabetes mellitus	13	
Trauma	12	28
Other diseases	19	3
None	8	43

[a] More than one predisposing factor existed in some patients.
(Data from Kelly et al.,[1] and Nelson et al.[2])

TABLE 2. Frequency of HLA-B27 in Patients with Arthritis After Infectious Diarrhea

Group	Infecting Pathogens: Shigella	Yersinia	Salmonella
Control	7[a]	14	10
No arthritis		15	8
Arthritis	80	88	69

[a] Values are percentages of the groups expressing HLA-B27.
(Data from Calin et al.,[13] Aho et al.,[14] and Hakansson et al.[15])

CLINICAL FEATURES

Site of Infection

The site of infection in cases with bacterial or suppurative arthritis is monarticular in 90 percent of children and adults.[1,2,4,17,18] The knee is the most commonly affected joint in both children and adults with bacterial arthritis as well as in infections with *Mycobacterium tuberculosis*[19] (Table 3). The hip is the next most commonly involved joint, with variation in the frequency of involvement of other joints. Adults tend to have more involvement of the shoulder, sternoclavicular, and sacroiliac joints, especially in parenteral drug abusers,[20,22] whereas children tend to have infection more commonly of the ankle and elbow.[2] The wrist and interphalangeal joints of the hand are infrequently involved with suppurative arthritis due to bacteria, although these joints are commonly involved in patients with infections with *N. gonorrhoeae*[8] and with *M. tuberculosis*.[19] Infectious arthritis of viral etiology (e.g., rubella) tends to involve multiple joints, with most having symptoms in the interphalangeal joints of the hands, the wrist, as well as the knees, ankles, and elbows[9,21] (Table 3).

TABLE 3. Frequency (Percentages) of Joint Involvement in Infectious Arthritis[a]

Joint	Bacterial (Suppurative): Children	Bacterial (Suppurative): Adults	Mycobacterial	Viral
Knee	41	48	24	60
Hip	23	24	20	4
Ankle	14	7	12	30
Elbow	12	11	8	20
Wrist	4	7	20	55
Shoulder	4	15	4	5
Interphalangeal and metacarpal	1.4	1	12	75
Sternoclavicular	0.4	8	0	0
Sacroiliac	0.4	2	0	0

[a] More than one joint may be involved, so the percentages exceed 100 percent.
(Data from refs. 1, 2, 4, 9, 17, 19, 20, 21.)

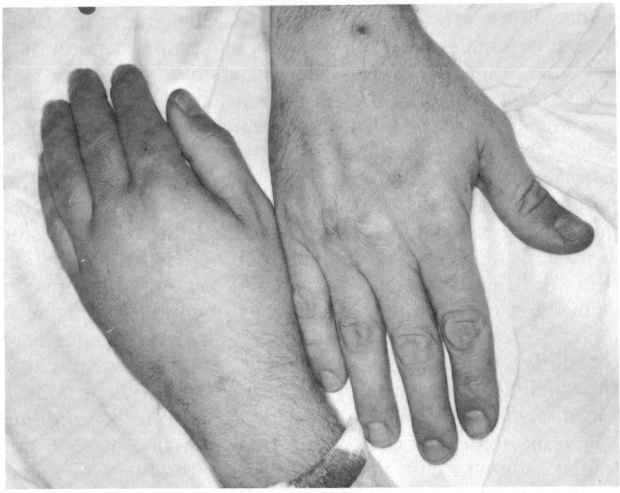

FIG. 1. Patient with chromic gonococcemia with swollen hand and skin lesions over dorsal surface of wrist. (Courtesy of *Current Prescribing*, April, 1979.)

Persons with bacterial (suppurative) arthritis generally have fever and symptoms in a single joint with pain on motion, limitation of motion, and swelling. The joints may vary from minimal tenderness to severe tenderness. Joint effusion can be demonstrated in 90 percent of the joints that can be examined easily. In 10 percent of persons, multiple joints may be involved with bacterial infection. Infections with mycobacteria or certain fungi such as *Sporothrix schenckii* may be so insidious and slow to evolve that an infection may not be considered.[19,23] A diagnosis of bacterial infection of hip joints is difficult since the symptoms may be minimal and effusions may be difficult to demonstrate.[5]

Inflammation of the tendon sheaths (tenosynovitis) occurs commonly with the disseminated gonococcal syndrome[8] (Fig. 1). Tenosynovitis also may be seen with other infections such as *Moraxella*, rubella, atypical mycobacteria, and sporotrichosis. Carpal tunnel syndrome (paresthesias of the hands), with or without joint symptoms, occurs with rubella, atypical mycobacteria, sporotrichosis, and histoplasmosis.

Septic bursitis is usually due to *Staphylococcus aureus* and more commonly follows local trauma.[24] The olecranon and prepatellar bursae are the usual sites. Occasionally, organisms of low pathogenicity cause chronic olecranon bursitis, such as nontuberculous *Mycobacterium*, *Prototheca*, and *Phialophora*.

LABORATORY FINDINGS

Patients with infectious arthritis, whether bacterial, viral, or mycobacterial, have an elevated erythrocyte sedimentation rate (ESR). The ESR is higher in those with bacterial infection and in those with an infection of long duration. Anemia may be noted, particularly in those with chronic infections or in those who develop infectious arthritis secondary to underlying joint disease such as rheumatoid arthritis. Children tend to have elevated white blood cell counts with a predominance of polymorphonuclear leukocytes, whereas many adults do not have an elevated peripheral blood leukocyte count.[1,2]

Joint fluid from monarticular bacterial arthritis generally appears turbid or purulent, although 10–20 percent have serosanguineous fluid. The joint leukocyte count is greater than 100,000/mm^3 in one-third to one-half, and most have a differential count of more than 90 percent polymorphonuclear leukocytes.[18] However, this finding is not specific for bacterial arthritis since many other joint conditions such as rheumatoid arthritis, rheumatic fever, and crystalline joint disease may be associated with a preponderance of polymorphonuclear leukocytes and, conversely, not all cases of bacterial infection have an elevated leukocyte count. Protein levels are generally elevated, but this has little specificity for joint infection. Although a low synovial fluid glucose content or a synovial fluid glucose content less than 40 mg/dl of the blood glucose is suggestive of suppurative arthritis,[5,17] this difference is valid only if the blood and synovial fluid specimens have been obtained simultaneously. Low joint fluid glucose concentrations have been found in only one-half of adult patients[25] and in an even smaller proportion of children with bacterial arthritis.[17] Other conditions are associated with a low joint fluid glucose value including rheumatoid arthritis; hence this test does not have the specificity of predictive value as a low cerebrospinal fluid glucose value does for bacterial meningitis. Viral arthritis may be associated with a modest elevation of the synovial fluid leukocyte count. In most instances the preponderant cell is mononuclear, although some cases with proven rubella arthritis have had a majority of polymorphonuclear leukocytes. In tuberculous arthritis, most patients had an elevated leukocyte count and a predominance of polymorphonuclear leukocytes.[26] A significantly decreased joint fluid glucose level was found in 61 percent. Leukocyte counts exceeding 1000/mm^3 are characteristic of staphylococcal bursitis.[24]

Smears of joint fluid stained for bacteria from persons with bacterial arthritis show the organisms in slightly over one-half of the cases.[5] The Gram stain can give false-positive results (positive test results not confirmed by a positive culture). The methylene blue stain is probably a more reliable stain. Both blood and joint fluid should be cultured aerobically and anaerobically. In addition, other appropriate cultures such as on spinal fluid should be done if there are central nervous system manifestations. Pharyngeal, rectal, and cervical or urethral cultures should be done if the disseminated gonococcal syndrome is considered. Blood cultures have been positive in 10–60 percent of the cases in adults and in 29 percent of children with bacterial arthritis.[1,4,17] Joint cultures are positive in up to 90 percent of those in whom a diagnosis of bacterial arthritis has been established and in 79 percent of those with tuberculosis.[26]

The most frequent roentgenographic abnormality in bacterial arthritis is distension of the joint capsule and soft tissue swelling in the adjacent space. However, these findings are not pathognomonic for infection. Destructive changes are rarely noted in bacterial infections save in those who are seen late (more than 2 weeks) in the course of infection, as with hip infection.[1] If the infection complicates rheumatoid arthritis, then cortical destruction and erosion is a more constant feature; however, these changes cannot be distinguished from rheumatoid arthritis without infection. Mycobacterial infection of the joint leads to joint space narrowing, metaphyseal and subchondral erosions, and cyst formation.[19] Viral infections rarely produce roentgenographic changes unless significant quantities of fluid are present and result in distension of the joint capsule.

PATHOLOGIC CHANGES

In experimental arthritis produced by the intra-articular injection of *Staphylococcus aureus* into rabbits, early pathologic changes were noted in the surface and in the matrix of the superficial zone of the articular surface by electron microscopy within 24 hours.[27] At this time, the joint cavity showed polymorphonuclear leukocytes, and lysosomal bodies were present in the synovial cells. By 3 days, the destruction of articular cartilage was more extensive and was even visible with light microscopy. The matrix appeared loose in the superficial zones, and degeneration of chondrocytes was noted in deeper zones. In chronic arthritis due to mycobacteria or fungi, histologic evidence of a granulomatous inflammation occurs with dense mononuclear inflammatory infiltrates consisting of lymphocytes.[26] Palisading of histiocytes may be detected around a foci of coagulation necrosis.[23,26] Organisms were demonstrated with special stain in only 19 percent with *M. tuberculosis* and rarely in fungal infections, but culture of the biopsy tissue was positive for the particular infecting organism.[23,26]

ETIOLOGIC AGENTS

Bacterial (Suppurative) Arthritis

The frequency of the etiologic agents that induce bacterial arthritis varies with age (Table 4). *Haemophilus influenzae* type b is the preponderant causative organism in children under 2 years of age. Although it is rarely seen after 5 years of age,[2,5] adults can develop septic arthritis with *H. influenzae* if they have immune defects.[28] In infants under 1 month of age, group B streptococci, gram-negative bacilli, and *S. aureus* are causative organisms. *Staphylococcus aureus* is the most frequent organism causing bacterial arthritis in children over 2 years of age[2,17] and is the causative organism in the vast majority of cases of suppurative arthritis in adults.[1,4,18] *Neisseria gonorrhoeae* is the preponderant cause of bacterial arthritis in adults under 30 years.[25] The frequency of streptococcal infections as a cause of bacterial arthritis is relatively constant from childhood through the adult years (13–17 percent). The most frequently isolated type in both children and adults is group A β-hemolytic streptococci; however, group B (in the neonate and adult diabetic), viridans streptococci, and microaerophilic and anaerobic streptococci have been isolated. *Streptococcus pneumoniae* is rarely encountered now as a cause of suppurative arthritis. It has been noted to be the causative organism of septic arthritis in children with sickle disease.[29] The course of suppurative arthritis, the frequency of multiple joint involvement, the sites of infection, and the laboratory abnormalities do not differ significantly with any of these major causative agents of bacterial arthritis.[25]

Infectious arthritis due to gram-negative bacilli (other than *H. influenzae*) as causative organisms is seen in 9–17 percent of the cases of infectious arthritis.[1,4,18,25] Most had either a chronic debilitating disease or a chronic arthritis in the infected joint along with an intercurrent urinary tract infection or had the clinical picture of gram-negative bacteremia.[30] Infection with these organisms was associated with a poor outcome since a large proportion of the patients died and most survivors developed significant flexion contractions, an ankylosing joint, or chronic effusions. Heroin addicts who develop septic arthritis are more likely to have *Pseudomonas* as the causative organism than any other group, with more frequent sternoclavicular and sacroiliac joint infections.[20] Septic arthritis due to *Salmonella* species occurs preponderantly in children but bears no association with sickle cell disease, unlike *Salmonella* osteomyelitis.

Gonococcal arthritis, one of the more commonly recognized features of disseminated gonococcal infections,[7,8] exists in either of two forms. (*1*) Patients have systemic symptoms with fever, shaking chills, skin lesion, and a polyarticular syndrome.

TABLE 4. Etiologic Agents as Causes of Bacterial (Suppurative) Arthritis (Percentages)

	Children		
Agent	*<5 Yr*	*>5 Yr*	*Adults*
Staphylococcus aureus	12	33	70
Haemophilus influenzae, type b	29	1	<1
Streptococcus sp[a]	12	13	17
Gram-negative bacilli	5	6	8
Anaerobic	0	1	<1
Neisseria	5	8	[b]
Other	2	5	0
Unknown	35	34	3

[a] Includes *Streptococcus pneumoniae*, groups A and B streptococci, viridans group streptococci, and microaerophilic and anaerobic streptococci.
[b] Excluded from most series of adult suppurative arthritis.
(Data from refs. 1, 4, 17, 18.)

Blood cultures are frequently positive, particularly if patients are seen within 2 days of the onset of symptoms, whereas synovial fluid cultures are rarely, if ever, positive. *N. gonorrhoeae* can be recovered if cultures of genital, rectal, and pharyngeal areas are done. The skin lesions begin as tiny erythematous papules, frequently petechiae, and may evolve to become vesicles or even be pustular (Fig. 1). These lesions are fairly transient and last 3–4 days. An occasional patient who fails to come to medical attention may have recurrent episodes of skin lesions and polyarthralgias for periods up to 3 months[8] (as in the case in Fig. 1). The organism is occasionally recovered from scrapings of the skin lesion, although more frequently organisms are recovered from blood. Other microorganisms to be considered in the differential diagnosis of patients with skin rash and arthritis include *Haemophilus influenzae, Moraxella osloensis, Streptobacillus moniliformis,* and *Neisseria meningitidis*. (*2*) Patients with gonococcal infection may also have a monarticular, suppurative joint infection with recovery of the organism from joint fluid. These patients may give a history of having had transient polyarthralgias before the monarticular arthritis developed and may even have a history of skin lesions; however, skin lesions are rarely present in those with a monarticular arthritis. Infection with *N. meningitidis* may mimic the disseminated gonococcemia syndrome with a high probability of greater than 100 skin lesions.[31] In addition, patients with meningococcemia may develop joint effusions 5–10 days after the onset of the infection. Sterile effusions are found in multiple joints and resolve rather rapidly regardless of antimicrobial therapy. An uncommon variety of meningococcal infection is chronic meningococcemia in which symptoms are present for more than a week without meningeal involvement.[10] These patients have low-grade fever; a rash that may be macular, papular, or petechial; joint involvement; and headache. Two-thirds of the patients have polyarthralgias, and one-third have arthritis with joint effusions. Infections with *Streptobacillus moniliformis* occur 2–3 days after rat bites with the onset of chills, a macular rash of the palms and soles, and arthralgias in large joints.[32] The organism, a pleomorphic gram-negative bacillus, can be grown in blood cultures but not from joint fluid. Intermittent attacks of a migratory polyarticular arthritis lasting weeks to months, usually in large joints, occur late in the disease course of many patients with Lyme disease.[33] This spirochetal infection transmitted by tick bite (Chapter 217) also rarely can result in a long-standing chronic arthritis of the knee joint.[33]

Obligate anaerobic bacteria rarely are the causative agents in bacterial arthritis, even when anaerobic cultures are performed routinely on joint fluid, but can result in a long-standing chronic arthritis of the knee joint.[34] The predominant obligate anaerobic bacteria causing septic arthritis in adults have been gram-negative cocci, especially after surgery.[34] *Bacteroides* species are less often encountered. The most frequent anaerobic arthritis in children is due to *Clostridium* species.[2]

Mycobacterial Infections

Chronic monarticular arthritis with a granulomatous reaction on pathologic examination may be caused by variety of organisms (Table 5). Mycobacterial infections of the joint are chronic, slowly progressive monarticular infections that may also involve the tendon sheaths, particularly the carpal tunnel area of the wrist. A granulomatous reactions of the synovium is seen pathologically, but organisms are rarely demonstrated save by appropriate culture of synovial tissue. Small particulate matter representing fibrinous deposits, called *rice bodies*, may be seen in synovial fluid or tissue with mycobacterial infections, brucellosis, and sporotrichosis.[19,23,35] Infections with *M. tuberculosis* principally involve the knee, followed by the hip, ankle, and wrist.[19] A number of nontuberculous mycobacteria produce infections of the joints (Table 5). *Mycobacterium kansasii* was the most common cause of monarticular synovitis seen in Dal-

TABLE 5. Infectious Causes of Chronic Monarticular Arthritis

Bacterial	
	Brucella sp.
Eubacteria	
	Mycobacterium tuberculosis
	M. kansasii
	M. marinum
	M. intracellulare
	M. fortuitum
	Nocardia asteroides
Fungi	
	Sporothrix schenckii
	Coccidioides immitis
	Blastomyces dermatitidis
	Candida albicans
	Pseudallescheria boydii

las, Texas.[36] This organism has a propensity to involve the wrist and hands and cause a flexor tenosynovitis, a carpal tunnel syndrome, and rarely olecranon bursitis.[36] *M. kansasii* may localize to a joint after trauma from a pulmonary focus. These patients do not usually have extra-articular infection. *Mycobacterium marinum* would be suspected in a patient with arthritis who develops the infection after exposure to tropical fish aquariums or marine life.[37] Synovial tissue from a patient with a chronic monarticular arthritis should be cultured for mycobacteria, observed at a few days (to recognize *M. fortuitum*, a rapid grower), and incubated at 30°C (*M. marinum* grows better at this temperature than at 37°C).

Fungal Arthritis

Sporothrix schenckii can cause infections of the joints.[23,38] The organism commonly infects the knee, the wrist, and the elbow. The ankle or small joints of the hand may be infected, but shoulders and hips are spared (Figs. 2 and 3). Sporotrichotic arthritis or tenosynovitis is not usually a sequel of cutaneous inoculation but may result from occult pulmonary infection. The course is progressive over months and years, usually without fever. With time, infection appears in contiguous bursae or bones as well as in distant joints. Diagnosis is by culture of fluid or tissue.

A chronic monarticular arthritis is seen with *Coccidioides immitis* with or without other evidence of disseminated infection.[39] The knee is the most frequently involved joint. The joint fluid may show either a polymorphonuclear or a lymphocytic cellular response, but smears and cultures are often negative. X-ray films show little evidence of bony destruction even after many months of clinical evidence. Diagnosis is made by culture of synovium. Patients' sera also have positive complement fixation responses with *Coccidioides* antigen.

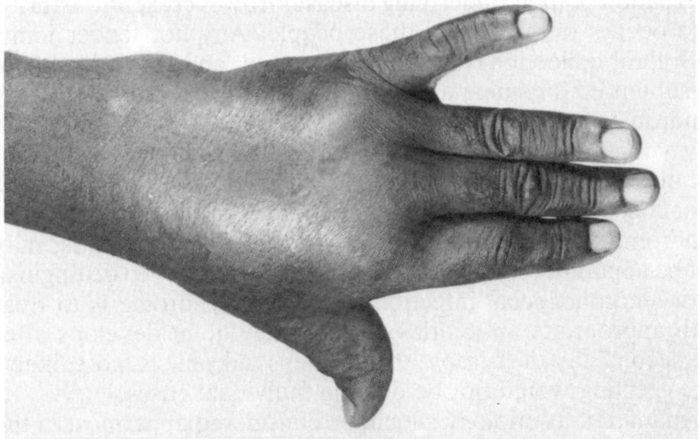

FIG. 2. Wrist of patient who had sporotrichosis of wrist and olecranon bursa. (Courtesy of *Current Prescribing*, April, 1979.)

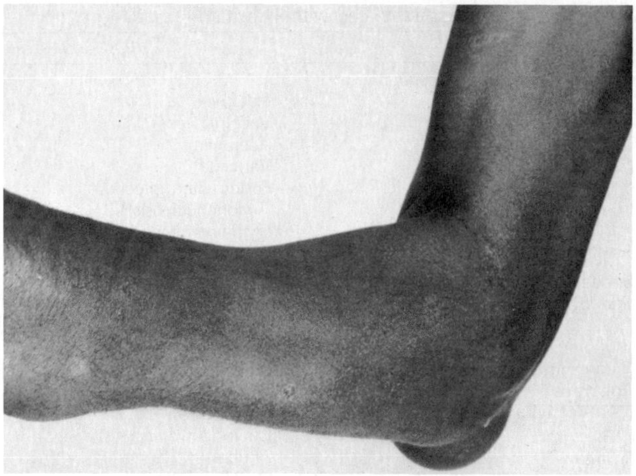

FIG. 3. Elbow of patient who had sporotrichosis of wrist and olecranon bursa. (Courtesy of *Current Prescribing*, April, 1979.)

Joint infection in patients with blastomycosis primarily spreads from osteomyelitis.[40] The diagnosis can be made by examination of synovial tissue and by appropriate culture of surgical material. Complement fixation tests are usually not helpful.

Infections of the joint with *Candida* species generally follows hematogenous spread of the organism, most frequently *Candida albicans*. Or the fungus may be introduced accidentally during intra-articular corticosteroid injection.[41] Synovial fluid shows a polymorphonuclear leukocytic response, and acute and chronic inflammatory cells are noted on microscopic examination. The knee is the most commonly involved joint, with hip, elbow, and other joints also noted. More than one joint may demonstrate infection. Migratory polyarthritis, usually in association with skin lesions or erythema nodosum and erythema multiforme, has been seen with acute histoplasmosis.[42] Carpal tunnel syndrome has also been noted in patients with disseminated histoplasmosis. *Pseudallescheria (Petriellidium) boydii* arthritis has occurred in several patients with penetrating trauma of the knee.

Viral Arthritis

Viral agents associated with symptoms and signs of arthritis are listed in Table 6. Arthritis is a reasonably frequent event and thus can be considered a common manifestation of infection with some agents such as rubella or mumps. Single or only a few cases have been reported with a number of other viruses, so arthritis occurs as an atypical manifestation of infection with these agents, for example, varicella, adenovirus, echovirus. Epidemic smallpox was associated with arthritis (with a frequency of 0.2–0.5 percent) exclusively in infants or children under 7 years of age.[43]

Patients with sporadic or epidemic hepatitis B have been noted to develop arthritis, frequently in association with urticaria.[44] The frequency of arthritis and urticaria is highly variable but was seen in 25 percent of the persons in one epidemic, with skin rash (urticaria, angioneurotic edema, and other erythematous reactions) in 42 percent of those who subsequently developed jaundice.[44] The joint and skin manifestations appear a few days to a few weeks before the onset of the jaundice, and in the great majority, the symptoms disappear with the onset of the jaundice.[45] The hands are most frequently involved. Joint effusions are scanty when present and reveal predominantly mononuclear cells. Hepatitis B antigen is frequently found in the serum at the time of the onset of the arthritis and has been detected in joint fluid in a few cases.[21] Circulating immune com-

TABLE 6. Viral Agents Associated with Arthritis

Group	Virus
Deoxyribonucleic acid viruses	
Poxvirus	Smallpox
	Vaccinia[a]
Adenovirus	Adenovirus[a]
Herpesvirus	Varicella[a]
	Epstein-Barr (infectious mononucleosis)[a]
Parvovirus	Erythema infectiosum
Hepadnavirus	Hepatitis B
Ribonucleic acid viruses	
Paramyxoviruses	Mumps
	Rubeola[a]
Orthomyxoviruses	Influenza[a]
Picornavirus	Echovirus[a]
Togavirus	
Alphavirus	Chikungunya
	O'nyong-nyong
	Sindbis
	Ockelbo disease
	Ross River virus
Rubivirus	Rubella
Arenavirus	Lymphocytic choriomeningitis virus

[a] Unusual manifestation of infection.

plexes containing immunoglobulin and complement components are detected in serum.[12] Joint symptoms may rarely persist up to 6 months, but no residual deformity or sequelae have been noted.

Arthritis occurs in association with mumps with a frequency of 0.44 percent and is seen more commonly in men.[9] The arthritis begins from 1 day before to 15 days after the onset of parotitis, with multiple large and small joints affected. Effusions are infrequent. Symptoms subside within 2 weeks, although arthritis may persist for up to 3 months.[46]

A number of alphaviruses of the togavirus family have arthritis as a frequent manifestation of the illness they cause. Chikungunya derives its name from its characteristic clinical finding (that which bends up). This disease is characterized by an abrupt onset of fever, chills, and severe incapacitating pain in the large joints, although hot, swollen joints are infrequently seen.[47] Maculopapular eruption occurred over the trunk and extensor surface of the extremities in 80 percent of those with the disease. A similar illness in Uganda in 1959 was given the name O'nyong-nyong fever (weakening of the joints).[48] The onset of O'nyong-nyong fever was also abrupt, with symmetric involvement of most of the large joints with excruciating pain. All eventually made a full recovery. Sindbis virus and Sindbis-related diseases such as Ockelbo disease in Sweden have been noted to have arthritis as a prominent manifestation of the illness.[49] In Australia, epidemics of polyarthritis with rash have been observed since 1928 that are due to the recently identified alphavirus, the Ross River agent.[50]

Arthritis due to rubella occurs principally in women.[9,21] The onset of the joint symptoms occurs either with the rash or within 3 days after the eruption. The small joints of the hand are most frequently involved, with knees, wrists, and ankles less commonly affected. Synovial fluid shows a predominance of mononuclear cells, and virus is rarely isolated from the joint fluid. The course is self-limited in most people, although symptoms will rarely last for longer than a month. Rubella vaccine induces joint symptoms with a frequency of 3 percent in children of both sexes but in 39 percent of susceptible postpubertal women.[51] The vaccine virus has rarely been recovered from synovial fluid, but persons with arthralgias or arthritis developed a significantly higher antibody titer than did those without joint reaction. Thus, the use of rubella vaccine in susceptible postpubertal women entails a risk of significant joint symptoms.

Lymphocytic choriomeningitis, caused by an arenavirus, was associated with arthritis in one outbreak among laboratory personnel.[11] Hence, the development of a severe influenza-like disease with headache and arthritis may be due to lymphocytic choriomeningitis virus rather than influenza, a disease in which arthritis is an uncommon complication. In outbreaks of epidemic erythema infectiosum, an infection caused by a parvovirus, a symmetric arthritis was noted in adults, particularly in women.[52]

Parasites

Joint manifestations are not a feature of any of the commonly recognized parasitic infections. However, in the Sepik district of Papua, New Guinea, arthritis in association with filarial infections was the most frequent cause of arthritis.[53] The knee was the most frequently involved joint and showed warmth, tenderness, and limitation of motion. Joint effusions were present in slightly less than one-half of the cases, and the fluid aspirated was creamy yellow. X-ray films showed no articular destruction, only soft tissue swelling. Microfilariae were present in the blood. The patients responded promptly to treatment with diethylcarbamazine, with improvement in the joint symptoms and loss of microfilariae in the blood.

APPROACH TO THE PATIENT

Differential Considerations

Any person with an acute monarticular arthritis should be suspected of having septic arthritis of bacterial etiology. However, a number of conditions may show a single joint involvement with effusions, including acute rheumatoid arthritis, gout, and chondrocalcinosis (pseudogout). In each of these conditions up to 90 percent of the synovial fluid cell count can demonstrate polymorphonuclear leukocytes. The synovial fluid glucose content may be diminished in rheumatoid arthritis and is not reliably diminished in bacterial arthritis. Hence, the ultimate diagnosis must be based on multiple studies including cultures of joint fluid and blood. Synovial fluid from any adult with monarticular arthritis should be examined for crystals, both for negatively birefringent (uric acid) and positively birefringent (calcium pyrophosphate) crystals. Simultaneous bacterial infection and crystalline joint disease has been reported.[54] Serologic studies including rheumatoid factor, LE cell and anti-nuclear antibody tests, and acute and convalescent studies for anti-streptolysin O (ASO) should be performed if more than one joint is affected. A small proportion of cases of suppurative arthritis (10 percent) do involve more than one joint. This may be particularly perplexing in the patient with rheumatoid arthritis since the involvement of a number of joints may herald an exacerbation of their underlying disease. However, septic arthritis also occurs frequently in these people. Any hot tender joints with fluid collections should be aspirated, and the fluid should be submitted for smear and culture. Gonococcal arthritis, Reiter syndrome, and acute rheumatic fever should be suspected in any young adult having fever and multiple joint involvement, although skin lesions are the clinical clue to the disseminated gonococcal syndrome. The other features of the triad of Reiter syndrome, the conjunctival manifestations and urethritis, may not be apparent initially. Frequently, the only way to distinguish between gonococcal infection and Reiter syndrome is to treat with appropriate antibiotics, and if a new joint develops after the second day of therapy, then Reiter syndrome is more likely. HLA testing would not be done in individual cases.

An infectious etiology should be considered uppermost in the differential diagnosis of any chronic monarticular arthritis, especially if tenosynovitis is present. The leading infectious cause is infection with nontuberculous mycobacteria, followed closely by *Sporothrix schenckii*. Infection with *M. tuberculosis* is less often seen today. In addition, Lyme arthritis should be considered if patient is from an endemic area.[33] A synovial biopsy should be done in any person with a chronic monarticular involvement whose synovial fluid cultures are negative, and the tissue should be cultured for fungus and acid-fast organisms. In Lyme arthritis, the infectious agent can be demonstrated by Dieterle silver stain in 25 percent, but all should have a diagnostic titer in a serum indirect immunofluorescent assay of 1:256 or greater.[33] Pathologic examination of the tissue and the culture results provide a clue to whether an infection or other rheumatic disease is the cause of chronic arthritis in most cases.

In any patient with an acute arthritis in whom a diagnosis of bacterial infection cannot be established and in whom other systemic manifestations consistent with a viral infection are present, a diagnosis of viral arthritis should be considered. Unfortunately, it is not usually possible to isolate virus from the joint fluid, so serologic confirmation of the infection is necessary using acute and convalescent sera. In general, the course is the major determinant in distinguishing between viral arthritis and rheumatic disorders such as adult Still's disease since the former has a self-limited course with no residual joint abnormalities.

Specific Antimicrobial Therapy

Most antimicrobial agents achieve therapeutic levels in the infected joint equal to or higher than serum levels.[55,56] Not only does intravenous administration lead to adequate levels of penicillin G, ampicillin, nafcillin, and cephalothin, but also adequate levels have been achieved after the oral administration of cloxacillin and penicillin V. However, borderline adequate levels of synovial fluid have been achieved with oral penicillin G, erythromycin,[56,57] and gentamicin. Thus, therapy with these latter antimicrobial agents must be followed carefully, and organisms must be subjected to in vivo testing. Intra-articular injection of antibiotics is not required, and in fact penicillin has induced a sterile synovitis after intra-articular injection.[4]

The appropriate antimicrobial therapy for bacterial arthritis varies with the age group. In very young infants (infants less than 1 month of age) organisms with widely varying antimicrobial susceptibilities may be the causative agent; empirical therapy must be directed at potential pathogens such as *S. aureus*, gram-negative organisms, and group B streptococci.[17] Initial therapy then would include a penicillinase-resistant synthetic penicillin such as nafcillin, 150 mg/kg/day, combined with gentamicin, 6 mg/kg/day.[17] Therapy would then be altered depending on the antimicrobial susceptibility of the infecting organism. Initial therapy for children under 5 years of age could also include a cephalosporin such as cefuroxime administered at a dose of 75 mg/kg/day.[58] The drug is useful because of the possibility of ampicillin-resistant *Haemophilus influenzae*. If *Haemophilus* is isolated and is β-lactamase-negative, then ampicillin can be substituted. For children over 5 years of age and for adults, initial therapy would be either nafcillin or cefuroxime unless the smear shows another organism. Since there are individual cases of streptococcal infections that do not appear to respond to the antistaphylococcal agents, if the Gram stain shows gram-positive cocci in chains or if the culture is positive for streptococci, then the patient's regimen should be switched to penicillin G intravenously. Initial therapy in all these cases should be with parenteral antibiotics. Oral antibiotics can be used later in the course with success, but adequacy of serum levels must be ensured.[58] If a person is allergic to penicillin, then alternative agents as vancomycin or clindamycin can be chosen.[17] Therapy for a renal dialysis patient with staphylococcal infection would be vancomycin, which can be given once a week to maintain adequate circulating levels. Therapy for gram-negative arthritis could include any third-generation cephalosporin, aztreonam, or imipenem-cilastatin, depending on susceptibility testing. The usual duration of therapy for suppurative arthritis is 2 weeks for *H. influenzae*, streptococci, or gram-negative cocci and 3 weeks for staphylocci or gram-negative bacilli.[59] In most cases, joint fluid cultures are negative within 7 days of therapy, but exceptions do occur.[60]

Recommended therapy for gonococcal arthritis is ceftriaxone 1.0 g i.v. or i.m. daily for 7–10 days. If the infecting organism is fully susceptible to penicillin or tetracycline, many patients who are improving after 3 days can be switched to amoxicillin 500 mg 4 times a day, doxycycline or tetracycline to complete a 7–10 day course.[(61,62)] Initiating therapy with a 3-day course of high dose intravenous penicillin is appropriate if the isolate is already known to be fully susceptible to penicillin. Arthritis due to Lyme disease agent can be treated successfully with penicillin, 20 million units daily for 10 days.[33]

Appropriate therapy for mycobacterial infection consists of isoniazid and rifampin for 9 months for *M. tuberculosis* and *M. kansasii* and rifampin and ethambutol for 6–12 weeks for *M. marinum*.[63,64] Treatment of other mycobacteria must be tailored to the results of in vitro susceptibility testing with a large number of agents since these organisms are relatively resistant to usually administered antituberculous drugs. Amphotericin B is the treatment of choice for arthritis due to fungi.[38–42] Intra-articular amphotericin B may benefit arthritis due to *S. schenckii*.[38] The proper duration and dose of amphotericin is not clearly established, although treatment periods of 6–10 weeks and a total dosage of 2 g or more have been used with some success.[23,38,41] Oral ketaconazole has proved useful in the chronic suppression of coccidioidal arthritis.[65]

Other Therapeutic Modalities

Most people with suppurative arthritis respond adequately to appropriate antimicrobial agents after an initial joint aspiration for diagnosis. Repeated needle aspiration for recurrent joint effusions has been used with success during the first 5–7 days of treatment.[66,67] If the volume of synovial fluid, the cell count, and the percentage of polymorphonuclear leukocytes decreases with each aspiration, then the combination of antimicrobial therapy and aspiration as needed should be adequate. Persistence of effusion beyond 7 days is evidence that surgical drainage is required.[66] Suppurative arthritis of the hip frequently requires surgical drainage since this joint is difficult to evacuate via needle aspiration.[1] There is no evidence that surgical drainage is required for persons with a suppurative arthritis in a joint with underlying joint disease since these patients do well with aspiration alone.[67] If open surgical drainage is performed, there is no evidence that continued irrigation of the joint after the drainage is of any value. Treatment with systemic antimicrobial agents should be continued for up to a week after open drainage, and the wound should be allowed to close by secondary closure.

In the usual case of septic arthritis, immobilization of the infected joint is not necessary, although weight bearing should be avoided until signs of inflammation and pain have disappeared. The joint should be maintained in the functional position, and passive motion may be instituted early, once the symptoms of pain have subsided. As the inflammation diminishes, active exercises may be instituted, and weight bearing may be permitted when all signs of inflammation have disappeared and no evidence of effusion is present.

Course of the Illness

Many persons with bacterial arthritis now recover with no long-term residual abnormalities.[5,67] The major determinants of a poor long-term response include (*1*) failure to recognize and to treat the infection within 7 days of onset,[5] (*2*) infection of the hip joint,[1] (*3*) infections with gram-negative bacilli, and age over 60 years.[18,30,59] The frequency of sequelae in children was shown to be 27 percent,[68] including slight limitation of movement, impairment of ambulation, and shortening of the extremity. These residua were more common with hip and ankle infection. In adults, up to 50 percent had limitation of motion or persistence of pain.[25] Infectious causes of chronic monarticular arthritis are occasionally associated with substantial residua even after maximal therapy.[23,36] Synovectomy has been combined with chemotherapy to achieve an inactive joint infection.[23,39]

REFERENCES

1. Kelly PJ, Martin WJ, Coventry MB. Bacterial (suppurative) arthritis in the adult. J Bone Joint Surg [Am]. 1970;52:1595–602.
2. Nelson JD, Koontz WC. Septic arthritis in infants and children: A review of 117 cases. Pediatrics. 1966;38:966–71.
3. Trueta J. The three types of acute haematogenous osteomyelitis. J Bone Joint Surg [Br]. 1959;41:671–80.
4. Argen RJ, Wilson CH Jr, Wood P. Suppurative arthritis. Arch Intern Med. 1966;117:661–6.
5. Ward JR, Atcheson SG. Infectious arthritis. Med Clin North Am. 1977;61:313–29.
6. Rimoin DLK, Wennberg JE. Acute septic arthritis complicating chronic rheumatoid arthritis. JAMA. 1966;196:617–21.
7. Keiser H, Ruben FL, Wolinsky E, et al. Clinical forms of gonococcal arthritis. N Engl J Med. 1968;279:234–40.
8. Holmes KK, Counts GW, Beaty HN. Disseminated gonococcal infection. Ann Intern Med. 1968;74:979–93.
9. Smith JW, Sanford JP. Viral arthritis. Ann Intern Med. 1967;67:651–9.
10. Kidd BL, Hart HH, Grigor RR. Clinical features of meningococcal arthritis: A report of four cases. Ann Rheum Dis. 1985;44:790–2.
11. Baum SG, Lewis AM Jr, Rowe WP, et al. Epidemic nonmeningitic lymphocytic-choriomeningitis-virus infection. N Engl J Med. 1966;274:934–6.
12. Wands JR, Mann E, Alpert E, et al. The pathogenesis of arthritis associated with acute hepatitis-B surface antigen–positive hepatitis: Complement activation and characterization of circulating immune complexes. J Clin Invest. 1975;55:930–6.
13. Calin A, Fries JF. An "experimental" epidemic of Reiter's syndrome revisited. Ann Intern Med. 1976;84:564–6.
14. Aho K, Ahvonen P, Lassus A, et al. HLA-27 in reactive arthritis. Arthritis Rheum. 1974;17:521–6.
15. Hakansson V, Low B, Eitren B, et al. HLA-27 and reactive arthritis in an outbreak of salmonellosis. Tissue Antigens. 1975;6:366–7.
16. Keat A. Reiter's syndrome and reactive arthritis in perspective. N Engl J Med. 1983;309:1606–15.
17. Jackson MA, Nelson JD. Etiology and medical management of acute suppurative bone and joint infections in pediatric patients. J Pediatr Orthop. 1982;2:313–23.
18. Cooper C, Cawley MID. Bacterial arthritis in an English health district: A 10 year review. Ann Rheum Dis. 1986;45:458–63.
19. Berney S, Goldstein M, Bishko F. Clinical and diagnostic features of tuberculous arthritis. Am J Med. 1972;53:36–42.
20. Gifford DB, Patzakis M, Ivler D, et al. Septic arthritis due to *Pseudomonas* in heroin addicts. J Bone Joint Surg [Am]. 1975;57:631–5.
21. Medical Staff Conference: Arthritis caused by viruses. Calif Med. 1973;119:38–44.
22. Gordon G, Kabins SA. Pyogenic sacroilitis. Am J Med. 1980;69:50–6.
23. Wilson DE, Mann JJ, Bennett JE, et al. Clinical features of extracutaneous sporotrichosis. Medicine (Baltimore). 1967;46:265–79.
24. Ho G Jr, Tice AD, Kaplan SR. Septic bursitis in the prepatellar and olecranon bursae. An analysis of 25 cases. Ann Intern Med. 1978;89:21–7.
25. Sharp JT, Lidsky MD, Duffy J, et al. Infectious arthritis. Arch Intern Med. 1979;139:1125–30.
26. Wallace R, Cohen AS. Tuberculous arthritis. A report of two cases with review of biopsy and synovial fluid findings. Am J Med. 1976;61:277–82.
27. Roy S, Bhawan J. Ultrastructure of articular cartilage in pyogenic arthritis. Arch Pathol. 1975;99:44–47.
28. Borenstein DG, Simon GL. *Haemophilus influenzae* septic arthritis in adults. A report of four cases and a review of the literature. Medicine (Baltimore). 1986;65:191–201.
29. Syrogiannopoulos GA, McCracken GH Jr, Nelson JD. Osteoarticular infections in children with sickle cell disease. Pediatrics. 1986;78:1090–6.
30. Goldenberg DL, Brandt KD, Cathcart ES, et al. Acute arthritis caused by gram-negative bacilli: A clinical characterization. Medicine (Baltimore). 1974;53:197–208.
31. Rompalo AM, Hook EW, Roberts PL, et al. The acute arthritis–dermatitis syndrome. The changing importance of *Neisseria gonorrhoeae* and *Neisseria meningitidis*. Arch Intern Med. 1987;147:281–3.
32. Roughgarden JW. Antimicrobial therapy of rat-bite fever. Arch Intern Med. 1965;116:39–54.
33. Goldings EA, Jericho J. Lyme disease. Clin Rheum Dis. 1986;12:343–67.
34. Fitzgerald RH Jr, Rosenblatt JE, Tenney JH. Anaerobic septic arthritis. Clin Orthop. 1982;164:141–8.
35. Kelly PJ, Martin WJ, Schirger MD, et al. Brucellosis of the bones and joints. JAMA. 1960;174:347–53.
36. Sutker WL, Lankford LL, Tompsett R. Granulomatous synovitis: The role of atypical mycobacteria. Rev Infect Dis. 1979;1:729–35.
37. Jolly HW Jr, Seabury JH. Infections with *Mycobacterium marinum*. Arch Dermatol. 1972;106:32–6.
38. Bayer AS, Scott VJ, Guze LB. Fungal arthritis. III. Sporotrichal arthritis. Semin Arthritis Rheum. 1979;9:66–74.
39. Bayer AS, Guze LB. Fungal arthritis. II. Coccidioidal synovitis: Clinical diagnostic, therapeutic, and prognostic considerations. Semin Arthritis Rheum. 1979;8:200–11.
40. Witorsch P, Utz JP. North American blastomycosis: A study of 40 patients. Medicine (Baltimore). 1968;47:169–200.
41. Bayer AS, Guze LB. Fungal arthritis. I. *Candida* arthritis: Diagnostic and prognostic implications and therapeutic considerations. Semin Arthritis Rheum. 1978;8:142–50.
42. Bayer AS, Choi C, Tilman DB, et al. Fungal arthritis. V. Cryptococcal and histoplasmal arthritis. Semin Arthritis Rheum. 1980;9:218–27.
43. Cockshott P, MacGregor M. Osteomyelitis variolosa. Q J Med. 1958;37:369–87.
44. Steigman AJ. Rashes and arthropathy in viral hepatitis. Mt. Sinai J Med. 1973;40:752–7.
45. Fernandez R, McCarty DJ. The arthritis of viral hepatitis. Ann Intern Med. 1971;74:207–11.
46. Gordon SC, Lauter CB. Mumps arthritis: A review of the literature. Rev Infect Dis. 1984;6:338–44.
47. Robinson MC. An epidemic of virus disease in Southern Province, Tanganyika Territory, in 1952–53. Trans R Soc Trop Med Hyg. 1955;49:28–32.
48. Shore H. O'nyong-nyong fever: An epidemic virus disease in East Africa. III. Some clinical and epidemiological observations in the North Province of Uganda. Trans R Soc Trop Med Hyg. 1961;55:361–73.
49. Niklasson B, Espmark A, Lundstrom J. Occurrence of arthralgia and specific IgM antibodies three to four years after Ockelbo disease. J Infect Dis. 1988;157:832–5.
50. Fraser JRE. Epidemic polyarthritis and Ross River virus disease. Clin Rheum Dis. 1986;12:369–88.
51. Lerman SJ, Nankervis GA, Heggie AD, et al. Immunologic response, virus excretion, and joint reactions with rubella vaccine. Ann Intern Med. 1971;74:67–73.
52. Reid DM, Brown T, Reid TMS, et al. Human parvovirus-associated arthritis: A clinical and laboratory description. Lancet 1985;1:422–5.
53. Salfield S. Filarial arthritis in the Sepik District of Papua New Guinea. Med J Aust. 1975;1:264–7.
54. Baer PA, Tenenbaum J, Fam AG, et al. Coexistent septic and crystal arthritis. Report of four cases and literature review. J Rheumatol. 1986;13:604–7.
55. Nelson JD. Antibiotic concentrations in septic joint effusions. N Engl J Med. 1971;284:349–53.
56. Parker RH, Schmid R. Antibacterial activity of synovial fluid during therapy of septic arthritis. Arthritis Rheum. 1971;14:96–104.
57. Chow A, Hecht R, Winters R. Gentamicin and carbenicillin penetration into the septic joint. N Engl J Med. 1971;285:178–9.
58. Nelson JD, Bucholz RW, Kusmiesz H, et al. Benefits and risks of sequential parenteral–oral cephalosporin therapy for suppurative bone and joint infections. J Pediatr Orthop. 1982;2:255–62.
59. Syrogiannopoulos GA, Nelson JD. Duration of antimicrobial therapy for acute suppurative osteoarticular infections. Lancet 1988;1:37–40.
60. Ho G Jr, Su EY. Therapy for septic arthritis. JAMA. 1982;247:797–800.
61. Treatment of sexually transmitted diseaese. Medical letter. 1988;30:5–10.
62. Bush LM, Boscia JA. Disseminated multiple antibiotic-resistant gonococcal infection: Needed changes in antimicrobial therapy. Ann Intern Med. 1987;107:692–3.
63. Dutt AK, Moers D, Stead WW. Short-course chemotherapy for extrapulmonary tuberculosis. Nine year's experience. Ann Intern Med. 1986;104:7–12.
64. Donta ST, Smith PW, Levitz RE, et al. Therapy of *Mycobacterium marinum* infections: Use of tetracyclines vs. rifampin. Arch Intern Med. 1986;146:902–4.
65. Catanzaro A, Einstein H, Levin B, et al. Ketoconazole for treatment of disseminated coccidioidomycosis. Ann Intern Med. 1982;96:436–40.
66. Schmid FR, Parker RH. Ongoing assessment of therapy in septic arthritis. Arthritis Rheum. 1969;12:529–34.
67. Goldenberg DL, Brandt KD, Cohen AS, et al. Treatment of septic arthritis. Arthritis Rheum. 1975;18:83–90.
68. Howard JG, Highgenboten CL, Nelson JD. Residual effects of septic arthritis in infancy and childhood. JAMA. 1976;236:932–5.

90. INFECTIONS WITH PROSTHESES IN BONES AND JOINTS

BARRY D. BRAUSE

Over the past 2 decades joint replacement surgery has become commonplace due to the magnificent success of these procedures in restoring function to disabled arthritic individuals. Initially, total prosthetic hip implantation techniques were devised. Subsequently, total knee replacement, total shoulder replacement, and total elbow replacement procedures using many of the same orthopedic principles became available. Patients receiving total joint replacements number in the hundreds of thousands each year worldwide, and virtually millions of people have indwelling prosthetic articulations. One to five percent of indwelling prostheses becomes infected; this is a calamity for the patient and is associated with significant morbidity and occasionally death. Prosthesis removal, which usually is necessary to treat these infections, produces large skeletal defects, shortening of the extremity, and severe functional impairment. The health care cost of treating septic prosthetic articulations has been estimated conservatively at 40–80 million dollars per year in the United States alone.[1] The patient faces protracted hospitalization, sizable financial expense, and potentially renewed disability.

PATHOGENESIS

Certain patient populations have been identified as predisposed toward infection of their prosthetic joints including those with prior surgery at the site of the prosthesis, rheumatoid arthritis, corticosteroid therapy, diabetes mellitus, poor nutritional status, obesity, and extremely advanced age.[2,3] Infection usually occurs in osseous tissue adjacent to the foreign body. Since most prostheses are cemented in place with polymethylmethacrylate, infection develops at the bone–cement interface. Sepsis involving cementless prostheses develops in the bone contiguous with the metallic alloy.

Prosthetic joints become infected by two different pathogenetic routes: locally introduced and hematogenous types of osteomyelitis. The locally introduced form of infection is the result of wound sepsis contiguous to the prosthesis or operative contamination. Any factor or event that delays wound healing increases the risk of infection. Ischemic necrosis, infected wound hematomas, wound infection (with or without identifiable cellulitis), and suture abscesses are common preceding events for joint replacement sepsis. During the early postimplantation period when these superficial infections develop, the fascial layers have not yet healed, and the deep, periprosthesis tissue is not protected by the usual physical barriers. Generally these infections are caused by a single pathogen, but polymicrobial sepsis with as many as five different organisms is also observed. *Staphylococcus epidermidis* is the most common etiologic agent in this clinical setting. Infrequently, latent foci of chronic, quiescent osteomyelitis are reactivated by the disruption of tissue associated with implantation surgery. Although bone cultures at the time of the joint replacement operation are sterile, old *Staphylococcus aureus* and *Mycobacterium tuberculosis* infections can recrudesce postoperatively.

Any bacteremia can induce infection of a total joint replacement by the hematogenous route.[4–6] Dentogingival infections and manipulations are known causes of viridans streptococcal and anaerobic (*Peptococcus, Peptostreptococcus*) infections in prostheses. Pyogenic skin processes can cause staphylococcal (*S. aureus, S. epidermidis*) and streptococcal (groups A, B, C, and G streptococci) infections of joint replacements. Genitourinary and gastrointestinal tract procedures or infections are associated with gram-negative bacillary, enterococcal, and anaerobic infections of prostheses. Twenty to forty percent of prosthetic joint infections arise by the hematogenous route, the remainder being of the locally introduced type.

TABLE 1. Bacteriology of Prosthetic Joint Infection

Pathogens	*Frequency (%)*
Staphylococci	53
S. epidermidis	28
S. aureus	25
Streptococci	20
β-Hemolytic streptococci	12
Viridans streptococci	8
Gram-negative aerobic bacilli	20
Anaerobes	7

The frequency of specific microorganisms etiologic in prosthetic joint sepsis varies among the published studies, but a general view of the spectrum of this bacteriology as well as the prominence of certain microbial groups is seen in Table 1. Staphylococci (*S. epidermidis* and *S. aureus*) are the principal causative agents, aerobic streptococci and gram-negative bacilli are each responsible for approximately 20 percent, and anaerobes represent 5–10 percent of these infections. The spectrum of microbial agents capable of causing prosthetic joint infection is unlimited and includes organisms ordinarily considered "contaminants" of cultures such as corynebacteria (aerobic diphtheroides), propionibacteria (anaerobic diphtheroids), and members of the *Bacillus* genus. Rarely have infections with fungi (particularly *Candida*) and mycobacteria been described.

As foreign bodies, the indwelling metallic prosthesis and the polymethylmethacrylate cement, which binds the metal alloy to adjacent bone, predispose both joint space and osseous tissue to septic processes. Foreign substances contribute to local sepsis experimentally by decreasing the quantity of bacteria necessary to establish infection and by permitting pathogens to persist on their avascular surface, sequestered from circulating immunologic defenses (leukocytes, antibodies and complement) as well as systemic antibiotics.[3,7] Polymethylmethacrylate cement appears to predispose toward infection to an extent beyond that of other inert foreign substances. The cement in unpolymerized form has been shown to inhibit phagocytic, lymphocytic, and complement function in vitro.[8,9] The polymerization process itself appears to enhance the risk of infection, possibly due to the substantial heat generated by this in vivo reaction.[8] In an effort to provide total joint replacement without polymethylmethacrylate, cementless prostheses have been designed. These devices have textured surfaces to provide fixation by the growth of adjacent bone into the "porous" interface of the prosthesis. The performance and durability of this new form of arthroplasty is uncertain.

Host responses to methylmethacrylate also may play a role in the pathogenesis of infection. Fibronectin, a connective tissue and plasma glycoprotein, appears to enhance *S. aureus* adherence to polymethylmethacrylate in vivo and thus may contribute to the occurrence of sepsis.[10] Microbial products may assist the development and persistence of infection in association with foreign substances. In the presence of prosthetic devices, many bacteria elaborate a fibrous exopolysaccharide material called *glycocalyx*. Organisms can grow within this matrix and form thick biofilms that are protected at least in part from host defense mechanisms[2,11] (see Chapter 2).

CLINICAL PRESENTATION

Prosthetic joint sepsis produces the cardinal symptoms of inflammation with a wide spectrum of severity. Most patients

TABLE 2. Presenting Symptoms of Prosthetic Joint Infection

Symptom	*Frequency (%)*
Joint pain	95
Fever	43
Periarticular swelling	38
Wound or cutaneous sinus drainage	32

present with a long indolent course characterized by a progressive increase in joint pain and occasionally the formation of cutaneous draining sinuses but no fever, soft tissue swelling, or systemic toxicity. Others present with an acute, fulminant illness with high fever, severe joint pain, local swelling, and erythema. The frequencies of these presenting symptoms are listed in Table 2.[12]

The pattern of clinical presentation is determined largely by three factors: (*1*) the virulence of the infecting pathogen, (*2*) the nature of the host tissue in which the microorganism grows, and (*3*) the route of infection. *Staphylococcus aureus* is a particularly virulent pathogen in this setting and usually produces a fulminant infection (occasionally with septic shock). β-Hemolytic streptococci and aerobic gram-negative bacilli are also capable of causing this clinical picture. Alternatively, the relatively avirulent but tenacious *S. epidermidis* is consistently associated with an indolent course. Characteristics of the involved tissue can influence the type of presentation on the basis of their support of microbial growth. Wound hematomas (as well as seromas and hemarthroses), fresh operative wounds, ischemic wounds, and tissues in diabetic and steroid-treated patients all enhance the ability of bacteria to multiply rapidly in expansive tissue planes. These factors promote the development of a more fulminant infection when a large inoculum of bacteria is allowed access to deep tissue compartments during surgery or in a slowly healing wound postoperatively. The hematogenous route of infection theoretically seeds the bone–cement interface with a relatively small number of organisms. When a blood-borne infection arises in a prosthetic joint several months or years after implantation surgery, the fully healed connective tissue often is capable of restricting the septic process to a relatively small but critical focus at the bone–cement interface. Joint pain is the principal symptom of deep tissue infection irrespective of the mode of presentation and suggests either acute inflammation of periarticular tissue or loosening of the prosthesis due to subacute erosion of bone at the bone–cement interface.

DIAGNOSIS

The clinical manifestations previously described (i.e., joint pain, swelling, erythema, and warmth) all reflect an underlying inflammatory process in the surrounding tissues but are not specific for infection. When a painful prosthesis is accompanied by a fever or purulent drainage from overlying cutaneous sinuses, infection may be presumed, pending further confirmatory tests. However, in the vast preponderance of cases, infection must be differentiated from aseptic and mechanical problems (e.g., hemarthrosis, gout, bland loosening, and dislocation), which are more common causes of pain and inflammatory symptoms in these patients.

Constant joint pain is suggestive of infection, whereas mechanical loosening commonly causes pain only with motion and weight bearing.[2] Plain x-ray films can reveal (*1*) abnormal lucencies greater than 2 mm in width at the bone–cement interface, (*2*) changes in the position of prosthetic components, (*3*) cement fractures, (*4*) periosteal reaction, or (*5*) motion of components on stress views. In addition, the intra-articular injection of dye (arthrography) may reveal abnormal communications between the joint space and multiple defects in the bone–cement interface. These radiologic abnormalities (Fig. 1) are found in 50 percent of septic prostheses. They are generally related to the duration of infection since it may require 3–6 months to manifest such changes. When both distal and proximal components of a prosthetic joint demonstrate radiographic pathology, sepsis is a more likely than is simple mechanical loosening. However, these changes seen on x-ray films are not specific for infection because they are also seen frequently with aseptic processes.

Radioisotopic scans with technetium diphosphonate demonstrate increased uptake in areas of bone with enhanced blood supply or increased metabolic activity. Increased technetium uptake is seen routinely around normal prostheses for 6 months after arthroplasty. Positive scan findings after this period are abnormal and reflect inflammation and possible loosening but not specifically infection of the implant. Sequential technetium-gallium bone scanning is also nondiagnostic due to unacceptable sensitivity (66 percent) and specificity (81 percent).[13] Indium-labeled leukocyte scanning, although very sensitive, also provides only nonspecific results.[14] Therefore normal or negative technetium or indium leukocyte scan findings can be considered strong evidence against the presence of infection, but they are not definitive in establishing the diagnosis. Elevated peripheral white blood cell counts and erythrocyte sedimentation rates, although suggestive, also are inadequate in diagnosing sepsis in this clinical setting.

The specific diagnosis of joint replacement infection is de-

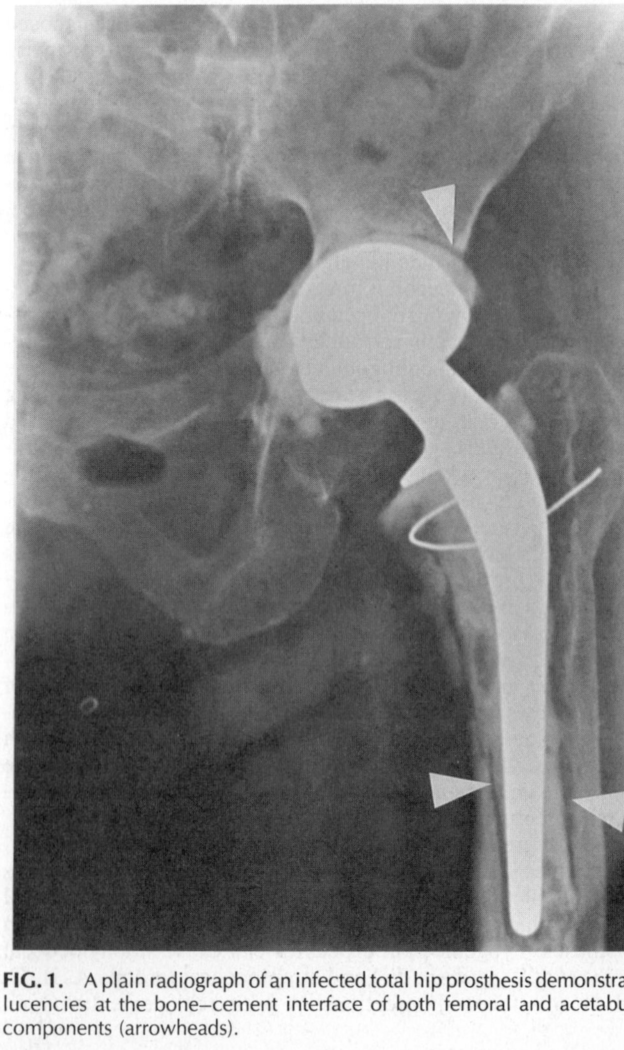

FIG. 1. A plain radiograph of an infected total hip prosthesis demonstrates lucencies at the bone–cement interface of both femoral and acetabular components (arrowheads).

pendent, in large part, upon isolation of the pathogen by aspiration of joint fluid or by culture of tissue obtained at arthrotomy.[15] Analysis of joint fluid often reveals a high leukocyte count (mainly polymorphonuclear cells), a high protein content, and a low glucose concentration. However the changes are only variably present and are neither prerequisites for making the diagnosis of joint replacement infection nor specific for this entity. Histopathologic examination of periprosthetic tissue frequently reveals an infiltration of polymorphonuclear leukocytes indicative of an acute inflammatory reaction, but this parameter is positive in only 55 percent of infected patients and also may not be sufficiently specific. Therefore the single observation that delineates the presence of implant infection is isolation of the pathogen by arthrocentesis or surgical débridement.

Since fastidious microorganisms, including anaerobes, may be etiologic agents in prosthetic arthroplasty infections, multiple specimens should be obtained and rapidly cultured in appropriate media. Arthrocentesis demonstrates the pathogen in 85–98 percent of cases.[15,16] Gram stain is positive in 32 percent. Fluoroscopic guidance and arthrography are useful in documenting accurate needle placement. When difficulty is encountered in obtaining intra-articular fluid, irrigation with sterile normal saline (without antiseptic preservative additives) can be used to provide the necessary fluid for culture. When initial cultures reveal a relatively avirulent organism (*S. epidermidis*, corynebacteria, propionibacteria, *Bacillus* sp.), a second aspirate should be considered to reconfirm the bacteriologic diagnosis and to eliminate the possibility that the isolate is artifactual. Operative cultures are definitively diagnostic; therefore the patient should not receive antimicrobial therapy for several weeks before the procedure. Multiple specimens of tissue and fluid should be submitted for culture. The results of these microbiologic techniques should confirm the presence and nature of the infection as well as allow for optimal treatment. In the uncommon circumstance when the clinical suggestion of sepsis is strong but the cultures are sterile, fastidious organisms (particularly anaerobes) should be suspected. In order to design efficacious and the least toxic antimicrobial therapy the patient's infecting strain of bacteria must be available for in vitro evaluation as described later in this chapter.

THERAPY

Successful treatment of a total joint arthroplasty infection depends upon extensive and meticulous surgical débridement and effective antimicrobial therapy. Simple surgical drainage (with retention of the prosthesis in situ) followed by a nonstandardized, finite course of antibiotic therapy has been only 20 percent successful.[17] In response to this 80 percent failure rate, two different approaches to more effective treatment of prosthetic joint infection have evolved over the past decade. Complete removal of all foreign materials (metallic prosthesis and cement) is an essential component of both regimens.

The most successful protocol incorporates standardized antimicrobial therapy with a two-stage surgical procedure. Removal of the prosthesis and cement is followed by a 6-week course of bactericidal antibiotic therapy chosen on the basis of in vitro susceptibility studies. Reimplantation is performed at the conclusion of the 6-week antibiotic course. With this protocol a 90 percent success rate has been achieved in total hip replacement infections, and a 97 percent success rate has been obtained in total knee replacement infections.[18–20] The success of this regimen relies on thorough débridement techniques and effective antimicrobial therapy. In this manner, both gram-positive bacteria (including multidrug-resistant staphylococci and enterococci) as well as gram-negative bacteria (including *Pseudomonas aeruginosa*) can be eliminated if the specific sensitivities of each isolate allow eradication. The empirical selection of a 6-week duration of antibiotic therapy may be critical for efficacy. Others have employed a similar approach to therapy but only a 2-week course of antibiotic treatment before reinsertion of the prosthesis.[21] With this protocol the pathogen was eradicated in only 79 percent of the cases, and only 35 percent of the patients obtained good function in the new prosthesis.

The alternative method of treatment involves metallic joint and cement extraction with immediate reimplantation of a new prosthesis in a one-stage surgical procedure (exchange operation) accompanied by nonstandardized antimicrobial therapy. Methylmethacrylate cement impregnated with an antibiotic (usually gentamicin or tobramycin) is employed during reimplantation. The antimicrobial agent leaches out from the hardened plastic to produce variable but high initial release as well as protracted diffusion of antibiotic into surrounding tissues at the bone–cement interface.[22] The protocol is effective in 70–80 percent of cases.[23–25] When using repeated exchange operations (in the 20–30 percent failure group) incorporating antibiotic-laden cement, the success rate is increased to 90 percent.[24] It has been suggested that this mode of therapy is applicable only to infections with the less virulent microorganisms since high failure rates are observed when *S. aureus* or gram-negative bacilli are the pathogens.[26] Systemic antibiotics are administered rarely and without standardization in this regimen. Moreover, the selection of an aminoglycoside as a component in the recementing phase of these operations may not have reflected the susceptibility of the pathogen being treated.

Future therapeutic approaches will likely include the most efficacious parts of these two protocols: combining the specific, standardized 6-week antibiotic regimen and two-stage prosthesis removal-reimplantation surgery with the incorporation of antibiotic-impregnated cement during arthroplasty reinsertion. In those clinical situations in which adequate antimicrobial potency cannot be achieved, arthrodesis or resection arthroplasty is recommended rather than attempting prosthesis reimplantation. However, with the advent of antibiotic-impregnated cement even these difficult cases may be candidates for another total joint arthroplasty.

SUPPRESSIVE ANTIBIOTIC THERAPY

Although removal of the implanted prosthesis is necessary to eradicate deep infection associated with these devices, this therapeutic approach is not always available. Occasionally surgical excision is contraindicated due to medical and surgical conditions or patient refusal. Since it is likely that the pathogen will be able to persist at the undébrided bone–cement interface despite high-dose, finite systemic antimicrobial therapy, lifelong oral antibiotic treatment can be considered to suppress the infection and retain the usefulness of the total joint replacement. In selected cases in which (*1*) prosthesis removal is not possible, (*2*) the pathogen is relatively avirulent, (*3*) the pathogen is exquisitely sensitive to an orally absorbed antibiotic, (*4*) the patient can tolerate an appropriate oral antibiotic, and (*5*) the prosthesis is not loose, suppressive oral antimicrobial therapy may be of value. Preliminary observations suggest that this form of therapy is effective only when all of these five criteria are fulfilled. Successful retention of the functioning arthroplasty has been seen in 63 percent of patients in this unusual clinical setting. The suppressive approach is not without risk. Serial radiographs are needed over the course of treatment to monitor for progressive bone resorption at the bone–cement interface that could reduce the success of any future revision surgery. Despite continual antibiotic therapy the localized septic process could extend into adjacent tissue compartments or become a systemic infection. Moreover, the patient would be subjected to the potential side effects of chronic antibiotic administration.

PREVENTION OF JOINT PROSTHESIS INFECTION

In view of the catastrophic effects of prosthetic arthroplasty infection, prevention of these septic processes is of prime importance. In anticipation of elective total joint replacement surgery, the patient should be evaluated for the presence of pyogenic dentogingival pathology, obstructive uropathy, and dermatologic conditions that might predispose to infection and bacteremia. Strong consideration should be given to reducing the risks represented by these factors (i.e., dental extraction, prostatic resection, control of dermatitis) before insertion of the prosthesis. Perioperative antibiotic prophylaxis has been shown to effectively reduce deep wound infection in total joint replacement surgery.[27] Oxacillin or cefazolin are commonly administered as antistaphylococcal agents immediately before the operation and for 1–2 days thereafter. Filtered laminar airflow systems in the operating room further reduce infection rates, especially when whole-body, exhaust-ventilated suits are worn by the operating team.[28,29]

For patients with indwelling joint prostheses, early recognition and prompt therapy for infection in any location is critical to reduce the risk of seeding the joint implant hematogenously. Situations likely to cause bacteremia should be avoided. The use of prophylactic antibiotics in anticipation of bacteremic events (i.e., dental surgery, cystoscopy, colonoscopic biopsy, surgical procedures on infected or contaminated tissues) has been suggested on the same empirical basis upon which endocarditis prophylaxis is recommended.[3,5] This approach to prevention is controversial at the present time, and no data are available to determine the adequacy or the cost-effectiveness of such measures. Clinical decisions regarding prophylactic antibiotics for expected bacteremias in patients with prosthetic joints should be made on an individual basis.

REFERENCES

1. Salvati EA, Small RD, Brause BD, et al. Infections associated with orthopedic devices. In: Sugarman B, Young EJ, eds. Infections Associated with Prosthetic Devices. Boca Raton, FL: CRC Press; 1984:181–218.
2. Gristina AG, Kolkin J. Total joint replacement and sepsis. J Bone Joint Surg [Am] 1983;65:128–34.
3. Brause BD. Infections associated with prosthetic joints. Clin Rheum Dis. 1986;12:523–36.
4. Ahlberg A, Carlsson AS, Lindberg L. Hematogenous infection in total joint replacement. Clin Orthop. 1978;137:69–75.
5. Lattimer GL, Keblish PA, Dickson TB, et al. Hematogenous infection in total joint replacement. JAMA. 1979;242:2213–4.
6. Lindqvist C, Slatis P. Dental bacteremia—a neglected cause of arthroplasty infections? Acta Orthop Scand. 1985;56:506–8.
7. Petty W, Spanier S, Shuster JJ, et al. The influence of skeletal implants on incidence of infection. J Bone Joint Surg [Am]. 1985;67:1236–44.
8. Petty W. The effect of methylmethacrylate on bacterial inhibiting properties of normal human serum. Clin Orthop. 1978;132:266–77.
9. Petty W. The effect of methylmethacrylate on bacterial phagocytosis and killing by human polymorphonuclear leukocytes. J Bone Joint Surg [Am]. 1978;60:752–7.
10. Vaudaux P, Suzuki R, Waldvogel FA, et al. Foreign-body infection: Role of fibronectin as a ligand for the adherence of *Staphylococcus aureus*. J Infect Dis. 1984;150:546–53.
11. Costerton JW, Irvin RT, Cheng K-J. The bacterial glycocalyx in nature and disease. Annu Rev Microbiol 1981;35:299–324.
12. Inman JN, Gallegos KV, Brause BD, et al. Clinical and microbial features of prosthetic joint infection. Am J Med. 1984;77:47–53.
13. Merkel KD, Brown ML, Fitzgerald RH. Sequential technetium-99m HMDP-gallium-67 citrate imaging for the evaluation of infection in the painful prosthesis. J Nucl Med. 1986;27:1413–7.
14. Pring DJ, Henderson RG, Rivett AG, et al. Autologous granulocyte scanning of painful prosthetic joints. J Bone Joint Surg [Br]. 1986;68:647–52.
15. O'Neill DA, Harris WH. Failed total hip replacement: Assessment by plain radiographs, arthrograms and aspiration of the hip joint. J Bone Joint Surg [Am]. 1984;66:540–6.
16. Eftehar NS. Wound infection complicating total hip joint arthroplasty. Orthop Rev. 1979;8:49–64.
17. Fitzgerald RH, Nolan DR, Ilstrup DM, et al. Deep wound sepsis following total hip arthroplasty. J Bone Joint Surg [Am]. 1977;59:847–55.
18. Callaghan JJ, Salvati EA, Brause BD, et al. Reimplantation for salvage of the infected hip. In: The Hip: Proceedings of the 14th Open Scientific Meeting of The Hip Society. St Louis: CV Mosby; 1986:65–94.
19. Insall JN, Thompson FM, Brause BD. Two-stage reimplantation for the salvage of infected total knee arthroplasty. J Bone Joint Surg [Am] 1983;65:1087–98.
20. Salvati EA, Chekofsky KM, Brause BD, et al. Reimplantation in infection. Clin Orthop. 1982;170:62–75.
21. Rand JA, Bryan RS. Reimplantation for the salvage of an infected total knee arthroplasty. J Bone Joint Surg [Am]. 1983;65:1081–6.
22. Trippel SB. Antibiotic-impregnated cement in total joint arthroplasty. J Bone Joint Surg [Am]. 1986;68:1297–302.
23. Buchholz HW, Elson RA, Lodenkamper H. The infected joint implant. In: McKibbin B, ed. Recent Advances in Orthopedics. Edinburgh: Churchill Livingstone; 1979:139–61.
24. Buchholz HW, Elson R, Engelbrecht E. Management of deep infection of total hip replacement. J Bone Joint Surg [Br]. 1981;63:342–53.
25. Carlsson AS, Josefsson G, Lindberg L. Revision with gentamicin-impregnated cement for deep infection in total hip arthroplasties. J Bone Joint Surg [Am]. 1978;60:1059–64.
26. Fitzgerald RH, Jones DR. Hip implant infection. Am J Med. 1986;78(Suppl 6B):225–8.
27. Norden C. A critical review of antibiotic prophylaxis in orthopedic surgery. Rev Infect Dis. 1983;5:928–32.
28. Lidwell O, Lowbury E, Whyte E. Effect of ultraclean air in operating rooms on deep sepsis in the joint after total hip or total knee replacement. Br Med J. 1982;285:10–4.
29. Salvati EA, Robinson RP, Zeno SM, et al. Infection rates after 3175 total hip and total knee replacements performed with and without a horizontal unidirectional filtered air-flow system. J Bone Joint Surg [Am]. 1982;64:525–35.

91. OSTEOMYELITIS

CARL W. NORDEN

Osteomyelitis continues to pose difficulties both in diagnosis and management and causes serious morbidity and, less frequently, mortality. Antibiotics have significantly altered the mortality and outcome of osteomyelitis, but chronic disease still occurs as a sequela. There are differences of opinion about the choice of antibiotic, the duration of treatment, the type of surgical intervention needed, and the effect of these factors on prognosis.

PATHOPHYSIOLOGY AND PATHOLOGY

Osteomyelitis may develop in any bone of the body. However, the predisposition of the disease for certain bones can be better understood after reviewing its structure. Bone is a metabolically active tissue with high rates of synthesis and resorption, processes that depend on an adequate vascular supply. Acute hematogenous osteomyelitis usually involves rapidly growing bone and characteristically affects the metaphysis of long bones. The anatomy of the vasculature in this area provides some explanation for this specific localization of bacteria. The capillary ramifications of the nutrient arteries supplying bone make sharp loops in the area of the epiphyseal growth plates and enter a system of sinusoidal veins connected with the venous network of the medullary cavity. The afferent loops of these metaphyseal capillaries lack phagocytic lining cells, and the efferent loops contain functionally inactive phagocytic cells. In the loops of the capillaries, flow becomes considerably slower and more turbulent. The capillary loops adjacent to the epiphyseal growth plates are essentially end-artery branches of the nutrient artery, and obstruction of these vessels results in areas of avascular necrosis.

In the prepubescent person, infection presumably starts in the metaphyseal sinusoidal veins, is contained by the growth plate, and spreads laterally where it breaks through the cortex and lifts the loose periosteum to result in a subperiosteal collection. In adults, the periosteum is firmly attached to the underlying bone, and because of this, subperiosteal abscess formation and intense periosteal proliferation are less frequently seen. Once infection has started, it provokes an acute suppurative response that contributes to necrosis of tissue, breakdown of bone, and removal of calcium. Infection may extend to neighboring bony structures through the Haversian and Volkmann canals, thereby shutting off the vascular supply and causing the death of more bone. At this point, the chronic phase of osteomyelitis may be established as large segments of avascular bone separate and form sequestra. There is also frequently deposition of new bone, an involucrum, under the elevated periosteum.

MANIFESTATIONS OF OSTEOMYELITIS

In any consideration of bone infections, it is logical to divide them into three main types: osteomyelitis resulting from hematogenous spread of infection, osteomyelitis that is secondary to a contiguous focus of infection, and osteomyelitis associated with vascular insufficiency (see Table 1 for a summary of the features of each). Other specific clinical situations and problems can then be considered.

Hematogenous Osteomyelitis

Age Distribution. Although classically described as a disease of children, hematogenous osteomyelitis is being reported with increased frequency in older age groups. One form, involving the vertebrae, is commonly a disease of individuals over the age of 50.

Bones Involved. Most frequently involved are the long bones of the lower extremities and the humerus (Fig. 1). The vertebrae are often the sites of infection in adults. Multiple bone involvement may occur in up to 15 percent of the patients.

Bacteriology. In most cases of acute hematogenous osteomyelitis, a determined diagnostic effort results in the identification of an etiologic agent. The most useful procedures for recovery of the etiologic agent are bone biopsies, blood cultures, and cultures of draining pus. *Staphylococcus aureus* has been the most common agent, but gram-negative bacilli (*Escherichia coli, Klebsiella, Salmonella, Proteus,* and *Pseudomonas*) are being found with increasing frequency.

Clinical Features. The classic presentation of acute hematogenous osteomyelitis in children is that of an abrupt onset of high fever, systemic toxicity, and physical findings of local suppuration about the involved bone. In adults, such a classic picture is less frequently seen. About one-half of the patients may have symptoms of pain, swelling, chills, and fever for less than 3 weeks before admission. Other patients may have had vague symptoms for 1 or 2 months with few constitutional complaints; the major complaint is pain in the involved limb. Drainage is an infrequent occurrence.

If chronic osteomyelitis supervenes, systemic signs such as toxicity and high fever are relatively uncommon. Local tenderness, swelling, and erythema are less frequent than in acute osteomyelitis. Drainage from a sinus tract is often the herald of an exacerbation of chronic osteomyelitis.

Laboratory Data. Sedimentation rates and white blood cell counts are frequently elevated, although the latter rarely exceed 15,000/mm^3. The magnitude of these values is of little help in predicting the outcome of disease.

Osteomyelitis Secondary to a Contiguous Focus of Infection

This form of osteomyelitis represents a direct infection of bone from an exogenous source or the spread of infection from a nearby infected focus. The most common precipitating factor is postoperative infection such as that after open reduction of fractures. Nonsurgically induced infections develop from soft tissue infections, infected teeth, or infected sinuses (Fig. 2). After animal bites, spread of locally inoculated organisms may occur with consequent development of osteomyelitis (most commonly due to *Pasteurella multocida*).

Age Distribution. Most cases of this type of osteomyelitis are seen in patients over the age of 50, presumably because the precipitating factors such as hip fractures or neurosurgery occur more frequently in older persons.

Bones Involved. Although any bone in the body may be involved, the long bones of the lower extremity (femur and tibia) are most frequently involved since these are often the site of fracture and open reduction. Pressure sores (decubitus ulcers) may overlie a focus of osteomyelitis. The diagnosis is not always easy and frequently requires a combination of x-ray films, bone scans, and bone biopsy for histologic examination. Culture of bone biopsy samples usually discloses anaerobic bacteria, gram-negative bacilli, or both. The diagnosis of osteomyelitis must be strongly considered if a pressure sore does not respond to local therapy.[1]

The skull and mandible are also frequent sites of osteomyelitis after neurosurgery, oral surgery, or dental infections. Sternal osteomyelitis is an uncommon but highly morbid complication of median sternotomy incisions for cardiac surgery. Mediastin-

TABLE 1. Major Types of Osteomyelitis

Feature	*Hematogenous*	*Secondary to Contiguous Focus of Infection*	*Due to Vascular Insufficiency*
Age distribution (yr)	Peaks at 1–20 and ≥50	≥50	≥50
Bones involved	Long bones Vertebrae	Femur, tibia, skull, mandible	Feet
Precipitating factors	Trauma (?) Bacteremia	Surgery Soft-tissue infections	Diabetes mellitus Peripheral vascular disease
Bacteriology	Usually only one organism *S. aureus* Gram-negative organisms	Often mixed infection *S. aureus* Gram-negative organisms Anaerobic organisms	Usually mixed infections *S. aureus* or *epidermidis* Streptococci Gram-negative organisms Anaerobic organisms
Episode Major clinical findings	Initial Fever Local tenderness Local swelling Limitation of motion	Initial Fever Erythema Swelling Heat	Initial and Recurrent Pain Swelling Erythema Drainage Ulceration
	Recurrent Drainage	Recurrent Drainage Sinus	

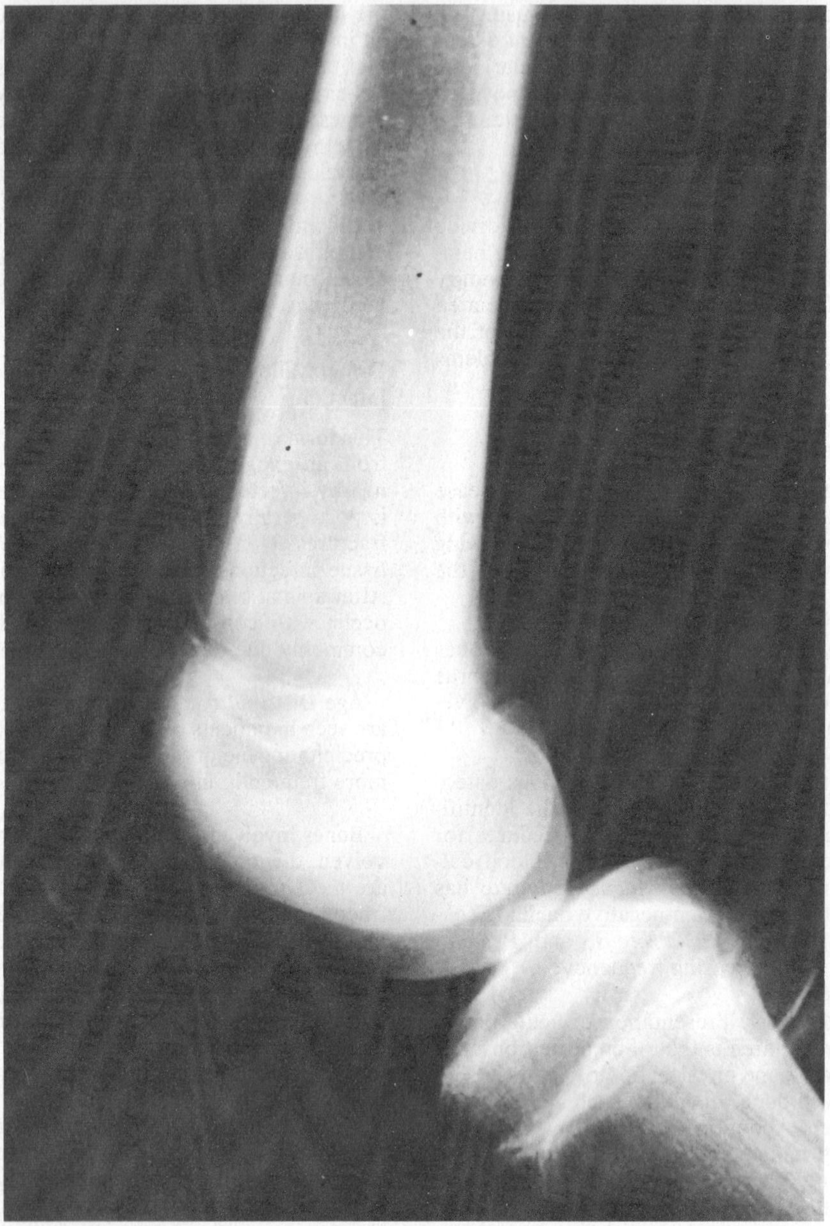

FIG. 1. Chronic hematogenous osteomyelitis. The patient is a 15-year-old boy with a 1 month history of pain in his leg, fever, and a swollen knee. Arthrocentesis revealed purulent but sterile fluid. At surgery, pus, which grew *S. aureus* when cultured, was curetted from the bone cavity. Full recovery followed intensive antibiotic therapy, with total disappearance of the lytic lesion.

itis regularly accompanies sternal infection. Initial manifestations include fever, leukocytosis, and erythema of the wound. With time, bone dissolution at the sternal edges leads to sternal instability despite the presence of sutures. Gram-positive and gram-negative bacteria as well as atypical mycobacteria are etiologic agents in this disease. Cure almost always requires reoperation for irrigation of the mediastinum and débridement of necrotic sternum.[2] When most of the sternum must be resected, closure is delayed until bilateral pectoralis muscle flaps can be placed over the wound.

Bacteriology. Unlike hematogenous osteomyelitis where a single organism is usually responsible, osteomyelitis secondary to a contiguous focus of infection is often associated with more than one species of bacteria. *Staphylococcus aureus* is still the most common infecting organism, but it is frequently found as part of a mixed infection. The value of culturing sinus tract drainage, even if it is purulent, is open to question.

A study comparing cultures of sinus tracts with cultures of operative specimens from patients with chronic osteomyelitis revealed that less than half the sinus tract cultures contained the operative pathogen. Isolation of *S. aureus* from sinus tracts correlated to some degree with the finding of this organism in bone; in contrast, isolation of bacteria other than *S. aureus* from sinus tracts had a low likelihood of predicting the pathogen isolated from bone.[3]

Clinical Signs. In the initial episodes, fever, swelling, and erythema are seen in approximately one-half of the cases. During recurrences, sinus formation and drainage are the two major presenting signs, and patients generally show fewer systemic signs in recurrences than in initial episodes.

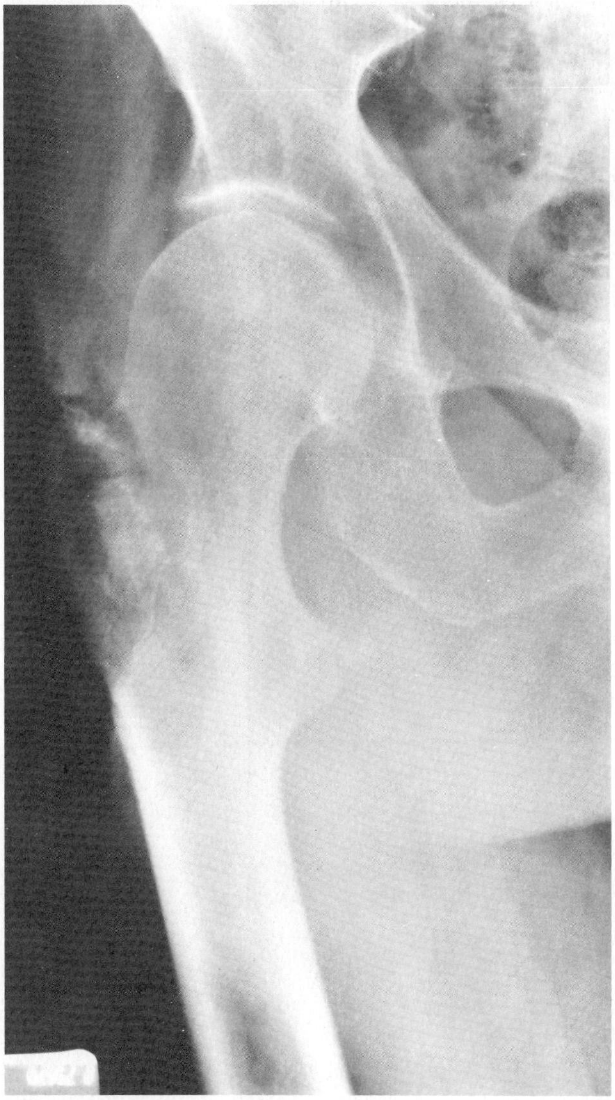

FIG. 2. Osteomyelitis secondary to a contiguous focus of infection. The patient is a debilitated 76-year-old man with a large decubitus ulcer overlying the right greater trochanter. Cultures of pus revealed mixed anaerobic–aerobic infection. An x-ray film reveals a soft-tissue defect as well as irregular loss of bone around the region of the greater trochanter.

Osteomyelitis Associated with Vascular Insufficiency

Patients with osteomyelitis associated with vascular insufficiency present difficult problems of management. Such patients nearly always have diabetes or severe atherosclerosis.

Age Distribution. Most patients are between 50 and 70 years old and have had diabetes mellitus from 2 to more than 10 years before infection occurs.

Bones Involved. The toes or other small bones of the feet are usually affected.

Bacteriology. Most cultures obtained from either surgical specimens or from the wound will show several different species of organisms. Staphylococci are most commonly isolated, but gram-negative aerobic organisms and gram-positive and gram-negative anaerobic bacteria are also recovered frequently.[4]

Clinical Signs. Local symptoms dominate the picture, and few patients manifest systemic signs. Patients may have long-standing chronic draining ulcers on their toes or feet or may be admitted because of cellulitis manifested by pain, swelling, and redness of the lower extremity. Fever and septicemia are uncommon. Such patients usually have evidence of long-standing diabetes with neuropathy and retinopathy. Peripheral pulses may be palpable in the face of vascular insufficiency since this is a disease of small vessels.

SPECIFIC CLINICAL SITUATIONS

Vertebral Osteomyelitis

Vertebral osteomyelitis is a diagnostic pitfall for practicing physicians since it is often protean and subtle in its presenting manifestations.[5,6] The infection generally occurs in drug addicts, after trauma (often surgical), or after hematogenous spread from another focus of infection (usually the urinary tract). It is postulated that infection disseminates from the urinary tract to the vertebral column via the posterior venous plexus and the vertebral venous system (Batson's veins).

The infecting bacteria may be isolated from blood cultures or from material aspirated from the vertebral body, disk space, or adjacent areas. Although *S. aureus* continues to be the predominant organism, Enterobacteriaceae (presumably from the urinary tract) have been responsible with increasing frequency.

The clinical diagnosis is based on the finding of localized pain and tenderness over one or more vertebrae in patients with fever. Symptoms may be minimal, and the initial presentation may be only that of malaise and low back pain. Fever can be low grade or absent. However, about 10 percent of patients are bacteremic and acutely ill on admission. Perhaps the most useful laboratory test is the sedimentation rate; the finding of an elevated sedimentation rate in association with low back pain, with or without fever, should make one think of vertebral osteomyelitis. Conventional roentgenograms as well as bone scans can suggest the appropriate diagnosis (Fig. 3).

Complications of vertebral osteomyelitis include subluxation of the atlantoaxial joint (in cervical spine disease), abscesses and local extension of infection, and significant neurologic lesions. A spinal epidural abscess, most often caused by *S. aureus,* may occur secondary to osteomyelitis; the major neurologic manifestations include spinal ache, foot weakness, paraparesis, and paraplegia. Diagnosis by myelography, magnetic resonance imaging (MRI), or computed tomography (CT) scan with subsequent evacuation of pus from the epidural space is critical for full recovery of neurologic function.

Until recently, it was common practice to immobilize patients with vertebral osteomyelitis, usually in a body cast. Several reports now strongly suggest that antibiotic therapy with simple bed rest suffices to cure pyogenic vertebral osteomyelitis, that external stabilization is not needed, and that we should avoid the inconvenience and hazards of body casts.

Osteomyelitis Due to Gram-Negative Organisms

Because the clinical patterns of osteomyelitis due to gram-negative organisms are somewhat different from those described in previous sections, it is appropriate to discuss them separately. *Pseudomonas aeruginosa* was the most frequent pathogen in one series, although *Proteus, E. coli, Salmonella,* and *Klebsiella* spp. were also encountered.[7] *Brucella* spondylitis will not be discussed here. The femur was the most frequently involved bone, followed by infection of the metatarsals. Draining wounds were seen in over half the patients when first examined. About one-third of the patients had underlying diseases such as malignancy, alcoholism, or collagen-vascular disease, which may have contributed to their susceptibility to infection. Surgery or a breach of the skin as from a puncture wound was an antecedent factor in many patients with osteomyelitis due

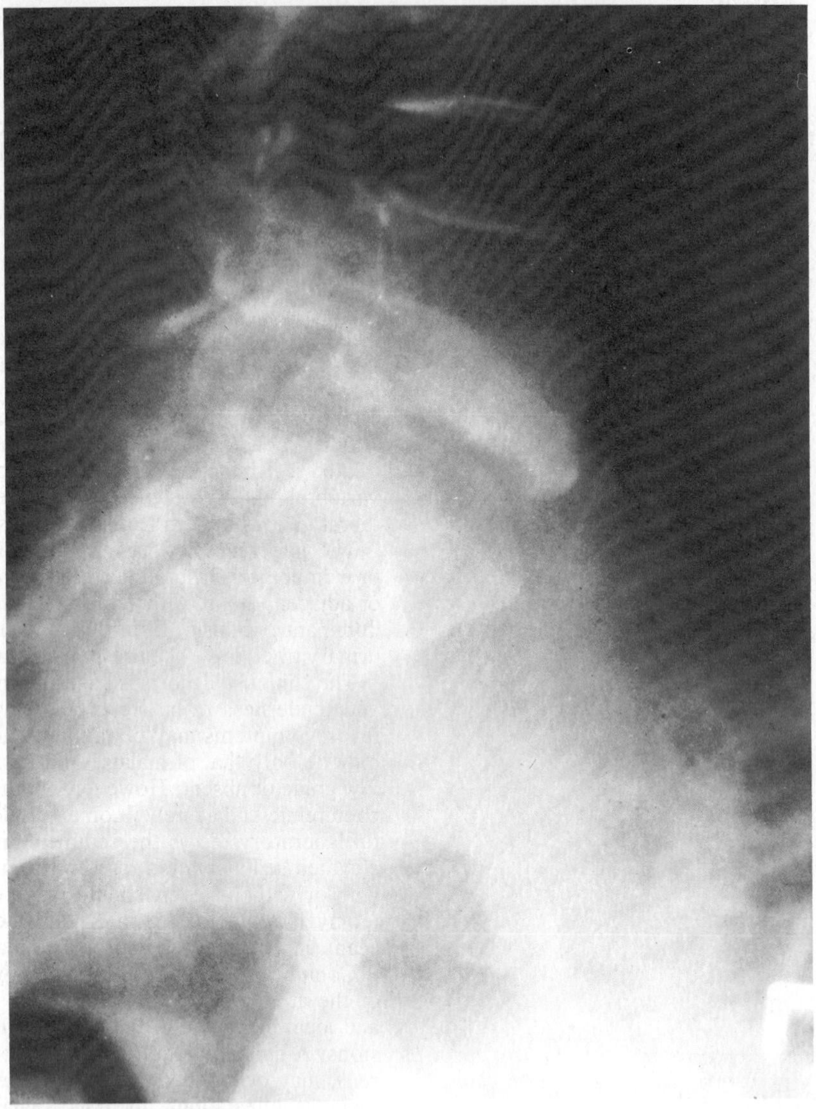

FIG. 3. Osteomyelitis involving vertebrae, in a 42-year-old man with postoperative infection of the fifth lumbar vertebral body. *Staphylococcus aureus* was recovered on biopsy. The tomogram reveals an irregular destructive process at the inferior surface of the L5 vertebral body as well as narrowing of the L5-S1 intervertebral space. With appropriate antibiotic therapy, the patient made an excellent recovery.

to *Pseudomonas*. Heroin addicts may also have osteomyelitis due to gram-negative organisms. Therapy for osteomyelitis caused by gram-negative organisms consists of appropriate antibiotic management as well as necessary surgical intervention. One of the difficulties with the treatment of gram-negative osteomyelitis has been that the minimal inhibitory concentrations (MICs) of gram-negative organisms are generally sufficiently high to make oral therapy, with its attendant lower levels of antibiotic in serum, less effective than similar oral therapy would be for osteomyelitis due to gram-positive organisms. Further, for organisms such as *P. aeruginosa,* there were no effective oral agents available. In one series, only half of the patients with osteomyelitis were successfully treated; this is a higher incidence of therapeutic failures than is generally reported for gram-positive organisms. It is possible that the use of quinolones may improve the prognosis for patients with osteomyelitis due to these organisms, but clinical trials will be required to verify this.[8,9]

Osteomyelitis Due to Anaerobic Organisms

Anaerobic organisms are found in osteomyelitis with some frequency and would probably be recovered more often if optimal techniques for isolation were used. In one series spanning 28 months, anaerobic bacteria were isolated from tissue obtained during débridement for osteomyelitis in 40 of 182 patients.[10] In 9, only anaerobic bacteria were recovered; in the rest, mixed aerobic–anaerobic infections were present. As a group, the patients in whom only anaerobes were isolated were older and had a short duration of symptoms (1 month or less in 7 of the 9), and in 7 the infection was associated with a metallic foreign body.

In a review of the literature, anaerobic osteomyelitis was found most frequently in long bones (40 percent) and skull and facial bones (27 percent).[11] The most common predisposing factors were previous fractures, diabetes, and human bites. *Bacteroides fragilis* and *Bacteroides melaninogenicus* were the anaerobes most frequently isolated. Suggested settings in which anaerobic osteomyelitis should be suspected include (*1*) hand infections after human bites, (*2*) infection of the pelvis after abdominal sepsis, (*3*) sacral osteomyelitis after decubitus ulcers, (*4*) osteomyelitis of the skull or facial bones, (*5*) chronic nonhealing indolent ulcers of the feet, (*6*) the presence of foul-smelling exudate, and (*7*) when there is a failure to grow bacteria from clinical specimens, particularly when the Gram stain has shown organisms. The role of anaerobes in cases of osteomyelitis that also yield aerobic organisms is unclear; whether they are primary pathogens or act synergistically with other bacteria remains to be determined. However, it seems wise to treat both the anaerobes and aerobes in mixed infections. Actinomycosis can cause osteomyelitis by the hematogenous route or by contiguous spread from lesions in the chest or abdomen. The diagnosis is made by a culture of deep tissue or by the demonstration of sulfur granules. Further details are given in Chapter 233.

Osteomyelitis Caused by Fungi

Hematogenous osteomyelitis is a frequent complication of blastomycosis and disseminated coccidioidomycosis. Both tend to present as indolent osteolytic lesions with pus in the contiguous soft tissue. Whereas osteomyelitis often accompanies sporotrichosis arthritis, the appearance on x-ray films is only a subtle decrease in trabeculation. *Candida* osteomyelitis is a rare, late complication of candidemia that usually presents as a single osteolytic lesion.[12]

Osteomyelitis in Hemodialysis Patients

Bacterial infections, usually staphylococcal, are common in hemodialysis patients in whom indwelling cannulae allow portals of bacterial entry. Osteomyelitis is a complication of chronic hemodialysis. Ribs and the thoracic vertebral column are the most common sites of involvement. Infection is probably hematogenous since most patients have prior bacteremias and the organisms infecting bone are the same as those found by blood culture. The diagnosis of osteomyelitis is usually made 12–72 months after the initiation of hemodialysis.

The patient may have a fever of unknown origin, the clinical and x-ray film signs may mimic those of renal osteodystrophy, and infection may not be recognized. Surgical intervention and antibiotic treatment can result in cure of the infection.

Osteomyelitis in Patients with Sickle Cell Disease

In a large series reviewing sickle cell disease and osteomyelitis, it was reported that 20 of 70 patients with complete hemoglobin defects had at least one hospitalization for the treatment of osteomyelitis during a 10-year study period.[13] In essentially all cases, the infecting organisms in patients with sickle cell disease were gram-negative rods. *Salmonella* sp. accounted for approximately 80 percent. In contrast, from the same hospital, records of 117 patients with osteomyelitis but with normal hemoglobin included only a single patient with *Salmonella* infection of the bone.

It is difficult to differentiate thrombotic marrow crisis from osteomyelitis in patients with sickle cell disease. In some children, there is a history of bone pain and fever that, after an interval of 5 days to 2 weeks, is followed by the onset of spiking fever, chills, and leukocytosis. Such a sequence is suggestive of osteomyelitis after a crisis. Children with sickle cell disease may have multiple sites of bone infection simultaneously. Frequently, because the symptoms may be insidious and mimic those of marrow crisis, early cultures of blood and stool offer the only clue to the correct diagnosis. Presumptive antibiotic therapy in children with sickle cell disease who are suspected of having osteomyelitis should include agents effective against *Salmonella* (generally ampicillin, a cephalosporin, or trimethoprim-sulfamethoxazole). X-ray films of patients appropriately treated will usually show complete healing of the changes of osteomyelitis.

Osteomyelitis in Heroin Addicts

One of the complications associated with drug addiction is osteomyelitis.[14] Generally, the clinical course is indolent, and fever is infrequent; sites of infection may be any bone including the vertebrae, pubis, and clavicles. The organisms causing infection generally reflect the spectrum of pathogens infecting addicts: staphylococci, gram-negative rods, and yeast. Primary infection of bone should be considered in narcotic addicts having localized pain. Roentgenographic changes may be initially absent, only to appear after several weeks, thus necessitating serial x-ray films. Surgical exploration is often required to make a bacteriologic diagnosis, particularly in view of the fact that the spectrum of organisms seen is much broader than that commonly associated with osteomyelitis.

Brodie's Abscess

Brodie's abscess is the name given to a chronic, localized bone abscess. While the more subacute cases may have fever, pain, and periosteal elevation, truly chronic cases are often afebrile and present with dull pain of weeks' to months' duration. The lesion is typically single and located near the metaphysis. About 75 percent of the patients reported were less than 25 years of age. The distal part of the tibia is the most common site. Surgical débridement is often curative, but antimicrobial therapy is also recommended.[15]

Gaucher's Disease

Patients with Gaucher's disease, particularly children, may develop all the signs and symptoms of acute bacterial osteomyelitis.[16] These bone crises have an acute onset of bone pain, usually over the tibia, that is often accompanied by high fever, leukocytosis, and an elevated sedimentation rate. The overlying skin may be warm and the area tender to palpation. Even the bone scan findings may be compatible with osteomyelitis. Although biopsy shows bone necrosis, the etiology is noninfectious. This entity of "pseudo-osteomyelitis" is important to recognize because bone biopsy is associated with a high incidence of chronic infection and persistent drainage from the operative site.[17]

Tuberculosis

Skeletal tuberculosis is presumably caused by dissemination of bacilli via the blood stream early in the course of the initial infection. In some cases, spread to bone appears to result from lymphatic drainage from another infected area such as the pleura or kidney. In both children and adults, skeletal involvement may be the only manifestation of systemic disease and, like the pulmonary form, may smolder for years before being discovered.

The basic lesion almost always is a combination of osteomyelitis and arthritis. An inflammatory reaction is followed by formation of granulation tissue that begins to erode and destroy cartilage and eventually cancellous bone, ultimately leading to demineralization and necrosis. The healing process involves deposition of fibrous tissue.

In adults, skeletal tuberculosis usually occurs in weight-bearing joints.[18] The spine is the most frequent site (Pott's disease) followed by the hip and the knee. Tuberculosis is the most common inflammatory process involving the ribs. More than one bone may be affected, and a patient presenting with multiple osteolytic lesions should have the diagnosis of widespread dissemination of bone tuberculosis considered.

Pain is generally the most common complaint. X-ray film evaluations should be followed by specimen collection and culture. Biopsy may be necessary to obtain tissue: a pathology report of granulomatous tissue compatible with tuberculosis is sufficient evidence to begin therapy since organisms may not be grown.

One of the most important radiologic distinctions is between tuberculous spondylitis and pyogenic infection of the spine. In tuberculosis, the first change noted in the spine is a slight narrowing of the intervertebral space. Later, adjacent vertebral bodies are destroyed with eventual collapse and formation of kyphosis and scoliosis (gibbus formation). Generally, pyogenic osteomyelitis involves the disk early and produces rapid sclerosis by 3 or 4 months, whereas tuberculous spondylitis moves more slowly, and the course can be measured over years.

Valuable clinical trials, carried out by the British Medical Research Council, have established that properly prescribed and adequately controlled chemotherapy is sufficient for the routine treatment of tuberculosis of the spine. Cases in which there are complications may need further measures, but for the uncomplicated case, immobilization, plaster jackets, and surgery are unnecessary. Chemotherapy with appropriate antituberculous drugs should provide adequate therapy.

Nontuberculous Mycobacterial Infections

Osteoarticular infections with nontuberculous mycobacteria fall into three distinct types: tenosynovitis, synovitis, and osteomyelitis. Multiple diverse species including *M. marinum, M. avium-intracellulare, M. fortuitum,* and *M. gordonae* have all been associated with infection. Many of these infections seem to respond well to surgery alone; the role of antituberculous therapy, particularly with organisms like *M. avium-intracellulare,* is not clear.[19]

DIAGNOSIS

Roentgenologic Observations

In most patients with hematogenous osteomyelitis, no changes on x-ray film are visible until 10 days after the onset of illness. Although roentgenographic bone changes are rather late events, deep soft tissue swelling and obliteration of the planes between muscles occur early and may provide the first diagnostic clue to the presence of osteomyelitis. The delay in roentgenographic bone changes is probably due to the time needed for more than 50 percent of the bone matrix to be removed before a lytic process can be visualized. Generally, changes of destruction precede new bone formation. In addition, periosteal reaction, cortical irregularity, demineralization, and sequestrum formation may be seen. Computed tomography may be of value for the study of the articular surface of bone and periarticular soft tissues, delineation of the extent of involvement, and demonstration of sequestra.[20] However, its use has not been compared systematically with that of either routine roentgenographic studies or radionuclide studies, and its role in the diagnosis and management of osteomyelitis is still unclear.

MRI with T1- and T2-weighted images is a technique that is currently under active investigation for the detection of inflammatory disease involving the musculoskeletal system. In vertebral osteomyelitis, MRI was as accurate and sensitive as radionuclide scanning in the detection of osteomyelitis. Although MRI can also be helpful in infection of the appendicular skeleton, it is unclear under what circumstances MRI can add significantly to other techniques in diagnosing bone infection.[21] It is probably better than radionuclide studies for differentiating soft tissue infection with periostitis from osteomyelitis. Its role in the immediate postoperative period in the presence of metallic implants is probably very limited. The current data base regarding MRI is small, and further studies of its role in the evaluation of inflammatory processes will be needed.[22]

Radionuclide Studies

The use of radionuclide scanning techniques has enhanced our ability to make an early diagnosis in cases of osteomyelitis.[23] Scanning agents are laid down in newly formed collagen; bone scan results are positive when there is either accelerated bone turnover or increased blood supply to the involved bone. Inflammatory processes, tumor, acute trauma with repair, synovitis, and arthritis may all give positive scan findings. The interpretation of a positive bone scan must depend on the clinical picture to distinguish between these different processes.

The most widely studied technique is technetium scanning, which is extremely sensitive and misses only a small percentage of infections in the musculoskeletal system. The major drawback to technetium scanning is specificity. Some workers feel that this can be improved by the three-phase bone scan, which allows some differentiation of osteomyelitis from soft tissue infection. The addition of gallium scans or indium-labeled white blood cell scintigraphy may be useful in patients with infection superimposed on previous surgery or trauma. In summary, it is fair to say that, although the more recent scanning techniques show promise for the identification of early osteomyelitis in patients with negative findings on x-ray films and technetium bone scanning, they remain expensive procedures whose precise sensitivity, specificity, and predictive value have not yet been firmly established.[23,24]

Microbiologic Studies

The importance of making a precise bacteriologic diagnosis of the infecting organism cannot be overemphasized. Since we are committing patients to prolonged courses of therapy and since there is no distinctive clinical or roentgenographic pattern by which we can make a precise diagnosis of the etiologic agents, it behooves the physician to do whatever tests are necessary to recover the responsible agent. In a comprehensive review of acute osteomyelitis in infants and children, bacteria were recovered in 85 percent of the episodes of osteomyelitis.[25] The frequency of positive cultures in relation to the sources of specimens in that same series was 57 percent for blood, 69 percent for needle aspirate of bone, 65 percent for bone pus obtained at surgery, 83 percent for joint fluid, and 100 percent for wound drainage. Comparable figures are not available for osteomyelitis cases in adults, but we would expect a similarly high percentage of recovery of bacteria for appropriate diagnostic procedures. Cultures for fungi and mycobacteria should be done when clinical suspicion of such infection exists.

Since osteomyelitis, in its chronic form, may persist for years despite antibiotic therapy, the question of the role of protoplasts (L-forms or cell wall-deficient forms) has been raised. Despite a careful search, no protoplasts were found in patients with osteomyelitis in one large series. There are well-documented reports of a few cases in which these forms were recovered. It would seem reasonable in a case of persistent osteomyelitis (particularly one previously treated with antibiotics) from which no bacteria have been recovered that cultures in appropriate hypertonic medium be performed to recover these fastidious forms.

TREATMENT

Antibiotics

Vital questions such as the optimal antibiotics to use, duration over which the agents should be administered, and importance of penetration of antibiotics into bone remain unanswered. Further, it is unlikely that answers will be forthcoming from clinical studies because of the tremendous number of variables involved in assessing the treatment of chronic osteomyelitis. Animal models that mimic the human disease offer some hope for providing rational guidelines.

"Levels" of different antibiotics in bone have been measured after antibiotic administration to patients undergoing surgery. It is difficult to compare the results of these studies since different assay techniques were used. Furthermore, many variables affect the uptake of antibiotics in bone tissue such as the vascularity, the presence of concomitant disease, and the anatomy of the bone chosen for study. Among the agents tested, clindamycin was found in a higher bone-to-serum ratio than were drugs such as methicillin, oxacillin, or cephalothin. Similar observation has been made in experimental animals. The clinical significance of "bone levels" is unknown; studies in experimental animals suggest that it is not necessarily a significant factor in predicting the success of therapy.[26]

When using a well-standardized technique, concentrations of methicillin, dicloxacillin, cephaloridine, or cefazolin were measured in pus and bone from children with osteomyelitis.[27] The penetration of the antibiotics into pus and bone was similar for the two penicillins and for the two cephalosporins despite the disparate protein-binding affinities of these drugs; both penicillins achieved higher bone-to-serum ratios than did the cephalosporins. These four agents attained tissue concentrations that were at least severalfold greater than the MIC values for the infecting *S. aureus* strains.

A model of chronic staphylococcal osteomyelitis in rabbits has been used to test various antimicrobial regimens.[28] Oxacillin, cephalothin, cephaloridine, lincomycin, and rifampin were all found to be associated with a significant number of failures to sterilize diseased bone when administered for 4 weeks. In contrast, it was found that the combinations of rifampin with an aminoglycoside or cephalothin or the combination of oxacillin with an aminoglycoside sterilized the bones of significantly more animals than these agents administered alone did. Because of the need to extrapolate these experimental data to the clinical situation, a controlled, multicenter trial was carried out in chronic staphylococcal osteomyelitis that compared nafcillin and rifampin to nafcillin alone. Although statistical significance was not reached, 80 percent of the patients receiving the two drugs had favorable responses with a minimum of a 2-year follow-up as compared with 50 percent of those receiving nafcillin alone.[29] These results suggest that the combination of nafcillin and rifampin is extremely effective in chronic staphylococcal osteomyelitis involving long bones and should be considered for refractory or difficult cases in particular.

A multicenter collaborative study was carried out to determine whether a standardized serum bactericidal test could be a predictor of therapeutic efficacy in acute and chronic osteomyelitis.[30] The authors evaluated 48 episodes of osteomyelitis (30 acute and 18 chronic) and concluded that patients with acute osteomyelitis should have serum bactericidal titers of 1:2 or greater at all times and that patients with chronic osteomyelitis should have serum bactericidal titers of 1:4 or greater at all times. In general, trough titers appeared to have better predictive value than do peak titers. The study was well done and carefully controlled, but certain caveats are in order. The number of treatment failures was small (four and six, respectively, in the acute and chronic patients), thus making interpretation of the predictive values of titers more difficult. It is my conclusion, based on the results of this study, that it is desirable to aim for a trough serum bactericidal titer of 1:2 or greater but that one must balance the potential toxicity of too high doses of drugs in attempting to obtain such level. I would recommend using these levels as a guide to therapy but not adhering to them rigidly.

Acute Osteomyelitis

The best measure of success of antibiotic therapy in acute osteomyelitis is the incidence of recurrent or chronic disease. In an excellent review of osteomyelitis in infants and children, Dich et al.[25] found a failure rate (defined as recurrent or chronic disease developing) of 19 percent in the patients who received antibiotic therapy for fewer than 21 days after the onset of illness. In contrast they found only 1 failure in 50 patients receiving antibiotics for more than 3 weeks. Their recommendations for the management of acute osteomyelitis should probably be followed until controlled studies indicate that other approaches would be as effective; similar recommendations seem appropriate for adults. They recommend immediate needle aspiration whenever osteomyelitis is suspected. If subperiosteal pus is not obtained, the needle is inserted into the bone, and if any amount of pus is obtained, the patient is taken to surgery for drainage. Antibiotic therapy is based on Gram stain and culture of aspirated material. Therapy is carried out with parenteral antibiotics in high dosage for 4 weeks; oral antibiotics are not subsequently administered. Other investigators have demonstrated that oral antimicrobial therapy after a brief course of parenterally administered drug has been successful in treating acute osteomyelitis.

Chronic Osteomyelitis

In contrast to these clear recommendations for the treatment of acute osteomyelitis, appropriate therapy for chronic osteomyelitis remains a conundrum. Since chronic osteomyelitis is associated with necrotic bone that may serve to sequester bacteria and because it is believed that the organisms are not rapidly multiplying but are relatively dormant, most feel that it is necessary to attain high levels of antibiotics over a prolonged period of time in the infected tissue. This logic has been translated into a recommendation for giving parenteral antibiotics for 1–2 months followed by oral antibiotics for another period of months.

The above recommendation has little hard data to support it. Furthermore, it may not be applicable to cases of chronic osteomyelitis caused by certain gram-negative organisms whose MIC is sufficiently high that orally administered antibiotics could not attain levels in serum or bone that would be adequate to inhibit the organism. Thus, the recommendation generally applies to staphylococcal osteomyelitis. Our present recommendation for chronic staphylococcal osteomyelitis is to establish the precise bacteriologic diagnosis by the culture of bone or pus and then to treat it with a penicillinase-resistant penicillin given intravenously for 4–6 weeks to be followed by an orally administered penicillinase-resistant penicillin for another 2 months. The addition of rifampin to a β-lactam antibiotic may be useful in recurrent or refractory staphylococcal osteomyelitis. Surgical intervention with removal of dead tissue and adequate débridement is an essential part of this therapy.

Because the administration of parenteral antibiotics for 4–6 weeks is expensive and time-consuming, there has been some effort to examine the outcome of treatment with orally administered antibiotics only. The most impressive data come from studies by Bell[31] who has used oral cloxacillin in doses of 5 g plus probenecid in doses of 2 g each day. Patients were treated for a minimum of 6 months and some as long as 1 year. Follow-up study has now continued in approximately 19 patients for 7–9 years with good results, that is, closure of sinuses and absence of clinical recurrences. These results, although highly encouraging, need confirmation before we can confidently recommend this approach. In an era of diagnosis-related groups (DRGs) and shortened hospitalizations, effort have been made to find ways to reduce the period of in-hospital treatment in patients with osteomyelitis. One approach has been to administer long-acting parenteral antimicrobial agents to outpatients; these have resulted in cost savings but paradoxically may increase the expense to patients unless third-party payers show an increased willingness and interest in paying for such programs.[32] Oral antimicrobial therapy with newer agents that may attain effective concentrations is also a promising approach; there needs to be further study with larger numbers of patients to be sure that such approaches are effective.[33]

Perfusion or Irrigation. Because of the difficulty of attaining adequate antibiotic concentrations in avascular necrotic bone, efforts have been made to deliver higher concentrations of antimicrobial agents to the infected area by special means. One such technique is regional perfusion of an extremity, similar to that used in the treatment of neoplasms. There are no controlled data to evaluate the efficacy of this form of treatment, and at present we cannot recommend it.

Another attempt to improve the results of treatment of chronic osteomyelitis involves postoperative irrigation with antibacterial solutions of the surgical wound. Once again, there are no controlled data to support the efficacy of this technique, and there is the potential hazard (often real based on personal experience) that irrigation itself may introduce superinfection with organisms resistant to the antimicrobial agents being used. Antibiotic-impregnated polymethylmethacrylate beads are being used with increased frequency for both the prevention and treatment of bone infections.[34] To date, most of the studies have been with aminoglycoside-impregnated bone cement or beads. There appears to be a paucity of controlled data comparing this approach with standard therapy; further studies are needed before this becomes an accepted method of treatment.

Other Therapeutic Measures. The role of surgery in the treatment of chronic osteomyelitis is an important one. The necessity for removing sequestra and necrotic tissue cannot be overemphasized. There are recent reports that microvascular techniques allowing transplantation of a muscle flap to distant areas have been used successfully in the management of chronic osteomyelitis in infected exposed bone.[35] Optimal management of chronic osteomyelitis is probably best achieved by a combined medical and surgical approach.

COMPLICATIONS

Secondary amyloidosis was once a frequent complication of osteomyelitis of long duration (and other chronic suppurative diseases) but appears to occur infrequently since the advent of antibiotics. The nephrotic syndrome, without secondary amyloidosis, has been reported in association with chronic osteomyelitis; renal biopsy specimens revealed membranoproliferative glomerulonephritis. Neither antibiotic treatment nor therapy with adrenal steroids proved beneficial.

Epidermoid carcinoma may arise in a draining sinus of chronic osteomyelitis with a latent period up to 30 years but frequently a much shorter period. Many of the signs such as pain, increased drainage, and increased bone destruction can occur with either carcinoma or infection alone, and the distinction may be difficult.

PROGNOSIS

The prognosis in acute osteomyelitis is good. The two major variables that affect the outcome are the duration of symptoms before antibiotic therapy is begun (patients generally do well if treated within 3–5 days after the onset of symptoms) and the duration of antibiotic therapy (in adequate dosages) of over 3 weeks. If these two conditions are met, the incidence of recurrent or chronic disease should be extremely low.

Once chronic osteomyelitis supervenes, the prognosis is significantly poorer. In one series, from the Mayo Clinic, of chronic osteomyelitis of hematogenous origin, 55 of 81 patients were treated successfully, 7 were improved, and 19 showed no improvement.[36] In the Massachusetts General Hospital series[37] treatment failure was reported in 13 of 18 cases with "recurrences of hematogenous osteomyelitis." It was also noted that the largest number of failures occurred in patients treated with "limited" antibiotic therapy (less than 4 weeks of parenterally administered antibiotics). Answers to the question "What is optimal therapy for chronic osteomyelitis?" should be forthcoming with further study and may help to improve the prognosis of this disease.

REFERENCES

1. Sugarman B, Hawes S, Musher D, et al. Osteomyelitis beneath pressure sores. Arch Intern Med. 1983;143:683–8.
2. Johnson P, Frederikson J, Sanders J, et al. Management of chronic sternal osteomyelitis. Ann Thorac Surg. 1985;40:69–73.
3. Mackowiak P, Jones S, Smith JW. Diagnostic value of sinus tract cultures in chronic osteomyelitis. JAMA. 1978;239:2772–5.
4. Wheat LJ, Allen SD, Henry M, et al. Diabetic foot infections. Bacteriologic analysis. Arch Intern Med. 1986;146:1935–40.
5. Sapico F, Montgomerie J. Pyogenic vertebral osteomyelitis: Report of nine cases and review of the literature. Rev Infect Dis. 1979;1:754–76.
6. Silverthorn KG, Gillespie WJ. Pyogenic spinal osteomyelitis: A review of 61 cases. NZ Med J. 1986;99:62–5.
7. Meyers B, Berson B, Gilbert M, et al. Clinical patterns of osteomyelitis due to gram-negative bacteria. Arch Intern Med. 1973;131:228–33.
8. Lesse A, Freer C, Salata R, et al. Oral ciprofloxacin therapy for gram-negative bacillary osteomyelitis. Am J Med. 1987;82(Suppl 4A):247–55.
9. Greenberg R, Tice A, Marsh P, et al. Randomized trial of ciprofloxacin compared with other antimicrobial therapy in the treatment of osteomyelitis. Am J Med. 1987;82(Suppl 4A):266–9.
10. Hall B, Fitzgerald R, Rosenblatt J. Anaerobic osteomyelitis. J Bone Joint Surg [Am]. 1983;65:30–5.
11. Raff M, Melo J. Anaerobic osteomyelitis. Medicine (Baltimore). 1978;57:83–103.
12. Gathe J Jr, Harris R, Garland B, et al. *Candida* osteomyelitis. Report of 5 cases and review of the literature. Am J Med. 1987;82:927–37.
13. Engh C, Hughes J, Abrams R, et al: Osteomyelitis in the patient with sickle cell disease. J Bone Joint Surg [Am]. 1971;53:1–15.
14. Chandresekar P, Narula A. Bone and joint infections in intravenous drug abusers. Rev Infect Dis. 1986;8:904–11.
15. Miller W, Murphy W, Gilula L. Brodie abscess: Reappraisal. Radiology 1979;132:15–23.
16. Beighton P, Goldblatt J, Sacks S. Bone involvement in Gaucher disease. In: Desnick RJ, Gatt S, Grabowski GA, eds. Gaucher Disease: A Century of Delineation and Research. New York: Alan R Liss; 1982:107–109.
17. Noyes FR, Smith WS. Bone crises and chronic osteomyelitis in Gaucher's disease. Clin Orthop. 1971;79:132–40.
18. Davidson P, Horowitz I. Skeletal tuberculosis. Am J Med. 1970;48:77–4.
19. Marchevsky A, Damsker B, Green S, et al. The clinicopathological spectrum of non-tuberculous mycobacterial osteoarticular infection. J Bone Joint Surg [Am]. 1985;67:925–9.
20. Azouz E. Computed tomography in bone and joint infections. J Can Assoc Radiol. 1981;32:102–6.
21. Tang J, Gold R, Bassett L, et al. Musculoskeletal infection of the extremities: Evaluation with MR imaging. Radiology 1988;166:205–9.
22. Modic M, Pflanze W, Feiglin D, et al. Magnetic resonance imaging of musculoskeletal infections. Radiol Clin North Am. 1986;24:247–58.
23. Wheat J. Diagnostic strategies in osteomyelitis. Am J Med. 1985;78(Suppl 6B):218–24.
24. Merkel K, Fitzgerald RH Jr, Brown M. Scintigraphic evaluation in musculoskeletal sepsis. Orthop Clin North Am. 1984;15:401–16.
25. Dich V, Nelson J, Haltalin K. Osteomyelitis in infants in children. Am J Dis Child. 1975;129:1273–8.
26. Norden C. Experimental osteomyelitis II. Therapeutic trials and measurement of antibiotic levels in bone. J Infect Dis. 1971;124:565–71.
27. Tetzlaff T, Howard J, McCracken G, et al. Antibiotic concentrations in pus and bone of children with osteomyelitis. J Pediatr. 1978;92:135–40.
28. Norden C. Experimental osteomyelitis IV. Therapeutic trials with rifampin alone and in combination with gentamicin, sisomicin, and cephalothin. J Infect Dis. 1975;132:493–9.
29. Norden C, Bryant R, Palmer D, et al. Chronic osteomyelitis caused by *Staphylococcus aureus*: Controlled clinicial trial of nafcillin therapy and nafcillin-rifampin therapy. South Med J. 1986;79:947–51.
30. Weinstein M, Stratton C, Hawley HB, et al. Multicenter collaborative evaluation of a standardized serum bactericidal test as a predictor of therapeutic efficacy in acute and chronic osteomyelitis. Am J Med. 1987;83:218–22.
31. Bell S. Further observations on the value of oral penicillins in chronic staphylococcal osteomyelitis. Med J Aust. 1976;2:591–3.
32. Eisenberg J, Kitz D. Savings from outpatient antibiotic therapy for osteomyelitis. Economic analysis of a therapeutic strategy. JAMA. 1986;255:1584–8.
33. Black J, Hunt TL, Godley PJ, et al. Oral antimicrobial therapy for adults with osteomyelitis or septic arthritis. J Infect Dis. 1987;155:968–72.
34. Seligson D. Antibiotic-impregnated beads in orthopedic infectious problems. J Ky Med Assoc. 1984;82:25–9.
35. Fitzgerald RH Jr, Ruttle P, Arnold P, et al. Local muscle flaps in the treatment of chronic osteomyelitis. J Bone Joint Surg [Am]. 1985;67:175–85.
36. Kelly P, Wikowski C, Washington J. Comparison of gram-negative bacillary and staphylococcal osteomyelitis of the femur and tibia. Clin Orthop 1973;96:70–5.
37. Waldvogel R, Medoff G, Swartz M. Osteomyelitis: A review of clinical features, therapeutic considerations, and unusual aspects. N Engl J Med. 1970;282:198–206.

SECTION M. DISEASES OF THE REPRODUCTIVE ORGANS AND SEXUALLY TRANSMITTED DISEASES

92. SKIN AND MUCOUS MEMBRANE LESIONS

MICHAEL F. REIN

The skin of the genital area is subject to many of the same diseases that affect other areas of the body. Wilson[1] provides an extensive list of nonvenereal and noninfectious conditions that can involve the genital epithelium alone or as part of the more generalized disease process. Among adults, sexually transmitted diseases are a frequent cause of genital lesions, and a sympathetically obtained sexual history and diligent search for extragenital manifestations of sexually transmitted diseases should be a part of the initial work-up.

HISTORY

Age

Candida albicans and herpes simplex can infect the neonatal genitalia, and herpetic vulvitis occurs occasionally in young children as the initial manifestation of exposure to the virus. Molluscum contagiosum is a common pediatric infection that only occasionally involves the genitalia, probably by autoinfection. Among adults, the sexually transmitted infections are considerably more common, but the presence of sexually transmitted lesions such as herpes genitalis,[2] condylomata accuminata,[3–5] and *exclusively* genital molluscum contagiosum[6] in a child should prompt an evaluation for sexual abuse.

Sexual History

Exposure to multiple partners increases the risk of sexually acquired infection. Orogenital contact can inoculate sexually transmitted pathogens into the oral or pharyngeal mucosa.[7–9] Receptive anal intercourse predisposes to perianal, anal, and rectal infection.[8–11] A history of genital symptoms or recent treatment of a sexual partner may be helpful diagnostically. Specific sexual practices such as particularly vigorous coitus or masturbation[12] or a history of being bitten by a sexual partner should be sought.

Incubation Period

We can occasionally estimate the incubation period for sexually transmitted infection by obtaining a history of a single sexual contact or specific exposure to a new partner. Genital lesions developing within hours of sexual exposure suggest trauma or allergy.[1,12–14] Localized penile edema occurring within hours of vigorous coitus has been reported.[12] The swelling decreased spontaneously, and no specific therapy was required. Incubation periods of less than 24 hours are occasionally noted in chancroid.[15,16] Some patients experience reactivation of herpes genitalis within 12 hours after coitus.[10,17] Somewhat longer incubation periods of 2–5 days are usually seen with chancroid[15,16] and most cases of herpes genitalis.[10,17] Although the mean incubation period for primary genital herpes is about 6 days,[10,17] clinical manifestations may follow infection by as much as 2–3 weeks for both these diseases. An incubation period of 1–3 weeks is usually seen with syphilis,[9] 4–12 weeks with venereal warts,[11] and about 4 weeks for pubic lice[18] and scabies (Chapters 269 and 270). The incubation period for molluscum contagiosum is not well documented and may range from 2 to 26 weeks.[19,20] The incubation periods for donovanosis is poorly defined[15] but in recent series averages around 2 weeks.[21,22] The incubation period for syphilis[9] ranges from 1 to 12 weeks, and for genital warts, it is about 2–3 months.[11]

Residence and Travel

Chancroid and lymphogranuloma venereum are considerably more common in Africa and the Far East than in the United States.[15] Outbreaks of chancroid have occurred recently in the United States,[23] but in general the disease accounts for only about 1 percent of genital ulcers in North America and Europe.[24–27] On the other hand, chancroid was diagnosed in from 40 percent to 90 percent of patients with genital ulcerations in some African and Indian series,[25,28–32] and the relative prevalence of genital herpes infection was correspondingly reduced. Donovanosis is endemic in India, New Guinea, the West Indies, and some parts of Africa and South America, but it is now rare in the United States.[15,21,22,33]

Use of Antibiotics

Antibiotics and other drugs have been reported to cause fixed drug eruptions that occasionally involve the genitalia.[1,34,35] The tetracyclines, commonly used in the treatment of genital infections, are incriminated with particular frequency.[35] Antibiotics may predispose to the development of candidiasis and may alter or completely eliminate the lesions of syphilis.[36]

Underlying Diseases

Immunodeficiency states predispose to a variety of genital lesions. Balanitis due to *Candida* occurs in neutropenic patients,[37] and balanitis caused by gram-negative bacteria[38] is seen in patients wearing condom catheters. The acquired immunodeficiency syndrome (AIDS) is associated with chronic necrotizing and recurrent genital[39] and perianal[40] herpes simplex virus (HSV) infections.

Mode of Onset and Course

Because lesions often change over time, a history of the initial manifestation may be crucial to making the diagnosis. Thus, the patient with genital ulcerations who can state with surety that the lesions began as vesicles has helped to make a diagnosis of herpes genitalis. Vesicles often rupture quickly so that this stage of the lesions goes unnoticed by women.[17] A prodrome of local paresthesia preceding the appearance of lesions is reported by 50–90 percent of patients with recurrent genital herpes.[8,17,41] Venereal warts and molluscum contagiosum may remain relatively static for long periods of time after their initial appearance. The lesions of syphilis often last for many weeks and then heal without antibiotic intervention.[9] Pearly penile papules are a completely benign condition appearing in single or multiple rows around the penile corona at puberty.[42]

A recurrence of the lesions at intervals strongly suggests genital herpes. The rate of recurrence varies strikingly among individuals, but the average rate of recurrence among patients genitally infected with HSV type 2 is 0.33 per month, whereas genital infections with HSV type 1 recur at an average rate of but 0.02 per month.[43] Indeed, whereas 90 percent of patients with type 2 genital infections report a recurrence within a year, recurrences are experienced by only 25 percent of the patients genitally infected with HSV type 1.

Pain

Although the syphilitic chancre is usually described as nontender, up to 30 percent of the patients with primary syphilis describe either pain or tenderness of the lesions.[36] The relative indolence of the lesions of donovanosis[15,33,44] sometimes results in long delays before the patient seeks medical attention. Pain usually accompanies the lesions of chancroid,[15,45] herpes genitalis,[8,17] tularemia,[46,47] and amebiasis.[48–50]

Pruritis

Itching is associated with herpes genitalis and is described by 50–90 percent of patients with recurrent disease,[8,17,41] particularly in the prodromal period. Pruritus accompanies 90 percent of infestations with pubic lice,[18] and severe itching increased by warming the skin, either in bed or when taking a bath, suggests scabies. Although *severe* pruritis is uncommon in secondary syphilis,[9] 42 percent of patients describe at least mild itching.[51] Itching also characterizes candidal balanitis, which is observed occasionally in male sexual partners of women with vulvovaginal candidiasis.[52,53]

Vaginal Discharge

Many infectious vaginitides are associated with vulvar lesions. The vulvovaginitis syndrome is discussed in Chapter 95.

Fever

Fever is described in 5–8 percent of the patients with secondary syphilis[9,51] and in many patients with disseminated gonococcal infection.[54,55] Fever accompanies primary herpes genitalis in 70 percent of women and 40 percent of men but is uncommon in recurrent disease.[8,17,41]

Other

Sacral root neurologic symptoms suggest herpes,[8,17] and a urethral discharge suggests gonorrhea or, rarely, Reiter syndrome (Chapter 95).

MORPHOLOGIC CHARACTERISTICS OF GENITAL LESIONS

Careful examination of the entire genital area is essential and will be facilitated by a good light source and a hand lens. A differential diagnosis can often be made on the basis of the morphologic characteristics of genital lesions, but variations from the typical morphologic features and clinical overlap among the various diseases are unfortunately common.[36,56,57] A clinical differential diagnosis of genital ulcers is perhaps the most difficult[30,56,58] with the most common error involving the overdiagnosis of chancroid.[26] Nonetheless, the morphologic characteristics of genital lesions often supply the first and most important clue to their cause. Table 1 provides a morphologic classification of genital lesions but can serve only as a rough guide.

TABLE 1. Morphologic Classification of Genital Lesions

Ulcers	Vesicles
Herpes genitalis	Herpes genitalis
Syphilis	Crusts
Trauma	Scabies
Chancroid	Herpes genitalis
Lymphogranuloma venereum	Miscellaneous lesions
Tularemia	Nits: crabs
Behçet's syndrome	Hypertrophic: donovanosis
Malignancy	Diffuse inflammation: drug reaction, candidiasis, trauma
Histoplasmosis	Linear tracks: scabies
Donovanosis (granuloma inguinale)	Reddish flecks: crab excreta
Candidiasis	Maculae caeruleae (sky blue spots): crabs
Mycobacterioses	Crepitus: anaerobes[62]
Amebiasis	
Fixed drug eruption	
Gonorrhea[29]	
Trichomoniasis[27]	
Papules	
Venereal warts	
Scabies	
Molluscum contagiosum	
Syphilis	
Pearly penile papules	
Candidiasis	

Genital Ulcers

As noted earlier, the causes of genital ulcers vary markedly in different parts of the world.[24,25,28–32] Because of the relative rarity of chancroid in the United States and its similarities to herpes simplex genital infection, we should regard a clinical diagnosis of chancroid with some suspicion.[56] Rare causes of destructive penile ulcerations include tuberculosis[59–62] and amebiasis.[48–50]

Number. The classic chancre of primary syphilis is a single lesion[9] (Figs. 1 and 2); however, in some series, almost half of the patients with proven primary syphilis had more than one

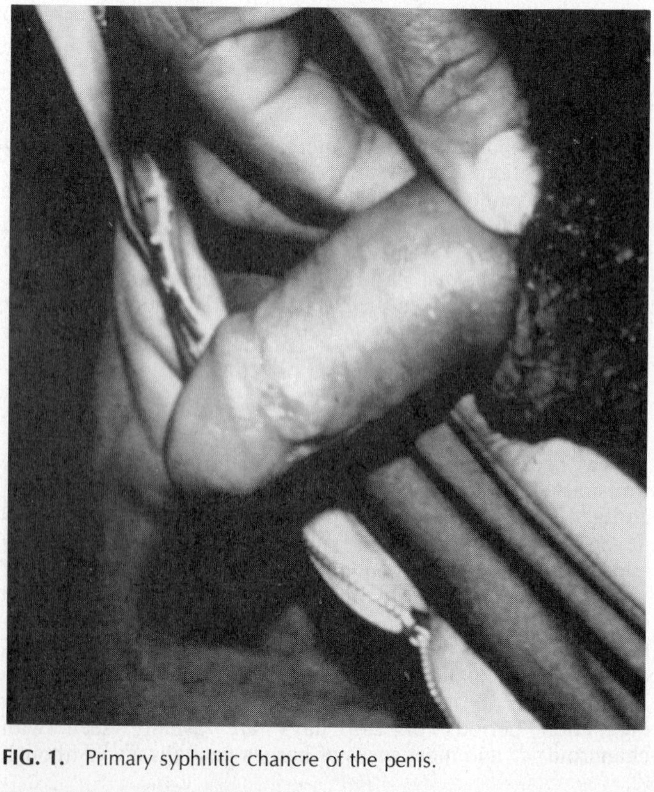

FIG. 1. Primary syphilitic chancre of the penis.

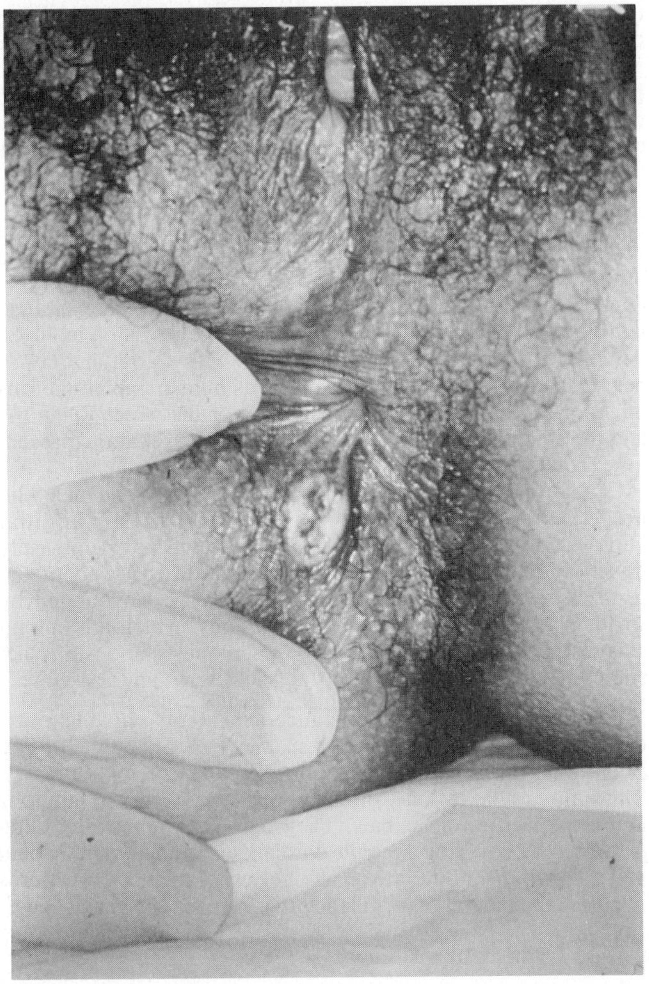

FIG. 2. Primary syphilitic chancre of the perineum.

penile ulcer.[27,36] Chancroid is usually said to be present as multiple ulcerations, yet in some series 40–70 percent of the affected men had but a single lesion.[45,63] The genital lesion of tick-borne tularemia is single.[46] Herpes genitalis characteristically produces multiple ulcerations in groups surrounded by an erythematous border (Fig. 3).[8,17,41] The vagina per se is involved in only 4 percent of cases.[8,17,36] Although the multiple lesions of syphilis and herpes are generally of uniform size, the lesions of chancroid may vary in an individual patient.[15] A rare cause of recurrent, multiple, genital ulcerations in the United States is Behçet syndrome,[64] an inflammatory disease of unknown cause that usually also involves the oral, conjunctival, and synovial membranes. Behçet's ulcers involve the scrotum and vulva more frequently than they do the penis, anus, and vagina, and scars from previous episodes may be present.[64] Ulcers are rarely observed in vulvovaginal or penile[24] candidiasis. Intravaginal ulcers may follow tampon use,[65] but infectious and neoplastic causes must be ruled out in these cases.

Tenderness. Tenderness on palpation may be extreme with herpes genitalis,[8,17] and chancroid[15,45] is present in 30 percent of syphilitic chancres[36] and characterizes tularemia.[46] Even massive ulcerated lesions of donovanosis are nontender.[15,33]

Ulcer Base. The lesions of chancroid are usually ragged and have a necrotic base.[15,30,45] On the other hand, syphilitic and herpetic ulcers are relatively clean (Figs. 1–3). The ulcers of Behçet syndrome often have a yellow, necrotic base.[64] Donovanosis produces ulcers with granulation tissue at the base yielding a beefy red lesion that often becomes exuberantly hypertrophic and produces large, friable, ulcerated masses projecting above the skin.[15,33]

Ulcer Edge. The ulcers of chancroid are characteristically undermined, but the edge is not indurated.[15,16,45,30,66] An indurated lesion is highly suggestive of syphilis[9,27] (and some rare conditions[60]), and occurs in 92 percent of the infected patients.[36] An erythematous border is seen both with herpes[8,17] and with chancroid.[15,45] The border of the lesion in donovanosis is often a stark white, which is characteristic of no other genital infection.[44] Lesions of donovanosis also often manifest a thickening of the edge that yields a rolled appearance.[33]

Serpiginous lesions, progressing in one area as they heal in another, are characteristic of donovanosis[15,33] and less so of chancroid.[15]

Genital Papules

Careful examination of the papules with the aid of a hand lens often yields an immediate etiologic diagnosis. Papules may be the transient, initial state of a variety of genital infections including syphilis.[36] scabies,[67] lymphogranuloma venereum,[68] chancroid,[15] and herpes.[8,17] Early condylomata accuminata usually appear as simple papules and can be identified when the hand lens reveals the beginning of a verrucous cap or tiny blood vessels at the base.

Pearly penile papules are normal and occur in 8–25 percent of men.[42] They are found more commonly in uncircumcised men

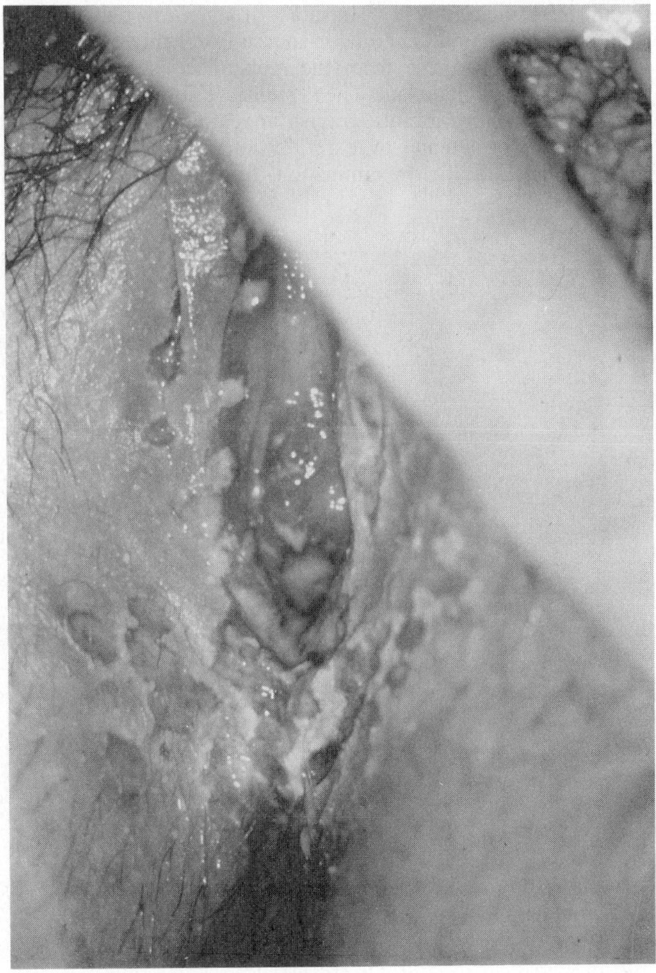

FIG. 3. Herpes (HSV-II) of the vulva.

and present as one or more rows of grayish white or pink papules along the corona or in the coronal sulcus. They usually appear at puberty and are of no pathologic significance. Patients concerned about venereal disease will occasionally notice the lesions and will seek medical attention. Although the histologic appearance is characteristic, biopsy is rarely warranted because the diagnosis can be made clinically.

Umbilication. The hand lens will reveal tiny umbilications at the vertex of the lesions of molluscum contagiosum[19,20] (Fig. 4, Chapter 116). The umbilications often appear to contain keratin plugs. These 1 to 5 mm papules occur singly or in small clusters on the penile shaft, glans, labia majora, thighs, and buttocks. In children, the disease is nonvenereally acquired and usually affects the trunk and extremities. The lesions are nonpruritic and may coalesce to form larger masses.[19,20] Squeezing expresses caseous material from the umbilication. Curettage easily removes the entire lesion and leaves a shallow, slightly hemorrhagic ulceration that heals without scarring. If the diagnosis is in doubt, a papule may be removed by curetting and crushed between two microscope slides. Wright or Giemsa stains reveal cells distended by intracytoplasmic inclusions (Chapter 116).

Verrucous papules suggest a diagnosis of condylomata acuminata (venereal warts). The lesions are usually multiple and may show a satelliting phenomenon wherein a larger wart is surrounded by smaller lesions. Stalked or sessile, the warts can be found anywhere on the external genitalia and in the vagina or on the cervix. Perianal warts in women may occur as a result of the spread from a genital focus. Perianal condylomas in men are associated with receptive anal intercourse,[10,11,69] and such men should be evaluated for intra-anal warts[19] and other anorectal infections as well.[70] In moist areas warts may become relatively elongated. The major source of diagnostic difficulty is differentiating these from the moist lesions of secondary syphilis, condylomata lata. The syphilitic lesions tend to be flatter and often have a more grayish appearance.[9] A differential diagnosis is best made by carefully abrading the lesions and performing a darkfield examination, for condylomata lata are teeming with spirochetes. Unfortunately, anaerobic spirochetes occasionally superinfect condylomata accuminata and may give an initial appearance of darkfield positivity. Venereal warts, particularly flat warts of the cervix, are strongly associated with cervical intraepithelial neoplasia and cancer[71] (Chapter 123), and culposcopy or biopsy may be indicated for suspicious lesions.

Although acetic acid applications have long been used to identify subclinical papillomavirus infections of the cervix and vagina, the technique has recently been employed to detect otherwise invisible lesions in men.[72–76] Acetic acid, 3–5%, is applied to the penis for 3–5 minutes, and the skin is examined with the colposcope. Flat, white lesions are revealed in 40–80 percent of the male partners of women with warts, and 60–80 percent of such lesions are identified as human papillomavirus infection by biopsy.[72–76] The accuracy of histologic diagnosis and the significance of "acetowhite" lesions are, at the present time, somewhat controversial.

Candidal balanitis occurs in up to 10 percent of the men who are the sexual partners of women with candidal vulvovaginitis[52,53] and is usually manifestated as an intensely pruritic papular lesion of the glans, foreskin, or shaft of the penis. The raised erythematous area may be surrounded by small, discrete papules, or satellite lesions, which are helpful diagnostically. Similar papular or papulopustular lesions accompany candidal infection of the groin, scrotum, and vulva.

Crusted Lesions. Herpetic ulcers heal by crusting over. Crusts are also characteristic of scabies (see Chapter 270, Fig. 2) and may be accompanied by moist papules[37] and burrows. These threadlike lesions, often stippled, may be 1–10 mm long and are specific for scabies. They may be dramatically demonstrated by covering a papule with ink (as from a fountain pen) and then wiping it off, with an alcohol swab. In about two-thirds of cases, the burrow, now filled with ink, is readily visualized.[77]

Diffuse Erythematous Lesions

Superficial infection with tinea or *Candida* may cause diffusely erythematous, intensely pruritic lesions of the genitalia and

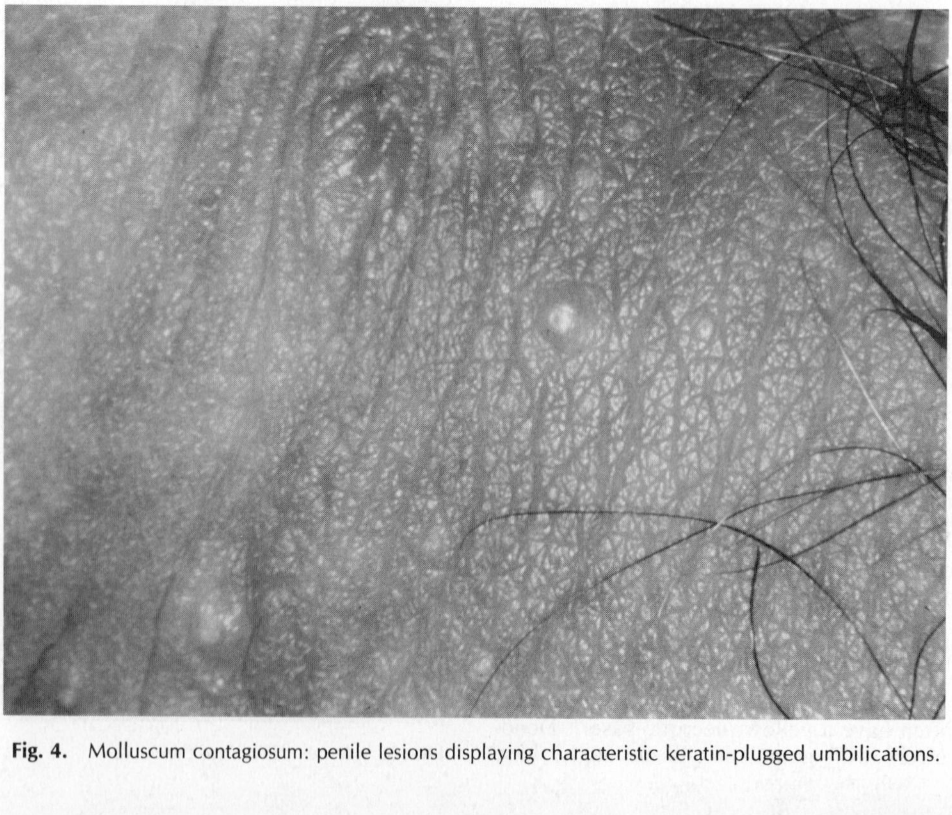

Fig. 4. Molluscum contagiosum: penile lesions displaying characteristic keratin-plugged umbilications.

groin area. Candidal lesions are often more intensely erythematous, whereas lesions caused by tinea are usually somewhat brown and may show central clearing. Involvement of the scrotum or the appearance of small papules or pustules beyond the main border of the lesion suggests candidal infection.

Group B streptococci have caused balanitis.[78] *Gardnerella vaginalis* is also felt to cause some cases of balanitis in uncircumcized men[79] in whom it is associated with the same fishy odor that characterizes bacterial vaginosis. Likewise, the condition responds to metronidazole.

Pubic Hair

Crab lice are usually manifested in very small numbers, an average infestation consisting of fewer than 10.[80] The lice are, however, observed in 97 percent of infested patients who have not treated themselves before seeking medical attention.[18] Examination of the pubic hair with a hand lens reveals them as gray-brown creatures climbing along the shafts or partially buried at the bases. They are found in perianal hair in about 50 percent of patients and in abdominal hair in about 17 percent of patients.[18] If the organisms themselves are not observed, the diagnosis can be made in 80 percent of patients by recognizing the eggs or nits, 0.5 mm ovoids adherent to the hair shafts, and a careful examination may reveal tiny reddish spots of louse excreta at the base of the hair in about 15 percent of patients.[18] Crab bites sometimes result in round to oval, 0.5–1.5 mm, bluish red macules called maculae caeruleae or sky blue spots.[18,81]

EXTRAGENITAL DERMATOLOGIC MANIFESTATIONS OF SEXUALLY TRANSMITTED DISEASES

Patients should be questioned about orogenital and receptive anal practices since these may result in direct inoculation of sexually transmitted pathogens into extragenital sites. Additionally, sexually transmitted infections may disseminate and result in secondary extragenital manifestations.

Mouth

Direct inoculation of sexually transmitted viruses can result in oral lesions. Intraoral condylomata accuminata are reported,[7] and lesions resemble those of the genital mucous membranes. Herpes simplex has been transmitted from the genital tract to the mouth and vice versa.[8,17,43] Genital lesions produced by HSV type 1 are indistinguishable from those produced by type 2. Likewise, oral inoculation can result in fever blisters, a primary gingivostomatitis, or a herpangina-like picture,[8,17,82] with clusters of vesicles and ulcers on the hard palate.

Although the oral mucosa is generally resistant to gonococcal infection, occasional cases of gonococcal stomatitis, presumably resulting from the direct inoculation, have been reported.[83] Chancres of the lip, buccal mucous membranes, gingiva, and tonsils are becoming relatively more common. They are usually painless and may be difficult to diagnose because normal oral spirochetes confound the darkfield examination.[9] Disseminated infections may also affect the mouth. Mucous patches occur in about 20 percent of patients with secondary syphilis[9,51] and appear on the oral mucous membranes and the tongue as painless, relatively clean, shallow ulcerations, often with a yellow or gray base and a small amount of surrounding erythema.[9] Palatal petechiae may accompany gonococcal bacteremia. Recurrent oral and genital ulcers suggest Behçet syndrome.[64]

Anorectum

A similar spectrum of diseases affects the rectal mucosa.[70] Perianal warts[10,11,69] and herpetic lesions[40,84] are seen in homosexual men who practice receptive anal intercourse. Both types of lesions can involve women in the same manner, but in women they may also have extended to the anus from a primary genital focus. Among patients with AIDS, herpetic proctitis may be chronic and relentlessly destructive.[40] Destructive perianal lesions occasionally result from amebiasis in endemic areas.[85]

Other Skin

The generalized rash of secondary syphilis frequently involves the genitalia. In fact, a generalized eruption sparing the genital area and the oral mucous membranes is unlikely to be syphilis.[9] The rash is highly variable, and the differential diagnosis is challenging.[51,57] One should consider secondary syphilis in the differential diagnosis of any generalized, relatively indolent eruption, particularly if the palms and soles are involved, if there is accompanying generalized lymphadenopathy (70–86 percent), or if there is a patchy hair loss.[9,51] The lesions are usually macular, maculopapular (70 percent), or papulosquamous[9,51] and symmetrically distributed. Markedly pruritic or vesicular lesions in an adult are unlikely to be syphilis.

About 33–50 percent of the patients with disseminated gonococcal infections will have small numbers of skin lesions, usually found on the distal portions of the extremities and occasionally involving the palms and the soles. The lesions are relatively pleomorphic and may be macular, maculopapular, petechial, vesicular, pustular, or necrotic.[55] The typical lesion is an erythematous or hemorrhagic spot 2–5 mm in diameter that is surmounted by a gray pustule, sometimes displaying a small eschar in its center.[54] The lesions of subacute meningococcemia may be similar and represent an important differential diagnosis.

The interdigital webs, wrists, and ankles are often involved with scabies.[86] Secondary papular lesions, thought to occur as a hypersensitivity phenomenon, may occur on the abdomen or the pelvic girdle area. Burrows, described above, are pathognomonic of scabies.[77] Maculae caerulae (see above) often occur on the anterior and lateral portions of the abdomen and thorax.[81]

Patients with AIDS may demonstrate a variety of skin lesions, including Kaposi sarcoma, at some distance from sexual orifices (Chapter 108).

Herpes genitalis involves the thigh or buttock in some 15 percent of infected women.[87,88]

LABORATORY EXAMINATIONS

Sufficiently accurate etiologic diagnoses can often be made on the basis of clinical examination when the lesions are typical. In many situations, particularly in the etiologic diagnosis of genital ulcers, laboratory examination is required.

Direct Microscopic Examinations

Any ulcerated genital lesion or hypertrophic lesion in a moist area may be examined by darkfield microscopy. Gloves must be worn. The lesion is cleaned with a dry gauze pad and is then abraded with gauze until some blood is seen. The blood is blotted until bleeding ceases, and a small amount of serous fluid is expressed by squeezing the edges of the lesion. A drop of this material may be picked up directly on a glass coverslip, which is then inverted on a microscope slide and is examined for characteristic motile spirochetes with darkfield illumination.

The diagnosis of chancroid is sometimes confirmed by cleaning the lesion with gauze and swabbing material from the undermined edge. Gram staining of this material sometimes reveals chains of streptobacilli suggestive of *Haemophilus ducreyi*,[45] but the smear technique has a low sensitivity and specificity, and is not useful in a clinical setting.[29,32,63,89]

A smear of material from the base of a freshly ruptured vesicle may be stained with Wright or Giemsa stains and examined for multinucleated giant cells that are diagnostic of herpes infection.[8,17] This Tzanck test is not generally helpful, however, because the presence of vesicles is essentially diagnostic of herpetic infection and the test is insensitive on genital ulcers, being positive in fewer than 40 percent of culture-proven cases.[90] Several recent developments appear likely to improve rapid diagnostic capabilities. Monoclonal antibodies will detect herpes viral antigens in material from 75 percent of herpetic lesions by direct examination with fluorescence microscopy,[91,92] and the technique also differentiates type 1 virus from type 2. DNA hybridization with radiolabeled probes has identified HSV in 80 percent of lesions.[93,94]

Bits of tissue from a hypertrophic lesion may be crushed between microscope slides, treated with Wright or Giemsa stains and examined for the characteristic intracytoplasmic bacterial inclusions of donovanosis.[15,21,22,33]

Papular lesions may be scraped, crushed, stained with a variety of agents, and examined for the balloonlike cells of molluscum contagiosum.[20] Heating such scrapings with 10% potassium hydroxide will destroy the squamous elements and may reveal tinea, *Candida*, or the mite or larvae of scabies.[67] Mixing scrapings with mineral oil rather than potassium hydroxide may have an advantage in the diagnosis of scabies, for unlike potassium hydroxide, mineral oil preserves mite fecal pellets and motility.[94a]

Scrapings or aspirations of the peripheral lesions of disseminated gonococcal infection reveal the organisms only infrequently by Gram stain but may be subjected to immunofluorescent microscopy, which will be diagnostic in about half the cases.[55,95]

Serologic Tests

Serologic tests are occasionally misleading in the diagnosis of syphilis. From 20 to 30 percent of the patients with a chancre, particularly if the lesion has just appeared, will have nonreactive nontreponemal tests for syphilis.[96–98] About 10–17 percent of the patients may have a reactive fluorescent treponemal antibody absorption (FTA-ABS) test even if the nontreponemal tests (e.g., Venereal Disease Research Laboratory [VDRL], rapid plasma reagin [RPR], automated reagin test [ART]) (see Chapter 213) are nonreactive.[96–98] The clinician may therefore wish to obtain an FTA-ABS test on patients with suspicious genital lesions, even if the nontreponemal test result is negative. In many areas, the microhemagglutination test for *Treponema pallidum* antibodies (MHA-TP) has replaced the more demanding FTA-ABS as the confirmatory treponemal test. The tests are not entirely equivalent since the MHA-TP is only about 89 percent sensitive in primary syphilis and will therefore miss about 10 percent of cases that would be detected by the FTA-ABS.[98] The vast majority of patients will have positive nontreponemal test findings within the week after the appearance of the chancre, and repeated serologic testing and darkfield examination may be necessary to make the diagnosis.

The sensitivity of nontreponemal and treponemal tests is almost 100 percent in secondary syphilis. Thus, a negative serologic examination essentially rules out this diagnosis.[96,98]

Serologic testing has almost no current role in the routine clinical diagnosis of genital HSV infection[17,94,99] because of cross-reactions resulting from highly prevalent herpes simplex type 1 infections. Serologic tests for chancroid and donovanosis are not available.

Culture

Tissue culture for herpes simplex is the most sensitive way to diagnose this infection. It is 70 percent sensitive in lesions that have ruptured and formed ulcers even in initial infections when cytologic findings are negative. Once the lesions have crusted over, however, sensitivity of the culture is reduced to about 30 percent.[100] The sensitivity is lower in recurrent disease, dropping to 30 percent in ulcers and to less than 20 percent in crusted lesions.[92]

The edge of a clean lesion may be cultured for *H. ducreyi*.[103] The medium employed dramatically affects sensitivity,[103] which is, even under the best circumstances, probably no higher than 80 percent.[30,31,63,103] Material from the lesion suspected of being molluscum contagiosum may be inoculated into tissue culture, and a cytopathic effect may be observed (Chapter 115). Culture for the agent of donovanosis is unreliable and not generally available.[33]

INITIAL APPROACH TO THERAPY

So diverse are the causes of the lesions in the genital area that initial therapy must be based on highly presumptive or definitive etiologic diagnosis. In most cases, it is possible to delay therapy until such a diagnosis has been reached. When dealing with multiple infections, it is important to avoid the situation in which treatment for one infection interferes with the diagnosis of another. Thus, if one is treating gonorrhea in the presence of a suspicious genital lesion, spectinomycin may be the treatment of choice because it does not interfere with the subsequent darkfield or serologic diagnosis of syphilis.

REFERENCES

1. Wilson JF. The nonvenereal diseases of the genitals: Their differentiation from venereal lesions. Med Clin North Am. 1964;48:787.
2. Hibbard RA. Herpetic vulvovaginitis and child abuse. Am J Dis Child. 1985;139:542–5.
3. Schachner L, Hankin DE. Assessing child abuse in childhood condyloma accuminatum. J Am Acad Dermatol. 1985;12:157–60.
4. Shelton TB, Jerkins GR, Noe HN. Condylomata accuminata in the pediatric patient. J Urol. 1986;135:548–9.
5. Bender ME. New concepts of condyloma accuminata in children. Arch Dermatol. 1986;122:1121–4.
6. Bargman H, Schachner L, Hankin D. Is genital molluscum contagiosum a cutaneous manifestation of sexual abuse in children? J Am Acad Dermatol. 1986;14:847–9.
7. Choukass NC, Toto PD. Condyloma accuminatum of the oral cavity. Oral Surg. 1982;54:480.
8. Corey L, Adams HG, Brown ZA, et al. Genital herpes simplex infection: Clinical manifestations, course, and complications. Ann Intern Med. 1983;98:958.
9. Stokes JH, Beerman H, Ingraham NR. Modern Clinical Syphilology. 3rd ed. Philadelphia: WB Saunders; 1944.
10. Carr G, William DC. Anal warts in a population of gay men in New York City. Sex Transm Dis. 1977;4:56.
11. Oriel JD. Genital warts. Sex Transm Dis. 1981;8:326.
12. Wilde H, Canby JP. Penile venereal edema. Arch Dermatol. 1973;108:263.
13. Fried FA. Glans penis dermatitis after treatment of wife's vaginitis. JAMA. 1981;245:2532.
14. Gochfeld M, Burger J. Sexual transmission of nickel and poison oak contact dermatitis. Lancet. 1983;1:589.
15. Hart G. Chancroid, Donovanosis, Lymphogranuloma Venereum. DHEW publication (CDC) 75-8302. 1975.
16. Fiumara NJ. A guide to lesions of the penis. Hosp Med. March: 1970.
17. Pazin GJ. Management of oral and genital herpes simplex virus infections: Diagnosis and treatment. DM 1986;32:725–824.
18. Chapel TA, Katta T, Kuszmar T, et al. Pediculosis pubis in a clinic for sexually transmitted diseases. Sex Transm Dis. 1979;6:257.
19. Margolis S. Genital warts and molluscum contagiosum. Urol Clin North Am. 1984;11:163–70.
20. Brown ST, Nalley JF, Kraus SJ. Molluscum contagiosum. Sex Transm Dis. 1981;8:227.
21. Sehgal VN, Shyam Prasad AL. Donovanosis: Current concepts. Int J Dermatol. 1986;25:8–16.
22. Rosen T, Tschen JA, Ramsdell W, et al. Granuloma inguinale. J Am Acad Dermatol. 1984;433–7.
23. Blackmore CA, Limpakarnjanarat K, Rigau-Perez JG, et al. An outbreak of chancroid in Orange County, California: Descriptive epidemiology and disease control measures. J Infect Dis. 1985;151:840–4.
24. Chapel T, Brown WJ, Jeffries C, et al. The microbiological flora of penile ulcerations. J Infect Dis. 1978;137:50.
25. Meheus A, Van Dyck E, Ursi JP, et al. Etiology of genital ulcerations in Swaziland. Sex Transm Dis. 1983;10:33.
26. Sturm AW, Stolting GJ, Cormane RH, et al. Clinical and microbiological evaluation of 46 episodes of genital ulceration. Genitourin Med. 1987;63:98–101.
27. Diaz-Mitoma F, Benningen G, Slutchuk M, et al. Etiology of nonvesicular genital ulcers in Winnipeg. Sex Transm Dis. 1987;14:33–6.

28. Nsanze H, Fast MV, D'Costa LJ. Genital ulcers in Kenya: Clinical and laboratory study. Br J Vener Dis. 1981;57:378.
29. Cooradia YM, Kharsany A, Hoosen A. The microbial aetiology of genital ulcers in black men in Durban, South Africa. Genitourin Med. 1985;61:266–9.
30. Plummer FA, D'Costa LJ, Nsanze H, et al. Clinical and microbiologic studies of genital ulcers in Kenyan women. Sex Transm Dis. 1985;12:193–7.
31. Fast MV, D'Costa LJ, Nsanze H, et al. The clinical diagnosis of genital ulcer disease in men in the tropics. Sex Transm Dis. 1984;11:72–6.
32. Sehgal VN, Prasad ALS. Chancroid or chancroidal ulcers. Dermatologica. 1985;170:136–41.
33. Kuberski T. Granuloma inguinale (donovanosis). Sex Transm Dis. 1980;7:29.
34. Talbot MD. Fixed genital drug eruption. Practitioner. 1980;224:823.
35. Dodds PR, Chi T-N. Balanitis as a fixed drug eruption to tetracycline. J Urol. 1981;133:1044–5.
36. Chapel TA. The variability of syphilitic chancres. Sex Transm Dis. 1978; 5:68.
37. Morrissey R, Xavier A, Nguyen N, et al. Invasive candidal balanitis due to a condom catheter in a neutropenic patient. South Med J. 1985;78:1247–9.
38. Manian FA, Alford RH. Nosocomial infectious balanoposthitis in neutropenic patients. South Med J. 1987;80:909–11.
39. Maier JA, Bergman A, Ross MG. Acquired immunodeficiency syndrome manifested by chronic primary genital herpes. Am J Obstet Gynecol. 1986;155:756–8.
40. Siegal FP, Lopez C, Hammer GS, et al. Severe acquired immunodeficiency in male homosexuals manifested by chronic perianal herpes simplex lesions. N Engl J Med. 1981;305:1439–44.
41. Guinan ME, MacCalman J, Kern ER, et al. The course of untreated recurrent genital herpes simplex infection in 27 women. N Engl J Med. 1981;304:759.
42. Rehbein HM. Pearly penile papules: Incidence. Cutis. 1977;19:54.
43. Lafferty WE, Coombs RW, Benedetti J, et al. Recurrences after oral and genital herpes simplex virus infection. Influence of site of infection and viral type. N Engl J Med. 1987;316:1444–9.
44. D'Aunoy R, Von Hamm E. Granuloma inguinale. Am J Trop Med. 1937;17:747.
45. Asin J. Chancroid: A report of 1402 cases. Am J Syph Gonorr Vener Dis. 1952;36:483.
46. Dienst FT. Tularemia: A perusal of 339 cases. J La State Med Soc. 1963;115:114.
47. Evans ME, Gregory DW, Schaffner W, et al. Tularemia: A 30 year experience with 88 cases. Medicine (Baltimore). 1985;64:251–69.
48. Parkash S, Ramakrishnan K, Ananthakrishnan N, et al. Amoebic ulcer of the penis. Postgrad Med J. 1982;58:375.
49. Veliath AJ, Bansal R, Sankaran V, et al. Genital amebiasis. Int J Gynaecol Obstet. 1987;25:249–56.
50. O'Leary RK, Posen J. Amoebiasis of the penis. S Afr Med J. 1984;65:113–6.
51. Chapel TA. The signs and symptoms of secondary syphilis. Sex Transm Dis. 1980;7:161.
52. Oriel JD, Partridge BM, Denny MJ, et al. Genital yeast infections. Br Med J. 1972;4:761.
53. Diddle AW. Oral contraceptive medication and vulvovaginal candidiasis. Obstet Gynecol. 1969;34:373.
54. Holmes KK, Counts GW, Beaty HN. Disseminated gonococcal infection. Ann Intern Med. 1971;74:979.
55. Masi AT, Eisenstein BI. Disseminated gonococcal infection (DGI) and gonococcal arthritis (GCA): II. Clinical manifestations, diagnosis, complications, treatment, and prevention. Semin Arthritis Rheum. 1981;10:173.
56. Chapel TA, Brown WJ, Jeffries C, et al. How reliable is the morphologic diagnosis of penile ulcerations? Sex Transm Dis. 1977;4:150.
57. Chapel TA. Physician recognition of the signs and symptoms of secondary syphilis. JAMA. 1981;246:250.
58. Verdich J. *Hemophilus ducreyi* infection resembling granuloma inguinale. Acta Derm Venereol (Stokh). 1984;64:452–5.
59. Vekataramaiah NR, van Raalte JA, Dutta SN. Tuberculous ulcer of the penis. Postgrad Med J. 1982;58:59.
60. Nishigori C, Taniguchi S, Hayakawa M, et al. Penis tuberculosis: Papulonecrotic tuberculosis on the glans penis. Dermatologica. 1986;172:93–7.
61. Kumar B, Skarma VK. Papulonecrotic tuberculids on glans penis. Dermatologica. 1987;174:151–3.
62. Carroll PR, Cattolica EV, Turzan CW, et al. Necrotizing soft-tissue infections of the perineum and genitalia. Etiology and early reconstruction. West J Med. 1986;144:174–8.
63. D'Costa LJ, Bowmer I, Nsanze H, et al. Advances in the diagnosis and management of chancroid. Sex Transm Dis. 1986;13:189–91.
64. Shimizu T, Ehrlich GE, Inaba G, et al. Behçet disease (Behçet syndrome). Semin Arthritis Rheum. 1979;8:223.
65. Weissberg SM, Dodson MG. Recurrent vaginal and cervical ulcers associated with tampon use. JAMA. 1983;250:1430.
66. Kraus SJ. Evaluation and management of acute genital ulcers in sexually active patients. Urol Clin North Am. 1984;11:155–62.
67. Shelley WB, Wood MG. Larval papule as a sign of scabies. JAMA. 1976;236:1144.
68. Schachter J, Dawson CR, Human Chlamydial Infection. Littleton, MA: PSG Publishing; 1978:45.
69. Oriel JD. Genital warts. Sex Transm Dis. 1977;4:153.
70. Quinn TC, Stamm WE, Goodell SE, et al. The polymicrobial origin of intestinal infections in homosexual men. N Engl J Med. 1983;309:576.
71. Campion MJ, Singer A, Clarkson PK, et al. Increased risk of cervical neoplasia in consorts of men with penile condylomata accuminata. Lancet. 1985;1:943–6.
72. Rosemberg SK. Subclinical papilloma viral infection of male genitalia. Urology. 1985;26:554–7.
73. Sand PK, Baven LW, Blischke PA, et al. Evaluation of male consorts of women with genital human papilloma virus infection. Obstet Gynecol. 1986;68:679–81.
74. Schultz RE, Skelton HG. Value of acetic acid screening for flat genital condylomata in men. J Urol. 1988;139:777–9.
75. Sedlack TV, Cunnane M, Carpiniello V. Colposcopy in the diagnosis of penile condyloma. Am J Obstet Gynecol. 1986;154:494–6.
76. Krebs H-B, Schneider V. Human papillomavirus-associated lesions of the penis: Colposcopy, cytology, and histology. Obstet Gynecol. 1987;70:299–304.
77. Woodley D, Saurat JH. The burrow ink test and the scabies mite. J Am Acad Dermatol. 1981;4:715.
78. Lucks DA, Venezio FR, Lakin CM. Balanitis caused by group B streptococcus. J Urol. 1986;135:1015.
79. Burdge DR, Bowie WR, Chow A. *Gardnerella vaginalis*-associated balanoposthitis. Sex Transm Dis. 1986;13:159–62.
80. Ackerman A. Crabs: The resurgence of *Phthirus pubis*. N Engl J Med. 1968;278:950.
81. Miller RA. Maculae ceruleae. Int J Dermatol. 1986;25:383–4.
82. Chang TW. Herpetic angina following orogenital exposure. J Am Vener Dis Assoc. 1975;1:163.
83. Jamsky RJ, Christen AG. Oral gonococcal infections. Oral Surg. 1982;53:358.
84. Goodell SE, Quinn TC, Mkrtichian PA-C, et al. Herpes simplex virus proctitis in homosexual men. Clinical, sigmoidoscopic and histopathological features. N Engl J Med. 1983;308:868.
85. deLeon JC. Cutaneous amebiasis. In: Padilla y Padilla CA, Padilla GM eds. Amebiasis in Man. Springfield, IL: Charles C Thomas; 1974:110.
86. Burkhart CG. Scabies: An epidemiologic reassessment. Ann Intern Med. 1983;98:498.
87. Weisman K, Secher L, Hjorth N. Recurrent genital herpes on the buttocks: "Herpes disciformis". Cutis. 1987;40:166–8.
88. Wickett WH, Miller RD. Sites of multiple lesions in recurrent genital herpes. Am Fam Physician. 1985;32:145–52.
89. Nsanze H, Fast MV, D'Costa LJ, et al. Genital ulcers in Kenya: Clinical and laboratory study. Br J Vener Dis. 1981;57:378.
90. Brown ST, Jaffe HW, Zaidi A, et al. Sensitivity and specificity of diagnostic tests for genital infection with *Herpesvirus hominis*. Sex Transm Dis. 1979;6:10.
91. Goldstein LC, Corey L, McDougall JK, et al. Monoclonal antibodies to herpes simplex viruses: Use in antigenic typing and rapid diagnosis. J Infect Dis. 1983;47:829.
92. Lafferty WE, Krofft S, Remington M, et al. Diagnosis of herpes simplex virus by direct immunofluorescence and viral isolation from samples of external genital lesions in a high prevalence population. J Clin Microbiol. 1987;25:323–6.
93. Redfield DC, Richman DD, Albanil S, et al. Detection of herpes simplex virus in clinical specimens by DNA hybridization. Diagn Microbiol Infect Dis. 1983;1:117.
94. Corey L. Laboratory diagnosis of herpes simplex virus infections. Principles guiding the development of rapid diagnostic tests. Diagn Microbiol Infect Dis. 1986;4(Suppl):111–9.
94a. Austin VH, Topham EB. Mineral oil versus KOH for *Sarcoptes*. J Am Acad Dermatol. 1982;7:555.
95. Tronca E, Handsfield HH, Wiesner PJ, et al. Demonstration of *Neisseria gonorrhoeae* with fluorescent antibody in patients with disseminated gonococcal infection. J Infect Dis. 1974;129:583.
96. Deacon WE, Lucas JB, Price EV. Fluorescent treponemal antibody absorption (FTA-ABS) test for syphilis. JAMA. 1966;198:624.
97. Duncan W, Knox J, Wende R. The FTA-ABS test in darkfield positive primary syphilis. JAMA. 1974;228:859.
98. Larsen SA, Hambie EA, Pettit DE, et al. Specificity, sensitivity, and reproducibility among the fluorescent treponemal antibody absorption test, the microhemagglutination assay for *Treponema pallidum* antibodies, and the hemagglutination treponemal test for syphilis. J Clin Microbiol. 1981;14:441.
99. Corey L, Holmes KK. Genital herpes simplex virus infections: Current concepts in diagnosis, therapy, and prevention. Ann Intern Med. 1983;98:973.
100. Moseley RC, Corey L, Benjamin D, et al. Comparison of viral isolation, direct immunofluorescence, and indirect immunoperoxidase techniques for detection of genital herpes simplex virus infection. J Clin Microbiol. 1981;13:913.
101. Hammond GW, Lian CJ, Witt JC, et al. Comparison of specimen collection and laboratory techniques for isolation of *Hemophilus ducreyi*. J Clin Microbiol. 1978;7:39.
102. Nobre GN. Identification of *Hemophilus ducreyi* in the clinical laboratory. J Med Microbiol. 1982;15:243.
103. Nsanze H, Plummer FA, Maggwa AB, et al. Comparison of media for the primary isolation of *Haemophilus ducreyi*. Sex Transm Dis. 1984;11:6–9.

93. INGUINAL ADENOPATHY

MICHAEL F. REIN

Inguinal and femoral adenopathies may be asymptomatic but more commonly produce noticeable pain, stiffness, or swelling in the groin. These symptoms may be the initial manifestation of an inflammatory or neoplastic process that will eventually involve many other groups of lymph nodes. Isolated inguinofemoral adenopathy usually results from infection or neoplasm of the external genitalia or lower extremities, but processes arising in the lower portion of the abdomen or internal genitalia occasionally involve these nodes, and conditions other than adenopathy may be manifested as swellings around the inguinal ligament.

CONDITIONS PRODUCING A MASS IN THE GROIN

The etiologic spectrum varies markedly with the age, general life-style (e.g., urban or rural), sexual practices, and geographic location of the patient population.

Sexually Transmitted Diseases

Among sexually active people, genital infections are common causes of inguinofemoral adenopathy. The inguinal nodes drain the distal part of the urethra in both sexes. It must be remembered that the proximal portion of the vagina and cervix are drained by deep inguinal and iliac nodes, and women with primary infections of the proximal aspect of the vagina and cervix do not manifest superficial inguinal or femoral adenopathy. Tender inguinal adenopathy has been reported in up to 40 percent of the patients with acute gonococcal urethritis,[1] but it is felt by most observers to occur less often and followed only 5 percent of experimentally induced infections.[2] The mechanism is unclear, but in two cases gonococci were isolated from aspirates of an inguinal node.[2,3] It is interesting that in both of these cases the precipitating urethral infection was asymptomatic. Similar adenopathy appears to accompany only about 1 percent of the cases of nongonococcal urethritis.[1] With either infection, the nodes are usually discrete and not fixed to the overlying skin.

Relatively painless and usually bilateral,[4] inguinal adenopathy (satellite bubo) appears in 50–70 percent of the cases of primary syphilis.[5] Nodes usually become enlarged about 7 days after the appearance of the chancre. The examiner usually palpates a chain of nodes rather than a single node, and these are discrete, firm, and freely movable. Suppuration is extremly rare.

Relatively tender adenopathy affects 80 percent of the patients with primary herpes genitalis and is seen in 20 percent of men and 30 percent of the women who have recurrent herpes.[4] The adenopathy is described as lasting about 9–14 days in patients with primary infection and 7–9 days in patients with recurrent infection.[6] The diagnosis is generally made on the basis of the characteristic skin lesions (Chapter 118). Occasionally, the adenopathy actually precedes the appearence of skin lesions.[7] Herpetic inguinal lymphadenopathy has been described in elderly patients with immunologic impairments.[8]

Tender buboes are observed in 25–60 percent of the patients with chancroid. Adenopathy is noted by only about one-third of patients at the time of initial presentation[9] with the ulcer but appears in most 7–10 days later. It is frequently unilateral and is often accompanied by reddening of the overlying skin. Outbreaks of chancroid have occurred in California.[10] The disease is edemic in Southeast Asia, Africa, and other tropical and subtropical regions. Its painful ulcers may be confused with herpes genitalis, but they are usually larger and have a more ragged appearance.[11]

The initial genital lesion of lymphogranuloma venereum (LGV) is unnoticed by 70–95 percent of the patients,[11–13] and inguinal adenopathy is the most common initial complaint. Unilateral in 70 percent of the cases, it is initially noted as a stiffness or aching in the groin 2–6 weeks after the infecting sexual contact.[11–13] The nodes become matted and attached to the overlying skin, which is said to develop a purplish color.[11] If untreated, the nodes frequently suppurate in 7–10 days[13] and rupture, and chronic lymphadenopathy develops in about 5 percent of the patients.[11–12] Lymphogranuloma venereum is uncommon in the United States, with fewer than 1000 civilian cases reported each year,[14–15] but it must be considered in the differential diagnosis of inguinal adenopathy without an obvious primary source.

Generalized lymphadenopathy is a frequent manifestation of infection with human immunodeficiency virus (HIV). The involved nodes are usually nontender and chronically enlarged (see Chapter 108).

Nonvenereal Infections

Streptococci and staphylococci are frequent causes of inguinal lymphadenitis in children and not uncommon causes in adults.[16–18] Although extension from the lower extremity is the most likely route of infection of the glands, the primary site often escapes detection. If the infection does not respond to antibiotics, the nodes are likely to suppurate and require surgical intervention. Pneumococcal[19] and even yersinial[20] inguinal adenopathies have been described in adults. In all cases, the nodes were fluctuant. Sexual transmission of these pathogens has been considered in some cases.

Cat-scratch disease (Chapter 228), the specific agent of which appears to be a bacillus, results in tender and poorly defined lymph nodes draining an area scratched by a domestic cat. A history of the cat scratch is obtained in somewhat more than half of the infected patients,[21] and the adenopathy appears 1–9 weeks after the initial injury. Inguinal or femoral nodes are involved in 10–25 percent of the patients,[22,23] and the adenopathy is bilateral in about 2 percent of the cases.[21–23] The adenopathy characteristically lasts for 2–4 months, and 12–33 percent of the nodes will suppurate. The skin test antigen is not generally available, and the diagnosis is often assumed on the basis of a consistent history, characteristic histopathology of excised lymph nodes,[24] and the absence of alternative diagnoses.

Isolated, painful, inguinal or femoral adenopathy is the most common manifestation of bubonic plague. About 25 percent of the patients exhibit inguinal and about 40 percent femoral adenopathy.[25] One-fourth of the patients complain of obvious pain in the groin preceding the swelling, and the adenopathy may be accompanied by erythema and edema of the overlying skin (Chapter 207). Patients are often systemically ill and have a leukocytosis with increased numbers of immature leukocytes.

Although rabbit-associated tularemia usually involves the nodes of the upper extremity, tick-borne infections frequently produce inguinal adenopathy, which is observed in 20–50 percent of the cases overall[26,27] and is more common in adults than in children.[26] The tick prefers warm moist areas, and the initial lesion, which may be pustular, crusted, or ulcerated, is often found on the scrotum or penis or in the groin itself.[28] The lesion may be very subtle and is absent in the so-called glandular form of the disease. Affected nodes are enlarged and tender and are usually firm, discrete, and not attached to the overlying skin. Along the lymphatic channels proximal to the site of inoculation, one may observe occasional nodules that mimic sporotrichosis. The peripheral white blood cell count is low, normal, or elevated, and the differential count is usually normal. Tick-borne disease occurs most frequently in the warm months.[27]

Enlargement of inguinal or femoral nodes occurs in 8 percent of the patients with brucellosis,[29] but other groups of nodes are always involved simultaneously. The nodes are often tender.

Typical and atypical mycobacteria rarely produce isolated inguinal adenopathy in children and adults.[30] Cervical nodes are involved far more frequently.[31,32] Early on, the affected nodes are discrete, firm, and movable, but later they become matted together and may undergo caseous necrosis and drain through the overlying skin to form chronic sinuses.

Infectious mononucleosis is rarely manifested as isolated inguinofemoral adenopathy.[33] Other groups of nodes are likely to be involved later in the course of the disease. Likewise, toxoplasmosis, which characteristically results in generalized lymphadenopathy, involves the inguinal nodes in 10–20 percent of cases[34,35] and presents as isolated inguinal adenopathy in perhaps 1 percent of the infections.[34]

Onchocerciasis produces inguinal lymphadenopathy and a loss of local elastic fibers that may be so pronounced as to create sacs that droop over the thigh yielding so-called hanging groin.[36] In African onchocerciasis the nodes themselves are usually atrophic and contain microfilariae, whereas the Arabian form (sowda) has hyperplastic nodes in which microfilariae have only recently been described.[37] Usually only single groups of nodes are involved.

Intravenous drug use may be associated with regional lymphadenopathy.[38] Addicts making use of veins on the foot or leg may have isolated inguinal or femoral lymphadenopathy that is usually relatively indolent. The observation of needle tracks is helpful diagnostically. Repeated minor infections of the feet can lead to the development of chronic indolent lymphadenopathy, which is more common in people who habitually go barefoot.[39] Malignancy arising in the genital tract[40,41] or lower extremities[42] or of an unknown primary[43] may metastasize to inguinal nodes and produce nontender adenopathy, and lymphoma is manifested as inguinal adenopathy in about 10 percent of patients.[44]

Conditions Mimicking Inguinal Adenopathy

Abscesses of the skin or soft tissue overlying the groin may produce a tender mass inviting confusion with inguinal adenopathy. Such infection may arise in a hair follicle. The mass cannot be moved independently of the overlying skin, and the examiner may be able to press his fingers behind the mass to establish its separation from the inguinal or femoral lymphatic chains. Such local infection may, however, elicit true local lymphadenopathy to confuse the picture. An intra-abdominal abscess such as a psoas abscess from tuberculous spondylitis occasionally points through the groin area or dissects into the inguinal canal. An inguinal or femoral hernia may also be manifested as a mass in the groin, but its softness and variation with respiration usually suggest its identity. A hematoma or pseudoaneurysm sometimes presents as a groin mass. Ultrasonography or computed tomography (CT) helps to distinguish these conditions from true adenopathy.

Donovanosis (granuloma inguinale), a sexually transmitted infection extremely rare in the United States, produces granulomatous lesions in the groin that may be confused with true adenopathy (Chapter 227). Genital lesions are common, but 3 percent of the cases have only inguinal involvement.[45] The initial inguinal mass or pseudobubo is indolent and doughy. It is clearly superficial and fixed to the overlying intact skin.[46] Genital and groin lesions break down into ulcerations and exuberant growths of beefy granulation tissue.[11,47] The diagnosis is based on biopsy specimens of the lesions (Chapter 227). Although not primrily a disease of the lymphatics, inguinal and femoral nodes may become secondarily involved.[48]

APPROACH TO THE PATIENT WITH INGUINAL ADENOPATHY

The initial work-up is aimed at detecting infection of the external and internal genitalia, infection of the lower extremities, and involvement of other groups of lymph nodes.

History

Age. Among children under the age of 10 years, staphylococci and streptococci are numerically significant causes of inguinal adenopathy.[16] Once the patient enters the age of sexual activity, sexually transmitted infections are more likely. Malignancy is somewht more likely in elderly patients.

Occupation. Brucellosis should be considered in patients having dairy- or farm animal-related occupations. Patients with outdoor occupations are at greater risk for tick-borne tularemia.

Residence. Plague is extremely rare in patients who have not lived in or passed through endemic areas in the southwestern United States or in Southeast Asia. Chancroid is prevalent in many areas of African and Asia. Tropical causes of inguinal adenopthy must be considered if residence in appropriate areas is documented.

Duration. Because painless adenopathy may go unnoticed, the patient's history is a minimum estimate of the duration of an indolent process. Most infections produce a relatively acute enlargement of the affected nodes, but fungal and mycobacterial infections, cat-scratch disease, and neoplastic processes are more often relatively chronic. Persistent swelling may result from diverse acute processes, and gradually increasing indolent adenopathy may accompany repeated minor injuries to the lower extremities.

Pain. Pain or tenderness accompanies many acute infections and is characteristic of brucellosis,[29] tularemia,[28,49] yersinial inguinal lymphadenitis,[20] chancroid,[11] herpes genitalis,[6] gonorrhea,[1–3] cat-scratch disease,[21,22] and infection with pyogenic cocci.[16,19] Tenderness is often less pronounced with LGV[11–13] and is unusual in nodes involved by syphilis,[50,51] lymphoma,[44] or other malignancies.[40–43]

Trauma. A history of nonspecific trauma to the lower extremity may be useful. A definite history of a cat scratch suggests cat-scratch disease, but such a history is obtained in only 50 percent of the affected patients.[21–23] Bites by domestic animals frequently result in regional adenopathy and may suggest infection with *Pasturella multocida* (Chapter 206).

Genital Lesions. The history of a painless papule or ulcer of the external genitalia that has disappeared is consistent with LGV but is reported by fewer than 25 percent of the infected patients.[11–15] An indurated, indolent, genital ulcer that heals spontaneously is also suggestive of syphilis.[5] For most other genital infections, lesions and adenopathy are concurrent and will be discussed as part of the physical examination.

Genital Discharge. This history directs attention toward infectious urethritis or cervicitis including gonococcal, nonspecific, and herpetic. Urethritis and cervicitis may be asymptomatic. Adenopathy rarely accompanies trichomoniasis or vulvovaginal candidiasis.

Sexual History. A history of prior sexually transmitted disease increases the probability that the patient currently suffers from a genital infection. A history of new or multiple sexual partners or of genital symptoms among sexual partners also points toward sexually transmitted infection as the cause of the patient's adenopathy. A history of male homosexual contacts increases concern regarding the acquired immunodeficiency syndrome (AIDS) (Chapter 106).

Drug Abuse. The intravenous or subcutaneous administration of drugs into the lower extremity can result in progressive inguinal adenopathy even in the absence of acute infectious episodes.[38] Intravenous drug abusers are at increased risk for infection with HIV. Recently, syphilis has recrudesced in heterosexual populations in association with the use of cocaine.[52]

Examination of the Nodes

Bilaterality. The satellite bubo of syphilis is usually bilateral,[5] as is the adenopathy associated with chancroid[11] and herpes genitalis.[6] Bilaterality is observed in one-third of the patients with LGV[11–14] and in some patients with gonorrhea.[1] Bilateral adenopathy directs attention away from disease processes of the lower extremities but has been reported rarely in cat-scratch disease.[21–23]

Tenderness has essentially the same diagnostic significance as pain.

Firmness. Firm nodes accompany most acute inflammatory processes and are of little differential diagnostic value. Hard nodes are characteristic of lymphoma and other malignancies.

If unchecked, many acute inflammatory adenopathies will result in fluctuance, which is particularly characteristic of plague[25] and other yersinial infections,[20] pyogenic cocci,[16–19] cat-scratch disease[21,23] and LGV.[11–14] It occurs in from 25[28] to 50 percent[49] of the patients with tularemia. It is rare in infectious mononucleosis,[33] syphilis,[5] and herpes genitalis.[6–8]

Matting together of nodes may accompany any intense inflammatory process but is rare in syphilis.[5]

Sign of the Groove. Inguinal adenopathy above and below Poupart's ligament gives the appearance of a single lymphoid mass bisected by a groove. This phenomenon is observed in 15–20 percent of the patients with LGV[12,13] and is highly suggestive but not diagnostic of this infection.[11–13] It has been reported with lymphoma[44] and can probably be seen with adenopathy of other causes.

Color. Redness of the skin overlying the nodes is frequently observed in chancroid[11] and tularemia[49] and less frequently with plague.[25] It has been described in mycobacterial infection[30] but is distinctly unusual with syphilis[5] and viral infections. A purple tinge in the skin overlying the affected nodes has been described in some cases of LGV[11] but is also seen in metastatic melanoma[42] and rarely in other conditions.[53]

Associated Findings

Urethral Discharge. Urethritis is almost invaribly sexually transmitted. Gonorrhea is more frequently associated with inguinal adenopathy than is nongonococcal urethritis.[1–3] Urethral discharge accompanies a few cases of LGV, presumably on the basis of an intraurethral primary lesion.[12]

Genital Lesions (Chapter 92). Groups of vesicles in the genital area are diagnostic of herpes genitalis. Early in the disease, the vesicles are sometimes observed to be umbilicated, and they quickly rupture to form groups of painful shallow ulcers,[6] which in dry skin sites heal by crusting. In primary herpetic infection, the lesions usually precede the adenopathy by 1–2 weeks,[6] although the reverse is occasionally true.[7] A history of recurrent vesicles in the same area or a prodrome of local paresthesia 6–12 hours before the eruption supports the diagnosis of recurrent disease. Observing one or two larger, ragged ulcers is more suggestive of chancroid.[11] A single painless ulcer with an indurated border suggests syphilis.[5] A single pustular or crusted lesion or a tender, shallow ulcer may be seen in tularemia.[28] A papule, sometimes slightly eroded, often initiates LGV but is observed in fewer than 50 percent of men and only very rarely in women.[11–13]

Lesions of the Lower Extremity. The lesions of herpes genitalis and syphilis may appear in the inguinal area. Chancroid may also involve the thigh and characteristically produces a "kissing lesion" immediately opposed to a similar lesion on the shaft of the penis.[11] Trauma to the lower extremity, including animal bites and splinters, are helpful diagnostically, particularly if there is local inflammation or if lymphatic streaking can be observed proximal to the lesion. Animal bites (Chapter 80) raise the possibility of infection with *P. multocida* (Chapter 206). A peripheral lesion of tularemia can be very small and may be missed by all but the most careful examination. It may be crusted or pustular or be manifested as the shallow ulcer giving the name to the ulceroglandular form of the disease that makes up 50–80 percent of the cases.[28] Careful examination of the interdigital spaces is important. Needle tracks should not be overlooked.[38]

Lymphangitis. Erythema and tenderness over lymphatic channels may accompany any acute infection. A series of nodules appearing along the course of the lymphatic channels suggests sporotrichosis but has also been reported in tularemia.[28] In either case the nodules may break down. Nontender, firm inflammation of the lymphatic channels, particularly in the penis, may be associated with syphilis and is referred to as *pipestem lymphangitis*.[5]

Coincident adenopathy at distant sites should be assiduously sought. Its presence changes the etiologic spectrum.

Laboratory Investigations

Peripheral leukocytosis is a regular feature of plague and is usually accompanied by an increased number of immature neutrophils.[25] Peripheral leukocytosis is also common with staphylococcal and streptococcal infections but is found only variably with other conditions. A high percentage of atypical lymphocytes supports a diagnosis of infectious mononucleosis, and bizzare forms may suggest lymphoma.

The diagnosis of herpes genitalis can usually be made clinically but may be confirmed with the Tzanck test. An intact vesicle is unroofed, and material from the base is smeared on a microscope slide and stained with Giemsa or Wright stain or with methylene blue. The preparation is observed under low (100×) and high (400×) power for the presence of multinucleated giant cells diagnostic of infection with a herpes group virus. The Tzanck test is insensitive on lesions that have spontaneously ruptured to become shallow ulcers,[54] and the diagnosis is best made in these cases by isolating the virus from a swab of the lesion.[55–57] Monoclonal antibodies can be used to identify herpesvirus in direct smears from lesions and, although less sensitive than culture is, may enable a rapid, specific diagnosis.[55–57] Once the lesions have crusted over, the virus can be recovered only with difficulty,[56] but by this time, the adenopathy should be resolving. Other techniques such as enzyme-linked immunosorbent assay (ELISA) and DNA hybridization offer promise.[55]

Ulcerated lesions for which an alternative diagnosis is not obvious should be subjected to darkfield examination for *Treponema pallidum* (Chapter 213).

A Gram-stained smear of an ulcerated lesion will occasionally reveal short gram-negative rods, sometimes in a parallel array resembling a school of fish. This finding is highly suggestive of chancroid but is seen in relatively few cases.[9] The edge of the lesion is the best site for obtaining this material. Fluid from the edge of the lesion can be cultured for *Haemophilus ducreyi*; however, the organism is quite fastidious.[9]

Urethral discharge (Chapter 94) should be stained with Gram stain and examined for the presence of gram-negative, cell-associated diplococci, which diagnose gonorrhea. The presence of neutrophils alone indicates nongonococcal urethritis. A urethral swab should be taken from asymptomatic men, and Gram staining will reveal gonococci in about two-thirds of the infected patients (Chapter 190). A urethral swab should be cultured for *Neisseria gonorrhoeae* before initiating therapy.

Before the development of effective antimicrobial chemotherapy, aspiration of enlarged nodes often resulted in sinus formation. The risk is now very small, and needle aspiration may reveal the cause if other diagnostic maneuvers have failed. This procedure is contraindicated if the inguinal mass may be an incarcerated hernia or aneurysm. Ultrasonography may help to resolve such questions. Fluctuant areas, if present, are appropriate targets. The overlying skin should be prepared with an iodophore that is allowed to dry and is washed off with alcohol. The skin may be infiltrated with a small amount of a local anesthetic agent, or it may be numbed with an ethyl chloride spray. Frequently, the approach producing the least total discomfort is to perform the aspiration without prior anesthesia. The femoral artery should be located by palpation and studiously avoided. A 21 gauge needle on a 6 ml syringe is introduced briskly through the skin and into the node. The plunger should be drawn back in an attempt to aspirate pus. If syphilis is suspected, the needle is plunged in various directions within the node while suction is applied to the syringe.[5] Material recovered from nonfluctuant nodes should be examined by darkfield microscopy. A good specimen contains about 10 lymphocytes per oil-immersion field and reveals spirochetes in about 95 percent of the cases of syphilis.[5] Pus from fluctuant nodes should be stained with Gram stain and examined for pyogenic cocci. Wayson stain will diagnose plague with a sensitivity of 60–85 percent.[25] The aspirate should be cultured for gonococci, pyogenic cocci, and *H. ducreyi*.[9]

If no material is obtained from a fluctuant node, the syringe may be disconnected from the needle and replaced with another containing a small amount of saline free of bacteriostatic agents. This saline is introduced into the node, reaspirated into the syringe, and processed as above. In general, surgical incision and drainage of the nodes should be avoided.

Serologic tests for plague, tularemia, and brucellosis are available but generally confirm a diagnosis only in retrospect. Serologic tests for syphilis are almost always positive in patients with inguinal adenopathy,[5,50,58] and a nonreactive fluorescent treponemal antibody absorption (FTA-ABS) test essentially rules out syphilis. The microhemagglutination test for *T. pallidum* (MHA-TP) is somewhat less sensitive in primary syphilis. The complement fixation test with chlamydial antigen will show a high ($\geq$1:32) or rising titer in 95 percent of the patients with LGV.[11–13] The test is sometimes positive in the presence of other chlamydial infections such as psittacosis, nongonococcal urethritis, or trachoma, but a negative examination with acute and convalescent sera rules out LGV. The older Frei test, an intradermal test with chlamydial antigen, is much less sensitive, and the antigen is no longer available. Serologic tests are useful in the diagnosis of toxoplasmosis.[59]

Eventually, biopsy may be necessary to establish a diagnosis. Few pathologic features are differentially diagnostic in acute infection. Noncaseating granulomas are frequently observed and may be seen with gonorrhea,[2] LGV,[11–13,58] and syphilis.[51] Langhans-type giant cells may be seen with LGV and syphilis and are not specific for mycobacterial infection. Stellate microabscesses are described in LGV[11–13] but can also be seen in other conditions including syphilis.[51] Highly suggestive of syphilis is the finding of fibrosis of the capsule and pericapsular tissues and phlebitis or endarteritis.[51] The combination of follicular hyperplasia, granulomas with giant cells, and microabscesses in the same specimen is highly suggestive of cat-scratch disease.[24] Follicular and sinusoidal hyperplasia and packing of the sinusoids with monomorphologic round cells are seen in nodes from patients with AIDS.[60]

In an unselected series of node biopsy specimens in general hospital admissions, 71 percent of inguinal nodes showed inflammatory disease, 21 percent showed carcinoma, and 8 percent showed lymphoma.[61]

Initial Therapeutic Approach

If a specific diagnosis can be made initially, the patient should, of course, be treated with the agent having the narrowest spectrum and the least toxicity. Systemically ill patients should be hospitalized. If there is a suspicion of plague or tularemia, initial therapy should include coverage for these diseases, probably with streptomycin. Treatment of indolent, slowly progressive, inguinal adenopathy may await the results of laboratory investigations. If plague and tularemia are not considerations and the patient is sexually active, initial therapy with ceftriaxone, 250 mg im, followed by erythromycin, 500 mg orally four times a day, will adequately cover gonorrhea, most cases of syphilis, nongonococcal urethritis, chancroid, LGV, and staphylococcal and streptococcal infections. Close follow-up study is required while the definitive diagnosis is awaited. Substantiation of an accurate diagnosis may lead to more appropriate therapy.

REFERENCES

1. Akers WA. Tender inguinal lymph nodes and gonococcal urethritis. Milit Med. 1972;137:107.
2. Dahl R, Dans PE. Gonococcal lymphadenitis. Arch Intern Med. 1974;134:1116.
3. DeHertogh DA, Murcia ES. Gonococcal inguinal lymphadenitis. Arch Intern Med. 1984;144:391.
4. Drusin LM. Syphilis: Clinical manifestations, diagnosis, and treatment. Urol Clin North Am. 1984;11:121–30.
5. Stokes JH, Beerman H, Ingraham NR. Modern Clinical Syphilology. 3rd ed. Philadelphia: WB Saunders; 1944.
6. Corey L, Adams HG, Brown ZA, et al. Genital herpes simplex virus infections: Clinical manifestations, course, and complications. Ann Intern Med. 1983;98:958.
7. Taxy JB. Herpes simplex lymphadenitis. An unusual presentation with necrosis and viral particles. Arch Pathol Lab Med. 1985;109:1043–4.
8. Epstein JL, Ambinder R, Kuhajada FP, et al. Localized herpes simplex lymphadenitis. Am J Clin Pathol. 1986;86:444–8.
9. D'Costa LJ, Bowmer I, Nsanze H, et al. Advances in the diagnosis and management of chancroid. Sex Transm Dis. 1986;3:189–91.
10. Blackmore CA, Limpokarnjanaratk, Rigau-Perez JG, et al. An outbreak of chancroid in Orange County, California: Descriptive epidemiology and disease control measures. J Infect Dis. 1985;151:840–4.
11. Hart G. Chancroid, Donovanosis, Lymphogranuloma Venereum. Atlanta: US DHEW; 1974.
12. Schachter J, Dawson CR: Human Chlamydial Infection. Littleton, MA: PSG Publishing; 1978:45.
13. Thorsteinsson SB. Lymphogranuloma venereum: Review of clinical manifestations, epidemiology, diagnosis, and treatment. Scand J Infect Dis. 1982;32(suppl):127.
14. McLelland BA, Anderson PC Lymphogranuloma venereum: Outbreak in a university community. JAMA. 1976;235:56.
15. Schachter J, Dawson CR. Lymphogranuloma venereum (Letter). JAMA. 1976;236:915.
16. Scobie WG. Acute suppurative adenitis in children: A review of 964 cases. Scott Med J. 1969;14:352.
17. Pattman RS. Two unusual manifestations of infection with *Staphylococcus aureus* presenting to a clinic for sexually transmitted diseases. Br J Clin Pract. 1983;37:228–9.
18. Ho DD, Murata GH. Streptococcal lymphadenitis in homosexual men with chronic lymphadenopathy. Am J Med. 1984;77:151–3.
19. Lebowitz AS, Tierno PM. Suppurative pneumococcal inguinal adenitis. NY State J Med. 1985;85:509–10.
20. Zimmerman RS, Hamilton JD. *Yersinia enterocolitica* inguinal lymphdenitis. Diagn Microbiol Infect Dis. 1986;5:265–8.
21. Spaulding WB, Hennessy JN. Cat scratch disease: A study of 83 cases. Am J Med. 1960;28:504.
22. Margileth AM. Cat scratch disease: Nonbacterial regional lymphadenitis. Pediatrics. 1968;42:803.

23. Carithers HA. Cat-scratch disease. An overview based on a study of 1200 patients. Am J Dis Child. 1985;139:1124–33.
24. Campbell JAH. Cat scratch disease Pathol Annu. 1977;12:277.
25. Butler T, Bell WR, Linh NN, et al. *Yersinia pestis* infection in Vietnam: 1. Clinical and hematologic aspects. J Infect Dis. 1974;129:578.
26. Jacobs RF, Condrey YM, Yamauchi T. Tularemia in adults and children: A changing presentation. Pediatrics. 1985;76:818–22.
27. Evans ME, Gregory DW, Schoffner W, et al. Tularemia: A 30 year experience with 88 cases. Medicine (Baltimore). 1985;64:251–69.
28. Dienst FT. Tularemia: A perusal of 339 cases. J La State Med Soc. 1963;115:114.
29. Bloomfield AL. Enlargement of superficial lymph nodes in brucella infection. Am Rev Tuberc. 1942;45:741.
30. Andringa CL, Cherry JD. Bilateral inguinal adenitis due to a nonphotochromogenic atypical mycobacterium: Report of a case. JAMA. 1966;198:785.
31. Spark RP, Fried MC, Bean CK, et al. Nontuberculous mycobacterial adenitis of childhood. The ten-year experience at a community hospital. Am J Dis Child. 1988;142a;106–8.
32. Martin T, Hoeppner VH, Ring ED. Superficial mycobacterial lymphadenitis in Saskatchewan. Can Med Assoc J. 1988;138:431–4.
33. Wechsler HF, Rosenblum AH, Sills CT. Infectious mononucleosis: Report of an epidemic in an army post. Ann Intern Med. 1946;25:113.
34. McCabe RE, Brooks RG, Dorfman RF, et al. Clinical spectrum in 107 cases of toxoplasmic lymphdenopathy. Rev Infect Dis. 1987;9:754–74.
35. Rafaty FM. Cervial adenopathy secondary to toxoplasmosis. Arch Otolaryngol. 1977;103:547–9.
36. Gibson DW, Connor DH. Onchocercal lymphadenitis: Clinicopathological study of 34 patients. Trans Soc Trop Med Hyg. 1978;72:137–54.
37. Abdel-Hameed AA, Voah MS, Schacher JF, et al. Lymphadenitis in sowda. Trop Geogr Med. 1987;39:73–6.
38. Geller SA, Stimmel B. Diagnostic confusion from lymphatic lesions in heroin addicts. Ann Intern Med. 1973;78:703.
39. Wapinick S, MacKintosh M, Mauchaza B. Shoelessness, enlarged femoral lymph nodes and femoral hernia: A possible association. Am J Surg. 1973;126:108.
40. Stein M, Steiner M, Suprun H, et al. Inguinal lymph node metasteses from testicular tumor. J Urol. 1985;134:144–5.
41. Sedlis A, Homasley H, Bundy BN, et al. Positive groin lymph nodes in superficial squamous cell vulvar cancer. A Gynecologic Oncology Group Study. Am J Obstet Gynecol. 1987;156:1159–64.
42. Singletary SE, Shallenbergen R, Guinee VF, et al. Melonoma with metasteses to regional axillary or inguinal lymph nodes: Prognostic factors and results of surgical treatment in 714 patients. South Med J. 1988;81:5–9.
43. Guarischi A, Keane TJ, Elhakim T. Metastatic inguinal nodes from an unknown primary neoplasm. A review of 56 cases. Cancer. 1987;59:572–7.
44. Murphy JF, Fred HL. Infectious lymphadenitis or lymphoma? Seven lessons. JAMA. 1976;235:742.
45. Lal S, Nicholas C. Epidemiological and clinical features in 165 cases of granuloma inguinale. Br J Vener Dis. 1970;47:461.
46. Davis CM. Granuloma inguinale: A clinical, histological and ultrastructural study. JAMA. 1970;211:632.
47. Sehgal VN, Shyam Prasad AL. Donovanosis: Current concepts. Int J Dermatol. 1986;25:8–16.
48. Greenblatt RB, Dienst RB, Pund ER, et al. Experimental and clinical granuloma inguinale. JAMA. 1939;113:1109.
49. Simpson SM. Tularemia: Histology, Pathology, Diagnosis, and Treatment. New York: Paul B Hoeber; 1929:67.
50. Bergstrom JF, Navin JJ. Luetic lymphadenitis: Lymphographic manifestations simulating lymphoma. Radiology. 1973;106:287.
51. Hartsock RJ, Halling LW, King FM. Luetic lymphadenitis: A clinical and histologic study of 20 cases. Am J Clin Pathol 1970;53:304.
52. Centers for Disease Control. Recommendations for diagnosing and treating syphilis in HIV-infected patients. MMWR. 1988;37:600–8.
53. Rheaume T, Robertson DI, Urbanski SJ, et al. Inguinal intranodal blue nevus: A case report. Can J Surg. 1986;29:282–3.
54. Brown ST, Jaffe HW, Zaidi A, et al. Sensitivity and specificity of diagnostic tests for genital infection with Herpesvirus hominis. Sex Transm Dis. 1979;6:10.
55. Corey L. Laboratory diagnosis of herpes simplex virus infections. Principles guiding the development of rapid diagnostic tests. Diagn Microbiol Infect Dis. 1986;4(Suppl):115.
56. Lafferty WE, Kroft S, Remington M, et al. Diagnosis of herpes simplex virus by direct immunofluorescence and viral isolation from samples of external genital lesions. J Clin Microbiol. 1987;25:323–6.
57. Goldstein LC, Corey L, McDougall JK, et al. Monoclonal antibodies to herpes simplex viruses: Use in antigenic typing and rapid diagnosis. J Infect Dis. 1983;47:829.
58. King FM. Case for diagnosis: Syphilitic lymphadenitis. Milit Med. 1972;137:155.
59. Brooks RG, McCabe RE, Remington JS. Role of serology in the diagnosis of toxoplasmic lymphadenopathy. Rev Infect Dis. 1987;9:1055–62.
60. Guarda LA, Buttler JJ, Mansell P, et al. Lymphdenopathy in homosexual men: Morbid anatomy with clinical and immunologic correlations. Am J Clin Pathol. 1983;79:559.
61. Lee Y-TN, Terry R, Lukes RJ: Biopsy of peripheral lymph nodes. Am Surg. 1982;48:536.

94. URETHRITIS

MICHAEL F. REIN

Urethritis affects an estimated 4 million American men each year.[1] The symptoms range from the trivial and often overlooked to the disabling. Urethral discharge is more frequently recognized by men than by women. It may be apparent at all times during the day and may be present in sufficient quantity to stain undergarments, or it may be so scanty that it is noted only on arising as a small bead of moisture or crust at the meatus. It may be completely clear, mucopurulent, or frankly purulent, and it may be white, yellow, green, or brown. Some patients complain only of a deviation of the first morning urine stream. Occasionally, urethral discharge comes to the attention of the patient through the observation of mucous strands in the urine specimen.

The urine stream transiently eliminates most inflammatory discharges; thus, scanty discharges are best observed on arising before the passage of any urine. Micturation immediately preceding urethral examination may completely eliminate signs of infection.

The discomfort of urethritis can take several forms. Dysuria is common, and men variously localize it to the meatus, the distal portion of the penis, or anywhere along the shaft. Discomfort is sometimes increased by the acidity or solute content of the urine and, therefore, may be most marked during the passage of a concentrated first morning urine. Dysuria may be increased in the presence of irritants such as alcohol, which is an observation that sometimes leads the patient to attribute his disease to the ingestion of specific foods or fluids. Discomfort may persist between micturations and is perceived as pain, itching, frequency, urgency, or a feeling of heaviness in the genitals. Women may complain of dysuria, but urethral pain between micturations is uncommon.

Discomfort only during ejaculation, deep pelvic pain, or pain radiating to the back is infrequent in uncomplicated urethritis and suggests prostatitis or inflammation involving other portions of the urogenital tract such as the epididymis. Hematuria, particularly if painless, or blood in the ejaculate are uncommon in urethritis.[2] The persistence of symptoms after cure of urethritis demands a thorough urologic evaluation.[2]

EXAMINATION OF THE URETHRA

Men should stand before the seated examiner so that the external genitalia are approximately eye level. A good light source is essential. The patient should lower his pants and underwear so the entire genital area may be observed. The underwear may reveal stains of dried discharge, which suggest that it is being produced in large amounts. This observation is particularly useful if the patient has recently urinated.

The patient is preferably examined at least 2 hours after his last micturation. If advised to restrict his fluids during the day preceding the examination, he may be able to present for evaluation before passing his first urine of the day, which sometimes permits the recovery of very small amounts of discharge.[3]

The entire genital area should be carefully examined since other sexually transmitted infections are relatively common in patients with urethritis. Inguinal adenopathy should be sought, and tenderness should be noted. The skin of the entire pubic area, scrotum, groin, and penis should be examined for lesions, and the hair should be examined for nits. The testes and the spermatic cords should be palpated for masses or tenderness. The foreskin should be completely retracted and the glans examined. The urethral meatus is examined for dried crusts, redness, and spontaneous discharge. If no discharge is present, the urethra should be gently stripped by placing the gloved thumb along the ventral surface of the base of the penis and the forefinger on the dorsum and then applying gentle pressure. The examiner's hand is moved slowly toward the meatus. This will frequently expell a discharge that may be collected on a swab for examination as described below.

If no discharge is delivered by this maneuver, the third and fourth fingers should be used to grip the penis lightly, just behind the glans. The thumb and forefinger can then spread open the meatus to examine for urethral redness or the presence of small amounts of discharge. Unless the patient has recently urinated or has been in a state of sexual arousal, virtually no fluid should be expressible from the urethra or observed by spreading the meatus.

If expressed material cannot be collected at the meatus, a specimen must be recovered from inside the urethra. This is best accomplished with a calcium alginate urethral or nasopharyngeal swab.[4] The swab should be inserted gently at least 2 cm into the urethra while taking care not to attempt to force the tip past an obstruction. The patient should be warned that the examination is uncomfortable; also, the insertion and removal of the swab should be accomplished as quickly as possible. Occasional patients will tolerate the examination better if they are supine. If additional specimens are required for multiple examinations or cultures, separate swabs should be used while taking care to insert each at least 1 cm deeper than that preceding it.

Regular cotton swabs should not be used for urethral examination, because their larger diameter makes insertion extremely uncomfortable and because of the possibility that the cotton or the wooden shaft may be toxic to some fastidious pathogens. A small platinum loop is effective, but it must be sterilized in a flame and carefully cooled between uses.

A woman's urethra is best examined when she is in the lithotomy position. The entire genital area should be examined for lesions, and the vagina should be examined as described in Chapter 95. The urethral meatus may be directly visualized, and the urethra may be gently stripped by placing the gloved finger inside the vagina and gently moving it along the urethra. A calcium alginate swab may be inserted a short distance within the meatus to obtain a urethral specimen.

EXAMINATION OF THE URETHRAL SPECIMEN

A swab that contains material from the urethra should be rolled across a clean microscope slide. Rolling rather than streaking the swab brings all its surfaces into contact with the slide and better preserves cellular morphologic characteristics. The material may be air-dried and fixed by gentle heating or by rinsing with methanol. Gram staining of urethral material is particularly useful in the work-up of urethritis and the specimen should be examined by using the oil-immersion objective. Specimens obtained from within the urethra generally reveal urethral epithelial cells. When recovered from near the meatus, these are typical squamous cells with a very large cytoplasmic/nuclear ratio, or when obtained from further within the urethra, they are cuboidal epithelial cells, which are smaller and have relatively larger, less dense nuclei.

Urethral material from patients with acute urethritis will contain polymorphonuclear neutrophils (PMNs). The area of the smear that contains most PMNs should be sought. More than four PMNs per oil-immersion microscopic field is always abnormal and is seen in 60–90 percent of all patients with acute symptomatic urethritis.[4–6] However, 16–50 percent of all men with documented urethral infection will not show four PMNs in maximally dense oil-immersion fields.[7–12] The number of PMNs in the smear is reduced by recent micturation[13]; also, there often is considerable observer variation in the number of PMNs detected in a single specimen.[14] Thus, although purulent discharges may reveal sheets of PMNs, the minimal number of these cells that indicate disease is not known. In general, the presence of even rare PMNs suggests infection, particularly in the patient who has urethral symptoms or who is found to have a small amount of discharge on examination.

The distal centimeter of the urethra is colonized by normal skin or introital flora. One usually will observe a variety of gram-positive and gram-negative organisms that have no particular significance. Of great diagnostic value, however, is the presence of typical gram-negative, "intracellular" diplococci (Fig. 1). These organisms are not randomly distributed among the cells but are seen in large numbers in a few PMNs. They will be observed in more than 95 percent of all symptomatic patients with gonococcal urethritis and in fewer than 2 percent of all symptomatic men who cannot be shown to have gonorrhea by culture.[15–17] Some strains of *Neisseria gonorrhoeae* are inhibited by the concentrations of vancomycin that usually are employed in selective isolation media; these organisms will not be recovered by standard culture techniques. Extracellular diplococci indicate gonorrhea in only 10–29 percent of all cases, and this predictive value is even further reduced in populations with a low prevalence of gonorrhea.[17,18] A shortcoming of the Gram-stained smear is that it cannot diagnose coincidental nongonococcal urethritis (NGU) in the presence of gonorrhea. Although a smear that does not reveal gram-negative intracellular diplococci strongly suggests NGU, a smear revealing these organisms does not rule out NGU.

In men with adequate amounts of urethral discharge, one can use commercially available kits to test for the presence of gonococcal oxidase. Experience with the technique is limited; however, preliminary data suggest a sensitivity of 96 percent but a specificity of only 85 percent.[19] Furthermore, the Gram stain provides information on the degree of inflammation present. Limulus lysate assays for gonococcal endotoxin, although greater than 95 percent sensitive and specific,[20] are of limited clinical utility because many patients have inadequate amounts of discharge.[21]

Candida may be recognized as gram-positive or beaded, oval bodies about 3 × 6 μm. Observing small numbers of yeast cells does not prove a candidial etiology for the urethritis since *Candida* may be recovered from normal patients, particularly if they are uncircumcised.

Trichomonads are very difficult to identify on Gram-stained smears.

Urethral material may be mixed with a small amount of saline and observed as a wet mount with the substage condenser racked down or the substage diaphragm partially closed. Motile trichomonads occasionally are observed but are rarely seen unless the examination is carried out before the first voiding. A positive wet mount diagnoses trichomoniasis, but the wet mount will be negative (even under ideal circumstances) in 10–50 percent of infected men.[22,23]

After the patient's urethra has been carefully examined, he may be asked to provide a divided urine specimen. The patient delivers the first 10 ml of urine into one container and the remainder of the urine specimen into a second. Mucous strands in the first fraction that clear in the second portion suggest urethritis. Equal aliquots of the fractions may be centrifuged and the sediments examined as wet mounts. Observing more white blood cells in the initial than in the second fraction suggests urethritis, while observing equal numbers of white cells in both fractions suggests cystitis or infection higher in the urinary tract.[2,3] A total of more than 15 white blood cells in five 400× microscopic fields of the sediment from the initial fraction strongly suggests urethritis,[4,7,10] but the minimum significant number of white blood cells is unknown. More than 10 PMNs per high-power field have been observed in 90 percent of all men with chlamydial urethritis,[7] and *N. gonorrhoeae* or *Chlamydia trachomatis* can be recovered from 90 percent of men

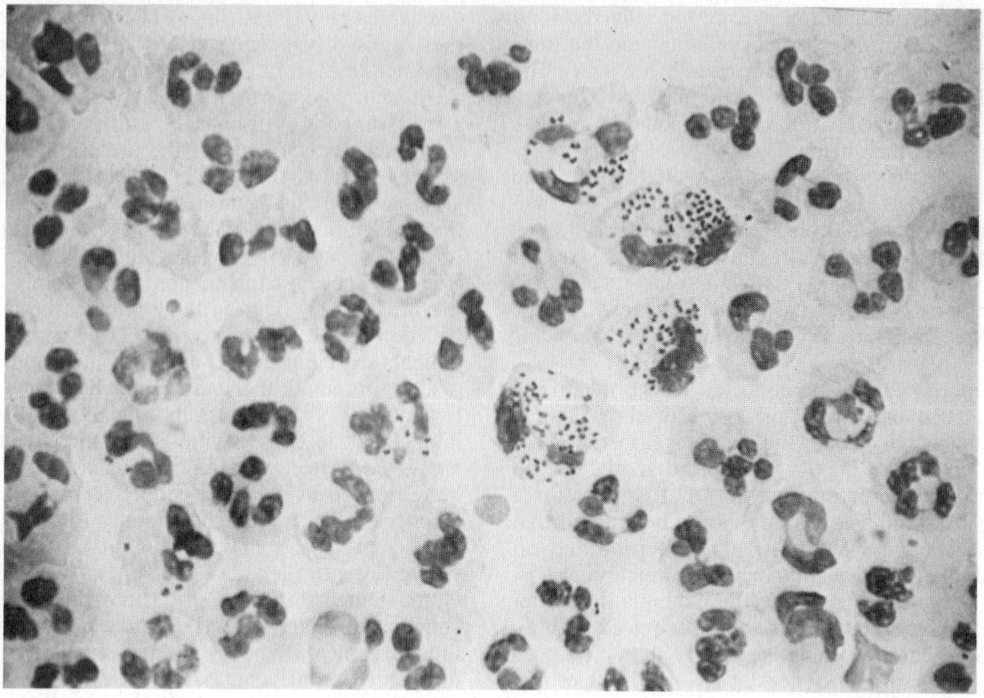

FIG. 1. Gram stain of urethral exudate from a man with gonorrhea. Several neutrophils contain many gram-negative cell-associated diplococci.

demonstrating this level of pyuria.[24] White blood cells or mucous strands in the initial urine fraction provide no clue to the etiology of the urethritis. If the urine specimen is a first morning micturation, motile trichomonads may be observed in the sediment from almost 80 percent of infected men, and they are recovered by culture in 95 percent of the cases.[13] Trichomonads are infrequently recovered from patients who have already voided during the day.

Material recovered from the urethra can be cultured with appropriate media for *N. gonorrhoeae* and *Trichomonas vaginalis*. Culture systems for *C. trachomatis* are becoming more generally available and less costly. Enzyme-linked immunosorbent assay (ELISA) and immunofluorescence techniques for identifying *C. trachomatis* in genital specimens have been developed (see Chapter 158) and are changing our approach to these infections. Their sensitivity in urethritis, however, may be as low as 70 percent.[25] Cultures for *Ureaplasma urealyticum* are less frequently performed; also, their interpretation is complicated by the high prevalence of colonization in asymptomatic, sexually active people. Although present in the distal urethra, normal skin flora (such as *Staphylococcus epidermidis*, α-hemolytic streptococci, and propionibacteria), normal vaginal flora (such as *Candida albicans*, lactobacilli, and *Escherichia coli*), and other organisms (such as *Gardnerella vaginalis*) are of no diagnostic significance.[26,27]

NONINFECTIOUS URETHRITIS

So psychically important is the genital tract that trivial symptoms often receive patients' frightened attention. The "worried well" make up a significant fraction of men who are seen in venereal disease clinics and in private practices. Sympathetic questioning as to why the patient thinks he has contracted a genital infection may reveal guilt over an act such as masturbation, which does not put the patient at significant risk of infection. The urethral specimen in these cases usually reveals normal epithelial cells and no white blood cells. Some patients confuse dried remnants of semen with inflammatory discharge. Microscopic examination again fails to reveal inflammatory cells, but spermatozoa may be recognized on the Gram stain as gram-positive ovoids whose coloration fades gradually toward the achrosomal cap or may be recognized on the wet mount. However, the physician must remember that symptoms and signs of true urethritis can be trivial and that microscopic examination may miss minimal inflammation, particularly if the patient has recently voided. Symptomatic patients with negative examinations should be asked to return in several days, by which time the symptoms may have resolved or examination may provide a diagnosis. An occasional patient who complains of a discharge is really suffering from urinary incontinence.

Chronic irritation of the urethra can elicit a clear, mucoid discharge. Occasional patients, concerned that they may have contracted a venereal disease, vigorously strip the urethra looking for a discharge. After several days of this, a clear discharge obligingly appears that may contain a few white blood cells. A history of vigorous urethral stripping is helpful diagnostically. Patients treated for other forms of urethritis should be cautioned not to examine themselves too vigorously for fear that such a traumatic discharge may confuse the clinical picture. Very rarely, patients will insert foreign bodies into the urethra and produce a discharge that may be blood-tinged.[28] This sort of self-abuse should be considered in retarded or psychotic individuals.

A heavy precipitation of crystals in the urine can suggest a discharge, and the presence of large amounts of crystalline material or calculous gravel may produce urinary discomfort. The intermittent nature of pain associated with the passage of gravel or the obvious presence of crystals on microscopic examination of the urine sediment usually confirms this diagnosis. White blood cells may be present.

Urethritis may accompany noninfectious systemic diseases such as Stevens-Johnson syndrome or Wegener's granulomatosis.

Chemicals may irritate the urethra, and alcohol has long been known to produce mild dysuria. The ingestion of alcohol during the treatment for gonorrhea was at one time thought to be responsible for the syndrome of postgonococcal urethritis discussed later, although it is now known to have an infectious etiology. An occasional patient may develop urethral symptoms on contact with vaginal chemicals used by a sexual partner. The history of discomfort immediately after sexual contact may be suggestive. This uncommon condition should be diagnosed only after other etiologies have been excluded. Shampoos and other bath products have produced urethritis in children.[29]

INFECTIOUS URETHRITIS

Gonococcal and Nongonococcal Urethritis

The major single specific etiology of acute urethritis is *Neisseria gonorrhoeae*. Urethral inflammation of all other etiologies is referred to collectively as NGU. As with gonorrhea, most cases of NGU are sexually acquired; also, over the past 15 years, the incidence of both infections has increased. NGU is twice as common as gonorrhea in the United States and in much of the developed world as well.[30–32] In some underdeveloped areas, however, gonorrhea accounts for 80 percent of the cases of acute urethritis. As with many other sexually transmitted diseases (STDs) gonococcal and nongonococcal urethritis have an increased incidence during the summer months,[31,32] presumably because of a seasonal increase in sexual activity. Although a number of reports have suggested that the incidence of NGU is increasing more rapidly than is that of gonorrhea, such conclusions must be viewed with caution. Public interest has focused on NGU, and patients may now be more likely to seek medical attention for mild genital symptoms than they had been in the past.[30] Indeed, except in Great Britain, the ratio of NGU to gonorrhea has remained relatively stable over the past decade.[30]

The ratio of nongonococcal to gonococcal urethritis has been thought to be greater among groups with higher socioeconomic status.[33] This differential distribution is most likely related to differences in health care behavior, with wealthier and better educated individuals more likely to seek medical care for milder symptoms. There are, however, some studies suggesting that blacks are more susceptible than are whites to gonococcal infection.[30]

Compared with gonorrhea, NGU is relatively less prevalent among homosexual than among heterosexual men with urethritis. Examining consecutive men attending an STD clinic, Stamm and colleagues recovered gonococci from 12 percent of heterosexual and 25 percent of homosexual men, whereas they recovered chlamydia from 14 percent of heterosexual but only 5 percent of homosexual men.[9]

Historically, there has been considerable interest in the possible contribution of circumcision in the epidemiology of STD. Such studies are difficult to interpret because certain behavioral factors are associated with circumcision.[34] The presence of a foreskin may mask a urethral discharge and delay patients from presenting for evaluation, but other roles remain speculative.[34]

The spectrum of gonorrhea differs from that of NGU, but there is sufficient clinical overlap so that an accurate differential diagnosis must be based on microscopic examination of the urethral specimen. Seventy-five percent of men acquiring urethral gonorrhea develop symptoms within 4 days[3] and 80–90 percent within 2 weeks.[30,35,36] The incubation period for NGU is much more variable and is often longer, usually between 7 and 14 days, but incubation periods ranging from 2 to 35 days have been described,[30,33,35] and almost 50 percent of the men with NGU developed urethral symptoms within 4 days.[3,30,35] Thus, an incubation period of less than 1 week is not a reliable factor in the differential diagnosis.[3,30,35,37] The incubation period of either infection can be prolonged by the ingestion of subcurative doses of antibiotics.[38]

The urethral discharge is described as frankly purulent in three-quarters of the patients with gonorrhea but in only 11–33 percent of the patients with NGU.[15,33,39] A purulent discharge issuing from the meatus without stripping the urethra correlates strongly with the diagnosis of gonorrhea but is also seen in 4 percent of patients with NGU.[15,39] Mucopurulent discharge, consisting of thin cloudy fluid or mucoid fluid with purulent flecks, is seen in about 50 percent of the patients with NGU but in only 25 percent of the patients with symptomatic gonorrhea.[15,39] The discharge is completely clear and moderately viscid in 10–50 percent of the patients with NGU, principally those who are minimally symptomatic, but in only 4 percent of symptomatic patients with gonorrhea.[15,39,40] A differential diagnosis on the basis of the clinical characteristics of the urethral discharge is unreliable and yields a correct diagnosis in only 73 percent of all cases, even under optimal circumstances.[39] Microscopic examination always should be part of the initial evaluation.

Dysuria has been described in 53–75 percent of the patients with NGU and in 73–88 percent of the patients wiht symptomatic gonorrhea.[15,41] Only about 10 percent of the patients complaining of dysuria without discharge have gonorrhea; the remainder suffer from NGU.[15] A combination of dysuria and discharge is seen in 71 percent of the patients with gonococcal urethritis but in only 38 percent of the patients with NGU. Thus, the combination of discharge and dysuria is associated with gonorrhea, while the appearance of one without the other is more frequently seen with NGU. The association is insufficiently specific for a differential diagnosis. Urethral discomfort may mimic cystitis in men and women and result in urinary frequency and urgency.

Symptoms of gonorrhea often begin abruptly, and the patient may remember the specific time of day when they were first noted. Nongonococcal urethritis usually has a less acute onset, with symptoms increasing over several days. A urethral discharge may appear days in advance of dysuria; the symptoms may wax and wane, even to the point of transiently disappearing before the patient seeks therapy. The mildness and variability of the symptoms may erroneously convince the patient with NGU that he does not have a significant disease; such patients often delay seeking medical attention.[15,41]

The symptoms of infectious urethritis will, in most cases, resolve even if the patient remains untreated. Ninety-five percent of untreated patients with acute gonogoccal urethritis will be free of symptoms 6 months after contracting the disease,[36] and the symptoms of NGU gradually subside over a period of 1–3 months in 30–70 percent of the patients.[42] How many of these asymptomatic patients remain infected and potentially infectious is unknown. Untreated gonococcal urethrits may subside to a chronic state characterized by little or no urethral discomfort and a small amount of mucoid discharge called "gleet." This discharge contains small numbers of gonococci and PMNs.

So great are the clinical overlaps between nongonococcal and gonococcal urethritis that a differential diagnosis should not be made on clinical grounds alone. A Gram-stained smear of urethral discharge material will reveal typical, gram-negative, "intracellular" diplococci in about 95 percent of the cases of gonococcal urethritis and will be negative in about 97 percent of the patients with NGU.[15–17] Thus, in a population in which about 50 percent of the acute urethritis is gonococcal, a positive Gram stain suggests gonorrhea, and a negative Gram stain suggests NGU with 98 percent accuracy.[15,17] The observation of typically shaped *extracellular* diplococci diagnoses gonorrhea with an accuracy of 10–30 percent.[17,18] The Gram stain is equivocal in about 15 percent of cases.[15] Other techniques for diagnosing gonococcal urethritis are described above.[19–21]

The sensitivity of the culture for *N. gonorrhoeae* is less than 100 percent, partly because some gonococci are inhibited by the vancomycin concentrations used in selective media. The chances of isolating the organism are further reduced if the patient has recently taken antibiotics or if there is a delay in processing the culture. Thus, it seems likely that most of the few patients with positive Gram stains and negative cultures actually have gonorrhea. In most cases of acute symptomatic urethritis it is unnecessary to culturally confirm a Gram stain diagnostic of gonorrhea. It must be remembered that the Gram stain will be negative in as many as 5 percent of such patients who have gonorrhea, so a Gram stain suggestive of NGU should be confirmed with a culture, although therapy need not be delayed until the results are known. The Gram stain cannot be used to make a diagnosis of simultaneous NGU in the presence of gonorrhea. Because of the frequency with which trichomonads may be missed with direct microscopic techniques, patients in whom trichomonal urethritis is suspected should be evaluated by culture as well as by wet mount.

There is no doubt that urethritis is sexually transmitted. It occurs most frequently during the ages of peak sexual activity and in groups with a high prevalence of other STDs. It is found with increased frequency in persons with a history of other sexually transmitted genital infections.[30,33] It frequently follows sexual exposure to a new partner and is (except as a part of some systemic conditions) almost never seen in virgins. As the etiologic agents of urethritis have been defined, they have been isolated with high frequency from the female and homosexual male sexual partners of infected men where, however, they usually are carried asymptomatically.

Recognizing urethritis as an STD is important for several practical reasons. It allows one to define a population at very high risk for carrying the agents, namely, the sexual partners of infected patients. The prevalence of colonization with these agents is sufficiently high among sexual partners to justify their treatment on epidemiologic grounds, even if they are asymptomatic. Many episodes of recurrent NGU are terminated only by the treatment of an asymptomatic sexual partner of the infected patient. Since persons with one STD are at increased risk for others, it is important to screen patients with urethritis for other STDs.

Etiology of NGU

The organism most clearly associated with nongonococcal urethritis, *Chlamydia trachomatis*, is discussed in detail in Chapter 158. This obligate intracellular parasite causes 30–50 percent of the cases of NGU.[7,26,31,43,44] *Chlamydia trachomatis* is sensitive to several drugs, including the tetracyclines, sulfonamides, and erythromycin. Significantly, it is not reliably eradicated by penicillins, cephalosporins, or spectinomycin in doses used in the treatment of uncomplicated gonorrhea.

Chlamydiae are not recovered from at least 50 percent of the men with NGU. Although the clinical features of *Chlamydia*-negative NGU are very similar to those of *Chlamydia*-positive NGU,[30,45] some workers have suggested that less discharge is produced in patients who are positive for *Chlamydia* than in those who are not, and the mean incubation period may be slightly shorter.[30,45]

The agents responsible for *Chlamydia*-negative NGU remain to some extent unidentified. *Ureaplasma urealyticum*, formerly known as the T-strain mycoplasma, has been recovered from 81 percent of the men with *Chlamydia*-negative NGU, which is significantly higher than the 60 percent isolation rate from asymptomatic controls.[26,46] Furthermore, *U. urealyticum* can be recovered in larger numbers from men with *Chlamydia*-negative NGU than from control subjects.[46–48] Supporting the hypothesis that these free-living agents (see Chapter 163) cause some cases of NGU is the observation that sulfa drugs or rifampin, to which the organisms are insensitive, fail to cure most patients with *Chlamydia*-negative NGU.[49,50] Conversely, spectinomycin, which is active against ureaplasmas but inactive against *Chlamydia*, cures patients with NGU from whom only *U. urealyticum* has been isolated.[49] Additional support comes from experiments in which two investigators inoculated themselves with ureaplasmas; both developed NGU.[51] Further, some patients with NGU show rises in IgM and IgG antibody titers against *U. urealyticum*.[52] *Mycoplasma hominis* is not a cause of NGU,[53,54] but a new mycoplasma, christened *M. genitalum*, has been recovered from a few patients with NGU[55] and shown to cause inflammation in the urethras of experimental animals.[56,57]

As with *Chlamydia*, the ureaplasmas are susceptible to erythromycin and, usually, tetracyclines—the agents that have been most successful in treating NGU. Some patients, however, are infected with tetracycline-resistant *U. urealyticum*[5,58–61]; about 20 percent of such patients are not cured by tetracycline therapy. Sixteen percent of men with NGU do not carry either *C. trachomatis* or *U. urealyticum*,[49,50,62,63] and it would not be surprising if other agents were in the future identified as causes of NGU. Patients with nonchlamydial, nonureaplasmal NGU have a higher recurrence rate after therapy than do men with chlamydial urethritis.[50,62,63]

Uncommon Causes of Nongonococcal Urethritis

Dysuria is described by 83 percent of women and 44 percent of men with primary herpes simplex genital infection. Some men notice a clear, mucoid discharge that seems disproportionately mild when compared with the amount of dysuria that they experience. Herpes simplex virus (HSV) is recovered from the urethras of about 80 percent of women and 30 percent of men with primary infection, and HSV must be regarded as a cause of some cases of NGU. Urethral involvement is less common in recurrent disease, and dysuria is described by only 27 percent of women and 9 percent of men.[64]

Trichomonas vaginalis has been isolated from 3–15 percent of the patients with NGU,[22,23,27] and it causes a small percentage of the cases. The syndrome is not clinically distinguishable from NGU of other etiologies, although the discharge often is so scant that it may be noticed only as a small bead at the meatus on arising in the morning.

Pre-existing urethral stricture, particularly in the presence of other infectious agents, may (it is said) produce a urethritis-like syndrome. Urethral infection with gram-negative rods can occur in patients with phimosis or with urethral trauma after instrumentation or indwelling catheterization.[65] Periurethral abscesses may occur in this setting. Somewhat fewer than 3 percent of the cases are due to infection higher up in the urinary tract. Syphilis, with an endourethral chancre, occasionally may be manifested as a urethral discharge. Intraurethral condylomata acuminata occasionally cause a urethral discharge.

A few investigators have attributed some cases of NGU to *Clostridium difficile, Branhamella catarrhalis, Haemophilus influenzae, Neisseria meningitidis*, corynebacteria, *Gardnerella vaginalis*, various anaerobes including bacteroides[66,67] and fusobacteria,[66,67] adenoviruses,[68] and shistosomes. These observations, however, are uncontrolled for the presence of such important pathogens as *C. trachomatis* and *U. urealyticum* and must be considered unproven. Indeed, other studies have recovered corynebacteria and *G. vaginalis* less frequently from patients with NGU than from asymptomatic controls.[26,46] Rhinosporidial infection produces a nonvenereal urethritis that is manifested as a friable, meatal mass and is seen primarily on the Indian subcontinent.[69]

POSTGONOCOCCAL URETHRITIS

Some patients who are correctly treated for acute gonococcal urethritis experience prompt resolution followed in a few days by a recurrence of symptoms—usually a mucoid or mucopurulent discharge and sometimes mild dysuria. Other patients may note that their symptoms never entirely disappeared and, after initial rapid improvement, stabilized at a low level. This syndrome is referred to as postgonococcal urethritis (PGU) and should be suspected if signs, symptoms, or laboratory evidence of urethritis is found 4–7 days after completing therapy for gonorrhea.[70,71] It is a manifestation of double urethral infection. The gonococcus and the agents of NGU are extremely prevalent in sexually active populations, and they are carried simultaneously and asymptomatically by many women. Male sexual partners of these women acquire both agents during the same sexual exposure. In the presence of gonorrhea, coincident NGU cannot be diagnosed by Gram stain. β-Lactam therapy eradicates the gonococci (eliminating the symptoms of gonorrhea), but it usually leaves the agents of NGU. When the incubation period of NGU is exceeded, the patient experiences a recurrence or persistance of milder symptoms that is consistent with the latter infection.

Although originally thought to result from the consumption of alcohol or other irritants during therapy for gonorrhea, PGU is now well established as a dual infection. *Chlamydia trachomatis* has been recovered from 11–50 percent of men with gonorrhea[43]; 75–100 percent of patients with gonorrhea who are also culture-positive for *Chlamydia* will develop PGU if their gonorrhea is treated with an agent that does not eradicate *Chlamydia*.[70–74] *Chlamydia trachomatis* can be recovered from almost 50 percent of the patients with PGU, which is similar to the recovery rate in NGU. Postgonococcal urethritis, however, also develops in 20–50 percent of the patients with gonorrhea, even if *Chlamydia* is also not recovered[70,71,73]; some of these cases appear to be associated with ureaplasmal infection.[71] As one might expect, if gonorrhea is treated with a regimen active against the agents of NGU, the incidence of PGU is lower.[74–76]

Patients suffering persistence or recurrence of urethral symptoms after therapy for acute gonococcal urethritis may indeed have PGU, but the physician also should remember the possibilities of gonococcal reinfection or frank treatment failure. The patient who is having recurrent urethritis must be treated like a new patient to differentiate gonococcal from nongonococcal infections.

ASYMPTOMATIC URETHRAL INFECTION

Many patients without specific complaints that are referable to the urethra will be found to have signs of urethritis on physical examination; sexually transmitted pathogens can be recovered from some patients who have neither symptoms nor signs of urethritis. Infected adolescents are less likely to complain of urethral symptoms than are adults.[77]

The importance of asymptomatic urethral gonococcal infection in men is well recognized.[78] Prolonged asymptomatic urethral carriage of gonococci occurs in about 2–3 percent of newly infected men[78]; however, since these men do not seek treatment, the prevalence of asymptomatic urethral infections in many populations is distinctly higher than 3 percent and may have considerable epidemiologic significance. Random screening of asymptomatic populations is unrewarding[78] except in high-risk populations.[79] Most cases of asymptomatic urethral infection are detected when gonorrhea is diagnosed in female sexual partners or if complications subsequently develop in the infected man. Asymptomatic urethral infection, therefore, is particularly prevalent among the male sexual partners of women who develop symptomatic complications of gonorrhea or where gonorrhea is detected by screening.[78] Up to 40 percent of the asymptomatic sexual partners of women with disseminated gonococcal infection or pelvic inflammatory disease are found to be infected[78]; 60 percent of the infected men may be asymptomatic. Asymptomatic urethral infection also is prevalent among men with the gonococcal dermatitis–arthritis syndrome.[78] Asymptomatic gonorrhea may be diagnosed by a Gram stain of urethral material collected on a swab with a sensitivity of about 70 percent.[78]

Part of the controversy over the etiologic role of *Ureaplasma urealyticum* is its recovery from 59 percent of sexually active, asymptomatic men attending venereal disease clinics.[26,46] *Chlamydia trachomatis* is recovered from about 3 percent of such men.[26,46] Most men harboring trichomonads are asymptomatic[22] and represent an important vector of infection.

Asymptomatic urethritis in many cases can be rapidly detected by observing PMNs in material recovered from the urethra with a swab or loop. About 25 percent of asymptomatic men with four or more PMNs per oil-immersion microscopic field were found to carry *C. trachomatis* in their urethras.[80]

Because of the frequency of asymptomatic, sexually transmitted urethral infections in men, asymptomatic sexual partners of infected women or homosexual men should always be evaluated. Since immediate diagnostic techniques are of relatively low sensitivity, such men should probably be treated at the time of their initial presentation (epidemiologic treatment).

URETHRAL SYMDROME AND RELATED DISEASES OF WOMEN

Dysuria, frequency, urgency, and nocturia are frequent symptoms of bacterial cystitis in women. A similar syndrome occurs in women who do not have classic bacterial infection of the lower urinary tract. Such women are said to have the acute urethral syndrome.[81] The usual work-up for bacterial urinary tract infection is unrewarding because fewer than 10^5 organisms are recovered from each milliliter of urine. The urine sediment contains PMNs, and the symptoms frequently respond to antimicrobial therapy. Some of these patients appear to suffer from bacterial cystitis, although bacteria are recovered from the urine in smaller than traditional numbers.[81,82] Other patients' symptoms, however, appear to be related to urethritis rather than to cystitis. *Escherichia coli* sometimes apparently causes urethritis in the absence of cystitis.[83] When ordinary bacterial pathogens associated with urinary tract infections are not isolated (even in small numbers), the condition appears to be due to sexually transmitted agents.[81,82]

Neisseria gonorrhoeae can affect the urethra in women as it does in men, and it occasionally causes the urethral syndrome.[84] Gently stripping the urethra may deliver a purulent discharge that with a Gram stain will reveal typical gram-negative, cell-associated diplococci. The Gram-stained smear from the female urethra has a sensitivity of about 50 percent for gonorrhea.[85] About three-quarters of these women also will have gonococci recoverable from the endocervix.[84] The syndrome responds to standard therapy for uncomplicated anogenital gonorrhea (see Chapter 190).

Chlamydia trachomatis is frequently recovered from women with dysuria, frequency, and pyuria.[81,82] Indeed, urinary tract symptoms are described by 53 percent of women from whom *C. trachomatis* is isolated from the urethra.[86,87] This association suggests that, in some cases, the urethral syndrome is the clinical manifestation of NGU in women. If such patients are initially treated with antimicrobial agents that are active against chlamydiae (e.g. tetracyclines, sulfonamides, sulfamethoxazole-trimethoprim [SMX-TMP]), their symptoms are likely to respond. Relapses, however, are frequent and may reflect reinfection from an asymptomatic male sexual partner. *Ureaplasma urealyticum* has not been statistically associated with the urethral syndrome[81,82,86–88] except among women with $>10^3$ organisms/ml and pyuria.[89] The acute urethral syndrome, which is associated with pyuria, must be differentiated from the chronic urethral syndrome. The latter is not associated with pyuria and responds poorly to antimicrobial therapy.[90–93] It may require traditional treatments such as dilation.[82]

Dysuria is a common complaint of women with trichomoniasis. The parasite is recovered from the urethra and periurethral glands of over 90 percent of women with the infestation (Chapter 258) and is associated with pyuria.[94] Dysuria also may result from vulvar irritation such as that accompanying vaginal candidiasis. It is far less common in patients with *G. vaginalis*-associated vaginitis.

The urethral syndrome has been treated with steroids[82] or

with surgery, particularly when it is seen in postmenopausal women. Among sexually active women, however, gonococcal infection should be ruled out; NGU or trichomoniasis should be considered before other therapies are tried.

Chlamydia trachomatis can be recovered from the endocervix of 45–90 percent of the sexual partners of infected men[31,42,78,95–97] and from the urethra alone in about 15–25 percent of these women.[86,94,98,99] Although infected women usually are asymptomatic, the organism is far from benign (see Chapter 158). Chlamydial infection can be documented in almost 50 percent of the women with hypertrophic or ulcerative cervicitis who are attending a VD clinic. Indeed, cervical abnormalities, often mild, may be seen in 80 percent of the women from whom *C. trachomatis* is recovered. *Chlamydia trachomatis* may be a cause of acute salpingitis and bartholinitis. In addition, babies born to infected women may develop chlamydial ophthalmia neonatorum or pneumonia, and asymptomatic women undoubtedly are a reservoir for recurrent NGU. The carriage of ureaplasmas has been linked to infertility, although the causal nature of the relationship is controversial.[53,54,100] These considerations support the routine treatment of female sexual partners of men with NGU.

COMPLICATIONS OF URETHRITIS

Both *Neisseria gonorrhoeae* and *Chlamydia trachomatis* have been identified as causes of acute epididymitis among sexually active men.[101,102] In 20–30 percent of the men with NGU prostatic involvement is documented; however, it is usually asymptomatic[5,103] and responds to standard treatments. The role of chlamydia in the development of clinical prostatitis remains controversial. The organism has been recovered from 2 to 56 percent of men with subacute or chronic prostatitis,[104–106] and the condition appears to respond to treatment with tetracyclines. The role of *Ureaplasma urealyticum* is even more controversial. The organism has been associated with prostatitis in some series[53,107] but not in others.[54] An association with male infertility and abnormal semen specimens has been described, but it also is regarded as controversial.[54,100,107] Stricture may follow gonococcal or nongonococcal urethritis. *Chlamydia trachomatis* can infect the conjunctiva (Chapter 158). Also, an oculogenital syndrome consisting of NGU and conjunctivitis may be seen in about 4 percent of the patients with NGU[108,109]; it responds to standard therapy with tetracyclines and must be differentiated from Reiter syndrome.

THERAPY

Specific forms of urethritis including chlamydial and ureaplasmal infections, gonorrhea, trichomoniasis, and syphilis should be treated as discussed in the appropriate chapters in Part III. As a syndrome, NGU has been treated with a variety of regimens, but a tetracycline (to which *C. trachomatis* and most *U. urealyticum* strains are both sensitive) probably is the drug of choice. Treatment for 7 days will cure 65–94 percent of the patients.[8,9,44,49,50,62,70,110–113] Although longer treatment for 14–21 days has been tried, there is little convincing evidence that full-dose regimens exceeding 7 days have any additional benefits.[42,63,111] Although in the interval immediately after therapy there may be some difference in relapse rate, after 6 weeks from the initiation of therapy, relapse rates appear to be about the same with therapy of either duration. Tetracycline hydrochloride may be administered in doses of 500 mg four times a day,[8,9,44,49,50,62,70,110–113] which appears superior to 250 mg four times a day.[111,113] The patient should be instructed to take the drug on an empty stomach and not accompanied by milk or antacids. Alternatively, doxycycline can be administered in a dose of 100 mg orally twice daily for 7 days.[114,115] This drug is highly effective and well tolerated by patients; however, its use is limited by cost and by an increased tendency to produce photosensitivity reactions. Minocycline has no apparent advantages over doxycycline, and it produces dizziness in many patients.[63,116]

Erythromycin is as effective as tetracycline,[8,117] and it may be of particular use in the pregnant patient for whom tetracycline is relatively contraindicated. It is active against tetracycline-resistent ureaplasmas.[5,61] Erythromycin has the additional theoretic advantage of producing higher prostatic levels than tetracycline hydrochloride does, and it may be of use in the retreatment of patients whose symptoms are relieved by tetracycline but return after therapy is completed. Such patients may have a prostatic focus of infection that is not cured by tetracycline.[8,118] A few anecdotal cases support this use of erythromycin. Gastrointestinal discomfort is an unfortunately common adverse effect of erythromycin therapy. Instead, patients who are not tolerating a dose of 500 mg four times daily for 7 days might be treated with 250 mg four times daily, a regimen that is almost as effective in NGU.[8,117]

Sulfa drugs (e.g., sulfisoxazole, 500 mg orally four times daily for 10 days) can be used to treat chlamydial NGU,[117] but they are ineffective in *Chlamydia*-negative infection.[49,115] Although SMX-TMP (two tablets twice daily) is more effective, it is not as good as tetracycline.[115,119]

Even if untreated, the symptoms of nongonococcal urethritis will resolve within 2 weeks in 14–30 percent of the patients[110,120]; up to 70 percent of the patients will have a complete resolution of symptoms within 6 months.[42] Resolution of symptoms does not, of course, mean that the infection is cured. Such asymptomatic patients may remain infected and infectious. Conversely, the inflammatory response accompanying NGU may take some time to resolve, even after the pathogens have been eliminated.[51]

During treatment, the symptoms of NGU frequently resolve before the patient has completed his therapy. Patients should be cautioned to complete the entire course of antibiotics since a relapse is considerably more common if therapy is aborted. To differentiate reliably a relapse from reinfection and to protect sexual partners, patients undergoing treatment for urethritis should refrain from coitus until post-treatment reexamination documents cure.

The treatment of women carrying the agents of NGU is the same as for men. Erythromycin may fail to eradicate ureaplasmas from the vagina, possibly in part because vaginal acidity interferes with the action of the drug.[59]

Because coincident chlamydial infection is very common in men with gonorrhea, the Centers for Disease Control have suggested that uncomplicated gonococcal urethritis should be treated with a combined regimen consisting of a single dose of a suitable β-lactam antibiotic followed by 7 days of tetracycline hydrochloride (500 mg orally four times daily), doxycycline hyclate (100 mg orally twice daily), or erythromycin (500 mg orally four times daily). This regimen has the advantage of providing effective single-dose therapy for gonorrhea and effective therapy for coincident, undiagnosed NGU.[121] Its disadvantages include increased cost, potential for adverse reactions, and the need to delay post-treatment tests of cure cultures for gonorrhea until after the completion of tetracycline therapy. The combination, however, may be of increasing importance because an increase in gonococcal resistance to tetracycline has been accompanied by a decreased effectiveness of tetracycline regimens for this disease. In the past, tetracycline regimens for NGU were at least 95 percent effective in uncomplicated gonococcal infections as well. At present, however, it probably is more prudent to use the combined regimen for urethritis of undetermined etiology. The failure of patients to complete a multidose tetracycline regimen has been a major concern, and it also influences the choice of therapy.[1,122]

Patients who are being treated for urethritis should be examined for other STDs and should be tested serologically for syphilis at the initial visit.

An initial work-up for trichomoniasis probably is not indicated in most routine settings since the infection accounts for only about 3–5 percent of the cases.[22] Additionally, direct microscopic examination of a urethral specimen usually is unrewarding unless the patient can be seen before first morning micturation. If the patient's urethritis has not been cured by previous antibacterial therapy or if symptoms or signs in the sexual partner suggest trichomonal infection, the patient's urine sediment can be examined as a wet mount or can be cultured on suitable media. Observation of motile trichomonads in the urine is an indication for therapy.

Patients treated for gonorrhea should return at least 3 days after completing therapy and should have a urethral specimen recultured to document cure because insufficient therapy may eliminate the symptoms without eradicating the pathogen in up to 50 percent of patients.[123] Men treated for nongonococcal urethritis should be reexamined to document the disappearance of urethral inflammation. One should probably wait for several weeks after completion of therapy before performing a test of cure for chlamydial infection. The sensitivity of the immunofluorescence or ELISA technique in this setting is undefined.

Patients initially treated for NGU whose symptoms are not eliminated by tetracycline should be suspected of having infection with *Trichomonas* or tetracycline-resistant *Ureaplasma*.[5,58,59,61] Because these infections may be impossible to differentiate clinically, such patients may be empirically treated with a single 2 g dose of metronidazole followed by erythromycin, 500 mg orally four times daily for 7 days. It is, of course, important that their sexual partners be treated with the same regimen.

Some men report that their urethral symptoms disappeared while they were taking tetracycline but reappeared days to weeks after completing therapy. Such recurrences are seen in about 20 percent of patients with chlamydial NGU and in about 40 percent of patients with nonchlamydial infection. Among NGU patients from whom neither chlamydiae nor ureaplasmas are isolated, the recurrence rate is greater than 50 percent.[50,62,63] Eighty percent of recurrent NGU occurs in patients in whom neither organism is initially recovered,[63] and 70–80 percent of men with recurrent NGU are culture-negative for both organisms at the time of recurrence.[85]

Men with recurrent disease should be questioned closely about the possibility of reexposure, and attention should be given to ensuring simultaneous treatment of all sexual partners. If reexposure is likely, the patient may be retreated with the initial tetracycline regimen. If the patient has not been reexposed, a recurrence of urethritis suggests the possibility that some pathogens remained in a relatively antibiotic protected site. Such men are sometimes cured by retreating them with a 3- to 6-week course of tetracycline.[85,124,125] Prostatic involvement is common in NGU. It is possible that some men may have a prostatic focus of infection that is not eradicated by treatment with tetracycline because it penetrates rather poorly into the prostate gland.[62] Men with repeated relapses occasionally are successfully treated with a 3- to 6-week course of doxycycline or erythromycin, which are active against *Chlamydia* and *Ureaplasma* and achieve better prostatic levels than does tetracycline hydrochloride. Patients whose relapses are not eliminated by these maneuvers should be referred for urologic evaluation to rule out anatomic abnormalities.[118,124] Such men most likely are not infected with *Chlamydia* or *Ureaplasma*. About one-quarter will be found to have a partial obstruction to urine flow, and about half of these will have urethral strictures.[118] They and their sexual partners do not appear to be at significant risk for complications.[125] Long-term antimicrobial suppression is useful in this setting.[125]

Sexual partners of patients with sexually transmitted urethritis should be treated simultaneously. Asymptomatic male sexual partners of women known to have gonorrhea or trichomoniasis should be treated even if direct microscopic examinations are negative. Sexual partners of men with gonococcal, nongonococcal, or trichomonal urethritis should be treated at the initial visit. A woman who has been the sexual partner of a man with urethritis of undetermined etiology should be treated with a regimen that is effective against gonococci, chlamydiae, and ureaplasmas. The combined β-lactam/tetracycline regimen described above is suitable in nonpregnant women. Erythromycin may be substituted for tetracycline in pregnancy.

REITER SYNDROME

Some cases of nongonococcal urethritis appear as one element of Reiter syndrome, which also includes arthritis, uveitis, and often, lesions of the skin and mucous membranes. The syndrome complicates 1–2 percent of the cases of NGU[124,126–128] and is felt to be the most common peripheral inflammatory arthritis in young men.[129] Its pathogenesis is unclear, but it probably represents an abnormal host response to any of a number of infections.[130] The idiosyncratic nature of the host's response is supported by a strong correlation between the development of Reiter syndrome and the presence of the HLA-B27 histocompatibility antigen. This antigen has been found in 60–96 percent of the patients with Reiter syndrome,[128,129,131,132] and it also has been related to uveitis and sacroileitis.[128] Although possibly providing a clue to pathogenesis, its diagnostic value has been questioned.[133]

The inciting infection is of two types. Reiter syndrome may follow sexually transmitted urethritis, and most cases in North American and Europe seem to occur in sexually active young people.[134,135] Many cases occur after contact with a new partner, and some cases have been epidemiologically linked.[128,136] In one series, 9 percent of cases followed gonococcal urethritis, although 50 percent of these patients subsequently developed PGU.[137] *Chlamydia trachomatis* has been impicated in the pathogenesis of Reiter syndrome[138] since it has been recovered from the urethras of 16–44 percent of the patients with Reiter syndrome and from 69 percent of those men who had signs of urogenital inflammation at the time of examination.[135,139,140] In addition, antibodies to *Chlamydia* have been detected in 46–67 percent and cell-mediated immunity in 72 percent of patients with Reiter syndrome.[130,140,141] Chlamydial antigens have been identified in synovial membranes,[142] and chlamydial elementary bodies have been observed in joint fluid[143] in a few patients. The significance of these recent observations is not yet defined, but the failure of antichlamydial therapy to influence the course of disease argues against it.

Reiter syndrome also follows bacterial gastroenteritis and has been described after infection with *Salmonella, Shigella, Yersinia,* and *Campylobacter*[127–129,131,137,144–148] and after antibiotic-associated colitis.[149] Postdysenteric Reiter syndrome has occurred in 0.24–1.50 percent of the patients after epidemics of gastrointestinal infection[145,147]; it is considerably more common among patients who are HLA-B27–positive. Antibodies reacting with *Yersinia* proteins occur in the sera of many patients with Reiter syndrome.[150]

Clinically, Reiter syndrome after genital infection is indistinguishable from that following bacterial gastroenteritis; indeed, 12–80 percent of the patients with postdysenteric Reiter syndrome have genital symptoms.[128,151] The age- and sex-specific attack rates, however, are different; 94–99 percent of the cases of Reiter syndrome after sexually transmitted infections occur in men. However, a much larger fraction—up to 10 percent—of the cases of postdysenteric Reiter syndrome occur in women.[134,147,152,153] It also is reported in sexually inactive children.[134,146]

Clinical Features

Nongonococcal urethritis is the initial manifestation in 80 percent of the patients.[128,129] As with other forms of nongonococcal urethritis, it usually occurs 7–14 days after sexual exposure.[128] The urethritis may be mild and may be unnoticed by the patient,[127] and it may be detectable only by physical examination performed before the first micturation. Gonococcal urethritis sometimes sets the stage for Reiter syndrome.[137] The discharge may be purulent or mucopurulent, and patients may or may not complain of dysuria. Accompanying prostatitis has been described by some authors.[127,129,151,153] If present, it usually is asymptomatic. Cystitis without urethritis is also reported and may be a common manifestation, particularly in women.[151] Cervicitis is associated with Reiter syndrome[154] and may represent female genital infection with the inciting microorganism.

The other features of Reiter syndrome develop 1–5 weeks after the onset of urethritis.[151] Arthritis begins within 4 weeks of the onset of urethritis in four-fifths of patients,[127,128] but it precedes urethritis in about 15 percent.[134] The knees are the most frequently involved, followed by the ankles and small joints of the feet. Sacroileitis, either symmetric[151] or more frequently asymmetric,[134,146,153] may develop later in up to two-thirds of patients.[151] It is more frequent in patients with the HLA-B27 antigen.[146] Ankylosing spondylitis, which occurs in only about 1 percent of the general population, complicates one-quarter to one-third of the cases of Reiter syndrome[128,132,146,155]; also, back pain is reported by 60 percent of all patients.[129] Ninety percent of patients with the HLA-B27 antigen who develop Reiter syndrome develop ankylosing spondylitis,[155,156] which is rare in patients without the antigen.[156] Spurring of the calcaneus may be seen in up to one-quarter of the patients with Reiter syndrome[134,153] and may produce heel pain. A dactylitis resulting in sausage-shaped swelling of the digits is also characteristic.[134] Arthritis is the most persistent feature of the syndrome and may last for 2–6 months after other manifestations have disappeared.[134,151]

Mild bilateral conjunctivitis, iritis, or uveitis is sometimes present but often lasts for only a few days.[127,151,153,157] It is occasionally accompanied by a purulent discharge or frank keratitis.[151,157] Unlike the conjunctivitis caused by direct infection with *Chlamydia trachomatis*, the inflamed conjunctivae in Reiter syndrome do not manifest follicular hypertrophy.

Dermatologic manifestations affect 50 percent of the patients.[127–129] The initial lesions are waxy papules, which often display a central yellow spot and occur most frequently on the soles and palms[151] and with decreasing frequency on the nails, scrotum, scalp, and trunk.[127] The papules epithelialize and thicken to produce keratoderma blenorrhagicum in about 10–25 percent of the patients.[129,154] Circinate balanitis is usually painless and occurs in about 25–40 percnet of all patients.[128,129,151] Circinate and ulcerative vulvitis also are described.[158] Painless erosions on the dorsum of the tongue and fauces occur most commonly with the initial episode and less frequently with recurrences.[153,154]

Incomplete Reiter syndrome consisting of urethritis and arthritis or arthritis alone has been reported.[129,144,159]

The initial episode of Reiter syndrome usually lasts for 2–6 months, but episodes lasting for 1 year have been described.[129,151,153] Most patients feel completely well after the attack subsides, but the disease recurs in 35–70 percent of the patients[128,129,134,153,155] at a rate of about 15 percent in each 5-year period after the initial attack.[160] During recurrences, the genital symptoms are usually less marked and may be entirely absent.[161,162] About 60–80 percent of the patients will have active disease 15–20 years after the initial episode,[125,129,132,155,160] with the risk of residuals being somewhat higher among patients with the HLA-B27 antigen.[163] Almost 50 percent of the affected patients develop some degree of permanent disability.[132,155]

Rare complications of Reiter syndrome include pericarditis,[154] myocarditis,[151] first-degree atrioventricular block,[153,164] and aortic insufficiency.[132,153] Thrombophlebitis, radiculitis,[154] and myelopathy[165] are occasionally described.

Laboratory Features

Anemia is common,[129] and the erythrocyte sedimentation rate is elevated in about 50 percent of the patients.[134,154] Fluid recovered at the same time from different joints is often different.[151] Synovial fluid may contain 1000–200,000 white blood cells, more than two-thirds of which are PMNs.[151] Complement levels in the fluid are generally elevated, which allows differentiation from rheumatoid arthritis,[146] and the glucose is low in about 50 percent of the joints.[151] Synovial biopsy specimens reveal infiltration by PMNs.[154]

Therapy

Treatment of Reiter syndrome is quite controversial. Because of the possibility that the inciting infection may be sexually transmitted NGU, treatment with tetracycline for 7 days is recommended[127,154] and has been said by some to reduce or eliminate the urethritis.[166] Others, however, have seen no effect on the arthritis or on the overall course of the disease.[154–161] The relative safety of oral tetracycline and the frequency with which chalmydiae are isolated from patients with Reiter syndrome makes a course of tetracycline reasonable.

Nonsteroidal anti-inflammatory drugs, particularly phenylbutazone given as 400–600 mg/day in divided doses, probably is the most effective treatment.[129] Indomethacin or tolmetin are favored by some workers,[167] and all of these are superior to salicylates or corticosteroids. Cytotoxic agents may be of value in recalcitrant cases.[167]

REFERENCES

1. Braun P, Sherman H, Komaroff AL. Urethritis in men: Benefits, risks, and costs of alternative strategies of management. Sex Transm Dis. 1982;9:188.
2. Amarasuriya KL. Haematuria presenting in outpatients attending a department of genitourinary medicine. Br J Vener Dis. 1979;55:214.
3. Swartz SL. Diagnosis of nongonococcal urethritis. In: Hobson D, Holmes KK, eds. Nongonococcal Urethritis and Related Infections. Lake Placid, NY: American Society for Microbiology; 1976:15.
4. Bowie WR. Comparison of the Gram stain and first-voided urine sediment in the diagnosis of urethritis. Sex Transm Dis. 1978;5:39.
5. Root TE, Edwards LD, Spengler PJ. Nongonococcal urethritis: A survey of clinical and laboratory features. Sex Trasnm Dis. 1980;7:59.
6. Swartz SL, Kraus SJ, Herrmann KL, et al. Diagnosis and etiology of nongonococcal urethritis. J Infect Dis. 1978;138:445.
7. Desai K, Robson HG. Comparison of the Gram-stained urethral smear and first-voided urine sediment in the diagnosis of nongonococcal urethritis. Sex Transm Dis. 1982;9:21.
8. Scheibel JH, Kristensen JK, Hentzler B, et al. Treatment of chlamydial urethritis in men and *Chlamydia trachomatis* positive female partners: Comparison of erythromycin and tetracycline in treatment courses of one week. Sex Transm Dis. 1982;9:128.
9. Stamm WE, Koutsky LA, Benedetti JK, et al. *Chlamydia trachomatis* urethral infections in men: Prevalence, risk factors, and clinical manifestations. Ann Intern Med. 1984;100:47.
10. Perera SA. Use of the Kova-Slide II with grid and uncentrifuged segmented urine specimens in the diagnosis of nongonococcal urethritis: A quantitative technique. Sex Transm Dis. 1985;12:14.
11. Veeravahu M, Smyth RW, Clay JC. Detection of leukocyte esterase in urine: A new screening test for nongonococcal urethritis compared with two microscopic methods. Sex Transm Dis. 1987;14:180.
12. Perera SAB, Jones C, Srikantha V, et al. Leukocyte esterase test as rapid screen for non-gonococcal urethritis. Genitourin Med. 1987;63:380–3.
13. Simmons PD. Evaluation of the early morning smear investigation. Br J Vener Dis. 1978;54:128.
14. Willcox JR, Adler MW, Belsey EM. Observer variation in the interpretation of Gram stained urethral smears. Br J Vener Dis. 1981;57:134.
15. Jacobs NF, Kraus SJ. Gonococcal and nongonococcal urethritis in men: Clinical and laboratory differentiation. Ann Intern Med. 1975;82:7.
16. Kraus SJ. Semiquantitation of urethral polymorphonuclear leukocytes as objective evidence of nongonococcal urethritis. Sex Transm Dis. 1982;9:52.
17. Goodhart ME, Ogden J, Zaidi AA, et al. Factors affecting the performance of smear and culture tests for the detection of *Neisseria gonorrhoeae*. Sex Transm Dis. 1982;9:63.
18. Kleris GS, Arnold AJ. Differential diagnosis of urethritis: Predictive value and therapeutic implications of the urethral smear. Sex Transm Dis. 1981;8:110.

19. Janda WH, Jackson T. Evaluation of Gonodecton for the presumptive diagnosis of gonococcal urethritis in men. J Clin Microbiol. 1985;21:143.
20. Prior RB, Spagna VA. Improved utility of Gonoscreen, a limulus amoebocyte lysate assay, in the evaluation of urethral discharges in men. J Clin Microbiol. 1985;22:141.
21. Judson FN, Werness BA, Shahan MR. Lack of utility of a limulus amoebocyte lysate assay in the diagnosis of urethral discharges in men. J Clin Microbiol. 1985;21:152.
22. Krieger JN. Urologic aspects of trichomoniasis. Invest Urol. 1981;18:412.
23. Kuberski T. *Trichomonas vaginalis* associated with nongonococcal urethritis and prostatitis. Sex Transm Dis. 1981;7:135.
24. Adger H, Shafer MA, Sweet RL, et al. Screening for *Chlamydia trachomatis* and *Neisseria gonorrhoeae* in adolescent males: Value of first catch urine examination. Lancet. 1984;2:944.
25. Chernsky MA, Mahony JB, Castriciano S, et al. Detection of *Chlamydia trachomatis* antigens by enzyme immunoassay and immunofluorescence in genital specimens from symptomatic and asymptomatic men and women. J Infect Dis. 1986;154:41.
26. Bowie WR, Pollock HM, Forsyth PS, et al. Bacteriology of the urethra in normal men and men with nongonococcal urethritis. J Clin Microbiol. 1977;6:482.
27. Wong JL, Hines PA, Brasher MD. The etiology of nongonococcal urethritis in men attending a venereal disease clinic. Sex Transm Dis. 1977;4:4.
28. Bacci M. Masturbation injury resulting from intraurethral introduction of spaghetti. Am J Forensic Med Pathol. 1986;7:254.
29. Rogers WB. Shampoo urethritis. Am J Dis Child. 1985;139:748.
30. McCutchen JA. Epidemiology of venereal urethritis: Comparison of gonorrhea and nongonococcal urethritis. Rev Infect Dis. 1984;6:669.
31. Judson FN. Epidemiology and control of nongonococcal urethritis and genital chlamydial infections: A revoew. Sex Transm Dis. 1981;8:117.
32. Wright RA, Judson FN. Relative and seasonal incidences of the sexually transmitted diseases: A two-year statistical review. Br J Vener Dis. 1978;54:433.
33. McChesney JA, Zedd A, King H, et al. Acute urethritis in male college students. JAMA. 1973;226:37.
34. Smith GL, Greenup R, Takafuji ET. Circumcision as a risk factor for urethritis in racial groups. Am J Public Health. 1987;77:452.
35. Boyd JT, Csonka GW, Oates JK. Epidemiology of nonspecific urethritis. Br J Vener Dis. 1958;34:40.
36. Holmes KK. Gonococcal infection: Clinical, epidemiologic and laboratory perspectives. Adv Intern Med. 1974;19:259.
37. Schofield CBS. Some factors affecting the incubation period and duration of symptoms of urethritis in men. Br J Vener Dis. 1982;58:184.
38. Harrison WO, Hooper R, Wiesner PJ, et al. Minocycline given after exposure to prevent gonorrhea. N Engl J Med. 1979;300:1074.
39. Rothenberg R, Judson FN. The clinical diagnosis of urethral discharge. Sex Transm Dis. 1983;10:24.
40. Lee Y-H, Rosner B, Alpert S, et al. Clinical and microbiological investigation of men with urethritis. J Infect Dis. 1978;158:798.
41. Volk J, Kraus SJ. Nongonococcal urethritis: A venereal disease as prevalent as epidemic gonorrhea. Arch Intern Med. 1974;134:511.
42. Oriel JD. Treatment of nongonococcal urethritis. In: Hobson D, Holmes KK, eds. Nongonococcal Urethritis and Related Infections. Lake Placid, NY: American Society for Microbiology; 1976:38.
43. Johannisson G, Lowhagin GB, Nilsson S. *Chlamydia trachomatis* and urethritis in men. Scand J Infect Dis. [Suppl] 1982;32:87.
44. Handsfield HH, Alexander ER, Wang S-P, et al. Differences in the therapeutic response of chlamydia-positive and chlamydia-negative forms of nongonococcal urethritis. J Am Vener Dis Assoc. 1976;2:5.
45. Jacobs NF, Arum ES, Kraus SJ. Nongonococcal urethritis: The role of *Chlamydia trachomatis*. Ann Intern Med. 1977;86:313.
46. Bowie WR, Wang SP, Alexander ER, et al. Etiology of non-gonococcal urethritis: Evidence for *Chlamydia trachomatis* and *Ureaplasma urealyticum*. J Clin Invest. 1977;59:735.
47. Viarengo J, Hebrant F, Piot P. *Ureaplasma urealyticum* in urethra of healthy men. Br J Vener Dis. 1980;56:169.
48. Hunter JM, Smith IW, Peutherer JF, et al. *Chlamydia trachomatis* and *Ureaplasma urealyticum* in men attending a sexually transmitted diseases clinic. Br J Vener Dis. 1981;57:130.
49. Bowie WR, Floyd JF, Miller Y, et al. Differential response of chlamydial and ureaplasma-associated urethritis to sulfafurazole (sulfisoxazole) and aminocyclitols. Lancet. 1976;2:1276.
50. Coufalike ED, Taylor-Robinson D, Csonka GW. Treatment of nongonococcal urethritis or the rifampicin as a means of defining the role of *Ureaplasma urealyticum*. Br J Vener Dis. 1979;55:36.
51. Taylor-Robinson D, Csonka GW, Prentice MJ. Human intraurethral inoculation of ureaplasmas. Q J Med. 1977;46:309.
52. Brown MB, Cassel GH, Taylor-Robinson D. Measurement of antibody to *Ureaplasma urealyticum* by an enzyme-linked immunoassay and detection of antibody responses in patients with nongonococcal urethritis. J Clin Microbiol. 1983;17:288.
53. Cassell GH, Cole BC. Mycoplasmas as agents of human disease. N Engl J Med. 1981;304:80.
54. Taylor-Robinson D, McCormack WM. The genital mycoplasmas. N Engl J Med. 1980;302:1003,1063.
55. Tully JG, Cole RM, Taylor-Robinson D, et al. A newly discovered mycoplasma in the human urogenital tract. Lancet. 1981;1:1288.
56. Taylor-Robinson D, Furr PM, Hetherington CM. The pathogenicity of a newly discovered human mycoplasma (Strain G37) for the genital tract of marmosets. J Hug (Lond). 1982;89:449.
57. Taylor-Robinson D, Tully JG, Barile MF. Urethral infection in male chimpanzees produced experimentally by *Mycoplasma genitalium*. Br J Exp Pathol. 1985;66:95.
58. Magalhaes M. Persistent nongonococcal urethritis associated with a minocycline-resistant strain of *Ureaplasma urealyticum*. Sex Transm Dis. 1983;10:151.
59. Arya OP, Pratt BC. Persistent urethritis due to *Ureaplasma urealyticum* in conjugal or stable partnerships. Genitourin Med. 1986;62:329.
60. Magalhaes M, Veras A. Minocycline resistance among clinical isolates of *Ureaplasma urealyticum*. J Infect Dis. 1984;149:117.
61. Stimson JB, Hale J, Bowie WK, et al. Tetracycline-resistant *Ureaplasma urealyticum*: A cause of persistent nongonococcal urethritis. Ann Intern Med. 1981;94:192.
62. Bowie WR. Urethritis and infections of the lower urogenital tract. Urol Clin North Am. 1980;7:17.
63. Bowie WR, Alexander ER, Stimson JB, et al. Therapy for non-gonococcal urethritis: double blind, randomized-comparison of two doses and two durations of minocycline. Ann Intern Med. 1981;95:306.
64. Corey L, Adams HG, Brown ZA, et al. Genital herpes simplex virus infection: Clinical manifestations, course, and complications. Ann Intern Med. 1983;98:958.
65. Nacey JN, Tulloch AGS, Ferguson AF. Catheter-induced urethritis: A comparison between latex and silicone catheters in a prospective clinical trial. Br J Urol. 1985;57:325.
66. Fontaine EAR, Bryant TN, Taylor-Robinson D, et al. A numerical toxonomic study of anaerobic gram-negative bacilli classified as *Bacteroides ureolyticus* isolated from patients with nongonococcal urethritis. J Gen Microbiol. 1986;132:3137.
67. Fontaine EA, Borriello SP, Taylor-Robinson D, et al. Characteristics of a gram negative anaerobe isolated from men with nongonococcal urethritis. J Med Microbiol. 1984;17:129.
68. Harnett GB, Phillips PA, Gollors MM. Association of genital adenovirus infection with urethritis in men. Med J Aust. 1984;141:337.
69. Sasidharan K, Subramonian P, Moni VN, et al. Urethral rhinosporidiosis. Analysis of 27 cases. Br J Urol. 1987;59:66.
70. Arya OP, Mallinson H, Pareek SS, et al. Postgonococcal cervicitis and postgonococcal urethritis: A study of their epidemiologic correlation and the role of *chlamydia trachomatis* in their etiology. Br J Vener Dis. 1981;57:395.
71. Bowie WR, Alexander ER, Holmes KK. Etiologies of post-gonococcal urethritis in homosexual and heterosexual men: Roles of *Chlamydia trachomatis* and *Ureaplasma urealyticum*. Sex Transm Dis. 1978;5:151.
72. Terho P. *Chlamydia trachomatis* in gonococcal and non-gonococcal urethritis. Br J Vener Dis. 1978;54:326.
73. Oriel JD, Ridgway GL, Reeve P, et al. The lack of effect of ampicillin plus probenecid given for genital infections with *Neusseria gonorrhoeae* on associated infections with *Chlamydia trachomatis*. J Infect Dis. 1976;133:568.
74. Stamm WE, Guinan ME, Johnson C, et al. Effect of treatment regimens for *Neisseria gonorrhoeae* on simultaneous infection with *Chlamydia trachomatis*. N Engl J Med. 1984;310:545.
75. Patrone P, Negosanti M, Ghetti P, et al. A combined treatment in prevention of postgonococcal urethritis. Dermatologica. 1984;168:300.
76. Holmes KK, Johnson DW, Floyd TM, et al. Studies of venereal disease: II observations on the incidence, etiology, and treatment of the postgonococcal urethritis syndrome. JAMA. 1967;202:467.
77. Chambers CV, Shafer M-A, Adger H, et al. Microflora of the urethra in adolescent boys: Relationships to sexual activity and nongonococcal urethritis. J Pediatr. 1987;110:314.
78. Handsfield HH, Lipman TO, Harnisch JP, et al. Asymptomatic gonorrhea in men: Diagnosis, natural course, prevalence, and significance. N Engl J Med. 1974;290:117.
79. Smith JA, Linder CW, Jay MS, et al. Isolation of *Neisseria gonorrhoeae* from the urethra of asymptomatic adolescent males. Clin Pediatr (Phila). 1986;25:566.
80. Swartz SL, Kraus SJ. Persistent urethral leukocytosis and asymptomatic chlamydial urethritis. J Infect Dis. 1979;140:614.
81. Stamm WE. Etiology and management of the acute urethral syndrome. Sex Transm Dis. 1981;8:235.
82. Stamm WE, Wagner KF, Amsel R, et al. Causes of the acute urethral syndrome in women. N Engl J Med. 1980;303:409.
83. Fihn SD, Johnson C, Stamm WE. *Escherichia coli* urethritis in women with symptoms of acute urinary tract infection. J Infect Dis. 1988;1:196.
84. Curran JW. Gonorrhea and the urethral syndrome. Sex Transm Dis. 1977;4:119.
85. Goh BT, Varia KB, Aylifte PF, et al. Diagnosis of gonorrhea by gram stained smears and cultures in men and women: Role of the urethral smear. Sex Transm Dis. 1985;12:135.
86. Paavonen J. *Chlamydia trachomatis*-induced urethritis in female partners of men with nongonococcal urethritis. Sex Transm Dis. 1979;6:69.
87. Paavonen J, Vesterinen E. *Chlamydia trachomatis* in cervicitis and urethritis in women. Scand J Infect Dis [Suppl]. 1982;32:45.
88. Hunter JM, Young H, Harris AB. Genitourinary infection with *Ureaplasma*

urealyticum in women attending a sexually transmitted disease clinic. Br J Vener Dis. 1981;57:338.
89. Stamm WE, Running K, Hale J, et al. Etiologic role of *Mycoplasma hominis* and *Ureaplasma urealyticum* in women with the acute urethral syndrome. Sex Transm. Dis. 1983;10:318.
90. Fihn SD, Stamm WE. The urethral syndrome. Semin Urol. 1983;1:121.
91. Latham RH, Stamm WE. Urethral syndrome in women. Urol Clin North Am. 1984;11:95.
92. Scotti RJ, Ostergard DR. The urethral syndrome. Clin Obstet Gynecol. 1984;27:515.
93. Bump RC, Copeland WE Jr. Urethral isolation of the genital mycoplasmas and *Chlamydia trachomatis* in women with chronic urologic complaints. Am J Obstet Gynecol. 1985;152:38.
94. Feldman RG, Johnson AL, Schober PC, et al. Aetiology of urinary symptoms in sexually active women. Genitourin Med. 1986;62:333.
95. Ghadirian FD, Robson HG. *Chlamydia trachomatis* genital infections. Br J Vener Dis. 1979;55:415.
96. Paavonen J, Karsa M, Sackku P, et al. Examination of men with nongonococcal urethritis and their sexual partners for *Chlamydia trachomatis* and *Ureaplasma urealyticum*. Sex Transm Dis. 1978;5:93.
97. Thelin I, Mardh P-A. Contact tracing in genital chlamydial infection. Scand J Infect Dis. [Suppl]. 1982;32:163.
98. Johannisson G, Lowhagen G-B, Lycke E. Genital *Chlamydia trachomatis* infection in women. Obstet Gynecol. 1980;56:671.
99. Wallin JE, Thompson SE, Zaidi A, et al. Urethritis in women attending an STD clinic. Br J Vener Dis. 1981;57:50.
100. Toth A, Lesser ML, Brooks C, et al. Subsequent pregnancies among 161 couples treated for T-mycoplasma genital-tract infection. N Engl J Med. 1983;308:505.
101. Berger RE. Acute epididymitis. Sex Transm Dis. 1981;8:286.
102. Berger RE, Alexander ER, Harnish JP, et al. Etiology and therapy of acute epididymitis: Prospective study of 50 cases. J Urol. 1979; 121:750.
103. Holmes KK, Handsfield HH, Wang S-P, et al. Etiology of nongonococcal urethritis. N Engl J Med. 1975;292:1199.
104. Bruce AW, Chadwick P, Willett WS, et al. The role of chlamydiae in genitourinary disease. J Urol. 1982;126:625.
105. Mardh PA, Ripa KT, Colleen S, et al. Role of *Chlamydia trachomatis* in nonacute prostatitis. Br J Vener Dis. 1978;54:330.
106. Nilsson S, Johannisson G, Lycke E. Isolation of *Chlamydia trachomatis* from the urethra and from prostatic fluid in men with signs and symptoms of acute urethritis. Acta Derm Venereol (Stockh). 1981;61:456.
107. Cassell GH, Younger JB, Brown MB, et al. Microbiologic study of infertile women at the time of diagnostic laparoscopy: Association of *Ureaplasma urealyticum* with a defined subpopulation. N Engl J Med. 1983;308:502.
108. Mordhorst CH. Clinical epidemiology of oculogenital chlamydial infections. In: Hobson D, Holmes KK, eds. Nongonococcal Urethritis and Related Infections. Lake Placid, NY: American Society for Microbiology; 1976:126.
109. Ronnerstam R, Persson K. Chlamydial eye infections in adults. Scand J Infect Dis [Suppl]. 1982;32:111.
110. Holmes KK, Johnson DW, Floyd TM. Studies of venereal disease: III. Double-blind comparison of tetracycline hydrochloride and placebo in treatment of nongonococcal urethritis. JAMA. 1967;201:474.
111. Arya OP, Alergant CD, Annels EH, et al. Management of nonspecific urethritis in men: Evaluation of six treatment regimens and effect of other factors including alcohol and sexual intercourse. Br J Vener Dis. 1978;54:414.
112. Thambar IV, Simmons PD, Thin RN, et al. Double-blind comparison of two regimens in the treatment of nongonococcal urethritis: Seven-day vs 21-day courses of triple tetracycline (Deteclo). Br J Vener Dis. 1979;55:284.
113. Bowie WR, Yu JS, Fawcett A, et al. Tetracycline in nongonococcal urethritis. Comparison of 2 g and 1 g daily for seven days. Br J Vener Dis. 1980;56:332.
114. Juvakowski T, Lauharanta J, Kanerva L, et al. One-week treatment of chlamydia-positive urethritis with doxycycline and tetracycline chloride in males. Acta Derm Venereol (Stockh). 1981;61:273.
115. Lassus A, Juvakoski T. Treatment of uncomplicated genital *Chlamydia trachomatis* infections in males. Scand J Infect Dis [Suppl]. 1982;32:169.
116. Oriel JD, Ridgway GL. Comparison of tetracycline and minocycline in the treatment of nongonococcal urethritis. Br J Vener Dis. 1983;59:245.
117. Bowie WR, Manzon LM, Borrie-Hume CJ. Efficacy of treatment regimens for lower urogenital *Chlamydia trachomatis* infection of women. Am J Obstet Gynecol. 1982;142:125.
118. Krieger JN, Hooton TM, Brust PJ, et al. Evaluation of chronic urethritis: Defining the role for endoscopic procedures. Arch Intern Med. 1988;148:703.
119. Willcox RR, Sparrow RW. Cotrimoxazole in the treatment of nongonococcal urethritis. Acta Derm Venereol (Stockh). 1974;54:317.
120. Willcox RR. "Triple tetracycline" in the treatment of nongonococcal urethritis in males. Br J Vener Dis. 1972;48:137.
121. Centers for Disease Control. Sexually transmitted diseases treatment guidelines, 1985. MMWR. 1985;34(Suppl 4):1.
122. Jordan WC. Doxycycline vs tetracycline in the treatment of men with gonorrhea: The compliance factor. Sex Transm Dis. 1981;8:105.
123. Schmid GP, Johnson RE, Brenner ER, et al. Symptomatic response to therapy of men with gonococcal urethritis: Do all need posttreatment cultures? Sex Transm Dis. 1987;14:37.
124. Kaufman RE, Wiesner PJ. Current concepts: Nonspecific urethritis. N Engl J Med. 1974;291:1175.
125. Berger RE. Recurrent nongonococcal urethritis. JAMA. 1983;249:409.
126. Csonka GW. Course of Reiter''s disease. Br Med J. 1958;1:1088.
127. Morton RS. Reiter's disease. Practitioner. 1972;209:631.
128. Keat A. Reiter's syndrome and reactive arthritis in perspective. N Engl J Med. 1983;309:1606.
129. Arnett FC Jr. Reiter's syndrome. Johns Hopkins Med J. 1982;150:39.
130. Ford DK, daRoza DM, Schulzer M. The specificity of synovial mononuclear cell-responses to microbiological antigens in Reiter's syndrome. J Rheumatol. 1982;9:561.
131. Lehman DH. Postdysenteric Reiter's syndrome. West J Med. 1977;126:405.
132. Sairanen E, Paronen I, Mahonen H. Reiter's syndrome: A followup study. Acta Med Scand. 1969;185:57.
132. Kahn M, Kahn M. Diagnostic value of HLA-B27 testing in ankylosing spondylitis and Reiter's syndrome. Ann Intern Med. 1982;96:70.
134. Hawkes JG. Clinical and diagnostic features of Reiter's disease: A followup study of 39 patients. NZ Med J. 1973;78:347.
135. Kousa M, Saikku P, Richmond S, et al. Frequent association of chlamydial infection with Reiter's syndrome. Sex Transm Dis. 1978;5:57.
136. Rustin MHA, Wedzicha JA, Keat AC, et al. Sexually transmitted arthritis? Two informative cases. J Rheumatol. 1982;9:646.
137. Leirisalo M, Skylv G, Kousa M, et al. Followup study on patients with Reiter's disease and reactive arthritis with special reference to HLA-B27. Arthritis Rheum. 1982;25:249.
138. Editorial. Is Reiter's syndrome caused by chlamydia? Lancet. 1985;1:317.
139. Keat AC, Thomas BJ, Taylor-Robinson D, et al. Evidence of *Chlamydia trachomatis* infection in sexually acquired reactive arthritis. Ann Rheum Dis. 1980;39:431.
140. Kousa M. Evidence of chlamydial involvement in the development of arthritis. Scand J Infect Dis [Suppl]. 1982;32:116.
141. Inman RD, Johnston MEA, Chici B, et al. Immunochemical analysis of immune response to *Chlamydia trachomatis* in Reiter's syndrome and nonspecific urethritis. Clin Exp Immunol. 1987;69:246.
142. Schumacher HR Jr, Cherian PV, Sieck M, et al. Ultrastructural identification of chlamydial antigens in synovial membrane in acute Reiter's syndrome (Abstract 115). Arthritis Rheum. 1986;29(Suppl 4):531.
143. Keat A, Thomas B, Dixey J, et al. *Chlamydia trachomatis* and reactive arthritis: The missing link. Lancet. 1987;1:72.
144. Jones RAK. Reiter's disease after *Salmonella typhimurium* enteritis. Br Med J. 1977;1:1391.
145. Noer HR. An "experimental" epidemic of Reiter's syndrome. JAMA. 1966;197:693.
146. Calin A. Reiter's syndrome. Med Clin North Am. 1977;61:365.
147. Paronon E. Reiter's disease: A study of 244 cases observed in Finland. Acta Med Scand. 1948;131(Suppl 212):1.
148. Urman JD, Zurier RB, Rothfield NF. Reiter's syndrome associated with *Campylobacter fetus* infection. Ann Intern Med. 1977;86:444.
149. Puddey I. Reiter's syndrome following antibiotic associated colitis. Aust NZ J Med. 1982;12:292.
150. Kobayashi S, Ogasawara M, Maeda K, et al. Antibodies against *Yersinia enterocolitica* in patients with Reiter's syndrome. J Lab Clin Med. 1985;105:380.
151. Weinberger HW, Ropes MW, Kulka JP, et al. Reiter's syndrome, clinical and pathologic observations. Medicine (Baltimore). 1962;41:35–91.
152. Smith DL, Bennett RM, Regan MG. Reiter's disease in women. Arthritis Rheum. 1980;23:335.
153. Good AE. Reiter's disease. Postgrad Med. 1977;61:153.
154. Catterall RD. Reiter's disease. In: Danielsson D, Juhlin L, Mardh P-A, eds. Genital Infections and Their Complications. Stockholm: Almquist & Widsell; 1975:205.
155. Marks JS, Holt PJL. The natural history of Reiter's disease—21 years of observations. Q J Med. 1986;60:685.
156. Morris R, Metzger AL, Bluestone R, et al. HL-A W27—a clue to the diagnosis and pathogenesis of Reiter's syndrome. N Engl J Med. 1974;290:554.
157. Mark DB, McCulley JB. Reiter's keratitis. Arch Ophthalmol. 1982;100:781.
158. Daunt SO, Kotowski KE, O'Reilly AP, et al. Ulcerative vulvitis in Reiter's syndrome. Br J Vener Dis. 1982;58:405.
159. Arnett FC, McClusley OE, Schacter BZ, et al. Incomplete Reiter's disease: Discriminating features and HL-A W27 in diagnosis. Ann Intern Med. 1976;84:8.
160. Csonka GW. Recurrent attacks in Reiter's disease. Arthritis Rheum. 1960;3:164.
161. Catterall RD. The role of microbiol infection in Reiter's syndrome. In: Dumonde DC, ed. Infection and Immunology in the Rheumatic Diseases. Oxford: Blackwell Scientific Publications; 1976:147.
162. Butler J, Russell AS, Percy JS, et al. A followup study of 48 patients with Reiter's syndrome. Am J Med. 1979;67:808.
163. Calin A, Fried JF. An "experimental" epidemic of Reiter's syndrome revisited. Ann Intern Med. 1976;84:564.
164. Ruppert GB, Lindsay J, Barth WF. Cardiac conduction abnormalities in Reiter's syndrome. Am J Med. 1982;73:335.
165. Montanaro A, Bennett RM. Myelopathy in Reiter's disease. J Rheumatol. 1984;11:540.
166. Ford DK. Reiter's syndrome: Current concepts of etiology and pathogenesis. In: Hobson D, Holmes KK, eds. Nongonococcal Urethritis and Related Infection. Lake Placid, NY: American Society for Microbiology; 1976:64.
167. Editorial. Treating Reiter's syndrome. Lancet. 1987;2:1125.

95. VULVOVAGINITIS AND CERVICITIS

MICHAEL F. REIN

THE NORMAL VAGINA

Under the influence of estrogens, the vaginal epithelium becomes cornified and supports a prodigious microbial flora. This adult microenvironment may develop transiently in neonates because of transplacentally acquired maternal estrogens[1] but resolves within several weeks as they are metabolized. The prepubescent vagina supports a flora rich in anaerobic bacteria, in particular, more *Bacteroides* species than are commonly found in the adult.[2] *Staphylococcus epidermidis* is frequently recovered,[2] and yeasts and *Gardnerella vaginalis* are isolated from 10 percent.[2,3] The vagina again matures in the immediate premenarchal period. In its mature state the vagina is colonized by a variety of bacteria,[4–8] primarily obligate and facultative anaerobes. More than 10^5 lactobacilli/ml of vaginal material are recovered from three-quarters and viridans streptococci and *Staphylococcus epidermidis* from almost half of asymptomatic women of childbearing age. Surprisingly, 10^5 *Bacteroides* were recovered from only one-sixth of these women[4,5,7,8] and *Gardnerella vaginalis* from 30–90 percent.[9,10] *Staphylococcus aureus* is recovered from the vaginas of only about 5 percent of healthy women.[11] Pregnancy has little effect on the distribution of most of the bacteria,[6,7] although the flora varies slightly during the menstrual cycle. Yeasts are carried by about 15–20 percent of healthy women.[12] With the onset of sexual activity, statistically significant increases are observed in the prevalence of *G. vaginalis*, lactobacilli, mycoplasmas, and ureaplasmas, but the prevalences of group B streptococci, *S. aureus*, and yeasts are not significantly altered.[13] It is of interest that ureaplasmas and *G. vaginalis* are recovered from 20–25 percent of young women who have not commenced sexual activity.[13]

Although our descriptive knowledge of vaginal microbiology has increased, our understanding of the factors controlling the flora remains primitive.[14] Specific and nonspecific vaginal host defenses have been catalogued, but again, their precise significance is unclear.[15]

Mucoid endocervical secretions combine with sloughed vaginal epithelial cells and normal bacteria to form a physiologic vaginal discharge. This material is usually unnoticed but may produce symptomatic "leukorrhea." It is often increased during pregnancy or with the use of oral contraceptives.

VULVOVAGINITIS

Vulvovaginitis is a common clinical syndrome and is diagnosed in more than one-quarter of women attending sexually transmitted disease clinics.[16] Treatment should be based on a specific etiologic diagnosis that can usually be made at the time of the initial evaluation.[17]

Candidiasis

The archaic term *moniliasis* should be discarded.[18] *Candida albicans* is isolated from about 80 percent of cases of vulvovaginal candidiasis, and other species of *Candida* account for about 15 percent.[19] *Candida tropicalis* infections may be associated with a higher rate of recurrence after standard treatments.[20] *Torulopsis glabrata* accounts for 3–16 percent of vaginal yeast isolates.[9,19] Symptomatic vaginitis caused by this organism is not distinguished from that caused by other *Candida* species in terms of clinical features or response to therapy,[21,22] and it is not dealt with separately.

Vulvovaginal candidiasis (VC) accounts for about one-third of vaginitis cases seen in private practice.[23] Some workers have estimated that 75 percent of adult women suffer at least one episode of VC during their lifetimes.[12] Yeast carried vaginally in small numbers and producing no symptoms may be considered part of the normal vaginal flora. If conditions in the vagina change so as to give the yeast an advantage over competing normal vaginal bacteria, VC may result. Inhibition of normal bacterial flora by broad-spectrum antibiotics favors the growth of yeasts. Thus yeasts were isolated from about 10 percent of women before but from 30 percent of women after 2- to 3-week courses of various tetracyclines.[9] Vulvovaginal candidiasis is said to follow 6–8 percent of single doses and 26 percent of 1-week courses of metronidazole.[24]

Overgrowth of yeasts is apparently favored by high estrogen levels. Vulvovaginal candidiasis is more common in pregnancy; it occurs in 10 percent of first-trimester women and 36–55 percent of women in their third trimesters.[9] Symptomatic disease has eventually developed in 60–90 percent of pregnant carriers, and old inoculation studies confirm the increased susceptibility of pregnant women.[9] Some nonpregnant women note recurrent or increasing symptoms preceding each menstrual period. The association with oral contraceptives surprisingly remains somewhat controversial.[9] The prevalence of vaginal carriage of *Candida* is higher among users of oral contraceptives than among women using other methods of birth control, and the percentage of these women developing symptoms is about the same in both groups.[25] Sequential regimens seem to predispose less than does a combination tablet.[9,26] Small series and anecdotal reports suggest that some patients with recurrent VC can be cured only when oral contraceptives are discontinued.[9] The mechanism of estrogenic predisposition is unclear, although some investigators have suggested that increased vaginal glycogen stores may play a role[9] or that estrogens influence vaginal pH in a way that makes the milieu more hospitable to the fungi.[12] An estrogen receptor in the cytosol of *C. albicans* suggests a possible direct effect of gestational hormones on the organism.[27] This mechanism has also been adduced to explain the association of VC with poorly controlled diabetes melitus.

It has been suggested that tight, insulating clothing predisposes to VC by increasing vulvar warmth and moisture. In a prospective study, a higher prevalence of candidal carriage and higher concentrations of organisms were found among women wearing tight rather than loose clothing.[28–30] Impaired immunity also predisposes to VC, and severe, refractory disease plagues women with the acquired immunodeficiency syndrome (AIDS).[31]

The mechanism by which *Candida* produces disease is not well defined. Strains isolated from symptomatic women are not demonstrably different in the laboratory than are isolates from asymptomatic carriers.[32] Filamentous forms (hyphae and pseudohyphae) are associated with active disease.[18] Pseudohyphae have been observed to penetrate vaginal epithelial cells[33] and are more adherent to cells than are blastospores.[34] Adherence appears to be an important pathogenic feature of *Candida* species,[35] and sublethal concentrations of antifungals may ameliorate disease by reducing adherence.[36]

The severity of symptoms in VC is not directly related to the number of yeasts present.[9] Indeed, very small numbers of yeasts may be present in vaginal material recovered from highly symptomatic women.[9,25]

Patients with candidal vulvovaginitis generally complain of perivaginal pruritus, often with little or no discharge. Dysuria is occasionally noted and is likely to be perceived as vulvar rather than urethral. The labia may be pale or erythematous, and excoriations may be noted. Tiny satellite papules or papulopustules just beyond the main area of erythema are helpful diagnostically. The vaginal walls may be erythematous. Candidal discharge is classically thick and adherent and contains curds. It may, however, be thin and loose and thus resemble the discharges of other vaginitides.

The vaginal pH is generally normal (approximately 4.5) in women with VC[37–39] in contrast to trichomoniasis or bacterial vaginosis. Thus, demonstrating a normal pH (see below) in a woman with signs and symptoms of vaginitis suggests that she has candidiasis rather than one of the other infections. The addition of 10% KOH to vaginal discharge on a slide or in the speculum (see below) fails to elicit a fishy odor in most women with VC. Such an odor (a positive "whiff test") suggests other infections.

An attempt should be made to demonstrate the organism on a wet mount of vaginal discharge. Although classic descriptions and most textbook pictures suggest that extensive tangles of filamentous forms can be seen, many patients in fact carry only small numbers of yeasts. Indeed, direct microscopic examination fails to reval fungi in 30–50 percent of infected women,[12,40,41] and a presumptive diagnosis must occasionally be made on other grounds with confirmation by culture or by antigen detection tests.[42] The discharge usually contains relatively few polymorphonuclear neutrophils.

Because many women carry yeasts in their vaginas, the examining physician faces a problem in interpretation: can a patient's vaginitis be attributed to the small number of yeasts present in her vagina, or has the vaginitis another etiology with the *Candida* present only by coincidence? Candidal vulvovaginitis should be diagnosed only after careful consideration of the total clinical picture of the history, physical examination, and laboratory data. Simultaneous infection with other organisms is not rare.

Vulvovaginal candidiasis is usually treated with the topical application of an antifungal agent. The striking variety of available drugs and regimens attests to the difficulty often encountered in satisfactorily managing this infection.[43]

Commercially available preparations are characterized by high patient acceptability and safety in pregnancy. Most of the commercially available drugs are polyenes (e.g., candicidin, which is no longer available in the United States, and nystatin) or imidazoles (e.g., clotrimazole, miconazole, butoconozole, terconazole, and econazole). They are available in a variety of forms including creams, tablets, and coated tampons.[39] It is difficult to compare therapies directly because of the variety of protocols used in various studies. Odds reviewed studies published through 1975 and concluded that in general imidazoles cured about 90 percent of patients and were superior to polyenes, which cured about 80 percent.[44] He could find no significant difference between delivery systems consisting of creams or vaginal tablets. More recent reviews generally support Odds' observations.[9,43]

Current interest centers on shorter courses of therapy. Seven days of treatment with miconazole cream yields cure rates ranging from 80 to 94 percent, results that are not significantly different from those obtained by the older 14-day regimen,[9] and a currently recommended therapy consists of a 100 mg intravaginal dose nightly for 7 nights. Tampons coated with 100 mg of miconazole are available in Europe.[39] Intravaginal treatment with 100 mg of clotrimazole for 6 or 7 days has produced cure rates of 88–94 percent.[9] Recent studies support the use of 200 mg of clotrimazole or miconazole or 100 mg of butoconazole inserted daily for 3 days, which produces approximately equivalent cure rates,[45–51] although some reviews suggest marginally better results with 7 days of therapy.[45] Because patients' compliance is likely to be better, it seems reasonable to recommend the 3-day regimen. Econazole is not currently marketed in the United States but produces effects roughly equivalent to those seen with clotrimazole. Mild systemic symptoms have followed its topical use.[43]

A few studies have examined the efficacy of single-dose treatments with larger amounts of imidazoles such as 500 mg of clotrimazole.[46,47,52,53] Such regimens may be preferred for the sake of convenience in the treatment of mild infections. Cure rates obtained in some studies have not quite matched those obtained with longer courses. Treatment in pregnancy is more often unsuccessful, and the longer-course regimens may be preferred in this setting.

Nystatin is a polyene that has been used in the United States for many years in a regimen consisting of one 100,000 unit tablet inserted intravaginally daily for 14 days. Although older series suggested a cure rate of about 80 percent,[44] recent studies have yielded cure rates in excess of 90 percent, approximately equivalent to those obtained with the imidazoles.[9] It must be remembered, however, that treatment with nystatin requires 2 weeks as compared with shorter-course regimens now recommended for the imidazoles.

Ketoconazole is an orally administered and well-absorbed imidazole of great value in treatment of systemic mycoses. A number of different regimens have been found effective in the treatment of VC.[9,54–56] Results do not appear to be substantially superior to those obtained with topical regimens, and the clinician must carefully consider the need for systemic therapy for VC in view of the potential toxicities of ketoconazole (see Chapter 33). Other orally absorbed imidazoles such as itraconazole and fluconazole may also have a future therapeutic role.[57]

Gentian violet, a classic treatment, has a low patient acceptability because it stains clothing. Povidone-iodine cures about 65 percent of patients.[58] It should probably be avoided in pregnancy because absorption of iodine might suppress fetal thyroid development.[59] In a single study, treatment with 600 mg of boric acid powder in gelatin capsules inserted intravaginally each evening for 14 days cured 92 percent of women.[60] Treatment of VC with various lactobacillus preparations has long been recommended in published anecdotes and in the lay press. Theoretically acting by restoring a normal bacterial flora that can successfully compete with yeasts, these regimens have not be evaluated in well-controlled trials.

Recurrent Infection. When patients treated for VC are recultured 3–6 weeks after the completion of therapy, a sizable proportion are found once again to harbor the yeasts. Results from a large number of studies[9,52,57,61] suggest a late recolonization rate of 21 ± 12 percent (mean ± SD), which is largely independent of the regimen used and often precedes symptomatic recurrence by 1–2 months.[54]

Recurrent symptomatic infection is a major problem. The mechanisms of recurrence remain obscure, but what is known has recently been analyzed by Sobel and colleagues.[12] Techniques for subspeciation of *Candida* are useful tools that will increase our understanding.[62,63] Such analyses suggest that about 40 percent of women with recurrent disease are demonstrably infected with new strains of *Candida*.[19] Obviously, women whose recurrence is associated with reappearance of the same strain might have suffered either recurrence or reinfection. The source of reinfection is poorly defined. Sexual transmission may be implicated in some cases. About 15 percent of women associate recurrences with sexual contact.[12] Yeasts are carried by 5 to 26 percent of male partners,[12,19] and 80 percent of the female partners of infected men are vaginally colonized.[12] Conjugal partners always carry the same strain.[12] Simultaneous treatment of male partners can delay symptomatic recurrence,[54] although the effect on vaginal recolonization is minimal.[54,57] Reinfection from contaminated douche equipment has also been proposed.[12]

Vaginal reinfection from a persistent rectal focus has been alleged, but support for this contention is weak. Admittedly, 40–70 percent of women with VC have positive rectal cultures, and 80 percent of doubly colonized women carry the same strain in rectal and vaginal sites,[12,19,64] but simultaneous treatment of a rectal focus with oral nystatin[65,66] or systemic ketoconazole[54–56] does not significantly lower recolonization or recurrence rates over vaginal therapy alone. One large recent study, however, suggests a benefit of oral nystatin,[67] with decreased colonization and symptomatic relapse rates during a relatively short 3–7 week follow-up period. The study population is not well defined but does not appear to have been specifically composed of women with frequently recurring disease. Care must be taken in interpreting these results. Whether certain individual women might benefit from coincident gastrointestinal therapy is unclear.

Endogenous vaginal relapse from small numbers of yeasts that survive chemotherapy has also been suggested. Intracellular residence may protect some fungal cells from antimycotic agents.[12,19] Small numbers of yeasts would certainly be invisible on wet mount and even by culture,[12] so early post-treatment evauation might erroneously suggest a cure.

As Lossick has remarked, the frequency with which *Candida* is carried asymptomatically suggests that mere reinoculation of yeasts is not an adequate cause of symptomatic recurrence.[68] Host susceptibility must also play a role. In addition to the risk factors described above, some women with recurrent VC appear to be mildly zinc deficient[69] or have defective cell-mediated immunity to yeasts.[70] The significance of these findings is unclear. Tolerance may be induced by chronic infection rather than acting as its cause.[12]

If our lack of understanding is dispiriting, our lack of effective therapy for recurrent VC is dramatically frustrating to patients and clinicians. One should attempt to reduce or eliminate the aforementioned risk factors. Short courses of antifungal therapy administered on the 5th–11th days of the menstrual cycle may reduce the rate of recurrence,[71] but such treatment rapidly becomes oppressively expensive. Simultaneous treatment of a rectal focus with oral nystatin or systemic treatment with ketoconazole does not significantly reduce the relapse rate.[56,65,66] Continuous treatment with ketoconazole, 100 mg orally per day, prevents recurrences but only for the duration of treatment.[55] Intermittent treatment at the time of menses permitted breakthrough recurrences in about one-quarter of the women.[54,55] In some cases of frequently recurrent VC, a switch to lower doses or to sequential oral contraceptives or even a discontinuance of oral contraceptives may be indicated. Oral glucose tolerance tests in such women have very low yield and are not routinely recommended.[12] Rarely, examination of sexual partners may reveal candidal balanitis, which could conceivably be a source of exogeneous reinfection.

The contribution of sexual transmission to vaginal candidiasis is apparently considerably smaller than for other forms of vaginitis. Balanitis, however, has been reported in 3–10 percent of the male sexual partners of women with candidal vulvovaginitis, and this condition is clearly sexually transmitted.[12,25,37,72] It responds to antifungal creams or ointments and treatment of the involved women. Some men develop pruritus within minutes of sexual contact. Symptoms usually resolve by the following day, and the syndrome may result from hypersensitivity to a partner's vaginal yeast.[12]

Trichomoniasis

Estimates based on the amount of metronidazole sold in this country suggest that 3 million Americans are infected with *Trichomonas vaginalis* each year. The disease is almost always sexually acquired and usually produces a combination of vaginal discharge and vulvovaginal irritation. About 25 percent of the women carrying trichomonads are asymptomatic, and the parasite has been recovered from up to 5 percent of sexually active asymptomatic women in Great Britain. The infection is discussed in detail in Chapter 258, to which the reader is referred.

Bacterial Vaginosis

Many young women with vulvovaginal signs or symptoms are not infected with *T. vaginalis* or *C. albicans*. Such women have been said to have "nonspecific vaginitis." This is an unfortunate term because it suggests an unknown etiology or a collection of undifferentiated diseases. Indeed, most of these women appear to have a specific condition first described by Gardner and Dukes in 1955, [73] and the condition is now usually referred to (perhaps unfortunately from the linguistic standpoint) as bacterial vaginosis (BV).[74] Inflammation and perivaginal irritation are often considerably milder than in trichomoniasis or candidiasis. Dysuria and dyspareunia are correspondingly rare. Affected women are sexually active and often complain predominantly of vaginal odor. This odor is described as "fishy" in the textbooks more frequently than by the patients. About 90 percent of patients also notice a mild to moderate discharge. Abdominal discomfort is occasionally present, but it is usually mild and should prompt evaluation for coincident infections including salpingitis.

Discharge is often present at the introitus and visible on the labia minora. The labia and vulva are generally not erythematous or edematous. On speculum examination the vaginal walls usually appear uninflamed. The vagina often contains a grayish, thin, homogeneous discharge manifesting small bubbles. This discharge differs from normal, physiologic discharge in that the latter has a floccular appearance and bubbles are absent. Although the discharge may be heavy enough to pool in the posterior fornix, it is usually present in smaller amounts. In some patients, the discharge may be so slight that it does not conspicuously pool. Because it is relatively thin but adherent to the vaginal walls, it is often apparent only as an increased light reflex. A distinct, pungent odor may be noted by the examiner.

The endocervix is unaffected by the process, and cervical discharge should be physiologic and therefore mucoid. The presence of a purulent cervical discharge or frank cervicitis is not rare but results from coincident gonococcal, chlamydial, or herpetic infection.[75] Abnormalities on bimanual examination are distinctly unusual and should prompt a search for other pathologic processes.

Other vaginal infections may closely resemble BV; an accurate differential diagnosis depends on laboratory examination of the genital specimen. The pH of vaginal discharge is elevated above the normal of 4.5 in about 90 percent of women with BV.[73,76,77] Although the pH may also be elevated in trichomoniasis, it is usually normal in vulvovaginal candidiasis. A vaginal pH ≥ 6 strongly suggests infection.[78] If 10% KOH is added to vaginal discharge samples either in the speculum blade or on a microscope slide, a distinctively pungent, fishy odor is generated.[8,9,76,79–81] This positive "whiff test" has been used as part of the case definition of BV by some workers and has been found to be positive in about 70 percent of cases in other series.[76,80] The accuracy of this test appears to improve with experience,[81] but the test is also positive in some patients with trichomoniasis, and its predictive value is therefore limited in populations with a high prevalence of the protozoal infection.

Bacterial vaginosis is perhaps most easily differentiated from trichomoniasis on the basis of direct microscopic examination of vaginal discharge. A wet mount of the discharge from patients with BV reveals clue cells, which are vaginal epithelial cells studded with tiny coccobacilli. These organisms are best appreciated at the edges of the cell (Fig. 1) but may be dense enough partially to obscure the nucleus. Not all cells in the specimen are clue cells, but some clue cells are seen in over 90 percent of patients with BV.[81,82] Predominant bacterial flora can also be assessed on a wet mount slide. In healthy women, the predominant morphotype is a large rod (presumably *Lactobacillus* species). In the discharge from a patient with BV, these rods have been completely supplanted by clumps of coccoba-

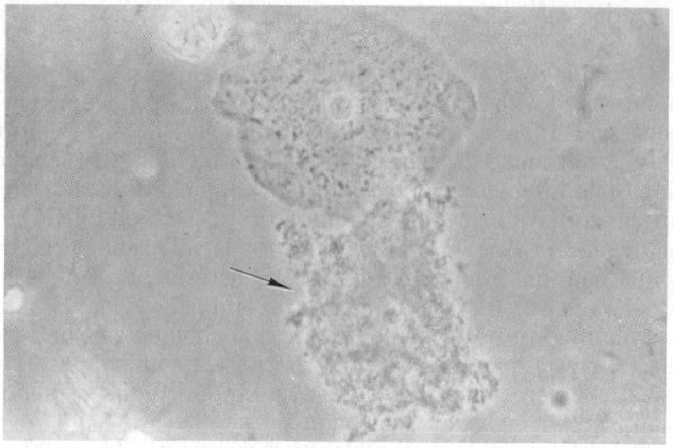

FIG. 1. A wet mount of vaginal discharge from a patient with bacterial vaginosis shows a normal epithelial cell (above) and a clue cell (below, arrow). (Phase microscopy, ×400)

cilli. Similar discrimination can be made on the basis of a Gram stain of the vaginal discharge.[9] Discharge in BV contrains few polymorphonuclear neutrophils (PMNs). This may in part explain the absence of the green or yellow color that frequently characterizes the discharge in trichomoniasis. About one PMN per epithelial cell is considered normal in a vaginal wet mount. Finding increased numbers of PMNs in a patient with BV suggests the presence of a second inflammatory process, often coincidental cervicitis.[75]

Culture for *Gardnerella vaginalis* is easily accomplished on a variety of media (Chapter 202). The organism is isolated from 98 percent of women with BV,[81] but also is recovered in smaller numbers[82] from up to 70 percent of some populations of asymptomatic women,[2,3,9,10,13,83,84] and its presence does not therefore prove that the patient has BV.[84] Thin-layer chromatography, gas–liquid chromatography, and enzyme assays can be used to diagnose BV by identifying specific bacterial products.[9,77,85,86] These techniques are not routinely available, but provide insight into the pathophysiology of BV.

Amsel et al.[81] suggest that the clinician look for a pH greater than 4.5; homogeneous, white, adherent vaginal discharge; a positive whiff test; and clue cells. Finding any three of these four signs strongly supports the diagnosis of BV, although an abnormal discharge, an elevated pH, and a positive whiff test often accompany trichomoniasis as well. The final diagnosis and decision to treat depends, however, on a complete evaluation of the patient. An isolated finding of clue cells in asymptomatic women does not demand treatment.

Pathophysiology. Microscopic examination of vaginal discharge in BV characteristically reveals a predominant flora of coccobacilli. On the basis of morphology this organism was originally called *Haemophilus vaginalis*[73] It has been transferred to its own genus and is now called *Gardnerella* in honor of Dr. Gardner's initial observations (Chapter 203).[87]

Several observations suggest a less than straightforward relationship between *G. vaginalis* and BV. Although Gardner and Dukes regularly produced BV by inoculating fresh vaginal discharge from patients into the vaginas of healthy recipients, inoculation of pure cultures of *G. vaginalis* was far less likely to produce disease.[73] In addition, *G. vaginalis* is isolated from 30–70 percent of asymptomatic women,[2,3,9,10,13,81,83,84] and only 50 percent of women with heavy vaginal colonization by *G. vaginalis* actually have BV.[84] Finally, the in vitro sensitivity of *G. vaginalis* to antimicrobial agents does not match the effectiveness of these agents in clinical disease. Metronidazole is highly effective therapy for BV[76,79,88–92] despite the fact that *G. vaginalis* is relatively resistant to the drug in vitro.[76,90,93]

An explanation for all these observations is that *G. vaginalis* is not the single cause of BV. There is considerable experimental support for the hypotheseis that BV is actually a synergistic infection involving not only *G. vaginalis* but certain anaerobic bacteria as well.[8,9,76,77,80,86,92,94] Various *Bacteroides* species other than *B. fragilis* and various peptococci are principally involved. Asymptomatic carriers of *G. vaginalis* might lack the anaerobic synergants. Pure cultures of *G. vaginalis* would not be able to produce clinical disease in patients lacking the other necessary bacteria, but the vaginal discharge from symptomatic women would be expected to contain all the necessary bacterial components. Drugs relatively inactive against *G. vaginalis* might still cure the disease if they acted against the other bacteria, and metronidazole is highly active against most strict anaerobes. The characteristic odor of BV is due to various aromatic amines such as putrescine and cadaverine, which are produced by anaerobes but not by *G. vaginalis*.[77] These aromatic diamines are volatilized at basic pH, which explains the positive whiff test associated with this infection.

Mycoplasmas are isolated from the vaginas of many women with BV.[13,14,95,96] A role in the production of BV has not been established.

Treatment. Many studies[76,79,88–92,97–100] have now shown that BV is most successfully treated with metronidazole, 500 mg orally twice daily or 250 mg orally three times daily for 7 days. Cure rates of over 90 pecent are reported. Most studies suggest that single doses of metronidazole are inadequate,[9,89–91,97–101] but tinidazole, a nitroimidazole with a longer half life that is available in Europe, cured 80 percent of patients after a single 2 g administration.[102] Ampicillin is highly active in vitro against *G. vaginalis*, with minimum inhibitory concentrations (MICs) of less than 2 μg/ml for most strains.[9,92,98] BV has been treated with 500 mg of ampicillin administered four times daily for 7 days. Although some studies have yielded a cure rate of about 90 percent,[82,92] others have yielded cure rates of only 40–70 percent.[76,88] Amoxicillin in the same doses is minimally if at all superior.[91,92] The inferiority of ampicillin to metronidazole probably derives in part from its inactivation by penicillinase elaborated by *Bacteroides* species in the vagina[76,92]; however, the combination of amoxicillin with clavulanic acid is still inferior to metronidazole.[91] Ampicillin or amoxicillin treatment blocks recolonization of the vagina by normal lactobacilli, whereas metronidazole does not.[92] Recolonization with lactobacilli may be part of the recovery process from BV. A recent study suggests that clindamycin, 300 mg orally, twice daily for 7 days, is effective therapy for BV.[102a]

The value of oral cephalosporins for BV remains controversial. Gardner and Dukes praise them anecdotally,[73,103] as do other workers. Indeed, cephalexin, 500 mg taken four times daily for 1 week, has cured some women whose disease relapsed after repeated treatments with metronidazole. Oral therapy with tetracyclines or erythromycin has been disappointing.[9]

Topical therapy with clindamycin cream is under investigation and appears promising. Sulfanilamide-aminacrine-allantoin and providone-iodine have unacceptably low cure rates.[9] Triple sulfa preparations have been used topically for some decades, but small series suggest that the compounds are ineffective.[76,104] Topical therapy with yogurt does not work.[105]

Although BV behaves epidemiologically as if it were a sexually transmitted disease, there are no data supporting the need to treat asymptomatic male sexual partners initially.[9] *Gardnerella vaginalis* is recovered from the urethras of 80 percent of the male sexual partners of women with BV,[76] and recolonization with the organism is far more common in women reexposed to untreated male partners than to those who are not.[76] Some women suffer from frequently relapsing disease that can be controlled only by the simultaneous treatment of male sexual partners. These men carry *G. vaginalis*, and it is unclear whether they should be treated with metronidazole or ampicillin.

Asymptomatic carriage of *G. vaginalis* is common and need not be treated.

Other Infections with G. vaginalis. *Gardnerella vaginalis* has been identified in urine obtained by suprapubic aspiration from pregnant women, but the organisms are usually present in very small numbers, and pyuria is distinctly unusual.[106] Urinary tract infection in a man, a possible perinephric abscess in a transplanted kidney, and balanoposthitis have all been reported.[9] *Gardnerella vaginalis* has been carried asymptomatically in the urethras of sexually active men, but it is not associated with nongonoccal urethritis.

Gardnerella vaginalis and the associated anaerobic bacteria and mycoplasmas are frequently isolated from the endometrium and blood of patients with postpartum fever and endometritis.[95,107–111] Premature labor has been associated with BV.[109]

Curved Anaerobic Rods. Considerable recent interest concerns vaginitis associated with motile, curved anaerobic rods that are gram-negative or gram-variable.[112–118] These organisms, classified in the new genus *Mobiluncus,*[119] are sensitive to ampicillin, but some species are relatively resistant to metronidazole.[114,117] The precise pathogenic role of these organisms remains to be elucidated.

Staphylococci. *Staphylococcus aureus* is recovered from the vaginas of only about 5 percent of healthy women.[11] The organism is isolated, however, from most women with menstruation-associated toxic shock syndrome.[120,121] (Chapter 173). Frank vaginitis with a vaginal discharge has been observed in about one-third to three-quarters of these women, and a history of vaginitis is associated with an increased incidence of toxic shock syndrome.[122] The disease is usually characterized by vulvar edema and vulvar and vaginal erythema.[121] A vaginal discharge, purulent but often scanty, is observed in about one-quarter to one-third of these patients.[120,121] Vaginal ulceration was noted in about 7 percent of these women.[121] The pathogenesis of the vaginitis is not entirely understood. Toxic shock syndrome is manifested as a polymucositis, and vaginitis is also reported in about one-third of women who have nonmenstrual toxic shock syndrome, sometimes with the staphylococcal source at sites other than the vagina. Thus, the vaginitis may reflect direct infection or may be a secondary effect of staphylococcal toxin. The ulcerations sometimes observed may result from tampon use, with which toxic shock syndrome is associated (see below).

Foreign Body Vaginitis. Secondary anaerobic infections may be associated with foreign bodies in the vagina. In adults, the most common of these are the forgotten vaginal tampon and various contraceptive devices such as the diaphragm, cervical cap, or a condom that has slipped off during coitus. Objects apparently used in masturbation are occasionally implicated.[123] In children and the mentally incompetent, a variety of objects may be found.[1] These infections often produce an intensely foul odor, and the discharge is usually scanty and contains small amounts of blood. Therapy often requires only the removal of the offending object, but oral metronidazole may speed recovery.

Tampon use has been observed to affect the vaginal mucosa.[124–127] Extended tampon use, particularly of superabsorbent tampons, may produce local drying and peeling of the vaginal mucosa and result in frank ulceration of the vaginal wall and exocervix. Tampon fibers have been observed within ulcerations.[126] Microscopic ulcers have been noted in up to one-fifth of women using tampons,[123] and larger lesions are occasionally observed.[125,127] Ulceration may be associated with vaginal bleeding and pain on insertion of the tampons. Because of possible confusion with other ulcerating vaginal diseases including malignancy, a thorough work-up is essential.[127]

Herpes Simplex Virus. The adult vaginal epithelium is relatively resistant to herpetic infection. Vaginal lesions have been observed in only about 4 percent of infected women.[128,129] Fourteen percent of women with primary genital herpes developed vulvovaginal candidiasis during the second week of infection.[128,129] Treatment of these secondary infections, however, must be done carefully because the topical antifungal miconazole cream appears to be associated with delayed healing of genital herpetic lesions.[130] Indeed, the application of any occulsive preparation to herpetic lesions should probably be avoided,[128,129] and oral ketoconazole might be useful in this setting.

Other Specific Infections

True vaginal infections with other specific agents such as *Mycobacterium tuberculosis*, salmonellae, Enterobacteriaceae, actinomycetes, and schistosomes are rare and usually occur in patients with underlying diseases or who are systemically ill. Group A streptococcal vaginitis has been described in children aged 3–5 years old. It is manifested as a blood-tinged discharge, "firey red" vaginal mucosae, and dysuria. A Gram stain is usually negative, and the disease responds promptly to penicillin G.[131]

Pre-existing lesions due to other diseases may become secondarily infected with a mixed anaerobic flora of fusobacteria and spirochetes. Such "fusospirochetal" infections can progress rapidly. Metronidazole, 250 mg orally three times daily, is recommended therapy.

Pinworms are an occasional cause of perivaginal itching, especially in children.[1] Perianal pruritus that becomes worse at night may suggest this diagnosis. True vaginal infestation has been described.[132]

Neisseria gonorrhoeae and *C. trachomatis* can cause frank vaginitis in prepubescent girls.[133]

"Doderlein cytolysis", a condition characterized by irritative symptoms exacerbating in the premenstrual interval and theoretically caused by microbially induced hyperacidity, is poorly substantiated. It is said to result from an overgrowth of lactobacilli and to respond to alkalinizing douches.[134]

Noninfectious Vulvovaginitis

Genital neoplasm may produce an abnormal vaginal discharge. Such conditions are more common in older women and are usually manifested by the gradual onset of a thin, often foul-smelling discharge that may be blood tinged.

In postmenopausal women, the absence of estrogen stimulation results in atrophy of the vaginal epithelium, which may lead to an atrophic vaginitis. The vaginal walls become secondarily infected with a number of different organisms, but treatment of the primery disease often requires estrogenic supplementation.

Occasional cases of vulvovaginal inflammation from chemicals including deodorant sprays[135] and allergic reactions to semen[136] and nickel[137] have been reported.

Desquamative or purulent vaginitis is characterized by a vaginal discharge containing large numbers of polymorphonuclear neutrophils. The etiology and therapy of the condition are unknown, but lichen planus should be considered in the differential diagnosis.[138,139]

Conditions Imitating Vulvovaginitis

Physiologic or normal vaginal discharge is sometimes referred to as leukorrhea and generally consists of cervical mucus combined with desquamated vaginal epithelial cells. This material passes through the vaginal introitus where it is noted by the patient as a vaginal discharge. Neonates may have a transient physiologic discharge until transplacentally acquired maternal estrogens are metabolized. In the adult, the output of the endocervical glands is highly responsive to hormonal levels and sometimes increases at the time of ovulation or in the immediate premenstrual period. Oral contraceptives may increase the cervical component, and women sometimes note a new discharge when they start to use these agents. This leukorrhea may cause considerable concern since it often begins coincidentally with first sexual exposures, thus raising the specter of venereal disease. Physiologic discharge accounted for 10 percent of women attending a private practice with vaginal complaints.[23] It may be heavy enough to stain underwear and may dry to a brown residue, which patients sometimes associate with infectious vaginitis. Unlike most infections, it is usually not associated with perineal burning or pruritus, dyspareunia, or dysuria, but odor is sometimes described.[140] Abdominal pain does not occur unless another process is present. Microscopic examination reveals normal vaginal flora and few polymorphonuclear neutrophils (PMNs). More than one PMN per epithelial cell is unusual in physiologic vaginal discharge.

Infectious cervicitis due to any of several different organisms may result in an inflammatory cervical discharge that passes through the vagina. This condition is discussed in a later section of this chapter.

A variety of inflammatory diseases confined to the perineum may produce symptoms suggesting vaginitis to the patient. The lesions of herpes genitalis or chancroid produce considerable perineal discomfort. Intertrigo may result in burning, an unpleasant odor, and staining of underwear. Infection of Bartholin's glands and Skene's glands sometimes produce perineal discomfort and a discharge and is dealt with in a later section of this chapter. Inflammatory diseases of the rectum occasionally result in a discharge that suggests vaginitis to the patient. Dysuria may be a symptom of urinary tract infection.

Of particular interest is a condition referred to as focal vulvitis or vestibular adenitis.[141,142] Affected women suffer vulvar pain and significant dyspareunia. They frequently undergo repeated treatments for vulvovaginal candidiasis, and they are often thought to be neurotic. Physical examination reveals rather subtle but exquisitely tender, erythematous patches, usually along the posterior portion of the introital ring. Biopsy demonstrates nonspecific inflammation of vestibular glands. Current therapy is surgical excision of the affected areas. An infectious etiology has not been demonstrated.

Vaginitis emphasematosa is an uncommon condition in which the vaginal walls contain submucosal, gas-filled cysts.[143] The exocervix too may be involved.[144] This benign condition is frequently associated with trichomoniasis.

Obstruction of the pelvic nodes is a rare cause of lymphatic weeping of the vagina. Massive lymphedema of the lower extremities usually accompanies this finding, and the diagnosis is not difficult.

There are small numbers of women who complain of vaginal discharge, discomfort, or odor without any objective findings.[145] Such women may be motivated by a neurotic fear of uncleanliness, guilt concerning sexual activities (or a desire to avoid them), or anxiety about venereal disease whether or not sexual exposure has actually taken place. These patients have often sought advice from numerous physicians and have symptoms that have failed to respond to a variety of standard therapies. They require careful and complete medical evaluation. The diagnosis of "worried well" must not be made without a thorough examination for physical disease. Women with psychosomatic complaints may respond to a careful and sympathetic explanation of the results of the examination and psychotherapy.[145]

Scabies, pediculosis, or enterobiasis may produce intense perivaginal itching and soreness.

APPROACH TO THE PATIENT WITH VAGINAL COMPLAINTS

History

The etiologic diagnosis of vaginitis depends on a careful evaluation of the history, physical examination, and immediate laboratory tests. Historical features are relatively nonspecific,[9] but they may direct clinical suspicion toward certain causes.

Age. Neonates can acquire trichomonal or candidal vulvovaginitis during passage through an infected birth canal, an argument for treating these infections in pregnant women before term. Neonatal vaginal thrush responds promptly to topical antifungal medications such as nystatin.[1] Neonatal trichomoniasis often does not require specific therapy and disappears when the estrogens are metabolized.[146] Thereafter, any vaginal discharge is abnormal and should prompt a vigorous search for disease. Immediately before menarche, physiologic discharge may reappear. Prepubescent vaginal epithelium is not cornified, and the entire vagina is susceptible to infection with *Neisseria gonorrhoeae* or *Chlamydia trachomatis*. Gonococcal vulvovaginitis often causes profuse vaginal discharge, and the rectum is almost always involved. Vaginal candidiasis is extremely rare in prepubescent girls.[147] A diagnosis of sexually transmitted disease in a young girl should raise the suspicion of child abuse, although some agents have been transmitted to children in the absence of frank sexual contact.

Patients in the sexually active years are more likely to have a sexually transmitted disease. Genital neoplasia is more common among older women, and postmenopausal women are more likely to have atrophic vaginitis.

Mode of Onset. An abrupt and identifiable time of onset of symptoms suggests infection. Vaginal discharge associated with neoplasia, estrogen depletion, or a foreign body often has a subacute onset with symptoms progressing over a period of weeks. Symptoms beginning during or immediately after the menstrual period are somewhat suggestive of trichomoniasis, and a premenstrual onset more frequently accompanies candidiasis.

Quantity of Discharge. The amount of discharge is highly variable in all conditions. Patients with candidiasis often have scanty discharge or note no discharge at all. Atrophic or neoplastic discharges are commonly scanty unless infection has supervened.

Perineal Irritation. Physiologic discharge is rarely associated with perineal discomfort. Pruritus with a scanty or absent discharge is frequently seen in candidiasis and less commonly with trichomoniasis. Perineal discomfort is an infrequent complaint in BV. Severe episodic perineal pain sometimes preventing urination is strongly suggestive of herpes genitalis, which affects the labia but usually spares the vagina per se.[128,129] Chronic discomfort, often interfering with sexual activity, should prompt consideration of focal vulvitis.[141,142]

Odor. An unpleasant odor accompanies many vaginal infections and sometimes physiologic discharge as well.[140] Vaginal odor in the absence of other symptoms is the initial complaint in many cases of BV. A feculent odor may accompany anaerobic superinfection of genital lesions or may be noted in the presence of a foreign body.

Abdominal Pain. Abdominal discomfort is rare in uncomplicated vulvovaginitis except for occasional cases of trichomoniasis. Women complaining of abdominal pain should be examined carefully for evidence of coincidental infections including cystitis and pelvic inflammatory disease.

Sexual History. Exposure to a new sexual partner increases the likelihood of sexually transmitted disease. A history of genital symptoms in a sexual partner is helpful diagnostically. The commencement of oral contraceptive use may be associated with increased physiologic discharge. The use of tampons, particularly the prolonged use of superabsorbent tampons, may be associated with ulcerative vaginitis.[124–127]

Other Diseases. Diabetes, AIDS,[31] malignancy and treatment thereof, and possibly hypoparathyroidism increase the risk of candidal vaginitis. Diseases known to impair host defenses may predispose to otherwise rare infections. Other diseases may be treated with drugs that predispose to vaginal infection.

Medication. Systemic or local medication may influence the spectrum of vaginal infection. Antibiotics, particularly tetracyclines and ampicillin, are active against much of the normal bacterial flora of the vagina, and their use predisposes to candidal vaginitis. Metronidazole is active against vaginal anaerobes and also predisposes to candidal infection, but less frequently than with many other antimicrobials. Low doses of many antibiotics can interfere with the isolation of *N. gonorrhoeae* and possibly *G. vaginalis*. Low-dose antibiotics may result in the development of atypical syphilitic chancres or may eliminate the primary stage of syphilis entirely.

Patients taking corticosteroids or oral contraceptives are at increased risk for developing candidal vaginitis. Oral contraceptive use may also be associated with the development of a physiologic vaginal discharge.

Local medication including vaginal douches may produce a chemical vaginitis, but douching immediately before examination may make etiologic diagnosis difficult.

Examination of the Female Genitalia

With the patient supine on the examining table, the pubic hair should be examined for the presence of crab lice or nits. The inguinofemoral areas are palpated for adenopathy. Superpubic and lower abdominal tenderness or masses are sought by palpation.

With the patient in the lithotomy position, the labia and the perineum should be examined for erythema, lichenification, excoriation, and discrete lesions. Diffuse perineal erythema may accompany trichomoniasis or candidiasis. Diffuse reddening with small satellite lesions, usually papular or papulopustular, suggests candiadiasis. The degree of perineal irritation is quite variable with all infectioins, but severe perivaginal irritation is uncommon with BV. Labial edema may accompany severe irritation.

Careful examination of all the extravaginal surfaces may reveal lesions of herpes genitalis, syphilis, condyloma accuminatum, molluscum contagiosum, scabies (which are discussed in Chapter 92) or focal vulvitis. Even though the patient's chief complaint may strongly suggest a true vaginitis, examination of the external genitalia for coincident infections is very important because multiple, coexistent sexually transmitted diseases are common.

By spreading the labia with the gloved hand, the urethral meatus is examined. The urethra may be gently stripped with the finger placed inside the introitus. Urethral discharge is not a common finding, but if delivered, such material should be examined microscopically and cultured. The introitus and the internal surfaces of the labia minora should be examined for lesions.

Vaginal discharge is sometimes observed on the labia or actually running out onto the perineum. Such copius discharge is usually associated with trichomoniasis but may accompany other infections.

If the patient has had a hysterectomy, a calcium alginate urethral swab should be inserted gently into the urethra and recovered material inoculated for gonococcal culture. This is unnecessary if the cervix is present since gonococci are more often recovered from the cervix than from the urethra. The urethra is frequently the only site from which *C. trachomatis* can be recovered.

A vaginal speculum moistened with warm water is gently inserted. In the presence of severe herpes genitalis or, occasionally, trichomoniasis, insertion of the speculum may be impossible because of the patient's discomfort. In such a case, a preliminary diagnosis is sometimes made from material recovered on a cotton swab gently inserted into the vagina.

After the speculum has been inserted, the vaginal walls are examined. Candidal or trichomonal vaginitis is often accompanied by erythema of the vaginal walls. The degree of erythema, however, is often very difficult to assess in an individual patient. Punctate hemorrhages of the vaginal walls strongly suggest trichomoniasis. A diffuse sheen, manifested by an increased light reflex, may be caused by thin discharge adhering to the walls. This is seen most frequently with BV but may accompany other infections. Fingerlike projections within the vagina may be condylomata accuminata, but these must be differentiated from hymenal tags. The latter are normal but are usually found only near the introitus.

The surface of the cervix may be inflamed. Punctate hemorrhages are rarely observed in patients with severe trichomoniasis (strawberry cervix), and ulcerations may be present with herpetic cervicitis. Mucoid material is normally observed at the cervical os and is present in increased amounts in women taking oral contraceptives. A normal cervical discharge may be clear or white. A purulent or mucopurulent discharge is associated with infectious cervicitis, primarily chlamydial, gonococcal, or herpetic.

Bimanual examination for adnexal tenderness and masses should be a part of the examination. Adnexal tenderness is uncommon with local vaginal infections and suggests salpingitis; palpation of abnormal adnexal mass may indicate a tuboovarian abscess or ectopic pregnancy and requires prompt gynecologic or surgical consultation.

The anus should be examined for the presence of discharge, chancres, or condylomata. A glove used in vaginal examination should never be introduced into the rectum since this may inoculate the rectum with gonococci, chlamydia, or herpes simplex virus.

Other Bedside Evaluation. After the speculum is withdrawn, the pH of vaginal secretions can be determined by inserting a strip of indicator paper in the material collected in the lower lip of the speculum. We have found nitrazine paper with a pH range of 4.5–7.0 to be useful. A normal pH of 4.5 is seen in most patients with vulvovaginal candidiasis, whereas a pH elevated to 5.0 or above is associated with BV and trichomoniasis.

If several drops of 10% KOH then added to the material on the speculum elicit a pungent, fishy, aminelike odor, this would constitute a positive "whiff test." The whiff test is positive in more than 90 percent of patients with BV and in many patients with trichomoniasis. It is negative in women with vulvovaginal candidiasis. The whiff test may also be performed on a slide that has been prepared for KOH microscopic examination.

Laboratory Examination

A wet mount is of greatest value in the differential diagnosis of a vaginal discharge, and the specimen may be prepared in several ways. A swab of vaginal discharge may be agitated in a tube containing about 1 ml of normal saline. One drop of the resulting suspension is put on a microscope slide, and a coverslip is applied. Alternatively, the examiner may place a drop of saline on the slide and mix in a loopful of vaginal material, after which a coverslip is applied. The slide is examined initially under low power on a brightfield microscope with the substage condenser racked down or with the substage diaphragm closed down to increase the contrast. Phase-contrast microscopy is becoming more widely available in clinical settings and provides an excellent means of examining vaginal wet mounts.

The relative numbers of epithelial cells and polymorphonuclear neutrophils (PMNs) should be noted. PMNs are present in physiologic endocervical discharge[148] that collects in the vagina, so small numbers of PMNs may be observed in the vaginal material recovered from healthy women. A finding of more than one PMN per epithelial cell should raise the examiner's suspicion of cervical or vaginal inflammation. Observing relatively few PMNs, however, does not rule out vaginal infection. Vaginal candidiasis often produces a discharge containing small numbers of PMNs.[38] The relative absence of PMNs is characteristic of the discharge of BV.[9] In fact, finding many PMN in the vaginal discharge of a patient with BV should prompt the examiner to search for simultaneous infection such as trichomoniasis, gonorrhea, or chlamydial cervicitis.

Large clumps of pseudohyphae suggest vaginal candidiasis, but the examiner often sees only moderate or even very small numbers of yeasts in this condition. Indeed, some patients with vulvovaginal candidiasis have organisms identified only by culture. The wet preparation should be scanned for motile trichomonads.

The wet mount should then be observed under high power (×400). Normal squamous epithelial cells have transparent cytoplasm and small nuclei. Epithelial cells covered with tiny coccobacillary forms (Fig. 1) are called "clue cells" and are associated with BV. Clue cells are best recognized by observing the edges of epithelial cells, which may be obscured by the adherent coccobacilli. Some cells are so heavily encrusted that the nuclei are obscured. Trichomonads are best be recognized by their characteristic twitching motility (Fig. 2). The flagella and undulating membrane may be observed by carefully focusing the microscope and adjusting the light source. Trichomonad motility is improved by gently warming the preparation. Unfortunately, the wet mount is negative in about 30 percent of the women with trichomoniasis (Chapter 258), and a negative wet mount does not rule out this infection, particularly in relatively asymptomatic women. A negative wet mount should be confirmed with a culture. Small numbers of *Candida* are frequently observed and do not necessarily indicate that the patient's vaginitis is of candidal etiology. Large numbers of *Candida*, frequent budding, and the presence of pseudohyphae add strength to the contention that *Candida* is the etiologic agent.

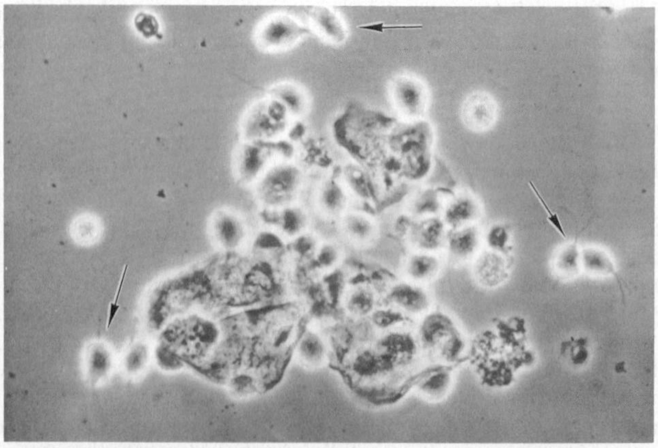

FIG. 2. A wet mount of vaginal discharge from a patient with trichomonal vaginitis shows epithelial cells, neutrophils, and trichomonads (arrows). (Phase microscopy, ×400)

The bacterial flora can often be assessed on the wet mount. Normal vaginal flora consist primarily of rods. In BV, the predominant flora is tiny coccobacilli.

Spermatozoa may be observed as long as 10 days after the last coitus. Motile sperm suggests sexual contact within the preceding 24 hours.[149]

Combining a drop of 10% or 20% KOH with the vaginal material on a microscope slide, applying a coverslip, and gently heating destroy epithelial cells and most microbial flora, leaving fungal elements behind. The potassium hydroxide preparation cannot be used for a microscopic diagnosis of trichomoniasis or BV, but elaboration of a fishy odor from the slide suggests these infections.

A Gram stain of vaginal material is generally less useful for the differential diagnosis than the wet mount. Normal vaginal flora consists primarily of gram-positive rods, which are presumably lactobacilli. In BV the normal flora is replaced by sheets of gram-variable coccobacilli, which may often be seen overlying the surface of epithelial cells. Small numbers of *Candida* are occasionally observed as dense, gram-positive ovoids, but the Gram stain is positive in fewer than one-third of the women from whom *Candida* can be cultured.[40] Women with active vaginal candidiasis often have large numbers of budding yeasts and pseudohyphae recognizable as thick gram-positive or beaded tubes. The Gram stain of vaginal material should not be used for the diagnosis of gonorrhea or trichomoniasis. Trichomonads are recognized only with difficulty on a Gram stain, and gonorrhea is a cervicitis rather than vaginitis in the adult.

Material recovered from the endocervix can be Gram stained. Cervical discharge always contains moderate numbers of PMNs, and their presence is not necessarily an indication of specific inflammation.[148] Large numbers of PMNs indicate cervicitis. Gram-negative, intracellular diplococci accurately diagnose gonorrhea (see Chapter 190), but extracellular diplococci are of no significance since nonpathogenic *Neisseria* is part of the normal flora of the female genital tract. Unfortunately, the cervical Gram stain is positive in only about one-half of the women with cervical gonorrhea, and a negative Gram stain does not rule out the infection.[40] Trichomonads are only infrequently found in the endocervix, and cervical material should not be used to examine for trichomoniasis. Cervical material recovered from women at risk should be cultured for *N. gonorrhoeae* and evaluated for *C. trachomatis*. The Papanicolaou smear may reveal *T. vaginalis* or clue cells, but neither of these findings is sufficiently sensitive for a negative result to rule out infection. Direct staining of cervical specimens using the Giemsa or Papanicolaou methods is insufficiently sensitive for the diagnosis of chlamydial cervicitis (Chapter 158).

CERVICITIS

Under the influence of estrogens, the normal vaginal epithelium cornifies and becomes relatively resistant to infection with a number of pathogens. The endocervix, however, is lined with columnar epithelium, which remains susceptible to many of these infections. Therefore, the examiner frequently finds infectious cervicitis in the absence of vaginitis and vice versa. Studies of the etiology of cervicitis have been hampered by the lack of a reliable definition of the syndrome.[74,150,151] Erythema around the cervical os may indicate infection or may merely represent cervical *erosion* or *eversion*, terms applied to the migration of endocervical epithelium over the surface of the cervix. Such lesions are usually symmetric about the os and are not particularly friable. They are more common in women taking oral contraceptives, and it may be impossible on clinical grounds alone to differentiate these from true infection. *Hypertrophic cervicitis*, on the other hand, is manifested as an intensely erythematous, raised, irregular lesion that bleeds easily.[75,150–152] Normal cervical discharge is clear and mucoid. Purulent or mucopurulent discharge is associated with gonococcal or chlamydial infection.[75,153–155] The color and quality of the cervical discharge can be assessed by obtaining endocervical material on a swab and comparing its consistency and color against a well-illuminated sheet of white paper or cloth. Polymorphonuclear neutrophils are normally present in the endocervix,[148] but abnormally increased numbers can be detected crudely on a Gram stain of endocervical material. After the exocervix has been cleaned off, a swab is inserted into the cervix and gently rotated, and the recovered material is applied to a microscope slide by rolling the swab over an area about 1 × 2 cm. The specimen is then Gram stained. Observing more than 10 polymorphonuclear neutrophils per oil-immersion field in the densest portion of the slide correlates statistically with the presence of gonococci or chlamydiae,[75,154,156] but the sensitivity and positive predictive value of the observation are far too low for a definitive diagnosis.

Specific Etiologies of Acute Cervicitis

The clinical features of specific cervical infections overlap too much to permit an accurate etiologic diagnosis without laboratory assistance.[75,150,157] Multiple infections are common[157] and may be missed if the diagnosis is attempted on clinical grounds alone.

Acute gonococcal cervicitis has been known for hundreds of years. The endocervix is the site from which gonococci are most frequently isolated in women with uncomplicated gonococcal infections. In typical cases the cervical os is reddened and productive of a purulent discharge.[158] A Gram stain of this material reveals typical gram-negative cell-associated diplococci in only about one-half of the infected women[40] (Fig. 3), and a negative Gram stain must never be used as an argument against treating women for uncomplicated gonorrhea. Examination for gonococcal cervicitis must include an appropriate culture. The sensitivity of the endocervical culture is disputed but is generally held to be on the order of 90 percent. Most women with uncomplicated gonococcal cervicitis are asymptomatic, but about one-third note vaginal discharge.[148,158]

Chlamydia trachomatis can be recovered from the endocervix of 60–90 percent of the sexual partners of men with chlamydial urethritis.[148,150–152,159,160] Cervical abnormalities, often subtle, have been observed in 80–90 percent of chlamydiae-positive women.[148,150–152,159,160] Most of these women are asymptomatic, but about one-third note a discharge from the vagina[148] that actually originates in the inflamed cervix. Chlamydiae have been isolated from 50–90 percent of sexually active patients with hypertrophic cervicitis.[148] Only 19–32 percent of women with chlamydial cervical infection manifest hypertrophic cervicitis, and only about 30 percent have a mucopurulent or purulent cervical discharge.[148,150,151,153,161] On examination 20–70 percent[153,161] of women have a completely normal cervix. Therefore, physical examination is never adequate to exclude chlamydial infection, similar to the situation with gonococcal cervicitis. Because chlamydiae are isolated from over 40–50 percent of the female partners of men with chlamydial nongonoccal urethritis, female partners should be epidemiologically treated even before the diagnosis of chlamydial infection is confirmed by laboratory techniques.

Chlamydiae can be identified in cervical specimens from 75 to 95 percent of infected women by using immunofluoresence microscopy.[153,161–163] An enzyme immunoassay is also about

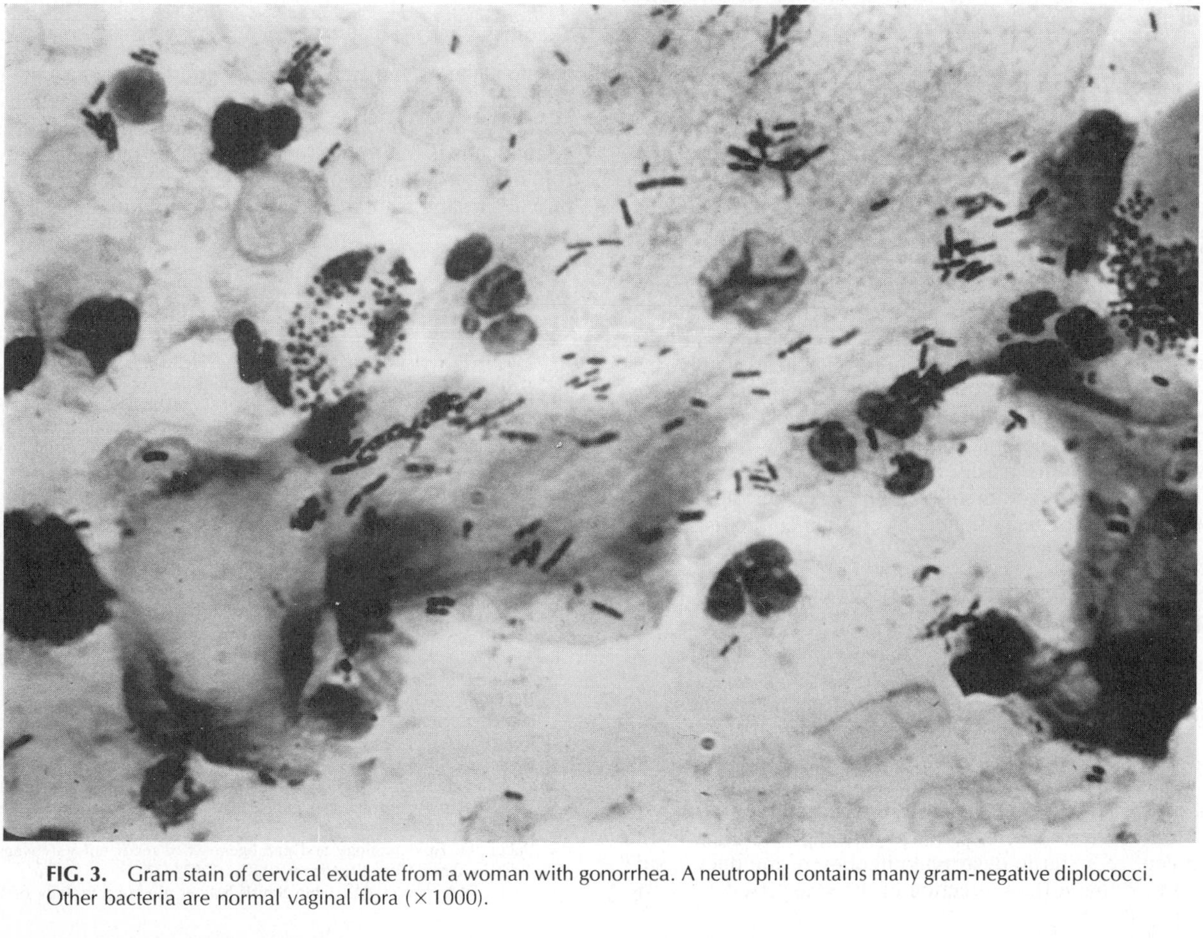

FIG. 3. Gram stain of cervical exudate from a woman with gonorrhea. A neutrophil contains many gram-negative diplococci. Other bacteria are normal vaginal flora (×1000).

80–90 percent sensitive in women.[136] The lower cost of these culture-independent tests has made selective screening for chlamydiae advisable in certain populations.[164] Routine cervical cytology is not useful because of its low sensitivity.[153,161,165] Colposcopy has revealed a typical follicular appearance in most cases and may be useful diagnostically.[166,167]

Herpes simplex virus is isolated from the cervix in 88 percent of women with primary infection but only from 12 percent of women with recurrent herpetic infection.[128,129] Cervicitis may be present without external lesions. Cervicitis is seen on physical examination in about 90 percent of culture-positive women.[128,129] The cervix usually displays diffuse friability and less frequently, frank ulcers or necrosis.[108] Cervical discharge is usually mucoid, but it is occasionally mucopurulent, and in one series, herpetic cervical infection caused 8 percent of cases of mucopurulent cervicitis.[75] Affected patients may have lower abdominal pain, but inguinal adenopathy is rare unless the disease is accompanied by lesions of the external genitalia.[168] The diagnosis may be made cytologically by observing multinucleated giant cells, often with intranuclear inclusions.[169] In the presence of severe necrosis, however, cellular architecture is so distorted that cytologic examination becomes insensitive, and the diagnosis is best made by recovering the virus in tissue culture or by immunofluorescent staining.[170]

Cancer of the cervix behaves epidemiologically as if it is a sexually transmitted disease.[171] A variety of sexually transmitted agents causing cervical infection have been more or less strongly associated with cervical malignancy. These include herpes simplex virus[128,129,171] and *Chlamydia trachomatis,*[166,167] but the strongest association has been established for some types of human papillomavirus[172] (see Chapter 123).

Other organisms occasionally considered causes of cervicitis include adenovirus,[173] type C viruses,[174] cytomegalovirus,[175] *Enterobius vermicularis,*[176] *Mycobacterium tuberculosis,*[177] group B streptococci,[178] and actinomycetes,[179] the last usually in association with the use of intrauterine contraceptive devices.

Therapeutic Approach to Cervicitis

Specifically diagnosed gonococcal cervicitis should be treated as recommended in Chapter 190. Because 30–60 percent of women with gonococcal cervicitis also have chlamydial infection, simultaneous treatment for both infections is advised when gonorrhea is diagnosed.[180] Cervicitis in patients who are the sexual partners of men with nongonococcal urethritis should be treated with tetracycline, 500 mg orally four times daily; doxycycline, 100 mg orally twice daily; or erythromycin, 500 mg orally four times daily, each for 7 days. Because none of these regimens can still be assumed to cure gonorrhea reliably, cervicitis of unknown etiology should probably be treated with one of the aforementioned regimens plus antigonococcal therapy such as ceftriaxone, 250 mg im. Therapy for cervicitis due to herpes simplex is discussed in Chapter 118. A variety of douches have been recommended in the past, but there are no data supporting their use in acute or chronic cervicitis.

INFECTIONS OF BARTHOLIN'S AND SKENE'S GLANDS

Bartholinitis

In the adult, Bartholin's gland is a 1 cm structure on each side of the vagina near the base of the labia minora. The healthy gland is not palpable and nontender. A 2 cm long duct lined with columnar epithelium opens on the inner surface of the labia minora at the junction of the posterior and middle thirds. Inflammation of the duct can produce blockage resulting in the development of a sterile cyst, and infection of the duct is said to be more common than infection of the gland itself.[181,182] Infection of the gland behind a blocked duct can result in the development of a Bartholin's gland abscess.

The frequency with which specific organisms infect Bartholin's glands is unclear. Early writers felt that clinically significant bartholinitis accompanied 2–50 percent of gonococcal infections.[181–183] Rees recovered gonococci from the glands of 28 percent of the women with gonorrhea, most of whom were asymptomatic,[182] but Lee et al. recovered gonococci from only 12 percent of a series of patients with Bartholin's gland abscess.[184] Gonococcal bartholinitis is usually asymptomatic, but about 1 in 5 women has a palpable enlargement or tenderness of the glands, and 1 in 20 has edema.[182] The examiner should attempt to palpate the glands during the pelvic examination. If material can be expressed from the duct opening, it should be examined with the Gram stain, and it should be cultured.

Chlamydia trachomatis is an apparent cause of bartholinitis,[185] although its incidence is undefined. Infection with normal genital flora is also significant. Single or mixed species of anaerobes have been recovered from up to 90 percent of the infected glands.[184,186–188] *Escherichia coli* and *Proteus mirabilis* are also frequently recovered.[184,186,188,189] *Staphylococcus aureus* is apparently a rare cause of abscess, but streptococci are frequently isolated.[184,186,190]

Lee et al. recovered *Ureaplasma urealyticum* from two-thirds of Bartholin's gland abscesses.[184] Occasionally, herpes genitalis involves the duct and produces a recurrent but transient swelling of the gland.

Bartholinitis accompanying gonococcal infection can be treated like acute gonorrhea,[182] although some workers have recommended repeating the treatment daily for 3 days.[181] The optimal initial therapy for bartholinitis of uncertain etiology is not known. A tetracycline, in doses adequate for chlamydial infection, and metronidazole might be considered. A failure of bartholinitis to respond to antibiotic therapy may require surgical drainage of the abscess.[191]

Skenitis

Skene's glands are small structures that empty into the urethra. Dysuria is the usual complaint of patients with infection of these glands,[181] and sometimes a bead of pus can be expressed. The gonococcus is felt to produce some cases of skenitis,[181] but the role of other potential pathogens has not been determined. Empirical therapy similar to that for bartholinitis may be tried.

REFERENCES

1. Lang WR. Pediatric vaginitis. N Engl J Med. 1955;253:1153.
2. Hammerschlag MR, Alpert S, Onderdonk AB, et al. Anaerobic microflora of the vagina in children. Am J Obstet Gynecol. 1978;131:853–60.
3. Hammerschlag MR, Alpert S, Rosner I, et al. Microbiology of the vagina in children: Normal and potentially pathogenic organisms. Pediatrics. 1978;62:57–62.
4. Levison ME, Corman LC, Carrington ER, et al. Quantitative microflora o the vagina. Am J Obstet Gynecol. 1977;127:80.
5. Tashjian JH, Coulam CB, Washington JA. Vaginal flora in asymptomatic women. Mayo Clin Proc. 1976;51:557.
6. Brown WJ. Variations in the bacterial flora: A preliminary report. Ann Intern Med. 1982;96:131.
7. Larsen B, Galask RP. Vaginal microbial flora: Composition and influences of host physiology. Ann Intern Med. 1982;96(Suppl 6):926.
8. Spiegel CA, Amsel R, Eschenbach D, et al. Anaerobic bacteria in nonspecific vaginitis. N Engl J Med. 1980;303:601.
9. Rein MF, Holmes KK. "Nonspecific vaginitis," vulvovaginal candidiasis, and trichomoniasis. In: Remington JS, Swartz MN, eds. Current Clinical Topics in Infectious Diseases. v. 4. New York: McGraw-Hill; 1983:281.
10. Easmon CSF, Ison CA. *Gardnerella vaginalis*. Lancet. 1983;2:343.
11. Guinan ME, Dan BB, Guidotti RJ, et al. Vaginal colonization with *Staphylococcus aureus* in healthy women: A review of four studies. Ann Intern Med. 1982;94:944.
12. Sobel JD. Epidemiology and pathogenesis of recurrent vulvovaginial candidiasis. Am J Obstet Gynecol. 1985;152:924–35.
13. Shafer MA, Sweet RL, Ohm-Smith MJ, et al. Microbiology of the lower

gential tract in postmenarchal adolescent girls: Differences in sexual activity, contraception, and presence of nonspecific vaginitis. J Pediatr. 1985;107:974–81.
14. Hill GB, Eschenbach DA, Holmes KK. Bacteriology of the vaginia. Scand J Urol Nephrol. 1984;18(Suppl 86):23–80.
15. Cohen MS, Black JR, Proctor RA, et al. Host defenses and the vaginal mucosa: A reevaluation. Scand J Urol Nephrol. 1984;8(Suppl 86):13–22.
16. Centers for Disease Control. Nonreported sexually transmitted diseases. MMWR. 1979;28:61.
17. Sweet RL. Importance of differential diagnosis in acute vaginitis. Am J Obstet Gynecol. 1985;152:921–3.
18. Odds FC. *Candida* and Candidiosis. Baltimore: University Park Press; 1979:4.
19. O'Connor MI, Sobel JD. Epidemiology of recurrent vulvovaginal candidiasis: Identification and strain differentiation of *Candida albicans*. J Infect Dis. 1986;154:358–63.
20. Horowitz BJ, Edelstein SW, Lippman L. *Candida tropicalis* vulvovaginitis. Obstet Gynecol. 1985;66:229–32.
21. Clark JFJ, Faggett T, Peters B, et al. Ulcerative vaginitis due to *Torulopsis glabrata*: A case report. J Natl Med Assoc. 1978;70:913.
22. Boquet-Jimenez E, San Cristobal AA. Cytologic and microbiologic aspects of vaginal torulopsis. Acta Cytol (Baltimore). 1978;22:331.
23. Fleury FJ. Adult vaginitis. Clin Obstet Gynecol. 1981;24:407.
24. Heary FJ. Recurrent *Candida* vulvovaginitis. Chemotherapy. 1982;28(Suppl 1):48–50.
25. Oriel JD, Partridge BM, Denny MJ, et al. Genital yeast infections. Br Med J. 1972;4:761.
26. Jackson JL III, Spain WT. Comparative study of combined and sequential anti-ovulatory therapy on vaginal moniliasis. Am J Obstet Gynecol. 1968;101:1134.
27. Powell BL, Frey CL, Drutz DJ. Estrogen receptor in *Candida albicans*. A possible explanation for hormonal influences in vaginal candidiasis (Abstract 751). In: Proceedings of the 23rd 23 ICAAC. Las Vegas, 1983.
28. Elegbe IA, Botu M. A preliminary study on dressing patterns and incidence of candidiasis. Am J Public Health. 1982;72:176.
29. Elgebe IA, Elgebe I. Quantitative relationships of *Candida albicans* infections and dressing patterns in Nigerian women. Am J Public Health. 1983;73:450–2.
30. Heidrich FE, Berg AO, Bergman JJ. Clothing factors and vaginitis. J Family Pract. 1984;19:491–4.
31. Rhoads JL, Wright DC, Redfield RR, et al. Chronic vaginal candidiasis in women with human immunodeficiency virus infection. JAMA. 1987;257:3105–9.
32. Odds FC. Genital candidosis. Clin Exp Dermatol. 1982;7:345–54.
33. Garcia-Tamayo J, Castillo G, Martinez AJ. Human genital candidiasis: Histochemistry, scanning and transmission electron microscopy. Acta Cytol (Baltimore). 1982;26:7.
34. Kimura LH, Pearsall NH. Relationship between germination of *Candida albicans* and increased adherence to human buccal epithelial cells. Infect Immun. 1980;28:464.
35. King RD, Lee JC, Morris AL. Adherence of *Candida albicans* and other *Candida* species to mucosal epithelial cells. Infect Immun. 1980;27:667.
36. Sobel JD, Muller G. Ketoconazole in the prevention of experimental candidal vaginitis. Antimicrob Agents Chemother. 1984;25:281–2.
37. Drake SM, Evans BA, Gerken A. Vaginal pH and microflora related to yeast infections and treatment. Br J Vener Dis. 1980;56:107.
38. Peeters F, Snauwaert R, Segers J, et al. Observation on candidal vaginitis: Vaginal pH, microbiology. Am J Obstet Gynecol. 1972;112:80.
39. Baldson MJ. Comparison of miconazole-coated tampons with clotrimazole vaginal tablets in the treatment of vaginal candidosis. Br J Vener Dis. 1981;57:275.
40. Rothenberg RB, Simm R, Chipperfield E, et al. Efficacy of selected diagnostic tests for sexually transmitted diseases. JAMA. 1976;235:49.
41. Pattman RS. Evaluation of a culture in the diagnosis of vaginal candidosis. Br J Vener Dis. 1981;57:67.
42. Rajakumar R, Lacey CJN, Evans EGV, et al. Use of a slide latex agglutination test for rapid diagnosis of vaginal candidosis. Genitourin Med. 1987;63:192–5.
43. Anonymous. Terconazole for candida vaginitis. Med Lett Drugs Ther. 1988;30:118–9.
44. Odds FC. Cure and relapse with antifungal therapy. Proc R Soc Med. 1977;70(Suppl 4):24.
45. Weisberg M. Treatment of vaginal candidiasis in pregnant women. Clin Ther. 1986;8:563–7.
46. Lebherz T, Guess E, Wolfson N. Efficacy of single- venous multiple-dose clotrimazole therapy in the management of vulvovaginal candidiasis. Am J Obstet Gynecol. 1985;152:965–7.
47. Heary F, Hughes D, Floyd R. Therapeutic results obtained in vaginal mycoses after single-dose treatment with 500 mg clotrimazole vaginal tablets. Am J Obstet Gynecol. 1985;152:968–70.
48. Anonymous. Butoconazole for vulvovaginal candidiasis. Med Lett Drugs Ther. 1986;28:68.
49. Loendersloot EW, Goormans E, Wiesenhann E, et al. Efficacy and tolerability of single-dose versus six-day treatment of candidal vulvovaginitis with vaginal tablets of clotrimazole. Am J Obstet Gynecol. 1985;152:953–5.
50. Bradbeer CS, Mayhew SR, Barlow D. Butoconazole and miconazole in treating vaginal candidiasis. Genitourin Med. 1985;61:270–2.
51. Droegemueller W, Adamson DG, Brown D, et al. Three-day treatment with butoconazole nitrate for vulvovaginal candidiasis. Obstet Gynecol. 1984;64:530–4.
52. Cohen L. Single dose treatment of vaginal candidosis: Comparison of clotrimazole and isoconazole. Br J Vener Dis. 1984;60:42–4.
53. Milson I, Forssman L. Treatment of vaginal candidosis with a single 500 mg clotrimazole pessary. Br J Vener Dis. 1982;58:124.
54. Sobel JD. Management of recurrent vulvovaginal candidiasis with intermittent ketoconazole prophylaxis. Obstet Gynecol. 1985;65:435–40.
55. Sobel JD. Recurrent vulvovaginal candidiasis. A prospective study of the efficacy of maintenance ketoconazole therapy. N Engl J Med. 1986;315:1455–8.
56. Eschenbach DA, Hummel D, Gravett MG. Recurrent and persistant vulvovaginal candidiasis: Treatment with ketoconazole. Obstet Gynecol. 1985;66:248–54.
57. Calderón-Márquez JJ. Itraconzole in the treatment of vaginal candidosis and the effect of treatment of the sexual partner. Rev Infect Dis. 1987;9(Suppl 1):143–5.
58. Clayton YM. Antifungal drugs in current use: A review. Proc R Soc Med. 1977;70(Suppl 4):15.
59. Vorherr H, Vorherr UF, Mehta P, et al. Vaginal absorption of povidone-iodine. JAMA. 1980;244:2628.
60. van Slyke KK, Michel VP, Rein MF. Treatment of vulvovaginal candidiasis with boric acid powder. Am J Obstet Gynecol. 1981;141:145.
61. Cohen L. Is more than one application of an antifungal necessary in the treatment of acute vaginal candidiasis. Am J Obstet Gynecol. 1985;152:961–4.
62. Odds FC, Abbott AB. A simple system for the presumptive identification of *Candida albicans* and differentiation of strains within the species. Sabouraudia. 1980;18:301–17.
63. Odds FC, Abbott AB. Modification and extension of tests for differentiation of *Candida* species and strains. Sabouraudia. 1983;21:79–81.
64. Hill LVH, Embil JA. Vaginits: Current microbiological and clinical concepts. Can Med Assoc J. 1986;134:3221–31.
65. Milne JD, Warnock DW. Effect of simultaneous oral and vaginal treatment on the rate of cure and relapse in vaginal candidosis. Br J Vener Dis. 1979;55:362.
66. Velupillai S, Thin RN. Treatment of vulvovaginal yeast infection with nystatin. Practitioner. 1977;219:897.
67. Nystatin Multicenter Study Group. Therapy of candidal vaginitis: The effect of eliminating intestinal *Candida*. Am J Obstet Gynecol. 1986;155:651–5.
68. Lossick JG. Sexually transmitted vaginitis. Semin Adolesc Med. 1985;2:131–42.
69. Edman J, Sobel JD, Taylor ML. Zinc status in women with recurrent vulvovaginal candidiasis. Am J Obstet Gynecol. 1986;155:1082–5.
70. Witkin SS, Yu IR, Ledger WJ. Inhibition of *Candida albicans*-induced lymphocyte proliferation by lymphocytes and sera from women with recurrent vaginitis. Am J Obstet Gynecol. 1983;147:809–11.
71. Davidson F, Mould RF. Recurrent genital candidosis in women and the effect of intermittent prophylactic treatment. Br J Vener Dis. 1978;54:176.
72. Waugh MA. Clinical presentation of candidal balanitis—its differential diagnosis and treatment. Chemotherapy. 1982;28(Suppl 1):56–60.
73. Gardner HL, Dukes CD. *Haemophilus vaginalis* vaginitis: A newly defined specific infection previously classified "non-specific" vaginitis. Am J Obstet Gynecol. 1955;69:962.
74. Mårdh PA, Taylor-Robinson D, eds. Bacterial vaginosis. Scand J Urol Nephrol. 1984;18(Suppl 86):1–270.
75. Brunham RC, Paavonen J, Stevens CE, et al. Mucopurulent cervicitis—the ignored counterpart in women of urethritis in men. N Engl J Med. 1984;311:1–6.
76. Phiefer TA, Forsyth PS, Durfee MA, et al. Nonspecific vaginitis: Role of *Haemophilus vaginalis* and treatment with metronidazole. N Engl J Med. 1978;298:1429.
77. Chen KCS, Forsyth PS, Buchanan TM, et al. Amine content of vaginal fluid from untreated and treated patients with nonspecific vaginitis. J Clin Invest. 1979;63:828.
78. Hanna NF, Taylor-Robinson D, Kalodiki-Karamanoli M, et al. The relation between vaginal pH and the microbiological status in vaginitis. Br J Obstet Gynaecol. 1985;92:1267–71.
79. Baldson MJ, Taylor GE, Pead L, et al. *Corynebacterium vaginale* and vaginitis: A controlled trial of treatment. Lancet. 1980;1:501.
80. Vontver LA, Eschenbach DA. The role of *Gardnerella vaginalis* in nonspecific vaginitis. Clin Obstet Gynecol. 1981;24:439.
81. Amsel R, Totten PA, Spiegel CA, et al. Nonspecific vaginitis: Diagnostic criteria and microbial and epidemiological associations. Am J Med. 1983;74:14.
82. Bhattycharyya MN, Jones BM. *Haemophilus vaginalis* infection: Diagnosis and treatment. J Reprod Med. 1980;24:71.
83. Ratnam S, Fitzgerald BL. Semiquantitative culture of *Gardnerella vaginalis* in laboratory determination of nonspecific vaginitis. J Clin Microbiol. 1983;18:344.
84. Totten PA, Amsel R, Hale J, et al. Selective differential human blood bilayer media for isolation of *Gardnerella* (*Haemophilus*) *vaginalis*. J Clin Microbiol. 1982;15:141–7.
85. Thomason JL, Gelbart SM, Wilcoski LM. Proline aminopeptidase activity as a rapid diagnostic test to confirm bacterial vaginosis. Obstet Gynecol. 1988;71:607–71.

86. Chen KCS, Amsel R, Eschenbach DA, et al. Biochemical diagnosis of vaginitis: Determination of diamines in vaginal fluid. J Infect Dis. 1982;145:337.
87. Greenwood JR, Picket MJ. Transfer of *Haemophilus vaginalis* to a new genus, *Gardnerella: G. vaginalis* (Gardner and Dukes) comb. nov. Int J Syst Bacteriol. 1980;30:170.
88. Malouf M, Fortier M, Morin G, et al. Treatment of *Hemophilus vaginalis* vaginitis. Obstet Gynecol. 1980;57:711.
89. Monhanty KC, Deighton R. Comparison of 2 g single dose of metronidazole, nimorazole and tinidazole in the treatment of vaginitis associated with *Gardnerella vaginalis*. J Antimicrob Chemother. 1987;19:393–9.
90. Mohanty KC, Deighton R. Comparison of two different metronidazole regimens in the treatment of *Gardnerella vaginalis* infection with or without trichomoniasis. J Antimicrob Chemother. 1985;16:799–803.
91. van der Meijden WI, Piot P, Loriaux SM, et al. Amoxycillin, amoxycillin-clavulanic acid and metronidazole in the treatment of clue cell positive discharge. A comparative clinical and laboratory study. J Antimicrob Chemother. 1987;20:735–42.
92. Amsel R, Critchlow CW, Spiegel CA, et al. Comparison of metronidazole, ampicillin, and amoxicillin for treatment of bacterial vaginosis (nonspecific vaginitis): Possible explanation for the greater efficacy of metronidazole. In: Finegold S, ed. United States Metronidazole Conference. Proceedings from a Symposium, Tarpon Springs, Florida, February 18–20, 1982. New York: Biomedical Information Corp; 1982:225.
93. Shanker S, Munro R. Sensitivity of *Gardnerella vaginalis* to metabolites of metronidazole and tinidazole. Lancet. 1982;1:167.
94. Taylor E, Blackwell AL, Barlow D, et al. *Gardnerella vaginalis*, anaerobes, and vaginal discharge. Lancet. 1982;1:1376.
95. Eschenbach DA, Gravett MG, Chen KCS, et al. Bacterial vaginosis during pregnancy: An association with prematurity and postpartum complications. Scand J Urol Nephrol. 1984;18(Suppl 86):213–22.
96. Paavonen J, Miettinen A, Stevens CE, et al. *Mycoplasma hominis* in nonspecific vaginitis. Sex Transm Dis. 1983;10:271–5.
97. Swedberg J, Steiner JF, Deiss F, et al. Comparison of single-dose vs. one-week course of metronidazole for symptomatic bacterial vaginosis. JAMA. 1985;254:1046–9.
98. Alawattegama AB, Jones BM, Kinghorn GR, et al. Single-dose versus seven-day metronidazole in *Gardnerella vaginalis* associated non-specific vaginitis. Lancet. 1984;1:1355–7.
99. Eschenbach DA, Critchlow CW, Watkins H, et al. A dose-duration study of metronidazole for the treatment of nonspecific vaginosis. Scand J Infect Dis. 1983;40(Suppl):73–6.
100. Jones BM, Geary I, Alawattegama AB, et al. *In vitro* and *in vivo* activity of metronidazole against *Gardnerella vaginalis*, *Bacteroides* spp. and *Mobiluncus* spp. in bacterial vaginosis. J Antimicrob Chemother. 1985;16:189–97.
101. Ison CA, Taylor RFH, Link C, et al. Local treatment for bacterial vaginosis. Br Med J. [Clin Res] 1987;295:886.
102. Bardi M, Maneti G, Mattioni D, et al. Metronidazole for nonspecific vaginitis. Lancet. 1980;1:1029.
102a. Greaves WL, Chungafung J, Morris B, et al. Clindamycin versus metronidazole in the treatment of bacterial vaginosis. Obstet Gynecol. 1988;72:799–802.
103. Garnder HL. *Hemophilus vaginalis* vaginitis after twenty-five years. Am J Obstet Gynecol. 1980;137:385–92.
104. Piot P, Van Dyck E, Godts P, et al. A placebo-controlled, double blind comparison of tinidazole and triple sulfonamide cream for the treatment of nonspecific vaginitis. Am J Obstet Gynecol. 1983;147:85–9.
105. Fredicsson B, Englund K, Weintraub L, et al. Ecological treatment of bacterial vaginosis. Lancet. 1987;1:276.
106. McDowall DRM, Buchanan JD, Fairley KF, et al. Anaerobic and other fastidious microorganisms in asymptomatic bacteriuria in pregnant women. J Infect Dis. 1981;144:114.
107. Rosene K, Eschenbach DA, Tompkins LS, et al. Polymicrobial early postpartum endometritis with facultative and anaerobic bacteria, genital mycoplasmas, and *Chlamydia trachomatis*: Treatment with piperacillin or cefoxitin. J Infect Dis. 1986;153:1028–37.
108. Lamey JR, Eschenbach DA, Mitchell SH, et al. Isolation of mycoplasmas and bacteria from the blood of postpartum women. Am J Obstet Gynecol. 1982;143:104–12.
109. Gravett MG, Hummel DH, Eschenbach DA, et al. Preterm labor associated with subclinical amniotic fluid infection and with bacterial vaginosis. Obstet Gynecol. 1986;67:229–37.
110. Venkataramani TK, Rathbun HK. *Corynebacterium vaginale* (*Hemophilus vaginalis*) bacteremia: Clinical study of 29 cases. Johns Hopkins Med J. 1976;139:93.
111. Reimer LG, Reller LB. *Gardnerella vaginalis* bacteremia: A review of 30 cases. Obstet Gynecol. 1984;65:170–2.
112. Darieux R, Dublanchet A. Les "vibrions" anaerobics des leucorrhees. I: Technique d'isolement et sensibilite aux antibiotiques. Med Mal Infect. 1980;10:109.
113. Sprott MS, Pattman RS, Ingham HR, et al. Anaerobic curved rods in vaginitis. Lancet. 1982;1:54.
114. Hjelm E, Hallen A, Forsum U, et al. Motile anaerobic curved rods in nonspecific vaginitis. Eur J Sex Transm Dis. 1982;1:9.
115. Spiegel CA, Eschenbach DA, Amsel R, et al. Curved anaerobic bacteria in bacterial vaginosis and their response to antimicrobial therapy. J Infect Dis. 1983;148:817.
116. Thomason JL, Schreckenberger PC, Spellacy WN, et al. Clinical and microbiological characterization of patients with nonspecific vaginosis associated with motile, curved anaerobic rods. J Infect Dis. 1984;149:801–9.
117. Spiegel CA. New developments in the etiology and pathogenesis of bacterial vaginosis. Adv Exp Med Biol. 1987;224:127–34.
118. Thomason JL and the Working Group. Diagnosis of infection with anaerobic cervical rods. Scan J Urol Neophrol. 1984;18(Suppl 86):261–2.
119. Spiegel CA, Roberts, M. *Mobiluncus* gen nov, *Mobiluncus curtisii* subspecies *curtisii* sp. nov., *Mobiluncus curtisii* subspecies *holmesii* subsp. nov., and *Mobiluncus mulieris* sp. nov; curved rods from the human vagina. Int J Syst Bacteriol. 1984;34:177–184.
120. Shands KN, Schmid GP, Dan BB, et al. Toxic shock syndrome in menstruating women: Association with tampon use and *Staphylococcus aureus* and clinical features in 52 cases. N Engl J Med. 1980;303:1436.
121. Tofte RW, Williams DN. Clinical and laboratory manifestations of toxic shock syndrome. Ann Intern Med. 1982;96:843.
122. Lanes SF, Poole C, Dreyer NA. Toxic shock syndrome, contraceptive methods, and vaginitis. Am J Obstet Gynecol. 1986;154:989–91.
123. Zaaijman JD, deBeer J. An unusual vaginal foreign body. S. Afr Med J. 1982;61:33.
124. Friedrich EG, Siegesmund KA. Tampon associated vaginal ulcerations. Obstet Gynecol. 1980;55:149.
125. Friedrich EG. Tampon effects on vaginal health. Clin Obstet Gynecol. 1981;24:295.
126. Jimerson SD, Becker JD. Vaginal ulcers associated with tampon usage. Obstet Gynecol. 1980;56:97.
127. Weissberg SM, Dodson MG. Recurrent vaginal and cervical ulcers associated with tampon use. JAMA. 1983;250:1430.
128. Corey L, Adams HG, Brown AZ, et al. Genital herpes simplex virus infections: Clinical manifestations, course, and complications. Ann Intern Med. 1983;98:958.
129. Pazin GH. Management of oral and genital herpes simplex viral infections: Diagnosis and treatment. DM. 1986;32:725–824.
130. Corey L, Holmes KK. The use of 2-deoxy-D-glucose for genital herpes. JAMA. 1980;243:29.
131. Ginsburg CM. Group A streptococcal vaginitis in children. Pediatr Infect Dis. 1982;1:36.
132. Symmers WStC. Pathology of oxyuriasis. Arch Pathol. 1950;50:475.
133. Dump RC. *Chlamydia trachomatis* as a cause of prepubertal vaginitis. Obstet Gynecol. 1985;65:384–8.
134. Cibley LF, Cibley LJ. Diagnostic considerations in vulvovaginal candidiasis. J Reprod Med. 1986;31(Suppl 7):648–9.
135. Fisher AA. Allergic reactions to feminine hygiene sprays. Arch Dermatol. 1973;108:801.
136. Chang T. Familial allergic seminal vulvovaginitis. Am J Obstet Gynecol. 1976;126:442.
137. Gochfeld M, Burger J. Sexual transmission of nickel and poison oak contact dermatitis. Lancet. 1983;1:589.
138. Gardner HL. Desquamative inflammatory vaginitis: A newly defined entity. Am J Obstet Gynecol. 1968;102:1102–5.
139. Edwards L, Friedrich EG. Desquamative vaginitis: Lichen planus in disguise. Obstet Gynecol. 1988;71:832–6.
140. Huggins GR, Preti G. Vaginal odors and secretions. Clin Obstet Gynecol. 1981;24:355.
141. Friedrich EG. The vulvar vestibule. J Reprod Med. 1983;28:773–7.
142. Peckham BM, Maki DG, Patterson JJ, et al. Focal vulvitis: A characteristic syndrome and cause of dyspareunia. Features, natural history, and management. Am J Obstet Gynecol. 1986;154:855–64.
143. Kramer K, Jobón H. Vaginitis emphasematosa. Arch Pathol Lab Med. 1987;111:746–9.
144. McCallion JS, Parkin DE. Emphasematous vaginitis masquerading as carcinoma of the cervix. Case report. Br J Obstet Gynecol. 1988;95:309–11.
145. Dodson MG, Friedrich EG. Psychosomatic vulvovaginitis. Obstet Gynecol. 1978;51(Suppl):23.
146. Al-Saliki FL, Curran JP, Wong J-S. Neonatal *Trichomonas vaginalis*: Report of three cases and review of the literature. Pediatrics. 1974;53:196.
147. Paradise JE, Campos JM, Friedman HM, et al. Vulvovaginitis in premenarchal girls: Clinical features and diagnostic evaluation. Pediatrics. 1982;70:193.
148. Rees E, Tait IA, Hobson D, et al. Chlamydia in relation to cervical infection and pelvic inflammatory disease. In: Hobson D, Holmes KK, eds. Nongonococcal Urethritis and Related Infections. Lake Placid, NY: American Society for Microbiology; 1976.
149. Silverman EM, Silverman AG. Persistence of spermatozoa in the lower genital tracts of women. JAMA. 1978;240:1875.
150. Tait IA, Rees E, Hobson D, et al. Chlamydial infection of the cervix in contacts of men with non-gonococcal urethritis. Br J Vener Dis. 1980;56:37.
151. Mardh P-A, Moller BR, Paavonen J. Chlamydial infection of the female genital tract with emphasis on pelvic inflammatory disease. A review of Scandinavian studies. Sex Transm Dis. 1981;8:140.
152. Paavonen J, Vesterinen E. *Chlamydia trachomatis* in cervicitis and urethritis in women. Scand J Infect Dis. 1982;32(Suppl):45.
153. Spence MR, Barbacci M, Kappus E, et al. A correlative study of Papanicolaou smear, fluorescent antibody, and culture for the diagnosis of *Chlamydia trachomatis*. Obstet Gynecol. 1986:68:691–5.
154. Paavonen J, Critchlow CW, DeRouen T, et al. Etiology of cervical inflammation. Am J Obstet Gynecol. 1986;154:556–64.

155. Harrison HR, Costin M, Meder JB, et al. Cervical *Chlamydia trachomatis* infection in university women: Relationship to history, contraception, ectopy, and cervicitis. Am J Obstet Gynecol. 1985;153:224–51.
156. Moscicki B, Shafer MA, Millstein SG, et al. The use and limitations of endocervical Gram stains and mucopurulent cervicitis as predictors for *Chlamydia trachomatis* in female adolescents. Am J Obstet Gynecol. 1987;157:65–71.
157. Wentworth BB, Bonin P, Holmes KK, et al. Isolation of viruses, bacteria and other organisms from venereal disease clinic patients: Methodology and problems associated with multiple isolations. Health Lab Sci. 1973;10:75.
158. Curran JW, Rendtorff RC, Chandler RW, et al. Female gonorrhea: Its relationship to abnormal uterine bleeding, urinary tract symptoms and cervicitis. Obstet Gynecol. 1975;45:195.
159. Hilton AL, Richmond SJ, Milne JD, et al. Chlamydia A in the female genital tract. Br J Vener Dis. 1974;50:1.
160. Oriel JD, Powis PA, Reeve P, et al. Chlamydial infection of the cervix. Br J Vener Dis. 1974;50:11.
161. Quinn TC, Gupta PK, Burkman RT. Detection of *Chlamydia trachomatis* cervical infections: A comparison of Papanicolaou and immunofluorescent staining with cell cultures. Am J Obstet Gynecol. 1987;157:394–9.
162. Stamm WE, Harrison HR, Alexander ER, et al. Diagnosis of *Chlamydia trachomatis* infections by direct immunofluorescence staining of genital secretions: A multicenter trial. Ann Intern Med. 1984;101:638–42.
163. Hipp SS, Han V, Murphy D. Assessment of enzyme immunoassay and immunofluorescence tests for detection of *Chlamydia trachomatis*. J Clin Microbiol. 1987;25:1983–92.
164. Phillps RS, Aronson MD, Taylor WC, et al. Should tests for *Chlamydia trachomatis* cervical infection be done during routine gynecological visits? An analysis of the costs of alternative strategies. Ann Intern Med. 1987;107:188–94.
165. Purola E, Paavonen J. Routine cytology as a diagnostic aid in chlamydial cervicitis. Scand J Infect Dis. 1982;32(Suppl):55.
166. Hare MJ, Toone E, Taylor-Robinson D, et al. Follicular cervicitis: Colposcopic appearances and association with *Chlamydia trachomatis*. Br J Obstet Gynecol. 1981;88:174.
167. Paavonen J, Vesterinen E, Meyer B, et al. Colposcopic and histological findings in cervical chlamydial infection. Obstet Gynecol. 1982;59:712.
168. Willcox RR. Necrotic cervicitis due to primary infection with the virus of herpes simplex. Br Med J. 1968;1:610.
169. Morse AR, Coleman DV, Gardner SD. An evaluation of cytology in the diagnosis of herpes simplex virus infection and cytomegalovirus infection of the cervix uteri. J Obstet Gynecol Br Commonwealth. 1974;81:393.
170. Corey L. Laboratory diagnosis of herpes simplex virus infections. Principles guiding the development of rapid diagnostic tests. Diagn Microbiol Infect Dis. 1986;4(Suppl):1115–95.
171. Aurelian L. The "viruses of love" and cancer. Am J Med Tech. 1974;40:496.
172. Pfister H. Relationship of papillomaviruses to anogenital cancer. Obstet Gynecol. Clin North Am. 1987;14:349–62.
173. Laverty CR, Russell P, Black J, et al. Adenovirus infection of the cervix. Acta Cytol (Baltimore). 1977;21:114.
174. Marquart K-H, Cunderlik VN. Oncornavirus-like particles in biopsy material from a glandular erosion of the human uterine cervix. Acta Cytol (Baltimore). 1976;29:335.
175. Deppisch LM. Cytomegalovirus inclusion body endocervicitis: Significance of CMV inclusions in endocervical biopsies. Mt. Sinai J Med. 1981;48:418.
176. Wong JV, Becker SN. *Enterobius vermicularis* ova in routine cervicovaginal smears. Light a scanning electron microscopic observations. Acta Cytol (Baltimore). 1982;26:484.
177. Tang LCH. Postmenopausal tuberculous cervicitis. Acta Obstet Gynecol Scand. 1986;65:279–81.
178. Buttigieg G. Cervicitis and urethritis caused by group B streptococcus: Case report. Genitourin Med. 1985;61:343–4.
179. Mao K, Guillebaud J. Influence of removal of intrauterine contraceptive devices on colonization of the cervix by *Actinomyces*-like organisms. Contraception. 1984;30:535–44.
180. Washington AE, Browner WS, Korenbrot CC. Cost-effectiveness of combined treatment for endocervical gonorrhea. Considering coinfection with *Chlamydia trachomatis*. JAMA. 1987;257:2056–60.
181. Morton RS. Gonorrhea. London: WB Saunders; 1977:108.
182. Rees E: Gonococcal bartholinitis. Br J Vener Dis. 1967;43:150.
183. Norris CC: Gonorrhea in Women. Philadelphia; WB Saunders; 1913:202.
184. Lee Y-H, Rankin JS, Alpert S, et al. Microbiological Investigation of Bartholin's gland abscesses and cysts. Am J Obstet Gynecol. 1977;129:150.
185. Davies JA, Rees E, Hobson D, et al. Isolation of *Chlamydia trachomatis* from Bartholin's duct. Br J Vener Dis. 1978;54:409.
186. Swensen RM. Anaerobic bacteria in infections of the female genital tract. In: Balows A, DeHaan RM, Dowell VR, et al., eds. Anaerobic Bacteria Role in Disease. Springfield, IL: Charles C Thomas, 1974.
187. Swenson RM, Michaelson TC, Dayl MJ, et al. Anaerobic bacterial infections of the female genital tract. Obstet Gynecol. 1973;42:538.
188. Kubitz R, Hoffman K. Bartholin's gland abscess in an infant. A case report. J Reprod Med. 1986;31:67–9.
189. Carson GD, Smith LP. *Escherichia coli* endotoxic shock complicating Bartholin's gland abscess. Can Med Assoc J. 1980;122:1397.
190. Morton BD, McCarthy LR. Bartholinitis: An unusual etiologic agent. Obstet Gynecol. 1980;55(Suppl):97.
191. Azzan BB. Bartholin's cyst and abscess: A review of treatment of 53 cases. Br J Clin Pract. 1978;32:101.

96. INFECTIONS OF THE FEMALE PELVIS

WILLIAM J. LEDGER

In most soft tissue infections of the female, multiple bacterial species are recovered, and frequently some or all of these organisms are anaerobes. In recent years, there has been increasing awareness of the importance of *Chlamydia trachomatis* in many of these pelvic infections.

PATHOGENESIS

Animal model studies of peritoneal infection have suggested a biphasic response to massive bacterial contamination of bowel flora,[1] with early-onset peritonitis and septicemia with gram-negative aerobic organisms, followed later by intra-abdominal abscess formation with anaerobic bacteria.[2] The significance of any animal model evaluation is only as great as the parallel with human experience, and it is clear that early-onset septicemia and late-onset abscess formation are recognizable clinical syndromes. The only variation from the animal model seen in female patients with infections of the pelvis is the frequency (25 percent or more) of anaerobic bacteria and gram-positive aerobic blood stream isolates in early-onset bacteremia.[3–5]

Microbiology

The diagnostic microbiology laboratory can be very helpful in the management of these women. However, the laboratory report will only be as good as the specimen submitted by the physician. Since there is an abundant normal anaerobic flora on the surface of the mucous membranes of the lower genital tract, a surface swab of the vagina or endocervix is not acceptable for the evaluation of cases of deep pelvic infections such as postabortion infection, postpartum endomyometritis, or salpingo-oophoritis. Sheathed containers can be used to obtain specimens from the endometrial cavity.[6] Needle sampling of the peritoneal cavity or direct aspiration of an abscess yields good material for the laboratory to isolate anaerobic bacteria (Fig. 1). This sample can be transported to the laboratory for processing in an air-free container, such as the syringe in which it is collected. Since serious infections usually occur late at night, either the laboratory should provide 24-hour coverage or the physician should be taught to plate the specimens directly and to incubate the plates in an anaerobic environment.[7] Agar dilution testing of gram-negative anaerobes is required for antibiotic sensitivity testing. This is important because it has been

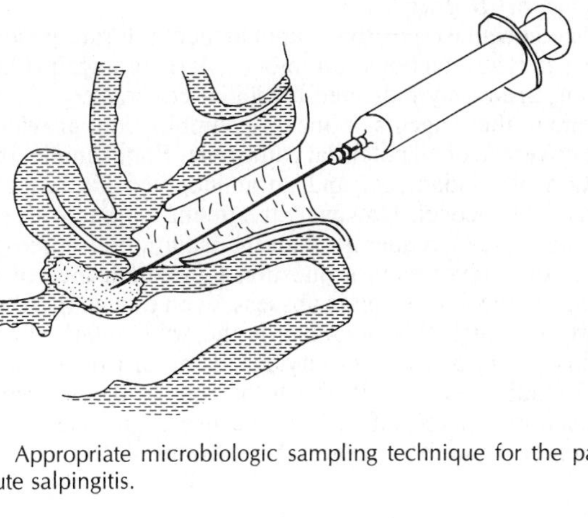

FIG. 1. Appropriate microbiologic sampling technique for the patient with acute salpingitis.

reported that the antibiotic susceptibility of *Bacteroides fragilis* varies considerably from institution to institution.[8] There has been increasing concern about the role of chlamydia in salpingitis in the United States. The inability to grow this organism from peritoneal fluid samples[9] has led to a new use of the endometrial biopsy to obtain the culture for this organism.[10] Tissue culture isolation systems are not available in all hospitals, but monoclonal antibody testing for *Chlamydia* is a feasible technique for all laboratories. Although not as specific as tissue culture (i.e., some positive tests are not culture positive), the test has good sensitivity.

The selection of antibiotics for the patient with a soft tissue pelvic infection should be guided by an awareness of the organisms frequently involved. Most patients are young, with intact hose defense mechanisms. Few have serious underlying diseases that require multiple hospital admissions or stays in nursing homes. As a result, resistant organisms are seldom a problem. Instead, more common gram-negative aerobic organisms, such as *Escherichia coli*, are usually isolated, in addition to anaerobes, *Chlamydia* strains, and enterococci.

Antibiotics

The aminoglycosides, cephalosporins, and penicillins, are used to treat the most common infections seen by obstetrician-gynecologists. The choice of antibiotic should be based upon the recent antibiotic susceptibility patterns of such organisms in the hospital, because the patterns of gram-negative aerobic antibiotic susceptibility vary from hospital to hospital. Aminoglycoside dosage should be based upon an accurate assessment of the patient's age and weight, on frequent studies of renal function, and on peak and trough antibiotic levels to assess the individual patient's response. Since most obstetric-gynecologic patients are young with good renal function, the major problem with aminoglycosides is underdosing. Despite this, aminoglycoside failures are few.[11]

For treatment of anaerobic organisms, additional antibiotics should be considered. In addition to gram-positive anaerobes, including peptostreptococci and clostridia, the major concern is gram-negative anaerobic rods. These include *B. fragilis, B. melaninogenicus, B. bivius, B. disiens*, and *Fusobacterium* strains. Clindamycin and metronidazole, have been approved by the Food and Drug Administration (FDA) for use in these situations. Newer penicillins given in high doses intravenously are effective against a high percentage of anaerobes. These include carbenicillin, ticarcillin, piperacillin, mezlocillin, and azlocillin. In addition, penicillins such as ticarcillin or ampicillin, with an added β-lactamase inhibitor, clavulanate, or sulbactam, are also effective. Cefoxitin, a cephamycin, and cefotetan have significant activity against anaerobes, including *B. fragilis*, and are useful agents in the treatment of pelvic infections. Metronidazole is the most bactericidal agent in laboratory tests against *B. fragilis*.

Since coagulase-positive staphylococci are rarely isolated in female pelvic infections, antibiotics, targeted against such organisms are rarely indicated for initial coverage.

None of these agents, alone or incombination, provides complete coverage of all potential pathogens. For example, the combination of clindamycin and an aminoglycoside is ineffective against enterococci. However, treatment failures with this regimen occur less frequently than the isolation of enterococci.[12] Thus, some investigators question the significance of enterococci as pathogens in pelvic abscess, even though there are case reports in which this organism is the sole isolate.[13] Cephalosporins do not possess activity against enterococci.[14] More detailed studies seem to establish the role of these streptococci in hospital-acquired infections, because cephalosporins are so frequently prescribed in the United States.[15]

An important consideration in the treatment of female pelvic infections is the development of abscesses. Patients with a pelvic abscess often require operative intervention for cure. However, some patients with a pelvic abscess will respond to medical treatment alone. Treatment with antibiotics is the important first step toward cure. The problem for the clinician is the patient who fails to respond to systemic antibiotics. In the past, physicians assumed that patients who failed medical treatment had antibiotic-resistant organisms at the site of infection; in such patients, other antibiotics were tried before resorting to operative intervention. In women with a suspected pelvic abscess, the physician should use antibiotics that are effective against gram-negative anaerobes from the beginning of therapy. If this is done and there is no clinical response, operative drainage or removal is necessary. One study of multiple-antibiotic therapy for the treatment of serious pelvic infections documented 40 patients who failed to respond and who required some form of operative intervention. In only 2 of these 40 women were the bacteria recovered from the abscess resistant in vitro to the antibiotics used.[16] In these cases, continued spiking fevers were not due to antibiotic resistance but to the unique environment of the abscess, which inhibited antibiotic effectiveness. Imaging techniques have been helpful in the management of the patient with a persistent fever. Ultrasound can demonstrate the presence of a fluid-filled mass, but in some cases, it will not differentiate an inflammatory cyst from an abscess. Computed tomography scanning and magnetic resonance imaging usually give better resolution of the pelvic findings and can guide directed needle aspiration of abscesses.[17] Clinical observation is important. Patient deterioration in the form of tachycardia, hypotension, or tachypnea may indicate loss of integrity of the abscess capsule with intra-abdominal leaking. In the face of these signs of clinical deterioration, continued physician dependence upon medical therapy is not in the patient's best interests. If the decision is made to operate, the least extensive operation compatible with cure should be used. If the abscess is amenable to extraperitoneal drainage, this alone should suffice. If not, operative extirpation will be necessary.

HOSPITAL-ACQUIRED INFECTIONS

Postpartum Endomyometritis

It is surprising that infection of the uterus is an infrequent postpartum event, since so many factors that can contribute to infection are present in abundance. The lower genital tract (i.e., the vagina and endocervix) has a heavy flora of bacteria, many of which can be pathogenic. During the course of every observed labor, many internal examinations are performed, each of which forces some bacteria above the endocervical canal into the uterus. In many women, invasive indwelling monitoring equipment consisting of a fetal scalp electrode and an intra-amniotic catheter will be used for many hours. Delivery, either vaginally or by cesarean section, is nearly always accompanied by tissue trauma, operative repair with the use of suture, a foreign material, and blood loss of 1–2 units even in uncomplicated cases. The combination of bacterial contamination and compromise of local host defense mechanisms by these operative procedures yields a high probability of a postpartum uterine infection. The observation that such infections occur in only a minority of women is evidence of the usual adequacy of host defense mechanisms in normal young patients with healthy tissues.

There are a number of recognized events that lower the risk of maternal postpartum infection. There is a remarkable change in the bacterial flora of the lower genital tract during the course of pregnancy; anaerobic organisms, particularly gram-negative ones, decrease late in pregnancy.[18] Amniotic fluid studies demonstrate increasing antibacterial activity as term approaches, which may be due in part to the activity of lysozymes,[19] β-lysin,[20] transferrin,[21] immunoglobulins,[22] peroxidase,[23] and another antibacterial substance,[24] which rises progressively until the 40th week of gestation, when a secondary fall is again seen.[24–27] The useful efficiency of these local host defense mechanisms in clearing the uterus of bacteria has been demonstrated by Spore et al.,[28] who found no bacteria in the uterine cavity at the time of elective tubal ligation postpartum. Normal women with no clinical evidence of infection have elevated white blood cell counts during pregnancy, labor, and the puerperium.[29] In addition, there is evidence of increased white blood cell activity, manifested by a higher percentage of women free of infection who have an elevated number of nitroblue tetrazolium dye-positive leukocytes.[29]

There are a number of factors that probably increase the risk of a postpartum uterine infection. In recent years, invasive monitoring techniques have been widely used in obstetrics. These techniques undoubtedly increase the risk of infection, but the degree of risk seems to be small. An increased risk can be demonstrated in middle-class private patients[30] but not in patients of the lower socioeconomic classes.[31] The percentage of women in the latter category who develop an infection after vaginal delivery is less than 4 percent. This is not the case among women undergoing cesarean section, which is more commonly performed for fetal indications than in the past. The infection rate is higher and the infections are more serious than those in women who have delivered vaginally.[32] Any analysis of infection in postpartum women is difficult because of the multiplicity of factors involved. The length of labor, invasive monitoring, ruptured membranes, number of vaginal examinations, and so on may be less important than the socioeconomic status of the patient. Major differences have been noted in an institution whose patients have different socioeconomic backgrounds.[31]

The organsms involved in postpartum uterine, pelvic, and abdominal wound infections are often found in the lower genital tract of asymptomatic patients. The most frequent isolates include aerobes such as *E. coli, Klebsiella* spp., group B β-hemolytic streptococci, enterococci, and anaerobes such as peptostreptococci, *B. fragilis, B. bivius*, and *B. disiens*. In most situations, the clinical diagnosis of an infection will be made before culture reports are available, and the initial antibiotic prescription must be made empirically. The selection of antibiotic agents before the receipt of culture reports should focus on the most commonly isolated bacteria. *Chlamydia trachomatis* should not be considered normal flora. It is involved in many cases of late postpartum endomyometritis.[33] A number of other pathogenic organsms are also occasionally associated with serious illness in this setting. These include group A β-hemolytic streptococci and the coagulase-positive staphylococci. Since these are uncommon isolates, they should not be a primary consideration when ordering the initial antibiotic postpartum.

Antibiotic therapy for the postpartum patient with a soft tisue infection is empiric and is not based on a prospective study documenting the best therapeutic approach. Data obtained from hospital surveillance are helpful.[34] Following vaginal delivery, I recommend a single antibiotic, either cefoxitin or a newer penicillin, in patients with no evidence of a urinary tract infection.

Two categories of patients who have undergone vaginal delivery have a more serious prognosis. First, women with extensive extrauterine soft tissue infection after pudendal or paracervical block anesthesia have complicated and protracted courses.[35] The most important early clinical sign is the patient's refusal to walk because of severe pain with any leg movement and the discovery on physical examination of a partially flexed lower extremity that is painful with any passive movement. Although these infections have been associated with the isolation of multiple organisms, anaerobes seem particularly important because of the clinical success seen when metronidazole was used.[36] Another rare but life-threatening infection is synergistic necrotizing fascitis that follows vaginal delivery and episiotomy repair.[37] Because of the rapid progression of gangrene and the risk of death, early operative débridement is critical.

The most serious postpartum infections occur in women who have undergone a cesarean section. Current clinical strategy employs antibiotics effective against gram-negative aerobes and anaerobes. This strategy is based upon the results of a comparison of a penicillin-gentamicin combination to clindamycin-gentamicin in postpartum cesarean section patients who developed clinical evidence of an endomyometritis.[12] The results demonstrate the clear superiority of the clindamycin-gentamicin regimen, with less protracted clinical courses and fewer maternal complications. These results indicate that early coverage of anaerobes, particularly *B. fragilis*, yields excellent results in postpartum cesarean section patients. Good results have also been achieved with cephalosporins, including cefoxitin, cefotetan, and the penicillins, including carbenicillin, ticarcillin, piperacillin, mezlocillin, and ampicillin with sulbactam added. Metronidazole has not been widely used in the United States because of theoretical concerns about the exposure of the breast-feeding baby to this agent.

Another approach to the problem of serious postpartum infection after cesarean section is the use of preventive antibiotics. Many of the factors that increase the infection rate in cesarean section seem amenable to systemic antibiotic prophylaxis. The surgical field at the time of cesarean section is usually contaminated with bacteria.[38] A number of prospective studies of antibiotic prophylaxis in cesarean section have been performed. In general, the reports have been enthusiastic. Such prophylaxis is a standard form of treatment for the patient in labor who requires this operation.

Operative strategies play an important role in both the prevention and treatment of pelvic infection after cesarean section. Techniques in the operating room on the patient in labor may alter the postoperative course of morbidity. One form of preventive operative therapy is the extraperitoneal approach at the time of the initial operation.[39] This does not eliminate postpartum infection, but it does eliminate intraperitoneal infection. The major drawbacks are the relative lack of experience with this operative technique in most medical centers and the awareness that the majority of patients can be safely managed without it.

Operative therapy for serious postpartum infections is uncommon, but it can be important for cure. In women who have developed a pelvic abscess, operative drainage or removal is imperative if antibiotic treatment fails. The decision concerning the approach is based on the location of the abscess. If extraperitoneal drainage can be easily accomplished, drainage will usually suffice. If the abscess is high in the pelvis, laparotomy with removal of the infected tissue is indicated. Laparotomy is the most frequently used therapeutic approach at present.

POSTOPERATIVE SOFT TISSUE GYNECOLOGIC INFECTIONS

A number of factors are involved in postoperative soft tissue gynecologic infections. Bacterial contamination occurs if the vagina is part of the operative field. This is the case with both vaginal and abdominal hysterectomy despite thorough preoperative cleansing of the vagina to remove the abundant normal flora. At least part of this subsequent bacterial contamination comes from the resident bacterial flora of the endocervix, which will not be eliminated by the usual surface preparation techniques. Some patients undergoing hysterectomy are more at risk than others for postoperative infections. In a nationwide evaluation of over 12,000 women undergoing hysterectomy, it was noted that blacks had a higher incidence of postoperative fever and received antibiotics more frequently than whites.[40] Whether these differences were related to the socioeconmic status of the population or to the presence of a population risk factor such as sickle cell trait is not known. In addition, many different evaluations have documented populations at risk for a postoperative pelvic abscess. These include premenopausal women who undergo vaginal hysterectomy,[41] particularly when the operation is performed on the clinic service.[42] It is not known whether the increased number of abscesses seen in these young women in the era before antibiotic prophylaxis was due to differences in the bacterial flora present in the lower genital tract; difficulty in obtaining hemostasis when performing vaginal hysterectomy in the more vascular pelvis of premenopausal women; or recurrent postoperative ovulation, which breaks the protective surface and exposes the interior of the ovary to the risk of infection. Whatever the mechanism, the premenopausal woman undergoing vaginal hysterectomy is at increased risk for a postoperative adnexal abscess. Although this has occurred much less frequently since the introduction of prophylactic antibiotics, these abscesses are still seen in premenopausal women.[43] The microorganisms involved in these infections are similar to those previously noted in the discussion of postpartum infections.

Antibiotic therapy for postoperative pelvic infections is empiric, since no prospective studies have been done. In view of the results of an experimental study[2] and clinical observations, early antibiotic coverage of gram-negative aerobes and of all anaerobes seems important. The use of prophylactic preoperative antibiotics have become routine in many situations, a subject that is discussed in Chapter 285.

The operative management of an established postoperative pelvic infection is very important for cure in the occasional patient who does not respond to antibiotic treatment. The basic management is drainage or removal of an infected, purulent collection. One diagnostic ritual in the evaluation of the febrile postoperative patient is the search by physical examination for an infected collection that can be drained. After hysterectomy, an uncommon infection is a vaginal cuff collection. If present, adequate drainage is easily accomplished and usually yields a cure. Other febrile patients seen a week or more postoperatively may have a pelvic abscess. The decision about the appropriate approach to these abscesses is based upon their location. If they are bulging into the vagina, vaginal drainage can easily be accomplished, with good therapeutic results.[44] If the abscess is high in the pelvic cavity and is not amenable to extraperitoneal drainage, laparotomy with removal of the abscess is necessary for cure.[41–43] These active therapeutic measures are important, for such pelvic abscesses can rupture into the peritoneal cavity, resulting in life-threatening illness and death.[41]

COMMUNITY-ACQUIRED INFECTIONS

The Infected Abortion

There have been dramatic changes in the past two decades in the clinical presentation of infected abortion in the United States. There has been a remarkable drop in the frequency of this syndrome. Of even greater significance is the decrease in the severity of the infections seen in this clinical population.[32] Before these changes occurred, septic abortion with endotoxic shock, as well as life-threatening myometritis due to *Clostridium perfringens*, were commonplace. The reasons for this dramatic change in clinical presentation were not due solely to better methods of therapy for the symptomatic patient. Instead, vast changes in health care delivery have had a major impact on this problem. More widespread availability of better methods of contraception to women from all social classes has decreased the number of women with unwanted pregnancies. The greatest impact occurred when restrictions on pregnancy termination in the hospital were lifted nationwide in the early 1970s. A poor woman with an unwanted pregnancy was no longer forced to seek the services of unskilled nonmedical personnel to terminate the pregnancy. The results were immediately apparent in urban hospitals, as both infected abortions and serious infection decreased.

The cornerstone of therapy for the patient with an infected abortion is the surgical removal of retained products of conception. Chow et al.[45] demonstrated that curettage was more beneficial than systemic antibiotics in the control of abortion-related infections. These products of conception are a nidus of continuing infection, and treatment with systemic antibiotics alone can be ineffective. There are also other situations in which operative intervention can be lifesaving. A syndrome of life-threatening sepsis in spontaneous mid-first trimester abortion has been reported in women wearing a large Dalkon Shield,[46] and at least part of the problem is continual bacterial seeding caused by the the heavily contaminated multifilamented tail.[47] Operative removal of this source of contamination may prove to be crucial for a clinical cure. Other situations include more extensive uterine damage in which the pelvic infection cannot be controlled by systemic antibiotics and curettage. This was not uncommon when necrosis-producing substances were used to induce abortion and an infection with potentially lethal agents like *Cl. perfringens* was established. In these women, surgical removal of the pelvic organs may be necessary for cure.

Antibiotic therapy for the patient with an infected abortion is usually empiric. Few prospective studies have been done, and those reported contain small numbers of patients. The best microbiologic study of women with an infected abortion was reported by Rotheram and Schick.[48] They found a high incidence of anaerobic organism bacteremia and suggested that an appropriate antibiotic strategy should include coverage of anaerobes, particularly *B. fragilis*. This is probably not necessary for all patients. In another study of a small number of patients, good results were noted when antibiotic coverage specifically for *B. fragilis* was not used as primary therapy.[49] This has been our clinical impression and probably reflects the overriding importance of curettage in therapy. In the infected abortion patient with septic shock, we recommend treatment for anaerobic organisms, as well as for the gram-negative aerobes usually associated with shock, since the septic shock syndrome can occur in women with anaerobic bacteremia.[50]

Salpingo-Oophoritis

A rational approach to patients with this infection is presented in Figure 2. The major grouping on the right focuses on the small percentage of the total population who are potential candidates for surgery. This is the smallest group in numbers, but these women with acute abdominal findings suggestive of an intraperitoneal abscess rupture have the most serious prognosis. Warning signs include upper abdominal rigidity and rebound, tenderness, tachycardia, and free pus on peritoneal aspiration. Although antibiotic coverage of aerobic and anaerobic organisms is important, immediate operative intervention with extirpation of the infected tissue and thorough peritoneal toilet is necessary for survival and cure.[51] Fortunately, this is a rare clinical picture. A more common event, although it is still found in a minority of the patients with salpingitis, is the presence of a pelvic mass. This may be a pelvic abscess that will eventually require operative intervention, either drainage or removal for cure. Since *B. fragilis* is frequently involved in pelvic abscesses, it is important to provide antibiotic coverage for this anaerobe from the onset of therapy.[52] Clinically, less than half of the

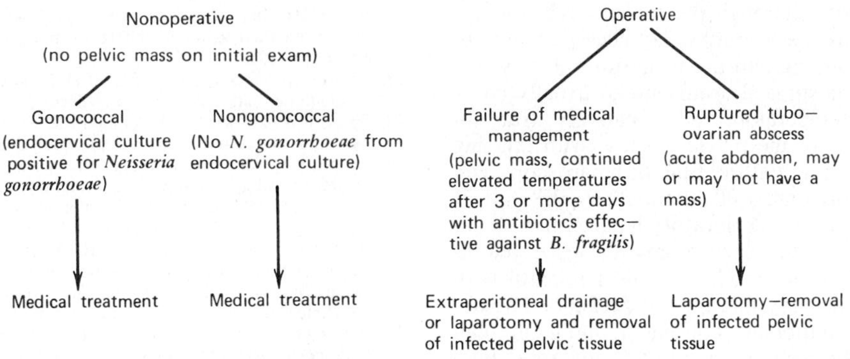

FIG. 2. Clinical classification of salpingo-oophoritis.

patients with a pelvic mass will require an operation.[53] Some abscesses are cured medically, and often the palpated mass is an inflammatory response to the infection rather than an abscess.

The majority of patients with salpingitis have neither a pelvic mass nor evidence suggesting an intraperitoneal accident. These women can be classified as having gonococcal or nongonococcal salpingitis. The physician should suspect gonococcal salpingitis in a woman with the first clinical episode of salpingitis, particularly when the symptoms occur with or just after menses and when the temperature is above 38°C. The key to this classification is the recovery of *Neisseria gonorrhoeae* from the endocervical culture. Obviously, this information will not be available at the onset of therapy, so the clinician should make a judgment based upon the Gram stain findings of an endocervical smear. Eschenbach et al.[54] found a good correlation between positive Gram stains and cultures positive for *N. gonorrhoeae*. In their study, approximately one-third of the women who had positive cultures did not have a positive smear, but all the women with a positive smear had positive cultures. The designation of gonococcal salpingitis has clinical significance. These women have a more favorable response to antibiotics than those with nongonococcal salpingitis.[55] They become afebrile more rapidly than women with nongonococcal salpingitis, seem less likely to develop a pelvic abscess during antibiotic therapy, and are more likely to be free of tubal damage after treatment. Since many men have positive cultures and are symptom free, it is important to culture and to treat the sexual partners of women with positive cultures.

Risk factors have been associated with either an increased frequency or an increased severity of infection. These risks have been assigned on the basis of clinical observations or by a case control method, but not by prospective study. An increased frequency of salpingo-oophoritis among women who use in intrauterine device for contraception has been reported in a number of studies.[56,57] The highest rate of pelvic infection has been noted in young nulliparous women.[58] In addition to the increased frequency of infection with an intrauterine device, there is evidence that the presentation of infection varies among intrauterine device users. Serious pelvic infections due to *Actinomyces bovis* have been reported among intrauterine device wearers.[59] These organisms can be detected on the cytology smear of women using this form of contraception, and these changes disappear when the intrauterine device is removed.[60] Another new phenomenon is the observation of unilateral tuboovarian abscesses among patients who use intrauterine devices. Although one study indicated that this finding only occurred in women who have used this method,[61] unilateral abscess in women who had never used this contraceptive has been reported.[62] Nevertheless, there was a greater than expected number of patients with unilateral pelvic abscess among intrauterine device wearers, and this was particularly true for those women with a Dalkon Shield in place. A strong clinical impression has been that infections are more severe among patients using an intrauterine device, but one prospective evaluation did not show this correlation.[16] The patient who has had salpingitis is more likely to have other episodes in the future. The mechanism is not known. It may reflect either changes in host defense mechanisms or simply exposure of these patients to sexual partners who reinfect them.

The antibiotic therapy of salpingo-oophoritis should have a number of goals. There should be a rapid clinical response without pelvic abscess formation, and the patient should have a pelvis free of adhesions or tubal abnormalities in which fertility is possible, since each episode of salpingitis increases the risk of infertility.[58,63] Unfortunately, few data are available on the long-term follow-up and subsequent fertility of women with salpingitis.

A number of treatment regimens can be used in the patient with salpingitis. The recommendations of the Centers for Disease Control are noted in Table 1.[64]

A few patients with salpingo-oophoritis require operative intervention for cure. In some instances, the decision to operate is relatively easy. The woman with a ruptured tuboovarian abscess has an operative emergency and requires immediate pel-

TABLE 1. Combination Regimens with Broad Activity Against Major Pathogens in Pelvic Inflammatory Disease

Regimen A (preferred when *Neisseria gonorrhoeae* or *Chlamydia trachomatis* is suspected as the primary pathogen):

Doxycycline: 100 mg IV twice a day
Plus
Cefoxitin: 2 g IV four times a day

Continue drugs IV for at least 4 days and for at least 48 hours after the patient improves (defervescence, decreased symptoms and signs). Then continue doxycycline, 100 mg by mouth twice a day, to complete 10–14 days of total therapy.

Regimen B (preferred when facultative gram-negative bacilli or anaerobes are suspected as the primary pathogens):

Clindamycin: 900 mg IV three times a day
Mixed in same infusion with
Gentamicin: 2 mg/kg IV

followed by 1.5 mg/kg, three times a day, for patients with normal renal function. Serum gentamicin levels should be monitored and dose or dose interval adjusted to maintain a gentamicin serum level of 5–10 μg/ml 30 minutes postadministration. Continue drugs IV for at least 4 days and at least 48 hours after the patient improves. Then continue clindamycin, 450 mg, by mouth four times a day, to complete 10–14 days of therapy.

Ambulatory Regimen

When the patient is not hospitalized, the following regimen is recommended:

Ceftriaxone: 250 mg IM in one dose
plus
Doxycycline: 100 mg by mouth twice a day for 10–14 days

(Data from Centers for Disease Control.[64])

vic tissue extirpation, plus thorough peritoneal cavity lavage for cure. Such patients are seen rarely today. The patient with a large pelvic abscess pointing into the posterior cul de sac is an excellent candidate for surgical drainage and usually has a rapid defervescence of temperature.[44] Alternatively, transabdominal needle aspiration of the pelvic abscess with imaging guidance[17] or needle aspiration at the time of laparoscopy can be done.[65] Both procedures are well tolerated by the patient and involve less morbidity than exploratory laparotomy. A patient who has had an exploratory laparotomy for suspected intraperitoneal rupture and is found to have acute salpingitis with no abscess formation is an easy therapeutic decision. The abdomen should be closed, antibiotics continued, and a cure can be expected. Antibiotics reduce the number of anaerobic bacteria in a model that simulates an abscess.[52] Since one therapeutic goal of antibiotic therapy is to eliminate anaerobic organisms at the site of infection, the use of antibiotics effective against anaerobes is indicated. A decision to operate should be made only when there is no response to this therapy.

REFERENCES

1. Weinstein WM, Onderdonk AB, Bartlett JG, et al. Experimental intra-abdominal abscesses in rats: Development of an experimental model. Infect Immun. 1974;10:1250.
2. Weinstein WM, Onderdonk AB, Bartlett JG, et al: Antimicrobial therapy of experimental intra-abdominal sepsis. J Infect Dis. 1975;132:282.
3. Ledger WJ, Norman M, Gee C, et al. Bacteremia on an obstetric-gynecologic service. Am J Obstet Gynecol. 1975;121:205.
4. Blanco JD, Gibbs RS, Castaneda YS. Bacteremia in obstetrics: Clinical course. Obstet Gynecol. 1981;58:621.
5. Bryan CS, Reynolds KL, Moore, EE. Bacteremia in obstetrics and gynecology. Obstet Gynecol. 1984;64:2.
6. Kauppel RA, Scerbo JC, Dzink J, et al. Quantitative transcervical uterine cultures with a new device. Obstet Gynecol. 1981;57:243.
7. Ledger WJ, Gee CL, Pollin P, et al. The use of pre-reduced media and portable jars for the collection of anaerobic organisms from clinical sites. Am J Obstet Gynecol. 1966;125:677.
8. Cuchoral GJ Jr, Tally FP, Jacobus NV, et al. Susceptibility of the *Bacteroides fragilis* group in the United States: Analysis by site of isolation. Antimicrob Agents Chemother. 1988;32:717.
9. Sweet RL, Mill J, Hadley KW, et al. Use of laparoscopy to determine the microbiologic etiology of acute salpingitis. Am J Obstet Gynecol. 1979;134:68.
10. Sweet RL, Schachter J, Robbie MO. Failure of beta-lactam antibiotics to eradicate *Chlamydia trachomatis* from the endometrium of patients with acute salpingitis despite apparent clinical cure. JAMA. 1983;250:2641.
11. Wood CA, Norton DR, Kohlhepp SJ, et al. The influence of tobramycin dosage regimens on nephrotoxicity-ototoxicity and antibacterial efficacy in a rat model of subcutaneous abscess. J Infect Dis. 1988;158:13.
12. Di Zerega G, Yonekura L, Roy S, et al. A comparison of clindamycin, gentamicin, and penicillin-gentamicin in the treatment of postcesarean endomyometritis. Am J Obstet Gynecol. 1979;134:238.
13. Gibbs RS, Listwa HM, Dreskin RB. A pure enterococcal abscess after cesarean section. J Reprod Med. 1977;19:17.
14. Moellering RC Jr, Enteroccal infections in patients treated with moxalactam. Rev Infect Dis. 1982;4:S708.
15. Terpenning MS, Zervos MJ, Schaberg DR, et al. Enterococcal infections: An increasing problem in hospitalized patients. Infect Cont Hosp Epidemiol 1988;9:457.
16. Ledger WJ, Moore DE, Lowensohn RI, et al. A fever index evaluation of chloramphenicol or clindamycin in patients with serious pelvic infections. Obstet Gynecol. 1977;50:523.
17. Gerzol SG, Robbins AH, Johnson WC, et al. Percutaneous catheter drainage of abdominal abscesses. N Engl J Med. 1981;305:653.
18. Goplerud CP, Ohm MJ, Galask RP. Aerobic and anaerobic flora of the cervix during pregnancy and the puerperium. Am J Obstet Gynecol. 1976;126:858.
19. Cherry SH, Filler M, Harvey H. Lysozyme content of amniotic fluid. Am J Obstet Gynecol. 1973;116:639.
20. Ford LC, Delange RJ, Lebherz TB. Identification of a bactericidal factor (B-lysin) in amniotic fluid at 40 weeks gestation. Am J Obstet Gynecol. 1977;127:788.
21. Larsen B, Synder IS, Galask RP. Transferrin concentration in human amniotic fluid. Am J Obstet Gynecol. 1973;117:952.
22. Cederqvist LL, Ewol LC, Bonsnas RW, et al. Detectability and pattern of immunoglobulins in normal amniotic fluid throughout gestation. Am J Obstet Gynecol. 1978;130:220.
23. Larsen B, Galask RP, Synder IS. Muramidase and peroxidase activity of human amniotic fluid. Obstet Gynecol. 1974;44:219.
24. Larson JW, Goldkrand JW, Hanson TM, et al. Intrauterine infection on an obstetric service. Obstet Gynecol. 1974;43:838.
25. Florman AL, Teubner D. Enhancement of bacterial growth in amniotic fluid by meconium. J Pediatr. 1969;74:111.
26. Blanco JD, Gibbs RS, Krebs, LF, et al. The association between the absence of amniotic fluid bacterial inhibitory activity and intra-amniotic infection. Am J Gynecol. 1982;143:749.
27. Tafari N, Ross SM, Naeye RL, et al. Failure of bacterial growth inhibition by amniotic fluid. Am J Obstet Gynecol. 1977;128:187.
28. Spore WW, Moskal PA, Nakamura RM, et al. The bacteriology of the postpartum oviducts and endometrium. Am J Obstet Gynecol. 1970;107:572.
29. Ledger WJ, Nakamura RM. Measurement of infectious disease morbidity in obstetrics and gynecology. Clin Obstet Gynecol. 1976;19:195.
30. Perloe M, Curet LB. The effect of internal fetal monitoring on cesarian section morbidity. Obstet Gynecol. 1979;53:354.
31. Anstey JT, Sheldon GW, Blythe JG. Infectious morbidity after primary cesarean section in a private institution. Am J Obstet Gynecol. 1980;136:205.
32. Ledger WJ, Kriewall TJ, Gee C. The fever index. A technic for evaluating the clinical response to bacteremia. Obstet Gynecol. 1975;45:603.
33. Wager GP, Martin DH, Koutsky L, et al. Puerperal infectious morbidity: Relationship to route of delivery and to antepartum *Chlamydia trachomatis* infection. Am J Obstet Gynecol. 1980;138:1028.
34. Ledger WJ, Reite AM, Headington JT. A system for infectious disease surveillance on an obstetric service. Obstet Gynecol. 1971;37:769.
35. Hibbard LT, Snyder EN, McVann RE. Subgluteal and retropsoal infection in obstetric practice Obstet Gynecol. 1972;39:172.
36. Ledger WJ, Lewis W, Golde S, et al. The use of metronidazole in obstetric and gynecologic infections. In: Finegold SM, McFadzean JA, Roe FJC, eds. Metronidazole. Princeton, N.J.: Excerpta Medica; 1977:353.
37. Golde S, Ledger WJ. Necrotizing fasciitis in postpartum patients. A report of four cases. Obstet Gynecol. 1977;50:670.
38. Wong R, Gee C, Ledger WJ. Prophylactic use of cefazolin in monitored patients undergoing cesarean section. Obstet Gynecol. 1978;51:407.
39. Imig JR, Perkins RP. Extraperitoneal cesarean section: A new need for old skills. Am J Obstet Gynecol. 1976;125:51.
40. Ledger WJ, Child M. The hospital care of patients undergoing hysterectomy. An analysis of 12,026 women from the Professional Activity Study. Am J Obstet Gynecol. 1973;117:423.
41. Ledger WJ, Campbell C, Willson JR. Postoperative adnexal infection. Obstet Gynecol. 1968;31:83.
42. Willson JR, Black JR. Ovarian abscess. Am J Obstet Gynecol. 1964;90:34.
43. Livengood CH III, Addison WA. Adnexal abscess as a delayed complication of vaginal hysterectomy. Am J Obstet Gynecol. 1982;143:596.
44. Rubenstein PR, Mishell DR, Ledger WJ. Colpotomy drainage of pelvic abscess. Obstet Gynecol. 1976;48:142.
45. Chow AW, Marshall JR, Guze LB. A double-blind study comparison of clindamycin with penicillin plus chloramphenicol in treatment of septic abortions. J Infect Dis. 1977;135:S35.
46. Christian CD. Maternal deaths associated with an intrauterine device. Am J Obstet Gynecol. 1974;119:441.
47. Tatum HJ, Schmidt FH, Phillips D, et al. The Dalkon Shield controversy. Structural and bacteriological studies of IUD tails. JAMA. 1975;231:711.
48. Rotheram EB, Schick SF. Nonclostridial anaerobic bacteria in septic shock. Am J Med. 1969;46:80.
49. Ostergard DR. Comparison of two antibiotic regimens in the treatment of septic abortion. Obstet Gynecol. 1970;36:473.
50. Ledger WJ, Gee CL, Lewis WP, et al. Comparison of clindamycin and chloramphenicol in treatment of serious infections of the female genital tract. J Infect Dis. 1977;135:S30.
51. Collins CG, Nix FG, Cerha HT. Ruptured tubo-ovarian abscess. Am J Obstet Gynecol 1956;72:820.
52. Bartlett JG, Recent developments in the management of anaerobic infections. Rev Infect Dis. 1983;5:235.
53. Ledger WJ. Selection of antimicrobial agents for the treatment of infections of the female genital tract. Rev Infect Dis. 1983;5:S98.
54. Eschenbach DA, Buchanan TM, Pollock HM, et al. Polymicrobial etiology of acute pelvic inflammatory disease. N Engl J Med. 1975;293:166.
55. Cunningham FG, Hauth JC, Strong JD, et al. Tetracyclines or penicillin-ampicillin for pelvic inflammatory disease. N Engl J Med. 1977;296:1380.
56. Westrom L, Bangtsson L, Mardh P. The risk of developing pelvic inflammatory disease in women using intrauterine devices as compared to non-users. Lancet. 1976;2:221.
57. Osser S, Liedholm P, Sjobert NO. Risk of PID among users of intrauterine devices, irrespective of previous pregnancy. Am J Obstet Gynecol. 1980;138:864.
58. Westrom L. Incidence, prevalence and trends of PID and its consequences in industrialized countries. Am J Obstet Gynecol. 1980;138:880.
59. Schiffer MA, Elquezobal A, Sultana M, et al. Actinomycosis infections associated with IUCD's Obstet Gynecol. 1975;45:67.
60. Gupta PK, Hollander SH, Frost JK. Actinomycetes in cervicovaginal smears. An associated with IUD usage. Acta Cytol. 1976;20:295.
61. Taylor ES, McMille JH, Greer BF, et al. The IUD and tubo-ovarian abscess. Am J Obstet Gynecol. 1975;123:338.
62. Golde SH, Israel R, Ledger WJ. Unilateral tubo-ovarian abscess. A distinct entity. Am J Obstet Gynecol. 1977;127:802.
63. Westrom L. Effects of acute PID on fertility. Am J Obstet Gynecol. 1975;121:707.
64. Centers for Disease Control. STO Treatment Guidelines 1987. MMWR. 1987;36(Suppl 55).
65. Henry-Sacket J, Soler A, Wilfredo V. Laparoscopic treatment of tubo-ovarian abscess. J Reprod Med. 1984;29:579.

97. PROSTATITIS, EPIDIDYMITIS, AND ORCHITIS

JOHN N. KRIEGER

ANATOMY AND PHYSIOLOGY OF THE TESTES AND MALE ACCESSORY SEX ORGANS

The testicle has two functional components, seminiferous tubules and interstitial cells. Sperm production is the primary function of the seminiferous tubules. Interstitial cells, located between the seminiferous tubules, are primarily responsible for hormone production. After spermatogenesis spermatozoa are transported from the testis into the epididymis (Fig. 1). Sperm then move into the vas deferens, a muscular tube approximately 12 inches long that is easily palpable in the scrotum. Fructose from the seminal vesicles is the major energy source for ejaculated sperm. In addition, the seminal vesicles provide a number of proteins that cause coagulation of the ejaculate. Liquification of the semen occurs within 5–30 minutes after ejaculation as a result of proteolytic enzymes from the prostate.[1]

HOST DEFENSES OF THE MALE LOWER UROGENITAL TRACT

Organisms ascend via the urethra to cause most infections of the urogenital ducts and accessory sex organs.[2] Thus, mechanical factors such as the flushing action of micturition and ejaculation should provide some protection against infection, although the relative significance of such defenses is unclear.

A zinc-containing polypeptide known as the prostatic antibacterial factor is the most important antimicrobial substance secreted by the prostate.[2,3] Men with well-documented chronic bacterial prostatitis have significantly lower levels of zinc in their prostatic fluid than do healthy men, but their serum zinc levels are within normal limits.[3] It is unclear whether reduced zinc concentrations precede the development of prostatic infection or represent a secretory dysfunction resulting from such infections. Prostatic secretions of patients with bacterial prostatitis contain high concentrations of immunoglobulins.[4,5] Several studies have demonstrated antigen-specific antibody coating of bacteria isolated from the lower urinary tracts of patients with prostatitis syndromes. The antigen-specific antibody response in prostatic secretions (predominately secretory IgA) is significantly greater than is the serologic response.[5]

The presence of leukocytes is characteristic of many conditions of the male lower urinary tract, including prostatitis.[6] Phagocytosis of abnormal sperm by leukocytes in some infertile men with pyosemina has been observed.

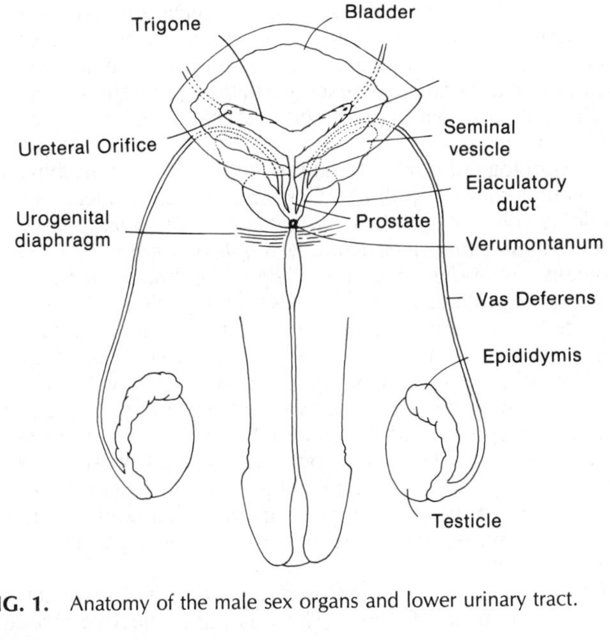

FIG. 1. Anatomy of the male sex organs and lower urinary tract.

PROSTATITIS

Classification of Prostatitis

The term *prostatitis* is employed clinically to describe a large group of adult men with a variety of complaints referable to the lower urogenital tract and perineum.[2,7] It has been estimated that 50 percent of men will experience symptoms of prostatitis at some time in their lives.[2] It is of critical importance to distinguish patients with lower urinary tract complaints associated with bacteriuria, such as patients who may have bacterial prostatitis, from the larger number of patients without bacteriuria. Further classification of patients with prostatitis depends on careful bacteriologic assessment of the lower urinary tract that is based on sequential urine cultures obtained during micturition[7,8] (Table 1). On the basis of results of lower urinary tract localization, men with prostatitis syndromes may be classified into four major groups: acute bacterial prostatitis, chronic bacterial prostatitis, nonbacterial prostatitis, and prostatodynia[7] (Table 2). In addition, rare patients develop granulomatous prostatitis.

Bacterial prostatitis is a frequent diagnosis in general clinical practice, but well-documented bacterial infections of the prostate, whether acute or chronic, are uncommon.[2,5] The great majority of patients with a diagnosis of prostatitis are adult men with perineal, lower back, or lower abdominal pain; urinary discomfort; or ejaculatory complaints. Most of these patients have no history of bacteriuria, and there is little objective evidence of bacterial infection of the prostate. Thus, most patients with prostatitis may be classified in the groups of nonbacterial prostatitis or prostatodynia, conditions about which there are few firm data to base therapeutic decisions.

Acute Bacterial Prostatitis. Acute bacterial prostatitis is usually not a subtle or difficult diagnosis. Patients complain of symptoms associated with lower urinary tract infection such as urinary frequency and dysuria. Patients may also experience lower urinary tract obstruction due to acute edema of the prostate. Signs of systemic toxicity are common. On physical examination patients may have a high temperature and lower abdominal or suprapubic discomfort due to bladder infection. The rectal examination is frequently impressive, with an exquisitely

TABLE 1. Lower Urinary Tract Localization Using Segmented Urine Cultures[a]

Specimen	*Symbol*	*Description*
Voided bladder 1	VB_1	Initial 5–10 ml of urinary stream
Voided bladder 2	VB_2	Midstream specimen
Expressed prostatic secretions	EPS	Secretions expressed from prostate by digital massage after midstream specimen
Voided bladder 3	VB_3	First 5–10 ml of urinary stream immediately after prostatic massage

[a] Unequivocal diagnosis of bacterial prostatitis requires that the colony count in the VB_3 specimen greatly exceed the count in the VB_1 specimen, preferably by at least 10-fold.[2,8] Many patients who have chronic bacterial prostatitis, however, harbor only small numbers of bacteria in their prostates. In such patients, direct culture of the prostatic secretions is particularly useful. Microscopic examination of the EPS is useful for identifying white blood cells and "oval fat bodies," large lipid-laden macrophages characteristic of the prostatic inflammatory response.[2,7]

TABLE 2. Classification of Prostatitis Syndromes on the Basis of Lower Urinary Tract Localization Studies

Condition	*Bacteriuria*[a]	*Infection Localized to Prostate*[b]	*Inflammatory Response in EPS*[c]	*Abnormal Rectal Examination of Prostate*[d]	*Systemic Illness*[e]
Acute bacterial prostatitis	+	+	+	+	+
Chronic bacterial prostatitis	+	+	+	−	−
"Nonbacterial" prostatitis	−	−	+	−	−
Prostatodynia	−	−	−	−	−

[a] Documented with an identical organism that is shown to localize to a prostatic focus when the midstream urine culture is negative.
[b] Refer to the text for diagnostic criteria.
[c] Prostatic secretions containing ≥ 12 WBC/HPF in a patient with no objective evidence of urethritis.
[d] Abnormal findings include exquisite tenderness and swelling that may be associated with signs of lower urinary tract obstruction.
[e] Systemic findings frequently include fever and rigors and may include signs of bacteremia.

tender, tense prostate on palpation. Urinalysis is abnormal, with evidence of pyuria, and cultures are positive. Bacteremia may be present spontaneously or may result from overly vigorous rectal examinations.

Results of antimicrobial therapy for acute bacterial prostatitis are often dramatic. Many drugs that do not penetrate into the prostate under normal conditions are effective in acute bacterial prostatitis.[2] Thus, drugs that would be appropriate in patients with bacteremia caused by Enterobacteriaceae, pseudomonads, and enterococci should be administered once specimens have been obtained for urine and blood cultures. General measures are also indicated including hydration, analgesics, and bed rest. The most important complications of acute bacterial prostatitis include prostatic abscess, prostatic infarction, chronic bacterial prostatitis, and granulomatous prostatitis.

Chronic Bacterial Prostatitis. Chronic bacterial prostatitis is an important cause of bacterial persistence in the male lower urinary tract. Patients characteristically experience recurrent bacterial urinary tract infections caused by the same organism.[2] Patients are generally asymptomatic between episodes of bladder bacteriuria. The prostate gland is usually normal on either rectal or endoscopic evaluation. Thus, careful lower urinary tract localization studies are the cornerstone on which to base a diagnosis of chronic bacterial prostatitis.[8] Diagnosis of chronic bacterial prostatitis based solely on symptoms, the number of leuckoytes in expressed prostatic secretions, or the use of prostate biopsy specimens is inadequate.

Gram-negative rods (Enterobacteriaceae or pseudomonads) are by far the most important pathogens in chronic bacterial prostatitis. Gram-positive cocci such as *Enterococcus faecalis* or, perhaps, *Staphylococcus saprophyticus,* may be the etiologic organisms in a few cases. Reports implicating many other organisms are generally difficult to evaluate due to methodologic problems with case definition or a lack of documentation of bacteriuria by the alleged pathogen.

Medical management is effective in curing or suppressing bacterial infections of the prostate. Trimethoprim has two useful characteristics: it achieves good levels in the prostatic parenchyma and is effective against most of the common bacterial pathogens.[2] Available studies have most commonly employed the combination of trimethoprim and sulfamethoxazole for the treatment of patients with well-documented chronic bacterial prostatitis. Long treatment courses result in symptomatic and bacteriologic cure in approximately one-third of patients, symptomatic improvement while receiving therapy in approximately one-third of patients who relapse after the drug therapy is stopped, and no improvement in the remaining patients.[9] Many other orally administered antimicrobial agents have been used for the treatment of patients with chronic bacterial prostatitis. Most of these studies are hampered by imprecise case definitions, a lack of sufficient microbiologic documentation or follow-up, or an abundance of patients infected with organisms generally considered urethral contaminants. In early studies, several of the new quinolones have shown promise as agents for the treatment of chronic bacterial prostatitis.[10–11]

Bacteria isolated from patients with chronic bacterial prostatitis, even after multiple episodes of symptomatic bacteriuria and prolonged courses of antibiotics, are generally antibiotic-sensitive strains.[2,9] Several findings may explain the disappointing results of antibiotic therapy including poor diffusion of most drugs into the prostatic parenchyma, changes in prostatic fluid pH level that are associated with infection, and infected calculi that may serve as persistent foci for bacteria.[9,13]

Patients with chronic bacterial prostatitis who are not cured may be rendered asymptomatic by long-term, suppressive treatment. Since patients are usually asymptomatic between episodes of bacteriuria, the goal of suppressive therapy is to prevent symptomatic episodes despite the persistence of bacteria in the prostate. Very low doses of agents such as penicillin, tetracycline, nitrofurantoin, nalidixic acid, or trimethoprim-sulfamethoxazole are remarkably effective in preventing episodes of symptomatic bladder infection in patients with chronic bacterial prostatitis.[2]

Nonbacterial Prostatitis and Prostatodynia. Patients with nonbacterial prostatitis and prostatodynia have no history of bacteriuria and lack objective evidence of bacterial infection of their prostatic secretions on careful lower urinary tract localization studies (Table 2).[7] Such patients may complain of a variety of perineal and pelvic symptoms. Pain or vague discomfort is common and may be suprapubic, infrapubic, scrotal, or inguinal in location. The discomfort may be described as either continuous or spasmodic and is commonly described as a "dull ache." Occasional patients complain of increased urinary frequency or dysuria, and ejaculatory complaints are not infrequent. Systemic symptoms or signs are absent. Physical examination is generally unremarkable.

Nonbacterial prostatitis and prostatodynia are distinguished by microscopic examination of the expressed prostatic secretions. Patients with nonbacterial prostatitis have objective evidence of an inflammatory response in their prostatic secretions, while patients with prostatodynia have no evidence of inflammation.

The etiology of nonbacterial prostatitis and prostatodynia remains uncertain. Mardh and Colleen found no evidence for an etiologic role for *Neisseria gonorrhoeae, Trichomonas vaginalis, Ureaplasma urealyticum, Mycoplasma hominis, Candida albicans,* anaerobic bacteria, *Chlamydia trachomatis,* or viruses in these syndromes.[14,15] However, other researchers have reported that many patients with "subacute or chronic prostatitis" are infected with *C. trachomatis*[16] or *U. urealyticum.*[17–19] The techniques, control groups, and findings in these later studies have been questioned by other workers.[2,20] Some workers have proposed that nonbacterial prostatitis is not an infectious disease.[21,22] In poorly controlled studies, prostaglandins, autoimmunity, psychological abnormalities, neuromuscular dysfunction of the bladder neck or urogenital diaphragm, and allergy to environmental agents have all been suggested as etiologic factors.

Current therapy for symptomatic patients with nonbacterial prostatitis is unsatisfactory. There is little objective evidence that patients with nonbacterial prostatitis or prostatodynia benefit from empirical antimicrobial therapy.

Granulomatous Prostatitis. Granulomatous prostatitis is a characteristic histologic reaction of the prostate to a variety of insults, with granulomas containing lipid-laden histiocytes, plasma cells, and scattered giant cells. In most cases granulomatous prostatitis follows an episode of acute bacterial prostatitis.[23,24] There are also a number of specific infectious causes of granulomatous reaction by the prostate. Tuberculous prostatitis is usually secondary to tuberculosis elsewhere in the genital tract.[25,26] Most patients have no symptoms referable to prostatic infection. On biopsy the granulomas may contain typical Langhans giant cells and may be associated with caseous necrosis. Such infections are most often caused by *Mycobacterium tuberculosis* but have also been reported to be caused by atypical mycobacteria.[27] Prostatitis may be secondary to systemic involvement with many of the deep mycoses.[28] Most cases of mycotic prostatitis reported have been associated with blastomycosis,[28] coccidioidomycosis,[29] and cryptococcosis.[30] However, paracoccidioidomycosis occasionally involves the prostate.[28] Other reported causes of granulomatous prostatitis include actinomycosis, candidiasis, syphilis, brucellosis, and sacral herpes zoster.[23]

Granulomatous prostatitis is most important in the differential diagnosis of an indurated, firm, or nodular prostate. The rectal examination of such patients raises the suspicion of prostatic carcinoma. Biopsy is usually necessary for diagnosis, and it is important that appropriate stains be used for the detection of specific etiologic agents.

Prostatic Abscess

Prostatic abscess is a rare complication in patients who receive appropriate treatment for acute bacterial prostatitis.[31] Most prostatic abscesses occur in patients with diabetes, in immunocompromised patients, and in patients who have not received appropriate therapy for acute prostatitis. The presence of a foreign body or urinary tract obstruction are other predisposing factors. In the past, *N. gonorrhoeae* was a common pathogen, but most cases are now caused by the common uropathogens. Infection generally occurs by the ascending route. On occasion, *Staphylococcus aureus* is the pathogen, which suggests the possibility of hematogenous infection. Patients are usually febrile with irritative voiding symptoms, and they may have signs of urosepsis. Thus, the clinical presentation closely resembles that of acute bacterial prostatitis. Classically, the abscess presents as a fluctuant area in the prostate that can be palpated during rectal examination. However, the presentation may be more subtle. The use of ultrasonography[32] or computed tomography[33] of the pelvis is helpful for confirming the diagnosis or in patients with equivocal clinical findings. Treatment includes draining the abscess, via either a perineal or transurethral route in addition to appropriate antimicrobial therapy.

EPIDIDYMITIS

Epididymitis is an inflammatory reaction of the epididymis to a variety of infectious agents or to local trauma. Epididymitis is common, accounting for over 600,000 visits to physicians per year in the United States. Acute epididymitis is responsible for more days lost from military service than any other disease and is responsible for 20 percent of urologic admissions in military populations.[35]

Patients with epididymitis usually complain of painful swelling of the scrotum. The onset may be acute over 1 or 2 days or more gradual and is often associated with dysuria or irritative lower urinary tract symptoms. Many patients have a urethral discharge.[34] Specific attention should be directed to eliciting a past history of genitourinary tract disease or sexual exposure. Some patients may have only a nonspecific finding of fever or other signs of infection. This is particularly frequent in hospitalized patients who have recent urinary tract manipulation and may be obtunded by medication.

Tender swelling, frequently accompanied by erythema, generally unilateral, may be noted primarily in the posterior aspect of the scrotum. If the patient is examined early in the course of the disease, the swelling may be localized to one portion of the epididymitis. Later, involvement of the ipsilateral testis is frequent, producing an epididymo-orchitis, and it may be difficult to distinguish the testicle from the epididymis within the inflammatory mass. Scrotal examination commonly reveals the presence of a hydrocele caused by the secretion of inflammatory fluid between the layers of the tunica vaginalis. Urethral discharge may be apparent on inspection or stripping of the urethra.

There are two common types of epididymitis, nonspecific bacterial epididymitis and sexually transmitted epididymitis. In addition, epididymitis may occur rarely after genital trauma or with disseminated infections.

Classification of Epididymitis

Nonspecific Bacterial Epididymitis. The most common cause of epididymitis in men over 35 years old is infection with coliform or *Pseudomonas* species.[34,36] In most series, gram-negative aerobic-rods caused over two-thirds of cases of bacterial epididymitis.[34,36,37] However, gram-positive cocci are also important pathogens and were the most common organisms in some reports.[39]

Many patients who develop bacterial epididymitis have underlying urologic pathology or have a history of recent genitourinary tract manipulation.[34,36] The development of epididymitis after surgery or urethral catheterization may occur weeks or rarely months after the manipulation. Epididymitis is particularly likely in patients who undergo urinary tract surgery or instrumentation while they are bacteriuric. Acute and chronic bacterial prostatitis are other important predisposing conditions for the development of bacterial epididymitis.

Bacterial epididymitis may be an important focus of organisms causing bacteremia and local morbidity in patients with indwelling transurethral catheters. Genitourinary tract complications of acute bacterial epididymitis include testicular infarction, scrotal abscess, pyozele, a chronic draining scrotal sinus, chronic epididymitis, and infertility.[39,40]

Tuberculous epididymitis generally occurs after involvement of the prostate and seminal vesicles.[25] There is characteristic scrotal swelling with "beadlike" enlargement of the vas deferens. Chronic draining scrotal sinuses may be present. The systemic mycoses may rarely cause epididymitis; blastomycosis is the most common pathogen.

Medical management is appropriate for most patients with bacterial epididymitis. Initial empirical treatment with agents appropriate for both gram-negative rods and gram-positive cocci should be initiated pending urine culture and sensitivity results. Nonspecific measures such as bed rest, scrotal elevation analgesics, and local ice packs are helpful. Surgery may be necessary for complications of acute epididymal infections.

Sexually Transmitted Epididymitis. Sexually transmitted epididymitis is the most common type of epididymitis in young men. *C. trachomatis* and *N. gonorrhoeae* are the major pathogens in this population. Chlamydiae have recently been identified as the most common cause of epididymitis in younger, sexually active populations.[41,42] Such patients were formerly considered to have "idiopathic," nonspecific epididymitis. Berger et al. documented infections with *C. trachomatis* in 17 of 34 cases of epididymitis in patients less than 35 years old and only 1 of 16 cases of epididymitis in patients older than 35. Patients with chlamydial epididymitis frequently did not complain of urethral discharge. However, 11 of 17 patients with epididymitis caused by chlamydiae had demonstrable discharge, usually the scant, watery discharge characteristic of nonspecific urethritis. The median interval from the last sexual exposure was 10 days and ranged from 1 to 45 days. Thus, patients may carry chlamydiae for long periods before the development of overt epididymitis.

Before the availability of penicillin, it was estimated that epididymitis occurred in 10–30 percent of men with gonococcal urethritis.[40] In more recent studies, *N. gonorrhoeae* was identified as the cause of acute epididymitis in 16 percent of cases in military populations[43] and in 21 percent of cases of epididymitis in civilians less than 35 years old.[34] Many patients with gonococcal epididymitis do not have a history of urethral discharge, and a discharge may be demonstrable in only 50 percent of such patients.

Underlying genitourinary tract abnormalities are uncommon in this population. Diagnosis depends on a high index of clinical suspicion, evaluation for presence of urethritis (which may be asymptomatic), and appropriate cultures. Specific antibiotic therapy, generally employing drugs appropriate for both chlamydiae and gonococci (i.e., tetracycline, 500 mg po four times daily for at least 10 days), is the most important aspect of treatment.[44] Patients should be evaluated for other sexually transmitted pathogens, and treatment of sexual partners is important. In general, a complete urologic work-up is not indicated for patients with uncomplicated sexually transmitted epididymitis. Complications of sexually transmitted epididymitis include abscess formation, testicular infarction, chronic epididymitis, and infertility.

ORCHITIS

Orchitis is significantly less common than is either prostatitis or epididymitis. Orchitis differs from infections of the male accessory sex glands in two important respects: blood-borne dissemination is the major route of infection, and viruses are clearly implicated as important pathogens.

Classification of Orchitis

Viral Orchitis. Viral infections, particularly mumps, are associated with most cases of orchitis. Although mumps rarely causes orchitis in prepubertal boys, orchitis occurs in approximately 20 percent of postpubertal patients with mumps.[45] Testicular pain and swelling usually begin 4 to 6 days after the onset of parotitis but may occur without parotid involvement. Orchitis is unilateral in approximately 70 percent of cases. Contralateral testicular swelling may occur 1 to 9 days after involvement of the first side. The clinical course is variable and ranges from mild testicular discomfort and swelling to severe testicular pain and marked swelling accompanied by nausea, vomiting, prostration, high fever, and constitutional symptoms. Epididymitis and inflammation of the spermatic cord may be noted on physical examination. Resolution of mild cases may occur in 4 or 5 days. More severe cases usually resolve in 3 to 4 weeks. Approximately one-half of the involved testes undergo some degree of atrophy. In older series, sterility was reported in 25 percent of patients with bilateral disease. However, more recent studies have found that mumps orchitis seldom results in infertility.[45] Coxsackie B virus produces a disease that clinically and histologically resembles mumps orchitis.

Bacterial Orchitis. With the exception of viral diseases, acute genitourinary tract infections involving only the testis are distinctly unusual. Pyogenic bacterial orchitis usually occurs as a consequence of the contiguous spread from an inflammatory process in the epididymis to cause an epididymo-orchitis. Thus, most cases of pyogenic orchitis are caused by *Escherichia coli, Klebsiella pneumoniae, Pseudomonas aeruginosa,* staphylococci, or streptococci. Occasionally, acute orchitis may be caused by other organisms as a result of metastatic seeding.

The patient with pyogenic orchitis appears acutely ill with a high fever and marked discomfort and swelling of the involved testicle. Generally the pain is described as radiating to the inguinal canal and is frequently accompanied by nausea and vomiting. On examination, there is usually an acute hydrocele, and the testis is swollen and exquisitely tender. The overlying scrotal skin is generally erythematous and edematous. Complications of pyogenic bacterial orchitis include testicular infarction, abscess formation, and pyocele of the scrotum. Surgery is usually required for treatment of these conditions. Orchitis can be caused by tuberculosis and blastomycosis, but by extension from the epididymis. Involvement of the testicle without palpable abnormality in the adjacent epididymis has rarely been observed with these agents.

REFERENCES

1. Jenkins AD, Turner TT, Howards SS. Physiology of the male reproductive system. Urol Clin North Am. 1978;5:437.
2. Stamey TA: Pathogenesis and Treatment of Urinary Tract Infections. Baltimore: Williams & Wilkins; 1980:1, 342.
3. Fair WR, Couch J, Wehner N. Prostatic antibacterial factor: Identity and significance. Urology. 1976;7:169.
4. Shortliffe LMD, Wehner N, Stamey TA. Use of solid-phase radioimmunoassay and formalin-fixed whole bacterial antigen in the detection of antigen-specific immunoglobulin in prostatic fluid. J Clin Invest. 1981;67:780.
5. Fowler JE Jr, Mariano M. Immunologic response of the prostate to bacteriuria and bacterial prostatitis: II. Antigen specific immumoglobulin in prostatic flud. J Urol. 1982;128:165.
6. Schaeffer AJ, Wendel EF, Dunn JK, et al. Prevalence and significance of prostatic inflammation. J Urol. 1981;125:215.
7. Drach GW, Meares EM, Fair WR, et al. Classification of benign diseases associated with prostatic pain: Prostatitis or prostatodynia? J Urol. 1978;120:266.
8. Meares EM, Stamey TA. Bacteriologic localization patterns in bacterial prostatitis and urethritis. Invest Urol. 1968;5:492.
9. Fair WR, Crane DB, Schiller N, et al. Re-appraisal of treatment in chronic bacterial prostatitis. J Urol. 1979;121:437.
10. Weidner W, Schiefer HG. Treatment of bacterial prostatitis with ciprofloxacin: Results of a one-year follow-up study. Am J Med. 1987;82(Suppl 4A):280.
11. Comhaire FH. Concentration of pefloxacine in split ejaculates of patients with chronic male accessory gland infection. J Urol. 1987;138:828.
12. Malinverni R, Glausser MP. Comparative studies of fluoroquinolones in the treatment of urinary tract infections. Rev Infect Dis. 1988;10(Suppl 1):153.
13. Eykyn S, Bultitude MI, Mayo ME, et al. Prostatitic calculi as a source of recurrent bacteriuria in the male. Br J Urol. 1974;46:527.
14. Mardh PA, Colleen S. Search for uro-genital tract infections in patients with symptoms of prostatitis. Scand J Urol Nephrol. 1975;9:8.
15. Mardh PA, Ripa KT, Colleen S et al. Role of *Chlamydia trachomatis* in nonacute prostatitis. Br J Vener Dis. 1978;54:330.
16. Weidner W, Arens M, Krauss H, et al. *Chlamydia trachomatis* in "abacterial" prostatitis: Microbiological cytological, and serological studies. Urol Int. 1983;38:146.
17. Weidner W, Brunner H, Krause W. Quantitative culture of *Ureaplasma urealyticum* in patients with chronic prostatitis or prostatosis. J Urol. 1980;124:622.
18. Poletti F, Medici MC, Alinovi A, et al. Isolation of *Chlamydia trachomatis* from the prostatic cells in patients affected by nonacute abacterial prostatitis. J Urol. 1985;134:691.
19. Schacter J. Is *Chlamydia trachomatis* a cause of prostatitis? J Urol 1985;134:711.
20. Taylor-Robinson D. The role of chlamydiae in genitourinary disease (Letter). J Urol. 1982;128:156.
21. Segura JW, Opitz JL, Green LF. Prostatosis prostatitis or pelvic floor tension myalgia? J Urol. 1979;122:168.
22. Nilsson JK, Colleen S, Mardh PA. Relationship between psychological and laboratory findings in patients with symptoms of non-acute prostatitis. In: Danielsson D, Juhlin L, Mardh PA, eds. Genital Infections and Their Complications. Stockholm: Almquist and Wiksell; 1975:133.
23. Kreiger JN. Prostatitis syndromes: Pathophysiology, differential diagnosis and treatment. Sex Transm Dis. 1984;11:100.
24. O'Dea MJ, Hunting DB, Greene LF. Nonspecific granulomatous prostatitis. J Urol 1977;118:58.
25. Venema RJ, Lattimer JK. Genital tuberculosis in the male. J Urol. 1957;78:65.
26. Simon HB. Genitourinary tuberculosis: Clinical features in a general hospital population. Am J Med. 1977;63:410.
27. Brooker WJ, Aufderheide AC. Genitourinary tract infections due to atypical mycobacteria. J Urol. 1980;124:242.
28. Schwarz J: Mycotic prostatitis. Urology. 1982;19:1.

29. Price MJ, Lewis EL, Carmalt JE. Coccidioidomycosis of prostate gland. Urology. 1982;19:653.
30. Hinchley WW, Someren A. Cryptococcal prostatitis. Am J Clin Pathol. 1981;75:257.
31. Meares EM Jr. Postatic Abscess. J Urol. 1986;136:1281.
32. Suago H, Takiuchi H, Sakurai T. Transrectal longitudinal ultrasonography of prostatic abscess. J Urol. 1986;136:1316.
33. Vaccaro JA, Belville WD, Kiesling VJ Jr, et al. Prostatic abscesses: Computerized tomography scanning as an aid to diagnosis and treatment. J Urol 1986;136:1318.
34. Berger RE, Alexander ER, Harnisch JP, et al. Etiology, manifestations and therapy of acute epididymitis: Prospective study of 50 cases. J Urol. 1979;121:750.
35. Bormel P: Current concepts on the etiology and treatment of epididymitis. Med Bull US Army, Europe. 1963;20:332.
36. Berger RE, Alexander ER, Monda GD, et al. *Chlamydia trachomatis* as a cause of acute "idiopathic" epididymitis. N Engl J Med. 1978;298:301.
37. Mittemeyer BT, Lennox KW, Borski AA. Epididymitis—a review of 610 cases. J Urol. 1966;95:390.
38. Witherington R, Harper WM IV. The surgical management of acute bacterial epididymitis with emphasis on epididymotomy. J Urol. 1982;128:722.
39. Nilsson S, Obrant KD, Persson PS: Changes in the testes parenchyma caused by acute nonspecific epididymitis. Fertil Steril. 1968;19:748.
40. Nickel WR, Plumb RT. Other infections and inflammations of the external genitalis. In: Harrison JH, Gittes RF, Perlmutter AD, et al, eds. Campbell's Urology. v. 1. ed 4. Philadelphia: WB Saunders; 1978:640.
41. Shapiro FR, Breschi LC: Acute epididymitis in Viet Nam. Review of 52 cases. Milit Med. 1973;138:643.
42. Harnisch JP, Berger RE, Alexander ER, et al. Aetiology of acute epididymitis. Lancet. 1977;1:819.
43. Watson RA. Gonorrhea and acute epididymitis. Milit Med. 1979;144:785.
44. Drotman PD. Epidemiology and treatment of epididymitis. Rev Infect Dis. 1982;4(Suppl):788.
45. Beard CM, Benson RC, Kelalis PP, et al. The incidence and outcome of mumps orchitis in Rochester, Minn. Mayo, 1935–1974. Mayo Clin Proc. 1977;52:3.

SECTION N. EYE INFECTIONS

98. CONJUNCTIVITIS

PETER J. McDONNELL
W. RICHARD GREEN

The most common eye disease in the Western Hemisphere is conjunctivitis. The normal flora of the conjunctiva, various sources of infection in conjunctivitis, and factors important in the resistance of the conjunctiva to infections have been well described.[1–15]

ETIOLOGIC AGENTS

The numerous agents that may cause conjunctivitis are listed in Table 1.

CLINICAL MANIFESTATIONS

The most obvious clinical manifestation of conjunctivitis is hyperemia of the conjunctiva. The dilatation and congestion of the vessels are greater near the periphery of the bulbar conjunctiva and become less marked as the limbus is approached.

The presence of secretion is almost always a feature of conjunctivitis. This is due to an exudation of inflammatory cells and a fibrin-rich edematous fluid from the blood, and the exudate is combined with denuded epithelial cells and mucus. The secretion may be purulent, mucopurulent, fibrinous, or serosanguineous, depending on the cause and severity of the disease. When the exudate dries, the eyelids may stick together.

Conjunctival edema (chemosis) may be present in parts of the conjunctiva that are freely movable over the globe and lids. The normal transparency of the conjunctiva may be lost, and it may appear thickened due to the infiltration of the tissues with leukocytes. If there is diffuse leukocytic infiltration of the conjunctival stroma, with hyperplasia of the overlying epithelium, papillae form. A papilla contains a central blood vessel in its core. This vessel branches on the surface of the papilla. Papillae usually occur in the tarsal conjunctiva. The conjunctiva may have a velvety appearance from numerous small papillae. When large, the papillae have the appearance of cobblestone excrescences. This is unusual in acute infectious conjunctivitis but more common in allergic and chronic conjunctivitis.

Normal conjunctiva has an occasional follicle in its substantia propria, especially in the fornices. In some forms of conjunctivitis, a follicular reaction may predominate. Follicles and papillae may be differentiated clinically because follicles resemble white grains whereas papillae are red with a central vascular tuft.

Membrane formation is also seen in some cases of conjunctivitis. This membrane consists of a superficial fibrinous layer connected to subconjunctival granulation tissue. When this membrane is excised, a raw bleeding surface is exposed.

The cornea is sometimes involved in viral conjunctivitis, and this may lead to photophobia, grittiness, and pain.

The various forms of conjunctivitis have many of the aforementioned signs and symptoms in common, with none having pathognomonic features. A morphologic diagnosis is rarely possible unless there are associated corneal changes (e.g., in epidemic keratoconjunctivitis or herpes simplex keratoconjunctivitis).

BACTERIAL CONJUNCTIVITIS

Bacterial conjunctivitis is the most common type of infectious conjunctivitis.

In adults, the most common bacterial isolates from an acute conjunctivitis are *Streptococcus pneumoniae, Staphylococcus aureus*, and *Staphylococcus epidermidis*. The role of the latter two organisms in causation is, however, disputed.[16–18]

In children, the chief organisms causing acute conjunctivitis are *Haemophilus influenzae, Streptococcus pneumoniae*, and perhaps *Staphylococcus aureus*.[19–21]

The bacterial etiology of chronic bacterial conjunctivitis is less well defined.

Anaerobic bacteria have been isolated from conjunctivitis patients in association with aerobic organisms thought to be the cause of the conjunctivitis.[19] The same organisms have been isolated in immunodeficient patients, in whom acute and chronic conjunctivitis are more common than in normal patients.[22] Table 1 identifies bacteria that probably have been responsible for conjunctivitides.

TABLE 1. Etiologic Agents of Conjunctivitis

Bacteria
Streptococcus
Staphylococcus aureus
Haemophilus influenzae
Neisseria gonorrhoeae
Haemophilus aegyptius (Koch-Weeks)
Haemophilus ducreyi
Neisseria meningitidis
Streptococci of the viridans group
Proteus vulgaris
Morax-Axenfeld (*Moraxella lacunata*)
Corynebacterium diphtheriae
Mycobacterium tuberculosis
Francisella tularensis
Treponema pallidum
Branhamella catarrhalis
Shigella flexneri
Yersinia enterocolitica
Staphylococcus epidermidis
Acinetobacter calcoaceticus var. *anitratus*
Aeromonas hydrophila
Peptostreptococcus
Propionibacterium
Cat scratch bacillus
Viruses
Adenoviridae
Poxviruses (variola, vaccinia, molluscum contagiosum)
Herpesviruses (herpes simplex, varicella-zoster, Epstein-Barr virus)
Papillomaviruses (papilloma virus)
Influenza
Paramyxoviruses (measles, mumps, Newcastle disease virus)
Picornaviruses (echovirus, enterovirus, coxsackievirus, and poliovirus)
Chlamydia trachomatis
Fungi
Candida sp.
Sporothrix schenckii
Rhinosporidium seeberi
Parasites
Onchocerca volvulus
Loa loa
Wuchereria bancrofti
Oestrus ovis (myiasis)

The significance of most studies of bacterial cultures during conjunctivitis remains to be explored. However, there seems little argument that bacterial and viral conjunctivitis may be mistakenly identified clinically one for the other, and that few bacterial conjunctivitides have pathognomonic features that identify their cause.[16]

The cause of epidemics of bacterial conjunctivitis has been better established, for example, *Streptococcus pneumoniae*.[23]

Of special interest is gonococcal conjunctivitis, in which the conjunctiva is markedly injected and chemotic, with a profuse purulent discharge.[24] The eyelids become swollen and difficult to open. Serious complications of untreated gonococcal conjunctivitis may include corneal ulceration and subsequent perforation. Sometimes gonococcal conjunctivitis has a prolonged asymptomatic course, in a manner similar to some of the genital infections.[25]

Membrane formation may be seen in any severe infection of the conjunctiva, but it is typically present in infections with streptococci and *Corynebacterium diphtheriae*. These membranes may lead to a spectrum of changes from fine corneal scarring to obliteration of the fornices. In contrast to most other types of conjunctivitis, pain is a common symptom with *C. diphtheriae* infection. Diphtheritic conjunctivitis does not occur as the sole manifestation of diphtheria, and so other manifestations of the disease should be sought.

Moraxella lacunata produces a localized "angular" conjunctivitis associated with fissuring and dermatitis of the external canthi and a scanty conjunctival discharge.

Certain nonpyogenic organisms (*Mycobacterium tuberculosis, Francisella tularensis, Treponema pallidum*) produce an atypical clinical picture characterized by unilateral conjunctival nodules that tend to ulcerate. Moderate localized conjunctival injection, minimal discharge, and a palpable preauricular lymph node on the affected side are present.

The pleomorphic gram-negative cat-scratch disease bacillus, first identified in lymph nodes,[26] produces a unilateral follicular conjunctivitis associated with prominent enlargement of the ipsilateral preauricular lymph node.[27] *Yersinia* infection has been implicated[28] in a syndrome similar to Reiter syndrome and consisting of a self-limited conjunctivitis, acute myalgia, fever, gastrointestinal symptoms, and a prolonged anterior uveitis, polyarthritis, sacroiliitis, and HLA-B27 association. Similar syndrome complexes were seen within family groups. *Yersinia entercolitica* has also been associated with an isolated conjunctivitis.[29]

Haemophilus ducreyi,[30] *Pasteurella multocida*,[31] *Francisella tularensis*,[32] *Neisseria meningitidis*,[33] streptococci,[34] *Acinetobacter calcoaceticus* (*Herellea vaginicola*),[35] and *Aeromonas hydrophila*[36] have caused isolated cases of acute conjunctivitis.

VIRAL CONJUNCTIVITIS

Viral conjunctivitis is fairly common, causing 20 percent of nonepidemic cases of conjunctivitis in one study in children[20] and 14 percent of adult patients in another study.[16] The morphology of associated corneal changes, the time course, systemic involvement, and epidemic characteristics will usually permit identification that the conjunctivitis is of viral origin. The actual causative virus usually cannot be implicated by ocular morphologic characteristics alone but requires cultures and serologic studies. Most viral conjunctivitides are self-limited and highly contagious, with low morbidity. The discharge is usually watery rather than purulent. A generalized conjunctival injection, moderate tearing, and mild itching are present. Follicle formation may be prominent. Preauricular lymphadenopathy is common, and occasionally the conjunctivitis is associated with an upper respiratory tract infection.

Adenoviruses are responsible for the most frequent epidemics of viral conjunctivitis in the United States.

Serotypes of adenoviruses typically associated with pharyngoconjunctival fever (PCF) are 3 and 7, with occasional involvement by types 1, 2, 4, 5, 6, 8, and 14. The clinical complex of pharyngitis, fever, and conjunctivitis, inferior forniceal follicles, and rarely, keratitis may help identify this conjunctivitis. Spontaneous resolution within 1 to 2 weeks is the rule.[37]

Epidemic keratoconjunctivitis (EKC) has most commonly resulted from infection with serotype 8, but types 2, 3, 4, 7, 9, 10, 11, 14, 16, 19, and 29 have been reported.[38–45] The clinical picture includes pharyngitis, preauricular lymphadenopathy, and follicular conjunctivitis, and there is a 7- to 10-day incubation period with a 5- to 12-day interval before characteristic (but inconsistent) corneal subepithelial infiltrates develop. These epidemics are sometimes propagated by eye health care personnel. Despite a wide spectrum of symptoms ranging from severe photophobia to mild irritation only, this disease is usually self-limited and is rarely associated with visual loss from corneal changes.[46,47] Occasional reports have described raised intraocular pressure[48] and chronic keratitis and a Stevens-Johnson syndrome[49] as a result of epidemic keratoconjunctivitis. Chronic adenovirus conjunctivitis has been reported.[50,51]

Reports of recent epidemics in Florida have emphasized the emergence of a picornavirus as a factor in epidemic hemorrhagic conjunctivitis (EHC) in the United States. Previous reports have been mainly from Africa.[52,53] Enterovirus, type 70, coxsackievirus A24, and adenovirus 11 have all resulted in a similar clinical picture[54–60] (Fig. 1). This consists of bilateral follicular conjunctivitis of sudden onset, with (rarely) corneal changes and systemic symptoms, a short (4–5 day) symptomatic course, and bulbar conjunctival hemorrhages.[62] Spontaneous resolution with low morbidity is the usual course, although occasional reports have described Bell's palsy, radiculomyelitis,

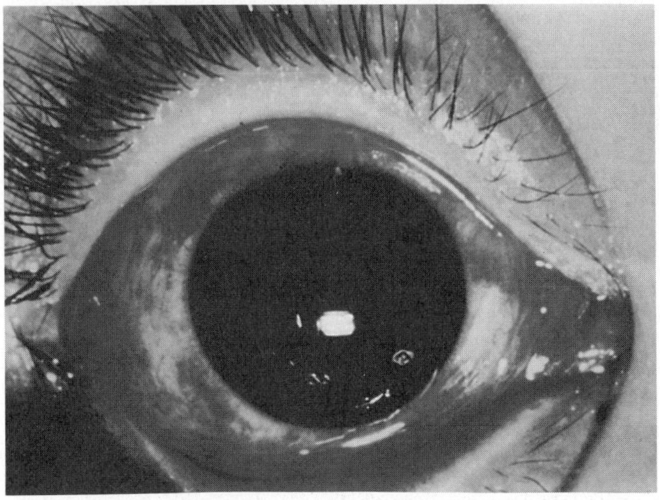

FIG. 1. Acute hemorrhagic conjunctivitis due to enterovirus 70. (From Kono et al,[61] with permission.)

cranial nerve palsies, and other types of central nervous system involvement.[63–66]

Ocular infection with vaccinia virus occurs when the virus is accidentally transferred from the site of medical inoculation to the eye. Vesicles appear on the lid margin,[67] and a conjunctivitis may follow. Conjunctivitis without lid lesions has also been reported.[68]

Molluscum contagiosum virus produces small, waxy, elevated lid-margin tumors with umbilicated centers that are associated with a chronic follicular conjunctivitis caused by the toxic effect of shed incomplete virions.[69]

Herpes simplex virus, types 1 and 2, varicella-zoster virus, and the Epstein-Barr virus can cause conjunctivitis.[70,71] Herpes simplex is responsible for the majority of cases of nonepidemic follicular conjunctivitis in young children.[72] Vesicular lid lesions and preauricular adenopathy may be present, and transient keratitis may be noted. The conjunctivitis is self-limited and is rarely associated with significant morbidity.

In patients with chickenpox, papules may develop on the lids and conjunctiva and at the limbus during the infection. These papules may become pustules and ulcerate. Vesicles may be found on the conjunctiva, particularly on the semilunar fold. Four percent of patients with chickenpox have conjunctival and corneal manifestations.[73] In herpes zoster ophthalmicus, a follicular conjunctivitis with regional adenopathy rarely occurs. In less than 5 percent of patients with infectious mononucleosis, a mild conjunctivitis is present.[74,75]

Human papillomavirus may produce lesions on the tarsal and bulbar conjunctivae and on the lid margin. A catarrhal conjunctivitis may result, and the cornea may show multiple punctate erosions. The presence of viral antigen and DNA sequences in some dysplastic epithelial lesions of the conjunctiva has raised concern that the virus may have a role in the development of conjunctival epithelial malignancies, similar to its suspected role in the female genital tract.[76]

Congenital rubella is associated with numerous ocular abnormalities.[77,78] Epidemic rubella in young children has produced a follicular conjunctivitis associated with occasional corneal epithelial changes.

The influenza viruses often cause catarrhal conjunctivitis and occasionally an acute follicular conjunctivitis. This ocular manifestation of influenza has been reported in both 48 percent[79] and 60 percent[80] of patients.

Infections due to the measles (rubeola) virus may be associated with mild paralimbal conjunctival epithelial erosion; the epithelia contain measles antigens that develop during the prodrome before the skin rash.[81] An epithelial keratitis with photophobia may occur after the skin rash occurs. Koplik's spots may be found on the semilunar fold.[82]

Conjunctivitis occurs rarely with mumps.[83] Newcastle disease virus (which causes a fatal pneumoencephalitis in fowl) may produce a self-limited, unilateral follicular conjunctivitis in humans.[84] Echo 11[85] and polio virus[86] have occasionally been described as a cause of follicular conjunctivitis.

Parinaud oculoglandular syndrome is a clinical complex of conjunctivitis, prominent preauricular lymphadenopathy, and a febrile illness with various possible causes, including infectious mononucleosis[87] and cat-scratch fever,[88] syphilis, tuberculosis, and sarcoidosis.

CHLAMYDIAL CONJUNCTIVITIS

Trachoma, one of the leading causes of blindness in the world,[89,90] is caused by a chlamydial organism that has a low infectivity. In the United States, the disease is largely confined to certain Native American populations that are characterized by poverty and poor communal hygiene. Repeated infections appear necessary to establish clinical trachoma. The conjunctivitis is characterized by a follicular reaction in the superior tarsal conjunctiva that is often associated with a concurrent papillary response. As follicles resolve, they appear to be replaced with fine subconjunctival scars. The degree of scarring seems to be related to the intensity of the follicular response and also to the presence of secondary bacterial infection. The subconjunctival scarring may in time lead to distortion of the tarsal plate and result in trichiasis.

Also associated with trachoma is the development of a superior limbic pannus with opacification of the corneal stroma and neovascularization. Follicles may occur in the limbus, and when these resolve, a clear depression persists (Herbert's pit).

Inclusion conjunctivitis is a fairly common infection caused by *Chlamydia trachomatis* that is venereally transmitted.[91,92] Since an infant may acquire the organism during his passage through the birth canal, it is one of the causes of ophthalmia neonatorum. Because the conjunctiva in the newborn does not form follicles, the injected appearance of this conjunctivitis in newborns is nonspecific. In adults, numerous papillae and follicles form on the tarsal conjunctiva and are more pronounced on the lower. The disease is usually bilateral, and the discharge is often profuse. Inclusion conjunctivitis is differentiated from trachoma by two important features: (*1*) corneal scarring rarely occurs in inclusion conjunctivitis; and (*2*) in trachoma the upper tarsal conjunctiva is more involved than the lower, although occasionally inclusion conjunctivitis may take on the characteristics of trachoma and various corneal changes have been described in inclusion conjunctivitis. Associated urethritis and cervicitis is common.[93]

Conjunctivitis is a rare manifestation of systemic lymphogranuloma venereum that is caused by certain immunotypes (L-1, L-2, L-3) of *C. trachomatis*. Moderate unilateral conjunctival injection, slight conjunctival discharge, and extreme edema of the upper and lower lids are present. In addition, ipsilateral preauricular, parotid, and submaxillary lymphadenopathy is present.[94] Types A, B, Ba, and C have been most commonly found in hyperendemic areas of trachoma.

OPHTHALMIA NEONATORUM

The incidence of acute conjunctivitis of the newborn (ophthalmia neonatorum) is reported to be as high as 12 percent of all newborns.[95] It has been most commonly the result of mild chemical irritation after ocular silver nitrate prophylaxis. This self-limited conjunctivitis appears within the first 24 hours, and it lasts 1–2 days. However, chlamydial conjunctivitis is becoming much more common, with an incidence of approximately 2.8 percent of all births at one clinic and occurring in more than

35 percent of the infants who are born to mothers with proven chlamydial cervicitis.[96] This has been substantiated by other studies.[97,98] The onset generally occurs within 5 to 19 days, with no pathologic features except for an association with other systemic chlamydial infections such as pneumonia and otitis media.[99,100] It has been suggested that the organism in these cases gains entry to the neonate through the conjunctival mucosa. There have been reports of occasional cases of chlamydial conjunctivitis in infants delivered by cesarean section.[101]

Bacterial conjunctivitis is most often the result of *Staphylococcus aureus* infection, with *Streptococcus pneumoniae* and *Haemophilus influenzae* the next most common.[102,103] There are no pathognomonic features of these infections, and they may occur as early as 24 hours after birth. Streptococcal infections may be associated with acute dacryocystitis of the newborn, and *Pseudomonas* sp. have been reported as an occasional cause.[104] Cases of staphylococcal "scalded skin" syndrome have been attributed to primary staphylococcal conjunctivitis.[105] *H. influenzae* conjunctivitis has been implicated in neonatal meningitis. *Shigella flexneri* has caused ethmoiditis and conjunctivitis.[106] *Branhamella catarhalis* is being more frequently diagnosed[107–109] and has been confused with true gonococcal ophthalmia neonatorum.

The prevailing incidence of gonococcal ophthalmia neonatorum is not known, but it is usually seen 1–2 days after birth and is characterized by a florid course and the threat of corneal ulceration and perforation. Recent cases of penicillin-resistant strains[110,111] and occasional cases with a deceptively mild course have made diagnosis and management more difficult.[112]

Infants born to mothers with herpes simplex virus cervicitis may develop a conjunctivitis within a few days of birth. The conjunctivitis is usually self-limited but may be associated with corneal epithelial changes and, rarely, stromal keratitis.

OTHER INFECTIVE AND NONINFECTIVE CONJUNCTIVITIDES

Ophthalmomyiasis,[113] nematode,[114] and trematode[115] infections have been described. Conjunctival inflammation (chemosis and injection and discharge) is seen as a result of many noninfectious conditions, but particularly as an allergic mucosal response. The agents responsible include drugs and devices such as hard and soft contact lenses,[116,117] contact lens sterilizing solutions (usually the preservative thiomerasol)[118,119] that cause giant papillary conjunctivitis, prostheses,[120,121] topical timolol,[122] atropine, antiviral agents, and other drugs,[123–127] cosmetics,[128] and external allergens that cause vernal keratoconjunctivitis.[129] Conjunctivitis may occur as a response to toxic agents such as gentian violet,[130] latex,[131] and ultraviolet irradiation.[132–134] Phlyctenular keratoconjunctivitis has occurred in patients with increased tuberculin sensitivity[135] and staphylococcal hypersensitivity.[136]

The exact causes of numerous other conditions with fairly specific clinical features have not been identified. These include keratoconjunctivitis sicca, superior limbic keratoconjunctivitis, ligneous conjunctivitis, mucocutaneous lymph node syndrome, and Reiter syndrome. Immune-mediated conjunctivitis has been implicated in mucous membrane pemphigoid[137] and in the conjunctivitis associated with graft-vs.-host disease in bone marrow transplant patients.[138]

DIFFERENTIAL DIAGNOSIS

Other serious, sight-threatening conditions that present as "red eye" may superficially resemble a conjunctivitis. The points of difference are highlighted in Table 2. Chronic, unilateral conjunctivitis in which a specific diagnosis is not made should alert the physician to the possibility of a meibomian gland carcinoma.[139]

TABLE 2. Comparison of Conjunctivitis and Other Conditions

Characteristic	*Conjunctivitis*	*Uveitis*	*Acute Angle-Closure Glaucoma*
Prominent symptoms	Discharge, irritation	Photophobia, visual loss	Pain, visual loss
Vision	Usually normal	Normal and occasionally decreased	Markedly reduced
Ocular injection	Conjunctival injection generalized	Paralimbal injection (ciliary flush)	Paralimbal injection
Cornea	Usually clear	Usually clear	Edematous and cloudy
Pupil	Normal	May be normal or small	Usually middilated, irregular, and immobile
Intraocular pressure	Normal	Normal or slightly elevated	Markedly elevated

LABORATORY INVESTIGATIONS

Mild conjunctivitis is rarely investigated, and it usually is treated empirically. Reports differ on the value of culturing suspected bacterial conjunctivitis.[140,141] Scrapings of the superior and inferior tarsal conjunctiva may be taken (after the administration of proparacaine HCl, 0.5%) for smears and cultures in a manner similar to that described in Chapter 99. Cultures are usually taken from both conjunctival sacs and separately from both lids in suspected conjunctivitis.[142] Chlamydial cultures are taken with a dry calcium alginate swab, which is then placed in chlamydial culture medium.

All cases of suspected ophthalmia neonatorum should have cultures and smears performed for bacteria, chlamydia, and herpes simplex virus. Acute and convalescent serologic tests for adenovirus and picornavirus may help in diagnosing epidemic conjunctivitis, but these are generally not required because of the self-limited nature of the infection, the nonspecific treatment available, and the diagnostic characteristics of the epidemic features. Serodiagnostic testing of tears in serum by using microimmunofluorescent tests has been described for patients with *C. trachomatis* inclusion conjunctivitis.[143] Serologic testing for SS-A and SS-B autoantibodies has assisted in the early diagnosis of keratoconjunctivitis sicca that is a prodrome of Sjögren syndrome.[144]

In a conjunctival scraping from a normal healthy eye, epithelial cells and occasional goblet cells are present. In acute bacterial infection, the scraping shows large numbers of neutrophils. Bacteria may be present within or outside leukocytes. In chronic bacterial infections, there is a decrease in neutrophils and an increase in lymphocytes and large mononuclear cells. In viral conjunctivitis, lymphocytes and monocytes are predominant. In herpes simplex infections, multinucleated epithelial cells may be seen. In chlamydial infections, a mixed inflammatory cell population (polymorphonuclear leukocytes and lymphocytes) is present, and basophilic intracytoplasmic inclusion bodies may be seen in epithelial cells; the latter finding is common in children and less common in adults. Immunofluorescent techniques promise to provide more sensitivity in identification. In allergic conjunctivitis, scrapings characteristically reveal eosinophils.[145] They are found in greatest abundance in vernal conjunctivitis. Between attacks of vernal conjunctivitis, mast cells and no eosinophils are seen.

Scrapings from patients with keratoconjunctivitis sicca and superior limbic keratoconjunctivitis reveal keratinized epithelial cells or condensed chromatin patterns when using the Papanicolaou staining technique.[146]

Impression cytology may offer an alternative to the conjunctival scraping method.[147] Immunoelectron microscopy and immunofluorescent techniques may aid in diagnosing viral conjunctivitis.[148,149]

TREATMENT

Most types of mild bacterial conjunctivitis and most types of viral conjunctivitis are self-limited, benign conditions that require no treatment. Topical gentamicin or tobramycin[150] for gram-negative rod infections; and erythromycin, bacitracin, chloramphenicol, or neomycin/polymixin for gram-positive infections, given every 2–4 hours for 7–10 days, are usually effective.[18,141] Often an organism reported to be resistant to a specific antibiotic in the laboratory will respond to that antibiotic clinically because of the high concentrations achievable in the tear film by topical application.

Gonococcal conjunctivitis requires urgent therapy with parenteral penicillin, topical penicillin, and frequent instillations of normal saline. Penicillinase-producing *Neisseria gonorrhoeae* (PPNG) require systemic ceftriaxone or another third generation cephalosporin. A single intramuscular dose of 125 mg of ceftriaxone resulted in a 100 percent cure rate for gonococcal ophthalmia neonatorum without the need for concomitant topical therapy.[151]

Herpes simplex virus conjunctivitis may be treated with topical trifluridine every 2 hours for 7 days, although this condition is usually benign and self-limited.

Adult inclusion conjunctivitis requires a 3-week course of either erythromycin or sulfamethoxazole and trimethoprim orally, supplemented with topical tetracycline ointment or erythromycin drops. A similar therapy is effective in treating trachoma, but prevention of reinfection and bacterial superinfection are equally important.

The place of interferon and interferon inducers in treating viral conjunctivitis remains conjectural.

Allergic and immune-mediated conjunctivitis responds best to topical corticosteroids, of which prednisolone acetate, 1%, is the most potent. The long-term use of topical steroids may be associated with glaucoma and cataracts, whereas short-term use may accelerate herpes simplex epithelial keratitis. Nonsteroidal anti-inflammatory agents such as aspirin[152] and cromolyn sodium[153,154] are becoming increasingly useful.

PROPHYLAXIS OF OPHTHALMIA NEONATORUM

There is considerable debate over the relative efficacy of 1% silver nitrate vs. topical antibiotics such as 0.5% erythromycin or 1% tetracyclines. Silver nitrate is still extremely effective, particularly against gonococcal infection, but it has little impact on the increasing incidence of chlamydial infections. Topical erythromycin seems the most effective agent in preventing this infection.[155] In infants born to mothers with known genital chlamydial infection, the routine use of erythromycin ointment will eliminate chlamydial conjunctivitis, but systemic erythromycin estolate is preferred to prevent nasopharyngeal colonization.[156,157]

Children born to mothers with known gonococcal genital infections should be treated with parenteral penicillin or ceftriaxone, depending on susceptibility.

REFERENCES

1. Allansmith MR, Ostler HB, Butterworth M. Concomitance of bacteria in various areas of the eye. Arch Ophthalmol. 1969;82:37.
2. Lucic H. Bacteriology of the normal conjunctival sac. Am J Ophthalmol. 1927;10:829.
3. Khorazo D, Thompson R. The bacterial flora of the normal conjunctiva. Am J Ophthalmol. 1935;18:1114.
4. Gowen GH. Source of staphylococci on normal conjunctiva of human eye. Am J Ophthalmol. 1934;17:36.
5. Locatcher-Khorazo D, Benham RW, Silva-Hunter M. Incidence of fungi from clinically healthy eyes of 508 young people 10–18 years of age and in 1347 adults 19–80 years of age. In: Locatcher-Khorazo D, Seegal BC, eds. Microbiology of the Eye. St Louis: CV Mosby; 1972;213.
6. Hammeke JC, Ellis PP. Mycotic flora of the conjunctiva. Am J Ophthalmol. 1960;49:1174.
7. Williamson J, Gordon AM, Wood R, et al. Fungal flora of the conjunctival sac in health and disease: Influence of topical and systemic steroids. Br J Ophthalmol. 1968;52:127.
8. Nema HV, Ahuja OP, Bal A, et al. Mycotic flora of the conjunctiva. Am J Ophthalmol. 1966;62:968.
9. Locatcher-Khorazo D, Guiterrez E. Eye infections following cataract extraction, with special reference to the role of *Staphylococcus aureus*. Am J Ophthalmol. 1956;41:981.
10. Allen HF, Mangiaracine AB. Bacterial endophthalmitis after cataract extraction. II. Incidence in 36,000 consecutive operations, with special reference to preoperative topical antibiotics. Trans Am Acad Ophthalmol Otolaryngol. 1973;77:581.
11. McMeel JW, Wapner JM. Infections and retina surgery. I. Bacteriologic contamination during scleral buckling surgery. Arch Ophthalmol. 1965;74:42.
12. Howard HJ. Role of the epithelial cell in conjunctival and corneal infections. Am J Ophthalmol. 1924;7:909.
13. Halbert SP, Locatcher-Khorazo D, Sonn-Kazar C, et al. Further studies on the incidence of antibiotic-producing microorganisms of the ocular flora. Arch Ophthalmol. 1957;58:66.
14. Halbert SP, Swick LS. Antibiotic-producing bacteria of the ocular flora. Am J Ophthalmol. 1952;35(5 Pt 2):73.
15. Halbert SP, Swick LS, Sonn C, et al. Ocular antibiotic-producing bacteria in normal eyes and in conjunctivitis. Arch Ophthalmol. 1954;51:7.
16. Leibowitz HM, Pratt MV, Flagstad IJ, et al. Human conjunctivitis. A diagnostic evaluation. Arch Ophthalmol. 1976;94:1747.
17. Brook I, Pettit TH, Martin WJ, et al. Anaerobic and aerobic bacteriology of acute conjunctivitis. Ann Ophthalmol. 1979;11:389.
18. Seal DV, Barrett SP, McGill JI. Aetiology and treatment of acute bacterial infection of the external eye. Br J Ophthalmol. 1982;66:357.
19. Brook I. Anaerobic and aerobic bacterial flora of acute conjunctivitis in children. Arch Ophthalmol. 1980;98:833.
20. Gigliotti F, Williams WT, Hayden FG, et al. Etiology of acute conjunctivitis in children. J Pediatr. 1981;98:531.
21. Levin RM, Ticknor W, Jordan C, et al. Etiology of conjunctiviits. J Pediatr. 1981;99:831.
22. Friedlaender MH, Masi RJ, Osumoto M, et al. Ocular microbial flora in immunodeficient patients. Arch Ophthalmol. 1980;98:1211.
23. Shayegani M, Parsons LM, Gibbons WE Jr, et al. Characterization of nontypable *Streptococcus pneumoniae*-like organisms isolated from outbreaks of conjunctivitis. J Clin Microbiol. 1982;16:8.
24. Valenton MJ, Abendanio R. Gonorrhea conjunctivitis. Can J Ophthalmol. 1973;8:421.
25. Tight RR. Gonococcal conjunctivitis. JAMA. 1982;247:2499.
26. English CK, Wear DJ, Margileth AM, et al. Cat-scratch disease, isolation and culture of the bacterial agent. JAMA. 1988;259:1347–52.
27. Wear DJ, Malaty RH, Zimmerman LE, et al. Cat scratch disease bacilli in the conjunctiva of patients with Parinaud's oculoglandular syndrome. Ophthalmology. 1985;92:1282–7.
28. Saari KM, Laitinen O, Leirisalo M, et al. Ocular inflammation associated with Yersinia infection. Am J Ophthalmol. 1980;89:84.
29. Crichton EP. Suppurative conjunctivitis caused by *Yersinia enterocolitica*. Can Med J. 1978;118:22.
30. Gregory JE, Henderson RW, Smith R. Conjunctivitis due to *Haemophilus ducreyi* infection. Br J Vener Dis. 1980;56:414.
31. Eschete ML, Rambin ED, West BC. *Clostridium pseudotetanicum* bacteremia in a patient with *Pasteurella multocida* conjunctivitis. J Clin Microbiol. 1978;8:509.
32. Guerrant RL, Humphries MK, Butler JE, et al. Tickborne oculoglandular tularemia. Case report and review of seasonal and vectorial associations in 106 cases. Arch Intern Med. 1976;136:811.
33. Brook I, Bateman JB, Pettit TH. Meningococcal conjunctivitis. Arch Ophthalmol. 1979;97:890.
34. Cohn H, Mondino BJ, Brown SI, et al. Marginal corneal ulcers with acute beta streptococcal conjunctivitis and chronic dacryocystitis. Am J Ophthalmol. 1979;87:541.
35. Abel R, Shulman J, Boyle GL, et al. Herellea vaginicola and ocular infections. Ann Ophthalmol. 1975;7:1485.
36. Smith JA. Ocular *Aeromonas hydrophila*. Am J Ophthalmol. 1980;89:449.
37. Bell JA, Rowe WP, Engler JI, et al. Pharyngoconjunctival fever: Epidemiological studies of a recently recognized disease entity. JAMA. 1955;175:1083.
38. O'Day DM, Guyer B, Hierholzer JC, et al. Clinical and laboratory evaluation of epidemic keratoconjunctivitis due to adenovirus types 8 and 19. Am J Ophthalmol. 1976;81:207.
39. Aoki K, Kato M, Ohtsuka H, et al. Clinical and aetiological study of adenoviral conjunctivitis, with special reference to adenovirus types 4 and 19 infections. Br J Ophthalmol. 1982;66:776.
40. Tullo AB, Higgins PG. An outbreak of adenovirus type 14 conjunctivitis. Br J Ophthalmol. 1980;64:489.
41. D'Angelo LJ, Hierholzer JC, Holman RC, et al. Epidemic keratoconjunctivitis caused by adenovirus type 8: Epidemiologic and laboratory aspects of a large outbreak. Am J Epidemiol. 1981;113:44.
42. Darougar S, Pearce R, Gibson JA, et al. Adenovirus type 21 keratoconjunctivitis. Br J Ophthalmol. 1978;62:836.
43. Taylor JW, Chandler JW, Cooney MK. Conjunctivitis due to adenovirus type 19. J Clin Microbiol. 1978;8:209.

44. Schaap GJP, deJong JC, van Bijsterveld OP, et al. A new intermediate adenovirus type causing conjunctivitis. Arch Ophthalmol. 1979;97:2336.
45. Newland JC, Cooney MK. Characteristics of an adenovirus type 19 conjunctivitis isolate and evidence for a subgroup associated with epidemic conjunctivitis. Infect Immun. 1978;21:303.
46. Beale AJ, Doane F, Ornsby HL. Studies on adenovirus infections of the eye in Toronto. Am J Ophthalmol. 1957;43:26.
47. Boniuk M, Phillips CA, Hines MJ, et al. Adenovirus infections of the conjunctiva and cornea. Trans Am Acad Ophthalmol Ortolaryngol. 1966;70:1016.
48. Hara J, Ishibashi T, Fujimoto F, et al. Adenovirus type 10 keratoconjunctivitis with increased intraocular pressure. Am J Ophthalmol. 1980;90:481.
49. Kiernan JP, Schanzlin DJ, Leveille AS. Stevens-Johnson syndrome associated with adenovirus conjunctivitis. Am J Ophthalmol. 1981;92:543.
50. Pettit TH, Holland GN. Chronic keratoconjunctivitis associated with ocular adenovirus infection. Am J Ophthalmol. 1979;88:748.
51. Darougar S, Quinlan MP, Gibson JA, et al. Epidemic keratoconjunctivitis and chronic papillary conjunctivitis in London due to adenovirus type 19. Br J Ophthalmol. 1977;61:76.
52. Epidemiology: Acute haemorrhagic conjunctivitis. Br Med J. 1982;284:833.
53. Hoffman M. Acute haemorrhagic conjunctivitis. S Afr Med J. 1982;62:311.
54. Christopher S, Theogaraj S, Godbole S, et al. An epidemic of acute hemorrhagic conjunctivitis due to coxsackievirus A24. J Infect Dis. 1982;146:16.
55. Langford MP, Stanton GJ, Barber JC, et al. Early-appearing antiviral activity in human tears during a case of picornavirus epidemic conjunctivitis. J Infect Dis. 1979;139:653.
56. Goh KT, Doraisingham S, Yin-Murphy M. An epidemic of acute conjunctivitis caused by enterovirus-70 in Singapore in 1980. Southeast Asian J Trop Med Public Health. 1981;12:473.
57. Hatch MH, Malison MD, Palmer EL. Isolation of enterovirus 70 from patients with acute hemorrhagic conjunctivitis in Key West, Florida. N Engl J Med. 1981;305:1648.
58. Kono R, Miyamura K, Yamazaki S, et al. Seroepidemiologic studies of acute hemorrhagic conjunctivitis virus (enterovirus type 70) in West Africa. II. Studies with human sera collected in West African countries other than Ghana. Am J Epidemol. 1981;114:274.
59. Bernard KW, Hierholzer JC, Dugan JB, et al. Acute hemorrhagic conjunctivitis in Southeast Asian refugees arriving in the United States: Isolation of enterovirus 70. Am J Trop Med Hyg. 1982;31:541.
60. Minami K, Otatsume S, Mingle JAA, et al. Seroepidemiologic studies of acute hemorrhagic conjunctivitis virus (enterovirus type 70) in West Africa. I. Studies with human sera from Ghana collected eight years after the first outbreak. Am J Epidemiol. 1981;114:267.
61. Kono R, Uchida Y. Acute hemorrhagic conjunctivitis. Ophthalmol Dig. 1977;39(April):14.
62. Wolken SH. Acute hemorrhagic conjunctivitis. Surv Ophthalmol. 1974;19:71.
63. Wadia NH, Wadia PN, Katrak SM, et al. Neurological manifestations of acute haemorrhagic conjunctivitis. Lancet. 1981;2:528.
64. Thakur LC. Cranial nerve paralyses associated with acute haemorrhagic conjunctivitis. Lancet. 1981;2:584.
65. Katiyar BC, Surendra M, Singh RB, et al. Neurological syndromes after acute epidemic conjunctivitis. Lancet. 1981;2:866.
66. John TJ, Christopher S, Abraham J. Neurological manifestation of acute haemorrhagic conjunctivitis due to enterovirus 70. Lancet. 1981;2:1283.
67. Bybee JD, Phillips CA, Ory EM, et al. Vaccinia of the eyelid. JAMA. 1967;199:126.
68. Croffead GW, Harrison SW. Vaccinia conjunctivitis. Am J Ophthalmol. 1962;53:531.
69. Denis J, Chauvaud D, Savoldelli M, et al. Fine structure of palpebral molluscum contagiosum and its secondary conjunctival lesions. Graefe Arch Ophthalmol. 1978;208:207.
70. North RD. Presumptive viral keratoconjunctivitis, mononucleosis, and the oncogenic viruses. Int Ophthalmol Clin. 1975;15:211.
71. Darougar S, Hunter PA, Viswalingam M, et al. Acute follicular conjunctivitis and keratoconjunctivitis due to herpes simplex virus in London. Br J Ophthalmol. 1978;62:843.
72. Jones BR. The management of ocular herpes. Trans Ophthalmol Soc UK. 1959;79:425.
73. Stucchi CA, Bianchi G. Complications oculaires graves post-varicelleuses chez l'adulte. Ophthalmologica. 1970;161:108.
74. Carter RL, Penman HG. Infectious Mononucleosis. Oxford: Blackwell Scientific Publications; 1969.
75. Wilhelmus KR. Ocular involvement in infectious mononucleosis. Am J Ophthalmol. 1981;91:117.
76. McDonnell JM, McDonnell PJ, Green WR, et al. Demonstration of papillomavirus capsid antigen in human conjunctival neoplasia. Arch Ophthalmol. 1986;104:1801.
77. Roy FH, Hiatt RL, Korones SB, et al. Ocular manifestations of congenital rubella syndrome. Arch Ophthalmol. 1966;75:601.
78. Hara J, Fujimoto F, Ishibashi T, et al. Ocular manifestations of the 1976 rubella epidemic in Japan. Am J Ophthalmol. 1979;87:642.
79. Holland WW. A clinical study of influenza in the Royal Air Force. Lancet. 1957;2:840.
80. Jordan WS Jr, Denny FW Jr, Badger GF, et al. A study of illness in a group of Cleveland families. Am J Hyg. 1958;68:190.
81. Nommensen FE, Dekkers NWHM. Detection of measles antigen in conjunctival epithelial lesions staining by lissamine green during measles virus infection. J Med Virol. 1981;7:157.
82. Deckard PS, Bergstrom TJ. Rubeola keratitis. Ophthalmology. 1981;88:810.
83. Riffenburgh RS. Ocular manifestations of mumps. Arch Ophthalmol. 1961;66:739.
84. Lippman O. Human conjunctivitis due to the Newcastle-disease virus of fowls. Am J Ophthalmol. 1952;35:1021.
85. Spalton DJ, Palmer S, Logan LC. Echo 11 conjunctivitis. Br J Ophthalmol. 1980;64:487.
86. Kasova V, John J, Koza J, et al. Poliovirus type 3 keratoconjunctivitis. J Infect Dis. 1980;42:292.
87. Meisler DM, Bosworth DE, Krachmer JH. Ocular infectious mononucleosis manifested as Parinaud's oculoglandular syndrome. Am J Ophthalmol. 1981;92:722.
88. Loftus MJ, Sweeney G, Goldberg MH. Parinaud oculoglandular syndrome and cat-scratch fever. J Oral Surg. 1980;38:218.
89. Schachter J, Dawson CR. Human Chlamydial Infections. Littleton, MA: PSG Publishing; 1978.
90. Darougar S. Chlamydial ocular infection. J Antimicrob Chemother. 1981;8:350.
91. Schacter J. Chlamydial infections. N Engl J Med. 1978;298:428.
92. Holmes KK. The Chlamydia epidemic. JAMA. 1981;245:1718.
93. Stenson S. Adult inclusion conjunctivitis. Clinical characteristics and corneal changes. Arch Ophthalmol. 1981;99:605.
94. Macnie JP. Ocular lymphogranuloma venereum. Arch Ophthalmol. 1941;25:255.
95. Pierce JM, Ward ME, Seal DV. Ophthalmia neonatorum in the 1980s: Incidence, aetiology and treatment. Br J Ophthalmol. 1982;66:728.
96. Schachter J, Holt J, Goodner E, et al. Prospective study of chlamydial infection in neonates. Lancet. 1979;2:377.
97. Heggie AD, Lumicao GG, Stuart LA, et al. *Chlamydia trachomatis* infection in mothers and infants. A prospective study. Am J Dis Child. 1981;135:507.
98. Persson K, Ronnerstam R, Svanberg L, et al. Maternal and infantile infection with *Chlamydia* in a Swedish population. Acta Paediatr Scand. 1981;70:101.
99. Schachter J, Lum L, Goodnig CA, et al. Pneumonitis following inclusion blennorrhea. J Pediatr. 1975;87:779.
100. Beem MO, Saxon EM. Respiratory-tract colonization and a distinctive pneumonia syndrome in infants infected with *Chlamydia trachomatis*. N Engl J Med. 1977;296:306.
101. Givner LB, Rennels MB, Woodward CL, et al. *Chlamydia trachomatis* infection in infant delivered by cesarean section. Pediatrics. 1981;68:420.
102. Stenson S, Newman R, Fedukowicz H. Conjunctivitis in the newborn: Observations on incidence, cause, and prophylaxis. Ann Ophthalmol. 1981;13:329.
103. Cohen KL, McCarthy LR. *Haemophilus influenzae* ophthalmia neonatorum. Arch Ophthalmol. 1980;98:1214.
104. Cole GF, Davies DP, Austin DJ. *Pseudomonas* ophthalmia neonatorum: A cause of blindness. Br Med J. 1980;281:440.
105. Fox KR, Golomb HS. Staphylococcal ophthalmia neonatorum and the staphylococcal scalded skin syndrome. Am J Ophthalmol. 1979;88:1052.
106. Overton ME, Heath JD, Stapleton FB. Conjunctivitis and ethmoiditis due to *Shigella flexneri* in an infant. Clin Pediatr (Phila). 1981;20:231.
107. Garvey RJP, Reed TAG. Ophthalmia neonatorum due to *Branhamella* (*Niesseria) catarrhalis*. Case reports. Br J Vener Dis. 1981;57:346.
108. Spark RP, Dahlberg PW, LaBelle JW. Pseudogonococcal ophthalmia neonatorum. *Branhamella* (*Neisseria*) *catarrhalis* conjunctivitis. Am J Clin Pathol. 1979;72:471.
109. Lue YA, Simms DH, Ubriani R, et al. Ophthalmia neonatorum caused by penicillin-resistant *Branhamella catarrhalis*. NY State J Med. 1981;81:1775.
110. Pang R, Teh LB, Rajan VS. Gonococcal ophthalmia neonatorum caused by beta-lactamase–producing *Neisseria gonorrhoeae*. Br Med J. 1979;280:380.
111. Dunlop EMC, Rodin P, Seth AD, et al. Ophthalmia neonatorum due to beta-lactamase–producing gonococci. Br Med J. 1980;281:483.
112. Podgore JK, Holmes KK. Ocular gonococcal infection with minimal or no inflammatory response. JAMA. 1981;246:242.
113. Wong D. External ophthalmomyiasis caused by the sheep bot *Oestrus ovis*. Br J Ophthalmol. 1982;66:786.
114. Ashton N, Cook C. Allergic granulomatous nodules of the eyelid and conjunctiva. The XXXV Edward Jackson Memorial Lecture. Am J Ophthalmol. 1979;87:1.
115. Mimori T, Hirai H, Kifune T, et al. *Philophthalmus* sp. (Trematoda) in a human eye. Am J Trop Med Hyg. 1982;31:859.
116. Stenson S. Superior limbic keratoconjunctivitis associated with soft contact lens wear. Arch Ophthalmol. 1983;101:402.
117. Allansmith MR, Baird RS, Greiner JV. Vernal conjunctivitis and contact lens–associated giant papillary conjunctivitis compared and contrasted. Am J Ophthalmol. 1979;87:544.
118. Binder PS, Rasmussen RM, Gordon M. Keratoconjunctivitis and soft contact lens solutions. Arch Ophthalmol. 1981;99:87.
119. Wright P, Mackie I. Preservative-related problems in soft contact lens wearers. Trans Ophthalmol Soc UK. 1982;102:3.
120. Srinivasan RB, Jakobiet FA, Iwamoto T, et al. Giant papillary conjunctivitis with ocular prostheses. Arch Ophthalmol. 1979;97:892.
121. Meisler DM, Krachmer JH, Goeken JA. An immunopathologic study of giant papillary conjunctivitis associated with an ocular prosthesis. Am J Ophthalmol. 1981;92:368.

122. Baldone JA, Hankin JS, Zimmerman TJ. Allergic conjunctivitis associated with timolol therapy in an adult. Ann Ophthalmol. 1982;14:364.
123. Vizel M, Oster MW. Ocular side effects of cancer chemotherapy. Cancer. 1982;49:1999.
124. Ostler HB. Acute chemotic reaction to cromolyn. Arch Ophthalmol. 1982;100:412.
125. Umez-Eronini EM. Conjunctivitis due to ketoprofen. Lancet. 1978;2:737.
126. Flach AJ, Peterson JS, Mathias CGT. Photosensitivity to topically applied sulfisoxazole ointment. Evidence for a phototoxic reaction. Arch Ophthalmol. 1982;100:1286.
127. Wilson FM II. Adverse external ocular effects of topical ophthalmic medications. Surv Ophthalmol. 1979;24:57.
128. Jacobson JH. Blepharitis and secondary conjunctivitis. Am J Ophthalmol. 1980;89:609.
129. Neumann E, Gutman MJ, Blumenkrantz N, et a. A review of 400 cases of vernal conjunctivitis. Am J Ophthalmol. 1959;47:166.
130. Parker WT, Binder PS. Gentian violet keratoconjunctivitis. Am J Ophthalmol. 1979;87:340.
131. Biedner BZ, Sachs U, Witztum A. *Euphorbia peplus* latex keratoconjunctivitis. Ann Ophthalmol. 1981;13:739.
132. Backman HA. The effects of PUVA on the eye. Am J Optom Physiol Opt. 1982;59:86.
133. Halperin W, Altman R, Black K, et al. Conjunctivitis and skin erythema. Outbreak caused by a damaged high-intensity lamp. JAMA. 1978;240:1980.
134. Rose RC, Parker RL. Erythema and conjunctivitis. Outbreak caused by inadvertent exposure to ultraviolet light. JAMA. 1979;242:1155.
135. Philip RN, Comstock GW, Shelton JH. Phlyctenular keratoconjunctivitis among Eskimos in southern Alaska: I. Epidemiologic characteristics. Am Rev Respir Dis. 1965;91:171.
136. Ostler HB, Lanier JD. Phlyctenular keratoconjunctivitis with special reference to the staphylococcal type. Trans Pac Coast Otoophthalmol Soc Annu Meet. 1974;55:237.
137. Mondino BJ, Brown SI, Lempert S, et al. The acute manifestations of ocular cicatricial pemphigoid: Diagnosis and treatment. Ophthalmology. 1979;86:543.
138. Hirst LW, Jabs DA, Tutschka PJ, et al. The eye in bone marrow transplantation. I. Clinical Study. Arch Ophthalmol. 1983;101:580.
139. Perlman E, McMahon RT. Sebaceous gland carcinoma of the eyelid. Am J Ophthalmol. 1978;86:699.
140. Stenson S, Newman R, Fedukowicz H. Laboratory studies in acute conjunctivitis. Arch Ophthalmol. 1982;100:1275.
141. Leibowitz HM, Pratt MV, Flagstad IJ, et al. Human conjunctivitis. II. Treatment. Arch Ophthalmol. 1976;94:1752.
142. Jones DB, Liesegang TJ, Robinson NM. Laboratory diagnosis of ocular infections. Cumitech. 1980;13:1.
143. Darougar S, Treharne JD, Minassian D, et al. Rapid serological test for diagnosis of chlamydial ocular infections. Br J Ophthalmol. 1978;62:503.
144. Forstot SL, Forstot JZ, Peebles CL, et al. Serologic studies in patients with keratoconjunctivitis sicca. Arch Ophthalmol. 1981;99:888.
145. Abelson MB, Madiwale N, Weston JH. Conjunctival eosinophils in allergic ocular disease. Arch Ophthalmol. 1983;101:555.
146. Wander AH, Masukawa T. Unusual appearance of condensed chromatin in conjunctival cells in superior limbic keratoconjunctivitis. Lancet. 1981;2:42.
147. Hershenfeld S, Kazdan JJ, Mancer K, et al. Impression cytology in conjunctivitis. Can J Ophthalmol. 1981;16:76.
148. Rodrigues MR, Leennette DA, Arentsen JJ, et al. Methods for rapid detection of human ocular viral infections. Ophthalmology. 1979;86:452.
149. Van Rij G, Klepper L, Peperkamp E, et al. Immune electron microscopy and a cultural test in the diagnosis of adenovirus ocular infection. Br J Ophthalmol. 1982;66:317.
150. Liebowitz HM, Hyndiuk RA, Smolin GR, et al. Tobramycin in external eye disease. A double-masked study vs gentamicin. Curr Eye Res. 1981;1:259.
151. Laga M, Naamara W, Brunham RC, et al. Single-dose therapy of gonococcal ophthalmia neonatorum with ceftriaxone. N Engl J Med. 1986;315:1382.
152. Abelson MB, Butrus SI, Weston JH. Aspirin therapy in vernal conjunctivitis. Am J Ophthalmol. 1983;95:502.
153. Foster CS, Duncan J. Randomized clinical trial of topically administered cromolyn sodium for vernal keratoconjunctivits. Am J Ophthalmol. 1980;90:175.
154. Friday GA, Biglan AW, Hiles DA, et al. Treatment of ragweed allergic conjunctivitis with cromolyn sodium 4% ophthalmic solution. Am J Ophthalmol. 1983;95:169.
155. Hammerschlag MR, Chandler JW, Alexander ER, et al. Erythromycin ointment for ocular prophylaxis of neonatal chlamydial infection. JAMA. 1980;244:2291.
156. Patamasucon P, Rettig PJ, Faust KL, et al. Oral versus topical erythromycin therapies for chlamydial conjunctivitis. Am J Dis Child. 1982;136:817.
157. Rees E, Tait A, Hobson D, et al. Persistence of chlamydial infection after treatment for neonatal conjunctivitis. Arch Dis Child. 1981;56:193.

99. KERATITIS

PETER J. McDONNELL
W. RICHARD GREEN

Keratitis or inflammation of the cornea may be produced by infectious organisms or by noninfectious stimuli such as trauma, hypersensitivity, and other immune-mediated reactions. Since the corneal epithelium and conjunctival epithelium are continuous, forming the ocular surface, agents causing conjunctival disease may also affect the cornea. Before most infectious agents and some mediators of the immune reaction can invade the corneal stroma, a defect in the ocular surface must be present. This defect may be caused by various kinds of external trauma, including trauma from contact lenses, trichiasis, entropion, or abnormal lid margins, or chronic surface problems such as dry eyes, exposure, or neurogenic corneal anesthesia. Systemic diseases such as diabetes mellitus or immunodeficiency states decrease the corneal host resistance when the ocular surface has been broached by one of the above mechanisms.

Any corneal inflammation should be considered potentially sight threatening, and it requires prompt management. Corneal perforation and loss of the eye can occur within 24 hours after a severe inflammatory episode or infection by organisms such as *Pseudomonas aeruginosa* or *Staphylococcus aureus*. Even minor corneal ulcers in the visual axis can cause severe visual loss.

ETIOLOGIC AGENTS

The various etiologic agents known to cause keratitis are listed in Table 1.

Clinical Manifestations

The most common symptom of inflammatory lesions of the cornea is pain. The movement of the eyelids over the cornea increases the pain. The examination of such patients is greatly facilitated by first instilling a drop of topical anesthetic on the eye (preferably proparacaine hydrochloride, 0.5%).

Unlike conjunctival infections, a keratitis is usually accompanied by a variable decrease in vision. Discharge, which is a distinctive feature of conjunctivitis, is generally absent in patients with keratitis unless a purulent bacterial corneal ulcer is present. Reflex tearing, photophobia, and blepharospasm are common.

Since the cornea is normally avascular, the clinical appearance of an inflammatory reaction in the cornea is different from that in other tissues. After a noxious agent enters the cornea, inflammatory cells enter the cornea from dilated limbal vessels (ciliary flush) and from the tear film. The first sign of keratitis is therefore a subtle loss of corneal transparency, localized or generalized, and frequently a localized epithelial defect that is observed best with a cobalt light after instillation of fluorescein. The most important result of the inflammatory reaction with invasion by any of the agents in Table 1 is a loss of corneal substance (ulcer formation), which may rapidly lead to perforation if untreated or to a corneal scar (leukoma) even if successful therapy is initiated promptly.

In severe keratitis there is frequently an invasion of the cornea by blood vessels. After the inflammation subsides, residual empty blood channels (ghost vessels) that are not visible to the naked eye may be the only evidence of a previous inflammatory condition.

Some degree of corneal edema accompanies almost all inflammatory conditions of the cornea, leading to a loss of corneal transparency and a decrease in vision. Edema fluid may also

TABLE 1. Some Infectious Agents That Cause Keratitis

Bacteria
- Gram-positive cocci
  - *Staphylococcus aureus*
  - *Staphylococcus epidermidis*
  - *Streptococcus pneumoniae*
  - Streptococci of the viridans group
  - *Streptococcus pyogenes* (group A)
  - *Enterococcus (Streptococcus) faecalis*
  - *Peptostreptococcus*
- Gram-negative bacilli
  - *Pseudomonas aeruginosa, P. mallei, P. fluorescens, P. pseudomallei, P. acidovorans, P. stutzeri*
  - *Proteus mirabilis*
  - *Morganella moragnii*
  - *Klebsiella pneumoniae*
  - *Serratia marcescens*
  - *Escherichia coli*
  - *Aeromonas hydrophila*
  - Cat-scratch bacillus
- Gram-negative coccobacilli
  - *Moraxella lacunata, M. nonliquefaciens*
  - *Acinetobacter calcoaceticus*
  - *Pasteurella multocida*
  - *Neisseria gonorrhoeae*
  - *Branhamella catarrhalis*
- Gram-positive bacilli
  - *Bacillus coagulans, B. laterosporus, B. cereus, B. licheniformis, B. brevis*
  - *Corynebacterium diphtheriae*
  - *Clostridium perfringens, C tetani*
- Spirochetes
  - *Treponema pallidum*
- Mycobacteria
  - *Mycobacterium tuberculosis, M. fortuitum, M. chelonae*
- Actinomycetes
  - *Nocardia* sp.

Chlamydia
  - *Chlamydia trachomatis*

Viruses
- Herpes simplex
- Adenovirus
- Varicella-zoster virus
- Epstein-Barr virus
- Poxviruses (variola, vaccinia, molluscum contagiosum)
- Rubeola (measles)

Fungi
- *Acremonium* sp.
- Fusarium
- *Bipolaris* sp.
- *Candida* sp.
- *Aspergillus* sp.
- *Pseudallescheria boydii*
- *Penicillium*
- *Paecilomyces*
- *Neurospora*
- *Phialophora*
- *Curvularia*

Parasites
- *Onchocerca volvulus*
- *Acanthamoeba polyphaga, A. castellanii*
- *Leishmania brasiliensis*
- *Trypanosoma* spp.

accumulate under the corneal epithelium and form bullae that cause severe "foreign body" pain when they rupture.

An associated intraocular inflammation is common. Early changes may be seen only by slit-lamp examination (flare and cells). Severe inflammation may lead to a layering of fibrin and white blood cells in the inferior portion of the anterior chamber (hypopyon) by gravity. The aqueous and vitreous remain sterile in most microbial corneal ulcers until a late stage, when infective endophthalmitis may occur.

BACTERIAL KERATITIS

Bacterial keratitis accounts for approximately 65–90 percent of all microbial corneal infections.[1–3] In the United States the most common infecting organisms are *Staphylococcus aureus, Streptococcus pneumoniae, Pseudomonas aeruginosa,* and *Moraxella. Staphylococcus aureus, S. pneumoniae,* and *P. aeruginosa* by themselves account for more than 80 percent of all bacterial corneal ulcers. The clinical appearance of various bacterial ulcers does *not* usually provide a basis for specific diagnosis. The prevalence of organisms incriminated in corneal ulcers has changed little during the last 10 years. Any apparent changes that have occurred result from improved isolation techniques from the cornea, an increase in the population of patients who are systemically immunosuppressed, an increase in topical steroid administration, and an increase in the use of soft contact lenses,[4–6] especially for extended wear. There have been occasional cases as a result or organ-cultured and M-K medium–stored corneal buttons used for corneal transplantation.[7] A geographic variation in causes of microbial keratitis has also been noted. The inoculation of the organisms into the corneal stroma may occur via obvious exogenous penetrating trauma (cat-scratch bacillus[8]), through intact corneal epithelium (*Neisseria gonorrhoeae, Listeria, Corynebacterium diphtheriae,* and *Haemophilis aegypticus*), or more often via inapparent minor corneal epithelial abrasions such as from contaminated mascara.[9,10]

Strains of staphylococci causing extensive corneal ulcers are the same ones that are found as inhabitants in other noninfected parts of the body.[11,12] Paralimbal corneal ulcers found in association with conjunctival cultures that are positive for staphylococci have been thought to be due to toxins or hypersensitivity reactions to these bacteria. *Staphylococcus epidermidis* and streptococci can cause corneal ulceration, usually in an immunocompromised host and occasionally in association with chronic dacryocystitis,[13] in which a peripheral ulcer may occur that is similar in appearance to the staphylococcal hypersensitivity ulcer described above.[14] A toxic factor (exopeptidase) has been implicated in the pathogenesis of corneal ulceration caused by *S. pneumoniae.*[15]

Pseudomonas aeruginosa is recognized for its particularly swift course to perforation because of its proteolytic enzyme production,[16] which degrades the corneal stroma. In comatose patients with corneal exposure and tracheostomies colonized by *P. aeruginosa,* the danger of corneal infection is greatly increased.[17] Unusual extension of the corneal ulcer into the sclera has been reported.[18,19] Other *Pseudomonas* species such as *P. acidovorans* and *P. stutzeri,* have caused corneal ulcers with a less malignant course.[20] Corneal ulcers due to *Morganella morganii* may be clinically indistinguishable from those *Pseudomonas* ulcers. *Serratia marcescens* corneal ulcers have been associated with contact lens wear[21] and contaminated eyedrops.[22] *Moraxella* ulcers have been described in debilitated alcoholic patients in whom the organism is also frequently a nasopharyngeal commensual[23] and in otherwise well patients when chronic ocular surface disease is present.[24] The infrequency of isolation of this bacterium may perhaps be explained by its fastidious nature in culture and the inhibitory topical anesthetic agents used to obtain the corneal cultures.

Neisseria gonorrhoeae may cause a keratitis during an episode of untreated or inadequately treated conjunctivitis. It is one of the few organisms that can penetrate an intact corneal epithelium. It is essential that the presence of the gonococcus be verified by culture because *Acinetobacter,* which is morphologically identical to the gonococcus and is penicillin resistant, can cause corneal perforation.

Gram-positive aerobic bacilli are widespread in nature and are of low virulence. They produce infections of the cornea when host resistance is lowered.[25] *Corynebacterium diphtheriae* may penetrate an intact corneal epithelium to produce a keratitis.[26]

Primary tuberculous keratitis is now extremely rare.

Atypical mycobacteria (*Mycobacterium fortuitum* and *M. chelonae*) are known to cause a keratitis.[27,28] These corneal ulcers usually follow removal of a foreign body and have a slow, progressive course without much anterior chamber reaction.

The incidence of ocular lesions of leprosy varies from about 15 percent of the patients with tuberculoid leprosy to about 100 percent of the patients with long-standing lepromatous leprosy.[29–31] Many other bacteria have been involved in corneal ulcers, including *Azobacter,*[32] *Branhamella catarrhalis,*[33] *Aeromonas hydrophila,*[34] *Pasteurella multocida,*[35] *Clostridium perfringens,*[36] *Bacillus licheniformis,*[37] *B. thuringiensis,*[38] and anaerobic streptococci.[39] Polymicrobial keratitis was seen in about 8 percent of one series of bacterial and fungal ulcers and is associated with the use of therapeutic soft "bandage" contact lenses in diseased corneas.

VIRAL KERATITIS

About 20 percent of infants born with herpes simplex virus types I or II infections have ocular changes.[40] Seven percent will have keratitis with either punctate keratopathy, dendritic ulcers, or disciform keratitis. Of these, 30 percent are infected by herpes simplex, type I. Keratouveitis may occasionally be present at the time of birth. Prophylactic silver nitrate use is not uniformly successful in preventing ocular disease in neonates born to infected mothers. Atypically, the primary keratitis may present as subepithelial dendritic opacities.[41] Morphologically the lesions of herpes simplex, types I and II, are identical.

Ocular herpes simplex acquired during childhood usually presents as a follicular conjunctivitis and is frequently undiagnosed. Transient epithelial lesions are common. However, very similar changes to those described below in adults may also be encountered.[42]

In adults with documented previous corneal herpetic infection, the recurrence rates are approximately 25 percent within 12 months of the last attack and 33 percent within 24 months.[43] Another study suggested a 40 percent recurrence rate for all cases of corneal epithelial herpes and a 25 percent recurrence rate in the form of stromal disease or keratouveitis.[44] Six percent developed visual loss secondary to stromal scarring.

The pattern of epithelial disease is either *dendritic* or *geographic,* with active viral replication in the ulcer margin in the epithelium. The geographic type is notable for a prolonged course. Both diseases are known to heal spontaneously within 10 to 14 days in 80 percent of cases. Stromal involvement is usually seen in recurrent attacks, and the cornea has not been conclusively shown to harbor active viral particles. This form of the disease (*disciform keratitis*) is thought to be an immune-mediated reaction. This process frequently leads to some stromal scarring, commonly with thinning and occasionally with perforation. An associated *uveitis* is common. Recurrent ocular herpes simplex is thought to result from reactivation of latent herpes in the trigeminal ganglion and centripetal spread to the eye.[45,46] Active virus has not been isolated from the lacrimal gland, tears, cornea, or iris between episodes. Corneal hypoesthesia,[47] which worsens with repeated attacks, is present.

The pattern of disease is different in immunosuppressed patients.[48,49] They may have bilateral corneal involvement, which is seen in only 5 percent of other patients, and may also have extensive and multiple lesions on the cornea and conjunctiva. These lesions tend to persist or recur with topical antiviral therapy until immunosuppressive therapy is reduced.

Some of the factors that may precipitate recurrent episodes are exposure to sunlight, menstruation, psychiatric disturbances, and fever.[50] Acute illnesses may temporarily suppress the immune mechanisms, and the most common cause of a unilateral red eye in a hospitalized patient is herpes simplex keratitis. The exact mechanisms involved are unknown. Topical and systemic steroids and immunosuppressive agents may provoke recurrences in corneal epithelium, and they enhance replication in established lesions.[51]

The subepithelial corneal opacities occurring in epidemic keratoconjunctivitis caused by an adenovirus probably represent an immune phenomenon. These opacities tend to appear 10–14 days after symptoms commence. The natural course of the corneal lesions is resolution over 2–3 weeks, although patients may be very photophobic during this period. The lesions tend to clear dramatically with the use of topical steroids, with occasional reappearance when the steroid therapy is discontinued.[52]

In about 10 percent of the patients with herpes zoster infections the ophthalmic division of the trigeminal nerve is involved. The various ocular manifestations include vesicles on the lid and conjunctiva, iridocyclitis, secondary glaucoma, ophthalmoplegia, neuroretinitis, optic neuritis, and retinal vascular occlusion.[53,54] Corneal findings include decreased corneal sensation, epithelial and subepithelial punctate keratitis, dendritic figures, disciform keratitis, segmental keratitis, and corneal vascularization. The corneal disease may occur after the skin eruption is healed, and it can be prolonged.[55] Visual loss may result from peripheral and central stromal involvement.[56]

In varicella infections (chickenpox), ocular involvement is usually limited to the appearance of vesicles on the lids, conjunctiva, and limbus. Superficial punctate keratitis, interstitial and disciform keratitis, and uveitis have also been reported.[57] Epithelial dendritic figures that are identical to those seen in herpes zoster keratitis may occur immediately or up to several months after the skin eruption.[58]

Vaccinia infections of the eye occur from accidental autoinoculation.[59] Corneal complications occur in one-third of the patients with ocular vaccinia, and they consist of superficial punctate keratitis, epithelial ulcers, and (rarely) disciform keratitis. The epithelial ulcers may superficially resemble herpetic keratitis.[60,61]

The keratitis that is occasionally associated with measles (rubeola) infections causes punctate or dendritic epithelial defects in the cornea.[62] In one adult population study, all rubeola patients had epithelial keratitis that followed a benign course.[63] The changing immune status of the population after vaccination programs is changing the pattern of the clinical disease—from a childhood illness to an adult disease and perhaps a different ocular expression of measles infection. In developing countries, vitamin A deficiency and malnutrition sometimes makes measles keratitis a blinding disease with secondary bacterial infection and perforation of the globe.

Infectious mononucleosis has been associated with a peripheral nummular interstitial keratitis with a benign course.[64] More recently, ring-shaped granular anterior stromal opacities have been associated with Epstein-Barr viral infection.[65]

There have been occasional reported cases of Jacob-Kreutzfeldt disease[66] and rabies transmission[67] by the use of infected donor tissue in corneal transplantation. Human immunodeficiency virus (HIV) has been demonstrated to be present within corneal epithelium.[68] Donor corneas from such patients should never be used.

OTHER CAUSES OF KERATITIS

In one series of culture-positive corneal ulcers,[3] approximately 35 percent were of fungal origin, whereas another study found 20 percent to have a fungal origin.[1] While the incidence appeared to be related to geographic location, with higher rates in Florida and decreased incidence in northern states, seasonal fluctuations were not remarkable. Although 35 genera have been associated with corneal ulcers, *Fusarium solani* is the most common offending agent and has been isolated in up to 65 percent of cases.[69–71] *Aspergillus*[72] and *Candida* are also commonly isolated.[73] More rarely, *Acremonium* and *Curvularia* may be found. An antecedent vegetable injury may have occurred, and the use of broad-spectrum topical antibiotics and steroids has been implicated in the development of fungal ulcers. In patients with local ocular surface abnormalities—such as with dry eyes, extended-wear contact lens use, exposure keratitis, and previous herpes simplex keratitis or with systemic immunosuppression—infection with *Candida* is more common. The morphology of a fungal ulcer is not pathognomonic, but a torpid course, prominent hypopyon, and stromal infiltrates surrounded by satellite lesions are signs suggestive of fungal etiology.

Nocardia[74] and *Bacterionema matruchotii*[75] are rare causes of corneal ulcers, and the lesions are indistinguishable from those of a fungal origin. Cases have been reported of corneal ulcers from infection with *Pullularia,*[76] *Helminthosporium,*[77] *Rhodotorula,*[75] *Scedosporium,*[79] *Phialophora bubakii,*[80] and *Tritirachium roseum.*[81]

Parasitic infestations in certain parts of the world are major causes of blindness. Sclerosing keratitis and stromal opacification occur from invasion of the corneal stroma by microfilariae of *Onchocerca volvulus.*[82–85] Leishmania may produce a similar keratitis.[85]

Corneal changes secondary to trachoma conjunctivitis are a major cause of worldwide blindness.[86] In developed countries, sexually transmitted *Chlamydia trachomatis* infection may mimic the morphology of true trachoma.

Acanthamoeba is being recognized more often as a cause of recalcitrant keratitis, frequently leading to a loss of vision or the eye.[87] Patients who develop infection with this organism often have a history of contact lens wear (using a homemade saline solution) or exposure to soil or standing water.[88] Extreme pain and a ring infiltrate in the cornea should suggest the diagnosis.

Perhaps the most common cause of keratitis is thought to be from a hypersensitivity reaction to the exotoxin of *Staphylococcus.* Typically, inferior punctate epithelial defects that stain with fluorescein dye, marginal corneal infiltrates, and ulcers are manifestations of this allergy. Histologically, lymphocytes and plasma cells are present in peripheral cornea, but the cornea is free of organisms.

Ring ulcers of the cornea may give the appearance of coalesced marginal ulcers. They are more dangerous to the eye than are the usual marginal ulcers because they may lead to total corneal destruction. Their cause is uncertain, but they are sometimes associated with acute systemic diseases such as influenza, bacillary dysentery, brucellosis, gonococcal arthritis, dengue fever, herpes zoster ophthalmicus, diabetes mellitus, and hookworm infestation. They may also be associated with a number of autoimmune diseases such as periarteritis nodosa, rheumatoid arthritis,[89] Wegener's granulomatosis,[90] systemic lupus erythematosus, and giant cell arteritis.[91]

The two major types of interstitial keratitis encountered clinically are due to syphilis and tuberculosis. About 90 percent of all the cases of interstitial keratitis are caused by congenital syphilis. Mycobacteria other than *M. tuberculosis* rarely cause a similar keratitis. The best explanation for the occurrence of interstitial keratitis in these two main conditions is as a host-immune response rather than an active microbial infection.

Ocular involvement with syphilis may be acquired or congenital. The chancre of acquired primary syphilis has been reported to have occurred in the conjunctiva.[92] Among patients with acquired secondary syphilis the incidence of ocular complications is 4.5 percent.[93] These include papulosquamous lesions of the skin of the lids, temporary loss of the eyebrows, diffuse papillary conjunctivitis, scleroconjunctivitis,[92] interstitial keratitis, iritis, chorioretinitis,[94,95] and optic[96] and retrobulbar neuritis.[97] The most common eye lesion in secondary syphilis is iridocyclitis, which accounts for about 75 percent of all the eye lesions of the early acquired disease.[98] The diagnosis here is not difficult because in almost all cases there are other manifestations of early syphilis. Iritis may also develop as a complication of antisyphilitic therapy in the Jarisch-Herxheimer reaction.

Interstitial keratitis is a rare complication of acquired primary or secondary syphilis. Fewer than 3 percent of all cases of interstitial keratitis occur in acquired syphilis. In acquired late syphilis, gummas of the conjunctiva, lids, sclera, cornea, iris, ciliary body, and orbit are rare occurrences. The most common ocular inflammatory lesion of late acquired syphilis is iridocyclitis.[99]

There are two clinical forms of congenital syphilis: infantile, or early, and tardive, or late. Interstitial keratitis occurs rarely in early congenital syphilis.[92] However, it is the most common lesion of late congenital syphilis and occurs in about 52 percent of untreated patients. It typically occurs in the early teens, with most of the cases occurring in patients between the ages of 5 and 20 years. In the acute stage the patients have decreased visual acuity, photophobia, pain, blepharospasm, and lacrimation. The corneal stroma becomes hazy within a few days and has a ground-glass appearance, with marked reduction in vision. A severe iridocyclitis is present in the early stages. Over a period of months, new vessels grow into the corneal stroma from the limbus at all levels. When the vessels meet in the center of the cornea, there is a dramatic regression of the disease; the corneal infiltrates are resorbed, and the vessels are partially obliterated. The final visual prognosis in these patients is surprisingly good. Seventy percent have 20/20 to 20/100 acuity, and only ten percent have poorer than 20/200 acuity.[92]

The most common mechanical cause of keratitis is a foreign body embedded in the cornea. Corneal exposure from improper lid closure may also result in keratitis. This occurs in patients with Bell's palsy and proptosis due to Graves disease and in comatose patients. Trichiasis secondary to abnormal lid structure (e.g., entropion) may cause a keratitis.

A severe liquefactive keratitis may develop secondarily to decreased tear production, which may be idiopathic[100,101] or due to decreased corneal sensation after local corneal disease (e.g., herpes zoster infection), to neurologic lesions of the ophthalmic division of the trigeminal nerve, or to medullary infarction. This problem is greatly compounded when associated with inadequate lid closure. Rarely, superficial or deep keratitis may be associated with dermatoses and/or systemic conditions, including ichthyosis, epidermal nevus syndrome, anhydrotic ectodermal dysplasia, pulmonary and plantar hyperkeratosis, and tyrosinemia.[102] Isolated epithelial keratitis of unknown etiology such as Thygeson's migratory keratitis occurs infrequently.[103]

The association of Reiter syndrome and a keratitis with stromal infiltrates needs to be further investigated.[104] Finally, one of the major causes of blindness in the third-world countries is xerophthalmia, in which vitamin A deficiency results in corneal opacification and stromal liquefaction and leads to perforation.[105]

LABORATORY FEATURES

Because the morphologic features of corneal ulcers and keratitis are rarely pathognomonic, great emphasis must be placed on adequate laboratory work-up of suspected cases. The possibility of rapid progression to perforation requires early scrapings of the ulcer for smears and cultures. Methods for culture taking vary considerably but may be summarized by the following: (*1*) scrapings with a heat-sterilized Kimura platinum spatula (with or without the use of topical proparacaine hydrochloride, 0.5%), transferred to glass slides for Gram, Giemsa, periodic acid–Schiff (PAS), and methenamine silver stains; (*2*) multiple inoculations with the Kimura spatula on blood agar held at room temperature and at 37°C, chocolate agar, thioglycolate or Schaedler broth or brain–heart infusion, Sabouraud agar, and a reduced blood agar in an anaerobic environment. Special cultures may require non-nutrient agar or media for culturing mycobacteria. In most cases, concomitant cultures of the conjunctiva and lid, on the involved and uninvolved eye, are frequently taken to ascertain the person's flora and to assist in assessing the significance of positive corneal cultures taken from the ulcer. The type and number of positive cultures needed to support a microbial diagnosis are still unsettled.[106–108] Negative cultures obtained from scrapings as described above, in the face of a suspicious corneal ulcer, should lead to a superficial keratectomy or corneal biopsy specimens taken in the operating room under microscopic control. These may prove positive when superficial scrapings were previously negative since fungi and acanthamoebae are characteristically deep in corneal parenchyma and conspicuously absent on the surface.[109]

Viral keratitis does not often require culture, and the diagnosis is sustained by the morphology of the lesions. Careful débridement of the corneal epithelium and transfer to viral transport media will usually suffice to grow herpes simplex virus, types I and II, and adenovirus. Herpes zoster virus is rarely isolated from corneal lesions. In doubtful cases, transmission electron microscopy may occasionally be helpful in establishing the viral etiology.[110]

The limulus lysate assay has been used in the diagnosis of corneal ulcers when gram-negative organisms are suspected.[111] Sensitivity testing should proceed according to the usual laboratory techniques, although laboratory sensitivity testing of fungi remains unsatisfactory.

TREATMENT

Early specific therapy is the prime requisite for successful management of corneal ulcers. Because of the rapid evolution to perforation of some ulcers and the visual loss by central corneal scarring, most patients with bacterial keratitis with significant ulceration should be hospitalized. There are several methods of antibiotic therapy. These include topical antibiotic drops and ointment, subconjunctival injection, continuous lavage, and parenteral administration.

Topical antibiotics in solution are preferred over ointments because hospital pharmacies can readily prepare highly concentrated solutions by using commercially available ocular lubricants and parenteral antibiotic preparations.[112]

Subconjunctival administration of antibiotics, although painful, provides a higher transient peak concentration of drug within the corneal stroma than is usually obtainable with topical therapy.[113]

Continuous lavage of the cornea with antibiotic solutions has been described.[114] The advantages of this method are the increased drug levels obtained within the aqueous humor[115] and the lack of dependence on nursing personnel for frequent drop instillations.

Parenteral (intramuscular or intravenous) administration of antibiotics is reserved for deep corneal ulcers with impending perforation. The choice of antibiotics is dictated by the Gram-stained smears and then is modified according to culture results. Initial broad-spectrum antibiotic cover with a cephalosporin and gentamicin is commonly advocated.[116]

Supportive therapy in the treatment of infectious keratitis consists of cycloplegics, enzyme inhibitors, therapeutic soft contact lenses, and topical steroids. Since a severe anterior chamber reaction may occur with a bacterial keratitis, cycloplegics should be used to prevent the formation of synechiae and to relieve the discomfort of ciliary spasm.

If corneal ulceration is marked, the temporary use of a therapeutic soft contact lens or "bandage" lens may facilitate stromal repair and promote reepithelialization by protecting the corneal surface from the mechanical trauma of lid movement. Topical medication may be continued after the contact lens insertion.

The use of topical corticosteroids in the management of bacterial keratitis is a controversial issue. It has been suggested that steroids in conjunction with specific antibacterial therapy minimize the inflammatory sequelae of bacterial keratitis.[114,115]

The treatment of the epithelial keratitis in herpes simplex infections consists of simple débridement of the epithelium[117] and use of an antiviral agent; this is effective in most cases of corneal dendritic ulcers. Extensive involvement, central lesions, geographic lesions, or resistant lesions are usually treated with a 10-day course of antiviral agents. Trifluridine and acyclovir are the preferred agents because of their lower corneal toxicity.[118] The use of corticosteroids is contraindicated in isolated epithelial herpes. Herpetic uveitis may resolve spontaneously, but most ophthalmologists would use cycloplegia and topical corticosteroids to reduce the damaging effect of prolonged stromal and anterior chamber inflammation. The use of an antiviral "umbrella" while the patient is being administered corticosteroids to prevent the recurrence of epithelial herpes is still widely debated.[119,120] Other methods of therapy such as topical interferon[121] and cryotherapy have been used. Uncontrolled herpetic stromal keratitis and secondary stromal scarring may require corneal transplantation.[122,123]

Epidemic keratocon junctivitis rarely requires more therapy than mild cycloplegics and antibiotic cover. Severe photophobia, incapacitating irritation, and decreased vision during the acute episodes may be relieved with use of topical corticosteroids. It is unclear whether their use prolongs the course of the disease.

Stromal keratitis caused by herpes zoster will frequently require corticosteroids to reduce the inflammatory response and resultant corneal destruction, although some authors have suggested that the use of the steroids alone has a deleterious effect on this keratitis.[120,124]

Fungal ulcers require the prolonged use of topical antifungal therapy and occasionally parenteral therapy. Topical natamycin, 5%, is a valuable addition to ocular therapy.[71] Topical miconazole (10 mg/ml) and fluocytosine, 1%, and amphotericin B drops (1 mg/ml) may occasionally be used, although the latter has definite epithelial toxicity.[107,108]

Resistant fungal ulcers may require the use of parenteral amphotericin B, flucytosine, or ketoconazole.[125] Corneal transplantation or conjunctival flaps may be needed to stabilize the eye. The addition of corticosteroids to therapy when a response to the antifungal agent has been observed remains controversial, but it may help to reduce corneal destruction caused by host response.

Nocardia asteroides has been reported to respond to topical and parenteral sulfadiazine administration.[74]

Currently recommended medical therapy for *Acanthamoeba* keratitis includes topical propamadine isethionate, dibromopropamadine isethionate, and neomycin. Although one patient has been successfully treated medically,[126] most cases require corneal transplantation and medical therapy to eradicate the infection.

The drug management of onchocerciasis is changing, with the recent addition of ivermectin as the therapeutic agent of choice.[127]

Since syphilitic interstitial keratitis is a manifestation of an immune phenomenon, specific antiluetic therapy does not greatly affect the course of the acute inflammation. However, therapy reduces the chances of recurrence from 27 percent in untreated cases to 3.6 percent in treated cases. Treatment also reduces the likelihood of bilateral ocular involvement. Topical steroids are used during the acute stages of the keratitis to avoid severe postinflammatory sequelae.[92]

Noninfected corneal ulcers with associated destruction of the stroma may require systemic immunosuppressive[128] or other supportive therapy, including corneal transplantation or tissue adhesive application.[129] Corneal changes in xerophthalmia can be reversed by topical or systemic vitamin A administration[130] if given early enough.

Foreign bodies embedded in the cornea are removed with a metal spud. This is usually followed by the use of a topical antibiotic, a cycloplegic, and patching of the eye. In exposure keratitis the lids may be taped. Artificial tears, topical ointments at night, and hydrophilic lenses are useful. In neuroparalytic keratitis, short-term taping of the eyelids usually is followed by partial tarsorraphy or a conjunctival flap.

REFERENCES

1. Jones DB. Polymicrobial keratitis. Trans Am Ophthalmol Soc. 1981;79:153.
2. Asbell P, Stenson S. Ulcerative keratitis. Survey of 30 years' laboratory experience. Arch Ophthalmol. 1982;100:77.
3. Liesegang TJ, Forster RK. Spectrum of microbial keratitis in south Florida. Am J Ophthalmol. 1980;90:38.
4. Eichenbaum JW, Feldstein M, Podos SM. Extended-wear aphakic soft contact lenses and corneal ulcers. Br J Ophthalmol. 1982;66:663.
5. Wilson LA, Schlitzer RL, Ahearn DG. *Pseudomonas* corneal ulcers associated with soft contact-lens wear. Am J Ophthalmol. 1981;92:546.
6. Krachmer JH, Purcell JJ. Bacterial corneal ulcers in cosmetic soft contact lens wearers. Arch Ophthalmol. 1978;96:57.
7. Escapini H Jr, Olson RJ, Kaufman HE. Donor cornea contamination with McCarey-Kaufman medium preservation. Am J Ophthalmol. 1979;88:59.
8. Udell IJ, Kelly CG, Wolf TC, et al. Cat scratch keratitis. Ophthalmology. 1987;94(Suppl):124.
9. Wilson LA, Ahearn DG. *Pseudomonas* induced corneal ulcers associated with contaminated eye mascaras. Am J Ophthalmol. 1977;84:112.
10. Reid FR, Wood TO. *Pseudomonas* corneal ulcer. The causative role of contaminated eye cosmetics. Arch Ophthalmol. 1979;97:1640.
11. Locatcher-Khorazo D, Butierrez E. Bacteriophage typing of *Staphylococcus aureus:* A study of normal, infected eyes and environment. Arch Ophthalmol. 1960;63:774.
12. Locatcher-Khorazo D, Sullivan N, Gutierrez E. *Staphylococcus aureus* isolated from normal and infected eyes: Phage types and sensitivity to antibacterial agents. Arch Ophthalmol. 1967;77:370.
13. Kim HB, Ostler HB. Marginal corneal ulcer due to β-*Streptococcus*. Arch Ophthalmol. 1977;95:454.
14. Cohn H, Mondino BJ, Brown SI, et al. Marginal corneal ulcers with acute beta streptococcal conjunctivitis and chronic dacryocystitis. Am J Ophthalmol. 1979;87:541.
15. Johnson MK, Allen JH. Ocular toxin of the pneumococcus. Am J Ophthalmol. 1971;72:175.
16. Brown SI, Bloomfield SE, Wai-Fong IT. The cornea-destroying enzyme of *Pseudomonas aeruginosa*. Invest Ophthalmol. 1974;13:174.
17. Hutton WL, Sexton RR. Atypical *Pseudomonas* corneal ulcers in semicomatose patients. Am J Ophthalmol. 1972;73:37.
18. Codere F, Brownstein S, Jackson WB. *Pseudomonas aeruginosa* scleritis. Am J Ophthalmol. 1981;91:706.
19. Raber IM, Laibson PR, Kurz GH, et al. *Pseudomonas* corneoscleral ulcers. Am J Ophthalmol. 1981;92:353.
20. Brinser JH, Torczynski E. Unusual *Pseudomonas* corneal ulcers. Am J Ophthalmol. 1977;84:462.
21. Lass JH, Haaf J, Foster CS, et al. Visual outcome in eight cases of *Serratia marcescens* keratitis. Am J Ophthalmol. 1981;92:384.
22. Templeton WC, Eiferman RA, Snyder JW, et al. *Serratia keratitis* transmitted by contaminated eyedroppers. Am J Ophthalmol. 1982;93:723.
23. Baum J, Fedukowicz HB, Jordan A. A survey of *Moraxella* corneal ulcers in a derelict population. Am J Ophthalmol. 1980;90:476.
24. Cobo LM, Coster DJ, Peacock J. *Moraxella* keratitis in a nonalcoholic population. Br J Ophthalmol. 1981;65:683.
25. van Bijsterveld OP, Richards RD. *Bacillus* infections of the cornea. Arch Ophthalmol. 1965;74:91.
26. Chandler JW, Milam DF. Diphtheria corneal ulcers. Arch Ophthalmol. 1978;96:53.
27. Turner L, Stinson I. *Mycobacterium fortuitum* as a cause of corneal ulcer. Am J Ophthalmol. 1965;60:329.
28. Meisler DM, Friedlaender MH, Okumoto M. *Mycobacterium chelonei* keratitis. Am J Ophthalmol. 1982;94:398.
29. Allen JH, Byers JL. The pathology of ocular leprosy. I. Cornea. Arch Ophthalmol. 1960;64:216.
30. Elliott DC. An interpetation of the ocular manifestations of leprosy. Ann NY Acad Sci. 1951;54:84.
31. Pillat A. Leprosy bacilli in the scraping from the diseased cornea in a leper, and comments on keratitis punctata superficialis leprosa. Arch Ophthalmol. 1930;3:306.
32. Liesegang TJ, Jones DB, Robinson NM. *Azotobacter* keratitis. Arch Ophthalmol. 1981;99:1587.
33. Wilhelmus KR, Peacock J, Coster DJ. *Branhamella* keratitis. Br J Ophthalmol. 1980;64:892.
34. Feaster FT, Nisbet RM, Barber JC. *Aeromonas hydrophilia* corneal ulcer. Am J Ophthalmol. 1978;85:114.
35. Purcell JJ, Krachmer JH. Corneal ulcer caused by *Pasteurella multocida*. Am J Ophthalmol. 1977;83:540.
36. Stern GA, Hodes BL, Stock EL. *Clostridium perfringens* corneal ulcer. Arch Ophthalmol. 1979;97:661.
37. Tabbara KF, Tarabay N. *Bacillus licheniformis* corneal ulcer. Am J Ophthalmol. 1979;87:717.
38. Samples JR, Buettner H. Corneal ulcer caused by a biologic insecticide (*Bacillus thuringiensis*). Am J Ophthalmol. 1983;95:258.
39. Ostler HB, Okumoto M. Anaerobic streptococcal corneal ulcer. Am J Ophthalmol. 1976;81:518.
40. Nahmias AJ, Visintine AM, Caldwell DR, et al. Eye infections with herpes simplex viruses in neonates. Surv Ophthalmol. 1976;21:100.
41. Stern GA, Zam ZS, Gutgesell VJ. Primary herpes simplex subepithelial dendritic keratitis. Am J Ophthalmol. 1981;91:496.
42. Poirier RH. Herpetic ocular infections of childhood. Arch Ophthalmol. 1980;98:704.
43. Shuster JJ, Kaufman HE, Nesburn AB. Statistical analysis of the rate of recurrence of herpesvirus ocular epithelial disease. Am J Ophthalmol. 1981;91:328.
44. Wilhelmus KR, Coster DJ, Donovan HC, et al. Prognostic indicators of herpetic keratitis. Analysis of a five-year observation period after corneal ulceration. Arch Ophthalmol. 1981;99:1578.
45. Stevens JG, Nesburn AB, Cook M. Latent herpes simplex virus recovered from trigeminal ganglia of rabbits with recurrent eye infection. Nature. 1972;235:216.
46. Baringer J, Swoveland P. Recovery of herpes simplex virus from human trigeminal ganglions. N Engl J Med. 1973;288:648.
47. Norn MS. Dendritic (herpetic) keratitis. IV. Follow-up examination of corneal sensitivity. Acta Ophthalmol. 1970;48:383.
48. Bloomfield SE, Lopez C. Herpes infections in the immunosuppressed host. Ophthalmology. 1980;87:1226.
49. Howcroft MJ, Breslin CW. Herpes simplex keratitis in renal transplant recipients. Can Med Assoc J. 1981;124:292.
50. Cleobury JF, Skinner GRB, Thouless ME, et al. Association between psychopathic disorder and serum antibody to herpes simplex virus (type 1). Br Med J. 1971;261:438.
51. Patterson A, Jones BR. Management of ocular herpes. Trans Ophthalmol Soc UK. 1967;87:59.
52. Theodore FH. Allergic keratitis. In: King JH, McTigue JW, eds: The Cornea World Congress. Washington, DC: Butterworths; 1965;197.
53. Womack LW, Liesegang TJ. Complications of herpes zoster ophthalmicus. Arch Ophthalmol. 1983;101:42.
54. Hedges TR III, Albert DM. The progression of the ocular abnormalities of herpes zoster. Histopathologic observations of nine cases. Ophthalmology. 1982;89:165.
55. Edgerton AE. Herpes zoster ophthalmicus: Report of cases and review of literature. Arch Ophthalmol. 1945;34:40.
56. Mondino BJ, Brown SI, Mondzelewski JP. Peripheral corneal ulcers with herpes zoster ophthalmicus. Am J Ophthalmol. 1978;86:611.
57. Strachman J. Uveitis associated with chickenpox. J Pediatr. 1955;46:327.
58. Uchida Y, Kaneko M, Hayashi K. Varicella dendritic keratitis. Am J Ophthalmol. 1980;89:259.
59. Frampton G, Smith C. Primary vaccinia of the eyelid. Br J Ophthalmol. 1952;36:214.
60. Bedell AJ. Multiple vaccination of the eyelids. Trans Am Ophthalmol Soc. 1919:17, 273.
61. Darrell RW, Vrabec F. Vaccinia virus infection of the rabbit cornea. Arch Ophthalmol. 1971;86:568.
62. Sachs U, Marcus M. Bilateral herpetic keratitis during measles. Am J Ophthalmol. 1981;91:796.
63. Deckard PS, Bergstrom TJ. Rubeola keratitis. Ophthalmology. 1981;88:810.
64. Pinnolis M, McCulley JP, Urman JD. Nummular keratitis associated with infectious mononucleosis. Am J Ophthalmol. 1980;89:791.
65. Matoba AY, Wilhemus KR, Jones DB. Epstein-Barr viral stromal keratitis. Ophthalmology. 1986;93:746–51.
66. Manuelidis EE, Angelo JN, Gorgacz EJ, et al. Experimental Creutzfeldt-Jakob disease transmitted via the eye with infected cornea. N Engl J Med. 1977;296:1334.
67. Houff SA, Burton RC, Wilson RW, et al. Human-to-human transmission of rabies virus by corneal transplant. N Engl J Med. 1979;300:603.
68. Salahuddin SZ, Palestine AG, Heck E, et al. Isolation of the human T-cell leukemia/lymphotrophic virus type III from the cornea. Am J Ophthalmol. 1986;101:149–52.
69. Jones BR, Richards AB, Morgan G. Direct fungal infection of the eye in Britain. Trans Ophthalmol Soc UK. 1969;89:727.
70. DeVoe AG, Silva-Hutner M. Fungal infections of the eye. In: Locatcher-Khorazo D, Seegal BC, eds. Microbiology of the Eye. St Louis; CV Mosby; 1972;208.
71. Jones DB, Forster RK, Rebell G. *Fusarium solani* keratitis treated with natamycin (pimaricin): 18 consecutive cases. Arch Ophthalmol. 1972;88:147.
72. Searl SS, Udel IJ, Sadun A, et al. *Aspergillus* keratitis with intraocular invasion. Ophthalmology. 1981;88:1244.
73. Polack FM, Kaufman HE, Newmark E. Keratomycosis: Medical and surgical treatment. Arch Ophthalmol. 1971;85:410.
74. Hirst LW, Harrison GK, Merz WG, et al. *Nocardia asteroides* keratitis. Br J Ophthalmol. 1979;63:449.
75. Wilhelmus KR, Robinson NM, Jones DB. *Bacterionema matruchotii* ocular infections. Am J Ophthalmol. 1979;87:143.
76. Jones FR, Christensen GR. *Pullularia* corneal ulcer. Arch Ophthalmol. 1974;92:529.
77. Krachmer JH, Anderson RL, Binder PS, et al. Helminthosporium corneal ulcers. Am J Ophthalmol. 1978;85:66.
78. Francois J, Rijsselaere. Corneal infections by rhodotorula. Ophthalmologica. 1979;178:241.
79. Zapater RC, Albesi EJ. Corneal monosporiosis. A review and report of 1 case. Ophthalmologica. 1979;178:142.
80. Eiferman RA, Snyder JW, Barbee JV Jr. Corneal chromomycosis. Am J Ophthalmol. 1982;95:255.
81. Rodrigues MM, Laibson P, Kaplan W. Exogenous corneal ulcer caused by *Tritirachium roseum*. Am J Ophthalmol. 1979;80:804.

82. Taylor HR. Treatment of onchocerciasis in the 1980s Postgrad Doctor Afr. 1983;5:74.
83. Buck AA, ed. Onchocerciasis: Symptomatology, pathology, diagnosis. Geneva: World Health Organization; 1974.
84. Gibson DW, Heggie C, Connor DH. Clinical and pathologic aspects of onchocerciasis. Pathol Ann. 1980;15:195.
85. Roizenblatt J. Interstitial keratitis caused by American (mucocutaneous) leishmaniasis. Am J Ophthalmol. 1979;87:175.
86. Dawson CR, Jones BR, Tarizzo ML. Guide to trachoma control in programmes for the prevention of blindness. Geneva: World Health Organization; 1981.
87. Ma P, Willaert E, Juechter KB, et al. A case of keratitis due to *Acanthamoeba* in New York, New York, and features of 10 cases. J Infect Dis. 1981;143:662.
88. Mannis MJ, Tamaro R, Roth AM, et al. *Acanthamoeba* sclerokeratitis. Determining diagnostic criteria. Arch Ophthalmol. 1986;104:1313–17.
89. Eiferman RA, Carothers DJ, Yankeelow JA. Peripheral rheumatoid ulceration and evidence for conjunctival collagenase production. Am J Ophthalmol. 1979;87:703.
90. Austin P, Green WR, Sallyer DC, et al. Peripheral corneal degeneration and occlusive vasculitis in Wegener's granulomatosis. Am J Ophthalmol. 1978;85:311.
91. Gerstle CC, Friedman AH. Marginal corneal ulceration (limbal guttering) as a presenting sign of temporal arteritis. Ophthalmology. 1980;87:1173.
92. Duke-Elder S. System of Ophthalmology. v. 8. Diseases of the Outer Eye. St Louis: CV Mosby; 1965;237, 239, 539, 828, 829, 1032.
93. Woods AC. Syphilis of the eye. Am J Syph Gonor Vener Dis. 1943;27:133.
94. Ballantyne AJ, Michaelson IC: Textbook of the Fundus of the Eye. Baltimore: Williams & Wilkins; 1962;564.
95. Knapp A. Bilateral circumpapillary chorioretinitis with detachment of the retina in syphilis. Trans Am Acad Ophthalmol Otolaryngol. 1920;25:132.
96. Stokes JH, Beerman H, Ingraham NR. Modern Clinical Syphilology. Philadelphia: WB Saunders; 1949:59.
97. Carrol FD. Retrobulbar neuritis. Arch Ophthalmol. 1940;24:44.
98. Hogan MJ, Zimmerman LE, eds. Ophthalmic Pathology. 3rd ed. Philadelphia: WB Saunders; 1968;397.
99. Moore JE. Syphilitic iritis. Am J Ophthalmol. 1931;14:110.
100. Krachmer JH, Laibson PR. Corneal thinning and perforation in Sjögren's syndrome. Am J Ophthalmol. 1974;78:917.
101. Pfister RR, Murphy GE. Corneal ulceration and perforation associated with Sjögren's syndrome. Arch Ophthalmol. 1980;98:89.
102. Charlton KH, Binder PS, Wozniak L, et al. Pseudodendritic keratitis and systemic tyrosinemia. Ophthalmology. 1981;88:355.
103. Tabbara KF, Ostler HB, Dawson C, et al. Thygeson's superficial punctate keratitis. Ophthalmology. 1981;88:75.
104. Mark DB, McCulley JB. Reiter's keratitis. Arch Ophthalmol. 1982;100:781.
105. Sommer A, Tarwotjo I, Hussaini G, et al. Incidence, prevalence, and scale of blinding malnutrition. Lancet. 1981;1:1407.
106. Jones DB, Liesgang TJ, Robinson NM. Laboratory diagnosis of ocular infections. Cumitech 13. 1981.
107. Forster RK, Rebell G. The diagnosis and management of keratomycoses. II. Medical and surgical management. Arch Ophthalmol. 1975;93:1134.
108. Jones DB. Decision-making in the management of microbial keratitis. Ophthalmology. 1981;88:814.
109. Naumann G, Green WR, Zimmerman LE. Mycotic keratitis. A histopathologic study of 73 cases. Am J Ophthalmol. 1967;64:668–82.
110. Boerner CF, Lee FK, Wichliffe CL, et al. Electron microscopy for the diagnosis of ocular viral infections. Ophthalmology. 1981;88:1377.
111. Wolters RW, Jorgensen JH, Calzada E, et al. Limulus lysate assay for early detection of certain gram-negative corneal infections. Arch Ophthalmol. 1979;97:875.
112. Chaudhuri PR, Godfrey B. Treatment of bacterial corneal ulcers with concentrated antibiotic eye drops. Trans Ophthalmol Soc UK. 1982;102:11.
113. Baum J, Barza M. Topical vs subconjunctival treatment of bacterial corneal ulcers. Ophthalmology. 1983;90:162.
114. Aronson SB, Moore TE Jr, O'Day DM. The effects of structural alteration on anterior ocular inflammation. Am J Ophthalmol. 1970;70:886.
115. Golden B, Fingerman LH, Allen HF. *Pseudomonas* corneal ulcers in contact lens wearers. Arch Ophthalmol. 1971;85:543.
116. Baum JL. Initial therapy of suspected microbial corneal ulcers: I. Broad antibiotic therapy based on prevalence of organisms. Surv Ophthalmol. 1979;24:97.
117. Wilhelmus KR, Coster DJ, Jones Br. Acyclovir and debridement in the treatment of ulcerative herpetic keratitis. Am J Ophthalmol. 1981;91:323.
118. LaLau C, Oosterhuis A, Versteeg J, et al. Acyclovir and trifluorothymidine in herpetic keratitis: A multicentre trial. Br J Ophthalmol. 1982;66:506.
119. Jones BR, Falcon MG, Williams HP, et al. Symposium on herpes simplex eye disease. Objectives in therapy of herpetic eye disease. Trans Ophthalmol Soc UK. 1977;97:305.
120. Ostler HB. The management of ocular herpesvirus infections. Surv Ophthalmol. 1976;21:136.
121. Jones BR, Coster DJ, Falcon MG, et al. Topical therapy of ulcerative herpetic keratitis with human inteferon. Lancet. 1976;2:128.
122. Cobo LM, Coster DJ, Rice NSC, et al. Prognosis and management of corneal transplantation for herpetic keratitis. Arch Ophthalmol. 1980;98:1755.
123. Foster CS, Duncan J. Penetrating keratoplasty for herpes simplex keratitis. Am J Ophthalmol. 1981;92:336.
124. Bergaust B, Westby RK. Zoster ophthalmicus: Local treatment with cortisone. Acta Ophthalmol. 1967;45:787.
125. Ishibashi Y. Oral ketoconazole therapy for keratomycosis. Am J Ophthalmol. 1983;95:342.
126. Wright P, Worhurst D, Jones BR. *Acanthamoeba* keratitis successfully treated medically. Br J Ophthalmol. 1985;69:778–82.
127. White AT, Newland HS, Taylor HR, et al. Controlled trial and dose-finding study of ivermectin for treatment of onchocerciasis. J Infect Dis. 1987;156:463–70.
128. Foster CS. Immunosuppressive therapy for external ocular inflammatory disease. Ophthalmology. 1980;87:140.
129. Kenyon KR. Decision-making in the therapy of external eye disease. Noninfected corneal ulcers. Ophthalmology. 1982;89:44.
130. Sommer A. Nutritional Blindness: Xerophthalmia and Keratomalacia. New York: Oxford University Press; 1982

100. ENDOPHTHALMITIS

PETER J. McDONNELL
W. RICHARD GREEN

Endophthalmitis is defined as an inflammatory process that involves an ocular cavity and adjacent structures and may be classified according to the type of etiologic agent, the mode of entry, and the location within the eye. Infectious etiologic agents include bacteria, fungi, viruses, protozoa, and parasites (Table 1). The infectious agent may be introduced directly into the eye as in cases of surgical and nonsurgical trauma or may reach the eye by hematogenous spread from a distant site of infection. Noninfectious stimuli causing endophthalmitis in-

TABLE 1. Infectious Agents That Cause Endophthalmitis

Bacteria	Fungi
Aerobic	*Acremonium (Cephalosporium)* species
Gram-positive cocci	*Aspergillus* species
Staphylococcus aureus, S. epidermidis	*Blastomyces dermatitidis*
Streptococcus pneumoniae, other species of *Streptococcus*	*Candida* species
Gram-positive bacilli	*Cladosporium* species
Bacillus cereus, B. subtilis, other *Bacillus* species	*Coccidioides immitis*
Corynebacterium pseudodiphtheriticum (*C. hofmannii*), *C. xerosis*, other *Corynebacterium* species	*Cryptococcus neoformans*
Listeria monocytogenes	*Exophiala jeanselmei*
Gram-negative cocci	*Fusarium* species
Neisseria meningitidis	*Graphium* species
Gram-negative bacilli	*Histoplasma capsulatum*
Acinetobacter species	*Mucor* species
Alcaligenes faecalis	*Neurospora sitophila*
Enterobacter species	*Rhizopus* species
Escherichia coli	*Paecilomyces* species
Flavobacterium meningosepticum	*Penicillium* species
Haemophilis influenzae	*Pseudallescheria (Petriellidium) boydii (Scedosporium apiospermum)*
Klebsiella species	*Sporothrix schenckii*
Moraxella species	*Torulopsis glabrata*
Proteus species	*Trichosporon* species
Pseudomonas aeruginosa	*Volutella* species
Salmonella typhimurium	Viruses
Serratia marcescens	Herpes simplex virus
Anaerobic	Herpes zoster virus
Clostridium species	Cytomegalovirus
Propionibacterium acnes	Rubella
Spirochetes	Rubeola
Treponema pallidum	Parasites
Higher bacteria	*Onchocerca volvulus*
Actinomyces israelii	*Taenia solium* (cysticercosis)
Mycobacterium tuberculosis, M. leprae, M. avium-intracellulare	*Toxocara canis* and *cati*
Nocardia species	*Toxoplasma gondii*

clude retained lens material, foreign materials introduced at the time of surgery, blood, and intraocular neoplasms. The inflammatory process may be localized to specific tissues within the eye or may involve the intraocular contents in a generalized fashion. When the episclera participates significantly in the inflammatory process, a panophthalmitis is said to be present. Pain, especially on movement of the eye, is a prominent feature of panophthalmitis.

BACTERIAL ENDOPHTHALMITIS

Bacteria are the most common infectious agents that cause endophthalmitis. Typically, a bacterial endophthalmitis develops suddenly and progresses rapidly.[1,2] The symptoms and signs become manifested in the first 24 to 48 hours after surgical or nonsurgical trauma. If, in the early postoperative period, the patient complains of increasing pain with progressive blurred vision and exhibits any unexpected degree of hyperemia, chemosis, lid edema, corneal edema, and anterior-chamber and vitreous reaction, bacterial endophthalmitis should be strongly suspected. Careful slit-lamp examination and direct or indirect ophthalmoscopy are necessary if the earliest signs of endophthalmitis are to be detected.

Bacterial endophthalmitis usually occurs as a complication of ocular surgery. The usefulness of prophylactic antibiotics topically or subconjunctivally, before, during, or after surgery, remains unproven, although preoperative topical antibiotics are widely used.[3–6] It should be emphasized that the ocular surface microflora are responsible for the majority of infections and probably gain access to the eye during surgery. *Staphylococcus aureus* is responsible for 50 percent of the cases of endophthalmitis after cataract extraction.[5] Infections due to *S. aureus* and *Pseudomonas* are usually manifested in a fulminating fashion in the early postoperative period. Virtually any bacterial microorganism, including those previously considered saprophytic, may cause endophthalmitis[7–25] (Table 1).

The incidence of endophthalmitis after cataract extraction varies from 0.078 percent[5,26] to 0.496 percent[6] and 0.533 percent,[27] and it occurs in 0.2 percent of cases after penetrating keratoplasties.[28] Contamination of intraocular lenses has produced isolated endophthalmitis.[29–31] Short-term storage of corneal buttons in McCarey-Kaufman media[32] has resulted in endophthalmitis.

Bacterial endophthalmitis may follow surgical procedures for glaucoma,[33–35] retinal detachment,[36] strabismus,[37] pterygia,[38] myopia,[39] and corneal transplantation.[32,40] Postoperative complications such as wound leaks,[41] unplanned filtering blebs,[42,43] vitreous wick syndromes,[44] deep sutures, epithelial ingrowth, and retained lens material[45] may predispose to bacterial endophthalmitis. An incidence of 1.2–9 percent has been reported for late endophthalmitis in patients who have had glaucoma procedures.[46,34] The use of contact lenses in patients with inadvertent postoperative blebs may lead to endophthalmitis.[42] Recently, persistent low-grade infections with organisms of low virulence such as *Propionibacterium acnes* have been recognized to cause chronic inflammation after cataract extraction.[47]

Bacterial endophthalmitis is surprisingly rare after penetrating nonsurgical trauma.[48–50] *Bacillus* species are most commonly isolated in this setting.[51] The development of systemic tetanus has been reported after penetrating ocular trauma.[52,53]

If there is a sudden onset of endophthalmitis in an unoperated nontraumatized eye, hematogenous spread from a distant focus of infection should be suspected.[54–60] The clinical picture is similar to that seen in postoperative bacterial endophthalmitis except that the posterior segment of the eye is usually involved and the patients are usually extremely ill and often immunologically compromised.[57,61–63] Dental procedures have occasionally preceded the developement of bacterial endophthalmitis.[64,65] Neonates and women in the puerperal period may also occasionally develop endogenous endophthalmitis.[66–68] The most common features are decreased visual acuity, pain, hypopyon or severe anterior uveitis, and conjunctival hyperemia. Within hours, a focal chorioretinitis occurs. Vitreous infection and finally an acute panophthalmitis may follow. Endophthalmitis may also occur as a result of progressive severe bacterial corneal ulceration.

In hematogenous bacterial endophthalmitis, a septic focus is usually apparent before intraocular inflammation occurs. In a review[60] of 20 such cases, meningitis, abdominal infection, endocarditis, pneumonia, otitis media, breast abscess, paronychia, pharyngitis, and lymphangitis were implicated as septic foci. The etiologic agent was the pneumococcus in 30 percent of the cases. Meningococci and staphylococci were each responsible for 15 percent of the cases. Since the etiologic agents are usually of low virulence in subacute bacterial endocarditis, ocular findings may be minimal. Conjunctival and retinal hemorrhages are the most frequent findings. Retinal hemorrhages that have white centers called *Roth spots* may represent septic retinitis. These lesions are characteristic but not pathognomonic of subacute bacterial endocarditis. Hemorrhages with white centers due to the accumulation of platelets and fibrin may be seen in other diseases. Bacterial endophthalmitis due to *Bacillus cereus* has been reported after transfusion with contaminated blood and in heroin addicts. Various agents including *Haemophilus influenzae, Streptococcus,* and *Neisseria meningitidis* have been implicated in unilateral and bilateral endophthalmitis associated with meningitis.[58,59,70]

In miliary tuberculosis, small elevated yellow-white choroidal nodules with indistinct borders may be seen.[71] Tuberculous retinitis and endophthalmitis have been observed.[72]

In congenital syphilis the severe chorioretinitis leads to extensive chorioretinal scarring with a variety of patterns.[72]

In secondary and late-acquired syphilis, iridocyclitis is the most frequent ocular finding.[73] Other inflammatory features include retinal vasculitis, phlebitis, periarteritis, panuveitis, "posterior uveitis," multifocal choroiditis, chorioretinitis, papillitis, and neuroretinitis.[72]

Nocardia asteroides is a higher bacteria. Disseminated nocardiosis occurs via hematogenous spread from a pulmonary lesion. There have been 11 reported cases of intraocular involvement. With ocular involvement, the patients complain of blurred vision and pain. On fundus examination, central or paracentral foci of necrotizing chorioretinitis are seen.[74,75] A vitreous abscess may occasionally occur. Of the 14 reported cases with intraocular involvement, 3 occurred after surgery or trauma, 1 occurred after carotid endarterectomy, and 10 were associated with systemic diseases and reduced immune competence.[72]

In Whipple's disease, macrophages with phagocytosed bacilli in varying stages of breakdown may be present in the vitreous cavity and retina.[76]

MYCOTIC ENDOPHTHALMITIS

The incidence of systemic mycotic infections has increased markedly in the past 3 decades. This increase is thought to be related in part to the widespread use of antibiotics, corticosteroids, chemotherapy, and immunosuppressive therapy; to an increased addictive drug usage[77–82]; and to hyperalimentation.[83–85]

Fungi generally considered to be saprophytes can cause endophthalmitis. Over 20 different fungal agents have been isolated from cases of intraocular mycoses.[86]

Fungal endophthalmitis may occur from exogenous and endogenous sources. Exogenous sources include extension of a fungal corneal ulcer and surgical or nonsurgical trauma,[87] including outbreaks of fungal endophthalmitis due to contaminated ophthalmic irrigation solutions.[88]

The main difference between bacterial and fungal endophthalmitis after trauma or surgery is the time of onset of symptoms and signs. Typically in a fungal endophthalmitis, there is a greater delay in the onset of symptoms and signs than in a bacterial endophthalmitis. After intraocular surgery, there may be a lapse of several weeks before the onset of ocular pain, ciliary injection, and signs of a nonspecific uveitis. On slit-lamp examination, a localized gray-white area may be seen in the anterior vitreous adjacent to the pupillary border. A transient hypopyon may occur, and additional satellite lesions occur in the anterior vitreous. In rare instances, the site of infection and abscess formation may occur in the anterior chamber, usually near the chamber angle.

The incidence of fungal endophthalmitis after cataract surgery is very low. In one series of 36,000 cataract extractions, only two cases of infection were reported.[89] However, epidemic fungal endophthalmitis has occurred after intraocular lens implantation[90,91] and in isolated cases after retinal reattachment surgery[92] and penetrating keratoplasty using cryopreserved or organ-icultured tissue.[93,94] Fungi isolated postoperatively have included *Volutella* species,[95] *Neurospora sitophila,*[96] *Scedosporium apiospermum,*[97] *Candida parapsilosis,*[98] *Trichosporon cutaneum,*[99] *Paecilomyces lilacinus,*[90,100] *Acremonium* (*Cephalosporium*),[94] and *Torulopsis glabrata*[93] (Table 1).

After penetrating nonsurgical trauma, signs of fungal endophthalmitis may develop in an indolent fashion many weeks later.[101–103] Extension of fungal corneal ulcer may also lead to endophthalmitis.[104,105]

In hematogenous fungal endophthalmitis, the ocular involvement may be the first or only manifestation. Evidence of nonocular foci of metastatic fungal disease may not be present. Of 133 patients who died after fungemia, 14 (10.5 percent) were found to have ocular involvement (11 with *Candida,* 2 with *Aspergillus,* and 1 with *Cryptococcus*).[106] Reduction of vision is the usual initial symptom. At first, only a slight preretinal vitreous haze may be seen. Within a few days, fluffy white balls of exudate occur in the vitreous just anterior to the retina. The degree of inflammation may vary from a localized abscess to a total endophthalmitis. Chorioretinal or vitreoretinal scarring may result in a severe reduction of vision or even loss of the eye.

Candida albicans is the most frequently reported cause of endogenous fungal endophthalmitis[107–113] (Chapter 234). There has been an impressive increase in *Candida* endophthalmitis over the last 3 or 4 decades, which is only partly accounted for by increased clinical suspicion and improved culture techniques.[114] Although intravenous drug addiction clearly has contributed to the problem, the major causal factor appears to be the extensive use of intravascular catheters.[80,83–85]

In a review of 100 reported cases of *Candida* endophthalmitis, it was determined that 85 patients had received broad-spectrum antibiotic therapy, 17 patients had received corticosteroids, and 8 patients had received both concurrently.[114] Fifty-three patients had undergone abdominal, thoracic, or cardiac surgery within a short time preceding the development of candidiasis. One-quarter of the abdominal procedures were performed for malignancy. Nine patients had diabetes mellitus, and six were alcoholics with cirrhosis of the liver. Blood cultures were positive in 41 patients, and urine cultures were positive in 25 patients. In 14 cases, culture of material from intravenous catheter tips yielded *Candida*.

There is an average delay of 18 days between the time a positive culture for *Candida* is obtained and the onset of ocular symptoms.[114] Blurred vision, pain, and ciliary injection may occur. A casual diagnosis of conjunctivitis or, in comatose patients, of exposure keratitis may be made. All too often, symptoms are reported late because the patient is comatose, on a respirator, or gravely ill. Periodic funduscopic examinations are indicated in patients with known or suspected candidemia. The earliest lesion is a small, yellow-white retinal exudate that may be mistaken for a lesion of diabetes mellitus, acute leukemia, or systemic lupus erythematosus. This early lesion, which may be unilateral or bilateral, may resolve spontaneously or progress slowly to a vitreous abscess. As extension to the vitreous occurs, margins of the lesion become hazy, the vitreous becomes progressively clouded, and one or more balls of yellowish white exudate protrude into the vitreous. Although the ciliary body or iris may on occasion be the site of an initial lesion, extension to the anterior chamber is usually a late finding.[115] Prognosis for the return of normal visual acuity in an eye with a *Candida* vitreous abscess is guarded despite appropriate therapy.[107–109] Recognition of an early funduscopic lesion may not only preserve vision but may provide useful evidence of disseminated candidiasis. In one autopsy series of 15 cases with *Candida* endophthalmitis, 13 had *Candida* in other organs.[108]

Twenty-two cases of endophthalmitis due to *Aspergillus* have been reported or presented.[72,114] Of these, 14 patients had underlying systemic debilitating conditions. Antibiotics, corticosteroids, and immunosuppressive therapy, alone or in combination, were used in about one-half the patients before the onset of infection. Intravenous injection of illicit drugs is another cause.[77,82] The most common sign is an iridocyclitis or a vitritis with associated yellow-white retinal lesions. Retinal hemorrhages, hypopyon, scleritis, and panophthalmitis are also seen. Endophthalmitis due to *Aspergillus* has also been observed after accidental and surgical trauma.[116]

Cryptococcal infection usually involves the central nervous system. Ocular manifestations include papilledema, nystagmus, extraocular muscle paresis, and optic atrophy.[117] Intraocular involvement may occur as a complication of disseminated cryptococcosis or as the sole manifestation. The most common ocular symptom is blurred vision. Intraocular signs include uveitis, papilledema, retinal hemorrhages, exudates, and detachment. Discrete yellow choroidal or chorioretinal lesions may be seen. As with other fungal infections, cryptococcosis tends to occur in patients with lymphomas or other disorders of the reticuloendothelial system and in patients receiving long-term corticosteroid therapy (Chapter 240).

Pulmonary infection is the most common systemic manifestation of coccidioidomycosis (Chapter 243). Hematogenous spread usually leads to bone or skin lesions. Coccidioidomycosis tends to occur in otherwise healthy persons. Ocular symptoms include blurred vision, pain, and photophobia. Multiple yellow-white chorioretinal lesions that are 0.1 to 0.5 optic disk diameter in size are present, often with pigmented borders. Juxtapapillary chorioretinal lesions, retinal exudates,[118] recurrent uveitis,[119,120] secondary glaucoma, perivascular sheathing, and serous retinal detachment overlying a lesion in the macular area have been reported.[121,122] In a 1980 study, 4 of 10 consecutive patients with chronic pulmonary and disseminated disease had chorioretinal involvement.[118]

The usual form of ocular involvement with *Sporothrix schenckii* is a lid or conjunctival nodule. With intraocular sporotrichosis, the most common presenting sign is anterior uveitis.[114,123] Of 22 reported cases of sporotrichosis,[72] 18 were endogenous. A lid or conjunctival lesion was present in 4 patients. In eight patients there was no evidence of systemic sporotrichosis or other ocular lesions.

Lid lesions are the most common ocular manifestations of North American blastomycosis. In the rare patient with intraocular involvement, blurred vision and pain may occur. An anterior uveitis and secondary glaucoma can be present.[124] Yellow nodules on the iris and yellow-white posterior fundus lesions may also be seen. Of the six cases of intraocular blastomycosis reported, endophthalmitis was observed in three, an iritis or iridocyclitis in two, and bilateral choroiditis in one.

In mucormycosis, the orbit is involved by direct extension from infection of the sinuses. No cases of hematogenous *Mucor* endophthalmitis have been reported.[114] In craniofacial mucormycosis, however, eyes examined histopathologically have shown changes varying from normal to panophthalmitis with ophthalmic artery and central retinal artery occlusion or thrombosis.[125]

Presumably during the course of unrecognized systemic histoplasmosis, multifocal choroiditis may occur scattered throughout the fundus, in the peripapillary area, and sometimes in the macular area.[72] The lesions heal with variable chorioretinal scarring. This pattern of chorioretinal scars is the principal basis on which the diagnosis of the ocular histoplasmosis syndrome is made. Clinical diagnosis is enhanced by corroborative evidence of a previous infection such a pulmonary calcification and a positive histoplasmin skin test response. Years later, macular and, sometimes, lesions at other sites may become "active." Such activity is due to leakage and hemorrhage from choroidal neovascularization tissue that extends to the scar. This sequence of change may threaten vision. The mechanism by which the macular lesion develops neovascularization and its sequelae are unknown. Recurrent low-grade inflammation, presumably related to residual organisms or *Histoplasma* antigen, may play a role. It has been shown that argon laser photocoagulation of vision-threatening macular lesions can significantly reduce the risk of visual loss.[126] *Histoplasma* organisms have been identified in eyes in 13 cases.[127] In an additional case, positive indirect immunofluorescence to *Histoplasma* antigen was observed. Of the 14 eyes with organisms present, 6 were said to have had the features of the ocular histoplasmosis syndrome. In the other eight cases, ocular involvement was associated with systemic histoplasmosis.

VIRAL INFECTIONS

Herpes Simplex

In herpes simplex keratitis, generally from herpes simplex virus, type 1, intraocular inflammation in the form of a persistent nongranulomatous iridocyclitis is often present. Occasionally, an iridocyclitis is seen in the absence of keratitis. In a few cases, herpes simplex virus has been isolated from the aqueous humor.[128]

The intraocular inflammation from herpes simplex is usually located in the anterior segment of the eye. However, posterior involvement has been documented,[129–132] especially in the newborn,[128,133–135] usually as a result of herpes simplex virus type 2 infection. Large patches of yellowish white retinal exudates accompanying perivascular and vitreous inflammatory infiltrates are present. The posterior pole of the fundus is usually more extensively involved than is the periphery. When the lesions heal, sharply circumscribed punched-out chorioretinal scars that may be confused with toxoplasmic scars are seen.

Histopathologically, areas of retinal necrosis are present.[76] Inflammatory cells are noted in the vitreous and choroid adjacent to these areas of necrosis. By electron microscopy, viral particles consistent with herpes simplex virus are present in the retinal pigment epithelium,[136] retinal ganglion cell, and inner nuclear layers.[137]

Varicella-Zoster Virus

Herpes zoster keratitis is commonly followed by iridocyclitis. A diffuse choroiditis may occur. The characteristic histopathologic feature of ocular herpes zoster infection is a chronic nongranulomatous infiltration around posterior ciliary nerves and vessels.[72] Occlusive vasculitis may lead to iris and ciliary body necrosis and anterior chamber hemorrhage. A perivasculitis and vasculitis of retinal vessels may lead to hemorrhagic retinopathy. Viral inclusions have been described in the necrotizing retinopathy of herpes zoster ophthalmicus.[138] An optic neuritis may occur secondary to a periarteritis.[139] Varicella-zoster virus is at least one cause of the acute retinal necrosis syndrome.[76,140]

In varicella infections, uveitis may develop either during the acutely infectious stage or during convalescence.

Cytomegalovirus

Congenital cytomegalovirus infection is a well-recognized cause of chorioretinitis[141] and occurs in 23–29 percent of the neonates with the disease.[142] Iritis, cataracts, and optic atrophy may also accompany congenital infection.

Symptomatic acquired cytomegalovirus infection in adults is uncommon.[143–145] It may occur in patients receiving chemotherapy for acute leukemia and malignant lymphomas.[146] However, most frequently it occurs in patients with the acquired immunodeficiency syndrome (AIDS) and in patients receiving immunosuppressive therapy after renal transplantation.[143,147–152] Patients usually complain of blurred vision and scotomas. Initially, this visual impairment is mild; but with progression of the disease, severe and permanent visual loss occurs. Ocular pain is usually not present. Fundus examination reveals retinal edema, scattered intraretinal hemorrhages, yellow-white exudates, vessel attenuation, and sheathing.[76] The picture of a branch vein occlusion or a necrotizing vasculitis may be simulated.[152] As the initial lesions heal, retinal and pigment epithelial atrophy occurs. Adjacent areas of active infection may be seen to progress through the same exudative, hemorrhagic, and atrophic stages.[147] The appearance of the fundus is quite distinctive and is the first clinical manifestation of systemic viral infection in the majority of cases.[144] Therefore, it is recommended that regular ophthalmoscopic examinations be performed in all organ transplant recipients.[144,153]

Rubeola and Rubella

Measles (rubeola) retinopathy (maculopathy) occurs 6–12 days after the skin rash and is clinically manifested by acute blindness. It may or may not accompany measles encephalitis. In the early stages, retinal edema, attenuated vessels, and a stellate macular figure are seen in the fundus.[76] In the later stages of the disease, there is frequently a return of useful vision and the occurrence of a secondary pigmentary retinopathy that may have a salt-and-pepper appearance.[154]

Subacute sclerosing panencephalitis (SSPE) is a progressive, invariably fatal disease caused by the measles virus, and it appears years after an attack of clinical measles. Chorioretinitis is a common ocular complication occurring in about 30 percent of the cases.[155] Optic atrophy, papilledema, and cortical blindness may also occur.[156]

The ocular complications of rubella virus infection include congenital cataracts, glaucoma, and a pigmentary retinopathy.[157]

PARASITIC ENDOPHTHALMITIS

Toxoplasma gondii is a protozoan that causes retinochoroiditis.[76] Since the *Toxoplasma* are found primarily in an area of coagulative necrosis of the retina, with a secondary granulomatous choroiditis, the term *retinochoroiditis* is applied to the ocular lesion.

Ocular involvement is present in both the congenital and acquired forms of the disease. A retinochoroiditis usually affecting the macula is present in 80 percent of the patients with congenital toxoplasmosis. The eye is rarely affected in the acquired form of the disease, but it has been suggested that almost all cases of ocular toxoplasmosis are congenital.[158]

In the active stage, the fundus lesion is whitish yellow, with indistinct borders and an overlying hazy vitreous. In recurrent disease, an active focus of inflammation is present at the border of an area of an inactive healed scar of retinochoroiditis. An iridocyclitis is usually present, and posterior vitreous detachment with vitreous precipitates on its detached surface is common. As the activity of the retinochoroiditis subsides, its color changes from yellowish white to gray, and the vitreous haze recedes. Glaucoma, cataract, vitreous hemorrhage, and retinal detachment are possible complications.

The nematode *Toxocara* is the most common parasitic cause of endophthalmitis.[159,160] The second-stage larva of this nematode is responsible for both endophthalmitis and visceral larva migrans. The average age of patients affected is 7.5 years, with a range of 2 to 31 years. Children become infected by the ingestion of ova present is soil contaminated with the excrement of dogs or cats. Nematode endophthalmitis has been diagnosed in 2 percent of 1000 eyes enucleated in children under 15 years of age[161] and is thought to be responsible for 10 percent of the cases of uveitis in children.[162]

The infestation may present as a diffuse chronic endophthalmitis, as a posterior-pole granuloma, or as a peripheral granuloma in a quiet eye[163]; a cloudy vitreous, cyclitic membrane, and posterior synechiae may be present. A *Toxocara* granuloma is typically white and hemispheric, with a diameter roughly equal to or bigger than the disk. It is primarily located in the retina. It may be present at the macula or at the periphery of the fundus. Other ocular manifestations of *Toxocara* infestation include a localized vitreous abscess, papillitis,[164] pars planitis, iridocyclitis, hypopyon,[165] preretinal and vitreous hemorrhages, and very rarely, central retinal artery occlusion.[166] In the presence of systemic disease (visceral larva migrans), ocular involvement is rare. Nematode granulomas in the eye have often been confused with retinoblastoma, and the differential diagnosis is important.

Diffuse unilateral neuroretinitis (DUSN) is a syndrome characterized by a loss of vision, vitritis, papillitis, and recurrent crops of gray-white retina lesions; the syndrome progresses to optic atrophy, retinal vessel narrowing, and diffuse pigmentary changes. DUSN may be caused by at least two different nematodes.[167]

Ocular infestation with *Cysticercus cellulosae* may occur in 13 percent[168] of patients with cysticercosis (Chapter 264). The parasite may be found in the vitreous cavity or in the subchoroidal space.[169] Ocular inflammation and charactistic retinal tracks may be seen with fly larvae (myiasis).[170] Onchocerciasis (river blindness) is usually manifested in the eye as keratitis, but iridocyclitis, glaucoma, and choroiditis also may occur (Chapter 262).

NONINFECTIOUS ENDOPHTHALMITIS

Other intraocular inflammatory syndromes such as sympathetic ophthalmia, idiopathic uveitis, and pars planitis may be confused with the previously described infectious diseases. Sterile endophthalmitis has resulted from surgical chemical contamination of the intraocular contents by starch particles[171] and from probable ethylene oxide/polymer by-products of the intraocular lens sterilization process.[172]

LABORATORY FINDINGS

Rapid and accurate diagnosis of the etiologic agent is essential if useful vision is to be salvaged in bacterial endophthalmitis. The site from which material is obtained for smears and cultures is important. Conjunctival cultures are inadequate and misleading in bacterial endophthalmitis. The anterior chamber, vitreous cavity, wound abscesses, and wound dehiscenses are the sites from which material should be cultured.[173–175]

All cases of traumatic and postsurgical endophthalmitis should have aqueous and vitreous aspiration for cultures and smears. In a study of 140 cases of endophthalmitis, an agent was isolated by vitreous and aqueous tap in 78 cases. In 27 of these, the organism was isolated from the vitreous alone, with a negative aqueous culture.[173] The vitreous specimen should be specially prepared for cytology,[176] and centrifugal cytology may be helpful.[177]

Material from each site should be separately stained with Gram, Giemsa, periodic acid–Schiff (PAS), and methenamine silver stains and should be cultured on blood and chocolate agar, thioglycollate media, or Schaedler broth or brain–heart infusion, Sabouraud agar, and on reduced blood agar kept in an anaerobic environment.[178] Vitreous irrigate material from vitrectomy can be centrifuged and smeared or can be passed through a Millipore filter, which can be stained and cultured. The limulus lysate test on aqueous and vitreous material may help in the rapid detection of gram-negative endophthalmitis.[179] Vitreous glucose estimations have been used to differentiate sterile from bacterial endophthalmitis. In patients with leukokoria and suspected nematode endophthalmitis, aqueous cytology revealing eosinophils and normal lactate dehydrogenase levels[180] may prevent enucleation as a result of a misdiagnosis of retinoblastoma. Enzyme-linked immunosorbent assay (ELISA) testing of aqueous humor material may aid in the diagnosis.[181,182]

TREATMENT

Effective therapy for endophthalmitis requires a low threshold of suspicion for diagnosing endophthalmitis of infective origin, early diagnostic aspirates, and immediate broad-spectrum antibiotic cover, followed by appropriate therapy to reduce the host immune and anti-inflammatory response and modification of the antibiotic therapy in view of culture results.[173,174,183,184] Animal and human studies demonstrate that the visual outcome is greatly influenced by the virulence of the etiologic agent. *Staphylococcus epidermidis* endophthalmitis, which appears to be increasing in frequency, responds well to relatively conservative therapy with topical, subconjunctival, and intravenous antibiotics together with corticosteroids.[174,185]

Unfortunately, reliable and rapid diagnosis of the organism involved remains difficult. Destruction of the eye by virulent organisms such as *Pseudomonas aeruginosa* and *Staphylococcus aureus* may occur within 24 hours, so aggressive therapy appears warranted if the type of organism is in doubt. There is no consensus, however, on what constitutes aggressive therapy. It may include early vitrectomy[186–189]; intravitreal antibiotics (gentamicin, cefazolin)[190]; early systemic, topical, and perhaps intravitreal corticosteroids[174]; and intravenous broad-spectrum antibiotics such as a third-generation cephalosporin. In cases of post-traumatic endophthalmitis, intravitreal and systemic clindamycin therapy should be added because of the risk of *Bacillus cereus* endophthalmitis.[191] Successful eradication of *Propionibacterium acnes* infection may require removal of all residual lens material by using vitrectomy instrumentation combined with intravitreal antibiotic therapy.[47]

The rationale for the use of early corticosteroids as an addition to therapy is based on the recognition of the visually destructive secondary processes that can occur after the successful inflammatory and immune response mounted by the host in response to the causative organism. Unlike various infections elsewhere, successful elimination of the organism is not the only criterion of successful treatment of endophthalmitis. If vision is to be retained, control of the inflammatory and immune response is crucial.

Data on the choice of antibiotics, route of administration and the degree of intraocular penetration of the antibiotics has been obtained from animal studies only. The results of these studies are not necessarily to be extrapolated to human endophthalmitis.

Therapy for suspected fungal endophthalmitis is more difficult still, with commonly a delay in diagnosis, and less information is available on the pharmacokinetics and sensitivity testing with the preferred antifungal agents. Currently, the combined use of topical natamycin, oral flucytosine, intravenous amphotericin B, and possibly intraocular amphotericin B is recommended.[192] This should be combined with a vitrectomy of any intravitreal abscess formation. The use of corticosteroids, either orally or intravitreally, together with antifungal agents remains extremely controversial.

Candida endophthalmitis appears to be best treated with intravenous amphotericin B.[114,193] As the retinal lesions resolve, scarring is a common occurrence. Once vitreous invasion is present, significant intraocular morbidity occurs despite treatment. Vitreous organization and vitreous traction leading to retinal detachment may occur.[109]

Candida endophthalmitis not involving the vitreous has been noted to rarely resolve spontaneously without antifungal treatment.[83] Presumably, these patients have relatively intact immunologic systems.

Combined therapy with amphotericin B and flucytosine appears to provide a syngergistic effect in vitro. This combination has been reported to be successful in the treatment of endogenous and postsurgical *Candida* endophthalmitis.[194] Pars plana vitrectomy is both a diagnostic and therapeutic modality that may be used in the management of *Candida* endophthalmitis. It facilitates diagnosis by making tissue available for culture and microscopic evaluation.[176] It plays a therapeutic role by removing replicating fungi in the vitreous body, by improving the diffusion of systematically administered antifungal agents into the vitreous cavity, and by preventing future vitreoretinal traction.[195] Because of toxicity, the place of intravitreal amphotericin B is unclear,[196–198] but 5–10 μg of amphotericin B have been injected into the vitreous with some success.

Intravenous amphotericin B successfully eradicates sytemic aspergillosis, but organisms usually remain in the eye[199] in endogenous *Aspergillus* endophthalmitis. Successful treatment of endogenous *Aspergillus* endophthalmitis has been accomplished in only two instances that combined surgical removal of infected vitreous and antifungal agents.[76,77]

Of five patients who received amphotericin B for cryptococcal endophthalmitis, two were successfully treated.[200,201]

Of 12 patients with endophthalmitis secondary to *Coccidioides immitis*[114] were treated with amphotericin B. There was dramatic improvement in both systemic and ocular disease manifestations in two patients.

In the ocular histoplasmosis syndrome, systemic steroids have been repoted to be of some value in treating the early stage of serous and/or hemorrhagic detachment of the retina and/or retinal pigment epithelium that occurs in an old macular scar.[202] Corticosteroids do not activate any latent histoplasmosis in such patients, nor is antifungal therapy of benefit in patients with this syndrome. In almost all instances, there is no evidence of actively replicating fungal organisms in these lesions, and the photocoagulation of macular lesions not involving the fovea has been proved to reduce the risk of visual loss.[126]

Topical corticosteroids and atropine are the mainstay of therapy for herpetic keratouveitis. The usefulness of an antiviral "umbrella" to prevent the recurrence of epithelial herpetic disease remains unproven. Acyclovir has been shown to be effective in the treatment of retinitis associated with varicella-zoster virus.[140,203] Herpetic retinitis may also may also be treated with short courses of systemic corticosteroids.[128]

Herpes zoster iridocyclitis is best treated with topical corticosteroids and cycloplegia. The role of acyclovir in the management of this condition is unclear.

In the treatment of cytomegalovirus infection in adults, early reduction or discontinuation of immunosuppressive therapy, if possible, should help in limiting the progression of the ocular and systemic infection.[204] Ganciclovir is an effective means of therapy for cytomegalovirus retinitis, but it must be given chronically to prevent reactivation.[205]

In the treatment of ocular toxoplasmosis, mydriatics, topical corticosteroids, systemic and/or periocular depot administration of corticosteroids, pyrimethamine, and triple sulfonamides have been recommended.[206] Some authorities only treat cases with extensive involvement or those in which the macula is threatened. Experimental studies in mice have shown that clindamycin may destroy encysted forms of the parasite in chronically infected tissues, and it has been combined with sulfadiazine to treat human ocular toxoplasmosis.[207]

To prevent ocular toxocariasis, prophylaxis should include avoidance of eating dirt and handling of puppies that have not been dewormed. Thiabendazole is effective in the treatment of visceral larva migrans. However, intraocular inflammation develops when the *Toxocara* larvae die within the eye. Therefore, systemic or periocular injection of corticosteroids is the usual therapy of choice.[160,208] Removal of the encysted larvae by vitrectomy may offer a solution.[209,210] Diethylcarbamazine treatment of onchocerciasis may cause intense ocular inflammation due to the death of microfilariae. Ocular corticosteroids are often administered to ameliorate this complication. Less inflammation may result if ivermectin is used to treat onchocerciasis.[211]

Intensive topical and systemic steroids most effectively treat the sterile endophthalmitis induced by intraocular lens sterilizing methods and other chemical agents.

REFERENCES

1. Forster RK. Etiology and diagnosis of bacterial postoperative endophthalmitis. Ophthalmology. 1978;85:320.
2. Theodore FH. Etiology and diagnosis of fungal postoperative endophthalmitis. Ophthalmology. 1978;85:327.
3. Allen HF. Prevention of postoperative endophthalmitis. Ophthalmology. 1978;85:386.
4. Binder PS, Abel R Jr, Bellows R. Postoperative bacterial endophthalmitis. Section II. Ann Ophthalmol. 1976;6:1129.
5. Allen HF, Mangiaracine AB. Bacterial endophthalmitis after cataract extraction. II. Incidence in 36,000 consecutive operations with special reference to preoperative topical antibiotics. Arch Ophthalmol. 1974;91:3.
6. Christy NE, Lall P. Postoperative endophthalmitis following cataract surgery. Effects of subconjunctival antibiotics and other factors. Arch Ophthalmol. 1973;90:361.
7. Brinser JH, Hess JB. Meningococcal endophthalmitis without meningitis. Can J Ophthalmol. 1981;16:100.
8. Wassermann HE. Avian tuberculosis endophthalmitis. Arch Ophthalmol. 1973;89:321.
9. Ebright JR, Lentino JR, Juni E. Endophthalmitis caused by *Moraxella nonliquefaciens*. Am J Clin Pathol. 1982;77:362.
10. Salceda SR, Lapuz J, Vizconde R. *Serratia marcescens* endophthalmitis. Arch Ophthalmol. 1973;89:163.
11. Bigger JF, Miltzer G, Mandell A, et al. *Serratia marcescens* endophthalmitis. Am J Ophthalmol. 1971;72:1102.
12. Oesterle CS, Kronenberg HA, Peyman GA. Endophthalmitis caused by an *Erwinia* species. Arch Ophthalmol. 1977;95:824.
13. Peyman GA, Vastine DW, Diamond JG. Vitrectomy and intraocular gentamicin management of *Herellea* endophthalmitis after incomplete phacoemulsification. Am J Ophthalmol. 1975;80:764.
14. Wahl JW. *Vibrio* endophthalmitis. Arch Ophthalmol. 1974;91:423.
15. Smolin G. *Proteus* endophthalmitis. Arch Ophthalmol. 1974;91:419.
16. Tabbara KF, Juffali F, Matossian RM. *Bacillus laterosporus* endophthalmitis. Arch Ophthalmol. 1977;95:2187.
17. Snead JW, Stern WH, Whitcher JP, et al. *Listeria monocytogenes* endophthalmitis. Am J Ophthalmol. 1977;84:337.
18. Friedman E, Peyman GA, May DR. Endophthalmitis caused by *Propionibacterium acnes*. Can J Ophthalmol. 1978;13:50.
19. Hanscom T, Maxwell WA. *Corynebacterium* endophthalmitis. Laboratory studies and report of a case treated by vitrectomy. Arch Ophthalmol. 1979;97:500.
20. Ballen PH, Loffredo FR, Painter B. *Listeria* endophthalmitis. Arch Ophthalmol. 1979;97:101.
21. Abbott, RL, Forster RK, Rebell G. *Listeria monocytogenes* endophthalmitis with a black hypopyon. Am J Ophthalmol. 1978;86:715.
22. Cooperman EW, Friedman AH. Exogenous *Moraxella liquefaciens* endophthalmitis. Ophthalmologica. 1975;171:177.
23. O'Day DM, Smith RS, Gregg CR, et al. The problem of *Bacillus* species infection, with special emphasis on the virulence of *Bacillus cereus*. Ophthalmology. 1981;88:833.
24. Bagnarello AG, Berlin AJ, Weinstein AJ, et al. *Listeria monocytogenes* endophthalmitis. Arch Ophthalmol. 1977;95:1004.
25. Werner EB, Herschorn BR. Exogenous endophthalmitis. Am J Ophthalmol. 1983;95:123.
26. Allen HF. Symposium: Postoperative endophthalmitis. Introduction: Incidence and etiology. Ophthalmology. 1978;85:317.
27. Fahmy JA. Endophthalmitis following cataract extraction. A study of 24 cases in 4,498 operations. Acta Ophthalmol. 1975;53:522.
28. Leveille AS, McMullan D, Cavanagh HD. Endophthalmitis following penetrating keratoplasty. Ophthalmology. 1983;90:38.

29. Zaidman GW, Mondino BJ. Postoperative pseudophakic bacterial endophthalmitis. Am J Ophthalmol. 1982;93:218.
30. Schanzlin DJ, Goldberg DB, Brown SI. *Staphylococcus epidermidis* endophthalmitis following intraocular lens implantation. Br J Ophthalmol. 1980;64:684.
31. Gerding DN, Poley BJ, Hal WH, et al. Treatment of *Pseudomonas* endophthalmitis associated with prosthetic intraocular lens implantation. Am J Ophthalmol. 1979;88:902.
32. Shaw EL, Aquavella JV. Pneumococcal endophthalmitis following grafting of corneal tissue from a (cadaver) kidney donor. Ann Ophthalmol. 1977;9:435.
33. Hattenhauer JM, Lipsich MP. Late endophthalmitis after filtering surgery. Am J Ophthalmol. 1971;72:1097.
34. Kanski JJ: Treatment of late endophthalmitis associated with filtering blebs. Arch Ophthalmol. 1974;91:339.
35. Freedman J, Gupta M, Bunke A. Endophthalmitis after trabeculectomy. Arch Ophthalmol. 1978;96:1017.
36. Pusin SM, Green WR, Tasman W, et al. Simultaneous bacterial endophthalmitis and sympathetic uveitis after retinal detachment surgery. Am J Ophthalmol. 1976;81:57.
37. Salamon SM, Friberg TR, Luxenberg MN. Endophthalmitis after strabismus surgery. Am J Ophthalmol. 1982;93:39.
38. Tarr KH, Constable IJ. *Pseudomonas* endophthalmitis associated with scleral necrosis. Br J Ophthalmol. 1980;64:676.
39. Gelender H, Flynn HW, Mandelbaum SH. Bacterial endophthalmitis resulting from radial keratotomy. Am J Ophthalmol. 1982;93:323.
40. LeFrancois M, Baum JL. *Flavobacterium* endophthalmitis following keratoplasty. Use of a tissue culture medium-stored cornea. Arch Ophthalmol. 1976;94:1907.
41. Gelender H. Bacterial endophthalmitis following cutting of sutures after cataract surgery. Am J Ophthalmol. 1982;94:528.
42. Bellows AR, McCulley JP. Endophthalmitis in aphakic patients with unplanned filtering blebs wearing contact lenses. Ophthalmology. 1981;88:839.
43. Swan KC, Campbell L. Unintentional filtration following cataract surgery. Arch Ophthalmol. 1964;71:43.
44. Ruiz, RS, Teeters VW. The vitreous wick syndrome. A late complication following cataract extraction. Am J Ophthalmol. 1970;70:483.
45. Allen HF. Recent advances in aseptic surgical technique. Trans Am Acad Ophthalmol Otolaryngol. 1960;64:493.
46. Sugar HS, Zekman T. Late infection of filtering conjunctival scar. Am J Ophthalmol. 1971;72:1097.
47. Meisler DM, Palestine AG, Vastine DW, et al. Chronic *Propionibacterium* endophthalmitis after extracapsular cataract extraction and intraocular lens implantation. Am J Ophthalmol. 1986;102:733.
48. Mason GI, Peyman GA, Jampol LM, et al. Peptostreptococcal endophthalmitis with a relapsing course. Arch Ophthalmol. 1978;96:1813.
49. Mason GI, Bottone EJ, Podos SM. Traumatic endophthalmitis caused by an *Erwinia* species. Am J Ophthalmol. 1976;82:709.
50. Lass JH, Thoft RA, Bellows AR, et al. Exogenous *Nocardia asteroides* endophthalmitis associated with malignant glaucoma. Ann Ophthalmol. 1981;13:317.
51. Affeldt JC, Flynn HW, Forster RK, et al. Microbial endophthalmitis resulting from ocular trauma. Ophthalmol. 1987;94:407.
52. Wetzel JO. Tetanus following eye injury. Report of a case: Review of literature. Am J Ophthalmol. 1942;25:933.
53. Muddappa TM, Rao RNS. Ocular tetanus. Indian J Ophthalmol. 1982;30:163.
54. Burns CL. Bilateral endophthalmitis in acute bacterial endocarditis. Am J Ophthalmol. 1979;88:809.
55. Jensen AD, Naidoff MA. Bilateral meningococcal endophthalmitis. Arch Ophthalmol. 1973;90:396.
56. Shammas HF. Endogenous *E. coli* endophthalmitis. Surv Ophthalmol. 1977;21:429.
57. Weinstein JM, Elliott J, Tilford RH. Metastatic endophthalmitis due to *Salmonella typhimurium*. Arch Ophthalmol. 1982;100:293.
58. Taylor JRW, Cibis GW, Hamtil LW. Endophthalmitis complicating *Haemophilus influenzae* type B meningitis. Arch Ophthalmol. 1980;98:324.
59. Hull DS, Patipa M, Cox F. Metastatic endophthalmitis: A complication of meningococcal meningitis. Ann Ophthalmol. 1982;14:29.
60. Gamel JW, Allansmith MR. Metastatic staphylococcal endophthalmitis presenting as chronic iridocyclitis. Am J Ophthalmol. 1974;77:454.
61. Rogers SJ, Johnson BL. Endogenous *Nocardia* endophthalmitis: Report of a case in a patient treated for lymphocytic lymphoma. Ann Ophthalmol. 1977;9:1123.
62. Nigrin J, Tyrrell DIJ, Jackson FL, et al. *Listeria monocytogenes* endophthalmitis in an immune-suppressed host. Can Med Assoc J. 1977;116:1378.
63. Bloomfield SE, David DS, Cheigh JS, et al. Endophthalmitis following staphylococcal sepsis in renal failure patients. Arch Intern Med. 1978;138:706.
64. Folk JC, Lobes LA Jr. Bacterial endophthalmitis and traumatic hyphema resulting from ocular injuries during dental procedures. Can J Ophthalmol. 1981;16:151.
65. May DR, Peyman GA, Raichand M, et al. Metastatic *Peptostreptococcus intermedius* endophthalmitis after a dental procedure. Am J Ophthalmol. 1978;85:662.
66. Weintraub MI, Otto RN. Pneumococcal meningitis and endophthalmitis in a newborn. JAMA. 1972;219:1763.
67. Berger BB. Endophthalmitis complicating neonatal group B streptococcal septicemia. Am J Ophthalmol. 1981;92:681.
68. Jain MR, Sharma HR. Puerperal sepsis leading to bilateral fulminating purulent endophthalmitis with tenonitis. Br J Ophthalmol. 1973;57:698.
69. Kerkenezov N. Panophthalmitis after a blood transfusion. Responsible organism *Bacillus cereus*. Br J Ophthalmol. 1953;37:632.
70. McLendon BF, Bron AJ, Mitchell CJ. *Streptococcus suis* type II (group R) as a cause of endophthalmitis. Br J Ophthalmol. 1978;62:729.
71. Massaro D, Katz S, Sachs M. Choroidal tubercles: A clue to hematogenous tubercles. *Ann Intern Med*. 1964;60:231.
72. Green WR. Uvea. In Spencer WH, ed. Ophthalmic Pathology. An Atlas and Textbook. v. 5. Philadelphia: WB Saunders; 1985:1352–2071.
73. Moore JE. Syphilitic iritis: A study of 249 patients. Am J Ophthalmol. 1931;14:110.
74. Jampol LM, Strauch BS, Albert DM. Intraocular nocardiosis. Am J Ophthalmol. 1973;76:568.
75. Meyer SL, Front RL, Shaver RP. Intraocular nocardiosis. Report of three cases. Arch Ophthalmol. 1970;83:536.
76. Green WR. Retina. In: Spencer WH, ed. Ophthalmic Pathology. An Atlas and Textbook. v. 2. Philadelphia: WB Saunders; 1985:589–1291.
77. Doft BH, Clarkson JG, Febell G, et al. Endogenous *Aspergillus* endophthalmitis in drug abusers. Arch Ophthalmol. 1980;98:859.
78. Elliott JH, O'Day DM, Gutow GS, et al. Mycotic endophthalmitis in drug abusers. Am J Ophthalmol. 1979;98:66.
79. Getnick RA, Rodrigues MM. Endogenous fungal endophthalmitis in a drug addict. Am J Ophthalmol. 1974;77:680.
80. Aguilar GL, Blumenkrantz MS, Egbert PR, et al. *Candida* endophthalmitis after intravenous drug abuse. Arch Ophthalmol. 1979;97:96.
81. Sugar HS, Mandell GH, Shalev J. Metastatic endophthalmitis associated with injection of addictive drugs. Am J Ophthalmol. 1971;71:1055.
82. Michelson JB, Freedman SD, Boyden DG. *Aspergillus* endophthalmitis in a drug abuser. Ann Ophthalmol. 1982;14:1051.
83. Dellon AL, Stark WJ, Chretien PB. Spontaneous resolution of endogenous *Candida* endophthalmitis complicating intravenous hyperalimentation. Am J Ophthalmol. 1978;79:648.
84. Henderson DK, Edwards JE, Montgomerie JZ. Hematogenous *Candida* endophthalmitis in patients receiving parenteral hyperalimentation fluids. J Infect Dis. 1981;143:655.
85. Freeman JB, Davis PL, MacLean LD. *Candida* endophthalmitis associated with intravenous hyperalimentation. Arch Surg. 1974;108:237.
86. François J, Rysselaere M. Oculomycoses. Springfield, MA: Charles C Thomas; 1972.
87. Fine BS, Zimmerman LE. Exogenous intraocular fungus infections: With particular reference to complications of intraocular surgery. Am J Ophthalmol. 1959;48:151.
88. McCray E, Rampell N, Solomon SL, et al. Outbreak of *Candida parapsilosis* endophthalmitis after cataract extraction and intraocular lens implantation. J Clin Microbiol. 1986;24:625.
89. Allen HF. Amphotericin B and exogenous mycotic endophthalmitis after cataract extraction. Arch Ophthalmol. 1972;88:640.
90. Pettit TH, Olson RJ, Foos RY, et al. Fungal endophthalmitis following intraocular lens implantation. Arch Ophthalmol. 1980;98:1025.
91. O'Day DM. Fungal endophthalmitis caused by *Paecilomyces lilacinus* after intraocular lens implantation. Am J Ophthalmol. 1977;83:130.
92. Landott E, Zuccoli A. Mycotic endophthalmitis after retinal surgery. Ophthalmologica. 1970;161:237.
93. Larsen PA, Lindstrom RL, Doughman DJ. *Torulopsis glabrata* endophthalmitis after keratoplasty with an organ-cultured cornea. Arch Ophthalmol. 1978;96:1019.
94. Rao GN, Aquavella JV. *Cephalosporium* endophthalmitis following penetrating keratoplasty. Ophthalmic Surg. 1979;10:34.
95. Foster JBJ, Almeda E, Liltman ML, et al. Some intraocular and conjunctival effects of amphotericin B in man and the rabbit. Arch Ophthalmol. 1958;60:555.
96. Theodore FH, Littman ML, Almeda E. Endophthalmitis following cataract extraction: Due to *Neurospora sitophila*, a so-called nonpathogenic fungus. Am J Ophthalmol. 1962;53:35.
97. Glassman MI, Henkind P, Alture-Werker E. *Monosporium apiospermum* endophthalmitis. Am J Ophthalmol. 1973;76:821.
98. Rosen R, Friedman AH. Successfully treated postoperative. *Candida parakrusei* endophthalmitis. Am J Ophthalmol. 1973;76:574.
99. Sheikh HA, Mahgoub S, Badi K. Postoperative endophthalmitis due to *Trichosporon cutaneum*. Br J Ophthalmol. 1974;58:591.
100. Miller GR, Rebell G, Magoon RC, et al. Intravitreal antimycotic therapy and the cure of mycotic endophthalmitis caused by a *Paecilomyces lilacinus* contaminated pseudophakos. Ophthalmic Surg. 1978;9:54.
101. Searl SS, Udell IJ, Sadun A, et al. *Aspergillus keratitis* with intraocular invasion. Ophthalmology. 1981;88:1244.
102. Rodrigues MM, MacLeod D. Exogenous fungal endophthalmitis caused by *Paecilomyces*. Am J Ophthalmol. 1975;79:687.
103. Elliott ID, Halde C, Shapiro J. Keratitis and endophthalmitis caused by *Petriellidium boydii*. Am J Ophthalmol. 1977;83:16.
104. Rowsey JJ, Acers TE, Smith DL, et al. *Fusarium oxysporum* endophthalmitis. Arch Ophthalmol. 1979;97:103.
105. Apostol JG, Meyer SL. *Graphium* endophthalmitis. Am J Ophthalmol. 1972;73:566.

106. McDonnell PJ, McDonnell JM, Brown RH, et al. Ocular involvement in patients with fungal infections. Ophthalmology. 1985;92:706.
107. Fishman LS, Griffin JR, Sapico FL, et al. Hematogenous *Candida* endophthalmitis: A complication of candidemia. N Engl J Med. 1972;286:675.
108. Griffin JR, Pettit TH, Fishman LS, et al. Bloodborne *Candida* endophthalmitis: A clinical and pathological study of 21 cases. Arch Ophthalmol. 1973;88:450.
109. Michelson PE, Stark WJ, Reeser F, et al. Endogenous *Candida* endophthalmitis: Report of 13 cases of 16 from the literature. In: Smith ME, ed. International Ophthalmology Clinics: Ocular Pathology. v. 2. Boston: Little, Brown; 1971:125.
110. Edwards JE Jr, Foos RY, Montgomerie JF, et al. Ocular manifestations of *Candida* septicemia: Review of seventy-six cases of hematogenous *Candida* endopthalmitis. Medicine (Baltimore). 1974;53:47.
111. Michelson PE, Rupp R, Efthimiadis B. Endogenous *Candida* endophthalmitis leading to bilateral corneal perforation. Am J Ophthalmol. 1975;80:800.
112. Cantrill HL, Rodman WP, Ramsay RC, et al. Postpartum *Candida* endophthalmitis JAMA. 1980;243:1163.
113. Baley JE, Annabele WL, Kliegman RM: *Candida* endophthalmitis in the premature infant. J Pediatr. 1981;98:458.
114. Clarkson JG, Green WR. Endogenous fungal endophthalmitis. In: Duane TD, ed. Clinical Ophthalmology. v. 4. Hagerstown, MD: Harper & Row, 1976.
115. Meyers BR, Lieberman TW, Ferry AP. *Candida* endophthalmitis complicating candidemia. Ann Intern Med. 1973;79:647.
116. Roney P, Barr CC, Chun CH, et al. Exogenous *Aspergillus* endophthalmitis. Rev Infect Dis. 1986;8:955.
117. Okun E, Butler WT. Ophthalmologic complications of cryptococcal meningitis. Arch Ophthalmol. 1964;71:52.
118. Blumenkranz MS, Stevens DS. Endogenous coccidioidal endophthalmitis. Ophthalmology 1980;87:974.
119. Bell R, Font RL. Granulomatous anterior uveitis caused by *Coccidioides immitis*. Am J Ophthalmol. 1972;74:93.
120. Cutler JE, Binder PS, Paul TO, et al. Metastatic coccidioidal endophthalmitis. Arch Ophthalmol. 1978;96:689.
121. Rainin EA, Little HL. Ocular coccidioidomycosis: A clinico-pathological case report. Trans Am Acad Ophthalmol Otolaryngol. 1972;76:645.
122. Glasgow BJ, Brown HH, Foos RV. Miliary retinitis in coccidioidomycosis. Am J Ophthalmol. 1987;104:24.
123. Cassady JR, Foerster HC. *Sporotrichum schenckii* endophthalmitis. Arch Ophthalmol. 1977;85:71.
124. Font RL, Spaulding AB, Green WR. Endogenous mycotic panophthalmitis caused by *Blastomyces dermatitidis*. Arch Ophthalmol. 1967;77:217.
125. Straatsma BR, Zimmerman LE, Gass JDM. Phycomycosis: A clinicopathologic study of fifty-one cases. Lab Invest. 1962;2:963.
126. Macular Photocoagulation Study Group. Argon laser photocoagulation for ocular histoplasmosis: Results of a randomized clinical trial. Arch Ophthalmol. 1983;101:1347.
127. Scholz R, Green WR, Kutys R, et al. *Histoplasma capsulatum* in the eye. Ophthalmology. 1984;91:1100.
128. Pavan-Langston D, Brockhurst RJ. Herpes simplex panuveitis. Arch Ophthalmol. 1969;81:783.
129. Bloom JN, Katz JI, Kaufman HE. Herpes simplex retinitis and encephalitis in an adult. Arch Ophthalmol. 1964;95:1798.
130. Cibis GW, Flynn JT, David EB. Herpes simplex retinitis. Arch Ophthalmol. 1978;96:299.
131. Partamian LG, Morse PH, Klein HZ. Herpes simplex type 1 retinitis in an adult with systemic herpes zoster. Am J Ophthalmol. 1981;92:215.
132. Uninsky E, Jampol LM, Kaufman S, et al. Disseminated herpes simplex infection with retinitis in a renal allograft recipient. Ophthalmology 1983;90:175.
133. Nahmias AJ, Hagler WS. Ocular manifestations of herpes simplex in the newborn (neonatal ocular herpes). In: Boniuk M, ed. Rubella and Other Intraocular Viral Diseases in Infancy. International Ophthalmology Clinics. v. 12. 1972:191.
134. Cibis A, Burde RM. Herpes simplex virus–induced congenital cataracts. Arch Ophthalmol. 1971;85:220.
135. Yanoff M, Allman FI, Fine BS. Congenital herpes simplex virus, type 2, bacterial endophthalmitis. Trans Am Ophthalmol Soc. 1977;75:325.
136. Minckler DS, McLean EB, Shaw CM, et al. *Herpesvirus hominis* encephalitis and retinitis. Arch Ophthalmol. 1976;94:89.
137. Cibis GW, Flynn JT, Davis EB. Herpes simplex retinitis. Arch Ophthalmol. 1978;94:299.
138. Schwartz JN, Cashwell F, Hawkins HK, et al. Necrotizing retinopathy with herpes zoster ophthalmicus: A light and electron microscopic study. Arch Pathol Lab Med. 1976;100:386.
139. Bartlett RE, Mumma CS, Irvine AR. Herpes zoster ophthalmicus with bilateral hemorrhagic retinopathy. Am J Ophthalmol. 1951;34:45.
140. Culbertson WW, Blumenkranz MS, Pepose JS, et al. Varicella zoster virus is a cause of the acute retinal necrosis syndrome. Ophthalmology. 1986;93:559.
141. Boniuk I. The cytomegaloviruses and the eye. Int Ophthalmol Clin. 1979;12:169.
142. Lonn LI. Neonatal cytomegalic inclusion disease chorioretinitis. Arch Ophthalmol. 1972;88:434.
143. deVenecia G, Zu Rhein GM, Pratt MV, et al. Cytomegalovirus retinitis in adults: A clinical, histopathologic, and ultrastructural study. Arch Ophthalmol. 1971;86:44.
144. Murray HW, Knox DL, Green WR, et al. Cytomegalovirus retinitis in adults: A manifestation of disseminated viral infection. Am J Ophthalmol. 1977;63:574.
145. Egbert PR, Pollard RB, Gallagher JG, et al. Cytomegalovirus retinitis in immunosuppressed hosts. II. Ocular manifestations. Ann Intern Med. 1980;93:664.
146. Smith ME. Retinal involvement in adult cytomegalic inclusion disease. Arch Ophthalmol. 1964;72:44.
147. Aaberg TM, Cesarz TJ, Rytel MW. Correlation of virology and clinical course of cytomegalovirus retinitis. Am J Ophthalmol. 1972;74:407.
148. Porter R. Acute necrotizing retinitis in a patient receiving immunosupressive therapy. Br J Ophthalmol. 1972;36:555.
149. Wyhinny GJ, Apple DJ, Guastella FR, et al. Adult cytomegalic inclusion retinitis. Am J Ophthalmol. 1973;76:773.
150. Newman NM, Mandel MR, Gullett J, et al. Clinical and histologic findings in opportunistic ocular infections. Arch Ophthalmol. 1983;101:396.
151. Holland GN, Gottlieb MS, Yee RD, et al. Ocular disorders associated with a new severe acquired cellular immunodeficiency syndrome. Am J Ophthalmol. 1982;93:393.
152. Astle JN, Ellis PP. Ocular complications in renal transplant patients. Ann Ophthalmol. 1974;6:1269.
153. Porter R, Crombie Al, Gardner PS, et al. Incidence of ocular complications in patients undergoing renal transplantation. Br Med J. 1972;3:133.
154. Scheie HG, Morse PH. Rubeola retinopathy. Arch Ophthalmol. 1972;88:341.
155. Robb RM, Walters GV. Ophthalmic manifestations of subacute sclerosing panencephalitis. Arch Ophthalmol. 1970;83:426.
156. La Piana FG, Tso MOM, Jenis EH. The retinal lesions of subacute sclerosing panencephalitis. Ann Ophthalmol. 1974;6:603.
157. Krill AE. Retinal disease of rubella. Arch Ophthalmol. 1967;77:445.
158. Perkins ES. Ocular toxoplasmosis. Br J Ophthalmol. 1973;57:1.
159. Molk R. Ocular toxocariasis: A review of the literature. Ann Ophthalmol. 1983;15:216.
160. Shields JA. Ocular toxocariasis. A review. Surv Ophthalmol. 1984;28:361.
161. Leopold IH. Is the dog really man's best friend? Am J Ophthalmol. 1965;59:717.
162. Perkins ES. Pattern of uveitis in children. Br J Opthalmol. 1966;50:169.
163. Wilkinson CP, Welch RB: Intraocular *Toxocara*. Am J Ophthalmol. 1971;71:921.
164. Bird AC, Smith JL, Curtin VT. Nematode optic neuritis. Am J Ophthalmol. 1970;69:72.
165. Smith PH, Greer CH. Unusual presentation of ocular *Toxocara* infestation. Br J Ophthalmol. 1971;55:317.
166. Schlaegel TF Jr, Knox DL. Uveitis and parasitoses. In: Duane TD, ed. Clinical Ophthalmology. v. 4. Hagerstown, MD: Harper & Row; 1976.
167. Gass JDM, Braunstein RA. Further observations concerning the diffuse unilateral subacute neuroretinitis syndrome. Arch Ophthalmol. 1983;101:1689.
168. Malik SRK, Gupta AK, Chounhry S. Ocular cysticercosis. Am J Ophthalmol. 1968;66:1168.
169. Topilow HW, Yimoyines DJ, Freeman HM, et al. Bilateral multifocal intraocular cysticercosis. Ophthalmology. 1981;88:1166.
170. Rapoza PA, Michels RG, Semeraro RJ, et al. Vitrectomy for excision of intraocular larva (*Hypoderma* species). Retina. 1986;6:99–104.
171. Aronson SB. Starch endophthalmitis. Am J Ophthalmol. 1972;73:570.
172. Stark WJ, Rosenblum P, Maumenee AE, et al. Postoperative inflammatory reactions to intraocular lenses sterilized with ethylene-oxide. Ophthalmology. 1980;87:385.
173. Forster RK, Zachary IG, Cottingham AJ Jr, et al. Further observations on the diagnosis, cause, and treatment of endophthalmitis. Am J Ophthalmol. 1976;81:52.
174. Forster RK, Abbott RL, Gelender H. Management of infectious endophthalmitis. Ophthalmology. 1980;87:313.
175. Engel HM, Green WR, Michels RG, et al. Diagnostic vitrectomy. Retina. 1981;1:121.
176. Engel H, de la Cruz ZC, Jimenes-Abalahin LD, et al. Cytopreparatory techniques for eye fluid specimens obtained by vitrectomy. Acta Cytol (Baltimore). 1982;26:551.
177. Stulting RD, Leif RC, Clarkson JG, et al. Centrifugal cytology of ocular fluids. Arch Ophthalmol. 1982;100:822.
178. Jones DB, Liesegang TJ, Robinson NM. Laboratory diagnosis of ocular infections. Cumitech. 1981;13:16.
179. Ellison AC. The limulus lysate test. A rapid test for diagnosis of *Pseudomonas* keratitis or endophthalmitis. Arch Ophthalmol. 1978;96:1268.
180. Shields JA, Lerner HA, Felberg NT. Aqueous cytology and enzymes in nematode endophthalmitis. Am J Ophthalmol. 1977;84:319.
181. Felberg NT, Shields JA, Federman JL. Antibody to *Toxocara canis* in the aqueous humor. Arch Ophthalmol. 1981;99:1563.
182. Searl SS, Moazed K, Albert DM, et al. Ocular toxocariasis presenting as leukocoria in a patient with low ELISA titer to *Toxocara canis*. Ophthalmology. 1981;88:1302.
183. Forster RK. Endophthalmitis. Diagnostic cultures and visual results. Arch Ophthalmol. 1974;92:387.
184. Baum JL. The treatment of bacterial endophthalmitis. Ophthalmology. 1978;83:350.
185. O'Day DM, Jones DB, Patrinely J, et al. *Staphylococcus epidermidis* en-

dophthalmitis. Visual outcome following noninvasive therapy. Ophthalmology. 1982;89:354.
186. Eichenbaum DM, Jaffe NS, Clayman HM, et al. Pars plana vitrectomy as a primary treatment for acute bacterial endophthalmitis. Am J Ophthalmol. 1978;86:167.
187. Diamond JG. Intraocular management of endophthalmitis. A systematic approach. Arch Ophthalmol. 1981;99:96.
188. Algvere P, Alanko H, Dickhoff K, et al. Pars plana vitrectomy in the management of intraocular inflammation. Acta Ophthalmol. 1981;59:727.
189. Peyman GA, Raichand M, Bennett TO. Management of endophthalmitis with pars plana vitrectomy. Br J Ophthalmol. 1980;64:474.
190. Baum J, Peyman GA, Barza M. Intravitreal administration of antibiotic in the treatment of bacterial endophthalmitis. III. Consensus. Surv Ophthalmol. 1982;26:204.
191. Schemmer GB, Dricke WJ. Post Traumatic *Bacillus cereus* endophthalmitis. Arch Ophthalmol. 1987;105:342.
192. Jones DB. Therapy of postsurgical fungal endophthalmitis. Ophthalmology. 1978;85:357.
193. Blumenkranz MS, Stevens DA. Therapy of endogenous fungal endophthalmitis. Miconazole or amphotericin B for coccidioidal and candidal infection. Arch Ophthalmol. 1980;98:1216.
194. Jones DB. Therapy of postsurgical fungal endophthalmitis. Ophthalmology. 1978;85:357.
195. Snip RC, Michels RG. Pars plana vitrectomy in the management of endogenous *Candida* endophthalmitis. Am J Ophthalmol. 1976;82:699.
196. Perraut LE Jr, Perraut LE, Bleiman B, et al. Successful treatment of *Candida albicans* endophthalmitis with intravitreal amphotericin B. Arch Ophthalmol. 1981;99:1565.
197. Axelrod AJ, Peyman GA, Apple DJ. Toxicity of intravitreal injection of amphotericin B. Am J Ophthalmol. 1973;76:578.
198. Souri EN, Green WR. Intravitreal amphotericin B toxicity. Am J Ophthalmol. 1974;78:77.
199. Naidoff MA, Green WR. Endogenous *Aspergillus* endophthalmitis occurring after kidney transplant. Am J Ophthalmol. 1975;79:502.
200. Grieco MH, Freilich DB, Louria DB. Diagnosis of cryptococcal uveitis with hypertonic media. Am J Ophthalmol. 1971;72:171.
201. Cameron ME, Harrison A. Ocular cryptococcosis in Australia: With a report of two further cases. Med J Austr. 1970;1:935.
202. Schlaegel TF Jr. Recent advances in uveitis. Ann Ophthalmol. 1972;4:525.
203. Jabs DA, Schachat AP, Liss R, et al. Presumed varicella zoster retinitis in immunocompromised patients. Retina. 1987;7:9.
204. Dorfman LJ. Cytomegalovirus encephalitis in adults. Neurology (Minn). 1973;23:136.
205. Henderly DE, Freeman WR, Causey DM, et al. Cytomegalovirus retinitis and response to therapy with ganciclovir. Ophthalmology. 1987;94:425.
206. Schlaegel TF Jr. Toxoplasmosis. In: Duane TD, ed. Clinical Ophthalmology. v. 4. Hagerstown, MD: Harper & Row; 1976:12.
207. Tabbara KF, O'Connor GR. Treatment of ocular toxoplasmosis with clindamycin and sulfadiazine. Ophthalmology. 1980;87:129.
208. Byers B, Kimura SJ. Uveitis after death of a larva in the vitreous cavity. Am J Ophthalmol. 1974;77:63.
209. Belmont JB, Irvine A, Benson W, et al. Vitrectomy in ocular toxocariasis. Arch Ophthalmol. 1982;100:1912.
210. Grand MG, Roper-Hall G. Pars Plana vitrectomy for ocular toxocariasis. Retina. 1981;1:258.
211. White AT, Newland HS, Taylor HR, et al. Controlled trial and dose-finding study of ivermectin for treatment of onchocerciasis. J Infect Dis. 1987;156:463.

101. PERIOCULAR INFECTIONS

L. NEAL FREEMAN
W. RICHARD GREEN

When considering infections involving periocular structures, the anatomic areas of concern are the eyelids, the components of the lacrimal apparatus, the orbit, and the paranasal and cavernous sinuses.

EYELIDS

Inflammations affecting the eyelids are commonly seen in an ophthalmologic practice. They include marginal blepharitis, hordeola (or sties), and chalazia. The eyelids show signs of inflammation very readily because the overlying skin is thin and the subcutaneous layer is composed of loose strands of connective tissue without fat. Bacteria are responsible for most infections of the eyelids, with *Staphylococcus* being the most common cause.[1]

The term *blepharitis* refers to inflammation of the lid margins and is usually chronic and bilateral. There are two main types: staphylococcal and seborrheic. The chief symptoms in both types are irritation of the eyes, a burning sensation, and itching of the lid margins.

Staphylococcal blepharitis is usually chronic and is manifested by hyperemia and small ulcerations of the lid margins, crusted exudate in the form of dry scales around the base of the lashes, and loss of the lashes. Although *Staphylococcus aureus* is the organism most commonly responsible, *Staphylococcus epidermidis* is increasingly being recognized as a cause of marginal blepharitis. Exotoxins elaborated by these bacteria may cause nonspecific conjunctivitis, inferior punctuate epithelial keratitis, and peripheral corneal infiltrates.[2] Associated seborrhea of the scalp and brows may be found. Acne rosacea is associated with a chronic blepharitis and occasional keratitis. Mascara use has been implicated in some cases of blepharitis.[3]

A *hordeolum* is a common acute purulent infection of the glands of the eyelids that is usually caused by *Staphylococcus*. Depending on the glands affected, a hordeolum can be classified into two types—internal and external.

An internal hordeolum is an infection of the meibomian glands, which are modified sebaceous glands located within the connective tissue tarsal plate of the lid. Hordeola may be associated with diffuse lid swelling, erythema, and tenderness. They may point toward the skin or the conjunctival surface of the lid.

An external hordeolum (or sty) is an infection of the glands of Zeis, which are small sebaceous glands connected with the follicles of the eyelashes, and the glands of Moll, which are apocrine sweat glands in the skin of the lid. External hordeola are smaller and more superficial than internal hordeola. They are discrete, elevated, erythematous tender pustules and point toward the skin surface of the lid, usually near the margin.

A *chalazion* is a nontender, sterile, chronic granulomatous inflammation of a meibomian gland and has a tendency to recur. It presents as a lid nodule and may begin with inflammation and tenderness similar to a hordeolum. However, a fully developed chalazion is differentiated from a hordeolum by the absence of acute inflammatory signs. If a chalazion becomes secondarily infected, signs of acute inflammation are evident. The majority of these lesions point toward the conjunctival surface of the lid, and they may be large enough to press on the globe and distort vision or be a cosmetic blemish. Since sebaceous gland carcinoma of the lid may be confused clinically with a chalazion, any recurrent chalazion should be examined histopathologically. The main histopathologic feature of a chalazion is a chronic granulomatous inflammatory reaction centered around clear spaces. These spaces represent areas of lipid material that are dissolved out during processing of the tissue.

If a chalazion ruptures through the tarsal conjunctiva, there may be an outgrowth of granulation tissue that results in a rapidly enlarging, painless, polypoid mass called a granuloma pyogenicum. Histopathologically it is composed of capillaries in a radiating pattern and is separated by a loose connective tissue with an acute and chronic inflammatory cell infiltrate.

Blepharitis and dermatitis may also be caused by molluscum contagiosum, herpes simplex virus,[4] *Pseudomonas*,[5] *Proteus mirabilis*,[6] and *Moraxella*[7] and may be secondary to contact allergies caused by agents such as cosmetics[8] and eye drops. The role of the hair follicle mites *Demodex folliculorum* and *D. brevis* in disease of the lids is unclear.[9–11] *Phthirus pubis* (pubic lice) may cause an irritating bloody blepharitis and is commonly transmitted as a venereal disease.[12]

LACRIMAL APPARATUS

The lacrimal apparatus has two major functions. The main lacrimal gland (located anteriorly in the superotemporal quadrant of the orbit) and the accessory lacrimal glands of Krause and Wolfring (located in the conjunctiva) produce the aqueous component of the tear film. The lacrimal puncta, the superior and inferior canaliculi, the common canaliculus, the lacrimal sac, and the nasolacrimal duct are concerned with the drainage of tears from the conjunctival cul-de-sac and tear lake to the nasal cavity. Pathologic processes affecting the main and the accessory lacrimal glands result in diminished tear production, whereas those affecting the lacrimal drainage apparatus cause obstruction resulting in epiphora (or "tearing").

Canaliculitis is a low-grade chronic inflammation in the canaliculi, that is usually due to infection from the anaerobic, gram-positive filamentous organisms *Actinomyces* or *Arachnia propionica*.[13] Other organisms that may be responsible include *Pityrosporum pachydermatis*,[14] *Fusobacterium*,[15] *Enterobacter cloacae*,[16] *Nocardia asteroides, Candida albicans,* and *Aspergillus niger*.[17] Viruses implicated in canaliculitis include herpes simplex,[18–20] herpes zoster,[18,19] and vaccinia.[19] Inflammation leads to obstruction of the lumen of the canaliculus,[21] which results in epiphora, chronic conjunctivitis, and a tender swollen nasal lid margin that may go undiagnosed for years. Typically, the punctum has a slightly distended appearance. In cases due to *Arachnia*, a gritty sensation is felt when the canaliculus is probed.

Dacryocystitis is inflammation of the lacrimal sac. It is clinically useful to divide dacryocystitis into chronic and acute forms. Chronic dacryocystitis is usually caused by a single site of partial or complete obstruction within the lacrimal sac or within the nasolacrimal duct. The infection is usually the result and not the cause of obstruction.

There are many causes of obstruction. In about 5 percent of all newborns the distal end of the nasolacrimal duct is not patent at birth, but in most cases there is spontaneous opening of the duct during the first few days or weeks of life.[22,23]

True congenital lacrimal sac mucoceles are uncommon and may require early probing.[24] Trauma causing fractures in the nasoethmoid region may obstruct the drainage system at the junction of the lacrimal sac and the nasolacrimal duct. Infection of the lacrimal sac by *Aspergillus, Candida albicans,* or *Actinomyces* may occur. With partial or complete obstruction of the nasolacrimal duct, a laminated concretion (dacryolith) may develop in the lacrimal sac and often is associated with bacterial and fungal infections.[25] Benign and malignant tumors of the lacrimal sac may cause obstruction of the outflow system. Obstruction in the area of the sac–duct junction from a silicone implant used for an orbital floor fracture repair has been reported; a chronic dacryocystitis developed.[26] Foreign bodies such as wood or cilia are rare causes of obstruction of the drainage apparatus.

Streptococcus pneumoniae is most commonly isolated from cases of chronic dacryocystitis. However, a mixed infection with *Staphylococcus, Streptococcus,* and *Pseudomonas aeruginosa* can occur, Sarcoidosis[27,28] and *Chlamydia trachomatis*[29] may cause a chronic recurrent dacryocystitis.

Epiphora is usually the only clinical finding in patients with chronic dacryocystitis. On palpation of the tear sac area, a mucoid discharge may be expressed through the lacrimal puncta.

Acute dacryocystitis occurs when both the proximal and distal ends of the drainage system become partially or totally obstructed. The obstruction may be due to trauma, dacryoliths acting as ball valves, or the flare-up of a chronic dacryocystitis or lacrimal sac sarcoidosis. The major symptom in patients with acute dacryocystitis is pain in the tear sac area. Erythema and swelling of the lacrimal sac area, a purulent discharge, and epiphora are signs of acute dacryocystitis. On palpation, tenderness in the tear sac area is present, and purulent material can be expressed in a retrograde fashion through the lacrimal puncta. A serious complication of acute dacryocystitis is orbital cellulitis (see below).[30,31] This occurs if the inflammatory process involving the lacrimal sac spreads posterior to the orbital septum; this is more likely in older patients with attenuated septa.[30] Marginal corneal ulcers have been described in β-streptococcal dacryocystitis.[32]

The common pathogens in acute dacryocystitis are *Staphylococcus aureus* and *Haemophilus influenzae* in children.[30]

Histopathologic study of bone from the area adjacent to the lacrimal sac showed normal bone in approximately one-half of patients undergoing dacryocystorhinostomy for acute or chronic dacryocystitis in a recent study. The other half of the bone samples revealed evidence of bone remodeling or woven bone, but no inflammation was present. The periosteum of the lacrimal fossa may help prevent bony changes in dacryocystitis.[33]

Dacryoadenitis refers to inflammation of the main lacrimal gland. Acute bacterial infections of the gland are uncommon. Infection may occur from an exogenous site on the skin, or the gland may be seeded during a bacteremia. Local trauma is a predisposing factor. The palpebral lobe of the gland is more frequently involved than is the orbital lobe.[34] Pyogenic bacteria such as *Staphylococcus aureus* and streptococci are often implicated as causes. Rarely, gonococcal bacteremia may result in an acute dacryoadenitis. *Cysticercus cellulosae* dacryoadenitis has been reported.[35] Viral infections of the lacrimal gland cause acute inflammation and usually occur in children. The two viral diseases that most often involve the gland are mumps[36] and infectious mononucleosis.[37] Clinically inapparent infection of the lacrimal gland may occur with cytomegalovirus, coxsackievirus A, echoviruses, or herpes zoster virus infections.[38] Patients with acute dacryoadenitis complain of severe pain in the lacrimal gland region, and signs of inflammation including erythema of overlying skin, swelling, and tenderness on palpation of this region are noted. Ocular motility defects such as combined abduction and elevation deficiency or isolated abduction deficiency may be seen.[34,39] In some cases (particularly in children), fever and leukocytosis occur.[38]

Chronic infections of the lacrimal gland may occur in tuberculosis,[40] syphilis, leprosy, and schistosomiasis.[41] Clinically, painless enlargement of one or both lacrimal glands may occur, and signs of acute inflammation are not present. Similar clinical features may be present in sarcoidosis.[42]

Fungal infections that may involve the lacrimal gland include blastomycosis, histoplasmosis, nocardiosis, and sporotrichosis.[38]

ORBIT AND CAVERNOUS SINUS

Orbital cellulitis is an acute infection of the orbital contents. It is most commonly caused by bacteria, although it may be caused by fungi in debilitated patients. It is a serious infection because of the risk of visual loss and the possibility of posterior spread to involve the cavernous sinus, which may lead to thrombosis and death.

There are many causes of orbital cellulitis. Most cases occur by spread from contiguous structures such as the paranasal sinuses. The potentially serious nature of this condition is frequently underestimated.[43] Any of the sinuses may be involved. The lamina papyracea separating the ethmoid air cells from the orbit is thin and may permit the spread of infection. Congenital or traumatic breaks may further compromise this barrier. Additionally, the anterior and posterior ethmoidal foramina allow communication between the sinus and orbit. The bones separating the frontal and maxillary sinuses from the orbit are also thin. In children, since the ethmoid sinuses are the first to pneumatize, ethmoiditis is the most common source.[45–48] In one large series, 84 percent of the children with orbital cellulitis had roentgenographic evidence of sinusitis. This sinusitis was bilateral in almost half the cases.[49] In adults, a frontal sinusitis is a common cause.

Direct inoculation of organisms may occur after puncture wounds to the orbit when they perforate the orbital septum. Retained orbital foreign bodies are another source of infection.[50] Orbital cellulitis may occur as a complication of orbital fractures, even in the absence of adjacent sinusitis.[51] Certain surgical procedures can rarely cause orbital infections. These include exploration for orbital tumors, retinal reattachment procedures, and strabismus operations.[52,53] Foreign materials such as sutures, encircling ocular bands, and sponges may serve as the nidus in postoperative orbital infections, and such materials must be removed to eliminate the infection. Acute dacryocystitis[30,51,54] or posterior perforation of the lacrimal sac during therapeutic probing may result in orbital cellulitis. Rare cases from bites by house pets and rats have been reported.[55] Dental and intracranial infections may extend into the orbit and produce an orbital cellulitis.

In adults, infection of the orbit by blood-borne bacterial metastases from a distant site is extremely rare. In children, however, orbital cellulitis may develop secondarily to a bacteremia caused by *Haemophilus influenzae*.[47] *Enterococcus (Streptococcus) faecalis* causing a bacteremia with the subsequent development of orbital cellulitis has also been reported.[56] Systemic diseases that may result in orbital infection include influenza, subacute bacterial endocarditis, scarlet fever, vaccinia, herpes simplex, and herpes zoster.[44] In newborns, intrauterine infections have been implicated in the causation of orbital cellulitis.[57] Anaerobes are frequently present in cases of chronic sinusitis and should be suspected in orbital cellulitis associated with long-standing sinus disease. Multiple anaerobic strains may be found.[58,59] Trauma with resultant inoculation of earthen material is a cause of orbital cellulitis due to *Clostridium perfringens*.[60]

The bacteria most commonly causing orbital cellulitis are *Staphylococcus aureus, Streptococcus pyogenes,* and *Streptococcus pneumoniae*.[47,48] Of these, *Staphylococcus* is the most common etiologic agent. However, given the variability of organisms found on the skin and conjunctiva and from foreign bodies, a mixed infection is usual. In children under 5 years of age, *H. influenzae* is the most common cause.[61] Anaerobic organisms found in infected paranasal sinuses can also cause orbital cellulitis.[58] If crepitation is present, the possibility of cellulitis secondary to clostridial organisms should be considered.[62,63] In patients receiving immunosuppressive drugs, atypical mycobacteria may rarely cause orbital cellulitis.[64]

Regardless of the source of the infection, many of the symptoms and signs of orbital cellulitis are distinctive. However, in some cases it may be difficult to establish an early diagnosis. For example, after severe injuries, hemorrhage and edema in the lids and orbit may prevent early recognition of the signs of infection. Likewise, nonseptic inflammation after intraorbital surgical procedures often mimics bacterial cellulitis by the presence of lid edema, chemosis, orbital edema, and restricted ocular motion. These factors may cause a delay in diagnosis. Therefore, it is imperative that the clinician maintain a high index of suspicion of the possibility of infection in such cases. After trauma, symptoms and signs of orbital cellulitis usually begin within 48 to 72 hours. However, occasionally a retained intraorbital foreign body may reveal signs of infection only several months later.

Fever, lid edema, and rhinorrhea are the most frequent early signs. They are followed by orbital pain, tenderness on palpation of the lids, and headache. Vision is usually normal during the early stages. As the infection progresses, the lids acquire a dark red discoloration and increased warmth. Conjunctival hyperemia, chemosis, and proptosis follow. The direction of proptosis may help to indicate the primary site of involvement in the orbit. There is limitation of ocular motility, with pain on attempted motion and increased resistance to retropulsion of the globe. Increased intraocular pressure, reduced corneal sensation, congestion of retinal veins, and chorioretinal striae may be present later in the course of the infection. In severe cases of orbital cellulitis, gangrene and sloughing of the lids have been reported.[65] Acute infarction of the choroid and retina from involvement of the posterior ciliary vessels and ophthalmic artery may rarely occur.[66] A leukocytosis with a WBC count greater than 15,000/mm^3 is usually present.

A different clinical course is seen in "posterior" orbital cellulitis.[67] These patients manifest an orbital apex syndrome in which profound visual loss and ophthalmoplegia develop with minimal external inflammatory signs.[67–69] This condition occurs as a result of contiguous spread into the orbit from an adjacent sphenoidal and/or ethmoidal sinusitis. The cause of visual loss in posterior orbital cellulitis is probably vascular compromise, but vasculitis of the optic nerve vasculature may also be of etiologic importance.[67,68] In the few cases reported, the visual loss has been almost uniformly irreversible. Posterior orbital cellulitis is less common than is orbital cellulitis; this is probably because of the thicker bony barrier and the more firmly attached periosteum of the posterior orbit.[67]

Preseptal and postseptal (orbital) cellulitis secondary to paranasal sinusitis may be classified into five clinical stages.[70] In the first stage (preseptal cellulitis), bacteria are not present within the orbit, but inflammatory orbital edema produced by the proximity of a suppurative sinusitis is present. During the second stage there is direct extension through bone, with infiltration of the orbital contents by bacteria and inflammatory cells. The third stage occurs after the infection has extended beneath bone, thereby leading to formation of a subperiosteal abscess. The fourth stage is reached when the infection within the orbit consolidates as an abscess. This may be clinically verifiable by the subcutaneous induration of the lids, as mentioned above, and by fluctuance in the orbit that is detectable on retropulsion of the globe. This is quite unlike the usual loss of resiliency and the difficulty in retropulsion that accompanies orbital cellulitis without abscess formation. Occasionally, the abscess may rupture through the orbital septum and present beneath the skin of the lid.[71] The fifth, or final, stage is that of cavernous sinus thrombosis.

Before antibiotics became available, about 19 percent of the patients with orbital cellulitis died of intracranial complications. About 20 percent of the patients were blinded in the involved eye, and an additional 13 percent suffered some visual loss from the infection.[72] Additional complications include osteomyelitis, strabismus, an afferent pupillary defect, a chronic draining sinus, and a scarred upper eyelid.[73] With antibiotic therapy, the prognosis in cases of orbital cellulitis has markedly improved.

Tuberculous involvement of the orbit is very rare, occurs by a hematogenous route, and is unassociated with miliary tuberculosis.[74] The patients are apparently healthy, without pulmonary disease or other signs of systemic tuberculosis.

Syphilitic gummas in the orbit are rare. They may occur in the extraocular muscles, the orbital nerves, and the optic nerve.[75]

The two most common fungal infections causing orbital infection are mucormycosis (Chapter 237) and aspergillosis (Chapter 236). Conditions predisposing to orbital mucormycosis and the clinical and pathologic features of the infection have been well described.[76–81]

The *Aspergillus* organism is an opportunistic fungus that is common in the air of many localities. The infection develops in a sinus and rarely spreads to the orbit.[82,83] Chronic sinus aspergillosis usually occurs in persons who are 40–60 years of age and who have a chronically obstructed sinus due to allergic diathesis, a deviated nasal septum, or nasal polyps. There appears to be a geographic factor related to humidity.[84] A similar syndrome produced by *Bipolaris, Curvularia,* and *Drechslera* species appears to be geographically disperse. Orbital infection with these fungi in the normal host is a slowly progressive, granulomatous, fibrosing disease. Thus, patients may be asymptomatic for extended periods of time, and the duration of symptoms may range from several months to 16 years. The chief symptoms and signs are ocular pain, decreased vision, and unilateral proptosis. The fibrosing nature of the granulomatous inflammation in the orbit may cause optic nerve damage with optic disk swelling, venous engorgement, and central retinal artery occlusion. Other signs of inflammation—such as lid edema, chemosis, fever, and leukocytosis—are usually absent.

Aspergillosis in the sinus of an immunosuppressed patient is typically an acute infection resembling mucormycosis.[83] As a third clinical form, *Aspergillus* may form a fungus ball in a chronically obstructed maxillary sinus without invading the sinus lining.

Orbital infections caused by other fungi[85–88] and parasites[76,89–96] are rare.

The nematode *Trichinella spiralis* may invade the extraocular muscles and result in periorbital edema and pain on movement of the eyes.[92]

Orbital inflammation may be due to a wide variety of noninfectious causes. The differential diagnosis of orbital inflammation has been well reviewed.[97]

Cavernous sinus thrombosis may be difficult to distinguish from mucormycosis and orbital cellulitis. Most often, cavernous sinus thrombosis results from blood-borne infection from the face, nasal cavity, paranasal sinuses, and ear.[98,99] It may also occur as a rare complication of orbital cellulitis.[100,101] Evidence of orbital infection was found in all of six cases of cavernous sinus thrombosis that came to autopsy in one series.[102] This suggests that although orbital cellulitis often occurs without involvement of the cavernous sinus most cases of cavernous sinus thrombosis will have coinvolvement of the orbit.[103] Aseptic thrombosis of the sinus is uncommon, and it usually follows surgical and/or nonsurgical trauma.[104]

The symptoms and signs of cavernous sinus thrombosis are graver than those of orbital cellulitis. The early onset of internal and external ophthalmoplegia is a suggestive feature. Decreased sensation about the eye, indicating involvement of the trigeminal nerve, and signs of bilaterality with paretic muscles in the contralateral eye are strong evidence of cavernous sinus thrombosis. Altered consciousness and other signs of meningitis indicate the seriousness of this clinical entity.

LABORATORY FEATURES

Patients with blepharitis may often be more symptomatic than the clinical findings seem to warrant. In such cases, bacteriologic culture of the lid margins may reveal a dense population of *Staphylococcus*.

In canaliculitis from *Arachnia* the recovery of concretions is diagnostic. Gram stain will demonstrate gram-positive filamentous organisms. Fluorescein-labeled antisera may aid in diagnosis.[13] Cultures should be obtained for confirmation, but the organisms may be difficult to isolate.[13]

When obstruction of the lacrimal drainage system is suspected, several procedures are available to evaluate its patency. When the drainage apparatus is fully patent, 2% fluorescein dye instilled in the conjunctival sac may usually be collected on a nasal applicator passed beneath the inferior turbinate (Jones I test). If no dye is recovered, the fornices are irrigated to remove residual fluorescein. The nasolacrimal sac is then cannulated and irrigated with saline (Jones II test). If dye is recovered with the Jones II test when none could be recovered with the Jones I test, a partial nasolacrimal duct obstruction is probably present. Probing of the lacrimal passages may provide information regarding the site of the obstruction.

Several other techniques have been devised to assess the patency and status of the lacrimal drainage system. Thermography, a process by which body surface temperatures are recorded in the form of thermal images, has been used to study lacrimal system obstructions and inflammations.[105,106] Inflammation induces hyperthermia, and canaliculitis and acute dacryocystitis may be demonstrated by comparisons to a normal contralateral side. Radiographic studies that have been used to evaluate the patency of the drainage system include plain film dacryocystography with contrast injection (distension dacryocystography), macrodacryocystography, scintillography, and tomography (including computed tomography).[107–109] Computed tomography of the outflow system after topical instillation of a contrast agent is useful as a physiologic test with good anatomic resolution.[109]

In cases of orbital cellulitis, the isolation of the causative agent is often difficult because external drainage is often absent, aspiration of fluid from the orbit is contraindicated (unless an abscess is present), and results of efforts to isolate organisms in periorbital and orbital cellulitis are variable. The assistance of an otolaryngologist is essential in the management of this infection because infectious sinusitis is the most common cause of orbital cellulitis. Careful clinical examination of the sinuses with microbiologic investigation of purulent material obtained from the nasopharynx, nasal mucosa, and conjunctiva is important. Blood cultures are essential and are most likely to be positive in children under 5 years of age with periorbital cellulitis associated with an upper respiratory tract infection.[48] Microbiologic investigation should consist of Gram and PAS stains and inoculation of blood agar, chocolate agar, Sabouraud agar and thioglycollate broth, and reduced blood agar in an anaerobic environment.

Ultrasonography is useful in the diagnosis of orbital cellulitis and orbital abscess. B-scan ultrasound may indicate fingerlike clear areas in the retrobulbar space in cases of cellulitis, and an abscess may be manifested as an area of low or medium reflectivity.[44] Plain orbital and sinus films are helpful in these cases and may show sinus opacification, air–fluid levels, bony abnormalities, or foreign bodies.

Computed tomography (CT) is the technique providing the most important information in patients with suspected orbital cellulitis with or without abcess formation.[44,110] Studies with and without contrast agent with multiple sections and views should be obtained when feasible. A correlation of CT findings with the clinical stages of orbital cellulitis mentioned previously has been recently proposed.[110] In stage II disease (orbital cellulitis without abcess), a low-density fluid collection is present between the periosteum and the adjacent rectus muscle. In stage III (subperiosteal abcess), the periosteum is elevated and the rectus muscle displaced by an abscess defined by an enhancing periosteal border. An orbital abscess (stage IV) is manifested by a homogeneous, heterogeneous, or ringlike mass within the orbital space.[111] CT will also delineate sinus and bony abnormalities and most orbital foreign bodies. Orbital venography may show attenuation of the superior ophthalmic vein from increased orbital pressure, which is compatible with cellulitis.

In cases of suspected cavernous sinus thrombosis, any of a number of diagnostic studies may be helpful. Carotid arteriography is of diagnostic usefulness, but is potentially dangerous. Orbital venography is effective in the region of the cavernous sinus, and modification of this technique by digital subtraction has also been used to diagnose thrombosis.[112] Contrast-enhanced computed tomography has been beneficial in some cases of cavernous sinus thrombosis.[103,113,114] It has recently been suggested that high-field magnetic resonance imaging may be the neuroimaging modality of choice in cases of suspected cavernous sinus thrombosis.[115] The cerebrospinal fluid will often show pleocytosis with an abundance of polymorphonuclear cells and an increased protein level.[103] Cultures of the cerebrospinal fluid, although, are often negative in cases of cavernous sinus thrombosis. Blood cultures are usually positive.[116]

In cases of mucormycosis, positive cultures are often difficult to obtain, and the diagnosis is usually made by histologic examination of excised tissue. Otolaryngologic consultation is necessary, and a biopsy and scraping samples from any necrotic area of the nasal mucosa or palate are essential. On tissue sections, nonseptate branching hyphae that are large (6–20 μm wide) and irregularly thick are found. A mainly acute suppurative inflammatory response is usually seen, although sometimes a granulomatous response is present at the sites of thrombosis and in surrounding necrotic tissues.

TREATMENT

In staphylococcal blepharitis, the use of a topical antibiotic (bacitracin, sulfacetamide, or erythromycin) or antibiotics/steroid combination ointment and lid scrubs with or without diluted shampoo applied to the lid margins may decrease lid inflammation.[117] Resistant cases or those associated with acne rosacea may benefit from the long-term, low-dose use of oral tetracyclines. Topical steroid drops are occasionally used to decrease ocular surface inflammation.

Any internal or external hordeolum should be treated with topical antibiotics and warm compresses until the inflammation subsides. The use of systemic antibiotics is rarely indicated, and surgical drainage is rarely required.

Because most chalazia seldom subside spontaneously and they show chronic or subacute inflammation, surgical curettage and excision may be done on chalazia. However, simple observation is reasonable because they tend to decrease in size with time. The use of intralesional corticosteroids has been suggested. *Phthirus pubis* may be treated by manual epilation of involved lashes together with the use of gamma benzene hexachloride shampoo on the body hair of the patient and that of other family members and sexual contacts.[12] In more widely involved cases, the application of a pediculocide—such as yellow mercuric oxide twice a day for a week, 0.25% physostigmine ointment twice a day for 10 days, or 20% fluorescein topically—may be used.[118]

The value of topical antiviral ointment to treat ulcerative herpes simplex blepharitis is unclear, although a short course of trifluridine or vidarabine ointment is reasonable in an effort to prevent inoculation of the ocular surface with herpes simplex virus.

Antibiotic irrigation of the canaliculi combined with topical antibiotic eyedrops is useful in the treatment of canaliculitis. Penicillin G (160,000 units/ml as an irrigant, 60,000 units/ml as drops) is used for *Arachnia* and *Actinomyces;* amphotericin B (1–5 mg/ml) is used against *Candida* and *Aspergillus*.[17] Systemic penicillin, erythromycin, or cephalosporins should be part of the treatment regimen in cases due to *Arachnia*.[17,119] When concretions are present, they should be removed by canaliculotomy and curettage. The canaliculus should then be reconstructed; silicone intubation may be needed.[120] Cases of canalicular obstruction associated with herpes simplex virus infection may require surgical intervention more frequently than in cases caused by bacteria. A possible explanation is that, in the situation with herpes, the epithelial lining of the canaliculi is damaged with resultant adherence of the subepithelial layers with scar formation. In the cases of bacterial infection, however, the epithelium remains intact, and the obstruction is due to edema, which is more reversible.[20]

Parents of infants with nasolacrimal duct obstruction should be taught to firmly massage the lacrimal sac area several times daily. Topical antibiotic eyedrops may be used for lid mattering. If symptoms persist for 6–8 months, the lacrimal drainage apparatus should be irrigated and probed. Probing is more successful in cases of lacrimal duct obstruction due to membranous obstruction than in cases due to narrowing of the duct. If probing is unsuccessful, repeat probing is done a few months later. Silicone intubation of the drainage apparatus is performed if the repeat probing also fails to succeed.[23]

In adults with acute dacryocystitis, treatment with warm compresses and systemic antibiotics should be given. If β-hemolytic streptococci are isolated or suspected, oral penicillin is used.[17] Staphylococci are best treated with a penicillinase-resistant penicillin.[17,30] After the acute infection is controlled, the patient should be taught to perform digital massage of the lacrimal sac, and topical antibiotic drops should be used. If epiphora persists, a dacryocystorhinostomy is performed in most cases to obtain adequate tear drainage.

Bacterial dacryoadenitis is treated with systemic antibiotics. If an orbital abscess forms, surgical drainage is necessary.

In treating orbital cellulitis, intravenous antibiotics and decongestion of the paranasal sinuses are vital. The bacterial agents most commonly responsible for this infection were mentioned above. In adults, nafcillin or oxacillin (1.5 g) every 4 hours should be the initial therapy. In cases of penicillin allergy, cefotaxime (if the allergic response was nonanaphylactic), clindamycin, chloramphenicol, or vancomycin may be substituted.[73,121] Because *H. influenzae* is the most common cause of orbital cellulitis in young children, ampicillin (200 mg/kg/day in divided doses) should be given intravenously along with nafcillin or oxacillin (100 mg/kg/day). If *H. influenzae* is isolated, it should be tested for sensitivity to ampicillin. A third-generation cephalosporin, such as cefotaxime or ceftriaxone, or chloramphenicol (100 mg/kg/day) is used in cases of suspected or confirmed resistance to ampicillin.[70,121,122] Methods of sinus decongestion include nasal sprays, oral decongestants, and oral antihistamines. If the sinusitis persists, surgical drainage of the sinuses should be performed. If the infection progresses and the clinical situation deteriorates despite adequate intravenous antibiotic therapy, it is probably due to the development of a subperiosteal or orbital abscess, and surgical drainage is imperative.[46–48] Material obtained from such drainage should have the complete microbiologic evaluation mentioned previously. In cases of radiographically suspected subperiosteal abscess that seem to be responding to conservative measures, surgery may be deferred, but inflammatory signs may persist much longer than in those patients treated by drainage.[110,123,124]

If the management of patients with orbital mucormycosis is to be successful, the combined efforts of internists, mycologists, otolaryngologists, and ophthalmologists are essential. The underlying disease, for example, diabetic ketoacidosis, should be treated. Intravenous amphotericin B is of value if begun early in the disease.[125,126] The drug may also be injected directly into the involved orbital, paranasal, or pharyngeal tissues, although the value of this type of regional therapy has not been proved.[127] Surgical débridement of devitalized tissue is extremely important. Frequently the involved eye may need to be sacrificed to obtain adequate orbital débridement.

In the treatment of chronic orbital aspergillosis, surgical excision appears to be the best method. Amphotericin B is only of ancillary help.

Cavernous sinus thrombosis is treated with high-dose intravenous antibiotics. Corticosteroids have been used successfully in this entity.[103,128] The role of anticoagulants is still unclear.[98,129,130]

REFERENCES

1. Smolin G, Okumoto M. Staphylococcal blepharitis. Arch Ophthalmol. 1977;95:812.
2. Valenton MJ, Okumoto M. Toxin-producing strains of *Staphylococcus epidermidis* (*albus*). Isolates from patients with staphylococcic blepharoconjunctivitis. Arch Ophthalmol. 1973;89:186.
3. Wilson LA, Julian AJ, Ahearn DG. The survival and growth of microorganisms in mascara during use. Am J Ophthalmol. 1975;79:596.
4. Egerer I, Stary A. Erosive-ulcerative herpes simplex blepharitis. Arch Ophthalmol. 1980;98:1760.
5. Rosenoff SH, Wolfe ML, Chabner BA. *Pseudomonas* blepharoconjunctivitis. A complication of combination chemotherapy. Arch Ophthalmol. 1974;90:490.
6. Parunovic A. *Proteus mirabilis* causing necrotic inflammation of the eyelid. Am J Ophthalmol. 1973;76:543.

7. van Bijsterveld OP. The incidence of *Moraxella* on mucous membranes and the skin. Am J Ophthalmol. 1972;74:72.
8. van Ketel WG, Liem DH. Eyelid dermatitis from nickel contaminated cosmetics. Contact Dermatitis. 1981;4:217.
9. Rufli T, Mumcuoglu Y. The hair follicle mites *Demodex folliculorum* and *Demodex brevis:* Biology and medical importance. A review. Dermatologica. 1981;162:1.
10. Roth AM. *Demodex folliculorum* in hair follicles of eyelid skin. Ann Ophthalmol. 1979;11:37.
11. Gutgesell VJ, Stern GA, Hood CI. Histopathology of meibomian gland dysfunction. Am J Ophthalmol. 1982;94:383.
12. Couth JM, Green WR, Hirst LW, et al. Diagnosing and treating *Phthirus pubis palpebrarum*. Surv Ophthalmol. 1982;26:219.
13. Hirst LW, Merz WB, Kaufmann CS, et al. *Actinomyces/Arachnia* lacrimal canaliculitis. Cornea. 1982;1:259.
14. Romano A, Segal E, Blumenthal M. Canaliculitis with isolation of *Pityrosporum pachydermatis*. Br. J Ophthalmol. 1978;62:732
15. Weinberg RJ, Sartoris MJ, Buerger GF Jr, et al. *Fusobacterium* in presumed *Actinomyces* canaliculitis. Am J Ophthalmol. 1977;84:371
16. Chumbley LC. Canaliculitis caused by *Enterobacter cloacae:* Report of a case. Br J Ophthalmol. 1984;68:364–6.
17. Starr MB. Lacrimal drainage system infections. In: Smith BC, Della Rocca RC, Nesi FA, et al, eds. Ophthalmic Plastic and Reconstructive Surgery. St Louis: CV Mosby; 1987:947–5.
18. Bouzas A. Canalicular inflammation in ophthalmic cases of herpes zoster and herpes simplex. Am J Ophthalmol. 1965;60:713–6.
19. Bouzas AG. Virus aetiology of certain cases of lacrimal obstruction. Br J Ophthalmol. 1973;57:849–51.
20. Harris GJ, Hyndiuk RA, Fox MJ, et al. Herpetic canalicular obstruction. Arch Ophthalmol. 1981;99:282–3.
21. Wolter JR. *Pityrosporum* species associated with dacryoliths in obstructive dacryocystitis. Am J Ophthalmol. 1977;84:806.
22. Korchmaros I, Szalay E. Cannula-probing combined with nasal procedure for dacryocystitis neonatorum. Acta Ophthalmol. 1978;56:357.
23. Kushner BJ. Congenital nasolacrimal system obstruction. Arch Ophthalmol. 1982;100:597.
24. Weinstein GS, Biglan AW, Patterson JH. Congenital lacrimal sac mucoceles. Am J Ophthalmol. 1982;94:106.
25. Berlin AJ, Rath R, Rich L. Lacrimal system dacryoliths. Ophthalmic Surg. 1980;11:435.
26. Mauriello JA, Fiore PM, Kotch M. Dacryocystitis—late complication of orbital floor fracture repair with implant. Ophthalmology. 1987;94:248–50.
27. Harris GJ, Williams GA, Clarke GP. Sarcoidosis of the lacrimal sac. Arch Ophthalmol. 1981;99:1198.
28. Coleman SL, Brull S, Green WR. Sarcoid of the lacrimal sac and surrounding area. Arch Ophthalmol. 1972;88:645.
29. Bahnasawi SA, Abdalla MI, Ghaly AF, et al. Trachoma of the lacrimal sac. Bull Ophthalmol Soc Egypt. 1976;69:619.
30. Hurwitz JJ, Rodgers KJA. Management of acquired dacryocystitis. Can J Ophthalmol. 1983;18:213–6.
31. Ahrens-Palumbo MJ, Ballen PH. Primary dacryocystitis causing orbital cellulitis. Ann Ophthalmol. 1982;14:600.
32. Cohn H, Mondino BJ, Brown SI, et al. Marginal corneal ulcers with acute beta streptococcal conjunctivitis and chronic dacryocystitis. Am J Ophthalmol. 1979;87:541.
33. Hinton P, Hurwitz JJ, Cruickshank B. Nasolacrimal bone changes in diseases of the lacrimal drainage system. Ophthalmic Surg. 1984;15:516–21.
34. Ulman S, Sergott R. Abduction deficit secondary to presumed bacterial dacryoadenitis. Arch Ophthalmol. 1986;104:1127–8.
35. Sen DK. Acute suppurative dacryoadenitis caused by a *Cysticercus cellulosa*. J Pediatr Ophthalmol Strabismus. 1982;19:100.
36. Riffenburgh RS. Ocular manifestations of mumps. Arch Ophthalmol. 1961;56:739.
37. Jones BR. Lacrimal disease associated with infectious mononucleosis. Trans Ophthalmol Soc UK. 1955;75:101.
38. Jakobiec FA, Jones IS. Orbital inflammations. In: Duane TD, ed. Clinical Ophthalmology. v. 2. Philadelphia: Harper & Row; 1987:65.
39. Duke-Elder S. The ocular adnexa. In: Duke-Elder S, ed. System of Ophthalmology. v. 13. St. Louis: CV Mosby; 1974:601.
40. Baghdassarian SA, Zakharia H, Asdourian KK. Report of a case of bilateral caseous tuberculous dacryoadenitis. Am J Ophthalmol. 1972;74:744.
41. Jakobiec FA, Gess L, Zimmerman LE. Granulomatous dacryoadenitis caused by *Schistosoma haematobium*. Arch Ophthalmol. 1977;95:278.
42. Obernauf CD, Shaw HE, Sydnor CJ, et al. Sarcoidosis and its ophthalmic manifestations. Am J Ophthalmol. 1978;86:648.
43. Check WA. Many misjudge severity of orbital cellulitis. JAMA. 1982;247:1236.
44. Hornblass A, Herschorn BJ, Stern K, et al. Orbital abcess. Surv Ophthalmol. 1984;29:169–78.
45. Macy JI, Mandelbaum SH, Minckler DS. Orbital cellulitis. Ophthalmology. 1980;87:1309.
46. Brook I, Friedman EM, Rodriguez WJ, et al. Complications of sinusitis in children. Pediatrics. 1980;66:568.
47. Noel LP, Clark WN, Peacocke TA. Periorbital and orbital cellulitis in childhood. Can J Ophthalmol. 1981;16:178.
48. Weiss A, Friendly D, Eglin K, et al. Bacterial periorbital and orbital cellulitis in childhood. Ophthalmology. 1983;90:195.
49. Watters EC, Wallar PH, Hiles DA, et al. Acute orbital cellulitis. Arch Ophthalmol. 1976;94:785–8.
50. Ferguson EC III. Deep wooden foreign bodies of the orbit: A report of two cases. Trans Am Acad Ophthalmol Otolaryngol. 1970;74:778.
51. Goldfarb MS, Hoffman DS, Rosenberg S. Orbital cellulitis and orbital fractures. Ann Ophthalmol. 1987;19:97–9.
52. Von Noorden GK. Orbital cellulitis following extraocular muscle surgery. Am J Ophthalmol. 1972;74:627.
53. Wilson ME, Paul TO. Orbital cellulitis following strabismus surgery. Ophthalmic Surg. 1987;18:92–4.
54. Allen MV, Cohen KL, Grimson BS. Orbital cellulitis secondary to dacryocystitis following blepharoplasty. Ann Ophthalmol. 1985;17:498–9.
55. Diwan R, Sen DK, Sood GC. Rat bite orbital cellulitis. Br J Ophthalmol. 1970;54:211.
56. Biedner BZ, Marmur U, Yassur Y. *Streptococcus faecalis* orbital cellulitis. Ann Ophthalmol. 1986;18:194–5.
57. Appalanarasayya K, Murthy ASR, Viswanath CK, et al. Proptosis in a newborn due to orbital infection: Case report. Int Surg. 1971;55:149.
58. Frederick J, Braude AL. Anaerobic infection of the paranasal sinuses. N Engl J Med. 1974;290:135.
59. Partamian LG, Jay WM, Fritz KJ. Anaerobic orbital cellulitis. Ann Ophthalmol. 1983;15:123–6.
60. Crock GW, Heriot WJ, Janakiraman P, et al. Gas gangrene infection of the eyes and orbits. Br J Ophthalmol. 1985;69:143–8.
61. Londer L, Nelson DL. Orbital cellulitis due to *Haemophilus influenzae*. Arch Ophthalmol. 1974;91:89.
62. Gorbach SL, Bartlett JG. Anaerobic infections. Part I. N Engl J Med. 1974;290:1177.
63. Sevel D, Tobias B, Sellars SL, et al. Gas in the orbit associated with orbital cellulitis and paranasal sinusitis. Br J Ophthalmol. 1973;57:133.
64. Levine RA. Infection of the orbit by an atypical mycobacterium. Arch Ophthalmol. 1969;82:608.
65. Ross J, Kohlhepp PA. Gangrene of the eyelids. Ann Ophthalmol. 1973;5:84.
66. El-Shewy TM. Acute infarction of the choroid and retina: A complication of orbital cellulitis. Br J Ophthalmol. 1973;57:204.
67. Slavin ML, Glaser JS. Acute severe irreversible visual loss with sphenoethmoiditis—"posterior" orbital cellulitis. Arch Ophthalmol. 1987;105:345–8.
68. Kjoer I. A case of orbital apex syndrome in collateral pansinusitis. Acta Ophthalmol. 1945;23:357–66.
69. Jarrett WH, Gutman FA. Ocular complications of infection in the paranasal sinuses. Arch Ophthalmol. 1969;81:683–8.
70. Chandler JR, Langenbrunner DJ, Stevens ER. The pathogenesis of orbital complications in acute sinusitis. Laryngoscope. 1970;80:1414–28.
71. Sen DK. Surgical treatment of "collar-stud" orbital abscess. Int Surg. 1970;54:379.
72. Birch-Hirshfield, cited by Duke-Elder S. The ocular adnexa. In: Textbook of Ophthalmology. v. 5. St Louis: CV Mosby; 1952:5420–44.
73. Bergin DJ, Wright JE. Orbital cellulitis. Br J Ophthalmol. 1986;70:174–8.
74. Mortada A. Tuberculoma of the orbit and lacrimal gland. Br J Ophthalmol. 1971;55:565.
75. Whitfield R, Wirotsko E. Ocular syphilis. In: Locatcher-Khorazo D, Seegal BC, eds. Microbiology of the Eye. St Louis: CV Mosby; 1972:322.
76. Jakobiec FA. Orbital infections. In: Spencer WH, ed. Ophthalmic Pathology: An Atlas and Textbook. 3rd ed. Philadelphia: WB Saunders; 1986:2812–31.
77. Gass JDM. Ocular manifestations of acute mucormycosis. Arch Ophthalmol. 1961;65:226.
78. Baum JL. Rhino-orbital mucormycosis occurring in an otherwise apparently healthy individual. Am J Ophthalmol. 1967;63:335.
79. Hale LM. Orbital-cerebral phycomycosis: Report of a case and a review of the disease in infants. Arch Ophthalmol. 1971;86:39.
80. Blodi FC, Hannah FT, Wadsworth JAC. Lethal orbitocerebral phycomycosis in otherwise healthy children. Am J Ophthalmol. 1969;67:698.
81. Straatsma BR, Zimmerman LE, Gass JDM. Phycomycosis: A clinico-pathologic study of fifty-one cases. Lab Invest. 1962;11:963.
82. Green WR, Font RL, Zimmerman LE. Aspergillosis of the orbit: Report of ten cases and review of the literature. Arch Ophthalmol. 1969;82:302.
83. Houle TV, Ellis PP. Aspergillosis of the orbit with immunosuppressive therapy. Surv Ophthalmol. 1975;20:35.
84. Miloshev B, Davidson CM, Gentles JC, et al. Aspergilloma of the paranasal sinuses and orbit in northern Sudanese. Lancet. 1966;1:746.
85. Morris FH Jr, Spock A: Intracranial aneurysm secondary to mycotic orbital and sinus infection: Report of a case implicating *Penicillium* as an opportunistic fungus. Am J Ophthalmol. 1969;68:14.
86. Olurin O, Lucas AO, Oyediran ABO. Orbital histoplasmosis due to *Histoplasma duboisii*. Am J Ophthalmol. 1969;68:14.
87. Vida L, Moel SA. Systemic North American blastomycosis with orbital involvement. Am J Ophthalmol. 1974;77:240.
88. Streeten BW, Rabuzzi DD, Jones DB. Sporotrichosis of the orbital margin. Am J Ophthalmol. 1974;77:750.
89. Baghdassarian SA, Zakheria H. Report of three cases of hydatid cyst of the orbit. Am J Ophthalmol. 1971;71:1081.
90. Mehra KS, Banerjee C, Somani PN, et al. Hydatid cyst in orbit. Acta Ophthalmol. 1965;43:761.
91. Talib H. Orbital hydatid cyst in Iraq. Br J Surg. 1972;59:391.

92. Kagan IG. Trichinosis: A review of biologic, serologic and immunologic aspects. J Infect Dis. 1960;107:65.
93. Hamed HH. Orbital affection with *Cysticercus cellulosae*. Bull Ophthalmol Soc Egypt. 1968;61:253.
94. Jones BR. Inflammatory pseudotumors of the orbit: A probable case of microfilarial granuloma of the orbit. Trans Ophthalmol Soc UK. 1970;90:299.
95. Mathur SP, Makhija JM. Invasion of the orbit by maggots. Br J Ophthalmol. 1967;51:406.
96. Wood TR, Slight JR. Bilateral orbital myiasis. Arch Ophthalmol. 1970;84:692.
97. Blodi FC. Orbital inflammations. Symposium on diseases and surgery of the lids, lacrimal apparatus, and orbit. Trans New Orleans Acad Ophthalmol. 1982:1–17.
98. Clune JP. Septic thrombosis within the cavernous chamber: Review of the literature with recent advances in diagnosis and treatment. Am J Ophthalmol. 1963;56:33.
99. Yarington CR Jr. The prognosis and treatment of cavernous sinus thrombosis: A review of 878 cases in the literature. Ann Otol Rhinol Layngol. 1961;70:263.
100. Price CD, Hameroff SB, Richards RD. Cavernous sinus thrombosis and orbital cellulitis. South Med J. 1971;64:1243.
101. Bell RW. Orbital cellulitis and cavernous sinus thrombosis caused by rhabdomyosarcoma of the middle ear. Ann Ophthalmol. 1972;4:1090.
102. Walsh FB. Ocular signs of thrombosis of the intracranial sinuses. Arch Ophthalmol. 1937;17:46.
103. Clifford-Jones RE, Ellis CJK, Stevens JM, et al. Cavernous sinus thrombosis. J Neurol Neurosurg Psychiatry. 1982;45:1092.
104. Geggel HS, Isenberg SJ. Cavernous sinus thrombosis as a cause of unilateral blindness. Ann Ophthalmol. 1982;14:569.
105. Raflo GT, Chart P, Hurwitz JJ. Thermographic evaluation of the human lacrimal drainage system. Ophthalmic Surg. 1982;13:119–24.
106. Rosenstock T, Chart P, Hurwitz JJ. Inflammation of the lacrimal drainage system—assessment by thermography. Ophthalmic Surg. 1983;14:229–37.
107. Galloway JE, Kavic TA, Raflo GT. Digital subtraction macrodacryocystography: A new method of lacrimal system imaging. Ophthalmology 1984;91:956.
108. Rossomondo RM, Carlton WH, Trueblood JH, et al. A new method of evaluating lacrimal drainage. Arch Ophthalmol. 1972;88:523.
109. Freeman LN, Zinreich SJ, Iliff NT. Radiography of the lacrimal system using topical CT dacryocystography (Abstract). Ophthalmology 1987;94:142.
110. Eustis HS, Amstrong DC, Buncic JR, et al. Staging of orbital cellulitis in children: Computed tomography characteristics and treatment guidelines. J Pediatr Ophthalmol. Strabismus 1986;23:246–51.
111. Harr DL, Quencer RM, Abrams GW. Computed tomography and ultrasound in the evaluation of orbital infection and pseudotumor. Radiology. 1982;152:395.
112. Fiandaca MS, Spector RH, Hartmann TM, et al. Unilateral septic cavernous sinus thrombosis—a case report with digital orbital venographic documentation. J Clin Neuro-ophthalmol. 1986;6:35–8.
113. Kline LB, Acker JD, Post MJD, et al. The cavernous sinus: A computed tomographic study. Am J Neurol Radiol. 2:299, 1981.
114. Lew D, Southwick FS, Montgomery WW, et al. Sphenoid sinusitis: A review of 30 cases. N Engl J Med. 1983;309:1149.
115. Savino PJ, Grossman RI, Schatz NJ, et al. High-field magnetic resonance imaging in the diagnosis of cavernous sinus thrombosis. Arch Neurol. 1986;43:1081–2.
116. Taylor PJ. Cavernous sinus thrombophlebitis. Br J Ophthalmol. 1957;41:228–37.
117. Aragones JV. The treatment of blepharitis: A controlled double blind study of combination therapy. Ann Ophthalmol. 1973;5:49.
118. Mathew M, D'Souza P, Mehta DK. A new treatment of pthiriasis palpebrarum. Ann Ophthalmol. 1982;14:439.
119. Seal DV, McGill J, Flanagan D. Lacrimal canaliculitis due to *Arachnia (Actinomyces) propionica*. Br J Ophthalmol. 1981;65:10–13.
120. Campbell CB, Flanagan JC, Schaefer AJ. Acquired lacrimal disorders. In: Smith BC, Della Rocca RC, Nesi FA, eds. Ophthalmic Plastic and Reconstructive Surgery. St Louis: CV Mosby; 1987:956.
121. Krohel G. Orbital cellulitis and abscess. In: Fraunfelder F, Roy H, eds. Current Ocular Therapy. 2nd ed. Philadelphia: WB Saunders; 1985:451.
122. Gutman L. Appropriate antibiotics in orbital cellulitis. Arch Ophthalmol. 1977;95:170.
123. Tannenbaum M, Tenzel J, Byrne SF, et al. Medical management of orbital abscess. Surv Ophthalmol. 1985;30:211–2.
124. Gold SC, Arrigg PG, Hedges TR. Computed tomography in the management of acute orbital cellulitis. Ophthalmic Surg. 1987;18:753–6.
125. Best M, Obstbaum SA, Friedman B, et al. Survival in orbital phycomycosis. Am J Ophthalmol. 1971;71:1078.
126. Bullock JD, Jampol LM, Fezza AJ. Two cases of orbital phycomycosis with recovery. Am J Ophthalmol. 1974;78:811.
127. Jones DB. Microbial preseptal and orbital cellulitis. In: Duane TD, ed. Clinical Ophthalmology. v. 4. Hagerstown, MD: Harper & Row; 1976:17.
128. Solomon OD, Moses L, Volk M. Steroid therapy in cavernous sinus thrombosis. Am J Ophthalmol. 1962;54:1122–5.
129. Parsons M. Intracranial venous thrombosis. Postgrad Med J. 1967; 43:409–14.
130. Lyons C. Treatment of staphylococcal cavernous sinus thrombophlebitis with heparin and chemotherapy. Ann Surg. 1941;113:113–7.

SECTION O. HEPATITIS

102. ACUTE VIRAL HEPATITIS

JAY H. HOOFNAGLE

Acute viral hepatitis is a common and serious infectious disease caused by several viral agents and marked by necrosis and inflammation of the liver. This disease was traditionally separated into two types: type A, or infectious hepatitis caused by the hepatitis A virus (HAV), and type B, or serum hepatitis caused by the hepatitis B virus (HBV).[1] In the last 25 years it has become clear that there are many agents that cause acute viral hepatitis. At present, five hepatitis virus agents have been identified: HAV[2]; HBV[3,4]; the hepatitis delta virus[5,6]; a parenterally transmitted, classic non-A, non-B hepatitis agent[7,8]; and an enterically transmitted, epidemic non-A, non-B hepatitis agent.[9,10] The five forms of acute viral hepatitis are similar clinically, but the agents that cause them are quite distinct.

Hepatitis A, B, delta, and the two forms of non-A, non-B hepatitis are primary infectious diseases of the liver; their main manifestations are those of hepatocellular necrosis and hepatic inflammation, and there is little evidence to suggest that they infect other organs to a major extent. Several other viral agents can secondarily affect the liver and induce a viral hepatitis-like syndrome. The most important of these agents are the Epstein-Barr virus (EBV) and cytomegalovirus (CMV); however, liver disease also can occur with infections with herpes simplex viruses; varicella-zoster virus; measles, rubella, rubeola, and coxsackie B viruses; and adenoviruses. While these agents can cause diagnostic confusion by producing some degree of liver inflammation and dysfunction, they are not considered to be primary causes of acute or chronic viral hepatitis.

Acute viral hepatitis is a common disease. Yearly estimates from the U.S. Centers for Disease Control suggest that the incidence of acute viral hepatitis has been rising slowly over the last 20 years.[11] During 1985, there were approximately 60,000 cases of viral hepatitis reported, among which an estimated 29 percent were due to hepatitis A, 44 percent to hepatitis B, and 27 percent to non-A, non-B hepatitis. These reports suggest that the annual incidence of acute viral hepatitis in the United States is 0.25 per 1000 population. This is clearly an underestimate.

Attempts at quantifying the degree of underreporting of viral hepatitis[12] have suggested that the true incidence is five to eight times that reported each year (thus 1–2 per 1000 population). Indeed, the use of serologic markers for evidence of previous HAV and HBV infections reveals that by the age of 50 years, 70 percent of middle-class white Americans have had HAV infection and 7 percent have had HBV infection.[13] These prevalences of antibody markers are higher among lower socioeconomic groups and among foreign-born U.S. citizens.

Acute viral hepatitis is a serious disease. The mortality rate for icteric viral hepatitis overall is approximately 1 percent. The mortality rate of acute hepatitis is higher in older persons, and some of the variation in the reported mortality rates of this disease relates to the age of the affected patients. In addition, fulminant cases occur more commonly in delta hepatitis than in the other forms of acute viral hepatitis. In various outbreaks of delta hepatitis, the mortality rate has been reported to be between 2 and 20 percent.[6,14] Finally, the epidemic form of non-A, non-B hepatitis has a striking characteristic of a high mortality rate (~10 percent) in pregnant women.[10]

In addition to mortality from the acute disease, viral hepatitis also has serious sequelae including chronic liver disease and cirrhosis, polyarteritis nodosa, cryoglobulinemia, glomerulonephritis, aplastic anemia, and hepatocellular carcinoma.[15–17] In the United States and Western Europe, chronic viral hepatitis is probably the second most frequent cause of cirrhosis, second only to alcohol abuse. The chronic forms of hepatitis B, delta hepatitis, and non-A, non-B hepatitis are frequent causes of terminal liver disease for which hepatic transplantation is performed. On a worldwide scale, chronic hepatitis B infection is the most important cause of cirrhosis and is a major cause of cancer mortality. It is estimated that 5 percent of the world's population has chronic HBV infection (the chronic carrier state) and up to 40 percent of these persons may ultimately develop hepatocellular carcinoma.[18]

The many advances that have been made in understanding viral hepatitis during the past 25 years are just now being translated into means of preventing and treating this disease. Serologic markers have been developed for all five forms of viral hepatitis and promise to have a major effect in preventing post-transfusion hepatitis and defining the epidemiology, natural history, and means of controlling sporadic viral hepatitis. A highly effective hepatitis B vaccine made from plasma has been available since 1982 and a "second-generation," recombinant hepatitis B vaccine since 1986.[19] Recently, experimental vaccines against hepatitis A have been developed and are being evaluated in selected human populations. Therapies for chronic viral hepatitis have been developed and are now under investigation as treatment for acute hepatitis. Such advances hold promise for the ultimate goal of controlling this common and serious infection.

CLINICAL MANIFESTATIONS

Symptoms

Acute viral hepatitis is such a sufficiently distinct clinical syndrome that it usually poses no difficult in diagnosis. It is conveniently separated into four stages: incubation period, preicteric phase, icteric phase, and convalescence. The timing and major symptoms of each of these stages are shown diagrammatically in Figure 1.

The incubation period of acute viral hepatitis varies from as short as a few weeks to as long as 6 months. The incubation period of type A hepatitis averages 30 days (range, 15–45 days), that of type B hepatitis averages 70 days (range, 30–180 days), that of classic non-A, non-B hepatitis averages 50 days (range, 15–150 days), and that of epidemic non-A, non-B hepatitis averages 40 days (range, 15–60 days). The incubation period of delta hepatitis has not been well documented. Because delta hepatitis invariably occurs in conjunction with type B hepatitis, its incubation period probably is similar.

The initial symptoms of acute hepatitis are nonspecific; in the typical case, the patient develops malaise and weakness, followed shortly by anorexia, intermittent nausea, vomiting, and a vague, dull, right upper quadrant pain. These symptoms of the preicteric phase usually last 3–10 days. The onset of jaundice and/or dark urine then ushers in the icteric phase. It is these symptoms that usually bring the patient to the doctor—the iatrogenic stimulus. The duration of icterus is, of course, quite variable; but, it usually lasts 1–3 weeks. In the average case, the patient often will begin to feel better quite soon after jaundice appears; the appetitie returns, nausea abates, and a sense of well-being returns, even while jaundice persists. Ma-

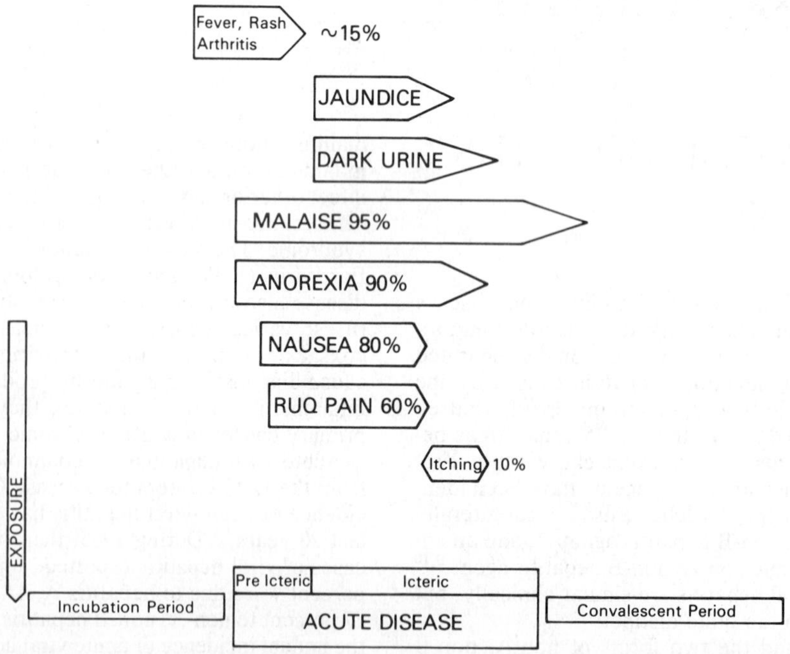

FIG. 1. The course of acute viral hepatitis. The timing and frequency of the major symptoms of viral hepatitis are shown.

laise usually is the last symptom to disappear, often concurrent with or shortly before jaundice clears.

While this may represent the "typical" case, one must stress that such cases probably represent a minority of hepatitis virus infections. The most characteristic feature of viral hepatitis is the variability of clinical expression. Icteric cases (which, for convenience, can be defined as those with a bilirubin level of ≥2.5 mg/dl, the approximate level at which jaundice can be visually detected) account for only 20–50 percent of hepatitis virus infections. The remainder pass unnoticed, without symptoms or with such mild and few symptoms that they are dismissed as inconsequential ("indigestion" or "the flu"). The spectrum of hepatitis virus infections ranges from inapparent to anicteric (but symptomatic) to icteric to fulminant. Any discussion of the clinical manifestations of viral hepatitis must take into account that only a part of this spectrum is being described.

The *onset* of viral hepatitis either can be sudden (most typical of type A hepatitis) or insidious (more typical of type B or non-A, non-B hepatitis), but it usually can be dated quite well. *Malaise* is no doubt the earliest, most common (~95 percent) and reliable symptom of this disease. It is variously reported as weakness, lethargy, easy fatigability, drowsiness, or just feeling low or ill. It usually is the first symptom to appear and the last to leave. *Anorexia* is almost as frequent (~90 percent) as malaise in symptomatic viral hepatitis, but it typically is one of the first symptoms to abate. It also assumes several forms—lack of desire for food, change in food preferences, easy satiety, or the provocation of nausea, indigestion, or abdominal pain by smell, taste, or ingestion of food. The end result is decreased food intake; weight loss of 5–20 lb (2–10 kg) is common during viral hepatitis. A loss of the taste for cigarettes is another form of the anorexia or dysgeusia of acute hepatitis. While it is said to be typical of acute viral hepatitis, this symptom actually is characteristic of any acute liver disease. *Nausea* and vomiting occur in about 80 percent of the patients with symptomatic viral hepatitis. The nausea is typically intermittent and rarely intractable. Nausea, as with malaise, may be absent early in the day and then appear and worsen as the day progresses. Abdominal *pain* can accompany acute viral hepatitis (~60 percent), and it usually consists of a dull, right upper quadrant, aching discomfort. It usually is not severe and is unaffected by meals, antacids, stool patterns, or position.

At least 25 percent of the patients with viral hepatitis describe the onset of their disease as an "influenza-like" illness with weakness, headaches, myalgias, chilliness, and fever. This onset is most common with type A hepatitis. The *headaches* are generalized, dull, and mild to moderate. *Fever*, if present, is low grade. In some instances, symptoms of an upper respiratory infection such as a sore throat and cough may be present. These symptoms are short-lived (1–3 days) and are replaced by the more typical symptoms of anorexia, nausea, and then jaundice. Fever, in particular, rarely persists into the icteric phase. Jaundice with high fever is *not* characteristic of viral hepatitis.

A smaller percentage of patients with acute hepatitis (5–10 percent) experience a "serum sickness-like syndrome" at the onset of their illness.[20] This consist of a triad of symptoms—fever, rash, and arthritis. This syndrome occurs during the preicteric phase and almost invariably will resolve dramatically with the onset of jaundice. *Fever* is usual but not invariable. The *rash* is typically urticarial, with pruritic hives appearing and disappearing in a largely peripheral distribution. More exanthem-like macular-papular lesions can also occur as well as fleeting irregular patches of erythema. The *arthritis* is mild to moderate, nondeforming, polyarticular, migratory. Major joints involved are the elbows, wrists, knees, and small joints of the hands. Arthralgias probably are more common than frank arthritis. This syndrome is most common with type B hepatitis, but it also has been reported in type A and in non-A, non-B hepatitis. It probably is a manifestation of immune complex (virus/antibody) deposition. In children with type B hepatitis, a condition perhaps related to this syndrome has been described—papular acrodermatitis (Gianotti's disease).[21] Isolated reports of other manifestations such as Raynaud's phenomenon, bullous formation, and erythema nodosum also have been described in acute hepatitis (but are rare).

Jaundice and dark urine are the most distinctive symptoms of this disease, but they can be unreliable. Many patients (and some physicians) may not recognize scleral icterus, even with a serum bilirubin level as high as 10 mg/dl. *Dark urine* often is more noticeable than scleral icterus, because the urine can turn dark before the icterus is visible. Dark urine also is helpful in indicating that the jaundice is accompanied by conjugated (direct) hyperbilirubinemia (not found with jaundice due to hemolysis or Gilbert syndrome). While jaundice and dark urine usually occur after a 4- to 10-day preicteric phase, some patients have jaundice only and deny any prodrome of malaise, anorexia, or nausea. Light stools also can occur with the jaundice of viral hepatitis, reflecting the absence of bile pigments being added to the intestinal contents. The lightening of stool color in viral hepatitis, however, usually is not as great as in obstructive jaundice, and white or chalky stools are uncommon. Persons with prominent jaundice will also often complain of *pruritus*. Approximately 40 percent of jaundiced patients will complain of itching at the peak of icterus or sometime into convalescence.

Diarrhea or *constipation* can occur during acute viral hepatitis, but they usually are not prominent. These changes in bowel habits may reflect changes in activity or diet rather than an effect of the viral infection.

Fulminant viral hepatitis is defined by the appearance of symptoms and signs of hepatic failure or encephalopathy during the course of viral hepatitis. Fulminant hepatic failure can occur at any time—early or late—during the course of the disease. The first symptoms usually are *lethargy*, *somnolence*, and a *change in personality*. There may be abnormal behavior with an unexpected display of sexual or aggressive activity or a subtle change in personality with untidiness, mild confusion, or a loss of the usual inhibitions. Patients may be excited, euphoric, and unruly. These symptoms are followed in more severe cases by *stupor* and then *coma*.

Physical Findings

The physical findings in acute viral hepatitis are few. In general, the patient may appear acutely but not chronically ill. Acute hepatitis, by and large, is a disease of the healthy; wasting or undernutrition are not part of this disease. The patient usually is afebrile. Vital signs are normal, although bradycardia can occur when significant hyperbilirubinemia is present. Icterus can be detected if the billirubin level exceeds 2.5–3.0 mg/dl. It is seen most easily in the sclera or under the tongue. In light-skinned people, the skin may have a yellowish hue. Natural light is mandatory in assessing mild degrees of jaundice. Also, a deliberate search for icterus should be included in the physician's evaluation of every ill patient.

The abdomen appears grossly normal. Bowel sounds are present. Palpation often demonstrates an enlarged and slightly tender liver. However, in acute viral hepatitis, the liver usually is only modestly enlarged (9–13 cm in breadth by percussion), and its edge is smooth, regular, and firm (not flabby or hard). Tenderness can be elicited by direct palpation of the edge or by gentle percussion of the lower ribs with the fist (comparing the right with the left side). A spleen tip is felt in 5–25 percent of the patients. Signs of portal hypertension (ascites, edema, prominent splenomegaly, abdominal venous patterns) are not seen in acute hepatitis except in late, severe disease (as with subacute hepatic necrosis). The rest of the examination is rarely helpful. Adenopathy, if present, is not prominent.

There are several skin findings in acute viral hepatitis. Vascular spiders often are found in light-skinned persons, but they are few and small. Excoriations will occur with severe pruritus. Multiple forearm venipuncture marks can suggest drug addiction, a common source of hepatitis virus infection. Patients with the serum sickness-like syndrome will have urticaria or a mild, fleeting erythematous rash and (occasionally) red, warm, and tender joints. Finally, acne-prone persons may exhibit an exacerbation of this condition with acute hepatitis, especially during recovery.

When fulminant hepatitis supervenes, signs of hepatic encephalopathy appear. These consist of lethargy, somnolence, untidiness, confusion, forgetfulness, and then stupor and full coma. Typical of hepatic encephalopathy is asterixis—the asynchronous irregular flapping of the forcibly dorsiflexed, outstretched hands. In stage I coma, mild mental changes are present, but asterixis is minimal or absent. Stage II coma is marked by worsening of mental changes and definite asterixis. In stage III coma, the patient develops stupor and semicoma but can still be roused. With stage IV coma, the patient no longer is arousable, and there may or may not be a response to deep pain stimuli. Patients with hepatic failure may demonstrate other neurologic signs—flapping of the tongue, involuntary movements, long-tract signs, and decerebrate posturing. They also may demonstrate the sweetish smell of fetor hepaticus.

Laboratory Findings

While the symptoms and signs of acute viral hepatitis are frequently nonspecific or vague, laboratory findings are quite characteristic. The typical ranges of key serum enzyme and bilirubin levels in acute viral hepatitis and other common liver diseases are shown in Figure 2. Most distinctive of viral hepatitis are the dramatic elevations in the *aminotransferases*—asparate aminotransferase (AST, SGOT) and alanine aminotransferase (ALT, SGPT). In acute viral hepatitis, concentrations of the two aminotransferases are both elevated (usually greater than eight times normal when jaundice appears) and to the same degree.[22] The ALT level is the most important because this serum enzyme is quite specific for liver injury (it also may be slightly elevated in muscle disease). In acute hepatitis, the ALT level usually is as high or higher than the AST (although above 20–40 times normal this distinction is less reliable). The *alkaline phosphatase* and other serum enzyme levels that denote biliary obstruction or cholestasis (leucine aminopeptidase, 5′-nucleotidase) are only mildly elevated (one to three times normal). The *lactic dehydrogenase* (LDH) concentration usually is mildly elevated in acute viral hepatitis (one to three times normal). The *creatine phosphokinase* (CPK) level, which is elevated in muscle and heart injury, is normal in viral hepatitis. Indeed, the dramatic elevation of both AST and ALT levels, with only mild elevation in alkaline phosphatase and LDH levels, is virtually diagnostic of "acute hepatitis" or "acute necroinflammatory disease of the liver." Given this enzyme pattern, one need then only to resolve whether this acute hepatitis is due to a hepatitis virus, a hepatotoxic drug, a toxin, or a nonspecific liver injury (anoxia, shock, or severe heart failure).

The AST and ALT levels become abnormal during the late incubation period of this disease. They are invariably abnormal once symptoms occur, usually rise during the preicteric phase, and peak early in the icteric phase. With recovery, the aminotransferase levels quickly fall but almost always remain slightly abnormal for several weeks after the jaundice and symptoms have abated.

The *bilirubin* level is variably elevated in icteric viral hepatitis. This elevation involves both the direct and indirect fractions, with the ratio being approximately 1:1. Disproportionate elevations in direct bilirubin concentration suggest cholestasis, whereas the preponderance of indirect bilirubin (≥80 percent)

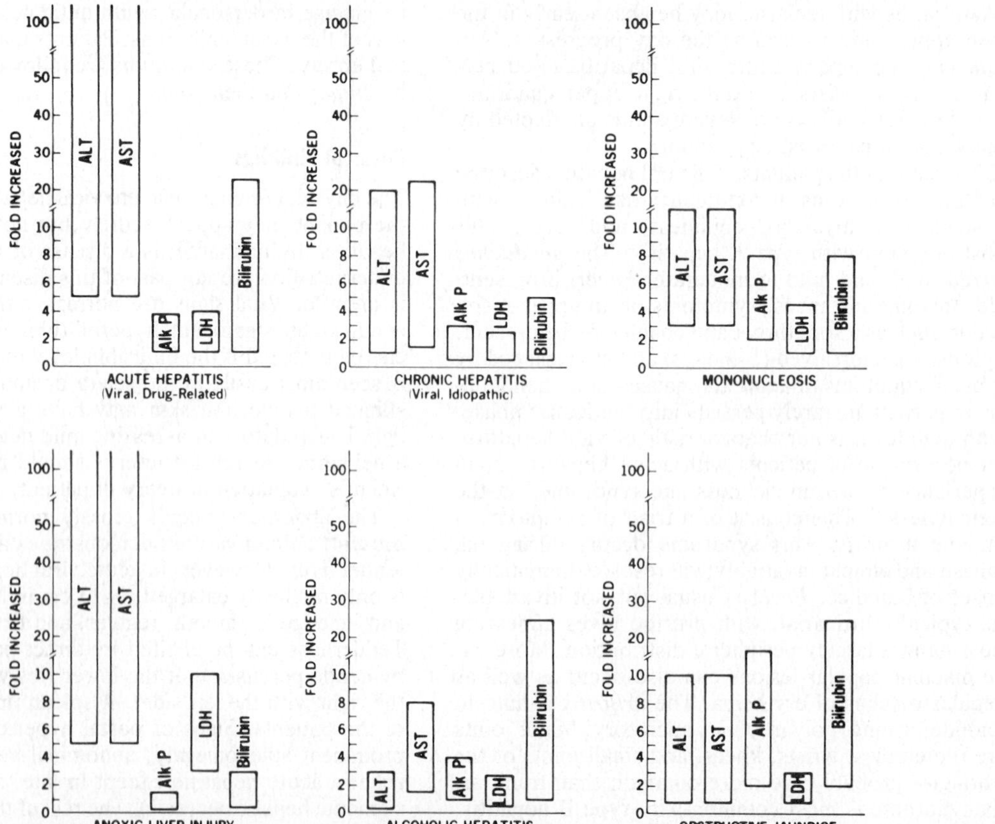

FIG. 2. The range of elevation of key serum enzyme levels in acute viral hepatitis, and other common liver diseases. ALT: alanine aminotransferase; AST: asparate aminotransferase; Alk P: alkaline phosphate; LDH: lactic dehydrogenase.

suggests hemolysis. Persons with underlying hemolytic states (glucose-6-phosphate dehydrogenase [G6PD] deficiency or thalassemia minor) may suffer accelerated hemolysis with many viral infections and especially viral hepatitis.[23] These persons may become markedly jaundiced and yet have relatively mild symptoms and aminotransferase level elevations.

The *prothrombin time* generally is normal in typical acute viral hepatitis, but it is invariably elevated in fulminant hepatitis. Abnormalities in the prothrombin time are the most reliable indicators of prognosis in acute hepatitis. Any elevation should be regarded as a serious sign. The *partial thromboplastin time* is not as sensitive or reliable a measure as the prothrombin time. Assays for the separate liver-synthesized coagulation factors (e.g., factors V, VII, and X) may be more sensitive and reliable measures of liver dysfunction than the prothrombin time. However, they are technically demanding and expensive, and their relative advantages have yet to be proved.

The *serum albumin* and *globulin* levels usually are normal in acute viral hepatitis. While the serum albumin level may fall and the serum globulin level may rise slightly during the course of the disease, this pattern of low albumin and high globulin levels should point once more toward a diagnosis of chronic liver disease.

Other laboratory test results rarely are abnormal. *Hemoglobin* and hematocrit values remain normal (decreased values should suggest hemolysis, chronic liver disease, or unrelated anemia). A *white blood cell count* is either normal or slightly low. A mild lymphocytosis can occur. The *platelet count* remains normal except with fulminant hepatitis, in which case disseminated intravascular coagulation can supervene.

Patients with acute viral hepatitis often develop low levels of anti-DNA and smooth muscle antibodies (SMA). Biologic false-positive VDRL test reactions are rare. Tests for other "autoantibodies" (rheumatoid factor, antinuclear antibody, lupus erythematosus phenomenon, and so on) usually are negative or normal. The sedimentation rate is normal or minimally elevated. Serum *complement* levels can be depressed in the preicteric phase of illness, especially in those patients with the serum sickness-like syndrome of polyarthritis, fever, and rash.[20] Serum *immunoglobulin* levels usually are normal except in type A hepatitis, in which case the serum IgM level may double during the course of the disease.

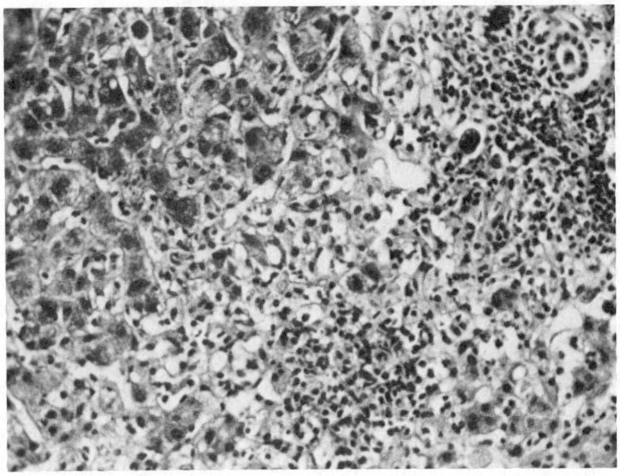

FIG. 3. Liver biopsy specimen from a patient with acute viral hepatitis. Note the lobular disarray, the occurrence of eosinophilic degeneration, free hyaline bodies, and spotty hepatocellular necrosis and the prominent mononuclear cell infiltrates in the portal zone and areas of parenchyma. (H&E, ×240) (Photomicrograph courtesy of Dr. Kamal Ishak, Washington, DC:AFIP negative No. 65-12490.)

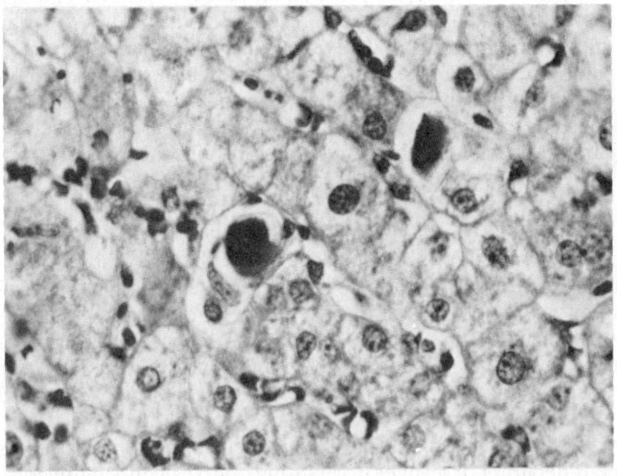

FIG. 4. The free hyaline body and eosinophilic generation typical of acute viral hepatitis. (H&E, ×660) (Photomicrograph courtesy of Dr. Kamal Ishak, Washington, DC:AFIP negative No. 68-8127.)

Pathologic Findings

The clinical history and pattern of serum enzyme levels in acute viral hepatitis are sufficiently characteristic that a percutaneous liver biopsy specimen is rarely necessary for diagnosis. However, when several possible causes of acute liver disease are present or when therapy is a consideration, a liver biopsy specimen can be helpful. The typical liver biopsy findings of acute viral hepatitis are the following: (*1*) lobular disarray, (*2*) ballooning and eosinophilic degeneration, (*3*) liver cell necrosis, (*4*) mononuclear cell infiltration of the parenchyma and portal tracts, and (*5*) variable degrees of cholestasis.[24] These changes are diffuse and generalized; therefore, sampling error from needle biopsy usually is not a problem. Lobular disarray refers to a loss of the orderly pattern of hepatic sinusoidal cords, the result of widespread anisocytosis, liver cell degeneration, regeneration, or death (Fig. 3). Liver cells demonstrate two forms of degeneration: ballooning degeneration (in which there is swelling of the liver cell and rarefaction of the cytoplasm) and eosinophilic degeneration (in which the cell shrinks and becomes a deeper red and more angular). The end result of eosinophilic degeneration is the free hyaline body (Fig. 4). There also may be "smudging" of hepatocytes with indistinctness of cell outline as well as cell "dropout"—with or without associated inflammatory cell reaction. Küpffer cells appear to be more numerous and enlarged. Areas of lymphocytic infiltration are common both in the parenchyma and in portal tracts. Polymorphonuclear leukocytes are not numerous. A few plasma cells and eosinophils may be found, but a prominence of portal tract plasma cells suggests chronic hepatitis; also, unusual numbers of eosinophils suggest drug addiction or a drug-related hepatitis. Cholestasis (bile staining of liver cells and bile "plugs") may be seen on liver biopsy specimens and generally correspond in degree to the height of the serum bilirubin level. The portal bile ducts, however, usually appear to be normal.

In typical viral hepatitis, cell necrosis is spotty and focal. More severe hepatitis may be accompanied by coalescent or bridging necrosis (between portal zones or from portal zones to central veins), multilobular necrosis, or massive necrosis.[24,25] Bridging necrosis found during acute viral hepatitis indicates a serious lesion that can progress to postnecrotic cirrhosis. Multilobular or massive necrosis is seen in severe and fulminant disease.

Fluorescence and electron microscopy of liver biopsy specimens in acute viral hepatitis rarely is helpful. Viral antigens and particles can be found in liver tissue during type A, type

B, and delta hepatitides. However, the techniques to detect these antigens in tissue are less sensitive and far more difficult than are the available serologic tests for viral antigens and antibodies in serum.[26]

DIFFERENTIAL DIAGNOSIS

Diseases that need to be excluded in the differential diagnosis of acute viral hepatitis are not so much other infectious diseases as other forms of liver disease (e.g., alcoholic hepatitis, cholecystitis, and Gilbert syndrome). The first step in the differential diagnosis should be the demonstration that acute necroinflammatory disease (acute hepatitis) is present. This distinction is based largely on the pattern of serum enzyme concentrations—dramatic elevations in aminotransferase levels with mild elevations in the alkaline phosphatase level. The second step in the differential diagnosis should be the exclusion of the nonviral causes of acute hepatitis. These include bacterial infections (pneumococcal pneumonia, leptospirosis), various drugs (acetaminophen, isoniazid), toxins (carbon tetrachloride), and nonspecific injury (shock, heart failure). These types of acute hepatitis usually can be excluded by a careful history with some support from laboratory data. Finally, with viral hepatitis diagnosed, the third step should be the identification of the responsible viral agent and the source of infection. Most cases of acute viral hepatitis are caused by one of five agents: HAV, HBV, delta, and the agents of non-A, non-B hepatitis. The diseases that these agents cause are quite similar. They overlap so much in symptoms and severity that they cannot be distinguished on clinical grounds, by biochemical tests, or even by liver biopsy findings. Fortunately, specific serologic assays and (in certain circumstances) typical epidemiologic features can separate and identify these five types of viral hepatitis.

Type A Hepatitis

Hepatitis A has certain clinical features that may help to distinguish it from other forms of acute viral hepatitis. In general, it is an acute self-limited disease. Type A hepatitis characteristically has an acute, sudden, influenza-like onset with a prominence of myalgia, headache, fever, and malaise.[1,27,28] This type of onset is less common with type B, delta, and non-A, non-B hepatitides, which tend to have a more gradual, insidious onset. Type A hepatitis usually is not as severe or as long lasting as type B hepatitis. However, a relapsing course occurs more commonly in hepatitis A than in other forms.[29] Furthermore, a prolonged cholestasis appearing late in the acute phase and lasting for several months is most typical of hepatitis A.[30] Both of these unusual forms of hepatitis A are often benign; the mortality rate of hepatitis A is low (~2/1000),[28] and the disease ultimately resolves. Hepatitis A does not lead to a chronic hepatitis or a carrier state.[31]

Epidemiologic features can be helpful in distinguishing hepatitis A from other forms of viral hepatitis.[11,32] Type A hepatitis is spread predominantly by the fecal–oral route. It is highly contagious and spreads rapidly. Type A hepatitis can occur in outbreaks that may have an identifiable point source (often a person in the incubation period of acute disease). Type A hepatitis has been shown to be spread (*1*) by contaminated water, milk, or food[33]; (*2*) after a breakdrown in the usual sanitary conditions or after floods or natural disasters[34]; (*3*) by the ingestion of raw or undercooked shellfish (oysters, clams, and mussels) from contaminated waters[34]; (*4*) during travel to areas of the world with poor hygienic conditions where hepatitis A is endemic[35]; (*5*) in institutionalized children and adults[1]; and (*6*) after exposure to recently imported chimpanzees or apes.[36]

Three other epidemiologic sources have recently been shown to be important in the spread of hepatitis A: exposure to children in day care centers,[32,37] male homosexuality,[38] and intravenous drug addiction.[11,32] Day care centers can serve as sources of outbreaks of hepatitis A—especially when there are children who are still not toilet trained in the centers. Male homosexuals have a high incidence of hepatitis A that probably is related to high degrees of promiscuity and practices of oral–anal and genital–anal intercourse. Drug addicts have recently been found to have a high incidence of hepatitis A, which may relate more to socioeconomic and hygienic standards than to the repeated parenteral exposures that occur with drug abuse. Yet, despite all these epidemiologic features, hepatitis A may be difficult to distinguish from other forms of viral hepatitis, and some cases occur without any known point source of infection. Blood transfusion is a very rare mode of transmission of hepatitis A.[11]

Unless hepatitis occurs as a part of a clear-cut epidemic with a definable incubation period, it usually is not possible to reliably diagnose hepatitis A without specific serologic assays. The serologic course of a typical case of hepatitis A is shown in Figure 5. Hepatitis A virus (HAV) and hepatitis A antigen can be detected in the stool during both the incubation period and early symptomatic phase of illness. Levels of virus in stool usually are decreasing and no longer may be detectable at the time of the onset of jaundice. Antibody to HAV (anti-HAV) is detectable in serum by the time of the onset of disease. Initially, the anti-HAV consists of both IgG and IgM class antibodies. After 3–12 months, IgM anti-HAV disappears, whereas IgG anti-HAV persists in high titer. Indeed, IgG anti-HAV seems to be long lasting and is associated with lifelong immunity. The diagnosis of acute hepatitis A can be made by the finding of IgM anti-HAV in a patient with either clinical symptoms or biochemical evidence of acute hepatitis.[39] Immunoassays are now available for IgM anti-HAV and for total anti-HAV. These assays allow for both diagnosis (IgM anti-HAV) as well as assessment of immunity (total anti-HAV) to hepatitis A.

Several research assays such as radioimmunoassay for hepatitis A antigen in serum and stool,[2] identification of virion HAV RNA in serum and stool,[29] direct culture of HAV in susceptible cell lines, and assay for neutralizing anti-HAV[28] have proved to be invaluable in study of the biology, natural history, and pathogenesis of hepatitis A but are not generally available for use in routine clinical settings.

Type B Hepatitis

Type B hepatitis appears to be a more serious disease than type A hepatitis, and it has a definite propensity to chronicity. It usually has a more insidious onset and a more prolonged course than type A hepatitis. In the individual case, however, type B

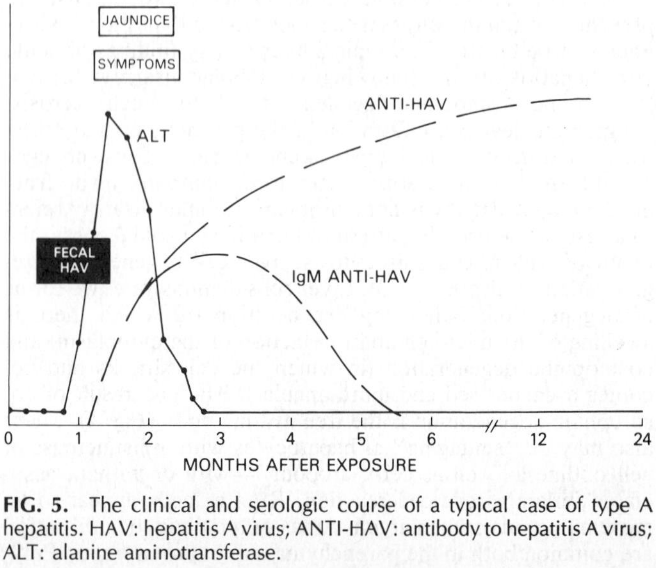

FIG. 5. The clinical and serologic course of a typical case of type A hepatitis. HAV: hepatitis A virus; ANTI-HAV: antibody to hepatitis A virus; ALT: alanine aminotransferase.

hepatitis cannot be distinguished from type A hepatitis or from non-A, non-B hepatitis on clinical grounds alone. The occurrence of the serum sickness-like syndrome of fever, rash, and polyarthritis during the preicteric phase favors the diagnosis of type B hepatitis (but also occurs in non-A, non-B hepatitis).

Epidemiologic features can strongly suggest hepatitis B virus (HBV) infection. This disease has a long incubation period (40–180 days) and is more likely to occur as sporadic rather than epidemic hepatitis.[1] It is spread predominantly by the parenteral route. Thus, type B hepatitis often occurs in persons with exposure to blood or blood products (multiply transfused patients, hemophiliacs, renal dialysis, and oncology ward patients), with exposure to contaminated needles and syringes (medical personnel with accidental needlesticks, drug addicts), with multiple sexual contacts (homosexuals, prostitutes, the sexually active),[40] and with exposure to saliva or other potentially infectious excreta (children in institutions for the mentally retarded).[1]

However, these same epidemiologic features also can be found in cases of non-A, non-B hepatitis and (occasionally) also in type A hepatitis. In at least 50 percent of acute type B hepatitis cases, no history of parenteral exposure is uncovered. Whether these cases were acquired by "nonparenteral" routes or by inapparent parenteral routes is not known.

The diagnosis of type B hepatitis should rest on specific serologic testing, with the finding of hepatitis B surface antigen (HBsAg) in the serum during the acute disease (Fig. 6). HBsAg appears in the serum during the incubation period 2–7 weeks before the onset of symptoms. It usually persists in the blood throughout the illness and disappears with convalescence.[41,42] Almost all patients (95 percent) will be HBsAg-positive at the onset of symptoms and jaundice. In some patients, however, HBsAg is cleared rapidly and may be absent by the time the patient is tested. In this situation, tests for antibody must be used to make this diagnosis. Antibody to HBsAg (anti-HBs) usually arises during convalescence from type B hepatitis and, indeed, may not be detectable for some time into the recovery phase. Antibody to hepatitis B core antigen (anti-HBc) is a more reliable marker of HBV infection and usually appears at or about the time of onset of symptoms. Sensitive and specific immunoassays are now available for assaying both anti-HBs and anti-HBc. However, neither of these assays are particulary helpful in the serodiagnosis of acute type B hepatitis. Both anti-HBs and anti-HBc are long-lived. The finding of either of these antibodies in the serum of a patient with acute hepatitis does not prove that the disease is due to HBV infection. Recently, immunoassays for IgM anti-HBc have been developed that promise to be of some help in the diagnosis of type B hepatitis. IgM anti-HBc arises early in the illness of patients with acute type B hepatitis, but it rapidly decreases in titer and no longer may be detectable 6–24 months after the illness.[43] Both false-positive and false-negative results can occur with the IgM anti-HBc test, but they are rare.

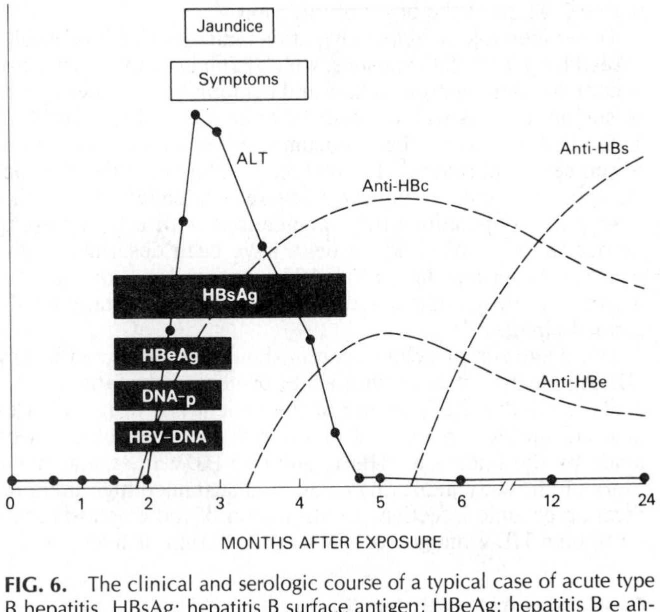

FIG. 6. The clinical and serologic course of a typical case of acute type B hepatitis. HBsAg: hepatitis B surface antigen; HBeAg: hepatitis B e antigen; DNA-p: DNA polymerase; HBV-DNA: hepatitis B virus DNA; ALT: alanine aminotransferase; Anti-HBc: antibody to hepatitis B core antigen; anti-HBe: antibody to HBeAg; anti-HBs: antibody to HBsAg.

Patients with acute type B hepatitis also develop hepatitis B e–antigen (HBeAg) as well as direct markers for the presence of HBV in serum such as HBV-DNA (as detected by molecular hybridization) and DNA polymerase (the endogenous polymerase of this virus). These are markers of active viral replication and are detected early in the course of acute hepatitis. By the peak of clinical illness and jaundice, levels of HBV in serum usually are decreasing or absent. Indeed, the seroconversion from HBeAg to antibody to HBeAg (anti-HBe) can be considered a favorable serologic sign indicating that the height of the viral replication has passed and that the infection is on the wane.

From 5 to 10 percent of patients with HBV infection do not clear HBsAg but become HBsAg carriers.[1,42] These people typically have mild, often anicteric and asymptomatic disease, which may explain why most chronic HBsAg carriers do not give a history of acute hepatitis. As many as 0.2–1.0 percent of adults in the United States are chronic HBsAg carriers. The prevalence of the carrier state is even higher in "high-risk" populations such as male homosexuals (6 percent), iv drug abusers (7 percent), hemophiliacs (7 percent), and renal dialysis patients (2–15 percent).[42] Most chronic HBsAg carriers are asymptomatic of their infection and have minimal or no accompanying liver injury.

The development of the chronic HBsAg carrier state as a result of symptomatic acute viral hepatitis is not common, but it does occur. Progression to a chronic carrier state should be suspected if the patient remains HBeAg-positive or if HBsAg titers do not decrease for more than 8 weeks after the onset of illness.[41]

The presence of the chronic HBsAg carrier state also can create diagnostic confusion in the serodiagnosis of acute viral hepatitis. A patient with acute viral hepatitis who is HBsAg-positive does not necessarily have acute type B hepatitis; the patient may be a chronic HBsAg carrier and have a superimposed and unrelated form of acute liver injury. This possibility is not as unlikely as it may seem. People who are at high risk for developing type B hepatitis and, therefore, the chronic HBsAg carrier state often are at high risk for developing other forms of acute viral hepatitis. Indeed, delta hepatitis represents just this phenomenon of an acute viral hepatitis being superimposed on the chronic HBsAg carrier state.[6] In this situation, testing for IgM anti-HBc can be helpful. This marker of acute type B hepatitis should be absent if the patient is a chronic HBsAg carrier with another form of acute hepatocellular injury.[43]

Delta Hepatitis

The delta agent was discovered in 1977 by Rizzetto and coworkers from Turin, Italy.[5] Subsequently, delta hepatitis has been shown to be caused by the delta hepatitis virus (HDV), an incomplete RNA virus that requires HBsAg for replication.[6,44] Delta infection occurs only in patients who have HBsAg in their serum and thus have either acute or chronic HBV infection. In the United States and Western Europe, delta hepatitis occurs most commonly in persons who have multiple parenteral exposures such as iv drug addicts, hemophiliacs, and persons who have multiple transfusions.[44] Delta infection is uncommon in medical care workers and male homosexuals. There are several areas of the world with a high prevalence of delta infection among carriers in the general population, including the Amazon Basin in South America, Central Africa, southern Italy, and Middle Eastern countries. Why delta infection became established among HBsAg carriers in those areas of the world and not in others such as China and Southeast Asia (where hepatitis B is very common) is not known.

Acute delta infection occurs in two forms depending upon the state of the underlying HBV infection: (*1*) as a coinfection in which acute delta hepatitis occurs simultaneously with acute hepatitis B (Fig. 7) and (*2*) as a superinfection in which acute delta hepatitis is superimposed upon chronic hepatitis B (Fig. 8).[45] Delta antigen can sometimes be detected in the serum during the early phase of acute delta hepatitis; with the disappearance of antigen, anti-HDV arises.[46] However, the appearance of anti-HDV may be delayed, short-lived, and low in titer. Thus, many patients with acute delta hepatitis will test negative for anti-HDV during the acute illness and will only become positive in convalescence and then only in low titer. A radioimmunoassay for anti-HDV is commercially available,[47] but anti-HDV tests are not always reliable for the diagnosis of acute HDV infection.

Most patients with acute delta coinfection recover; as the hepatitis B resolves and HBsAg is cleared from the serum, the HDV infection also resolves. Thus, fewer than 5 percent of cases of acute delta coinfection result in chronic delta hepatitis. In contrast, most patients with acute delta superinfection are left with chronic delta hepatitis; because HBsAg persists, the HDV infection can persist. More than 70 percent of cases of delta superinfection result in chronic hepatitis (Fig. 8).[46] The diagnosis of chronic is easier than that of acute delta hepatitis; high titers of anti-HDV (>1:100 by commerical radioimmunoassay) indicate ongoing delta infection. Furthermore, patients with chronic delta hepatitis will have HDV antigen in the liver and persistence of IgM anti-HDV in serum.[46] HDV antigen is readily detectable in liver when using immunoperoxidase techniques.

Recently, two new research assays have provided new information regarding the natural history and biology of HDV infection: tests of HDV antigen in serum and liver by using Western blotting (immunoblotting)[48] and tests for HDV RNA in serum and liver by using molecular hybridization with a cloned cDNA or RNA ("riboprobe").[49] The finding of HDV antigen or RNA in serum is a direct demonstration of the presence of virus and documents active viral replication. Hepatitis D virus antigen and RNA are typically present transiently during the early phases of acute delta hepatitis and for prolonged periods in chronic delta hepatitis. The sensitivity of these assays is still not well documented; only 50–80 percent of patients with chronic delta hepatitis (as shown by the presence of delta antigen in liver by immunoperoxidase) have detectable HDV antigen or RNA in their serum.

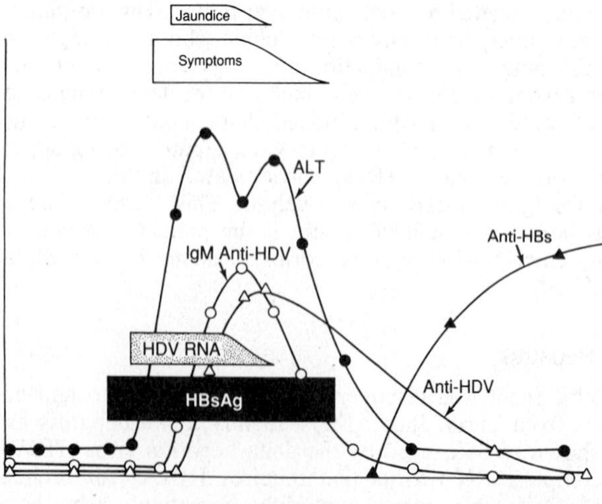

FIG. 7. The clinical and serologic course of a typical case of acute delta coinfection. ALT: alanine aminotransferase; HDV: hepatitis delta virus; HBsAg: hepatitis B surface antigen; anti-HBs: antibody to HBsAg; anti-HDV: antibody to HDV.

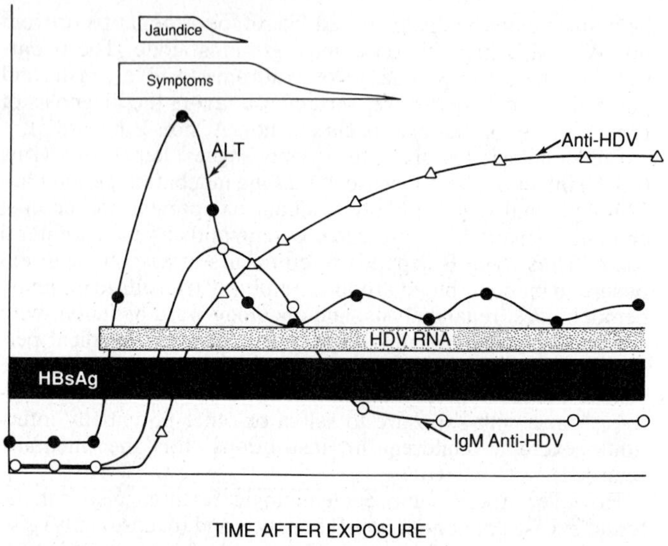

FIG. 8. The clinical and serologic course of a typical case of acute delta superinfection that leads to chronic delta hepatitis. ALT: alanine aminotransferase; HDV: hepatitis delta virus; HBsAg: hepatitis B surface antigen; Anti-HDV: antibody to HDV.

Clinically, delta hepatitis tends to be a severe illness. Acute delta hepatitis has a mortality of 2–20 percent.[44] The illness also often has a biphasic and protracted course. Chronic delta hepatitis is also a severe illness and is more likely to result in serious morbidity or mortality than is chronic hepatitis B alone or non-A, non-B hepatitis. In large series, 60–70 percent of patients with chronic delta hepatitis eventually developed cirrhosis, and most of these patients died of liver disease.[50] The progression to cirrhosis usually takes 10–15 years, but it can be quite rapid, within 2 years of the onset of infection.[44]

The epidemiology of delta hepatitis indicates that it is usually spread by parenteral exposure, which explains why this disease is common among drug addicts and hemophiliacs. Other modes of spread are less well defined. In some areas of the world intrafamilial spread has been documented as well as spread between sexual partners.[51] Interestingly, delta hepatitis often occurs in indolent, prolonged, severe epidemics that strike susceptible populations (i.e., populations with a high HBsAg carrier rate).[14] Epidemics of delta have been described in the Amazon basin and in central Africa, as well as among communities of drug addicts and institutionalized, mentally handicapped children.[44]

The diagnosis of delta hepatitis should be suspected in any HBsAg-positive patient with acute or chronic hepatitis, especially if the disease is severe or the patient is a drug addict or has had multiple parenteral exposures. The diagnosis can be made by the finding of HBsAg and anti-HDV in serum: rising titers of antibody indicating acute, and sustained high titers indicating chronic infection. Confirmation of the diagnosis rests on finding HDV antigen or RNA in the serum or liver.

Classic Non-A, Non-B Hepatitis

Non-A, non-B hepatitis is defined as an acute or chronic viral hepatitis-like syndrome in which serologic evidence of HAV or

HBV infection does not appear and no other cause of liver injury is apparent.[52,53] Despite attempts to identify the non-A, non-B hepatitis agent by many investigators during the last 15 years, the etiologic agent of non-A, non-B hepatitis has remained elusive, and the diagnosis is still made by the exclusion of other causes. Fortunately, this situation may soon change. In 1988, Houghton and coworkers from the Chiron Corporation in California announced the identification and cloning of a viral genome that appeared to be related to the agent of classic, parenterally transmitted non-A, non-B hepatitis.[8] By using molecular biologic techniques they developed a radioimmunoassay for antibody to this agent, which they have called the hepatitis C virus (HCV). Preliminary and as yet unpublished data indicated that this assay for anti-HCV successfully identified 50–90 percent of cases of acute and chronic non-A, non-B hepatitis.

Non-A, non-B hepatitis is a form of serum hepatitis. It is the most common cause of post-transfusion hepatitis and is commonly spread by the parenteral route,[52] the disease being frequent among dialysis patients, hemophiliacs, drug addicts, and medical care workers. This disease also occurs sporadically and without obvious parenteral exposure. In recent U.S. surveys, non-A, non-B hepatitis was considered to be the cause of 20–40 percent of cases of sporadic acute viral hepatitis.[32,53,54] Furthermore, analysis of the incidence of non-A, non-B hepatitis resulting from blood transfusion has indicated that as many as 1 percent of American blood donors harbor the agent of non-A, non-B hepatitis.[52] Thus, non-A, non-B hepatitis must be spread by intrafamilial, intimate, or sexual exposure, although proof of such transmission had yet to be demonstrated.

Clinically, non-A, non-B hepatitis is similar to hepatitis B. Approximately 25 percent of cases of acute disease are icteric, and the death rate is less than 1 percent.[52] Non-A, non-B hepatitis has several distinctive clinical and biochemical characteristics. On the average, non-A, non-B hepatitis has a more indolent and prolonged course than hepatitis B does. Serum aminotransferases often fluctuate widely and peak at levels (10–20 times normal) somewhat lower than those in hepatitis B (20–50 times normal) (Fig. 9). Non-A, non-B hepatitis also tends to have an insidious onset and a protracted, relapsing course.

Perhaps the most distinctive feature of non-A, non-B hepatitis is its propensity to progress to chronic hepatitis. In prospective studies, 50–70 percent of persons with acute non-A, non-B hepatitis have been left with biochemical evidence of chronic hepatitis.[52,55] Furthermore, the chronicity rate tends to be just as high after sporadic as after transfusion-related non-A, non-B hepatitis.[54] Chronic non-A, non-B hepatitis tends to be indolent and often silent. However, long-term follow-up studies of patients with this disease have shown that 20–25 percent ultimately develop cirrhosis of the liver.[55] It is often with the development of end-stage liver disease that symptoms first appear. Chronic non-A, non-B hepatitis is one of the major causes of cirrhosis in the United States and ranks as one of the most common indications for liver transplantation in adults.

Advances in knowledge about non-A, non-B hepatitis have been stymied by the lack of a sensitive and specific serologic assay for this infection. The recent development of an assay for anti-HCV promises to correct this lack. Preliminary data indicate that the classic non-A, non-B hepatitis agent (HCV) is a medium-sized (30–60 nm) RNA virus that is present in the blood in acute and chronic infections in low titer. This virus particle has not been visualized, but the genome has been cloned and characterized as a 10.5 kilobase [kb], single-stranded (+) RNA that produces a single polyprotein. Antibody to HCV (anti-HCV) can be detected with immunoassays using an expressed protein from the cDNA clone of this viral genome. Anti-HCV was detected in most cases of non-A, non-B hepatitis. However, the antibody arose rather late in the course of acute disease, often during convalescence. This feature made anti-HCV testing an unreliable diagnostic marker for non-A, non-B hepatitis during the acute illness. Anti-HCV testing was, however, quite reliable in identifying cases of chronic non-A, non-B hepatitis. Preliminary results showed that anti-HCV was detected in 80–90 percent of pedigreed cases of chronic non-A, non-B hepatitis. It follows from these results that screening of donor blood for anti-HCV may identify most infectious donors and make post-transfusion non-A, non-B hepatitis as rare as post-transfusion hepatitis B. Further information regarding these assays for anti-HCV is eagerly awaited, as is the commercial availability of this antibody test.

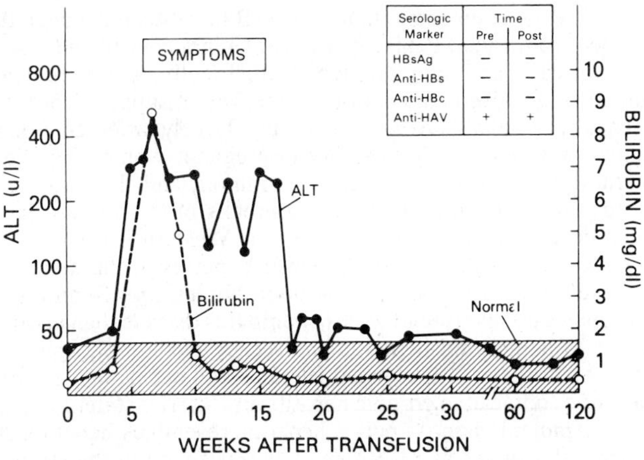

FIG. 9. The clinical and serologic course of a typical case of post-transfusion non-A, non-B hepatitis. ALT: alanine aminotransferase; HBsAg: hepatitis B surface antigen; Anti-HBs: antibody to HBsAg; Anti-HBc: antibody to hepatitis B core antigen; Anti-HAV: antibody to hepatitis A virus.

Epidemic Non-A, Non-B Hepatitis

Not all cases of non-A, non-B hepatitis are associated with parenteral exposure. In recent years, several large outbreaks of viral hepatitis linked to water contamination have been shown to be unrelated to either HBV or HAV infection.[10,56,57] These outbreaks have been studied extensively and shown to be caused by a non-A, non-B hepatitis agent that is distinct from the classic, parenterally transmitted form of disease (Table 1). This disease has been referred to as "epidemic" or "enterally transmitted" non-A, non-B hepatitis. The identification of the virus by immune electron microscopy,[9] the development of serologic assays for antibody to this agent,[58,59] and the announcement that the genome of the virus has been cloned indicate that this agent is distinct from HCV and warrants being referred to as hepatitis E virus (HEV).

TABLE 1. Comparison of Classic and Epidemic Non-A, Non-B Hepatitis

Feature	*Classic*	*Epidemic*
Mode of spread	Parenteral	Enteral
Pattern of spread	Endemic Exposure to blood	Epidemics Water contamination
Viral agent	Unknown	Unknown
Genome	RNA	RNA
Size	30–60 nm	27–34 nm
Location	Serum	Stool
Similarity	HBV-like	HAV-like
Incubation period		
Mean (range)	50 (20–90) days	40 (15–60) days
Mortality	<1%	<1%, but higher in pregnant women
Chronicity	50–70%	None

(Data from Refs. 3, 7, 54–57.)

Outbreaks of epidemic non-A, non-B hepatitis have been described from India, Pakistan, Russia, China, central and northern Africa, Peru, and Mexico.[10] Most outbreaks have been linked to fecal contamination of the water supply. The outbreaks were distinctive in that they largely affected young adults and had a high mortality in pregnant women.[57,58] Secondary cases in families were uncommon, and the outbreaks were generally self-limited. No outbreaks of this disease have been described in the United States or Western Europe.

Clinically, epidemic non-A, non-B hepatitis is characterized as a self-limited disease that is often cholestatic. Serum aminotransferase levels tend to be lower in this disease than in other forms of acute viral hepatitis and serum alkaline phosphatase somewhat higher.[57] Prolonged jaundice can occur, but this disease does not lead to chronic hepatitis or a carrier state. In many ways, epidemic non-A, non-B hepatitis resembles hepatitis A.

The HEV is a small RNA virus that is found in the stool of patients during the incubation period and early acute phase of illness.[9,58] Evidently, the amount of HEV shedding in stool is not as great as the amount of HAV shedding that occurs in hepatitis A. These features may explain why secondary spread of epidemic non-A, non-B hepatitis is uncommon.

Antibody to HEV (anti-HEV) can be detected by immune electron microscopy or by the inhibition of immunofluorescence detection of HEV antigen in hepatocyte cytoplasm.[58,59] Both techniques are cumbersome but have shown that this antibody develops early during the course of illness. Cases of hepatitis associated with large-scale epidemics of non-A, non-B hepatitis have invariably demonstrated the development of anti-HEV. In contrast, none of a large number of cases of sporadic non-A, non-B hepatitis from the United States have demonstrated anti-HEV reactivity. These preliminary results suggest that epidemic non-A, non-B hepatitis, which may be the most common cause of jaundice and acute hepatitis in the underdeveloped world, is a very rare cause of hepatitis in the United States.

Serodiagnosis of Acute Viral Hepatitis

A guide to the serodiagnosis of acute viral hepatitis is given in Table 2. Patients with acute hepatitis should be tested for IgM anti-HAV and HBsAg. The presence of IgM anti-HAV establishes the diagnosis of hepatitis A. The presence of HBsAg suggests the diagnosis of hepatitis B, but two further tests may be helpful to confirm the diagnosis: IgM anti-HBc and anti-HDV. The presence of IgM anti-HBc confirms the diagnosis of *acute* hepatitis B; its absence suggests that the patient is actually a chronic carrier of HBsAg and that the hepatitis is either due to an exacerbation of the underlying chronic hepatitis B or due to superinfection with another hepatitis agent. The presence of anti-HDV suggests the diagnosis of delta hepatitis, although it is not conclusive and does not indicate whether the delta infection is resolved or ongoing, acute or chronic. The titer of anti-HDV can help to separate acute (rising titers) or chronic delta hepatitis (sustained high titers).

Non-A, non-B hepatitis is marked by the absence of IgM anti-HAV, HBsAg, and IgM anti-HBc, but other causes should also be excluded before the diagnosis is made (see below). Tests for anti-HCV and anti-HEV are not currently available. Anti-HCV testing is likely to become a valuable adjunct to serologic diagnosis, but it may not be particularly reliable during the acute illness and may require retesting in convalescence. Anti-HEV testing is rarely necessary because epidemic non-A, non-B hepatitis is uncommon in the United States and can usually be suggested by epidemiologic features such as occurrence in an epidemic or travel to an endemic area.

A careful history and physical examination are of prime importance in diagnosis of the form of viral hepatitis. Often, epidemiologic features or a history of exposure to hepatitis will provide the necessary confirmation of the diagnosis, especially if tests for IgM anti-HAV and HBsAg are negative. Research tests may also be helpful in special situations by providing definitive evidence of the type of hepatitis. These confirmatory research tests include molecular hybridization assays for HAV RNA, HBV DNA and HDV RNA in serum or liver tissue as well as more conventional immunoassays for HAV, HBV, or HDV antigens in liver biopsy samples. Nevertheless, use of the standard, commercially available serologic tests and a careful clinical history should indicate the accurate diagnosis in more than 90 percent of cases of acute hepatitis.

TABLE 2. Serodiagnosis of Acute Viral Hepatitis

IgM Anti-HAV	*HBsAg*	*IgM Anti-HBc*	*Interpretation*
+	−	−	Acute hepatitis A
−	+ (or −)	+	Acute hepatitis B
−	+	−	Chronic hepatitis B[a]
−	−	−	Non-A, non-B hepatitis

[a] In this situation, delta hepatitis should be considered.

Chronic Hepatitis

Chronic hepatitis with an acute exacerbation can mimic acute viral hepatitis and can represent a significant problem in the differential diagnosis. This is best demonstrated for HBsAg-positive chronic hepatitis. These patients occasionally can be asymptomatic, except for recurrent bouts of jaundice and symptoms of hepatitis that can occur with almost seasonal regularity. Several features should suggest the presence of chronic hepatitis. These include previous bouts of hepatitis or jaundice, a prolonged and indolent preicteric phase of disease, protracted and only mild-to-moderate elevations in aminotransferase and serum bilirubin levels (Fig. 2), and increased globulin and decreased serum albumin levels. In most instances the presence of HBsAg with absence of IgM anti-HBc confirms the diagnosis of chronic infection. In the final analysis, however, differentiation requires the test of time. The persistence of symptoms or abnormal serum enzyme levels for more than 6 months indicates chronic hepatitis. A liver biopsy specimen usually can be helpful if it demonstrates chronic hepatitis with fibrosis or with ground-glass cells. However, it may not clearly differentiate acute from chronic hepatitis at the height of an acute exacerbation. Other features of chronic hepatitis will be discussed in the next chapter.

Acute Hepatitis Due to Other Viruses

Several other common viral infections can secondarily affect the liver and can cause an acute hepatitis-like picture. The liver disease associated with these infections usually is mild, self-limited, subclinical, and overshadowed by the other symptoms in these diseases.

Of prime importance as a secondary cause of viral hepatitis is the Epstein-Barr virus (EBV), the agent of heterophile-positive infectious mononucleosis. When sought, mild elevations in serum aminotransferase levels (two to five times normal) are very common in acute mononucleosis. This syndrome should offer no diagnostic confusion with acute viral hepatitis; the liver disease is mild and subclinical. However, on rare occasions, EBV infection can be manifested as acute icteric hepatitis without the usual symptoms of mononucleosis.[22] Physical examination may reveal little or no evidence of pharyngitis or lymphadenopathy. Several features of the hepatitis should suggest that it is due to EBV infection. First, fever (which usually is not prominent in acute viral hepatitis) is prominent and persistent in mononucleosis. High fever lasting into the icteric phase should suggest infectious mononucleosis. Second, the serum enzyme levels in mononucleosis are not entirely typical of those in acute viral hepatitis. The alkaline phosphatase and LDH levels usually are higher than expected from the degree of jaundice and aminotransferase elevation (Fig. 2). Most suggestive, however, is the presence of a significant lymphocytosis (>50 percent) with atypical lymphocytes (>20 percent). Without this, hepatitis cannot be readily ascribed to EBV infection. Finally, the mononucleosis slide test or heterophile antibody is usually but not invariably reactive. Absolute confirmation of infectious mononucleosis rests on the appearance of anti-EBV or on a fourfold rise in titer when tested on paired sera. Because most adults have anti-EBV, a single positive specimen is not meaningful. Liver biopsy findings in acute mononucleosis hepatitis are quite characteristic but add little. A diagnosis of acute hepatitis as being due to infectious mononucleosis requires only a typical pattern of serum enzyme levels, atypical lymphocytosis, and a positive heterophile test.

Much of what is said about EBV-related hepatitis can be repeated for the cytomegalovirus (CMV). However, the role of CMV infection in causing a hepatitis in adults still is subject to debate, especially as it relates to post-transfusion hepatitis.[55,60,61] The problem centers on relating changes in anti-CMV titers and/or excretion of the virus to an episode of hepatitis. Such changes can occur in totally asymptomatic patients and are frequent after blood transfusions (regardless of the occurrence of hepatitis).[60] There is no doubt that primary CMV infection can cause a heterophile-negative mononucleosis syndrome that frequently is accompanied by hepatosplenomegaly and minor elevations of serum aminotransferase levels.[61] Whether CMV can induce a purely hepatitis-like syndrome is unclear. If it can, it probably is rare in adults. The diagnosis rests either on the finding of atypical lymphocytosis with acute liver injury, the absence of heterophile antibody, and the appearance or titer rise of anti-CMV (without anti-EBV rise) or on the excretion of the virus in urine or oropharyngeal secretions.

Several other common human viruses (including rubella rubeola, and mumps viruses; and coxsackie B virus) can induce mild abnormalities in liver enzymes.[62] These changes are not common and rarely are accompanied by jaundice. In the immunosuppressed host, however, several usually benign viruses can cause a disseminated infection, part of which may be hepatic involvement. Chief among these are the herpes simplex virus, CMV, and the varicella-zoster virus.[60–63] These are all herpesviruses that are ubiquitous and common benign infections in humans. In the patient with poor host defenses, dissemination with these viruses can occur. Hepatic necrosis, marked elevations in the serum aminotransferase levels, icterus, and even death from hepatic failure have been described. In the immunosuppressed or the immunoincompetent host with fulminant hepatic failure, a search for these viruses should be made. Liver biopsy specimens may demonstrate inclusion bodies and/or intranuclear herpesvirus particles. These viruses, however, are not common causes of sporadic acute hepatitis in the otherwise healthy host.

One more virus that is responsible for severe hepatic failure should be mentioned as a rare cause of acute viral hepatitis—yellow fever virus. Yellow fever has not been reported in the United States for over 40 years. It is, however, still enzootic in Central America, South America, and central Africa. Clinically, it is marked by a short incubation period (3–7 days), severe hepatitis with high aminotransferase level elevations, and a high mortality (approximately 20 percent).[64] It need be considered only in the recent traveler to enzootic areas who has not received adequate immunization. The diagnosis is made by isolating the virus from the blood, by finding a significant rise in antibody titers on paired sera, or by characteristic pathologic findings in the liver.

Hepatitis Due to Nonviral Infectious Diseases

Elevations in serum enzyme levels and liver dysfunction can occur with many nonviral infectious diseases due to bacteria, mycobacteria, rickettsia, and fungi. Thus jaundice with mild elevations in aminotransferase and alkaline phosphatase levels (two to five times normal) can be seen with several types of sepsis as well as with pneumococcal pneumonia.[22,65] Furthermore, minor elevations of liver enzyme levels without jaundice often are seen with many severe infections that usually do not primarily involve the liver—pulmonary and miliary tuberculosis,[66] brucellosis, tularemia, plague, gram-negative sepsis, legionnaires' disease, and so on. Liver biopsy specimens usually show nonspecific changes and focal areas of necrosis. However, at times (as in miliary tuberculosis), a liver biopsy specimen can be very helpful in establishing the primary diagnosis.

Three nonviral infectious agents that can produce an acute hepatitis-like syndrome deserve special note: syphilis, leptospirosis, and Q fever. Early syphilis, either primary or early secondary, can be accompanied by significant serum aminotransferase level elevations (three to eight times normal).[67] Jaundice, however, is rare, and the chancre of primary syphilis or the rash of secondary syphilis should be present. The liver enzyme tests, as in mononucleosis hepatitis, show atypically high elevations of alkaline phosphatase levels (four to eight times normal) when compared with the extent of aminotransferase abnormalities. Diagnosis is established by the finding of a reactive VDRL and fluorescent treponemal antibody (FTA) as well as by the typical clinical setting and response to treatment.

Leptospirosis is a well-known but rare cause of jaundice and hepatitis in the United States. The disease is caused by at least 15 serotypes of *Leptospira interrogans*.[59] The serotypes that are responsible for most of the infections in this country are (*1*) *icterohemorrhagiae* (30–40 percent), which is enzootic in rats; (*2*) *canicola* (30 percent), enzootic in dogs; and (*3*) *pomona* (10–20 percent), enzootic in cattle and swine. The history usually points to exposure to these animals or their urine (lake water, swimming holes). The clinical manifestations include malaise, fever, chills, severe myalgias, and headache.[68] Later symptoms of cough, sputum production, prostration, and hepatic and renal involvement appear. Hepatic involvement is most common with the serotype *icterohemorrhagiae*. Evaluation may demonstrate fever, prostration, severe muscle tenderness, hepatosplenomegaly, and pneumonitis. Laboratory abnormalities include leukocytosis and a left shift in the differential count. The urinalysis may show albuminuria, casts, and white and red blood cells. In severe cases, the urine output falls, and the blood urea nitrogen level rises; central nervous system manifestations and pneumonitis also may appear. Liver function tests reveal jaundice that is often out of proportion to the degree of serum enzyme level elevations. As with the jaundice of pneumococcal pneumonia,[65] the jaundice in leptospirosis appears to be a result of a defect in bilirubin excretion, rather than the result of hepatic necrosis.[68] The diagnosis is made by finding a high titer or a significant rise in leptospiral agglutinins. It is unclear whether early antibiotic treatment ameliorates this disease. A differential diagnosis from typical acute viral hepatitis usually is not difficult.

Q fever is the third nonviral infectious disease that may be mistaken for acute viral hepatitis. This rare disease is caused by the rickettsial agent *Coxiella brunetti*. In this disease, as in leptospirosis, constitutional symptoms are prominent with fever, chills, and pneumonitis. Overt jaundice occurs in only about 5 percent of the cases, although subclinical hepatic involvement is quite common. In rare cases, hepatitis without pneumonitis occurs, and a differentiation from acute viral hepatitis may be difficult.[69] Epidemiologic features should reveal exposure to farm or wild animals (cows, goats, sheep). Clinically, persistent fever, pneumonitis, and prostration are more prominent than in viral hepatitis. Liver function tests reveal jaundice with only mild elevations in aminotransferase levels (two to five times normal) and sometimes marked elevations in the alkaline phosphatase concentration. The diagnosis is made by demonstration of a rise in agglutination titers against *C. burnetii* in paired sera. As in leptospirosis, early antibiotic treatment has not been found to be helpful in this rickettsial disease.

Drug-Related Acute Hepatitis

The major differential diagnosis in acute hepatitis is between viral and drug-related hepatitis. Every patient with hepatitis should be questioned carefully about all medications that he uses and should be specifically asked about "over-the-counter" products. Drug-related acute liver injury is not nearly as common as acute viral hepatitis, but it often is much more serious and is a prominent cause of fulminant hepatic failure.[70] Many drugs and toxins have been shown to induce hepatic injury, but few have actually been repeatedly implicated as causing an acute hepatitis-like syndrome. The major common medications available in the United States that are associated with significant hepatotoxicity are listed in Table 3 by the type of injury usually seen and with an approximate incidence. This is not an exhaustive list. Any patient who develops hepatitis while taking a drug that is a known or potential hepatotoxin should have treatment with the medication stopped until the full clinical picture can be evaluated. The most serious mistake that can be made in caring for patients with acute hepatitis injury is to underestimate the role of drugs and to continue administering them in the face of acute hepatitis. The suspicion of drug-induced liver injury should be the greatest when epidemiologic features are not absolutely typical of acute viral hepatitis (e.g., in the elderly, in patients with underlying diseases, and in patients who develop fulminant hepatitis). However, even when epidemiologic features are appropriate for acute viral hepatitis, the role of drugs should not be dismissed: the renal dialysis patient taking methyldopa or the drug addict receiving isoniazid who develop acute hepatitis should have treatment with these medications stopped until adequate evaluation dismisses their role.

Some of the most commonly encountered causes of drug-related acute hepatitis are aspirin, acetaminophen, isoniazid, rifampin, phenytoin, and the anesthetic halothane. *Aspirin* (acetylsalicylic acid) can cause dramatic elevations in serum enzyme levels (two to five times normal), but it rarely causes jaundice. Aspirin hepatotoxicity seems to occur only with a high maintenance dosage, usually with serum salicylate levels of 20 mg/dl or greater. Characteristically, the biochemical abnormalities subside rapidly on withdrawing the drug. *Acetaminophen* (paracetamol) regularly causes severe hepatic necrosis similar to acute viral hepatitis when taken in large amounts (especially >15 g), as with a suicide attempt. Acetaminophen overdose seems to be becoming a more popular method of suicide and has become a major cause of fulminant hepatic failure both in the United States and England. The liver disease appears 2–5 days after the overdose. Interestingly, the liver injury can be averted if the patient is treated within 10 hours of the overdose with large doses of glutathione precursors (cysteamine, methionine, *N*-acetyl cysteine). Liver injury from the chronic use of acetaminophen in high doses also has been described.[71] Unexplained fulminant hepatitis should lead the physician to consider an acetaminophen overdose, the history of which the patient

TABLE 3. Common Causes of Drug-Related Liver Injury

Agent Class	*Agent*	*Frequency of Occurrence*[a]	*Type of Injury*
Analgesic	Acetaminophen	Dose-related	Hepatitis
	Aspirin	Dose-related	Hepatitis
Anesthetic	Halothane	Rare (0.01–0.1%)	Hepatitis
	Methoxyflurane	Rare	Hepatitis
Antiarthritic	Allopurinol	Rare	Granuloma/hepatitis
	Indomethacin	Very rare	Hepatitis
	Phenylbutazone	Rare	Granuloma/mixed
Antibacterial	Carbenicillin	Low[b]	Hepatitis
	Erythromycin estolate	Low	Cholestasis
	Nitrofurantoin	Rare	Mixed
	Oxacillin	Rare	Hepatitis
	Sulfonamides/sulfones	Rare	Hepatitis
	Tetracycline	Dose-related	Steatosis/necrosis
Antifungal	Ketoconazole	Rare	Hepatitis
Antineoplastic	Azathioprine	Rare[b]	Cholestasis
	6-Mercaptopurine	Common[b] (10–35%)	Hepatitis
	Methotrexate	Dose-related	Fibrosis
	Mithromycin	Rare[b]	Necrosis
Antituberculosis	Isoniazid	Low (1%)	Hepatitis
	Para-aminosalicylic acid	Low (0.1–1%)	Hepatitis
	Rifampin	Low	Hepatitis
Cardiovascular	Methyldopa	Low	Hepatitis
	Quinidine	Rare	Granuloma/hepatitis
	Thiazides	Very rare	Mixed
	Amiodarone	Low (1–3%)	Steatosis/necrosis
Endocrinologic	17-Alkylated androgens	Dose-related	Cholestasis
	Chlorpromamide	Rare	Cholestasis
	Oral contraceptives	Rare	Cholestasis
	Propylthiouracil	Rare	Hepatitis
	Tolbutamide	Very rare	Cholestasis
Neuro- and psychopharmacologic	Dantrolene	Low (1–2%)	Hepatitis
	Monoamine oxidase inhibitors	Low	Hepatitis
	Phenothiazines	Low (1–2%)	Cholestasis
	Phenytoin	Rare	Hepatitis
	Valproic acid	Low (1–2%)	Steatosis/necrosis

[a] The frequency of occurrence is an estimate from the literature[70]: common ≃ >2 percent, low ≃ 0.1–2 percent, rare <0.1 percent, very rare = isolated case reports only.
[b] Dose-related to some degree.

may have denied. Both *isoniazid* and *rifampin* have been implicated in causing an acute hepatitis-like syndrome; both have been associated with fulminant hepatic failure. Rifampin hepatic injury usually has its onset within the first weeks of therapy, whereas isoniazid hepatotoxicity is most common after 1–2 months of therapy. The incidence of isoniazid hepatotoxicity is approximately 1 percent, but it is definitely higher in older age groups and approaches 10 percent in patients over the age of 40. Treatment with these drugs should be discontinued if symptoms of hepatitis or jaundice appear or if aminotransferase levels are persistently elevated more than five times normal. Phenytoin can cause an acute hepatitis, usually within 1–6 weeks of starting the medication and associated with other manifestations of hypersensitivity such as fever, rash, lymphadenopathy, and eosinophilia. It has a mortality of approximately 10 percent. Therapy with this drug should be stopped in any patient showing evidence of acute hepatitis. The anesthetic agents *halothane* and *methoxyflurane* perhaps are the most controversial drugs incriminated in causing acute hepatic necrosis. A recent cooperative study on halothane-induced hepatitis suggested that approximately 1/10,000 patients given this anesthetic for the first time and 1/1000 given it more than once develop fulminant hepatic necrosis.[72] While halothane-induced hepatitis is rare, it nevertheless is a significant cause of death from hepatic failure. Clinically, halothane-related jaundice appears within 3–14 days of its use and resembles an acute, severe viral hepatitis. Fever is very characteristic early in the course; many patients have an accompanying leukocytosis and eosinophilia. Halothane-induced hepatitis usually is not confused with post-transfusion hepatitis because of its early onset after surgery and anesthesia.

Many other medications have been implicated or cited as causes of acute hepatic injury. Every agent that a person with acute hepatitis is taking should be held in suspicion. The suspicion of drug-induced liver injury should weigh heavily in the performance of a liver biopsy procedure. In many situations, liver biopsy findings can help to identify the cause of hepatic injury and can aid in the future use of the implicated drugs.

Anoxic Liver Injury

A syndrome resembling acute viral hepatitis can occur after anoxic injury to the liver due to a period of hypotension, severe left- or right-sided heart failure, or cardiopulmonary arrest.[73] The clinical and historical features usually can distinguish this nonspecific type of liver injury from acute viral hepatitis. However, in some cases, no clear history of an anoxic episode is obtained, or the patient is brought to the hospital comatose and unable to give an adequate history. In these situations, a diagnosis usually can be made on the basis of serum enzymes. Within hours of an anoxic episode, there are marked elevations of aminotransferase levels into the range seen with acute viral hepatitis (Fig. 2). The alkaline phosphatase level remains only minimally elevated or is normal. The LDH level, conversely, is dramatically elevated (as is the CPK level), and it may be most helpful in suggesting this diagnosis. Most typical of anoxic liver injury, however, is the rapid resolution of these enzyme abnormalities. The aminotransferase levels often decrease by half each day and can fall from 50–100 times elevated to normal within a week. Jaundice is uncommon and mild; it generally occurs several days after injury. In some cases, aminotransferase levels remain elevated to two to five times normal for 5–14 days after the injury, in which case differentiation from acute viral hepatitis may be difficult and may require a liver biopsy procedure (which will show a bland centrozonal necrosis). While a liver biopsy specimen is diagnostic, it generally is not needed for the diagnosis when the clinical history and pattern of enzyme levels are typical.

Alcoholic Liver Disease

Alcohol abuse is the most common cause of serious liver disease in the United States. Alcoholic liver disease (i.e., fatty liver, alcoholic hepatitis, and Laennec cirrhosis) usually can be readily differentiated from acute viral hepatitis by history and biochemical tests. Acute alcoholic hepatitis is the syndrome that, perhaps, is most easily confused with viral hepatitis. These patients have the gradual and imprecisely dated onset of malaise, anorexia, weight loss, nausea and vomiting, fever, chills, abdominal swelling, and jaundice or dark urine. The history of alcohol intake should suggest the diagnosis, but many patients conceal or underestimate the amount of alcohol they consume. The lower limit of alcohol intake said to lead to alcoholic liver disease is 80 g/day—the equivalent to a half-pint of 86 proof whiskey, four conventional "cocktails," five to six cans (12 oz) of beer, or 1 quart of wine each day.[70,74] Alcoholic liver disease is rarely manifested until after 10 or more years of excessive drinking.

Clinically, the patient usually appears chronically ill and typically is older than the average patient with viral hepatitis. Fever and tachycardia are common. Examination may reveal evidence of *chronic* liver disease and alcohol abuse that is not seen with acute viral hepatitis—wasting, parotid enlargement, palmar erythema, vascular spiders, gynecomastia, testicular atrophy, significant hepatomegaly, and signs of portal hypertension (ascites, edema, splenomegaly, and prominent abdominal veins). The laboratory data are most helpful.[22] The white blood cell count is usually elevated with a left shift. The hematocrit may be slightly decreased, and the red blood cell indices reveal macrocytosis (with or without folate deficiency). Liver function tests reveal hyperbilirubinemia and typically a low albumin level and a prolonged prothrombin time. The aminotransferase values are most characteristic (Fig. 2) in that the AST levels almost always are elevated, but rarely more than eight times normal. Furthermore, the AST level is elevated out of proportion to the ALT level (which can be slightly elevated, normal, or even low). Thus, the aminotransferase levels in alcoholic hepatitis differ greatly from those in viral hepatitis—not only in the degree of elevation but also by the relative elevation of the AST to the ALT level. The alkaline phosphatase level can be quite variable in alcoholic liver disease and sometimes is quite high. The LDH values are variable. If the clinical and biochemical pictures are unclear, acute alcoholic hepatitis can be readily diagnosed by a liver biopsy procedure, which is also helpful in judging the severity of liver injury and in gauging the prognosis.

Cholestatic Liver Disease

Cholestatic liver disease refers to a host of diseases marked by bile retention. Cholestasis can be due either to extrahepatic biliary obstruction (from gallstones, stricture, pancreatitis, or cancer) or to intrahepatic causes (from primary biliary cirrhosis, several childhood cholestatic syndromes, and drug-induced cholestasis from phenothiazines or methyltestosterone). These patients have the nonspecific symptoms of acute liver disease with jaundice, but the differentiation from acute viral hepatitis rarely is difficult. In general, signs and symptoms of cholestasis are prominent; the degree of jaundice, lightening of stools, and itching overshadow the amount of anorexia or malaise. Laboratory data are confirmatory and show modest abnormalities in aminotransferase levels but marked elevations in alkaline phosphatase levels (Fig. 2). Gallstone obstruction perhaps most closely mimics acute viral hepatitis, with its typical manifestation being fever, chills, malaise, right upper quadrant pain, nausea, vomiting, jaundice, and dark urine. Fever is prominent and often hectic, thus pointing away from viral hepatitis. Furthermore, the liver usually is quite tender, and there may be signs of localized peritonitis. Leukocytosis and a left shift usually are present; although aminotransferase levels can be quite high (up to 10–15 times normal), the alkaline phosphatase level usually is also markedly elevated.

Other Liver Diseases

Few other causes of jaundice pose a problem in the differential diagnosis of acute hepatitis. Rare causes of an acute hepatitis-like syndrome include Wilson's disease,[75] sickle cell crisis,[76] acute Budd-Chiari syndrome or veno-occlusive disease,[77] and massive replacement of the liver by tumor.[78] These causes usually are associated with a fulminant or severe hepatitis. Patients with hemolytic anemia may have vague nonspecific symptoms and jaundice, but the urine will have no bilirubin, and the aminotransferase levels will be normal. Patients with congenital disorders of bilirubin metabolism (Gilbert and Dubin-Johnson syndromes) may become notably jaundiced, especially during intercurrent viral illnesses, but serum enzyme levels should be normal.

Patients who are found, on routine blood tests (either during a screening test or during evaluation for other problems), to have abnormal aminotransferase levels sometimes are suspected of having anicteric or preicteric acute viral hepatitis. Actually, such patients with asymptomatic elevations in aminotransferase levels are far more likely to have chronic liver disease, and their evaluation should proceed with that in mind.

MANAGEMENT

Supportive Care

There is no specific therapy for acute viral hepatitis. Good management consists of supportive measures, relief of symptoms, and avoidance of further injury.

Hospitalization. Most patients with acute viral hepatitis do not require hospitalization. Little can be done for most patients in the hospital that is not available at home; also, for many, hospitalization is a heavy emotional and financial burden. However, several factors should be weighed when deciding not to hospitalize the patient with acute hepatitis. Home care should be reserved for patients who have only mild to moderate symptoms, who have someone at home to care for and feed them, and who can return for regular medical evaluation without difficulty. Hospitalization is advisable in any patient whose prothrombin time shows any prolongation or who has any clinical evidence of hepatic failure. The duration of hospitalization, of course, will vary with the severity of illness. Once symptoms have abated, the patient usually can be discharged to continue convalescence at home. There is no need to continue hospitalization until laboratory test values return to normal.

Rest. Bed rest should be prescribed for patients with acute viral hepatitis during the period of symptoms. However, the bed rest should not be absolute; use of the bathroom and periods of being up each day should be encouraged. Traditionally, it has been recommended that bed rest be continued until recovery is complete and liver function test values have returned to normal. While most patients are willing to remain at bed rest for the duration of the symptoms, most—and especially the young—will be anxious to return to normal activity once the symptoms abate. Indeed, controlled studies have shown that after the symptoms have cleared normal activity and even strenuous exercise does not slow recovery, induce relapses, or predispose to chronic liver disease.[79] It is unnecessarily restrictive to insist on bed rest until the aminotransferase levels return to normal or until HBsAg is negative. A gradual return to activity with monitoring of liver function test values is warranted once the symptoms have abated. Relapses of symptoms should be treated with a return to bed rest.

Alcohol. Alcohol traditionally has been prohibited not only during the acute illness but also for an extended period into convalescence. However, there are no data to suggest that moderate alcohol intake leads to a worsening of acute hepatitis or predisposes to chronic hepatitis. While it is prudent to advise abstinence during the acute symptomatic phase of viral hepatitis, the recommendation of total abstinence for 6–12 months after viral hepatitis is unnecessarily strict.

Diet. There is little evidence that any dietary regimen has any effect on the course of acute hepatitis. A generally nutritious diet should be encouraged. During the symptomatic phase, patients frequently are anorexic and may have distinct likes and dislikes. The person with anorexia cannot be forced to eat; however, some encouragement can come from the use of frequent small feedings and a diet low in fat but high in carbohydrates. Forced or nasogastric tube feedings should be avoided.

Drugs. Most medications are best avoided during acute hepatitis. Antibiotics are not indicated. Immune serum globulin has no effect. No single drug has yet been shown to significantly shorten or to ameliorate the course of the disease. Symptomatic therapy for nausea, pain, or sleeplessness may be needed at times. Antiemetics can be helpful, but chlorpromazine (because of its potential to cause intrahepatic cholestasis) should be avoided. Among analgesics, acetaminophen is preferable to aspirin (because of its effects on platelet function and the gastric mucosa) and codeine or morphine derivatives (because of their sedative effects). Sedatives should not be used at all, if possible. Mild sleeping medications such as triazolam or flurazepam often have been prescribed without incident, but they should not be considered routine. Previous data have suggested that estrogens might worsen the course of typical acute viral hepatitis; however, prospective studies of women with acute viral hepatitis who were taking oral contraceptives have failed to support this.[80] Nevertheless, it is advisable that treatment with all but the most necessary medications be discontinued during the acute phase of viral hepatitis. Vitamins often are given but have not been shown to be beneficial in patients with acute hepatitis. If the prothrombin time is prolonged, a trial of vitamin K (1–5 mg im) can be given. The administration of vitamin K, however, will have little or no effect on the prothrombin time in typical viral hepatitis unless there has been prolonged cholestasis.

Treatment

There are no specific therapies for acute viral hepatitis. Corticosteroids have not been shown to shorten the course or to aid in the healing of acute viral hepatitis.[81,82] Indeed, some studies have indicated that corticosteroids may predispose to more prolonged illness, more relapses, and more chronic liver disease.[82] Corticosteroids are definitely not indicated for the typical case of acute viral hepatitis.

Corticosteroids have sometimes been recommended for two situations in acute viral hepatitis: fulminant hepatic failure and cholestatic hepatitis. In prolonged cholestasis after acute viral hepatitis, corticosteroids can decrease serum bilirubin levels and ameliorate symptoms of fatigue and itching. The use of corticosteroids in this situation, however, should be limited to cases of hepatitis A in which the possibility of transition to chronic hepatitis is not present. In fulminant hepatitis, corticosteroids are often used, frequently because no other options are available. However, controlled clinical trials have failed to demonstrate any benefit of corticosteroids in acute viral hepatitis, and some have indicated that the adverse side effects of high doses of corticosteroids outweigh their potential benefit.[82]

Antiviral medications that have shown promise as therapy in chronic viral hepatitis[83,84] also hold promise as therapy for acute disease. So far, the only studies of antiviral treatment in severe acute viral hepatitis have been nonrandomized trials in small numbers of patients. In a study from Israel,[85] five patients with fulminant hepatitis were treated with interferon-α, and three survived, which led the authors to suggest that antiviral therapy might be helpful in a subset of patients with severe or fulminant hepatitis. However, in a later study from Spain,[86] only 2 of 12 patients with fulminant hepatitis B or delta who were treated with high doses of parenteral interferon-α survived, thus indicating that this medication is unlikely to be of benefit in reversing fulminant viral hepatitis.[86] Nevertheless, the possible role of interferon-α or other antiviral agents in typical acute or in severe hepatitis deserves further evaluation. The absence of a beneficial effect of therapy in fulminant hepatitis does not necessarily indicate that the therapy will have no effect in patients with less advanced or severe hepatic injury.

Monitoring

Monitoring during acute viral hepatitis should be regular and specific. While the patient is hospitalized, a daily check on major symptoms is important. The patient should be examined for the degree of icterus, liver size, and the presence of asterixis or other evidence of hepatic encephalopathy. The ALT, AST, alkaline phosphatase, and bilirubin levels and the prothrombin time should be monitored once or twice a week during hospitalization and every 1–2 weeks thereafter until they return to normal. Initially, the patient should be tested for HBsAg. If positive, the test is best repeated every 1–2 months until HBsAg disappears. The continued presence of HBsAg 4–6 months after acute viral hepatitis indicates the establishment of the chronic HBsAg carrier state. Other specialized testing of liver function or structure such as bromosulfophthalein retention, indocyanine green excretion, ultrasonography, computed tomography (CT), and liver–spleen radionuclide scanning are not helpful, nor are they needed in acute viral hepatitis.

A percutaneous liver biopsy specimen in acute viral hepatitis may well establish the diagnosis, but generally it is not necessary. However, in two situations, liver biopsy is indicated: (*1*) when the diagnosis is in doubt; if diagnostic confusion remains despite clinical, biochemical, and serologic data; if more than one explanation of acute liver injury exists; or if drug-related acute hepatitis is a possibility; and (*2*) when therapy is being considered.

Fulminant Viral Hepatitis

The management of fulminant viral hepatitis should begin with its early recognition. The initial signs and symptoms of hepatic encephalopathy may be subtle (nightmares, slight changes in personality, restlessness) or dramatic (unexpected aggressive physical or sexual activity). It is important to recognize these signs for what they are and not respond to them by using sedative or physical restraints.

At the first sign of encephalopathy, vigorous management should be started.[85] This should include bed rest, a low-protein diet (20–30 g/day), the administration of enemas to cleanse the bowel, and the use of oral neomycin (1.0–1.5 g every 6 hours) or lactulose (30–60 cc in sorbitol every 2–6 hours until loose stools are achieved). Treatment with all sedatives should be stopped. With deepening coma, the patient may require iv fluids, a central venous pressure line, a nasogastric tube, and a urinary bladder catheter. Coagulation defects may require correction with the use of freshly frozen plasma (the coagulation factor concentrates such as fibrinogen and prothrombin complex should not be used). The patient should be carefully monitored for gastrointestinal bleeding. Cimetidine (300–500 mg iv every 6 hours) or vigorous antacid therapy may be begun to help prevent upper gastrointestinal bleeding. Most important is careful attention to all the details of "routine" medical management (fluid and electrolyte balance, acid-base balance, pulmonary toilet, iv and bladder catheter care, skin care, and monitoring for signs of blood loss or superinfection). Corticosteroids may be used as outlined above. More aggressive approaches such as exchange transfusions, "total body washout," charcoal hemoperfusion, cross-circulation with a human or baboon liver, and immunotherapy with antibody to HBsAg each have had their advocates, but none has been repeatedly shown to be more effective than "conventional" medical management is.

The most promising new therapy for fulminant hepatic failure is emergency hepatic transplantation.[87,88] Since the early 1980s and the introduction of cyclosporine A as an immunosuppressive agent, liver transplantation has become a successful and well-accepted approach to severe liver disease. At present, 1200–1500 liver transplants are done yearly in the United States in 40–50 different medical centers. Approximately 7 percent of patients undergo liver transplantation for fulminant or subacute hepatic failure. The 1- to 2-year survival rates have ranged between 60 and 90 percent.[87]

The major reason to avoid liver transplantation in fulminant hepatic failure is the possibility of spontaneous recovery. The survival rate of patients with fulminant hepatitis in stage III–IV coma averages 20–30 percent. Features that predict a poor outcome include age (either less than 10 or greater than 40 years), non-A, non-B hepatitis or medications as a cause of the liver injury, and a prothrombin time greater than 50 seconds.[89] The decision for transplantation needs to be made before severe complications supervene, in particular decerebration, after which recovery is unlikely even with liver transplantation. Interestingly, the cause of liver injury usually does not recur in the transplanted liver[90]: hepatitis B causing fulminant hepatitis rarely infects the new liver. Thus, at the first sign of hepatic failure, the physician should refer the patient with acute viral hepatitis to a liver transplant center. The criteria for transplantation in fulminant hepatitis are currently changing, and the decision for organ transplantation should be made by a team of physicians with experience in treating fulminant hepatic failure.

Prevention

Specifics of prevention in viral hepatitis will be presented in later chapters. Management of needlestick injuries in hospital employees is discussed in Chapters 282 and 283. Certain nonspecific measures regarding the patient with acute hepatitis should be stressed here.

If the patient is hospitalized, he should be placed in a private room with separate toilet facilities. The major reason for such isolation is to prevent the spread of type A hepatitis. Even with lax precautions, such spread is very rare; most patients with type A hepatitis are no longer excreting virus once they have become symptomatic. Nevertheless, there are exceptions, and isolation is prudent. Secretions and blood products should be handled with care. Gowns, masks, and gloves are not necessary, but a prominent sign reading "needle and blood precautions" is appropriate. Labeling of blood specimens, as from a patient with hepatitis, is a common practice. It should be stressed, however, that all blood from any patient should be handled as if potentially infectious.

If at home, the patient should be advised about care in personal hygiene—use of a private bathroom, if possible, and careful hand washing. Attention also should be paid to blood and blood products and the handling of cuts and lacerations.

Recommendations regarding the prevention of acute hepatitis are governed by the type of viral hepatitis that is being considered. In the case of acute type A hepatitis, all family members and close personal contacts should receive immune serum globulin (ISG) at a dosage of 2–5 ml im as soon as possible after exposure. Office, factory, and school contacts do not need to be treated. Immune serum globulin can be given for up to 4 weeks after exposure, but it probably is only effective if given within 7–14 days. In the case of acute type B hepatitis, prophylaxis only needs to be provided for "regular" sexual contacts. The best form of protection is argued. Hepatitis B immune globulin (HBIG) at a dosage of 5 ml im as soon as possible and again 1 month later has been the conventional recommendation in this situation. However, the efficacy of HBIG in preventing the sexual spread of acute type B hepatitis has not been well proved.[91] In addition, there is now evidence that postexposure immunization with HBV vaccine can attentuate or prevent acute type B hepatitis.[92,93] In view of this, a practical approach is the administration of one injection of HBIG and the simultaneous initiation of vaccination. Vaccine should be given in 20 μg amounts (0.5–1.0 cc) im as soon as possible and then 1 month and 6 months later. In the case of acute delta hepatitis, the recommendations are the same as for type B hepatitis. Prevention of type B hepatitis also will prevent delta hepatitis. In the case of non-A, non-B hepatitis, there is little or no information concerning the efficacy of any mode of prevention. Prophylaxis probably is unnecessary, except for household contacts. Sexual partners may be at highest risk. Because ISG is inexpensive and safe and may have some effect in preventing icteric disease, it often is recommended for the regular sexual contacts of patients with acute non-A, non-B hepatitis.

There often is a delay between the diagnosis of acute viral hepatitis and the identification of whether the disease is due to type A, type B, delta, or non-A, non-B hepatitis. Indeed, serologic testing sometimes is not available. The recommendations given above require that the prophylaxis of family and intimate contacts of patients be postponed until the results of serologic testing are known. A simplified approach to prophylaxis is to administer ISG immediately to all family, household, and intimate contacts and to begin HBV vaccination of the sexual contact(s) if the disease is subsequently shown to be type B (or delta) hepatitis. This schema could be modified if the hepatitis is obviously not due to HAV (e.g., post-transfusion hepatitis). This approach is appealing because of its simplicity and also because the titers of anti-HBs (the protective antibody in type B hepatitis) in standard preparations of ISG have been increasing over the past 10–15 years.[91] Thus, ISG that is currently being produced may be partially effective in preventing type B hepatitis.

Finally, it should be stressed that viral hepatitis is a reportable disease. Once the diagnosis is verified and serologic testing data are available, they should be reported to the local or state department of health.

REFERENCES

1. Krugman S, Giles JP, Viral hepatitis. New light on an old disease. JAMA. 1970;212:1019.
2,. Feinstone SM, Kapikian AZ, Purcell RH. Hepatitis A: Detection by immune electron microscopy of a virus-like antigen associated with acute illness. Science. 1973;182:1026.
3. Blumberg BS, Alter HJ, Visnich S. A "new" antigen in leukemia sera. JAMA. 1965;191:541.
4. Tiollais P, Pourcel C, Dejean A. The hepatitis B virus. Nature. 1985;317:489.
5. Rizzetto M, Canese MG, Arico S, et al. Immunofluorescence detection of a new antigen–antibody system (δ/anti-δ) associated with hepatitis B virus in liver and serum of HBsAg carriers. Gut. 1977;18:997.
6. Rizzetto M. The delta agent. Hepatology. 1983;3:729.
7. Feinstone SM, Kapikian AZ, Purcell RH, et al. Transfusion-associated hepatitis not due to viral hepatitis type A or B. N Engl J Med. 1975;292:767.
8. Houghton M, Wiener J, Rutter WJ, et al. Non-A, non-B agent. News conference. 1988.
9. Balayan MS, Andjaparidze AG, Savinskaya SS, et al. Evidence for a virus in non-A/non-B hepatitis transmitted via the fecal oral route. Intervirology. 1983;20:23.
10. Gust ID, Purcell RH. Waterbourne non-A, non-B hepatitis. J Infect Dis. 1987;156:630.
11. Centers for Disease Control. Hepatitis surveillance report. No. 51:13, 1987.
12. Koff RS, Chalmers TC, Culhane PO, et al. Underreporting of viral hepatitis. Gastroenterology. 1973;64:1194.
13. Szmuness W, Dienstag JL, Purcell RH, et al. Distribution of antibody to hepatitis A antigen in urban adult populations. N Engl J Med. 1976;295:755.
14. Hadler SC, de Monzon M, Ponzetto A, et al. An epidemic of severe hepatitis due to delta virus infection in Yucpa Indians of Venezuela. Ann Intern Med. 1984;100:339.
15. Hoofnagle JH, Shafritz DA, Popper H. Chronic type B hepatitis and the "healthy" HBsAg carrier state. Hepatology. 1987;7:758.
16. Zeldis JB, Dienstag JL, Gale RP. Aplastic anemia and non-A, non-B hepatitis. Am J Med. 1983;74:64.
17. Beasley RP, Hwang LY, Lin CC, et al. Hepatocellular carcinoma and hepatitis B virus. A prospective study of 22,707 men in Taiwan. Lancet. 1981;2:1129.
18. Beasley RP. Hepatitis B virus as the etiologic agent in hepatocellular carcinoma—epidemiologic considerations. Hepatology. 1982;2(Suppl):21.
19. Stevens CE, Taylor PE. Hepatitis B vaccine: Issues, recommendations, and new developments. Semin Liver Dis. 1986;6:23.
20. Alpert E, Isselbacher KJ, Schur PH. The pathogenesis of arthritis associated with viral hepatitis. N Engl J Med. 1971;285:185.
21. Gianotti F. Hepatitis B antigen in papular acrodermatitis of children. Br Med J. 1974;3:169.
22. Zimmerman HG. The differential diagnosis of jaundice. Med Clin North Am. 1968;52:1417.
23. Salen G, Goldstein F, Haurani F, et al. Acute hemolytic anemia complicating viral hepatitis in patients with glucose-6-phosphate dehydrogenase deficiency. Ann Intern Med. 1966;65:1210.
24. Ishak KG. Light microscopic morphology of viral hepatitis. Am J Clin Pathol. 1976;65:787.
25. Boyer JL, Klatskin G. Pattern of necrosis in acute viral hepatitis. Prognostic value of bridging (subacute hepatic necrosis). N Engl J Med. 1970;283:1063.
26. Mathiesen LR, Fauerholt L, Moller Am, et al. Immunofluorescence studies for hepatitis A virus and hepatitis B surface and core antigen in liver biopsies from patients with acute viral hepatitis. Gastroenterology. 1979;77:623.
27. Boggs JD, Melnick JL, Conrad ME, et al. Viral hepatitis, clinical and tissue culture studies. JAMA. 1970;214:1041.
28. Lemon S. Type A viral hepatitis. New developments in an old disease. N Engl J Med. 1985;313:1059.
29. Sjogren MH, Tanno H, Fay O, et al. Hepatitis A virus in stool during clinical relapse. Ann Intern Med. 1987;106:221.
30. Gordon SC, Reddy KR, Schiff L, et al. Prolonged intrahepatic cholestasis secondary to acute hepatitis A. Ann Intern Med. 1984;101:635.
31. Rakela A, Redeker AF, Edwards VM, et al. Hepatitis A virus infection in fulminant hepatitis and chronic active hepatitis. Gastroenterology. 1978;74:879.
32. Francis DP, Hadler SC, Prendergast TJ, et al. Occurrence of hepatitis A, B, and non-A, non-B hepatitis in the United States—CDC Sentinel County hepatitis study I. Am J Med. 1984;76:69.
33. Dienstag JL, Routenberg JA, Purcell Rh, et al. Foodhandler-associated outbreak of hepatitis type A. An immune electron microscopic study. Ann Intern Med. 1975;83:647.
34. Mackowiak PA, Caraway CT, Portnoy EL. Oyster-associated hepatitis. Lessons from the Louisiana experience. Am J Epidemiol. 1976;103:181.
35. Woodson RD, Clinton JJ. Hepatitis prophylaxis abroad. Effectiveness of immune serum globulin in protecting Peace Corps volunteers. JAMA. 1968;109:1053.
36. Pattison CP, Maynard JE, Bryan JS. Subhuman primate-associated hepatitis. J Infect Dis. 1975;132:478.
37. Hadler SC, Erben JJ, Francis DP, et al. Risk factors for hepatitis A in daycare centers. J Infect Dis. 1982;145:255.
38. Corey L, Holmes KK. Sexual transmission of hepatitis A in homosexual men. Incidence and mechanism. N Engl J Med. 1980;302:435.
39. Decker RH, Kosakowski SM, Vanderbilt AS, et al. Diagnosis of acute hepatitis A by Havab-M, a direct radioimmunoassay for IgM anti-HAV. Am J Clin Pathol. 1981;76:140.
40. Szmuness W, Much MI, Prince AM, et al. On the role of sexual behavior in the spread of hepatitis B infection. Ann Intern Med. 1975;83:489.
41. Krugman S, Overby LR, Mushahwar IK, et al. Viral hepatitis type B. Studies on the natural history and prevention reexamined. N Engl J Med. 1979;300:101.
42. Hoofnagle JH, Seeff LB, Bales ZB, et al. Serologic responses in type B hepatitis. In: Vyas GN, Cohen SN, Schmid R, eds. Viral Hepatitis. Philadelphia: Franklin Institute Press; 1978:219–44.
43. Chau KH, Hargie MP, Decker RH, et al. Serodiagnosis of recent hepatitis B infection by IgM class anti-HBc. Hepatology. 1983;3:142.
44. Rizzetto M, Gerin JL, Purcell RH, eds. Hepatitis Delta Virus and Its Infection. New York: Alan R Liss; 1987.
45. Hoofnagle JH. Type D hepatitis. JAMA. 1989;261:1321.
46. Farci P, Gerin JL, Aragona M, et al. Diagnostic and prognostic significance of the IgM antibody to the hepatitis delta virus. JAMA. 1986;255:1443.
47. Mushawar IK, Decker RH. Prevalence of delta antigen and antidelta detected by immunoassays in various HBsAg positive populations. In: Vyas GN, Dienstag JL, Hoofnagle JH, eds. Viral Hepatitis and Liver Disease. Orlando, FL: Grune & Stratton; 1984:617.
48. Bergmann KF, Gerin JL. Antigens of hepatitis delta virus in the liver and serum of humans and animals. J Infect Dis. 1986;514:702.

49. Smedile A, Baroudy BM, Bergmann KF, et al. Clinical significance of HDV RNA in HDV disease. In: Rizzetto M, Gerin JL, Purcell RH, eds. Hepatitis Delta Virus and Its Infection. New York: Alan R. Liss; 1987:231–4.
50. Rizzetto M, Verme G, Recchia S, et al. Chronic HBsAg hepatitis with intrahepatic expression of delta antigen. An active and progressive disease unresponsive to immunosuppressive treatment. Ann Intern Med. 1983;98:437.
51. Rocca G, Poli G, Gerardo P, et al. Familial clustering of delta infection. In: Verme G, Bonino F, Rizzetto M, eds. Viral Hepatitis and Delta Infection. New York: Alan R Liss; 1984:133–7.
52. Dienstag JL. Non-A, non-B hepatitis. I. Recognition, epidemiology, and clinical features. Gastroenterology. 1983;85:439.
53. Dienstag JL. Non-A, non-B hepatitis. II. Experimental transmission, putative virus agents and markers, and prevention. Gastroenterology. 1983;85:743.
54. Alter MJ, Gerety RJ, Smallwood LA, et al. Sporadic non-A, non-B hepatitis: Frequency and epidemiology in an urban U.S. population. J Infect Dis. 1982;145:886.
55. Alter HJ, Hoofnagle JH. Non-A, non-B. Observations on the first decade. In: Vyas GN, Dienstag JL, Hoofnagle JH, eds. Viral Hepatitis and Liver Disease. Orlando, FL: Grune & Stratton; 1984:345–55.
56. Wong DC, Purcell RH, Sreenivasan MA, et al. Epidemic and endemic hepatitis in India: Evidence for non-A/non-B hepatitis virus etiology. Lancet. 1980;2:876.
57. Khuroo SM. Study of an epidemic of non-A, non-B hepatitis. Possibility of another human hepatitis virus distinct from post-transfusion non-A, non-B type. Am J Med. 1980;68:818.
58. Kane MA, Bradley DW, Shrestha SM, et al. Epidemic non-A, non-B hepatitis in Nepal: Recovery of a possible etiologic agent and transmission studies in marmoset. JAMA. 1984;252:3140.
59. Kraczynski K, Bradley DW, Kane MA. Virus associated antigen of epidemic non-A, non-B hepatitis and specific antibodies in outbreaks and in sporadic cases of NANB hepatitis. Hepatology. 1988;8:1223.
60. Purcell RH, Walsh JH, Holland PV, et al. Seroepidemiological studies of transfusion-associated hepatitis. J Infect Dis. 1981;123:406.
61. Lamb SG, Stern H. Cytomegaolovirus hepatitis. Lancet. 1966;2:1003.
62. Gavish D, Kleinman Y, Morag A, et al. Hepatitis and jaundice associated with measles in young adults. Arch Intern Med. 1983;143:674.
63. Shalev-Zimels H, Weizman Z, Lotan C, et al. Extent of measles hepatitis in various ages. Hepatology. 1988;8:1138.
64. Francis TI, Moore DL, Edington GM, et al. A clinicopathological study of human yellow fever. Bull WHO. 1972;46:659.
65. Zimmerman HG, Fang M, Utili R, et al. Jaundice due to bacterial infection. Gastroenterology. 1979;77:362.
66. Bowry S, Chan CH, Weiss H, et al. Hepatic involvement in pulmonary tuberculosis. Histologic and functional characteristics. Am Rev Respir Dis. 1970;101:941.
67. Lee RV, Thornton GF, Conn HO. Liver disease associated with secondary syphilis. N Engl J Med. 1971;284:1423.
68. Heath CW Jr, Alexander AD, Galton MM. Leptospirosis in the United States. Analysis of 483 cases in man, 1949–1961. N Engl J Med. 1965;273:857.
69. Bernstein M, Edmondson HA, Barhour BH. The liver lesion in Q fever. Clinical and pathologic features. Arch Intern Med. 1965;116:491.
70. Zimmerman HJ. Hepatotoxicity. The Adverse Effects of Drugs and Other Chemicals on the Liver. New York: Appleton-Century-Crofts; 1978.
71. Johnson GK, Tolman KG. Chronic liver disease and acetaminophen. Ann Intern Med. 1977;87:302.
72. Subcommittee on the National Halothane Study of the Committee on Anesthesia. Possible association between halothane anesthesia and postoperative hepatic necrosis. JAMA. 1966;197:775.
73. Bynum TE, Boinoit JK, Maddrey WC. Ischemic hepatitis. Am J Dig Dis. 1979;24:129.
74. Lieber CS. Biochemical and molecular basis of alcohol-induced injury to the liver and other tissues. N Engl J Med. 1988;319:1639.
75. Roche-Sicot J, Benhamou JP. Acute intravascular hemolysis and acute liver failure associated as a first manifestation of Wilson's disease. Ann Intern Med. 1977;86:301.
76. Rosenblate HJ, Eisenstein R, Halmes AW. The liver in sickle cell anemia. Arch Pathol Lab Med. 1970;90:235.
77. Parker RGF. Occlusion of the hepatic veins in man. Medicine (Baltimore). 1959;38:369.
78. Harrison HB, Middleton HM III, Crosby JH, et al. Fulminant hepatic failure. An unusual presentation of metastatic liver disease. Gastroenterology. 1981;80:820.
79. Repsher LH, Freebern RK. Effects of early and vigorous exercise on recovery from infectious hepatitis. N Engl J Med. 1969;281:1393.
80. Schweitzer IL, Weiner JM, McPeak CM, et al. Oral contraceptives in acute viral hepatitis. JAMA. 1975;233:979.
81. Blum AI, Stutz R, Haemmerli UP, et al. A fortuitously controlled study of steroid therapy in acute viral hepatitis. I. Acute disease. Am J Med. 1969;47:82.
82. Gregory PB, Knauer CM, Miller R, et al. Steroid therapy in severe viral hepatitis. N Engl J Med. 1976;294:681.
83. Sherlock S, Thomas HC. Treatment of chronic hepatitis due to hepatitis B virus. Lancet. 1985;2:1343.
84. Hoofnagle JH, Mullen KD, Jones DB, et al. Treatment of chronic non-A, non-B hepatitis with recombinant human alpha interferon. N Engl J Med. 1986;315:1575.
85. Levin S, Hahn T. Interferon system in acute viral hepatitis. Lancet. 1982;1:592.
86. Sanchez-Tapias JM, Mas A, Costa J, et al. Recombinant alpha 2c interferon therapy in fulminant viral hepatitis. J Hepatol. 1987;5:205.
87. Peleman RR, Gavaler JS, Van Thiel DH, et al. Liver transplantation for acute and subacute hepatic failure. Hepatology. 1985;5:1045.
88. Vickers C, Neuberger J, Buckels J, et al. Transplantation of the liver in adults and children with fulminant hepatic failure. J Hepatol. 1988;7:143.
89. Bernuau J, Gordeau A, Poynard T, et al. Multivariate analysis of prognostic factors in fulminant hepatitis. Hepatology. 1986;6:648.
90. Auslander MO, Gitnick GL. Vigorous medical management of acute fulminant hepatitis. Arch Intern Med. 1977;137:599.
91. Seeff LB, Hoofnagle JH. Immunoprophylaxis of viral hepatitis. Gastroenterology. 1979;77:161.
92. Center for Disease Control. Post-exposure prophylaxis of hepatitis B. Ann Intern Med. 1984;101:351.
93. Beasley RP, Hwang LY, Lee GC, et al. Prevention of perinatally transmitted hepatitis B virus infections with hepatitis B immune globulin and hepatitis B vaccine. Lancet. 1983;2:1099.

103. CHRONIC HEPATITIS

SHALOM Z. HIRSCHMAN

Chronic hepatitis is defined as an abnormality in liver function that persists for 6 or more months.[1] Two broad classes of chronic hepatitis have been established through the study of liver histology, i.e., chronic persistent hepatitis and chronic active hepatitis (Table 1).[2] The former is most often a benign entity requiring no therapy, while the latter frequently leads to hepatic cirrhosis. The histologic separation of the two is by no means always clear, and the total clinical status of the patient must be considered in arriving at a diagnosis.[3]

CHRONIC PERSISTENT HEPATITIS

The overall architecture of the liver is usually normal in patients with chronic persistent hepatitis. The portal triads may be normal or moderately increased in size and contain an inflammatory cell infiltrate consisting mainly of lymphocytes and mononuclear cells (Fig. 1). Most important, the limiting plate of liver cells between portal zones and the lobule is intact (Fig. 1). Even if necrosis of these cells is present, it is not extensive. Minimal collections of inflammatory cells or foci of parenchymal cell necrosis may be present in the lobule. Piecemeal necrosis, that is, the destruction of liver cells at an interface between par-

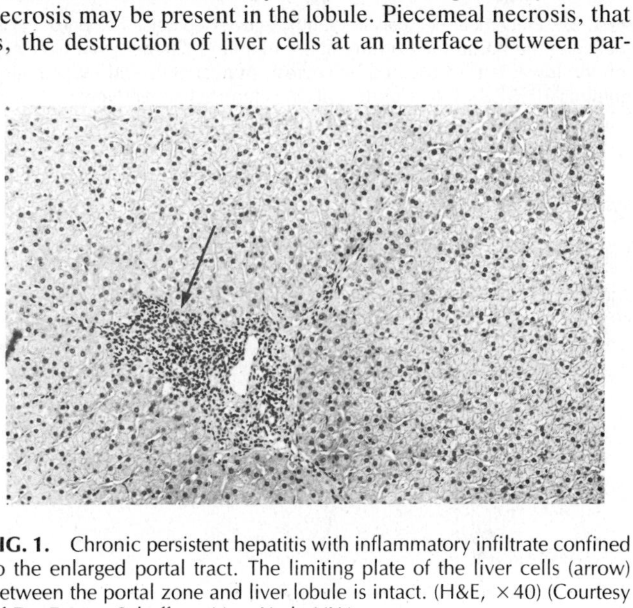

FIG. 1. Chronic persistent hepatitis with inflammatory infiltrate confined to the enlarged portal tract. The limiting plate of the liver cells (arrow) between the portal zone and liver lobule is intact. (H&E, ×40) (Courtesy of Dr. Fenton Schaffner, New York, NY.)

TABLE 1. Chronic Hepatitis

Type	Etiology	Histology	Prognosis	Therapy
Chronic persistent hepatitis	Hepatitis B virus; non-A, non-B virus(es) Drugs Unknown cause	Unresolved hepatitis with minimal periportal inflammation and no necrosis of the liver plate	Benign	Periodic reassessment
Chronic active hepatitis	Hepatitis B virus Non-A, non-B hepatitis virus(es) Autoimmune Drugs	With no cirrhosis Portal piecemeal necrosis and inflammation Bridging hepatic necrosis Periportal piecemeal necrosis with bridging hepatic necrosis With cirrhosis	Results in liver failure	Corticosteroid and/or azathioprine for autoimmune hepatitis

enchyma and connective tissue, together with a predominantly lymphocytic plasma cell infiltrate is not seen. Although the abnormalities of chronic persistent hepatisis may remain for many years, the prognosis for eventual complete recovery is excellent.

CHRONIC ACTIVE HEPATITIS

Chronic active hepatitis, formerly called chronic aggressive hepatitis as defined by an international group of hepatologists,[4] is a chronic inflammatory and fibrosing liver lesion of varied etiology and variable histologic features. The features common to all untreated cases are piecemeal necrosis together with new fiber formation and lymphocytic infiltration of portal tracts and lobules (Fig. 2). Other infiltrating cells, including neutrophils, may also be found, and features of acute hepatitis such as spotty necrosis (hepatocytolysis) may be superimposed. Passive septa formed by collapse after bridging (Fig. 3) or multilobular liver cell necrosis may be present. Cirrhosis is not a necessary defining criterion but can develop (Fig. 4). Liver cell regeneration is seen in chronic active hepatitis, and the borderline between chronic active hepatitis and cirrhosis in the more severe cases is not sharp. The severity of chronic active hepatitis varies with the degree of piecemeal and confluent necrosis and the density of the inflammatory infiltrate.

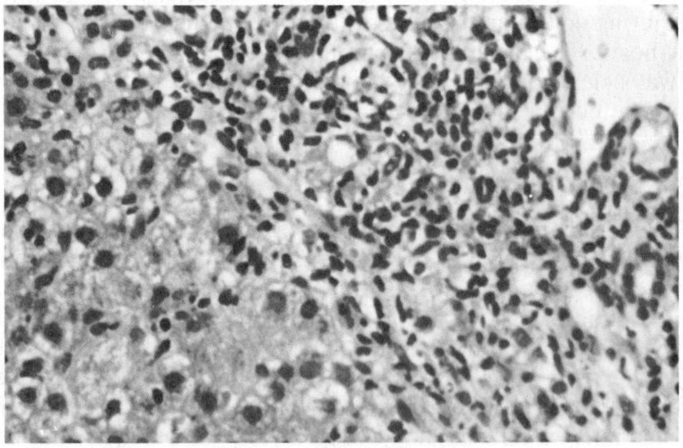

FIG. 2. Piecemeal necrosis in chronic active hepatitis. The border zone between the portal tract on the upper right and parenchymal liver cells on the lower left is obscured by necrosis of liver cells and inflammatory infiltrate. (H&E, ×250) (Courtesy of Dr. Fenton Schaffner, New York, NY.)

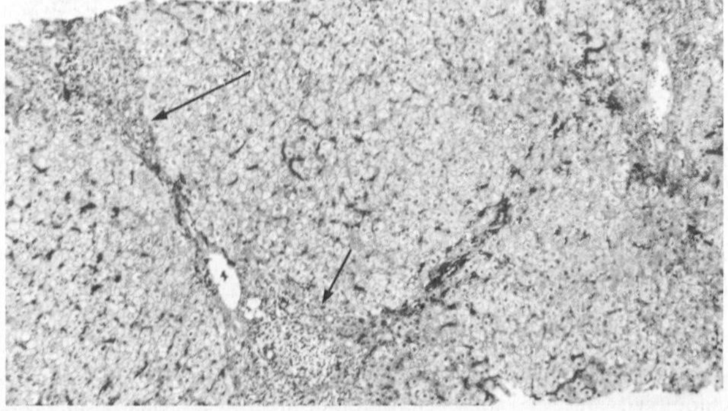

FIG. 3. Chronic active hepatitis with bridging necrosis (arrows) dissecting lobular parenchyma. (H&E, ×40) (Courtesy of Dr. Fenton Schaffner, New York, NY.)

Piecemeal necrosis is a major characteristic of chronic active hepatitis (Fig. 2). The process may be seen either at the edges of portal tracts or the septa of cirrhotic liver or at the margins of septa resulting from collapse after confluent necrosis. Therefore, it is not necessarily confined to the periportal areas of hepatic lobules. The inflammatory infiltrate contains lymphocytes and plasma cells; polymorphonuclear leukocytes may also be present. The lymphocytes are closely associated with hepatocytes, and within the lymphoid infiltrate, hepatocytes may be seen singly or in groups. At the advancing edge of piecemeal necrosis, the liver cells show hydropic swelling and are at times arranged in abnormal configuration such as liver cell rosettes.

Several histologic subgroups of chronic active hepatitis have been defined. These have been conveniently divided into those with or without morphologic evidence of cirrhosis.

Chronic Active Hepatitis without Evidence of Cirrhosis

This subgroup of chronic active hepatitis is characterized by either a portal inflammatory infiltrate with substantial necrosis of the limiting plate of lvier cells (Fig. 2), bridging necrosis (Fig. 3) that interconnects between the two portal triads or with a central vein, or both. The portal triads are swollen with inflammatory infiltrate consisting mainly of lymphocytes and plasmacytes. The limiting plate of liver cells is destroyed to a variable degree by cell necrosis occurring in irregular fashion (piecemeal necrosis). Inflammatory infiltrates extend from the portal triads into the lobules and form septa that are often associated with increases in collagen. With more extensive necrosis, cell collapse extends between portal triads or between portal triads and central veins to create recognizable necrotic and inflammatory bridges known as bridging hepatic necrosis (Fig. 3). This portal–central or portal–portal bridging type of parenchymal cell necrosis was originally termed *subacute hepatic necrosis*[5] or *subacute hepatitis*.[6]

Chronic Active Hepatitis with Evidence of Cirrhosis

In this type of histologic pattern of chronic active hepatitis, the cirrhosis is usually quite active, and regenerating nodules and fibrosis coexist with areas of more recent parenchymal cell necrosis and collapse (Fig. 4). The cell necrosis may be piecemeal, bridging, or multilobular in pattern. Bridging fibrosis, repre-

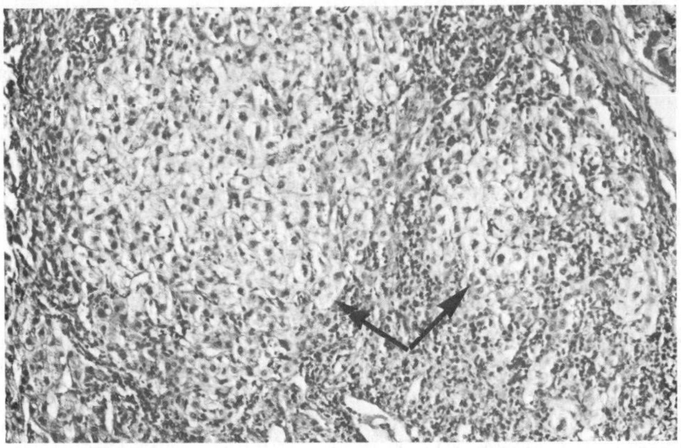

FIG. 4. Chronic active hepatitis with a transition to cirrhosis and the formation of two adjacent nodules (arrows) of liver cells. (H&E, ×100) (Coutesy of Dr. Fenton Schaffner, New York, NY.)

senting the final stage int he progression of necrotic lesions with condensation of reticulin fibers and an increase in fibrosis, may also be present.

Most workers believe that piecemeal necrosis is the most important pathologic process in the development of chronic active hepatitis.[4] However, attention also has been drawn to the nonhomogeneous nature of liver cell damage, to focal hepatocytolysis with inflammatory cell infiltration, and to unevenly distributed regeneration as important features. Bridging hepatic necrosis was considered by some to be the most important lesion in the development of chronic active hepatitis.[5,7] Undoubtedly, all these processes, including piecemeal necrosis, bridging hepatic necrosis, and focal hepatocytolysis and regeneration, are involved in the pathogenesis of chronic active hepatitis and cirrhosis. Confluent necrosis alone is usually followed by healing, leaving either a scarred or a substantially normal liver. This is well documented in the complete recovery of some patients from severe necrotizing acute hepatitis and from nonfatal hepatic necrosis due to shock, carbon tetrachloride, or acetaminophen. In these situations, inflammatory infiltration is usually slight, and piecemeal necrosis is absent. Chronic hepatitis due to hepatitis B virus (HBV) and the non-A, non-B type cannot be distinguished histopathologically unless hepatocytes containing hepatitis B surface antigen (HBsAg) are demonstrated.[8]

CLINICAL PRESENTATIONS OF CHRONIC PERSISTENT HEPATITIS

The clinical presentation usually does not differentiate the patient with chronic persistent hepatitis from the patient with chronic active hepatitis. The patient with chronic persistent hepatitis may complain of fatigue, and jaundice may be present. As a general rule symptoms in patients with chronic persistent hepatitis tend to be mild, and features of cirrhosis do not develop.

CLINICAL PRESENTATIONS OF CHRONIC ACTIVE HEPATITIS

Symptoms and Signs

The patient usually complains of a slow onset of increasing fatigue and fluctuating jaundice. Fatigue is a very important symptom and usually increases in the afternoon and evening. Amenorrhea is common. Examination of the patient shows malnutrition, and arachnoid nevi (spiders) may be found on the upper part of the body. Hepatosplenomegaly may be present. Features of cirrhosis such as hepatic encephalopathy, edema, ascites, and bleeding esophageal varices develop late in the advanced stage of the disease. However, the process may be quite insidious, and cirrhosis may develop in patients without significant symptoms or an antecedent history of jaundice. Therefore, liver biopsy is necessary in asymptomatic patients with chronic abnormalities in liver function.

Biochemical Abnormalities

The biochemical abnormalities are quite variable. The serum bilirubin level may or may not be elevated. The serum glutamic oxaloacetic transaminase (SGOT) and serum glutamic pyruvic transaminase (SGPT) levels are usually increased to at least five times the normal values. The serum alkaline phosphatase and γ-glutamyl transpeptidase values are also increased to at least twice normal. The serum γ-globulin concentration is usually elevated and is of polyclonal type. Serum albumin levels remain within normal limits until the late stage of the disease.

The biochemical abnormalities cannot be used to differentiate chronic persistent from chronic active hepatitis, although elevation of the γ-globulin level is much more common in the latter. In addition, serum bile acid concentrations are more likely to be elevated in patients with chronic active hepatitis than in patients with chronic persistent hepatitis.[9,10]

Immunologic Abnormalities

Patients with chronic active hepatitis due to HBV infection show a selective sensitization of peripheral blood T lymphocytes to hepatitis B core antigen (HBcAg). The specific proliferation was limited to the CD4+ cells.[11] The percentage of resting T cells expressing HLA class II antigens is higher in patients with chronic hepatitis than in controls.[12] Chronic HBsAg carriers have increased proportions of suppressor/cytotoxic T cells in their peripheral blood.[13] Liver damage in hepatitis B appears to be due to a loss of hepatocytes replicating virus rather than a cytotoxic effect of the virus itself.[14]

There is a reduction in γ-interferon production by peripheral blood mononuclear cells of patients with chronic liver disease.[15] Some hepatitis B carriers have a reduced capacity to produce both α- and γ-interferon.[16] No serum interferon was detected in patients with acute or chronic hepatitis when compared with controls.[17]

ETIOLOGY OF CHRONIC HEPATITIS

Chronic Active Hepatitis Associated with Hepatitis B Virus

Chronic active hepatitis is an important complication of HBV infection. Positive serologic tests for HBsAg have been observed in a substantial percentage of patients with chronic active hepatitis, ranging from 10 to 67 percent of the cases. After acute hepatitis B infection, approximately 80 percent of the patients recover completely, and 20 percent develop chronic hepatitis. Of the latter, about 15 percent have chronic persistent hepatitis, and 5 percent have chronic active hepatitis. Only about 2.5 percent of patients progress to cirrhosis. Non-A, non-B acute hepatitis also seems to carry a definite risk for the development of chronic active hepatitis.[18] On the other hand, epidemiologic studies have not demonstrated a risk for the development of chronic active hepatitis after hepatitis A virus (HAV) infection.[19]

Factors Indicating Risk for Chronic Active Hepatitis B

Several factors are useful in pointing to a greater risk of chronicity (Table 2). Clinically, the type of acute attack of HBV infection is helpful in indicating possible progression to chronicity.[20] The patient with an explosive onset of acute hepatitis and deep jaundice usually recovers completely. Survivors of fulminant viral hepatitis rarely progress to chronic disease de-

TABLE 2. Factors Indicating Increased Risk of Chronic Hepatitis B

Age: infants and elderly	
Sex: males	
Insidious and mild acute hepatitis B	
Immunosuppression	
Increased exposure to hepatitis B virus (drug addicts, homosexuals, health workers and renal dialysis units, multiple blood transfusions)	
Geographic location: Mediterranean area, China, Africa	
Persistence of serum	HBsAg
	HBcAg
	DNA polymerase
	HBeAg
Chronic delta virus infection	
Absence of serum	Anti-HBe
	Anti-Hbs
Genetic: ?HLA-B8	

spite the extreme hepatic necrosis during the acute illness. These patients appear to have normal immunologic mechanisms that can clear the virus. Similarly, cholestatic acute viral hepatitis, despite deep jaundice, rarely progresses to chronic hepatitis. In contrast, the patient with an insidious onset with mild prodromal symptoms, slight or even absent jaundice, and continued fatigue seems more likely to slip into chronic disease. Patients receiving immunosuppressive therapy or corticosteroids during the acute attack may also have an increased risk of developing chronic hepatitis.

The very young and very old are at greater risk of developing chronic hepatitis. This may be related to impaired cellular immunity that may be present both in the elderly and in the very young. Men are more often affected than are women during epidemics of hepatitis B infection. Thus, chronic hepatitis B is a disease that predominantly affects men, usually in the 30- to 50-year age range.

Serologic markers for delta hepatitis virus in patients with chronic hepatitis B infection are associated with symptomatic chronic disease and chronic hepatitis.[21,22] Moreover, patients with serologic markers for delta hepatitis more often progress from chronic hepatitis B to cirrhosis.[23] Persistent IgM antibodies to delta antigen indicate chronic delta virus infection.[24]

Patients with acute hepatitis B infection who suffer from chronic diseases that depress immunologic competence such as patients with renal failure, neoplastic disease, or renal transplantation are at particular risk of chronic hepatitis. Persons continually exposed to HBV are also at risk. Health workers such as physicians and laboratory personnel, drug addicts, and homosexuals are at risk. Both patients and personnel in dialysis units are at great risk of exposure. HBV infection is more prevalent in certain geographic areas such as the Mediterranean area, China, and Africa. Patients receiving multiple blood transfusions are also at greater risk of hepatitis developing.

The presence of HBsAg in liver cells of biopsy specimens can be suspected by the ground glass appearance of the cytoplasm. The presence of HBsAg can be confirmed by the orcein stain of Shikata and colleagues[25] or preferably by the presence of cytoplasmic immunofluorescence using anti-HBs. Hepatitis B core antigen (HBcAg) can be identified in the nucleus of the liver cell by immunofluorescent staining. Core particles of HBV with diameters of 27 nm can also be visualized in the nuclei of hepatocytes by electron microscopy.

Patients with persistent HBsAg, HBcAg, and DNA polymerase activity in serum after an acute attack of HBV infection are at greater risk of developing chronic hepatitis. Circulating immune complexes containing HBsAg and IgM usually disappear within 4 weeks of the onset of hepatitis B. Persistence of such complexes after the early phase of acute viral hepatitis B is a predictor of progression to chronic disease.[26] Patients with persistent e antigen (HBeAg) and without anti-HBe appear to be at greater risk of progressing to chronic active hepatitis.[27–29] Patients who develop chronic active hepatitis tend to have persistent anti-HBc in their serum and often have no detectable anti-HBs. HBeAg is present particularly in chronic active and chronic persistent hepatitis. Anti-HBe is found in healthy carriers and in patients with cirrhosis and hepatocellular carcinoma.[30] Most patients who recover without sequelae from acute HBV infection develop anti-HBc before anti-HBs, and the anti-HBc disappears more quickly. Anti-HBs titers fall slowly over the subsequent years. HBeAg, HBcAg, and DNA polymerase appear early in acute disease and disappear rather quickly in those who recover completely.

Many patients with chronic-type B hepatitis eventually undergo a spontaneous remission in clinical and biochemical evidence of active disease, which is usually indicated by the disappearance of HBeAg, HBcAg, and DNA polymerase. Patients who remain HBeAg-positive continue to have elevated aminotransferase levels.[31]

There is some evidence that chronic active hepatitis is more apt to develop in patients who have had acute HBV infection and who are of HLA type B8.[32] Thus, there appears to be a genetic predisposition to development of chronic active hepatitis after acute HBV infection.

By using a radiolabeled 50-base oligonucleotide complementary with the measles virus gene encoding the nucleocapsid as a probe, Robertson and coworkers[33] identified a persistent measles virus genome in the lymphocytes of 12 of 18 patients with autoimmune chronic active hepatitis. These findings raise the possibility that persistent measles virus infection may be a cause of autoimmune chronic active hepatitis. Indeed, the persistence of the measles genome in these patients was correlated with high levels of antibodies to measles.

Clinical Presentation of Chronic Hepatitis B

Chronic hepatitis B may be recognized as unresolved acute viral hepatitis, with persistent abnormalities in lvier function, particularly when HBsAg positivity continues for more than 3 months. About one-half of the patients have established liver disease or a positive test for serum HBsAg. The serum bilirubin, transaminase, and γ-globulin levels are moderately increased, but jaundice is rarely severe. Smooth muscle antibody is most often absent and if present is of low titer. Antimitochondrial antibody is usually absent. Histologic liver sections show the classic features of chronic active hepatitis.

Autoimmune Chronic Hepatitis

Despite documented virus- and drug-related chronic hepatitis, the cause of most chronic cases remains obscure. Chronic active hepatitis of unknown etiology is more commonly associated with autoimmune phenomena including hypergammaglobulinemia, antinuclear factor, a positive lupus erythematosus (LE) cell test, and other serologic tests that suggest an underlying abnormality of the immune response. Chronic active hepatitis has often been described in young women who have arthralgia, amenorrhea, signs of hypercortisolism, and high levels of immunoglobulins.[34] The disease has variously been termed *lupoid hepatitis, plasma cell hepatitis, Waldenström's chronic active hepatitis*, and *active juvenile cirrhosis*. The disease is strongly associated with other clinical manifestations believed to be related to autoimmunity including ulcerative colitis, diabetes mellitus, Coombs-positive hemolytic anemia, pericarditis and myocarditis, pleurisy, pulmonary infiltrations, glomerulitis, renal tubular acidosis, thyroiditis, thrombocytopenic purpura, nondeforming migratory arthritis, leg ulcers, acne and other skin lesions, fibrosing alveolitis, and neurologic lesions.[1] This multisystem involvement indicates that there is a more generalized disorder of immune function. Suppressor T-cell activity is decreased especially in hepatitis B-negative chronic active hepatitis.[35–37] However, increased prostaglandin-producing suppressor cell activity was found in both hepatitis B-positive and

B-negative chronic active hepatitis.[38] Patients with "autoimmune" or hepatitis B-negative chronic hepatitis more often have autoantibodies to liver-specific protein (LSP).[39,40] There is also evidence that genetic factors may determine the type of immune response in patients with chronic hepatitis. The incidence of HLA-A1 and -8 is as high as 70 percent in some of these patients,[41] and there is an increased incidence of antimitochondrial antibodies and other serologic abnormalities in first-degree relatives including an association with familial hypergammaglobulinemia.[1] The clinical characteristics of chronic "autoimmune" hepatitis are compared with those of chronic hepatitis B in Table 3.

Autoimmune hepatitis commonly affects women between the ages of 15 and 25 years and recurs about the time of menopause. Illness often begins insidiously but may resemble acute viral hepatitis in onset. Fever is present in those who are acutely ill. Arachnoid nevi are often present, as is hepatosplenomegaly. Skin striae, acne, and moon face are common. Serologic tests show a positive antinuclear factor in more than 50 percent of cases and smooth muscle antibody in about 67 percent. The serum γ-globulin is quite high, and LE cells are present in about 15 percent of cases. Thrombocytopenia and leukopenia are frequent even before the onset of portal hypertension. The prothrombin time may be prolonged even in the early stages of the disease. Liver biopsy specimen shows histologic evidence of chronic active hepatitis. This type of chronic active hepatitis is most amenable to therapy, and the prognosis currently is very good.

Drug-Related Chronic Hepatitis

Drugs are increasingly implicated in both acute and chronic hepatitis. Chronic hepatitis may result from a direct hepatotoxic effect of the drug or drug metabolite or from an idiosyncratic drug allergy directed toward hepatic tissue. Drugs that are most commonly associated with chronic hepatitis include methotrexate, acetylsalicylic acid, isoniazid, α-methyldopa, and oxyphenacetin. Prolonged administration of nitrofurantoin also has been associated with hepatic necrosis and chronic active hepatitis.[42,43] Abnormalities in liver function often improve after withdrawal of the drug. The clinical and histologic characteristics of drug-related chronic hepatitis are frequently indistinguishable from other forms of chronic hepatitis when eosinophilia or extrahepatic manifestations of drug allergy are absent. In such instances, it is often difficult to establish a relationship between chronic liver disease and the drug.

Oxyphenacetin, found in some laxatives, is no longer used in the United States and was the first drug to be associated with chronic active hepatitis. Isoniazid, used in the treatment of tuberculosis, has been associated with the picture of chronic active hepatitis and may result in fatal disease. α-Methyldopa is used in the treatment of hypertension, and severe, even fatal hepatitis has been reported with this drug; the acute hepatitis may progress to chronic active hepatitis. Thus, it is important to take an accurate history of drug usage in all patients with chronic active hepatitis.

Isoniazid can lead to serious hepatotoxic disease resulting in death.[44] About one-half of the cases are recognized during the first 2 months of therapy and the other half up to a period of 1 year. Hepatic injury presenting after 2 months of therapy is more likely to prove fatal. Approximately 50 percent of the patients have gastrointestinal complaints including anorexia, nausea, vomiting, and abdominal distress. About 40 percent of the patients complain of symptoms suggestive of "viral" illness either with or without gastrointestinal complaints, and the remaining 10 percent have jaundice. Fever is rarely observed, and hepatomegaly is seen in about a third of the patients. Serum transaminase and alkaline phosphatase levels are usually elevated. Marked hyperbilirubinemia is generally associated with more severe disease and a poorer prognosis. Histologic examination of the liver shows hepatocellular damage. Most often the liver cellular structure resembles that of acute viral hepatitis with ballooning degeneration, sinusoidal acidophilic bodies, and focal necrosis. Some patients show bridging hepatic necrosis. A histologic picture resembling chronic active hepatitis is seen in about 10 percent of the patients. Most patients respond to discontinuing isoniazid therapy.

Methyldopa can also lead to liver cellular patterns resembling that of chronic active hepatitis.[45] Nausea, vomiting, and fatigue begin within 1 to 2 weeks after drug administration. Jaundice supervenes if the therapy is continued. The serum transaminase levels are elevated. Liver biopsy specimens show a predominantly mononuclear infiltrate in the portal triads. The LE cell preparation and the anti–smooth muscle antibody test may be positive. The hepatitis resolves when the drug is removed, although residual fibrosis due to extensive cell necrosis may be present.

TABLE 3. Clinical Characteristics of Chronic Active Hepatitis

Characteristic	*Autoimmune*	*Hepatitis B*
Predominant sex	Female	Male
Age	15–25; menopause	Older adults; neonates
Serum HBsAg	Negative	Usually positive
Serum HBcAg	Negative	May be positive
Serum hepatitis B DNA polymerase	Negative	May be positive
Serum HBeAg	Negative	May be positive
Serum γ-globulin	Markedly increased	Normal or moderately increased
Smooth muscle antibody	High	Absent or low
Associated autoimmune disease	Common	Uncommon
Frequent HLA type	A1, A8	B8
Response to immunosuppressive therapy	Good	Poor

DIFFERENTIAL DIAGNOSIS OF CHRONIC ACTIVE HEPATITIS

The differential diagnosis of chronic hepatitis includes prolonged viral hepatitis, primary biliary cirrhosis, alcoholic liver disease, pericholangitis with inflammatory bowel disease, Wilson's disease (hepatolenticular degeneration), granulomatous hepatitis, and α_1-antitrypsin deficiency.

Prolonged Viral Hepatitis

It is often difficult to distinguish relapsing or unresolved acute hepatitis from which recovery will be complete from chronic hepatitis. Needle liver biopsy is mandatory, but at times the interpretation can be difficult. In instances where the diagnosis is doubtful, several needle biopsies may be required to elucidate the nature of the disease.

Primary Biliary Cirrhosis

Primary biliary cirrhosis, a chronic obstructive, granulomatous cholangitis, usually is seen in middle-aged women with a predominant cholestasis and marked pruritus.[46] Antimitochondrial antibody is usually present in high titer, and the serum IgM level is raised in 80 percent of patients. Histologic sections of the liver show inflammation of the bile ductules with lymphocytes and plasma cells. Granulomas are found next to damaged intrahepatic bile ductules and in lymph nodes outside the liver, hepatic hilum, omentum, and lungs, especially in early stages of the disease.

Alcoholic Liver Disease

Patients with alcoholic liver disease tend to be older. There is a history of the chronic use of large amounts of alcohol, and the patient shows many arachnoid nevi. Histologic sections of the liver show fatty infiltration, Mallory's hyaline bodies, and a central zonal type of liver damage.

Pericholangitis with Inflammatory Bowel Disease

Inflammatory bowel disease including ulcerative colitis, granulomatous colitis, and regional enteritis may be complicated by pericholangitis. The serum globulin levels are usually normal, and the alkaline phosphatase level is very elevated. Liver biopsy specimens show a portal zone of inflammation, especially around the bile ducts. Anti-smooth muscle and anti-mitochondrial antibodies are usually absent.

Wilson's Disease

Patients with this disease may have all the typical features of chronic active hepatitis, often with ascites or with acute hemolysis.[47] There may be a history of parental consanguinity or a familial history of liver disease. Examination of the cornea by slit lamp may show Kaiser-Fleischer rings indicating copper deposition. The serum ceruloplasmin levels are low, and the serum copper level is high. Urinary copper and the copper content of the liver are also high. The disease can be treated with D-penicillamine and a low-copper diet.

Granulomatous Hepatitis

The presentation of granulomatous hepatitis often may be confused with chronic active hepatitis (see Chapter 104).

α_1-Antitrypsin Deficiency

α_1-Antitrypsin is a glycoprotein with a molecular weight of 50,000 that occupies the α_1-globulin position on standard serum protein electrophoresis.[48] The electrophoretic phenotype, called the protease inhibitor (Pi) type, is determined by codominant genes. In most populations 85 percent are PiM, containing about 2.2 mg/ml of serum α_1-antitrypsin. Serum protease inhibitor concentrations of 1.8 mg/ml or less are found in Pi types ZZ, SZ, (−) null, S (−), and Z (−), the first two being more common. These patients develop familial emphysema beginning early in life. There is an increased prevalence of the MZ phenotype in patients with α_1-antitrypsin deficiency and chronic active hepatitis or cryptogenic cirrhosis.[49] Neonatal hepatitis and cirrhosis also are associated with α_1-antitrypsin deficiency. Although these patients usually have neonatal jaundice progressing to cholestasis during childhood, chronic active hepatitis has been reported.[50] The diagnosis can be made by measuring the concentration of α_1-antitrypsin in the serum.

TREATMENT OF CHRONIC PERSISTENT HEPATITIS

It is generally agreed that chronic persistent hepatitis is a benign disease that does not evolve into cirrhosis, although hepatic inflammation may be present for many years. Therefore, steroid and immunosuppressive therapy is not used in this condition. Unfortunately, most cases of chronic persistent hepatitis have been observed only for short periods of time, so the ultimate prognosis of such patients cannot be certain. Therefore, these patients must be reexamined periodically. Repeat liver biopsy may be necessary to establish a definitive diagnosis.

TREATMENT OF CHRONIC ACTIVE HEPATITIS

Chronic active hepatitis is a progressive disease that often responds to corticosteroid therapy with improvement in liver function and reduction in mortality. However, there is evidence that the prognosis of patients with chronic active hepatitis depends on the specific etiology of the liver disease and the type of liver lesion.[51–53] Patients with periportal piecemeal necrosis without bridging necrosis or fibrosis respond well to corticosteroid therapy and do not progress to cirrhosis. On the other hand, patients with bridging necrosis or multilobular necrosis have a high incidence of progression to cirrhosis even with corticosteroid therapy. Moreover, patients with an active stage of cirrhosis on liver biopsy are more likely to be refractory to steroid therapy and relapse more frequently when steroid treatment is withdrawn. There is also increasing evidence that patients with chronic active hepatitis after HBV infection with chronic carriage of HBsAg are more refractory to corticosteroid therapy, and indeed, the lesions may worsen with such therapy. Prednisolone was found to have a deleterious effect in patients with HBsAg-positive chronic active hepatitis.[54,55] Immunosuppressive therapy appears to favor the replication of HBV in patients with HBsAg-positive chronic active hepatitis.[56–58]

There is general agreement that patients with autoimmune chronic active hepatitis respond well to corticosteroid therapy and that the prognosis is quite good. These patients lose their feelings of fatigue, the menses return, and liver function test findings become normal. The hepatic lesions are arrested. Prednisolone therapy significantly improves survival by reducing mortality in the early active phase of hepatitis B-negative chronic active hepatitis.[59] However, clinical deterioration can occur unpredictably after cessation of corticosteroid therapy.[60]

Most treatment regimens use prednisone or prednisolone. The choice of whom to treat or not to treat is often quite difficulte. Moreover, the type of therapy must be individualized with each patient. Generally, the initial dose of prednisone or prednisolone is 30–50 mg/day for 1 week with reduction over the following weeks to a maintenance dose of 10–20 mg/day. The maintenance dose is adjusted so that the patient is asymptomatic and liver function test results are relatively normal. Alternate-day prednisone therapy has also been used in an attempt to minimize side effects. However, such therapy cannot be used in every patient because the liver cells may not respond.

Liver biopsy and liver function tests should be performed before beginning corticosteroid therapy. Clinical examination and follow-up liver function tests should then be done at approximately monthly intervals. Liver biopsy should be repeated by 6 months to determine the effect of therapy on liver histology.

Azathioprine has been added to prednisone in those patients who do not respond or in those patients who have side effects with larger doses of prednisone and the dose must be reduced.[53] In such cases, azathioprine has often been effective. White blood cell counts should be checked at regular intervals in patients receiving azathioprine. The drug may be teratogenic and should not be given to pregnant patients. Moreover, when used as long-term therapy, the drug has been associated with the development of neoplasms in patients with renal transplants. Azathioprine is used usually at a dose of 50–100 mg/day.

A satisfactory remission is characterized by the absence of symptoms, normal serum globulin levels, and normal or minimally elevated transaminase levels. Histologic liver sections show no evidence of piecemeal necrosis or other signs of active hepatitis. Almost 90 percent of the patients who respond should achieve a clinical and biochemical remission after about a year and a half of therapy, whereas only 60 percent show a histologic remission. Relapse is uncommon after a full clinical and biochemical remission of 6 months' duration. In most patients the total duration of therapy is at least 2 years, and in many it is much longer.

In addition to immunosuppressive therapy patients should be urged to eat a balanced diet and to obtain adequate amounts of rest and sleep, and they should be given an individualized exercise program to promote a general sense of well-being. Failure of immunosuppressive therapy occurs in about 20 percent of the patients, and these may develop liver failure. In such patients, the dose of prednisone and azathioprine is increased in the hope of inducing a remission.

Several experimental modalities of therapy have been applied to patients with chronic active hepatitis B. Early studies indicated that the combination of human leukocyte interferon with vidarabine showed some promise in eliminating viral replication in chronic hepatitis B infection[61]; the use of vidarabine monophosphate (ara-AMP) administered intramuscularly allowed outpatient therapy.[62,63] Recombinant α-interferon administered to patients with chronic hepatitis B mediated a decrease in serum viral DNA polymerase activity.[64] It appears that a major effect of α-interferon on immunoregulation in patients with chronic type B hepatitis is the inhibition of late stages of B-cell differentiation into immunoglobuline-producing and -secreting plasma cells.[65] However, the results of a more recent large randomized study did not support the use of ara-AMP and human leukocyte interferon in chronic persistent or chronic active hepatitis B.[66]

Acyclovir does not appear to inhibit the replication of HBV.[67,68] However, patients with chronic HBV infection had greater decreases in serum viral DNA polymerase and HBeAg when treated with interferon and acyclovir in combination than when treated with either agent alone.[69] Suramin, an inhibitor of retroviral DNA polymerases, is not useful in treating chronic hepatitis B.[70] There have been reports, as yet unconfirmed, that cianidanol may be useful in treating HBeAg-positive chronic active hepatitis.[71] Long-term therapy with the immune modulator levamisole showed a trend toward normalization of serum aminotransferase activities and suppression of viral replication in patients with chronic hepatitis B.[72] Recombinant interleukin-2 (r-IL2) decreased serum viral DNA polymerase activity and resulted in a loss of serum HBeAg in two of five patients.[73]

Prolonged treatment of chronic non-A, non-B hepatitis with recombinant α-interferon resulted in a sustained improvement in serum aminotransferase levels.[74] Three patients with hypogammaglobulinemia given α-interferon for chronic non-A, non-B hepatitis showed striking decreases in serum aminotransferase levels after the start of each course of therapy.[75] Further studies are needed to define the role, if any, of α-intereferon in therapy for non-A, non-B hepatitis.

REFERENCES

1. Sherlock S. Chronic hepatitis. Gut. 1974;15:581.
2. DeGroote J, Desmet VJ, Gedigk P, et al. A classification of chronic hepatitis. Lancet. 1968;2:626.
3. Boyer JL. Chronic hepatitis: A perspective on classification and determinants of prognosis. Gastroenterology. 1976;70:1161.
4. Bianchi CC, Mulligan R, Sherlock S. Controlled prospective trial of corticosteroid therapy in active chronic hepatitis. Q J med. 1971;40:159.
5. Boyer JL, Klatskin G. Pattern of necrosis in acute viral hepatitis: Prognostic value of bridging (subacute hepatic necrosis). N Engl J Med. 1970;283:1063.
6. Tisdale WA. Subacute hepatitis. N Engl J Med. 1963;268:85.
7. Ware AJ, Eigenbrodt EH, Combes B. Prognostic significance of subacute hepatic necrosis in acute hepatitis. Gastroenterology. 1975;68:519.
8. Thorne CH, Higgins GR, Ulrich TR, et al. A histologic comparison of hepatitis B with non-A, non-B chronic active hepatitis. Arch Pathol Lab Med. 1982;106:433.
9. Jones MB, Weinstock S, Koretz RL, et al. Clinical value of serum bile acid levels in chronic hepatitis. Dig Dis Sci. 1981;26:978.
10. Monroe PS, Baker AL, Schneider JF, et al. The aminopyrine breath test and serum bile acids reflect histologic severity in chronic hepatitis. Hepatology. 1982;2:317.
11. Ferrari C, Penna A, Sansoni P, et al. Selective sensitization of peripheral blood T lymphocytes to hepatitis B core antigen in patients with chronic active hepatitis type B. Clin Exp Immunol. 1986;66:497.
12. Scudeletti M, Indiveri F, Pierri I, et al. T cells from patients with chronic liver diseases: Abnormalities on PHA-induced expression of HLA class II antigens and in autologous mixed-lymphocyte reactions. Cell Immunol. 1986;102:227.
13. Alexander GJ, Mondelli M, Naumor NV, et al. Functional characterization of peripheral blood lymphocytes in chronic HBsAg carriers. Clin Exp Immunol. 1986;63:498.
14. Chu CM, Karayiannis P, Fowler MJ, et al. Natural history of chronic hepatitis B virus infection in Taiwan: Studies of hepatitis B virus DNA in serum. Hepatology. 1985;5:431.
15. Fuji A, Kakumu S, Ohtani Y, et al. Interferon-gamma production by peripheral blood mononuclear cells of patients with chronic liver disease. Hepatology. 1987;7:577.
16. Ikeda T, Lever AM, Thomas HC. Evidence for a deficiency of interferon production in patients with chronic hepatitis B virus infection acquired in adult life. Hepatology. 1986;6:962.
17. Pieovino M, Aguet M, Huber M, et al. Absence of detectable serum interferon in acute and chronic viral hepatitis. Hepatology. 1986;6:645.
18. Hoofnagle JH, Garety RJ, Tabor E, et al. Transmission of non-A, non-B hepatitis. Ann Intern Med. 1977;87:14.
19. Dienstag JL, Ezmuness W, Stevens CE, et al. Hepatitis A virus infection: New insights from seroepidemiologic studies. J Infect Dis. 1978;137:328.
20. Sherlock S. Predicting progression of acute type B hepatitis to chronicity. Lancet. 1976;2:354.
21. Shields MT, Czaja AJ, Taswell HF, et al. Frequency and significance of delta antibody in acute and chronic hepatitis B. A United States experience. Gastroenterology. 1985;89:1230.
22. Hadziyannis SJ, Sherman M, Lieberman HM, et al. Liver disease activity and hepatitis B virus replication in chronic delta antigen–positive hepatitis B virus carriers. Hepatology. 1985;5:544.
23. Fattovich G, Boscaro S, Noventa F, et al. Influence of hepatitis delta virus infection on progression to cirrhosis in chronic hepatitis type B. J Infect Dis. 1987;155:931.
24. Aragona M, Macagno S, Caredda F, et al. Serological response to the hepatitis delta virus in hepatitis D. Lancet 1987;1:478.
25. Shikata T, Uzawa T, Yoshiwara N, et al. Staining methods of Australia antigen in paraffin sections: Detection of cytoplasmic inclusion bodies. Jpn J Exp Med. 1974;44:25.
26. Careoda F, de Fravebis R, D'Arminio Monforte A, et al. Persistence of circulating HBsAg/IgM complexes in acute viral hepatitis, type B: An early marker of chronic evolution. Lancet. 1982;2:358.
27. Nielsen JO, Dietrichson O, Juhl E. Incidence and meaning of the "e" determinant among hepatitis B antigen positive patients with acute and chronic liver disease. Lancet. 1974;2:913.
28. Vogten AJM, Schalm SW, Sumemrskill WHJ, et al. Behavior of e antigen and antibody during chronic active liver disease: Relation to HB antigen-antibody system and prognosis. Lancet. 1976;2:126.
29. Trepo CG, Magnius LO, Schaefer RA, et al. Detection of e antigen and antibody: Correlations with hepatitis B surface and hepatitis B core antigens, live disease, and outcome in hepatitis B infections. Gastroenterology. 1976;71:804.
30. Viola LA, Barrison IG, Coleman JC, et al. The HBe antigen-antibody system and its relationship to clinical and laboratory findings in 100 chronic HBsAg carriers in Great Britain. J Med Virol. 1981;8:169.
31. Hoofnagle JH, Dusheiko GM, Seeff LB, et al. Seroconversion from hepatitis B e antigen to antibody in chronic type B hepatitis. Ann Intern Med. 1981;94:744.
32. Page AR, Sharp HL, Greenberg LJ, et al. Genetic analysis of patients with chronic active hepatitis. J Clin Invest. 1975;56:530..
33. Robertson DAG, Guy EC, Zhang SL, et al. Persistent measles virus genome in autoimmune chronic active hepatitis. Lancet. 1987;2:9–11.
34. Sherlock S. Waldenstrom's chronic active hepatitis. Acta Med Scand. 1966;445(suppl):426.
35. Tremolada F, Fattovich G, Panebianco G, et al. Suppressor cell activity in viral and non-viral chronic active hepatitis. Clin Exp Immunol. 1980;40:89.
36. Nonomura A, Tanino M, Kurumaya H, et al. Disordered immunoregulatory functions in patients with chronic active hepatitis. Clin Exp Immunol. 1982;47:595.
37. Carella G, Chatenoud L, Degos F, et al. Regulatory T cell-subset imbalance in chronic active hepatitis. J Clin Immunol. 1982;2:93.
38. Krawitt EL, Albertini RJ, Webb DD, et al. Immune regulation and HLA types in chronic hepatitis. Hepatology. 1981;1:300.
39. Manns M, Meyer zum Buschenfelde KH, Hutteroth TH, et al. Detection and characterization of liver membrane autoantibodies in chronic active hepatitis by solid-phase radioimmunoassay. Clin Exp Immunol. 1980;42:263.
40. Meliconi R, Baraldini M, Stefanini GF, et al. Antibodies against human liver-specific protein (LSP) in acute and chronic viral hepatitis types A, and B and non-A, non-B. Clin Exp Immunol. 1981;46:382.
41. MacKay IR, Morris PJ. Association of autoimmune chronic active hepatitis with HL-A1,8. Lancet. 1972;2:793.
42. Sharp JR, Ishak KG, Zimmerman JH. Chronic active hepatitis and severe hepatic necrosis associated with nitrofurantoin. Ann Intern Med. 1980;92:14.
43. Black M, Rabin L, Schatz N. Nitrofurantoin-induced chronic active hepatitis. Ann Intern Med. 1980;92:62.
44. Black M, Mitchell JR, Zimmerman HJ, et al. Isoniazid-associated hepatitis in 114 patients. Gastroenterology. 1975;69:289.
45. Maddrey WC, Boitnott JK. Severe hepatitis from methyldopa. Gastroenterology. 1975;68:351.
46. Sherlock S. Primary biliary cirrhosis. Mt Sinai J Med. 1977;44:790.
47. Sternleib I, Scheinberg IH. Chronic hepatitis as a first manifestation of Wilson's disease. Ann Intern Med. 1972;76:59.
48. Norum RA, Kearn AG, Briscoe WA, et al. Alpha-1-antitrypsin and disease. Mt Sinai J Med. 1977;44:827.
49. Hodges JR, Millward-Sadler GH, Barbatis C, et al. Heterozygous MZ alpha-1-antitrypsin deficiency in adults with chronic active hepatitis and cryptogenic cirrhosis. N Engl J Med. 1981;304:557.
50. Fisher RL, Taylor L, Sherlock S. Alpha-1-antitrypsin deficiency in liver disease: The extent of the problem. Gastroenterology. 1976;71:651.
51. Cook GC, Mulligan R, Sherlock S. Controlled prospective trial of corticosteroid therapy in active chronic hepatitis. Q J Med. 1971;40:159.

52. Soloway RD, Summerskill WHJ, Baggenstoss AH, et al. Clinical, biochemical and histological remission of severe chronic active liver disease: A controlled trial of treatments and an early prognosis. Gastroenterology. 1972;63:820.
53. Summerskill WHJ, Korman MG, Ammon HV, et al. Prednisone for chronic active liver disease: Dose titration, standard and combination with azothioprine compared. Gut. 1975;16:876.
54. Lam KC, Lai CL, Trepo C, et al. Deleterious effect of prednisolone in HBsAg-positive chronic active hepatitis. N Engl J Med. 1981;304:380.
55. Hoofnagle JH, Davis GL, Pappas SC, et al. A short course of prednisolone in chronic type B hepatitis. Report of a randomized, double-blind, placebo controlled trial. Ann Intern Med. 1986;104:12.
56. Weller IV, Bassendine MF, Murray AK, et al. Effects of prednisolone/azathioprine in chronic hepatitis B viral infection. Gut. 1980;23:650.
57. Sagnelli E, Manzillo G, Maio G, et al. Serum levels of hepatitis B surface and core antigens during immunosuppressive treatment of HBsAg-positive chronic active hepatitis. Lancet. 1980;2:395.
58. Sherlock S, Thomas HC. Treatment of chronic hepatitis due to hepatitis B virus. Lancet. 1985;2:1343.
59. Kirk AP, Jain S, Pocock S, et al. Late results of the Royal Free Hospital prospective controlled trial of prednisolone therapy in hepatitis B surface antigen negative chronic active hepatitis. Gut. 1980;21:78.
60. Czaja AJ, Ludwig J, Baggenstoss AA, et al. Corticosteroid-treated chronic active hepatitis in remission: Uncertain prognosis of chronic persistent hepatitis. N Engl J Med. 1981;304:5.
61. Scullard GH, Pollard RB, Smith JL, et al. Antiviral treatment of chronic hepatitis B virus infection. I. Changes in viral markers with interferon combined with adenine arabinoside. J Infect Dis. 1981;143:772.
62. Smith CI, Kitchen LW, Scullard GH, et al. Vidarabine monophosphate and human leukocyte interferon in chronic hepatitis B infection. JAMA. 1982;247:2261.
63. Weller IV, Bassendine MF, Craxi A, et al. Successful treatment of HBs and HBeAg positive chronic liver disease: Prolonged inhibition of viral replication by highly soluble adenine arabinoside 5′-monomphosphate(ARA-AMP). Gut. 1982;23:717.
64. Eisenberg M, Rosno S, Garcia G, et al. Preliminary trial of recombinant fibroblast interferon in chronic hepatitis B virus infection. Antimicrob Agents Chemother. 1986;29:122.
65. Peters H, Walling DM, Kelly K, et al. Immunologic effects of interferon-alpha in man: Treatment with human recombinant interferon-alpha suppresses in vitro immunoglobulin production in patients with chronic type B hepatitis. J Immunol. 1986;137:3147.
66. Garcia G, Smith CI, Weisberg JI, et al. Adenine arabinoside monophosphate (vidarabine phosphate) in combination with human leukocyte interferon in the treatment of chronic hepatitis B. A randomized, double-blind, placebo controlled trial. Ann Intern Med. 1987;107:278.
67. Smith CI, Scullard GH, Gregory PB, et al. Preliminary studies of acyclovir in chronic hepatitis B. Am J Med. 1982;73:267.
68. Alexander GJ, Fagan EA, Hegarty JE, et al. Controlled trial of acyclovir in chronic hepatitis B virus infection. J Med Virol. 1987;21:81.
69. Schalm SW, Heytink RA, van Buuren HR, et al. Acyclovir enhances the antiviral effect of interferon in chronic hepatitis B. Lancet. 1985;2:358.
70. Loke RH, Anderson MG, Coleman JC, et al. Suramin treatment for chronic active hepatitis B—toxic and ineffective. J Med Virol. 1987;21:97.
71. Suzuki H, Yamamoto S, Hirayama C, et al. Cianidanol therpay for HBe-antigen–positive chronic hepatitis: A multicenter, double blind study. Liver. 1986;6:35.
72. Fattovich G, Brollo L, Pontisso P, et al. Levamisole therapy in chronic type B hepatitis. Results of a double-blind randomized trial. Gastroenterology. 1986;91:692.
73. Nishioka M, Kagawa H, Shirai M, et al. Effects of human recombinant interleukin 2 in patients with chronic hepatitis B: A preliminary report. Am J Gastroenterol. 1987;82:438.
74. Hoofnagle JH, Muller KD, Jones DB, et al. Treatment of chronic non-A, non-B hepatitis with recombinant human alpha interferon. A preliminary report. N Engl J Med. 1986;315:1575.
75. Thomson BJ, Doran M, Lever AM, et al. Alpha-interferon therapy for non-A, non-B hepatitis transmitted by gammoglobulin replacement therapy. Lancet. 1987;1:539.

104. GRANULOMATOUS HEPATITIS

ANTHONY S. FAUCI
GARY S. HOFFMAN

Granulomas in the liver are histopathologic manifestations of a broad range of disease processes that may be of diverse etiologies, both infectious and noninfectious. They do not represent a distinct disease; also, in and of themselves, they rarely are diagnostic of a particular disease entity since their etiology is seldom determined purely on histologic criteria.[1] Most often (74 percent), they reflect a systemic granulomatous disease. Less frequently (21 percent), they represent a process that primarily is neither a systemic granulomatous nor a hepatic disease; only rarely (4 percent) do they represent an isolated hepatic disease.[1] In this regard, the demonstration of hepatic granulomas may serve to confirm documented underlying disease, or it may present a diagnostic challenge requiring an organized and directed approach in determining its underlying etiology. Since the histopathologic features of granulomas resulting from infectious and noninfectious etiologies may be identical and since the treatment regimens (particularly corticosteroids) used in diseases with hepatic granulomata of noninfectious etiologies are directly contraindicated in most disorders of infectious etiologies, it is imperative to appreciate the intricacies of this clinicopathologic process.

PATHOPHYSIOLOGIC MECHANISMS OF GRANULOMA FORMATION

It is now fairly well established that granulomas form by a stepwise series of events that include the migration of monocyte–macrophages into an area of inflammatory or immunologic reactivity and the transformation of these cells into epithelioid cells, which may remain as such or may fuse to form the characteristic multinucleated giant cells.[2–5] The morphologic changes that impart an epithelial-like appearance to the macrophage are accompanied by functional changes. The macrophage–phagocyte becomes a nonphagocytic epithelioid cell having increased organelles for enzyme and other protein synthesis and secretion.[6,7] The persistence of incompletely degraded foreign matter in tissues represents one type of stimulus for such cellular transformation. An example is found in tuberculosis, the clinically most common microbial cause of granulomata. It has been demonstrated that mycobacterial lipids persist within the macrophage and trigger its transformation.[8] Although this is an excellent example of persistence of microbial intracellular antigen-enhancing granuloma formation, persistent extracellular stimuli such as schistosome eggs lead to similar responses.[7] In addition, nonmicrobial particles may also stimulate granuloma formation (e.g., silica, metal salts), although in these examples nonimmunologic mechanisms appear to activate macrophages.

It is quite clear that undegraded materials are not the only stimuli of epithelioid cell transformation and granuloma formation since antigen persistence cannot adequately explain many of the granulomatous responses of hypersensitivity etiology.[3] Pure foreign body granulomas in which antigen persistence triggers the reaction fall on one end of the spectrum, and pure hypersensitivity responses in which it is highly unlikely that antigen persistence is operable forms the other end of the spectrum.[9] In the latter circumstance, sensitized lymphocytes on exposure to antigen (which, in many cases, is soluble) amplify the immune response by release of mediators. Monocyte–macrophages accumulate, most likely in response to mediators, and subsequently undergo transformation as described above. In experimental animals, cyclosporine A has been demonstrated to markedly reduce the granulomatous response induced with a variety of mycobacterial agents.[6] This observation suggests that, at least in this setting, granuloma formation is highly dependent upon T-lymphocyte mediators that may inhibit migration and cause activation of macrophages (e.g., γ-interferon).[10,11]

Most infectious diseases in which granulomas occur constitute an overlap of mechanisms since microbes can serve both as a foreign body and as an antigen for an immunologic response. In addition, immune complexes made up of host antibody and microbial or nonmicrobial antigen may, under certain circumstances, stimulate granuloma formation. Finally,

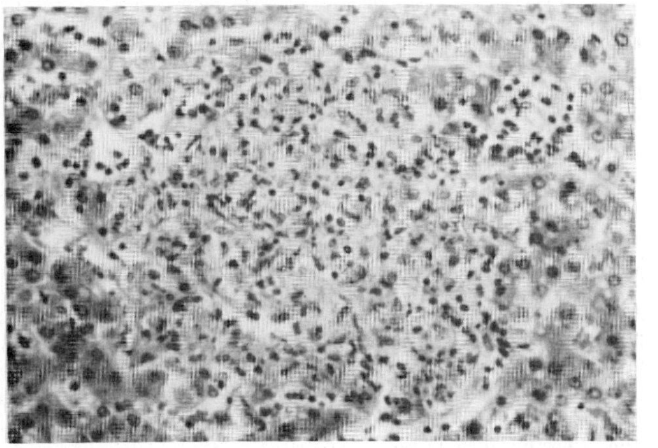

FIG. 1. Liver biopsy specimen from a patient with disseminated histoplasmosis. A typical granuloma is shown with epithelioid cells and mononuclear cell infiltration. (H&E, ×220)

certain T-lymphocyte neoplasms may secrete soluble factors that activate macrophages,[12] an alternative mechanism for granuloma formation in diseases such as lymphomatoid granulomatosis.[13]

The liver serves as a particularly susceptible target organ for granuloma formation. It is an extremely large organ rich in reticuloendothelial cells. In addition to their phagocytic ability, certain of these cells possess receptors such as those for the Fc portion of immunoglobulin,[14] thus allowing for nonspecific (as well as a degree of immunologically specific) clearance of circulting antigens, unopsonized and opsonized microorganisms, and immune complexes. It is clear then why hepatic granulomas are found in such a high proportion of diseases with systemic granulomatous responses and why a liver biopsy specimen provides such a high-yield source of diagnostic tissue in such diseases (Fig. 1).

Histopathologically, hepatic granulomas are characterized by the presence of generally discrete nodular infiltrates of epithelioid cells interspersed with greater or lesser degrees of mononuclear cells. The epithelioid cells usually are compactly arranged and may merge to form typical multinucleated giant cells. However, the presence of these giant cells is not necessary to make the diagnosis of a granulomatous reaction. This histopathologic picture of hepatic granulomas is clearly distinguishable from portal triaditis, which is more commonly seen in a number of inflammatory conditions and which is characterized by the infiltration of mononuclear cells as well as granulocytes around the portal tract areas. Thus, it is not strictly correct to term granulomatous hepatitis a true "hepatitis" since classic inflammatory responses are rarely seen and, as will be discussed below, significant hepatocellular dysfunction is rare.[15,16]

DISEASES CHARACTERIZED BY HEPATIC GRANULOMAS

Infectious Diseases

Infectious diseases clearly are the most common underlying causes of granulomas in general and of hepatic granulomas in particular.[17–19] Table 1 lists some of the various types of infectious diseases that may be associated with granulomas in the liver. Tuberculosis continues to lead the list as the most common infectious disease cause of hepatic granulomas.[17–19] Even when one considers all causes of hepatic granulomas (infectious and noninfectious), tuberculosis still ranks very high in incidence. In Klatskin's series[1] of 433 patients with documented granulomatous diseases in other organs, tuberculosis ranked

TABLE 1. Infectious Disease Causes of Granulomatous Hepatitis

Bacterial
Mycobacteriosis
Tuberculous
Nontuberculous
Lepromatous leprosy
Brucellosis (*Brucella abortus*)
Tularemia
Granuloma inguinale
Melioidosis
Listeriosis
Fungal
Histoplasmosis
Coccidioidomycosis
Candidiasis
Viral
Cytomegalovirus
Infectious mononucleosis
Viral hepatitis
Parasitic
Schistosomiasis (*Schistosoma mansoni*)
Visceral larva migrans (*Toxocara canis* or *catis*)
Fascioliasis (*Fasciola hepatica*)
Capillaria hepatica
Rickettsial
Q fever (*Coxiella burnetii*)
Spirochetal
Syphilis

second to sarcoidosis in the incidence of demonstrable hepatic granulomas. Of 164 tuberculous patients 70 had granulomas on liver biopsy specimens. Caseating granulomas are the classic findings in tuberculosis. However, noncaseating granulomas also are quite common in tuberculous hepatic involvement. In one series reporting noncaseating granulomas of infectious and noninfectious etiology in 50 liver biopsy specimens, tuberculosis again ranked second to sarcoidosis and accounted for 10 percent of the total.[20] In other studies of hepatic granulomas unrestricted in regard to the presence or absence of caseous changes, fewer than 15 percent of patients found to have tuberculosis had caseous necrosis in the liver.[21,22] Certain consistent findings emerge from various series on the diagnostic import of liver biopsy specimens in patients who ultimately are proved to have tuberculosis. Thirty-one percent of the patients with "isolated" active pulmonary tuberculosis were shown to have hepatic granulomas.[1] In series of patients with documented pulmonary and extrapulmonary tuberculosis (exclusive of miliary involvement), 70–80 percent had hepatic granulomas.[1,23] In cases of miliary tuberculosis, greater than 90 percent of the patients will have hepatic granulomas.[1,24] There is no question that the tubercule bacillus can be demonstrated by appropriate staining techniques as well as by culture from liver biopsy specimens.[23–26] Yet, when one looks at all cases of hepatic granulomas associated with tuberculosis of any extent, this demonstration is rather uncommon.[27,28] However, in a series of 23 liver biopsies in documented miliary tuberculosis, 43 percent either had a positive culture or smear.[24]

Other mycobacterial infections that may cause hepatic granulomas are disseminated atypical mycobacterial disease,[29] lepromatous leprosy,[30] and BCG-osis after Calmette-Guérin bacillus (BCG) vaccination, immunotherapy for neoplasms, or intravesical therapy in the treatment of bladder cancer.[31–33] It is noteworthy that, in the hepatic granulomas associated with lepromatous leprosy, organisms are plentiful and can be easily demonstrated within Küpffer cells.[30] It is of interest that granulomatous tissue reactions rarely are found; if present, they are poorly formed in the *Mycobacterium avium-intracellulare* infections that are commonly seen in patients with acquired immunodeficiency syndrome (AIDS).[34] This is likely due to the fact that these patients have markedly suppressed inducer–helper T-lymphocyte numbers and function,[35] which is required for the immunologic component of the granulomatous response to mycobacteria.

Brucellosis is quite commonly associated with hepatic granulomas.[35] In infections with *Brucella abortus*, the granulomas are well formed and discrete. Infection with *Brucella suis* and *Brucella melitensis* results in less distinct changes in the liver, which may be manifested merely as isolated areas of necrosis.[28,36]

Although tularemia often is cited as one of the bacterial diseases that can lead to hepatic granulomas, in reality this is not the case. Classic well-formed granulomas with multinucleated giant cells are seldom seen in this disease. The most common finding is scattered necrotic nodules with neutrophil infiltration.[37]

Other uncommon bacterial causes of hepatic granulomas are granuloma inguinale,[39] melioidosis,[39] and disseminated infection with *Listeria monocytogenes*, particularly in a rare syndrome in neonates called miliary granulomatosis or granulomatosis infantisepticum.[40]

Fungi are another common cause of hepatic granulomas. Depending on the reported series and geographic location, they may be the most common infectious disease cause, surpassing even tuberculosis in some individual reports.[20] In the United States, disseminated histoplasmosis is the most common of the fungal etiologies of hepatic granulomas. A hepatic biopsy specimen is a more fruitful source of diagnostic tissue in histoplasmosis as compared with tuberculosis.[41] In a prospective study of 26 patients with disseminated histoplasmosis at the National Institutes of Health, 21 of 26 patients had liver function abnormalities; in the 8 in whom liver biopsy specimens were obtained, 5 had granulomas.[42] Furthermore, *Histoplasma* was cultured from four of the eight biopsy specimens and was demonstrated by staining techniques in three of the four cultured specimens.

Other disseminated mycotic infections such as coccidioidomycosis, candidiasis, and aspergillosis rarely may cause hepatic granulomas. However, the other organ system manifestations of these diseases in their disseminated form far overshadow the hepatic granulomas when present. For the most part, the finding of hepatic granulomas in this setting adds little to an already obvious clinicopathologic setting.

It is now well established that viral infections may cause hepatic granulomas. Cytomegalovirus and infectious mononucleosis,[1] in particular, have been associated with granulomatous hepatitis. In addition, in a large biopsy series of hepatitis of various causes, granulomas were demonstrated in the liver biopsy specimens of 2 percent of the patients with acute viral hepatitis and 12 percent of the patients with chronic active hepatitis.[1]

It is uncertain whether influenza virus may cause granulomatous hepatitis. There has been an association of influenza B infection and granulomatous hepatitis,[43] but the two may have been unrelated.[17]

Several parasites encountered throughout the world may cause hepatic granulomas.[17,44] Of particular importance are schistosomiasis (resulting from *Schistosoma mansoni*) and visceral larva migrans (caused by *Toxocara canis* or *Toxocara cati*). Granuloma formation in these disorders most likely results from a deposition of eggs in the liver, with a subsequent combination foreign body reaction to the eggs themselves and a cell-mediated or delayed hypersensitivity reaction to antigenic determinants of the parasite. Another potential cause of parasite-related granulomatous reaction in the liver is fascioliasis caused by the liver fluke *Fasciola hepatica*.

Of the rickettsioses, *Coxiella burnettii*, which is the agent causing Q fever, most often is associated with granulomatous hepatitis.[45,46] Q fever is not associated with an exanthem (characteristic of the other rickettsioses); in some cases, it may present with a clinical syndrome identical to viral hepatitis. Thus, the finding of granulomas on a liver biopsy specimen in such a clinical setting should suggest Q fever as part of the differential diagnosis.

The liver may be involved in secondary and tertiary syphilis. During the era when late syphilis was much more common than it is at present, variable degrees of hepatic involvement were frequently seen. Hepatic gummas and hepar lobatum are the typical changes of late syphilitic liver involvement, and interstitial hepatitis is the typical finding in congenital syphilis.[28] Well-formed granulomas, however, are not characteristic but may be found in certain cases.

Noninfectious Diseases

Among diseases in which a diagnosis is ultimately made, sarcoidosis is the most common noninfectious disease cause of hepatic granulomas[1,17]; in addition, it is the most common cause—infectious and noninfectious—of noncaseating hepatic granulomas.[20] It is the histopathologic prototype of the classic noncaseating granuloma.

Other noninfectious disease causes of granulomatous hepatitis are listed in Table 2 and have been reviewed in detail elsewhere.[46–48] Of particular interest in this group, with regard to infectious diseases, are erythema nodosum and chronic granulomatous disease (CGD) of childhood.

Erythema nodosum is a hypersensitivity manifestation of several different clinical entities that is characterized predominantly by tender subcutaneous nodules over the anterior surface of the lower extremities beneath the knees and (occasionally) elsewhere.[49] It can be associated with granulomatous hepatitis as part of the syndrome complex itself. In addition, some of the infectious disease entities with which it is associated (e.g., tuberculosis, coccidioidomycosis, histoplasmosis, and lepromatous leprosy), in and of themselves, can cause hepatic granulomas; this makes the diagnostic approach even more complex when hepatic granulomas are found in erythema nodosum.

In up to 29 percent of patients with hepatic granulomas, medications have been suspected causes. Granulomas are said to always be noncaseating and often contain large numbers of eosinophils (>5–10 per granuloma), a finding that would be very unusual in tuberculosis or sarcoidosis. In a minority of cases, drug-induced granulomas may be found in extrahepatic sites such as lymph nodes and bone marrow. Eosinophilic granulomas may also occur in schistosomiasis, visceral larva migrans, Hodgkin's disease, and histoplasmosis. In the absence of these disorders, the question of drug-induced disease should be considered.[50] The terms "probable" and "possible" have been applied to drug-suspected cases when the withdrawal of a drug has been associated with resolution of symptoms, normalization of liver function test results (if these had been abnormal), and diminution or absence of granulomas in a repeat liver biopsy specimen. A "definite" diagnosis of drug-induced disease would require the demonstration of recurrent abnormalities

TABLE 2. Noninfectious Disease Causes of Granulomatous Hepatitis

Sarcoidosis
Hypersensitivity diseases
Erythema nodosum
Berylliosis
Hypersensitivity drug reactions
Primary liver disease
Primary biliary cirrhosis
Rarely, others such as Laennec's cirrhosis, postnecrotic cirrhosis, alcoholic hepatitis, or chronic active hepatitis
Neoplasms
Hodgkin's disease and, rarely, other lymphomas and solid tumors
Host defense defects
Chronic granulomatous disease of childhood
Immune deficiencies (hypogammaglobulinemia)
Others
Temporal arteritis—polymyalgia rheumatica syndrome
Allergic granulomatosis
Idiopathic granulomatous hepatitis
Ulcerative colitis
Crohn's disease

after reinstitution of the suspected agent. Both moral and legal considerations should discourage intentional manipulations to establish such definite relationships unless the medication in question was considered essential and another with similar properties, but chemically unrelated, was not available. Since it is conceivable that many different medications may play a role in granuloma formation, it would be judicious to discontinue treatment with any nonessential drugs and follow the patient's clinical course and, when indicated, hepatic histopathology up to 8 weeks later before a diagnosis of either sarcoidosis or idiopathic granulomatous hepatitis is considered.

Patients with the host defense defect of CGD frequently have disseminated granulomas with a predominance of liver involvement.[51] It is felt that the mechanism of granuloma formation in this disease is an intracellular persistence of microorganisms or their products that is related to the well-established microbial killing defect. This triggers the epithelioid cell transformation with subsequent granuloma formation as described above. Granulomas persist in these patients, and it is difficult to recover microorganisms from the liver tissue. Hence, although the syndrome of CGD is not an infectious disease per se, the granulomatous reaction results from an inability to normally handle a variety of microorganisms.

Hodgkin's disease and other lymphomas are recognized as the most common malignancies associated with hepatic granulomas. Although other tumors (renal cell, rectal, nasopharyngeal, and primary hepatocellular carcinoma) have also been noted to share this association, those examples are not as well documented.[22,48,50] Further confusion is added by the observation that malignancies related to hepatic granulomas may not become apparent until months or even several years after the initial evaluation. Preliminary data have suggested that individuals who later (4–40 months) demonstrate lymphomas are more likely to have at initial presentation (*1*) prolonged (>4 weeks) unexplained fevers, (*2*) liver or (*3*) spleen size extending more than 4 cm below the costal margins, and (*4*) eosinophilia of greater than 4 percent of the peripheral white blood cell count. The presence of any two of these features had an 80 percent specificity in distinguishing hepatic granulomas and lymphoma from other causes of such hepatic abnormalities. The sensitivity of having at least two of four features for lymphoma was 100 percent.[52]

Another interesting and perplexing category of granulomatous hepatitis is that group of patients in whom the etiology of the granulomatous reaction remains unknown despite extensive diagnostic investigation.[53] In various series, this group of idiopathic granulomatous hepatitis ranged to as high as 36 percent of the cases with documented hepatic granulomas.[17,19,27,30] In addition, in a group of 72 patients with hepatic granulomas whose underlying disease did not appear to be hepatic or granulomatous in nature, 37 of these remained undiagnosed.[1] These patients do not have extra-abdominal granulomas, and other criteria for sarcoidosis are absent.[44] This group probably represents hypersensitivity states that are clinically and histopathologically reflected primarily in the liver, with the responsible antigen remaining unidentified.

GRANULOMATOUS HEPATITIS AND FEVER

Fever is a major manifestation in most cases of granulomatous hepatitis. In fact, in one large series, over 40 percent of the patients with hepatic granulomas had fevers of unknown origin.[17] This is not difficult to understand when one considers the current theories on the pathogenesis of fever. It has been demonstrated that the final common mediators of fever are proteins called endogenous pyrogens, which are synthesized by phagocytic cells of the host. On release from these cells, these pyrogens act on specific neurons of the anterior hypothalamus–preoptic region of the brain, with resulting elevation of body temperature.[54] The liver is rich in phagocytic Küpffer cells, which are highly efficient producers of endogenous pyrogen.[54] Triggering of these cells by antigens, immune complexes, or microorganisms in the pathogenesis of granuloma formation can potentially lead to the release of pyrogen. This is of particular relevance in the diagnostic challenge of granulomatous hepatitis with regard to infectious disease etiologies. On the one hand, an infectious agent that may be the underlying cause of the hepatic granulomas can cause fever; conversely, the hepatic granulomas, whether resulting from infectious or noninfectious causes, can of themselves be the sources of fever. Finally, it has been recently demonstrated that the pyrogen molecule is, in fact, identical to interleukin-1, which is secreted by monocyte–macrophages and which is critically involved in the activation of T lymphocytes.[55] This observation lends further support to the complex relationship among immunologic reactions, granuloma formation, and the presence of a febrile response.

DIAGNOSTIC APPROACH TO HEPATIC GRANULOMAS

Hepatic granulomas really are quite common and may be found in up to 10 percent of specimens from liver biopsy procedures performed in general hospitals.[17] Although laparotomy with a biopsy specimen of a substantial amount of tissue is the obvious highest-yield approach, it is now clear that percutaneous needle biopsy is a safe and efficient procedure for obtaining tissue for diagnostic and extent-of-disease work-up as well as for follow-up of the clinical course and therapeutic response. In particular, its value in certain circumstances in the diagnostic approach to fevers of unknown origin is well established.[56] Once hepatic granulomas have been histologically demonstrated and the underlying diagnosis is still not established, a stepwise diagnostic approach should be undertaken. Bearing in mind that infectious diseases are the leading causes of all types of hepatic granulomas, bacterial, fungal, and mycobacterial cultures should be performed. In addition, special staining techniques should be applied to histologic sections, and appropriate skin tests and diagnostic serologic tests should be used. Also, viral infections such as cytomegalovirus and infectious mononucleosis infrequently may cause granulomatous hepatitis (Table 1). The diagnostic culture yield of tissue for the recovery of virus is so low that the diagnosis, when suspected, can be best made on clinical and serologic grounds.

If infectious disease causes have been ruled out and the diagnosis is still unknown, an orderly diagnostic approach that includes clinical, histopathologic, serologic, and radiologic parameters should be used to rule out other noninfectious disease causes (Table 2). Recently provided (within 6 months) medications should be suspected and treatment with all nonessential medications discontinued. If after this diagnostic approach one is still left with a diagnosis of granulomatous hepatitis of unknown etiology, then careful follow-up, subsequent reevaluation, and (in some cases) empirical therapy (discussed below) are indicated.

There may be specific laboratory abnormalities associated with various diseases in which granulomatous hepatitis may be a manifestation.[13,20,53] However, the laboratory abnormalities usually associated with hepatic granulomas as such are generally nonspecific. The erythrocyte sedimentation rate is almost invariably elevated. Liver function test findings may be completely normal or, in most cases, mildly abnormal. Increased serum levels of alkaline phosphatase and transaminase are frequent abnormalities. Hyperbilirubinemia is most unusual except in cases of primary biliary cirrhosis. Mild hyperglobulinemia may be found, and prothrombin elevations are unusual.

TREATMENT OF GRANULOMATOUS HEPATITIS

When the underlying cause of the granulomatous hepatitis is known, treatment obviously should be directed toward that etiology, whether infectious or noninfectious. The disappearance of granulomas usually parallels the therapeutic response of the underlying disease. After successful therapy for the underlying disease, there usually is little if any histopathologic residue of the granulomas.[47,53]

In the clincal setting where one has ruled out as far as possible infectious and other causes of granulomatous hepatitis and where the diagnosis of idiopathic granulomatous hepatitis remains, corticosteroids often lead to clinical and histopathologic improvement.[53] Since the obvious danger in this situation is to administer corticosteroids to a patient with an underlying, but undetectable infection (particularly tuberculosis), there is a place for empirical antituberculous therapy. Several cases of what appeared to be granulomatous hepatitis in which tuberculosis could not be demonstrated responded to antituberculous drugs. Conversely, occasional patients who have lacked evidence for tuberculosis and were treated with steroids for idiopathic granulomatous hepatitis have died of disseminated tuberculosis.[22] Due to these observations, it is recommended that all patients with granulomatous hepatitis in whom an etiology cannot be established should be given an empirical trial of two-drug antituberculous therapy. If a clinical response is seen, the drugs are continued for the usual recommended course. If no clinical response is seen after 2 months, corticosteroids are added. If the patient is tuberculin skin test–positive, a single drug (isoniazid) should be continued with the corticosteroid. Therapeutic responses should be monitored by clinical and laboratory parameters as well as by repeat liver biopsy procedures every 6–12 months. Once improvement occurs, it is highly recommended to attempt to convert the therapeutic regimen to alternate-day corticosteroids since granulomatous hepatitis can be controlled quite adequately in many patients with alternate-day corticosteroid regimens.[53]

REFERENCES

1. Klatskin G. Hepatic granulomata: Problems in interpretation. Ann NY Acad Sci. 1976;278:427.
2. Silverman L, Shorter RG. Histogenesis of the multinucleated giant cell. Lab Invest. 1963;12:985.
3. Epstein WL. Granulomatous hypersensitivity. Prog Allergy. 1967;11:36.
4. Epstein WL, Krasnobrod H. The origin of epithelioid cells in experimental granulomas of man. Lab Invest. 1968;18:190.
5. Gillman T, Wright LJ. Probable in vivo origin of multinucleated giant cells from circulating mononuclears. Nature. 1963;209:263.
6. Muller-Hermelink HK, Kaiserling E, Sonntag HG. Modulation of epitheloid cell granuloma formation to apathogenic mycobacteria by cyclosporin A. Pathol Res Pract. 1982;175:80.
7. Williams GT, Williams WJ. Granulomatous inflammation—a review. J Clin Pathol. 1983;36:723.
8. Rich AR. The Pathogenesis of Tuberculosis. Springfield, IL: Charles C Thomas; 1951:13.
9. Warren KS. Granulomatous inflammation. In: Lepow IH, Ward PW, eds. Inflammation: Mechanisms and Control. New York: Academic Press; 1972:203.
10. Weinberg JB, Hobbs MM, Misukonis MA. Recombinant human γ-interferon induces human monocyte polykaryon formation. Proc Natl Acad Sci USA 1984;81:4554.
11. Block CM, Catterall JR, Remington JS. In vivo and in vitro activation of alveolar macrophges by recombinant interferon-γ. J Immunol. 1987;138:491.
12. Simrell CR, Crabtree GR, Cossman J, et al. Stimulation of phagocytosis by a T cell lymphoma derived lymphokine. In: Vitetta E, Fox CF, eds. B and T Cell Tumors: Biological and Clinical Aspects. UCLA Symposia on Molecular and Cellular Biology. v. 24. New York: Academic Press; 1982:247.
13. Fauci AS, Haynes BF, Costa J, et al. Lymphomatoid granulomatosis. Prospective clinical and therapeutic experience over 10 years. N Engl J Med. 1982;306:68.
14. Atkinson JP, Frank MM. Studies on the in vivo antibody and complement in the immune clearance and destruction of erythrocytes in man. J Clin Invest. 1974;54:339.
15. Sherlock S. Hepatic granulomas. In: Sherlock S, ed. Diseases of the Liver and Biliary System, ed 5. Oxford, Blackwell Scientific Publications; 1975:598.
16. Harrington PT, Gutierrez JJ, Ramirez-Ronda CH, et al. Granulomatous hepatitis. Rev Infect Dis. 1982;4:638.
17. Guckian JC, Perry JE. Granulomatous hepatitis. An analysis of 63 cases and review of the literature. Ann Intern Med. 1969;65:1081.
18. Gold J, Wigderson A, Leiman E, et al. Report of a case with review of the literature. Gastroenterology. 1957;33:113.
19. Bowry S, Chan CH, Weiss H, et al. Hepatic involvement in pulmonary tuberculosis. Histologic and functional characteristics. Am Rev Respir Dis. 1970;101:941.
20. Mir-Madjlessi SH, Farmer RG, Hawk WA. Granulomatous hepatitis. A review of 50 cases. Am J Gastroenterol. 1973;60:122.
21. Irani SK, Dobbins WO III. Hepatic granulomas: A review of 73 patients from one hospital and survey of the literature. J Clin Gastroenterol. 1979;1:131.
22. Cunningham D, Mills PR, Quigley EMM, et al. Hepatic granulomas: Experience over a 10-year period in West of Scotland. Q J Med. 1982;51:162.
23. Korn RJ, Kellow WF, Heller P, et al. Hepatic involvement in extrapulmonary tuberculosis. Histologic and functional characteristics. Am J Med. 1959;27:60.
24. Cucin RL, Coleman M, Eckardt JJ, et al. The diagnosis of miliary tuberculosis: Utility of peripheral blood abnormalities, bone marrow and liver needle biopsy. J Chronic Dis. 1973;26:355.
25. Healey RJ, Leff AH, Rosenak BD. Needle biopsy in tuberculosis of the liver, with culture of acid-fast bacilli. Am J Dig Dis. 1959;4:638.
26. Rumball JM, Baum GL. Liver biopsy culture in the diagnosis of miliary tuberculosis: A case report. Gastroenterology. 1952;22:124.
27. Wagoner GP, Anton AT, Gall EA, et al. Needle biopsy of the liver. VII. Experiences with hepatic granulomas. Gastroenterology. 1953;25:487.
28. Rubin E. Interpretation of the liver biopsy. Diagnostic criteria. Gastroenterology. 1963;45:400.
29. Koenig MG, Collins RD, Heyssel RM. Disseminated mycobacteriosis caused by Battey type mycobacteria. Ann Intern Med. 1966;64:145.
30. Browne SG. The liver in leprosy: A review. W Afr Med J. 1964;13:35.
31. Marans HY, Bekirov HM. Granulomatous hepatitis following intravesical bacillus Calmette-Guerin therapy for bladder carcinoma. J Urol. 1987;137:111.
32. Hunt JS, Silverstein MJ, Spark FC, et al. Granulomatous hepatitis: A complication of BCG immunotherapy. Lancet. 1973;2:820.
33. Bodurtha A, Kim YH, Laucius JF, et al. Hepatic granulomas and other hepatic lesions associated with BCG immunotherapy for cancer. Am J Clin Pathol. 1974;61:714.
34. Greene JB, Sidhu GS, Lewin S, et al. *Mycobacterium avium-intracellulare*: A cause of disseminated life-threatening infection in homosexuals and drug abusers. Ann Intern Med. 1982;97:539.
35. Fauci AS. The syndrome of Kaposi's sarcoma-opportunisitc infections: An epidemiolologically restricted disorder of immunoregulation. Ann Intern Med. 1982;96:777.
36. Spink WW, Hoffbauer FW, Walher WW, et al. Histopathology of the liver in human brucellosis. J Lab Clin Med. 1949;34:40.
37. Foshay L. Tularemia: A summary of certain aspects of the disease including methods for early diagnosis and the results of serum treatment in 600 patients. Medicine (Baltimore). 1940;19:1.
38. Lyford J III, Johnson RW Jr, Blackman S, et al. Pathologic findings in a fatal case of disseminated granuloma inguinale with miliary bone and joint involvement. Bull Johns Hopkins Hosp. 1946;79:349.
39. Borchardt KA, Stansifer P, Albano PM. Osteomyelitis due to *Pseudomonas pseudomallei*. JAMA. 1966;196:660.
40. Ray CJ, Wedgewood RJ. Neonatal listeriosis; six case reports and a review of the literature. Pediatrics. 1964;34:378.
41. Schiff L. The clinical value of needle biopsy of the liver. Ann Intern Med. 1951;34:948.
42. Smith JW, Utz JP. Progressive disseminated histoplasmosis. A prospective study of 26 patients. Ann Intern Med. 1972;76:557.
43. Klatskin G, Yesner R. Hepatic manifestations of sarcoidosis and other granulomatous diseases. Yale J Biol Med. 1950;23:207.
44. Marcial Rojas RA. Helminthic diseases. In: Schiff L, ed. Diseases of the Liver. ed 2. Philadelphia: JB Lippincott; 1963:800.
45. Dupont HL, Hornick RB, Levin HS, et al. Q fever hepatitis. Ann Intern Med. 1971;74:198.
46. Travis LB, Travis WD, Li C-Y, et al. Q fever: A clinicopathologic study of five cases. Arch Pathol Lab Med 1986;110:1017.
47. Fauci AS, Wolff SM. Granulomatous hepatitis. In: Popper H, Schaffner F, eds. Progress in Liver Diseases. v. 5. New York: Grune & Stratton; 1976:609.
48. Anderson CS, Nicholls J, Rowland R, et al. Hepatic granulomas: A 15-year experience in the Royal Adelaide Hospital. Med J Aust. 1988;148:71.
49. Epstein WL. Erythema nodosum. In: Samter M, ed. Immunological Diseases. v. 2. Boston: Little, Brown; 1971:944.
50. McMaster KR III, Hennigar GR. Drug-induced granulomatous hepatitis. Lab Invest. 1981;44:61.
51. Good RA, Quie PG, Windhorst DB, et al. Fatal (chronic) granulomatous disease of childhood: A hereditary defect of leukocyte function. Semin Hematol. 1968;5:215.
52. Aderka D, Kraus M, Weinberger A, et al. Parameters which can differentiate patients with "idiopathic" from patients with lymphoma-induced liver granulomas. Am J Gastroenterol. 1985;80:1004.
53. Simon HB, Wolff SM. Granulomatous hepatitis and prolonged fever of unknown origin: A study of 13 patients. Medicine (Baltimore). 1973;52:1.
54. Dinarello CA, Wolff SM. Exogenous and endogenous pyrogen. In: Brazier MAB, Coceani F, eds. Brain Dysfunction in Infantile Febrile Convulsions. v. 2. New York: Raven Press; 1976:117.
55. Oppenheim JJ, Gery I. Interleukin 1 is more than an interleukin. Immunol Today. 1982;3:113.
56. Wolff SM, Simon HB. Granulomatous hepatitis and prolonged fever of unknown origin. Trans Am Clin Climatol Assoc. 1973;84:149.

SECTION P. ACQUIRED IMMUNODEFICIENCY SYNDROME

105. INTRODUCTION

R. GORDON DOUGLAS, JR.

Acquired immunodeficiency syndrome (AIDS) was first recognized in 1981. Since then, modern science has discovered its cause as a novel retrovirus known as human immunodeficiency virus (HIV), defined the nature of the immune defect, developed tests to detect antibodies to determine the presence of infection and to screen blood and blood products for HIV, and developed a specific antiviral treatment that, although not a cure, significantly prolongs life. Research progress continues at a great rate. More is being learned about the basic properties and behavior of the virus as well as the immune defects. Such research is yielding new ideas for chemotherapeutic agents, immunologic stimulators and modifiers, and potential vaccines, and clinical trials to test these agents are under way.

Despite these remarkable accomplishments, the epidemic progresses unchecked, resulting in enormous demands on health care facilities and health care providers. Clinicians have had to learn to cope with new, difficult, and confusing opportunistic infections. Yet advances in the treatment and prevention of these illnesses have benefited many AIDS victims.

What appears to have happened with AIDS is the rapid introduction of an infectious agent into an immunologically naive population. In this case, the virus probably originated from primates in central Africa and has rapidly adapted to humans.[1] History of such introductions of new infectious agents to naive populations indicates the prospect for a devastating outcome: for example, influenza in 1918, bubonic plague in the 14th century, measles in island populations.[2,3] This bleak outlook for mankind is further supported by the failure of antibody that is neutralizing in vitro to be protective in vivo in humans or chimpanzees. Despite these dismal predictions, in the developed world, the disease is difficult to transmit from person to person and thus is restricted primarily to certain population groups, namely, male homosexuals or bisexuals and intravenous drug abusers (IVDA). It is this epidemiologic restriction that limits the magnitude of the epidemic. With time, the primary epidemic population has shifted from homosexuals and bisexuals to the IVDA population, mostly due to modification of behavior on the part of the former groups. Further, antibody testing has virtually eliminated transfusion of blood and blood products as a source of HIV infection.

The concentration of AIDS in these groups and the very skewed geographic distribution of cases in the United States has led to a mixed public reaction to recognition of the importance of the disease and, consequently, to public support for health care and research.

Increasing the controversies surrounding the disease are concerns related to the Federal Drug Administration's lengthy approval process for new drugs and the issue of confidentiality of HIV antibody testing—who should and should not be tested and who has a right to know the results. Vaccine development produces several concerns of its own. For example, candidate vaccines will convert an individual from seronegative to seropositive for HIV with all the attendant risks, such as uninsurability and possible loss of job, housing, and schooling.

Infectious disease specialists have felt the brunt of the epidemic.[4,5] They are often asked to be the role models and standard-bearers for professional behavior. They have shouldered much of the responsibility for the health care of AIDS victims and for performance of the clinical investigations related to specific antiviral agents and immunomodulators versus HIV, treatment for opportunistic infections, and vaccine development.[6,7]

Thus, major textbooks of infectious diseases must present comprehensive, up-to-date material related to all aspects of AIDS and HIV infection. AIDS was not mentioned in the first edition of this text published in 1979. In the second edition, published in 1985, only one short chapter was devoted to AIDS. For the present edition, the section on AIDS was completely reorganized and rewritten. AIDS is treated as a syndrome, as is proper, and thus most of the material related to AIDS appears in Part II, "Syndromes," with separate chapters on Epidemiology (Chapter 106), Immunology (Chapter 107), Clinical Manifestations (Chapter 108), Detection of HIV Infections (Chapter 109), Therapy (Chapter 110), and Vaccines (Chapter 111). The chapter concerning Human Immunodeficiency Virus (HIV) (Chapter 147) appears in Part III, in the section on Retroviridae. Also in keeping with the organization of the book, the chapter on HIV in the health care setting (Chapter 283) appears in the section in Part IV dealing with nosocomial infections. Other sections of the book contain important information on AIDS. For example, the section on anti-infective therapy in Part I discusses antiviral agents versus HIV and drugs used to treat opportunistic infections. Specific organisms that opportunistically infect patients with AIDS are discussed in the relevant chapters of Part III.

REFERENCES

1. Gallo RC. HIV—the cause of AIDS: An overview on its biology, mechanisms of disease induction, and our attempts to control it. J Acquired Immune Deficiency Syn. 1988;1:521–35.
2. Ludmerer KM. Patients Beyond the Pale: Historical View. Fifth Conference on Health Policy, Cornell University Medical College. 1989;1:1–20.
3. Sigerist HE. Civilization and Disease. New York: Cornell University Press; 1943:112–7.
4. Loewy EH. Duties, fears and physicians. Social Sci Med. 1986;22:1364.
5. Zuger A, Miles SH. Physicians, AIDS, and occupational risk. JAMA. 1987;258:1924–5.
6. Ada GL. Prospects for HIV vaccines. J Acquired Immune Deficiency Syn. 1988;1:295–303.
7. Oberg B. Antiviral therapy. J Acquired Immune Deficiency Syn. 1988;1:257–66.

106. EPIDEMIOLOGY AND PREVENTION OF AIDS AND HIV INFECTION

MARY E. CHAMBERLAND
JAMES W. CURRAN

Acquired immunodeficiency syndrome (AIDS) is the most severe manifestation of a clinical spectrum of illness after infection with a retrovirus, human immunodeficiency virus (HIV).

The syndrome is defined by the development of serious opportunistic infections, neoplasms, or other life-threatening manifestations resulting from progressive HIV-induced immunosuppression. AIDS was first recognized in mid-1981 when unusual clusters of *Pneumocystis carinii* pneumonia and Kaposi sarcoma were reported in young, previously healthy homosexual men in New York City, Los Angeles, and San Francisco.[1,2] The subsequent documentation of cases among persons with hemophilia, blood transfusion recipients, and heterosexual iv drug abusers and their sex partners suggested that a transmissible agent was the primary cause of the immunologic defects characteristic of AIDS.[3] In 1983, more than 2 years after the first reports of AIDS, a cytopathic retrovirus was isolated from persons with AIDS and associated conditions such as chronic lymphadenopathy.[4–6]

SURVEILLANCE AND REPORTING OF AIDS

All 50 states require AIDS cases to be reported. Surveillance of AIDS cases has been ongoing in the United States since 1981. In 1981, before the etiology of AIDS was known and a specific diagnostic test was available, the Centers for Disease Control (CDC) developed a surveillance case definition.[7] The initial case definition included a limited number of specific opportunistic diseases diagnosed by reliable methods in patients with no other known causes of immunodeficiency. Although the surveillance definition excluded other less severe manifestations of illness, it was highly specific, uniformly interpreted, and permitted a consistent evaluation of trends of severe underlying immunodeficiency caused by what was then an unknown agent. The definition was adopted worldwide for surveillance of AIDS in all industrialized nations.

The discovery of HIV as the cause of AIDS and the subsequent development of serologic tests to detect HIV resulted in an increased appreciation of the spectrum of HIV-associated clinical and immunologic manifestations. In addition, a review of death certificates in 1985 in four cities showed that reported AIDS cases underestimated the actual incidence of AIDS-related deaths: 13 percent of deaths were attributed to *P. carinii* pneumonia, Kaposi sarcoma, and other opportunistic diseases that had been diagnosed without the recommended rigorous histologic or cultural techniques required to meet the surveillance definition.[8] To more completely and effectively monitor serious HIV-associated morbidity, the original case definition was modified in 1985 and again in September 1987.[9,10] The 1987 revision incorporated a broader range of AIDS-indicative diseases, most notably HIV encephalopathy and wasting syndrome; included patients whose indicator diseases were diagnosed presumptively, without confirmatory laboratory evidence of the opportunistic disease; and took advantage of the increasing use of HIV diagnostic tests to further improve the sensitivity and specificity of the definition (Table 1).

TABLE 1. Revised Surveillance Case Definition for AIDS, Centers for Disease Control, September 1987

I. Indicator diseases diagnosed definitively in the absence of other causes of immunodeficiency and laboratory tests for HIV
   - Candidiasis of the esophagus, trachea, bronchi, or lungs
   - *Cryptococcus*, extrapulmonary
   - Cryptosporidiosis with diarrhea >1 mon
   - Cytomegalovirus disease exclusive of liver, spleen, or lymph nodes in patients >1 mon of age.
   - Herpes simplex virus infection causing a mucocutaneous ulcer >1 mon or bronchitis, pneumonitis, or esophagitis in patients >1 mon of age
   - Kaposi sarcoma in patients <60 yr of age
   - Lymphoma of the brain (primary) in patients <60 yr of age
   - Lymphoid interstitial pneumonia and/or pulmonary lymphoid hyperplasia in patients <13 yr of age
   - *Mycobacterium avium* complex or *M. kansasii* disease, disseminated
   - *Pneumocystis carinii* pneumonia
   - Progressive multifocal leukoencephalopathy
   - Toxoplasmosis of the brain in patients >1 mon of age

II. Indicator diseases diagnosed definitively regardless of other causes of immunodeficiency and laboratory evidence of HIV present
   - All indicator diseases listed in Section I
   - Bacterial infections, recurrent or multiple, in patients <13 yr of age that are caused by *Haemophilus*, *Streptococcus*, or other pyogenic bacteria
   - Coccidioidomycosis, disseminated
   - HIV encephalopathy
   - Histoplasmosis, disseminated
   - Isosporiasis with diarrhea >1 mon
   - Kaposi sarcoma at any age
   - Primary lymphoma of the brain at any age
   - Non-Hodgkin's lymphoma of B cell or unknown immunologic phenotype including small noncleaved lymphoma or immunoblastic sarcoma
   - Mycobacterial disease exclusive of *M. tuberculosis*, disseminated
   - *M. tuberculosis*, extrapulmonary
   - *Salmonella* septicemia, recurrent
   - HIV wasting syndrome

III. Indicator diseases diagnosed presumptively with laboratory evidence of HIV infection
   - Candidiasis, esophageal
   - Cytomegalovirus retinitis with loss of vision
   - Kaposi sarcoma
   - Lymphoid interstitial pneumonia and/or pulmonary lymphoid hyperplasia in patients <13 yr of age
   - Mycobacterial disease, disseminated
   - *Pneumocystis carinii* pneumonia
   - Toxoplasmosis, brain, in patients >1 mo of age

IV. Indicator diseases diagnosed definitively in the absence of other causes of immunodeficiency and negative laboratory tests results for HIV
   - *Pneumocystis carinii* pneumonia
   - Other indicator diseases listed in Section I and a T-helper/inducer (CD4) lymphocyte count <400/mm^3

The impact of the 1987 revision on the reported number of AIDS cases will depend on the use and reporting of HIV antibody tests and employment of presumptive methods to diagnose the indicator diseases.[11] These factors are likely to vary with geographic location, hospital size, patients' socioeconomic status and/or method of payment, physicians' clinical experience, and availability of HIV testing. In the first 8 months after implementation of the September 1987 revised case definition, 17,969 AIDS cases were reported to the CDC, of which 2279 (13 percent) were diagnosed presumptively and 2944 (16 percent) involved indicator diseases (such as wasting syndrome or HIV encephalopathy) that met the revised criteria only. During this period, New York and California accounted for 45 percent of reported AIDS cases that met the pre-1987 case definition but only 24 percent of cases that met the 1987 revision. Cases reported in heterosexual iv drug abusers were more likely than those in exclusively homosexual or bisexual men to fulfill only 1987 criteria (44 vs 22 percent). A higher proportion of blacks (36 percent) and Hispanics (35 percent) than whites (24 percent) met the new definition categories of presumptive diagnoses, HIV encephalopathy, and HIV wasting syndrome.

Several studies have documented high levels of case reporting,[8,12,13] but the timeliness of reporting to state and local health departments and to the CDC has diminished somewhat, given the increasing number of case reports.[14] In 1987, the median and mean intervals between diagnosis and report were 2.9 and 4.8 months respectively, with 80 percent of cases reported within 6 months of diagnosis.

AIDS IN ADULTS

Incidence of AIDS in the United States

As of May 1988, 60,000 cases of AIDS in adults were reported in the United States. The number of cases has increased rapidly over time. The first 15,000 cases were reported over a 54-month period between June 1981 and November 1985. In contrast, the fourth quartile of 15,000 cases was reported over a 6-month period between November 1987 and May 1988. Based on an empirical mathematic model, 80,000 AIDS cases are projected to be diagnosed in 1992 alone, and the cumulative number of diagnosed cases is estimated to total 365,000 by the end of 1992

(Fig. 1).[15] These projections do not take into account AIDS cases that are never diagnosed or reported to the CDC and other HIV-related illnesses and deaths that do not meet the 1987 surveillance case definition. Factors that may alter the projected course of the epidemic include the development of effective therapeutic modalities and intervention and prevention efforts to reduce HIV transmission.

Transmission Groups

For surveillance purposes, AIDS cases are classified into a hierarchy of mutually exclusive risk or transmission groups (Table 2). Patients with more than one risk factor are ordered in the highest ranking transmission group. Of the first 60,000 reported cases, 13 percent of patients with AIDS had two or more reported risk factors for infection. The largest overlaps occurred in homosexual/bisexual men and iv drug abusers (4445 patients) and among heterosexual iv drug abusers and persons with heterosexual sex partners in risk groups (971 patients).

Since 1981, cases in homosexual and bisexual men have consistently represented the largest proportion (63 percent). However, the proportion of homosexual and bisexual men decreased from 66 percent of the third quartile of 15,000 cases (reported between February 1987 and October 1987) to 56 percent of the fourth quartile of cases (reported between November 1987 and May 1988). This declining trend was similar for homosexual and bisexual men who abused iv drugs as well. There has been a corresponding increase in the proportion of AIDS cases attributable to iv drug abuse by heterosexuals. When analyses are restricted to patients meeting only the pre-1987 case definition, there are no significant changes in the proportion of cases in homosexual men and iv drug abusers, which suggests that diagnostic and reporting practices involving the use of HIV antibody tests and presumptive diagnostic methods vary by transmission group and need to be considered when evaluating trend data.

The proportion of cases in persons with hemophilia or other coagulation disorders requiring iv administration of clotting factors has remained stable at 1 percent. Recipients of transfused blood or blood components account for 3 percent of all AIDS cases. While there has been a small but steady increase in the proportion of transfusion-associated cases, from 2 percent of the first quartile of 15,000 cases to 3 percent of the fourth quartile of cases, all but a few of these cases reflect transmission from blood products received before screening for HIV antibody was available.[16] Because of the long period from the date of transfusion to the development of AIDS, additional transfusion-associated cases will be diagnosed and reported.[17,18]

Heterosexual transmission cases comprise persons who report either specific heterosexual contact with a person with or at increased risk for HIV infection or persons who were born in areas such as Haiti or central Africa where heterosexual transmission is a major route of HIV infection. Of the 2468 persons in the heterosexual transmission category, 1464 (59 percent) reported contact with a specific at-risk partner, and 1004 (41 percent) were born in Haiti or central Africa. While the overall proportion of heterosexually acquired AIDS cases has remained constant at 4 percent, there has been a striking change in the composition of this group over time. Of the 594 heterosexual transmission cases reported between June 1981 and November 1985 in the first quartile of 15,000 cases, 378 (64 percent) were in persons of Haitian or central African origin. In contrast, only 208 (31 percent) of the 668 heterosexual transmission cases in the fourth quartile were in persons from Haiti or central-Africa. The decline in cases among Haitians may reflect a concomitant decline in immigration to the United States.[19] The vast majority of Haitians in the United States immigrated before 1978. However, 75,000–150,000 additional Haitians entered the United States between 1978 and 1981. Since 1981, immigration has declined to the pre-1978 rate of 6,000–9,000 persons per year. Most AIDS cases in Haitians in the United States have occurred in relatively recent immigrants, thus suggesting that

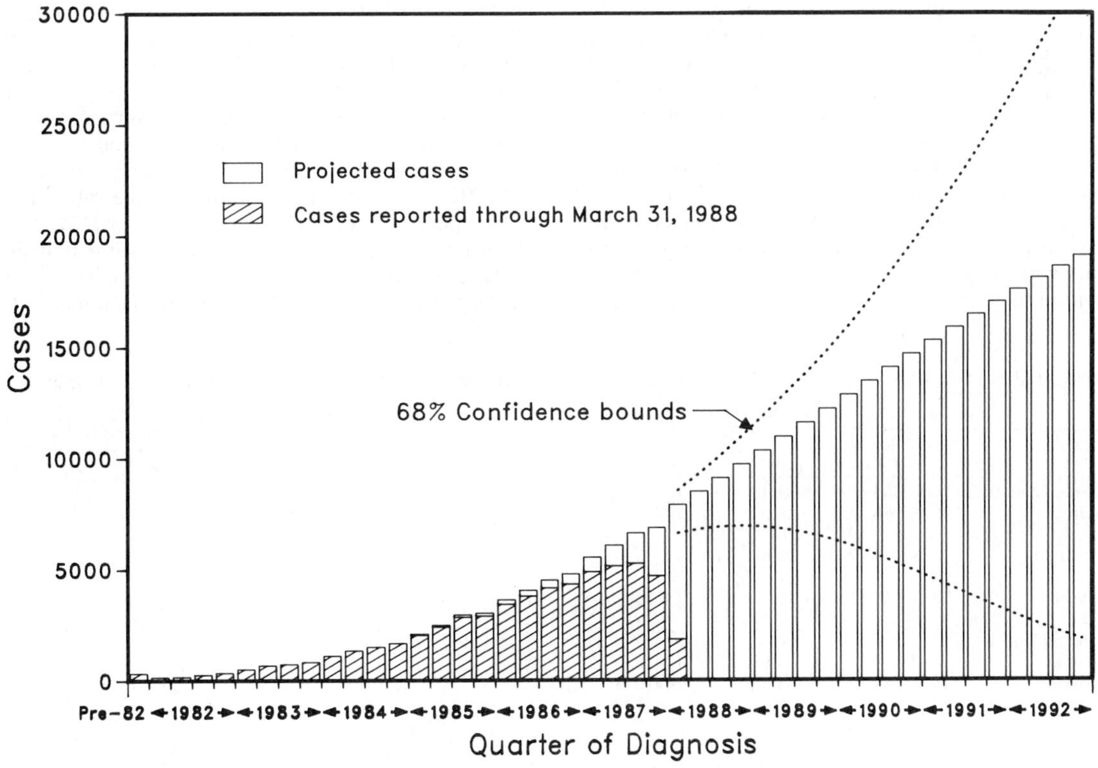

FIG. 1. Reported and projected incidence of AIDS in the United States by quarter year of diagnosis through 1992. The projections are based on a statistical extrapolation from cases reported to the CDC through March 1988 and diagnosed through June 1987.

TABLE 2. Distribution of Adults with AIDS by Transmission Group for Each Quartile of 15,000 Reported Cases[a]

	Reported Cases (%)				
Transmission Group	*First 15,000*	*Second 15,000*	*Third 15,000*	*Fourth 15,000*	*Total*
Homosexual/bisexual man	65	66	66	56	63
Heterosexual iv drug abuser	18	17	15	24	19
Homosexual man and iv drug abuser	8	8	8	7	7
Hemophilia/coagulation disorder	1	1	1	1	1
Heterosexual transmission					
Heterosexual contact	1	2	3	3	2
Born in country with high incidence of heterosexual transmission	3	2	1	1	2
Transfusion recipient	2	2	3	3	3
Undetermined	2	2	3	5	3

[a] The first quartile of 15,000 cases was reported between June 1981 and November 1985, the second 15,000 between December 1985 and January 1987, the third 15,000 between February 1987 and October 1987, and the fourth 15,000 between November 1987 and May 1988.

HIV infection was acquired before leaving Haiti and that AIDS was relatively uncommon in Haiti until the late 1970s.[19,20] Studies of Haitians with AIDS have shown that most are heterosexual men and women often with a history of sexually transmitted diseases (STDs), sexual contact with female prostitutes, or multiple heterosexual partners—findings that suggest acquisition of HIV through heterosexual contact.[20,21]

The index partners for 70 percent of patients with heterosexually acquired AIDS (exclusive of persons born in Haiti or central Africa) are iv drug abusers. In addition, 12 percent of the partners are bisexual men (female patients only), 3 percent were born in Haiti or central Africa, and 3 percent have received blood or blood components; for 12 percent the risk of the partner is unreported or under investigation.

Overall, 3 percent of all AIDS cases have no risk factor reported and are classified as undetermined. When follow-up information is available, risk factors can be identified for over 70 percent of these patients, and they are reclassified into the appropriate transmission categories.[22] As of May 1988, 1880 patients were classified in the undetermined category: 16 percent could not be reclassified after follow-up investigation; 20 percent had died, refused to be interviewed, or were lost to follow-up; and 64 percent were still under investigation. The proportion of AIDS patients with undertermined risk has increased from 2 percent of the first 15,000 cases to 5 percent of the most recently reported 15,000 cases. However, 92 percent of the cases reported in the last quartile are still under investigation; other risk factors for HIV infection will be identified for most of these persons when investigations have been completed, thus lowering this proportion.[22] The race/ethnicity and gender of AIDS patients with an undetermined risk are demographically distinctive within the U.S. population (Table 3), which suggests that they probably represent a mixture of persons who either have risk factors that they are unwilling to report or are sex partners of persons in risk groups.[22–25] The possibility of infection through heterosexual contact can be inferred from follow-up investigations of patients with undetermined risk: nearly 40 percent report a history of STDs, and one-third of interviewed men give a history of heterosexual contact with a prostitute.[22]

Demographic Characteristics

Eighty-nine percent of adults with AIDS are 20–49 years of age; only 10 percent are older than 49 years. Transfusion recipients have the highest mean and median ages (53.9 and 58.0 years, respectively), similar to that of all recipients of blood transfusions in the United States (Table 3).

Overall, 59 percent of reported AIDS cases are in white persons, 26 percent in blacks, and 14 percent in Hispanics (Table 3). The racial/ethnic group distribution of AIDS patients has been affected by the 1987 revision of the case definition: the proportion of cases in whites decreased from 63 percent of the third quartile of 15,000 cases to 54 percent of the fourth quartile of cases. The proportion of cases among blacks and Hispanics increased commensurately during this period from 36 to 45 percent. This is consistent with the observed change in the proportion of cases among homosexual and bisexual men and iv drug abusers. Blacks and Hispanics have higher relative risks of AIDS than do whites (defined as the ratio of the number of cases per million population of blacks or Hispanics to the number of cases per million population of whites) in all transmission categories except hemophilia and associated coagulation disorders in which the relative risk for black men is 0.5 [26,27] Black

TABLE 3. Demographic Characteristics of the First 60,000 Adults with AIDS Reported in the United States, by Transmission Group

		Age at Diagnosis (yrs)		*Sex (%)*		*Race/Ethnicity (%)*			
Transmission Group	*No. Cases*	*Mean*	*Range*	*Male*	*Female*	*White*	*Black*	*Hispanic*	*Other*
Homosexual/bisexual man	38,055	37.1	13–80	100	0	74	15	10	1
Heterosexual iv drug abuser	11,086	35.3	15–72	78	22	19	51	29	1
Homosexual man and iv drug abuser	4,445	34.0	15–75	100	0	62	24	13	1
Hemophilia/coagulation disorder	588	35.7	13–86	96	4	85	6	7	2
Heterosexual transmission									
Heterosexual contact	1,464	34.9	15–78	22	78	29	48	22	1
Born in country with high incidence of heterosexual transmission	1,004	33.2	16–73	78	22	<1	99	1	0
Transfusion recipient	1,478	53.9	13–90	65	35	74	15	8	3
Undetermined	1,880	39.9	17–85	79	21	37	40	21	2
Total	60,000	36.9	13–90	92	8	59	26	14	1
U.S. population				49	52	80	12	6	2

women are 13.4 times and Hispanic women 9.5 times more likely than are white women to have AIDS. The disproportionate incidence rates of AIDS among black and Hispanic women as compared with white women are most striking for those who report iv drug abuse (18.9 and 10.0 times greater than whites, respectively) or heterosexual contact with a male iv drug abuser (20.2 and 20.5 times greater). The risk of AIDS in exclusively homosexual men without a history of iv drug abuse is 1.4 and 1.8 times greater in black and Hispanic men, respectively, than in white men. For bisexual men with AIDS, the relative risks are higher (3.9 and 2.9 in blacks and Hispanics, respectively). In contrast, heterosexual black and Hispanic men who report iv drug abuse are each 20 times more likely than white heterosexual men are to have AIDS.

Men account for 92 percent of all AIDS cases, which reflects the large number of cases in homosexual and bisexual men and male iv drug abusers (Table 3). However, there has been a small but significant increase from 1981 to 1988 in the proportion of women with AIDS, from 7 percent of the first 15,000 reported cases to 10 percent of the most recent 15,000 cases reported. Heterosexual contact is the only transmission group with a predominance of women. The smaller number of men with heterosexually acquired AIDS is undoubtedly partly due to the much smaller reservoir of infection in women and the possible lower efficiency of female-to-male transmission.[28,29]

Geographic Distribution of Cases

The first reports of AIDS were clustered among homosexual men and iv drug abusers residing in major metropolitan areas on the east and west coasts.[30] Since then, cases of AIDS have been reported from all 50 states, the District of Columbia, Puerto Rico, the Virgin Islands, and Guam. Although five states—New York, California, Florida, Texas, and New Jersey—have reported most cases (68 percent), there has been a steady decrease in the proportion of cases from these states from 75 percent of the first quartile of 15,000 cases to 63 percent of the fourth quartile. This trend is primarily due to the more rapid increase in the number of cases reported from the remaining 45 states. In general, the cumulative reported incidence of AIDS by state roughly parallels the prevalence of HIV infection in military recruits, with the sex-adjusted prevalence of HIV in recruit applicants through March 1988 3–10 times higher than the cumulative incidence of reported AIDS (Fig. 2).

The distribution of cases by state of residence varies among the transmission groups. Nearly half the AIDS cases in homosexual or bisexual men have been reported from California and New York. Sixty-seven percent of cases in heterosexual iv drug abusers have been reported from New Jersey and New York; in contrast these two states account for 32 percent of AIDS cases overall. Most patients who acquired AIDS through heterosexual contact with an iv drug abuser also have been from New York and New Jersey. Florida and New York account for three-fourths of heterosexually acquired AIDS cases in persons born outside the United States, primarily in Haiti. AIDS patients with hemophilia or who received transfusions are distributed throughout the United States. These geographic patterns reflect the rapidity and magnitude of the introduction of HIV into various susceptible populations.

Opportunistic Diseases

The most frequently reported opportunistic disease among adults with AIDS is *P. carinii* pneumonia (62 percent) followed by Kaposi sarcoma (17 percent), esophageal or bronchial candidiasis (15 percent), extrapulmonary cryptococcosis (7 percent), disseminated *Mycobacterium avium* complex (5 percent), cytomegalovirus disease (5 percent), HIV wasting syndrome (4 percent), herpes simplex (4 percent), toxoplasmosis of the brain (4 percent), chronic cryptosporidiosis (3 percent), HIV encephalopathy (2 percent), non-Hodgkin's lymphoma (2 percent), extrapulmonary tuberculosis (1 percent), and other disseminated mycobacterial diseases (1 percent). Other opportunistic infections or cancers that have been reported in fewer than 1 percent of all AIDS patient are disseminated histoplasmosis, cytomegalovirus retinitis, progressive multifocal leukoencephalopathy, primary lymphoma of the brain, recurrent *Salmonella* septicemia, chronic isosporiasis, and disseminated coccidioidomycosis. The reported frequency of each of these opportunistic diseases represents a minimum estimate of the actual incidence among AIDS patients since there is substantial underreporting of opportunistic diseases diagnosed after the initial case report to the CDC. For example, only 5 percent of AIDS patients reported to the CDC have a diagnosis of disseminated *M. avium* complex; in contrast, in one series of 71 AIDS patients, 24 (34 percent) developed infection secondary to *M. avium* complex at some point in the course of their illness.[31]

P. carinii pneumonia is the most commonly reported opportunistic infection overall and for every transmission group (Table 4). When analyzed by year of diagnosis, the percentage of AIDS patients initially presenting with *P. carinii* pneumonia has increased from 31 percent in 1981 to 72 percent in 1988. The reason for this increase is unknown but does not appear to be related to changes in the distribution of cases by transmission group, race/ethnicity, geographic location, or the use of presumptive diagnostic measures.[32]

One of the strongest associations between a particular disease and the various transmission categories is the high frequency of Kaposi sarcoma in homosexual and bisexual men. Kaposi sarcoma accounts for nearly eight times the proportion of cases reported in homosexual and bisexual men when compared with heterosexual iv drug abusers. In heterosexuals, Kaposi sarcoma is most frequently reported for persons born in other countries (predominantly Haitians) and persons classified in the undetermined group. The reason for the relatively higher frequency of Kaposi sarcoma in homosexual men is unknown. The use of nitrite inhalants by homosexual men has been proposed as a possible cofactor in the development of Kaposi sarcoma. While nitrites may have some immunosuppressive effects that theoretically could result in increased susceptibility to infection or malignancy,[33,34] nitrite use has been inconsistently associated with Kaposi sarcoma and HIV infection in homosexual men.[35–40] Similarly, cytomegalovirus has also been suggested as a cofactor in the etiology of Kaposi sarcoma.[41–43] While many homosexual men have serologic evidence of cytomegalovirus infection, not all develop Kaposi sarcoma. In addition, a cohort study of HIV-infected homosexual men demonstrated no association between Kaposi sarcoma and elevated cytomegalovirus antibody titer.[44] When analyzed by year of diagnosis, the percentage of AIDS patients initially presenting with Kaposi sarcoma has decreased from 28 percent in 1981 to 9 percent in 1988. This decline was observed in every transmission group with the exception of heterosexual contact cases (exclusive of persons born in Haiti or Central Africa) and transfusion-associated cases. Studies in San Francisco suggest that the decline in Kaposi sarcoma is not secondary to diagnostic bias or selective underreporting of Kaposi sarcoma.[45] The proportional decrease in new cases of AIDS with Kaposi sarcoma suggests the possibility of a concomitant decrease in exposure to a cofactor necessary for the development of Kaposi sarcoma. However, none of several cofactors evaluated in a cohort of homosexual men in San Francisco were associated with the diagnosis of Kaposi sarcoma, including a history of STDs, enteric infections, iv drug use, and specific sexual practices.[45]

Since many HIV-associated infections result from the endogenous reactivation of previously acquired pathogens,[46,47] geographic residence and the associated higher prevalence of asymptomatic infection with certain pathogens influences the frequency of reported opportunistic infections. For example,

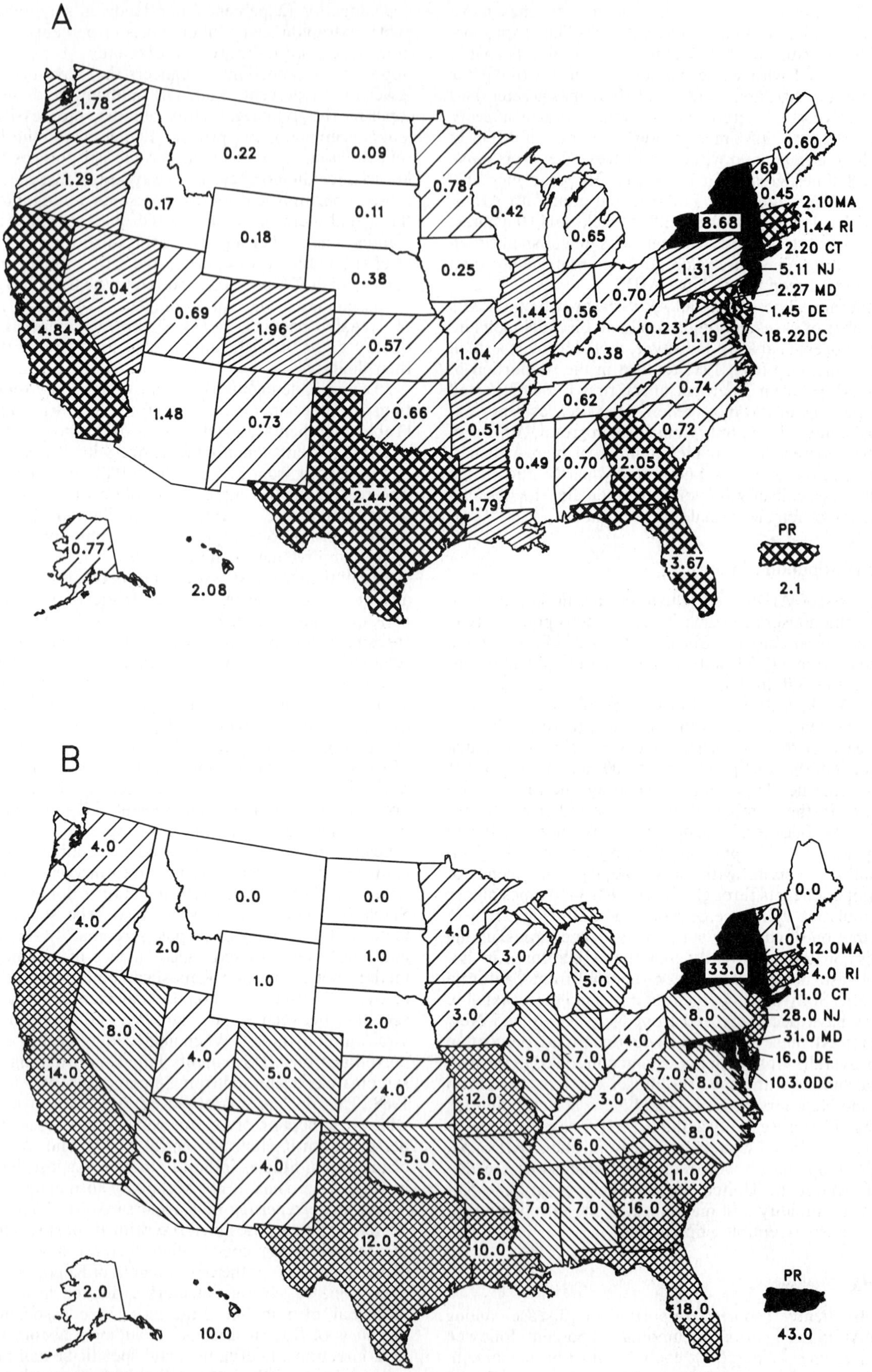

Source: Department of Defense

FIG. 2. **(A)** Reported cumulative incidence rates of AIDS as of May 1988, and **(B)** HIV seroprevalence rates in U.S. military recruit applicants, by state, from November 1985 through March 1988. Rates are per 10,000 population; military recruit applicant data are sex adjusted.

TABLE 4. Distribution of Selected Opportunistic Diseases by Transmission Group for the First 60,000 Adults with AIDS, United States

		Opportunistic Disease (%)[a]									
Transmission Group	*No. Cases*	Pneumocystis carinii *Pneumonia*	*Kaposi Sarcoma*	*Esophageal or Bronchial Candidiasis*	*Extrapulmonary Cryptococcosis*	*Disseminated* Mycobacterium avium	*Cytomegalovirus disease*	*Herpes Simplex*	*Cryptosporidiosis*	*Toxoplasmosis*	*Extrapulmonary Tuberculosis*
Homosexual/bisexual man	38,055	63	23	12	6	5	5	4	3	3	1
Heterosexual iv drug abuser	11,086	60	3	19	9	4	2	3	1	5	2
Homosexual man and iv drug abuser	4,445	59	20	16	8	6	5	5	3	4	2
Hemophilia/coagulation disorder	588	62	1	23	9	5	4	2	3	3	1
Heterosexual transmission											
Heterosexual contact	1,464	69	2	19	6	4	4	5	3	4	2
Born in country with high incidence of heterosexual transmission	1,004	44	7	19	11	3	4	5	4	15	8
Transfusion recipient	1,478	63	3	24	7	4	6	3	2	4	1
Undetermined	1,880	64	7	17	8	4	5	4	3	5	2

[a] Row percentages may total more than 100 percent because some patients had more than one disease.

the proportion of Haitian-born adults with AIDS and toxoplasmosis and disseminated tuberculosis is five and six times higher, respectively, than in non-Haitian-born adults. Similarly, disseminated histoplasmosis is diagnosed and reported more frequently in AIDS patients residing in the Mississippi valley states, while disseminated coccidioidomycosis is more common among AIDS patients residing in Arizona than in all other states.[32]

Several reports have noted a significant increase in tuberculosis associated with HIV infection.[48–50] In New York City, AIDS patients with and without tuberculosis were similiar in median age at AIDS diagnosis (34 compared with 36 years) and in sex (predominantly male).[50] However, AIDS patients with tuberculosis were more likely to be non-Haitian black, Haitian, Hispanic, and iv drug abusers than AIDS patients without tuberculosis.

Mortality of Patients with AIDS

Fifty-nine percent of the first 60,000 patients with AIDS are reported to have died. Reported fatalities increase as time from diagnosis of AIDS increases, with 31 percent of patients reported to have died within 1 year of diagnosis and 56 and 76 percent reported to have died 2 and 3 years, respectively, after diagnosis. However, reporting of deaths is known to be incomplete. In one study, when intensive follow-up was undertaken of 147 persons with AIDS who were not reported to have died after 3 years, 31 percent had died, 30 percent were lost to follow-up, and 39 percent were alive.[51] Factors that may influence survival include type of opportunistic disease at diagnosis, age, race/ethnicity, sex, mode of HIV transmission, and specific antiviral therapy (e.g., zidovudine [AZT]). Longer survival has been consistently associated with the diagnosis of Kaposi sarcoma.[51–55] Reported median survival times for patients with only Kaposi sarcoma range from 11 to 25 months as compared with 7–13 months for patients with Kaposi sarcoma and other opportunistic infections and 7–13 months for persons with opportunistic infections but not Kaposi sarcoma.[52–55] In patients with Kaposi sarcoma, younger age at diagnosis, no other opportunistic diseases, and earlier stages of clinical illness, as manifested by immunologic parameters, have been correlated with a more favorable prognosis.[51–56]

One measure of the impact of premature mortality is the years of potential life lost before the age of 65 (YPLL). This measure emphasizes deaths of children and young adults, whereas crude mortality statistics represent all deaths, which largely occur among the elderly. The leading causes of YPLL have changed only minimally from 1979 to 1986, except for AIDS. Fewer than five AIDS deaths were retrospectively identified in 1979, but by 1986 AIDS had become the eighth leading cause of YPLL in the United States.[57] The impact of AIDS on patterns of premature death is particularly important in areas such as New York City and San Francisco where AIDS has been the leading cause of YPLL for single men aged 25–44 since 1984.[58] AIDS is the leading cause of death for men aged 30–39 years and for women aged 25–29 years in New York City.[59,60] In New York City, mortality rates secondary to AIDS differ significantly by race/ethnicity: for black and Hispanic men, mortality rates as compared with white males are 1.6 and 1.5 times higher, respectively.[59] Black and Hispanic women have mortality rates 6.0 and 5.2 times higher than white women do.

AIDS IN CHILDREN

Less than $1\frac{1}{2}$ years after AIDS was first recognized in adults the first cases of unexplained immunodeficiency were reported in children.[61–64] For national reporting, pediatric cases of AIDS include children less than 13 years of age who have an illness characterized by essentially the same range of "indicator" diseases as adults with AIDS (Table 1). Two important exceptions are the inclusion of recurrent bacterial infections and lymphoid interstitial pneumonia and/or pulmonary lymphoid hyperplasia (LIP/PLH complex) affecting a child less than 13 years of age. Toxoplasmosis, herpes simplex virus infection, and cytomegalovirus disease must be diagnosed after 1 month of age.

As of May 1988, the first 1000 cases of AIDS in children were reported in the United States. The date of initial infection with HIV can be estimated for most children as either the year of birth for those with perinatally acquired infection or the year of transfusion for those who acquired HIV through blood transfusions. For perinatally acquired cases, the earliest year of birth is 1977; the first reported transfusion of blood that transmitted HIV to a child was administered in 1977 (Fig. 3).

Children born to mothers known to be infected with HIV or at increased risk for infection account for approximately three-quarters of reported cases. Of these mothers 72 percent were iv drug abusers or had sexual contact with an iv drug abuser, 19 percent acquired their infection through heterosexual contact with infected men other than iv drug abusers, 3 percent had a history of a blood transfusion, and 6 percent had AIDS or infection with HIV, but the specific route of transmission was unreported. Risk factors for the remaining children include receipt of transfusion (14 percent) and hemophilia (6 percent); 4 percent had an undetermined risk. When follow-up information is available, most children who are initially reported with an undetermined risk are reclassified; in one study, half of those reclassified had mothers who used iv drugs or were partners of men who used iv drugs.[65]

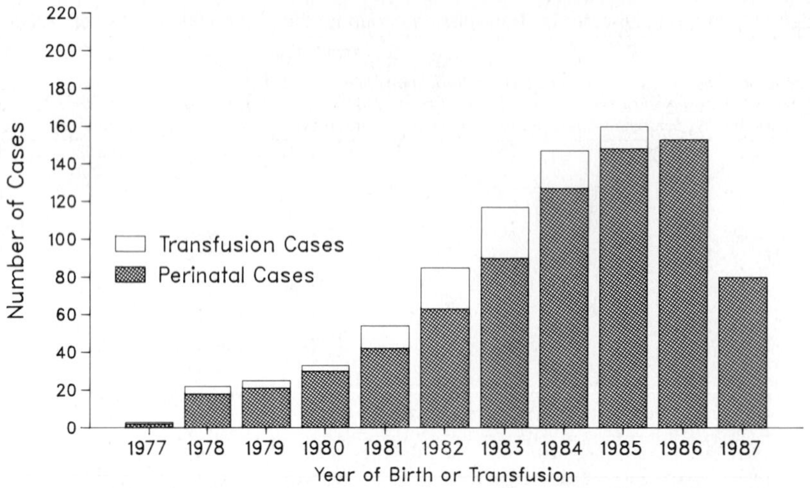

FIG. 3. Children in the United States with AIDS reported through May 1988 by year of birth for perinatally acquired cases and by year of transfusion for transfusion-acquired cases.

Most reported cases of AIDS in children are initially diagnosed at less than 2 years of age (64 percent), with 24 percent less than 6 months of age; only 11 percent are older than 5 years. Children with hemophilia have the highest mean and median ages (8.7 and 9.1 years, respectively).

The demographic characteristics of children with AIDS are very similar to those of heterosexual adult patients with AIDS: 53 percent are black, 22 percent are Hispanic and 23 percent are white. The cumulative incidence rates in black and Hispanic children are 11.2 and 7.4 times the rate for white children, with the highest rates of AIDS reported for transmission categories associated with iv drug abuse. For children whose mothers are iv drug abusers, the rates for blacks and Hispanics are 24.3 and 17.0 times greater than that for whites, respectively, and for children whose mothers have sex partners who are iv drug abusers, 17.2 and 17.9 times greater, respectively. The racial/ethnic distribution of children with AIDS varies by transmission group: of the 771 children who acquired AIDS perinatally, 84 percent were black or Hispanic as compared with 43 percent of 135 children with transfusion-associated AIDS and 23 percent of children with hemophilia. The racial/ethnic distribution of children with an undetermined risk is nearly identical to that of children with perinatally acquired infection.

There is an equal distribution by sex for perinatal cases and cases with an undetermined risk. Males are overrepresented in hemophilic children (95 percent) and transfusion recipients (62 percent). The sex distribution of transfusion-acquired cases is similar to that of all transfused infants in the United States in that more male than female infants receive transfusions.[66]

AIDS in children has been reported from 40 states, the District of Columbia, and Puerto Rico. Four states—New York, California, Florida, and New Jersey—have reported most of the cases (64 percent). However, there has been an increase in the proportion of children with AIDS residing in states other than these four, from 27 percent of the first 250 cases (which were reported over a 3-year period) to 41 percent of the most recent 250 cases (reported over a 6-month period). The geographic distribution of perinatally acquired cases is similar to that for women with AIDS in that 69 percent were reported from New York, New Jersey, Florida, and California as compared with 44 percent of the transfusion-acquired cases and 33 percent of hemophilia-associated cases in children.

Overall, 59 percent of children with AIDS are reported to have died. However, reported death rates vary significantly by age: 71 percent of infants younger than 1 year at diagnosis are reported to have died as compared with 51 percent of children older than 1 year. Similar to adult AIDS cases, mortality data are underreported in children with AIDS; actual fatality rates for reported cases are undoubtedly much higher. The length of survival is likely influenced by age at diagnosis and by type of opportunistic disease at initial presentation. The reported median survival time for infants (4.0 months) is significantly less than for children older than 1 year (11.2 months). Children with *P. carinii* pneumonia have been reported to have shorter survival times, while children with lymphocytic interstitial pneumonitis have been reported to live longer.[67]

MODES OF TRANSMISSION

HIV is transmitted almost exclusively through sexual contact, parenteral exposure to blood or blood products, and perinatally from infected mothers to their infants.

Sexual Transmission

Sexual transmission is the predominant mode of HIV transmission throughout the world. In general, the risk of acquiring HIV infection through a single sexual contact depends on several factors including specific sex practices, the infectivity of the source partner, the susceptibility of the recipient partner, and possibly the viral strain.[68] As the prevalence of infection in the population increases, the likelihood of encountering an infected partner also increases.

Homosexual and bisexual men, the population in the United States in whom AIDS was first recognized, have continued to account for most U.S. AIDS cases. Multiple epidemiologic studies have identified specific risk factors associated with HIV infection in homosexual men, including increased number of sex partners, receptive anal intercourse, and other practices associated with rectal trauma such as "fisting" and douching.[35–39,69–72] While no sexual activities involving exposure to semen or blood have been shown to be without risk, the precise risk of specific sexual activities, such as fellatio, is difficult to ascertain because most homosexual men report engaging in multiple sex practices. Nonetheless, several reports suggest that the risks of HIV transmission that are associated with insertive anal intercourse and oral intercourse are less than that associated with receptive anal intercourse.[38,39,71–74]

Two instances of female-to-female transmission of HIV have been reported after traumatic sex practices.[75,76]

Bidirectional heterosexual transmission of HIV infection is well documented, but the relative efficiency of male-to-female as compared with female-to-male transmission is not clearly established.[77–85] The approximate 1:1 sex ratio of cases in Africa has been cited as evidence of equal bidirectional efficiency. Actually, the male-to-female ratio of AIDS and HIV infection in many African areas varies by age, e.g., in Kinshasa, Zaire, for persons 20–29 years, the male-to-female ratio of AIDS case rates is 1:2.7; for those 30–39 years, 1.3:1; and for those 40–49 years, 4.2:1.[86,87] These sex and age distributions are similar to other STDs both in industrialized and developing countries where disease incidence and associated morbidity are higher among younger women. Other factors related to HIV infection and transmission among heterosexuals of African or Haitian descent include high rates of concurrent STDs, particularly those causing genital ulceration, large numbers of different heterosexual partners, and to a lesser extent, the possibility of parenteral exposures to contaminated needles.[20,21,85–90]

The highest reported rates of heterosexual transmission of HIV have been reported for the partners of infected iv drug abusers and persons born in Haiti or central Africa, although the duration of unprotected sexual contact has not been adequately controlled for in all studies.[14] The difference in these rates may reflect biologic factors such as concurrent infections in either the index patient or the partner, behavioral factors such as unreported drug abuse by the partner, or varying levels of infectivity in the source patient over the course of infection. Epidemiologic and laboratory data suggest that infectivity may be related to the source partner's clinical stage of infection. In a prospective study of infected hemophilic men and their female sex partners, transmission of HIV was associated with the development of severe immunodeficiency in the men, as manifested by very low numbers of T4 cells.[91] This is consistent with the observation that the ability to isolate HIV in vitro significantly increases as the number of T-helper cells declines and the clinical course advances.[92]

Most heterosexual transmission of HIV occurs through penile–vaginal contact, but in two studies receptive anal intercourse was associated with an increased risk of transmission between heterosexual partners.[82,93] Transmission of HIV has been reported after a single heterosexual contact,[84] but other studies have reported no evidence of heterosexual transmission even after hundreds of contacts.[77,80–84]

Case–control studies of homosexual men have documented an association between HIV infection and STDs such as syphilis, gonorrhea, and genital herpes.[35,36,38,39,70,72] STDs reflect, in part, a sexually active life-style that usually includes large numbers of sex partners. In addition, STDs may play a direct role in facilitating HIV transmission by disrupting genital epithelium. Additional studies of homosexual men show an association between syphilis and herpes simplex virus type 2 and HIV infection that is independent of the number of partners and specific sex practices.[94,95] Similarly, genital ulcer disease, particularly chancroid, has been associated with HIV infection in both heterosexual men and female prostitutes in Kenya.[88,90,96–98] Given these data, the recent increases in primary and secondary syphilis and chancroid in heterosexual men and women in the United States are of concern.[99]

Parenteral Exposure to Blood or Blood Products

Among iv drug abusers, HIV is transmitted by parenteral exposure to HIV-contaminated needles and other equipment used for injection. Specific risk factors that have been associated with HIV seropositivity include duration of iv drug use since 1978, needle sharing, number of persons with whom needles are shared, number of injections, median number of injections in "shooting galleries," and residence in an area with a high prevalence of HIV infection.[100–102]

AIDS in persons with hemophilia and recipients of transfusions has clearly implicated blood as a major vehicle of HIV transmission. Whole blood, blood cellular components, plasma, and clotting factors have transmitted HIV.[103,104] Several epidemiologic and laboratory studies have shown that recipients of other products prepared from blood or plasma including hepatitis B immune globulin, immune serum globulin, $Rh_o(D)$ immune globulin, and hepatitis B vaccine have not developed serologic evidence of HIV infection.[105–107] These products are prepared by using one of several fractionation processes that are effective in removing and inactivating HIV.[108]

The likelihood of becoming infected with HIV after receiving a single-donor blood product documented to be HIV-seropositive approaches 100 percent.[109] Investigation of donors of blood given to patients who later developed AIDS has often identified a donor infected with HIV and/or at high risk for AIDS.[103,110] Because many donors are asymptomatic at donation, effective screening of blood for transfusion depends on the use of serologic tests to detect HIV antibody. It has been estimated that between 1978 and 1984, before the implementation of HIV antibody testing of donated blood, as many as 29,000 transfusion recipients in the United States received a unit of blood infected with HIV and that approximately 12,000 are still alive.[18] Serologic screening of blood for HIV and donor deferral procedures have vastly reduced transmission of HIV by transfusion. The rare exception is recently infected donors who have not yet developed detectable HIV antibody. The rate of such transmission by HIV-seronegative blood has been estimated to be 26 per 1 million transfusions in the United States.[16]

The risk of HIV infection for patients with hemophilia who receive concentrated clotting factors composed of blood components from potentially thousands of donors was substantial before 1984–1985.[111] This risk has been reduced to a very low level with the implementation of heat treatment of clotting factor concentrates, HIV antibody testing of donated blood, and donor deferral procedures.[112]

Transmission of HIV has also been linked to recipients of organs, tissues, and semen from donors at increased risk for or documented to have HIV infection.[113–115] The U.S. Public Health Service has recommended that potential donors of organs, tissues, or semen be screened for HIV antibody and that organs from HIV-seropositive donors not be used for transplantation except under extremely unusual circumstances and with informed consent.[114,116]

Parenteral, nonintact skin, and mucous membrane exposures to blood have infrequently resulted in occupationally acquired HIV infections in health care workers.[117] Data from several prospective surveillance projects of health care workers indicate that the risk of seroconversion after needlestick exposures to blood from HIV-infected patients is less than 1 percent and that the level of risk associated with the exposure of nonintact skin or mucous membranes is far less.[117–120] In one study, 179 health care workers reported 2703 cutaneous exposures to HIV-infected blood; none of these workers became infected with HIV.[121] The increasing number of persons being treated for HIV-associated illnesses makes it likely that more health care workers will encounter patients and laboratory specimens infected with HIV. The risk of transmission can be minimized if health care workers adhere to published recommendations and use universal precautions when caring for all patients.[122–124]

Perinatal Transmission

HIV can be transmitted from an infected woman to her fetus or newborn in the following ways: antepartum through the maternal circulation, during delivery through exposure to blood or other infected fluids, and postpartum through breast-feeding. The occurrence of intrauterine infection is supported by the detection of HIV in fetal tissues[125,126] and the isolation of HIV from cord blood.[127] The isolation of HIV from breast milk[128] as well as several case reports of breast-feeding mothers who became infected after delivery and subsequently transmitted HIV to their infants indicate that breast-feeding can transmit HIV.[129–131]

Precise estimates of the frequency of perinatal transmission are lacking because of the unavailability of a reliable method to detect HIV infection in newborn infants. Prospective studies indicate perinatal transmission rates ranging from 23 to 45 percent.[132–136] Preliminary data suggest that the risk of perinatal transmission increases with the progression of HIV-associated immunosuppression and disease in the mother.[127,137]

Other Modes of Transmission

Sexual contact, exposure to blood, and perinatal transmission are the major modes of HIV infection, but there is concern that alternate, albeit rare, modes of transmission exist.[138,139] HIV has been isolated from blood,[4–6] semen,[140] vaginal secretions,[141,142] the uterine cervix,[143] saliva,[144–146] breast milk,[128] tears,[147] urine,[146] cerebrospinal fluid,[146,148] alveolar fluid,[149] and amniotic fluid.[150] However, isolation of virus from a body fluid does not necessarily implicate that body fluid as an important source of infection. For example, although virus has been isolated from saliva, it is recovered much less frequently from saliva than from blood.[145,146] Additionally, in vitro laboratory data indicate that both whole saliva and saliva filtrates contain components that inactivate HIV.[151] Contact with HIV-contaminated saliva has occurred through human bites and in the health care setting. A case report of two siblings infected with HIV suggested a bite as the route of transmission for the previously uninfected sibling.[152] Because the bite did not break the skin or result in bleeding, the precise mode of transmission remains unclear. Fifteen other persons have been reported who did not become infected with HIV after a human bite from a person known to be infected with HIV.[153,154] More than 100 health care workers have been followed prospectively after parenteral, mucous membrane, or nonintact skin exposure to the saliva of HIV-infected persons, and none have become infected with HIV.[117–121] Over 1800 dental professionals have been evaluated in other studies, and only one dentist without a history of behavioral risk factors for AIDS was HIV-seropositive.[155–157] The infected dentist reported several needlestick injuries and trauma to his hands and did not routinely wear gloves when providing dental care; whether saliva or blood was the mode of transmission cannot be determined.[155] Thus, epidemiologic evidence has not conclusively documented transmission of HIV by saliva and suggests that the risk of HIV infection after such extensive exposure to saliva, if present at all, is extremely low.[139]

To examine the risk of HIV transmission through casual contact, more than 700 nonsexual household contacts of both adults and children with HIV infection have been evaluated.[78,80,81,84,138,139,158–160] Many of these household members shared bathroom and kitchen facilities including toilets, baths, and eating utensils with the AIDS patient. In addition, close personal interaction frequently occurred, including hugging and kissing on the cheek and lips. No transmission of HIV has been documented exclusive of sex partners, children both to infected mothers, and persons who themselves had risk factors for AIDS.

Laboratory and epidemiologic studies have failed to demonstrate either replication of HIV within insects or transmission of HIV through biting or bloodsucking insects.[161,162] The role of insect-mediated HIV infection was evaluated in a case–control study of residents in Belle Glade, Florida; HIV infection was not associated with either epidemiologic or laboratory evidence of exposure to mosquitoes, as measured by the presence of antibodies to five arboviruses.[163] Furthermore, HIV infection was not detected in any adults older than 60 years or in children aged 2–10 years. The high rate of HIV infection in this community appears to be the result of transmission through sexual contact and iv drug abuse and not insect vectors. Additional studies in Haiti and Africa have failed to establish an association between the presence of dengue or malaria antibodies and HIV.[164,165]

HIV INFECTION OTHER THAN AIDS

Spectrum and Progression of HIV Infection

Patients infected with HIV may present with a spectrum of clinical manifestations ranging from asymptomatic infection to severe immunodeficiency associated with serious secondary infections, neoplasms, and other conditions.[165a]

Various systems have been proposed to classify the manifestations of HIV infection in both children and adults (Tables 5 and 6).[166–169] Staging criteria generally include serologic evidence of HIV infection; the presence or absence of clinical signs and symptoms of disease; and various immunologic parameters such as T-helper (T4) lymphopenia, decreased T-helper/T-suppressor (T4/T8) ratio, and evidence of cutaneous anergy. These systems have both clinical and public health applications including disease surveillance and reporting, design and analysis of epidemiologic studies, development and implementation of prevention and control strategies, formulation of health policy and strategy, and facilitation of scientific communication regarding HIV infection.[170]

An acute, mononucleosis-like illness has been described in association with initial infection with the virus.[171–172a] Features of this illness include fever, lymphadenopathy, sweats, myalgia, arthralgia, rash, malaise, lethargy, sore throat, anorexia, nausea, vomiting, headaches, photophobia, and diarrhea. *Candida* esophagitis during the acute retroviral illness has also been reported.[173] The rate of symptomatic primary HIV infection is difficult to determine because symptoms tend to be nonspecific, may cause little discomfort, pass largely unnoticed by the patient, and are often assessed retrospectively. For example, of 54 HIV-infected transfusion recipients, only 13 (24 percent) recalled an illness compatible with the acute retroviral syndrome.[174] Among patients with well characterized exposures to HIV and compatible symptoms, the interval between exposure

TABLE 5. Centers for Disease Control Classification Systems for Human Immunodeficiency Virus

I.	Classification system for HIV infection in adults
Group I.	Acute infection
Group II.	Asymptomatic infection
Group III.	Persistent generalized lymphadenopathy
Group IV.	Other diseases
Subgroup A.	Constitutional disease including HIV wasting syndrome in the CDC surveillance definition for AIDS
Subgroup B.	Neurologic disease including HIV encephalopathy in the CDC surveillance definition for AIDS
Subgroup C.	Secondary infectious diseases
Category C-1.	Specified secondary infectious diseases in the CDC surveillance definition for AIDS
Category C-2.	Other specified secondary infectious diseases
Subgroup D.	Secondary cancers in the CDC surveillance definition for AIDS
Subgroup E.	Other conditions
II.	Classification system for HIV infection in children under 13 years of age
Class P-0.	Indeterminate infection
Class P-1.	Asymptomatic infection
Subclass A.	Normal immune function
Subclass B.	Abnormal immune function
Subclass C.	Immune function not tested
Class P-2.	Symptomatic infection
Subclass A.	Nonspecific findings
Subclass B.	Progressive neurologic disease including HIV encephalopathy in the CDC surveillance definition for AIDS
Subclass C.	Lymphoid interstitial pneumonitis in the CDC surveillance definition for AIDS
Subclass D.	Secondary infectious diseases
Category D-1.	Specified secondary infectious diseases in the CDC surveillance definition for AIDS
Category D-2.	Recurrent serious bacterial infections in the CDC surveillance definition for AIDS
Category D-3.	Other specified secondary infectious diseases
Subclass E.	Secondary cancers
Category E-1.	Specified secondary cancers in the CDC surveillance definition for AIDS
Category E-2.	Other cancers possibly secondary to HIV infection
Subclass F.	Other diseases possibly due to HIV infection

(Modified from refs. 168 and 169.)

TABLE 6. The Walter Reed Staging Classification for HIV Infection in Adults

Stage	HIV Antibody and/or Virus Isolation	Clinic Lymphadenopathy	T-Helper Cells/mm^3	Cutaneous Anergy	Thrush	Opportunistic Infection
0	−	−	>400	Normal	−	−
1	+[a]	−	>400	Normal	−	−
2	+[a]	+[a]	>400	Normal	−	−
3	+[a]	+/−	<400[a]	Normal	−	−
4	+[a]	+/−	<400[a]	Partial[a]	−	−
5	+[a]	+/−	<400	Complete and/or	+[a]	−
6	+[a]	+/−	<400	Partail or complete	+/−	+[a]

[a] Essential criteria for assignment to each stage.
(Modified from Redfield et al.,[167] with permission.)

and symptomatic illness ranges from 6 to 58 days (Horsburgh CR Jr: Unpublished data, 1988).

Observations in persons with primary HIV infection indicate that HIV antigen can be detected within 1–4 weeks, followed by the development of HIV anti-core (p24) and anti-envelope antibodies (gp41).[171,172,175–176b] HIV antibodies usually develop within 3–12 weeks of the infection and evidence suggests that infection with HIV is persistent and lifelong. In one study, the virus was isolated from 22 (96 percent) of 25 blood donors who had been infected for 1–4 years.[110] Virus has been recovered from some homosexual men as long as 6 years after the initial detection of HIV antibody.[177] Loss of serologically detectable antibodies to HIV is rare in asymptomatic, latently infected persons. In a longitudinal study of 1000 HIV-seropositive homosexual men without AIDS, serologic tests for HIV antibody for 4 men (0.4 percent) apparently reverted from positive to negative, although polymerase chain reaction (gene amplification) assays demonstrated HIV provirus in all 4.[178] Long-term follow-up will be required to determine whether serologic reexpression of HIV occurs and whether clinical evidence of infection develops.

The period of time between the initial infection with HIV and the development of AIDS is usually long. While the risk for disease progression increases with the duration of infection, the risk is not uniform over time. Typically, a low rate of disease progression is observed in the first few years after infection. Of 6700 homosexual and bisexual men enrolled from 1978 to 1980 for studies of hepatitis B in San Francisco, 70 percent are estimated to be infected with HIV.[179] For a sample of 184 men from this study who had known dates of seroconversion, the cumulative proportion who have developed AIDS after 10 years is 48 percent.[180] Fewer than 5 percent were diagnosed with AIDS in the first 2 years after infection, however. In studies of persons with hemophilia, the rate of disease progression to AIDS is similar to that reported for homosexual men. For hemophilic persons followed 7 years after HIV seroconversion, the actuarial AIDS incidence is 22 percent.[180–181a] Transfusion recipients may have a more rapid rate of progression to AIDS. In one study, 23 percent of 71 transfusion recipients followed for a median of 4 years developed AIDS.[182]

The average period of time between infection with HIV and the development of AIDS is underestimated from such follow-up studies because persons with longer incubation periods who have not yet become ill are selectively excluded from analysis. To adjust for this limitation, various mathematic models have been developed. When using a model-based approach, the mean incubation period for both homosexual men and for adults with transfusion-associated AIDS is estimated to be approximately 8 years[183,183a] In contast, the calculated mean incubation period for infants with transfusion-mediate infection is 2 years.[183,184]

Prevalence and Incidence of HIV Infection

Because of the long incubation period, surveillance data for AIDS cannot be used to accurately monitor the incidence of HIV infection. The Public Health Service estimated in 1988 that approximately 1–1.5 million persons were infected with HIV in the United States.[185] The highest rates of infection are concentrated among persons known to be at an increased risk.

Reported HIV seroprevalence rates in homosexual and bisexual men range from 10 percent to as high as 70 percent, with most between 20 and 50 percent.[185] While the prevalence of HIV infection among iv drug abusers varies more widely, consistently high rates (usually > 50 percent) have been reported from New York, New Jersey, and Puerto Rico.[185] In contrast, the prevalence of HIV infection in hemophilic persons varies according to the severity of disease and tends to be uniformly distributed throughout the country. Overall, approximately 70 percent of persons with hemophilia A (factor VIII deficiency) and 35 percent of persons with hemophilia B (factor IX deficiency) are seropositive.[185]

Female prostitutes are at risk of HIV infection because of iv drug abuse and multiple sex partners. In a multicenter study of prostitutes in various settings in selected cities, 65 (10 percent) of 670 women had antibody to HIV.[186] Seroprevalence rates for HIV ranged from 0 percent of prescreened prostitutes in southern Nevada who were seen at STD clinics to 69 percent of prostitutes being treated for drug addition in northern New Jersey. Among prostitutes who were studied, the major risk factor for HIV infection was iv drug abuse. In a study of prostitutes in southern Florida in 1987, 37 (41 percent) of 90 inner-city prostitutes were HIV antibody-positive, including 29 (46 percent) of 63 women who abused iv drugs and 8 (30 percent) of 27 women who denied abusing iv drugs.[187] These data indicate that female prostitutes are at high risk for HIV infection and represent a potential source for heterosexual transmission.

Few specific data are available on the transmission of HIV among heterosexuals in the United States who are not the direct sex partners of iv drug abusers or other persons at high risk. The level of HIV infection in persons attending STD clinics who do not acknowledge homosexual contact, iv drug abuse, or sexual contact with persons at high risk varies, depending on the method used to ascertain risk history (i.e., self-administered questionnaire vs. in-person interview), the population being tested, and geographic location. In surveys conducted in three cities, seroprevalence rates in persons who did not report any high-risk behavior ranged from 2.7 percent of men and 1.8 percent of women in Baltimore[188] to 1.4 percent of men and 0.4 percent of women in New York City[189] and 0.2 percent of men and 0 percent women in Denver.[190] A survey of 602 parturient women in New York City identified 12 (2 percent) who were infected with HIV; 5 of the 12 women had no identified risk factors.[191] These studies suggest that patients at perinatal or STD clinics, particularly those located in areas where HIV seroprevalence is high among iv drug abusers, represent a group at increased risk for HIV infection. Beginning in 1988, a comprehensive family of HIV surveys and a national household-based seroprevalence survey will be undertaken by the U.S. Public Health Service in collaboration with local and state health departments and other agencies.[192] This surveillance approach will help monitor the levels and trends of HIV infection in the United States.

HIVseroprevalence data are more extensive from blood donors and military recruit applicants. Because these two populations are screened to select out homosexual men, iv drug abusers, and persons with hemophilia, the observed prevalence of HIV infection in these groups is much lower than the actual prevalence in the general population. For these same reasons, the relative proportion of unrecognized heterosexual and unexplained transmission will probably be higher in those who are seropositive for HIV. Among blood donors, 0.020 percent of 12.6 million American Red Cross blood donations collected between April 1985 and May 1987 were seropositive for HIV.[185] The overall level decreased from 0.035 percent in mid-1985 to 0.012 percent in mid-1987, primarily as a result of eliminating previously identified seropositive persons from the donor pool. Among first-time donors, who provide a measure of the prevalence of infection in the geographic area from which they are drawn, the level of HIV seropositivity averaged 0.043 percent during 1985–1987.[185] The overall prevalence of HIV infection among military recruits remained relatively stable at 0.15 percent between October 1985 and September 1987 and decreased slightly between October 1987 and March 1988.[185a] Among active-duty U.S. Army personnel who were tested more than once for HIV, 7.7 per 10,000 per year became infected since their initial test.[185]

HIV antibody prevalence for childbearing women has been ascertained by blinded surveys of blood samples collected on filter paper from newborns for routine metabolic assays such as phenylketonuria. These surveys provide unbiased population-based estimates of HIV infection in women bearing children. In Massachusetts, of over 30,000 specimens tested, 81 (0.3 percent) were confirmed as HIV-positive.[193] The prevalence of HIV infection varied by type and location of the hospital and ranged from 8.0 per 1000 in inner-city hospitals to 0.9 per 1000 in suburban and rural hospitals. In New York, HIV seroprevalence rates ascertained by this method were 1.6 percent in New York City and 0.2 percent for the remainder of the state.[194]

AIDS AND HIV INFECTION OUTSIDE THE UNITED STATES

Soon after the initial reports of AIDS in the United States, similar cases were identified in Europe.[195] Most of the initial European patients were homosexual and bisexual males. By early 1983, cases were recognized in Caribbean and central African expatriates residing in Europe.[195,196] Studies in Haiti and central Africa confirmed that homosexuality and iv drug abuse did not appear to be common risk factors in these patients.[21,88,89,197] These studies and the approximately equal proportion of cases among men and women suggested the occurrence of heterosexual transmission.[86–89]

The origin and global dissemination of HIV infection is of considerable interest. Antibodies to HIV have been detected in stored serum specimens obtained as early as 1959 in Zaire[198] and 1963 in Burkina Faso.[199] These observations suggest that sporadic cases of AIDS and HIV infection antedated the recognized epidemic in Africa as well as in the United States and other areas.[200] In retrospect, clinical evidence of the syndrome was not recognized with any regularity in Africa until the late 1970s and early 1980s when increases in several opportunistic infections and cancers were documented, including esophageal candidiasis,[197] unusually severe Kaposi sarcoma,[201] as well as wasting syndrome or "slim disease."[202]

Through May 1988, 96,433 cases of AIDS were reported to the World Health Organization (WHO).[203] However, WHO estimates that as many as 150,000 cases of AIDS may have occurred worldwide through 1987.[204] Precise enumeration of the number of AIDS cases is not possible, particularly in developing countries, because of the inability to obtain definitive diagnostic studies including HIV antibody tests and the absence of formalized disease surveillance and reporting systems. A systematic, hospital-based program of surveillance was initiated in Kinshasa, Zaire, in 1984 that used a modified version of the CDC surveillance case definition.[86] Even though the ability to diagnose many opportunistic diseases in this setting (most notably *P. carinii* pneumonia) was limited, an incidence rate of 55–100 per 100,000 Kinshasa residents was calculated. This was similar to the incidence rate of 82–100 per 100,000 calculated for recent Haitian entrants into the United States that same year.[19,58]

While similar modes of transmission exist worldwide, their geographic distribution and relative importance vary considerably. In western Europe, North America, Australia, New Zealand, and parts of South America, homosexual and bisexual men and iv drug abusers initially exposed to the virus in the mid-1970s or early 1980s remain the predominantly affected population group.[204,205] In Africa, the Caribbean, and some areas of South America, heterosexual sexual transmission, perinatal transmission, and receipt of HIV-infected blood are the primary modes of infection. Significant rates of HIV infection have been documented among women of childbearing age: between 3 and 11 percent of pregnant women in some urban areas of central and East Africa are seropositive.[127,132,206–208] Prostitutes studied in central and East Africa have also had high rates of HIV seroprevalence reported.[90,96,197] A retrospective, longitudinal seroepidemiologic study of prostitutes in Nairobi documented a steady increase in HIV seroprevalence from 4 percent in 1981 to 61 percent in 1985.[90] A concomitant rise in seroprevalence occurred in men treated for chancroid at a Nairobi STD clinic: 0 percent in 1981 to 15 percent in 1985. High rates of HIV infection in heterosexuals in these areas have resulted in a substantial and growing burden of perinatally acquired HIV infection in infants.[127,132,206–208]

In Kinshasa, Zaire, treatment of malaria-associated anemia with blood transfusions is an important factor in the exposure of children to HIV infection. In one hospital alone, an estimated 561 transfusions of HIV-seropositive blood were given to children with malaria over a 1-year period.[165] Receipt of injections and scarifications have been inconsistently associated with HIV infection,[206,209] the role of these and other nonsexual cultural practices in the transmission of HIV is not clear.[210]

HIV-2

A second retrovirus, HIV-2, has been isolated and associated with the development of serious opportunistic diseases that are clinically indistinguishable from AIDS caused by HIV-1. HIV-1 and HIV-2 are genetically and immunologically distinct. HIV-2 has only 40 percent DNA homology with HIV-1.[211] Serologic screening tests for HIV-1 antibodies have been estimated to detect 42–96 percent of HIV-2 infections.[212] While serum samples reactive to antigens of both viruses have been reported, this dual seropositivity is most often secondary to cross-reactivity of HIV-1-positive serum with HIV-2 antigens.[213,214]

Most cases of HIV-2 infection have been reported from countries in West Africa, but several well-documented cases have also been reported in Europeans and in West Africans residing in Europe and the United States.[213,215,216] Although the reported spectrum of disease is as broad as that for HIV-1-associated infection, the relative pathogenicity of the two viruses is unknown. Most persons infected with HIV-2 in West Africa have not progressed to develop AIDS.[217] Preliminary epidemiologic studies indicate that the modes of HIV-2 transmission are the same as those of HIV-1.[213,217]

PREVENTION OF AIDS AND HIV INFECTION IN THE COMMUNITY

In the absence of vaccines and only a limited number of effective antiviral agents or other therapeutic modalities, prevention of HIV infection must be based on strategies that interrupt sexual, blood-borne, and perinatal transmission of the virus.[218] Such strategies must be grounded in an understanding of the epidemiology of HIV infection. Application of such epidemiologic information is therefore critical in the design, implementation, and evaluation of prevention efforts.[219]

Prevention of Transmission

The risk of sexual transmission of HIV can be completely eliminated by either abstention from sexual activity or participation in a mutually monogamous relationship with an uninfected person. Other approaches that will reduce (but not completely eliminate) the risk of transmission include reduction of number of sex partners and efforts to minimize the likelihood of genital or oral mucous membrane exposure to blood, semen, saliva, cervical secretions, and vaginal secretions during intercourse.[220] The correct and consistent use of condoms and possibly condoms in conjunction with spermicides can reduce transmission of HIV by preventing exposure to infectious secretions and lesions. Laboratory testing has demonstrated latex condoms to be effective mechanical barriers to HIV as well as a number of other sexually transmitted pathogens.[221] Epidemiologic studies suggest that the usage of condoms may be associated with a reduction in acquisition of HIV from sexual partners either known to have AIDS or at increased risk of infection.[81,222] Most condom failures result from incorrect use, but breakage does occur.[221]

Examination of trends in self-reported sexual behaviors among homosexual and bisexual men point to significant reductions in certain high-risk behaviors such as the number of nonsteady partners and insertive anal intercourse.[223,224] Declining rates of rectal and pharyngeal gonorrhea among males in New York City and, more importantly, reductions in incident HIV infections among men in San Francisco provide additional evidence that the sexual transmission of HIV can be reduced.[225–266a] Comparable data to suggest significant changes in sexual behavior by heterosexual men and women in response to AIDS are not available. There is ample evidence that, while both homosexual and heterosexual persons are generally aware of the risk of sexually acquired HIV infection, many continue not to take precautions to protect themselves against AIDS and other STDs.[70,81,99,223,224,226–228]

Prevention of HIV infection through transmission by blood and blood products depends on deferral of blood and plasma donation by persons at increased risk for HIV infection, serologic screening of donated blood and plasma for HIV antibody, and heat treatment of clotting factor concentrates.[112,229–232] These measures have vastly reduced transmission of HIV by blood and blood products in the United States and other industrialized nations.[16,233] Although there is evidence that high-risk donors are voluntarily refraining from donation,[234] follow-up of seropositive donors has shown that most have a risk factor for HIV infection.[16,232,235,236] Therefore, additional strategies to reduce the already very low incidence of HIV transmission by blood or plasma transfusion need to focus on learning why some persons at risk for HIV infection continue to donate blood, improving educational programs to dissuade such persons from donating, and implementing more sensitive serologic assays to detect HIV as they become available.[16,233]

Strategies to prevent the transmission of HIV through iv drug abuse need to be tailored specifically to three target groups: (*1*) persons who have not yet begun iv drug abuse; (*2*) persons who are willing to enter treatment programs to eliminate iv drug use; and (*3*) persons who are unwilling to enter treatment.[237] A creative blend of educational, therapeutic, and law enforcement approaches and a substantial amount of resources will be required for each target group. The Presidential Commission on the HIV Epidemic has recommended that prevention and treatment of iv drug abuse must be a national priority and that treatment capacity must be greatly expanded in the United States.[238] Data are limited but indicate that many current abusers are aware of the risk associated with injection, and that some have decreased their risk by reduced needle sharing, increased procurement of sterile needles, and increased needle cleaning practices.[237,239]

Primary prevention of perinatally acquired HIV infection should center on routine, voluntary counseling and HIV antibody testing of childbearing age women in settings where HIV prevalence is moderate to high (e.g., 0.5 percent or higher) and in women with identified risks for HIV infection.[240] Women at increased risk for HIV infection include those who have used iv drugs; engaged in prostitution; had sex partners who were infected or at risk for HIV infection because they were bisexual, iv drug abusers, or hemophilic; lived in communities or were born in countries where there is a known or suspected high prevalence of infection in women; or received a blood transfusion before blood was being screened for HIV antibody but after HIV infection occurred (e.g., in the United States from 1978 to 1985). Because a substantial proportion of women may not initially acknowledge high-risk behavior or not have complete knowledge of the infection status of their partners, routine HIV counseling and testing must be considered a standard of care in areas of high prevalence (e.g., 0.5 percent or higher) and not be reserved for those women with self-reported risk histories.[191]

HIV-infected women should be advised to avoid pregnancy in view of the significant probability that they will transmit HIV to their unborn children[132–136] and the possibility that pregnancy may accelerate the progression of their HIV disease.[241,242] To avoid postnatal transmission to a child who may not be infected, breast-feeding is not recommended for HIV-infected women living in countries where alternative and effective infant nutrition is widely available.[243] In developing countries where the risk of infant mortality is significantly higher for bottle-fed than for breast-fed infants, the documented benefits of breast-feeding need to be weighed against the risk of transmission of HIV through breast-feeding.[244,245] In such settings, the WHO recommended in 1987 that breast-feeding should remain the feeding method of choice, even for HIV-infected mothers.[244]

In many developed countries, the effective treatment of iv drug abuse remains an essential adjunct to preventing perinatal transmission of HIV because mothers of most children with perinatally acquired AIDS either abuse iv drugs themselves or are the sex partners of men who do.

Counseling and HIV Antibody Testing

Counseling and HIV antibody testing programs are important to facilitate behavioral changes needed to prevent HIV transmission. The U.S. Public Health Service, in consultation with other public health agencies, has formulated guidelines for counseling and testing for HIV antibody.[240] Specific population groups or settings in which testing is recommended include the following:

- Persons who seek treatment for an STD
- IV-drug abusers
- Persons who consider themselves at risk
- Women of childbearing age with identifiable risks for HIV infection
- Persons planning marriage
- Persons undergoing medical evaluation or treatment for selected clinical conditions that may indicate underlying HIV infection such as generalized lymphadenopathy; unexplained dementia; unexplained fever, diarrhea, weight loss; diseases such as tuberculosis, generalized herpes, and chronic candidiasis
- Persons admitted to hospitals to determine HIV seroprevalence in age groups at highest risk for infection

Persons in correctional systems
Prostitutes
Other health care settings where the prevalence of unsuspected HIV infection is moderate to high.

The U.S. Public Health Service, the Presidential Commission, and the American Medical Association have recommended that partner notification and/or contact tracing of HIV-infected persons should be incorporated in HIV prevention, counseling, and testing programs.[238,240,246] In addition, these guidelines stress the need for ensuring quality performance of laboratory tests for HIV through employment of trained personnel, establishment of quality controls, and participation in performance evaluation systems. Confidentiality and avoidance of discrimination toward persons who test seropositive must be ensured.

Preliminary studies indicate that antibody testing and counseling may have useful public health outcomes in terms of reductions in high-risk behavior in persons tested. However, such testing is often accompanied by adverse psychological consequences such as anxiety and depression.[247–249]

CONCLUSION

HIV infection and AIDS are now major causes of morbidity and mortality in the United States and other areas of the world. Although the basic epidemiology of the disease and its modes of transmission have been established, important questions remain regarding the incidence and prevalence of HIV infection, the efficiency of transmission and the role of cofactors in facilitating transmission of HIV, the natural history of infection in various population groups, and the effectiveness of various prevention strategies. In addition to the clinical and epidemiologic aspects of the epidemic, its economic impact is substantial—in terms of both the cost of providing medical and psychosocial services and losses incurred from disability and premature death. The control and prevention of HIV infection will require a coordinated, sustained, and costly global commitment that will extend into the next century.

REFERENCES

1. *Pneumocystis* pneumonia—Los Angeles. MMWR. 1981;30:250–2.
2. Kaposi's sarcoma and *Pneumocystis* pneumonia among homosexual men—New York City and California. MMWR. 1981;30:305–8.
3. Curran JW. AIDS—two years later (Editorial). N Engl J Med. 1983;309:609–11.
4. Barre-Sinoussi F, Chermann JC, Rey F, et al. Isolation of a T-lymphotropic retrovirus from a patient at risk for acquired immune deficiency syndrome (AIDS). Science. 1983;220:868–71.
5. Gallo RC, Salahuddin SZ, Popovic M, et al. Frequent detection and isolation of cytopathic retroviruses (HTLV-III) from patients with AIDS and at risk for AIDS. Science. 1984;224:500–3.
6. Levy JA, Hoffman AD, Kramer SM, et al. Isolation of lymphocytopathic retroviruses from San Francisco patients with AIDS. Science. 1984;225:840–2.
7. Update on acquire immune deficiency syndrome (AIDS)—United States. MMWR. 1982;31:507–14.
8. Hardy AM, Starcher ET II, Morgan WM, et al. Review of death certificates to assess completeness of AIDS case reporting. Public Health Rep. 1987;102:386–91.
9. Revision of the case definition of acquired immunodeficiency syndrome for national reporting—United States. MMWR. 1985;34:373–5.
10. Revision of the CDC surveillance case definition for acquired immunodeficiency syndrome. MMWR. 1987;36(Suppl 1):1–15.
11. Starcher ET II, Biel JK, Castano RR, et al. The impact of presumptively diagnosed opportunistic infections and cancers on national reporting of AIDS (Abstract) In: Proceedings of the Third International Conference on AIDS, June 1–5, 1987. Washington, DC: The U.S. Department of Health and Human Services and the WHO; 1987:125.
12. Chamberland ME, Allen JR, Monroe JM, et al. Acquired immunodeficiency syndrome in New York City. Evaluation of an active surveillance system. JAMA. 1985;254:383–7.
13. Rauch, KJ, Rutherford GW, Badran C, et al. Surveillance of acquired immunodeficiency syndrome in San Francisco: Evaluation of the completeness of reporting (Abstract). In: Proceedings of the International Conference on AIDS, June 23–25, 1986. Paris: The U.S. Department of Health and Human Services and the WHO; 1986:152.
14. Curran JW, Jaffe HW, Hardy AM, et al. Epidemiology of HIV infection and AIDS in the United States. Science. 1988;239:610–6.
15. Report of the Second Public Health Service AIDS Prevention and Control Meeting. Public Health Rep. 1989;103:10–8.
16. Ward JW, Holmberg SD, Allen JR, et al. Transmission of human immunodeficiency virus (HIV) by blood transfusions screened as negative for HIV antibody. N Engl J Med. 1988;318:473–8.
17. Peterman TA, Jaffe HW, Feorino PM, et al. Transfusion-associated acquired immunodeficiency syndrome in the United States. JAMA 1985;254:2913–17.
18. Peterman TA, Lui K-J, Lawrence DN, et al. Estimating the risks of transfusion-associated acquired immune deficiency syndrome and human immunodeficiency virus infection. Transfusion. 1987;27:371–4.
19. Hardy AM, Allen JR, Morgan WM, et al. The incidence rate of acquired immunodeficiency syndrome in selected populations. JAMA. 1985;253:215–20.
20. The Collaborative Study Group of AIDS in Haitian-Americans. Risk factors for AIDS among Haitians residing in the United States. Evidence of heterosexual transmission. JAMA. 1987;257:635–9.
21. Pape JW, Liautaud B, Thomas F, et al. The acquired immunodeficiency syndrome in Haiti. Ann Intern Med. 1985;103:674–8.
22. Castro KG, Lifson AR, White CR, et al. Investigations of AIDS patients with no previously identified risk factors. JAMA. 1988;259:1338–42.
23. Chamberland ME, Castro KG, Haverkos HW, et al. Acquired immunodeficiency syndrome in the United States: An analysis of cases outside high-incidence groups. Ann Intern Med. 1984;101:617–23.
24. Lekatsas AM, Walker J, O'Donnell R, et al. Identification of risk in persons with AIDS in New York City: When is "no risk" without risk? (Abstract). In: Proceedings of the Internationl Conference on AIDS, June 23–25, 1986. Paris: L'Association pour la Recherche sur les Déficits Immunitaire Viro-Induits (ARDIVI); 1986:151.
25. Potterat JJ, Phillips L, Muth JB. Lying to military physicians about risk factors for HIV infections (Letter). JAMA. 1987;257:1727.
26. Acquired immunodeficiency syndrome (AIDS) among blacks and Hispanics—United States. MMWR. 1986;35:655–8, 663–6.
27. Selik RM, Castro KG, Pappaioanou M. Racial/ethnic differences in the risk of AIDS in the United States. Am J Public Health. 1988;78:1539–45.
28. Guinan ME, Hardy A. Epidemiology of AIDS in women in the United States. 1981 through 1986. JAMA. 1987;257:2039–42.
29. Chamberland ME, Dondero TJ Jr. Heterosexually acquired infection with human immunodeficiency virus (HIV). A view from the III International Conference on AIDS (Editorial). Ann Intern Med. 1987;107:763–6.
30. Jaffe HW, Bregman DJ, Selik RM. Acquired immune deficiency syndrome in the United States: The first 1,000 cases. J Infect Dis. 1983;148:339–45.
31. Agins B, Spicehandler D, Della-Latta P, et al. *M. avium-intracellulare* infection in AIDS (Abstract). In: Proceedings and abstracts of the 24th Interscience Conference on Antimicrobial Agents and Chemotherapy, October 8–10, 1984. Washington, DC: The American Society for Microbiology; 1984:229.
32. Selik RM, Starcher ET, Curran JW. Opportunistic diseases reported in AIDS patients: Frequencies, associations, and trends. AIDS. 1987;1:175–82.
33. Newell GR, Adams SC, Mansell PWA, et al. Toxicity, immunosuppressive effects and carcinogenic potential of volatile nitrites: Possible relationship to Kaposi's sarcoma. Pharmacotherapy. 1984;4:284–91.
34. Goedert JJ, Neuland CY, Wallen WC, et al. Amyl nitrite may alter T lymphocytes in homosexual men. Lancet. 1982;1:412–6.
35. Marmor M, Friedman-Kien AE, Laubenstein L, et al. Risk factors for Kaposi's sarcoma in homosexual men. Lancet. 1982;1:1083–7.
36. Jaffe HW, Choi K, Thomas PA, et al. National case–control study of Kaposi's sarcoma and *Pneumocystis carinii* pneumonia in homosexual men: Part 1, epidemiologic results. Ann Intern Med. 1983;99:145–51.
37. Melbye M, Biggar RJ, Ebbeson P, et al. Seroepidemiology of HTLV-III antibody in Danish homosexual men: Prevalence, transmission, and disease outcome. Br Med J. 1984;289:573–5.
38. Darrow WW, Echenberg DF, Jaffe HW, et al. Risk factors for human immunodeficiency virus (HIV) infections in homosexual men. Am J Public Health. 1987;77:479–83.
39. Moss AR, Osmond D, Bacchetti P, et al. Risk factors for AIDS and HIV seropositivity in homosexual men. Am J Epidemiol. 1987;125:1035–47.
40. Haverkos HW, Pinsky PF, Drotman DP, et al. Disease manifestion among homosexual men with acquired immunodeficiency syndrome: A possible role of nitrites in Kaposi's sarcoma. Sex Transm Dis. 1985;12:203–8.
41. Giraldo G, Beth E, Huang E-S. Kaposi's sarcoma and its relationship to cytomegalovirus (CMV). III. CMV DNA and CMV early antigens in Kaposi's sarcoma. Int J Cancer. 1980;26:23–9.
42. Drew WL, Mintz L, Miner RC, et al. Prevalence of cytomegalovirus infection in homoosexual men. J Infect Dis. 1981;143:188–92.
43. Drew WL, Conant MA, Miner RC, et al. Cytomegalovirus and Kaposi's sarcoma in young homosexual men. Lancet. 1982;2:125–7.
44. Polk BF, Fox R, Brookmeyer R, et al. Predictors of the acquired immunodeficiency syndrome developing in a cohort of seropositive homosexual men. N Engl J Med. 1987;316:61–6.
45. Lifson AR, Darrow WW, O'Malley PM, et al. Decline in Kaposi's sarcoma among homosexual and bisexual men and analysis for cofactors (Abstract). In: Proceedings of the Fourth International Conference on AIDS, Book 1,

June 12–16, 1988. Stockholm: The Swedish Ministry of Health and Social Affairs; 1988:290.
46. Blaser MJ, Cohn DL. Opportunistic infections in patients with AIDS: Clues to the epidemiology of AIDS and the relative virulence of pathogens. Rev Infect Dis. 1986;8:21–30.
47. Glatt AE, Chirgwin K, Landesman SH. Treatment of infections associated with human immunodeficiency virus. N Engl J Med. 1988:318:1439–48.
48. Tuberculosis and acquired immunodeficiency syndrome—Florida. MMWR. 1986;35:587–90.
49. Tuberculosis and AIDS—Connecticut. MMWR. 1987;36:133–5.
50. Tuberculosis and acquired immunodeficiency syndrome—New York City. MMWR. 1987;36:785–90, 795.
51. The Long-Term Survivor Collaborative Study Group, Hardy AM. Characterization of long-term survivors (LTS) of AIDS (Abstract). In: Proceedings and abstracts of the 27th Interscience Conference on Antimicrobial Agents and Chemotherapy, October 4–7, 1987. New York: The American Society for Microbiology; 1987:98.
52. Bacchetti P, Osmond D, Chaisson RE, et al. Survival patterns in San Francisco AIDS patients (Abstract). In: Proceedings and abstracts of the 27th Interscience Conference on Antimicrobial Agents and Chemotherapy, October 4–7, 1987. New York: The American Society for Microbiology; 1987:98.
53. Moss AR, McCallum G, Volberding PA, et al. Mortality associated with mode of presentation in the acquired immune deficiency syndrome. JNCI. 1984;73:1281–4.
54. Marasca G, McEvoy M. Length of survival of patients with acquired immune deficiency syndrome in the United Kingdom. Br Med J. 1986;292:1727–9.
55. Rothenberg R, Woelfel M, Stoneburner R, et al. Survival with the acquired immunodeficiency syndrome. Experience with 5833 cases in New York City. N Engl J Med. 1987;317:1297–302.
56. Vadhan-Raj S, Wong G, Gnecco C, et al. Immunological variables as predictors of prognosis in patients with Kaposi's sarcoma and the acquired immunodeficiency syndrome. Cancer Res. 1986;46:417–25.
57. Changes in premature mortality—United States, 1979–1986. MMWR. 1986;37:47–8.
58. Curran JW, Morgan WM, Hardy AM, et al. The epidemiology of AIDS: Current status and future prospects. Science. 1985;229:1352–7.
59. Kristal AR. The impact of the acquired immunodeficiency syndrome on patterns of premature death in New York City. JAMA. 1986;255:2306–10.
60. Chiasson MA, Fleisher E, Petrus D, et al. Epidemiologic characteristics of women with AIDS in New York City (Abstract). In: Proceedings of the Third International Conference on AIDS, June 1–5, 1987. Washington DC: The U.S. Department of Health and Human Services and the WHO; 1987:174.
61. Unexplained immunodeficiency and opportunistic infections in infants—New York, New Jersey, California. MMWR. 1982:31:665–7.
62. Oleske J, Minnefor A, Cooper R, et al. Immune deficiency syndrome in children. JAMA. 1983;249:2345–9.
63. Rubinstein A, Sicklick M, Gupta A, et al. Acquired immunodeficiency with reversed T4/T8 ratios in infants born to promiscuous and drug-addicted mothers. JAMA. 1983;249:2350–6.
64. Thomas PA, Jaffe HW, Spira TJ, et al. Unexplained immunodeficiency in children. A surveillance report. JAMA. 1984;252:639–44.
65. Lifson AR, Rogers MF, White C, et al. Unrecognized modes of transmission of HIV: Acquired immunodeficiency syndrome in children reported without risk factors. Pediatr Infect Dis. 1987;6:292–3.
66. Friedman BA, Burns TL, Schork MA. A study of national trends in transfusion practice. Ann Arbor: The University of Michigan Medical School and School of Public Health; 1980:1–283.
67. Thomas PA, O'Donnell RE, Lessner L. Survival analysis of children reported with AIDS in New York City, 1982–1986 (Abstract). In: Proceedings of the Third International Conference on AIDS, June 1–5, 1987. Washington, DC: The U.S. Department of Health and Human Services and the WHO; 1987:75.
68. Peterman TA, Curran JW. Sexual transmission of human immunodeficiency virus. JAMA. 1986;256:2222–6.
69. Goedert JJ, Sarngadharan MG, Biggar RJ, et al. Determinants of retrovirus (HTLV-III) antibody and immunodeficiency conditions in homosexual men. Lancet. 1984;2:711–6.
70. Stevens CE, Taylor PE, Zang EA, et al. Human T-cell lymphotropic virus type III infection in a cohort of homosexual men in New York City. JAMA. 1986;255:2167–72.
71. Winkelstein W, Lyman DM, Padian N, et al. Sexual practices and risk of infection by the human immunodeficiiency virus. The San Francisco Men's Health Study. JAMA. 1987;257:321–5.
72. Kingsley LA, Detels R, Kaslow R, et al. Risk factors for seroconversion to human immunodeficiency virus among male homosexuals. Results from the Multicenter AIDS Cohort Study. Lancet 1987;1:345–9.
73. Mayer KH, DeGruttola V. Human immunodeficiency virus and oral intercourse (Letter). Ann Intern Med. 1987;107:428–9.
74. Lyman D, Winkelstein W, Ascher M, et al. Minimal risk of transmission of AIDS-associated retrovirus infection by oral-genital contact (Letter). JAMA. 1986;255:1703.
75. Marmor M, Weiss LR, Lyden M, et al. Possible female-to-female transmission of human immunodeficiency virus (Letter). Ann Intern Med. 1986;105:969.
76. Monzon OT, Capellan JMB. Female-to-female transmission of HIV (Letter). Lancet. 1987;2:40–1.
77. Kreiss JK, Kitchen LW, Prince HE, et al. Antibody to human T-lymphotropic virus type III in wives of hemophiliacs. Evidence for heterosexual transmission. Ann Intern Med. 1985;102:623–6.
78. Redfield RR, Markham PD, Salahuddin SZ, et al. Frequent transmission of HTLV-III among spouses of patients with AIDS-related complex and AIDS. JAMA. 1985;253:1571–3.
79. Allain J-P. Prevalence of HTLV-III/LAV antibodies in patients with hemophilia and in their sexual partners in France (Letter). N Engl J Med. 1986;315:517–8.
80. Jason JM, McDougal JS, Dixon G, et al. HTLV-III/LAV antibody and immune status of household contacts and sexual partners of persons with hemophilia. JAMA. 1986;255:212–5.
81. Fischl MA, Dickinson GM, Scott GB, et al. Evaluation of heterosexual partners, children, and household contacts of adults with AIDS. JAMA. 1987;257:640–4.
82. Padian N, Wiley J, Winkelstein W. Male-to-female transmission of human immunodeficiency virus (HIV): Current results, infectivity rates, and San Francisco population seroprevalence estimates (Abstract). In: Proceedings of the Third International Conference on AIDS, June 1–5, 1987. Washington, DC: The U.S. Department of Health and Human Services and the WHO; 1987:171.
83. Smiley L, White GC II, Macik G, et al. Transmission of human immunodeficiency virus from hemophiliacs to their sexual partners: Role of parenteral exposures (Abstract). In: Proceedings of the Third International Conference on AIDS, June 1–5, 1987. Washington, DC: 1987:23.
84. Peterman TA, Stoneburner RL, Allen JR, et al. Risk of human immunodeficiency virus transmission from heterosexual adults with transfusion-associated infections. JAMA. 1988;259:55–8.
85. Padian NS. Heterosexual transmission of acquired immunodeficiency syndrome: International perspectives and national projections. Rev Infect Dis. 1987;9:947–60.
86. Mann JM, Francis H, Quinn T, et al. Surveillance for AIDS in a central African city. Kinshasa, Zaire. JAMA. 1986;255:3255–9.
87. Quinn TC, Mann JM, Curran JW, et al. AIDS in Africa: An epidemiologic paradigm. Science. 1986;234:955–63.
88. Piot P, Quinn TC, Taelman H, et al. Acquired immunodeficiency syndrome in a heterosexual population in Zaire. Lancet. 1984;2:65–9.
89. Clumeck N, Van de Perre P, Carael M, et al. Heterosexual promiscuity among African patients with AIDS (Letter). N Engl J Med. 1985;313:182.
90. Piot P, Plummer FA, Rey M-A, et al. Retrospective seroepidemiology of AIDS virus infection in Nairobi populations. J Infect Dis. 1987;155:1108–12.
91. Goedert JJ, Eyster ME, Biggar RJ. Heterosexual transmission of human immunodeficiency virus (HIV): Association with severe T4-cell depletion in male hemophiliacs (Abstract). In: Proceedings of the Third International Conference on AIDS, June 1–5, 1987. Washington, DC: The U.S. Department of Health and Human Services and the WHO; 1987:106.
92. Redfield RR, Wright DC, Khan NC, et al. Correlation of HIV isolation rate and stage of infection (Abstract). In: Proceedings of the Third International Conference on AIDS, June 1–5, 1987. Washington, DC: The U.S. Department of Health and Human Services and the WHO; 1987:180.
93. Steigbigel NH, Maude DW, Feiner CJ, et al. Heterosexual transmission of infection and disease by the human immunodeficiency virus (HIV) (Abstract). In: Proceedings of the Third International Conference on AIDS, June 1–5, 1987. Washington, DC: The U.S. Department of Health and Human Services and the WHO; 1987:106.
94. Handsfield HH, Ashley RL, Rompalo AM, et al. Association of anogenital ulcer disease with human immunodeficiency virus infection in homosexual men (Abstract). In: Proceedings of the Third International Conference on AIDS, June 1–5, 1987. Washington, DC: The U.S. Department of Health and Human Services and the WHO; 1987:206.
95. Holmberg SD, Stewart JA, Gerber AR, et al. Prior herpes simplex virus type 2 infection as a risk factor for HIV infection. JAMA. 1988;259:1048–50.
96. Kreiss JK, Koech D, Plummer FA, et al. AIDS virus infection in Nairobi prostitutes. Spread of the epidemic to East Africa. N Engl J Med. 1986;314:414–8.
97. Greenblatt RM, Lukehart SL, Plummer FA, et al. Genital ulceration as a risk factor for human immunodeficiency virus infection in Kenya (Abstract). In: Proceediings of the Third International Conference on AIDS, June 1–5, 1987. Washington, DC: The U.S. Department of Health and Human Services and the WHO; 1987:174.
98. Cameron DW, Plummer FA, Simonsen JN, et al. Female to male heterosexual transmission of HIV infection in Nairobi (Abstract). In: Proceedings of the Third International Conference on AIDS, June 1–5, 1987. Washington, DC: The U.S. Department of Health and Human Services and the WHO; 1987:25.
99. Increases in primary and secondary syphilis—United States. MMWR. 1987:36:393–7.
100. Schoenbaum EE, Selwyn PA, Klein RS, et al. Prevalence of and risk factors associated with HTLV-III/LAV antibodies among intravenous drug abusers in methadone program in New York City (Abstract). In: Proceedings of the International Conference on AIDS, June 23–35, 1986. Paris: L'Association pour la Recherche sur les Déficits Immunitaire Viro-Induits (ARDIVI); 1986:111.
101. Weiss SH, Ginzberg HM, Altman R, et al. Risk factors of HTLV-III/LAV infection and the development of AIDS among drug abusers (DA) (Abstract). In: Proceedings of the International Conference on AIDS, June 23–25, 1986.

Paris: L'Association pour la Recherche sur les Déficits Immunitaire Viro-Induits (ARDIVI); 1986:124.
102. Chaisson RE, Moss AR, Onishi R, et al. Human immunodeficiency virus infection in heterosexual intravenous drug users in San Francisco. Am J Public Health. 1987;77:169–72.
103. Curran JW, Lawrence DN, Jaffe H, et al. Acquired immunodeficiency syndrome (AIDS) associated with transfusions. N Engl J Med. 1984;310:69–75.
104. Evatt BL, Ramsey RB, Lawrence DN, et al. The acquired immunodeficiency syndrome in patients with hemophilia. Ann Intern Med. 1984;100:499–504.
105. Safety of therapeutic immune globulin preparations with respect to transmission of human T-lymphotropic virus type III/lymphadenopathy-associated virus infection. MMWR. 1986;35:231–3.
106. Lack of transmission of human immunodeficiency virus through $Rh_0(D)$ immune globulin (human). MMWR. 1987;36:728–9.
107. Hepatitis B vaccine: Evidence confirming lack of AIDS transmission. MMWR. 1984;33:685–7.
108. Wells MA, Wittek AE, Epstein JS, et al. Inactivation and partition of human T-cell lymphotrophic virus, type III, during ethanol fractionation of plasma. Transfusion. 1986;26:210–3.
109. Ward JW, Deppe DA, Samson S, et al. Risk of human immunodeficiency virus infection from blood donors who later developed the acquired immunodeficiency syndrome. Ann Intern Med. 1987;106:61–2.
110. Feorino PM, Jaffe HW, Palmer E, et al. Transfusion-associated acquired immunodeficiency syndrome. Evidence for persistent infection in blood donors. N Engl J Med. 1985;312:1293–6.
111. Stehr-Green JK, Holman RC, Jason JM, et al. Hemophilia-associated AIDS in the United States, 1981 to September 1987. Am J Public Health. 1988;78:439–42.
112. Survey of non-U.S. hemophilia treatment centers for HIV seroconversions following therapy with heat-treated factor concentrates. MMWR. 1987;36:121–4.
113. L'age-Stehr J, Schwarz A, Offermann G, et al. HTLV-III infection in kidney transplant recipients (Letter). Lancet. 1985;2:1361–2.
114. Human immunodeficiency virus infection transmitted from an organ donor screened for HIV antibody—North Carolina. MMWR. 1987;36:306–8.
115. Stewart GJ, Tyler JPP, Cunningham AL, et al. Transmission of human T-cell lymphotropic virus type III (HTLV-III) by artificial insemination by donor. Lancet. 1985;2:581–5.
116. Testing donors of organs, tissues, and semen for antibody to human T-lymphotropic virus type III/lymphadenopathy-associated virus. MMWR. 1985;34:294.
117. Update: Acquired immunodeficiency syndrome and human immunodeficiency virus infection among health-care workers. MMWR. 1988;37:229–34,239.
118. Marcus R and The CDC Cooperative Needlestick Surveillance Group. Surveillance of health care workers exposed to blood from patients infected with the human immunodeficiency virus. N Engl J Med. 1988;319:118–23.
119. Henderson DK, Saah AJ, Zak BJ, et al. Risk of nosocomial infection with human T-cell lymphotropic virus type III/lymphadenopathy-associated virus in a large cohort of intensively exposed health care workers. Ann Intern Med. 1986;104:644–7.
120. Gerberding JL, Bryant-LeBlanc CE, Nelson K, et al. Risk of transmitting the human immunodeficiency virus, cytomegalovirus, and hepatitis B virus to health care workers exposed to patients with AIDS and AIDS-related conditions. J Infect Dis. 1987;156:1–8.
121. Henderson DK, Fahey BJ, Willy ME. Frequency and intensity of cutaneous exposures to blood and body fluids among health care providers in a referral hospital (Abstract). In: Proceedings of the Fourth International Conference on AIDS, Book 1, June 12–16, 1988. Stockholm: The Swedish Ministry of Health and Social Affairs; 1988:480.
122. 1988 agent summary statement for human immunodeficiency virus and report on laboratory-acquired infection with human immunodeficiency virus. MMWR. 1988;37(Suppl 4):1–22.
123. Recommendations for prevention of HIV transmission in health-care settings. MMWR. 1987:36(Suppl 2):1–18.
124. Update: Universal precautions for prevention of transmission of human immunodeficiency virus, hepatitis B virus, and other bloodborne pathogens in health-care settings. MMWR. 1988;37:377–82, 387–8.
125. Jovaisas E, Koch MA, Shafer A, et al. LAV/HTLV-III in 20-week fetus (Letter). Lancet. 1985;2:1129.
126. Lapointe N, Michaud J, Pekovic D, et al. Transplacental transmission of HTLV-III virus (Letter). N Engl J Med. 1985;312:1325–6.
127. Nzilambi N, Ryder RW, Behets F, et al. Perinatal HIV transmission in two African hospitals (Abstract). In: Proceedings of the Third International Conference on AIDS, June 1–5, 1987. Washington, DC: The U.S. Department of Health and Human Services and the WHO; 1987:158.
128. Thiry L, Sprecher-Goldberger S, Jonckheer T, et al. Isolation of AIDS virus from cell-free breast milk of three healthy virus carriers (Letter). Lancet. 1985;2:891–2.
129. Ziegler JB, Stewart GJ, Penny R, et al. Breast feeding and transmission of HIV from mother to infant (Abstract). In: Proceedings of the Fourth International Conference on AIDS, Book 1, June 12–16, 1988. Stockholm: The Swedish Ministry of Health and Social Affairs; 1988:339.
130. Colebunders R, Kapita B, Nekwei W, et al. Breastfeeding and transmission of HIV (Letter). Lancet. 1988;2:1487.
131. Weinbreck F, Loustaud V, Denis F, et al. Postnatal transmission of HIV infection. Lancet. 1988;1:482.
132. Ryder RW, Rayfield M, Quinn T, et al. Transplacental HIV transmission in African newborns (Abstract). In: Proceedings of the Fourth International Conference on AIDS, Book 1, June 12–16, 1988. Stockholm: The Swedish Ministry of Health and Social Affairs; 1988:345.
133. The European Collaborative Study. Mother-to-child transmission of HIV infection. Lancet. 1988;2:1039–43.
134. Blanche S, Rouzioux C, Tricoire J, et al. Prospective study on newborns of HIV seropositive women (Abstract). In: Proceedings of the Fourth International Conference on AIDS, Book 1, June 12–16, 1988. Stockholm: The Swedish Ministry of Health and Social Affairs; 1988:434.
135. Scott G, Hutto C, Mastrucci T, et al. Probability of perinatal infections in infants of HIV-1 positive mothers (Abstract). In: Proceedings of the Fourth International Conference on AIDS, Book 2, June 12–16, 1988. Stockholm: The Swedish Ministry of Health and Social Affairs; 1988:292.
136. Mendez H, Willoughby A, Hittelman J, et al. Infants of HIV seropositive (SP) women and their seronegative (SN) controls (Abstract). In: Proceedings of the Fourth International Conference on AIDS, Book 2, June 12–16, 1988. Stockholm: The Swedish Ministry of Health and Social Affairs; 1988:295.
137. Mok JQ, Giaquinto C, De Rossi A, et al. Infants born to mothers seropositive for human immunodeficiency virus. Preliminary findings from a multicentre European study. Lancet. 1987;1:1164–8.
138. Friedland GH, Klein RS. Transmission of the human immunodeficiency virus. N Engl J Med. 1987;317:1125–35.
139. Lifson AR. Do alternate modes for transmission of human immunodeficiency virus exist? A review. JAMA. 1988;259:1353–6.
140. Zagury D, Bernard J, Leibowitch J, et al. HTLV-III in cells cultured from semen of two patients with AIDS. Science. 1984;226:449–51.
141. Vogt MW, Witt DJ, Craven DE, et al. Isolation of HTLV-III/LAV from cervical secretions of women at risk for AIDS. Lancet. 1986;1:525–7.
142. Wofsy CB, Cohen JB, Hauer LB, et al. Isolation of AIDS-associated retrovirus from genital secretions of women with antibodies to the virus. Lancet. 1986;1:527–9.
143. Pomerantz RJ, de la Monte SM, Donegan SP, et al. Human immunodeficiency virus (HIV) infection of the uterine cervix. Ann Intern Med. 1988;108:321–7.
144. Groopman JE, Salahuddin SZ, Sarngadharan MG, et al. HTLV-III in saliva of people with AIDS-related complex and healthy homosexual men at risk for AIDS. Science. 1984;226:447–9.
145. Ho DD, Byington RE, Schooley RT, et al. Infrequency of isolation of HTLV-III virus from saliva in AIDS (Letter). N Engl J Med. 1985;313:1606.
146. Levy JA, Kaminsky LS, Morrow WJW, et al. Infection by the retrovirus associated with the acquired immunodeficiency syndrome. Clinical, biological, and molecular features. Ann Intern Med. 1985;103:694–9.
147. Fujikawa LS, Salahuddin SZ, Palestine AG, et al. Isolation of human T-lymphotropic virus type III from the tears of a patient with the acquired immunodeficiency syndrome. Lancet. 1985;2:529–30.
148. Ho DD, Rota TR, Schooley RT, et al. Isolation of HTLV-III from cerebrospinal fluid and neural tissues of patients with neurologic syndromes related to the acquired immunodeficiency syndrome. N Engl J Med. 1985;313:1493–7.
149. Ziza J-M, Brun-Vezinet F, Venet A, et al. Lymphadenopathy-associated virus isolated from bronchoalveolar lavage fluid in AIDS-related complex with lymphoid interstitial pneumonitis (Letter). N Engl J Med. 1985; 313:183.
150. Mundy DC, Schinazi RF, Gerber AR, et al. Human immunodeficiency virus isolated from amniotic fluid (Letter). Lancet. 1987;2:459–60.
151. Fultz PN. Components of saliva inactivate human immunodeficiency virus (Letter). Lancet. 1986;2:1215.
152. Wahn V, Kramer HH, Voit T, et al. Horizontal transmission of HIV infection between two siblings (Letter). Lancet. 1986;2:694.
153. Rogers MF, White CR, Sanders R. Can children transmit HTLV-III/LAV infection? (Abstract). In: Proceedings and abstracts of the 26th Interscience Conference on Antimicrobial Agents and Chemotherapy, September 28–October 1, 1986. New Orleans: The American Society for Microbiology; 1986:284.
154. Tsoukas C, Hadjis T, Theberge L, et al. Risk of transmission fo HTLV-III/LAV from human bites (Abstract). In: Proceedings of the International Conference on AIDS, June 23–25, 1986, Paris: L'Association pour la Recherche sur les Déficits Immunitaire Viro-Induits (ARDIVI); 1986:125.
155. Klein RS, Phelan JA, Freeman K, et al. Low occupational risk of human immunodeficiency virus infection among dental professionals. N Engl J Med. 1988;318:86–90.
156. Flynn NM, Pollet SM, Van Horne JR, et al. Absence of HIV antibody among dental professionals exposed to infected patients. West J Med. 1987;146:439–42.
157. Gerberding JL, Nelson K, Greenspan D, et al. Risk to dental professionals (DP) from occupational exposure to human immunodeficiency virus (HIV): Followup (Abstract). In: Proceedings and abstracts of the 27th Interscience Conference on Antimicrobial Agents and Chemotherapy, October 4–7, 1987. New York: The American Society for Microbiology; 1987:219.
158. Berthier A, Chamaret S, Fauchet R, et al. Transmissibility of human immunodeficiency virus in haemophilic and non-haemophilic children living in a private school in France. Lancet. 1986;2:598–601.
159. Mann JM, Quinn TC, Francis H, et al. Prevalence of HTLV-III/LAV in household contacts of patients with confirmed AIDS and controls in Kinshasa, Zaire. JAMA. 1986;256:721–4.
160. Friedland GH, Kahl P, Feiner C, et al. The effect of AIDS diagnosis upon

close personal interaction among family members of AIDS patients (Abstract). In: Proceedings of the Third International Conference on AIDS, June 1–5, 1987. Washington, DC: The U.S. Department of Health and Human Services and the WHO; 1987;196.
161. Srinivasan A, York D, Bohan C. Lack of HIV replication in arthropod cells (Letter). Lancet. 1987;1:1094–5.
162. Miike L. Do insects transmit AIDS? Washington, DC: Health Program, Office of Technology Assessment, U.S. Congress; 1987:1–43.
163. Castro KG, Lieb S, Jaffe HW, et al. Transmission of HIV in Belle Glade, Florida: Lessons for other communities in the United States. Science. 1988;239:193–7.
164. Pape JW, Stanback ME, Pamphile M, et al. Pattern of HIV infection in Haiti: 1977–1986 (Abstract). In: Proceedings of the Third International Conference on AIDS, June 1–5, 1987. Washington, DC: The U.S. Department of Health and Human Services and the WHO; 1987:6.
165. Greenberg AE, Nguyen-Dinh P, Mann JM, et al. The association between malaria, blood transfusions, and HIV seropositivity in a pediatric population in Kinshasa, Zaire. JAMA. 1988;259:545–9.
165a. Stoneburner RL, Des Jarlais DC, Benezra D, et al. A larger spectrum of severe HIV-I related disease in intravenous drug users in New York City. Science. 1988;242:916–9.
166. Haverkos HW, Gotlieb MS, Killen JY, et al. Classification of HTLV-III/LAV-related diseases (Letter). J Infect Dis. 1985;152:1095.
167. Redfield RR, Wright DC, Tramont EA. The Walter Reed staging classification for HTLV-III/LAV infection. N Engl J Med. 1986;314:131–2.
168. Classification system for human T-lymphotropic virus type III/lymphadenopathy-associated virus infections. MMWR. 1986;35:334–9.
169. Classification system for human immunodeficiency virus (HIV) infection in children under 13 years of age. MMWR. 1987;36:225–36.
170. Solomon SL, Curran JW. Public health applications of a classification system for human immunodeficiency virus infection (Editorial). Ann Intern Med. 1987;106:319–21.
171. Ho DD, Sarngadharan MG, Resnick L, et al. Primary human T-lymphotropic virus type III infection. Ann Intern Med. 1985;103:880–3.
172. Cooper DA, Gold J, Maclean P, et al. Acute AIDS retrovirus infection. Definition of a clinical illness associated with seroconversion. Lancet. 1985;1:537–40.
172a. Tindall B, Barker S, Donovan B, et al. Characterization of the acute clinical illness associated with human immunodeficiency virus infection. Arch Intern Med. 1988;148:945–9.
173. Pedersen C, Gerstoft J, Lindhardt BO, et al. *Candida* esophagitis associated with acute human immunodeficiency virus infection (Letter). J Infect Dis. 1987;156:529–30.
174. Ward JW, Deppe D, Perkins H, et al. Risk of disease in recipients of blood from donors later found infected with human immunodeficiency virus (HIV) (Abstract). In: Proceedings of the Third International Conference on AIDS, June 1–5, 1987. Washington, DC: The U.S. Department of Health and Human Services and the WHO; 1987:2.
175. Allain J-P, Laurian Y, Paul DA, et al. Serological markers in early stages of human immunodeficiency virus infection in haemophiliacs. Lancet. 1986;2:1233–6.
176. Gaines H, von Sydow M, Sonnerborg A, et al. Antibody response in primary human immunodeficiency virus infection. Lancet. 1987;1:1249–53.
176a. Simmonds P, Lainson FAL, Cuthbert R, et al. HIV antigen and antibody detection: Variable responses to infection in the Edinburgh haemophiliac cohort. Br Med J. 1988;296:593–8.
176b. Ward JW, Schable C, Dickinson GM, et al. Acute human immunodeficiency virus (HIV) infection: Antigen detection and seroconversion in immunosuppressed patients. Transplantation. In press.
177. Jaffe HW, Feorino PM, Darrow WW, et al. Persistent infection with human T-lymphotropic virus type III/lymphadenopathy-associated virus in apparently healthy homosexual men. Ann Intern Med. 1985;102:627–8.
178. Farzadegan H, Polis MA, Wolinsky SM, et al. Loss of human immunodeficiency virus type 1 (HIV-1) antibodies with evidence of viral infection in asymptomatic homosexual men. A report from the Multicenter AIDS Cohort Study. Ann Intern Med. 1988;108:785–90.
179. Hessol NA, Rutherford GW, Lifson AR, et al. The natural history of HIV infection in a cohort of homosexual and bisexual men: A decade of follow-up (Abstract). In: Proceedings of the Fourth International Conference on AIDS, Book 1, June 12–16, 1988. Stockholm: The Swedish Ministry of Health and Social Affairs; 1988:283.
180. Lifson AR, Rutherford GW, Jaffe HW. The natural history of human immunodeficiency virus infection. J Infect Dis. 1988;158:1360–7.
181. Eyster ME, Goedert JJ. Predictive value of T4 cell count and HIV antigen in antibody positive hemophiliacs (Abstract). In: Proceedings of the Fourth International Conference on AIDS, Book 2, June 12–16, 1988. Stockholm: The Swedish Ministry of Health and Social Affairs; 1988:365.
181a. Jason J, Lui K-J, Ragni MV, et al. Risk of developing AIDS in HIV-infected cohorts of hemophilic and homosexual men. JAMA. In press.
182. Ward J, Perkins H, Pepkowitz S, et al. Dose response or strain variation may influence disease progression in HIV-infected blood recipients (Abstract). In: Proceedings of the Fourth International Conference on AIDS, Book 2, June 12–16, 1988. Stockholm: The Swedish Ministry of Health and Social Affairs; 1988:352.
183. Medley GF, Anderson RM, Cox DR, et al. Incubation period of AIDS in patients infected via blood transfusion. Nature. 1987;328:719–21.
183a. Lui K-J, Darrow WW, Rutherford GW III. A model-based estimate of the mean incubation period for AIDS in homosexual men. Science. 1988; 240:1333–5.
184. Lui K-J, Peterman TA, Lawrence DN, et al. A model-based approach to characterize the incubation period of paediatric transfusion-associated acquired immunodeficiency syndrome. Stat Med. 1988;7:395–401.
185. Human immunodeficiency virus infection in the United States: A review of current knowledge. MMWR. 1987;36(Suppl 6):1–48.
185a. Trends in human immunodeficiency virus infection among civilian applicants for military service—United States, October 1985–March 1988. MMWR. 1988;37:677–9.
186. Darrow WW, Cohen JB, French J, et al. Multicenter study of HIV antibody in U.S. prostitutes (Abstract). In: Proceedings of the Third International Conference on AIDS, June 1–5, 1987. Washington, DC: The U.S. Department of Health and Human Services and the WHO; 1987:105.
187. Fischl MA, Dickinson GM, Flanagan S, et al. Human immunodeficiency virus (HIV) among female prostitutes in south Florida (Abstract). In: Proceedings of the Third International Conference on AIDS, June 1–5, 1987. Washington, DC: The U.S. Department of Health and Human Services and the WHO; 1987:105.
188. Quinn TC, Glasser D, Cannon RO, et al. Human immunodeficiency virus infection among patients attending clinics for sexually transmitted diseases. N Engl J Med. 1988;318:197–203.
189. Stoneburner RL, Chiasson MA, Lifson AR, et al. HIV-1 infection in persons attending a sexually transmitted disease clinic in New York City (Abstract). In: Proceedings of the Fourth International Conference on AIDS, Book 1, June 12–16, 1988. Stockholm: The Swedish Ministry of Health and Social Affairs; 1988:377.
190. Judson FN, Douglas J, Cohn D. HIV seroprevalence in heterosexual men and women, Denver Metro STD Clinic, 1985–1987 (Abstract). In: Proceedings of the Fourth International Conference on AIDS, Book 1, June 12–16, 1988. Stockholm: The Swedish Ministry of Health and Social Affairs; 1988:263.
191. Landesman S, Minkoff H, Holman S, et al. Serosurvey of human immunodeficiency virus infection in parturients. Implications for human immunodeficiency virus testing programs of pregnant women. JAMA. 1987;258:2701–3.
192. Dondero TJ Jr, Pappaioanou M, Curran JW. Monitoring the levels and trends of HIV infection: The Public Health Service's HIV surveillance program. Public Health Rep. 1988;103:213–20.
193. Hoff R, Berardi VP, Weiblen BJ, et al. Seroprevalence of human immunodeficiency virus among childbearing women. Estimation by testing samples of blood from newborns. N Engl J Med. 1988;318:525–30.
194. Quarterly report to the Domestic Policy Council on the prevalence and rate of spread of HIV and AIDS in the United States. MMWR. 1988;37:223–6.
195. Update: Acquired immunodeficiency syndrome—Europe. MMWR. 1984;33:607–9.
196. Clumeck N, Sonnet, J, Taelman H, et al. Acquired immunodeficiency syndrome in African patients. N Engl J Med 1984;310:492–7.
197. Van de Perre P, Rouvroy D, Lepage P, et al. Acquired immunodeficiency syndrome in Rwanda. Lancet. 1984;2:62–5.
198. Nahmias AJ, Weiss J, Yao X, et al. Evidence for human infection with an HTLV III/LAV-like virus in central Africa, 1959 (Letter). Lancet. 1986;1:1279–80.
199. Epstein JS, Moffitt AL, Mayner RE, et al. Antibodies reactive with HTLV-III found in freezer-banked sera from children in West Africa (Abstract). In Proceedings and abstracts of the 25th Interscience Conference on Antimicrobial Agents and Chemotherapy, September 29–October 1, 1985. Minneapolis: The American Society for Microbiology; 1985:130.
200. Huminer D, Rosenfeld JB, Pitlik SD. AIDS in the pre-AIDS era. Rev Infect Dis. 1987;9:1102–8.
201. Bayley AC. Aggressive Kaposi's sarcoma in Zambia, 1983. Lancet. 1984;1:1318–20.
202. Serwadda D, Mugerwa RD, Sewankambo NK, et al. Slim disease: A new disease in Uganda and its association with HTLV-III infection. Lancet. 1985;2:849–52.
203. World Health Organization. Acquired immunodeficiency syndrome (AIDS)—data as at 31 May 1988. Weekly Epidemiol Rec. 1988;63:173–4.
204. Piot P, Plummer FA, Mhalu FS, et al. AIDS: An international perspective. Science. 1988;239:573–9.
205. Holmberg SD, Curran JW. The epidemiology of HIV infection in industrialized nations. In: Holmes KK, Mardh P-A, Sparling PF, et al., eds. Sexually Transmitted Diseases. 2nd ed. New York: McGraw-Hill; In press.
206. Mann JM, Francis H, Davachi F, et al. Risk factors for human immunodeficiency virus seropositivity among children 1–24 months old in Kinshasa, Zaire. Lancet. 1986;2:654–7.
207. Francis H, Lubaki N, Duma MP, et al. Immunologic profiles of mothers in perinatal transmission of HIV infection (Abstract). In: Proceedings of the Third International Conference on AIDS, June 1–5, 1987. Washington, DC: The U.S. Department of Health and Human Services and the WHO; 1987:214.
208. Braddick M, Kreiss J, Embree J, et al. Vertical transmission of HIV in Nairobi (Abstract). In Proceedings of the Fourth International Conference on AIDS, Book 1, June 12–16, 1988. Stockholm: The Swedish Ministry of Health and Social Affairs; 1988:346.
209. N'Galy B, Ryder R, Bila K, et al. Human immunodeficiency virus infection among employees in an African hospital. N Engl J Med. 1988;319: 1123–7.

210. Hrdy DB. Cultural practices contributing to the transmission of human immunodeficiency virus in Africa. Rev Infect Dis. 1987;9:1109–19.
211. Guyader M, Emerman M, Sonigo P, et al. Genome organization and transactivation of the human immunodeficiency virus type 2. Nature. 1987;326:662–9.
212. Denis F, Leonard G, Mounier M, et al. Efficacy of five enzyme immunoassays for antibody to HIV in detecting to HTLV-IV (Letter). Lancet. 1987;1:324–5.
213. AIDS due to HIV-2 infection—New Jersey. MMWR. 1988;37:33–5.
214. Foucault C, Lopez O, Jourdan G, et al. Double HIV-1 and HIV-2 seropositivity among blood donors (Letter). Lancet. 1987;2:165–6.
215. Brun-Vezinet F, Rey MA, Katlama C, et al. Lymphadenopathy-associated virus type 2 in AIDS and AIDS-related complex. Clinical and virological features in four patients. Lancet. 1987;1:128–32.
216. Clavel F, Mansinho K, Chamaret S, et al. Human immunodeficiency virus type 2 infection associated with AIDS in West Africa. N Engl J Med. 1987;316:1180–5.
217. Horsburgh CR Jr, Holmberg SD. The global distribution of human immunodeficiency virus type 2 (HIV-2) infection. Transfusion. 1988;28:192–5.
218. Francis DP, Chin J. The prevention of acquired immunodeficiency syndrome in the United States. An objective strategy for medicine, public health, business, and the community. JAMA. 1987;257:1357–66.
219. Allen JR, Curran JW. Prevention of AIDS and HIV infection: Needs and priorities for epidemiologic research. Am J Public Health. 1988;78:381–6.
220. Additional recommendations to reduce sexual and drug abuse-related transmission of human T-lymphotropic virus type III/lymphadenopathy-associated virus. MMWR. 1986;35:152–5.
221. Condoms for prevention of sexually transmitted diseases. MMWR. 1988;37:133–7.
222. Mann J, Quinn TC, Piot P, et al. Condom use and HIV infection among prostitutes in Zaire (Letter). N Engl J Med. 1987;316:345.
223. Self-reported changes in sexual behaviors among homosexual and bisexual men from the San Francisco City Clinic Cohort. MMWR. 1987;36:187–9.
224. Martin JL. The impact of AIDS on gay male sexual behavior patterns in New York City. Am J Public Health. 1987;77:578–81.
225. Declining rates of rectal and pharyngeal gonorrhea among males—New York City. MMWR. 1984;33:295–7.
226. Winkelstein W Jr, Samuel M, Padian NS, et al. The San Francisco Men's Health Study: III. Reduction in human immunodeficiency virus transmission among homosexual/bisexual men, 1982–86. Am J Public Health. 1987; 77:685–9.
226a. Winkelstein W Jr, Wiley JA, Padian NS, et al. The San Francisco Men's Health Study: Continued decline in HIV seroconversion rates among homosexual/bisexual men. Am J Public Health. 1988;78:1472–4.
227. Positive HTLV-III/LAV antibody results from sexually active female members of social/sexual clubs—Minnesota. MMWR. 1986;35;697–9.
228. HIV infection and pregnancies in sexual partners of HIV-seropositive hemophilic men—United States. MMWR. 1987;36:593–5.
229. Prevention of acquired immune deficiency syndrome (AIDS): Report of inter-agency recommendations. MMWR. 1983;32:101–3.
230. Provisional Public Health Service inter-agency recommendations for screening donated blood and plasma for antibody to the virus causing acquired immunodeficiency syndrome. MMWR. 1985;34:1–5.
231. Update: Revised Public Health Service definition of persons who should refrain from donating blood and plasma—United States. MMWR. 1985;34:547–8.
232. Ward JW, Grindon AJ, Feorino PM, et al. Laboratory and epidemiologic evaluation of an enzyme immunoassay for antibodies to HTLV-III. JAMA. 1986;256:357–61.
233. Zuck TF. Greetings—a final look back with comments about a policy of a zero-risk blood supply (Editorial). Transfusion. 1987;27:447–8.
234. Grindon A. Efficacy of voluntary self-deferral of donors at high risk of AIDS (Abstract). Transfusion. 1984;24:434.
235. Rabkin CS, Van Devanter N, Ewing WE, et al. Risk factors for antibody to HIV in New York blood donors: Validation of AIDS risk classification and of confidential donor self-exclusion at the time of donation (Abstract). In: Proceedings of the Third International Conference on AIDS, June 1–5, 1987. Washington, DC: The U.S. Department of Health and Human Services and the WHO; 1987:103.
236. Ward JW, Kleinman JH, Douglas DK, et al. Epidemiologic characteristics of blood donors with antibody to human immunodeficiency virus. Transfusion. 1988;28:298–301.
237. Des Jarlais DC, Friedman SR. Editorial review. HIV infection among intravenous drug users: Epidemiology and risk reduction. AIDS. 1987;1:67–76.
238. Report of the Presidential Commission on the Human Immunodeficiency Virus Epidemic. Submitted to the President of the United States, June 24, 1988. Washington, DC: U.S. Government Printing Office; 1988:1–201.
239. Des Jarlais DC, Friedman SR, Hopkins W. Risk reduction for the acquired immunodeficiency syndrome among intravenous drug users. Ann Intern Med. 1985;103:755–9.
240. Public Health Service guidelines for counseling and antibody testing to prevent HIV infection and AIDS. MMWR. 1987;36:509–15.
241. Scott GB, Fischl MA, Klimas N, et al. Mothers of infants with the acquired immunodeficiency syndrome. Evidence for both symptomatic and asymptomatic carriers. JAMA. 1985;253:363–6.
242. Minkoff HL. Care of pregnant women infected with human immunodeficiency virus. JAMA. 1987;258:2714–7.
243. Recommendations for assisting in the prevention of perinatal transmission of human T-lymphotropic virus type III/lymphadenopathy-associated virus and acquired immunodeficiency syndrome. MMWR. 1985;34:721–6,731–2.
244. World Health Organization. Breast-feeding/breast milk and human immunodeficiency virus (HIV). Weekly Epidemiol Rec. 1987;62:245–6.
245. Oxtoby MJ. Breast milk and human immunodeficiency virus: placing the issues in broader perspective. Pediatr Infect Dis J. 1988;7:825–35.
246. Abraham L. AIDS contact tracing, prison testing stir debate. American Medical News 1988 July 8/15:4.
247. Coates TJ, Morin SF, McKusick L. Behavioral consequences of AIDS antibody testing among gay men (Letter). JAMA. 1987;258:1889.
248. McCusker J, Stoddard AM, Mayer KH, et al. Effects of HIV antibody test knowledge on subsequent sexual behaviors in a cohort of homosexually active men. Am J Public Health. 1988;78:462–7.
249. Casadonte PP, Des Jarlais D, Smith T, et al. Psychological and behavioral impact of learning HTLV-III/LAV antibody test results (Abstract). In: Proceedings of the International Conference on AIDS, June 23–25, 1986. Paris: L'Association pour la Recherche sur les Déficits Immunitaire Viro-Induits (ARDIVI); 1986:163.

107. IMMUNOLOGY OF AIDS AND HIV INFECTION

MARGARET A. HAMBURG
SCOTT KOENIG
ANTHONY S. FAUCI

A remarkable recent development in the field of infectious diseases has been the relatively sudden appearance and rapid spread of the acquired immune deficiency syndrome (AIDS). Infection with the human immunodeficiency virus (HIV), the etiologic agent of AIDS, results in a wide range of immunologic abnormalities involving a variety of immunopathogenic mechanisms. While patients with AIDS may share certain laboratory and clinical features in common with other disorders caused by defects in the immune system—particularly those with primary immunodeficiencies such as the severe combined immunodeficiencies (SCID)—the pathophysiology and spectrum of clinical manifestations associated with HIV infection and AIDS is quite unique.[1–6]

HIV infection can occur through sexual contact, infected blood, or blood products, and from mother to infant. The clinical syndrome of AIDS follows infection with HIV after a variable, often prolonged, period of time. Although multiple components of the immune system are at least indirectly affected in individuals with HIV infection, it is the impairment of T-cell mediated responses that appears to produce the most significant clinical consequences. Because the T4 cell is pivotally involved in virtually all immune responses, a major host defense defect results from T4 cell depletion and renders the body highly susceptible to "opportunistic" infections and unusual neoplasms.[1–9] Moreover, the pathogens for these opportunistic infections may alter immune function independent of HIV.[10] The long and variable latent period from initial infection to symptomatic disease is a demonstration of the fact that despite rapid cytopathicity of HIV for T lymphocytes in vitro,[11,12] the virus can persist in cells in a state of low-level or latent infection for prolonged periods in vivo. In addition, it has been demonstrated that cells of the monocyte/macrophage lineage, including bone marrow precursor cells, can be infected without cyytopathic effects and may serve as a reservoir for HIV in the body.[13] HIV also has a tropism for the brain leading to neuropsychiatric abnormalities. While components of the host immune system respond to infection with HIV, these responses appear to be minimally protective against HIV infection or disease progression.

This chapter will examine these characteristics of HIV infection and the range of mechanisms—many of which remain to be fully elucidated—whereby HIV relentlessly compromises and ultimately destroys the immune system and produces central nervous system disease.

THE ETIOLOGIC AGENT

In order to understand the pathogenic mechanisms and immune response to HIV infection, it is important to examine the infectious agent (see also Chapter 147). HIV is an RNA retrovirus belonging to the lentivirus family.[14–16] Two major forms of HIV have been described in humans, HIV-1[17–20] and HIV-2.[21–25] HIV-1 is the more common form and has been studied fairly extensively. Most current knowledge regarding immunologic changes associated with AIDS has derived from studies of individuals infected with HIV-1, which is widely disseminated throughout the world. HIV-2 shares serologic reactivity and polynucleotide sequence homology with simian immunodeficiency virus (SIV),[22,26] which produces disease in a limited number of simian species.

The HIV Genome

As visualized by electron microscopy, the mature virion has a dense cylindrical core that encases two molecules of the viral RNA (see also Chapter 147). A spherical lipid envelope, acquired as the virion buds from the surface of an infected cell, surrounds the central core. The HIV proviral genome measures approximately 10 kilobases in length.[27] It consists of three structural genes, *gag, pol*, and *env*, located between shorter segments called long terminal repeat (LTR) sequences. The *gag* gene codes for components of the viral core, *pol* codes for the viral enzymes involved in replication (reverse transcriptase, a protease, and integrase), and *env* codes for the internal and external envelope proteins. Adjacent to or within the LTR segments are the genes coding for the regulatory proteins required for HIV replication. Other genes identified in the HIV-1 genome include *tat* (transactivator), *rev* (regulator of expression of virion proteins), *vif* (virion infectivity factor), *nef* (negative factor), *vpr* (viral protein R), and *vpu* (viral protein U).[28] The expression of these genes has significant impact on the immunopathogenic mechanisms of the virus.

IMMUNOPATHOGENIC MECHANISMS OF HIV INFECTION

It has been clearly established that infection with HIV results in selective defects in immune function. The most prominent feature of the immunopathogenesis of HIV infection–AIDS is depletion of the T4 (helper–inducer) subset of T lymphocytes. Multiple other arms of the immune system are at least indirectly affected, and a wide spectrum of immunologic abnormalities has been observed to accompany HIV infection.

HIV and CD4 as Receptor

From an immunopathogenic perspective, a critical structural feature of HIV appears to be the outer envelope. It has been well documented that the glycoprotein portion, gp120, interacts avidly and specifically with the CD4 molecule, which is expressed predominantly on the T4 cells and acts as a high-affinity receptor for HIV.[12,29,30] In fact, the gp120 portion of HIV has the capability of specifically binding to the CD4 molecule with an affinity that is greater than that for the CD4 molecule's natural ligand, the class II major histocompatibility complex (MHC) molecule.[12,29,30] In vitro studies have demonstrated that monoclonal antibodies to the CD4 molecule could prevent infection.[12,29] Furthermore, certain epitopes of the CD4 molecule appear more essential to viral binding.[31] In one study, various antibodies to CD4 manifested differential capacities for blocking infection.[31] In a more recent report, synthetic CD4 peptide fragments were used as competitive blockers and demonstrated markedly different abilities to inhibit HIV infection and cytopathicity.[32]

A number of other experiments have also shown convincingly that the initial step in HIV infection is the binding of the virus to a cellular receptor such as the CD4 molecule. One such demonstration comes from studies in which cells from the human HELA line were transfected with the cloned CD4 gene, resulting in the expression of the CD4 protein and consequent susceptibility to infection by HIV.[33] By contrast, murine cells made to express the human CD4 molecule could not be infected with HIV. Nonetheless, those cells could support HIV replication following transfection with the HIV genome, suggesting that other mechanisms may facilitate HIV entry. Some researchers have proposed that the HLA-DR molecule may provide another receptor mechanism for HIV entry into cells. In this regard, it has been shown that HLA-DR expression decreases transiently after viral exposure. This occurs in association with a more persistent decline in CD4 expression from those same cells.[34] Further study is currently being directed at the characterization of the role of HLA-DR in the infective process.

Since the binding of the virus to a cellular receptor is a crucial step in HIV infection, virtually any cell expressing the CD4 surface molecule may be a target for infection. In addition to the T4 cell, which represents a major target cell for HIV infection, cells of the monocyte–macrophage lineage and others are capable of binding and becoming infected with HIV.[35–40] After binding to the CD4 molecule, the virus is internalized, uncoated, and, through the action of viral reverse transcriptase, the virion RNA is transcribed into DNA. This can then exist either in an unintegrated form or as a provirus integrated into the cellular DNA. Following integration of provirus, the infection may enter a latent phase within the host cell until cellular activation occurs. Once the infected cell is activated, the proviral DNA transcribes viral genomic RNA and messenger RNA. Subsequent protein synthesis, processing, and viral assembly leads ultimately to the budding of the mature virion from the surface of the cell[41] (Fig. 1).

T-Cell Abnormalities

One of the earliest laboratory abnormalities recognized in AIDS patients was a striking depletion of T4 lymphocytes, characterized not only by an overall reduction in lymphocyte numbers, but also a marked alteration in the ratio of T4 to T8 cells in the circulating T-lymphocyte pool.[1] This depression of the T4/T8 ratio and depletion of the T4 population correlates to some degree with severity of disease, particularly at the extremes of the spectrum. HIV-infected but asymptomatic individuals tend to have higher T4 counts than patients with frank disease.[42] Although not absolute, low T4 cell counts (less than 200/mm^3) in HIV-seropositive individuals often portends imminent development of full-blown AIDS with an opportunistic infection.[43–45] However, there is marked variation in the rate of depletion of T4 cells among HIV-infected individuals. Following an initial drop in number, many individuals maintain relatively normal or slightly lower than normal levels of T4 cells for prolonged periods of time, often followed by a precipitous decline. The rapid fall in T4 cells may coincide with notable increases in circulating p24 antigen (Lane HC, unpublished data.) Other patients may experience a continual, progressive decline in CD4+ cells, with a rapid and unfavorable clinical course.[46,47] A recent study indicates that virulence of HIV may increase in the later stages of disease progression.[48]

Alterations in the numbers of CD8+, or suppressor T cells,

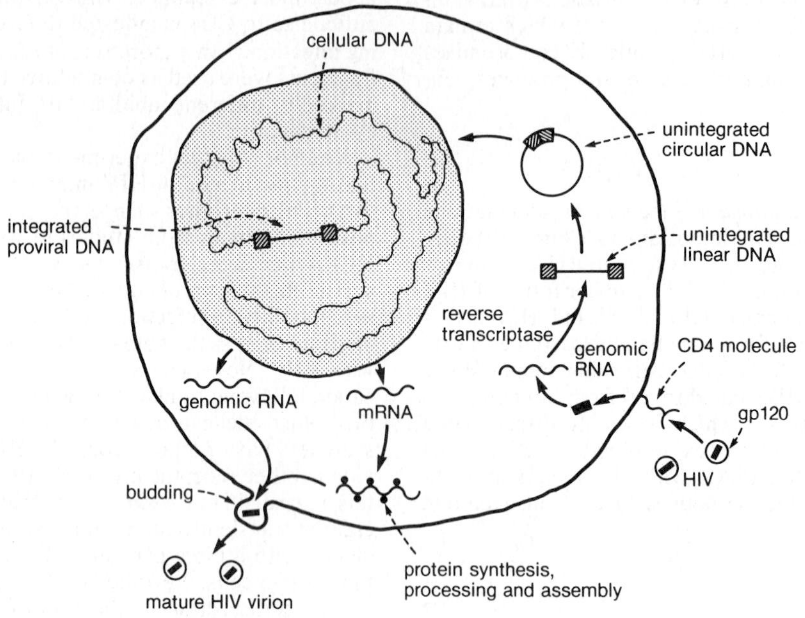

FIG. 1. Schematic diagram of the life cycle of HIV. (From Fauci,[41] with permission.)

have also been noted with HIV infection. Early in the course of HIV infection, many healthy HIV-seropositive individuals, as well as those with lymphadenopathy syndromes, were found to have measurable increases in CD8+ cells. Expansion of the CD8+ cell population may reflect the instigation of cytotoxic responses against HIV or other pathogens. An alternative explanation is that CD8+ suppressor cells may be stimulated to down-modulate other immune responses, such as the polyclonal activation of B cells found in seropositive patients. Interestingly, it has been observed that HIV can be more easily isolated from peripheral blood cultures of seropositive individuals if the CD8+ cells were removed; addition of the CD8+ cells back into the culture suppressed HIV propagation.[49] Although conclusive evidence is lacking, it would seem likely that the CD8+ population may act, at least in part, to suppress HIV replication in vivo, even in symptomatic patients.

Later in the course of disease, AIDS patients with opportunistic infection are often depleted of virtually all lymphoid cells, including the CD8+ population.[42] The mechanism for this depletion remains to be clarified.

Cytopathic Mechanisms of T4 Cell Depletion. The mechanisms by which HIV actually destroys the cells it infects remain unknown. Compared with most other retroviruses, an unusual feature of HIV infection is the accumulation of large amounts of unintegrated viral DNA in the infected cells.[50] When such a phenomenon does occur in other retroviral systems, it is generally associated with a significant cytopathic effect.[50] Such a process has been proposed to be responsible for the cytopathic effects of HIV, although no experimental evidence has yet to directly implicate the finding of unintegrated viral DNA in HIV cytotoxicity.

Another proposed mechanism for the cytopathic effect of HIV on CD4+ cells is the production and budding off from the cell surface of large amounts of virus with a resulting massive increase in cell membrane permeability and eventual cell lysis.[50a] Others have suggested that the cytopathic effects of HIV are a function of the density of the CD4 molecule on the surface of cells. This was proposed in conjunction with the observation that the cell lines with the highest CD4 density appeared to be the most susceptible to cell death. It was speculated that complexing of CD4 with the envelope protein of HIV in the cytoplasm might be cytopathic for cells.[51,52] Such a hypothesis, however, is not supported by recent evidence that there are marked cytopathic effects of HIV even in cell lines that express only modest amounts of CD4 on their surface membrane (Rabson AB, unpublished data). A potentially important mode of T-cell destruction studied in vitro involves syncytia formation. Following HIV infection of CD4+ cells and integration of the viral genome, the HIV envelope glycoprotein is expressed on the surface of the cell. Uninfected T4 cells, with CD4 molecules on their surface that can serve as potential receptors for the virus or for envelope proteins, may bind to those infected cells and lead to the formation of multinucleated giant cells (syncytia)[53–56] (Fig. 2). Multinucleated giant cells have been observed in lymph nodes[57] and brain specimens[58] from HIV-infected patients, but it is uncertain whether they form as result of cell fusion. While syncytia formation has been proposed as a mechanism of HIV cytopathicity in vivo, there is considerable debate as to whether or not it plays a major role.

In addition to the possible direct cytopathic effects of HIV discussed above, other indirect mechanisms almost certainly contribute to the depletion of T4 lymphocytes in vivo. Immune-mediated responses may play an important role.[59,60] For example, HIV-infected cells expressing viral antigens on their surface may be eliminated by HLA-restricted and -unrestricted cytotoxic cells as part of routine immune surveillance. Arguing somewhat against this explanation, the use of fluoresceinated antibodies against viral encoded proteins and in situ hybridization techniques to detect cells expressing viral proteins or mRNA has demonstrated that only an extremely small percentage (perhaps 1 in 100,000) of T4 cells in the peripheral blood of HIV-infected individuals expresses viral proteins at any given time.[61] Given the normal turnover of T lymphocytes in the body, it would seem possible for the T-cell pool to compensate for such a seemingly low rate of destruction.[41] However, impaired maturation of stem cells coupled with progressive depletion may make this proposal feasible (see below). Also, if a large proportion of cells is latently infected, significant cell losses could occur due to viral persistence, reactivation of latent virus, and progressive dissemination to uninfected cells over time. The development of the polymerase chain reaction

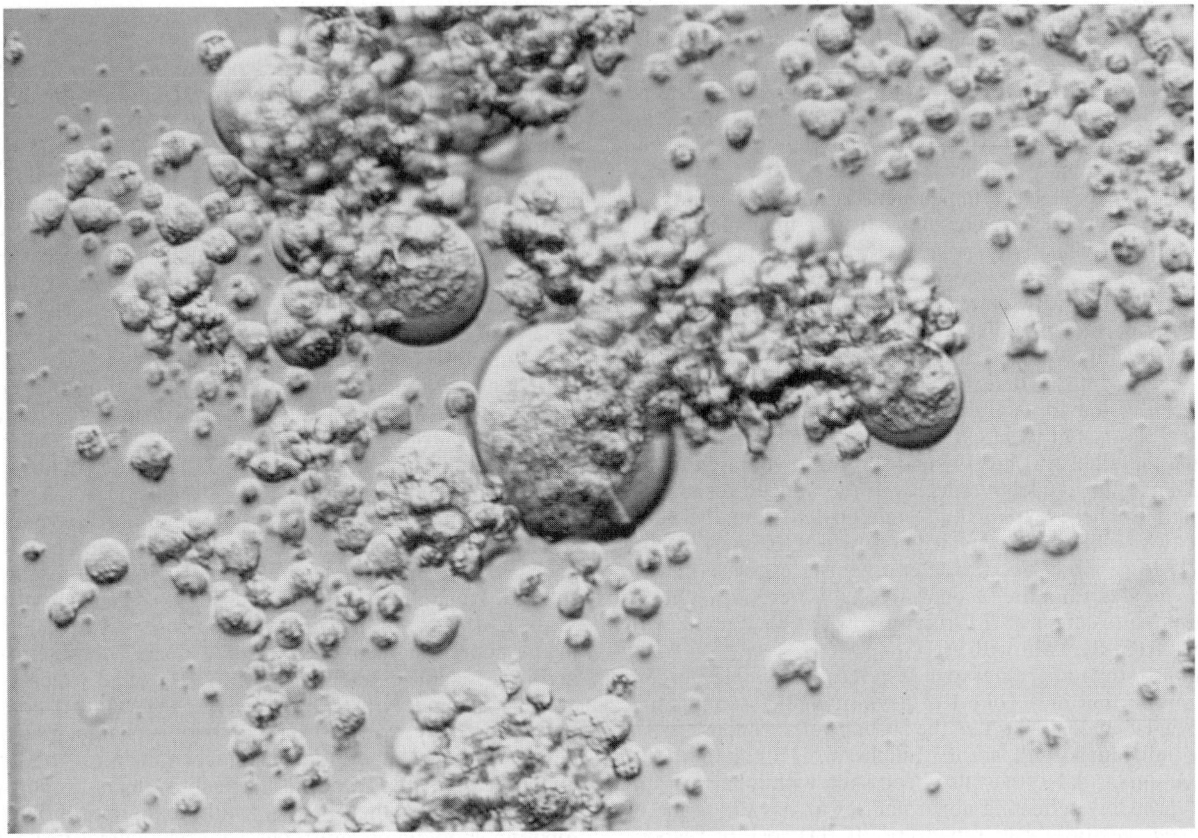

FIG. 2 Photomicrograph of syncytia formation between HIV-infected cells and uninfected CD4+ cells. (Courtesy of Dr. Cecil Fox, Bethesda, MD.)

(PCR) technique—a selective DNA amplification approach that enables direct detection of exceedingly small amounts of proviral DNA—may help shed new light on this area.[62]

Additional mechanisms underlying lymphodepletion may involve concomitant failure of hematopoietic organs to produce mature cells. For example, HIV might infect a T4 cell precursor or stem cell, leading to an inability to regenerate depleted lymphocytes. In this regard, it has been demonstrated that AIDS patients have a decreased capacity to generate T-cell colonies.[63] Furthermore, colony formation of granulocytes–macrophages (CFU-GM) and erythrocytes (BFU-E) from bone marrow of AIDS patients is inhibited when cultured in the presence of their sera. It is possible to isolate HIV from some of those cultures.[64]

Recent studies indicate that HIV can infect certain bone marrow cells. These infectible cells belong to the myelomonocytic cell lineage that develops into monocytes–macrophages. These studies found that HIV can propagate and remain within those bone marrow cells. Thus these cells may represent important reservoirs of HIV in the body.[13]

Emerging evidence suggests that autoimmune phenomena may be partially responsible for the cytopathic effects and T4 cell depletion associated with HIV infection. An autoimmune process may be induced through the interaction of the CD4 molecule with HIV envelope proteins; the binding of free HIV envelope proteins to the CD4 molecule on uninfected cells may result in the immune system responding to these cells as nonself,[65] with consequent elimination by immune clearance or by antibody-dependent cellular toxicity (ADCC).[66] Another autoimmune theory involves immune system clearance of cells bearing the class II MHC molecule.[60] This theory derives from the fact that the CD4 molecule on the T4 cell recognizes and binds a portion of the class II MHC molecule. Because the HIV envelope binds to the CD4 molecule as well, it may mimic the configuration of a portion of the class II MHC antigen. It is conceivable that an immune response—either antibodies or cytotoxic lymphocytes—directed against the envelope proteins may result in a cross-reactive response against class II MHC-bearing cells as well as an anti-idiotypic response against cells expressing CD4.[60] Recent data indicate that T4 cells can process and present antigens, such as gp120, in conjunction with class II MHC molecules in a CD4-mediated process. Thus CD4+ T cells may be targeted for destruction by gp120-specific cytotoxic cells via a CD4-dependent autocytolytic mechanism.[67,68] To what degree, if any, such phenomena play a role in the cytopathicity of HIV infection is unclear at present.

Functional Impairment of CD4+ Lymphocytes. Although quantitative depletion of CD4+ lymphocytes is the most prominent immunologic abnormality in HIV-infected individuals, there is growing evidence that HIV can cause a qualitative or functional impairment of immune cells in the absence of a cytopathic effect. Unfractionated peripheral blood mononuclear cells (PBMC) from AIDS patients manifest profound decreases in responses to mitogens, alloantigens, and soluble antigens.[69–71] The degree of these functional changes is variable, but depression of T-cell function appears more pronounced in AIDS patients with opportunistic infections than in individuals with other HIV-related conditions.[42]

When unfractionated PBMC from uninfected individuals and from AIDS patients were stimulated with common mitogens such as pokeweed, concanavalin A (con A), and phytohemagglutinin (PHA), the cells from AIDS patients consistently demonstrated a diminution of response. Depresssed mitogenic responses by PBMC of AIDS patients could be restored by increasing the absolute number of CD4+ lymphocytes so that cultures from both control and AIDS patients contained equivalent numbers of such cells.[70,72] This indicates that this functional T-cell defect is intimately related to the depletion of CD4 cells. By contrast, reconstituting PBMC from AIDS patients to normal proportions of CD4 cells did not result in the restoration of an absent response to tetanus toxoid (TT) antigen, suggesting that antigen-responsive CD4 cells are either selectively depleted or, in fact, functionally impaired.

Evidence for a selective impairment in antigen responsiveness during HIV infection comes from a number of sources. Cutaneous hypersensitivity responses, which depend on the subset of CD4 cells that recognizes and responds to soluble antigen, are selectively deficient in AIDS patients.[69] Correspondingly, purified populations of these CD4 lymphocytes from AIDS patients also do not proliferate normally to soluble antigen in vitro.[69] This defect does not appear to be due to an abnormality of the antigen-presenting cells necessary for such responses. Studies of identical twins, in which one sibling had AIDS and the other was healthy and seronegative, provide further evidence for a selective defect in the antigen-responsive CD4 cells. In these experiments, monocytes from the seronegative twin, when cocultured with his own autologous T cells, were able to generate good proliferative TT responses. However, monocytes from the seronegative twin were incapable of reconstituting a defective TT response when cocultured with CD4 cells from the twin with AIDS.[73]

In another study of proliferative responses to soluble antigen, a large proportion of a cohort of asymptomatic, seropositive homosexual men demonstrated the absence of a response to TT even in individuals with normal numbers of circulating CD4 cells.[73] A similar defect has also been seen with other test antigens,[74] probably reflecting abnormalities across the scope of the antigen-specific T-cell repertoire. If this loss of responsiveness simply reflected the depletion of antigen-responsive cells, one would expect a cumulative quantitative loss of most of the CD4 cells, which was not the case. This finding strongly supports the contribution of a functional impairment of CD4 lymphocytes in the abnormal antigen responses. Because the decreased response to soluble antigen appears early in the course of HIV infection, even in those individuals with total lymphocyte numbers above 1000 cells/mm^3,[69] a functional impairment of T4 cells may represent a critical initial step in the progressive immune defects seen with HIV infection.

There is evidence of functional abnormalities of T4 cells caused by exposure to HIV without the development of a productive or cytopathic infection. In one series of experiments, exposure of PBMC stimulated in vitro with a soluble antigen to noncytopathic concentrations of HIV resulted in a marked inhibition of response to soluble antigen and a lesser inhibition of mitogen response.[75] Other studies have shown that certain purified subunits of HIV, particularly gp120 envelope protein, could inhibit antigen-specific responses when exposed to lymphocytes, even though they would be incapable of producing infection.[76]

Several potential mechanisms could explain this impairment of T4 cell function by exposure to HIV, but not actual infection of the cell. Antigen-specific responses of T4 cells require the interaction of the CD4 molecule expressed on the surface of the T4 cell with the class II MHC molecule of the antigen-presenting cell as part of the presentation of processed antigen to the CD3-Ti antigen receptor complex on the T4 cell.[77] It is conceivable that since the HIV envelope binds avidly to the CD4 molecule on the T4 cell,[12,29,30] this could interfere with the normal interaction of the CD4 molecule with the class II MHC molecule on the antigen-presenting cell.[77,78] Responses of T4 cells to mitogens are not critically dependent on the CD4–class II MHC molecule interaction.[73] The cellular activation pathway of mitogen stimulation could bypass this step, inducing an essentially normal proliferative response in cells rendered refractory to antigenic stimulation. This would be consistent with the observations noted earlier of normal mitogen responses under certain circumstances in which a selective defect in antigen responses is seen.[69]

Another hypothesis is that exposure of T cells to HIV or its products might cause a postreceptor signal transduction defect that mitogen, but not antigen, can at least partially override. Since the triggering of cells by soluble antigens and mitogens occurs through different pathways,[79] it is possible that the virus-induced block in T-cell function occurs following ligand binding to the CD4 molecule and may offer an explanation of the discrepancy between suppression of antigen responses as opposed to mitogen responses.[69] It has recently been observed that HIV-infected T cells have a defect in the calcium mobilization necessary for activation when stimulated through the CD3-Ti complex but not through the CD2 pathway.[80]

IL-2 has an important role in the generation of T-cell activation and response. A functional defect in IL-2 gene expression may contribute to the antigen-specific defect that requires IL-2 for amplification of response in cells displaying a noncytopathic infection with HIV.[41]

In addition to the deficiencies noted in proliferative responses to antigen, AIDS patients demonstrate impaired cytotoxic responses. For instance, depressed HLA class I-restricted cytotoxic T-lymphocyte (CTL) responses against cytomegalovirus (CMV) and influenza have been observed in patients early in the course of their disease.[74,81–83] This depressed function involves responses mediated by CD8+ cells, which typically are not infected with HIV, suggesting that another component must be involved. Class I CTL activity is characteristically dependent on the intact T4-cell inducer function. The observed impairment of this response no doubt reflects T-cell dysfunction. This implies that the reconstitution of appropriate T4 cell function should ameliorate this cytotoxic defect if the effector function of CD8+ cells is intact. Supporting this notion, in vitro T-cell-mediated cytotoxicity to CMV was restored with the addition of IL-2, possibly by bypassing the usual CD4+ inductive signals.[84] Correspondingly, CD8+ cytotoxic responses against alloantigens appear to be relatively preserved in AIDS patients. CD4+ cells are not considered necessary for induction of those alloreactive responses.[85]

Role of Monocytes–Macrophages

Infection. It is now well established that monocytes and macrophages can be infected with HIV and thus play an important role in the pathogenesis of HIV infection.[35–40] The virus can infect cells of the monocyte–macrophage lineage through attachment to the CD4 molecule expressed on the surface of certain subsets of the cells, or via phagocytic engulfment.[35–40] Virus can be isolated from these cells in the blood and various organs of HIV-infected individuals.[39,40] An important difference in HIV infection of monocytes–macrophages and T lymphocytes is that the monocyte is relatively refractory to the cytopathic effects of the virus. Not only can the virus survive within cells of the monocyte–macrophage lineage, but it can replicate within the cell. Electron micrographs demonstrate that the replicating virions bud inward into intracytoplasmic vesicles and thus can remain sequestered from immune surveillance by the host.[86] A critical implication of this phenomenon is that the monocyte–macrophage has the potential to harbor the virus and serve as a reservoir of infection in the host. Persistence of HIV infection in monocytes may help to partially explain the inability of an HIV-specific immune response to clear the body of virus. Furthermore, because monocytes–macrophages circulate, these cells may be responsible for disseminating the virus to various parts of the body, including the brain, the lung, and perhaps the bone marrow.

Functional Abnormalities. There is a growing appreciation of the major role played by monocytes–macrophages in the propagation and pathogenesis of HIV infection. The ability of

HIV to infect and persist within cells of the monocyte–macrophage lineage has been well documented, and was discussed above. Although many monocyte activities appear to be preserved in AIDS patients, a number of functional abnormalities of these cells have also been reported, including defective chemotaxis and killing of certain organisms.[87–89] Certain of these abnormalities may reflect direct infection of monocytes by HIV. However, given the relatively low number of infected circulating monocytes, it is more likely that multiple influences are at work. Many of the functional defects observed in monocyte function may reflect deficient inductive signals from CD4 cells. For example, γ-interferon produced by normal CD4 cells is capable of reconstituting certain defective functions of monocytes,[90] although following prolonged courses of intravenous γ-interferon, impaired monocyte respiratory burst activity persists in these AIDS patients.[91]

Chemotaxis is the monocyte function most frequently observed to be impaired in HIV-infected patients,[87,89] but this defect is not necessarily specific for HIV infection, since many patients chronically ill from other viral and malignant disorders also have depressed chemotactic responses. Reports from many studies indicate that a range of functions appears to remain intact in monocytes derived from HIV-infected patients. These include phagocytic activity,[92] ADDC,[89] tumoricidal activity, cytotoxicity against *Toxoplasma gondii* and *Chlamydia psittaci* in response to γ-interferon,[90] and fungicidal activity against *Aspergillus fumigatus, Cryptococcus neoformans*, and *Thermoascus crustaceus*,[92] as well as *Candida*.[93]

Macrophages from AIDS patients also appear to function reasonably well in soluble antigen presentation, in both syngeneic and class II MHC-compatible systems. Minimal abnormalities have been observed in soluble antigen presentation by circulating monocytes in a syngeneic system using highly enriched cell populations derived from healthy identical twins.[73] Similar results have been found by others using class II MHC-compatible presenting cells,[94] although one report indicates decreased expression of class II antigens on monocytes of patients with AIDS.[95] Compared with normal individuals, a higher proportion of HIV-infected lymphadenopathy patients demonstrated a low proliferative response to anti-T3 antibody. This could be augmented by the addition of normal allogeneic macrophages, suggesting a defect of accessory cell function in this T-cell dependent response.[89]

HIV infection may directly and/or indirectly influence secretion of monokines such as IL-1 and tumor necrosis factor (TNF, formerly called cachectin).[41] Although it has generally been felt that IL-1 production and secretion by monocytes was relatively preserved,[96,97] some findings suggest that inhibitors of IL-1 may be present in the circulation of AIDS patients.[97] These issues, and their clinical significance, require further clarification.

Related Pathogenic Effects. HIV INFECTION OF THE BRAIN. It is well established that HIV can cause brain disease, ranging from asymptomatic infection to meningoencephalitis and dementia.[98] Neuropsychiatric manifestations occur to a greater or lesser degree in about 60 percent of HIV-infected patients.[98] Circulating infected monocytes may be responsible for the initiation of infection in the brain. Brain tissue studies demonstrate that the predominant cell type infected with HIV is the monocyte–macrophage.[40]

Pathologic findings from patients with AIDS-related dementia complex suggest several potential indirect mechanisms of brain tissue damage in which infected monocytes–macrophages may play a role. Infected monocytes–macrophages may release chemotactic factors that lead to the infiltration of the brain with inflammatory cells.[98] Alternatively, activated and infected macrophages may release factors toxic for the growth of neurons and may stimulate reactive glial cell growth. Reactive glial cells have been found in intimate contact with macrophages in the brains of AIDS patients.[99] Glial cells, which sometimes express CD4 molecules and under certain circumstances bind virus, may be permissive for HIV replication.[100,101] Infected macrophages may be the primary source of HIV for these cells. However, there is little evidence of infection in neurons, oligodendrocytes, or astrocytes.[40,99]

It has been observed in vitro that the HIV envelope protein can inhibit neuronal growth. A putative nerve growth factor, neuroleukin, has been implicated in this process.[102] One proposed pathogenic mechanism involves a partial sequence homology between HIV gp120 and neuroleukin and suggests that the HIV envelope could compete for binding to the growth factor receptor on neurons[103] and inhibit neuroleukin-induced neuronal growth. Whether infected macrophages in the central nervous system release high concentrations of viral envelope that is inhibitory to neuron growth in vivo is unclear at present.

HIV INFECTION OF BONE MARROW CELLS. HIV-infected individuals manifest a wide range of hematologic abnormalities, including leukopenia, anemia, and thrombocytopenia, as well as myelodysplasia.[104,105] The presence of these hematologic disorders led researchers to examine the possible role of HIV infection of bone marrow progenitor cells; a major obstacle to the study of HIV infection of human bone marrow, however, has been the inability to obtain purified bone marrow precursor cells devoid of mature T lymphocytes. Using a newly developed cell fractionation technique, researchers have been able to show infection in vitro of monocytic progenitor cells with HIV.[13] Virus production in these cells occurs predominantly intracellularly, producing minimal cytopathic effect and displaying intracellular budding of virus particles into cytoplasmic vesicles rather than from the surface of the cell membrane. Electron microscopic analysis reveals that the virus load in these cells can be of such magnitude that, in many instances, entire regions of cytoplasm are replaced with mature virions. The extent to which HIV-infected bone marrow cells contribute to the hematologic abnormalities observed in AIDS patients is uncertain at present.

HIV INFECTION OF OTHER CELL TYPES. Other cell types capable of infection with HIV include Langerhans cells of the skin,[106] endothelial cells,[107] colorectal cells,[108] cervical cells,[109] retinal cells,[110] pulmonary macrophages,[38] and transformed B cells.[111] Some but not all of these cell types have been shown to express CD4 mRNA or protein. The physiologic significance and contribution of HIV infection in these cells to the pathogenesis and clinical manifestations of AIDS remains to be determined.

Other Immunologic Abnormalities

B-Cell Involvement. B-cell function and humoral immunity is markedly abnormal in patients with AIDS. Beyond the consequences of deficient CD4+ T-helper cells in initiating specific antibody production, intrinsic B-cell physiology and activity is abnormal in HIV-infected individuals. AIDS patients characteristically develop polyclonal B-cell activation, manifested by hypergammaglobulinemia, spontaneous B-cell proliferation, and increased spontaneous secretion of immunoglobulin in vitro.[1,2,112–117] In symptomatic individuals, serum levels of IgG, IgA, and IgD are elevated,[112–114,118] with more variable changes noted in IgM. Generally IgM levels appear to be relatively normal in adults with AIDS,[116] although IgM hypergammaglobulinemia is frequently noted in pediatric AIDS.[116]

In contrast to the increased spontaneous activity noted in B cells from AIDS patients, antigen-specific and -nonspecific B-cell responses are impaired.[112] In vitro proliferative responses to antigens and mitogens are decreased, as are pokeweed mitogen (PWM)-induced immunoglobulin synthesis.[115] In vivo responses to primary and secondary immunizations of AIDS patients are poor, with reduced specific antibody production shown to both protein and polysaccharide antigens.[112,116] An inability to mount an adequate IgM response to antigenic challenge is an obvious and clinically significant humoral defect.

Consequences of this are most severe in HIV-infected infants and children who have not previously been exposed to a variety of pathogenic bacterial organisms and must rely on an initial IgM response for immune protection.[119] Certain adult AIDS patients also appear to have an increased susceptibility to certain pyogenic bacteria, which probably reflects defective humoral responses.[120]

The polyclonal hyperactivity of the B-cell limb of the immune response in AIDS patients no doubt reflects multiple factors. Several well-established polyclonal B-cell activators such as Epstein-Barr virus (EBV) and cytomegalovirus are frequently found to coinfect this patient population and may contribute to such hyperactivity.[117,124]

Increased spontaneous transformation of B cells of AIDS patients by EBV in vitro has been reported and is thought to reflect impaired T-cell and natural killer (NK)-cell surveillance,[121] not necessarily related to intrinsic B-cell dysfunction. This phenomenon may be associated with the increased incidence of B-cell lymphomas observed in AIDS patients. It is important to note, however, that despite the ability of HIV to infect EBV-transformed cells in vitro, there is no evidence of HIV integration in the B-cell lymphomas of AIDS patients.[122] The high incidence of these lymphomas in AIDS patients may be associated with increased transformation by EBV and may simply reflect the high incidence of coinfection with EBV in these individuals.

The mechanisms of B-cell dysfunction in HIV infection remain somewhat poorly understood. There is no current indication that nontransformed B cells can be infected with HIV, nor have HIV-infected B cells been identified in HIV-seropositive individuals. Despite the apparent inability of HIV to infect these cells directly, the effects of viral proteins on B-cell activity may account for some of the observed in vivo changes. Both intact infectious HIV and disrupted viral particles induce polyclonal activation of normal B cells with proliferative responses and immunoglobulin synthesis comparable to that of other B-cell mitogens.[117,121,123] Whether these responses reflect direct effects solely on B cells, or whether they require T cells to secrete soluble factors or to "present" concentrated virions, remains to be resolved.

In addition to the stimulatory effects of viral particles on B cells, HIV has been found to suppress EBV-induced immunoglobulin production by purified B cells.[124] The mechanism of this process is unclear, but because EBV is mitogenic for B cells in the absence of T cells or accessory cells, it raises the possibility of a direct effect of HIV on B cells.

Natural Killer Cell Impairment. A group of phenotypically distinct cell types associated with the functional properties of NK cells are included in this classification. The majority of these cells composes a relatively small circulating population of large granular lymphocytes (LGL) and bear CD16 on their surface. A smaller circulating population of CD16 cells expressing the product of the γ-δ-T-cell receptor gene have also been shown to have NK cell activity.[125] These NK cells are capable of killing virally infected cells, tumor cells, and allogeneic cells. They are thought to have a central role in immunosurveillance against viral infections and spontaneously developing tumors.

The number of circulating NK cells does not appear to be significantly decreased with HIV infection, even in those patients who have developed AIDS. These cells bind normally to their target cells[126]; however, compared with uninfected individuals, their cytotoxic capability is diminished.[126,127] Using lysis of tumor cell lines as a standard of NK activity, NK cell function measured in unfractionated populations of mononuclear cells from AIDS patients has been found to be depressed as compared with healthy seronegative controls.[84,126–130] NK function can be enhanced or restored to normal levels when activated by IL-2, concanavalin A, or phorbol ester and calcium ionophore.[126,131] Thus, NK cells from AIDS patients appear to be intrinsically able to perform their cytolytic function once activated, but manifest a postbinding or "triggering" defect that interferes with the normal pathway for delivery of a transmembrane signal for activation when in contact with an appropriate target.[132]

Other Immune Factors

A number of other factors have been proposed to account for some of the immune defects seen in AIDS patients. In addition to hypergammaglobulinemia,[111] circulating autoantibodies[133–137] and circulating immune complexes have been detected in AIDS patients.[138,139] The clinical consequences of an elevation in circulating immune complexes are unclear but may have relevance to certain symptoms such as arthritis, nephritis, and thrombocytopenia, which are sometimes seen in HIV-infected individuals.

Elevated levels of acid-labile α-interferon,[140,141] α-1-thymosin,[142] and β-2-microglobulin[143] have been reported in patients with AIDS but are of unknown clinical significance. Antibodies to α-1-thymosin appear to cross react with p17 and may be effective in viral neutralization.[144]

HIV Variation and Possible Selective Cell Tropism

An important topic for current debate in the virology of AIDS concerns whether or not individuals can harbor several forms of HIV, manifesting different selective tropisms for particular cell types in vivo. In the laboratory it has been documented that some HIV isolates obtained from brain and lung of AIDS patients exhibit selective tropism for monocytes and are capable of only feeble infection of T cells.[39] Conversely, peripheral blood HIV isolates that were passaged in vitro through T cells were unable to infect monocytes. Recent studies from another group support these observations of differential cell tropisms using a culture system that enhances the growth of macrophages in vitro. Of particular interest is that CD4 could not be detected on the surface of these monocytes, suggesting that another receptor or mechanism may allow viral entry into monocytes.[86]

Another group reported dual infection of the central nervous system by HIV isolates with distinct cellular tropisms.[145] These two structurally dissimilar viruses were obtained from frontal cortex tissue and cerebrospinal fluid (CSF) of a patient with encephalopathy. In contrast to the other studies, both of these viral isolates were passaged in lectin-stimulated lymphocytes. Following this, the viral isolate from the cortex infected macrophages as well, whereas the CSF-derived isolate infected glioma cells but not macrophages.

The nature, control, and ultimate significance of HIV variation and selective cell tropism are not yet fully understood. The selective cell tropisms observed in viral isolates may be coded by genes for viral-specific envelope sequences or by acquisition of a receptor from the host cell membrane during the process of budding. Molecular cloning of these biologically different isolates should provide future insight into this issue.

ACTIVATION OF LATENT HIV INFECTION

Significant gaps exist in the present understanding of the events that surround the progression of illness in HIV-infected individuals from asymptomatic infection to immunosuppression and full-blown AIDS. Recent clinical observations suggest that early in the course of infection with HIV, rising levels of the HIV structural protein, p24, can be detected in patients. With the onset of antibody production against the virus, these levels generally decline. This p24 antigenemia is felt to reflect active viral replication, and it is interesting to note that during the period of asymptomatic infection, small intermittent bursts of p24 antigenemia that usually return to baseline may be detected. However, late in the course of infection, the HIV-infected individual may manifest sustained p24 antigenemia (Lane HC, unpublished data). These rising levels of p24 antigen have important prognostic implications for the development of AIDS, although the mechanisms and triggers underlying this phenomenon are not understood.

It has been observed in vitro that while inactivated cells can be infected with HIV, productive infection requires an activation signal. Virus isolation from HIV-infected patients requires the stimulation of PBMC cultures. Early experiments demonstrated that HIV replication could be induced in latently infected cells following exposure of the cells to PHA.[11,14] However, for the HIV-infected individual, exposure to antigenic stimuli is much more likely to have physiologic relevance than exposure to mitogens. When similar experiments were undertaken using specific antigenic stimuli, it was demonstrated that PBMC that had been activated by antigen (such as the soluble antigens TT and keyhole impact hemocyanin [KLH]) prior to exposure to HIV were 10 to 100 times more susceptible to viral replication than PBMC that had been preincubated without antigen.[75]

Heterologous viruses represent one possible source of antigenic stimulation to which HIV-infected individuals may be exposed during the course of their infection. There is reason to suspect that concurrent infections with viral pathogens such as cytomegalovirus, Epstein-Barr virus, hepatitis B, and herpes simplex virus could activate latent HIV and induce viral expression in those individuals infected with HIV.[146] It has been shown in vitro that HIV expression can be up-regulated in cells following transfection with heterologous viruses.[147,148] More recently, it has been shown that HIV reverse transcriptase activity increases when a full-length infectious HIV clone is cotransfected with heterologous viral DNAs.[149]

In addition to mitogens, antigens, and coinfecting viruses, normal physiologic stimuli such as cytokines appear to play a role in the induction of productive HIV infection from a latent or low-level chronic infection. Studies using chronically infected cell lines indicate that exposure to a variety of cytokines, including granulocyte–macrophage-colony stimulating factor (GM-CSF) and particularly TNF-α, can produce physiologic cellular inductive signals with consequent upregulation of HIV infection. Further investigation of this phenomenon suggests that enhanced HIV expression by cytokines reflects induction of the promotor region of HIV by the transactivating effect of a DNA binding protein (Rubson A, personal communication). Full understanding of the mechanisms of activation of latent HIV infection will be essential in attempting to develop strategies to limit progression of HIV-induced disease.

IMMUNE RESPONSES TO HIV

Once diagnosed with AIDS, the life expectancy of an individual is approximately 2 years or less, depending on the initial clinical manifestations and response to treatment. The availability of the antiretroviral agent azidothymidine (AZT)—the only drug presently approved for the treatment of AIDS—has led to modest but significant increases in life span for those who can tolerate its potentially toxic side effects.[150] New agents under development may improve prospects for the future. Investigations into the nature and course of the immune response to HIV infection offer some insight into approaches to prevention and control of the relentless progression of HIV infection.

Multiple conditions can influence the outcome of an individual's exposure to HIV and the clinical sequelae of HIV infection. Factors such as the route of viral entry, the integrity of skin and other protective barriers to entry, the size of the viral inoculum, the virulence of the viral isolate, the presence of coinfecting pathogens, the number of contacts, the nutritional state, and the response of the immune system of the exposed individual may all determine whether or not that individual will become infected with HIV or manifest symptoms. Interestingly, there are reports of individuals with documented exposure to HIV, such as the wives of HIV-infected hemophiliacs, who remain uninfected, even after multiple contacts, while others with similar exposure seroconvert rapidly.[151] A resistance to infection based on HLA association has been looked for but not found. One study reported a relationship between an individual's group-specific component (Gc) type and resistance or susceptibility to infection and ultimate progression of disease.[152] However, subsequent studies did not corroborate this initial observation.[153,154]

The best available evidence indicates that infection with HIV leads to viral DNA integration and lifelong chronic infection of lymphocytes, monocytes, and other cells expressing the CD4 surface molecule. Seropositivity, reflecting the production of antibodies to HIV, develops approximately 3 to 12 weeks following infection and persists thereafter. Characteristically, there is a variable but relatively long period of time from initial infection to the development of AIDS. What proportion of infected individuals will develop AIDS over an extended time period remains undetermined. Current estimates indicate that approximately 37 percent of HIV-seropositive individuals will develop an AIDS-associated condition within 7 years of infection.[155] Unless an effective therapy is developed, it may well be the case that virtually all of those infected with HIV will ultimately die from AIDS. Despite a few isolated reports of asymptomatic seropositive individuals reverting to a seronegative state, reexamination of those cases using the newly developed gene amplification technique of polymerase chain reaction (PCR) suggests that those individuals remain latently infected with HIV.[156]

The conditions influencing disease course and clinical sequelae following HIV infection are unclear. Many factors similar to those bearing on initial susceptibility to infection may also influence the postinfectious course; such factors include the virulence of a particular viral isolate, the size of the initial inoculum, or the type and nature of other pathogens coinfecting individuals. Undoubtedly, a major determinant of clinical outcome in an individual is the capacity of their immune system to contain or eliminate the virus. The conditions necessary for development of effective immunity in an exposed or infected individual have not been established.

Many different responses, involving multiple limbs of the immune system, may participate in the body's attempt to mount a protective immune response to HIV. Humoral responses would include the production of neutralizing and cytolytic antibodies. Activation of the complement cascade may occur, with resultant killing of free and cell-bound virions. The development of cell-mediated responses, such as cytotoxic T cells, antibody-dependent cytotoxicity, and NK cell activity, may play an even more critical role in providing immune protection against HIV.

Neutralizing Antibodies

For virtually all individuals, HIV infection is associated with humoral immune response that produces antibodies to multiple viral proteins[157,158] but appears inadequate in preventing HIV propagation and clinical progression. Low titers of antibodies with neutralizing capacity have been detected in seropositive individuals at all stages of clinical disease. However, the finding of neutralizing antibodies in roughly equivalent levels in both AIDS patients and healthy seropositive individuals suggests that their presence may have little clinical significance. In several studies, no clear correlation of the in vitro effects of such neutralizing antibodies with clinical course or ability to prevent disease could be determined.[159–162]

The specificity of neutralizing antibody—determined by the ability of sera to inhibit viral isolates—may be type-specific (responding only to a restricted range of closely related strains) or group-specific (responding to a broad, heterogenous group of viral isolates). The potential specificity differences for neutralizing antibodies results from the diversity found within the HIV envelope, where variable regions demonstrating less than 50 percent homology among HIV strains are interposed with sequences that are more highly conserved.

Attempts to stimulate neutralizing antibody production experimentally with a variety of recombinant and purified proteins have been successful in both uninfected animals and humans.[163,164] Glycosylation of these proteins does not appear to be necessary to induce antibodies with neutralizing capability, although theoretically it may yield some qualitative advantages.[165,166] However, not all of the experimentally induced antibodies are neutralizing. For example, antibodies generated against the amino-terminal half of gp120 and gp41 envelope protein components could bind but not neutralize HIV.[165]

The specificity of neutralizing antibody has been examined in animal models as well as in individuals infected with HIV. This area of research has important implications for the feasibility of and approach to developing a successful vaccine against HIV. Most neutralizing antibody responses that have been generated in animal models by immunization with envelope protein appear to be type-specific. For example, in one recent study, antibody produced in response to immunization with envelope from the HIV-1 III-B strain could not neutralize the HIV-1 RF strain, and vice versa.[167] However, using other immunogenic epitopes of HIV, it may be possible to generate group-specific responses. Support for this comes from recent work in a rabbit model, which demonstrated that a peptide within a conserved portion of the envelope region could generate a group-specific neutralizing response against both HIV-1 III-B and HIV-1 RF isolates.[168] Studies in humans indicate the appearance of both patterns of neutralizing activity, but neither seems to confer a particular protective advantage to the individual.

In addition, there may be an important dichotomy in the regions that can induce antibody formation and T-cell proliferation. Virally induced antibodies found in sera from HIV-exposed patients reacted strongly with recombinant proteins from the carboxy terminus of gp120, but only bound weakly to proteins from the amino terminus. Conversely, T cells from those same patients demonstrated marked proliferative responses to the gp120 amino-terminus proteins, but poor response to the carboxy-terminus gp120.[169] Found within a conserved region of gp120, a specific sequence has been demonstrated to stimulate T-helper cell responses in mice immunized with HIV envelope proteins.[167] This sequence portion of the HIV envelope was predicted to be immunogenic based on the location within amphipathic α-helical regions. Cells from mice that were immunized with purified envelope proteins showed proliferative responses to a 16-residue synthetic peptide derived from that epitope.[167] However, the study did not determine whether neutralizing antibodies were produced to this peptide.

There is a concern that even if high-titered neutralizing antibodies could be stimulated in uninfected individuals, the very nature of HIV may hinder full and persistent protection against infection. It has been well demonstrated that a biologic property of HIV is easy and rapid mutation, resulting in the frequent creation of new strains.[19] There appears to be strong selective pressures for inducing changes within the envelope regions in particular. Neutralizing antibodies may in fact hasten this selection process, a phenomenon noted in vitro for HIV[170] and seen in vivo in other lentiviral diseases.[171] In a study of chimpanzees immunized with purified gp120, neutralizing antibodies were formed in response to immunization, but despite this, the animals became infected after challenge with HIV.[172] Ethical considerations clearly preclude direct investigation into the ability of neutralizing antibody to confer protection in human subjects against challenge with HIV, but accumulated evidence suggests that neutralizing antibodies have only a limited role in inhibiting HIV propagation and clinical progression of disease. There is no evidence to support the notion that the presence of neutralizing antibody to HIV could be protective for the uninfected individual exposed to HIV.

Cell-Mediated Cytotoxicity

The development of cellular cytotoxic immune responses may play a more critical role than neutralizing antibody formation in providing protection against HIV and other retroviruses. In a murine system using the Friend leukemia virus, it has been demonstrated that animals that developed cell-mediated cytotoxic responses to HIV along with neutralizing antibodies were protected against the development of leukemia following viral challenge, whereas animals that developed only neutralizing antibodies succumbed to leukemia.[173] The nature and scope of cellular immune responses in HIV infection is the subject of considerable current investigation. Protective cell-mediated responses against HIV may include ADCC, CTL, and NK cell responses.

Antibody-Dependent Cellular Cytotoxicity

ADCC may prove to be a key feature of the immune response to HIV. It has been shown that sera from HIV-seropositive individuals can mediate ADCC activity in vitro.[174–176] Some studies suggest that the level of this activity may correlate roughly with the clinical condition of the individual; sera derived from individuals with AIDS demonstrate less activity as compared with those of healthy seropositives.[174] However, this decrease in ADCC activity may simply reflect a more global defect in immune function in clinically advanced disease. One study attempted to compare ADCC specific antibody titer and anti-HIV antibody titer as measured by the ELISA assay, but no correlation was evident.[176] Presence or absence of antibody to a particular viral protein may be more critical than total anti-HIV antibody titers. ADCC activity appears to correlate best with the presence of antibodies to HIV envelope protein, although antibodies directed against other viral proteins may be involved as well. In one fairly recent report, ADCC activity was undetectable when anti-envelope activity was absent[176] but was present in sera without anti-p24 activity. The relationship of ADCC activity to anti-p24 activity is somewhat unclear, however, given an earlier study indicating that ADCC activity correlated best with anti-p24 activity.[174] In another study, although ADCC activity was not specifically examined, it was shown in a cohort of healthy seropositive homosexual men followed over a 3-year period that those individuals who remained healthy also demonstrated substantially greater anti-p24 activity.[177] No significant difference in neutralizing activity was observed between those who became symptomatic and those who remained healthy. Large-scale, careful examination of sera from HIV-infected individuals, looking at both neutralizing antibodies and ADCC activity, should be done—either prospectively or retrospectively—and correlated with clinical progression. In this manner, important insights may be gained into the potential components of effective immune response to HIV.

Natural Killer Cells

As mentioned earlier, natural killer cells appear to participate in the host elimination of HIV-infected cells. Several different cell phenotypes may be involved in this response, including those that express CD16 and Leu19. In addition, certain T cells, those with the γ-δ-T-cell receptor rearrangement in particular, may be involved in the lysis of HIV-infected cells in an MHC-unrestricted manner.[178] Large granular lymphocytes (LGLs) are the predominant cells containing NK activity. Purified populations of LGLs from seronegative individuals have been shown to mediate a small cytolytic response against HIV-infected targets. This response could be markedly augmented by culture in the presence of IL-2.[179] A similar enhancement of HLA-unrestricted cytotoxic activity was found when unfractionated cells from both seronegative and seropositive individuals were cultured in the presence of IL-2.[83] It has been demonstrated that the majority of HIV envelope-specific cytoxicity in the peripheral blood of HIV-seropositive individuals is HLA-unrestricted and mediated by cells expressing CD16.[180] The activity of these cells appeared to correlate with the patient's clinical status in that the healthier individuals demonstrated greater activity. Since cells that bear CD16 can participate in either NK-mediated lysis or ADCC activity, a portion of these cells may effect lysis through an ADCC-dependent mechanism.

Cytotoxic T Cells

T cells with cytotoxic activities have been detected in the circulation and lungs of HIV-infected individuals, and, with a variety of different assay systems, have been demonstrated to lyse target cells expressing HIV or HIV-associated proteins. An important area of current research concerns the delineation of the antigens recognized by cytotoxic T lymphocytes in infected individuals, as well as attempts to further characterize the cytotoxic effector cell population and the nature of the cytotoxic response to HIV proteins.

One group has reported the presence of CTL to HIV envelope and *gag* proteins in PBMC from HIV-infected individuals, using target cells infected with a recombinant vaccinia virus expressing HIV proteins.[181] These peripheral blood cells could lyse envelope- and *gag*-expressing targets that were either MHC class I- or class II-matched to the effector cells. It was later reported that PBMC from HIV-seropositive individuals could lyse target cells expressing the *pol* gene product and reverse transcriptase. In most patients this cytotoxic response could be blocked with antibody to CD8 or CD3.[182] CTL activity was present in all seropositive patients studied, including those with ARC and AIDS, and some features of HLA restriction were noted.[183] Other investigators have reported similar activity in a large proportion of healthy HIV-seropositive individuals studied, some patients with ARC, and rare AIDS patients with Kaposi sarcoma, but not in those AIDS patients with opportunistic infections.[184] This activity did not appear to be HLA class I-restricted. Another group studying anti-envelope responses following in vitro priming, reported finding low but statistically significant HLA class I-restricted CTL in some seropositive individuals.[185] In another study using a somewhat different approach, cytotoxic cell lines were generated from the bronchiolar lavage fluids from HIV-infected patients with interstitial pneumonitis. These cells were able to lyse macrophages infected with HIV, as well as target cells expressing envelope HLA class I-matched proteins. Further study demonstrated that these cytotoxic cells expressed CD8, and the response appeared to be HLA-A2-restricted in the individuals tested.[186]

In an animal model of HIV immune response, peripheral blood cells obtained from chimpanzees immunized with recombinant vaccinia viruses expressing HIV envelope proteins demonstrated proliferative responses to purified whole and envelope proteins.[185] Cells cloned from these immunized chimpanzees were cytotoxic for target cells infected with vaccinia virus expressing the recombinant envelope protein. However, these cytotoxic cells proved to be CD4+.

Efforts to characterize further the cell types involved in the cytolytic response to HIV clearly indicate that several cell types may be involved in the process. Using envelope-expressing targets derived from HIV isolates with envelope regions differing by at least 21 percent, it has been demonstrated that a group-specific cytotoxic response against envelope proteins is present in the majority of seropositive individuals. Recent evidence indicates that such a group-specific response against envelope-expressing target cells can be MHC-restricted.[178]

It remains to be determined whether both class I and class II HIV-specific CTL activity is generated in the course of natural infection and with immunization with recombinant proteins, and whether the CTL process confers any protection to the uninfected and immunized host.

CONCLUSIONS

In the relatively short period of time since this new disease entity was established and the causal virus discovered, an extraordinary amount of information has been gained about HIV, the pathogenesis of infection, and the immune response to the virus. Laboratory studies of HIV and the cells it infects are providing important insights into how the virus produces disease. Virtually the entire HIV genome has now been deciphered and the function of the major viral proteins determined. Infection with HIV can result in a complex array of immunopathogenic effects (Fig. 3). While the precise mechanisms whereby HIV infection leads to the immunosuppression and clinical manifestations characteristic of the disorder are complex and incompletely understood, it is evident that the depletion and functional impairment of T4 lymphocytes plays a central role. Defects in these cells—which occupy a prominent position in all the body's major defense mechanisms—produce consequential abnormalities in other immune effector cells, including B cells, T cells, and monocytes.

Many critically important but as yet poorly understood functional changes occur early in the course of HIV infection, often preceding significant losses of T4 lymphocytes. The mechanisms of T4 lymphocyte loss in vivo remain to be clarified, although virally induced cytotoxic and fusogenic processes along with autoimmune phenomena all appear to be contributors. In addition, cells of the monocyte–macrophage lineage may play an important role in the initiation and propagation of HIV infection and may serve as a reservoir of infection in the host. Experimentally, activation of HIV from latent or low-level chronic infection to productive infection may occur through mitogens, antigens, other infections, or through cytokines involved in the normal immune response. These represent potential mechanisms by which HIV infection in individuals can progress from an asymptomatic state to clinical AIDS. It is also evident that HIV infection of a given cell can result in modulation of expression of certain cellular genes and thereby has the potential to compound immunoregulatory abnormalities. Clearly, a greater understanding of these complex issues will be essential in developing effective treatment strategies for HIV infection and AIDS.

Further knowledge of protective immune responses to HIV will be critical to efforts to prevent infection or limit the clinical progression of disease. Major gaps persist in understanding the nature of protective immunity against HIV, including the relationship between the quantity and type of antibody produced and an individual's clinical status, as well as the role of cell-mediated immunity. Development of an effective vaccine against HIV will depend upon such information. Major efforts are currently under way, and the first candidate vaccines are being tested in humans in the United States and Africa.[187] However, given the long latency for development of AIDS in seropositive individuals, as well as the myriad ethical complexities of large-scale trials of an AIDS vaccine in humans, determining the efficacy of a vaccine may prove difficult.

Although devastating in its consequences, the discovery of HIV and its role in the development of AIDS and AIDS-related conditions has opened up exciting new avenues of research. Concerted efforts to elucidate the immunopathogenesis and immune response to HIV should ultimately lead to successful strategies to combat HIV-induced disease and will have important, broader implications for understanding the mechanisms of normal and aberrant regulation of the human immune system.

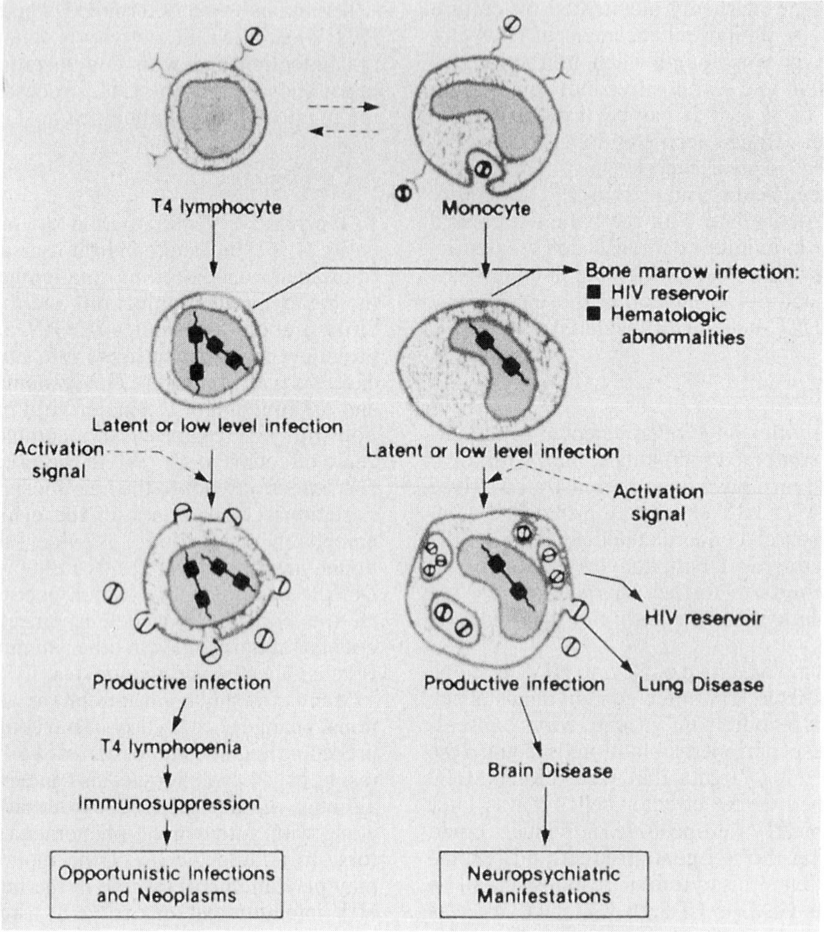

FIG. 3. Schematic diagram of the pathogenic mechanisms of HIV infection.

REFERENCES

1. Gottlieb MS, Schroff R, Schanker HM, et al. *Pneumocystis carinii* pneumonia and mucosal candidiasis in previously healthy homosexual men: evidence of a new acquired cellular immunodeficiency. N Engl J Med. 1981;305:1425–1.
2. Masur H, Michelis MA, Greene JB, et al. An outbreak of community-acquired *Pneumocystis carinii* pneumonia: initial manifestation of cellular immune dysfunction. N Engl J Med. 1981;305:1431–8.
3. Siegel FP, Lopez C, Hammer GS, et al. Severe acquired immunodeficiency in male homosexuals, manifested by chronic perianal ulcerative herpes simplex lesions. N Engl J Med. 1981;305:1439–4.
4. Centers for Disease Control. Acquired immunodeficiency syndrome weekly surveillance report, September 19, 1988. Centers for Disease Control, Atlanta, GA.
5. Public Health Service, DHHS. Quarterly report to the domestic policy council on the prevalence and rate of spread of HIV in the United States, July, 1988. Centers for Disease Control, Atlanta, GA.
6. Piot P, Plummer FA, Mhalu FS, et al. AIDS: an international perspective. Science. 1988;239:573–9.
7. Fauci AS, Masur H, Gelmann EP, et al. The acquired immunodeficiency syndrome: an update. Ann Intern Med. 1985;102:800–3.
8. Poon MC, Landay A, Prasthofer EF, et al. Acquired immunodeficiency syndrome with *Pneumocystis carinii* pneumonia and *Mycobacterium avium-intracellulare* infection in a previously healthy patient with classic hemophilia. Ann Intern Med. 1983;98:287–90.
9. Hymesk, Cheung T, Greene JB, et al. Kaposi's sarcoma in homosexual men: a report of eight cases. Lancet. 1981;2:598–600.
10. Reinherz E, O'Brien C, Rosenthal P, et al. The cellular basis for viral-induced immunodeficiency: analysis by monoclonal antibodies. J Immunol. 1980;125:1264–4.
11. Klatzmann D, Barré-Sinoussi F, Nugeyre MT, et al. Selective tropism of lymphadenopathy associated virus (LAV) for helper-inducer T lymphocytes. Science. 1984;225:59–63.
12. Dalgleish AG, Beverly CL, Clapham PR, et al. The CD4 (T4) antigen is an essential component of the receptor for the AIDS retrovirus. Nature. 1984;312:763–7.
13. Folks, TM, Kessler, SW, Orenstein, JM, et al. Infection and replication of human immunodeficiency virus-1 (HIV-1) in highly purified progenitor cells from normal human bone marrow. Science. 1988;242:919–22.
14. Gallo RC, Salahuddin SZ, Popovic M, et al. Frequent detection and isolation of cytopathic retrovirus (HTLV-III) from patients with AIDS and at risk for AIDS. Science. 1984;224:500–3.
15. Levy JA, Hoffman AD, Kramer SM, et al. Isolation of lymphocytopathic retroviruses from San Francisco patients with AIDS. Science. 1984;225:840–2.
16. Coffin J, Haase A, Levy JA, et al. Human immunodeficiency viruses. Science. 1986;232:697.
17. Barré-Sinoussi F, Chermann JC, Rey F, et al. Isolation of a T lymphotropic retrovirus from a patient at risk for acquired immune deficiency syndrome (AIDS). Science. 1983;220:868–71.
18. Popovic M, Sarngadharan MG, Read E, et al. Detection, isolation, and continuous production of cytopathic retroviruses (HTLV-III) from patients with AIDS and pre-AIDS. Science. 1984;224:497–500.
19. Fisher AG, Ensoli B, Looney D, et al. Biologically diverse molecular variants within a single HIV-1 isolate. Nature. 1988;334:444–7.
20. Benn S, Rutledge R, Folks T, et al. Genomic heterogeneity of AIDS retroviral isolates from North American and Zaire. Science. 1985;230:949.
21. Brun-Vezinet F, Rey MA, Katlama C, et al. Lymphadenopathy-associated virus type 2 in AIDS and AIDS-related complex. Lancet. 1987;1:128–32.
22. Clavel F, Guyader M, Guetard D, et al. Molecular cloning and polymorphism of the human immune deficiency virus type 2. Nature. 1986;324:691–5.
23. Horsburgh CR, Holmberg SD. The global distribution of human immunodeficiency virus type 2 (HIV-2). Infection. 1988;28:192–5.
24. Clavel F, Mansinho K, Chamaret S, et al. Human immunodeficiency virus type 2 infection associated with AIDS in West Africa. N Engl J Med. 1987;316:1180–5.
25. Public Health Service, DHHS. AIDS due to HIV-2 infection—New Jersey. MMWR. 1988;37:33–5.
26. Letvin N, Daniel MD, Sengal PK, et al. Induction of AIDS-like disease in

macaque monkeys with T-cell tropic retrovirus STLV-III. Science. 1985;230:71–3.
27. Rabson AB, Martin MA. Molecular organization of the AIDS retrovirus. Cell. 1985;40:477–80.
28. Gallo R, Wong-Staal F, Montagnier L, et al. HIV/HTLV gene nomenclature. Nature. 1988;333:504.
29. Klatzmann D, Champagne E, Charmaret S, et al. T-lymphocyte T4 molecule behaves as the receptor for human retrovirus LAV. Nature. 1984;312:767–8.
30. McDougal JS, Kennedy MS, Sligh JM, et al. Binding of HTLV-III/LAV to T4+ T cells by a complex of the 110 K viral protein and the T4 molecule. Science. 1985;231:382–5.
31. Sattentau QJ, Dalgleish AG, Weiss RA, et al. Epitopes of the CD4 antigen and HIV infection. Science. 1986;234:1120.
32. Lifson JD, Hwang KM, Nara PL, et al. Synthetic CD4 peptide derivatives that inhibit HIV infection and cytopathicity. Science. 1988;241:712–6.
33. Maddon PJ, Dagleish AG, McDougal JS, et al. The T4 gene encodes the AIDS virus receptor and is expressed in the immune system and the brain. Cell. 1986;47:333–8.
34. Mann DL, Lesane F, Blattner WA, et al. HLA-DR is involved in the HIV receptor (Abstract). In: III International Conference on Acquired Immunodeficiency Syndrome (AIDS). Washington, DC: U.S. Department of Health and Human Services. 1987;209.
35. Levy JA, Shimabukuro J, McHugh T, et al. AIDS-associated retrovirus (ARV) can productively infect other cells besides human T helper cells. Virology. 1985;147:441–8.
36. Ho DD, Rota TR, Hirsch MS. Infection of monocyte/macrophages by human T lymphotropic virus type III. J Clin Invest. 1986;77:1712–5.
37. Nicholson JKA, Cross GD, Callaway CS, et al. In vitro infection of human monocytes with human T-lymphotropic virus type III/lymphadenopathy-associated virus (HTLV-III/LAV). J Immunol. 1986;137:323–9.
38. Salahuddin SZ, Rose RM, Groopman JE, et al. Human T lymphotropic virus type II infection by human alveolar macrophages. Blood. 1986;68:281–4.
39. Gartner S, Markovits P, Markovits DM, et al. The role of mononuclear phagocytes in HTLV-III/ALV infection. Science. 1986;233:215–24.
40. Koenig S, Gendelman HE, Orenstein JM, et al. Detection of AIDS virus in macrophages in brain tissue from AIDS patients with encephalopathy. Science. 1986;233:1089–193.
41. Fauci AS. The human immunodeficiency virus: infectivity and mechanisms of pathogenesis. Science. 1988;239:617–22.
42. Lane HC, Masur H, Gelmann EP, et al. Correlation between immunologic function and clinical subpopulations of patients with the acquired immune deficiency syndrome. Am J Med. 1985;78:417–22.
43. Mittelman, Wong G, Safai B, et al. Analysis of T cell subsets in different clinical subgroups of patients with the acquired immune deficiency syndrome. Am J Med. 1985;78:951–6.
44. Polk BF, Fox R, Bookmeyer R, et al. Predictors of the acquired immunodeficiency syndrome developing in a cohort of seropositive homosexual men. N Engl J Med. 1987;316:61–6.
45. Goedert JJ, Bigga RJ, Melbye M, et al. Effect of T4 count and cofactors on the incidence of AIDS in homosexual men infected with human immunodeficiency virus. JAMA. 1987;257:331–4.
46. Kaplan JA, Spira TJ, Fishbein DB, et al. Lymphadenopathy syndrome in homosexual men: evidence for continuing risk of developing the acquired immunodeficiency syndrome. JAMA. 1987;257:335–7.
47. Fahey JL, Giorgi J, Martinez-Maza O, et al. Immune pathogenesis of AIDS and related syndromes. Ann Inst Pasteur Immunol. 1987;138:245–52.
48. Cheng-Mayer C, Seto D, Tateno M, et al. Biologic features of HIV-1 that correlate with virulence in the host. Science. 1988;240:80–2.
49. Walker CM, Moody DJ, Stites DP, et al. $CD8^+$ lymphocytes can control HIV infection in vitro by suppressing virus replication. Virology. 1986;234:1563.
50. Rabson, AB. The molecular biology of HIV infection: clues for possible therapy. In: Levy JA, ed. AIDS Pathogenesis and Treatment. New York: Marcel Dekker; 1988.
50a. Leonard R, Zagury D, Desportes I, et al. Cytopathic effect of human immunodeficiency virus in T4 cells is linked to the last stage of virus infection. Proc Natl Acad Sci USA. 1988;85:3570–4.
51. Hoxie JA, Alpers JD, Rackowski JL, et al. Alterations in T4 (CD4) protein and mRNA synthesis in cells infected with HIV. Science. 1986;234:1123–7.
52. Asjö B, Ivhed I, Gidlund M, et al. Susceptibility to infection by the human immunodeficiency virus (HIV) correlates with T4 expression in a parental monocytoid cell line and its subclones. Virology. 1987;157:359–65.
53. Sodrowski J, Goh WC, Rosen C, et al. Role of the HTLV-III/LAV envelope in syncytium formation and cytopathicity. Nature. 1986;322:470–4.
54. Lifson JD, Reyes, McGrath MS, et al. AIDS retrovirus induced cytopathology: giant cell formation and involvement of CD4 antigen. Science. 1986;232:1123–7.
55. Lifson JD, Feinberg MB, Reyes GR, et al. Induction of CD4-dependent cell fusion by the HTLV-III/LAV envelope glycoprotein. Nature. 1986;323:725–8.
56. Yoffe B, Lewis DE, Petrie BL, et al. Fusion as a mediator of cytolysis in mixtures of uninfected CD4+ lymphocytes and cells infected by human immunodeficiency virus. Proc Natl Acad Sci USA. 1987;84:1429–33.
57. Ewing EP, Chandler FW, Spira TJ, et al. Primary lymph node pathology in AIDS and AIDS-related lymphadenopathy. Arch Pathol Lab Med. 1985;109:977.
58. Epstein LG, Sharer LR, Joshi VV, et al. Progressive encephalopathy in children with acquired immune deficiency syndrome. Annal Neurol. 1985;17:488–96.
59. Klatzmann D, Montagnier L. Approaches to AIDS therapy. Nature. 1986;319:10–1.
60. Ziegler JL, Stites DP. Hypothesis: AIDS is an autoimmune disease directed at the immune system and triggered by a lymphotropic retrovirus. Clin Immunol Immunopathol. 1986;41:305–13.
61. Harper ME, Marselle LM, Gallo RC, et al. Detection of lymphocytes expressing human T-lymphotropic virus type III in lymph nodes and peripheral blood from infected individual by *in situ* hybridization. Pro Natl Acad Sci USA. 1986;83:772–6.
62. Ou CY, Kwok S, Mitchell SW, et al. DNA amplification for direct detection of HIV-1 in DNA of peripheral blood mononuclear cells. Science. 1988;239:295–7.
63. Winkelstein A, Klein RS, Evans TL, et al. Defective in vitro T cell colony formation in the acquired immunodeficiency syndrome. J Immunol. 1985;134:151–6.
64. Donahue RE, Johnson MM, Zon LI, et al. Suppression of in vitro haematopoiesis following human immunodeficiency virus infection. Nature. 1987;326:200–5.
65. Klatzmann D, Gluckman JC. HIV infection: facts and hypotheses. Immunol Today. 1986;7:291–6.
66. Katz JD, Nishanian P, Mitsuyasu R, et al. Antibody-dependent cellular cytotoxicity (ADCC)-mediated destruction of human immunodeficiency virus (HIV)-coated CD4+ T lymphocytes by acquired immunodeficiency syndrome (AIDS) effector cells. Clin Immunol. 1988;8:453–8.
67. Siliciano RF, Lawton T, Knall C, et al. Analysis of host-virus interactions in AIDS with anti-gp120 T cell clones: effect of HIV sequence variation and a mechanism for CD4+ cell depletion. Cell. 1988;54:561–6.
68. Lanzavecchia A, Roosnek E, Gregory T, et al. T cells can represent antigens such as HIV gp120 targeted to their own surface molecules. Nature. 1988;334:530.
69. Lane HC, Depper JM, Greene WC, et al. Qualitative analysis of immune function in patients with the acquired immunodeficiency syndrome. N Engl J Med. 1985;313:79–84.
70. Smolen JS, Bettelheim P, Köller U, et al. Deficiency of the autologous mixed lymphocyte reaction in patients with classic hemophilia treated with commercial factor VIII concentrate. J Clin Invest. 1985;75:1828–34.
71. Gupta S, Gillis S, Thornton M, et al. Autologous mixed lymphocyte reaction in man. XIV. Deficiency of the autologous mixed lymphocyte reaction in acquired immune deficiency syndrome (AIDS) and AIDS related complex (ARC). In vitro effect of purified interleukin-1 and interleukin-2. Clin Exp Immunol. 1984;58:395–401.
72. Lane HC, Fauci AS. Immunologic reconstitution in the acquired immunodeficiency syndrome. Ann Intern Med. 1985;103:714–8.
73. Fauci AS. AIDS: immunopathogenic mechanisms and research strategies. Clin Res. 1987;35:503–10.
74. Shearer GM, Salahuddin SZ, Markham PD, et al. Prospective study of cytotoxic T lymphocyte responses to influenza and antibodies to human T lymphotropic virus-III in homosexual men. J Clin Invest. 1985;76:1699–704.
75. Margolick JB, Volkman DJ, Folks TM, et al. Amplification of HTLV-III/LAV infection by antigen-induced activation of T cells and direct suppression by virus of lymphocyte blastogenic responses. J Immunol. 1987;138:1719–23.
76. Shalaby MR, Krowka JF, Gregory TJ, et al. The effects of human immunodeficiency virus recombinant envelope glycoprotein on immune cell functions in vitro. Cell Immunol. 1987;110:140–8.
77. Gay D, Maddon P, Sekaly R, et al. Functional interaction between human T-cell protein CD4 and the major histocompatibility complex HLA-DR antigen. Nature. 1987;626–9.
78. Doyle C, Strominger JL. Interaction between CD4 and class II MHC molecules mediates cell adhesion. Nature. 1987;330:256–9.
79. Alcover A, Ramarli D, Richardson NE, et al. Functional and molecular aspects of human T lymphocyte activation via T3-T1 and T11 pathways. Immunol Rev. 1987;95:5–6.
80. Linette GP, Hartzmann RJ, et al. HIV-1-infected T cells show a selective signaling defect after perturbation of CD3/antigen receptor. Science. 1988;241:573–576.
81. Shearer GM, Payne SM, Joseph LJ, et al. Functional T lymphocyte immune deficiency in a population of homosexual men who do not exhibit symptoms of acquired immune deficiency syndrome. J Clin Invest. 1984;74:496.
82. Sheridan JF, Aurelian L, Donnenberg AD, et al. Cell-mediated immunity of cytomegalovirus (CMV) and herpes simplex virus (HSV) antigens in the acquired immune deficiency syndrome: interleukin-1 and interleukin-2 modify in vitro responses. J Clin Immunol. 1984;4:304.
83. Rook AH, Manischewitz JD, Frederick WR, et al. Deficient, HLA-restricted, cytomegalovirus-specific cytotoxic T cells and natural killer cells in patients with the acquired immunodeficiency syndrome. J Infect Dis. 1985;152:627–8.
84. Rook AH, Masur H, Lane HC, et al. Interleukin-2 enhances the depressed natural killer and cytomegalovirus-specific cytotoxic activities of lymphocytes from patients with the acquired immune deficiency syndrome. J Clin Invest. 1983;72:398–403.

85. Mizuochi T, Goldberg H, Rosenberg AS, et al. Both L3T4$^+$ and Lyt-2$^+$ helper cells initiate cytotoxic T lymphocyte responses against allogeneic major histocompatibility antigens but not against trinitrophenyl-modified self. J Exp Med. 1985;162:427–33.
86. Gendelman HE, Orenstein JM, Martin MA, et al. Efficient isolation and propagation of human immunodeficiency virus on recombinant colony- stimulating factor 1-treated monocytes. J Exp Med. 1988;167:1428–31.
87. Smith PD, Ohura K, Masur H, et al. Monocyte function in the acquired immune deficiency syndrome. J Clin Invest. 1984;74:2121–8.
88. Prince HE, Moody DJ, Shubin BI, et al. Defective monocyte function in acquired immune deficiency syndrome (AIDS): evidence from a monocyte-dependent T-cell proliferative system. J Clin Immunol. 1985;5:21–5.
89. Poli G, Bottazzi B, Acero R, et al. Monocyte function in intravenous drug abusers with lymphadenopathy syndrome and in patients with acquired immunodeficiency syndrome: selective impairment of chemotaxis. Clin Exp Immunol. 1985;62:136–42.
90. Murray HW, Rubin BY, Masur H, et al. Impaired production of lymphokines and immune (gamma) interferon in the acquired immunodeficiency syndrome. N Engl J Med. 1984;310:883–9.
91. Pennington JE, Groopman JE, Small GJ, et al. Effect of intravenous recombinant gamma interferon in the respiratory burst of blood monocytes from patients with AIDS. J Infect Dis. 1986;153:609–12.
92. Washburn RG, Tuazon CU, Bennett JE. Phagocytic and fungicidal activity of monocytes from patients with acquired immunodeficiency syndrome. J Infect Dis. 1985;151:565.
93. Estevez ME, Ballart IJ, Diez RA, et al. Early defect of phagocytic cell function in subjects at risk for acquired immunodeficiency syndrome. Scand J Immunol. 1986;24:215–21.
94. Hofmann B, Odum N, Jakobsen BK. Immunological studies in the acquired immunodeficiency syndrome. Scand J Immunol. 1986;23:669–78.
95. Heagy W, Kelley VE, Strom TB, et al. Decreased expression of human class II antigens on monocytes from patients with acquired immune deficiency syndrome. J Clin Invest. 1984;74:2089–96.
96. Kleinerman ES, Ceccorulli LM, Zwelling LA, et al. Activation of monocyte-mediated tumoricidal activity in patients with acquired immunodeficiency syndrome. J Clin Oncol. 1985;3:1005–12.
97. Enk C, Gerstoft J, Moller S, et al. Interleukin 1 activity in the acquired immunodeficiency syndrome. Scand J Immunol. 1986;23:491–7.
98. Price RW, Brew B, Sidtis J, et al. The brain in AIDS: central nervous system HIV-1 infection and AIDS dementia complex. Science. 1988;239:586–92.
99. Gyorkey JF, Melnick JL, Gyorkey P. Human immunodeficiency virus in brain biopsies of patients with AIDS and progressive encephalopathy. J Infect Dis. 1987;155:870–6.
100. Dewhurst S, Bresser J, Stevenson M, et al. Susceptibility of human glial cells to infection with human immunodeficiency virus (HIV). FEBS Lett. 1987;213:138–43.
101. Chiodi F, Fuerstenberg S, Gidlund M, et al. Infection of brain-derived cells with the human immunodeficiency virus. J Virol. 1987;93:1244–7.
102. Gurney ME, Apatof BR, Spear GT, et al. Neuroleukin: a lymphokine product of lectin-stimulated T cells. Science. 1986;234:574–81.
103. Lee MR, Ho DD, Gurney ME. Functional interaction and partial homology between human immunodeficiency virus and neuroleukin. Science. 1987;237:1047–51.
104. Spivak JL, Bender BS, Quinn TC. Hematologic abnormalities in the acquired immune deficiency syndrome. Am J Med. 1984;77:224–8.
105. Delacretaz F, Perey L, Schmidt PM, et al. Histopathology of bone marrow in human immunodeficiency virus infection. Virchows Arch [A]. 1987; 411:543–51.
106. Belsito DV, Sanchez MR, Baer RL, et al. Reduced Langerhan's cell Ia antigen and ATPase activity in patients with the acquired immunodeficiency syndrome. N Engl J Med. 1984;310:1279–82.
107. Tschler E, Groh V, Popvic M, et al. Epidermal Langerhans cells—a target for HTLV-III/LAV infection. J Invest Dermatol. 1987;88:233–7.
108. Adachi A, Koenig S, Gendelman HE, et al. Productive, persistent infection of human colorectal cell lines with human immunodeficiency virus. J Virol. 1987;61:209–13.
109. Pomerantz RJ, de la Monte SM, Donegan SP, et al. Human immunodeficiency virus (HIV) infection of the uterine cervix. Ann Intern Med. 1988;108:321–7.
110. Pomerantz RJ, Kuritzkes DR, De La Monte SM, et al. Infection of the retina by human immunodeficiency virus type 1. N Engl J Med. 1987;317:1643–7.
111. Montagnier L, Gruest J, Chamaret S, et al. Adaption of lymphadenopathy associated virus (LAV) to replication in EBV-transformed B lymphoblastoid cell lines. Science. 1984;225:63–6.
112. Lane HC, Masur H, Edgar LC, et al. Abnormalities of B-cell activation and immunoregulation in patients with the acquired immunodeficiency syndrome. N Engl J Med. 1983;309:453–8.
113. Chess Q, Daniels J, North E, et al. Serum immunoglobulin elevations in the acquired immunodeficiency syndrome (AIDS): IgG, IgA, IgM, and IgD. Diagn Immunol. 1984;148–53.
114. Papadopoulos NM, Frieri M. The presence of immunoglobulin D in endocrine disorders and diseases of immunoregulation, including the acquired immunodeficiency syndrome. Clin Immunol Immunopathol. 1984;132:248–52.
115. Anderson KC, Boyd AW, Fisher DC, et al. Isolation and functional analysis of human B cell populations. J Immunol. 1985;134:820–7.
116. Pahwa SG, Quilop MTJ, Lange M, et al. Defective B-lymphocyte function in homosexual men in relation to the acquired immunodeficiency syndrome. Ann Intern Med. 1984;101:757–63.
117. Pahwa S, Pahwa R, Saxinger C, et al. Influence of the human T-lymphotropic virus/lymphadenopathy-associated virus on functions of human lymphocytes: evidence of immunosuppressive effects and polyclonal B cell activation by banded viral preparation. Proc Natl Acad Sci USA. 1985;82:8198–202.
118. Ammann AJ, Abrams D, Conant M, et al. Acquired immune dysfunction in homosexual men: immunologic profiles. Clin Immunol Immunopathol. 1983;27:315–52.
119. Ammann AJ, Schiffman G, Abrams D, et al. B-cell immunodeficiency in acquired immune deficiency syndrome. JAMA. 1984;251:1447–9.
120. Polsky B, Gold JWM, Whimbey E, et al. Bacterial pneumonia in patients with the acquired immunodeficiency syndrome. Ann Intern Med. 1986; 104:38–41.
121. Yarchoan R, Redfield RR, Broder S. Mechanisms of B cell activation in patients with acquired immunodeficiency syndrome and related disorders. J Clin Invest. 1985;78:439–47.
122. Pelicci PG, Knowles DM, Arlin ZA, et al. Multiple monoclonal B-cell expansions and c-myc oncogene rearrangements in AIDS-related lymphoproliferative disorders: implications for lymphomagenesis. J Exp Med. 1986;164:2049–60.
123. Schnittman SM, Lane HC, Higgins SE, et al. Direct polyclonal activation of human B lymphocytes by the acquired immune deficiency syndrome virus. Science. 1986;233:1084–6.
124. Pahwa S, Pahwa R, Good RA, et al. Stimulatory and inhibitory influences of human immunodeficiency virus on normal B lymphocytes. Proc Natl Acad Sci USA. 1986;83:9124–8.
125. Borst J, van de Griend RJ, van Oostveen JW, et al. A T-cell receptor γ/CD3 complex found on cloned functional lymphocytes. Nature. 1987;325:683–8.
126. Rook AH, Hooks JJ, Quinnan GV, et al. Interleukin 2 enhances the natural killer cell activity of acquired immunodeficiency syndrome patients through a γ-interferon-independent mechanism. J Immunol. 1985;134:1503–7.
127. Reddy MM, Chinoy P, Grieco MH. Differential effects of interferon-α_2 and interleukin-2 on natural killer cell activity in patients with acquired immune deficiency syndrome. J Biol Response Mod. 1984;3:379–86.
128. Lew F, Tsang P, Solomon S, et al. Natural killer cell function and modulation of α-IFN and IL-2 in AIDS patients and prodromal subjects. Clin Lab Immunol. 1984;14:115–21.
129. Creemers PC, Stark DF, Boyko WJ. Evaluation of natural killer cell activity in patients with persistent generalized lymphadenopathy and acquired immunodeficiency syndrome. Clin Immunol Immunopathol. 1985;36:141–50.
130. Hersh EM, Gutterman JU, Spector S, et al. Impaired in vitro interferon, blastogenic, and natural killer cell responses to viral stimulation in acquired immune deficiency syndrome. Cancer Res. 1985;45:406–10.
131. Bonavida B, Katz J, Gottlieb M. Mechanism of defective NK cell activity in patients with acquired immunodeficiency syndrome (AIDS) and AIDS-related complex. J Immunol. 1986;137:1157–63.
132. Katzman M, Lederman MM. Defective postbinding lysis underlies the impaired natural killer activity in factor VIII-treated, human T lymphotropic virus type III seropositive hemophiliacs. J Clin Invest. 1986;77:1057–62.
133. Pollack MS, Callaway C, LeBlanc D, et al. Lymphocytotoxic antibodies to non-HLA antigens in the sera of patients with acquired immunodeficiency syndrome (AIDS). In: Cohen E, Singal DP, eds. Non-HLA antigens in Health, Aging, and Malignancy. New York: Alan R. Liss; 1983: 209–13.
134. Kloster BE, Tomar RH, Spira TJ. Lymphocytotoxic antibodies in the acquired immune deficiency syndrome (AIDS). Clin Immunol Immunopathol. 1984;30:330–5.
135. Williams RC Jr, Masur H, Spira TJ. Lymphocyte-reactive antibodies in acquired immune deficiency syndrome. J Clin Immunol. 1984;4:118–23.
136. Dorsett B, Cronin W, Chuma V, et al. Anti-lymphocyte antibodies in patients with the acquired immune deficiency syndrome. Am J Med. 1985;78:621–6.
137. Tomar RH, John PA, Hennig AK, et al. Cellular targets of antilymphocyte antibodies in AIDS and LAS. Clin Immunol Immunopathol. 1985;37:37–47.
138. McDougal JS, Hubbard M, Nicholson JKA. Immune complexes in the acquired immunodeficiency syndrome (AIDS). J Clin Immunol. 1985;5:130–8.
139. Gupta S, Licorish K. Circulating immune complexes in AIDS. N Engl J Med. 1984;310:1530–1.
140. DeStefano E, Friedman RM, Friedman-Kien AE, et al. Acid-labile human leukocyte interferon in homosexual men with Kaposi's sarcoma and lymphadenopathy. J Infect Dis. 1982;146:451–5.
141. Buimovici-Klein E, Lange M, Klein RJ, et al. Long-term follow-up of serum-interferon and its acid-stability in a group of homosexual men. *AIDS Research*. 1986:99–108.
142. Hersh EM, Reuben JM, Rios A, et al. Elevated serum thymosin alpha$_1$ levels associated with evidence of immune dysregulation in male homosexuals with a history of infectious diseases or Kaposi's sarcoma. N Engl J Med. 1983;308:45.
143. Bhalla RB. Abnormally high concentrations of beta 2 microglobulin in acquired immunodeficiency syndrome (AIDS) patients. Clin Chem. 1983;29:1560.
144. Sarin PS, Sun DK, Thornton AH, et al. Neutralization of HTLV-III/LAV replication by anti-serum to thymosin α_1. Science. 1986;232:1135–7.
145. Koyanagi Y, Miles S, Mitsuyasu RT, et al. Dual infection of the central

nervous system by AIDS viruses with distinct cellular tropisms. Science. 1987;236:819–22.
146. Gendelman HE, Phelps W, Feigenbaum L, et al. Transactivation of the human immunodeficiency virus terminal repeat sequence by DNA viruses. Proc Natl Acad Sci USA. 1986;83:9759–63.
147. Mosca JD, Bednarik DP, Raj NBK, et al. Herpes simplex virus type-1 can reactivate transcription of latent human immunodeficiency virus. Nature. 1987;325:67–70.
148. Davis MG, Kenney SC, Kamine J, et al. Immediate-early gene region of human cytomegalovirus transactivates the promotor of human immunodeficiency virus. Proc Natl Acad Sci USA. 1987;84:8642–6.
149. Ostrove JM, Leonard J, Weck KE, et al. Activation of the human immunodeficiency virus by herpes simplex virus by type 1. J Virol. 1987;61:3726–32.
150. Broder S, Fauci AS. Progress in the development of drug therapies for AIDS. Public Health Rep. May-June 1988;103:224–8.
151. Smiley ML, White II GC, Becherer P, et al. Transmission of human immunodeficiency virus to sexual partners of hemophiliacs. Am J Hematol. 1988;28:27–32.
152. Eales LJ, Ke N, Parkin JM, et al. Genetic factors in susceptibility to HIV infection and to HIV related diseases: variation in Gc subtypes. Lancet. 1987;1:999–1002.
153. Gilles K, Louie L, Newman B, et al. Genetic susceptibility to AIDS: absence of an association with group-specific component. N Engl J Med. 1987; 317:630–41.
154. Daiger SP, Brewton GW, Rios AA, et al. Letter. N Engl J Med. 1987;17:631–2.
155. Curran JW, Jaffe HW, Hardy AM, et al. Epidemiology of HIV infection and AIDS in the United States. Science. 1988;239:610–6.
156. Farzadegan H, Polis MA, Wolinsky SM, et al. Loss of HIV-1 antibodies with evidence of viral infection in asymptomatic homosexual men. Ann Intern Med. 1988;108:785–90.
157. Sarngadharan MF, Veronese FM, Lee S, et al. Immunological properties recognized by sera of patients with AIDS and AIDS-related complex and of asymptomatic carriers of HTLV-III infection. Cancer Res. 1985;45:4574–7.
158. Montagnier L, Clavel F, Kurst B, et al. Identification and antigenicity of the major envelope glycoprotein of lymphadenopathy-associated virus. Virology. 1985;141:283–9.
159. Robert-Guroff M, Brown M, Gallo RC. HTLV-III-neutralizing antibodies in patients with AIDS and AIDS-related complex. Nature. 1985;316:72–4.
160. Weiss RA, Clapham PR, Cheingsong-Popov R, et al. Neutralization of human T-lymphotropic virus type III by sera of AIDS and AIDS-risk patients. Nature. 1985;316:69–72.
161. Weiss RA, Clapham PR, Weber JN, et al. Variable and conserved neutralization antigens of human immunodeficiency virus. Nature. 1986;324:572.
162. Matthews TJ, Langlois AJ, Robey WG, et al. Restricted neutralization of divergent human T-lymphotropic virus type III isolates by antibodies to the major envelope glycoprotein. Proc Natl Acad Sci USA. 1986;83:9709–13.
163. Lasky LA, Groopman JE, Fennie CW, et al. Neutralization of the AIDS retrovirus by antibodies to a recombinant envelope glycoprotein. Science. 1986;233:209–12.
164. Zagury D, Bernard J, Cheynier R, et al. A group specific anamnestic immune reaction against HIV-1 induced by a candidate vaccine against AIDS. Nature. 1988;332:728–31.
165. Putney SD, Matthews TJ, Robey WG, et al. HTLV-III/LAV-neutralizing antibodies to an *E. coli*-produced fragment of the virus envelope. Science. 1986;234:1392–5.
166. Krohn K, Robey WG, Putney S, et al. Specific cellular immune response and neutralizing antibodies in goats immunized with native or recombinant envelope proteins derived from human T-lymphotropic virus type III_B and in human immunodeficiency virus-infected men. Proc Natl Acad Sci USA. 1987;84:4994–8.
167. Cease KB, Margalit H, Cornette JL, et al. Helper T-cell antigenic site identification in the acquired immunodeficiency syndrome virus gp120 envelope protein and induction of immunity in mice to the native protein using a 16-residue synthetic peptide. Proc Natl Acad Sci USA. 1987;84:249–53.
168. Ho DD, Kaplan JC, Rackauskas IE, et al. Second conserved domain of gp120 is important for HIV infectivity and antibody neutralization. Science. 1988;239(4843):1021–3.
169. Ahearne PM, Matthews TJ, Lyerly HK, et al. Cellular immune response to viral peptides in patients exposed to HIV. AIDS Res Hum Retroviruses. 1988;4:259–67.
170. Robert-Guroff M, Reitz MS, Robey WG, et al. In vitro generation of an HTLV-III variant by neutralizing antibody. J Immunol. 1986;137:3306–9.
171. Montelaro RC, Parakh B, Orrego A, et al. Antigenic variation during persistent infection by equine infectious anemia virus, a retrovirus. J Biol Chem. 1984;259:10539–44.
172. Prince AM, Horowitz B, Baker L, et al. Failure of an HIV immune globulin to protect chimpanzees against experimental challenge with HIV. Proc Natl Acad Sci US. 1988;85:6944–8.
173. Earl P, Moss B, Morrison RP, et al. T-lymphocyte priming and protection against Friend leukemia by vaccinia-retrovirus env gene recombinant. Science. 1986;234:728–31.
174. Rook AH, Lane HC, Folks T, et al. Sera from HTLV-III/LAV antibody-positive individuals mediate antibody-dependent cellular cytotoxicity against HTLV-III/LAV-infected T cells. J Immunol. 1987;138:1064–7.
175. Ojo-Amaize EA, Nishanian P, Keith DE, et al. Antibodies to human immunodeficiency virus in human sera induce cell-mediated lysis of human immunodeficiency virus-infected cells. J Immunol. 1987;139:2458.
176. Ljunggren K, Böttiger B, Biberfeld G, et al. Antibody-dependent cellular cytotoxicity-inducing antibodies against human immunodeficiency virus. J Immunol. 1987;139:2263.
177. Weber JN, Clapham, Weiss RA, et al. Human immunodeficiency virus infection in two cohorts of homosexual men: neutralizing sera and association of anti-gag antibody with prognosis. Lancet. 1987;1:119.
178. Koenig S, Earl P, Powell D, et al. Group specific, major histocompatibility complex class I restricted cytotoxic responses to human immunodeficiency virus-1 envelope proteins by cloned peripheral blood T cells from an HIV infected individual. Proc Natl Acad Sci USA. 1988;85:8638–42.
179. Ruscetti FW, Mikovits JA, Kalyanaraman VS, et al. Analysis of effector mechanism against HTLV-1 and HTLV-III/LAV infected lymphoid cells. J Immunol. 1986;136:3619–24.
180. Weinhold KJ, Lyerly HK, Matthews TJ, et al. Cellular anti-GP120 cytolytic reactivities in HIV-1 seropositive individuals. Lancet. 1988;1:902–905.
181. Walker BD, Chakrabarti S, Moss B, et al. HIV-specific cytotoxic T lymphocytes in seropositive individuals. Nature. 1987;328:345–8.
182. Walker BD, Flexner C, Paradis TJ, et al. HIV-1 reverse transcriptase is a target for cytotoxic T lymphocytes in infected individuals. Science. 1988;240:64–66.
183. Quinnan GV. Detection of HLA restricted human immunodeficiency virus (HIV) envelope antigen-specific cytotoxic lymphocytes (CTL) [Abstract]. In: III International Conference on Acquired Immunodeficiency Syndrome (AIDS). Washington, DC: U.S. Department of Health and Human Services; 1987:59.
184. Koenig S, Earl P, Powell D, et al. Cytotoxic T cells directed against target cells expressing HIV-1 proteins [Abstract]. In: III International Conference on Acquired Immunodeficiency Syndrome (AIDS). Washington, DC: U.S. Department of Health and Human Services; 1987:59.
185. Zarling JM, Eichberg JW, Moran PA, et al. Proliferative and cytotoxic T cells to AIDS virus glycoproteins in chimpanzees immunized with a recombinant vaccinia virus expressing AIDS virus envelope glycoproteins. J Immunol. 1987;139:988–90.
186. Plata F, Autran B, Pedroza Martins L, et al. AIDS virus-specific cytotoxic T lymphocytes in lung disorders. Nature. 1987;328:348.
187. Koff WC, Hoth DF. Development and testing of AIDS vaccines. Science. 1988;241:426–32.

108. CLINICAL MANIFESTATIONS OF HIV INFECTION

RICHARD E. CHAISSON
PAUL A. VOLBERDING

Infection with the human immunodeficiency virus (HIV) results in a wide range of clinical consequences from asymptomatic carriage to life-threatening opportunistic infections and malignancies. The disease state called acquired immunodeficiency syndrome (AIDS) is at the terminal stage of this axis when the infected host can no longer control opportunistic organisms or malignancies that rarely cause illness in immunocompetent individuals. In persons infected with HIV, the sequential decline and ablation of cell-mediated immunity result in diverse manifestations of opportunistic disease. Those manifestations may vary according to the individual's age, race, geographic location, and behavioral history. This chapter will review the clinical features of HIV infection from the acquisition of the virus to death with AIDS and discuss the classification and evaluation of HIV-related syndromes.

HISTORY

Disease caused by HIV-induced immunosuppression was first described in late 1980 and early 1981 when physicians in Los

Angeles, New York, and San Francisco observed opportunistic infections in homosexual men.[1–4] Simultaneously, an outbreak of Kaposi sarcoma, a previously rare malignancy, was reported in young homosexual men from the same three cities.[5,6] These patients also had a selective defect in cell-mediated immunity that was manifested by low numbers of CD4+ T lymphocytes and the development of opportunistic infections.

That opportunistic diseases occurred in homosexual men who had been healthy previously suggested that immunodeficiency developed because of an acquired rather than a congenital trait. In 1982, the Centers for Disease Control (CDC) developed a case definition, based on the clinical, immunologic, and epidemiologic features of the first clusters of cases, for what was called the acquired immunodeficiency syndrome[7] (AIDS). AIDS was defined as the occurrence of a reliably diagnosed disease at least moderately indicative of underlying cellular immunodeficiency in a person without a condition known to be associated with an increased incidence of diseases related to cellular immunodeficiency.[6,8] AIDs became a reportable condition in 1983. Soon after the initial case reports of AIDS, additional cases were observed in persons other than homosexual men. In 1981 and 1982, heterosexual intravenous drug users and immigrants from Haiti were reported to have AIDS.[2,9–12] AIDS cases in hemophiliacs, recipients of blood transfusions, and Africans were also soon reported.[13,14]

While the groups of persons at risk for AIDS expanded, clinicans noted an increasing spectrum of clinical manifestations of AIDS-associated immunodeficiency. Unexplained generalized lymphadenopathy, idiopathic thrombocytopenia, oral candidiasis, herpes zoster, and a constitutional wasting syndrome were observed in persons from AIDS risk groups who had deficits in cellular immunity.[15–19] The term *AIDS-related complex* (ARC) was coined in 1984 to describe the symptoms of immunodeficiency recognized with increasing frequency in persons at risk for AIDS.[20] In 1982–1983, several investigators postulated an asymptomatic carrier state of the AIDS agent in healthy homosexual men, heterosexual partners of iv drug users, and Haitians who were noted to have laboratory evidence of impaired cellular immunity.[21] As discussed elsewhere, HIV was first described in 1983 by Barre-Sinoussi et al.[22] Gallo and coworkers and Levy and associates[23,24] confirmed the pathogenic nature and continuous culture of HIV in 1983–1984. Serologic tests to identify persons infected with HIV were developed shortly thereafter, and this allowed large serologic surveys of risk group members to estimate the number of individuals infected with the virus and to delineate the spectrum of HIV-associated diseases. The CDC expanded its case definition of AIDS in 1985 and again in 1987 (Table 1) to accommodate the increased number of manifestations of impaired cellular immunity that had become associated with chronic HIV infection.[7,25,26] The World Health Organization also promulgated a case definition for AIDS for use in developing countries that lacked sophisticated diagnostic resources (Table 2).[27] As the epidemic continues to grow and additional cases are observed, the list of diseases recognized as complications of HIV infection will undoubtedly be modified.

TABLE 1. CDC Surveillance Case Definition for AIDS

Diseases diagnosed definitively without confirmation of HIV infection in patients without other causes of immunodeficiency
Candidiasis of the esophagus, trachea, bronchi, or lungs
Cryptococcosis, extrapulmonary
Cryptosporidiosis >1 mon duration
Cytomegalovirus (CMV) infection of any organ except the liver, spleen, or lymph nodes in patients >1 mon old
Herpes simplex infection, mucocutaneous (>1 mon duration) or of the bronchi, lungs, or esophagus in patients? 1 mon duration
Kaposi sarcoma in patients <60 yr old
Primary CNS lymphoma in patients <60 yr old
Lymphoid interstitial pneumonitis (LIP) and/or pulmonary lymphoid hyperplasia (PLH) in patients <13 yr old
Mycobacterium avium complex or *M. kansasii* disseminated
Pneumocystis carinii pneumonia
Progressive multifocal leukoencephalopathy
Toxoplasmosis of the brain in patients >1 mon old
Diseases diagnosed definitively with confirmation of HIV infection
Multiple or recurrent pyogenic bacterial infections in patients <13 yr old
Coccidioidomycosis, disseminated
Histoplasmosis, disseminated
Isosporiasis >1 mon duration
Kaposi sarcoma, any age
Primary CNS lymphoma, any age
Non-Hodgkin's lymphoma (small, noncleaved lymphoma; Burkitt or non-Burkitt type; or immunoblastic sarcoma)
Mycobacterial disease other than *M. tuberculosis*, disseminated
M. tuberculosis, extrapulmonary
Salmonella septicemia, recurrent
Diseases diagnosed presumptively with confirmation of HIV infection
Candidiasis of the esophagus
CMV retinitis
Kaposi sarcoma
LIP/PLH in patients <13 yr old
Disseminated mycobacterial disease (not cultured)
Pneumocystis carinii pneumonia
Toxoplasmosis of the brain in patients >1 mon old
HIV encephalopathy
HIV wasting syndrome

(From Centers for Disease Control.[25])

TABLE 2. World Health Organization Adult Case Definition for AIDS

Major signs[a]
>10% weight loss
Diarrhea >1 mon duration
Fever >1 mon duration
Minor signs[a]
Cough >1 mon duration
General pruritic dermatitis
Recurrent herpes zoster
Oropharyngeal candidiasis
Progressive, disseminated herpes simplex
Generalized lymphadenopathy
Diagnostic of AIDS
Cryptococcal meningitis
Disseminated Kaposi sarcoma

[a] The presence of at least two major signs and one minor sign is diagnostic of AIDS.
(From World Health Organization,[27] with permission.)

CLASSIFICATION OF HIV INFECTION AND RELATED DISEASES

HIV is a pathogen that causes a variety of specific and nonspecific defects in immune function that result in diverse clinical consequences. AIDS, the end stage of HIV infection, currently affects only a small proportion of persons infected with HIV. HIV infection therefore represents the underlying disease process and will probably result in serious immunologic and clinical consequences (discussed below). While individuals who are HIV infected but asymptomatic should not be classified as being ill, they do have a chronic and progressive disease that may result ultimately in significant impairment and/or death.

Several systems to classify HIV infection and disease have been proposed.[26,29] The CDC bases its classification system for HIV infection on clinical manifestations. HIV-infected persons are placed into four categories: group I, acute infection; group II, asymptomatic seropositive; group III, persistent generalized lymphadenopathy; and group IV, symptomatic HIV disease (Table 3). Although clinically based, the CDC system has several drawbacks. The system is hierarchic (persons in a higher category are presumed to have more advanced disease); however, the categories do not reflect disease progression. A number of prospective studies have shown, for instance, that persistent, generalized lymphadenopathy (group III) is not associated with a greater degree of immunopathology or an increased risk of developing AIDS or other opportunistic processes than is asymptomatic infection without lymphadenopathy (group II).[30] Moreover, some manifestations of group IV (e.g., aseptic meningitis, subgroup IVB), may be early mani-

TABLE 3. CDC Classification System of HIV Infection

Group I. Acute infection
Group II. Asymtomatic infection
Group III. Persistent generalized lymphadenopathy
Group IV. Other diseases
- Subgroup A. Constitutional disease
- Subgroup B. Neurologic disease
- Subgroup C. Secondary infections diseases
  - Category C-1. Specified secondary infections diseases listed in the CDC surveillance definition for AIDS[a]
  - Category C-2. Other specified secondary infections diseases
- Subgroup D. Secondary cancers
- Subgroup E. Other conditions

[a] Includes those patients whose clinical presentation fulfills the definition of AIDS used by the CDC for national reporting.

festations of HIV infection and unrelated to its subsequent course.[31] Most importantly, the CDC system contains no prognostic variables and cannot be used to predict future immunologic deterioration and progression of the disease. The system has proved useful for surveillance and administrative purposes and has fostered the concept that an individual with HIV infection can be considered to have AIDS-related illness without manifesting life-threatening opportunistic diseases.

The Walter Reed (WR) staging system for HIV infection (Table 4) classifies patients on the basis of CD4 lymphocyte counts, skin test responsiveness, and the presence of lymphadenopathy, oral candidiasis, and opportunistic infections. The stages of the WR system are hierarchic, and they roughly parallel the natural history of HIV in infected individuals. This system is limited by several factors. While the predictive value of both CD4 lymphocyte counts and oral candidiasis have been established, cutaneous anergy and lymphadenopathy have not attained similar prognostic importance. The strata of CD4 cell counts used in the WR system may not be sensitive enough to give precise prognostic information. The system requires that skin tests be performed routinely—a practice that is often clinically cumbersome and impractical in managing large numbers of patients. As many as 30–70 percent of HIV-seropositives cannot be placed into WR stages because they have >400 CD4+ cells but are anergic.[32,33] The Walter Reed system must be prospectively evaluated before it is recommended for widespread application. Adding other laboratory markers of immunosuppression, discussed below, may strengthen the Walter Reed system.

We prefer to classify HIV-infected patients according to clinical and prognostic parameters (Table 5). Clinical outcomes can be categorized relative to acquiring the infection as early, middle, or late complications. Prognostic variables are laboratory measures that assess the degree of immunopathology caused by HIV and predict subsequent clinical deterioration and disease progression. Those laboratory markers are discussed below.

DIAGNOSIS OF HIV INFECTION

The diagnosis of HIV infection (see also Chapter 109) is best accomplished by detecting specific antibodies against viral antigens serologically. Directly detecting viral antigens and cocultivating the virus in cell culture are also possible; however, the former is relatively insensitive, and the latter is very expensive. Other diagnostic tests are being developed, including the use of polymerase chain reaction assays and other methods for detecting the viral genome. Use of the enzyme-linked immunosorbant assay (ELISA) for HIV antibodies, however, is the most sensitive, efficient, and practical way to diagnose HIV infection.

Detecting anti-HIV antibodies by ELISA is highly sensitive (>99 percent) and specific (95–99 percent). As with any diagnostic test, the predictive value of a positive test result depends on the prevalence of infected persons in the population being tested. A number of conditions including collagen-vascular diseases, chronic hepatitis, malaria, and certain HLA phenotypes have been associated with false-positive results on ELISA. The use of assays with recombinant antigens, which do not require culture in human cell lines, may significantly reduce the proportion of false-positive results. The cost-effectiveness of recombinant ELISA testing has not been demonstrated. Serum samples that are reactive by ELISA should be retested; repeatedly positive specimens should then be confirmed with a

TABLE 4. Walter Reed Staging System for HIV Disease

Stage	*HIV (Antibody/Antigen)*	*Lymphadenopathy*	*CD4+ Lymphocytes/mm³*	*Skin Tests*	*Thrush*	*Opportunistic Infection*
WR 0	−	−	>400	NL	−	−
WR 1	+	−	>400	NL	−	−
WR 2	+	+	>400	NL	−	−
WR 3	+	±	<400	NL	−	−
WR 4	+	±	<400	Partial anergy	−	−
WR 5	+	±	<400	Complete anergy	+	−
WR 6	+	±	<400	Complete anergy	+	+

Abbreviations: NL: normal.
(From Redfield et al.,[29] with permission.)

TABLE 5. Staging of HIV Disease

Stage	*Clinical*	*T4*	*p24Ag*	*β_2-Microglobulin*	*Hct*
Acute	Mononucleosis-like illness	Normal	+	Normal	Normal
Early	Asymptomatic or Persistent generalized lymphadenopathy Aseptic meningitis Dermatologic manifestations	>400	−	Normal	Normal
Middle	Asymptomatic or Persistent generalized lymphadenopathy Thrush Hairy leukoplakia Idiopathic thrombocytopenic purpura, etc.	200–400	±	Moderately high	Normal or low
Late	Opportunistic infections Malignancy Wasting Dementia	<200	±	High	Low

highly specific test such as an immunofluorescence assay (IFA) or a Western blot (WB). Other specific methods such as radioimmunoprecipitation assay are not practical for routine use in clinical laboratories. When confirmed reactive by IFA or WB, specimens should be considered true positives. Individuals positive by these tests should be informed that they are infected with HIV, counseled about the implications of HIV infection, and advised to eliminate behaviors that might result in transmitting the virus to others. Medical screening and follow-up should be offered to all HIV-seropositives.

The serologic response to HIV infection is shown in Figure 1. Shortly after exposure to the virus, a period of viremia and p24 antigenemia occurs. Antigenemia generally occurs within 2 weeks of exposure and lasts for several weeks. Both IgM and IgG antibodies to core (p24) and envelope (gp41, gp120) antigens develop 1–3 months after exposure, although longer periods of seroconversion have been documented. As a rule, infection with HIV and seropositivity for antibodies are lifelong. Rare cases of seroreversion (loss of specific antibodies after a period of antibody positivity) have been reported.[34] However, all four persons who seroreverted had HIV genome detected by polymerase chain reaction (in peripheral blood mononuclear cells).

Months to years after seroconversion, a significant proportion of HIV-infected individuals begin to lose antibodies to core antigens, although antibodies to envelope antigens, reverse transcriptase, and regulatory proteins remain. Most such individuals then develop core antigenemia; a minority may have antigen detected in the cerebrospinal fluid (CSF). Developing antigenemia presumably reflects an antigen-excess state, with anti-core antibodies consumed in immune complexes. This excess of antigen may signal increasing replication of the virus and carries a poor prognosis.

HIV antibody testing should be performed only for a valid medical or public health purpose. Patients being tested for HIV antibody should be told why they are being tested and should give consent for the procedure. Some states require written, informed consent before testing. Like all medical data, HIV antibody test results should be kept confidential; unauthorized disclosure should be vigorously avoided.

NATURAL HISTORY OF HIV INFECTION

The number of asymptomatic carriers of HIV far exceeds the number of persons with late complications or with AIDS. A number of studies have focused on the rate at which infected individuals progress to clinical disease and death. Initial reports indicated that fewer than 5 percent of seropositive individuals developed AIDS during several years of follow-up. Goedert and coworkers evaluated five small cohorts of HIV-seropositives and found 3-year progression rates of 5–36 percent.[35] Larger prospective studies now show that the rate of progression is high and grows as the length of time from infection increases.[36–38]

The rate at which AIDS develops in seropositive persons has been estimated by several studies to be approximately 4–10 percent per year of infection, with a low incidence in the first several years and an inflection upwards in the incidence curve thereafter. Eyster and colleagues studied a group of 85 hemophiliacs for whom seroconversion dates were known for a median of 4.5 years.[39] They found an actuarial rate of progression to AIDS at 18 percent 6 years after infection. Adults had a significantly higher progression rate (34 percent at 6 years) than did hemophiliacs less than 22 years old (10 percent at 6 years). The San Francisco Department of Public Health and the CDC have studied a cohort of 132 homosexual men in whom serconversion dates are known for a median of 8 years.[36,40] In this group, the actuarial progression rate to AIDS at 9 years was 42 percent; an additional 32 percent developed symptomatic conditions (ARC) that are not AIDS defining by surveillance criteria. Both of these studies, although small, show an increasing incidence of AIDS as the infection persists.

Studies of prevalent HIV infections have shown similar rates of progression to AIDS. Moss and associates followed 288 HIV-seropositive homosexual men for 3 years; they estimated that the median duration of infection was 6 years.[38] The 3-year actuarial rate of progression to AIDS was 22 percent; an additional 19 percent developed ARC (oral candidiasis, hairy leukoplakia, chronic diarrhea, or persistent constitutional symptoms). Moreover, the projected rate of progression to AIDS is 50 percent and to ARC is 25 percent at 6 years (or 9 years from infection) by extrapolating from predictors of progression at 3 years. Long-term projections of disease progression show that most seropositive subjects will develop illness in the 10–15 years after infection.[41]

Clinical and laboratory findings may help predict how the disease develops in seropositive subjects. Oral candidiasis (thrush), itself an opportunistic infection, is an early clinical marker of immunosuppression and heralds the development of AIDS in many patients.[42] Carne and colleagues studied 100 homosexual men with generalized lymphadenopathy and found that the risk of developing AIDS over an 18-month period increased 12-fold for subjects with thrush when compared with subjects without this finding.[43] Hairy leukoplakia, an opportunistic infection associated with Epstein-Barr virus (EBV), also predicts the development of AIDS. Greenspan et al. found that a referred population of homosexual men with hairy leukoplakia had an actuarial progression rate to opportunistic infection of 48 percent at 16 months and 83 percent at 31 months.[44] Dermatomal or disseminated outbreaks of herpes zoster appear

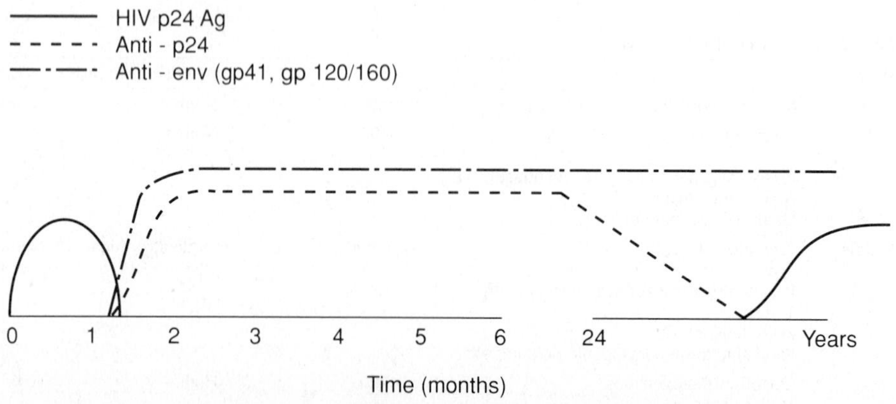

FIG. 1. Serologic response to HIV infection.

to be associated with the HIV infection, per se, but not with the progressive development of AIDS. One study of 112 homosexual men in New York City who had had an episode of shingles between 1980 and 1986 found that 73 percent had developed AIDS 6 years after the outbreak.[45] This finding, however, probably reflects an incubation period of HIV before full-blown AIDS symptoms developed. Prospective studies of seropositive homosexual men have failed to confirm zoster as a risk factor for progression to immunodeficiency. Generalized lymphadenopathy has also been proposed as a predictor of progression to AIDS, but prospective studies have failed to confirm this. One study found that average CD4+ lymphocyte counts were higher in homosexual men with lymphadenopathy than in seropositives without enlarged nodes.[30]

A number of laboratory tests have correlated progressive immunodeficiency and the development of AIDS.[46] CD4+ lymphocyte counts, a specific test for HIV-induced immunopathology, have sensitively predicted the development of AIDS and ARC. Goedert et al. found that CD4 cell counts $<300/mm^3$ were associated with a progression rate of 18.5 cases/100 person-years in seropositive homosexual men as compared with 1.5 cases/100 person-years for men with >550 CD4 cells/mm^3.[47] Polk and associates also showed that the development of AIDS was associated with a CD4 cell count of less than 300/mm^3 during a 15-month period of follow-up.[48] Moss and coworkers associated a baseline CD4 cell count of 200/mm^3 or less with a 3-year progression rate to AIDS of 89 percent; the rate for those with baseline CD4 counts of 200–400/mm^3 was 46 percent, and those with more than 400 cells/mm^3 had a 15 percent progression rate (Table 6).[38] Other studies have shown similar findings. Several studies have focused on the ratio of CD4 to CD8 cells and have shown higher rates of progression in individuals with ratios of less than 0.6.[48] Most studies find no independent association with the CD4:CD8 ratio when it is controlled for CD4 count. Likewise, the absolute number of CD8 cells falls in advanced infection with HIV and does not independently predict outcome. Other cell determinations that predict the development of AIDS in a seropositive individual include a total lymphocyte count of less than 1000, a total white blood cell count of less than 4000, a hematocrit of less than 40, and a low proportion of lymphocytes with the CD4 phenotype, regardless of the total CD4 count.[38,43]

As discussed earlier, the presence of HIV core antigen in the serum reflects either recent infection or an antigen-excess state from unchecked viral replication. In chronically infected subjects, HIV antigenemia is associated with a high rate of disease progression. Moss et al. compared initially antigenemic subjects with antigen-negative subjects. Of the antigenemic subjects 59 percent developed AIDS, and 30 percent developed ARC in 3 years as compared with 16 and 17 percent, respectively, for antigen-negative subjects.[38] Approximately 7 percent of antigen-negative subjects became antigenemic annually. Allain and coworkers showed that in hemophiliacs HIV antigenemia was a better predictor of progression to disease than was the CD4 cell count.[49] DeWolf and associates also found a higher rate of disease progression in antigenemic homosexual men in Amsterdam.[50] Conversely, Polk et al. reported that the rate of disease progression was higher in subjects who had lower titers of HIV antibody by ELISA,[48] a finding that probably reflects the loss of anti-core antibodies in persons with advanced disease. Weber and colleagues associated the loss of anti-p24 with the development of AIDS in a cohort of infected homosexual men.[51] Moss et al. found, however, that the absence of p24 antibodies did not predict disease progression independently of p24 antigen.

Levels of serum β_2-microglobulin, a low-molecular-weight immunoglobulin that forms the light chain of the class I major histocompatibility center (MHC) receptor, are elevated in HIV infection, particularly in subjects with advanced disease. A β_2-microglobulin level greater than 5 μg/ml was associated with a 3-year actuarial rate of AIDS of 69 percent in one study.[38] Subjects with a β_2-microglobulin level greater than 5 μg/ml had a seventeenfold greater hazard for developing AIDS than did seropositive subjects with normal levels. Both cytomegalovirus (CMV) infection and acid-labile interferon-α (INF-α) induce the synthesis of β_2-microglobulin. High titers of anti-CMV antibodies and acid-labile, INF-α have also been shown to predict disease activity in seropositive subjects.[48,52]

A number of researchers have extensively studied behavioral factors as predictors of disease progression; however, no convincing evidence has been found that individuals decrease the risk of becoming ill by modifying their behavior. In vitro, HIV replication can be induced by coinfection with herpesviruses. It has been theorized that in vivo exposure to potentially activating pathogens such as herpes simplex virus (HSV) or syphilis may lead to a greater degree of viral replication. Large prospective studies have not associated sexual activities, a history of sexually transmitted diseases, or exposure to specific infectious agent(s) with disease progression.[53] Epidemiologic cohort studies detect such influences poorly, however, and as a result, it is prudent to advise seropositive individuals to avoid other sexually transmitted diseases. Similarly, inactivated-virus vaccines stimulate and activate CD4 cells and, theoretically, may increase viral replication.[54] The use of influenza and pneumococcal vaccines in adults with HIV infection carries the same theoretic risk, but no in vivo evidence of harm exists.[55]

Antigenic stimulation by foreign proteins contaminating unsterile hypodermic needles (such as those used by iv drug users to inject drugs) may also increase the rate of progression of disease in seropositive drug users. DesJarlais et al. studied declines in CD4 cell counts in 163 HIV-infected drug users and found that subjects who continued to inject drugs had a greater loss of cells than did those who were abstinent.[56] While it is again prudent to advise seropositive addicts to avoid drug injection or needle sharing, the decline in CD4 cell counts during a very short period of follow-up cannot be assumed to reflect differential rates of developing AIDS. Continued drug injection, particularly cocaine injection, increases the risk of non-AIDS-associated infections such as absesses and endocarditis.[57]

Striking racial differences in the prevalence of AIDS and HIV infection, particularly among iv drug users, has led some investigators to speculate that genetic factors may lead to higher rates in acquiring the disease. Studies of HIV infection in drug users, however, suggest that racial differences are largely behavioral.[58] A widely reported study by Eales and associates in London stated that allelic differences in the group-specific pro-

TABLE 6. Predictors of Progression to AIDS in HIV Seropositive Homosexual Men

Variable	*Category*	*3-Year Rate of Progression[a] (%)*	*Relative Hazard*
CD4+ lymphocyte count	<200/mm^3	87	13.4
	200–400/mm^3	46	3.6
	>400/mm^3	16	1.0
CD4+ lymphocyte proportion (of total lymphocytes)	<25%	48	5.1
	≥25%	12	1.0
HIV p24 antigen	Positive	59	4.6
	Negative	15	1.0
Anti-p24 antibody	Negative	43	3.2
	Positive	16	1.0
β-2 microglobulin	>5 μg/ml	69	16.9
	3.1–5 μg/ml	33	4.5
	≤3 μg/ml	12	1.0
Hemoglobin	<13.5 g/dl	50	4.5
	≥13.5 g/dl	21	1.0

[a] Actuarial progression rate by product-limit method
(From Moss et al.,[38] with permission.)

tein (GC) predicted both HIV infection and the development of AIDS in infected subjects.[59] These investigators later retracted their findings and blamed malfunctioning laboratory equipment for generating erroneous data.[59a] The predilection of Kaposi sarcoma (KS) for certain racial and ethnic groups suggests a genetic predisposition that may explain the occurrence of KS in some persons with HIV infection. An early study found that KS was associated with the HLA-DR5 phenotype, but this finding has not been confirmed for other groups. Nevertheless, genetic differences in susceptibility to HIV infection or disease may exist.

Biologic differences in disease progression do exist. Age is an important factor in the rate at which AIDS develops in seropositive subjects. Eyster et al. reported that disease progression was three- to fivefold higher in adult hemophiliacs with HIV infection when compared with subjects under 21 years old.[39] Moss and associates observed a relative hazard of 2.2 for developing AIDS, independent of the CD4 cell count, in seropositive homosexual men over 35 years old.[38] Bacchetti et al. studied the first 500 AIDS cases in San Francisco and found that patients over the age of 40 had significantly shorter survival than did patients 20–39 years old.[60] This difference was most pronounced for patients with an initial diagnosis of Kaposi sarcoma. While immunocompetence is known to decline with senescence, the striking differences in disease progression and mortality by age are poorly understood.

Acute Retroviral Syndrome

In 1985 Cooper and colleagues in Australia identified an acute mononucleosis-like syndrome in 11 of 12 homosexual men who became antibody-positive for HIV antibodies.[61] Similar reports of a characteristic syndrome occurring in all AIDS risk groups, including health care workers exposed to accidental parenteral inoculation of HIV, were soon published.[62] The CDC classification system lists the acute retroviral syndrome as category I of HIV disease.

The incidence of the acute retroviral syndrome is not precisely known. Retrospective studies of homosexual men infected with HIV find a low prevalence of seroconversion illness.[63,64] A prospective study of homosexual men showed a 55 percent incidence of a mononucleosis-like illness in 22 subjects who become antibody-positive as compared with 21 percent in 44 nonconverting controls.[65] Other studies show a higher incidence of the syndrome. In a follow-up study to the report of Cooper et al., Tindall and associates evaluated 39 homosexual men known to have become antibody-positive and found that 36 (92 percent) recalled an illness consistent with the acute retroviral syndrome during the time when their tests showed seroconversion.[66] Forty percent of a seronegative control group also reported a mononucleosis-like illness, however. Most health care workers with occupational acquisition of HIV had the acute retroviral syndrome after exposure.[62,68] Overall, this syndrome is probably underreported and underdiagnosed; its true incidence may be between one-third and two-thirds of all persons who acquire HIV infection.

The clinical features of the acute retroviral syndrome are nonspecific and variable. The onset of the illness ranges from 1 to 6 weeks after exposure to the virus. Fever, sweats, malaise, myalgias, anorexia, nausea, diarrhea, and a nonexudative pharyngitis are prominent symptoms.[69,70] Many patients report headaches, photophobia, and meningismus. One-quarter to one-half of patients may have a truncal exanthem that may be maculopapular, roseola-like, or urticarial.[71] In addition to aseptic meningitis, neurologic symptoms occur in a minority of patients and may include encephalitis, peripheral neuropathy, and an acute, ascending polyneuropathy (Guillain-Barré syndrome).[72–77] Physical examination frequently reveals cervical, occipital, or axillary lymphadenopathy; rash; and less commonly, hepatosplenomegaly. Oral aphthous ulcerations have been reported in several cases; these may involve the esophagus. Oral and esophageal candidiasis during the seroconversion illness has been reported.[78] The remainder of the physical examination is usually unremarkable.

Laboratory evaluation of patients with the syndrome reveals a reduced total lymphocyte count, elevated sedimentation rate, negative heterophil-antibody test, and elevated transaminase and alkaline phosphatase levels.[66,79,80] When lymphocyte phenotyping is performed, a characteristic pattern is observed.[81] Initially, the total lymphocyte count decreases with a normal ratio of CD4 to CD8 T lymphocytes. Within several weeks, both the CD4 and CD8 cell populations begin to increase. The rise in CD8 cell numbers is relatively greater than is that in CD4 cells, and the CD4:CD8 ratio is inverted. In the weeks that follow, the CD8 cell population increases rather markedly. The total lymphocyte count also increases, and atypical lymphocytes may be seen on the peripheral smear. The ratio of CD4:CD8 cells usually remains inverted as the acute illness resolves (primarily due to excess numbers of CD8 cells). In patients with neurologic symptoms, cerebrospinal fluid may show a lymphocytic pleocytosis with normal levels of protein and glucose.[76,82]

Serologic studies of patients with the acute illness may be useful in making an early diagnosis. HIV core (p24) antigen may be detected in the serum and cerebrospinal fluid of patients with primary infection within 2 weeks of exposure, often coincidently with the onset of symptoms.[69,83] Antigenemia can persist for several weeks or months and generally resolves when antibodies to p24 are produced in sufficient quantity to form complexes with free antigen. The ELISA for HIV antibodies remains negative for an average of 2–3 months despite the appearance of specific antibodies on a Western blot of the patient's serum. Anti-p24 appears on the Western blot shortly before seroconversion is detected by ELISA and the appearance of antibodies to other antigens.[84] Prolonged seronegative, antigen-positive states have been reported, although the frequency of these states is not known.[85] Most investigators have observed seroconversion within several months of acute illness and the appearance of antigenemia.

The differential diagnosis of the acute retroviral syndrome includes a number of other illnesses: infectious mononucleosis; other viral infections such as influenza, measles, rubella, and herpes simplex; and secondary syphilis. Evaluation of patients presenting with an illness consistent with acute retroviral infection should include a careful history to elicit risks for HIV infection, laboratory tests to rule out mononucleosis and syphilis, HIV antibody and antigen tests, and complete blood counts and differential. Sera should be saved so that acute and convalescent titers of HIV and other viral antibodies can be performed.

Therapy for primary HIV infection is symptomatic and supportive. Fever, myalgias, and headaches may be treated with acetaminophen or nonsteroidal anti-inflammatory drugs. Bed rest and hydration may be necessary. Specific antiviral therapy has been proposed as postexposure prophylaxis for persons with known HIV exposures; however, the therapy is likely to be less effective after clinical symptoms appear than as an immediate intervention.

Persistent Generalized Lymphadenopathy

Infection with HIV is associated with a high prevalence of generalized lymphadenopathy, often beginning with the acute retroviral syndrome. In the early 1980s, clinicians in New York and San Francisco recognized persistent generalized lymphadenopathy (PGL) and suggested a prodromal state to the development of AIDS in homosexual men who were otherwise healthy.[15,16,86] The syndrome of PGL was defined as the presence of two or more extrainguinal sites of lymphadenopathy for a minimum of 3–6 months for which no other explanation could be found. Biopsy specimens of lymph nodes from such patients usually revealed a follicular hyperplasia without specific pathogens. An increasing proportion of these patients developed AIDS over time, thus linking PGL and AIDS before HIV was discovered.[87]

After becoming antibody-positive, approximately 50–70 percent of infected individuals develop PGL. The most frequently involved node groups are the posterior and anterior cervical, submandibular, occipital, and axillary chains; epitrochlear and femoral nodes may also be enlarged. Mediastinal and hilar adenopathy are not characteristic of the syndrome; however, abdominal computed tomography (CT) often reveals enlarged mesenteric and retroperitoneal adenopathy in HIV-infected persons. Although first described in homosexual men, PGL appears to occur with equal frequency in all infected groups. The natural history of PGL does not differ significantly from that of the HIV infection itself, although the CDC defines PGL as a separate category in its classification system for HIV disease (category III). Persistent generalized lymphadenopathy is a very sensitive marker of HIV infection: this finding in an individual who has no other reason for lymphadenopathy should prompt an evaluation for HIV, including HIV serologic testing.

Physical examination usually reveals symmetric, mobile, rubbery, lymph nodes ranging from 0.5 to 2 cm and distributed as previously described. Pain and tenderness are uncommon. Localized (i.e., asymmetric) adenopathy and rapid nodal enlargement are not characteristic and suggest an infectious or malignant process. The remainder of the physical examination is often unremarkable, although other complications of HIV infection may be found such as thrush or hairy leukoplakia. Laboratory evaluation is generally unrewarding, with the exception of HIV serology and T-cell subset phenotyping.

The differential diagnosis of PGL includes HIV infection and a wide variety of other processes that are associated with generalized lymphadenopathy: sarcoid, secondary syphilis, and Hodgkin's disease, for example. In patients with HIV infection, lymphadenopathy may also be caused by mycobacterial infections, Kaposi sarcoma, and lymphoma.[88] If not already known, the HIV serostatus should be determined with the patient's consent. Many patients who assume that they are infected with HIV decline to undergo serologic testing, although this preference is changing as both the knowledge of the natural history and the treatment of HIV advance. Aspiration of lymph nodes usually reveals benign cells.[89] Biopsy specimens show follicular hyperplasia, with the normal architecture distorted by greatly expanded germinal centers composed of B lymphocytes. The peripheral blood may also show a B-cell lymphocytosis and a polyclonal gammopathy.

Management of lymphadenopathy in a patient with known or suspected HIV infection should include node aspiration or biopsy in certain circumstances. Patients who may have been previously infected with *Mycobacterium tuberculosis* (e.g., iv drug users and persons from developing countries) have an increased risk of tuberculous adenitis and should be evaluated by aspiration or biopsy. A purified protein derivative (PPD) test should be administered to all patients. In addition, the presence of constitutional symptoms such as fever and weight loss with PGL merits a work-up to rule out lymphoma or opportunistic infection.[90,91] Likewise, localized or rapidly enlarging lymphadenopathy suggests an underlying infection or malignancy and should be evaluated by needle aspiration or biopsy. Fine-needle aspiration by an experienced pathologist is an acceptable alternative to biopsy and identifies infections and lymphomas very sensitively.[89,90] Follow-up biopsies for immunocytologic studies may need to be performed when a lymphoma is diagnosed by needle aspiration.

Most patients with PGL require no invasive evaluation and can be managed expectantly for the occurrence of other AIDS-related manifestations.

Immune Thrombocytopenia and Hematologic Manifestations

Thrombocytopenia was identified early in the AIDS epidemic in persons with high-risk groups. In homosexual men, thrombocytopenia was often diagnosed simultaneously with lymphadenopathy, while isolated thrombocytopenia was reported in iv drug users from the New York area. Prospective studies of persons with HIV infection now indicate that 5–15 percent of HIV-seropositives may have persistent thrombocytopenia (platelet count, $<100{,}000/mm^3$; a smaller proportion have platelet counts $<50{,}000/mm^3$). The natural history of HIV infection does not appear to differ in persons with immune thrombocytopenia and in nonthrombocytopenic persons, and specific risk factors for developing immune thrombocytopenia have not been identified.

HIV-related immune thrombocytopenia may be manifested by easy bruising, petechiae, bleeding gums, and prolonged bleeding from minor cuts and abrasions. Most patients are asymptomatic and are found to have low platelet counts incidently during routine clinical evaluation. More severe bleeding complications such as gastrointestinal (GI) hemorrhage or cerebrovascular bleeding are very rare. Platelet counts typically remain low for months to years, although platelet counts increase in some patients as HIV disease advances.

The pathophysiology of immune thrombocytopenia has been studied in both homosexual men and drug users, and the primary mechanism of disease has been identified as the peripheral destruction of platelets. Examination of the bone marrow usually shows normal or increased production of megakaryocytes and erythroid hyperplasia. Deposition of immune complexes on platelets has been postulated as one mechanism of destruction. Investigation of homosexual men with HIV-related immune thrombocytopenia showed the presence of a specific platelet membrane antigen against which antibodies were directed.[92] The same antigen and antibodies were also found, however, in HIV-infected controls without immune thrombocytopenia. Splenomegaly is often found on physical examination and is frequently present when abdominal CT scans are performed.[93]

A limited differential diagnosis of isolated thrombocytopenia in an HIV-infected person includes drug-induced thrombocytopenia, particularly in heroin addicts and alcoholics, consumptive thrombocytopenia, or splenic sequestration. Some patients with thrombocytopenia may also present with leukopenia or anemia. The presence of constitutional symptoms and pancytopenia suggests an opportunistic infection, particularly disseminated mycobacterial or fungal infection, or a lymphoma. Patients with these clinical findings should undergo bone marrow aspiration and biopsy, with appropriate stains and cultures. Isolated immune thrombocytopenia in an HIV-infected person can be managed expectantly by advising the patient to avoid aspirin and drugs that may exacerbate thrombocytopenia. Managing drugs associated with thrombocytopenia (e.g., rifampin) depends on the need for the drug and the degree of thrombocytopenia. If the patient does not have significant bleeding and maintains a platelet count above $20{,}000/mm^3$, the medication can be continued with close observation. If an alternative agent can be reasonably substituted, this should be done. Some patients with advanced HIV disease who are taking azidothymidine (AZT) may present with pancytopenia. While AZT is clearly associated with anemia and leukopenia, it does not cause thrombocytopenia; in fact, it significantly increases platelet counts in most patients.[94] This finding should be evaluated with appropriate diagnostic studies.

Other Hematologic Manifestations

HIV infection is associated with other abnormalities of the blood. Thrombotic thrombocytopenic purpura (TTP) has been reported in a small number of persons with HIV disease, and its clinical features appear to be similar to other populations. Intravascular hemolysis and thrombocytopenia are pronounced. The prevalence of TTP appears to be extremely low, and it is unclear whether HIV itself or another infectious agent is responsible for TTP in HIV-infected patients.

Anemia is a prominent feature of HIV disease. Most patients with advanced disease, particularly those with opportunistic infections, have a normochromic, normocytic anemia. The anemia is generally mild (hemoglobin content, 11–14 g/dl) and nonprogressive, although patients with a history of multiple opportunistic infections may have a hemoglobin level as low as 8–9 g/dl. Anemia is caused by a number of factors. HIV may infect erythroid precursors in the bone marrow[95] and inhibit the production of red cells; however, AIDS patients with anemia usually show normal myeloid and erythroid precursors and adequate iron stores upon aspiration and biopsy of the bone marrow. Sequestration of red cells in the spleen and, to a lesser extent, the liver may contribute to the anemia. Concurrent opportunistic infections or malignancies frequently depress the hematocrit value. Suppression of erythropoietin production may also affect red cell production.

The differential diagnosis of anemia in a person with HIV disease should include blood loss, infiltration of the bone marrow by opportunistic pathogens (e.g., *Mycobacterium avium* complex, *Histoplasma capsulatum*), malignancy, and drug toxicity. Depression of all cell lines suggests opportunistic disease, whereas isolated, mild anemia is most often associated with HIV. Bone marrow biopsy is not usually indicated in the latter situation. Although HIV-induced anemia generally does not require specific therapy, a low hematocrit predicts disease progression in asymptomatic HIV-seropositives.[38]

Constitutional Disease

Prolonged infection with HIV is often completely asymptomatic; however, a minority of patients complain of nonspecific constitutional symptoms in the months or years after primary infection. Patients commonly complain of being easily fatigued and report the need to reduce their normal activities somewhat. Debilitating fatigue is uncommon in the early years of infection. Low-grade fevers (temperature, <38°C), occasional night sweats, and intermittent diarrhea are also reported. The exact incidence of these findings is not known, and attributing them solely to HIV infection may be mistaken. The differential diagnosis of these findings includes intercurrent minor illnesses and psychological disorders. Anxiety and depression are common responses to knowledge or suspicion of HIV infection.[96] Many patients infected with HIV may have underlying psychiatric conditions. Intravenous drug users, in particular, have a high prevalence of affective disorders that may result in somatic complaints. Moreover, the physical effects of opiates and withdrawal from stimulants such as cocaine and amphetamines cause fatigue and other constitutional symptoms.

In patients with more advanced HIV disease and severe depletion of CD4+ cells, constitutional disease may primarily reflect immunosuppression or may herald the onset of opportunistic infections or malignancies. For example, the prodrome of *P. carinii* pneumonia (PCP) often consists of a month or more of fevers, weight loss, and fatigue before respiratory complaints develop. Disseminated mycobacterial infections typically cause fatigue, fever, night sweats, and diarrhea. In African patients with HIV infection, a wasting illness termed "slim disease" has been described.[97] These patients have debilitating fatigue, fevers, sweats, protracted diarrhea, and severe weight loss. Opportunistic or conventional pathogens are not revealed upon evaluation, but the patients waste away and die of severe malnutrition and terminal secondary infections. This illness has been encountered in developed countries as well, but far less commonly than in Africa—a pattern that suggests underdiagnosis of opportunistic diseases in Africa. One study of African patients with enteropathic slim disease found that most (16/22) had enteric pathogens or microsporidia found when a thorough evaluation was performed.[97a] In the United States, the CDC considers that an individual has AIDS when he has an unexplained constitutional disease for more than 1 month with a temperature greater than 38.3°C, diarrhea, and a loss of more than 10 percent of baseline body weight in the presence of HIV infection.[25]

Patients with progressive constitutional symptoms should be evaluated carefully for opportunistic pathogens. A history of respiratory, neurologic, gastrointestinal, and dermatologic symptoms should be elicited and a thorough physical examination completed. The skin may reveal characteristic lesions of Kaposi sarcoma or localized viral or bacterial infections. The oral cavity may show thrush (a finding extremely common in *P. carinii* pneumonia), hairy leukoplakia, oral Kaposi sarcoma, or other opportunistic processes. Asymmetric adenopathy should prompt an evaluation as outlined above. The chest findings are often normal, although rales or rhonchi indicating pulmonary infection may be heard. Abdominal examination may reveal hepatosplenomegaly or tenderness, particularly in the presence of retroperitoneal adenopathy. A rectal examination may show perirectal ulceration, vesicles, or erythema. A careful neurologic examination may identify evidence of global or focal neurologic impairment.

Laboratory evaluation should include a complete blood count, chemistry panel, and determination of T-cell subsets (if recent values are not available). An elevated erythrocyte sedimentation rate (ESR) is a sensitive, although nonspecific finding. A chest radiograph may reveal infiltrates, even though respiratory complaints are absent. When diarrhea is present, the stool should be evaluated as discussed below. Some clinicians find whole-body gallium scanning useful to evaluate systemic symptoms in HIV-infected patients because a focal uptake of gallium can identify clinically occult sites of opportunistic infection. Often, however, gallium may be taken up in the spleen and the transverse colon although a specific diagnosis is never reached. A physician should ascribe severe constitutional symptoms to HIV-induced wasting syndrome and diagnose AIDS *only* after a thorough evaluation.

Oral Disease

Abnormalities of the oral cavity occur throughout the course of HIV infection. Primary HIV infection has been associated with severe aphthous stomatitis and with oropharyngeal and esophageal candidiasis.[78] As the infection progresses and immunologic impairment proceeds, numerous oral complications arise. In the late stages of disease, oral manifestations are universal and frequently severe.[98,100]

Oral Candidiasis. *Candida* infections of the hard and soft palates, buccal mucosa, tongue, pharynx, and hypopharynx are observed frequently. Contrary to systemic *Candida* infections, which appear to result from defects in phagocyte function and number, mucosal candidal infections result from impaired cellular immunity. The incidence of candidiasis increases with progressive cellular immunodeficiency, particularly as CD4+ lymphocyte counts fall below 200–300/mm^3. Since oral candidiasis itself is an opportunistic infection, it predicts the disease progression and development of other AIDS-related infections.

A variety of manifestations of candidiasis have been described in HIV-infected patients. The most common form is thrush (pseudomembranous candidiasis). Characteristic cottage cheese plaques that can be removed with a tongue blade are seen on the soft palate, tonsils, and buccal mucosa. Less often, thrush involves the lateral and posterior aspects of the tongue, the hard palate, and the hypopharynx. *Candida* infection can produce flat, erythematous plaques distributed in the same way as the pseudomembranous form of the disease, but without the characteristic white exudate. This atrophic form of candidiasis is underdiagnosed because many clinicians are unfamiliar with its appearance. *Candida* can also cause a nonscrapable white plaque similar to hairy leukoplakia (see below). This hypertrophic form of disease may involve the lateral border of the tongue, the palate, and the buccal mucosa.

The diagnosis of candidiasis is frequently made on the basis of physical examination alone. A KOH preparation of scraped material from a plaque is diagnostic and can be performed easily in most clinical settings. Cultures for *Candida* are rarely necessary. Biopsy specimen of oral lesions can distinguish various forms of leukoplakia. A therapeutic trial of antifungal agents can also help to establish a diagnosis. *Candida* infection of the corners of the mouth (angular cheilitis) can cause pain, fissures, and difficulty opening the mouth. Physical examination, KOH preparation, and the response to antifungal therapy establish the diagnosis.

Hairy Leukoplakia. Originally described in 1984 by Greenspan et al., hairy leukoplakia (HL) is a raised, white lesion of the oral mucosa that is unique to HIV infection.[101] The lesion was initially described in homosexual men; it has subsequently been observed in all other groups of persons at risk for HIV infection.[102] Hairy leukoplakia appears asymptomatically when immunodeficiency has progressed to an advanced stage. In one prospective study of patients referred for evaluation of HL, the actuarial rate of progression to an AIDS-defining opportunistic infection was 85 percent at 2 years.[44] Other studies have shown a less dramatic (although substantial) rate of progression to AIDS after the diagnosis of HL.

The cause of HL is not completely understood, but it appears to be related to the replication of Epstein-Barr virus (EBV) in the epithelium of keratinized cells on the surface of the tongue and buccal mucosa.[104] Other herpesviruses have also been isolated from cultures of biopsied lesions; however, their role in the pathogenesis of HL is unclear. HIV is not routinely cultured from specimens and is not found with DNA probes. The diagnosis of HL is established by visual inspection, failure of the lesion to scrape off with a tongue blade, failure to respond to antifungal therapy, and by biopsy material or scrapings in which EBV can be identified.[104] Hairy leukoplakia is usually asymptomatic, although large lesions may impair taste, hinder eating, and cause discomfort.

Severe gingivitis and periodontitis have been observed in patients with HIV disease.[98] The onset of symptoms is often insidious but may be abrupt. Pain is often severe; patients may note foul breath, bleeding gums, and loosening of teeth. Physical examination may reveal a bright red marginal line on the gingiva, necrosis and ulceration of interdental papillae, gingival erosion, exfoliation of enamel, and loose teeth. The etiology of gingivitis and periodontitis is unclear. Mixed cultures of aerobic and anaerobic flora have been obtained from gingival biopsy samples. More severe, ulcerating gingivitis can be caused by infections with gram-negative bacilli, particularly *Klebsiella pneumoniae* and *Enterobacter cloacae*. Infections tend to be chronic, but topical antiseptic agents or metronidazole therapy may control some cases.

Peripheral Neuropathy

In most patients with AIDS, the peripheral nervous system is involved, and 20–40 percent of patients may have symptomatic peripheral nerve disease.[105,106] Symptoms may occur at any time during the course of HIV infection. Each stage of the infection is associated with specific neuropathies, as outlined in Table 7. The most common peripheral neuropathy, a distal, predominantly sensory polyneuropathy, accounts for at least 50 percent of cases.[107] Patients with this neuropathy usually complain of chronic, symmetric, painful dysesthesias in a stocking distribution, particularly in the soles; numbness; and (less often) weakness. Some patients feel pain when lightly touched. Sensory deficits, decreased or absent ankle jerks, and weakness may also be observed on examination, and patellar reflexes may be brisk. Electromyography shows a combined sensory and motor neuropathy consistent with demyelination in the lower extremities. Nerve biopsy may reveal axonal degeneration. Distal, sensory neuropathy is most often found in patients with advanced symptomatic HIV disease.

TABLE 7. Peripheral Neuropathies in HIV Disease by Stage

Disorder	*Seropositive*	*ARC*	*AIDS*
Guillain-Barre Syndrome	—————	———→	
Chronic inflammatory demyelinating polyneuropathy	—————	—————	———→
Multiple mononeuropathy		—————	———→
Sensory neuropathy		—————	———→

Abbreviation: ARC: AIDS-related complex.
(Adapted from McArthur,[106] with permission.)

Chronic inflammatory demyelinating polyneuropathy (CIDP), the second most common peripheral neuropathy, tends to occur before other clinical manifestations of HIV develop.[108,109] Acute, inflammatory, demyelinating polyneuropathy (Guillain-Barré syndrome) is also reported early in the course of HIV disease. Patients report motor weakness that occurs acutely or gradually and have minimal sensory complaints. Weakness and areflexia are often noted on examination; a CSF pleocytosis is often present and the CSF protein level elevated. Nerve biopsy shows mononuclear cell infiltration and demyelination. The clinical course may wax and wane, and some patients recover spontaneously. Inflammatory demyelinating polyneuropathies may be associated with CMV infection, although the etiology may be autoimmune.[110]

Other rarer neuropathies include multiple mononeuropathy, possibly associated with vasculitis, herpesvirus and CMV radiculitis, and neuropathies of vitamin deficiency.

Musculoskeletal Complications

Polymyositis complicates HIV infection in a small number of patients.[111,112] Clinical features include myalgias, weakness of the proximal muscles, muscle tenderness, wasting, and fatigue. Creatinine kinase and other muscles enzyme concentrations are usually elevated, and electrophysiologic studies are consistent with a myopathy. Biopsies reveal muscle fiber necrosis and inflammatory infiltrates. Recent reports suggest that patients taking zidovudine (AZT) may be at increased risk for myopathy, although this not not been proved in prospective studies.[113]

Several reports have postulated the existence of an HIV-associated arthropathy.[114,115] Defining a specific arthropathy caused by HIV is difficult because many patients with HIV infection are already at increased risk for inflammatory joint disease. Intravenous drug users, for example, may develop septic arthritis caused by pyogenic bacteria, particularly *Staphylacoccus aureus*. Homosexual men may have increased risk of gonococcal arthritis or reactive arthritis associated with genital or gastrointestinal tract infections (Reiter syndrome). In patients with HIV infection, immune complex deposition or hepatitis B infection may also contribute to arthritis. HIV-associated arthropathy probably does exist since retrovirally induced arthritis is seen in other species.

Rheumatologic complications of HIV are highly prevalent. One prospective study of patients with HIV infection found that 71 percent had rheumatic manifestations (Table 8).[116] Arthralgias, arthritis, Reiter syndrome, and an oligoarticular painful syndrome were the most common findings. Arthralgias were intermittent and involved primarily the knees, shoulders, ankles, and elbows. Arthritis in HIV-seropositive patients may be due to a variety of conventional causes, or it may be unexplained and associated temporally with AIDS-related opportunistic infections. In the latter case, a painful mono- or oli-

TABLE 8. Frequency of Rheumatologic Manifestations in 101 Patients with HIV Disease

Manifestation	*Patients (%)*
Arthralgias	35
Arthritis	12
Reiter syndrome	10
Painful articular syndrome	10
Psoriatic arthritis	2
Polymyositis	2
Vasculitis	1
Total	71

(From Berman et al.,[116] with permission.)

goarticular inflammatory arthritis is present, often affecting the large joints.[114–116] The arthritis is nondeforming and nonerosive.

Aspirating the synovial fluid is generally unremarkable, and synovial biopsy specimens show mononuclear cell infiltrates. HIV has been cultured from the synovial fluid of one patient, although the meaning of this finding is not clear. The erythrocyte sedimentation rate may be elevated; other studies are nonspecific. Some patients may be HLA-B27–positive. In one series, a precipitating infection was detected in only 3 of 13 patients, although 7 additional patients had diarrhea and/or urethritis of undetermined etiology.[114]

The clinical course is often progressive. Some patients show little response to anti-inflammatory drugs, and most clinicians are reluctant to use cytotoxic or immunosuppresive drugs in such patients.

Reiter syndrome in HIV-infected persons can be particularly severe. Patients with this syndrome are usually HLA-B27–positive and present with an asymmetric oligoarticular arthritis and sacroiliitis with a variety of extra-articular signs and symptoms.[117] Reiter syndrome may occur in advanced HIV infection because of yet-unexplained immunologic mechanisms or the susceptibility of this population to infections with arthritogenic agents. Managing these patients clinically is difficult because the symptoms may not respond to nonsteroidal anti-inflammatory agents.

Berman et al. have described a painful articular syndrome in patients with advanced HIV infection.[116] This syndrome is characterized by excrutiating, oligo- or monoarticular pain that starts abruptly and resolves in several hours to 1 day. Physical examination of the joints is negative. The cause of this syndrome is not known, and it has not been widely reported.

Other rheumatic manifestations of HIV that have been reported include psoriatic arthritis, sicca syndrome, and vasculitis.[118] Prospective studies of populations of HIV-infected persons are necessary to further delineate the spectrum of HIV-associated musculoskeletal conditions.

Cutaneous Manifestations

Dermatologic consequences of HIV infection include primary cutaneous opportunistic infections and malignancies (that may also disseminate to the viscera) and systemic, opportunistic diseases with skin involvement. Examples of the former include Kaposi sarcoma (discussed subsequently) and dermatophytoses; the latter are exemplified by herpesvirus infections, syphilis, and fungal infections such as cryptococcosis.

Viral Infections of the Skin and Mucus Membranes. A wide range of viruses involve the skin in HIV-immunosuppressed patients. Herpesviruses in particular cause frequent morbidity in patients with advanced HIV disease. Serology documents previous infection with HSV-2 in more than 90 percent of homosexual men with HIV infection; it is less prevalent in other AIDS risk group members.[229] While HSV-2 recurs frequently even in nonimmunosuppressed hosts, it occurs frequently and for prolonged periods in patients with HIV infection. The CDC considers chronic mucocutaneous HSV-2 disease (<1 month) diagnostic of AIDS by its surveillance criteria. HSV-2, a common pathogen of the sacral root dermatomes, often causes outbreaks in the buttocks, perineum, scrotum or vulva, and the shaft and glans of the penis. Characteristic lesions of herpes appear first as painful erythematous papules; later they vesiculate and ulcerate, and in superinfection, pustules may form. Chronic ulcers may become granulated and bloody. Herpes proctitis is associated with severe rectal pain, fever, tenesmus, and obstipation. External lesions may be absent, and the diagnosis is established by anoscopic or sigmoidoscopic examination and cultures. Giant perirectal ulcers that yield thymidine kinase–resistant strains of HSV-2 have been reported in patients who were previously treated with acyclovir. Herpes simplex virus infections are diagnosed by the typical appearance and distribution of the lesions and culture. Tzanck preparations may show giant cells, which suggests HSV infection. Some physicians base their diagnoses on how patients respond to an empirical trial of acyclovir. Orolabial HSV infections in HIV-infected persons may be caused by either HSV-1 or HSV-2. While primary infections may occur after patients acquire HIV, recurrences are more common. Often, a prodrome of tingling and pain precedes the appearance of painful vesicles and ulcers. Lesions may be found on the lips, buccal mucosa, gingiva, soft palate, uvula, and tongue. Herpes simplex virus disease may recur chronically in patients with advanced immunosuppression.

In persons with HIV infection, varicella-zoster virus (shingles) often reactivates. As a result, the virus has been proposed as a marker of disease progression.[230] Prospective clinical trials have failed, however, to associate shingles and the subsequent development of AIDS. Dermatomal outbreaks are most common, and a substantial proportion of patients may have several dermatomes involved. Shingles is often characterized by radicular pain and itching several days before erythematous papules appear, and vesiculation occurs within several days. Lesions are often extremely pruritic, and excoriation with secondary bacterial infection commonly occurs. Over a period of 4–7 days lesions form bullae and crust and begin to heal, although some patients have zoster chronically. Cranial and thoracic dermatomes, followed by lumbar and sacral roots, are most often involved. Outbreaks along the ophthalmic branch of the trigeminal nerve may result in corneal involvement and lead to scarring and opacification that impair vision. Varicella-zoster virus appears to disseminate less often in patients with HIV infection than in other immunosuppressed patients. A substantial proportion of patients may experience post-herpetic scarring and pain. Although considered extremely rare before AIDS, recurrences of zoster have been reported from a number of patients with HIV infection. Chronic or nonremitting zoster has also been observed.

Molluscum contagiosum, a cutaneous poxvirus infection, is seen more often in HIV-infected persons than in other populations. The agent is transmitted by sexual or other close contact; reactivation of remote infection may cause outbreaks in immunosuppressed hosts. Molluscum lesions are small, firm papules with a pearly white surface distributed on the face, trunk, or genital areas. The lesions are usually painless and can be differentiated from herpetic lesions by the absence of erythema and the smaller size and resolution of lesions without ulcerating or crusting. Molluscum lesions can become superinfected with bacteria if they become excoriated, but otherwise they do not cause complications. Liquid nitrogen is used effectively to treat this condition.

LATE SYNDROMES

Gastrointestinal Syndromes

As HIV infection progresses, diseases of the gastrointestinal tract occur with greater frequency. Virtually every component of the gut represents a potential site of pathologic involvement.[119] Functional alimentation and nutrition are deranged, and this poses an additional burden on patients. Besides opportunistic disease resulting from HIV-induced immunodeficiency, persons with AIDS may have more common gastrointestinal problems exacerbated by advanced systemic illness. Therefore, clinicians evaluating gastrointestinal complaints in HIV-infected patients must consider conventional gut pathology.

Esophageal Disease. Several specific agents cause esophageal pathology in HIV infection. Esophagitis secondary to infections by *Candida*, cytomegalovirus, and herpes simplex viruses are the most common opportunistic manifestations of HIV disease in the upper GI tract.[120–123] In approximately 3 percent of AIDS cases in the United States, esophageal candidiasis is the presenting AIDS diagnosis. Other esophageal infections are less common. The subsequent development of esophageal disease after another index AIDS diagnosis is not unusual.

These processes most commonly present with odynophagia, often associated with persistent or intermittent retrosternal pain, nausea, anorexia, and weight loss. Dysphagia without pain is also encountered and may be associated with opportunistic infection, particularly esophageal candidiasis. The duration of symptoms may be brief or prolonged, and other manifestations of immunodeficiency often coincide. In particular, the finding of oral candidiasis in a patient with odynophagia strongly suggests esophageal involvement. While one site of another pathogen (e.g., CMV retinitis) may suggest a secondary esophageal process with the same organism, multiple etiologies of diverse organ system disease in AIDS is remarkably common.

Evaluation of patients with symptoms of esophagitis begins with a careful physical examination. The finding of oropharyngeal candidiasis strongly suggests esophageal candidiasis, and physicians may elect a trial of antifungal therapy. If symptoms resolve, the diagnosis can be established empirically. In patients who do not have oral thrush or who fail to respond to empirical antifungal therapy, upper gastrointestinal contrast radiography may show characteristic abnormalities that suggest a specific diagnosis. *Candida* esophagitis is associated with a classic pattern of diffuse ulcerations and plaques that creates a cobblestone appearance. Cytomegalovirus esophagitis frequently causes numerous, large, shallow ulcerations, although single ulcers are also reported. Herpes simplex infection of the esophagus usually produces multiple, deep ulcers. Esophageal endoscopy is a highly sensitive procedure to establish a diagnosis in patients with odynophagia or dysphagia. Friable cheesy plaques that may be easily removed with biopsy forceps are characteristic in candidal esophagitis, while diffuse erythematous ulcers are more common in viral esophagitis.[119] Lesions should be biopsied and tissue sections prepared for histopathologic stains to identify viral inclusion bodies or invasive yeast forms. Cultures for fungi and viruses should also be obtained from biopsy specimens. The yield of contrast radiography and of endoscopy with biopsy and culture are extremely high; additional diagnostic manuevers are not usually required. Additional pathology that may be found in evaluating esophageal symptoms in HIV-infected patients includes reflux esophagitis, esophageal Kaposi sarcoma, lymphoma, carcinoma, or peptic ulcer disease.

Disorders of the Stomach, Small Bowel, and Hepatobiliary System. As with esophageal diseases in HIV-infected patients, gastric disease may be opportunistic or may be unrelated to immunodeficiency. Common complaints include nausea, early satiety, anorexia, vomiting, hematemesis, and abdominal pain. Esophageal pathology may also involve the stomach. Cytomegalovirus gastritis has been described alone or associated with esophageal CMV ulcers. Cytomegalovirus gastritis causes an intense inflammatory response, ulceration, enlargement of ruggal folds, and edema. Cytomegalovirus gastritis may appear on a radiograph to be a mass lesion engulfing the entire stomach. Gastric Kaposi sarcoma is a common complication of cutaneous KS and is often asymptomatic.[124] The GI tract is the organ system most involved in visceral KS, and gastric lesions may occur in 25 percent of patients who undergo endoscopy. Occasionally, gastrointestinal KS may be associated with nausea, early satiety, severe pain, and gastrointestinal hemorrhage.

Barium contrast radiographs aid in evaluating an HIV-seropositive patient with gastric symptoms. They may show typical abnormalities such as duodenal ulcers, gastroesophageal reflux, or gastritis. Patients with a history of alcohol abuse may develop any of the upper GI complications of chronic alcoholism. When radiographic studies suggest non–AIDS-related pathology, standard therapy should be offered. If no response is observed, further diagnostic procedures are warranted. Upper GI contrast radiographs may reveal specific lesions consistent with an opportunistic process. Gastric KS appears in radiographs as an ulcerated, target lesion with underlying submucosal masses.

Definitive diagnoses of upper GI pathology may be made by endoscopic observation, biopsy, and culture. Kaposi sarcoma typically appears as a violet-blue submucosal mass without mucosal ulceration or bleeding. Biopsy of these lesions results in a histologic diagnosis in only about one-third of the cases—presumably because of the nonmucosal location of the tumor.[119] When other KS lesions are histologically confirmed, observing characteristic lesions on endoscopy is sufficient to make a diagnosis. Gastric lymphomas are diagnosed by endoscopic biopsy with histologic and immunohistochemical stains. Like KS, AIDS-related lymphomas are almost always multifocal, so a biopsy of the most accessible lesion can establish a diagnosis. Gastric ulcers and mass lesions should be sent for viral culture, and standard histologic stains should be performed to identify viral inclusion bodies.

Acalculous cholecystitis has been associated with both *Cryptosporidium* and CMV infections.[125,126] The usual presentation is postprandial pain, fever, right upper quadrant pain and tenderness, and an elevated alkaline phosphatase level. Ultrasonography or computed tomography may reveal typical findings of cholecystitis as well as a thickened gallbladder wall and obliteration of the bladder lumen. On histologic study, Cryptosporidia have been seen in the gallbladder mucosa, as have CMV inclusions.

Papillary stenosis and sclerosing cholangitis have been documented in a growing proportion of AIDS patients who present with right upper quadrant pain and tenderness, fever, and an elevated alkaline phosphatase level.[127,128] Dilatation of intrahepatic and extrahepatic ducts is noted on ultrasonography, and papillary stricture is frequently observed. In 75 percent of the patients studied, Cello and coworkers reported that endoscopic retrograde cholangiopancreatography identified cholangitis, ductal sclerosis, isolated papillary stenosis, or a combination of these findings.[119] Papillary stenosis was associated with *Cryptosporidium* or CMV in almost one-half of the cases. Jacobson et al. found that 12 of 36 patients with CMV end-organ disease had cholestatic liver enzyme abnormalities, and one-third of those undergoing ultrasound had biliary dilatation.[129] A significantly higher proportion of AIDS patients with CMV cultured from the blood have elevated liver enzymes than patients with negative blood cultures. Endoscopic sphincterotomy may significantly relieve pain and normalize the alkaline phosphatase level in patients with sclerosing cholangitis.

Liver disease in AIDS patients is extremely common.[130–132] It may result from previous injury (e.g., hepatitis B infection, non-A, non-B hepatitis, or alcoholic liver disease) or HIV disease. Right upper quadrant pain, hepatomegaly, and elevated liver function test values are the common presenting features. Both *M. avium* complex (MAC) and Kaposi sarcoma are frequently found in the liver. In one series, KS was the most common postmortem diagnosis, and MAC was the most frequently identified pathogen when a percutaneous liver biopsy was performed.[132] Forty percent of biopsies and autopsies demonstrated HIV-related pathologies. In addition to MAC and KS, other diagnoses included lymphoma, tuberculosis (TB), CMV infection, and viral hepatitis. Alcohol-related pathology was also commonly identified. Frequently, patients whose clinical findings suggest liver disease may be diagnosed on the basis of noninvasive tests or biopsies of other organs. When a primary hepatic process appears likely or when other diagnostic procedures fail to reveal a cause of the symptoms, percutaneous liver biopsy is indicated. Specimens should undergo standard histologic and microbiologic staining and should be cultured for viruses, fungi, and mycobacteria. Hepatotoxicity of drugs used to treat HIV-related disorders should also be considered when evaluating patients with liver dysfunction. Rarer causes of infiltrative liver disease in patients with HIV disease include hepatic pneumocystosis, leishmaniasis, histoplasmosis, and other fungal infections.

Enterocolitis. Small and large bowel infections and disease processes may cause symptoms in association with HIV infection. Table 9 lists the principal causes of lower gastrointestinal tract disease in patients with AIDS. A variety of infectious agents may produce diarrhea, abdominal cramping, and pain, and they may be managed less readily by a host with HIV-induced immunosuppression. Before the AIDS epidemic, both symptomatic and asymptomatic gastrointestinal infections were found to be prevalent in homosexual men. Asymptomatic carriage of some pathogens has also been observed in patients with HIV infection and AIDS.[133] The incidence of gastroenteritis in patients with HIV infection is high, and some specific infections (e.g., *Salmonella*, *Cryptosporidium*, *Isospora*, CMV, *Microsporidia*) have been found to occur more frequently in AIDS patients.

Small bowel infections generally produce bloating, nausea, cramping, and profuse diarrhea and may be associated with significant weight loss. Colitis and proctitis more often cause lower quadrant cramping and pain, urgency, tenesmus, and smaller, more frequent stools. Distinguishing small bowel infections and colitis clinically may be difficult, however, and some infections may cause a panenteritis. The differential diagnosis of enterocolitis includes bacteria (such as *Salmonella*, *Shigella*, *Campylobacter*, mycobacteria) protozoa (such as *Entamoeba histolytica*, *Giardia lamblia*, *Cryptosporidium*, *Isospora*), and cytomegalovirus. In addition, *Clostridium difficile*-associated colitis may be more common in patients with HIV disease, particularly in those who have previously received antimicrobial therapy.

TABLE 9. Lower Gastrointestinal Tract Disease in Patients with HIV Infection

Causes of enterocolitis
Bacteria
Campylovacter jejuni and other spp.
Salmonella spp.
Shigella flexneri
Mycobacterium avium-complex
Clostridium difficile (toxin)
Parasites
Cryptosporidium spp.
Entamoeba histolytica
Giardia lamblia
Isospora spp.
Viral
Cytomegalovirus
HIV (?)
Causes of proctocolitis
Bacteria
Chlamydia trachomatis
Neisseria gonorrhoeae
Treponema pallidum
Viral
Herpes simplex

Patients with AIDS and diarrhea frequently have an enteric pathogen that is identified when stool studies are performed. Infectious agents have been found in 55–85 percent of AIDS patients who present with diarrhea[134]; from 10 to 40 percent of AIDS patients without diarrhea are infected with an enteric pathogen.[133] Asymptomatic HIV-seropositive patients also carry intestinal pathogens at a high rate. Treatable pathogens are found in about one-half of patients studied. Cytomegalovirus and *Cryptosporidium* are the most often identified enteric pathogens in symptomatic patients; next are *Giardia*, *Salmonella*, *Campylobacter* and *C. difficile*. More extensive, invasive diagnostic evaluations probably yield a higher number of pathogens.

Renal Disease

Renal abnormalities have been described in a variety of patients with AIDS, but it is still debated whether a specific AIDS-associated nephropathy (AAN) exists. Ascribing renal dysfunction to HIV infection or AIDS is problematic because some AIDS patients have a high risk for renal disease. Intravenous drug use, hepatitis B infection, fluid and electrolyte disorders, therapy with nephrotoxic drugs, and concomitant opportunistic infections and malignancies are all associated with renal dysfunction. In 1984, Rao and colleagues reported on 11 AIDS patients who had renal disease.[135] The patients were characterized clinically by proteinuria and mildly elevated serum creatinine levels and pathologically by focal and segmental glomerulosclerosis. While this entity is similar to heroin-associated nephropathy, only one-half of the patients studied gave a history of iv drug use. In a review of 75 consecutive AIDS patients in Miami, 43 percent of the patients had proteinuria >0.5 g/24 hr; 9 percent had >3 g/24 hr.[136] In 36 autopsied patients, 17 (47 percent) had renal pathology, 5 had focal glomerulosclerosis, and 12 had mesangial proliferation. A subsequent review of the same patient population found that patients with a history of iv drug use had the highest incidence of renal disease; however, Haitians, homosexual men, and children with perinatally acquired HIV infection also developed proteinuria and glomerulosclerosis.[137] In another series of patients, renal disease was observed in 13 of 32 patients and included focal glomerulosclerosis, mesangial proliferation, and glomerulonephritis.[138] Renal disorders developed in association with fungal infections, disseminated *Mycobacterium avium-intracellulare* infection, hypotension, and the use of nephrotoxic drugs (such as aminoglycosides or amphotericin B). AIDS-associated nephropathy appears more frequently in the eastern United States where large numbers of iv drug users with AIDS are found. Large numbers of patients followed in San Francisco and other cities have not had as much kidney involvement as those seen in New York and Miami. Moreover, AAN is more commonly reported in blacks than in other racial groups, which suggests a biologic susceptibility to this disorder. Further prospective studies of how HIV-seropositives develop renal disease are needed.

Renal dysfunction in AIDS patients is usually diagnosed incidently when patients present with opportunistic infections. Asymptomatic proteinuria, up to 5 g/day, is often the initial finding, and the serum creatinine level is often normal or only mildly elevated. The albumin concentration is almost always low (as is true for most AIDS patients with opportunistic infections), and the blood pressure is usually normal. Renal biopsy most often shows focal and segmental glomerulosclerosis with tubular dilatation and atrophy, fibrosis, and a mononuclear cell infiltrate. Immunofluorescence studies often reveal deposits of IgM and C3, and electron micropsy shows electron-dense mesangial deposits and mesangial hypocellularity. One report of intranuclear and intracytoplasmic inclusion bodies, which suggest a viral etiology of renal pathology, has been published.

The clinical course of AAN progresses quickly, usually because many other opportunistic processes occur simultaneously. Rao et al.[135] originally reported death with renal failure in 8 of 11 patients with AAN in less than 4 months. Since AAN is diagnosed late in the course of HIV disease, it is difficult to determine the effect of renal dysfunction on survival. Rao and associates have also reported on 18 patients who developed AIDS while receiving hemodialysis for end-stage renal disease. They survived a median of 1 month beyond their AIDS diagnosis.[139] Other centers have also reported that patients with AIDS responded poorly to maintenance by hemodialysis.[140] Activating the cellular immune system through chronic dialysis may accelerate HIV pathology. On the other hand, AIDS patients who have acute renal failure from a reversible insult (such as hypotension or nephrotoxic drugs) respond to conservative measures and the brief use of hemodialysis.

Pulmonary Disease

Opportunistic pulmonary diseases are the most common cause of acute illness and death in patients with HIV infection.[141] In the United States, approximately 65 percent of AIDS-defining illnesses are pulmonary opportunistic infections; most of these are *P. carinii* pneumonia (PCP). Moreover, pulmonary diseases (such as PCP) are assuming a greater role in the clinical spectrum of AIDS as the relative prevalence of Kaposi sarcoma as an AIDS-defining diagnosis decreases.[142] Before the AIDS epidemic, PCP was a rare opportunistic pathogen encountered in patients with severe malnutrition, hematologic malignancies, and iatrogenic immunosuppression. As of June 1989, approximately 55,000 AIDS patients in the United States had had an index AIDS diagnosis of PCP. It has been estimated that an additional 16,000–18,000 patients had PCP as a secondary AIDS diagnosis not reported to public health authorities. Reports of the prevalence of PCP in AIDS patients are substantially lower in developing countries than in industrial nations; however, significant underdiagnosis and underreporting of PCP may be caused by the lack of sophisticated diagnostic facilities.

The multiple etiologies of pulmonary disease in patients with HIV infection are listed in Table 10. In addition to *P. carinii*, other common infectious agents that cause pneumonitis in AIDS are mycobacteria (particularly *M. tuberculosis*), fungi (such as *Cryptococcus*), encapsulated bacteria, cytomegalovirus, and possibly HIV itself.[143,144] Kaposi sarcoma is found frequently in the lungs of patients with mucocutaneous lesions and is associated with an accelerated clinical course.[145] The differential diagnosis of respiratory complaints in an HIV-seropositive patient is quite extensive. Patients with known or suspected HIV infection who present with pulmonary symptoms should be expeditiously evaluated with reliable diagnostic procedures to achieve a specific diagnosis so that therapy can be initiated as soon as possible. Empirical antimicrobial therapy is often appropriate while the diagnostic evaluation proceeds.

TABLE 10. Pulmonary Complications of AIDS

Protozoa
Pneumocystis carinii
Bacteria
Mycobacterium tuberculosis
Mycobacterium avium-intracellulare
Streptococcus pneumoniae
Haemophilus influenzae
Legionella pneumophila
Nocardia asteroides
Fungi
Cryptococcus neoformans
Histoplasma capsulatum
Coccidioides immitis
Candida albicans
Viruses
Cytomegalovirus
? Human immunodeficiency virus
Tumors
Kaposi sarcoma
Non-Hodgkin's lymphoma
Nonspecific pneumonitis
? Human immunodeficiency virus

A clinical history is useful in evaluating patients who may have AIDS-related pulmonary disease. In AIDS patients (as opposed to other immunocompromised hosts), PCP often has an insidious onset.[146] Patients have a constitutional prodrome of fevers, night sweats, weight loss, and oral candidiasis for weeks followed by increasing respiratory distress—with shortness of breath at first on exertion and finally dyspnea at rest. Approximately 80 percent of patients with PCP note a dry cough, and many report retrosternal irritation on deep breathing. About 5–10 percent of patients with PCP may initially deny respiratory symptoms. These same symptoms may occur in patients with other pulmonary pathogens. Bacterial pneumonias in HIV-seropositive individuals tend to have a more abrupt and severe onset.[147,148,149] In one study, the median duration of symptoms for AIDS patients with pneumonia caused by *H. influenzae* and *S. pneumoniae* was 5 days vs. 21 days in patients with PCP.[150] Seventy percent of patients with bacterial pneumonia may report pleuritic chest pain (uncommon in PCP), and most have a fever, a productive cough, and progressive dyspnea. Patients with cryptococcal pneumonitis generally have disseminated disease and may have a paucity of pulmonary complaints.

Tuberculosis in HIV-seropositive patients most often presents as pulmonary disease and often has an accelerated clinical course.[151,152] In patients already diagnosed as having AIDS, tuberculosis may be a multiorgan, disseminated disease and may present as a systemic illness. Pulmonary Kaposi sarcoma may be a primary lesion but most commonly occurs in patients with extensive tumor(s) elsewhere.[145] Respiratory symptoms tend to progress slowly at first, and constitutional symptoms may be minimal. Upper respiratory tract infections are common in AIDS patients and are most often remarkable for pronounced cough without dyspnea.

A variety of upper respiratory tract symptoms and signs may be elicited. Rales are often detected in patients with PCP and other opportunistic infections. Bacterial pneumonias tend to be focal and may result in localized findings of consolidation on auscultation. Pulmonary Kaposi sarcoma is frequently associated with pleural effusions that are detected by dullness to percussion and diminished breath sounds at the lung bases. Many patients will have normal chest examination findings despite the presence of active pulmonary infection or malignancy. Physical examination may be of limited value to establish a specific diagnosis, and all patients with respiratory symptoms should undergo further diagnostic work-up as outlined below.

Figure 2 shows the diagnostic algorithm employed in the authors' institutions to evaluate patients with suspected AIDS-related pulmonary disease. The protocol has proved to be efficient, cost-effective, and reliable in expeditiously diagnosing both hospitalized and ambulatory patients. A chest radiograph is performed initially. It may be read as normal or have one or more of the following abnormalities: interstitial infiltrates, focal infiltrate with or without cavitation, pleural effusion, intrathoracic adenopathy, or nodules (Table 11). Although 5–10 percent of patients with proven PCP may present with normal chest film findings, PCP is most often associated with interstitial infiltrates.[153] Since a patient with diffuse infiltrates probably has PCP, immediate specific tests for *P. carinii* are indicated. In most institutions, initial pulmonary specimens are obtained by induction of sputum with an ultrasonic nebulizer.[154–156] Patients whose respiratory symptoms are due to PCP, tuberculosis, fungal disease, nonspecific pneumonitis, upper respiratory disease, severe anemia, and other conditions may, however, have normal chest films. Since PCP is less likely in patients with normal chest films, a nonspecific but noninvasive evaluation is useful. Arterial oxygen tension is useful to screen for PCP, although the arterial PaO_2 is both insensitive and nonspecific. Determining the PaO_2 does assess a patient's need for supplemental

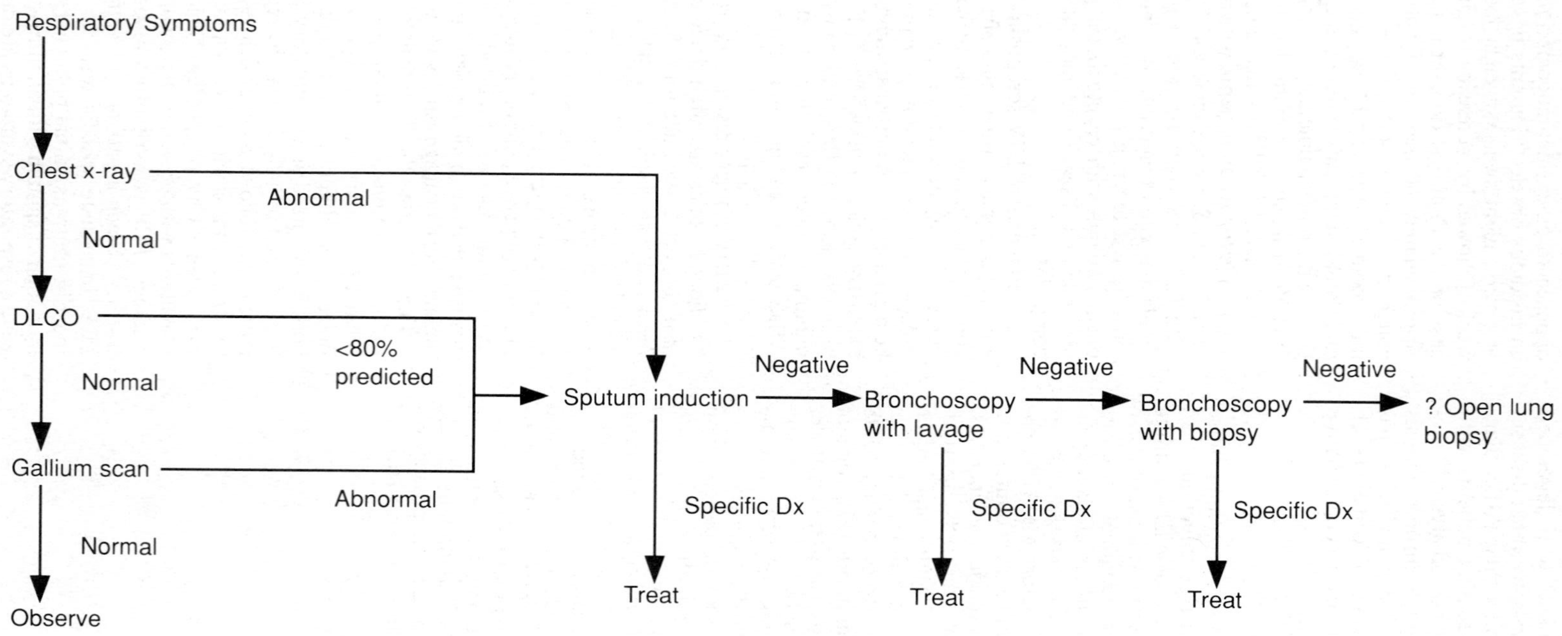

FIG. 2. Algorithm for evaluating pulmonary disease in patients with HIV.

TABLE 11. Chest Radiographic Findings in AIDS Patients with Respiratory Disease

CXR Pattern	*Illnesses*
Normal	No disease *Pneumocystis carinii* pneumonia Disseminated fungal infection
Focal infiltrate	Pyogenic pneumonia Tuberculosis Cryptococcal pneumonia *Pneumocystis carinii* pneumonia
Pleural effusion	Kaposi sarcoma Pyogenic pnumonia Tuberculosis
Mediastinal adenopathy	Tuberculosis/Mycobacterium avium complex Lymphoma
Interstitial infiltrate	*Pneumocystis carinii* pneumonitis Tuberculosis Lymphocytic interstitial pneumonia Nonspecific pneumonitis Pyogenic pneumonia

oxygen. Arterial blood gases have been evaluated in patients after exercise to screen patients with normal chest radiographs for PCP. The baseline A-aO_2 gradient is compared with the gradient after 3 minutes of exercise.[131] Recruitment of underventilated areas of the lungs during exercise normally decreases the A-aO_2 gradient; however, the A-aO_2 gradient often increases in patients with PCP. This procedure is about 80 percent sensitive, but it is not widely used, primarily because of its inconvenience. Determining the diffusing capacity of carbon monoxide (DLCO) provides a very sensitive test for PCP. Of patients with PCP, 95 percent have a DLCO of less than 80 percent of the predicted value (corrected for hemoglobin). In one study, the mean DLCO for patients with PCP was 62 percent of the predicted value.[156a] This test is nonspecific, however; in the same study, patients without PCP had an average DLCO that was 72 percent of the predicted value. Other abnormalities of pulmonary function are frequently encountered in patients with PCP, including a decreased total lung capacity and vital capacity. These maneuvers are less sensitive than is the DLCO. Patients who present with an abnormal DLCO should be evaluated specifically for *P. carinii*.

Gallium lung scanning is also used to evaluate pulmonary disease in patients with HIV infection.[157] Patients receive an injection of 5–8 mCu of ^{67}Ga and undergo scintigraphic scanning 48 and/or 72 hours later. Scans may be interpreted by qualitative or semiquantitative methods. Typically, PCP results in a diffuse uptake of gallium in the lungs. Any pulmonary uptake is abnormal and should prompt additional specific studies to diagnose pulmonary infection. Gallium scanning, like pulmonary function testing, is nonspecific, and PCP should never be diagnosed on the basis of a positive gallium scan alone.

Examination of induced sputum is now widely used initially to identify *P. carinii*. Specimens should be collected and processed properly, and only well-trained laboratory personnel should review stained specimens to identify organisms. Table 12 describes how to obtain and prepare samples of induced sputum. An ultrasonic nebulizer and 3% to 5% saline solution are essential, as is processing of the sputum specimen with a mucolytic agent. A number of reagents may be used to stain *P. carinii*. A modified Giemsa stain (Dif-Quik), silver methenamine, and toluidine blue O have all produced good results. Silver methenamine, which stains *P. carinii* cysts, may be less sensitive than trophozoite stains are (such as Giemsa). In institutions with staff experienced in the procedure, the overall sensitivity of sputum induction is about 80 percent. Obtaining a second sample of induced sputum may increase the yield and reduce the need for subsequent bronchoscopy from patients with initially negative results. Both direct and indirect immunofluorescence assays (IFA) have recently been developed; they may increase the sensitivity of sputum induction to nearly 90 percent.[155] False-positive results may be obtained with IFA however. Additional studies are required to determine the specificity of these assays. A sample of sputum that is obviously purulent should have a Gram stain and bacterial culture, and antibacterial therapy is appropriate. Laboratories should also perform acid-fast smears and mycobacterial cultures on induced sputum, especially where tuberculosis is more prevalent. Fungal and viral cultures of induced sputum may also be performed, particularly if *P. carinii* is found and subsequent bronchoscopy will not be performed. The yield for these tests, however, is low.

TABLE 12. Method for Sputum Induction

Patient preparation	
	Overnight fast
	Thorough mouth cleansing with saline
	Inhalation of 3% saline from ultrasonic nebulizer
Specimen preparation	
	Digestion (dithiothreitol)
	Centrifugation
	Smear, air-dry, and heat fix
	Giemsa, silver methanamine, or fluorescent antibody stain

Since the negative predictive value of sputum induction is no more than 60 percent, patients who do not have a pathogen identified by this method should undergo a bronchoscopic procedure to establish a diagnosis. Fiber-optic bronchoscopy is an effective, low-morbidity procedure that has a high yield for diagnosing pulmonary pathogens in patients with HIV infection.[158–161] The combination of bronchoalveolar lavage (BAL) and transbronchial biopsy has a diagnostic yield of >95 percent for all pathogens in AIDS patients, and its yield is 100 percent for *P. carinii*. Bronchoalveolar lavage alone has a sensitivity of 85–95 percent and can be performed safely in most patients with suspected PCP. Brush biopsies are not sensitive and are not taken in many institutions. In the our institutions, BAL alone is performed initially. Centrifuged specimens are stained with Giemsa, silver methenamine, and an AFB stain and are also cultured for mycobacteria and fungi. When this procedure does not establish a diagnosis, a repeat bronchoscopic examination is performed, and BAL and transbronchial biopsies are done. Six biopsies of the right lower lobe are generally taken—again without fluoroscopic guidance—unless a focal abnormality is present on the chest radiograph. Fresh biopsy material is examined by touch imprints. Formalin-fixed specimens are stained with hematoxylin and eosin (H&E), Giemsa, acid-fast stains, and silver methenamine. Performance of transbronchial biopsy is not recommended for patients who require mechanical ventilation or have an uncorrectable coagulopathy, although BAL may be performed in such instances. Bronchoalveolar lavage can result in hypoxemia transiently after the procedure. A transbronchial biopsy results in pneumothorax in about 10 percent of patients, at least 50 percent of whom require tube thoracostomy for reexpansion.

Although open lung biopsy (OLB) was previously considered the gold standard for diagnosing PCP, its use is now restricted to several unusual circumstances in patients with HIV-related pulmonary disease. Rarely, a patient with progressive respiratory impairment will have a nondiagnostic sputum induction and bronchoscopy or will have a coagulopathy that contraindicates transbronchial biopsy. Such patients may benefit from OLB.

The serologic diagnosis of PCP has been evaluated in patients who have undergone bone marrow transplant. Neither anti-*P. carinii* antibodies nor *P. carinii* antigen were sensitive or specific in diagnosing PCP. Serologic studies of this population have proved unhelpful: the prevalence of *P. carinii* antibodies is relatively high, and the antibody titers may not increase significantly after the disease is reactivated.

Specific Pathogens. PNEUMOCYSTIS CARINII. *Pneumocystis carinii* (see Chapter 256) is generally considered to be a protozoon, although recent studies suggest that it may be more closely related to fungi.[163] Infection with *P. carinii* is common early in life and does not generally result in symptomatic disease in immunocompetent hosts. Patients with chronic HIV infection develop disease caused by *P. carinii* very frequently—principally an intra-alveolar pneumonitis. *Pneumocystis carinii* pneumonia often presents as a slowly progressive pneumonitis associated with fever, sweats, weight loss, increasing cough, and dyspnea. Kovacs and colleagues compared patients with AIDS-related PCP with patients with PCP and other types of immunodeficiency.[146] The median duration of symptoms was prolonged in the AIDS group (28 vs. 5 days in non-AIDS patients), and AIDS patients with PCP tended to have less fever, a lower respiratory rate, and a higher arterial PO_2. Similar studies by other authors have confirmed the difference between AIDS and non-AIDS PCP. The longer prodrome of PCP in AIDS patients may reflect a better host response to *P. carinii* or may be secondary to other infectious processes (e.g., CMV, mycobacteria, or HIV itself).

Pathologically, PCP causes air space consolidation because a protein-rich exudate consisting of numerous *P. carinii* trophozoites fills the alevoli and causes intrapulmonary right-to-left shunting and arterial hypoxemia. Alveolar membranes become thickened, and parenchymal inflammation, edema, and fibrosis occur. Patients with advanced PCP may have what physiologically appears to be the adult respiratory distress syndrome. Alveolar capillaries leak solutes into the air spaces, pulmonary fluids increase and worsen the shunting of pulmonary capillary blood flow, and arterial hypoxemia increases. Hughes has proposed a histopathologic staging system for PCP in adults that reflects the natural progression of pneumonitis caused by the organism.[164] In stage 1 (early infection), scattered *P. carinii* cysts can be seen in the alveolar wall, but no inflammatory response is evident. Neither autopsy nor biopsy materials for asymptomatic HIV-infected patients have demonstrated that this stage of the disease is common before patients develop symptomatic PCP. Stage 2 is marked by an increase in the number of *P. carinii* cysts in the alveolar wall, alveolar septal inflammation, and desquamation of alveolar cells into the lumen. In addition, *P. carinii* trophozoites can be seen by electron microscopy. In stage 3, alveolar hypertrophy occurs along with a mononuclear cell infiltration and extensive alveolar desquamation; numerous *P. carinii* cysts and trophozoites are found in pulmonary macrophages. After acute PCP is resolved, *P. carinii* cysts or trophozoites may be found in up to 60 percent of patients, although it is not known whether the organisms are viable. Over time the recovery of *P. carinii* declines. Alveolar hypertrophy, interstitial fibrosis, and nonspecific inflammation may be found on biopsy or at autopsy. Approximately 20–25 percent of patients with an initial episode of PCP die acutely—a proportion that has not changed significantly over the course of the epidemic. A study conducted at the National Institutes of Health suggests that early mortality can be predicted by histopathologic findings when the lungs are biopsied.[165] Patients with more extensive edema, fibrosis, and inflammation (stage 3 disease) have a significantly higher mortality rate than do those with less severe disease. Consequently, earlier diagnosis and treatment may improve survival of the first episode of PCP. Patients dying of respiratory failure due to PCP are frequently found to have additional pathogens in the lungs at autopsy (most commonly CMV), but how other infections contribute to the morbidity of PCP is not yet known.

Although most patients with disease caused by *P. carinii* appear to have pneumonitis alone, several reports of extrapulmonary pneumocystosis have been published.[166–169] *Pneumocystis carinii* has been identified in specimens obtained from the middle ear, mastoid, retina, liver, lymph nodes, spleen, and bone marrow. More extensive extrapulmonary dissemination has been reported in patients without HIV infection. How *P. carinii* disseminates and how prevalent extrapulmonary disease is in patients with PCP are both unknown (although the prevalence is felt to be low). Autopsies of patients dying of AIDS only occasionally have identified *P. carinii* outside the lungs.[170]

MYCOBACTERIA. Both tuberculosis and atypical mycobacterial disease (see Chapters 229 and 231) are common manifestations of chronic HIV infection. Disease caused by *M. tuberculosis* may occur early in the course of HIV-induced immunosuppression.[171] Infections with the generally avirulent, atypical organisms (e.g., *M. avium* complex) probably manifest later severe immunodeficiency. Other mycobacteria that cause disease in AIDS patients are *M. kansasii*, *M. xenopi*, *M. cheloni*, *M. gordonae*, and *M. bovis*.[172–174]

In HIV disease, tuberculosis may be the initial manifestation of immunodeficiency in patients who were previously infected with *M. tuberculosis*.[175] Tuberculosis appears more frequently in populations that have an increased risk of the disease, particularly iv drug users, blacks, and Hispanics in the United States and residents of developing countries where tuberculosis may emerge as the predominant AIDS-related opportunistic infection.[176] In Miami, approximately 60 percent of Haitian AIDS patients have tuberculosis.[151] At a tuberculosis sanitorium in Zaire, 33 percent of those with pulmonary tuberculosis were infected with HIV.[177]

In the United States, tuberculosis has recently become more prevalent, primarily because of the HIV epidemic.[178] The number of cases of tuberculosis rose from 1985 to 1986 by 2.6 percent, with New York City reporting the largest increase. Demographically, tuberculosis increased in both sexes, in people aged 25–44, and in blacks and Hispanics. AIDS and tuberculosis registries in New York, San Francisco, and Florida have been matched and reveal that between 2 and 10 percent of AIDS patients have tuberculosis.[179,180] Studies in Miami and San Francisco show that approximately 30 percent of individuals newly diagnosed with tuberculosis have HIV infection[171,181]; most patients had no other clinical evidence of AIDS.

Clinical features of tuberculosis in AIDS patients vary with the degree of immunosuppression. Most patients appear to have been infected previously with *M. tuberculosis*, and the infection is reactivated by progressive immunodeficiency. These patients may have tuberculosis months to years before the diagnosis of AIDS. The pattern of tuberculosis in these individuals is typical of the reactivation seen in other populations; characteristic pulmonary symptoms and clinical findings are the rule. Most patients (60–80 percent), despite moderately severe CD4 lymphopenia, respond to intradermal tuberculin. Chest radiographs show localized or diffuse lung abnormalities in half of the patients. Tuberculosis most commonly affects the pulmonary system, although 20–40 percent of patients may have extrapulmonary disease concomitantly. Tuberculosis is diagnosed by examinating pulmonary specimens with stains for acid-fast organisms and by culture for mycobacteria. Clinicians should employ the diagnostic algorithm for pulmonary disease described above. In some patients with AIDS, tuberculosis may appear as a late opportunistic complication coinciding with or following other opportunistic diseases.[182–184] Clinically, this type of tuberculosis often differs from early reactivation. Constitutional symptoms are more pronounced; chest radiographic findings are usually atypical, with diffuse infiltrates and intrathoracic adenopathy predominant; a response to tuberculin testing occurs at a rate of only 30–40 percent; and extrapulmonary dissemination is found in 50–70 percent of the cases.[175] The lungs remain the site where the organism is most frequently isolated and an important source to spread the infection to other susceptible individuals.

The pathology of tuberculosis in HIV-infected persons reflects the stage of immunosuppression at which disease occurs. In patients whose earlier TB is reactivated, well-formed granulomas may be found on biopsy or autopsy. A brisk inflammatory response is reflected in localized pulmonary symptoms, radiographic infiltrates, and tuberculin reactivity. As immunosuppression advances, pathologic findings become more atypical, and poorly formed granulomas without caseation may be found. Although tuberculosis responds excellently to chemotherapy, the overall prognosis for patients infected with TB and AIDS is very poor. In one study, the median survival rate was 6 months.[179] Most patients, however, die of other opportunistic diseases.

Early in the AIDS epidemic, clinicians recognized infections caused by nontuberculous mycobacteria as complications of HIV-induced immunosuppression. In 1981–1982 investigators found high-grade, disseminated infections with *M. avium* complex in patients with AIDS.[185,186] Approximately 4 percent of AIDS cases have nontuberculous mycobacterial infections as an index AIDS diagnosis[187]; 97 percent are caused by *M. avium* complex, and 3 percent are due to *M. kansasii*, *M. xenopi*, *M. gordonae*, and others.[187] As many as 25–50 percent of AIDS patients may subsequently develop nontuberculous mycobacterial disease. It may be difficult to diagnose *M. avium* complex (MAC) while patients are alive; autopsy series show that over 50 percent of these infections may be clinically undetected.[170,188] Nontuberculous mycobacterial disease appears to be equally prevalent in males and females, in all age groups, and in different geographic regions. *Mycobacterium avium* complex, a common environmental saprophyte, may be acquired orally or inhaled. In several studies, researchers have isolated MAC in the respiratory system before its dissemination in 50–75 percent of the cases.[189–191] Others have reported little association between colonization in the respiratory tract and subsequent systemic spread. One study found numerous mycobacteria in macrophages of the lamina propria in the small bowel—a finding consistent with acquiring the gastrointestinal infection.[192] Since nontuberculous mycobacteria are distributed uniformly among different risk groups, the disease caused by MAC is probably a new infection rather than a previous infection reactivated.

In AIDS patients, nontuberculous mycobacterial disease is characterized pathologically by continuous bacteremia, with as many as 10^4 to 10^5 colony-forming-units per milliliter of blood.[193,194] *Mycobacterium avium* complex can infect numerous organs: bone marrow, liver, spleen, gut, lymph nodes, lungs, skin, brain, adrenals, and kidneys. There is little histologic response despite relatively large numbers of organisms. Granulomas, when present, are usually poorly formed. Some studies suggest that MAC disease may be associated with abnormal levels of lymphokines and the dysfunction of macrophages rather than the intrinsic loss of helper-inducer T lymphocytes.[195] In infected patients, macrophages may be packed with organisms that have not been killed in the cells themselves with antimicrobial therapy. Mycobacteremia may fail to clear because of impaired host defenses or because of intrinsic resistance to these agents.[198] How MAC infection contributes to AIDS mortality is not known. One study suggested that survival improved when MAC disease was treated.[199] The study was, however, prone to significant lead-time bias because cases were diagnosed earlier in their clinical course than historical controls. One study followed 161 patients from the date PCP was diagnosed; they found that those who had or subsequently developed MAC infection had a marginally longer median survival rate than did patients without MAC.[191] This finding probably reflects an increased incidence of MAC over time, with longer survivors most likely to acquire the organism. Several autopsy series have found MAC postmortem in a large proportion of subjects; however, in one series (where cause of death was listed), only 1 of 36 (3 percent) AIDS deaths was attributed to MAC.[170] It appears that nontuberculous mycobacterial infections mark severe, cellular immunodeficiency associated with an extremely poor prognosis, but they may not directly affect survival.

In patients with PCP, recovery of MAC from pulmonary specimens is often an incidental finding, and most patients recover with anti-*Pneumocystis* therapy alone. Abundant clinical data, however, show significant morbidity from MAC. A minority of patients, may have respiratory tract disease caused by MAC alone, an infection that results in diffuse pulmonary infiltrates, arterial hypoxemia, and progressive pulmonary deterioration.[200] Clinicians should evaluate patients carefully for other pulmonary pathogens before ascribing respiratory findings to MAC.

Mycobacterium avium complex disease most commonly presents as a systemic illness with fevers, night sweats, fatigue, and weight loss. Gastrointestinal symptoms such as abdominal pain and persistent diarrhea are also often reported. Patients usually appear emaciated and have generalized lymphadenopathy and other findings associated with immunodeficiency (e.g., oral candidiasis). Abdominal examination may show diffuse tenderness and hepatosplenomegaly. Laboratory evaulation is usually nonspecific, although anemia and leukopenia are usually pronounced. Computed tomography scans of the abdomen may show marked hepatosplenomegaly and diffuse lymphadenopathy (often with central attenuation). The bowel wall is often thickened—consistent with an inflammatory colitis. Gallium scans may show intense colonic uptake. Biopsy or autopsy specimens of the colon show acute and chronic inflammation and numerous acid-fast bacilli in the mucosa and submucosa. Concurrent infections with *Cryptosporidium*, CMV, and other pathogens may be found. The small bowel may also be involved and result in a histologic appearance similar to Whipple's disease and the chronic diarrhea syndrome. *Mycobacterium avium* complex has been found in enlarged periportal lymph nodes in patients whose extrahepatic bile ducts were extrinsically obstructed. *Mycobacterium avium* complex has also been found in the adrenals of patients with acute adrenal insufficiency (although CMV is most often associated with this clinical entity), in brain abscesses and in the bone biopsy of patients with osteomyelitis.

PYOGENIC BACTERIA. Infections with pyogenic bacteria occur more frequently in patients with HIV disease, particularly in children and iv drug users. The incidence of bacterial pneumonia, for example, is increased greatly in HIV-seropositive iv drug users when compared with seronegative controls.[201] Encapsulated bacteria (particularly *Streptococcus pneumoniae* and *Haemophilus influenzae*) are the most common pathogens.[202] Table 13 lists bacteria that cause serious infections in HIV-infected persons.

In HIV-infected patients, bacterial infections involve primarily the skin, lungs, sinuses, and middle ear. Children appear to have a high prevalence of otitis media and pneumonia caused by *S. pneumoniae* and *H. influenzae*. In adults, pyogenic infections are manifested most commonly as skin and soft tissue infections, sinusitis, and pneumonia. Persistent impetigo, furunculosis, folliculitis, and skin abscesses in adults with HIV infection; streptococci and *Staphylococcus aureus* are usually responsible. In patients with HIV infection, sinusitis may be

TABLE 13. Bacteria Causing Serious Infections in Patients with HIV Infection

	Organism	Site(s) of Disease
Gram-positive	*Streptococcus pneumoniae*	Lung, sinuses, blood
	Streptococcus spp.	Lung
	Staphylococcus aureus	Skin, blood, lung, perineum
	Listeria monocytogenes	Meninges, blood
	Nocardia asteroides	Lung, brain
Gram-negative	*Haemophilus influenzae*	Lung, blood
	Haemophilus spp.	Lung
	Branhamella catarrhalis	Lung
	Salmonella spp.	Gut, blood, brain
	Shigella spp.	Gut
	Campylobacter spp.	Gut
	Legionella pneumophila	Lung
Spirochetes	*Treponema pallidum*	Skin, meninges, brain

caused by *S. pneumoniae*, *H. influenzae* other or *Haemophilus* species, *Branhamella catarrhalis*, or other organisms. The clinical presentation is often subacute; congestion, cough, and headache are the most prominent symptoms. Sinus tenderness is uncommon, but sinus x-ray films frequently reveal sinus thickening and air–fluid levels within the paranasal sinuses. Aspirating the sinus fluids may be both diagnostic and therapeutic.

Bacterial pneumonias (discussed earlier) present as clinically distinct from PCP. Bacterial pneumonia may occur more frequently in iv drug users, cigarette smokers, and children with HIV infection and bacterial bronchitis, more commonly in the HIV-infected population. Patients usually complain of a chronic cough with scant sputum production and minimal dyspnea. Evaluation reveals rhonchi or wheezes, and chest films are normal. Sputum Gram staining may show polymorphonucleocytes (PMNs) and gram-positive diplococci or gram-negative coccobacillary organisms. Although bronchitis is rarely associated with bacteremia, bacterial pneumonias in AIDS patients are often bacteremic. Up to 80 percent of patients with *S. pneumoniae* pneumonia and 25 percent of patients with *H. influenzae* pneumonia have bacteremia.[148,202,203] Infection may be more difficult to eradicate in these patients, and relapses after appropriate therapy are common.

Reports suggest that bacteremia occurs more frequently in patients with advanced HIV disease. One report found 22 cases of *Staphylococcus aureus* bacteremia in patients with AIDS or advanced HIV disease.[204] Six of those patients had intravenous catheters in place. Many physicians have reported a high rate of catheter-related sepsis in AIDS patients, particularly those with central venous lines who are receiving intravenous therapy at home. The organisms responsible for catheter-related sepsis are predominantly *S. aureus* or *epidermidis*; gram-negative bacilli are encountered less frequently. Why the risk of infection increases is not known: AIDS patients may be more likely to employ inadequate hygienic techniques than are other patient groups with indwelling venous catheters, and host mechanisms that control integumental defense may be impaired. Patients with HIV infection who have a central venous catheter should receive careful instructions on how to control infection, adequate nursing supervision, and medical follow-up.

Neurologic Complications

HIV is a neurotrophic virus with a variety of clinical manifestations in the central and peripheral nervous systems.[206] Numerous neurologic opportunistic infections occur in AIDS patients in addition to the direct, immunologic sequelae of HIV infection, so the neurologic complications of HIV infection can best be considered primary and secondary consequences.

Aseptic Meningitis. When HIV directly infects the central nervous system, several distinct clinical syndromes result. In approximately 25 percent of the cases, an aseptic meningitis characterizes the acute retroviral syndrome (described previously). Although cranial neuropathies have been reported, meningeal signs may be minimal and laboratory evaluation remarkable for only a slight CSF pleocytosis and elevation of the CSF protein.[207,208] Culture of CSF may reveal HIV, and free viral core antigen may be detected.[209–211] Seroconversion can result in the intrathecal production of anti-HIV antibodies. Patients with this presentation may wax and wane clinically for months. HIV-related meningitis was reported in one series of 14 patients who presented no evidence of recently acquiring HIV.[207] The symptoms that prompted evaluation lasted from 10 days to more than 10 months. Signs of immunodeficiency were found in eight cases (57 percent). A mild CSF pleocytosis was noted in all patients, and both CSF protein levels and opening pressure were elevated in five patients. Eighty percent of patients tested had positive HIV cultures. A CSF pleocytosis, detection of HIV antigen, and viral cocultivation can also be found in asymptomatic HIV-seropositive patients, however, so attributing meningitis in HIV-infected persons to HIV itself is speculative.

HIV Encephalopathy. A progressive neurologic syndrome (now termed HIV encephalopathy) can be caused when HIV infects the central nervous system (CNS) white matter. Ninety percent of patients with AIDS have cognitive, affective, and psychomotor abnormalities[213]; patients with less advanced opportunistic disease have a lower frequency of these abnormalities. A study of asymptomatic, seropositive subjects found no encephalopathic abnormalities before overt clinical opportunistic disease developed elsewhere. HIV-encephalopathy can be divided into two phases, early and late, and each has a distinct clinical presentation. In early HIV encephalopathy, the major symptoms are memory loss, impaired concentration, and mental slowness. Patients also demonstrate affective symptoms, apathy, behavior change, and motor complaints. Patients with early HIV encephalopathy may have hyperreflexia, hypertonia, frontal-release signs, tremor, psychomotor slowing, ataxia, and abnormal results of mental status examination. Laboratory evaluation is essential to rule out opportunistic infection, tumor, or other causes of mental status changes. In 70–90 percent of patients, CT scans of the head show generalized atrophy that is usually inconsistent with the patient's age.[214] Magnetic resonance imaging (MRI) also shows cerebral atrophy, often with marked abnormalities of the subcortical white matter and an increased signal intensity that is distributed multifocally. Magnetic resonance image scanning is more specific but less sensitive than CT scanning.[214] A slight CSF pleocytosis is found in a minority of individuals and normal glucose and elevated CSF protein levels (primarily CSF IgG) in more than half of the patients. Oligoclonal bands may be present in a small proportion of subjects tested. HIV isolation and antigen detection assays may be positive, although these tests are both nonspecific and insensitive for predicting and diagnosing HIV encephalopathy. Other diagnostic test findings, e.g., electroencephalography (EEG), may be abnormal but have not been adequately evaluated to be helpful.

Late HIV encephalopathy is a more fulminant process. Patients present with marked cognitive abnormalities, memory loss, behavioral change, and significant, psychomotor impairment. Profound weakness, neglect, tremor, seizures, and psychosis may also be noted. Computed tomography and MRI scanning findings are often more severely abnormal; extreme cerebral atrophy and white matter changes are common. Other diagnostic studies are used to rule out opportunistic infections. A clinical diagnosis of HIV encephalopathy is made by excluding other causes of encephalopathy and documenting HIV infection. Characteristic findings on history and examination, suggestive radiographic or imaging findings, and the absence of space-occupying lesions, opportunistic pathogens, or intoxicating drugs all support the diagnosis. Brain biopsy has been performed in some patients with results consistent with autopsy findings; however, the yield of brain biopsy in reaching a treatable diagnosis is very low in the absence of localizing lesions by noninvasive imaging studies. Consequently, routine biopsy cannot be recommended. In children infected with HIV, CNS involvement appears very frequently. It can be manifested by a failure to thrive, cognitive deficits, abnormalities of muscle tone, and paraparesis. Seizures have been reported occasionally as a late complication in both children and adults.

In the brains of patients with HIV encephalopathy, pathologic findings are varied. Seventy-five percent of patients had cerebral atrophy that was most pronounced in the frontal and temporal lobes. Almost all patients have gliosis and focal necrosis. Microglial nodules of macrophages, lymphocytes, and microglia are reported in up to 70 percent of patients. Demyelination and myelin pallor are common; focal perivascular myelin rarefaction or demyelination and vacuolation are also frequently noted. The basal ganglia are commonly involved. Multinucleated giant cells, produced by direct HIV infection in the brain, can be found scattered throughout the cerebral cortex and white matter. Perivascular and leptomeningeal inflammation may also be found.

Intracranial Mass Lesions. Central nervous system dysfunction from intracranial mass lesions is a late complication of HIV disease. Processes associated with mass lesions of the brain are listed in Table 14. Cerebral toxoplasmosis is the most common cause of intracranial masses in patients with AIDS, followed by CNS lymphoma, progressive multifocal leukoencephalopathy (PML), and other infectious agents (e.g., *M. tuberculosis*, *Cryptococcus*, *Candida*). As many as 10 percent of biopsied or autopsied intracranial masses have nondiagnostic histopathology.[214] In many cases, neither the clinical presentation nor the neuroradiologic appearance of CNS lesions permits a definitive diagnosis. Patients with opportunistic CNS disease may present with a variety of signs and symptoms. Headache may occur in one-third to three-quarters of patients and altered sensorium in 50–90 percent. Incoordination, ataxia, hemiparesis, and cranial neuropathies are present in fewer than 25 percent of patients with intracranial mass lesions.[215] The radiographic appearance of various CNS lesions may be distinct but not pathognomonic. A diagnosis of CNS disease is challenging without examining tissue. However, because brain biopsy is not always feasible, empiric therapy for toxoplasmosis is warranted in selected patients. A clinical response establishes the diagnosis reliably (see below). Figure 3 presents a diagnostic algorithm for evaluating patients with HIV infection and suspected intracranial mass lesions.

Patients who present with clinical findings suggestive of intracranial pathology should be evaluated with a brain imaging study. Both CT and MRI have been shown to be sensitive for assessing CNS disease in HIV infection. Double-dose, delayed-contrast CT scanning identifies ring-enhancing abscesses and other mass lesions more sensitively than do single-dose studies. Lesions are typically hypodense with surrounding edema and may have a mass effect. Characteristically, abscesses are enhanced by contrast in tuberculoma, cryptococcoma, nocardiosis, and pyogenic brain abscesses. A lack of enhancement is more often associated with PML and lymphomas. Multiple

TABLE 14. Causes of Intracranial Mass Lesions in AIDS

Infections
Toxoplasma gondii
Progressive multifocal leukoencephaly (JC virus)
M. tuberculosis
Cryptococcus neoformans
Nocardia asteroides
Histoplasma capsulatum
Cytomegalovirus
Herpes simplex virus
Human immunodeficiency virus
Candida albicans
Neoplasms
Primary CNS lymphoma
Metastatic lymphoma
Kaposi sarcoma
Unidentified
Nonspecific gliosis

ring-enhancing lesions are the sine qua non of toxoplasmosis; however, many toxoplasmic abscesses are not detected by CT scanning. Therefore, the appearance of a single ring-enhancing lesion by CT does not rule out toxoplasmosis. Toxoplasmosis is frequently associated with bilateral lesions, and most patients have basal ganglia involvement.[214] Lesions are often small (1–3 cm) and hemorrhage rare. Progressive multifocal leukoencephalopathy is a demyelinating disease that results in diffuse, nonenhancing, hemispheric, white matter lesions without edema or mass effect. Primary CNS lymphoma usually produces single, hyperdense lesions that enhance unevenly. Multiple lesions may be found in some patients, particularly in serial studies of untreated individuals. CT scanning may have normal findings, or it may reveal cerebral atrophy. Up to one-half of patients with HIV encephalopathy and a substantial proportion of patients with other CNS pathology may have atrophy. In patients with HIV infection, normal CT scan results do not rule out CNS disease. If clinical findings suggest intracranial mass lesions, a negative CT scan should be followed by an MRI scan. High–field strength, T 2-weighted MRI scans are more sensitive than CT scans are in detecting cerebral abscesses and other CNS pathology.[216] Magnetic resonance imaging often reveals multiple high-intensity target lesions (which suggest toxoplas-

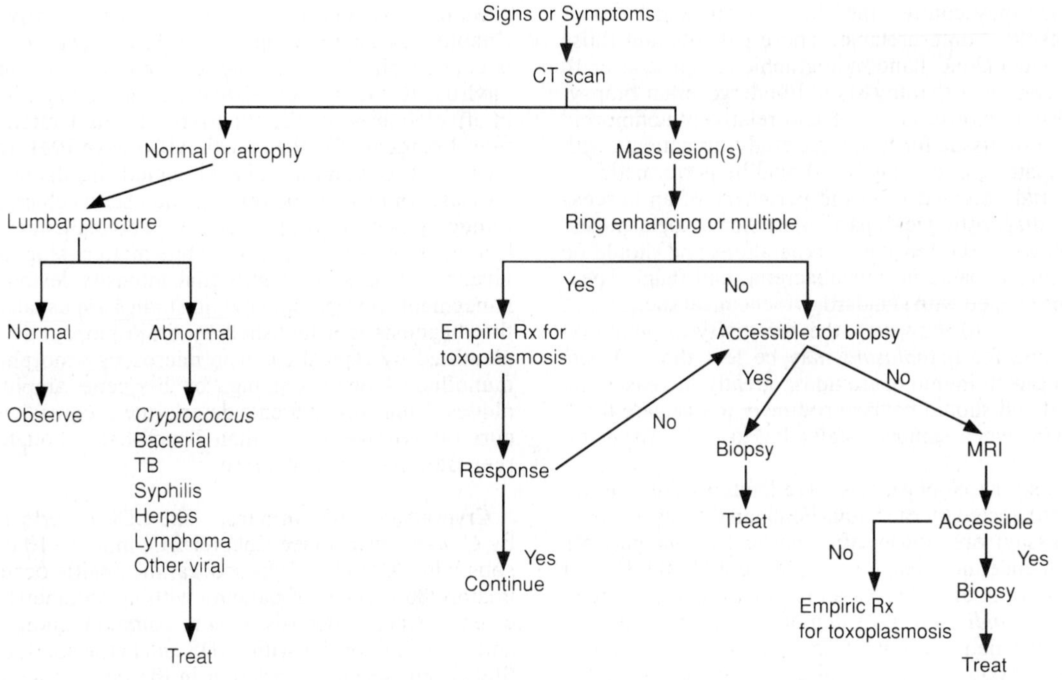

FIG. 3. Algorithm for evaluating neurologic abnormalities in patients with HIV.

mosis) when the CT scan shows only a single ring-enhancing lesion. Magnetic resonance image scanning also reveals lesions in the basal ganglia in virtually all patients with toxoplasmosis. When multiple lesions and basal ganglia lesions are absent in MRI scanning, this finding strongly suggests a diagnosis other than toxoplasmosis. Progressive multifocal leukoencephalopathy characteristically causes hemispheric, white matter lesions; on MRI scans, multiple, high-signal, nonenhancing white matter lesions are found. Solitary lesions on MRI scans may be CNS lymphomas, cryptococcomas, tuberculomas, or viral encephalitides.

Patients with suspected CNS mass lesions can first be evaluated with a CT scan. If the scan reveals no mass effect, a lumbar puncture can be performed. Cerebrospinal fluid should be sent for a cell count and differential; protein and glucose determination; cryptococcal antigen assay; bacterial, mycobacterial, viral, and fungal culture; cytology; and VDRL testing. *Toxoplasma* serology may be peformed; however, it is nonspecific and insensitive and should not be relied on to determine treatment options.[217] If the CT scan findings are normal or show only atrophy and no alternative diagnosis is established by clinical examination or laboratory studies, an MRI scan should be performed. Similarly, if the CT scan finds only a single focal lesion and biopsy of the lesion is not feasible (e.g., a basal ganglion lesion), MRI scanning should be performed. Previously, focal lesions on the CT or MRI scan of an immunocompromised patient required a brain biopsy to make a specific diagnosis. In recent years, empirical anti-*Toxoplasma* therapy has been accepted as an alternative to biopsy in selected patients because a growing number of AIDS patients have intracranial masses and among such patients toxoplasmosis is prevalent. Patients who may be empirically treated include the following:

1. Patients who have typical CT or MRI scan findings (multiple ring-enhancing lesions) and consistent clinical presentation
2. Patients with no lesion accessible for biopsy
3. Patients who refuse biopsy.

Empirical therapy is not indicated for patients with a single lesion detected by MRI scan; patients with tuberculosis, cryptococcosis, other fungal infection, or malignancy at an anatomic site outside the CNS; or patients allergic to anti-*Toxoplasma* drugs. Empirical treatment should be avoided in patients with mass effect who require steroid therapy because the response to steroids alone may confuse the clinical picture and render later biopsy results uninterpretable. These patients and those who have not had a clinical and radiographic response after 10 to 14 days of empirical therapy should undergo brain biopsy. Stereotactic needle biopsy is a safe and relatively nonmorbid way to obtain brain tissue for histologic study. In patients with impending herniation, open biopsies should be performed.

Biopsy material obtained from the periphery of an abscess has the highest diagnostic yield, particularly for toxoplasmosis. Fresh tissue may be used for touch preparations and should be cultured for viruses, bacteria, mycobacteria, and fungi. Specimens should be stained with standard cytochemical stains (e.g., hematoxylin and eosin); however, the sensitivity of hematoxylin-eosin staining for *toxoplasma* may be less than 50 percent.[218] Staining with immunoperoxidase greatly increases the diagnostic yield and should be used routinely to evaluate brain biopsy specimens when standard stains fail to make a specific diagnosis.

Serologic tests for toxoplasmosis have limited value. Serum IgG antibodies (detected by the Sabin-Feldman dye test or hemagglutination assay) are nonspecific, particularly in patients from areas with endemic *Toxoplasma* infections. In the United States 30–50 percent of AIDS patients have previously been infected with *T. gondii* and have demonstrable antibodies.[219] At the Memorial Sloan Kettering Cancer Center, one-third of the IgG-positive AIDS patients studied later developed CNS toxoplasmosis.[219] Conversely, IgG-negative patients with biopsy-confirmed CNS toxoplasmosis have been reported.[213,220] In patients with AIDS, increases in baseline IgG titers indicate active toxoplasmosis unreliably.[222] IgM antibody levels against *Toxoplasma* are frequently increased in nonimmunosuppressed patients with acute toxoplasmosis but are rarely elevated in AIDS-related, reactivated disease.[223–225] The intrathecal production of anti-*Toxoplasma* IgG has been proposed as a relatively sensitive and specific test that suggests CNS toxoplasmosis when positive (ratio >1). This method is limited clinically because treatment often must be given long before test results are available. Moreover, this technique has not been sufficiently assessed to determine its sensitivity and specificity. Consequently, treatment decisions should not be based on serologic test results alone.

Specific Etiologies of Opportunistic CNS Disease. TOXOPLASMOSIS. Toxoplasmosis (see Chapter 255) causes most intracranial mass lesions in AIDS patients. CNS toxoplasmosis is the index diagnosis of AIDS in approximately 2 percent of patients in the United States, and it occurs as a secondary diagnosis in an additional 2–5 percent.[226] In geographic areas where the underlying prevalence of remote infection with *T. gondii* is high (e.g., France, Haiti), cerebral toxoplasmosis among AIDS patients is very prevalent. Of those AIDS patients who have mass lesions revealed by CT head scans, 50–70 percent have toxoplasmosis.[214]

Central nervous system toxoplasmosis presents as a global encephalitis with altered mental status in up to 75 percent of patients. Fifty percent of patients report headaches, although those headaches are not typically severe. About 50 percent may have focal neurologic signs (i.e., seizure, hemiparesis, or ataxia); fewer than 50 percent may have fever. Symptoms often have a subscute onset—over a period of days to several weeks—with a median of 22 days in one series.[206] Pathologically, toxoplasmosis results in a diffuse encephalitis with focal areas of intense inflammation and necrosis. Abscesses show acute and chronic inflammation and infiltration by PMNs, lymphocytes, and histiocytes. The abscess centers are necrotic, with scant organisms. On the periphery of an abscess, numerous *T. gondii* tachyzoites may be found, while cyst forms can be seen in non-necrotic tissue. In small vessels surrounding abscesses, vasculitis may be present; reactive astrocytosis is seen adjacently.

PROGRESSIVE MULTIFOCAL LEUKOENCEPHALOPATHY. PML (see Chapter 124), a demyelinating disease of cerebral white matter, is characterized by multiple, discrete foci of disease. A papovavirus, JC virus, is consistently identified in oligodendrocytes in affected areas of the syndrome. In the United States, fewer than 1 percent of patients with AIDS have PML reported to the CDC.[226] The symptoms of PML include headache, ataxia, hemiparesis, confusion, and other mental status changes. Computed tomography scans most often reveal nonenhancing, low-density lesions of the periventricular white matter. Magnetic resonance imaging scans show high-signal intensity lesions without enhancement. Cerebrospinal fluid studies are usually unrevealing; the diagnosis is established by brain biopsy. JC virus can be identified by typical electron microscopy morphology, by immunofluorescence staining, or by gene amplification techniques. Clinically, patients deteriorate progressively. Death occurs on average in less than 3 months, although spontaneous remission has been reported.[228]

Cryptococcus neoformans. The CDC reports disease caused by *C. neoformans* (see Chapter 241) in up to 10 percent of persons with AIDS.[231] Cryptococcal meningitis occurs in approximately 80 percent of patients with symptomatic cryptococcal disease. Cryptococcosis is more common among iv drug users and ethnic minorities with AIDS and in the south-central United States. No seasonal variation in the occurrence of cryptococcosis has been reported. A number of other clinical syndromes including pneumonitis, multiple skin lesions resembling molluscum contagiosum, fungemia, and prostatitis may also be seen. Cryptococcal meningitis often presents clinically with nonspecific symptoms. Eighty percent of patients complain only of fever, night sweats, malaise, and a dull headache.[232] Severe headache, photophobia, meningismus, and an altered sensorium occur in 2–20 percent of patients. Focal neurologic complaints such as seizures, cranial nerve abnormalities, or hemiparesis are rare. Many patients may have only low-grade fever. Other symptoms may be elicited retrospectively after cryptococcosis is diagnosed. Clinicians need to be vigilant to detect cryptococcal disease early in its course before it disseminates and fulminant disease develops.

The diagnosis of cryptococcal meningitis is made by detecting cryptococcal antigen and growth of *Cryptococcus* in the cerebrospinal fluid. Patients with suspected cryptococcal meningitis should be carefully examed neurologically and ophthalmologically. If no focal neurologic abnormalities are noted and papilledema is absent, a lumbar puncture may be performed with small risk of complication. If neurologic abnormalities or altered sensorium are noted, a CT scan of the head should be obtained before performing a lumbar puncture. In many institutions, clinicians perform CT scanning on all patients before a lumbar puncture. The CSF findings of cryptococcal meningitis in AIDS is usually benign, with a pleocytosis of 5–50 mononuclear cells/mm^3, slightly elevated protein levels, and a normal glucose concentration. India ink examination reveals organisms in 50–90 percent of cases, and the cryptococcal antigen is positive in more than 95 percent of patients. Cultures of the CSF are invariably positive in primary disease but may be negative in patients who are relapsing from previously treated cryptococcosis. A rising antigen titer in the CSF strongly suggests relapse in this setting, particularly if the lysis-centrifugation technique is used.

Cryptococcal infections are acquired by inhaling the organism into the lungs. The primary pulmonary infection is often asymptomatic, even in immunodeficient hosts; however, cryptococcal pneumonia does occur in patients with advanced HIV infection. The clinical features of cryptococcal pneumonia include the insidious onset of fever, night sweats, malaise, cough, and dyspnea. The radiograph may show focal lobar infiltrates, sometimes with cavitation. Examination of induced sputum (using silver methenamine stain) may show yeast. Bronchoalveolar lavage fluid and transbronchial biopsy specimens may also show yeast, and cultures may yield *C. neoformans*. Cryptococcal antigenemia is present variably, and fungal blood cultures may grow *Cryptococcus*.

Other extraneural sites of disease are less common in AIDS patients with cryptococcosis. Fungemia is present in >80 percent of patients with cryptococcal meningitis, but other organs are not usually involved. The organism has been found in the bone marrow, liver, spleen, kidneys, skin, and other organs, and it may compromise organ function in some cases.

Cytomegalovirus. Cytomegalovirus (see Chapter 120) is ubiquitous in patients with HIV infection and causes serious morbidity in AIDS. Cytomegalovirus is transmitted by the same routes as HIV, and almost all patients with sexually acquired HIV infection are also infected with CMV. Like other herpesviruses, CMV may infect cells latently and reactivate when host defenses are impaired. Asymptomatic CMV viruria and viremia may be found in more than 50 percent of patients with AIDS,[233] but whether this predicts the subsequent development of CMV disease is uncertain. Ultimately, between 2 and 10 percent of AIDS patients have organs involved with CMV, and most AIDS patients autopsied have evidence of CMV infection.[170]

CMV RETINITIS. The eye is the end organ most often involved in CMV disease.[234] Cytomegalovirus retinitis is the index diagnosis of AIDS in 1–2 percent of patients and occurs subsequently in 4–6 percent. The onset of CMV retinitis may be insidious or rapid. Patients complain of painless, progressive visual loss, blurring, and "floaters." Cytomegalovirus retinitis usually presents unilaterally, although it may subsequently progress to the contralateral retina. Funduscopic examination of the involved eye typically reveals coalescing white exudates in a vascular pattern with surrounding hemorrhage and edema.

Often, lesions are peripheral initially, involve the fovea later, and result in visual loss. Retinal detachment may occur as a late complication.

Patients complaining of ocular symptoms should undergo a thorough ophthalmologic examination. The differential diagnosis of retinal lesions includes cotton wool spots, ischemic retinopathy, Roth spots, and toxoplasmic retinitis. Cotton wool spots are very prevalent in patients with AIDS but do not appear to predict the development of other retinal disease. The cotton-wool spots are distributed in a vascular pattern similar to CMV, but do not have the irregular pattern of exudate and hemorrhage that is characteristic of CMV retinitis. Similarly, *Toxoplasma* retinitis shows discrete, rounded, pale exudates. Autopsy studies of persons dying with CMV retinitis have shown retinal necrosis, hemorrhage, and mononuclear cell infiltration. Cytomegalovirus (but not HIV) DNA and RNA can be detected in affected cells. An ophthalmologist or other highly trained observer can make a premortem diagnosis by visually inspecting the lesions. Cultures of the blood and urine yield CMV in 80–100 percent of cases, respectively. At autopsy, one quarter of patients with CMV retinitis may also have CMV encephalitis.[234a]

MALIGNANCIES IN THE HIV-INFECTED PATIENT

Along with opportunistic infections and clinical problems directly attributed to HIV itself, malignant neoplasms are frequent causes of severe morbidity and mortality. The recognition and management of these cancers are key components of comprehensive AIDS care, and research into their etiology and pathogenesis is expected to shed additional light on oncogenesis in non–HIV-infected patients.

Early Reports of AIDS-Related Cancers

Cases of Kaposi sarcoma (KS) in young homosexual men in the early 1980s helped alert the medical community to the AIDS epidemic. Before this, KS had been a rare and relatively indolent cutaneous neoplasm of elderly men in the United States and elsewhere[235] and also an endemic malignancy in parts of central Africa.[236–238] Additionally, KS had been reported as a complication of exogenous corticosteroids taken to prevent organ transplant rejection.[239–245] Although an interesting disease because of these unusual geographic patterns and postulated associations with CMV infection[246,247] and iatrogenic immune suppression, KS was not a clinically significant problem in the United States.

In 1980 several cases of KS were diagnosed in homosexual men in New York, and these and similar cases from California were described in a series of reports in 1981 and 1982.[248–250] Several aspects of these cases were distinctly unusual (Table 15). First, they affected a much younger population than prior ("classic") KS in the United States, Second, the tumor was much more aggressive, with early and wide dissemination the rule. Finally, the patients often had the same spectrum of unusual infections being diagnosed simultaneously in other homosexual men but had no known reason for immune deficiency. The combination of these striking findings in similar "risk" populations soon led to the recognition of a common underlying disorder, AIDS.

The second malignancy recognized as part of the AIDS epidemic was non-Hodgkins lymphoma (NHL). Sporadic cases of NHL of CNS origin in individuals with other manifestations of AIDS resulted in the early inclusion of this cancer in AIDS surveillance definitions.[251–253] Subsequently, NHL of peripheral origin was also reported in association with AIDS.[254–264] Since 1984, NHL in both sites has become increasingly common, and its clinical appearance, biology, and management have been the subject of several reviews and ongoing clinical trials. The severe clinical problems caused by NHL make it, like KS, an important disease for the clinician to understand.

In addition to KS and NHL, an increasing variety of other cancers have been diagnosed in HIV-infected individuals. Although less common than KS and NHL and less clearly linked causally to HIV infection, these tumors may also offer insight into the relationship between HIV, immune deficiency, and oncogenesis. While the wide variety of these cancers and their relative rarity precludes extensive discussion in this chapter, their diagnosis should be considered when clinically appropriate.

Epidemiology of AIDS-Related Malignancies—Kaposi Sarcoma

Kaposi sarcoma (KS) is, by far, the most common neoplasm in HIV-infected patients.[265–267] Overall, 9 percent of all AIDS cases reported to the CDC have been initially diagnosed with KS as compared with <1 percent with NHL, the next most common cancer. Many more patients develop KS or lymphoma later in their disease course. Kaposi sarcoma is, in fact, one of the most common clinical manifestations of HIV-disease, and as mentioned, its increased incidence was an early indicator of the AIDS epidemic.

Kaposi sarcoma, for reasons still unclear, disproportionately affects HIV-infected male homosexuals.[265–268] In the first several years of the epidemic, for example, 47 percent of newly diagnosed AIDS cases in homosexual and bisexual men had KS as compared with 3.9 percent in intravenous drug users.[269] Kaposi sarcoma is rare in all heterosexuals with HIV disease except black Africans.[270,271] In Africa, KS is more common and clinically more aggressive in the HIV-infected population when compared with reports before the HIV epidemic.[272–276] While precise incidence figures are not available, KS does seem more common in African AIDS patients than in other groups of heterosexuals.[277,278] Kaposi sarcoma in children with AIDS has been reported but is rare.[279] Recent work suggests that even when adjusted for risk-group category KS may be more common in whites than blacks.[280]

Adding even more to the interest in KS are studies showing that it is an epidemiologic "moving target." For example, its incidence in homosexual men is clearly decreasing in the United States.[281,282] Compared with initial rates of 36 percent of AIDS cases at diagnosis, more recent work now shows a 6 percent incidence of KS.[269]

Not only is the incidence of KS declining, but its mortality rate also appears to be worsening. In a preliminary study from San Francisco the median duration of survival for a group of KS patients diagnosed in 1982–1983 was 24 months, while a cohort diagnosed from 1984 to 1986 had a 14-month median survival.[283] In this study, HIV p24 antigen was more frequently detectable in the more recent group (76 vs. 43 percent, $p = .03$), which suggests that KS had been diagnosed at a later point in the course of the HIV infection.

Explanations for the unusual epidemiologic profile of KS in the AIDS epidemic are yet being developed.[284] The relative restriction to homosexuals has been speculated secondary to recreational drug use[285,286] or to a second, as yet unidentified sexually transmitted virus. Either theory could at least partially explain the change in KS incidence (decreasing exposure to a second "cofactor"), but neither clarifies the more rapid disease course now being seen.

Ideally, information from epidemiology studies could contribute to our knowledge of the pathogenesis of KS, but this is not yet the case. No recreational drug used primarily by homosexual men, including the inhaled nitrites once popular, have been clearly shown to be carcinogenic or particularly immunosuppressive. Similarly, despite some early speculation, no coincident "KS virus" has been found. Recent work points to HIV-induced endothelial growth factors as potentially involved in KS formation, but to date this theory is not reconciled with the complex and variable epidemiology of KS in different HIV-infected populations.

Clinical Appearance and Pathophysiology of Kaposi Sarcoma in HIV Infection. Kaposi sarcoma (Table 15) is considered by most an endothelial neoplasm of either capillary or lymphatic origin.[287–289] Histologically, the tumor is typified by a proliferation of vascular structures, often with large malignant-appearing endothelial cells, set against a background of a bland proliferation of spindle-shaped cells and extravasated erythrocytes.[236,290–294] Efforts to establish KS cell lines in culture have made little headway,[295,296] and direct tumor transplants to immunodeficient animals have been unsuccessful. This and the not uncommonly indolent clinical behavior have led to speculation that KS is not in the truest sense a malignancy at all but rather a striking benign cellular proliferation[297] in response to some circulating "growth factor."

Laboratory support for a KS growth factor comes from the preliminary work of Dr. Robert Gallo. Here, inoculation of immunodeficient mice with cells cultured from human KS tumors led to the appearance of vascular tumors in the mouse. Interestingly, however, these tumors were of murine rather than human genetic origin.[295,296]

The clinical pattern of KS is usually not difficult to recognize and can be somewhat predicted from the histologic appearance. Kaposi sarcoma lesions are typically nodular, pigmented, and initially asymptomatic. Size varies from several millimeters to confluent tumor plaques 5–10 cm in diameter. Violaceous to red pigmentation is common, but KS in dark-skinned persons may be nearly black, and occasionally patients irrespective of race have subcutaneous lesions that are nonpigmented. Nodularity of KS lesions is typical, and even small lesions are usually palpable. Many areas of the body can be affected by KS, although some are rarely involved. For example, KS is frequently seen on the skin and in the oral cavity, and while the soles are one of the most common KS sites, the tumor rarely affects the palms.[249,298–308]

Kaposi sarcoma is a multicentric tumor, and numerous lesions can appear simultaneously in widely scattered areas of the body. Kaposi sarcoma in the HIV-infected patient, unlike most other KS populations, often involves visceral structures.[309] Kaposi sarcoma in the gastrointestinal tract is seen in almost 50 percent of cases, most commonly in the stomach, duodenum, and rectum. Another important visceral site of KS is the lung. Both sites will be discussed below.

The lymphatic endothelial origin postulated for KS is often reflected in the gross clinical appearance of the disease. Linearity of lesions following cutaneous lymphatic drainage patterns is particularly common across the chest and back. Lymphedema, often out of proportion to the visible extent of tumor,

TABLE 15. Kaposi Sarcoma in AIDS—Distinguishing Characteristics

Extent of disease	Unlike "traditional" KS, AIDS/KS is *rarely* limited to a single anatomic region
Site of involvement	The head and neck are common primary sites (including the face, oral cavity)
Visceral involvement	Common, rarely symptomatic except for pulmonary KS, which is *rapidly* fatal
Opportunistic infections	Almost uniform during the course of disease; usual cause of death
Social problems	The stigma of AIDS is exacerbated by visible lesions

is seen in some patients and usually affects either the lower extremities or face. In extreme cases, lymphedema of the lower portion of the body to the level of the diagphragm is observed.

Gastrointestinal Kaposi Sarcoma. The GI tract is the most common visceral site of KS.[310–313] As many as 50 percent of patients with KS have lesions in the GI tract even early in the course of their disease. Gastrointestinal KS is seldom symptomatic and is rarely if ever fatal. In some cases, however, GI KS can cause intestinal obstruction, bleeding, or enteropathy. Essentially, any segment of the GI tract may be involved with KS, although the stomach and duodenum are most commonly affected.[314]

The diagnosis of GI KS is most often made by the endoscopic visualization of typical lesions.[311,315] Endoscopy is not routinely recommended in all KS patients and should be reserved for those with GI symptoms. Radiographic visualization of KS is possible, with contrast studies showing raised, smooth, rounded intraluminal masses. The diagnostic accuracy of these studies, however, is not as high as with endoscopy.[316,317]

On endoscopy, KS lesions are nodular and raised and appear highly vascular. As with cutaneous lesions, they vary in size from several millimeters to several centimeters in diameter. Any number may be present, but confluent tumor masses are unusual. Despite their ready visualization, GI KS lesions are not easily diagnosed by biopsy because the tumor is subcutaneous, beyond the depth of the biopsy forceps in 77 percent of cases.[315] If biopsy confirmation is considered essential for patient management, a higher yield may be achieved with loop biopsy technique (Cello J, personal communication, 1988).

Pulmonary KS. Pulmonary parenchymal involvement by KS is less commonly recognized than gastrointestinal spread is but, when present, is more often symptomatic.[318–321] In fact, the general principle that KS, even in the HIV-infected patient, is not directly fatal is not true with symptomatic pulmonary disease where the median duration of survival is approximately 3 months.[319]

The symptoms of pulmonary KS, described in several reviews,[318–320,322] usually consist of dyspnea, a severe but minimally productive cough, chest tightness, and less commonly, fever. These symptoms clearly overlap with those of *Pneumocystis carinii* and CMV and mycobacterial pneumonias, which are the main diseases to be considered in a differential diagnosis.

The diagnosis of pulmonary KS is to some degree one of exclusion, particularly of PCP. The chest x-ray findings in pulmonary KS tend to show a more nodular pattern with less even infiltration than is typical of PCP. Pleural effusions are also more suggestive of pulmonary KS. These effusions are frequently bloody, but cytologic examination is usually nondiagnostic. Pulmonary gallium scan can provide useful information in some cases, generally showing no uptake in patients with pulmonary KS in contrast to those with infectious pneumonias.[322,323]

Bronchoscopy provides the strongest evidence of pulmonary KS. Although the pulmonary parenchyma is the principle site of disease, in most cases endobronchial lesions are easily visualized by an experienced bronchoscopist. Lesions are several millimeters or more in diameter and appear redder and more vascular than cutaneous KS lesions are. Biopsy is relatively contraindicated because of possible hemorrhage, but transbronchial biopsy has been used to diagnose KS in some cases. Patients with pulmonary KS almost always have extensive cutaneous KS as well, although primary pulmonary KS has been reported.[318,324] At any rate, the presence of typical pulmonary symptoms and diagnostic tests in the absence of an infectious pneumonia should be considered adequate to warrant management for pulmonary KS.

Diagnosis of Cutaneous Kaposi Sarcoma. A clinician should, with some experience, have no difficulty in recognizing typical cutaneous KS lesions, but biopsy confirmation should be obtained, particularly if this information will be used to make an initial AIDS diagnosis. A punch biopsy (ideally ≥4 mm in diameter) is usually sufficient. The biopsy can be safely performed in an outpatient setting with local anesthesia. Despite the vascular nature of KS, hemorrhage is rarely encountered. While KS has been diagnosed from fine-needle aspiration cytology specimens, this technique is almost certainly less sensitive and specific, and its use should be limited.

Oral Kaposi Sarcoma. The oral cavity is an extremely common site of KS.[302,325,326] In as many as one-third of patients this represents the first site of disease, while it appears later in the course of KS in many others. Intraoral lesions are most common on the hard palate but are not uncommon on the posterior pharyngeal wall or the gingiva.[327] The tongue is an uncommon site of KS, and the buccal mucosa is almost always spared.

The appearance of oral KS is typical and similar to cutaneous disease. Lesions on the hard palate, however, are often not palpable and are blue to violet in color. Biopsy (usually by an oral surgeon) can be performed, and this should be done if other, more easily sampled cutaneous lesions are not present.[307,328]

Intraoral KS is generally asymptomatic until late in the disease course. Then, the lesions can become bulky, with superficial necrosis leading to pain, bleeding, and occasionally difficulty in swallowing. Gingival KS can additionally contribute to the periodontal disease seen in many AIDS patients.

Staging, Clinical Course, and Management of Kaposi Sarcoma. PROGNOSTIC FACTORS/STAGING Staging of KS (Table 16) by estimates of tumor burden have been proposed by several groups.[306,329] Usually, KS in these systems is categorized by the number, size, appearance, site of involvement, and the rate of growth. Although most experienced clinicians are convinced that KS patients can be divided into those with "minimal" tumor burden and those with "advanced" KS, no common definitions have been accepted. This is problematic for the individual patient and practitioner who would like more precise information available to better discuss the prognosis and plan therapy, but it is of even more concern for the design and comparison of clinical investigations.

Admitting limitations, some broad staging guidelines of KS extent can be proposed. Patients with "few" lesions (for example, <25), those without known visceral or intraoral disease, and those with an established history of "slow" tumor growth are judged more stable than are those patients with many lesions or with any extracutaneous involvement. Similarly, patients with a history of minimal increase in lesion size or number over a several month period (not an uncommon observation at the time of actual biopsy) have a better prognosis than do patients in whom new lesions are rapidly appearing. Some feel that the prognosis is improved when the lesions are geographically con-

TABLE 16. Prognostic Variables in Kaposi Sarcoma

Predicts Indolent Course	*Predicts Aggressive Course*
Few lesions (<25)	Many KS lesions
Low rate of growth	Rapid appearance of new lesions
No visceral KS identified	Intraoral or visceral lesions
No fevers, drenching night sweats, or weight loss	One or more constitutional symptoms
No prior opportunistic infection	One prior or concurrent opportunistic infection
Absolute CD4+ count, >400/mm^3	CD4+ cell count, <200/mm^3
Normal ESR	ESR, >40 mm/hr
HIV p24 antigen not detectible	HIV p24 detectable
Normal β_2-microglobulin	β_2-microglobulin, >5
Normal blood counts	Leukopenia or anemia present

fined to one body area, for example, the skin of one extremity, No firm data exist to support this, however. Certainly, the prognosis is worsened if visceral KS is diagnosed. The median duration of survival is less than 4 months, for example, in patients with pulmonary KS. While the effect of gastrointestinal and intraoral KS on survival duration is less clear, disease in these sites is also felt to imply a worsened prognosis.

Along with estimates of KS tumor burden, it is known that the symptomatic status of the patient is important in the prognosis. Similar to Hodgkin's and non-Hodgkin's lymphoma, KS patients with chronic systemic symptoms such as unexplained fevers, night sweats, and weight loss have a decrease in median survival duration.[330] Also, this effect is cumulative, and the prognosis is additionally limited in patients with multiple constitutional symptoms. Whether one or more specific symptoms have a greater impact is now being investigated.

A final means of staging KS involves laboratory tests grouped into those of general value an those specifically estimating HIV burden and/or immunologic impairment.[298,300,331,332] Survival duration is decreased in patients with severe anemia or neutropenia or with erythrocyte sedimentation rates above 40 mm/hr. Abnormalities in serum chemistry test results have not been shown to be of independent value, although elevated serum globulin levels are common in KS as in other HIV-infected patients.

Probably the strongest laboratory predictors of outcome in KS are likely to be those that are more directly involved in HIV and its immune effects. HIV p24 antigen, for example, if present in AIDS patients in detectable concentrations, implies a poor prognosis,[333] which is also correlated with severe depression in the number of circulating CD4+ cells. This general observation is likely to hold true in patients with KS. Similar speculations can be made for other markers such as β_2-microglobulin.

As with other methods of staging KS, laboratory abnormalities are often closely correlated with other poor prognostic markers. Rather than enabling the clinician or clinical investigator to precisely define the stage of disease or prognosis, all staging information must be taken into account. It is, from a clinical practice standpoint, probably adequate to group KS patients into those with a reasonably high likelihood of a 1-year survival without secondary opportunistic infections or rampant KS growth and into others where these clinical events are much more probable. Using this information, the clinician can better advise the patient concerning opportunistic infection prophylaxis and the need for specific antineoplastic therapy. A summary of the prognostic and staging variables discussed is shown in Table 16.

INITIAL EVALUATION OF THE PATIENT WITH KAPOSI SARCOMA. The goals of an initial evaluation of a patient with suspected KS vary depending on the patients' prior health status. If KS represents the initial AIDS-defining process, biopsy is essential. If, on the other hand, the patient has had prior opportunistic infections and if the KS is not likely to require treatment either because of poor baseline prognosis or because the extent of KS is still minimal, biopsy may not be required, especially if the lesion sites are on visible skin or are intraoral.

The initial evaluation can, overall, be divided into those tests that would be performed in any new AIDS patient to estimate viral burden and immune damage and to rule out opportunistic infections. The specific application of these tests to the new KS patient is to estimate the prognosis and plan treatment. To this end, a careful examination of the entire body surface is essential, with recording of the number, size, site, and general appearance of visible KS lesions. Photography of selected areas can be useful for later establishing progression or response to treatment. The examination should include a digital rectal exam to palpate possible KS lesions and a careful examination of the pharynx to identify intraoral KS lesions on the palate, posterior oral pharynx, or gingiva. Routine gastrointestinal endoscopy is not recommended unless indicated for specific symptomatology.

The initial (and each subsequent) medical history should inquire about the constitutional symptoms discussed previously and about any symptoms potentially related to opportunistic infections. Because these are often the cause of death in patients with KS,[334] their diagnosis, prophylaxis, and treatment must be considered at *all* times by treating physicians.

Laboratory studies in the KS patient should include a complete blood count, determination of the ESR, and a routine chemistry panel. As with all parts of the spectrum of HIV disease, HIV infection must be established with HIV antibody tests, and all patients should be tested for serologic evidence of syphilis and active hepatitis B infection. HIV status can be additionally evaluated with an HIV p24 antigen and indirectly with β_2-microglobulin determination. Immunologic testing should include T-lymphocyte subset testing with enumeration of CD4+ and CD8+ populations. Given recent evidence, these can probably be expressed most accurately as their percentages of the total T-lymphocyte population, although following their absolute number (a further calculated estimate) is more commonly used.[298,300] The use of skin testing for delayed hypersensitivity reactivity is advocated by some groups but is probably of limited additional value when compared with the other tests discussed.

As soon as the results of the initial examination are available, the patient should be informed of the results. This discussion should attempt to give the patient a better sense of the disease prognosis to help further decision making. Specific counseling should address the need for considering antiretroviral therapy and the importance of recognizing, treating, and if possible, preventing opportunistic infections. The options for treating the KS directly should also be frankly reviewed. This discussion should, of course, include the possibility of not treating the KS per se if that seems an option and should also address the common concerns about the visible nature of KS and the fear that antineoplastic treatment—particularly chemotherapy and radiation therapy—may cause further immune impairment or may further compromise the ability to tolerate zidovudine administration.

Therapy for Kaposi Sarcoma. Although perhaps less dramatic than progress in antiretroviral drug development, research in the treatment of KS has improved overall patient care. Kaposi sarcoma therapy (Table 17) currently reflects the growing realization that the tumor, which while not a true malignancy according to some definitions,[297] has a heterogeneous natural history ranging from indolent to rapidly fatal that takes place against a backdrop of progressive HIV-induced immune depletion. Thus, recent reports include both local treatments and increasingly aggressive chemotherapy regimens as well as attempts to combine antineoplastic drugs with agents of antiviral potential such as zidovudine. These approaches are summarized in Table 17, which stresses the individualization of treatment based on the patient's estimated prognosis.

LOCAL THERAPY. Many patients experience more problems from individual lesions than from their overall disease. This is especially common in patients with bulky intraoral KS, those with scattered facial lesions, and those with lesions in areas subjected to recurrent minor trauma (e.g., the ankle). Surgical excision or local radiation therapy remain good options for some of these situations, and increasingly, topical or intralesional treatments are also being evaluated. Radiation therapy rapidly shrinks individual KS lesions and is also frequently administered to somewhat broader areas of the body to control plaques of coalesced lesions or to reduce KS-associated lymphedema.[335–344] Although tumor responses to relatively low doses of radiation therapy (2000–3000 rads) are gratifying, local toxicity remains a problem for some patients. Particularly common

TABLE 17. Guidelines for Kaposi Sarcoma Treatment

Patient Status	*Options*
Favorable prognostic indicators[a]	Expectant observation Alternating single-agent chemotherapy such as vinblastine/vincristine Interferon-α with or without zidovudine Experimental treatment trials
Unfavorable prognostic indicators[a]	Early initiation of therapy Alternating vincristine/vinblastine chemotherapy Other single-agent chemotherapy (e.g., Adriamycin) Combination chemotherapy (e.g., Adriamycin, bleomycin, vincristine)
Local tumor problems	Radiation therapy Topical liquid nitrogen Intralesional dilute vinblastine Surgical excision

[a] See Table 15.

are moderate to severe mucositis from radiating large intraoral KS lesions and cutaneous erythema from radiating larger lesions on the feet. These local toxicities are temporary and, in the case of intraoral mucositis, can be reduced by scrupulous attention to oral hygiene and control of minor infections such as with *Candida albicans*.

Intralesional or topical treatments being investigated for KS include some that are not directly antineoplastic in the usual sense such as cryotherapy with liquid nitrogen or topical applications of dinitrochlorobenzene (DNCB). Other local treatments include injections of intralesional tumor necrosis factor or dilute vinblastine, agents that are presumably directly active on the tumor cells.

One observation only now being actively studied is that agents that cause a local inflammatory reaction can lead to KS regression. The most straightforward of these is the topical application of liquid nitrogen. This therapy (personal communication, Alvin Friedman-Kien, 1988) consists of applying liquid nitrogen by a cotton applicator to the lesion until a "halo" of surrounding erythema is observed. A mild inflammation results, and the lesion flattens as this resolves. Larger lesions may require repeated applications at approximately 2-week intervals. Small lesions may completely disappear with this therapy; larger ones may leave a residual hemosiderin "tattoo."

A similar result has been reported with injections of small volumes of dilute vinblastine directly into the KS lesion.[345] Here, a 0.2 mg/cc solution of sterile vinblastine is prepared and injected through a fine-gauge needle placed perpendicular to the skin surface in the center of small KS lesions. Larger lesions (>1 cm) may require two or more such injections at separate sites. Sufficient volume is injected into the lesion (usually less than 0.5 cc). Because of the low dose, multiple lesions can be treated simultaneously. As with liquid nitrogen application, a mild inflammatory reaction ensues, but cutaneous ulcerations are not common, and small lesions typically heal without scarring. Therapy can be repeated every 2 weeks if required. This therapy has also been applied to intraoral lesions, but these, if extensive, are probably best treated with radiation therapy even considering the frequent mucositis seen in HIV-infected patients with this therapy.

Other local therapies under investigation include intralesional injections of recombinant tumor necrosis factor.[346] This is supposedly directly cytotoxic to the KS lesion. Because even local injections of tumor necrosis factor have led to systemic side effects, this therapy is currently considered appropriate for experimental uses only. Similarly, groups are investigating intralesional injections of interferon-α, an agent recently approved for systemic use in KS.

SYSTEMIC CHEMOTHERAPY. Even early in the AIDS epidemic, recognition of the variable natural history of KS and the many uncertainties of staging led to concern that overly aggressive chemotherapy—particularly the use of combinations of agents—might be inappropriate in some patients. Awareness of the underlying immune deficiency caused fears of the immunologic toxicity resulting from the aggressive use of cytotoxic drugs. Thus, most subsequent efforts were directed at single-agent chemotherapy—giving this more frequently but in lower doses or in alternating regimens with other single-agent therapy. This direction has been of value; single-agent chemotherapy with vinblastine alone[347] at a dose of 4–8 mg weekly or alternated with vincristine[348] at 1–2 mg/dose is considered by many as a standard for HIV-related KS, especially if the disease is relatively indolent. Recently, equal or increased activity has been shown for single-agent Adriamycin given in attenuated doses (10–30 mg total dose) intravenously every 1–2 weeks.[349] In a study of the National Institute of Allergy and Infectious Diseases (NIAID)-supported AIDS Clinical Trials Group, for example, Adriamycin therapy administered weekly at a dose of 15 mg/m^2 resulted in a 16 percent partial remission in a group of 32 previously untreated patients. Also, vincristine as a single-drug treatment regimen is used for KS patients who are thrombocytopenic. This regimen has a high response rate—over 50 percent—with acceptable neurotoxicity.[350]

Although concern about immune toxicity is still appropriate, more information suggests that some combination chemotherapy can be used safely.[351,352] The group of KS patients with rapidly progressing and often fatal disease may, in fact, benefit from these more aggressive chemotherapeutic approaches. Gill et al. have reported recently that a combination of Adriamycin, bleomycin, and vincristine results in rapid and often complete KS responses with no apparent increase in expected rates of opportunistic infections. Doses of each agent are as follows: Adriamycin, 20 mg/m^2; bleomycin, 10 mg/m^2; vincristine, 1.4 mg/m^2, all given intravenously every other week.[353] Because of the cardiac, pulmonary, and neurologic toxicities of these agents, this regimen should probably be reserved for patients with poor overall prognoses. Its use should be accompanied by careful monitoring of toxicities.

INTERFERON-α. Systemic recombinant interferon-α has an established level of activity in treating HIV-related KS and recently earned Food and Drug Administration (FDA) approval for this indication. Objective response rates of approximately 40 percent can be expected and are even higher in selected patients with a more favorable overall prognosis.[354–358] The doses used have varied widely in reported trials, but daily doses of greater than 10 million units may be required for the optimum antineoplastic effect. The major predictor of poor response in several studies is the presence of chronic constitutional symptoms or a prior AIDS diagnosis when therapy with interferon is initiated. The drawbacks to single-agent interferon-α therapy are the side effects seen with the high doses required and the need for parenteral injection. Toxicities are primarily subjective—fever, malaise, nausea—but neutropenia is not uncommon, and central nervous system effects including confusion are also seen.

Recent studies in New York and Miami (again, supported by the NIAID AIDS Clinical Trials Group) show antineoplastic activity with low doses (9–18 million units) of recombinant or lymphoblastoid interferon-α along with low doses (100 mg every 4 hours) of zidovudine.[359–361] Hematologic toxicity was seen in these studies but was considered moderate and usually manageable by the investigators. Although this combination employs drugs readily available by prescription in the United States, physicians might be advised to await publication of final study results to permit a more detailed assessment of the attendant risks and benefits.

CHEMOTHERAPY WITH ZIDOVUDINE. Although carefully designed clinical trials of cytotoxic chemotherapy combined with zidovudine are not yet reported, considerable clinical experience has been collected that suggests that this will be difficult to administer. This is unfortunate because the rationale of this combination is attractive considering the dual problems of KS and the underlying HIV infection. Both zidovudine and many cytotoxic regimens used in KS induce some degree of myelosuppression, which is expected to be at least additive when these drugs are combined. Because of a lack of published investigation, no firm guidelines can be provided; however, in general, it seems prudent to maintain patients on a regimen of zidovudine as long as possible to achieve the expected survival benefit. Kaposi sarcoma can then be managed either by increasing the use of local therapies or by the use of non–marrow-toxic agents such as bleomycin and/or vincristine.

Antibiotic Prophylaxis of Opportunistic Infections. It is clear that most KS patients die not of their tumor but of opportunistic infections.[334] In the United States the most common of these is *Pneumocystis carinii* pneumonia. Recent studies show that this infection can be largely prevented by the use of appropriate antibiotics. In a Miami study by Fischl et al.[362] oral trimethoprim-sulfamethoxazole, when tolerated, completely prevented PCP in KS patients, whereas a concurrent group had an incidence of 53 percent without prophylaxis. The toxicity of this prophylaxis was reduced in the investigators' opinion by the inclusion of 5 mg/day of oral leucovorin. Still, 17 percent of subjects experienced toxicity including rash and myelosuppression, which required discontinuation of treatment.

Another attractive option for PCP prophylaxis is pentamidine isethionate given as an inhaled aerosol.[362–364] Although careful prospective results of clinical trials have not been published, this form of prophylaxis may avoid the problems of side effects common with trimethoprim-sulfamethoxazole.

Non-Hodgkin's Lymphoma

The second most common HIV-associated malignancy, non-Hodgkin's lymphoma (NHL), bears little epidemiologic resemblance to KS. Non-Hodgkin's lymphoma is less frequent than KS is; it is seen in <1 percent of reported cases of AIDS in the United States, but is not seemingly restricted to any specific risk group. Nor does the relative frequency of diagnosed NHL seem to be changing, although the absolute number of cases is increasing with the epidemic.[255,261,365]

The pathogenesis of HIV-associated NHL is unknown but is the subject of active laboratory investigation, although some of the tumor's biologic characteristics are understood.[366] Non-Hodgkin's lymphoma in AIDS is a B-lymphocyte neoplasm of unfavorable histologic grade.[260] Most are either large cell, undifferentiated, or immunoblastic types with a clinical presentation and natural history that matches their highly malignant pathologic appearance. No single cytogenetic abnormality has been found, but several different gene rearrangements have been reported.[367–369] A relationship to EBV has been proposed, but again, laboratory studies have been inconclusive, with EBV-related DNA sequences found in some, but not all specimens from several tumor sites in a single affected individual.[370]

Non-Hodgkin's lymphoma in HIV can be present in single or multiple sites, and the clinical problems are determined, in part, by areas of involvement, by the rate of tumor growth, and by the presence or absence of underlying or pre-existing HIV-related opportunistic infections. Malignant lymphocytes are often found in the peripheral blood of NHL patients with HIV, but it is uncommon for the lymphoma to present without easily identifiable solid tumor masses.

Central Nervous System Non-Hodgkin's Lymphoma. Non-Hodgkin's lymphoma occurring in the CNS in AIDS patients was recognized early in the epidemic, well before the peripheral lymphomas were reported, and thus the early CDC surveillance definitions of AIDS included NHL only of CNS origin.[253,371–373]

Central nervous system lymphomas cause the array of clinical problems expected from space-occupying intracranial masses, but these tumors have been surprisingly difficult to diagnose.[252,374] In part, diagnosis is difficult because of the other CNS processes that are more common in HIV infection, especially *Toxoplasma* encephalitis. In several autopsy series, CNS lymphomas have been surprisingly frequent, further attesting to the need to consider them in differential diagnoses and obtain a brain biopsy to establish the diagnosis.

Patients with NHL in the CNS may complain of motor deficits, but others present with cranial neuropathies, headache, or seizures, and frequently some combination of these are present. The onset of symptoms is usually rapid, and death can occur quickly in the absence of therapy.

The diagnosis of CNS NHL relies on a combination of suggestive imaging studies and brain biopsy. Either CT or MRI head scanning are commonly employed, but MRI is probaby a more sensitive test. In contrast to toxoplasmosis, NHL usually presents with a single mass lesion, but tumors occurring along the base of the skull can be missed by imaging. A brain biopsy must be used to finally establish the NHL diagnosis, especially if an empirical course of therapy for toxoplasmosis fails to rapidly (1–2 weeks) lead to a decrease in mass size. Examination of the CSF is not of significant value and should be deferred until large intracranial mass lesions are excluded by imaging studies.

Peripheral Non-Hodgkin's Lymphoma. The clinical presentation of NHL outside the CNS is highly varied because essentially any organ can be affected. In contrast to NHL in non–HIV-infected patients, extralymphatic disease is extremely common, with 63 percent of patients having stage IV disease.[253,254,260,263,375] Also, NHL in the HIV-infected group presents with disease in sites otherwise rarely seen. These have included primary lymphoma in the liver, common bile duct, rectum, soft tissue, duodenum, and lung.[254,376,377]

The clinical course and prognosis of NHL in the HIV infected is not surprising considering the tumor's aggressive histology. Patients often have fulminant disease progression, even developing the tumor lysis syndrome before initiation of therapy due to rapid tumor cell turnover. The prognosis of NHL in HIV infection is extremely grave. In several reports from Los Angeles, New York, and San Francisco, the median survival from diagnosis was <12 months.[254,255,364] Markers of prognosis include histologic type and stage as with the non–HIV-infected patient, but the most important factor is whether or nor the lymphoma represents the patient's first HIV-induced opportunistic disease. Patients with a prior history of AIDS have a median survival of 3 months as compared with 12 months for those initially diagnosed with AIDS on the basis of the lymphoma.[254] In fact, some would generally discourage treatment for patients with a prior AIDS diagnosis because of the poor prognosis and limited ability to tolerate the aggressive chemotherapy otherwise essential to control the lymphoma.

The relationship between persistent generalized lymphadenopathy (PGL) and NHL has been widely discussed but is still quite unclear. It is obvious that in some HIV-infected individuals B-cell proliferation results in diffuse and persisting lymph node enlargment. Occasionally, NHL arises in patients with PGL, but it is not certain that the factors responsible for PGL are the same as those causing the malignant proliferation. What is clear is that the usual caveats against biopsying nodes in patients with PGL need revision if one nodal group is rapidly enlarging. Because this is often due to NHL, immediate biopsy is essential.[378,379]

The diagnosis of NHL should ideally be made by histologic examination of tissue obtained by incisional or excisional biopsy. This permits a more accurate assessment of histologic type for special stains and immunologic subtyping. It may be possible, however, to make an adequate diagnosis from needle aspiration cytology, and this may be required if the patient's clinical condition is critical or deteriorating rapidly.[378] Because the disease is so often widespread, the initial clinical evaluation of the NHL patient should include imaging of the head, chest, and abdomen[380,381]; bone marrow aspiration and biopsy; and lumbar puncture. Once staging is completed, therapy, if it is to be recommended, should be initiated promptly and should be coordinated by an oncologist experienced with these extremely complex patients.

Therapy for HIV-Related Non-Hodgkin's Lymphoma. Therapy for HIV-related NHL is still under active investigation. If therapy is to be employed (potentially excluding those with extremely poor prognoses), an aggressive regimen must be used to achieve acceptable complete response rates. However, because patients with HIV infection have a limited bone marrow reserve, the clinician is frequently faced with the dilemma of selecting a regimen and dose of chemotherapy that controls the tumor without precipitating death from secondary infections. For NHL confined to the CNS, these questions are less urgent since primary therapy usually consists of whole brain radiation with intrathecal chemotherapy.[373]

CHEMOTHERAPY FOR NON-HODGKIN'S LYMPHOMA IN HIV-INFECTED PATIENTS. Few definite guidelines are possible for the treatment of HIV-related NHL. As with all aggressive lymphomas, the use of combinations of drugs is essential. In most reports, cyclophosphamide has been the primary agent,[254,260,263,382] however, because of the compromised marrow reserve at least one investigator favors an attenuated dose at the beginning and subsequent dose escalation. Older combinations such as Cytoxan, Adriamycin, vincristine, and prednisone (CHOP) are often avoided because their relatively prolonged dosing intervals may allow rapid tumor growth between cycles. Most clinicians favor attenuated doses of aggressive regimens such as M-BACOD (methotrexate, leucovorin rescue, bleomycin, doxorubicin, cyclophosphamide, vincristine, and dexamethasone (M-BACOD); methotrexate with leucovorin rescue, doxorubin, cyclophosphamide, vincristine, prednisone, and bleomycin (MACOP-B); cyclophosphamide, vincristine, prednisone, bleomycin, doxorubicin, and procarbazine (COP-BLAM); or cyclophosphamide, vincristine, methotrexate with leucovorin rescue, and cytarabine (COMLA). Even these general guidelines, however, should not be accepted as established because further clinical trials are clearly needed.

Drug regimens for peripheral NHL must include intrathecal therapy, which can be relatively brief in the absence of identified CNS involvement. Specific guidelines are available in recent clinical reviews from Los Angeles[262,382] and San Francisco.[254]

The newer areas of therapy such as the use of zidovudine to treat the concomitant HIV infection and hematopoietic hormones such as granulocyte colony-stimulating factor (G-CSF) and granulocyte-macrophage colony-stimulating factor (GM-CSF) to permit more aggressive lymphoma chemotherapy are especially relevant to the treatment of HIV-related NHL. Zidovudine, because of its associated myelotoxicity, should, in general, be avoided in the early chemotherapy of HIV-related NHL. Most clinicians would consider it more critical to attain a complete tumor response but would then try to combine zidovudine in standard doses with any ongoing maintenance chemotherapy.

One group of studies just being initiated are designed to use the hematopoietic hormone GM-CSF to ameliorate the myelotoxicity of aggressive chemotherapy in HIV-associated NHL. This drug has already shown a remarkable activity in elevating peripheral leukocyte counts in chemotherapy for other cancers, and it is hoped that positive results will be forthcoming in HIV-related NHL.

A final area of NHL therapy deserving attention is the prophylaxis of opportunistic infections. Even more than in KS, these are a frequent cause of mortality for patients with NHL.[254]

TABLE 18. Cancers in the HIV Epidemic

Incidence increased:
Kaposi sarcoma
CNS non-Hodgkin's lymphoma
Peripheral non-Hodgkin's lymphoma
Cases reported
Hodgkin's lymphoma
Squamous carcinoma
Small cell carcinoma
Testicular cancer
Basal cell cancer
Melanoma
Anticipated relationship:
Hepatocellular carcinoma

Although no controlled series have been published, it would seem advisable to use prophylactic aerosolized pentamidine, thus avoiding the additional myelotoxicity of trimethoprim-sulfamethoxazole. Clinicians should follow the results of ongoing clinical trials in this area closely, but 300 mg of pentamidine delivered monthly by a Respigard II nebulizer is recommended.

Other Cancers in HIV Infection

In addition to those cancers described with a presumed etiologic relationship to HIV, many other neoplasms have been reported in HIV-infected subjects (Table 18). In some, the number of reports begin to suggest an etiologic relationship while in others the connection is uncertain. Irrespective of the causal role of HIV, there is a suspicion that the natural history of tumors and their response to therapy may be affected by the HIV infection.

One tumor relatively commonly seen in HIV is Hodgkin's lymphoma.[383–393] Although Hodgkin's disease has been commonly reported in HIV-infected patients, several studies have not shown it to occur at a higher than expected frequency. When seen with HIV infection, however, Hodgkin's disease tends to be more advanced and responds less completely to therapy. Most centers still attempt "curative" chemotherapy; however, the meaning of "cure" is uncertain given the HIV infection status. Thus some have suggested using less aggressive chemotherapy designed primarily to control rather than cure the malignancy. No recent findings have changed this recommendation, and large-scale clinical trials are not yet underway. Until more is known, these patients should be treated with conventional regimens such as melphalan, vincristine, procarbazine, and prednisone (MOPP) or this alternating with Adriamycin, bleomycin, vincristine, and dacarbazine (ABVD). As with NHL, PCP prophylaxis should be considered due to a high risk of opportunistic infections.

Other cancers reported in HIV-infected individuals include malignant melanoma,[393] squamous cell carcinomas,[394–396] testicular cancers of all histologies,[397–399] small cell carcinomas,[394–396] basal cell cancers,[400,401] carcinoid tumors,[402] liposarcoma,[403] and colonic adenocarcinoma.[404] Each of these has been seen in insufficient numbers to draw any strong inference as to etiology, but a growing clinical impression is that their natural history is also more aggressive.

REFERENCES

1. Gottlieb MS, Schroff R, Schanker HM, et al. *Pneumocystis carinii* pneumonia and mucosal candidiasis in previously healthy homosexual men: Evidence of a new acquired cellular immunodeficiency. N Engl J Med. 1981;305:1425–31.
2. Masur H, Michelis MA, Greene JB, et al. An outbreak of community-acquired *Pneumocystis carinii* pneumonia: Initial manifestation of cellular immune dysfunction. N Engl J Med. 198;305:1431–8.
3. Siegal FP, Lopez C, Hammer GS, et al. Severe acquired immunodeficiency in male homosexuals manifested by chronic perianal ulcerative herpes simplex lesions. N Engl J Med. 1981;305:1431–8.
4. Follansbee SE, Busch DF, Wofsy CB, et al. An outbreak of *Pneumocystis carinii* pneumonia in homosexual men. Ann Intern Med. 1982;96:705–13.

5. Centers for Disease Control. Kaposi's sarcoma and *Pneumocystis pneumonia* among homosexual men—New York City and California. MMWR. 1982;30:305–8.
6. Centers for Disease Control. Opportunistic infections and Kaposi's sarcoma among Haitians in the United States. MMWR. 1982;31:353–61.
7. Centers for Disease Control. Update on acquired immunodeficiency syndrome (AIDS)—United States. MMWR. 1982;31:507–14.
8. Centers for Disease Control. Update: Acquired immunodeficiency syndrome—United States. MMWR. 1985;34:245–8.
9. Pape JW, Liautaud B, Thomas F, et al. Characteristics of the acquired immunodeficiency syndrome (AIDS) in Haiti. N Engl J Med. 1983;309:945–50.
10. Pape JW, Liautaud B, Thomas F, et al. The acquired immunodeficiency syndrome in Haiti. Ann Intern Med. 1985;103:674–8.
11. Malebranche R, Annoux E, Guerin JM, et al. AIDS with severe gastrointestinal manifestations in Haiti. Lancet. 1983;2:873–8.
12. Centers for Disease Control. *Pneumocystis carinii* pneumonia among persons with hemophilia A. MMWR. 1982;31:365–7.
13. Centers for Disease Control. Update on acquired immune deficiency syndrome (AIDS) among patients with hemophilia A. MMWR. 1982;31:644–6,52.
14. Centers for Disease Control. Possible transfusion-associated acquired immune deficiency syndrome AIDS—California. MMWR. 1982;31:652–4.
15. Abrams DI, Lewis BJ, Beckstead JP, et al. Persistent diffuse lymphadenopathy in homosexual men: Endpoint or prodrome? Ann Intern Med. 1984;100:801–8.
16. Abrams DI. Lymphadenopathy syndrome in male homosexuals. In: Gallin JI, Fauci AS, eds. Acquired Immunodeficiency Syndrome. Advances in Host Defense Mechanisms. v. 5. New York: Raven Press, 1985:75–97.
17. Morris L, Distenfeld A, Amorosi E, et al. Autoimmune thrombocytopenic purpura in homosexual men. Ann Intern Med. 1982;96:714–7.
18. Walsh CM, Nardi MA, Karpatkin S. On the mechanism of thrombocytopenic purpora in sexually active homosexual men. N Engl J Med. 1984;311:635–9.
19. Abrams DI, Volberding PA, Linker CA, et al. Immune thrombocytopenic purpura in homosexual men: Clinical manifestations and treatment results (Abstract). Blood. 1983;62:1082.
20. Abrams DI. AIDS-related conditions. Clin Immunol Allergy. 1986;6:581.
21. Harris C, Small CB, Klein RS, et al. Immunodeficiency in female sexual partners of men with the acquired immunodeficiency syndrome. N Engl J Med. 1984;308:1181–4.
22. Barre-Sinoussi F, Chermann JC, Rey F, et al. Isolation of a T-lymphotropic retrovirus from a patient at risk for acquired immunodeficiency syndrome (AIDS). Science. 1983;220:868–71.
23. Gallo RC, Salahudin SZ, Popovic M, et al. Frequent detection and isolation of cytopathic retroviruses (HTLV-III) from patients with AIDS and at risk for AIDS. Science. 1984;224:500–3.
24. Levy JA, Hoffman AD, Kramer SD, et al. Isolation of lymphocytopathic retrovirus from San Francisco patients with AIDS. Science. 1984;225:840–2.
25. Centers for Disease Control. Revision of the CDC surveillance case definition for acquired immunodeficiency syndrome. MMWR. 1987;36(Suppl):1.
26. Centers for Disease Control. Current trends: Classification system for human T lymphotropic virus type III/lymphadenopathy associated virus infections. MMWR. 1986;35:334–39.
27. World Health Organization. Acquired immunodeficiency syndrome (AIDS). Weekly Epidemiol Rec 1986;61:69–73.
28. Centers for Disease Control. Current trends: Classification system for human T lymphotropic virus type III/lymphadenopathy associated virus infections. MMWR. 1986;35:334–39.
29. Redfield RR, Wright DC, Tramont EC: The Walter Reed staging classification for HTLV-III/LAV infection. N Engl J Med. 1986;314:131–2.
30. Osmond D, Chaisson RE, Moss AR, et al. Lymphadenopathy in asymptomatic patients seropositive for HIV. New Engl J Med. 1987;317:246.
31. McArthur JC, Johnson RT. Primary infection with human immunodeficiency virus. In: Rosenblum ML, Levy RM, Bredesen DE, et al., eds. AIDS and the Nervous System. New York: Raven Press; 1988.
32. MacDonnell KB, Chmiel JS, Goldsmith J, et al. Prognostic usefulness of the Walter Reed staging classification for HIV infection. J AIDS. 1988;1:367–74.
33. Terragna A, Dodi F, Anselmo M, et al. The Walter Reed staging classification in the follow-up of HIV infection. N Engl J Med. 1986;315:1355–6.
34. Farzadagen H, Polis MA, Wolinsky SM, et al. Loss of human immunodeficiency virus type 1 (HIV-1) antibodies with evidence of viral infection in asymptomatic homosexual men: A report from the multicenter AIDS cohort study. Ann Intern Med. 1988;108:785–790.
35. Goedert JJ, Biggar RJ, Weiss SH, et al. Three-year incidence of AIDS in five cohorts of HTLV-III-infected risk group members. Science. 1986;231:992–5.
36. Jaffe HW, Darrow WW, Echenberg DF, et al. The acquired immunodeficiency syndrome in a cohort of homosexual men: A six year follow-up study. Ann Intern Med. 1985;103:210–4.
37. Melbye M, Biggar RJ, Ebbesen P, et al. Long-term HTLV-III seropositive homosexual men without AIDS develop measurable immunologic and clinical abnormalities: A longitudinal study. Ann Intern Med. 1986;104:496–500.
38. Moss AR, Bacchetti P, Osmond D, et al. Seropositivity for HIV and the development of AIDS or ARC: Three year follow-up of the San Francisco General Hospital cohort. Br Med J. 1988;296:745–50.
39. Eyster ME, Gail MH, Ballard JO, et al. Natural history of human immunodeficiency virus infections in hemophiliacs: Effects of T-cell subsets, platelet counts and age. Ann Intern Med. 1987;107:1–6.
40. Hessol NA, Rutherford GW, Lifson AR, et al. The natural history of HIV infection in homosexual and bisexual men: a decade of followup. (Abstract 4096) Proceedings of the 4th International Conference on AIDS. Stockholm, Sweden, June 12–16, 1988.
41. Bacchetti P, Moss AR. The incubation period of AIDS in San Francisco. Nature. In press.
42. Klein RS, Harris CA, Small CB, et al. Oral candidiasis in high-risk patients as the initial manifestation of the acquired immunodeficiency syndrome. N Engl J Med. 1984;311:354–8.
43. Carne CA, Weller IVD, Loveday C, et al. From persistent generalized lymphadenopathy to AIDS: Who will progress? Br Med J. 1987;294:868–9.
44. Greenspan D, Greenspan JS, Hearst NG, et al. Relation of oral hairy leukoplakia to infection with the human immunodeficiency virus and the risk of developing AIDS. J Infect Dis. 1987;155:475.
45. Melbye M, Grossman RJ, Goedert JJ, et al. Risk of AIDS after herpes zoster. Lancet. 1987;1:728–30.
46. Moss AR. Predicting progression to AIDS. Br Med J. 1988;297:1067–8.
47. Goedert JJ, Bigga RJ, Melbye M, et al. Effect of T4 count and cofactors on the incidence of AIDS in homosexual men infected with human immunodeficiency virus. JAMA. 1987;257:331–4.
48. Polk BF, Fox R, Brookmeyer R, et al. Predictors of the acquired immunodeficiency syndrome developing in a cohort of seropositive homosexual men. N Engl J Med. 1987;316:61–6.
49. Allain J-P. Laurian Y, Paul DA, et al. Long-term evaluation of HIV antigen and antibodies to p24 and gp41 in patients with hemophilia. N Engl J Med. 1987;317:1114–21.
50. De Wolf F, Goudsmit J, Paul DA, et al. Risk of AIDS related complex and AIDS in homosexual men with persistent antigenemia. Br Med J. 1987;295:569–72.
51. Weber JN, Clapham PR, Weiss RA, et al. Human immunodeficiency virus infection in two cohorts of homosexual men: Neutralising sera and association of anti-*gag* antibody with prognosis. Lancet. 1987;1:119–21.
52. Eyster ME, Goedert JJ, Poon MC, et al. Acid-labile interferon: A possible preclinical marker for the acquired immunodeficiency syndrome in hemophilia. N Engl J Med. 1983;309:583–6.
53. Holmberg SD, Gerber AR, Stewart JA, et al. Herpesviruses as co-factors in AIDS (Letter). Lancet. 1988;2:746–7.
54. Oxtoby MS, Mvula M, Ryder R, et al. Measles and measles immunization in African children with human immunodeficiency virus (Abstract 1353). In Proceedings of the 28th Inter Science Conference on Antimicrobial Agents and Chemotherapy. Am Soc Microbiol, Washington, DC: American Society for Microbiology; 1988.
55. Nelson KE, Clements ML, Miotti P, et al. The influence of human immunodeficiency virus (HIV) infection on antibody responses to influenza vaccines. Ann Intern Med. 1988;109:383–8.
56. DesJarlais DC, Friedman SR, Marmor M, et al. HTLV-III/LAV-associated disease progression and co-factors in a cohort of IV drug users. AIDS. 1987;1:105–11.
57. Chambers HF, Morris DL, Tauber MG, et al. Cocaine use and the risk of endocarditis in intravenous drug users. Ann Intern Med. 1987;106:833–6.
58. Chaisson RE, Bacchetti P, Osmond D, et al. Cocaine use and HIV infection in intravenous drug users in San Francisco. JAMA. 1989;261:561–65.
59. Eales LS, Nye KE, Parkin SM, et al. Association of different allelic forms of group specific component with susceptibility to and clinical manifestation of human immunodeficiency virus infection. Lancet. 1987;1:999–1002.
59a. Eales LJ, Nye KE, Pinching AJ. Group-specific component and AIDS: erroneous data. Lancet. 1988;1:936.
60. Bacchetti P, Osmond D, Chaisson RE, et al. Patterns of survival in the acquired immunodeficiency syndrome. J Infect Dis. 1988;157:1044–7.
61. Cooper DA, Gold J, MacLean P, et al. Acute AIDS retrovirus infection. Definition of a clinical illness associated with seroconversion. Lancet. 1985;1:537–40.
62. Anonymous. Needlestick transmission of HTLV-III from a patient infected in Africa. Lancet. 1984;2:1376–7.
63. Moss AR, Osmond D, Bacchetti P, et al. Risk factors for AIDS and HIV seropositivity in homosexual men. Am J Epidemiol 1987;125:1035–47.
64. Jaffe HW, Hardy AM, Morgan WM, et al. The acquired immunodeficiency syndrome in gay men. Ann Intern Med. 1985;103:662–4.
65. Fox R, Eldred LJ, Fuchs EJ, et al. Clinical manifestations of acute infection with human immunodeficiency virus in a cohort of gay men. AIDS. 1987;1:35–8.
66. Tindall B, Barker S, Donovan B, et al. Characteristics of the acute clinical illness associated with human immunodeficiency virus infection. Arch Intern Med. 1988:148(4):945–49.
67. Pyun KH, Ochs HD, Dufford MTW, et al. Perinatal infection with human immunodeficiency virus. Specific antibody responses by the neonate. N Engl J Med. 1987;317:611–4.
68. Stricof RL, Morse DL. HTLV-III/LAV seroconversion following a deep intramuscular needlestick injury. N Engl J Med. 1986;314:1115.
69. Kessler HA, Blaauw B, Spear J, et al. Diagnosis of human immunodeficiency virus infection in seronegative homosexuals presenting with an acute viral syndrome. JAMA. 1987;258:1196–9.

70. Valle S-L. Febrile pharyngitis as the primary sign of HIV infection in a cluster of cases linked by sexual contact. Scand J Infect Dis. 1987;19:13–7.
71. Rustin MHA, Ridely CM, Smith MD, et al. The acute exanthem associated with seroconversion to human T-cell lymphotropic virus III in a homosexual man. J Infect Dis. 1986;12:161–3.
72. Carne CA, Tedder RS, Smith A, et al. Acute encephalopathy coincident with seroconversion for anti-HTLV-III. Lancet. 1985;2:1206–8.
73. Denning DW, Anderson J, Rudge P, et al. Acute myelopathy associated with primary infection with human immunodeficiency virus. Br Med J. 1987;294:143–4.
74. Elder G, Dalakas M, Pezeshkpour G, et al. Ataxic neuropathy due to ganglioneuritis after probable acute human immunodeficiency virus infection. Lancet. 1986;2:1275–6.
75. Farthing C, Gazzard B: Acute illnesses associated with HTLV-III seroconversion. Lancet. 1985;1:935–6.
76. Ho DD, Sarngadharan MG, Resnick L, et al. Primary human T-lymphotropic virus type III infection. Ann Intern Med. 1985;103:880–3.
77. Piette AM, Tusseau F, Vignon D, et al. Acute neuropathy coincident with seroconversion for anti-LAV/HTLV-III. Lancet. 1986;1:852.
78. Podzamczer D, Casanova A, Santa-Maria P, et al. Esophageal candidiasis in the diagnosis of HIV-infected patients. JAMA. 1988;259:1328–9.
79. Cooper DA, Imrie AA, Penny R. Antibody response to human immunodeficiency virus after primary infection. J Infect Dis. 1987;155:1113–8.
80. Cooper DA, Tindall B, Wilson E, et al. Characterization of T lymphocyte responses during primary HIV infection. J Infect Dis. 1988;157(5):889–96.
81. Cooper DA, Tindall B, Wilson EJ, et al. Characterization of T lymphocyte responses during primary infection with human immunodeficiency virus. J Infect Dis. 1988;157:889–96.
82. Goudsmit J, De Wolf F, Paul DA, et al. Expression of human immunodeficiency virus antigen (HIV-Ag) in serum and cerebrospinal fluid during acute and chronic infection. Lancet. 1986;2:177–80.
83. Allain J-P, Laurian Y, Paul DA, et al. Serological markers in early stages of human immunodeficiency virus infection in hemophiliacs. Lancet. 1986;2:1233–6.
84. Gaines H, Sonnerborg A, Czajkowski J, et al. Antibody response in primary human immunodeficiency virus infection. Lancet. 1987;1249–53.
85. Ranki A, Valle S-L, Krohn M, et al. Long latency period precedes overt seroconversion in sexually transmitted human-immunodeficiency-virus infection. Lancet. 1987;2:589–93.
86. Metroka CE, Cunningham-Rundles S, Pollack MS, et al. Persistent generalized lymphadenopathy in homosexual men. Ann Intern Med. 1983;99:585.
87. Abrams DI, Kirn DH, Feigal DW, et al. Lymphadenopathy: Update of a 60 month prospective study (Abstract). In: Proceedings of the III International Conference on AIDS. Washington, DC:USDH and WHO; 1987:118.
88. Hewlett D, Duncanson FP, Jagadha V, et al. Lymphadenopathy in an inner-city population consisting principally of intravenous drug abusers with suspected acquired immunodeficiency syndrome. Am Respir Rev Dis. 1988;137:1275–9.
89. Bottles K, McPhaul LW, Volberding P. Fine-needle aspiration biopsy of patients with the acquired immunodeficiency syndrome (AIDS): Experience in an outpatient clinic. Ann Intern Med. 1988;108:42–5.
90. Hales M, Bottles K, Miller T. Diagnosis of Kaposi's sarcoma by fine-needle aspiration biopsy. Am J Clin Pathol. 1987;88:20–5.
91. Abrams DI. AIDS-related lymphadenopathy: The role of biopsy. J Clin Oncol. 1986;4:126–7.
92. Stricker RB, Abrams DI, Corash L, et al. Target platelet antigen in homosexual men with immune thrombocytopenia. N Engl J Med. 1985;313:1375–80.
93. Federle MP, Megibow AJ, Naidich DP, eds. Radiology of AIDS. New York: Raven Press; 1988.
94. The Swiss Group for Clinical Studies on AIDS, Luthy R, Chairman. Zidovudine for the treatment of thrombocytopenia associated with human immunodeficiency virus (HIV): A prospective study. Ann Intern Med. 1988;109:718–21.
95. Folks TM, Kessler SW, Orenstein JM, et al. Infection and replication of HIV-1 in purified progenitor cells of normal human bone marrow. Science. 1988;242:919–22.
96. Ochitill HN, Dilley JW. Neuropsychiatric aspects of acquired immunodeficiency syndrome. In: Rosenblum ML, Levy RM, Bredesen DE, eds. AIDS and the Nervous System. New York: Raven Press; 1988.
97. Serwadda D, Mugerwa RD, Sewankambo NK, et al. Slim disease: A new disease in Uganda and its association with HTLV-III infection. Lancet. 1985;2:1849.
97a. Sewankambo N, Mugerwa R, Goodgame R, et al. Enteropathic AIDS in Uganda: An endoscopic, histologic and microbiologic study. AIDS. 1987;1:9–14.
98. Greenspan D, et al., eds. AIDS and the Dental Team. Copenhagen; 1986.
99. Greenspan JS, Greenspan D, Winkler JR. Diagnosis and management of the oral manifestations of HIV infection and AIDS. Infect Dis Clin N Am. 1988;2:373–85.
100. Greenspan JS, Greenspan D, Winkler JR. Diagnosis and management of the oral manifestations of HIV infection and AIDS. In: Sande ME, Volberding PA, eds. The Medical Management of AIDS. Philadelphia: WB Saunders Co; 1988:127–40.
101. Greenspan D, Greenspan JS, Conant M, et al. Oral "hairy" leukoplakia in male homosexuals: Evidence of association with both papillomavirus and a herpes-group virus. Lancet. 1984;2:831–4.
102. Greenspan D, Hollander H, Freidman-Kein A, et al. Oral hairy leukoplakia in two women, a haemophiliac, and a transfusion recipient. Lancet. 1986;2:978–9.
103. Jaffe HW, Darrow WW, Echenberg DF, et al. The acquired immunodeficiency syndrome in a cohort of homosexual men: A six year follow-up study. Ann Intern Med. 1985;103:210.
104. Greenspan JS, Greenspan D, Lennette ET, et al. Replication of Epstein-Barr virus within the epithelial cells of oral "hairy" leukoplakia and AIDS-associated lesion. N Engl J Med. 1985;313:1564–71.
105. Levy RM, Bredesen DE, Rosenblum ML. Neurological manifestations of the acquired immunodeficiency syndrome (AIDS): Experience at UCSF and review of the literature. J Neurosurg. 1985;62:475.
106. McArthur JC. Neurologic manifestations of AIDS. Medicine (Baltimore). 1987;66:407–37.
107. Cornblath DR, McArthur JC. Predominantly sensory neuropathy in patients with AIDS and AIDS-related complex. Neurology (NY). 1988;38: 794–6.
108. Cornblath DR, McArthur JC, Kennedy PG, et al. Inflammatory demylinating peripheral neuropathies associated with human T-cell lymphotrophic virus type III infection. Ann Neurol. 1987;21:32–40.
109. Lipkin WI, Parry G, Kiprov D, et al. Inflammatory neuropathy in homosexual men with lymphadenopathy. Neurology (NY). 1985;35:1479–83.
110. Bredesen DE, et al. Inflammatory polyradiculoneuropathy with culture of cytomegalovirus from nerve. Neurology (NY). In press.
111. Dalakas MC, Pezeshkpour GH, Gnavall M, et al. Polymyositis associated with AIDS retrovirus. JAMA. 1986;256:2381–3.
112. Simpson DM, Beuder AN. HTLV-II-associated myopathy. Neurology (NY). 1987;37(Suppl):319.
113. Helbert M, Fletcher T, Peddle B, et al. Zidovudine-associated myopathy. Lancet. 1988;2:689–90.
114. Forster SM, Seeifert MH, Keat AC, et al. Inflammatory joint disease and human immunodeficiency virus infection. Br Med J. 1988;296:1625–7.
115. Rynes RI, Goldenberg DL, DiGiacomo R, et al. Acquired immunodeficiency syndrome-associated arthritis. Am J Med. 1988;84:810–6.
116. Berman A, Espinoza LR, Diaz JD, et al. Rheumatic manifestations of human immunodeficiency virus infection. Am J Med. 1988;85:59–64.
117. Winchester R, Bernstein DH, Fischer HD, et al. The co-occurrence of Rieter's syndrome and acquired immunodeficiency. Ann Intern Med. 1987;106:19–26.
118. Couderc LJ, D'Agay MF, Danon F, et al. Sicca complex and infection with human immunodeficiency virus. Arch Intern Med. 1987;147:898–901.
119. Cello JP. Gastrointestinal manifestations of HIV infection. Infect Dis Clin North Am. 1988;2:387–96.
120. Freedman PG, Weiner BC, Balthazan ES. Cytomegalovirus esophagogastritis in a patient with acquired immunodeficiency syndrome. Am J Gastroenterol. 1985;80:434–7.
121. Rabeneck L, Boyko WJ, McLean DM, et al. Unusual esophageal ulcers containing enveloped virus-like particles in homosexual men. Gastroenterology. 1986;90:1882.
122. St Onge G, Bezahler GH. Giant esophageal ulcer associated with cytomegalovirus. Gastroenterology. 1983;83:127.
123. Tavitian A, Raufman JP, Rosenthal LE. Oral candidiasis as a marker for esophageal candidiasis in the acquired immunodeficiency syndrome. Ann Intern Med. 1986;104:54.
124. Friedman SL, Wright TL, Altman DF. Gastrointestinal KS in patients with acquired immunodeficiency syndrome: Endoscopic and autopsy findings. Gastroenterology. 1985;89:102–8.
125. Blumberg RS, Kelsey P, Perrone T, et al. Cytomegalovirus- and *Cryptosporidium*-associated acalculous gangrenous cholecystitis. Am J Med. 1984;76:1118.
126. Kavin H, Jonas RB, Chowdhury L, et al. Acalculous cholecystitis and cytomegalovirus infection in the acquired immunodeficiency syndrome. Ann Intern Med. 1986;104:53.
127. Margulis SJ, Honig CL, Soave R, et al. Biliary tract obstruction in the acquired immunodeficiency syndrome. Ann Intern Med. 1986;105:207.
128. Schneiderman DJ, Cello JP, Laing FC. Papillary stenosis and sclerosing cholangitis in the acquired immunodeficiency syndrome. Ann Intern Med. 1987;106:546.
129. Jacobson MA, Cello JP, Sande MA. Cholestasis and disseminated cytogalovirus disease in patients with acquired immunodeficiency syndrome. Am J Med. 1987;84:218–24.
130. Glasgow BJ, Anders K, Layfield LJ, et al. Clinical and pathologic finding of the liver in the acquired immune deficiency syndrome. Am J Clin Pathol. 1985;83:582.
131. Lebovics E, Thung SN, Schaffner F, et al. The liver in the acquired immunodeficiency syndrome: A clinical and histologic study. Hepatology. 1985;5:293.
132. Schneiderman DJ, Arenson DM, Cello JP, et al. Hepatic disease in patients with acquired immune deficiency syndrome (AIDS). Hepatology. 1987;7:925.
133. Laughon BE, Druckman DA, Vernon A, et al. Prevalence of enteric pathogens in homosexual men with and without AIDS. Gastroenterology. 1988;94:984–93.
134. Smith PD, Lane HC, Gill VJ, et al. Intestinal infections in patients with the acquired immunodeficiency syndrome (AIDS). Etiology and response to therapy. Ann Intern Med. 1988;108:328–33.
135. Rao TKS, Filippone EJ, Nicastri AD, et al. Associated focal and segmental

glomerulosclerosis in the acquired immunodeficiency syndrome. N Engl J Med. 1984;310:669–73.
136. Pardo V, Aldana M, Colton RM, et al. Glomerular lesions in the acquired immunodeficiency syndrome. Ann Intern Med. 1984;101:429–34.
137. Pardo V, Meneses R, Ossa L, et al. AIDS-related glomerulopathy: Occurrence in specific risk groups. Kidney Int. 1987;31:1167–73.
138. Gardenswartz MH, Lerner CW, Seligson GR, et al. Renal disease in patients with AIDS: A clinicopathologic study. Clin Nephrol. 1984;21:197–204.
139. Rao TKS, Friedman EA, Nicastri AD. The types of renal disease in the acquired immunodeficiency syndrome. N Engl J Med. 1987;316:1062–8.
140. Ortiz C, Meneses R, Jaffe D, et al. Outcome of patients with human immunodeficiency virus on maintenance hemodialysis. Kidney Int. 1988;34:248–53.
141. Hopewell PC, Luce JM. Pulmonary involvement in the acquired immunodeficiency syndrome. Chest. 1984;87:104–12.
142. Selik R, Curran JW. Frequency of opportunistic infections in AIDS. AIDS. 1987;1:175–82.
143. Murray JF, Felton CP, Garay SM et al. Pulmonary complications of the acquired immunodeficiency syndrome: Report of a National Heart, Lung and Blood Institute Workshop. N Engl J Med. 1984;310:1682–8.
144. Stover DE, White DA, Romano PA, et al. Spectrum of pulmonary diseases associated with the acquired immunodeficiency syndrome. Am J Med. 1985;78:429–37.
145. Ognibene FP, Steis RG, Macher AM, et al. Kaposi's sarcoma causing pulmonary infiltrates and respiratory failure in the acquired immunodeficiency syndrome. Ann Intern Med. 1985;102:471–5.
146. Kovacs JA, Hiemenz JW, Macher AM, et al. *Pneumocystis carinii* pneumonia: A comparison between patients with the acquired immunodeficiency syndrome and patients with other immunodeficiencies. Ann Intern Med. 1984;100:663–71.
147. Simberkoff MS, El-Sadr W, Schiffman G. *Streptococcus pneumoniae* infections and bacteremia in patients with acquired immune deficiency syndrome, with report of a pneumococcal vaccine failure. Am Rev Respir Dis. 1984;145:837–40.
148. Polsky B, Gold JWM, Whimbey E, et al. Bacterial pneumonia in patients with the acquired immunodeficiency syndrome. Ann Intern Med. 1986;104:38–41.
149. Chaisson RE. Infections due to encapsulated bacteria, *Salmonella, Shigella* and *Campylobacter* (medical management of AIDS). Infect Dis Clin North Am. 1988;2:475–84.
150. Gerberding JL, Krieger J, Sande MA. Recurrent bactermic infection with *S. pneumoniae* in patients with AIDS virus (AV) infection (Abstract 443). In: Proceedings of the 26th ICAAC. Washington, DC: American Society for Microbiology; 1986.
151. Pitchenik AE, Cole C, Russell BW, et al. Tuberculosis, atypical mycobacteriosis and the acquired immunodeficiency syndrome among Haitian and non-Haitian patients in South Florida. Ann Intern Med. 1984;101:641–5.
152. Chaisson RE, Schecter GF, Theuer CP, et al. Tuberculosis in patients with the acquired immunodeficiency syndrome: Clinical features, response to therapy and outcome. Am Rev Respir Dis. 1987;136:570–4.
153. Goodman PC, Broaddus VC, Hopewell PC. Chest radiographic patterns in the acquired immunodeficiency syndrome. Am Rev Respir Dis. 1984;129:36.
154. Bigby TD, Margolskee D, Curtis JL, et al. The usefulness of induced sputum in the diagnosis of *Pneumocystis carinii* pneumonia in patients with the acquired immunodeficiency syndrome. Am Rev Respir Dis. 1986;133:515–8.
155. Kovacs JA, Ng VL, Masur H, et al. Diagnosis of *Pneumocystis carinii* pneumonia: Improved detection in sputum with use of monoclonal antibodies. N Engl J Med. 1988;318:589–93.
156. Pitchenik AE, Ganjei P, Torres A, et al. Sputum examination for the diagnosis of Pneumocystis carinii pneumonia in the acquired immunodeficiency syndrome. Am Rev Resp Dis. 1986;133:226–9.
156a. Curtis J, Goodman P, Hopewell PC. Noninvasive tests in the diagnostic evaluation for P. carinii pneumonia in patients with or suspected of having AIDS. Am Rev Resp Dis. 1986;132:A182.
157. Coleman DL, Hattner RS, Luce JM, et al. Correlation between gallium lung scans and fiberoptic bronchoscopy in patients with suspected *Pneumocystis carinii* pneumonia and the acquired immunodeficiency syndrome. Am Rev Respir Dis. 1984;130:1155–9.
158. Coleman DL, Dodek PM, Luce JM, et al. Diagnostic utility of fiberoptic bronchoscopy in patients with *Pneumocystis carinii* pneumonia and the acquired immunodeficiency syndrome. Am Rev Respir Dis. 1983;128:795–9.
159. Ognibene FP, Shelhamer S, Gill V, et al. The diagnosis of *Pneumocystis carinii* pneumonia in patients with the acquired immunodeficiency syndrome using subsegmental bronchoalveolar lavage. Am Rev Respir Dis. 1984;130:659–62.
160. Stover DE, White DA, Romano PA, et al. Diagnosis of pulmonary disease in acquired immunodeficiency syndrome (AIDS): Role of bronchoscopy and bronchoalveolar lavage. Am Rev Respir Dis. 1984;102:747–52.
161. Broaddus C, Dake MD, Stulbarg MS, et al. Bronchoalveolar lavage and transbronchial biopsy for the diagnosis of pulmonary infections in the acquired immunodeficiency syndrome. Ann Intern Med. 1985;102:747–52.
162. Milligan SA, Luce JM, Golden J, et al. Transbronchial biopsy without fluoroscopy in patients with diffuse roentgenographic infiltrates and the acquired immunodeficiency syndrome. Am Rev Respir Dis. 1988;137:486–8.
163. Edman JC, Kovacs JA, Masur H, et al. Ribosomal RNA sequence shows *Pneumocystis carinii* to be a member of the fungi. Nature. 1988;334:519–22.
164. Hughes WT. *Pneumocystis carinii.* Boca Raton, FL: CRC Press; 1987.
165. Brenner M, Ognibene FP, Lack EE, et al. Prognostic factors and life expectancy of acquired immunodeficiency syndrome patients with *Pneumocystis carinii* pneumoniae. Am Rev Respir Dis. 1987;136:1199–206.
166. Gherman CR, Ward RR, Basis ML: *Pneumocystis carinii* otitis media and mastoiditis as the initial manifestation of the acquired immunodeficiency syndrome. Am J Med. 1988;85:250–2.
167. Pilon A, Echols RM, Celo JS, et al. Disseminated *Pneumocystis carinii* infection in AIDS. N Engl J Med. 1987;316:1410–1.
168. Grimes MM, LaPook JD, Bar MH, et al. Disseminated *Pneumocystis carinii* infection in a patient with acquired immunodeficiency syndrome. Hum Pathol. 1987;18:307–8.
169. Schinella RA, Breda SD, Hammerschlag PE. Otic infection due to *Pneumocytis carinii* in an apparently healthy man with antibody to the human immunodeficiency virus. Ann Intern Med. 1987;106:399–400.
170. Welch K, Finkbeiner W, Alpers CE, et al. Autopsy findings in the acquired immune deficiency syndrome. JAMA. 1984;252:1152–9.
171. Theuer CP, Chaisson RE, Schecter GF, et al. Human immunodeficiency virus infection in tuberculosis patients in San Francisco (Abstract). Am Rev Respir Dis. 1988;137:121.
172. Horsburgh CR, Selik RA. Mycobacterial infections in patients with AIDS. Am Rev Respir Dis. 1989. In press.
173. Sherer R, Sable R, Sonnenburg M, et al. Disseminated infection with *Mycobacterium kansasii* in the acquired immunodeficiency syndrome. Ann Intern Med. 1986;105:710–2.
174. Chan J, McKitrick JC, Klein RS. *Mycobacterium gordonae* in the acquired immunodeficiency syndrome. Ann Intern Med. 1984;101:400.
175. Chaisson RE, Slutkin G. Tuberculosis in patients with human immunodeficiency virus infection. J Infect Dis. 1989;159:96–100.
176. Selwyn PA, Hartel D, Lewis VA, et al. A prospective study of the risk of tuberculosis among intravenous drug users with human immunodeficiency virus infection. New Engl J Med. 1989;320:545–50.
177. Mann J, Snider DE Jr, Francis H, et al. Association between HTLV-III/LAV infection and tuberculosis in Zaire (Letter). JAMA. 1986;256:346.
178. Centers for Disease Control. Tuberculosis, final data—United States, 1986. MMWR. 1988;36:817–20.
179. Chaisson RE, Schecter GF, Theuer CP, et al. Tuberculosis in patients with the acquired immunodeficiency syndrome: Clinical features, response to therapy, and survival. Am Rev Respir Dis. 1987;136:570–4.
180. Tuberculosis and acquired immunodeficiency syndrome—New York City. MMWR. 1987;36:785–95.
181. Pitchenik AE, Burr J, Suarez M, et al. Human T-cell lymphotrophic virus III (HTLV-III) seropositivity and related disease among 71 consecutive patients in whom tuberculosis was diagnosed. Am Rev Respir Dis. 1987;135:875–90.
182. Sunderam G, McDonald RJ, Maniatis T, et al. Tuberculosis as a manifestation of the acquired immunodeficiency syndrome. JAMA. 1986;256:362–6.
183. Louie E, Rice LB, Holzman RS. Tuberculosis in non-Haitian patients with acquired immunodeficiency syndrome. Chest. 1986;90:542–5.
184. Handwerger S, Mildvan D, Senie R, et al. Tuberculosis and the acquired immunodeficiency syndrome at a New York City Hospital: 1978–1985. Chest. 1987;91:176–80.
185. Greene JB, Sidhu GS, Lewis S, et al. *Mycobacterium avium-intracellulare:* A cause of disseminated life-threatening infection in homosexuals and drug abusers. Ann Intern Med. 1982;97:539–46.
186. Macher AM, Kovacs JA, Gill V, et al. Bacteremia due to *Mycobacterium avium-intracellulare* in the acquired immunodeficiency syndrome. Ann Intern Med. 1983;99:782–5.
187. Horsburgh CR, Selik RM. The epidemiology of disseminated nontuberculous mycobacterial infection in AIDS. Am Rev Respir Dis. 1989;139:4–7.
188. Wilkes MS, Fortin AH, Felix JC, et al. Value of necropsy in acquired immunodeficiency syndrome. Lancet. 1988;2:85–8.
189. Mess TP. *Mycobacterium avium* complex isolated from the lung only, does it disseminate? (Abstract WP217). In: Proceedings of the III International Conference on AIDS. Washington, DC, June 1–5, 1987.
190. Tenholder MF, Moser RJ, Tellis CJ. Mycobacteria other than tuberculosis: Pulmonary involvement in patients with acquired immunodeficiency syndrome. Arch Intern Med. 1988;148:953–5.
191. Demopulos P, Sande MA, Bryant C, et al. Influence of *Mycobacterium avium-intracellulare* infection on morbidity and survival in patients with *Pneumocystis carinii* pneumonia and the acquired immunodeficiency syndrome (Abstract 745). In: Proceedings of the 25th Interscience Conference on Antimicrobial Agents and Chemotherapy. Washington, DC: American Society for Microbiology; 1985.
192. Hawkins CC, Gold JWM, Whimbey E, et al. *Mycobacterium avium* complex infections in patients with the acquired immunodeficiency syndrome. Ann Intern Med. 1986;105:184–8.
193. Jacobson MA. Mycobacterial diseases: Tuberculosis and *Mycobacterium avium* complex. Infect Dis Clin North Am 1988;2:465–74.
194. Young LS. *Mycobacterium avium* complex infection. J Infect Dis. 1988;157:863–7.
195. Bermudez LE, Young LS. Interaction between macrophages and *M. avium complex* (MAC) from AIDS patients (Abstract D129). In: Proceedings of the Annual Meeting of the American Society for Microbiology. Washington, DC: American Society for Microbiology; 1986.
196. Beutler B. The presence of cachectin/tumor necrosis factor in human disease states. Am J Med. 1988;85:287–8.

197. Lahdevirta J, Maury CPJ, Teppo AM, et al. Elevated levels of circulating cachetin/tumor necrosis factor in patients with acquired immunodeficiency syndrome. Am J Med. 1988;85:289–91.
198. Yajko DM, Nassos PS, Hadley WK. Therapeutic implications of inhibition versus killing of *Mycobacterium avium* complex by antimicrobial agents. Antimicrob Agents Chemother. 1987;31:117–20.
199. Agins B, Spicehandler D, Zuger A, et al. *M. avium*-complex (MAC) infections in AIDS: Significance of respiratory isolates and therapy (Abstract 746). In: Proceedings of the 25th Interscience Conference on Antimicrobial Agents and Chemotherapy. Washington, DC: American Society for Microbiology; 1985.
200. Packer SJ, Cesario T, Williams JH Jr. *Mycobacterium avium* complex infection presenting an endobronchial lesions on immunosuppressed patients. Ann Intern Med. 1988;109:389–93.
201. Selwyn PA, Feingold AR, Hartel D, et al. Increased of bacterial pneumonia in HIV-infected intravenous drug abusers without AIDS. AIDS. 1988;2:267–72.
202. Schlamm HT, Yancovitz SR. *Haemophilus influenzae* pneumonia in young adults with AIDS, ARC or risk of AIDS. Am J Med. 1989;86:11–14.
203. Gerberding JL, Kreiger J, Sande MA. Recurrent bacteremic infection with *S. pneumoniae* in patients with AIDS virus (AV) infection (Abstract 443). In: Proceedings of the 26th Interscience Conference on Antimicrobial Agents and Chemotherapy. Washington, DC: American Society for Microbiology; 1986:177.
204. Jacobson MA, Gellermann H, Chambers H. *Staphylococcus aureus* bacteria and recurrent staphylococcal infection in patients with acquired immunodeficiency syndrome and AIDS-related complex. Am J Med. 1988;85:172–6.
205. Jacobson MA, Gellermann H, Chambers H. *Staphylococcus aureus* bacteremia amd recurrent staphylococcal infection in patients with acquired immunodeficiency syndrome and AIDS-related complex. Am J Med. 1988;85:172–6.
206. Levy RM, Bredesen DE, Rosenblum ML. Neurological manifestations of the acquired immunodeficiency syndrome (AIDS): Experience of UCSF and review of the literature. J Neurosurg. 1985;62:75–95.
207. Hollander H, Stringari S. Human immunodeficiency virus-associated meningitis. Clinical course and correlations. Am J Med. 1987;83:813–16.
208. Hollander H, Levy JA. Neurologic abnormalities and recovery of human immunodeficiency virus from cerebrospinal fluid. Ann Intern Med. 1987;106:692.
209. Levy JA, Shimabukuro J, Hollander H, et al. Isolation of AIDS-associated retroviruses from cerebrospinal fluid and brain of patients with neurological symptoms. Lancet. 1985;2:586–8.
210. Goudsmit J, deWolf F, Paul DA, et al. Expression of human immunodeficiency virus antigen (HIV-Ag) in serum and cerebrospinal fluid during acute and chronic infection. Lancet. 1986;2:177.
211. Goudsmit J, Wolters EC, Bakker M, et al. Intrathecal synthesis of antibodies to HTLV-III in patients without AIDS or AIDS related complex. Br Med J. 1986;292:1231.
212. Hollander H, Stringari. Human immunodeficiency virus-associated meningitis. Clinical course and correlations. Am J Med. 1987;83:813–6.
213. McArthur JC. Neurologic manifestations of AIDS. Medicine (Baltimore). 1987;66:407–37.
214. De la Paz R, Enzmann D. Neuroradiology of the acquired immunodeficiency syndrome. In: Rosenblum ML, Levy RM, Bredesen DE, eds. AIDS and the Nervous System. New York: Raven Press; 1988.
215. Levy RM, Bredesen DE. Central nervous system dysfunction in acquired immunodeficiency syndrome. In: Rosenblum ML, Levy RM, Bredesen DE, eds. AIDS and the Nervous System. New York: Raven Press, 1988.
216. Levy RM, Mills CM, Posin JP, et al. The superiority of cranial magnetic resonance imaging to computed tomographic (CT) brain scans for the diagnosis of cerebral lesions in patients with AIDS (Abstract 146). In: Proceedings of the Second International Conference on AIDS. Paris, June 23–25, 1986.
217. Potasman I, Resnick L, Luft BJ, et al. Intrathecal production of antibodies against *T. gondii* in patients with toxoplasmic encephalitis and AIDS. Ann Intern Med. 1988;108:49–51.
218. Luft BJ, Brooks RG, Conley FK. Toxoplasmic encephalitis in patients with acquired immune deficiency syndrome. JAMA. 1984;252:913–7.
219. Grant IH, Gold JWM, Armstrong D. Risk of CNS toxoplasmosis in patients with acquired immune deficiency syndrome (Abstract 441). Proc 26th ICAAC Washington, DC: American Society for Microbiology; 1986.
220. Leoung GS, Mills J, Hadley WK, et al. Cerebral toxoplasmosis (CNS-T) in AIDS patients: Clinical presentation with laboratory, radiographic and histologic correlations (Abstract). In: Proceedings of the First International Conference on AIDS. Atlanta, Georgia, April 14–17, 1985.
221. McArthur JC. Neurologic manifestations of AIDS. Medicine (Baltimore). 1987;66:407–37.
222. Snider WD, Simpson DM, Nielson S, et al. Neurologic complications of the acquired immunodeficiency syndrome: Analysis of 50 patients. Ann Neurol. 1983;14:403–14.
223. Anonymous: Toxoplasmosis diagnosis and immunodeficiency. Lancet. 1984;1:605.
224. McCabe RE, Gibbons D, Brookes RG, et al. Agglutination test for diagnosis of toxoplasmosis in AIDS. Lancet. 1983;2:680.
225. Wong B, Gold JWM, Brown AE, et al. Central-nervous-system toxoplasmosis in homosexual men and parenteral drug abusers. Ann Intern Med. 1984;100:36–42.
226. Levy RM, Janssen RS, Bush TJ, et al. Neuroepidemiology of acquired immunodeficiency syndrome. In: Rosenblum ML, Levy RM, Bredesen DE, eds. AIDS and the Nervous System. New York: Raven Press; 1988:13–27.
227. Levy RM, Bredesen DE, Rosenblum ML. Neurological manifestations of the acquired immunodeficiency syndrome (AIDS): Experience at UCSF and review of the literature. J Neurosurg. 1985;62:475–95.
228. Berger JR, Mucke L. Neurologic recovery and prolonged survival in progressive multifocal leukoencephalopathy with HIV infection. In: Proceedings of the Third International Conference on AIDS. Washington, DC, June 1–5, 1987.
229. Rogers MF, Morens DM, Stewart JA, et al. National case control study of Kaposi's sarcoma and *Pneumocystis carinii* pneumonia in homosexual men. Part 2. Laboratory results. Ann Intern Med. 1983;99:151–8.
230. Friedman-Kien AE, Lafleur FL, Gendler E, et al. Herpes zoster: A possible early clinical sign for development of acquired immunodeficiency syndrome in high-risk individuals. J Am Acad Dermatol. 1986;14:1023–8.
231. Horsburgh CR, Selik R. Extrapulmonary cryptococcosis (CC) in AIDS patients: Risk factors and association with decreased survival (Abstract 564). In: Proceedings of the 28th Interscience Conference on Antimicrobial Agents and Chemotherapy. Microbiology, Washington, DC: American Society for Microbiology; 1988:207.
232. Kovacs JA, Kovacs AA, Polis M, et al. Cryptococcosis in the acquired immunodeficiency syndrome. Ann Intern Med. 1985;103:533–8.
233. Quinnan GV, Masur H, Rook AH, et al. Herpesvirus infections in the acquired immune deficiency syndrome. JAMA. 1984;252:72–7.
234. Jacobson MA, Mills J. Serious cytomegalovirus disease in acquired immunodeficiency syndrome (AIDS). Clinical findings, diagnoses, and treatment. Ann Intern Med. 1988;108:585–94.
234a. Pepose JS, Holland GN, Nestor MSA, et al. Acquired immune deficiency syndrome: pathogenic mechanisms of ocular disease. Ophthalmology. 1985;92:472–84.
235. Safai B, Good RA. Kaposi's sarcoma: A review and recent developments. Clin Bull. 1980;10:62–8.
236. Templeton AC. Kaposi's sarcoma. Pathol Annu. 1981;16:315–36.
237. Hutt MSR. The epidemiology of Kaposi's sarcoma. Antibiot Chemother. 1981;29:3–8.
238. Taylor JF, Templeton AC, Vogel CL, et al. Kaposi's sarcoma in Uganda: A clinico-pathological study. Int J Cancer. 1971;8:122–35.
239. Zisbrod Z, Haimov M, Schanzer H, et al. Kaposi's sarcoma after kidney transplantation. Transplantation. 1980;30:383–4.
240. Myers BD, Kessler E, Levi J, et al. Kaposi's sarcoma in kidney transplant recipients. Arch Intern Med. 1974;133:307–11.
241. Penn I. Kaposi's sarcoma in immunosuppressed patients. J Clin Lab Immunol. 1983;12:1–10.
242. Little PJ, Al Khader A, Farthing CF, et al. Kaposi's sarcoma in a patient after renal transplantation. Postgrad Med J. 1983;59:325–6.
243. Meyers AM, Rice GC, Kaye S, et al. Kaposi's sarcoma in an immunosuppressed renal allograft recipient. S Afr Med J. 1976;50:1299–300.
244. Stribling J, Weitzner S, Smith GV. Kaposi's sarcoma in renal allograft recipients. Cancer. 1978;42:442–6.
245. Klepp O, Dahi O, Stenwig JT. Association of Kaposi's sarcoma and prior immunosuppressive therapy. Cancer. 1978;42:2626–30.
246. Giraldo G, Beth E, Huang E-S. Kaposi's sarcoma and its relationship to cytomegalovirus (CMV) III. CMV DNA and CMV early antigens in Kaposi's sarcoma. Int J Cancer. 1980;26:23–9.
247. Giraldo G, Beth E, Coeur P, et al. Kaposi's sarcoma: A new model in the search for viruses associated with human malignancies. JNCI. 1972;49:1495–507.
248. Urmacher C, Myskowski P, Ochoa M, et al. Outbreak of Kaposi's sarcoma with cytomegalovirus infection in young homosexual men. Am J Med. 1982;72:569–75.
249. Friedman-Kien AE, Laubenstein LJ, Rubinstein P, et al. Disseminated Kaposi's sarcoma in homosexual men. Ann Intern Med. 1982;96:693–700.
250. Friedman-Kien AE. Kaposi's sarcoma and *Pneumocystis* pneumonia among homosexual men—New York City and California. MMWR. 1981;30:305–8.
251. Editor. Revision of the case definition of acquired immunodeficiency syndrome for national reporting—United States. N Engl J Med. 1987;34:373–5.
252. Levy RM, Pons VG, Rosenblum ML. Central nervous system mass lesions in the acquired immunodeficiency syndrome (AIDS). J Neurosurg. 1984;61:9–16.
253. Rosenblum ML, Levy RM, Bredesen DE, et al. Primary central nervous system lymphomas in patients with AIDS. Ann Neurol. 1988;23(Suppl):13–6.
254. Kaplan LD. AIDS-associated lymphomas. Infect Dis Clin North Am. 1988;2:525–32.
255. Ioachim HL, Cooper MC, Hellman GC. Lymphomas in men at high risk for acquired immune deficiency syndrome (AIDS). Cancer. 1985;56:2831–42.
256. Hoffken G, Kramer A, Dienemann B, et al. Malignant tumors other than Kaposi's sarcoma in persons at high risk for AIDS (Abstract). Tumor Biol. 1987;286.
258. Monfardini S, Italian Cooperative Group for AIDS-Related tumors. Malignant lymphomas in patients with or at risk for AIDS in Italy. JNCI. 1988;80:855–60.
259. Nasr SA, Brynes RK, Garrison CP, et al. Peripheral T-cell lymphoma in a

patient with acquired immune deficiency syndrome. Cancer. 1988;61:947–51.
260. Di Carlo EF, Amberson JB, Metroka CE, et al. Malignant lymphomas and the acquired immunodeficiency syndrome (Abstract). Arch Pathol Lab Med. 1986;110:1012–6.
261. Ziegler JL, Beckstead JA, Volberding PA, et al. Non-Hodgkin's lymphoma in 90 homosexual men. N Engl J Med. 1984;311:565–70.
262. Kreiss JK, Kitchen LW, Prince HE, et al. Antibody to human T-lymphotropic virus type III in wives of hemophiliacs. Ann Intern Med. 1985;102:623–6.
263. Levine AM, Gill PS, Meyer PR, et al. Retrovirus and malignant lymphoma in homosexual men. JAMA. 1985;254:1921–5.
264. Ahmed T, Wormser GP, Stahl RE, et al. Malignant lymphomas in a population at risk for acquired immune deficiency syndrome. Cancer. 1987;60:719–23.
265. Levine AM. Non-Hodgkin's lymphomas and other malignancies in the acquired immune deficiency syndrome. Semin Oncol. 1987;14:34–9.
266. Haverkos HW, Drotman DP. Prevalence of Kaposi's sarcoma among patients with AIDS. N Engl J Med. 1985;312:1518.
267. Rogers MF, Morens DM, Stewart JA, et al. National case-control study of Kaposi's sarcoma and *Pneumocystis carinii* pneumonia in homosexual men: Part 2, laboratory results. Ann Intern Med. 1983;99:151–8.
268. Jaffe HW, Keewhan C, Thomas P, et al. National case-control study of Kaposi's sarcoma and *Pneumocystis carinii* pneumonia in homosexual men: Part 1, epidemiologic results. Ann Intern Med. 1983;99:145–51.
269. DeJarlais DC, Marmor M, Thomas P, et al. Kaposi's sarcoma among four different AIDS risk groups. Lancet. 1988;1:1119.
270. Jaffe HW, Bregman D, Selik RM. Acquired immune deficiency syndrome in the United States: The first 1,000 cases. J Infect Dis. 1983;148:339–45.
271. Cohn DL, Judson FN. Absence of Kaposi's sarcoma in hemophiliacs with the acquired immunodeficiency syndrome. Ann Intern Med. 1984;101:401.
272. Garrett TJ, Lange M, Ashford A, et al. Kaposi's sarcoma in heterosexual intravenous drug users. Cancer. 1985;55:1146–8.
273. Van de Perre P, Lepage P, Kestelyn P, et al. Acquired immunodeficiency syndrome in Rwanda. Lancet. 1984;2:62–5.
274. Kestens L, Melbye M, Biggar RJ, et al. Endemic African Kaposi's sarcoma is not associated with immunodeficiency. Int J Cancer. 1985;36:49–54.
275. Bayley AC, Cheingsong-Popov R, Dalgleish AG, et al. HTLV-III serology distinguishes atypical and endemic Kaposi's sarcoma in Africa. Lancet. 1985;359–61.
276. Downing RG, Eglin RP, Bayley AC. African Kaposi's sarcoma and AIDS. Lancet. 1984;478–80.
277. Bayley AC. Aggressive Kaposi's sarcoma in Zambia, 1983. Lancet. 1988;1318–22.
278. Montgomery AB, Luce JM, Turner J, et al. Aerosolised pentamidine as sole therapy for *Pneumocystis carinii* pneumonia in patients with acquired immunodeficiency syndrome. Lancet. 1987;480–3.
279. Safai B. Pathophysiology and epidemiology of epidemic Kaposi's sarcoma. Semin Oncol. 1987;14:7–12.
280. Buck BE, Scott GB, Valdes-Dapena M, et al. Kaposi's sarcoma in two infants with acquired immune deficiency syndrome. J Pediatr. 1983;103:911–3.
281. Haverkos HW, Amsel Z, Drotman DP, et al. Kaposi's sarcoma in homosexual men with AIDS, by race. Lancet. 1988;1075.
282. Drew WL, Mills J, Hauer LB, et al. Declining prevalence of Kaposi's sarcoma in homosexual AIDS patients paralleled by fall in cytomegalovirus transmission. Lancet. 1988;66.
283. Declines in proportion of Kaposi's sarcoma among cases of AIDS in multiple risk groups in New York City. Lancet. 1987;1024.
284. Volberding PA, Kusick P, Feigal DW. HIV antigenemia at diagnosis with Kaposi's sarcoma: Predictors of shortened survival (Abstract). In: Proceedings of the Fourth International Conference on AIDS. 1988:136.
285. Marmor M, Laubenstein LJ, William DC, et al. Risk factors for Kaposi's sarcoma in homosexual men. Lancet. 1982;1083–6.
286. Haverkos HW. Factors associated with the pathogenesis of AIDS. J Infect Dis. 1987;156:251–7.
287. Newell GR, Mansell PWA, Spitz MR, et al. Volatile nitrites use and adverse effects related to the current epidemic of the acquired immune deficiency syndrome. Am J Med. 1985;78:811–6.
288. Hashimoto H, Muller H, Falk S, et al. Histogenesis of Kaposi's sarcoma associated with AIDS: A histologic, immunohistochemical and enzyme histochemical study. Pathol Res Pract. 1987;182:658–68.
289. Nadji M, Morales AR, Ziegles-Weissman J, et al. Kaposi's sarcoma: Immunohistologic evidence for an endothelial origin. Arch Pathol Lab Med. 1981;105:274–5.
290. Beckstead JH, Wood GS, Fletcher V. Evidence for the origin of Kaposi's sarcoma from lymphatic endothelium. Am J Pathol. 1985;119:294–300.
291. Dorfman RF. Kaposi's sarcoma revisited. Hum Pathol. 1984;15:1013–7.
292. McNutt NS, Fletcher V, Conant MA. Early lesions of Kaposi's sarcoma in homosexual men. Am J Pathol. 1983;111:62–77.
293. Jones RR, Spaull J, Spry C, et al. Histogenesis of Kaposi's sarcoma in patients with and without acquired immune deficiency syndrome (AIDS). J Clin Pathol. 1986;39:742–9.
294. Green TL, Beckstead JH, Lozada-Nur F, et al. Histopathologic spectrum of oral Kaposi's sarcoma. Oral Surg. 1984;58:306–14.
295. Lesbordes JL, Martin PMV, Ravisse P, et al. Clinical and histopathological aspects of Kaposi's sarcoma in Africa: Relationship with HIV serology. 1988;139:197–203.
296. Nakamura S, Salahuddin SZ, Biberfeld P, et al. Kaposi's sarcoma cells: Long-term culture with growth factor from retrovirus-infected CD4 T cells. Science. 1988;242:426–30.
297. Salahuddin SZ, Nakamura S, Biberfeld P, et al. Angiogenic properties of Kaposi's sarcoma-derived cells after long-term culture in vitro. Science. 1988;242:430–3.
298. Costa J, Rabson AS. Generalised Kaposi's sarcoma is not a neoplasm. Lancet. 1983;58.
299. Mitsuyasu RT. Clinical variants and staging of Kaposi's sarcoma. Semin Oncol. 1987;14:13–8.
300. Safai B, Sarngadharan MG, Koziner B, et al. Spectrum of Kaposi's sarcoma in the epidemic of AIDS. Cancer Res. 1985;45(Suppl):4646–8.
301. Vadhan-Raj S, Wong G, Gnecco C, et al. Immunological variables as predictors of prognosis in patients with Kaposi's sarcoma and the acquired immunodeficiency syndrome. Cancer Res. 1986;46:417–25.
302. Rawlinson KF, Zubrow AB, Harris MA, et al. Disseminated Kaposi's sarcoma in pregnancy: A manifestation of acquired immune deficiency syndrome. Obstet Gynecol 1984;63(Suppl):2–6.
303. Patow CA, Steis R, Longo DL, et al. Kaposi's sarcoma of the head and neck in the acquired immune deficiency syndrome. Otolaryngology. 1984;92:255–60.
304. Real FX, Oettgen HF, Krown SE. Kaposi's sarcoma and the acquired immunodeficiency syndrome: Treatment with high and low doses of recombinant leukocyte A interferon. J Clin Oncol. 1986;4:544–51.
305. Hymes KB, Greene JB, Marcus A, et al. Kaposi's sarcoma in homosexual men—a report of eight cases. Lancet. 1981;598–600.
306. Seftel AD, Sadick NS, Waldbaum RS. Kaposi's sarcoma of the penis in a patient with the acquired immune deficiency syndrome. J Urol. 1986;136:673–5.
307. Mitsuyasu RT, Taylor J, Glaspy J, et al. Heterogeneity of epidemic Kaposi's sarcoma. Cancer. 1986;57:1657–61.
308. Lumerman H, Freedman PD, Kerpel SM, et al. Oral Kaposi's sarcoma: A clinicopathologic study of 23 homosexual and bisexual men from the New York metropolitan area. Oral Surg. 1988;65:711–6.
309. Gnepp DR, Chandler W, Hyams V. Primary Kaposi's sarcoma of the head and neck. Ann Intern Med. 1984;100:107–14.
310. Moskowitz LB, Hensley GT, Gould EW, et al. Frequency and anatomic distribution of lymphadenopathic Kaposi's sarcoma in the acquired immunodeficiency syndrome: An autopsy series. Hum Pathol. 1985;16:447–56.
311. Lustbader I, Sherman A. Primary gastrointestinal Kaposi's sarcoma in a patient with acquired immune deficiency syndrome. Am J Gastroenterol. 1987;82:894–5.
312. Rose HS, Balthazar EJ, Megibow AJ, et al. Alimentary tract involvement in Kaposi sarcoma: Radiographic and endoscopic findings in 25 homosexual men. AJR. 1982;139:661–6.
313. Scott LF, Wright TL, Altman DF. Gastrointestinal Kaposi's sarcoma in patients with acquired immunodeficiency syndrome. Gastroenterology. 1988;89:102–8.
314. Dworkin B, Wormser GP, Rosenthal WS, et al. Gastrointestinal manifestations of the acquired immunodeficiency syndrome: A review of 22 cases. Am J Gastroenterol. 1985;80:774–8.
315. Barrison IG, Foster S, Harris JW, et al. Upper gastrointestinal Kaposi's sarcoma in patients positive for HIV antibody without cutaneous disease. Br Med J. 1988;296:92–3.
316. Friedman SL, Wright TL, Altman DF. Gastrointestinal Kaposi's sarcoma in patients with acquired immunodeficiency syndrome. Gastroenterology. 1985;89:102–8.
317. Federle MP. A radiologist looks at AIDS: Imaging evaluation based on symptom complexes. Radiology. 1988;166:553–62.
318. Frager DH, Frager JD, Brandt LJ, et al. Gastrointestinal complications of AIDS: Radiologic features. Radiology. 1986;158:597–603.
319. Rucker L, Meador J. Kaposi's sarcoma presenting as homogeneous pulmonary infiltrates in a patient with acquired immunodeficiency syndrome. West J Med. 1985;142:831–3.
320. Ognibene FP, Steis RG, Macher AM, et al. Kaposi's sarcoma causing pulmonary infiltrates and respiratory failure in the acquired immunodeficiency syndrome. Ann Intern Med. 1985;102:471–5.
321. Caray SM, Belenko M, Fazzini E, et al. Pulmonary manifestations of Kaposi's sarcoma. Chest. 1987;91:39–43.
322. Meduri GU, Stover D, Lee M, et al. Pulmonary Kaposi's sarcoma in the acquired immune deficiency syndrome. Am J Med. 1986;81:11–8.
323. Kaplan LD, Hopewell PC, Jaffe HW, et al. Kaposi's sarcoma involving the lung in patients with the acquired immunodeficiency syndrome. J AIDS. 1988;1:23–30.
324. Nash G, Fligiel S. Kaposi's sarcoma presenting as pulmonary disease in the acquired immunodeficiency syndrome: Diagnosis by lung biopsy. Hum Pathol. 1984;15:999–1001.
325. Kornfeld H, Axelrod JL. Pulmonary presentation of Kaposi's sarcoma in a homosexual patient. Am Rev Respir Dis. 1983;127:248–9.
326. Keeney K, Abaza NA, Tidwel O, et al. Oral Kaposi's sarcoma in acquired immune deficiency syndrome. J Oral Maxillofac Surg. 1987;45:815–21.
327. Lozada F, Silverman S, Migliorati CA, et al. Oral manifestations of tumor and opportunistic infections in the acquired immunodeficiency syndrome (AIDS): Findings in 53 homosexual men with Kaposi's sarcoma. Oral Surg. 1983;56:491–4.
328. Emery CD, Wall SD, Federle MP, et al. Pharyngeal Kaposi's sarcoma in patients with AIDS.; AJR. 1986;147:919–22.

329. Green TL, Beckstead JH, Lozada-Nur F, et al. Histopathologic spectrum of oral Kaposi's sarcoma. Oral Surg. 1984;58:306–14.
330. Krigel RL, Laubenstein LJ, Muggia FM. Kaposi's sarcoma: A new staging classification. Cancer Treat Rep. 1983;67:531–4.
331. Volberding PA. The role of chemotherapy for epidemic Kaposi's sarcoma. Semin Oncol. 1987;16(Suppl 3):23–6.
332. Taylor J, Afrasiabi R, Fahey JL, et al. Prognostically significant classification of immune changes in AIDS with Kaposi's sarcoma. Blood. 1986;67:666–71.
333. Lane HC, Masur H, Gelmann EP, et al. Correlation between immunologic function and clinical subpopulations of patients with the acquired immune deficiency syndrome. Am J Med. 1985;78:417–22.
334. Moss AR. Predicting who will progress to AIDS. Br Med J. 1988;297:1067–8.
335. Moss AR, McCallum G, Volberding PA, et al. Mortality associated with mode of presentation in the acquired immune deficiency syndrome. JNCI. 1984;73:1281–4.
336. El-Akkad S, Bull CA, El-Senoussi MA, et al. Kaposi's sarcoma and its management by radiotherapy. Arch Dermatol. 1986;122:1396–9.
337. Holecek MJ, Harwood AR. Radiotherapy of Kaposi's sarcoma. Cancer. 1978;41:1733–8.
338. Hill DR. The role of radiotherapy for epidemic Kaposi's sarcoma. Semin Oncol. 1987;14:19–22.
339. Groopman JE. AIDS-related Kaposi's sarcoma: Therapeutic modalities. Semin Hematol. 1987;24:5–8.
340. Cooper JS, Fried PR. Treatment of aggressive epidemic Kaposi's sarcoma of the conjunctiva by radiotherapy. Arch Ophthalmol. 1988;106:20–1.
341. Cooper JS, Fried PR, Laubenstein LJ. Initial observations of the effect of radiotherapy on epidemic Kaposi's sarcoma. JAMA. 1984;252:934–5.
342. Volberding PA. Therapy of Kaposi's sarcoma in AIDS. Semin Oncol. 1984;11:60–7.
343. Harris JW, Reed TA. Kaposi's sarcoma in AIDS: The role of radiation therapy. Front Radiat Ther Oncol. 1985;19:126–32.
344. Nisce LZ, Safai B, Poussin-Rosillo H. Once weekly total and subtotal skin electron beam therapy for Kaposi's sarcoma. Cancer. 1981;47:640–4.
345. Nobler MP, Leddy ME, Huh SH. The impact of palliative irradiation on the management of patients with acquired immune deficiency syndrome. J Clin Oncol. 1987;5:107–12.
346. Brambilla L, Boneschi V, Beretta G, et al. Intralesional chemotherapy for Kaposi's sarcoma. Dermatology. 1984;169:149–55.
347. Kahn J, Kaplan LD, Jaffe HW, et al. Intralesional recombinant tumor necrosis factor for AIDS related Kaposi's sarcoma (Abstract). In: Proceedings of the Fourth International Conference on AIDS. Washington, DC: Bio-Data Publishers; 1988:324.
348. Volberding PA, Abrams DI, Conant MA, et al. Vinblastine therapy for Kaposi's sarcoma in the acquired immunodeficiency syndrome. Ann Intern Med. 1985;103:335–8.
349. Kaplan LD, Abrams DI, Volberding PA. Treatment of Kaposi's sarcoma in acquired immunodeficiency syndrome with an alternating vincristine vinblastine regimen. Cancer Treat Rep. 1986;70:1121–2.
350. Fischl MA, Krown S, O'Boyle K, et al. Weekly doxorubicin in the treatment of patients with AIDS-related Kaposi's sarcoma (Abstract). In: Proceedings of the Fourth International Conference on AIDS. Washington, DC: Bio-Data Publishers; 1988:202.
351. Mintzer DM, Real FX, Jovino L, et al. Treatment of Kaposi's sarcoma and thrombocytopenia with vincristine in patients with the acquired immunodeficiency syndrome. Ann Intern Med. 1985;102:200–2.
352. Laubenstein LJ, Krigel RL, Odajnyk CM, et al. Treatment of epidemic Kaposi's sarcoma with etoposide or a combination of doxorubicin, bleomycin, and vinblastine. J Clin Oncol. 1984;2:1115–20.
353. Gill PS, Krailo MD, Slater L, et al. Results of a randomized trial of ABV (Adriamycin, bleomycin, vincristine) vs an advanced epidemic Kaposi's sarcoma. (Abstract). In: Proceedings of the Fourth International Conference on AIDS. Washington, DC: Bio-Data Publishers; 1988:323.
354. Flepp, M, Tauber MG, Luthy R, et al. Kaposi's sarcoma in AIDS patients: Long-term treatment with recombinant interferon alpha-2A and chemotherapy. Klin Wochenschr. 1988;66:437–42.
355. Gelmann EP, Preble OT, Steis R, et al. Human lymphoblastoid interferon treatment of Kaposi's sarcoma in the acquired immune deficiency syndrome. Am J Med. 1985;78:737–41.
356. Krown SE, Real FX, Cunningham-Rundles S, et al. Preliminary observations on the effect of recombinant leukocyte A interferon in homosexual men with Kaposi's sarcoma. N Engl J Med. 1983;308:1071–6.
357. Redfield RR, Markham PD, Salshuddin SZ, et al. Frequent transmission of HTLV-III among spouses of patients with AIDS-related complex and AIDS. JAMA. 1985;253:1571–3.
358. Rios A, Mansell PWA, Newell GR, et al. Treatment of acquired immunodeficiency syndrome-related Kaposi's sarcoma with lymphoblastoid interferon. J Clin Oncol. 1985;3:506–12.
359. Krigel RL, Slywotzky CM, Lonberg M, et al. Treatment of epidemic Kaposi's sarcoma with a combination of interferon-alpha 2b and etoposide. J Biol Response Mod. 1988;7:359–64.
360. Krown SE, Bundow D, Tong WP, et al. Interferon-alpha plus azidothymidine (AZT) in AIDS-associated Kaposi's sarcoma (KS). J Interferon Res. 1987;7:688–9.
361. Krown S, Bundow D, Gansbacher B, et al. Interferon-alpha plus zidovudine: A phase I trial in AIDS-associated Kaposi's sarcoma (KS) (Abstract). In: Proceedings of the Fourth International Conference on AIDS. Washington, DC: Bio-Data Publishers; 1988:173.
362. Fischl MA, Dickinson GM, LaVoie L. Safety and efficacy of sulfamethoxazole and trimethoprim chemoprophylaxis for *Pneumocystis carinii* pneumonia in AIDS. JAMA. 1988;259:1185–9.
363. Girard PM, Brun-Pascaud M, Farinotti, R, et al. Pentamidine aerosol in prophylaxis and treatment of murine *Pneumocystis carinii* pneumonia (Abstract). Antimicrob Agents Chemother. 1987;31:978–81.
364. Lowery S, Fallat R, Feigal DW, et al. Changing patterns of *Pneumocystis carinii* pneumonia (PCP) on pentamidine aerosol prophylaxis (Abstract). In: Proceedings of the Fourth International Conference on AIDS. Washington, DC: Bio-Data Publishers; 1988:419.
365. Levine AM. Non-Hodgkin's lymphomas and other malignancies in the acquired immune deficiency syndrome. Semin Oncol. 1987;14:34–9.
366. Biggar RJ, Horm J, Lubin JH, et al. Cancer trends in a population at risk of acquired immunodeficiency syndrome. JNCI. 1985;74:793–7.
367. Rechavi B, Ben-Bassat B, Berkowicy M, et al. Molecular analysis of Burkitt's leukemia in two hemophilic brothers with AIDS. Blood. 1987;70:1713–7.
368. Groopman JE, Sullivan JL, Mulder C, et al. Pathogenesis of B cell lymphoma in a patient with AIDS. Blood. 1986;67:612–5.
369. Lippman SM, Volk JR, Spier CM, et al. Clonal ambiguity of human immunodeficiency virus-associated lymphomas. Arch Pathol Lab Med. 1988;112:128–32.
370. Subar M, Neri A, Inghirami G, et al. Frequent c-*myc* oncogene activation and infrequent presence of Epstein-Barr virus genome in AIDS-associated lymphoma. Blood. 1988;72:667–71.
371. Loeffler JS, Ervin TJ, Mauch P, et al. Primary lymphomas of the central nervous system: Patterns of failure and factors that influence survival. J Clin Oncol. 1985;3:490–4.
372. Elkin CM, Leon E, Grenell SL, et al. Intracranial lesions in the acquired immunodeficiency syndrome. JAMA. 1985;253:393–6.
373. So YT, Beckstead JH, Davis RL. Primary central nervous system lymphoma in acquired immune deficiency syndrome: A clinical and pathological study (Abstract). Ann Neurol. 1986;20:566–72.
374. Levy RM, Bredesen DE, Rosenblum ML. Neurologic manifestations of the acquired immunodeficiency syndrome (AIDS): Experience at UCSF and review of the literature. J Neurosurg. 1985;62:475–95.
375. Knowles DM, Chamulak GA, Subar M, et al. Lymphoid neoplasia associated with the acquired immunodeficiency syndrome (AIDS). Ann Intern Med. 1988;108:744–53.
376. Ioachim HL, Weinstein MA, Robbins RD, et al. Primary anorectal lymphoma: A new manifestation of the acquired immune deficiency syndrome (AIDS). Cancer. 1987;60:1449–53.
377. Caccamo D, Pervez NK, Marchevsky A. Primary lymphoma of the liver in the acquired immunodeficiency syndrome. Arch Pathol Lab Med. 1986;110:553–5.
378. Bottles K, McPhaul LW, Volberding PA. Fine needle aspiration biopsy of patients with acquired immunodeficiency syndrome (AIDS): Experience in an outpatient clinic. Ann Intern Med. 1988;108:42–5.
379. Abrams DI, Kaplan LD, McGrath MS, et al. AIDS-related benign lymphadenopathy and malignant lymphoma: Clinical aspects and virology interactions. AIDS Res. 1986;2:131–40.
380. Jeffrey RB, Nyberg DA, Bottles K, et al. Abdominal CT in acquired immunodeficiency syndrome. AJR. 1986;146:7–13.
381. Nyberg DA, Jeffrey RB, Federle MP, et al. AIDS-related lymphomas: Evaluation by abdominal CT. Radiology. 1986;159:59–63.
382. Gill PS, Levine AM, Krailo MD, et al. AIDS-related malignant lymphoma: Results of prospective treatment trials. J Clin Oncol. 1987;5:1322–8.
383. Schoeppel SL, Hoppe RT, Dorfman RF, et al. Hodgkin's disease in homosexual men with generalized lymphadenopathy. Ann Intern Med. 1985;102:68–70.
384. Robert NJ, Schneiderman H. Hodgkin's disease and the acquired immunodeficiency syndrome. Ann Intern Med. 1984;100:142–3.
385. Ioachim HL, Cooper MC, Hellman GC. Hodgkin's disease and the acquired immunodeficiency syndrome. Ann Intern Med. 1984;101:876–7.
386. Unger PD, Strauchen JA. Hodgkin's disease in AIDS complex patients. Cancer. 1986;4:821–5.
387. Baer DM, Anderson ET, Wilkinson LS. Acquired immune deficiency syndrome in homosexual men with Hodgkin's disease. Am J Med. 1986;80:738–40.
388. Gongora-Biachi RA, Gonzalez-Martinez P, Bastarrachea-Ortiz J. Hodgkin's disease as the initial manifestation of acquired immunodeficiency syndrome. Ann Intern Med. 1987;107:112.
389. Mitsuyasu RT, Coman MF, Sun NCJ. Simultaneous occurrence of Hodgkin's disease and Kaposi's sarcoma in a patient with the acquired immune deficiency syndrome. Ann J Med. 1986;80:954–8.
390. Picard O, De Gramont A, Krulik M, et al. Rectal Hodgkin disease and the acquired immunodeficiency syndrome. Ann Intern Med. 1987;106:775.
391. Unger PD, Strauchen JA. Hodgkin's disease in AIDS complex patients. Cancer. 1986;58:821–5.
392. Robert NJ, Scheiderman H. Hodgkin's disease and the acquired immunodeficiency syndrome. Ann Intern Med. 1988;101:142–43.
393. Krause W, Mittag H, Gieler U, et al. A case of malignant melanoma in AIDS-related complex. Arch Dermatol. 1987;123:867–8.
394. Frager DH, Wolf EL, Competiello LS, et al. Squamous cell carcinoma of the esophagus in patients with acquired immunodeficiency syndrome. Gastrointest Radiol. 1988;13:358–60.

395. Kaplan MJ, Sabio H, Waneba HJ, et al. Squamous cell carcinoma in the immunosuppressed patient: Fanconi's anemia. Laryngoscope. 1985;95:771–5.
396. Enck RE. Squamous cell cancers and the acquired immunodeficiency syndrome. Ann Intern Med. 1987;106:773.
397. Tessler AN, Catanese A. AIDS and germ cell tumors of testis. Urology. 1987;203–4.
398. Logothetis CJ, Newell GR, Samuels ML. Testicular cancer in homosexual men with cellular immune deficiency: Report of 2 cases. J Urol. 1985;133:484–6.
399. Quang TN, Beuzeboc P, Lurie A, et al. Cancer du testicule chez deux homosexuels avec anticorps anti HIV. Ann Med Interne (Paris). 1987;138:233–40.
400. Slazinski L, Stall JR, Mathews CR. Basal cell carcinoma in a man with acquired immunodeficiency syndrome. J Am Acad Derm. 1984;11:140–1.
401. Sitz KV, Keppen M, Fohnson DF. Metastatic basal cell carcinoma in acquired immunodeficiency syndrome-related complex (Abstract). JAMA. 1987;257:340–3.
402. Weitberg AB, Mayer KH, Miller ME, et al. Dysplastic carcinoid tumor and AIDS-related complex. N Engl J Med. 1986;314:1455.
403. Grieger T, Carl M, Liebert H, et al. Mediastinal liposarcoma in a patient infected with the human immunodeficiency virus. Am J Med. 1988;84:366.
404. Cappell MSl, Yao F, Cho KC. Colonic adenocarcinoma associated with the acquired immune deficiency syndrome. Cancer. 1988;62:617–9.

109. DETECTION OF HIV-1 INFECTION

CHARLES J. SCHLEUPNER

In 1983–1984 as the isolation of human immunodeficiency virus (HIV-1) was first reported, serologic tests were described that recognized antibodies to HIV-1 in the sera of patients with the acquired immunodeficiency syndrome (AIDS).[1–7] The first assay for screening blood donors became licensed for commercial use on March 2, 1985, when blood centers initiated screening of all donated blood for antibody to HIV-1.[8] The "first generation" of these enzyme immunoassays (EIAs) were adaptations of assays using antigens derived from lysed HIV-1-infected cell cultures.[6] They were designed for sensitivity of detection of HIV infection; the EIA gained specificity only upon repeated testing with positive results and "confirmatory" evaluation with Western blot (WB). The test was clearly successful at its primary purpose, making the blood supply safer.[8,9]

To prevent individuals in high-risk groups from using blood banks for diagnostic testing (thereby increasing the risk of contamination of the blood supply), alternate test sites were also established where patients in high-risk groups could have EIA evaluations (and WB if indicated) performed anonymously or confidentially and without charge after appropriate counseling. Therefore, continued self-deferral of high-risk donors was facilitated.[10]

Through counseling, another goal of EIA testing for antibody to HIV-1 evolved, i.e., prevention of infection or spread thereof to others. In December 1985, the Centers for Disease Control (CDC) extended its recommendation for EIA testing to pregnant women and women who might become pregnant while being at high risk for HIV-1 infection.[11] In the spring of 1986, serologic testing was additionally recommended for persons attending sexually transmissible disease (STD) clinics and clinics for prostitutes and intravenous drug abusers.[12] Testing was further advised for recipients of transfusions between 1978 and 1985 and all patients with tuberculosis.[13]

At the same time that the target high-risk populations for diagnostic testing were being extended, the limitations of the "first-generation" EIAs were acknowledged; the rate of false positivity was high in low-risk populations (80–90 percent), which resulted in an unnecessary reduction in the sources of the nation's blood supply and unwarranted emotional stress for individuals receiving such erroneous information.[14–16] With the purpose of increasing the specificity of both screening and confirmatory tests, EIAs using specific HIV-1 proteins produced by recombinant technology were developed.[17] With the application of these assays together with the development of an EIA for HIV core antigen,[18–20] the use of serologic assays has been extended to include a better understanding of the pathogenesis of HIV-1 infection, evaluation of the success of therapy, and definition of the strategies for earlier initiation of therapy.[21,22]

SEROLOGIC RESPONSE TO HIV INFECTION

The serologic response to HIV is best understood by an appreciation of the major protein products of the viral genome (see Chapter 147). The temporal course of the appearance of serum HIV antigen and antibodies to several viral proteins is shown in Figure 1. After infection, p24 antigen is the first serologic marker to be detected.[23,24] The appearance of antibody to p24 is temporally associated with falling p24 antigen levels and with immune complexes of these reactants.[18,23,25–27] Antibodies to the carboxy terminal envelope cleavage product (gp41) of gp160 are often detectable before anti-p24 (Fig. 1) by WB, competitive EIA using recombinant antigens (CIA-RA), or radioimmunoprecipitation (RIPA).[23,28] Months or years after the development of antibodies to both the core and envelope proteins, the core antigen may reappear (Fig. 1); this is usually coincident with the loss of anti-p24 and correlates with the development of AIDS.[19,22,29–35]

HIV-1 ANTIBODY ASSAYS

Enzyme Immunoassays

All seven licensed "first-generation" EIAs for the detection of antibody to HIV-1 use virus derived from lysed cell cultures.[36–38] All kits use the human T-cell leukemia/lymphoma virus (HTLV-III) strain of HIV-1, except for the Genetic Systems assay, which uses the lymphadenopathy-associated virus (LAV) strain. The cell source of HIV-1 varies according to each manufacturer. The Abbott, Dupont, Electronucleonics (ENI), Organon-Teknika, Cellular Products, and Ortho kits use the H-9 cell line. Genetic Systems uses the CEM-F line.[38,39] (The Organon-Teknika kit is an improved version of what was formerly the Litton EIA.) The partially purified virus is bound to a microtiter well or to a latex or a polystyrene-coated metal bead (the solid phase; Table 1). Most EIAs are indirect; viral antigen is exposed to a patient specimen (serum, cerebrospinal fluid [CSF], other body fluid) and incubated to allow antigen–antibody binding. The solid phase is then washed to remove unbound immunoglobulin and is exposed to an enzyme-labeled anti-human globulin (e.g., horseradish peroxidase or alkaline phosphatase). After binding has occurred, these complexes are exposed to a substrate for the attached enzyme to allow a colorimetric reaction to occur, which is proportional to the amount of bound anti-HIV-1 globulin in the patient specimen. Both strongly and weakly reactive controls as well as negative con-

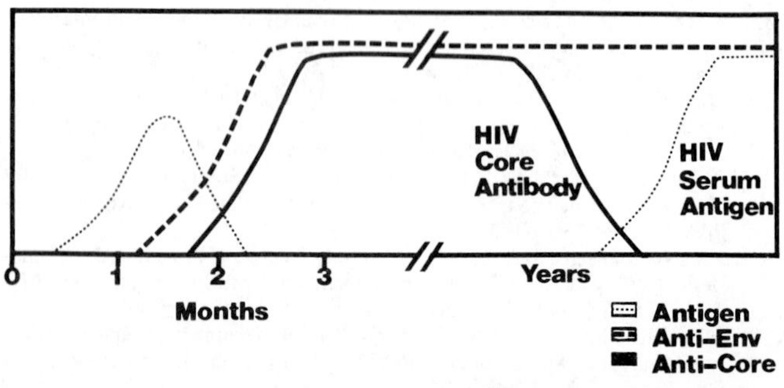

FIG. 1. Chronology of HIV-1 infection defined by the presence of core (p24) antigen and antibodies to core protein and envelope (gp41) glycoprotein. (Courtesy of Abbott Diagnostics Division, Abbott Laboratories, North Chicago, IL.)

TABLE 1. Summary of Methodology for Six Commonly Used Screening EIAs for HIV-1 Antibody

Features	*ABB*	*DU*	*ENI*	*GS*	*OT*	*OR*
Viral antigen source						
HTLV-III	X	X	X		X	X
LAV				X		
H-9 cell line	X	X	X		X	X
CEM-F cell line				X		
Antigen-coated beads	X				X	
Latex	X					
Plastic-coated ferrous metal					X	
Antigen-coated wells		X	X	X		X
Assay performed in						
Microtiter plate		X	X	X	X	X
Test tube	X					
Anti-human IgG						
Peroxidase conjugated	X		X	X	X	X
Alkaline phosphatase conjugated		X				
Substrate						
O-phenylenediamine	X		X			X
Para-nitrophenyl-phosphate		X				
2,2′-Azino-di-[3-ethylbenzthiazoline sulfonate]					X	
Tetramethylbenzidine				X		
Total test time (hr)	4.4	2.5	2.0	3.0	3.0	3.0

Abbreviations: ABB: Abbott; DU: Dupont; ENI: Electronucleonics; GS: Genetic Systems; OT: Oganon/Teknika; OR: Ortho Diagnostics.

trols are run in parallel on each occasion that unknown sera are assayed. Some more recent kits use a competitive inhibition enzyme immunoassay. In the latter assay, the color reaction is inversely proportional to the amount of bound anti-HIV-1 globulin in the patient specimen. An EIA assay takes up to 4 hours to perform (Table 1).

With either indirect or competitive EIA, the optical density (OD) of each unknown (individual or paired) and each control is measured at the optimal wavelength for substrate absorption after undergoing the colorimetric reaction. A cutoff OD is then calculated by using negative and/or positive control values (the equation varies with each kit), and a ratio of sample to cutoff OD is calculated. For the indirect or "sandwich" EIA, values ≥ 1.0 are considered positive; for the competitive EIA, values <1.0 are positive. These EIAs are usually performed with serum, but an EIA has been reported to detect HIV-1 antibodies in saliva with a sensitivity equal to that in serum.[40]

Burke et al. have shown that OD readings vary with the intensity of various WB banding patterns.[41] While the Abbott EIA has greatest sensitivity for antibodies to gp41 and the polymerase gene products, the Dupont, ENI, and Litton EIAs are more sensitive for antibodies to the gag (core) proteins.[41] This has relevance to the sensitivity of each EIA for HIV-1 antibody during various stages of infection; for example, during AIDS when anti-p24 has usually disappeared, the latter EIAs may be less sensitive for detecting infection due to their greater sensitivity for p24 antibody. Cooper et al. have compared four EIAs for their ability to identify infection during acute HIV-1 illness[42]; the ENI assay was the most sensitive for early diagnosis, while the Abbott EIA was the least.

If a blood or plasma collection center or a referral laboratory detects HIV-1 antibody by EIA in a plasma or serum sample, a repeat EIA is performed on a second specimen (Fig. 2). If the repeated assay is positive, a confirmatory test is ordered (usually a WB), and the donor or patient is notified. If the repeated test is negative, a different EIA should be performed.[8] In either case, the unit of blood or plasma is discarded, and the donor is referred to a private physician, a health department, or an alternate testing site for evaluation and counseling. For specimens indeterminate by WB analysis, a repeat specimen obtained in 2–3 months should be evaluated, and/or the specimen can be examined by another confirmatory test method (e.g., RIPA).

Because the EIA for anti-HIV-1 has been used for serologic evaluation of high-risk populations in addition to volunteer blood donors,[15,16,38] any discussion of the validity of test results must take into account the population tested and its overall seropositivity rate. In blood donor populations, initial reports of the performance of the screening "first-generation" EIA (usually the Abbott test) showed positive predictive values of 3.8–27.3 percent.[9,43] These predictive values varied depending on the EIA OD reactivity, with low positive OD values being associated with greater degrees of false positivity.[43–45] Other early studies compared various EIA tests against the same sera, usually from a group of patients with a spectrum of risk for HIV-1 infection.[46–49] While the Abbott and the Wellcome Diagnostics EIAs were usually among the most sensitive, the Abbott assay had the highest false-positive rate among low-risk groups (i.e., blood donors), followed by the Organon, Dupont, and Litton assays. The sensitivity and specificity for most man-

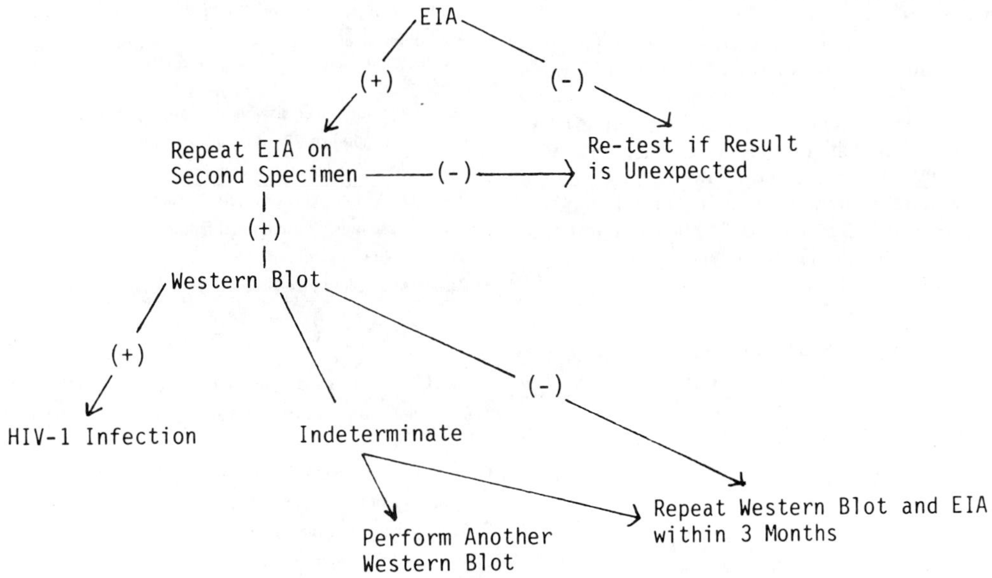

FIG. 2. An algorithm for the management of HIV-1 serologic results.

ufacturers' assays were 97.2–100 percent and 99.6–100 percent, respectively, when using sera from patients in high-risk groups,[47] except for one report of low specificity for the Abbott test in this risk group.[50]

Subsequent reports have evaluated the Genetic Systems EIA, along with the others mentioned previously, by using sera from a similar spectrum of patients.[28,44,45,51] The Genetic Systems EIA repeatedly ranked best in these studies in terms of sensitivity, specificity, and reproducibility. The most recent studies, some using EIA assays with more purified disrupted viral antigens, further confirm the excellence of the Genetic Systems and the new, improved Organon-Teknika EIAs.[34,52–54] A number of recent studies have also pointed out the relevance of the distribution of positive and negative OD values above and below the cutoff to differentiate true positive from negative results.[44,53,54] It is evident that an EIA with many OD determinations clustered around the OD cutoff will be subject to more false-positive and/or negative results (e.g., Litton, ENI, and Ortho).[44,53,54] A recent CDC survey of health department and American Red Cross laboratories identified similar problems with specimens having OD results around cutoff values.[55] It was noteworthy that, despite a confirmation of higher false-positive rates with the Abbott EIA, 80–85 percent of laboratories reported using this assay; another 3–8 percent of laboratories reported using the ENI or Organon-Teknika kits. Schwartz et al. recently discussed arguments for varying the OD cutoff values defining positive and negative specimens.[56] Since a rise of the OD cutoff of the noncompetitive EIA increases the specificity at the cost of sensitivity, these authors argued for raising cutoff values when these tests are being used for diagnostic rather than screening purposes. Future experience will determine whether such variations of definition of reactive specimens are warranted.

Variations of specificity and positive predictive value are codependent upon the prevalence of HIV-1 infection in the population tested, as shown in Table 2. For any laboratory test, methodologic error, regardless of source, occurs with a relatively fixed frequency; therefore, for each population tested, regardless of risk for HIV-1 infection, the number of false-positives per 1000 tests will be approximately the same. However, in a low-risk population (with few true positives), the number of false-positives will be a much greater percentage of those called positive than for the high-risk population. Therefore, the positive predictive value of such a screening test in a low-risk population may only be 10%, while it would be as high as 97.3% in a high-risk population.[15,16] This is anticipated since these screening EIAs were designed for optimum sensitivity at the expense of specificity.[15]

The relevance of false positivity in a low-risk population is apparent from American Red Cross data[9,39] (Table 3). Among 2.58 million volunteer blood donors, only 3.5 percent of initially positive EIAs and only 13 percent of repeatedly reactive EIAs were reactive by WB.[39] This high prevalence of false positivity in low-risk groups brings into focus the relatively high cost of identifying one truly infected person in such a population, estimated conservatively to be $35,000 to $40,000 per infected person (for example, if all hospital admissions underwent mandatory screening annually).

TABLE 2. Example of Problems with the HIV-1 Antibody EIA When Applied to High- and Low-Risk Populations

Assay Result	*High-Risk Population*	*Low-Risk Population*
No. tested	10,000	10,000
Percentage positive	10%	0.3%
Total no. positive	1000	30
No. false-positives[a]	27	27
No. true positives	973	3
Positive predictive value	973/1000 (97.3%)	3/30 (10%)

[a] False-positives due to intrinsic methodologic inaccuracies, regardless of the population tested.

TABLE 3. Correlation between EIA and Western Blot Positivity for 2.58 Million American Red Cross Blood Donors

	Blood Donor Results	
Assay Result	*Number*	*Percent*
EIA, initially positive	25,800	1
Repeat EIA positive	6966	0.27
WB positive	903	0.035
Positive predictive values		
Initial EIA	—	3.5
Repeat EIA	—	13

The false-positive and false-negative results obtained with EIAs are due to a variety of clinical and technical variables.[57] It has been noted that heat-inactivated sera (treated to enhance laboratory safety) cause false-positive reactions with the Abbott EIA.[48,58,59] Sera with rapid plasma reagin (RPR) reactivity have also been reported to cause false-positive EIAs for HIV-1 antibody only with the Abbott kit; the false-positive rate with RPR-positive sera when using the most recent viral lysate Abbott EIA has been reduced to approximately 3 percent.[60] Other factors are also associated with erroneous results, as noted in Tables 4 and 5.[38,43,49,61–71] By far the most important cause of false positivity is cross-reacting antibodies in serum to HLA class II antigens present in HIV-1 preparations harvested from H-9 cells.[43,61–65] The Genetic Systems and Wellcome assays avoid this problem by use of CEM-F cells for virus propogation; this cell line lacks such HLA reactivity[53,56] (Table 1). While too insensitive to assay for HIV-2 antibodies, anti-HIV-1 EIAs, especially competitive EIAs, can be falsely positive due to cross-reacting core antibodies with HIV-2.[72]

Using WB and the Dupont EIA, Tribe et al. have also recognized some sera that are repeatedly reactive by EIA but nonreactive by WB blot criteria due to their EIA reactivity with gag proteins of HIV-1.[73] These sera react predominantly with p15/p17 and less frequently with p24, but they lack anti-env reactivity. Such individuals must be excluded from blood donation until the reasons for this continued reactivity are clarified (e.g., cross-reactivity with other [retro] viruses or tissue proteins).

Despite the foregoing comments, the probability of a false-positive result after the complete testing sequence (Fig. 2) has been estimated to be 1–5 per 100,000 persons screened.[13] Per-

TABLE 4. Causes of False-Positive EIA Reactions to HIV-1

Antibody against smooth muscle, parietal cell, mitochondrial, nuclear, leukocyte, and T-cell antigens; anti-HAV-IgM and anti-HBc-IgM
Antibodies against class II leukocyte antigens (HLA-DR4, -DQw3) present on H-9 cells (more frequently observed in multiparous women, multiply transfused patients)
Severe alcoholic liver disease, primary biliary cirrhosis, sclerosing cholangitis
Heat inactivation or RPR positivity of serum tested (Abott EIA only)
Hematologic malignancies, lymphoma
Acute DNA viral infections, HIV-2 infection
Renal transplants, chronic renal failure
Stevens-Johnson syndrome
Passively acquired HIV-1 antibody (hepatitis B immunoglobulin)

TABLE 5. Causes of False-Negative EIA Reactions to HIV-1

Incubation period or acute disease before seroconversion ("window-period")
Malignancy
Intensive or long-term immunosuppressive therapy
Replacement transfusion
Bone marrow transplantation
Kits that detect antibody to p24 primarily
B-cell dysfunction

haps more important from a clinical perspective, estimates of the false-negative rate of EIAs for HIV-1 antibody range from 1 in 40,000 to 1 in 1 million.[74] The causes of such false negativity are presented in Table 5. This problem has been recently reviewed with regard to the transfusion-related transmission of HIV-1.[75]

The most recently developed "second-generation" EIAs for antibody to HIV-1 use polypeptide antigens of the HIV-1 core and envelope that are produced by recombinant DNA technology. None is yet licensed, apparently due to the lack of acceptance by regulatory agencies of recombinant proteins for the detection of antibody. While Dupont, Cambridge Bioscience, and Smith Kline Bioscience Laboratories are developing similar assays, Abbott has produced a competitive enzyme immunoassay (CIA-RA) using recombinant HIV-1 antigens (p24 and gp41) individually and an indirect EIA combining these two proteins (Envacore); each has been evaluated for screening and confirmatory purposes. The inital report with CIA-RAs demonstrated sensitivity superior to both "first-generation" (viral lysate antigen) EIAs and WB.[23] Subsequent studies confirmed this initial impression and demonstrated greater specificity for CIA-RA.[34,35,50,76]

Other authors reported similarly enhanced sensitivity and specificity for the Cambridge Bioscience assay (recombinant envelope protein only) and another recombinant EIA for HIV-1 antibody.[17,77,78] These studies noted that the enhanced sensitivity of such recombinant protein assays for antibody were dependent to a significant extent upon the presence of envelope-patterned peptides, including both gp160 and gp41,[17,35,38,77,78] since antibodies to gp160/120 and gp41 develop before anti-p24 and remain after anti-p24 disappears.[23,35,38]

Some theoretic limitations of these recombinant protein assays include (*1*) the lack of glycosylation of env proteins, which may limit interactions with serum antibodies, and (*2*) limited cross-reactions with HIV-1 variants (e.g., HIV-2).[17,38] These assays retain the limitations of all antibody assays in that they fail to detect p24 antigen before antibody seroconversion.[17] Their advantages are significant, however, including safety, reproducibility of antigen content, and lack of contaminating cellular proteins that cause false positivity.[38] Due to their technical ease, assays for antibody to individual recombinant antigens may be useful as (or replace) confirmatory tests such as WB.[38]

Western Blot

The WB was developed as a method for separating proteins obtained from HIV-1 harvested from cell lysates and thereby analyzing sera for antibody content to these specific proteins. HIV-1 is allowed to replicate in continuous lymphoid cell lines, usually HUT-78 (H-9) cells. Cells are lysed to release viral and precursor proteins; virus is then partially purified by centrifugation[29,79,80] (Fig. 3). The viral protein is then electrophoresed in polyacrylamide gel. The lower-molecular-weight proteins (p17, p24) migrate farther in the gel, with the higher-molecular-weight proteins (gp160/120) remaining near the origin. The proteins are then blotted (or transferred) to nitrocellulose paper electrophoretically, and the paper is dried and cut into strips (or lanes) of approximately 5 mm width. The strips are subsequently exposed to a dilution of patient serum, washed, and incubated with anti-human IgG labeled with an enzyme that produces a colored band upon exposure to its substrate. Molecular weight standards as well as positive and negative control sera are incorporated into each assay. This reference WB technique is performed according to the Towbin method[80]; Figure 4 depicts test strips developed by using the Dupont licensed WB kit, which provides nitrocellulose paper strips with pre-electrophoresed disrupted viral proteins blotted onto the strips.

The WB has the advantage over nonrecombinant EIAs that antibodies to individual viral proteins can be assayed. The WB is more sensitive for the assay of anti-p24 than anti-gp41 since the latter glycosolated proteins do not transfer as well to nitrocellulose paper.[23,37,45,51] Western blot is also less sensitive for the detection of antibody to gp160/120 than are other confirmatory assays (e.g., RIPA) because of less resolving power. This is due to clumping of higher-molecular-weight antigens at the origin.[28,45] During the spectrum of HIV-1 infection, WB is insensitive during early HIV-1 infection (similar to EIA due to lack of anti-p24 and/or anti-gp41) and in patients with AIDS (due to a loss of anti-p24 late in disease).[28,29,51]

The definition of a positive WB result has been in a state of flux for some time. In addition to the cumbersome nature of the assay, which allows for the possibility of multiple technical errors, the test is also subjective in interpretation (reading the presence or absence of faint bands). The CDC has variably

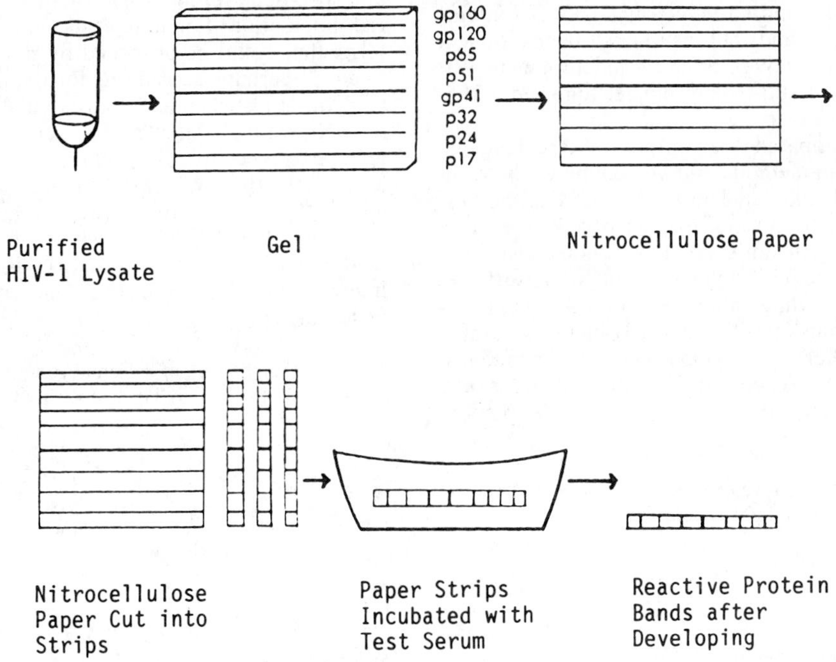

FIG. 3. Western blot procedure in diagramatic format. (Modified from Griffith et al.,[79] with permission.)

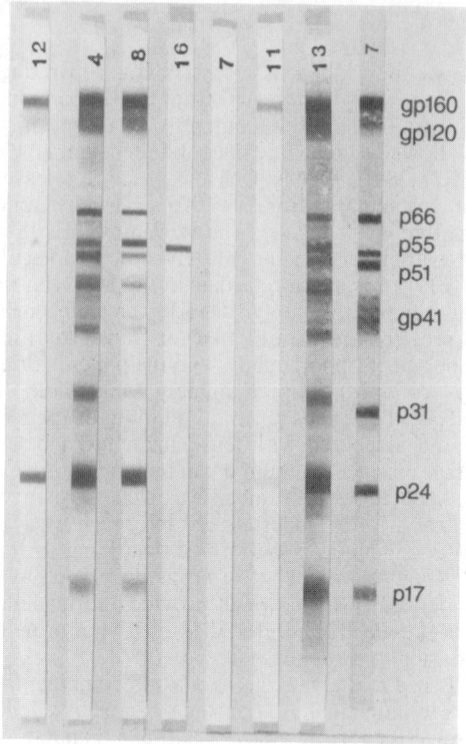

FIG. 4. Typical Western blot result using the Dupont immunoblot kit. Number 12 is indeterminate serum; numbers 4, 8, and 13 are positive sera; numbers 7 (middle), 11, and 16 are negative sera; and number 7 (right) is a positive control.

called WB with anti-p24 or anti-gp41 bands positive.[36,37] The licensed Dupont kit defines the presence of anti-p24, either anti-gp41 or gp160, and anti-p31 as a positive test[36,37,56,57]; the American Red Cross uses a similar definition,[56] while the U.S. Army accepts the presence of either anti-gp41 or both anti-p24 and anti-p55 bands.[57,81] Most recently, the Association of State and Territorial Public Health Laboratory Directors published recommended guidelines.[82] A *reactive* WB must contain two of three major bands of diagnostic significance (anti-gp160/120, anti-gp41, anti-p24); a *nonreactive* WB is defined as one without any HIV-1-specific bands, and an *indeterminate* WB contains one or more viral specific bands but insufficient bands to meet the definition of reactive (above). Such an indeterminate WB should be repeated and, if still indeterminate, followed with a repeat blot in 2–3 months (Fig 2).

A recent report has compared three different WB techniques, one similar to the Towbin method and two commercially available kits, Bio-Rad and Dupont.[83] The Dupont kit had the best sensitivity (dilutional reactivity) and specificity (lack of reaction with cellular and subcellular antisera). It was noted that antibodies to HLA class I cellular antigens tend to cause false-positive anti-gp41 bands, while antibodies to HLA class II antigens primarily caused false-positive anti-p31 bands; a parallel WB of uninfected H-9 cellular proteins was recommended to detect these false-positive reactions. Unexplained occasional anti-HIV-1 gag protein bands (falsely positive) were also noted by these authors[83] and others,[34,81,84,85] as has been noted for EIAs.[73] Overall, false-positive WB results are estimated to occur no more frequently than 1 in 20,000[37]; the potential cross-reacting antibodies are noted in Table 6.[81,84,85] Their false positivity is determined by a negative RIPA or immunofluorescence assay.

False-negative reactions by WB occur usually very early after HIV-1 infection or late after the development of AIDS.[28,29,36,37,51] HIV-1 culture positivity has been noted in WB-negative patients.[37,43,71,86,87] In conjunction with serial EIA determinations, the false-negative rate of WB for blood donors is estimated to be 1 in 250,000.[37] Should the prevalence of HIV-2 infection increase in the United States, it may become necessary to incorporate both HIV-1 and HIV-2 antigens in both EIA and WB assays because these viruses only cross react with antibodies to p24.[37]

TABLE 6. Causes of False-Positive Western Blot Reactions to HIV-1 Antigens (gag, env, and pol Proteins)

Cross reactions with
Normal human ribonucleoproteins
Other human retroviruses
Antibody to mitochondrial, nuclear, T-cell, and leukocyte antigens
Antibodies to HLA antigens (classes I and II)
Globulins produced during polyclonal gammopathy

Indirect Immunofluorescence Assay

The indirect immunofluorescence assay (IFA) is a rapid and reliable supplemental test using uninfected and HIV-1-infected H-9 (or HUT-78) cells in the logarithmic growth phase. The cells are air-dried and fixed to a fluorescent glass microscope slide.[37] A small quantity of a 1:10–1:20 test serum dilution is applied to each well, incubated to allow antibody to react with antigen, washed, and air-dried. Subsequently, anti-human IgG labeled with fluorescein isothiocyanate is applied to each well, followed again by incubation, washing, drying, and mounting. The use of known positive and negative control sera with both infected and uninfected cells in each assay allow for correction due to nonspecific fluorescence. Specimens are evaluated for fluorescence intensity, the percentage of fluorescent cells, and the fluorescent pattern; each test serum is determined to be qualitatively positive or negative but may be quantitatively assayed by the use of serial dilutions. Through the use of anti-human globulin specific for IgM, this immunoglobulin response can be also differentiated.

The IgM and IgG antibody responses to acute HIV-1 infection can be detected by IFA earlier than other currently available antibody assays[42] (Table 7). Sandstrom et al. found excellent overall agreement of IFA results with those of WB for both low- and high-risk populations; IFA was also shown to be more sensitive than EIA.[88] Others have suggested similar sensitivity and specificity for high-risk patients.[29,89–91] However, for a low-risk population, Lennette et al. noted nonspecific staining patterns that could be absorbed by noninfected HUT-78 cell antigens,[91] perhaps accounting for the false-positives reported by Carlson et al. when a similar population was screened by IFA in their study.[92] Most authors concur that IFA requires less technical expertise, is quicker to perform (<2 hours), and is less costly than WB, while being equally sensitive and specific.[89–91] Infrequently, however, false-negative assays have been identified.[87,88] The sensitivity of IFA may vary according to the cell line in which the virus is grown.[28] Generally, IFA interpretation is subjective and requires an experienced observer.[37]

TABLE 7. Comparison of IFA and Western Blot: Day of Acute Illness When Initially Positive for Indicated Antibody

	Day of Illness According to Test	
Antibody	*IFA*	*WB (8)*[a]
IgM	5 (5)	—
IgG	11 (6)[a]	—
p24/gp41	—	24
p55	—	40
p68	—	57
p34	—	71

[a] The number of patients evaluated are in parentheses.
(From Cooper et al.,[42] with permission.)

Radioimmunoprecipitation Assay

The radioimmunoprecipitation assay is a research technique confined to laboratories capable of propagation of HIV-1 in cell culture. The virus is grown in H-9 cells to logarithmic growth and then exposed to a radiolabeled amino acid or other substance that allows isotopic incorporation in or transfer to viral proteins.[37,93] Cells are subsequently lysed, thereby releasing labeled viral proteins. Cell lysates are exposed to test serum, the IgG content of which has been previously bound to the "Fc" receptors of protein A coated Sepharose beads. The immunoprecipitates are then eluted from the beads and separated electrophoretically on polyacrylamide gels, as for WB. The HIV-1 antigen–antibody complexes are detected in the gel by autoradiography (due to isotopic labeling); the bands are similar to those of WB except that the gp160 and gp120 bands are better separated and defined.[28,37,45,51,93]

RIPA is more sensitive than WB for the detection of antibodies to the higher-molecular-weight proteins of HIV-1; due to this sensitivity, gp 160/120 antibodies may be detected with RIPA before anti-p24 or anti-gp41, thereby potentially allowing for earlier detection of seroconversion.[28,51,93] In contrast, RIPA has been found to be less sensitive than WB at detecting antibodies to p24 in most studies,[28,51] while one group reported greater sensitivity for anti-p24 by RIPA as compared with WB.[93] Generally, RIPA is more sensitive late during HIV-1 infection when WB may revert to negativity.[51] Few false-positives have been detected,[28,34] and RIPA is usually negative among blood donors when WB may be falsely reactive with anti-p24 bands.[28,93] There are rare false-negatives by RIPA.[51,87] RIPA has also been applied to the detection of salivary antibodies.[94]

Overall, RIPA is slightly more sensitive and specific than WB and, therefore, can be used to supplement WB assays when the results are indeterminate.[28,37] Theoretic reasons for the advantages of this assay include (*1*) retention of three-dimensional structure by soluble proteins, which allows for more specific antibody binding; (*2*) greater multivalent binding by antibody in a liquid medium, thereby increasing sensitivity; and (*3*) the formation of more stable antigen–antibody complexes in a soluble phase, thereby detecting low-avidity antibodies.[93] Despite these advantages, whether real or theoretic, RIPA will remain a supplemental test confined to research laboratories due to its being labor intensive, expensive, and requiring the use of HIV-1-infected cell lines and radioisotopes.

Latex Agglutination

For developing countries many of the screening tests described above are not practical due to lack of needed equipment, biohazard containment facilities, sufficient skilled technicians and/or sufficient financial resources. Furthermore, current EIAs are recognized to give a high rate of false positivity with African sera,[95] possibly due to cross-reactivity with other retroviruses.[39,72] Riggin et al. have reported the development of a rapid latex agglutination (LA) assay using recombinant envelope antigen (CBre3) to detect HIV-1 antibodies.[96] This antigen incorporates the immunodominant regions of gp120 and gp41 and has been used by others for a recombinant EIA.[17,77] Riggin et al. showed complete agreement of LA with WB and only one discordant result with EIA among 211 serum specimens (95 positive by WB and EIA)[96]; most positive specimens were strongly reactive by LA and easy to interpret. Similar results have been reported by others with this Cambridge Bioscience kit when using sera from 300 African patients[52] and 2820 sera from many areas of the globe (the Carribean, Africa, North and South America, and Europe).[97] Van de Perre et al. did note a need to dilute sera for the LA test to avoid a prozone phenomenon causing false-negative results[52]; these authors believed that LA results did not require confirmation. Quinn et al. cautioned about the need for positive and negative LA controls and a trained observer due to the subjective determination of reactivity with LA.[97] The need for such training, its limited shelf life, and need for refrigeration of reagents may unfortunately limit the use of LA in developing countries.[98] The LA does appear to be an excellent screening (and possibly confirmatory) assay for future use. However, its applicability to low-risk population screening (e.g., blood donors) requires evaluation due to anticipated increases in rates of false positivity.

Other Antibody Tests

Van de Perre et al. have described a dipstick screening test for HIV-1 antibodies.[52] An HIV-1-infected H-9 cell lysate is coated onto a polystyrene stick, which is then reacted with test serum and immunoenzymatic reagents modified from an EIA. The color reaction is observer visible after three 15-minute incubations. This assay was 98 percent sensitive but suffered from false positivity (90 percent specific). Confirmation of results was needed when using the dipstick as a screen. Its low cost and lack of equipment requirements may make this assay applicable as a screening test in developing countries.

A rapid dot immunobinding assay for HIV-1 antibodies has been described recently for screening purposes.[99,100] The lysate of HIV-1-infected cells[100] or a recombinant HIV-1 envelope polypeptide is spotted onto nitrocellulose paper and reacted with test sera; this is followed by typical EIA immunoenzymatic reactions resulting in the development of color. The color intensity is judged as positive or negative by the observer when compared with both positive and negative controls.[101] The test has the advantage of being simple, rapid (30 minutes), stable, and requiring no equipment, but it is subject to observer variability. It also does not detect HIV-1 antibodies to defined viral antigens. The assay was sensitive and specific when compared with the Genetic Systems EIA and WB. It may have applicability in developing countries.

The most recent development regarding screening for HIV-1 infection uses the patient's own blood, with autologous red cell agglutination being a positive test.[102] A nonagglutinating murine monoclonal antibody was made to human red blood cells; to this monoclonal antibody was bound a synthetic peptide containing the immunoreactive portion of gp41. The addition to this monoclonal antibody–peptide complex results in binding of the antibody to red blood cells and agglutination if HIV-1 envelope antibodies are present in the patient's blood. This assay can be performed with 0.01 ml of the patient's blood and takes 2 minutes. The sensitivity reported was 98 percent for patients with AIDS; a false-positive rate of 0.1 percent with sera from healthy blood donors was noted, as compared with a 0.2 percent rate when using the Genetic Systems EIA on the same samples. This assay, pending the results of further tests, may have major applications as a screening test in the future, especially considering its simplicity and speed.

A confirmatory technique has been recently described and marketed, although not licensed for clinical use, that incorporates recombinant HIV-1 antigens with a protein electrophoretic immunoblot technique.[103] In this Chiron immunoblot, recombinant p24, p31, gp41, and gp120 are electrophoresed and blotted onto nitrocellulose sheets, which are cut into strips. These strips are sold in kits similar to the Dupont WB kit. Controls include an antibody-negative serum and two sera with high and low levels of antibody. With this kit, the bands are sharp, well separated, and defined; this assay also requires less reaction time with the patient's serum than the WB.[103] Data on the sensitivity and specificity of this assay are lacking. Calarco et al. reported on the sequence in which antibodies appear during acute HIV-1 infection when using this recombinant technology, i.e., antibodies to gp41 and/or p24, followed by anti-p31, and finally anti-gp120.[103]

Hofbauer et al. have reported on a similar recombinant envelope (gp41) immunoblot.[104] This recombinant blot was easier to read than was the WB when using viral lysate. This assay detected anti-gp41 before anti-p24 was detected by the conventional WB, lacked any false-positives, and was more sensitive than either the conventional WB or IFA. Further studies are needed to define the use of these recombinant antigen immunoblots in the diagnosis of HIV-1 infection.

Some virologists consider the ability of serum to neutralize the infectivity of a virus to be a reference serologic test. With HIV-1, this is a tedious assay requiring its culture in H-9 cells and is confined to laboratories with stringent biohazard capabilities. There are few reports of the assay of neutralizing antibody. Several authors have reported the association of neutralizing antibody with a lack of symptoms and the progression to symptomatic HIV-1 infection with a loss of such antibodies.[105,106] Weber et al. did show a similar trend but were unable to associate neutralizing antibody with anti-p24 activity.[32] The complexity of the assay will limit its application and availability in the future.

HIV-1 ANTIGEN DETECTION

The detection of the p24 antigen in serum and CSF has become important for experimental protocols in the diagnosis and treatment of HIV-1 infection since the Abbott EIA became available in 1986 (for research use only). A Genetic Systems antigen EIA is also currently available for research use, while Dupont and Coulter have similar assays in development or pending licensure.

The detection of the p24 antigen viral marker differs from antibody detection in two ways: (*1*) only low antigen concentrations are present, and (*2*) p24 forms immune complexes with its antibody that are not detected by the antigen assay. The EIA for p24 antigen only detects free antigen in excess of antibody, and this implies the presence of active viral replication.

With this indirect EIA for p24 antigen, the test specimen is incubated overnight with polystyrene beads or in a microtiter well coated with polyclonal HIV-1 antibody. After rinsing, the bead or well is allowed to react with rabbit or goat anti-HIV-1. After rinsing, the bead or well is then exposed to an enzyme-linked anti-rabbit or anti-goat immunoglobulin. The substrate is added to allow the color to develop, after which absorbance is measured. The OD is proportional to the amount of antigen present, with the limit of detection for the assay being between 50 and 100 pg/ml.[18,30] The entire assay consumes 24–30 hours.[37]

For a specimen that is repeatedly reactive, the specificity of the assay must be confirmed by the use of a blocking ("neutralizing") antibody.[37,82] The specimen as well as positive and negative controls are incubated with reference human sera with or without antibody to HIV-1 and then reassayed for the presence of detectable p24 antigen. Specificity is confirmed by a concomitant reduction (50 percent or greater) in OD with the specimen exposed to human anti-HIV-1 or by an OD of the non-neutralized specimen equal to or greater than the cutoff value.[37] Including repetition and the blocking assay, confirmation of a positive p24 antigen assay may take 3–4 days.

The major advantages of this assay over viral culture include working with noninfectious HIV-1 antigen and the lack of HLA determinants contaminating the antigen preparation used in the former assay. A major disadvantage is the complexity and duration of the assay itself, especially when coupled with confirmatory tests. Additionally, this assay is not a screening test and must be used in conjunction with an antibody assay.

Suggested uses for the antigen assay are (*1*) detection of HIV-1 in cell culture, (*2*) prediction of disease progression (by the reappearance of p24), (*3*) monitoring antiviral therapy, and (*4*) assessing the HIV-1 infection status of neonates born to seropositive mothers.[82,107] Cerebrospinal fluid can also be assayed for p24 to provide evidence for HIV-1 central nervous system involvement.[19]

TABLE 8. Correlation of the Clinical Status of HIV-1 Infection with p24 Antigen Detection

Clinical Status	*Percentage with p24 Antigenemia*
Asymptomatic	4
AIDS-related complex	56
AIDS	70

(From Kenny et al.,[113] with permission.)

During acute infection, p24 antigenemia precedes seroconversion, usually resolves within 2–3 weeks as antibodies to p24 appear,[18,25,27,108–110] but may persist for 6–14 months before seroconversion.[24,25] However, during early infection, antigen detection is not as sensitive as viral culture.[111] Additionally, while detection of p24 antigen has been shown to correlate with virus culture positivity, the antigen assay is an insensitive test for infection due to its usual negativity during asymptomatic illness when patients remain culture-positive.[37,112] Its sensitivity improves as HIV-1-related disease develops[113] (Table 8). As the infection progresses clinically with the development of AIDS, p24 antibodies decline, and p24 antigen reappears.[19,22,27,30,31,110,112–114]

The specificity of p24 antigen positivity by EIA is very good since Stute found only a 0.43 percent false positivity rate among volunteer blood donors.[115] Such specificity provides a rationale for including p24 antigen testing with antibody screening of all blood donors in the future.

The p24 antigen assay has been useful for following HIV-1-infected patients receiving azidothymidine (AZT).[20,116] During therapy, falling p24 levels have correlated with diminished symptoms, rising CD4 cell counts, and a better prognosis. Before therapy, a high serum antigen concentration has correlated with a poor prognosis.[116]

In addition to the detection of soluble antigen in serum, HIV-1 antigens have also been detected on the surface of peripheral blood lymphocytes from HIV-1-infected patients by direct and indirect immunofluorescence.[117]

HIV-1 DETECTION

Viral Culture

The in vitro propagation of HIV-1 was initially reported in 1983 and was followed by improvements in culture techniques by other researchers.[3–5] While the virus was initially identified in cell culture by electron microscopy,[2] most laboratories today detect HIV-1 indirectly by assaying for reverse transcriptase (RT) activity in cell culture supernatants. This enzyme is produced by HIV-1-infected cells in large quantities. Interestingly, the lack of universal culture positivity among patients with HIV-1 seropositivity may be at least partially attributable to the presence of an inhibitor of RT.[118] Reverse transcriptase activity is not specific for HIV-1 since it is also produced by other retroviruses.[119] More specific indirect assays for the presence of HIV-1 in cell culture have been described, including HIV-1 antigen (p24) detection in culture supernatants by EIA,[21,37,120–122] antigen detection by a dot immunoenzymatic binding assay,[123] and a radioimmunoassay (RIA) designed for antigen detection in cell culture.[121]

Each of these indirect methods of viral detection requires HIV-1 culture, which is cumbersome, costly, and time-consuming (weeks) and exposes personnel to an infectious risk.[37] A typical HIV-1 culture requires (*1*) separation of peripheral blood mononuclear cells (PBMC) from other blood components, (*2*) incubation of patient PBMC with PBMC from a HIV-1-seronegative donor for several weeks in the presence of interleukin-2 and phytohemagglutinin, and (*3*) once- or twice-weekly assay of supernatants from these cultures for RT activity or p24 antigen.[3–5,37] In culture supernatants, antigen detection is more sensitive and positive earlier than the RT assay for HIV-1[21,37,120,122,124]; 60–94 percent of supernatants are positive by the p24 detection assay at day 10 of culture as compared with 20–25 percent by the RT assay. The RIA and EIA are equally sensitive.[121] Technically, however, antigen detection has numerous advantages over RIA and the RT assay.[37,120–122]

The clinical indications for HIV-1 culture are similar to those for p24 antigen detection, but culture is the more sensitive technique. Cultures may be used to assess strain virulence (proportional to the rate of replication), viral inoculum (inversely proportional to the time of culture positivity), and efficacy of therapy.[37] However, due to the many technical difficulties with HIV-1 culture, it will remain confined to a limited number of laboratories.[37,82]

DNA Probes

A recently used alternative method for the detection of HIV-1 in culture-negative patients is molecular hybridization using DNA-probes and peripheral blood nonlymphoid mononuclear cells.[24,37] Previous attempts at direct detection of the HIV-1 circular proviral genome in the host cell nucleus with hybridization were quite insensitive.[37] To enhance sensitivity, subsequent attempts have relied upon amplification of the virus in host cells before hybridization by cocultivation in vitro[125] or by oligonucleotide probes of DNA extracted from mononuclear cells and blotted on nitrocellulose.[37,124] These probes of subgenomic size are made by inserting fragments of the HIV-1 genome into plasmids, by allowing the plasmids to replicate, and then by extracting the subgenomic fragments from the plasmids.[124] These fragments are then isotopically labeled. DNA is extracted from a patient's mononuclear cells and blotted onto nitrocellulose paper. Hybridization is then attempted with the blotted cellular DNA extract and the labeled subgenomic HIV-1 DNA fragments. Blots are subsequently washed, dried, and exposed to film for the detection of hybridized, labeled DNA. Such hybridization assays have been shown to be at least as sensitive and specific as HIV-1 culture.[24,124] The method is time-consuming and technically difficult but faster and easier than culture.[124] As few as 1 in 10,000 PBMC may express HIV-1 RNA by hybridization.[125]

Much excitement has been generated by the development of far more sensitive amplification techniques for the detection of as little as one genome of nonreplicating HIV-1 in mononuclear cells; these techniques may totally circumvent the need for HIV-1 culture in the future.[125] Molecular hybridization without amplification requires an actively replicating HIV-1 infection. The polymerase chain reaction (PCR) involves annealing two short DNA chains to the viral genome after DNA denaturation, one onto each strand of the HIV-1 proviral DNA. This template-directed replication of the HIV-1 genome is initiated by the addition of DNA polymerase; the products of this replication serve as templates for repeated cycles (up to 25) of denaturation, annealing, and replication until there are sufficient numbers of oligonucleotides to be detected by a complementary, labeled oligonucleotide DNA probe. This technique has the capability of detecting latent HIV-1 infection in the nonreplicative state in patients who are seronegative.[126–128] This assay takes about 1 day to complete.

Potential applications for the PCR include (*1*) identification of all HIV-1-infected blood donors; (*2*) confirmation of the diagnosis of HIV-1 infection, especially when false-positive screening and/or confirmatory tests are suspected; (*3*) identification of seronegative infected patients; (*4*) early diagnosis of infection before seroconversion; and (*5*) confirmation of infection in newborns. Until further simplifications of the PCR assay are developed and cost reduced, broad applicability will not be feasible, however. While hybridization and PCR technologies hold great promise, they are not currently recommended for general use.[82]

TABLE 9. Population Groups Currently Screened for HIV-1 Antibody

Mandatory
Blood donors
Federal prisoners
Military recruits and active duty personnel
Foreign service officers
Aliens seeking immigration
With consent
Patients in STD clinics, prostitutes
Intravenous drug users
Women of childbearing age with a recognized risk for HIV-1 infection
Persons planning marriage (in a few states)
Hospital admissions in high-risk groups

TABLE 10. Considerations for Determining Justification for Mandatory Screening Programs for Antibody to HIV

The population selected should have a reservoir of infected persons so that disproportionate numbers of uninfected persons do not have to submit to intrusive testing
The population must pose a significant risk of communication of infection
Knowledge of results should allow for the reduction of transmission
Benefits must outweigh the ill effects of testing
No less intrusive/restrictive alternatives are available

(From Gostin et al.,[133] with permission.)

APPLICATION OF HIV-1 ANTIBODY SCREENING

Since the screening EIA became available in March 1985, much discussion and debate have ensued among the public and among legal and health care professionals as to the appropriateness of broad-based screening programs for HIV-1 antibody. Arguments have been presented for and against premarital and preoperative mandatory screening as well as screening employees in the workplace.[129–131] Issues of ethics, confidentiality, and informed consent have been raised.[132–135] Appropriate hospital policies have been debated.[136,137] At present, in the United States, the population groups undergoing mandatory and voluntary screening are defined in Table 9. Proposed justifications for mandatory screening are enumerated in Table 10. As the sensitivity and especially the specificity of the current means for diagnosing HIV-1 infection improve,[56] screening tests for HIV-1 infection will gain broader applicability.

REFERENCES

1. Centers for Disease Control. Prevention of acquired immunodeficiency syndrome (AIDS): Report of inter-agency recommendations. MMWR. 1984;32:101–3.
2. Barre-Sinoussi F, Chermann JC, Rey F, et al. Isolation of a T-lymphotropic retrovirus from a patient at risk for acquired immune deficiency syndrome (AIDS). Science. 1983;220:868–71.
3. Popovic M, Sarngadharan MG, Read E, et al. Detection, isolation, and continuous production of cytopathic retroviruses (HTLV-III) from patients with AIDS and pre-AIDS. Science. 1984;224:497–500.
4. Gallo RC, Salahuddin SZ, Popovic M, et al. Frequent detection and isolation of cytopathic retroviruses (HTLV-III) from patients with AIDS and at risk for AIDS. Science. 1984;224:500–2.
5. Levy JA, Hoffman AD, Kramer SM, et al. Isolation of lymphocytopathic retroviruses from San Francisco patients with AIDS. Science. 1984;225:840–2.
6. Sarngadharan MG, Popovic M, Bruch L, et al. Antibodies reactive with human T-lymphotropic retroviruses (HTLV-III) in serum of patients with AIDS. Science. 1984;224:506–8.
7. Brun-Vezinet F, Barre-Sinoussi F, et al. Detection of IgG antibodies to lymphadenopathy-associated virus in patients with AIDS or lymphadenopathy syndrome. Lancet. 1984;1:1253–6.
8. Centers for Disease Control. Provisional Public Health Service inter-agency recommendations for screening donated blood and plasma for antibody to the virus causing acquired immunodeficiency syndrome. MMWR. 1985;34:1–5.
9. Schorr JB, Berkowitz A, et al. Prevalence of HTLV-III antibody in American blood donors. N Engl J Med. 1985;313:384–5.

10. Centers for Disease Control. Human T-lymphotropic virus type III/lymphadenopathy-associated virus antibody testing at alternate sites. MMWR. 1986;35:284–7.
11. Centers for Disease Control. Recommendations for assisting in the prevention of perinatal transmission of human T-lymphotropic virus type III/lymphadenopathy-associated virus and acquired immunodeficiency syndrome. MMWR. 1985;34:721–6,731–3.
12. Centers for Disease Control. Additional recommendations to reduce sexual and drug abuse-related transmission of human T-lymphotropic virus type III/lymphadenopathy-associated virus. MMWR. 1986;35:152–5.
13. Centers for Disease Control. Perspectives in disease prevention and health promotion: Public Health Service guidelines for counseling and antibody testing to prevent HIV infection and AIDS. MMWR. 1987;36:509–15.
14. Weiss SH, Goedert JJ, et al. Screening test for HTLV-III (AIDS agent) antibodies; specificity, sensitivity, and applications. JAMA. 1985;253:221–5.
15. Carlson JR, Bryant ML, et al. AIDS serology testing in low and high risk groups. JAMA. 1985;253:3405–8.
16. Sivak SL, Wormser GP. Predictive value of a screening test for antibodies to HTLV-III. Am J Clin Pathol. 1986;85:700–3.
17. Burke DS, Brandt BL, et al. Diagnosis of human immunodeficiency virus infection by immunoassay using a molecularly cloned and expressed virus envelope polypeptide; comparison to Western blot on 2707 consecutive serum samples. Ann Intern Med. 1987;671–6.
18. Goudsmit J, Paul DA, et al. Expression of human immunodeficiency virus antigen (HIV-Ag) in serum and cerebrospinal fluid during acute and chronic infection. Lancet. 1986;2:177–80.
19. Lange JMA, Paul DA, et al. Persistent HIV antigenaemia and decline of HIV core antibodies associated with transition to AIDS. Br Med J. 1986;293:1459–62.
20. Chaisson RE, Allain JP, et al. Significant changes in HIV antigen level in the serum of patients treated with azidothymidine. N Engl J Med. 1986;315:1610–11.
21. Diggs JL. Testing for HIV antigen. Infect Control Hosp Epidemiol. 1988;9:353–4.
22. Allain JP, Laurian Y, et al. Long-term evaluation of HIV antigen and antibodies to p24 and gp41 in patients with hemophilia. N Engl J Med. 1987;317:1114–21.
23. Allain JP, Laurian Y, et al. Serological markers in early stages of human immunodeficiency virus infection in haemophiliacs. Lancet. 1986;2:1233–6.
24. Ranki A, Krohn M, et al. Long latency precedes overt seroconversion in sexually transmitted human-immunodeficiency-virus infection. Lancet. 1987;1:589–93.
25. Simmonds P, Lainson FAL, et al. HIV antigen and antibody detection: Variable responses to infection in the Edinburgh haemophiliac cohort. Br Med J. 1988;296:593–8.
26. Cooper DA, Tindall B, et al. Characterization of T lymphocyte responses during primary infection with human immunodeficiency virus. J Infect Dis. 1988;157:889–96.
27. Von Sydow M, Gaines H, et al. Antigen detection in primary HIV infection. Br Med J. 1988;296:238–40.
28. Gaines H, Sonnerborg A, et al. Antibody response in primary human immunodeficiency virus infection. Lancet. 1987;1:1249–53.
29. Pan LZ, Cheng-Mayer C, Levy JA. Patterns of antibody response in individuals infected with the human immunodeficiency virus. J Infect Dis. 1987;155:626–32.
30. Goudsmit J, Lange JMA, et al. Antigenemia and antibody titers to core and envelope antigens in AIDS, AIDS-related complex, and subclinical human immunodeficiency virus infection. J Infect Dis. 1987;155:558–60.
31. Mayer KH, Falk LA, et al. Correlation of enzyme-linked immunosorbent assays for serum human immunodeficiency virus antigen and antibodies to recombinant viral proteins with subsequent clinical outcomes in a cohort of asymptomatic homosexual men. Am J Med. 1987;83:208–12.
32. Weber JN, Weiss RA, et al. Human immunodeficiency virus infection in two cohorts of homosexual men: Neutralising sera and association of anti-gag antibody with prognosis. Lancet. 1987;1:119–21.
33. Schupbach J, Haller O, et al. Antibodies to HTLV-III in Swiss patients with AIDS and pre-AIDS and in groups at risk for AIDS. N Engl J Med. 1985;312:265–70.
34. Lelie PN, Reesink HW, Huisman H. Evaluation of three second-generation and three confirmatory assays for antibodies to human immunodeficiency virus. Vox Sang. 1988;54:84–91.
35. Dawson GJ, Heller JS, et al. Reliable detection of individuals seropositive for the human immunodeficiency virus (HIV) by competitive immunoassays using *Escherichia coli*-expressed HIV structural proteins. J Infect Dis. 1988;157:149–55.
36. Steckelberg JM, Cockerill FR. Serologic testing for human immunodeficiency virus antibodies. Mayo Clin Proc. 1988;63:373–80.
37. Jackson JB, Balfour HH Jr. Practical diagnostic testing for human immunodeficiency virus. Clin Microbiol Rev. 1988;1:124–38.
38. Allain JP, Hojvat S. Development in HIV serology. In: de la Maza LM, Peterson EM, eds. Proceedings of the 1987 International Symposium on Medical Virology. Anaheim, CA. Amsterdam: Elsevier Science Publishing; 1987:315–30.
39. Houn HY, Pappas AA, Walker EM Jr. Status of current clinical tests for human immunodeficiency virus (HIV): Applications and limitations. Ann Clin Lab Sci. 1987;17:279–85.
40. Parry JV, Perry KR, Mortimer PP. Sensitive assays for viral antibodies in saliva: An alternative to tests on serum. Lancet. 1987;2:72–5.
41. Burke DS, Redfield RR, et al. Variations in Western blot banding patterns of human T-cell lymphotropic virus type III/lymphadenopathy-associated virus. J Clin Microbiol. 1987;25:81–4.
42. Cooper DA, Imrie AA, et al. Antibody response to human immunodeficiency virus after primary infection. J Infect Dis. 1987;155:1113–8.
43. Ward JW, Grindon AJ, et al. Laboratory and epidemiologic evaluation of an enzyme immunoassay for antibodies to HTLV-III. JAMA. 1986;256:357–61.
44. Nishanian P, Taylor JMG, et al. Significance of quantitative enzyme-linked immunosorbent assay (ELISA) results in evaluation of three ELISAs and Western blot tests for detection of antibodies to human immunodeficiency virus in a high risk population. J Clin Microbiol. 1987;25:395–400.
45. Handsfield HH, Wandell M, et al. Screening and diagnostic performance of enzyme immunoassay for antibody to lymphadenopathy-associated virus. J Clin Microbiol. 1987;25:879–84.
46. Voeller B. Evaluation of eight ELISA kits for the detection of anti-LAV/HTLV-III antibodies. Lancet. 1986;1:1152–3.
47. Reesink HW, Huisman JG, et al. Evaluation of six enzyme immunoassays for antibody against human immunodeficiency virus. Lancet. 1986;2:483–6.
48. Evans RP, Shanson DC, Mortimer PP. Clinical evaluation of Abbott and Wellcome enzyme linked immunosorbent assays for detection of serum antibodies to human immunodeficiency virus (HIV). J Clin Pathol. 1987;40:552–5.
49. Burkhardt U, Mertens Th, Eggers HJ. Comparison of two commercially available anti-HIV ELISAs: Abbott HTLV III EIA and Du Pont HTLV III-ELISA. J Med Virol. 1987;23:217–24.
50. Deinhardt F, Eberle J, Gurtler L. Sensitivity and specificity of eight commercial and one recombinant anti-HIV ELISA tests. Lancet. 1987;1:40.
51. Saah AJ, Farzadegan H, et al. Detection of early antibodies in human immunodeficiency virus infection by enzyme-linked immunosorbent assay, Western blot, and radioimmunoprecipitation. J Clin Microbiol. 1987;25:1605–10.
52. Van De Perre P, Nzaramba D, et al. Comparison of six serological assays for human immunodeficiency virus antibody detection in developing countries. J Clin Microbiol. 1988;26:552–6.
53. Ozanne G, Fauvel M. Performance and reliability of five commercial enzyme-linked immunosorbent assay kits in screening for anti-human immunodeficiency virus antibody in high-risk subjects. J Clin Microbiol. 1988;26:1496–500.
54. Engle JC, Schleupner CJ. Performance evaluation of six commercially available enzyme linked immunosorbent assays kits for antibody to human immunodeficiency virus (Abstract). In: de la Maza LM, Peterson EM, eds. Proceedings of the 1987 International Symposium on Medical Virology. Anaheim, CA. Amsterdam: Elsevier Science Publishing; 1987:357.
55. Taylor RN, Przybyszewski VA. Summary of the Centers for Disease Control human immunodeficiency virus (HIV) performance evaluation surveys for 1985 and 1986. Am J Clin Pathol. 1988;89:1–13.
56. Schwartz JS, Dans PE, Kinosian BP. Human immunodeficiency virus test evaluation, performance, and use. JAMA. 1988;259:2574–9.
57. Centers for Disease Control. Update: Serologic testing for antibody to human immunodeficiency virus. MMWR. 1988;36:833–45.
58. Van Den Akker R, Hekker AC, Osterhaus ADME. Heat inactivation of serum may interfere with HTLV-III/LAV serology. Lancet. 1985;2:672.
59. Jungkind DL, DiRenzo SA, Young SJ. Effect of using heat-inactivated serum with the Abbott human T-cell lymphotropic virus type III antibody test. J Clin Microbiol. 1986;23:381–2.
60. Kvinesdal B, Pedersen NS. False-positive HIV antibody tests in RPR-reactive patients. JAMA. 1988;260:923–4.
61. Kuhnl P, Seidl S, Holzberger G. HLA DR4 antibodies cause positive HTLV-III antibody ELISA results. Lancet. 1985;1:1222–3.
62. Ameglio F, Dolei A, et al. Antibodies reactive with nonpolymorphic epitopes on HLA molecules interfere in screening tests for the human immunodeficiency virus. J Infect Dis. 1987;156:1034–5.
63. Wartick MG, McCarroll DR, Wiltbank TB. A second discriminator for biological false positive results in enzyme-linked immunosorbent assays for antibodies to human immunodeficiency virus (HTLV-III/LAV). Transfusion. 1987;27:109–11.
64. Blanton M, Balakrishnan K, et al. HLA antibodies in blood donors with reactive screening tests for antibody to the immunodeficiency virus. Transfusion. 1987;27:118–9.
65. Smith DM, Dewhurst S, et al. False-positive enzyme-linked immunosorbent assay reactions for antibody to human immunodeficiency virus in a population of midwestern patients with congenital bleeding disorders. Transfusion. 1987;127:112.
66. Mendenhall CL, Roselle GA, et al. False positive tests for HTLV-III antibodies in alcoholic patients with hepatitis. N Engl J Med. 1986;314:921–2.
67. Marlink RG, Allain JS, et al. Low sensitivity of ELISA testing in early HIV infection. N Engl J Med. 1986;315:1549.
68. Biberfeld G, Bredberg-Raden U, et al. Blood donor sera with false-positive Western blot reactions to human immunodeficiency virus. Lancet. 1986;2:289–91.
69. Albersheim SG, Smyth JA, et al. Passively acquired human immunodeficiency virus seropositivity in a neonate after hepatitis B immunoglobulin. J Pediatr. 1988;112:915–6.

70. Saag MS, Britz J. Asymptomatic blood donor with a false-positive HTLV-III western blot. N Engl J Med. 1986;314:118.
71. Goetz DW, Hall SE, et al. Pediatric acquired immunodeficiency syndrome with negative human immunodeficiency virus antibody response by enzyme-linked immunosorbent assay and Western blot. Pediatrics. 1988;81:356–9.
72. Denis F, Leonard G, et al. Comparison of 10 enzyme immunoassays for detection of antibody to human immunodeficiency virus type 2 in West African sera. J Clin Microbiol. 1988;26:1000–4.
73. Tribe DE, Reed DL, et al. Antibodies reactive with human immunodeficiency virus gag-coded antigens (gag reactive only) are a major cause of enzyme-linked immunosorbent assay reactivity in a blood donor population. J Clin Microbiol. 1988;26:641–7.
74. Hickman M, Mortimer JY, Rawlinson VI. Donor screening for HIV: How many false negatives? Lancet. 1988;1:1221.
75. Ward JW, Holmberg SD, et al. Transmission of human immunodeficiency virus (HIV) by blood transfusions screened as negative for HIV antibody. N Engl J Med. 1988;318:473–8.
76. Navarro MDR, Pineda JA, et al. Recombinant EIA for anti-HIV testing is more specific than conventional EIA. Vox Sang. 1988;54:62–3.
77. Thorn RM, Beltz GA, et al. Enzyme immunoassay using a novel recombinant polypeptide to detect human immunodeficiency virus env antibody. J Clin Microbiol. 1987;25:1207–12.
78. Gnann JW Jr, Schwimmbeck PL, et al. Diagnosis of AIDS by using a 12-amino acid peptide representing an immunodominant epitope of the human immunodeficiency virus. J Infect Dis. 1987;156:261–7.
79. Griffith BP, Ferguson D, Landry ML. Detection of antibodies to human immunodeficiency virus: Principles, use and interpretation. VA Practitioner. 1988;5:50–61.
80. Towbin H, Staehelin T, et al. Electrophoretic transfer of proteins from polacrylamide gels to nitrocellulose sheets: Procedure and some applications. Proc Natl Acad Sci USA. 1979;76:4350–4.
81. Burke DS, Redfield RR. False-positive Western blot tests for antibodies to HTLV-III. JAMA. 1986;256:347.
82. Hausler WJ Jr. Report of the Third Consensus Conference on HIV Testing sponsored by the Association of State and Territorial Public Health Laboratory Directors. Infect Control Hosp Epidemiol. 1988;9:345–9.
83. Blomberg J, Klasse PJ. Specificities and sensitivities of three systems for determination of antibodies to human immunodeficiency virus by electrophoretic immunoblotting. J Clin Microbiol. 1988;26:106–10.
84. Mathex D, Leibovitch J, et al. LAV/HTLV-III seroconversion and disease in hemophiliacs treated in France. N Engl J Med. 1986;314:118–9.
85. Courouce AM, Muller JY, Richard D. False-positive Western blot reactions to human immunodeficiency virus in blood donors. Lancet. 1986;2:921–2.
86. Salahuddin SZ, Groopman JE, Markham PD, et al. HTLV-III in symptom-free seronegative persons. Lancet. 1984;2:1418–20.
87. Groopman JE, Hartzband PI, et al. Antibody seronegative human T-lymphotropic virus type III (HTLV-III)-infected patients with acquired immunodeficiency syndrome or related disorders. Blood. 1985;66:742–4.
88. Sandstrom EG, Schooley RT, et al. Detection of human anti-HTLV-III antibodies by indirect immunofluorescence using fixed cells. Transfusion. 1985;25:308–12.
89. Gallo D, Diggs JL, et al. Comparison of detection of antibody to the acquired immune deficiency syndrome virus by enzyme immunoassay, immunofluorescence, and Western blot methods. J Clin Microbiol. 1986;23:1049–51.
90. Hedenskog M, Dewhurst S, et al. Testing for antibodies to AIDS-associated retrovirus (HTLV-III/LAV) by indirect fixed cell immunofluorescence: Specificity, sensitivity, and applications. J Med Virol. 1986;19:325–34.
91. Lennette ET, Karpatkin S, Levy JA. Indirect immunofluorescence assay for antibodies to human immunodeficiency virus. J Clin Microbiol. 1987;25:199–202.
92. Carlson JR, Yee J, et al. Comparison of indirect immunofluorescence and Western blot for detection of anti-human immunodeficiency virus antibodies. J Clin Microbiol. 1987;25:494–7.
93. Tersmette M, Lelie PN, et al. Confirmation of HIV seropositivity: Comparison of a novel radioimmunoprecipitation assay to immunoblotting and virus culture. J Med Virol. 1988;24:109–16.
94. Archibald DW, Zon LI, et al. Salivary antibodies as a means of detecting human T cell lymphotropic virus type III/lymphadenopathy-associated virus infection. J Clin Microbiol. 1986;24:873–5.
95. Biggar RJ, Gigase PL, et al. ELISA HTLV retrovirus antibody reactivity associated with malaria and immune complexes in healthy Africans. Lancet. 1985;2:520–3.
96. Riggin CH, Beltz GA, et al. Detection of antibodies to human immunodeficiency virus by latex agglutination with recombinant antigen. J Clin Microbiol. 1987;25:1772–3.
97. Quinn TC, Riggin CH, et al. Rapid latex agglutination assay using recombinant envelope polypeptide for the detection of antibody to the HIV. JAMA. 1988;260:510–3.
98. Heyward WL, Curran JW. Rapid screening tests for HIV infection. JAMA. 1988;260:542.
99. Carlson JR, Yee JL, et al. Rapid, easy, and economical screening test for antibodies to human immunodeficiency virus. Lancet. 1987;1:361–2.
100. Heberling RL, Kalter SS, et al. Dot immunobinding assay compared with enzyme-linked immunosorbent assay for rapid and specific detection of retrovirus antibody induced by human or simian acquired immunodeficiency syndrome. J Clin Microbiol. 1988;26:765–7.
101. Heberling RL, Kalter SS. Rapid dot-immunobinding assay on nitrocellulose for viral antibodies. J Clin Microbiol. 1986;23:109–13.
102. Kemp BE, Rylatt DB, et al. Autologous red cell agglutination assay for HIV-1 antibodies: Simplified test with whole blood. Science. 1988;241:1352–4.
103. Calarco TL, Polito AJ, et al. Nitrocellulose cellulose strip ELISA for antibodies to human immunodeficiency virus employing recombinant antigens. In: de la Maza LM, Peterson EM, eds. Proceedings of the 1987 International Symposium on Medical Virology. Anaheim, CA. Amsterdam: Elsevier Science Publishing; 1987:293–314.
104. Hofbauer JM, Schulz TF, et al. Comparison of Western blot (immunoblot) based on recombinant-derived p41 with conventional tests for serodiagnosis of human immunodeficiency virus infections. J Clin Microbiol. 1988;26:116–20.
105. Anderson KC, Gorgone BC, et al. Transfusion-acquired human immunodeficiency virus infection among immunocompromised persons. Ann Intern Med. 1986;105:519–27.
106. Robert-Guroff M, Brown M, Gallo RC. HTLV-III-neutralizing antibodies in patients with AIDS and AIDS-related complex. Nature. 1985;316:72–4.
107. Borkowsky W, Paul D, et al. Human-immunodeficiency-virus infections in infants negative for anti-HIV by enzyme-linked immunoassay. Lancet. 1987;1:1168–71.
108. Kessler HA, Blaauw B, et al. Diagnosis of human immunodeficiency virus infection in seronegative homosexuals presenting with an acute viral syndrome. JAMA. 1987;258:1196–9.
109. Wall RA, Denning DW, Amos A. HIV antigenaemia in acute HIV infection. Lancet. 1987;1:566.
110. Goudsmit J, Paul DA. Circulation of HIV antigen in blood according to stage of infection, risk group, age and geographic origin. Epidemiol Infect. 1987;99:701–10.
111. Gaines H, Albert J, et al. HIV antigenaemia and virus isolation from plasma during primary HIV infection. Lancet. 1987;1:1317–8.
112. Wittek AE, Phelan MA, et al. Detection of human immunodeficiency virus core protein in plasma by enzyme immunoassay. Ann Intern Med. 1987;107:286–92.
113. Kenny C, Parkin J, et al. HIV antigen testing. Lancet. 1987;1:565–6.
114. Lange J, Goudsmit J. Decline of antibody reactivity to HIV core protein secondary to increased production of HIV antigen. Lancet. 1987;1:488.
115. Stute R. HIV antigen detection in routine blood donor screening. Lancet. 1987;1:566.
116. Jackson GG, Paul DA, et al. Human immunodeficiency virus (HIV) antigenemia (p24) in the acquired immunodeficiency syndrome (AIDS) and the effect of treatment with Zidovudine (AZT). Ann Intern Med. 1988;108:175–80.
117. Pekovic DD, Chausseau JP, et al. Detection of HTLV-III/LAV antigens in peripheral blood lymphocytes from patients with AIDS. Arch Virol. 1986;91:11–9.
118. Sano K, Lee MH, et al. Antibody that inhibits human immunodeficiency virus reverse transcriptase and association with inability to isolate virus. J Clin Microbiol. 1987;25:2415–7.
119. Poiesz BJ, Ruscetti FW, et al. Detection and isolation of type C retrovirus particles from fresh and cultured lymphocytes of a patient with cutaneous T-cell lymphoma. Proc Natl Acad Sci USA. 1980;77:7415–9.
120. Viscidi R, Farzadegan H, et al. Enzyme immunoassay for detection of human immunodeficiency virus antigens in cell cultures. J Clin Microbiol. 1988;26:453–8.
121. Gupta P, Balachandran R, et al. Detection of human immunodeficiency virus by reverse transcriptase assay, antigen capture assay, and radioimmunoassay. J Clin Microbiol. 1987;25:1122–5.
122. Feorino P, Forrester B, et al. Comparison of antigen assay and reverse transcriptase assay for detecting human immunodeficiency virus in culture. J Clin Microbiol. 1987;25:2344–6.
123. Blumberg RS, Hartshorn KL, et al. Dot immunobinding assay for detection of human immunodeficiency virus-associated antigens. J Clin Microbiol. 1987;25:1989–92.
124. Richman DD, McCutchan JA, Spector SA. Detecting human immunodeficiency virus RNA in peripheral blood mononuclear cells by nucleic acid hybridization. J Infect Dis. 1987;156:823–7.
125. Ou CY, Kwok S, et al. DNA amplification for direct detection of HIV-1 in DNA of peripheral blood mononuclear cells. Science. 1988;239:295–7.
126. Farzadegan H, Polis MA, et al. Loss of human immunodeficiency virus type 1 (HIV-1) antibodies with evidence of viral infection in asymptomatic homosexual men. Ann Intern Med. 1988;108:785–90.
127. DeRossi A, Amadori A, et al. Polymerase chain reaction and in-vitro antibody production for early diagnosis of paediatric HIV infection. Lancet. 1988;2:278.
128. Loche M, Mach B. Identification of HIV-infected seronegative individuals by a direct diagnostic test based on hybridization to amplified viral DNA. Lancet. 1988;2:418–21.
129. Cleary PD, Barry MJ, et al. Compulsory premarital screening for the human immunodeficiency virus; technical and public health considerations. JAMA. 1987;258:1757–62.
130. Hagan MD, Meyer KB, Pauker SG. Routine preoperative screening for HIV; does the risk to the surgeon outweigh the risk to the patient? JAMA. 1988;259:1357–9.
131. HIV testing in the workplace (Editorial). Lancet. 1988;2:199–200.
132. Bayer R, Levine C, Wolf SM. HIV antibody screening: An ethical framework for evaluating proposed programs. JAMA. 1986;256:1768–74.

133. Gostin L, Curran WC. AIDS screening, confidentiality, and the duty to warn. Am J Public Health. 1987;77:361–5.
134. Dixon RE. Sacred secrets: Confidentiality, informed consent, and diagnostic testing in the AIDS era. Infect Control Hosp Epidemiol. 1988;9:187–8.
135. Sherer R. Physician use of the HIV antibody test; the need for consent, counseling, confidentiality, and caution. JAMA. 1988;259:264–5.
136. Eickhoff TC. Hospital policies on HIV antibody testing. JAMA. 1988;259:1861–2.
137. Henry K, Willenbring K, Crossley K. Human immunodeficiency virus antibody testing: A description of practices and policies at US infectious disease-teaching hospitals and Minnesota hospitals. JAMA. 1988;259:1819–22.

110. THERAPY FOR AIDS

HENRY MASUR

Experience in the United States with the first 80,000 cases of the acquired immunodeficiency syndrome (AIDS) from 1979 to 1988 has clearly demonstrated that the quality and duration of patient survival are dismal. The 1-year survival rate for AIDS patients in New York City (1981–1985) was less than 45 percent for patients initially presenting with *Pneumocystis* pneumonia, less than 72 percent for patients initially presenting with Kaposi sarcoma, and less than 39 percent for patients presenting with other AIDS-defining illnesses.[1] One-year survival probabilities for the first 500 patients in San Francisco, calculated by different techniques, were no better.[2] In addition to the duration of patient survival being distressingly short, the quality of patient survival has usually been poor as manifested by decreasing performance scores and repeated needs for inpatient or outpatient medical interventions. The development of an effective antiretroviral drug, zidovudine (also known as azidothymidine or AZT), has been a major advance in the management of AIDS patients since its chronic administration clearly decreases the number (and probably the severity) of life-threatening illnesses and prolongs survival. Zidovudine is not a cure for AIDS, however, since patients chronically treated with this drug continue to develop serious tumors and infections and die prematurely.

Until more effective antiretroviral and immunomodulating agents can be developed, the management of AIDS patients will have to rely on zidovudine and on strategies that either prevent or more effectively treat the severe and life-threatening processes that are caused by the human immunodeficiency virus (HIV) itself, by immunologically mediated processes, or by opportunistic infections and tumors.[3] Autopsy studies suggest that almost 90 percent of life-threatening illnesses and deaths have been due to opportunistic infections.[4–6] Thus, a major focus in the management of HIV-infected patients must be placed on infectious processes. An increasing amount of data indicate that aggressive efforts to prevent opportunistic infections and aggressive efforts to diagnose complications expeditiously and intervene with therapy early can improve the prognosis for patients with this epidemic disease.

Some clinicians and patients question the utility of expending resources and subjecting patients to uncomfortable procedures and therapies when the underlying retroviral process is inevitably fatal.[7] The goals for the management of AIDS patients should be no different, however, from goals for the management of other incurable diseases such as cancer or atherosclerosis: to improve the quality and duration of survival in a manner that is reasonable in terms of the individual patient's wishes, a realistic assessment of the immediate prognosis, and the medical resources that are available. Experience is accumulating that shows that some patients with AIDS clearly benefit from surgical procedures, ventilatory support, and prolonged intensive care and survive for many months outside the hospital after such events.[7–9] Clinicians need considerable knowledge about the natural history of HIV infection, its complications, and the patient's wishes in order to make such decisions rationally.

THERAPY FOR UNDERLYING RETROVIRAL DISEASE

Since the clinical manifestations of AIDS are a direct consequence of HIV or the consequences of the effect of this virus on immune response, the most logical therapeutic strategy against AIDS would be to eradicate the HIV and to restore immune function to normal levels. During the 1980s, there has been an explosion in knowledge about the immunopathogenesis of AIDS. A variety of logical therapeutic strategies have been proposed, and many antiretroviral and immunomodulating agents with promising in vitro properties have been identified (Table 1). It is important to recognize that in vitro activity is not synonymous with clinical efficacy and safety. Before any therapeutic agent is introduced into standard clinical practice, there must be convincing demonstration that the new agent has therapeutic activity and is safe. In addition, advantage over existing therapy in terms of enhanced efficacy, decreased toxicity, decreased cost, or increased convenience of administration are desirable. Although many new agents are highly promising, as of May 1989 zidovudine was the only drug among the antiretroviral agents that had unequivocally been demonstrated to provide objective clinical benefit to HIV-infected patients (interferon-α has antiretroviral activity, but the only proven clinical benefit to date is its activity against Kaposi sarcoma, hairy cell leukemia, and papillomavirus infections). It is important for clinicians to avoid being influenced to use a drug solely because of aggressive advocacy by the drug's sponsor or enthusiastic interest on the part of patient groups.

In assessing antiretroviral and immunomodulating agents, a variety of laboratory assays are currently being used such as HIV cultures of circulating mononuclear cells, serum p24 antigen levels, drug levels, and the peripheral CD4-positive lymphocyte number.[10–12] The utility of any of these markers for predicting efficacy or avoiding toxicity is currently being assessed. The optimal laboratory parameters to follow are likely to change rapidly as technology becomes increasingly sophisticated. The ultimate criteria for the efficacy of any agent are not laboratory parameters, however, but are objective clinical markers showing improved quality or duration of survival.

Zidovudine (AZT) inhibits HIV replication in vitro at concentrations greater than 0.1 μmol (greater than 0.37 μg/ml), while uninfected lymphocytes or bone marrow progenitor cells are inhibited by concentrations of about 0.9 μmol[13–15] (see also Chapter 34). Zidovudine has little or no known direct activity against the common opportunistic pathogens associated with

TABLE 1. Examples of Antiretroviral and Immunomodulating Agents Undergoing Clinical Trials as Therapy for AIDS

Antiretroviral Agents	*Immunomodulating Agents*
Zidovudine (AZT)	Interferon-α
Dideoxycytidine (DDC)	Interferon-γ
Dideoxyinosine (DDI)	Interleukin-2 (IL-2)
Dideoxyadenosine (DDA)	Interferon-β
3′-deoxy-2′,3′-didehydrothymidine (D4T)	Isoprinosine
	Ampligen
AL721	Granulocyte-macrophage colony–stimulating factor
Interferon-α	
Dextran sulfate	Tumor necrosis factor
Intravenous immunoglobulin	Methionine enkephalin
Soluble CD4	Imreg
Antisense oligonucleosides	AS101
Ribavirin	

AIDS. Zidovudine is converted by a cellular thymidine kinase to a monophosphate form and ultimately into a triphosphate form that inhibits HIV reverse transcriptase about 100 times more effectively than mammalian polymerases. Zidovudine is available as an oral drug and as an investigational intravenous preparation. The oral drug is rapidly absorbed. Chronic administration of 250 mg every 4 hours results in peak and trough levels of 0.62 and 0.16 μg/ml, respectively.[15–17] The mean half-life is about 1 hour, and metabolism occurs primarily by hepatic glucuronidation, with total urinary recovery of about 90 percent. The drug penetrates the blood-brain barrier. Antiviral concentrations can be obtained in cerebrospinal fluid (CSF) when oral doses of 200–250 mg q4h are given.[15]

A multicenter, placebo-controlled trial of zidovudine (250 mg orally every 4 hours) was completed in 1986 with 282 patients who had either AIDS (first episode of *Pneumocystis* pneumonia within the preceding 120 days) or symptomatic AIDS-related complex (ARC).[16,17] Significant differences between the zidovudine- and placebo-treated patients were found in terms of the occurrences of opportunistic infections and deaths in both the AIDS and ARC patients. In the placebo-treated group, 19 patients died as compared with only 1 who was treated with zidovudine, and 45 opportunistic infections occurred in the placebo-treated group as compared with 24 opportunistic infections in the zidovudine-treated group.

Indicators of improved general clinical status such as increased body weight and higher Karnofsky performance status were also noted in zidovudine recipients. Psychometric testing demonstrated that zidovudine-treated patients showed significant cognitive improvement when compared with placebo-treated patients.[18,19] This improvement was often noted during the first 1–3 weeks of therapy. On the basis of this trial, zidovudine was licensed by the Food and Drug Administration for the management of patients with HIV infection who have a history of confirmed *Pneumocystis* pneumonia or who are symptomatic and have an absolute peripheral CD4 lymphocyte count of less than 200/mm^3 before therapy is initiated. The dose recommended was 200 mg orally six times per day.

The beneficial effects of zidovudine appear to persist beyond the 6-month period of observation reported in the initial trial, but opportunistic infections and deaths do continue to occur.[20,21] The magnitude of the benefit after the initial 6 months of therapy needs to be more clearly defined. A review of compassionate plea data suggests that sustained benefit is less likely in patients who did not start their zidovudine within 120 days of their episode of *Pneumocystis* pneumonia or in patients with very low peripheral CD4 lymphocyte counts.[20] Preliminary results of one large study of zidovudine for patients who have had a recent episode of *Pneumocystis* pneumonia suggest that, if specific anti-*Pneumocystis* therapy is not administered, a second episode of *Pneumocystis* pneumonia will occur in about 30 percent of patients still taking zidovudine after 6 months and 60 percent of patients still taking zidovudine after 12 months.

Zidovudine also has been shown to have benefit for HIV-infected patients with thrombocytopenia. All 10 patients in one study demonstrated elevations in platelet counts that averaged 54,000/mm^3.[22] Zidovudine may thus be preferable to other treatment modalities for severe HIV-related thrombocytopenia.[22,23] Zidovudine also appears to decrease the size of enlarged lymph nodes, liver, and spleen. Whether such decreases in organomegaly correlate with increased survival remains to be determined. Preliminary studies suggest that zidovudine does not have a major effect on Kaposi sarcoma lesions.

Whether zidovudine produces clinical benefit for other HIV-infected patient populations is not yet certain. It is logical to consider the possibility that zidovudine could improve the quality or duration of survival for asymptomatic patients with high peripheral CD4 lymphocyte counts, patients with Kaposi sarcoma and high or low peripheral CD4-positive lymphocyte counts, or patients with recent sexual or percutaneous or mucosal exposure to HIV. Such studies have not yet been completed and analyzed, however, and thus there are currently no data on which to base treatment recommendations for these patient groups.

The clinical benefit that zidovudine provides for patients with symptomatic AIDS or ARC does not clearly correlate with objective immunologic improvement. Peripheral CD4-positive lymphocyte counts may peak after a month of zidovudine therapy; they rise an average of 90/mm^3 in AIDS patients and 98/mm^3 in ARC patients.[16] The increase persists for only 16–20 weeks in AIDS patients. These modest increases may be more sustained in ARC patients. Other studies assessing patients with better initial immune function have been unable to demonstrate any benefit of zidovudine in terms of CD4-positive lymphocyte counts. Serum IgG and IgM levels diminish during zidovudine therapy, however, which suggests that zidovudine may influence polyclonal B-cell activation.

Zidovudine does have a measurable effect on HIV activity. Serum p24 antigen levels, a marker of the *gag* gene product, decrease during the initial 2–4 weeks of therapy in most antigen-positive patients.[10–12] Most HIV-infected patients remain culture-positive for HIV during zidovudine therapy even if they convert their serum p24 antigen from positive to negative (many HIV-infected patients have no measurable p24 antigen in their serum, however, during long periods of serial study). This suggests that zidovudine induces a decrease in active viral replication as manifested by a decrease in p24 antigen but that the drug has no effect on latent or slowly replicating virus. It may also be that zidovudine has only incomplete or intermittent antiviral activity. It is important to note that some patients who show an initial antiviral response may manifest rising serum p24 levels after many months of zidovudine therapy. Whether this represents the development of drug resistance or an alteration in zidovudine pharmacokinetics over time remains to be determined.

Zidovudine therapy has been associated with considerable toxicity.[17] Nausea, myalgias, insomnia, and severe headaches were reported substantially more often in zidovudine-treated patients as compared with the placebo-treated group in the initial controlled trial.[17] Occasionally these symptoms can be so severe that dose reduction or discontinuation of zidovudine therapy is necessary. Confusion, anxiety, and tremulousness can also occur, especially when high doses of zidovudine are used.[17,19,20] Zidovudine can also produce a bluish pigmentation in the nail beds of black patients.

The major toxicity of zidovudine is hematologic suppression.[17,20,21] A dose-dependent anemia is the most common effect recognized. During the second week of therapy, a macrocytosis is initially seen. In the initial placebo-controlled zidovudine trial, a 50 percent decrease in the hemoglobin level was seen in 8.4 percent of zidovudine-treated patients as compared with 0.7 percent of control patients.[17] Transfusions were administered to 31 percent of zidovudine recipients but only 11 percent of placebo recipients. Transfusions are usually necessary 6–15 weeks after the initiation of zidovudine therapy. Zidovudine appears to cause anemia by a direct effect on the bone marrow: erythroid hypoplasia or pure red cell aplasia are usually seen without peripheral evidence of hemolysis.[24] Serum erythropoietin levels are usually elevated.[24] A fall in reticulocyte count is usually the earliest predictor of toxicity. Interestingly, those patients who develop a markedly increased mean corpuscular volume are usually those patients who are less likely to develop substantial anemia and require transfusions. Many clinicians provide patients receiving zidovudine with enough transfusions to maintain their hemoglobin levels above 100 g/liter.

Leukopenia and granulocytopenia are also common occurrences in patients treated with zidovudine. A 50 percent decrease in neutrophil counts was seen in 52 percent of zidovudine-treated patients as compared with 10 percent of controls.[17] Complications of granulocytopenia are rarely seen. Thrombocytopenia is not a frequent occurrence due to zidovudine. Platelet counts usually rise even when initial values are above 100,000/mm^3. Toxicity required 45 percent of patients in the placebo-controlled trial to have their dose of zidovudine reduced or suspended.[17] There is little information about the efficacy of doses lower than 200–250 mg orally five times per day, although some European experience suggests that 250 mg orally four times per day has an antiviral effect.[22] It seems logical to use reduced doses of zidovudine rather than no drug at all if full doses cannot be tolerated while further studies are in progress. When the dose of zidovudine is reduced or terminated, an acute meningoencephalitis characterized by fever, headache, and confusion has been reported.[25] This syndrome appears to occur more commonly in patients who had neurologic dysfunction before the institution of zidovudine. This syndrome may remit spontaneously after 5–7 days, although one patient with this syndrome died. How often this syndrome occurs in the setting of a dose reduction is unknown. It has been suggested that the concurrent use of zidovudine and acetaminophen may predispose to toxicity. Patients who have low hemoglobin levels, low CD4 counts, low serum B_{12} levels, and constitutional symptoms are the subpopulation most likely to develop toxicity. Whether acetaminophen really predisposes to toxicity or whether patients who take acetaminophen are those who have symptoms attributable to severe HIV disease for which they coincidentally take acetaminophen has not been delineated. The recommendation to avoid acetaminophen while taking zidovudine is thus based on suggestive but inconclusive evidence.

There are very few data to date concerning how various drugs interact with zidovudine in terms of altering efficacy, toxicity, or pharmacokinetics. Many drugs used to treat opportunistic infections or tumors such as ganciclovir, trimethoprim-sulfamethoxazole, pentamidine, flucytosine, or cyclophosphamide have hematologic toxicities that may be difficult to distinguish from the toxicities of zidovudine or that may produce toxicities that are additive to those of zidovudine. Moreover, drugs such as amphotericin that may alter renal function or drugs such as flucytosine or phenytoin (Dilantin) that may alter hepatic function could alter zidovudine pharmacokinetics. Clinicians need to be aware of these potential interactions when managing HIV-infected patients who are receiving multiple drugs.

An expanding spectrum of agents with antiretroviral properties are being introduced into clinical trials (Table 1). None of these agents other than zidovudine has been proved to produce improved patient longevity. Certain nucleoside analogues such as dideoxycytidine appear to produce decreases in serum p24 antigen levels, although the toxicities of dideoxycytidine require that modifications from the doses used in initial trials be made. Recombinant interferon-α has been shown to reduce serum p24 antigen levels as well as the size of Kaposi sarcoma lesions in two small trials, especially in patients with relatively high CD4 counts.[26,27] Improved immunologic status was not observed to occur. Larger studies with longer follow-up are needed to determine whether recombinant interferon-α can prolong survival. Fatigue, myalgia, weight loss, hepatitis, thrombocytopenia, and leukopenia can occur with the interferon regimens employed in these studies. A reversible cardiomyopathy has also been reported.

OPPORTUNISTIC INFECTIONS

As indicated in Table 2, most opportunistic pathogens that cause disease in HIV-infected patients can be successfully treated with available anti-infective agents.[3,28] The opportunistic pathogens commonly seen in HIV-infected patients can be categorized into two groups: those that may respond to conventional or experimental drugs but have a high likelihood of recurring or relapsing when therapy is discontinued and those for which no therapy currently appears to be effective. The successful management of those opportunistic infections that are treatable depends on (*1*) prompt diagnosis and initiation of therapy before the clinical syndrome is severe, (*2*) recognition that a poor response to therapy may indicate that a pathogen other than the one initially identified may have been present or may have developed subsequently and requires additional therapy, and (*3*) recognition that some therapies must be lifelong to prevent relapses or recurrences.

TABLE 2. Therapy for Common Opportunistic Pathogens in HIV-Infected Patients

Pathogens that may respond to therapy but frequently recur or relapse
Pneumocystis carinii
Toxoplasma gondii
Isospora belli
Leishmania donovani
Herpes simplex virus
Varicella-zoster virus
Cytomegalovirus
Candida species
Cryptococcus neoformans
Histoplasma capsulatum
Coccidioides immitis
Salmonella species
Campylobacter species
Shigella species
Mycobacterium tuberculosis
Streptococcus pneumoniae
Pathogens for which no therapy currently appears to be effective
Cryptosproridia
Epstein-Barr virus
Microsporidia
Mycobacterium avium-intracellulare

The management of opportunistic infections in HIV-infected patients differs from management in other patient populations because the natural history of specific processes like *Pneumocystis* pneumonia or cryptococcal meningitis is different from non-AIDS patients, because the tolerance of HIV-infected patients for therapeutic agents such as trimethoprim-sulfamethoxazole or flucytosine may be less than for other patient populations, and because consideration must be given to interactions between the drugs directed against opportunistic pathogens and drugs directed against HIV itself or the immune defect or associated tumors such as the potential interaction between ganciclovir and zidovudine or the potential interaction between interferon-α and zidovudine. When feasible, specific therapy (Table 3) for an identified pathogen is preferable to empirical therapy due to the predilection of AIDS patients to have adverse drug reactions and the prospect that drug interactions may present management problems for a population that is often taking many drugs chronically.

PNEUMOCYSTIS PNEUMONIA

The likelihood that an AIDS patient will survive an episode of *Pneumocystis* pneumonia (see also Chapter 256) depends on the severity of pulmonary dysfunction at the time therapy is initiated, the patient's ability to tolerate available regimens, and the severity of the patient's immunologic dysfunction. A poor prognosis correlates with an alveolar–arterial gradient greater than 30 mmHg, a severely abnormal chest radiograph, a high number of organisms detected on lavage or biopsy, and an episode that is the second or greater episode rather than a first episode of *Pneumocystis* pneumonia.[29] Thus any drug therapy is more likely to be successful if the patient is having a first episode of *Pneumocystis* pneumonia, if therapy is started at a time when pulmonary dysfunction is mild, and if other severe opportunistic infections are absent. Patients who have been receiving the full recommended dose of zidovudine for at least 6 weeks also appear to have a better prognosis.

TABLE 3. Therapy for Frequent Infectious Diseases in AIDS Patients

Clinical Disease	*Drug*	*Usual Daily Adult Dose*	*Interval between Divided Doses*	*Route*	*Minimum Duration*[a]
Protozoa					
Pneumocystis pneumonia	Trimethoprim-sulfamethoxazole	15–20 mg/kg trimethoprim with 75–100 mg/kg sulfamethoxazole	q6–8h	iv, po	14–21 days
	or Pentamidine isethionate	3–4 mg/kg	qd	iv	14–21 days
	or Trimethoprim-dapsone	1200 mg trimethoprim with 100 mg dapsone	trimethoprim q6h, dapsone qd	po	14–21 days
Toxoplasmosis	Pyrimethamine	75 mg once, then 25 mg	qd	po	28 days
	and Sulfadiazine	4 g	q6h	po	28 days
Cryptosporidiosis	None	—	—	—	—
Fungi					
Oral thrush (*Candida*)	Nystatin or	3 × 10[6] units	q4h	po	7–10 days
	Ketoconazole	400 mg	q12h	po	7–10 days
Candida esophagitis	Amphotericin B	0.6 mg/kg	qd	iv	7–10 days
	or Ketoconazole	400 mg	q12h	po	7–10 days
Cryptococcosis	Amphotericin B with or without	0.4 mg/kg	qd	iv	42 days
	Flucytosine	150 mg/kg	q6h	po, iv	42 days
Isosporiasis	Trimethoprim	640 mg	q6h	po	7–10 days
	and Sulfamethoxazole	3200 mg	q6h	po	7–10 days
Viruses					
Mucocutaneous herpes simplex	Acyclovir	15 mg/kg	q8h	iv, po	7 days
Disseminated herpes zoster	Acyclovir	30 mg/kg	q8h	iv	7 days
CMV	Ganciclovir or	10 mg/kg	q12h	iv	21 days
	Foscarnet	180 mg/kg	q8h	iv	21 days
Bacteria					
Mycobacterium avium-intracellulare	None	—	—	—	—
Mycobacterium tuberculosis	INH and	300 mg	q24h	po, im	9 mon
	Rifampin and	600 mg	q24h	po, iv	9 mon
	Ethambutol	15 mg/kg	q24h	po	9 mon

[a] Before the maintenance regimen.

Trimethoprim-sulfamethoxazole and parenteral pentamidine isethionate are effective agents for the treatment of *Pneumocystis* pneumonia in AIDS patients.[30,31] The survival rate for all patients treated with these two regimens is about 75 percent. The survival rate for certain AIDS populations such as patients with first episodes of *Pneumocystis* pneumonia, no serious concomitant opportunistic infections, and an alveolar–arterial gradient less than 30 mmHg is probably better than 90 percent.[29–31] Intravenous trimethoprim-sulfamethoxazole, oral trimethoprim-sulfamethoxazole, oral trimethoprim-dapsone, and parenteral pentamidine are all probably equally effective. Oral trimethoprim-sulfamethoxazole is the regimen of choice for most clinicians because of the convenience of administration, the high degree of efficacy, and the manageability of associated toxicities. There is no clear reason to prefer intravenous over oral trimethoprim-sulfamethoxazole in compliant patients with no obvious gastrointestinal dysfunction. Monitoring serum drug concentrations is probably more useful for managing toxicity than for maximizing efficacy. Peak serum sulfamethoxazole levels should probably be maintained at 100–150 μg/ml. The major disadvantages of trimethoprim-sulfamethoxazole and parenteral pentamidine are that they are less than 100 percent effective and adverse reactions are frequent.[30–32] Adverse reactions can occur in 50–100 percent of AIDS patients treated with trimethoprim-sulfamethoxazole or parenteral pentamidine. Because adverse reactions are so common and because *Pneumocystis* is responsible for only about 40–60 percent of the pulmonary syndromes that present in this population, empirical therapy is less desirable than is the establishment of a specific diagnosis followed by the institution of specific therapy.

For trimethoprim-sulfamethoxazole, common adverse reactions include skin rash, granulocytopenia, transaminase elevations, nephritis, nausea, and vomiting (see Chapter 29). These adverse reactions do not invariably require discontinuation of trimethoprim-sulfamethoxazole therapy.[33] The skin rashes, which commonly occur between the 8th and 12th days of therapy, may be limited in extent and associated with a degree of pruritus that the patient can tolerate for 21 days. Life-threatening mucocutaneous sloughing such as the Stevens-Johnson syndrome are extraordinarily rare in AIDS patients, although a few fatal cases have been reported. Thus, the development of a rash associated with trimethoprim-sulfamethoxazole therapy is not necessarily an indication to discontinue this drug regimen. Granulocytopenia appears to be a dose-related phenomenon that may resolve partially or completely if the dose of trimethoprim-sulfamethoxazole is reduced by 25 percent.[33] Granulocytopenia only rarely responds to leucovorin administration. Nausea and vomiting can be troublesome complications of trimethoprim-sulfamethoxazole therapy: severe nausea may be due to very high sulfonamide levels and may improve if the dose is reduced. Clinical hepatitis is less often a clinically important complication of trimethoprim-sulfamethoxazole therapy. Transaminase levels may fluctuate until therapy is stopped; however, at which time they usually return promptly to baseline values. Overall, adverse reactions have in the past required discontinuation of trimethoprim-sulfamethoxazole therapy in about 25 percent of cases. Although it has not been proved by a prospective study, adverse reactions can probably be reduced without sacrificing efficacy by lowering the recommended dose of trimethoprim-sulfamethoxazole from trimethoprim, 20 mg/kg/day, with sulfamethoxazole, 100 mg/kg/day, to trimethoprim, 15 mg/kg/day, with sulfamethoxazole, 75 mg/kg/day.[33]

Parenteral pentamidine is effective therapy for *Pneumocystis* pneumonia (see Chapter 36). This regimen is inconvenient to administer, however, and the adverse reactions associated with it can be life-threatening. Renal dysfunction, hypoglycemia, hyperglycemia, granulocytopenia, and hypotension are reported in 10–50 percent of patients.[30,31,33] For many years pentamidine was administered intramuscularly because early reports had described fatal hypotension when the drug was given intravenously. Intramuscular administration of pentamidine is no longer recommended except in unusual circumstances, however, because the intramuscular injections are often associated with painful sterile abscesses that can also become superinfected. Moreover, the hypotension originally associated with intravenous pentamidine was probably related to the rate of infusion. When pentamidine is administered over a 60-minute period in 100–150 ml of dextrose in water, clinically important hypotension is unusual. The renal dysfunction associated with pentamidine can be severe. If the serum creatinine level rises by more than 1.0–2.0 mg/dl, strong consideration should be given to withholding therapy for a few days or switching to an alternative agent. Hypoglycemia can be a life-threatening complication of pentamidine therapy and occurs at any juncture during therapy or after therapy has been completed.[34] Hypoglycemia occurs more frequently in patients who also develop renal dysfunction due to pentamidine. The unpredictability of the hypoglycemia adds an element of danger to the inpatient or outpatient use of this drug. Life-threatening hypoglycemia is sufficiently uncommon, however, that this effective agent is still recommended for trimethoprim-sulfamethoxazole–intolerant or trimethoprim-dapsone intolerant patients. Toxicity may be reduced without sacrificing efficacy by lowering the dose of parenteral pentamidine from 4 to 3 mg/kg/day.[33,35]

The relapse rate after conventional therapy with trimethoprim-sulfamethoxazole or parenteral pentamidine is about 60 percent per 12 months for AIDS patients receiving zidovudine but no specific anti-*Pneumocystis* prophylaxis. The likelihood of a relapse cannot be predicted from clinical features of an episode or the rate of response to acute therapy. Every patient who completes a course of therapy for *Pneumocystis* pneumonia and every patient whose CD4 count is less than 200/mm^3, especially those with oral candidiasis or fever, should receive anti-*Pneumocystis* prophylaxis.

There are several investigational therapies that show promise for the treatment of *Pneumocystis* pneumonia in AIDS patients. Aerosolized pentamidine isethionate has been used successfully to treat some patients with mild to moderately severe disease.[35,36] Since *Pneumocystis* is almost always confined to the lungs, this therapy has the virtue of delivering high concentrations of drug to the target organ with little systemic absorption and little serious toxicity when compared with intravenous administrations. The delivery of pentamidine to the lungs depends on the particle size generated by the specific nebulizer used as well as the tubing length, the baffles, and the patient's ventilatory pattern. Aerosol delivery may not provide optimal drug concentrations in the upper lobes. Since this delivery system was designed to avoid substantial serum concentrations of pentamidine, it will also be important to determine whether extrapulmonary *Pneumocystis* becomes a substantially more common occurrence in patients treated only by the aerosol route. Cases of disseminated *Pneumocystis* infection with involvement of multiple visceral organs, skin, and lymph nodes have been reported in patients who were receiving aerosol pentamidine prophylaxis and in patients who had been receiving no prophylaxis at all. Toxicity of aerosolized pentamidine has been uncommon and consists primarily of reversible bronchospasm, especially in smokers. Hypoglycemia has also been reported. Where aerosolized pentamidine will fit into the anti-*Pneumocystis* armamentarium remains to be determined by controlled trials comparing this promising therapy with conventional approaches.

Dapsone (100 mg po qd) plus trimethoprim (5 mg/kg po q6h or 300 mg po q6h) appears to be as effective as trimethoprim-sulfamethoxazole but less toxic in limited experience.[37] Skin rashes are very common among AIDS patients treated with dapsone, but a 21-day course of therapy can usually be completed without interruption. This regimen may therefore be preferable to trimethoprim-sulfamethoxazole because of the reduced toxicity. Dapsone alone has some efficacy when 100 mg po qd is used for 21 days, but higher doses may be necessary to achieve a satisfactory response rate. Whether higher doses would be well tolerated remains to be determined.

Trimetrexate is a potent inhibitor of dihydrofolate reductase that is effective therapy against *Pneumocystis* pneumonia when used either alone (30–45 mg/m^2 iv qd) or in combination with a sulfonamide.[38] Since trimetrexate inhibits the dihydrofolate reductase of human cells as well as the enzyme of *Pneumocystis*, it must be given in conjunction with high-dose leucovorin (20 mg/kg iv or po q6h), which rescues mammalian cells without diminishing the anti-*Pneumocystis* effect. Trimetrexate appears to be well tolerated. Reversible leukopenia is its major adverse effect. The efficacy of trimetrexate as compared with trimethoprim-sulfamethoxazole is being assessed by controlled trials. It remains to be documented whether or not any very potent dihydrofolate reductase inhibitor such as trimetrexate (or piritrexim, a structurally similar compound) can be as effective as a combination regimen that includes a dihydrofolate reductase inhibitor plus a sulfonamide or sulfone. At this juncture it is uncertain to what extent the sulfonamide contributes to efficacy when dihydrofolate reductase inhibitors are used in conjunction with sulfonamides in regimens such as trimethoprim-sulfamethoxazole, pyrimethamine-sulfadiazine, or trimetrexate-sulfadiazine. The relapse rate after trimetrexate therapy is high: 40–60 percent of patients relapse within the first 60 days if no prophylactic regimen is employed.

Difluoromethylornithine (DFMO), an inhibitor of polyamine synthesis, and primaquine-clindamycin have been used to treat AIDS patients with *Pneumocystis* pneumonia, but there are currently inadequate data to assess their potential roles. Corticosteroids have been advocated as an adjunct to conventional anti-*Pneumocystis* agents for patients who present with substantial pulmonary dysfunction, but the results of trials comparing such a regimen to conventional therapies are not yet available.[39]

When an AIDS patient with *Pneumocystis* pneumonia fails to improve when receiving conventional therapy, there are no controlled data to indicate what modifications in therapy are optimal. The mean time to improvement for AIDS patients treated with conventional therapy is 5–6 days, so patients should probably not be considered therapeutic failures until they have received 7–10 days of therapy.[30,31] Clinicians often feel compelled to alter therapy earlier, however, especially if the patient is deteriorating rapidly. If a patient has not improved after 7–10 days of therapy, a repeat diagnostic procedure should be considered to determine whether another treatable pathogen is present. Bronchoscopy with transbronchial biopsies is the procedure of choice since lung tissue is usually necessary to assess the presence of cytomegalovirus (CMV) or perhaps fungal diseases, which are the major diagnostic considerations. *Pneumocystis* will usually be present in lavage or tissue for at least 3–4 weeks after initiating therapy even in patients who respond promptly, so their presence after 7–10 days of therapy does not necessarily imply ineffective therapy. The presence of extensive intra-alveolar exudate after 7–10 days of therapy is probably a more ominous sign. Open lung biopsy should rarely be necessary to supplement bronchoalveolar lavage and transbronchial biopsy given the very high yield of bronchoscopy for most treatable infections. Kaposi sarcoma of the lung is one treatable process that is difficult or impossible to reliably diagnose from transbronchial biopsy specimens. Nodular lesions on chest computed axial tomography (CAT) scan, progressing skin lesions, and the presence of a bloody pleural effusion may be helpful clues.[40]

If *Pneumocystis* is the only identifiable cause of the pulmonary dysfunction after 7–10 days of therapy and the patient has failed to improve, there are several therapeutic alternatives: (*1*) switch from trimethoprim-sulfamethoxazole to parenteral pentamidine or vice versa, (*2*) add corticosteroids to conventional therapy, (*3*) switch to trimetrexate, (*4*) switch to difluoromethylornithine, or (*5*) switch to clindamycin-primaquine. Each of these approaches has been demonstrated to be successful in some cases. A controlled trial is needed to determine the best approach. Whether AIDS patients with *Pneumocystis* pneumonia should be aggressively supported with intensive care, mechanical ventilation, or other interventions is a controversial issue.[7–9] The most reasonable approach would appear to be to individualize each patient in terms of how many days of therapy have been received, what therapeutic alternatives are available, what concomitant processes are present, what the patient's wishes are, and what resources are available. There is published literature indicating that AIDS patients with *Pneumocystis* pneumonia can survive intubation and mechanical ventilation and lead independent lives for several months after hospital discharge.[7–9] The best candidates for intensive care and mechanical ventilation would be those patients presenting with an initial episode of *Pneumocystis* pneumonia and no other serious opportunistic processes, those who have received less than 7 days of therapy, and those who have clearly articulated a desire for aggressive support.

The prevention of *Pneumocystis* pneumonia is a major priority given the high frequency of this life-threatening infection among AIDS patients (at least 65 percent will have one or more episodes) and the high likelihood for a second episode if no prophylaxis is administered after the first episode (about 60 percent over a period of 12 months even if chronic zidovudine therapy is given). Candidate patients especially well-suited for prophylaxis include those who have had an episode of *Pneumocystis* pneumonia (secondary prophylaxis) and those HIV-positive patients who have fewer than 200 circulating CD4-positive cells/mm^3 (primary prophylaxis), especially those with oral candidiasis or fever. The only placebo-controlled trial of prophylaxis for AIDS patients has demonstrated that trimethoprim, 160 mg, with sulfamethoxazole, 800 mg po q12h, plus leucovorin, 5 mg po qd, is highly effective as primary prophylaxis.[41] Adverse reactions occurred in 27 percent of treated patients, but prophylaxis had to be discontinued because of toxicity in only 17 percent. Whether other trimethoprim-sulfamethoxazole regimens employing fewer doses per week would be equally effective (in pediatric cancer patients 3 consecutive days per week are as effective as 7 days per week) remains to be determined. Aerosolized pentamidine is used widely for prophylaxis. Preliminary assessment of ongoing trials suggests a high degree of efficacy and low toxicity when pentamidine is administered according to protocol. How often the *Pneumocystis* disease that does occur during aerosolized pentamidine prophylaxis will be atypical, extrapulmonary, or difficult to treat remains to be determined. Other drugs with potential as prophylactic agents include dapsone, dapsone plus trimethoprim, or pyrimethamine plus sulfadoxine.

TOXOPLASMA GONDII

When an HIV-infected patient with substantial immunodeficiency presents with a space-occupying cerebral lesion that involves gray matter, the differential diagnosis primarily includes toxoplasmosis (see Chapters 36 and 255) and lymphoma.[42–46] Fungal, mycobacterial, and viral processes present as space-occupying lesions only rarely, and progressive multifocal leukoencephalopathy should primarily involve white matter. The definitive diagnostic study (i.e., brain biopsy) has some morbidity associated with it, and the diagnostic yield is often only 50 percent if toxoplasmosis is the etiology. The cysts and tachyzoites of *T. gondii* can be very difficult to recognize in fragments of necrotic brain tissue, and even several small needle biopsy samples may miss the area that has abundant organisms. Since toxoplasmosis is the only common etiology for gray matter lesions that clearly benefits from therapy and because brain needle biopsy has diagnostic limitations, empirical therapy with pyrimethamine (75 mg po the first day followed by 25 mg po qd) and sulfadiazine (1–2 g po q6h) is reasonable. Some clinicians use higher doses of both drugs, but there is no clear evidence that higher doses are more effective, and they almost certainly produce more toxicity. If there is not unequivocal improvement by clinical and radiologic criteria within 14–21 days, a biopsy should be performed to establish whether the etiology is an infectious or neoplastic process other than toxoplasmosis.[42–44] Corticosteroids to reduce inflammation may be necessary in patients with substantial or progressive neurologic dysfunction or signs of increased intracranial pressure. The administration of corticosteroids may make evaluation of the clinical and radiologic response to specific therapy difficult since the observed improvement may be solely due to corticosteroid therapy and may be unrelated to the anti-*Toxoplasma* regimen employed. Chronic antiseizure medication should routinely be instituted. For patients who do respond, anti-*Toxoplasma* therapy should be continued for life since relapses do occur in the same sites as those presenting initially if therapy is discontinued, even after 8–12 months.[44] Whether the chronic suppressive regimen will be as effective if both pyrimethamine and sulfadiazine are not included at full doses remains to be demonstrated.

Treatment failures are very unusual for patients with toxoplasmosis who are able to tolerate both pyrimethamine and sulfadiazine.[45] Radiologically proven failures in patients who are unequivocally taking their drugs should raise the possibility that toxoplasmosis is not the correct diagnosis. Adverse reactions to sulfadiazine (leukopenia, rash, elevated transaminase level, nausea, nephritis) and to pyrimethamine (leukopenia, thrombocytopenia) are common. The leukopenia often will not respond to leucovorin therapy, although a short course of leucovorin (10–20 mg po or iv q6h) should be attempted. There are no alternative regimens that are clearly effective for patients who cannot tolerate both pyrimethamine and sulfadiazine. Alternatives that are currently being assessed include higher doses of pyrimethamine alone (50–150 mg po qd with or without leucovorin), clindamycin, clindamycin plus pyrimethamine, dapsone plus pyrimethamine, trimetrexate, and spiramycin. Clindamycin (intravenous three times daily) plus pyrimethamine has been effective in some patients and is currently the most promising alternative to pyrimethamine and sulfadiazine. Oral clindamycin plus pyrimethamine may not be as effective as intravenous clindamycin plus pyrimethamine.

HERPES SIMPLEX AND VARICELLA-ZOSTER VIRUS INFECTIONS

Acyclovir (200 mg po q4h) is very effective therapy for herpes simplex viral perirectal lesions, proctitis, oral lesions, digital lesions, and esophagitis (see Chapters 34, 118, and 119).[47] Disseminated herpes simplex viral infections almost never occur in HIV-infected patients. Intravenous therapy is rarely necessary unless the patient has a major gastrointestinal disorder that prevents oral absorption. Topical acyclovir has not been demonstrated to be effective in AIDS patients. Acyclovir-resistant disease or acyclovir-resistant isolates have been very uncommon. The response of herpes simplex lesions is usually prompt and occurs within 3–10 days. Therapy should continue until the lesions are crusted over or epithelialized. Relapses occur with high frequency. If relapses occur quickly or often, therapy may have to be continuous for life. Whether daily doses lower than those used for therapy would be adequate prophylaxis has not been determined. Some therapeutic benefits of the combination of zidovudine plus acyclovir have been suggested but need to be confirmed in larger trials.

Dermatomal herpes zoster does not usually need to be treated in HIV-infected patients because dissemination of the virus has rarely followed.[48] Local involvement in more than one dermatome is seen. Even when extensive disseminated cutaneous lesions have been observed, however, clinically apparent visceral disease has rarely been documented. Whether acyclovir therapy has any role in hastening the crusting of lesions or in preventing recurrences in HIV-infected patients is not known. Patients with persistent or recurrent lesions or zoster ophthalmicus might be logical candidates for high-dose oral acyclovir (400–800 mg po q4h). Whether acyclovir is beneficial in decreasing the severity or duration of post-herpetic neuralgia has not been determined. Corticosteroid therapy to prevent post-herpetic neuralgia is not recommended in AIDS patients because of the potentially adverse effect of corticosteroids on immune function and on Kaposi sarcoma activity.

CYTOMEGALOVIRUS

Cytomegalovirus infection (see Chapters 34 and 120) is almost universal among HIV-infected patients as assessed by serology. HIV-infected patients with fewer than 100–200 circulating CD4 cells are often viremic and viruric with CMV, but only a few of these patients develop specific organ damage that needs to be treated. Retinitis is the most commonly recognized disorder caused by CMV.[49] Cytomegalovirus retinitis has the potential to rapidly involve the macula and optic disk and result in visual impairment and ultimately in blindness. When lesions are recognized close to the macula or disk or when extensive lesions are present, therapy is warranted. Whether patients benefit from prompt treatment of peripheral lesions rather than close observation until the lesions progress remains to be determined. Cytomegalovirus retinitis responds to either ganciclovir (DHPG) administered at a dose of 5 mg/kg iv q12h or foscarnet (phosphonoformate) at 60 mg/kg iv q8h.[49–56] Empirical therapy without a specific histologic or virologic diagnosis is reasonable since obtaining retinal or vitreous material for examination is risky (detached retinas or secondary infection may result), the ophthalmologic appearance of CMV retinitis is quite characteristic to an experienced ophthalmologist, and CMV causes almost all the retinitis that occurs in HIV-infected patients.[57] The response to ganciclovir is quite prompt. New lesions or progressive disease may be identified during the first 7 days of therapy and do not necessarily imply a poor response. Considerable improvement in inflammation, edema, and hemorrhage will be recognized in responders before the end of 21 days of therapy. Without maintenance suppressive therapy, relapse at the same site as the initial lesions and at new sites almost invariably occurs within a few weeks or months. Maintenance regimens using ganciclovir, 5–6 mg/kg iv qd 5–7 days per week, are often administered, but these regimens seem only to prolong the interval until relapse. They do not prevent relapses from occurring. At the time of relapse, patients will usually respond to reinstitution of ganciclovir, 5 mg/kg iv q12h. Ganciclovir's major toxicity is bone marrow suppression with neutropenia and thrombocytopenia. Confusion, nausea, vomiting, transaminase elevation, and inhibition of spermatogenesis also occur. Some AIDS patients will be unable to tolerate parenteral ganciclovir therapy. Intravitreal injections of ganciclovir have been assessed in a few hundred patients. This therapy appears to be effective and relatively safe, although retinal detachment resulting from repeated injections is a concern.[54] When patients with sight threatening CMV lesions become neutropenic due to ganciclovir, the clinician and patient must often make a choice between saving vision and accepting neutropenia. When neutropenia occurs during ganciclovir therapy, other infectious, neoplastic, immunologic, and drug-related causes of the neutropenia should be sought. Alternatively, another therapy such as intravitreal ganciclovir or parenteral foscarnet may be tried. Foscarnet has in vitro and clinical antiviral activity against CMV.[55,56] It also has activity against HIV. This drug is nephrotoxic but not bone marrow toxic. Its efficacy, as determined in much more limited trials, appears to be generally similar to that of ganciclovir. Acyclovir, even in high doses, has not convincingly been shown to have anti-CMV activity.

Esophagitis, enteritis, colitis, and pneumonitis are life-threatening syndromes caused by CMV that have been documented to respond to ganciclovir therapy.[50,51,53,58,59] For these syndromes, a specific diagnosis should be established by histology since the syndromes are indistinguishable from those caused by other pathogens if clinical criteria alone are used. Culture of CMV from tissue or secretions or excretions is probably too nonspecific to be used as a basis for therapy.

For patients with esophagitis, colitis, or rectal ulcers, improvement in clinical symptoms is usually noted during the first week of therapy. Improved performance status and increased weight is often noted, especially if therapy results in less dysphagia or less diarrhea. There is considerably less experience with ganciclovir therapy for CMV pneumonia. There are reports of successful therapy for CMV pneumonia in a patient with AIDS.[50] There is no consensus about the specific criteria for establishing the diagnosis, however, and some patients who failed ganciclovir therapy had very severe lung damage before ganciclovir treatment was started. Ganciclovir therapy alone has not been reported to be effective in bone marrow transplant recipients unless immune serum globulin or hyperimmune globulin is given concurrently.[60,61] How often ganciclovir will be effective in AIDS patients either alone or in conjunction with immunoglobulin remains to be determined.

EPSTEIN BARR VIRUS

Epstein Barr virus (EBV) (see Chapter 121) can be cultivated from the oropharynx and peripheral mononuclear cells of a substantial proportion of AIDS patients. This virus has been implicated in the pathogenesis of hairy leukoplakia and may have a role in the pathogenesis of nonspecific pneumonitis, lymphadenopathy, lymphoma, fever, or wasting. There is insufficient evidence to warrant specific therapy for EBV at this point, nor is there a drug that would clearly be effective.

PROGRESSIVE MULTIFOCAL LEUKOENCEPHALOPATHY

Progressive multifocal leukoencephalopathy (see Chapter 124) is caused by JC and SV-40 viruses. No therapy is known to be effective. Management should consist of early diagnosis so that arrangements for appropriate supportive care can be made.

CANDIDA SPECIES

Stomatitis, esophagitis, vaginitis, and proctitis due to *Candida* species (see Chapters 33 and 235) will respond to topical therapy (nystatin or clotrimazole), oral therapy (ketoconazole or fluconazole), or intravenous therapy (amphotericin B).[62,63] Ketoconazole (200 mg po q12h) is often the most convenient regimen, although the longer half-life for the investigational agent fluconazole may make this agent more convenient. There is usually no urgency to institute amphotericin B for any of these disorders: esophagitis is rarely associated with bleeding, perforation, fungemia, or disseminated fungal disease. Stomatitis, esophagitis, and proctitis often recur when therapy is discontinued. Ketoconazole administration may thus have to be continued for life. Occasional patients who do not respond to topical or oral therapy, especially those who are extremely debilitated or immunosuppressed, may respond to amphotericin B.

Disseminated candidiasis is not a common occurrence in AIDS patients unless they are receiving drug therapy that makes them neutropenic (especially cytotoxic antineoplastic therapy) or they have an infected intravenous catheter. Treatment is similar to that in other patient populations, with particular attention directed at removing infected intravenous lines or discontinuing therapies that may be producing neutropenia.

CRYPTOCOCCUS NEOFORMANS, HISTOPLASMA CAPSULATUM, COCCIDIOIDES IMMITIS

Cryptococcosis (see Chapters 241, 242, 244, and 33) is very difficult to cure in patients with AIDS. Even among those responding to therapy, relapse is usual.[64–66] Isolation of *Cryptococcus neoformans* from any body fluid is diagnostic and should prompt a careful assessment to determine the extent of dissemination. Culture of CSF, blood, and urine as well as a determination of the serum and CSF antigen titers are useful. The lysis–centrifugation technique is superior to other methods for isolating *C. neoformans* from blood.

The therapy of choice for cryptococcosis in AIDS is amphotericin B, 0.4–0.6 mg/kg daily or double that dose on alternate days. It is not known in this group of patients whether flucytosine can be used to permit a reduced dose of amphotericin B. The common occurrence of worsening hepatic or bone marrow function during flucytosine therapy makes this drug difficult to use in AIDS patients.

Almost all patients with cryptococcosis are switched from intensive to long-term, intermittent amphotericin B at some point in therapy, but that point remains to be defined, as does the optimum maintenance regimen.[64–66] One strategy is to continue daily or alternate-day therapy until at least 2.0–2.5 g of amphotericin B have been received and until cultures have become negative. At that juncture, treatment with amphotericin B, 1.0 mg/kg one to three times per week, is often chosen. It is probably unrealistic to continue intensive therapy until the CSF smears and antigen titers are negative because that goal is rarely attainable.

Oral fluconazole is being evaluated in a multicenter trial for maintenance suppressive therapy in cryptococcal meningitis. There is early evidence that this drug may be useful not only in the maintenance but also in acute treatment of some patients with cryptococcosis.[67–69]

Disseminated histoplasmosis in AIDS patients has not responded to ketoconazole and has often relapsed after treatment with amphotericin B.[70,71] Maintenance daily ketoconazole or weekly intravenous amphotericin B has been used to prevent relapse. Disseminated coccidioidomycoses in AIDS patients have proved difficult to control even with amphotericin B.[72]

MYCOBACTERIUM SPECIES

Mycobacterium avium-intracellulare (see Chapters 32, 229, and 231) is a common pathogen among HIV-infected patients, but what role this organism plays in contributing to morbidity or mortality is uncertain. A variety of antimicrobial agents have some activity against *Mycobacterium avium-intracellulare*, including ansamycin (rifabutin), clofazimine, imipenem, various quinolones, amikacin, cycloserine, pyrazinamide, and ethambutol.[73–75] Isoniazid and rifampin rarely have in vitro activity. There has been no convincing in vivo evidence that any antimicrobial regimen has clinical or microbiologic effect.[75–77] All therapeutic regimens must therefore be considered to be experimental.

Mycobacterium tuberculosis isolates from AIDS patients appear to be identical to isolates from other patients in terms of susceptibility to antimicrobacterial drugs. A regimen of isoniazid (300 mg po qd), rifampin (600 mg po qd), and ethambutol (15 mg/kg/day po) for 9 months (and a minimum of 6 months after cultures become negative) is recommended, although lifelong therapy may be more prudent.[78]

ENTERIC PATHOGENS: SALMONELLA SPECIES, SHIGELLA SPECIES, CAMPYLOBACTER SPECIES, ENTAMEBA HISTOLYTICA, GIARDIA LAMBLIA, CRYPTOSPORIDIA, ISOSPORA BELLI, MICROSPORIDIA

When *Salmonella* species, *Shigella* species, and *Campylobacter* species cause persistent diarrhea, severe diarrhea, or bacteremic disease, therapy is indicated. The antimicrobial susceptibility of these pathogens does not appear to differ from that in other patients.[79–82] Appropriate antibiotic therapy will usually control the bacteremia or diarrhea, but eradication of the organism can often not be accomplished. Chronic suppressive regimens with quinolones, trimethoprim-sulfamethoxazole, erythromycin, or ampicillin may be necessary (depending on the specific isolate), often in conjunction with antimotility drugs.

Amebiasis and giardiasis in AIDS patients do not appear to be associated with any more severe disease than that seen in HIV-negative homosexual men. Therapy can thus follow routine guidelines.

Cryptosporidia can cause severe gastrointestinal or biliary disease, but there is no specific therapy for it (see Chapter 261). Spiramycin does not appear to be effective. Antimotility drugs are often useful. Total parenteral nutrition may benefit patients who are becoming debilitated due to severe diarrhea if the patient and health care team deem this type of intervention to be appropriate.

Isospora belli (see Chapter 260) responds to trimethoprim-sulfamethoxazole (trimethoprim, 160 mg, plus sulfamethoxazole, 800 mg po q6h for 7–10 days), but the relapse rate is high and necessitates chronic suppression with trimethoprim-sulfamethoxazole.[83,84] Metronidazole, quinacrine, or pyrimethamine may be alternatives for patients with severe intolerance to trimethoprim-sulfamethoxazole.

TREPONEMA PALLIDUM

Syphilis is often recognized in HIV-infected patients either because of characteristic lesions of primary or secondary disease or because a screening serology for *T. pallidum* (see also Chapter 213) is positive. It is becoming increasingly apparent that, in patients with primary and secondary syphilis, central nervous system involvement is more common than was previously thought.[85,86] As many as 40 percent of patients with primary or secondary syphilis will have serologic or microbiologic evidence of *T. pallidum* in their cerebrospinal fluid regardless of their HIV status if careful diagnostic studies are employed.[83] It is also becoming increasingly apparent that, in HIV-infected patients with primary, secondary, or latent syphilis, a single dose of 2.4 mIU benzathine penicillin may be inadequate to cure the central nervous system or to prevent systemic relapses as measured by subsequent rises in serum VDRL titers. The optimal treatment for HIV-infected patients with early or latent syphilis is not established: procaine penicillin (1.2 mIU daily for 10–14 days) may be preferred over serial doses of benzathine penicillin (2.4 mIU every week for 3 or 4 weeks).[87]

KAPOSI SARCOMA

Although Kaposi sarcoma can often involve extensive areas of skin and mucous membranes on physical examination and although postmortem examination may reveal many visceral lesions, Kaposi sarcoma does not directly cause death in most patients with this tumor.[4–6] Kaposi sarcoma can cause cosmetically unpleasant lesions such as those on the face or hands, and Kaposi sarcoma can cause painful lesions such as those overlying joints or on the sole of the feet. Kaposi sarcoma lesions can also become impressively extensive. Most patients with Kaposi sarcoma ultimately die of opportunistic infections. Thus a major principal of therapy for this tumor is to avoid potentially toxic therapeutic modalities until the bulk of the tumor is extensive or until a vital organ is compromised.

When patients have individual lesions that are unattractive or painful or when lymphatic obstruction causes extensive lower extremity edema, radiation therapy may be beneficial.[88,89] Kaposi sarcoma lesions tend to recur despite intensive radiation therapy. When the oropharynx is radiated, mucositis seems to be especially common.

When cutaneous Kaposi sarcoma is extensive, recombinant interferon-α therapy (10–30 million units/m^2 im, iv, or sc qd) can be useful, especially for patients with circulating CD4 counts greater than 100–200/mm^3.[90–92] Objective tumor responses can be seen in 4–8 weeks, with maximal responses in 12–24 weeks. Late initial responses after many months of therapy occasionally occur. Tumor response may persist for over 1 year, especially when maintenance therapy is given. Because the tumor response is not rapid, interferon-α therapy is not desirable for urgent, life-threatening situations. Adverse effects of interferon-α include confusion, fatigue, myalgias, leukopenia, thrombocytopenia, hepatitis, and cardiomyopathy.

Kaposi sarcoma can cause life-threatening disease by obstructing a vital structure such as the larynx, bronchus, biliary tract, or bowel. Kaposi sarcoma can occasionally infiltrate a vital organ such as the lung and cause fatal hypoxemia. In these life-threatening situations, either radiation therapy or cytotoxic chemotherapy is necessary to produce a rapid and substantial response. The optimal mode of therapy depends on the location and extent of tumor. In appropriate clinical settings, short-term palliation of life-threatening symptoms rather than long-term survival is the therapeutic goal, and thus the immunosuppressive nature of some therapies is not the overriding concern. A variety of chemotherapeutic regimens have been used with some success including vinblastine; etoposide; vincristine; vincristine and vinblastine; vinblastine and bleomycin; doxorubicin, bleomycin, and vincristine.[93,94] The optimal drug regimen for specific situations has not been determined.

Lymphomas of the Hodgkin, non-Hodgkin, and Burkitt types generally are associated with short patient survival regardless of the therapeutic modality chosen. A variety of cytotoxic regimens and irradiation have been used in order to reduce tumor size or palliate specific syndromes such as neurologic dysfunction caused by central nervous system lesions. The response rate has been lower in AIDS patients than in non-AIDS patients, and relapses have been prompt and frequent.[46,95] Whether any regimen prolongs survival and which regimen is optimal have not yet been determined. Patients die as a direct result of lymphoma, as a result of AIDS-related infections, and as a result of chemotherapy-associated infections.

REFERENCES

1. Rothenberg R, Woelfel M, Stoneburner R, et al. Survival with the acquired immunodeficiency syndrome: Experience with 5833 cases in New York City. N Engl J Med. 1987;317:1297–302.
2. Bacchetti P, Osmond D, Chaisson RE, et al. Survival patterns of the first 500 patients with AIDS in San Francisco. J Infect Dis. 1988;157:1044–7.
3. Sande MA, Volberding PA, eds. The Medical Management of AIDS. Philadelphia: WB Saunders; 1988.
4. Moskowitz L, Hensley GT, Chen JC, et al. Immediate causes of death in acquired immunodeficiency syndrome. Arch Pathol Lab Med. 1985;109:735–8.
5. Niedt GW, Schinella RA. Acquired immunodeficiency syndrome. Clinicopathologic study of 56 autopsies. Arch Pathol Lab Med. 1985;109:727–34.
6. Welch K, Finkbeiner W, Alpers C, et al. Autopsy findings in the acquired immune deficiency syndrome. JAMA. 1984;252:1152–9.
7. Lo B, Raffin TA, Cohen NH, et al. Ethical dilemmas about intensive care for patients with AIDS. Rev Infect Dis. 1987;9:1163–7.
8. El Sadr W, Simberkoff M. Survival and prognostic factors in severe *Pneumocystis carinii* pneumonia requiring mechanical ventilation. Am Rev Respir Dis. 1988;137:1264–7.
9. Rogers PL, Lane HC, Henderson DK, et al. Admissions of AIDS patients to a medical intensive care unit: Cause and outcome. Crit Care Med. 1989;17:113–7.
10. Jackson GG, Paul DA, Falk LA, et al. Human immunodeficiency virus (HIV) antigenemia (p24) in the acquired immunodeficiency syndrome and the effect of treatment with zidovudine (AZT). Ann Intern Med. 1988;108:175–80.
11. De Wolf F, Gaudsmit J, DeGans J, et al. Effect of zidovudine on serum human immunodeficiency virus antigen levels in symptom free subjects. Lancet. 1988;1:373–6.
12. Chaisson RE, Leuther MD, Allain JP, et al. Effect of zidovudine on serum human immunodeficiency virus core antigen levels. Arch Intern Med. 1988;148:2151–3.
13. Mitsuya H, Weinhold KJ, Furman PA, et al. 3′-Azido-3′-deoxythymidine (BW A509U): An antiviral agent that inhibits the infectivity and cytopathic effect of human T lymphotropic virus type III 1 (lymphadenopathy associated virus) in vitro. Proc Natl Acad Sci USA. 1985;82:7096–100.
14. Sommadossi JP, Carlisle R. Toxicity of 3′-azido-3′-deoxythymidine and 9-(1,3-dihydroxy-2-propoxymethyl) guanine for normal human hematopoietic progenitor cells in vitro. Antimicrob Agents Chemother. 1987;31:452–4.
15. Hirsch MS. Azidothymidine. AIDS commentary. J Infect Dis. 1988;157:427–30.
16. Fischl MA, Richman DD, Grieco MH, et al. The efficacy of azidothymidine (AZT) in the treatment of patients with AIDS and AIDS-related complex. N Engl J Med. 1987;317:185–202.
17. Richman DD, Fischl MA, Grieco MH, et al. The toxicity of azidothymidine (AZT) in the treatment of patients with AIDS and AIDS related complex. A double blind, placebo controlled trial. N Engl J Med. 1987;317:192–7.
18. Schmitt FA, Bigley JW, McKinnis R, et al. Neuropsychologic outcome of zidovudine (AZT) treatment of patients with AIDS and AIDS related complex. N Engl J Med. 1988;319:1573–8.
19. Pizzo PE, Eddy J, Falloon J, et al. Effect of continuous intravenous infusion of zidovudine (AZT) in children with symptomatic HIV infection. N Engl J Med. 1988;319:889–96.
20. Creagh-Kirk T, Doi P, Andrews E, et al. Survival experience among patients with AIDS receiving zidovudine: Follow-up of patients in a compassionate plea program. JAMA. 1988;260:3009–15.
21. Dournon E, Matheron S, Rozenbaum W, et al. Effects of zidovudine in 365 consecutive patients with AIDS or AIDS related complex. Lancet. 1988;2:1297–302.
22. The Swiss Group for Clinical Studies on the Acquired Immunodeficiency Syndrome (AIDS). Zidovudine for the treatment of thrombocytopenia associated with human immunodeficiency virus. Ann Intern Med. 1988;109:718–21.
23. Pottage JC, Benson CA, Spear JB, et al. Treatment of human immunodeficiency virus related thrombocytopenia with zidovudine. JAMA. 1988;260:3045–8.
24. Walker RE, Parker RI, Kovacs JA, et al. Anemia and erythropoiesis in patients with acquired immunodeficiency syndrome (AIDS) and Kaposi sarcoma treated with zidovudine. Ann Intern Med. 1988;108:372–6.
25. Helbert M, Peddle B, Kocsis A, et al. Acute meningoencephalitis on dose reduction of zidovudine. Lancet. 1988;1:1249–52.
26. Lane HC, Kovacs JA, Feinberg J, et al. Antiretroviral effects of interferon-alpha in AIDS associated Kaposi's sarcoma. Lancet. 1988;2:1218–22.
27. De Wit R, Schattenkerk JKME, Boucher CAB, et al. Clinical and virologic effects of high dose recombinant interferon alpha in disseminated AIDS related Kaposi's sarcoma. Lancet. 1988;2:1214–7.
28. Glatt AE, Chirgwin K, Landesman SH. Treatment of infections associated with human immunodeficiency virus. Current concepts. N Engl J Med. 1988;3189:1439–48.
29. Brenner M, Ognibene FP, Lack EE, et al. Prognostic factors and life expectancy of acquired immunodeficiency syndrome patients with *Pneumocystis carinii* pneumonia. Am Rev Respir Dis. 1987;136:1199–206.
30. Kovacs JA, Hiemenz JW, Macher AM, et al. *Pneumocystis carinii* pneumonia: A comparison between patients with the acquired immunodeficiency syndrome and patients with other immunodeficiencies. Ann Intern Med. 1984;100:663–71.
31. Wharton JM, Coleman DL, Wofsy CB, et al. Trimethoprim-sulfamethoxazole or pentamidine for *Pneumocystis carinii* pneumonia in the acquired immunodeficiency syndrome. A prospective randomized trial. Ann Intern Med. 1986;195:37–44.
32. Gordin FM, Simon GL, Wofsy CB, et al. Adverse reactions to trimethoprim-sulfamethoxazole in patients with the acquired immunodeficiency syndrome. Ann Intern Med. 1984;100:495–9.
33. Sattler FR, Cowan R, Nielsen DM, et al. Trimethoprim-sulfamethoxazole versus pentamidine for therapy of *Pneumocystis* pneumonia: A prospective non crossover study in patients with AIDS. Ann Intern Med. 1988;109:280–7.
34. Waskin H, Stehr-Green JK, Helmick CG, et al. Risk factors for hypoglycemia associated with pentamidine therapy for *Pneumocystis* pneumonia. JAMA. 1988;260:345–7.
35. Conte JE Jr, Hollander H, Golden JA. Inhaled or reduced dose intravenous pentamidine for *Pneumocystis carinii* pneumonia. A pilot study. Ann Intern Med. 1987;107:495–8.

36. Montgomery AB, Debs RJ, Luce JM, et al. Aerosolised pentamidine as sole therapy for *Pneumocystis carinii* pneumonia in patients with acquired immunodeficiency syndrome. Lancet. 1987;2:480–3.
37. Leoung GS, Mills J, Hopewell PC, et al. Dapsone-trimethoprim for *Pneumocystis carinii* pneumonia in the acquired immunodeficiency syndrome. Ann Intern Med. 1986;105:45–8.
38. Allegra CJ, Chabner BA, Tuazon CU, et al. Trimetrexate for the treatment of *Pneumocystis carinii* pneumonia in patients with acquired immunodeficiency syndrome. N Engl J Med. 1987;317:978–85.
39. MacFadden DK, Edelson JD, Hyland RH, et al. Corticosteroids as adjunctive therapy in treatment of *Pneumocystis carinii* pneumonia in patients with acquired immunodeficiency syndrome. Lancet. 1987;1:1477–9.
40. Ognibene FP, Steis RG, Macher AM, et al. Kaposi's sarcoma causing pulmonary infiltrates and respiratory failure in the acquired immunodeficiency syndrome. Ann Intern Med. 1985;102:471–5.
41. Fischl M, Dickinson GM, LaVoie L. Safety and efficacy of sulfamethoxazole and trimethoprim chemoprophylaxis for *Pneumocystis carinii* pneumonia in AIDS. JAMA. 1988;259:1185–9.
42. Navia BA, Petito CK, Gold JWM, et al. Cerebral toxoplasmosis complicating the acquired immune deficiency syndrome: Clinical and neuropathological findings in 27 patients. Ann Neurol. 1986;19:224–38.
43. Luft BJ, Remington JS. Toxoplasmic encephalitis. AIDS commentary. J Infect Dis. 1988;157:1–6.
44. Wanke C, Tuazon CU, Kovacs JA, et al. *Toxoplasma* encephalitis in patients with acquired immune deficiency syndrome: Diagnosis and response to therapy. Am J Trop Med Hyg. 1987;36:509–16.
45. Leport C, Raffi F, Matheron S, et al. Treatment of central nervous system toxoplasmosis with pyrimethamine/sulfadiazine combination in 35 patients with acquired immunodeficiency syndrome. Efficacy of long term continuous therapy. Am J Med. 1988;84:94–100.
46. So YT, Beckstead JH, Davis RL. Primary central nervous system lymphoma in acquired immunodeficiency syndrome: A clinical and pathological study. Ann Neurol. 1986;20:566–72.
47. Kalb RE, Grossman ME. Chronic perianal herpes simplex in immunocompromised hosts. Am J Med. 1986;80:486–90.
48. Melbye M, Grossman RJ, Goedert JS, et al. Risk of AIDS after herpes zoster. Lancet. 1987;1:728–31.
49. Jacobson MA, Mills J. Serious cytomegalovirus disease in the acquired immunodeficiency syndrome (AIDS): Clinical findings, diagnosis, and treatment. Ann Intern Med. 1988;108:585–94.
50. Masur H, Lane HC, Palestine A, et al. Effect of 9-(1,3-dihydroxy-2-propoxymethyl) guanine on serious cytomegalovirus disease in eight immunosuppressed homosexual men. Ann Intern Med. 1986;104:41–4.
51. Laskin OL, Stahl-Bayliss CM, Kalman CM, et al. Use of ganciclovir to treat serious cytomegalovirus infections in patients with AIDS. J Infect Dis. 1987;155:323–7.
52. Felsenstein D, D'Amico DJ, Hirsch MS, et al. Treatment of cytomegalovirus retinitis with 9-[(2-hydroxy-2-(hydroxymethyl)ethoxymethyl)] guanine. Ann Intern Med. 1985;103:377–80.
53. Collaborative DHPG Treatment Study Group. Treatment of serious cytomegalovirus infections with 9-(1,3-dihydroxy-2-propoxymethyl) guanine in patients with AIDS and other immunodeficiencies. N Engl J Med 1986;314:801–5.
54. Henry K, Cantrill H, Fletcher C, et al. Use of intravitreal ganciclovir (dihydroxy propoxy methyl guanine) for cytomegalovirus retinitis in a patient with AIDS. Am J Ophthalmol. 1987;103:17–23.
55. Jacobson MA, O'Donnell JJ, Mills J. Tolerance and efficacy of intermittent intravenous foscarnet therapy for cytomegalovirus retinitis in AIDS patients (Abstract 7179). In: Proceedings of the Fourth International Conference on AIDS. Stockholm: 1988.
56. Walmsley SL, Chew E, Read SE, et al. Treatment of cytomegalovirus retinitis with trisodium phosphonoformate hexahydrate (foscarnet). J Infect Dis. 1988;157:569–72.
57. Bloom JN, Palestine AG. The diagnosis of cytomegalovirus retinitis. Ann Intern Med. 1988;109:963–9.
58. Chachoua A, Dieterich D, Krasinski K, et al. 9-(1,3-2-Propoxymethyl) guanine (ganciclovir) in the treatment of cytomegalovirus gastrointestinal disease with the acquired immunodeficiency syndrome. Ann Intern Med. 1987;107:133–7.
59. Mansell P, Roston K, Hoy J, et al. Treatment of CMV infections in patients with AIDS or following bone marrow transplantation with DHPG (Abstract). In: Proceedings of the International Conference on AIDS. Paris: 1986:62.
60. Reed EC, Bowden RA, Dandliker PS, et al. Treatment of cytomegalovirus pneumonia with gancyclovir and intravenous cytomegalovirus immunoglobulin in patients with bone marrow transplants. Ann Intern Med. 1988;109:783–8.
61. Emanuel D, Cunningham I, Jules-Elysee K, et al. Cytomegalovirus pneumonia after bone marrow transplantation successfully treated with the combination of gancyclovir and high dose intravenous immune globulin. Ann Intern Med. 1988;109:777–82.
62. Klein RS, Harris CA, Small CB, et al. Oral candidiasis in high-risk patients as the initial manifestation of the acquired immunodeficiency syndrome. N Engl J Med. 1984;311:354–8.
63. Rhoads JL, Wright DC, Redfield RR, et al. Chronic vaginal candidiasis in women with human immunodeficiency virus infection. JAMA. 1987;257:3105–7.
64. Dismukes WE. Cryptococcal meningitis in patients with AIDS. J Infect Dis. 1988;157:624–8.
65. Zuger A, Louie E, Holzman RS, et al. Cryptococcal disease in patients with the acquired immunodeficiency syndrome: Diagnostic features and outcome of treatment. Ann Intern Med. 1986;104:234–40.
66. Kovacs JA, Kovacs AA, Polis M. Cryptococcosis in the acquired immunodeficiency syndrome. Ann Intern Med. 1985;103:533–8.
67. Byrne WR, Wajszczuk CP. Cryptococcal meningitis in the acquired immunodeficiency syndrome (AIDS); Successful treatment with fluconazole after failure of amphotericin B. Ann Intern Med. 1988;108:384–5.
68. Stern JJ, Hartman BJ, Sharkey P, et al. Oral fluconazole therapy for patients with acquired immunodeficiency syndrome and cryptococcosis: Experience with 22 patients. Am J Med. 1988;85:477–80.
69. Sugar AM, Saunders C. Oral fluconazole as suppressive therapy of disseminated *Cryptococcus* in patients with acquired immunodeficiency syndrome. Am J Med. 1988;85:481–9.
70. Wheat IJ, Slama TG, Zeckel ML. Histoplasmosis in the acquired immune deficiency syndrome. Am J Med. 1985;78:203–10.
71. Johnson PC, Khardori N, Najjor AF, et al. Progressive disseminated histoplasmosis in patients with acquired immunodeficiency syndrome. Am J Med. 1988;85:152–8.
72. Bronnimann DA, Adam RD, Galgiani JN. Coccidioidomycosis in the acquired immunodeficiency syndrome. Ann Intern Med. 1987;106:372–9.
73. Young LS. *Mycobacterium avium* complex infection. AIDS commentary. J Infect Dis. 1988;157:863–7.
74. Inderlied CB, Young LS, Yamada JK. Determination of in vitro susceptibility of *Mycobacterium avium* complex isolates to antimycobacterial agents by various methods. Antimicrob Agents Chemother. 1987;31:1697–702.
75. Agins BD, Berman DS, Spicehandler D, et al. Effect of combined therapy with ansamycin, clofazimine, ethambutol, and isoniazid for *Mycobacterium avium* infection in patients with AIDS. J Infect Dis. 1989;159:784–7.
76. Masur H, Tuazon CU, Gill V, et al. Effect of combined clofazimine and ansamycin therapy of *Mycobacterium avium-Mycobacterium intracellulare* bacteremia in patients with AIDS. J Infect Dis. 1985;151:523–7.
77. Hawkins CC, Gold JWM, Whimbey E. *Mycobacterium avium* complex infections in patients with the acquired immunodeficiency syndrome. Ann Intern Med. 1986;105:184–8.
78. American Thoracic Society, Centers for Disease Control. Mycobacterioses and the acquired immunodeficiency syndrome. Am Rev Resp Dis. 1987;136:492–6.
79. Schroeder S, Sande MA, Root RK, et al. Incidence of salmonellosis in patients with AIDS. J Infect Dis. 1987;156:998–1002.
80. Perlman DM, Ampel NM, Schifman RB, et al. Persistent *Campylobacter jejuni* infections in patients infected with human immunodeficiency virus (HIV). Ann Intern Med. 1988;108:540–6.
81. Sperber SJ, Schleupner CJ. Salmonellosis during infection with human immunodeficiency virus. Rev Infect Dis. 1987;9:925–34.
82. Smith PD, Lane HC, Gill VJ, et al. Intestinal infections in patients with acquired immunodeficiency syndrome: Etiology and response to therapy. Ann Intern Med. 1988;108:328–33.
83. DeHovitz JA, Pape JW, Boncy M, Johnson WD Jr. Clinical manifestations and therapy of isospora belli infection in patients with the acquired immunodeficiency syndrome. N Engl J Med. 1986;315:87–90.
84. Pape JW, Verdier R, Johnson WD. Treatment and prophylaxis of *Isospora belli* infection in patients with the acquired immunodeficiency syndrome. N Engl J Med. 1989;320:1044–7.
85. Johns DR, Tierney M, Felsenstein D. Alteration in the natural history of neurosyphilis by concurrent infection with human immunodeficiency virus. N Engl J Med. 1987;315:1569–72.
86. Lukehart SA, Hook EW, Baker-Zander SA, et al. Invasion of the central nervous system by *Treponema pallidum*: Implications for diagnosis and treatment. Ann Intern Med. 1988;109:855–62.
87. Musher D. How much penicillin cures early syphilis? Ann Intern Med. 1988;109:849–51.
88. Chak LY, Gill PS, Levine A, et al. Radiation therapy for acquired immunodeficiency syndrome-related Kaposi's sarcoma. J Clin Oncol. 1988;6:863–7.
89. Cooper JS, Eried PR. Defining the role of radiation therapy in the management of epidemic Kaposi's sarcoma. Int J Radiat Oncol Biol Phys. 1987;13:35–9.
90. Volberding PA, Mitsuyasu RT, Golando JP, Spiegel RJ. Treatment of Kaposi's sarcoma with interferon alfa-2b (Intron A). Cancer. 1987;59:620–5.
91. Groopman JE, Gottlieb MS, Goodman J. Recombinant alpha-2 interferon therapy for Kaposi's sarcoma associated with the acquired immunodeficiency syndrome. Ann Intern Med. 1984;100:671–6.
92. Oettgen HF, Safai B. Preliminary observations on the effect of recombinant leukocyte A interferon in homosexual men with Kaposi's sarcoma. N Engl J Med. 1983;308:1071.
93. Volberding PA, Abrams DI, Conant M. Vinblastine therapy for Kaposi's sarcoma in the acquired immunodeficiency syndrome. Ann Intern Med. 1985;103:335–8.
94. Kaplan L, Abrams D, Volberding P. Treatment of Kaposi's sarcoma in acquired immunodeficiency syndrome with an alternating vincristine-vinblastine regimen. Cancer Treat Rep. 1986;70:1121–2.
95. Gill PS, Levine PM, Krailo M, et al. AIDS related malignant lymphoma: Results of prospective treatment trials. J Clin Oncol. 1987;5:1322–8.

111. AIDS VACCINES

MARY LOU CLEMENTS

Since human immunodeficiency virus type 1 (HIV-1) can be incorporated into the human genome and persist there in a dormant state for an indefinite period, it is unlikely that antiviral treatment will ever eradicate the virus in an infected person. For this reason, an effective vaccine is the only foreseeable intervention to prevent HIV-1 transmission, infection, and disease. Recent advances in molecular biology, immunology, and biochemistry have made it possible to develop and produce new vaccines and approaches for immunization against HIV-1 infection. The fact that most or all HIV-infected individuals will eventually develop the acquired immunodeficiency syndrome (AIDS) makes it necessary to design a vaccine that will not only protect against disease but will prevent HIV-1 infection. Such a goal will undoubtedly be difficult to achieve since none of the current, highly effective vaccines have been able to provide complete protection against virus infection. Moreover, the paucity of knowledge of the immune correlates of protection against HIV-1 infection, the high mutation rate of HIV-1 strains, and the potential for immunopathogenicity of HIV-1 viral products and immune enhancement all pose special challenges to the goal to develop and evaluate an effective HIV-1 vaccine. Several obstacles and strategies for HIV-1 vaccine development that have been reviewed elsewhere are discussed in this chapter.[1–11]

ISSUES RELATED TO VACCINE DEVELOPMENT

Genetic Variation

One potential obstacle in the development of an effective HIV-1 vaccine is the high mutation rate of HIV-1 strains that results in considerable genetic diversity of HIV-1 isolates and immunologically different subtypes.[12–18] Several constant and variable domains that contain antigenic sites that evoke neutralizing antibodies to HIV-1 have been identified in the envelope glycoprotein 120 (gp120).[19–24] The most substantial variation among HIV-1 isolates is located in the NH_2 terminal region (referred to as the hypervariable region) of gp120.[25] Differences in amino acid content in this region range from 3 to 30 percent in U.S. isolates[13,14,21] and up to 50 percent in African isolates.[13,16,26] Such sequence variations in the envelope gene of HIV-1 may be an important feature that enables the virus to escape host immune surveillance mechanisms.[14,25,27] For lentiviruses related to HIV-1 such as visna virus, there is evidence that progressive changes in the envelope gene lead to changes in envelope antigenicity and the inability for antibodies to effectively neutralize subsequent virus variants.[28] This could pose a particular problem for vaccine development since an effective vaccine to prevent HIV-1 infection would need to elicit an immune response against a number of HIV-1 strains or subtypes.[18]

Mode of HIV-1 Transmission

An effective vaccine strategy must take into account whether HIV-1 infection is transmitted by virus-infected cells, free virus particles, or both.[7] Since HIV-1 infection is likely to be transmitted by virus-infected cells as well as by free virus particles, it is unlikely that humoral antibody alone will be able to protect a person against dormant or proviral forms of HIV-1 that are hidden in lymphocytes or macrophages. In this case, other forms of immunity, such as cell-mediated cytotoxic reactions, will be required for killing virus-infected cells before or after they express viral proteins.

Correlates of Immunity

Much of the current understanding of the immune responses to HIV-1 is derived from responses of individuals who have already been infected with HIV-1 and who are at various stages of the clinical spectrum.[29–31] Other factors are likely to influence the outcome of an HIV-1 infection including the route of virus entry, the size of the virus inoculation, the virulence of the infecting virus and of subsequent progeny viruses,[17] the presence of coinfecting pathogens, the duration of infection, the underlying nutritional and immunologic status of the individual, the age and sex of the person, and possibly genetic factors.

Most individuals infected with HIV-1 develop a variety of humoral and cell-mediated immune responses to HIV-1 in the face of persistent viral replication or latency.

Neutralizing Antibody. Neutralizing antibody that blocks or restricts viral replication is an important correlate of protective immunity for many viral diseases.[31a] Vaccines that stimulate the production of neutralizing antibodies have been shown to be highly effective in preventing such diseases as hepatitis B, polio, and influenza.[31a] Neutralizing antibodies to HIV-1 appear to be directed primarily against the viral envelope of gp120,[18,20–22,29] but they may also be directed to some extent against the core (gag) protein.[32]

Low levels of antibodies with neutralizing activity have been detected in serum of HIV-1-seropositive individuals at all stages of clinical infection.[29–31,33] Some studies have reported a correlation between the ability of a patient's serum to neutralize HIV-1 in vitro and disease status,[22,29–31] but others have not.[21,33] This suggests that the presence of neutralizing antibody per se does not fully protect HIV-1-infected individuals against the development of disease. The levels of neutralizing activity detected may have been influenced in part by the sensitivity of the assay employed and a general decline in immune competence of infected individuals with progressive disease.

The relevance of titers of neutralizing antibody to protective immunity is not known. Cats with weak neutralizing antibody titers of only 1:2 to 1:8 to the retrovirus feline leukemia virus were able to resist virus challenge.[34] However, a recent study conducted in chimpanzees by Prince and coworkers failed to demonstrate any protective effect of high-titered neutralizing antibody against intravenous challenge with a 400 ($TCID_{50}$) tissue culture infectious dose of HIV-1.[35] It is possible that the high challenge dose may have overwhelmed any protective effect of neutralizing antibody.

The high rate of mutation among HIV-1 strains resulting in genomic heterogeneity within the *env* gene that encodes for gp120 poses a significant problem since neutralizing antibodies induced in animals against gp120 derived from HIV-1-infected cells appear to be type specific.[18,20,21,36] A key question is whether an antigen representing conserved epitopes from a single virus type will induce antibodies that will neutralize less related variants. If so, the design of effective polyvalent synthetic HIV-1 vaccines may depend on the selection of conserved regions of gp120 that contain neutralizing epitopes.[18,36]

Cell-Mediated Immune Responses. Relatively little is known about which cell-mediated immune responses might provide protection against HIV-1 infection or disease. In a murine retrovirus system, mice that developed cell-mediated cytotoxic responses to Friend murine leukemia virus were protected against leukemia, whereas those that developed only neutralizing antibody died.[37] This observation and studies in other viral systems suggest that cellular anti-HIV-1 immune responses may be required to destroy HIV-1-infected cells and restrict virus replication.[38,39]

ANTIBODY-DEPENDENT CELLULAR CYTOTOXICITY. One of the immune responses against murine or feline retroviruses is antibody-dependent, cell-mediated cytotoxicity (ADCC) directed against virus-infected cells.[40–43] ADCC killing depends on effector cells with Fc receptors for immunoglobulin (Ig) that bind and kill Ig-coated target cells that express viral gene products. Antibodies active in ADCC are present in serum from patients infected with HIV-1.[44–48] Also, there is evidence that sera from healthy HIV-1-seropositive individuals mediate higher levels of ADCC activity as compared with sera obtained from subjects with AIDS.[44,48] This suggests that ADCC may represent a protective immune response, or as with cytomegalovirus,[38] it may be important for recovery from viral infection.

Protective immunity in animals against disease with passively administered antibodies has been induced 1 month after virus inoculation with Friend murine leukemia virus or feline leukemia virus.[43,49–51] This suggests that serum antibody with potent ADCC activity might help control cell-to-cell spread of the virus by killing HIV-1-infected cells early in the infection. ADCC might also contribute to host surveillance against residual virus-infected cells that remain dormant but could emerge and express viral protein on their cell surface at a later time.[47,48]

Different studies suggest that the location of the determinant for ADCC activity is within the transmembrane gp41,[45] the gp120,[41,47] or the p24[44] protein.

NATURAL KILLER CYTOLYTIC ACTIVITY. One study demonstrated that HIV-1-infected peripheral blood mononuclear cells that mediated HLA-unrestricted natural killer (NK) cytolytic activity appeared to be higher in healthy HIV-1-infected individuals than in those with AIDS.[46] This suggests that NK cells may also be important in early infection.

CYTOTOXIC T-CELL ACTIVITY. Cytotoxic T lymphocytes specific for HIV-1 proteins, including the envelope and gag proteins and those with reverse transcriptase activity, have been detected in HIV-1-seropositive persons.[52–54] Weinhold and colleagues[54] detected cell-mediated cytotoxicity (CMC) against autologous target cells bearing the HIV-1 gp120 envelope protein in HIV-1-seropositive patients but not in HIV-1-seronegative individuals. Healthy HIV-1-infected persons had the highest CMC, whereas those with the AIDS-related compex (ARC) or AIDS showed progressively less reactivity. The gp120-specific cytolysis appeared to be mediated by non-T-cell effectors that resembled NK cells phenotypically. CMC was not restricted by the major histocompatibility complex and was highly augmented by interleukin-2 (IL-2). Whether all or part of CMC might be antibody dependent is not known. A totally antibody-independent lytic mechanism would require induction of a specific receptor, whereas antibody-dependent lysis would make use of existing antibodies that are capable of interacting with resident cells bearing Fc receptors.[54]

Cytotoxic cells, with their inherent ability to recognize and lyse virally infected cells, could limit cell-to-cell spread. On the other hand, they could cause a deleterious immune response if the HIV-1 vaccine is not fully protective. For example, when gp120 is liberated from cells during viral replication, it could bind to normal CD4-bearing cells and make them targets for lympholysis mediated by HIV-1 gp120 effector cells. Studies by Plata and coworkers[55] suggest that CD8-positive T lymphocytes with cytotoxic activities induce local inflammation in the lungs by their interaction with HIV-1-infected macrophages.

COMPLEMENT-MEDIATED CYTOTOXIC ANTIBODY. It is important to determine which components of the immunologic responses protect chimpanzees that have been infected with HIV-1 against the development of disease. One immunologic difference between HIV-1-infected humans and inoculated chimpanzees that has been noted is the development of complement-mediated cytotoxic antibody (ACC) for HIV-1 cells in chimpanzees but not in humans, despite the presence of a high titer of broadly reactive neutralizing antibodies in both species.[56] The pre-existence of broadly reactive ACC and neutralizing antibody ready to kill a cell that has just begun to express virus might be important in preventing or eliminating disease.

Secretory Mucosal Immunity. Secretory antibodies in the mucosal secretions are important mediators of protection in other viral diseases,[57] but their role in protective immunity against HIV-1 replication and infection is not known. Several investigators have found secretory IgA in blood, saliva, and other mucosal fluids of HIV-1 patients with AIDS and ARC.[58] To protect against sexually transmitted HIV-1 infection, an effective AIDS vaccine may need to stimulate secretory immunity to prevent viral entry and replication through mucosal sites.

Risks of Immunopathology

No experiments to date have indicated that HIV-1 vaccine candidates using HIV envelope or core proteins as antigens cause toxic effects in animals[59] or in humans. However, some experts have expressed concern that immunization with vaccine preparations that contain certain viral proteins of HIV-1 might cause immunosuppression and immunopathology.[59–63]

Several regions within the envelope protein of HIV-1 bind with high affinity to CD4 lymphocytes.[64,65] The binding of the gp120 vaccine component could mask epitopes of CD4 that would otherwise function in immunologic recognition.[66] In addition, it has been suggested that HIV-1 envelope proteins such as gp41 are partly responsible for T-cell loss and the decline in function that occurs with AIDS.[67–69] Similar immunodeficiencies that occur after infection with murine and feline leukemia virus are ascribed to the transmembrane protein.[70] Viral gp41 or a factor related to this protein may also be partially responsible for in vivo impairment of monocyte chemotaxis or the ability of monocytes to migrate to the foci of inflammation.[70]

Anti-CD4 antibodies and HIV-1 gp120 share binding sites on the CD4 molecule,[71] and anti-CD4 antibodies may mimic gp120.[63] Since CD4 serves as a receptor for both HIV-1 and class II histocompatibility molecules, an immune response to HIV-1 might result in a cross-reactive response against class II bearing cells and an idiotypic response against cells expressing CD4.[41,63] Such autoimmune mechanisms may be involved in CD4 depletion with AIDS. This suggests that HIV-1-seronegative persons vaccinated against HIV-1 might be subject to more severe disease if the vaccine is not protective and they become infected with HIV-1.[63]

Structural homologies have been identified between HIV-1 proteins and the following endogenously produced regulatory proteins: HIV-1 gag (core) protein and thymosin α_1,[32] gp120 and neuroleukin,[72] and gp41 and IL-2.[73] These relationships raise the question about whether an antibody response to HIV-1 proteins will cross react with lymphoid and thymic epithelial cells involved in the production of these peptides.[59] Clearly, evidence of these toxic effects should be sought in extensive animal testing of vaccine candidates before they are evaluated in humans.

Immune Enhancement

The phenomenon of immune enhancement has been associated with vaccination against dengue[74] and is of theoretic concern with HIV-1 vaccines.[62,62a] Robinson and coworkers have identified heat-stable and heat-labile factors in the serum of HIV-infected patients that in combination appear to enhance HIV-1 infection in vitro. The enhancing activity appears to be related to antibody (possibly to viral protein) and activation of the alternate pathway of complement.[75] Data in vitro and in vivo suggest that the alternate pathway of complement is chronically activated in patients with ARC more than in those with lymphadenopathy syndrome.[76] Thus, high HIV-1-enhancing activity mediated by antibodies may result in a depletion of complement and worsening of disease. HIV-1 vaccine candidates should be evaluated for their ability to stimulate antibody formation that enhances infection.

PRECLINICAL TESTS

Before a candidate AIDS vaccine is evaluated in humans, a number of tests to assess the safety, toxicity, and immunogenicity of the vaccine are usually conducted in vitro, in small animals, and subsequently in primates.[1,7]

In Vitro Tests

A major constraint in the development and evaluation of AIDS vaccines is the lack of uniform reference reagents and standardized methods to assess neutralization titers, cell-mediated immune responses, and immunopathogenicity of vaccine candidates.[7] Several methods have been used to measure neutralizing antibodies to HIV-1, and all are subject to technical limitations.[3,77] One approach involves inoculating cell cultures with HIV-1 and subsequently quantitating the virus production by detecting reverse transcriptase activity or core antigen.[29,78] Another, more sensitive and convenient method involves the use of vesicular stomatitis virus to form pseudotype viruses with envelopes bearing HIV-1 antigens and then monitoring their cytopathic effect.[33] Other methods measure cytolytic effects of HIV-1 in human T-cell leukemia/lymphoma virus-1 (HTLV-1)-infected cell lines.[21,79] The relevance of antibodies for the neutralization of HIV-1 as measured by each of these tests is not clear. More recently, a plaque reduction microassay to measure neutralizing antibodies was developed.[80] This assay, which measures the percent reduction of giant cells (syncytia formation) in the presence of test serum, may be more sensitive than are the other assays.

Tests in Animals

Another major problem in the development of a safe, effective AIDS vaccine is the lack of relevant animal models to evaluate whether immunization with a candidate AIDS vaccine will prevent HIV-1 infection and development of disease.[7] Candidate HIV-1 vaccines are generally administered to small animals (e.g., mice, guinea pigs, and rabbits) initially to determine whether they stimulate the production of neutralizing antibodies in serum and other immune responses to the HIV-1.[7]

The chimpanzee is the only animal model that can be readily infected with HIV-1.[81–84] After intravenous inoculation with HIV-1, virus can be recovered from peripheral mononuclear cells, and HIV-1-specific immune responses can be detected in the blood.[81,82] However, with few exceptions, infected chimpanzees, some of whom have been followed for as long as 5 years, remain clinically and immunologically well in contrast to HIV-1-infected humans, who develop AIDS.[81,82] These issues together with their endangered status, limited availability, and cost make the use of chimpanzees for screening of AIDS vaccines problematic.[3,77,85,86] For these reasons, many experts question the validity of the chimpanzee model for human AIDS vaccine.[77,85,86] Yet others believe that a candidate HIV-1 vaccine should demonstrate an ability to induce protective immunity in chimpanzees before the vaccine is tested in humans.[7,77,87] Since many of the chimpanzees designated for AIDS vaccine testing have already been infected with hepatitis B or non-A, non-B viruses, it is possible that those chimpanzees that are infected with another infectious agent may have an altered immune response to an HIV-1 vaccination, challenge, or both.

To date, there has been no standardization of the protocols for vaccination (i.e., number of doses, spacing of doses) or for virus challenge (i.e., dose and route of virus inoculation, cell-free vs. cell-associated virus inoculum, or homologous versus heterologous challenge) in chimpanzees or other animals. As yet, chimpanzees previously immunized with various prototype AIDS vaccines and subsequently challenged with HIV-1 have not been protected against virus infection.[2,85,87] However, the challenge doses used have been as high as 300,000 HIV-1 tissue culture infectious doses ($TCID_{50}$) and all challenges to date have been given intravenously. Experimental HIV-1 infection resulting from virus challenge that employs such high doses and the intravenous route of transmission probably does not mimic human HIV-1 infection transmitted by sexual activity.

An alternate animal model is the rhesus macaque monkey, which can be persistently infected with simian immunodeficiency virus (SIV).[7,85,88–90] SIV rapidly induces an immune deficiency syndrome remarkably similar to AIDS, with wasting, opportunistic infections, and a high fatality rate.[89] Studies in the SIV system may provide insights about the role of cell-mediated immune responses and neutralizing antibody in protection against virus infection and the development of simian AIDS. Prototype vaccine candidates can also be developed in the SIV system and tested for safety and efficacy in macaques. Whether genetic and biologic differences between the two viruses and their hosts will limit the usefulness of this model for vaccine screening is not known.

Lentiviruses, which are genetically and biologically similar to HIV-1, have been isolated from household cats, domestic cattle, and several other ungulate (hoofed) mammals.[91–93] The availability of cats and cattle in contrast to primates and the ability of these lentiviruses to induce disease after infection make them potential animal models for the evaluation of vaccines applicable to HIV-1. Animal studies with ungulate and feline retroviruses may also provide insights about host-specific immunologic responses and vaccine-induced immune enhancement to retrovirus infections. One study in which goats were immunized with inactivated caprine arthritis-encephalitis virus suggested that a vaccine-enhanced immune response to CAEV virus caused severe destructive arthritis.[94]

VACCINE APPROACHES

An ideal vaccine should possess all of the antigens capable of protecting against infection with HIV-1 and its antigenic variants but not cause the harmful immunologic effects that occur with natural infection. In addition, the vaccine should be easily administered, inexpensive, stable, and readily available. Several vaccine approaches are listed in Table 1.

The most common approach used to develop an HIV-1 vaccine is to employ protein subunits of the virus that are produced by genetic engineering and recombinant DNA methods. This approach offers several advantages[65]: (*1*) recombinant proteins are safe to prepare, and no genetic material is used for vaccination; (*2*) purified recombinant proteins can be more efficiently produced than can purified native viral proteins obtained from virus-infected cells; and (*3*) synthetic peptides can be prepared that bear neutralizing epitopes representing a spectrum of envelope sequences.

There are also several concerns with the subunit approach for an HIV-1 vaccine. First, a single viral protein such as the envelope might not be immunogenic enough because the antigen may not be presented or structurally configured to be recog-

TABLE 1. Potential HIV-1 Vaccine Approaches

Immunization of HIV-1–seronegative persons
Subunit preparations:
Recombinant envelope glycoproteins (gp120, gp160)
Native envelope glycoproteins
Synthetic envelope peptides
Synthetic core proteins
Live non-HIV virus recombinants (vaccinia or adenovirus)
Inactivated (killed) HIV-1 vaccine
Live attenuated (nonpathogenic) HIV-1 strains
Anti-idiotypes
Passive immunization
Immunization of HIV-1–seropositive persons
Inactivated HIV-1 virus vaccine
Hyperimmunization with non–HIV-1 vaccines

nized by the host immune system. Second, a subunit vaccine may protect against only one strain rather than against multiple variants. Thus, a combination of antigens rather than a single peptide or protein may be required to stimulate protective immunity.[7]

Subunit Vaccines: Recombinant Envelope Proteins

The HIV-1 envelope protein is a 160 kD glycosylated protein (gp160) that is composed of a gp120 external glycoprotein and a gp41 transmembrane protein.[95–97] The envelope glycoprotein is an accessible target for antibody-directed neutralization and cytotoxic immunity because of its location on the outer surface of the virus.[20,65,95–101] On the basis of animal retroviral models[102–104] it may be possible to prevent primary virus infection with a vaccine incorporating all or part of the envelope gp120 and, to a lesser extent, the transmembrane gp41. One approach to constructing such a vaccine is to clone the appropriate gene sequences of envelope glycoproteins and to express these proteins through genetic engineering techniques in eukaryotic (mammalian, insect, or yeast) or prokaryotic (*Escherichia coli*) cell cultures.[5,7,41,65,100,105–108] Such recombinant glycoproteins have induced neutralizing antibodies in animals and in vitro against the homologous virus but not against less related HIV-1 variants.[7,20,21,97,98,100] This suggested that an effective gp120 vaccine might need to incorporate envelope proteins or peptides containing selected sequences from the variable regions of different isolates to provide group-specific neutralizing antibodies.

Native gp120 is heavily glycosylated.[101] However, recombinant envelope proteins lacking natural sugar residues appear to be effective immunogens since these sugars are not required for the induction of neutralizing antibodies.[7,65] Krohn and colleagues[109] have shown that gp120 also contains an immunogenic T-cell epitope that will evoke a group-specific cellular immune response.

A recombinant gp120 envelope vaccine preparation expressed in Chinese hamster ovary cells stimulated neutralizing antibodies in rabbits and guinea pigs,[99,108] but it failed to protect chimpanzees against experimental challenge with HIV-1[109a] and has not been tested in humans. The first vaccine preparation that has been evaluated in humans in the United States is a recombinant envelope gp160 gene product.[105,106,108] The HIV-1 gp160 gene was inserted into the baculovirus genome, and the recombinant baculovirus was cultured in an insect cell line from which the gp160 was extracted and purified.[105,108] The vaccine stimulated neutralizing antibodies but no toxic reactions in animals.[2] This subunit envelope protein vaccine prototype does appear to elicit immunologic responses in humans,[2] but the functional significance of these antibodies is not yet known.

Subunit Vaccines: Native Proteins

Another subunit approach is to isolate and purify natural gp120 envelope glycoprotein from cells infected with HIV-1.[7,9] Goats, horses, rhesus monkeys, and chimpanzees immunized with native gp120 developed low to moderate titers of neutralizing antibodies but no toxic reactions.[7,109,110] However, the production of native HIV-1 products is hazardous for laboratory workers.

Subunit Vaccines: Synthetic Envelope Peptides

Another subunit approach involves the chemical synthesis of peptide segments of HIV-1 protein, and it has the advantage that large quantities of peptide antigens without other contaminating material can be produced.[111–113] To be effective immunogens, synthetic peptides or polypeptides must incorporate the amino acid sequences that are important for binding or cellular attachment and for inducing neutralizing antibody, cellular reactivity, or both.[111] Synthetic peptides must also be presented in the appropriate steric configuration so that they will be accessible to antibodies and B cells and T cells will recognize the different antigenic determinants on the molecules.[113–115] Several methods can be used to predict the amino acid sequences that contain epitopes from conserved regions of different isolates that are recognized by both B and T cells.[114,115] Since synthetic peptides are weak immunogens, they will require appropriate adjuvants and delivery systems and possibly need a carrier molecule before they can be used as a potent vaccine.[116]

Non-neutralizing domains should be excluded since they could sterically hinder critical epitopes or elicit blocking antibodies and interfere with the action of neutralizing antibodies.[74] In addition, coating of HIV-1 by non-neutralizing antibodies could lead to enhancement of virus uptake by Fc receptor–bearing cells such as monocytes and macrophages,[62a] as has been reported for dengue virus.[74] This may be important since human monocytes and macrophages are capable of supporting HIV-1 replication.[117]

Immunogenic peptide products include C21E, peptide sequences 732–735, and PB1. Antibodies against a conserved part of the central region of gp120, referred to as C21E, have been shown to block virus replication and mediate ADCC.[24] Peptide sequences 735–752 mimic epitopes found in native HIV-1 transmembrane gp41.[109] PB1, a 180 amino acid peptide of gp120 expressed in *E. coli*, elicited high titers of cross-neutralizing antibody in goats.[109]

Subunit Vaccine: Synthetic Core Proteins

Yet another approach is to use a synthetic protein (p17) that is part of the core proteins of HIV-1.[32] There is evidence in humans that HIV-1-infected persons who remain asymptomatic have higher titers of antibodies to p24 (the core protein) than do those who manifested AIDS or ARC.[118,119] An antiserum prepared against a naturally occurring peptide from the thymus gland, thymosin α_1, which is similar in amino acid composition to the (core) protein of HIV-1, weakly neutralized HIV-1 and blocked its replication in H9 cells in vitro.[32] In addition, a synthetic p17 protein induced neutralizing antibodies in rabbits.[32] Since the core region is highly conserved among HIV-1 isolates, a vaccine directed against this protein might overcome the problem of genetic drift of HIV-1 strains.

Live Virus Recombinants

In another approach, genes encoding for the HIV-1 envelope protein can be inserted in a non-HIV-1, which then serves as a vehicle for producing the HIV-1 protein. Vectors used for this purpose include vaccinia virus, the virus used for smallpox vaccine,[120–123] and an attenuated adenovirus that is used to immunize army recruits against respiratory disease caused by adenovirus.[124]

Buller and colleagues[125] constructed thymidine kinase–negative (tk−) vaccinia virus recombinants by inserting a variety of DNA coding sequences into the thymidine kinase gene of vaccinia virus and demonstrated that the tk− recombinants were less pathogenic for mice than was wild-type virus. This genetic modification attenuated the vaccinia virus, as evidenced by a reduction in its ability to initiate and maintain a viremia.[125] Moreover, with the insertion of foreign genes into the thymidine kinase gene, reversion of tk− to tk+ virus is unlikely to occur.

Several investigators have inserted cloned genes encoding HIV-1 envelope gp120 or gp160 from the HIV-1 into the DNA of vaccinia.[121,122] Chakrabarti and coworkers demonstrated that the envelope protein expressed by a gp160-recombinant vaccinia virus reacted by immunoprecipitation with sera from unrelated AIDS patients and that a single inoculation with purified recombinant HIV-1 vaccinia induced antibodies to gp120 in mice.[122]

Several studies have demonstrated that primates immunized

with a recombinant vaccinia virus expressing the complete HIV gp160 envelope gene developed cell-mediated immune responses to HIV-1 envelope glycoproteins.[121,126,127] In one study, the chimpanzees were subsequently challenged with a 100 tissue culture infectious dose ($TCID_{50}$) of HIV-1.[2] The results indicated that prior immunization with the HIV-1 gp160–vaccinia recombinant had primed the immune system of the chimpanzees for developing neutralizing antibodies to HIV-1 envelope proteins but did not prevent HIV-1 infection.[2]

Zagury and others conducted a small trial in Zaire to determine the safety and immunogenicity of an HIV-1 gp160–vaccinia recombinant virus in healthy HIV-1-seronegative adult volunteers.[128,129] Twelve volunteers were inoculated intradermally with recombinant vaccinia virus that expressed the complete gp160 envelope protein of the HTLV-III_B strain of HIV-1. No adverse effects or immune defects were detected after immunization. The vaccine induced antibodies to vaccinia and a low level of neutralizing antibodies to HTLV-III_B antigens. About 3 months after the primary vaccination, one vaccinated individual was boosted with intravenously administered, paraldehyde-fixed autologous cells that had been infected in vitro with the HTLV-III_B gp160–vaccinia virus recombinant. He was boosted again 10 and 12 months after primary vaccination with a gp160 preparation derived from an HTLV-III_B clone by using a hybrid vaccinia virus/bacteriophage T7 expression system.[129] This complicated immunization induced neutralizing antibodies against two divergent HIV-1 strains that persisted for over a year after the original vaccination and elicited group-specific, cell-mediated immune responses and cell-mediated cytotoxicity against infected T4 cells. Since these results were observed in only one individual, they should be viewed with caution. Nevertheless, this trial demonstrated for the first time that group-specific cell-mediated and humoral immune responses to vaccination against HIV-1 can be induced in humans. This vaccination approach is not feasible for use on a larger scale unless another method for boosting can be used to replace the autologous vaccinia virus recombinant–infected cells.[129] Another trial with a vaccinia recombinant expressing the genes for HIV gp160 has been initiated in the United States.[2,130]

The low cost, ease of administration, and high degree of stability under field conditions make this type of vaccine approach attractive for use in developing countries.[120] However, there are several possible disadvantages to this approach. Infrequent (but severe) complications that have been associated with smallpox vaccination include generalized vaccinia, encephalitis, vaccinia necrosum, and accidental self-inoculation.[131] The ability of the vaccinia virus to produce a progressive infection in immunodeficient individuals is a serious risk,[131] and a reaction of this type in an asymptomatic man infected with HIV-1 was recently reported.[132] Of special concern is the use of vaccinia–HIV-1 recombinants in persons who may have contact with immunosuppressed, HIV-1-infected persons since transmission of vaccinia virus infection from a vaccinated individual to an unvaccinated person can occur.

It may be possible to further attenuate the vaccinia virus by incorporating the gene for a lymphokine such as IL-2 into its genome.[133] IL-2 is secreted by CD4 lymphocytes in response to antigenic stimulation and is important for the activation of specific and nonspecific immune responses.[133] Ramshaw and colleagues showed that thymic nude mice infected with the vaccinia–IL-2 recombinant cleared their virus infection rapidly whereas mice infected with the unaltered vaccinia strain developed progressive vaccinia disease.[134] This suggests that live virus vaccines that express IL-2 might minimize or eliminate the complications associated with inadvertent transmission of vaccine virus to immunodeficient persons. Concomitant expression of IL-2 or other lymphokines with HIV-1 antigens in live recombinant vaccines may be particularly important for the wide-scale use of an HIV-1–vaccinia recombinant vaccine in populations where HIV-1 is endemic and prior screening is not practical.[134]

Killed Virus Vaccine

To prepare a safe whole HIV-1 vaccine, it will be necessary to destroy (inactivate) the infectivity of the virus by disrupting the function of the viral nucleic acid but preserving the functional activity of the relevant protective antigens.[135] Inactivation of the virus can be accomplished by the use of formalin, psoralen, B propriolactone, irradiation, or heat.

Protection against retroviral disease has been induced by inactivated virus vaccines in animal studies.[136] Immunization of rhesus monkeys with formalin-inactivated whole SIV, type C, retrovirus containing the adjuvant threonyl muramyl dipeptide provided full protection against intravenous challenge with a heterologous (type D) retrovirus.[136] However, in other trials, inactivated type C SIV vaccine given with immune stimulatory complexes (ISCOMS) or threonyl muranyl dipeptides failed to protect rhesus monkeys or macaques against intravenous challenge with a homologous rhesus SIV.[86] In another study an inactivated whole SIV (type C) vaccine with an adjuvant appeared to partially protect macaques against experimental challenge with homologous SIV administered intramuscularly 1 week after the fifth immunization (R. Derrosier et al., manuscript in preparation). After challenge, two of six vaccinated macaques remained clinically and immunologically well, with no evidence of viremia or anamnestic antibody response, whereas all seven unvaccinated challenged macaques became infected and most died. Additional studies are needed to further investigate the protective capability of inactivated SIV and HIV-1 vaccines.

Immunization of HIV-1-Seropositive Individuals

Another approach has been taken by Salk and others[135,139] in an attempt to protect persons already infected with HIV-1 and to prevent infants born to HIV-1-infected mothers from developing AIDS. The rationale for this strategy is based on the long incubation period between HIV-1 infection and the development of disease.[137,138] This suggests that a postinfection intervention, like that for hepatitis B virus infection,[140] might be feasible to prevent the progression of immunologic disease in healthy HIV-1 carriers and, possibly, to halt deterioration in symptomatic carriers whose disease is not far advanced. This would be accomplished by inducing cytotoxic mechanisms to destroy HIV-1 and HIV-1 antigen-producing cells.[135] If successful, HIV-1 would remain as a latent infection in a proviral form within infected cells. Also, immunized HIV-1 carriers might have a reduced ability to transmit the infection. The availability of an effective intervention for HIV-1-seropositive individuals could increase voluntary HIV-1 testing, identification of cases, and the opportunity to initiate early treatment of infected persons.[135]

A postexposure vaccine trial with killed SIV is being conducted in rhesus monkeys.[139] Also, a small trial with an HIV-1 preparation inactivated by γ-irradiation has been initiated in HIV-1-seropositive persons in California.[135,139] Yet another postinfection trial in which 10 patients with AIDS are receiving their own infected cells and inactivated HIV-1 is being conducted in Zaire.[139]

Nonpathogenic Variants

It is possible to produce genetically engineered nonpathogenic variants by rendering them unable to replicate but able to express all other antigens.[141] A mutant of HIV-1 (designated X10-1) that has a deletion of a 200 base pair segment spanning the last 14 base pairs of the envelope gene and the 3′ *orf* genes was able to replicate in and infect cells but did not kill normal human

T cells in vitro.[141] Such a noncytopathic mutant might be used to make an inactivated virus vaccine that would be less likely to cause disease than would a vaccine prepared from a pathogenic virus.

Anti-idiotype

HIV-1 isolates appear to use CD4 as a receptor.[142] Thus, one approach to vaccines to prevent HIV-1 infection is to generate an antibody-based vaccine, such as an anti-CD4 idiotype vaccine that would mimic the CD4 antigen and bind to HIV-1 envelope glycoprotein.[143,144] Koprowski and colleagues immunized mice with a protein from the HIV-1.[7,144] They then immunized mice with the first antibody (Ab1) and induced the animals to make a second antibody (Ab2) whose binding site resembled the original antigen from the HIV-1. Subsequently, Ab2 was used as an antigen to induce mice to make a third generation of antibodies (Ab3) that should bind to the HIV-1. Thus, Ab3 would mimic the CD4 receptor for the HIV-1.[143] Such anti-idiotype vaccines might induce a broadly reactive response, and no infectious material or antigens from HIV-1 would be used.[144]

One monoclonal anti-idiotype raised against a monoclonal antibody (Leu3a) to CD4 in mice reacted with gp120 in Western blot analysis and partly neutralized one HIV-1 isolate.[145] Dalgleish and colleagues[143] showed that a repeated-dose regimen in mice stimulated polyclonal anti-idiotypic antibodies that neutralized three different isolates of HIV-1 and one isolate of HIV-2. This suggests that this approach might overcome the diversity in HIV-1 isolates.

Immunizing with an anti-CD4 preparation could be harmful since anti-idiotype antibodies to CD4 could block CD4 epitopes on T cells that are responsible for helper activity.[146] Immunosuppression in mice has been observed when large quantities of anti-CD4 were given,[147] but it is hoped that the low quantities of anti-CD4 needed to induce an anti-idiotype response against HIV-1 would not be immunosuppressive.[143,146]

PASSIVE IMMUNOTHERAPY

Passive immunotherapy has been suggested as a way to prevent HIV-1 infection in infants born to HIV-1-infected mothers and to prevent the development of ARC and AIDS in HIV-1-infected persons. Preliminary studies were conducted by Prince and colleagues with anti-HIV-1 globulin extracted from HIV-1-infected individuals.[35] The serum was fractionated and purified to inactivate HIV-1. One unimmunized chimpanzee and four chimpanzees immunized with serum (1 or 10 ml/kg of body weight) containing high titers of neutralizing antibody were challenged with 400 tissue culture infectious doses of HIV-1. All of the chimpanzees became infected; the high-titered anti-HIV-1 globulin preparation did not alter the incubation period between the virus challenge and manifestation of viremia or seroconversion. However, it is possible that the dose employed for challenge may have overwhelmed any protective effect of neutralizing antibody. Studies using a lower dose of virus for challenge should answer the question about what role if any neutralizing antibody plays in the prevention of HIV-1 infection or progression of disease.

HYPERIMMUNIZATION

One brief report suggested that chronic nonspecific hyperimmunization may ameliorate symptoms of HIV-1 infection.[148] In this study, four HIV-1-infected patients who received inactivated polio vaccine subcutaneously three times a week for 3–12 months experienced improvement or resolution of their symptoms of fatigue, lymphadenopathy, or thrush. A potential risk associated with this approach is that antigenic stimulation by non-HIV-1 immunogens might accelerate virus expression in CD4+ lymphocytes and result in their destruction.[149]

ADJUVANTS

A suitable adjuvant is needed to augment and prolong the immune response of HIV-1 vaccine antigens without causing side effects.[116,150,151] Adjuvants appear to work by at least two mechanisms[116]: (*1*) by slowing the excretion of antigen and thereby extending the time of interaction between antigen and antigen-presenting cells and (*2*) by attracting immunocompetent cells to the site of injection and possibly by directing antigen to T-cell-containing areas in regional lymph nodes. Aluminum salt compounds are the only adjuvants licensed by the Federal Drug Administration. While aluminum salts are generally safe and induce humoral immunity,[116,150] more potent adjuvants that elicit cell-mediated immunity are needed for HIV-1 vaccine preparations. Other new potential adjuvants include muramyl dipeptides, which can be used with viral antigens (administered by the parenteral or oral routes), synthetic peptides, and nonpyrogenic subunits of lipopolysaccharides.[116,151,152] When muramyl dipeptide is administered in liposomes or is made lipophilic by the addition of glycerol mycolate,[153] it markedly increases cell-mediated immunity.[154]

Liposomes, concentric spheres consisting of phospholipid bilayers separated by aqueous compartments, have been used effectively as carriers of diphtheria toxoid proteins and other antigens.[152] Liposomes are a potentially promising vehicle for HIV-1 vaccine antigens since liposome–antigen complexes appear to elicit both humoral and cell-mediated immunity.[116,155] The potency of these complexes can be increased by the inclusion of bacterial lipopolysaccharides[156] or muramyl dipeptides[154,157] within the liposomes.

Another promising adjuvant system consists of immune-stimulating complexes (ISCOMS), which are matrices composed of quil A, an extract from the bark of the *Quillaja sonponaria molina* tree.[158–160] ISCOMS are composed of subunits of about 12 nm each that are held together by hydrophobic interactions between the matrix, lipids, and amphipathic antigens.[158,159] ISCOM-bound antigens stimulate an immune response that is generally 10-fold higher when compared with the same antigen packaged in a micelle or in a virus particle.[158,160] Potent cell-mediated immune responses have been elicited after parenteral immunization of monkeys with ISCOMS containing cytomegalovirus antigens and after inoculation with ISCOMS containing hepatitis B surface antigen.[160–162] Furthermore, ISCOMS containing gp120 from feline leukemia virus induced both neutralizing antibody and protective immunity in cats when compared with vaccines consisting of whole killed virus, which failed to induce neutralizing antibody or protective immunity.[34] Vaccine candidates incorporating HIV-1 envelope proteins or synthetic peptides in ISCOMS appear to be safe and immunogenic in gibbons and apes.[163] After repeated immunizations with HIV-1 protein products p17, p41, and gp120 incorporated into ISCOMS, antibodies to all of the proteins were induced in several animal species.[163] However, this ISCOM preparation only stimulated a low level of neutralizing activity against the homologous HIV-1, possibly because it did not contain enough gp120.[163]

CLINICAL TRIALS IN HUMANS

Human trials of four candidate AIDS vaccines have already been initiated in the United States, England, and Africa, with the expectation that they will provide useful information about the safety of and immune response to HIV-1 immunogens in humans.[2] In general, the clinical trials will be carried out in three phases to assess the safety and immunogenicity of candidate vaccines.[1,3,10,85] In phase I trials, different doses of vaccine are generally evaluated in about 10–30 healthy adults per dose group in a double-blinded, placebo-controlled, dose-escalating manner. If the vaccine is found to be safe and sufficiently immunogenic, phase II trials would then be conducted to evaluate the safety and immunogenicity of the vaccine candidate in larger numbers of persons, approximately 40–80 persons per dose. Information regarding the optimal dose and interval between booster doses will be sought from phase I and II trials, each of which will take 1 to 2 years to complete. Only after a vaccine has been shown to be safe and highly immunogenic will it be considered for phase III efficacy testing in humans.

To assess the tolerability and reactogenicity of the vaccine, local and systemic reactions and a variety of laboratory and immunologic parameters of recipients of HIV-1 vaccine will be compared with those of placebo recipients. In one phase I HIV-1 gp160 vaccine trial, yeast-derived recombinant hepatitis B vaccine was used as a control in addition to a placebo so that variations in certain test results (e.g., numbers of CD4+ cells) that might occur after immunization with a recombinant protein could be differentiated from those that might be due specifically to vaccination with the HIV-1 recombinant protein.[75,108] The determination of which group of adults should be selected for vaccine trials will depend to some extent on the phase of the trial and type of vaccine to be evaluated.[1,3,10,85] In general, there are two reasons for selecting persons at low risk for acquiring HIV-1 infection for phase I trials (and possibly for phase II trials) instead of persons at high risk. First, persons at high risk may already be infected with HIV-1 before vaccination or may become infected during the vaccine trial. If this happens, it would be difficult to distinguish their immune responses to the vaccine from those resulting from intercurrent HIV-1 infection. Second, since persons at high risk for acquiring HIV-1 infection are often infected with other agents, they may respond differently to the HIV-1 vaccine than do persons not infected with other agents.[164]

Populations at high risk for HIV-1 infection should be targeted for phase III vaccine efficacy trials.[1,3,10] The sample size required to assess vaccine efficacy will depend on the current incidence of infection and the confidence levels sought to signify significant protection from infection. Finding an adequate volunteer population for phase III vaccine efficacy studies will be difficult.[10,85] It is possible that by the time of the phase III trials the homosexual risk group will have an incidence of infection too low for participation in a vaccine trial. The number of sexual partners of hemophiliacs constitute too small a group to study. Other high-risk populations such as intravenous drug users and prostitutes may not be compliant with the long-term follow-up (7–10 years) required to assess protection against disease. It is possible that trials to determine vaccine efficacy may have to be targeted for populations in Africa where the incidence of HIV-1 infection remains high.[3,10]

ETHICAL ISSUES

Special ethical considerations must be taken into account in the design and conduct of HIV-1 vaccine trials.[1,3,10,165] The consent form not only must clearly state all of the risks associated with the vaccine candidate, but it must educate the volunteer about how to reduce the risk of acquiring HIV-1 infection. In addition, all volunteers who participate in AIDS vaccine trials must be counseled about how to avoid becoming infected with HIV-1. The counseling itself may lower the overall rate of infection in both the unvaccinated control group and the vaccinees and thus increase the amount of time required to determine the efficacy of a vaccine.

Maintenance of strict confidentiality of the study participants throughout these trials is of utmost importance since the volunteers who might be identified as members of high-risk groups could be subjected to discrimination or abuse.[1,165] Of paramount concern is the fact that persons immunized with HIV-1 vaccine candidates who mount an immune response may test positive for HIV-1 antibody by the enzyme-linked immunosorbent assay (ELISA) used for screening.[1,3,10,165] It is possible that persons who seroconvert after receiving an HIV-1 vaccine preparation may not be able to travel to foreign countries where HIV-1 testing is required by immigration, donate blood, enter the miltary or foreign service, or obtain a marriage license or health and life insurance.[1,3,10,165] Clearly, the risks of social and economic hazards associated with HIV-1 seroconversion have already had a negative impact on recruitment efforts for AIDS vaccine trials.

The urgent need to control the transmission of HIV-1 has fueled efforts to develop HIV-1 vaccines. The application of modern molecular biotechnology and the identification of the specific function of amino acid sequences and peptides of HIV-1 proteins has made the task of vaccine development somewhat less formidable.[9] The need to expedite the development of an effective HIV-1 vaccine warrants the evaluation of different vaccine strategies simultaneously.[5] Finally, the issue of potential liability for producers of HIV-1 vaccines and those who conduct the clinical trials is a problem that could block the eventual availability of an HIV-1 vaccine and, therefore, needs to be resolved.[7,166]

REFERENCES

1. Koff WC, Hoth DF. Development and testing of AIDS vaccines. Science. 1988;241:426–32.
2. Barnes DM. Obstacles to an AIDS vaccine. Science. 1988;240:719–21.
3. Homsy J, Steimer K, Kaslow R. Towards an AIDS vaccine: Challenges and prospects. Immunol Today. 1987;8:193–7.
4. Purdy BD, Plaisance KI. Current concepts in clinical therapeutics: Immunologic treatment of human immunodeficiency virus infections. Clin Pharmacol. 1987;6:851–65.
5. Dreesman GR, Eichberg JW, Chanh TC, et al. Use of vaccination in prevention of HIV infection. In: AIDS. Acquired Immunodeficiency Syndrome and Other Manifestations of HIV Infections. Park Ridge, NJ: Noyes Publications; 1987:1037–52.
6. Fischinger PJ, Gallo RC, Bolognesi DP. Toward a vaccine against AIDS: Rationale and current progress. Mt Sinai J Med. 1986;53:639–47.
7. Barnes DM. Strategies for an AIDS vaccine. Science. 1986;233:1149–53.
8. Vogt M, Hirsch MS. Prospects for the prevention and therapy of infections with the human immunodeficiency virus. Rev Infect Dis. 1986;8:991–1000.
9. Fischinger PJ, Robey WG, Koprowski H, et al. Current status and strategies for vaccines against diseases induced by human T-cell lymphotropic retroviruses (HTLV-1, -II, -III). Cancer Res. 1985;45(Suppl):4694–9.
10. Francis DP, Petricciani JC. The prospects for and pathways toward a vaccine for AIDS. N Engl J Med. 1985;313:1586–90.
11. Hunsmann G. Subunit vaccines against exogenous retroviruses: Overview and perspectives. Cancer Res. 1985;45(Suppl):4691–3.
12. Wong-Staal F, Shaw GM, Hahn BH, et al. Genomic diversity of human T-lymphotropic virus type III (HTLV-III). Science. 1985;229:759–62.
13. Benn S, Rutledge R, Folks T, et al. Genomic heterogeneity of AIDS retroviral isolates from North America and Zaire. Science. 1985;230:949–51.
14. Starcich BR, Hahn BH, Shaw GM, et al. Identification and characterization of conserved and variable regions in the envelope gene of HTLV-III/LAV, the retrovirus of AIDS. Cell. 1986;45:637–48.
15. Hahn BH, Shaw GM, Taylor ME, et al. Genetic variation in HTLV-III/LAV over time in patients with AIDS or at risk for AIDS. Science. 1986;232:1548–53.
16. Willey RL, Rutledge RA, Dias S, et al. Identification of conserved and divergent domains within the envelope gene of the acquired immunodeficiency syndrome retrovirus. Proc Natl Acad Sci USA. 1986;83:5038–42.
17. Cheng-Mayer C, Seto D, Tateno M, et al. Biologic features of HIV-1 that correlate with virulence in the host. Science. 1988;240:80–2.
18. Cheng-Mayer C, Homsy J, Evans LA, et al. Identification of human immunodeficiency virus subtypes with distinct patterns of sensitivity to serum neutralization. Proc Natl Acad Sci USA. 1988;85:2815–9.
19. Barin F, McLane MF, Allan JS, et al. Virus envelope protein of HTLV-III represents major target antigen for antibodies in AIDS patients. Science. 1985;228:1094–6.
20. Matthews TJ, Langlois AJ, Robey WG, et al. Restricted neutralization of divergent human T-lymphotropic virus type III isolates by antibodies to the major envelope glycoprotein. Proc Natl Acad Sci USA. 1986;83:9709–13.
21. Weiss RA, Clapham PR, Weber JN, et al. Variable and conserved neutralization antigens of human immunodeficiency virus. Nature. 1986;324:572–5.
22. Ho DD, Sarngadharan MG, Hirsch MS, et al. Human immunodeficiency virus neutralizing antibodies recognize several conserved domains on the envelope glycoproteins. J Virol. 1987;61:2024–8.

23. Modrow S, Hahn BH, Shaw GM, et al. Computer-assisted analysis of envelope protein sequences of seven human immunodeficiency virus isolates: Prediction of antigenic epitopes in conserved and variable regions. J Virol. 1987;61:570–8.
24. Ho DD, Kaplan JC, Rackauskas IE, et al. Second conserved domain of gp120 is important for HIV infectivity and antibody neutralization. Science. 1988;239:1021–3.
25. Hahn BH, Gonda MA, Shaw GM, et al. Genomic diversity of the acquired immune deficiency syndrome virus HTLV-III: Different viruses exhibit greatest divergence in their envelope genes. Proc Natl Acad Sci USA. 1985;82:4813–7.
26. Alizon M, Wain-Hobson S, Montagnier L, et al. Genetic variability of the AIDS virus: Nucleotide sequence analysis of two isolates from African patients. Cell. 1986;45:63–74.
27. Sanchez-Pescador R, Power MD, Barr PJ, et al. Nucleotide sequence and expression of an AIDS-associated retrovirus (ARV-2). Science. 1985;227:484–92.
28. Clements JE, Pedersen FS, Narayan O, et al. Genomic changes associated with antigenic variation of visna virus during persistent infection. Proc Natl Acad Sci USA. 1980;77:4454–8.
29. Robert-Guroff M, Brown M, Gallo RC. HTLV-III–neutralizing antibodies in patients with AIDS and AIDS-related complex. Nature. 1985;316:72–4.
30. Robert-Guroff M, Oleske JM, Connor EM, et al. Relationship between HTLV-III neutralizing antibody and clinical status of pediatric acquired immunodeficiency syndrome (AIDS) and AIDS-related complex cases. Pediatr Res. 1987;21:547–50.
31. Ranki A, Weiss SH, Sirkka-Liisa V, et al. Neutralizing antibodies in HIV (HTLV-III) infection: Correlation with clinical outcome and antibody response against different viral proteins. Clin Exp Immunol. 1987;69:231–9.
31a. Murphy BR, Chanock RM. Immunization against viruses. In: Fields BN, Knipe DN, Chanock RM, et al., eds. Virology. New York: Raven Press; 1985:349–70.
32. Sarin PS, Sun DK, Thornton AH, et al. Neutralization of HTLV-III/LAV replication by antiserum to thymosin α1. Science. 1986;232:1135–7.
33. Weiss RA, Clapham PR, Cheingson-Popov R, et al. Neutralization of human T-lymphotropic virus type III by sera of AIDS and AIDS-risk patients. Nature. 1985;316:69–72.
34. Osterhaus A, Weijer K, Uytdehagg F, et al. Induction of protective immune response in cats by vaccination with feline leukemia virus ISCOM. J Immunol. 1985;135:591–6.
35. Prince AM, Horowitz B, Baker L, et al. Failure of a human immunodeficiency virus (HIV) immune globulin to protect chimpanzees against experimental challenge with HIV. Proc Natl Acad Sci USA. 1988;85:6944–8.
36. Palker TJ, Clark ME, Langlois AJ, et al. Type-specific neutralization of the human immunodeficiency virus with antibodies to *env*-encoded synthetic peptides. Proc Natl Acad Sci USA. 1988;85:1932–6.
37. Earl PL, Moss B, Morrison RP, et al. T-lymphocyte priming and protection against Friend leukemia by vaccinia-retrovirus env gene recombinant. Science. 1986;234:728–31.
38. Quinnan GV, Kirmani N, Rook AH, et al. HLA-restricted T-lymphocyte and non T-lymphocyte cytotoxic responses correlate with recovery from cytomegalovirus infection in bone-marrow-transplant recipients. N Engl J Med. 1982;307:7–13.
39. Yap KL, Braciale TJ, Ada GL. Role of T-cell function in recovery from murine influenza infection. Cell. 1979;43:341–51.
40. Tam MR, Green WR, Nowinski RC. Cytotoxic activities of monoclonal antibodies against the envelope proteins of murine leukemia virus. Cancer Res. 1980;40:3850–3.
41. Lyerly HK, Matthews TJ, Langlois AJ, et al. Human T-cell lymphotropic virus IIIB glycoprotein [gp120] bound to CD4 determinants on normal lymphocytes and expressed by infected cells serves as target for immune attack. Proc Natl Acad Sci USA. 1987;84:4601–5.
42. Grant CK, Essex M, Pedersen NC, et al. Lysis of feline lymphoma cells by complement-dependent antibodies in feline leukemia virus contact cats. Correlation of lysis and antibodies to feline oncornavirus-associated cell membrane antigen. JNCI. 1978;60:161–6.
43. Matthews TJ, Weinhold KJ, Langlois AJ, et al. Immunologic control of a retrovirus-associated murine adenocarcinoma. VI. Augmentation of antibody-dependent killing following quantitative and qualitative changes in host peritoneal cells. JNCI. 1985;75:703–8.
44. Rook AH, Lane HC, Folks T, et al. Sera from HTLV-III/LAV antibody–positive individuals mediate antibody-dependent cellular cytotoxicity against HTLV-III/LAV–infected T cells. J Immunol. 1987;138:1064–7.
45. Blumberg RS, Paradis T, Hartshorn KL, et al. Antibody-dependent cell-mediated cytotoxicity against cells infected with the human immunodeficiency virus. J Infect Dis. 1987;156:878–84.
46. Ojo-amaize EA, Nishanian P, Keith DE Jr, et al. Antibodies to human immunodeficiency virus in human sera induce cell-mediated lysis of human immunodeficiency virus–infected cells. J Immunol. 1987;139:2458–63.
47. Spickett GP, Dalgleish AG. Cellular immunology of HIV-infection. Clin Exp Immunol. 1988;71:1–7.
48. Ljunggren K, Bottiger B, Biberfeld G, et al. Antibody-dependent cellular cytotoxicity-inducing antibodies against human immunodeficiency virus. J Immunol. 1987;139:2263–7.
49. DeNoronha F, Schafer W, Essex M, et al. Influence of antisera to oncornavirus glycoprotein (gp 71) on infections of cats with feline leukemia virus. Virology. 1978;85:617–21.
50. Schwarz H, Ihle JN, Wecker E, et al. Properties of mouse leukemia viruses. XVII. Factors required for successful treatment of spontaneous AKR leukemia by antibodies against gp71. Virology. 1981;111:568–78.
51. Ward EC, Iglehart JD, Weinhold KJ, et al. Immunotherapy of a murine leukemia virus–infected, chemically induced murine sarcoma with antiviral antibodies. JNCI. 1982;69:509–14.
52. Walker BD, Chakrabarti S, Moss B, et al. HIV-specific cytotoxic T lymphocytes in seropositive individuals. Nature. 1987;328:345–7.
53. Walker BD, Flexner C, Paradis TJ, et al. HIV-1 reverse transcriptase is a target for cytotoxic T lymphocytes in infected individuals. Science. 1988;240:64–6.
54. Weinhold KJ, Lyerly HK, Matthews TJ, et al. Cellular anti-gp120 cytolytic reactivities in HIV-1 seropositive individuals. Lancet. 1988;1:902–5.
55. Plata F, Autran B, Martins LP, et al. AIDS virus–specific cytotoxic T lymphocytes in lung disorders. Nature. 1987;328:348–51.
56. Nara PL, Robey WG, Gonda MA, et al. Absence of cytotoxic antibody to human immunodeficiency virus–infected cells in humans and its induction in animals after infection or immunization with purified envelope glycoprotein gp120. Proc Natl Acad Sci USA. 1987;84:3797–801.
57. Ogra PL, Karzon DT. Distribution of poliovirus antibody in serum, nasopharynx and alimentary tract following segmental immunization of lower alimentary tract with poliovaccine. J Immunol. 1968;102:1423–30.
58. Archibald DW, Barr CE, Torosian JP, et al. Secretory IgA antibodies to human immunodeficiency virus in the parotid saliva of patients with AIDS and AIDS-related complex. J Infect Dis. 1987;155:793–6.
59. Barnes DM. Solo actions of AIDS virus coat. Science. 1987;237:971–3.
60. del Guercio P, Zanetti M. The CD4 molecule, the human immunodeficiency virus and anti-idiotypic antibodies. Immunol Today. 1987;8:204–5.
61. Ellrodt A, Le Bras P. The hidden dangers of AIDS vaccination. Nature. 1987;325:765.
62. Robinson WE Jr, Montefiori DC, Mitchell WM. Antibody-dependent enhancement of human immunodeficiency virus type 1 infection. Lancet. 1988;1:790–4.
62a. Takeda A, Tuazon CU, Ennis FA. Antibody-enhanced infection by HIV-1 via Fc receptor-mediated entry. Science. 1988;242:580–3.
63. Martinez AC, Marcos MAR, de la Hera A, et al. Immunological consequences of HIV infection: Advantage of being low responder casts doubts on vaccine development. Lancet. 1988;1:454–7.
64. Dalgleish AG, Beverley PCL, Clapham PR, et al. The CD4 (T4) antigen is an essential component of the receptor for the AIDS retrovirus. Nature. 1984;312:763–7.
65. Putney SD, Matthews TJ, Robey WG, et al. HTLV-III/LAV–neutralizing antibodies to an *E. coli*–produced fragment of the virus envelope. Science. 1986;234:1392–5.
66. Lasky LA, Nakamura G, Smith JH, et al. Delineation of a region of the human immunodeficiency virus type 1 (HIV-1) gp120 glycoprotein critical for interaction with the CD4 receptor. Cell. 1987;50:975–85.
67. Lifson JD, Feinberg MB, Reyes GR, et al. Induction of CD4-dependent cell fusion by the HTLV-III/LAV envelope glycoprotein. Nature. 1986;323:725–8.
68. Sodroski J, Goh WC, Rosen C, et al. Role of the HTLV-III/LAV envelope in syncytium formation and cytopathicity. Nature. 1986;322:470–4.
69. Tas M, Drexhage HA, Goudsmit J. A monocyte chemotaxis inhibiting factor in serum of HIV infected men shares epitopes with the HIV transmembrane protein gp41. Clin Exp Immunol. 1988;71:13–8.
70. Mathes LE, Olsen RG, Hedebrand LC. Immunosuppressive properties of a virion polypeptide, a 15,000-dalton protein, from feline leukemia virus. Cancer Res. 1979;39:950–5.
71. McDougal JS, Mawle A, Cort SP, et al. Cellular tropism of the human retrovirus HTLV-III/LAV. I. Role of the T cell activation and expression of the T4 antigen. J Immunol. 1985;135:3151–62.
72. Gurney ME, Apatoff BR, Spear GT, et al. Neuroleukin: A lymphokine product of lectin-stimulated T cells. Science. 1986;234:574–81.
73. Reiher WE, Blalock JE, Brunck TK. Sequence homology between acquired immunodeficiency syndrome virus envelope protein and interleukin 2. Proc Natl Acad Sci USA. 1988;83:9188–92.
74. Halsted SB, O'Rourke EJ. Dengue viruses and mononuclear phagocytes. I. Infection enhancement by non-neutralizing antibody. J Exp Med. 1977; 146:201–17.
75. Anonymous. First AIDS vaccine to enter clinical trials. Innovations. 1987;2:1,7.
76. Perricone R, Fontana L, DeCarolis C, et al. Evidence for activation of complement in patients with AIDS related complex (ARC) and/or lymphadenopathy syndrome (LAS). Clin Exp Immunol. 1987;70:500–7.
77. Barnes DM. The challenge of testing potential AIDS vaccines. Science. 1986;233:1151.
78. Wittek AE, Phelan MA, Wells MA, et al. Detection of human immunodeficiency virus core protein in plasma by enzyme immunoassay. Association of antigenemia with symptomatic disease and T-helper cell depletion. Ann Intern Med. 1987;107:286–92.
79. Harada S, Koyanagi Y, Yamamoto N. Infection of HTLV-III/LAV in HTLV-1-carrying cells MT-2 and MT-4 and application in a plaque assay. Science. 1985;229:563–6.
80. Vujcic LK, Shepp DH, Klutch M, et al. Use of sensitive neutralization assay to measure the prevalence of antibodies to the human immunodeficiency virus. J Infect Dis. 1988;157:1047–50.
81. Fultz PN, McClure HM, Swenson RB, et al. Persistent infection of chim-

panzees with human T-lymphotropic virus type III/lymphadenopathy-associated virus: A potential model for acquired immunodeficiency syndrome. J Virol. 1986;58:116–24.
82. Nara PL, Robey WG, Arthur LO, et al. Persistent infection of chimpanzees with human immunodeficiency virus: Serological responses and properties of reisolated viruses. J Virol. 1987;61:3173–80.
83. Alter JH, Eichberg JW, Masur H, et al. Transmission of HTLV-III infection from human plasma to chimpanzees: An animal model for AIDS. Science. 1984;226:549–52.
84. Gajdusek DC, Gibbs CJ, Rodgers-Johnson P, et al. Infection of chimpanzees by human T-lymphotropic retroviruses in brain and other tissues from AIDS patients. Lancet. 1985;1:55–6.
85. Barnes DM. Broad issues debated at AIDS vaccine workshop. Science. 1987;236:255.
86. Newmark P. Problems with AIDS vaccines. Nature. 1986;324:304–5.
87. Barnes D. AIDS vaccine trial OKed. Science. 1987;237:973.
88. Daniel MD, Letvin NL, King NW, et al. Isolation of T-cell tropic HTLV-III-like retrovirus from macaques. Science. 1985;228:1201–4.
89. Letvin NL, Daniel MD, Sehgal PK, et al. Induction of AIDS-like disease in macaque monkeys with T-cell tropic retrovirus STLV-III. Science. 1985;230:71–3.
90. Bryant ML, Yamamoto J, Luciw P, et al. Molecular comparison of retroviruses associated with human and simian AIDS. Hematol Oncol. 1985;3:187–97.
91. Gonda MA, Wong-Staal F, Gallo RC. Sequence homology and morphologic similarity of HTLV-III and visna virus, a pathogenic lentivirus. Science. 1985;227:173–7.
92. Pedersen NC, Ho EW, Brown ML, et al. Isolation of a T-lymphotropic virus from domestic cats with an immunodeficiency-like syndrome. Science. 1987;235:790–3.
93. Gonda MA, Braun MJ, Carter SG, et al. Characterization and molecular cloning of a bovine lentivirus related to human immunodeficiency virus. Nature. 1987;330:388–91.
94. McGuire TC, Adams DS, Johnson GC, et al. Challenge exposure of vaccinated or persistently infected goats. Am J Vet Res. 1986;47:537–40.
95. Allan JS, Coltigan JE, Barin F, et al. Major glycoprotein antigens that induce antibodies in AIDS patients are encoded by HTLV-III. Science. 1985;228:1091–4.
96. Veronese FD, DeVico AL, Copeland TD, et al. Characterization of gp41 as the transmembrane protein coded by the HTLV-III/LAV envelope gene. Science. 1985;229:1402–5.
97. Robey WG, Safai B, Oroszlan S, et al. Characterization of envelope and core structural gene products of HTLV-III with sera from AIDS patients. Science. 1985;228:593–5.
98. Robey WG, Arthur LO, Matthews TJ, et al. Prospect for prevention of human immunodeficiency virus infection: Purified 120-kDa envelope glycoprotein induces neutralizing antibody. Proc Natl Acad Sci USA. 1986;83:7023–7.
99. Lasky LA, Groopman JE, Fennie CW, et al. Neutralization of the AIDS retrovirus by antibodies to a recombinant envelope glycoprotein. Science. 1986;233:209–12.
100. Crowl R, Ganguly K, Gordon M, et al. HTLV-III env gene products synthesized in *E. coli* are recognized by antibodies present in the sera of AIDS patients. Cell. 1985;41:979–86.
101. Ratner L, Gallo RC, Wong-Staal F. HTLV-III, LAV, ARV are variants of the same AIDS virus. Nature. 1985;313:636–7.
102. Lewis MG, Mathes LE, Olson RG. Protection against feline leukemia by vaccination with a subunit vaccine. Infect Immun. 1981;34:888–94.
103. Onuma M, Hodatsu T, Yamamoto S, et al. Protection by vaccination against bovine leukemia virus infection in sheep. Am J Vet Res. 1984;45:1212–5.
104. Hunsmann G, Schneider J, Schulz A. Immunoprevention of Friend virus-induced erythroleukemia by vaccination with viral envelope glycoprotein complexes. Virology. 1981;113:602–12.
105. Jasny BR. Insect viruses invade biotechnology. Science. 1987;238:1653.
106. Rusche JR, Lynn DL, Robert-Guroff M, et al. Humoral immune response to the entire human immunodeficiency virus envelope glycoprotein made in insect cells. Proc Natl Acad Sci USA. 1987;84:6924–8.
107. Chang NT, Chanda PK, Barone AD, et al. Expression in *Escherichia coli* of open reading frame gene segments of HTLV-III. Science. 1985;228:93–6.
108. Wright K. AIDS protein made. Nature. 1986;319:525.
109. Krohn K, Robey WG, Putney S, et al. Specific cellular immune response and neutralizing antibodies in goats immunized with native or recombinant envelope proteins derived from human T-lymphotropic virus type III_B and in human immunodeficiency virus-infected men. Proc Natl Acad Sci USA. 1987;84:4994–8.
109a. Berman PW, Groopman JE, Gregory T, et al. Human immunodeficiency virus type 1 challenge of chimpanzees immunized with recombinant envelope glycoprotein gp120. Proc Natl Acad Sci USA. 1988;85:5200–4.
110. Arthur LO, Pyle SW, Nara PL, et al. Serological responses in chimpanzees inoculated with human immunodeficiency virus glycoprotein (gp120) subunit vaccine. Proc Natl Acad Sci USA. 1987;84:8583–7.
111. Cease KB, Margalit H, Cornette JL, et al. Helper T-cell antigenic site identification in the acquired immunodeficiency syndrome virus gp120 envelope protein and induction of immunity in mice to the native protein using a 16-residue synthetic peptide. Proc Natl Acad Sci USA. 1987;84:4249–53.
112. Kennedy RC, Henkel RD, Pauletti D, et al. Antiserum to a synthetic peptide recognizes the HTLV-III envelope glycoprotein. Science. 1986;231:1556–1559.
113. Steward MW, Howard CR. Synthetic peptides: A next generation of vaccines? Immunol Today. 1987;8:51–7.
114. Hopp TP, Woods KR. Prediction of protein antigenic determinants from amino acid sequences. Proc Natl Acad Sci USA. 1981;78:3824–8.
115. DeLisi C, Berzofsky JA. T-cell antigenic sites tend to be amphipathic structures. Proc Natl Acad Sci USA. 1985;82:7048–52.
116. Warren HS, Vogel FR, Chedid LA. Current status of immunological adjuvants. Annu Rev Immunol. 1986;4:369–88.
117. Gartner S, Markovits P, Markovitz DM, et al. The role of mononuclear phagocytes in HTLV-III/LAV infection. Science. 1986;233:215–9.
118. Weber JN, Clapham PR, Weiss RA, et al. Human immunodeficiency virus infection in two cohorts of homosexual men: Neutralising sera and association of anti-gag antibody with prognosis. Lancet. 1987;1:119–22.
119. Groopman JE, Chen FW, Hope JA, et al. Serological characterization of HTLV-III infection in AIDS and related disorders. J Infect Dis. 1986;153:736–42.
120. Brown F, Schild GC, Ada GL. Recombinant vaccinia viruses as vaccines. Nature. 1986;319:549–50.
121. Hu S-L, Kosowski SG, Dalrymple JM. Expression of AIDS virus envelope gene in recombinant vaccinia viruses. Nature. 1986;320:537–40.
122. Chakrabarti S, Robert-Guroff M, Wong-Staal F, et al. Expression of the HTLV-III envelope gene by a recombinant vaccinia virus. Nature. 1986;320:535–7.
123. Moss B, Flexner C. Vaccinia virus expression vectors. Annu Rev Immunol. 1987;5:305–24.
124. Davis AR, Kostek B, Mason BB, et al. Expression of hepatitis B surface antigen with a recombinant adenovirus. Proc Natl Acad Sci USA. 1985;82:7560–4.
125. Buller RML, Smith GL, Cremer K, et al. Decreased virulence of recombinant vaccinia virus expression vectors is associated with a thymidine kinase-negative phenotype. Nature. 1985;317:813–5.
126. Hu S-L, Fultz PN, McClure HM, et al. Effect of immunization with a vaccinia-HIV *env* recombinant on HIV infection of chimpanzees. Nature. 1987;328:721–3.
127. Zarling JM, Morton W, Moran PA, et al. T-cell responses to human AIDS virus in macaques immunized with recombinant vaccinia viruses. Nature. 1986;323:344–6.
128. Zagury D, Leonard R, Fouchard M, et al. Immunization against AIDS in humans. Nature. 1987;326:249–50.
129. Zagury D, Bernard J, Cheynier R, et al. A group specific anamnestic immune reaction against HIV-1 induced by a candidate vaccine against AIDS. Nature. 1988;332:728–31.
130. Ezzell C. Another AIDS vaccine. Nature. 1987;328:509.
131. Chapter 7. Developments in vaccination and control between 1900 and 1966. In: Fenner F, Henderson DA, Arita I, et al, eds. Smallpox and Its Eradication. Geneva: World Health Organization; 1988:277–314.
132. Redfield RR, Wright DC, James WD, et al. Disseminated vaccinia in a military recruit with human immunodeficiency virus (HIV) disease. N Engl J Med. 1987;316:673–6.
133. Flexner C, Hugin A, Moss B. Prevention of vaccinia virus infection in immunodeficient mice by vector-directed IL-2 expression. Nature. 1987;330:259–62.
134. Ramshaw IA, Andrew ME, Phillips SM, et al. Recovery of immunodeficient mice from a vaccinia virus/IL-2 recombinant infection. Nature. 1987;329:545–6.
135. Salk J. Prospects for the control of AIDS by immunizing seropositive individuals. Nature. 1987;327:473–6.
136. Marx PA, Pedersen NC, Lerche NW, et al. Prevention of simian acquired immune deficiency syndrome with a formalin-inactivated type D retrovirus vaccine. J Virol. 1986;60:431–5.
137. Ranki A, Krohn M, Allain JP, et al. Long latency precedes overt seroconversion in sexually transmitted human-immunodeficiency-virus infection. Lancet. 1987;2:589–93.
138. Francis DP, Jaffe HW, Fultz PN, et al. The natural history of infection with the lymphadenopathy-associated virus human T-lymphotropic virus type III. Ann Intern Med. 1985;103:719–22.
139. Ezzell C. Killed HIV treatment in clinical trials. Nature. 1988;332:668.
140. Szmuness W, Stevens CE, Harley EJ, et al. Hepatitis B vaccine. Demonstration of efficacy in a controlled clinical trial in a high risk population in the United States. N Engl J Med. 1980;303:833–41.
141. Fisher AG, Ratner L, Mitsuya H, et al. Infectious mutants of HTLV-III with changes in the 3′ region and markedly reduced cytopathic effects. Science. 1986;233:655–9.
142. Klatzmann D, Champagne E, Chamaret S, et al. T-lymphocyte T4 molecule behaves as the receptor for human retrovirus. Nature. 1984;312:767–8.
143. Dalgleish AG, Thomson BJ, Chanh TC, et al. Neutralisation of HIV isolates by anti-idiotypic antibodies which mimic the T4(CD4) epitope: A potential AIDS vaccine. Lancet. 1987;2:1047–50.
144. Koprowski H. Unconventional vaccines: Immunization with anti-idiotype antibody against viral disease. Cancer Res. 1985;45(Suppl):4689–90.
145. Chanh TC, Dreesman GR, Kennedy RC. Monoclonal antiidiotypic antibody mimics the CD4 receptor and binds human immunodeficiency virus. Proc Natl Acad Sci USA. 1987;84:3891–5.
146. Dalgleish AG. The T4 molecule. Immunol Today. 1986;7:142–4.

147. Benjamin RJ, Waldmann H. Introduction of tolerance by monoclonal antibody therapy. Nature. 1986;320:449–51.
148. Pitts FN Jr, Allen RE, Haraszti JS, et al. Improvement of four patients with HIV-1 related symptoms after hyperimmunization with killed poliomyelitis (Salk) vaccine. Clin Immunol Immunopathol. 1988;46:167–8.
149. Kehrl JH, Fauci AS. Activation of human B lymphocytes after immunization with pneumococcal polysaccharides. J Clin Invest. 1983;71:1032–40.
150. Edelman R. Vaccine adjuvants. Rev Infect Dis. 1980;2:370–83.
151. Chedid L, Audibert F, Lefrancier P, et al. Modulation of the immune response by a synthetic adjuvant and analogs. Proc Natl Acad Sci USA. 1976;73:2472–5.
152. Allison AC, Gregoriadis G. Liposomes as immunological adjuvants. Nature. 1974;252:252.
153. Parant M, Audibert F, Chedid L, et al. Immunostimulant activities of a lipophilic muramyl dipeptide derivative and of desmuramyl peptidolipid analogs. Infect Immun. 1980;27:826–31.
154. Masek K, Zaoral M, Jezek J, et al. Immunoadjuvant activity of synthetic *N*-acetylmuramyl dipeptide. Experimentia. 1978;34:1363–4.
155. Sanchez Y, Ionescu-Matiu I, Dreesman GR, et al. Humoral and cellular immunity to hepatitis B virus–derived antigens: Comparative activity of Freund complete adjuvant, alum and liposomes. Infect Immun. 1980;30:728.
156. Desiderio JV, Campbell SG. Immunization against experimental murine salmonellosis with liposome-associated O-antigen. Infect Immun. 1985; 48:658–63.
157. Jolivet M, Sache E, Audibert F. Biological studies of lipophilic MDP derivatives incorporated into liposomes. Immunol Commun. 1981;10:511–22.
158. Morein B. The iscom antigen–presenting system. Nature. 1988;332:287–88.
159. Morein B, Sundquist B, Hoglund S, et al. Iscom, a novel structure for antigenic presentation of membrane proteins from enveloped viruses. Nature. 1984;308:457–60.
160. Morein B, Lovgren K, Hoglund S, et al. Iscom: An immune stimulating complex. Immunol Today. 1987;8:333–8.
161. Wahren B, Nordlund S, Akesson A, et al. Monocyte and ISCOM enhancement of cell-mediated response to cytomegalovirus. Med Microbiol Immunol. 1987;176:13–9.
162. Howard CR, Sundquist B, Allen J, et al. Preparation and properties of immune-stimulating complexes containing hepatitis B virus surface antigen. J Virol. 1987;68:2281–9.
163. Newmark P. Human and monkey virus puzzles. Nature. 1987;327:458.
164. Nabel GJ, Rice SA, Knipe DM, et al. Alternative mechanisms for activation of human immunodeficiency virus enhancer in T cells. Science. 1988;239:1299–302.
165. Walters L. Ethical issues in the prevention and treatment of HIV infection and AIDS. Science. 1988;239:597–603.
166. Barnes DM. Will an AIDS vaccine bankrupt the company that makes it? Science. 1986;223:1035.

INFECTIOUS DISEASES AND THEIR ETIOLOGIC AGENTS

PART III

SECTION A. VIRAL DISEASES

112. INTRODUCTION TO VIRUSES AND VIRAL DISEASES

KENNETH L. TYLER
BERNARD N. FIELDS

HISTORY

The history of virology encompasses virtually the entire time span of recorded history.[1] Viral diseases have the distinction of being among both the oldest recorded human diseases (e.g., rabies, polio) as well as some of the most recently described (acquired immunodeficiency syndrome [AIDS]). The tempo of advances in the history of virology began to accelerate during the nineteenth century. First, careful clinical observations led to the identification and differentiation of a number of viral illnesses (e.g., smallpox from chickenpox and measles from rubella). Second, this improved clinical definition of illnesses combined with improvements in pathologic techniques and methods, exemplified by Virchow, allowed the pathologic substrate of many viral diseases to be identified. Finally, the work of Pasteur ushered in the systematic use of laboratory animals to study the pathogenesis of disease.

As the nineteenth century ended and the twentieth century began, the first viruses were identified. Beijerinck identified tobacco mosaic virus and Loeffler and Frosch discovered foot and mouth disease virus. This was quickly followed by the discovery of the first human disease-causing virus, yellow fever virus, and the seminal work on the pathogenesis of yellow fever by Walter Reed and the Army Yellow Fever Commission.[2] By the end of the 1930s tumor viruses, bacteriophages, influenza viruses, mumps, and many arboviruses had been identified. This process of discovery has continued unabated through the present, with the human immunodeficiency (HIV) and human T-cell lymphotropic viruses being the most recent additions to the catalog of human disease-causing viruses.

In the 1940s, using bacteriophages as a model, Delbruck, Luria, and others established many of the basic principles of microbial genetics and molecular biology and identified the major events in the viral growth cycle.[3,4] The pioneering experiments of Avery and associates on the transformation of pneumococcal types, which established that DNA was the genetic material,[5] set the stage for the experiments by Hershey and Chase[6] showing that the genetic material of bacteriophages was also DNA. In the late 1940s, Enders and colleagues grew poliovirus in tissue culture.[7] This work led to the subsequent development of both formalin-inactivated (Salk) and live attenuated (Sabin) vaccines for polio[8,9] and ushered in the modern era of virology.

Technical advances such as the development of electron microscopy, ultracentrifugation, and techniques for the electrophoresis of nucleic acids and proteins set the stage for improved understanding of viral structure and for a detailed biochemical analysis of purified virion components and their biologic properties.

In the modern era the use of x-ray crystallography has allowed structural definition of viruses and their components at a near-atomic level. By using the techniques of molecular biology, the entire genomes of many viruses have been sequenced. Monoclonal antibodies have enabled specific domains on viral proteins to be defined with a precision previously impossible. These techniques and others are already being applied to the development of new strategies for the diagnosis of viral illness and the design of effective antiviral therapy. For example, the polymerase chain reaction (PCR) technique allows small amounts of nucleic acid, for example, the integrated DNA of a retrovirus such as HIV that is present in some circulating host cells, to be dramatically amplified, which greatly facilitates its subsequent detection. Techniques such as this may prove to be greatly superior to conventional serologic approaches to diagnosis of viral diseases. Among the challenges for the future will be the application of these powerful new techniques to expand our understanding at the molecular level of how viruses interact with target cells to alter function, how the interaction of viruses and cells within a living host produce disease, and how events in the infected host result in the transmission of disease and the maintenance of infectious viruses in the environment. Improved understanding of these aspects of viral infection should lead to new approaches to the diagnosis, prevention, and cure of viral diseases.

VIRUS STRUCTURE AND CLASSIFICATION

The first classification of viruses as a group distinct from other microorganisms was based almost exclusively on their ability to pass through filters of a small pore size (''filterable agents''). Initial subdivisions were based primarily on pathologic properties such as specific organ tropism (e.g., enteroviruses) or on common epidemiologic features such as tranmission by arthropod vectors (e.g., arboviruses). Since the 1950s classification has depended predominantly on morphologic and physicochemical criteria.[10] More recently, the availability of an increasing body of knowledge concerning the nucleic acid properties of many viral genomes has led to attempts to reorganize classification along lines of genetic relatedness. The key constituents of current classification systems are (*1*) the type and structure of the viral nucleic acid and the strategy used in its replication, (*2*) the type of symmetry of the virus capsid (helical vs. icosahedral), and (*3*) the presence or absence of an envelope (see Table 1). Each of these features will be discussed in more detail in subsequent sections.

Much of our current knowledge about viral structure has been gained from the examination of electron micrographs of negatively stained viral particles (virions). The use of high-resolution x-ray crystallographic techniques has recently provided views of viral structure at the atomic level. Identification of key structural motifs such as receptor binding sites or immunodominant domains can provide the framework for beginning to understand structural features involved in virus–cell interactions.

The genetic information of viruses is encoded in nucleic acids, which occurs in individual viral families in a wide variety of forms and sizes (Table 1 and Fig. 1). The nucleic acid may be composed of either RNA or DNA. Its size can range from 10^6 daltons in small viruses such as the Parvoviridae to $>200 \times 10^6$ daltons in complex viruses such as the Poxviridae. The genomes of the smallest viruses probably encode only three or four unique proteins, whereas those of the largest viruses may encode several hundred proteins. The DNA and RNA can occur in either single- or double-stranded forms and can be either circular (i.e., closed) or linear (i.e., open ended) in shape. Viruses with linear RNA may have either a single piece of nucleic acid

TABLE 1. Classification of Viruses

Family	*Example*	*Type of Nucleis Acid*	*Genome Size (Kilobases or Kilobase Pairs)*	*Envelope*	*Capsid Symmetry*
Picornaviridae	Poliovirus	SS (+) RNA	7.2–8.4	No	I
Caliciviridae	Norwalk virus	SS (+) RNA	8	No	I
Togaviridae	Rubella virus	SS (+) RNA	12	Yes	I
Flaviviridae	Yellow fever virus	SS (+) RNA	10	Yes	Unk
Coronaviridae	Coronaviruses	SS (+) RNA	16–21	Yes	H
Rhabdoviridae	Rabies virus	SS (−) RNA	13–16	Yes	H
Filoviridae	Marburg virus	SS (−) RNA	13	Yes	H
Paramyxoviridae	Measles virus	SS (−) RNA	16–20	Yes	H
Orthomyxoviridae	Influenza viruses	8 SS (−) RNA segments[a]	14	Yes	H
Bunyaviridae	California encephalitis virus	3 circular SS (−) RNA segments	13–21	Yes	H
Arenaviridae	Lymphocytic choriomeningitis virus	2 circular SS (−) RNA segments	10–14	Yes	H
Reoviridae	Rotaviruses	10–12 DS RNA[2] segments	16–27	No	I
Retroviridae	HIV-1	2 identical SS (+) RNA segments	3–9	Yes	I—capsid H—nucleocapsid (probable)
Hepadnaviridae	Hepatitis B	DS DNA with SS portions	3	Yes	Unk
Parvoviridae	Human parvovirus B-19	SS (+) or (−) DNA	5	No	I
Papoviridae	JC virus	Circular DS DNA	8	No	I
Adenoviridae	Human adenoviruses	DS DNA	36–38	No	I
Herpesviridae	Herpes simplex virus	DS DNA	120–220	Yes	I
Poxviridae	Vaccinia	DS DNA with covalently closed ends	130–280	No	Complex

Abbreviations: DS: double stranded; SS: single stranded; (+): message sense; (−): anti-message sense; I: icosahedral; H: helical; Unk: unknown.
(From Murphy,[10] with permission.)
[a] Influenza C: seven segments.
[b] Reovirus, orbivurus: 10 segments; rotavirus: 11 segments; Colorado tick fever: 12 segments.

or a variable number of segments. The number of RNA segments can vary in number from as few as 2 (Arenaviridae) to as many as 12 (some Reoviridae).

The viral nucleic acid is packaged in a protein coat (capsid) that is composed of multiple, nearly identical repeating protein subunits (capsomeres). The combination of the viral nucleic acid and the surrounding protein capsid is often referred to as the nucleocapsid (Fig. 2). A number of general principles have emerged from studies of virus structure.[13,14] First, in almost all cases the capsid is composed of a repeating series of structurally similar subunits, each of which is in turn composed of at most only a few different proteins. The parsimonious use of structural proteins in a repetitive motif minimizes the amount of the viral genome that must be committed to encode the capsid components. The use of only a few different types of proteins and the repetition of subunits also leads to structural arrangements of virus capsids with symmetric features. All but the most complex viruses exhibit one of two types of capsid symmetry (Table 1). In helically symmetric viruses the repeating protein subunits of the capsid are bound periodically along the helical spiral formed by the viral nucleic acid. Interestingly, all animal viruses that show this type of symmetry have RNA genomes.

The second major type of capsid symmetry is icosahedral. Viruses with this type of symmetry typically have a nearly spherical shape, with twofold, threefold, and fivefold axes of rotational symmetry. The nucleic acid, which can be either DNA or RNA, is tightly packed inside the spherical core and is also intimately associated with specific viral capsid proteins, although the details of this interaction are not as well understood as they are for helically symmetric viruses.

The use of repeating subunits with symmetric protein–protein interactions undoubtedly facilitates the assembly of the viral capsid. In most cases this appears to be an autocatalytic process that occurs spontaneously under the appropriate physiologic conditions. In some viruses such as the bacteriophages, assembly of the capsid may proceed through a series of intermediates or subassemblies, each of which seems to nucleate the addition of subsequent components in the sequence.

One of the most poorly understood aspects of viral assembly is the process that ensures that the viral nucleic acid is correctly packaged into the capsid. In the case of helically symmetric viruses there may be an initiation site on the nucleic acid to which the initial capsomere subunit binds, triggering the addition of subsequent subunits. In preparations of many icosahedral viruses, it is not uncommon to find empty capsids (i.e., capsids lacking nucleic acid), which indicates that assembly may proceed to completion without a requirement for the presence of the viral genome.

In some viruses the nucleocapsid is surrounded by a lipid envelope acquired as the virus particle buds from host cell cytoplasmic or nuclear membranes or the endoplasmic reticulum. Into this lipid bilayer are inserted virally encoded proteins (e.g., the hemagglutinin [HA] and neuraminidase [NM] of influenza), which are exposed on the outside of the virus particle. These viral proteins typically contain a glycosylated hydrophilic external portion and internally positioned hydrophobic domains that span the lipid membrane and serve to anchor the proteins. In some cases another viral protein may associate with the internal (cytoplasmic) surface of the lipid envelope where it can interact with the cytoplasmic domains of the envelope glycoproteins. These matrix (M) proteins may play a role in directing the insertion of viral glycoproteins into host cell membranes, in stabilizing the interaction between these proteins and the lipid envelope, or in facilitating viral budding.

Viruses belonging to the family Reoviridae, which includes the human rotaviruses, have an outer protein shell that surrounds the nucleocapsid. The mechanisms by which the two capsids are assembled in proper relationship to each other remains to be identified.

VIRUS–CELL INTERACTIONS

The interaction between a virus and a target cell begins with attachment of the virus particle to the cell surface.[15] This process is initiated by a random collision between a virus particle and the cell surface. Tighter binding is facilitated by appropriate ionic and pH conditions in the extracellular milieu. Attachment may involve the interaction between specific proteins on the

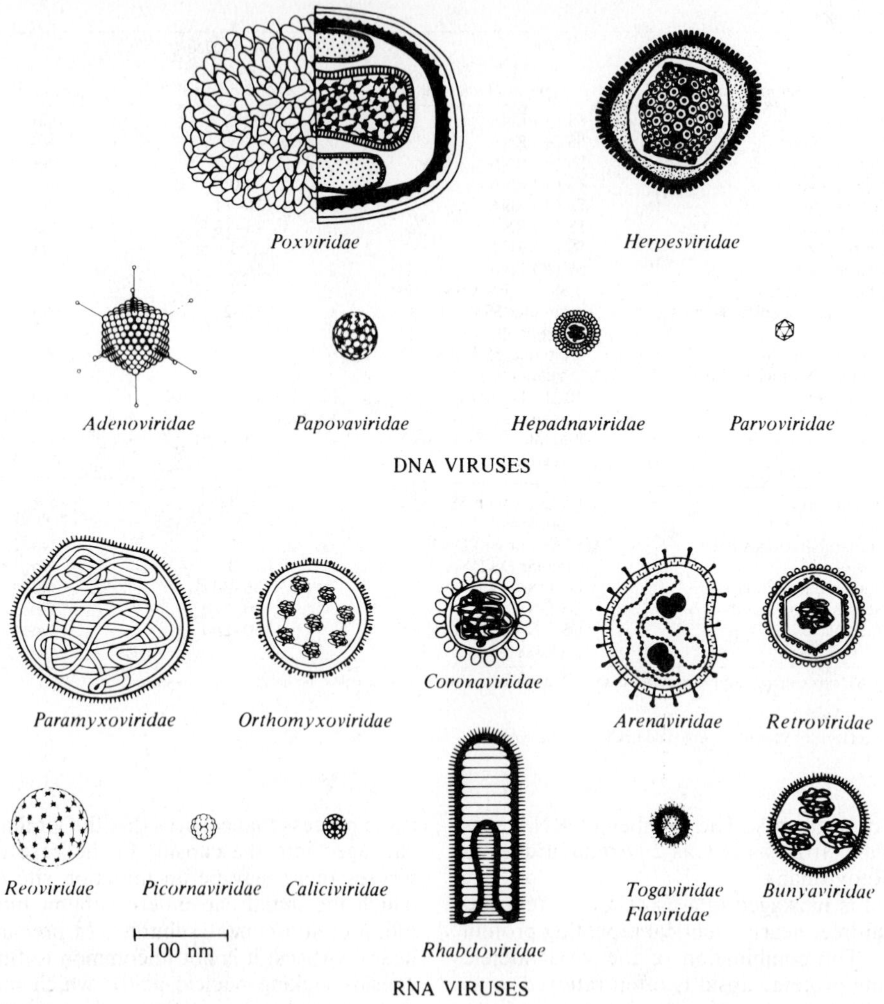

FIG. 1. Diagrams illustrating the general sizes and shapes of animal viruses belonging to families known to be pathogenic to humans. (From White et al.,[11] with permission.)

viral surface (virion attachment protein [VAP]) and specific receptors in the target cell membrane. The nature of the VAP has been identified for a number of viruses. In the case of enveloped viruses the VAP is typically one of the envelope glycoproteins such as the HA glycoprotein of influenza. Outer capsid proteins typically serve as the VAPs for nonenveloped viruses. For some viruses more then one surface protein may be involved in receptor binding.

Using high resolution x-ray crystallography it has been possible to obtain detailed views of the three-dimensional structure of the VAPs of a number of viruses including influenza and several of the picornaviruses (polio, rhino, mengo, encephalomyocarditis [EMC], Theiler).[16–20] The receptor binding domain of the flu HA is located at the distal end of its globular head (Fig. 3). The receptor-binding sites of the picornaviruses appear to take the form of depressions or indentations in the surface topology of the virion. These depressions can take the form of ''pits'' (mengovirus), ''canyons'' (rhinovirus), or ''valleys'' (poliovirus) and are clearly visible on electron density maps of the virus particles.

One of the most dynamic areas of current research in virology deals with the identification of viral receptors on host cells. A number of putative viral receptors have now been identified (Table 2); however, in many cases considerable controversy concerning these identifications still exists.

A number of important principles have emerged from studies of VAPs and host cell receptors. First, cells presumably did not evolve with viral receptors on their surfaces. Instead, viruses have adapted to ''parasitize'' host-cell surface molecules designed to subserve a variety of normal cellular functions. These may either be highly specialized proteins with somewhat limited distribution such as neurotransmitters, hormones, and complement receptors or may be more ubiquitous components of cellular membranes such as sialoglycoproteins or phospholipids. Second, it appears that some viruses may use more then one type of host cell receptor or possibly both specific receptor-mediated and other nonspecific pathways to enter cells. Finally, it has been frequently demonstrated that not all cells carrying the receptor for a particular virus can be productively infected by that virus. Therefore, although receptor binding may be a first step in the interaction between viruses and cells, subsequent events in the viral life cycle must also be successfully completed for productive infection to occur.

Once attachment has occurred, the virus must penetrate the plasma membrane of the cell, and then the capsid must undergo a series of conformational changes (uncoating) that prepares the virus for subsequent replication. Many enveloped and nonenveloped viruses penetrate cells through a process analogous to the receptor-mediated endocytosis of nonviral ligands such as hormones, growth factors, and toxins[23–25] (Fig. 4). In this schema viral–receptor complexes aggregate at distinct sites on the plasma membrane where specialized pits lined with the protein clathrin (''clathrin-coated pits'') occur. These pits then invaginate to form coated vesicles, which are subsequently uncoated and form endosomes. The acidic pH of the interior of endosomes may trigger pH-dependent conformational changes

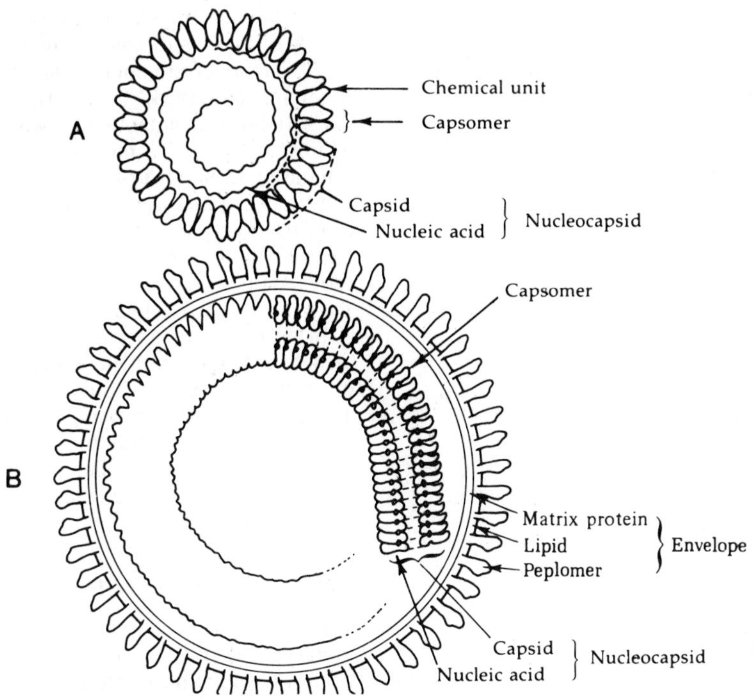

FIG. 2. Schematic diagrams of the structure of a nonenveloped icosahedral virus (**A**) and an enveloped helical virus (**B**). (Modified from Caspar et al.,[12] with permission.)

TABLE 2. Putative Viral Receptors

Virus	*Receptor*
Cytomegalovirus	β_2-Microglobulin/MHC
Encephalomyocarditis virus	Glycophorin A (RBCS)
Epstein-Barr virus	C3d receptor (CR2)
Human immunodeficiency virus	CD4 (T4 antigen)
Influenza virus	Glycophorin A (RBCS)
	Sialic acid
Lactate dehydrogenase–elevating virus	Ia
Rabies virus	Acetylcholine receptor
Reovirus type 3 (Dearing)	β-adrenergic–related receptor
	Glycophorin A (RBCS)
Semliki Forest virus	HLA, H-2 antigens
Sendai virus	Sialic acid
Vaccinia virus	Epidermal growth factor receptor
Vesicular stomatitis virus	Phospho- or glycolipids

(Data from Crowell et al.[21] and Marsh et al.[22])

in specific viral proteins. These conformational changes may uncover protein domains capable of mediating fusion between the viral envelope or capsid and the endosomal membrane, thereby allowing escape of the viral nucleocapsid into the cytoplasm. Endosomal vesicles may subsequently fuse with lysosomes. Proteolytic enzymes present in lysosomes may also trigger partial digestion of viral capsid proteins, which leads to activation of viral transcription.

Viruses may also enter cells through nonendocytic pathways such as direct translocation across the plasma membrane. For some enveloped viruses this may be mediated by direct fusion of the viral envelope with the outer membrane of target cells with subsequent entry of the nucleocapsid into the cytoplasm.[26]

Once a virus has successfully entered a target cell, it must replicate both its genome and the associated structural and nonstructural proteins. A discussion of the many strategies of replication used by different families of viruses is beyond the scope of this chapter (see Fields and Knipe[27]). However, certain basic principles are worth noting. First, there is no enzymatic mechanism in host cells to replicate RNA from an RNA template (i.e., no RNA-dependent RNA polymerases). Second, the host cell enzymes for making mRNA from DNA are all located in the nucleus and are therefore not accessible to DNA viruses whose replication is exclusively cytoplasmic.

There are two basic replication strategies used by single-stranded RNA viruses. If the genomic RNA is (+)sense it can serve directly as messenger RNA. For example, after infection of target cells with picornaviruses such as poliovirus, the viral genomic RNA serves directly as messenger RNA and is translated on target cell ribosomes into a large polyprotein. This protein is subsequently cleaved into several smaller proteins. One of these proteins is a RNA-dependent RNA polymerase, which serves to replicate the viral RNA. A different strategy is required for viruses with (−)sense genomic RNA since this RNA cannot serve directly as mRNA. These viruses all contain an RNA-dependent RNA polymerase that transcribes a (+)sense RNA segment from the original (−)sense genomic RNAs. These (+)sense RNAs can serve both as mRNAs and as templates for the replication of more genomic (−)sense RNAs.

RNA viruses belonging to the family Reoviridae have a segmented double-stranded RNA genome. These viruses contain a double-stranded RNA–single-stranded RNA polymerase that allows the production of (+)sense single-stranded RNA from the double-stranded RNA segments by using the (−)sense strand as a template. The reovirus (+)sense RNAs are capped at their 5′-terminal end by virally encoded enzymes and then extruded from the viral core through a channel formed by the core spike protein and serve as mRNAs. The (+)sense RNAs also serve as the templates for the viral polymerase to make (−)sense RNA segments that can then anneal with the complementary (+)sense strands to form new genomic double-standed RNAs.

Perhaps the most intriguing RNA replicative strategy is that used by the retroviruses. The viral genomic RNA is (+)sense and single stranded. However, unlike the case with the picornaviruses, it does not serve directly as mRNA. It is transcribed into DNA through the operation of a virally encoded RNA-dependent DNA polymerase ("reverse transcriptase"). The virally encoded DNA is then translocated into the host cell nu-

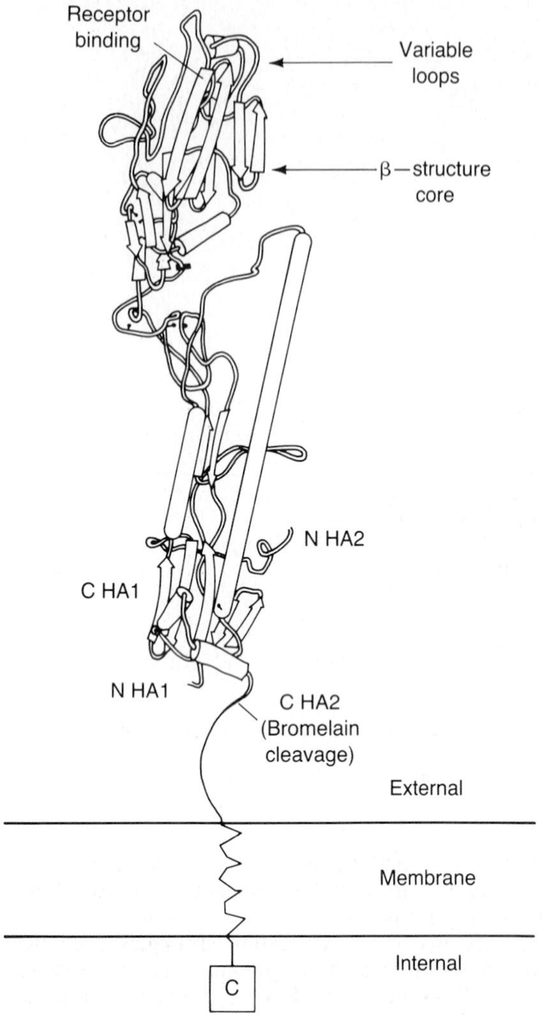

FIG. 3. The hemagglutinin (HA) of influenza virus. Arrows represent β-strands and cylinders, α-helices. The location of the receptor binding site is indicated. (Modified from Wilson,[17] with permission.)

cleus where it becomes integrated into the chromosomal DNA of the host ("provirus"). Transcription of this integrated DNA then falls under the control of the same transcriptase enzymes used by the host to replicate its own DNA. This transcription produces both mRNAs that encode viral proteins and genomic-length RNAs for packaging into progeny virions. The factors that govern whether this integrated viral DNA remains latent and untranscribed or is actively transcribed to produce progeny virions remains one of the unsolved mysteries of viral replication.

Viruses whose genomes are in the form of DNA did not have to develop as complex replicative strategies as those outlined above for RNA viruses. These viruses, which typically replicate in the nucleus of target cells, can use host cell enzymes for the production of mRNA from their DNA. In most cases, as exemplified by the herpesviruses, the viral mRNA encodes a DNA polymerase that serves to replicate the viral genomic DNA. A further degree of complexity is added by the fact that some DNA viruses can remain latent in the host. Unlike the case with retroviruses, the viral DNA does not typically integrate into host cell chromosomes but instead exists in episomal form. The factors that govern the reactivation from latency to active infection are currently the subject of active investigation.[28,29]

Knowledge of the replicative strategies of viruses has provided insights into critical steps in the viral life cycle that can serve as potential targets for antiviral therapy (see Shannon[30]). For example, drugs can be designed that interfere with the capacity of viruses to bind to their target cell receptors or to successfully undergo penetration-uncoating once receptor attachment has occurred. Two currently available antiviral agents, rimantadine and amantadine, which are effective in prophylaxis against influenza A infections, probably act by inhibiting viral uncoating in target cells. Steps involved in the transcription of the viral genome are another obvious target for antiviral therapy. A number of currently available (acylovir, vidarabine) and experimental (phosphonoformic acid, bromovinyldeoxyuridine) antiherpesvirus agents act, at least in part, by inhibiting the viral DNA polymerase.

In the future, a better understanding of viral replicative strategies will undoubtedly pave the way for the design and testing of a multitude of novel antiviral agents. One of the most exciting approaches to this problem will be to use high resolution x-ray crystallography to study the interaction between antiviral drugs and virions at the molecular level.[31] As more viral structures are solved, this approach may allow the design of highly specific antiviral agents.

VIRUS–HOST INTERACTION

One of the most fundamental challenges in virology is trying to integrate lessons learned from the study of virus–cell interaction in tissue culture into a conception of how viruses interact with an intact living host in order to produce the signs and symptoms of disease. The process by which a virus produces disease in an animal host is referred to as *pathogenesis*. The capacity of a virus to produce illness or death in susceptible animals is referred to as *virulence*, and it is often measured in terms of the amount of virus required to kill or cause infection in 50 percent of a cohort of mice infected under defined conditions. Pathogenesis and virulence were initially defined in largely descriptive terms. Specific stages in the pathogenesis of particular viral infections were identified and their associated pathologic substrates defined. More recently it has been possible, in some cases, to begin to identify the role played by specific viral genes and the proteins they encode at specific stages in viral pathogenesis and the importance of specific viral genes in determining viral virulence. The goal for future studies of pathogenesis will be to continue to define at a genetic and molecular level viral components involved at discrete steps in disease production.

The first step in the process of virus–host interaction is exposure of a susceptible host to infectious virus under conditions that are propitious for transmission.[32] The infecting virus may be present in respiratory droplets or aerosols, in fecally contaminated food or water, or in a body fluid or tissue (e.g., blood, saliva, urine, semen, or a transplanted organ) to which the susceptible host is exposed. In some cases the virus is inoculated directly into the host through the bite of an insect or animal vector or through the use of a sullied needle.

Infection can also be transmitted vertically, from a mother to her fetus or newborn child, through virus carried in the germ cell line, virus that has infected the placenta or maternal birth canal, or virus in maternal milk. In some cases acute viral infection results from the reactivation of endogenous latent virus that had previously lain dormant in the host (e.g., shingles, recurrent herpes labialis or genitalis), rather than from de novo exposure to exogenous virus.

One of the most important routes of transmission of infection to a susceptible host is through infected respiratory droplets or aerosols. A simple cough can generate up to 10,000 small potentially infectious aerosol particles and a sneeze, nearly 2 million! The distribution of these particles depends on a variety of ambient environmental factors, the most important of which are probably temperature, humidity, and air currents. Amother critical factor is particle size. In general, smaller particles remain airborne longer than do larger ones. Airborne particles are inspired through the nasopharynx, after which their ultimate fate

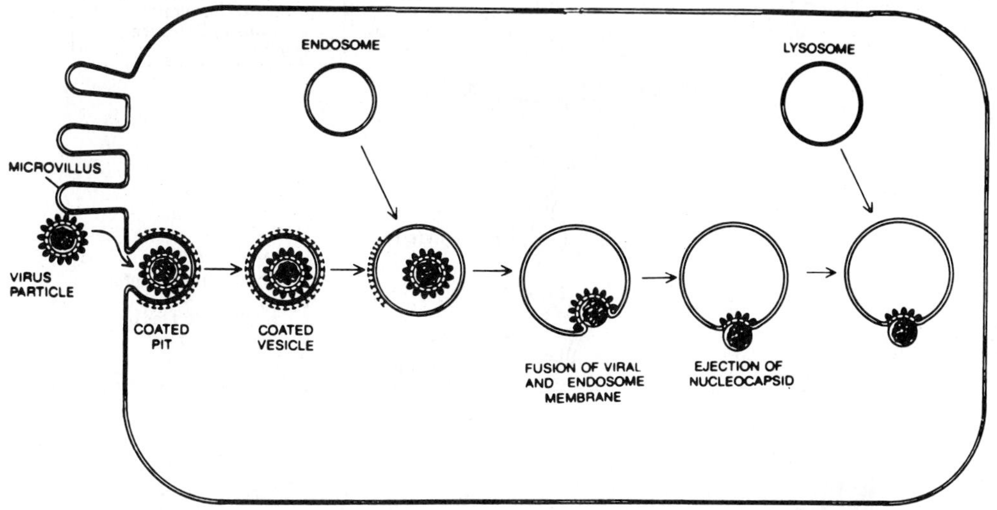

FIG. 4. Pathway of viral entry into cells. (Modified from Simons et al.,[25] with permission.)

depends largely on their size. Larger particles (>6 μm) are generally trapped in the nasal turbinates, whereas smaller particles may find their way into the tracheae and the bronchi of the upper respiratory tract or the alveolar spaces of the lower respiratory tract.

A second common route of viral transmission is through "fecal–oral" spread. Food, water, or hands contaminated by infected fecal material can allow the entry of virus via the mouth into the upper gastrointestinal (GI) tract. Once a virus has reached the upper GI tract, it faces a formidable physicochemical environment. Gastric juice is extremely acidic, at times approaching pH 2.0. Bile and proteolytic enzymes secreted from the gallbladder and pancreas enter the duodenum. The intestinal epithelial cells are covered by a carpet of mucous secreted by adjacent goblet cells. Secretory immunoglobulin (IgA) as well as non-immunoglobulin-inhibitory substances are also present.

The physicochemical environment of the GI tract essentially mandates that viruses infecting via this route have certain prescribed physical properties. They must be acid stable to survive transit through the stomach. Since bile salts are extremely destructive of the lipids present in viral envelopes, most enteric viruses are also nonenveloped. Finally, many viruses infecting via the GI tract have become adapted so that partial proteolytic digestion, rather than inhibiting viral infectivity, may actually be a necessary first step in the viral replicative cycle. This appears to be the case during rotavirus infection in which partial proteolytic digestion of the viral outer capsid actually enhances viral infectivity.

The lumens of the GI, respiratory, and genitourinary tracts can be considered extensions of the external environment. In order to produce systemic disease, a virus must cross the mucosal barrier that separates these luminal compartments from the host's parenchymal tissues. Studies with reovirus have illustrated a strategy by which, after entry into the GI tract, viruses can invade the host, by crossing mucosal barriers, thereby initiating systemic infection.[33,34] After oral inoculation of mice, reovirions adhere to the surface of intestinal microfold cells (M cells) that overlie collections of intestinal lymphoid tissue (Peyer's patches). In electron micrographs, virions can be followed sequentially as they are transported within vesicles from the luminal to the abluminal surface of M cells. Virions subsequently appear within Peyer's patches and, in the case of reovirus type 1, can subsequently spread to regional lymph nodes and to extraintestinal lymphoid organs such as the spleen. Although the use of M cells to transport virus has only been specifically described for reoviruses, it would appear likely that this represents a more ubiquitous pathway for invasion of the host from the GI tract by enteric viruses.

Once a virus has entered the host via respiratory, GI, or genitourinary routes or through direct inoculation, it may either produce a local infection or spread from its site of entry to distant target organs to produce systemic disease (Fig. 5). Examples of localized infections in which viral entry, primary replication, and tissue tropism all occur at the same anatomic site include the upper and lower respiratory infections caused by the rhinoviruses and the myxoviruses, the enteric illness produced by rotaviruses, and the dermatologic diseases produced by papillomavirus (warts) and paravaccinia virus (milker's nodules). Conversely, enteroviruses (e.g., poliovirus) must spread from the GI tract to the central nervous system (CNS) to produce meningitis, encephalitis, or poliomyelitis. Measles and varicella enter the host through the respiratory tract but then spread to the skin to produce exanthemal lesions and often to visceral organs as well.

The primary pathways of spread used by viruses to reach target organs are through the lymphatic system, through the blood stream, or through nerves. Rabies virus, herpes simplex and simiae, varicella-zoster virus, bornavirus, and the scrapie agent all spread via nerves.[35] A number of viruses including rabies have been shown to accumulate at the neuromuscular junctions after inoculation and subsequent multiplication in skeletal muscle. In the case of rabies it has been suggested that the acetylcholine receptor (AChR) may serve as a viral receptor that enables virus to enter the distal axon terminals of motor neurons.[36,37] Interestingly, the major envelope glycoprotein of rabies (G protein) has areas of amino acid sequence similarity with certain snake neurotoxins that are known to also bind to the AChR.[38] Herpes simplex virus also appears to enter nerve cells via receptors that are located primarily at synaptic endings rather than on the nerve cell body.[39] Spread of both of these viruses to the CNS can be inhibited by interruption of the appropriate nerves or by chemical agents that inhibit axonal transport.[40–42]

Certain strains of poliovirus can also be shown to spread through nerves to reach the CNS in infected animals, although the importance of neural spread in human infection has never been conclusively established.[42–45] Studies of the kinetics of the neural spread of herpes, rabies, and polio suggest that the neural spread of these viruses is probably due to fast axonal transport. Recent studies of the neural spread of reovirus type 3 (Dearing) also indicate that this virus spreads to the CNS via nerves.[48] By using selective pharmacologic inhibitors of either fast or

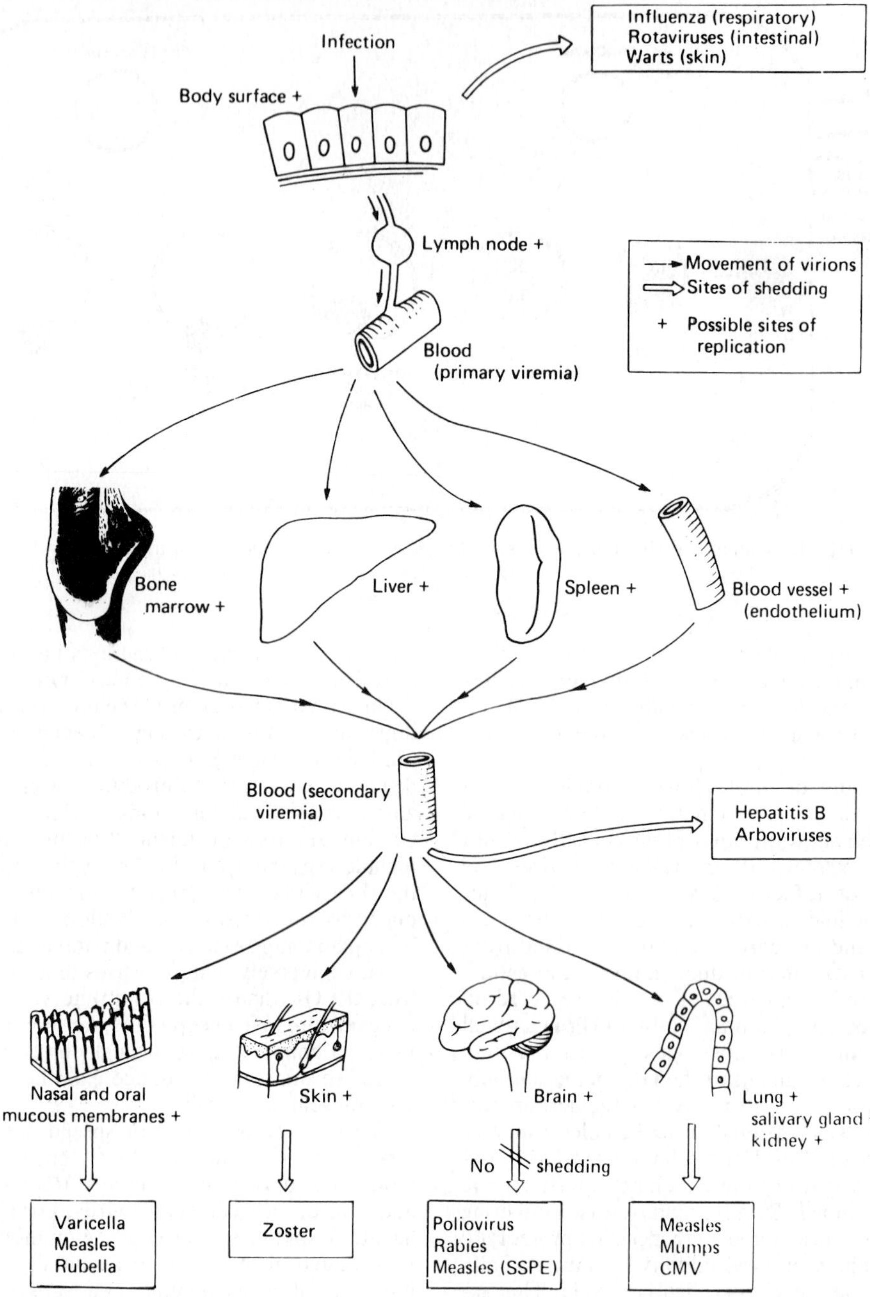

FIG. 5. The spread of virus through the body in human viral infections. Also shown are potential sites for shedding of virus, with examples of diseases in which that route of excretion is important. (Modified from Mims et al.,[32] with permission.)

slow axonal transport it was shown that the spread of reovirus type 3 is also mediated by the microtubule-associated system of fast axonal transport. Kinetic studies of the spread of the scrapie agent to the CNS after peripheral inoculation, or within the CNS after intracerebral or intraocular inoculation, suggest that this agent also travels via nerves.[47,48] The rate of spread was extremely slow which suggests that this agent may actually use the intermediate filament-associated system of slow axonal transport rather then the microtubule-based system of fast axonal transport.

A second major pathway for the spread of viruses from their site of primary replication to distant target tissues is through the blood stream.[32] In some cases virus may enter the blood stream directly, as when a patient is transfused with contaminated blood or blood products or when an addict uses a dirty needle for injecting drugs. More commonly, virus enters the blood stream after replication at some primary site. Important sites of primary replication include Peyer's patches and mesenteric lymph nodes for enteric viruses, epithelial and alveolar cells for respiratory viruses, and skeletal muscle, subcutaneous tissues, and brown fat for togaviruses and some enteroviruses.

Classic studies by Fenner with mousepox suggested that an initial low-titer viremia ("primary viremia") served to seed virus to a variety of organs where a period of further replication led to a much larger high-titer viremia ("secondary viremia") that served to disseminate virus to target organs.[49] It is often exceedingly difficult to identify "primary" and "secondary" viremias in naturally occurring viral infections; however, multiplication of many viruses in reticuloendothelial organs (liver, spleen, lymph nodes, bone marrow), muscle, fat, and even vascular endothelial cells often plays an important role in maintaining viremia.

A virus that reaches the blood stream may travel either free in the plasma (e.g., picornaviruses, togaviruses) or in association with specific cellular elements.[32] A number of viruses are known to travel in association with macrophages (e.g., lentiviruses including HIV) and lymphocytes (e.g., Epstein-Barr virus, HIV). Although many viruses have the capacity to agglutinate red cells in vitro (hemagglutination), only in exceptional cases (e.g., Colorado tick fever virus) have red cells been shown to be important in transporting virus.

The maintenance of viremia appears to depend on the interplay between factors contributing to the maintenance of viremia (e.g., continued virus replication) and host mechanisms designed to remove virus from the circulation ("clearance") or inactivate circulating virus (e.g., neutralizing antibody). A number of factors have been identified that can alter the outcome of these events.[32] In general, the larger the viral particle, the more efficiently it is cleared. Studies of the clearance of reoviruses from the circulation indicate that the outer capsid protein sigma-1 plays a role in determining the pattern of clearance of these viruses and that this pattern can be altered by the presence of antibody bound to the virion.[50] This type of study suggests that the nature of specific components of the virion, especially those present on the outer surface, may be important in determining patterns of clearance in the infected host. Inhibition of the capacity of cells in the host reticuloendothelial system (RES) to phagocytose circulating viruses can also lead to prolongation and magnification of the viremic state. This can be accomplished experimentally by giving animals compounds such as silica or thorotrast, which are avidly phagocytosed by RES cells and seem to "block" their capacity to subsequently clear circulating virus.

Little is known about how specific viral genes and the proteins they encode determine the pathways used by viruses to spread from their site of entry in the host to the ultimate target tissues. Recent experiments with reoviruses have provided some insights into how viruses "choose" between blood-borne and neural routes of spread.[46] Reovirus type 1 (Lang) spreads via the blood stream, and reovirus type 3 (Dearing) spreads via nerves to reach the spinal cord after intramuscular inoculation. By using reovirus reassortants containing different combinations of genes derived from these two parents it was shown that a single viral gene encoding a surface (outer capsid) protein determines the pattern of spread used by these viruses. Studies using intertypic recombinants between herpes simplex virus types 1 and 2 have also identified specific regions in the genome of herpes simplex virus that are important in determining the neural spread of these viruses.[51,52] The region of the genome initially identified as important in determining the capacity of herpes simplex type 1 to spread via nerves from the eye to the brain (0.31–0.44 m.u.) was rather large and encoded a number of proteins (including the DNA polymerase, the major nucleocapsid protein, an immediate early DNA binding protein [ICP8], and a major envelope glycoprotein, gB). Subsequent studies strongly suggest that it is the gene encoding the DNA polymerase that is important,[52] although the mechanism of action remains obscure. Interestingly, studies comparing the neuroinvasiveness of two strains of herpes simplex type 1 identified an overlapping region of the genome (0.25–0.53 m.u.) as critical for neuroinvasiveness.[53] Thus, as illustrated by both reoviruses and herpesviruses, there is evidence that the nature of the pathways used by viruses to spread in the infected host is genetically determined.

It is important to recognize that viruses are not limited to using only a single route of spread. Varicella-zoster virus, for example, is believed to spread from its site of initial entry in the host through the respiratory tract to the skin via the blood stream. Infection of the skin produces the characteristic exanthem of chickenpox. The virus subsequently travels retrogradely up the distal terminals of sensory neurons to reach the dorsal root ganglia where it remains latent. Reactivation of virus from the latent state results in transport of virus down the sensory nerve axon to produce zoster (shingles).[54] Polioviruses represent another example of viruses that appear capable of spreading via both neural and hematogenous routes. Polioviruses are generally believed to travel from the GI tract to the CNS via the blood stream, although the alternative suggestion that they may travel via autonomic nerves in the gut to reach the brain stem and spinal cord has never been conclusively excluded.[55,56] Once the virus reaches the CNS, axonal transport appears to be its major route of dissemination.[45]

In a series of papers nearly 30 years ago, Holland and McLaren suggested that the capacity of poliovirus to injure specific tissues while sparing others during acute poliomyelitis paralleled the capacity of homogenates of these tissues to bind poliovirus in vitro.[57] They also suggested that several types of cells that were not naturally susceptible to infection with poliovirus would support a single cycle of viral replication if transfected with poliovirus RNA. These studies helped establish the principle that the presence or absence of receptors on specific cells was a major determinant of the capacity of viruses to selectively infect and injure these cells ("tropism").

It is important to recognize that the interaction between virion attachment proteins and host cell receptors is not the only determinant of tropism. Obviously, in order for a virus to infect a specific population of cells it must first reach these cells. The route of entry and pathway of spread used by a virus to infect the host can therefore profoundly influence tropism.[58] It is commonly recognized that a wide variety of host factors can dramatically affect the ultimate tropism of a virus. These can include the age, immune status, genetic composition, and nutritional state of the host. Examples of age-related susceptibility and/or resistance to viral infection abound. Similarly, the pathogenesis of viral infection differs markedly in an immune as compared with a nonimmune host. The basis for genetic determinants of viral susceptibility are extremely complex.[59] Studies with inbred strains of mice suggest that a variety of different mechanisms for genetic-related variations in susceptibility exist. These may involve differences in immune responses, the induction of antiviral mediators such as interferon, the presence or absence of genes encoding viral receptors, and in the case of certain retroviruses, the existence of defective endogenous proviruses in the genome. In many cases, although the existence of genetic factors that determine susceptibility is clear, their mechanism of action remains unknown. Nutritional factors such as starvation or malnutrition may act by altering the host's immune responsiveness or through yet unidentified modes of action.

It is important to recognize that the events, including receptor binding, that bring a virus into contact with susceptible cells in target tissues are merely the first steps along a pathway that may lead to replication of viral genomes and production of progeny virions. As discussed in the section dealing with virus–cell interactions, a complex series of events are initiated by virus attachment to host cell receptors. It is necessary for all of these events to proceed successfully for infectious progeny virions to be produced.

An important recent development in understanding viral tropism has been the recognition that some viruses contain elements in their genome that act to stimulate the transcription of specific sets of viral genes in a tissue-specific fashion.[60] Enhancers are one of the most important tissue-specific genetic elements. Enhancers are short strings of nucleotides, often repeated in tandem, that act in a position- and orientation-independent fashion to stimulate the transcription of specific sets of viral genes. In some cases these enhancers are "promiscuous," that is, they seem to be active in virtually all types of cells. Other enhancers show exquisite tissue specificity. For example, the JC virus promoter–enhancer region seems to be specifically active in human cultured fetal glial cells but not in HeLa or CV-1 cells.[61] This correlates well with the capacity of this virus, under certain circumstances, to produce a disease known as progressive multifocal leukoencephalopathy (PML) in which permissive infection is limited to oligodendroglia in the CNS.

One of the most exciting technological advances in molecular biology has been the development of transgenic mice. Transgenic mice are produced when a fertilized mouse egg is microinjected with foreign DNA and this DNA becomes incorporated into the somatic cell line as the embryo matures. Transgenic mice have been produced that contain the enhancer regions of SV40, JC virus, and more recently portions of the genome of the human immunodeficiency virus (HIV-1).[62,63] Studying the tissue-specific pattern of viral gene expression in these mice has provided a valuable method to investigate and identify tissue-specific elements in the genomes of these viruses.

In a simplified sense, viral virulence reflects the capacity of a virus to successfully complete these stages and subsequently injure or kill the host. One of the most important areas of recent research in viral pathogenesis has been to try to identify the role played by specific viral genes and the proteins they encode in determining viral virulence. It has been possible to identify specific "virulence determinants" in the genomes of a number of types of viruses including the togaviruses, bunyaviruses, reoviruses, herpesviruses, rhabdoviruses, myxoviruses, and picornaviruses. Although the nature of these virulence determinants varies for each viral group, a common theme is for the involved protein(s) to be viral surface proteins and frequently to include the virion cell attachment protein (e.g., the G glycoprotein of rabies, the sigma-1 protein of reovirus, the HA of influenza).

One of the important continuing themes in the study of viral–host interactions will be the further definition at a molecular and genetic level of the role played by individual viral genes and the proteins they encode at specific stages in the pathogenesis of an increasing number of viral infections. These studies will be complemented by studies designed to identify precise cellular targets, such as receptors, that are involved in viral–host interactions. One can predict that, as viral–host interactions are understood at an increasingly basic level, this will pave the way toward new strategies for preventing or treating viral diseases.

VIRUS–ENVIRONMENT INTERACTIONS

For a virus to propagate itself in nature, the outcome of virus–host interaction must be the shedding of infectious virus into the environment in a manner that optimizes the possibility for infection of subsequent susceptible hosts (Fig. 6). As discussed earlier, infectious virus may be shed from an infected host through a variety of mediums. Virus may be expelled from the respiratory tract in the form of aerosols generated by coughing or sneezing. Virus may be contained in saliva and transmitted through biting or intimate personal contact. Virus contained in feces may contaminate food or water that is subsequently ingested. Virus in semen or genital secretions may be transmitted during sexual intercourse. Each of these modes of transmission requires that virus be stable (i.e., remain infectious) under specific defined environmental conditions. Largely because of the obvious implications of this information for the inactivation and sterilization of viruses or virally infected material, the effects of temperature, pH, and of a variety of chemical and physical agents on the infectivity of a number of viruses has been extensively investigated. For example, polioviruses are resistant to inactivation by ether, chloroform, bile, detergents, and acidic pH but are quite susceptible to heat, dessication, ultraviolet (UV) irradiation, formalin, and chlorine. However, it was not until recently that it became possible to begin to correlate the susceptibility of viruses to specific agents of this type with specific aspects of their structural composition. In the case of poliovirus, many of the conditions that inactivate the virus (e.g., heating, UV irradiation, high pH) seem to result in a loss or alteration of the outer capsid protein VP4.[65] This in turn may create a "hole" in the viral capsid that allows the viral RNA to leak out. Obviously particles lacking RNA ("empty capsids") will not be infectious. Extensive studies of the effects of a variety of chemical and physical inactivating agents on the inactivation of reoviruses of different serotypes indicate that the surface proteins of the virus appear to play a critical role in determining the relative susceptibility of these viruses to inactivation.[66] The outer capsid protein sigma-1 was important in determining susceptibility to alkaline pH and guanidine, the outer capsid protein sigma-3 in determining susceptibility to sodium dodecyl sulfate (SDS) and high temperature, and the outer capsid protein mu-lc in determining sensitivity to phenol and ethanol. It is easy to appreciate how some

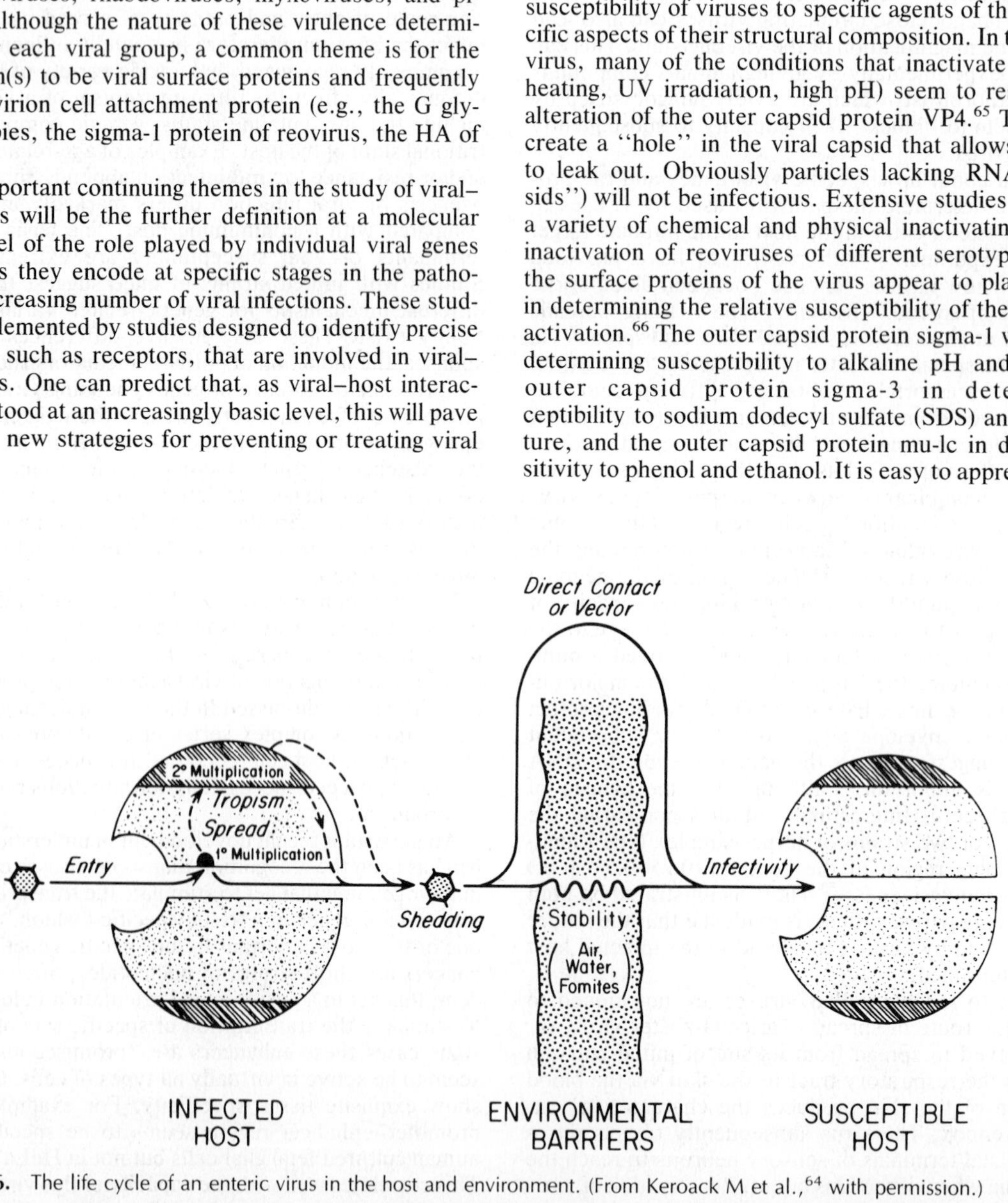

FIG. 6. The life cycle of an enteric virus in the host and environment. (From Keroack M et al.,[64] with permission.)

of the physical and chemical manipulations correlated with viral structure (e.g., temperature and pH sensitivity) may have direct relevance to understanding how viruses survive in the environment.

The future direction of research on how viruses interact with the environment will focus in part on defining in better detail, for a variety of viral systems, how specific structural components of virions determine the stability of these particles in defined physicochemical settings. This type of knowledge should be directly applicable to improving understanding of key factors in virion structure and chemistry that allow viruses to survive in the environment. This in turn may allow for better methods of decontamination of virally infected materials and for the design of public health strategies that will serve to interrupt the cycle of virus transmission through the environment.

REFERENCES

1. Waterson AP, Wilkinson L. An Introduction to the History of Virology. London: Cambridge University Press; 1978.
2. Reed W. Recent researches concerning the etiology, propagation and prevention of yellow fever by the United States Army Commission. J Hyg 1902;2:101–19.
3. Delbruck M. The growth of bacteriophage and lysis of the host. J Gen Physiol. 1940;23:643.
4. Luria SE. Bacteriophage: An essay on virus reproduction. Science. 1950; 111:507–11.
5. Avery OT, MacLeod CM, McCarty M. Studies on the chemical nature of the substance inducing transformation of pneumococcal types. Induction of transformation by a desoxyribonucleic acid fraction isolated from pneumococcus type III. J Exp Med. 1944;79:137–58.
6. Hershey AD, Chase M. Independent functions of viral protein and nucleic acid in the growth of bacteriophage. J Gen Physiol. 1952;36:39–56.
7. Enders JF, Weller TH, Robbins FC. Cultivation of the Lansing strain of poliomyelitis virus in cultures of various human embryonic tissues. Science. 1949;109:85–7.
8. Salk JE, Bennett BL, Lewis LJ, et al. Studies in human subjects on active immunization against poliomyelitis. I. A preliminary report of experiments in progress. JAMA. 1953;151:1081–98.
9. Sabin AB, Boulger LR. History of Sabin attenuated poliovirus oral live vaccine strains. J Biol Stand. 1973;1:115–8.
10. Murphy FA. Virus taxonomy. In: Fields BN, Knipe DM, eds. Fundamental Virology. New York: Raven Press; 1986:7–25.
11. White DO, Fenner FJ. Medical Virology. 3rd ed. San Diego: Academic Press, 1986.
12. Caspar D, Dulbecco R, Klug A, et al. Proposals. Cold Spring Harbor Symp Quant Biol. 1962;27:49.
13. Harrison S. Principles of virus structure. In: Fields BN, Knipe DM, eds. Fundamental Virology. New York: Raven Press; 1986:27–44.
14. Wiley DC. Viral membranes. In: Fields BN, Knipe DM, eds. Fundamental Virology. New York: Raven Press; 1986:45–67.
15. Lonberg-Holm K. Attachment of animal viruses to cells: An introduction. In: Lonberg-Holm K, Philipson L, eds.: Virus Receptors. part 2. London: Chapman & Hall; 1981:3–20.
16. Wilson IA, Skehel JJ, Wiley DC. Structure of the haemagglutinin membrane glycoprotein of influenza virus at 3 angstrom resolution. Nature. 1981; 289:366–73.
17. Wilson IA. The three-dimensional structures of surface antigens from animal viruses. In: Notkins AL, Oldstone MBA, eds. Concepts in Viral Pathogenesis II. New York: Springer Publishing; 1986:15–24.
18. Hogle JM, Chow M, Filman DJ. Three dimensional structure of poliovirus at 2.9 angstrom resolution. Science. 1985;229:1358–65.
19. Rossmann MG, Arnold E, Erickson JW, et al. Structure of a human common cold virus and functional relationship to other picornaviruses. Nature. 1985;317:145–53.
20. Luo M, Vriend G, Kamer G, et al. The atomic structure of Mengo virus at 3 angstrom resolution. Science. 1987;235:182–91.
21. Crowell RL, Hsu K-HL. Isolation of cellular receptors for viruses. In: Notkins AL, Oldstone MBA, eds. Concepts in Viral Pathogenesis II. New York, Springer Publishing; 1986:117–25.
22. Marsh M, Helenius A. Virus entry into animal cells. Adv Virus Res. 1988. In press.
23. Goldstein JL, Anderson RW, Brown MS. Coated pits, coated vesicles, and receptor mediated endocytosis. Nature. 1979;21:679–85.
24. Helenius A, Kartenbeck J, Simons K, et al. On the entry of Semliki Forest virus into BHK-21 cells. J Cell Biol. 1980;84:404–20.
25. Simons K, Garoff H, Helenius A. How an animal virus gets into and out of its host cell. Sci Am. 1982;246:58–66.
26. White J, Killian M, Helenius A. Membrane fusion proteins of enveloped animal viruses. Q Rev Biophys. 1981;16:151–95.
27. Fields BN, Knipe DM, eds. Fundamental Virology. New York: Raven Press; 1986.
28. Deatly AM, Spivack JG, Lavi E, et al. RNA from an immediate early region of the type 1 herpes simplex virus genome is present in the trigeminal ganglia of latently infected mice. Proc Natl Acad Sci USA. 1987;84:3204–8.
29. Stevens JG, Wagner EK, Devi-Rao GB, et al. RNA complementary to a herpesvirus alpha gene mRNA is prominent in latently infected neurons. Science. 1987;235:1056–9.
30. Shannon WM. Mechanisms of action and pharmacology: Chemical Agents. In: Galasso GJ, Merigan TC, Buchanan RA, eds. Antiviral Agents and Viral Diseases of Man. 3rd ed. New York: Raven Press; 1984:55–121.
31. Smith TJ, Kremer MJ, Luo M, et al. The site of attachment in human rhinovirus 14 for antiviral agents that inhibit uncoating. Science. 1986;233:1286–93.
32. Mims CA, White DO. Viral Pathogenesis and Immunology. Oxford: Blackwell Scientific Publications; 1984.
33. Wolf JL, Rubin DH, Finberg R, et al. Intestinal M cells: A pathway for entry of reovirus into the host. Science. 1981;212:471–2.
34. Wolf JL, Kauffman RS, Finberg R, et al. Determinants of reovirus interaction with the intestinal M cells and absorptive cells of murine intestine. Gastroenterology. 1983;85:291–300.
35. Johnson RT: Viral Infections of the Nervous System. New York: Raven Press; 1982:37–60.
36. Lentz TL, Burrage TG, Smith AL, et al. Is the acetylcholine receptor a rabies virus receptor? Science. 1982;215:182–4.
37. Burrage TG, Tignor GH, Smith AL. Rabies virus binding at neuromuscular junctions. Virus Res. 1985;2:273–89.
38. Lentz TL, Wilson PT, Hawrot E, et al. Amino acid sequence similarity between rabies virus glycoprotein and snake venom curaremimetic neurotoxins. Science. 1984;226:847–8.
39. Ziegler RJ, Herman RE. Peripheral infection in culture of rat sensory neurons by herpes simplex virus. Infect Immun. 1980;28:620.
40. Tsiang H. Evidence for intraaxonal transport of fixed and street rabies virus. J Neuropathol Exp Neurol. 1979;38:286–97.
41. Lycke E, Tsiang H. Rabies virus infection of cultured rat sensory neurons. J Viol. 1987;61:2733–41.
42. Kristensson K, Lycke E, Sjostrand J. Spread of herpes simplex virus in peripheral nerves. Acta Neuropathol (Berl). 1971;17:44–53.
43. Howe HA, Bodian DB. Neural Mechanisms of Poliomyelitis. New York: Commonwealth Fund; 1942.
44. Nathanson N, Bodian D. Experimental poliomyelitis following intramuscular virus injection. I. The effect of neural block on a neurotropic and a pantropic strain. Bull J Hopkins Hosp. 1961;108:308–33.
45. Jubelt B, Narayan O, Johnson RT. Pathogenesis of human poliovirus infection in mice. II. Age-dependency of paralysis. J Neuropathol Exp Neurol. 1980;39:149–59.
46. Tyler KL, McPhee DA, Fields BN. Distinct pathways of viral spread in the host determined by the reovirus S1 gene segment. Science. 1986;233:770–4.
47. Fraser H. Neuronal spread of scrapie agent and targeting of lesions within the retino-tectal pathway. Nature. 1982;295:149–50.
48. Kimberlin RH, Walker CA. Pathogenesis of mouse scrapie: Evidence for neural spread of infection to the CNS. J Gen Virol. 1980;51:183–7.
49. Fenner F. The pathogenesis of acute exanthems. Lancet. 1948;2:915.
50. Verdin EM, Lynn SP, Fields BN, et al. Uptake of reovirus serotype 1 by the lungs from the bloodstream is mediated by the viral hemagglutinin. J Virol. 1988;62:545–51.
51. Oakes JE, Gray WL, Lausch RN. Herpes simplex virus type 1 DNA sequences which direct spread of virus from the cornea to central nervous system. Virology. 1986;150:513–7.
52. Day SP, Lausch RN, Oakes JE. Evidence that the gene for herpes virus type 1 DNA polymerase accounts for the capacity of an intertypic recombinant to spread from eye to central nervous system. Virology. 1988;163:166–73.
53. Thompson RL, Cook ML, Devi-Rao GB, et al. Functional and molecular analysis of the avirulent wild-type herpes simplex virus type 1 strain KOS. J Virol. 1986;58:203–11.
54. Gelb LD. Varicella-zoster virus. In: Fields BN, ed. Virology. New York: Raven Press; 1985:591–627.
55. Bodian D. Poliomyelitis: Pathogenesis and histopathology. In: Rivers TM, Horsfall FL, eds. Viral and Rickettsial Infections of Man. 3rd ed. Philadelphia: JB Lippincott; 1959:479–518.
56. Sabin AB. Paralytic poliomyelitis: Old dogmas and new perspectives. Rev Infect Dis. 1981;3:543–64.
57. Holland JJ. Receptor affinities as major determinants of enterovirus tissue tropisms in humans. Virology. 1961;15:312–26.
58. Tyler KL. Host and viral factors that influence viral neurotropism. Trends Neurosci. 1987;10:455–60,492–7.
59. Rosenstreich DL, Weinblatt AC, O'Brien AD. Genetic control of resistance to infection in mice. CRC Crit Rev Immunol. 1982;3:263–300.
60. Khoury G, Gruss P. Enhancer elements. Cell. 1983;33:313–4.
61. Kenney S, Natarajan V, Strike D, et al. JC virus enhancer–promoter active in human brain cells. Science. 1984;226:1337–9.
62. Palmiter R, Chen H, Messing A, et al. SV40 enhancer and large-T-antigen are instrumental in development of choroid plexus tumors in transgenic mice. Nature. 1985;316:457–60.
63. Small J, Scangos G, Cork L, et al. The early region of human papovavirus JC induces dysmyelination in transgenic mice. Cell. 1986;46:13–8.
64. Keroack M, Bassel-Duby R, Fields B, et al. Genetic alterations in reovirus and their impact on host and environment. In: Fields BN, Martin MA, Kamely D, eds. Genetically Altered Virus and the Environment. Cold Spring Harbor, NY: Cold Spring Harbor Laboratory; 1985.

65. Rueckert R. Picornaviruses and their replication. In: Fields BN, ed. Virology. New York: Raven Press; 1985:705–38.
66. Drayna D, Fields BN. Biochemical studies on the mechanism of chemical and physical inactivation of reovirus. J Gen Virol. 1982;63:161–70.

DNA VIRUSES

Poxviridae

113. INTRODUCTION

JOHN M. NEFF

The pox viruses are a complex group of viruses whose classification is based primarily on the morphology of the virion and the viral nucleic acid.[1] This group of viruses represents the largest of all viruses. These viruses replicate in cytoplasm, rather than in the nucleus of cells, and by this characteristic differ from most other DNA viruses. The genomes of these agents are virtually homologous along 25–62 percent of the length of the internal segment.[2] The virus particles are asymmetric and brick-shaped, with round corners, and are very resistant to chemical and physical inactivation. They contain double-stranded DNA and have specific enzymes not found in other DNA viruses that allow them to replicate in the cytoplasm. Within the cytoplasm, they produce eosinophilic inclusions called *Guanieri bodies*. Originally, the pox viruses were classified according to their capability to produce vesicular skin lesions or cytoplasmic inclusion bodies. Since 1966, with the establishment of the International Committee on the Nomenclature of Viruses, the classification of these viruses has depended on the large shape of the virion and the presence of a large single linear molecule of double-stranded DNA.[3] The accepted classification of poxviruses of vertebrates is as follows: family: Poxviridae; subfamily: Chordopoxvirinae; genera: *Orthopoxvirus, Avipoxvirus* (fowlpox), *Capripoxvirus* (sheep pox), *Leporipoxvirus* (myxoma), *Parapoxvirus* (milker's nodule), *Suipoxvirus* (swinepox), unclassified (molluscum contagiosum, tanapox).

The genus *Orthopoxvirus* includes at least nine different species that are generally very homogeneous. They are the causative agents for vaccinia, variola, cowpox, monkeypox, ectromelia, camelpox, taterapox, raccoonpox, and Uasin Gishu disease.

The two major viruses of the *Orthopoxvirus* genus, vaccinia and variola, are closely related and have similar chemical and physical characteristics. Morphologically, they cannot be distinguished. The viral surface is composed of tubular structures surrounding a central nucleoid with a dense dumbbell-shaped core. On either side of the nucleoid core, inside the viral coat, is an elliptical body that gives the virion an appearance of central swelling.[2]

The virions are generally resistant to drying agents and many disinfectants. They may maintain infectivity for months at room temperature and for years below −20°C. They can be inactivated by autoclaving, by heating at 60°C for 10 minutes, and by the chlorine preparations, formaldehyde, iodophores, and quaternary ammonium compounds.[4]

The vaccinia and variola viruses share common antigens. Infection produces hemagglutination-inhibition (HAI) and neutralizing (N) antibodies. Because of the close antigenic similarity of these viruses, routine serologic testing is, in general, not useful in distinguishing variola infection from vaccinia infection or the different strains of variola from each other.[5] The enzyme-linked immunosorbent assay (ELISA) technique and radioimmunoassay have provided more sensitive differentiation between the antibodies produced by infection with these agents, as well as among the other viruses that make up the *Orthopoxvirus* genus group.[6,7] The monoclonal antibody technique may provide an even more specific differentiation.[8]

REFERENCES

1. Fenner F, Henderson DA, Arita L, et al. Smallpox and Its Eradication. Geneva: World Health Organization; 1988:69–103.
2. Dales S, Pogo BGT. Biology of poxviruses. Virol Monogr 1981;18:1.
3. Matthews REF. A Critical Appraisal of Viral Taxonomy, Boca Raton, Fla: CRC Press; 1983.
4. WHO Technical Report Series, No 283, WHO Expert Committee on Smallpox, First Report. Geneva: World Health Organization; 1964.
5. Bedson HS, Dumbell KR. Smallpox and vaccinia. Br Med Bull 1967;23:119.
6. Marennikova SS, Malceva NN, Habahpaseva NA. ELISA: A simple test for detecting and differentiating antibodies to closely related orthopoxviruses. Bull WHO 1981;59(3):365.
7. Walls HH, Ziegler DW, Nakano JH. Characterization of antibodies to orthopoxviruses in human sera by radioimmunoassay. Bull WHO 1981;59(2):253.
8. Kitamoto N, Tanimoto S, Hiroi K, et al. Monoclonal antibodies to cowpox virus: Polypeptide analyses of several major antigens. J Gen Virol 1987;68:239–46.

114. VACCINIA VIRUS (COWPOX)

JOHN M. NEFF

Little is known about the origins of vaccinia virus.[1] The virus was used for vaccination before there was any ability to characterize it or standardize its use. Vaccinia itself now has no natural host. One plausible theory of origin is that it derived from the cowpox virus, but in the early nineteenth century it was gradually transformed into the current virus as a result of person-to-person vaccination.

Edward Jenner, in his "Inquiry into the Causes and Effects of the Variolae Vaccinae" in 1798, was the first to observe that pustular material from the lesions of cowpox, when inoculated into humans, protected them from infection with smallpox.[2] Following Jenner's work, Woodville and Pearson of the Smallpox Hospital in London experimented extensively with this technique and distributed vaccination material to many physicians throughout England. The practice of vaccination then spread throughout the world and has been directly responsible for eradication of smallpox.[3]

VACCINES AND VACCINATION TECHNIQUES

Several years ago, many vaccine strains were in use, and there was much uncertainty about the protective value or risk of a given vaccine. Under the leadership of the World Health Organization (WHO), the use of strains was reduced generally to the derivatives of one of three strains: Elstree strain (Lister Institute), the EM63 strain (Moscow Research Institute of Virus Preparation), and the New York Board of Health strain.[4] WHO also established standards for production and use.[5] In general, smallpox vaccines are produced from a seed virus propagated on the skin of calves and then processed to eliminate bacterial contamination. The final vaccine is stored in liquid form or as a freeze-dried preparation. The latter preparations may maintain their titer even after incubation at 37°C for 4 weeks.[4] With the development of freeze-dried vaccines, it has been possible to distribute standard vaccines to remote and temperate countries throughout the world without loss of titer.

To pass WHO standards, a vaccine should be able to produce major reactions in 95 percent of the primary vaccinees and in 90 percent of those who were vaccinated more than 10 years previously. To obtain such results, most vaccines should have a titer of at least 10^8 pock-forming units per milliliter.

Vaccinations should be made over the deltoid region of the upper arm. The preferred method of vaccination is to use a bifurcated needle that has been dipped into the vaccine. The needle is then held perpendicular to the skin and pressed in and out 5 times for primary vaccinees and 15 times for revaccinees. Pressure should be sufficient to produce a trace of blood on the skin. Successful vaccination produces a major response in both primary vaccinees and revaccinees. A *major* response is defined by WHO as a "pustular lesion or an area of definite induration or congestion surrounding a central lesion (scab or ulcer) 6–8 days after vaccination." Any other response is called *equivocal*.[4]

Primary vaccinees in general demonstrate a vesicle within 3–5 days after vaccination. This becomes pustular and reaches its maximum size approximately 9 days after vaccination. The lesion forms a scab and ultimately leaves a small circular scar approximately 1 cm in diameter. Revaccinations yield variable results, ranging from an accelerated reaction, which become vesicular within 1–2 days after vaccination, to lesions that are very similar to primary reactions. Usually revaccinations do not result in scar formation even in remote revaccinees.

IMMUNITY RESULTING FROM VACCINATION

After vaccination there is local replication of virus. There also may be some replication of virus in the regional lymph nodes. Viremia, however, has not been demonstrated in uncomplicated vaccinations using modern, standardized vaccines.[6] Protection against smallpox that results from vaccination is probably due to both T and B cell-mediated antibodies. The dermal reaction that results from revaccination is a rough measurement of T-cell function and the circulating antibodies of B-cell function. The dermal evidence of immunity and circulating antibodies can be demonstrated within 4–5 days and increases up to 4 weeks after vaccination.[7,8] Circulating antibodies may persist for years after vaccination, and the dermal response after vaccination may demonstrate evidence of modification for up to 20 years. Although a primary vaccinee may rarely demonstrate seroconversion without a dermal response, the absence of a primary take and a following scar is considered to be an inadequate response to immunization.[4,9]

Successful vaccination is highly protective against smallpox even though the exact factors responsible for this protection have not been accurately defined. In general, protection against smallpox is nearly 100 percent for the first 1–3 years after vaccination. Persons who have not been vaccinated within 3 years may acquire smallpox on exposure, but this is a modified and nonfatal form of the disease. This modification can occur for up to 20 years after vaccination. After 20 years, there is very little remaining protection from vaccination.[4]

PASSIVE IMMUNITY

Hyperimmune vaccinial gamma globulin obtained from recent revaccinees is probably effective in reducing the incidence and severity of smallpox in intimate family contacts of an index case. If administered shortly after exposure and simultaneously with vaccination, there is limited evidence indicating that the resulting morbidity and mortality from smallpox will be less than would be expected in those who receive only a vaccination.[10]

COMPLICATIONS RESULTING FROM VACCINATION

In the majority of situations, primary vaccination results in modified swelling and tenderness at the site of vaccination, some regional lymphadenopathy, and occasionally a low-grade fever at the peak of the dermal response. At times, the pustular lesion itself may be as large as 4 cm but usually does not exceed 2 cm in diameter. Occasionally, abnormal reactions occur that may be mild or may be severe enough to result in fatality. Complications that result from vaccination have been broadly classified into (*1*) central nervous system, (*2*) dermal, and (*3*) other.[11,12]

Central Nervous System Complications

The principal central nervous system complication that results from vaccination is a postinfectious encephalitis,[13–24] which is similar to the encephalitis that occurs after measles and a few other acute viral illnesses. The vaccinia virus cannot be isolated from the central nervous system lesions. Most cases occur 1–2 weeks after vaccination, and the signs and symptoms are those of a generalized encephalitis. There also may be spinal cord signs when there is transverse myelitis or, rarely, focal neurologic signs. Routine diagnostic tests are of little help, except to rule out other possible causes of the illness. Treatment is supportive and symptomatic. The extent and severity of residual neurologic problems depend on the severity and location of the original lesions. Mortality is generally in the range of 10–30 percent. There is no known predilection for this disorder.[18]

The reported incidence of this disease has varied considerably from country to country, and the explanation for this variance has not been absolutely clear.[19] The incidence of this complication in the United States, where the New York Board of Health strain was used, was a little more than 1 in 100,000 primary vaccinees. This incidence was slightly higher when vaccination occurred before the first birthday. Similar rates have been observed in Great Britain, where the Elstree strain was used.[13] Although some countries have reported a higher incidence of this complication in adult primary vaccinees, as compared with children, this has not been observed either in the United States or in Great Britain.

Dermal Complications

The most frequent complications reported after smallpox vaccination are dermal. These can be roughly classified as those that are associated with an underlying illness and those that are not.[11,25,26] The former include vaccinia necrosum, or progressive vaccinia, and eczema vaccinatum; the latter, accidental infection, generalized vaccinia, and erythematous urticarial eruptions.

Vaccinia Necrosum. Vaccinia necrosum is the most severe complication occurring after smallpox vaccination.[27–31] It invariably results when a person with an immunologic deficiency is inadvertently vaccinated. The disease is insidious. The lesion begins as a normal vaccination but continues to progress, and in fatal cases shows no evidence of resolution. Paradoxically, the patient initially may have no systemic signs, no regional lymphadenopathy or erythema, but only progressive necrosis at the site of vaccination. As the disease continues, the patient develops metastatic lesions throughout the body. Vaccinia virus can easily be isolated from any of the lesions.

Eczema Vaccinatum. Patients with atropic dermatitis are unusually susceptible to two viral infections—herpes simplex and vaccinia. In both infections the clinical picture, Kaposi's varicellaform eruption, is similar, and the syndrome can be distinguished only by the history and viral isolation. Eczema vaccinatum is the clinical result of local spread and/or dissemination of vaccinia virus infections in such persons[32–34] (Dr. J. M. Neff, unpublished data). The complication may be a result of inadvertent vaccination or of intimate contact with a recently vaccinated person.

The treatment of eczema vaccinatum is to administer vaccinia immune globulin (VIG) in the therapeutic dose of 0.6 cc/kg/24 hr, repeated daily until no new lesions appear.

Accidental Infection. Not uncommonly, a healthy person may acquire vaccinial lesions accidentally as a result of either autoinoculation at the time of vaccination or intimate body contact with a person who had been recently vaccinated.[14,15] These lesions almost always occur in primary vaccinees. They are identical to a primary vaccination and are self-limited. When autoinoculation occurs, it is generally a coprimary reaction on a mucous membrane, the palpebral margins of the eyelid (ocular vaccinia), the nose, mouth, or anus.[35,36]

Generalized Vaccinia. *Generalized vaccinia* is a nonspecific term that is used to describe a vesicular rash that develops after vaccination. If cases of eczema vaccination and vaccinia necrosum (illnesses that truly represent a generalized vaccinia) are excluded, it is extremely rare to document a generalized, systemic viral dissemination resulting from vaccination. On the other hand, it is not uncommon to see, at about 7–12 days after vaccination, a patient who develops a rash characterized by multiple small vesicular lesions, each with an erythematous base.[14,15,25,26,32] The patient is nontoxic and often afebrile. Vaccinia virus cannot be isolated from the blood or the peripheral lesions. These cases have often been reported as generalized vaccinia. They occur in primary vaccinees and are seen most frequently in children vaccinated before their first birthday. The etiology is not known, and there is no specific treatment.

Erythematous Urticarial Eruptions. There are several erythematous rashes similar to enterovirus- or roseola-like rashes that are frequently observed 7–12 days after vaccination.[37] These are self-limited reactions lasting no more than a few days. The patients are not acutely ill and require no specific treatment. The pathogenesis is unknown.

Other Complications

Many other complications of vaccinations have been reported. These include myocarditis, thrombocytopenia, arthritis, and pericarditis. There also have been cases of malignant melanoma occurring in vaccination scars, as well as reports of acute erythema nodosum leprosum or lepra reactions after vaccination of patients with lepromatous leprosy.[11,38]

Three more frequent but still rare reactions should be noted: (*1*) bullous erythema multiforma, (*2*) overwhelming viremia resulting in sudden death in infancy, and (*3*) fetal vaccinia.

Further Attenuated Vaccines

Two strains that have been tested most widely have been those that were derived from the CV-1 and CV-2 strains of Rivers. In the United States the CV-1 strain has been studied most thoroughly.[39] It was found to be safe when administered to over 1000 eczematous children as a preimmunizing agent.[40] In healthy children, it has also been demonstrated to be more attenuated than standard calf lymph vaccine, and it may not provide full protection against smallpox. Since the successful eradication of smallpox, vaccination has not been performed frequently on a worldwide basis. Fortunately, the resulting complications have become rare.

There may, however, be new situations that could result in more frequent use of vaccinia and in a reappearance of complications. The first is the continuation of vaccination of military personnel because of the concern of biologic warfare.[41] This potential risk has been demonstrated in a report of disseminated vaccinia occurring in a military recruit who was immunologically impaired because of a concurrent infection with human immunodeficiency virus (HIV).[42] The second potential risk is from the use of new, experimental recombinant live virus vaccines.[43] In these vaccines, vaccinia is used as the biologic carrier for immunizing genes. Extensive work has already been done in this field, recombining vaccinia with genes for several other immunizing agents, including respiratory syncytial virus (RSV), HIV, parainfluenza, rotavirus, malaria, hepatitis B, and herpes simplex viruses.[44–49] Vaccinia is an ideal agent for such recombinant research because of its large size and extraordinary stability. This may be an important advance allowing the simultaneous delivery of several immunizing antigens through one vehicle. This agent, because of its stability, ease of storage, and mode of delivery, can be used in areas of the world where the use of other vaccines may not be practical. Vaccinia is also being used experimentally in a melanoma oncolysate to stimulate the production of antimelanoma antibodies in high-risk melanoma patients.[50] On a very preliminary basis, it has also been used as treatment for a patient with IgA multiple myeloma.[51]

This ongoing experimental use of vaccinia virus will require knowledge and evaluation of its immunogenic characteristics and its complications as an immunizing agent and as a recombinant.

REFERENCES

1. Baxby D. The origins of vaccinia virus. J Infect Dis. 1977;136:453.
2. Downie AW. Jenner's cowpox inoculation. Br Med J. 1951;2:251.
3. Dixon CW. Smallpox. London: Churchill Livingstone; 1962:249.
4. WHO Technical Report, Series No 493, WHO Expert Committee on Smallpox Eradication, Second Report. Geneva: World Health Organization; 1972.
5. WHO Technical Report, Series No 323, WHO Expert Group on Requirements for Biological Substances. Geneva: World Health Organization; 1965.
6. Glattner RJ, Norman JO, Hays FM, et al. Antibody response to cutaneous inoculation with vaccinia virus: Viremia and viruria in vacc children. J Pediatr. 1964;64:839.
7. Pincus WB, Flick JA. The role of hypersensitivity in the pathogenesis of vaccinia virus infection in humans. J Pediatr. 1963;62:57.
8. Wulff H, Chin TDY, Wenner HA. Serological responses of children after primary vaccination and revaccination against smallpox. Am J Epidemiol. 1969;90:312.
9. Pincus WB, Flick JA. Successful vaccinia infection without a local lesion. Am J Public Health. 1963;53:898.
10. Kempe CH, Bowles C, Meiklejohn G, et al. The use of vaccinia hyperimmune gamma globulin in the prophylaxis of smallpox. Bull WHO. 1961;25:41.
11. Lane JM, Millar JD, Neff JM. Smallpox and smallpox vaccination policy. Ann Rev Med. 1971;22:251.
12. Kempe CH. Studies on smallpox and complications of smallpox vaccination. Pediatrics. 1960;26:176.
13. Conybeare ET. Illness attributed to smallpox vaccination during 1951–60. Part II. Illness reported as affecting the central nervous system. Monthly Bull Ministry Health Public Health Lab Serv. 1964;23:150.
14. Neff JM, Lane JM, Pert JH, et al. Complications of smallpox vaccination, I National Survey in the United States, 1963. N Engl J Med. 1967;276:125.
15. Lane JM, Ruben FL, Neff JM, et al. Complications of smallpox vaccination 1968. National Surveillance in the United States. N Engl J Med. 1969;281:1201.
16. de Vries E. Postvaccinial Perivenous Encephalitis. Amsterdam: Elsevier; 1960.
17. Scott TFM. Postinfectious and vaccinial encephalitis. Med Clin North Am. 1967;51:701.
18. Keuter EJW. Predisposition of Post Vaccinial Encephalitis. Amsterdam: Elsevier; 1969.
19. Stuart G. Memorandum on post-vaccinial encephalitis. Bull WHO. 1947;1:36.
20. Nanning W. Prophylactic effect of antivaccinia gamma-globulin against post-vaccinial encephalitis. Bull WHO. 1962;27:317.
21. Noordaan J van der, Dekking F, Posthuma J, et al. Primary vaccination with an attenuated strain of vaccinia virus. Arch Gesamte Virusforsch. 1967;22:210.
22. Ehrengut W, Ehrengut-Lang J. Non-infectious smallpox vaccine in the prophylaxis of postvaccinial encephalitis. Int Symp Smallpox Vaccine, Bilthoven. 1972;19:319.
23. Polak MF. Complication of smallpox vaccination in the Netherlands 1959–1970. Int Symp Smallpox Vaccine, Bilthoven. 1972;19:235.
24. Berger K, Heinrich W. Decrease of postvaccinial deaths in Austria and in-

troduction of less pathogenic virus strain. Int Symp Smallpox Vaccine, Bilthoven. 1972;19:119.
25. Sarkany I, Caron GA. Cutaneous complications of smallpox vaccination. Trans St John Hosp Dermatol Soc. 1963;48:163.
26. Conybeare ET. Illness attributed to smallpox vaccination during 1951–60. Part I. Illnesses reported as "generalized vaccinia." Monthly Bull Ministry Health Public Health Lab Serv. 1964;23:126.
27. Fulginiti VA, Kempe CH, Hathaway WE, et al. Progressive vaccinia in immunologically deficient individuals. In: Bergsma D, ed. Birth Defects: Immune Deficiency Diseases of Man. v. 4. New York: The National Foundation—The March of Dimes; 1968:129.
28. Rosen FS, Janeway CA. The gamma globulins. III. The antibody deficiency syndrome. N Engl J Med. 1966;275:709.
29. O'Connell CJ, Karzon DT, Barron AL. Progressive vaccinia with normal antibodies. Ann Intern Med. 1964;60:282.
30. Lane JM, Ruben FL, Abrutyn E, et al. Deaths attributed to smallpox vaccination 1959 to 1966, 1968. JAMA. 1970;212:441.
31. Neff JM, Lane JM. Vaccinia necrosum following smallpox vaccination for chronic herpetic ulcers. JAMA. 1970;213:123.
32. Lane JM, Ruben FL, Neff JM, et al. Complications of smallpox vaccination, 1968 II. Results of ten statewide surveys. J Infect Dis. 1970;122:303.
33. Copeman PWM, Wallace HJ. Eczema vaccinatum. Br Med J. 1964;2:5415, 902.
34. Rachelefsky GS, Opelz G, Mickey R. Defective T cell function in atopic dermatitis. J Allergy Clin Immunol. 1976;57:569.
35. Ruben FL, Lane JM. Ocular vaccinia, an epidemiologic analysis of 348 cases. Arch Ophthalmol. 1970;84:45.
36. Fulginiti VA, Winograd LA, Jackson M, et al. Therapy of experimental vaccinial keratitis: Effect of idoxuridine and VIG. Arch Ophthalmol (Chicago). 1965;74:539.
37. Neff JM, Drachman RH. Complications of smallpox vaccination 1968. Surveillance in a comprehensive care clinic. Pediatrics. 1972;50:481.
38. Conybeare ET. Illness attributed to smallpox vaccination during 1951–60. Part III. Fatal illnesses reported as associated with vaccination (but not as generalized vaccinia or as post-vaccinial encephalomyelitis). Monthly Bull Ministry Health Public Health Lab Serv. 1964;23:182.
39. Galasso GJ, Karzon DT, Katz SL, et al, eds. Clinical and serological study of four smallpox vaccines comparing variations of dose and routes of administration. J Infect Dis. 1977;135:131.
40. Kempe CH, Fulginiti V, Minamitani M, et al. Smallpox vaccination of eczematous patients with a strain of attenuated live vaccinia (CVI-78). Pediatrics. 1968;42:980.
41. Halsey NA, Henderson DA. HIV infection and immunization against other agents. N Engl J Med. 1987;316:683–5.
42. Redfield RR, Wright DC, James WD, et al. Disseminated vaccinia in a military recruit with human immunodeficiency virus disease. N Engl J Med. 1987;316:673–6.
43. Quinnan GV. Vaccinia vectors for vaccine antigens. Proceedings of the Workshop on Vaccinia Viruses as Vectors for Vaccine Antigens, Held November 13–14, 1984, in Chevy Chase, Maryland. New York: Elsevier; 1985.
44. Stott EJ, Taylor G, Ball LA, et al. Immune and histopathological responses in animals vaccinated with recombinant vaccinia viruses that express individual genes of human respiratory syncytial virus. J Virol. 1987;61:3855–61.
45. Spriggs MK, Murphy BR, Prince GA, et al. Expression of the F and HN glycoproteins of human parainfluenza virus type B by recombinant vaccinia virus: Contribution of the individual proteins to host immunity. J Virol. 1987;61:3416–23.
46. Mackett M. Vaccinia virus recombinants: Potential vaccines. Acta Trop (Basel). 1987;445(Suppl 12):94–7.
47. Andrew ME, Boyle DB, Coupar BE, et al. Vaccinia virus recombinants expressing the SA 11 rotavirus VP7 glycoprotein gene induce serotype-specific neutralizing antibodies. J Virol. 1987;61:1054–60.
48. Langford CJ. Live viruses for the delivery of malaria vaccines. Papua New Guinea Med J. 1986;29:103–8.
49. Hu SL, Kosowski SG, Dalrymple JM. Expression of AIDS virus envelope gene for recombinant vaccinia virus. Nature. 1986;320:537–40.
50. Hersey P, Edwards A, Coates A, et al. Evidence that treatment with vaccinia melanoma cell lysates may improve survival of patients with Stage II melanoma. Cancer Immunol Immunother. 1987;25:257–65.
51. Kawa A, Arakawa S. The effect of attenuated vaccinia virus as strain on multiple myeloma; a case report. Jpn J Exp Med. 1987;57:79–81.

115. VARIOLA (SMALLPOX) AND MONKEYPOX VIRUSES

JOHN M. NEFF

Although a great deal is known about the chemical and biologic properties of vaccinia virus, the study of variola virus has been limited because of the obvious laboratory hazards involved. Where comparative studies have been possible, very similar characteristics between the two viruses have been found. Therefore, what has been noted about the morphology and biochemistry of vaccinia also applies to variola. The differences between variola and vaccinia lie in their predilection for certain hosts and their different growth characteristics in the laboratory.[1] Whereas vaccinia virus infects a wide range of hosts, variola infection is limited to humans and, under certain circumstances, to monkeys. In the laboratory, the two viruses can be distinguished by the appearance of the pock lesions formed on the chorioallantoic membrane of the chick embryo.[2] The pocks caused by variola are small and gray-white, while those caused by vaccinia are large and sometimes hemorrhagic. The two viruses can also be distinguished by their different growth characteristics in tissue culture.

There are at least two different strains of variola virus. The most virulent strain causes variola major, with a mortality of 20–50 percent. Variola minor, or alastrim, has a mortality of less than 1 percent. These two strains can easily be distinguished by their temperature-sensitive growth characteristics on the chorioallantoic membrane.

LABORATORY DIAGNOSIS OF SMALLPOX

One of the most important factors in the control of smallpox was the availability of rapid diagnostic techniques that differentiated smallpox from other vesicular illnesses.[2] The two techniques that are most commonly used are electron microscopy and gel diffusion. In both tests, vesicular scrapings are used. By using the electron microscope the pox virus particles can be distinguished from herpes or chickenpox. In situations where this technique is not available, variola viral particles, Guarnieri bodies, may be seen under light microscopy after staining by the Gispens method. Gel diffusion tests the vesicular fluid antigen against known hyperimmune vaccinia antiserum. It is not as sensitive as the electron microscope or as direct virus isolation on the chorioallantoic membrane. It is, however, a good, rapid diagnostic tool in a laboratory where an electron microscope is not available.[3,4] None of these tests help to distinguish vaccinia from variola. For this differentiation, the growth characteristics on the chorioallantoic membrane, mentioned above, are used.

CLINICAL ILLNESS

Variola no longer exists in an indigenous state in nature since the implementation of the successful worldwide eradication program. The last reported case was in Somalia in October 1977.[5] In 1980 the World Health Organization (WHO) Global Commission for the Certification of Smallpox Eradication officially declared that smallpox eradication had been achieved throughout the world.[6] Since 1977, there have been no indigenous cases of variola despite extensive surveillance.

The history, epidemiology, and clinical manifestations of smallpox have been well documented. The best of the most recent summaries can be found in the 1988 WHO publication *Smallpox and Its Eradication*.[7] Clinically, smallpox is a homogeneous illness that begins after an incubation period of 12 days, with a prodromal period of 2–4 days during which the virus can easily be isolated from the blood. The ensuing rash progresses in a uniform pattern as follows: maculopapules to vesicles to pustules and scabs over 1–2 weeks. The rash follows a centrifugal pattern. The progress of the disease may vary anywhere from death, occurring before the appearance of any rash in its most fulminant form, to a discrete form following a full course to recovery. Except when the disease appears in its toxic or vaccinio-modified form, it is easily diagnosed.

Smallpox is a relatively noncontagious disease requiring close contact for spread. It can easily be contained by careful identification and vaccination of contacts.

MONKEYPOX

Monkeypox is the only other member of the *Orthopoxvirus* species that has any significant clinical application to humans (Ref. 7, pp. 1287–1311). This virus creates a vesicular illness in monkeys that is very similar to variola. It occurs mostly in monkeys from the tropical rain forests of western and central Africa, and has infected humans sporadically in this same area. When the illness occurs in humans, it produces a vesicular rash very much like variola and generally does not pass on to other generations. This occurs occasionally, however, and there is one report of its spread through four generations.[8] WHO is carefully investigating all sporadic cases of monkeypox and has an active surveillance program in the geographic area where monkeypox is likely to occur. Most of the cases by far have occurred in Zaire, where 331 cases in a population of 5 million were identified in 3 years. It is considered to be a rare disease in humans (Ref. 7, pp. 1310–11).

It is unlikely that any of the other orthopoxviruses will cause any significant pathologic disease in humans. There is no natural reservoir of variola, and it is extremely unlikely that the genomes of any of the other orthopoxviruses will alter in nature to a form that infects and persists in humans. The only credible source of variola is from infection in a laboratory where the virus is stored.[9] At present, only two such laboratories in the world contain the virus (Ref. 1, pp. 1338–41). If for any reason this virus were once again introduced to humans, the resulting disease could be easily contained by vaccination of identified contacts. Control depends on the early recognition of a case and knowledge of its clinical and epidemiologic characteristics.

REFERENCES

1. Bedson HS, Dumbell KR. Smallpox and vaccinia. Br Med Bull. 1967;23:119.
2. World Health Organization: Guide to the Laboratory Diagnosis of Smallpox for Smallpox Eradication Programs. Geneva: World Health Organization; 1969.
3. Mitra AC, Sarkar SK, Mukherjee MK, et al. Evaluation of the precipitation-in-gel reaction in the diagnosis of smallpox. Bull WHO. 1973;49:555.
4. Nakano JH. Evaluation of virological laboratory methods in smallpox diagnosis. Bull WHO. 1973;48:529.
5. Deria A, Jezek Z, Markvart K, et al. The world's last endemic case of smallpox. Bull WHO. 1980;58:279–83.
6. WHO Declaration of global eradication of smallpox. Weekly Epidemiol Rec. 1980;55:145–52.
7. Fenner F, Henderson DA, Arita I, et al. Smallpox and Its Eradication. Geneva: World Health Organization; 1988.
8. Jezek Z, Arita I, Mutombo M, et al. Four generations of probably person to person transmission of human monkeypox. Am J Epidemiol. 1986;123:1004–12.
9. Dumbell K. What should be done about smallpox virus? Lancet. 1987;2:957–8.

116. PARAPOXVIRUSES AND MOLLUSCUM CONTAGIOSUM AND TANAPOX VIRUSES

JOHN M. NEFF

Within the Poxviridae family there are a few other viruses, other than the orthopoxvirus genus, that produce diseases in humans. They are the unclassified molluscum contagiosum and tanapox viruses, and the milker's node virus and bovine pustular stomatitis virus (orf) of the parapoxvirus genus.[1]

MOLLUSCUM CONTAGIOSUM

Molluscum contagiosum is a benign human disease that occurs worldwide and may be spread by close human contact including sexual intercourse. The disease is characterized by small firm umbilicated papules that are present on exposed epithelial surface areas of children or the genital areas of adults. The lesions resolve spontaneously without significant associated systemic symptoms. The virus has not been cultivated. Electron microscopy studies, however, have revealed a virus indistinguishable from other poxviruses.[2,3]

Recently, molluscum contagiosum has occurred as an opportunistic infection in patients with the acquired immune deficieny synrome (AIDS). Clinically the presentation is the same as described in healthy people except that the lesions may not resolve spontaneously but instead may continue to increase in size, number, and severity. Diagnosis is confirmed by histologic and electron microscopic examination.[4]

TANAPOX VIRUS

The tanapox virus is the source of a recently identified disease occurring in humans along the Tana river in Kenya and in Zaire. This disease is similar to monkeypox.[5]

MILKER'S NODE VIRUS

Milker's node virus produces a cutaneous disease in cattle that may be transmitted to humans through intimate contact. The disease in cattle is manifested by vesicular lesions of the udder or teets and in humans by watery, painless small nodules on exposed surfaces. The lesions in humans are self-limited, with complete recovery in 4–8 weeks. The immunity does not last. The virus has been isolated in primary fetal bovine kidney culture but cannot be serially propagated in continuous human cell lines. By electron microscopy the virus particles have typical poxvirus morphology.

BOVINE PUSTULAR STOMATITIS

Bovine pustular stomatitis virus (orf) causes watery papillomatous lesions on the cornea and mucous membranes of lambs. When humans are infected by close contact, a single lesion develops at the site of an abrasion. The lesion evolves into a hyperplastic nodular mass. The viral particles observed by electron microscopy are large, but instead of having the typical poxivrus brick shape, they are ovoid. None of these viruses provide any cross-immunity with the vaccinia or cowpox viruses.

REFERENCES

1. Fenner F, Henderson DA, Arita I, et al. Smallpox and Its Eradication. Geneva: World Health Organization; 1988:1288.
2. Postlethwaite R. Molluscum contagiosum. A review. Arch Environ Health 1970;21:432–52.
3. Fenner F, Henderson DA, Arita I, et al. Smallpox and Its Eradication. Geneva: World Health Organization; 1988:1317–18.
4. Katzman M, Carey JT, Elmets CA, et al. Molluscum contagiosum and the acquired immunodeficiency syndrome: Clinical and immunological details of two cases. Br J Dermatol. 1987;116:131–38.
5. Jezek Z. Arita I, Szczeniowski M, et al. Human tanapox in Zaire: Clinical and epidemiological observations on cases confirmed by laboratory studies. Bull WHO. 1985;63:1027–35.

Herpesviridae

117. INTRODUCTION TO HERPESVIRIDAE

STEPHEN E. STRAUS

The members of the Herpesviridae family are large, DNA-containing, enveloped viruses. Nearly 80 known herpesviruses infect a broad spectrum of the animal kingdom. Six human viruses are recognized (Table 1). Numerous herpesviruses infect new- or old-world monkeys, one of which is a rare cause of disease in humans. Well-characterized examples of other herpesviruses that do not infect humans include the channel catfish virus, Marek's disease virus of chickens, and several economically important viruses of horses, pigs, and cattle.[1–5]

CLASSIFICATION

The herpesviruses may be classified into three subfamilies according to virus host range and other biologic properties (Table 1). The α-herpesviruses grow rapidly in a wide range of tissues and efficiently destroy their host cells. The β-herpesviruses grow slowly and only in limited types of cells. Members of the γ-herpesvirus subfamily, almost without exception, grow slowly in or immortalize lymphoid cells of their natural hosts.

STRUCTURE

All herpesviruses are large particles (150–250 nm) that are composed of four fundamental structural elements (Fig. 1) that, moving inwardly, include a trilaminar outer envelope, the tegument, the nucleocapsid, and an internal core consisting of proteins and the viral genome.[7–10]

The envelope is derived from portions of the nuclear and cytoplasmic membranes that are pinched off as the developing particle traverses the nucleus into the cytoplasm and eventually exits the cell. In the process, viral glycoproteins that had been inserted into the cellular membranes are captured, with the end result that they project outward from the virion envelope.

The envelope glycoproteins of herpesviruses exhibit a number of biologic properties, some obvious and some obscure.[11] Certain of the glycoproteins such as glycoproteins B and D of herpes simplex viruses 1 and 2 are probably responsible for the binding and penetration of virions into cells.[11,12] Others, such as the herpes simpiex virus 1 and 2 glycoproteins E, are Fc receptors, while glycoprotein C has C3b-binding activity.[13,14] The cell surface receptors to which herpesvirus glycoproteins must bind to initiate infection are generally not known except for Epstein-Barr virus, which binds to the cellular C3d complement receptor.[15] Antibodies to most herpesvirus envelope glycoproteins neutralize virus infectivity, presumably by interfering with receptor binding.

The virion tegument consists of a seemingly amorphous assemblage of one or more virus-encoded proteins that may be important for initiating the viral replicative cycle within susceptible cells.

Herpesvirus nucleocapsids are approximately 100 nm in diameter and consist of 162 discrete protein capsomeres in an icosapentahedral array with 5:3:2 symmetry. The nucleocapsids contain viral DNAs that for all herpesviruses are linear double-stranded DNA molecules. Herpesvirus DNAs are structurally organized into a variety of complicated patterns depending upon the relative number, size, and position of repeated sequences. For example, herpes simplex viruses 1 and 2 possess two major, virtually uninterrupted expanses of unique DNA sequences. Each of these unique sequences is flanked by repeated sequences[16] (Fig. 2). For some herpesviruses the unique sequences can be inverted, one relative to the other, during the course of replication. Each virion contains one of the possible isomeric forms of the genome. All isomers of herpesvirus DNAs appear to be infectious. Although many herpesvirus DNAs are similarly organized, most show little sequence homology. By DNA hybridization, herpes simplex viruses 1 and 2 can be shown to share long stretches of homologous DNA (>50 percent overall relatedness). Most of the other viruses possess only scattered regions of DNA homology such that there is a weak (<5 percent) overall sequence relatedness that can be demonstrated only by using relatively nonstringent DNA hybridization conditions.

As herpesviruses spread serially through the community, minor mutations gradually accrue in their DNA sequences. Ultimately, these minor changes can be detected by sensitive molecular techniques such as restriction endonuclease cleavage analysis. The virus strain recovered from one person is generally indistinguishable from that of the person from whom the virus was acquired. Viruses from individuals who have not been in contact with one another are readily distinguished by endonuclease analysis. This powerful molecular epidemiologic tool has aided in our understanding of herpesvirus spread and reactivation.

Herpesvirus DNA sequences are used very efficiently, expressing sufficient numbers of RNAs to encode 70 to over 100 distinct proteins. The viral RNAs are transcribed from both strands of the genome in a generally nonoverlapping manner, with very few noncoding regions.

VIRUS REPLICATION

Herpesvirus replication is a carefully regulated, multistep process.[17] Shortly after infection a small number of genes is tran-

TABLE 1. Classification and Structure of Herpesviridae That Infect Humans

Common Name	Other Designation	Subfamily	Genome Size (MW × 106)	No. of Genome Isomers	Genome Type[a]	Guanine-Plus-Cytosine Content (%)
Human viruses						
Herpes simplex virus type 1	Human herpesvirus 1	α	96	4	1	67
Herpes simplex virus type 2	Human herpesvirus 2	α	96	4	1	69
Varicella-zoster virus	Human herpesvirus 3	α	80	2	2	46
Epstein-Barr virus	Human herpesvirus 4	γ	114	1	3	59
Cytomegalovirus	Human herpesvirus 5	β	145	1	1	57
B-lymphotropic virus	Human herpesvirus 6	γ	~115	?	?	46
Simian viruses						
Herpes B virus	Herpesvirus simiae	α	~105	?	?	74

Abbreviation: MW: molecular weight.
[a] Genomic arrangements are shown in Figure 2.

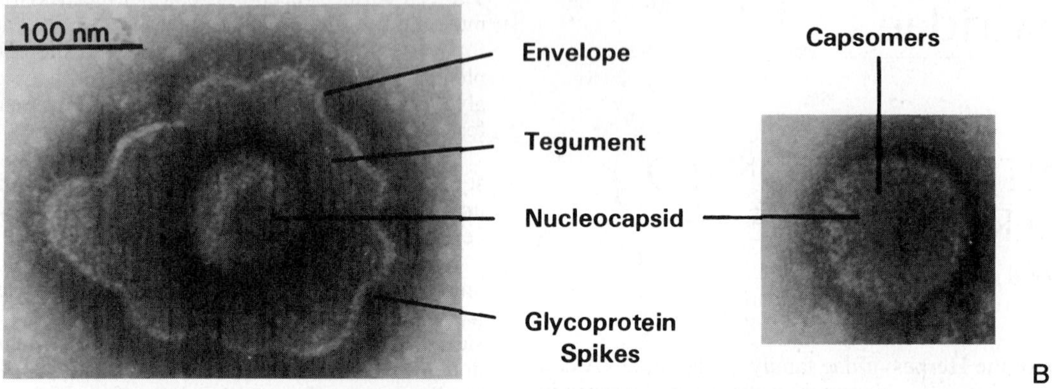

FIG. 1. Electron micrographs of varicella-zoster virus negatively stained with phosphotungstic acid. (×40,000) **(A)** The complete enveloped virion. **(B)** A purified viral nucleocapsid. (From Straus,[6] with permission.)

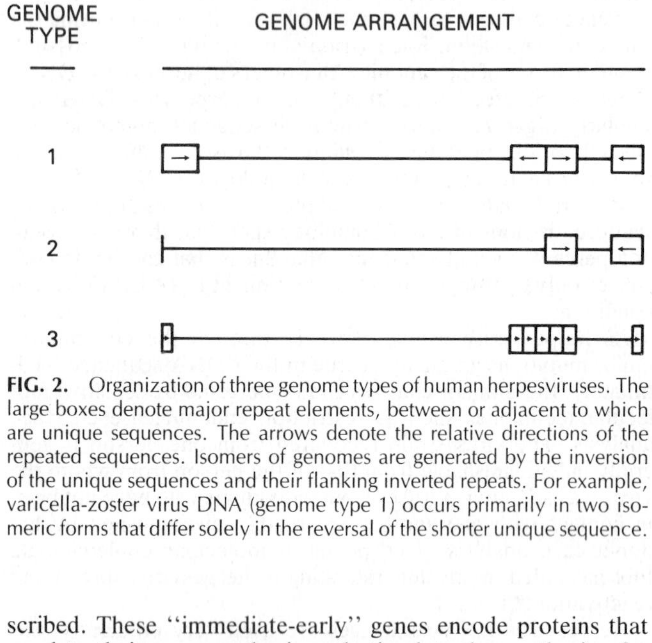

FIG. 2. Organization of three genome types of human herpesviruses. The large boxes denote major repeat elements, between or adjacent to which are unique sequences. The arrows denote the relative directions of the repeated sequences. Isomers of genomes are generated by the inversion of the unique sequences and their flanking inverted repeats. For example, varicella-zoster virus DNA (genome type 1) occurs primarily in two isomeric forms that differ solely in the reversal of the shorter unique sequence.

scribed. These "immediate-early" genes encode proteins that regulate their own synthesis and stimulate the synthesis of a second, larger wave of proteins from the "early" genes of the virus. Herpesvirus early proteins are involved in genome replication. The best characterized of these include the deoxypyrimidine (thymidine) kinases, DNA polymerases, ribonucleotide reductases, exonucleases, etc.

The precise manner in which herpesvirus DNA is replicated is not known, but the existence of terminal repeat sequences implies that circularization of the genome may be involved. There is evidence with some herpesviruses that progeny DNA molecules are generated continuously by a rolling circle mechanism.[18] Newly synthesized multimers of the genome are then cleaved appropriately and packaged.

After DNA replication the bulk of herpesvirus genes are expressed. These "late" gene products are incorporated into or aid in the assembly of progeny virions. New particles bud out of their host cells and promptly infect contiguous susceptible cells.

TROPISM

Herpesviruses vary widely in their abilities to infect different types of cells, a feature that is considered in classifying the virus into subfamilies (Table 1). For example, herpes simplex viruses grow readily in epithelial cells and fibroblasts of humans, monkeys, rabbits, mice, and many other animals. Varicella-zoster virus grows best in human epithelial cells and fibroblasts. In cell culture cytomegalovirus grows well only in human fibroblasts. Epstein-Barr virus can be cultivated only in B-lymphocytes.

The relative breadth of a herpesvirus' host range, however, is of more than taxonomic importance; it is highly predictive of the tissues that are clinically infected by the virus. Thus, the diseases associated with the lymphotropic herpesviruses are predominantly lymphoproliferative ones. In contrast, the herpesviruses that replicate readily in tissues of epithelial origin are primarily associated with mucocutaneous infections.

LATENCY

All herpesviruses induce lifelong latent infection in their natural hosts. The process of virus latency is still incompletely understood, but some of the key questions regarding its nature have been resolved in the past few years. It is clear that for any herpesvirus latency occurs within small numbers of very specific types of cells (Table 2). Latent herpes simplex viruses and Epstein-Barr virus genomes are carried extrachromosomally.[19,20] Integrated copies of the genome also exist for some viruses such as Epstein-Barr virus.[21]

There had been a long-standing debate as to whether latent herpesvirus genomes are totally quiescent or whether viral genes are expressed. Compelling data from studies of Epstein-Barr virus in lymphoid cell lines and of herpes simplex virus within ganglion neuronal cells indicate that the latent state is characterized by a vigorous expression of selected viral genes. Up to six Epstein-Barr virus genes are expressed as proteins displayed on the cell surface or within the nucleus of virus-immortalized cell lines.[22] A single region of the herpes simplex virus genome was recently shown to be active in latently infected ganglia.[23] Analyses of the selected herpesvirus genes that remain active suggest that they are regulatory in nature and may be serving to maintain the virus in its latent state.

TRANSFORMATION

Another biologic attribute of most herpesviruses is the ability to transform cells. Some of the viruses transform only cells of animals different from their natural hosts, while others transform their hosts' cells as well. The relevance of transformation that is observed to occur only in laboratory-derived model systems is uncertain. Thus, the ability of herpes simplex virus type 1 or 2, cytomegalovirus, or parts of their genomes to transform cells in culture may be clinically meaningless.[24] In fact, there remains no definitive evidence linking these herpesviruses to

TABLE 2. Features of Productive, Latent, and Transforming Herpesvirus Infections of Humans

Virus	*Typical Primary Infections*	*Typical Recurrent Infections*	*Infection in the Compromised Host*	*Sites of Latency*	*Association with Human Cancers*
Herpes simplex virus 1	Gingivostomatitis Keratoconjunctivitis Cutaneous herpes Genital herpes Encephalitis	Herpes labialis Keratoconjunctivitis Cutaneous herpes Encephalitis	Gingivostomatitis Keratoconjunctivitis Cutaneous herpes Esophagitis Pneumonitis Hepatitis, etc.	Sensory nerve ganglia	Squamous carcinoma of the oropharynx??
Herpes simplex virus 2	Genital herpes Cutaneous herpes Gingivostomatitis Meningoencephalitis Neonatal herpes	Genital herpes Cutaneous herpes	Genital herpes Cutaneous herpes Disseminated infection	Sensory nerve ganglia	Cervical cancer?
Varicella-zoster virus	Varicella	Dermatomal zoster	Disseminated infection	Sensory nerve ganglia	None
Cytomegalovirus	Mononucleosis Hepatitis Congenital cytomegalic inclusion disease	?	Hepatitis Retinitis Pneumonitis Encephalitis Colitis, etc.	Monocytes? Neutrophils? Lymphocytes?	Kaposi sarcoma?
Epstein-Barr virus	Mononucleosis Hepatitis Encephalitis	?	Lymphoproliferative syndromes	B lymphocytes, salivary glands	African-type Burkitt's lymphoma Nasopharyngeal carcinoma
Human herpesvirus type 6	?	?	?	Lymphocytes?	Rare B cell lymphomas?
Simian herpes B virus	Mucocutaneous lesions Encephalitis	?	?	Sensory nerve ganglia?	?

cancer. An active search for the effects of related virus sequences in human neoplasms should continue nonetheless.

To date, only lymphotropic herpesviruses are proved to be tumorigenic; most lead to lymphoproliferative malignancies.[25] Epstein-Barr virus, however, is also associated with naospharyngeal carcinoma and rare other carcinomas as well. Viral gene expression in cell lines transformed by lymphotropic herpesviruses is closely regulated but may differ from that typical of latent infection. In vivo, specific mechanisms must be engaged to prevent completion of the virus replicative cycle and to foil immune surveillance of virally induced tumors.

EPIDEMIOLOGY AND TRANSMISSION

Herpesviruses are fragile and do not survive for prolonged periods in the environment. As such, transmission generally requires the inoculation of a virus-containing fresh body fluid of an infected person directly into the susceptible tissues of a previously uninfected person. Susceptible sites include oral, ocular, genital, or anal mucosa, the respiratory tract, and the blood stream. Herpesviruses do not penetrate keratinized skin efficiently.

The six herpesviruses whose modes of transmission to humans are understood are acquired predominantly by intimate contact (Table 3). Direct contact with infected lesions transfers herpes simplex, varicella-zoster, and herpes B viruses.[26] Sexual intercourse and oral–genital contact transmit herpes simplex viruses and cytomegalovirus.[27] The major vehicle for Epstein-Barr virus is probably infected saliva; however, the recent identification of this virus in exfoliated cervical cells suggests that it may also be sexually transmitted.[28–30]

Given the prolonged intimate contact between mother and baby during pregnancy and delivery, it is not surprising that all of the human herpesviruses cause congenital and neonatal infections; those associated with cytomegalovirus are the most prevalent.[27] Some herpesviruses can be transmitted without person-to-person contact. For example, varicella can result from inhalation of infectious aerosols.[31] Cytomegalovirus and Epstein-Barr virus can also be transmitted by blood transfusion and transplantation.[27,29]

Herpesviruses are ubiquitous, and few humans escape being infected by them. Behaviors that promote the exchange of body fluids increase the risk of acquiring every herpesvirus (Table 3). The viruses are transmitted by individuals in whom active virus replication is occurring either during the course of their own primary infections or during reactivation infections. Some of those who transmit herpesviruses are symptomatic, but many are asymptomatic.

Except for the varicella-zoster virus infections, most herpesvirus infections are transmitted asymptomatically. Over the course of a lifetime, episodes of asymptomatic shedding of herpesviruses probably exceed those of symptomatic shedding, and thus there may be more opportunities to transmit these viruses asymptomatically than symptomatically. With herpes simplex viruses, asymptomatic reactivation and shedding of virus occurs on about $\frac{1}{2}$–1 percent of days.[26] Epstein-Barr virus shedding rates are much higher, exceeding 20 percent of the days in normal seropositive individuals.[31]

The likelihood of transmission depends on the quantity of virus shed. There are indications that the titer of virus recoverable during symptomatic infections greatly exceeds that of asymptomatic infections. The net result of these factors is that both symptomatic and asymptomatic infections contribute substantially to rates of herpesvirus transmission. The best data are available for genital herpes infections. Between one-half to three-fourths of infections are acquired from asymptomatic sexual partners.[32] It is likely that an even greater proportion of Epstein-Barr virus infections are transmitted asymptomatically.

PATHOGENESIS

Herpesviruses induce disease in three manners: by direct destruction of tissues, by provoking immunopathologic responses, and by facilitating neoplastic transformation.

Mucocutaneous herpes simplex virus, varicella-zoster virus, and herpesvirus simiae infections represent the direct consequences of tissue destruction by replicating virus. Visceral infections with these viruses or with cytomegalovirus, such as encephalitis, pneumonitis, retinitis, and hepatitis, also reflect virus-induced cytopathogenicity.

Certain complications of herpesvirus infections, however, such as erythema multiforme, hemolytic anemia, and thrombocytopenia are primarily immune mediated.[33,34] Whether the neurologic complications of varicella and zoster are also im-

TABLE 3. Transmission and Seroepidemiology of Herpesviruses That Infect Humans.

	Modes of Transmission				*Seroprevalence (%) (United States)*		
Virus	*Perinatal*	*Blood Products*	*Intimate Contact*	*Aerosol*	*Normal Children*	*Normal Adults*	*Groups or Activities with Higher Risk of Infection*
Herpes simplex virus 1	+	–	+	–	20–40	50–70	Frequent intimate contact
Herpes simplex virus 2	+	–	+	–	0–5	20–50	Frequent intimate contact
Varicella-zoster virus	+	–	+	+	50–75	85–95	Children in day care
Cytomegalovirus	+	+	+	–	10–30	40–70	Children in day care Promiscuous gay men Transplant or blood recipients
Epstein-Barr virus	+	+	+	–	10–30	60–90	Frequent intimate contact
Human herpesvirus type 6	?	?	?	?	10–60?	20–80?	Cellular immune deficiency states
Simian herpes B	?	–	+	–	0	<1	Monkey handlers

Abbreviations: +: well-recognized association; –: rare or no association; ?: inadequate data.

TABLE 4. Clinical Syndromes Associated with Herpesviruses

Syndrome	*Herpes Simplex Virus 1*	*Herpes Simplex Virus 2*	*Varicella-Zoster Virus*	*Cytomegalovirus*	*Epstein-Barr Virus*	*Herpesvirus Simiae*
Gingivostomatitis	+	+				+
Genital lesions	+	+	+			+
Cutaneous lesions	+	+	+			+
Keratoconjunctivitis	+	+	+			+
Retinitis	+			+		
Esophagitis	+	+	+	+		
Pneumonitis	+	+	+	+	+	
Hepatitis	+	+	+	+	+	
Myopericarditis			+	+	+	
Meningitis		+	+			
Encephalitis	+	+	+	+	+	+
Myelitis	+	+	+			+
Erythema multiforme	+	+	+			
Arthritis			+		+	
Hemolytic anemia			+	+	+	
Leukopenia			+	+	+	
Thrombocytopenia			+	+	+	
Mononucleosis				+	+	
Lymphoma					+	

TABLE 5. Available Means to Prevent or Treat Herpesvirus Infections

Virus	*Host*	*Indication*	*Prevention*	*Treatment*
Herpes simplex virus 1	Any	Primary mucocutaneous infection	Avoid contact	None or po acyclovir
	Normal	Recurrent mucocutaneous infection	Avoid UV exposure	None
	Immune compromised	Any syndrome	None	iv or po acyclovir
	Any	Visceral infection	None	iv acyclovir
Herpex simplex virus 2	Any	Primary mucocutaneous infection	Avoid contact	po or iv acyclovir
	Any	Recurrent mucocutaneous infection	None	po or iv acyclovir
	Neonate	Visceral infection	Avoid contact	iv acyclovir
Varicella-zoster virus	Normal	Varicella	Vaccine?	None
	Immune compromised		Varicella-Zoster immune globulin Vaccine	iv acyclovir
	Normal	Zoster	None	None, or po acyclovir
	Immune compromised		None	po or iv acyclovir or none
Cytomegalovirus	Normal	Any syndrome	None	None
	Immune compromised	Visceral infection	Seronegative donor tissues and blood Specific immune globulin?, acyclovir?	Ganciclovir?
Epstein-Barr virus	Normal	Infectious mononucleosis	None	None, steroids in selected cases
	Immune compromised	Any infection	None	None, or acyclovir?
Human herpesvirus type 6	Any	Any infection	?	?
Herpesvirus simiae	Any	Any infection	Avoid infected monkeys	Acyclovir?, ganciclovir?

mune mediated has been widely debated. Because encephalitis, transverse myelitis, and cranial nerve palsies typically arise as the cutaneous component of varicella-zoster infection is resolving, these neurologic problems are often considered to be immune mediated.[35] Isolated instances in which the virus or its constituents have been detected in the involved central nervous system tissues, however, suggest that the virus itself can directly contribute to neurologic disease in some settings.[36]

It is very likely that most of the clinical manifestations of Epstein-Barr virus infection, including the hematologic and neurologic complications, are immunopathologically mediated. Except in the setting of severe congenital or acquired cellular immune deficiency disorders, only a minute fraction of the cells that infiltrate the lymph nodes, liver, and spleen during primary Epstein-Barr virus infection are actually virus-infected B lymphocytes.[37] Most represent reactive T cells of diverse types. It is for this reason that corticosteroids have a role in the management of some severe complications of Epstein-Barr virus infection and, conversely, that the potent antiviral drug acyclovir is not useful in the treatment of acute infectious mononucleosis.[38,39]

While the association of Epstein-Barr virus with certain B-cell lymphomas and nasopharyngeal carcinoma is well known, the role this virus plays in tumorigenesis is not. Most recent hypotheses assume Epstein-Barr virus to confer growth advantages on cells, thereby increasing opportunities for spontaneous chromosomal translocations or other potentially transforming events to occur and to allow tumor cells to escape immune surveillance.[40]

DIAGNOSIS

Most herpesvirus infections can be diagnosed clinically, but there are several situations in which specific tests are helpful. Laboratory confirmation of a herpesvirus infection helps to exclude other similar illnesses, may allay anxiety, guides counseling and treatment, and can be used to identify drug-resistant viruses.

A practical example of the value of confirmatory testing is genital herpes, the diagnosis of which often implies recurrent discomfort and chronic psychological and social distress. It would be unfair and inappropriate to casually render this diagnosis, recommend behavioral modification, and prescribe acyclovir. Another example of the value of testing is recurrent zosteriform eruptions, which are frequently misdiagnosed as repeated zoster outbreaks rather than as recurrent cutaneous herpes simplex virus infections.[41] Timely proof of the diagnosis in herpes simplex encephalitis, neonatal herpes, cytomegalovirus pneumonia, and other life-threatening infections permits the most efficient use of clinical resources and avoids the hazards and expense of ceaseless empiricism.

Acute herpes simplex virus, varicella-zoster virus, and herpesvirus simiae infections are best diagnosed by isolation of the virus in culture.[42–44] Serologic tests for these viruses are predominantly used to confirm recent or past infections. Diagnoses of Epstein-Barr virus infections, however, are most often confirmed serologically, isolation methods being too cumbersome or expensive for routine use.[45] Cytomegalovirus infections are often diagnosed serologically, but there is an increased effort to detect the virus in clinical specimens, particularly with relatively rapid methods.[46] Once a diagnosis has been made, serial serologic determinations are of little value in considering chronic or recurrent virus activity.

CLINICAL SYNDROMES

Herpesviruses cause a wide spectrum of clinical disease (Table 4). These can be grouped into mucocutaneous, visceral, central nervous system, and reactive syndromes. These infections are covered in detail in Chapters 118, 119, 120, and 121. Human infections with two other viruses warrant a more thorough review here.

Herpesvirus simiae infections are too rare to define their full spectrum. This virus is enzootic in macaques. Of rhesus monkeys in captivity, 30–80 percent are seropositive and experience recurrent symptomatic and asymptomatic infections that closely resemble those caused in humans by herpes simplex viruses. During periods of stress, as in handling or shipping, rhesus monkeys show high rates of virus shedding.[47] Monkey handlers bitten or scratched by infectious animals are at risk of acquiring the virus. Fortunately such infections have been documented rarely. As of 1988 only about 30 symptomatic human infections were recorded. Over two-thirds developed progressive mucocutaneous disease and fatal encephalitis. A recent outbreak involving four cases of symptomatic infection was particularly instructive in revealing that human-to-human transmission occurs via direct contact and that acyclovir suppresses mild infections.[48] Continued surveillance of the survivors of that outbreak revealed evidence of periodic asymptomatic reactivation and shedding of herpesvirus simiae.

Herpesvirus type 6 infection has not as yet been firmly linked to specific disease entities. Preliminary data suggest that it may be associated with exanthem subitum (roseola infantum) and a mononucleosis-like illness.[49] Herpesvirus type 6 is recovered from peripheral blood mononuclear cells by cocultivation in human umbilical cord blood lymphocytes.[50] Virus is most readily recovered from patients with lymphoproliferative malignancies and the acquired immunodeficiency syndrome (AIDS). It grows in B and T lymphocytes and in a few special nonlymphoid cell lines as well.[51] Unlike Epstein-Barr virus, infected lymphocytes are destroyed rather than immortalized. However, herpesvirus type 6 DNA has been detected by hybridization in B-cell lymphomas arising in immunocompromised individuals. Herpesvirus type 6 infections are common; most healthy children and adults possess antibodies to this virus.

PREVENTION AND TREATMENT

Rapid progress has been made over the last few years in the prevention and treatment of some herpesvirus infections (Table 5). A live varicella vaccine has been proved efficacious and is currently under consideration for licensure.[53,54] Varicella-zoster immune globulin is now widely available, albeit expensive.[55] Studies of cytomegalovirus-specific immune globulin, plasma, and vaccines are underway.[56,57]

Acyclovir is the major antiviral drug in use today and has proven indications for the treatment of several mucocutaneous and visceral herpesvirus infections.[58–60] Ganciclovir, a more toxic analogue of acyclovir, is being evaluated for the treatment of life-threatening cytomegalovirus infections in immunocompromised patients.[61] Its efficacy for arresting sight-threatening cytomegalovirus retinitis in patients with AIDS is already evident.[62]

REFERENCES

1. Roizman B, Batterson W. Herpesviruses and their replication. In: Fields BN, Knipe, DM, Chanock RM, et al., eds. Virology. New York: Raven Press; 1985:497–526.
2. Roizman B, ed. The Herpesviruses. v. 1. New York: Plenum; 1982.
3. Roizman B, ed. The Herpesviruses. v. 2. New York: Plenum; 1983.
4. Roizman B, ed. The Herpesviruses. v. 3. New York: Plenum; 1985.
5. Roizman B, Lopez C, eds. Immunobiology and Prophylaxis of Human Herpesvirus Infections. New York: Plenum; 1984.
6. Straus SE, Ostrove JM, Inchauspe G, et al. Varicella zoster virus infections: Biology, natural history, treatment, and prevention. Ann Intern Med. 1988;108:221.
7. Wildy P, Russell WC, Horne RW. The morphology of herpes virus. Virology. 1960;12:204.
8. Epstein MA. Observations on the mode of release of herpes virus from infected HeLa cells. J Cell Biol. 1962;12:589.
9. Ben-Porat T, Kaplan AS. Studies on the biogenesis of herpesvirus envelope. Nature. 1972;235:165.

10. Roizman B, Furlong D. The replication of herpesviruses. In: Fraenkel-Conrat H, Wagner RR, eds. Comprehensive Virology. v. 3. New York: Plenum; 1974:229–403.
11. Spear P. Herpesviruses. In: Blough HA, Tiffany JM, eds. Cell Membranes and Viral Envelopes. v. 2. New York: Academic Press; 1980:709–750.
12. Highlander SL, Sutherland SL, Gage PJ, et al. Neutralizing monoclonal antibodies specific for herpes simplex vires glycoprotein D inhibit virus penetration. J Virol. 1987;61:3356.
13. Baucke RB, Spear PG. Membrane proteins specified by herpes simplex virus. V. Identification of an Fc-binding glycoprotein. J Virol. 1979;32:779.
14. Friedman HM, Cohen GH, Eisenberg RJ, et al. Glycoprotein C of HSV-1 functions as a C3b receptor on infected endothelial cells. Nature. 1984;309:633.
15. Frade R, Barel M, Ehlin-Henriksson B, et al. gp140, the C3d receptor of human B lymphocytes, is also the Epstein-Barr virus receptor. Proc Natl Acad Sci USA. 1985;82:1490.
16. Roizman B. The structure and isomerization of herpes simplex virus genomes. Cell. 1979;16:481.
17. Jones PC, Roizman B. Regulation of herpesvirus macromolecular synthesis. VIII. The transcription program consists of three phases during which transcription and accumulation of RNA in the cytoplasm are regulated. J Virol. 1979;31:299.
18. Ben-Porat T, Tokazewski S. Replication of herpesvirus DNA. II. Sedimentation characteristics of newly synthesized DNA. Virology. 1977;79:292.
19. Mellerick DM, Fraser NW. Physical state of the latent herpes simplex virus genome in a mouse model system: Evidence suggesting an episomal state. Virology. 1987;158:265.
20. Adams A, Lindahl T. Epstein-Barr virus genomes with properties of circular DNA molecules in carrier cells. Proc Natl Acad Sci USA. 1975;72:1477.
21. Adams A, Lindahl T, Klein G. Linear associations between cellular DNA and EBV DNA in a human lymphoblastoid cell line. Proc Natl Acad Sci USA. 1973;70:2888.
22. Dambaugh T, Hennessy K, Fennewald S, et al. The virus genome and its expression in latent infections. In: Epstein MA, Achong BG, eds. The Epstein-Barr Virus: Recent Advances. v. 1. London: William Heinemann; 1986:13–46.
23. Stevens JG, Wagner EK, Devi-Rao GB, et al. RNA complementary to a herpes virus α gene mRNA is prominent in latently infected neurons. Science. 1987;235:1056.
24. Tevethia MJ. Transforming potential of herpes simplex viruses and human cytomegalovirus. In: Roizman B, ed. The Herpesviruses. v. 3. New York: Plenum; 1982:257–314.
25. Magrath I. Infectious mononucleosis and malignant neoplasia. In: Schlossberg D, ed. Infectious Mononucleosis. New York: Praeger Publishers; 1983:225–77.
26. Whitley RJ. Epidemiology of herpes simplex viruses. In: Roizman B, ed. The Herpesviruses. v. 3. New York: Plenum; 1982:1–44.
27. Naraqi S. Cytomegaloviruses. In: Belshe RB, ed. Textbook of Human Virology. Littleton, MA: PSG Publishing; 1984:887–928.
28. Chang RS, Lewis JP, Abildgaard CF. Prevalence of oropharyngeal excretors of leukocyte transforming agents among a human population. N Engl J Med. 1973;289:1325.
29. Fleisher GR. Epidemiology and pathogenesis. In: Schlossberg D, ed. Infectious Mononucleosis. New York: Praeger Publishers; 1983:15–47.
30. Sixbey JW, Lemon SM, Pagano JS. A second site for Epstein-Barr virus shedding: The uterine cervix. Lancet. 1986;2:1122.
31. Leclair JM, Zaia JA, Levin MJ, et al. Airborne transmission of chickenpox in a hospital. N Engl J Med. 1980;302:450.
32. Mertz GJ, Schmidt O, Jourden JL, et al. Frequency of acquisition of first-episode genital infection with herpes simplex virus from symptomatic and asymptomatic source contacts. Sex Transm Dis. 1985;12:33.
33. Oorton PW, Huff JC, Tonnesen MG, et al. Detection of a herpes simplex viral antigen in skin lesions of erythema multiforme. Ann Intern Med. 1984;101:48.
34. Harris AI, Meyer RJ, Brody EA. Cytomegalovirus-induced thrombocytopenia and hemolysis in an adult. Ann Intern Med. 1975;83:670.
35. Johnson R, Milbourne PE. Central nervous system complications of chickenpox. Can Med Assoc J. 1970;102:831.
36. Ryder JW, Croen K, Kleinschmidt-DeMasters BK, et al. Progressive encephalitis three months after resolution of cutaneous zoster in a patient with AIDS. Ann Neurol. 1985;19:182.
37. Rocchi G, DeFelici A, Ragona G, et al. Quantitative evaluation of Epstein-Barr virus infected mononuclear peripheral blood leukocytes in infectious mononucleosis. N Engl J Med. 1972;296:132.
38. Bender DE. The value of corticosteroids in the treatment of infectious mononucleosis. JAMA. 1967;199:529.
39. Andersson J, Britton S, Ernberg I, et al. Effect of acyclovir on infectious mononucleosis: A double-blind placebo-controlled study. J Infect Dis. 1986;153:283.
40. Erikson J, Finan J, Nowell PC, et al. Translocation of immunoglobulin V_H genes in Burkitt's lymphoma. Proc Natl Acad Sci USA. 1982;79:5611.
41. Kalman CM, Laskin OL. Herpes zoster and zosteriform herpes simplex virus infections in immunocompetent adults. Am J Med. 1986;81:775.
42. Straus SE, Rooney JF, Sever JL, et al. Herpes simplex virus infection: Biology, treatment, and prevention. Ann Intern Med. 1985;103:404.
43. Straus SE, Ostrove JM, Inchauspe G, et al. Varicella-zoster virus infections: Biology, natural history, treatment, and prevention. Ann Intern Med. 1988;108:221.
44. Kalter SS, Hilliard JK, Heberling RL. The differential diagnosis of herpesvirus infections in man and animals. Dev Biol Stand. 1982;52:101.
45. Henle W, Henle GE, Horwitz CA. Epstein-Barr virus specific diagnostic tests in infectious mononucleosis. Hum Pathol. 1974;5:551.
46. Gleaves CA, Smith RF, Shuster EA, et al. Comparison of standard tube and shell vial cell culture techniques for the detection of cytomegaloviruses in clinical specimens. J Clin Microbiol. 1985;21:217.
47. Palmer AE. B-virus, herpesvirus simiae: Historical perspective. J Med Primatol. 1987;16:99.
48. Centers for Disease Control. B-virus infection in humans. Pensacola, Florida. MMWR. 1987;36:209.
49. Yamanishi K, Okuno T, Shiraki K, et al. Identification of human herpesvirus type-6 as a causal agent for exanthan subitum. Lancet; 1988;1:1005.
50. Salahuddin SZ, Ablashi DV, Markham PD, et al. Isolation of a new virus, HBLV, in patients with lymphoproliferative disorders. Science. 1986;234:596.
51. Ablashi DV, Salahuddin SZ, Josephs SF, et al. Human B-lymphotropic herpesviruses (HBLV) in human cell lines. Nature. 1987;329:207.
52. Josephs SF, Buchbinder A, Streicher HZ, et al. Detection of human B-lymphotropic virus (human herpesvirus 6) sequences in B cell leukemia. Leukemia. 1988;2:132.
53. Weibel RE, Neff BJ, Kuter BJ, et al. Live attenuated varicella virus vaccine: Efficacy trial in healthy children. N Engl J Med. 1984;310:1409.
54. Gershon AA, Steinberg SP, Gelb L. Live attenuated varicella vaccine use in immunocompromised children and adults. Pediatrics. 1986;78:757.
55. Centers for Disease Control. Varicella-zoster immune globulin for the prevention of chickenpox: Recommendations of the Immunization Practices Advisory Committee. Ann Intern Med. 1984;100:859.
56. Winston DJ, Pollard RB, Winston GH, et al. Cytomegalovirus immune plasma in bone marrow transplant recipients. Ann Intern Med. 1982;97:11.
57. Starr SF, Glazer JP, Friedman HM, et al. Specific cellular and humoral immunity after immunization with live Towne strain cytomegalovirus vaccine. J Infect Dis. 1981;143:585.
58. Mitchell CD, Bean B, Gentry SR, et al. Acyclovir therapy for mucocutaneous herpes simplex infections in immunocompromised patients. Lancet 1981;1:1389.
59. Corey L, Fife KH, Benedetti JK, et al. Intravenous acyclovir for the treatment of primary genital herpes. Ann Intern Med. 1983;98:914.
60. Straus SE, Takiff HE, Seidlin M, et al. Suppression of frequently recurring genital herpes: A placebo-controlled double-blind trial of oral acyclovir. N Engl J Med. 1984;310:1545.
61. Masur H, Lane HC, Palestine A, et al. Effect of 9-(1,3-dihydroxy-2-propoxymethyl) guanine on serious cytomegalovirus disease in eight homosexual men. Ann Intern Med. 1986;104:41.
62. Collaborative DHPG Treatment Study Group. Treatment of serious cytomegalovirus infections with 9-(1,3-dihydroxy-2-propoxymethyl) guanine in patients with AIDS and other immunodeficiencies. N Engl J Med. 1986;314:801.

118. HERPES SIMPLEX VIRUS

MARTIN S. HIRSCH

Herpes simplex virus (HSV) infections are among the most common maladies affecting humans. Often they are annoying and troublesome; occasionally they are life-threatening. The term *herpes* is derived from the Greek word meaning to creep, and clinical descriptions of herpes labialis go back to the time of Hippocrates.[1] Astruc, physician to the king of France, is credited with the first description of genital herpes in 1736.[2] Between 1910 and 1920, the infectious nature of herpes lesions was demonstrated by producing corneal lesions in rabbits with material derived from herpes keratitis and labialis.[3] As techniques for isolating and characterizing the virus became more simplified and serologic procedures were developed, our understanding of the HSV clinical spectrum has greatly expanded. Studies during the past two decades have brought insights into the molecular biology of HSV,[4,5] the mechanisms of HSV latency and recurrence,[6–9] and the first successful approaches to therapy for certain types of HSV infections.[10,11]

DESCRIPTION OF THE PATHOGEN

Herpes simplex virus (herpesvirus hominis) shares many properties with other members of the herpesvirus groups, which in humans includes varicella-zoster, cytomegalovirus, Epstein-Barr virus, and human herpesvirus type 6. The members of this group have an internal core containing double-stranded DNA, an icosahedral capsid with 162 hollow capsomeres, and a lipid-containing laminated membrane or envelope. The overall diameters of enveloped herpesviruses are 150–200 nm. Replication occurs primarily within the cell nucleus and is completed by the addition of protein envelopes as the virus passes through the nuclear membrane. Complete virus replication is associated with lysis of the productive cell. All members of the human herpesvirus group can also establish latent states within certain types of cells they infect, although the physical nature of the viruses during periods of latency is unclear.

The most commonly used means of separating HSV from other members of the herpesvirus group are antigenic analyses and definition of biologic properties, for example, host range and types of cytopathologic changes. Herpes simplex virus may also be differentiated by neutralization kinetics, polypeptide analysis, DNA base composition, or molecular hybridization characteristics.[12]

Within recent years, further subdivision of HSV into specific types has become possible (Table 1). Although the most readily apparent differences between HSV-1 and HSV-2 are in their clinical and epidemiologic patterns, they can also be separated by a variety of biochemical and biologic characteristics. Among these are the pock size on chick embryo chorioallantoic membranes, the ability to form plaques in chick embryo cultures, the ability to induce syncytial giant cells in cell cultures, neurotropism in mice, sensitivity to heparin or temperature change in cell culture, and the base composition of their DNA.[12,13–15]

The development of monoclonal antibody and restriction enzyme technologies have permitted an even finer definition of variations among individual HSV isolates.[16–20] It is now clear that HSV-1 and HSV-2 share certain glycoprotein antigens (e.g., gB) and differ with respect to others (e.g., gG). Serologic differentiation between HSV-1 and HSV-2 infections can be readily made by detection of type-specific gG antibodies. Moreover, recognition of ever more subtle differences among isolates by DNA analysis has introduced a new field of medical investigation, that of molecular epidemiology.[16–18]

EPIDEMIOLOGY

Herpes simplex viruses have a worldwide distribution. Even remote Brazilian Indian tribes are infected with these agents.[21] There are no known animal vectors for HSV, and although experimental animals can easily be infected, humans appear to be the only natural reservoir. Direct contact, with transmission through infected secretions, is the principal mode of spread. HSV-1 is transmitted primarily by contact with oral secretions and HSV-2 by contact with genital secretions. Transmission can occur both from overtly infected persons or from asymptomatic excretors, although virus titers are higher in persons with active lesions and thus transmissability may be greater. Approximately 0.65–15 percent of the adults may be excreting HSV-1 or HSV-2 at any given time depending on the population studied.[22–25] For example, since shedding of HSV-2 is related to sexual activity, prostitutes may have unusually high rates of excretion.[25]

There does not appear to be a marked seasonal or sexual variation in the incidence of overt infection, but rates of infection are inversely related to socioeconomic status.[26–28] Only 30–50 percent of the adults in higher socioeconomic groups have HSV antibodies, whereas in lower socioeconomic groups, the rates are 80–100 percent, probably reflecting more crowded living conditions among the latter populations. The age-related patterns of infection are different for HSV-1 and HSV-2. HSV-1 antibodies rapidly rise during childhood. By puberty, nearly all members of lower socioeconomic groups have been infected; the incidence in higher socioeconomic groups is somewhat lower. In contrast, the major period of infection with HSV-2 follows puberty and is related to venereal transmission between the ages of 14–29. The frequency of HSV-2 antibodies among populations varies from approximately 3 percent in nuns to 70 percent in prostitutes.[25,27]

Spread of HSV-1 infection from oral secretions to other skin areas is a hazard of certain occupations such as dentists, respiratory care unit personnel, and wrestlers.[29,30] Laboratory-acquired and nosocomial outbreaks in hospital personnel or in neonatal nurseries have been reported.[16,31,32] Transmission of HSV-2 to other skin sites can occur among infants born to mothers having genital infections. Anal and perianal infections with HSV-2 are common among sexually active male homosexual populations.[33,34] Autoinoculation from genital areas to other sites including hands, thighs, and buttocks is not uncommon. With changing sexual mores and increasing oral–genital contact, some studies have reported an increasing incidence of genital HSV-1 and oral HSV-2 infections.[35,36]

Recurrent infection occurs frequently with both HSV-1 and HSV-2. Most recurrences are secondary to the endogenous reactivation of virus rather than exogenous reinfection[37] and occur despite the presence of circulating antiviral antibodies. Recurrent infections of the lips or perioral areas occur in 20–40 percent of the population.[38,39] HSV-2 oral–labial lesions recur less frequently than do HSV-1 lesions.[40] Recurrences vary in frequency from more than one attack per month (5–25 percent) to less than one attack every 6 months (10–65 percent).[39,41] The precipitating factors may be stereotyped for any given person and yet vary considerably among individuals. They include sunlight, fever, local trauma, trigeminal nerve manipulation, menstruation, and emotional stress. Recurrent HSV keratitis is less common; it has been estimated that 5 percent of all people attending ophthalmologic clinics have ocular HSV infections; of these, 25–50 percent have a recurrence within 2 years.[42,43] The frequency of genital recurrences depends on a variety of factors including sex, HSV type, and both the presence and titer of neutralizing antibody.[44] HSV-1 genital lesions recur less frequently than do HSV-2 lesions, and recurrences develop more frequently in men than in women. Overall recurrence rates approximate 60–90 percent of those with initial episodes. Although most recurrences are related to reactivation, reinfection accounts for occasional episodes.[37]

TABLE 1. Differences between HSV-1 and HSV-2[a]

Characteristics	*HSV-1*	*HSV-2*
Urogenital infections	−(10–30%)	+(70–90%)
Nongenital infections		
Labialis	+(80–90%)	−(10–20%)
Keratitis	+	−
Whitlow (hand)	+	+
Encephalitis (adult)	+	−
Neonatal infection	−(~30%)	+(~70%)
Transmission	Primarily nongenital	Primarily genital
Mice–genital or intramuscular	Less neurotropic	More neutropic
Pock size on chorioallantoic membranes	Small	Large
Plaques in chick embryo monolayers	−	+
Temperature sensitivity (40°C)	−	+
Heparin sensitivity	+	−
Syncytium formation in human embryonic kidney cells	−	+

[a] Antigenic differences between HSV-1 and HSV-2 can be detected by a variety of serologic techniques including immunofluorescence, immunoperoxidation, microneutralization, and enzyme-linked immmunoadsorption.

PATHOGENESIS

On entry into skin sites, HSV replicates locally in parabasal and intermediate epithelial cells, which results in the lysis of infected cells and the instigation of a local inflammatory response.

This series of events results in the characteristic lesion of superficial HSV infection, that is, a thin-walled vesicle on an inflammatory base. Multinucleated cells are formed with ballooning degeneration, marked edema, and characteristic Cowdry type A intranuclear inclusions. Such lesions are indistinguishable from those caused by varicella-zoster virus. Lymphatics and regional lymph nodes draining the site of primary infection become involved. Further virus replication may result in viremia and visceral dissemination, depending on the immune competence of the host. In murine models the maturity of macrophages at the site of local infection helps determine whether virus remains localized or disseminates.[45] Subsequently, other host defense mechanisms, for example, the production of interferons, natural killer cells, protective antibodies, and sensitized killer lymphocytes, are elicited to prevent the spread of infection.[46,47] It is unclear whether similar mechanisms operate in humans, although infants with immature immune mechanisms as well as immunosuppressed or malnourished children and adults are more likely to disseminate their infections. Depression of cell-mediated immune mechanisms appears to be more closely associated with severe HSV infections than does alteration in humoral immunity.[48] Viremia can be demonstrated in malnourished children with widespread infection, in certain immunosuppressed adults, and occasionally in immunologically intact persons.[49–52] Viremic spread may result in the infection of multiple visceral organs including the liver, lung, and central nervous system.

After primary infection, HSV may become latent within sensory nerve ganglion sites via travel along sensory nerve pathways.[6–9] Once within the ganglion, viral DNA and possibly some mRNA transcripts can be localized within neurons, although the intracellular form of the HSV DNA is unclear. Various immunologic and biochemical theories of HSV latency and reactivation have been proposed but remain unproven.[8,9,11,53,54] Reactivated virus or viral genetic information appears to spread peripherally by sensory nerves as well. The neuron appears to be unique in that production of fully infectious virus does not result in cell lysis. It is possible that only early viral products are produced within the neuron and that the final viral replicative assembly takes place in epithelial cells. Once HSV has traveled to cutaneous sites, further spread is from cell to cell, and limitation of spread results from the activation of humoral and cellular immune mechanisms, perhaps acting through the local production of interferon.[46,47]

Latency has been demonstrated in humans within trigeminal, sacral, and vagal ganglia.[67,55,56] Reactivation depends on the integrity of the anterior root and peripheral nerve pathways. A curious observation is that all areas supplied by a latently infected nerve are not equally involved and that recurrences usually develop in the vicinity of the primary infection. However, latent infections have not been demonstrated at skin sites themselves.[57] It is possible that other sites of HSV latency will be uncovered since intermittent oral or genital secretion and leukocyte carriage have been demonstrated.

A variety of humoral and cell-mediated immune mechanisms are recruited in response to primary and recurrent HSV infections including the production of various types of antibodies, the production of interferon, the activation of macrophages, the induction of T-lymphocyte–mediated reactivity, and the development of both natural killer cell and antibody dependent lymphocyte cytotoxicity. The relative roles of these mechanisms in the limitation of HSV infection are unclear.

CLINICAL MANIFESTATIONS

Primary Infections

Primary HSV-1 infection is frequently asymptomatic but may present as gingivostomatitis and pharyngitis most commonly in children under the age of 5 years but occasionally in older persons. Incubation periods range from 2 to 12 days and are followed by fever and sore throat with pharyngeal edema and erythema. Shortly after its onset, small vesicles develop on the pharyngeal and oral mucosa; these rapidly ulcerate and increase in number, often involving the soft palate, buccal mucosa, tongue, and floor of the mouth. Gums are tender and bleed easily, and lesions may extend to the lips and cheeks (Fig. 1). Fever and toxicity may persist for many days, and the patient complains of severe mouth pain. Breath is fetid, and cervical adenopathy is present. In children, dehydration may result from poor intake, drooling, and fever. In college-aged persons, primary HSV infection often presents as a posterior pharyngitis or tonsilitis.[58] Included in the age-related differential diagnosis are streptococcal or diphtheritic pharyngitis, herpangina, aphthous stomatitis, Stevens-Johnson syndrome, Vincent's infection, and infectious mononucleosis. The severe systemic symptoms, diffuse intraoral involvement, and the lack of other mucous membrane lesions usually cause little problem in recognizing the disease in children. The disease generally runs its course in 10–14 days with no sequelae, although cervical adenopathy may persist for several weeks. Autoinoculation of other sites, particularly the fingers in young children, is not uncommon.

Herpes simplex virus infections of the eye are usually caused by HSV-1.[59,60] Primary infections may be manifested by a unilateral follicular conjunctivitis with regional adenopathy and/or a blepharitis with vesicles on the lid margin. Photophobia, chemosis, excessive tearing, and edema of the eyelids may be present. Some patients develop dendritic figures (Fig. 2) or coarse, punctate, epithelial opacities. If disease is limited to the conjunctiva, healing takes place within 2–3 weeks. However, if systemic symptoms and signs of stromal involvement are

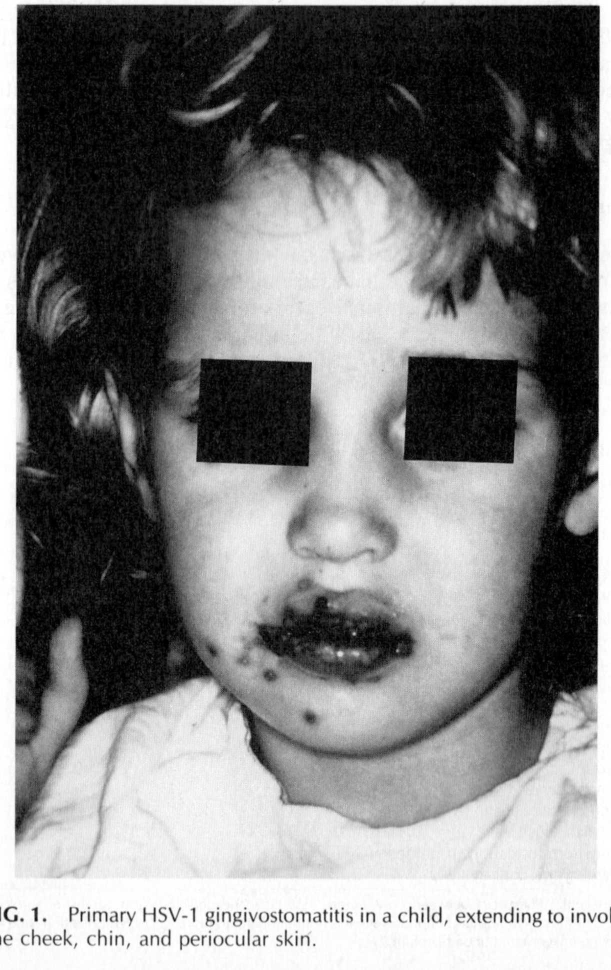

FIG. 1. Primary HSV-1 gingivostomatitis in a child, extending to involve the cheek, chin, and periocular skin.

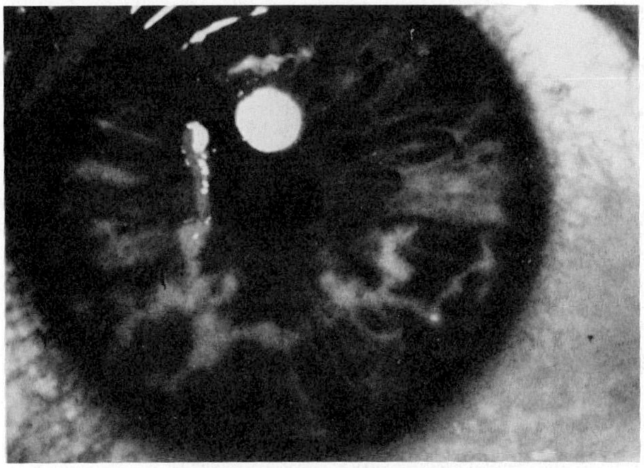

FIG. 2. HSV-1 dendritic keratitis. (From Pavan-Langston,[61] with permission.)

present, the healing phase may be delayed. Spontaneous healing of the conjunctiva and cornea is usually complete.

Primary genital infection is most common in adolescents and in young adults and is usually (in 70–95 percent of the cases) caused by HSV-2. Incubation periods are 2–7 days. In men, vesicular lesions on an erythematous base usually appear on the glans penis or the penile shaft. In the female, lesions may involve the vulva, perineum, buttocks, cervix, and vagina and are frequently accompanied by a vaginal discharge (Fig. 3). Extragenital lesions occur during the course of primary infection in 10–20 percent of patients.[44] Primary infection in both sexes may be associated with fever, malaise, anorexia, and tender bilateral inguinal adenopathy. Although vesicular lesions may persist for several days in men, in women they rapidly ulcerate and become covered by a grayish white exudate. Such lesions may be exquisitely tender, and urethral involvement may result in dysuria or urinary retention. Herpetic sacral radiculomyelitis accompanying genital infection may also lead to urinary retention, neuralgias, and obstipation; in such patients a loss of anal tone, diminished bulbocavernosus reflex, and cystometrographic evidence of lower motor neuron dysfunction can sometimes be demonstrated.[62] Lesions of primary genital herpes may persist for several weeks before healing is complete. Previous HSV-1 infection may reduce the severity and duration of a first episode of genital herpes. In the diagnosis of genital herpes, other venereal infections such as chancroid or syphilis, erosions secondary to excoriation, genital manifestations of Behçet syndrome or erythema multiforme, and local moniliasis must all be distinguished.

Although primary infections are usually in perioral, ocular, or genital areas, any skin site may be initially involved. Primary HSV skin infections may be extensive and mimic herpes zoster, although a dermatomal distribution is not usually maintained and the pain is less severe. Primary finger infections (whitlows) may be misdiagnosed as pyogenic paronychiae and may be unnecessarily incised. Usually only one digit is involved, initially with intense itching or pain, and is followed by one or many deep vesicles that may coalesce (Fig. 4). Systemic complaints and intense local pain are frequently present, and neuralgia and axillary adenopathy may occur. If not incised, healing gradually takes place over a period of 2–3 weeks; if incised, secondary bacterial infection may develop and delay healing. Among medical, paramedical, or dental personnel, whitlows are commonly caused by HSV-1, whereas in the general community they are more commonly secondary to infection with HSV-2.[63]

Primary perianal and anal HSV-2 infection is becoming increasingly well recognized, particularly in male homosexuals.[34] Pain is the primary symptom, with itching, tenesmus, and discharge also noted. Systemic complaints of fever, chills, malaise, headache, difficulty in urinating, and sacral paresthesias may be present. On examination, vesicles and ulcerations may be seen in perianal and sometimes in anal areas. They may become confluent and result in a grayish ulcerating cryptitis surrounded by a red edematous mucosa. Bilateral inguinal adenopathy is common. The course is generally self-limited unless bacterial infection supervenes, with healing occurring in 1–3 weeks. However, in the setting of the acquired immunodeficiency syndrome (AIDS), herpes proctitis may be prolonged and progressive.[33]

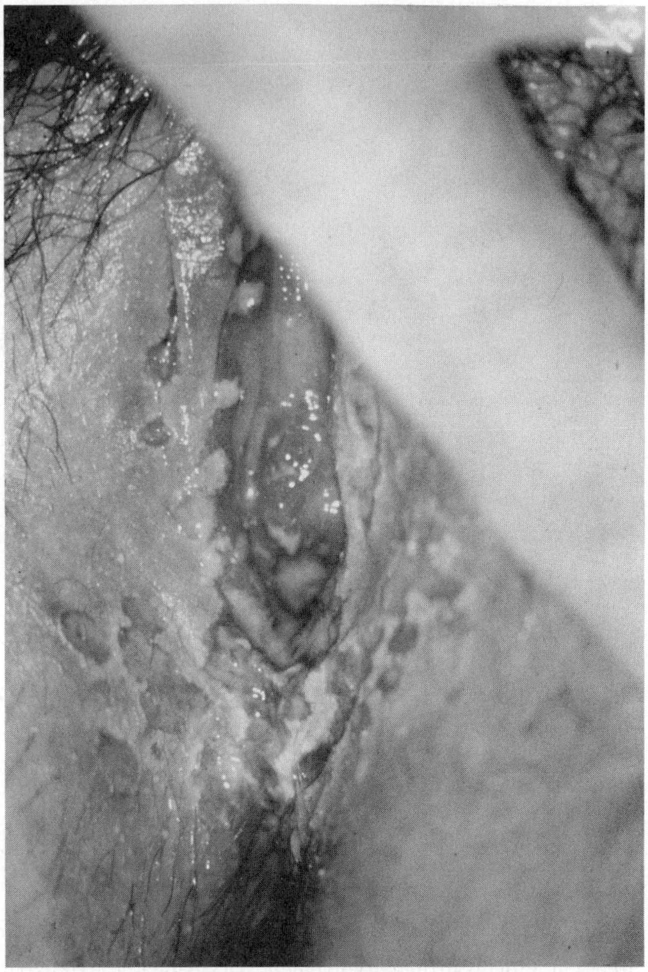

FIG. 3. Herpes (HSV-2) of the vulva.

Recurrent Infections

Recurrent herpes labialis is frequently heralded by prodromal symptoms (pain, burning, tingling, or itching) generally lasting for less than 6 hours but occasionally as long as 24–48 hours.[39,41] Vesicles appear most commonly at the vermillion border of the outer lip and are associated with considerable pain. The lower lip is more frequently involved, although individual patients may have stereotyped lesions at similar sites during each recurrence. The lesion area is usually less than 100 mm^2, and lesions progress from the vesicle to the ulcer/crust stage within 48 hours. Pain is most severe within the first 24 hours after the appearance of lesions. Healing is generally complete within 8–10 days. Rarely, recurrences may occur in the mouth or on the nose, chin, or cheek. Systemic complaints do not usually accompany recurrent herpes labialis, although local adenopathy may occur.

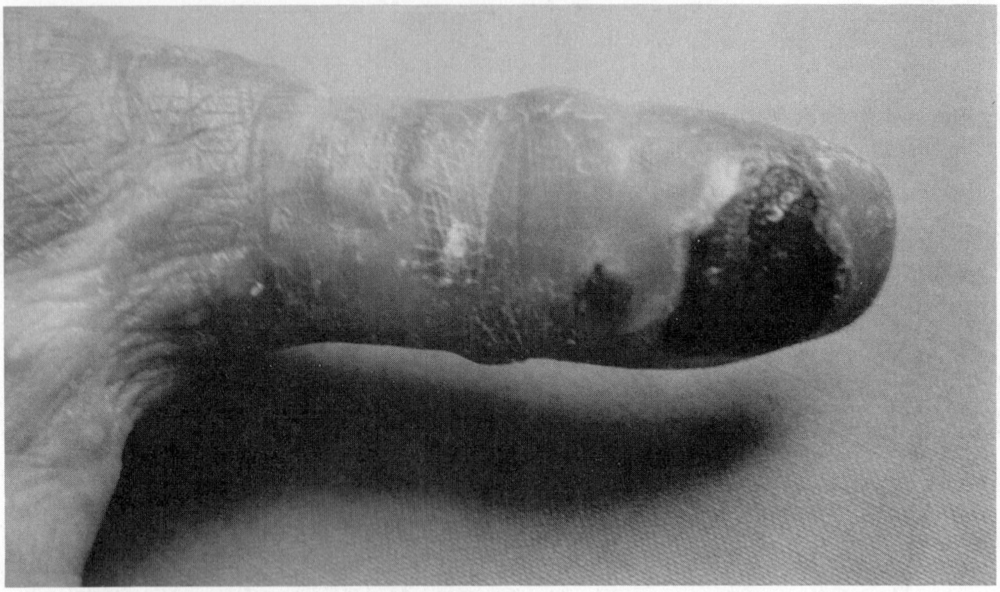

FIG. 4. Ulcerated herpetic whitlow in a respiratory care nurse. Her uncovered thumb had been used on a suction device to remove secretions from the mouth of a patient with herpes labialis. Secondary vesicles are seen at the base of the thumb.

Ocular infection may recur as keratitis, blepharitis, or keratoconjunctivitis. Recurrent keratitis is usually unilateral but is rarely (in 2–6 percent of the cases) bilateral. Two main types of keratitis may develop: dendritic ulceration or stromal involvement. Branching dendritic ulcers that stain with fluorescein are virtually diagnostic (Fig. 1) and are often accompanied by a loss in corneal sensation. Visual acuity may be decreased because the ulcers frequently involve the pupillary portion of the cornea. They may be accompanied by minimal anterior opacification or deep stroma involvement. Occasionally, extensive ameboid corneal ulcers may evolve, particularly if topical steroids have been applied. Superficial keratitis usually heals, but recurrent infection may lead to deep stromal involvement and uveitis, which may in part be mediated by hypersensitivity reactions to viral or altered cellular antigens.[64] A gradual diminution in visual acuity takes place, and individual attacks may last for several months with the formation of dense scars, corneal thinning, and neovascularization. Permanent visual loss may result, and rarely, rupture of the globe develops.

Recurrent genital lesions in both sexes are generally associated with less severe systemic symptoms and less extensive local involvement than are primary attacks. A prodrome of tenderness, itching, burning or tingling is often noted for several hours before a recurrence. Lesions in women are most often noted on the labia minora, labia majora, and perineum and less commonly on the mons pubis or buttocks.[65] Lesions in men are most often found on the glans or penile shaft. In women recurrences tend to be more severe.[44] Healing generally occurs in 6–10 days.[65,66] Virus shedding diminishes more slowly in women and can occur between recurrences in both sexes.[66,67] Occasionally, genital recurrences are associated with headache and even with aseptic meningitis.[68] Urethral stricture and labial fusion have also been reported after recurrent genital infections.

Recurrent HSV-1 or HSV-2 infections may develop on extremities; occasionally such lesions are associated with severe local neuralgia.[69,70] Local edema and lymphangitis may also occur during recurrences on extremities.

Complications

Encephalitis. Herpes simplex encephalitis is a rare complication of herpetic infection and yet is one of the most common acute sporadic viral diseases of the brain in the United States.[71–74] Estimates of its frequency range from several hundred to several thousand cases per year. Beyond the neonatal period, HSV-1 is the principal causal agent. Although little is known about the pathogenesis of HSV-1 encephalitis in humans, the virus is believed to spread by neural routes into the brain during either primary or recurrent infection.[18,74,75] Temporal lobes are the principal target areas of the virus, and a necrotizing hemorrhagic encephalitis results.

Herpes simplex encephalitis occurs at all ages, in both sexes, and in all seasons. The clinical course may begin suddenly or after a brief influenza-like prodrome. Headache, fever, behavioral disorders, speech difficulties, and focal seizures are prominent features; olfactory hallucinations may be present. Cerebrospinal fluid examination is variable but frequently shows a moderate pleocytosis with mononuclear and polymorphonuclear leukocytes; protein levels are slightly elevated, and glucose is generally normal. Infectious virus is rarely present in cerebrospinal fluid during encephalitis, and brain biopsy with appropriate histologic and cultural techniques is currently the most reliable way to make the diagnosis.[70–73] Although various antibody and antigen assays may provide adjunctive information,[74,76] they are not sensitive enough to provide a sufficiently early diagnosis. Herpes simplex virus encephalitis must be distinguished from other forms of viral encephalitis, tuberculous and fungal meningitis, brain abscesses, cerebrovascular accidents, and brain tumors. It is often helpful to identify the involved brain area by electroencephalography (EEG), magnetic resonance imaging (MRI), or computerized axial tomography so that biopsies can be appropriately localized. Of these, MRI and EEG may provide the earliest evidence of localization.[73,77] The course in untreated patients is usually one of rapid deterioration over several days that progresses to coma and death. Mortality in untreated biopsy-proven cases is 60–80 percent, and fewer than 10 percent of the patients are left without significant neurologic sequelae.[70–72]

Neonatal Infections. Involvement of the newborn with HSV can range from a mild localized infection to a fatal disseminated one. The incidence of neonatal HSV infection has been estimated to be between 1 in 2500 and 1 in 10,000 live births and is higher in premature than in full-term infants.[77–79] Most infections result from the retrograde spread of HSV-2 secondary to maternal genital infection or via passage of the infant through an infected maternal genital tract. The use of fetal monitor scalp electrodes may increase the risk of transmission.[80] The overall risk of serious neonatal infection has been estimated to be 40–50 percent after primary maternal infection and ≤8 percent after recurrent infection.[78] Primary infection during pregnancy may also lead to abortion, premature labor, skin lesions, chorioretinitis, microcephaly, or uterine growth retardation.[79] Both primary and recurrent infections during pregnancy may be asymptomatic with unsuspected viral shedding.[81] Rarely, nosocomial nursery infection may occur.[16,31,32]

Congenital infection may be recognized at birth along with jaundice, hepatosplenomegaly, a bleeding diathesis, central nervous system anomalies such as microcephaly or microphthalmia, seizures, irritability, temperature instability, chorioretinitis, and skin vesicles. In the absence of vesicles, congenital HSV infection may be difficult to distinguish from similar syndromes caused by rubella, cytomegalovirus, or *Toxoplasma*. In contrast, neonatal infection appears several days to several weeks after birth and may mimic neonatal sepsis. Often, infection occurs in the setting of prematurity. Vesicles may or may not be present, and conjunctivitis may be the first observed abnormality. Neurologic signs often predominate; seizures, cranial nerve palsies, lethargy, and coma may develop. The neurologic morbidity associated with neonatal HSV-2 infection is greater than that with HSV-1 infection.[82] A cerebrospinal fluid pleocytosis with increased protein and normal glucose levels is observed. Although some children with relatively localized disease apparently recover without significant sequelae, many develop severe complications such as destructive encephalitis or disseminated intravascular coagulation. Hepatic and adrenal necrosis may occur in fatal cases. The mortality of untreated neonatal infections is related to the type of illness, disseminated disease having the highest mortality (approximately 85 percent) and localized disease of the skin, eye, or mouth having virtually no mortalities.

Compromised Host. Patients compromised by immunodeficiency or immunosuppression, by malnutrition, or by disorders of skin integrity (e.g., burns, eczema) are at greater risk of developing severe HSV infections.

The renal, cardiac, or bone marrow transplant recipient frequently excretes HSV-1 in throat washings during the first few weeks after grafting.[48,83–86] Often these infections are asymptomatic, but occasionally they are particularly severe and persist for weeks to months (Fig. 5); they may spread down the respiratory or gastrointestinal tracts and result in tracheobronchitis, pneumonia, or esophagitis.[87] It appears that such severe infections are related to iatrogenic suppression of cell-mediated immunity early after transplantation.[49,85,86] Patients with hematologic and lymphoreticular neoplasms and children with congenital thymic disorders also may develop unusually severe, chronic, or progressive mucocutaneous HSV infection.[88,89] HSV infection during pregnancy[90,91] or in geriatric populations[92] may on rare occasions be associated with disseminated disease involving visceral organs, particularly the liver. Such disseminated disease is perhaps secondary to relative T-lymphocyte immunodeficiency states that occur with aging or during pregnancy. Instrumentation of debilitated patients with devices such as nasogastric tubes appears to facilitate spread. Herpetic esophagitis has been found to occur in approximately 25 percent of unselected autopsied patients, most of whom had nasogastric tubes in place shortly before death.[93] Herpetic esophageal ulcers are sometimes asymptomatic but may be associated with odynophagia, gastrointestinal bleeding, and diffusely scattered shallow ulcers on double-contrast esophagograms.[94]

Severe HSV infections are a prominent feature of AIDS.[33] Progressive HSV perianal ulcers, colitis, esophagitis, pneumonia, and a variety of neurologic disorders have been observed in patients with AIDS.

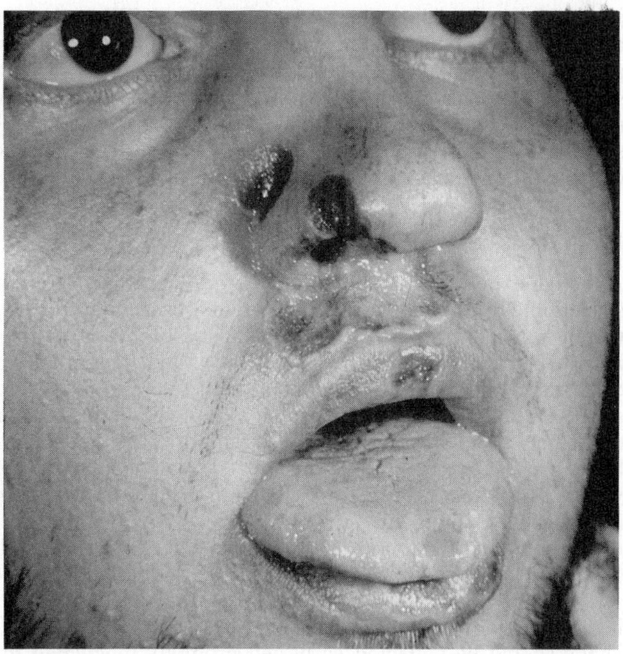

FIG. 5. Progressive HSV-1 infection of a renal transplant patient involving lip, tongue, and nose. The infection spread to involve trachea and lungs, resulting in fatal hemorrhagic pneumonitis.

Burn wound infections with HSV are becoming increasing well recognized.[95] Erosive, discolored, or vesicular areas in partially healing burns are suspicious of herpes simplex infection and should be cultured, or biopsies should be done. Occasionally HSV in burn patients disseminates to other skin areas, to the upper and lower respiratory tract, or to visceral organs. Patients with a variety of other skin disorders, for example, eczema, pemphigus, Darier's disease, or Sézary syndrome may also be unable to effectively localize their infections, thereby resulting in widespread cutaneous spread (eczema herpeticum, Kaposi varicelliform eruption).[96–98] These infections may recur and disseminate to visceral organs.[98]

Relationship to Other Diseases

Erythema Multiforme. Allergic cutaneous and mucous membrane disorders may accompany or follow acute HSV infections.[99–102] Up to 75 percent of all cases of erythema multiforme are regularly preceded by an attack of herpes simplex. Both HSV-1 and HSV-2 may be involved, and the cutaneous manifestations range from mild to severe (Stevens-Johnson syndrome) and may be recurrent. Inactivated HSV antigens injected intradermally into persons subject to erythema multiforme have induced such attacks,[99] and HSV antigen has been identified in skin biopsy specimens from affected lesions.[102]

Cancer. Many series, although not all, have indicated that patients with cervical carcinoma have a higher incidence and higher titers of HSV-2 antibodies than do matched controls.[103,104] These findings may reflect an earlier age of first intercourse and multiple sexual partners. Attempts to demonstrate infectious virus, viral antigens, or viral DNA sequences in cervical carcinoma cells have given contradictory results.[105,106]

Idiopathic Neurologic Syndromes. Herpes simplex virus infections have been implicated as possible factors involved in the pathogenesis of various neurologic disorders of unknown etiology including idiopathic facial paralysis (Bell's palsy), multiple sclerosis, atypical pain syndromes, ascending myelitis, trigeminal neuralgia, and temporal lobe epilepsy.[56,107–111] The associations are based on the known predilection of HSV for nerve tissue, on serologic studies, and on the occasional observations of temporal relationships between attacks of herpes labialis or genitalis and attacks of the neurologic syndrome.

DIAGNOSIS

Although experimental animals and embryonated eggs are both susceptible to infection with HSV strains, tissue cultures have largely replaced these hosts for diagnostic purposes. Primary human embryonic kidney, rabbit kidney, and human amnion cells readily support the replication of HSV. Continuous cell strains or cell lines of human diploid origin and certain continuous monkey kidney cell lines also support HSV replication, but to a lesser extent. Cytopathic effects usually appear rapidly, within 24–48 hours if the virus inoculum is high. Cells become rounded and clump, with rapid progression of cytopathic effects throughout the cell monolayer. Ballooning degeneration and the formation of multinucleated syncytial giant cells may be observed, particularly with HSV-2 isolates. Vesicles contain their highest titers of virus within the first 24–48 hours,[41] and specimens should be collected early and promptly inoculated into tissue cultures. If a delay is unavoidable, specimens can be stored in appropriate carrying medium at 4–9°C for a few hours, but for longer periods they should be stored at −70°C. Typing of isolates can be accomplished by using a variety of serologic techniques including immunofluorescence or microneutralization[112,113] or by certain biologic properties, for example, temperature or heparin sensitivity.[14,15] When tissue specimens such as neural ganglia are being studied for the presence of virus, tissue explantation or cell cocultivation techniques have proved useful in facilitating virus isolation.

The recent development of monoclonal antibodies to individual herpes virus antigens should allow for the more precise identification and typing of HSV isolates.[19,20,114,115] HSV-1 and HSV-2 have both type-specific and cross-reactive antigens that are useful for both grouping and type discrimination. Moreover, the cloning of herpes DNA fragments in recombinant bacteria may permit the production of probes to identify herpes genomes in the absence of infectious virus.[115]

For a rapid diagnosis of skin or mucous membrane lesions, scrapings from suspect lesions may be smeared, fixed with ethanol or methanol, and stained with Giemsa or Wright preparation. The presence of multinucleated giant cells indicates infection with HSV or varicella-zoster virus (Fig. 6). When using cytologic techniques, e.g., the Papanicolaou cervicovaginal stain or the Paragon multiple stain, intranuclear inclusions may also be seen.[116] Alternatively, such material can be examined for herpes antigens by immunofluorescent techniques or for virus particles by electron microscopy.

Serologic techniques may be helpful in diagnosing primary HSV infections but are rarely of value in recurrent infections. A variety of assays have been used including neutralization, complement fixation, passive hemagglutination, indirect immunofluorescence, radioimmunoassay, complement-mediated cytolysis, and antibody-dependent cellular cytolysis. During primary infections, a fourfold or greater rise in titer is observed between acute and convalescent sera. In recurrent infections such rises may or may not be observed.

Measurement of IgM HSV antibodies in infants may be helpful in the diagnosis of neonatal infection.[117] Such antibodies usually appear within the first 4 weeks of life in infected infants and persist for many months. Measurement of IgM antibodies in older persons has not proved useful in separating primary from recurrent infections.

Approaches to detect specific HSV antigens or antibodies to them by immunoblotting techniques in cerebrospinal fluid are under study. Such techniques may circumvent the need for invasive procedures such as brain biopsy to make the diagnosis of herpes encephalitis.[76,118]

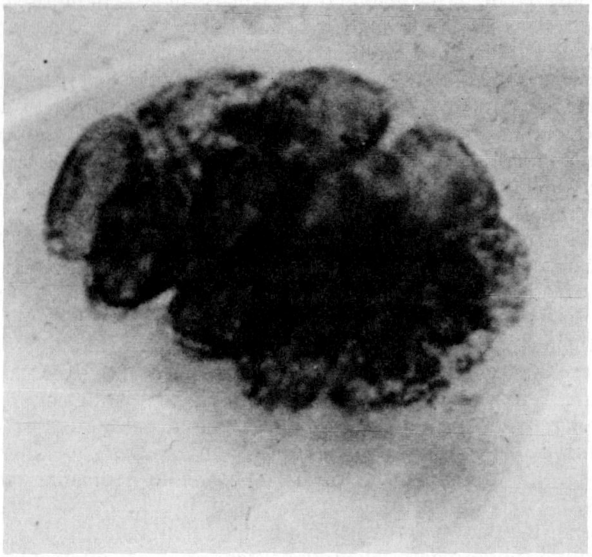

FIG. 6. Scraping of a vesicle base, stained with Giemsa preparation (Tzanck smear), showing a multinucleated giant cell indicative of infection with herpes simplex or varicella-zoster virus.

Studies of cell-mediated immunity in HSV infection are still in their infancy. Some observers have noted diminished lymphocyte proliferation to herpes virus antigens and a reduced production of certain lymphokines in association with recurrences.[49,119–121] However, these assays have not yet reached the stage of clinical usefulness.

PREVENTION AND TREATMENT

A number of nucleoside derivatives interfere with the synthesis of HSV DNA. Some of these (idoxuridine, trifluorothymidine, vidarabine) are useful in and licensed for the topical treatment of herpes keratitis[122] (see also Chapters 34 and 99). Vidarabine and acyclovir are also useful for systemic HSV infections. None of these agents affects latent virus.

Vidarabine (9-β-D-arabinofuranosyladenine) has shown efficacy in both herpes simplex encephalitis and neonatal herpes infection. In herpes encephalitis, placebo-controlled double-blind studies indicate that vidarabine, in intravenous doses of 15 mg/kg/day for 10 days, can reduce both mortality and morbidity.[71,72] The age and level of consciousness at entry are important variables in determining the outcome; patients under the age of 30 with higher levels of consciousness do better.

Controlled trials also indicate that vidarabine can lower the mortality from neonatal HSV infections.[123] In infants with central nervous system or disseminated disease, fatalities were reduced from 74 to 38 percent. Subsequent studies suggest that newborns tolerate higher doses of vidarabine than do older people and that progression from localized skin involvement to central nervous system disease is less when doses of 30 mg/kg/day for 10 days are employed. Topical vidarabine is also effective for the treatment of herpes simplex keratitis[124] but not for therapy for cutaneous infections.[125,126]

The most common adverse effects of intravenous vidarabine have been gastrointestinal and neurologic. Tremors, paresthesias, ataxia, and seizures may appear several days after the onset of therapy but are usually reversible. Pre-existing renal or hepatic disease may predispose patients to vidarabine neurotoxicity. The drug should be used cautiously in patients with renal insufficiency, with dose reductions of at least 25 percent.

The development of acyclovir, 9-(2-hydroxyethoxy methyl) guanine, represents a major advance in antiherpes therapy. Infection of cells with HSV results in the induction of a viral thymidine kinase that phosphorylates acyclovir to a monophosphate form. This is subsequently converted to acyclovir triphosphate by cellular enzymes. Acyclovir triphosphate is a potent inhibitor of HSV DNA polymerase and has little cellular toxicity.

Acyclovir is available in three formulations in the United States—a topical 5% ointment, an intravenous form, and an oral form. All three preparations are useful in the treatment of primary genital herpes.[127–131] The oral formulation is recommended for most uses (200 mg five times daily for 10 days). Acyclovir has only a modest effect on recurrent genital herpes attacks and does not appear to influence subsequent recurrences[132]; it is thus not recommended for therapy for most episodes of recurrent herpes in the immunologically competent host. In individuals subject to frequent and severe recurrences, suppression or prophylaxis with oral acyclovir may be indicated.[133,134] In patients whose recurrences are associated with severe complications such as erythema multiforme, recurrent aseptic meningitis, or eczema herpeticum, suppression is also of benefit. Oral administration appears safe and effective when used continuously for up to 1 year. Daily suppressive regimens (200 mg three to four times a day) are more effective than are intermittent regimens.[135,136]

The use of acyclovir in oral–labial HSV infections has been less extensively studied. Anecdotal reports suggest its use in primary attacks, but it is not generally recommended for recurrent herpes labialis.

In the immunocompromised host, acyclovir is useful as both treatment and suppression of recurrent mucocutaneous HSV lesions.[136–142] For the treatment of acute episodes, virus shedding, local symptoms, e.g., pain, and time to healing can be reduced by intravenous or oral regimens (e.g., 400 mg five times per day). Acyclovir is also useful in the prevention of herpetic recurrences in immunocompromised hosts including transplant recipients, leukemics undergoing induction chemotherapy, and patients with AIDS. Regimens of 200–400 mg two to five times per day have been satisfactory in preventing recurrences among seropositive patients.

Parenteral acyclovir is indicated for disseminated or central nervous system HSV infections. In patients with biopsy-proven HSV encephalitis, acyclovir was compared with vidarabine and found to be superior in reducing mortality (54 vs 28 percent, $p = .008$). Acyclovir in a dose of 10 mg/kg every 8 hours is recommended.[143] In newborns with disseminated HSV infections, acyclovir and vidarabine appear equivalent (R. J. Whitley, unpublished observations).

Acyclovir has little acute toxicity. Drug-related neurotoxicity (disorientation, hallucinations, tremors, ataxia, seizures) has been described rarely, and reversible renal dysfunction may follow a rapid bolus infusion.

A concern with respect to chronic acyclovir treatment is the possible development of resistant mutants of HSV. Mutants may have thymidine kinase with altered substrate specificity, lack thymidine kinase, or have DNA polymerase with altered substrate specificity.[144] Thymidine kinase–deficient (TK-) mutants have been isolated from immunocompromised patients, both in the presence and in the absence of acyclovir. Most of these have not been associated with progressive disease. However, acyclovir-resistant pathogenic isolates are becoming increasingly associated with progressive disease,[145,146] and it is possible that resistance will become a major problem in the years ahead. A number of other agents have received attention in the treatment of HSV infections including interferons and phosphonoformate, but none of these agents has been licensed for use in herpes infections. These agents may be useful for the treatment of infections resulting from TK-, acyclovir-resistant mutants.[147]

Experimental vaccines against HSV have shown promise in animal models,[148] and some are undergoing human trials. It is unlikely, however, that a human HSV will be generally available in the near future.

Attempts at prophylaxis have also been directed toward avoiding contact with infected lesions. Medical and dental personnel should be strongly encouraged to avoid direct contact with potentially infectious lesions by wearing gloves. Patients with extensive herpetic lesions, for example, eczema herpeticum, should be isolated. The use of condoms is recommended to prevent genital spread when one sexual partner has active lesions or a history of recurrent genital infections.

The prevention of neonatal disease in the offspring of mothers with genital infection presents special problems.[78–80] Although sufficient data have not yet been accumulated, it appears that if clinically apparent cervical infection is detected at parturition before membrane rupture, cesarean section is recommended. However, if membrane rupture has occurred, it is doubtful whether cesarean section is safer than vaginal delivery is, although rapid delivery by either route is clearly indicated to lessen the exposure of the infant. If clinical examination is negative at parturition, vaginal delivery appears safe. However, close monitoring of infants born to seropositive women is essential, with early intervention if illness develops during the first weeks of life.

REFERENCES

1. Wildy P. Herpes: History and classification. In: Kaplan AS, ed: The Herpesviruses. New York: Academic Press; 1973:1.
2. Hutifield DC. History of herpes genitalis. Br J Vener Dis. 1966;42:263.
3. Lowenstein A. Aetiologische untersuchungen uber den fieberhaften Herpes. Munch Med Wochenschr. 1919;66:768.
4. Roizman B. The structure and isomerization of herpes simplex virus genomes. Cell. 1979;16:481.
5. Schaffer PA. Molecular genetics of herpes simplex viruses. In: Nahmias AJ, Dowdle WR, Schinazi RF, eds. The Human Herpesviruses: An Interdisciplinary Approach. New York: Elsevier Science Publishing; 1981:55.
6. Bastian FO, Rabson AS, Yee CL, et al. Herpesvirus hominis: Isolation from human trigeminal ganglion. Science. 1972;178:306.
7. Baringer JR, Swoveland P. Recovery of herpes-simplex virus from human trigeminal ganglions. N Engl J Med. 1973;288:648.
8. Stevens JG, Wagner EK, Dovi-Rao GB, et al. RNA complementary to a herpesvirus and gene in RNA is prominent in latently infected neurons. Science. 1987;236:1056.
9. Openshaw H, Sekizawa T, Wohlenberg C, et al. The role of immunity in latency and reactivation of herpes simplex viruses. In: Nahmias AJ, Dowdle WR, Schinazi RF, eds. The Human Herpesviruses: An Interdisciplinary Approach. New York: Elsevier Science Publishing; 1981:289.
10. Hirsch MS, Schooley RT. Treatment of herpes virus infections. N Engl J Med. 1983;309:963,1034.
11. Corey L, Spear PG. Infections with herpes simplex viruses. N Engl J Med. 1986;314:686,749.
12. Gentry GA, Randal CC. The physical and chemical properties of the herpesviruses. In: Kaplan AS, ed. The Herpesviruses. New York: Academic Press; 1973:45.
13. Nahmias AJ, Josey WE. Epidemiology of herpes simplex viruses 1 and 2. In: Evans A, ed. Viral Infections of Humans: Epidemiology and Control. 2nd ed. New York: Plenum; 1982:351.
14. Nordlund JJ, Anderson C, Hsiung GD. The use of temperature sensitivity and selective cell culture systems for differentiation of herpes simplex virus types 1 and 2 in a clinical laboratory. Proc Soc Exp Biol Med. 1977;155:118.
15. Marks-Hellman S, Ho M. Use of biological characteristics to type herpesvirus hominis types 1 and 2 in diagnostic laboratories. J Clin Microbiol. 1976;3:277.
16. Buchman TG, Roizman B, Adams G, et al. Restriction endonuclease fingerprinting of herpes simplex virus DNA: A novel epidemiological tool applied to a nosocomial outbreak. *J Infect Dis.* 1978;138:488.
17. Hammer SM, Buchman TG, D'Angelo LJ, et al. Temporal cluster of herpes simplex encephalitis: Investigation by restriction endonuclease cleavage of viral DNA. J Infect Dis. 1980;141:436.
18. Whitley R, Lakeman AD, Nahmias A, et al. DNA restriction-enzyme analysis of herpes simplex virus isolates obtained from patients with encephalitis. N Engl J Med. 1982;307:1060.
19. Showalter SD, Zweig M, Hampar B. Monoclonal antibodies to herpes simplex virus type 1 proteins, including the immediate early protein ICP 4. Infect Immun. 1981;34:684.
20. Pereira L, Dondero DV, Gallo D, et al. Serological analysis of herpes simplex virus types 1 and 2 with monoclonal antibodies. Infect Immun. 1982;35:363.
21. Black FL. Infectious diseases in primitive societies. Science. 1975;187:515.

22. Douglas RG Jr, Couch RB. A prospective study of chronic herpes simplex virus infection and recurrent herpes labialis in humans. J Immunol. 1970;104:289.
23. Centifanto YM, Drylie DM, Deardourff SL, et al. Herpes type 2 in the male genitourinary tract. Science. 1972;178:318.
24. Bolognese RJ, Corson SL, Fuccillo DA, et al. Herpesvirus hominis type II infections in asymptomatic pregnant women. Obstet Gynecol. 1976;48:507.
25. Duenas A, Adam E, Melnick JL, et al. Herpesvirus type 2 in a prostitute population. Am J Epidemiol. 1972;95:483.
26. Buddingh GJ, Schrum DI, Lanier JC, et al. Studies on the natural history of herpes simplex infection. Pediatrics. 1953;11:595.
27. Nahmias AJ, Josey WE, Naib AM, et al. Antibodies to herpesvirus hominis types 1 and 2 in humans. I. Patients with genital herpetic infections. Am J Epidemiol. 1970;91:539.
28. Rawls WE, Campione-Piccardo J. Epidemiology of herpes simplex virus type 1 and type 2 infections. In: Nahmias AJ, Dowdle WR, Schinazi RF, eds. The Human Herpesviruses: An Interdisciplinary Approach. New York: Elsevier Science Publishing; 1981:137.
29. Rosato FE, Rosato EF, Plotkin SA. Herpetic paronychia: An occupational hazard of medical personnel. N Engl J Med. 1970;283:804.
30. Selling B, Kibrick S. An outbreak of herpes simplex among wrestlers (herpes gladiatorum). N Engl J Med. 1964;270:979.
31. Hale BD, Rendtorff RC, Walker LC, et al. Epidemic herpetic stomatitis in an orphanage nursery. JAMA. 1963;183:1068.
32. Francis DP, Herrmann KL, MacMahon JR, et al: Nosocomial and maternally acquired herpesvirus hominis infections. Am J Dis Child. 1975;129:889.
33. Siegal FP, Lopez C, Hammer GS, et al. Severe acquired immunodeficiency in male homosexuals manifested by chronic perianal ulcerative herpes simplex lesions. N Engl J Med. 1981;305:1439.
34. Goodell SE, Quinn TC, Mkrtichian E, et al. Herpes simplex virus proctitis in homosexual men. Clinical, sigmoidoscopic, and histopathological features. N Engl J Med. 1983;308:868.
35. Chang TW. Genital herpes and type 1 herpesvirus hominis. JAMA. 1977;238:155.
36. Wolontis S, Jeanson S. Correlation of herpes simplex virus type 1 and 2 with clinical features of infection. J Infect Dis. 1977;135:28.
37. Buchman TG, Roizman B, Nahmias AJ. Demonstration of exogenous genital reinfection with herpes simplex virus type 2 by restriction endonuclease fingerprinting of viral DNA. J Infect Dis. 1979;140:295.
38. Embil JA, Stephens RG, Manuel FR. Prevalence of recurrent herpes labialis and aphthous ulcers among young adults on six continents. Can Med Assoc J. 1975;113:627.
39. Young SK, Rowe NH, Buchanan RA. A clinical study for the control of facial mucocutaneous herpes virus infections. 1. Characteristics of natural history in a professional school population. Oral Surg. 1976;41:498.
40. Lafferty WE, Coombs RW, Benedetti J, et al. Recurrences after oral and genital herpes infection and viral type. N Engl J Med. 1987;316:1444.
41. Spruance SL, Overall JC Jr, Kern ER, et al. The natural history of recurrent herpes simplex labialis: Implications for antiviral therapy. N Engl J Med. 1977;297:69.
42. Kaufman HE, Brown DC, Ellison ED. Herpes virus in the lacrimal gland, conjunctiva, and cornea of man: A chronic infection. Am J Ophthalmol. 1968;65:32.
43. Carroll JM, Martola EL, Laibson PR, et al. The recurrence of herpetic keratitis following idoxuridine therapy. Am J Ophthalmol 1967;63:103.
44. Corey L, Adams H, Brown Z, et al. Genital herpes simplex virus infections: Clinical manifestations, course, and complications. Ann Intern Med. 1983;98:958.
45. Hirsch MS, Zisman B, Allison AC. Macrophages and age-dependent resistance to herpes simplex virus in mice. J Immunol. 1970;104:1160.
46. Notkins AL. Interferon as a mediator of cellular immunity in viral infections. In: Notkins AL, ed. Viral Immunology and Immunopathology. New York: Academic Press; 1975:149.
47. Lopez C. Resistance to herpes simplex virus–type 1 (HSV-1). Curr Top Microbiol Immunol. 1981;92:15.
48. Hirsch MS. Herpesgroup virus infections in the compromised host. In: Rubin RH, Young LS, eds. Clinical Approach to Infection in the Immunocompromised Host. 2nd ed. New York: Plenum; 1988:347.
49. Rand KH, Rasmussen LE, Pollard RB, et al. Cellular immunity and herpesvirus infections in cardiac-transplant patients. N Engl J Med. 1977;296:1372.
50. Becker WB, Kipps A, McKenzie D. Disseminated herpes simplex virus infection—its pathogenesis based on virological and pathological studies in 33 cases. Am J Dis Child. 1968;115:1.
51. Naraqi S, Jackson GG, Jonasson OM. Viremia with herpes simplex type 1 in adults: Four nonfatal cases, one with features of chicken pox. Ann Intern Med. 1976;85:165.
52. Craig C, Nahmias A. Different patterns of neurologic involvement with herpes simplex virus types 1 and 2: Isolation of herpes simplex virus type 2 from the buffy coat of two adults with meningitis. J Infect Dis. 1973;127:365.
53. Galloway DA, Fenoglio C, Shevchuk M, et al. Detection of herpes simplex RNA in human sensory ganglia. Virology. 1979;95:265.
54. Puga A, Cantin EM, Wohlenberg C, et al. Different sizes of restriction endonuclease fragments from the terminal repetitions of the herpes simplex type 1 genome latent in trigeminal ganglia of mice. J Gen Virol. 1984;65:347.
55. Baringer JR. Recovery of herpes simplex virus from human sacral ganglions. N Engl J Med. 1974;291:828.
56. Warren KG, Gilden DH, Brown SM, et al. Isolation of herpes simplex virus from human trigeminal ganglia, including ganglia from one patient with multiple sclerosis. Lancet. 1977;2:637.
57. Rustigian R, Smulow JB, Tye M, et al. Studies on latent infection of skin and oral mucosa in individuals with recurrent herpes simplex. J Invest Dermatol. 1966;47:218.
58. Glezen WP, Fernald GW, Lohr JA. Acute respiratory disease of university students with special reference to the etiologic role of herpesvirus hominis. Am J Epidemiol. 1975;101:111.
59. Binder PA. Herpes simplex keratitis. Surv Ophthalmol. 1977;21:313.
60. Ostler HB. Herpes simplex: The primary infection. Surv Ophthalmol. 1976;21:91.
61. Pavan-Langston D, ed. Ocular Viral Disease. v. 15. Boston: Little, Brown; 1975;19–36.
62. Caplan LR, Kleeman FJ, Berg S. Urinary retention probably secondary to herpes genitalis. N Engl J Med. 1977;297:920.
63. Glogau R, Hanna L, Jawetz E. Herpetic whitlow as part of genital virus infection. J Infect Dis. 1977;136:689.
64. O'Connor GR. Recurrent herpes simplex uveitis in humans. Surv Ophthalmol. 1976;21:165.
65. Guinan ME, MacCalman J, Kern ER, et al. The course of untreated recurrent genital herpes simplex infections in 27 women. N Engl J Med. 1981;304:759.
66. Vontver LA, Reeves WC, Rattray M, et al. Clinical course and diagnosis of genital herpes simplex virus infection and evaluation of topical surfactant therapy. Am J Obstet Gynecol. 1979;133:548.
67. Adam E, Dreesman GE, Kaufman RH, et al. Asymptomatic virus shedding after herpes genitalis. Am J Obstet Gynecol. 1980;137:827.
68. Hevron JE JR. Herpes simplex virus type 2 meningitis. Obstet Gynecol. 1977;49:622.
69. Layzer RB. Neuralgia in recurrent herpes simplex. Arch Neurol. 1974;31:233.
70. Hinthorn DR, Baker LH, Romig DA. Recurrent conjugal neuralgia caused by herpesvirus hominis type 2. JAMA. 1976;236:587.
71. Whitley RJ, Soong S-J, Dolin R, et al. Adenine arabinoside therapy of biopsy-proved herpes simplex encephalitis. NIAID collaborative antiviral study. N Engl J Med. 1977;297:289.
72. Whitley RH, Soong S-J, Hirsch MS, et al. Herpes simplex encephalitis. Vidarabine therapy and diagnostic problems. N Engl J Med. 1981;304:313.
73. Whitley RJ, Soong S-J, Linneman C Jr, et al. Herpes simplex encephalitis. Clinical assessment. JAMA. 1982;247:317.
74. Nahmias AJ, Whitley RJ, Visintine AM, et al. Herpes simplex virus encephalitis: Laboratory evaluations and their diagnostic significance. J Infect Dis. 1982;145:829.
75. Ojeda V. Fatal herpes simplex encephalitis with demonstration of virus in the olfactory pathway. Pathology. 1980;12:429.
76. Lakeman FD, Koga J, Whitley RJ. Detection of antigen to herpes simplex virus in cerebrospinal fluid from patients with herpes simplex encephalitis. J Infect Dis. 1987;155:1172.
77. Schroth G, Gawehn J, Thron A, et al. Early diagnosis of herpes simplex encephalitis by MRI. Neurology (NY). 1987;37:179.
78. Brown ZA, Vontver LA, Benedetti J, et al. Effects on infants of first episode of genital herpes during pregnancy. N Engl J Med. 1987;317:1246.
79. Hulto C, Arvin A, Jacobs R, et al. Intrauterine herpes simplex virus infections. J Pediatr. 1987;110:97.
80. Kaye EM, Dooling EC. Neonatal herpes simplex meningoencephalitis associated with fetal monitor scalp electrodes. Neurology (NY). 1981;31:1045.
81. Prober CG, Hensleigh PA, Boucher FD, et al. Use of routine viral cultures at delivery to identify neonates exposed to herpes simplex virus. N Engl J Med. 1988;318:887.
82. Corey L, Whitley RJ, Stone EF, et al. Difference between herpes simplex virus type 1 and type 2 neonatal encephalitis in neurological outcome. Lancet. 1988;1:1.
83. Montgomerie JZ, Croxson MC, Becroft DMO, et al. Herpes simplex virus infection after renal transplantation. Lancet. 1969;2:867.
84. Korsager B, Spencer ES, Mordhorst CH, et al. Herpes virus hominis infections in renal transplant recipients. Scand J Infect Dis. 1975;7:11.
85. Pass RF, Whitley RJ, Whelchel JD, et al. Identification of patients with increased risk of infection with herpes simplex virus after renal transplantation. J Infect Dis. 1979;140:487.
86. Meyers JD, Fluornoy N, Thomas ED. Infection with herpes simplex virus and cell-mediated immunity after marrow transplant. J Infect Dis. 1980;142:338.
87. Ramsey PG, Fife KH, Hackman RC, et al. Herpes simplex virus pneumonia: Clinical, virologic, and pathologic features in 20 patients. Ann Intern Med. 1982;97:813.
88. Muller SA, Herrmann EC Jr, Winkelmann RD. Herpes simplex infections in hematologic malignancies. Am J Med. 1972;52:102.
89. Buss DH, Scharyj M. Herpes virus infection of the esophagus and other visceral organs in adults: Incidence and clinical significance. Am J Med. 1979;66:457.
90. Young EJ, Killam AP, Greene JF Jr. Disseminated herpesvirus infection: Association with primary genital herpes in pregnancy. JAMA. 1976;235:2731.
91. Hillard P, Seeds J, Cefalo R. Disseminated herpes simplex in pregnancy: Two cases and a review. Obstet Gynecol Surv. 1982;37:449.

92. Eron L, Kosinski K, Hirsch MS. Hepatitis in an adult caused by herpes simplex virus type 1. Gastroenterology. 1976;71:500.
93. Nash G, Ross JS. Herpetic esophagitis: A common cause of esophageal ulceration. Hum Pathol. 1974;5:339.
94. Agha FP, Lee HH, Nostrant TT. Herpetic esophagitis; a diagnostic challenge in immunocompromised patients. Am J Gastroenterol. 1986;8:246.
95. Foley FD, Greenwald KA, Nash G, et al. Herpesvirus infection in burned patients. N Engl J Med. 1970;282:652.
96. Pugh RCB, Dudgeon JA, Bodian M. Kaposi's varicelliform eruption (eczema herpeticum) with typical and atypical visceral necrosis. J Pathol Bacteriol. 1955;69:67.
97. Hazen PG, Bennett-Eppes R. Eczema herpeticum caused by herpesvirus type 2. A case in a patient with Darier disease. Arch Dermatol. 1977;113:1085.
98. Orenstein JM, Castadot MJ, Wilens SL. Fatal herpes hepatitis associated with pemphigus vulgaris and steroids in an adult. Hum Pathol. 1974;5:489.
99. Shelley WB. Herpes simplex virus as a cause of erythema multiforme. JAMA. 1967;201:153.
100. Bean SF, Quezada RK. Recurrent oral erythema multiforme: Clinical experience with 11 patients. JAMA. 1983;249:2810.
101. Britz M, Sibulkin D. Recurrent erythema multiforme and herpes genitalis (type 2). JAMA. 1975;233:812.
102. Orton PW, Huff JC, Tonnesen MG, et al. Detection of a herpes viral antigen in skin lesions of erythema multiforme. Ann Intern Med. 1984;101:48.
103. Rawls WE, Garfield CH, Seth P, et al. Serological and epidemiological considerations of the role of herpes simplex virus type 2 in cervical cancer. Cancer Res. 1976;36:829.
104. Nahmias AJ, Josey WE, Oleske JM. Epidemiology of cervical cancer. In: Evans A, ed. Viral Infections of Humans: Epidemiology and Control. New York: Plenum; 1975:501.
105. Aurelian L, Kessler II, Rosenshein NB, et al. Viruses and gynecologic cancers: Herpesvirus protein (ICP 10/AG-4), a cervical tumor antigen that fulfills the criteria for a marker of carcinogenicity. Cancer. 1981;48:455.
106. Galloway DA, McDougall JK. The oncogenic potential of herpes simplex viruses: Evidence for a "hit and run" mechanism. Nature. 1983;302:21.
107. Finelli PF. Herpes simplex virus and the human nervous system: Current concepts and review. Milit Med. 1975;140:765.
108. Ellison GW. Multiple sclerosis: A fever blister of the brain. Lancet. 1974;2:664.
109. Krohel GB, Richardson JR, Farelli DF. Herpes simplex neuropathy. Neurology (NY). 1976;26:596.
110. Adour KK, Hilsinger RL Jr, Byl FM. Herpes simplex polyganglionitis. Otolaryngol Head Neck Surg. 1980;88:270.
111. Vahlne A, Edström S, Arstila P, et al. Bell's palsy and herpes simplex virus. Arch Otolaryngol. 1981;107:79.
112. Hanna L, Keshishyan H, Jawetz E, et al. Diagnosis of herpesvirus hominis infections in a general hospital laboratory. J Clin Microbiol. 1975;1:318.
113. Corey L. Laboratory diagnosis of herpes simplex virus infections. Principles guiding the development of rapid diagnostic tests. Diag Microbiol Infect Dis. 1986;4:1115.
114. Goldstein LC, Corey L, McDougall JK, et al. Monoclonal antibodies to herpes simplex viruses: Use in antigenic typing and rapid diagnosis. J Infect Dis. 1983;147:829.
115. Goldin AL, Sandri-Goldin RM, Levine M, et al. Cloning of herpes simplex virus type 1 sequences representing the whole genome. J Virol. 1981;38:50.
116. Barr RJ, Herten J, Graham JH. Rapid method for Tzanck preparation. JAMA. 1977;237:119.
117. Nahmias AJ, Dowdle WR, Josey WE, et al. Newborn infection with herpesvirus hominis types 1 and 2. J Pediatr. 1970;17:185.
118. Kahlon J, Chatterjee S, Lakeman FD, et al. Detection of antibodies to herpes simplex virus in the cerebrospinal fluid of patients with herpes simplex encephalitis. J Infect Dis. 1987;155:38.
119. Kirchner H, Schwenteck M, Northoff H, et al. Defective in vitro lymphoproliferative responses to herpes simplex virus in patients with frequently recurring herpes infections during disease-free intervals. Clin Immunol Immunopathol. 1978;11:267.
120. Arvin AM, Pollard RB, Rasmussen LE, et al. Cellular and humoral immunity in the pathogenesis of recurrent herpes viral infections in patients with lymphoma. J Clin Invest. 1980;65:869.
121. Sheriden JF, Donnenberg AD, Aurelian L, et al. Immunity to herpes simplex virus type 2. IV. Imparied lymphokine production during recrudescence correlates with an imbalance in T lymphocyte subsets. J Immunol. 1982;129:326.
122. Pavan-Langston D. Herpetic diseases. In: Smolin G, Thoft R, eds. The Cornea—Scientific Foundations and Clinical Practice. Boston: Little, Brown; 1983:178.
123. Whitley RJ, Nahmias AJ, Soong SJ, et al. Vidarabine therapy of neonatal herpes simplex virus infection. Pediatrics. 1980;66:495.
124. Pavan-Langston D, Buchanan RA. Vidarabine therapy of simple and IUD-complicated herpetic keratitis. Trans Am Acad Ophthalmol Otolaryngol. 1976;81:813.
125. Goodman EL, Luby JP, Johnson MT. Prospective double-blind evaluation of topical adenine arabinoside in male herpes progenitalis. Antimicrob Agents Chemother. 1975;8:693.
126. Adams HG, Benson EA, Alexander ER. Genital herpetic infection in men and women: Clinical course and effect of topical application of adenine arabinoside. J Infect Dis. 1976;133(Suppl):151.
127. Corey L, Nahmias AJ, Guinan ME, et al. A trial of topical acyclovir in genital herpes simplex virus infections. N Engl J Med. 1982;306:1313.
128. Reichman RC, Badger GJ, Guinan ME, et al. Topically administered acyclovir in the treatment of recurrent herpes simplex genitalis: A controlled trial. J Infect Dis. 1983;147:336.
129. Mindel A, Adler MW, Sutherland S, et al. Intravenous acyclovir treatment for primary genital herpes. Lancet. 1982;1:697.
130. Nilsen AE, Aasen T, Halsos AM, et al. Efficacy of oral acyclovir in treatment of initial and recurrent genital herpes. Lancet. 1982;2:571.
131. Bryson YJ, Dillon M, Lovett M, et al. Treatment of first episodes of genital herpes simplex virus infection with oral acyclovir. A randomized double-blind controlled trial in normal subjects. N Engl J Med. 1983;308:916.
132. Reichman RC, Badger GJ, Mertz GJ, et al. Treatment of recurrent genital herpes simplex infections with oral acyclovir: A controlled trial. JAMA. 1984;251:2103.
133. Straus SE, Takiff HE, Seidlin M, et al. Suppression of frequently recurring genital herpes: A placebo-controlled trial of oral acyclovir. N Engl Med. 1983;310:1545.
134. Douglas JM, Critchlow C, Benedetti J, et al. Prevention of recurrent genital herpes simplex infection with daily oral acyclovir: A double-blind trial. N Engl J Med. 1984;310:1551.
135. Straus SE, Seidlin M, Takiff HE, et al. Double-blind comparison of weekly and daily regimens of oral acyclovir for suppression of recurrent genital herpes. Antiviral Res. 1986;6:151.
136. Gold D, Corey L. Acyclovir prophylaxis for herpes simplex virus infection. Antimicrob Agents Chemother. 1987;31:361.
137. Saral R, Burns WH, Laskin OL, et al. Acyclovir prophylaxis of herpes-simplex-virus infections: A randomized, double-blind controlled trial in bone-marrow-transplant recipients. N Engl J Med. 1981;305:63.
138. Wade JC, Newton B, McLaren C, et al. Intravenous acyclovir to treat mucocutaneous herpes simplex virus infection after marrow transplantation. Ann Intern Med. 1982;96:265.
139. Meyers JD, Wade JC, Mitchell CD, et al. Multicenter collaborative trial of intravenous acyclovir for treatment of mucocutaneous herpes simplex virus infection in the immunocompromised host. Am J Med. 1982;73(1A):229.
140. Whitley RJ, Levin M, Barton N, et al. Infections caused by herpes simplex virus in the immunocompromised host: Natural history and topical acyclovir therapy. J Infect Dis. 1984;150:323.
141. Shepp DH, Newton BA, Dandliker PS, et al. Oral acyclovir therapy for mucocutaneous herpes simplex virus infections in immunocompromised marrow transplant recipients. Ann Intern Med. 1985;102:783.
142. Conant MA. Prophylactic and suppressive treatment with acyclovir and the management of herpes in patients with acquired immunodeficiency syndrome. J Am Acad Dermatol. 1988;18:186.
143. Whitley RJ, Alford CA, Hirsch MS, et al. Vidarabine versus acyclovir therapy in herpes simplex encephalitis. N Engl J Med. 1986;314:144.
144. Crumpacker C. Resistance of herpes viruses to nucleoside analogues—mechanisms and clinical importance. In: Mills J, Corey L, ed. Antiviral Chemotherapy—New Directions for Clinical Application and Research. New York: Elsevier Science Publishing; 1986:226.
145. Erlich KS, Mills J, Chatis P, et al. Acyclovir resistant herpes simplex virus infections in patients with the acquired immunodeficiency syndrome. N Engl J Med. 1989;320:293.
146. Mirsch MS, Schooley RT. Resistance to antiviral drugs: The end of innocence. N Engl J Med. 1989;320:313.
147. Chatis PA, Miller CH, Schrager LE, et al. Successful treatment with foscarnet of an acyclovir-resistant mucotaneous infection with herpes simplex virus in a patient with acquired immunodeficiency syndrome. N Engl J Med. 1989;320:297.
148. Rooney JF, Wohlenberg C, Cremer KJ, et al. Immunization with a vaccinia virus recombinant expressing herpes simplex virus type I glycoprotein D: Long-term protection and effect of revaccination. J Virol. 1988;62:1530.

119. VARICELLA-ZOSTER VIRUS

RICHARD J. WHITLEY

Varicella-zoster virus (VZV) causes two distinct clinical diseases. Varicella, or more commonly chickenpox, is the primary infection and results from exposure of a susceptible individual to the virus. Chickenpox is ubiquitous and extremely contagious, but for the most part, it is a benign illness characterized by a generalized exanthematous rash. It occurs seasonally and in epidemics. Recurrence of infection results in the more localized phenomenon known as herpes zoster, often referred to as shingles, a common infection among the elderly. As of this date, there is no licensed vaccine for the prevention of chickenpox in the United States, although a promising candidate is under review of the Bureau of Biologics. Infection caused by VZV remains of medical significance. It is estimated that between 300,000 and 500,000 individuals seek medical care for chickenpox, with nearly half of these patients requiring a second office appointment. Similarly, it is estimated that herpes zoster accounts for over 1.5 million physician visits per year and that most of these individuals require follow-up medical care.

HISTORY

Shingles has been recognized since ancient times as a unique clinical entity because of the dermatomal vesicular rash; however, chickenpox was often confused with smallpox.[1] In 1875, Steiner successfully transmitted VZV by inoculation of the vesicular fluid from an individual suffering from chickenpox to "volunteers."[2] The infectious nature of VZV was further defined by von Bokay, who observed chickenpox in individuals who had close contact with others suffering from herpes zoster.[3,4] He correctly described the mean incubation period for the development of chickenpox in susceptible patients as well as the average range in days. Kundratitz in 1925 showed that the inoculation of vesicular fluid from patients with herpes zoster into susceptible individuals resulted in chickenpox.[5] Similar observations were reported by Bruusgaard[6] and others,[7] and in 1943 Garland suggested that herpes zoster was the consequence of the reactivation of latent VZV.[8]

Since early in the twentieth century, similarities in the histopathologic findings of skin lesions and in epidemiologic and immunologic studies indicated that varicella and herpes zoster were caused by the same agent.[9,10] Tyzzer described the histopathology of skin lesions resulting from VZV infections and noted the development of intranuclear inclusions and multinucleated giant cells.[11] These descriptions came from histologic studies performed on serial skin biopsy specimens that were obtained over the first week of illness. The histopathologic descriptions were amplified by Lipschutz in 1921 for herpes zoster.[12]

Isolation of VZV in 1958 permitted a definition of the biology of this virus.[10] Viral isolates from patients with chickenpox and herpes zoster demonstrated similar alterations in tissue culture, specifically the appearance of eosinophilic intranuclear inclusions and multinucleated giant cells. These findings are virtually identical to those encountered with clinically available biopsy material. Taken together these data provided a universal acceptance that both diseases were caused by VZV. By 1958, Weller and colleagues had been able to establish that there were no differences between the viral agents isolated from patients with these two clinical entities from either a biologic or immunologic standpoint.[10,13–15]

Later studies proved their identity by rigorous biochemical methods.[16] More recently, viral DNA from a patient with chickenpox who subsequently developed herpes zoster was examined by restriction endonuclease analyses, and the molecular identity of these two viruses was verified.[17,18]

PATHOGEN AND REPLICATION

Varicella-zoster virus is a member of the Herpesviridae and shares structural characteristics with other members of the family. The virus has icosahedral symmetry containing centrally located double-stranded DNA with a surrounding envelope. The total size of the virus is approximately 150–200 nm and has a lipid-containing envelope with glycoprotein spikes.[17] The naked capsid has a diameter of approximately 90–95 nm.[19–21] The DNA contains 125,000 base pairs or approximately 80 megadaltons and encodes approximately 75 proteins. The organization of the viral genome is similar to other herpesviruses. There are unique long (U_l)—105 kilobases—and unique short (U_s)—5.2 kilobases—regions of the viral genome. Each unique sequence contains terminal repeat sequences. With replication, the U_s region can invert upon itself and result in two isomeric forms, as recently reviewed.[22]

Five families of VZV glycoproteins (gp) have been identified, gp I, gp II, gp III, gp IV, and gp V. Viral infectivity can be neutralized by monoclonal antibodies directed against gp I, gp II, and gp III. These glycoproteins have been the subject of intense investigative interest because they represent the primary marker for both humoral and cell-mediated immunity.

Only enveloped virions are infectious; this may account for the lability of VZV. Furthermore, the envelope is sensitive to detergent, ether, and air drying.

Varicella-zoster virus is highly cell associated and spreads from cell to cell by direct contact. Virus can be isolated in a variety of continuous and discontinuous cell culture systems of human and simian origin. Approximately 8–10 hours after infection, virus-specific immunofluorescence can be detected in the cells immediately adjacent to the initial focus of infection. This parallels the microscopic observation of the radial spread of cytopathology.[23,24] Electron microscopic studies demonstrate the appearance of immature viral particles within 12 hours of the onset of infection. As with herpes simplex, the naked capsids acquire their envelope at the nuclear membrane, being released into the perinuclear space where large vacoules are formed.[19,25] Infectious virus is then spread to adjacent cells after fusion of plasma membranes.

EPIDEMIOLOGY OF VARICELLA-ZOSTER VIRUS INFECTIONS

Chickenpox

Humans are the only known reservoir for VZV. Chickenpox follows exposure of the susceptible or seronegative individual to VZV and represents the primary form of infection. Although it is assumed that the virus is spread by the respiratory route and replicates in the nasopharynx or upper respiratory tract, retrieval of virus from individuals incubating VZV has been uncommon. Chickenpox is a common infection of childhood and involves both sexes equally and individuals of all races. To a certain extent the virus is endemic in the population at large; however, it becomes epidemic among susceptible individuals during seasonal periods, namely, late winter and early spring. It is estimated that 3 million cases occur each year.[26] Intimate contact appears to be the key determinant for transmission. Overall, chickenpox is a disease of childhood because 90 percent of cases occur in children less than 3 years of age. Typically, the virus is introduced into the susceptible school-age or preschool child. In a study by Wells and Holla, 61 of 67 susceptible children in kindergarten through the fourth grade contracted chickenpox.[27] Approximately 10 percent of individuals over the age of 15 years are considered susceptible to VZV infection. The incubation period of chickenpox, namely, the time interval between exposure of a susceptible person to an infected individual, the index case, and the development of a vesicular rash in generally regarded as 14–15 days, but disease can appear within a range of 10–20 days.[28,29] Secondary attack rates in susceptible siblings within a household are defined as between 70 and 90 percent.[30] Patients are infectious for a period of approximately 48 hours before the period of vesicle formation and generally 4–5 days therefore until all vesicles are crusted.

While chickenpox exists worldwide in children, it should be noted that it occurs more frequently in adults resident in tropical regions than in other geographic areas. Stokes noted a higher incidence of chickenpox among soldiers during World War II where the incidence was 1.41 and 2.27 per 1,000 individuals annually. These data contrast with the United States where the rates were approximately one-half.[31]

Herpes Zoster

The epidemiology of herpes zoster is somewhat different. Varicella-zoster virus characteristically becomes latent after primary infection. It is presumed that VZV establishes latency within the dorsal root ganglia. Reactivation leads to herpes zoster, a sporadic disease. Histopathologic examination of the nerve route after infection with VZV demonstrates characteristics indicative of VZV infection. In those individuals who die after recent herpes zoster infection, an examination of the dorsal root ganglia reveals satellitosis, lymphocytic infiltration in the nerve route, and degeneration of the ganglia cells.[32,33] Intranuclear inclusions can be found within the ganglia cells. Although it is possible to demonstrate the presence of VZV by electronmicroscopy, it is not possible to isolate this virus in cultures, usually from explant dorsal root ganglia, as has been done after herpes simplex virus infection. The biologic mechanism by which VZV establishes latency remains a mystery at this time.

Herpes zoster is a disease that occurs at all ages, but it will afflict about 10 percent or more of the population overall, mainly among the elderly.[34,35] Herpes zoster, known also as shingles, occurs in individuals who are seropositive for VZV or, more specifically, in individuals who have had prior chickenpox. Reactivation appears dependent upon a balance between virus and host factors. Most patients who develop herpes zoster have no history exposure to other individuals with VZV infection at the time of the appearance of lesions. The highest incidence of disease varies between 5 and 10 cases per 1000 for individuals over the sixth decade of life.[13] It has been recognized that approximately 4 percent of patients will suffer a second episode of herpes zoster. Notably, a rare patient will even experience a third episode. In a 7-year study performed by McGregor the annualized rate of herpes zoster was 4.8 per 1000 patients, with three-fourths of those patient being over the age of 45 years.[36] Individuals who are immunocompromised have a higher incidence of both chickenpox and shingles.[37–40]

Herpes zoster has occurred within the first 2 years of life in children born to women who have had chickenpox during pregnancy. These particular cases likely reflect in utero chickenpox with reactivation early in life.

PATHOGENESIS

The pathogenesis of VZV infection that results in chickenpox reflects the natural history of the disease. It occurs in susceptible individuals who are exposed to virus after intimate contact. The appearance of a diffuse vesicular rash has been well studied from a pathologic standpoint. Histopathologic findings in human VZV infection, whether chickenpox or herpes zoster, are virtually identical. The vesicles involve the corium and dermis. As viral replication progresses, the epithelial cells undergo degenerative changes characterized by ballooning, with the subsequent appearance of multinucleated giant cells and prominent eosinophilic intranuclear inclusions, as noted previously from early reports of the disease. Under unusual circumstances, necrosis and hemorrhage may appear in the upper portion of the dermis. As the vesicle evolves, the collected fluid becomes cloudy as a consequence of the appearance of polymorphonuclear leukocytes, degenerated cells, and fibrin. Ultimately, the vesicles either rupture and release the infectious fluid or gradually become reabsorbed.

Transmission is likely by the respiratory route, followed by localized replication at an undefined site, which leads to seeding of the reticuloendothelial system and, ultimately, viremia. The occurrence of viremia in patients with chickenpox is supported by the diffuse and scattered nature of the skin lesions and can be verified in selected cases by the recovery of virus from the blood.[41] As noted, the mechanism of the reactivation of VZV that results in herpes zoster is unknown.

CLINICAL MANIFESTATIONS

Chickenpox

The medical importance of chickenpox should be stressed. There are approximately 100 deaths per year in the United States from this infection. For the normal child, mortality is less than 2 per 100,000 cases. This risk increases by over 15-fold for adults. Chickenpox presents with a rash, low-grade fever, and malaise. A prodrom of symptoms may occur 1–2 days before the onset of the exanthem in a few patients. For the most part, chickenpox in the immunocompetent child is a benign illness associated with lassitude and a temperature of 100–103°F of only 3–5 days' duration. Constitutional symptoms that develop after the onset of rash include malaise, pruritus, anorexia, and listlessness. These symptoms gradually resolve as the illness abates. The skin manifestations, the hallmark of infection, consist of maculopapules, vesicles, and scabs in varying stages of evolution. The lesions initially contain clear vesicular fluid, but over a very short period of time they pustulate and scab. Most lesions are small, having an erythematous base with a diameter of 5 mm to as large as 12–13 mm. The lesions can be round or oval, with central umbilication occurring as healing progresses. The lesions themselves have often been referred to as "dew drop-like" during the early stages of formation. If they do not rupture within a few hours, the contents will rapidly become purulent in appearance. The lesions appear on the trunk and face and rapidly spread centripally to involve other areas of the body. Successive crops of lesions generally appear over a period of 2–4 days. Thus early in the disease, the hallmark of the infection is the appearance of lesions at all stages, as noted previously. The lesions can also be found on the mucosa of the oropharynx and even the vagina; however, these sites are less common overall. It is customary for the crust to completely fall off within 1–2 weeks after the onset of infection and leave a slightly depressed area of skin.

Immunocompromised children, particularly those with leukemia, have more numerous lesions, often with a hemorrhagic base. Healing takes nearly three times longer in this population.[37] These children are at greater risk for visceral complications, which occur in 30–50 percent of cases and can be fatal in as many as 15 percent of cases. A notable complication of cutaneous lesions is secondary bacterial infection—often in association with gram-positive organisms. Infection in the neutropenic host can be systemic.

Noncutaneous sites of involvement after chickenpox most frequently involve the central nervous system and are manifested as acute cerebellar ataxia or encephalitis.[26,42,43] Cerebellar ataxia has been estimated to occur in 1 in 4,000 cases for children less than 15 years of age. Cerebellar ataxia can appear as late as 21 days after the onset of rash. It is more common, however, for acute cerebellar ataxia to present within a week of the onset of the exanthem. An extensive review of Underwood of 120 cases demonstrated that ataxia, vomiting, altered speech, fever, vertigo, and tremor were all common on physical examination.[44] Cerebrospinal fluid from these patients often demonstrates lymphocytosis and elevated levels of cerebrospinal fluid protein. This is usually a benign complication in children, and resolution occurs within 2–4 weeks.

A more serious central nervous system complication is encephalitis, which can be life-threatening in adults. Encephalitis is reported to occur in 0.1–0.2 percent of individuals suffering from the disease.[45] Underwood's review reveals this illness to be characterized by depression in the level of consciousness with progressive headaches vomiting, altered thought patterns, fever, and frequent seizures.[44] The duration of disease in these patients is at least 2 weeks. Some patients suffer from progressive neurologic deterioration leading to death. Mortality in these patients has been estimated to vary between 5 and 20 percent, and neurologic sequelae have been detected in as many as 15 percent of survivors.

A neurologic complication of note is the late appearance of cerebral angiitis after zoster ophthalmicus. This problem has been noted in several patients and defined to be progressive, with mortality being exceedingly high. Other nervous system manifestations of chickenpox include meningitis, transverse myelitis, and Reye syndrome.

A serious and life-threatening complication is the appearance of varicella pneumonitis, a complication that occurs more commonly in adults and in the immunocompromised host.[26,42,46] In adults, it is estimated to occur in 1 in 400 cases of infection and, not infrequently, in the absence of clinical symptoms. It generally appears 3–5 days into the course of illness and is associated with tachypnea, cough, dyspnea, and fever. Chest radiographs usually reveal nodular or interstitial pneumonitis.

In a prospective study of male military personnel, radiographic abnormalities were detected in nearly 16 percent of enlisted men who developed varicella, yet only one-quarter of these individuals had evidence of cough.[47] Only 10 percent of those with radiographic abnormalities developed evidence of tachypnea, thus indicating that asymptomatic pneumonitis may exist more commonly than was initially predicted. Other non-cutaneous and non-neurologic sites of involvement include the appearance of myocarditis, nephritis, bleeding diatheses, and hepatitis.

Perinatal varicella is associated with a high death rate when maternal disease develops 5 days before delivery or 48 hours postpartum.[48,49] In large part, this is the consequence of the newborn not receiving protective transplacental antibodies and the immaturity of the immune system. It has been reported that under such circumstances the mortality is as high as 30 percent. These children have been reported to have progressive disease involving visceral organs, especially the lung. The outcome in these children has been summarized by Brunell.[50] Congenital varicella with clinical manifestations at birth is uncommon, but it has been characterized by skin scarring, hypoplastic extremities, eye abnormalities, and evidence of central nervous system impairment.[51]

It should be noted that varicella has been associated epidemiologically with the development of Reye syndrome.[52] The syndrome begins in the later stages of varicella with vomiting, followed by restlessness, irritability, and a progressive decrease in the level of consciousness, all associated with progressive cerebral edema. The encephalopathy is associated with elevated levels of ammonia, a bleeding diathesis, hyperglycemia, and elevated transaminase levels.[53] The recent association between the administration of aspirin as an antipyretic and the development of Reye syndrome would indicate a statistical association between these two entities. Therefore, aspirin is contraindicated for individuals with varicella infection.

Chickenpox in the Immunocompromised Patient. Chickenpox in the immunocompromised child or adult poses significant hazards of morbidity and mortality. As noted previously, the duration of healing of cutaneous lesions can be extended by a minimum of threefold. However, a more important problem is the progressive involvement of visceral organs. Data from a variety of immunocompromised patient populations indicate a broad spectrum of disease in individuals with lymphoproliferative malignancies and solid tumors vs. bone marrow transplant recipients. In studies at St. Jude's by Feldman and colleagues, approximately one-third of children developed progressive disease with involvement of multiple organs, including the lungs, liver, and central nervous system.[54] Most of these children, 20 percent of all of those who acquire chickenpox, developed pneumonitis within the first week after the onset of infection. Mortality in this patient population has been thought to approximate 15–18 percent.[54–56] Those individuals with lymphoproliferative malignancies who require continuous chemotherapy appear to be at the greatest risk for visceral involvement.

In individuals undergoing bone marrow transplantation, the incidence of VZV infections over the first year has been estimated to be 30 percent by 1 year post-transplant. Eighty percent of these infections occurred within the first 9 months after transplantation, and 45 percent of these patients had cutaneous or visceral dissemination. Overall, 23 deaths occurred in one prospective series.[57] Risk factors identified for the acquisition of VZV infection included an age between 10 and 29 years, a diagnosis other than chronic myelogenous leukemia, the post-transplant use of anti-thymocyte globulin, allogenic transplant, and acute or chronic graft-vs.-host disease. Notably, graft-vs.-host disease increases the probability of visceral dissemination significantly.

Herpes Zoster

Herpes zoster, or shingles, is characterized by a unilateral vesicular eruption with a dermatomal distribution. Thoracic and lumbar dermatomes are most commonly involved; however, the ophthalmic branch of the trigeminal nerve can lead to zoster ophthalmicus, a sight-threatening complication. Generally, the onset of disease is heralded by pain within the dermatome that precedes the lesions by 48–72 hours. Early in the disease course erythematous, macropapular lesions will appear that rapidly evolve into a vesicular rash. Vesicles may coalesce to form bullous lesions. In the normal host, these lesions continue to form over a period of 3–5 days, with the total duration of disease being 10–15 days. However, it may take as long as 1 month before the skin returns to normal.

Unusual cutaneous manifestations of herpes zoster, in addition to zoster ophthalmicus, include the involvement of the maxillary or mandibular branch of the trigeminal nerve, which results in intraoral involvement with lesions of the pallet, tonsillar fossa, floor of the mouth, and tongue. When the geniculate ganglion is involved, the Ramsay Hunt syndrome may occur, with pain and vesicles in the external auditory meatus, loss of taste in the anterior two-thirds of the tongue, and ipsilateral facial palsy.

No known factors are responsible for the precipitation of the events of herpes zoster. If herpes zoster occurs in the child, the course is generally benign and not associated with progressive pain or discomfort. In the adult, systemic manifestations include those mainly associated with pain, as noted below.

The most significant clinical manifestations of herpes zoster is the associated acute neuritis and, later, post-herpetic neuralgia. Post-herpetic neuralgia, while uncommon in young individuals, may occur in as many as 25–50 percent of patients over the age of 50 years.[58–60] It is estimated that as many as 50 percent of individuals over 50 years of age will have pain considered debilitating that persists for over 1 month.

Extracutaneous sites of involvement include the central nervous system with the appearance of meningoencephalitis or encephalitis. The clinical manifestations are similar to that of other viral infections of the central nervous system. However, a rare manifestation of central nervous system involvement by herpes zoster is gramulomatous angiitis, usually involving the internal carotid artery. It should be noted that involvement of the central nervous system with cutaneous herpes zoster probably is more common than is recognized clinically. Invariably, patients who undergo cerebrospinal fluid examination for other reasons during episodes of shingles are found to have evidence of pleocytosis without elevated cerebrospinal fluid protein levels. These patients are without signs of meningeal irritation and infrequently complain of headaches.

Classically, VZV infection involves dorsal root ganglia. Motor paralysis can occur as a consequence of the involvement of the anterior horn cells in a manner similar to that encountered with polio. Patients with involvement of the anterior horn cells are particularly prone to excruciating pain. Other neuromuscular disorders associated with herpes zoster include transverse myelitis[61] and myositis.[62,63]

Herpes zoster in the immunocompromised host is more severe than in the normal individual. Lesion formation continues for up to 2 weeks, and scabbing may not take place until 3–4 weeks into the disease course.[40] Patients with lymphoproliferative malignancies are at risk for cutaneous dissemination and visceral involvement, including varicella pneumonitis, hepatitis, and meningoencephalitis. However, even in the immunocompromised patient disseminated herpes zoster is rarely fatal.

It should be noted that a new clinical manifestation of herpes zoster has become apparent in recent years. Chronic herpes zoster may also occur in the immunocompromised host, particularly those individuals with a diagnosis of human immunodeficiency virus infection. Individuals have sustained new lesion formation with an absence of healing of the existing lesions. These syndromes can be particularly debilitating and, interestingly, have been associated with the isolation of a VSV isolate resistant to acyclovir.

DIAGNOSIS

The diagnosis of both chickenpox and shingles is usually made by history and physical examination. In the latter part of the twentieth century, the differential diagnosis of varicella and herpes zoster is less confusing than it was 20–30 years ago. Smallpox or disseminated vaccinia were confused with varicella because of the similar appearance of the cutaneous lesions. Now with the worldwide eradication of smallpox and the discontinuation of vaccination, these disease entities no longer confuse the clinical diagnosis. For the most part, the characteristic skin rash with evidence of lesions in all stages of development provide the clinical diagnosis of infection. The presence of pruritus, pain, and low-grade fever are sufficient to establish a diagnosis of chickenpox. The localization of a vesicular rash makes the diagnosis of herpes zoster highly likely; however, other viral infections can masquerade as this disease.

Impetigo and varicella can be confused clinically. While impetigo is usually caused by the group A β-hemolytic streptococcus, it will follow an abrasion of the skin or inoculation of bacteria at the site of the skin break and lead to small vesicles in the surrounding area. There may or may not be systemic signs of disease unless the skin affliction is associated with progressive cellulitis or secondary bacteremia. Unroofing of these lesions and careful Gram staining of the scraping of the base of the lesion should reveal evidence of gram-positive cocci in chains, which is suggestive of the streptococcus, or gram-positive cocci in clusters, which is suggestive of staphylococcus, a less common cause of vesicular skin lesions. Obviously, the treatment modality for these diseases are distinctly different from that used in the management of chickenpox and would require the administration of an appropriate antibiotic.

In a smaller number of cases, disseminated vascular lesions can be caused by herpes simplex virus. In these children, disseminated herpes simplex virus infection usually is a consequence of an underlying skin disease such as atopic dermatitis or eczema. In this situation an unequivocal diagnosis can only be confirmed by isolation of the offending pathogen in an appropriate tissue culture system.

More recently, it has been recognized that disseminated enteroviral infections, particularly those caused by group A coxsackievirus, can provide widespread distal vesicular lesions. These rashes are more commonly morbilliform in nature with a hemorrhagic component rather than a vesicular or vesiculopustular appearance. Generally these diseases occur during late summer and early fall and are associated with lesions of the oropharynx, palms, and soles. This latter finding is most helpful in distinguishing enteroviral disease.

Unilateral vesicular lesions in the dermatomal pattern should immediately lead the clinician to suspect a diagnosis of shingles. It has been reported that herpes simplex virus infections and coxsackievirus infections can masquerade as dermatoma vesicular lesions. In such situations, diagnostic viral cultures remain the best method for determining the etiology of infection. Confirmation of the diagnosis is possible through the isolation of VZV in susceptible tissue culture cell lines or by the demonstration of either seroconversion or seroboosting when using standard antibody assays and employing both acute and convalescent specimens. A Tzanck smear, performed by scraping the base of the lesion, may demonstrate multinucleated giant cells. Direct immunofluorescence staining of cells from the skin base or the detection of viral antigens by other assays can be used, although most of these procedures are only performed by research groups at the present time. Useful antibody assays include immune adherence hemagglutination, fluorescence antibody to membrane antigen (FAMA) or enzyme-linked immunoabsorbent assays (ELISA).[64]

THERAPY

The medical management of chickenpox and shingles in the normal host is directed toward avoiding known complications. For chickenpox, hygiene is important including bathing, astringent soaks, and closely cropped fingernails to avoid a source for secondary bacterial infection associated with the pruritic skin lesions. Pruritus can be decreased with topical dressing or the administration of antipruritic drugs. Aluminum acetate or Burrow solution soaks for the management of herpes zoster can be both soothing and cleansing. Acetaminophen should be used to reduce fever in the child suffering from chickenpox because of the association between aspirin and the appearance of Reye syndrome.

At the present time, the treatment of chickenpox and herpes zoster in the normal host does not entail the administration of either antiviral drugs or corticosteroids. The latter has been suggested to be useful for decreasing both acute neuritis and the frequency of post-herpetic neuralgia; however, these data are controversial. In the immunocompromised host or with the appearance of visceral complications in the normal host such as varicella pneumonitis, the deployment of either acyclovir or vidarabine may be of value.[65–68] Although commonly believed to be superior, acyclovir is not licensed for use in VZV infections. Vidarabine has been extensively studied for the treatment of both chickenpox and herpes zoster in the immunocompromised host. In studies of vidarabine for chickenpox therapy in immunosuppressed children at a dosage of 10 mg/kg/day of body weight given intravenously over a period of 12 hours the duration of lesion formation was decreased from 5.6 to 3.8 days, and the frequency of visceral complications decreased from 8 of 13 to 1 of 8. Furthermore, there were two study deaths in the placebo recipients. Both the duration of lesion formation and the decreased frequency of visceral dissemination were statistically superior in the treated group as compared with the counterpart placebo recipients. In two studies of vidarabine therapy for localized and disseminated zoster in the immunocompromised host, it was possible to demonstrate slowing of new lesion formation and clearance of virus from lesions as well as a decreased time to total healing. Visceral complications were decreased from 58 to 14 in placebo recipients and from 63 to 5 in treated patients, with a parallel decrease in visceral complications from 11 to 3 patients in each of the respective groups. These outcome events were statistically significantly accelerated for treated as compared with placebo recipients. Furthermore, there was a suggestion from these studies that improvement of both acute pain and resolution of chronic pain were enhanced in the treated as compared with the placebo recipients. The dosage is 10 mg/kg/day administered once daily intravenously over a period of 12 hours at a concentration of 0.5 mg of standard intravenous fluids.

More recently, acyclovir has been evaluated in controlled studies for all herpesvirus infections. Acyclovir is a guanine derivative that was a degree of selectivity for the inhibition of VZV replication that is predicated on its selected phosphorylation and activation by virus-coded thymidine kinase and, then, its selective inhibition of the viral DNA polymerase. It is estimated that the concentration of acyclovir required to inhibit VZV replication in vitro varies between 2.1 and 6.3 μM, a concentration easily achieved after the intravenous administration of medication.[69] It should be noted, however, that such concentrations are not easily achieved after even high-dose administration of oral acyclovir. Studies of acyclovir administered at 500 mg/m^2 every 8 hours vs. placebo indicate acceleration of healing in adults with localized infection as evidenced by the decreased frequency of visceral disease. However, it was not apparent from the original controlled study that the value of acyclovir would be unequivocal for the management of zoster in targeted patient populations.

One controlled study has indicated that acyclovir appears to be superior for therapy for localized zoster in bone marrow transplant patients when compared with vidarabine.[70] The decreased frequency of complications when acyclovir is used has led to its deployment by many physicians, even though it is not licensed for therapy for VZV infections in the immunocompromised host at the present time. The recommended dosage for acyclovir is from 5 to 10 mg/kg administered every 8 hours or, as suggested by some, 500 mg/m^2 every 8 hours, especially for children.

Management of varicella pneumonitis and other complications requires excellent supportive nursing care in addition to evaluating, on an individual basis, the potential for antiviral therapy. The management of acute neuritis and/or post-herpetic neuralgia can be particularly problematic. It requires the judicious use of analgesics ranging from non-narcotic to narcotic derivatives and may include the deployment of such drugs as amitriptyline hydrochloride and fluphenazine hydrochloride.

PREVENTION

In the normal host, prophylaxis and treatment of chickenpox are of little relevance since the disease is usually benign. Transmission of infection can be prevented by isolation of the infected patient (see Chapter 277). It is important to recognize that patients who require hospitalization because of varicella are a source of nosocomial infection within the hospital environment. Because approximately 10 percent of adults are seronegative, the risks in the medical care environment can be extremely high. Those most likely to become infected are nurses and medical personnel providing care to the infected individuals. Airflow can be documented as a means of transmission of infection from one area to another in the hospital environment.

In the immunocompromised host who has not been previously exposed to chickenpox, the deployment of varicella immune globulin (VZIG) and varicella-zoster immune plasma (ZIP) have been shown to be useful for both prevention and/or amelioration of symptomatic chickenpox is high-risk individuals.[71–74] VZIG should be administered to the immunodeficient patient under 15 years of age who has a negative or unknown history of chickenpox, who has not been vaccinated against VZV, or who has had contact in the household with a playmate or in a shared hospital room for more than 1 hour. It should also be administered to the newborn whose mother had an onset of chickenpox less than 5 days before delivery or 48 hours postpartum. The use of VZIG for susceptible individuals over 15 must be evaluated on an individual basis.

A vaccine is being developed for the prevention of chickenpox in the immunocompromised and normal hosts.[75–81] Although licensed in Japan, this vaccine remains experimental in the United States and is under review by the Bureau of Biologics. Studies performed to date indicate a high probability of protection after vaccination.

The Oka strain of VZV has been developed by Takahashi and colleagues in Japan and studied as a vaccine extensively in both the normal and leukemic child. In immunocompromised children, serologic evidence of host response after vaccination has been achieved in between 89 and 100 percent of vaccinated individuals. These studies now have encompassed well over 1000 patients. Vaccine-induced rash, however, is not uncommon and occurs in varied percentages of patients from approximately 6 percent to as high as 47 percent. The factor most predictive of the appearance of rash is the degree of immunosuppression. Specifically, for children with acute lymphoblastic leukemia, the likelihood of rash can be as high as 40–50 percent. The subsequent occurrence of natural varicella after community exposure is decreased in the larger control studies and averaging 8–16 percent. The occurrence of herpes zoster after vaccination does not seem to pose a major risk at the present time.

Similar studies have been performed in normal children, with total numbers well in excess of 1000 individuals as recently reviewed.[22] In these studies the appearance of antibody responses was higher than in the immunocompromised host and varied between 94 and 100 percent. Vaccine-induced rash was far less common in these individuals and occurred at a frequency of 0.5 percent to approximately 19 percent overall, with the subsequent appearance of varicella after community exposure averaging between 1 and 5 percent. Theoretically, this vaccine might be useful for boosting immunity in older individuals as a mechanism to prevent herpes zoster infection; however, this hypothesis remains to be tested. It should be noted that the subsequent development of herpes zoster is not increased in vaccine recipients.[82]

REFERENCES

1. Gordon JE, Meader FM. The period of infectivity and serum prevention of chickenpox. JAMA. 1929;93:2013.
2. Steiner P. Zur Inokulation der Varicellen. Wein Med Wochenschr. 1875;25:306.
3. von Bokay J. Das Auftreten der Schafblattern uter besonderen Umstanden. Unger Arch Med. 1892;1:159.
4. von Bokay J. Uberden atiologischen zusammenhang der varizellen mit gewissen fallen von herpes zoster. Wein Klin Wochenschr. 1909;22:1323.
5. Kundratitz K. Experimentelle ubertragungen von herpes zoster auf menschen und die beziehungen von herpes zoster zu varicellen. Z Kinderheilkd. 1925;39:379.
6. Brunsgaard E. The mutual relation between zoster and varicella. Br J Dermatol Syph. 1932;44:1.
7. School Epidemics Committee of Great Britian. Epidemics in Schools. Medical Research Council. Special Report Series, No. 227. London: His Majesty's Stationery Office; 1938.
8. Garland J. Varicella following exposure to herpes zoster. N Engl J Med. 1943;228:336.
9. Seiler HE. A study of herpes zoster particularly in its relationship to chickenpox. J Hyg. 1949;47:253–62.
10. Weller TH, Witton HM. The etiologic agents of varicella and herpes zoster: Serologic studies with the viruses as propagated in vitro. J Exp Med. 1958;228:336–7.
11. Tyzzer EE. The histology of the skin lesions in varicella. Philippine J Sci. 1906;1:349.
12. Lipschutz B. Untersuchengen uber die Atiologies der Krankheiten der Herpesgruppe (Herpes Zoster, Herpes Genitalis, Herpes Febrilis). Arch Dermatol Syph. 1921;136:428.
13. Weller TH. Serial propagation in vitro of agents producing inclusion bodies derived from varicella and herpes zoster. Proc Soc Exp Biol Med. 1953;83:340–6.
14. Weller TH, Coons AH. Fluorescent antibody studies with agents of varicella and herpes zoster propagated in vitro. Proc Soc Exp Biol Med. 1954;86:789.
15. Weller TH, Stoddard MB. Intranuclear inclusion bodies in cultures of human tissue inoculated with varicella vesicle fluid. J Immunol. 1952;68:311.
16. Davison AJ, Scott JE. The complete DNA sequence of varicella-zoster virus. J Gen Virol. 1986;67:1759–816.
17. Sawyer MH, Ostrove JM, Felser JM, et al. Mapping of the varicella zoster virus deoxypyrimidine kinase gene and preliminary identification of its transcript. Virology. 1986;149:1–9.

18. Dumas AM, Geelen JL, Mares W, et al. Infectivity and molecular weight of varicella-zoster virus DNA. J Gen Virol. 1980;47:233–5.
19. Achong BC, Meurisse EV. Observations on the fine structure and replication of varicella virus in cultivated human amnion cells. J Gen Virol. 1968;3:305.
20. Almeida JD, Howatson AF, Williams MG. Morphology of varicella (chickenpox) virus. Virology. 1962;16:353.
21. Tournier P, Cathala F, Bernhard W. Ultrastructure et developpement intracellulaire du virus de la varicelle. Observe ou microscope electronique Presse Med. 1957;65:1229.
22. Straus SE, Ostrove JM, Inchauspe G. Varicella-zoster virus infections: Biology, natural history, treatment and prevention. Ann Intern Med. 1988;108:221–37.
23. Rapp F, Vanderslice D. Spread of zoster virus in human embryonic lung cells and the inhibitory effect of idoxyuridine. Virology. 1964;22:321.
24. Vaczi L, Geder L, Koller M, et al. Influence of temperature on the multiplication of varicella virus. Acta Microbiol Acad Sci Hung. 1963;10:109.
25. Grose C, Perrotta DM, Brunell PA, et al. Cell-free varicella-zoster virus in cultured human melanoma cells. J Gen Virol. 1979;43:15.
26. Preblud SR. Varicella: Complications and costs. Pediatrics. 1986;78:728–35.
27. Wells MW, Holla WA. Ventilation in the flow of measles and chickenpox through a community. JAMA. 1950;142:1337.
28. Preblud SR, Orenstein WA, Bart KJ. Varicella: Clinical manifestations, epidemiology, and health impact in children. Pediatr Infect Dis. 1984;3:505–9.
29. Hope-Simpson RE. Infectiousness of communicable diseases in the household (measles, chickenpox, and mumps). Lancet. 1952;2:549.
30. Ross AH. Modification of chicken pox in family contacts by administration of gamma globulin. N Engl J Med. 1962;267:369–76.
31. Strokes J Jr. Chickenpox. Communicable diseases transmitted chiefly through respiratory and alimentary tracts. In: Preventive Medicine in World War II. v. 4. Washington, DC: Department of the Army;1958:55.
32. Bastain FO, Rabson AS, Yee CL, et al. Herpesvirus varicellae: Isolated from human dorsal root ganglia. Arch Pathol. 1974;97:331.
33. Esiri MM, Tomlinson AH. Herpes zoster; Demonstration of virus in trigeminal nerve and ganglion by immunofluorescence and electron microscopy. J Neurol Sci. 1972;15:35.
34. Ragozzino MW, Melton LJ III, Kurland LT, et al. Population-based study of herpes zoster and its sequelae. Medicine (Baltimore). 1982;51:310–6.
35. Hope-Simpson RE. The nature of herpes zoster: A long-term study and a new hypothesis. Proc R Soc Med. 1965;58:9.
36. McGregor RM. Herpes zoster, chickenpox, and cancer in general practice. Br Med J.1957;1:84.
37. Feldman S, Hughes WT, Daniel CB. Varicella in children with cancer; Seventy-seven cases. Pediatrics. 1975;56:388–97.
38. Arvin AM, Pollard RB, Rasmussen LE, et al. Cellular and humoral immunity in the pathogenesis of recurrent herpes viral infections in patients with lymphoma. J Clin Invest. 1980;68:869–78.
39. Locksley RM, Flournoy N, Sullivan KM, et al. Infection with varicella zoster virus after marrow transplantation. J Infect Dis. 1985; 152:1172–81.
40. Whitley RJ. Varicella-zoster infections. In: Galasso G, Merigan T, Buchanan R, eds. Antiviral Agents and Viral Infections of Man. New York: Raven Press; 1984:517–41.
41. Asano Y, Itakura N, Hiroishi Y, et al. Viremia is present in incubation period in nonimmunocompromised children with varicella. J Pediatr. 1985;106:69–71.
42. Fleisher G, Henry W, McSorley M, et al. Life-threatening complications of varicella. Am J Dis Child. 1981;135:896–9.
43. Johnson R, Milbourne PE. Central nervous system manifestations of chickenpox. Can Med Assoc J. 1970;102:831–4.
44. Underwood EA. The neurological complications of varicella: A clinical and epidemiological study. Br J Child Dis. 1935;32:83,177,241.
45. Johnson R, Milbourn PE. Central nervous system manifestations of chickenpox. Can Med J 1970;102:831.
46. Triebwasser JH, Harrie RE, Bryant RE, et al. Varicella pneumonia in adults: Report of seven cases and a review of literature. Medicine (Baltimore). 1967;46:409–23.
47. Ward JR, Bishop B. Varicella arthritis. JAMA. 1970;212:1954.
48. Brunell PA. Fetal and neonatal varicella zoster infections. Semin Perinatol. 1983;7:47–56.
49. Preblud SR, Bregman DJ, Vernon LL. Deaths from varicella in infants. Pediatr Infect Dis. 1985;4:503–7.
50. Brunell PA. Placental transfer of varicella-zoster antibody. Pediatrics. 1966;38:1034.
51. Paryani SG, Arvin AM. Intrauterine infection with varicella zoster virus after maternal varicella. N Engl J Med. 1986;314:1542–6.
52. Linnemann CC, Shea L, Partin JC, et al. Reye's syndrome: Epidemiologic and viral studies. Am J Epidemiol. 1975;101:517.
53. Hilty MD, Romshe CA, Delamater PV. Reye's syndrome and hyperaminoacidemia. J Pediatr. 1974;84:362.
54. Feldman S, Hughes WT, Daniel CB. Varicella in children with cancer. Seventy-seven cases. Pediatrics. 1975;56:388.
55. Arvin AM, Kushner JH, Feldman S, et al. Human leukocyte interferon for treatment of varicella in children with cancer. N Engl J Med. 1982;306:761.
56. Whitley RJ, Soong SJ, Dolin R, et al. Early vidarabine therapy to control the complications of herpes zoster in immunosuppressed patients. N Engl J Med. 1982;307–971.
57. Loxley RM, Flournoy N, Sullivan KM, et al. Infection with varicella-zoster virus after marrow transplantation. J Infect Dis. 1985;6:1172–81.
58. deMoragas JM, Kierland RR. The outcome of patients with herpes zoster. Arch Dermatol. 1957;73:193–6.
59. Watson PN, Evans RJ. Postherpetic neuralgia; A review. Arch Neurol. 1986;43:836–40.
60. Esmann V, Kroon S, Petersblund NA, et al. Prednisolone does not prevent post-herpetic neuralgia. Lancet. 1987;2:126–9.
61. Hogan EL, Krigman MR. Herpes zoster myelitis. Arch Neurol. 1973;29:309.
62. Norris FH, Dramov B, Calder CD, et al. Virus-like particles in myositis accompanying herpes zoster. Arch Neurol. 1969;21:25.
63. Rubin D, Fusfeld RD. Muscle paralysis in herpes zoster. Calif Med. 1965;103:261.
64. Forghani B, Schmidt NJ, Dennis J. Antibody assays for varicella-zoster virus; comparison of enzyme immunoassay with neutralization, immune adherence hemagglutination and complement fixation. J Clin Microbiol. 1978;8:545–52.
65. Whitley RJ, Hilty M, Haynes R, et al. Vidarabine therapy of varicella in immunosuppressed patients. J Pediatr. 1982;101:125–31.
66. Prober CG, Kirk LE, Keeney RE. Acyclovir therapy of chickenpox in immunosuppressed children: A collaborative study. J Pediatr. 1982;101:622–5.
67. Whitley RJ, Chien LT, Dolin R, et al. Adenine arabinoside therapy of herpes zoster in immunosuppressed patients. N Engl J Med. 1982;307:971–5.
68. Balfour HH Jr, Bean B, Laskin OL, et al. Acyclovir halts progression of herpes zoster in immunocompromised patients. N Engl J Med. 1983;308:1448–53.
70. Shepp DH, Dandliker PS, Meyers JD. Treatment of varicella zoster virus infection in severely immunocompromised patients: A randomized comparison of acyclovir and vidarabine. N Engl J Med. 1986;314:208–12.
71. Brunell PA, Ross A, Miller H, et al. Prevention of varicella by zoster immune globulin. N Engl J Med. 1969;280:1191–4.
72. Gershon AA, Steinberg S, Brunell PA. Zoster immune globulin: A further assessment. N Engl J Med. 1969;280:1191–4.
73. Zaia JA, Levin MJ, Preblud SR, et al. Evaluation of varicella zoster immune globulin: Protection of immunosuppressed children after household exposure to varicella. J Infect Dis. 1983;147:737–43.
74. Centers for Disease Control. Varicella zoster immune globulin for the prevention of chickenpox: Recommendations of the immunization practices advisory committee. Ann Intern Med. 1984;100:859–65.
75. Takahashi M, Otsuka T, Okuno Y, et al. Live vaccine used to prevent the spread of varicella in children in hospital. Lancet. 1974;2:1288–90.
76. Gershon AA, Steinberg SP, Gelb L. Live attenuated varicella vaccine use in immunocompromised children and adults. Pediatrics. 1986;78:757–62.
77. Takahashi M. Clinical overview of varicella vaccine: Development and early studies. Pediatrics. 1986;78:736–41.
78. Yabuuchi H, Baba K, Tsuda N, et al. A live varicella vaccine in a pediatric community. Biken J. 1984;27:43–9.
79. Horiuchi K. Chickenpox vaccination of healthy children: Immunological and clinical responses and protective effect in 1978–1982. Biken J. 1984;27:37–8.
80. Weibel RE, Neff BJ, Kutter BJ, et al. Live attenuated varicella virus vaccine: Efficacy trial in healthy children. N Engl J Med. 1984;310:1409–15.
81. Asano Y, Nagai T, Miyata T, et al. Long-term protective immunity of recipients of the OKA strain of live varicella vaccine. Pediatrics. 1985;75:667–71.
82. Lawrence R, Gershon AA, Holzman R, et al. The risk of zoster after vaccination in children with leukemia. N Engl J Med. 1988;318:543–8.

120. CYTOMEGALOVIRUS

MONTO HO

Cytomegalovirus (CMV) causes a number of protean disease syndromes in pediatric and adult medicine. It exemplifies a characteristic of many infectious agents. Infection is common and reaches most of the population, while associated disease is a relatively exceptional event. In newborns it causes a congenital syndrome that may at times be fatal. In normal immunocompetent subjects, it is a recognized cause of CMV mononucleosis. But it is among various groups of the immunosuppressed such as the immature neonate, the recipients of organ transplants, and in acquired immunodeficiency syndrome (AIDS) that CMV causes its most significant disease syndromes. Infection and diseases caused by CMV are still relatively refractory to both prevention and therapy.

CMV shares with other herpesviruses the unique capacity to remain latent in tissues after recovery of the host from an acute infection. "Once infected, always infected." Hence they are "opportunists" par excellence because they are frequently already in hosts waiting to be activated when they become immunosuppressed. But immunosuppression alone does not explain all aspects of CMV disease. Why do some apparently normal people get CMV mononucleosis instead of the usual asymptomatic infection? We now know that most perinatal as well as congenital infections are also asymptomatic. Occasionally, though, a baby born with CMV will present with the fulminant congenital disease. Others may develop subtle disabilities later in life. Why is this?

The distinction between primary and secondary infections should be clearly understood. The first occurs in the seronegative immunologic "virgin," while secondary infection represents activation of a latent infection or reinfection or a seropositive "immune" person. Secondary infection is not a problem with virus infections that do not become latent or when acquired immunity is almost absolute. Clinical disease may result from either primary or secondary infection by CMV, although primary infections usually cause more severe disease.

In this chapter, emphasis is placed on up-to-date developments and clinical relevance. To understand the diseases caused by the virus, virologic, epidemiologic, and pathogenetic aspects are discussed first. For more details, Ho's monograph[1] may be consulted.

DESCRIPTION OF THE PATHOGEN

The Agent and Its History

In 1881 Ribbert[2] first noted large "protozoan-like" cells in the kidney of a stillborn. By 1932, 25 cases of cytomegalic inclusion disease were described. Farber and Wolbach[3] found by postmortem examination that 12 percent of the submaxillary glands from 183 infants who died of various causes had intranuclear and cytoplasmic inclusions, thus suggesting that the infection was not a rare event.

The modern virologic era began with the isolation of murine CMV in mouse cell culture by Smith.[4] Later, the isolation of human CMV was accomplished independently by Smith,[5] Rowe et al.,[6] and Weller et al.[7]

The term *cytomegalovirus* was coined by Weller et al.[8] to replace *salivary gland virus* or *cytomegalic inclusion disease virus*. Klemola and Kaariainen[9] first described recognizable CMV infection and disease in a normal, healthy adult. Later it was found that CMV mononucleosis can occur sporadically and also after blood[10] and leukocyte transfusions.[11]

The site of latency of CMV is not precisely known, but it probably includes at least the circulating peripheral mononuclear and possibly polymorphonuclear leukocyte.[12,13] In normal seropositive individuals lymphocytes have been found when using an immediate early antigen probe, to be abortively infected by CMV by in situ hybridization.[14] These infected cells do not ordinarily produce virus. This finding may explain why blood and organs have been found to transmit CMV, although we still do not understand how an abortive infection is triggered into a productive cycle.

One unproven characteristic of human CMV is its possible oncogenicity. All members of the herpesvirus group are candidate oncogenic agents, but the evidence for Epstein-Barr virus (EBV) is the strongest. The association of CMV with Kaposi's sarcoma is based on the epidemiologic finding that CMV infection is more common in African patients with Kaposi's sarcoma,[15] and the finding by some investigators that low copy numbers of CMV genomes are present in cells of Kaposi's sarcoma.[16]

Laboratory Diagnosis

The diagnosis of CMV infection in children and adults and in healthy or immunosuppressed persons requires laboratory confirmation and cannot be made on clinical grounds alone.

The first useful laboratory test was reported by Fetterman,[17] who found large, inclusion-bearing cells in the urine sediment. This test is diagnostic when positive but may be falsely negative in viruric patients. It is less valuable after the newborn period.

The laboratory diagnosis of CMV infection depends on either isolation of the virus or demonstration of a serologic rise. The sensitivity and precision of both approaches is generally good.

More recent technical developments include the use of monoclonal antibodies to early antigens to detect infected cells in tissue specimens[18] and the use of labeled, cloned, viral nucleic acid probes to detect virus DNA or RNA in specimens by nucleic acid hybridization.[19,20] The main advantage of these techniques is rapidity. Hybridization methods have been applied to both the clinical specimens such as buffy coat, or tissue specimens. So far they are adjunctive methods and have not supplanted cultural methods.

Cultivation of Cytomegalovirus

Human CMV cannot be readily grown in any experimental animal.[21] It, however, is easily cultured on human fibroblast cultures. The one drawback is the time needed to develop cytopathology. Ordinarily this may take 1–4 weeks, but the time required has also been shortened to 48 hours by the use of cytospin and monoclonal antibody to detect cytopathology before it becomes visible.[22] The typical cytopathology of CMV is usually sufficiently characteristic for identification in the laboratory without further serologic confirmation. When in doubt, antigen may be prepared from the virus for identification by the complement fixation (CF) test using known antiserum.[21]

When present, CMV may be readily isolated from urine, mouth swabs, buffy coat, cervical swabs, or other tissues obtained from biopsies or at postmortem examination. Virus is demonstrable in patients even if they have circulating neutralizing antibodies.

Ordinarily, CMV is not detectable in normal adults. The exceptions are females who may carry the virus in the cervix and males, particularly homosexual males, who may carry CMV in semen. The presence of CMV in the throat, urine, and blood by culture is usually abnormal. It is, however, important to note additional circumstances under which CMV may be chronically carried. Anyone who is recovering from an acute infection may carry CMV in the urine, throat, and occasionally blood for months. Patients with congenital or perinatal infection and immunosuppressed patients with transplants or human immunodeficiency virus (HIV) infection and AIDS are often chronic virus carriers for years. The meaning of isolating the virus from such patients requires careful interpretation.

Serology of Cytomegalovirus

Like herpes simplex virus, strains of CMV have enough genomic variation so that they may be "fingerprinted" after digestion with restriction endonucleases. There is, however, still enough DNA homology among different strains to suggest that, for diagnostic purposes, only one serotype of human CMV exists. The problem is more complex in understanding immunity to CMV since serologic distinctions on the basis of neutralization or other biologically meaningful measures may be present. The CF antigen of AD169 is more broadly reactive than are antigens of other strains and has been extensively used in epidemiologic and clinical studies. The CF test itself is no longer widely used because of its relative lack of sensitivity.

Compared with the CF test, the indirect fluorescent antibody (IFA) and the anti-complement immunofluorescent (ACIF) tests are more sensitive.[23,24] In primary infections, titers by IFA and ACIF tests are higher and become positive earlier than do the corresponding CF titers, at times by as much as 1–2 months. The ACIF test is superior because there is less nonspecific fluorescence.[23]

Many other tests are on the market, largely because fluorescence microscopy is cumbersome. These are the indirect hemagglutination test, radioimmunoassay, latex agglutination, automated immunofluorescence, and various versions of the enzyme-linked immunosorbent assay (ELISA). By and large the same antigens are used as in the older CF and fluorescence tests. Each one must be checked out against the reliable older ones. At times, the lower level of sensitivity (i.e., whether a test is positive or negative) is unknown or unreliable. This information may be essential to evaluate the immune and risk status before pregnancies and organ transplantation. A diagnosis of infection by serology requires either an elevation of antibody titer or its conversion from negative to positive. Samples of serum before and after an illness are essential. When they are not available, the presence of IgM antibody against CMV is a useful but not completely reliable indication of an acute infection. IgM titers may not be positive during an active infection (false-negative), or they may persist for such a long time that it may not be diagnostic (false-positive). For example IgM titers has been found to be elevated in asymptomatic homosexuals.

EPIDEMIOLOGY OF CYTOMEGALOVIRUS INFECTIONS

Incidence and Prevalence of Infections

Studies of the prevalence of antibody against CMV in sera of the general population show that infection with this virus is widespread and usually inapparent. Depending on the socioeconomic condition of the population, the prevalence of antibodies in adults ranges from 40 to 100 percent.[25] It is lower in Europe, Australia, and parts of North America, while it is significantly higher in developing areas such as Africa and Southeast Asia. There is a wide range in various parts of the United States. For example, it is 45 percent in Albany, NY, and 79 percent in Houston.

Analysis of studies on age-related incidence rate of infection suggests that there is at least one and perhaps two periods of increased infection during a life span. The first is the perinatal period. In some countries, such as Japan, Thailand, Guatemala, and Finland (a mix of economically advanced and developing countries), perinatal infection as demonstrated by viruria during the first year of life is 36–56 percent.[1] Infection increases slowly throughout childhood after the first year. The second major spurt, particularly in countries with more susceptible seronegative subjects, is during the reproductive ages and is presumably accounted for by sexual activity (see below). Babies and children become infected in a number of ways. One source of infection is passage through a contaminated uterine cervix during birth. A second mechanism is transmission from human milk by breast-feeding or from banked milk.[26] CMV has been found in the milk of seropositive women.[27] A third mechanism of infection is transmission from other children in the newborn nursery,[28] in day care centers,[29] and probably among children within the family.[30] Infected children tend to carry the virus for long periods of time in the respiratory tract and in urine.[31] Other adults in the family are probably negligible sources of virus since healthy adults usually do not shed virus in the urine or respiratory tract.

Transmission by Blood

Kaariainen et al.[10] implicated blood transfusions in the transmission of CMV. Henle et al.[32] suggested that the risk was proportional to the number of units transfused, estimated as 5–12 percent per unit. Prince et al.[33] found that 31 of 152 patients who received 1269 units of blood subsequently seroconverted. They estimated an overall risk of 2.4 seroconversions per 100 units transfused. The risk of infection may also be estimated by primary infection (seroconversion or virus isolation) in children receiving blood. Armstrong et al.[34] studied a group of 93 seronegative children undergoing open heart surgery who received a mean of 3.9 units. Nine (9.7 percent) of this group subsequently became infected with CMV. This infection rate is consistent with a model of transmission by blood transfusion with a risk not greater than 2.7 percent per unit of blood, which is consistent with the findings of a number of other studies before 1980.[1] However, more recent studies evaluating large numbers of seronegative transfusion recipients show significantly less CMV infection.[35] Infection is usually asymptomatic, but symptomatic infection in well children and adults is a definite hazard with multiple transfusion after trauma or invasive surgery. It may also occur after the transfusion of granulocytes.[11] The risk of infection is decreased by using cryopreserved blood, leukocyte-poor blood, or blood from seronegative donors.[1]

The seronegative neonate who is immature at birth is at markedly greater risk for developing significant CMV disease from as little as 100 ml blood. Fifty percent of primary infections may be serious or fatal. CMV infection in such infants has been prevented by using blood from seronegative donors.[36]

Attempts to culture CMV from blood donors despite a clear indication that it must be present is usually unsuccessful.[1] The explanation is that CMV genomes are latently present in blood leukocytes but remain unexpressed in normal healthy seropositive individuals.[14] Presumably they are activated when transfused to a recipient, particularly if immunologically immature or deficient. Chou and colleagues[37] reported that if the recipient is HLA matched with the donor activation occurs much more frequently, perhaps because of better survival of infected cells.

Transmission by Sex

Two potential sources of venereal transmission of CMV are virus in the uterine cervix and in semen. The frequency of CMV infection of the cervix varies with age, socioeconomic class, sexual promiscuity, and parity. About 1–2 percent of women having routine medical examinations in private practice in this country carry the virus in the cervix.[1] In Taiwan, however, 18 percent of a nonpromiscuous female population carried the virus.[38] The cause of this marked discrepancy is unclear, and it is unknown how women acquire the virus at this site. On the other hand in a study of 347 young women attending a sexually transmitted disease (STD) clinic in Seattle, 34 percent of seropositive women over 21 years of age shed CMV in the cervix. The frequency of colonization was positively correlated with the number of sex partners and younger age of first sexual intercourse.[39] There is no direct evidence that virus in the cervix comes from sexual intercourse or that it can be transmitted by sexual intercourse. However, these data suggest that the uterine cervix is either constantly reinfected by sexual intercourse or that cervical carriage established at an early age persists. The role of pregnancy is discussed below. Indirect evidence of transmission by heterosexual sex comes from small outbreaks of CMV mononucleosis among sex partners in a university community. In one report, two males were presumably infected by a woman who was carrying the virus in the uterine cervix.[40]

CMV may also be found in high titers in the semen of both heterosexual and homosexual males.[41] How the virus gets there and the reasons for its persistence, just as in the case of the virus in the uterine cervix, is also unknown. Possibly, semen may carry CMV for only short periods after an active infection unless repeated infection takes place or chronic infection is facilitated by early age of infection or by immunosuppression. While there are no comparable data from heterosexual males, sperm carriage in homosexual males has been shown to be a reflection of sexual activity. CMV could be isolated from asymptomatic homosexual males, most frequently from semen, in 35–42 percent of the cases irrespective of whether they were HIV-positive.[42] The presence of CMV has been correlated with younger age of the subject (≤24), passive anal sex, and large numbers of sex partners.

Most homosexual males in this country have been infected with CMV. Those who are not become rapidly infected when followed prospectively.[43] What is even more striking, however, is that past infections continue to be active. Although CMV is carried in many other body fluids (urine, saliva, and blood), the high carriage frequency in semen in the healthy homosexual and its association with passive anal intercourse and the number of partners suggests that, as in the case of HIV infection,[44] CMV may be readily transmitted by infected sperm during anal intercourse.

Cervical Infection during Pregnancy and Perinatal Transmission

CMV in the uterine cervix is not only a potential source of venereal transmission to a sexual partner but also to a neonate during passage through the birth canal. Numazaki et al.[45] first reported from Japan an increased rate of cervical infection in the later stages of pregnancy. Similar results were found by Montgomery et al.[46] and by the Alabama group.[47]

The three studies covering 987 pregnant women are summarized in Table 1. All three found an increasing prevalence of infection progressing from the first (0–2 percent) to the second (6–10 percent) and third trimesters (11–28 percent). The three groups represent different populations. The Japanese group represents a nonpromiscuous middle-class population that was 85 percent CMV-seropositive. The Alabama group was also a high prevalence group (89 percent seropositive), but it was a young sexually promiscuous group with a 10 percent rate of gonorrhea. Montgomery et al.[46] studied 125 middle-class white and black pregnant women and 71 Navaho Indians.

High cervical CMV excretion during the third trimester of pregnancy suggests that the neonate is at risk during the process of birth. Reynolds et al.[48] showed this clearly. Only 2 (4 percent) of 50 babies born of nonsecretors became infected. In contrast, 12.5 percent of babies born to mothers who secreted CMV from the cervix only during the first or second trimester became infected, and 37 percent of the babies born of third-trimester excretors became infected. The infection rate of babies whose mothers shed virus postpartum and who were presumably shedding at birth rose to 57 percent. None of the babies of urine shedders were infected. About 5 percent of all live births in the Alabama population from a low socioeconomic stratum were perinatally infected.

Perinatal infection is usually diagnosed in a neonate who does not show evidence of infection at birth but becomes viruric 4–8 weeks after birth when the virus acquired during birth has replicated. Perinatal infections are usually asymptomatic, and no late deleterious effects have been described. They may be difficult to distinguish from infections acquired during birth, particularly if the child is first seen some months after birth.

TABLE 1. Cervical CMV Infection during Pregnancy

Source	Infection in Trimester: First	Second	Third	Overall Infection
Numazaki et al.[45]	0/30[a] (0%)	6/62 (9.7%)	17/61 (27.9%)	23/153 (15.0%)
Montgomery et al.[46]	1/43 (2%)	6/83 (7.2%)	6/49 (12.2%)	13/175 (7.4%)
Stagno et al.[47]	3/183 (1.6%)[b]	22/359 (6.1%)	42/371 (11.3%)	63/659 (9.6%)
Total infected/tested	4/256	34/504	65/481	99/987
Percentage infected	1.6	6.7	13.5	10.0

[a] Represents number of positive patients per number of patients tested.
[b] Number infected per number of specimens tested.

Congenital Infections in Infants of Nonimmune Mothers. Intrauterine or congenital infection by CMV occurs in between 0.5 and 2.2 percent of all live births.[49] Although less frequent than perinatal infection, congenital or intrauterine infections are important because most serious CMV disease syndromes in the neonate may be attributed to this type of infection. The diagnosis of congenital infection is most reliably demonstrated by viruria within the first week after birth. The presence of IgM-type antibodies against CMV in the cord serum is helpful but neither completely sensitive or specific.

The majority of clinically apparent congenital infections have occurred in infants of primiparous mothers who had a primary infection during pregnancy.[1] Such infections may be diagnosed by a change in antibody titer against CMV from negative to positive or by an IgM antibody test. The radioimmune IgM assay is reportedly both *sensitive* and *specific*.[50] The risk of intrauterine infection after primary infections can only be documented in large prospective studies in which mothers are followed throughout pregnancy. A number of such studies are summarized in Table 2.

Monif et al.[51] followed 664 pregnant women whose CF titers were less than 1:8 at bimonthly intervals. Two primary infections were documented in the second trimester. They were associated with two infants with elevated IgM in their cord serum, viruria, and multiple stigmata of congenital infection. Two cases of seroconversion occurred during the third trimester. Both mothers produced infants with elevated IgM in cord serum and viruria at birth. They were otherwise healthy. In this study, there was 100 percent correlation between primary CMV infection in the mother and congenital infection in the baby.

Stern and Tucker[52] studied 1040 pregnant women in London; 56 percent of the white and 90 percent of the Asian women were seropositive. Primary infection detected by the CF test occurred in 8 (3 percent) of 254 whites and 3 (19 percent) of 16 Asian women. About 45 percent of the offspring (5 of 11) had viruria at birth. One mentally retarded child was infected during the second trimester. Nankervis et al.[53] identified a total of 8 primary infections among over 3000 pregnant women. Four infected babies were produced; all were viruric but clinically healthy. Stagno et al.[54] followed 3712 pregnant women from both upper and lower socioeconomic strata from Alabama. Of 21 primary infections among 1382 seronegative mothers, there were 11 congenital infections, of whom 3 were symptomatic. These reports indicate that intrauterine infection after primary CMV infection is high (24 of 44, 55 percent). The rate of primary infection did not vary significantly with the socioeconomic status or immune status of the population. In these series, it was 0.52 percent. The rate of intrauterine CMV infection (24 in 8416 pregnancies) resulting from primary infections was 0.3 percent, of whom 25 percent (6 of 44) were symptomatic. It appears that primary infection at any stage of pregnancy presents a risk, but Stagno and Whitley[55] believe that infection during the first half of pregnancy produces more disease.

Congenital Infection of Infants of Immune Mothers. Stagno et al.[54] also reported 20 (0.5 percent) babies with congenital infections from 2330 mothers who were immune or seropositive. This type of congenital infection occurred more frequently in mothers of the lower socioeconomic group, who had a high prevalence of past infection. However, none of the 20 babies was symptomatic, although other workers have found that symptomatic congenital infection may occasionally result from infection in an immune mother.[56] There are also scattered reports of congenital disease in consecutive pregnancies, but as expected, these too are rare.[1] There seems no doubt, however, that immunity in the mother protects the baby from the disease.

Summarizing the above, it appears that several natural mechanisms exist in a population of immune mothers that facilitate CMV infections in the newborn, most or all of which are asymptomatic in nature and may be considered a form of natural live

TABLE 2. Risk of Congenital CMV Infection after Primary Infection of Mothers during Pregnancy

			Primary Infection in Mothers		*Congenital Infection in Babies*		*Symptomatic Babies*	
Authors	*Number Pregnancies*	*Trimester*	*Number*	*Percentage*[a]	*Number*	*Percentage*[b]	*Number*	*Percentage*[c]
Monif et al.[51]	664	1st	0	0	0		0	
		2nd	2	0.3	2	100	2	100
		3rd	2	0.3	2	100	0	0
Stern and Tucker[52]	1040	1st	2	0.19	2	100	0	100
		2nd	4	0.38	2	50	1	50
		3rd	5	0.48	1	20	0	0
Nankervis et al[53]	3000	1st	1	0.03	0	0	0	
		2nd	4	0.13	1	25	0	0
		3rd	3	0.1	3	100	0	0
Stagno et al.[54]	3712	All	21	0.57	11	52	3	27
Total	8416		44	0.52	24	55	6	25

[a] Percentage of primary infection in the total number of pregnancies.
[b] Percentage of congenital infections in offspring after primary infection in mothers.
[c] Percentage of congenital infections in offspring who showed stigmata of disease.

immunization. A small number of these infections arise transplacentally, and significant numbers are perinatal infections from CMV carried in the cervix during the later stages of pregnancy and perinatal infection from CMV in breast milk. The baby is protected from hazards of this ''live immunization'' by antibodies passively transferred from the mother and is rarely symptomatic. The noenate who gets CMV disease is one whose mother is not immune. Such infants are at particular risk if their mothers get a primary infection during pregnancy.

Cytomegalovirus Infection in the Immunosuppressed (Transplant Group)

It is remarkable that after organ transplantation most if not all patients develop CMV infection. This has been shown in all types of major transplantations such as renal, liver, heart, heart–lung, and bone marrow transplants (see also Chapters 290, 291, 292). For example, in 15 studies of 1145 patients the rate of infections after renal transplants as determined by serologic rise or isolation of the virus from the blood, urine, or throat varies from 52 to 100 percent with a mean of 71 percent.[1] The infection rate was significantly higher in those who were seropositive before organ transplantation (85 percent) and lower in seronegative recipients (53 percent).

For the development of primary infection, exposure to a source of virus is necessary. Theoretically, the virus may come from a contaminated environment such as intensive care units or dialysis centers or from infected contacts. In fact, the most important sources are transplanted tissues or organs and, to a lesser degree, transfused blood. In contrast, secondary infection may occur in anyone who is seropositive and latently infected.

Donated Organ or Tissue as a Source of Infection. As in the case of blood, attempts to isolate CMV from organs have failed; still, CMV may be transmitted by any major transplant. There are two types of evidence for this. The first type is epidemiologic. In the case of kidney transplantations, Ho et al.[57] and Betts et al.[58] noted that primary infections developed in 83 percent of seronegative recipients who received kidneys from seropositive donors, while very few of those who received kidneys from seronegative donors became infected. Besides incriminating the donated organ as the vehicle of infection, such data suggest that primary infection may be largely prevented if one uses organs from seronegative donors. This type of evidence is also available for heart, bone marrow, and liver transplantation (for details, see Chapters 291 and 292).

Role of Immunosuppressive Drugs. The most important factor accounting for reactivations of CMV infections is the iatrogenic immunosuppression essential for maintenance of the graft.[59] Cytotoxic drugs such as cyclophosphamide or azathioprine alone can reactivate a latent CMV infection but do not produce disease.[60] Corticosteroids play a subsidiary role. They continue to be used with all types of immunosuppressive regimes in moderate doses. It has been pointed out that CMV disease has decreased when compared with the time when corticosteroids were used in much higher doses as an adjunct to azathioprine.[61] Corticosteroids alone, which were used before the introduction of cytotoxic drugs, were insufficient to enhance CMV infection.

The addition of anti-lymphocyte serum to a combination of azathioprine and prednisone has reportedly been shown to increase the morbidity due to CMV infection.

Since 1981 cyclosporine has gradually supplanted azathioprine as the primary immunosuppressive agent. Its superiority has made possible a marked increase in the number and types of transplant operations. A controlled study in which renal transplant patients received either azathioprine and prednisone or cyclosporine and prednisone showed that infection and morbidity from CMV was comparable in both groups.[62] We also showed that, besides immunosuppression, the type of transplantations was also important in determining CMV morbidity. Liver, heart, and heart–lung transplant recipients had more morbidity due to CMV than did kidney recipients.[63,64]

Immunosuppression may be complicated in the future by the introduction of new agents or the use of multiple agents in an attempt to reduce the toxicity of cyclosporine due to excess or prolonged use. Each novel regimen will have to be evaluated for its effect on CMV infection. This includes the anti-lymphocyte serums and azathioprine. Polyclonal and monoclonal anti-lymphocyte serums have also been used for the treatment of rejections in addition to classic steroids. We showed, for example, that the OKT3 antiserum used to treat rejection in liver transplant patients increased the frequency of severe CMV diseases such as hepatitis and dissemination.[65]

Usually, immunosuppression does not inhibit the development of CMV antibodies. Rarely, in very severe infections, antibody production is inhibited.[66]

Effect of Allograft Reactions. Two types of allograft reactions may occur after organ transplantation, the host-vs.-graft (HvG) reaction and the graft-vs.-host (GvH) reaction. Depending on genetic compatibility and the transplant involved, one or both reactions may occur. Both reactions have been shown in experimental animals to affect virus infections. After C3H mice chronically infected with murine CMV received skin allografts from histoincompatible BALB/c donors, which produced an HvG reaction, CMV titers were increased in the spleen and kidneys.[67] Mouse CMV infection was also enhanced in the same model of infection under stimulation of a GvH reaction brought on by the administration of multiple doses of parental splenocytes to F_1(DBA/2 × C3H/he) recipients.[68]

One sees the most severe and lethal form of CMV disease, interstitial pneumonia, after bone marrow transplantation. Meyers et al.[69] showed that after patients who had leukemia or aplastic anemias were given *bone marrow transplants* those undergoing a GvH reaction were associated with CMV infection. GvH disease was significantly more common among patients with (82 percent) than among those without (27 percent) CMV interstitial pneumonia. Of patients with GvH disease 66 percent (27 of 41) developed interstitial pneumonia as compared with only 14 percent (6 of 44) of patients without GvH disease. Thus GvH reaction, of which a target organ may be the lung, is an important cofactor for CMV disease. The precise immunopathologic reaction underlying CMV interstitial pneumonia in marrow transplant recipients is still unknown, but its existence is underscored by the failure of antiviral therapy in this condition.[69a]

The evidence that an HvG reaction enhances CMV infection in humans is less clear-cut. CMV pneumonia is more common after heart–lung transplantation than after heart or renal transplantation.[64] Severe CMV hepatitis is a special problem after liver transplantation.[70] In both cases, the target organ of CMV disease is a cadaver allograft in which tissue mismatching is common and varying degrees of allograft reactions are expected to be present (see Chapter 292).

Cytomegalovirus Infection in the Immunosuppressed (Malignancies)

The frequency and morbidity of CMV infection in patients with malignancies is not as high as after major organ transplantation. Even patients with immunosuppressive malignancies (such as Hodgkin's lymphoma) or who are receiving immunosuppressive chemotherapy are not sufficiently immunosuppressed for a long enough period to get in trouble from a reactivation infection. Also, the primary complication of chemotherapy, neutropenia, does not appear to be a major risk factor for CMV infection. Finally, unless transfused many times, the patient with cancer does not have a ready outside source of virus for a primary infection.

That patients with malignancies may be infected by CMV may be documented in many ways. In early studies, evidence of increased infection was found in postmortem studies; by cultures of urine, throat, or blood; or by serologic studies. Before 1965, CMV disease in adults was primarily described in patients with chronic debilitating diseases, especially hematologic malignancies.[71] Since then, with the advent of chemotherapy, particularly in leukemias, CMV infections have been more frequently described. For example, Bodey et al.[72] report from the National Cancer Institute that, before 1962, 3 percent of autopsies on patients with acute leukemias showed CMV disease but, in 1962–1963, 15 percent of such patients were similarly afflicted. Some reports indicate higher CMV infection in leukemic children as measured by virurias.[1]

The significance of this is difficult to evaluate in children without controls. Henson et al.[73] followed 88 leukemic children of a mean age of 7.3 years for a mean period of 8.2 months. Evidence of infection over this time period was seen in 24 patients (27 percent) as measured by repeated urine and throat cultures. No serologic rise was observed in 16 of the virus excretors. Some had disseminated disease, and they had serologic rises. Infected patients had more pneumonitis and fever than did uninfected patients. Other findings coincident with a serologic rise were parotitis, prostatitis, upper respiratory infection, and hepatitis. Thus, in an individual patient, it is difficult to determine the etiologic role of CMV for such manifestations. Frequently infection occurred without clinical manifestations. More epidemiologic and clinical follow-up studies are needed in adults and in patients with other types of malignancies.

Cytomegalovirus Infection in the Immunosuppressed (AIDS and HIV Infection)

There is an intimate relationship between CMV and HIV infection. With progressive immunosuppression as a result of HIV infection, CMV activity increases. As stated above, 30–40 percent of homosexuals actively shed CMV in semen or urine irrespective of whether they are HIV-positive.[42] Of those infected, 95 percent have at one time or another elevated IgM titers against CMV, which suggests active infection. Such infection probably represents both activation of latent infections by one or more endogenous strains as well as superinfection by additional strains from repeated exposure.[74] Viremia usually remains absent in asymptomatic HIV-infected individuals,[75] while in progressive AIDS-related complex (ARC) patients and all patients with AIDS (Kaposi's sarcoma and/or opportunistic infections) viremia was present. As in the case of transplant recipients,[63] viremia is usually present in symptomatic CMV disease.

Since active CMV infection is present in most advanced HIV infections irrespective of whether CMV produces any symptoms, laboratory diagnosis of significant infection or disease is difficult. Serology is not helpful since primary infections are unusual and many have persistent IgM antibodies. Culturing the virus in urine, throat, semen, or even blood may not help. A sine qua non for the attribution of a clinical syndrome to CMV is the demonstration of local pathology characteristic of CMV infection or isolation or demonstration of the virus or viral activity at a local site. Even so, if CMV is present with other microbial agents such as *Pneumocystis carinii, Mycobacterium avium-intracellulare*, or HIV, which may be the actual cause of local pathology, the pathogenic role of the CMV may not be ascertained.

CLINICAL MANIFESTATIONS

Disease in Children

As already pointed out, symptoms occur in less than a quarter of the congenitally infected. The classic fulminant congenital cytomegalic inclusion disease (CID) is characterized by jaundice, hepatosplenomegaly, a petechial rash, and multiple system and organ involvement.[1] Microcephaly, motor disability, chorioretinitis, and cerebral calcifications are also seen.[76] The involvement of the central nervous system, the inner ear, and the choroid of the eye appears to be unique for congenital infection.

Clinically, immediately at birth or shortly thereafter, there is an onset of lethargy, respiratory distress, and convulsive seizures. The patient may die at any time from a few days to a few weeks. Most of the patients described in the earlier literature expired shortly after birth. Infants were later found to survive. Hemorrhagic phenomena, jaundice, and hepatosplenomegaly may subside after a variable period. However neurologic sequelae such as microcephaly, mental retardation, and motor disability may become apparent only later and are also the least likely to clear.

A large number of extraneural organ defects have also been associated with congenital infection. It should be noted, however, that most of the disease manifestations in congenital infection are associated with direct and active inflammation secondary to virus invasion or possibly immunologic reactions. Indirect interference with organ development, well documented in the case of rubella, is not evident in most cases of CMV infection.

The picture of postnatally acquired CMV disease is different from CID. Diffuse visceral or central nervous system involvement is rarely observed. When clinical manifestations are apparent, they may resemble some aspect of CMV mononucleosis. Mononucleosis itself may be absent, although it may occur, even in very young children.[9] Serious disease, however, can result from exchange transfusions.[36] Outbreaks of CMV infection have been described in neonatal intensive care units, where the seronegative, poorly developed infant may be at particular risk.[28]

Infants may also demonstrate prolonged respiratory disease such as pharyngitis, bronchitis, pneumonia, and croup. The association of CMV with pertussus is evident from the older literature. Olson and associates[30] noted that children with respiratory infection more frequently carried CMV in the upper respiratory tract. It is difficult to distinguish the precise etiologic role of CMV in such cases.

Subtle Sequelae of Neonatal Infections

Both perinatal and intrauterine CMV infections may be completely asymptomatic. So far no immediate or long-term abnormalities have been described in perinatally infected children. However, they may not have been followed long enough in sufficient numbers to rule out development of subtle abnormalities. In contrast, there is ample documentation of subtle sequelae after inapparent intrauterine infections.

In 8644 neonates from a higher socioeconomic class Hanshaw et al.[77] identified 53 with IgM antibodies against CMV in cord blood (1 in 163, 0.6 percent). One was stillborn, and one had clinical disease and died at 48 hours. Forty-four were evaluated at 3.5–7.0 years of age. The mean IQ of the group was 103, which was lower than matched controls. The predicted school failure rate, based on IQ and behavioral, neurologic, and auditory data, was 2.7 times that of controls matched for socioeconomic status. Five of forty (13 percent) had severe bilateral hearing loss, and three had profound deafness. This would go far to explain the estimated 1 in 1000 incidence of unexplained profound deafness in children. A more recent prospective controlled study showed that in the absence of hearing loss a lower IQ is not a late sequela of congenital infection.[78]

Stagno et al.[79] reported from Alabama on the incidence of sensorineural hearing loss in neonatal CMV infection in three types of neonatal CMV infection. There were 59 patients with congenital or intrauterine infection, 8 of whom were symptomatic at birth. Twenty-one had perinatal CMV infection, none of whom developed hearing loss. Late-onset hearing loss developed in 17 percent of all congenital and 14 percent of all subclinical congenital CMV infections. Pathologic studies in two patients showed virus in cells of the organ of Corti and in neurons of the spiral ganglia. Rare cells with typical intranuclear inclusions were seen in the cochlea. A third patient studied at postmortem examination had disseminated symptomatic disease but no evidence of viral infection in the inner ear.

The insidious nature of this problem was that (*1*) hearing loss could not be predicted by the severity of infection or the height of IgM levels at birth; (*2*) it may be progressive, and estimates so far may be minimal; and (*3*) the subtlety of the defect makes evaluation of preventive measures such as the use of vaccines difficult. Possibly an immune mechanism underlies its pathogenesis.

In contrast, eye pathology corresponds roughly to the severity of infection. It was found in 8 of 43 patients with congenital CMV infection. Five of the eight patients (63 percent) who were symptomatically infected had lesions. None with perinatal infections had pathologic eye changes.

Cytomegalovirus-Induced Mononucleosis and Disease Manifestations in Normal Adults

CMV-induced mononucleosis is clinically difficult to distinguish from infectious or EBV-induced mononucleosis. Fever is usually a dominant problem. There is relative and absolute lymphocytosis with abundant atypical lymphocytes. These may appear relatively late in the course of the disease, at times 1–2 weeks after the onset of fever. Relative well-being and paucity of findings are characteristic. CMV mononucleosis should be suspected in any case of mononucleosis in which the heterophile–agglutinin test is negative and in patients with fever of unknown origin. The prognosis is usually excellent.

Like EBV-induced mononucleosis, CMV mononucleosis may occur sporadically without any traceable source. The most important identifiable source is blood. In older children and adults, the probability of being infected by a unit of blood is around 3 percent or less.[34,35] Hence a large number of units transfused may present a proportionately greater risk. CMV is a cause of postoperative pyrexia. It should be considered along with other causes of postoperative sepsis, especially when large amounts of blood have been transfused.

Sexual or intimate contact with an infected person is undoubtedly important in the transmission of the virus. A history of such contact, however, is rarely obtained in an individual case.

The clinical features of this disease are described in a 8-year prospective study of 494 cases of mononucleosis by the Finnish group.[80] Most (79 percent) had positive heterophile–agglutinins and had EBV infection. Among 73 patients over 15 years of age with a negative response, 33 (45 percent) had CMV infection. When the first serum was taken 3–20 days after the onset of disease, 11 of 19 such patients were seronegative ($\leq$1:4) and developed a rise in CF antibodies. Peak titers were reached 4–7 weeks after the onset. Viruria was present in 10 of 12 tested. From this it appears that CMV mononucleosis usually represents primary infections in previously seronegative persons.

The age range was 18–66, the median age being 29, which is higher than is the susceptible age for EBV-induced mononucleosis. All patients were febrile, with fever lasting from 9 to 35 days with a mean of 19 days. Lymphocytosis varied from 55 to 86 percent, with 12–55 percent of the total leukocytes being atypical lymphocytes. Tonsillitis or pharyngitis is rare.

Enlargement of lymph nodes and the spleen is usually not striking but may occur. Mild elevations of liver function test results are a regular feature and an important aid to diagnosis. However, severe hepatitis or jaundice is unusual although chemical hepatitis is common.

In both CMV- and EBV-induced mononucleosis, there may be laboratory evidence of transient immunologic aberrations. For example, the appearance of mixed cryoglobulins, cold agglutinins, rheumatoid factor, and antinuclear and anticomplementary activity has been described.[80]

Most sporadic symptomatic cases represent primary infection in healthy subjects. However, secondary or reactivation infections may cause mononucleosis in the immunosuppressed, although it has been noted that atypical lymphocytosis per se is less apparent in such patients.

A number of complications or associated findings may occur more or less uncommonly with CMV infections, occasionally as the presenting syndrome, even in immunocompetent subjects.

Interstitial pneumonitis, a hallmark of CMV disease in the transplant patient may occur in CMV-induced mononucleosis. In the Finnish series, it was found in 2 of 33 patients.[81] These are primarily radiographic findings that eventually clear. This is in striking contrast to the life-threatening pneumonitis one sees in the immunosuppressed (see below). They may be different pathogenetically.

Hepatitis may be an initial asymptomatic sign of CMV infection. Symptomatic hepatitis occurs only rarely in immunocompetent subjects. Carter[82] described a 21-year-old immunocompetent man suspected of infectious hepatitis who had an enlarged and tender liver. Atypical lymphocytes were not seen. CMV was isolated from the urine, and there was a rise in CF antibodies.

Granulomatous hepatitis may also occasionally occur in healthy adults as an initial problem or accompanying mononucleosis.[83] There may be malaise, nausea, vomiting, and up to 50 percent atypical lymphocytes in the peripheral blood smear. CMV may be isolated from the throat, and there is an appropriate serologic rise. A percutaneous liver biopsy specimen shows resolving hepatitis, mononuclear infiltrates in portal areas, and scattered microscopic granulomas with giant cells. The patient usually recovers completely. These are important cases because one does not usually think of CMV when granulomas are found in the liver.

The *Guillain-Barré* syndrome is now a well-recognized and not uncommon complication of CMV-induced mononucleosis. Leonard and Tobin[84] described 9 patients with polyneuritis characterized by sensory and motor weakness in the extremities. Cranial nerve involvement was common, and 4 patients had to be treated in the respiratory unit. Sensation recovered before motor impairment, and complete recovery took about 3 months. There is no indication that immunosuppressed patients are more prone to this complication.

Schmitz and Enders[85] detected 10 cases of CMV infection in a series of 94 cases of Guillain-Barré syndrome (about 10 percent). They point out that the CF antibody titer is frequently already elevated by the time the patient is first seen within 1 week after onset and that no further diagnostic rise is observed. On the other hand, the IgM immunofluorescent antibody titer was high in 9 of 10 patients in the initial specimen, and all 10 showed a diagnostic decline at discharge. Six patients had to be cared for in the respiratory unit, but all recovered. The spinal fluids showed typically elevated protein levels and few cells. All patients had atypical lymphocytes.

Meningoencephalitis has been described in some cases of CMV infection in the immunocompetent.[86] It is usually associated with CMV-induced mononucleosis. These patients may have sensory and motor weaknesses that may be difficult to distinguish from polyradiculopathy. However, there may be severe headaches, photophobia, and pyramidal tract signs, and the spinal fluid may show mild mononuclear pleocytosis. It is not known whether this picture of "aseptic" meningoencephalitis is directly due to viral invasion or due to an allergic reaction.

Myocarditis has been described as a complication of CMV-induced mononucleosis. Tiula and Leinikki[87] reported that, in three of eight cases of mononucleosis, inversion of T waves was found in several leads by ECG examination. They described a 14-year-old boy with serologic evidence of CMV infection who died with evidence of hepatitis, myocarditis, and consumptive coagulopathy. Virus was found in the lungs at autopsy. Waris et al.[88] described a 43-year-old previously healthy woman who developed myocarditis, heart failure, encephalitis, hepatitis, and adrenal insufficiency. Evidence of CMV was found in the adrenals at autopsy. In general, myocardial involvement is rare in congenital CMV disease.

Thrombocytopenia and *hemolytic anemia* are well recognized in congenital CMV disease. They may also occur as a complication of CMV-induced mononucleosis in adults. Chanarin and Walford[89] described a 33-year-old man with CMV-induced mononucleosis who had generalized purpura and bleeding gums. His platelet count was 500/mm^3; hemoglobin, 3.6 g/dl; and reticulocyte count, 1.2 percent. There was serologic evidence of CMV infection and viruria. The patient recovered after treatment with prednisone.

Harris et al.[90] described a 26-year-old man with CMV infection who in addition to thrombocytopenia and purpura had red cells whose life span was decreased and an elevated reticulocyte count.

Petechial rashes may be observed in congenital CMV diseases. Rubelliform or maculopacular rashes may occur in CMV-induced mononucleosis with or without the administration of ampicillin.[91] Vesicular lesions are distinctly unusual in congenital or acquired CMV infection. Muller-Stamou et al.[92] described an unusual case of a 40-year-old man who developed generalized epidermolysis 8 weeks after the onset of hepatitis. He had viruria and viremia.

Clinical Aspects of Cytomegalovirus Infection in the Immunosuppressed

CMV infection is frequently asymptomatic, even in the immunosuppressed, but it may also produce protean clinical manifestations. A febrile mononucleosis indistinguishable from the disease in the nonsuppressed appears to be the most common clinical presentation. But in other immunosuppressed patients more extensive organ involvement, rarely seen in the healthy subjects, may be evident. Knowledge of the diverse pathologic spectrum due to CMV in adults has significantly increased since the discovery of AIDS. CMV can cause pneumonitis, hepatitis, gastrointestinal ulcerations, retinitis, encephalopathy, and endocrine disturbances. These are described below. Very often the precise role of CMV and other competing pathogens is difficult to ascertain. There is clear indication in AIDS that the degree of morbidity and its extensiveness is determined by the degree of suppression of CD4 lymphocytes.

In the *transplant recipient*, two factors determine the degree of morbidity due to CMV. The first is the degree and type of immunosuppression. Deaths due to CMV infection may be related to the use of anti-thymocyte globulin.[93] The second is the type of organ transplantation. Morbidity due to CMV is lowest in kidney transplantation and highest in bone marrow transplantation (see Chapters 291 and 292).

Suwansirikul et al.[94] and Betts et al.[95] reported the clinical and laboratory findings on a total of 154 renal transplant patients with CMV infection. Primary infections were significantly more symptomatic, but only 19 percent of the secondary infections were febrile. In the series of Suwansirikul et al.,[94] 13 of 18 primary infections were associated with at least two of the following: fever, leukopenia, atypical lymphocytes, lymphocytosis, hepatosplenomegaly, myalgia, or arthralgia.

Betts et al.[95] found elevations of hepatic enzyme (SGOT) levels in 10 of 16 (63 percent) primary infections. Five had pneumonia. A striking feature of their series was that primary infections occurred mainly in younger recipients who received parental kidneys. They also found that rejection occurred in 4 of 16 patients with primary infection. Twenty-four seronegative patients who received kidneys from seronegative donors and remained uninfected did not reject them. This is one of the few studies that shows clearly that CMV infection may increase rejection.

An important indirect effect of primary CMV infection is an increase in both serious fungal and bacterial infections after renal and cardiac transplantation.[96] This is the clinical significance of the known nonspecific immunosuppressive effect of CMV infection.[97]

Interstitial Pneumonia. Next to fever and mononucleosis, the most common manifestation of CMV infection in the compromised host is pneumonitis. It has been described in the immunocompetent host but is more common in the immunosuppressed.[1] The pneumonitis is more likely to show an interstitial rather than alveolar pattern, but nodules or cavities may be seen on x-ray films. Association with pneumocystis may be striking. This is particularly true in the case of AIDS. CMV pneumonia may range from asymptomatic virus shedding to rapidly fatal pneumonia. Respiratory complaints were present usually less than 2 weeks. Consistently, fever, nonproductive cough, and dyspnea associated with hypoxia were observed. Hypoxia is a poor prognostic sign. Most who required respiratory assistance expired. The severity and lethality of CMV pneumonia probably varies in different types of patients and varying degrees of immunosuppression. This has been best studied in interstitial pneumonia after bone marrow transplantation and where the lung may be a target for a GvH reaction. Eighty-four percent died.[98] In a much smaller series of renal transplant patients, 48 percent died.[99]

Hepatitis. CMV infection in its mildest symptomatic form is usually associated with chemical hepatitis and elevation of serum hepatic enzyme levels. Jaundice and hyperbilirubinemia are distinctly unusual. We have rarely seen clinically significant CMV hepatitis in patients after renal transplantation. However, this has been described in other centers, perhaps as a complication of more severe immunosuppression from using anti-lymphocyte globulin. Aldrete et al.[100] reported gastrointestinal and hepatic complications affecting 126 patients after renal transplantation. Hepatic dysfunction occurred in 22 percent of the patients. Severe hepatitis was seen in seven, from all of whom CMV was isolated in the blood, urine, sputum, or feces. Autopsies on five of these patients revealed evidence of CMV in the liver.

However, even in centers where it is not seen in renal and other types of transplantations, CMV hepatitis has become an important general problem after liver transplantation in both adults and children.[70,101] Like most other severe CMV diseases in transplant recipients, it is more common after primary infection. It is also associated with grafting a liver from a CMV-seropositive donor.[65] Recognition of this is partly due to the frequent practice of protocol liver biopsy to manage rejection in the first months after transplantation. However, it is not just a matter of recognition because all cases had clinical hepatitis characterized by prolonged fever, bilirubinemia, and elevated enzyme concentrations. Liver failure due to CMV hepatitis requiring retransplantation has also been seen. The most important management problem is to distinguish between rejection and CMV hepatitis. This differential diagnosis can only be made by a study of the biopsy specimen.[101] It is important to make this differential diagnosis because rejection is treated by increasing immunosuppression while CMV infection may be helped by decreasing immunosuppression and instituting antiviral therapy.

Cytomegalovirus Disease of the Gastrointestinal Tract. The etiologic role of CMV is frequently difficult to evaluate because CMV may be a fellow-traveling "opportunist." This is particularly true of CMV in the gastrointestinal tract. CMV has, for example, been suspected to play a role in acute idiopathic ulcerative colitis[102] and in gastric ulcers occurring in a patient with CMV mononucleosis.[103] The evidence for a causal relationship is often weak.

In contrast to the above and despite the difficult of diagnosis, there is little doubt now that CMV may cause important and at times lethal gastrointestinal syndromes in the immunosuppressed. Transplant patients may develop gastrointestinal hemorrhages or perforation that may be traced to submucosal ulcerations anywhere in the gastrointestinal tract from the esophagus to the rectum.[1,99] Patients with AIDS and CMV colitis may present with explosive watery diarrhea. Occasionally there may also be hematochezia. Fever is common, and other intestinal pathogens such as cryptosporidia or *Mycobacterium avium-intracellulare* may be present at the same time. By endoscopy, there may be plaquelike pseudomembranes, multiple erosions and serpigenous ulcers,[104] or lesions resembling Kaposi's sarcoma.[105] Perforation and gangrene has been described, although CMV may not be the sole cause. CMV may be demonstrated by a culture of specimens or biopsy material, or there may be typical inclusion bodies in the submucosal endothelium[105] or mucosal crypts.[104]

Besides the gastrointestinal tract itself, CMV is known to involve both the acinar and islet components of the pancreas,[1] and it can be seen in acute pancreatitis in an AIDS patient.[106] Cholecystitis has been associated with finding CMV in the bile duct, the gall bladder, and the biliary tree.[106,107]

Cytomogalovirus Retinitis. Chorioretinitis is a well-recognized finding in congenital CMV infections. It is usually not acquired postnatally in children, and it is quite rare in immunocompetent subjects. Foerster[108] described CMV retinitis in an enucleated eye of a 59-year-old woman with no apparent underlying disease or immunosuppression. CMV retinitis is usually a manifestation of severe immunosuppression. It is seen in transplant patients, in cancer patients receiving immunosuppressive drugs,[109] and particularly in patients with AIDS.[110] In the transplant recipient, unlike the acute infection that usually occurs regularly 2–6 months after organ transplantation, CMV retinitis may occur at any time. It is in AIDS that we see the full scope of the devastating effects of CMV retinitis.

Nonspecific complaints of blurred vision, scotoma, and decreased visual activity are the most frequent ophthalmologic symptoms. Visual impairment is usually progressive and irreversible, particularly with central retinal involvement. Blindness in one or both eyes is the expected result. The disease, however, may also be asymptomatic or discovered only at autopsy.

CMV retinitis has a characteristic funduscopic and pathologic appearance (Fig. 1). Initially, white granular necrotic patches develop that may be superimposed with patches of flame-shaped intraretinal hemorrhages. Pathologic examination shows extensive necrosis and disruption of all layers of the sensory retina and pigment epithelium. Wyhinny et al.[111] pointed out that in adult CMV retinitis the lesions are restricted by Bruch's membrane and do not extend to the choroid.

Retinitis is often a sign of active systemic infection, frequently of disseminated nature. The diagnosis may be made on the basis of the distinctive ophthalmologic picture and laboratory evidence of CMV systemic infection. The virus has been cultured from the aqueous or vitreous humor,[112] although this is not essential for the diagnosis.

Meningoencephalitis and Encephalopathy. The most devastating component of congenital CID is its destructive effect

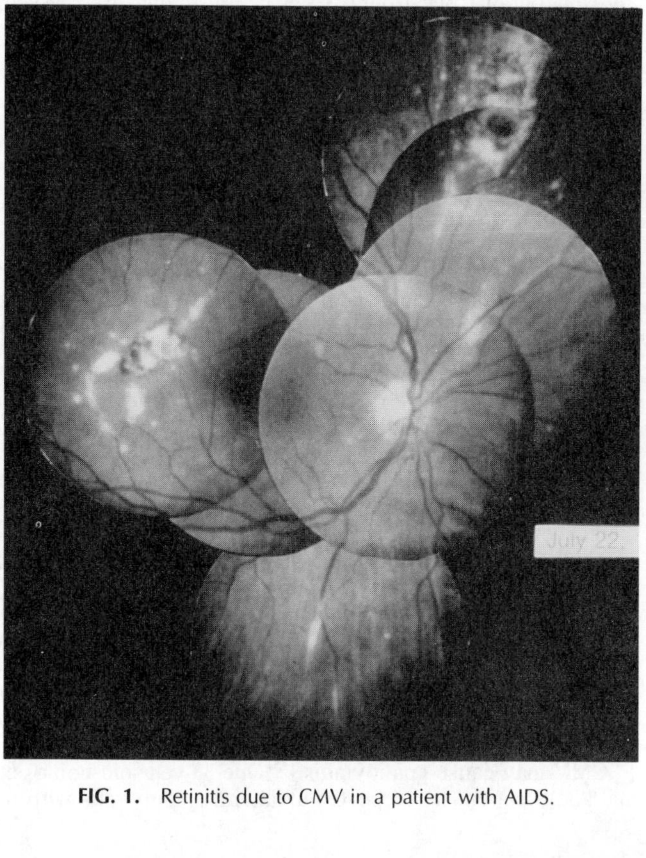

FIG. 1. Retinitis due to CMV in a patient with AIDS.

on the central nervous system. The severely brain-damaged infant may have periventricular calcifications, microcephaly, seizures, and spastic quadriplegia. About half of symptomatic congenital infections have some degree of central nervous system disease.[1] Asymptomatic ones may suffer late neurologic sequelae, the most important being neurosensory deafness (see above).

However, in postnatal life, the affinity of CMV for the central nervous system is much reduced, even in the immunosuppressed. When it has been found, its pathogenetic role is not always clear-cut. Rare cases of meningoencephalitis in immunocompetent individuals have been described. In two cases described by Phillips et al.,[113] the virus was isolated from a brain biopsy specimen and cerebrospinal fluid (CSF) as well as from urine. Both had headaches and minor CSF pleocytosis. Microglial and astrocyte proliferation with satellitosis of neurons and focal neuronal degeneration was found. Both patients recovered. Occasional cases of CMV encephalopathy have also been described in immunosuppressed transplant patients. The characteristic lesion is also microglial nodules, at times associated with cells that rarely have intranuclear inclusions.[114] However, it is in HIV infection and in AIDS that CMV has presented many neurologic complications, many of which remain to be clarified.

About 40 percent of patients with AIDS develop neurologic signs and symptoms. At postmortem examination, even more (78 percent) have pathologic changes in the central nervous system.[115–117] However, very likely the most common clinical central nervous system syndrome is due to HIV itself and is now subsumed under the term *AIDS dementia complex*.[117,118] This complex includes much of the pathology earlier ascribed to CMV such as the "subacute encephalitis" described by some authors.[115] The role of CMV in AIDS dementia complex is probably secondary.[118] The complex is associated with confusion, progressive dementia, and often, weakness and paresis. It is, however, possible that some cases are due to CMV, although when both HIV and CMV are present in the same lesion, it will be difficult to sort them out.

Other pathologic processes attributed to CMV and supported by isolation of CMV from CSF or neural tissues are CMV-induced demyelinating lesions associated with microglial nodules and lymphocyte infiltration in the brain[119] or spinal cord.[120] Clinically these cases would be difficult to distinguish from the HIV dementia and encephalitis complex, except for patients with radiculomyelitis, ascending myelitis, and necrotizing spinal lesions,[116] which may be more uniquely attributed to CMV.

Endocrinopathies and Glandular Involvement. The involvement of various endocrine organs as a part of disseminated CMV infection is well known, but clinical endocrinopathies were rare until the advent of AIDS. Diabetes mellitus may occur after congenital infection[121] and perhaps secondary to pancreatitis in an adult.[122] A case of acute CMV pancreatitis with histologic proof was described in a transplant patient.[123] A case of adrenal insufficiency in a healthy subject without pathologic proof is mentioned above.[88] Adrenalitis due to CMV is a common finding in AIDS patients. Of 41 autopsy cases, 21 showed cortical as well as medullary lesions.[124] However, no definite clinical evidence of adrenal cortical insufficiency was available even though hypotension and hyponatremia were common findings.

We have seen an AIDS patient who had CMV in his blood and CSF, who had CMV retinitis, and who developed adrenal insufficiency proven by a lack of adrenocorticotropic hormone (ACTH) stimulation. He also had diabetes insipidus controlled with vasopressin. I am not aware of any report of pathologic evidence of involvement of the posterior pituitary gland.

CMV may cause epididymitis.[125] One 33-year-old homosexual AIDS patient had repeated unilateral epididymitis with fevers that was resistant to antibiotics and treated with epididymectomy. Intracytoplasmic inclusions were seen in ductal epithelial cells.

Other related involvement by CMV in immunosuppressed adults includes a number of pathologic findings without clear clinical involvement: CMV oophoritis[126,127] and infection of the thyroid.[128] Two AIDS patients were described to have hypercalcemia, suppressed parathyroid activity, and disseminated CMV.[129]

TREATMENT AND PREVENTION OF CYTOMEGALOVIRUS INFECTIONS

Treatment

Specific treatment of systemic virus diseases until recently has been largely experimental. Putative antivirals were frequently not effective enough or too toxic. With the development of a series of promising nucleosides, specific therapy for infection with the herpesviruses is now an achievable goal. Unfortunately, CMV seems to be an unusually recalcitrant member of this group of viruses and is much more difficult to treat than is herpes simplex or varicella-zoster virus.

The treatment of a chronic viral infection in the immunosuppressed presents special problems. As in bacterial infections where the efficacy of certain antibiotics may be depressed because of the lack of critical host defenses essential for optimum effect of the drug, antivirals may have diminished effectiveness or may only be virus suppressive as long as they are administered. When they are removed, the infection reappears. Concurrent infections from other causes may complicate the picture. Compromised renal or other organ function may alter pharmacodynamics. The frequent bone marrow-suppressive or immunosuppressive properties of an antiviral agent itself may also complicate already considerable toxicity.

Interferon, a natural cytokine previously made in human leukocytes but now available as a recombinant product, can suppress CMV but is of questionable clinical usefulness. Hirsch et al.[130] reported that 3×10^6 units of α-interferon administered two to three times per week for 14 weeks after renal transplantation did not reduce infectivity, but morbidity among the infected was 5 percent (1/20) in the treated group while it was 32 percent (7/22) in the controls. This is a marginal benefit. α-Interferon was not effective for prophylaxis against CMV in bone marrow recipients.[131] It was also without therapeutic effect either alone or with other antivirals in the treatment of CMV pneumonia after bone marrow transplantation.[132]

Neither adenine-arabinoside (ara-A, vidarabine), or acyclovir, two FDA-approved nucleoside antivirals effective against herpes simplex and varicella-zoster viruses, can cure CMV infections.[133] However, high dose acyclovir (1500 mg/m^2 per day) was recently reported to reduce prophylactically CMV infections and disease in marrow recipients.[133a]

Ganciclovir. Ganciclovir is 10–100 times more effective than is acyclovir against herpes simplex and CMV infections.[134] Clinical trials in patients with CMV retinitis are encouraging. For example, one study involved 8 patients where 14 of 16 eyes showed active retinitis. When given 5 mg/kg intravenously two to three times a day for 3 weeks, 8 of 14 eyes with retinitis showed better than 90 percent resolution.[135,136] Blood and urine cultures for CMV became negative 1–4 weeks after the onset of therapy. However, all patients relapsed clinically and virologically 2–5 weeks after the cessation of therapy.

The response of other types of serious CMV disease was varied. If treatment was started early and if the patient survived long enough to benefit from treatment, efficacy was observed. For example, 30 of 40 patients with CMV gastrointestinal infection improved clinically, and a virologic response was seen in 32. Those who did not respond included eight who died within

INDEX

Page numbers in *italic* indicate tables and figures.